PRINCIPLES OF
SURGERY

PRINCIPLES OF SURGERY

EDITOR-IN-CHIEF

Seymour I. Schwartz, M.D.
Professor of Surgery
University of Rochester School of Medicine and Dentistry

ASSOCIATE EDITORS

G. Tom Shires, M.D.
Professor and Chairman
Department of Surgery
Cornell University Medical College

Frank C. Spencer, M.D.
Professor and Director
Department of Surgery
New York University School of Medicine

Edward H. Storer, M.D.
Professor of Surgery
Yale University School of Medicine

THIRD EDITION
©1979

McGRAW-HILL BOOK COMPANY
New York   St. Louis   San Francisco   Auckland   Bogotá   Düsseldorf
Johannesburg   London   Madrid   Mexico   Montreal   New Delhi
Panama   Paris   São Paulo   Singapore   Sydney   Tokyo   Toronto

NOTICE

Medicine is an ever-changing science. As new research and clinical experience broaden our knowledge, changes in treatment and drug therapy are required. The editors and the publisher of this work have made every effort to ensure that the drug dosage schedules herein are accurate and in accord with the standards accepted at the time of publication. Readers are advised, however, to check the product information sheet included in the package of each drug they plan to administer to be certain that changes have not been made in the recommended dose or in the contraindications for administration. This recommendation is of particular importance in regard to new or infrequently used drugs.

To students of surgery,
at all levels,
in their quest for knowledge

PRINCIPLES OF SURGERY

1 2 3 4 5 6 7 8 9 0 DODO 7 8 3 2 1 0 9 8

This book was set in Times Roman by York Graphic Services, Inc.
The editors were J. Dereck Jeffers, Stuart D. Boynton,
and Bob Leap; the designer was Barbara Ellwood;
the production supervisor was Robert C. Pedersen.
New drawings were done by J & R Services, Inc.
The cover was designed by Nicholas Krenitsky.
R. R. Donnelley & Sons Company was printer and binder.

Library of Congress Cataloging in Publication Data

Main entry under title:

Principles of surgery.

    Bibliography: p.
    Includes index.
    1. Surgery. I. Schwartz, Seymour I.
[DNLM: 1. Surgery. W0100.3 P957]
RD31.P88 1979b   617   78-13763
ISBN 0-07-055735-7

LC CIP DATA (2 vol ed.)

RD31.P88 1979   617   78-6763
ISBN 0-07-055736-5

Contents

List of Contributors

James T. Adams, M.D.
Professor of Surgery, University of Rochester School of Medicine and Dentistry

R. Peter Altman, M.D.
Associate Professor of Surgery, George Washington University; Senior Attending Surgeon, Children's Hospital National Medical Center

Kathryn D. Anderson, M.D.
Assistant Professor of Surgery, George Washington University; Senior Attending Surgeon, Children's Hospital National Medical Center

Richard M. Bergland, M.D.
Associate Professor of Neurosurgery, Harvard; Chief, Division of Neurosurgery, Beth Israel Hospital

George H. Bornside, Ph.D.
Professor of Surgical Research and Microbiology, Louisiana State University School of Medicine

Thomas J. Brobyn, M.D.
Clinical Assistant Professor of Plastic Surgery, Thomas Jefferson University; Associate Chief of Plastic Surgery, Chesnut Hill Hospital

Lester R. Bryant, M.D.
Professor and Chairman, Department of Surgery, East Tennessee State University

Peter C. Canizaro, M.D.
Associate Professor of Surgery, Cornell University Medical College

C. James Carrico, M.D.
Professor of Surgery, University of Washington School of Medicine

Robert A. Chase, M.D.
Professor, Department of Surgery, Stanford University School of Medicine

Isidore Cohn, Jr., M.D.
Professor and Chairman, Department of Surgery, Louisiana State University School of Medicine

William F. Collins, Jr., M.D.
Professor and Chairman, Section of Neurological Surgery, Yale University School of Medicine

Robert E. Condon, M.D.
Professor of Surgery, The Medical College of Wisconsin

Lester M. Cramer, M.D.
Clinical Professor of Plastic Surgery, University of Colorado Medical Center; Chief of Plastic Surgery, Chesnut Hill Hospital

Joseph N. Cunningham, M.D.
Associate Professor, Department of Surgery, New York University School of Medicine

P. William Curreri, M.D.
Professor of Surgery and Director, Burn Center, The New York Hospital—Cornell Medical Center

Louis R. M. Del Guercio, M.D.
Professor and Chairman, Department of Surgery, New York Medical College

James A. DeWeese, M.D.
Professor of Surgery, University of Rochester School of Medicine and Dentistry

J. Herbert Dietz, Jr., M.D.
Associate Professor of Rehabilitation (Surgery), Cornell University Medical College; Chief, Rehabilitation Service (Surgery), Memorial Sloan-Kettering Cancer Center

Robert B. Duthie, M.D., M.B.
Nuffield Professor of Orthopedic Surgery, Nuffield Orthopedic Center, Oxford, England

F. Henry Ellis, Jr., M.D., Ph.D.
Chairman, Department of Thoracic and Cardiovascular Surgery, Lahey Clinic Foundation and New England Deaconess Hospital; Associate Clinical Professor of Surgery, Harvard Medical School

John E. Foker, M.D.
Assistant Professor of Surgery, University of Minnesota

John H. Foster, M.D.
Professor of Surgery, Vanderbilt University School of Medicine

Irwin N. Frank, M.D.
Professor of Surgery, Urology Division, University of Rochester School of Medicine and Dentistry

Donald S. Gann, M.D.
Professor of Surgery, The Johns Hopkins School of Medicine; Director of Emergency Medicine, Johns Hopkins Hospital

Adolph H. Giesecke, Jr., M.D.
Professor and Chairman, Department of Anesthesiology, The University of Texas Southwestern Medical School at Dallas

Stanley M. Goldberg, M.D.
Clinical Professor of Surgery, Director and Head, Division of Colon and Rectal Surgery, Department of Surgery, University of Minnesota Health Sciences Center

Nicholas M. Greene, M.D.
Professor, Department of Anesthesiology, Yale University School of Medicine

Timothy S. Harrison, M.D.
Professor of Surgery and Physiology, The Milton S. Hershey Medical Center, The Pennsylvania State University

Charles M. Haskell, M.D.
Associate Professor of Medicine and Surgery, Department of Medicine, UCLA School of Medicine, University of California at Los Angeles

Arthur L. Herbst, M.D.
Professor and Chairman, Department of Obstetrics and Gynecology, The University of Chicago

Franklin T. Hoaglund, M.D.
Professor and Chairman, Department of Orthopedic Surgery, University of Vermont College of Medicine

Anthony M. Imparato, M.D.
Professor of Clinical Surgery, New York University School of Medicine

E. R. Johnson, M.D.
Associate Professor of Physical Medicine and Rehabilitation, The University of Texas Southwestern Medical School at Dallas

Robert F. Jones, M.D.
Professor of Surgery, University of Washington School of Medicine

Ronald C. Jones, M.D.
Professor of Surgery, The University of Texas Southwestern Medical School at Dallas

Edwin L. Kaplan, M.D.
Professor of Surgery, Pritzker School of Medicine, University of Chicago

James F. Lee, M.D.
Professor of Anesthesiology, The University of Texas, Southwestern Medical School at Dallas

Richard R. Lower, M.D.
Professor and Chairman, Division of Thoracic and Cardiac Surgery, Medical College of Virginia

Robert N. McClelland, M.D.
Professor of Surgery, The University of Texas Southwestern Medical School at Dallas

Donald F. McDonald, M.D.
Professor, Division of Urology, University of Texas Medical Branch at Galveston

René B. Menguy, M.D.
Professor of Surgery, University of Rochester School of Medicine and Dentistry

Calvin Morgan, M.D.
Clinical Assistant Professor of Surgery, East Tennessee State University

Donald L. Morton, M.D.
Professor of Surgery and Chief, Divisions General Surgery and Oncology, UCLA School of Medicine, University of California at Los Angeles

John H. Morton, M.D.
Professor of Surgery, University of Rochester School of Medicine and Dentistry

John S. Najarian, M.D.
Professor and Chairman, Department of Surgery, University of Minnesota Health Sciences Center

Santhat Nivatvongs, M.D.
Assistant Professor, Division of Colon and Rectal Surgery, Department of Surgery, University of Minnesota Health Sciences Center

W. Spencer Payne, M.D.
Professor of Surgery, Mayo Medical School, Mayo Graduate School of Medicine, Consultant Section of Thoracic, Cardiovascular and General Surgery in the Mayo Clinic and Mayo Foundation

Erle E. Peacock, Jr., M.D.
Professor of Surgery, Plastic Surgery Section, Tulane University School of Medicine

Malcolm O. Perry, M.D.
Professor of Surgery and Chief, Division of Vascular Surgery, Cornell University Medical College

Judson G. Randolph, M.D.
Professor of Surgery, George Washington University; Surgeon-in-Chief, Children's Hospital, National Medical Center

Benjamin F. Rush, Jr., M.D.
Professor and Chairman, Department of Surgery, College of Medicine and Dentistry of New Jersey at Newark

Howard A. Rusk, M.D.
Professor of Rehabilitation Medicine, New York
University School of Medicine

Seymour I. Schwartz, M.D.
Professor of Surgery, University of Rochester School of
Medicine and Dentistry

G. Tom Shires, M.D.
Professor and Chairman, Department of Surgery,
Cornell University Medical College

William Silen, M.D.
Chief of Surgery, Beth Israel Hospital; Professor of
Surgery, Harvard Medical School

Richard L. Simmons, M.D.
Professor of Surgery and Microbiology, Department of
Surgery, University of Minnesota Health Sciences
Center

William H. Snyder, III, M.D.
Associate Professor of Surgery, The University of Texas
Southwestern Medical School at Dallas

Frank C. Sparks, M.D.
Professor and Chairman, Department of Surgery,
University of Connecticut Health Center, School of
Medicine

Dennis D. Spencer, M.D.
Assistant Professor, Section of Neurosurgery, Yale
University School of Medicine

Frank C. Spencer, M.D.
Professor and Director, Department of Surgery, New
York University School of Medicine

Edward H. Storer, M.D.
Professor of Surgery, Yale University School of
Medicine

Erwin R. Thal, M.D.
Associate Professor of Surgery, The University of Texas
Southwestern Medical School at Dallas

Donald R. Tredway, M.D., Ph.D.
Associate Professor and Chief, Section of Reproductive
Endocrinology, Department of Obstetrics and
Gynecology, The University of Chicago

Howard Ulfelder, M.D.
Joe V. Meigs Professor of Gynecology, Harvard Medical
School

Joan L. Venes, M.D.
Associate Professor, Section of Neurosurgery, Yale
University School of Medicine

Franklin C. Wagner, Jr., M.D.
Associate Professor, Section of Neurosurgery, Yale
University School of Medicine

Preface
to the Third Edition

The science of surgery continues to expand and change at a rate which makes only the title of a textbook immutable. The editors remain devoted to the concept of a *modern* source of information and therefore offer this third edition as evidence of their concern. The third edition of *Principles of Surgery* maintains its consistent format, while reflecting the changes which have evolved over the past five years.

There are 15 new authors and approximately 35 percent of the text has been altered. Chapters which were rewritten by new authors include: Endocrine and Metabolic Responses to Injury; Shock; Burns; Chest Wall, Pleura, Lung, and Mediastinum; Peritonitis and Intraabdominal Abscesses, Pituitary and Adrenal; Pediatric Surgery; and Urology. All other chapters have been extensively revised and updated. Each of the chapters in the "Basic Considerations" section have undergone major change—particularly those concerned with oncology and transplantation—reflecting the explosion of knowledge in these areas. The specific organ system chapters have been revised with an emphasis on newly introduced diagnostic techniques and current consensus of opinion regarding management. The References of each chapter have been brought up to date.

The editors wish to thank the readers for their past reception of our efforts, and offer the present work as a statement of our appreciation in the hopes that the third edition serves the same purpose as its two predecessors and is equally well received.

Seymour I. Schwartz

Acknowledgments

The editors appreciate the efforts of all the contributors whose expertise, lucid presentation, and promptness have eased our task. This statement is an expression of particular thanks to Ms. Wendy Husser, Administrative Assistant, who devoted her intellectual energies throughout the entire development of this edition. Finally, once again, the four editors would like to acknowledge the patience, cooperation, and sacrifice on the part of our families, permitting us uncompromised devotion to this project which has now extended over twelve years.

Seymour I. Schwartz

Preface to the First Edition

The raison d'etre for a new textbook in a discipline which has been served by standard works for many years was the Editorial Board's initial conviction that a distinct need for a modern approach in the dissemination of surgical knowledge existed. As incoming chapters were reviewed, both the need and satisfaction became increasingly apparent and, at the completion, we felt a sense of excitement at having the opportunity to contribute to the education of modern and future students concerned with the care of surgical patients.

The recent explosion of factual knowledge has emphasized the need for a presentation which would provide the student an opportunity to assimilate pertinent facts in a logical fashion. This would then permit correlation, synthesis of concepts, and eventual extrapolation to specific situations. The physiologic bases for diseases are therefore emphasized and the manifestations and diagnostic studies are considered as a reflection of pathophysiology. Therapy then becomes logical in this schema and the necessity to regurgitate facts is minimized. In appreciation of the impact which Harrison's *Principles of Internal Medicine* has had, the clinical manifestations of the disease processes are considered in detail for each area. Since the operative procedure represents the one element in the therapeutic armentarium unique to the surgeon, the indications, important technical considerations, and complications receive appropriate emphasis. While we appreciate that a textbook cannot hope to incorporate an atlas of surgical procedures, we have provided the student a single book which will satisfy the sequential demands in the care and considerations of surgical patients.

The ultimate goal of the Editorial Board has been to collate a book which is deserving of the adjective "modern." We have therefore selected as authors dynamic and active contributors to their particular fields. The *au courant* concept is hopefully apparent throughout the entire work and is exemplified by appropriate emphasis on diseases of modern surgical interest, such as trauma, transplantation, and the recently appreciated importance of rehabilitation. Cardiovascular surgery is presented in keeping with the exponential strides recently achieved.

There are two major subdivisions to the text. In the first twelve chapters, subjects that transcend several organ systems are presented. The second portion of the book represents a consideration of specific organ systems and surgical specialties.

Throughout the text, the authors have addressed themselves to a sophisticated audience, regarding the medical student as a graduate student, incorporating material generally sought after by the surgeon in training and presenting information appropriate for the continuing education of the practicing surgeon. The need for a text such as we have envisioned is great and the goal admittedly high. It is our hope that this effort fulfills the expressed demands.

Seymour I. Schwartz

Chapter 1

Endocrine and Metabolic Responses to Injury

by Donald S. Gann

Injury comes in so many variegated forms that it is no small wonder that response to injury may also be quite variable. There are, however, endocrine and metabolic changes that are common to many kinds of injury and that, when taken together, constitute one aspect of the body's response to trauma. These responses are sometimes greatly modified by anesthesia, by fluid and electrolyte replacement, by transfusion, and by other surgical and anesthetic iatrogens, so that identical injuries produced, on the one hand, by an automobile accident and, on the other, during a planned and controlled operation under general anesthesia may lead to courses which vary considerably either in magnitude or direction of response.

Furthermore, adaptation to certain kinds of injury may occur—e.g., to Noble-Collip drum shock or hemorrhagic shock in the rat, altitude hypoxia and poisons in man—thus increasing an already marked individual variation in response. As will be seen later, such adaptations may lead either to attenuated or to enhanced response to a subsequent insult.

In this initial chapter consideration will be given to some of the factors producing the changes consequent upon injury, to the mechanisms through which they are known or thought to act, and to the changes themselves. Some specific examples will be given to illustrate patient management problems related to trauma, together with their suggested solutions.

STIMULI INDUCING CHANGE

Once an injury has been incurred, a series of endocrine and metabolic events follow. Although it is clear that the neuroendocrine response to injury involves changes in the secretion of a large number of hormones, most of the studies of the details of this response have focused on changes in the secretion of ACTH and of cortisol. Accordingly, the mechanisms controlling secretion of these hormones are emphasized in this section. It seems likely that the neural mechanisms subserving control of other hormones involved in the neuroendocrine response are analogous to those subserving control of ACTH. Our own finding that every central nervous area receiving afferent signals from cardiovascular receptors signaling changes in blood volume is in turn involved in control of ACTH implies that the same areas must share in part in the

Fig. 1-1. Adrenocortical response to a burn following section of the cord at the level of C_7. A burn below the level of section produced no increase in the adrenocorticosteroid secretion over the control values. Five units of ACTH given intravenously produced an immediate marked rise in adrenocortical output. With the dog under Nembutal anesthesia a burn of the left hind leg leg produced no significant increase in adrenocorticosteroid output. In contrast, a burn of the neck above the level of cord section produced a marked and immediate increase in adrenocortical secretion. (*From D. M. Hume and R. H. Egdahl, Ann Surg, 150:697, 1959.*)

control of several hormones. Such a sharing provides a neural basis for a coordinated multihormonal response.

AFFERENT NERVE STIMULI FROM THE INJURED AREA. This is a major factor in the initiation of many of the endocrine changes that follow injury, particularly those related to increased ACTH and cortisol secretion. Abdominal laparotomy, burns, or severe trauma in dogs failed to

Fig. 1-2. Comparison of the adrenal venous blood 17-hydroxy-corticosteroid (17-OHCS) response to a gastric operation in a patient with spinal cord transection at T_4 with that seen in a normal patient. The paraplegic patient fails to release endogenous ACTH in response to the operation but shows a marked rise in adrenal 17-OHCS secretion following ACTH. The normal patient shows a maximal secretion of 17-OHCS in response to the operation, and no further increase is seen with ACTH. (*From D. M. Hume et al., Surgery, 52:174, 1962.*)

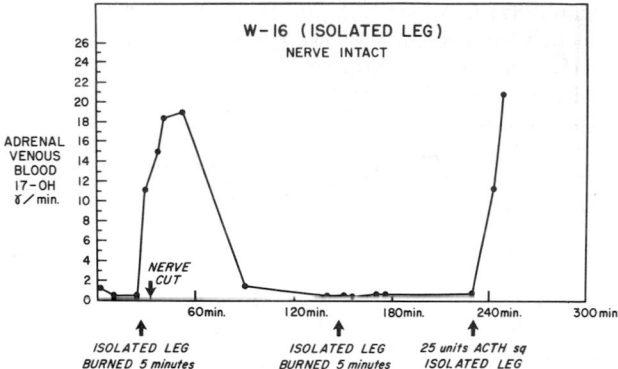

Fig. 1-3. Effect of limb denervation on ACTH secretion following trauma. The hind leg has been isolated so that it is attached to the body only by one artery, one vein, and one nerve. The burn of the isolated leg produces a marked and immediate response in adrenal venous blood corticosteroid secretion. During the height of the response the nerve was cut, and the secretion dropped rather promptly to control levels. A second burn of the same leg now produced no adrenocortical response. ACTH injected subcutaneously into the isolated leg produced a prompt and marked increase in adrenocorticosteroid secretion. (*From D. M. Hume and R. H. Egdahl, Ann Surg, 150:697, 1959.*)

produce an increased ACTH release if the traumatized area had been denervated so that afferent impulses from it failed to reach the brain. Trauma to the area which remained innervated continued to produce a normal response. This absence of increased ACTH release was also shown to be true for paraplegic or quadriplegic patients undergoing traumatic plastic or orthopedic procedures in the denervated area, or abdominal laparotomy for gastric resection (Figs. 1-1 and 1-2). Egdahl performed an ingenious experiment which confirmed these observations. In a series of dogs he divided the skin, muscle, and bone of one hind leg, thus isolating it from the body except for the femoral artery, vein, and nerve. Trauma to the innervated portion of the leg continued to evoke an increased secretion of ACTH and cortisol. The nerve was then divided, leaving the artery and vein intact. Following this, trauma no longer produced an increased secretion of ACTH (Fig. 1-3).

HEMORRHAGE AND HYPOVOLEMIA. The most prominent characteristic of trauma is a loss of circulating body fluids. Naturally, many severe injuries are accompanied by hemorrhage and thus direct loss of blood. In addition, as pointed out by Blalock, there is a sequestration of fluids in an injured region with formation of a so-called "third space." This sequestration leads to a loss of extracellular fluid available for exchange and thus to further hypovolemia. The cardiovascular system, acting through receptors in the atria and arteries (baroreceptors), exerts a tonic, inhibitory influence over the release of certain hormones which may be controlled either directly through the central nervous system or through peripheral sympathetic nerves. When blood volume decreases, the extent of cardiovascular inhibition of nervous function decreases. As the inhibition is released, there is direct central neural stimulation of the secretion of ACTH, vasopressin (ADH), and growth hormone (GH) from the anterior and posterior pituitary gland. Furthermore, with the release of inhibition, sympathetic neural activity increases and there is thus enhanced secretion of epinephrine and norepinephrine from the adrenal medulla, of renin from the kidney, and of glucagon from the pancreas. The same sympathetic stimulation or circulating catecholamines may inhibit release of insulin from the pancreas. The effect of hemorrhage on secretion of cortisol is shown in Fig. 1-4. This multihormonal response to hypovolemia is entirely analogous to the reflex changes in myocardial contractility, heart rate, and peripheral resistance which occur in response to the classic baroreceptor reflex in the presence of hypovolemia. In addition, changes in renal hemodynamics brought about by sympathetic stimulation may lead to changes in the renal handling of salt and water on a nonhormonal basis. These changes are further augmented by the secretion of aldosterone, stimulated by the renin angiotensin system, and by vasopressin. These changes are discussed below.

LOCAL WOUND FACTORS. As indicated above, afferent nerve impulses are required to convey signals from a wounded area to initiate direct release of hormones. Thus it might appear that local wound factors are unimportant in the metabolic response to injury. However, this does not appear to be the case, although local changes in a wounded area seem to evolve more slowly than do afferent signals conveyed over nerves. The blood sequestered in an injured area, together with decreased tissue perfusion brought about by local vascular injury and by edema, leads to local acidosis and results in the movement of potassium out of cells. In the presence of infection, bacterial toxins also accumulate in the wound area. Furthermore, the synthesis of kinins and prostaglandins may be accelerated in the presence of acidosis. With the return of adequate perfusion to the injured areas, these factors may be washed into the general circulation, where they may potentiate or initiate portions of the response to injury. Finally, there may be specific neuroendocrine responses to injury of critical areas such as the heart, great vessels, or brain.

SHOCK. When, as a consequence of severe hypovolemia, bacterial toxins, or myocardial infarction, or for any other reason, tissue perfusion drops to shock levels, profound metabolic disturbances occur. The decrease in tissue perfusion is made worse by direct damage to vital organs, particularly the brain, liver, heart, lungs, and kidneys. Until shock becomes profound, the chain of events set in motion by hypovolemia may appear first, followed then by changes due to organ failure and acidosis.

CHANGES IN BLOOD pH. Severe acidosis may be produced by some types of trauma including bacterial infection, prolonged shock, open heart surgical procedures with the pump-oxygenator, operations on diabetics who are out of control, temporary respiratory and cardiac arrest, and ingestion of acid, to name but a few. Acidosis itself interferes further with cellular function, and if compensatory mechanisms are blocked or if the change occurs too rapidly, death may supervene. Alkalosis also may occur with trauma, particularly in patients who are on gastric suction or those with cirrhosis, who are frequently alkalotic when they go to the operating room. The development of marked alkalosis is sometimes seen in patients who are

Fig. 1-4. Following a hemorrhage of 30 ml/kg, secretion of cortisol (measured as 17-OHCS) increases rapidly to rates equal to that elicited by a supramaximal dose of ACTH. Increased secretion of cortisol is sustained in the presence of this degree of hypovolemia.

hyperventilated or those overtreated with bicarbonate. In addition, pain may induce hyperventilation and thus lead to alkalosis. A marked change of pH in either direction from normal may be hazardous or even fatal to the patient. Respiratory alkalosis may convert rapidly and catastrophically to metabolic acidosis.

INFECTION. Bacterial endotoxin is capable of providing direct hypothalamic stimulation with attendant release of ACTH, epinephrine, norepinephrine, ADH, and GH (Fig. 1-5). In addition to this, of course, severe infection has profound influences on the cardiovascular system and can, if unchecked, lead to shock and ultimately to renal, hepatic, cardiac, and cerebral failure and to death.

ANESTHESIA AND OTHER DRUGS. Anesthesia has an effect upon the endocrine system, the cardiovascular system, the pulmonary and renal systems, the brain, and in fact the entire metabolism of the body. Depending upon the anesthetic agent employed, it may depress or abolish certain of the endocrine responses or else stimulate or augment them. It may produce a relative hypoxia or improve oxygenation. It may produce vasodilatation or vasoconstriction, stimulate the heart or depress it. Almost all anesthetic agents, however, depress hepatic function to a greater or lesser degree. No operative trauma ought to be thought of without a consideration of the particular anesthetic agent employed, as well as the depth and duration of anesthesia.

Morphine and Nembutal tend to depress hypothalamic stimulation of ACTH and GH release, but this depression can be overcome by operative trauma. They also depress respiration and gastrointestinal motility. Atropine produces tachycardia and decreases salivary gland activity. Antihy-

Fig. 1-5. Effects of endotoxin on 17-OHCS and epinephrine secretion. A. In the normal dog, a small dose of endotoxin produces a marked increase in the adrenal venous blood secretion of 17-OHCS, with almost no increase in the adrenal medullary output of epinephrine. A larger dose of endotoxin produces an increase both in 17-OHCS and epinephrine secretion in the adrenal venous blood. B. When the same experiment is repeated in the dog with section of the spinal cord, the endotoxin again produces a marked increase in the secretion of adrenal venous blood 17-OHCS, but now there is no increase at all in epinephrine secretion.

The experiments in A and B demonstrate that endotoxin acts at the level of the hypothalamus to stimulate the release of ACTH and also to stimulate the cells controlling the secretion of epinephrine via the spinal cord and sympathetic nerves. When the cord is cut, although the hypothalamic effect of endotoxin on ACTH release is retained, impulses can no longer pass down the cord and into the sympathetic nerves to bring about a release of epinephrine. (*From R. H. Egdahl, J Clin Invest, 38:1120, 1959.*)

pertensive drugs may lead to a marked hypotension with the induction of anesthesia, and many other commonly used drugs may have important effects in altering the response to injury.

CENTRAL NERVOUS SYSTEM INJURY. The endocrine and metabolic responses to injury may be greatly altered

if the central nervous system itself is injured. Thus the patient who is in a coma from a head injury may respond very differently to a severe injury elsewhere in the body than he would without an associated head injury. Head injury can produce diabetes insipidus, abnormal salt metabolism, inappropriate secretion of ADH, depressed pulmonary and cardiac action, or arrest, shock, and death. The patient whose spinal cord is transected may have tremendous vasodilatation of the vessels in the lower part of the body and cannot compensate for blood loss. In addition, as noted above, the patient will not respond to severe trauma below the level of cord section with an increased ACTH secretion.

EMOTIONAL TRAUMA. The emotional trauma of an injury may either inhibit or stimulate the endocrine response, although it usually does the latter. The effect of emotional trauma on endocrine secretion was originally demonstrated by Harris, who showed indirect evidence for an increased adrenocortical secretion in rabbits who were restrained. It was subsequently demonstrated by Ganong et al. that a tremendous rise in adrenal venous blood corticosteroid output accompanied restraint in nervous dogs (Fig. 1-6).

Everyone is familiar with the effect which emotional factors have on epinephrine release (sweating, tachycardia, dry mouth, pallor, intestinal motility, blood pressure, etc.). This factor may contribute to some of the differences between the effects of injury in the conscious state versus those of the same type of injury in the anesthetized patient.

ANOXIA. Anoxia caused, for example, by a pneumothorax due to a penetrating wound or a flail chest with rib fractures may produce profound change through tissue hypoxia. It is a strong stimulant to release of catecholamines and of ACTH.

IMMOBILIZATION. Immobilization leads to metabolic change by muscle wasting and mobilization of skeletal calcium and phosphorus. Bed rest reduces the secretion of renin, aldosterone, and to some extent epinephrine and norepinephrine. It promotes thrombosis in the deep veins of the pelvis and lower extremities.

STARVATION. Many types of severe trauma are accompanied by a negative nitrogen balance. This negative balance is augmented by starvation. Inadequate intake of vitamins and calories may produce considerable metabolic change, particularly if starvation is present over a long period of time.

HYPOGLYCEMIA. Hypoglycemia is a potent stimulus to the hypothalamic centers controlling the secretion of ACTH, GH, epinephrine, and norepinephrine. If it is persistent and profound, it will produce marked interference with central nervous system activity.

ENVIRONMENTAL TEMPERATURE CHANGES AND FEVER. If the trauma has a thermal component, profound general changes can be brought about by heat or cold alone. A hot or cold environment produces striking change in skin circulation with concomitant compensatory changes in other parts of the body. Heat and cold by themselves can each produce changes in the output of many hormones, including ACTH, cortisol, aldosterone, ADH, epinephrine, norepinephrine, thyroxine, and others. Respiration may be increased, fluid and electrolyte losses occur, and many other changes may ensue (Fig. 1-7). Fever increases catabolism, oxygen consumption, cardiac work, and water and salt loss. Ambient temperature alterations were shown by Redding and Mueller to have a profound effect on survival following tourniquet shock.

POISONS. Some injuries are accompanied by the addition of poisons, which may act locally or systemically. The bite of a poisonous snake is an example in which the local and general changes wrought by the injury itself are minor compared with those caused by the poison. Crush injury may be accompanied by the release of methemoglobin. Toxic bacterial products occur in injury associated with infections. Various other poisons, such as methyl alcohol, may have been ingested prior to the injury, giving rise to widespread metabolic changes.

WITHDRAWAL SYMPTOMS. The injured patient may be an alcoholic, and the early postoperative course may be complicated by the severe withdrawal symptoms of delirium tremens with its profound metabolic complications. The same may be said of narcotic withdrawal, or even withdrawal of commonly used drugs, such as insulin—for example, in patients who are unconscious and not known to be diabetics.

Fig. 1-7. Effects of hypothermia on ACTH and 17-OHCS secretion. *A.* The plasma ACTH levels and adrenal venous blood 17-OHCS output in a dog traumatized under ether anesthesia and then subjected to hypothermia. There is a marked depression of corticosteroid secretion during hypothermia with an increase again after rewarming. Blood ACTH, which is elevated before the induction of hypothermia, becomes too low to measure during hypothermia and is again easily detected after rewarming. *B.* Epinephrine, norepinephrine, and corticosteroid secretion in the adrenal venous blood of a dog traumatized under ether anesthesia before, during, and after induction of hypothermia. A marked decrease in epinephrine and norepinephrine output occurs during hypothermia, while a marked increase in the secretion of these substances is seen on rewarming. The output of 17-OHCS follows a similar pattern. (*From D. M. Hume and R. H. Egdahl, Ann NY Acad Sci, 80:435, 1959.*)

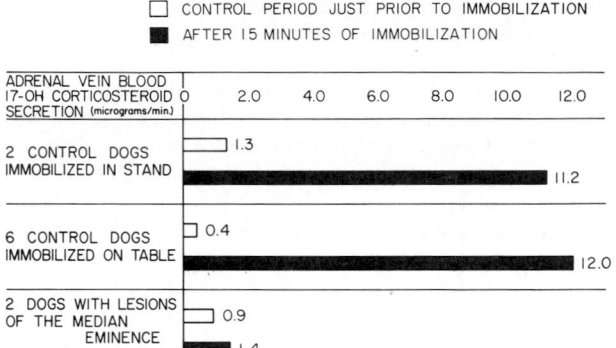

Fig. 1-6. Effect of forced immobilization on adrenal venous blood 17-OHCS secretion. This is shown in two groups of control dogs. Fifteen minutes after the introduction of the restraint there is an output of adrenal venous blood 17-OHCS secretion equivalent to that seen during major operative trauma as a consequence of the emotional stress of forced immobilization in untrained dogs. Lesions of the median eminence abolish this response, indicating that it is mediated by the hypothalamus. (*From W. F. Ganong et al., Fed Proc, 14:54, 1955.*)

ANAPHYLAXIS. Under some circumstances the overreactive response of the body to the injury can be much more devastating than the injury itself. A typical example of this is a bee sting in a patient who is hypersensitive to bee stings. Under these circumstances a bee sting may produce shock, coma, and death, the devastating chain of events occurring because of the body's pathologic hypersensitivity response to the antigen.

Thus it may be seen that there are many stimuli producing their effects through many different pathways in different kinds of trauma. Very frequently there are several stimuli to endocrine and metabolic change working simultaneously in the same patient.

ADRENAL CORTICOSTEROID OUTPUT AND BLOOD ACTH LEVELS IN HYPOTHERMIA

ADRENAL SYMPATHIN AND CORTICOSTEROID OUTPUT IN HYPOTHERMIA

CENTRAL NERVOUS SYSTEM AND ENDOCRINE CHANGES

As indicated above, the principal signals to initiate the endocrine response to injury are those of hypovolemia and of pain. The hormonal response is diffuse, including increased release of ACTH, cortisol, growth hormone, epinephrine, norepinephrine, glucagon, renin, and aldosterone. In each case the prompt initiation of hormonal release depends upon a reflex activated by afferent nerves. Although the reflex initiation of increased sympathetic activity may take place at the level of the medulla or spinal cord, it appears that even for these reflexes hypothalamic coordination is involved, as it is in the control of the release of the anterior pituitary hormones. The precise pathways from afferent nerve endings to the hypothalamus have been studied in detail only for ACTH and to some extent for vasopressin. However, where they are available, data for the control of other hormones seem analogous; and it is highly likely that the afferent pathways are shared to a considerable extent, providing a basis for coordinated neuroendocrine response to injury.

The central pathways have been best delineated for the neural control of ACTH in response to hypovolemia. The principal afferent receptors lie in the right atrium (Fig. 1-8) and in the carotid arteries. The afferent nerves converge on the lateral solitary nucleus and related structures in the dorsolateral medulla. From this point, they project without synapsing to the nuclei of the coeruleus complex in the dorsal pons, with medial projections to the tegmental and raphe nuclei. From this point, they project, apparently again without synapsing, to the hypothalamus in three principal pathways, two stimulatory and one inhibitory. A dorsal stimulatory pathway courses through the dorsal longitudinal fasciculus to end in the dorsal hypothalamus, including the paraventricular nucleus. A ventral stimulatory pathway courses through the ventral tegmental area of the midbrain to enter the medial forebrain bundle and terminate in the anteroventral hypothalamic nuclei, including the suprachiasmatic and ventromedial nuclei. The intermediate inhibitory pathway passes up the central tegmental tract to terminate in the posterior hypothalamic area. These stimulatory and inhibitory signals then converge on the medial basal hypothalamus to control release of corticotropin-releasing factor, the agent which controls pituitary release of ACTH, from the median eminence. These multiple pathways provide a basis for the observation of different degrees of steroid suppressibility in response to small and large hemorrhage, as discussed below.

In the case of pain transmission, neurophysiologic studies have not been coordinated with endocrine ones, but it is possible to piece together a likely pattern. In this case, afferent pain endings in the tissues synapse first in the substantia gelatinosa of the dorsal horn of the spinal cord. From here, fibers pass up the spinothalamic tract to terminate in the gigantocellular tegmental field of the medulla and pons. The degree of interaction at the pontine level with volume signals is unclear at present, but fibers appear to pass from the pontine level to the hypothalamus along the same pathways described above, with a major projection to the anteroventral hypothalamus through the medial forebrain bundle and a possible additional projection above the dorsal longitudinal fasciculus as well. There is no evidence at this time that the inhibitory pathway is involved in the control of ACTH release in response to pain.

Within the hypothalamus, specific nuclei control the release of releasing factors, which in turn govern the secretion of various anterior pituitary hormones or sympathetic activity, but there is clear overlap of function. For example, the posterior hypothalamic area is involved in the control of ACTH and of descending sympathetic activity. The paraventricular nucleus is involved in the control of vasopressin, of oxytocin, and of ACTH. The ventromedial nucleus is involved in the control of growth hormone and of ACTH. The supraoptic nucleus has been shown to be active in the control of vasopressin and oxytocin. The suprachiasmatic nucleus appears to control ACTH release and to contain corticotropin-releasing factor, but it has been shown to effect secretion of gonadotropins as well (Fig. 1-9). Hypothalamic control of the anterior pituitary is accomplished by secretion of neurohormones onto capillary loops in the median eminence (Fig. 1-10). Although this view focuses on the role of the hypothalamus in neuroendocrine control, it is clear that this region of the brain

Fig. 1-8. Secretion of cortisol (F) after supramaximal doses of ACTH (stippled bars) and after sequential hemorrhages of 5 ml/kg in a dog with an inflatable balloon in the right atrium. Inflation of the balloon prevents the response to small hemorrhage, indicating mediation of this response by right atrial receptors. (*From G. L. Cryer and D. S. Gann, Am J Physiol, 227:325, 1974.*)

Fig. 1-9. Horizontal view through the median eminence. This indicates some of the relationships of the supraoptic nucleus (SON) and the tuberal nucleus to the hypophyseoportal blood vessels. The laterally placed axons of the supraoptic nucleus concerned with the production and release of ADH travel down into the posterior lobe (PL), as shown in the diagram. The more mediad placed cells of the suprachiasmatic nucleus (SC) terminate in the anterior portion of the median eminence on the hypophyseoportal capillaries. A lesion made at the point indicated by A will abolish the ACTH response to trauma without producing diabetes insipidus. A lesion made at the point indicated by B will produce diabetes insipidus without interfering with ACTH release. If a lesion is made at the level indicated by A but is somewhat larger, extending laterally, it will produce both diabetes insipidus and a failure of ACTH release in response to trauma. The cells of the tuberal nucleus which control gonadotropin release terminate in the posterior part of the median eminence on capillary loops of the posterior portion of the hypophyseoportal system. Their action is unaffected by lesions located either at A or B.

is important in the coordination of other autonomic functions as well in the control of other hormones which appear to be less affected by injury.

Modulation of Neuroendocrine Response

CORTISOL FEEDBACK

As indicated above, injury leads to the increased secretion of ACTH and of cortisol. Elevated plasma levels of cortisol lead in turn to inhibition of further release of ACTH. This effect is exerted primarily through action within the central nervous system, although there is almost certainly some direct effect on the pituitary gland as well. Thus one would expect to see diminished secretion of ACTH and cortisol after a second stimulus. Under appropriate circumstances this is the case (Fig. 1-11). This feedback effect takes approximately 90 minutes to work in most species studied. As indicated below, however, this feedback effect is not usually seen with respect to cortisol because of

potentiation. However, increased plasma levels of cortisol also lead to inhibition of release of vasopressin, growth hormone, and prolactin. Thus the feedback effect of cortisol may be general and may extend far beyond the control of ACTH release per se. The coordinated neuroendocrine response that is an important feature of host defense against injury may be disrupted by recent previous injury. This feature is especially important, since for most patients who have been traumatized, surgery may constitute a second injury, often taking place just at the time when cortisol feedback might be expected to have its principal effect on

Fig. 1-10. Sagittal section of the hypothalamus and pituitary of the dog. A. The brain has been injected with India ink to show the vascular supply. The open area above is the third ventricle, while the clear area with the capillary loops is the median eminence. A portion of the posterior lobe is shown to the right, and the anterior lobe is the dark area to the left and below. At the extreme left, superiorly, is the optic chiasm. Connections can be seen between the vessels of the posterior lobe of the pituitary and the capillary loops in the median eminence. The capillary loops transmitting the hormones controlling gonadotropin secretion to the anterior lobe are in the extreme upper right hand corner of the picture, while those controlling ACTH and TSH secretion are in the anterior portion of the median eminence. B. High-powered view of the median eminence superiorly and the anterior lobe below. The optic chiasm is to the right, but out of view. The capillary loops may be seen projecting up into the median eminence and then descending down into the anterior pituitary.

the neuroendocrine response to the surgical intervention. Feedback inhibition of ACTH release can under appropriate circumstances be demonstrated for most stimuli, including pain, tissue trauma, and small hemorrhage. However, the response to some stimuli cannot be inhibited by even very high plasma levels of cortisol. The most common physiologic insult which cannot be suppressed by cortisol is large hemorrhage, although the response to intestinal traction also appears to be insuppressible by cortisol. In the presence of significant hypovolemia, ACTH release will

Fig. 1-11. Effects of two successive hemorrhages of 10 ml/kg, of reinfusion of shed blood, and of ACTH on secretion of cortisol. The response to the second hemorrhage 90 minutes after the first is attenuated, a reflection of cortisol feedback. Adrenal responsiveness to ACTH is maintained. (*From D. S. Gann et al., Am J Physiol, 232:R5, 1977.*)

Fig. 1-12. Effect of two successive rapid hemorrhages (10 ml/kg/45 seconds) on secretion of cortisol in a dog whose blood volume had been previously expanded by dextran so that hemorrhage would not lead to hypovolemia. The initial response, to rate of hemorrhage, is small and there is no significant cortisol feedback. The response to the second identical hemorrhage 90 minutes later is increased, an indication of physiologic facilitation. (*From D. S. Gann et al., Am J Physiol, 232:R5, 1977.*)

Dog #200

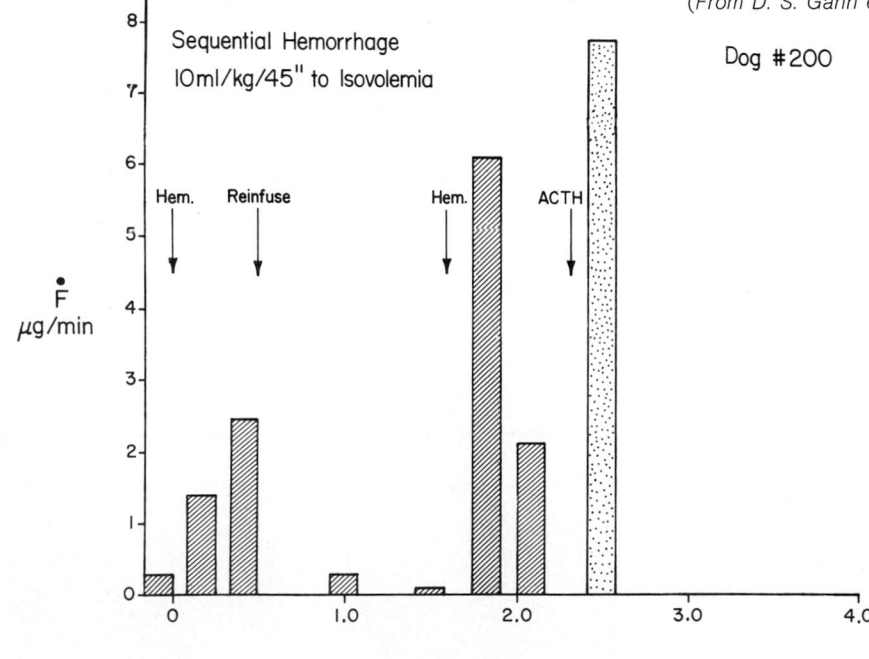

persist until blood volume is restored. Thus hypovolemia seems to hold a preferential position among the various stimuli to ACTH release. The question of whether or not cortisol may suppress the release of hormones other than ACTH in the presence of hypovolemia has not been studied.

PHYSIOLOGIC FACILITATION

Under most circumstances, the adrenocortical response to a second stimulus appears unchanged from that to an initial stimulus. Because the feedback effect described above might be expected to inhibit this second response, the lack of inhibition has been ascribed to a physiologic facilitation. Under appropriate circumstances this facilitation can be demonstrated, provided that the initial stimulus is small enough to prevent high levels of cortisol (Fig. 1-12). The facilitation mechanism also appears to take 60 to 90 minutes and appears to be of sufficient magnitude to offset the feedback effect under most circumstances. The sites of action of facilitative mechanisms are not yet clear, but some data suggest that the adrenal cortex has an enhanced sensitivity to ACTH. There are also suggestions that this increased sensitivity is controlled by the central nervous system through a mechanism independent of ACTH release. Physiologic facilitation has also been observed in the adrenal medullary response to injury. In this case there is not only increased secretion of catecholamines but increased activity of several enzymes involved in catecholamine biosynthesis, including tyrosine hydroxylase. This effect appears to be mediated by increased corticosteroids as well as by increased nervous activity, since it is prevented by hypophysectomy. Cortisol, and possibly a history of increased sympathetic activity, appears to increase release of other hormones under sympathetic control, including glucagon and renin. Thus physiologic facilitation may lead to further imbalance among hormonal responses resulting from repeated injury. Again, the pattern of response to a second injury may be different from the response to the first.

Hormones with Generally Increased Secretion in Trauma

ACTH—CORTISOL

Most types of trauma are characterized by an increased secretion of ACTH and thus of cortisol. A more profound response is seen when the magnitude of the trauma is great, when infection, hemorrhage, and emotional trauma are present, and when stimulating anesthetic agents such as ether are used. The response may be diminished or abolished by cord section or by preexisting pituitary or adrenal disease (Figs. 1-13–1-16).

ADRENAL INSUFFICIENCY The prolonged administration of corticosteroids partially inhibits ACTH, as described under Cortisol Feedback, and leads to decreased adrenal stimulation, atrophy, and finally very little production of corticosteroid. If the adrenal is sufficiently atrophic, even a large dose of ACTH will fail to arouse the adrenal cortex acutely to produce an increased output of

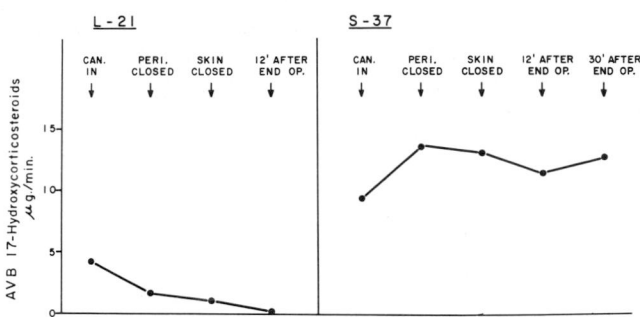

Fig. 1-13. Effects of anterior median eminence lesion on 17-OHCS secretion with operative trauma. Adrenal venous blood corticosteroid secretion in response to operative trauma. At the left are the values obtained in a dog with a lesion of the anterior median eminence. At the right are the values obtained in a normal control animal. A very minimal response was seen in the animal with the hypothalamic lesion, and the values declined during the course of the operation. In contrast, there was an excellent response in the normal animal which continued throughout the operative and immediate postoperative period. This illustrates the importance of the hypothalamus to the release of ACTH in response to trauma. (*From D. M. Hume, "Reticular Formation of the Brain," p. 231, Little, Brown and Company, Boston, 1958.*)

corticosteroids. Patients who have been on steroid administration for long periods of time, whose adrenal has become atrophic, and who are not given corticosteroids to support them during an operation have sometimes died because of the failure of cortisol release from an adrenal rendered temporarily inactive by atrophy. Patients should be questioned for a history of corticosteroid therapy. If acute adrenal insufficiency occurs, the most prominent features are fever and hypotension.

Fig. 1-14. Effect of anterior median eminence lesion on 17-OHCS and ACTH secretion during laparotomy: the adrenal venous blood 17-OHCS secretion and the blood ACTH level in response to operative trauma in normal dogs contrasted to dogs with lesions of the anterior median eminence. The solid bars represent mean values and the vertical lines the range of values. It may be seen that the animals with hypothalamic lesions show a markedly reduced pituitary and adrenal response to trauma. (*From D. M. Hume, "Reticular Formation of the Brain," p. 231, Little, Brown and Company, Boston, 1958.*)

Fig. 1-15. Effect of nerve impulses from injured area on 17-OHCS secretion. This experiment was performed on an animal with a unilateral adrenalectomy and a cannula placed in the adrenal vein of the opposite side. The animal was put to sleep under Nembutal anesthesia, and after a series of base-line measurements a snare around the medial end of the adrenal view was pulled up so that all of the secretion of the only remaining adrenal drained to the outside over a period of 20 minutes. This had the effect of suddenly stopping all adrenal secretion into the blood of the animal, but this sudden hypoadrenalism did not produce a stimulus to ACTH release or increase in the secretion of 17-OHCS. After releasing the snare again, and following a suitable control period, the experiment was repeated exactly as before except that this time after the control period and the pulling up of the snare the animal was suddenly severely traumatized. Within 2 minutes there was a marked increase in adrenal venous blood 17-OHCS secretion. This indicates that the release of ACTH in response to trauma is not brought about as a consequence of a sudden diminution in blood levels of 17-OHCS but is instead stimulated by nervous impulses originating in the injured area.

Similarly, if a patient with unsuspected adrenal insufficiency is inadvertently operated upon without being supported with exogenous corticosteroids, death is likely to ensue. Thus cortisol is necessary for the normal response in trauma. Severe adrenal insufficiency (Addison's disease) is more fully discussed in the section on the adrenal (see Chap. 37). For purposes of the present discussion it is important to recognize that severe insufficiency may be seen in several forms. It may first be noted in the immediate newborn period, when it occurs as part of the adrenogenital syndrome. It is particularly hard to recognize in males, who, unlike females, do not show any physical stigmata of the syndrome. In females, the syndrome may be suspected because of enlargement of the clitoris. Adrenal insufficiency in the infant may be manifested by fever, weight loss, vomiting, hyponatremia, shock, and marked salt loss in the urine. These symptoms usually appear in the first week after birth but sometimes do not become manifest for 5 or 6 weeks. The disease is caused by an enzymatic defect in the adrenal cortex which leads to failure of hydroxylation at the C_{11}, C_{20}, or C_{21} positions. Addison's disease is particularly apt to occur when the defect is in C_{20} or C_{21} hydroxylation. A C_{20} block produces a general deficiency of corticosteroids. No survivals have ever been reported. A C_{21} defect with Addison's disease can be successfully treated if recognized (Fig. 1-17).

If chronic adrenal insufficiency is present prior to the time of surgical treatment and is unrecognized, death is likely to occur within a matter of hours after operation has begun. Typically, chronic adrenal insufficiency is characterized by pigmentation, weakness, weight loss, hypotension, easy fatigability, nausea, vomiting, abdominal pain, hypoglycemia, hyponatremia, and hyperkalemia. Opera-

Fig. 1-16. Comparison of 17-OHCS increases following surgical procedures and ACTH injection. A. The response to cholecystectomy in an eighty-two-year-old patient. There is a marked increase in the level of plasma 17-OHCS during the operative procedure which rapidly returns to normal levels on the day after operation. The response to operative trauma is not quite as high as the response to an injection of ACTH. B. The plasma 17-OHCS response to a vagotomy and subtotal gastrectomy. There is a marked increase in the levels of 17-OHCS on the operative day, the values returning to normal the day after operation. The peak response was even greater than that seen with ACTH. This operation was of somewhat greater magnitude than the cholecystectomy shown in A.

CORTISOL

Fig. 1-17. Steroid nucleus showing, in the circles, three of the defects which may be seen with congenital adrenal hyperplasia. A defect located at *A* produces hypertension, one located at *B* produces severe salt wasting and hypotension, and one located at *C* is usually fatal.

Table 1-1. DAILY SECRETION RATES OF HORMONES

Compound	Mean 24-hr secretion rate
Cortisol, mg	15–30
Corticosterone, mg	2–5
Aldosterone, μg	50–150
Dehydroepiandrosterone, mg.	15–30
Androstenedione, mg	0–10
Hydroxyandrostenedione, mg	0–10
Progesterone, mg	0.4–0.8
Pregnenolone, mg	0.5–0.8
17-OH pregnenolone, mg.	0.2–0.4
Estradiol, mg	Trace

SOURCE: From P. H. Forsham, The Adrenal Cortex, in R. H. Williams (ed.); "Textbook of Endocrinology," p. 287, W. B. Saunders Company, Philadelphia, 1968.

tive intervention will precipitate an acute Addisonian crisis leading to death if treatment is not promptly instituted.

A semiacute type of adrenal insufficiency occurs when the adrenal damage takes place at the time of, or shortly after, the operative event. This has occasionally been seen in patients who were given heparin and developed bilateral adrenal hemorrhages in the postoperative period, and of course it occurs automatically when the operation is a bilateral adrenalectomy. Here, however, exogenous corticosteroids are administered to compensate for the failure of endogenous secretion. If the condition is unrecognized, the patients tend to get along fairly well for 3 or 4 days, after which increasing difficulties develop which may lead

to severe hyponatremia, hypoglycemia, and death if untreated.

The hormones secreted by the adrenal cortex are shown in Fig. 1-18, and their relative secretion rates are shown in Table 1-1 and Fig. 1-19. The adrenal androgens and estrogens seem relatively unimportant in the response to trauma, but cortisol and aldosterone are of the utmost importance. A diagram showing the pathways for the control of secretion of cortisol may be seen in Fig. 1-20. The degradation of cortisol takes place by reduction (A-ring reduction) to tetrahydrocortisol and conjugation with glucuronic acid or sulfuric acid. When these steps have taken place, the cortisol becomes highly water-soluble and can be readily excreted in urine. Since the liver is responsible for

Fig. 1-18. Principal steroids secreted by the adrenal cortex.

GLUCOCORTICOIDS　　MINERALOCORTICOIDS　　ANDROGENS　　ESTROGEN　　PROGESTIN

CORTISOL　　ALDOSTERONE　　ANDROSTENEDIONE　　ESTRADIOL　　PROGESTERONE

CORTICOSTERONE　　DEHYDROEPIANDROSTERONE　　II-B HYDROXYANDRO-STENEDIONE　　PREGNENOLONE

17α –HYDROXYPREGNENOLONE

Fig. 1-19. Adrenal venous blood glucocorticoid secretion in man during operative trauma, at rest, and after an injection of ACTH. The principal glucocorticoid is cortisol (compound F), and the second is corticosterone (compound B). Only small amounts of cortisone (compound E and compound S) are secreted. (*From D. M. Hume et al., Surgery, 52:174, 1962.*)

reduction and conjugation of corticosteroids, severe liver disease may interfere with this step, and the level of blood conjugates may be very low. The kidney is responsible for excreting the greater part of the conjugated cortisol, so that the presence of kidney disease permits extremely high levels of the conjugates to build up in the bloodstream. The reduced and conjugated corticosteroid is no longer biologically effective.

Despite the obvious demonstration that an increased secretion of cortisol occurs in response to almost all types of trauma, that cortisol is necessary for the organism to withstand trauma successfully, and that patients with unrecognized adrenal insufficiency die following trauma whereas patients with bilateral adrenalectomy can tolerate trauma if given exogenous cortisol, adrenal insufficiency is rarely the cause of death after injury.

Fig. 1-20. Control of ACTH and cortisol. The cardiovascular system signals atrial and arterial receptors by means of pressures ($\bar{P}_{at}$ and $\bar{P}_a$), and atrial volume and rate of change of that volume (V, V̇). Signals are first processed in the nuclei of the solitary tract (NTS) and then ascend to the hypothalamus for control of CRF. Both ACTH and cortisol (F) are distributed, bound, and metabolized (D, B, M), and the results of these processes establish the plasma concentrations. Cortisol feedback may inhibit release of ACTH at hypothalamic and pituitary sites. Cortisol acts with other hormones to increase blood volume. Other stimuli reach the hypothalamus as shown.

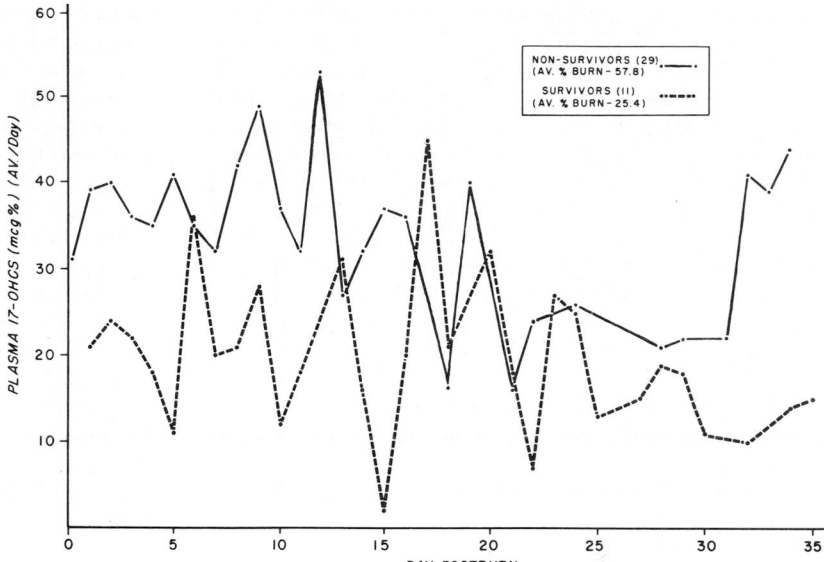

Fig. 1-21. Plasma 17-OHCS values in burn patients. It may be seen that the values in those patients who ultimately recovered gradually declined during the postburn period, whereas those patients who did not survive had higher values at first and later showed gradually increasing values up to the time of death.

It was demonstrated by Ingle that adrenalectomized animals traumatized while on a constant dose of corticosteroids showed some of the metabolic changes formerly ascribed to an *increased* secretion of these hormones, and this effect has been termed by him the "permissive" action of corticosteroids. Recent observations in our own laboratory indicate that restitution of blood volume required *increased* cortisol, so that the permissive action cannot be the sole explanation of the effect of cortisol in trauma. However, paraplegic patients, who fail to respond to operative trauma with an increased secretion of cortisol, generally tolerate the operative procedure well. These seeming paradoxes may be explained, at least in part, in the following ways:

In severe trauma, hepatic conjugation of corticosteroids into the inactive form may be reduced, so that larger amounts of unconjugated (active) corticosteroids are suddenly available even though the rate of infusion or secretion remains constant. The secretion of cortisol in the paraplegic remains low despite trauma because of the absence of afferent nerve impulses, but it can still increase if uncompensated hemorrhage or infection supervenes or if hypothalamic stimulation results from hypoglycemia or an excitatory anesthetic agent. Finally, an operative trauma is far better tolerated in patients whose body cells have not been deprived of the adrenal corticosteroids preoperatively than in those in whom preexisting deficiency is present. For this reason the patient who has adrenal insufficiency because of Addison's disease will tolerate the immediate operative event less well than a normal patient whose adrenals are removed without his being given cortisol or one whose adrenals are suppressed by prolonged corticosteroid administration which is stopped abruptly at operation. Nevertheless it should be emphasized that when in the past bilateral adrenalectomy was attempted in patients prior to the availability of cortisone, it was universally fatal, and hypophysectomy without corticosteroid support was likewise accompanied by an increased mortality.

However, in the absence of corticosteroid administration, hypophysectomy is tolerated far better than adrenalectomy.

Adrenal exhaustion, which was once thought to occur following prolonged trauma, probably never occurs. Most patients who die following injury, sepsis, burns, infection and other forms of severe prolonged trauma die with very high blood levels of corticosteroids (Fig. 1-21). In fact the very existence of continued high levels of plasma corticosteroids in the severely burned patient is usually a bad prognostic sign, suggesting that the trauma of burns is continuing and severe (Figs. 1-21 and 1-22). Nonetheless there is an occasional burned patient who shows evidences of adrenal insufficiency; there is an occasional patient in whom it develops in response to bilateral adrenal hemor-

Fig. 1-22. Relationship between plasma 17-OHCS and percentage of burn. It may be seen that the more severe the burn, the higher in general were the plasma 17-OHCS values.

rhage due to anticoagulant therapy; and there is an occasional patient in whom prolonged corticosteroid administration or preexisting Addison's disease has been unrecognized at the time of operation. Since the operative event is so apt to be fatal under these circumstances and since excellent replacement therapy is now available, adrenal insufficiency becomes an important and preventable cause of postoperative demise, despite its rarity. The causes and manifestations of adrenal insufficiency are dealt with further in the chapter on the adrenal (Chap. 37).

The Waterhouse-Friderichsen syndrome, which consists of bilateral adrenal hemorrhage in patients, usually children, with meningococcal septicemia, was originally thought to produce death as a consequence of adrenal failure. When death occurs in this condition, however, it occurs very rapidly and is due to the meningococcal septicemia—the adrenal hemorrhage occurring as a terminal complication and an almost incidental finding. These patients die with elevated blood cortisol levels.

When the patient has been found to have adrenal insufficiency, replacement therapy is given. While orally or intravenously administered cortisol is effective almost at once, intramuscularly administered cortisol acetate is slowly absorbed and does not become maximally effective until 12 to 18 hours after administration. Initial therapy therefore always should be intravenous and should consist of 100 to 200 mg of cortisol as the 21-hemisuccinate or phosphate. These two conjugates are lysed quickly in blood.

RENIN

Most traumatic events lead to increased secretion of renin from the cells of the juxtaglomerular apparatus of the renal afferent arterioles. The secretion of renin is under the control of multiple factors. The principal factors that

lead to increased secretion of renin are increased sympathetic stimulation of the juxtaglomerular cells through a beta adrenergic mechanism, decreased renal arterial perfusion pressure, and decreased delivery of sodium chloride to the macula densa (a collection of modified distal tubular cells which have a constant proximity to the juxtaglomerular apparatus of the afferent arteriole) of the distal tubule. Following trauma, all three of these factors may stimulate increased secretion of renin as sympathetic nervous activity is increased, as arterial pressure falls, and as renal mechanisms for conservation of sodium and water in the proximal tubule come into effect. The principal factors leading to inhibition of renin release are angiotensin II, vasopressin, and potassium. Again, the plasma levels of all these factors are elevated after trauma, but in general the stimulatory factors outweigh the inhibitory ones. Renin released into the circulation acts as an enzyme to convert angiotensinogen (a hepatic α_2-globulin) to angiotensin I. The latter is converted by an enzyme to the active form angiotensin II, an octapeptide. The converting enzyme appears to have its major activity in the lung but is present in other tissues as well. Angiotensin II stimulates the adrenal cortex to secrete aldosterone. It is also the most potent hyperten-

Fig. 1-23. Signal flow in the control of secretion of aldosterone (+, stimulation; −, inhibition). *RF*, reticular formation; *C*, corticotropin-releasing factor; *NTS*, nucleus tractus solitarius; *VMC*, vasomotor center; *SNS*, sympathetic nervous system; *BV*, blood volume; *BP*, blood pressure; *MAP*, mean arterial pressure; *Na DELIV.*, sodium delivery; *MD*, macula densa; *JG*, juxtaglomerular apparatus; *TBW*, total body water; *DOC*, desoxycorticosterone; *B*, corticosterone; *18-OH-B*, 18-hydroxycorticosterone; *ECF*, extracellular fluid. (*From T. S. Harrison, D. S. Gann, A. J. Edis, and R. H. Egdahl, "Surgical Disorders of the Adrenal Gland," p. 13, Grune & Stratton, New York, 1975.*)

sive agent known. In addition, angiotensin acts to increase the secretion of vasopressin and of ACTH from the pituitary to constrict the veins, thus decreasing vascular compliance, and to limit excretion of sodium and water by decreasing glomerular filtration.

ALDOSTERONE

The increased secretion of aldosterone seen in response to injury results from increased stimulation of the zona glomerulosa of the adrenal cortex by three factors: angiotensin II, ACTH, and potassium. As indicated previously, the levels of all three of these factors are elevated in injury. The effect of angiotensin II is certainly more potent than that of ACTH in stimulating secretion of aldosterone in the chronic state, but both factors appear important in the acute response of the adrenal cortex to hypovolemia. The control of aldosterone synthesis and secretion is illustrated in Fig. 1-23. Aldosterone acts on the distal nephron to increase reabsorption of sodium, in part together with chloride and water and in part in exchange for potassium and hydrogen. The latter effect is critical for life, since it is the principal mechanism by which the kidney may excrete the potassium and acid which build up in severe trauma.

EPINEPHRINE AND NOREPINEPHRINE

Epinephrine and norepinephrine are both secreted in response to trauma, although the amounts of these substances secreted during operative trauma depend to a considerable extent on the anesthesia employed. Ether, for example, is a strong stimulus to epinephrine release, whereas Nembutal inhibits it almost entirely. The increased secretion of epinephrine and norepinephrine is quite short-lived and is usually limited to the day of trauma unless the injury is a very severe and continuing one. During operative trauma, with the anesthetic agents commonly employed, there is a greater total secretion of norepinephrine than of epinephrine. This is probably because the entire source of epinephrine is from the adrenal medulla, whereas norepinephrine is also secreted from the sympathetic nerve endings. There is a greater secretion of epinephrine in the adrenal venous blood than of norepinephrine, though this is not striking (Fig. 1-24).

Epinephrine and norepinephrine both increase cardiac output and elevate the blood pressure; epinephrine stimulates glycogenolysis and lipolysis and inhibits release of insulin. Increased secretion of the catecholamines is brought about both by changes in blood volume and by afferent sensory impulses. Cells in the posterior hypothalamus are stimulated and send impulses down through the parabrachial region of the pons to the lateral reticular nucleus of the medulla. From this point, impulses travel down the cord to the intermediolateral cell columns and out into the sympathetic efferents. Adrenal medullary secretory activity is brought about through the splanchnic sympathetics. Denervation of the adrenal stops the secretion of catecholamines in the adrenal venous blood. Some noxious stimuli, such as endotoxin, can act directly upon the hypothalamic sympathetic control centers to produce epinephrine and norepinephrine release (see Fig. 1-5). Hypoglycemia is also a stimulus to epinephrine and nor-

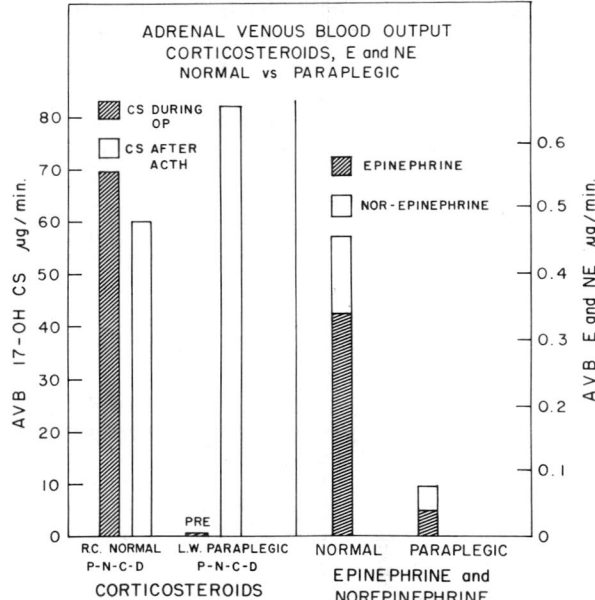

Fig. 1-24. Adrenal venous blood corticosteroids, epinephrine, and norepinephrine in normal versus paraplegic patients. It may be seen that the intraoperative production of 17-OHCS in the paraplegic patient was so low as to be nearly unmeasurable whereas after the injection of ACTH it rose promptly to a very high level. The secretion of epinephrine and norepinephrine too was greatly reduced in paraplegic patients.

epinephrine release. This apparently acts at a hypothalamic level. Although histamine in large doses is a potent stimulus to epinephrine release, it is doubtful whether the amounts of histamine released physiologically play any role in the increased secretion of catecholamines seen in response to trauma.

VASOPRESSIN (ANTIDIURETIC HORMONE, ADH)

Most trauma is accompanied by an increased secretion of ADH brought about by afferent neural stimuli impinging upon the hypothalamus. Stimulation of the supraoptic and paraventricular nuclei leads to a release of ADH from the posterior pituitary. Hypovolemia is also a potent stimulus to ADH release, acting through receptors and pathways similar to those controlling secretion of ACTH. Vasopressin acts on the distal tubule and collecting duct to increase water reabsorption and also has an important role in effecting splanchnic vasoconstriction. In the presence of increased vasopressin, administration of water without salt will lead to dilutional hyponatremia and, in the extreme, to water intoxication.

With head injury two additional peculiarities in ADH secretion sometimes occur. The first of these is called *inappropriate ADH secretion*. This is a term given to excessive secretion of ADH beyond that needed to promote homeostasis. The ADH secretion continues after the initial period of damage and produces a low urinary output with high osmolarity and a profound dilutional hyponatremia (see Chap. 42). The converse phenomenon of diabetes insipidus is sometimes seen with head injury, particularly basilar skull fractures. This may be either temporary or permanent and results from damage to the supraoptico-hypophyseal system. It may cause severe dehydration or even death in patients with head injury and coma who are given tube feedings. Since the patient is comatose, he cannot express thirst, and a continued excessive polyuria dehydrates him, leading to hypernatremia. This is compounded by the use of tube feedings high in sodium, small protein fractions, and glucose, which thus combines an excessive sodium load with an osmotic diuresis, further dehydrating the patient.

GROWTH HORMONE (GH)

The hypothalamic mechanisms controlling release of growth hormone involve both stimulation and inhibition. Pituitary release of growth hormone is stimulated by growth-hormone-releasing factor, coming principally from the ventromedial, arcuate, and perhaps dorsomedial nuclei. The growth-hormone-inhibiting hormone, somatostatin, comes principally from the preoptic area and from the amygdala. The release of growth hormone is promoted by hypoglycemia and also especially by blood loss and tissue injury. Meyer and Knobil found hemorrhage to be a potent stimulus to growth-hormone release in monkeys, and Carey et al. found war wounds to be strong stimuli to growth-hormone release in man. Carey et al. postulated that the elevated levels of plasma amino acid that were seen in injury were responsible for the increase in GH secretion. This seems unlikely, however, as plasma amino acid levels usually are not elevated in injury, and arginine concentration, which is the best stimulus to GH release, decreases. Growth hormone may act in trauma to increase glucose levels by opposing the action of insulin, by promoting gluconeogenesis, by promoting the synthesis of certain specific proteins, and by promoting lipolysis.

GLUCAGON

Glucagon is a diabetogenic hormone made by the alpha cells of the pancreatic islets. A glucagonlike substance is also made in the upper small intestine. Glucagon secretion is stimulated by hypoglycemia and by sympathetic stimulation acting directly on the alpha cell. There is increasing interest in the role of glucagon in the metabolism of injury. Some of its effects are listed in Tables 1-2 and 1-3.

Glucagon is a marked stimulus to lipolysis, increasing cyclic adenosine monophosphate (cyclic AMP) in fat, which in turn increases the activity of the lipolytic enzyme that hydrolyzes triglyceride to fatty acid and glycerol. The elevated free fatty acid levels stimulate gluconeogenesis, but glucagon has a direct effect on gluconeogenesis as well. Glucagon also promotes glycogenolysis through cyclic AMP activation of phosphorylase.

The main results of increased glucagon secretion in trauma are to produce increases in blood glucose through stimulation of glycogenolysis, gluconeogenesis, and lipolysis. Glucagon also promotes ketogenesis and ureagenesis and decreases lipoprotein release, but these effects are less striking than those relating to glucose and fat mobilization.

Glucagon also produces ionotropic cardiovascular effects when given to patients or animals in shock. These effects consist of an increase in cardiac output and stroke volume,

and a decrease in peripheral vascular resistance despite β-receptor blockade. To what degree these effects are part of the physiologic response to injury is unknown.

Hormones with Unaltered or Decreased Secretion in Trauma

TSH—THYROXIN

Because there is a hypermetabolic state in the immediate postoperative or posttraumatic period, it was originally thought that TSH secretion led to increased thyroid activity. More recent studies seem to indicate that this is not so. Although the presence of thyroid hormone is necessary for the normal functioning of organs in response to a traumatic stress, an increased secretion is apparently not necessary to meet this challenge, and release of thyroid hormones may actually decrease after trauma.

INSULIN

Insulin secretion is not usually increased in response to trauma. Epinephrine, which is, inhibits the release of insulin, and many factors are working to produce an elevation of the blood sugar level and to make carbohydrate available. The administration of glucose intravenously may call forth an insulin secretion, but there is a relatively diabetic glucose tolerance curve in the immediate posttraumatic period. The relative hypoinsulinism of trauma augments the hyperglycemia, gluconeogenesis, decreased amino acid

Table 1-2. REPORTED EFFECTS OF GLUCAGON ON ISOLATED LIVER

Process	Change	Involvement of cyclic AMP
Glycogenolysis	Increase	Yes
Phosphorylase	Increase	Yes
Gluconeogenesis	Increase	Yes
Glycogen synthesis	Decrease	Yes
Glycogen synthetase	Decrease	Yes
Ureogenesis	Increase	Yes
Protein synthesis	Decrease (?)	?
Protein breakdown	Increase (?)	?
Ketogenesis	Increase	Yes
Lipolysis	Increase	Yes
Amino acid uptake	Increase	Yes
Tyrosine aminotransferase	Increase	Yes
p-Pyruvate carboxykinase	Increase	Yes
Lysosome activation	Increase	?
K⁺ release	Increase	Yes
Ca⁺⁺ release	Increase	Yes
Mitochondrial pyruvate uptake .	Increase	?
Krebs cycle	Increase	?
Transamination	Increase	?
Lipoprotein release	Decrease	Yes

SOURCE: J. H. Exton, M. Vi, S. B. Lewis, and C. R. Park, Mechanism of Glucagon Activation of Gluconeogenesis, in H. D. Soling and B. Willms (eds.), "Regulation of Gluconeogenesis," p. 160, Academic Press, Inc., New York, 1971.

Table 1-3. SOME METABOLIC EFFECTS OF HORMONES WITH GENERALLY INCREASED SECRETION IN TRAUMA

	Proteolysis (in muscle)	Gluconeogenesis (in liver & kidney)	Glycolysis Muscle	Glycolysis Adipose tissue	Glycogenolysis Liver	Glycogenolysis Muscle	Lipolysis (adipose tissue, liver, muscle)	Insulin antagonism	Insulin secretion	Sodium retention	Potassium loss	Water retention
ACTH-cortisol	+++	+++	0	0	....	0	++	++	++	++	++	0
Renin-aldosterone	....	....	..	....	....	......	....	......	......	+++	+++	++
Epinephrine, norepinephrine	+	++*	0	++	++++	++	++++*	+++	0	+	0	+
ADH	....	....	..	++	....	......	....	......	......	......	......	++++
Growth hormone	0	+	0	++	....	......	++*	+	+++			
Glucagon	++	+++*	0	....	++†	......	+++*	++	+++			

*Only in the presence of the adrenal corticosteroids.
†By stimulating catecholamine secretion.

uptake, and lipolysis stimulated by epinephrine, ACTH, cortisol, GH, and glucagon.

FSH-LH AND SEX HORMONE SECRETION

No increased secretion of FSH or LH occurs in response to trauma, and there is some evidence to indicate that the secretion of these substances may even be inhibited somewhat during this period. Menstrual periods may be missed in the immediate postoperative period but may also occur on schedule or early. The emotional response to the trauma may to some extent influence cyclic activity. It is much more common to note amenorrhea in patients with chronic renal failure, however, than in the otherwise healthy woman who undergoes a severe trauma.

There are few data on the secretion of androgens of either testicular or adrenal origin in the posttraumatic period. No good data indicate whether or not adrenal androgens are increased following trauma. In the immediate posttrauma period there is only a very modest increase in urinary 17-ketosteroids.

Goals of Endocrine Changes

Survival after injury depends critically upon continued delivery of oxygen and nutrients to the brain and heart. The initial trend toward cardiovascular stabilization in the presence of hypovolemia is brought about by baroreflex increase in sympathetic nervous activity. The resulting increase in peripheral vasoconstriction may be augmented by the actions of angiotensin II, vasopressin, and circulating catecholamines. The increase in myocardial contractility may be augmented by circulating epinephrine and glucagon. Other hormonal changes also seem organized to promote the restitution of blood volume and thus cardiovascular stabilization. Increased secretion of cortisol, glucagon, and probably growth hormone appear to be required to bring about the prompt increase in extracellular osmolality that follows volume loss and that promotes the movement of fluids from the cells to the interstitium to

Fig. 1-25. The neuroendocrine response to injury (pain, hemorrhage, and ECF loss) viewed as a homeostatic reflex organized for the control of blood volume and for cardiovascular stabilization. In response to volume loss the inhibition of the central nervous system (CNS) by the cardiovascular system (CVS) is released, leading to increased activity of the sympathetic nervous system (SNS) and to the endocrine changes described in the text. The autonomic and multihormonal reflexes are coordinated for the restitution of blood volume and for cardiovascular stability. (*From D. S. Gann, Ann NY Acad Sci, 297:591, 1977.*)

promote restitution of blood volume on protein, as discussed below. Many of the detrimental metabolic consequences of injury follow upon this immediate and homeostatic hormonally induced change in plasma osmolality. The renal effects of hormones increased after injury also tend to support the restitution of blood volume by limiting renal loss of salt and water. In the absence of such conservative mechanisms, homeostatic increases in blood volume would be negated by continuing renal loss. Thus the actions of the catecholamines in promoting salt and water reabsorption in the proximal tubule and of aldosterone and vasopressin in promoting reabsorption of salt and water in the distal nephron can again be viewed in terms of circulatory support. As indicated previously, the release of many of these hormones can be brought about by tissue injury per se. Such reflexly induced release of hormones may anticipate the hormonal response to loss of plasma volume. Most of these anticipatory responses can be inhibited by increased cortisol, whereas severe hypovolemia leads to a responsive ACTH release which is not cortisol-suppressible. Thus the general hormonal response to injury can be viewed in one sense as part of a cardiovascular reflex aimed at restitution of blood volume and ultimate stabilization of the cardiovascular system, as shown diagrammatically in Fig. 1-25. Some of these effects are brought about by the metabolic effects outlined in Table 1-3.

One may summarize the endocrine changes which occur in response to injury by saying that they seem to be directed toward water and salt conservation, blood pressure maintenance, gluconeogenesis, glycolysis, general mobilization of carbohydrate, lipolysis, the outpouring of hormones essential for cell life, and the providing of ready energy to the muscles, heart, and brain.

METABOLIC CHANGES

Following a severe injury there is marked tissue wasting and weight loss. This is partly due to semistarvation and partly to the extreme catabolism which occurs in the immediate postinjury period. The intensity and duration of the catabolic period depends upon the severity of the injury and on whether or not the injury is protracted by sepsis and other serious complications. The protein loss is far greater in healthy young men than in elderly patients, women, or children (Fig. 1-26), but it can be greatly decreased by the administration of amino acids and calories intravenously.

The metabolic changes which accompany trauma depend not only upon the intensity and duration of the injury but upon the presence or absence of shock, the degree of anoxia, the type of repair solutions administered to the patient, and the success or failure of the body in adapting itself to the injury. In order to understand the metabolic response to injury it becomes necessary to examine the energy sources available to the body, the effect of starvation and hyperalimentation, the changes produced by increased hormone secretion, and the adaptive mechanisms essential to recovery from profound injury.

Energy Metabolism

Energy is stored in the body in the form of carbohydrate (glycogen), protein, and fat (triglycerides). Glycogen is stored in muscle and liver in combination with water and electrolytes, so that 1 Gm of glycogen yields only 1 or 2 kcal instead of the 4 kcal found in 1 Gm of dry carbohydrate. Protein is stored primarily in muscle, and, like carbohydrate, in combination with water. Therefore, muscles are only one-quarter to one-fifth protein. Furthermore, body protein is not designed primarily as a source of fuel, but performs other important functions in the form of enzymes, plasma protein, structural protein, cardiac and skeletal muscle, etc. Ingested protein beyond that needed to replenish body stores is metabolized, the nitrogen is excreted as urea, and the calories thus created are expended or, if unneeded, stored as fat.

Lipid is not stored in combination with water, and body fat therefore yields lipid contents as high as 90 percent of total weight. One gram of body fat thus provides nearly the full 9.4 kcal present in one gram of pure triglyceride.

Table 1-4 is modified from a concise and lucid review by Cahill on the metabolic effects of starvation in man. It may be seen that extracellular fluids and muscle and liver glycogen make very small contributions to the body energy pool when compared to muscle protein, and especially to fat—the major energy depot. During starvation man attempts to conserve protein by burning fat instead, and to preserve muscle and liver glycogen by accelerating gluconeogenesis. Cahill did not list plasma protein as a potential source of fuel, because in simple, short-term starvation the body is able to replenish plasma protein at a rate equal to its degradation. Plasma protein can probably be used as fuel, however, as demonstrated by the experiments of Allen et al., in which puppies were maintained and grew while receiving protein only in the form of intravenous plasma. With prolonged fasting in the face of trauma and marked catabolism, endogenous plasma proteins are burned, and the liver is incapable of synthesizing albumin at a rate equal to its loss, necessitating the replacement of plasma proteins from exogenous sources. Red blood cells probably are consumed as well. It is extremely important, therefore, to administer amino acids, albumin, plasma, or whole blood to surgical patients who are in a catabolic state and unable to eat, not only to replace plasma protein and blood lost externally or to the third space but also that which is burned as fuel.

With acute trauma, anoxia, and exercise muscle and liver glycogen are used as emergency fuels, and with severe or prolonged injury muscle protein is used as well, unless attempts are made to conserve it by the vigorous intravenous administration of protein or amino acids, and calories.

Starvation

An understanding of the metabolic changes seen following injury in man requires a consideration of the effects of starvation, which may accompany injury of a progressive or long-term nature. These are shown in Figs. 1-27 and 1-28. Glucose is derived from glycogenolysis of liver glycogen and from gluconeogenesis. The new glucose formed from gluconeogenesis derives in part from amino acids and in part from glycerol, which comes from the triglycerides of body fat. In the early fasting state, shown in Fig. 1-27 and in Table 1-5, a 70-kg man would be expected to make about 16 Gm of new glucose from glycerol and about 43 Gm from muscle protein for a total of 59 Gm a day. In addition to this he would obtain 85 Gm of glucose from glycogen breakdown and 36 Gm from recycled glucose, for a total of 180 Gm a day. Whereas the brain normally completely metabolizes glucose to carbon dioxide and water, other glycolytic tissues such as peripheral nerve, erythrocytes, leukocytes, bone marrow, renal medulla, and to a lesser extent normal muscle metabolize glucose mainly by converting it to lactate and pyruvate. These substances are released into the bloodstream and carried back to the liver and kidney, where they are remade into glucose, thus contributing to the total available glucose without creating any net gain of glucose. This process is known as the *Cori cycle;* its effect is to provide energy for the peripheral tissues by the anaerobic glycolysis of glucose, while the energy thus given up is regained in the liver by the reconversion of lactate into glucose utilizing energy derived from the oxidation of fat (Fig. 1-29). The entire process of gluconeogenesis requires energy, and this energy is sup-

Table 1-4. FUEL COMPOSITION OF NORMAL 70-kg MAN

Fuel	Kilograms	Calories
Tissues:		
Fat (adipose triglyceride)	15.0	141,000
Protein (mainly muscle)	6.0	24,000
Glycogen (muscle)	0.150	600
Glycogen (liver).	0.075	300
Total	. . . . . .	165,900
Circulating fuels:		
Glucose (extracellular fluid) . . .	0.020	80
Free fatty acids (plasma)	0.0003	3
Triglycerides (plasma)	0.003	30
Plasma proteins	0.210	840
Total	. . . . . .	953

SOURCE: Adapted from G. F. Cahill, Jr., *N Eng J Med,* **282**:668, 1970.

Table 1-5. GLUCOSE AVAILABLE IN EARLY STARVATION STATE IN A 70-kg MAN

Origin	Amount of glucose, Gm/24 hr
New glucose (gluconeogenesis):	
Fat (glycerol)	16
Protein	43
Stored or recycled glucose:	
Glycogen	85
Recycled glucose	36
Total	180

Fig. 1-26. A comparison of the nitrogen excretion in a burned woman and a burned man illustrating the far greater catabolism and nitrogen loss in the man. *A.* Twenty-eight-year-old white man with 55 percent burn. *B.* Thirty-one-year-old white woman with 55 percent burn.

plied by the oxidation of fatty acids. By means of the Cori cycle the amount of glucose that has to be supplied from protein breakdown is limited.

Whereas the brain and the other glycolytic tissues depend directly upon glucose for their energy, the rest of the organism derives its energy from fat, in the form of either fatty acids or ketone bodies created by the partial oxidation of fatty acids to acetoacetate or β-hydroxybutyrate. Although these tissues, especially muscle, readily utilize glucose in the presence of insulin in the nonfasting state or with vigorous exercise or anoxia, they abandon glucose metabolism during starvation, thus helping to conserve body protein.

The liver derives its energy from fatty acid oxidation in two stages: The partial oxidation of fatty acids to acetyl coenzyme A (acetyl CoA), and the terminal combustion of the acetate in the tricarboxylic acid cycle (Krebs cycle). About one-third of the total energy in fat is ordinarily derived from the first stage, but in starvation ketosis the first stage provides the major portion of the liver's energy, since the function of the tricarboxylic acid cycle is diminished and acetyl CoA is disposed of in the circulation as

acetoacetate and β-hydroxybutyrate. Ketogenesis generally, though not always, parallels the rate of gluconeogenesis.

In prolonged fasting rather profound changes in metabolism occur, as shown in Table 1-6 and in Fig. 1-28. It is apparent that liver and muscle glycogen cannot continue to supply glucose at all, since the total body store is only 225 Gm and this would be exhausted in a few days. Furthermore, body protein cannot continue to be converted to glucose at the rate of 75 Gm a day, since in about a month this would deplete the total body protein beyond the level which would permit survival. It thus becomes apparent that diminished utilization of glucose and sparing of body protein is essential for the survival of prolonged starvation.

If the brain is the one organ which needs glucose normally, it must either reduce its fuel consumption or substi-

NITROGEN METABOLISM FOLLOWING THERMAL INJURY

Fig. 1-26. Continued.

tute another fuel, or the body must make glucose directly from fatty acids, which it cannot do, since the enzymes required for this are not found in animals.

Owen and coworkers found that on prolonged fasting the ketone bodies, acetoacetate and β-hydroxybutyrate, replaced glucose as the predominant fuel for brain metabolism. This change of fuels by the brain did not produce any deficits in the function of the brain or change in the electroencephalogram. The amount of glucose completely utilized by the brain drops from 144 Gm to 30 Gm a day, 14 of the 44 Gm presented to the brain being recycled through the Cori cycle. The blood ketones are capable of being utilized by the brain in part because they, like glu-cose, are water-soluble and readily penetrate the blood-brain barrier.

The body not only manages to conserve protein, but also maintains almost normal levels of blood glucose, glycerol, amino acids, lactate, and pyruvate. The blood levels of free fatty acids and ketones are of course markedly increased.

One other striking change that occurs in prolonged fasting is a shift from the liver to the kidney of gluconeogenesis from protein sources. The liver continues to make glucose by recycling lactate and pyruvate, and it also continues gluconeogenesis from glycerol. Almost all of the gluconeogenesis from amino acids, however, takes place in the kidney, where there is a stoichiometric relation between ammoniogenesis and gluconeogenesis. The ammoniogenesis is required to maintain acid homoeostasis by titrating the ketone acids lost in the urine.

While there is only a slight change in concentration of total amino acids during starvation, there are striking changes in the values for individual amino acids. Glycine increases during starvation; valine, leucine, and isoleucine increase briefly and then decrease, arghine falls progressively; and lysine does not change at all. Alanine falls progressively, decreasing to less than one-third of the fed level. Alanine is the principal amino acid utilized by the liver for gluconeogenesis, and it is the decrease of alanine during fasting which limits gluconeogenesis in the liver.

Table 1-6. GLUCOSE AVAILABLE IN LATE STARVATION STATE IN A 70-kg MAN

Origin	Amount of glucose, Gm/24 hr
New glucose (gluconeogenesis):	
Fat (glycerol)	18
Protein	12
Stored or recycled glucose:	
Glycogen	0
Recycled glucose	50
Total	80

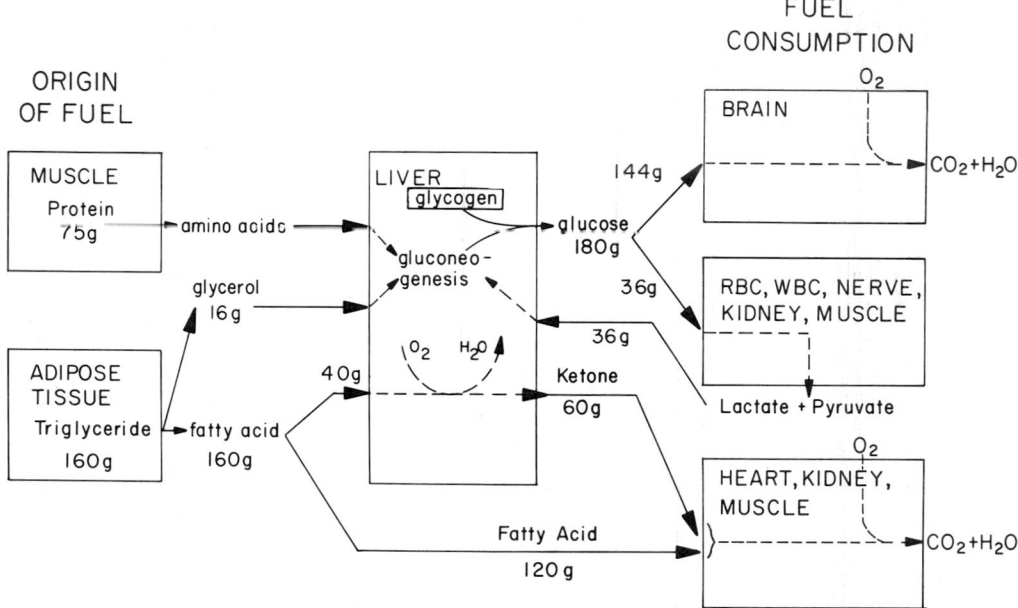

FASTING MAN
(24 hours, basal : ~1800 calories)

Fig. 1-27. Scheme of fuel metabolism in a normal, fasted man. The two primary fuel sources are muscle protein and fat. The brain oxidizes glucose completely, the glycolyzers break down glucose by anaerobic metabolism into lactate and pyruvate, which are remade in the liver into glucose, and the rest of the body burns fatty acids and ketones. (*Adapted from G. F. Cahill, N Engl J Med, 282:668, 1970.*)

Alanine comes from muscle protein and also may be synthesized from pyruvate, as shown in Fig. 1-29.

ROLE OF THE HORMONES IN ALTERED METABOLISM OF STARVATION

The presence of cortisol is essential for a normal rate of gluconeogenesis, and this hormone participates in the hyperglycemia which occurs in the early posttraumatic period. The administration of large doses of cortisol analogues to fasting subjects did not result in an increased rate of nitrogen excretion, however.

GH likewise fails to increase daily nitrogen excretion in fasting subjects but elevates the level of insulin and blood glucose. Dwarfs having a congenital lack of growth hormones were found to be capable of mobilizing fatty acids and excreting nitrogen at rates similar to those observed in normal persons of the same size.

There is a marked rise in circulating glucagon in patients fasting for 2 or 3 days. Glucagon not only increases glycogenolysis in the liver but also increases gluconeogenesis, directly opposing insulin in this regard. Glucagon appears to have a role in regulating the level of circulating amino acids. The near absence of glucagon in totally pancreatectomized subjects may be the reason that such patients require less insulin to affect homeostasis than do most severely ill diabetics.

Insulin has at least two important effects on the regulation of fuel sources: it increases the rate of synthesis of triglycerides in adipose tissue, in which it opposes the catecholamines, ACTH, and glucagon; and it increases amino acid uptake by muscle and protein synthesis in which it appears to be opposed by glucagon and cortisol. Insulin, therefore, not only impedes fatty acid release but impedes amino acid release from muscle as well.

The hypothalamus controls all the hormones regulating glucose production, including glucagon and insulin. In addition, it contains an appetite-satiety center which is presumably responsive to the blood glucose level, and has been said by Conway et al. to regulate lipolysis in response to changes in glucose levels.

Gamble demonstrated many years ago that small amounts of administered glucose were capable of decreasing the excretion of nitrogen in the urine; this concept has recently been challenged by Blackburn et al. The classic concept is to maintain that the daily administration of 100 Gm of glucose given intravenously spares the proteolysis of about 50 Gm of protein. This effect presumably results from the increased secretion of insulin brought about by the elevated glucose level which in turn inhibits muscle proteolysis. The need for gluconeogenesis by the liver is no longer present, since the administered glucose takes care of the brain's need. Ketogenesis also ceases, and the rest of the body continues to utilize free fatty acids.

Clearly it is important to spare protein breakdown in the starved injured patient, since protein breakdown leads to muscle wasting, ineffective coughing, pneumonia, impaired wound repair, poor resistance to infection, and diminished synthesis of enzymes and plasma proteins. Blackburn et al. contend that they were unable to achieve nitrogen balance in fasting patients given an amino acid solution intravenously in combination with 100 Gm of glucose every 24 hours whereas they were able to achieve

Fig. 1-28. Scheme of fuel metabolism after 5 or 6 weeks of starvation. Liver glycogen sources are depleted, there is a diminished utilization of muscle protein, the brain is burning ketones, and gluconeogenesis from amino acids is taking place primarily in the kidney. (*Adapted from G. F. Cahill, N Engl J Med, 282:668, 1970.*)

Fig. 1-29. The Cori cycle (top) provides for a transfer of energy from the liver to the periphery. Glucose gives up energy in the periphery by anaerobic glycolysis to lactate and pyruvate. The latter are then remade into glucose in the liver, utilizing energy derived by the metabolism of fatty acids. In the glucose-to-alanine-to-glucose cycle (bottom) described by Felig et al., glucose is metabolized to pyruvate in muscle; pyruvate is then converted to alanine, which is transported to the liver, where it is remade into glucose.

nitrogen balance in those patients given the same amount of amino acids without any added glucose. Their explanation is that the administration of glucose increases the output of insulin, which in turn exerts an antilipolytic effect which decreases the mobilization of fatty acids and makes it necessary to continue using muscle protein as a source of energy. By giving protein without glucose the insulin level remained low, and there was an increased mobilization of body fat with an associated ketosis, thus leading to a use of body fat as the energy source and sparing protein. Positive nitrogen balance could be achieved by administering 90 Gm of amino acid/day without any other caloric source. Although it may be true that small amounts of glucose, even in the presence of protein administration, may not lead to optimal utilization of body fat as an energy source, it is certainly true that the administration of hyperalimentation mixtures containing protein hydrolysates or amino acids in conjunction with an adequate caloric intake supplied by hypertonic glucose provides optimal protein sparing and improves wound healing and resistance to infection.

Metabolic Effects of Injury

The effects of trauma and sepsis on body metabolism are summarized in Table 1-7 and Fig. 1-30. In contrast to starvation, injury produces (1) hyperglycemia, unless the injury is overwhelming and fatal; (2) marked fatty acid mobilization and elevation of plasma free fatty acids; (3) a striking catabolism of muscle protein beyond that needed as a source for energy, in contrast to late starvation, where protein conservation is seen; (4) an increase in the synthesis of urea and the so-called "acute-phase reactants" (AP reactants) (Table 1-8); and (5) an increased extracellular osmolality.

Oxygen consumption is not increased in ordinary elective operations, but it is increased by as much as 25 percent after multiple fractures, and with severe sepsis may increase by 50 percent. Burns increase oxygen consumption by as much as 100 percent, partly because of sepsis and partly because of the break in the epidermis producing evaporative water loss which requires enormous expenditures of energy.

Carbohydrate Metabolism

The early elevation of blood glucose level after most types of injury is brought about primarily by the catecholamines and to a lesser extent by glucagon, cortisol, and growth hormone. There is an initial increase in hepatic glycogenolysis and an inhibition of insulin production. The elevated blood levels are also a consequence of enhancement of gluconeogenesis, brought about by cortisol and glucagon, and to a lesser extent by the catecholamines and GH. Cortisol also impedes the entry of glycolytic intermediates into the pentose shunt and into the tricarboxylic acid cycle, thus favoring increased release of glucose into blood. The increased plasma fatty acid concentrations also stimu-

Table 1-7. EFFECT OF TRAUMA ON CARBOHYDRATE, FAT, AND PROTEIN METABOLISM

Charge	Cause	Charge	Cause

Carbohydrate:
  Early hyperglycemia
	Increased glycogenolysis produced principally by CA* and to lesser extent by glucagon.
	Increased gluconeogenesis produced by increased fatty acid level and by 17-OHCS and GH.
	Insulin inhibition produced by CA, glucagon, 17-OHCS and GH.
		Triglycerides: no change
		
		Rise in β-hydroxybutyrate/acetoacetate ratio blood, liver, kidney, etc., in profound shock or sepsis
		Protein:
		  Muscle:
			In trauma there is an increased ability to remove excess lipids from bloodstream, thus compensating for increased fat mobilization.
			Hypoxia.

Hyperglycemia and glucose intolerance during convalescence	Moderate injury: insulin intolerance with decreased ability to oxidize glucose and block of conversion of pyruvate to two-carbon fragments. Severe injury: no change or an increase in rate oxidation glucose, but marked increase in glucose production.	Markedly increased catabolism Decreased protein synthesis	17-OHCS and glucagon promote catabolism muscle proteins to amino acids and inhibit protein synthesis. Starvation also leads to protein breakdown. Some breakdown due direct trauma, wound loss, etc. Protein catabolism above that needed for energy alone supplies carbohydrate intermediates, and is required to maintain level of circulating amino acids. Inhibition of increased insulin secretion. Insulin has an anabolic effect.
Hypoglycemia seen in profound shock or sepsis	Glycogen depletion. Utilization of glucose at rate faster than gluconeogenesis can provide it. Defect in gluconeogenesis.		

Table 1-7. Continued

Charge	Cause	Charge	Cause
Rise in lactate/pyruvate ratio in blood and tissue in profound shock or sepsis	Hypoxia, producing a block in conversion of pyruvate to acetyl CoA, rise in lactic acid level, and progressive tissue deficit of ATP.	Liver and kidney proteins: Increased turnover of protein, but no protein depletion	Increased protein synthesis involves largely "export" proteins like albumin and acute-phase (AP) reactants but probably involves intrinsic protein as well.
Fat: Fatty acid mobilization Elevated FFA plasma	CA and glucagon increase cyclic AMP in fat, thus increasing activity of lipolytic enzyme which hydrolyzes triglyceride to fatty acids and glycerol. GH and 17-OHCS have similar but much weaker effect. Insulin especially, and prostaglandins and metabolites (glucose, lactate, pyruvate, ketone bodies) to a lesser extent have opposite effect.		Whereas in starvation there may be a decrease in liver and kidney protein, in injury the 17-OHCS produces a preferential increase in catabolism of muscle protein, which leads to an increased synthesis of protein in liver and kidney—mainly through alanine release from muscle protein.
Elevation liver ketones	Moderate injury: FFA mobilization produces an increase in hepatic fatty acid oxidation to ketones. Glucagon stimulates this. Severe injury: Inhibition of liver citrate synthase due to ischemia, prevents acetyl CoA from entering tricarboxylic acid cycle, thus diverting it to synthesis of ketone bodies.	Plasma proteins: Increased catabolism Probably increased synthesis of albumin as well, but masked by catabolism γ-Globulin increased	Plasma proteins participate in protein catabolism seen in trauma. Liver increases synthesis of "export" proteins. γ-globulin increased by antibody production in response to sepsis.
Blood ketones unchanged or slightly elevated	Ketone metabolism unimpaired, some excess excreted urine.	Plasma amino acids: Decreased somewhat as gluconeogenesis uses up substrates; subsequently total kept fairly constant, although some glucogenic amino acids (such as alanine) tend to fail while lysine does not change at all and glycine rises	Exact mechanism unknown, though balance between insulin (which decreases amino acid release from muscle and decreases gluconeogenesis) and glucagon and 17-OHCS (which increase amino acid release from muscle and increase gluconeogenesis) plays an important regulatory role. If amino acids are infused at rates in excess of energy needs, the excess will be converted to fat and the nitrogen excreted in the urine, while the plasma level remains constant.
Lipoproteins: cholesterol falls	Cause unknown; related to albumin level; may be due to starvation, or to glucagon.		
		Urea: Urea synthesis greatly increased Urea excretion in urine greatly increased Plasma urea increased due to increased production; further increased if renal failure present	Increased deamination of alanine in liver to provide substrate for increased gluconeogenesis makes nitrogen available to the liver for synthesis into urea.
		AP reactants: Increased synthesis	Reason unknown.

*CA: catecholamines (epinephrine and norepinephrine).
17-OHCS: glucocorticoids (cortisol and corticosterone principally).
GH: growth hormone.
FFA: free fatty acids.

Fig. 1-30. Hypothetic scheme of rates of substrate flow in a traumatized individual excreting 40 Gm of nitrogen/day. Presumably reparative tissues are glucose utilizers, but the amount of glucose terminally combusted to carbon dioxide and that metabolized to lactate would depend both on the maturity of the tissue (presence of mitochondria) and on adequate perfusion and oxygenation. Fat still provides the bulk of the calories. (*From G. F. Cahill et al., in C. L. Fox, Jr., and G. G. Nahas [eds.]: "Body Fluid Replacement in the Surgical Patient," p. 286, Grune & Stratton, Inc., New York, 1970.*)

late gluconeogenesis, and the presence of available substrate, especially alanine, provides an additional stimulus to this reaction.

The presence of hyperglycemia provides a ready source of energy to the brain and thus may be important to early survival. Starvation reduces the ability of the body to tolerate shock. The administration of glucose prolongs survival after shock, as shown by Drucker and his colleagues in hypovolemic dogs and Berk and his associates in endotoxin shock. McNamara and his colleagues demonstrated that patients in hypovolemic shock who were resuscitated in the usual manner and at the same time received either 50% glucose, 25% mannitol, or 3% saline solution in equal total osmolar doses had a much greater increase in blood pressure and pulse pressure when they received glucose than with either of the other two agents. However, because of the different concentrations of the solutions, they may have induced different rates of leakage of protein into the interstitium. It appears quite possible that, as suggested by Järhult and by ourselves, the principal homeostatic significance of increased plasma glucose may be the resulting osmotic transfer of fluids, leading to restitution of blood volume.

While hemorrhagic shock has been found by some workers to be associated both with hyperglycemia and an

Table 1-8. ACUTE-PHASE (AP) REACTANTS

Haptoglobin
Fibrinogen
Ceruloplasmin
Seromucoid fraction
C-reactive protein
α_2-AP globulin
α_1-Acid glycoprotein
α_1-Antitrypsin

elevated insulin level, others have claimed that insulin levels are low. All agree, however, that there are elevated levels of anti-insulin hormones and that there is both a glucose intolerance and insulin resistance after injury.

During the recovery phase there continues to be a diabeticlike glucose tolerance curve which is more marked after severe injury. There is an insulin intolerance and a decrease in the ability to oxidize glucose. Drucker has demonstrated a partial block in the metabolic conversion of pyruvate to two-carbon fragments.

In profound shock or sepsis hypoglycemia may be present. This is due to depletion of glycogen stores and the utilization of glucose at a rate faster than gluconeogenesis can provide it. It is also due to a defect in gluconeogenesis. There may be a rise in the lactate/pyruvate ratio due to hypoxia, which produces a block in the conversion of pyruvate to acetyl CoA, a rise in the lactic acid level, and a progressive tissue deficit of adenosine triphosphate (ATP).

Fat Metabolism

Fat is the main energy source in trauma, as in starvation. The catecholamines, glucagon, ACTH, and GH increase cyclic AMP in fat, thus increasing the activity of the lipolytic enzyme which hydrolyzes triglyceride to fatty acid and glycerol. Lipolysis induced by these hormones requires the presence of cortisol.

The glycerol provides substrate for gluconeogenesis. The fatty acids are burned in the liver to supply energy for gluconeogenesis, and in the periphery to supply energy directly.

Liver ketone levels are elevated as a result of the increase in free fatty acids and the influence of glucagon. In very severe injury the level of ketones is further increased because of inhibition of liver citrate synthase, which prevents acetyl CoA from entering the tricarboxylic acid cycle, thus diverting it to the synthesis of ketone bodies.

In profound shock and sepsis there is a rise in the ratio of β-hydoxybutyrate to acetoacetate in blood, liver, kidney and other tissues as a consequence of hypoxia. As indicated above, the ketone bodies may provide an important source of energy to the brain. They may also contribute to the rise in extracellular osmolality.

Protein Metabolism

The daily intake of protein for a healthy young adult is usually about 80 to 120 Gm, or 13 to 20 Gm of nitrogen. Of this quantity of nitrogen about 2 to 3 Gm/day is lost in the stool and 11 to 17 Gm in the urine. Urinary nitrogen excretion increases greatly after injury, rising to as much as 30 to 50 Gm/day following severe trauma. This is nearly all in the form of urea nitrogen. In the patient with anuria or one whose kidneys have been removed preparatory to transplantation, operative trauma produces a very rapid rise in blood urea nitrogen (BUN) in comparison to that seen between dialyses in the nontraumatized state (Fig. 1-31).

The increase in nitrogen excretion begins shortly after injury, reaches a peak about the first week, and may continue for 3 to 7 weeks. In elective operative procedures the negative nitrogen balance is rapidly reversed, but in the burned patient the negative balance may be prolonged for a very considerable period of time. During this time the patient may lose 50 to 75 lb of weight. In the early postinjury period protein may be lost from the body surface if there is a large open or burned area, into the peritoneal cavity if there is peritonitis or ascites, into edema fluid if there is an extensive crush injury or burn, in tissue slough and necrotic muscle, and into areas where blood has been sequestered, or lost to the body economy.

The source of the great urinary protein loss is still not entirely certain. In studies of burned rats Levenson and his colleagues have demonstrated that the incorporation of labeled nitrogen in tissue protein was equal to, or greater than, that seen in the control animals, which means that they were synthesizing protein at the same time that they were losing large quantities of nitrogen in the urine. Therefore simple catabolism of body protein was not the only source for urinary nitrogen loss.

In a subsequent series of experiments it was found that the protein content of the liver and other active organs changed very little after burns whereas the muscle, which had a rather slow turnover rate, lost enough protein to

Fig. 1-31. Comparison of dialysis in patients with minimal and severe catabolism. *A*. Chronic dialysis in an anephric patient with very little catabolism, taking 2 Gm of protein/kg body weight daily. Note the slow rise in BUN and creatinine levels between dialyses despite high protein intakes. *B*. Dialysis in a patient with multiple fractures and acute tubular necrosis on no protein intake. Note the rapid rise in BUN and creatinine levels associated with marked catabolism. The patient recovered completely.

account for most of the urinary nitrogen loss. These experiments suggested that the integrity of the vital organs was maintained at the expense of skeletal muscle. Munro and Chalmers found that in rats fed on a protein-free diet until they were depleted negative nitrogen balance failed to develop after injury, and they hypothesized that the protein lost after injury was storage protein. If storage protein is largely muscle protein, this would account for the far greater protein loss seen in muscular young men than in women or debilitated elderly patients (see Fig. 1-20). It has also been noted by Browne and Schenker and by Howard et al. that if the patient has repeated injuries in close succession, the protein loss is less with each succeeding injury, perhaps because the storage protein has been wiped out by the previous trauma (Fig. 1-32). The striking muscle protein catabolism seen in trauma is far in excess of that

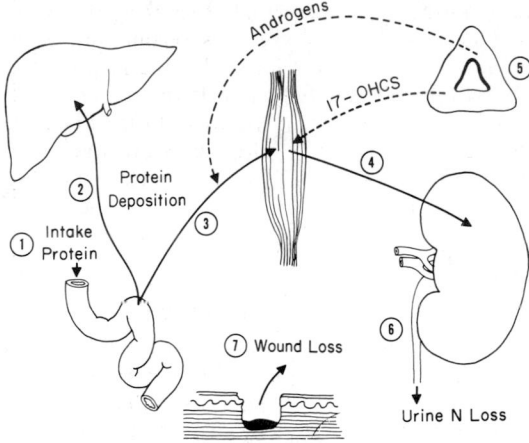

Fig. 1-32. Protein storage and catabolism. Protein may be preferentially deposited in the liver while it is being catabolized from muscle stores. Its catabolism is increased by glucocorticoids and decreased by insulin and adrenal androgens.

needed to supply energy. The magnitude of this response is related to the magnitude of the injury.

Protein contribution to the normal caloric requirement is in the range of 12 to 15 percent of the total, while Duke observed that this remained approximately 15 percent in most surgical conditions and did not rise much above 20 percent even with major increases in nitrogen excretion after extensive injury. Thus the major weight loss seen after surgery is not primarily the result of protein breakdown as a means of obtaining extra fuel. Although it has been claimed by Blackburn et al. that injury inhibits the mobilization and oxidation of fat from adipose tissue as a fuel source, Carlson and other investigators have shown that free fatty acids are readily mobilized in injury. They have even raised the question of whether excessive mobilization of fatty acids may sometimes occur.

The protein loss after injury does not result from impaired protein synthesis. Furthermore the protein loss occurs primarily from muscle, there being no decrease in the protein content of the liver and kidneys. Increased cortisol and glucagon and decreased insulin all limit the ability of muscle to take up amino acids. As catabolism of muscle continues, while anabolism is limited by these hormonal changes, there is a net release of amino acids from muscle cells. As mentioned earlier, alanine is the principal amino acid released from muscle, and this amino acid is the principal gluconeogenic precursor in the liver. Felig et al. have suggested that a cycle similar to the Cori cycle of glucose to lactate to glucose may be achieved through glucose to alanine to glucose. This cycle then provides a source for gluconeogenesis. Branched-chain amino acids are also lost from muscle, and their plasma concentration may increase for 2 hours to weeks after trauma. Increased concentrations of amino acids thus may contribute to the hyperosmolality of trauma.

There is some evidence that the increased nitrogen metabolism may be related to the need for carbohydrate intermediates via gluconeogenesis, rather than to the total energy needs of the body as indicated by its oxygen con-

sumption. This evidence as summarized by Kinney et al. is as follows: (1) the caloric contribution of protein to the fuel mixture of normal and injured man is rather small; (2) two-carbon fragments are readily available from adipose tissue and are utilized as the major energy source in most tissues after injury; (3) the body has a continuous requirement for carbohydrate intermediates for synthetic purposes, for which deamination of amino acids is the primary endogenous source; and (4) fatty acids cannot directly yield a net gain of carbohydrate intermediates, glucose, or glycogen.

Carbohydrate intermediates are used for the synthesis of nonessential amino acids, glycogen, glucose, and tricarboxylic acid cycle intermediates. As a by-product of the increased gluconeogenesis of trauma, there is an increased synthesis of urea, which is made from nitrogen stripped from alanine and other glucogenic amino acids as their carbon remains are used in the formation of glucose (Fig. 1-31).

The plasma proteins undergo increased catabolism, but there is an increased synthesis of albumin as well. γ-Globulin is likewise increased, presumably by antibody production against microorganisms. The total plasma amino acids decrease somewhat, but individual amino acids may increase or decrease depending on their utility as gluconeogenic substrates.

Acute-phase-reactant proteins (AP reactants) (Table 1-8) are those protein components of plasma whose concentration is significantly increased in the acute phase of trauma or inflammation. All these contain 5 to 20 percent carbohydrate in the molecule, and all are synthesized exclusively in the liver. An article by Koj summarizes our current knowledge of them.

Although most of the AP reactants are present normally and show an increased response to trauma, at least two of them, C-reactive protein in man and rabbit and α_2-AP globulin in the rat, do not appear to be present in healthy animals but appear only after injury. In some forms of trauma there may be an increase in the rate of synthesis of albumin as well as AP reactants, but because in severe trauma there is a marked increase in catabolism of albumin, the increased synthesis is not apparent. Increased synthesis of albumin is stimulated by cortisol and by growth hormone. However, this effect is not apparent for approximately 2 days, even after simple hemorrhage.

The AP-reactant glycoproteins appear at different time intervals after injury. C-reactive protein in man and α_2-AP globulin in rats respond most promptly, appearing in plasma soon after injury, while haptoglobin and fibrinogen appear 4 to 6 hours after, and seromucoid and ceruloplasmin reach maximal value several days after injury. The response of the various AP reactants to repeated injuries or to adrenalectomy or the administration of corticosteroids is very variable. Some of the AP reactants are inhibited and others are stimulated by adrenalectomy.

Presumably the AP reactants are of some benefit to the injured organism. Fibrinogen apparently improves clotting, and haptoglobins may help to prevent damage to the kidneys by binding hemoglobin released as a consequence of the injury. Other AP reactants may bind toxic products or inactivate lyzosomal enzymes whose release triggers production of toxins.

Restitution of Blood Volume

The restitution of blood volume in hypovolemia occurs in two major phases. The first phase is initiated by the fall in capillary pressure associated with hypotension and augmented by sympathetically mediated arteriolar vasoconstriction. In the presence of decreased capillary pressure, essentially protein-free fluid moves from the interstitium to the capillaries, leading to restitution of 20 to 50 percent of the lost volume. However, this fluid transfer leads to a fall in interstitial pressure and in capillary oncotic pressure, leading to the development of a pseudosteady state in which further restitution of blood volume is impossible. As shown first by Cope and Litwin, further restitution of blood volume depends upon restitution of plasma protein, primarily albumin. This second phase of blood volume restitution cannot depend upon the synthesis of new albumin, for, as indicated above, this does not occur for at least 2 days. Albumin loss from the circulation may be retarded in the presence of vasoconstriction, particularly of the splanchnic circulation, but this cannot account entirely for protein restitution. Thus the major source of albumin for blood volume restitution in the second phase must be the interstitium itself. The movement of protein from the interstitium to the circulation, either up the lymphatics or across the semipermeable capillary membranes, depends almost entirely upon interstitial pressure. Since the compliance of the interstitium is fixed, interstitial pressure can be increased only by the movement of fluid into the interstitium, primarily from cells. The movement of fluid between cells and interstitium is controlled exclusively by the osmotic gradient across the cell membrane. Because of this fact, the increased extracellular osmolality which occurs in the presence of injury and hypovolemia is critical for the second phase of blood volume restitution. As indicated above, the extracellular osmolality increases as a result of various metabolic effects of the hormones that are increased after injury. It depends critically upon increased concentrations of cortisol, but preliminary evidence has implicated glucagon, epinephrine, and growth hormone in this response as well. Both the extent and the duration of increased osmolality are functions of the extent of hypovolemia or injury, as shown by Boyd and Mansberger and by ourselves. The role of extracellular hyperosmolality and the ensuing second phase of restitution of blood volume appears critical in cardiovascular stabilization after injury. Its absence may account at least in part for the peculiar sensitivity to injury of patients with adrenal insufficiency. Of course, once hormonal changes have been initiated, the effects of the hormones will not cease merely because hormonal secretion is turned off by replacement of blood volume. Thus, once the metabolic effects of injury have begun, therapeutic or endogenous restitution of blood volume may lessen the severity of the metabolic consequences but cannot prevent them. In one sense, however, the protein loss, fat mobilization, and hypoglycemia and carbohydrate depletion of injury may be viewed as late

metabolic consequences of an initial attempt by the body to restore blood volume through this second phase of restitution. In this phase, the neuroendocrine response to injury induces a set of metabolic effects that serve to increase extracellular osmolality. Fluid then shifts from cells to interstitium, increasing interstitial pressure and thus leading directly to movement of fluid and protein into the vascular compartment.

Wound Healing

Wound healing is discussed in detail in Chap. 8. Many factors affect wound healing, chief among them being local factors of hematoma, dehiscence, infection, edema, blood supply, location, and extent. The administration of antibiotics can improve wound healing by decreasing sepsis, and the correction of clotting defects can promote healing by preventing hemorrhage in the wound. Various systemic metabolic factors are involved in wound healing.

Ascorbic acid is essential for collagen synthesis, and thus plays an important role in the healing of wounds. Cognizance is customarily taken of this by the intravenous administration of large doses of ascorbic acid after operation. It has been demonstrated by Levenson and his associates that injuries are accompanied by a decrease in plasma ascorbic acid concentration and by similar changes in thiamine and nicotinamide. This is associated with a decrease in urinary excretion of these substances. A decrease in the urinary excretion of riboflavin is also seen. It was found that the decrease in plasma ascorbic acid constituted a true physiologic scurvy and that this could be reversed by the administration of large doses of ascorbic acid, 500 to 2,000 mg daily. Sullivan and Eisenstein have noted ascorbic acid depletion during hemodialysis corrected by adding ascorbate to the dialysate concentrate.

There are considerable recent data on the effects of the fat-soluble vitamins on wound healing. Certain types of trauma are accompanied by a decrease in blood and hepatic concentrations of vitamin A. Chernov et al. reported that vitamin A depletion following thermal injury is associated with stress ulcers. Restoration of serum vitamin A levels markedly reduced the risk of ulceration. Hutcher et al. showed that vitamin A reduced the incidence of steroid-induced gastric ulcers. Collagen synthesis and wound healing are suppressed by corticosteroids, but collagen synthesis and tensile strength can be returned to normal by vitamin A administration, as shown by Hunt and his colleagues, and by Stein and Keiser. When steroids are used for immunosuppression, it was shown by Cohen and Cohen that vitamin A must be used with caution because it exerts an adjuvant-like effect and antagonizes steroid-induced immunosuppression.

It may be necessary to administer vitamin K in prolonged starvation, mild liver damage, biliary fistulas, or other circumstances in which intestinal absorption of this vitamin is chronically reduced. In the absence of preexisting vitamin K deficiency its acute depletion in trauma is not generally a problem. The same may be said for vitamin D, which is stored in the body for long periods of time. Although the role of trace metals in wound repair and metabolism awaits clearer definition, there is increasing evidence that zinc and copper are essential for normal healing. Hsu and Hsu have shown that zinc is necessary for both epithelialization and collagen synthesis. Cohen et al. have recently noted that zinc-depleted burned patients have decreased taste acuity and an associated anorexia, which is corrected by zinc repletion. While zinc depletion interferes with wound healing, this process cannot be speeded up by giving zinc to individuals with normal levels.

Abnormal wound healing in copper deficiency is detailed in Carnes' review. Copper is essential for lysyl oxidase, the enzyme that cross-links collagen. Drugs such as D-penicillamine which bind copper and block aldehyde cross-link sites will subsequently diminish collage cross linking and inhibit wound healing. They may be clinically useful in the treatment of diseases characterized by over-abundant collagen deposition, such as cirrhosis, esophageal stricture, or keloids. D-Penicillamine has been clinically used by Harris and Sjoerdama for patients with scleroderma to inhibit skin collagen deposition.

Although various substances have been claimed to accelerate normal wound healing, there are no scientific data to show that cartilage extracts, vitamins, or metals accelerate healing in a normal healing wound.

The oxygen tension of the healing wound is said by Hunt and others to be directly related to the rate of healing. In the wound the oxygen reaches the area of injury by diffusion, and as the blood P_{O_2} is increased by breathing oxygen, the oxygen available in the wound is greater, and wound healing is accelerated. This is said to be because increases in wound P_{O_2} levels have three effects: (1) to increase the rate at which fibroblasts reproduce, (2) to increase the rate at which fibroblasts synthesize collagen, and (3) to increase the rate at which epithelial cells reproduce.

The studies of wound oxygen concentrations seem to give validity to the use of hyperbaric oxygen in the treatment of chronically unhealed wounds, supporting the claims that it improves wound healing.

Therapeutic Considerations

NUTRITIONAL SUPPLEMENTATION

The parenteral nutritional supplementation of the surgical patient has for many years included glucose solutions and blood and blood products, with abortive attempts to introduce amino acids intravenously to produce a positive nitrogen balance, and fat solutions to provide concentrated calories. In recent years, with the advent of parenteral "hyperalimentation" utilizing concentrated glucose and amino acid solutions introduced through an intraatrial catheter via the subclavian vein, there has been a plethora of papers devoted to the advantages and hazards of such therapy. Intravenous fat (Intralipid) was developed in Sweden and has received extensive experimental trial in this country. It seems to be a useful source of calories and of essential fatty acids.

Greenstein and his colleagues in 1960 produced a nutri-

tionally complete water-soluble liquid diet which when administered orally to rats maintained them for long periods without any detectable deficiencies. The diet contained 18 crystalline amino acids (9 essential and 9 non-essential), the water-soluble vitamins, the trace metals (Mg, Fe, Mn, Cu, Co, Zn) Na, K, Ca, ethyl linoleate, and sometimes vitamins A and D. Diets which did not include a linoleic acid source produced signs of essential fatty acid deficiency (scaling of skin, failure to grow well, occasionally cachexia).

Terry and his colleagues in 1948 first demonstrated that it was possible to maintain dogs for prolonged periods of time solely on oral glucose and parenteral plasma. The plasma proteins contributed to body tissue protein and did not produce a urinary nitrogen loss, but in fact decreased the urinary nitrogen loss seen in fasting. Total parenteral alimentation in dogs was described by Meng and Early in 1949. Allen et al. in 1956 used intravenously given plasma as the only protein source for littermate puppies and were able to obtain growth rates equivalent to those seen when the same amount of protein was given orally. Stemmer et al. republished these results 10 years later.

To Dudrick and his colleagues belongs the credit for pushing studies on parenteral hyperalimentation with amino acid and concentrated carbohydrate mixtures. In 1967–1968 these investigators demonstrated that it was possible to achieve normal growth in puppies supported entirely by intravenous feedings. The feedings consisted of amino acids, glucose, vitamins, Na, K, Ca, Cl, HPO_4, and trace metals with or without the addition of fat. They also reported 30 patients fed exclusively by vein for 10 to 200 days, using amino acids, 20% glucose, electrolytes, trace metals, and vitamins. Positive nitrogen balance was achieved, and the patients demonstrated better wound healing, weight gain, and increased strength and activity.

It seems clear that parenteral hyperalimentation is unnecessary for short-term surgical problems but is of great value for patients with long-term problems or for malnourished patients prior to surgery. It has also proved useful for putting the bowel at rest in severe diarrheal states such as ulcerative colitis and granulomatous colitis, and for maintaining patients with the short bowel syndrome.

The requirements for total parenteral alimentation solutions are given in Table 1-9. The amino acids may be supplied by any of the solutions shown in Table 1-10.

Table 1-9. REQUIREMENTS FOR PROLONGED INTRAVENOUS TOTAL ALIMENTATION

Essential amino acids
Possibly alanine and some other nonessential
    amino acids
Glucose
Na, K, Ca
Vitamins
Trace metals (Zn, Cu, Cr, Co,
    Mg, Mn, I, Fe)
Cl and HPO_4
Plasma or albumin
Linoleic acid

Table 1-10. AMINO ACID SOURCES FOR
INTRAVENOUS ALIMENTATION

Protein hydrolysates
Crystalline amino acid mixtures
Essential amino acids only
Plasma
Plasmanate
Albumin
Whole blood

Protein hydrolysates differ from mixtures of crystalline amino acids primarily by virtue of their contamination with trace elements and peptides, and (except for Aminosol) their content of phosphate (Table 1-11). The essential amino acids are listed in Table 1-12. The amino acid content of two of the commonly used commercial solutions are shown in Table 1-13, and a composition in which they are often administered is shown in Table 1-14.

Mixtures containing only the essential amino acids are used for patients with uremia or hepatic failure. In 1956 Rose and Dekker showed in rats that urea could be used for synthesis of nonessential amino acids when essential amino acids were supplied in the diet. This led to the clinical use by Giordano and by Giovannetti and Maggiore of similar diets for patients with uremia. The use of a parenteral essential amino acid–hypertonic glucose mixture has been described by Dudrick and his coworkers and others for surgical patients with renal failure and inability to eat. The blood urea nitrogen level falls, or remains stable after dialysis, and hyperphosphatemia, hypocalcemia, and acidosis are spontaneously reversed. Protein synthesis occurs, presumably from the metabolism of urea nitrogen. More recently, Walser and his associates have shown that administration of α-keto analogues of essential amino acids will lead to biosynthesis of those amino acids, in association with falls in plasma urea, ammonia, and glutamine concentrations. Infusion of the keto acids in starving subjects demonstrated a prolonged nitrogen-sparing effect. The possible usefulness of the keto acids after injury has not been evaluated at this time.

In liver failure the administration of protein hydrolysates is contraindicated because of their high ammonia content. Concentrated glucose solutions can be administered using the techniques of hyperalimentation. Although mixtures containing only essential amino acids can sometimes be used, their effect on hepatic encephalopathy is unpredictable. It is preferable to use albumin, which is capable of directly entering into body protein tissues without deamination or increasing ammonia levels. Furthermore, the albumin exerts an oncotic force which helps to mobilize and excrete ascitic and edema fluid.

There are various well-known complications that occur with intravenous hyperalimentation. These can be divided into catheter problems—which include pneumothorax, sepsis, subclavian artery injury, or air or fat embolization—and metabolic problems. Chief among the metabolic problems is hyperglycemic, hyperosmolar dehydration usually secondary to too rapid administration, to too concentrated glucose solutions, to latent diabetes, or to administration during a state of glucose intolerance such as one sees soon after severe trauma or during continued sepsis. Reactive hypoglycemia also can be seen if the fluid is suddenly stopped, particularly if insulin has been used.

Table 1-12. ESSENTIAL AMINO ACIDS

Leucine	Threonine
Valine	Methionine
Lysine	Histidine
Isoleucine	Tryptophan
Phenylalanine	

Table 1-13. AMINO ACID CONTENT OF TWO
COMMONLY USED PARENTERAL
AMINO ACID SOLUTIONS

Amigen (casein hydrolysate)

Essential	Nonessential
Leucine	Glutamic acid
Valine	Proline
Lysine	Serine
Isoleucine	Aspartic acid
Phenylalanine	Alanine
Threonine	Arginine
Methionine	Tyrosine
Histidine	Hydroxyproline
Tryptophan	Glycine
	Cystine

Freamine (synthetic amino acids)

Essential	Nonessential
Leucine	Alanine
Valine	Arginine
Lysine	Proline
Isoleucine	Serine
Phenylalanine	Cysteine
Threonine	Glycine
Methionine	
Histidine	
Tryptophan	

Table 1-11. PHOSPHATE CONTENT OF AMINO
ACID SOLUTIONS

Amino acid solution	Percent	Phosphate, mEq/L
Protein hydrolysate:		
Amigen	5	30
CPH	5	11
Hyprotigen	5	13
Aminosol	5	0
Crystalline amino acid:		
Cutter	8	0
Freamine	8.5	0
Freamine-E	5.25	0

Table 1-14. COMPOSITION OF AMINO ACID–SUGAR SOLUTIONS COMMONLY ADMINISTERED

Amigen, 800 (5% Amigen; 12.5% fructose, 2.4% alcohol)

Protein, Gm	37.4
Nitrogen, Gm	5.54
Calories	800
Na, mEq	35
K, mEq	19
Ca, mEq	5
Mg, mEq	2
Cl, mEq	20
HPO₄, mEq	30

Freamine

Dextrose, Gm	250
Nitrogen, Gm	4.17
Calories	900
Na, mEq	23.6
K, mEq	40
Mg, mEq	5
Cl, mEq	35
Acetate, mEq	52
ZnSO₄, mEq	2.5

Five other metabolic complications are seen occasionally with long-term hyperalimentation. The first of these is an excessive plasma level of amino acids beyond that which the body can metabolize. This produces impairment of brain function, and stimulation of insulin secretion. The effect of excess aminoacidemia can be ameliorated in part by the concomitant administration of large amounts of carbohydrate.

The second complication is a metabolic hyperchloremic acidosis produced only by the synthetic amino acid mixtures. Heird and his colleagues ascribe this to the catabolism of positively charged amino acids. This problem is not seen with the hydrolysates because they have sufficient negatively charged amino acids and peptides to offset the hydrogen ion release by the cationic amino acids.

The third complication is hypophosphatemia, which occurs when fibrin hydrolysates or crystalline amino acids are used without added phosphate (Table 1-11). This can be corrected by adding Ca and P to the solutions.

The fourth complication is deficiency of essential fatty acids. Fatty acid deficiency was first described in animals by Burr and Burr in 1929. Pensler and his colleagues described the first clinical case in 1971. The essential defect

Table 1-15. ESSENTIAL FATTY ACID DEFICIENCY

Fall in:
    Linoleic
    Arachidonic
    8,11,14-Eicosatetraenaic
Rise in:
    Palmitoleic
    Oleic
    5,8,11-Eicosatetraenoic

is a decrease in plasma linoleic, arachidonic, and linolenic acids, with an increase in oleic, palmitoleic, and 5,8,11-eicosatetraenoic acids. It is characterized clinically by scaly skin, itching, poor wound healing, weakness, lethargy, and thrombocytopenia. The thrombocytopenia appears to be due to a failure of separation of megakaryocyte buds.

Linoleic acid is the key essential acid, since arachidonic acid can be synthesized from it, and it has not been established whether linolenic acid is essential (Table 1-15). Although it has been recommended that patients on long-term hyperalimentation receive plasma on a weekly basis for its essential fatty acid content, it is doubtful whether this supplies enough linoleic acid to prevent the development of fatty acid deficiency. Intravenous fat in the form of Intralipid will correct the defect, but this substance is still available in this country only on an experimental basis.

The fifth complication is deficiency of trace elements. Although trace elements have often been added to pediatric hyperalimentation mixtures, they are not routinely added to mixtures for adults. The trace elements thought to be important are listed in Table 1-16. The administration of amino acid mixtures without trace elements led to the development of copper deficiency in one of our patients. This was characterized by dryness of the skin, weakness, and anemia, associated with a very low serum copper level. The symptoms were corrected by the intravenous administration of copper. As plasma and plasmanate contain trace elements, the periodic administration of plasma may prevent the development of deficiencies.

Alcohol, a component of some hyperalimentation solutions, probably should not be used. It potentiates ketosis, increases metabolic acidosis, uncouples oxidative phosphorylation (thus increasing oxygen consumption without energy production), depolarizes nerves, and may produce sedation and mild inebriation in children.

Fructose, also a component of some solutions, appears definitely inferior to glucose. It increases uric acid, lactic acid, amino acids, and bilirubin. The latter effect is apparently due to hepatic cell injury by fructose, which also increases the serum glutamic oxaloacetic transaminase (SGOT).

The elements are now available for the production of an ideal parenteral alimentation solution tailored to the individual patient. Long-term home hyperalimentation has

Table 1-16. TRACE METALS PRESENT IN ENZYMES

Metal	*Enzymes*
Iron	Cytochromes, peroxidases
Copper	Tyrosinase, ascorbic oxidase
Zinc	Peptidase, carbonic anhydrase
Magnesium	Phosphatases, kinases
Maganese	Kinases, peptidases, arginase
Molybdenum	Xanthine oxidase, nitrate reductase
Cobalt	Vitamin B₁₂ coenzyme complexes
Potassium	Pyruvic kinase, β-methyl aspartase

SOURCE: Conn and Stumpf, "Outlines of Biochemistry," 3d ed., p. 233, John Wiley & Sons, Inc., New York, 1972.

been started, and a completely closed portable system has been devised. Provided the use of hyperalimentation solutions is not extended to patients who could do better without them and precautions are taken to avoid the complications, it will provide an exciting and important contribution to the care of the surgical patient.

COMPONENT THERAPY

Component therapy is a term for the intravenous administration of blood components, or substitutes for these components, instead of whole blood in order to create an intravenous mixture that offers some particular advantage over whole blood. To some extent this advantage may simply be that of greater availability, as for example reconstituted blood over fresh blood, but in some circumstances it may actually do a better job.

OXYGEN TRANSPORT. Traumatized patients may develop a shift of the oxygen dissociation curve to the left as a consequence primarily of alkalosis and lowered erythrocyte 2,3-diphosphoglycerate (2,3-DPG) levels. The reduced DPG level interferes with the ability of the red cell to give up its oxygen to the tissues. Old banked blood contains red cells with low 2,3-DPG content, and multiple transfusions of such blood tend to contribute to tissue anoxia. One may improve tissue oxygenation by correcting alkalosis or by providing erythrocytes high in 2,3-DPG content. Experiments have been made with free hemoglobin solutions and with chemical substitutes for hemoglobin.

Frozen erythrocytes are high in 2,3-DPG, in contrast to blood banked in the usual fashion, and have the advantage over fresh whole blood of not containing white cells (which are antigenic) and being far less likely to transmit hepatitis virus.

Free hemoglobin can also be used as an oxygen carrier. Although myoglobin produces renal damage, hemoglobin does not. Hemoglobin contaminated with red cell stroma produces a consumption coagulopathy, and pure hemoglobin produces anticoagulation as a result of reduced plasma factor VIII and factor V activity. Absorption with aluminum hydroxide was shown by Moss and his colleagues to remove the anticoagulant activity.

Fluorocarbons have been under investigation as an oxygen transport system, and there has been a recent symposium published on this subject. Clark and Galan first demonstrated that mice could be given liquid ventilation with an oxygenated fluorocarbon fluid at atmospheric pressure. Modell and his colleagues were able to ventilate dogs for 8 hours on liquid fluorocarbons with survival. Acidosis tends to develop because of poor CO_2 diffusion; however, mechanical hyperventilation produces pulmonary edema, and the chemicals themselves produce alveolitis, atelectasis, perivascular hemorrhage, and other lung changes.

Geyer and his coworkers have been able to replace almost all the erythrocytes in rats with emulsified perfluorochemicals and keep them alive on 50% oxygen for hours. It was found by Sloviter and his colleagues, however, that these substances produced a progressive anoxia and death in most laboratory animals, although frogs and mice could live several days with their erythrocytes replaced by circulating fluorocarbons. At least part of the damage caused by the perfluorochemicals is related to the fact that they produce pronounced platelet agglutination and microemboli, not prevented by heparin. Geyer has not confirmed these results and has shown that under some circumstances, increased numbers of platelets enter the circulation during perfusion.

While hemoglobin substitutes are an intriguing possibility, they do not yet seem to be serious contenders with red cells, or even free hemoglobin, for the honor of carrying the oxygen around the body. However, advances in this field are proceeding rapidly, and important progress is to be anticipated.

CLOTTING COMPONENTS. The clinically useful clotting components consist of fresh frozen plasma, cryoprecipitate, concentrates of factors II, VII, IX, X, antihemophilic globulin, platelet packs, and fibrinogen.

Fresh frozen plasma can be used to replenish the factors contributing to the prothrombin time and in bleeding patients in hepatic failure whose prothrombin times are low. It has the advantage over banked blood that it contains some labile factor V, which is characteristically low in liver failure and absent from banked blood, and the disadvantage that it contains no platelets. It is used in plasmapheresis for hepatic coma, where it is combined with the patient's own erythrocytes, and therefore it can be used for patients with rare blood types for whom the acquisition of multiple units of fresh whole blood might be difficult. Fresh frozen plasma is also useful for patients undergoing operations who develop bleeding tendencies secondary to deficiencies of clotting factors.

Cryoprecipitate contains factor VIII and some fibrinogen, while antihemophilic globulin contains only concentrated factor VIII. Both are used for hemophiliacs with factor VIII deficiency for whom replacement is desired.

Preparations containing factors II, VII, IX, and X (Konyne, Proplex) are used to treat Christmas disease.

Platelet packs are used to administer platelets to patients with hypersplenism, thrombocytopenic purpura, massive transfusions, and other deficiency states where thrombocytopenia can be demonstrated to be contributing to the bleeding disorder.

Fibrinogen is the specific therapy for patients with bleeding due to the presence of excessive amounts of fibrinolysin. It may be combined with steroids and EACA (ε-amino caproic acid).

PLASMA SUBSTITUTES. The risk of hepatitis from pooled plasma is so great that most hospitals have stopped using this preparation entirely. There is, of course, a significant risk from single blood or plasma transfusions, too, and for this reason transfusions or plasma infusions should never be given without a specific important indication. Apart from the administration of fresh frozen plasma discussed above, there is almost never a reason to administer plasma.

Ringer's lactate solution is, more or less, plasma without the plasma proteins, i.e., the immunoglobulins (IgG, IgA, IgM), albumin, fibrinogen, and the prothrombin-related clotting factors. The combination of Ringer's lactate solution (sometimes with modifications of the electrolyte content) and albumin makes a very satisfactory plasma substitute. Albumin itself is the therapy of choice in cirrhosis, not only because it replaces a specific loss, provides oncotic pull, and helps to promote diuresis, but also because its amino acids can enter muscle protein without deamination to create toxic nitrogen fragments. Furthermore hepatitis is not transmitted by albumin preparations.

Plasmanate is plasma with the clotting factors removed. It is made up as 5% protein in saline solution, and contains 88% albumin and 12% globulins. It is nearly free of hepatitis transmission.

The administration of fibrinogen to traumatized patients is seldom necessary, because there is an increased hepatic synthesis of fibrinogen in response to injury. It may be necessary, however, in patients with increased fibrinolysin.

ALIMENTATION MIXTURES. Special alimentation mixtures, discussed earlier in this chapter, offer a variety of combinations to fit the circumstances. Apart from hyperalimentation in severe, sustained, or septic trauma, the single most dramatic effect is that of essential amino acid mixtures in renal failure. This type of therapy makes possible the administration of amino acids which are not metabolized to release nitrogen but which are used in muscle synthesis—thus not contributing to urea formation—and in the presence of hypertonic glucose, even inducing the body to burn urea.

COMPONENT BLOOD. Frozen red cells are at present the best oxygen carrier available. Added to Ringer's lactate solution and albumin, they make a very acceptable blood substitute for patients not requiring clotting factors. Fresh frozen plasma is the best source of clotting factors but is the first component to introduce a risk of hepatitis. Platelet packs complete the clotting constituents, with the exception of fibrinogen which is needed only in the presence of excess fibrinolysins.

Apart from the leukocytes, which are specifically contraindicated in patients awaiting renal transplantation, and the ready availability of the constituents, there is no advantage attributable to component blood over fresh blood, which itself has the advantage of being cheaper and easier to prepare.

ACID-BASE BALANCE AND WATER AND ELECTROLYTE METABOLISM

Alkalosis

Attention has been directed to the development of alkalosis after trauma or operative insult. Some of the mechanisms involved have been summarized by Lyons and Moore, who find that alkalosis is observed more frequently than acidosis in patients with mild to moderate trauma who have not deteriorated to the point of severe renal circulatory or pulmonary decompensation. The criteria used by these writers to describe changes in acid-base balance are reproduced in Table 1-17, since they provide a handy guide for discussion of this subject. It was found that 64 percent of 105 patients operated upon developed

alkalosis on at least one determination in the postoperative period. Of the 67 patients in whom alkalosis developed, 29 demonstrated this change after open heart operations, 19 after ventilatory assistance, 8 had alkalosis from chronic pulmonary disease, 5 had so-called "residual posttraumatic alkalosis," and 6 had miscellaneous forms of alkalosis. It is of significance that the open heart surgical patients received 9 to 18 Gm of tris buffer routinely in the first few hours after bypass and were hyperventilated after operation. These pH changes were therefore not so much the consequence of trauma as of overenthusiastic use of the measures taken for the prevention of acidosis. Among the patients with ventilatory alkalosis only those with pulmonary disease had elevated buffer base values. Extreme hypocapnic alkalosis occasionally developed in patients with normal lungs.

Lyons and Moore point out that it is important to prevent severe alkalosis in the surgical patient because of its potential hazards and that by the same token it might be well to avoid creating it by the injudicious use of administered base or hyperventilation. Among the dangers listed by these writers was the production of tissue hypoxia through the effect of alkalosis on the oxygen-hemoglobin dissociation curve and on vasomotor tone. The rise in blood lactate level which accompanies respiratory alkalosis sets the stage for severe metabolic acidosis should hypocapnia suddenly yield to hypoventilation or hypoperfusion. Alkalosis tends to produce hypocalcemia and hypokalemia, and the latter may be extremely dangerous to the patient receiving digitalis or to patients who already have hypokalemia. Hypocapnic vasoconstriction tends to produce a reduced cerebral blood flow.

One of the mechanisms for the development of alkalosis is pulmonary arteriovenous shunting, which occurs in patients with cirrhosis or atelectasis. Patients with cirrhosis frequently have hypokalemia and a metabolic alkalosis to begin with, and this is further complicated by the respiratory alkalosis which develops as a consequence of the shunting. The shunting that occurs in atelectasis permits venous blood to traverse the pulmonary bed unoxygenated. The resultant hypoxia increases ventilation, thereby blowing off carbon dioxide and producing respiratory alkalosis.

Atelectasis can produce hyperventilation even in the absence of hypoxia by stimulation of the Hering-Breuer reflexes, whereas hypoxemia produces hyperventilation by stimulating the aortic and carotid body chemoreceptors. Furthermore a reduction in blood flow to the chemoreceptor bodies will stimulate hyperventilation, since these receptors extract oxygen from the blood rapidly and extensively. Thus respiration may be stimulated during hypotension and decreased cardiac output even though the arterial blood is adequately oxygenated. This, then, may be another mechanism for the production of respiratory alkalosis in surgical patients. Three of the patients described by Lyons and Moore had a metabolic alkalosis, one from overtreatment of diabetic acidosis and the others from gastrointestinal obstruction and vomiting.

Lactic acid accumulation occurs with hyperventilation and can be prevented by adding carbon dioxide to the

Table 1-17. COMPARISON OF SYSTEMS OF NOMENCLATURE USED TO DESCRIBE DISTURBANCES OF NEUTRALITY REGULATION*

Disturbance in conventional terms	pH (units)	$[H^+]$ (mEq/ L)	P_{CO_2} (mm Hg)	Standard HCO_3^- (mM/ L)	Actual HCO_3^- (mM/ L)	CO_2 content (mM/ L)	CO_2 combining power† (mM/ L)	Buffer base (mM/L) Hemoglobin (Gm %) 10	15	20	Buffer base deviation (mM/L) Hemoglobin (Gm %) 10	15	20
Normal.	7.40	39.8	40.0	23.9	23.9	25.1	25.1	45.7	48.0	50.1	0.0	0.0	0.0
Uncompensated respiratory alkalosis	7.53	29.5	25.0	23.9	20.2	20.9	22.9	45.0	48.0	50.9	− 0.7	0.0	+ 0.8
Uncompensated metabolic alkalosis	7.53	29.3	40.0	32.5	32.5	33.7	33.7	55.7	58.0	60.1	+10.0	+ 10.0	+10.0
Mixed respiratory and metabolic alkalosis	7.68	24.0	25.0	32.5	28.5	29.3	31.2	55.1	58.0	61.0	+ 9.4	+10.0	+10.9
Uncompensated respiratory acidosis	7.31	48.9	55.0	23.9	26.8	28.4	26.7	46.5	48.0	49.4	+ 0.8	0.0	− 0.7
Uncompensated metabolic acidosis	7.24	57.2	40.0	16.7	16.7	17.9	17.7	36.1	38.0	39.7	− 9.6	−10.0	−10.4
Mixed respiratory and metabolic acidosis	7.16	68.4	55.0	16.7	19.2	20.8	19.2	36.7	38.0	39.1	− 9.0	−10.0	−11.0
Mixed respiratory alkalosis and metabolic acidosis	7.40	39.8	25.0	18.4	15.0	15.7	17.5	37.7	41.5	43.1	− 8.0	− 7.5	− 7.0
Mixed respiratory acidosis and metabolic alkalosis.	7.40	39.8	55.0	30.0	32.9	34.6	32.7	53.3	55.0	56.5	+ 7.6	+ 7.0	+ 6.4
Respiratory alkalosis with metabolic compensation	7.47	34.2	25.0	21.0	17.4	18.2	20.2	41.4	44.2	47.0	− 4.3	− 3.8	− 3.1
Metabolic alkalosis with respiratory compensation‡	7.47	34.2	50.0	32.5	34.8	36.3	35.0	56.2	58.0	59.7	+10.5	+10.0	+ 9.6
Respiratory acidosis with metabolic compensation	7.35	44.3	55.0	26.5	29.5	31.3	29.7	49.7	51.3	52.8	+ 4.0	+ 3.3	+ 2.7
Metabolic acidosis with respiratory compensation	7.35	44.3	25.0	16.7	13.5	14.2	16.0	35.4	38.0	40.4	−10.3	−10.0	− 9.7

*Actual bicarbonate obtained from Henderson-Hasselbalch equation with $pK^1 = 6.10$. Buffer base, buffer base deviation, standard bicarbonate, and CO_2 combining power obtained from Siggaard-Andersen blood acid-base curve and alignment nomograms. Equilibration temperature = 38°C, oxyhemoglobin saturation = 100 percent and hemoglobin = 15 Gm percent unless otherwise indicated.

†Expressed as total CO_2 of anaerobically collected separated plasma or serum.

‡Some deny the clinical existence of this disturbance. Other studies indicate that respiratory compensation does occur but is weaker than the compensation accompanying metabolic acidosis.

SOURCE: J. H. Lyons, Jr., and F. D. Moore, *Surgery,* **60**:93, 1966.

inspired gas mixture. It is apparently dependent upon the reduction of carbon dioxide tension P_{CO_2} rather than the associated change in pH. Its exact mechanism is not known but may be related to the effect of hypocapnia on carbohydrate metabolism. If hyperventilation is suddenly stopped, the P_{CO_2} may rise more rapidly than the accumulated lactate can be cleared from the blood, leading to an acute metabolic acidosis. This is worsened by the accumulation of lactic acid of hypoxic origin.

The effects of alkalosis on ionized calcium and on potassium are important to myocardial irritability. It is claimed by Lyons and Moore that alkalosis generally promotes the renal excretion of sodium bicarbonate and an alkaline urine but that in the posttraumatic period this mechanism is blocked by adrenal cortical activity. This produces increased renal potassium loss and, acutely, aciduria. Administration of potassium and chloride permits the correction of the alkalosis. Chronic alkalosis cannot be corrected in the absence of exogenous potassium and chloride. These factors are of special importance in the management of the patient with pyloric obstruction.

Acidosis

Many articles have called attention to the development of acidosis in response to injury or operative trauma. Some of the patients alluded to above would have been acidotic had it not been for their vigorous treatment pushing them over into alkalosis.

BLOOD TRANSFUSION. Blood transfusion may produce either alkalosis or acidosis. Since citrated blood is intrinsically acid by virtue of the citric acid anticoagulant, it produces a metabolic acidosis upon rapid, massive infusion that persists until the fixed acid is metabolized. A standard acid citrate dextrose (ACD) solution also contains about 17 mEq of trisodium citrate per unit of blood, however. As the citrate is catabolized, sodium ions are released to the cation pool of the body and are balanced by newly formed bicarbonate. If renal bicarbonate excretion is inhibited, as it is following trauma, an "addition" metabolic alkalosis results. It takes about 135 mEq of sodium citrate, or the amount contained in 8 units of blood, to produce a discernible alkalosis. In the presence of hepatic impairment, whether brought about by preexisting disease, hypotension, hypoxia, or hypothermia, citrate metabolism is delayed, and transfusion acidosis then becomes more prominent. Transfusion alkalosis is postponed or never appears.

SHOCK. Severe shock, whether bacterial or hypovolemic, tends to produce acidosis. The mechanism for this is decreased tissue perfusion secondary to hypotension compounded by the release of catecholamines in response to hemorrhage, which further produces tissue anoxia by vasospasm. Arteriovenous shunting may increase further the hypoperfusion of tissues. Acidosis also increases coagulability of the blood and may produce capillary thrombosis. If the condition is allowed to persist, cellular death and terminal acidosis result. Hardaway and others have suggested that this condition can be reversed by the simultaneous administration of vasodilators to open up the arterioles together with blood or other fluid to maintain effective circulating blood volume. The increased blood flow to the organs improves tissue oxygenation and decreases the likelihood of capillary thrombosis. The acidosis can be further corrected by the administration of bicarbonate or other base.

Wilson et al. have used phenoxybenzamine, an α-adrenergic antagonist, in 19 patients with shock refractory to conventional treatment. The patients received doses varying between 0.2 and 2 mg/kg of body weight. This was administered over a 5-minute period in patients who were in pulmonary edema and over a 60-minute period in patients who were less severely ill. Large volumes of fluid were needed to maintain blood pressure, and attempts were made to correct acid-base changes when needed. The cardiac output increased in 8 of 9 patients studied, and urine output increased in 7 of 19. The use of vasodilators, or of vasoactive drugs of any kind, in patients with shock is waning in popularity, although phenoxybenzamine unquestionably improves renal cortical blood flow. This effect can be achieved equally well with dopamine, which also provides circulatory support. However, fluid and blood replacement, monitoring of venous pressure and blood gases, adequate ventilation, and treatment of sepsis remain the primary modalities for the treatment of shock.

The accumulation of lactic acid accounts in part for the progressive acidosis of shock, as shown by Broder and Weil. Likelihood of survival of patients in profound shock could be estimated by the levels of excess lactate in the blood. When it was less than 1 mM/liter, 82 percent survived; when it was 2 mM/liter, 60 percent survived; and when it was 2 to 4 mM/liter, only 26 percent survived. If the excess lactate was ever over 3 mM/liter, a fatal outcome could not be averted.

Boyd et al. have shown that nonlactate solutes may also accumulate in shock and that their accumulation indicates a poor prognosis. The presence of these substances, most of which have not been identified, may be demonstrated by measuring serum osmolality and then calculating by a formula using sodium, glucose, and blood urea nitrogen levels. The difference between the measured and calculated osmolality is called the *osmolal discriminant*, and it is only partly accounted for by lactic acid levels. If the osmo-

lality and the osmolal discriminant remain high after treatment, the prognosis is grave. The lactic acid concentration is also high in this group, of course.

MacLean and his coworkers reported studies on 56 patients in shock. These patients were divided into two groups according to whether the central venous pressure was above or below normal prior to treatment and were further subdivided into those patients who were alkalotic or normal and those who were frankly acidotic. The patients were treated with isoproterenol (2 μg/minute) combined with blood and saline solution, which produced an increase in cardiac output and blood pressure with a decline in central venous pressure and in arterial blood lactate.

If the patient was normovolemic before the onset of septic shock, the manifestations included hyperventilation, respiratory alkalosis, high cardiac index, elevated central venous pressure, low peripheral resistance, increased blood volume, hypotension, oliguria, warm, dry extremities, and arterial blood lactate accumulation. If this syndrome was recognized while the patient was still alkalotic, he responded to therapy designed to maintain the cardiac output at even higher levels. In contrast, if the patient was hypovolemic at the onset of sepsis, the clinical picture consisted of low central venous pressure, low cardiac output, high peripheral resistance, and cold, cyanotic extremities. These patients were also initially alkalotic and responded to treatment consisting of volume replacement and surgical procedures. If, however, they were not seen until they were acidotic, a low fixed output persisted and a high mortality rate ensued.

Acidosis is the result of shock, not the cause of it. Prevention or correction of acidosis seldom influences survival in hypovolemic shock. On the other hand, restoring fluid volume without correcting the acidosis does favorably influence the outcome. Severe acidosis (pH below 7.1) occurs in exhaustive exercise and in diabetic acidosis without producing shock, with good cardiac performance and ultimate recovery. The important thing is to remove the cause of the acidosis, not to treat the acidosis per se.

More patients with a normal or alkalotic pH survived than those with acidosis. In fact, of 18 patients with acidosis only 1 survived the shock episode, and none survived subsequently, whereas 33 of 48 who were normal or alkalotic survived the shock episode. It is postulated that in bacteremic shock hyperventilation occurs, leading to respiratory alkalosis. If the patient does not respond to treatment, a continued depression of tissue perfusion leads to the accumulation of large amounts of lactate with acidosis and death.

Bergentz and Brief showed that the development of refractory oligemic shock in dogs was accompanied by the production of acidosis and that the administration of a buffer prevented acidosis as well as the development of refractory shock. An identical volume of a concentrated sodium chloride solution also usually prevented the development of refractory shock without correcting the acidosis. It was felt that the improvement noted with hypertonic solutions was due to a redistribution of fluids from the intracellular to the extracellular space, thus perhaps preventing cellular swelling and promoting an expansion of the extracellular fluid volume. As noted above, expansion of the extracellular fluid volume leads to increased movement of albumin into the plasma and thus to sustained increased blood volume. Improved tissue perfusion might be expected to result.

CARDIAC ARREST. Chazan and his coworkers studied 22 patients during cardiac arrest and found that 10 had predominantly respiratory acidosis and 8 had metabolic acidosis. Most patients with a metabolic acidosis had had a myocardial infarction and had an arterial pH of 7.15 to 7.35. These patients appeared to be benefited by sodium bicarbonate with or without hyperventilation. In the 10 patients with respiratory acidosis, who were chiefly patients with pulmonary problems, the pH was 6.86 to 7.09 in 8. Hypercapnia was prevalent, alkalitherapy seemed less effective, and improved ventilation appeared to be the major therapeutic objective. Recent studies by Bishop and Weisfeldt suggest, in fact, that bicarbonate solutions may worsen the acidosis of cardiac arrest, and that they should not be used in this condition unless effective hyperventilation to remove CO_2 can be achieved. Acidosis tends to develop during cardiac arrest, because the cardiac index is markedly reduced during resuscitation by closed-chest massage; and this results in decreased tissue perfusion, hypoxia, anaerobic metabolism, and the production of lactic acid. In addition, many of the patients may be inadequately ventilated, causing a rise in P_{CO_2} and the development of respiratory acidosis. Only 2 patients in the group of 22 survived and left the hospital, although several others recovered temporarily, only to die later. In 4 patients, the acidosis could not be definitely classified as either metabolic or respiratory.

BURNS. Peaston demonstrated that although there is a paucity of information on acid-base disturbances in burn patients, acidosis is a frequent finding in these patients. He studied 14 consecutive unselected patients admitted to a regional burn unit and expressed the severity of acidosis in terms of the base deficit, after the method of Siggaard-Andersen et al., obtained by interpolation from the Siggaard-Andersen nomogram. Significant respiratory alkalosis was assumed when the arterial P_{CO_2} was below 30 mm Hg. Uncompensated acidosis was said to be present when the arterial pH fell below 7.35. It was found that 12 of the 14 patients had a base deficit at some stage after thermal injury and that in 7 of these the metabolic acidosis was maximal on admission and in 3 others within 24 hours of admission. The maximal degree of acidosis was found to correlate closely with the total extent of the body burn surface area. The severe degrees of base deficit observed were usually compensated by respiratory alkalosis. Acidosis was treated by the administration of sodium bicarbonate in doses as great as 400 mEq over 24 hours, or 2,750 mEq over a period of 11 days. The acidosis could not be attributed to the liberal use of normal saline solution, because in many patients it was maximal on admission before the patients had received any saline solution. It was felt that because of the unfavorable effect of acidosis on renal function the prompt correction of acidosis in the burn patient would help to prevent acute renal failure.

EFFECTS OF ACIDOSIS. Acidosis has profound effects on the cardiovascular system, producing a decreased myocardial contractility, a decreased response of the myocardium and peripheral vasculature to catecholamines, and a predisposition to cardiac arrhythmias. Acidosis predisposes to acute renal failure. Furthermore, it increases respiratory work.

Greenberg and Kittle have studied the effect of pH and P_{CO_2} changes on coronary blood flow and cardiac output, and find that both are increased by elevations of P_{CO_2} and that they are further increased by an elevation of pH. Thus both are increased in respiratory acidosis and metabolic alkalosis (particularly the latter), and both are reduced in metabolic acidosis and respiratory alkalosis.

Huckabee reported a series of 9 patients who had a syndrome of hyperpnea, tachypnea, and dyspnea with weakness and fatigue progressing to stupor and finally death. All these patients had acidosis characterized by a low serum bicarbonate level and a high value of unmeasured anion in the serum electrolyte pattern which turned out to be lactate. This group of patients had nothing else in common except for a very high level of lactic acidosis, which appeared to be due to widespread tissue hypoxia. This again illustrates the lethal nature of uncorrected acidosis.

A Problem in Acid-Base Balance. Figure 1-33 presents some of the findings from a very interesting patient who progressed from presumed metabolic acidosis to respiratory acidosis to respiratory alkalosis to metabolic alkalosis, all within a 24-hour period. This fourteen-year-old boy who had a large pheochromocytoma of the left adrenal was operated upon under general anesthesia, and the pheochromocytoma was removed. Within minutes after the last vein was tied off, the patient's blood pressure fell precipitously, and a severe bradycardia, hypotension, pulmonary edema, and cardiac arrest developed despite the administration of norepinephrine and all other attempts to support his blood pressure and cardiac action. It became necessary to open his chest in order to restore a cardiac beat, and there was a considerable period of hypotension and hypoxia, which almost certainly must have led to metabolic acidosis, although no measurements were made at this precise time.

When the operation was completed, the patient was removed to the recovery room, where because of continued poor ventilation and pulmonary edema he was placed on a respirator. He failed to regain consciousness, and it was then discovered that the respirator was defective. A blood pH taken at this time was 7.02, and the patient was found to have a profound respiratory acidosis. When the respirator was noted to be defective, the patient was placed on a manual bag and breathed vigorously. His respiration was further improved by placing him on a volume respirator, which lowered his P_{CO_2} from 72 to 26 and raised his pH to 7.54. A profound respiratory alkalosis then developed with a pH of 7.74, a P_{CO_2} of 33, and a potassium level of 2.3 mEq/L. At this point carpopedal spasm developed, and the respirator was stopped. Because of the alkalosis and because he had been receiving dexamethasone, large amounts of urinary potassium were lost. A spot check

Fig. 1-33. Acid-base abnormalities in a patient with pheochromocytoma. The patient had a cardiac arrest on the operating table associated with peripheral vasoconstriction, overtransfusion with blood, tissue hypoxia, and pulmonary edema. It was necessary to open his chest to restore effective cardiac activity. During this time a severe metabolic acidosis was presumed to have developed, and the patient was given sodium bicarbonate intravenously. After getting his heart started again, the patient was maintained on intravenously administered norepinephrine and was returned to the recovery room and placed on a respirator. The respirator proved to be defective, producing a very severe hypoxia and a marked respiratory acidosis with a P_{CO_2} of 72. The patient's pH at this time was 7.02. When it was discovered that the respirator was defective, the patient was shifted to a manual bag, and this quickly brought the P_{CO_2} down, at which time the patient was placed on a volume respirator. This ventilated him so well that a rather marked respiratory alkalosis developed, with a pH of 7.74. Carpopedal spasm developed, and the respirator was discontinued. Subsequent to this a mild metabolic alkalosis developed, partly as a consequence of the administration of corticosteroids, and large amounts of potassium were lost in the urine, a rather significant hypokalemia developing. This was corrected by the administration of large amounts of potassium chloride intravenously, and the patient ultimately recovered completely.

showed 83 mEq/L of potassium in the urine, while the sodium concentration was 11 mEq/L. The marked potassium loss continued, and an acid urine developed. The pH, which had fallen to 7.42, rose to 7.51, with a P_{CO_2} of 250 (on oxygen), a P_{CO_2} of 41, a carbon dioxide level of 30, and a potassium level of 2.5 mEq/L in spite of the administration of large amounts of potassium intravenously. At this point an uncompensated metabolic alkalosis appeared to have developed. Still larger amounts of potassium were administered, and the dose of dexamethasone was reduced. He went on to make an uneventful recovery.

It is important to note that at times it may be necessary to administer very much larger doses of potassium than one is accustomed to give. Several cases of this type, all of them diabetics, were collected by Pullen et al., in which potassium was administered in doses of up to 860 mEq in 24 hours.

Water and Electrolyte Metabolism

Although it is axiomatic that the response to injury or operation depends upon the utilization and type of anesthetic agent, the preinjury state of the patient, the type of injury, and the particular fluid and electrolyte solutions used in the patient's treatment, nevertheless some generalizations can be made to serve as a frame of reference for the infinite variations produced by the factors just mentioned.

SODIUM METABOLISM

In the normal steady state, human beings excrete a quantity of sodium in the urine equal to the intake. In general, this quantity ranges between 60 and 100 mEq. Following injury, urinary sodium excretion falls to nearly zero, a direct consequence of the hormonal response to injury. If hypovolemia is severe and shock is present, there may also be a decrease in glomerular filtration in response to a fall in perfusion pressure. Filtration may also fall as a result of the action of angiotensin II, as described above. In the absence of any changes in glomerular filtration, however, nearly total sodium conservation is evident. Several mechanisms combine to produce this effect. Renal sympathetic nervous activity is enhanced in response to the injury itself, as well as in response to hypovolemia. In part, this sympathetic activity serves to maintain glomerular filtration in the presence of decreased total renal blood flow. However, as the fraction of blood which is filtered increases, the fraction that is contributed to peritubular blood flow in the renal cortex decreases. Since the glomerulus is nearly impermeable to protein, this change in filtration fraction results in an increase in protein concentration in the peritubular capillary perfusing the proximal tubule. The resulting rise in peritubular oncotic pressure results in increased net transfer of water and accompanying sodium bicarbonate and sodium chloride from the proximal tubule back into the blood. This process may be further enhanced by a direct action of sympathetic nerves on sodium reabsorption and by decrease in a circulating natriuretic hormone. The net effect of these mechanisms is that a decreased proportion of filtered fluid is delivered to the loop of Henle. The reabsorption of sodium chloride in the loop of Henle is critical for the maintenance of medullary hyperosmolality, however, so that in the presence of enhanced proximal tubular reabsorption of sodium and sustained medullary blood flow, medullary osmolality falls. This fall in medullary hyperosmolality leads to a defect in urinary concentrating ability, so that more urine must be excreted to eliminate the same amount of solute. Gann and Wright have shown that in postoperative patients, expansion of the extracellular fluid can reverse the defect in sodium excretion and in concentrating ability, suggesting that hypovolemia, presumably as a result of sequestration of fluid in the third space, is the principal mechanism involved (Fig. 1-34). However, they also demonstrated that even if extracellular fluid volume is maintained, injury leads to the conservation mechanisms outlined.

Sodium that escapes reabsorption in the proximal tubule and in the loop of Henle is in general captured in the distal tubule and collecting duct under the influence of aldosterone. In the distal tubule, sodium is reabsorbed together with chloride and water to maintain osmotic equilibrium. In the collecting duct, however, sodium is reabsorbed in exchange for potassium and hydrogen, providing the principal mechanism for potassium excretion. If insufficient sodium is delivered to this site in the nephron, accumulated potassium and hydrogen cannot be excreted adequately and hyperkalemia and acidosis may ensue. Since

Fig. 1-34. Decreased extracellular fluid volume leads to sodium retention, reflected as decreased rate of sodium excretion ($U_{Na}V$). Since the increased reabsorption occurs in the proximal tubule, less sodium is delivered to the medulla and the urine cannot be concentrated maximally. Decreased urine osmolality (Uosm) and free water reabsorption ($T^c_{H_2O}$) follow despite administration of vasopressin. In this dog, the ECF was depleted 20 percent by intraperitoneal lavage with hypertonic glucose between two solute diureses. The latter allowed testing over a range of osmolar clearances (Cosm). (*From D. S. Gann and H. K. Wright, J Surg Res, 6:196, 1966.*)

both potassium and acid accumulate in injury, maintained delivery of sodium to the most distal portions of the nephron and maintained urinary excretion are critical to the prevention of life-threatening hyperkalemia and acidosis.

WATER EXCRETION

One of the most constant responses to injury of all types is the release of vasopressin. This hormone produces oliguria unless specific steps are taken to overcome it. It was originally suggested that oliguria was a normal accompaniment of surgical trauma and that it did no particular harm. It is certainly reasonably well tolerated in most types of mild to moderate surgical trauma, but it is a potentially harmful condition in two ways: the first is that it predisposes to acute tubular necrosis in patients with severe trauma in whom hypovolemia and hypotension are apt to occur, and the second is that it sets the stage for the development of water intoxication if large amounts of non-solute-containing fluids are given to the patient before, during, or immediately after the operative event.

The increased ADH activity persists for 3 to 5 days postoperatively, depending upon the severity of the trauma, and it is a very common event to see patients who have undergone rather severe operative trauma eliminate their water load with a very brisk diuresis, sometimes ranging up to 200 or 300 ml/hour on the third or fourth postoperative day.

Measurements of vasopressin levels in surgical patients were made by Moran et al.; they found that the night before the operation the blood level of ADH was 0.6 μU/ml of whole blood, while just prior to the induction of anesthesia the value had risen to 1.7 μU, apparently as a consequence of the standard practice of withholding fluids the night before the surgical procedure. The rise was greatest in those patients who had been placed on nasogastric suction. Adequate fluid replacement prior to the induction of anesthesia reduced these values to 0.7 μU/ml. The start of the operation was delayed for up to 40 minutes to note the effect of anesthesia per se on ADH levels. Anesthesia produced a slight increase in ADH levels, but this could be completely offset by the rapid administration of parenteral fluid, which led instead of falling ADH levels. The value for the anesthetic period was therefore 1.4 μU/ml, which was similar to that of the preinduction period.

The anesthetic agents used were halothane, Pentothal, methoxyflurane, and nitrous oxide. If the operation was performed under epidural anesthesia, no response to the abdominal incision was noted. In patients operated on under general anesthesia an increased output of ADH occurred within 5 minutes, and in all patients this increase occurred once traction was applied to the viscera innervated outside the area of effective block. A very minor response to skin incision alone took place, but a tenfold increase occurred when the incision was rapidly carried through all layers of the abdominal wall and traction was applied to the viscera.

The responses occurring during the intermediate portion of the operation were very variable. Sometimes the ADH level rose to a plateau which was maintained throughout the procedure, and at other times it simply rose and fell according to visceral traction. Levels as high as 40 to 150 μU/ml occurred during visceral traction. The magnitude of response was related generally to the magnitude of the procedure. Levels of the sort observed are capable of producing a temporary complete cessation of urine flow. In two patients with high ADH values the creatinine clearance decreased 50 percent, whereas in a patient with a much smaller response there was no change in the creatinine clearance.

The postoperative period was characterized by two phases: the first phase began shortly after skin closure, lasted 6 to 12 hours, and was characterized by a plateau of moderately increased ADH output; this period was followed by a gradual decrease of ADH levels until normal levels were reached on the fourth or fifth postoperative day. In cases of lesser magnitude the return to normal levels occurred by the second postoperative day. The high levels of ADH could be correlated very well with a low urinary output, while the falloff in ADH levels corresponded with diuresis. While hydration was capable of suppressing the increased output of ADH preoperatively and during anesthesia alone, it was not capable of suppressing the elevated levels of ADH seen during operation and in the postoperative period.

The unopposed output of vasopressin leads to water retention, concentrated urine, and oliguria. If water is administered without salt to patients with high levels of ADH, hyponatremia will result. Maximum urine concentration often will not occur, however, because of limited medullary hyperosmolality, as discussed above. Wright and Gann showed that if the extracellular fluid volume was expanded in patients demonstrating postoperative antidiuresis, a dilute urine could be produced. These findings suggest strongly that volume expansion corrected the diuresis by inhibiting secretion of vasopressin and suggested, in addition, that hypovolemia dominates among the various stimuli to secretion of vasopressin as a result of injury or surgery.

Insensible Water Loss

Insensible water losses have been said by Hayes to be about the same after as before injury and of the order of 750 ml/m²/day. This would be an insensible water loss of about 1,300 ml/day, which seems excessively high. Gump and Kinney report a loss of about 2 ml/m²/hour, which comes to about 860 ml/day. Actually it is more frequently in the order of 500 ml/day. We have had an opportunity to carry a large number of patients through operative procedures in the complete absence of all renal tissue. Unless there are excessive losses into the wound or an exceptionally high fever, the patients are maintained in equilibrium on about 500 ml/day. Increased losses can occur in the presence of hyperventilation or fever, and huge losses occur from the skin wounds of burned patients and from the lungs of those with tracheostomies.

HYDRATION. It was shown by Hume and Egdahl that acute anuria after kidney transplantation in dogs could be prevented by sufficient hydration of the donor prior to and during operation in order to provide a brisk diuresis of the donor kidney before its removal. The same principle has been applied to renal homotransplantation in man. Barry and Malloy have stressed the value of preventing oliguria in the surgical patient by means of sustained hydration. These writers showed that at all concentrations of halothane anesthesia studied renal plasma flow, glomerular filtration rate, and urine flow were significantly depressed in fluid-restricted subjects. In contrast these measurements were normal in hydrated subjects, except when very high concentrations of halothane were used. The hydrated group was given a 0.3% saline solution. Sodium excretion in the hydrated and dehydrated groups were the same, but urine osmolality exceeded serum osmolality in all dehydrated subjects, whereas urine osmolality was considerably lower in the hydrated subjects.

During surgical procedures some sequestration of fluid occurs in the operative area (the so-called "third space"), and this produces a reduction in central circulatory volume which leads to a fall in renal blood flow. Renal blood flow can be restored to normal by the prompt administration of fluid, but if the deficit in central circulatory volume is allowed to persist beyond certain critical limits, the ability of renal circulation to respond promptly to restoration is lost. This reduction in central circulatory volume produces stimulation of the volume receptors, thus leading to the release of vasoconstrictor substances such as angiotensin II and catecholamines. This produces a further decrease in renal blood flow which may be resistant to change. Oliguria can be prevented by the routine administration of 1,000 to 1,500 ml of a balanced salt solution in the 2- to 3-hour period prior to the beginning of anesthesia or by the administration of mannitol during the operative event. Since solute diuresis leads to further loss of salt and water, mannitol should be given in 0.45% saline solution to prevent hyponatremia and hypovolemia, as suggested by Gann, Wright, and Newsome. It is very important that the diuresis be established before the introduction of anesthesia.

Postoperative Patterns

The two patterns that are perhaps most frequently seen in the postoperative patient are illustrated in Figs. 1-35 and 1-36. The first is that of a mild to moderate dilutional hyponatremia with hyperkalemia. This is primarily brought about by ADH secretion plus overhydration of the patient with non-salt-containing fluids. The potassium level may be elevated by the movement of potassium out of cells as a result of protein catabolism, by breakdown of red cells in a wound, or as a result of administration of old blood. This may pose a serious threat if renal function is impaired.

This response is made much worse if the trauma is severe and prolonged or if the patient has had a chronic wasting illness prior to operation. Other factors which make the response worse are starvation, which in itself can produce hyponatremia, preexisting renal impairment, which predisposes to a further elevation of potassium level and depression of sodium level, cardiac disease with edema, preexisting hyponatremia, a pronounced shift of sodium into the cell with severe trauma, and episodes of hypotension during the operation which may further im-

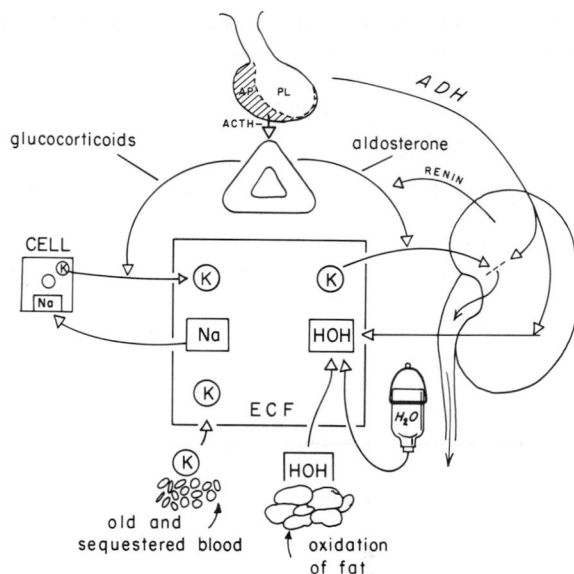

Fig. 1-35. Pattern of hyponatremia in the postoperative patient. Solute is diluted principally by excessive administration of water without salt. In addition, in severe trauma sodium will move into cells in exchange for potassium. The hyperkalemia may be further aggravated by acidosis, by the action of cortisol, and by the breakdown of blood and may be opposed by the action of aldosterone. The dilution may be aggravated by the oxidation of fat and sugar.

Fig. 1-36. Pattern of hypokalemic alkalosis in the postoperative patient. This is most commonly seen in patients who have been on gastric suction and who are alkalotic at the time of operation. The alkalosis produces an additional potassium loss in the urine. Hyperventilation increases the alkalosis and promotes further potassium loss. The administration of sodium bicarbonate, sometimes given in circumstances thought likely to produce acidosis, may further increase the alkalosis. These events then conspire to produce a severe hypokalemic alkalosis which, if renal function is good, may be made worse by the action of the corticosteroids in promoting potassium excretion.

pair renal function. If a marked diuresis is induced by mannitol, this may produce considerable sodium diuresis and add to the hyponatremia if non-sodium-containing repair solutions are used. The cardiac patient needs sodium therapy postoperatively, even though he has an elevated total body sodium. Calcium can also be used but may potentiate digitalis effect if the potassium level remains high. These changes can be prevented or minimized by the use of sodium chloride-containing solutions in the preoperative, operative, and postoperative periods, and by the avoidance of potassium-containing solutions during periods of decreased renal perfusion or when such perfusion is uncertain, as during major surgery.

The second pattern is one of hypokalemic alkalosis. This is classically seen in the patient with an obstructing duodenal ulcer on gastric suction. The alkalosis created by the loss of hydrogen ion from the stomach produces marked urinary potassium loss. This condition is made worse by starvation; the intravenous administration of fluids without potassium; the administration of chlorothiazide diuretics; the administration of corticosteroids; the presence of diarrhea or a fistula; hyperventilation alkalosis; the preoperative existence of certain diseases, such as severe liver disease, where hypokalemia may frequently be present; the administration of sodium bicarbonate or tris buffer, particularly to open heart patients on extracorporeal circulation; or the presence of chronic pulmonary disease, where pulmonary arteriovenous shunts produce hypoxia and a secondary stimulus to hypocapnia. These changes can be prevented by avoidance of the factors listed above, which intensify the response, and by the administration of potassium-containing fluids as needed in the postoperative period. Chloride ion is a critical factor in the repair of hypokalemic alkalosis. In particular the restoration of acquired deficits prior to operation when possible helps to prevent development of these changes.

OXYGEN TRANSPORT

Certain organic phosphates in erythrocytes interact with deoxygenated hemoglobin, thereby altering the affinity of hemoglobin for oxygen. The most abundant of these phosphates in man is 2,3-DPG, the erythrocyte concentration of which has an inverse relationship to the affinity of hemoglobin for oxygen.

Blood stored in ACD at $4°C$ shows a progressive loss of 2,3-DPG, and after 15 days there is almost none at all. This shifts the oxyhemoglobin dissociation curve strikingly to the left. If such blood is infused into patients, it has a diminished ability to give up oxygen to the tissues.

There are other factors which lower erythrocyte 2,3-DPG levels and produce tissue anoxia. These include (1) acidosis, (2) alkalosis, (3) hypophosphatemia (especially seen with hyperalimentation with synthetic amino acids without added phosphate), (4) septic shock, and (5) trauma without hypotension.

Hemorrhagic shock in patients or baboons usually does not alter red cell 2,3-DPG levels, but resuscitation with old banked blood does. Less severe trauma is usually associated with respiratory alkalosis, and this may depress 2,3-DPG levels and reduce tissue oxygenation. Severe shock with acidosis or septic shock reduces 2,3-DPG and interferes with tissue oxygenation.

Hyperalimentation with essential amino acid solutions not containing added phosphate leads to severe hypophosphatemia, which in turn reduces erythrocyte 2,3-DPG and ATP levels and increases red cell avidity for oxygen, leading to tissue hypoxia.

Increases in erythrocyte 2,3-DPG occurs at high altitudes, with chronic anemia, and in congestive heart failure.

Changes in erythrocyte 2,3-DPG levels were not observed by Naylor and his colleagues in rhesus monkeys subjected either to endotoxin or hypovolemic shock.

In clinical settings, the use of old banked blood, marked alkalosis, septic shock, and hyperalimentation are the circumstances in which depressed erythrocyte 2,3-DPG levels are usually seen. All these except septic shock are easily reversed. The administration of fresh or frozen blood, correction of alkalosis, and addition of phosphate to hyperalimentation mixtures solve the other problems.

IMMUNOLOGIC PROTECTIVE MECHANISMS

After injury there is an acute fall in lymphocytes, an increase in polymorphonuclear leukocytes, and a transient suppression of the reticuloendothelial system (RES). Although some of these effects may be produced by cortisol, the decrease in immunologic competence occurs after injury in the absence of increased steroids, as shown by Munster and his colleagues.

Immediately after a severe trauma there is a surge of neuroendocrine activity designed to counteract the early effects of the injury, an event obviously of paramount importance to the survival of the organism. If the individual survives, this surge diminishes in favor of the mechanisms of orderly repair, and protein and fat repletion. If the injury is complicated by sepsis or repeated traumatic insult, there will be a continuous neuroendocrine stimulus, and cortisol levels will generally remain elevated right up to the point of death. The lymphocyte and eosinophil counts remain low, and cellular immunity continues to be suppressed.

Stetson showed that most of the effects of endotoxin could be produced by antigen-antibody complexes, and Pillemer and his colleagues showed that gram-negative bacterial endotoxins could activate complement. Weil and Spink noted a marked resemblance between endotoxin shock and anaphylactic shock. Schumer and his colleagues investigated the thesis that endotoxin shock was produced by antigen-antibody complexes and complement, which combined to produce an anaphylactic reaction, and found that corticosteroids exerted a protective effect by decreasing either complement or complement fixation. Schumer has recently demonstrated the efficacy of corticosteroid therapy in septic shock in man. While this may not be the sole explanation for the production of endotoxin shock or the beneficial effect of pharmacologic doses of corticosteroids, it seems likely that antigen-antibody complexes and complement play an important role in the production of this type of shock.

Polymorphonuclear leukocytes and platelets are increased in numbers by cortisol, so that although the lymphatic system is suppressed, the bone marrow is generally stimulated. The RES, like the lymphatic system, is suppressed early after severe injury, at which time there is an increased susceptibility to shock and infection. Later there is a recovery and even hyperactivity of the RES. These patterns of activity are frequently correlated with plasma cortisol, but the correlation may be accidental and is certainly not necessary.

The RES plays a role in resistance to certain types of shock which is quite apart from its antibacterial role. Stimulation of the RES by estrogen, choline, or zymosan increases phagocytic function and also increases the resistance to trauma. Adaptation to repeated trauma is accompanied by a marked hypertrophy and hyperfunction of the RES.

The RES aids in clearing away fibrin and other coagulation debris, and RES blockade leads to intravascular fibrin deposition and renal corticol necrosis. It also leads to increased susceptibility to shock.

In hemorrhagic shock the RES cell is said by Bell and his colleagues to undergo lysosomal disruption, a change which may lead to autolysis and RES failure.

Distant trauma increases the rate of wound or peritoneal infection in response to a bacterial inoculum. This is said by Hawley to be counteracted by dextran, which works by diminishing blood viscosity. The increased blood viscosity which normally accompanies trauma interferes with tissue perfusion and oxygenation, and thus increases susceptibility to infection.

Thus the obvious effects of trauma upon the immune system vary with the time after injury, the type of trauma, and the particular segment of the immune system which is studied. There are still many gaps in our knowledge of the response of the immune defense mechanisms to injury, and further work needs to be done to clarify this relationship.

ORGAN SYSTEM CHANGES

Cardiovascular Function

SURGERY. Many of the cardiovascular changes in severe trauma and shock have already been described. Clowes and Del Guercio followed the cardiac response in a series of patients before, during, and after operation. During operation the cardiac output fell an average of 33 percent from the preoperative level, mainly because of a decrease in stroke volume. This was accompanied by an elevation of central venous pressure. Immediately after the operation, following endotracheal extubation, the cardiac output rose on the average to 130 percent of the preoperative value and remained at somewhat elevated levels for the first postoperative week. This elevation of cardiac output after the end of the operation was characteristic of thoracic procedures but was not seen following abdominal laparotomy. Patients who died during the postoperative period

never achieved circulatory flows comparable to their preoperative levels.

BURNS. Berk and his colleagues studied eight severely burned patients and found a characteristic pattern consisting of a decrease in cardiac output with normal blood pressure and increased total peripheral resistance. The oxygen consumption was increased with a high arteriovenous oxygen difference, resulting from the low total cardiac flows. The central blood volume was increased, and central venous pressure showed no evidence of hypovolemia.

SHOCK. MacLean and Duff found that septic shock in dogs and man was accompanied by a fall in cardiac output, arterial pressure, and central venous pressure. In dogs, treatment with isoproterenol, blood, and hyperbaric oxygen restored cardiac output and decreased peripheral resistance but did not improve survival. In patients there was generally an increased peripheral resistance associated with hemorrhagic shock. Transfusion and isoproterenol restored venous pressure, cardiac output, and blood pressure to or toward normal and decreased peripheral resistance. Survival seems to have been favorably influenced by this treatment.

Wilson and coworkers evaluated the data in 31 patients in shock. Those in septic shock had a higher cardiac output and lower peripheral resistance than those in hypovolemic or cardiac shock, where the peripheral resistance was always high. No survival was noted in the septic shock group unless cardiac output was at least 2 liters/m^2/minute. It was stressed that although vasodilators, such as phenoxybenzamine, might be of value when peripheral resistance was increased, their use in patients with decreased peripheral resistance was of no definite benefit and might be deleterious.

Severe trauma is thus characterized by a decreased cardiac output and often an increased peripheral resistance. Tissue arteriovenous shunts may open up, partly as a consequence of epinephrine release, thus increasing venous oxygenation and further intensifying tissue anoxia. This increases acidosis and additionally reduces cardiac output.

The use of phenoxybenzamine in certain patients in septic shock to overcome some of the unfavorable cardiovascular changes has been championed by Hardaway and his associates. Before administering phenoxybenzamine the patients had been treated with volume replacement, antibiotics, correction of acid-base imbalances, corticosteroids, and vasopressors, with progressive deterioration on this regimen. It is emphasized that vasodilators should be used only when preceded by fluid volume replacement to the point of an elevated central venous or pulmonary artery pressure. At this time, when the cardiac index is low and peripheral resistance high, phenoxybenzamine may produce a dramatic increase in cardiac index, fall in peripheral resistance, and brisk diuresis (Fig. 1-37). Respiratory insufficiency, which is usually present, must be corrected and treatment instituted for sepsis and defects in coagulation. Apart from its peripheral effect of vasodilatation and improved tissue perfusion, phenoxybenzamine is believed to improve cardiac performance by direct inotropic action on the myocardium, vasodilating effect on

Fig. 1-37. Effect of phenoxybenzamine in septicemic shock. After raising the central venous pressure with colloids and after the failure of other modalities of treatment, phenoxybenzamine produced a rise of blood pressure, a fall in central venous pressure, a fall in peripheral resistance, an increase in cardiac index, a fall in pulse, an increase in stroke volume, and a marked increase in urinary output. (*From R. M. Hardaway et al., JAMA, 199:779, 1967.*)

the coronary vessels and myocardial microvasculature, and relief of postcapillary pulmonary vasoconstriction with increased venous return to the left side of the heart. Most patients in septic shock, however, have peripheral vaso-dilatation, at least in the early and intermediate stages, and a hyperdynamic state. Therefore, the popularity of vasodilators has declined.

The cause of cardiac failure in shock, particularly in septic shock, is still being hotly debated. However, there is general agreement that septic shock induces initially a hyperdynamic state with a high cardiac output and a low peripheral resistance, unless the patient has previously had a reduced blood volume. Although those findings might be explained by arteriovenous shunting in the peripheral tissues or by defective oxygen transfer to the tissues as a consequence of the low erythrocyte 2,3-DPG levels known to be present in septic shock, Wright and his coworkers have developed evidence to suggest that there is instead a primary failure of the peripheral tissues in septic shock

to extract oxygen, and that the hyperdynamic state results as a compensatory mechanism.

After a period of time the hyperdynamic state gives way to deterioration of cardiac function and ultimately cardiac failure and death. During the period of deterioration of function Cann and his coworkers found that ouabain was the only agent they tested which was capable of improving myocardial function. Coalson and her colleagues, however, found that digoxin treatment provided functional protection for the heart and prevented the mitochondrial changes produced in the myocardium by endotoxin.

Interest has recently been renewed in the concept that there is a circulatory factor present in shock, particularly endotoxin shock, which is a specific myocardial depressant, and that this agent is responsible for the failure of the heart in septic shock. Attar et al. believe that plasma kallikreins are partly responsible for this effect. These are proteolytic enzymes activated by Hageman factor which release bradykinin from its precursor. The kallikreins were found to be increased in shock, and were assumed to release bradykinin, thus producing hypotension.

Solis and Downing, Lefer et al., Glenn and Lefer, and Wagensteen and his colleagues have written a series of papers reviving the concept that MDF is the primary agent producing myocardial depression in shock, particularly septic shock. MDF is a small peptide produced in the pancreas by the action of lysosomal proteases released during shock. They feel that the primary event in any type of shock is splanchnic hypoperfusion which then releases lysosomal hydrolases, primarily from the pancreas, giving rise to MDF, which in turn exerts strong negative inotropic effect on the heart.

Goodyer and his colleagues have shown that the canine myocardium, which usually extracts pyruvate from coronary blood, produces pyruvate in hemorrhagic shock, even when the ventricular function is still well preserved. The coronary sinus oxygen saturation falls below 20 percent at a time when the cardiac function is still quite good, and this may be responsible for the early abnormality in pyruvate metabolism, and the late impairment in contractile function. They feel that some factor present in the blood after 1 hour of shock may give rise to this change in oxygenation and in pyruvate metabolism and that their data generally support the concept of an MDF of some type. Low norepinephrine levels have been observed in the myocardium in shock by Hiott and Richardson, but the reduced myocardial effort could not be related to the levels of norepinephrine.

In the later stages of endotoxin shock there is universal agreement that cardiac failure supervenes. Hinshaw and his coworkers have noted a characteristic elevation of left ventricular end-diastolic pressure, decreased maximal change in the left ventricular pressure, and the need for a positive inotropic agent to drive the heart through an imposed after-load performance curve. Only slight improvement was noted with beta-adrenergic stimulatory agents.

Greenfield et al. and Hinshaw et al. have demonstrated normal myocardial performance in the early phases of endotoxin shock, and no adverse effects on cardiac work or metabolism during cross circulation with animals in the intermediate or late stages. These experiments did not, therefore, substantiate a primary role for MDF in endotoxin shock.

Levinson and Hume carried out exchange transfusions in animals and in four patients in refractory shock. In the animal experiments this procedure proved to be much more effective than administration of corticosteroids, isoproterenol, or Ringer's lactate solution. The four patients showed improvement in cardiac output, mean arterial pressure, urine output, and arterial pH—although all ultimately died. It was postulated that the exchange transfusions might have washed out substances interfering with cardiac function, including vasoactive polypeptides, histamine, serotonin, catecholamines, or MDF. The exchange also added erythrocytes containing normal amounts of 2,3-DPG to replace those with the depressed 2,3-DPG levels seen in septic shock, thus perhaps improving tissue oxygenation.

It is obvious that the question of the primacy of MDFs in septic shock has not yet been answered.

ANESTHESIA. Baez and Orkin studied the effect of various anesthetic agents on microcirculation and concluded that with cyclopropane anesthesia the compensatory mechanisms of vasomotion, epinephrine reactivity, and overall blood flow are well maintained whereas with ether these compensatory reactions, initially enhanced, are then depressed below normal. Halothane sustained compensatory vascular patterns until late in the course of observation. Methoxyflurane depressed compensatory mechanisms early. It was felt that these experiments confirmed the clinical observations of the utility of cyclopropane and halothane in shock.

Pulmonary Function

ANESTHESIA AND SURGERY. Hypoxia and hypercapnia following operation may be due to the continuing effects of anesthesia and muscle relaxants, together with the development of atelectasis. Significant decreases in pulmonary diffusion have been found following all types of operations, lasting as long as 5 days following operation. The ventilation perfusion defect or pulmonary arteriovenous shunting may involve 25 percent of the total pulmonary blood flow. This produces a considerable degree of hypoxia.

The work of breathing, which normally requires 1 to 2 percent of the cardiac output, may require as much as 30 to 50 percent of the total cardiac output after operation or trauma. Assisted respiration produces a decrease in oxygen consumption and cardiac output.

Anesthesia and surgical procedures alter respiration by depressing the pulmonary reflexes and the central nervous system response, thus depressing the patient's desire to breathe. This is true of both preoperative and postoperative medications, the general anesthetic agent, and of course the muscle relaxants. Patients may occasionally have very severe reactions to a muscle relaxant, so that

they will not breathe on their own for several hours after the end of the operation. Respiratory excursion is also interfered with by spinal and epidural anesthesia and by disruption of the thorax, abdomen, or the respiratory tract itself. Secretions collect in the bronchial tree because of difficulty in coughing and moving, and this gives rise to atelectasis. Pulmonary arteriovenous shunts may be operative in atelectasis and in patients with cirrhosis, and profound acid-base changes may result as a consequence of hyperventilation or of prolonged cardiopulmonary bypass.

Peters and Hedgpeth have shown that an increase in airway resistance and pulmonary vascular resistance both cause increased respiratory work. They also lead to ventilation perfusion incoordination by changing the time constants for ventilation of the various areas of the lung. This causes more work. The increased respiratory work then leads to further acidosis in a vicious cycle, since acidosis leads to pulmonary vasoconstriction and further sensitizes the lung to vasoconstriction due to hypoxia. Metabolic acidosis superimposed on respiratory acidosis retards the increased cardiac output associated ordinarily with respiratory acidosis. Metabolic acidosis increases pulmonary vascular resistance, thus increasing respiratory work. Acidosis also leads to movement of potassium ion out of muscle cells, decreasing excitability and potentiating further the vicious cycle.

Prophylaxis. In an attempt to determine whether postoperative pulmonary complications can be prevented by the use of isoproterenol and intermittent positive pressure breathing (IPPB), Anderson and his colleagues studied 160 control patients and 42 patients receiving IPPB and isoproterenol. A very significant reduction in postoperative complications was encountered in the treated group. Roe has also urged the wider use of airway moisture, expectorants, tracheal aspiration, bronchoscopy, and tracheostomy as prophylaxis against pulmonary complications in postoperative patients. Should endotracheal intubation be required, effective prophylaxis against atelectasis and shunting is best achieved by constant positive pressure breathing (CPPB), together with maintained elevation of positive end-expiratory pressure (PEEP). The PEEP must be low enough to prevent decreased venous return.

High-Output Respiratory Failure. Burke and his coworkers have described the syndrome of high-output respiratory failure as that type of respiratory failure characterized by inability to produce adequate tissue oxygenation, and later carbon dioxide excretion, despite an initially increased gas exchange. In a study of 21 patients this type of failure frequently was associated with severe peritonitis or ileus. No deaths were directly attributable to the high-output failure. The syndrome of high-output respiratory failure may be suspected by persistent elevation of pulse and respiration with a normal blood pressure in an anxious exhausted patient. It is confirmed by a depressed arterial oxygen saturation. Previous lung disease, obesity, smoking, or severe debility predispose to it. Tracheostomy and assisted respiration may have to be used to treat it.

Nash and his coworkers have described a pulmonary lesion associated with oxygen therapy and artificial ventilation in 70 patients who died after prolonged artificial ventilation. These patients all showed characteristic pulmonary changes consisting of heavy, beefy, and edematous lungs. Microscopically these showed an early exudative phase characterized by congestion, alveolar edema, intraalveolar hemorrhage, and a fibrin exudate, with formation of prominent hyaline membranes without any associated inflammatory component. A late proliferative phase was characterized by marked aveolar and interlobular septal edema, fibroblastic proliferation with early fibrosis, and prominent hyperplasia of the lining cells. These changes were not related to the duration of the ventilation but to high concentrations of inspired oxygen. It was felt that patients should receive inspired oxygen concentration sufficient to ensure normal or nearly normal arterial oxygen tension and that this should be reduced as soon as blood-gas measurements show that reduction can be accomplished safely.

SHOCK. Cook and Webb have studied the pulmonary changes in shock and found that there was a rise in transpulmonary vascular pressure and a great increase in pulmonary vascular resistance which persisted for several hours after the shock was corrected. There was congestive atelectasis, recruitment of pulmonary vascular segments, and alveolar capillary dilatation, suggesting venous constriction. Ventilation increased while compliance decreased, indicating a diminished gas exchange with increased ventilatory work. Veith and his coworkers found that shock and transfusion produced an initial active arteriolar vasoconstriction followed by secondary vasodilatation, congestion, hemorrhage, and edema. These changes may help to explain the frequent pulmonary complications accompanying hemorrhagic shock.

POSTTRAUMATIC PULMONARY INSUFFICIENCY. There has been a great deal of interest recently in the lung changes that occur in severe trauma not involving the thorax. The condition has often been called "shock lung," but as shock alone does not actually produce it, it is probably best called the *posttraumatic pulmonary insufficiency syndrome.* There are several different etiologic factors—some or all of them operative in each case. Among the factors most frequently incriminated in the syndrome are (1) oxygen therapy, (2) loss of pulmonary surfactant, (3) alveolar collapse, (4) platelet aggregate emboli induced by trauma, (5) platelet aggregates and other debris in infused blood, (6) viable immunologically competent leukocytes in fresh blood, (7) pump oxygenators, (8) fat emboli, (9) pulmonary arteriovenous shunting, (10) sepsis, endotoxin, (11) vomiting and aspiration, (12) fluid overload, and (13) vasoactive substances released into the pulmonary circulation.

Blaisdell and his colleagues have shown that microemboli of various types are probably a factor in most patients with the pulmonary insufficiency syndrome. Platelet microemboli tend to develop in vivo after hemorrhage and as a consequence of endotoxemia. They also develop in banked blood and increase as the storage period is extended, and in pump-oxygenator systems. They are caused by an increase in platelet adhesiveness. Micropore filters have been developed to remove the emboli from infused blood.

Nahas and his colleagues have claimed that viable leukocytes infused in fresh blood can mount a graft versus host reaction in the lung. This can be avoided by the use of frozen red cells. Fat emboli occur not only from bone marrow injury, but also from the reesterification of fatty acids mobilized by the catecholamines and glucagon.

Oxygen toxicity is capable of producing fatal pulmonary damage. When oxygen concentrations of 70 to 100% are used with respirators for prolonged periods of time (giving P_{O_2} values above 350 mm Hg), there is damage to the endothelial cells, with interstitial edema, hyaline membrane deposition, alveolar epithelial cell hypertrophy and desquamation, and alveolar hemorrhage. Arteriovenous shunting and hypoxemia result from this. These are similar to changes seen in the posttraumatic lung.

Sepsis is a major factor in the lung changes seen after trauma. The bacteria may be filtered out by the lung following their embolization from a distant site, they may enter directly through the airway, or they may affect the lungs by means of endotoxins. Endotoxin produces damage to pulmonary capillaries, thus initiating the changes of the pulmonary insufficiency syndrome.

Probably the most important cause of the lung changes of trauma is the loss of pulmonary surfactant with alveolar collapse, focal atelectases, decreased compliance, arteriovenous shunting, and interstitial edema.

Hypothalamic hypoxia is thought to contribute to the development of the syndrome by producing autonomically mediated pulmonary venular spasms leading to interstitial edema, intraalveolar hemorrhage, surfactant neutralization by plasma, hyaline membranes, and alveolar atelectasis.

The hypocapnia that normally develops as a consequence of the postinjury hyperventilation is thought by Trimble and associates to be an important etiologic agent in the production of pulmonary insufficiency. Hypocapnia is said to induce bronchoconstriction, and the alkalosis produced by blowing off carbon dioxide affects blood flow to the lung and unfavorably affects oxyhemoglobin dissociation. The addition of carbon dioxide to the inspired air is said to improve oxygenation and other parameters of pulmonary physiology.

Vomiting and aspirating stomach contents or blood and fluid overloading are contributing factors to the development of lung lesions after trauma.

The lysis of platelet aggregates and resulting reactions lead to release of serotonin, bradykinin, and prostaglandins (especially $F_{2\alpha}$) into the pulmonary circulation. Venular constriction and bronchoconstriction may result, leading in turn to interstitial movement of fluid and colloid, to a diffusion block for O_2, and thus to increased shunting.

The treatment and/or prevention of the pulmonary insufficiency syndrome consists of (1) the use of micropore filters for infused blood, (2) the avoidance of blood with viable leukocytes, (3) the treatment of sepsis, (4) the avoidance of aspiration or fluid overloading by administering corticosteroids if aspiration occurs and diuretics for fluid overloads, (5) the use of corticosteroids for massive fat embolization, (6) the use of oxygen mixtures of 45% or less, (7) the determination of serial blood gases, (8) the use of a volume respirator which "sighs" periodically, and especially (9) the application of continuous positive pressure to provide 6 cm water pressure at the end of expiration or, more appropriately, a level of PEEP that does not lead to a fall in arterial pressure. This helps to correct the alveolar collapse brought about by loss of surfactant.

The question of whether resuscitation with noncolloidal fluids is more damaging to the lung than if colloids had been used is still largely unresolved. While the functional differences between these two repair solutions is slight, there are more ultrastructural lung changes when noncolloids are used than when albumin is used.

The use of a membrane oxygenator and extracorporeal heart-lung machine for a severe case of pulmonary failure has been said by Hill and his colleagues to have resulted in survival. This may be an important therapeutic modality in the future.

The effects of the pulmonary insufficiency syndrome are to produce a progressive hypoxemia with arteriovenous shunting, acidosis, hypercapnia, interstitial edema, and sepsis, with stiff, beefy, heavy, wet lungs and, ultimately, death.

Hepatic Function

DRUGS AND ANESTHETIC AGENTS. Hepatic function may be depressed by many drugs and anesthetic agents administered to the patient prior to or during surgical procedures. If the liver is not diseased and the degree of trauma not too severe, these minor changes in function usually pass unnoticed and do not prove to be of any clinical significance. If the patient has cirrhosis or other liver damage, some of the commonly used drugs and virtually all the anesthetic agents may produce a depression of hepatic function which, because of inability of the damaged liver to detoxify them, leads to a profound generalized effect. Among these drugs are morphine, which may precipitate coma in patients with cirrhosis, and paraldehyde, which may produce a profound sleep or even death in such patients. This is also true of the barbiturates which are metabolized by the liver. Other drugs may interfere with bilirubin metabolism, such as the sulfonamides, which inhibit plasma binding; flavaspidic acid, which interferes with bilirubin transport through the cell; novobiocin, which interferes with glucuronide conjugation; cholecystographic media, which compete with the conjugated bilirubin for excretion into the biliary canaliculus; and methyltestosterone or chlorpromazine, which interfere with the excretion of the bilirubin into the canaliculus. In most instances these reactions are reversible. Direct hepatic toxicity sometimes results from the tetracyclines, particularly in malnutrition or pregnancy, ferrous sulfate, 6-mercaptopurine, methotrexate, and 5-fluoro-2-deoxyuridine. Cinchophen and iproniazid may cause a hepatitis-like reaction.

A great deal of debate has occurred over the effect of the anesthetic agent halothane as a hepatotoxin. Severe reactions and even death can occur occasionally with halothane anesthesia, although fortunately these reactions are rare. They usually depend upon a personal individual sensitivity and almost always occur only when anesthesia has been administered twice for separate operations. It is therefore probably not wise to repeat halothane anesthesia within 6 months. Some of the antituberculosis drugs may cause a hypersensitivity reaction; chief among this group is para-aminosalicylate. Chlorpropamide and tolbutamide can also cause this reaction.

If hepatic reserve is decreased, as it may be in severe cirrhosis, very minor trauma or brief anesthesia can precipitate hepatic failure, coma, and even death.

SHOCK. In severe trauma and shock there is an increased Bromsulphalein (BSP) retention, increased serum bilirubin, increased prothrombin time, decreased fibrinogen, increased SGOT, increased blood ammonia, and decreased urea formation. Glycogen stores are depleted, and lactate acid accumulates. Ketonemia follows and ultimately gives way to low blood ketone levels as hepatic function is further impaired. Blood amino acid nitrogen level rises. Impairment of enzyme systems occurs, and the liver content of high-energy stores such as ATP, ADP, thiamine pyrophosphate (TPP), and flavin adenine dinucleotide (FAD) as well as phosphocreatinine becomes depleted. CoA and succinate oxidase are reduced. There is a reduced capacity for aerobic metabolism.

Damage to the liver has been implicated as one of the causes of irreversibility in shock. It has been postulated that the inability of the liver to detoxify injurious agents released in shock is responsible for the trend toward irreversibility. Actually most of the experiments suggesting this possibility have been carried out in the dog, although differences in the splanchnic circulation and regular hepatic infection with microorganisms make this animal a poor model for the human system. The liver does seem to protect somewhat against intestinal ischemic shock. There is some depression of the RES of the liver in profound shock.

Holden and his coworkers carried out an electron microscopic study of the liver of the rat in shock. After 2 hours of shock there was a distortion of the endoplasmic reticulum, depletion of the glycogen granules, disorganization and swelling of the mitochondria, and in some cells an increase in the number and size of bodies thought to be lysosomes. Hypoxia produced by an atmosphere of 93% nitrous oxide and 7% oxygen for 1 hour failed to produce similar changes. It was suggested that the ultrastructural and biochemical changes observed in hypovolemic shock were not solely the result of cellular hypoxia but rather the result of the combined effects of cellular hypoxia, the neuroendocrine response to hypovolemia, and the altered physiochemical composition of extracellular fluid (ECF) resulting from diminished capillary perfusion.

A study of liver cell lysosomes in traumatic, ischemic, and endotoxin shock by Janoff showed that there was a disruption of lysosomes and the release of their contained enzymes in free active form in the liver of shocked animals. It was felt that the activation of lysosomal hydrolases within cells and their release into the circulation might play an important role in exacerbating tissue injury and accelerating the development of irreversible shock. In those animals rendered tolerant of shock or pretreated with cortisone there was a stabilization of lysosomes, and it was felt that this effect might constitute an important component of the resistance of such animals to shock. The exacerbating effect of reticuloendothelial blocking colloids on the lethality of shock procedures may be due in part to a direct action of these agents on lysosomes.

Blair and his colleagues have performed electron microscopic studies of the liver in shock and found that there was progressive hepatocellular damage during the first hour, characterized by reduction in glycogen, increased prominence of smooth endoplasmic reticulum, swelling of mitochondria, and a disarrangement of the rough endoplasmic reticulum. After 3 hours of shock there was a progressive increase in secondary lysosomes, and by $4\frac{1}{2}$ hours there was a marked prominence of secondary lysosomes which was related to the irreversible shock state. Clermont et al. demonstrated an increase in lysosomal enzyme acid phosphatase content of hepatic blood, lymph, and bile after the second hour of shock.

In addition to the changes in lysosomes, there is a decrease in cell transmembrane potential difference, a decrease in cyclic AMP, and a decrease in the energy-producing capabilities of mitochondria. The energy availability of the cell is dependent upon mitochondrial respiration, which in turn may be controlled by ATP-dependent membrane transport. Baue and his coworkers demonstrated that hepatic ATP-dependent membrane transport was progressively activated in shock, leading to increased sodium and decreased potassium in the mitochondria, with decreased mitochondrial respiration and energy depletion.

Patients with hepatic failure may have a buildup in the blood of substances profoundly toxic to cells throughout the body. Thus hepatic coma eventuates from the effect of these substances on the brain, oliguria appears as a consequence of their action on the kidney, and hypotension results from a depressed cardiac output as a consequence of a toxic effect on the myocardium. Further depression of hepatic function itself may also take place. These effects sometimes can be dramatically reversed by exchange transfusion, in which the toxic substances are washed out of the bloodstream as the patient's blood is replaced by large quantities of fresh donor blood. Fortunately, hepatic reserve in the normal patient is so great that liver failure is seldom a problem in severe trauma.

Gastrointestinal Function

The gastrointestinal changes in trauma range from the mild syndrome of ileus and temporary loss of appetite following intestinal operations, and mucosal changes in the intestinal tract brought about by shock, to stress ulcers of the stomach and duodenum.

SHOCK. Gurd has studied the metabolic and functional changes in the intestine in shock. He found that in dogs

with irreversible shock there was a profound depression of oxygen uptake by the intestine after retransfusion, despite a return of mesenteric blood flow to normal. This was in spite of the fact that oxygen consumption in the liver and limbs returned for a time to normal, as did the cardiac output. Studies with ^{32}P showed a depression of oxidative phosphorylation and nucleotide synthesis in the mucosa of the small intestine of these animals after retransfusion, while full recovery of these processes was noted in the liver. Hemorrhagic necrosis of the bowel was often seen in dogs and could be protected against by the injection of Trasylol, a trypsin inhibitor, into the lumen of the bowel. Hemorrhagic necrosis of this sort is seldom seen in man, where the amount of trypsin present in the intestinal chyme is far less than in dogs, but has been reported in cases of severe shock.

A higher metabolic activity was observed in bowel washed free of its fecal content, suggesting that contact with feces has a deleterious effect on cellular metabolism in ischemic anoxia. After curare was placed in the lumen, the bowel demonstrated an increased permeability in the metabolically depressed mucosa. If the pancreatic ducts were ligated 48 hours before the shock state was induced, hemorrhagic necrosis was prevented.

It could be demonstrated that the mucin coat over the villi was lost at the moment when signs of irreversibility appeared in hypovolemia. In time mucin production ceased. The first areas to lose the mucin coat were the tips of the villi. The loss of mucin permitted damage to the cells by trypsin and led to the development of hemorrhagic necrosis.

There is a striking species difference between the intestinal changes seen in shock in dogs and those in primates. In dogs endotoxin shock produces mesenteric vasoconstriction, intestinal ischemia, and epithelial necrosis, while in primates Barton and his colleagues found that endotoxemia was associated with a normal mesenteric blood flow, a fall in mesenteric vascular resistance, and no gross changes in the intestine. Hypovolemic shock in dogs characteristically produces intense mesenteric vasoconstriction, with diffuse necrosis of the epithelium. In primates mesenteric blood flow was decreased and vascular resistance was increased, but no lesions of the intestine were produced. Vyden and Corday, however, showed that in man gastrointestinal necrosis was sometimes seen in acute myocardial infarction, and that superior mesenteric artery blood flow fell under these circumstances. Drucker and his colleagues have reported a group of patients with hemorrhagic necrosis of the intestine and have suggested that the lesions were produced by anoxia brought about by decreased perfusion and vasospasm.

Intraluminal mucosal nutrients were shown to protect the mucosa of the ischemic bowel from necrosis. Chiu et al. achieved protection by using intraluminal glucose, and Bounous et al. by an elemental diet. This protection was thought to be afforded by direct utilization of the substrate by the mucosa.

In hypovolemic shock Cook and associates have shown that the intestine becomes a secretory rather than absorptive organ and that there can be huge fluid losses into the intestinal lumen.

In experiments on dogs in hemorrhagic shock the intestine has often been implicated as the cause of irreversibility due to the absorption of toxins from the ischemic intestine. This was first thought to be due to bacteria which escaped from the bowel lumen into the circulation as a consequence of ischemic destruction of the intestinal mucosal barrier. However, bacteremia is not found in standard irreversible shock, and Lillehei and coworkers have shown that pretreatment of the dogs with oral neomycin and other antibiotics to the point of sterilization of the stool cultures does not influence the result of hemorrhagic shock. The course prior to death and the hemorrhagic necrosis of the intestinal mucosa at autopsy do not differ in treated dogs from other dogs not receiving oral antibiotics.

Moreover, Zweifach and coworkers found no increased survival from shock in germ-free rats, and Carter and Einheber have shown that intestinal ischemia produced by occluding the superior mesenteric artery in germ-free rats was acutely lethal and there was no significant difference in survival times of germ-free, contaminated germ-free, and normal control rats. The mucosal destruction in dogs is considerably greater than in man, and this is apparently related in part to loss of protecting mucin and the presence of trypsin and other proteolytic enzymes.

Goodman and Osborn have discussed the problem of acute gastric ulceration and its diverse origins. In the neurogenic ulcer seen after head injury there is frequent perforation from esophagogastromalacia, whereas stress ulcers seen with shock rarely perforate. Corticosteroid ulcers are usually antral and respond to antacids, whereas stress ulcers are superficial linear fundic erosions unaffected by antacids and not associated with increased acid production. Postburn ulcers are located in the depths of rugal folds of the fundus as well as the duodenum, are round and deep, and may show bacterial colonies in the base.

Robert and coworkers and Menguy and Masters have shown that steroid ulcers are due to a loss of mucin protection of the epithelium, and Hutcher and his colleagues found that vitamin A prevented steroid ulcers by restoring mucin production. Stress ulcers show relatively little deficit in mucin, however, although Lev and his coworkers found some reduction. The main etiologic factor in stress ulcers is probably mucosal ischemia. Sepsis, in some unknown way, greatly increases the likelihood of the development of stress ulcers.

Intraluminal nutrients protect against stress ulceration, as shown by Voitk, and hyperalimentation does also; hypoglycemia and starvation increase the likelihood of ulceration.

Renal Function

As mentioned earlier in this section, renal function is generally depressed in operative trauma as a result of dehydration of the patient prior to operation, the cardiac depression produced by some anesthetic agents, the hypotension that may occur with blood loss, and the neuroendocrine effects on renal handling of salt and water. Renal function can usually be preserved at normal levels during operative trauma with proper hydration of the patient prior to operation, the avoidance of hypotension by the prompt replacement of blood loss, the monitoring of venous pressure, and the administration of mannitol to maintain an osmotic diuresis.

SHOCK. Severe shock may produce acute tubular necrosis or even cortical necrosis, with temporary or permanent renal failure. The treatment of this condition is considered in Chap. 40. It is now generally felt that the severely injured patient with acute tubular necrosis and severe oliguria or anuria should be treated with repetitive hemodialysis or peritoneal dialysis very early in the course of the renal insufficiency in order to ensure a smoother convalescence and to help prevent death from the complications of anuria. It is recognized that hyperkalemia is not the only indication for dialysis in renal shutdown, and the severely injured patient generally catabolizes tissue at such a rapid rate that early dialysis is mandatory to prevent demise. We have had occasion to dialyze patients within 48 hours of severe injury.

When cardiac output and aortic pressure are reduced experimentally by cardiogenic shock to 50 percent of normal, renal blood flow is 75 percent of normal, whereas similar conditions of cardiac function produced by hemorrhagic shock lead to renal blood flow that is 10 percent of normal. Gorfinkel and his colleagues conclude that this is a reflection of the intense renal vasoconstriction seen with hemorrhagic shock.

Severe oliguria and renal failure may occur in shock due to gram-negative septicemia. Under these circumstances renal function can often be restored by the administration of plasma until the venous pressure is at the upper limits of normal, of phenoxybenzamine to overcome peripheral vasoconstriction and improve renal plasma flow, and of mannitol to induce diuresis. More recently, dopamine has proved useful in producing vasodilation and maintained glomerular filtration; it may be used with furosemide to produce a natriuresis and diuresis. As with mannitol, this regimen requires care in replacing fluid volume to prevent secondary renal shutdown. In the traumatized patient who has become overly treated with fluids and who is edematous or in pulmonary edema, furosemide alone has been extremely valuable in promoting diuresis.

Staphylococcal toxin can produce shock and a profound depression of renal function consisting of reduction in total and effective renal plasma flow with congestion and secondary ischemia of the peripheral cortical zone. The free-water clearance falls, and the percentage of filtered sodium in the urine increases.

The depression of renal function in patients with severe shock differed in the survivors and nonsurvivors in a study by Strauch and coworkers in that the sodium and chloride clearances of the survivors reached levels of 1.2 to 1.4 ml/minute, whereas the values never exceeded 0.4 ml/minute in the nonsurvivors. There was a severe depression of glomerular filtration rate and urea clearance in all patients, but whereas this was transient in survivors, it was progressive in nonsurvivors.

Other aspects of renal function in trauma and shock have been considered in the preceding sections.

GENERAL CONSIDERATIONS

The foregoing discussion of the endocrine and metabolic response to injury has perhaps demonstrated that there are many gaps in our knowledge and that many areas of controversy still remain. The degree to which the body is able to compensate for injury is astonishing, although at times the compensating mechanisms may work to the patient's disadvantage.

Therapeutic trends which have perhaps excited the most interest among surgeons recently include the protection of renal function by hydration and osmotic diuresis; the monitoring of central venous pressure and left atrial pressure as an aid in the assessment of fluid replacement and cardiac action; the swing away from the use of vasoconstrictors in shock to the use of blood volume replacement, maintenance of normal venous pressure, and control of sepsis; the use of intravenously administered bicarbonate to correct situations in which acidosis is known to occur; the correction of clotting defects with specific coagulation agents and fresh blood; an appreciation of the lung problems associated with injury and their correction with proper respirators; the electronic monitoring of blood pressure and other vital parameters; the more exact determination of antibiotic sensitivity of microorganisms; the realization that complete intravenous therapy can be given to patients who are forced to undergo long periods of starvation by the administration of protein and calories; and the frequent measurement of blood gases and fluid and electrolyte flux to determine the pattern of the endocrine and metabolic response to injury. This chapter simply serves as an introduction to some of these subjects, most of which will be covered in more detail in other portions of the book.

References

Stimuli Inducing Change

Baertschi, A. J., Ward, D. G., and Gann, D. S.: Role of Atrial Receptors in the Control of ACTH, *Am J Physiol,* **231:**692, 1976.

Brown, R. S., Mohr, P. A., Carey, J. S., and Shoemaker, W. C.: Cardiovascular Changes after Cranial Cerebral Injury and Increased Intracranial Pressure, *Surg Gynecol Obstet,* **125:**1205, 1967.

Bursten, B., and Russ, J. J.: Preoperative Psychological State and Corticosteroid Levels of Surgical Patients, *Psychosom Med,* **27:**309, 1965.

Cryer, G. L., and Gann, D. S.: Right Atrial Receptors Mediate the Adrenocortical Response to Hemorrhage, *Am J Physiol,* **225:**1345, 1973.

Dallman, M. F., and Yates, F. E.: Anatomical and Functional Mapping of Central Neural Input and Feedback Pathways of the Adrenocortical System, *Mem Soc Endocrinol,* **17:**39, 1968.

Davis, J., Morrill, R., Fawcett, J., Upton, V., Bondy, P. K., and Spiro, H. M.: Apprehension and Elevated Serum Cortisol Levels, *J Psychosom Res,* **6:**83, 1962.

Gann, D. S.: Carotid Vascular Receptors and the Control of Adrenal Corticosteroid Secretion, *Am J Physiol,* **211:**193, 1966.

——— and Cryer, G. L.: Models of Adrenal Cortical Control, *Adv Biomed Eng,* **2:**1, 1972.

——— and Egdahl, R. H.: Responses of Adrenal Corticosteroid Secretion to Hypotension and Hypovolemia, *J Clin Invest,* **44:**1, 1965.

Ganong, W. F., Gold, N. I., and Hume, D. M.: The Effect of Hypothalamic Lesions on the Plasma 17-Hydroxycorticosteroid Response to Immobilization in the Dog, *Fed Proc,* **14:**54, 1955.

Gerich, J. E., Charles, M. A., and Grodsky, G. M.: Regulation of Pancreatic Insulin and Glucagon Secretion, *Annu Rev Physiol,* **38:**353, 1976.

Harris, G. W.: "Neural Control of the Pituitary Gland," Edward Arnold (Publishers) Ltd., London, 1955.

Hume, D. M.: The Method of Hypothalamic Regulation of Pituitary and Adrenal Secretion in Response to Trauma, in S. Curri and L. Martini (eds.), "Pathophysiologia Diencephalica," p. 217, Springer-Verlag OHG, Vienna, 1958.

Noble, R. L.: The Development of Resistance by Rats and Guinea-pigs to Amounts of Trauma Usually Fatal, *Am J Physiol,* **138:**346, 1943.

——— and Collip, J. B.: A Quantitative Method for the Production of Experimental Traumatic Shock without Hemorrhage in Unanaesthetized Animals, *Q J Exp Physiol,* **31:**187, 1942.

Redding, M., and Mueller, C. B.: Effect of Ambient Temperature upon Responses to Hypovolemic Insult in the Unanesthetized, Unrestrained Albino Rat. *Surgery,* **64:**110, 1968.

Central Nervous System and Endocrine Changes

Bowman, H. M., Cowan, D., Kovach, G., Jr., and Hook, J. B.: Renal Effects of Glucagon in Rhesus Monkeys during Hypovolemia, *Surg Gynecol Obstet,* **134:**937, 1972.

Carey, L. C., Cloutier, C. T., and Lowery, B. D.: Growth Hormone and Adrenal Cortical Response to Shock and Trauma in the Human, *Ann Surg,* **174:**451, 1971.

———, Lowery, B. D., and Cloutier, C. T.: Blood Sugar and Insulin Response of Humans in Shock, *Ann Surg,* **172:**342, 1970.

Cerchio, G. M., Moss, G. S., Popovich, P. A., Butler, E., and Siegel, D. C.: Serum Insulin and Growth Hormone Response to Hemorrhagic Shock, *Endocrinology,* **88:**138, 1971.

Cooper, C. E., and Nelson, D. H.: ACTH Levels in Plasma in Preoperative and Surgically Stressed Patients, *J Clin Invest,* **41:**1599, 1962.

Dallman, M. F., and Jones, M. T.: Corticosteroid Feedback Control of Stress-Induced ACTH Secretion, in A. Brodish and E. S. Redgate (eds.), "Brain-Pituitary-Adrenal Interrelationships," p. 176, Karger, Basel, 1973.

Egdahl, R. H.: Pituitary-Adrenal Response following Trauma to the Isolated Leg, *Surgery,* **46:**9, 1959.

Exton, J. H., Ui, M., Lewis, S. B., and Park, C. R.: Mechanism of

Glucagon Activation of Gluconeogenesis, in H. D. Soling and B. Willms (eds.), "Regulation of Gluconeogenesis," p. 160, Academic Press, Inc., New York, 1971.

Frohlich, J., and Wieland, O.: Dissociation of Gluconeogenic and Ketogenic Action of Glucagon in the Perfused Rat Liver, in H. D. Soling and B. Willms (eds.), "Regulation of Gluconeogenesis," p. 179, Academic Press, Inc., New York, 1971.

Gann, D. S.: Parameters of the Stimulus Initiating the Adrenocortical Response to Hemorrhage, *Ann NY Acad Sci,* **156:**740, 1969.

———: Endocrine Control of Plasma Protein and Volume, *Surg Clin North Am,* **56:**1135, 1976.

———, Baertschi, A. J., Ward, D. G., and Pirkle, J. C., Jr.: Homeostasis of Blood Volume through Hemodynamic Control of ACTH and Cortisol, Endocrinology—Proc V Int'l Congr Endocrinol, in V. H. T. James (ed.), *Excerpta Medica,* vol. 1, p. 245, Amsterdam, 1976.

——— and Cryer, G. L.: Feedback Control of ACTH Secretion by Cortisol, in "Brain-Pituitary-Adrenal Interrelationships," *op. cit.,* p. 197.

———, ———, and Pirkle, J. C., Jr.: Physiological Inhibition and Facilitation of Adrenocortical Response to Hemorrhage, *Am J Physiol,* **232:**R5, 1977.

———, Ward, D. G., Baertschi, A. J., Carlson, D. E., and Maran, J. W.: Neural Control of ACTH Release in Response to Hemorrhage, *Ann NY Acad Sci,* **297:**447, 1977.

Genuth, P., and Lebovitz, H. E.: Stimulation of Insulin Release by Corticotropin, *Endocrinology,* **76:**1093, 1965.

Grizzle, W. E., Dallman, M. F., Schramm, L. P., and Gann, D. S.: Inhibitory and Facilitatory Hypothalamic Areas Mediating ACTH Release in the Cat, *Endocrinology,* **95:**1430, 1974.

———, Johnson, R. N., Schramm, L. P., and Gann, D. S.: Hypothalamic Cells in an Area Mediating ACTH Release Respond to Right Atrial Stretch, *Am J Physiol,* **228:**1039, 1975.

Guillen, J., and Pappas, G.: Improved Cardiovascular Effects of Glucagon in Dogs with Endotoxin Shock, *Ann Surg,* **175:**535, 1972.

Halmagyi, D. F. J., Gillett, D. J., Lazarus, L., and Young, J. D.: Blood Glucose and Serum Insulin in Reversible Post Hemorrhagic Shock, *J Trauma,* **6:**623, 1966.

Henneman, D. H., and Henneman, P. H.: Effects of Human Growth Hormone on Levels of Blood and Urinary Carbohydrate and Fat Metabolites in Man, *J Clin Invest,* **39:**1239, 1960.

Herman, A. H., Mack, E., and Egdahl, R. H.: The Relationship of Adrenal Perfusion to Corticosteroid Secretion in Prolonged Hemorrhagic Shock, *Surg Gynecol Obstet,* **132:**795, 1971.

Hiebert, J. M., Soeldner, J. S., and Egdahl, R. H.: Altered Insulin and Glucose Metabolism Produced by Epinephrine during Hemorrhagic Shock in the Primate, *Surgery,* **74,** 1973.

Hume, D. M.: Hypothalamic Localization for the Control of Various Endocrine Secretions, in H. H. Jasper et al. (eds.), "International Symposium; Reticular Formation of the Brain," p. 231, Little, Brown and Company, Boston, 1958.

———, Bell, C. C., Jr., and Bartter, F.: Direct Measurement of Adrenal Secretion during Operative Trauma and Convalescence, *Surgery,* **52:**174, 1962.

——— and Egdahl, R. H.: Effect of Hypothermia and of Cold Exposure on Adrenal Cortical and Medullary Secretion, *Ann NY Acad Sci,* **80:**435, 1959.

——— and ———: The Importance of the Brain in the Endocrine Response to Injury, *Ann Surg,* **150:**697, 1959.

——— and Nelson, D. H.: Adrenal Cortical Function in Surgical Shock, *Surg Forum,* **5:**568, 1955.

———, ———, and Miller, D. W.: Blood and Urinary 17-Hydroxycorticosteroids in Patients with Severe Burns, *Ann Surg,* **143:**316, 1956.

Ingle, D. J.: Permissive Action of Hormones, *J Clin Endocrinol Metab,* **14:**1272, 1954.

Jones, M. T., Hillhowe, E., and Burden, J.: Secretion of Corticotropin-Releasing Hormone in Vitro, in L. Martini and W. F. Ganong (eds.), *Frontiers in Neuroendocrinology,* **4:**195, 1976.

Kaneto, A., Kajinuma, H. and Kosaka, K.: Effect of Splanchnic Nerve Stimulation on Glucagon and Insulin Output in the Dog, *Endocrinology,* **96:**143, 1975.

Krulich, L., and McCann, S. M.: Influence of Stress on the Growth Hormone (GH) Content of the Pituitary of the Rat, *Proc Soc Exp Biol Med,* **122:**612, 1966.

Kuetnansky, R., and Mikulaj, L.: Adrenal and Urinary Catecholamines in Rats during Adaptation to Repeated Immobilization Stress, *Endocrinology,* **87:**738, 1970.

———, Weise, V. K., and Kopin, I. J.: Effect of Dibutyryl Cyclic-AMP on Adrenal Catecholamine Synthesizing Enzymes in Repeatedly Immobilized Hypophysectomized Rats, *Endocrinology,* **89:**50, 1971.

Madden, J. J., Jr., Ludewig, R. M., and Wangensteen, S. L.: Failure of Glucagon in Experimental Hemorrhagic Shock, *Am J Surg,* **122:**502, 1971.

Martin, J. B.: Brain Regulation of Growth Hormone Secretion, in *Frontiers in Neuroendocrinology, op. cit.,* **5:**129, 1976.

Meyer, W., and Knobil, E.: Growth Hormone Secretion in the Unanesthetized Rhesus Monkey in Response to Noxious Stimuli, *Endocrinology,* **80:**163, 1967.

Moran, W. H., Jr., Miltenberger, F. W., Shuayb, W. A., and Zimmerman, B.: Relationship of Antidiuretic Hormone Secretion to Surgical Stress, *Surgery,* **56:**99, 1964.

Moss, G. S., Cerchio, G., Siegel, D. C., Reed, P. C., Cochin, A., and Fresquez, V.: Decline in Pancreatic Insulin Release during Hemorrhagic Shock in the Baboon, *Ann Surg,* **175:**210, 1972.

Newsome, H. H., Jr.: Pituitary-Adrenal Responsiveness in Surgical Patients on Acute and Chronic Corticosteroid Therapy, *Surgery,* **74,** 1973.

——— and Manalan, S. A.: Plasma Cortisol and Cortisone Concentrations following Postoperative Adrenal Steroid Replacement, *Surgery,* **73:**429, 1973.

Parmley, W. W., Gleck, G., and Sonnenblick, E. H.: Cardiovascular Effects of Glucagon in Man, *N Engl J Med,* **279:**12, 1968.

Price, H. L., Linde, H. W., Jones, R. E., Black, G. W., and Price, M. L.: Sympatho-adrenal Responses to General Anesthesia in Man and Their Relation to Hemodynamics, *Anesthesiology,* **20:**563, 1959.

Sachs, H., Share, L., Osinchak, J., and Carpi, A.: Capacity of the Neurohypophysis to Release Vasopressin, *Endocrinology,* **81:**755, 1967.

Samols, E., Tyler, J., Megyesi, C., and Marks, V.: Immunochemical Glucagon in Human Pancreas, Gut, and Plasma, *Lancet,* **2:**727, 1966.

Unger, R. H., Ohneda, A., Valverde, I., Eisentraut, A. M., and Exton, J.: Characterization of the Responses of Circulating Glucagon-like Immunoreactivity to Intraduodenal and Intravenous Administration of Glucose, *J Clin Invest,* **47:**48, 1968.

VanderWall, D. A., Stowe, N. T., Spangenberg, R., and Hook, J. B.: Effect of Glucagon in Hemorrhagic Shock, *J Surg Oncol,* **2:**177, 1970.

Von Euler, U. S.: Adrenal Medullary Secretion and Its Neural Control, in L. Martini and W. F. Ganong (eds.), "Neuroendocrinology," vol. II, Academic Press, Inc., New York, 1967.

Ward, D. G., and Gann, D. S.: Inhibitory and Facilitatory Areas of the Rostral Pons Mediating ACTH Release in the Cat, *Endocrinology,* **99:**1220, 1976.

———, Grizzle, W. E., and Gann, D. S.: Inhibitory and Facilitatory Areas of the Dorsal Medulla Mediating ACTH Release in the Cat, *Endocrinology,* **99:**1213, 1976.

Webb, W. R., Degerli, I. U., Hardy, J. D., and Unal, M.: Cardiovascular Responses in Adrenal Insufficiency, *Surgery,* **58:**273, 1965.

Wilmore, D. W., Long, J. M., Mason, A. D., Shreen, R. W., and Pruitt, B. A.: Catecholamines: Mediator of the Hypermetabolic Responses to Thermal Injury, *Ann Surg,* **180:**653, 1974.

Metabolic Changes: General

Balegno, H. F., and Neuhaus, O. W.: Effect of Insulin on the Injury-stimulated Synthesis of Serum Albumin in the Rat, *Life Sci (II),* **9:**1039, 1970.

Baue, A. E.: Metabolic Abnormalities of Shock, *Surg Clin North Am,* **56:**1059, 1976.

Bauer, W. E., Vigas, S. N. M., Haist, R. E., and Drucker, W. R.: Insulin Response during Hypovolemic Shock, *Surgery,* **66:**80, 1969.

Blackburn, G. L., Flatt, J. P., Clowes, G. H. A., O'Donnell, T. F., and Hensle, T. E.: Protein Sparing Therapy during Periods of Starvation with Sepsis or Trauma, *Ann Surg,* **177:**588, 1973.

Cahill, G. F., Jr.: Starvation in Man, *N Engl J Med,* **282:**668, 1970.

Carey, L. C., Cloutier, C. T., and Lowery, B. D.: Growth Hormone and Adrenal Cortical Response to Shock and Trauma in the Human, *Ann Surg,* **174:**451, 1971.

Clowes, G. H. A., Jr., O'Donnell, T. F., Blackburn, G. C., and Maki, T. N.: Energy Metabolism and Proteolysis in Traumatized and Septic Man, *Surg Clin North Am,* **56:**1169, 1976.

Conway, M. J., Goodner, C. J., and Werrbach, J. H.: Studies of Substrate Regulation in Fasting: II. Effect of Infusion of Glucose into the Carotid Artery upon Fasting Lipolysis in the Baboon, *J Clin Invest,* **48:**1349, 1969.

Cuthbertson, D., and Tilstone, W. D.: Metabolism during the Post-Injury Period, *Adv Clin Chem,* **12:**1, 1969.

Dale, G., Young, G., Latner, A. L., Goode, A., Tweedle, D., and Johnson, I. D. A.: The Effect of Surgical Operation on Venous Plasma Free Amino Acids, *Surgery,* **81:**295, 1977.

Drucker, W. R., Craig, J., Kingsbury, B., Hofmann, N., and Woodward, H.: Citrate Metabolism during Surgery, *Arch Surg,* **85:**557, 1962.

Duke, J. H., Jr., Jorgensen, S. B., Broell, J. R., Long, C. L., and Kinney, J. M.: Contribution of Protein to Caloric Expenditure following Injury, *Surgery,* **68:**168, 1970.

Exton, J. H., Lewis, S. B., and Park, C. R.: Mechanism of Glucagon Activation of Gluconeogenesis, in H. D. Soling and B. Willms (eds.), "Regulation of Gluconeogenesis," p. 160, Academic Press, Inc., New York, 1971.

Felig, P., Marliss, E., Owen, O. E., and Cahill, G. F., Jr.: Role of Substrate in the Regulation of Hepatic Gluconeogenesis in Fasting Man, *Adv Enzyme Regul,* **7:**41, 1969.

———, Owen, O. E., Wahren, J., and Cahill, G. F., Jr.: Amino Acid Metabolism during Prolonged Starvation, *J Clin Invest,* **48:**584, 1969.

Frohlich, J., and Wieland, O.: Dissociation of Gluconeogenic and Ketogenic Action of Glucagon in the Perfused Rat Liver, in H. D. Soling and B. Willms (eds.), "Regulation of Gluconeogenesis," p. 179, Academic Press, Inc., New York, 1971.

Gump, F. E., Long, C. L., Killian, P., and Kinney, J. M.: Studies of Glucose Intolerance in Septic Injured Patients, *J Trauma,* **14:**378, 1974.

Halmagyi, D. F. J., Neering, I. R., Lazarus, L., Young, J. D., and Pullin, J.: Plasma Glucagon in Experimental Posthemorrhagic Shock, *J Trauma,* **9:**320, 1969.

Hanson, R. W., Patel, M. S., Reshef, L., and Ballard, F. J.: The Role of Pyruvate Carboxylase and *P*-Enolpyruvate Carboxykinase in Rat Adipose Tissue, in H. D. Soling and B. Willms (eds.), "Regulation of Gluconeogenesis," p. 255, Academic Press, Inc., New York, 1971.

Heath, D. F., and Threlfall, C. J.: The Interaction of Glycolysis, Gluconeogenesis and the Tricarboxylic Acid Cycle in Rat Liver in Vivo, *Biochem J,* **110:**337, 1968.

Howard, J. M.: Studies of the Absorption and Metabolism of Glucose following Injury: The Systemic Response to Injury, *Ann Surg,* **141:**321, 1955.

Kinney, J. M., Long, C. L., and Duke, J. H.: Carbohydrate and Nitrogen Metabolism after Injury, in R. Porter and J. Knight (eds.), "Energy: Metabolism in Trauma," p. 123, J. & A. Churchill, London, 1970.

Koj, A.: Synthesis and Turnover of Acute-Phase Reactants, in R. Porter and J. Knight (eds.), "Energy: Metabolism in Trauma," p. 79, J. & A. Churchill, London, 1970.

Levenson, S. M., Pulaski, E. J., and Del Guercio, L. R. M.: Metabolic Changes Associated with Injury, in Zimmerman, L. M., and Levine, R. (eds.), "Physiologic Principles of Surgery," W. B. Saunders Company, Philadelphia, 1964.

McNamara, J. J., Molot, M. D., Dunn, R. A., and Stremple, J. F.: Effect of Hypertonic Glucose in Hypovolemic Shock in Man, *Ann Surg,* **176:**247, 1972.

Mallette, L. E., Exton, J. H., and Park, C. R.: Control of Gluconeogenesis from Amino Acids in the Perfused Rat Liver, *J Biol Chem,* **244:**5713, 1969.

Moss, G. S., Cerchio, G. M., Siegel, D. C., Popovich, P. A., and Butler, E.: Serum Insulin Response in Hemorrhagic Shock in Baboons, *Surgery,* **68:**34, 1970.

Owen, O. E., Morgan, A. P., Kemp, H. G., Sullivan, J. M., Herrera, M. G., and Cahill, G. F., Jr.: Brain Metabolism during Fasting, *J Clin Invest,* **46:**1589, 1967.

Schumer, W., and Sperling, R.: Shock and Its Effect on the Cell, *JAMA,* **205:**215, 1968.

Soling, H. D., Willms, B., and Kleineke, J.: Regulation of Gluconeogenesis in Rat and Guinea Pig Liver, in H. D. Soling and B. Willms (eds.), "Regulation of Gluconeogenesis," p. 210, Academic Press, Inc., New York, 1971.

Stoner, H. B., and Threlfall, C. J. (eds.): "The Biochemical Response to Injury," Charles C Thomas, Publisher, Springfield, Ill., 1960.

Threlfall, C. J., and Stoner, H. B.: Carbohydrate Metabolism in Ischemic Shock, *Q J Exp Physiol,* **39:**1, 1954.

Vaidyanath, N., Birkhahn, R., Border, J. R., McMenamy, R. H., Oswald, G., Trietleg, G., and Yuan, T. F.: The Turnover of Amino Acids in Sepsis and Starvation: Effects of Glucose Infusion, *J Trauma,* **16:**125, 1976.

Wilmore, D. W.: Hormonal Responses and Their Effect on Metabolism, *Surg Clin North Am,* **56:**999, 1976.

Energy Metabolism

Kinney, J. M.: Energy Significance of Weight Loss, in G. S. M. Cowan, Jr., and W. L. Scheetz (eds.), "Intravenous Hyperalimentation" p. 84, Lea & Febiger, Philadelphia, 1972.

————, Long, C. L., and Duke, J. H.: Carbohydrate and Nitrogen Metabolism after Injury, in R. Porter and J. Knight (eds.), "Energy Metabolism in Trauma," p. 103, J. & A. Churchill, London, 1970.

————, ————, and ————: Energy Demands in the Surgical Patient, in C. L. Fox, Jr., and G. G. Nahos (eds.), "Body Fluid Replacement in Surgical Patient," Grune & Stratton, Inc., New York, 1970.

Mehlman, M. A., and Hanson, R. W., (eds.): "Energy Metabolism and the Regulation of Metabolic Processes in Mitochondria," Academic Press, Inc., New York, 1972.

Porter, R., and Knight, J. (eds.): "Energy Metabolism in Trauma," J. & A. Churchill, London, 1970.

Soling, H. D., and Willms, B. (eds.): "Regulation of Gluconcogenesis," Academic Press, Inc., New York, 1971.

Wilmore, D. W.: Energy Requirements of Seriously Burned Patients and the Influence of Caloric Intake in Their Metabolic Rate, in G. S. M. Cowan, Jr., and W. L. Scheetz (eds.), "Intravenous Hyperalimentation," p. 96, Lea & Febiger, Philadelphia, 1972.

Starvation

Cahill, G. F., Jr.: Starvation in Man, *N Engl J Med,* **282:**668, 1970.

———— and Aoki, T. T.: The Starvation State and Requirements of the Deficit Economy, in G. S. M. Cowan, Jr. and W. L. Scheetz (eds.), "Intravenous Hyperalimentation," p. 21, Lea & Febiger, Philadelphia, 1972.

————, Felig, P., and Marliss, E. B.: Some Physiological Principles of Parenteral Nutrition, in C. L. Fox, Jr., and G. G. Nahas (eds.), "Body Fluid Replacement in the Surgical Patient," p. 286, Grune & Stratton, New York, 1970.

Owen, O. E., Felig, P., Morgan, A. P., Wahren, J., and Cahill, G. F., Jr.: Liver and Kidney Metabolism during Prolonged Starvation, *J Clin Invest,* **48:**574, 1969.

————, Morgan, A. P., Kemp, H. G., Sullivan, J. M., Herrera, M. G., and Cahill, G. F., Jr.: Brain Metabolism during Fasting, *J Clin Invest,* **46:**1589, 1967.

Sapir, D. G., Owen, O. E., Pozefsky, L., and Walser, M.: Nitrogen Sparing Induced by a Mixture of Essential Amino Acids Given Chiefly as Their Keto-Analogues During Prolonged Starvation in Obese Subjects, *J Clin Invest,* **54:**974, 1974.

Saudek, C. D., and Felig, P.: The Metabolic Events of Starvation, *Am J Med,* **60:**117, 1976.

Carbohydrate Metabolism

Berk, J. L., Hagen, J. F., Beyer, W. H., and Gerber, M. J.: Hypoglycemia of Shock, *Ann Surg,* **171:**400, 1970.

Drucker, W. R.: Carbohydrate Metabolism: The Traumatized versus Normal States, in G. S. M. Cowan and W. L. Scheetz (eds.), "Intravenous Hyperalimentation," p. 55, Lea & Febiger, Philadelphia, 1972.

————, Schlatter, J. E., and Drucker, R. P.: Metabolic Factors Associated with Endotoxin-induced Tolerance for Hemorrhagic Shock, *Surgery,* **64:**75, 1968.

Giddings, A. E.: The Control of Plasma Glucose in the Surgical Patient, *Br J Surg,* **6:**787, 1974.

Green, H. N., and Stoner, H. B.: Effects of Injury on Carbohydrate Metabolism and Energy Transformation, *Br Med J,* **10:**38, 1955.

Jordan, G. L., Jr., Fischer, E. P., and Lefrak, E. A.: Glucose Metabolism in Traumatic Shock in the Human, *Ann Surg,* **175:**685, 1972.

McCoy, S., and Drucker, W. R.: Carbohydrate Metabolism, in W. F. Ballinger, J. A. Collins, W. R. Drucker, S. J. Dadrich, and R. Zeppa (eds.), "Manual of Surgical Nutrition," p. 13, W. B. Saunders Company, Philadelphia, 1975.

Pappova, E., Urbaschek, B., Heitmann, L., Oroz, M., Steit, O. E., Lemeunier, A., and Lundsgaard-Hansen, P.: Energy-rich Phosphates and Glucose Metabolism in Early Endotoxin Shock, *J Surg Res,* **11:**506, 1971.

Rayfield, E. J., Carnow, R. T., George, D. T., and Beisel, W. R.: Impaired Carbohydrate Metabolism during a Mild Viral Illness, *N Eng J Med,* **289:**618, 1975.

Schumer, W.: Metabolic Considerations in the Preoperative Evaluation of the Surgical Patient, *Surg Gynecol Obstet,* **121:**611, 1965.

————: Localization of the Energy Pathway Block in Shock, *Surgery,* 1974.

Taylor, F. H. L., Levenson, S. M., and Adams, M. A.: Abnormal Carbohydrate Metabolism in Human Thermal Burns, *N Engl J Med,* **231:**437, 1944.

Fat Metabolism

Barton, R. N.: Ketone Body Metabolism after Trauma, in R. Porter and J. Knight (eds.), *Ciba Found Symp Energy Metab Trauma,* 1970, p. 173.

Carlson, L. A.: Mobilization and Utilization of Lipids after Trauma: Relation to Caloric Homeostasis, in R. Porter and J. Knight (eds), *Ciba Found Symp Energy Metab Trauma,* 1970, p. 155.

————: Fat Metabolism, in G. S. M. Cowan and W. L. Scheetz, (eds.), "Intravenous Hyperalimentation," p. 68, Lea & Febiger, Philadelphia, 1972.

Coran, A. G., Cryer, P. E., Horwitz, D. L., and Herman, C. M.: The Metabolism of Fat and Carbohydrate during Hemorrhagic Shock in the Unanesthetized Subhuman Primate: Changes in Serum Levels of Free Fatty Acids, Total Lipids, Insulin, and Glucose, *Surgery,* **71:**465, 1972.

Evarts, C. M.: The Fat Embolism Syndrome: A Review, *Surg Clin North Am,* **50:**493, 1970.

Farago, G., Levene, R. A., Lau, T. S., and Drucker, W. R.: Availability of Lipid for Energy Metabolism during Hypovolemia, *Surg Forum,* **22:**7, 1971.

Hansen, O. H.: Fat Embolism and Post-traumatic Diabetes Insipidus, *Acta Chir Scand,* **136:**161, 1970.

Lyman, R. L.: Endocrine Influences on the Metabolism of Polyunsaturated Fatty Acids, *Prog Chem,* **9:**193, 1968.

McGarry, J. D., Wright, P. H., and Foster, D. W.: Hormonal Control of Ketogenesis: Rapid Activation of Hepatic Ketogenic Capacity in Fed Rats by Anti-Insulin Serum and Glucagon, *J Clin Invest,* **55:**1202, 1975.

McKee, A., and Russell, J. A.: Effect of Acute Hypophysectomy and Growth Hormone on FFA Mobilization, Nitrogen Excretion and Cardiac Glycogen in Fasting Rats, *Endocrinology,* **83:**1162, 1968.

McNamara, J. J., Molot, M., Dunn, R., Burran, E. L., and Stremple, J. F.: Lipid Metabolism after Trauma: Role in the Pathogenesis of Fat Embolism, *J Thorac Cardiovasc Surg,* **63:**968, 1972.

Masoro, E. J.: The Effect of Physical Injury on Lipid Metabolism, in H. B. Stoner and C. J. Threlfall (eds.), "The Biochemical Response to Injury," p. 175, Charles C Thomas, Publisher, Springfield, Ill., 1960.

———: Lipids and Lipid Metabolism, *Annu Rev Physiol,* **39:**301, 1977.

Moore, F. D., Haley, H. B., Bering, E. A., Jr., Brooks, L., and Edelman, I. S.: Further Observations on Total Body Water: II. Changes of Body Composition in Disease, *Surg Gynecol Obstet,* **95:**155, 1952.

Reichard, G. A., Owen, O. E., Huff, A. C., Paul, P., and Bortz, W. M.: Ketone-Body Production and Oxidation in Fasting Obese Humans, *J Clin Invest,* **53:**508, 1974.

Shafrir, E., and Steinberg, D.: The Essential Role of the Adrenal Cortex in the Response of Plasma Free Fatty Acids, Cholesterol, and Phospholipids to Epinephrine Injection, *J Clin Invest,* **39:**310, 1960.

Spergel, G., Bleicher, S. J., and Ertel, N. H.: Carbohydrate and Fat Metabolism in Patients with Pheochromocytoma, *N Engl J Med,* **278:**803, 1968.

Symbas, P. N., Abbott, O. A., and Ende, N.: Surgical Stress and Its Effects on Serum Cholesterol, *Surgery,* **61:**221, 1967.

Wadström, L. B.: Effect of Glucose Infusion on Plasma Lipids in Newly Operated Patients, *Acta Chir Scand,* **116:**395, 1958.

Wilmore, D. W.: Fat Metabolism, in W. F. Ballinger, J. A. Collins, W. R. Drucker, S. J. Dadrich, and R. Zeppa (eds.), "Manual of Surgical Nutrition," p. 33, W. B. Saunders Company, Philadelphia, 1975.

Protein Metabolism

Browne, J. S. L., and Schenker, V.: "Conferences on Metabolic Aspects of Convalescence Including Bone and Wound Healing: Transactions of Third Meeting," p. 162, Josiah Macy, Jr. Foundation Publications, New York, 1943.

Buse, M. G., and Reid, S. S.: Leacine: A Possible Regulator of Protein Turnover in Muscle, *J Clin Invest,* **56:**1250, 1975.

Cannon, P. R., Wissler, R. W., Woolride, R. L., and Benditt, E. P.: Relationship of Protein Deficiency to Surgical Infection, *Ann Surg,* **120:**514, 1944.

Clarke, H. C. M., Freeman, T., and Pryse-Phillips, W.: Serum Protein Changes after Injury, *Clin Sci,* **40:**337, 1971.

Costa, G., Ullrich, L., Kantor, F., and Holland, J. F.: Production of Elemental Nitrogen by Certain Mammals including Man, *Nature (Lond),* **218:**546, 1968.

Cuthbertson, D. P.: Further Observations on Disturbance of Metabolism Caused by Injury, with Particular Reference to Dietary Requirements of Fracture Cases, *Br J Surg,* **23:**505, 1936.

Davies, J. W. L., Bull, J. P., and Ricketts, C. R.: Catabolic Response to Injury, *Lancet,* **2:**320, 1971.

Flear, C. T. G., and Clarke, R.: The Influence of Blood Loss and Blood Transfusion upon Changes in the Metabolism of Water, Electrolytes and Nitrogen Following Civilian Trauma, *Clin Sci,* **14:**575, 1955.

Fleck, A.: Protein Metabolism after Injury, *Proc Nutr Soc,* **30:**152, 1971.

Fulks, R. M., Li, J. B., and Goldberg, A. L.: Effects of Insulin, Glucose and Amino Acids on Protein Turnover in Rat Diaphragm, *J Biol Chem,* **250:**290, 1975.

Hinton, P., Allison, S. P., Littlejohn, S., and Lloyd, J.: Insulin and Glucose to Reduce Catabolic Response to Injury in Burned Patients, *Lancet,* **1:**767, 1971.

Howard, J. E., Bingham, R. S., Jr., and Mason, R. E.: Studies on Convalescence: IV. Nitrogen and Mineral Balances during Starvation and Graduated Feeding in Healthy Young Males at Bed Rest, *Trans Assoc Am Physicians,* **59:**242, 1946.

Kekomaki, M., and Louhimo, I.: Observations on Plasma Amino Acid Concentrations during Haemorrhagic Shock in the Rabbit, *Ann Chir Gynaecol Fenn,* **60:**214, 1971.

Kukral, J. C., Riveron, E., Tiffany, J. C., Vaitys, S., and Barrett, B.: Plasma Protein Metabolism in Patients with Acute Surgical Peritonitis, *Am J Surg,* **113:**173, 1967.

Levenson, S. M., Howard, J. M., and Rosen, I. T.: Studies of the Plasma Amino Acids and Amino Conjugates in Patients with Severe Battle Wounds, *Surg Gynecol Obstet,* **101:**35, 1955.

——— and Watkin, D. M.: Protein Requirements in Injury and Certain Acute and Chronic Diseases, *Fed Proc,* **18:**1155, 1959.

Munro, H. N., and Allison, J. B. (eds.): "Mammalian Protein Metabolism," Academic Press, Inc., New York, 1964.

——— and Chalmers, M. I.: Fracture Metabolism at Different Levels of Protein Intake, *Br J Exp Pathol,* **26:**396, 1945.

Sherwin, R. S., Hendler, R. G., and Felig, P.: Effect of Ketone Infusions on Amino Acid and Nitrogen Metabolism in Man, *J Clin Invest,* **55:**1382, 1975.

Restitution of Blood Volume

Boyd, D. R., and Mansberger, A. R.: Serum Water and Osmolal Changes in Hemorrhagic Shock: An Experimental and Clinical Study, *Am Surg,* **34:**744, 1968.

Cope, O., and Litwin, S. B.: Contributions of the Lymphatic System to the Replenishment of the Plasma Volume Following a Hemorrhage, *Ann Surg,* **156:**655, 1962.

Deaux, E., and Kakolewski, J. W.: Emotionally Induced Increases in Effective Osmotic Pressure and Subsequent Thirst, *Science,* **169:**1226, 1970.

Gann, D. S.: Endocrine Control of Plasma Protein and Volume, *Surg Clin North Am,* **56:**1135, 1976.

——— and Pirkle, J. C., Jr.: Role of Cortisol in the Restitution of Blood Volume after Hemorrhage, *Am J Surg,* **130:**565, 1975.

Pirkle, J. C., Jr., and Gann, D. S.: Restitution of Blood Volume After Hemorrhage: Mathematical Description, *Am J Physiol,* **228:**821, 1975.

——— and ———: Restitution of Blood Volume after Hemorrhage: Role of the Adrenal Cortex, *Am J Physiol,* **230:**1683, 1976.

———— and ————: Pituitary and Adrenal Glands Are Required for Full Restitution of Blood Volume after Hemorrhage, *Fed Proc,* **35:**637, 1976.

Skillman, J. J., Amwad, H. K., and Moore, F. D.: Plasma Protein Kinetics of the Early Transcapillary Refill after Hemorrhage, *Surg Gynecol Obstet,* **125:**983, 1967.

Stewart, J. D., and Rourke, M. G.: Intracellular Fluid Loss in Hemorrhage, *J Clin Invest,* **15:**697, 1936.

Zollinger, R. M., Jr.: Plasma Volume and Protein Restoration after Hemorrhage: Role of the Left Thoracic Duct versus Transcapillary Refilling, *J Surg Res,* **12:**151, 1972.

Wound Healing

Azar, M. M., and Good, R. A.: The Inhibitory Effect of Vitamin A on Complement Levels and Tolerance Production, *J Immunol,* **106:**241, 1971.

Calloway, D. H., Grossman, M. I., Bowman, J., and Calhoun, W. K.: Effect of Previous Level of Protein Feeding on Wound Healing and on Metabolic Response to Injury, *Surgery,* **37:** 935, 1955.

Carnes, W. H.: Role of Copper in Connective Tissue Metabolism, *Fed Proc,* **30:**995, 1971.

Chernov, M. S., Halc, H. W., and Wood, M.: Prevention of Stress Ulcers, *Am J Surg,* **122:**674, 1971.

Cohen, B., and Cohen, I. K.: "Vitamin A: Adjuvant and Steroid Antagonist in the Immune Response," Plastic Surgery Research Council, St. Louis, May, 1973.

Cohen, I. K., Schechter, P. J., and Henkin, R. I.: Hypogeusia, Anorexia, and Altered Zinc Metabolism following Thermal Burn, *JAMA,* **223:**914, 1973.

Harris, E. D., and Sjoerdsma, A.: Effect of Penicillamine on Human Collagen and Its Possible Application in Treatment of Scleroderma, *Lancet,* **2:**996, 1966.

Hsu, T. H. S., and Hsu, J. M.: Zinc Deficiency and Epithelial Wound Repair: An Autoradiographic Study of 3H-Thymidine Incorporation, *Proc Soc Exp Biol Med,* **140:**157, 1972.

Hunt, T. K., Ehrlich, H. P., Garcia, J. A., and Dunphy, J. E.: Effect of Vitamin A on Reversing the Inhibitory Effect of Cortisone on Healing of Open Wounds in Animals and Man, *Ann Surg,* **170:**633, 1969.

————, Niinikoski, J., and Zederfeldt, B.: Role of Oxygen in Repair Processes, *Acta Chir Scand,* **138:**109, 1972.

Hutcher, N., Silverberg, S. G., and Lee, H. M.: The Effect of Vitamin A on the Formation of Steroid Induced Gastric Ulcers, *Surg Forum,* **22:**322, 1971.

Levenson, S. M., Green, R. W., Taylor, F. H. L., Robinson, P., Page, R. C., Johnson, R. E., and Lund, C. C.: Ascorbic Acid, Riboflavin, Thiamine, and Nicotinic Acid in Relation to Severe Injury, Hemorrhage and Infection in the Human, *Ann Surg,* **124:**840, 1946.

————, Pirani, C. L., Braasch, J. W., and Waterman, D. F,: The Effect of Thermal Burns on Wound Healing, *Surg Gynecol Obstet,* **99:**74, 1954.

————, Upjohn, H. L., Preston, J. A., and Steer, A.: Effect of Thermal Burns on Wound Healing, *Ann Surg,* **146:**357, 1957.

Niinikoski, J., Henghan, C., and Hunt, T. K.: Oxygen Tensions in Human Wounds, *J Surg Res,* **12:**77, 1972.

Quarantillo, E. P., Jr.: Effect of Supplemental Zinc on Wound Healing in Rats, *Am J Surg,* **121:**661, 1971.

Siegel, R. C., Pinnell, S. R., and Martin, G.: Cross-linking of Collagen and Elastin: Properties of Lysyl Oxidase, *Biochemistry,* **9:**4486, 1970.

Stein, H. D., and Keiser, H. R.: Collagen Metabolism in Granulating Wounds, *J Surg Res,* **11:**277, 1971.

Stephens, F. P., Hunt, T. K., Jawetz, E., Sonne, M., and Duphy, J. E.: Effect of Cortisone and Vitamin A on Wound Infection, *Am J Surg,* **121:**569, 1971.

Sullivan, J. F., and Eisenstein, A. B.: Ascorbic Acid Depletion during Hemodialysis. *JAMA,* **220:**1697, 1972.

Williamson, M. B., McCarthy, T. H., and Fromm, H. J.: Relation of Protein Nutrition to the Healing of Experimental Wounds, *Proc Soc Exp Biol Med,* **77:**302, 1951.

Udupa, K. N., Woessner, J. F., and Dunphy, J. E.: The Effect of Methionine on the Production of Mucopolysaccharides and Collagen in Healing Wounds of Protein-depleted Animals, *Surg Gynecol Obstet,* **102:**639, 1956.

Nutritional Supplementation

Abbott, W. E., Krieger, H., and Levey, S.: Postoperative Metabolic Changes in Relation to Nutritional Regimen, *Lancet,* **1:**704, 1958.

Abel, R. M., Beck, C. H., Jr., Abbott, W. M., Ryan, J. A., Jr., Barnett, G. O., and Fischer, J. E.: Improved Survival from Acute Renal Failure after Treatment with Intravenous Essential L-Amino Acids and Glucose, *N Engl J Med,* **288:**695, 1973.

Allen, J. G., Stemmer, E. A., and Head, L. R.: Similar Growth Rates of Littermate Puppies Maintained on Oral Protein with Those on the Same Quantity of Protein as Daily Intravenous Plasma for 99 Days as Only Protein Source, *Ann Surg,* **144:** 349, 1956.

Blackburn, G. L., and Bistrian, B. R.: Nutritional Care of the Injured and/or Septic Patient, *Surg Clin North Am,* **56:**1195, 1976.

Brennan, M. F., Goldman, M. H., O'Connell, R. C., Kundsin, R. B., and Moore, F. D.: Prolonged Parenteral Alimentation: Candida Growth and the Prevention of Candidemia by Amphotericin Installation, *Ann Surg,* **176:**265, 1972.

Burr, A. O. and Burr, M. M.: A New Deficiency Disease Produced by the Rigid Exclusion of Fat from the Diet, *J Biol Chem,* **82:**345, 1929.

Cahill, G. F., Jr., and Aoki, T. T.: The Starvation State and Requirements of the Deficit Economy, in G. S. M. Cowan, Jr., and W. L. Scheetz (eds.), "Intravenous Hyperalimentation," p. 20, Lea & Febiger, Philadelphia, 1972.

————, Felig, P., and Marliss, E. B.: Some Physiological Principles of Parenteral Nutrition, in C. L. Fox, Jr. and G. G. Nahas (eds.), "Body Fluid Replacement in the Surgical Patient," p. 286, Grune & Stratton, Inc., New York, 1970.

Caldwell, M. D., Jonnooon, H. T., and Othorsen, H. B, Jr.: Essential Fatty Acid Deficiency in an Infant Receiving Prolonged Parenteral Alimentation, *J Pediatr,* **81:**894, 1972.

Collins, F. D., Sinclair, A. J., and Royle, J. P.: Plasma Lipids in Human Linoleic Acid Deficiency, *Nutr Metabol,* **13:**150, 1971.

Cowan, G. S. M., Jr., and Scheetz, W. L. (eds.): "Intravenous Hyperalimentation," Lea & Febiger, Philadelphia, 1972.

Deitrick, J. E., Whedun, G. D., and Shorr, E.: Effects of Immobilization upon Various Metabolic and Physiologic Functions of Normal Men, *Am J Med,* **4:**3, 1948.

Dudrick, S. J., Wilmore, D. W., Vars, H. M., and Rhoads, J. E.: Long Term Total Parenteral Nutrition with Growth, Development and Positive Nitrogen Balance, *Surgery,* **64:**134, 1968.

———, MacFadyen, B. V., VanBuren, C. T., Ruberg, R. L., and Maynard, A. T.: Parenteral Hyperalimentation: Metabolic Problems and Solutions, *Ann Surg,* **176:**259, 1972.

———, Steiger, E., and Long, J. M.: Renal Failure in Surgical Patients: Treatment with Intravenous Essential Amino Acids and Hypertonic Glucose, *Surgery,* **68:**180, 1970.

———, ———, ———, Ruberg, R. L., Allen, T. R., Vars, H. M., and Rhoads, J. E.: General principles and techniques of intravenous hyperalimentation, in G. S. M. Cowan, Jr., and W. L. Scheetz (eds.), "Intravenous Hyperalimentation," p. 2, Lea & Febiger, Philadelphia, 1972.

Feller, I.: The Use of Plasma and Albumin in the Burned Patient, in C. L. Fox, Jr., and G. G. Nahas (eds.), "Body Fluid Replacement in the Surgical Patient," p. 153. Grune & Stratton, Inc., New York, 1970.

Fox, C. L., Jr., and Nahas, G. G. (eds.): "Body Fluid Replacement in the Surgical Patient," Grune & Stratton, Inc., New York, 1970.

Gann, D. S., and Robinson, H. B.: Salt, Water, and Vitamins, in W. F. Ballinger et al. (eds.), "Manual of Surgical Nutrition," p. 73, W. B. Saunders Company, Philadelphia, 1975.

Giordano, C.: Use of Exogenous and Endogenous Urea for Protein Synthesis in Normal and Uremic Subjects, *J Lab Clin Med,* **62:**321, 1963.

Giovannetti, S., and Maggiore, Q.: A Low Nitrogen Diet with Protein of High Biological Value for Severe Chronic Uremia, *Lancet,* **1:**1000, 1964.

Greenstein, J. P., Otey, M. C., Birnbaum, S. M., and Winitz, M.: Quantitative Nutritional Studies with Water-Soluble, Chemically Defined Diets: X. Formulation of a Nutritionally Complete Liquid Diet, *J Natl Cancer Inst,* **24:**211, 1960.

Hamilton, R. F., Davis, W. T., Stephenson, D. V., and McGee, D. F.: Effects of Parenteral Hyperalimentation on Upper Gastrointestinal Tract Secretions, *Arch Surg,* **102:**348, 1971.

Heird, W. C., Dell, R. B., Driscoll, J. M., Jr., Grebin, B., and Winters, R. W.: Metabolic Acidosis Resulting from Intravenous Alimentation Mixtures Containing Synthetic Amino Acids, *N Engl J Med,* **287:**943, 1972.

Holden, W. D., Krieger, H., Levey, S., and Abbott, W. E.: The Effect of Nutrition on Nitrogen Metabolism in the Surgical Patient, *Ann Surg,* **146:**563, 1957.

Holman, R. T.: Essential Fatty Acid Deficiency, *Prog Chem Toxicol,* **9:**279, 1968.

Host, W. H., Serlin, O., and Rush, B. F., Jr.: Hyperalimentation in Cirrhotic Patients, *Am J Surg,* **123:**57, 1972.

Jacobson, S., and Wretling, A.: The Use of Fat Emulsions for Complete Intravenous Nutrition, in C. L. Fox, Jr., and G. G. Nahas (eds.), "Body Fluid Replacement in the Surgical Patient," p. 334, Grune & Stratton, Inc., New York, 1970.

Kekomaki, M., Louhimo, I., Rahiala, E. L., and Suutarinen, T.: Comparison of Fructose and Glucose Solutions in the Treatment of Hypovolemic Shock in Rabbits, *Acta Chir Scand,* **138:**239, 1972.

Kinney, J. M., Long, C. L., and Duke, J. H., Jr.: Energy Demands in the Surgical Patient, in C. L. Fox and G. G. Nahas (eds.),

"Body Fluid Replacement in the Surgical Patient," p. 296, Grune & Stratton, Inc., New York, 1970.

Long, J. M., Dudrick, S. J., Steiger, E., Ruberg, R. L., and Allen, T. R.: Use of Intravenous Hyperalimentation in Patients with Renal or Liver Failure, in G. S. M. Cowan, Jr., and W. L. Scheetz (eds.), "Intravenous Hyperalimentation," p. 147, Lea & Febiger, Philadelphia, 1972.

Meng, H. C., and Early, F.: Study of Complete Parenteral Alimentation on Dogs, *J Lab Clin Med,* **34:**1121, 1949.

Munro, H. N.: Adaptation of Mammalian Protein Metabolism to Hyperalimentation, in G. S. M. Cowan, Jr., and W. L. Scheetz (eds.), "Intravenous Hyperalimentation," p. 34, Lea & Febiger, Philadelphia, 1972.

Ravdin, I. S., McNamee, H. G., Kamholz, J. H., and Rhoads, J. E.: Effect of Hypoproteinemia on Susceptibility to Shock Resulting from Hemorrhage, *Arch Surg,* **48:**491, 1944.

Rose, W. C., and Dekker, E. E.: Urea as a Source of Nitrogen for the Biosynthesis of Amino Acids, *J Biol Chem,* **223:**107, 1956.

Schumer, W.: High Calorie Solutions in Traumatized Patients, in C. L. Fox, Jr. and G. G. Nahas (eds.), "Body Fluid Replacement in the Surgical Patient, p. 326, Grune & Stratton, Inc., New York, 1970.

Scribbner, B. H., Cole, J. J., Christopher, P. H., Vizzo, J. E., Atkins, R. C., and Blagg, C. R.: Long Term Total Parenteral Nutrition: The Concept of an Artificial Gut, *JAMA,* **212:**457, 1970.

Stemmer, E. A., Allen, J. G., and Connolly, J. E.: Nutritional Value of Blood Plasma Protein: Growth in Puppies on Intravenous Diets of Plasma, Red Cells and Amino Acid, *Am Surg,* **32:**665, 1966.

———, ———, and ———: Value of Blood Plasma in Restoring Plasma Proteins in the Depleted Surgical Patient, *Am J Surg,* **112:**251, 1966.

Terry, R., Sandrock, W. E., Nye, R. E., and Whipple, G. H.: Parenteral Plasma Protein Maintains Nitrogen Equilibrium over Long Periods, *J Exp Med,* **87:**547, 1948.

Walser, M., Sapir, D. G., and Maddrey, W. C.: The Use of Alpha-Keto Analogues of Essential Amino Acids, in J. Fischer (ed.), "Total Parenteral Nutrition," Little, Brown and Company, Boston, 1976.

Whedon, G. D., Deitrick, J. E., and Shorr, E.: Modification of the Effects of Immobilization upon Metabolic Physiologic Functions of Normal Men by the Use of an Oscillating Bed, *Am J Med,* **6:**684, 1949.

Wilkinson, A. W.: Restriction of Fluid Intake after Partial Gastrectomy, *Lancet,* **2:**428, 1956.

Wilmore, D. W., Curreri, W., Spitzer, K. W., Spitzer, M. E., and Pruitt, B. A.: Supra-normal Dietary Intake in Thermally Injured Hypermetabolic Patients, *Surg Gynecol Obstet,* **132:**881, 1971.

Yuile, C. L., O'Dea, A. E., Lucas, F. V., and Whipple, G. H.: Plasma Protein Labeled with Lysine-E-D_{14}: Its Oral Feeding and Relating Protein Metabolism in the Dog, *J Exp Med,* **96:**247, 1952.

Component Therapy

Clark, I. C., Jr.: Symposium on Inert Organic Liquids for Biological Oxygen Transport, *Atlantic City, New Jersey, April 13, 1969, Fed Proc,* **29:**1698, 1970.

——— and Gollan, F.: Survival of Mammals Breathing Organic Liquids Equilibrated with Oxygen at Atmospheric Pressure, *Science,* **152:**1755, 1966.

Geyer, R. P.: Whole Animal Perfusion with Fluorocarbon Dispersions, *Fed Proc,* **29:**1758, 1970.

———: The Design of Artificial Blood Substitutes, in E. J. Ariens (ed.), "Drug Design," Academic Press, New York, 1976.

———, Monroe, R. G., and Taylor, K.: Survival of Rats Totally Perfused with a Fluorocarbon-Detergent Preparation, in J. Folkman, W. G. Hardison, L. E. Rudolf, and F. J. Veith (eds.), "Organ Perfusion and Preservation," p. 85, Appleton-Century-Crofts, New York, 1968.

Modell, J. H., Newby, E. J., and Ruiz, B. C.: Long Term Survival of Dogs after Breathing Oxygenated Fluorocarbon Liquid, *Fed Proc,* **29:**1731, 1970.

Moss, G. S.: Massive Transfusion of Frozen Processed Red Cells in Combat Casualties: Report of Three Cases, *Surgery,* **66:**1008, 1969.

———, Cochin, A., and DeWoskin, R.: "Pure" Hemoglobin Solution: Coagulability Changes Produced In Vitro, *Surgery,* **74,** 1973.

Patel, M. M., Patel, M. K., Szanto, P., Alrenga, D. P., and Long, D. M.: Ventilation with Synthetic Fluids, *Surg Clin North Am,* **51:**25, 1971.

Sloviter, H. A.: Erythrocyte Substitutes, *Med Clin North Am,* **54:**787, 1970.

———, Petkovic, M., Ogoshi, S., and Yamada, H.: Dispersed Fluorochemicals as Substitutes for Erythrocytes in Intact Animals, *J Appl Physiol,* **27:**666, 1969.

———, Yamada, H., and Ogoshi, S.: Some Effects of Intravenously Administered Dispersed Fluorochemicals in Animals, *Fed Proc,* **29:**1755, 1970.

Acid-Base Balance, Salt, and Water

Astrup, P., Jorgensen, K., Siggaard-Andersen, O., and Engel, K.: The Acid-Base Metabolism: A New Approach, *Lancet,* **1:**1035, 1960.

Barry, K. G., and Malloy, J. P.: Oliguric Renal Failure: Evaluation and Therapy by Intravenous Infusion of Mannitol, *JAMA,* **179:**510, 1962.

Bergentz, S.-E., and Brief, D. K.: The Effect of pH and Osmolality on the Production of Canine Hemorrhagic Shock, *Surgery,* **58:**412, 1965.

Bishop, R. L., and Weisfeldt, M. L.: Sodium Bicarbonate Administration during Cardiac Arrest, *JAMA,* **235:**506, 1976.

Blackburn, G. L., and Schloerb, P. R.: Intracellular Acid-Base Regulation in Hypoxia, *Arch Surg,* **93:**573, 1966.

Bleich, H. L., Tanner, R. L., and Schwartz, W. B.: The Induction of Metabolic Alkalosis by Correction of Potassium Deficiency, *J Clin Invest,* **45:**573, 1966.

Bradley, M. N.: Profound Shock Associated with Acidosis: Occurrence and Treatment, *Am Surg,* **30:**589, 1964.

Broder, G., and Weil, M. H.: Excess Lactate: Index of Reversibility of Shock in Human Patients, *Science,* **143:**1457, 1964.

Dudley, H. W., Boiling, H. R., Jr., and Moyer, C. A.: A Bioassay of Treatment of Hemorrhagic Shock: II. The Expansion of Volume Distribution of Extracellular Ions during Hemorrhagic Hypotension and Its Possible Relationship to Change in Physical-Chemical Properties of Extravascular-Extracellular Tissue, *Arch Surg,* **93:**556, 1966.

Chazan, J. A., Stenson, R., and Kurland, G. S.: Acidosis of Cardiac Arrest, *N Engl J Med,* **278:**360, 1968.

Collins, J. A.: Effect of Massive Blood Transfusions on Acid-Base Status of Combat Casualties in Vietnam, in C. L. Fox, Jr., and G. G. Nahas (eds.), "Body Fluid Replacement in the Surgical Patient," p. 72, Grune & Stratton, Inc., New York, 1970.

———, Simmons, R. L., James, P. M., Bredenberg, C. E., Anderson, R. W., and Heisterkamp, C. A.: Acid-Base Status of Seriously Wounded Combat Casualties: II. Resuscitation with Stored Blood, *Ann Surg,* **173:**6, 1971.

Crandall, W. B., and Stueck, G. H., Jr.: Acid-Base Balance in Surgical Patients: I. A Survey of 62 Selected Cases, *Ann Surg,* **149:**342, 1959.

Cunningham, J. N., Shires, G. T., and Wagner, Y.: Changes in Intracellular Sodium and Potassium Content of Red Blood Cells in Trauma and Shock, *Am J Surg,* **122:**650, 1971.

DeWardener, H. E.: The Control of Sodium Excretion, in J. Orloff and R. W. Berliner (eds.), "Handbook of Physiology," sec. 8, Renal Physiology, p. 721, American Physiological Society, Washington, 1973.

Dillion, J., Lynch, L. J., Jr., Myers, R., Butcher, H. R., Jr., and Moyer, C. A.: Bioassay of Treatment of Hemorrhagic Shock, *Arch Surg,* **93:**537, 1966.

Dudley, H. F., Boling, E. A., LeQuesne, L. P., and Moore, F. D.: Studies on Antidiuresis in Surgery: Effects of Anesthesia, Surgery and Posterior Pituitary Antidiuretic Hormone on Water Metabolism in Man, *Ann Surg,* **140:**354, 1954.

Earley, L. E., and Schrier, R. W.: Intrarenal Control of Sodium Excretion by Hemodynamic and Physical Factors, in J. Orloff and R. W. Berliner (eds.), "Handbook of Physiology," sec. 8, Renal Physiology, p. 677, American Physiological Society, Washington, 1973.

Eichenholz, A., Mulhausen, R. O., Anderson, W. E., and MacDonald, F. M.: Primary Hypocapnia: A Cause of Metabolic Acidosis, *J Appl Physiol,* **17:**283, 1962.

Flemma, R. J., and Young, W. G., Jr.: The Metabolic Effects of Mechanical Ventilation and Respiratory Alkalosis in Postoperative Patients, *Surgery,* **56:**36, 1964.

Gann, D. S., and Wright, H. K.: Augmentation of Sodium Excretion in Postoperative Patients by Expansion of the Extracellular Fluid Volume, *Surg Gynecol Obstet,* **118:**1024, 1964.

——— and ———: Effects of Trauma on Sodium Metabolism and Urinary Concentrating Ability, *J Surg Res,* **6:**93, 1965.

——— and ———: Increased Renal Sodium Reabsorption After Depletion of the Extracellular or Nitrovascular Fluid Volumes, *J Surg Res,* **6:**196, 1966.

———, ———, and Newsome, H. H.: Prevention of Sodium Depletion during Osmotic Diuresis, *Surg Gynecol Obstet,* **119:**265, 1964.

Gill, J. R., Jr.: The Role of the Sympathetic Nervous System in the Regulation of Sodium Excretion by the Kidney in W. F. Ganong and L. Martini (eds.), "Frontiers in Neuroendocrinology," p. 289, Oxford University Press, New York, 1969.

Greenberg, A. G., and Kittle, C. F.: The Effects of Acute Changes in Acid-Base Status on Coronary Blood Flow, *Surgery,* **64:**315, 1968.

Gruber, U. F., Smith, L. L., and Moore, F. D.: The Effect of Acute Addition Metabolic Alkalosis on the Cardiovascular Response of the Dog to Hemorrhage, *J Surg Res,* **3:**21, 1963.

Gump, F. E., and Kinney, J. M.: Measurement of Water Balance: A Guide to Surgical Care, *Surgery,* **64:**154, 1968.

Hardaway, R. M., James, P. M., Jr., Anderson, R. W., Bredenberg, C. E., and West, R. L.: Intensive Study and Treatment of Shock in Man, *JAMA,* **199:**779, 1967.

Heaton, F. W., Clark, C. G., and Coligher, J. C.: Magnesium Deficiency Complicating Intestinal Surgery, *Br J Surg,* **54:**41, 1967.

Hoye, R. C., Ketcham, A. S., and Berlin, N. I.: Total Red Cell and Plasma Volume Alterations Occurring with Extensive Surgery in Humans, *Surg Gynecol Obstet,* **123:**27, 1966.

Huckabee, W. E.: Abnormal Resting Blood Lactate: I. The Significance of Hyperlactalemia in Hospitalized Patients, *Am J Med,* **30:**833, 1961.

Kassirer, J. P., Berkman, P. M., Lawrenz, D. R., and Schwartz, W. B.: The Critical Role of Chloride in the Correction of Hypokalemic Alkalosis in Man, *Am J Med,* **38:**172, 1965.

Litwin, M. S., Smith, L. L., and Moore, F. D.: Metabolic Alkalosis following Massive Transfusion, *Surgery,* **45:**805, 1959.

Lyons, J. H., Jr., and Moore, F. D.: Posttraumatic Alkalosis: Incidence and Pathophysiology of Alkalosis in Surgery, *Surgery,* **60:**93, 1966.

MacLean, L. D., Mulligan, W. G., McLean, A. P. H., and Duff, J. H.: Patterns of Septic Shock in Man: A Detailed Study of 56 Patients, *Ann Surg,* **166:**543, 1967.

Peaston, M. J. T.: Metabolic Acidosis in Burns, *Br Med J,* **1:**809, 1968.

Pullen, H., Doig, A., and Lambie, A. T.: Intensive Intravenous Potassium Replacement Therapy, *Lancet,* **2:**809, 1967.

Rector, F. C., Jr., Bloomer, H. A., and Seldin, D. W.: Effect of Potassium Deficiency on the Reabsorption of Bicarbonate in the Proximal Tubule of the Rat Kidney, *J Clin Invest,* **43:**1976, 1964.

Robbins, H. S., and Dufrene, J. H.: Hyperkalemia in Anesthesia, *Pa Med,* **75:**77, 1972.

Schlobohm, R. M., and Holaday, D. A.: Prevention and Correction of Acidosis, in C. L. Fox, Jr., and G. G. Nahas (eds.), "Body Fluid Replacement in the Surgical Patient," p. 246, Grune & Stratton, Inc., New York, 1970.

Siggaard-Andersen, O.: The Acid-Base Status of Blood, *Scand J Clin Lab Invest,* **15**(*Suppl* 70):1, 1963.

Wacker, W. E. C., and Parisi, A. F.: Magnesium Metabolism, *N Engl J Med,* **278:**712, 1968.

Wright, H. K., and Gann, D. S.: Correction of the Force Water Defect in Postoperative Patients by Extracellular Fluid Volume Expansion, *Ann Surg,* **158:**70, 1963.

——— and ———: A Defect in Urinary Concentrating Ability during Postoperative Antidiuresis, *Surg Gynecol Obstet,* **121:**47, 1965.

Oxygen Transport

Benesch, R., and Benesch, R.: Intracellular Organic Phosphates as Regulators of Oxygen Release by Haemoglobin, *Nature, (Lond),* **221:**618, 1969.

Naylor, B. A., Welch, M. H., Shafer, A. W., and Cuenter, C. A.: Blood Affinity for Oxygen in Hemorrhagic and Endotoxic Shock, *J Appl Physiol,* **32:**829, 1972.

Plzak, L. F.: Hyperalimentation and the Oxy-hemoglobin Dissociation Curve, in G. S. M. Cowan, Jr., and W. L. Scheetz, (eds.)

"Intravenous Hyperalimentation," p. 196, Lea & Febiger, Philadelphia, 1972.

Proctor, H. J., Lentz, R. R., and Johnson, G., Jr.: Alterations in Baboon Erythrocyte 2,3-Diphosphoglycerate Concentration Associated with Hemorrhagic Shock and Resuscitation, *Ann Surg,* **174:**923, 1971.

Shoemaker, W. C., Boyd, D. R., Kim, S. I., Brown, R. S., Dreiling, D. A., and Kark, A. E.: Sequential Oxygen Transport and Acid-Base Changes after Trauma to the Unanesthetized Patient, *Surg Gynecol Obstet,* **132:**1033, 1971.

Sugerman, H., Miller, L. D., Oski, F. A., Diaco, J., Delivoria-Papadopoulos, M., and Davidson, D.: Decreased 2,3-Diphosphoglycerate (DPG) and Reduced Oxygen (O_2) Consumption in Septic Shock, *Clin Res,* **18:**418, 1970.

Travis, S. F., Sugerman, H. J., Ruberg, R. L., Dudrick, S. J., Delivoria-Papadopoulos, M. D., Miller, L. D., and Oski, F. A.: Alterations of Red Cell Poikilitic Intermediates and Oxygen Transport as a Consequence of Hypophosphatemia in Patients Receiving Intravenous Hyperalimentation, *N Engl J Med,* **285:**763, 1971.

Immunologic Protective Mechanisms

Bell, M. L., Herman, A. H., Egdahl, R. H., Smith, E. E., and Rutenburg, A. M.: Role of Lysosomal Disruption in the Development of Refractory Shock, *Surg Forum,* **21:**10, 1970.

Greyson, N. D., Rhodes, B. A., Buchanan, J. W., and Wagner, H. N., Jr.: Local Increases in Reticuloendothelial Function during Healing, *J Reticuloendothel Soc,* **11:**293, 1972.

Hawley, P. R.: The Role of Trauma in the Development of Peritonitis and the Protection Afforded by Intravenous Dextran Solutions, *Br J Surg,* **58:**305, 1971.

Liedberg, C. F.: Antibacterial Resistance in Burns: II. The Effect on Unspecific Humoral Defense Mechanisms, Phagocytosis and the Development of Bacteremia, *Acta Chir Scand,* **121:**351, 1961.

Munster, A. M., Eurenius, K., Mortensen, R. F., and Mason, A. D.: Ability of Splenic Lymphocytes from Injured Rats to Induce a Graft-versus-Host Reaction, *Transplantation,* **14:**106, 1972.

———, ———, Katz, R. M., Canales, L., Foley, F. D., and Mortensen, R. F.: Cell-mediated Immunity after Thermal Injury, *Ann Surg,* **177:**139, 1973.

Palmerio, C., and Fine, J.: The Nature of Resistance to Shock, *Arch Surg,* **98:**679, 1969.

Pillemer, L., Schoenberg, M. D., Blum, L., and Wurz, L.: Properdin System and Immunity: II. Interaction of the Properdin System with Polysaccharides, *Science,* **122:**545, 1955.

Schildt, B. E.: Function of the RES after Thermal and Mechanical Trauma in Mice, *Acta Chir Scand,* **136:**359, 1970.

——— and Low, H.: Relationship between Trauma, Plasma Corticosterone and Reticuloendothelial Function in Anaesthetized Mice, *Acta Endocrinol (Kbh),* **67:**141, 1971.

Schumer, W.: Steroids in the Treatment of Clinical Septic Shock, *Ann Surg,* **184:**333, 1976.

———, Erve, P. R., and Obernolte, R. P.: Mechanisms of Steroid Protection in Septic Shock, *Surgery,* **72:**119, 1972.

Stetson, C. A., Jr.: Studies on the Mechanism of the Shwartzman Phenomenon: Similarities between Reactions to Endotoxins and Certain Reactions of Bacterial Allergy, *J Exp Med,* **101:**421, 1955.

Weil, M. H. and Spink, W. W.: A Comparison of Shock Due to Endotoxin with Anaphylactic Shock, *J Lab Clin Med,* **50:**501, 1957.

Zweifach, B. W.: Relation of the RES to Natural and Acquired Resistance to Shock, in S. G. Hershey (ed.), "Shock," Little, Brown and Company, Boston, 1964.

———, Benacerraf, B., and Thomas, L.: The Relationship Between the Vascular Manifestations of Shock Produced by Endotoxin, Trauma, and Hemorrhage, *J Exp Med,* **106:**403, 1957.

Organ System Changes: General

Bock, K. D. (ed.): "Shock: Pathogenesis and Therapy: An International Symposium, Stockholm, 27th-30th June, 1961," Ciba Symposium, Springer-Verlag OHG, Berlin, 1962.

Hardaway, R. M.: The Problem of Acute Severe Trauma and Shock, *Surg Gynecol Obstet,* **133:**799, 1971.

Hershey, S. G. (ed.): "Shock," Little, Brown and Company, Boston, 1964.

Jacobson, E. D.: A Physiologic Approach to Shock, *N Engl J Med,* **278:**834, 1968.

Landy, M., and Braun, W. (eds.): Bacterial Endotoxins, *Proc Symp Inst Microbiol Rutgers State Univ,* New Brunswick, N.J., 1964.

Mills, L. C., and Moyer, J. H. (eds.): "Shock and Hypotension: Pathogenesis and Treatment: The 12th Hahnemann Symposium," Grune & Stratton, Inc., New York, 1965.

Cardiovascular Function

Anderson, R. W., James, P. M., Bredenberg, C. E., and Hardaway, R. M.: Phenoxybenzamine in Septic Shock, *Ann Surg,* **165:**341, 1967.

Attar, S., McLaughlin, J., Hanashiro, P., and Cowley, R. A.: The Kallikreins in Human Shock and Trauma, *Surg Forum,* **22:**11, 1971.

Baez, S., and Orkin, L. R.: Microcirculatory Effects of Anesthesia in Shock, in S. G. Hershey (ed.), "Shock," p. 207, Little, Brown and Company, Boston, 1964.

Berk, J. L., Hagen, J. F., Beyer, W. H., and Niazmand, R.: Effect of Epinephrine on Arteriovenous Shunts in Pathogenesis of Shock, *Surg Gynecol Obstet,* **124:**347, 1967.

Cann, M. S., Stevenson, T., Fiallos, E. E., and Thal, A. P.: Effect of Digitalis on Myocardial Contractility in Sepsis, *Surg Forum,* **22:**1, 1971.

Clowes, G. H. A., Jr., and Del Guercio, L. R. M.: Circulatory Response to Trauma of Surgical Operations, *Metabolism,* **9:**67, 1960.

Coalson, J. J., Woodruff, H. K., Greenfield, L. J., Guemter, C. A., and Hinshaw, L. B.: Effects of Digoxin on Myocardial Ultrastructure in Endotoxin Shock, *Surg Gynecol Obstet,* **135:**908, 1972.

Cohn, J. N.: Central Venous Pressure as Guide to Volume Expansion, *Ann Intern Med,* **66:**1283, 1967.

Duff, J. H., Malave, G., Peretz, D. I., Scott, H. M., and MacLean, L. D.: Hemodynamics of Septic Shock in Man and in the Dog, *Ann Surg,* **162:**161, 1965.

Glenn, T. M., Herlihy, B. L., Ferguson, W. W., and Lefer, A. M.: Protective Effect of Pancreatic Duct Ligation in Splanchnic Ischemia Shock, *Am J Physiol,* **222:**1278, 1972.

——— and Lefer, A. M.: Protective Effect of Thoracic Lymph Diversion in Hemorrhagic Shock, *Am J Physiol,* **219:**1305, 1970.

——— and ———: Significance of Splanchnic Proteases in the Production of a Toxic Factor in Hemorrhagic Shock, *Circ Res,* **29:**338, 1971.

Goodyer, A. V. N., Hammond, G. L., Gross, C. C., and Kabimba, J.: Myocardial Production of Pyruvate in Hemorrhagic Shock, *J Surg Res,* **11:**501, 1971.

Greenfield, L. J., McCurdy, J. R., Hinshaw, L. B., and Elkins, R. C.: Preservation of Myocardial Function during Cross-Circulation in Terminal Endotoxin Shock, *Surgery,* **72:**111, 1972.

Hardaway, R. M., James, P. M., Jr., Anderson, R. W., Bredenberg, C. E., and West, R. L.: Intensive Study and Treatment of Shock in Man, *JAMA,* **199:**779, 1967.

Hermreck, A. S., and Thal, A. P.: Mechanisms for the High Circulatory Requirements in Sepsis and Septic Shock, *Ann Surg,* **170:**677, 1969.

Hinshaw, L. B., Greenfield, L. J., Archer, L. T., and Guenter, C. A.: Effects of Endotoxin on Myocardial Hemodynamics, Performance, and Metabolism during Beta Adrenergic Blockade, *Proc Soc Exp Biol Med,* **137:**1217, 1971.

———, ———, Owen, S. E., Black, M. R., and Guenter, C. A.: Precipitation of Cardiac Failure in Endotoxin Shock, *Surg Gynecol Obstet,* **135:**39, 1972.

Hiott, D. W., and Richardson, J. A.: Cardiac Norepinephrine Levels and Contractile Force Responses with Hemorrhagic Shock, Acidosis and Sympathetic Stimulation, *Res Comm Chem Pathol Pharmacol,* **2:**429, 1971.

Huberty, J. R., Schwarz, R. H., and Emich, J. P., Jr.: Central Venous Pressure Monitoring, *Obstet Gynecol,* **30:**842, 1967.

Lefer, A. M., Cowgill, R., Marshall, F. F., Hall, L. M., and Brank, E. D.: Characterization of a Myocardial Depressant Factor Present in Hemorrhagic Shock, *Am J Physiol,* **213:**492, 1967.

Levinson, S. A., and Hume, D. M.: Effect of Exchange Transfusion with Fresh Whole Blood on Refractory Septic Shock, *Am Surg,* **38:**49, 1972.

Longerbeam, J. K., Vannix, R., Wagner, W., and Joergenson, E.: Central Venous Pressure Monitoring: Useful Guide to Fluid Therapy during Shock and Other Forms of Cardiovascular Stress, *Am J Surg,* **110:**220, 1965.

MacLean, L. D., and Duff, J. H.: Use of Central Venous Pressure as Guide to Volume Replacement in Shock, *Dis Chest,* **48:**199, 1965.

Martin, A. M., Jr., Hackel, D. B., Entman, M. L., Capp, M. P., and Spach, M. S.: Mechanisms in the Development of Myocardial Lesions in Hemorrhagic Shock, *Ann NY Acad Sci,* **156:**79, 1969.

Mundth, E. D., Wright, J. E. C., Wanibuchi, Y., and Austen, W. G.: Effect of Varying After-load and Epinephrine Levels on the Ischemic Survival Time of the Dog Heart, *Surg Forum,* **22:**133, 1971.

Osborn, J. J., Russon, J. C. A., Beaumont, J. O., Hill, J. D., Kerth, W. J., Popper, R. W., and Gerbode, F.: Respiratory Causes of Sudden Unexplained Arrhythmia in Post-Thoracotomy Patients, *Surgery,* **69:**24, 1971.

Rush, B. F., Jr., Rosenberg, J. C., and Spencer, F. C.: Effect of Dibenzyline Treatment on Cardiac Dynamics and Oxidative Metabolism in Hemorrhagic Shock, *Ann Surg,* **162:**1013, 1965.

Schumer, W.: Microcirculatory and Metabolic Effects of Dibenzyline in Oligemic Shock, *Surg Gynecol Obstet,* **123:**787, 1966.

Shires, G. T., Carrico, C. J., and Canizaro, P. C.: "Shock," W. B. Saunders Company, Philadelphia, 1973.

Solis, R. T., and Downing, S. E.: Effects of *E. Coli* Endotoxemia on Ventricular Performance, *Am J Physiol,* **211:**307, 1966.

Thal, A. P., Brown, E. B., Jr., Hermreck, A. S., and Bell, H. H.: "Shock: A Physiologic Basis for Treatment," Year Book Medical Publishers, Inc., Chicago, 1971.

Wangensteen, S. L., Geissinger, W. T., Lovett, W. L., Glenn, T. M., and Lefer, A. W.: Relationship between Splanchnic Blood Flow and a Myocardial Depressant Factor in Endotoxin Shock, *Surgery,* **69:**410, 1971.

Weil, M. H., Schubin, H., and Rusoff, L.: Fluid Repletion in Circulatory Shock: Central Venous Pressure and Other Practical Guides, *JAMA,* **192:**688, 1965.

Weinstein, L., and Klainer, A. S.: Septic Shock: Pathogenesis and Treatment: IV. Management of Emergencies, *N Engl J Med,* **274:**950, 1966.

Wilson, R. F., Jablonski, D. V., and Thal, A. P.: Usage of Dibenzyline in Clinical Shock, *Surgery,* **56:**172, 1964.

———, Thal, A. P., Kindling, P. H., Grifka, T., and Ackerman, E.: Hemodynamic Measurements in Septic Shock, *Arch Surg,* **91:**121, 1965.

Wright, C. J., Duff, J. H., McLean, A. P. H., and MacLean, L. D.: Regional Capillary Blood Flow and Oxygen Uptake in Severe Sepsis, *Surg Gynecol Obstet,* **132:**637, 1971.

Pulmonary Function

Anderson, W. H., Dossett, B. E., Jr., and Hamilton, G. L.: Prevention of Postoperative Pulmonary Complications: Use of Isoproterenol and Intermittent Positive Pressure Breathing on Inspiration, *JAMA,* **186:**763, 1963.

Ashbaugh, D. G., and Petty, T. L.: The Use of Corticosteroids in the Treatment of Respiratory Failure Associated with Massive Fat Embolism, *Surg Gynecol Obstet,* **123:**493, 1966.

———, ———, Bigelow, D. B., and Harris, T. M.: Continuous Positive-Pressure Breathing (CPPB) in Adult Respiratory Distress Syndrome, *J Thorac Cardiovasc Surg,* **57:**31, 1969.

———, Svitek, V., and Ambrose, P.: The Incidence and Effects of Particulate Aggregation and Microembolism in Pump-Oxygenator Systems, *J Thorac Cardiovasc Surg,* **55:**691, 1968.

Ayres, S. M., Mueller, H., Giannelli, S., Jr., Fleming, P., and Grace, W. J.: The Lung in Shock: Alveolar-Capillary Gas Exchange in the Shock Syndrome, *Am J Cardiol,* **26:**588, 1970.

Barber, R. E., Lee, J., and Hamilton, W. K.: Oxygen Toxicity in Man: Study in Patients with Irreversible Brain Damage, *N Engl J Med,* **283:**1498, 1970.

Barnes, R. W., and Merendino, K. A.: Post-traumatic Pulmonary Insufficiency Syndrome, *Surg Clin North Am,* **52:**625, 1972.

Bendixen, H. H., Hedley-Whyte, J., and Laver, M. B.: Impaired Oxygenation in Surgical Patients during General Anesthesia with Controlled Ventilation, *N Engl J Med,* **269:**991, 1963.

Bergofsky, E. H.: The Adult Acute Respiratory Insufficiency Syndrome following Nonthoracic Trauma: The Lung in Shock, *Am J Cardiol,* **26:**619, 1970.

Blaisdell, F. W., Lim, R. C., Jr., and Stallone, R. J.: The Mechanism of Pulmonary Damage following Traumatic Shock, *Surg Gynecol Obstet,* **130:**1, 1970.

——— and Lewis, F. R., Jr.: "Respiratory Distress Syndrome of Shock and Trauma," W. B. Saunders Company, Philadelphia, 1977.

Burke, J. F., Pontoppidan, H., and Welch, C. E.: High Output Respiratory Failure: An Important Cause of Death Ascribed to Peritonitis or Ileus, *Ann Surg,* **158:**581, 1963.

Calabresi, P., and Abelmann, W. H.: Porto-caval and Portopulmonary Anastomoses in Laennec's Cirrhosis and in Heart Failure, *J Clin Invest,* **36:**1257, 1957.

Carlson, L. A.: Lipid Mobilization in Trauma: Friend or Foe?, in A. P. Morgan (ed.), "Proceedings of Conference on Energy Metabolism and Body Fuel Utilization," p. 50, Harvard University Press, Cambridge, Mass., 1966.

Comroe, J. H., Jr., Forster, R. E., II, Du-Bois, A. B., Briscoe, W. A., and Carlsen, E.: "The Lung," Year Book Medical Publishers, Inc., Chicago, 1962.

Cook, W. A., and Webb, W. R.: Pulmonary Changes in Hemorrhagic Shock, *Surgery,* **64:**85, 1968.

Dowd, J., and Jenkins, L. C.: The Lung in Shock: A Review, *Can Anaesth Soc J,* **19:**309, 1972.

Eltringham, W. K., Schroder, R., Jenny, M., Matloff, J. M., and Zollinger, R. M., Jr.: Pulmonary Arteriovenous Admixture in Cardiac Surgical Patients, *Circulation,* **37, 38** (*Suppl* 2):207, 1968.

Geiger, J. P., and Gleichinsky, L.: Acute Pulmonary Insufficiency: Treatment in Vietnam Casualties, *Arch Surg,* **102:**400, 1971.

Hamilton, W. K.: Alterations in Pulmonary Functions, *JAMA,* **202:**116, 1967.

Hechtman, H. B., Weisel, R. D., and Berger, R. L.: Independence of Pulmonary Shunting and Pulmonary Edema, *Surgery,* **74,** 1973.

Hill, J. D., O'Brien, T. G., Murray, J. J., Dontigny, L., Bramson, M. L., Osborn, J. J., and Gerbode, F.: Prolonged Extracorporeal Oxygenation for Acute Post-traumatic Respiratory Failure (Shock-Lung Syndrome), *N Engl J Med,* **286:**629, 1972.

Hillen, G. P., Gaisford, W. D., and Jensen, C. G.: Pulmonary Changes in Treated and Untreated Hemorrhagic Shock, *Am J Surg,* **122:**639, 1971.

Hirsch, E. F., Fletcher, R., and Lucas, S.: Hemodynamic and Respiratory Changes Associated with Sepsis following Combat Trauma, *Ann Surg,* **174:**211, 1971.

Kumar, A., Falke, K. J., Gettin, B., Aldredge, C. F., Laver, M. B., Lowenstein, E., and Pontoppidan, H.: Continuous Positive-Pressure Ventilation in Acute Respiratory Failure: Effects on Hemodynamics and Lung Function, *N Engl J Med,* **283:**1430, 1970.

Lahdensuu, M.: Studies on Phospholipid Metabolism in the Lung and Alveolar Surfactant in Experimental Traumatic and Haemorrhagic Shock, *Ann Chir Gynaecol Fenn,* **60:**245, 1971.

Lawson, D. W., Defalco, A. J., Phelps, J. A., Bradley, B. E., and McClenathan, J. E.: Corticosteroids as Treatment for Aspiration of Gastric Contents: An Experimental Study, *Surgery,* **59:**845, 1966.

Levitsky, S., Annable, C. A., Park, B. S., Davis, A. L., and Thomas, P. A.: Depletion of Alveolar Surface Active Material by Transbronchial Plasma Irrigation of the Lung, *Ann Surg,* **173:**107, 1971.

McNamara, J. J., Melot, M. D., and Stremple, F. J.: Screen Filtration Pressure in Combat Casualties, *Ann Surg,* **172:**334, 1970.

Magilligan, D. J., Jr., Oleksyn, T. W., and Schwartz, S. I.: Pulmonary Intravascular and Extravascular Volumes in Hemorrhagic Shock and Fluid Replacement, *Surgery,* **72:**780, 1972.

Meagher, D. M., Piermattei, D. L., and Swan, H.: Platelet Aggregation during Progressive Hemorrhagic Shock in Pigs, *J Thorac Cardiovasc Surg,* **62:**823, 1971.

Moore, F. D., Lyons, J. H., Jr., Pierce, E. C., Morgan, A. P., Jr., Drinker, P. A., MacArthur, J. D., and Dammin, G. J.: "Posttraumatic Pulmonary Insufficiency," W. B. Saunders Company, Philadelphia, 1969.

Moseley, R. V., and Doty, D. B.: Physiologic Changes Due to Aspiration Pneumonitis, *Ann Surg,* **171:**73, 1970.

Moss, G., Staunton, C., and Stein, A. A.: Cerebral Hypoxia as the Primary Event in the Pathogenesis of the "Shock Lung Syndrome," *Surg Forum,* **22:**211, 1971.

Nahas, R. A., Melrose, D. G., Sykes, M. K., and Robinson, B.: Post-perfusion Lung Syndrome: Effect of Homologous Blood, *Lancet,* **2:**254, 1965.

———, ———, ———, and ———: Post-perfusion Lung Syndrome: Role of Circulatory Exclusion, *Lancet,* **2:**251, 1965.

Nash, G., Blennerhassett, J. B., and Pontoppidan, H.: Pulmonary Lesions Associated with Oxygen Therapy and Artificial Ventilation, *N Engl J Med,* **276:**368, 1967.

Pelter, L. F.: Fat Embolism: A Pulmonary Disease, *Surgery,* **62:**756, 1967.

Peters, R. M., and Hedgpeth, E. McG., Jr.: Acid-Base Balance and Respiratory Work, *J Thorac Cardiovasc Surg,* **52:**649, 1966.

———, Hilberman, M., Hogan, J. S., and Crawford, D. A.: Objective Indications for Respiration Therapy in Post-Trauma and Postoperative Patients, *Am J Surg,* **124:**262, 1972.

Powers, S. R., Jr., Mannal, R., Neclerio, M., English, M., Marr, C., Leather, R., Ueda, H., Williams, G., Custead, W., and Dutton, R.: Physiologic Consequences of Positive End-Expiratory Pressure (PEEP) Ventilation, *Ann Surg,* **178:**265, 1973.

Ratliff, N. B., Wilson, J. W., Mikat, E., Hackel, D. B., and Graham, T. C.: The Lung in Hemorrhagic Shock: IV. The Role of Neutrophilic Polymorphonuclear Leukocytes, *Am J Pathol,* **65:**325, 1971.

Robb, H. J., Margulis, R. R., and Jabs, C. M.: Role of Pulmonary Microembolism in the Hemodynamics of Endotoxin Shock, *Surg Gynecol Obstet,* **135:**777, 1972.

Robin, E. D.: Abnormalities of Acid-Base Regulation in Chronic Pulmonary Disease, with Special Reference to Hypercapnia and Extracellular Alkalosis, *N Engl J Med,* **268:**917, 1963.

Roe, B. B.: Prevention and Treatment of Respiratory Complications in Surgery, *N Engl J Med,* **163:**547, 1960.

Siegel, D. C., Cochin, A., and Moss, G. S. The Ventilatory Response to Hemorrhagic Shock and Resuscitation, *Surgery,* **72:**451, 1972.

———, Moss, G. S., Cochin, A., and DasGupta, T. K.: Pulmonary Changes following Treatment for Hemorrhagic Shock: Saline versus Colloid Infusion, *Surg Forum,* **21:**17, 1970.

Suter, P. M., Fairley, H. B., and Isenberg, M. D.: Optimum End-Expiratory Airway Pressure in Patients with Acute Pulmonary Failure, *N Engl J Med,* **297:**284, 1975.

Trimble, C., Smith, D. E., Rosenthal, M. H., and Fosburg, R. G.: Pathophysiologic Role of Hypocarbia in Post-Traumatic Pulmonary Insufficiency, *Am J Surg,* **122:**633, 1971.

Veith, F. J., Hagstrom, J. W. C., Panossian, A., Nehlsen, S. L.,

and Wilson, J. W.: Pulmonary Microcirculatory Response to Shock, Transfusion, and Pump-Oxygenator Procedures: A Unified Mechanism Underlying Pulmonary Damage, *Surgery,* **64:**95, 1968.

Hepatic Function

Ballinger, W. F., Vollenweider, H., and Montgomery, E. H.: The Response of the Canine Liver to Anaerobic Metabolism Induced by Hemorrhagic Shock, *Surg Gynecol Obstet,* **112:**19, 1961.

Baue, A. E., Wurth, M. A., and Sayeed, M. M.: The Dynamics of Altered ATP-dependent and ATP-yielding Cell Processes in Shock, *Surgery,* **72:**94, 1972.

Blair, O. M., Stenger, R. J., Hopkins, R. W., and Simeone, F. A.: Hepatocellular Ultrastructure in Dogs with Hypovolemic Shock, *Lab Invest,* **18:**172, 1968.

Bloom, W. L.: Changes in Blood Ketones during Hemorrhagic Shock in Rats, *Metabolism,* **10:**171, 1961.

——— and Ward, J. A.: Changes in Carbohydrate Metabolism during Blood Loss, Shock, and Anoxia, *Metabolism,* **10:**379, 1961.

Buxton, R. W., Haines, B. W., and Michaelis, M.: Effects of Hemorrhagic Shock upon Succinic Oxidation in Dog, Liver and Brain Slices, *Bull School Med Univ Maryland,* **46:**3, 1961.

Clermont, H. G., Williams, J. S., and Adams, J. T.: Liver Acid Phosphatase as a Measure of Hepatocyte Resistance to Hemorrhagic Shock, *Surgery,* **71:**868, 1972.

DePalma, R. G., Holden, W. D., and Robinson, A. V.: Fluid Therapy in Experimental Hemorrhagic Shock: Ultrastructural Effects in Liver and Muscle, *Ann Surg,* **175:**539, 1972.

Holden, W. D., DePalma, R. G., Drucker, W. R., and McKalen, A.: Ultrastructural Changes in Hemorrhagic Shock: Electron Microscopic Study of Liver, Kidney, and Striated Muscle, *Ann Surg,* **162:**517, 1965.

Janoff, A.: Alterations in Lysosomes (Intracellular Enzymes) during Shock: Effects of Preconditioning (Tolerance) and Protective Drugs, in S. G. Hershey (ed.), "Shock," p. 93, Little, Brown and Company, Boston, 1964.

Kekomaki, M., and Louhimo, I.: Blood Ammonium Concentration during Hemorrhagic Shock in the Rabbit, *Acta Chir Scand,* **137:**745, 1971.

Lavine, L., Harano, Y., and DePalma, R. G.: ATPase Activity and Palmitate Oxidation of Hepatic Mitochondria in Energy Production in Endotoxemia, *Surg Forum,* **22:**5, 1971.

Murray, J. F., Dawson, A. M., and Sherlock, S.: Circulatory Changes in Chronic Liver Disease, *Am J Med,* **24:**358, 1958.

Rutenburg, A. M., Bell, M. L., Butcher, R. W., Polgar, P., Dorn, B. D., and Egdahl, R. H.: Adenosine 3′,5′-Monophosphate Levels in Hemorrhagic Shock, *Ann Surg,* **174:**461, 1971.

Selkurt, E. E.: Role of Liver and Toxic Factors in Shock, in S. G. Hershey (ed.), "Shock," p. 34, Little, Brown and Company, Boston, 1964.

Sherlock, S.: Diseases of the Digestive System. Drugs and the Liver, *Br Med J,* **1:**227, 1968.

Shorthouse, W. C., and Fitch, L. B.: Hepatic Lesions of Hemorrhagic Shock, *Arch Surg,* **85:**492, 1962.

Smart, C. J., and Rowlands, S. D.: Oxygen Consumption and Hepatic Metabolism in Experimental Posthemorrhagic Shock, *Trauma,* **12:**327, 1972.

Wurth, M. A., Sayeed, M. M., and Baue, A. E.: (Na$^+$ + K$^+$)-ATPase Activity in the Liver with Hemorrhagic Shock, *Proc Soc Exp Biol Med*, **139:**1238, 1972.

Gastrointestinal Function

Abe, H., Carballo, J., Appert, H. E., and Howard, J. M.: The Release and Fate of the Intestinal Lysosomal Enzymes after Acute Ischemic Injury of the Intestine, *Surg Gynecol Obstet*, **135:**581, 1972.

Bacalzo, L. V., Jr., Parkins, F. M., Miller, L. D., and Parkins, W. M.: Effects of Prolonged Hypovolemic Shock on Jejunal Fluid and Sodium Transport, *Surg Gynecol Obstet*, **134:**399, 1972.

Barton, R. W., Reynolds, D. G., and Swan, K. G.: Mesenteric Circulatory Responses to Hemorrhagic Shock in the Baboon, *Ann Surg*, **175:**204, 1972.

Bounous, G.: Metabolic Changes in Intestinal Mucosa during Hemorrhagic Shock, *Can J Surg*, **8:**332, 1965.

———, McArdle, A. H., Hodges, D. M., Hampson, L. G., and Gurd, F. N.: Biosynthesis of Intestinal Mucin in Shock: Relationship to Tryptic Hemorrhagic Enteritis and Permeability to Curare, *Ann Surg*, **164:**13, 1966.

———, Sutherland, N. G., McArdle, A. H., and Gurd, F. N.: The Prophylactic Use of an "Elemental" Diet in Experimental Hemorrhagic Shock and Intestinal Ischemia, *Ann Surg*, **166:**312, 1967.

Carter, D., and Einheber, A.: Intestinal Ischemic Shock in Germ-free Animals, *Surg Gynecol Obstet*, **122:**66, 1966.

Chiu, C. J., Scott, H. J., and Gurd, F. N.: Volume Deficit Versus Toxic Absorption: A Study of Canine Shock after Mesenteric Arterial Occlusion, *Ann Surg*, **175:**479, 1972.

Clermont, H. G., and Williams, J. S.: Lymph Lysosomal Enzyme Acid Phosphatase in Hemorrhagic Shock, *Ann Surg*, **176:**90, 1972.

Cook, B. H., Wilson, E. R., Jr., and Taylor, A. E.: Intestinal Fluid Loss in Hemorrhagic Shock, *Am J Physiol*, **221:**1494, 1971.

DenBesten, L., and Hamza, K. N.: Effect of Bile Salts on Ionic Premeability of Canine Gastric Mucosa during Experimental Shock, *Gastroenterology*, **62:**417, 1972.

Drucker, W. R., Davis, J. H., Holden, W. D., and Reagan, J. R.: Hemorrhagic Necrosis of the Intestine, *Arch Surg*, **89:**42, 1964.

Fine, J.: Intestinal Circulation in Shock, *Gastroenterology*, **52:**454, 1967.

Fischer, R. P., and Stremple, J. F.: Stress Ulcers in Post-traumatic Renal Insufficiency in Patients from Vietnam, *Surg Gynecol Obstet*, **134:**790, 1972.

Goodier, T. E. W., Horwich, L., and Galloway, R. W.: Morphological Observations on Gastric Ulcers Treated with Carbonoxolone Sodium. *Gut*, **8:**544, 1967.

Goodman, A. A., and Osborne, M. P.: An Experimental Model and Clinical Definition of Stress Ulceration, *Surg Gynecol Obstet*, **134:**563, 1972.

Gurd, F. N.: Metabolic and Functional Changes in Intestine in Shock, *Am J Surg*, **110:**333, 1965.

——— and McClelland, R. N.: Trauma Workshop Report: The Gastrointestinal Tract in Trauma, *J Trauma*, **11:**1089, 1970.

Howerton, E. E., and Kolmen, S. N.: The Intestinal Tract as a Portal of Entry of Pseudomonas in Burned Rats, *J Trauma*, **12:**335, 1972.

Hutcher, N., Silverberg, S. G., and Lee, H. M.: The Effect of

Vitamin A on the Formation of Steroid Induced Gastric Ulcers, *Surg Forum*, **22:**322, 1971.

Lev, R., Molot, M. D., McNamara, J., and Stremple, J. F.: "Stress" Ulcers following War Wounds in Vietnam: A Morphologic and Histochemical Study, *Lab Invest*, **25:**491, 1971.

Lillehei, R. C., Longerbeam, J. K., Bloch, J. H., and Manax, W. G.: The Nature of Experimental Irreversible Shock with Its Clinical Application, in S. G. Hershey (ed.), "Shock," p. 139, Little, Brown and Company, Boston, 1964.

Menguy, R., and Masters, Y. F.: Effect of Cortisone on Mucoprotein Secretion by Gastric Antrum of Dogs: Pathogenesis of Steroid Ulcer, *Surgery*, **54:**19, 1963.

——— and ———: Influence of Parathyroid Extract on Gastric Mucosal Content of Mucus, *Gastroenterology*, **48:**342, 1965.

Ritchie, W. P., and Fischer, R. P.: Studies on the Pathogenesis of "Stress Ulcer": Electrical Potential Difference and Ionic Fluxes across Canine Gastric Mucosa during Hemorrhagic Shock, *J Surg Res*, **12:**173, 1972.

———, Roth, R. R., and Fischer, R. P.: Studies on the Pathogenesis of "Stress Ulcer": Effect of Hemorrhage, Transfusion, and Vagotomy in the Restrained Rat, *Surgery*, **71:**445, 1972.

Robert, A., Bayer, R. B., and Nezamis, J. E.: Gastric Mucus Content during Development of Ulcers in Fasting Rats, *Gastroenterology*, **45:**740, 1963.

——— and Nezamis, J. E.: Effect of Prednisolone on Gastric Mucus Content and on Ulcer Formation, *Proc Soc Exp Biol Med*, **114:**545, 1943.

Shirazi, S. S., DenBesten, L., and Hamza, K. N.: Absorption of Bile Salts from the Gastric Mucosa during Hemorrhagic Shock, *Proc Soc Exp Biol Med*, **140:**924, 1972.

Swan, K. G., Barton, R. W., and Reynolds, D. G.: Mesenteric Hemodynamics during Endotoxemia in the Baboon, *Gastroenterology*, **61:**872, 1971.

——— and Reynolds, D. G.: Blood Flow to the Liver and Spleen during Endotoxin Shock in the Baboon, *Surgery*, **72:**388, 1972.

Voitk, A. J., Chiu, C. J., and Gurd, F. N.: Prevention of Porcine Stress Ulcer following Hemorrhagic Shock with Elemental Diet, *Arch Surg*, **105:**473, 1972.

Vyden, J. K., and Corday, E.: The Effect of Cardiogenic Shock on the Superior Mesenteric Circulation, *Geriatrics*, **26:**85, 1971.

Wilmore, D. W., Dudrick, S. J., Dailey, J. M., and Vars, H. M.: The Role of Nutrition in the Adaptation of the Small Intestine after Massive Resection, *Surg Gynecol Obstet*, **132:**673, 1971.

Zweifach, W. B., Gordon, H. A., Wagner, M., and Reyniers, J. A.: Irreversible Shock in Germ-free Rats, *J Exp Med*, **107:**437 1958.

Renal Function

Barry, K. G., Mazze, R. I., and Schwartz, F. D.: Prevention of Surgical Oliguria and Renal-Hemodynamic Suppression by Sustained Hydration, *N Engl J Med*, **270:**1371, 1964.

Baxter, C., and Powers, S. R., Trauma Workshop Report: Kidney Response to Trauma, *J Trauma*, **10:**1072, 1970.

Blagg, C. R., and Parsons, F. M.: Earlier Dialysis and Anabolic Steroids in Acute Renal Failure, *Am Heart J*, **61:**287, 1961.

Boba, A., and Landmesser, C. M.: Renal Complications after Anesthesia and Operation, *Anesthesiology*, **22:**781, 1961.

Gorfinkel, H. J., Szidon, J. P., Hirsch, L. J., and Fishman, A. P.:

Renal Performance in Experimental Cardiogenic Shock, *Am J Physiol*, **222**:1260, 1972.

Habif, D. V., Paper, E. M., Fitzpatrick, H. F., Lowrance, P., Smythe, C. McC., and Bradley, S. E.: Renal and Hepatic Blood Flow, Glomerular Filtration Rate, and Urinary Output of Electrolytes during Cyclopropane, Ether, and Thiopental Anesthesia, Operation, and Immediate Postoperative Period, *Surgery*, **30**:241, 1951.

Hatcher, C. R., Jr., Gagnon, J. A., and Clark, R. W.: Effects of Hydration on Epinephrine-induced Renal Shut Down in Dogs, *Surg Forum*, **9**:106, 1958.

Jones, L. W., and Weil, M. H.: Water, Creatinine and Sodium Excretion following Circulatory Shock with Renal Failure, *Am J Med*, **51**:314, 1971.

Knuth, O. E., Wagenknecht, L. V., and Madsen, P. O.: The Effect of Various Treatments on Renal Function during Endotoxin Shock, *Invest Urol*, **9**:304, 1972.

Logan, A., Jose, P., Eisner, G., Lilienfield, L., and Slotkoff, L.: Intracortical Distribution of Renal Blood Flow in Hemorrhagic Shock in Dogs, *Circ Res*, **29**:257, 1971.

Mazze, R. I., Schwartz, F. D., Slocum, H. C., and Barry, K. G.: Renal Function during Anesthesia and Surgery. I. Effects of Halothane Anesthesia, *Anesthesiology*, **24**:279, 1963.

Merrill, J. P.: "The Treatment of Renal Failure," Grune & Stratton, Inc., New York, 1965.

Moyer, C. A.: Acute Temporary Changes in Renal Function Associated with Major Surgical Procedures, *Surgery*, **27**:198, 1950.

Mueller, C. G.: Mechanism and Use of Mannitol Diuresis in Major Surgery and in Trauma, *South Med J*, **59**:408, 1966.

Nagy, Z., Bencsath, P., Tornyai, K., and Vaslaki, L.: Arteriovenous Anastomoses in the Kidney: IX. Intrarenal Circulation During Tourniquet Shock, *Acta Physiol Acad Sci Hung*, **40**:121, 1971.

————, Meszaros, A., and Vaslaki, L.: Arterio-venous Anastomoses in the Kidney: X. Effect of Phenoxybenzamine on Intrarenal Circulation of Dogs in Tourniquet Shock, *Acta Physiol Acad Sci Hung*, **40**:129, 1971.

Parry, W. L., Schaefer, J. A., and Mueller, C. B.: Experimental Studies of Acute Renal Failure. I. Protective Effect of Mannitol, *J Urol*, **89**:1, 1963.

Selkurt, E. E.: Atropine Influence on Altered Hemodynamics of the Primate Kidney in Hemorrhagic Shock, *Proc Soc Exp Biol Med*, **138**:497, 1971.

————: Influence of Aortic Constriction on the Positive Free-Water Clearance of Primate Hemorrhagic Shock, *Proc Soc Exp Biol Med*, **140**:221, 1972.

Skinner, D. G., and Hayes, M. A.: Effect of Staphylococcic Toxin on Renal Function: Irreversible Shock, *Ann Surg*, **162**:161, 1965.

Strauch, M., McLaughlin, J. S., Mansberger, A., Young, J., Mendonca, P., Gray, K., and Cowley, R. A.: Effects of Septic Shock on Renal Function in Humans, *Ann Surg*, **165**:536, 1967.

Stremple, J. F., Ellison, E. H., and Carey, L. C.: Osmolar Diuresis: Success and/or Failure: A Collective Review, *Surgery*, **60**:924, 1966.

Tobian, L.: Renin-Angiotensin Mechanisms in Shock, in L. C. Mills and J. H. Moyer (eds.), "Shock and Hypotension: Pathogenesis and Treatment, The 12th Hahnemann Symposium," Grune & Stratton, Inc., New York, 1965.

Uldall, P. R., and Kerr, D. N. S., Post-traumatic Acute Renal Failure, *Br J Anaesth*, **44**:283, 1972.

Chapter 2

Fluid, Electrolyte, and Nutritional Management of the Surgical Patient

by G. Tom Shires and Peter C. Canizaro

One of the most critical aspects of patient care is management of the body composition of fluid and electrolytes. Most diseases, many injuries, and even operative trauma impose a great impact on the physiology of fluid and electrolytes within the body. These changes often exceed those brought about by acute lack of alimentation. There-fore, a thorough understanding of the metabolism of salt, water, and electrolytes and of certain metabolic responses is essential to the care of surgical patients.

An attempt will be made here to define the anatomy of body fluids and the physiologic principles governing function of fluids and electrolytes. In addition to these normal functions, a classification of derangements will be developed so that rational therapy may be described.

ANATOMY OF BODY FLUIDS

A prerequisite to the understanding of fluid and electrolyte management is knowledge of the extent and composition of the various body fluid compartments. Early attempts to define these compartments were relatively accurate, but a more precise definition has been obtained by many investigators through the use of isotope tracer techniques. The wide range of normal values is a function of body size, weight, and sex, but these compartments are relatively constant in size in the individual patient in the normal steady state. The figures used in this section, therefore, are approximate and presented as a percentage of body weight.

Total Body Water

Water constitutes between 50 and 70 percent of total body weight. Using deuterium oxide or tritiated water for measurement of total body water (TBW), the average normal value for young adult males is 60 percent of body weight and 50 percent for young adult females. A normal variation of ± 15 percent applies to both groups. The actual figure for each healthy individual is remarkably constant and is a function of several variables, including lean body mass and age. Since fat contains little water, the lean individual has a greater proportion of water to total body weight than the obese person. Thus, an extremely obese individual may have 25 to 30 percent less body water than a lean individual of the same weight. The lower percentage of total body water in females correlates well with a relatively large amount of subcutaneous adipose tissue and small muscle mass. Moore et al. have shown that total body water, as a percentage of total body weight, decreases steadily and significantly with age to a low of 52 and 47 percent in males and females respectively.

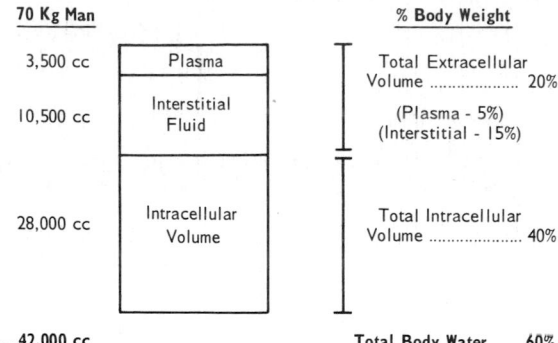

Fig. 2-1. Functional compartments of body fluids.

Conversely, the highest proportion of total body water to body weight is found in newborn infants, with a maximum of 75 to 80 percent. During the first several months following birth there is a gradual "physiologic" loss of body water as the infant adjusts to his environment. At one year of age, the total body water averages approximately 65 percent of the body weight and remains relatively constant throughout the remainder of infancy and childhood.

The water of the body is divided into three functional compartments (Fig. 2-1). The fluid within the body's diverse cell population, intracellular water, represents between 30 and 40 percent of the body weight. The extracellular water represents 20 percent of the body weight and is divided between the intravascular fluid, or plasma

(5 percent of body weight), and the interstitial, or extravascular, extracellular fluid (15 percent of body weight).

Intracellular Fluid

Measurement of intracellular fluid is determined indirectly by subtraction of the measured extracellular fluid from the measured total body water. The intracellular water is between 30 and 40 percent of the body weight, with the largest proportion in the skeletal muscle mass. Because of the smaller muscle mass in the female, the percentage of intracellular water is lower than in the male.

The chemical composition of the intracellular fluid is shown in Fig. 2-2, with potassium and magnesium the principal cations, and phosphates and proteins the principal anions. This is an approximation, since so few data concerning the intracellular fluid are available.

Extracellular Fluid

The total extracellular fluid volume represents approximately 20 percent of the body weight. The extracellular fluid compartment has two major subdivisions. The plasma volume comprises approximately 5 percent of the body weight in the normal adult. The interstitial, or extravascular, extracellular fluid volume, obtained by subtracting the plasma volume from the measured total extracellular fluid volume, comprises approximately 15 percent of the body weight.

The interstitial fluid is further complicated by having,

		PLASMA 154 mEq/l CATIONS	154 mEq/l ANIONS		INTERSTITIAL FLUID 153 mEq/l CATIONS	153 mEq/l ANIONS		INTRACELLULAR FLUID 200 mEq/l CATIONS	200 mEq/l ANIONS

Na^+ 142 Cl^- 103 Na^+ 144 Cl^- 114 K^+ 150 $HPO_4^{\equiv}$ } SO_4^{--} } 150

HCO_3^- 27

SO_4^{--} } PO_4^{---} } 3 HCO_3^- 30

SO_4^{--} 3 HCO_3^- 10

K^+ 4 PO_4^{---}

K^+ 4   Organic Acids 5 Mg^{++} 40   Protein 40

Ca^{++} 5   Organic Acids 5 Ca^{++} 3   Organic Acids 5

Mg^{++} 3   Protein 16 Mg^{++} 2   Proteins 1 Na^+ 10

PLASMA   **INTERSTITIAL FLUID**   **INTRACELLULAR FLUID**

Fig. 2-2. Chemical composition of body fluid compartments.

normally, a rapidly equilibrating, or functional, component, as well as several slower-equilibrating, or relatively nonfunctioning, components. The nonfunctioning components include connective tissue water as well as water that has been termed *transcellular,* which includes cerebrospinal and joint fluids. This nonfunctional component normally represents only 10 percent of the interstitial fluid volume (1 to 2 percent of body weight) and is not to be confused with the *relatively* nonfunctional extracellular fluid, often called a "third space," found in burns and soft tissue injuries.

The normal constituents of the extracellular fluid are shown in Fig. 2-2, with sodium the principal cation, and chloride and bicarbonate the principal anions. There are minor differences in ionic composition between the plasma and interstitial fluid occasioned by the difference in protein concentration. Because of the higher protein content (organic anions) of the plasma, the total concentration of cations is higher and the concentration of inorganic anions somewhat lower than in the interstitial fluid, as explained by the Gibbs-Donnan equilibrium equation.* For practical consideration, however, they may be considered equal. The total concentration of intracellular ions exceeds that of the extracellular compartment and would seem to violate the concept of osmolar equilibrium between the two compartments. This apparent discrepancy is due to the fact that the concentration of ions is expressed in milliequivalents (mEq) without regard to osmotic activity. In addition, some of the intracellular cations probably exist in undissociated form.

Osmotic Pressure

Relevant to a discussion of the complicated interactions between the various body fluid compartments is the definition of commonly used terms: The physiologic and chemical activity of electrolytes depend on (1) the *number of particles* present per unit volume [moles or millimoles (mM) per liter], (2) the *number of electric charges* per unit volume (equivalents or milliequivalents per liter), and (3) the *number of osmotically active particles,* or ions per unit volume [osmoles or milliosmoles (mO) per liter]. The use of the terms *grams* or *milligrams per 100 milliliters* expresses the weight of the electrolytes per unit volume but does not allow a physiologic comparison of the solutes in a solution.

A mole of a substance is the molecular weight of that substance in grams, and a millimole is that figure expressed in milligrams. For example, a mole of sodium chloride is 58 grams (Na—23, Cl—35), and a millimole is 58 milligrams. This expression, however, gives no direct information as to the number of osmotically active ions in solution or the electric charges that they carry.

The electrolytes of the body fluids then may be expressed in terms of chemical combining activity, or "equivalents." An equivalent of an ion is its atomic weight

expressed in grams divided by the valence, whereas a milliequivalent of an ion is that figure expressed in milligrams. In the case of univalent ions, a milliequivalent is the same as a millimole. However, in the case of divalent ions, such as calcium or magnesium, one millimole equals two milliequivalents. The importance of this expression is that a milliequivalent of any substance will combine chemically with a milliequivalent of any other substance; in any given solution, the number of milliequivalents of cations present is balanced by precisely the same number of milliequivalents of anions.

When the osmotic pressure of a solution is considered, it is more descriptive to employ the terms osmole and milliosmole. These terms refer to the actual number of osmotically active particles present in solution, but are not dependent on the chemical combining capacities of the substances. Thus, a millimole of sodium chloride, which dissociates nearly completely into sodium and chloride, contributes two milliosmoles, and one millimole of sodium sulfate (Na_2SO_4), which dissociates into three particles, contributes three milliosmoles. One millimole of an un-ionized substance such as glucose is equal to one milliosmole of the substance.

The differences in ionic composition between intracellular and extracellular fluid are maintained by the cell wall, which functions as a semipermeable membrane. The total number of osmotically active particles is 290 to 310 mO in each compartment. Although the total osmotic pressure of a fluid is the sum of the partial pressures contributed by each of the solutes in that fluid, the *effective* osmotic pressure is dependent on those substances which fail to pass through the pores of the semipermeable membrane. The dissolved proteins in the plasma, therefore, are primarily responsible for effective osmotic pressure between the plasma and the interstitial fluid compartments. This is frequently referred to as the *colloid osmotic pressure.* The effective osmotic pressure between the extracellular and intracellular fluid compartments would be contributed to by any substance that does not traverse the cell membranes freely. Thus sodium, which is the principal cation of the extracellular fluid, contributes a major portion of the osmotic pressure, but substances that fail to penetrate the cell membrane freely, such as glucose, also increase the effective osmotic pressure.

Since the cell membranes are completely permeable to water, the effective osmotic pressures in the two compartments are considered to be equal. Any condition that alters the effective osmotic pressure in either compartment will result in redistribution of water between the compartments. Thus, an increase in effective osmotic pressure in the extracellular fluid, which would occur most frequently as a result of increased sodium concentration, would cause a net transfer of water from the intracellular to the extracellular fluid compartment. This transfer of water would continue until the effective osmotic pressures in the two compartments were equal. Conversely, a decrease in the sodium concentration in the extracellular fluid will cause a transfer of water from the extracellular to the intracellular fluid compartment. However, depletion of the extracellular fluid volume without a change in the

---

*The product of the concentrations of any pair of diffusible cations and anions on one side of a semipermeable membrane will equal the product of the same pair of ions on the other side.

concentration of ions will not result in transfer of free water from the intracellular space.

Thus, the intracellular fluid shares in losses that involve a change in concentration or composition of the extracellular fluid but shares slowly in changes involving loss of isotonic volume alone. For practical consideration, most losses and gains of body fluid are directly from the extracellular compartment.

CLASSIFICATION OF BODY FLUID CHANGES

The disorders in fluid balance may be classified in three general categories: disturbances of (1) volume, (2) concentration, and (3) composition. Of primary importance is the concept that although these disturbances are interrelated, each is a separate entity.

If an isotonic salt solution is added to or lost from the body fluids, only the *volume* of the extracellular fluid is changed. The acute loss of an isotonic extracellular solution, such as intestinal juice, is followed by a significant decrease in the extracellular fluid volume and little, if any, change in the intracellular fluid volume. Fluid will not be transferred from the intracellular space to refill the depleted extracellular space as long as the osmolarity remains the same in the two compartments.

If water alone is added to or lost from the extracellular fluid, the *concentration* of osmotically active particles will change. Sodium ions account for 90 percent of the osmotically active particles in the extracellular fluid and generally reflect the tonicity of body fluid compartments. If the extracellular fluid is depleted of sodium, water will pass into the intracellular space until osmolarity is again equal in the two compartments.

The concentration of most other ions within the extracellular fluid compartment can be altered without significant change in the total number of osmotically active particles, thus producing only a *compositional* change. For instance, a rise of the serum potassium concentration from 4 to 8 mEq/L would have a significant effect on the myocardium, but it would not significantly change the effective osmotic pressure of the extracellular fluid compartment. Normally functioning kidneys minimize these changes considerably, particularly if the addition or loss of solute or water is gradual.

An internal loss of extracellular fluid into a nonfunctional space, such as the sequestration of isotonic fluid in a burn, peritonitis, ascites, or muscle trauma, is termed a *distributional* change. This transfer or functional loss of extracellular fluid internally may be extracellular (e.g., as in peritonitis) or intracellular (e.g., as in hemorrhagic shock). In any event, all distributional shifts or losses result in a contraction of the *functional* extracellular fluid space.

Volume Changes

Volume deficit or excess generally must be diagnosed by clinical examination of the patient. There are no readily available laboratory tests of benefit in the acute phase except measurement of the plasma volume. Changes secondary to long-standing derangements in volume, however, may be discernible by laboratory tests. For example, the blood urea nitrogen (BUN) level slowly rises with a long-standing extracellular fluid deficit of sufficient magnitude to reduce glomerular filtration. The concentration of serum sodium is *not* related to the volume status of extracellular fluid; a severe volume deficit may exist with a normal, low, or high serum sodium level.

VOLUME DEFICIT. Extracellular fluid volume deficit is by far the most common fluid disorder in the surgical patient. The loss of fluid is not water alone, but water and electrolytes in approximately the same proportion as that in which they exist in normal extracellular fluid. The most common disorders leading to an extracellular fluid volume deficit include losses of gastrointestinal fluids due to vomiting, nasogastric suction, diarrhea, and fistular drainage. Other common causes include sequestration of fluid in soft tissue injuries and infections, intraabdominal and retroperitoneal inflammatory processes, peritonitis, intestinal obstruction, and burns. The signs and symptoms of this state are easily recognized and are listed in Table 2-1. The central nervous system and cardiovascular signs occur early with acute rapid losses, whereas tissue signs may be absent until the deficit has existed for at least 24 hours. The central nervous system signs are similar to barbiturate intoxication and may be missed by the casual observer if the volume deficit is mild. The cardiovascular signs are secondary to a decrease in plasma volume and may be associated with varying degrees of hypotension in the patient with a severe extracellular fluid volume deficit. Skin turgor may be difficult to assess in the elderly patient or in the patient with recent weight loss and is not diagnostic in the absence of other confirmatory signs. The body temperature tends to vary with the environmental temperature. In a cool room, the patient may be slightly hypothermic and the febrile response to illness may be suppressed. This occurs frequently and can be very misleading during clinical evaluation of the septic patient. After partial correction of the volume deficit, the temperature will generally rise to the appropriate level.

VOLUME EXCESS. Extracellular fluid volume excess is generally iatrogenic or secondary to renal insufficiency. Both the plasma and interstitial fluid volumes are increased. In the healthy young adult, the signs are generally those of circulatory overload, manifested primarily in the pulmonary circulation, and of excessive fluid in other tissue (Table 2-1). In the elderly patient, congestive heart failure with pulmonary edema may develop rather quickly with a moderate volume excess.

Concentration Changes

Since the sodium ion is primarily responsible for the osmolarity of the extracellular fluid space, determination of the serum concentration of sodium generally indicates the tonicity of body fluids. Hyponatremia and hypernatremia can be diagnosed on clinical grounds (Table 2-2), but discernible signs and symptoms are not generally present until the changes are severe. Changes in concentration

Table 2-1. EXTRACELLULAR FLUID VOLUME

Type of sign	Deficit		Excess	
	Moderate	*Severe*	*Moderate*	*Severe*
Central nervous system	Sleepiness Apathy Slow responses Anorexia Cessation of usual activity	Decreased tendon re-flexes. Anesthesia distal ex-tremities Stupor Coma	None	None
Gastrointestinal	Progressive decrease in food consumption	Nausea, vomiting Refusal to eat Silent ileus and dis-tension	At surgery: Edema of stomach, colon, lesser and greater omenta and small bowel mesentary	
Cardiovascular	Orthostatic hypotension Tachycardia Collapsed veins Collapsing pulse	Cutaneous lividity Hypotension Distant heart sounds Cold extremities Absent peripheral pulses	Elevated venous pressure Distension of peripheral veins Increased cardiac output Loud heart sounds Functional murmurs Bounding pulse High pulse pressure Increased pulmonary 2d sound Gallop	Pulmonary edema
Tissue	Soft, small tongue with longitudial wrinkling Decreased skin turgor	Atonic muscles Sunken eyes	Subcutaneous pitting edema Basilar râles	Anasarca Moist râles Vomiting Diarrhea
Metabolic	Mild decrease temperature, 97–99°R	Marked decrease tem-perature, 95–98°R	None	None

should be noted early by appropriate laboratory tests and corrected promptly. Clinical signs of hyponatremia or hypernatremia tend to occur early and with greater severity if the rate of change in extracellular sodium concentration is very rapid.

HYPONATREMIA. Acute symptomatic hyponatremia (sodium less than 130 mEq/L) clinically is characterized by central nervous system signs of increased intracranial pressure and tissue signs of excessive intracellular water. There are no cardiovascular signs per se. The hypertension is probably induced by the rise in intracranial pressure, since the blood pressure generally returns to normal with the administration of hypertonic solutions of sodium salts. Of importance with severe hyponatremia is the relatively rapid development of oliguric renal failure, which may not be reversible if therapy is delayed.

Many hyponatremic states are asymptomatic until the serum sodium level falls below 120 mEq/L. One important exception is the patient with increased cerebrospinal fluid pressure, as following closed head injury, in whom mild hyponatremia may be extremely deleterious, even fatal, because of the progressive increase in intracellular water as the extracellular fluid osmolarity falls.

HYPERNATREMIA. Central nervous system and tissue signs, listed in Table 2-2, characterize acute symptomatic

hypernatremia. This is the only state in which dry, sticky mucous membranes are characteristic. This sign does not occur with pure extracellular fluid volume deficit alone, and may be misleading in the patient who breathes through his mouth. Body temperature is generally elevated and may approach a lethal level, as in the patient with heatstroke.

While volume changes occur frequently without a change in serum sodium, the reverse is not true. The disease states that cause a significant acute alteration in the serum sodium frequently produce a concomitant change in the extracellular fluid volume.

Mixed Volume and Concentration Abnormalities

Mixed volume and concentration abnormalities may develop as a consequence of the disease state or occasionally may result from inappropriate parenteral fluid therapy. Moyer noted that the clinical picture associated with a combination of fluid abnormalities will tend to be an algebraic composite of the signs and symptoms of each state. Like signs produced by both abnormalities will be additive, and opposing signs will tend to nullify one another. For example, the tendency for the body temperature

Table 2-2. ACUTE CHANGES IN OSMOLAR CONCENTRATION

Type of signs	Hyponatremia (water intoxication)		Hypernatremia (water deficit)	
Central nervous system	Moderate: Muscle twitching Hyperactive tendon reflexes Increased intra-cranial pressure (compensated phase)	Severe: Convulsions Loss of reflexes Increased intra-cranial pressure (decompensated phase)	Moderate: Restlessness Weakness	Severe: Delirium Maniacal be-havior
Cardiovascular	Changes in blood pressure and pulse secondary to increased intracranial pressure		Tachycardia Hypotension (if severe)	
Tissue	Salivation, lacrimation, watery diarrhea "Fingerprinting" of skin (sign of intracellular volume excess)		Decrease saliva and tears Dry and sticky mucous membranes Red, swollen tongue Skin flushed	
Renal	Oliguria progressing to anuria		Oliguria	
Metabolic	None		Fever	

to fall with an extracellular volume deficit may be counteracted by the tendency for it to rise with severe hypernatremia.

One of the more common mixed abnormalities is an extracellular fluid deficit and hyponatremia. This state is readily produced in the patient who continues to drink water while losing large volumes of gastrointestinal fluids. It may also occur in the postoperative period when gastrointestinal losses are replaced with only 5% dextrose in water or a hypotonic sodium solution. An extracellular volume deficit accompanied by hypernatremia may be produced by the loss of a large amount of hypotonic salt solution, such as sweat, in the absence of fluid intake.

The prolonged administration of excessive quantities of sodium salts with restricted water intake may result in an extracellular volume excess and hypernatremia. This may also occur when pure water losses (such as insensible loss of water from the skin and lungs) are replaced with sodium-containing solutions only. Similarly, the excessive administration of water or hypotonic salt solutions to the patient with oliguric renal failure may rapidly produce an extracellular volume excess and hyponatremia.

Normally functioning kidneys may minimize these changes to some extent and compensate for many of the errors associated with parenteral fluid administration. In contrast, the patient in anuric or oliguric renal failure is particularly prone to develop these mixed volume and osmolar concentration abnormalities. Fluid and electrolyte management in these patients, therefore, must be precise. Unfortunately, the fact that a patient with normal kidneys who develops a significant volume deficit may be in a state of "functional" renal failure is often not appreciated. As the volume deficit progresses, the glomerular filtration rate falls precipitously, and the kidneys' unique functions for

maintaining fluid homeostasis are lost. These changes may occur with only a mild volume deficit in the elderly patient with borderline renal function. In these elderly patients, the blood urea nitrogen level may rise higher than 100 mg/100 ml in response to the fluid deficit with a concomitant rise in the serum creatinine level. Fortunately, these changes are usually reversible with early and adequate correction of the extracellular fluid volume deficit.

Composition Changes

Compositional abnormalities of importance include changes in acid-base balance and concentration changes of potassium, calcium, and magnesium.

ACID-BASE BALANCE

The pH (the negative logarithm of the hydrogen ion concentration) of the body fluids is normally maintained within narrow limits in spite of the rather large load of acid produced endogenously as a by-product of body metabolism. The acids are neutralized efficiently by several buffer systems and subsequently excreted by the lungs and kidneys.

The important buffers include proteins and phosphates, which play a primary role in maintaining intracellular pH, and the bicarbonate–carbonic acid system, which operates principally in the extracellular fluid space. The proteins and hemoglobin have only minor influence in the extracellular fluid space, but the latter is of prime significance as a buffer in the red cell.

A buffer system consists of a weak acid or base and the salt of that acid or base. The buffering effect is the result of the formation of an amount of weak acid or base equivalent to the amount of strong acid or base added to the system. The resultant change in pH is considerably less than if the substance were added to water alone. Thus, inorganic acids (e.g., hydrochloric, sulfuric, phosphoric) and organic acids (e.g., lactic, pyruvic, keto acids) combine with base bicarbonate producing the sodium salt of the acid and carbonic acid:

$$HCL + NaHCO_3 \longrightarrow NaCl + H_2CO_3$$

The carbonic acid formed is then excreted via the lungs as CO_2. The inorganic acid anions are excreted by the kidneys with hydrogen or as ammonium salts. The organic acid anions generally are metabolized as the underlying disorder is corrected, although some renal excretion may occur with high levels.

The functions of the buffer systems are expressed in the Henderson-Hasselbalch equation, which defines the pH in terms of the ratio of the salt and acid. The pH of the extracellular fluid is defined primarily by the ratio of the amount of base bicarbonate (majority as sodium bicarbonate) to the amount of carbonic acid (related to the CO_2 content of alveolar air) present in the blood:

$$pH = pK + \log \frac{BHCO_3}{H_2CO_3} = \frac{27 \text{ mEq/L}}{1.33 \text{ mEq/L}} = \frac{20}{1} = 7.4$$

pK represents the dissociation constant of carbonic acid in the presence of base bicarbonate and by measurement is 6.1. At a body pH of 7.4, the ratio must be 20:1, as depicted. From a chemical standpoint, this is an inefficient buffer system, but the unusual property of CO_2 to behave as an acid or change to a neutral gas subsequently excreted by the lungs makes it quite efficient biologically.

As long as the 20:1 ratio is maintained, regardless of the absolute values, the pH will remain at 7.4. When an acid is added to the system, the concentration of bicarbonate (the numerator in the Henderson-Hasselbalch equation) will decrease. Ventilation will immediately increase to eliminate larger quantities of CO_2 with a subsequent decrease in the carbonic acid (the denominator in the Henderson-Hasselbalch equation) until the 20:1 ratio is reestablished. Slower, more complete compensation is effected by the kidneys with increased excretion of acid salts and retention of bicarbonate. The reverse will occur if an alkali is added to the system. Respiratory acidosis and alkalosis are produced by disturbances of ventilation, with an increase or decrease in the denominator and a resultant change of the 20:1 ratio. Compensation is primarily renal, with a retention of bicarbonate and increased excretion of acid salts in respiratory acidosis and the reverse process in respiratory alkalosis.

The four types of acid-base disturbances are listed in Table 2-3. Use of the CO_2 combining power (approximates the plasma bicarbonate) or CO_2 content (includes bicarbonate, carbonic acid, and dissolved CO_2) and knowledge of the patient's disease may allow an accurate diagnosis in the uncomplicated case. However, use of the CO_2 content or CO_2 combining power alone is generally inadequate as an index of acid-base balance. Both these tests principally reflect the level of plasma bicarbonate, since

Table 2-3. ACIDOSIS-ALKALOSIS

Type of acid-base disorder	Defect	Common causes	$\dfrac{BHCO_3}{H_2CO_3} = \dfrac{20}{1}$	Compensation
Respiratory acidosis	Retention of CO_2 (Decreased alveolar ventilation)	Depression of respiratory center—morphine, CNS injury Pulmonary disease—emphysema, pneumonia	↑ Denominator Ratio less than 20:1	Renal Retention of bicarbonate, excretion of acid salts, increased ammonia formation Chloride shift into red cells
Respiratory alkalosis	Excessive loss of CO_2 (Increased alveolar ventilation)	Hyperventilation: Emotional, severe pain, assisted ventilation, encephalitis	↓ Denominator Ratio greater than 20:1	Renal Excretion of bicarbonate, retention of acid salts, decreased ammonia formation
Metabolic acidosis	Retention of fixed acids or Loss of base bicarbonate	Diabetes, azotemia, lactic acid accumulation, starvation Diarrhea, small bowel fistulae	↓ Numerator Ratio less than 20:1	Pulmonary (rapid) Increase rate and depth of breathing Renal (slow) As in respiratory acidosis
Metabolic alkalosis	Loss of fixed acids Gain of base bicarbonate Potassium depletion	Vomiting or gastric suction with pyloric obstruction Excessive intake of bicarbonate Diuretics	↑ Numerator Ratio greater than 20:1	Pulmonary (rapid) Decrease rate and depth of breathing Renal (slow) As in respiratory alkalosis

dissolved CO_2 and carbonic acid contribute no more than a few millimoles under most circumstances. In the acute phase, therefore, respiratory acidosis or alkalosis may exist without any change in the CO_2 content; determinations of the pH and P_{CO_2} from a freshly drawn arterial blood sample are necessary for diagnosis. Thus, measurements of pH, bicarbonate concentration, and P_{CO_2} are required for a more complete understanding of the acid-base status in most patients (Table 2-4).

Unfortunately, more complex acid-base disturbances are frequently encountered. Combinations of respiratory and metabolic changes occur and may represent compensation for the initial acid-base disturbance or may indicate two or more coexisting primary disorders (e.g., a *primary* respiratory acidosis complicated by a *primary* metabolic acidosis or alkalosis).

Usually primary acid-base disturbances are compensated to some extent. A primary metabolic disturbance is initially compensated by changes in pulmonary ventilation, while respiratory disturbances are compensated by renal mechanisms. For example, the initial compensation for an acute metabolic acidosis is an increase in the rate and depth of breathing to lower the arterial P_{CO_2}. As pointed out by Astrup et al., the actual state of the acid-base disorder may be characterized by the degree of compensation—*not compensated* (early or compensatory mechanisms not functioning), *partially compensated* (pH has not returned to a normal value), *compensated,* or *overcompensated.*

As previously noted, a knowledge of the pH, bicarbonate concentration, and P_{CO_2} will allow an accurate diagnosis of most acid-base disturbances. However, the clinical interpretation of these measurements is associated with some inherent problems. Although the arterial P_{CO_2} is considered an accurate index of primary respiratory disturbances, changes in the level may represent compensation for a primary metabolic alteration. Thus, a depressed P_{CO_2} (below 40 mm Hg) is characteristic of respiratory alkalosis but also represents the normal compensatory response to a metabolic acidosis. Similarly, the level of plasma bicarbonate cannot be regarded exclusively as an index of metabolic disturbances. An elevated plasma bicarbonate level may indicate a primary metabolic alkalosis or a compensatory response to chronic respiratory acidosis.

In an effort to separate the respiratory and metabolic components of acid-base disorders, two other approaches have been introduced: in 1948 Singer and Hastings introduced the concept of *whole blood buffer base,* and later Astrup and his colleagues proposed the use of the *standard bicarbonate* and *base excess* values. The approach advocated by Astrup has been the more popular of the two, although both are attempts to quantify the metabolic, or nonrespiratory, component in an acid-base disturbance and separate it from the respiratory component.

The standard bicarbonate is defined as the concentration of bicarbonate in plasma, when whole blood with fully oxygenated hemoglobin has been equilibrated with CO_2 at a P_{CO_2} of 40 mm Hg at a temperature of 38°C. This value may be rapidly and accurately determined using the Astrup technique by measuring pH values at two known levels of P_{CO_2} and reading the standard bicarbonate directly from a nomogram. The normal mean value for standard bicarbonate is 24.5 mEq/L of plasma. As a measure of bicarbonate concentration in plasma, the standard bicarbonate is probably superior to both the CO_2 content and CO_2 combining power values, since the latter two determinations vary with the actual P_{CO_2} and oxygen saturation. Unfortunately, the standard bicarbonate, unlike the whole blood buffer base, does not indicate the total amount of surplus acid or base present, since the bicarbonate–carbonic acid system does not account for the entire buffering capacity of the blood. This information can be obtained by expressing the base content of the blood as *base excess* or *base deficit.* Base excess (or deficit) directly expresses the amount, in milliequivalents, of fixed base (or

Table 2-4. RESPIRATORY AND METABOLIC COMPONENTS OF ACID-BASE DISORDERS

| Type of acid-base disorder | Acute (uncompensated) | | | Chronic (partially compensated) | | |
	pH	P_{CO_2} (respiratory component)	Plasma HCO_3^-* (metabolic component)	pH	P_{CO_2} (respiratory component)	Plasma HCO_3^-* (metabolic component)
Respiratory acidosis...	↓↓	↑↑	N	↓	↑↑	↑
Respiratory alkalosis..	↑↑	↓↓	N	↑	↓↓	↓
Metabolic acidosis...	↓↓	N	↓↓	↓	↓	↓
Metabolic alkalosis..	↑↑	N	↑↑	↑	↑?	↑

*Measured as standard bicarbonate, whole blood buffer base, CO_2 content or CO_2 combining power. The *base excess value* is positive when the standard bicarbonate is above normal and negative when the standard bicarbonate is below normal.

fixed acid) added to each liter of blood. This value is obtained by multiplying the deviation of standard bicarbonate from the normal mean by a factor of 1.2. This factor corrects for the buffering capacity of the red cells and will vary slightly with changes in hemoglobin concentration. To avoid calculations, the base excess may be read directly from a nomogram. When the term *base excess* is used exclusively, the *positive* values represent the excess of base, and the *negative* values reflect the deficit of base (or excess of acid).*

In an excellent review of the Singer-Hastings and the Astrup systems, Schwartz and Relman state that neither system offers any advantage over the classic approach for the diagnosis of acid-base disorders. They question the validity of using an in vitro CO_2 titration curve as a measure of in vivo acid-base changes. Additionally, they note that the use of either of the two systems may be misleading in the analysis of chronic disorders. For example, a low pH with an elevated P_{CO_2}, a normal standard bicarbonate value, and a base excess value of zero are compatible with a diagnosis of primary uncompensated respiratory acidosis. After several hours or days, compensatory renal mechanisms would cause elevation of standard bicarbonate level above normal, resulting in a positive base excess value. This partially compensated respiratory acidosis, then, may be erroneously interpreted as a respiratory acidosis *plus* a metabolic alkalosis as indicated by a significant base excess.

Despite these shortcomings, either approach may be useful when properly interpreted as a single laboratory test. Other systems have been recommended, some with ingeniously devised nomograms, but all are subject to misinterpretation. Unfortunately, there are no shortcuts. Regardless of the methods used, the proper analysis of complex acid-base disorders requires a thorough knowledge of the clinical situation, good judgment, and a sound understanding of acid-base physiology.

RESPIRATORY ACIDOSIS. This condition is associated with retention of CO_2 secondary to decreased alveolar ventilation. The more common causes are listed in Table 2-3. Initially, the arterial P_{CO_2} is elevated (usually above 50 mm Hg), and the plasma bicarbonate concentration (measured as CO_2 combining power, CO_2 content, or standard bicarbonate) is normal. In the chronic form, the P_{CO_2} remains elevated, and the bicarbonate concentration rises as compensation occurs.

This problem may be particularly serious in the patient with chronic pulmonary disease in whom preexisting respiratory acidosis may be accentuated in the postoperative period. A number of conditions resulting in inadequate ventilation—airway obstruction, atelectasis, pneumonia, pleural effusion, hypoventilation due to the pain of upper abdominal incisions, or abdominal distension limiting diaphragmatic excursion— may exist singly or in combination to produce respiratory acidosis. Although restlessness, hy-

*The deficit or excess of base in the extracellular compartment can be estimated in milliequivalents by multiplying the negative or positive value for base excess, in milliequivalents per liter of blood, by 0.3 times the body weight in kilograms [Mellemgaard and Astrup].

pertension, and tachycardia in the immediate postoperative period may be due to pain, similar signs indicate inadequate ventilation with hypercapnia. The use of narcotics in this situation will compound the problem by further depressing respiration.

Management involves prompt correction of the pulmonary defect, when feasible, and measures to ensure adequate ventilation. Endotracheal intubation and mechanical ventilation are occasionally necessary to achieve this objective. Strict attention to tracheobronchial hygiene during the postoperative period is an important preventive measure in all patients, particularly those with chronic pulmonary disease. Encouraging deep breathing and coughing, using humidified air to prevent inspissation of secretions, and avoiding oversedation are all indicated.

RESPIRATORY ALKALOSIS. Respiratory alkalosis is a more common problem in the surgical patient than previously recognized. Hyperventilation due to apprehension, pain, hypoxia, central nervous system injury, and assisted ventilation are all common causes. Any of these conditions may cause a rapid depression of the arterial P_{CO_2} and elevation of the pH. The plasma bicarbonate concentration is normal in the acute phase, but falls with compensation if the condition persists.

Mild respiratory alkalosis secondary to hyperventilation during the operative procedure frequently occurs. This is of little consequence in the majority of patients and generally requires no therapy. One important exception is the patient with impaired cerebral blood flow from obstructive arterial disease (or during performance of carotid endarterectomy), in whom modest hypocapnia with cerebral vasoconstriction may cause irreparable damage.

The majority of patients who require ventilatory support in the postoperative period will develop varying degrees of respiratory alkalosis. This may be inadvertent, due to improper use of the mechanical respirator, or it may occur during attempts to raise the P_{O_2} in an hypoxic patient. Proper management of the patient on a mechanical ventilator requires frequent measurements of blood gases and appropriate corrections of the ventilatory pattern when indicated. The arterial P_{CO_2} should not be allowed to fall below 30 mm Hg, as serious complications may occur, particularly in the presence of a complicating hypokalemia or metabolic alkalosis. Generally, the P_{CO_2} can be maintained at an acceptable level by proper adjustments of the ventilatory rate and volume. Increasing the pulmonary dead space is of doubtful benefit, while adding 5 percent CO_2 to the inspired air is potentially dangerous and poorly tolerated by most patients.

The dangers of a severe respiratory alkalosis are those related to potassium depletion and include the development of ventricular arrhythmias and fibrillation, particularly in patients who are digitalized or have preexisting hypokalemia. Other complications include a shift of the oxygen dissociation curve to the left, which limits the ability of hemoglobin to unload oxygen at the tissue level except at low intracellular P_{O_2}, and the development of tetany and convulsions if the level of ionized calcium is significantly depressed. The development of hypokalemia may be quite sudden and is related to entry of potassium ions into the cells in exchange for hydrogen and an excessive urinary potassium loss in exchange for sodium. Severe and persistent respiratory alkalosis is often difficult to correct and may be associated with a poor prognosis because of the underlying cause of hyperventilation. Treatment is primarily directed toward preventing the condition by the proper use of mechanical respirators and correcting any preexisting potassium deficits.

METABOLIC ACIDOSIS. Metabolic acidosis results from the retention or gain of fixed acids (diabetic acidosis, lactic acidosis, azotemia) or the loss of base bicarbonate (diarrhea, small bowel fistula, renal insufficiency with inability to resorb bicarbonate). The excess of hydrogen ion results in lower pH and plasma bicarbonate concentration. The initial compensation is pulmonary, with an increase of the rate and depth of breathing and depression of the arterial P_{CO_2}.

Renal damage may interfere with the important role of the kidneys in the regulation of acid-base balance. The kidneys serve a vital function in this regard through the excretion of nitrogenous waste products and acid metabolites and the resorption of bicarbonates. If renal damage occurs and these functions are lost, metabolic acidosis develops rapidly and may be difficult to control.

With normal kidneys, metabolic acidosis may develop when the capacity of the kidneys for handling chlorides is exceeded. This is particularly common in patients who have excessive losses of alkaline gastrointestinal fluids (biliary, pancreatic, small bowel secretions) and are maintained on parenteral fluids for an extended period of time. Continued replacement of these losses with fluids having an inappropriate chloride/bicarbonate ratio, such as isotonic sodium chloride solution, will not correct the pH change; the use of a balanced salt solution, such as lactated Ringer's, is indicated.

One of the most common causes of severe metabolic acidosis in surgical patients is acute circulatory failure with accumulation of lactic acid. This is a reflection of tissue hypoxia due to inadequate perfusion, although it is only one of the manifestations of cellular dysfunction. Acute hemorrhagic shock may result in a rapid and profound drop in the pH, and attempts to raise the blood pressure with vasopressors will simply compound the problem. Similarly, attempts to correct the acidosis by the infusion of large quantities of sodium bicarbonate without restoration of flow are futile. Following restoration of adequate tissue perfusion by proper volume replacement, the lactic acid is quickly metabolized and the pH returned to normal. The use of lactated Ringer's solution to replace the extracellular fluid deficit incurred with hemorrhagic shock concomitant with administration of whole blood does not accentuate the lactic acidosis. Instead, there is a rapid decrease in the lactate level and return of pH toward normal, as opposed to the results when whole blood alone is used.

The indiscriminate use of sodium bicarbonate during the resuscitation of patients in hypovolemic shock is discouraged for several reasons. A mild metabolic alkalosis is a common finding following resuscitation, in part due to the alkalinizing effects of blood transfusions and the adminis-

tration of lactated Ringer's solution. After infusion (and partial restoration of hepatic blood flow), the citrate contained in the transfused blood and the lactate in lactated Ringer's solution are metabolized and bicarbonate is formed. The organic acidosis (lactic acid) that developed during the shock episode is rapidly cleared once adequate tissue perfusion is restored. Lactic acid production ceases, the hydrogen ion load is buffered and excreted via the lungs as CO_2, and the organic anion, lactate, is metabolized by the liver. If excessive quantities of sodium bicarbonate are administered simultaneously, severe metabolic alkalosis can result. An alkaline pH may be highly undesirable in this situation, particularly in patients with hypoxia or low fixed cardiac outputs, because it shifts the oxygen dissociation curve to the left. Other factors that tend to shift the oxygen dissociation curve to the left in this situation include the depressed level of erythrocyte 2,3-diphosphoglycerate in the transfused blood and the development of hypothermia. If the curve shifts far enough to the left, significant interference with oxygen unloading at the cellular level may occur.

The treatment of metabolic acidosis, therefore, should be directed toward correction of the underlying disorder when possible. Bicarbonate therapy properly may be reserved for the treatment of severe metabolic acidosis, particularly following cardiac arrest, when partial correction of the pH may be essential to restore myocardial function. However, recent studies indicate that the acidosis accompanying cardiac arrest is well compensated for a significant period of time if the patient is well ventilated and not previously acidotic. In addition, the administration of bicarbonate in the usual recommended doses may induce an acute and severe hypernatremia and hyperosmolarity. Thus bicarbonate should be used judiciously during cardiac arrest. Mattar et al. recommended that the initial dose of bicarbonate not exceed 50 ml of 7.5% solution (45 mEq $NaHCO_3$ containing 90 mO) and that the decision for additional doses be based on measurements of pH and P_{CO_2} when possible.

Similarly, pH correction of more protracted states of metabolic acidosis may be indicated but should be accomplished slowly. Frequent measurements of serum electrolytes and blood pH are the best guides to therapy, since a satisfactory formula to estimate the amount of alkali needed has not been devised.

METABOLIC ALKALOSIS. Metabolic alkalosis results from the loss of fixed acids or the gain of base bicarbonate and is aggravated by any preexisting potassium depletion. Both the pH and plasma bicarbonate concentration are elevated. Compensation for metabolic alkalosis is primarily by renal mechanisms, since respiratory compensation is generally small and cannot be detected in most patients. Rarely, hypercapnia may represent a compensatory response to metabolic alkalosis in patients without chronic pulmonary disease. When this is suspected, rapid reduction in P_{CO_2} by mechanical ventilation should be avoided. Rather, the P_{CO_2} will fall as the metabolic alkalosis is corrected.

The majority of patients with metabolic alkalosis have some degree of hypokalemia. Depletion of cellular potassium results in entry of hydrogen and sodium ions into the cells with resultant lowering of intracellular pH and an extracellular alkalosis. Metabolic alkalosis, in turn, results in excessive urinary potassium loss in exchange for sodium, which further accentuates the alkalosis. The dangers of metabolic alkalosis are the same as discussed with respiratory alkalosis.

An interesting and not infrequent problem in the surgical patient is hypochloremic, hypokalemic metabolic alkalosis resulting from persistent vomiting or gastric suction in the patient with pyloric obstruction. Unlike vomiting with an open pylorus (involving a loss of gastric, pancreatic, biliary, and intestinal secretions), this entity results in loss of fluid with high chloride and hydrogen ion concentration in relation to sodium. The loss of chloride causes accelerated loss of sodium and bicarbonate in the urine and partial compensation of the alkalosis. In addition, the alkalosis itself causes increased renal excretion of potassium. As the volume deficit progresses, potassium and hydrogen ions are excreted into the urine in increasing quantities in an attempt to conserve sodium, resulting in an uncompensated alkalosis and hypokalemia. The initially alkaline urine becomes acid after a period of time due to the hydrogen ion excretion ("paradoxic aciduria"). Proper management includes replacement of the extracellular fluid volume deficit with isotonic sodium chloride solution in addition to replacement of potassium. A severe potassium depletion is invariably present but may be overlooked due to concentration of the serum potassium by a severe volume deficit. However, volume repletion should be started and a good urine output obtained before potassium is administered.

Rarely, severe hypokalemic metabolic alkalosis in a patient with pyloric outlet obstruction may be refractory to standard therapy. This occurs most often in patients who also have severe hypochloremia and several liters of nasogastric drainage daily. In the past, the infusion of ammonium chloride or arginine hydrochloride was the usual method for increasing the level of nonvolatile acids. However, infusion of the first may produce ammonia toxicity, and the latter solution is no longer available commercially. Recently, the use of $0.1N$ to $0.2N$ hydrochloric acid has been shown to be safe and effective therapy for correction of severe, resistant metabolic alkalosis. The technique for infusion of hydrochloric acid, as described by Abouna et al., involves the preparation of an isotonic solution by the addition of 150 ml of $1N$ hydrochloric acid (300 mEq of hydrogen and chloride) to 1 liter of sterile water. The hydrochloric acid can be added to a liter of isotonic saline or 5% dextrose solution if desired. The infusion should be administered over a 6- to 24-hour period, with measurements of pH, P_{CO_2} and serum electrolytes every 4 to 6 hours. Generally, 1 or 2 liters of solution over a period of 24 hours is sufficient, although one should not hesitate to infuse additional hydrochloric acid when the need is based on appropriate clinical and laboratory evidence. Temporary control of the alkalosis with this method is usually successful, but underlying cause should be controlled as soon as possible.

The initial dose of hydrochloric acid solution can be roughly calculated from the estimated chloride or hydrogen ion deficit. The chloride deficit is calculated from the plasma chloride concentration and the chloride space (approximately 20 percent of body weight). The hydrogen ion deficit can be calculated from the plasma base excess and the hydrogen ion space (approximately 60 percent of total body weight). As an example, for a 70-kg patient with a metabolic alkalosis and a plasma chloride of 80 mEq/L the initial dose of hydrochloric acid is calculated as follows:

$$
\begin{aligned}
\text{Chloride deficit} &= (20\% \text{ of body weight}) \\
&\quad \times (\text{normal plasma chloride} \\
&\quad - \text{observed plasma chloride}) \\
&= (0.2 \times 70 \text{ kg}) \\
&\quad \times (103 \text{ mEq/L} - 80 \text{ mEq/L}) \\
&= 322 \text{ mEq}
\end{aligned}
$$

This amount of chloride (as hydrochloric acid) would be contained in approximately 2 liters of the solution described above. It is emphasized that while calculations of this type are helpful, close monitoring of pH and serum electrolytes is essential.

POTASSIUM ABNORMALITIES

The normal dietary intake of potassium is approximately 50 to 100 mEq daily, and in the absence of hypokalemia, the majority of this is excreted in the urine. Ninety-eight percent of the potassium in the body is located within the intracellular compartment at a concentration of approximately 150 mEq/L, and it is the major cation of intracellular water. Although the total extracellular potassium in a 70-kg male would approximate only 63 mEq (4.5 mEq/L × 14L), this small amount is critical to cardiac and neuromuscular function. In addition, the turnover rate in the extracellular fluid compartment may be extremely rapid.

The intracellular and extracellular distribution of potassium is influenced by many factors. Significant quantities of intracellular potassium are released into the extracellular space in response to severe injury or surgical stress, acidosis, and the catabolic state. A significant rise in serum potassium may occur in these states in the presence of oliguric or anuric renal failure, but dangerous hyperkalemia (greater than 6 mEq/L) is rarely encountered if renal function is normal. After severe trauma, however, normal or excessive urinary volumes may not reflect the ability of the kidney to clear solutes or to excrete potassium. (See the section High-Output Renal Failure.)

HYPERKALEMIA. The signs of a significant hyperkalemia are limited to the cardiovascular and gastrointestinal systems. The gastrointestinal symptoms include nausea, vomiting, intermittent intestinal colic, and diarrhea. The cardiovascular signs are apparent on the electrocardiogram initially, with high peaked T waves, widened QRS complex, and depressed ST segments. Disappearance of T waves, heart block, and diastolic cardiac arrest may develop with increasing levels of potassium.

Treatment of hyperkalemia consists of immediate measures to reduce the serum potassium level, withholding of exogenously administered potassium, and correction of the

Table 2-5. COMPOSITION OF GASTROINTESTINAL SECRETIONS

Type of secretion	Volume (ml/24 hr)	Na (mEq/L)	K (mEq/L)	Cl (mEq/L)	HCO₃ (mEq/L)
Salivary	1,500 (500–2,000)	10 (2–10)	26 (20–30)	10 (8–18)	30
Stomach	1,500 (100–4,000)	60 (9–116)	10 (0–32)	130 (8–154)	
Duodenum	(100–2,000)	140	5	80	
Ileum	3,000 (100–9,000)	140 (80–150)	5 (2–8)	104 (43–137)	30
Colon	. . . .	60	30	40	
Pancreas	. . . . (100–800)	140 (113–185)	5 (3–7)	75 (54–95)	115
Bile	. . . . (50–800)	145 (131–164)	5 (3–12)	100 (89–180)	35

underlying cause if possible. Temporary suppression of the myocardial effects of a sudden rapid rise of potassium level can be accomplished by the intravenous administration of a solution containing 80 mEq of sodium lactate, 100 ml of calcium gluconate, and 100 ml of 50% dextrose in water. The administration of dextrose stimulates the synthesis of glycogen, resulting in an uptake of potassium. Insulin may also be given, but it should be limited to 1 unit per 5 Gm or more of glucose, since rebound hypoglycemia may be fatal. The sodium lactate raises the pH and shifts potassium intracellularly, and the calcium gluconate tends to counteract the myocardial effects of hyperkalemia. Administration of this solution over a 2-hour period allows time to prepare for definitive removal of the excess potassium by hemodialysis or peritoneal dialysis. A slow rise of potassium level (less than 1 mEq/L/day) can be controlled by the use of cation-exchange resins, preferably in the sodium cycle,* administered by rectum in doses of 24 Gm every 12 hours. To prevent rapid absorption of water from the colon, 200 ml of 10% dextrose in water is used as the vehicle.

HYPOKALEMIA. The more common problem in the surgical patient is hypokalemia, which may occur as a result of (1) excessive renal excretion, (2) movement of potassium into cells, (3) prolonged administration of potassium-free parenteral fluids with continued obligatory renal loss of potassium (20 mEq/day or more), (4) parenteral hyperalimentation with inadequate potassium replacement, and (5) loss in gastrointestinal secretions.

Potassium plays an important role in the regulation of acid-base balance. Increased renal excretion occurs with both respiratory and metabolic alkalosis. Potassium is in competition with hydrogen ion for renal tubular excretion in exchange for sodium ion. Thus, in alkalosis, the increased potassium ion excretion in exchange for sodium ion permits hydrogen ion conservation. Hypokalemia itself may produce a metabolic alkalosis, since an increase in excretion of hydrogen ions occurs when the concentration of potassium in the tubular cell is low. In addition, movement of hydrogen ions into the cells as a consequence of potassium loss is partly responsible for the alkalosis. In metabolic acidosis the reverse process occurs, and the excess hydrogen ion exchanges for sodium with retention of greater amounts of potassium.

Renal tubular excretion of potassium ion is increased when large quantities of sodium are available for excretion. The more sodium ion available for resorption, the more potassium is exchanged for it in the lumen. Potassium requirements for prolonged or massive isotonic fluid volume replacement are increased, probably on this basis. The same mechanism may also explain the increased potassium ion excretion with steroid administration.

The renal excretion of potassium may be small when compared to the amount of potassium that may be lost in gastrointestinal secretions. The amount per liter in various types of gastrointestinal fluids is shown in Table 2-5. Although the average potassium concentration of some of these fluids is relatively low, significant hypokalemia will result if potassium-free fluids are used for replacement.

Hypokalemia also may be a serious problem in the patient maintained on intravenous hyperalimentation. Large quantities of supplemental potassium generally are necessary to restore depleted intracellular stores and to meet the requirements for tissue synthesis during the anabolic phase. (See the section Nutrition.)

In summary, most of the factors that tend to influence potassium metabolism result in excess excretion, and a tendency toward hypokalemia occurs frequently in the surgical patient except when shock or acidosis interferes with the normal renal handling of potassium.

The signs of potassium deficit are related to failure of normal contractility of skeletal, smooth, and cardiac muscle and include weakness that may progress to flaccid paralysis, diminished to absent tendon reflexes, and paralytic ileus. Sensitivity to digitalis with cardiac arrhythmias and electrocardiographic signs of low voltage, flattening of T waves, and depression of ST segments are characteristic. However, signs of potassium deficit may be masked

*Kayexalate.

by those of a severe extracellular fluid volume deficit. Repletion of the volume deficit may further aggravate the situation by lowering the serum potassium level secondary to dilution.

The treatment of hypokalemia involves, first, prevention of this state. In the replacement of gastrointestinal fluids, it is safe to replace the upper limits of loss, since an excess is readily handled by the patient with normal renal function. Potassium is available in 20-mEq and 40-mEq ampules for addition to intravenous fluids. No more than 40 mEq should be added to a liter of intravenous fluid, and the rate of administration should not exceed 40 mEq/hour unless the electrocardiogram is being monitored. In the absence of specific indications, potassium should not be given to the oliguric patient or during the first 24 hours following severe surgical stress or trauma.

CALCIUM ABNORMALITIES

The majority of the 1,000 to 1,200 Gm of body calcium in the average-sized adult is found in the bone in the form of phosphate and carbonate. Normal daily intake of calcium is between 1 and 3 Gm. Most of this is excreted via the gastrointestinal tract, and 200 mg or less is excreted in the urine daily. The normal serum level is between 9 and 11 mg/100 ml (depending on the individual laboratory's normal range), and approximately half of this is not ionized and is bound to plasma protein. An additional nonionized fraction (5 percent) is bound to other substances in the plasma and interstitial fluid, whereas the remaining 45 percent is the ionized portion that is responsible for neuromuscular stability. Determination of the plasma protein level, therefore, is essential for proper analysis of the serum calcium level. The ratio of ionized to nonionized calcium is also related to the pH; acidosis causes an increase in the ionized fraction, whereas alkalosis causes a decrease.

Disturbances of calcium metabolism generally are not a problem in the uncomplicated postoperative patient, with the exception of skeletal loss during prolonged immobilization. Routine administration of calcium to the surgical patient, therefore, is not needed in the absence of specific indications.

HYPOCALCEMIA. The symptoms of hypocalcemia (serum level less than 8 mg/100 ml) are numbness and tingling of the circumoral region and the tips of the fingers and toes. The signs are of neuromuscular origin and include hyperactive tendon reflexes, positive Chvostek's sign, muscle and abdominal cramps, tetany with carpopedal spasm, convulsions (with severe deficit), and prolongation of the Q-T interval on the electrocardiogram.

The common causes include acute pancreatitis, massive soft tissue infections (necrotizing fasciitis), acute and chronic renal failure, pancreatic and small intestinal fistulas, and hypoparathyroidism. Transient hypocalcemia is a frequent occurrence in the hyperparathyroid patient following removal of a parathyroid adenoma, owing to atrophy of the remaining glands. Asymptomatic hypocalcemia may occur with hypoproteinemia (normal ionized fraction), whereas symptoms may appear with a normal serum calcium level in a patient with severe alkalosis. The latter is due to a decrease in the physiologically active or ionized fraction of total serum calcium. Calcium levels also may fall with a severe depletion of magnesium.

Treatment is directed toward correction of the underlying cause with concomitant repletion of the deficit. Acute symptoms may be relieved by the intravenous administration of calcium gluconate or calcium chloride. Calcium lactate may be given orally, with or without supplemental vitamin D, in the patient requiring prolonged replacement. The routine administration of calcium during massive transfusions of blood remains controversial and reflects a paucity of studies where calcium *ion* levels are measured. In the majority of studies, calcium ion concentrations have been estimated from measured *total* serum calcium levels. Presently, available data indicate that the majority of patients receiving blood transfusions do not require calcium supplementation. The binding of ionized calcium by citrate is generally compensated for by the mobilization of calcium from body stores. For patients receiving blood as rapidly as 500 ml every 5 to 10 minutes, however, calcium administration is recommended. An appropriate dose, from the data of Moore, is 0.2 Gm of calcium chloride (2 ml of 10% calcium chloride solution), administered intravenously in a separate line, for every 500 ml of blood transfused. To avoid dangerous levels of hypercalcemia, this dose of calcium is recommended only while blood is being transfused at the rate noted above. Additionally, the total dose of calcium generally should not exceed 3 Gm unless there is objective evidence of hypocalcemia. Larger doses are rarely indicated, since there is some mobilization of calcium and citrate breakdown with release of calcium ion even with shock and inadequate peripheral perfusion. During massive transfusions, some attempt should be made to monitor the calcium level. A rough approximation of calcium ion concentration can be obtained by monitoring the Q-T interval on the ECG, although techniques for the rapid measurement of calcium ion concentration are now available.

HYPERCALCEMIA. The symptoms of hypercalcemia are rather vague and of gastrointestinal, renal, musculoskeletal, and central nervous system origin. The early manifestations of hypercalcemia include easy fatigue, lassitude, weakness of varying degree, anorexia, nausea, vomiting, and weight loss. With higher serum calcium levels, lassitude gives way to somnambulism, stupor, and finally coma. Other symptoms include severe headaches, pains in the back and extremities, thirst, polydypsia, and polyuria. The critical level for serum calcium is between 16 and 20 mg/100 ml, and unless treatment is instituted promptly, the symptoms may rapidly progress to death. The two major causes of hypercalcemia are hyperparathyroidism and cancer with bony metastasis. The latter is most frequently seen in the patient with metastatic breast cancer who is receiving estrogen therapy.

The treatment of acute hypercalcemia crisis is an emergency. Measures to lower the serum calcium level are instituted immediately while preparations are being made for more definitive treatment. Of particular importance is the rapid repletion of the associated extracellular fluid volume deficit, which will immediately lower the calcium level by dilution. Other measures which have been used and may be of temporary benefit include the use of a chelating agent (EDTA), steroids, sodium sulfate solution, and hemodialysis. Recently, intravenous mithromycin has been shown to reduce the serum calcium level in normocalcemic and hypercalcemic patients. The definitive treatment of acute hypercalcemic crisis in patients with hyperparathyroidism is immediate surgery.

Treatment of hypercalcemia in the patient with metastatic cancer is primarily that of prevention. The serum calcium level is checked frequently; if it is elevated, the patient is placed on a low-calcium diet, and measures to ensure adequate hydration are instituted.

MAGNESIUM ABNORMALITIES

The infrequent occurrence of magnesium deficiency and the previous lack of a rapid, precise technique for measurement of magnesium ion concentration accounts for the late appreciation of this entity. The total body content of magnesium in the average adult is approximately 2,000 mEq, about half of which is incorporated in bone and only slowly exchangeable. The distribution of magnesium is similar to that of potassium, the major portion being intracellular. Plasma magnesium concentration normally ranges between 1.5 and 2.5 mEq/L. The normal dietary intake of magnesium is approximately 20 mEq (240 mg) daily. The larger part is excreted in the feces, and the remainder in the urine. The kidneys show a remarkable ability to conserve magnesium; on a magnesium-free diet, renal excretion of this ion may be less than 1 mEq/day.

MAGNESIUM DEFICIENCY. Magnesium deficiency is known to occur with starvation, malabsorption syndromes, protracted losses of gastrointestinal fluid, and prolonged parenteral fluid therapy with magnesium-free solutions, and during parenteral hyperalimentation when inadequate quantities of magnesium have been added to the solutions. Other causes include acute pancreatitis, diabetic acidosis during treatment, primary aldosteronism, chronic alcoholism, and burns (late stage).

The magnesium ion is essential for proper function of most enzyme systems, and depletion is characterized by neuromuscular and central nervous system hyperactivity. The signs and symptoms are quite similar to those of calcium deficiency, including hyperactive tendon reflexes, muscle tremors, and tetany with a positive Chvostek sign. Progression to delirium and convulsions may occur with a severe deficit. A concomitant calcium deficiency occasionally is noted, particularly in those with clinical signs of tetany.

The diagnosis of magnesium deficiency depends on an awareness of the syndrome and clinical recognition of the symptoms. Laboratory confirmation is available but not reliable, as the syndrome may exist in the presence of a normal serum magnesium level. The possibility of magnesium deficiency should always be considered in the surgical patient who exhibits disturbed neuromuscular or cerebral activity in the postoperative period. This is particularly important in patients who have had protracted dysfunction of the gastrointestinal tract with long-term maintenance on parenteral fluids and in patients on parenteral hyperalimentation. Routine magnesium is always indicated in the management of these patients.

Treatment of magnesium deficiency is by the parenteral administration of magnesium sulfate or magnesium chloride solution. If renal function is normal, as much as 2 mEq of magnesium/kg of body weight can be administered in a day in the face of severe depletion. Magnesium sulfate (50% solution contains approximately 4 mEq of magnesium ion per milliliter) may be given intravenously or intramuscularly. The intravenous route is preferable for the initial treatment of a severe symptomatic deficit. The solution is prepared by the addition of 80 mEq of magnesium sulfate (20 ml of 50% solution) to a liter of intravenous fluid and is administered over a 4-hour period. If the patient is not symptomatic, the infusion should be given over a longer period of time. The possibility of acute magnesium toxicity should be kept in mind when giving this ion intravenously. When large doses are given, the heart rate, blood pressure, respiration, and ECG should be monitored closely for signs of magnesium toxicity, which could lead to cardiac arrest. It is advisable to have calcium chloride or calcium gluconate available to counteract any adverse effects of a rapidly rising plasma magnesium level.

Partial or complete relief of symptoms may follow this infusion as a result of increased concentration of magnesium ion in the extracellular fluid compartment, although continued replacement over a 1- to 3-week period is necessary to replenish the intracellular compartment. For this purpose and for the asymptomatic patient who is likely to have significant magnesium depletion, 10 to 20 mEq of 50% magnesium sulfate solution is given daily by the intramuscular route or in infusion fluids. When magnesium sulfate is used, it should be given in divided doses or at multiple sites, since the intramuscular injection of this salt is painful. Following complete repletion of intracellular magnesium and in the absence of abnormal loss, balance may be maintained by the administration of as little as 4 mEq of magnesium ion daily. The amount of magnesium supplementation required for patients on parenteral hyperalimentation varies but approximates 12 to 24 mEq daily.

Magnesium ion should not be given to the oliguric patient or in the presence of severe volume deficit unless actual magnesium depletion is demonstrated. If given to a patient with renal insufficiency, considerably smaller doses are used, and the patient is carefully observed for signs or symptoms of toxicity.

MAGNESIUM EXCESS. Symptomatic hypermagnesemia, although rare, is most commonly seen with severe renal insufficiency. Retention and accumulation of magnesium may occur in any patient with impaired glomerular or renal tubular function, and the presence of acidosis may rapidly compound the situation. Serum magnesium levels tend to parallel changes in potassium concentration in these cases. Therefore, magnesium levels should be carefully monitored in cases of acute and chronic renal failure and in selected patients with borderline renal function. Randall et al. have shown that in patients on ordinary dietary intakes of magnesium, increased serum concentrations of the ion do not occur until the glomerular filtration rate falls below 30 ml/minute. As noted by Henzel et al., however, magnesium-containing antacids and laxatives (milk of magnesia, epsom salts, Gelusil, Maalox) are commonly administered in quantities sufficient to produce toxic serum levels of magnesium where impaired renal function is present. Other conditions which may be associated with symptomatic hypermagnesemia include early-stage burns, massive trauma or surgical stress, severe extracellular volume deficit, and severe acidosis.

The early signs and symptoms include lethargy and weakness with progressive loss of deep tendon reflexes. Interference with cardiac conduction occurs with increasing levels of magnesium and changes in the electrocardiogram (increased P-R interval, widened QRS complex, and elevated T waves) resemble those seen with hyperkalemia. Somnolence leading to coma and muscular paralysis occur in the later stages, and death is usually caused by respiratory or cardiac arrest.

Treatment consists of immediate measures to lower the serum magnesium level by correcting any acidosis, replenishing any preexisting extracellular volume deficit, and withholding exogenously administered magnesium. Acute symptoms may be temporarily controlled by the slow intravenous administration of 5 to 10 mEq of calcium chloride or calcium gluconate. If elevated levels or symptoms persist, peritoneal dialysis or hemodialysis is indicated.

NORMAL EXCHANGE OF FLUID AND ELECTROLYTES

Knowledge of the basic principles governing both the internal and external exchanges of water and salt is mandatory for care of the patient undergoing major operative surgery. The stable internal fluid environment, which is maintained by the kidneys, brain, lungs, skin, and gastrointestinal tract, may be compromised by severe surgical stress or direct damage to any of these organs.

Water Exchange

The normal individual consumes an average of 2,000 to 2,500 ml water/day; approximately 1,500 ml water is taken by mouth, and the rest is extracted from solid food, either from the contents of the food or as the product of oxidation (Table 2-6). The daily water losses include 250 ml in stools, 800 to 1,500 ml as urine, and approximately 600 to 900 ml as insensible loss. A patient deprived of all external access to water must still excrete a minimum of 500 to 800 ml urine/day in order to excrete the products of catabolism, in addition to the mandatory insensible loss through the skin and lungs

Insensible loss of water occurs through the skin (75 percent) and the lungs (25 percent) and is increased by hypermetabolism, hyperventilation, and fever. The insensible water loss through the skin is not from evaporation of water from sweat glands but from water vapor formed

Table 2-6. WATER EXCHANGE (60–80 kg man)

Routes	Average daily volume, ml	Minimal, ml	Maximal, ml
H$_2$O gain:			
Sensible:			
Oral fluids	800–1,500	0	1,500/hr
Solid foods	500–700	0	1,500
Insensible:			
Water of oxidation . .	250	125	800
Water of solution . . .	0	0	500
H$_2$O loss:			
Sensible:			
Urine	800–1,500	300	1,400/hr (diabetes insipidus)
Intestinal	0–250	0	2,500/hr
Sweat	0	0	4,000/hr
Insensible:			
Lungs and skin	600–900	600–900	1,500

within the body and lost through the skin. With excessive heat production (or excessive environmental heat), the capacity for insensible loss through the skin is exceeded, and sweating occurs. These losses may, but seldom do, exceed 250 ml/day/degree of fever. An unhumidified tracheostomy with hyperventilation increases the loss through the lungs and results in a total insensible loss up to 1.5 liters/day.

A frequently overlooked source of gain is the water of solution, which is the water that holds carbohydrates and proteins in solution in the cell. Normally, gain of water from this source is zero, but after 4 to 5 days without food intake, the postoperative patient may begin to gain significant quantities of water (maximum 500 ml daily) from excessive cellular catabolism. The amount depends on the degree of trauma and the complications occurring postoperatively.

Salt Gain and Losses

In the normal individual, the salt intake per day varies between 50 and 90 mEq (3 to 5 Gm) as sodium chloride (Table 2-7). Balance is maintained primarily by the normal kidneys that excrete the excess salt. Under conditions of reduced intake or extrarenal losses, the normal kidney can reduce sodium excretion to less than 1 mEq/day within 24 hours after restriction. In the patient with salt-wasting kidneys, however, the loss may exceed 200 mEq/L of urine. Sweat represents a hypotonic loss of fluids with an average sodium concentration of 15 mEq/L in the acclimatized patient. In the unacclimatized individual, the sodium concentration in sweat may be 60 mEq/L or more. Insensible fluid lost from the skin and lungs, by definition, is pure water. For practical considerations then, normal losses may be relatively free of salt in the healthy individual with normal renal function.

The volume and composition of various types of gastrointestinal secretions are shown in Table 2-5. Gastrointesti-

Table 2-7. SODIUM (SALT) EXCHANGE
(60–80 kg man)

Sodium exchange	Average	Minimal	Maximal
Sodium gain:			
Diet	50–90 mEq/day	0	75–100 mEq/hr (oral)
Sodium loss:			
Skin (sweat) . .	10–60 mEq/day*	0	300 mEq/hr
Urine	10–80 mEq/day	<1 mEq/day†	110–200 mEq/L‡
Intestines . . .	0–20 mEq/day	0	300 mEq/hr

* Depending on the degree of acclimatization of the individual.
† With normal renal function.
‡ With renal salt wasting.

nal losses are usually isotonic or slightly hypotonic, although there is considerable variation in the composition. These should be replaced by an essentially isotonic salt solution. It is also important to reiterate that distributional or sequestration losses of extracellular fluid at any point in the operative or postoperative course also represent isotonic losses of salt and water.

FLUID AND ELECTROLYTE THERAPY

Parenteral Solutions

The composition of various parenteral fluids available for administration is shown in Table 2-8. There is sufficient variety to satisfy the majority of fluid requirements in the surgical patient. The proper choice of parenteral fluid in a given situation will correct the abnormalities but impose minimal demands on the kidneys.

A good available isotonic salt solution for replacing

Table 2-8. COMPOSITION OF PARENTERAL FLUIDS
Electrolyte content (mEq/L)

Solutions	Cations					Anions		
	Na	K	Ca	Mg	NH₄	Cl	HCO₃⁻	HPO₄⁻
Extracellular fluid.	142	4	5	3	.3	103	27	3
Lactated Ringer's	130	4	2.7	. . . .		109	28*	
0.9% sodium chloride (saline)	154	. . . .				154		
M/6 sodium lactate	167	. . . .				. . . .	167*	
M (molar) sodium lactate	1,000	. . . .				. . . .	1,000*	
3% sodium chloride	513	. . . .				513		
5% sodium chloride	855	. . . .				855		
0.9% ammonium chloride	. . . .				168	168		

* Present in solution as lactate which is converted to bicarbonate.

gastrointestinal losses and repairing preexisting volume deficits, in the absence of gross abnormalities of concentration and composition, is lactated Ringer's solution. This solution is "physiologic" and contains 130 mEq sodium balanced by 109 mEq chloride and 28 mEq lactate. This fluid has minimal effects on normal body fluid composition and pH even when infused in large quantities. The chief disadvantage of lactated Ringer's solution is the slight hyposmolarity with respect to sodium. Each liter of lactated Ringer's solution furnishes approximately 100 to 150 ml free water. This rarely presents a clinical problem if it is considered in calculating water replacement. The remainder of the solutions listed in Table 2-8 are used to correct specific defects. Choice of a particular fluid depends on the volume status of the patient and the type of concentration or compositional abnormality present.

Isotonic sodium chloride contains 154 mEq sodium and 154 mEq chloride/L. The high concentration of chloride above the normal serum concentration of 103 mEq/L imposes on the kidneys an appreciable load of excess chloride which cannot be rapidly excreted. Thus, a dilutional acidosis may develop.* This solution is ideal, however, for the initial correction of an extracellular fluid volume deficit in the presence of hyponatremia, hypochloremia, and metabolic alkalosis. In a similar situation with moderate metabolic acidosis, $M/6$ sodium lactate (167 mEq/L each of sodium and lactate) may be given. Another solution for this purpose can be made by adding one ampule of sodium bicarbonate (40 ml solution containing 40 mEq each of sodium and bicarbonate) to 1,000 ml lactated Ringer's solution.

Molar sodium lactate solution or 3 or 5% sodium chloride may be used to correct symptomatic hyponatremic states. The choice of anion (lactate or chloride) is determined by the accompanying acid-base derangement. The need for ammonium chloride solutions in the treatment of an uncompensated metabolic alkalosis is extremely rare. Indications for their use include very shallow or slow breathing with cyanosis or severe tetany. Following the correction of concentration or compositional abnormalities using specific repair solutions, a balanced salt solution is used to replenish the remaining volume deficit.

Preoperative Fluid Therapy

Preoperative evaluation and correction of existing fluid disorders is an integral part of surgical care. An orderly approach to these problems requires an understanding of the common fluid disturbances associated with surgical illness and adherence to a few simple guidelines. There are no shortcuts; close observation of the patient and frequent reevaluation of the clinical situation is the most rewarding approach.

The analysis of a fluid disorder may be facilitated by categorizing the abnormalities into *volume, concentration,*

* Infusion of a large volume of isotonic sodium chloride solution may induce or aggravate a preexisting acidosis by reducing the amount of base bicarbonate in the body relative to the carbonic acid content.

and *compositional* changes. Although some disease states produce characteristic changes in fluid balance, much confusion may be avoided by regarding each disturbance as a separate entity. For example, volume changes cannot be accurately predicted from a knowledge of the level of serum sodium, since an extracellular fluid volume deficit or excess may exist with a normal, low, or high sodium concentration. Similarly, any of the four primary acid-base disturbances may be associated with any combination of volume and concentration abnormalities.

CORRECTION OF VOLUME CHANGES

Changes in the volume of extracellular fluid are the most frequent and important abnormalities encountered in the surgical patient. Depletion of the extracellular fluid compartment without changes in concentration or composition is a common problem. The diagnosis of volume changes is made almost entirely on clinical grounds. The signs that will be present in an individual patient depend not only on the relative or absolute quantity of extracellular fluid which has been lost but also on the rapidity with which it is lost and the presence or absence of signs of associated disease.

Volume deficits in the surgical patient may result from external loss of fluids or from an internal redistribution of extracellular fluid into a nonfunctional compartment. Generally, it involves a combination of the two, but the internal redistribution is frequently overlooked.

The phenomenon of internal redistribution or translocation of extracellular fluid is peculiar to many surgical diseases; in the individual patient, the loss may be quite large. Although the concept of a "third space" is not new, it is generally considered only in relation to patients with massive ascites, burns, or crush injuries. Of more importance, however, is the "third space" loss into the peritoneum, the bowel wall, and other tissues with inflammatory lesions of the intraabdominal organs. The magnitude of these losses may not be fully appreciated without realization of the fact that the peritoneum alone has approximately 1 m² of surface area. A slight increase in thickness from sequestration of fluid, which would not be appreciated on casual observation, may result in a functional loss of several liters of fluid. Swelling of the bowel wall and mesentery and secretion of fluid into the lumen of the bowel will cause even larger losses. Similar deficits may occur with massive infection of the subcutaneous tissues (necrotizing fasciitis) or with severe crush injury.

These "parasitic" losses remain a part of the extracellular fluid space and may be measured as a slowly equilibrating volume. The term *nonfunctional* is used because the fluid is no longer able to participate in the normal functions of the extracellular fluid compartment and may just as well have been lost externally. Any transfer of intracellular fluid to the extracellular compartment for replenishment of the loss is insignificant in the acute phase. The patient with ascites may have an enormous total extracellular fluid volume although the functional component is severely depleted. The same is true of extensive inflammatory or obstructive lesions of the gastrointestinal tract, although the loss is not as obvious. These losses will

evoke the signs and symptoms of an extracellular fluid volume deficit with or without the concomitant external loss of fluids.

Exact quantification of these deficits is impossible and, at the present time, probably unnecessary. The defect can be estimated on the basis of the severity of the clinical signs. A mild deficit represents a loss of approximately 4 percent of body weight, a moderate loss is 6 to 8 percent of body weight, and a severe deficit is approximately 10 percent of body weight. It is important to reemphasize the fact that cardiovascular signs predominate when there is acute rapid loss of fluid from the extracellular fluid compartment with few or no tissue signs. In addition to the estimated deficit, fluids lost during the period of treatment must be replaced.

Fluid replacement should be started and changed according to the response of the patient noted on frequent clinical observation. Reliance on a formula or single clinical sign to determine adequacy of resuscitation is fraught with danger. Rather, reversal of the signs of the volume deficit, combined with stabilization of the blood pressure and pulse, and an hourly urine volume of 30 to 50 ml are used as general guidelines. An adequate hourly urine output, although usually a reliable index of volume replacement, may be totally misleading. The excessive administration of glucose (over 50 Gm in a 2- to 3-hour period) may result in osmotic diuresis, while an osmotic agent such as mannitol tends to produce urine at the expense of the vascular volume. Patients with chronic renal disease or incipient acute renal damage from shock and injury also may have inappropriately high urinary volumes. In addition, the rapid administration of salt solutions may transiently expand the intravascular volume, increase the glomerular filtration rate, and result in an immediate outpouring of urine, although the total extracellular fluid space remains quite depleted.

The choice of the proper fluid for replacement depends on the existence of concomitant concentration or compositional abnormalities. With pure extracellular fluid volume loss or when only minimal concentration or compositional abnormalities are present, the use of a balanced salt solution, such as lactated Ringer's, is desirable.

CORRECTION OF CONCENTRATION CHANGES

If severe *symptomatic* hyponatremia or hypernatremia complicates the volume loss, prompt correction of the concentration abnormality to the extent that symptoms are relieved is necessary. Volume replenishment then should be accomplished with slower correction of the remaining concentration abnormality. For immediate correction of severe hyponatremia, 5% sodium chloride solution or molar sodium lactate solution is used, depending on the patient's acid-base status. In any case, the sodium deficit can be estimated by multiplying the decrease in serum sodium concentration below normal (in milliequivalents per liter) *times* the liters of total body water. Total body water averages 60 percent of the body weight in young adult males and 50 percent in young adult females. Initially, up to one-half of the calculated amount of sodium may be administered slowly, followed by clinical and chemical reevaluation of the patient before any additional infusion of sodium salts.

> Example: A twenty-four-year-old female with symptomatic hyponatremia, weight = 60 kg, serum sodium = 120 mEq/L:
>
> Total body water = 60 kg × 0.50 = 30 liters
> Sodium deficit = (140 − 120 mEq/L) × 30 liters
>   = 600 mEq
>
> Half of this amount (300 mEq) could be given by slowly infusing approximately 350 ml 5% sodium chloride solution.

Note that this estimate is based on total body water, since the effective osmotic pressure in the extracellular compartment cannot be increased without increasing this function proportionately in the intracellular compartment. Although absolute reliance on any formula is undesirable, proper use of this estimate will allow a safe quantitative approximation of the sodium deficit. Generally, only a portion of the total deficit is replaced initially to relieve acute symptoms. Further correction is facilitated when renal function is restored by correction of the volume deficit. If the total calculated deficit were given rapidly, severe hypervolemia might occur particularly in patients with limited cardiac reserve. In practice, the infusion of small, successive increments of hypertonic saline solution with frequent evaluation of the clinical response and serum sodium concentration is recommended.

In the treatment of moderate hyponatremia with an associated volume deficit, volume replacement can be started immediately with concomitant correction of the serum sodium deficit. Isotonic sodium chloride solution (normal saline) is used initially in the presence of metabolic alkalosis, whereas $M/6$ sodium lactate is used to correct an associated acidosis. Only a few liters of these solutions may be necessary to correct the serum sodium concentration; the remainder of the volume deficit may be repaired with lactated Ringer's solution.

Treatment of hyponatremia associated with volume excess is by restriction of water. In the presence of severe symptomatic hyponatremia, a small amount of hypertonic salt solution may be infused cautiously to alleviate symptoms. As this will cause additional volume expansion, it is contraindicated in patients with limited cardiac reserve; peritoneal dialysis or hemodialysis is preferred in this situation.

For the correction of severe, symptomatic hypernatremia with an associated volume deficit, 5% dextrose in water may be infused slowly until symptoms are relieved. If the extracellular osmolarity is reduced too rapidly, however, convulsions and coma may result. For this reason, correction of hypernatremia concomitant with repletion of the volume deficit by half-strength sodium chloride or half-strength lactated Ringer's solution is safer in most cases. In the absence of a significant volume deficit, water should be administered cautiously since dangerous hypervolemia may result; constant observation and frequent determinations of the serum sodium concentration are indicated. The problem is somewhat simplified once a sufficient quantity of fluid has been given to permit renal excretion of the solute load.

RATE OF FLUID ADMINISTRATION. This varies considerably, depending on the severity and type of fluid disturbance, the presence of continuing losses, and the cardiac status. In general, the most severe volume deficits may be safely replaced initially with isotonic solutions at a rate of 2,000 ml/hour, reducing the rate as the fluid status improves. Constant observation by a physician is mandatory when the administration exceeds 1,000 ml/hour. At these rates, a significant portion may be lost as urinary output owing to a transient overexpansion of the plasma volume.

In elderly patients, associated cardiovascular disorders do not preclude correction of existing volume deficits, but they do require slower, more careful correction with constant monitoring of all functions including the central venous pressure. Hypertonic salt solutions should be given under close supervision, and the rate of administration generally should not exceed 100 to 150 ml/hour.

COMPOSITION AND MISCELLANEOUS CONSIDERATIONS

Correction of existing potassium deficits should be started *after* an adequate urine output is obtained, particularly in the patient with metabolic alkalosis since this may be secondary to or aggravated by potassium depletion. Potassium chloride is available in 20-mEq and 40-mEq ampules for addition to intravenous fluids. A maximum of 40 mEq of potassium chloride per hour may be safely administered to the adult of average size who is not severely depleted of extracellular fluid volume, in frank hypovolemic shock, or in established oliguric or high-output renal failure. The concentration of potassium chloride should not exceed 40 mEq/L of intravenous fluids, with rare exception, such as the treatment of digitalis intoxication during which the electrocardiogram must be constantly monitored. Calcium and magnesium rarely are needed during preoperative resuscitation, but should be given if any doubt exists, particularly to patients with massive subcutaneous infections, those with acute pancreatitis, and those who have been chronically starved.

Fluid abnormalities also must be suspected in the patient for whom an elective procedure is planned. Chronic illnesses frequently are associated with extracellular fluid volume deficits, and concentration and compositional changes are not uncommon. Correction of anemia and recognition of the fact that a contracted blood volume may exist in the chronically debilitated patient is of obvious importance. The choice of whole blood versus packed cells for correction of anemia depends on the volume status. If there is any question, 1 unit of packed cells may be given and the hemoglobin and hematocrit determined subsequently. The hemoglobin generally increases approximately 1.5 following the infusion of 250 ml of packed cells into the adult of average size. The increase will be significantly greater than 1.5 Gm/100 ml in the patient with a contracted intravascular volume, indicating the probable need for whole blood transfusions. If available, measurement of the blood volume is obviously more accurate.

Of additional importance is the prevention of volume depletion during the preoperative period. Prolonged periods of fluid restriction in preparation for various diagnostic procedures, and the use of cathartics and enemas for preparation of the bowel may cause a significant acute loss of extracellular fluid. Prompt recognition and treatment of these losses is necessary to prevent complications during the operative period.

Intraoperative Management of Fluids

If preoperative replacement of extracellular fluid volume has been incomplete, hypotension may develop promptly with the induction of anesthesia. This can be quite insidious, as the ability of the awake patient to compensate for mild volume deficit is revealed only when the compensatory mechanisms are abolished with anesthesia. This problem is prevented by maintaining base-line requirements and replacing abnormal losses of fluids and electrolytes by intravenous infusions in the preoperative period.

Blood lost during the operative procedure should be replaced steadily. It is usually unnecessary to replace blood loss of less than 500 ml, but after the loss has exceeded this, replacement should begin. The warnings against the use of a single transfusion during operation have been somewhat confusing. There may be a very definite need for a single-unit transfusion in the patient who loses between 500 and 1,000 ml of blood during operation.

In addition to blood losses during operation, there appear to be extracellular fluid losses during major operative procedures. Some of these, including edema from extensive dissection, collections within the lumen and wall of the small bowel, and accumulations of fluid in the peritoneal cavity, are clinically discernible and well recognized. They generally are felt to represent distributional shifts, in that the functional volume of extracellular fluid is reduced but not externally lost from the body. These functional losses are often referred to as "a parasitic loss of extracellular fluid," "a third space edema," or "a sequestration" of extracellular fluid. Another source of extracellular fluid loss during major operative trauma is the wound itself. This is a relatively smaller loss and very difficult to quantify except in extensive and major operative procedures.

At the beginning of this century, surgeons became aware that many changes occurred in urinary output, blood volume, and fluid and electrolyte composition during and after surgery. Assessment of these changes, however, awaited the development of analytic techniques and their application to patient studies. In the following 25 years, saline solutions in varying combinations were given to patients undergoing operation, often in excessive amounts. Work in the late 1930s and early 1940s by Moyer and by many others indicated that during and after operative procedures, saline and water solutions should be withheld

entirely, because most of the fluid administered was retained.

The possibility existed that the operative and postoperative retention of salt and water administered in relatively small amounts might simply be physiologic retention to replace a deficit of salt and water incurred by the operative procedure. Subsequent studies have revealed that functional extracellular fluid decreases with major abdominal operations, largely as sequestered loss into the operative site. This extracellular fluid volume deficit can be replaced during the operative procedure. These data have led to the conclusion that the need for an extracellular "mimic" in the form of balanced salt solution now can be clinically estimated. Intraoperative correction of the volume deficit with salt solution markedly reduces "postoperative salt intolerance," but is not intended to substitute for blood replacement. Rather, it is felt to be a physiologic supplement, or adjunct, to replace sequestered losses.

Thus, the pendulum has swung from indiscriminate use of salt solutions in the first quarter of this century to almost total withholding of fluid and electrolytes from surgical patients in the second quarter of the century; indications at present are that proper management lies somewhere between these two extremes. Some guidelines are necessary for the intraoperative administration of saline solutions as a "mimic" for the sequestered extracellular fluid. Since this varies from an almost imperceptible minimum to a high of approximately 3 liters during an uncomplicated procedure, quantification is extremely difficult with the presently available means of measuring functional extracellular fluid. Consequently, no accurate formula for intraoperative fluid administration can yet be derived. Some arbitrary but clinically useful guidelines are the following: (1) Blood should be replaced as lost, irrespective of any additional fluid and electrolyte therapy. (2) The replacement of extracellular fluid should begin during the operative procedure. Recent data reveal that if the operative replacement of extracellular fluid is delayed until the adrenal compensatory mechanisms have started to react to the operative trauma in the immediate postoperative period, dangerous overloads may be produced. (3) Balanced salt solution needed during operation is approximately $\frac{1}{2}$ to 1 liter/hour, but only to a maximum of 2 to 3 liters during a 4-hour major abdominal procedure, unless there are other measurable losses.

Using a similar fluid regimen, Thompson and associates reported experiences in a series of 670 patients undergoing major aortoiliac reconstructive procedures. In this group of patients, the average amount of Ringer's lactate solution administered was 3555 ml, giving an average intraoperative replacement of salt solution of 677 ml per hour of operative procedure. In the last 6 years of this study there were only two deaths in 298 operations, an operative mortality of 0.67 percent. Among the entire 670 patients, only two patients died of renal failure, an incidence of 0.3 percent. No patient died of pulmonary insufficiency. This extremely low incidence of renal failure, even in the presence of extensive operative trauma, is similar to the authors' data for major abdominal operative procedures.

Postoperative Management of Fluids

IMMEDIATE POSTOPERATIVE PERIOD

Orders for postoperative fluids are not written until the patient is in the recovery room and the fluid status has been assessed. Evaluation at this point should include a review of preoperative fluid status, the amount of fluid loss and gain during operation, and clinical examination of the patient with assessment of the vital signs and urinary output. Initial fluid orders are written to correct any *existing* deficit, followed by maintenance fluids for the remainder of the day. For the patient with complications who has received or lost large amounts of fluid, it is frequently difficult to estimate the fluid requirements for the ensuing 24 hours. In this situation, intravenous fluids are ordered 1 liter at a time and the patient checked frequently until the situation is clarified. Proper replacement of fluids during this relatively short period will facilitate subsequent fluid management.

Immediately after operation, extracellular fluid volume depletion may occur as a result of continued losses of fluid at the site of injury or operative trauma—for example, into the wall or lumen of the small intestine. Several liters of extracellular fluid may be slowly deposited in such areas within a few hours or more during the first day or so from the time of the injury. Unrecognized deficits of extracellular fluid volume during the early postoperative period are manifest primarily as circulatory instability. The signs of volume deficiency in other organ systems may be delayed for several hours with this type of fluid loss. Postoperative hypotension and tachycardia require prompt investigation, followed by appropriate therapy. The generally accepted adequate blood pressure of 90/60 and a pulse of less than 120 in postoperative patients may not be sufficient to prevent renal ischemia unless, in addition to lack of signs of shock, urine flow is adequate. Evaluation of the level of consciousness, pupillary size, airway patency, breathing patterns, pulse rate and volume, skin warmth, color, body temperature, and a 30- to 50-ml hourly urine output, combined with critical review of the operative procedure and the operative fluid management, usually is rewarding. Since operative trauma frequently involves loss or transfer of significant quantities of whole blood, plasma, or extracellular fluid which can be only grossly estimated, circulatory instability is most commonly caused by underestimated initial losses or insidious, concealed continued losses. Operative blood loss is usually estimated by the operating surgeon to be 15 to 40 percent less than the isotopically measured blood loss from that patient. In addition, several liters of extravascular, extracellular fluid can be sequestered in areas of injury and manifested only by oliguria and mild depression of the blood pressure with a rapid pulse. For a patient with circulatory instability, further volume replacement of an additional 1,000 ml isotonic salt solution, while determining whether continuing losses or other causes are present, often resolves the problem. Contributing causes must be vigorously pursued with all diagnostic aids before excessive volumes of fluid have been administered.

It is unnecessary and probably unwise to administer potassium during the first 24 hours postoperatively, unless a definite potassium deficit exists. This is particularly important for the patient subjected to prolonged operative trauma involving one or more episodes of hypotension and for the posttraumatic patient with hemorrhagic hypotension. Oliguric renal failure or the more insidious high-output renal failure may develop, and the administration of even a small quantity of potassium may be quite detrimental.

LATER POSTOPERATIVE PERIOD

The problem of volume management during the postoperative convalescent phase is one of accurate measurement and replacement of all losses. In the otherwise healthy individual, this involves the replacement of measured sensible losses, which are generally of gastrointestinal origin, and the estimation and replacement of insensible losses.

The insensible loss is usually relatively constant and will average 600 to 900 ml daily. This may be increased by hypermetabolism, hyperventilation, and fever to a maximum of approximately 1,500 ml daily. The estimated insensible loss is replaced with 5% dextrose in water. This loss may be partially offset by an insensible gain of water from excessive tissue catabolism in the complicated postoperative patient, particularly if associated with oliguric renal failure.

Approximately 1 liter of fluid should be given to replace that volume of urine required to excrete the catabolic end products of metabolism (800 to 1,000 ml/day). In the individual with normal renal function, this may be given as 5% dextrose in water, since the kidneys are able to conserve sodium with excretion of less than 1 mEq daily. It is probably unnecessary to stress the kidneys to this degree, however, and a small amount of salt solution may be given in addition to water to cover urinary loss. In the elderly patient with salt-losing kidneys or in patients with head injuries, an insidious hyponatremia may develop if urinary losses are replaced with water. Urinary sodium in these circumstances may exceed 100 mEq/L and result in a daily loss of significant amounts of sodium. Measurement of urinary sodium will facilitate accurate replacement.

Urine volume is not replaced on a milliliter-for-milliliter basis. A urinary output of 2,000 to 3,000 ml on a given day may simply represent diuresis of fluids given during surgery or may represent excessive fluid administration. If these large losses are completely replaced, the urine output will progressively increase, and this may logically progress to a unique situation resembling diabetes insipidus with urinary outputs in excess of 10 liters daily.

Sensible losses, by definition, can be measured or, as in the case of sweating, the amount can be estimated. Gastrointestinal losses are usually isotonic or slightly hypotonic, and they are replaced with an essentially isotonic salt solution. When the estimated loss is slightly above or below isotonicity, appropriate corrections can be made in the daily water administration, while isotonic salt solutions are used to replace these losses volume for volume. Sweating is not usually a problem except with the febrile patient in whom losses may, but seldom do, exceed 250 ml/day/degree of fever. Excessive sweating may, in addition, represent a considerable loss of sodium in the unacclimatized individual.

Determination of serum electrolyte levels is generally unnecessary in the patient with an uncomplicated post-operative course maintained on parenteral fluids for 2 to 3 days. A more prolonged period of parenteral replacement or one complicated by excessive fluid losses requires frequent determinations of the serum sodium, potassium, and chloride levels, and carbon dioxide combining power. Adjustments then can be made with intravenous fluids of appropriate composition. For example, gastrointestinal losses should be replaced with isotonic sodium chloride solution in a patient with hyponatremia, hypochloremia, and mild metabolic alkalosis, and this should be continued until these abnormalities are corrected. In the hyponatremic patient with obvious overload, the amount of water given is restricted. In the presence of hyponatremia and mild metabolic acidosis, $M/6$ sodium lactate or lactated Ringer's solution with added sodium bicarbonate may be used. In this way, severe concentration and compositional changes can be avoided while an adequate extracellular fluid volume is maintained by appropriate maintenance fluids.

Maintenance fluids are administered at a steady rate over an 18- to 24-hour period as the losses are incurred. If given over a shorter period of time, renal excretion of the excess salt and water may occur while the normal losses continue over the full 24-hour period. For the same reason, fluids of different composition are alternated, and additives to intravenous fluids (e.g., potassium chloride and antibiotics) are evenly distributed in the total volume of fluid given.

In summary, daily fluid orders should begin with an assessment of the patient's volume status and a check for possible concentration or compositional disorders as reflected by proper laboratory determinations. All measured and insensible losses are replaced with fluids of appropriate composition, allowing for any preexisting deficit or excess. The amount of potassium replacement is 40 mEq daily for renal excretion of potassium in addition to approximately 20 mEq/L for replacement of gastrointestinal losses. Inadequate replacement may prolong the usual postoperative ileus and contribute to the insidious development of a resistant metabolic alkalosis. Calcium and magnesium are replaced when needed, as previously discussed.

SPECIAL CONSIDERATIONS IN THE POSTOPERATIVE PATIENT

VOLUME EXCESSES. The administration of isotonic salt solutions in excess of volume losses (external or internal) may result in overexpansion of the extracellular fluid space. The otherwise normal person in a postoperative state tolerates an acute overexpansion extremely well. Excesses administered over a period of several days, however, will soon exceed the kidneys' ability to excrete sodium; since water losses continue, hypernatremia will ensue. Therefore, it is important to determine as accurately

as possible from intake and output records and serum sodium concentrations the actual needs of the patient managed over several postoperative days. Attention to the signs and symptoms of overload usually prevents this fluid abnormality. It arises most frequently with attempts to meet excessive volume losses that are not measurable, such as those occurring from incompletely controlled fistula drainage.

The earliest sign is a weight gain (when measurable) during the catabolic period, when the patient should be losing $\frac{1}{4}$ to $\frac{1}{2}$ lb/day. Heavy eyelids, hoarseness, or dyspnea on exertion may rapidly appear. Circulatory and pulmonary signs of overload appear late and represent a rather massive overload. Peripheral edema may be a sign, but it does not necessarily indicate volume excess. In the absence of additional evidence for volume overload, other causes for peripheral edema should be considered. Of particular importance is the fact that overexpansion of the *total* extracellular fluid may coexist with *depletion* of the functional extracellular fluid compartment. Central venous pressure measurements may be helpful during volume replacement but may be misleading, as a rapid rise may indicate an excessive rate of fluid administration or primary pump failure but it does not accurately establish volume status.

HYPONATREMIA. Significant postoperative alterations in serum sodium concentration are not frequently observed if the fluid resuscitation during operation has included adequate volumes of isotonic salt solutions. The kidneys retain the ability to excrete moderate excesses of salt water administered in the early postoperative period if functional extracellular fluid has been adequately replaced during the operative or immediate postoperative period. Previous studies of sodium balance have revealed that patients do excrete sodium after the functional deficit incurred by the shift of extracellular fluid has been replaced. Wright and Gann have demonstrated normal capacity to excrete water postoperatively when isotonic salt solutions are administered prior to a challenge with a water load. Thus, the commonly described hyponatremia associated with surgical procedures and traumatic injury is prevented by the replacement of extracellular fluid deficits. The daily maintenance of normal osmolarity is simplified by the replacement of observable losses of known sodium content.

Hyponatremia may easily occur when water is given to replace losses of sodium-containing fluids or when water administration consistently exceeds water losses. The latter may occur with oliguria or in association with decreased water loss through the skin and lungs, intracellular shifts of sodium, or the cellular release of excessive amounts of endogenous water. Severe or refractory hyponatremia, however, is difficult to produce if renal function remains normal.

Replacement of Sodium Losses with Water. A common error is replacement of gastrointestinal and other salt losses with only water or a hypotonic solution. Patients with head injury or with preexisting renal disease (loss of concentrating ability) may elaborate urine with a high salt concentration (50 to 200 mEq/L).

Progressive hyponatremia in the patient with head injury, despite adequate salt administration, is believed to be due to excessive secretion of antidiuretic hormone with consequent water retention. The loss of renal concentrating ability due to impairment of renal tubular function ("salt-wasting kidneys") is a common problem in elderly patients. This source of sodium loss is frequently not anticipated, since the blood urea nitrogen and creatinine levels usually fall within normal limits. Continued replacement of these urinary losses with water only eventually may result in symptomatic hyponatremia. The urine sodium concentration should be determined if the diagnosis is in doubt; with hyponatremia and normal renal function, the urine should be virtually free of sodium.

Decreased Urinary Volume. Oliguria, from whatever cause (prerenal or renal), reduces the daily water requirements if not corrected. Cellular catabolism and the metabolic acidosis produced by the retention of nitrogenous waste products increases the cellular release of water. Therefore, the gain of endogenous water decreases the total water requirement beyond that expected when the urinary volume is low.

Decreased Insensible Loss. Cutaneous vasoconstriction from any cause decreases both insensible and evaporative water loss by this route. This condition most commonly accompanies generalized hypothermia.

Endogenous Water Release. The patient maintained on intravenous fluids without adequate caloric intake will, between the fifth and tenth days, gain significant quantities of water (maximum, 500 ml daily) from excessive cellular catabolism, thus decreasing the quantity of exogenous water required per day.

Intracellular Shifts. Systemic bacterial sepsis is often accompanied by a precipitous drop in serum sodium concentration. This sudden change is poorly understood, but usually accompanies loss of extracellular fluid as either interstitial or intracellular sequestrations. This can be treated by withholding free water, restoring extracellular fluid volume, and initiating treatment of the sepsis.

Many hyponatremic states are asymptomatic until the serum sodium level falls below 120 mEq/L. This moderate asymptomatic hyponatremia, however, signifies inappropriate therapy or indicates the basic underlying condition. Symptomatic hyponatremia, or water intoxication, is difficult to produce if renal function is normal. Convulsions and apnea from uncorrected water excesses occur most often in children and elderly adults. Within the limits imposed by the circulatory apparatus, these deficits should be corrected by the administration of hypertonic salt solution to a serum sodium level above 130 mEq/L. Mild or moderate degrees of hyponatremia may be simply corrected by temporary restriction of water intake.

In the presence of hyperglycemia, determination of the glucose concentration is necessary to evaluate the significance of a depressed serum sodium level. Since glucose does not enter cells by passive diffusion, it exerts an osmotic force in the extracellular compartment. This contribution to osmotic pressure is normally small, but with an elevated glucose concentration, the increased osmotic pressure causes the transfer of cellular water into the extracellular compartment, resulting in a dilutional hypo-

natremia. Hyponatremia therefore may be observed when the total effective osmotic pressure in the extracellular compartment is normal or even above normal. In terms of tonicity, each 100 mg/100 ml rise in the blood glucose *above normal* is roughly equivalent to a 3 mEq/L rise in the serum sodium concentration. Consider a patient with a serum sodium concentration of 125 mEq/L and a blood glucose level of 500 mg/100 ml. The glucose level is approximately 400 mg/100 ml above normal, which is equivalent to a 12 mEq/L rise in the serum sodium level. Thus, $125 + 12 = 137$ mEq/L; the tonicity is normal despite the marked reduction in sodium concentration. In this instance, therapy is directed toward lowering the blood glucose level. The sodium concentration will return toward normal as the excess water leaves the extracellular compartment. In practice, a true sodium deficit may be secondary to the underlying disorder and must be corrected.

HYPERNATREMIA. Hypernatremia (serum sodium concentration above 150 mEq/L), although uncommon, is a dangerous abnormality. In contradistinction to decreased serum sodium concentration, hypernatremia is easily produced when renal function is normal. The extracellular fluid hyperosmolarity results in a shift of intracellular water from within the cell to the extracellular fluid compartment; in this situation, a high serum sodium level may indicate a significant deficit of total body water. In surgical patients hypernatremia arises most often from excessive or unexpected water losses, although it may result from use of salt-containing solutions to replace water losses. The following classification of water losses may be helpful in preventing and treating this abnormality.

Excessive Extrarenal Water Losses. With increased metabolism from any cause, but particularly associated with fever, the water loss through evaporation of sweat may reach several liters daily. Patients with tracheostomy in dry environments can (with excessive minute volume air exchange) lose as much as 1 to 1.5 liters of water/day by this route. Increased water evaporation from a granulating surface is of significant magnitude in the thermally injured patient, and losses may be as great as 3 to 5 liters/day.

Increased Renal Water Losses. Extremely large volumes of solute-poor urine may result from hypoxic damage to the distal tubules and collecting ducts or loss of antidiuretic hormone stimulation from damage to the central nervous system. In both instances, facultative water resorption is impaired. The former occurs in high-output renal failure; in our experience, this is the most common type of renal failure following severe injury or operative trauma. The latter occurs with extensive head injuries accompanied by temporary diabetes insipidus.

Solute Loading. High protein intake may produce an increased osmotic load of urea, which necessitates the excretion of large volumes of water. Hypernatremia, azotemia, and extracellular fluid volume deficits follow. In general, these can be prevented by an intake of 7 ml of water/Gm of dietary protein.

Excessive glucose administration results in the need for a large volume of water for excretion. Osmotic diuretics such as mannitol and urea also result in the obligatory excretion of a large volume of water as well as increasing urinary sodium losses. In addition, isotonic salt solutions, if used to replace pure water losses, rapidly produce hypernatremia.

HIGH-OUTPUT RENAL FAILURE. Acute renal insufficiency following trauma or surgical stress is a highly lethal complication. The diagnosis is classically based on persistent oliguria and chemical evidence of uremia after stabilization of the circulation. The clinical course is characterized by oliguria lasting from several days to several weeks, followed by a progressive rise in daily urine volume until both the excretory and concentrating functions of the kidney are gradually restored.

Uremia, occurring without a period of oliguria and accompanied by a daily urine volume greater than 1,000 to 1,500 ml/day, is a more frequent but less well recognized entity. Clinical experience and laboratory experiments suggest that high-output renal failure represents the renal response to a less severe or modified episode of renal injury than that required to produce classic oliguric renal failure. Its importance lies in the fact that it is a milder form of renal insufficiency and that realization of its presence, by serial measurement of blood urea nitrogen and serum electrolytes, permits intelligent chemical and fluid volume management with a much greater latitude because of the daily urine volume excretion. Normal extracellular fluid volume and normal serum sodium concentration, therefore, are quite easily maintained when accurate daily outputs of each are obtained and replaced accordingly. The sodium-containing fluids may be administered as lactate to control the mild metabolic acidosis that occurs. Severe acidosis may develop if isotonic losses from the gastrointestinal tract or renal excretion of sodium are replaced with sodium chloride.

The chief dangers of high-output renal failure are failure to recognize its existence because of normal output, and the intravenous administration of potassium salts. Good urinary output and gastrointestinal involvement requiring suction usually indicate the need for daily potassium replacement. With this type of renal failure, however, potassium intoxication may be produced. As little as 20 mEq of potassium chloride given intravenously may rapidly produce myocardial potassium intoxication requiring resin or hemodialysis treatment.

The typical course of high-output renal failure begins without a period of oliguria. The daily urine volumes are normal or greater than normal, often reaching levels of 3 to 5 liters/day while blood urea nitrogen is increasing. An attempt to decrease urine output by water restriction rapidly results in hypernatremia without a change in urine volume. On the average, urea nitrogen continues to increase for 8 to 12 days before a downward trend occurs. The blood/urine urea ratio is about 1:10 until a decrease occurs in the blood urea concentration.

Functionally, the lesion is characterized by a glomerular filtration rate of less than 20 percent of normal and complete resistance to vasopressin for 1 to 3 weeks after the blood urea nitrogen has declined. During the next 6 to 8 weeks, the glomerular filtration rate gradually rises, and the response to vasopressin becomes normal. The early recognition of high-output renal failure by serial blood determinations of blood urea nitrogen is important. Failure to recognize its presence may result in death from hyperkalemia, hypernatremia, or acidosis. As alluded to previously, it is unwise to administer potassium during the first 24 postoperative hours unless a definite potassium deficit exists. This is particularly important in the patient subjected to prolonged operative trauma involving one or more episodes of hypotension and in the patient with posttraumatic hemorrhagic hypotension.

NUTRITION IN THE SURGICAL PATIENT

The majority of patients undergoing elective surgical operations withstand the brief period of catabolism and starvation without noticeable difficulty. However, maintaining an adequate nutritional regimen may be of critical importance in managing seriously ill surgical patients with preexisting weight loss and depleted energy reserves. Between these two extremes are patients for whom nutritional support is not essential for life but may serve to shorten the postoperative recovery phase and minimize the number of complications. Not infrequently a patient may become ill or even die from complications secondary to starvation rather than the underlying disorder. Therefore, it is essential that the surgeon have a sound grasp of the fundamental metabolic changes associated with surgery, trauma, and sepsis and an awareness of the methods available to reverse or ameliorate these events.

Body Fuel Reserves

The body must mobilize appropriate nutrients from fuel reserves in order to withstand the necessary periods of partial or complete starvation and to meet the additional requirements imposed by surgery, trauma, or sepsis. The extent and availability of these reserves may be of critical importance for successful recovery from an illness. Available information concerning body fuel composition and the rate of fuel consumption in man has recently been reviewed by Cahill and is summarized below.

Carbohydrates, proteins, and fats are the three sources of fuel in man. Their relative contributions both by weight and caloric potential are illustrated in Fig. 2-3. Carbohydrate stores, primarily in the form of liver and muscle glycogen, are relatively small and could supply basal caloric requirements for less than 1 day. However, this relatively small quantity is absolutely essential in the emergency situation for the production of high-energy phosphates during anaerobic metabolism. Although glucose yields approximately 4 kcal/Gm, its storage as glycogen requires the addition of 1 or 2 Gm of intracellular water and electrolytes. Therefore, it yields only 1 or 2 kcal/Gm of wet weight.

Protein represents a considerably larger source of fuel, but, as emphasized by Cahill, every molecule of protein in the body has a specific purpose, such as an enzyme, a structural component, or a contractile protein in muscle. Thus, any protein loss represents loss of an essential function. Additionally, the amount of total body protein is

WEIGHT (Kg)		CALORIES
0.3	CARBOHYDRATE	1,200
6	PROTEIN	25,000
15	FAT	140,000

Fig. 2-3. Body fuel composition in the normal individual. (*From G. F. Cahill, Jr., Bull Am Coll Surg, 55:12, 1970.*)

relatively fixed in the normal healthy individual, and any additional protein is metabolized, the excess calories being stored as fat. Protein, like glycogen, represents an inefficient energy source relative to its wet weight, since it exists in an aqueous environment.

In contrast to glycogen and protein, fat is stored in a relatively anhydrous state. By weight, then, it is a relatively rich source of energy, supplying approximately 9 kcal/Gm. Most of the fat in the body serves as a readily available energy source; the few areas where fat serves a specific function (e.g., mechanical fat pads) are the last to be mobilized during starvation.

In summary, protein and fat are the only major sources of fuel. Total protein mass is relatively fixed in amount, and caloric excess or deficiency is met by an increase or decrease in the body's fat mass. Fat depots serve as sources of energy, protein stores represent *potential* sources of energy but only through the loss of some important function, and the small stores of carbohydrates are generally protected except for emergency use during anaerobic glycolysis.

Starvation

During the first several days of complete starvation, caloric needs are supplied by body fat and proteins; the small glycogen reserve is largely spared. Previous studies have shown an obligatory loss of approximately 10 to 15 grams of nitrogen daily in the urine during this period, indicating the utilization of approximately 60 to 90 grams of protein (each gram of nitrogen represents approximately 6.25 grams of muscle protein). The majority of this protein, which is largely derived from skeletal muscle, is converted to glucose in the liver by the process of gluconeogenesis; most of this endogenously produced glucose is used by the brain. The remainder is used by certain tissues such as red blood cells and leukocytes which convert the glucose to lactate and pyruvate. These are returned to the liver and resynthesized into glucose (the Cori cycle). This obligatory nitrogen loss, then, reflects the use of amino acids derived from muscle protein for gluconeogenesis to supply glucose to the brain. No patient, however, should be allowed to

starve completely. The administration of at least 100 Gm of glucose will obviate most of this gluconeogenesis and reduce the nitrogen loss by at least one-half—the well-known "protein-sparing effect" described by Gamble. Available evidence from Cahill indicates that this protein-sparing effect is regulated by insulin, which is released when exogenous glucose is infused for use by the brain. The slightly elevated insulin level reduces amino acid release from the muscle, amino acid extraction by the liver, and gluconeogenesis. In the diabetic with an absolute or relative lack of insulin, the infusion of glucose does not inhibit gluconeogenesis, and muscle breakdown to amino acids continues unabated. The liver derives its energy by oxidizing fatty acids to ketones, and the remainder of the body utilizes both fatty acids and ketones to meet caloric requirements. Generally a small quantity of the ketones is excreted into the urine.

If complete starvation continues for more than a few days, the obligatory nitrogen loss progressively decreases, as the brain begins to use fat as its fuel source. Unlike other body tissues, however, the brain cannot utilize free fatty acids, since they do not cross the blood-brain barrier. Instead, use of keto acids which are produced by the liver and readily cross the blood-brain barrier gradually displaces the use of glucose by the brain. After prolonged starvation, the net effect of this adaptation to ketone utilization is a protein-sparing effect with reduction of urinary nitrogen excretion to approximately 4 Gm/day. This 4 Gm of nitrogen represents approximately 25 Gm of protein, or about 100 Gm of lean wet muscle. Thus, the normal individual with an average supply of fat and muscle may survive total starvation for several months. Insulin again may be the signal for the reduction in muscle catabolism and gluconeogenesis (coincident with the increased use of keto acids by the brain), according to Cahill. However, changes in the blood level of alanine, which is quantitatively one of the more important amino acids, may also play a role. A fall in the blood level of this amino acid appears to decrease gluconeogenesis and glucose production by the liver.

Surgery, Trauma, Sepsis

The sequence of metabolic and endocrine events occasioned by surgery, trauma, or sepsis may be divided into several phases. As pointed out by Moore (1960), the magnitude of the changes and the duration of each phase vary considerably and are directly related to the severity of the injury.

CATABOLIC PHASE. This phase has also been termed the *adrenergic-corticoid phase* since it corresponds to the period during which changes induced by adrenergic and adrenal corticoid hormones are most striking. Immediately following surgery or trauma, there is a sudden increase in metabolic demands and urinary excretion of nitrogen beyond the levels associated with simple starvation. The patient generally cannot eat, cannot lower his metabolic rate, and cannot effectively alter the source of endogenous fuels to spare protein utilization. This is in distinct contrast to events in the normal individual subjected to prolonged starvation, where most body tissues use fat as their main source of fuel, thereby sparing protein. Trauma apparently results in a continued and excessive mobilization of protein; unfortunately, the administration of moderate amounts of glucose to these individuals produces little or no change in the rate of protein catabolism, although Blackburn has suggested that the administration of glucose-free crystalline amino acid solutions results in a decrease in urinary nitrogen excretion. During the hypermetabolic, reparative phase following injury, increased flow of glucose from the liver to the periphery has been documented by Wilmore and Dudrick. Simultaneously, increased Cori cycle activity is stimulated and three-carbon intermediates are converted back to glucose in the liver by pyruvate carboxylase and phosphoenolpyruvate carboxylase. Increased synthesis of these two enzymes occurs in the presence of elevated levels of glucagon, glucocorticoids, and catecholamines and low concentrations of insulin—the hormonal environment present during the catabolic phase of injury.

The extent of the negative nitrogen balance in these patients varies considerably and is largely related to the magnitude of the injury. In Fig. 2-4 daily net nitrogen losses during simple starvation with and without the administration of glucose are compared to losses sustained with moderate to severe surgical illness.

EARLY ANABOLIC PHASE. After several days or weeks, depending on the severity of injury, the body turns from a catabolic to an anabolic phase. This turning point, also known as the *corticoid-withdrawal phase*, is characterized by a sharp decline in nitrogen excretion and restoration of a positive potassium balance. Generally, this transition period lasts no more than a day or two.

The prolonged anabolic phase may last from a few weeks to a few months and generally coincides with the resumption of oral intake. Nitrogen balance is positive, indicating synthesis of proteins, and there is a rapid and progressive gain in weight and muscular strength. The patient is usually active, has an excellent appetite, and generally is discharged from the hospital at this point. Positive nitrogen balance reaches a maximum of approximately 4 Gm/day, which represents the synthesis of approximately 25 Gm of protein and the gain of over 100 Gm of lean body mass/day. The total amount of nitrogen gain will ultimately equal the amount lost during the catabolic phase, although the rate of gain will be much slower than the rate of initial loss.

LATE ANABOLIC PHASE. The final period of convalescence or the late anabolic phase may last from several weeks to several months after a severe injury. This phase is associated with the gradual gain of fatty tissue as the previously positive nitrogen balance declines toward normal. Weight gain is much slower during this phase because of the higher calorie content of fat and can be realized only if intake is in excess of caloric expenditure. In most individuals, the phase ends with a gradual return to the previously normal body weight. The patient who is partially immobilized during this period of time, however, may exhibit a marked gain in weight due to decreased energy expenditure.

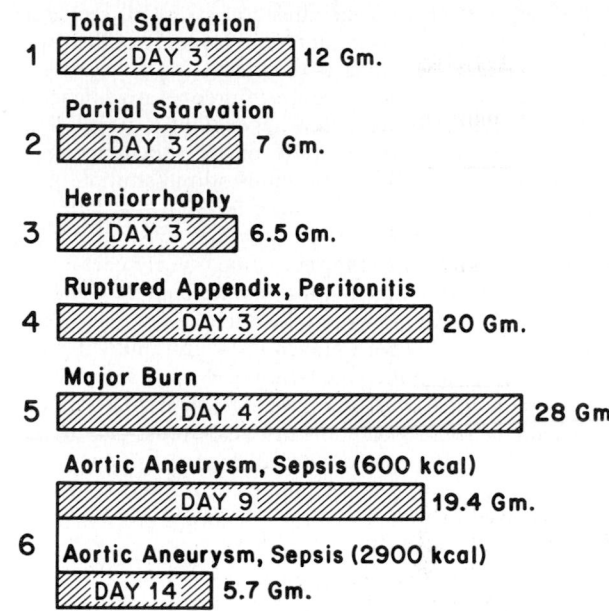

Fig. 2-4. The extent of negative nitrogen balance in adult patients during starvation alone and during various surgical illnesses associated with partial starvation. Note the difference in negative nitrogen balance in case 6 with low and high calorie parenteral supplementation. (*Cases 1 to 4 from W. D. Holden et al., Ann Surg, 146:563, 1957. Case 5 from J. M. Kinney, "Proceedings of a Conference on Energy Metabolism and Body Fuel Utilization," Harvard University Press, Cambridge, 1966. Case 6 from L. J. Lawson, Br J Surg, 52:795, 1965.*)

Base-Line Requirements

The normal caloric and protein requirements for individuals leading a sedentary life approximate 1 Gm of protein and 35 kcal/kg of body weight, or approximately 1400 kcal/m² of body surface area per day. These requirements, which have been recommended by the Food and Nutritional Board of the National Research Council, vary with age, sex, and the degree of daily activity.

These base-line requirements are totally inadequate for patients who have undergone surgery or who have suffered severe trauma or sepsis. The exact caloric and nitrogen requirements necessary to maintain an individual in balance after severe injury are unknown. However, guidelines for nutritional supplementation based on previous experimental data and clinical experience have been recommended. Moore has suggested that intakes in the region of 0.2 Gm of nitrogen/kg and 50 kcal/kg/day are necessary to maintain constant weight after moderate injury. Studies by Kinney suggest that a moderately positive caloric balance (1000 to 2000 kcal/day above resting expenditure) with a calorie-to-nitrogen ratio of approximately 150:200 may be appropriate for acutely ill surgical patients. Similarly, Dudrick et al. have noted that the average depleted or complicated major surgical patient requires between 2500 and 4000 kcal/day with approximately 12 to 24 Gm of nitrogen. These approximations are useful, although the quantity and composition of the nutrients must be tailored to meet individual needs.

The requirements for vitamins and essential trace minerals usually can be easily met in the average patient with an uncomplicated postoperative course, and vitamins usually are not given in the absence of preoperative deficiencies. The exception is vitamin C, essential for wound healing, which can be given orally or by subcutaneous or intravenous routes. The intravenous administration of vitamin C is associated with a large urinary loss, but since it is relatively nontoxic, large amounts (300 to 500 mg daily) can be given. Patients maintained on elemental diets or parenteral hyperalimentation require complete vitamin and mineral supplementation. Several commercial preparations are available for intravenous or intramuscular use, although most do not contain vitamin K and some do not contain vitamin B_{12} or folic acid. Supplemental essential trace minerals and essential fatty acids must also be administered to patients receiving all their nutrition via the parenteral route with hypertonic dextrose and crystalline amino acids.

Indications and Methods for Nutritional Support

The selection of patients who require partial or complete nutritional support has become increasingly important. The ability to provide complete nutritional support in the starving patient and to counteract the nitrogen losses in catabolic states with elemental diets or parenteral hyperalimentation represents a substantial contribution. However, it should be emphasized that the majority of surgical patients do not require special nutritional regimens. The reasonably well-nourished and otherwise healthy individual who undergoes an uncomplicated major surgical procedure has sufficient body fuel reserves to withstand the catabolic insult and partial starvation for at least 1 week. Adequate quantities of parenteral fluids with appropriate electrolyte composition and a minimum of 100 Gm of glucose daily to minimize protein catabolism will be all that is necessary in most patients. Assuming that the patient has a relatively uncomplicated postoperative course and resumes normal oral intake at the end of this period, elemental diets or parenteral hyperalimentation are unnecessary and probably inadvisable because of the associated risks. During the early anabolic phase, the patient must be provided with an adequate caloric intake of proper composition to meet the energy needs of the body and allow protein synthesis. A high calorie-to-nitrogen ratio (optimal ratio approximately 150 kcal/Gm nitrogen) and an adequate supply of vitamins and minerals are necessary for maximum anabolism during this period.

In contrast to this group, there is a small but significant number of surgical patients for whom an adequate nutritional regimen may be of critical importance for a successful outcome. This category includes preoperative patients who are chronically debilitated from their diseases or malnutrition and patients who have suffered trauma, sepsis, or surgical complications and cannot maintain an adequate caloric intake for any number of reasons.

The methods for partial or complete nutritional supplementation in the surgical patient fall into three general categories: Nasopharyngeal, gastrostomy, and jejunostomy tube feedings are appropriate routes for alimentation in patients who have a relatively normal gastrointestinal tract but cannot or will not eat. Elemental diets may be administered by similar routes when bulk and fat-free nutrients requiring minimal digestion are indicated. Finally, parenteral hyperalimentation may be used for supplementation in the patient with limited oral intake or, more commonly, for complete nutritional management in the absence of oral intake.

NASOPHARYNGEAL TUBE FEEDING

Nasopharyngeal feedings, preferably through small, soft silastic tubes, should be used only in alert patients who are unable or unwilling to eat normally for various reasons; it is contraindicated in most other cases. The foremost contraindication for nasopharyngeal tube feeding is unconsciousness or lack of protective laryngeal reflexes, which may result in fatal pulmonary complications due to tracheal aspiration of regurgitated gastric content. Even with a tracheostomy, it is inadvisable to feed mentally obtunded patients via nasopharyngeal tubes, since such feedings often can be recovered from tracheostomy suction, indicating continued aspiration of gastric content even around a snugly fitting tracheostomy tube. An inflated tracheostomy tube cuff might prevent this, but the required constant inflation is inadvisable since it may cause pressure necrosis of the trachea. Furthermore, the prolonged use of a nasopharyngeal tube may cause severe discomfort, nasopharyngeal and laryngeal pressure necrosis, and esophagitis with stricture.

Pharyngeal tube feedings are often indicated for patients with oropharyngeal tumor; irritation may be prevented by inserting the tube into the pyriform sinus, as recommended by Graham and Royster. This technique also allows concealment of the feeding tube under the patient's clothing.

The nasopharyngeal tube may allow feeding beyond dysfunctional gastric stomas and high gastrointestinal fistulas. In such cases, it may be possible to maintain nutrition without a jejunostomy tube until stomal dysfunction relents or the fistula heals. This may be done by passing a Cantor tube or, preferably, a small polyethylene feeding tube weighted with a rubber finger cot filled with 1 ml of mercury distal to the faulty stoma or fistula, as recommended by Bachrach and Tecimer. The polyethylene feeding tube is prepared by passing a #1 silk thread through the tube with a wire. The mercury-filled finger cot is tied to the silk thread distad and the thread fixed to the tube proximally. The tube is then inserted through the nose into the stomach, and the patient is positioned so that the mercury weight tends to lead the small tube well into the jejunum. When the tube reaches the proper position (as noted on x-ray after the injection of a small amount of water-soluble opaque medium), the silk string is released proximally, and peristalsis carries the mercury-weighted finger cot and thread distad until they are passed per rectum. Feedings are started after a few hours when the string has cleared the tube. This small, flexible plastic tube and mercury weight may be more readily introduced into the intestine than the bulkier, more rigid, long intestinal tubes and is more conducive to patient comfort.

Whenever dietary preparations are administered into the gastrointestinal tract via tubes, it is advisable to employ bedside infusion pumps to ensure a constant rate of delivery over each 24-hour period. The utilization of such pumps decreases the incidence of gastrointestinal side effects induced by too rapid delivery of hyperosmolar solutions, while at the same time allowing safer administration of larger daily volumes of nutrients, since gastric distension is minimized.

GASTROSTOMY TUBE FEEDING

The administration of blended food through a gastrostomy tube is a good method for feeding patients with a variety of chronic gastrointestinal lesions arising at or above the cardioesophageal junction. However, gastrostomy tube feedings are contraindicated for mentally obtunded patients with inadequate laryngeal reflexes. This feeding method should be used only in alert patients or in patients with total obstruction of the distal esophagus.

Generally, gastrostomies of the Stamm (serosa-lined, temporary) or modified Glassman (mucosa-lined, permanent) type are constructed. The feeding mixture may be ordinarily prepared food converted by a blender into a semiliquid. Hyperosmolarity of the feeding formula is not generally a problem as long as the pylorus is intact. The jejunostomy formula outlined below also may be used.

JEJUNOSTOMY TUBE FEEDING

Jejunostomy tube feedings are generally required for patients in whom nasopharyngeal or gastrostomy tube feedings are contraindicated, e.g., comatose patients or patients with high gastrointestinal fistulas or obstructions. The jejunostomy may be of the Roux en Y (permanent) or the Witzel (temporary) type. The latter is constructed by inserting a #18 French rubber catheter into the proximal jejunum approximately 12 in. distal to the ligament of Treitz. The wall of the jejunum is inverted over the tube for about 3 cm as it emerges from the bowel to create a serosa-lined tunnel which allows rapid sealing of the jejunal opening when the tube is removed. The tube may then be brought out through a stab wound in the left upper quadrant of the abdomen. The jejunum is sutured to the anterior abdominal wall at the point of tube entry to seal it from the peritoneal cavity.

If the jejunostomy tube is inadvertently removed, blind attempts at reinsertion are contraindicated. If discovered within a few hours, the tube may be reinserted under fluoroscopic control to be sure it is in the bowel before feedings are resumed. The patient is observed for signs of peritonitis for 12 to 18 hours after feedings are restarted. If there is any doubt about the position of the tube, it should be replaced surgically. Feedings are safely begun 12 to 18 hours after jejunostomy construction, even though peristalsis is not audible. A progressive regimen of feeding modified from that recommended by Zollinger is prefera-

Table 2-9. JEJUNOSTOMY FEEDING REGIMEN

1. 12–18 hours after jejunostomy—nothing.
2. First day—50 ml/hr × 20 of 5% dextrose/water.
3. Second day—100 ml/hr × 20 of 5% dextrose/water.
4. Third day—50 ml/hr × 20 of homogenized milk.
5. Fourth day—100 ml/2hr × 10 of homogenized milk.
6. Fifth day—180 ml/2hr × 10 of homogenized milk.
7. Sixth day—240 ml/2hr × 10 of homogenized milk.
8. Continue same regimen as on sixth day but add an additional half cup of powdered milk to each quart of homogenized milk daily until 1.5 cups per quart of homogenized milk is being used as feeding formula. Thereafter, give 240 ml of this mixture q. 2 h. × 10 daily. Feedings should begin at 6 A.M. and continue through 12 midnight. Additional water may be given between feedings when indicated.

ble (Table 2-9). The full-strength formula suitable for most patients is simply a mixture of 1.5 cups of powdered milk, 1 qt of homogenized milk, and 1 ml of Tween 40 (an emulsifying agent allowing better fat absorption). This mixture contains about 1 kcal/ml, and, when given in the final volume recommended in Table 2-9, provides about 2500 kcal, 140 Gm of protein, and adequate carbohydrates. The fat content represents less than 4 percent of the total. Polyvisol and Fer-in-sol, 0.6 ml each, are added once daily to the formula. Many of the more complex jejunostomy feedings are difficult to prepare, likely to spoil before use, too high in fat content, and excessively hyperosmolar, leading to a greater incidence of patient intolerance.

With proper care, about 85 percent of jejunostomy patients tolerate their feedings. Diarrhea is usually controlled if the concentration and volume of formula are temporarily reduced. Failing this, feeding is halted for a day, then resumed from the beginning of the feeding regimen, progressing somewhat more slowly than before. If mild diarrhea or cramping persists, a pulverized Lomotil tablet or 8 to 10 drops of tincture of belladonna may be given through the tube 30 minutes prior to formula infusion. At times it may be necessary to give 5 ml paregoric 15 to 30 minutes before the formula to control cramping and diarrhea, but this should be employed sparingly and for as short a period as possible. In many cases, symptoms are relieved if the rate and volume of infusion are reduced and cold formula avoided. Each feeding should be infused in about 20 minutes.

If the patient with a jejunostomy has a proximal bowel or biliary fistula draining more than 300 ml daily for prolonged periods, the fistular drainage may be collected by sump suction, cooled in an ice basin at bedside, and promptly refed in small increments throughout the day. To avoid jejunal overloading, the fistular fluid is refed between formula feedings. It is not advisable to refeed aspirated gastric juice, for this may cause jejunal irritation and profuse diarrhea. If the fistular drainage is profuse, it is usually not possible to refeed more than 2 liters/day, and fluid and electrolyte losses must be replaced by appropriate intravenous supplements. Additional water may be given with the feedings or administered between the feedings as indicated. Occasionally, an elemental diet, as discussed below, may be indicated when other jejunostomy formulas are not tolerated.

ELEMENTAL DIETS

Clinical experience with chemically formulated bulk-free elemental diets has been encouraging. These diets may be used for complete nutritional support or as dietary supplements for patients who are unable to eat or digest enough food to meet their energy requirements. They may be preferable to high-caloric parenteral feedings for patients who have at least part of the small bowel available for the absorption of simple sugars and amino acids. As outlined by Randall et al., elemental diets have been found useful for patients with depleted protein reserves secondary to gastrointestinal tract disease, such as ulcerative or granulomatous colitis and malabsorption syndrome, and for patients with only partial function of the gastrointestinal tract, such as the short bowel syndrome or gastric or small bowel fistulas with feeding distal to the fistula. The diets also have been used during preoperative bowel preparation and in place of ordinary jejunostomy feedings when the latter cannot be tolerated.

Elemental diets differ from conventional foods in that they are formulated synthetically out of known chemical nutrients, such as purified amino acids and simple carbohydrates. As commercially prepared, these diets also contain base-line electrolytes, water- and fat-soluble vitamins (except vitamin K), and trace minerals. They contain no bulk and therefore produce a minimum of residue. The compositions of three elemental diets which are currently

Table 2-10. ELEMENTAL DIETS*
Approximate composition per 1,800 ml†

	W-T low-residue Food	Vivonex-100	Vivonex-100 HN (high-nitrogen)
Kilocalories. . . .	1800	1800	1800
Carbohydrates Gm	408 (dextrin)	407 (glucose)	379
Protein, Gm . . .	39	37	75
Nitrogen, Gm . .	5.4	5.9	12
Fat, Gm	1.3	1.3	0.8
Sodium, mEq . .	100	104	60
Potassium, mEq	54	54	32
Chloride, mEq. .	151	128	94
Calcium, mEq . .	50	40	24
Magnesium mEq	33	13	17
Osmolality, mOsm/L	650	1175	844

*All diets contain standard fat and water-soluble vitamins for normal daily requirements (based on 2000 kcal) and essential trace minerals. Contain only minimal quantities of vitamin K, which should be supplemented to the full therapeutic level. Additional quantities of B vitamins and vitamin C should also be added.

†Six 80-Gm packets diluted with water to a total of 1,800 ml.
SOURCE: VIVONEX-100, Eaton Laboratories, Norwich, N.Y.; W-I Low Residue Food, Warren-Teed Pharmaceuticals, Inc., Columbus, Ohio.

available are shown in Table 2-10. The diets with lower protein content may be taken orally or by tube, while the diet with higher protein content is unpalatable and intended primarily for tube feeding. Unfortunately, patient acceptance of the flavored diets has been only fair, and they frequently must be given by tube.

The amount of elemental diet required to maintain weight and nitrogen balance varies with the individual patient. In severe catabolic states the standard diet often fails to achieve positive nitrogen balance. The following guidelines are based on those recommended by Randall. For oral feedings, the diets are made up in standard dilution (25% weight/volume) and provide 1 kcal/ml of solution. The solution is cooled and ingested in small amounts of 100 to 150 ml at a time. Approximately 2,000 ml or more may be taken in a day, providing approximately 2000 kcal and 40 Gm of protein. Depending on patient tolerance, the volume of diet may be increased as indicated.

Either the high- or low-protein diets may be used for intragastric or jejunostomy tube feedings initially. The diet is mixed at half the standard dilution (12.5% weight/volume or less) and administered continuously by pump or gravity drip at a rate of 40 to 50 ml/hour. Once the individual has adjusted to the diet, the concentration may be gradually increased to the standard dilution and the volume increased in small increments until the desired caloric and protein intake is achieved. The development of nausea, vomiting, or diarrhea is an indication to slow or stop the infusion for a short period of time. The feeding may then be restarted at a slower rate or at a lower concentration. Lomotil tablets, tincture of belladonna, or paregoric may be indicated to control diarrhea as discussed previously. Using the high-protein diet, as much as 3000 ml/day may be administered, providing approximately 3000 kcal and 20 Gm of nitrogen.

Careful attention to water and electrolyte balance is mandatory, particularly when large quantities of fluid are being lost through fistulas or other routes. Additional sodium and potassium may be added to the mixture (not to exceed a total of 100 mEq), although they should be given in intravenous fluids when larger quantities are needed. Water may be added to the mixture in the face of excessive pure water losses.

Complications include nausea, vomiting, and diarrhea which develop because of the high osmolarity of the diets. This generally can be controlled by decreasing the rate and/or concentration of the mixture. Hypertonic nonketotic coma may occur in the presence of excessive water losses or if the diets are administered at concentrations above those recommended. Hyperglycemia and glycosuria may occur in any severely ill patient, particularly latent diabetics, and insulin may be indicated. Aspiration is a constant threat with intragastric feedings; for this reason, this route should not be used in the absence of laryngeal reflexes or in mentally obtunded patients.

PARENTERAL ALIMENTATION

The parenteral route for nutritional supplementation when oral or tube feedings into the gastrointestinal tract are not feasible has been tried for several decades but until recently has fallen short of expectations. Parenteral infusion of 5% dextrose solutions is totally inadequate to meet caloric requirements within the limits of fluid tolerance, while the use of hypertonic solutions of dextrose, fructose, or invert sugar has been limited by a high incidence of thrombophlebitis. The use of plasma and blood for nutritional supplementation is mentioned only to be condemned; they are very expensive and inefficient sources of calories, and their administration is associated with an unnecessary number of complications. High-caloric solutions, such as ethyl alcohol (7 kcal/Gm) and fat (9 kcal/Gm) have found limited use.

Recently, Dudrick et al. have demonstrated the clinical practicality of providing complete nutritional needs for an extended period of time using high-caloric parenteral feedings. Parenteral hyperalimentation involves the continuous infusion of a hyperosmolar solution containing carbohydrates, proteins, and other necessary nutrients through an indwelling catheter inserted into the superior vena cava. In order to obtain the maximum benefit, the ratio of calories to nitrogen must be adequate (at least 100 to 150 kcal/Gm nitrogen) and the two materials must be infused simultaneously. When the sources of calories and nitrogen are given at different times, there is a significant decrease in nitrogen utilization. These nutrients can be given in quantities considerably greater than the basic caloric and nitrogen requirements, and this method has proved to be highly successful in achieving growth and development, positive nitrogen balance, and weight gain in a variety of clinical situations.

INDICATIONS FOR THE USE OF INTRAVENOUS HYPER-ALIMENTATION. The principal indications for parenteral hyperalimentation are found in seriously ill patients suffering from malnutrition, sepsis, or surgical or accidental trauma when use of the gastrointestinal tract for feedings is not possible. The safe and successful use of this regimen requires proper selection of patients with specific nutritional needs, experience with the technique, and an awareness of the associated complications. The number of reported complications has increased significantly since this technique has become more popular; it has been used in many instances either where it is not needed or where use of the gastrointestinal tract is more appropriate. For this reason, Dudrick et al. have recently outlined specific goals and indications for parenteral hyperalimentation, listed below:

1. Newborn infants with catastrophic gastrointestinal anomalies, such as tracheoesophageal fistula, gastroschisis, omphalocele, or massive intestinal atresia
2. Infants who fail to thrive nonspecifically or secondarily to gastrointestinal insufficiency associated with the short bowel syndrome, malabsorption, enzyme deficiency, meconium ileus, or idiopathic diarrhea
3. Adult patients with short-bowel syndrome secondary to massive small bowel resection or enteroenteric, enterocolic, enterovesical, or enterocutaneous fistulas
4. Patients with high alimentary tract obstructions without vascular compromise, secondary to achalasia, stricture, or neoplasia of the esophagus; gastric carcinoma; or pyloric obstruction
5. Surgical patients with prolonged paralytic ileus following major operations, multiple injuries, or blunt or open abdomi-

nal trauma, or patients with reflex ileus complicating various medical diseases
6. Patients with normal bowel length but with malabsorption secondary to sprue, hypoproteinemia, enzyme or pancreatic insufficiency, regional enteritis, or ulcerative colitis
7. Adult patients with functional gastrointestinal disorders such as esophageal dyskinesia following cerebral vascular accident, idiopathic diarrhea, psychogenic vomiting, anorexia nervosa, or hyperemesis gravidarum
8. Patients who cannot ingest food or who regurgitate and aspirate oral or tube feedings because of depressed or obtunded sensorium following severe metabolic derangements, neurologic disorders, intracranial surgery, or central nervous system trauma
9. Patients with excessive metabolic requirements secondary to severe trauma, such as extensive full-thickness burns, major fractures, or soft tissue injuries
10. Patients with granulomatous colitis, ulcerative colitis, and tuberculous enteritis, in which major portions of the absorptive mucosa are diseased
11. Paraplegics, quadriplegics, or debilitated patients with indolent decubitus ulcers in the pelvic areas, particularly when soilage and fecal contamination are a problem
12. Patients who will eventually require surgery but in whom prolonged progressive malnutrition has greatly increased the risk of operation
13. Patients in whom protein deficiency states are to be avoided, reduced, or corrected
14. Patients with potentially reversible acute renal failure, in whom marked catabolism results in the liberation of intracellular anions and cations, inducing hyperkalemia, hypermagnesemia, and hyperphosphatemia

Conditions *contraindicating* hyperalimentation include the following:

1. Lack of a specific goal for patient management, or where instead of extending a meaningful life, inevitable dying is prolonged.
2. Periods of cardiovascular instability or severe metabolic derangement requiring control or correction before attempting hypertonic intravenous feeding.
3. Feasible gastrointestinal tract feeding. In the vast majority of instances, this is the best route by which to provide nutrition.
4. Patients in good nutritional status, in whom only short-term parenteral nutrition support is required or anticipated.
5. Infants with less than 8 cm of small bowel, since virtually all have been unable to adapt sufficiently despite prolonged periods of parenteral nutrition. Intravenous hyperalimentation must be seriously questioned until bowel transplantation has been perfected for these neonates.
6. Patients who are irreversibly decerebrate or otherwise dehumanized.

INSERTION OF CENTRAL VENOUS INFUSION CATHETER. The successful use of intravenous hyperalimentation generally depends upon the proper placement and management of the central venous feeding catheter. A 16-gauge, 8- or 12-in. radiopaque catheter is introduced percutaneously through the subclavian or internal jugular vein and threaded into the superior vena cava. Although the technique for subclavian vein puncture advocated by Dudrick and others has been quite popular, the internal jugular approach as described by Jernigan et al. has been equally satisfactory (Figs. 2-5 and 2-6).

For insertion of the intravenous catheter through the subclavian vein, the patient is placed on his back in a 15° head-down position with a small pad placed between the

Fig. 2-5. Use of the subclavian vein for insertion of central venous catheter.

shoulder blades to allow the shoulders to drop posteriorly. This allows expansion of the subclavian vein and easier penetration. The skin is scrubbed with ether or acetone to defat the surface and then with an iodophor compound. Drapes are carefully placed, and *scrupulous* aseptic precautions are observed. Local anesthetic is infiltrated into the skin, subcutaneous tissue, and periosteum at the inferior border of the midpoint of the clavicle. A 2-in.-long, 14-gauge needle attached to a small syringe is inserted, beveled down through the wheal, and advanced toward the tip of the operator's finger, which is pressed well into the patient's suprasternal notch. The needle should hug the inferior clavicular surface and go over the first rib into the subclavian vein. With slight negative pressure applied to the syringe, entrance into the vein will be noted by the appearance of blood. The needle is advanced a few millimeters further to be sure that it is entirely within the lumen of the vein. The patient is asked to perform a Valsalva maneuver, or the thumb is held over the needle hub as the syringe is removed. A 16-gauge, 8- or 12-in. radiopaque catheter is then introduced through the needle and threaded into the superior vena cava. The needle is then withdrawn from the patient, and a small plastic splint is fitted over the junction of the catheter and needle to prevent catheter severance by the needle. The catheter is

Fig. 2-6. Use of internal jugular vein for insertion of central venous catheter.

connected to a sterile intravenous administration tubing, and a slow infusion is begun while the catheter is sewn to the skin with a small synthetic suture. Antibiotic ointment is applied around the entrance of the catheter into the skin, and an occlusive dressing is applied over it including the junction of the intravenous tubing with the catheter. A chest film is immediately obtained to confirm the position of the radiopaque catheter in the vena cava and to check for a possible pneumothorax.

Every 2 or 3 days, the intravenous tubing is changed, the catheter site is scrubbed as for an operative procedure, and antibiotic ointment and a new occlusive dressing are applied. In general, withdrawal or administration of blood through the catheter or the use of the catheter for central venous pressure measurements should be avoided, since the risk of contamination and catheter occlusion are significantly increased.

The use of the internal jugular approach has also been quite satisfactory and is probably the preferred technique for the pediatric age group. It is probably unwise, unless absolutely necessary, to place catheters into the inferior vena cava from the lower extremities because of the greater likelihood of sepsis and thromboembolic phenomena. Additionally, cut-down catheter insertions into the cephalic or basilic veins have not proved satisfactory.

PREPARATION AND ADMINISTRATION OF SOLUTIONS. The basic solution contains between 20% and 25% dextrose and between 3% and 5% crystalline amino acids in water. The solutions are usually prepared in the pharmacy from commercially available kits containing the component solutions and transfer apparatus. Preparation in the pharmacy under laminar flow reduces the incidence of bacterial contamination of the solution. Proper preparation with suitable quality control is absolutely essential to avoid septic complications.

Since the formulation of commercially available hyperalimentation solutions varies considerably with regard to amino acid and electrolyte concentration, it is imperative that the physician become thoroughly familiar with the levels of the components within the solution utilized. Only in this manner may additives, in the form of additional electrolytes, be rationally planned to meet specific metabolic needs of the patient.

For the average adult patient without significant cardiac, renal, or hepatic disease, a typical hyperalimentation solution would contain components as outlined in Table 2-11. One should recognize that the recommended concentrations of electrolytes are only estimates and that actual requirements may vary considerably between individual patients, dependent on routes of fluid and electrolyte loss, renal function, metabolic rate, cardiac function, and the underlying disease state.

Intravenous vitamin preparations should be added to each bottle of solution as recommended in Table 2-11. In addition, phytonadione (vitamin K_1) 10 mg and folic acid 5 mg should be administered intramuscularly once a week, since these are unstable in the hyperalimentation solution. Cyanocobalamin (vitamin B_{12}) 1000 μg is given by intramuscular injection once a month. Intramuscular administration of iron may be required for patients with iron

Table 2-11. CONSTITUENTS OF SOLUTION FOR
TOTAL PARENTERAL NUTRITION
(PARENTERAL HYPERALIMENTATION)

(*Volume: 1050; osmolarity: 1900 mO; total caloric value:
1030 kcal; nitrogen content: 6.3 Gm*)

Protein equivalent (as crystalline aminoacid)	39 Gm
Dextrose	250 Gm
Calcium	4.7 mEq
Magnesium	8 mEq
Potassium	39 mEq
Sodium	49 mEq
Acetate	36 mEq
Chloride	35 mEq
Phosphate	29 mEq
Vitamin B complex*	2 ml
Ascorbic acid*	500 mg

*One day a week, these additives should be replaced by a
multiple vitamin preparation containing: Vitamin A, 10,000 units;
Ergocalciferol, 1,000 units; Vitamin E, 5 units; Thiamine HCl,
50 mg; Riboflavin, 10 mg; Pyridoxine HCl, 15 mg; Niacinamide,
100 mg; Dexpanthenal, 25 mg; Ascorbic acid, 500 mg.

deficiency anemia. After 30 to 40 days, essential fatty acid
deficiency may become clinically apparent, manifested by
a dry, scaly dermatitis and loss of hair. Chemical confirmation is obtained by noting an increase in the triene to
tetraene ratio (>0.3) of total serum fatty acids. The syndrome may be prevented by weekly administration of a
soybean fat emulsion. Essential trace minerals may be
required after prolonged total parenteral nutrition and
may be supplied by 1 or 2 units of plasma each week.

The infusion is started at 1 to 2 liters/day in the average
adult and gradually increased to tolerance (3 to 4 liters/
day). Rarely, additional intravenous fluids and electrolytes
may be necessary with continued abnormal large losses of
fluids. The patient should be carefully monitored for development of electrolyte, volume, acid-base, and septic
complications. Vital signs and urinary output are regularly
observed, and the patient should be weighed daily. Frequent adjustments of the volume and composition of the
solutions are necessary during the course of therapy. Electrolytes are drawn daily until stable and every 2 or 3 days
thereafter, and the hemogram and blood urea nitrogen are
determined weekly.

The urine sugar level is checked every 6 hours and blood
sugar concentration at least once daily during the first few
days of the infusion and at frequent intervals thereafter.
Relative glucose intolerance may occur following initiation
of parenteral hyperalimentation, and blood sugar levels
may rise as high as 400 mg/100 ml or more. Subsequently,
blood sugar levels usually fall toward normal, urine sugar
levels become negative to 2+, and insulin is not required
in most cases. To avoid excessive glycosuria, the infusion
is maintained at a rate which will not allow urinary glucose
level to exceed a 3+ reaction. However, if blood sugar
levels remain elevated or urine sugar levels again become
3 or 4+, insulin (15 units) may be added to each liter of
solution. The rise in blood glucose concentration observed
after initiating a hyperalimentation program is generally
temporary, as the normal pancreas increases its output of

insulin in response to the continuous carbohydrate infusion. In patients with diabetes mellitus, additional crystalline insulin may be required.

The administration of adequate amounts of potassium
is essential to achieve positive nitrogen balance and replace
depleted intracellular stores. In addition, a significant shift
of potassium ion from the extracellular to the intracellular
space may take place because of the large glucose infusion,
with resultant hypokalemia, metabolic alkalosis, and poor
glucose utilization. In some cases as much as 240 mEq of
potassium ion daily may be required. Hypokalemia may
cause glycosuria, which would be treated with potassium,
not insulin. Thus, before giving insulin, the serum potassium level must be checked to avoid compounding the
hypokalemia.

Often the blood urea nitrogen level rises, even in patients with normal renal function, but azotemia is not a
contraindication to giving the solution if the elevation is
moderate, does not continue to rise sharply, and does
not rise over approximately 80 mg/100 ml. Wilmore and
Dudrick, Abel, and Fischer have demonstrated the safety
and efficacy of parenteral hyperalimentation in patients
with renal failure and some forms of hepatic disease. For
this purpose, special solutions of amino acids are required.
Solutions for patients with acute renal failure contain 40 to
50% dextrose (to provide maximum caloric intake while
restricting the volume of water infused) and only essential
l-amino acids, which are efficiently utilized for protein
synthesis. Solutions designed for patients with hepatic
failure contain increased concentrations of branched-chain
amino acids and decreased levels of the aromatic amino
acids.

There is usually a delay of about a week before weight
gain and positive nitrogen balance become apparent; the
patient then may gain as much as $\frac{1}{2}$ to 1 lb daily. After
several days, one frequently notes marked improvement in
the patient's general appearance and healing of previously
indolent wounds and intestinal fistulas. Dramatic recovery
often ensues, whereas formerly death from inanition inexorably occurred.

FAT EMULSIONS. Recently a 10% fat emulsion, derived
from soybean oil (Intralipid), has been marketed. The
emulsion may be administered without many of the severe
side effects previously observed after infusion of cotton-
seed oil emulsions two decades ago. The use of fat as an
adjunctive nutrient prevents the development of essential
fatty acid deficiency. In addition, the emulsion is not hypertonic and therefore may be delivered via a peripheral
vein. A solution providing a source of nitrogen (5% crystalline amino acid) should be simultaneously infused. Fat
emulsions may not be premixed with amino acid solutions,
since the emulsion becomes unstable. Therefore the solutions are delivered via separate tubing joined together by a
Y connector at the intravenous catheter. Patients with
abnormal fat transport or metabolism, diabetes mellitus,
liver disease, coagulopathy, or serious pulmonary disease
should not receive fat emulsions, since inadequate clearance of fat from the bloodstream, additional hepatic or
pulmonary dysfunction, or clinical hypocoagulability may
be induced. Most investigators advise limitation of admin-

istered fat emulsion in adults to between 1.5 and 2.0 gm/kg body weight per day. Therefore caloric requirements of patients with major burns, severe trauma, and extensive surgical procedures cannot be met by the administration of fat emulsions alone. Furthermore, Long has recently demonstrated that infusion of fat is not as efficient in sparing protein as an isocaloric quantity of carbohydrate.

COMPLICATIONS. One of the more common and serious complications associated with long-term parenteral feeding is sepsis secondary to contamination of the solution, administration tubing, or the central venous catheter. This problem occurs more frequently in patients with systemic sepsis and in many cases is due to hematogenous seeding of the catheter with bacteria. More often, however, it is due to failure to observe strict aseptic precautions during preparation and administration of the solutions. One of the earliest signs of systemic sepsis may be the sudden development of glucose intolerance in a patient who previously has been maintained on parenteral hyperalimentation without difficulty. When this occurs or if fever develops without obvious cause, the solution and intravenous tubing are replaced. Other causes of fever should also be investigated; if fever persists, the infusion catheter should be removed and cultured. Antibiotics may be appropriate at this point in some cases. The catheter may be replaced in the opposite subclavian vein or into one of the internal jugular veins and the infusion restarted. In general, however, it is probably advisable to wait a short period of time before reinserting the catheter.

Other complications related to catheter placement include the development of pneumothorax, hemothorax, or hydrothorax; subclavian artery injury; cardiac arrhythmias if the catheter is placed into the atrium or the ventricle; air embolism or catheter embolism; and, rarely, cardiac perforation with tamponade. Thrombophlebitis or thrombosis of the superior vena cava has been an exceptionally rare complication. All these complications may be avoided by strict adherence to the techniques previously outlined.

Hyperosmolar nonketotic hyperglycemia may develop with normal rates of infusion in patients with impaired glucose tolerance or in any patient if the hypertonic solutions are administered too rapidly. This is a particularly common complication in latent diabetics and in patients following severe surgical stress or trauma. If blood and urine sugar concentrations are not monitored frequently, the blood sugar level may become markedly elevated with ensuing weakness, lethargy, and eventual coma. Treatment of the condition consists of volume replacement with correction of electrolyte abnormalities and the administration of insulin. This particularly serious complication can be avoided with careful attention to daily fluid balance and frequent determinations of urine and blood sugar levels and serum electrolyte content.

A number of volume, concentration, and compositional abnormalities may also develop, but these are largely avoided by careful attention to the details of patient management. This is particularly important for elderly patients and for patients with significant cardiovascular, renal, or hepatic disorders. Changes in the volume and composition of the administered solutions are often necessary to avoid complications. Additionally, the use of parenteral hyperalimentation in pediatric patients requires knowledge of the specific nutritional requirements of this age group and the special precautions that should be observed.

References

Fluid and Electrolyte Therapy

Abouna, G. M., Veazey, P. R., and Terry, D. B.: Intravenous Infusion of Hydrochloric Acid for Treatment of Severe Metabolic Alkalosis, *Surgery,* **75:**194, 1974.

Andersen, O. S., and Engel, K.: A New Acid-Base Nomogram: An Improved Method for the Calculation of the Relevent Blood Acid-Base Data, *Scand J Clin Lab Invest,* **12:**177, 1960.

Astrup, P., Jorgensen, K., Andersen, O. S., and Engel, K.: The Acid-Base Metabolism: A New Approach, *Lancet,* **1:**1035, 1960.

Bartlett, W. C.: Acute Hyperparathyroid Crisis, *Am J Surg,* **114:**796, 1967.

Baxter, C. R., Zedlitz, W. H., and Shires, G. T.: High-Output Acute Renal Failure Complicating Traumatic Injury, *J Trauma,* **4:**467, 1964.

Bishop, R. L., and Weisfeldt, M. L.: Sodium Bicarbonate Administration during Cardiac Arrest: Effect on Arterial pH, P_{CO_2} and Osmolality, *JAMA,* **235:**506, 1976.

Canizaro, P. C., Nelson, J., and Hennessy, J.: Alterations in Oxygen Transport, in G. T. Shires, C. J. Carrico, and P. C. Canizaro, "Shock," W. B. Saunders Company, Philadelphia, vol. XIII, 1973.

———, Prager, M. D., and Shires, G. T.: The Infusion of Ringer's Lactate Solution during Shock, *Am J Surg,* **122:**494, 1971.

Collins, J. A.: Problems Associated with the Massive Transfusion of Stored Blood, *Surgery,* **75:**274, 1974.

Cooper, N., Brazier, J. R., Hottenrott, C., Mulder, D. G., Maloney, J. V., and Buckberg, C. D.: Myocardial Depression Following Citrated Blood Transfusion, *Arch Surg,* **107:**756, 1973.

Elias, E. G., and Evans, J. T.: Hypercalcemic Crisis in Neoplastic Diseases: Management with Mithramycin, *Surgery,* **71:**631, 1972.

Harken, A. H., Gabel, R. A., Fencl, V., and Moore, F. D.: Hydrochloric Acid in the Correction of Metabolic Acidosis, *Arch Surg,* **110:**819, 1975.

Henzel, J. H., DeWeese, M. S., and Ridenhour, G.: Significance of Magnesium and Zinc Metabolism in the Surgical Patient. I. Magnesium, *Arch Surg,* **95:**974, 1967.

Jenkins, M. T., and Beck, G. P.: Differential Diagnosis of Hypotension Occurring during Anesthesia and Surgery, *Clin Anesthiol,* **3:**106, 1963.

Mattar, J. A., Weil, M. H., Shubin, H., and Stein, L.: Cardiac Arrest in the Critically Ill. II. Hyperosmolal States Following Cardiac Arrest, *Am J Med,* **56:**162, 1974.

McClelland, R. N., Shires, G. T., Baxter, C. R., Coln, C. D., and Carrico, C. J.: Balanced Salt Solution in the Treatment of Hemorrhagic Shock: Studies in Dogs, *JAMA,* **199:**830, 1967.

Mellemgaard, K., and Astrup, P.: The Quantitative Determination of Surplus Amounts of Acid or Base in the Human Body, *Scand J Clin Lab Invest,* **12:**187, 1960.

Mengoli, L. R.: Excerpts from the History of Postoperative Fluid Therapy, *Am J Surg,* **121:**311, 1971.

Moncrief, J. A., and Mason, A. D.: Water Vapor Loss in the Burned Patient, *Surg Forum,* **13:**38, 1962.

Moore, F. D., Olesen, K. H., McMurrey, J. D., Parker, H. V., Ball, M. R., and Boyden, C. M.: "Body Cell Mass and Its Supporting Environment: Body Composition in Health and Disease," W. B. Saunders Company, Philadelphia, 1963.

Moyer, C. A.: "Fluid Balance." Year Book Medical Publishers, Inc., Chicago, 1954.

Randall, R. E., Jr., Cohen, M. D., Spray, C. C., Jr., and Rossmeisl, E. C.: Hypermagnesemia in Renal Failure: Etiology and Toxic Manifestations, *Ann Intern Med,* **61:**73, 1964.

Schwarz, W. B., and Relman, A. S.: A Critique of the Parameters Used in the Evaluation of Acid-Base Disorders, *N Engl J Med,* **268:**1382, 1963.

Shavelle, H. S., and Parke, R.: Postoperative Alkalosis and Acute Renal Failure: Rationale for the Use of Hydrochloric Acid, *Surgery,* **78:**439, 1975.

Shires, G. T., Cunningham, J. N., Baker, C. R. F., Reeder, S. F., Illner, H., Wagner, I. Y., and Maher, J.: Alterations in Cellular Membrane Function During Hemorrhagic Shock in Primates, *Ann Surg,* **176:**288, 1972.

————, and Holman, V.: Dilutional Acidosis, *Ann Intern Med,* **28:**551, 1948.

————, and Jackson, D. E.: Postoperative Salt Tolerance, *Arch Surg,* **84:**703, 1962.

————, Williams, J., and Brown, F.: Acute Changes in Extracellular Fluids Associated with Major Surgical Procedures, *Ann Surg,* **154:**803, 1961.

Singer, R. B., and Hastings, A. B.: An Improved Clinical Method for the Estimation of Disturbances of the Acid-Base Balance of Human Blood, *Medicine,* **27:**223, 1948.

Thompson, J. E., Vollman, R. W., Austin, D. J., and Kartchner, M. M.: Prevention of Hypotensive and Renal Complications of Aortic Surgery Using Balanced Salt Solution, *Ann Surg,* **167:**767, 1968.

Tuller, M. A., and Mehdi, F.: Compensatory Hypoventilation and Hypercapnia in Primary Metabolic Alkalosis, *Am J Med,* **50:**281, 1971.

Wright, H. K., and Gann, D. S.: Correction of Defect in Free Water Excretion in Postoperative Patients by Extracellular Fluid Volume Expansion, *Ann Surg,* **158:**70, 1963.

Nutrition

Ballinger, W. F., Collins, J. A., Drucker, W. R., Dudrick, S. J., and Zeppa, R.: "Manual of Surgical Nutrition," W. B. Saunders Company, Philadelphia, 1975.

Boles, T., and Zollinger, R. M.: Critical Evaluation of Jejunostomy, *Arch Surg,* **65:**358, 1952.

Bury, K. D., Stephens, R. V., and Randall, H. T.: Use of a Chemically Defined, Liquid, Elemental Diet for Nutritional Management of Fistulas of the Alimentary Tract, *Am J Surg,* **121:**174, 1971.

Cahill, G. F., Jr.: Body Fuels and Their Metabolism, *Bull Am Coll Surg,* **55:**12, 1970.

Cuthbertson, D. P.: The Disturbance of Metabolism Produce by Bony and Non-bony Injury, with Notes on Certain Abnormal Conditions of Bone, *Biochem J,* **24:**1244, 1930.

Dudrick, S. J., Groff, D. B., and Wilmore, D. W.: Long-Term Venous Catheterization in Infants, *Surg Gynecol Obstet,* **129:**805, 1969.

————, Steiger, E., and Long, J. M.: Renal Failure in Surgical Patients: Treatment with Intravenous Essential Amino Acids and Hypertonic Glucose, *Surgery,* **68:**180, 1970.

————, ————, ————, Ruberg, R. L., Allen, T. R., Vars, H. M., and Rhoads, J. E.: General Principles and Techniques of Intravenous Hyperalimentation, in G. S. M. Cowan, Jr., and W. L. Scheetz (eds.), "Intravenous Hyperalimentation," Lea & Febiger, Philadelphia, 1972.

————, Wilmore, D. W., Vars, H. M., and Rhoads, J. E.: Long-Term Parenteral Nutrition with Growth, Development, and Positive Nitrogen Balance, *Surgery,* **64:**134, 1968.

Felig, P., Pozefsky, T., Marliss, E., and Cahill, G. F., Jr.: Alanine: Key Role in Gluconeogenesis, *Science,* **167:**1003, 1970.

Fischer, J. E.: "Total Parenteral Nutrition," Little, Brown and Company, Boston, 1976.

Graham, W. P., and Royster, H. P.: Simplified Cervical Esophagostomy for Long-Term Extraoral Feeding, *Surg Gynecol Obstet,* **125:**127, 1967.

Gump, F. E., Kinney, J. M., and Price, J. B., Jr.: Energy Metabolism in Surgical Patients: Oxygen Consumption and Blood Flow, *J Surg Res,* **10:**613, 1970.

Jernigan, W. R., Gardner, W. C., Mahr, M. M., and Milburn, J. L.: Use of the Internal Jugular Vein for Placement of Central Venous Catheter, *Surg Gynecol Obstet,* **130:**520, 1970.

Kinney, J. M.: A Consideration of Energy Exchange in Human Trauma, *Bull NY Acad Med,* **36:**617, 1960.

Long, J. M., Wilmore, D. W., Mason, A. D., Jr., and Pruitt, B. A., Jr.: Effect of Carbohydrate and Fat Intake on Nitrogen Excretion during Total Intravenous Feeding, *Ann Surg,* **185:**417, 1977.

McDougal, W. S., Wilmore, D. W., and Pruitt, B. A., Jr.: Glucose-Dependent Hepatic Membrane Transport in Nonbacteremic and Bacteremic Thermally Injured Patients, *J Surg Res,* **22:**697, 1977.

McMinn, R. M. H.: "Tissue Repair," Academic Press, Inc., New York, 1969.

Moore, F. D.: "Metabolic Care of the Surgical Patient," W. B. Saunders Company, Philadelphia, 1960.

White, P. L., and Nagy, M. E.: "Total Parenteral Nutrition," Publishing Sciences Group, Inc., Acton, Mass., 1974.

Wilmore, D. W., and Dudrick, S. J.: Treatment of Acute Renal Failure with Intravenous Essential L-amino Acids, *Arch Surg,* **99:**669, 1969.

Winters, R. W., and Hasselmeyer, E. G.: "Intravenous Nutrition in the High Risk Infant," John Wiley & Sons, New York, 1975.

Chapter 3

Hemostasis, Surgical Bleeding, and Transfusion

by Seymour I. Schwartz

Few events in clinical medicine are so ominous as the failure of hemostasis. For the surgeon, few failures in normal physiology are potentially so catastrophic. Disruption in normal hemostasis often can be anticipated, just as the physiologic failure usually can be identified and corrected. In this chapter the reader will become acquainted with the events of normal hemostasis. Advances in understanding in this area have come largely from the laboratory, not the clinic. As a consequence of this and because of the complex nature of some of the events involved, disproportionate emphasis often is placed upon the laboratory in attempting to solve what, primarily, are clinical problems. We shall try to provide a background whereby the problems encountered can be solved by careful evaluation of the patient and judicious use of the laboratory. A desired by-product will be the evolution of logical therapeutic programs. These may include methods for local control of bleeding, replacement for the loss of circulating blood volume, and selective transfusion of physiologic products necessary to provide normal hemostasis.

BIOLOGY OF NORMAL HEMOSTASIS

Cessation of blood flow from an injured vessel, the cumulative phenomenon we call hemostasis, occurs as a result of many events. Blood coagulation frequently is equated with hemostasis. Coagulation is not, however, always the central or most important factor. Clinical testimony to this heresy is supplied by the patient with congenital afibrinogenemia. This illness, characterized in the laboratory by incoagulability of the blood, may present clinically as a relatively minor hemostatic problem. This paradox is explained by the important role of the platelets, which, in this setting, are able to function in a near-normal manner because of the trace amount of fibrinogen present on their surface.

The accomplishment of hemostasis depends, to a variable degree, on the clinical condition of the patient, the nature of insult to the blood vessel, the type of vessel or vessels injured, the anatomic site of injury, the coagulation mechanism, and fibrinolytic activity. A lateral incision in a small artery may remain open because of physical forces and can be associated with extensive and continued bleeding. By contrast, a complete transection of a similar-sized vessel, as Hunter demonstrated centuries ago, contracts to the extent that the bleeding may cease spontaneously. Illustrative of the importance of anatomic site of injury is the fact that bleeding from a small venule ruptured by trauma in the thigh of a healthy athlete may be negligible because of the support of surrounding muscle. Bleeding from a similar vessel due to trauma of the nasal mucosa may be extensive in the same individual. An elderly person with atrophy of the subcutaneous connective tissue or a patient who has received corticosteroid therapy for a long time may sustain a large ecchymosis from minor trauma to the dorsum of the hand, while a younger person might note no change secondary to comparable trauma at the same site. Normal hemostasis, then, results from the interplay of multiple factors. A gross defect in one function or a lesser defect involving multiple functions usually

Fig. 3-1. Schematic representation of hemostasis.

HEMOSTASIS

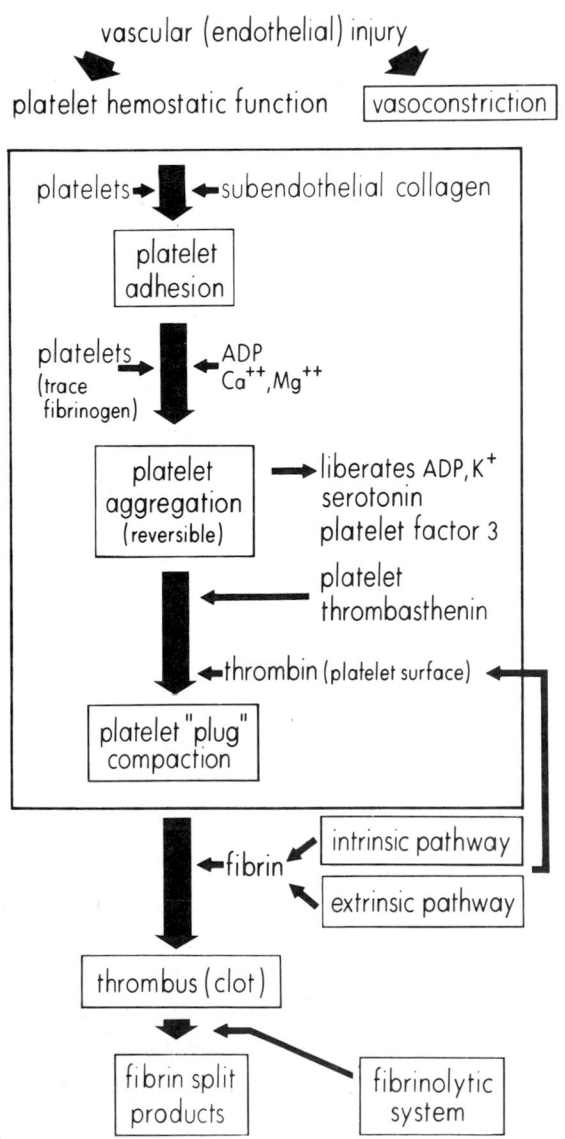

proves necessary to effect significant bleeding. Description of the events of normal hemostasis will permit consideration of the points at which failure may occur and also provides an opportunity to correlate laboratory tests with their physiologic counterparts.

VASCULAR RESPONSE. The initial vascular response to injury, even at the capillary level, is that of vasoconstriction. Experimental observation has demonstrated that adherence of endothelial cell to endothelial cell, with obliteration of microdefects, may, in itself, be sufficient to effect hemostasis. Whether vasoconstriction of these small vessels is neurogenically or humorally mediated remains unsettled. Human platelets normally carry vasoactive amines, some of which are liberated at the site of injury. The initial vasoconstriction described, however, occurs prior to platelet adherence at the site of injury. Animal experiments demonstrate that when platelets have been depleted of serotonin in vivo and vascular injury has been produced, vasoconstriction still occurs.

Patients with a mild bleeding disorder have been described in whom the only laboratory abnormality is a prolonged bleeding time. Capillary microscopy in certain of these patients reveals that the capillary loops do not constrict following injury. A capillary structural defect has been postulated, and support for this concept is provided by the observation that, even in the absence of trauma, the capillary loops are dilated and tortuous.

PLATELET FUNCTION. In less than 15 seconds following vascular injury, platelets (Fig. 3-1) adhere to the injured margins of the vessels. For many years it was believed that the platelets adhered directly to the injured endothelial cells. More recently, phase microscopy and electron microscopic observations have revealed that this early platelet adherence is to subendothelial collagen fibrils. The mechanism of attraction between collagen fibrils and platelets has not been defined, nor has the physiologic significance clearly been established. Two types of observations suggest that the platelet-collagen interaction is important. Quick demonstrated that the bleeding time, fastidiously performed, may be lengthened in patients taking aspirin. Platelet-rich plasma derived from patients taking aspirin demonstrates an impairment of the platelet-collagen reaction in vitro. The second observation, related to the first, is that of Vigliano and Horowitz. These writers described a patient with multiple myeloma and hemorrhagic tendency in whom the principal laboratory abnormality was impairment of the collagen-platelet interaction.

Within seconds of the collagen-platelet response, platelets begin to adhere to one another at the site of injury. The initial aggregation is loose. The loose aggregates may be fragmented and dispersed by the pressure of blood issuing from tiny arterioles. This platelet aggregation is thought to occur as a result of a platelet-ADP (adenosinediphosphate) interaction. Gaarder et al. initially demonstrated that ADP, added in minute amounts, results in rapid platelet aggregate formation in whole blood or platelet-rich plasma. Trace amounts of calcium or magnesium are necessary for this reaction. Interestingly, and probably significantly, heparin does not interfere with this reaction. The maintenance of normal hemostasis in the heparinized patient may well be explained by the platelets' ability to aggregate loosely at sites of minimal trauma, even when the blood is relatively incoagulable.

A relatively rare clinical entity, thrombasthenia of the Glanzmann type, may represent a naturally occurring failure of hemostasis at this level. Platelets from such patients fail to aggregate in the presence of ADP. This is not their only abnormality of platelet function, for blood clots from these patients also display poor retraction. The platelets lack fibrinogen, and it is possible that all these abnormalities are related.

Following the formation of the loose platelet aggregate the mass of platelets begins to compact. When observed microscopically, the platelets lose their individual identity and begin to fuse with one another. The platelet granules concentrate toward the center of the platelet, and fibrin strands now can be identified scattered throughout the platelet mass. These changes are described as viscous metamorphosis and have a biochemical counterpart. During compaction the platelets, normally rich in adenosinetriphosphate (ATP), suffer a drop in content of this energy-rich compound and liberate ADP. Potassium and serotonin, normally present in platelets, also are liberated at this time. Platelet factor 3 (phospholipid) is made available for the clotting process, but a small amount probably becomes available earlier. Platelet factor 3 is a normal component within the platelet membrane as well as in certain of the platelet granules.

The events initiating these morphologic and biochemical processes have not been established with certainty. Probably trace amounts of the enzyme thrombin are formed at the surface of the platelet. All the necessary plasma factors are present in the immediate plasmatic environment of the platelet. All the observed platelet changes can be produced in vitro by the addition of trace amounts of thrombin. Indirect experimental data suggest that this also occurs in vivo.

The events culminating in the compaction of the loose platelet aggregate into a "platelet plug" seem to correspond to what we measure with the bleeding time. Failure of any of the early events described above can result in lengthening of the bleeding time.

Approximately 15 percent of human platelet protein is contractile. This material is called *thrombosthenin*. It is very similar to muscle actomyosin and is an ATPase. Compaction of the platelet plug is credited to the contractile protein, which participates in the biochemical events as well. The platelets' responses to thrombin end in destruction of the platelets as intact cells. The sequential changes in the platelets have been described as preaggregation, aggregation, thrombocytorrhexis, and thrombocytolysis.

The platelet is equipped to enhance its function in many ways. Laboratory studies have demonstrated that platelets are capable of liberating enough ADP during hydrolysis of the energy-rich ATP to supply their own stimulus for the ADP aggregation. Interestingly, ADP aggregation is facilitated by amines which also are liberated from the platelets early in their hemostatic function. The serotonin which is released may induce vascular constriction in the immediate area. While evidence for the importance of

serotonin in normal hemostasis is lacking, its presence is provocative.

BLOOD COAGULATION. Until this point in the hemostatic process, the role of blood coagulation has been inferential and invoked only to explain the initiation of viscous metamorphosis by the platelets. Microscopic clotting, assumed to take place at the platelet surface, is thought to evolve through the effects of tissue thromboplastin on the plasma procoagulant substances at the platelet surface. Reliance on the concept of a *tissue* thromboplastin leading to microscopic clotting at the platelet surface, rather than an *intrinsic* thromboplastin, is explained by the normal platelet function and bleeding time with defects in intrinsic thromboplastin formation.

The complex series of reactions that ultimately leads to the transformation of the soluble protein fibrinogen to the insoluble fibrin clot constitutes the process of coagulation. Failure at any one of the stages may manifest itself as a potential bleeding disorder. The importance of blood coagulation has been appreciated since antiquity. Allowable exceptions to the covenant of circumcision demanded by the Old Testament are described in the Babylonian Talmud. While our understanding of blood clotting has become somewhat more precise since that time, a degree of faith remains requisite in the student of the hemostatic process. Nowhere is this better demonstrated than in the earliest step in the coagulation process, activation of factor XII.

Factor XII (Hageman factor) deficiency results in lengthening of the whole blood clotting time. Despite this gross laboratory abnormality, the deficiency is not associated with significant hemostatic problems. A patient named Hageman, the first patient demonstrated to have this deficiency, underwent gastrectomy without bleeding complication. Interestingly, the same patient succumbed to complications of thromboembolic disease many years later.

The concept of the blood coagulation mechanism representing a "waterfall," or "cascade," phenomenon was developed simultaneously and independently by Davie and Ratnoff and by Macfarlane (Fig. 3-2). These writers view the activation of factor XII as the initiation of the coagulation sequence. In vitro studies demonstrate that activation of factor XII is accomplished by virtually any nonendothelial surface. The activated factor XII, which differs from the inactive form in certain physicochemical features, has enzymatic properties. The substrate for activated factor XII is believed to be factor XI (plasma thromboplastin antecedent, PTA). Factor XI seemingly can be changed to its activated form without depending upon activated factor XII. This could explain the absence of hemostatic problems in patients with factor XII deficiency.

Deficiency of factor XI clinically is associated with a mild bleeding disorder known as *Rosenthal's syndrome*. This is inherited as an incompletely recessive autosomal trait. Factor XI behaves as an enzyme when activated either by factor XII or by some unexplained process. Factor IX (Christmas factor, plasma thromboplastin component, PTC) serves as the substrate for activated factor XI. This step requires the presence of ionized calcium. Deficiency of factor IX is characterized clinically by the disorder known as *Christmas disease, PTC deficiency,* or *hemophilia B.* This sex-linked recessive trait will be discussed later in the chapter.

Activated factor IX is believed to have enzymatic activity interacting with its specific substrate factor VIII (antihemophilic factor, AHF). The effect of factor IX upon factor VIII requires the presence of phospholipid (platelet factor 3) as well as ionized calcium. Although the phospholipid normally is contributed by the platelets, it is clear from in vitro studies that other tissues may serve as a source. Under pathologic circumstances, such as massive intravascular hemolysis, it is possible that the phospholipid can be derived from the red blood cell membrane. Inherited deficiency of factor VIII clinically is represented by classical hemophilia, or hemophilia A.

The events in blood coagulation described until this point are relatively time-consuming. The steps leading to the activation of factor VIII probably consume 90 percent of the time that is required for blood to clot grossly. Accordingly, defects within this portion of the clotting sequence are characterized by prolonged whole blood clotting time when severe or by abnormalities in other test systems which relate to this slower phase of blood coagulation.

Activated factor VIII is believed to use factor X (Stuart-Prower factor) as its substrate. Factor X deficiency is a rare but potentially serious disorder which may manifest laboratory abnormalities characteristic of both the earlier and later phases of blood coagulation. Thus, severe deficiency of factor X may result in a prolonged whole blood clotting time and impaired prothrombin consumption. Such a deficiency also invariably will prolong the one-stage *prothrombin time.* Activated factor X appears to act upon, or act with, factor V (proaccelerin). When this stage is completed, the activator *prothrombinase* has evolved. In the presence of ionized calcium, prothrombinase will split the prothrombin molecule (factor II) to form the smaller molecular species thrombin. Figure 3-2 schematically depicts the foregoing discussion. Examples of each of the clinical deficiencies will be discussed subsequently.

Normal hemostasis also requires the integrity of the extrinsic system of blood coagulation (Fig. 3-3). This pathway of blood coagulation takes origin with the interaction of tissue lipoprotein (tissue thromboplastin) and factor VII (proconvertin). Factor X then is activated, and the sequence continues as previously described for the intrinsic system. The formation of the platelet hemostatic plug, described earlier, is believed to be triggered by the effect of thrombin on the platelet surface. An explanation for this early appearance of a trace amount of thrombin, too soon to be explained by the more leisurely intrinsic pathway of blood coagulation, is the "shortcut" provided by tissue thromboplastin and factor VII as the extrinsic clotting system.

The in vitro equivalent of the extrinsic pathway is the one-stage prothrombin determination. In this test an extrinsic source of tissue lipoprotein and calcium is added

Fig. 3-2. "Waterfall" phenomenon: intrinsic pathway for the formation of thrombin. The inhibitors of various steps and the alterations induced by thrombin in antihemophilic factor and proaccelerin are omitted from the diagram. (*From C. R. M. Prentice and O. D. Ratnoff, Semin Hematol, 4:93, 1967.*)

to plasma. Deficiencies in factor VII, factor X, factor V, or fibrinogen will lengthen the clotting time in this test. Since delays in clotting in this test are measured in seconds, it is clear that defects in this portion of the process will not noticeably lengthen the whole blood clotting time. The range of normal for the whole blood clotting time is appreciable, and even a substantial lengthening of the prothrombin time would be obscured within the variability of the whole blood clotting time.

The role of thrombin in the hemostatic mechanism has been the focus of much study. Thrombin probably serves as an initiator of the biochemical and functional platelet changes early in normal hemostasis. It has the ability to enhance strikingly the activation of certain of the blood clotting factors, e.g., factor V, factor VIII, and factor XIII (fibrin-stabilizing factor). The key position occupied by thrombin is emphasized further by our clinical approach to anticoagulation. On one hand the coumarin drugs are used to impair synthesis of those precursors that will lead to thrombin generation, while on the other hand the efficacy of heparin is its ability to impair or interfere with the effect of thrombin on fibrinogen.

The chemistry of the thrombin-fibrinogen reaction now is well characterized. Thrombin enzymatically cleaves two pairs of peptide chains from the fibrinogen molecule. The action of thrombin on fibrinogen ends at that point. Thereafter, the soluble fibrinogen monomers, which are the fibrinogen molecules minus the two pairs of peptide chains, unite by hydrogen bonding. This is a loose chemical bond that is easily separated. The weak formation is converted to a stable one through the enzymatic activity of factor XIII, fibrin-stabilizing factor. This enzyme probably works by facilitating conversion of sulfhydryl groups to disulfide bonds.

Inherited and acquired hemostatic abnormalities have been identified for these steps. Impaired organization of the fibrin monomers occurs in dysglobulinemic states, and the faulty clot structure has been blamed for the bleeding tendency. Congenital and acquired deficiencies of factor XIII have been described. Of interest to the surgeon is the repeated observation of impaired wound healing in patients with factor XIII deficiency. In vitro studies have suggested that fibroblasts grown on a medium lacking factor XIII show faulty organization, and it is possible that the biologic importance of factor XIII lies outside the immediate realm of hemostasis.

CLOT DISSOLUTION. Fibrinolysis (Fig. 3-4) is the mechanism by which dissolution of blood clots occurs. Although fibrinolysis is not necessarily part of the hemostatic mechanism, excessive fibrinolysis may cause failure of hemostasis. The process of clot dissolution is as complex as the clotting system itself but is not yet as thoroughly understood. The enzyme plasmin, which is derived from a precursor plasma protein (plasminogen), is essential to the mechanism of fibrinolysis. Under the influence of kinases, which may be blood activators, tissue activators, streptokinase, or urokinase, the precursor plasma protein (plasminogen) is converted into an enzyme with proteolytic activity (plasmin). There is some question as to whether the kinases act directly on plasminogen or transform a

Fig. 3-3. Extrinsic pathway for the formation of thrombin. Inhibitors of the various steps and alterations induced by thrombin in proaccelerin are omitted from the diagram. (*From C. R. M. Prentice and O. D. Ratnoff, Semin Hematol, 4:93, 1967.*)

proactivator in the human plasma into an activator, which in turn converts plasminogen into plasmin. While fibrin is its preferred substrate, plasmin also can digest fibrinogen, factor V, and factor VIII. The fibrinolytic system can be activated in many ways, including by activated factor XII. It is likely that fibrinolysis progresses at the same time that the blood-clotting process itself is being activated. The initiation of fibrinolysis may arise from tissue sources, vascular endothelium representing a particularly likely possibility. Ischemia is a potent stimulator of the activation of the fibrinolytic system.

What Sherry has viewed as "physiologic proteolysis" results from the natural affinity of plasminogen for fibrin. The latter adsorbs the former during clot formation. The plasminogen then is in position to attack only the fibrin to which it is adsorbed, a locally controlled form of fibrinolysis resulting. On the other hand, pathologic proteolysis may occur when plasminogen free in the plasma is activated. The activated plasminogen may then attack other coagulant proteins as well.

The failure of hemostasis related to excessive activation or ineffective inactivation of the fibrinolytic system is due to several factors. The smaller fragments of fibrin liberated by proteolysis may interfere with normal platelet aggrega-

Fig. 3-4. Fibrinolytic system.

FIBRINOLYTIC SYSTEM

tion. The larger fibrin fragments are incorporated into the clot in lieu of normal fibrin monomers and create an unstable clot. When proteolysis is excessive, other plasma clotting factors also serve as substrates for protein digestion. Human blood normally has a high content of antiplasmin, which inhibits plasminogen activation, and platelets are also believed to possess an antifibrinolytic property.

TESTS OF HEMOSTASIS AND BLOOD COAGULATION

BLEEDING TIME. This is the time required for bleeding to cease after a standard skin incision has been made. The bleeding time probably corresponds to that time required for compaction of the platelet plug in the hemostatic process described above.

With the Duke technique, a clean 2- or 3-mm incision is made with a #11 Bard-Parker blade in the most dependent portion of the earlobe. A piece of filter paper is held below the wound, but not touching it, to catch each drop of blood as it forms and falls. The paper is held so that each drop strikes the margin of the filter paper serially. In this way, a permanent record of the bleeding time can be obtained and, if desired, entered in the patient's chart. The wound itself should not be disturbed, since this may prolong the bleeding time. When blood flow ceases, the time lapse following incision is recorded as the bleeding time. The upper limits of normal vary but probably should not exceed $3\frac{1}{2}$ minutes. The Ivy technique requires the placement of a blood pressure cuff above the elbow with inflation to 40 mm Hg pressure. A standard 5-mm incision is made to a depth of 2 mm on the volar surface of the forearm, taking care to avoid any obvious venules in the skin. Pressure within the cuff is maintained while a piece of filter paper is employed to touch the drops of blood carefully as they form. Once again, the wound must not be disturbed. With this method, a normal upper limit of 5 minutes is accepted. If the above tests are equivocal, an incision made through a template slit method of Mielke et al. will provide a more accurate result.

In our experience, abnormalities of bleeding time usually are fairly clear-cut. The bleeding time usually is normal in patients with a platelet count greater than 75,000/mm³. Patients with a qualitative platelet abnormality (thrombocytopathia or thrombasthenia), patients with defective capillaries as described earlier in this chapter, or patients with von Willebrand's disease all may have prolonged bleeding time. Aspirin ingested within 1 week will affect the results. Bleeding times as prolonged as 24 minutes have been related to aspirin alone.

RUMPEL-LEEDE (TOURNIQUET) TEST. This test, to our view, has little clinical application today. It is designed to estimate capillary fragility. A blood pressure cuff is applied to the upper arm and inflated to a pressure midway between diastolic and systolic pressure. The pressure is maintained at that level for a maximum of 5 minutes—less if many petechiae appear on the forearm before that time. Semiquantification of capillary fragility is obtained by counting the number of petechiae seen within a predetermined area, which should be at some distance from the blood pressure cuff. The antecubital space is not used, for some normal individuals will show petechiae in this area. No more than 2 to 4 petechiae should be seen in a circle of 2.5 cm diameter.

The test need not be performed on patients known to have a low platelet count or prolonged bleeding time. The demonstration of capillary fragility will not contribute to the diagnosis in such circumstances. Rather, it results in some discomfort to the patient, and the petechiae merely serve as a frightening reminder that something is grossly abnormal. The test characteristically is abnormal when thrombocytopenia is present, but this may be determined readily by inspection of the blood smear or a direct platelet count. It also may be abnormal in the group of patients with prolonged bleeding time as well as in elderly patients with poor tissue turgor. Severe vitamin C deficiency also may result in a positive tourniquet test.

PLATELET ESTIMATION AND COUNT. Thrombocytopenia is the most common abnormality of hemostasis encountered in the surgical patient. Microscopic examination of a properly stained blood smear can provide much information about such patients. When an area where the red blood cells display their customary central pallor and where few of the red blood cells overlap one another is examined, 15 to 20 platelets per oil immersion field should be noted. If the blood is not anticoagulated before the smear is prepared, as many as half of these may be in clumps of three or four platelets. A well-stained blood smear that fails to display more than three or four platelets in at least every other oil immersion field can be considered significantly thrombocytopenic. In this situation, the patient's platelet count generally is less than 75,000/mm³. Blood smears which must be searched because platelets appear in only every four or five oil immersion fields usually represent platelet counts of fewer than 40,000/mm³. If cover slip smears have been prepared, the cover slips always should be mounted as matched pairs. Platelets occasionally stick to one of the cover slips, and examination of both will obviate a false impression of thrombocytopenia. Lightly stained blood smears may appear thrombocytopenic in that the platelets are not prominent enough to attract the examiner's attention.

Inspection of the blood smear has the other obvious advantage of permitting the examiner to identify additional pathologic features which may have meaning in the care of the patient. The presence of nucleated red blood cells or abnormal white cells can provide information important to the diagnosis. The presence of giant platelets or large fragments of megakaryocyte cytoplasm also will alert the examiner to possible pathologic platelet function.

Direct enumeration of blood platelets can be accomplished quite accurately. The most reliable microscopic method is that described by Brecher and Cronkite, employing the phase contrast microscope. With this method, normal values ranging from 160,000 to 350,000/mm³ are obtained. Electronic particle counters recently have been adapted for platelet counting. The degree of precision matches that obtained by phase contrast microscopy. *Spontaneous* bleeding only rarely can be related to thrombocytopenia with platelet counts greater than 50,000/mm³. Platelet counts of 60,000 to 70,000/mm³ usually are sufficient to provide adequate hemostasis following trauma or surgical procedures if other hemostatic factors are normal.

CLOT RETRACTION. Normal platelet function is responsible for retraction of the clot, but this gross phenomenon has no clear function in hemostasis. The macroscopic event, however, may well have its microscopic equivalent in the compaction of the platelet plug.

Semiquantification of this platelet function can be obtained. If an applicator stick, string, or partially straightened paper clip is suspended in 5 ml of freshly drawn blood and the blood permitted to clot undisturbed about this object, the clot can be removed 1 hour following coagulation and the serum that has been expressed from the clot measured. Clot retraction then can be expressed as a percentage of the serum related to the original volume of blood. With blood of normal hematocrit, the usual range is 40 percent or slightly higher. Normally, clot retraction in a test tube is complete within 3 or 4 hours at room temperature. A rough relationship exists between the platelet count and clot retraction. Significant thrombocytopenia can exist in the presence of normal clot retraction, since the clot will retract well if the platelet count is slightly less than 100,000/mm³.

OTHER TESTS OF PLATELET FUNCTION. The ability of the platelets to liberate platelet factor 3 (phospholipid), essential in tiny amounts at several stages of the blood-clotting process (Fig. 3-2), also can be measured. Impairment of platelet factor 3 release has been reported in conditions described as *thrombocytopathia*. This defect can represent a primary disease entity, but similar impairment has been described as a secondary phenomenon in uremia and liver disease. Whether the impairment plays a functional role, for example, in the bleeding associated with uremia, remains uncertain. The inability of the platelet to make platelet factor 3 available for the clotting process may be a part of a more fundamental surface membrane abnormality.

The role of ADP in platelet aggregation during hemostasis has been mentioned earlier. The ability of platelets to aggregate in plasma upon the addition of ADP serves as another test of platelet function. Failure of platelets to aggregate following the addition of ADP is seen in patients with the Glanzmann type of thrombasthenia and also, artifactually, when anticoagulants, such as EDTA, which tightly bind divalent cations, are used.

The ability of platelets to adhere to a standardized glass bead column also has been used as a measure of platelet function. This test, refined by Salzman, is reported to be grossly abnormal in patients with von Willebrand's disease. The test requires meticulous preparation of the glass bead column and, while of great interest, does not yet enjoy total acceptance.

WHOLE BLOOD COAGULATION TIME. This test is of historical interest as a diagnostic aid but is quite insensitive as a detector of coagulation defects. The most commonly employed method is a modification of the Lee-White method, in which venous blood is removed by clean venipuncture and 1-ml volumes are delivered into each of three tubes. The first tube is tilted every 30 seconds until no flow of blood is observed. A similar procedure is carried out sequentially on the second and third tubes. The clotting time is taken as the elapsed time from the drawing of blood until coagulation is observed in the third tube.

The coagulation time of blood so studied is influenced by many factors. Several of these relate to the amount of surface activation occurring during the procedure. The smaller the amount of blood relative to the size of the tube, the greater the surface contact and activation. If the tube is tilted more frequently than every 30 seconds, surface activation also is increased. If the venipuncture has not been made cleanly, even minute amounts of tissue juice (tissue thromboplastin) may accelerate the clotting time. To obviate the latter a two-syringe technique may be used. Following successful venipuncture, 1 or 2 ml of blood is drawn into the first syringe, which is carefully disconnected while the needle is held in place and the second syringe attached. Blood is then drawn into the second syringe and provides the sample for the determination. When 1 ml of blood is added, with care to avoid bubbling, to 3 to 10 mm inner diameter clean glass test tubes, the normal range for clotting in the third tube is between 9 and 14 minutes. For practical purposes, only severe deficiencies of factors VIII, IX, XI, XII, and rarely X will be detected by this method. The sensitivity of the test can be increased by employing silicone-coated syringes and clotting tubes or by using plastic syringes and plastic (Lusteroid) tubes. When the latter are employed, the normal clotting time is up to 40 minutes. The test performed with untreated glassware finds its principal use in the control of patients receiving anticoagulation treatment with heparin.

ONE-STAGE PROTHROMBIN TIME (QUICK TEST). This test measures the speed of the events described earlier as the extrinsic pathway of blood coagulation. A tissue source of procoagulant, ideally derived from acetone-dehydrated rabbit brain, as described by Quick, is added with calcium to an aliquot of citrated plasma and the clotting time determined. The laboratory should establish a normal dilution curve and normal values daily. The 100 percent value using the method of Quick should be 15 seconds. Using other sources of tissue thromboplastin, the 100 percent value may be as low as 11 seconds. The prothrombin time will be prolonged in the presence of even minute amounts of heparin. The presence of heparin, by its antithrombin action, will artificially prolong the clotting time of the mixture so that it appears that the prothrombin complex is low, Accordingly, an accurate prothrombin determination cannot be carried out in a patient receiving anticoagulation treatment with heparin until the heparin has disappeared from the plasma. This should be at least 5 hours following the last intravenous dose.

The use of tissue procoagulants in the test eliminates the roles of factors VIII, IX, XI, XII, and platelets. Properly done, the test will detect deficiencies of factors II, V, VII, X, and fibrinogen. The one-stage prothrombin time is the preferred method of controlling anticoagulation with the coumarin and indandione drugs.

PARTIAL THROMBOPLASTIN TIME (PTT). The partial thromboplastin time technically is a variant of the one-stage prothrombin time but provides broader information. The tissue source of procoagulant, commercially available, is extracted and refined so that the in vitro clotting system now is sensitive to factors VIII, IX, XI, XII, as well as the factors normally detected by the one-stage prothrombin time. The range of normal with this test varies with the product used. Each laboratory should establish a normal dilution curve daily, and the patient's plasma must be compared with a normal control.

The partial thromboplastin time, when used in conjunction with the one-stage prothrombin time, can help to place a clotting defect in the first or second stage of the clotting process. If the partial thromboplastin time is prolonged and the one-stage prothrombin time is normal, factors VIII, IX, XI, or XII may be deficient. If the partial thromboplastin time is normal and the one-stage prothrombin time is prolonged, a single or multiple deficiency of factors II, V, VII, or X or of fibrinogen may be present. The partial thromboplastin time also is abnormal in the presence of circulating anticoagulants or during heparin administration. The sensitivity of the test is such that only extremely mild cases of factor VIII or IX deficiency may be missed. In one study of over 600 patients with clotting abnormalities, only two mild abnormalities failed to be detected with this test.

THROMBIN TIME. The test is of value in detecting qualitative abnormalities in fibrinogen, in the detection of circulating anticoagulants and inhibitors of fibrin polymerization. The clotting time of the patient's plasma is measured following the addition of a standard amount of thrombin to a fixed volume of plasma. Controls of normal plasma must be run in parallel. Failure of the clot to form, in the absence of circulating inhibitors such as heparin, is consistent with severe diminution of fibrinogen, usually well below 100 mg/100 ml.

THROMBOPLASTIN GENERATION TEST (TGT). The development of this test permitted a distinction of deficiencies in the hemophilia family of diseases without requiring use of plasma from patients with known abnormalities. The thromboplastin generation test, or modification of it, has been used with success in performing assays of specific clotting factors of the first stage. In most laboratories in this country, the test has been replaced by the partial thromboplastin time test, or variations of it. The thromboplastin generation test has facilitated understanding of current concepts in blood coagulation and continues to be used with success in Great Britain, where it was developed. Preparation of the reagents can be time-consuming, and the test must be done with great precision in order to be reproducible.

TESTS OF FIBRINOLYSIS. The most gross and earliest determination of fibrinolysis was that of observing the whole blood clot for dissolution. Normally, this may not occur for 48 hours or more. When fibrinolysis is a significant factor in hemostatic failure, dissolution of the whole blood clot is observed in 2 hours or less. The test has the disadvantage of being time-consuming in a circumstance where time may be of the essence. In addition, a false impression of increased fibrinolytic activity may be gained from clots formed in patients with high hematocrits or in thrombocytopenia, where red cells may fall away from the clot. The euglobulin clot lysis time and dilute whole blood or plasma clot lysis time are more sensitive indices and permit more rapid evaluation of fibrinolysis.

OTHER TESTS OF HEMOSTASIS. Specific assays of all the known clotting factors now can be performed. The most popular of these assays are based upon modification of the partial thromboplastin time. The accuracy of these tests varies somewhat, but, on the average, the more accurate values are obtained when the factors are significantly reduced. Imprecision usually is found at the higher, clinically less important levels. These tests prove to be of significant clinical value but require an experienced laboratory staff.

Relatively simple tests permit identification of circulating anticoagulants. The simplest of these are based on the retardation of clotting of normal recalcified plasma by varying mixtures of the test plasma. The sensitivity of such tests usually can be increased by incubating the test plasma with the normal plasma for 30 minutes at body temperature prior to recalcification.

The *thrombotest,* devised by Owren, employs a refined tissue procoagulant which seems a little less sensitive than that used for the partial thromboplastin time but slightly more sensitive than that used for the standard one-stage prothrombin time. It has been credited with being more sensitive to factor X deficiency than the one-stage prothrombin time. While its developers have used it extensively, most laboratories will find the Quick one-stage prothrombin time test suitable.

The *thromboelastogram* is a graphic representation of clotting obtained by employing a special instrument, the thromboelastograph. The record obtained provides information about the clotting time, the speed of fibrin polymerization, and the strength and tendency toward dissolution of the clot. The instrument has provided information of research value but has not, in our experience, greatly aided the studies of clinical problems.

EVALUATION OF THE SURGICAL PATIENT AS A HEMOSTATIC RISK

General Considerations

Every patient viewed as a candidate for surgical treatment should be evaluated in terms of the risk of bleeding. The realities of time and economics dictate how exhaustive the approach to a given patient will be. For the patient requiring surgical intervention on an elective basis several points can be emphasized. The nondirective, open-ended patient interview has proved of value in many diagnostic settings. Direct questioning, however, is required to elicit most hints of a bleeding tendency.

The history should determine if circumcision was accompanied by unusual bleeding, since such bleeding is a frequent occurrence in patients who have inherited hemostatic problems. Hemophilic infants have been circumcised, however, without bleeding when the circumcision was performed immediately following delivery. Sufficient factor VIII may be supplied by transplacental transfer. The dental history can be of great significance. Many patients with inherited bleeding disorders may have bleeding with eruption of the teeth or bleeding after extraction. In the case of the hemophiliac, bleeding may begin hours after extraction and continue to be a problem for several days. The patient with a bleeding disorder, either acquired or inherited, who does not bleed after tonsillectomy sufficiently to require reexploration or transfusion is rare. It also is unusual for the patient with a hemorrhagic diathesis to have hematemesis, epistaxis, or hemoptysis without some other hemorrhagic manifestation. The gastrointestinal tract has been regarded as an area of poor resistance in patients with hemostatic difficulties, but isolated gastrointestinal bleeding, *in the absence of bleeding or bruising tendency elsewhere,* usually is not associated with generalized hemostatic failure. More often, it may be related to local disease or associated with lesions such as hereditary hemorrhagic telangiectasia. Excessive menstrual flow, rather than intermenstrual bleeding, is a common complaint in patients with generalized hemostatic problems. It is not infrequent for such a patient, usually with thrombocytopenia, to be subjected to uterine curettage. Such an oversight can result in catastrophic complications. A detailed history of drug ingestion is essential, and it is wise to specify products by name. The patient may not regard aspirin, tranquilizers, and other pharmacologic agents which can affect the hemostatic process as drugs.

Special emphasis must be made of the family history. It is not enough to question the health of siblings and parents. Appreciation of simple genetic principles, such as the sex-linked recessive mode of transmission of some of the more serious clotting disorders, requires that we inquire into the health of grandparents, occasionally great grandparents, and certainly uncles and cousins. Patterns for the genetic transmission of hemorrhagic disorders are presented later in this chapter.

Certain findings on the physical examination should alert the examiner to the possibility of a hemostatic problem. The entire body should be inspected for ecchymoses or petechiae. These lesions are likely to appear at pressure points, where snug foundation garments are worn, or under belts or garters. Purpuric lesions are characteristically spontaneous in origin, often multiple, and frequently bilateral. The lesions of senile purpura are most common on forearms and hands, where tissue support is loose, while lesions of Henoch-Schönlein purpura generally are distributed over the buttocks, backs of the legs, elbows, and ankles. Spider angiomas are suggestive of liver disease. While not related, they may be associated with reduction in the prothrombin complex. Lesions characteristic of hereditary hemorrhagic telangiectasia are often found on the lips, under the fingernails, or around the anus. Examination of these areas is indicated in patients with gastrointestinal bleeding. When inspecting the skin, the site of a recent venipuncture should be evaluated for petechiae, ecchymoses, or hematoma.

Widespread lymph node enlargement, the presence of an enlarged liver or spleen, may suggest the possibility of reticuloendothelial disease. Jaundice, hepatomegaly, ascites, distended abdominal veins, and splenomegaly may be stigmata of liver disease. Again, these may be associated with a significant reduction in the level of the prothrombin complex.

Evaluation of the Unsuspected Bleeder

The surest method of identifying an unsuspected bleeder is to obtain a complete history and perform a thorough physical examination. The ideal laboratory test to detect these patients has yet to be described. The single most productive laboratory procedure, unquestionably, is the examination of the peripheral blood smear. Since thrombocytopenia is the most common abnormality resulting in failure of hemostasis and is so easily identified by simple inspection of a well-stained blood smear, the importance of this examination cannot be overemphasized. Other important information derived from examination of the blood smear has already been described.

Measurement of the bleeding time is an imperfect screening test. When abnormal, one must heed its warning. When normal, as it frequently is in a variety of serious hemostatic disorders, little confidence should be derived. Regrettably, this test historically has been coupled with the whole blood clotting time as a screening battery for the detection of hemostatic defects. The limitations of the whole blood clotting time as a diagnostic screening test also have been noted earlier. Fully one-third of patients affected by blood-clotting disorders that theoretically might be identified by this test will be missed. Observation of the clot retraction is another time-honored test which is not recommended for reliable screening. Platelet counts as low as 60,000 to 70,000/mm^3 can result in respectable clot retraction. Significant thrombocytopenia may go undetected if one relies too heavily on this test. Its one virtue is its simplicity.

Simple tests with reliability are available. The partial thromboplastin time, performed with care and with normal controls, is of sufficient sensitivity that abnormalities likely to result in life-endangering bleeding at operation are unlikely to be missed. The partial thromboplastin time will detect not only those abnormalities that would be identified by the whole blood clotting time but also those abnormalities characterized by defects in the prothrombin complex. The Quick one-stage prothrombin time also is a simple and accurate test which will identify abnormalities of factors V, VII, and X and prothrombin (factor II). When used in conjunction with the partial thromboplastin time, it can separate an abnormality into problems of the first stage (hemophilia group) and those of the second stage (prothrombin complex). For screening related to problems of fibrinolysis, as in patients with metastatic prostatic carcinoma or pancreatic disease, the dilute whole blood or plasma clot lysis tests are applicable.

Evaluation of the Suspected Potential Bleeder

The patient who is suspected of having hemostatic dysfunction requires a more comprehensive evaluation. This includes a particularly detailed history, a thorough physical examination, and more complete study in the laboratory. Accordingly, time must be set aside to permit these efforts. These can usually be done on an outpatient basis, or if the patient is already hospitalized and scheduled for operation, scheduling of the case should permit time for the necessary evaluations. If suspicion of an abnormality is based on family history, every effort should be made to study other members of the family. If suspicion is based on previous bleeding following surgical treatment, every effort should be made to obtain the old hospital records, since they may provide important information. When the question of bleeding related to drug administration has been raised, identification of the drug through prescription files in pharmacies and obtaining the medications for inspection may be helpful.

If the history of drug exposure or the physical findings of petechiae or mucous membrane bleeding suggest the possibility of thrombocytopenia, in addition to the examination of the blood smear, direct platelet counting should be performed. Bleeding times should be determined using the template technique. Drug-related immunologic forms of thrombocytopenia can be evaluated with the clot retraction inhibition test. This takes advantage of the fact that antibody may remain in the patient's serum for 4 to 6 months. An aliquot of the patient's serum together with an aliquot of a saturated solution of the suspected drug are clotted together with an aliquot of the patient's blood. If the platelets are immunologically damaged in the presence of the drug, the clot retraction is inhibited. The use of appropriate normal controls is imperative. More detailed observations, such as the platelets' ability to aggregate in their native plasma following the addition of ADP, and measurements of platelet factor 3 release also can be performed.

If a blood coagulation defect is suspected, a combination of tests can help place the defect (Table 3-1). If the partial thromboplastin time is abnormal and the one-stage prothrombin time is normal, the defect is almost certainly in the first stage of clotting. One then has the option of

performing mixing and matching studies or, more desirably, specific clotting factor assays. The former require samples of plasma from patients with proved abnormalities. One then tests the patient in question by determining if a small amount of the patient's plasma will correct the abnormality of the known deficient sample in vitro. Such tests can give reliable qualitative results in terms of establishing a specific diagnosis. Assays for individual blood-clotting factors can be performed by many laboratories. In addition to the specificity of the test, quantitative values are obtained, permitting estimation of the severity of the disease process. The specific assays are of particular value in controlling the transfusion program of affected patients undergoing surgical treatment.

Evaluation of the Patient Who Begins to Bleed during or after Surgical Procedures

The patient who bleeds excessively during or shortly following surgical procedures is an emergency problem. The approach to this difficult situation must be prompt and well organized. Generally, bleeding at the time of operation ultimately is identified as being due to, singly or in combination, (1) ineffective local hemostasis, (2) complications of blood transfusion, (3) a previously present but unsuspected hemostatic defect, (4) sepsis, (5) induced fibrinolysis or defibrination.

Bleeding from one site only, such as the surgical wound, usually is not due to a generalized hemostatic defect. The patient who manifests bleeding at the primary incisional site, for example, but not at the site of a stab wound where drains have been placed or the patient who is bleeding from a thoracotomy wound but not at all from his tracheostomy site is more likely to have a local problem than a generalized defect. One exception to this generalization should be noted: Occasionally following prostatic surgical treatment excessive bleeding from the prostatic bed is noted. The plasminogen activator present in prostatic tissue is activated by the urokinase normally present in the

Table 3-1. DIAGNOSIS OF INHERITED DISORDERS OF COAGULATION

Deficient factor	Bleeding time	One-stage prothrombin time	Partial thromboplastin time	Thrombin time	Fibrinogen time	Platelet adhesiveness
I (fibrinogen)	Long or normal	Long	Long	Long	Low	Normal
II	Normal	Long	Long	Normal	Normal	Normal
V	Normal	Long	Long	Normal	Normal	Normal
VII	Normal	Long	Normal	Normal	Normal	Normal
VIII	Normal	Normal	Long	Normal	Normal	Normal
IX	Normal	Normal	Long	Normal	Normal	Normal
X	Normal	Long	Long	Normal	Normal	Normal
XI	Normal	Normal	Long	Normal	Normal	Normal
XII	Normal	Normal	Long	Normal	Normal	Normal
XIII	Normal	Normal	Normal	Normal	Normal	Normal
Von Willebrand's disease	Long	Normal	Long	Normal	Normal	Low

SOURCE: E. W. Salzman, Hemorrhagic disorders, in J. M. Kinney, R. H. Egdahl, and G. D. Zuidema (eds.), "Manual of Preoperative and Postoperative Care," p. 157, W. B. Saunders Company, Philadelphia, 1971.

urine as it washes over the raw prostatic bed. Increased fibrinolysis occurs locally on the raw surface of the wound, and bleeding is aggravated. This is a failure of local hemostasis based, not on any mechanical problem, but rather on the increased activation of the local fibrinolytic process. A 24- to 48-hour period of interruption of this plasminogen activation by the administration of ε-aminocaproic acid (ε-ACA) usually suffices to still the blood loss.

Although one may be reasonably certain on clinical grounds that surgical bleeding is related to local problems, laboratory investigation must be confirmatory. Prompt examination of the blood smear to determine the number of platelets and an actual platelet count if the smear is not clear-cut should be done. A partial thromboplastin time, one-stage prothrombin time, and thrombin clotting time all can be determined within minutes. Correct interpretation of the results should confirm the clinical impression or identify the exceptional problem.

Complications of blood transfusion are an occasional cause of hemostatic failure. Massive blood transfusion with banked blood is a well-documented cause of thrombocytopenia. Most patients who receive 10 units or more of banked blood within a period of 24 hours will be measurably thrombocytopenic, but usually not sufficiently so to result in hemostatic failure. Patients who receive 14 units or more of banked blood in a period of 24 hours or less invariably will be significantly thrombocytopenic and may have frank bleeding as a result. *The patient in whom signs of hemostatic failure develop during or following operation when large quantities of banked blood have been used should be assumed to be thrombocytopenic until demonstrated otherwise.* Treatment consists of supplying fresh platelets in the form of platelet concentrates or, if volume is also required, as fresh platelet-rich plasma. Following transfusion of 10 units of banked blood, prophylactic administration of fresh platelet packs is appropriate.

Another cause of hemostatic failure involving transfusion is that of the hemolytic transfusion reaction. This complication, usually so readily detected in the conscious patient, can be difficult to recognize in the anesthetized patient. The characteristic chilly sensation, muscle ache, backache, headache, and ultimate hemoglobinuria will not be evident. The first hint to the experienced surgeon that the patient is undergoing hemolytic transfusion reaction may be progressive failure of hemostasis. Tissues in the operative field which have previously been dry begin to ooze.

The pathogenesis of this bleeding is not perfectly established, but several probable causes have been suggested. The release of ADP from the hemolyzed red cells may be sufficient to cause platelet aggregation, and the platelet clumps then are swept out of the circulation. Red blood cells also are a rich source of the procoagulant platelet factor 3 (phospholipid) necessary at several stages of blood coagulation. Release of these substances during hemolytic transfusion reaction may result in progression of the clotting mechanism and intravascular defibrination. In addition, the fibrinolytic mechanism may be triggered by the intravascular clotting. Both defibrination and fibrinolysis have been documented clinically and experimentally following hemolytic transfusion reaction. Their incidence is low but must be considered when the clinical events are consistent. The bleeding problem associated with hemolytic transfusion reaction should be considered due to thrombocytopenia until other laboratory measures suggest defibrination or fibrinolysis.

Transfusion purpura, which has been described in detail by Shulman and associates, is an uncommon but interesting cause of thrombocytopenia and associated bleeding following transfusion. In this circumstance, the donor platelets are of the uncommon Pl^{A1} group. These platelets sensitize the recipient, who makes antibody to the foreign platelet antigen. The foreign platelet antigen does not completely disappear from the recipient circulation but seems to attach to the recipient's own platelets. The antibody, which attains a sufficient titer within 6 or 7 days following the sensitizing transfusion, then destroys the recipient's own platelets. The resultant thrombocytopenia and bleeding may continue for several weeks. This uncommon cause of thrombocytopenia should be considered if bleeding follows transfusion by 5 or 6 days. Platelet transfusions are of little help in the management of this syndrome, since the new donor platelets usually are subject to the binding of antigen and damage from the antibody. Corticosteroids may be of some help in reducing the bleeding tendency. Posttransfusion purpura is self-limited, and the passage of several weeks inevitably leads to subsidence of the problem.

The patient with a hemostatic defect which manifests itself first during surgical treatment is likely to have other evidence of bleeding, such as ecchymoses at the sites of injection or venipunctures, and bloody drainage from nasogastric tubes or bladder catheters.

A hemostatic defect may be imposed iatrogenically during surgical treatment employing extracorporeal bypass. Many etiologic factors may be involved, but the most commonly implicated is the introduction of heparin into the circulation. Bleeding after discontinuation of extracorporeal bypass may be due to inadequate neutralization of heparin with protamine sulfate. Since both protamine sulfate and Polybrene are themselves anticoagulants when large doses are used, it is possible that bleeding was caused by these drugs. This is a rare occurrence. Rapid tests can be performed in vitro by adding small amounts of protamine sulfate to see if the clotting time is shortened. Other abnormalities attributed to extracorporeal circulation are defibrination and fibrinolysis. Fibrinolytic activity is often increased. These changes usually are related to the duration of pumping. We are impressed by the *lack* of clinical bleeding in the patients with laboratory evidence of fibrinolysis. Thrombocytopenia, hypofibrinogenemia, and reduction in factors V and VIII have been demonstrated. The thrombocytopenia usually is not severe, and the platelet count generally remains above 50,000/mm^3. Evaluation of the patient with intraoperative or postoperative bleeding suspected of being due to hemostatic defect follows the same course previously outlined for preoperative evaluation of these patients.

At times, an operation performed in a patient with sepsis is attended by continued bleeding. Severe hemorrhagic disorders due to thrombocytopenia have occurred consequent to gram-negative sepsis. The pathogenesis of endotoxin-induced thrombocytopenia has been studied in detail, and it is suggested that a labile factor, possibly factor V, is necessary for this interaction. Defibrination and hemostatic failure also may occur with meningococcemia, *Clostridium welchii* sepsis and staphylococcal sepsis. Hemolysis appears to be one mechanism in sepsis leading to defibrination.

The appearance of pathologic fibrinolysis during surgical treatment is an uncommon but potentially serious event. It can occur subsequent to shock, following intravascular defibrination, and in association with operation on tissues rich in activators of the fibrinolytic mechanism. These include pancreas, prostate, and lung. Defibrination also can occur as a consequence of hemolytic transfusion reaction and sepsis.

The thrombin time can be of value in detecting abnormalities in fibrinogen. When fibrinolysis is a significant factor, dissolution of the whole blood clot is observed in 2 hours or less, but the euglobulin clot lysis and dilute whole blood clot lysis are more sensitive indices and permit more rapid evaluation.

CLINICAL HEMOSTATIC DEFECTS

Inheritance

The importance of a detailed family history in the evaluation of the patient with a possible hemostatic defect has been emphasized. The sensible use of this information requires an understanding of genetic principles and knowledge of the specific genetic features of the hemostatic disorders.

The modes of inheritance of hemostatic disorders, with few rare exceptions, are three in type: (1) autosomal dominant, (2) autosomal recessive, and (3) sex-linked recessive. The 46 chromosomes of man consist of 22 autosomal pairs, plus a pair of sex chromosomes, the X and Y. Since one chromosome of each of the 22 autosomal pairs normally is derived from each parent, any gene inherited as a part of an autosomal chromosome normally will occur with equal frequency among males and females. Each child of a parent carrying an autosomal dominant gene has one chance in two of inheriting that trait. The most common hemostatic disorder transmitted by the autosomal dominant mode is von Willebrand's disease. Hereditary hemorrhagic telangiectasia and factor XI deficiency also appear to be transmitted in this fashion.

A normal individual should transmit no disease to his progeny. Occasionally, in a pedigree with an autosomal dominant gene, an *apparently* normal person may transmit disease to his or her child. The parent clearly carried the gene, which clinically expressed no defect. Explanation of this phenomenon is not at hand. The gene activity in the parent is referred to as "incompletely penetrant."

In inherited hemostatic disorders, the difference in clinical expression between dominant and recessive genes is a graded one rather than an "all-or-none" phenomenon. The heterozygous individual with an autosomal recessive trait may have a measurable deficiency of the factor governed by that gene, but no clinical disease. In order to demonstrate clinical expression of disease, the individual must be homozygous. This appears to be the case, for example, in factor X deficiency. The homozygote with clinical disease, as described by Hougie, has less than 5% of factor X activity, while heterozygotes have levels ranging from 21 to 50%. Since the presumed heterozygotes within the same pedigree vary in factor X activity, it is convenient to suggest that the gene shows variable expression. Other hemostatic disorders probably inherited in this mode are factor V, factor VII, and factor I deficiencies. This mode of transmission could be regarded as incompletely dominant inheritance, rather than incompletely recessive, depending upon one's view. Since these traits are not very common, it is difficult to resolve this problem.

Sex-linked recessive inheritance governs true hemophilia (factor VIII deficiency) and factor IX deficiency (Christmas disease). The genes for these diseases are recessive in expression and are carried on the female (X) chromosome. When paired with the normal X chromosome (the female carrier state), clinical disease is not present. When the affected X chromosome is paired with the normal male (Y) chromosome, clinical disease is expressed.

Theoretically, with the "graded" expression, the female carrier should be detectable in the laboratory. In fact, since the range of factor VIII activity normally is so broad, most female carriers *appear* to fall in the low-normal range. Estimates vary, but possibly as many as 50 percent of female carriers can be identified. Although the sex-linked recessive mode of inheritance has been confirmed repeatedly in true hemophilia, it seems likely that an *autosomal* gene also may influence factor VIII activity. This probability is emphasized by the autosomal dominant mode of inheritance of von Willebrand's disease, characterized by low factor VIII activity, and also by the patterns of variation in factor VIII activity among individuals within the same normal family and among different normal families.

Despite the lack of complete understanding of genetic determinants in hemostatic disorders, detailed consideration of the family history facilitates accurate diagnosis.

Factor VIII Deficiency (Classical Hemophilia)

Classical hemophilia (hemophilia A) is a disease of males. The failure to synthesize normal factor VIII activity is inherited as a sex-linked recessive trait. Incidence of the disease is approximately 1:25,000 population, and the clinical manifestations can be extremely variable.

CLINICAL MANIFESTATIONS. Characteristically, the severity of clinical manifestations is related to the degree of deficiency of factor VIII. Spontaneous bleeding and severe complications are the rule when virtually no factor VIII can be detected in the plasma. When plasma factor VIII concentrations are in the range of 25%, the patient may have no spontaneous bleeding yet may bleed severely with trauma or surgical treatment. Typically, members of the same pedigree with true hemophilia will have approximately the same degree of clinical manifestations.

While the severely affected patient may bleed during early infancy, significant bleeding typically is noted first when the child is a toddler. At that time, in addition to the classic bleeding into joints, bleeding may occur at other sites. Epistaxis and hematuria may be noted. Bleeding which is life-threatening may follow injury to the tongue or frenulum. We have seen tracheal compression following tonsillar infection and retropharyngeal bleeding. Vascular and neural compromise may occur in relation to pressure secondary to bleeding into a soft tissue closed space. Equinus contracture deformity may be seen in severely hemophilic patients secondary to bleeding into the calf. Volkmann's contracture of the forearm and flexion contractures of the knees and elbows are also disabling sequelae of deep soft tissue bleeding.

Hemarthrosis is the most characteristic orthopedic problem. Bleeding into the joint may cause few symptoms until distension of the joint capsule occurs. Muscle spasm and pain around the joint arise from involvement of periarticular structures. A large hemarthrosis generally is manifested by a tender, swollen, warm, and painful joint. These signs may mimic infection. The same orthopedic problems are noted in association with severe factor IX deficiency (Christmas disease).

Retroperitoneal bleeding may follow lifting of a heavy object or strenuous exercise. Signs of posterior peritoneal irritation and spasm of the iliopsoas suggest the diagnosis. Hypovolemic shock may occur, since the amount of blood loss that can take place in this setting is enormous. The potential space in the retroperitoneal area readily accommodates several liters of blood in the adult. An intramural hematoma within the intestine also can pose problems of differential diagnosis. The clinical manifestations of nausea and vomiting, crampy abdominal pain, and signs of peritoneal irritation mimic those of appendicitis. Fever and leukocytosis may be noted. Roentgenograms of the abdomen may fail to reveal an abnormality or may display a modest amount of ileus. Upper gastrointestinal examination may demonstrate a uniform thickening of mucosal folds which has been described as a "picket fence" or "stack of coins" appearance (Fig. 3-5). Intramural hematomas of the intestine occur with other hemostatic disorders and, therefore, should be considered when any patient with a hemostatic problem presents with findings suggesting an acute intraabdominal process.

TREATMENT. This requires an appreciation of the transfusion therapy necessary to correct factor VIII deficiency as well as the application of specific surgical principles.

Replacement Therapy. The plasma concentration of factor VIII necessary for maintenance of hemostatic integrity is normally quite small. Patients with as little as 2 to 3% of factor VIII activity usually do not bleed spontaneously. Once serious bleeding begins, however, a much higher level of factor VIII activity, probably approaching 30%, is necessary to achieve hemostasis.

Following transfusion, the plasma level of factor VIII

Fig. 3-5. Upper gastrointestinal roentgenogram of patient with "acquired hemophilia." Note thickening of mucosal folds indicative of an intramural hematoma. The spontaneous bleeding in this patient was ascribed to powerful circulating anticoagulant to factor VIII.

in vivo depends upon the potency of the administered preparation and the survival of the infused factor VIII. Many formulas have been developed as a guide to replacement. These should not be used in a cookbook fashion. We view laboratory control of the level of factor VIII as extremely important. This is particularly pertinent since the amount of factor VIII in individual aliquots of frozen plasma and cryoprecipitate varies considerably.

Following administration of a given dose of factor VIII, approximately one-half of the initial posttransfusion activity disappears from the plasma in 4 hours. This early disappearance is thought to be due, in large part, to diffusion from the intravascular space. The period of equilibration extends for as long as 8 hours, at which time only about one-quarter of the initial level remains in the circulating blood. From that time on, the slope of disap-

Fig. 3-6. Schematic representation of in vivo decay of a single dose of factor VIII. (*From N. R. Shulman, Mod Treat, 5:61, 1968.*)

in different lesions. Remembering the loss from the circulation, one-half the initial dose would need to be supplied every 12 hours. The use of fresh plasma in such a circumstance would require a volume that is excessive. Factor VIII concentrates now available circumvent this problem. Cryoprecipitate concentrates of factor VIII can be regarded as containing 9.6 units/ml. The amount of material to be given can be computed from the formula

$$\frac{\text{Patient's weight (kg)} \times \text{desired rise of factor VIII (\% average normal)}}{\text{Total units of factor VIII in dose}} = R$$

where *R* is a factor which is fairly constant for any given type of material and represents the rise of factor VIII obtained in the patient's plasma for every unit of transfused factor VIII per kg of the patient's body weight. Half that amount is subsequently administered every 12 hours to maintain a safe level. A promising factor VIII concentrate prepared as a glycine precipitate also is available. Concentrations as high as 70 or 80 units/ml are obtainable, simplifying the management of the hemophilic patient. Regardless of the preparation employed, continued laboratory assessment of circulating factor VIII level is an important element in the control of these patients.

Following major surgical treatment of the hemophiliac, transfusion replacement of factor VIII should be continued for at least 10 days. Wounds should be well healed and all drains removed prior to the termination of therapy. If sutures remain, transfusion should be reinstituted prior to their removal.

The virus of homologous serum hepatitis is transmitted by the various concentrates of plasma. Whether the new glycine precipitates are free of this virus remains to be demonstrated. Other complications of replacement therapy include the appearance of inhibitors of factor VIII, which may arise in the hemophiliacs who have had transfusion.

pearance is less steep (Fig. 3-6). Twenty-four hours after a given dose, no more than 7 to 8% of administered factor VIII activity remains within the circulation.

One unit of factor VIII activity is considered that amount present in 1 ml of normal plasma. Actually, fresh frozen plasma contains 0.60 units/ml. Theoretically, in a patient with 0% activity, to achieve an initial post-transfusion level of 60% of normal, using fresh plasma, a volume of plasma equal to 60% of the patient's estimated plasma volume would have to be administered. Table 3-2 shows approximate levels of factor VIII required for hemostasis

Table 3-2. APPROXIMATE LEVELS OF FACTOR VIII REQUIRED FOR HAEMOSTASIS IN DIFFERENT LESIONS

Lesion	Level of factor VIII desired in patient's blood immediately after transfusion (% average normal)	Dose of factor VIII (units/kg body weight)[a]
Minor spontaneous haemarthrosis and muscle haematomas	15–20 (0–5)	10–15
Severe haemarthrosis and muscle haematomas, haematomas in dangerous situations	20–40 (5–10)	15–20
Major surgery	80–100 (or less if transfusion given 8-hourly or 6-hourly)	40–50

Figures in parentheses are the approximate levels to which factor VIII will have fallen 24 hours after dose.

[a] 1 unit of factor VIII is the amount present in 1 ml of fresh average normal citrated plasma.

SOURCE: Clinics in Haematology, vol. 5, no. 1, February 1976. C. R. Rizza "Coagulation Factor Therapy," p. 113–133.

These inhibitors have been characterized as antibodies of the γ G variety. They tend to diminish in several weeks if further transfusion is not employed. Laboratory search for these factors should be carried out in every hemophilic patient who is considered a candidate for elective surgical treatment, as their presence enormously complicates transfusion management.

Adjunctive Management. Treatment of soft tissue bleeding is directed at the prevention of airway obstruction and vascular and neural damage. These are accomplished best by the administration of sufficient factor VIII. Bed rest and cold packs can be of some assistance. In general, results of fasciotomy to relieve pressure have varied from disappointing to disastrous. The occasional development of large cysts has resulted in sufficient deformity and disability to require amputation.

The primary treatment of hemophilic hemarthrosis is directed at maintaining full range of motion and minimal destruction of the cartilage. Aspiration of blood from the hemophilic joint is not uniformly endorsed, and when regarded as necessary, it should be considered a major surgical event. Elevation of factor VIII level by transfusion is necessary. The procedure should be carried out in the operating room under strict sterile precautions. In most instances, aspiration is not required, and the combination of factor VIII replacement and local cold packing proves sufficient. Physiotherapy plays a critical role and should consist of *active* exercises, since the patient is unlikely to move the extremity to a point where bleeding will recur. Passive exercises often result in recurrence of bleeding. The reader is referred to the review by Curtiss for details of orthopedic management.

The management of intramural intestinal hematoma and retroperitoneal bleeding is predicated on appropriate transfusion therapy and avoidance of surgical treatment. It is to be emphasized that even when a relatively minor procedure, such as tracheostomy, is performed, the plasma level of factor VIII should be raised above 25 to 30%. Since dental hygiene usually is poor in hemophilic patients, dental and oral surgical treatment frequently are necessary. The same principles of transfusion therapy pertain, and the procedures should be delegated to well-trained personnel working where optimal care can be provided.

Recently, the question of transplantation of the spleen as therapy for hemophilia has been raised. Norman and associates have suggested that the spleen may be a site of factor VIII synthesis and/or storage. Also, it has been reported that the spleen is receptive to circulating factor VIII–trophic substance in the plasma of human hemophiliacs. In hemophilic dogs receiving heterotrophic splenic transplants, factor VIII levels were increased thirtyfold, to levels more than that required to prevent spontaneous bleeding. In an independent study, Webster and associates reported dissimilar results and an absence of significant effect on factor VIII. They warned against clinical applicability of this procedure. This concern has been reinforced by one subsequent clinical case of splenic transplantation in a human being, with continued postoperative bleeding and splenic infarction necessitating removal of the transplanted spleen.

Von Willebrand's Disease (Pseudohemophilia)

Von Willebrand's disease occurs as commonly as true hemophilia. The increasing recognition is related to more reliable factor VIII assays. This hereditary disorder of hemostasis is transmitted as an autosomally dominant trait and, accordingly, appears in consecutive generations with males and females equally affected. The disease is characterized by a diminution of the level of factor VIII activity. The reduction of factor VIII activity usually is not as great as that seen in classical hemophilia. Also unlike classical hemophilia, where factor VIII activity remains constant, in the patient with von Willebrand's disease variation in the level of circulating factor VIII activity may be noted. Characteristically, these patients also have a prolonged bleeding time, but this is less constant than the factor VIII reduction. A given patient may have an abnormal bleeding time on one occasion and a normal bleeding time on another. Abnormalities of platelet adhesiveness in vitro, using Salzman's method, also have been described. Von Willebrand's disease can be distinguished from classical hemophilia by two findings: the level of factor VIII antigen is disproportionately lower than that of factor VIII, and ristocetin fails to cause platelet aggregation.

CLINICAL MANIFESTATIONS. The manifestations of bleeding usually are mild and often overlooked until trauma or the stress of surgical treatment makes them apparent. A careful clinical history is, therefore, of great importance in these patients. Spontaneous manifestations often are limited to bleeding into the skin or mild mucous membrane bleeding. Epistaxis and menorrhagia have been relatively common in our personal experience. Serious bleeding following dental extractions and tonsillectomy also are not uncommon. Fatal bleeding from the gastrointestinal tract has been described.

TREATMENT. The typical patient with von Willebrand's disease will produce factor VIII activity in response to transfusion of modest amounts of fresh frozen plasma, cryoprecipitate, or other factor VIII concentrates. This is unlike the classical hemophiliac in whom factor VIII concentration rises only in proportion to the amount of that substance actually transfused. In von Willebrand's disease, some 4 to 6 hours following transfusion an increase in circulating factor VIII activity to the range of five to eight times that which could be ascribed to transfusion alone is noted. This apparent synthesis continues for approximately 24 hours. Exceptions to this characteristic response recently have been described.

When a patient with von Willebrand's disease is scheduled to undergo surgical treatment, plasma transfusion should be instituted at least 48 hours prior to the operative procedure. In this manner, it can be determined whether the patient will respond to infusion with appearance of factor VIII activity. If factor VIII activity is not generated, a more ambitious program of transfusion is necessary to sustain the patient through the operative and postoperative period. In most patients, infusion of 10 ml of plasma/kg of body weight/24 hours will ensure hemostatically effective levels of factor VIII. Duration of treatment should be the same as that described for the patient with classical hemophilia.

Factor IX Deficiency (Christmas Disease)

Factor IX deficiency clinically is indistinguishable from factor VIII deficiency. These two entities were considered a single disease until 1952, when their unique deficiencies were documented. The incidence of factor IX deficiency is approximately 1:100,000 population.

TREATMENT. Factor IX, although not in the prothrombin complex, is dependent upon vitamin K for its synthesis in the liver. It is present in banked blood, plasma, and serum. Initially, the rate of disappearance of factor IX from the circulation is more rapid than that of factor VIII, but subsequently factor IX has a slower disappearance rate (Fig. 3-7). Half of the factor IX which is present 5 or 6 hours following transfusion remains after 24 hours. An infusion of plasma containing factor IX raises the recipient's factor IX level less than would be predicted. The extravascular space into which factor IX distributes itself may be larger than the distribution space for factor VIII. The longer survival of factor IX helps compensate for its more rapid initial disappearance following transfusion. Accordingly, a dose of 15 ml of plasma/kg of body weight administered over a 1- or 2-hour period 6 hours or more prior to operation usually serves to raise the plasma level to a suitable point. Half that volume then is administered every 12 hours as long as clinical indications require. An alternative method of treatment is that of administering 60 ml of plasma/kg over a 10- to 20-hour period 24 hours prior to anticipated surgical treatment and repeating doses of 7 ml/kg every 12 hours.

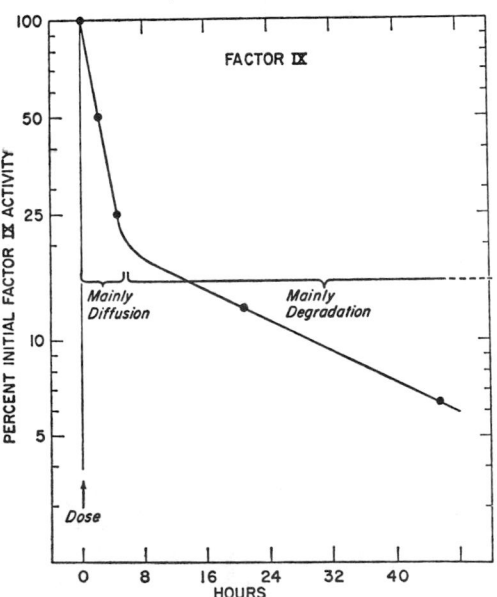

Fig. 3-7. Schematic representation of in vivo decay of a single dose of factor IX. (*From N. R. Shulman, Mod Treat, 5:61, 1968.*)

It should be emphasized that the patient with a mild factor IX deficiency, like the patient with a mild factor VIII deficiency, can bleed massively with surgical treatment and requires planned replacement therapy. There are now several preparations of factor IX concentrate available for replacement therapy.

Factor XI (PTA) Deficiency (Rosenthal's Syndrome)

This uncommon and relatively mild disorder is inherited in an autosomally dominant fashion. Without careful laboratory testing, the affected males and females may be confused with von Willebrand's disease patients. A majority of patients are of Jewish ancestry.

Epistaxis is a common spontaneous clinical manifestation. The disease usually is recognized as a result of bleeding during and after operation. The bleeding usually is minor. Some patients have undergone major procedures without significant hemorrhage.

TREATMENT. Factor XI actually may gain in potency during storage, so that plasma is a suitable therapeutic medium. This factor disappears slowly from the circulation, and its biologic half-life may be as long as 48 hours. An initial dose of 10 ml of plasma/kg of body weight can be given 6 or 8 hours prior to anticipated surgical treatment, followed by a maintenance dose of 5 ml/kg administered every 24 hours. Therapy usually can be discontinued several days earlier than with patients with more serious hemostatic disorders.

Factor V (Proaccelerin) Deficiency (Parahemophilia)

This extremely rare deficiency usually is associated with mild bleeding, but serious bleeding may be encountered. The disease is transmitted as an autosomal recessive trait and is found in males and females alike. Only patients who presumably inherit the gene from both parents seem to be bleeders.

Factor V is synthesized in the liver but differs from prothrombin and factors VII, IX, and X in that factor V synthesis is not dependent upon vitamin K or inhibited by the administration of the coumarin drugs. Patients with severe parenchymal liver disease may be deficient in factor V.

TREATMENT. Excessive bleeding may occur at the time of operation, usually in patients who have levels of less than 1% of normal factor V concentration. No more than 25% of normal activity is necessary for hemostasis during operative procedures. This level can be achieved by administering 15 ml of fresh or freshly frozen plasma per kg of body weight 12 hours prior to operation. The administration of 7 to 10 ml/kg every 24 hours will suffice to maintain hemostasis until healing has occurred. Once again, it is wise to administer the factor at the time of suture removal. Factor V, also known as labile factor, loses its activity during storage. Only fresh plasma or plasma freshly frozen is applicable as therapy.

Factor VII (Proconvertin) Deficiency

Factor VII (stable factor) deficiency is an uncommon but not rare disease. Mild clinical manifestations are the rule. The deficiency is inherited as an autosomal gene of "intermediate penetrance." The homozygous state results in significant deficiency and may be associated with serious bleeding. In these patients, spontaneous epistaxis, genitourinary and gastrointestinal bleeding, and even hemarthroses, may be seen. The heterozygotes have minimal, if any, clinical manifestations.

Factor VII, like factors II, IX, and X, requires vitamin K for synthesis. The synthesis is blocked by coumarin administration. Coumarin inhibition of synthesis is reversed by vitamin K administration. The administration of vitamin K to patients *congenitally* deficient in these activities will *not* result in synthesis and increased plasma levels.

As is also true for factor V–deficient patients and in patients with deficiencies of factors II and X, the one-stage prothrombin time is prolonged in patients with factor VII deficiency. Since factor VII is active only in the "extrinsic" blood-clotting system, deficient patients have a normal prothrombin consumption test. In contrast, patients with factor X deficiency have abnormal prothrombin consumption, significant prothrombin remaining in the serum 1 hour after coagulation. Another laboratory distinction between factor VII and factor X deficiency can be made by the use of the Stypven time test. Factor X is necessary for the effect of this viper venom in blood coagulation, while factor VII is not. Accordingly, the factor VII–deficient patient has a normal Stypven time.

TREATMENT. The biologic half-life of factor VII probably is the briefest of any of the blood-clotting factors. The initial half-life, thought to be due to equilibration between the intravascular and extravascular compartments, probably is no more than 30 minutes. The remainder of the disappearance time presumably represents catabolism and is estimated at between 5 and 6 hours. Despite this relatively rapid disappearance, the transfusion management of patients with factor VII deficiency is not a great problem. Factor VII levels of less than 4 to 5% of normal are necessary before significant bleeding occurs. Even at these low levels of plasma activity, replacement transfusion is not always necessary for surgical procedures. Although the one-stage prothrombin time recognizes deficiency of factor VII, this test is not an effective guide to the treatment of factor VII–deficient patients. The test is markedly abnormal at factor VII levels at which the deficient patient may not bleed. Transfusion of banked plasma, 10 ml/kg of body weight, on the day of the operation, followed by half that amount daily for the next 5 or 6 days, provides adequate factor VII for hemostasis during major surgical treatment.

Factor X (Stuart-Prower) Deficiency

This relatively rare deficiency is inherited as an autosomal recessive trait and has been described in amyloido-sis. Clinically, affected patients are homozygotes, while the heterozygotes are clinically well and only minimally affected. The latter may demonstrate mild abnormalities with the one-stage prothrombin test and the thromboplastin generation test.

TREATMENT. Little experience has been acquired in the surgical management of patients with factor X deficiency. Plasma levels of 15% of normal have proved sufficient to prevent significant bleeding following dental extractions. Plasma transfusion experiments in patients with factor X deficiency have demonstrated an 8- to 10-hour first-phase disappearance time of half the administered activity, followed by a disappearance time estimated at 40 hours. Applying these data, plasma levels of 15% or greater could be achieved by infusing 15 to 20 ml of normal plasma per kg of body weight initially, followed by half that amount per 24 hours for 5 days. It is always prudent to give an additional infusion at the time of removal of the operative sutures.

Inherited Hypoprothrombinemia (Factor II Deficiency)

This deficiency, inherited as an autosomal recessive trait, is perhaps the most rare of the inherited disorders of hemostasis. The prothrombin levels reported in affected patients have averaged about 10% of normal. Although the level of prothrombin activity required for hemostasis following surgical treatment is not precisely established, it seems likely that a level of 15% of normal is effective.

TREATMENT. The disappearance time of prothrombin from the intravascular compartment approximates that of factor X. An initial equilibration time of 9 hours has been estimated, followed by a much slower disappearance of activity with another half-life of up to 3 days. Stored plasma contains factor II. Surgical treatment without faulty hemostasis should be possible in affected patients if an initial plasma infusion of 15 ml/kg of body weight is administered 12 to 24 hours prior to the scheduled operation. This can be followed by an infusion of half this amount once daily until healing has occurred.

When the transfusion programs outlined above for deficiency of the prothrombin group of factors (factors II, V, VII, and X) are employed, the one-stage prothrombin time does not return to normal. Rather, a one-stage prothrombin time slightly less than twice the control value is achieved. This is sufficient to result in normal hemostasis. Of the four "prothrombin" factors, only factor V must be provided as fresh or freshly frozen plasma. Stored plasma is equally effective as therapy for factors II, VII, and X.

Inherited Fibrinogen Abnormalities

For nearly 50 years following the first description of a patient with congenital afibrinogenemia, this rare abnormality was considered the only inherited defect involving fibrinogen. More recently, families with qualitatively abnormal fibrinogen have been identified. These latter patients have varied in their clinical manifestations as well as in laboratory features.

Congenital afibrinogenemia is ascribed to an autosomal recessive mode of inheritance. The parents of patients with this entity usually have normal concentrations of fibrinogen. The affected individuals presumably are homozygous for the trait. Plasma fibrinogen levels of less that 5 mg/100 ml are usual, and, occasionally, immunochemical methods have been necessary to identify even trace amounts of fibrinogen in the plasma of these patients. The deficiency, however, usually is less of a clinical problem than classical hemophilia. Severely affected infants have bled following sectioning of the umbilical cord. More often the clinical manifestations include bleeding following lacerations, purpura, epistaxis, and bleeding following loss of deciduous teeth. The characteristic laboratory defect is the failure of the blood to clot in vitro, even following the addition of thrombin.

Less profound inherited deficiencies of fibrinogen have been observed. The bleeding usually is more modest, and therefore the treatment requires proportionately smaller amounts of fibrinogen concentrate or plasma. Patients with "dysfibrinogenemia" are uncommon. The characteristic abnormality is the retarded rate of clotting upon the addition of thrombin ("thrombin time"). Interestingly, thrombotic disease as well as bleeding disorders have been described in this heterogeneous group of patients. Although surgical experience with this type of patient has been negligible, the administration of normal fibrinogen should serve to diminish the hemorrhagic aspect of the problem.

TREATMENT. Approximately one-half of the transfused fibrinogen given to a deficient patient disappears from the intravascular compartment within the first 24 hours after administration. Following this, the biologic half-life is 3 days or more. The disappearance of fibrinogen is no more rapid in deficient patients than when fibrinogen is transfused into normal subjects, thus suggesting that accelerated fibrinogen catabolism is not a pathogenic mechanism. Although the hemostatically optimal level of fibrinogen is not known, a level of close to 100 mg/100 ml usually permits normal hemostasis. The patient's fibrinogen level should be raised above this prior to major surgical treatment. The volume of normal plasma necessary to accomplish this could sometimes exceed 50 ml/kg of body weight initially. Fibrinogen replacement has been made substantially easier by increasing the use of concentrates. A dose of 1 Gm of fibrinogen/10 kg/day has proved adequate. Approximately one-fifth of this then is administered daily following the initial loading dose. A substantial risk of homologous serum hepatitis is incurred when fibrinogen fractions are used. These concentrates are prepared from pooled plasma. The hepatitis risk can be reduced by using the cryoprecipitate preparation described for the treatment of hemophilia. Approximately one-half of the fibrinogen in the initial plasma is available in the precipitate. A 60-kg patient requires the precipitate obtained from approximately 25 units of plasma as a loading dose.

Acquired Hypofibrinogenemia

DEFIBRINATION SYNDROME

The largest proportion of patients with fibrinogen-related problems of surgical concern are in this group. The fibrinogen deficiency rarely is an isolated defect, as thrombocytopenia and factors II, V, and VIII deficiencies of variable severity usually accompany this state.

The majority of patients with acquired hypofibrinogenemia suffer from intravascular coagulation, more properly known as *defibrination syndrome* or *consumptive coagulopathy,* and it is to this group of patients that the term *disseminated intravascular coagulation* (DIC) has been applied. The syndrome, now recognized with increasing frequency, is caused by the introduction of thromboplastic materials into the circulation. Because this material is found in most tissues, many disease processes may activate the coagulation system. The hemorrhagic disasters of the perinatal period, e.g., retained dead fetus, premature separation of the placenta, and amniotic fluid embolus, primarily are due to this pathophysiologic mechanism. The hemorrhagic state following hemolytic transfusion reaction is also related to this process. Defibrination has been observed as a complication of extracorporeal circulation, disseminated carcinoma, lymphomas, thrombotic thrombocytopenia, rickettsial infection, snakebite, and shock. Release of thromboplastic material has long been a recognized complication of gram-negative sepsis and has been attributed to the effects of circulating endotoxin on platelets. More recently, it has been recognized that septicemia due to gram-positive organisms may also be associated with DIC.

The differentiation between DIC with secondary protective fibrinolysis from primary fibrinolytic states can be extremely difficult, as the thrombin time, which many consider to be the most useful single test in establishing the presence of significant DIC or fibrinolysis, is prolonged in both cases. The salient differentiating features are that DIC is more common and is associated with an increased amount of cold insoluble fibrinogen (cryofibrinogen) and, most important, thrombocytopenia.

TREATMENT. The most important facets of treatment are relieving the patient's primary medical or surgical problem and maintaining adequate capillary flow. The use of intravenous fluids to maintain volume and, at times, vasodilators to open the arterioles is indicated. If blood flow deficiency is related to inability of a damaged heart to pump, the use of drugs such as digitalis or Isuprel may be indicated. Viscosity may be affected by an increased hematocrit, and, therefore, a plasma expander may be beneficial.

In the past heparin has been regarded as the treatment of choice, since it provides the most direct interference with the coagulation process. However, there has been little evidence of success associated with this form of therapy. Administration of fibrinogen should be limited, since it may result in further intravascular coagulation, and the use of ϵ-aminocaproic acid to inhibit secondary fibrinolysis is contraindicated, since uncontrolled disseminated intravascular coagulation may result.

FIBRINOLYSIS

The acquired hypofibrinogenemic state in the surgical patient also can be due to pathologic fibrinolysis. This may occur in patients with metastatic prostatic carcinoma, shock, sepsis, hypoxia, neoplasia, cirrhosis, and portal hypertension.

The pathogenesis of this bleeding disorder is complex. Secondary to shock or hypoxia, a release of excessive plasminogen activator into the circulation occurs. This is thought to be endogenous kinases which can be released from vascular endothelium and other tissues. Pharmacologic activation of plasminogen also occurs with pyrogens, epinephrine, nicotinic acid, and acetylcholine. Electric shock and pneumoencephalopathy have also been reported to cause activation. Patients with cirrhosis and portal hypertension have a diminished ability to clear normal amounts of plasminogen activator from the blood.

In addition to the reduction in levels of plasma fibrinogen, diminution of factors V and VIII also occurs, since they also serve as substrates for the enzyme plasmin. Thrombocytopenia is not an accompaniment of the purely fibrinolytic state. Polymerization of fibrin monomers, a step in normal fibrin formation, is interfered with by the proteolytic residue of fibrinogen and fibrin. The fibrin and fibrinogen breakdown products usually disappear from the circulation in a matter of hours. The biologic half-life of the interfering products has been estimated at approximately 9 hours.

Streptokinase and urokinase have been used to induce therapeutic fibrinolysis, but enthusiasm for these drugs as treatment for venous thrombosis, pulmonary embolism, and clotted hemothorax is not widespread. As there is a limited endogenous supply of activator available, it is soon exhausted by the injections, and later injections fail to achieve the desired effect. Also, treatment with these drugs is frequently accompanied by chills and fever. Excessive bleeding has been noted in almost half the patients treated, and anemia has appeared beyond that anticipated by the amount of bleeding. At present, results of urokinase therapy for deep venous thrombosis should be regarded as encouraging but not conclusive.

TREATMENT. The successful treatment of the underlying disorder usually is followed by rapid spontaneous recovery, since the severity of fibrinolytic bleeding is dependent upon the concentration of breakdown products in the circulation. ε-Aminocaproic acid, a synthetic amino acid, interferes with fibrinolysis by inhibiting plasminogen activation. The drug may be administered intravenously or orally. An initial dose of 5 Gm for the average-sized adult is followed by another 5 Gm every 4 to 6 hours until the hemorrhagic state subsides. Treatment rarely is required for more than 2 or 3 days. Just as the administration of ε-aminocaproic acid to a patient with consumptive coagulopathy is potentially dangerous, the administration of heparin to the patient who has a primary pathologic fibrinolysis is fraught with danger. Thus, fine clinical judgment and reliable laboratories are needed to avoid therapeutic complications. Restraint in definitive treatment of both fibrinolysis and consumptive coagulopathy is recommended, while measures designed to reverse the shock and stabilize the patient are emphasized.

Thrombocytopenia

Thrombocytopenia, as stated earlier, is the most common abnormality of hemostasis resulting in bleeding in the surgical patient. A wide variety of diseases can lead to reduction in platelet count and purpuric bleeding. Thrombocytopenia may be primary and idiopathic (idiopathic thrombocytopenic purpura, or ITP) or secondary and symptomatic (lupus erythematosus, drug reaction, or portal hypertension). The lack of platelets may be associated with megakaryocytes in the bone marrow (ITP, congestive splenomegaly) or with absence of megakaryocytes (leukemia, following cytotoxic therapy).

Microscopic examination of a properly stained blood smear should suggest the diagnosis. The presence and extent of thrombocytopenia can be defined precisely by a quantitative platelet count. In general, 60,000 to 70,000 platelets per cubic millimeter are adequate for normal hemostasis, but often a poor correlation between bleeding and the platelet count is noted. The bleeding time may be prolonged with marked thrombocytopenia or, less commonly, with qualitative platelet abnormality. Clot retraction usually is abnormal when the platelet count is below 70,000. Thrombocytopenia obviously can exist in the presence of normal clot retraction. In patients with thrombocytopenia, the clotting time and one-stage prothrombin time are normal.

The numerous etiologic bases of thrombocytopenia create a therapeutic challenge for the surgeon. The problems can be reduced to manageable proportions by attempting to define the pathophysiology of the thrombocytopenic state. The patient whose bone marrow is replaced by leukemia, metastatic tumor, or fibrous tissue and is therefore not producing platelets will not benefit from splenectomy. If an immune mechanism is responsible for the thrombocytopenia, it is important to determine if this is related to an extrinsic stimulus, drug, or infection. If drug-related, the thrombocytopenia will correct itself within days to weeks of discontinuation of the medication. If thrombocytopenia is secondary to bacteremia, the repair usually occurs in a day or two. If thrombocytopenia is related to viral infection, the return of platelets may not take place for 3 weeks or longer. Occasionally, severe thrombocytopenia and bleeding are secondary to vitamin B_{12} or folic acid deficiency and are associated with a megaloblastic bone marrow. This may occur 2 or 3 years following total gastrectomy or in association with severe intestinal malabsorption. In either case, supplying the appropriate nutrient will correct the thrombocytopenia within 2 or 3 days. Thrombocytopenia has recently been reported in association with acute alcoholism in the noncirrhotic patient. The marrow megakaryocytes are normal, and the platelet count returns to normal 5 to 7 days after the alcohol intake ceases.

If the thrombocytopenia is associated with splenomegaly

and megakaryocytes remain in the marrow, removal of the spleen offers a good chance for relief of thrombocytopenia.

TREATMENT. Treatment must be based upon consideration of the patient at hand. Management of the thrombocytopenic patient takes one of four forms, separately or in combination. These include (1) careful observation alone, (2) steroid therapy, (3) splenectomy, and (4) transfusion therapy.

Careful observation, a form of management, is neglected too often in our anxiety to do something for the patient. This approach is applicable in the patient with chronic thrombocytopenia (75,000 to 85,000 platelets per cubic millimeter) and no bleeding symptoms or signs. The patient with drug-induced, immune-related thrombocytopenia or postinfectious thrombocytopenia also requires only careful observation if there is no significant bleeding.

Corticosteroid therapy is appropriate for the patient with thrombocytopenia who is having significant bleeding but is known to have a self-limited process. Although neither firm experimental data nor properly controlled clinical observations are available, a strong impression exists that corticosteroid administration to the thrombocytopenic patient reduces the bleeding tendency. This seems to be true even if there is no increase in the number of platelets in the peripheral blood. Corticosteroid administration to the patient with ITP can result in a partial or complete, temporary or permanent, remission. The incidence of success varies with the clinic. The most enthusiastic clinics do not report much more than 65 percent remission, either temporary or complete. Our experience suggests a figure of 50 percent or less, with fewer than 25 percent complete and permanent. The role of steroids in chronic ITP is to facilitate the management of acute bleeding episodes and to permit the scheduling of operations on a semielective basis.

Treatment of acute ITP is discussed in Chap. 33. Our approach is as follows: The patient is given 40 mg of prednisone daily in divided doses. If no return of platelets is noted after 4 weeks, the dose of prednisone is doubled. If no return of platelets occurs in 4 weeks with the higher dose, the patient then is considered a candidate for splenectomy. Should the platelets return during the course of prednisone treatment, the dose is decreased in a stepwise fashion over a 4- to 6-week period. If relapse occurs, the patient is considered a candidate for splenectomy rather than retreatment with steroids.

In certain patients, splenectomy may be considered because of relative contraindications to continued steroid therapy, e.g., an active peptic ulcer, serious psychologic changes, and diabetes in which difficulty of control is related to the steroid therapy.

Emergency splenectomy for ITP usually is limited to the patient who presents with central nervous system bleeding. If this is the case, the patient is given 200 mg of intravenous hydrocortisone immediately, and an intravenous infusion of 100 mg of hydrocortisone in 5% dextrose and water is administered over each 6-hour period. Platelet-rich plasma or platelet concentrates are administered preoperatively and during operation. Blood transfusions should consist of fresh whole blood. The platelet preparations and hydro-cortisone are continued postoperatively until the platelets return. Remission occurs in 65 to 70 percent of patients, usually within 3 to 4 days. Occasionally, return of platelets occurs more slowly, over 10 to 14 days.

To rapidly increase the platelet count in surgical patients with thrombocytopenia, particularly that which is associated with massive bleeding and replacement with banked blood, platelet packs are advised. Special platelet transfusion sets are used to reduce loss of platelets due to adherence. For the average patient an administration of 1×10^{11} platelets/m^2 of body surface area will increase circulating platelets by 12×10^9/l. Fever, infection, hepatosplenomegaly, and the presence of antiplatelet alloantibodies will decrease the effectiveness of platelet transfusion.

Recently it has been shown that normal survival of platelets can be obtained with platelets prepared and stored with agitation at room temperature for 72 hours. It has also been demonstrated that these stored concentrates are capable of producing satisfactory posttransfusion elevations in thrombocytopenic patients. Aster et al. have shown that the hemostatic effectiveness of platelets stored at 4°C for 24 hours is equivalent to that of fresh platelets and superior to that of platelets stored at room temperature.

In patients refractory to standard platelet transfusions, the use of HL-A–compatible platelets coupled with special processors has proved effective. Platelet aggregometry has been applied to screening for potential donors. When these refined techniques are not available, in most instances members of the family will provide suitable donors for otherwise refractory patients.

Myeloproliferative Diseases

POLYCYTHEMIA VERA

Surgical treatment of the patient with polycythemia vera is complicated by distinctly increased morbidity and mortality. This is particularly true for the untreated patient but also applies, to some extent, to the patient who has been treated successfully. Spontaneous thrombosis is a complication of polycythemia vera and can be explained, in part, by increased blood viscosity, increased platelet count, and increased tendency toward stasis. Paradoxically, a significant tendency to spontaneous hemorrhage also is noted in these patients. Approximately one-third of patients with polycythemia vera have some form of hemorrhagic complaint at the time of initial diagnosis. The tendency to bleed usually is a function of an excessively high platelet count. Patients with spontaneous bleeding characteristically have a platelet count of 1.5 million per cubic millimeter or greater. The bleeding time may be prolonged. Evidence has been offered that the platelets in these patients may be qualitatively defective. Despite intensive study, the seeming paradox of hemorrhagic tendency accompanied by thrombocytosis is poorly understood.

The polycythemic patient with marked thrombocytosis is a major surgical risk. Operation should be considered only for the most grave surgical emergency. If possible, operation should be deferred until medical management has returned the blood volume, hematocrit, and hemostatic process to normal.

TREATMENT. Thrombocytosis can be reduced by the careful administration of alkylating agents such as busulfan or chlorambucil. These measures are time-consuming. Surgical procedure should be delayed weeks to months following institution of treatment. Ideally, the hematocrit should be kept below 48 percent and the platelet count less than 400,000 per cubic millimeter. The blood volume also can be reduced more rapidly by phlebotomy. Prior to operation, a thorough laboratory investigation of hemostatic function should be conducted. Any gross defect, such as deficiency of vitamin K–dependent factors or low plasma fibrinogen values, should be investigated and corrected when possible. When surgical treatment is judged imperative in these patients, the erythremic state should be reduced by phlebotomy. Operation, at all times, must be performed fastidiously. Postoperative fibrinolysis also has been known to occur, further complicating the postoperative course.

In one series reported from a clinic with considerable experience, 46 percent of polycythemic patients undergoing major procedures had complications at the time of operation or during the postoperative course, and a 16 percent mortality was associated with the surgical procedures. Significantly, 80 percent of the deaths were encountered in patients on whom operations were performed while the disease was not under control. In operations on patients in whom hematocrit and platelet count had been reduced prior to operation the mortality and incidence of complications decreased. Hemorrhage is the most common complication occurring during or following operation and accounts for greater than two-thirds of the deaths. Thrombosis, either venous or arterial, is the next most frequent complication. Infection also is surprisingly common, occurring in approximately 20 percent of patients.

MYELOID METAPLASIA

Myeloid metaplasia frequently represents part of the natural history of polycythemia vera. Approximately 50 percent of patients with myeloid metaplasia are postpolycythemic, while in the remainder the condition apparently occurs as a separate, possibly related, disease entity. Myeloid metaplasia is characterized by many of the features of polycythemia vera. Splenomegaly usually is more prominent and may be massive. Laboratory features include leukocytosis, which may be severe, or, at times, severe leukopenia. Young myeloid forms may be present. Platelets may be strikingly increased in number, but thrombocytopenia also may be present. The latter is usually characteristic of the patient who has myelofibrosis rather than a hyperplastic bone marrow. Examination of the peripheral blood smear may reveal large, bizarre platelets, fragments of megakaryocyte nuclei, occasional nucleated red cells, and bizarre variations in red cell shape. Evidence suggesting qualitative platelet abnormalities has been described. This is considered as a factor in bleeding in some myeloid metaplasia patients. Abnormalities of platelet factor 3 release have been demonstrated, as have abnormalities in platelet aggregation with ADP.

The morbidity rate following surgical treatment in patients with myeloid metaplasia has been reported as high as 68 percent in a small series. The mortality rate in the same experience was greater than 42 percent. Relatively innocuous surgical procedures have been accompanied by nearly uncontrollable bleeding. Spontaneous bleeding from esophageal varices in patients with myeloid metaplasia and massive splenomegaly also has been reported. Preparation for an operation is similar to that described for polycythemia vera.

Other Diseases Associated with Increased Risk of Bleeding

A number of illnesses not primarily characterized by hemostatic failure may be associated with increased risk of bleeding. These diseases frequently involve organs of formation or synthesis of products essential to hemostasis. Diseases such as leukemia, lymphoma, or multiple myeloma may lead to thrombocytopenia because of the replacement of the megakaryocytes in the bone marrow. Illnesses resulting in severe impairment of hepatic function may limit synthesis of plasma factors essential to normal coagulation. The patient with advanced cirrhosis may be lacking in factors of the prothrombin complex (II, V, VII, X), as well as factor XIII.

Illnesses increasing the removal of products essential to hemostasis also occur. Representative of this problem is the patient with splenomegaly in whom sequestration and removal of platelets proceeds at an abnormally rapid rate. Accelerated removal of plasma factors necessary for coagulation has been mentioned in the discussion of the consumptive coagulopathies. The reciprocal of the latter problem has been identified in the case of the patients with cirrhosis and portal hypertension who fail to clear the activators of fibrinolysis from the circulation. This results in a longer biologic survival of these activators and attendant increased fibrinolytic activity.

Some illnesses are characterized by the production of substances which interfere with the normal hemostatic mechanism. These diseases are associated with the production of abnormal proteins which may coat the platelets, as in macroglobulinemia, or bind with certain of the normal blood-clotting factors, as in multiple myeloma or in states associated with the production of cryoglobulin.

Certain diseases may be associated with multiple hemostatic defects. These may include qualitative and quantitative platelet problems, vascular abnormalities, and impaired metabolism and excretion of administered anticoagulant. Any combination of these problems may be noted in patients with renal failure and uremia. The most common problem in this group of patients is thrombocytopenia concurrent with qualitative platelet defects which parallel the degree of azotemia. The hemostatic problems of patients with severe liver disease may be multiple. Major hemorrhagic episodes in these patients usually are accompanied by significant thrombocytopenia, but this is rarely the sole cause. Deficiencies of the coagulation factors normally synthesized in the liver may be present, and increased fibrinolysis also may be evident.

Iatrogenic disorders may result from the administration of drugs which directly or indirectly influence the hemostatic process. Agents which may damage or inhibit the bone marrow include alkylating agents used in malignant disease, antibiotics, such as chloramphenicol, or antibiotics which occasionally result in immunologic removal of platelets, e.g., penicillin, ristocetin, streptomycin. In the idiosyncratic patient, a wide variety of agents may precipitate immune responses leading to platelet removal, e.g., quinidine, quinine, chlorothiazides. Vasculitis and purpura may follow the use of sulfonamides. Salicylates and phenylbutazone may interfere with the platelet-collagen reaction early in the hemostatic process.

TREATMENT. The management of the patient with liver disease is discussed in Chap. 30. Transfusion with freshly drawn whole blood or freshly prepared platelet-rich plasma may be necessary. When thrombocytopenia is significant, the administration of corticosteroids may diminish the bleeding tendency, even though the platelet count is not raised. Bleeding encountered in patients with bone marrow replacement or bone marrow destruction is thrombocytopenic in origin. The use of whole fresh blood, fresh platelet-rich plasma, or fresh platelet concentrates is indicated for control of acute bleeding episodes. Corticosteroids also have been helpful in this situation. Patients with dysproteinemia and attendant bleeding are particularly difficult to manage. Generally, surgical treatment should be deferred until the basic disease is ameliorated and the production of abnormal protein is diminished. In some instances, diminution of the hemorrhagic potential has been accomplished by intensive plasmapheresis with reduction in the level of the abnormal circulating protein.

Anticoagulation and Bleeding

Spontaneous bleeding may be a complication of anticoagulant therapy with either heparin or the coumarin and indandione derivatives. An exaggerated response to oral anticoagulants may occur if dietary vitamin K is inadequate. The anticoagulant effect of coumarin is consistently reduced in patients receiving barbiturates, and increased coumarin requirements have also been documented in patients receiving contraceptives, other estrogen-containing compounds, corticosteroids, and ACTH. Therefore, reduced anticoagulant dosage should be anticipated following discontinuance of any of these drugs. Medications known to increase the effect of oral anticoagulants include phenylbutazone, the cholesterol-lowering agent clofibrate, anabolic steroids (norethandrolone), D-thyroxine, glucagon, quinidine, and a variety of antibiotics.

The history is all-important in recognizing these patients. Questioning should be specific. The patient should be asked if he is presently taking drugs to "thin out" his blood or prevent clotting. Unexplained bleeding in medical and paramedical personnel occasionally is due to surreptitious anticoagulation. The onset of hematuria or melena in the patient receiving anticoagulants should be investigated, since it has been shown that anticoagulants may unmask underlying tumors. Patients with bleeding secondary to anticoagulation may present with only epistaxis, gastro-intestinal hemorrhage, or hematuria. Physical examination, however, almost always reveals other signs of bleeding such as ecchymoses, petechiae, or hematoma. Bleeding secondary to anticoagulation is not an uncommon cause of rectus sheath hematoma, simulating appendicitis, and intramural intestinal or retroperitoneal hematoma.

Surgical intervention may prove necessary in patients receiving anticoagulant therapy. The typical example is the patient with rheumatic heart disease receiving long-term anticoagulation because of repeated arterial emboli, who then is seen subsequent to a critical embolic episode. Increasing experience suggests that surgical treatment can be undertaken without discontinuing the anticoagulant program. The risk of thrombotic complications reportedly is increased when anticoagulant therapy is discontinued suddenly. If so, this may not be related to what has been called the "rebound phenomena" but may represent an event in a patient who has an underlying thrombotic tendency. When the clotting time is less than 25 minutes in the heparinized patient or when the prothrombin time is greater that 20% of normal in a patient on coumarin, reversal of anticoagulant therapy may not be necessary. Meticulous surgical technique is mandatory, and the patients must be observed closely.

Certain surgical procedures should not be performed in the face of anticoagulation. In sites where even minor bleeding can cause great morbidity, e.g., the central nervous system and the eye, anticoagulants should be discontinued and, if necessary, reversed. Because of the added problem of local fibrinolysis, prostatic surgical treatment should not be carried out in a patient on anticoagulants. Procedures requiring blind needle introduction should be avoided. Deaths have been reported following sympathetic block for peripheral vascular disease in patients receiving anticoagulation. Splenoportography has a markedly increased morbidity in patients in whom prothrombin times are less than 30% and who are thrombocytopenic.

Emergency operation occasionally is necessary in patients who have been heparinized as treatment for deep venous thrombosis. Reversal of heparinization may be desirable. The patient with repeated episodes of pulmonary embolization while fully heparinized is an example. Reversal of heparinization also can be a problem in cardiac surgical procedures employing extracorporeal circulation. The anticoagulant effect of heparin can be rapidly counteracted with protamine sulfate when the heparin has been given intravenously. Protamine sulfate also is administered intravenously. Theoretically, 1.28 mg should neutralize 1 mg of heparin. In fact, 1 milligram of protamine may be given for each milligram of heparin, provided the intravenous heparin was not given more than 2 hours previously. Protamine sulfate in large doses also has an anticoagulant activity. The formation of both extrinsic and intrinsic prothrombinase can be retarded, prolonging the one-stage prothrombin time test and the partial thromboplastin time test. Some patients exhibit the phenomenon of "heparin rebound" following apparently adequate heparin neutralization with protamine. Prolongation of the clotting time again recurs after adequate postoperative antagonism of the heparin. This can contribute to postoperative bleeding. In our experience, this is the major cause of "unexplained" postoperative bleeding following extracorporeal cardiac bypass surgical procedures. Activation of fibrinolysis and thrombocytopenia may also contribute to this problem.

Bleeding infrequently is related to hypoprothrombinemia if the prothrombin concentration is greater than 15%. We have successfully resected a ruptured aortic aneurysm and inserted a prosthetic graft in a patient with a prothrombin concentration at this level. Excessive bleeding was not encountered.

In the elective surgical patient receiving coumarin therapy adequately effecting anticoagulation, the drug can be discontinued several days prior to operation, and the prothrombin concentration then checked. A level greater than 50% is considered safe. If emergency surgical treatment is required, parenteral injection of vitamin K_1 can be used. Since the reversal effect may take 6 hours, transfusion of whole blood or, preferably, freshly frozen plasma may be required. Parenteral administration of vitamin K also is indicated in elective surgical treatment of patients with biliary obstruction, malabsorption, and hypoprothrombinemia. The drug should result in a normal prothrombin time. In contrast, if the hypoprothrombinemia is related to hepatocellular dysfunction, vitamin K therapy is ineffective and should not be prolonged over a week if no response is noted. Vitamin K is an oxidant, and one must be aware that patients with red cell enzyme deficiencies may sustain hemolysis following its administration.

LOCAL HEMOSTASIS

Surgical bleeding, even when alarmingly excessive, is usually caused by ineffective local hemostasis. The goal of local hemostasis is to prevent the flow of blood from incised or transected blood vessels. This may be accomplished by interrupting the flow of blood to the involved area or by direct closure of the blood vessel wall defect. The techniques may be classified as mechanical, thermal, or chemical.

Mechanical Procedures

The oldest mechanical device to effect closure of a bleeding point or to prevent blood from entering the area of disruption is digital pressure. When pressure is applied to an artery proximal to an area of bleeding, profuse bleeding is reduced, permitting more definitive action. The Pringle maneuver of occluding the hepatic artery in the hepatoduodenal ligament as a method of controlling bleeding from a transected cystic artery or from the surface of the liver is a classic example. Direct digital pressure over a bleeding site, such as a lateral rent in the interior vena cava, is also effective. The finger has the advantage of being the least traumatic vascular hemostat. All clamps, including the so-called atraumatic vascular clamps, do result in damage to the intimal wall of the blood vessel. The obvious disadvantage of digital pressure is that it cannot be used permanently.

The hemostat also represents a temporary mechanical device to stem bleeding. In smaller and noncritical vessels, the trauma and adjacent tissue necrosis associated with the application of a hemostat are of little consequence. These minor disadvantages are outweighed by the mechanical advantage that the instrument offers to subsequent ligation. When bleeding occurs from a vessel which should be preserved, relatively atraumatic hemostats should be employed to limit the extent of intimal damage and subsequent thrombosis.

In general, a ligature replaces the hemostat as a permanent method of effecting hemostasis in a single vessel. When a vessel is transected, a simple ligature usually is sufficient. For large arteries with pulsation and longitudinal motion, transfixion suture to prevent slipping is indicated. When the bleeding site is from a lateral defect in the blood vessel wall, suture ligatures are required. The adventitia and media constitute the major holding forces within the walls of large vessels, and therefore multiple fine sutures are preferable to fewer larger sutures.

Historically, Aulus Cornelius Celsus devised the use of ligatures in 100 A.D. Because of the strong influence of Galen, who was inclined to cautery, this method did not gain popularity. Paré, in 1552, rediscovered the principle of ligature. In 1800, Physick used absorbable sutures of buckskin and parchment. In 1858, Simpson introduced the wire suture, and in 1881 Lister employed chromic catgut. Halsted, in the early 1900s, emphasized the importance of incorporating as little tissue as possible in the suture and indicated the advantages of silk. In 1911, Cushing reported on the use of silver clips to effect hemostasis in delicate vessels in critical areas. Recently, a wide variety of staples made of different metals, which are relatively inert in tissue, have been employed. The advantages of stapling are speed, accuracy, minimal tissue trauma, and the ability to effect hemostasis in otherwise inaccessible areas. Staples have not replaced the ligature, since they are less reliable and harder to apply to larger vessels.

All sutures represent foreign material, and the selection is based on the characteristics of the material and the state of the wound. Nonabsorbable sutures, such as silk, polyethylene, and wire, evoke less tissue reaction than absorbable materials, such as catgut. The latter are preferable, however, in the face of overt infection. The presence of nonabsorbable material in an infected wound can lead to extrusion or sinus tract formation. Wire is the least reactive of the nonabsorbable sutures but the most difficult to handle. Monofilament wire and coated sutures have an advantage over multifilament sutures in the presence of infection. The latter tend to fragment and permit sinus formation due to the interstices.

Diffuse bleeding from multiple transected vessels may be controlled by mechanical techniques which employ pressure directly over the bleeding area, pressure at a distance, or generalized pressure. These techniques are based on the premise that as pressure and flow are decreased in the area of vascular disruption, a clot will occur. Pressure at a distance was effected by application of tourniquets and other pressure devices at pressure points proximal to bleeding sites as a standard procedure by military surgeons in the seventeenth century. Now it is generally felt that direct pressure is preferable and is not attended by the danger of tissue necrosis associated with prolonged use of tourniquets. In our present aerospace age, gravitational suits have been employed to create generalized pressure and to decrease temporarily bleeding from rupture of major intraabdominal vessels.

Direct pressure applied by means of packs affords the best method of controlling diffuse bleeding from large areas. At times, hemostatic chemical materials, such as oxidized cellulose, are incorporated in the packing. Rarely is it necessary to leave a pack at the bleeding site and remove it at a second sitting. If this is done, several days should elapse before removal, and the possibility of recurrent bleeding should be anticipated. The question as to whether hot wet packs or cold wet packs should be applied has been investigated. Unless the heat is so great as to denature protein, it may actually increase bleeding, whereas cold packs promote hemostasis by inducing vascular spasm and increasing endothelial adhesiveness. Bleeding from cut bone may be controlled by packing beeswax in the area. This material effects pressure and is relatively nonirritative to the body.

Thermal Agents

Galen's favoring of cautery influenced medicine for 1,500 years, until the teachings of Paré were appreciated. The use of cautery was revitalized in 1928, when Cushing and Bovie applied this technique for effecting hemostasis of delicate vessels in recessed areas, such as the brain. Heat achieves hemostasis by denaturation of protein, which results in coagulation of large areas of tissue. With actual cautery, heat is transmitted from the instrument by conduction directly to the tissue, whereas with electrocautery, heating occurs by induction from an alternating-current source.

When electrocautery is employed, the amplitude setting should be high enough to produce prompt coagulation but not so high as to set up an arc between the tissue and the cautery tip. This avoids burns outside the operative field and prevents exit of current through electrocardiographic leads or other monitoring devices. A negative plate should be placed beneath the patient whenever cautery is employed to avoid severe skin burns. The advantage of cautery is that it saves time, whereas the disadvantage is that more tissue is necrosed than with precise ligature. Certain anesthetic agents cannot be used with electrocautery because of the hazard of explosion.

A direct current can also result in electrical hemostasis. Since the protein moieties and cellular elements of blood have a negative surface charge, they are attracted to the positive pole, where a thrombus is formed. Direct currents in the 20- to 100-ma range have been applied to control diffuse bleeding from large serous surfaces. High-power argon-laser treatment has been applied successfully to the control of bleeding from superficial erosions.

At the other end of the thermal spectrum, cooling has been applied to control bleeding, particularly from the mucosa of the esophagus and stomach. Generalized hypo-thermia is of little avail, since, in order to reduce the blood flow to visceral organs, the systemic temperature must be brought down to the level of 35°C. At this point shivering and ventricular fibrillation may be encountered. Thrombocytopenia may also be a consequence of generalized cooling. Direct cooling is effective and acts by increasing the local intravascular hematocrit and decreasing blood flow by vasoconstriction. A variety of gastric balloons and cooling devices have been employed locally to cool the stomach and distal esophagus as treatment for bleeding esophagogastric varices and gastritis.

Extreme cooling, i.e., cryogenic surgery, has been applicable particularly in neurosurgery. Temperature ranges of −20 to −180°C are used, and freezing occurs around the tip of the cannula within 5 seconds. At temperatures of −20°C or below, the tissue, capillaries, small arterioles, and venules undergo cryogenic necrosis. This is caused by dehydration and denaturation of lipid molecules. The muscular walls of large arteries are an exception. Although the major arteries and blood may be frozen solid, the blood contained in these vessels does not clot. When thawing occurs, normal circulation is resumed.

Chemical Agents

Chemical agents vary in their hemostatic action. Some are vasoconstrictive, while others have coagulant properties. Still others are relatively inert but possess hygroscopic properties which increase their bulk and aid in plugging disrupted blood vessels.

Epinephrine, applied topically, induces vasoconstriction, but extensive application can result in considerable absorption and systemic effects. The drug generally is used on oozing sites in mucosal areas, during tonsillectomy, for example.

Historically, skeletal muscle was one of the first materials with locally hemostatic properties to be employed, its use having been introduced by Cushing in 1911. Shortly thereafter, hemostatic fibrin was manufactured. The properties required for local hemostatic materials include handling ease, rapid absorption, nonirritation, and hemostatic action independent of the general clotting mechanism. The most widely used of the commercially available materials are gelatin foam (Gelfoam), oxidized cellulose (Oxycel), and oxidized regenerated cellulose (Surgicel). All these materials act, in part, by transmitting pressure against the wound surface, and the interstices provide a scaffold on which the clot can organize.

Gelfoam is made from animal skin gelatin which has been denatured. In itself, Gelfoam has no intrinsic hemostatic action, but it can be used in combination with topical thrombin, for which it serves as an absorbable carrier. Its main hemostatic activity is related to the contact between blood and the large surface area of the sponge and to the pressure exerted by the weight of the sponge and absorbed blood. Prior to application of Gelfoam, the sponge should be moistened in saline or thrombin solution, and all the air should be removed from the interstices.

Oxycel and Surgicel are altered cellulose materials capable of reacting chemically with blood and producing a sticky mass which functions as an artificial clot. These substances are relatively inert and are removed by liquefaction in 1 week to 1 month. They should be dry when they are applied. Like Gelfoam, these materials are nontoxic and relatively nonirritating but are somewhat detrimental to wound healing and require phagocytosis to be removed. Surgicel has been shown to have an antibacterial effect.

Recently, adhesive chemicals have been developed to literally cement bleeding sites. One example is methyl-2-cyanoacrilate (Eastman 9-10), which is a rapidly polymerizing substance. These agents have little toxicity but do evoke a marked inflammatory response. Aneurysms have been reported subsequent to the application of cements to major blood vessels. Methyl-2-cyanoacrilate has been applied to the surface of the liver for hemostasis with reported success. Another local approach to the problem of bleeding from a large area is the application of tanned collagen sponge, which functions as a collagenous framework. This encourages the invasion and proliferation of fibroblasts while applying constant pressure against the wound to effect hemostatic action. Microcrystalline collagen has been shown to be more effective than other materials as a topical hemostatic agent.

TRANSFUSION

Background

In 1967, the tercentenarial anniversary of the transfusion of blood into human beings was celebrated. In June of 1667, Jean Baptiste Denis and a surgeon, Emmerez, transfused blood from a sheep into a fifteen-year-old boy who had been bled many times as treatment for fever. The patient apparently improved, and a successful experience was reported simultaneously in another patient. Because of two subsequent deaths associated with transfusion from animals to man, criminal charges were brought against Denis. In April of 1668, further transfusions in man were forbidden unless approved by the Faculty of Medicine in Paris. It was not until the nineteenth century that human blood was recognized as the only appropriate replacement. In 1900, Landsteiner and his associates introduced the concept of blood grouping and identified the major A, B and O groups. In 1939, the Rh group was recognized. Numerous other groups have been uncovered since that time. Development of sensitive cross-matching procedures took place in the 1940s, and with the impetus of World War II blood transfusion became a common procedure. The introduction of various preservative solutions, such as acid citrate dextrose (ACD) and citrate-phosphate-dextrose (CPD), contributed to the development of blood banking.

As the scope of surgery has expanded, the requirement for larger amounts of blood for transfusion has increased. Approximately 14 percent of all patients operated upon, exclusive of procedures performed in the outpatient department or emergency area, are transfused. Of 604 adults who received blood at a university medical center in association with surgical treatment, 125 required over 5,000 ml.

The record administration in this hospital in a patient who survived was 100 units within a 36-hour period. The logistics of the problem have resulted in modernization of transfusion practices, including the use of plasma expanders and component therapy. Preservation of blood and its constituents has been achieved by freezing. Cadaver blood has been used in large amounts in the U.S.S.R.

Characteristics of Blood and Replacement Therapy

BLOOD

Blood has been described as a vehicular organ which perfuses all other organs. It provides transportation of oxygen to satisfy the metabolic demands and removes the by-product carbon dioxide. Blood also transports chemical nutriments for, and waste products from, metabolic activity. Homeostatic governors, including hormones, coagulation factors, and antibodies, are carried to and from appropriate sites within the fluid portion of the blood. Red blood cells, with their oxygen-carrying capacity, white blood cells, which function in body defense processes, and platelets, which contribute to the hemostatic process, comprise the formed elements.

REPLACEMENT THERAPY

BANKED WHOLE BLOOD. Whole blood generally is collected in CPD solution and stored at 4°C. Such blood is considered suitable for administration any time up to 21 days of storage. Following this period, at least 70 percent of the transfused erythrocytes remain in the circulation 24 hours posttransfusion and are viable. Normal survival of red blood cells is 110 to 120 days. Sixty days after transfusion, approximately 52 percent of the cells will survive if the transfusion uses fresh blood. Fifty percent will survive if the transfusion is with CPD blood stored 14 days. In contrast, only 25 percent of erythrocytes survive at 60 days if the transfusion utilized blood stored for 28 days in CPD. The major loss occurs in the first 24 hours after transfusion, and subsequent to that time the survival slope for red cells from fresh blood and stored blood is identical.

Banked blood is a poor source of platelets, since they lose their ability to survive transfusion after 24 hours of storage. Among the clotting factors, factor II (prothrombin), factor VII, factor IX, and factor XI are stable in banked blood. Factor V is not stable in banked blood, while factor VIII also deteriorates during storage.

During the storage of whole blood, red cell metabolism and plasma protein degradation results in certain chemical changes in the plasma (Table 3-3). Lactic acid increases from 20 to 150 mg/100 ml, an amount which is insignificant in terms of transfusion at the end of 28 days. The pH decreases from 7 to 6.68 within 21 days. Little change in the sodium occurs, but the potassium concentration rises steadily to 32 mEq at the end of 21 days. This must be considered when transfusing patients with anuria, oliguria, or hyperkalemia. In these cases, fresh whole blood obviously is preferable. The ammonia concentration also rises steadily during storage from 50 to 680 μg at the end of

Table 3-3. CHARACTERISTICS OF PLASMA STORED IN
ACD SOLUTION AT $4 \pm 1°C$

Constituents	Unit value	Days stored				
		0	7	14	21	28
Dextrose	mg/100 ml	350	300	245	210	190
Lactic acid	mg/100 ml	20	70	120	140	150
Inorganic phosphate.	mg/100 ml	1.8	4.5	6.6	9.0	9.5
pH*		7.0	6.85	6.77	6.68	6.65
Hemoglobin	mg/100 ml	0–10	25	50	100	150
Sodium	mEq/L	150	148	145	142	140
Potassium	mEq/L	3–4	12	24	32	40
Ammonia	µg/100 ml	50	260	470	680	

*Determined with glass electrode.
SOURCE: From M. M. Strumia, W. H. Crosby, J. G. Gibson II, T. J. Greenwalt, and J. R. Krevans, "General Principles of Blood Transfusion," J. B. Lippincott Company, Philadelphia, 1963.

21 days. This may be of significance for the patient with hepatic disease. The hemolysis which occurs during storage for 21 days is insignificant, since lysis of only about 1 percent of the red cells occurs and the free hemoglobin is rapidly cleared from the circulation following transfusion.

Typing and Cross Matching. In selecting blood for transfusion, serologic compatibility is established routinely for the recipients' and donors' A, B, O, and Rh groups. Cross matching between the donors' red cells and recipients' sera (the "major" cross match) is performed. The donor sera and recipient cells ("minor" cross match) also are checked. As a rule, Rh-negative recipients should be transfused only with Rh-negative blood. Since this group represents 15 percent of the donor population, the supply may be limited. If the recipient is an elderly male who has not been transfused previously, the transfusion of Rh-positive blood is reasonable if Rh-negative blood is unavailable. Anti-Rh antibodies form in several weeks of transfusion. If further transfusions are needed within a few days, more Rh-positive blood can be used. Rh-positive blood should not be transfused to Rh-negative females who are capable of childbearing. Administration of hyperimmune anti-Rh globulin to Rh-negative women shortly after Rh sensitization largely eliminates Rh disease in subsequent offspring. This promising observation may serve as a model to facilitate transfusions. At present, however, type-specific transfusions remain the basis for therapy. Any Rh-negative woman who has borne children may have been sensitized during pregnancy.

A variety of cell-serum interactions may be detected by careful cross matching. Incompatibility may be due to the fact that either the donor or recipient has been wrongly grouped. An interaction may be caused by a difference in a subgroup, e.g., a donor who is A_1 and a recipient who is A_2 with anti-A_1 in the serum. Interactions may also be due to other naturally occurring antibodies such as anti-P_1 or anti-Le.

In the patient who is receiving repeated transfusions,

serum drawn not more than 24 hours prior to cross matching should be utilized for matching with cells of the donor. The recipient cells used for the minor cross match also should be relatively fresh. Antigenic potency for certain blood groups is lost after several days of storage, and failure to detect minor incompatibility can result. Emergency blood transfusion can be performed with group O blood. If it is known that the prospective recipient is group AB, group A blood is preferable. The O donor blood should have low titers of anti-A and anti-B. Such emergency cases are extremely rare with the exception of battlefield casualties, and it should be possible to wait 45 minutes, during which time the patient's group can be determined and type-specific blood used. The use of plasma expanders in the meantime makes this particularly possible.

When the blood of multiple donors is to be transfused, such as in the case of extracorporeal circulatory procedures, the question arises as to whether all samples should be cross-matched with each other. In determining compatibility, screening is performed in the usual fashion. Major and minor cross matches are performed. Cold agglutinin titer of the recipient serum should be determined if hypothermia is to be employed. In patients with malignant lymphoma and leukemia cryoglobulins may be present, and the blood should be administered at room temperature. If these antibodies are present in high titer, hypothermia may be contraindicated.

In patients with thalassemia and, more particularly, with acquired hemolytic anemia, typing and cross matching may be difficult, and sufficient time should be allotted during the preoperative period to accumulate blood that may be required during the operation. Cross matching should always be carried out prior to the administration of dextran, since dextran interferes with the typing procedure.

FRESH WHOLE BLOOD. This refers to blood which is administered within 24 hours of its donation. In the patient who requires platelets, the blood must be transfused within

6 hours of donation. As noted earlier, such fresh blood also is a potential source of factors V and VIII.

PACKED RED CELLS AND FROZEN RED CELLS. Concentrated suspensions of red cells can be prepared by removing most of the supernatant plasma citrate from the blood following settling of the cells or centrifugation. A small amount of plasma citrate is left, so that the packed cell volume is approximately 70%.

The use of frozen red blood cells represents a recent addition to the transfusion armamentarium. The preparation is time-consuming and requires the addition of glycerol to assure uniform rate of intracellular crystal formation during freezing. At thawing, the cells are washed to remove the glycerol. An advantage of frozen red cells is that their use markedly reduces the risk of infusing hepatitis virus or antigens to which the patient has been previously sensitized. Either packed or frozen red cells are applicable in the treatment of anemia without hypovolemia. The use of packed red cells reduces the danger of circulatory overload. Reactions secondary to allergens in plasma to which the recipient is sensitive also can be minimized.

LEUKOCYTE AND PLATELET-POOR RED CELLS. These are prepared by aspirating the buffy coat and supernatant plasma, following slow centrifugation or settling. The red cells then are washed with sterile isotonic solution. The preparation is time-consuming and increases the possibility of bacterial contamination. This should be done only for patients with demonstrated hypersensitivity to either leukocytes or platelets (buffy coat reactions). Usually this syndrome is manifest by fever, chilly sensations, and urticaria in the absence of hemolysis.

PLATELET-RICH PLASMA AND PLATELET CONCENTRATES. The indications for platelet transfusion are as follows: thrombocytopenia due to massive blood loss and replacement with stored blood, thrombocytopenia due to inadequate platelet production, thrombocytopenia due to platelet destruction, and qualitative platelet disorders. The preparations should be used within 6 hours of blood donation. One unit of platelet-rich plasma has a volume of approximately 200 ml. The recovery of platelets in the recipient usually is no more than 60 percent of those present in the donor blood. The platelet concentrate consists of platelets prepared from a unit of platelet-rich plasma. These are resuspended in 30 ml of fluid and should be administered without a filter. The platelet concentrate has the advantage of obviating circulatory overload. Both preparations may harbor the hepatitis virus and account for allergic reactions similar to those due to whole blood. When treating thrombocytopenic bleeding or preparing thrombocytopenic patients for surgery, it is advisable to elevate the platelet levels to the range of 50,000 to 100,000/mm^3 in order to provide continued protection. The development of isoimmunity remains one of the most important factors limiting the usefulness of platelet transfusion. Isoantibodies are demonstrable in about 5 percent of patients after 1 to 10 transfusions, 20 percent after 10 to 20 transfusions, and 80 percent after more than 100 transfusions. The use of HL-A–compatible platelets addresses this problem.

POOLED PLASMA. Plasma prepared from pooled blood is associated with a high incidence of hepatitis. Some investigators suggest that this may be reduced by storage at 31.6°C for 6 months. Banked plasma has been used to treat certain coagulation defects. Frozen plasma prepared from freshly donated blood or fresh plasma is necessary to provide factors V and VIII. The other plasma clotting factors are present in banked preparations. The use of plasma for therapy in patients with hypovolemia rarely is indicated. Ringer's lactate or buffered saline solution, administered in amounts two to three times the estimated blood loss, is effective in an emergency and is associated with fewer complications. Dextran or a combination of Ringer's lactate solution and normal human serum albumin are preferred for rapid plasma expansion. Commercially available dextran preparations probably should not be administered in amounts exceeding 1 liter/day, since prolongation of bleeding time and hemorrhage can occur. Low-molecular-weight dextran, i.e., molecular weight of 30,000 to 40,000, has achieved recent popularity because it possesses a higher colloidal pressure than plasma and effects some reversal of erythrocyte agglutination.

CONCENTRATES. *Antihemophilic concentrates* are prepared from plasma and are available for the treatment of factor VIII deficiency. Some of these concentrates are twenty to thirty times as potent as an equal volume of fresh-frozen plasma. The simplest factor VIII concentrate, described initially by Pool and Shannon, is the plasma cryoprecipitate. Plasma is frozen rapidly by immersion of the plastic container in a dry ice–acetone mixture. The frozen plasma is thawed slowly (18 hours) at refrigerator temperature (4°C), and a sticky precipitate is found clinging to the bag. The thawed liquid plasma is expressed, and the precipitate, containing the bulk of the initial factor VIII activity, can be dissolved in 10 ml of sterile saline solution, pooled with other units if desired, and administered. *Desiccated human fibrinogen* is commercially available. The preparation is made from plasma pooled from many donors and carries a risk of transmitting the virus of hepatitis. *Albumin* also has been concentrated, so that 25 Gm may be administered and provide the osmotic equivalent of 500 ml of plasma. The advantage of albumin is that it is a hepatitis-free product. Salt-poor albumin is available for patients with sodium retention.

Indications for Replacement of Blood or Its Elements

VOLUME REPLACEMENT. The most common indication for blood transfusion in diseases of surgical interest is the replenishment of the circulating blood volume. It is difficult to evaluate the volume deficit accurately.

A variety of techniques employing dyes or isotopically tagged colloids have been introduced to determine the blood volume more precisely. Values for "normal blood volume" are variable, and the techniques are relatively inaccurate when there is a rapidly changing situation, such as hemorrhage. Chronically ill and elderly patients may have a diminution of blood volume. In patients with cardiac decompensation, the blood volume may be greater than normal. Many patients with chronically reduced blood volume are well accommodated to that volume. Blood volume, in itself, does not serve as an absolute indication for transfusion. Measurement of hemoglobin or hematocrit also is used to interpret blood loss. This is misleading in the face of acute blood loss, since the hematocrit may be normal in spite of a severely contracted blood volume. Ebert et al. showed that after a healthy adult male lost approximately 1,000 ml of blood rapidly, the venous hematocrit fell only 3 percent during the first hour, 5 percent at 24 hours, 6 percent at 48 hours, and 8 percent at 72 hours, thus indicating the time required for the body to restore blood volume.

A healthy person can lose 430 ml in 20 minutes with only minor effects on the circulation and little change in blood pressure or pulse, as evidenced by the normal blood donor. The normal person may lose 1 liter of blood rapidly without a fall in blood pressure as long as he remains supine. About 40% of blood volume, or 2 liters of blood, usually is lost before significant hypotension develops. Loss of blood may be evaluated in the operating room by estimating the amount of blood in the wound and on the drapes and by weighing sponges. The loss determined by weighing sponges is only about 70% of true loss.

IMPROVEMENT IN OXYGEN-CARRYING CAPACITY. This is primarily a function of the red cell. When anemia can be treated by specific therapy, transfusion should be withheld. Acute anemias, such as hemolytic anemia, are more disabling physiologically than chronic anemia, since most patients with chronic anemia have undergone an adjustment to the situation. In pregnancy, there is a moderate drop in hematocrit, and transfusions are not indicated to correct the physiologic anemia of pregnancy prior to surgical treatment. The correction of chronic anemia prior to surgical treatment, though often performed, is difficult to justify, and there is no indication that anemia predisposes to wound dehiscence. Peskin and associates have described a stroma-free hemoglobin solution which has the ability to carry and exchange oxygen and, in experimental animals, has demonstrated no toxicity. Blood volume may be replaced with dextran solution or Ringer's lactate solution with a reduction of the hemoglobin to levels below 10 Gm and little demonstrable change in the effects of a reduction in oxygen-carrying capacity or the capacity to remove metabolic gaseous by-products.

REPLACEMENT OF CLOTTING FACTORS. Transfusion of platelets and/or proteins contributing to coagulation may be indicated in specific patients either prior to or during operation. In the treatment of certain hemorrhagic conditions, it is to be appreciated that the clotting defects may be multiple and the injection of substitutes and extracts may be less effective than transfusion of fresh blood. Treatment with clotting factors requires an accurate diagnosis of the hemorrhagic disease with an appreciation of the changes which occur in the biologic properties of the factors during storage and the biologic effects and quantitative changes which occur after injection.

When transfusion with fibrinogen is deemed necessary, a plasma level greater than 100 mg/ml should be maintained. The hypofibrinogenemia encountered during surgi-cal treatment is frequently related to excessive consumption. Adequate levels of fibrinogen frequently will return within hours without replacement therapy if the precipitating cause is corrected. Deficiency of factor V, per se, is relatively rare; although transfusion will increase the level, there is suggestion that the biologic half-life is short and may not exceed 12 hours.

Hypoprothrombinemia and deficiency of factor VII in patients on anticoagulant therapy can be reversed with injection of vitamin K_1. In patients who are deficient in prothrombin, such as those with cirrhosis, and who require surgical treatment, transfusion with banked blood may effect immediate benefit.

Transfusion therapy for patients with hemophilia subjected to trauma or surgical procedures requires sufficient quantities to raise and maintain the level of factor VIII in the plasma to above 30% of normal. Transfusion of small amounts of factor VIII is not justified. If a life-threatening situation exists, large amounts must be used. The factor IX–deficient patient subjected to surgery or trauma also requires levels of 20 to 30% for secure hemostasis. Such levels are difficult to attain with plasma infusions despite the stability of factor IX in stored plasma. Fortunately, factor IX concentrates now being tested offer considerable promise. The biologic half-life of factor IX is appreciably longer than that of factor VIII.

Usually, the hemostatic mechanism is not markedly altered with platelet counts greater than 50,000. If thrombocytopenia is more pronounced, however, the transfusion of fresh platelets may be indicated to prevent or treat active bleeding. The life span of freshly infused platelets is only about 10 days, and in some instances the recipient represents a hostile environment, and the survival is reduced to several hours.

SELECTIVE THERAPY

Johnson and Greenwalt have pointed out that less than 50 years ago we were concerned with making blood transfusions easier to administer while presently we are searching for arguments with which to discourage the administration of unnecessary transfusions and methods to place transfusion on a more logical basis. If the patient has severe anemia and hypovolemia, which are usually associated with massive hemorrhage, whole blood represents the treatment of choice, and ordinary banked blood generally can be used. An alternative to this approach is a combination of packed red cells plus a plasma volume expander. Operative blood losses of 1,000 to 1,500 ml may be replaced without untoward difficulty using Ringer's lactate or buffered saline solution. When anemia exists without hypovolemia, packed red cells represent the treatment of choice. This can be accomplished with the standard packed cells or with frozen cells, which, although presently expensive, provide a method of storage for many years, avoid the complication of hepatitis, and reduce the incidence of fever, chills, and allergic reactions. The use of packed red cells is particularly applicable in patients with severe anemia who have diminished cardiac reserve or hypervolemia.

Thrombocytopenic bleeding is treated with platelet con-

Table 3-4. REPLACEMENT OF CLOTTING FACTORS

Factors	Normal level	Life span in vivo ($\frac{1}{2}$ life)	Fate during coagulation	Level required for safe hemostasis	Stability in ACD bank blood (4°)	Ideal agent for replacing deficit
I (fibrinogen)	200–400 mg/ 100 ml	72 hr	Consumed	60–100 mg/ 100 ml	Very stable	Bank blood; concentrated fibrinogen
II (prothrombin)	20 mg/100 ml (100%)	72 hr	Consumed	15–20%	Stable	Bank blood; concentrated preparation
V (proaccelerin, accelerator globulin labile factor)	100%	36 hr	Consumed	5–20%	Labile (40% at 1 week)	Frozen fresh plasma; blood under 7 days
VII (proconvertin, serum prothrombin conversion accelerator [SPCA] stable factor)	100%	5 hr	Survives	5–30%	Stable	Bank blood; concentrated preparation
VIII (antihemophilic factor [AHF], antihemophilic globulin, [AHG]	100% (50–150)	6–12 hr	Consumed	30%	Labile (20–40% at 1 week)	Fresh frozen plasma; concentrated AHF; cryoprecipitate
IX (Christmas factor, plasma thromboplastin component [PTC], hemophilia B factor)	100%	24 hr	Survives	20–30%	Stable	Fresh frozen plasma, bank blood, concentrated preparation
X (Stuart-Prower factor)	100%	40 hr	Survives	15–20%	Stable	Bank blood; concentrated preparation
XI (plasma thromboplastin antecedent [PTA])	100%	Probably 40–80 hr	Survives	10%	Probably stable	Bank blood
XII (Hageman factor)	100%	Unknown	Survives	Deficit produces no bleeding tendency	Stable	Replacement not required
XIII (fibrinase, fibrin-stabilizing factor [FSF])	100%	4–7 days	Survives	Probably less than 1%	Stable	Bank blood
Platelets	150,000–400,000/ mm³	8–11 days	Consumed	60,000–100,000/ mm³	Very labile (40% at 20 hr; 0 at 48 hr)	Fresh blood or plasma; fresh platelet concentrate (not frozen plasma)

SOURCE: E. W. Salzman, Hemorrhagic disorders, in J. M. Kinney, R. H. Egdahl, and G. D. Zuidema (eds.), "Manual of Preoperative and Postoperative Care," p. 157, W. B. Saunders Company, Philadelphia, 1971.

centrates or platelet-rich plasma (Table 3-4). Deficiencies of factors VII, IX, X, or XI unaccompanied by anemia can be treated with stored plasma or any plasma preparation. If patients with these defects are undergoing elective or emergency surgical treatment, stored blood may be preferable. Factor V deficiency requires fresh frozen plasma or fresh whole blood as therapy. Hemophilia without severe anemia should be treated with factor VIII concentrate or fresh frozen plasma as an alternative. If there is an accompanying severe anemia, the preferable treatment is packed red cells with either factor VIII concentrate or fresh frozen plasma, but fresh blood administered shortly after collection may be used. Congenital hypofibrinogenemia should be treated with whole blood or fibrinogen from small donor pools, while acute acquired hypofibrinogenemia requires, in addition to fibrinogen or whole blood, treatment of the underlying problem, i.e., heparin for defibrination and ε aminocaproic acid for fibrinolysis.

SPECIFIC INDICATIONS

SINGLE-UNIT TRANSFUSION. There has been a general trend toward condemning all single-unit transfusion on surgical services. As has been previously mentioned, they are usually uncalled for. However, the Committee on Blood of the American Medical Association found it necessary to oppose this trend, pointing out that it is a poor practice to order 2 units of blood to escape criticism for using a single unit, and an appropriate volume of blood should be given whenever transfusion is required.

MASSIVE TRANSFUSION. The term *massive transfusion* implies a single transfusion greater than 2,500 ml or 5,000 ml transfused over a period of 24 hours. The approximate percentages of *original* blood volume remaining after varying degrees of hemorrhage and transfusion are shown in Table 3-5. A variety of problems may attend the use of massive transfusion. Dilutional thrombocytopenia, impaired platelet function, and deficiencies of factors V, VIII, and XI may occur. The acid load present in stored blood may have an additive effect in a patient with preexisting acidosis. Routine alkalinization is not advisable, since this could have an adverse effect on the oxyhemoglobin dissociation curve and presents an additional sodium load to a compromised patient. The increased potassium content of multiple units of stored blood does not provide clinical effects unless the patient is severely oliguric.

Table 3-5. PERCENTAGE OF ORIGINAL BLOOD VOLUME REMAINING
IN A PATIENT WITH A 5-LITRE BLOOD VOLUME TRANSFUSED WITH
500-ML UNITS

	Magnitude of hemorrhage and transfusion		
Situation*	1 Blood volume (10 units)	2 Blood volumes (20 units)	3 Blood volumes (30 units)
Best	37%	14%	5%
Usual	25–30%	10%	3–4%
Worst	18%	3%	0.4%

*The "best" situation requires simultaneous and equal replacement during hemorrhage; the "worst" situation means initial loss of one-half blood volume not replaced until the hemorrhage has stopped.

SOURCE: After Collins.

Citrate toxicity may be associated with massive transfusion, particularly in young children and patients with severe hypotension or liver disease. This is related to an excessive binding of ionized calcium and is usually corrected by spontaneous mobilization of calcium from bone. The availability of a calcium ion–sensing electrode should provide a base for intelligent calcium therapy and avoidance of iatrogenic hypercalcemia. The function of hemoglobin is altered by storage in that the concentration of 2,3-DPG (diphosphoglyceric acid) falls to a negligible level by the third week. This results in an increased affinity of the red blood cells for oxygen and a less efficient oxygen delivery system. The shift to CPD blood has a favorable consequence in that 2,3-DPG remains at normal levels for 1 week. Collins has shown that in itself reduction of 2,3-DPG may not have a significant effect but when combined with acute anemia may be an important factor.

When large transfusions are administered, a heat exchanger may be used to warm the blood, since hypothermia may cause a decrease in cardiac rate and output and a reduction in the blood pH. Warming the blood significantly decreases the frequency of intraoperative cardiac arrest.

The use of blood from many donors increases the possibility of hemolytic transfusion reaction due to incompatibility. This can be reduced by screening each potential donor in the pool and eliminating those who show possible incompatibility. Paradoxically, patients who survive a massive transfusion do not have a high probability of developing isoantibodies subsequently, and the risk is no greater than that from a single transfusion. The risk of homologous serum hepatitis increases progressively with each succeeding unit.

EXTRACORPOREAL CIRCULATION. Fresh, heparinized blood generally has been used for open heart operations and other applications of extracorporeal circulation in order to decrease the danger of citrate effect. Subsequent to the procedure, the excess heparin is usually neutralized with protamine. Johnson and Greenwalt indicate that their experience with over 2,000 replacement transfusions demonstrates that this can be performed adequately with ACD blood which is less than 5 days old and modified by the addition of heparin and calcium. Prior to its use, the ACD blood is heparinized with 20 to 25 mg/unit and treated with 500 to 600 mg of calcium chloride/unit. When treated ACD blood is compared with heparinized blood, the pH of the former is lower during the first few minutes of perfusion, and the platelet counts are significantly lower 10 minutes after perfusion. By the end of perfusion there is no difference in the two series. A variety of physiologic compatible fluids, such as Ringer's lactate solution, buffered saline solution, and dextran, may be applied to prime the pump during extracorporeal circulation and reduce the need for blood.

Methods of Administering Blood

ROUTINE ADMINISTRATION. The rate of transfusion depends upon the patient's status. Usually, 5 ml/minute is administered for 1 minute, following which 10 to 20 ml/min may be administered to complete routine transfusion. When marked oligemia is being treated, the first 500 ml may be given within 10 minutes, and the second 500 ml may be given equally rapidly in most cases. Cold blood may be used for this amount, but when larger amounts are administered, warm blood is desirable.

The gauge of the needle is a critical factor in the rate of flow. Flow also is determined by the height at which the bottle is suspended. In patients with peripheral circulatory failure, the veins may be constricted with resultant increased resistance to flow, necessitating raising of the bottle. Positive pressure may be applied by some form of rotary pump or fingers which compress the tubing of the transfusion set and drive the blood onward. If plastic bags have been used as containers for the blood, they may be surrounded with a blood pressure cuff and pressure applied. Air pumped into the transfusion bottle has been used extensively as a method of increasing pressure, but this technique is associated with a definite danger of air embolism.

When large transfusions are administered, it is important not to overload the circulation, and the use of central venous pressure monitoring is particularly pertinent. There is no practical advantage in the use of intraarterial transfusion as compared with the intravenous route in the treatment of oligemia. It has been shown that coronary flow and systemic arterial pressure respond as rapidly and to the same extent whether the blood is administered intravenously or intraarterially. The theoretical advantage of intraarterial infusion for patients in whom the blood cannot pass from the venous to the arterial side of the circulation because of cardiac arrest or ineffective ventricular contraction is offset by the delay in setting up an intraarterial transfusion.

OTHER METHODS. Blood may be instilled intraperitoneally or into the medullary cavity of the sternum and long bones. Intrasternal and intramedullary transfusion may be painful, and the rate of administration is limited. Approximately 90 percent of red cells injected intraperitoneally enter the circulation, but uptake is not complete for at least a week, and therefore the method is not suitable when immediate transfusion is required.

In 1934, Tiber reported 123 autotransfusions using intraperitoneal blood in patients with ruptured ectopic gestation. There was only one death. This technique has also been applied to patients with ruptured livers and spleens. Blood is suctioned gently from the peritoneal cavity and then reinfused after passing through a filter. A transient increase in free hemoglobin and thrombocytopenia results, but red blood cell survival is normal.

Complications

HEMOLYTIC REACTIONS. Hemolytic reactions due to incompatibility of A, B, O, and Rh groups or many other independent systems may result from errors in the laboratory of a clerical or technical nature or the administration of the wrong blood at the time of transfusion. Hemolytic reactions are characterized by intravascular destruction of red blood cells and consequent hemoglobinemia and hemoglobinuria. Circulating haptoglobin is capable of binding 100 mg of hemoglobin/100 ml of plasma, and the complex is cleared by the reticuloendothelial system. When the binding capacity is exceeded, free hemoglobin circulates, and the heme is released and combines with albumin to form methemalbumin. When free hemoglobin exceeds 25 mg/100 ml of plasma, some is excreted in the urine, but in most subjects hemoglobinuria occurs when the total plasma level exceeds 150 mg/100 ml. The renal lesions which may occur consist of tubular necrosis and precipitation of hemoglobin within the tubules.

Clinical Manifestations. There is an increased hazard in patients with a previous transfusion reaction. If the patient is awake, the most common symptoms are the sensation of heat and pain along the vein into which the blood is being transfused, flushing of the face, pain in the lumbar region, and constricting pain in the chest. The patient may experience chills, fever, and respiratory distress, hypotension, and tachycardia from amounts as small as 50 ml. In patients who are anesthetized and undergoing operation, the two signs which may call attention are abnormal bleeding and continued hypotension despite adequate replacement. Abnormal bleeding may be related to the fact that thromboplastic substances are released as the cells are

lysed. The mortality and morbidity resulting from hemolytic reactions is high if the patient receives a full unit of incompatible blood. Acute hemorrhagic diatheses occur in 8 to 30 percent of patients. There is a sudden fall in the platelet count, an increase in fibrinolytic activity, and consumption of coagulation factors, especially V and VIII, due to disseminated intravascular clotting.

Rudowski reported the following incidences of clinical manifestations in a large series with hemolytic posttransfusion reactions: oliguria, 58 percent; hemoglobinuria, 56 percent; arterial hypotension, 50 percent; jaundice, 40 percent; nausea and vomiting, 30 percent; flank pain, 25 percent; cyanosis and hypothermia, 22 percent; dyspnea, 20 percent; chills, 18 percent; diffuse bleeding, 16 percent; neurologic signs, 10 percent; and allergic reaction, 6 percent. The laboratory criteria are hemoglobinuria with a concentration of free hemoglobin over 5 mg/100 ml, a serum haptoglobin level below 50 mg/100 ml, and serologic criteria to show antigen incompatibility of the donor and recipient blood. The simplest clinical diagnostic test is insertion of a bladder catheter and evaluation of the color and volume of the excreted urine, since hemoglobinuria and oliguria are the most characteristic signs.

Treatment. If a transfusion reaction is suspected, the transfusion should be stopped immediately, and a sample of the recipient's blood should be drawn and sent along with the suspected unit to the blood bank for comparison with the pretransfusion samples. The residual blood from the transfusion should be cultured, and the serum bilirubin should be determined in the recipient. Each gram of hemoglobin is converted to about 40 mg of bilirubin. The hemolytic reaction is characterized by an increase in the indirect reacting fraction.

A Foley catheter should be inserted, and the hourly urine output recorded. Since renal toxicity is affected by the rate of urinary excretion and the pH and since alkalinizing the urine prevents precipitation of hemoglobin within the tubules, attempts are made to initiate diuresis and alkalinize the urine. This can be accomplished with 100 ml of 20% mannitol plus 45 mEq of bicarbonate. If marked oliguria or anuria occurs, the fluid intake and potassium intake are restricted, and the patient is treated as a case of renal shutdown. In some instances, dialysis is required. Following recovery from oliguria or anuria, diuresis is often copious and may be associated with significant losses of potassium and sodium which require replacement.

ALLERGIC REACTIONS. These are relatively frequent, occurring in about 1 percent of transfusions. Reactions are usually mild and are manifested by urticaria and fever. In rare instances, the reaction may be severe enough to cause anaphylactic shock. Allergic reactions are caused by transfusion of antibodies from hypersensitive donors or the transfusion of antigens to which the recipient is hypersensitive. Reactions may occur following the administration of whole blood, packed red cells, plasma, and antihemophilic factor. Treatment consists of antihistamines, epinephrine, and steroids, depending on the severity of the reaction.

BACTERIAL SEPSIS. Bacterial contamination of infused

blood is rare and may be acquired either from the contents of the container or the skin of the donor. Gram-negative organisms, which are capable of growth at 4°C, are the most common cause. Clinical manifestations include fever, chills, abdominal cramps, vomiting, and diarrhea. There may be hemorrhagic manifestations and increased bleeding if the patient is undergoing surgical treatment. In some instances, bacterial toxins can produce profound shock. If the diagnosis is suspected, the transfusion should be discontinued and the blood cultured. Emergency treatment includes adrenergic blocking agents, oxygen, antibiotics, and, in some cases, judicious transfusion.

EMBOLISM. Although air embolism has been reported as a complication of intravenous transfusion, healthy animals tolerate large amounts of air injected intravenously at a rapid rate. In experimental animals, the minimal lethal dose averages 7.5 ml/kg, and the mortality rate accompanying this amount of air injection can be halved by placing the animal on the left side at the time of injection. This displaces the air away from the outflow tract in the right ventricle. It has been suggested that the normal adult generally will tolerate an embolism of 200 ml of air. Smaller amounts, however, can cause alarming signs and may be fatal. The most common method of producing air embolism during transfusion is by injecting air under pressure into the container in order to increase rate of flow. Manifestations of venous air embolism include a rise in venous pressure and cyanosis, a "mill wheel" murmur heard over the precordium, hypotension, tachycardia, and syncope. Death usually is related to primary respiratory failure. Treatment consists of placing the patient on the left side in a head-down position with the feet up. Arterial air embolism is manifested by dizziness and fainting, loss of consciousness, and convulsions. Air may be visible in the retinal arteries, and bubbles of air may flow from transected vessels.

Plastic tubes used for transfusion also have embolized after they have broken off within the vein. Plastic tubes have passed into the right atrium and the pulmonary artery, resulting in death. Embolized catheters have been removed successfully.

THROMBOPHLEBITIS. Prolonged infusions into peripheral veins using either needles, cannulae, or plastic tubes are associated with superficial venous thrombosis. Intravenous infusions which last more than 8 hours are more likely to be followed by thrombophlebitis. There is an increased incidence in the lower limb as compared to upper limb infusions. Treatment consists of discontinuation of the infusion and local compressing. Embolism from superficial thrombophlebitis of this nature is extremely rare.

OVERTRANSFUSION AND PULMONARY EDEMA. Overloading the circulation is a complication which is avoidable. It may occur with rapid infusion of blood, plasma expanders, and other fluids, particularly in patients with heart disease. The central venous pressure should be monitored in these patients and whenever large amounts of fluid are administered in order to prevent this complication.

Circulatory overloading is manifested by a rise in the venous pressure, dyspnea, and cough. Râles generally can be heard at the bases of the lung. Treatment consists of stopping the infusion, placing the patient in a sitting position, and, occasionally, venous section for removal of blood.

Although acute pulmonary edema occurs more frequently following large transfusions, it has been reported in patients receiving small transfusions. A syndrome which can be confused with pulmonary edema consists of postoperative hypoxia seen in patients who have undergone cardiac surgical treatment and extracorporeal bypass procedures. A damaging factor apparently is carried by the perfusing blood, and immature plasma cells are found in the interalveolar tissue. The lesion represents an immune response to homologous blood. The incidence is reduced by employing the hemodilution technique of pump priming.

TRANSMISSION OF DISEASE. Malaria, Chagas' disease, brucellosis, and syphilis can be transmitted by blood transfusion. Positive serologic tests for syphilis may result 20 days after transfusion from donors with positive reactions.

Viral Hepatitis. Viral hepatitis is the most important disease transmitted by transfusion of blood components. Included in the general term are viral hepatitis A (formerly called infective hepatitis) and viral hepatitis B (formerly called serum hepatitis). The main clinical difference in the two types is in the incubation period, type A having an incubation of 15 to 50 days and type B 30 to 160 days. A serologic marker for either infection with or carriage of the virus of type B hepatitis is detectable. This serum antigen was formerly called Australian antigen but is now known as hepatitis B surface antigen (HB_sAg). A serum antigen specific for type A hepatitis has not been precisely defined.

In recipients who receive transfusions of an average of 2 units of blood, an incidence of hepatitis of approximately 0.5 percent has been reported. The clinical manifestations of hepatitis include lethargy and anorexia as part of anicteric disease, icterus, and chronic liver disease. HB_sAg persists in about 35 percent of patients who develop serum hepatitis of type B. The risk of hepatitis is definitely diminished by freezing the red cells in plasma. There is no risk from human serum albumin and other plasma protein fractions.

Krugman et al. have reported that immune serum globulin is effective in preventing type A hepatitis but inconsistent in regard to type B. Accidental self-inoculation with material which is definitely known to contain HB_sAg or the transfusion of blood which is HB_sAg-positive constitutes an indication for the immediate use of human specific immunoglobulin (HSI) anti-HB_sAg. The dosage is empirical, but the presently recommended dose is 0.5 IgG given by deep intramuscular injection. Another situation in which the HSI anti-HB_sAg may be of value is in chronic renal dialysis units.

References

General

Biggs, R. P., and Macfarlane, R. G.: "Human Blood Coagulation and Its Disorders," 3d ed., F. A. Davis Company, Philadelphia, 1962.

Hougie, C.: "Fundamentals of Blood Coagulation in Clinical Medicine," McGraw-Hill Book Company, New York, 1963.

Quick, A. J.: "Hemorrhagic Diseases and Thrombosis," Lea & Febiger, Philadelphia, 1966.

Ratnoff, O. D.: "Bleeding Syndromes," Charles C Thomas, Publisher, Springfield, Ill., 1960.

Ulin, A. W., and Gollub, S. S. (eds.): "Surgical Bleeding: Handbook for Medicine, Surgery, and Specialties," McGraw-Hill Book Company, New York, 1966.

Wintrobe, M. M.: "Clinical Hematology," Lea & Febiger, Philadelphia, 1967.

Biology of Normal Hemostasis

Astrup, T.: "Connective Tissue, Thrombosis, and Atherosclerosis," Academic Press, Inc., New York, 1959.

Davie, E. W., and Ratnoff, O. D.: Waterfall Sequence for Intrinsic Blood Clotting, *Science,* **145:**1310, 1964.

Gaarder, A., Jonsen, J., Laland, S., Hellem, A., and Owren, P. A.: Adenosine Diphosphate in Red Cells as a Factor in the Adhesiveness of Human Blood Platelets, *Nature (Lond),* **192:**531, 1961.

Macfarlane, R. G.: Enzyme Cascade in the Blood Clotting Mechanism and Its Function as a Biochemical Amplifier, *Nature (Lond),* **202:**498, 1964.

Quick, A. J.: Effect of Aspirin on the Bleeding Time, *Fed Proc,* **25:**498, 1966.

Rodman, N. F.: The Morphologic Basis of Platelet Function, in K. M. Brinkhous, R. W. Shermer, and F. K. Mostofi (eds.), "The Platelet," The Williams & Wilkins Company, Baltimore, 1971.

Sherry, S.: Present Concept of the Fibrinolytic System, *Ser Haemat,* **7:**70, 1965.

Vigliano, E. M., and Horowitz, H. I.: Bleeding Syndrome in a Patient with IGA Myeloma: Interaction of Protein and Connective Tissue, *Blood,* **29:**823, 1967.

Weiss, H. J.: Platelet Physiology and Abnormalities of Platelet Function, *N Engl J Med,* **293:**531, 1975.

—— Platelet Physiology and Abnormalities of Platelet Function, *N Engl J Med,* **293:**580, 1975.

Tests of Hemostasis and Blood Coagulation

Brecher, G., and Cronkite, E. P.: Morphology and Enumeration of Blood Platelets, *J Appl Physiol,* **3:**365, 1950.

Budtz-Olsen, A. E.: "Clot Retraction," Charles C Thomas, Publisher, Springfield, Ill., 1951.

Bull, B. S.: A Semiautomatic Micro Sample Dilutor, *Am J Clin Pathol,* **47:**549, 1967.

Cartwright, G. E.: "Diagnostic Laboratory Hematology," 4th ed., Grune & Stratton, Inc., New York, 1968.

DeNicola, P.: "Thromboelastography," Charles C Thomas, Publisher, Springfield, Ill., 1957.

Didisheim, P.: Screening Tests for Bleeding Disorders, *Am J Clin Path,* **47:**622, 1967.

Duke, W. W.: The Relation of Blood Platelets to Hemorrhagic Disease: Description of a Method for Determining the Bleeding Time and Coagulation Time, and Report of Three Cases of Hemorrhagic Disease Relieved by Transfusion, *JAMA,* **55:**1185, 1910.

Jim, R. T. S.: A Study of the Plasma Thrombin Time, *J Lab Clin Med,* **50:**45, 1957.

Lee, R. I., and White, P. D.: A Clinical Study of the Coagulation Time of Blood, *Am J Med Sci,* **145:**495, 1923.

Margolius, A., Jr., Jackson, D. P., and Ratnoff, O. D.: Circulating Anticoagulants: A Study of 40 Cases and a Review of the Literature, *Medicine (Baltimore),* **40:**145, 1961.

Mielke, C. H., Kaneshiro, M. M., Weiner, J. M., and Rapaport, S. I.: The Standardized Normal Ivy Bleeding Time and Its Prolongation by Aspirin. *Blood,* **34:**204, 1969.

Nye, S. W., Graham, J. B., and Brinkhous, K. M.: The Partial Thromboplastin Time as a Screening Test for the Detection of Latent Bleeders, *Am J Med Sci,* **243:**279, 1962.

Owren, P. A.: Thrombotest: A New Method for Controlling Anticoagulant Therapy, *Lancet,* **2:**754, 1959.

Quick, A. J.: Clinical Interpretation of the One-Stage Prothrombin Time, *Circulation,* **24:**1422, 1961.

Salzman, E. W.: Measurement of Platelet Adhesiveness: A Sample In Vitro Technique Demonstrating an Abnormality in von Willebrand's Disease, *J Lab Clin Med,* **62:**724, 1963.

Evaluation of the Surgical Patient as a Hemostatic Risk

Biggs, R., and Macfarlane, R. G.: "Human Blood Coagulation and Its Disorders," 3d ed., F. A. Davis Company, Philadelphia, 1962.

Hougie, C.: "Fundamentals of Blood Coagulation in Clinical Medicine," McGraw-Hill Book Company, New York, 1963.

Shulman, N. R., Aster, R. H., Leitner, A., and Hiller, M. C.: Immunoreactions Involving Platelets. V. Posttransfusion Purpura Due to Complement-fixing Antibody against Genetically Controlled Platelet Antigen: Proposed Mechanism for Thrombocytopenia and Its Relevance, in "Autoimmunity," The Year Book Medical Publishers, Inc., Chicago, 1962–1963.

Clinical Hemostatic Defects

Aster, R. H., Becker, G. A., Hamid, M., and Calvert, D. N.: Storage of Platelet Concentrates at 4°C; Use of Refrigerated Platelet Concentrates in the Treatment of Hemorrhage in Thrombocytopenic Patients, in M. G. Baldini and S. Ebbe (eds.), "Platelets: Production, Function, Transfusion, and Storage," Grune & Stratton, Inc., New York, 1974.

Baldini, M.: Idiopathic Thrombocytopenic Purpura, *N Engl J Med,* **274:**1245, 1966.

Biggs, R., and Macfarlane, R. G.: "Human Blood Coagulation and Its Disorders," 3d ed., F. A. Davis Company, Philadelphia, 1962.

Breckenridge, R. T., and Ratnoff, O. D.: Therapy of Hereditary Disorders of Blood Coagulation, *Mod Treat,* **5:**39, 1968.

Curtiss, P. H., Jr.: Orthopedic Management of Patients with Hereditary Disorders of Blood Coagulation, *Mod Treat,* **5:**84, 1968.

Griner, P. F.: Drug Effects on Oral Anticoagulants, in R. L. Weed (ed.), "Hematology for Internists," Little, Brown and Company, Boston, 1971.

Hardaway, R. M., III: Disseminated Intravascular Coagulation, *Thromb Diath Haemorrh [Suppl],* **56:**207, 1971.

Hoak, J. C., and Koepke, J. A.: Platelet transfusions, in "Clinics in Hematology," W. B. Saunders Company, Philadelphia, 1976.

Hougie, C.: "Fundamentals of Blood Coagulation in Clinical Medicine," McGraw-Hill Book Company, New York, 1963.

Hoyer, L. W.: Disseminated Intravascular Coagulation, in R. L.

Weed (ed.), "Hematology for Internists," Little, Brown and Company, Boston, 1971.

Klingensmith, W.: Surgical Implications of Hemorrhage during Anticoagulant Therapy, *Surg Gynecol Obstet,* **125:**1333, 1967.

Norman, J. C., Covelli, V. H. and Sise, H. S.: Experimental Transplantation of the Spleen for Classical Hemophilia: A Rationale and Long-Term Results, *Bibl Haematol,* **34:**187, 1970.

Prentice, C. R. M., and Ratnoff, O. D.: Genetic Disorders of Blood Coagulation, *Semin Hematol,* **4:**93, 1967.

Ratnoff, O. D.: Hereditary Disorders of Hemostasis, in J. B. Stanbury, J. B. Wyngaarden, and D. S. Fredrickson, "The Metabolic Basis of Inherited Disease," 2d ed., McGraw-Hill Book Company, New York, 1966.

———: An approach to the Diagnosis of Disorders of Hemostasis, *Mod Treat,* **5:**11, 1968.

Rizza, C. R.: Coagulation Factor Therapy, in "Clinics in Hematology," W. B. Saunders Company, Philadelphia, 1976.

Schwartz, S. I.: Myeloproliferative Disorders. *Ann Surg,* **182**(4):464, 1975.

Sherry, S.: Urokinase, *Ann Intern Med,* **69:**415, 1968.

Shulman, N. R.: Surgical Care of Patients with Hereditary Disorders of Blood Coagulation, *Mod Treat,* **5:**61, 1968.

Smith, W. W.: Bleeding Disorders in Surgical Patients, *Monogr Surg Sci,* **1:**3, 1964.

Stableforth, P., Hughes, J., Wilson, E., and Dormandy, K.: The von Willebrand Syndrome, *Br J Haematol,* **29:**605, 1975.

Wasserman, L. R., and Gilbert, H. S.: Polycythemia Vera and Myeloid Metaplasia, in A. W. Ulin and S. S. Gollub (eds.), "Surgical Bleeding: Handbook for Medicine, Surgery, and Specialties," McGraw-Hill Book Company, New York, 1966.

Webster, W. P., Zukoski, C. F., Hutchin, P., Reddick, R. L., Mandel, S. R., and Penick, G. D.: Plasma Factor VIII Synthesis and Control as Revealed by Canine Organ Transplantation, *Amer J Physiol,* **220:**1147, 1971.

Yankee, R. A.: HL-A Antigens and Platelet Therapy, in M. G. Baldini and S. Ebbe (eds.), "Platelets: Production, Function, Transfusion, and Storage," Grune & Stratton, Inc., New York, 1974.

Local Hemostasis

Abbott, W., and Austen, W. G.: The Effectiveness and Mechanism of Collagen-Induced Topical Hemostasis, *Surgery,* **78:**723, 1975.

Cushing, H.: The Control of Bleeding in Operations for Brain Tumor, *Ann Surg,* **54:**1, 1911.

Hait, M. R.: Microcrystalline Collagen: A New Hemostatic Agent, *Am J Surg,* **120:**330, 1970.

Halsted, W. S.: The Employment of Fine Silk in Preference to Catgut and the Advantages of Transfixing Tissues and Vessels in Controlling Hemorrhage, *JAMA,* **60:**1119, 1913.

Hinman, F., and Babcock, K. O.: Local Reaction to Oxidized Cellulose and Gelatin Hemostatic Agents in Experimentally Contaminated Renal Wounds, *Surgery,* **26:**633, 1949.

Jenkins, H. P., and Clarke, J. S.: Gelatin Sponge: A New Hemostatic Substance, *Arch Surg,* **51:**253, 1945.

Just-Viera, J. O., Puron-Del Aquila, R., and Yeager, G. H.: Control of Hemorrhage from the Liver without the Use of Sutures or Clamps: Preliminary Report, *Am Surg,* **28:**11, 1962.

Lindstrom, P. A.: Complications from the Use of Absorbable Sponges, *Arch Surg,* **73:**133, 1956.

Ravitch, M. M., Steichen, F. M., Fishbein, R. H., Knowles, P. W., and Weil, P.: Clinical Experiences with the Soviet Mechanical Bronchus Stapler (UKB-25), *J Thorac Cardiovasc Surg,* **47:**446, 1964.

Sawyer, P. N., and Wesolowski, S. A.: Electrical Hemostasis, in Conference on Bleeding in the Surgical Patient, *Ann NY Acad Sci,* **115:**455, 1964.

Schechter, D. S.: History of the Evolution of Methods of Hemostasis and the Study of Blood Coagulation, in A. W. Ulin and S. S. Gollub (eds.), "Surgical Bleeding: Handbook for Medicine, Surgery, and Specialties," McGraw-Hill Book Company, New York, 1966.

Schwartz, S. I., Muyshondt, E., and Penn, I.: Isotopic Evaluation of Bioelectric Factors Affecting Thrombogenesis, in Philip N. Sawyer (ed.), "Biophysical Mechanisms in Vascular Homeostasis and Intravascular Thrombosis," Appleton-Century Crofts, Inc., New York, 1965.

Silverstein, F. E., Auth, D. C., Rubin, C. E., and Protell, R. L.: High Power Argon Lazer Treatment Via Standard Endoscope. I. A Preliminary Study of Efficacy in Control of Experimental Erosive Bleeding, *Gastroenterology,* **71:**558, 1976.

Waltz, J. M., and Cooper, I. S.: Cryogenic Surgery, in A. W. Ulin and S. S. Gollub (eds.), "Surgical Bleeding: Handbook for Medicine, Surgery, and Specialties," McGraw-Hill Book Company, New York, 1966.

Wangensteen, S. L., Orahood, R. C., Voorhees, A. B., Smith, R. B., III, and Healey, W. V.: Intragastric Cooling in the Management of Hemorrhage from the Upper Gastrointestinal Tract, *Am J Surg,* **105:**401, 1963.

Willman, V. L., and Hanlon, C. R.: The Influence of Temperature on Surface Bleeding: Favorable Effects of Local Hypothermia, *Ann Surg,* **143:**660, 1956.

Transfusion

Aggeler, P. M.: Physiological Basis for Transfusion Therapy in Hemorrhagic Disorders: A Critical Review, *Transfusion,* **1:**71, 1961.

American Medical Association Committee on Blood: Single Unit Transfusions, *JAMA,* **189:**955, 1964.

Barry, K. G., and Crosby, W. H.: The Prevention and Treatment of Renal Failure following Transfusion Reactions, *Transfusion,* **3:**34, 1963.

Bennett, S. H., Geelhoed, G. W., Gralnick, H. R., and Hoye, R. C.: Effects of Autotransfusion on Blood Elements, *Am J Surg,* **125:**273, 1973.

Blakeley, W. R., Bennett, L. R., and Maloney, J. V., Jr.: An Evaluation of Preoperative Blood Volume Determination in the Debilitated Surgical Patient, *Surg Gynecol Obstet,* **115:**257, 1962.

Braude, A. I.: Transfusion Reactions from Contaminated Blood: Their Recognition and Treatment, *N Engl J Med,* **258:**1289, 1958.

Brzica, S. M., Pineda, A. A., and Taswell, H. F.: Autologous Blood Transfusion, *Mayo Clin Proc,* **51:**723, 1976.

Bunker, J. P., Stetson, J. B., Coe, R. C., Grillo, H. C., and Murphy, A. J.: Citric Acid Intoxication, *JAMA,* **157:**1361, 1955.

Caceres, E., and Whittembury, G.: Evaluation of Blood Losses during Surgical Operations: Comparison of the Gravimetric Method with the Blood Volume Determination, *Surgery,* **45:**681, 1959.

Carter, J. F. B.: Reduction in Thrombophlebitis by Limiting Duration of Intravenous Infusions, *Lancet,* **2:**20, 1951.

Case, R. B., Sarnoff, S. J., Waithe, P. E., and Sarnoff, L. C.: Intra-arterial and Intravenous Blood Infusions in Hemorrhagic Shock: Comparison of Effects on Coronary Blood Flow and Arterial Pressure, *JAMA,* **152:**208, 1953.

Chaplin, H., Jr., Brittingham, T. E., and Cassell, M.: Methods for Preparation of Suspensions of Buffy Coat–poor Red Blood Cells for Transfusion, including a Report of 50 Transfusions of Suspensions of Buffy Coat–poor Red Blood Cells Prepared by a Dextran Sedimentation Method, *Am J Clin Pathol,* **31:**373, 1959.

Collins, J. A.: Massive Blood Transfusions, in "Clinics in Hematology," W. B. Saunders Company, Philadelphia, 1976.

Durant, T. M., Oppenheimer, M. J., Lynch, P. R., Ascanio, G., and Webber, D.: Body Position in Relation to Venous Air Embolism: A Roentgenologic Study, *Am J Med Sci,* **277:**509, 1954.

Ebert, R. V., Stead, E. A., and Gibson, J. G.: Response of Normal Subjects to Acute Blood Loss, with Special Reference to the Mechanism of Restoration of Blood Volume, *Arch Intern Med,* **68:**578, 1941.

Gollub, S., and Bailey, C. P.: Management of Major Surgical Blood Loss without Transfusion, *JAMA,* **198:**1171, 1966.

Grady, G. F., Chalmers, T. C., and the Boston Inter-Hospital Liver Group: Risk of Post-transfusion Viral Hepatitis, *N Engl J Med,* **271:**337, 1964.

Grossman, E. B., Stewart, S. G., and Stokes, J. S., Jr.: Post-transfusion Hepatitis in Battle Casualties: A Study of Its Prophylaxis by Means of Human Immune Serum Globulin, *JAMA,* **129:**991, 1945.

Hoff, H. E., and Guillemin, R.: The Tercentenary of Transfusion in Man, *Cardiovasc Res Cent Bull,* **6:**47, 1967.

Holland, P. V., Rubinson, R. M., Morrow, A. G., and Schmidt, P. J.: Gamma Globulin in the Prophylaxis of Post-transfusion Hepatitis, *JAMA,* **196:**471, 1966.

Howland, W. S., Schweizer, O., and Boyan, O. P.: The Effect of Buffering on the Mortality of Massive Blood Replacement, *Surg Gynecol Obstet,* **121:**777, 1965.

Huggins, C. E: Frozen Blood: Principles of Practical Preservation, *Monogr Surg Sci,* **3:**133, 1966.

Ingram, G. I. C.: The Bleeding Complications of Blood Transfusion, *Transfusion,* **5:**1, 1965.

Johnson, S. A., and Greenwalt, T. J.: "Coagulation and Transfusion in Clinical Medicine," Little, Brown and Company, Boston, 1965.

Katz, R., Rodriguez, J., and Ward, R.: Posttransfusion Hepatitis: Effect of Modified Gamma-Globulin Added to Blood In Vitro, *N Engl J Med,* **285:**925, 1971.

Kliman, A.: Complications of Massive Blood Replacement, *N Y State J Med,* **65:**239, 1965.

Krevans, J. R., and Jackson, D. P.: Hemorrhagic Disorder following Massive Whole Blood Transfusions, *JAMA,* **159:**171, 1955.

Krugman, S., Giles, J. P., and Hammond, J.: Viral Hepatitis, Type B (MS-2 Strain): Prevention with Specific Hepatitis B Immune Serum Globulin, *JAMA,* **218:**1665, 1971.

Lalich, J. J., and Schwartz, S. I.: The Role of Aciduria in the Development of Hemoglobinuric Nephrosis in Dehydrated Rabbits, *J Exp Med,* **92:**11, 1950.

Langdell, R. D., Adelson, E., Furth, F. W., and Crosby, W. H.: Dextran and Prolonged Bleeding Time: Results of a Sixty-Gram, One-Liter Infusion Given to One Hundred and Sixty-three Normal Human Subjects, *JAMA,* **162:**346, 1958.

Lehane, D., Kwantes, C. M. S., Upward, M. G., and Thomson, D. R.: Homologous Serum Jaundice, *Br Med J,* **2:**572, 1949.

Luscher, E. F.: Biochemical Basis of Platelet Function, in K. M. Brinkhous, R. W. Shermer, and F. K. Mostofi (eds.), "The Platelet," The Williams & Wilkins Company, Baltimore, 1971.

MacCallum, F. O., McFarlan, A. M., Miles, J. A. R., Pollock, M. R., and Wilson, C.: Infective Hepatitis: Studies in E. Anglia during the Period 1943–7, *Med Res Counc Spec Rep Ser* (*Lond*), no. **273,** 1951.

Macon, W. L., and Pories, W. J.: The Effect of Iron Deficiency Anemia on Wound Healing, *Surgery,* **69:**792, 1971.

Maloney, J. V., Jr., Smythe, C. McC., Gilmore, J. P., and Handford, S. W.: Intra-arterial and Intravenous Transfusion, *Surg Gynecol Obstet,* **97:**529, 1953.

McNair, T. J., and Dudley, H. A. F.: The Local Complications of Intravenous Therapy, *Lancet,* **2:**365, 1959.

Med Lett Drugs Ther, vol. 9, no. 22, issue 230, Nov. 3, 1967.

Mollison, P. L.: "Blood Transfusion in Clinical Medicine," 4th ed., F. A. Davis Company, Philadelphia, 1967.

Morton, J. H.: Surgical Transfusion Practices, 1967, *Surgery,* **65:**407, 1969.

Moyer, C.: "Conference on Blood Groups and Blood Transfusion," Better Bellevue Association, New York, 1967.

Perrault, R., Jackson, J. R., Martin-Villar, J., and Smiley, R. K.: Experience with the Use of Frozen Blood, *Can Med Assoc J,* **96:**1504, 1967.

Peskin, G. W., O'Brien, K., and Rabiner, S. F.: Stroma-free Hemoglobin Solution: The "Ideal" Blood Substitute? *Surgery,* **66:**185, 1969.

Phillipps, E., and Fleischner, F. G.: Pulmonary Edema in the Course of a Blood Transfusion without Overloading the Circulation, *Dis Chest,* **50:**619, 1966.

Pruitt, B. A., Jr., Moncrief, J. A., and Mason, A. D., Jr.: Efficacy of Buffered Saline as the Sole Replacement Fluid following Acute Measured Hemorrhage in Man, *J Trauma,* **7:**767, 1967.

Reece, R. L., and Beckett, R. S.: Epidemiology of Single-Unit Transfusion: A One-Year Experience in a Community Hospital, *JAMA,* **195:**801, 1966.

Rigor, B., Bosomworth, P., and Rush, B. F., Jr.: Replacement of Operative Blood Loss of More than One Liter with Hartmann's Solution, *JAMA,* **203:**399, 1968.

Rudowski, W. J.: Complications Associated with Blood Transfusion, in M. Allgower, S.-F. Bergentz, R. Y. Calne, and U. F. Gruber (eds.), "Progress in Surgery," S. Karger, New York, 1971.

Schwartz, S. I., Adams, J. T., and Bauman, A. W.: Splenectomy for Hematologic Disorders, *Curr Probl Surg,* The Year Book Medical Publishers, Inc., Chicago, May, 1971.

Shields, C. E., Dennis, L. H., Eichelberger, J. W., and Conrad, M. E.: The Rapid Infusion of Large Quantities of ACD Adenine Solution into Humans, *Transfusion,* **7**:133, 1967.

Shires, T., Coln, D., Carrico, J., and Lightfoot, S.: Fluid Therapy in Hemorrhagic Shock, *Arch Surg,* **88**:688, 1964.

Strumia, M. M., Crosby, W. H., Gibson, J. G., II, Greenwalt, T. J., and Krevans, J. R.: "General Principles of Blood Transfusion," J. B. Lippincott Company, Philadelphia, 1963.

Tiber, L. J.: Ruptured Ectopic Pregnancy, *Calif Med,* **41**:16, 1934.

Tocantis, L. M., and O'Neill, J. F.: Infusion of Blood and Other Fluids into the General Circulation via the Bone Marrow: Technique and Results, *Surg Gynecol Obstet,* **73**:281, 1941.

Transfusion of Blood Components, *Med Lett Drugs Ther,* **9**:85, 1967.

Wallace, J.: Blood Transfusion and Transmissible Disease, in "Clinics in Hematology," W. B. Saunders Company, Philadelphia, 1976.

Wallace, J. M., and Henry, J. B.: Isoimmunization after Massive Transfusion for Open Heart Surgery, *Transfusion,* **5**:153, 1965.

Walter, C. W.: Blood Donors, Blood and Transfusion, in J. M. Kinney, R. H. Egdahl, and G. D. Zuidema (eds.), "Manual of Preoperative and Postoperative Care," W. B. Saunders Company, Philadelphia, 1971.

Waterman, D. F., Birkhill, F. R., Pirani, C. L., and Levenson, S. M.: The Healing of Wounds in the Presence of Anemia, *Surgery,* **31**:821, 1952.

Wilson, R. F., Bassett, J. S., and Walt, A. J.: Five Years Experience with Massive Blood Transfusions, *JAMA,* **194**:851, 1965.

Young, L. E.: Complications of Blood Transfusion, *Ann Intern Med,* **61**:136, 1964.

Chapter 4

Shock

by **G. Tom Shires, Peter C. Canizaro, and C. James Carrico**

CLINICAL MANIFESTATIONS OF SHOCK

Classification; Clinical and Physiologic Manifestations of Shock

DEFINITION AND WORKING CLASSIFICATION

The scope of modern medicine is increasing steadily. As understanding of physiologic and biochemical derangements is broadened, so is the horizon of possibilities for the relief of illness. As more seriously ill patients are presented, the symptom complex of shock is more frequently encountered by the physician.

Although shock has been recognized for over 100 years, a clear definition and dissection of this complex and devastating state has emerged only slowly. Many attempts have been made over the years to define adequately the entity known as shock. In 1872 the elder Gross defined shock as a "manifestation of the rude unhinging of the machinery of life." Although the accuracy of this definition is unquestioned, it is obviously far from precise. In 1942 Wiggers, on the basis of an exhaustive examination of available evidence at that time, offered the definition: "Shock is a syndrome resulting from a depression of many functions, but in which reduction of the effective circulating blood volume is of basic importance, and in which impairment of the circulation steadily progresses until it eventuates in a state of irreversible circulatory failure." Blalock offered the definition in 1940: "Shock is a peripheral circulatory failure, resulting from a discrepancy in the size of the vascular bed and the volume of the intravascular fluid." A more modern definition has been devised by Simeone, who stated that shock may be defined as "a clinical condition characterized by signs and symptoms which arise when the cardiac output is insufficient to fill the arterial tree with blood under sufficient pressure to provide organs and tissues with adequate blood flow."

Shock of all forms appears to be invariably related to inadequate tissue perfusion. The low-flow state in vital organs seems to be the final common denominator in all forms of shock.

For purposes of a working clinical classification, the etiologic classification offered by Blalock in 1934 is still a useful and functional one. Blalock suggested four categories:

1. Hematogenic (oligemic)
2. Neurogenic (caused primarily by nervous influences)
3. Vasogenic (initially decreased vascular resistance and increased vascular capacity)
4. Cardiogenic
    a. Failure of the heart as a pump
    b. Unclassified category (including diminished cardiac output from various causes)

It is now clear that shock invariably results from one or more of four separate but interrelated dysfunctions, involving (1) the pump (heart), (2) the fluid which is pumped (blood volume), (3) the arteriolar resistance vessels, and

(4) the capacity of the venous vessels. These dysfunctions may be correlated as follows with Blalock's etiologic classification:

1. Cardiogenic shock implies failure of the heart as a pump and may be brought about by primary myocardial dysfunction from myocardial infarction, serious cardiac arrhythmias, or a variety of causes resulting in myocardial depression; or by miscellaneous causes, including mechanical restriction of cardiac function or venous obstruction such as occurs in the mediastinum with tension pneumothorax, vena cava obstruction, or cardiac tamponade.

2. Reduction in blood volume may take the form of loss of whole blood, of plasma, or of extracellular fluid in the extravascular space or a combination of these three.

3. Changes in arterial resistance or venous capacity may be brought about by specific disorders. A decrease in resistance may result from spinal anesthesia or from neurogenic reflexes, as in acute pain, or may accompany the end stages of hypovolemic shock. Septic shock may produce changes in peripheral arterial resistance and in venous capacity, as well as peripheral arteriovenous shunting.

Therapy of shock will obviously revolve around the etiologic type or combination of types of shock present in a given patient who has undergone trauma.

CLINICAL MANIFESTATIONS

The signs and symptoms of hypovolemic shock, when they are well established, are classic and usually easy to recognize. Most of the signs of clinical shock are characteristic of low peripheral blood flow and are contributed to by the effects of excess adrenosympathetic activity. The signs and symptoms of human shock, according to the severity of the shock, were well described by Beecher et al., as summarized in Table 4-1.

On first inspection the patient in shock presents an anxious, tired expression, which early is that of restlessness and anxiety and later becomes a picture of apathy or exhaustion. Typically, the skin feels cool and is pale and mottled, and there is evidence of decreased capillary flow exhibited by easy blanching of the skin, particularly the nail beds.

There are varying discrepancies in the classic picture of shock. In neurogenic shock, particularly that in response to spinal anesthesia, the pulse rate is normal or, more often, decreased; the pulse pressure is wide, and the pulse feels strong rather than weak. The rapid pulse characteristic of early hemorrhagic or wound shock may be absent, even if the patient has lost blood rapidly. This is also true if the position is supine or prone, in which case a rapid pulse may not appear until the patient is moved or elevated to a sitting position. The varying clinical picture in septic shock is discussed subsequently.

In observing a large number of patients in hemorrhagic hypovolemic shock, one sees remarkably varied but typical responses of the sensorium to the shock episode. Most young, healthy patients who sustain wound or hemorrhagic shock, when seen early after the wounding, will appear to be restless and anxious and give the appearance of great fear. Shortly after being seen by a physician and started on treatment, this restlessness frequently gives way to great apathy and the patient appears sleepy. When aroused, he may complain of weakness or of a chilly sensation, although he does not actually have a chill. If blood loss is unchecked, the patient's apathy and sleepiness will rapidly progress into coma. In treating a large number of accident victims, it has been our experience that a patient who has bled into frank coma from which he cannot be aroused, resulting simply from blood loss alone (unassociated with other injuries such as brain damage), has usually sustained lethal blood loss. This sign usually indicates rapid massive hemorrhage for which compensations are inadequate to maintain sufficient cerebral blood flow to sustain consciousness.

Another characteristic of the wounded person, described

Table 4-1. GRADING OF SHOCK

| Degree of shock | Blood pressure (approx.) | Skin | | | | Thirst | Mental state |
		Pulse quality	Temperature	Color	Circulation (response to pressure blanching)		
None	Normal	Normal	Normal	Normal	Normal	Normal	Clear and distressed
Slight	To 20% increase	Normal	Cool	Pale	Definite slowing	Normal	Clear and distressed
Moderate	Decreased 20–40%	Definite decrease in volume	Cool	Pale	Definite slowing	Definite	Clear and some apathy unless stimulated
Severe	Decreased 40% to nonrecordable	Weak to imperceptible	Cold	Ashen to cyanotic (mottling)	Very sluggish	Severe	Apathetic to comatose, little distress except thirst

SOURCE: H. K. Beecher, F. A. Simeone, C. H. Burnett, S. L. Shapiro, E. R. Sullivan, and T. B. Mallory, The Internal State of the Severely Wounded Man on Entry to the Most Forward Hospital, *Surgery*, **22:**672, 1947.

by many investigators, is thirst. Thirst seems to be a characteristic of the injured person and is found in most emergency room patients brought in acutely ill from trauma with or without shock. The studies carried out to elucidate the nature of the thirst are many and varied. Most of these patients have intense adrenal medullary stimulation from trauma, not necessarily accompanied by shock. Consequently caution must be used in allowing water, since dangerous water intoxication may be induced by this intense stimulus to imbibe liquids in the face of altered renal function.

Another characteristic of the patient in hemorrhagic shock is the low peripheral venous pressure, manifested on inspection by empty peripheral veins. Indeed, the starting of a simple intravenous infusion in a patient in hemorrhagic shock can be quite difficult. Obviously there are exceptions, such as shock due to cardiac tamponade, in which there is restriction to inflow of blood to the right side of the heart. In this instance the peripheral veins, including the neck veins, are distended.

Nausea and vomiting from hypovolemic shock are common. It is true that other causes should be sought for, but shock alone may be first manifested in this manner.

Another classic finding in hemorrhagic hypovolemia is a fall in body "core" temperature. Whether this is due to a lowered metabolic rate or to lower perfusion in areas where body temperature is measured is debatable.

PHYSIOLOGIC CHANGES

BLOOD PRESSURE. Arterial blood pressure is normally maintained by the cardiac output and the peripheral vascular resistance. Thus, when the cardiac output is reduced because of loss of intravascular volume, the blood pressure may remain normal so long as the total peripheral vascular resistance can be increased to compensate for the reduction in cardiac output. The vascular resistance varies for different organs and in different parts of the same organ, depending on the local conditions that determine the state of vasoconstriction or vasodilatation at the time of the loss of intravascular volume. An example of the differential increase in peripheral resistance with reduction in cardiac output is seen in the change in distributional total blood flow to organs such as the heart and the brain, as opposed to that of most other organs which are not essential for immediate survival. In hemorrhagic shock the heart may receive 25 percent of the total cardiac output, as opposed to the normal 5 to 8 percent. The great increase in peripheral resistance in such organs as the skin and the kidney causes significant reduction in flow in these organs while providing a lifesaving diversion of the cardiac output to the brain and the heart. Consequently the blood pressure may not fall until the reduction in cardiac output or loss of blood volume is so great that the adaptive homeostatic mechanisms can no longer compensate for the reduced volume. As the deficit continues, however, there is a progressive hypotension.

PULSE RATE. Characteristically, reduction of the volume in the vascular tree is associated with tachycardia. A fall in pressure within the great vessels results in excitation of the adrenosympathetic division of the autonomic nervous system and, simultaneously, inhibition of the vagal-medullary center (Marey's reflex). Consequently, with hemorrhage or loss of circulating blood volume, the resulting fall in arterial blood pressure should cause an increase in heart rate.

This compensatory mechanism, however, is variable in its effectiveness. Obviously, the degree of loss of intravascular volume, the amount of reduction in venous return, and other variables such as ventricular function may markedly influence the ability of Marey's reflex to compensate for the reduction in blood volume. Work with slow hemorrhage in normal healthy volunteers by Shenkin et al. has shown that, as long as the supine position is maintained, as much as 1000 ml of blood may be lost without significant increase in pulse rate. Similarly, the pacemaker system of the heart within the sinoatrial node is obviously influenced by other stimuli, such as fear and anxiety, that may also accompany the trauma producing the loss of intravascular volume.

Consequently, during the course of observation and treatment of shock, changes in pulse rate are of value only when followed over an extended period. Change in pulse rate may indicate response to therapy once other external sources that may have changed cardiac rate are diminished or removed.

VASOCONSTRICTION. Increase in peripheral vascular resistance by production of peripheral vasoconstriction rapidly becomes maximal in an effort to compensate for the reduced cardiac output. Vascular resistance can be measured only indirectly in human beings and in animals. There is good evidence that early disproportionate reduction in vascular resistance in the heart occurs while there is still little change in vascular resistance in many organs. Subsequently, maximal vasoconstriction occurs in the skin, kidneys, liver, and finally, the brain. Concomitantly, there is generalized constriction of the veins in response to reduction in intravascular volume. Venoconstriction is a necessary homeostatic mechanism, since over half the total blood volume may be contained within the venous tree.

These vascular responses to hemorrhage are immediate and striking. Within seconds following the onset of hemorrhage there are unequivocal signs of sympathetic and adrenal activation. Serum catecholamine levels show prompt elevation, indicative of action of the adrenal medullary function. The adrenal cortical and pituitary hormones also show prompt increase in serum levels following shock. Many of the clinical signs associated with shock are simply signs of response of the sympathetic and adrenal medullary system to the insult sustained by the organism.

HEMODILUTION. All the responses to reduction of intravascular volume eventually result in decreased flow to tissues and initiation of compensatory mechanisms directed at correction of the low-flow state. One such compensation is movement of fluid into the circulation, resulting in hemodilution. This fluid, commonly known as extracellular fluid, has the composition of plasma but a lower protein content.

It is now clear, however, that the hematocrit reading, or hemoglobin concentration, in shock is simply an index of the balance between the amount of whole blood or plasma lost and the amount of extravascular extracellular fluid gained. For example, in hemorrhagic hypovolemia there is generally progressive hemodilution, which increases with the severity of the shock state. Obviously, in this circumstance there has been a greater movement of fluid from the extravascular to the intravascular space with progression of the shock. This is in contradistinction to shock associated with loss of intravascular volume due primarily to plasma loss. High-hematocrit shock may occur with massive losses of plasma and extravascular extracellular fluid, such as is associated with peritonitis, burns, large areas of soft tissue infection, and the crush syndrome.

The mechanism of hemodilution following hemorrhage is probably on the basis of the Starling hypothesis: that is, the reduction in hydrostatic pressure in the capillaries because of hypotension and arterial and arteriolar vasoconstriction results in a shift of the pressure gradient to favor the passage of fluid from the tissue extracellular space into the intravascular capillary bed.

It is worthy of note that the studies of Carey et al. do not demonstrate a significant reduction in serum protein content in patients following hemorrhagic shock and resuscitation.

BIOCHEMICAL CHANGES

The biochemically measurable changes that occur as a response to the stress invoked by shock fall into three fairly well-defined categories. These are (1) the changes invoked by the pituitary-adrenal response to stress, (2) the changes brought about by a net reduction in organ perfusion imposed by a low rate of blood flow, and (3) the changes brought about by failing function within specific organs.

PITUITARY-ADRENAL. The immediate effects seen from adrenosympathetic activity are those associated with high circulating epinephrine levels. Characteristically, these include eosinopenia and lymphocytopenia along with thrombocytopenia. This doubtless represents the laboratory reflection of increased circulating epinephrine that can be measured and has been found to be elevated as an early response to shock. These changes are nonspecific and are found early in a patient with shock or severe trauma. The phenomena usually disappear rapidly. Other evidences of the pituitary and hormonal response to shock are seen in the well-known stress reaction or metabolic responses so well described by Moore. These include a striking negative nitrogen balance and retention of sodium and water, as well as a notable increase in the excretion of potassium.

LOW-FLOW STATE. Those changes incident to the low rate of blood flow during shock are now becoming better understood. More evidence is accumulating to support the observation that, as a result of a decreased blood flow or low rate of perfusion, there is a reduction in oxygen delivered to the vital organs and, consequently, a mandatory change in metabolism from aerobic to anaerobic. In the switch from aerobic to anaerobic metabolism, energy made available by the oxidation of glucose is greatly reduced during shock. The most striking example of a shift in metabolism is the production of lactic acid as the end product instead of the normal aerobic end product, carbon dioxide. This is reflected in a metabolic acidosis with a reduction in the carbon dioxide–combining power of the blood. The available buffer base is progressively decreased by combining with the increased lactic acid, and the respiratory compensation that occurs early in the course of hemorrhagic shock is frequently inadequate. Consequently the progressive decline in pH toward a striking acidosis is thereby hastened. Indeed, in several studies the ability of animals as well as human beings to recover from shock has been found to correlate rather closely with the degree of lactic acid production and the decrease in the alkali reserve and pH of the blood.

In some cases determination of blood pH may not accurately reflect changes in pH at the cellular level. After the induction of hemorrhagic shock in experimental animals, skeletal muscle surface pH changes precede those in blood, and minimal changes may be masked by the efficient blood buffer systems. Lactate and excess lactate levels correlate well with the clinical impression of the depth of shock, but the injuries producing the shock state have a much greater bearing on ultimate prognosis.

Drucker has pointed out that there is a consistent elevation of the blood sugar level in relation to the degree of blood loss and the severity of shock. This was earlier observed in battle casualties studied in World War II and has since been thoroughly confirmed by Simeone and others. It is Drucker's belief that this represents an increase in hepatic glycolysis in the change from aerobic or anaerobic metabolism, while Egdahl believes that there is decreased insulin secretion and decreased peripheral utilization of glucose.

Other evidences of failure of different parameters of cell metabolism have been presented by Thal, Schumer, Mela and Baue.

ORGAN FAILURE. The biochemical changes that appear incident to organ failure seem to be dependent in large part on the duration and severity of the shock. The changes in renal function induced by hypovolemia may vary from simple oliguria with a concentrated and acid urine to high-output renal failure with a urine of low specific gravity and high pH, or frank anuric renal failure. Similarly, the blood nonprotein nitrogen content depends on the degree of impairment in renal function. This may vary from slight or no retention of nitrogenous products to a steep and progressive rise that may require therapy.

Changes in ion concentration, including a rise of serum potassium, are dependent on many things, among them adrenal cortical response, the change in metabolism from aerobic to anaerobic with resultant release of potassium, and specific changes within tissues invoked by the shock. If renal function is maintained, the rise inevitably seen in serum potassium soon after the onset of shock is short-lived, in that the renal excretion of potassium is high during recovery from hemorrhagic shock. If renal function is impaired, the concentration of potassium and magnesium as well as creatine can rise to high levels in the serum.

PATHOPHYSIOLOGIC RESPONSES TO SHOCK

Experimental Studies of the Response of Extracellular Fluid

EARLY RESULTS

Hypovolemic shock is the most common form seen clinically and is also the form that has been studied most intensively both clinically and in the laboratory. Most of our own studies have been carried out using hypovolemic shock produced by external blood loss as the model. A method has been developed which allows the simultaneous measurement of total-body red cell mass with the use of ^{51}Cr-tagged red blood cells and total-body plasma volume with the use of ^{131}I-tagged and, later, ^{125}I-tagged human serum albumin. In addition, total-body extracellular fluid can be measured simultaneously with the use of ^{35}S-tagged sodium sulfate. The three isotopes are simultaneously injected intravenously, and with the use of appropriate energy-differentiating counting instruments, all three isotopes can be traced after equilibration. Volumes are then determined by the dilution principle, using multiple sampling.

In an early study the three volumes were measured; splenectomized dogs were then bled a sublethal, subshock amount of 10 percent of the measured blood volume. After hemorrhage the three volumes were again measured. The loss of the amount of red blood cells and plasma removed during the hemorrhage could be detected by the method described. It was shown that the decrease in extracellular fluid volume was only the amount lost as plasma removed during the hemorrhage.

By use of the same model, volumes were measured before and after hemorrhage of 25 percent of the measured blood volume. This hemorrhage was again sublethal but produced hypotension. In this group of animals also the loss of the amount of red blood cells and plasma removed could be detected. In addition, however, the functional extracellular fluid volume as measured by the ^{35}S-tagged sodium sulfate was found to have decreased by 18 to 26 percent of the original volume. Since there was no measurable external loss of ^{35}S sulfate, this reduction was presumed to be an internal redistribution of extracellular fluid. Subsequent studies of external bleeding of 35, 45, and even over 50 percent hemorrhage always produced the same reduction in functional extracellular fluid as long as the animal was in shock.

In subsequent studies, splenectomized dogs were subjected to "irreversible" hemorrhagic shock according to a modified method of Wiggers, which utilizes a reservoir. Return of shed blood in this severe preparation resulted in the return of blood pressure to near control levels, followed by a fall in blood pressure within 1 to 16 hours; death resulted in 80 percent of the dogs, i.e., a standard mortality rate.

In one group of animals the three volumes were measured and the dogs were then subjected to shock by the Wiggers method. The three volumes were remeasured by reinjection during the period of shock; then shed blood was returned. The decrease in blood volume was the amount which had been removed. Concurrently, the functional extracellular fluid exhibited a decided reduction. Immediately after the return of the shed blood, the red cell mass returned to essentially normal levels, as did the plasma volume; however, there remained a deficit of functional extracellular fluid. In dogs treated with shed blood plus plasma (10 ml/kg), the losses during shock were again similar. After therapy with plasma, plus return of shed blood, there was a return of blood volume to normal. There remained, however, a decrease in functional extracellular fluid volume.

Dogs treated with an extracellular "mimic," such as a balanced salt solution plus shed blood, had comparable losses during shock. As in the previous groups, the blood volume returned essentially to normal after treatment. But dogs treated with salt solution plus shed blood exhibited return of functional extracellular fluid volume to control levels.

In this study only 20 percent of those dogs treated with shed blood alone survived longer than 24 hours. When plasma was used in addition to whole blood as therapy, 30 percent of the dogs survived. Of the animals treated with lactated Ringer's solution plus shed blood, 70 percent survived (Fig. 4-1). The 80 percent mortality rate of a standard "irreversible" shock preparation was reduced to 30 percent by restoration of functional extracellular fluid volume in addition to return of shed blood.

All these early studies of the measurement of the functional extracellular fluid were based on volume distribution curves of sulfate measured for approximately 1 hour. At any point in the course of the curve there is a reduction in extracellular fluid in the untreated state of shock. Subsequent work has continued these volume distribution curves for many hours. In true untreated hemorrhagic shock there is a reduction in the total extracellular fluid, or final diluted volume of radiosulfate, when compared with preshock volumes (Fig. 4-2).

Even when a less severe shock preparation is used, there is still a reduction in early equilibrating extracellular fluid or early available extracellular fluid, whereas the total anatomic extracellular fluid may remain normal. Subsequent studies have shown that if shock is not of sufficient duration to produce reduction in both functional and total extracellular fluid, the reduction may be only in functional extracellular fluid. Furthermore, if therapy is instituted quickly and blood pressure is returned to normal, a long sulfate equilibration curve may fail to reveal the acute reduction which was corrected early.

Consequently, the current status of sulfate as a measure of the functional extracellular fluid must be interpreted as indicating that early sulfate volume measurement reveals functional or available extracellular fluid and that prolonged measurement of the volume distribution curves gives total extracellular fluid values. If therapy has been instituted or has been completed, then the reduction in

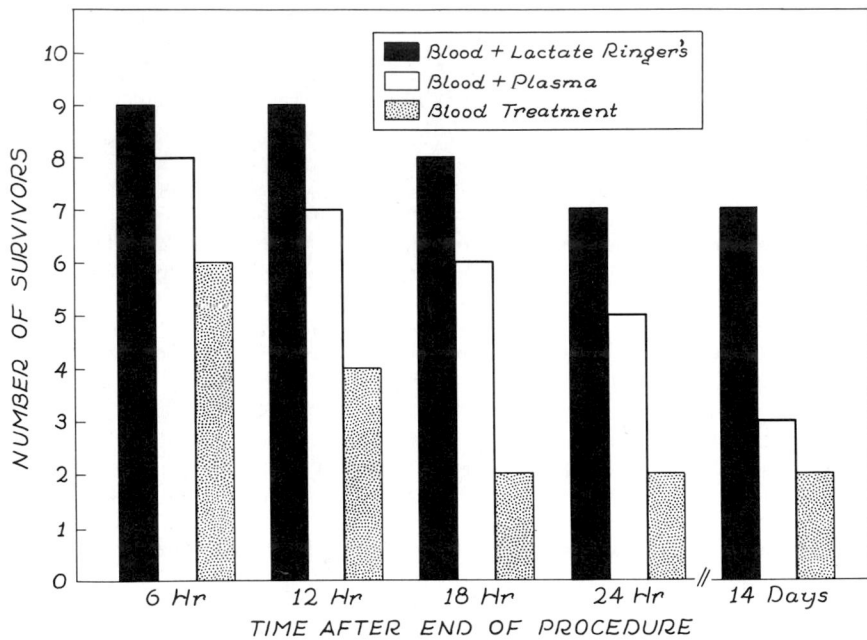

Fig. 4-1. Acute hemorrhagic shock: survival study.

total or even in the available extracellular fluid may not be measurable.

Unquestionably, some plasma, or transcapillary, refilling occurs in response to hemorrhage and to hemorrhagic shock. This response, however, is initially rather limited and, in severe hemorrhagic shock, is grossly inadequate to explain the reduction seen in interstitial fluid. Since there is no source for external loss, the question arose as to whether interstitial fluid might move into the cell mass in an isotonic fashion (Fig. 4-3).

CELLULAR STUDIES

Subsequently, studies of ion transport across the cell membrane were undertaken in order to determine the possibility of intracellular swelling in skeletal muscle in response to hemorrhagic shock. Using a Ling-Gerard ultramicroelectrode with glass tip diameter of less than 1μ (Fig. 4-4), intracellular transmembrane potential record-

Fig. 4-2. Radiosulfate equilibration curve: semilogarithmic plot, summary model.

ings were made. The electrode was modified to record intracellular transmembrane potentials in vivo before, during, and after shock (Fig. 4-5).

Skeletal muscle measurements in acute hemorrhagic shock demonstrate a constant and sustained fall in the normally negative intracellular transmembrane potential. This may represent a reduction in efficiency of the sodium pump induced by tissue hypoxia; it is present only during shock-producing hypotension. Additional studies in splenectomized dogs showed that changes in variables such as pH, P_{CO_2}, and bicarbonate do not influence the transmembrane potential in shock. Even with progressive metabolic acidosis and its subsequent correction, the potential still follows the blood pressure and shock state.

Studies have been reported which utilized the ultramicroelectrode measurement of transmembrane potential combined with direct aspiration of skeletal muscle interstitial fluid by a modification of the technique of Hagberg. Using this technique, it was found that as blood pressure fell and transmembrane potential was reduced, plasma potassium rose slowly during the shock period (Fig. 4-6). However, the directly aspirated interstitial fluid potassium during the same period of time rose to a height of more than 15 mEq/L of interstitial fluid. This explained where potassium, moving out of skeletal muscle cells, was being sequestered as sodium chloride and water moved into muscle cells.

Additional studies have been performed in primates which show essentially the same phenomenon (Fig. 4-7). These studies also reveal that this cellular membrane transport is a reversible phenomenon, i.e., once the shock state is treated, transmembrane potential recovers. Concomitant muscle biopsies show clearly that muscle cells gain sodium, water, and chloride while losing potassium.

NORMAL

VASCULAR TREE   INTERSTITIAL FLUID   CELL FLUID

HEMORRHAGIC SHOCK

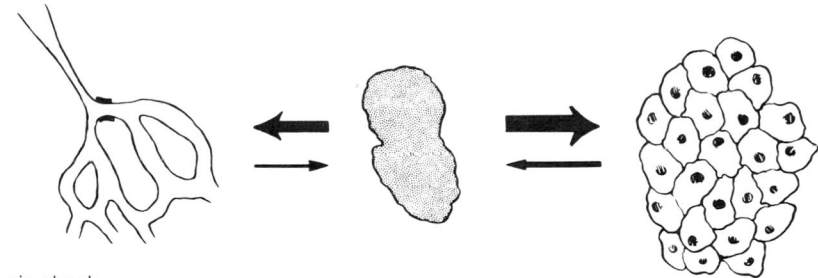

Fig. 4-3. Interstitial fluid response to hemorrhagic shock.

Fig. 4-4. Schematic of intracellular recording. (*From Ruch and Fulton,* eds., *Medical Physiology and Biophysics, 18th ed.,* W. B. Saunders Company, Philadelphia, 1960.)

Fig. 4-5. In vivo transmembrane potential measurement in rat skeletal muscle.

Thus the data reveal an isotonic swelling of skeletal muscle cells in response to shock injury (Fig. 4-8).

Studies in human beings reveal the same response to shock injury. Interesting corroborative changes in action potentials of single cells in skeletal muscles have been revealed in primates (Fig. 4-9). One study shows a decrease in resting membrane potential, a decrease in amplitude of action potential, and prolongation of both repolarization and depolarization times. Resuscitation quickly reversed these changes, except for repolarization time, which remained prolonged for several days. This confirms in vitro the alterations in intracellular sodium and potassium con-

centrations which were measured by skeletal muscle biopsy and resting membrane potential measurements.

INTERPRETATION

Concisely stated, reduction in extracellular fluid in reversible hemorrhagic shock can consistently be shown (1) with extracellular fluid markers that enter cells slowly or not at all in the shock state when (2) reinjection of the extracellular fluid markers is utilized in the shock state, (3) extracellular fluid markers or tracers are allowed sufficient time for equilibration, (4) shock measurements are obtained while hemorrhagic shock is sustained, and (5) the shock preparation is sufficiently severe and is maintained until there is a change in cellular membrane transport.

The data obtained from prior experiments support the use of transmembrane potential measurements as an accurate indicator of cellular alterations resulting from the low-flow state of hemorrhagic shock. Severe hypotension is associated with depression of transmembrane potential difference (PD) which is sustained in the presence of a continued shock state.

Transmembrane PD is generally agreed to be the result of either an electrogenic sodium pump (with active outward extrusion of sodium from muscle cells by a redox system) or a coupled sodium-potassium exchange pump with diffusion of sodium and potassium down their respective chemical gradients. In the latter theory the relative permeabilities of the membrane to the two ions must be considered and the potential interpreted on the basis of the Hodgkin-Katz-Goldman equation in which pNa^+ (relative permeability to sodium) is 0.01. Since permeability to potassium is assumed to be much greater than permeability to sodium in the cell membrane, the PD is essentially a potassium diffusion potential.

The present data thus suggest that skeletal muscle cells

Fig. 4-6. Changes in membrane potential and interstitial K^+ in rats with hemorrhagic shock.

Fig. 4-7. Changes in membrane potential and blood pressure in primates during hemorrhagic shock and after resuscitation.

may be a principal site of fluid and electrolyte sequestration after severe, prolonged hemorrhagic shock. Adjunctive studies by Grossman suggest that similar changes in the intracellular mass of neurons in the brain also occur in response to hypovolemic shock. Furthermore, an increase in the cellular water content of both cellular and connective tissue components following hemorrhagic shock has been demonstrated by Slonim and Stahl, and Fulton has suggested that connective tissue may be the site of some sodium and water sequestration.

The exact mechanism for the production of electrolyte changes as well as for the notable diminution in extracellular water which occurs after hemorrhagic shock is not

Fig. 4-8. Changes in membrane potential, extracellular water, and intracellular Na^+ in primates after resuscitation from hemorrhagic shock.

known. It appears that the changes may well represent a reduction in the efficiency of an active ionic pump mechanism or a selective increase in muscle cell membrane permeability to sodium, or both (Fig. 4-10).

With a reset membrane potential, extracellular fluid electrolyte concentrations are unchanged. Consequently, from the Nernst equation, intracellular Cl^- must rise from 3.5 to 10 mEq and intracellular Na^+ from 10 to 22 mEq. For transposition of these data to the previously cited measurements in hemorrhagic shock, a model is shown. This model shows a 10 percent isotonic swelling of muscle cells to explain the reduction in extracellular fluid measured in hemorrhagic shock. Studies are under way to determine the involvement of cell masses other than muscle during the course of hemorrhagic shock. One such study indicates that severe hemorrhagic shock of significant duration is associated with elevation of the internal sodium

Fig. 4-9. Action potentials in primates in hemorrhagic shock.

concentration of the red blood cells. The magnitude of these changes appears to be a function of both the severity and the duration of the shock process and seems to be well correlated with changes in clinical course when sequential sampling procedures are utilized.

There is a measurable reduction in extravascular extracellular fluid in response to sustained hemorrhagic shock. The cellular response to hypovolemic hypotension is characterized by a consistent change in active transport of ions. Evidence obtained directly from living cells indicates that sodium and water enter muscle cells, with resultant loss of cellular potassium to the extracellular fluid. The interstitial fluid holds the extruded potassium.

Replenishment of the depleted extracellular fluid counteracts these changes at the cellular level and is an important feature of therapy in patients with hypovolemic shock.

Renal Responses

The observation was made long ago that during severe shock, from any cause, renal function essentially stops in man. The kidneys, like the skin and the liver, share in the relative oligemia which is a rapid compensatory mechanism in shock to divert blood flow to those organs, such as the brain and the heart, most vital for maintaining life.

Consequently the relative oligemia suffered by the kidneys in response to shock is severe and immediate.

The development of oliguria and, indeed, even anuria is apparently a direct function of the severity and duration of the renal ischemia inevitably attendant on shock. In man, under normothermic conditions, normal kidneys will tolerate renal ischemia for periods varying from 15 minutes to a maximum of approximately 90 minutes. After this degree of ischemia, some functional and anatomic changes inevitably occur. With the use of hypothermia, the period of renal ischemia tolerated during hemorrhagic shock can be considerably prolonged.

SUBCLINICAL RENAL DAMAGE FOLLOWING INJURY AND SHOCK

In civilian and military practice, improved resuscitation with balanced electrolyte solution and blood and immediate corrective surgery have resulted in a great reduction in the incidence of primary oliguric renal failure. Recognition of nonoliguric renal failure as a less severe form of renal insufficiency suggested that graded renal damage might occur in association with systemic injury. Identification of patients with subclinical renal damage should be important in their postinjury care.

PATIENT STUDIES. A study was recently undertaken to determine the presence and degree of such renal damage during the early course of severely injured civilian patients. During the period of this study, 96,000 patients were treated in the emergency department, 988 of whom were admitted to the hospital for care of their injuries. Forty of the most severely injured were selected for continued care in a Trauma Research Unit after resuscitation and operative treatment of injuries. The criteria for inclusion in the study were hypotension following trauma and multiple long bone fractures.

All 40 patients showed generalized depression of renal function initially. Within 24 hours of admission, 30 demonstrated return of clearances to normal ranges. The patients were divided into groups according to blood urea nitrogen (BUN) values (Fig. 4-11). Group I, considered to show a characteristic renal response to trauma, was selected on the basis of BUN values continuously below 20 Gm/100 ml after the first hospital day. This group included 30 of the 40 patients. Eight patients with renal

Fig. 4-10. Theoretic transport mechanisms responsible for alterations in potential difference (P.D.) and fluid-electrolyte distribution in hemorrhagic shock.

Fig. 4-11. Renal function after trauma: blood urea nitrogen values.

Fig. 4-12. Renal function after trauma: glomerular filtration rate.

dysfunction (Group II) showed persistent moderate elevation of BUN values above 20 mg/100 ml. Two patients showed frank renal failure with rapidly progressing azotemia. One of these patients had sustained a gunshot wound of the renal vein and vena cava and had had the renal pedicle on the involved side clamped for one hour. The other patient, with a gunshot wound of the aortic bifurcation, represented failure of resuscitation. These two patients with renal failure are not considered in the subsequent comparisons between patients with the characteristic renal response (Group I) and those with renal dysfunction (Group II). Three patients with direct renal injury requiring suture or partial nephrectomy were included in Group I.

As would be expected on the basis of the selection criteria for the groups, glomerular filtration rate (GFR) was quite different for the two groups (Fig. 4-12). Urea clearance (C_{urea}), another clearance primarily related to filtration, was depressed in both groups initially, with a rapid return to and above normal in the characteristic group and a slow return toward normal in the dysfunction group. Urine/plasma (U/P) urea ratio and osmolar clearances (C_{osm}) were different in the two groups only subsequent to 12 hours after admission (Fig. 4-13).

Tubular resorption of water (TcH_2O) was significantly different in the two groups only at 18 and 24 hours after admission. The trend in Group I was toward excretion of free water while the trend in the dysfunction group was toward continued retention of free water. Cardiac output was not significantly different in the two groups.

Sodium clearances (C_{Na}) were similar in the two groups until after 12 hours following admission (Fig. 4-14). Subsequently C_{Na} fell in Group II. Postoperative sodium bal-

ance, represented as the difference between daily sodium intake and urinary sodium excretion, was different in the two groups. Group I showed positive sodium balance during day 1, balance during day 2, and negative balance during day 3. In Group II, the dysfunction group, increasing sodium retention occurred during each of the 3 days of the study.

There were no discernible differences between the two groups in age, type of injury, length of hypotensive episode, fluid administration, positive-pressure ventilation,

Fig. 4-13. Renal function after trauma: urine/plasma urea ratio.

Fig. 4-14. Renal function after trauma: sodium clearance.

nephrotic antibiotics, minute urine volume, blood volume, or arterial P_{O_2} and pH.

Discussion

Classic renal clearance techniques have been used infrequently in surgical patients, partly because of errors inherent in the methods. All renal clearances are urine flow–sensitive. An increase in urine flow leads to a decrease in mean urine transit time. Consequently new filtrate washes out tubular and collecting system contents at a more rapid rate, yielding a factitiously high clearance. Conversely, a decrease in urine flow may lead to a factitiously low clearance. Errors in clearance measurements can be minimized by using constant mechanical infusion, long collection periods, and bladder washes. The long collection periods may obscure fluctuations during the period, but they provide accurate mean clearances.

In the normal human kidney, GFR may promptly increase 30 percent above basal level during diuresis. In the above-mentioned study, GFR was measured without fluid loading, yet six of the patients in Group I showed a GFR above 150 ml/minute, suggesting the presence of postinjury stimuli in the patients tending to increase GFR maximally. The patients with renal dysfunction (Group II) were presumably subject to similar stimuli but were unable to respond with any elevation in GFR because of renal damage or persistent nervous or humoral influences affecting GFR.

Endogenous creatinine clearance (C_{cr}) in both groups was always higher than GFR. Notable variation in C_{cr} in the injured patient was noted by Ladd, who concluded that endogenous C_{cr} was unsuitable for evaluation of GFR in battle casualties. Creatinine as determined by the Jaffe reaction overestimates the true creatinine in plasma, and since creatinine is secreted in human beings, the usual

agreement of endogenous C_{cr} with inulin or iothalamate ^{125}I clearance is coincidental. Twofold and threefold increases in endogenous C_{cr} occur in association with the changes in muscle metabolism following severe trauma. Apparently normal values for C_{cr} may lead to a false sense of security when, in fact, the GFR may be reduced by a factor of 2 or 3 in the severely injured patient.

Muscle metabolism is profoundly altered in the injured patient, resulting in increased loads of creatinine and creatine presented to the kidney. In the early postinjury period, many patients had metabolic changes similar to those found in patients placed on a high protein diet. Even with increases in urea nitrogen load from tissue injury, multiple transfusions, and gluconeogenesis, these patients did not undergo azotemia and creatinemia. Azotemia and creatinemia are not inevitable consequences of severe tissue injury, and other factors are operative in the injured patient who exhibits such changes.

Flear and Clarke demonstrated that transfused patients lost less nitrogen in the period following injury than similarly injured nontransfused patients. It is not surprising that catabolism and nitrogen excretion are inversely related to the adequacy of resuscitative therapy. The patients with the greatest catabolic responses had sustained a more severe injury than the patients who did not demonstrate such changes. Flear and Clarke also demonstrated that transfused patients had negative sodium balances after the first postoperative day. Patients with the most severely damaged kidneys demonstrate positive free water clearances, as do septic patients, so care must be taken in interpreting the finding of positive free water clearances. The earliest possible restoration of circulating volume with electrolyte solution and blood, combined with definitive treatment of injuries, should decrease the degree of secondary systemic injury.

Trueta first described arterialization of rabbit renal venous blood secondary to stimuli which led to renal failure when prolonged. From these and other observations he developed a concept of renal arteriovenous shunting as a main factor in the development of posttraumatic renal failure. Recent technical improvements in determining internal intrarenal blood flow support his earlier observations. Padula et al. evaluated the effect of equiosmolar loads of mannitol, glucose, urea, and sodium chloride on an isolated dog kidney preparation. The administration of each agent was followed initially by a decrease in renal resistance and an increase in directly measured renal blood flow. The administration of mannitol, glucose, or urea alone was followed by a decrease in renal O_2 utilization, while the administration of sodium chloride was followed by an increase in O_2 consumption. An interpretation differing from that of the author's would consider the saline-induced increase in O_2 utilization indicative of internal redistribution of renal blood flow to ischemic cortical areas.

Small transient increases of GFR were apparent after administration of the diuretic in some patients. In view of the demonstrated slow improvement in GFR which occurs after resuscitation and injury repair, it is difficult to ascribe increases in GFR during this early hospital period to furosemide. Further study of changes in GFR after administration of furosemide is indicated, however, in view of reports suggesting a beneficial effect of furosemide on renal function.

C_{urea}, C_{cr}, C_{osm}, and U/P urea, U/P creatinine, and U/P osmolarity ratios have each been proposed as good clinical determinants of renal damage. Objections to the use of creatinine determinations alone have been noted above. Otherwise there is little to recommend any one of these tests over the others, since all relate filtration to some aspect of tubular function. Recognition of the need to measure at least one of the foregoing in urine and plasma simultaneously is important. U/P ratios approaching unity and clearances below 10 ml/minute are diagnostic of some form of renal failure. Attempted diuresis with volume replacement and ethacrynic acid or furosemide is indicated early in the course of patients with apparent posttraumatic renal failure.

A spectrum of secondary renal injury exists after severe trauma, varying from oliguric renal failure to transient depression of glomerular filtration and tubular function. Tissue trauma and multiple transfusions do not lead to azotemia in the injured patient with normal renal function. Conversely, even minimal persistent elevations of BUN are uniformly associated with significant renal dysfunction and sodium and water retention.

The more severely injured patient can be readily identified in the early postoperative phase by serial evaluation of the renal metabolism of urea or sodium. Identification of such patients should lead to meticulous supportive care, since the general metabolic reserve of the more severely injured patients is diminished and further insults are poorly tolerated.

HIGH-OUTPUT RENAL FAILURE

Posttraumatic acute renal insufficiency is well recognized as a highly lethal complication. The diagnosis is classically based on persistent oliguria and chemical evidence of uremia after stabilization of the circulation. The clinical course is characterized by oliguria of several days' to several weeks' duration, followed by a progressive rise in daily urine volume until both the excretory and concentrating functions of the kidney are gradually restored.

It is less well recognized that renal insufficiency may occur without an observed period of oliguria. This variant of renal insufficiency has been reported infrequently after burns, head injury, and soft tissue trauma. The reported cases are characterized by increasing azotemia, while the daily urine volume remains normal or increased. Many of these patients have an apparently inappropriate increase in urine volume, and the term *high-output renal failure* may best describe this entity, despite a theoretical objection. Until recently, this type of renal failure has not been noted frequently after trauma, nor has the clinical course been described in sufficient detail for recognition or management.

PATIENT STUDIES. A report is here presented to describe the clinical course of acute renal failure without oliguria, to emphasize the problems encountered in management, and to suggest renal ischemia as the basic causative mechanism (Fig. 4-15).

Fig. 4-15. High-output renal failure.

After severe abdominal trauma, the patients were in shock an average of 3.5 hours, the individual times varying from 1 to 6 hours. The average blood loss was 4.2 liters and average blood replacement 3.6 liters. The recorded blood loss was the amount measured at the time of operation. In most patients external bleeding was minimal. In addition to whole blood, they were given an average of 4 liters of Ringer's lactate solution per patient prior to and during the operative procedure.

After operation the diagnosis of renal failure was not immediately suspected, since urine volumes were above 30 ml/hour and few abnormalities were present in the initial values of blood urea nitrogen, potassium, sodium, carbon dioxide–combining power, and chlorides obtained on the first postoperative day.

In all cases not involving direct damage to the urinary tract, the urinalysis after operation showed specific gravities between 1.003 and 1.010, pH of 5.5 to 6.5, and urinary sediments containing at most a few red blood cells per high power field and an occasional cast. The urine:plasma ratio of urea nitrogen was found to be slightly less than 20:1.

The mean values of the daily urinary outputs for these patients can be seen in Fig. 4-16. On the day of operation the minimum urinary output was 730 ml. This represented the output for less than 12 hours in each case. There was a progressive increase in the mean urine volume for the first 6 to 8 days, reaching a height of 2350 ml and returning gradually to normal between the sixteenth and seventeenth days. The only low volumes were observed in an eight-year-old child with extensive blunt trauma requiring nephrectomy. The continued high output of 3 liters/day after the sixteenth day occurred in only one patient; the BUN in this patient did not return to normal for 37 days. The ranges denoted by the bars in Fig. 4-16 show the extremely high outputs in some patients compared to the relatively normal values in others during the period of azotemia. The highest urine volumes were found in patients with the highest BUN values.

Figure 4-17 shows a progressive rise of the mean BUN during the 6 to 8 days after injury and a gradual return to

Fig. 4-16. High-output renal failure: urine volumes.

normal between the sixteenth and eighteenth days. The serum creatinine levels paralleled the azotemia, the highest value being 6.8 mg/100 ml. In all patients the increasing BUN level was paralleled by an increasing daily urinary volume. Similarly, the stepwise decline in blood urea was paralleled by a decreasing urinary volume.

In Fig. 4-18 the average values and ranges of the serum potassium levels are shown. In most instances the initial values after operation were slightly below normal. In some the serum potassium levels were above 6 mEq/L by the second or third postoperative day, while the remaining patients showed a slow but sustained rise. All the accelerated rises resulted from intravenous administration of potassium salts (not more than 60 mEq/day). When the serum potassium reached 6 mEq/L, treatment with cation exchange resins was instituted. This proved effective in preventing further rises in serum K. An increase of serum potassium from 5.5 to 9.2 mEq/L was caused by the intravenous administration of 60 mEq of KCl in a 12-hour period. Extracorporeal hemodialysis was necessary to reduce the potassium intoxication that occurred. The bar graph represents the serum potassium levels resulting from the inability of the kidneys to excrete normal amounts of potassium and the administration of potassium salts, as well as the effective use of resins and the artificial kidney.

Moderately low values for the carbon dioxide–combining power were present for the first 4 or 5 days after injury and represent a mild to moderate metabolic acidosis. All isotonic losses were replaced with lactated Ringer's solution when acidosis persisted. In most patients the acidosis was well controlled by the administration of isotonic lactate solutions, which occasionally resulted in a mild metabolic alkalosis, although two patients had carbon dioxide–combining power values between 15 and 18 mEq/L despite lactate therapy and died on the tenth and twelfth postoperative days. After the eighth postoperative day carbon dioxide–combining powers were within a normal range without lactate administration. The serum chlorides did not show a reciprocal relationship to the carbon dioxide–combining powers.

Serum sodium determinations were made throughout the period of renal failure. The highest values of 150 to 154 mEq occurred during a trial of fluid restriction to determine whether the high urinary outputs were being induced by excessive administration of fluids. On these two occasions, hypernatremia was readily produced, indicating that the kidney was excreting a solute-poor urine.

Surviving patients were available for follow-up. Evaluation of renal function was carried out 1 to 1½ years after injury. Determinations of blood urea nitrogen, creatinine, sodium, potassium, carbon dioxide, and chloride were normal. Intravenous pyelography was normal. The lowest urinary concentration obtained was 1.020, and excretion of phenolsulfonphthalein (PSP) exceeded 30 percent in 30 minutes in all patients studied. Within 3 months both tubular and glomerular functions had returned to normal.

Fig. 4-17. High-output renal failure: blood urea nitrogen values.

*BUN normal on 37th p.o.d.

Autopsy was performed on patients who died. Microscopic examination of the kidneys from these patients showed regenerating patchy tubular necrosis. The damage in each instance was principally to the distal nephron; less severe changes were seen in the proximal segments.

A typical course of high-output renal failure shows an increasing urea nitrogen which parallels the increasing urine volume, a mild metabolic acidosis, and an acute hyperkalemia produced by the administration of potassium salts. Recognition of the disease entity permits control of these abnormalities.

ANIMAL STUDIES. Animal experiments using dogs were carried out to determine the modifying effect of hypothermia on renal ischemia. After contralateral nephrectomy, the remaining renal pedicle was clamped for 2 hours in each day.

As seen in Fig. 4-19, Group A consists of normothermic controls. Group B dogs had regional renal hypothermia produced by irrigation of the peritoneal cavity with cold saline solution. Group C dogs had profound renal hypothermia to 25°C produced by circulating cold saline solution continuously around the kidney. This cooling technique has been previously described.

The results show progressive azotemia and death in untreated animals that are not cooled (Group A). There was only transient elevation of the BUN when the kidneys were cooled to 25°C (Group C). In Group B, regional hypothermia, the BUN rose to an average height of 60 mg/100 ml by the sixth to tenth day and gradually returned to normal between the twelfth and sixteenth days.

Utilizing this same model in six dogs with exteriorized ureters, minimum urine volumes of 400 ml/day were obtained without an observed period of oliguria. Usually the

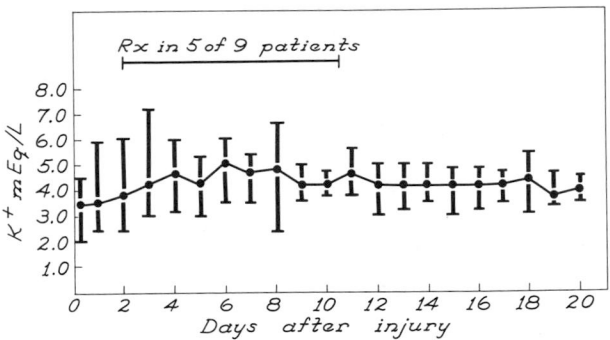

Fig. 4-18. High-output renal failure: serum potassium levels.

daily urine volume increased to between 600 and 900 ml/day before the BUN began to decline. Microscopic examination of these and six similarly treated animals, sacrificed between the fifth and tenth days, showed the tubular lesion to be confined principally to the distal tubules but with some proximal tubular involvement. These changes, both degenerative and regenerative, were scattered and irregular in distribution.

Consequently it can be seen that high-output renal failure in animals is an intermediate form of renal failure. With severe renal ischemia, unmodified oliguric renal failure inevitably resulted. When the kidney was protected with profound hypothermia, no significant renal failure resulted. On the other hand, with modest but practical protection to the kidney afforded by peritoneal sluicing with cold saline solution, moderate elevation of BUN associated with high urine volume was obtained. This protection resulted in recovery of the animal in each instance.

Fig. 4-19. Blood urea levels in dogs with renal ischemia, showing effect of hypothermia.

Discussion

Renal insufficiency without oliguria is important from the standpoint of recognition and clinical management of a variant of classic acute renal failure.

The clinical course of patients has been shown to be qualitatively the same as that occurring when oliguria is present. Quantitatively, however, these patients retain a limited ability to excrete acid products of metabolism, potassium, and urea. It is of primary importance that renal insufficiency of itself was not sufficient in terms of acidosis, uremia, potassium intoxication, or fluid volume control to cause death in this series.

The normal or high daily output of urine, although solute-poor, permits administration of fairly large quantities of water daily, in addition to replacement of isotonic salt losses such as those from gastrointestinal suction. The maintenance of normal extracellular fluid volume and normal serum sodium concentration is, therefore, easily accomplished when accurate daily outputs of each are obtained and losses are replaced accordingly. The quantity of fluids containing sodium may be administered as lactate to control the mild metabolic acidosis that occurs. The observations of Moore indicate that if the acidosis is not treated, it may become so severe as to become the outstanding abnormality in these cases.

The chief dangers of high-output renal failure are (1) failure to recognize the existence of renal failure because of normal output and (2) the administration of potassium salts intravenously. Good urinary output and gastrointestinal involvement requiring suction would usually indicate the need for daily replacement of potassium. When this type of renal failure exists, however, potassium intoxication may be produced. In the early patients studied, five of nine required therapy for hyperkalemia. One required emergency hemodialysis for control of excessively high serum potassium levels. It is important that the serum level be determined daily and prior to the administration of any potassium-containing solutions.

The factors involved in the production of acute renal failure following trauma are incompletely understood, but renal ischemia is of unquestioned importance. This concept implies that the ischemia produces damage to the nephrons, which results in failure of the kidneys to excrete urine. Diuresis is felt to represent the recovery phase. Allowing for the physiologic variation between individuals and between given degrees of renal ischemia, a spectrum of the length of the oliguric phase should occur. This has been well documented by Teschan and Mason. Presumably, a few cases of renal insufficiency without oliguria should occur. Although some theorize that renal failure without oliguria should be the most common type of renal failure observed, there is little documented support.

The frequency with which these cases occurred in relation to the small number of oliguric renal failures that were seen during the same period may represent differences in the therapy given during the ischemic episode. There are two outstanding differences in the therapy that we have routinely used. One is the administration of balanced salt solution along with whole blood in the resuscitation from hemorrhagic shock. It is well recognized that prolonged or severe extracellular fluid deficits are necessary for the production of renal failure in animals and may contribute to renal damage in man. The second difference in treatment is the use of renal hypothermia of a moderate degree to modify or prevent ischemic renal damage.

Clinical experience and laboratory experiments suggest that high-output renal failure represents the renal response to a less severe (or modified) episode of renal injury than that required to produce classic oliguric renal failure.

Pulmonary Responses

Acute respiratory failure following severe injury and critical illness has received increasing attention over the last decade. With advances in the management of hemorrhagic shock and support of circulatory and renal function in injured patients, it has become apparent that 1 to 2 percent of significantly injured patients develop acute respiratory failure in the postinjury period. Initially this lung injury was thought to be peculiar to the particular clinical situation. This is implied by such names as "shock lung" and "traumatic wet lung," which have been applied to acute respiratory insufficiency. It is now recognized that there are many similarities in the clinical presentation and the physiologic and pathologic findings of the pulmonary injury seen following a variety of insults. This has resulted in the concept that the lung has a limited number of ways of reacting to injury and that several different types of acute diffuse lung injury result in a similar pathophysiologic response. The common denominator of this response appears to be injury at the alveolar-capillary membrane, with resulting leakage of proteinaceous fluid from the intravascular space into the interstitium and subsequently into alveolar spaces. It has become acceptable to describe this entire spectrum of acute diffuse injury under the general term of *adult respiratory distress syndrome* (ARDS).

CLINICAL PRESENTATION. The syndrome of ARDS may occur under a variety of circumstances and result in a spectrum of clinical severity from mild dysfunction to progressive, eventually fatal, pulmonary failure. Fortunately, with proper management, the latter type is far less frequent than a milder type of abnormality.

For descriptive purposes the clinical picture can be divided into arbitrary stages. The first stage (injury, resuscitation, and alkalosis) immediately follows initial injury and is characterized by spontaneous hyperventilation with

Table 4-2. DIAGNOSTIC CRITERIA IN POST-INJURY PULMONARY INSUFFICIENCY

Major:
    Hypoxemia (unresponsive)
    Stiff lung (low compliance)
    Decreased resting volume (functional residual capacity)
    Diffuse interstitial pattern on x-ray
    Increased dead space ventilation
Minor:
    Increased cardiac output
    Hyperventilation
    Nonthoracic trauma

Table 4-3. BASIC TERMINOLOGY AND SYMBOLS

VO_2 . . . . Oxygen consumption
C.O. . . . . Cardiac output
VD/VT . . . . Physiologic dead space ventilation
                   as a fraction of tidal volume
Qs/Qt . . . . Venous admixture as a fraction of
                   total cardiac output
AaD . . . . Alveolar-arterial gradient
F_{IO_2} . . . . Fraction of inspired O_2
V/Q . . . . Ratio of ventilation to perfusion

hypocapnia, diminished pulmonary compliance, mixed metabolic and respiratory alkalosis, and a normal chest x-ray. After apparent stabilization of vital signs and adequate tissue perfusion, the patient enters Stage 2 (circulatory stability and beginning respiratory difficulty). This may persist for several hours to days. Persistent *hyperventilation,* progressive hypocapnia, increased cardiac output, progressive decrease in compliance, falling oxygenation, and increasing pulmonary shunt fraction all indicate that progressive pulmonary insufficiency will predominate in the subsequent clinical course. Recognition and therapeutic intervention at this point is believed to be extremely important. Stage 3 (progressive pulmonary insufficiency) and Stage 4 (terminal hypoxia with asystole) complete the syndrome.

The hallmarks of the clinical syndrome are

1. Hypoxemia which is relatively unresponsive to elevations of inspired oxygen concentration (indicating ventilation/perfusion imbalance and shunting).
2. Decreased pulmonary compliance (progressively increased airway pressure required to achieve adequate ventilation).
3. Chest x-ray changes, characteristically minimal in the early stages. With progression of the syndrome interstitial edema and diffuse infiltrates appear which may progress to widespread areas of consolidation.

Minor criteria for diagnosis include hyperventilation, increased cardiac output, and a history of nonthoracic trauma. The diagnostic criteria are summarized in Table 4-2.

MECHANISM. A review of a basic terminology is shown in Table 4-3.

The prominent derangements in pulmonary function associated with ARDS are (1) hypoxia which is unresponsive to increased inspired oxygen concentrations, (2) decreased pulmonary compliance (compliance defined as the amount of volume increase in the lungs obtained by a given change in pressure), which clinically appears as "stiff lungs," and (3) a fall in resting lung volume, specifically a fall in the functional residual capacity. The functional residual capacity, as shown in Fig. 4-20, is the amount of air remaining in the lungs after a normal expiration.

The possible causes of hypoxia (decreased arterial P_{O_2}) are shown in Table 4-4. All clinicians are familiar with

Table 4-4. CAUSES OF HYPOXEMIA

1. Hypoventilation
2. Diffusion defects
3. V/Q abnormalities
4. Shunting

Fig. 4-20. Lung volumes and capacities: *TLC,* total lung capacity; *VC,* vital capacity; *IC,* inspiratory capacity; *FRC,* functional residual capacity; *RV,* residual volume; *ERV,* expiratory reserve volume; *TV,* tidal volume; *IRV,* inspiratory reserve volume.

hypoventilation as a cause of hypoxia, as seen in the recovery room, but it is unlikely that hypoventilation is responsible for the hypoxia in this syndrome. Hypoventilation significant enough to result in hypoxia is associated with a rise in the P_{CO_2}. These patients, however, have an abnormally low P_{CO_2}.

Although diffusion defects can theoretically result from interstitial edema and thickening, they should respond to the administration of 100 percent oxygen. This is not the case in the patients in question, so diffusion defects alone would appear to be unlikely causes of the clinical syndrome.

Ventilation/perfusion inequalities could explain the hypoxia seen in these patients, and shunting represents the ultimate ventilation/perfusion abnormality. This statement deserves further explanation. Normally, there is autoregulation of ventilation and perfusion within the lung so that a balance exists between ventilation and perfusion of alveolar groups. When a group of alveoli become nonventilated or have decreased ventilation, compensatory mechanisms bring about a reflex decrease in blood supply to these alveoli. This, in its extreme, results in no ventilation and no perfusion to these alveolar units; thus no abnormality in terms of dead space ventilation or shunting occurs. The effects of loss of this normal balance or loss of compensatory mechanisms are shown in Fig. 4-21. On the left, alternations in blood flow are demonstrated. It can be seen that progressive decrease in blood flow with continued ventilation affects primarily carbon dioxide elimination. This can be defined as high ventilation/perfusion ratio and is usually reflected by increases in dead space ventilation. Such changes do not result in hypoxia. On the right side of Fig. 4-21 is shown the effect of reduction in ventilation while perfusion is maintained. It can be seen that progressive lowering of ventilation can result in hypoxia until the ultimate reduction, i.e., nonventilation, occurs. In theory, as long as any ventilation of the alveolus occurs, the hypoxia should be responsive to oxygen. This, then, is generally referred to as a ventilation/perfusion abnormality characterized by a low V/Q ratio. When alveolar collapse or nonventilation occurs for any reason, the hypoxia secondary to this is no longer responsive to oxygen; this is defined as a shunt.

Causes of pulmonary shunting are shown in Fig. 4-22.

PULMONARY GAS EXCHANGE
CONTRIBUTING FACTORS

Fig. 4-21. Diagrammatic representation of ventilation/perfusion ratio (V/Q) abnormalities.

Shunting normally takes place, to the extent of about 3 percent of the cardiac output, through both intrapulmonary and extrapulmonary routes. Although pathologic shunts occur from extrapulmonary causes, intrapulmonary shunting appears to be the problem in posttraumatic pulmonary insufficiency. Basically, there is perfusion of alveoli which are collapsed or for other reasons cannot be ventilated. The alveoli, for example, may be filled with secretions, exudate, blood, edema, or protein.

Whatever the cause, the clinical picture appears to result from a distortion of the normal ventilation/perfusion balance. This concept is shown in Fig. 4-23. In some areas of the lung there appears to be perfusion with poor ventilation; in other areas there is ventilation of nonperfused alveoli. This combination of abnormalities will produce decreased resting lung volume (functional residual capacity, or FRC), shunting, and increased dead space ventilation.

The common denominator producing the abnormalities

Fig. 4-22. Mechanisms of arteriovenous admixture in pulmonary shunting.

Fig. 4-23. Diagrammatic representation of mismatched ventilation and perfusion.

in ventilation and perfusion and other abnormalities seen in ARDS is thought to be injury to the alveolar-capillary membrane. This injury results in loss of integrity of the membrane, with increased permeability to albumin. The consequent leak of protein-rich fluid leads to *interstitial pulmonary edema* and decreased pulmonary compliance. With continued leakage, the alveolar units become fluid-filled and hypoxia (shunting) ensues. Thus the entire clinical picture of ventilation of poorly perfused segments (capillary injury), decreased compliance (interstitial edema), perfusion of poorly ventilated segments, and loss of lung volume (partially and completely fluid-filled alveoli) appears to result from capillary injury with a "capillary leak."

The majority of the causative factors listed in the next section cause such an alveolar-capillary injury.

ETIOLOGY. It appears likely that a variety of different injuries can produce a picture clinically indistinguishable from that described above. The most important of these are shown in Table 4-5.

Hemorrhagic Shock (Ischemic Pulmonary Injury). Pulmonary failure is commonly seen in severely injured patients, many of whom have been in shock. Initially, it was assumed that at least in part, the respiratory failure noted following injury was analogous to renal failure and was a result of ischemic injury to the lung. Support for this hypothesis came from early studies in animals and in human beings. Retrospective clinical reports implied a correlation between shock and pulmonary failure. Hemorrhage and congestion were noted in canine and human lungs after hemorrhagic shock and resuscitation. However, careful studies in dogs, primates, and other experimental animals, while demonstrating anatomic lesions of varying degree associated with hemorrhagic shock, do not demonstrate any measurable functional defect in the lung.

Table 4-5. POSSIBLE CAUSES OF ARDS
FOLLOWING INJURY

1. Ischemic pulmonary injury (?)	7. Fluid overload
2. Pulmonary infection	8. Oxygen toxicity
3. Systemic infection (sepsis)	9. Microatelectasis
4. Aspiration	10. Direct pulmonary injury
5. Fat embolism	11. Cerebral Injury
6. Microembolism	

Table 4-6. INCIDENCE OF PULMONARY
FAILURE AFTER INJURY

Group	Total no.	Significant pulmonary dysfunction	
		Number	Percent
All patients operated for trauma	978	21	2.1
Patients selected for study	49	21	43
Shock (all types)	28	11	39
No shock	21	10	48
Sepsis	10	8	80
No sepsis	39	13	33

Specifically, no significant or progressive hypoxia occurs. In fact, several studies have shown a decrease rather than an increase in pulmonary shunting in hemorrhagic shock. Adequate arterial oxygenation has been maintained during and up to several days following hypovolemic shock.

Only in extremely severe hemorrhagic shock preparations, lasting more than several hours, have preterminal decreases in arterial oxygen concentration been demonstrated. This is in contradistinction to sepsis and septic shock, in which hypoxia has been shown to occur regularly. Recent clinical studies have confirmed this finding. The highest incidence of pulmonary dysfunction is noted in those patients with sepsis, irrespective of the presence or absence of shock. The results of one prospective study are shown in Table 4-6. Thus, while hemorrhagic shock may compound other pulmonary injuries, it does not appear to be a primary cause of respiratory failure following trauma.

Pulmonary Infection. Pulmonary infection is eventually present in virtually all patients succumbing to respiratory insufficiency and usually becomes clinically apparent during the later stages of the syndrome. Although this can certainly compound the syndrome and produce further hypoxia and decreased compliance, it is probably a secondary event and not the initiating cause for the entire clinical picture. There is valid reason for concern about the role of ventilators and other respiratory equipment in the introduction of pulmonary infection. Without proper precautions, devices which are in line with the airway can be a source of bacteria. Pierce and his coworkers have shown that with appropriate measures this can be controlled so that the equipment used for respiratory assistance does not contribute to the incidence of bacterial pneumonia in patients.

Sepsis. Significant extrapulmonary infection with systemic sepsis appears to be a constant finding in a number of clinical studies of ARDS. In fact, acute respiratory failure may be the first manifestation of sepsis in a patient with burns, intracranial lesions, and pulmonary contusion. The syndrome of ARDS is rarely seen without severe sepsis. The concept that sepsis is an important causative agent is supported by a significant amount of laboratory evidence. A variety of septic insults, including injection of *Escherichia coli* endotoxin or live *E. coli* organisms and peritonitis-induced septicemia, produce significant derangements in pulmonary gas exchange.

The specific mechanism of septic lung damage is still speculative, but a number of factors appear to be operative:

1. Direct endothelial damage to the pulmonary capillaries with resultant loss of integrity and alveolar injury (see Mechanism)
2. Gross disturbances in the clotting mechanism as well as the release of a variety of vasoactive and bronchoconstrictive substances
3. Decrease in activity or amount of surfactant

Whatever the mechanism, available information supports the hypothesis that sepsis produces pronounced changes in vascular resistance, airway resistance, direct alveolar and vascular injury, interstitial and intraalveolar edema, hemorrhage, changes in surfactant, and progressive hypoxia. The association of sepsis and acute respiratory failure appears clear.

Aspiration. The syndrome produced by aspiration of gastric contents, blood, or mouth organisms with subsequent pneumonia can resemble the clinical picture described above. It would appear likely that in a small but significant number of patients, aspiration (recognized or unrecognized) occurs and may occasionally be the causative factor in posttraumatic pulmonary insufficiency.

Fat Embolism. A syndrome associated with multiple long bone fractures, which appears to be related to embolization of fat, can produce a clinical picture similar to that described above. Although mild x-ray differences may occur, these patients are difficult to distinguish from other patients with pulmonary insufficiency after injury. Fulminant fat embolism has been described in combat casualties. There is evidence that a more subtle form may occur in less severely injured patients, especially after significant soft tissue trauma and long-bone fractures. Again, the mechanism remains to be defined.

Microembolization. There is a growing body of evidence that microemboli of various sorts, with their attendant release of vasoactive substances, injury to pulmonary capillaries and adjacent alveoli, and hemodynamic effects can produce defects in pulmonary function. A number of theories are offered to explain the significance and source of such microscopic emboli.

One source of microemboli appears to be stored blood. Changes in screen filtration pressure due to particulate material in stored, banked blood have been reported. Several series have demonstrated a rough correlation between the number of transfusions and the incidence of pulmonary failure. The precise role of such filters remains to be established.

A second source of microemboli appears to be the formation of intravascular microaggregates. These have been demonstrated in the venous return following release of a cross-clamped aorta and following massive soft tissue injury. Recently they have been demonstrated in the venous effluent of limited nonhypotensive soft tissue injuries and in hypovolemic, nonhypotensive states. It now appears that arterial hypotension, hypovolemia, low-flow states, and trauma may all lead to the formation of microemboli. A third possible source of microembolism is disseminated intravascular coagulation.

In summary, many of these mechanisms appear to be operative in the trauma patient who develops pulmonary failure. However, the value of specific therapy in preventing or treating each entity has not been determined.

Fluid Overload. The role of fluid administration in the production of ARDS has created great controversy. It has been proposed that, in the severely injured patient, a point is reached at which maintenance of renal function and restoration of adequate tissue perfusion are gained at the cost of significant fluid overload to the detriment of pulmonary function.

Although there is little question regarding the deleterious effects of *massive* fluid overload, its role in the production of this syndrome remains questionable. Experimental animals massively transfused with balanced electrolyte solutions (amounts equivalent to 30 liters/hour in man) develop fulminant pulmonary edema. However, they respond briskly to assisted ventilation, and ventilatory therapy prevents hypoxia. Those that survive the insult clear the edema rapidly and do not develop the progressive pulmonary failure characteristic of the clinical syndrome. Similarly, clinical studies show no correlation between the amounts of fluids received and the development of pulmonary insufficiency.

While gross fluid overload is not desirable, excessive "drying out" of the lungs also may be dangerous. If excessive fluid restriction results in a fall of cardiac output, the degree of hypoxia resulting from any pulmonary damage will be compounded. At present the most reasonable course appears to be to maintain fluid balance as close to normal as possible.

An even more controversial subject is the administration of colloid versus electrolyte solutions in the production of the syndrome. If the pulmonary vasculature is normal, a fall in the serum oncotic pressure renders the lungs more susceptible to pulmonary edema. Some authors reason that if crystalloid solutions are used in resuscitation, a fall in oncotic pressure may occur and cause or compound a pulmonary abnormality. If this were the case, the administration of colloid might be potentially beneficial to these patients. Clinical reports on the use of colloid solutions in the therapy of this condition are scanty and the results difficult to evaluate. They do not conclusively demonstrate the clinical effectiveness of colloid or diuretic therapy in decreasing extravascular lung water and restoring normal serum oncotic pressure.

The available evidence implies that the pulmonary capillary membrane is abnormal in ARDS. Therefore colloids administered intravenously may gain access to the pulmonary interstitium and could potentially increase the interstitial oncotic pressure. This conceivably could compound the pulmonary problem in the healing phase.

Unfortunately, insufficient experimental data are available at present to resolve these conflicting hypotheses. A reliable experimental model of the syndrome is lacking. A large number of studies have evaluated pulmonary capillary permeability in hemorrhagic shock. Few changes in permeability or ultrastructural interstitial changes due to shock alone have been shown. This tends to support evidence that shock per se is not a primary factor in the etiology of this syndrome. Although large amounts of colloid have been shown to produce some changes in interstitial ultrastructure, no defect in oxygenation was produced. There is no significant difference in pulmonary function after resuscitation from hemorrhagic shock between crystalloid and colloid solution.

It is unlikely that the type of resuscitative fluid plays a primary role in the etiology of the syndrome. Hypervolemia produced by either type of fluid may produce pulmonary edema, but this responds quickly to standard treatment and should not be confused with the syndrome being described. Attempts at "drying out" the lung may be dangerous, because a decrease in cardiac output secondary to hypovolemia may compound any pulmonary functional defect present.

Oxygen Toxicity. Prolonged use of high oxygen concentrations can result in a clinical picture and pathologic findings identical to those seen in ARDS. Ventilation with high concentrations of oxygen is thought to poison cell enzyme systems and disrupt membrane integrity. It has also been shown to significantly reduce mucociliary clearance in the tracheobronchial tree. The critical level appears to be between 40% and 50% oxygen. There is also a time factor involved: the higher the oxygen tension, the less the time required to produce symptoms and evidence of damage. A conscientious attempt to keep inspired oxygen below these levels should prevent oxygen toxicity. It seems unlikely that oxygen toxicity is a major factor in the etiology of this syndrome, although it may compound the problem if oxygen is given in high concentrations for significant periods of time.

Microatelectasis. Microatelectasis can result from recumbency, sedation, operation, and anesthesia. Although not the primary factor responsible for the clinical picture, it may contribute to the hypoxia seen in these patients. Again, increased oxygen concentration increases the possibility of atelectasis.

Direct Pulmonary Injury. There is little doubt that direct pulmonary injury (pulmonary contusion) can produce the progressive syndrome previously outlined. Although many patients considered to have this syndrome are thought to have nonthoracic injury, unrecognized injury may well have occurred. A force applied to an animal's abdomen, comparable to that of a steering wheel blow received during a head-on collision, results in raising the diaphragm to the level of the second intercostal space posteriorly. Thus abdominal trauma may produce tremendous compressive pulmonary injury, which may not be immediately apparent.

Cerebral Injury. Massive head injury has been associated with acute pulmonary edema, and there is laboratory evidence of a cause-and-effect relationship. The progression of acute pulmonary edema to the clinical syndrome under discussion has not been established. A centrineurogenic basis for progressive pulmonary insufficiency has been proposed. There is some evidence that hypoxia in animals without direct head injury can produce the syndrome. The clinical significance of these observations has not been established.

TREATMENT. Therapeutic maneuvers could theoretically

Table 4-7. CONDITIONS INVOLVING GREATEST RISK FOR POSTINJURY RESPIRATORY FAILURE

1. Sepsis (systemic and pulmonary)
2. Massive soft tissue injury with or without long bone fractures
3. Direct pulmonary injury
4. Massive transfusion of whole blood
5. Aspiration of gastric contents

be directed at (1) manipulating pulmonary blood flow to increase the perfusion of well-ventilated units and decrease the perfusion of poorly ventilated units, (2) directly reducing the capillary leak by reversing the membrane injury, (3) indirectly reducing the interstitial edema, or (4) improving ventilation of poorly ventilated segments and preventing further alveolar filling or collapse. Often the one of these which is most practical and which is used clinically is the last. This involves using ventilatory support designed to support and increase alveolar volume.

The earlier in the course such therapy is applied, the more successful it is likely to be. Thus it is important to identify and closely monitor patients at high risk for developing ARDS after injury. Table 4-7 indicates patients in the high-risk category. Of these five groups, patients who have either systemic or pulmonary sepsis are most likely to develop acute respiratory failure. They should be admitted to an intensive care unit for repeated evaluation of pulmonary function.

Monitoring Pulmonary Functioning

Assessment of the adequacy of pulmonary function should begin immediately after injury in those patients at risk for developing ARDS. Endotracheal tubes inserted for airway control during surgery should not be removed prematurely. In many patients an additional 4 to 6 hours of intubation postoperatively will be sufficient to allow the physician to determine that ARDS is not a threat. Extubation should not be considered until adequate lung function

has been demonstrated (described below). If several days of intubation are contemplated, a nasotracheal tube may be substituted for the endotracheal tube in the operating room. This will allow for greater patient comfort and acceptance.

A prerequisite for optimal lung function is normal cardiovascular status. Hemodynamic monitoring, therefore, should be instituted routinely. This includes recording of heart rate, arterial pressure, electrocardiogram, central venous pressure, and pulmonary artery pressure if indicated. Serial body weight, intake and output balance, bacteriologic studies, coagulation profile, and chest x-rays are important data.

Monitoring of pulmonary function can be conveniently divided into three general areas: evaluation of oxygenation, ventilation, and lung-thorax mechanics. Table 4-8 details the most easily obtained tests and includes normal values. As a general principle, isolated determinations are not as valuable as serial measurements obtained at regular intervals. Hypoxemia is often detected in apparently normal patients who appear to be doing well clinically.

The partial pressure of oxygen in the arterial blood (Pa_{O_2}) is the hallmark of adequacy of oxygenation. This must be considered in the light of the inspired oxygen concentration (F_{IO_2}). A simple means of establishing a measurable relationship between Pa_{O_2} and F_{IO_2} is their ratio (Pa_{O_2}/F_{IO_2}). Ratios between 350 and 500 are considered adequate, while a value of less than 300 is definitely abnormal. This ratio provides the clinician with a gross estimate of the efficacy of oxygenation at the bedside during rapid changes in therapy. It appears to be most reliable when the F_{IO_2} is between 0.2 and 0.5.

The alveolar-arterial oxygen difference (AaD_{O_2}) may allow rapid differentiation of the cause of hypoxemia. Of the four causes of hypoxemia (hypoventilation, diffusion defects, ventilation/perfusion abnormalities, and pulmonary shunt), only the intrapulmonary shunt is theoretically

Table 4-8. ASSESSMENT OF PULMONARY FUNCTION

Function and measure	Acceptable result	Indication for therapy
Oxygenation: Partial pressure of oxygen, arterial blood (Pa_{O_2})	$Pa_{O_2}>90$ mm on 40% F_{IO_2}	<90 mmHg on 40% F_{IO_2} or decreasing
Ratio of partial pressure of oxygen, arterial blood, to fraction of inspired oxygen (Pa_{O_2}) . . . . Alveolar-arterial oxygen gradient	$Pa_{O_2}/F_{IO_2}>350$ 50–200 mmHg	<300 >200 mmHg or increasing
Ventilation: Partial pressure of carbon dioxide, arterial blood	35–40 mmHg	30 or decreasing
Minute volume	<12 liters/min	Increasing
Mechanics: Rate . . . . Effective compliance	12–25/min 50 ml/cm H_2O	>25 or increasing <50 or decreasing

refractory to O_2 administration. In general, this relationship holds true. However, the AaD_{O_2} is affected by cardiac output, O_2 consumption, the position of the hemoglobin/O_2 dissociation curve, and the magnitude of the pulmonary shunt. If the three other variables are constant, the AaD_{O_2} is a good reflection of the amount of pulmonary shunting. Characteristically, the patient with ARDS will have hypoxemia resistant to oxygen administration and therefore an elevated shunt fraction.

The adequacy of ventilation is determined by the arterial partial pressure of carbon dioxide (Pa_{CO_2}). By definition, hypoventilation occurs when the Pa_{CO_2} is elevated. Postinjury pulmonary failure is usually associated with hypocapnia (hyperventilation). Therefore the patient with a decrease in both Pa_{CO_2} and Pa_{O_2} probably has ARDS. Tidal volume (VT)—the amount of air breathed during one respiratory cycle—is another indication of the adequacy of ventilation. This is readily measured with a modestly priced respirometer. VT multiplied by the respiratory rate is called the *minute ventilation.* This value is easily derived but by itself is only a rough guide to adequate ventilation. In many postinjury patients, high minute ventilations are recorded. It is not established whether this is a compensatory response or an indicator of a pathologic condition.

The effective compliance (C_{eff}) may be quite valuable as an assessment of the ease of distensibility of lung and thoracic cage. This derived value is obtained by dividing the VT by the peak airway pressure. C_{eff} indicates the "stiffness" of the lungs, i.e., how difficult they are to ventilate (low C_{eff} means increased stiffness). A decreased C_{eff} may indicate increased extravascular lung water, airway constriction, or increased chest wall resistance (impaired bellows activity). Low values are usually found in patients with ARDS.

An adequate assessment of pulmonary function can be achieved by serial measurement of arterial blood gases, tidal volume, minute ventilation, and effective compliance. Several other monitoring devices have been advocated. The work of breathing is almost always increased in ARDS. This value is a measure of the mechanical cost of achieving adequate ventilation. The major disadvantage of this test is that it requires an intraesophageal balloon to measure transthoracic pressure and the availability of an analog computer for usable results. Although highly desirable, the measurement of the work of breathing is difficult in the critically ill patient.

Although sophisticated and expensive equipment is available to continuously monitor arterial and venous blood gases and other pulmonary function tests, it has not been shown to significantly improve patient survival.

Ventilatory Support

Indications. There are no universal guidelines for the institution of ventilatory support. The indications outlined in Table 4-7 have been found reliable in treating a large number of patients. The most common indication for beginning ventilatory therapy is hypoxemia. Initial management should be to increase the F_{IO_2} both as a diagnostic test and to temporarily relieve hypoxemia if the Pa_{O_2} is less than 65 mmHg. For effective therapy, control of the airway must be achieved. The most rapid and reliable way to do this is the insertion of an endotracheal or nasotracheal tube. Mechanical ventilation may then be applied. Since a defect in the matching of ventilation to perfusion is present, therapy is directed at maintaining ventilation to marginally ventilated alveoli and the recruiting collapsed or partially occluded alveoli. This will directly increase the FRC of the lungs.

Technique. The volume ventilator is the device most often chosen for the treatment of ARDS. The initial tidal volume setting may be 10 to 15 ml/kg body weight at a rate of 12 to 14 breaths per minute, with an inspiration:expiration ratio of 1:2. The ventilator is adjusted so that the patient can "trigger" additional ventilator breaths. This can be described as assisted mechanical ventilation (AMV). An F_{IO_2} of 0.4 should be applied initially and blood gas determinations used to indicate the efficacy of this treatment. Humidification of the inspired air via a heated nebulizer is essential to avoid drying airway secretions.

Blood gases are checked within 10 to 20 minutes of beginning respiratory treatment to determine the patient's response. If hypoxemia persists on 40% oxygen, increasing the VT still further may be warranted in an effort to increase the FRC. The effect of this maneuver is best assessed by following serial compliance changes. If the C_{eff} is improving, benefit from increased VT may be expected. If C_{eff} decreases with an increase in VT, too much volume is being given to the patient. Lower tidal volume ventilation will then be required to minimize the risk of complications of ventilatory therapy. The compliance curve is shaped somewhat like the Starling curve of cardiac function, i.e., a plateau is reached, after which any increase in volume is achieved only at the expense of a marked increase in airway pressure.

Alternate methods of mechanical ventilatory support are available. One which is being used more frequently is intermittent mandatory ventilation (IMV). This is a technique of mechanical ventilation which allows the patient to breathe spontaneously and at the same time to receive periodic support from the ventilator.

Acceptable levels of Pa_{O_2} are between 65 and 80 torr. If this cannot be achieved with the treatment outlined above, there are two alternatives: manipulation of F_{IO_2} and support of lung volume.

The F_{IO_2} may be increased to higher levels. Since pulmonary shunting is caused by continued perfusion of nonventilated alveoli, simply increasing the concentration of oxygen will have no significant effect on the shunt. In addition, washout of nitrogen from poorly ventilated alveoli will make them more susceptible to collapse, thus converting low V/Q areas to areas of shunt resulting in more atelectasis. Although there is still controversy over the role of O_2 toxicity in the genesis of ARDS (see above), the literature clearly indicates that prolonged use of high O_2 concentrations can produce a clinical picture similar to ARDS. A concentration of more than 50% O_2 is required to produce deleterious effects in patients with normal lungs, depending on the amount of time alveolar hyperoxia is maintained. The higher the O_2 concentrations, the less the time required to produce damage. Therefore every effort should be made to limit the F_{IO_2} to less than 0.5.

Since acceptable manipulation of the F_{IO_2} is limited, the second alternative is to recruit collapsed or partially collapsed alveoli with some modification of ventilatory therapy. This can be done by applying continuous positive end-expiratory pressure (PEEP) to the airway. PEEP may be achieved by either inserting an airflow resistance during expiration or using a ventilator with an end-expiratory plateau of positive pressure. Providing positive pressure throughout the respiratory cycle prevents alveolar and small airway collapse and may recruit lung units which were previously collapsed. The beneficial effects of this modality are (1) increased FRC, compliance, and Pa_{O_2}; (2) increased V/Q ratio (when initially low); (3) decreased pulmonary shunting; and (4) decreased mortality from ARDS.

Technique of PEEP. The commonly used volume ventilators have the capability of instituting PEEP without modifying the equipment. Although there is some controversy about the absolute level required, incremental increases in pressure are advocated. The usual beginning level is 5 cm H_2O of PEEP. Cardiorespiratory function is monitored after 10 to 15 minutes to assess the effects. If no beneficial effect is noted, further increases in PEEP follow in increments of 3 to 5 cm H_2O pressure.

There may be variable response to PEEP. While some patients respond with an immediate increase in Pa_{O_2}, others may not show improvement for $\frac{1}{2}$ to 1 hour or longer. Therefore absence of immediate response should not be interpreted as an absolute failure of PEEP. Each patient has a different but demonstrable optimal PEEP level which correlates well with the highest compliance. Thus a practical bedside monitor of the effectiveness of PEEP may be compliance.

Complications of PEEP. It has been shown that cardiac output may be decreased secondary to an increase in intrathoracic pressure and decreased venous return. This is usually significant only when the intravascular volume is decreased. Therefore fluids should be given to assure a normal volume status before beginning PEEP therapy. Monitoring of the pulmonary wedge pressure is valuable in the assessment of volume prior to and during the administration of PEEP. Cardiac output may also be measured to assure normal values.

Excessive pressure applied to the terminal airways may overdistend and rupture normal alveoli, leading to pneumothorax. This complication of PEEP is uncommon below 20 cm H_2O pressure.

Close attention to the effective compliance can prevent excessive airway and alveolar pressure being applied during PEEP therapy. PEEP is most beneficial when FRC is low initially. In patients with a high FRC from preexisting lung disease (Chronic Obstructive Pulmonary Disease), any level of PEEP may be detrimental. This can be deter-

mined only by closely monitoring the patient's response to treatment, noting compliance especially.

Control of Pa_{CO_2}. Hyperventilation is a common problem in patients who are being artificially ventilated. Hypocarbia has been shown to be deleterious to the cerebral circulation (vasoconstriction) and the pulmonary circulation. Therefore ventilatory therapy should be set to maintain normal levels of Pa_{CO_2}. With high tidal volume ventilation, a compensatory decrease in respiratory rate is necessary to maintain a normal Pa_{CO_2}. Increasing the inspired concentration of CO_2 or adding dead space have both been advocated as methods of increasing the Pa_{CO_2} but are rarely effective in patients with ARDS. Effective control of the Pa_{CO_2} requires heavy sedation or muscle relaxation and control of the patient's respiration. Decrease of the Pa_{CO_2} below 30 is an indication for instituting respiratory control.

Adjunctive Therapy during Mechanical Ventilation. Oxygen-carrying Capacity of Blood. Although the Pa_{O_2} can be increased by higher levels of F_{IO_2}, it is the red blood cell that carries almost all the O_2 to the tissues. One unit of packed red cells carries more O_2 than plasma exposed to pure O_2 at hyperbaric pressure. The hemoglobin (Hb) concentration should therefore be maintained at 12 to 14 Gm/100 ml. Attention should also be given to the acid-base status of the patient. Both acidosis and alkalosis produce shifts of the Hb/O_2 dissociation curve, which can affect the ability of Hb to off-load O_2 at the tissue level (see Alterations in Oxygen Transport, below).

Fluid Management. As noted in the discussion of the etiology of ARDS, there is much debate concerning proper fluid management. It is our opinion that maintenance of normal fluid balance is important. This will obviate any deleterious effects of hypovolemia on the Pa_{O_2} and minimize any decrease in cardiac output which may occur with PEEP administration.

Diuretics. Diuretics have been suggested as a means for reducing the amount of pulmonary edema. There is no study which has randomly and prospectively shown that diuretics are as effective as or more effective than ventilatory therapy alone in ARDS. It is reasonable to give small doses of furosemide *when hemodynamic studies indicate that fluid overload has occurred* (elevated pulmonary artery wedge pressure). No attempt should be made to "dry out" the patient by long-term administration of diuretics.

Steroids. There is no conclusive proof that pharmacologic doses of steroids should be part of the specific therapy of the ARDS syndrome, although data indicate that steroids may be effective in treating pulmonary fat embolism, septic shock, and aspiration of gastric acid.

Heparin. If intravascular coagulation is shown to be a problem in the postinjury patient with ARDS, appropriate heparin therapy may be of benefit. Heparin is associated with significant side effects and should not be used indiscriminately in the patient who has recently sustained a traumatic injury.

Antibiotics. Prophylactic use of broad-spectrum antibiotics has no place in the primary therapy of ARDS. Indiscriminate use of these agents may allow the emergence of resistant strains of bacteria, which are very difficult to treat. Many patients will already have been given antibiotics because of certain types of injury. Specific antibiotics are used to treat pulmonary sepsis. Their choice is determined by serial cultures of the sputum.

Ancillary Pulmonary Care. Patients treated in the intensive care unit tend to be bound to the bed by numerous tubes, wires, and catheters. Change in position then becomes a difficult problem. It has been shown, however, that significant improvement in oxygenation results from frequent position changes. Maintenance of one position is likely to compound pulmonary abnormalities.

Routine pulmonary toilet, suctioning with sterile technique, and attempts to prevent pulmonary infection are important. These must all be done on a routine basis.

Weaning from Ventilatory Therapy. The criteria for discontinuing ventilatory therapy are the obverse of the indications for its institution, i.e., return of pulmonary function tests to normal. The primary requisites for weaning from ventilatory therapy are a stable cardiovascular system and the absence of cardiac arrhythmias. Monitoring must therefore continue during the process. The patient with chronic obstructive lung disease should meet these same criteria. Objective criteria for weaning are shown in Table 4-9. The recommended steps in weaning are as follows:

1. The F_{IO_2} is decreased to as close to room air as possible as rapidly as possible.
2. A stepwise decrease (3 to 5 cm H_2O at a time) in the level of PEEP is begun until intermittent positive pressure breathing (IPPB) is tolerated.
3. The tidal volume is decreased to normal values.
4. The patient is weaned from the mechanical ventilator.
5. The tracheostomy tube is removed.

Arterial blood gases should be analyzed at frequent intervals after each stage of the weaning process to assure that the patient does not become hypoxemic or hypercapnic. Several hours should elapse between steps so that the process is not carried out too rapidly.

A relatively new concept in weaning is the introduction of intermittent mandatory ventilation (IMV). IMV allows the patient to gradually resume the work of breathing, in contrast to conventional weaning, in which the entire burden is put on the patient for increasing periods of time. The rate of IMV may be varied from 30 respirations to 1 (at a preset tidal volume) per minute. We have been unable to demonstrate its superiority in our patients. Some patients require a great deal of time to be successfully

Table 4-9. MINIMAL CRITERIA FOR WITHDRAWING VENTILATORY SUPPORT

1. Clinical stability
2. Inspiratory force < -15 torr
3. $Pa_{O_2} > 250$ torr ($F_{IO_2} = 1.0$) or equivalent oxygenation index
4. Dead space/tidal volume < 0.6
5. Vital capacity > 10 ml/kg

SOURCE: Adapted from T. W. Feeley and J. Hedley-Whyte, Weaning from Controlled Ventilation and Supplemental Oxygen, *N Engl J Med,* **292:**903, 1975.

weaned, particularly those with persistent sepsis and a severe catabolic state. Reeducation of the muscles of respiration may require repeated exercise by increasing the time off IPPB.

Once the patient is able to tolerate being off the ventilator, supplemental heated nebulized oxygen should be given by means of a T piece. If this is tolerable, the patient may be extubated or a fenestrated tracheostomy tube may be inserted. The supplemental O_2 may then be decreased over a period of several days to complete the weaning process.

Summary

The syndrome of acute pulmonary failure, as it occurs in the injured patient, has many possible causes. The definable causes are amenable to specific modes of therapy. The chief functional defect, hypoxemia unresponsive to increased F_{IO_2}, is treated with ventilatory therapy with or without PEEP on an empirical basis.

With early, aggressive ventilatory support, morbidity and mortality may be minimized. Adjunctive therapy may play a significant role when there are specific indications.

Alterations in Oxygen Transport

Cell hypoxia and eventually cell death may result from the complex changes induced by shock, regardless of the type, and restoration of delivery of oxygen to the tissues at an adequate concentration and pressure forms the basis for treatment. In the past, attention was directed primarily toward the factors affecting oxygen transport capability, including the concentration and partial pressure of oxygen in the inspired air, alveolar ventilation, ventilation/perfusion relationships, cardiac output, blood volume, and hemoglobin concentration. The demonstration that the level of organic phosphates in the red blood cell has a significant effect on the position of the oxygen/hemoglobin dissociation curve has served to focus attention on the processes responsible for release of oxygen at the tissue level. Because of the clinical implication of these findings, a knowledge of factors regulating both uptake and release of oxygen has assumed increasing importance in the care of critically ill patients.

OXYGEN TRANSPORT

The oxygen transport system consists of several component processes that function collectively to extract oxygen from inspired air and deliver it at a partial pressure sufficient to allow rapid diffusion from blood into the body cells. Each of the component processes has its own internal controls, and failure of any one may be compensated for by adjustments in the remainder of the system. The functions of the oxygen transport system are summarized in the following formula:

Oxygen consumption = arteriovenous oxygen difference
$$\times \frac{\text{cardiac output (liters/minute)}}{100}$$

The amount of oxygen in whole blood includes that bound to hemoglobin (1.38 ml O_2/Gm of hemoglobin) and a small amount dissolved in plasma (0.003 ml/mm of oxygen tension). The oxygen content of arterial (Ca_{O_2}) and venous blood CV_{O_2} are calculated by the formula

Oxygen content = (1.38 × Hb conc. × Hb sat.)

$$+ (0.003 \times P_{O_2})$$

Consider a person with a hemoglobin of 15 Gm/100 ml, an arterial oxygen tension of 100 mmHg, a venous oxygen tension of 40 mmHg, arterial and venous hemoglobin saturations of 97 and 75 percent respectively, and a cardiac output of 6 liters/minute. Substituting these values in the formulas above, arterial oxygen content is 20.4 vol%, venous oxygen content is 15.6 vol%, arteriovenous oxygen difference is 4.8 vol%, and oxygen consumption is 288 ml/minute.

Changes in any one of these factors are of variable significance regarding oxygen delivery. For instance, pulmonary gas exchange with 20% inspired oxygen concentration ($F_{I_{O_2}}$) normally produces an arterial oxygen tension (Pa_{O_2}) of approximately 100 mmHg, slightly less than average alveolar oxygen tension. Increasing the $F_{I_{O_2}}$ to 100% would raise Pa_{O_2} to approximately 650 mmHg. This would increase the amount of dissolved oxygen in the plasma from 0.3 to 2.0 vol% but would only increase the hemoglobin saturation from 97 to 100 percent. In contrast, even moderate changes in hemoglobin concentration or cardiac output have a strong influence on oxygen transport capability. A hemoglobin concentration of 10 Gm/100 ml (instead of 15) in the example above would reduce the oxygen-carrying capacity of the blood by one-third (Ca_{O_2} = 13.7 vol%). Coupled with a fall in cardiac output from 6 to 3 liters/minute, assuming that other variables remain unchanged, oxygen consumption theoretically would fall from 288 to 96 ml/minute. This is a not infrequent clinical occurrence, although oxygen consumption would be maintained at a higher level by adjustments in other parts of the system (e.g., increase of arteriovenous oxygen difference).

Therapy designed to improve tissue oxygenation, therefore, includes an evaluation of all factors affecting the oxygen transport system. Adjustment of inspired oxygen concentration and efforts to improve alveolar ventilation are of obvious importance; however, therapeutic attempts to maintain a normal hemoglobin concentration and cardiac output deserve special attention.

OXYGEN/HEMOGLOBIN DISSOCIATION CURVE

Another aspect of oxygen transport which deserves emphasis is the relationship between hemoglobin oxygen saturation and oxygen tension. The oxyhemoglobin dissociation curve describes hemoglobin affinity for oxygen, and its unusual sigmoid shape reflects the phenomenon of heme-heme interaction. Each of four heme groups in the hemoglobin molecule reacts with oxygen in a prescribed order, and uptake of an oxygen molecule by one heme group facilitates the oxygenation of the next heme group. The sigmoid configuration of this curve is particularly suitable for the uptake, transport, and subsequent release of oxygen. Since the upper portion of the dissociation

Fig. 4-24. Oxygen-hemoglobin dissociation curves in (A) normal, (B) rightward-shifted, and (C) leftward-shifted positions. The P_{50} value denotes the position of the curve along the horizontal axis and represents the oxygen tension (in mm Hg) necessary to saturate 50 percent of available hemoglobin with oxygen. Note that as the curve moves toward the left, the arteriovenous oxygen difference, (a-v̄) O_2, can be maintained only by decreasing venous oxygen tension. (*Adapted from S. D. Shappell and C. J. M. Lenfant, Anesthesiology, 37:127, 1972.*)

curve is relatively flat, oxygen loading by hemoglobin may remain relatively normal despite wide variations in the alveolar oxygen tension. As oxygenated blood traverses the peripheral capillary, however, P_{O_2} drops from approximately 100 to 40 mmHg, hemoglobin saturation falls from 97 to 75 percent, and the blood releases just over 22 percent of its oxygen load (Fig. 4-24). Since P_{O_2} values at the peripheral capillary level fall on the steep portion of the curve, significant changes in oxygen release are produced by only small alterations in oxygen tension.

The position of the oxyhemoglobin dissociation curve along the horizontal axis is characteristically termed the P_{50} value. This reflects the oxygen tension necessary to saturate 50 percent of the hemoglobin with oxygen; the normal value is approximately 27 mmHg.

The importance of positional changes of the curve is also related to its sigmoid shape. Within limits, rightward or leftward shifts have little effect on arterial oxygen saturation if Pa_{O_2} is above 80 mmHg. At the peripheral capillary level, however, even small shifts of the curve may be important. A rightward shift of the dissociation curve (P_{50} above 27 mmHg) indicates decreased hemoglobin affinity for oxygen, while a leftward shift (P_{50} below 27 mmHg) is associated with an increase of hemoglobin/oxygen affinity. Compared to the normally positioned curve, more oxygen is released at any given P_{O_2} with a rightward-shifted curve and less is released with a leftward shifted curve. Therefore, if arterial and venous oxygen tensions remain constant, arteriovenous oxygen difference increases with a rightward shift of the curve and decreases with a leftward shift (Fig. 4-25).

Fig. 4-25. Oxygen-hemoglobin dissociation curves similar to those in Fig. 4-24. Note that if arterial and venous oxygen tensions remain constant, arteriovenous oxygen difference decreases as the curve moves toward the left.

Changes in position of the oxygen/hemoglobin dissociation curve are significant in at least two respects. The transfer of oxygen from the blood to the sites of intracellular utilization is directly related to the oxygen pressure differential. Thus a rightward shift of the curve is theoretically advantageous, since an equivalent amount of oxygen is released at a higher P_{O_2} than with a leftward-positioned curve. (Note that in curve B of Fig. 4-24, half of the oxygen would be released at a P_{O_2} of 36 mmHg; in curve C, less than 10 percent of the oxygen would be released at the same P_{O_2}.) Secondly, the ability to maintain or enlarge the arteriovenous oxygen difference is dependent to some extent on the position of the curve. Normally, arterial hemoglobin saturation is near the upper limit and cannot be increased appreciably. Any enlargement of the arteriovenous oxygen difference necessitates reduction in venous hemoglobin saturation and venous oxygen tension Pv_{O_2}. As the curve moves to the left, maintenance of any given arteriovenous oxygen difference requires a progressive decrease in Pv_{O_2}. The fall in Pv_{O_2} is finally limited by the fact that a certain partial pressure is necessary for transfer of oxygen from the blood to the tissue cell. That level of oxygen pressure below which diffusion may be theoretically impaired and cellular function disturbed has been termed the "critical P_{O_2}."

Available data concerning the critical P_{O_2} are limited but suggest that it varies in individual organ systems and may depend on the level of activity of the tissues. Opitz and Snyder showed that oxygen uptake by the brain is impaired when venous oxygen tension falls below 20 to 25 mmHg, while Berne et al. indicated loss of myocardial function at oxygen tensions between 10 and 12 mmHg. With a leftward movement of the curve, therefore, maintaining or enlarging the arteriovenous oxygen difference is theoretically limited as the Pv_{O_2} approaches this critical level. Tissue oxygen delivery may be sustained in this

instance by other mechanisms, principally by increasing cardiac output.

During hypovolemic shock, cardiac output is low and relatively fixed. Normally, enlargement of arteriovenous oxygen difference will partially compensate for the diminished blood flow; however, the response may be totally inadequate with a leftward shift of the dissociation curve. Continued survival and maintenance of essential organ function may be obtained only by shunting blood from tissues that tolerate a limited period of severe hypoxia (skin, skeletal muscle) to organs that require high oxygen flow rates (brain, heart).

FACTORS INFLUENCING THE POSITION OF THE OXYGEN/HEMOGLOBIN DISSOCIATION CURVE

Attempts to ensure a normal or rightward-positioned dissociation curve may be essential during treatment of patients with low-flow states. Factors affecting the position of the curve have been summarized by Shappel and Lenfant and are outlined in Table 4-10. The main in vivo influences include changes in pH, temperature, partial pressure of carbon dioxide, and level of red blood cell organic phosphates. Changes in hydrogen ion concentration and temperature have predictable and instantaneous effects on the position of the curve, while P_{CO_2} exerts its influence both by changing pH and by a pH-independent effect. The quantitative effects of these influences on the dissociation curve have been reviewed in several excellent publications.

The position of the dissociation curve is also influenced by interaction of hemoglobin with organic phosphates in the red blood cell. Both ATP and 2,3-diphosphoglycerate (DPG) bind to hemoglobin and lower the affinity of hemoglobin for oxygen, i.e., shift the dissociation curve to the right. In a quantitative sense, DPG is the more important of the two phosphates and exerts an additional influence in the intact red blood cell by lowering intracellular pH via Donnan equilibrium. Significant concentrations of DPG are found only in the red blood cell, and DPG is present in a concentration approximately equimolar with that of hemoglobin. DPG is a product of erythrocyte glycolysis, formed via a branch of the Embden-Myerhof pathway by conversion of 1,3-DPG to 2,3-DPG, catalyzed by diphosphoglycerate mutase.

Erythrocyte DPG undergoes considerable changes in response to several stimuli, with parallel changes in the position of the dissociation curve. Investigations have revealed that hypoxia increases erythrocyte DPG in conditions such as exercise, anemia, exposure to high altitude, cardiac failure, and various pulmonary diseases. The concomitant rightward shifts of the dissociation curve are thought to represent significant compensatory responses, allowing release of more oxygen at a higher P_{O_2}.

The regulation of DPG synthesis is complex and as yet not fully clarified. Although numerous factors influence the level of DPG (Table 4-10), the principal *mechanism* for increasing or decreasing its concentration appears to be related to the level of hydrogen ions in the red cell. DPG concentration increases as the red blood cell pH rises and decreases as the pH falls. These changes are due, in part, to

Table 4-10. FACTORS THAT ALTER HEMOGLOBIN/OXYGEN AFFINITY

Increase P_{50}	Decrease P_{50}
By direct effect:	By direct effect:
Increased [H^+]	Decreased [H^+]
temperature	temperature
P_{CO_2}	P_{CO_2}
DPG, ATP	DPG, ATP
Hb conc.	Hb conc.
Ionic strength	Ionic strength
Abnormal hemoglobin	Abnormal hemoglobin
Aldosterone	Carboxyhemoglobin
	Methemoglobin
By increasing DPG:	By decreasing DPG:
Decreased [H^+]	Increased [H^+]
Thyroid hormone	Decreased thyroid hormone
Pyruvate kinase deficiency	Hexokinase deficiency
Increased inorganic phosphate	Decreased inorganic phosphate
Cortisol	Cell age (old)
Cell age (young)	

SOURCE: Adapted from S. D. Shappell and C. J. M. Lenfant, Adaptive, Genetic and Iatrogenic Alterations of the Oxyhemoglobin Dissociation Curve, *Anesthesiology,* **37:**127, 1971.

the differential effects of pH on the activity of two red cell enzymes, DPG mutase and phosphatase. For instance, alkalosis stimulates DPG synthesis by increasing DPG-mutase activity and reducing the breakdown of DPG by DPG-phosphatase. The rise in red cell pH may be secondary to elevation of whole blood pH or, as in hypoxic states, a relative increase in the amount of deoxyhemoglobin. The pH also influences DPG binding to hemoglobin and may affect other enzymes in the glycolytic cycle. The net effect of pH changes on DPG concentration, therefore, probably represents a combination of these (and other unknown) influences. It should be noted that the pH-induced changes in DPG concentration tend to counteract the direct pH effects on the curve via the Bohr effect. Therefore the immediate rightward shift of the curve secondary to acute acidosis is eventually offset by a pH-induced reduction in DPG concentration.

DPG synthesis is also responsive to hormonal influences and the level of inorganic phosphate. The phosphate level is directly related to DPG concentration, and maintenance of a normal inorganic phosphate level during intravenous hyperalimentation is necessary to prevent a reduction in the level of erythrocyte 2,3-DPG. Thyroid hormone acts directly to increase DPG synthesis, a fact which probably explains the elevated levels of this compound in hyperthyroid patients. Cortisol and aldosterone both shift the dissociation curve to the right, thereby decreasing hemoglobin/oxygen affinity. The effects of cortisol are probably secondary to direct stimulation of DPG synthesis. Hemoglobin/oxygen affinity also increases as the erythrocyte ages, presumably owing to a decreasing DPG concentration.

BLOOD TRANSFUSIONS, ERYTHROCYTE DPG, AND OXYGEN DELIVERY

The acceptability for transfusion of blood which has been stored in ACD (acid citrate dextrose) solution for up to 3 weeks is based on survival of at least 70 percent of the cells in the recipient's circulation. During this 3-week period, however, there is a rapid decline in erythrocyte DPG and a progressive increase in hemoglobin/oxygen affinity. Following transfusion, several hours are required for the DPG levels to return to normal. These findings suggest that oxygen delivery may be impaired after the administration of large quantities of stored blood and have led to a reevaluation of transfusion practices.

Several studies in both experimental animals and man have failed to show significant impairment of tissue oxygenation with markedly reduced levels of erythrocyte DPG and leftward shifts of the oxygen dissociation curve. Similar findings were noted in our study of 45 injured patients who received more than 5 units of whole blood stored in ACD solution during resuscitation and the subsequent operative procedure. Erythrocyte DPG levels were below normal in a majority of these patients and correlated well with the amount and storage time of the transfused blood. There were no consistent correlations, however, between DPG concentration and the measured parameters of oxygen delivery. This lack of correlation may be explained by two observations. First, the position of the dissociation curve cannot be reliably predicted from a knowledge of the DPG concentration alone. DPG represents only one of several factors that affect the curve, and the final P_{50} represents a composite of these influences. Normal or elevated P_{50} values noted in several patients with low DPG concentrations were probably due to other factors (e.g., pH and temperature) which tended to counteract the influence of DPG. A second observation is the lack of a consistent relationship between the P_{50} value and oxygen consumption. The majority of patients with leftward shifts of the dissociation curve had reasonably normal arteriovenous oxygen difference and oxygen consumption. Additionally, several of the patients with narrowed arteriovenous oxygen differences maintained oxygen delivery simply by increasing the cardiac output.

These findings do not imply that the position of the dissociation curve and the factors that influence it are unimportant. They do suggest that a person with reasonably intact cardiovascular and pulmonary systems is able to tolerate rather significant leftward shifts of the oxygen dissociation curve. The consequences may be quite different, however, in a patient with limited compensatory mechanisms and in some therapeutic regimens followed without understanding of their effects on the position of the curve. An example of this is shown in Fig. 4-26. Despite the sharp reduction in cardiac output following hemorrhage to a mean blood pressure of 50 mmHg, the control dog with a normal P_{50} value was able to maintain normal oxygen delivery by increasing the arteriovenous oxygen difference from 4.5 to 10.6 ml. In contrast the DPG-depleted dog was unable to expand the arteriovenous oxygen difference sufficiently (P_{50} value 15 mmHg). The problem was compounded by attempts to correct pH to normal by infusion of sodium bicarbonate solution. The dissociation curve moved further to the left (P_{50} value 8 mmHg), the hemoglobin concentration fell secondary to hemodilution, and oxygen consumption fell to near zero. Although extreme, the experimental conditions are not unlike those which may be found in the clinical setting.

In summary, available evidence suggests that changes in hemoglobin/oxygen affinity, as reflected by the position of the oxygen dissociation curve, may be important in several circumstances. The elevated DPG concentrations and rightward shifts of the dissociation curve observed in hypoxic states (pulmonary disease, cardiac failure, anemia, exposure to high altitude, and so on) probably represent compensatory responses that facilitate oxygen unloading in the tissue capillaries. Oxygenation can be maintained in these instances by other mechanisms (e.g., increasing cardiac output) but at greater expense to body economy.

Leftward shifts of the dissociation curve observed following transfusions of stored blood, acute alkalosis, hypothermia, and so forth are, at best, undesirable phenomena and may significantly impair oxygen unloading. Although leftward shifts are tolerated in many circumstances, maintenance of a normally positioned dissociation curve may be of singular importance in patients with hypoxia, anemia, or hypotension when compensatory responses are limited.

THERAPEUTIC IMPLICATIONS

Obtaining a sufficient quantity of fresh blood for resuscitation of the patient in hemorrhagic shock is difficult, and attempts are being made to find a suitable storage medium that will maintain the levels of organic phosphates in the red blood cells. At present, storage of blood in CPD (citrate phosphate dextrose) solution seems to be the most practical alternative. Survival of red blood cells is similar after transfusion of blood stored in either ACD or CPD solution. Compared to blood stored in ACD solution, however, blood stored in CPD media has a higher pH, and DPG and P_{50} are maintained at consistently higher levels. Conversion from ACD to CPD solution for blood storage is a simple matter for blood banks and has been accomplished in many areas. When large quantities of blood are administered, particularly in critically ill patients, some attention should be paid to the storage age of each unit of blood. If a significant portion of the blood administered has been stored for more than 7 to 10 days, every attempt should be made to obtain fresh blood for additional transfusion requirements. In our experience the institution of these simple changes, including conversion to CPD storage media, has been rewarding. The large reductions in DPG and P_{50} noted in the past are rarely seen today, even after massive transfusions.

Other factors that influence the position of the dissociation curve (Table 4-10) may also be important in the individual patient. For instance, the induction of respiratory alkalosis may produce an abrupt increase in hemoglobin/oxygen affinity. This is a common occurrence during operations and in patients requiring ventilatory assistance in the postoperative period; coupled with other factors that limit oxygen transport, the capacity to maintain tissue oxygenation may be sharply reduced. Similarly, the sudden correction of an acidosis, whether metabolic or respiratory, may have undesirable effects. In this regard the indiscriminate use of sodium bicarbonate during resuscitation of patients in hypovolemic shock is discouraged. The presence of a mild metabolic alkalosis is a common finding after resuscitation, owing in part to the alkalinizing effects of blood transfusions and the administration of lactated Ringer's solution. After infusion (and partial restoration of hepatic blood flow), the citrate and lactate contained in transfused blood and the lactate in lactated Ringer's solution are metabolized and bicarbonate is formed. If excessive quantities of sodium bicarbonate are administered simultaneously, a severe metabolic alkalosis may result. The alkaline pH may be highly undesirable, particularly in patients with hypoxia or low fixed cardiac output. Combined with other factors incident to blood replacement which increase hemoglobin/oxygen affinity (low DPG concentration and hypothermia), significant interference

Fig. 4-26. Effects of hemorrhagic shock and sodium bicarbonate infusion on oxygen consumption after exchange transfusion with fresh blood (dog A) and DPG-depleted blood (dog B). I, Control period; II, after exchange transfusion (DPG concentration 6.20 μM/ml RBC in dog B); III, after induction of hypotension; IV, continued hypotension and sodium bicarbonate infusion.

with oxygen unloading at the cellular level may occur.

The immediate and direct pH influences on the curve (via the Bohr effect) are eventually offset by reciprocal changes in DPG concentration. There is, however, a lag period of approximately 4 hours before any change in DPG concentration is noted, and the final level is not reached until 48 hours after induction of acidosis or alkalosis. The fact that the effects of sudden large changes in pH may persist for several hours should be considered during therapy. Correction of a metabolic acidosis, therefore, is properly directed toward correction of the underlying disorder. Bicarbonate therapy may be reserved for the treatment of severe metabolic acidosis, particularly following cardiac arrest, when *partial* correction of pH is essential to restore myocardial function. Similarly, pH correction in more protracted states of metabolic acidosis may be indicated but should be accomplished slowly.

Lowering body temperature also causes a leftward shift of the dissociation curve and an increase in hemoglobin/oxygen affinity, but any interference in oxygen delivery may be countered effectively by the hypothermia-induced reduction in metabolic requirements.

Rightward shifts of the curve are usually desirable and, unless extreme, rarely interfere with oxygen uptake in the lungs. Rightward shifts generally occur as a compensatory response to hypoxia, regardless of the cause. Nevertheless, in patients with severe arterial desaturation (exposure to high altitude, congestive failure, right-to-left cardiac shunts), any potential benefit from shifting the curve further to the right may be offset by interference with oxygen loading.

In a complex clinical setting, multiple factors that influence hemoglobin/oxygen affinity may be operative at any given time, and abrupt changes secondary to therapy or the disease process itself may occur. Evaluation of these multiple influences may be difficult, since few data concerning their cumulative effects are available. Nevertheless their *net* effect can be estimated by determining the position of the oxygen dissociation curve.

Techniques for constructing an oxygen dissociation curve are time-consuming and not readily available in most hospitals. For this reason we have developed a rapid, though less precise, method for estimating the position of the curve (the P_{50} value). Since the shape and slope of the curve do not change appreciably with changes in position, determination of a single point on the steep part of the slope should allow a rough estimate of the entire curve. To obviate the use of a tonometer, a single sample of venous blood is drawn anaerobically and the P_{O_2} and oxygen saturation are measured. (An arterial sample is unsuitable, since the values fall on the upper flat portion of the curve.) An estimated P_{50} value may then be obtained using the Severinghaus slide rule or a nomogram as depicted in Fig. 4-27. The nomogram represents a computer plot of a family of O_2 dissociation curves, using the correction factor for pH as suggested by Severinghaus. The point on the nomogram corresponding to the measured P_{O_2} and saturation values is found and traced to the line representing 50 percent oxygen saturation. This intersect represents the estimated P_{50}; the normal value is approximately 27 mmHg. A P_{50} above this level represents a rightward shift of the oxygen dissociation curve, while a lower value represents a leftward shift.

To test the validity of this technique, oxygen dissociation curves were constructed using a standard mixing technique on 50 occasions in 27 acutely ill patients. In each instance an estimated P_{50} was obtained from the nomogram using a single sample of venous blood drawn at the same time. Correlation between the two values was excellent (correlation coefficient .92).

Estimates of P_{50} have become routine in our care of critically ill patients. Combining this with measurements of both arterial and venous blood gases, a considerable amount of information may be obtained about the state of oxygenation and oxygen transport capability.

THERAPY OF SHOCK

Hypovolemic Shock

It is apparent from the previously described etiologic classification of shock that therapy will of necessity depend on detection of the causative mechanisms while providing support to the patient. Correction of the underlying causative factors can then be carried out. Consequently one sees again the usefulness of a practical clinical classification that includes (1) oligemic shock, (2) cardiogenic shock, and (3) shock caused by changes in peripheral resistance and

Fig. 4-27. Nomogram for estimation of P_{50} value (position of the oxygen-hemoglobin dissociation curve). The point on the nomogram corresponding to the measured P_{O_2} and saturation of a sample of venous blood is traced to the line representing 50 percent oxygen saturation. This intersect represents the estimated P_{50} (normal value approximately 27 mm Hg). In the example shown, the venous blood sample P_{O_2} is 39 mm Hg, the oxygen saturation 65 percent, and the P_{50} value 31 mm Hg (a rightward-positioned dissociation curve).

P_{50} NOMOGRAM

OXYHEMOGLOBIN (%)

OXYGEN TENSION (mm Hg)

capacity vessels (neurogenic shock and septic shock). In a patient who has undergone trauma, more than one causative factor may be operating. Once the diagnosis of shock has been made and supportive therapy begun, a diligent search can be made for the causative factor or factors.

Treatment of shock, therefore, can best be thought of in relation to the type of shock that is present. As pointed out earlier, the pathogenesis of hypovolemic hypotension is varied. Recognition of deficits of total body water and electrolytes is usually subtle, and correction requires specific therapy with crystalloid solutions. Reductions in the extracellular fluid volume (plasma and interstitial fluids) primarily, as in burns, peritonitis, and some forms of crush injury, are more easily recognized. Specific therapy should be started with electrolyte solutions and rarely may require the use of plasma or some source of protein. External blood loss as seen in lacerations should be corrected immediately, as fluid therapy is begun, with first-aid measures, including pressure tamponade. Surgical procedures may then be carried out. Similarly, an external loss, such as bleeding from a duodenal ulcer, should be treated with the usual measures, including decompression of the stomach, while supportive therapy is begun.

The only other immediate concern in addition to control of the causative wounds is maintenance of an open airway. Pulmonary insufficiency rarely occurs from shock alone, but concomitant injuries may include crush injuries of the chest, pneumothorax, hemothorax, or specific obstruction of the airway from injuries to the head and neck. In these circumstances adequate respiratory exchange must be restored promptly.

VOLUME. The treatment of hemorrhagic shock continues to be the adequate replacement of whole blood, since this is the fluid that has been lost. Early use of properly cross-matched, type-specific whole blood is still the primary therapy when shock is due to whole blood loss. When available, type-specific or Rh-negative "universal donor" type O blood with low anti-A titer can be administered.

Extracellular Fluid Replacement

An effective therapeutic regimen for the treatment of hemorrhagic shock has now been used successfully in several thousand patients, taking into account the previously described changes in the peripheral circulation and interstitial fluid.

When patients are admitted to the emergency room in hemorrhagic shock, a large-gauge needle or catheter is inserted into an appropriate vein (preferably in the arm) and an infusion of lactated Ringer's solution is begun immediately. At the same time, blood is drawn for typing and cross matching. The lactated Ringer's solution is run at a rapid rate so that in a period of 45 minutes between 1,000 and 2,000 ml of lactated Ringer's solution is given intravenously. This approach has several advantages.

The procedure is a highly effective therapeutic trial to determine the preexisting amount of blood loss or the presence of continuing blood loss. It is often observed that blood pressure will return to normal, become stable, and remain so in patients with severe hypotension after infusion of 1 or 2 liters of a balanced salt solution. When such a

response is correlated with measurements of red blood cell mass, plasma volume, and extracellular fluid volume, the preexisting blood loss is shown to be relatively minimal. If blood loss has been minimal and hemorrhage is not continuing, hemorrhagic hypotension can be alleviated simply by the infusion of a balanced salt solution.

If blood loss has been severe or hemorrhage is continuing, the elevation of blood pressure and decrease in pulse rate that occur with rapid intravenous infusion of lactated Ringer's solution is usually transient. When this occurs, whole blood that has been accurately typed and cross-matched is available and can be given immediately. Consequently, the initial use of the balanced salt solution allows time for accurate typing and cross-matching.

In view of the disparate reduction in the extravascular, extracellular fluid as demonstrated in animals and man, it is felt that even though blood is needed, as it is in the majority of patients admitted in hemorrhagic hypovolemia, alleviation of the reduction in functional extracellular fluid is desirable.

Lactated Ringer's solution as initial therapy, both from the standpoint of a therapeutic trial and as a therapeutic adjunct, is a procedure that has been found to be effective. This is understandable, since lactated Ringer's solution is isotonic, essentially free from side reactions, and virtually harmless from the standpoint of aggravation of other fluid and electrolyte imbalances that may be present.

Further, it appears that the use of a balanced salt solution in this fashion significantly reduces the requirement of whole blood in the patient with hemorrhagic hypotension. This is true not only from the standpoint of proper hemoglobin and hemoconcentrations following therapy, but also from the standpoint of prevention of, or recovery from, renal failure.

A concern that Ringer's lactate solution may aggravate the existing lactate acidosis when used to treat patients in shock has been expressed by several investigators, but previous studies in both experimental animals and patients do not support this view. The use of blood plus Ringer's lactate solution to treat hemorrhagic shock in experimental animals results in a more rapid return to normal of lactate, excess lactate, and pH than does treatment with return of shed blood alone. Recently, serial determinations of lactate, excess lactate, pH, and base excess have been obtained in 52 patients in hemorrhagic shock. All patients received Ringer's lactate solution in addition to whole blood during the period of resuscitation. There was a significant reduction in lactate and excess lactate levels and a return of pH and base excess values toward normal during the period of shock while Ringer's lactate solution was being infused. After resuscitation, all these values rapidly returned to normal levels.

Blood Transfusions. Blood transfusions have been discussed above under Blood Transfusions, Erythrocyte DPG, and Oxygen Delivery.

Hemoconcentration. For many years the belief was held that hemorrhage and shock were separate entities, because hemorrhage was not accompanied by hemoconcentration and shock invariably was. As shown in Fig. 4-28 and as described previously under Pathophysiologic Responses to

Fig. 4-28. Six possible results in shock cases, showing the fallacy of using hemoconcentration as the only guide to treatment. (*From H. N. Harkins, Surgery, 9:231, 1941.*)

Shock, the hemoconcentration is not a differentiating factor. The extent of concentration depends on the proportion of red blood cells and plasma lost in the hypovolemic episode, as well as on the compensatory adjustments that the interstitial fluid has been able to make to the intravascular volume reduction.

Blood Substitutes. In the absence of whole blood, many substances have been proposed as transient substitutes for the combination of red blood cells and plasma available in whole blood. The most popular and commonly used substitute has been human plasma. In some circumstances, e.g., battlefield conditions, plasma has been a highly serviceable substitute. Plasma carries with it the same risk of viral hepatitis that whole blood does. A unit of pooled plasma, however, carries a greater risk of harboring and transmitting the infective viral hepatitis than a unit of blood. As shown by Allen, storage of fresh plasma at room temperature for 6 to 8 months significantly reduces the attack rate and infectivity of the virus of infectious hepatitis. In any event, the administration of plasma carries with it some risk of hepatitis as well as the poorly understood antigen-antibody reactions that frequently occur from homologous plasma. Further, the volume of plasma required is such that for all practical purposes restoration of blood

volume is not generally feasible with plasma alone. Plasma contains no hemoglobin and, therefore, no oxygen-carrying capacity beyond that of any non-erythrocyte-containing liquid. (Physically dissolved oxygen in plasma constitutes only 0.3 percent by volume.)

It should be pointed out that volume replacement with plasma is rapidly equilibrated into the total extracellular fluid. The albumin that remains in the vascular tree is easily degraded at a rapid rate. Moore estimates that plasma dispersal from the intravascular to the extravascular phase may proceed at a rate approaching 500 ml, or 2 units, per hour. Therefore plasma or albumin as a blood volume substitute is transient at best.

A number of other substances have been proposed for transfusion in hemorrhagic shock since early in World War I, when solutions of acacia were used. Several excellent review articles are available which summarize the problems with all these artificial solutions. Suffice it to say that at present the only acceptable one of the entire group continues to be dextran. This substance has been shown to be effective clinically in the absence of a severe need for hemoglobin and its oxygen carrying capacity. Nevertheless, like all other plasma or blood substitutes, this substance still causes occasional severe antigen-antibody reactions and above all, regularly produces defects in the clotting mechanism. This has been shown in volunteers and patients when amounts of more than 1 liter of clinical dextran, with an average molecular weight of approximately 75,000, are used in man. The longest effect of dextran in maintaining an expanded plasma volume has been shown to be 24 to 48 hours. Low-molecular-weight dextran in the average range of 35,000 to 40,000 has recently received renewed interest because of data suggesting its ability to lower the viscosity of blood and possibly to prevent agglutination of erythrocytes during the low-flow state induced by hypovolemic shock. But work by Replogle indicates that the effect of low-molecular-weight dextran on blood viscosity is produced entirely by hemodilution or change in blood volume. When these parameters were controlled, no evidence of alterations in blood viscosity associated with infusions of low-molecular-weight dextran were observed. Although there are some theoretical advantages in using this plasma expander, investigative studies reveal serious clotting-mechanism defects with low-molecular-weight dextran, such as had been seen with the higher-molecular-weight dextrans.

POSITIONING. Positioning of the patient in shock has long been thought to be an adjunct in the treatment of hypovolemic shock. Most first-aid courses teach that the patient in shock should be placed in the head-down position. Although it is true that some forms of shock, particularly neurogenic shock, will respond to the head-down position, the effect of posture on the cerebral circulation in the face of true hypovolemia has not been defined. Frequently the patient with multiple trauma has sustained other injuries, within both the abdomen and the chest, so that the routine use of the Trendelenburg, or head-down, position may interfere with respiratory exchange far more than when the patient is left supine. The beneficial effect of the head-down position is probably the result of transient autotransfusion of pooled blood in the capacity or venous side of the peripheral circulation. This beneficial effect can be obtained easily by elevating both legs while maintaining the trunk and the remainder of the patient in the supine position. This is probably the preferable position, then, for the treatment of hypovolemic shock.

PULMONARY SUPPORT. In the past, most writings on the treatment of hypovolemic shock stated that breathing high oxygen concentrations is probably of little avail during a period of hypotension. These conclusions were based on the concept that the principal defect is in volume flow to tissues and decreased cardiac output. The oxygen saturation in the majority of patients with uncomplicated hypovolemic shock is generally normal, and the small increase in dissolved oxygen in the blood contributed by raising the P_{O_2} above this level is insignificant, particularly in the face of a markedly decreased cardiac output. This concept continues to be valid in terms of improvement of the shock state or tissue oxygenation itself. Nevertheless, in the small but significant group of patients in hypovolemic shock in whom the oxygen saturation is not normal, the *initial* use of increased oxygen concentrations may be extremely important, since the fall in cardiac output accompanying hemorrhagic shock has been shown to compound existing defects in oxygenation. This may occur in patients with preexisting defects, such as chronic obstructive lung dis-

ease, but more frequently problems in oxygenation arise directly from the patient's injury. Examples of this are a coexisting pneumothorax, pulmonary contusion, aspiration of gastric contents or blood, and larger obstructive problems. Thus, although oxygen is not routinely administered to patients in shock, if any doubt exists as to the possibility of one of these circumstances or as to the adequacy of oxygenation of arterial blood, the initial administration of oxygen until the injuries to the patient have been diligently assessed is certainly justified. If oxygen is to be administered to patients under these circumstances, it should be delivered through loose-fitting face masks designed for this purpose. If controlled airway is indicated for other reasons, an endotracheal tube is ideal. The use of nasal catheters, particularly those passed into the nasopharynx, is avoided because of potential complications of pharyngeal lacerations and gastric distension. Gastric rupture has been recorded secondary to such a catheter being inadvertently placed in the esophagus.

ANTIBIOTICS. Antibiotics were used in the treatment of hypovolemic shock for many years and were thought to exert a protective mechanism against the ravages of hypovolemia. Subsequent data fail to support this hypothesis. The use of antibiotics in patients who have open or potentially contaminated wounds, however, continues to be sound practice, when combined with good surgical debridement and care. Consequently the use of wide-spectrum antibiotics, as well as specific coverage against streptococci and staphylococci, is advisable as a preventive measure in the severely injured patient. Generally, penicillin is used in doses of 1 to 5 million units/24 hours, with parenteral administration of tetracycline in doses of 1 to 2 Gm for the first 24 hours. These are started immediately in patients who have sustained hypovolemic shock from trauma.

TREATMENT OF PAIN. Treatment of pain in the patient with hypovolemic shock is rarely a problem from the standpoint of shock itself. If, however, the causative injury produces severe pain, as in fracture, peritonitis, injury to the chest wall, and the like, control of pain becomes mandatory. Generally, when the patient is moved to the emergency facility where physicians and care are available, simple restorative measures, administration of intravenous fluids, passing of catheters, and so forth, will give reassurance. The need for analgesics is greatly reduced, since the need to allay fear and anxiety becomes markedly less. If, however, the patient continues to have severe pain, the observations made by Henry K. Beecher in World War II become extremely pertinent. Beecher pointed out that many battle casualties received morphine or other narcotic agents by subcutaneous administration early after wounding. Since these analgesics were not put into the circulation immediately, the pain continued and the patient ultimately received several doses that were not absorbed. Once effective therapy was begun for shock, the doses previously administered were absorbed and profound sedation resulted. As a result, the recommendation was made that small doses of narcotics be given *intravenously* for the management of pain in the patient with shock. This has been standard practice for 20 years and relieves pain without contributing significantly to the potentiation of the shock syndrome.

STEROIDS. Adrenocorticoid depletion was commonly regarded as a contributory factor in shock after it was learned that the presence of hypovolemic shock could in itself deplete the adrenal cortex of adrenocortical steroids. Subsequent studies, however, have shown that adrenocortical steroid production is stimulated maximally by the presence of hypovolemic shock. Steroid depletion with hypovolemic shock may possibly occur in the elderly patient or in patients who have specific adrenocortical diseases such as incipient Addison's disease, postadrenalectomy patients, or patients who have had adrenal suppression with exogenous adrenocortical steroids. In these specific instances the intravenous administration of hydrocortisone is desirable. In the general patient, with hypovolemic shock, however, administration of adrenocorticoids is probably not indicated.

DIGITALIS. Digitalis has been advocated in the treatment of hypovolemic shock. There is no doubt that in some patients, particularly elderly ones, the stress of hypovolemic shock will in itself induce or aggravate cardiac failure. In these patients, digitalis is found to be helpful. Over the years many have investigated the role of the heart as a cause of the irreversible form of hemorrhagic shock, but experimental data obtained in patients indicate that heart failure in response to hypovolemic shock is merely a terminal event. Further evidence of this is supplied by the fact that the central venous pressure does not rise except terminally in hypovolemic shock.

INTRAARTERIAL INFUSIONS. Intraarterial infusions were advocated for many years for the rapid replacement of intravascular volume in hypovolemic hypotension and shock. The weight of evidence at present, supplied by Hampson, Scott and Gurd, Harkins, and others, is that "the side of the circulation into which the blood is transfused is of no importance provided that the same rapid rate can be assured." Consequently the present-day usefulness of intraarterial transfusion resolves to a matter of convenience. If the operative procedure is in the area of a major artery, as in open-chest procedures, then a given quantity of blood may be delivered much faster via the intraarterial route. Otherwise no specific advantage seems to be offered by the arterial route of transfusion.

HYPOTHERMIA. Since the basic defect during shock is inadequate perfusion to tissues for maintenance of normal metabolism, a logical approach to supportive therapy would include some mechanism to lower the normal tissue metabolism. Hypothermia is available at present to lower metabolism. Experimental results in animals have demonstrated that induction of hypothermia prior to the onset of hemorrhagic shock will in fact protect against the lethality of the shock. Similarly, some experiments have shown that therapy of hemorrhagic shock with hypothermia has provided some beneficial effect. The available data for evaluation of hypothermia in human hypovolemic shock are meager. Since the induction of a hypothermic state is a serious undertaking, it is difficult to assess the effects on the

severely injured patient. Some available data would indicate that under some circumstances, hypothermia may be desirable. These circumstances need to be further elucidated and are probably concerned with the later stages of prolonged hypovolemic or possibly septic shock.

RENAL HYPOTHERMIA. Local or regional cooling is of proved benefit in protecting the kidney from damage during ischemic periods. The methods of local cooling previously described have been developed in an attempt to reduce postoperative renal complications induced by the total ischemia necessary during renal artery repair, heminephrectomy, or stone removal, as well as aorticorenal surgery. Of far more common occurrence are the renal ischemia and resultant renal damage occasioned by hemorrhagic or hypovolemic shock. Since the kidney is rendered ischemic even in mild hypovolemic shock, rapid lowering of intrarenal temperature should afford protection during the prolonged periods of ischemia.

The effective methods of introducing local renal hypothermia previously described are limited for optimal use in emergency situations by requiring (1) the additional operative trauma of mobilization of the kidney; (2) cumbersome special equipment that is not readily available or is difficult to sterilize and maintain; and (3) careful attention to prevent interference with other operative procedures within the abdominal cavity.

The open peritoneal cavity affords a large surface area for heat exchange. Jaeger found that the introduction of a large volume of cold isotonic solution into the closed peritoneal cavity of dogs resulted in a rapid decrease in body temperature. If intraabdominal organs, particularly the kidneys, which are apparently the most sensitive to hypoxia, can be effectively cooled by the direct introduction of cold solution, then a simple, expedient, practical method of cooling is readily available in every operating room. This consists of filling the open abdominal cavity with isotonic salt solution that has been cooled in the operating-room refrigerator (Fig. 4-29).

Experiments in animals were undertaken (1) to compare the temperatures obtained and the protection afforded the ischemic kidney by this method with that of direct surface hypothermia, (2) to evaluate the depth of cooling obtained in the ischemic versus the intact kidney, and (3) to determine the depth of cooling obtained in the kidney during hemorrhagic shock. A summary of the results of these experiments follows.

1. Figure 4-19 shows the degree of protection afforded by surface cooling as opposed to formal hypothermic perfusion, as described earlier; surface cooling provided significant protection from renal ischemia (100 percent survival rate). Lower intrarenal temperatures could be obtained by circulating coolant; however, the survival rate was lowered, probably because of the necessary extensive mobilization of the kidney.

2. A subsequent experimental study was designed to evaluate the effect of intact blood supply on the degree of hypothermia obtained by peritoneal cooling. The results of this study are shown in Fig. 4-30, and a comparison between esophageal temperatures and renal temperatures

Fig. 4-29. Technique of regional abdominal hypothermia.

with and without intact renal blood supply is also seen. These results demonstrate that there is some decrease in total body temperature, especially with intact blood supply to the kidneys, but that the intrarenal temperature even with intact blood flow is decreased at more than twice the rate of the general body temperature. Without blood flow, the depth of renal hypothermia achieved is three times that of the esophageal temperature as long as cooling is continued. An equally important observation is that the ischemic

kidney rewarms only slowly as compared to the kidney with intact blood supply.

3. The results of the third study to determine the depth of cooling obtained during hemorrhagic shock are shown in Fig. 4-31. The depth of hypothermia obtained is seen to be approximately the same as that in the intact kidneys, without hemorrhagic hypotension. Similarly, there was a

Fig. 4-30. Degrees of peritoneal hypothermia obtained in dogs by introduction of intraperitoneal iced saline solution at 2 to 3°C (left renal pedicle occluded).

Fig. 4-31. Degrees of peritoneal hypothermia obtained in dogs by introduction of intraperitoneal iced saline solution at 2 to 3°C after blood loss shock (renal pedicle not occluded).

concomitant lowering of the total body temperature to approximately 88°F. But after the chilled solution had been removed from the abdominal cavity, the intrarenal temperatures in the hypotensive animals continued to decline, reaching 75°F in 30 minutes. Despite this, the total body temperatures did not reach significantly lower levels.

The studies indicate that intrarenal temperatures of approximately 25°C should furnish good protection with only transient mild suppression of renal function. Certainly 20°C offers complete protection to the ischemic kidney for periods extending to 6 hours. The effective cooling of the kidney with an intact blood supply versus the ischemic kidney emphasizes the importance of blood supply in determining the rate and depth of cooling.

Studies were then made in patients on the basis of the animal experiments. It was felt that this type of hypothermia could be used in patients with safety and could be expected to produce a sustained lowering of intrarenal temperatures during hypovolemic hypotension. Intrarenal hypothermia in patients was produced by filling the abdominal cavity with 2 liters of refrigerated (3°C) isotonic salt solution. The salt solution was allowed to remain in contact with the peritoneal cavity for approximately 1 to 2 minutes. The bulk of this was removed by suction, and this was repeated several times, employing a total of 4 to 6 liters of the cold solution during a 5-minute period. Intrarenal temperatures were measured by sterilized needle prior to the induction of hypothermia and at intervals during and after cooling.

Figure 4-32 shows the intrarenal temperatures of 10 patients taken 5 minutes after the beginning of peritoneal hypothermia. It can be seen that in those patients who were normotensive there was minimal lowering of the renal temperature. On the other hand, in patients with modest

hypotension, intrarenal temperatures were lowered to 88 to 90°F, and in the severely hypotensive patient the intrarenal temperature in 5 minutes had reached the level of 78°F.

Figure 4-33 depicts three patients in whom intrarenal temperatures were measured prior to induction of renal hypothermia and at 1-minute intervals thereafter. As would be expected from the studies just presented, the rate of fall of intrarenal temperature was directly proportional to the degree of hypotension present at the time of cooling.

Esophageal temperatures were monitored. In general, the fall in esophageal temperature was approximately half the fall in intrarenal temperatures in the first 10 minutes. The lowest temperature reached was 88°F in two patients. No untoward effects were noted other than a modest fall in blood pressure (less than 10 mmHg diastolic) in normotensive patients. There were no changes in cardiac rate or rhythm during this procedure.

The animal experiments show that an intrarenal tem-

Fig. 4-32. Intrarenal temperatures in 10 patients 5 minutes after beginning of peritoneal hypothermia.

Fig. 4-33. Intrarenal temperatures of patients after induction of peritoneal hypothermia in relation to degree of hypotension.

perature of 28 to 30°C is easily attainable in the ischemic dog kidney by sluice-cooling of the peritoneal cavity. This moderate degree of hypothermia produced 100 percent survival, but with mild elevation of the BUN for a period of 12 to 15 days. All these animals excreted normal or increased amounts of urine.

The preliminary data suggest that cooling by means of peritoneal irrigation (1) produces sufficient lowering of intrarenal temperatures to afford protection to the kidney with decreased blood flow, (2) offers a rapid means of lowering total body temperature, and (3) should produce a decrease in intrarenal temperature in a kidney completely deprived of blood comparable to that obtained by other local techniques.

In the past the chief objection to peritoneal irrigation was the introduction of infection. Peritoneal dialysis for uremia has proved to be a safe procedure on a short-term basis, infection occurring only after prolonged use. In our experience the use of copious quantities of refrigerated salt solution in the operating room has been completely free from complications. Specifically, there have been no cases or peritonitis, abscess formation, wound disruption, or prolonged ileus in the patients studied.

VASOPRESSORS. In recent years the addition of substances that cause additional vasoconstriction in hypovolemic shock has been popular. These have been used largely because human blood pressure can usually be elevated somewhat by the addition of one of a series of pressor agents. Although it is true that blood pressure can be elevated, the objective in treating hypovolemic shock is to increase tissue perfusion. By the use of vasopressors, the blood pressure is raised by increasing peripheral vascular resistance and decreasing tissue perfusion. Therefore the injurious effects of shock may well be aggravated.

As experience has accumulated with the use of vasopressors, it is obvious that the alpha- and beta-stimulating functions of the vasopressors generally have a threefold action consisting of central inotropic and chronotropic effects and a peripheral vasoconstricting effect. In an evaluation of the comparative effects of a number of the cate-

cholamines, Waldhausen et al. demonstrated significant differences. Isoproterenol hydrochloride (Isuprel), levarterenol bitartrate (Levophed), epinephrine (Adrenalin), and phenylephrine hydrochloride (Neo-Synephrine) all produced a significant increase in contractility of the heart and an increase in heart rate. Isoproterenol had, in addition, a vasodilator effect on the peripheral vessels, while the other three amines were largely peripheral vasoconstrictors. Metaraminol (Aramine) produced a significant increase in myocardial contractility, further increasing the efficiency of the heart beat while the heart rate fell; this amine was also a moderate vasopressor. Of the drugs tested, phenylephrine showed the least efficient inotropic effect and was predominantly a peripheral vasopressor. Dopamine, a naturally occurring catecholamine biochemical precursor of norepinephrine, is similar to isoproterenol in exerting positive inotropic and chronotropic effects on the heart by stimulation of beta-adrenergic receptors. Because of its lower potential for causing tachyarrhythmias and its ability to enhance renal blood flow when infused at a dose below 30 μg/kg/minute, dopamine has virtually replaced isoproterenol as the agent of choice.

In 1923 Cannon condemned the use of vasopressors on this physiologic basis: "Damming the blood in the arterial portion of the circulation, when the organism is suffering primarily from a diminished quantity of blood flow, obviously does not improve the volume flow in the capillaries." In 1940 Blalock also condemned the use of vasopressors in treating shock. Recent studies have more clearly defined the hazards of using vasopressors in hypovolemic shock. Clowes and his associates demonstrated a sharp increase in the mortality of dogs rendered hypotensive by hemorrhage when norepinephrine was administered in sufficient doses to raise the blood pressure from 40 mmHg to 100 mmHg. Mortality in animals so treated was 64 percent compared with 33 percent in the untreated controls. Catchpole et al., using a drip of norepinephrine after 30 minutes of hypotension and again before reinfusion of shed blood, obtained no improvement in survival. Additionally, Hakstian, Hampson, and Gurd demonstrated no significant protection during hemorrhagic hypotension through the use of norepinephrine. On the other hand, studies by Lansing and Stevenson suggest that the use of norepinephrine for the maintenance of blood pressure and cardiac output *after* normovolemia has been restored may be advantageous. Simeone has similarly shown that the use of vasopressors after restoration of normal blood volume may be of some significant help if applied early. Probably the beneficial effects of these experimental studies can be related more properly to their inotropic effect on the heart than to their vasoconstrictor properties. This is especially true since these studies show benefit only after volume has been restored.

There is other available evidence that the administration of vasopressors during hypovolemia will reduce the already depleted plasma volume. Our own data tend to support this concept.

The use of vasopressors in hemorrhagic shock is rapidly disappearing. Suffice it to say that, as more and more data have become available, it is doubtful whether the use of vasopressors in the treatment of hypovolemic shock is ever warranted.

VASODILATORS. In 1948 Wiggers and his associates predicted that a significantly increased survival rate in animals treated with an adrenergic blocking agent and subjected to hemorrhagic shock would indicate the detrimental influence of protracted vasoconstriction in shock. Subsequently, in 1950, Remington and his associates reported an increased survival rate in dogs pretreated with Dibenamine before the induction of hemorrhagic shock. Zweifach, Baes, and Shorr similarly found that Diben-

amine protected rats against lethal-graded hemorrhage if the animals were pretreated, and Boba and Converse reported that ganglionic blocking agents increased the survival of experimentally shocked animals.

Webb et al. found that the administration of hydralazine during the hypovolemic hypotensive phase of experimental hemorrhagic shock was deleterious. In contrast, Hakstian, Hampson, and Gurd obtained 15 survivals out of 16 animals subjected to hemorrhagic shock and treated with hydralazine during the shock period. Collins, Jaffee, and Zahony reported survival in a study of 396 patients treated with chlorpromazine; 186 of these patients were treated after the onset of shock, and the survival rate was said to be twice that of the control group. Longerbeam, Lillehei, and Scott found that giving Dibenzyline (phenoxybenzamine) led to a remarkable improvement in the mortality rate of their animals. Thal recently reported encouraging results with Dibenzyline in the treatment of refractory normovolemic endotoxic shock (Fig. 4-34).

HEMODYNAMIC MEASUREMENTS. A patient in hemorrhagic or oligemic shock may rarely fail to respond to vigorous management as outlined above. Such a patient usually presents a complicated clinical picture. Frequently surgical procedures have been carried out for correction of the underlying causes of shock. Thus the problem is often compounded by massive fluid and blood administration, general anesthesia, and surgical trauma. At this point a comprehensive but rapid reevaluation of the patient must be carried out in order to institute effective therapy.

The basic defect underlying this "refractory shock" must be corrected. Possible causes are multiple: (1) continuing blood loss from the primary injury or disease or from another source, (2) inadequate replacement of fluids, (3) massive trauma and other derangements secondary to the trauma, especially cardiac tamponade and pneumothorax, (4) myocardial insufficiency either as a direct result

Fig. 4-34. Adrenergic mechanisms. (*From C. M. Lewis and M. H. Weil, JAMA, 208:1391, 1969. Copyright, 1969, American Medical Association.*)

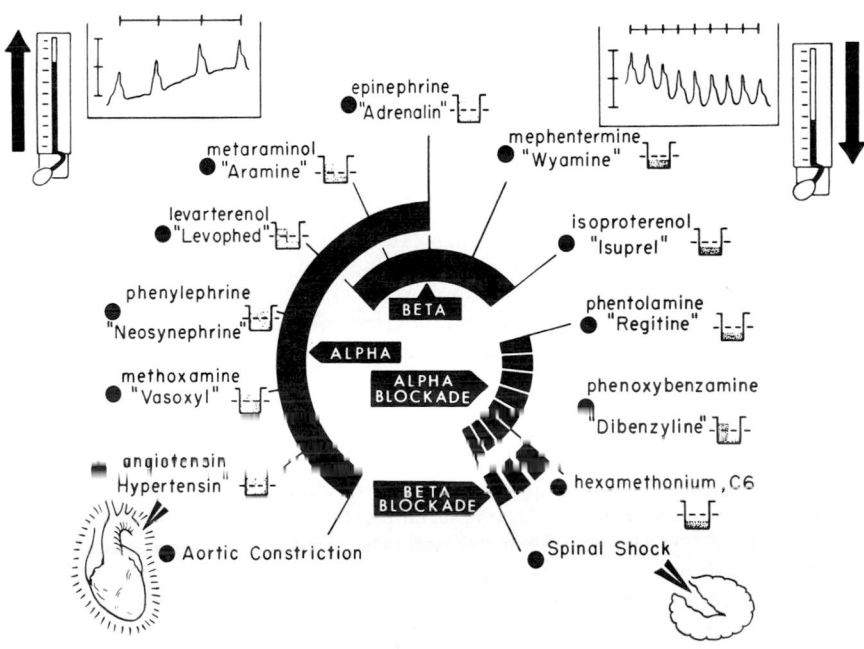

of inadequate perfusion for a prolonged period or secondary to anesthetic agents, and (5) even concomitant septic shock, as with intraperitoneal contamination from bowel perforation. The answers to this problem can best be obtained by careful clinical evaluation of the patient and evaluation of a few relatively simple hemodynamic parameters that may serve as a guide to satisfactory treatment (Chap. 13).

Cardiogenic Shock

In this form of shock the heart fails as a pump. Consequently primary therapy is directed toward the heart. Cardiac arrythmias, whatever their origin, should be treated promptly. Cardiac tamponade, if this is the cause, should be relieved by pericardiocentesis. When the origin of the pump failure is myocardial infarction or myocarditis, the primary therapy again is directed toward the myocardial damage. If the myocardial damage is sufficiently severe to produce reduction in blood pressure, and indeed in organ perfusion, to the point that organ functions begin to fail, drugs with positive inotropic action may be efficacious.

HEMODYNAMIC MEASUREMENTS

Hemodynamic measurements play an important role in the management of postoperative patients with this type of hypotension. As previously described, the classic findings are a central venous pressure that is elevated or rises briskly with fluid administration. This is accompanied by a cardiac output that is depressed and fails to respond to fluid administration. In evaluating postoperative hypotension, as after an extensive procedure in the elderly or especially after cardiac surgery, the measurement of hemodynamic parameters may be of great benefit in differentiating hypovolemic hypotension from hypotension due to depressed myocardial function.

When hemodynamic measurements suggestive of deficient pumping action are found, myocardial insufficiency is usually at fault. It should be stressed again, however, that this can be due to mechanical obstruction (e.g., cardiac tamponade or mediastinal compression in the injured patient or pulmonary embolism in the postoperative patient), and treatment directed at primary myocardial insufficiency can lead to unnecessary delay and catastrophic results. Although identification of abnormalities causing mechanical obstruction to venous return or myocardial function must rest largely on clinical grounds, hemodynamic measurements may be of some benefit in that one may find a slow increase in cardiac output and arterial blood pressure accompanying the rising venous pressure produced by rapid fluid administration. This is in contrast to the picture usually seen in pure myocardial insufficiency, in which the cardiac output frequently falls in the face of a rising venous pressure. The rise in cardiac output probably occurs because the rising venous pressure is partially effective in overcoming the obstruction and maintaining a nearer to normal cardiac filling.

It has been demonstrated that with myocardial injury and after cardiac surgery, differences in functional reserve of the two ventricles occur and the central venous pressure

alone loses a great deal of its reliability. Thus in these patients the use of pulmonary artery pressure, pulmonary wedge pressure, and, when feasible, left atrial pressure have their greatest value. Left atrial pressure (or left ventricular end-diastolic pressure) is not necessarily the same as right atrial pressure (or central venous pressure, or right ventricular end-diastolic pressure) under these circumstances.

In patients with low cardiac output from low blood volume who also have certain forms of heart disease, left atrial pressure may be considerably higher than right atrial pressure. Examples of such conditions are mitral stenosis and insufficiency, aortic stenosis and insufficiency, severe hypertension, and coronary artery disease. In such patients, unless one is actually measuring left atrial pressure, rapid infusion should probably be stopped when right atrial or central venous pressure reaches 12 mmHg (150 mm saline solution). The relation between changes in atrial pressure and changes in stroke volume or cardiac output at relatively high atrial pressures is not known. In most patients, however, when atrial pressures are about 15 mmHg (230 mm saline solution), further increases do not seem to increase cardiac output. Thus when central venous or right atrial pressure is less than 6 mmHg (80 mm saline solution), augmentation of blood volume is indicated. As the infusion proceeds, if central venous pressure rises rapidly and there is little evidence of increase in cardiac output, the infusion should probably be discontinued as being ineffective.

ABNORMALITIES IN CONTRACTILITY

In the condition in which there is low cardiac output and high atrial pressures and in which tamponade and ventricular outflow obstruction have been ruled out, there is probably an acute reduction of myocardial contractility. Treatment must therefore be directed toward improving contractility.

The drugs to be considered are

1. *Digitalis.* If time permits, digitalis is given, and digoxin is recommended. The estimated digitalizing dose given intravenously to a child or adult is 0.9 mg/m² of body surface area (1.5 mg for average adult). Half or two-thirds of this may be given initially intravenously. An effect can be seen in 10 to 20 minutes, and the peak effect is reached in about 2 hours. After 1 to 3 hours, if no contraindication develops and further effect is desired, an additional one-sixth of the estimated digitalizing dose is given. This may be repeated after another 2 to 3 hours. In less acute situations the same drug may be given orally; the digitalizing dose is then 1 mg/m². The estimated daily maintenance dose is one-quarter of the estimated digitalizing dose, usually given in divided doses.

2. *Catecholamines.* Isoproterenol has a specific chronotropic effect on cardiac muscle and theoretically is the drug of choice when one needs a prompt and potent agent. It also has a peripheral vasodilating effect which may produce increased hypotension in a patient in shock. Because of a tendency to produce tachycardia and ventricular irritability, isoproterenol is particularly useful when the pulse rate is slow. It is administered by slow intravenous infu-

sion drop by drop of a solution of 0.5 mg of isoproterenol in 250 ml of 5% glucose in water (2 μg/ml). The rate of infusion is regulated to obtain the desired hemodynamic effect.

Norepinephrine or epinephrine may be used when undue hypertension results from isoproterenol. They increase systemic venous tone and therefore can increase both right and left atrial pressures strikingly; thus caution is indicated, since pulmonary edema can result. These drugs are given intravenously by drop-by-drop infusion of a solution containing 4 mg in 250 ml of 5% glucose in water. Prior to treating patients with low cardiac output and high atrial pressures with these drugs on the basis that the cause is poor myocardial contractility, one must rule out pericardial tamponade. If high intrapericardial pressure exists in patients with high atrial and ventricular end-diastolic pressure, transmural pressure is low, and the poor output is due to end-diastolic ventricular volume and fiber length. The treatment is relief of the pericardial tamponade, which is about the only acute cause of high atrial pressures and small end-diastolic ventricular volume. A clinical analysis and chest x-ray are helpful in establishing the diagnosis. The presence of a paradoxic pulse should suggest strongly the presence of tamponade, and needle aspiration or open pericardiotomy is indicated.

3. *Ganglionic Blocking Agents.* Some patients with low cardiac output and high atrial pressures have relatively high arterial blood pressure. Systemic arteriolar resistance is high (*afterload-load* resisting shortening of myocardial sarcomeres). In these circumstances systolic left ventricular pressure is relatively high, as is systolic ventricular wall stress. Theoretically, reducing arterial blood pressure and systolic ventricular wall stress increases cardiac output. This can be done with an agent such as Arfonad. One should measure cardiac output before and during administration of this drug, and only if a significant increase in cardiac output has accompanied the decrease in arterial blood pressure should the drug be continued. Because of present uncertainties with the use of this drug (such as the effect on coronary, cerebral, liver, and renal blood flow) in this situation, it should be given only under special circumstances.

ABNORMALITIES IN RATE

Rapid ventricular rates (over 150 to 180 beats/minute) are usually deleterious to cardiac output. Ventricular end-diastolic pressure is small because of the short period of ventricular filling with tachycardia, and ventricular extensibility is probably decreased because ventricular relaxation is not complete by the end of the extremely short diastolic period. Both tend to reduce stroke volume more than can be compensated for by the rapid heart rate, and cardiac output falls. If atrial fibrillation is the cardiac mechanism, digoxin is the drug of choice. Atrial flutter is more difficult to treat but should likewise be treated with digoxin. If no progress has been achieved with the drug after two-thirds of the digitalizing dose has been given, electroversion should be considered. Atrial tachycardia and premature atrial contractions as causes of excessively rapid heart rates are still more difficult to treat. A continuous

intravenous infusion of a drug with pure peripheral vasoconstrictor properties may be helpful (Aramine, 500 mg in 500 ml of 5% glucose in water).

Premature ventricular contractions may on occasion cause fast ventricular rates. Their tendency to cause ventricular fibrillation is of even greater concern. Potassium chloride may be infused over a 10- to 20-minute period. If this is not effective or if the premature ventricular contractions are frequent, lidocaine (Xylocaine) should be given intravenously in a single injection of 50 mg. If further lidocaine is needed, a solution containing 2 mg/ml of lidocaine can be given continuously. If it is used excessively, central nervous system irritability and depression of myocardial contractility may result. If protection against premature ventricular contractions is needed later, Pronestyl (procainamide hydrochloride) can be given orally in doses of 250 to 500 mg every 3 hours.

Low output associated with ventricular rates of less than 60 to 70 beats/minute may occur in patients in whom cardiac performance is impaired. Because the myocardium is impaired, stroke volume cannot increase sufficiently to compensate for the slow rate. Regardless of whether the mechanism is sinus rhythm, atrial fibrillation with slow ventricular rate (too much digitalis or too little potassium), or complete atrioventricular dissociation, electrical pacing of the heart at a rate of 80 to 110 beats/minute is advantageous. If there is a sinus mechanism, atrial pacing is preferred. Otherwise, direct ventricular pacing is indicated.

MECHANICAL ASSISTANCE

Effective support for cardiogenic shock may eventually depend on mechanical assistance. Assistive devices are currently available in several centers. At present their use is restricted to patients who do not respond to more conventional therapy.

Neurogenic Shock

Neurogenic shock, or, by the older classification, "primary shock" is that form of shock which follows serious interference with the balance of vasodilator and vasoconstrictor influences to both arterioles and venules. This is the shock that is seen with clinical syncope, as with sudden exposure to unpleasant events such as the sight of blood, the hearing of bad tidings, or even the sudden onset of pain. Similarly, neurogenic shock is often observed with serious paralysis of vasomotor influences, as in high spinal anesthesia. The reflex interruption of nerve impulses also occurs with acute gastric dilatation.

The clinical picture of neurogenic shock is quite different from that classically seen in oligemic or hypovolemic shock. While the blood pressure may be extremely low, the pulse rate is usually slower than normal and is accompanied by dry, warm, and even flushed skin. Measurements made during neurogenic shock indicate a reduction in cardiac output, but this is accompanied by a decrease in resistance of arteriolar vessels as well as a decrease in the venous tone. Consequently there appears to be a normovolemic state with a greatly increased reservoir capacity in both arterioles and venules, thereby inducing a decreased venous return to the right side of the heart and subsequently a reduction in cardiac output.

If neurogenic shock is not corrected, a reduction of blood flow to the kidneys and damage to the brain result, and subsequently all the ravages of hypovolemic shock appear. Fortunately, treatment of neurogenic shock is usually obvious. Gastric dilatation can be rapidly treated with nasogastric suction. Shock in high spinal anesthesia can be treated effectively with a vasopressor such as ephedrine or phenylephrine (Neo-Synephrine), which will increase cardiac output as well as produce peripheral vasoconstriction. With the milder forms of neurogenic shock, such as fainting, simply removing the patient from the stimulus or relieving the pain will in itself be adequate therapy so that the vasoconstrictor nerves may regain the ability to maintain normal arteriolar and venous resistance.

There is rarely need for hemodynamic measurement in this usually benign and frequently self-limited form of hypotension. Correction of the underlying deficit usually results in prompt resumption of normal cardiovascular dynamics. The exception to this occurs when this form of shock results from injury, as with spinal cord transection from trauma. In this instance there may be significant loss of blood and extracellular fluid into the area of injury surrounding the cord and vertebral column. Considerable confusion can arise as to the relative need for fluid replacement, as opposed to the need for vasopressor drugs, under these circumstances. Similarly, if surgical intervention for any reason becomes necessary, hemodynamic measurements may be of great value in the management of these patients. In uncomplicated neurogenic shock, central venous pressure should be normal or slightly low, with a normal or elevated cardiac output. On the other hand, as hypovolemia ensues, central venous pressure decreases, as does cardiac output. Thus careful monitoring of central venous pressure may be of great aid. Fluid administration without vasopressors in this form of hypotension may produce a gradually rising arterial pressure and cardiac output without elevation of central venous pressure, by gradually "filling" the expanded vascular pool; therefore caution must be utilized during fluid administration.

In management of these patients balancing the two forms of therapy, slight volume overexpansion is much less deleterious than excessive vasopressor administration. The latter decreases organ perfusion in the presence of inadequate fluid replacement. Balance can best be obtained by maintaining a normal central venous pressure that rises slightly with rapid fluid administration (thus ensuring adequate volume) and using a vasopressor such as phenylephrine judiciously to support arterial pressure.

Septic Shock

During the past several years there has been a progressive increase in the incidence of shock secondary to sepsis, and the mortality rate remains in excess of 50 percent. This has occurred despite a better understanding of this entity, use of newer treatment regimens, and development of more potent antimicrobial agents. The most frequent causative organisms are gram-positive and gram-negative bacteria, although any agent capable of producing infection (including viruses, parasites, fungi, and rickettsiae) may initiate septic shock. Because of effective antibiotic control of most gram-positive infections, the majority of septic processes that result in shock are now caused by gram-negative bacteria. Among other causes, Altemeier and associates attribute this rising incidence of gram-negative sepsis to (1) the widespread use of antibiotics, with development of a reservoir of virulent and resistant organisms; (2) concentration in hospitals of large numbers of patients with established infections; (3) more extensive operations on elderly and poor-risk patients; (4) an increasing number of patients suffering from severe trauma; and (5) the use of steroids and immunosuppressive and anticancer agents.

GRAM-POSITIVE SEPSIS AND SHOCK

The shock state may be caused by gram-positive infections that produce massive fluid losses (necrotizing fasciitis) by dissemination of a potent exotoxin without evident bacteremia (*Clostridium perfringens, Clostridium tetani*) or, most often, by a fulminating infection from staphylococcus, streptococcus, or pneumococcus organisms. In the latter instance, shock is theoretically related to the release of exotoxins which many strains of staphylococcus and streptococcus (but not pneumococcus) are known to produce. The hemodynamic changes that occur are different from those seen in shock due to gram-negative organisms. Kwaan and Weil have noted hypotension of comparable severity in shock from both gram-positive and gram-negative infections, but their patients with gram-positive infections failed to show the other clinical manifestations of shock. Arterial resistance fell, but there was little or no reduction in cardiac output even with progressive hypotension. Urine flow was normal, sensorium clear, and perfusion of other organs was not grossly impaired, since neither acidosis nor a significant increase in serum lactic acid concentration appeared.

Treatment consists in the use of appropriate antibiotics, surgical drainage when indicated, and correction of any fluid volume deficit. A rapid and favorable response may be anticipated in many patients, and survival is substantially better than with gram-negative infections.

GRAM-NEGATIVE SEPSIS AND SHOCK

Gram-negative sepsis as a cause of shock is a more frequent and difficult problem. The highest incidence occurs during the seventh and eighth decades of life, and the response to treatment depends to a large extent on the age and previous health of the patient. There have been significant advances in the understanding of this entity, although much of the available information is still subject to controversy.

SOURCE. The most frequent source of gram-negative infections is the genitourinary system; almost half the patients have had an associated operation or instrumentation of the urinary tract. The second most frequent site of origin is the respiratory system, and many of the patients have an associated tracheostomy. Next in frequency is the alimentary system, with diseases such as peritonitis, intra-abdominal abscess, and biliary tract infections; and then diseases of the integumentary, including burns and soft tissue infections. Indwelling venous catheters for monitoring and hyperalimentation are an increasing source of contamination, particularly with prolonged use. The reproductive system continues to be a significant source of infection (principally from septic abortions and postpartum infections), although the incidence is variable, depending on the hospital population.

The severity of septic shock varies considerably and appears to be a time-dose phenomenon, depending on the type and site of infection. For instance, mild hypotension following instrumentation of the genitourinary tract may represent nothing more than a transient bacteremia which is self-limited or responds to minimal therapy. In contrast, the patient with necrotizing pneumonia or multiple intra-abdominal abscesses may have sepsis from an overwhelming number of organisms for a period of several days, and a much poorer prognosis. Similarly, the outlook is more favorable when the source of infection is accessible to surgical drainage, as in septic abortion, in which the infected products of conception can be removed readily. Variations in these factors must be considered when interpreting reported mortality rates and during the evaluation of new therapeutic regimens.

ASSOCIATED CONDITIONS. The presence of underlying disorders which limit cardiac, pulmonary, hepatic, or renal function increases the susceptibility to gram-negative infections and adversely affects the response to treatment. In Altemeier's reported series of 398 patients with gram-negative sepsis, almost half the patients had serious associated disease, including diabetes mellitus, malignant neoplasms, uremia, cirrhosis, burns, and malignant hematologic disorders. Of these conditions, cirrhosis of the liver appeared to have the most unfavorable prognosis. In addition, a small but significant number of patients were on corticosteroids or immunosuppressive agents, and corresponding mortality rates were 74 and 83 percent respectively.

BACTERIOLOGY. The common causative organisms are similar to those found in the human gastrointestinal tract and include (1) *E. coli;* (2) *Klebsiella aerobacter;* (3) *Proteus;* (4) *Pseudomonas;* and (5) *Bacteroides,* in order of decreasing frequency. Recently the *Klebsiella*-Enterobacteriaceae-*Serratia* groups have been isolated with increasing frequency, and many are resistant to more conventional antibiotics. It now appears that *Bacteroides* species may be the predominant organisms in the fecal flora. These anaerobic organisms are difficult to culture and may account for a far greater number of infections than was previously reported. The majority of infections are caused by a single gram-negative organism, although in 10 to 20 percent of cases more than one organism may be isolated. The isolates may be two or more gram-negative organisms or mixed cultures containing both gram-negative and gram-positive bacteria.

CLINICAL MANIFESTATIONS. Gram-negative infections are often recognized initially by the development of chills and elevated temperature above 101°F. The onset of shock may be abrupt and coincident with the signs and symptoms of sepsis or may occur several hours to days after recognition of an established infection. The complex hemodynamic abnormalities that follow are incompletely understood but are probably initiated by endotoxins from the cell walls of gram-negative bacteria. Intravenous injection of this lipopolysaccharide-protein complex into experimental animals will produce a shock state, but the hemodynamic responses vary in different animal species. The use of experimental animal models has contributed to our understanding of this entity, but direct extrapolation of the findings to human septic shock is difficult. A single injection of endotoxin into dogs causes pooling of blood in the splanchnic circulation, decreased venous return to the heart, reduction in cardiac output, and an abrupt fall in blood pressure. This initial response is transient and apparently due to hepatic venous outflow obstruction. Shortly thereafter the blood pressure rises toward normal but then slowly declines over the next several hours until death of the animal. This pattern is different from that seen in the subhuman primate and in human beings. Injection of *E. coli* endotoxin into human volunteers has been shown to produce (1) no response; (2) chills, fever, and vasoconstriction; or (3) peripheral vasodilation and a rise in cardiac output. These observations emphasize our lack of understanding of the effects of gram-negative infections and septicemia on the human circulation and the need for the development of more realistic experimental animal models.

Clinically, the shock state may be characterized by a primary adrenergic response, as seen in hypovolemic shock, with hypotension, peripheral vasoconstriction, and cold, clammy extremities. Earlier in the course, however, there may be an absence of adrenergic effects, with warm, dry extremities and decreased peripheral resistance. These diverse responses, presumably to the same stimulus, have led to a considerable amount of confusion over the clinical manifestations of septic shock, although a report by MacLean and associates tends to shed some light on this subject. They have noted two distinct hemodynamic patterns, depending on the volume status of the patient, and believe that the natural history of septic shock is one of progression from respiratory alkalosis to metabolic acidosis. A syndrome of early septic shock occurs in patients who are *normovolemic* prior to onset of sepsis and exhibit a hyperdynamic circulatory pattern characterized by (1) hypotension, (2) high cardiac output, (3) normal or increased blood volume, (4) normal or high central venous pressure, (5) low peripheral resistance, (6) warm, dry extremities, (7) hyperventilation, and (8) respiratory alkalosis. A typical patient with this pattern is the young, previously healthy person with a septic abortion. The high cardiac output is often associated with a decrease in oxygen utilization per unit flow, i.e., a narrowed arteriovenous oxygen difference. These findings can be explained by any of several mechanisms, but the two most likely possibilities are arteriovenous shunting and a primary cellular defect in the utilization of oxygen due to a direct effect of sepsis. Data by Wright et al. suggest a primary cellular defect as the most likely cause. In either case the presence of oliguria, altered sensorium, and blood lactate accumulation reflects the need for a further increase in flow despite the high cardiac output. MacLean suggests that treatment include measures to increase the cardiac output even more, combined with appropriate antibiotic therapy and early surgical drainage. In his series all but 4 of 28 patients with this hemodynamic pattern survived the episode of shock. If control of the infection is delayed or unsuccessful, the patient may pass into an acidotic phase with evidence of cellular damage (narrowing arteriovenous oxygen difference, decreasing oxygen consumption) and become refractory to further therapy.

In contrast, if septic shock develops in a patient who is *hypovolemic,* a hypodynamic pattern emerges characterized by (1) hypotension, (2) low cardiac output, (3) high peripheral resistance, (4) low central venous pressure, and (5) cold, cyanotic extremities. This response is typically seen in a patient with strangulation obstruction of the small bowel and a moderate to severe extracellular fluid and plasma volume deficit. If seen early, these patients are also alkalotic and will respond favorably to treatment. In the absence of overt cardiac failure, prompt volume replacement will often increase cardiac output, and a more favorable hyperdynamic circulation may develop. If therapy to combat sepsis is delayed or unsuccessful, the patient will inevitably have cardiac and circulatory failure, with a low fixed cardiac output and a resistant metabolic acidosis. At this point the patient may not be salvageable.

Our own experience in the treatment of septic shock tends to confirm MacLean's findings, although the presence of a metabolic acidosis has not necessarily been an ominous finding. We have seen several patients with hypodynamic and hyperdynamic circulatory patterns and metabolic acidosis in the early phase who have responded satisfactorily to therapy. The clinical picture may also be influenced by the patient's ability to meet the increased circulatory requirements imposed by sepsis. The elderly patient with limited cardiac reserve may be unable to increase cardiac output and enter the hyperdynamic phase, even with prompt volume replacement and measures designed to increase cardiac efficiency. In this instance the typical adrenergic response may persist, and the patient may rapidly succumb to the disease process.

The laboratory tests of value for diagnosis will depend to a large extent on the specific disease causing sepsis. Generally, the white blood cell count is appropriately elevated, but in debilitated and hypovolemic patients, those on immunosuppressive agents, and those with overwhelming sepsis, the white blood cell count may be normal or low. However, there is usually a noticeable left shift in the white blood cell differential, with many immature cell types. Recent work by Rowe et al. indicates that a falling platelet count may be an early and sensitive indicator of gram-negative septicemia in pediatric patients. It has been suggested that endotoxin reacts with platelets, producing platelet aggregates which are subsequently trapped in the microcirculation. They suggest that patients at risk for sepsis have serial platelet counts; a fall in the platelet count below 150,000 suggests the presence of gram-negative septicemia, and measures to find and eradicate the source should be undertaken. Rarely, a sudden fall in the platelet count may be a manifestation of disseminated intravascular coagulation (DIC), a syndrome known to be initiated by several stimuli, including endotoxin.

Progressive pulmonary insufficiency is characteristically seen in many patients with septic shock. Mild hypoxia with compensatory hyperventilation and respiratory alkalosis are commonly seen early in the course of shock in the absence of clinical or x-ray evidence of pulmonary disease. The arterial desaturation has been attributed to a variety of causes, including the presence of physiologic arteriovenous shunts in the pulmonary circulation secondary to perfusion of atelectatic or nonaerated alveoli. Regardless of the cause, the picture is frequently that of rapid deterioration of pulmonary function, development of patchy infiltrates which become confluent, superimposed bacterial infection, severe hypoxemia, and death.

Finally, it is worth emphasizing that development of mild hyperventilation, respiratory alkalosis, and an altered sensorium may be the earliest signs of gram-negative infection. This triad may precede the usual signs and symptoms of sepsis by several hours to several days. The exact cause is not known, although the condition is thought to represent a primary response to bacteremia. Early recognition of these findings, followed by a prompt search for the source of infection, may allow proper diagnosis prior to the onset of shock.

TREATMENT. The only effective way to reduce mortality in septic shock is by prompt recognition and treatment of the associated infection prior to the onset of shock. Once shock occurs, the control of infection by early surgical debridement or drainage and use of appropriate antibiotics represents *definitive* therapy. Other recommended measures, including fluid replacement, steroid administration, and the use of vasoactive drugs, represent *adjunctive* forms of therapy and are useful to prepare the patient prior to surgical intervention or to support the patient until the infectious process is controlled. This point deserves special emphasis, since death of the patient is inevitable if the infection cannot be adequately controlled.

As soon as gram-negative sepsis and shock are apparent, a prompt and thorough search for the source of infection is made while instituting other supportive measures. Because of the multiple complicating factors that may accompany endotoxemia, the patient is preferably treated in an intensive care unit. Careful monitoring of direct arterial pressure, central venous pressure (preferably pulmonary artery and pulmonary wedge pressures measured via a Swan-Ganz catheter), urine output, and arterial and central venous blood gases may be essential for proper management.

If the infectious process is amenable to drainage, operation is performed as soon as possible after initial stabilization of the patient's condition. In some cases surgical debridement or drainage of the infection must be accomplished before the patient will respond; this may be performed under local or general anesthesia. For example, a patient with ascending cholangitis and shock secondary to sepsis may respond temporarily to supportive treatment. Improvement may be short-lived, however, unless prompt drainage of the biliary tract is instituted. The importance of surgical drainage is emphasized by the experience of

MacLean et al. in their treatment of 53 patients. Forty-eight percent of their patients with infections amenable to surgical drainage survived, while only 23 percent of those not amenable to surgical treatment survived.

Antibiotic Therapy. The use of specific antibiotics based on appropriate cultures and sensitivity tests is desirable when possible. The results may not be available for several days, but useful information may be gained from previous wound and blood cultures obtained during an earlier phase of the septic process and Gram stains of appropriate material. Antibiotics must often be chosen, however, on the basis of the suspected organisms and their previous sensitivity patterns. These patterns are sufficiently diverse to preclude selection of a single antibiotic agent which will be effective against all the potential pathogens.

At present an effective combination of antibiotics in our hospital population when gastrointestinal tract organisms are suspected includes cephalothin (6 to 8 Gm/day intravenously in four to six divided doses) or penicillin (10 to 20 million units daily) and gentamicin (5 mg/kg/day). These are average adult doses and should be reduced after initial control of the infection and modified in any patient with impaired renal function. This combination is effective against a majority of gram-negative organisms, with the notable exception of *Bacteroides* species. If presence of these organisms is suspected, an antibiotic of known effectiveness (e.g., clindamycin or Chloromycetin) should be added to the regimen.

When culture and sensitivity reports are available, more specific antibiotic coverage may be initiated if the infection is not under control. Altemeier and associates reported a mortality rate of 54 percent from sepsis in patients receiving inappropriate antibiotics and 28 percent when appropriate antibiotics were given.

Fluid Replacement. Prompt correction of preexisting fluid deficits is essential. A majority of patients will incur fluid losses from the disease processes that initiate sepsis and shock. "Third space losses," with massive sequestration of plasma and extracellular fluid, are characteristic of many surgical conditions, including peritonitis, burns, strangulation obstruction of the bowel, and extensive soft tissue infections.

The type of fluid used will vary, although most "third space losses" are properly replaced with a balanced salt solution such as Ringer's lactate. Any deficits in red blood cell mass should be corrected by the administration of packed cells or whole blood in order to maintain optimal oxygen-carrying capacity of the blood. Large quantities of replacement fluids are often needed in order to maintain an effective circulating volume. However, a fine balance exists between the need for volume replacement and the harmful effects that fluid overload may have on lungs already injured by the septic process. In this regard, attempts to increase pulmonary capillary osmotic pressure by the infusion of large volumes of plasma or albumin, in the absence of a specific need, may be detrimental. Because of the increase in pulmonary capillary permeability associated with severe sepsis, the use of large quantities of colloid solutions may result in an increase in extravascular

pulmonary water. Careful replacement of "third space losses" with crystalloid solutions on the basis of patient response and continuous monitoring of the central venous or pulmonary artery and pulmonary wedge pressures are indicated.

Properly interpreted, the central venous pressure (CVP) will give a reliable estimate of the ability of the right side of the heart to pump the blood delivered to it. It is best used as an upper-limit guide; a rapid increase in central venous pressure, regardless of the initial level, may indicate that fluid is being administered too rapidly or that the heart is unable to handle additional volume. If central venous pressure is below 10 cm of water, fluids may be administered as rapidly as tolerated. If central venous pressure is above this level, fluids are still administered but at a slower rate of infusion. The central venous pressure may fall as blood pressure rises, owing to better perfusion of the coronary arteries and improved myocardial function. An abrupt rise in the central venous pressure or a fall in arterial pressure may indicate inability of the heart to respond, and the use of drugs that increase myocardial performance should be considered.

In many instances, measurement of the CVP alone during fluid resuscitation is not sufficient, since it gives no direct information regarding function of the left side of the heart. Insertion of a Swan-Ganz catheter (via a cutdown in an antecubital vein or by direct percutaneous insertion into the subclavian vein) for measurements of *both* pulmonary artery (PA) and pulmonary capillary wedge (PW) pressure, the latter a reflection of left ventricular end-diastolic pressure, is necessary. This is particularly true in patients on mechanical ventilation and positive end-expiratory pressure. Recently, Krausz et al. assessed the value of PWP monitoring during fluid resuscitation in patients in septic shock. In one group of patients the PW pressure prior to the administration of fluid was lower than the CVP, suggesting acute right ventricular failure due to increased pulmonary vascular resistance coexistent with relative hypovolemia. The intravenous administration of fluid in this group was accompanied by a significant rise in blood pressure and cardiac output without significant change in the pulse rate or the PA pressure. In a second group, the initial PW pressure was higher than the CVP, and signs of fluid overloading appeared after the administration of only a moderate amount of fluid without change in either blood pressure or cardiac output. Although not stated by the authors, the use of inotropic agents to improve myocardial performance may be indicated in the latter group of patients.

Many patients will respond favorably to fluid administration combined with prompt control of the infection with a rise in blood pressure, an increase in urine output, warming of the extremities, and clearing of the sensorium. In those instances no additional therapy may be indicated.

Steroids. The use of pharmacologic doses of corticosteroids in the treatment of septic shock is controversial but has become a common practice. There is no direct evidence that steroids are beneficial in these cases, although favorable responses, with improvement in cardiac, pulmonary, and renal functions and better survival rates, have been reported. Large doses of steroids are known to exert a modest inotropic effect on the heart and produce mild peripheral vasodilation. Although these salutary effects may be desirable, there are other, more potent drugs available with similar actions. Others have suggested that steroids protect the cell and its contents from the effects of endotoxin, for example, by stabilizing cellular and lysosomal membranes. In a recent prospective study of 172 consecutive patients in septic shock, Schumer noted a mortality rate of 10.4 percent in the steroid-treated patients, compared to a mortality rate of 38.4 percent in patients not receiving steroids. In a retrospective study of an additional 328 patients, the results were similar. Although impressive, evidence regarding the beneficial effects of steroids remains presumptive, because of many variables present in the clinical situation, including causes, associated conditions, and treatment.

Short-term, high-dose steroid therapy is associated with a minimal number of complications and is recommended in most cases that do not respond promptly to other measures. Steroids may be administered concomitant with volume replacement or reserved for use if the response to fluid administration is only temporary or produces a rapid rise in central venous pressure. Many dosage schedules have been recommended, and most stress the need for a large initial dose and cessation of therapy within 48 to 72 hours. Our current regimen is based on guidelines suggested by Lillehei. An initial dose of 15 to 30 mg/kg of body weight of methylprednisolone (or equivalent dose of dexamethasone) is given intravenously over a 5- to 10-minute period. The same dose may be repeated within 2 to 4 hours if the desired effects have not been achieved. If a beneficial response is obtained, additional injections are not given unless the effects are only short-lived. Used in this manner, there is rarely a need for more than two doses.

Vasoactive Drugs. Vasopressor drugs with prominent alpha-adrenergic effects are of limited value in treatment of this type of shock, since artificial attempts to maintain blood pressure without regard to flow are potentially harmful. Further, they are probably contraindicated in hypovolemic patients with increased peripheral resistance, in view of the known deleterious effects of prolonged vasoconstriction. Beneficial effects attributed to these agents are probably due to their inotropic effects on the heart, although better drugs are available for this purpose. Rarely, use of a vasoactive drug with mixed alpha- and beta-adrenergic effects (e.g., metaraminol) may be indicated in a patient with an elevated cardiac output and pronounced hypotension due to very low peripheral resistance. The increase in resistance (and slight increase in cardiac output) may produce a desired rise in blood pressure and improvement in flow.

Vasodilator drugs such as phenoxybenzamine have enjoyed some popularity, particularly when combined with additional fluid administration. Their use is based in part on improved survival of dogs when vasodilator drugs are given prior to the onset of endotoxic shock. These observations probably represent a specific canine response and cannot be directly extrapolated to human septic shock.

Vasodilator agents have also been used in conjunction with adrenergic agents (for their inotropic effects), but data on their usefulness are limited.

Since the heart is frequently unable to meet the increased circulatory demands of sepsis, the use of an inotropic agent such as isoproterenol or dopamine would seem ideal when volume replacement and other measures have failed to restore adequate circulation. Isoproterenol has potent inotropic and chronotropic effects on the heart and produces mild peripheral vasodilation. It is a relatively safe drug, but close observation of the patient is necessary, since severe tachycardia or cardiac arrhythmias may occur, particularly in digitalized patients. One or two milligrams of isoproterenol diluted in 500 ml of 5% dextrose in water may be administered by slow intravenous drip at a rate of 1 to 2 μg/minute, depending on the response. The infusion should be slowed or stopped completely if significant tachycardia or cardiac arrhythmias occur. In the absence of arrhythmias, a fall in blood pressure may result from the vasodilation induced by isoproterenol and indicates the need for additional volume replacement to maintain cardiac filling pressure. This combination may effectively restore blood flow even though systolic blood pressure remains less than 100 mmHg. The response is often temporary, but occasionally the infusion may be continued for 2 to 3 days without loss of effect or known deleterious effects. Dopamine, a naturally occurring catecholamine biochemical precursor of norepinephrine, is similar to isoproterenol in exerting positive inotropic and chronotropic effects on the heart by stimulation of beta-adrenergic receptors. Because of its lower potential for tachyarrhythmias and the ability to enhance renal blood flow when infused at a dose below 30 μg/kg/minute, dopamine has virtually replaced isoproterenol as the agent of choice.

In summary, a "polypharmacy" approach is discouraged, although proper selection and use of vasoactive drugs may offer needed support until infection can be controlled or eradicated. If eradication is not possible, response to any of these drugs is only temporary. Determination of cardiac output, combined with arterial, pulmonary artery, and pulmonary wedge pressure measurements can be of great benefit in establishing the nature of the hemodynamic alterations and evaluating responses to therapy.

Digitalis. Although Hinshaw et al. have shown that digitalis can prevent or reverse heart failure in septic animals, the clinical importance of this finding has yet to be established. We have not routinely administered digitalis to patients in septic shock in the absence of specific indications. Gram-negative sepsis and shock frequently occur in older patients with congestive failure or may precipitate cardiac failure in patients with limited cardiac reserve. In these instances digitalis can be administered cautiously in full doses, although toxicity may occur if the patient is hypokalemic or receiving isoproterenol.

Pulmonary Therapy. Many patients with sepsis and shock will develop significant pulmonary insufficiency and require maintenance of a controlled airway (via nasotracheal or endotracheal intubation) and assisted ventilation. (For a discussion of the adult respiratory distress syndrome as related to sepsis and the management of patients requiring ventilatory support, the reader is referred to the section Pulmonary Responses.)

Since inadequate tissue oxygenation is a consistent feature of shock, attention to all components of the oxygen transport system is essential (see the section Oxygen Transport). Efforts to maintain a normal or rightward-positioned oxygen/hemoglobin dissociation curve may be particularly important in view of reported reductions in red blood cell organic phosphates in late septic shock. The use of hyperbaric oxygen has also been suggested and would appear to be an ideal therapeutic approach. Limited experience with its use has been disappointing, however.

References

Clinical and Physiologic Manifestations of Shock

Baue, A. E., Wurth, M. A., and Sayeed, M. M.: The Dynamics of Altered ATP-dependent and ATP-yielding Cell Processes in Shock, *Surgery,* **72:**94, 1972.

Blalock, A.: Shock: Further Studies with Particular Reference to Effects of Hemorrhage, *Arch Surg,* **29:**837, 1937.

————: "Principles of Surgical Care, Shock and Other Problems," C. V. Mosby Company, St. Louis, 1940.

Canizaro, P. C., Prager, M. D., and Shires, G. T.: The Infusion of Ringer's Lactate Solution during Shock, *Am J Surg,* **122:**494, 1971.

Carey, L. C., Lowery, B. D., and Cloutier, C. T.: Treatment of Acidosis, *Curr Probl Surg,* January 1971, p. 37.

Cloutier, C. T., Lowery, B. D., and Carey, L. C.: The Effect of Hemodilutional Resuscitation on Serum Protein Levels in Humans in Hemorrhagic Shock, *J Trauma,* **9:**514, 1969.

Drucker, W. R., et al.: Metabolic Aspects of Hemorrhagic Shock: I. Changes in Intermediary Metabolism during Hemorrhage and Repletion of Blood, *Surg Forum,* **9:**49, 1959.

Gross, S. G.: "A System of Surgery: Pathological, Diagnostic, Therapeutic and Operative," Lea & Febiger, Philadelphia, 1872.

Hiebert, J. M., McCormick, J. M., and Egdahl, R. H.: Direct Measurement of Insulin Secretory Rate: Studies of Shocked Primates and Postoperative Patients, *Ann Surg,* **176:**296, 1972.

Lemieux, M. D., Smith, R. N., and Couch, N. P.: Surface pH and Redox Potential of Skeletal Muscle in Graded Hemorrhage, *Surgery,* **65:**457, 1969.

Mela, L. M., Miller, L. D., and Nicholas, G. G.: Influence of Cellular Acidosis and Altered Cation Concentrations on Shock-induced Mitochondrian Damage, *Surgery,* **72:**102, 1972.

Moore, F. D.: "Metabolic Care of the Surgical Patient," W. B. Saunders Company, Philadelphia, 1959.

Shenkin, H. S., et al.: On the Diagnosis of Hemorrhage in Man: A Study of Volunteers Bled Large Amounts, *Am J Med Sci,* **208:**421, 1944.

Shumer, W., Erve, P. R., and Obermolte, R. P.: Mechanisms of Steroid Protection in Septic Shock, *Surgery* 72:119, 1972

Simeone, F. A.: Shock, In "Christopher's Textbook of Surgery," p. 58, W. B. Saunders Company, Philadelphia, 1964.

Thal, A. P., and Wilson, R. F.: Shock, *Curr Probl Surg,* September 1965.

Watts, D. T.: Arterial Blood Epinephrine Levels during Hemorrhagic Hypotension in Dogs, *Am J Physiol,* **184:**271, 1956.

Wiggers, C. J.: Present Status of Shock Problem, *Physiol Rev,* **22:**74, 1942.

Response of Extracellular Fluid

Baue, A. E., Wurth, M. A., and Sayeed, M. M.: The Dynamics of Altered ATP-dependent and ATP-yielding Cell Processes in Shock, *Surgery,* **72:**94, 1972.

Campion, D. S., et al.: The Effect of Hemorrhagic Shock on Transmembrane Potential, *Surgery,* **66:**1051, 1969.

Conway, E. J.: Nature and Significance of Concentration Relations of Potassium and Sodium Ions in Skeletal Muscle, *Physiol Rev,* **37:**84, 1957.

Cunningham, J. N., Jr., Shires, G. T., and Wagner, Y.: Cellular Transport Defects in Hemorrhagic Shock, *Surgery,* **70:**215, 1971.

————, ————, and ————: Changes in Intracellular Sodium and Potassium Content of Red Blood Cells in Trauma and Shock, *Am J Surg,* November 1971, p. 650.

Fulton, R. L.: Absorption of Sodium and Water by Collagen during Hemorrhagic Shock, *Am Surg,* **172:**861, 1970.

Goldman, D. E.: Potential, Impedance and Rectification in Membranes, *J Physiol,* **27:**37, 1943.

Grossman, R.: Intracellular Potentials of Motor Cortex Neurons in Cerebral Ischemia, *Electroencephalogr Clin Neurophysiol,* **24:**291, 1968.

Hagberg, S., Haljamas, H., and Rockert, H.: Shock Reactions in Skeletal Muscle: III. The Electrolyte Content of Tissue Fluid and Blood Plasma before and after Induced Hemorrhagic Shock. *Ann Surg,* **168:**243, 1968.

Hodgkin, A. L., and Katz, B.: The Effect of Sodium Ions on the Electrical Activity of the Giant Axon of the Squid, *J Physiol,* **108:**37, 1949.

Ling, G., and Gerard, R. W.: The Normal Membrane Potential of Frog Sartorius Fibers, *J Cell Sci,* **34:**383, 1949.

Mela, L. M., Miller, L. D., and Nicholas, G. G.: Influence of Cellular Acidosis and Altered Cation Concentrations on Shock-induced Mitochondrian Damage, *Surgery,* **72:**102, 1972.

Middleton, E. S., Mathews, R., and Shires, G. T.: Radiosulphate as a Measure of the Extracellular Fluid in Acute Hemorrhagic Shock, *Ann Surg,* **170:**174, 1969.

Shires, G. T., et al.: Alterations in Cellular Membrane Function during Hemorrhagic Shock in Primates, *Ann Surg,* **176:**288, 1972.

————, Brown, F. T., Canizaro, P. C., and Somerville, N.: Distributional Changes in Extracellular Fluid during Acute Hemorrhagic Shock, *Surg Forum,* **11:**115, 1960.

————, and Carrico, C. J.: Current Status of the Shock Problem, *Curr Probl Surg,* March 1966.

————, ————, and Canizaro, P. C.: "Shock," Chap. 4, Pulmonary Responses, W. B. Saunders Company, Philadelphia, 1973.

————, Coln, D., Carrico, C. J., and Lightfoot, S.: Fluid Therapy in Hemorrhagic Shock, *Arch Surg,* 88:688, 1964

Slonim, M., and Stahl, W. M.: Sodium and Water Content of Connective versus Cellular Tissue Following Hemorrhage, *Surg Forum,* **19:**53, 1968.

Van Leeuwen, A. M.: Net Cation Equivalency (Base Building Power) of the Plasma Proteins, *Acta Med Scand [Suppl],* **422:**3-206, 1964.

Welt, L. G., Sachs, J. R., and McManus, T. J.: An Ion Transport Defect in Erythrocytes from Uremic Patients, *Trans Assoc Am Physicians,* **77:**169, 1964.

Wilde, W. S.: The Chloride Equilibrium in Muscle, *Am J Physiol,* **143:**666, 1945.

Renal Responses

Baker, C. F., Baxter, C. R., and Shires, G. T.: The Evaluation of Renal Function Following Severe Trauma, *J Trauma.* (In press.)

Baxter, C. R., Crenshaw, C. A., Lehman, I., and Shires, T.: A Practical Method of Renal Hypothermia, *J Trauma,* **3:**349, 1963.

———, and Maynard, D. R.: Prevention and Recognition of Surgical Renal Complications, *Clin Anesth,* **3:**322, 1968.

———, Zedlitz, W. H., and Shires, G. T.: High Output Acute Renal Failure Complicating Traumatic Injury, *J Trauma,* **4:**567, 1964.

Brun, C., and Munck, O.: "Acute Renal Failure in The Kidney," Ed: F. K. Mostofi and D. E. Smith, International Academy of Pathology Monograph, Williams & Wilkins, Baltimore.

Defalco, A. J., Mundth, E. D., Brettschneider, L., Jacobson, Y. G., and McClenathan, J. E.: A Possible Explanation for Transplantation Anuria, *Surg Gynecol Obstet,* **120:**748, 1965.

Doberneck, R. C., Schwartz, F. D., and Barry, K. G.: A Comparison of the Prophylactic Value of 20 Per Cent Mannitol, 4 Per Cent Urea, and 5 Per Cent Dextrose on the Effects of Renal Ischemia, *J Urol,* **89:**300, 1963.

Finckh, E. S.: The Failure of Experimental Renal Tubulonecrosis to Produce Oliguria in the Rat, *Australas Ann Med,* **9:**283, 1960.

Flear, C. T. G., and Clarke, R.: The Influence of Blood Loss and Blood Transfusion upon Changes in the Metabolism of Water, Electrolytes and Nitrogen following Civilian Trauma, *Clinical Science,* **14:**575, 1955.

Fudenberg, H., and Allen, F. H., Jr.: Transfusion Reactions in Absence of Demonstrable Incompatibility, *N Engl J Med,* **256:**1180, 1957.

Graber, I. G., and Sevitt, S.: Renal Function in Burned Patients and Its Relationship to Morphological Changes, *J Clin Pathol,* **12:**25, 1959.

Ladd, M.: "Battle Casualties in Korea," vol. 4, p. 193, U.S. Army Medical Service Graduate School, Walter Reed Army Medical Center, 1956.

Meroney, W. H., and Rubini, M. E.: Kidney Function during Acute Tubular Necrosis: Clinical Studies and Theory, *Metabolism,* **8:**1, 1959.

Moore, F. D.: "Metabolic Care of the Surgical Patient," W. B. Saunders Company, Philadelphia, 1959.

Munck, O.: Renal Blood Flow and Oxygen Consumption in Acute Renal Failure Measured by Use of Radioactive ^{85}Krypton, in Proc. 1st Int. Cong. Nephrol. Geneve/Evian 1960, p. 230, 1961.

Oliver, J., MacDowell, M., and Tracy, A.: The Pathogenesis of Acute Renal Failure Associated with Traumatic and Toxic Injury: Renal Ischemia: Nephrotoxic Damage and the Ischemuric Episode, *J Clin Invest,* **30:**1307, 1951.

Padula, R. T., Camishion, R. C., Magee, J. H., Noble, P. H., and Cowan, G. S. M.: Evaluation of the Protective Effect of Osmotic Diuretics, *Adv Surg Res,* **1:**177, 1969.

Phillips, R. A., and Hamilton, P. B.: Effect of 20, 60 and 120

Minutes of Renal Ischemia on Glomerular and Tubular Function, *Am J Physiol,* **152:**523, 1948.

Powers, S. R.: Maintenance of Renal Function Following Massive Trauma, *Trauma,* **10:**554, 1970.

———: Renal Response to Systemic Trauma, *Am J Surg,* **119:**603, 1970.

Sevitt, S.: Distal Tubular Necrosis with Little or No Oliguria, *J Clin Pathol,* **9:**12, 1956.

Tanner, G. A., and Selkurt, E. E.: Kidney Function in the Squirrel Monkey before and after Hemorrhagic Hypotension. *Am J Physiol,* **219:**597, 1970.

Taylor, W. H.: Management of Acute Renal Failure Following Surgical Operation and Head Injury, *Lancet,* **2:**703, 1957.

Teschan, P. E., et al.: Post-traumatic Renal Insufficiency in Military Casualties: I. Clinical Characteristics, *Am J Med,* **18:**172, 1955.

———, and Mason, A. D.: Reproducible Experimental Acute Renal Failure in Rats, *Clin Res,* **6:**155, 1958.

Wright, H. K., and Gann, D. S.: Correction of Defect in Free Water Excretion in Postoperative Patients by Extracellular Fluid Volume Expansion, *Ann Surg,* **158:**70, 1963.

Pulmonary Responses

Ashbaugh, D. G., Bigelow, D. B., Petty, T. L., and Levine, B. E.: Acute Respiratory Distress in Adults, *Lancet,* **2:**319, 1967.

Bates, D. V., Macklem, P. T., and Christie, R. V.: The Normal Lung: Physiology and Methods of Study, in "Respiratory Function in Disease," Chap. 2, W. B. Saunders Company, Philadelphia, 1971.

Baue, A. E.: The Pushmi-Pullyu Syndrome, *Surgery,* **72:**655, 1972.

Berman, I. R., and Ducker, T. B.: Pulmonary, Somatic and Splanchnic Circulatory Responses to Increased Intracranial Pressure, *Ann Surg,* **169:**210, 1969.

Blaisdell, F. W., and Lewis, F. R.: Etiologic Factors in the Respiratory Distress Syndrome, in "Respiratory Distress Syndrome of Shock and Trauma," W. B. Saunders Company, Philadelphia, 1977.

———, Lim, R. C., Jr., and Stallone, R. J.: The Mechanism of Pulmonary Damage following Traumatic Shock, *Surg Gynecol Obstet,* **130:**15, 1970.

Boyd, D. R.: Monitoring Patients with Post-Traumatic Pulmonary Insufficiency, *Surg Clin North Am,* **52:**31, 1972.

Bredenberg, C. E., et al.: Respiratory Failure in Shock, *Ann Surg,* **169:**392, 1969.

Buckberg, G. D., and Dowell, A. R.: The Effects of Hemorrhagic Shock and Pulmonary Ischemia on Lung Compliance and Structure in Baboons, *Surg Gynecol Obstet,* **131:**1065, 1970.

———, Lipman, C. A., Hahn, J. A., Smith, M. J., and Hennessen, J. A.: Pulmonary Changes following Hemorrhagic Shock and Resuscitation in Baboons, *J Thorac Cardiovasc Surg,* **59:**450, 1970.

Burford, T. H., and Burbank, B.: Traumatic Wet Lung: Observations on Certain Physiologic Fundamentals of Thoracic Trauma, *J Thorac Surg,* **14:**415, 1945.

Burke, J. F., Pontoppidan, H., and Welch, C. E.: High Output Respiratory Failure: An Important Cause of Death Ascribed to Peritonitis or Ileus, *Ann Surg,* **158:**581, 1963.

Burnham, S. C., Martin, W. E., and Cheney, F. W., Jr.: The Effects of Various Tidal Volumes on Gas Exchange in Pulmonary Edema, *Anesthesiology,* **37:**27, 1972.

Cafferata, H. T., Aggeler, P. M., Robinson, A. J., and Blaisdell, F. W.: Intravascular Coagulation in the Surgical Patient, *Am J Surg,* **118:**281, 1969.

Camerson, J. L., Anderson, R. P., and Zuidema, G. D.: Aspiration and Pneumonia: A Clinical and Experimental Review, *J Surg Res,* **7:**44, 1967.

Carey, L. C., Lowery, B. D., and Cloutier, C. T.: "Hemorrhagic Shock," Current Problems in Surgery, Monograph, January 1971.

Churchill, E. D.: Pulmonary Atelectasis: With Especial Reference to Massive Collapse of Lung, *Arch Surg,* **11:**489, 1925.

Clauss, R. H., Scalabrini, B. Y., Ray, J. F., II, and Reed, C. E.: Effects of Changing Body Position upon Improved Ventilation-Perfusion Relationships, *Circulation,* **37–38** (Suppl II): 214, 1968.

Clowes, G. H. A., Jr., et al.: Observations on the Pathogenesis of the Pneumonitis Associated with Severe Infections in Other Parts of the Body, *Ann Surg,* **167:**630, 1968.

———, Farrington, G. H., Zuschneid, W., Cossette, G. R., and Saravis, C.: Circulating Factors in the Etiology of Pulmonary Insufficiency and Right Heart Failure Accompanying Severe Sepsis (Peritonitis), *Ann Surg,* **171:**663, 1970.

Coalson, J. J., Hinshaw, L. B., and Guenter, C. A.: The Pulmonary Ultrastructure in Septic Shock, *Exp Mol Pathol,* **12:**84, 1970.

Collins, J. A.: The Causes of Progressive Pulmonary Insufficiency in Surgical Patients, *J Surg Res,* **9:**685, 1969.

———, et al.: Inapparent Hypoxemia in Casualties with Wounded Limbs: Pulmonary Fat Embolism? *Ann Surg,* **167:**511, 1968.

Comroe, J. H., Jr., Forster, R. E., II, Dubois, A. B., Briscoe, W. A., and Carlsen, E. (eds.): The Pulmonary Circulation and Ventilation/Blood Flow Ratios, in "The Lung: Clinical Physiology and Pulmonary Function Tests." Chicago, Year Book Medical Publishers, 1962.

Ducker, T. B.: Increased Intracranial Pressure and Pulmonary Edema: Part I. Clinical Study of 11 Patients, *J Neurosurg,* **28:**112, 1968.

Eaton, R. M.: Pulmonary Edema: Experimental Observation on Dogs Following Acute Peripheral Blood Loss, *J Thorac Surg,* **16:**668, 1947.

Eiseman, B., and Ashbaugh, D. G. (eds.): Pulmonary Effects of Nonthoracic Trauma: Proceedings of a Conference Conducted by the Committee on Trauma, Division of Medical Sciences, National Academy of Sciences–National Research Council, *J Trauma,* vol. 8, 1968.

Elliot, T. R., and Dingley, L. A.: Massive Collapse of the Lungs following Abdominal Operation, *Lancet,* **1:**1305, 1914.

Falke, K. J., et al.: Ventilation with End-Expiratory Pressure in Acute Lung Disease, *J Clin Invest,* **51:**2315, 1972.

Feeley, T. W., and Hedley-Whyte, J.: Weaning from Controlled Ventilation and Supplemental Oxygen, *N Engl J Med,* **292:**903, 1975.

Fleming, W. H., and Bowen, J. C.: The Use of Diuretics in the Treatment of Early Wet Lung Syndrome, *Ann Surg,* **175:**505, 1972.

Fulton, R. L., and Jones, C. E.: The Cause of Post-traumatic Pulmonary Insufficiency in Man, *Surg Gynecol Obstet,* **140:**179, 1975.

Geiger, J. P., and Gielchinsky, I.: Acute Pulmonary Insufficiency, *Arch Surg,* **102:**400, 1971.

Gerst, P. H., Rattenborg, C., and Holday, D. A.: The Effects of Hemorrhage on Pulmonary Circulation and Respiratory Gas Exchange, *J Clin Invest,* **38:**524, 1959.

Gotoh, F., Meyer, J., and Takagi, Y.: Cerebral Effects of Hyperventilation in Man, *Arch Neurol,* **12:**419, 1965.

Greenfield, L. J.: Pulmonary Dysfunction in Shock, in L. B. Hinshaw and B. G. Cox (eds.): "The Fundamental Mechanisms of Shock: Advances in Experimental Medicine and Biology," vol 23, p. 47, Plenum Press, New York, 1972.

Guenter, C. A., Firoica, V., and Hinshaw, L. B.: Cardiorespiratory and Metabolic Responses to Live E. coli and Endotoxin in the Monkey, *J Appl Physiol,* **26:**780, 1969.

Gump, F. E., Mashima, Y., Ferenczy, A., and Kinney, J. M.: Pre- and Postmortem Studies of Lung Fluids and Electrolytes, *J Trauma,* **11:**474, 1971.

Halmagyi, D. F. J., Goodman, A. H., Little, M. J., Kennedy, M., and Varga, D.: Portal Blood Flow and Oxygen Usage in Dogs after Hemorrhage, *Ann Surg,* **172:**284, 1970.

Hedden, M., and Miller, G. J.: Mendelson's Syndrome and Its Sequelae, *Can Anaesth Soc J,* **19:**351, 1972.

Henry, J. N., McArdle, A. H., Scott, H. J., and Gurd, F. N.: A Study of the Acute and Chronic Respiratory Pathophysiology of Hemorrhagic Shock, *J Thorac Cardiovasc Surg,* **54:**666, 1967.

Herndon, J. H., Riseborough, E. J., and Fischer, J. E.: Fat Embolism: A Review of Current Concepts, *J Trauma,* **11:**673, 1971.

Hill, J. D., et al.: Acute Respiratory Insufficiency: Treatment with Prolonged Extracorporeal Oxygenation, *J Thorac Cardiovasc Surg,* **64:**551, 1972.

Hillen, G. P., Gaisford, W. D., and Jensen, C. G.: Pulmonary Changes in Treated and Untreated Hemorrhagic Shock: I. Early Functional and Ultrastructural Alterations after Moderate Shock, *Am J Surg,* **122:**639, 1971.

Hinshaw, L. B., Emerson, T. E., Jr., and Reins, D. A.: Cardiovascular Responses of the Primate in Endotoxin Shock, *Am J Physiol,* **210:**335, 1966.

Hirsch, E. F., Fletcher, R., and Lucas, S.: Hemodynamic and Respiratory Changes Associated with Sepsis Following Combat Trauma, *Ann Surg,* **174:**211, 1971.

Holcroft, J. W., Trunkey, D. D., and Lim, R. C.: Further Analysis of Lung Water in Baboons Resuscitated from Hemorrhagic Shock, *J Surg Res,* **20:**291, 1976.

Horovitz, J. H., and Carrico, C. J.: Lung Colloid Permeability in Hemorrhagic Shock, *Surg Forum,* **23:**6, 1972.

———, ———, Maher, J., and Shires, G. T.: Pulmonary Shunt Determination: A Comparison between Oxygen Inhalation (Berggren) and Xenon-133 Methods, *J Lab Clin Med,* **78:**785, 1971.

———, ———, and Shires, G. T.: The Pulmonary Response to Major Injury, *Arch Surg,* **105:**699, 1974.

Huller, T., and Bazini, Y.: Blast Injuries of the Chest and Abdomen, *Arch Surg,* **100:**24, 1970.

Jenkins, M. T., Jones, R. F., Wilson, B., and Moyer, C. A.: Congestive Atelectasis: A Complication of the Intravenous Infusion of Fluids, *Ann Surg,* **100:**027, 1956.

Kafer, E. R.: Pulmonary Oxygen Toxicity: A Review of the Evidence for Acute and Chronic Oxygen Toxicity in Man, *Br J Anaesthiol,* **43:**687, 1971.

Keller, C. A., Schramel, R. J., Hyman, A. L., and Creech, O., Jr.: The Cause of Acute Congestive Lesions of the Lung, *J Thorac Cardiovasc Surg,* **53:**743, 1967.

Kim, S. I., Desai, J. M., and Shoemaker, W. C.: Sequential Respiratory Changes in an Experimental Hemorrhagic Shock Preparation Designed to Simulate Clinical Shock, *Ann Surg*, **170**:166, 1969.

Kuman, A., et al.: Continuous Positive-Pressure Ventilation in Acute Respiratory Failure: Effects on Hemodynamics and Lung Function, *N Engl J Med*, **283**:1430, 1970.

Laennec, R. T. H.: "De l'auscultation médiate ou traité du diagnostic des maladies des poumons et du coeur, fondé principalement sur ce nouveau moyen d'exploration," Paris, 1819.

Lande, A. J., et al.: Prolonged Cardio-Pulmonary Support with a Practical Membrane Oxygenator, *Trans Am Soc Artif Intern Organs*, **16**:352, 1970.

Levine, M., Gilbert, R., and Auchincloss, J. H., Jr.: A Comparison of the Effects of Signs, Large Tidal Volumes, and Positive End Expiratory Pressure in Assisted Ventilation, *Scand J Respir Dis*, **53**:101, 1972.

Lim, R. C., Jr., Blaisdell, F. W., Choy, S. H., Goodman, J. R., and Hall, A. D.: Pulmonary Microvascular Changes Following Regional Shock: A Clinical and Experimental Study, *Bull Soc Int Chir*, **1**:22, 1968.

Markello, R., Winter, P., and Olszowka, A.: Assessment of Ventilation-Perfusion Inequalities by Arterial-Alveolar Nitrogen Differences in Intensive-Care Patients, *Anesthesiology*, **37**:4, 1972.

Martin, A. M., Jr., Soloway, H. B., and Simmons, R. L.: Pathologic Anatomy of the Lungs Following Shock and Trauma, *J Trauma*, **8**:687, 1968.

McLaughlin, J. S.: Physiologic Consideration of Hypoxemia in Shock and Trauma, *Ann Surg*, **173**:667, 1971.

McNamara, J. J., Molot, M. D., and Stremple, J. F.: Screen Filtration Pressure in Combat Casualties, *Ann Surg*, **172**:334, 1970.

Meyer, J. A.: Mechanical Support of Respiration, *Surg Clin North Am*, **54**:(5):115, 1974.

Michenfelder, J., Fowler, W., and Theye, R.: CO_2 Levels and Pulmonary Shunting in Anesthetized Man, *J Appl Physiol*, **21**:1471, 1966.

Mills, M.: The Clinical Syndrome, *J Trauma*, **8**:651, 1968.

Monaco, V., et al.: Pulmonary Venous Admixture in Injured Patients, *J Trauma*, **12**:15, 1972.

Moore, F. D., et al.: "Post-Traumatic Pulmonary Insufficiency," W. B. Saunders Company, Philadelphia, 1969.

Moseley, R. V., and Doty, D. B.: Changes in the Filtration Characteristics of Stored Blood, *Ann Surg*, **171**:329, 1970.

Moss, G., Staunton, C., and Stein, A. A.: Cerebral Etiology of the "Shock Lung Syndrome," *J Trauma*, **12**:885, 1972.

Motsay, G. J., Alho, A. V., Schultz, L. S., Dietzman, R. H., and Lillehei, R. C.: Pulmonary Capillary Permeability in the Post-traumatic Pulmonary Insufficiency Syndrome: Comparison of Isogravimetric Capillary Pressures, *Ann Surg*, **173**:244, 1971.

Naimark, A., Dugard, A., and Rangno, R. E.: Regional Pulmonary Blood Flow and Gas Exchange in Hemorrhagic Shock, *J Appl Physiol*, **25**:301, 1968.

Nash, G., Bowen, J. A., and Langlinais, P. C.: "Respirator Lung": A Misnomer, *Arch Pathol*, **21**:234, 1971.

Neeley, W. A., et al.: Postoperative Respiratory Insufficiency: Physiological Studies with Therapeutic Implications, *Ann Surg*, **171**:679, 1970.

Nichols, R. T., Pearce, H. J., and Greenfield, L. J.: Effects of Experimental Pulmonary Contusion on Respiratory Exchange and Lung Mechanics, *Arch Surg*, **96**:723, 1968.

Olcott, C., Barber, R. E., and Blaisdell, F. W.: Diagnosis and Treatment of Respiratory Failure after Civilian Trauma, *Am J Surg*, **122**:260, 1971.

Pierce, A. K., et al.: Long-term Evaluation of Decontamination of Inhalation Therapy Equipment and the Occurrence of Necrotizing Pneumonia. *N Engl J Med*, **282**:528, 1970.

Pinardi, G., Leal, E., and Sallas Coll, A.: Vascular Permeability to Red Blood Cells and Protein in Hemorrhagic Shock, *Acta Physiol Lat Am*, **17**:175, 1967.

Pontoppidan, H., Geffin, B., and Lowenstein, E.: Acute Respiratory Failure in the Adult, *N Engl J Med*, **287**:690, 1972.

———, Laver, M. B., and Geffin, B.: Acute Respiratory Failure in the Surgical Patient, *Adv Surg*, **4**:163, 1970.

Powers, S. R., Jr.: The Use of Positive and Expiratory Pressure (PEEP) for Respiratory Support, *Surg Clin North Am*, **54**:1125, 1974.

———, et al.: Studies of Pulmonary Insufficiency in Non-thoracic Trauma, *J Trauma*, **12**:1, 1972.

Proctor, H. J., Ballantine, T. V. N., and Broussard, N. D.: An Analysis of Pulmonary Function Following Non-thoracic Trauma, with Recommendations for Therapy, *Ann Surg*, **172**:180, 1970.

Robin, E. D., Carey, L. C., Grenvik, A., Glauser, F., and Gaudio, R.: Capillary Leak Syndrome with Pulmonary Edema, *Arch Intern Med*, **130**:66, 1972.

Rosen, A. J.: Shock Lung: Fact or Fancy? *Surg Clin North Am*, **55**:613, 1975.

Rounthwaite, H. L., Scott, H. J., and Gurd, F. N.: Changes in the Pulmonary Circulation during Hemorrhagic Shock and Resuscitation, *Surg Forum*, **3**:454, 1952.

Said, S. I., et al.: Pulmonary Gas Exchange during Induction of Pulmonary Edema in Anesthetized Dogs, *J Appl Physiol*, **19**:403, 1964.

Schloerb, P. R., Hunt, P. T., Plummer, J. A., and Cage, G. K.: Pulmonary Edema after Replacement of Blood Loss by Electrolyte Solutions, *Surg Gynecol Obstet*, **135**:893, 1972.

Schon, G. R., Delphin, E. S., Millan, P. R., and Labat, R.: Relationship of Blood Substitutes to Pulmonary Changes and Volemia, *Ann Surg*, **173**:504, 1971.

Sealy, W. C., Ogino, S., Lesage, A. M., and Young, W. G., Jr.: Functional and Structural Changes in the Lungs in Hemorrhagic Shock, *Surg Gynecol Obstet*, **122**:754, 1966.

Shires, G. T., Carrico, C. J., and Canizaro, P. C.: "Shock," Chap. 4, Pulmonary Responses, W. B. Saunders Company, Philadelphia, 1973.

Siegel, D. C., Cochin, A., and Moss, G. S.: The Ventilatory Response to Hemorrhagic Shock and Resuscitation, *Surgery*, **72**:451, 1972.

———, Moss, G. S., Cochin, A., and Das Gupta, T. K.: Pulmonary Changes following Treatment for Hemorrhagic Shock: Saline versus Colloid Infusion, *Surg Forum*, **21**:17, 1970.

Simeone, F. A.: Shock, in "Christopher's Textbook of Surgery," 8th ed., Ed: Loyal Davis, p. 58, W. B. Saunders Company, Philadelphia, 1964.

Simmons, R. L., Martin, A. M., Jr., Heisterkamp, C. A., III, and Ducker, T. B.: Respiratory Insufficiency in Combat Casualties: II. Pulmonary Edema following Head Injury, *Ann Surg*, **170**:39, 1969.

Skillman, J. J., Parikh, B. M., and Tanenbaum, B. J.: Pulmonary Arteriovenous Admixture Improvement with Albumin and Diuresis, *Am J Surg,* **119:**450, 1970.

Sladen, A., Laver, M. B., and Pontoppidan, H.: Pulmonary Complications and Water Retention in Prolonged Mechanical Ventilation, *N Engl J Med,* **279:**448, 1968.

Stallone, R. J., Herbst, H., Blaisdell, F. W., and Murray, J. F.: Pulmonary Changes following Ischemia of the Lower Extremities and Their Treatment, *Am Rev Respir Dis,* **100:**813, 1969.

Staub, N. C.: Pathogenesis of Pulmonary Edema, *Am Rev Respir Dis,* **109:**358, 1974.

Sterling, G. M.: The Mechanism of Bronchoconstriction Due to Hypocapnia in Man, *Clin Sci,* **34:**277, 1968.

Sugg, W. F., et al.: Congestive Atelectasis: An Experimental Study, *Ann Surg,* **168:**234, 1968.

Swank, R. L.: Alteration of Blood on Storage: Measurement of Adhesiveness of "Aging" Platelets and Leukocytes and Their Removal by Filtration, *N Engl J Med,* **265:**728, 1961.

Sykes, M. P., Adams, A. P., Finlay, W. E. I., Wightman, A. E., and Munroe, J. P.: The Cardiorespiratory Effects of Haemorrhage and Overtransfusion in Dogs, *Br J Anaesthiol,* **42:**573, 1970.

Terzi, R. G., and Peters, R. M.: The Effect of Large Fluid Loads on Lung Mechanics and Work, *Ann Thorac Surg,* **6:**16, 1968.

Trimble, C., Smith, D. E., Rosenthal, M. H., and Fosburg, R. G.: Pathophysiologic Role of Hypocarbia in Post-traumatic Pulmonary Insufficiency, *Am J Surg,* **122:**633, 1971.

Wahrenbrock, E. A., Carrico, C. J., Amundsen, D. A., Trummer, M. J., and Severinghaus, J. W.: Increased Atelectatic Pulmonary Shunt during Hemorrhagic Shock in Dogs, *J Appl Physiol,* **29:**615, 1970.

———, ———, Schroeder, C. F., and Trummer, M. J.: The Effect of Posture on Pulmonary Function and Survival of Anesthetized Dogs, *J Surg Res,* **10:**13, 1970.

Wangensteen, O. D., Wittmers, L. E., and Johnson, J. A.: Permeability of the Mammalian Blood-Gas Barrier and Its Components, *Am J Physiol,* **216:**719, 1969.

Willwerth, B. M., Crawford, F. A., Young, W. G., Jr., and Sealy, W. C.: The Role of Functional Demand in the Development of Pulmonary Lesions during Hemorrhagic Shock, *J Thorac Cardiovasc Surg,* **54:**658, 1967.

Wilson, J. W.: Treatment or Prevention of Pulmonary Cellular Damage with Pharmacologic Doses of Corticosteroid, *Surg Gynecol Obstet,* **134:**675, 1972.

Wilson, R. F., Kafi, A., Asuncion, Z., and Walt, A. J.: Clinical Respiratory Failure after Shock or Trauma, *Arch Surg,* **98:**539, 1969.

Wyche, M. Q., Marshall, B. E., Mehall, S. L., and Schuetze, M. M.: Lung Function, Pulmonary Extravascular Water Volume and Hemodynamics in Early Hemorrhagic Shock in Anesthetized Dogs, *Ann Surg,* **174:**296, 1971.

Alterations in Oxygen Transport

Bellingham, A. J., Detter, J. C., and Lenfant, C.: Regulatory Mechanisms of Hemoglobin Oxygen Affinity in Acidosis and Alkalosis, *J Clin Invest,* **50:**700, 1971.

Benesch, R., and Benesch, R. E.: The Effect of Organic Phosphates from the Human Erythrocyte on the Allosteric Properties of Hemoglobin, *Biochem Biophys Res Commun,* **26:**162, 1967.

Berne, R. M., Blackman, J. R., and Gardner, T. H.: Hypoxemia and Coronary Blood Flow, *J Clin Invest,* **36:**1101, 1957.

Beutler, E., Meul, A., and Wood, L. A.: Depletion and Regeneration of 2,3-Diphosphoglyceric Acid in Stored Red Blood Cells, *Transfusion,* **9:**109, 1969.

Bowen, J. C., and Fleming, W. H.: Increased Oxyhemoglobin Affinity after Transfusion of Stored Blood, *Ann Surg,* **180:**760, 1974.

Canizaro, P. C., Nelson, J. L., Hennessy, J. L., and Bright, P. B.: A Technique for Estimating the Position of the Oxygen-Hemoglobin Dissociation Curve, *Ann Surg,* **180:**364, 1974.

Chaunutin, A., and Curnish, R. R.: Effect of Organic and Inorganic Phosphates on the Oxygen Equilibrium of Human Erythrocytes, *Arch Biochem Biophys,* **121:**96, 1967.

Dawson, R. B., Edinger, M. C., and Ellis, T. J.: Hemoglobin Function in Stored Blood, *J Lab Clin Med,* **77:**46, 1971.

Dennis, R. C., Vito, L., Weisel, R. D., Valeri, C. R., Berger, R. L., and Hechtman, H. B.: Improved Myocardial Performance Following High 2-3 Diphosphoglycerate Red Cell Transfusions, *Surgery,* **77:**741, 1975.

Duhm, J., Deuticke, B., and Gerlach, E.: Complete Restoration of Oxygen Transport Function and 2,3-Diphosphoglycerate Concentration in Stored Blood, *Transfusion,* **11:**147, 1971.

Harker, A. H.: The Surgical Significance of the Oxyhemoglobin Dissociation Curve, *Surg Gynecol Obstet,* **144:**935, 1977.

Lenfant, C., et al.: Effects of Altitude on Oxygen Binding by Hemoglobin and on Organic Phosphate Levels, *J Clin Invest,* **47:**2652, 1968.

———, Ways, P., and Aucutt, C.: Effect of Chronic Hypoxic Hypoxia on the O_2-Hb Dissociation Curve and Respiratory Gas Transport in Man, *Respir Physiol,* **7:**7, 1969.

McConn, R., and Del Guercio, L. R. M.: Respiratory Function of Blood in the Acutely Ill Patient and the Effect of Steroids, *Ann Surg,* **174:**436, 1971.

Opitz, E., and Schneider, M.: Über die Sauerstoffversorgung des Gehirns und den Mechanismus von Mangelverhungerung, *Ergeb Physiol,* **46:**126, 1950.

Oski, F. A., et al.: The *in vitro* Restoration of Red Cell 2,3-Diphosphoglycerate Levels in Banked Blood, *Blood,* **37:**52, 1971.

Pollock, T. W., et al.: *In vivo* Effect of Inosine, Pyruvate, and Phosphate (IPP) on Oxygen-Hemoglobin Affinity, *Fed Proc,* **30:**546, 1971.

Rice, C. L., Herman, C. M., Kiesow, L. A., Homer, L. D., and John, D. A.: Benefits from Improved Oxygen Delivery of Blood in Shock Therapy, *Surg Res,* **19:**193, 1975.

Severinghaus, J. W.: Blood Gas Calculator, *J Appl Physiol,* **21:**1108, 1966.

Shappell, S. D., and Lenfant, C. J. M.: Adaptive, Genetic, and Iatrogenic Alterations of the Oxyhemoglobin-Dissociation Curve, *Anesthesiology,* **37:**127, 1972.

Valeri, C. R., and Hirsch, N. M.: Restoration *in vivo* of Erythrocyte Adenosine Triphosphate, 2,3-Diphosphoglycerate, Potassium Ion, and Sodium Ion Concentrations Following the Transfusion of Acid-Citrate-Dextrose-Stored Human Red Blood Cells, *J Lab Clin Med,* **73:**722, 1969.

Therapy of Shock

Alican, F., Dalton, M. L., Jr., and Hardy, J. D.: Experimental Endotoxin Shock, *Am J Surg,* **103:**702, 1962.

Altemeier, W. A., Todd, J. C., and Inge, W. W.: Gramnegative Septicemia: A Growing Threat, *Ann Surg,* **166:**530, 1967.

Baue, A. E.: The Treatment of Septic Shock: A Problem Intensified by Advancing Science, *Surgery,* **65:**850, 1969.

Blair, E., Ollodart, R., Esmond, W. G., Attar, S., and Crowley, R. A.: Effect of Hyperbaric Oxygenation (OHP) on Bacteremic Shock, *Circulation,* **29** (Suppl I):135, 1964.

Carey, J. S., et al.: Cardiovascular Function in Shock; Responses to Volume Loading and Isoproterenol Infusion, *Circulation,* **35:**327, 1967.

Clermont, G., Williams, J. S., and Adams, J. T.: Steroid Effect on the Release of the Lysosomal Enzyme Acid Phosphatase in Shock, *Ann Surg,* **179:**917, 1974.

Duff, J. H., Malave, G., Pertz, D. I., Scott, H. M., and MacLean, L. D.: The Hemodynamics of Septic Shock in Man and in the Dog, *Surgery,* **58:**174, 1965.

Grollman, A.: "Cardiac Output of Man in Health and Disease," Charles C Thomas, Springfield, Ill., 1932.

Hinshaw, L. B., Archer, L. T., Black, M. R., Greenfield, L. J., and Guenter, C. A.: Prevention and Reversal of Myocardial Failure in Endotoxin Shock, *Surg Gynecol Obstet,* **136:**1, 1973.

Iampietro, P. F., Henshaw, L. B., and Brake, C. M.: Effect of an Adrenergic Blocking Agent on Vascular Alterations Associated with Endotoxin Shock, *Am J Physiol,* **204:**611, 1963.

Krausz, M. M., Perel, A., Eimerl, D., and Cotev, S.: Cardiopulmonary Effects of Volume Loading in Patients in Septic Shock, *Ann Surg,* **185:**429, 1977.

Kwaan, H. M., and Weil, M. H.: Differences in the Mechanism of Shock Caused by Bacterial Infections, *Surg Gynecol Obstet,* **128:**37, 1969.

Loeb, H. S., Winslow, E. B. J., Rahimtoola, S. H., Rosen, K. M., and Gunnar, R. M.: Acute Hemodynamic Effects of Dopamine in Patients with Shock, *Circulation,* **44:**163, 1971.

MacLean, L. D., Mulligan, W. G., MacLean, A. P. H., and Duff, J. H.: Patterns of Septic Shock in Man: A Detailed Study of 56 Patients, *Ann Surg,* **166:**543, 1967.

Motsay, G. J., Dietzman, R. H., Ersek, R. A., and Lillehei, R. C.: Hemodynamic Alterations and Results of Treatment in Patients with Gram-negative Septic Shock, *Surgery,* **67:**577, 1970.

Ollodart, R. M., Hawthorne, I., and Attar, S.: Studies in Experimental Endotoxemia in Man, *Am J Surg,* **113:**599, 1967.

Rowe, M. I., Buckner, D. M., and Newmark, S.: The Early Diagnosis of Gram-negative Septicemia in the Pediatric Surgical Patient, *Ann Surg,* **182:**280, 1975.

Schuler, J. J., Erve, P. R., and Schumer, W.: Glucocorticoid Effect on Hepatic Carbohydrate Metabolism in the Endotoxin-Shocked Monkey, *Ann Surg,* **183:**345, 1976.

Schumer, W.: Steroids in the Treatment of Clinical Septic Shock, *Ann Surg,* **184:**333, 1976.

———, and Nyhus, L. M.: "Corticosteroids in the Treatment of Shock," University of Illinois Press, Urbana, 1970.

Shubin, H., and Weil, M. H.: Bacterial Shock: A Serious Complication in Urological Practice, *JAMA,* **185:**850, 1963.

Spath, J. A., Gorczynski, R. J., and Lefer, A. M.: Possible Mechanisms of the Beneficial Action of Glucocorticoids in Circulatory Shock, *Surg Gynecol Obstet,* **137:**597, 1973.

Spink, W. W.: The Ecology of Human Septic Shock, in S. G. Hershey, L. R. M. Del Guercio, and R. McConn (eds.), "Septic Shock in Man," Little, Brown and Company, Boston, 1971.

Swan, H. J. C., et al.: Catheterization of the Heart in Man with Use of a Flow-Directed Balloon-Tipped Catheter, *N Engl J Med,* **283:**447, 1970.

Waldhausen, J. A., Kilman, J. W., and Abel, F. L.: Effects of Catecholamines on the Heart: Myocardial Contractility, Cardiac Efficiency, and Total Peripheral Resistance, *Arch Surg,* **91:**86, 1965.

Weil, M. H., Shubin, H., and Rosoff, L.: Fluid Repletion in Circulatory Shock: Central Venous Pressure and Other Practical Guides, *JAMA,* **192:**668, 1965.

Wilson, J. N., Grow, J. B., Demong, C. V., Prevedel, A. E., and Owens, J. C.: Central Venous Pressure in Optimal Blood Volume Maintenance, *Arch Surg,* **85:**563, 1962.

Wilson, R. F., and Fisher, R. R.: The Hemodynamic Effects of Massive Steroids in Clinical Shock, *Surg Gynecol Obstet,* **127:**769, 1968.

———, Sukhnanden, R., and Thal, A. P.: Combined Use of Norepinephrine and Dibenzyline in Clinical Shock, *Surg Forum,* **15:**30, 1964.

Wright, C. J., Duff, J. H., MacLean, A. P. H., and MacLean, L. D.: Regional Capillary Blood Flow and Oxygen Uptake in Severe Sepsis, *Surg Gynecol Obstet,* **132:**637, 1971.

Chapter 5

Infections

by Isidore Cohn, Jr. and George H. Bornside

INTRODUCTION

Infection is a dynamic process involving invasion of the body by pathogenic microorganisms and reaction of the tissues to organisms and their toxins. Soon after birth, a variety of microorganisms colonize the external and internal surfaces of the human body. This indigenous microflora usually does no harm; it produces no detectable pathologic effects in tissues and may be beneficial. Indeed, current research indicates that the normal intestinal flora functions as a barrier providing natural resistance against enteric infections with pathogens such as *Salmonella* and *Shigella* species. Infection evolves into overt disease only when the equilibrium between host and parasite is upset. Of the thousands of species of microorganisms in nature, only a few hundred are known to be pathogenic for man.

Current thinking concerning clinical disease resulting from host and parasite interrelationships recognizes the role of the general health of the host, his previous contact with infectious microorganisms, his past clinical history, and various insults (toxic, traumatic, or therapeutic) of nonmicrobial origin. When the host's resistance is lowered, the indigenous microflora can become involved in infectious disease. This presents a dilemma to both the clinician and the microbiologist, as it must be decided which of the several microorganisms usually isolated from a clinical specimen are involved in the patient's disease. There are very few pathogenic species which cause disease at all times. Most organisms found in and on man often are harmless but are capable of causing disease in patients who are elderly, very young, or debilitated (Table 5-1).

Despite 80 years of aseptic surgery and more than 40 years of experience with antimicrobial agents, the surgeon finds that infections are as great a problem now as in the past. But the etiologic agents have changed. Streptococci and pneumococci are no longer the captains of death, because they can be controlled by antibiotics. Staphylococci con-

Table 5-1. SOME INDIGENOUS MICROORGANISMS AND SOME INFECTIONS WITH WHICH THEY MAY BE INVOLVED

Microorganism	*Infection*
Aerobic or facultative:	
Achromobacter spp.	Bloodstream, burns, meningitis, urethritis
Acinetobacter spp.	Bloodstream, burns, meningitis, urethritis, pneumonia
Alcaligenes fecalis	Bloodstream, conjunctivitis, meningitis, respiratory tract, urinary tract
Candida albicans and other yeasts	Bacterial endocarditis, pneumonitis, septicemia, thrush, vulvovaginitis, candidiosis
Corynebacterium spp.	Bacterial endocarditis, lung abscesses
Enterobacteriaceae (*Escherichia, Klebsiella, Enterobacter, Proteus,* etc.)	Abscesses, bloodstream, meningitis, peritonitis, pneumonia, wounds, urinary tract, endocarditis, pyelonephritis, cystitis
Hemophilus spp.	Bronchitis, conjunctivitis, meningitis, urinary tract
Moraxella spp.	Conjunctivitis
Nocardia spp.	Nocardiosis
Pseudomonas spp.	Bloodstream, burns, meningitis, urinary tract, wounds
Staphylococcus aureus	Abscesses, pneumonia, wounds, pseudomembranous enterocolitis
Staphylococcus epidermidis	Bacterial endocarditis, septicemia, thrombophlebitis
Streptococcus fecalis	Bacterial endocarditis, bloodstream, urinary tract, wounds, peritonitis, meningitis
Streptococcus viridans	Bacterial endocarditis
Anaerobic:	
Actinomyces spp.	Actinomycosis
Bacteroides spp.	Abscesses, bacterial endocarditis, peritonitis
Clostridium spp.	Cellulitis, myonecrosis
Fusobacterium spp.	Abscesses, myonecrosis, bacteremia
Lactobacillus spp.	Bacterial endocarditis
Peptostreptococcus spp.	Abscesses, myonecrosis
Veillonella spp.	Bacterial endocarditis

tinue to cause nosocomial (hospital-acquired) infections, and those gram-negative bacteria usually considered nonpathogens, opportunists, or secondary invaders have become a major problem. Nosocomial infection results from the transmission of pathogens to a previously uninfected patient from a source in the hospital environment (cross infection). Alternatively, the pathogens may come from the patient himself (autoinfection). He may be a carrier of the pathogen or become colonized with virulent hospital strains during hospitalization. Many nosocomial infections have a iatrogenic basis (i.e., result from treatment by the physician and his professional collaborators). Frequent or prolonged use of supportive procedures such as indwelling venous or urinary catheters, tracheostomies, and equipment for postoperative respiratory care are responsible for most iatrogenic infections. Nosocomial infection causes morbidity, mortality, expense to the patient, and increasing malpractice liability for the surgeon and hospital.

A surgical infection is an infection which requires surgical treatment and has developed before, or as a complication of, surgical treatment. Thus, a postoperative wound infection is also a specific nosocomial infection. Surgical infections may be analyzed in relation to procedures in clean or contaminated fields, the anatomic site or system involved, and the pathophysiologic activities of the causative microorganisms (Table 5-2). The microorganisms commonly encountered in surgical infections are the staphylococci, streptococci, clostridia, bacteroides, and the enteric bacteria. Most surgical incisions are contaminated but not infected with normal skin flora (bacteria such as coagulase-negative staphylococci and anaerobic diphtheroids). However, traumatic wounds are usually contaminated if not yet infected, and operations on infected or "contaminated" tissue usually result in infection. Postoperative infections present a double hazard: First, the infection itself may result in toxemia or produce extensive tissue damage and perhaps septicemia. Second, the local effects of infection delay healing of the wound and may cause hemorrhage or disruption of the wound. In either case, the patient's hospitalization is extended.

GENERAL PRINCIPLES

Pathogenic species of bacteria have the capacity to invade and produce disease. However, disease is a biologic accident and represents a complex interaction between the microorganism and the host which occurs only under special circumstances. Healthy people may harbor pathogenic bacteria and yet be clinically unaffected. They are referred to as carriers of the particular pathogen. The healthy carrier of pathogenic microorganisms is the principal reservoir of most diseases. Although species such as *Staphylococcus aureus* and *Escherichia coli* are examples of pathogens, individual strains may be too feeble to cause infection. Feeble or noninvasive strains may cause infection if the resistance of the host is extremely low or if tremendous numbers of bacteria are introduced. Some bacteria which are nonpathogenic under ordinary conditions are opportunistic and may be pathogenic when the host-parasite

Table 5-2. CLASSIFICATION OF
SURGICAL INFECTIONS

I. Relative to final outcome
   A. Self-limiting infections: The patient recovers completely
      without medical or surgical treatment, or despite it (e.g.,
      a boil).
   B. Serious infections requiring treatment: The outcome de-
      pends largely on the nature of treatment, the time after
      outset that it is administered, and clinical judgment (e.g.,
      septicemia, pneumonia, empyema, primary peritonitis).
   C. Fulminating infections: These prove to be fatal or per-
      manently disabling (e.g., retroperitoneal cellulitis).
II. Relative to time of onset
   A. Anteoperative surgical infections: These include all infec-
      tions in which the microorganisms have gained entrance to
      the body before any operative procedure.
     1. Time and portal of entry are known—accidents.
     2. Time and portal of entry are not known—disease
        (infection) is established before the surgeon treats the
        patient.
   B. Operative surgical infections: These include all in which
      microorganisms gain entrance to the body during an opera-
      tive procedure or as an immediate result of it (i.e., sur-
      gery may be considered either directly or indirectly respon-
      sible for the development of infection).
     1. Preventable operative surgical infections—failure of the
        surgeon or operating-room personnel to adhere to the
        principles of sterile procedure and all accepted and ac-
        credited practices
     2. Nonpreventable operative surgical infections
        a. Pathogenic microorganisms already resident within
          body tissues (e.g., incision seeded with Staphylococcus
          aureus resident in ducts and glands of normal skin)
        b. Microorganisms from a deep focus of infection (e.g.,
          peritoneal abscess, lung abscess, etc.)
        c. Microorganisms resident on the surface of normal
          mucous membranes (e.g., intestinal tract, respiratory
          tract, genitourinary tract)
        d. Microorganisms on dust particles and borne by air
          currents
   C. Postoperative surgical infections: These are complications
      of the operation or the postoperative management of the
      patient
     1. Surgical wound infection
     2. Respiratory tract infection
     3. Urinary tract infection

SOURCE: Modified from F. L. Meleney, "Treatise on Surgical
Infections," Oxford University Press, New York, 1948.

equilibrium is upset, e.g., when normal flora is eliminated
by antibiotics or when incision makes available a new area
of the body. Antibiotic-resistant strains of Staphylococcus
aureus of specific phage types, which cause nosocomial
postoperative wound infections, may be endemic among
carrier personnel of a particular hospital. The patient may
become infected by direct contact with a carrier or may
become infected with a hospital staphylococcus with which
he has become colonized during hospitalization.

The term virulence refers to the tissue-invading powers
of a specific strain of a pathogen and is used in two different ways: First, virulence describes quantitatively the
smallest dose of a bacterial strain which will produce
disease in a specified host. This assessment is usually conducted in experimental animals and may have no relation
to human disease. Second, virulence describes an epi-

demiologic concept such as a given phage type of Staphylococcus aureus producing human disease more frequently
than another. In this situation, virulence is based on eco-
logic advantage in the external environment but may not
necessarily involve greater capacity to be virulent as measured by the critical dose of bacteria causing clinical infection.

A large infecting dose is favorable to the production of
bacterial disease, because only a small number of bacteria
may actually reach a favorable site in the host. A sudden
change to a different environment or to a new site may
injure most of the inoculum. Moreover, the defense mechanisms of the host often destroy a large proportion of the
invading organisms before they can become established.
The greater the number of bacteria introduced into the
host, the greater the amount of preformed toxins that will
be carried along. Preformed toxins may protect bacteria
from destruction during the period when they are adapting
to the new environment and are incapable of producing
additional toxin. The resistance of the host is shown in
his ability to keep bacteria out of the body initially and,
failing in this, to localize and destroy them. A healthy,
unbroken skin is the first line of resistance. Although mucous membranes are less resistant, even here minute breaks
usually provide for bacterial entry. It is then that active
defensive measures come into play. Primary defenses include the system of fixed phagocytic cells (i.e., the histiocytes of the reticuloendothelial system) and mobile phagocytes. These are aided by antibacterial substances in blood
plasma, lymph, and interstitial fluid, by physical barriers
to the spread of bacteria (i.e., ground substances, serous
and fibrous membranes), and by local and systemic reactions such as hyperemia, fever, and leukocytosis. Secondary defenses are dependent upon the presence of specific
antigenic stimuli (bacteria and bacterial products). The
antibodies formed in response to these antigens inhibit or
destroy bacteria, or neutralize their toxins. In the presence
of sufficient antibodies, the primary defenses are greatly
accelerated, bacteria are phagocytized and digested more
quickly than before, and the ability of serum to neutralize
bacterial toxins is increased many thousandfold. The presence of other disease may greatly reduce resistance to
microbial infection. For example, diabetes predisposes to
infection of the skin and the genitourinary tract. Influenza,
measles, and other viral infections markedly predispose to
secondary bacterial infections of the respiratory tract. Malignant disease, malnutrition, chronic alcoholism, or metabolic disease may interfere seriously with an individual's
resistance to infectious disease.

Bacteria cause disease by invading tissues and producing
toxins. Bacterial invasion leads to demonstrable damage
of host cells and tissues in the vicinity of the invasion,
whereas bacterial toxins are transported by the blood and
lymph to cause cytotoxic effects at sites removed from the
initial lesion. Species such as Streptococcus pyogenes are
both invasive and toxigenic. Staphylococcus aureus produces local damage but has little tendency to spread, although the local inflammatory response may be severe as
in the case of carbuncles. Clostridium tetani is almost solely
toxigenic. Generally, invasiveness and toxigenicity are not

completely separable, since invasion involves some degree of toxin production and toxigenicity requires some degree of bacterial multiplication. *Exotoxins* are specific, soluble, diffusible proteins produced by gram-positive bacteria as they multiply in a circumscribed area. Exotoxins lose their toxicity upon denaturation but retain much of their original antigenicity. Such modified exotoxins are called *toxoids*. Those prepared from *Clostridium tetani* are used to induce active immunity in man. The alpha toxin of *Clostridium perfringens* is a lecithinase which acts upon the membrane lipids of body cells and erythrocytes. *Endotoxins* are complex lipopolysaccharides of the bacterial cell wall produced by many gram-negative species. They are released only on partial or complete dissolution of the bacterial cell. Endotoxins are relatively heat-stable; many withstand temperatures of 60 to 100°C for 1 hour. They do not form toxoids. Their toxicity is associated with the phospholipid moiety of the molecule, whereas their antigenic determinants are associated with the polysaccharide moiety.

Diagnosis

The classic signs and symptoms of infection are redness, swelling, heat, and pain. Redness of the skin, due to intense hyperemia, is seen only in infections of the skin itself. Swelling accompanies infection unless the infection is confined to bone which cannot swell. Heat results from hyperemia and may be detected in the absence of redness. Pain is the most universal sign of infection. Along with pain goes tenderness, or pain to the touch, which is greatest over the area of maximal involvement. Loss of function is another sign of infection. It is brought about by reflex and by voluntary immobilization. The patient immobilizes the painful part in the most comfortable position he can find. For example, a finger with an infected tendon sheath is kept flexed. In peritonitis, the abdominal muscles are maintained in a state of tonic contraction to keep the inflamed peritoneum beneath from moving. Fever and tachycardia are additional, albeit nonspecific, signs of infection. Fever and chills indicate septicemia, while an elevated pulse rate is a sign of a toxic state.

Leukocytosis accompanies an acute bacterial infection more often than a viral infection. The more severe the infection, the greater is the leukocytosis. In most surgical infections, the total leukocyte count is only slightly or moderately elevated. However, a high leukocyte count ($35,000/mm^3$) occurs as a result of suppuration. The endotoxin released by gram-negative bacilli is thought to contribute to the production of high leukocyte counts. However, in the elderly, in the severely ill, and during therapy with antibiotic and immunosuppressive drugs, white cell counts may be normal or low. The leukopenia of overwhelming sepsis is probably due to exhaustion of the supply of leukocytes and to bone marrow depression. Although the total number of leukocytes is normal in some infections, there is a preponderance of immature granulocytes, which may be increased above 85 percent compared with the normal below 75 percent ("shift to the left"). A chronic infection may be evident only by fatigue, low-grade fever, and perhaps anemia. Moreover, massive pyogenic abscesses may occur without leukocytosis, fever, or tenderness.

Exudate from the area of infection should be examined for color, odor, and consistency. The microorganisms causing a surgical infection often may be seen microscopically on gram-stained smears. For each bacterial cell observed under the oil-immersion lens, there are approximately 10^5 similar organisms in each milliliter of exudate from which the smear was prepared. The staining and examination of slides are simple, rapid, inexpensive procedures which provide valuable and immediate information for the surgeon. Pus from deep-seated abscesses may be obtained by needle aspiration or at the time of definitive drainage. Exudate from surface infections may be examined directly. Specimens submitted to the bacteriologic laboratory should be collected before chemotherapy is begun and should be labeled adequately to identify the patient, the clinical diagnosis, and the nature and site of the specimen. The laboratory should be requested to do aerobic and anaerobic cultures and antibiotic-sensitivity tests. The surgeon must initiate treatment immediately upon clinical judgment, although the subsequent laboratory report will often enable him to make appropriate changes.

Biopsy is useful in establishing a diagnosis in granulomatous infections such as tuberculosis, syphilis, and mycoses. Additional sources of biopsy material are enlarged lymph nodes draining an area of infection or a sinus tract. Blood cultures are the single most definitive method of determining etiology in infectious disease and are often helpful in identifying the microorganisms causing surgical infection. Transient bacteremias accompany the early phase of many infections and may result from manipulation of infected or contaminated tissues (e.g., surgical incision of furuncles or abscesses, instrumentation of the genitourinary tract, and dental procedures). Bacteria usually enter the circulation via the lymphatic system. Consequently, when bacteria multiply at a site of local infection in tissues, the lymph drained from that area carries bacteria to the thoracic duct and eventually to the venous blood. However, a blood culture taken at the time of chill and fever may be negative for bacteria, as phagocytes promptly remove bacteria suddenly entering the bloodstream and chill and fever occur 30 to 90 minutes later. Thus, blood cultures should be taken at frequent intervals in a patient with febrile disease of unknown origin in an attempt to obtain blood before an expected chill and rise in temperature. A careful history and physical examination provide the basis for diagnosis and laboratory tests.

Surgical Therapy

It is necessary to distinguish between contamination and infection. Almost all wounds are contaminated with bacteria from the skin or from sources external to the patient. However, very few wounds become infected (i.e., exhibit disease manifested by inflammation, dehiscence, suppuration, and necrosis). The major clinical responses to wound infection are suppuration and invasion. Bacteria grow in the wound on substrates consisting of blood clots, lymph, leukocytes, and necrotic debris. Extension of the local inflammatory response to adjacent tissues is associated with a systemic reaction. The hazard of generalized infection is associated with all traumatic wounds. These and preoperative surgical infections are treated to overcome existing infection and to prevent postoperative infection. Local treatment consists of debridement of all necrotic or injured tissue, drainage of abscesses, removal of foreign bodies, and adjunctive therapy with antibiotics. Supportive measures governing the treatment of established surgical infections are bed rest, immobilization of the infected region, elevation to promote venous and lymphatic drainage, and relief of swelling and pain. Moist heat is applied to increase local blood supply, facilitate exudation, and hasten sloughing. The detailed management of wounds is discussed in Chap. 8 (Wound Healing and Wound Care).

Antibiotic Therapy

The adjunctive use of antibiotics in the treatment of infections is dependent upon an adequate blood supply and is most effective against acute infections such as cellulitis, septicemia, or peritonitis. Antibiotics have slight access to abscesses and penetrate by slow diffusion, if at all. In these situations, they should be used in conjunction with incision and drainage. Antibiotics are the primary treatment for acute spreading infections and should result in clinical improvement in 24 to 48 hours. Change to a more effective antibiotic may be based on the culture and sensitivity report.

Although clinical judgment frequently must be used to select an antibiotic and although the causative microorganism often is revealed on microscopic examination of a gram-stained smear of exudate or pus, the infecting microorganisms should be identified and antibiotic sensitivities determined by the laboratory. Accordingly, the specimen for culture (pus, exudate, blood, or urine) should be obtained before chemotherapy is begun. In severe infections, exudate can often be inoculated on a blood agar plate and antibiotic sensitivity discs positioned so that rapid, presumptive sensitivity information can be obtained after incubation overnight or for several hours. This crude procedure does not replace the official pure culture studies of all microorganisms isolated from the specimen.

Hyperbaric Therapy

Brummelkamp and associates in Amsterdam introduced the hyperbaric oxygen chamber for operative procedures. In 1963 they reported the first use of hyperbaric oxygen for gas-producing infections. Both the patient and medical personnel were placed in a room-sized chamber in which the air pressure was raised to three times that of the normal atmosphere (i.e., 2,280 mm Hg, or 3 atm absolute). For seven periods of 1½ hours during 3 days, the patient inhaled 100% oxygen from a face mask. This increased the normal oxygen tension in plasma, lymph, and tissue fluids about fifteen to twenty times. Dramatic clinical improvement was described in most patients within the first day. Roding and colleagues advise that "operations be limited to opening

the original wound and incising abscesses. Any further excision and removal of necrotic tissue can be done much later after clinical resolution. The advantage of postponement is that the operation can be performed in a dramatically improved patient who is no longer toxic." Large pressure chambers are available at only a few medical centers in the world and at special military and marine industrial facilities. In addition, much less expensive single-patient chambers are available and are also used to treat patients. Therapy with hyperbaric oxygen, antibiotics, and surgical debridement has been effective for clostridial myonecrosis. Hyperbaric oxygenation appears to reduce toxemia and diminish the amount of tissue requiring excision. However, gas-producing infection due to anaerobic streptococci, *Escherichia coli,* and *Klebsiella* species showed no improvement after exposure to high-pressure oxygen. The use of hyperbaric oxygen is advocated as an adjunct to the surgical treatment of clostridial infections. In cases of clostridial myonecrosis, all conventional means of treatment should be employed, including early surgical debridement and administration of antibiotics. The reliability of immediate surgical treatment and adjunctive antibiotic therapy remains unquestioned.

SOME COMMON SURGICAL INFECTIONS

Cellulitis is a nonsuppurative inflammation of the subcutaneous tissues extending along connective tissue planes and across intercellular spaces. There is widespread swelling, redness, and pain without definite localization. Central necrosis and suppuration may occur at a later stage. In severe infections, blebs and bullae form on the skin. Although a variety of aerobic and anaerobic bacteria produce cellulitis, the hemolytic streptococci are the classic etiologic agents. Treatment consists of antibiotic therapy and rest. Failure of the inflammatory swelling to subside after 48 to 72 hours of antibiotic therapy suggests that an abscess has developed, and that incision and drainage are needed.

Lymphangitis is an inflammation of lymphatic pathways which is usually visible as erythematous streaking of the skin. This is especially true in infections by hemolytic streptococci. Lymphangitis and the associated inflammatory swelling of lymph nodes (*lymphadenitis*) are a normal defense reaction against bacterial invasion and are frequently seen in the forearm of a patient with an infection of the hand or fingers. Most cases will respond to antibiotic therapy and rest.

Erysipelas is an acute spreading cellulitis and lymphangitis, usually caused by hemolytic streptococci which gain entrance through a break in the skin. There is a severe systemic as well as local reaction with abrupt onset, chills, fever, and prostration. The skin is red, swollen, and tender, and there is a distinct line of demarcation at the advancing margin of the infection. Erysipelas may develop on any cutaneous surface but commonly involves the face in a "butterfly lesion" over the nose and cheeks. Recurrent erysipelas in an extremity may lead to chronic lymphedema. Antibiotic therapy will usually halt the progress of the invasive infection, but the erythema disappears more slowly since it is a toxigenic consequence of bacterial invasion.

Infection in soft tissues is of paramount concern to the surgeon, and a variety of superficial infections will be discussed. An *abscess* is a localized collection of pus surrounded by an area of inflamed tissue in which hyperemia and infiltration of leukocytes is marked. A *furuncle*, or boil, is an abscess in a sweat gland or hair follicle. The inflammatory reaction is intense, leading to tissue necrosis and the formation of a central core. This is surrounded by a peripheral zone of cellulitis. An abscess beneath the corium of the skin is a *subepithelial abscess*. *Impetigo* is an acute contagious skin disease characterized by the formation of a series of intraepithelial abscesses. Gangrenous impetigo may occur as a complication in severe chronic debilitating diseases (e.g., chronic ulcerative colitis), and hemolytic streptococci and staphylococci can be cultured from the exudate. The lesions appear as multiple small pustules which extend and coalesce to form large areas of cutaneous gangrene and ulceration. Although management is similar to that of postoperative gangrene, favorable response is proportional to success in overcoming the primary disease.

A *carbuncle* is a multilocular suppurative extension of a furuncle into the subcutaneous tissues. The nape of the neck, dorsum of trunk, hands and digits, and hirsute portions of the chest and abdomen are apt to be involved. Individual compartments in a carbuncle are maintained through persistence of fascial attachments to the skin. As these numerous component locules rupture separately, individual fistulas appear. Most abscesses are caused by pyogenic cocci, usually *Staphylococcus aureus*. However, gram-negative bacilli and streptococci may be found coincidentally. Carbuncles may be more extensive than they appear and should be excised widely to prevent spread and to effect a cure. The wound contracts to a small scar, and a skin graft is not usually required.

The course of a furuncle is often self-limited and may require no specific therapy. However, furuncles can be serious and may become carbuncles. Large furuncles and abscesses should be incised and drained and the patient treated with antibiotics. Abscesses in the "dangerous" nasolabial area of the face bounded by the bridge of the nose and the angles of the mouth may become complicated by septic phlebitis with intracranial extension along the nasal veins to the cavernous sinus. The incidence of septic cavernous sinus thrombosis has declined since the introduction of antibiotics, and this lethal complication is now rare but unfortunately still occurs.

Bacteremia is defined as bacteria in the circulating blood with no indication of toxemia or other clinical manifestations. Bacteremia is usually transient and may last only a few moments, as the reticuloendothelial system localizes and destroys these organisms under favorable conditions. The normal individual probably experiences bacteremia, unknowingly, many times each year. This state follows dental procedures, major traumatic wounds, etc., and may be the means by which apparently isolated infections arise in internal organs, e.g., osteomyelitis, pyelonephritis (descending type), or subacute bacterial endocarditis.

Septicemia is a diffuse infection in which infectious bacteria and their toxins are present in the bloodstream. Septicemia may arise directly from the introduction of infecting organisms into the circulation but, as a rule, is secondary to a focus of infection within the body. The major routes by which bacteria reach the blood are (1) by direct extension and entrance into an open vessel, (2) by release of infected emboli following thrombosis of a blood vessel in an area of inflammation, (3) by discharge of infected lymph into the bloodstream following lymphangitis. Many specific diseases, e.g., typhoid fever and brucellosis, include a septicemic phase. In the absence of systemic disease, beta-hemolytic streptococci (*Streptococcus pyogenes*) are most frequently responsible. Septicemia caused by alpha-hemolytic streptococci (*Streptococcus viridans*) is usually a consequence of subacute bacterial endocarditis. The majority of bacteria that produce suppurative lesions may give rise to secondary septicemia. *Pyemia* is septicemia in which pyogenic microorganisms, most notably *Staphylococcus aureus*, and their toxins are carried in the bloodstream and sequentially initiate multiple focal abscesses in many parts of the body. Before the advent of chemotherapy, staphylococcic pyemia was almost always fatal; the mortality is still high. In *toxemia*, toxins are circulating in the blood, though the microorganism producing the toxin need not be. Toxemia is usually associated with infection by toxin-producing bacteria (e.g., the clostridia of gas gangrene and the diphtheria bacillus), but this is not always so. For example, botulinum toxin and staphylococcal enterotoxin may be ingested directly to cause a profound toxemia without true infection.

PRINCIPLES OF ANTIBIOTIC THERAPY

Basic Considerations

Chemotherapeutic agents act primarily upon the parasite and not upon the host. They include antibiotics and metabolic antagonists such as the sulfonamides. An antibiotic is a chemical compound derived from, or produced by, living organisms and capable, at low concentrations, of inhibiting the life processes of microorganisms. *Bacteriostatic* agents prevent the growth of bacteria but do not destroy them. The defense mechanisms of the body then eliminate the bacteria which are unable to multiply. If the defenses are insufficient or if the bacteriostatic drug is withdrawn prematurely, then the bacterial population will resurge, and the patient will suffer a relapse. *Bactericidal* agents actively kill bacteria and must be employed in patients whose defense mechanisms are impaired or altered by disease or immunosuppressive therapy. The distinction between bactericidal and bacteriostatic effects is sometimes relative to duration of therapy and dosage. Some drugs are bacteriostatic at low concentrations and bactericidal at high concentrations. With most bactericidal drugs, the rate of killing increases with concentration. Antibiotic agents exert their effects in a variety of ways (Table 5-3). They may inhibit the synthesis of the bacterial

Table 5-3. ANTIBIOTICS: MODES OF ACTION

Cellular site of inhibition	Bactericidal	Bacteriostatic
Cell wall synthesis . . .	Penicillins Cephalosporins Vancomycin Bacitracin	
Barrier function of cell membrane. . . .	Polymyxin B Colistin Amphotericin B	Nystatin
Protein synthesis in ribosome	Streptomycin Kanamycin Neomycin Gentamicin	Tetracyclines Chloramphenicol Erythromycin Lincomycin Clindamycin
DNA replication in chromosome	Griseofulvin	

cell wall and consequently interfere with the cell's osmotic defenses, or they may affect the barrier function of the cell membrane and cause loss of vital metabolites. An entirely different mode of action impairs the translation of genetic information and affects protein synthesis. Bacteriostatic drugs affect early stages of protein synthesis in the ribosome and result in an insufficiency, preventing growth and proliferation of bacteria without actually destroying them. However, bactericidal drugs cause the ribosome to miscode and consequently induce the manufacture of defective proteins or enzymes which poison the cell. Replication of deoxyribonucleic acid (DNA) in the chromosome at the level of the assembly of purine nucleotides may be affected by some antibiotics. Although their precise locus of action is not known, these drugs impede the replication of genetic information.

The addition of antibiotics to the armamentarium of the physician has revolutionized the practice of medicine, but has been a double-edged sword. It is pertinent to point out that the surgeon employs antibiotic drugs as adjunctive agents in the treatment of surgical infections, whereas the internist usually employs antibiotics as the primary treatment for medical infections. For the surgeon the aims of antibiotic therapy are much the same as those of surgical therapy, i.e., to control or eradicate bacterial infections acquired before or during hospitalization and to prevent infection from developing postoperatively. To obtain these goals, antibiotic agents are administered (1) systemically by either parenteral or oral routes, (2) preoperatively for preparation of the large intestine (intestinal antisepsis), or (3) locally by (*a*) topical irrigation, (*b*) topical application, (*c*) intraperitoneal, intrapleural, or intrathecal instillation or irrigation, and (*d*) intraluminal instillation into the large intestine. Antibacterial drugs may be administered preoperatively, peroperatively, and postoperatively to prevent infection (prophylaxis) or to treat already established infection.

The fundamental principles governing the use of antibiotics are (1) administration of an agent active against the infecting microorganism, (2) adequate contact between the drug and the infecting microbe, (3) absence of (or minimal) toxic side effects or complications, and (4) utilization of host defenses to augment antibacterial effects of the antibiotic. The specificity of the antibiotic for the infecting microorganism is based upon laboratory identification and antibiotic-sensitivity studies. Clinical judgment is called upon in serious, rapidly developing infections, such as gram-negative shock, to administer antibiotics known to be effective. However, cultures should be taken before antibiotic therapy is initiated, and the antibiotic changed, if necessary, when culture and antibiotic-sensitivity reports are available.

The antibiotic must come in contact with the infecting microorganism. In an acute, diffuse infection, blood flow into the area of infection will usually deliver adequate levels of systemic antibiotic. A spreading cellulitis with lymphangitis and lymphadenitis often responds within 24 hours to an appropriate antibiotic. However, since antibiotics cannot penetrate a thick-walled pyogenic abscess or an infected serous cavity, they should be used in conjunction with drainage of the abscess, debridement of necrotic tissue, and removal of any foreign bodies. These principles apply to every organ of the body. A spreading infection of the meninges responds to chemotherapy, but a brain abscess must be drained; a staphylococcal septicemia is treated by chemotherapy, but a pulp abscess of the fingertip must be drained.

The surgeon must be aware of toxic complications of antibiotics and should be prepared to treat them. Toxic effects range from minor skin rashes, drug fever, and gastrointestinal disturbances to renal tubular necrosis, loss of vision and hearing, irreversible blood dyscrasias, and anaphylactic shock. In addition, alterations in the normal flora of the body may occur in patients receiving prolonged antibiotic therapy. In most cases these changes produce no ill result, but in some the alterations of flora result in the rapid overgrowth of virulent, antibiotic-resistant bacteria which may have been present originally in small numbers (colonization). If the patient's general resistance to infection is depressed, a new infection may follow the antibiotic-induced alteration of flora (superinfection). The term *colonization* indicates an antibiotic-induced quantitative change in the resident microflora of the patient, a common consequence of antimicrobial therapy. There is no clinical evidence of secondary infection, and discontinuance of the antibiotic usually allows the normal flora to become reestablished. However, there is the risk that colonization will lead to superinfection, a clinical event which may be of great danger to the patient. The term *superinfection* usually refers to a new microbial disease induced by antibiotic therapy. Superinfection is most frequent with broad-spectrum antibiotics. Inhibition of the normal flora allows proliferation of species and strains of bacteria not inhibited by the antibiotic. Superinfection is often due to gram-negative bacilli and fungi which are more difficult to eradicate than are gram-positive streptococci and pneumococci. Superinfection may be fatal, usually occurs in elderly patients, and often follows therapy with aminoglycoside antibiotics (e.g., gentamicin and kanamycin) and other broad-spectrum drugs (either alone or in combination with penicillin). Clinical evidence of secondary infection (i.e., a rise in temperature, increased peripheral white blood cell count, and physical signs of a disease not present at the beginning of antibiotic therapy) indicates that colonization has progressed to superinfection. Serial superinfections with different antibiotic-resistant microbial species may occur in the same patient.

Secondary or opportunistic infections may also occur in patients with noninfectious diseases. For example, mycotic infections may develop in patients with lymphoma or leukemia. Deficiencies in host resistance as a result of disease (e.g., diabetes mellitus, hematopoietic disorders, renal failure, liver disease) or as a consequence of therapy with radiation, antimetabolites, or corticosteroids confer the potential for pathogenicity on many ordinary nonpathogenic microorganisms. Indwelling venous or urinary catheters also contribute to lowered host resistance. The term *suprainfection* designates a secondary infection unrelated to antibiotic therapy, and the term *antibiotic-induced suprainfection* describes secondary infections arising during treatment with antimicrobial agents.

Chemoprophylaxis

Prophylactic antibiotics are administered to an uninfected patient who is in jeopardy of acquiring a bacterial infection. There is controversy regarding prophylactic antibiotic therapy because prophylaxis has not been as valuable as therapeutic use. In surgical patients, prophylactic antibiotics are administered to treat contaminated wounds before infection occurs. However, the administration of antibiotic drugs cannot be substituted for sound surgical judgment and good surgical technique. Prophylactic antibiotic therapy has no place in clean operative procedures or in those carrying a minimal risk of sepsis, but it should be considered for traumatic injuries and severe burns and for operations in infected tissues or those associated with heavy contamination (e.g., operations involving the large intestine). An equally beneficial role for chemoprophylaxis is prior to operations on patients especially prone to infection because of malnutrition, impoverished blood supply, or preexisting infection remote from the operative site. The patient undergoing immunosuppressive therapy and/or requiring insertion of a permanent prosthetic device is particularly prone to infection.

Surgical wounds have been designated as "clean," "contaminated," or "dirty" depending upon the presence or absence of prior infection and contact with the interior of the respiratory, urinary, or gastrointestinal tracts. Traumatic wounds are generally grossly contaminated, whereas elective clean surgical procedures may be slightly contaminated during the operative procedure. Infection does not necessarily follow contamination, since host factors as well as microbial factors are involved. However, the greater the contamination, the greater the possibility of consequent infection. Accordingly, in surgery of traumatic wounds or in elective "contaminated" or "dirty" surgery, prophylaxis should be started before the operation so that adequate levels of antibiotic may be obtained in tissue and body fluids during the operative procedure. Bernard and Cole (1964) investigated the use of antibiotics administered

intramuscularly 1 to 2 hours prior to surgery, intravenously during the operation, and postoperatively when the patient was in the recovery room. They found a reduced incidence of postoperative infection (5 percent) with prophylactic treatment compared with administration of a placebo (25 percent). However, a prophylactic antibiotic regimen may not be successful if the drug is not effective against all potential pathogens or if the agent does not come in contact with susceptible pathogens at the site of infection. The antibiotic should be administered parenterally and in sufficient dosage to achieve high circulating blood levels. For treatment of patients with severe trauma, antibiotic therapy should be started prior to operation, as manipulation of wounds causes transient bacteremia.

Intestinal Antisepsis

The protocol for preoperative preparation of the large intestine includes the specific prophylactic use of antibiotics. Bacterial infection following elective colonic surgery results from unavoidable seeding of the wound with contents of the colon. This is manifested by intraabdominal abscesses and anastomotic disruption with resultant peritonitis and fistula formation. The ideal antibiotic agent for preoperative preparation of the colon has rapid bactericidal activity against pathogens in the gastrointestinal tract, minimal absorption, and the absence of undesirable or toxic side effects. The protocol we employ involves a 3-day period of hospitalization during which the patient is placed on a low-residue diet (some surgeons prefer a clear diet), given a cathartic and daily enemas, and administered a suitable chemotherapeutic agent for 72 hours. Although mechanical cleansing alone diminishes the volume of feces and, consequently, the total number of fecal bacteria, the remaining feces contain the usual large numbers of bacteria (on the order of 10^{11} bacteria per gram), and the potential for postoperative infections remains a major hazard. Therefore, although there is no uniform agreement, we feel that antibiotic therapy along with mechanical cleansing is essential for effective preoperative preparation of the large intestine. The antibiotics most frequently employed are kanamycin (1 Gm every hour for 4 hours, and then every 6 hours for a total of 72 hours) and Sulfathalidine-neomycin in combination (every hour for 4 hours, and then every 4 hours for a total of 72 hours). Nichols et al. employ a combination of neomycin and erythromycin base in a three-day cleansing protocol which differs in administering the antibiotic on the third day only. One gram of each is given at 1:00, 2:00, and 11:00 P.M.; the operation is scheduled for 8:00 A.M. Intestinal antisepsis has been shown to reduce the incidence of postoperative complications related to bacteria but does not protect against errors of surgical skill or judgment.

Intraperitoneal Antibiotic Therapy

The most frequent indications for the intraperitoneal instillation of antibiotics are perforated and gangrenous appendicitis, perforated peptic ulcer, gangrenous intestinal obstruction, traumatic perforation of the gastrointestinal tract at any level, intraabdominal abscess, and excessive spillage associated with elective colonic, gastric, or small bowel surgery. Intraperitoneally administered antibiotics may be useful in pelvic inflammatory disease, acute pancreatitis, major intraabdominal vascular procedures, closure of evisceration, and repair of large abdominal incisional hernias. To be effective for routine intraperitoneal instillation, the antibiotic must provide adequate control of endogenous enteric bacteria that may be expected in the peritoneal cavity, with minimal accompanying pain and local or systemic reaction. Since intraperitoneal antibiotics are usually administered to anesthetized patients, the possible synergistic activity of the antibiotic and the anesthetic agent must be considered. This danger may be avoided if the catheter is placed in the peritoneal cavity after the operation, but before the incision is completely closed, and antibiotic instilled after the patient has recovered from anesthesia. Neomycin is safe for intraperitoneal administration only when the dosage is carefully controlled. Clinical success and safety have been achieved with kanamycin and also with cephalothin. Multiple postoperative instillations of kanamycin in patients with peritonitis

reduce the incidence of wound infections and are more effective than a single instillation of the drug. The intraluminal administration of kanamycin into the colon to prevent perforation, slough, and leakage at the anastomosis has been recommended to support a colon anastomosis postoperatively.

ANTIMICROBIAL AGENTS

Antibiotics and chemotherapeutic agents which are currently useful in surgical practice are described briefly in this section. It is important to use an antibiotic agent for a sensitive microorganism and not to treat a particular disease. Precise antimicrobial therapy is based upon the laboratory culture and sensitivity report. Table 5-4 is a guide to the activities of antibiotics against microorganisms commonly involved in surgical infections. Table 5-5 summarizes the routes of administration and doses commonly employed. The selection of antibiotic and dosage for a specific infection depend upon clinical judgment, bacterial sensitivity tests, and awareness of the toxicity of the drug.

Table 5-4. ANTIBIOTICS USEFUL AGAINST MICROORGANISMS IN SURGICAL INFECTIONS

Microorganism	First choice	Alternate agents
Gram-positive cocci:		
Staphylococcus aureus		
Penicillinase-producing	Methicillin	Oxacillin, cloxacillin, cephalothin
Non-penicillinase-producing	Penicillin G	Erythromycin, cephalothin, kanamycin
Streptococcus pyogenes	Penicillin G	Erythromycin, cephalothin
Streptococcus pneumoniae	Penicillin G	Erythromycin, cephalothin
Streptococcus viridans	Penicillin G	Erythromycin, cephalothin
Streptococcus fecalis	Penicillin G + kanamycin	Ampicillin, kanamycin
Peptostreptococcus spp.	Penicillin G	Tetracycline
Gram-negative cocci:		
Neisseria gonorrhoeae	Penicillin G	Erythromycin, cephaloridine, kanamycin
Gram-positive rods:		
Clostridium spp.	Penicillin G	Tetracycline, erythromycin
Gram-negative rods:		
Acinetobacter calcoaceticus	Kanamycin	Gentamicin
Bacteroides fragilis	Clindamycin	Chloramphenicol, erythromycin
Bacteroides spp.	Penicillin G	Clindamycin, chloramphenicol, tetracycline
Escherichia coli	Kanamycin	Ampicillin, gentamicin, cephalothin
Fusobacterium spp.	Penicillin G	Clindamycin, chloramphenicol, tetracycline
Hemophilus influenzae	Ampicillin	Cephalothin, chloramphenicol
Klebsiella-Enterobacter-Serratia group	Gentamicin	Kanamycin, cephalothin, tetracycline
Proteus mirabilis	Ampicillin	Gentamicin, carbenicillin, cephalothin
Proteus spp. (indol-positive)	Kanamycin	Gentamicin, carbenicillin
Providencia spp.	Carbenicillin	Gentamicin, kanamycin
Pseudomonas aeruginosa	Gentamicin ($\pm$ carbenicillin)	Carbenicillin, amikacin, tobramycin
Salmonella spp.	Ampicillin	Chloramphenicol, tetracycline
Actinomycetes:		
Actinomyces israelii	Penicillin G ($\pm$ tetracycline)	Tetracycline, clindamycin, ampicillin
Nocardia spp.	Sulfadiazine (+ streptomycin)	Ampicillin
Fungi:		
Blastomyces dermatitidis	Amphotericin B	2-Hydroxystilbamidine
Candida albicans and other yeasts	Amphotericin B	5-Fluorocytosine, nystatin (oral or topical)
Coccidioides immitis	Amphotericin B	
Cryptococcus neoformans	Amphotericin B	5-Fluorocytosine
Histoplasma capsulatum	Amphotericin B	—
Mucor spp; *Rhizopus* spp; *Aspergillus* spp.	Amphotericin B	—
Paracoccidioides brasiliensis	Amphotericin B	—
Sporotrichum schenckii	Potassium iodide	Amphotericin B

Table 5-5. ROUTES OF ADMINISTRATION AND DAILY DOSAGE OF
ANTIBIOTICS COMMONLY USED IN ADULT SURGICAL PATIENTS

Drug (trade name)	Oral	Dose (grams per day)	
		Intramuscular	Intravenous
Aminoglycosides:			
Amikacin (Amikin)	. . . . .	1–1.5	1–1.5
Gentamicin (Garamycin)	. . . . . .	0.18–0.24	0.18–0.24
Kanamycin (Kantrex)	4–7*	0.5–1	0.5–1
Streptomycin	. . . . . .	1–2	Not recommended
Tobramycin (Nebcin)	. . . . . .	0.21–0.35	0.21–0.35
Cephalosporins:			
Cephalexin (Keflex)	1–4	. . . . .	. . . . .
Cephalothin (Keflin)	. . . . .	2–4	4–12
Cephaloridine (Loridine)	. . . . .	1–2	1–2
Chloramphenicol (Chloromycetin)	. . . . .	Not recommended	2–4
Clindamycin (Cleocin)	. . . . .	1.2–2.4	1.2–2.4
Erythromycin (Erythrocin)	1–2	0.2–0.6	1–4
Penicillin:			
Ampicillin (Amcill, Omnipen, Penbritin, Polycillin, Principen)	1–2	2–8	2–8
Carbenicillin (Geopen)	. . . . .	8–12	20–40
Cloxacillin (Tegopen)	4–6	. . . . .	. . . . .
Dicloxacillin (Dynapen, Pathocil, Veracillin)	2–3	. . . . .	. . . . .
Methicillin (Celbenin, Staphcillin)	. . . . .	4–6	4–24
Nafcillin (Nafcil, Unipen)	2–6	2–6	4–24
Oxacillin (Bactocill, Prostaphlin)	2–6	2–6	4–24
Penicillin G, potassium or sodium	0.5–2 million units/day	2–12 million units/day	4–20 million units/day
Tetracyclines:			
Doxycycline (Vibramycin)	0.1–0.2	. . . . .	. . . . .
Oxytetracycline (Terramycin)	1–2	0.2–0.8	1–2
Tetracycline (Achromycin, Panmycin, Sumycin, Tetracyn, Tetrex) . . .	1–2	0.2–0.8	1–2

*Intestinal antisepsis only.

The white blood cell count is important in evaluating the response to antibiotic treatment and the appearance of adverse reactions in patients with infections. Individual drugs will be considered in terms of mechanism of antimicrobial action, absorption, distribution, metabolic fate, excretion, toxicity, and indications for use.

Antibiotics Active against Gram-positive Microorganisms

Penicillin G (benzyl penicillin) is active against almost all gram-positive pathogens. If necessary, very large doses can be given to combat infections by bacterial species which may be moderately resistant. Penicillin is bactericidal for susceptible bacteria; it blocks the synthesis of bacterial cell walls. Penicillin G is well absorbed but is not suitable for oral administration, because it is destroyed by gastric acidity. Therefore, it is injected intramuscularly or intravenously and becomes distributed throughout the body within a few minutes following injection. Excretion is mainly by the renal tubules. Hypersensitivity to penicillin is an important problem; it is usually manifested as urticaria, but almost any type of allergic response may develop. Anaphylactic reactions may occur in the highly sensitized patient within minutes after an injection and will require subcutaneous epinephrine. Penicillin G is recom-

mended (provided hypersensitivity does not exist) for severe infections produced by beta-hemolytic streptococci, enterococci, pneumococci, gonococci, meningococci, clostridia, actinomycetes, and treponemata.

Penicillin V (phenoxymethyl penicillin) is a natural penicillin obtained when phenoxyacetic acid is the precursor during fermentation. It is acid-stable and may be administered orally. Penicillin V is more active than penicillin G against resistant staphylococci because it is more slowly destroyed by penicillinase; it is slightly less active against streptococci. Penicillin V is not indicated for infections involving the respiratory tract or the urinary tract.

The natural penicillins have been superseded by several semisynthetic penicillins prepared by adding side chains to the 6-aminopenicillanic acid nucleus. The semisynthetic penicillins combine one or more of the following advantages: (1) they are acid-resistant and suitable for oral use; (2) they exert prolonged action in the body; (3) they are resistant to penicillinase produced by *Staphylococcus aureus* and some gram-negative bacilli; and (4) they are active against gram-negative bacteria.

Methicillin (Staphcillin) is sensitive to acid but resistant to staphylococcal penicillinase. It must be administered parenterally, and it is rapidly excreted by the renal tubules. Methicillin is inactivated by penicillinase 100 times more slowly than is penicillin G but has only one-tenth the potency of penicillin G. Methicillin is also the preferred parenteral semisynthetic penicillin against streptococci, pneumococci, and gram-negative bacteria.

Oxacillin, cloxacillin, and *dicloxacillin* are semisynthetic isoxazolyl penicillins combining resistance to penicillinase with resistance to acid. They can be administered orally and are effective against streptococcal infections complicated by the presence of penicillinase-producing staphylococci. *Nafcillin* is also resistant to penicillinase and to acid. It may be used either orally or parenterally, but relatively low blood levels are obtained due to inactivation in the liver.

These penicillinase-resistant penicillins are effective, specific agents for treatment of serious staphylococcal infections, such as pneumonia, septicemia, wound infection, and infections occurring as a consequence of malignant diseases or cardiac, hepatic, or renal disease. Although methicillin has the lowest activity against staphylococci, 60 percent of the dose is free in the blood. On the other hand, the acid-resistant penicillins have higher antibacterial activity, but only 5 percent is free. Accordingly, adequate doses of any one of these penicillins will achieve similar effects, and initial treatment of a severe staphylococcal infection should always be with one of these penicillins (unless the staphylococcus has been shown to be sensitive to penicillin G). Concomitant administration of probenecid, which partially blocks tubular excretion of penicillins, may be used to double blood levels.

Cephalothin is one of a group of exceedingly useful antibiotics known as the cephalosporins, which are structually similar to the penicillins and may be used as alternative agents for therapy in patients allergic to penicillin. However, they are often given in excessively high doses for prolonged periods. Their use is unwarranted in infections which can be readily treated with less expensive agents (e.g., penicillin for pneumococcal pneumonia) and in surgical prophylaxis. Cephalothin is effective against staphylococci, streptococci (except enterococci), and pneumococci. Most strains of *Escherichia coli, Proteus mirabilis,* and *Klebsiella* species are susceptible. *Enterobacter aerogenes, Pseudomonas aeruginosa, Hemophilus influenzae,* and group D streptococci (enterococci) are resistant. Cephalosporin antibiotics, like the penicillins, are bactericidal and inhibit the synthesis of bacterial cell walls. Cephalothin must be administered parenterally, as it is not absorbed orally. Excretion is by the renal tubules. Intramuscular injections may be painful, and frequent injections are required if adequate levels of antibiotic are to be maintained. Phlebitis occurs with intravenous use; rashes are sometimes produced. Cephalothin may be administered to patients who are allergic to penicillin without danger of cross reaction, but sensitization to cephalothin itself may occur. The antibiotic is active against penicillin-resistant staphylococci. However, antibiotic-induced suprainfection with gram-negative bacilli or fungi can occur if indiscriminately large doses are used for 1 to 3 weeks. Cephalothin has a broader spectrum than ampicillin and is useful in treating urinary tract infections caused by sensitive enterobacteria.

Cephaloridine is a derivative similar to cephalothin both in its properties and indications for use. It is more stable in the body and is cleared more slowly. Renal toxicity has been encountered following large doses. Although it is not effective orally, there is little or no pain when it is injected intramuscularly. Cephaloridine is not a substitute for cephalothin, since staphylococci are not uniformly susceptible. Antibiotic-induced suprainfections have occurred.

Cephalexin is a semisynthetic cephalosporin which is almost completely absorbed after oral administration. Food delays absorption. Cephalexin is excreted in urine by glomerular filtration and tubular secretion. High urinary concentrations are obtained. Some cephalexin is excreted in the bile of patients with normal gallbladders. Diarrhea, vomiting, cramps, and hypersensitivity reactions have been observed. Cephalexin has been used for urinary tract infections due to *Escherichia coli, Proteus mirabilis,* and *Klebsiella* species. It appears to be about as effective as ampicillin for these infections. However, use of any cephalosporin as the sole drug in treating gram-negative sepsis without in vitro evidence of susceptibility is not good practice.

Vancomycin is active against gram-positive organisms only, and it is of clinical importance against staphylococci and streptococci. Microorganisms sensitive to vancomycin do not acquire resistance. The antibiotic is bactericidal; it inhibits the incorporation of amino acids into the bacterial cell wall and suppresses the growth of protoplasts. Vancomycin is not absorbed from the alimentary tract and is administered intravenously; intramuscular injections cause pain and necrosis. The antibiotic becomes widely distributed, but little is found in bile or spinal fluid. Excretion is by glomerular filtration, but this is delayed in patients with impaired renal function. Because of serious ototoxicity and nephrotoxicity, vancomycin should not be used in patients with renal insufficiency or in patients who have significant hearing loss. Antibiotic-induced suprainfections with fungi and gram-negative bacteria may appear during treatment. Thrombophlebitis, fever, and rashes occur. Vancomycin is now regarded as a reserve drug which may be valuable for the treatment of serious staphylococcal or streptococcal disease in patients allergic or nonresponsive to other antibiotics (penicillin G, methicillin, cephalothin).

Erythromycin is active against pneumococci, betahemolytic streptococci, enterococci, many staphylococci, gonococci (although less effective as an alternative agent than tetracycline), and clostridia. Erythromycin is bacteriostatic but may be bactericidal in high concentrations, inhibiting bacterial protein synthesis. Erythromycin may be administered orally or intravenously. Most strains of *Bacteroides* can be inhibited by the high levels of erythromycin attained in serum after parenteral injection. The antibiotic is uniformly distributed throughout the body and is excreted in the urine and bile. However, the major portion of the drug is broken down in the body. Erythromycin base is generally well tolerated but may cause some gastrointestinal disturbance (nausea, vomiting, diarrhea, flatulence). Erythromycin estolate (the propionyl ester) can produce hepatic disease during prolonged administration. For this reason the plain erythromycin base is recommended. Erythromycin may be used as an alternative to penicillin for hemolytic streptococcal, staphylococcal, or pneumococcal infections in patients allergic to penicillin and for elimination of *Corynebacterium diphtheriae* from the pharynx of carriers. Bacterial resistance to erythromycin is common during long-term treatment.

Lincomycin resembles erythromycin in its antibacterial activity against staphylococci, hemolytic streptococci, and pneumococci. Bacteroides and anaerobic cocci are also sensitive. Enterobacteria and enterococci are resistant. Lincomycin is bacteriostatic; it inhibits protein synthesis. The antibiotic is absorbed from the gastrointestinal tract, but food delays absorption. The drug may also be administered intramuscularly and intravenously; it becomes widely distributed, and significant levels occur in tissues and fluids. Therapeutic levels of lincomycin are found in bone. Excretion is primarily biliary; urine levels are low. Diarrhea and pseudomembranous colitis have been reported as adverse reactions to this antibiotic. Lincomycin is recommended for the treatment of both acute and chronic osteomyelitis. Although the antibiotic is effective against severe staphylococcal and streptococcal infections, these diseases are readily treated with semisynthetic penicillins. Lincomycin resistance is easily induced, and the antibiotic has cross resistance with erythromycin.

Clindamycin is a synthetically modified lincomycin (7-chloro-7-deoxylincomycin-HCl hydrate) which is more thoroughly absorbed and produces higher blood levels. Diarrhea and pseudomembranous colitis have been reported as adverse reactions to this antibiotic. Clindamycin is also more active against staphylococci and pneumococci and equally active against other species susceptible to lincomycin. The lincosamines (*lincomycin* and *clindamycin*) are, however, no more effective than the penicillins or erythromycin for treatment of infections caused by gram-positive aerobes or *Clostridium* species. They are second-line agents for treatment of staphylococcal infections (except chronic osteomyelitis), since they appear to be as effective as the penicillinase-resistant penicillins and cephalosporins. In staphylococcal infections their use should be limited primarily to patients allergic to the preferred drugs. Use of vancomycin should also be considered in serious staphylococcal infections. The lincosamines can sometimes produce an illness with features indistinguishable from idiopathic ulcerative colitis. However, lincomycin and clindamycin are especially effective in the treatment of abdominal and pelvic infections due to *Bacteroides fragilis*.

Bacitracin is a polypeptide antibiotic active against gram-positive bacteria and pathogenic *Neisseria* species, but inactive against common gram-negative bacilli. It is bactericidal, and inhibits bacterial cell wall synthesis by binding to the cell membrane. Therefore, unlike penicillin, bacitracin is active against protoplasts. The antibiotic is not absorbed orally or by the skin. After intramuscular injection, which causes painful infiltrates at the site of injection, much of the antibiotic is bound by tissues so that systemic absorption is limited. Bacitracin does not cross the blood-brain barrier. It is excreted by the kidneys, and glomerular and tublar damage may occur. Bacitracin has no place in the systemic treatment of clinical infections, but it is useful for irrigating wounds, infected joints, or abscess cavities. It is used topically with neomycin and polymyxin in treating superficial infections of the skin, infected wounds, and suppurative conjunctivitis.

Antibiotics Active against Some Gram-positive or Some Gram-negative Microorganisms or Both

Ampicillin is a semisynthetic penicillin which is slightly less active than benzyl penicillin against most gram-positive bacteria, is slightly more active against enterococci, and is destroyed by penicillinase. It is not indicated for staphylococcal infections. Ampicillin is recommended for the treatment of gram-negative infections due to *Escherichia coli, Proteus mirabilis,* and *Salmonella* and *Shigella* species. It is bactericidal and well absorbed when administered orally. Excretion is mainly renal, although some biliary excretion occurs. The toxicity of ampicillin is similar to that of penicillin G, but macular rashes are more frequent.

Carbenicillin is a semisynthetic, bactericidal penicillin; it may be used parenterally or orally. It is active against *Pseudomonas aeruginosa,* all species of *Proteus,* and some other enterobacteria, but it is inferior to benzyl penicillin against gram-positive bacteria. Synergism with gentamicin has been demonstrated, and combination therapy has been recommended because *Pseudomonas aeruginosa* may become resistant during treatment with carbenicillin alone. Carbenicillin is one of the few drugs effective for the treatment of systemic *Pseudomonas* infections. Very large doses for prolonged periods are required. Probenecid elevates serum levels twofold to fourfold and is a useful adjunct to therapy.

Polymyxin B and *colistin* (polymyxin E) are basic polypeptide antibiotics having similar structure and antibacterial activity. Most species of gram-negative bacilli are sensitive to polymyxin. The exceptions are *Proteus* species, and *Neisseria* species. All species of gram-positive bacteria and fungi are resistant. Both these antibiotics are bactericidal and disrupt the cell membranes of susceptible bacteria. They are not absorbed from the alimentary tract but are well absorbed following intramuscular injection. The polymyxins are nephrotoxic in the presence of renal disease and may be associated with respiratory arrest. Polymyxin B was formerly recommended for pseudomonal meningitis and pseudomonal endocarditis and was also useful in treating infection by most strains of *Escherichia coli* and *Klebsiella-Enterobacter*. Colistin was formerly recommended for treatment of systemic pseudomonal infections and for the same infections as those responsive to polymyxin. The introduction of broad-spectrum penicillins, cephalosporins, and aminoglycosides has, however, lessened the importance of polymyxins. In particular, the availability of gentamicin and carbenicillin, either separately or in combination, for the treatment of pseudomonal infections has practically eliminated the need for polymyxins in clinical medicine.

Chloramphenicol is a broad-spectrum antibiotic; it is bacteriostatic and inhibits protein synthesis by interfering with messenger ribonucleic acid (mRNA). It is well absorbed orally and parenterally. Excretion is mainly renal;

about 90 percent can be detected in urine as an inactive conjugate with glucuronic acid; only about 10 percent appears as active antibiotic. Two different lethal toxic effects are known: First, a rare total aplasia of the bone marrow with aplastic anemia may occur during treatment or as long as 4 months afterward. Second, because of deficiency in detoxifying enzymes, premature infants may accumulate sufficient free chloramphenicol to cause an acute and usually fatal circulatory collapse (gray syndrome). Minor toxic effects include soreness of the mouth from overgrowth of *Candida albicans* resulting from depression of normal flora due to antibiotic in the saliva, and optic neuritis in children with cystic fibrosis of the pancreas receiving treatment with chloramphenicol for pulmonary infection. Chloramphenicol should not be used for trivial infections or as a prophylactic agent to prevent bacterial infection. It is effective for typhoid fever and other severe *Salmonella* infections, but since most *Salmonella* infections will respond to ampicillin, chloramphenicol should be used only if the patient does not respond to ampicillin or is allergic to it. Chloramphenicol is recommended for patients who cannot tolerate tetracyclines and for those who have rickettsial disease, psittacosis, or lymphopathia venereum. It can be a life-saving drug in the treatment of patients with meningitis when penicillin cannot be administered. Chloramphenicol is the drug of choice in *Bacteroides* sepsis, in treatment of typhoid fever, and in severe infections such as *Hemophilus influenzae* in patients allergic to penicillin. Prolonged usage and repeated exposure should be avoided. Leukocyte counts with a differential should be taken daily, and therapy should be discontinued if leukopenia occurs.

The aminoglycosides include streptomycin, neomycin, paromomycin, kanamycin, gentamicin, tobramycin, and amikacin. They possess a wide range of bactericidal activity against gram-negative and gram-positive bacteria and mycobacteria. Bacteria acquire resistance to aminoglycosides slowly. There is little absorption from the alimentary tract and fairly slow renal excretion in unchanged form after intramuscular injection. This affords therapeutic levels for 6 to 8 hours. Aminoglycosides exhibit a high degree of mutual cross resistance, a strong dose-related tendency to damage the auditory branch of the eighth nerve, and some possibility of damage to the kidney.

Streptomycin is bactericidal and particularly active against *Mycobacterium tuberculosis,* gram-negative bacilli, and some strains of *Staphylococcus aureus.* However, the introduction of other aminoglycosides has relegated streptomycin to a minor role in the treatment of infections by gram-negative and gram-positive bacteria. Bactericidal effects usually occur during the phase of multiplication. There is damage to the cell membrane and also interference with protein synthesis by disorganizing the proper attachments of mRNA to ribosomes. Streptomycin usually is administered intramuscularly for systemic treatment. It is completely absorbed following parenteral injection, but it is absorbed poorly from the intestinal tract. Streptomycin is rapidly excreted in the urine. Streptomycin combined with isoniazid and p-aminosalicylic acid is indicated for the treatment of tuberculosis. Streptomycin with sulfadiazine is used to treat nocardiosis.

Neomycin is bactericidal; it is active against gram-negative enteric bacteria, some strains of staphylococci, and mycobacteria, but has limited usefulness because of its toxicity. Its major use is in ointments and solutions for topical application although skin sensitivity may occur. Following oral therapy, neomycin-resistant staphylococci are often found in the stool, and enteritis or even pseudomembranous enterocolitis may result. Neomycin inhibits absorption of oral penicillin V and has caused malabsorption of fat (with or without diarrhea). There is considerable risk of ototoxicity and nephrotoxicity when neomycin is given parenterally. Neomycin is used in treating patients with cirrhosis who have elevated levels of ammonia, and it is used in combination with other agents, such as sulfathalidine, bacitracin, erythromycin, or polymyxin B, for intestinal antisepsis prior to abdominal surgery. *Paromomycin* is similar to neomycin and kanamycin but generally administered orally. The main difference between paromomycin and other aminoglycosides is its direct activity against *Entamoeba histolytica.*

Kanamycin is bactericidal. It is rapidly absorbed after intramuscular injection and acts like streptomycin with regard to blood levels, distribution, and excretion. It is necessary to limit the dose in accordance with renal function; the length of treatment should be limited to 7 to 10 days. Kanamycin is the drug of choice in the management of septicemias due to gram-negative bacilli and is recognized as a second-line drug for treatment of tuberculosis in patients whose infecting mycobacteria are resistant to primary antituberculous drugs. Kanamycin is not absorbed from the gastrointestinal tract and can be used for preoperative intestinal antisepsis. Ototoxicity may occur; it is related to duration of therapy, blood level, and dosage greater than 15 mg/kg body weight/day. However, in patients with meningitis or other serious infections, temporary increases above this level may be necessary. Kanamycin continues to be valuable for the treatment of infections due to *Escherichia coli, Proteus* species, and some strains of the *Klebsiella-Enterobacter-Serratia* group.

Gentamicin is another bactericidal aminoglycoside. It is administered by intramuscular injection but is not absorbed orally. It is well-distributed in most highly vascular organs, and excretion is mainly renal. Gentamicin may exhibit nephrotoxicity and ototoxicity (affecting both vestibular and auditory branches of the eighth nerve), particularly in patients with any impairment of renal function. It should not be administered with streptomycin, kanamycin, colistin, polymyxin B, or vancomycin, as additional toxicity may result. Gentamicin is useful in treating bacteremia and severe soft tissue infections due to *Escherichia coli, Serratia marcescens,* and many *Proteus* species (but not *Proteus vulgaris*), and it is most effective in treatment of infections due to *Pseudomonas aeruginosa.* However, it is not recommended as an initial therapy of severe infections of unknown cause, because many gram-negative bacteria are resistant.

Tobramycin is virtually identical with gentamicin. *Amikacin* is a semisynthetic aminoglycoside derived from kanamycin and possesses attributes of both kanamycin and gentamicin. Parenteral aminoglycosides are among the most valuable agents available for the treatment of life-threatening infections by enteric gram-negative bacteria. Because of the emergence of resistant strains of *Pseudomonas, Proteus rettgeri, Providencia,* and *Serratia,* hospitals should select a single aminoglycoside antibiotic for primary use and hold the others in reserve for use against infections caused by resistant bacteria. The tetracyclines are a family of closely related antibiotics. Those now widely used are *tetracycline, oxytetracycline,* and *doxycycline.* There is no good evidence that tetracycline has any advantage over oxytetracycline in the treatment of disease or in the production of fewer side effects in the adult. Doxycycline possesses the advantage, because of its slower excretion, of requiring only one dose daily. Members of this group are broad-spectrum and active against those gram-positive species which are also sensitive to penicillin, against many gram-negative species which are not sensitive to penicillin, against *Treponema pallidum* and other treponemata, and against *Mycobacterium tuberculosis.* They also inhibit the growth of actinomycetes, rickettsiae, mycoplasma, and agents of the psittacosis–lymphogranuloma venerum–trachoma group of *Chlamydia.* The tetracyclines are bacteriostatic. They interfere with protein synthesis by inhibiting amino acid transfer from RNA to microsomal protein. Resistance may be due to decreased permeability to the antibiotic. A microorganism resistant to one tetracycline is equally resistant to the others. Tetracyclines are usually administered orally; they become distributed throughout the body and appear to have affinity for fast-growing tissues, such as liver, tumors, and new bone. They are slowly filtered by the renal glomeruli and are excreted in the urine unchanged. Some biliary excretion occurs. Tetracyclines are deposited in teeth during early stages of calcification, causing a yellow to brownish discoloration which is undesirable cosmetically. Therefore, tetracycline treatment should be avoided in early childhood except for imperative reasons or unless a short course will suffice. Liver damage has resulted from excessive doses. Replacement of suppressed normal flora by tetracycline-resistant microorganisms (antibiotic-induced suprainfection) causes gastrointestinal disturbance such as nausea, vomiting, diarrhea, and flatulence. Suprainfection with *Candida albicans* may produce soreness of the mouth and even thrush, which may spread to the pharynx and bronchi, or diarrhea and pruritus ani. Suprainfection with *Proteus* and *Pseudomonas* species resistant to tetracycline commonly produces diarrhea. Suprainfection with *Staphylococcus aureus* may produce a fatal staphylococcal enterocolitis. Tetracycline is effective against 50 percent of strains of *Bacteroides.* Tetracycline with penicillin is recommended for actinomycosis and, with sulfadiazine, for nocardiosis. If penicillin cannot be used, tetracycline is recommended for treatment of gonorrhea and syphilis.

Antifungal Antibiotics

Nystatin is effective in the treatment of candidosis. It is fungistatic and damages the fungal cell membrane by binding to sterol sites in it. The antibiotic is not absorbed from the gastrointestinal tract, skin, or mucosal surfaces. It is used to treat gastrointestinal candidosis, which may result as a complication of therapy with broad-spectrum antibiotics. Such antibiotic-induced suprainfection often disappears with discontinuance of the antibacterial therapy which provoked it. Nystatin is available in topical powders, creams, and ointments which may be useful in treating cutaneous and mucocutaneous candidosis. Nystatin tablets may be sucked for candida stomatitis; vaginal tablets are available for treatment of vaginal candidosis. Nystatin is harmless by local application. There have been rare cases of diarrhea, nausea, and vomiting after administration of large oral doses.

Griseofulvin has its greatest activity against dermatophytes and is useful in treating superficial dermatomycoses of skin, hair, or nails due to species of *Microsporum, Epidermophyton,* and *Trichophyton.* Griseofulvin is fungicidal, impairs synthesis of nucleic acids and protein, and breaks down intracellular membranes of dermatophytes but not of fungi causing systemic mycoses. The antibiotic is administered orally, and it is incorporated into liver, fat, keratin, and skeletal muscle. The antibiotic is well tolerated even during long courses of treatment, and toxic effects (skin reactions, gastric discomfort, and neurologic reactions) are uncommon and rarely severe. Griseofulvin has value in the systemic treatment of chronic fungal infection of the nails and hair. Cultures are needed to determine that skin lesions are not due to *Candida* or bacteria, as these are not improved by griseofulvin and may be exacerbated by the antibiotic.

Amphotericin B is the only antifungal antibiotic effective in the treatment of systemic mycotic infections. It binds to sterols, specifically ergosterol, and interferes with the permeability of the fungal cell wall. Amphotericin B is the drug of choice for treatment of systemic candidosis, mucormycosis, disseminated active histoplasmosis, cryptococcosis, coccidioidomycosis, and pulmonary sporotrichosis. Amphotericin is not appreciably absorbed from the gastrointestinal tract or the skin; it is administered intravenously or intrathecally, or instilled directly into the site of infection. Initial toxic effects commonly include fever, chills, nausea, vomiting, and headache. Toxic effects brought on by continued usage may include anemia, thrombophlebitis at the site of injection, hypokalemia, rise of blood urea and serum creatinine levels, and permanent damage to the kidney.

5-Fluorocytosine is a halogenated pyrimidine inhibiting nucleic acid synthesis in fungi; it is not metabolized by mammalian cells. This compound is effective in systemic cryptococcosis and candidosis and has been used after failure of therapy with amphotericin.

Sulfonamides

Introduced in 1935, the sulfonamides initiated the modern antibacterial chemotherapeutic revolution in medicine. Their use antedates that of the antibiotics by several years, since penicillin did not become available until 1941. The sulfonamides are valuable agents in the management of some infections, particularly urinary tract infections due to *Escherichia coli,* and can be employed for the prophylaxis of recurrences of rheumatic fever. Although one of these compounds, mafenide acetate (Sulfamylon), has an important use in the topical therapy of severe burn wounds, the value of the sulfonamides in the treatment of surgical infections is severely limited by their inactivation by pus. The sulfonamides are bacteriostatic and active against both gram-positive and gram-negative bacteria. The drugs are strongly antagonized by *p*-aminobenzoic acid (PABA), an essential intermediate in the synthesis of folic acid by bacterial cells, and act as competitive inhibitors. Bacteria sensitive to the sulfonamides are unable to utilize preformed folic acid in the body and must synthesize it themselves. Folic acid acts as a coenzyme in the transfer of fragments containing one carbon atom, which are involved in the synthesis of amino acids (such as methionine and serine), purine, and thymine. These compounds also inhibit the activity of sulfonamides, but unlike PABA they are noncompetitive inhibitors, and their effect is not reversed by increasing the concentration of drugs. Accordingly, pus, which is rich in amino acids and purines made available by the breakdown of cellular protein and nucleic acids, inactivates the sulfonamides.

Some of the sulfonamides of use in surgical practice are sulfadiazine, which is the preparation of choice in treating nocardiosis; phthalylsulfathiazole (Sulfathalidine), which is poorly absorbed from the gastrointestinal tract and is used in combination with neomycin for preoperative preparation of the large intestine; sulfisoxazole (Gantrisin) and sulfamethoxazole (Gantanol), which are used for treating urinary tract infections; and mafenide (Sulfamylon), which is applied topically and used to treat burn wound infections. Mafenide is not inhibited by the products of tissue necrosis but causes pain. Of comparable value in the treatment of burns is the silver salt of sulfadiazine (Silvadene), which does not cause pain on application and is free of major toxicity.

Except for nonabsorbable sulfonamides, orally administered sulfonamides are rapidly absorbed in the stomach and duodenum and become distributed in all tissues and fluids. The sulfonamides are bound to either serum albumin or to tissue proteins, and they are detoxified in the liver. Both the drug and its less active metabolites are excreted by glomerular filtration. Sensitivity to one sulfonamide frequently confers sensitivity to others. Toxic reactions limiting sulfonamide therapy range from nausea, vomiting, and dermatitis to crystalluria, renal injury, hepatic damage, and hematologic disorders.

STREPTOCOCCAL INFECTIONS

Streptococci form the dominant aerobic flora of the mouth and pharyngeal areas of man. They are gram-positive spherical or ovoid cells (rarely elongated into rods) arranged in pairs (short chains). Long chains are observed when the organism is cultured in fluid media. Although most species are aerobic or facultatively anaerobic, there are also species which are obligately anaerobic (e.g., *Peptostreptococcus putridus* and *Peptostreptococcus micros*) or microaerophilic. They may be divided into those which

produce a soluble hemolysin and those which do not. Aerobes producing a clear zone of hemolysis on blood agar (beta hemolysis) include most of the species associated with primary streptococcal infections in man and can be subdivided into 15 broad groups (Lancefield groups) which are identified by precipitin tests with group-specific antisera against specific carbohydrate haptens (C antigens) of the streptococci. Strains belonging to Lancefield group A (*Streptococcus pyogenes*) are responsible for over 90 percent of human streptococcal infections. These group A strains can be further subdivided for epidemiologic studies into Griffith types according to their surface protein antigens (M, T, and R) by capillary precipitin or slide agglutination tests.

Another group of streptococci produce an ill-defined zone of partial hemolysis having a green or brownish-green color (alpha hemolysis). These are strains of *Streptococcus viridans*. Streptococci which are without effect on blood agar (nonhemolytic) include the fecal enterococci (*Streptococcus fecalis*). Viridans and nonhemolytic streptococci are associated with chronic diseases or are nonpathogenic. *Streptococcus viridans* is part of the commensal flora of the mouth and throat and is dangerous in individuals with congenitally deformed or rheumatically damaged heart valves. It is the commonest cause of subacute bacterial endocarditis. *Streptococcus viridans* has been incriminated in apical tooth infections and is commonly found in carious teeth. Bacteremia frequently follows tooth extraction and even routine dental procedures. In otherwise healthy individuals the streptococci are rapidly removed from the circulation, but in those with heart lesions the organisms settle in or on the defective valves. Accordingly, patients with congenital or other valvular cardiac defects should be given penicillin prophylactically before and after any dental attention.

Nonhemolytic streptococci are always present in the colon and may be isolated from the terminal ileum and upper jejunum of 60 percent of surgical patients. These enterococci (*Streptococcus fecalis*) can cause suppurative lesions and urinary tract infections. In our hospital, enterococci are isolated from 12 percent of surgical wound infections and from 8 percent of urinary tract infections. Some strains of *Streptococcus fecalis* produce a true beta hemolysis; they belong to Lancefield group D.

Group A beta-hemolytic streptococci (*Streptococcus pyogenes*) are the principal causes of streptococcal pharyngitis, scarlet fever, and rheumatic fever. They also cause bacteremias following surgical procedures in patients with malignant disease. Groups B, C, D, F, and G are usually less virulent. Although group B streptococci are often isolated from patients with puerperal sepsis, with meningitis of the newborn, with diabetes mellitus, and/or with peripheral vascular insufficiency, they are also involved in pneumonias and infections of the male genitourinary tract. Since group C streptococci are part of the skin flora, they may be isolated from wounds and exudates more often than group B strains. The group G streptococci involved in infections usually originate in the genitourinary tract or skin, but they may also originate in the upper respiratory tract or gastrointestinal tract. We find streptococci in

4 percent of surgical wound infections and in 6 percent of nosocomial respiratory tract infections.

Streptococcus pyogenes is an invasive microorganism; it secretes two distinct hemolysins (streptolysins O and S) and several other products which aid in invasion. Streptolysin O is cardiotoxic and leukocidic and may be identical with leukocidin. Streptolysin S is a pure hemolysin responsible for beta hemolysis on blood agar plates. Hyaluronidase hydrolyzes hyaluronic acid and allows increased permeability of tissues. Streptokinase reduces fibrinolysis by activating the plasmin system. Streptodornase depolymerizes DNA. Erythrogenic toxin produces erythema when injected intradermally and is responsible for the punctate erythema of scarlet fever. The hyaluronidase and streptokinase produced by most strains of *Streptococcus pyogenes* are responsible for the spreading cellulitis (erysipelas) which is the typical streptococcal lesion. When abscess occurs, the pus is watery and often blood-stained due to the action of streptodornase and streptokinase, since the viscosity of pus is due to DNA and fibrin.

Erysipelas

Erysipelas is a spreading streptococcal cellulitis and lymphangitis with raised, sharply defined, irregular, reddish borders. The classic lesion of erysipelas is a "butterfly" erythema centered around the nose and extending onto both cheeks. Since erythrogenic toxin is produced in variable amounts by hemolytic streptococci, the development of cutaneous erythema is an inconstant manifestation of streptococcal infection. Minor skin abrasions and fissures predispose to these infections of the skin. The cutis is edematous and reddened, with a palpably raised border; the lesion is hot, tender, and painful. The systemic manifestations of erisipelas may be severe and suggest invasion via the lymphatics or bloodstream. Penicillin is usually effective against the invasive infection, but the erythema disappears more slowly.

Erysipeloid, a nonstreptococcal disease distinct from erysipelas, is a type of cutaneous cellulitis. Erysipeloid often is contracted after contamination of a cutaneous abrasion of the hand, particularly the fingers. The typical lesion is a violaceous nodule, often having a curved shape, which differs from that of erysipelas by its tendency to central clearing and the absence of suppuration. Human cases of erysipeloid may also occur as either a severe, generalized cutaneous disease or as septicemia with or without cutaneous involvement and often associated with endocarditis. Penicillin therapy is specific for most cases. Erysipeloid is due to infection by *Erysipelothrix rhusopathiae*, a grampositive, nonsporulating, facultative anaerobe in the family Corynebacteriaceae. Erysipelothrix infection is considered an occupational disease of abattoir workers, fish handlers, and others exposed to meat, poultry, and fish products.

Necrotizing Fasciitis

This is a life-threatening infection which may occur in only one or two patients a year in large city-county hospitals. The most significant manifestation of the infection is extensive necrosis of the superficial fascia with resultant widespread undermining of surrounding tissue and extreme systemic toxicity. The bacteria involved in about 90 percent of cases have usually been beta-hemolytic streptococci, coagulase-positive staphylococci, or both. Gramnegative enteric pathogens alone have been associated with about 10 percent of cases of necrotizing fasciitis. The disease appears to be a clinical entity and not a specific bacterial infection. It has been described previously as hemolytic or acute streptococcal gangrene, gangrenous or necrotizing erysipelas, suppurative fasciitis, and hospital gangrene. Although necrotizing fasciitis may develop following surgical procedures such as appendectomy, the majority of cases have occurred outside the hospital following minor trauma such as abrasions, cuts, bruises, boils, and insect bites on the extremities, particularly in individuals with diabetes and peripheral vascular disease. The chief diagnostic criterion for necrotizing fasciitis is superficial and widespread fascial necrosis. Cellulitis as well as edema (mild to massive) are present in most patients. The involved skin is pale red without distinct borders and with blisters or bullae. Pale red areas progress to a distinct purple. The diagnosis is confirmed by observation of (1) serosanguinous exudate; (2) swollen, stringy, dull gray, necrotic fascia with extensive undermining; and (3) a gram-stained smear of the pus or fluid.

TREATMENT. This consists of multiple linear incisions over the affected area. In an open wound, the extent of undermining can be ascertained by passing a sterile hemostat along the plane just superficial to the deep fascia. In simple cellulitis or erysipelas, the hemostat cannot be passed. Before operation, the patient should be given a full dose of systemic antibiotic(s) effective against both hemolytic streptococci and penicillinase-producing staphylococci. Therapy is continued postoperatively until the infection is controlled. Repeated debridement may be necessary if the patient continues to be febrile. With the appearance of clean granulation tissue after 5 to 10 days, the wound may be closed by skin graft or suture. Rea and Wyrick (1970) report a 30 percent mortality.

Peptostreptococci (anaerobic streptococci) are also pathogenic. They are normal inhabitants of the mouth, intestine, and vagina. They are abundant in the presence of poor oral hygiene, and aspiration into the lungs and sinuses may lead to putrid lung abscess, empyema, and sinusitis. Brain abscesses often develop as complications of chronic or acute infections of the lungs, sinuses, or ears. *Peptostreptococcus putridus* has been isolated from cases of puerperal sepsis, brain abscess, and infected wounds. *Nonclostridial crepitant anaerobic cellulitis* is due to peptostreptococci, whereas *synergistic necrotizing cellulitis* with widespread involvement of deeper tissues is caused by the symbiotic activity of peptostreptococci, aerobic gramnegative rods, and frequently bacteroides.

Streptococcal Myonecrosis

Anaerobic streptococci also can cause gas gangrene. Facultative streptococci and *Staphylococcus aureus* may also be isolated. *Streptococcal myonecrosis* resembles subacute clostridial gas gangrene and was not described until World War II. After an incubation period of 3 to 4 days, there is swelling, edema, and purulent wound exudate. These signs are followed by pain which rapidly becomes severe. Gas is present, and the infected muscle changes from pale and soft to bright red, striped with purple, and finally purple and gangrenous. The seropurulent discharge has a sour odor. In this disease, muscle is involved, in contrast to necrotizing fasciitis, in which the fascia is affected. Treatment consists of incision and drainage, antibiotic therapy, and supportive measures.

Progressive Synergistic Gangrene

Frank L. Meleney (1889–1963) established the importance of microaerophilic and anaerobic streptococci in special wound infections known as progressive synergistic gangrene and chronic burrowing ulcer. *Meleney's progressive synergistic gangrene* characteristically develops in sutured, infected thoracic or abdominal incisions or around a colostomy, ileostomy, or simple abrasion. The initial lesion is a small, painful, superficial ulcer which gradually spreads. The central ulcerated area is surrounded by a rim of gangrenous skin, which is in turn encircled by a zone of purple erythema blending into a surrounding area of bright, painful erythema. There is seropurulent discharge. Cultures taken from the outer edematous part of the lesion yield microaerophilic or anaerobic nonhemolytic streptococci. Cultures taken from the central ulcerated area yield *Staphylococcus aureus* and sometimes gram-negative bacilli, such as *Proteus* species. However, clinical cases of progressive synergistic gangrene from which anaerobic or microaerophilic streptococci could not be isolated have been reported. Treatment involves wide excision and therapy with penicillin or chloramphenicol. Corticosteroids have been employed to aid healing. Ledingham and Tehrani find that the problem in acute dermal gangrene following surgery, such as necrotizing fasciitis and progressive synergistic gangrene, is no longer any apparent specificity of invading bacteria but rather a vicious cycle of infection, local ischemia, and diminished host defense mechanisms.

Meleney's Ulcer

Chronic burrowing or undermining ulcer, often designated as *Meleney's ulcer,* is caused by a nonhemolytic anaerobic or microaerophilic streptococcus. The lesion begins as a small, superficial ulcer following trauma or surgery and may also originate from an infected lymph node or subcutaneous abscess. The ulcer is only mildly painful, and systemic reaction is minimal. Slow, progressive enlargement of the lesion occurs over months or years. Infection of subcutaneous tissue is associated with ulceration of the overlying skin. Cutaneous gangrene is absent, and the edges of the undermined skin roll inward. The periphery of the lesion is erythematous, and the advancing edge of the lesion is characterized by pain and tenderness. Meleney's ulcer occurs most frequently after incision of a lymph node in the neck, axilla, or groin and after opera-

tions on the genital and intestinal tracts. As the lesion spreads, multiple ulcers and sinuses develop, producing epithelial strands and undermined bridges of skin. Treatment consists of debridement, drainage of sinuses, penicillin therapy, and split-thickness skin grafts over denuded areas as soon as the wound appears clean.

Peptostreptococci, either in pure culture or mixed with bacteroides, are frequently involved in appendiceal abscesses, peritonitis, abdominal wall sepsis, perirectal abscesses, and superficial abscesses related to infections of pilonidal and sebaceous cysts. Most abscesses are treated successfully by incision and drainage, and penicillin therapy. Peptostreptococcal infections, including septicemias, commonly occur in the female pelvic area following septic abortion and postpartum sepsis.

STAPHYLOCOCCAL INFECTIONS

Staphylococci form part of the permanent bacterial flora of the normal skin and nasopharynx and may cause a variety of infections, often characterized by suppuration, ranging from mild, localized pustules to lethal septicemias. Surgical and traumatic wounds are particularly susceptible to purulent infection. In stained preparations of pus, staphylococci appear as spherical cells occurring singly, in pairs, or in small clusters. They are gram-positive and nonmotile, and produce no spores. Staphylococci are aerobic or facultatively anaerobic and grow on ordinary unenriched bacteriologic media. They may produce pigmentation varying from white, orange, or yellow to golden. Blood agar is often hemolyzed (beta hemolysis). Two species are of medical importance: *Staphylococcus aureus* and *Staphylococcus epidermidis* (formerly called *Staphylococcus albus*). *Staphylococcus aureus* is usually associated with disease, and will be discussed subsequently. On the other hand, *Staphylococcus epidermidis* usually has not been considered a pathogen, but it has become recognized as an important cause of opportunistic infection following surgical procedures in which foreign materials and prostheses are placed in the patient. *Staphylococcus epidermidis* causes endocarditis following open heart surgery and occasionally produces septicemia.

The criteria identifying staphylococci are colonial appearance on blood agar, Gram-stain reaction, microscopic morphologic features, production of coagulase, and fermentation of mannitol. *Staphylococcus aureus* is coagulase-positive and produces acid from mannitol. *Staphylococcus epidermidis* produces neither coagulase nor acid from mannitol. Filtrates of cultures of *Staphylococcus aureus* contain hemolysins, dermonecrotic and lethal factors, leukocidins, and enzymes. Strains of *Staphylococcus aureus* may be classified into groups on the basis of their susceptibility to various bacteriophages. Although phage typing of isolates is of value in epidemiologic investigations, it is not employed by the diagnostic laboratory for routine identification of clinical isolates.

Staphylococci are readily phagocytized by polymorphonuclear leukocytes, which may then be killed by the bacteria, presumably by their leukocidins. Although leukocidins, hemolysins, and coagulase are antigenic, antibodies to these antigens provide little or no protection. Since the antigenic components of staphylococci responsible for virulence are unknown, it has not been possible to make effective vaccines.

Staphylococcal infections in man depend upon many factors, including the type and number of staphylococci, the route of introduction, and the toxic substances produced by the staphylococci. Of equal importance are the susceptibility of the host, his previous exposure to specific strains, his general health and nutritional state, and the amount of trauma he has sustained. Factors such as toxemia, allergic reactions, starvation, and diabetes influence the onset and course of staphylococcal infections. Foreign body reaction as a consequence of sutures is an important factor in staphylococcal infection.

The skin is the most common site of staphylococcal infections. Lesions range from furuncles (boils) and carbuncles to surgical wound infections. Hospital-acquired staphylococcal infection by antibiotic-resistant strains reached epidemic proportion during the 1950s. The development and use of semisynthetic penicillinase-resistant penicillins has controlled these infections. However, the antibiotic-resistant staphylococci are endemic in hospitals and pose a continual threat to the patient. A rapidly spreading cellulitis is sometimes seen with staphylococcal infections and should be treated vigorously with an appropriate antibiotic. Often there is pain, swelling, induration, patchy discoloration of the skin, and fever. Cellulitis may occur at the site of a venipuncture for intravenous cannulation. Staphylococcal abscesses characteristically begin in hair follicles or small sebaceous glands. An indurated area of cellulitis undergoes central necrosis and formation of an abscess having thick, odorless, and yellow or greenish pus. Staphylococci are a primary cause of acute wound sepsis and are involved in postoperative infections of "clean" incised wounds. The source of the infecting microorganisms is frequently exogenous. Virulent, antibiotic-resistant, hospital strains of *Staphylococcus aureus* may be carried in the nares and on the hands of physicians and hospital personnel, and these may be newly colonized on the skin of the patient. The air in the operating room may bear microorganisms from the nasopharynx, skin, hair, and clothing of the surgical staff and of the patient. Accordingly, it is essential to maintain strict, rigid rules for asepsis in the operating room. At our hospital, coagulase-positive staphylococci are isolated from 8 percent of postoperative surgical wound infections and account for 5 percent of nosocomial infections.

Infected incisions should be opened widely and allowed to drain. Therapy with antistaphylococcal antibiotics should be initiated. Fulminating septicemias may arise from severe wound infections. The patient is ill with high fever, leukocytosis, toxemia, and evidence of irritation of the central nervous system. The mortality rate in fulminating untreated infections may be as high as 90 percent. If the infection persists, metastatic abscesses form in lungs, heart, kidneys, gallbladder, appendix, liver, peritoneum, and bone. Meningitis and brain abscesses hasten death.

Endocarditis is a frequent complication of staphylococcal septicemia. Staphylococcal pneumonia is another nosocomial postoperative infection. It may be severe and is often associated with a tracheostomy. In fatal cases, the major finding at autopsy is marked pulmonary edema with little destruction of tissue.

Staphylococcal Enteritis

Enteritis with a drug-resistant staphylococcus following oral administration of a broad-spectrum antibiotic was first described by Kramer in 1948. Generally, this disease is benign with mild to moderate symptoms including nausea, vomiting, diarrhea, abdominal distension, fever, and weakness, but may be fulminating and lead to septicemia and death. Discontinuance of the oral antibiotic usually leads to disappearance of symptoms. The prognosis is good so long as the intestinal mucosa remains intact.

Staphylococcal enterocolitis (*pseudomembranous enterocolitis*) is an acute inflammatory disease of the small and large intestine characterized by foci of epithelial necrosis and erosion of the mucosa. There is profuse, continuous diarrhea which soon becomes watery, contains desquamated, membranous patches, and often is greenish. The disease is a complication in debilitated surgical patients following therapy with broad-spectrum antibiotics. The use of neomycin in debilitated patients for preoperative intestinal antisepsis and for treatment of hepatic coma has resulted in staphylococcal enterocolitis. The major etiologic factors are suppression of normal gastrointestinal flora by a broad-spectrum antibiotic and acquisition of an enterotoxic strain of *Staphylococcus aureus* possessing multiple antibiotic-resistance. Secondary factors are debilitation and an empty small bowel (as a result of preoperative starvation). Although stool cultures from some patients yield a pure culture of *Staphylococcus aureus,* pseudomembranous enterocolitis may exist without culturable *Staphylococcus aureus.* Conversely, *Staphylococcus aureus may exist in pure culture in the intestine of a patient with the symptoms of enteritis but in the absence of a pseudomembrane.*

TREATMENT. Treatment consists of discontinuing previous antibiotics and employing a specific antistaphylococcal drug such as methicillin, hydration with intravenously administered fluids, replacement of electrolytes, intramuscular administration of corticosteroids, and attempts to reestablish a normal flora. The fulminating form of enterocolitis may be refractory to all forms of therapy and result in death.

Peptococci and Disease?

Both obligately anaerobic staphylococci (peptococci) and facultatively anaerobic staphylococci grow in anaerobic cultures. However, the facultatives (e.g., *Staphylococcus aureus*) can be subcultured aerobically and separated from the peptococci which grow anaerobically only. In contrast to the role of pure cultures of staphylococci in disease, the peptococci may be found in wound infections, abscesses, and septicemias in association with bacteroides, clostridia, aerobic gram-negative bacilli, and aerobic cocci. These bacterial groups are major components of the normal flora of the skin and mucous membranes and can exert a role in mixed infections when these sites are disturbed. Peptococci (e.g., *Peptococcus magnus* and *Peptococcus asaccharolyticus*) account for approximately 20 percent of anaerobes found in clinical specimens from surgical patients (Holland et al.). Nevertheless, the peptococci have slight, if any, propensity to produce disease and seem unable to cause progressive infection in laboratory animals. This apparent nonpathogenicity is shared by many anaerobic species from normal flora found in anaerobic infections and has led to speculation that the unitarian theory of infection which has evolved from the monumental work of Koch and Ehrlich (one microbe, one disease, one drug) does not explain all infectious disease (Gorbach and Bartlett).

CLOSTRIDIAL INFECTIONS

The clostridia are large, gram-positive, rod-shaped microorganisms. They are ubiquitous. *Clostridium perfringens* is more widespread than any other pathogen. Its principal habitats are the soil and the intestinal tract of man and animals. The most characteristic feature of clostridia is the presence of an oval, central, or subterminal spore. In the case of *Clostridium tetani,* the spore is spherical and terminally located and produces a characteristic drumstick appearance. The clostridia are obligate anaerobes and can be cultured only on media having a low oxidation-reduction potential. This may be achieved by employing fresh media incubated in an anaerobic atmosphere in specially designed jars or with liquid media exposed to the atmosphere, but containing added reducing agents (such as sodium thioglycolate, powdered iron, or chopped meat).

The lesions produced by the pathogenic clostridia are due to their exotoxins. Gas gangrene is a necrosis of tissue along with putrefaction and is usually caused by clostridia derived from the intestine or soil. The infection is localized but its systemic effects are far-reaching. Gas gangrene is rarely a pure culture infection. It usually involves *Clostridium perfringens* along with other clostridial species, such as *Clostridium novyi, Clostridium septicum, Clostridium bifermentans (sordelli),* sometimes *Clostridium tetani* and *Clostridium botulinum,* and often nonpathogenic but proteolytic *Clostridium sporogenes* and *Clostridium histolyticum.* In addition, gram-positive cocci and gram-negative enterobacteria are often present.

Clostridium perfringens is, nevertheless, the most important organism. Five types, A through F, have been described. They are differentiated on the basis of production of lethal toxins. All types produce alpha toxin, a lethal, necrotizing, hemolytic exotoxin, which is also a lecithinase. *Clostridium perfringens* type A produces the greatest amount of alpha toxin. In addition, some strains of type A produce variable amounts of hemolysin (theta toxin), collagenase (kappa toxin), hyaluronidase (mu toxin), and deoxyribonuclease (nu toxin).

Clostridial Wound Infection

MacLennan in 1962 described three types of anaerobic wound infection: simple contamination, clostridial cellulitis, and clostridial myonecrosis.

SIMPLE CONTAMINATION

Simple contamination of a wound by clostridia is common. It causes no discomfort to the patient and is of little concern to the surgeon. When anaerobes are digesting dead tissue, there may be a thin seropurulent exudate. If the necrotic material is removed, there will be no subsequent invasion of underlying tissues. The relatively common occurrence of clostridia in accidental wounds in the absence of anaerobic infection is probably due to the ubiquitous presence of these anaerobes and their spores. The absence of subsequent anaerobic infections is most likely due to unsuitable conditions for further multiplication of the contaminant and for toxin production. MacLennan estimated that between 10 and 30 percent of all severe civilian wounds were infected with spore-forming anaerobic bacilli. A high oxidation-reduction potential (Eh) due to the surrounding healthy tissues prevents colonization of the tissues. In the absence of treatment, however, cellulitis or myonecrosis may develop from the simple contamination, and the three types of anaerobic wound infection may be considered as ascending grades of severity.

CLOSTRIDIAL CELLULITIS

This is a gassy, crepitant infection involving necrotic tissue (killed by ischemia or trauma, but not by bacterial activity). Intact, healthy muscle is not invaded. The cellulitis is characterized as a foul, seropurulent infection of the depths and crevices of a wound. There is often local extension along fascial planes, but involvement of healthy muscle and marked toxemia are absent. Although *Clostridium perfringens* may be present, the predominant organisms are proteolytic and nontoxigenic clostridia, such as *Clostridium sporogenes* and *Clostridium tertium.* Clostridial cellulitis generally has a gradual onset; the incubation period is from 3 to 5 days; systemic effects are usually mild; there is no toxemia; the skin is rarely discolored; and there is little or no edema. This distinguishes the infection from gas gangrene. The spread of the cellulitis in the tissue spaces often has been rapid and extensive, necessitating immediate radical surgical drainage.

CLOSTRIDIAL MYONECROSIS (GAS GANGRENE)

This infection is rapid-spreading. It may be crepitant, or noncrepitant and edematous, mixed, or toxemic. The lesion also has been described as a "myositis," which is not as precise a term as is *myonecrosis.* The infection occurs in association with severe wounds of large muscle masses that have become contaminated with pathogenic clostridia, especially *Clostridium perfringens.* Such wounds are most commonly caused by the high-velocity missiles of modern warfare and by accidental trauma. Sometimes clostridial myonecrosis follows clean elective surgical procedures.

Many patients with clostridial myonecrosis harbor a variety of anaerobic as well as aerobic bacteria. In fatal cases it is rare for only a single species to be present. Clostridial myonecrosis is most likely to develop in wounds in which there has been extensive laceration or devitalization of thick muscle masses, such as the buttock, thigh, and shoulder. Associated with such trauma is impaired arterial supply to the limb or muscle group and gross contamination of the wound by soil, clothing, and other foreign bodies. These conditions provide an ideal substrate for the development of clostridia. In anoxic muscle glycolysis continues, and the oxidation-reduction potential (Eh) of the muscle falls. With the accumulation of lactate, alkaline reservoirs become depleted, and the pH also falls. As a consequence of lowered Eh and pH, the proteinases present and the amino acids produced not only lower the pH further but provide substrate for the growth of clostridia. Once bacterial growth is established and toxins and other products of bacterial metabolism accumulate, the invasion of uninjured tissue is promoted, and the anaerobic infection is established. The infection is further aided by the fact that neither phagocytes nor antibodies can enter the necrotic lesion. Gas gangrene is considered to have begun when the infecting pathogenic anaerobes have produced sufficient toxins to overcome local defenses. Gas gangrene is relatively infrequent in clinical practice. The overall incidence is less than 2 percent, although from 4 to 40 percent of wounds may be contaminated with clostridia.

TREATMENT. Early and adequate surgery is the most effective means of treating gas gangrene. Because of the rapid spread of the infection, a 24-hour delay in treatment may be fatal. The diagnosis of gas gangrene is based on clinical evidence. Multiple longitudinal incisions for decompression and drainage and surgical debridement usually arrest the disease. If not or if early diagnosis was not made, then amputation is necessary. Antibiotic therapy with penicillin G and tetracycline has been most effective as an adjunct to operative treatment. Antitoxin is of no value therapeutically or prophylactically and should not be used. Adjunctive hyperbaric oxygenation has been used with success.

Infections of the Gastrointestinal Tract

Clostridia are usually present among the mixed flora in peritonitis, appendicitis, and strangulation intestinal obstruction. Quantitatively, the most numerous flora in peritoneal and loop fluids of dogs with experimental strangulation intestinal obstruction are clostridia, coliforms, bacteriodes, and streptococci, in that order. Although it appears reasonable to assume that *Clostridium perfringens* actively participates in the pathophysiology of severe cases of appendicitis and acute cases of strangulated intestinal obstruction, direct clinical evidence is lacking. Experimental studies demonstrate that clostridial exotoxins contribute to the lethal activity of filter-sterilized strangulation fluids. However, this finding does not preclude a role for combinations of varying proportions of viable bacteria, bacterial endotoxins, and clostridial exotoxins. In biliary tract infections due to clostridia, acute emphysematous cholecystitis (gas gangrene of the gallbladder) and postcholecystectomy septicemia, it is generally believed that clostridia are transported to the liver from the gastrointestinal tract via the portal circulation and then excreted with the bile into the biliary tract. In postoperative gas gangrene of the abdominal wall, a rare complication of abdominal surgery, intestinal clostridia contaminate the abdominal wound at the time of operation. It occurs less often after operations on the stomach and duodenum than after those involving the lower intestinal tract. These infections are usually due to *Clostridium perfringens* and are fatal; they require awareness and early treatment. Gas gangrene of the abdominal wall must be distinguished from Meleney's progressive synergistic gangrene of the abdominal wall following drainage of appendiceal abscesses. Synergistic gangrene is a chronic, superficial progressive gangrene characterized by a slow, relentless progression, severe local symptoms, and absence of severe systemic symptoms. It is due to anaerobic cocci mixed with *Staphylococcus aureus, Streptococcus pyogenes, Pseudomonas aeruginosa,* or *Proteus* species.

Urogenital Infections

Postoperative infections due to *Clostridium perfringens* have occurred following procedures such as nephrectomy, lithotomy, and prostatectomy. Almost all uterine clostridial infections are due to *Clostridium perfringens.* They generally occur following criminal abortion and are rare following normal childbirth. Introduction of the organisms into the uterus is favored by instrumentation and manipulation. In modern obstetrics, the use of prophylactic antibiotic therapy and the wide use of cesarean section probably account for the decreasing frequency of this already rare form of uterine infection. In contrast, in cases of criminal abortion both endogenous and exogenous sources of contamination occur as the result of unskilled manipulations and the use of unsterile and unclean instruments and abortifacients. Once the interior of the puerperal or postabortal uterus has been contaminated, fragments of blood clot and necrotic tissue provide conditions favorable for multiplication of clostridia. Early diagnosis depends upon clinical recognition of such signs as jaundice, hypotension, tachycardia, shock, hemoglobinuria, uterine or perianal tenderness, and offensive vaginal discharge. The simplest method for the rapid detection of *Clostridium perfringens* is the demonstration of gram-positive rods with rounded ends in direct smears from the cervical os or canal. The treatment of uterine gas gangrene involves immediate chemotherapy, hyperbaric oxygenation, treatment of shock, hysterectomy, and management of renal failure. Penicillin is the antibiotic of choice.

Tetanus

This disease is a toxemia resulting from the growth of contaminating *Clostridium tetani* at a traumatized site and consequent production of exotoxin. In contrast to the clostridia of gas gangrene, *Clostridium tetani* is noninvasive, and neurotoxin is responsible for the symptoms of tetanus.

The conditions necessary for the development of tetanus are the presence of the organisms or spores in the wound and favorable anaerobic conditions for bacterial growth and the elaboration of exotoxin. The presence of *Clostridium tetani* in soil and in the intestine of man and animals ensures that accidental wounds are exposed to the risk of contamination at the time of injury. However, as with other clostridial infections, the mere presence of *Clostridium tetani* or its spores in a wound is not followed by tetanus, and the organism may be isolated from wounds in individuals who never develop tetanus. A low oxygen tension is necessary if *Clostridium tetani* is to grow. Currently, tetanus commonly follows mild injuries because the routine protective measures employed in severe cases are frequently omitted. The type of lesions leading to the development of tetanus are penetrating wounds due to splinters, thorns, rusty nails, and even dirty abrasions. In about 50 percent of cases, it is presumed that the wound was slight and healed before evidence of intoxication developed. Such mild injuries may not induce significant local anoxia, but they may be accompanied by other infections which lower the oxidation-reduction potential of the tissues to a point at which the spores of *Clostridium tetani* can germinate. For example, chronic ulcers of the leg, measles rash, boils, paronychia, and dental extractions have been implicated as modes of entry. In the United States, tetanus has become a disease primarily of adults. The median age of patients with nonneonatal tetanus varies from fifty-five to fifty-seven years; the median age for those dying from tetanus is from fifty-five to sixty years.

Currently, tetanus is seen in urban centers of the United States as a complication of narcotic addiction; *urban tetanus* has a mortality of 90 percent. *Tetanus neonatorum* results from contamination of the cut surface of the umbilical cord and is an important cause of infant mortality in developing countries where primitive unhygienic obstetric practices prevail. There is often continuous crying for hours followed by cessation of sucking and crying, convulsions, and fever. Severe spasm of the respiratory muscles is a common cause of death. *Postabortal tetanus* and *puerperal tetanus* result from unsterile manipulation or instrumentation of the genital tract. *Postoperative tetanus* sometimes follows elective surgical procedures, and is usually due to some breakdown in sterile technique, but it may also be caused by contamination from the patient's intestinal tract.

CLINICAL MANIFESTATIONS. The average incubation period for tetanus is from 7 to 10 days after injury, but it may range between 3 and 30 days. The incubation period is followed by the *period of onset*, that is, the time interval between the first symptom (usually trismus) and the onset of spasms. In severe cases reflex spasms may begin 12 hours after onset, in moderately severe cases after 2 to 3 days, and in milder cases after 5 or more days. In general, the shorter the periods of incubation and onset, the worse the prognosis. Even with modern treatment, the mortality rate is rarely less than 30 percent.

Trismus is the most common early symptom. It often is combined with pain and stiffness in the neck, back, and abdomen. Occasionally dysphagia appears first. These symptoms increase according to the severity of the attack. Twenty-four hours after the onset, a patient with a moderately severe attack has a characteristically anxious expression (*risus sardonicus*) in which the eyebrows and the corners of the mouth are drawn up. The muscles of the neck and trunk are rigid to varying degrees, and the back is usually slightly arched. The patient is usually comfortable except for occasional pain in the neck or back, which tends to be made worse by movement. Manipulation of a limb or palpation of any part of the body tends to increase muscular rigidity and may bring on cramplike pain. Initially, reflex spasms are brought on by external stimuli, such as moving the patient or knocking the bed, but later they occur spontaneously at regular and increasingly shorter intervals until the height of the disease is reached. Spasms often begin with a sudden jerk. Every muscle in the body is thrown into intense tonic contraction, the jaws are tightly clenched, the head is retracted, the back is arched, the chest and abdomen are fixed, and the limbs are usually extended. A severe spasm may stop respiration. Spasms may last a few seconds or several minutes. When spasms occur frequently, they lead to rapid exhaustion and sometimes to death from asphyxiation. Without spasms, mortality is low; with severe spasms, few survive. Aspiration pneumonia is a common contributory cause of death.

Less common manifestations of the disease include local contracture of muscles in the neighborhood of the wound: *local tetanus*. This may precede the more generalized forms of involvement. *Cephalic tetanus* is a manifestation in which irritation or paralysis of cranial nerves appears early and dominates the picture. The facial nerve is affected most often, but ophthalmoplegia from involvement of the ocular nerves and spasm or paralysis of the tongue from involvement of the hypoglossal nerve may develop. Trismus and dysphagia may also be present. This condition, which is a type of local tetanus, follows wounds of the head and face, and the symptoms often appear first on the injured side.

Severe tetanus is terrible and often fatal, but those who recover do so completely. The patient who has survived tetanus is not immune and, unless immunized, is susceptible to a second attack. *Recurrent tetanus* in the same patient has been reported. Apparently a sublethal amount of tetanus toxin is not sufficient to provide an adequate antigenic stimulus for the production of active immunity.

The diagnosis of tetanus is a clinical one with bacteriologic confirmation sometimes possible. Frequently the presumed lesion has been so slight that it is not detectable at the time when clinical tetanus develops.

IMMUNIZATION. Prophylaxis with tetanus toxoid is the best means of preventing tetanus. For active immunization of individuals seven years old or over, the initial dose is 0.5 ml aluminum phosphate adsorbed tetanus toxoid given intramuscularly, preferably in the left deltoid region, but it also may be given subcutaneously. This is repeated in 4 to 6 weeks, and a third injection is given in 6 to 12 months (or more). Only after this third injection is the basic series considered complete. For children six years old or under, diphtheria and tetanus toxoid combined with pertussis vaccine (DTP) is used. Delay in administering the second and third injections is not disadvantageous, and the series does not need to be restarted or repeated. Even after 25 years, a booster will rapidly recall complete active protection.

Following the initial dose of tetanus toxoid, nonimmunized individuals require approximately 30 days to acquire a safe antibody level (at least 0.01 I.U. of serum antitoxin per milliliter of blood). Patients are passively immunized in the interim by intramuscular administration of human hyperimmune globulin containing 250 units of tetanus antitoxin simultaneously with the toxoid. This protects for about 4 weeks. Passive immunization is not recommended for individuals who have received previous active immunization.

TREATMENT. Surgical care of wounds should be immediate. The most important features of surgical wound care are thorough cleansing and debridement. Foreign bodies and necrotic tissue can be massively contaminated with *Clostridium tetani* and establish wound conditions promoting growth and exotoxin production by *Clostridium tetani*. The wound should be left open until the patient has recovered from the convulsive stage of the disease. Antibiotic therapy with penicillin is effective against vegetative cells of *Clostridium tetani*. Oxytetracycline or chloramphenicol may be used if an allergy to penicillin exists. Antibiotics also are important as prophylaxis against respiratory infections, which are common in tetanus. Treatment of the patient with severe tetanus involves the use of muscle relaxants, sedation with Pentothal sodium, balance of fluid and electrolytes, control of respiratory secretions, and elimination of visceral stimuli such as distension of the urinary bladder and fecal impaction. A tracheostomy is performed if needed or when the period of onset is 1 day or less. Constant nursing care is required.

COMPLICATIONS. Tetanus is a particularly lethal disease, and death is generally due to respiratory arrest. Some complications of tetanus and its treatment are drug intoxication, especially from barbituates; bronchopneumonia or other pulmonary infection; compression fracture of vertebrae, especially the thoracic vertebrae; anemia; and exhaustion, which may be so severe as a result of repeated convulsions that the patient lapses into coma and expires. Before human tetanus immune globulin was available, the risk of anaphylaxis complicated the use of bovine or equine tetanus antitoxin.

PROPHYLAXIS. The Committee on Trauma of the American College of Surgeons recommends the following guidelines in management of the tetanus-prone wound:

I. General principles
  A. For each patient the attending physician must determine the adequate prophylaxis against tetanus.
  B. Meticulous surgical care, including removal of all devitalized tissue and foreign bodies, should be provided immediately for all wounds regardless of the active immunization status of the patient. Such care is an essential part of the prophylaxis against tetanus.
  C. Each patient with a wound should receive adsorbed tetanus toxoid intramuscularly at the time of injury, either as an initial immunizing dose or as a booster for previous immunization, unless he has received a booster or has completed his initial immunization series within the past 12 months. As the antigen concentration varies in different products, specific information on the volume of a single dose is provided on the label of the package.
  D. Need for passive immunization with homologous (human) tetanus immune globulin must be considered in relation to the characteristics of the wound, the conditions under which it was incurred, and the previous active immunization status of the patient.
  E. Every wounded patient should be given a written record of the immunization provided, and instructed to carry the record at all times and, if indicated, to complete active immunization. For precise tetanus prophylaxis, an accurate and immediately available history regarding previous active immunization against tetanus is required.
  F. Basic immunization with adsorbed toxoid requires three injections. A booster of adsorbed toxoid is indicated 10 years after the third injection or 10 years after an intervening wound booster.
II. Specific measures for patients with wounds
  A. For previously immunized individuals
    1. When the patient has been immunized within the past 10 years
      a. To the majority, give 0.5 ml of adsorbed tetanus toxoid as a booster unless it is certain that the patient has received a booster within the previous 12 months.
      b. To those with severe, neglected, and old (more than 24 hours) tetanus-prone wounds, give 0.5 ml of adsorbed toxoid unless it is certain that a booster was received within the previous 6 months.
    2. When the patient received active immunization more than 10 years previously and has not received a booster within the past 10 years
      a. To the majority, give 0.5 ml of adsorbed tetanus toxoid.
      b. To those with wounds which indicate an overwhelming possibility that tetanus might develop
        (1) Give 0.5 ml of adsorbed tetanus toxoid.
        (2) Give 250 units of tetanus immune globulin (human). Use different syringes, needles, and sites. For severe, neglected, or old wounds, 500 units of tetanus immune globulin (human) is advisable.
        (3) Consider administering oxytetracycline or penicillin prophylactically.
  B. For individuals not previously immunized
    1. With clean minor wounds in which tetanus is most likely, give 0.5 ml of adsorbed tetanus toxoid (initial immunizing dose).
    2. With all other wounds
      a. Give 0.5 ml of adsorbed tetanus toxoid (initial immunizing dose).
      b. Give 250 units of tetanus immune globulin (human). For severe, neglected, or old wounds, 500 units of tetanus immune globulin (human) is advisable.
      c. Consider administering oxytetracycline or penicillin prophylactically.

Medical students sometimes question on theoretical grounds the validity of administering toxoid and antitoxin (immune globulin) simultaneously to a previously unimmunized patient. The problem of interference during simultaneous active and passive immunization against tetanus has been studied quantitatively (Rubbo and Suri). There is some lowering of the antigenicity of toxoid, but the interference is not clinically significant if 250 units of tetanus immune globulin is injected. The antibody level in patients receiving immune globulin is protective for at least

4 weeks, and the second and third doses of toxoid produce an active antitoxin response. In addition, alum-adsorbed tetanus toxoid stimulates a quicker, higher, and more durable immunity than does plain toxoid because the aluminum in the preparation is an immunologic adjuvant. Use of the recommended adsorbed toxoid is, therefore, more reliable.

Wound Botulism

Botulism is an example of an intoxication resulting from the ingestion of exotoxin formed by *Clostridium botulinum* growing in improperly sterilized or inadequately preserved foods. Following gastrointestinal symptoms, botulism progresses to diplopia, blurred vision, and dysphagia and to a descending motor paralysis spreading to involve other cranial nerves and peripheral motor nerves. Although *C. botulinum* may be isolated from a wound as a simple contaminant, *wound botulism* occurs and is indicated by the presence of clinical signs of botulism. Thus wound botulism should be suspected in any patient with a wound who presents with clinical signs of descending paralysis and a negative food history. Therapy of the wound is routine; therapy of the botulism is supportive, with respiratory care and assisted ventilation if required. Equine trivalent antitoxin should be given after testing for sensitivity to equine serum.

INFECTIONS CAUSED BY GRAM-NEGATIVE BACILLI

The gram-negative bacilli of importance to surgery are for the most part indigenous to man and often found in the intestinal tract. They are non-spore-forming rods, and they may be aerobes, facultative anaerobes, or obligate anaerobes. The role of some gram-negative bacilli as primary pathogens has long been known, e.g., *Pseudomonas aeruginosa* and *Salmonella typhi*. Others have been recognized only rarely as primary pathogens in human beings, e.g., *Serratia marcescens* and *Enterobacter aerogenes* (formerly *Aerobacter aerogenes*). However, since the development of modern chemotherapy after World War II, the gram-negative bacilli have become increasingly important as causes of serious infection, particularly in hospitalized patients. Prior to the introduction of broad-spectrum antibiotics, the role of gram-negative bacilli as pathogens was usually overshadowed by the pneumococci, streptococci, and staphylococci. We now know that infection is most likely to occur when body defense mechanisms are either undeveloped or overtaxed, as in the case of infants and debilitated patients, and that therapeutic measures to combat one situation may provide an environment promoting the establishment of infection by almost any mixture of gram-negative bacilli. This situation prevails because of the great number of patients with impaired host defenses secondary to the use of multiple antibiotics, corticosteroids, immunosuppressive agents, antineoplastic drugs, and radiotherapy. Surgical procedures in which foreign bodies such as prosthetic valves or grafts are inserted appear to allow these less virulent species to become established and to produce infection. Indwelling venous and urethral catheters, endotracheal tubes and mechanical ventilators, peritoneal dialysis apparatus, and pump-oxygenators for extracorporeal circulation in cardiac surgery often serve as portals of entry for the gram-negative bacilli. The current taxonomic organization of gram-negative bacilli (aerobic, facultative, and anaerobic) is outlined in Table 5-6.

Aerobic and Facultative Bacteria

Pseudomonas aeruginosa is a strict aerobe; it is widely distributed and is frequently present in small numbers on healthy skin surfaces and in the normal intestinal flora of some individuals. *P. aeruginosa* is an opportunistic pathogen which can cause serious and lethal infections in debilitated or immunosuppressed patients, such as those with cancer, large burns, or cystic fibrosis, and is common in postoperative infections following the use of mechanical ventilators and indwelling urinary catheters. It is incriminated in primary infections such as meningitis resulting from lumbar puncture, traumatic injuries to the eye, and enteritis with associated bacteremia. Heroin addicts are subject to hematogenous pseudomonal osteomyelitis. Although *P. aeruginosa* is gram-negative and produces an endotoxin, its cell-wall lipopolysaccharides are not as toxic as those isolated from the enteric bacteria. It does, however, produce a variety of extracellular products that contribute to its pathogenicity, including hemolysins, proteases, an enterotoxin, and a heat-labile exotoxin. This exotoxin is more toxic than the other extracellular products or the endotoxin. *Pseudomonas* infections are treated with either gentamicin or carbenicillin, alone or in combination.

Escherichia coli is found in the intestinal tract of man and animals and is the predominant facultative commensal in the normal intestinal flora. Although more than 145

Table 5-6. TAXONOMY OF GRAM-NEGATIVE BACILLI

Family	Tribe	Genus
Pseudomonaceae. . . .	. . . .	*Pseudomonas*
Enterobacteriaceae. . .	Eschericheae	*Escherichia* (*E. coli*, including *Alkalescens-Dispar* group)
		Shigella
	Edwardsielliae	*Edwardsiella*
	Salmonelleae	*Salmonella*
		Arizona
		Citrobacter (including Bethesda-Ballerup group)
	Klebsielleae	*Klebsiella*
		Enterobacter (including *Hafnia*)
		Pectobacterium
		Serratia
	Proteae	*Proteus*
		Providencia
Bacteroidaceae	. . . .	*Bacteroides*
		Fusobacterium

different envelope capsular (K) antigens have been identified, the ability of a strain to be typed does not necessarily
denote pathogenicity or virulence. Nevertheless, certain
strains belonging to distinct antigenic types are *entero-
pathogenic,* others are *enterotoxigenic* by their capacity to
produce toxins, and others are *enteroinvasive* by their ability to penetrate mucosal cells. These strains produce diarrheal disease, especially in infants. Stool isolates may have
none, one, two, or all three of these pathogenic characteristics. *Escherichia coli* may produce meningitis, septicemia,
endocarditis, appendiceal abscess, peritonitis, septic
wounds, and pyogenic infections, chiefly urinary tract infections (pyelitis, cystitis, etc.) in pure culture or in association with fecal streptococci. *Escherichia coli* also has the
capacity to produce a potent endotoxin which enters the
circulation and induces shock. The antibiotic of choice in
the treatment of the patient seriously ill with *Escherichia
coli* sepsis is an aminoglycoside, such as kanamycin or
gentamicin.

The *Salmonella* species are a large group of enteric
pathogens transmitted via food and water. They cause
enteric fevers (particularly typhoid fever), gastroenteritis,
and septicemia. *Salmonella typhi* and *Salmonella enteritidis*
pass from the small intestine by way of the lymphatics to
the mesenteric glands. After multiplication there, they
invade the bloodstream via the thoracic duct. Complications which may result from this hematogenous dissemination include thrombophlebitis, lymphadenitis, pneumonia,
osteomyelitis, arthritis, endocarditis, and meningitis. Hemorrhage may occur from perforation of ulcers in lymphoid
tissue of the intestine. The specific surgical treatment for
perforation, i.e., simple closure or segmental resection, is
determined by the pathologic findings encountered at operation. Chloramphenicol has long been advocated in the
treatment of typhoid fever, but ampicillin is equally effective. Although postoperative wound infection due to *Salmonella typhi* is rare, recorded cases occur after gallbladder
surgery in patients who are unsuspected typhoid carriers.
Contaminated wound drainage and positive stools from
such patients are distinct hazards to other hospitalized
patients.

Before the introduction of modern chemotherapy,
gram-negative bacilli of the tribe Klebsielleae were rarely
noted as primary pathogens. However, along with other
gram-negative bacilli, they have assumed increasing importance as causes of serious hospital-acquired infections.
Klebsiella pneumoniae (Friedlander's bacillus) causes a
severe pneumonia having a propensity for debilitated (frequently alcoholic) patients. *Klebsiella* has also been implicated in endocarditis, septic thrombophlebitis, septicemia,
urinary tract infection, wound infection, crepitant cellulitis,
and myonecrosis. *Enterobacter aerogenes* (formerly *Aerobacter aerogenes*) is a commensal in the intestinal tract of
approximately 5 percent of healthy individuals. It has less
pathogenic potential than strains of *Klebsiella* but is commonly involved in hospital-acquired sepsis. *Serratia marcescens* is another species formerly considered to be nonpathogenic for man. Although it too has low virulence for
healthy individuals, it is now found primarily in hospitalized patients with some underlying disease. It may spread

like other "hospital bacteria," and infection may not always produce clinical symptoms. Classically, *Serratia marcescens* has been recognized by its ability to produce a
characteristic red pigment, and it has been thought to be an
obligate pigment producer. However, the majority of
strains of *Serratia marcescens* involved in hospital-acquired
infections are nonpigmented and often have been mistaken
for other enterobacteria. These nonchromogenic strains of
Serratia marcescens now can be identified by appropriate
biochemical tests. The *Klebsiella-Enterobacter-Serratia*
species are often isolated in mixed culture from sputum,
urine, blood, and wounds in which there are other potential pathogens such as streptococci, staphylococci, *Escherichia coli, Proteus* species, *Citrobacter* species, and *Pseudomonas aeruginosa.* Epidemiologic studies indicate that
the particular strains and types of the gram-negative species producing infection are nosocomial and acquired in
the intestinal tract of patients during hospitalization. They
are often highly drug-resistant, and the overall mortality
associated with bacteremia is approximately 50 percent.
The risk of bacteremia appears to be related to the underlying disease of the patient and the nature of his infection
(urinary tract, respiratory, wound infection, abscess, etc.).
Gentamicin is the antibiotic of choice in treatment of
infections caused by the *Klebsiella-Enterobacter-Serratia*
species. Kanamycin is a satisfactory alternate drug.

Gram-negative bacilli in the genera *Proteus* and *Providencia* also compete for prominence with the other aerobic
gram-negatives in infections. Rapid and abundant urease
production distinguishes *Proteus* from *Providencia.* These
organisms often occur in abscesses, in infected wounds,
and also in burns as one component of a mixed infection.
They are resistant to most antibiotics, and what was originally a mixed infection may be converted into a pure
proteus infection as a result of antibiotic therapy. Sepsis
due to indol-negative *Proteus* (*Proteus mirabilis*) is treated
with ampicillin, while that due to indol-positive species
(*Proteus vulgaris, P. morganii,* and *P. rettgeri*) is treated
with kanamycin or carbenicillin. *Providencia* species are
sensitive to carbenicillin. The genus *Acinetobacter* includes
gram-negative pleomorphic aerobes previously known by a
wide variety of names. *Acinetobacter calcoaceticus* var.
anitratus (formerly *Herellea vaginicola* and *Bacterium ani-
tratum*) and *Acinetobacter calcoaceticus* var. *lwoffi* (formerly *Mima polymorpha*) are opportunists capable of
causing therapy-potentiated infections in compromised
patients. Kanamycin or gentamicin constitute appropriate
therapy for these infections.

Anaerobic Bacteria

Obligately anaerobic bacteria, especially gram-negative
bacilli, are found as normal flora on skin and all mucous
membrane surfaces. They are by far the major component
of the normal flora. In the normal oral cavity, anaerobes
outnumber aerobes 10 to 1, and in the normal colon, 1000
to 1. When the mucous membrane barrier is disturbed by
disease, trauma, or surgical procedures, these bacteria can
invade adjacent tissue and may cause infection. In the
upper respiratory tract and lungs, the major anaerobic

pathogens are peptostreptococci, fusobacteria, and *Bacteroides melaninogenicus*. In intraabdominal infections, *Bacteroides fragilis* is the most frequent isolate; clostridia, peptostreptococci, and peptococci are also found. In infection of the female genital tract, the same anaerobes are also the principal pathogens. Although anaerobic infections often originate close to a mucosal surface, they may occur anywhere in the body as a result of direct or hematogenous spread. Clues to diagnosis include foul-smelling discharge, gas, necrotic tissue, abscess formation, and failure to obtain growth on aerobic culture despite the presence of organisms on Gram-stained direct smear. Anaerobes are associated with 90 percent of cases of intraabdominal abscess, 95 percent of appendiceal abscess, 90 percent of aspiration pneumonia, 95 percent of lung abscess, 85 percent of brain abscess, and 75 percent of upper tract female pelvic infections.

The bacteroides are obligately anaerobic, gram-negative, non-spore-forming bacilli. They are sometimes the only microorganisms found in clinical specimens but more often are found in association with other anaerobes and aerobes. Currently, human pathogens are assigned to the genus *Bacteroides* and the genus *Fusobacterium*. *Bacteroides* are rod-shaped cells with rounded ends and are sometimes coccobacillary; *Fusobacterium* may be bacilli with pointed ends or pleomorphic, filamentous forms with swellings and free, round bodies. Species causing infections in human beings are *Bacteroides fragilis, Bacteroides melaninogenicus, Fusobacterium fusiforme,* and *Fusobacterium necrophorus* (previously known as *Bacteroides fundiformis* and as *Sphaerophorus necrophorus*).

In circumstances such as chronic illness, malignant disease, surgical treatment, and cystoscopy, the bacteroides may invade the bloodstream to cause septicemia and penetrate tissue and organs to produce abscesses. The clinical spectrum of infections varies from superficial infections to deep abscesses with overwhelming bacteremia and shock. The gastrointestinal tract, especially the colon and appendix, appears to be the most frequent source of bacteroides infection. Gynecologic infections involve the vagina, uterus, and contiguous structures, and are related to malignancy of pelvic organs, septic abortions, and postpartum complications. Upper respiratory tract infections and those of the nasopharynx, mouth, and jaw (tonsillar and peritonsillar abscesses, chronic otitis media, and dentoalveolar abscesses) have become relatively uncommon since the widespread use of antibiotics (penicillin or tetracycline) for the treatment of undiagnosed pharyngitis. Brain abscesses are a well-known complication of these upper respiratory tract infections in which bacteroides are involved along with other microorganisms, such as anaerobic streptococci.

Bacteroides bacteremia is characterized by a spiking fever, jaundice, and leukocytosis. In the patient more than forty years old, it is associated with chronic debilitating disease, hypotension, and a high mortality. Bacteremias have followed primary infection in the gastrointestinal, pelvic, and pharyngeal areas, and may originate from thrombophlebitis in these sites of infection. An indication of *Bacteroides* infection is the presence of a foul-smelling exudate from wounds or abscesses which contain gram-negative forms but produce no growth on aerobic culture. There appears to be a disposition toward *Bacteroides* infection in patients with underlying malignant disease. Often these patients have undergone elective intestinal surgery after preoperative intestinal antisepsis. This suggests that changes in the normal intestinal flora may predispose to *Bacteroides* infection. Therefore, the surgeon should be alert to the possibility of *Bacteroides* infection. A changing pattern of pyogenic abscesses of the liver has been characterized by an increased incidence of *Bacteroides* as the pathogen.

Treatment of anaerobic infections consists of surgical drainage of abscesses, excision of necrotic tissue, and appropriate antibiotic therapy. This should be based upon the results of sensitivity tests, since anaerobes can be divided into two groups on the basis of antibiotic susceptibility tests, i.e., *Bacteroides fragilis* and all other anaerobes. Penicillin G is the drug of choice for virtually all anaerobic infections except those caused by *Bacteroides fragilis*, which require chloramphenicol or clindamycin. However, the efficacy of penicillin in some infections in which *Bacteroides fragilis* is present in mixed culture is due to its effectiveness against the other members of the mixed flora.

PSEUDOMYCOTIC INFECTIONS

Among the actinomycetes, *Actinomyces israelii* and *Nocardia asteroides* are isolated most frequently as human pathogens, although other species of each genus may also be implicated in human infections. Actinomycetes are true bacteria but traditionally have been studied and grouped with the fungi because of their resemblance to mycotic agents and their involvement in diseases resembling mycoses. Infections caused by these false fungi (pseudomyces) may be called pseudomycoses to separate them from true fungal infections. They will therefore be considered separately from the true mycoses.

Actinomycosis

Actinomyces israelii is a strict anaerobe present in normal oral flora. Actinomycosis is therefore an endogenous infection. There are three clinical types of actinomycosis: cervicofacial (the most common type), thoracic, and abdominal. A dense fibroblastic reaction is produced, and connective and granulation tissue tend to form a wall around the abscess. Wherever lesions occur, abscesses expand into contiguous tissue and form burrowing, tortuous sinuses to the outside, where they discharge pus and necrotic material. This pus contains dense clusters of organisms and hyphae appearing as macroscopic, yellow-brown "sulfur granules," which facilitate diagnosis when examined microscopically and cultured. Actinomycosis can be cured with massive doses of penicillin G or ampicillin. Tetracycline, lincomycin, and clindamycin are alternative agents. Surgical drainage of abscesses and aggressive resection of damaged tissue are important adjuncts to long-term chemotherapy.

Nocardiosis

Nocardia, in contrast to actinomycetes, are aerobic inhabitants of soil and are not part of the normal flora of man. *Nocardia asteroides* and *Nocardia brasiliensis,* opportunistic pathogens for man, are less acid-fast than mycobacteria, and their filaments tend to branch. Nocardiosis tends to be progressive and fatal but is a rare disease. Pulmonary infection arises from inhalation of the organisms, while subcutaneous abscesses (mycetomas) result from contamination of skin wounds, usually of the hands and feet of laborers. Massive doses of sulfonamides, e.g., sulfadiazine 6 to 8 Gm/day orally for at least 4 to 6 months, is the preferred therapy; ampicillin is an alternate agent. Drainage of empyema and abscesses is an important surgical adjunct to chemotherapy.

MYCOTIC INFECTIONS

The relation of the surgeon to mycotic infection has changed in recent years. The need for surgical treatment has diminished because of more effective modern chemotherapy. However, the long-term use of cytotoxic agents, corticosteroids, and antibacterial drugs for patients with leukemia and neoplasms has increased the incidence of opportunistic mycotic infections. Among the pathogenic fungi to be discussed, *Blastomyces dermatitidis, Paracoccidioides brasiliensis, Histoplasma capsulatum, Cryptococcus neoformans,* and even *Coccidioides immitis* are frank pathogens but may be opportunistic to the extent that they cause progressive infections in debilitated patients more frequently than in healthy ones. Definite opportunistic infections are caused by species of *Mucor, Rhizopus, Aspergillus,* and *Candida.* Fungal infection threatens any compromised hosts, such as severely burned patients and those with implanted prosthetic devices and transplanted organs. Some of the symptoms of mycotic disease are chronic skin or mucous membrane lesions, low-grade fever, weight loss, chronic pulmonary or meningeal involvement, hepatosplenomegaly, and lymphadenopathy. Mycotic disease should be suspected unless another cause

is clearly established. A mycosis may coexist with a lymphomatous disease, e.g., the association of histoplasmosis and cryptococcosis with Hodgkin's disease. A presumptive clinical diagnosis of a mycosis must be confirmed in the laboratory. Serologic tests are useful in reaching a presumptive diagnosis. The morphologic features of the fungus in tissue and culture are significant in identification.

The majority of patients with fungal infections seen by the physician have serious illness and present with typical symptoms of infection. Symptoms of pulmonary involvement frequently are present. Hematogenous dissemination of the disease produces manifestations such as tender swollen joints, draining subcutaneous abscesses, ulcerative lesions of the oropharynx, and meningitis. Many patients with systemic mycoses, as well as those with dermatophytoses, have skin lesions which are painful, itching, weeping, crusting, malodorous, and disfiguring. Fungi of ever-increasing importance as agents of infection in surgical patients are grouped in Table 5-7 according to the type of disease they cause and will be discussed in the order shown.

Blastomycosis (North American Blastomycosis)

Blastomyces dermatitidis is a dimorphic fungus; it grows in tissues and in culture at 37°C as a spherical thick-walled, single-budding yeast and in culture at room temperature as a mold. Lateral, rounded conidia borne along hyphae are presumably the infectious spores. Demonstration of non-encapsulated, thick-walled, multinucleate yeast cells in pus, sputum, or tissue sections and their subsequent laboratory culture establish the diagnosis. Blastomycosis usually begins in the lungs as a subacute respiratory infection (pulmonary form) which gradually increases in severity over a period of weeks or months and sometimes resembles tuberculosis or carcinoma. Frequently, during the course of infection, patients develop skin lesions. These may be the only apparent signs of blastomycosis. Pulmonary blastomycosis spreads hematogenously to establish focal destructive lesions in other parts of the body. Spreading, ulcerated, crusted skin lesions in particular arise as metastases from the primary pulmonary lesions. Cure has been

Table 5-7. MYCOSES IMPORTANT IN SURGICAL INFECTIONS

Type of disease	Mycosis	Representative fungus	Fungal morphology		
			Dimorphism	Infected tissue	Laboratory culture
Systemic	Blastomycosis	*Blastomyces dermatitidis*	Yes	Yeast	Mycelia
	Paracoccidioidomycosis	*Paracoccidioides brasiliensis*	Yes	Yeast	Mycelia
	Histoplasmosis	*Histoplasma capsulatum*	Yes	Yeast	Mycelia
	Coccidioidomycosis	*Coccidioides immitis*	Yes	Spherules	Mycelia
	Cryptococcosis	*Cryptococcus neoformans*	No	Yeast	Yeast
Subcutaneous	Sporotrichosis	*Sporotrichum schenckii*	Yes	Yeast	Mycelia
Systemic, particularly opportunistic . .	Phycomycosis	*Mucor corymbifera*	No	Mycelia	Mycelia
		Rhizopus oryzae	No	Mycelia	Mycelia
	Aspergillosis	*Aspergillus fumigatus*	No	Mycelia	Mycelia
	Candidosis	*Candida albicans*	Yes	Yeast and hyphae	Yeast and hyphae

effected in many cutaneous cases by 2-hydroxystilbami-dine. However, amphotericin B is indicated in treating all forms of blastomycosis. If surgery is indicated for diagnosis to rule out bronchogenic carcinoma, amphotericin is used both pre- and postoperatively to minimize operative spread.

Paracoccidioidomycosis (South American Blastomycosis)

Paracoccidioides brasiliensis is dimorphic and grows in tissue as a multiple-budding yeast, in contrast to the single-budding yeast in blastomycosis. Paracoccidioido-mycosis is characterized by primary pulmonary lesions with dissemination to visceral organs, by conspicuous ul-cerative granulomas of the buccal and nasal mucosa, and by generalized lymphangitis. In blastomycosis, visceral organs are *not* involved. Treatment with amphotericin B is usually effective.

Histoplasmosis

Histoplasma capsulatum is dimorphic; it appears charac-teristically in infected tissues as many, small, oval yeast cells packed within macrophages and reticuloendothelial cells; at room temperature it forms slowly growing mycelial colonies. This pathogen is present in soil, espe-cially that enriched by feces of birds and bats, and is endemic in the Mississippi and Ohio valleys and along the Appalachian mountains of the United States. Inhalation of conidia leads to pulmonary infection. The initial infection is mild and may be inapparent or may occur as a primary acute disease. Symptoms may include fever, cough, chest pain, dyspnea, and pleurisy with effusion. Localized pul-monary histoplasmosis resembles tuberculosis in its histo-pathology. In a few individuals the infection becomes progressive and widely disseminated and may simulate miliary tuberculosis. Disseminated histoplasmosis primar-ily involves the reticuloendothelial system in various tis-sues and organs and often coexists in individuals who have tuberculosis, leukemia, or Hodgkin's disease. Histoplas-mosis is treated with high doses of intravenous amphoteri-cin B. In chronic cavitary disease surgical resection should be performed, with amphotericin therapy given before and after surgery to reduce postoperative complications and avoid relapse.

Coccidioidomycosis

Coccidioides immitis is a somewhat different dimorphic fungus; it varies in structure between a hyphal form found in soil and a spherule or sporangium form found in in-fected tissues. The sporangia are thick-walled structures filled with globular endospores or sporangiospores. At maturity the sporangium bursts and releases hundreds of endospores, each of which can form a new sporangium in tissue. When sporangia are plated on Sabouraud agar, growth of the mycelial form occurs. Barrel-shaped arthro-spores are formed in the mycelium. These arthrospores are highly infectious and become airborne easily. The mycelial

(saprophytic) form is readily converted into the sporan-gium (parasitic) form in man. *Coccidioides immitis* is en-demic in the southwestern United States and adjacent Mexico, where it grows as a saprophyte in desert soils. Infection is established by inhalation of airborne arthro-spores.

About 60 percent of infected individuals remain asymp-tomatic but become skin-sensitive to coccidioidin. The acute and most common form of coccidioidomycosis re-sembles influenza. When confined to the lungs, the disease is usually self-limited and heals with scarring. However, a chronic, progressive, granulomatous disease occurs in fewer than 1 percent of infected individuals. Years may elapse between primary infection and the more serious disseminated disease. Patients with disseminated coccidi-oidomycosis appear to have some defect in their immune response to the fungus. The symptoms are similar to those seen in advancing tuberculosis. Any organ or tissue of the body may be involved. However, the infection shows pred-ilection for bone, skin, and subcutaneous tissue. This dis-ease is not contagious, since it is spread only by saprophytic arthrospores. The majority of patients with primary infec-tion recover without therapy or with only symptomatic care. Amphotericin B is used to treat disseminated coccidi-oidomycosis but is less effective than with blastomycosis, histoplasmosis, and cryptococcosis.

Cryptococcosis

Cryptococcus neoformans is *not dimorphic;* in both in-fected tissue and in culture it appears as encapsulated yeast cells. The yeast cells are thin-walled, but the large, clear polysaccharide capsules surrounding them are distinctive. *Cryptococcus neoformans* is found in dust and bird drop-pings. Inhalation of yeast cells is thought to initiate pulmo-nary infection, which may be inapparent or mild. There is little inflammatory response of invaded tissues. Cryptococ-cosis is a subacute or chronic mycotic infection most fre-quently involving tissues of the central nervous system but occasionally producing lesions in the lungs or skin. Cryp-tococcal meningitis is the most frequent form of dissemi-nated disease and mimics tuberculous meningitis, brain abscess, or brain tumor. Pulmonary lesions are usually found at autopsy. Many patients with pulmonary or der-mal cryptococcosis respond to therapy with 5-fluorocyto-sine. Surgical resection is indicated for both cavitary and nodular pulmonary disease. When diagnosis is established by surgery, therapy with amphotericin B is begun postop-eratively to avoid meningitis and recurrence. Amphotericin B is the drug of choice for cryptococcosis of the central nervous system. Cryptococcosis is an opportunistic mycosis in debilitated patients, particularly those with Hodgkin's disease or leukemia.

Sporotrichosis

Sporotrichum schenckii is dimorphic. When found in tissues or exudate stained by the periodic acid–Schiff tech-nique, this fungus appears as fusiform bodies or round budding cells, but these are rarely seen. When these materials are cultured on Sabouraud agar at room temperature, the mycelial form grows. Microscopically, hyphae are slender and septate, and conidia are individually attached by sterigmata to a common conidiophore. Hyphae are converted to the yeast form by injection into mice and by cultivation at 37°C on enriched media. Man becomes infected by accidental subcutaneous inoculation from thorns and splinters. Sporotrichosis is a chronic progressive infection of the skin and subcutaneous tissue which frequently begins as a primary lesion of the skin of the hand or forearm and secondarily involves lymphatic channels and lymph nodes draining the area, which become cord-like, resulting in a chain of ulcers. Generalized infection occurs in the compromised host by way of the blood, and any organ or tissue can be the site of lesions. Symptoms are then related to the region involved. Orally administered potassium iodide is specific in sporotrichosis and must be continued for several weeks after recovery seems complete. Intravenous amphotericin B is indicated for disseminated sporotrichosis. *Sporotrichum schenckii* has caused supra-infection in patients with underlying hematologic malignant disease who have been treated with antitumor agents and steroids.

Phycomycosis

Species of *Mucor* and *Rhizopus* are saprophytes common in nature and are *not dimorphic*. They can produce rapidly fatal disease when they invade the brain, lungs, or other organs of a compromised host. These fungi may also produce a superficial infection of the skin with occasional ulceration and granuloma or abscess formation. *Mucor* and *Rhizopus* are opportunistic and are held in check by normal serum factors which become diminished in individuals suffering from uncontrolled diabetes mellitus, blood dyscrasias, endocrine disturbances, malnutrition, and burns. Corticosteroid therapy and prolonged use of broad-spectrum antibiotics may also enhance susceptibility to phycomycosis. The local cutaneous lesions heal with proper hygiene and fungicides; extensive lesions may require debridement. Amphotericin B and correction of the underlying disease is the therapy for the acute form of phycomycosis. Amphotericin should be used to treat any patient not responding to other measures. Surgery should be considered for patients with pulmonary lesions not responsive to amphotericin.

Aspergillosis

Aspergillus has become an important pathogen in patients with impaired host defenses. These mycelial fungi are saprophytic and are not dimorphic but can cause local as well as disseminated disease. *Aspergillus fumigatus* is the most commonly reported species. Two forms of pulmonary aspergillosis are frequently seen: (1) pulmonary or bronchial aspergilloma (fungus ball), due to secondary invasion of a tuberculous or coccidioidal cavity, and (2) allergic bronchopulmonary aspergillosis. In the compromised host these may proceed to disseminated infection. Otomycosis is secondary to bacterial infection of the ear. The fungus grows on ear wax and macerated tissue. Systemic aspergillosis may complicate severe underlying diseases which are being treated with steroids, immunosuppressive drugs, or broad-spectrum antibiotics. Local superficial lesions often heal spontaneously with hygienic care. Localized abscesses and granulomas should be excised. Systemic infection requires treatment with amphotericin B. The prognosis in disseminated aspergillosis is poor; the patient often succumbs to the underlying disease.

Candidosis

Candida albicans is indigenous in man and is dimorphic; both yeast and mycelial forms are seen in infected tissue. *Candida albicans* affects mucous membranes and causes diseases ranging from thrush (oral candidosis) and vulvovaginal candidosis to systemic candidosis. The former are common medical problems, the latter an opportunistic infection of the compromised host. Patients with hemopoietic and lymphoreticular neoplasms, as well as those being treated with immunosuppressives, glucocorticoids, and broad-spectrum antibiotics, are particularly prone to systemic fungal infections. Patients with burns and those undergoing intravenous hyperalimentation are also prone to systemic candidosis. Candidal endocarditis, especially that due to *Candida parapsilosis,* is seen in drug addicts using intravenous heroin.

Thrush and other clinically distinctive candidal infections frequently result from antibacterial therapy, and discontinuance of the therapy will usually cause the antibiotic-induced suprainfection to disappear. Topical nystatin is effective in treating candidal infections of the skin, mouth, and vagina. Amphotericin B is the mainstay in treating systemic candidosis. Oral 5-fluorocytosine is considerably less toxic than amphotericin, but 50 percent of *Candida* strains are initially resistant.

SURGICAL ASEPSIS

Surgical asepsis, the prevention of the access of microorganisms to an operative wound, is achieved by methods designed to destroy bacteria or remove them from all objects coming in contact with the wound. Modern surgery is aseptic in the use of sterile instruments, sutures, and dressings and in the wearing of sterile caps, gowns, masks, and rubber gloves by the operating personnel. Although this is presently the extent of routine sterility in surgical asepsis, the technology of germ-free research is able to provide sterile flexible plastic isolation chambers in which neonates or antibiotic-decontaminated patients may be maintained in a sterile environment. Operations may be performed in "surgical" isolators cemented to the operative site of the patient. The surgeon makes his incision through the site of attachment of the isolator, and the operation may be conducted in the absence of all microorganisms. There is currently considerable interest in unidirectional (laminar) airflow systems as a less absolute means of limiting the number of bacteria to which a patient is exposed. These systems recirculate air through high-efficiency particulate air filters that assure unidirectional flow in either a downward or horizontal direction. However, the advantages or necessity of such systems in operating rooms are controversial, since there has not yet been substantial evidence to demonstrate their effectiveness in reducing postoperative infections. The Committee on Control of Operating Room Environment of the American College of Surgeons does not recommend laminar airflow for general use in operating rooms.

It is necessary to resort to the use of antiseptics to degerm the site of the operation on the patient's skin. The surgeon and operating-room personnel usually use soaps or detergents containing antiseptics for scrubbing their hands before donning gloves or else rinse in an antiseptic after the scrub. An *antiseptic* is a chemical agent which either kills pathogenic microorganisms or inhibits their growth so long as there is contact between agent and microbe. By custom as well as by federal law, the term "antiseptic" is reserved for agents applied to the body. The antiseptic may actually be a disinfectant used in dilute solutions to avoid damage to tissues. A *disinfectant* is a germicidal, chemical substance used on inanimate objects to kill pathogenic microorganisms but not necessarily all others. These germicidal agents are used to disinfect instruments and other equipment which cannot be exposed to heat. They are essential for good housekeeping practices in hospitals, where they are used to disinfect floors, fabrics, and excreta. The first step in any process of biologic decontamination is thorough mechanical cleansing with soap or detergent and water to remove all traces of blood, pus, proteins, and mucus before the antiseptic or disinfectant is employed.

Sterilization

Sterilization is the process of killing all microorganisms (bacteria, spores, viruses, mycotic agents, and parasites). It is the ultimate in disinfection. The practical criterion of sterility is the failure of microbial growth to appear on tests in suitable bacteriologic media. Sterilization can be achieved by either physical or chemical agents. *Steam under pressure* is the most reliable means of sterilizing surgical supplies because of its power of penetration, microbiologic efficiency, ease of control, and economy of operation. Application of steam under a pressure of 15 psi (pounds per square inch) for 15 to 45 minutes will destroy all forms of life. Free-flowing steam, like boiling water, has a temperature of 100°C, but the same steam under pressure of 15 psi exerts a temperature of 121°C. Steam gives up heat by condensing into water. Thus when a bundle containing surgical pads or sponges is sterilized, the steam contacts the outer layer. There a portion of it condenses into water and releases heat. The steam then penetrates to a second layer, where another portion condenses and gives up heat. The steam thus approaches the center of the package, layer after layer, until the whole package is sterilized. The time of exposure depends upon the size of the parcel and its wrappings. Sterilization by steam under pressure is carried out in an autoclave. A major caution to be recognized when operating an auto-

clave is that a mixture of air and steam has a lower temperature than does pure steam. Therefore, when air is present in the chamber, the killing power of the process is diminished in proportion to the amount of air present. Most autoclaves depend upon gravity displacement of air from the chamber and from within articles being sterilized. Thus, improperly packed and positioned articles in the autoclave may fail to become sterile even though all physical conditions of the run may be correct. A new development in autoclaves is the high-vacuum sterilizer. A vacuum pump is incorporated into the system, and a vacuum is pulled in the chamber at the beginning and end of the sterilizing cycle. There is a considerable shortening of the time needed for sterilization, as only 3 minutes are needed to achieve sterility rather than the 20 minutes on the regular systems. In addition, there appears to be less damage to rubber, fabrics, and sharp instruments because of reduced exposure to moisture. There is less danger of creating air pockets and less chance of the steam's failing to penetrate to the center of bundles. Materials emerge dry, and much greater tolerances in packing the chamber are afforded.

Dry-heat sterilization is commonly used for glassware, for items that are injured by moisture, and for materials that resist penetration by steam, such as talc, vaseline, fats, and oils. The process consists of baking the material to be sterilized in a hot-air oven. At a temperature of 121°C (250°F) it takes about 6 hours to sterilize glassware, but at 170°C (340°F) the time required is about 1 hour. *Gas sterilization* is practical with ethylene oxide, a gas employed as a sterilizing agent in specially designed chambers in which temperatures and humidity can be controlled and from which air can be evacuated. The killing action is slow, and an exposure period from 3 to 6 hours is needed. Sterilization employing ethylene oxide is used for delicate surgical instruments with optical lenses, for tubing and plastic parts of heart-lung machines and respirators, for prepacked commercial plastic products such as disposable syringes, and for blankets, pillows, and mattresses. Ethylene oxide is most reliable when applied to clean, dry surfaces that do not absorb the chemical. The gas dissolves in plastic, rubber, fabric, and leather, and chemical burns may occur when materials laden with ethylene oxide are applied to tissue. The dissolved chemical escapes from materials when they are exposed to air, and a minimum of 24 hours of aeration is necessary to ensure removal of the gas from sterilized articles. However, solid metal or glass items may be used immediately after sterilization. *Radiation sterilization* refers to ionizing radiation by cobalt 60 sources (γ-radiation) and by electron accelerators (high-energy electrons). It is currently used commercially to sterilize disposable hospital supplies, such as plastic hypodermic syringes and sutures. Radiation sterilization of heat-sensitive pharmaceuticals has been recommended.

Chemical sterilization is currently achieved with a 2% aqueous solution of glutaraldehyde. This compound is an effective disinfectant for surgical, anesthetic, and dental equipment, rubber and plastic mouthpieces, catheters, and other heat-sensitive hospital equipment. Either a buffered alkaline solution (Cidex) or a potentiated acid solution

(Sonacide) of glutaraldehyde may be used. They are equally bactericidal, sporicidal, and virucidal. Isopropyl alcohol may also be used for the chemical sterilization of instruments if they are first cleansed of all blood, pus, and body fluids. Only in the absence of spores is alcohol an effective sterilizing agent.

Degerming of Skin

Antiseptics incorporated into soaps are used for preoperative preparation of the skin at the operative site and for surgical hand scrubs by operating personnel. The bacteriologic content of normal skin consists of a resident flora, composed of coagulase-negative *Staphylococcus epidermidis* and anaerobic diphtheroides (e.g., *Propionibacterium acnes*), which reside on the surface of the skin, in hair follicles, and in the ducts of sebaceous glands. These bacteria can be diminished temporarily, but they cannot be permanently eradicated. They are not usually responsible for surgical infections. Superimposed upon the resident flora is a transient flora consisting of bacteria picked up as a result of temporary colonizing of the skin. In the hospital, this transient flora often consists of pathogens resistant to antibiotics and is likely to be composed of pathogenic strains of *Staphylococcus aureus* and gram-negative enterobacteria. Therefore, pathogenic bacteria on the hands of operating personnel at the time of operation must be removed by scrubbing and destroyed by an antiseptic agent. The patient's skin must be degermed in the area of operation prior to the incision. The most efficient method is a vigorous scrub with liquid soaps containing either hexachlorophene or an iodophor.

Hexachlorophene is a bisphenol which disinfects the skin slowly. Commercial preparations containing 3% hexachlorophene, a detergent, and liquid soap are used for surgical scrubbing. Over a period of days, regular use of these surgical soaps brings about a progressive decrease in the number of bacteria on and in the skin. The hexachlorophene leaves an active film, which is renewed with each scrubbing. Consequently, its antibacterial activity persists so long as one continues to wash with soap containing hexachlorophene. A single washing with ordinary soap removes the antibacterial film. Hexachlorophene is effective against gram-positive pathogens such as *Staphylococcus aureus,* but it is without activity against gram-negative bacteria, such as the pseudomonas and the enterobacteria. This fact should be seriously considered by anyone using hexachlorophene, since gram-negative bacteria are currently responsible for the majority of nosocomial infections.

Iodophors are organic complexes of iodine and a synthetic detergent. About 1% iodine is available in the formula, whose germicidal action results from the liberation of free iodine when the compound is diluted with water. The detergent in the complex enhances the bactericidal activity of the iodine. Advantages of iodophors are that they destroy both gram-positive and gram-negative bacterial cells, but not spores; they do not stain skin and clothing; and they do not produce allergic reactions. Iodophors have been incorporated into surgical scrub soaps for hands and for the operative site.

Other Surgical Antiseptics

No economical antiseptic or disinfectant is available to kill all microbial flora in a reasonable time at concentrations which will not irritate tissue or damage medical devices. However, there are several agents that have high reliability and low toxicity as surgical antiseptics. Among them are alcohol and iodine. The combination of inorganic iodine and alcohol, either as a tincture or as a mixture of 1% to 3% iodine with 70% ethyl or isopropyl alcohol, kills both gram-positive and gram-negative bacteria. Only a short contact time is needed, and the solution itself is not likely to be contaminated. Some patients, however, have adverse reactions to iodine, and most physicians hesitate to use this combination on mucous membranes or denuded skin. Aqueous iodophor solutions are available as an alternative. These also have a broad antimicrobic spectrum and are not likely to be contaminated, and they provoke adverse reaction less frequently than do inorganic tinctures of iodine. For patients sensitive to iodine, a thorough scrub with soap and water followed by a 2-minute scrub with 70% to 90% ethyl or isopropyl alcohol is effective surgical antisepsis. Isopropyl alcohol is slightly more effective than ethyl alcohol when used as a 70% solution and is less expensive and more readily obtained because it is not potable. As a group, alcohols exhibit many desirable features. They are bactericidal, have a cleansing action, and evaporate readily. They do not, however, kill spores, and the best one can hope to accomplish with alcohol is to reduce the number of viable bacteria and destroy pathogens which may be on the skin as transients.

Aqueous quaternary ammonium compounds such as benzalkonium chloride (Zephiran Chloride) are used diluted 1:750 for skin antisepsis for venipuncture and for disinfection of cystoscopes, bronchoscopes, and intravenous tubing. They are less expensive than many other products and are nontoxic and nonallergenic but *must* be used with caution. Although they are potent bactericides in vitro and are particularly active against gram-positive cocci, benzalkonium antiseptics have been implicated in nosocomial infections by resistant *Pseudomonas cepacia* and *Enterobacter* species which contaminate working solutions of these compounds. Accordingly, there are few applications for quaternary ammonium compounds in hospitals other than for environmental sanitation. Alternative surgical antiseptics such as iodine, iodophors, and alcohol have a broad antibacterial spectrum.

References

Introduction; General Principles; Surgical Infections

Alexander, J. W.: Emerging Concepts in the Control of Surgical Infections, *Surgery,* **75**:934, 1974.
American College of Surgeons, Committee on Control of Surgical

Infections: "Manual on Control of Surgical Infections," J. B. Lippincott Company, Philadelphia, 1976.

Brummelkamp, W. H., Boerema, I., and Hoogendyk, L.: Treatment of Clostridial Infections with Hyperbaric Oxygen Drenching: A Report of 26 Cases, *Lancet,* **1**:235, 1963.

Casaubon, J.-N., Dion, M. A., and Larbrisseau, A.: Septic Cavernous Sinus Thrombosis after Rhinoplasty, *Reconstr Surg,* **59**:119, 1977.

Dubos, R. J.: "Biochemical Determinants of Microbial Diseases," Harvard University Press, Cambridge, Mass., 1954.

Holland, J. A., Hill, G. B., Wolfe, W. G., Osterhout, S., Saltzman, H. A., and Brown, I. W.: Experimental and Clinical Experience with Hyperbaric Oxygen in the Treatment of Clostridial Myonecrosis, *Surgery,* **77**:75, 1975.

Meleney, F. L.: "Treatise on Surgical Infections," Oxford University Press, New York, 1948.

———: "Clinical Aspects and Treatment of Surgical Infections," W. B. Saunders Company, Philadelphia, 1949.

Noble, W. C., and Somerville, D. A.: "Microbiology of Human Skin," W. B. Saunders Company, Philadelphia, 1974.

Polk, H. C., Jr., and Stone, H. H. (eds.): "Hospital-acquired Infections in Surgery," University Park Press, Baltimore, 1977.

Pulaski, E. J.: Common Bacterial Infections: Pathophysiology and Clinical Management," W. B. Saunders Company, Philadelphia, 1964.

Roding, B., Groeneveld, P. H. A., and Boerema, I.: Ten Years of Experience in The Treatment of Gas Gangrene with Hyperbaric Oxygen, *Surg Gynecol Obstet,* **134**:579, 1972.

Rosebury, T.: "Microorganisms Indigenous to Man," McGraw-Hill Book Company, New York, 1962.

Slack, W. K., Hanson, G. C., and Chew, H. E. R.: Hyperbaric Oxygen in the Treatment of Gas Gangrene and Clostridial Infection: A Report of 40 Patients Treated in a Single-Person Hyperbaric Oxygen Chamber, *Br J Surg,* **56**:505, 1969.

Wangensteen, O. H., Wangensteen, S. D., and Klinger, C. F.: Surgical Cleanliness, Hospital Salubrity, and Surgical Statistics, Historically Considered, *Surgery,* **71**:477, 1972.

Basic Considerations of Antibiotic Therapy

Crofton, J.: Some Principles in the Chemotherapy of Bacterial Infections, *Br Med J,* **2**:137, 209, 1969.

Kabins, S.: Interactions among Antibiotics and Other Drugs, *JAMA,* **219**:206, 1972.

Kantor, H. S., and Shaw, W. V.: Microbial Suprainfection. Recognition and Management, *Med Clin North Am,* **55**:471, 1971.

Pratt, W. B.: "Fundamentals of Chemotherapy," Oxford University Press, New York, 1973.

Weinstein, L., and Musher, D. M.: Antibiotic-induced Suprainfection, *J Infect Dis,* **119**:662, 1969. (Editorial.)

Yale, C. E., and Peet, W. J.: Antibiotics in Colon Surgery, *Am J Surg,* **122**:787, 1971.

Chemoprophylaxis; Intestinal Antisepsis; Intraperitoneal Antibiotics

Bernard, H. R., and Cole, W. R.: The Prophylaxis of Surgical Infection: The Effect of Prophylactic Antimicrobial Drugs on the Incidence of Infection following Potentially Contaminated Operations, *Surgery,* **56**:151, 1964.

Bornside, G. H., and Cohn, I., Jr.: Stability of Normal Human

Fecal Flora During a Chemically Defined, Low Residue Diet, *Ann Surg,* **181**:58, 1975.

Burke, J. F.: Use of Preventive Antibiotics in Clinical Surgery, *Am Surg,* **39**:6, 1973.

Cohn, I., Jr.: "Intestinal Antisepsis," Charles C Thomas, Publisher, Springfield, Ill., 1968.

———: Intestinal Antisepsis, *Surg Gynec Obstet,* **130**:1006, 1970.

———, Langford, D., and Rives, J. D.: Antibiotic Support of Colon Anastomoses, *Surg Gynecol Obstet,* **104**:1, 1957.

DiVincenti, F. C., and Cohn, I., Jr.: Prolonged Administration of Intraperitoneal Kanamycin in the Treatment of Peritonitis, *Amer Surg,* **37**:177, 1971.

MacLean, L. D.: Prophylactic Antibiotic Therapy in Surgery, *Can J Surg,* **18**:243, 1975.

Nelson, J. L., Kuzman, J. H., and Cohn, I., Jr.: Intraperitoneal Lavage and Kanamycin for the Contaminated Abdomen, *Surg Clin North Am,* **55**:1391, 1975.

Nichols, R. L., Broido, P., Condon, R. E., Gorbach, S. L., and Nyhus, L. M.: Effect of Preoperative Neomycin-Erythromycin Intestinal Preparation on the Incidence of Infectious Complications Following Colon Surgery, *Ann Surg,* **178**:453, 1973.

———, and Condon, R. E.: Preoperative Preparation of the Colon, *Surg Gynecol Obstet,* **132**:323, 1971.

Smith, E. B.: A Rationale for Intraperitoneally Administered Antibiotic Therapy, *Surg Gynecol Obstet,* **143**:561, 1976.

Antimicrobial Agents

Garrod, L. P., Lambert, H. P., O'Grady, F., and Waterford, P. M.: "Antibiotic and Chemotherapy," 4th ed., Churchill Livingstone, Edinburgh, 1973.

Kagan, B. M. (ed.): "Antimicrobial Therapy," 2d ed., W. B. Saunders Company, Philadelphia, 1974.

Kucers, A., and Bennett, N. McK.: "The Use of Antibiotics: A Comprehensive Review with Clinical Emphasis," 2d ed., J. B. Lippincott Company, Philadelphia, 1975.

Smith, H.: "Antibiotics in Clinical Practice," 3d ed., University Park Press, Baltimore, 1977.

Streptococcal Infections

Abrams, J. S.: Role of Steroids in the Management of Phagedenic Ulcer, *Surgery,* **66**:297, 1969.

Altemeier, W. A., and Culbertson, W. R.: Acute Non-clostridial Crepitant Cellulitis, *Surg Gynecol Obstet,* **87**:206, 1948.

Armstrong, D., Blevins, A., Louria, D. B., Henkel, J. S., Moody, M. D., and Sukany, M.: Groups B, C, and G Streptococcal Infections in a Cancer Hospital, *Ann NY Acad Sci,* **174**:511, 1970.

Brewer, G. E., and Meleney, F. L.: Progressive Gangrenous Infection of the Skin and Subcutaneous Tissues, following Operation for Acute Perforative Appendicitis: A Study in Symbiosis, *Ann Surg,* **84**:438, 1926.

Grieco, M. H., and Sheldon, C.: *Erysipelothrix rhusopathiae, Ann NY Acad Sci,* **174**:523, 1970.

Ledingham, I. McA., and Tehrani, M. A.: Diagnosis, Clinical Course and Treatment of Acute Dermal Gangrene, *Br J Surg,* **62**:364, 1975.

MacLennan, J. D.: Streptococcal Infection of Muscle, *Lancet,* **1**:582, 1943.

Meleney, F. L., Friedman, S. T., and Harvey, H. D.: The Treatment of Progressive Bacterial Synergistic Gangrene with Penicillin, *Surgery,* **18:**423, 1945.

———, and Johnson, B. A.: Further Laboratory and Clinical Experiences in the Treatment of Chronic, Undermining, Burrowing Ulcers with Zinc Peroxide, *Surgery,* **1:**169, 1937.

Rea, W. J., and Wyrick, W. J., Jr.: Necrotizing Fasciitis, *Ann Surg,* **172:**957, 1970.

Stone, H. H., and Martin, J. D., Jr.: Synergistic Necrotizing Cellulitis, *Ann Surg,* **175:**702, 1972.

Strasberg, S. M., and Silver, M. S.: Hemolytic Streptococcus Gangrene: An Uncommon but Frequently Fatal Infection in the Antibiotic Era, *Am J Surg,* **115:**763, 1968.

Staphylococcal Infections

Altemeier, W. A., Hummel, R. P., and Hill, E. O.: Staphylococcal Enterocolitis following Antibiotic Therapy, *Ann Surg,* **157:**847, 1963.

Andriole, V. T., and Lyons, R. W.: Coagulase-negative Staphylococcus, *Ann NY Acad Sci,* **174:**533, 1970.

Elek, S. D.: "Staphylococcus Pyogenes and Its Relation to Disease," Livingstone Ltd., London, 1959.

Gorbach, S. L., and Bartlett, J. G.: Anaerobic Infections: Old Myths and New Realities, *J Infect Dis,* **130:**307, 1974. (Editorial.)

Hardaway, R. M., III, and McKay, D. G.: Pseudomembranous Enterocolitis: Are Antibiotics Wholly Responsible? *Arch Surg,* **78:**446, 1959.

Holland, J. W., Hill, E. O., and Altemeier, W. A.: Numbers and Types of Anaerobic Bacteria Isolated from Clinical Specimens since 1960, *J Clin Microbiol,* **5:**20, 1977.

Kramer, I. R. H.: Fatal Staphylococcal Enteritis Developing during Streptomycin Therapy by Mouth, *Lancet,* **2:**646, 1948.

Wilson, T. S., and Stuart, R. D.: *Staphylococcus albus* in Wound Infection and in Septicemia, *Can Med Assoc J,* **93:**8, 1965.

Clostridial Infections

Altemeier, W. A., and Fullen, W. D.: Prevention and Treatment of Gas Gangrene, *JAMA,* **217:**806, 1971.

Altemeier, W. A., and Hummel, R. P.: Treatment of Tetanus, *Surgery,* **60:**495, 1966.

Athavale, V. B., Pai, P. N., Fernandez, A., Patnekar, P. N., and Acharya, V. S.: Tetanus Neonatorium; Tetanus in Children, *Prog Drug Res,* **19:**189, 209, 1975.

Brooks, G. F., Buchanan, T. M., and Bennett, J. V.: Tetanus Toxoid Immunization of Adults: A Continuing Need, *Ann Intern Med,* **73:**603, 1970.

Cherubin, C. E.: Clinical Severity of Tetanus in Narcotic Addicts in New York City, *Arch Intern Med,* **121:**156, 1968.

Clay, R. C., and Bolton, J. W.: Tetanus Arising from Gangrenous Unperforated Small Intestine, *JAMA,* **187:**856, 1964.

DeJongh, D. S.: Postoperative Synergistic Gangrene, *JAMA,* **200:**227, 1967.

Dickinson, K. M., and Edgar, W. M.: Anaerobic Cellulitis of the Abdominal Wall after Prostatectomy and Orchidectomy, *Lancet,* **1:**1139, 1963.

Faust, R. A., Vickers, O. R., and Cohn, I., Jr.: Tetanus: 2,449 Cases in 68 Years at Charity Hospital, *J Trauma,* **16:**704, 1976.

Grainger, R. W., MacKenzie, D. A., and McLachlin, A. D.: Progressive Bacterial Synergistic Gangrene: Chronic Undermining Ulcer of Meleney, *Can J Surg,* **10:**439, 1967.

Isenberg, A. N.: *Clostridium welchii* Infection, *Arch Surg,* **92:**727, 1966.

Lowbury, E. J. L., and Lilly, H. A.: Contamination of Operating-Theatre Air with *Cl. tetani, Br Med J,* **2:**1334, 1958.

MacLennan, J. D.: The Histotoxic Clostridial Infections of Man, *Bacteriol Rev,* **26:**177, 1962.

McNally, M. J., and Crile, G., Jr.: Diagnosis and Treatment of Gas Gangrene of the Abdominal Wall, *Surg Gynecol Obstet,* **118:**1046, 1964.

Meleney, F. L.: Bacterial Synergism in Disease Processes: With a Confirmation of the Synergistic Bacterial Etiology of a Certain Type of Progressive Gangrene of the Abdominal Wall, *Ann Surg,* **94:**961, 1931.

Oakley, C. L.: Gas Gangrene, *Br Med Bull,* **10:**52, 1954.

Rubbo, S. D., and Suri, J. C.: Combined Active-Passive Immunization against Tetanus with Human Immune Globulin, *Med J Aust,* **2:**109, 1965.

Treadway, C. R., and Prange, A. J., Jr.: Tetanus Mimicking Psychophysiologic Reaction: Occurrence after Dental Extraction, *JAMA,* **200:**891, 1967.

Vakil, B. J., Singhal, B. S., Pandya, S. S., and Irani, P. F.: Cephalic Tetanus, *Prog Drug Res,* **19:**443, 1975.

Willis, A. T.: "Clostridia of Wound Infection," Butterworth Scientific Publications, London, 1969.

Aerobic Infections

Artenstein, M. S., and Sanford, J. P. (eds.): Symposium on *Pseudomonas aeruginosa, J Infect Dis,* Vol. 130, Suppl, November 1974.

DiGioa, R. A., Kane, J. G., and Parker, R. H.: Crepitant Cellulitis and Myonecrosis Caused by Klebsiella, *JAMA,* **237:**2097, 1977.

Forkner, C. E., Jr.: "Pseudomonas Aeruginosa Infections," Grune & Stratton, Inc., New York, 1960.

Kaul, B. K.: Operative Management of Typhoid Perforation in Children, *Int Surg,* **60:**407, 1975.

Reisig, G., and Schaffner, W.: Postoperative Detection of *Salmonella typhi, Arch Surg,* **104:**349, 1972.

Steinhauer, B. W., Eickhoff, T. C., Kislak, J. W., and Finland, M.: The *Klebsiella-Enterobacter-Serratia* Division: Chemical and Epidemiologic Characteristics, *Ann Intern Med,* **65:**1180, 1966.

Thong, M. L.: Acinetobacter Anitratus Infections in Man, *Aust NZ J Med,* **5:**435, 1975.

Wilkowske, C. J., Washington, J. A., II, Martin, W. J., and Ritts, R. E., Jr.: *Serratia marcescens:* Biochemical Characteristics, Antibiotic Susceptibility Patterns, and Clinical Significance, *JAMA,* **214:**2157, 1970.

Anaerobic Infections

Altemeier, W. A., Schowengerdt, C. G., and Whiteley, D. H.: Abscesses of the Liver: Surgical Considerations, *Arch Surg,* **101:**258, 1970.

Anderson, C. B., Marr, J. J., and Ballinger, W. F.: Anaerobic Infections in Surgery: Clinical Review, *Surgery,* **79:**313, 1976.

Finegold, S. M.: "Anaerobic Bacteria in Human Disease," Academic Press, New York, 1977.

Gorbach, S. L., and Bartlett, J. G.: Anaerobic Infections, *N Engl J Med,* **290:**1177, 1237, 1289, 1974.

Gorbach, S. L., and Bartlett, J. G. (eds.): The Role of Clindamycin in Anaerobic Bacterial Infections, *J Infect Dis,* Vol. 135, Suppl, March 1977. (Symposium.)

Holland, J. W., Hill, E. O., and Altemeier, W. A.: Numbers and Types of Anaerobic Bacteria Isolated from Clinical Specimens since 1960, *J Clin Microbiol,* **5:**20, 1977.

Leigh, D. A.: Wound Infections Due to *Bacteroides fragilis* Following Intestinal Surgery, *Br J Surg,* **62:**375, 1975.

Meyer, R. D., and Finegold, S. M.: Anaerobic Infections: Diagnosis and Treatment, *South Med J,* **69:**1178, 1976.

Sinkovics, J. G., and Smith, J. P.: Septicemia with Bacteroides in Patients with Malignant Disease, *Cancer,* **25:**663, 1970.

Stone, H. H., Kolb, L. D., and Geheber, C. E.: Incidence and Significance of Intraperitoneal Anaerobic Bacteria, *Ann Surg,* **181:**705, 1975.

Swenson, R. M., Lorber, B., Michaelson, T. C., and Spaulding, E. H.: The Bacteriology of Intra-abdominal Infections, *Arch Surg,* **109:**398, 1974.

Mycotic Infections

Bennett, J. E.: Chemotherapy of Systemic Mycoses, *N Engl J Med,* **290:**30, 323, 1974.

Bernhardt, H. E., Orlando, J. C., Benfield, J. R., Hirose, F. M., and Foos, R. Y.: Disseminated Candidiasis in Surgical Patients, *Surg Gynecol Obstet,* **134:**819, 1972.

Emmons, C. W., Binford, C. H., Utz, J. P., and Kwon-Chung, K. J.: "Medical Mycology," 3d ed., Lea & Febiger, Philadelphia, 1977.

MacMillan, B. G., Law, E. J., and Holder, I. A.: Experience with *Candida* Infections in the Burn Patient, *Arch Surg,* **104:**509, 1972.

Moss, E., and McQuown, A. L.: "Atlas of Medical Mycology," 3d ed., The Williams & Wilkins Company, Baltimore, 1969.

Nash, G., Foley, F. D., Goodwin, M. N., Jr., Bruck, H. M., Greenwald, K. A., and Pruitt, B. A., Jr.: Fungal Burn Wound Infection, *JAMA,* **215:**1664, 1971.

Nelson, A. R.: The Surgical Treatment of Pulmonary Coccidioidomycosis, *Curr Probl Surg,* October 1974.

Schroter, G. P. J., Temple, D. R., Husberg, B. S., Weil, R., III, and Starzl, T. E.: Cryptococcosis after Renal Transplantation, *Surgery,* **79:**268, 1976.

Surgical Asepsis

Block, S. S. (ed.): "Disinfection, Sterilization, and Preservation," 2d ed., Lea & Febiger, Philadelphia, 1977.

Bornside, G. H., Crowder, V. H., Jr., and Cohn, I., Jr.: A Bacteriological Evaluation of Surgical Scrubbing with Disposable Iodophor-Soap Impregnated Polyurethane Scrub Sponges, *Surgery,* **64:**743, 1968.

Collins, F. M., and Montalbine, V.: Mycobactericidal Activity of Glutaraldehyde Solutions, *J Clin Microbiol,* **4:**408, 1976.

Crowder, V. H., Jr., Bornside, G. H., and Cohn, I., Jr.: Bacteriological Comparison of Hexachlorophene and Polyvinylpyrrolidine-Iodine Surgical Scrub Soaps, *Am. Surg,* **33:**906, 1967.

Frank, M. J., and Schaffner, W.: Contaminated Aqueous Benzalkonium Chloride: An Unnecessary Hospital Infection Hazard, *JAMA,* **236:**2418, 1976.

Kaslow, R. A., Mackel, D. C., and Mallison, G. F.: Nosocomial Pseudobacteremia: Positive Blood Cultures Due to Contaminated Benzalkonium Antiseptic, *JAMA,* **236:**2407, 1976.

Levenson, S. M., Trexler, P. C., Malm, O. J., LaConte, M. L., Horowitz, R. E., and Moncrief, W. H.: A Plastic Isolator for Operating in a Sterile Environment, *Am J Surg,* **104:**891, 1962.

Trauma

by **G. Tom Shires**

GENERAL CONSIDERATIONS

(by G. Tom Shires and Ronald C. Jones)

The magnitude of the problem of trauma in the United States is probably not adequately appreciated. In this country trauma is the leading cause of death in the first three decades of life. It ranks overall as the fourth leading cause of death in the United States today; if arteriosclerosis is considered as a single entity, trauma is the third leading cause of death. Fifty million injuries occur annually in the United States, over ten million of them being disabling. Over 100,000 deaths occur each year from accidents. Automobile accidents alone kill more Americans each year than were lost during the entire Korean conflict. Unlike many serious disease entities in the United States, the incidence of and mortality from injuries are increasing each year.

Accident patients take up to 22 million hospital bed days a year in the United States—more than are needed to take care of the delivery of all the babies in a given year, more than are needed by all the heart patients, and four times more than are needed by all cancer patients. Even during wartime, deaths from accidents always exceed battle deaths. In World War II, United States battle deaths were 292,000; accidental civilian deaths during the same period in the United States alone were 450,000. And more military personnel die from accidents than from combat during a period of national involvement.

An attempt will be made in this chapter to cover certain principles related to injuries, as well as selected areas of bodily injury. The following discussions of certain specifics of the patient who has sustained trauma will, of necessity, omit several critical areas concerned with care of the traumatized patient. These related problems are being discussed elsewhere in the text and include related principles such as those of shock, cardiac arrest, transfusion problems, pulmonary ventilation, and surgical infections initiated by trauma. Other organ system injuries covered elsewhere include burns, injuries to central nervous system, thoracic trauma, and genitourinary trauma. Similarly, complications including renal failure and embolism are covered in detail in separate chapters.

Initial Resuscitation of the Severely Injured Patient

The patient with multiple injuries is best managed by one physician. When the responsibility is divided, evaluation of the patient's overall problems may be lacking, and complications may not be recognized for several hours.

PRIORITY BY INJURY

There are three categories of patients, according to immediacy of injury. The first group includes injuries which interfere with vital physiologic function and therefore immediately threaten life, such as obstruction of an airway or bleeding from a gunshot wound. The primary treatment is to establish an airway and control the bleeding. This type of patient may require surgical treatment for massive internal bleeding within 5 to 10 minutes following arrival in the emergency room. The operating room should be alerted when the patient is admitted to the emergency room, and no time is wasted in getting the patient into "operative" condition. Often the control of hemorrhage is dependent on a rapid thoracotomy or laparotomy to occlude injured major vessels.

A second group of patients are those with injuries which offer no immediate threat to life. These include patients who have received gunshot wounds, stab wounds, or blunt trauma to the chest and abdomen but whose vital signs are stable. The majority of injured patients are in this category. Although they will require surgical procedures within 1 to 2 hours, there is time for additional information to be obtained. Blood for typing and cross matching is drawn, and blood is made available if there is any possibility that the patient will require surgical intervention. If vital signs are stable, x-rays may be obtained to determine the course of the missile and the extent of possible associated injuries, such as fractures. Cystography and pyelography may be done to assess hematuria. Since patients with penetrating and blunt abdominal injuries may develop shock at any moment, a physician must be in constant attendance during all evaluations. Patients who suddenly go into shock are immediately taken to the operating room without additional diagnostic procedures.

The third group of patients are those whose injuries produce occult damage. This group is composed primarily of patients who have sustained blunt trauma to the abdomen which may or may not require surgical intervention and in whom the exact nature of the injury is not apparent. These patients usually have time for extensive laboratory studies, x-rays, and more complete physical examination. Surgical intervention in this group may be delayed hours or days, as with delayed rupture of the spleen.

Patients who are severely injured should be admitted to the emergency room in a trauma area equipped for emergency resuscitation. This room should contain such items as intravenous fluids, overhead operating-room light, oxygen, cardiac monitor and defibrillator, and a portable carriage which is suitable for an operating-room table in an emergency situation. A cabinet should be in the room containing a tracheostomy tray, closed chest drainage tray, venous section tray, closed-chest drainage bottle, intravenous fluids with tubing and needles, and syringes for four-quadrant abdominal paracentesis and pericardiocentesis. The cabinet shelf should have clearly visible labels under each tray or set of instruments. These trays and instruments should be kept in this trauma room and not in central supply, as a waiting period of even 5 minutes may prove fatal.

ADEQUATE AIRWAY. The first and most important emergency measure in the management of the severely injured patient is to establish an effective airway. A cabinet should be available at the head of the emergency room carriage in which a laryngoscope and cuffed endotracheal tubes of various sizes are available. Endotracheal intubation is a most rapid method of obtaining an adequate airway. Once an airway is established, a means of positive-pressure breathing should be available, such as an Ambu bag or an intermittent positive-pressure breathing machine. A cuffed endotracheal tube is desirable, so that positive-pressure breathing may be accomplished if needed in the resuscitation or in the administration of anesthesia. Either wall suction or a portable suction machine must be available in the trauma room to remove pulmonary secretions, foreign bodies, and, frequently, blood from the upper respiratory tract. When an endotracheal tube cannot readily be inserted, a tracheostomy may be done.

SHOCK AND HEMORRHAGE. Shock is usually controlled while the patient's airway is being cleared by another person. Internal hemorrhage will require immediate surgical intervention. Hypovolemic shock is best prevented or controlled by starting intravenous infusions in at least two extremities, using 18-gauge needles or cutdown catheters of comparable size. At least one upper extremity should be chosen for the intravenous infusion in the presence of abdominal wounds. If the inferior vena cava or one of its major tributaries is partially severed, the intravenous fluid may pour from the lower extremity into the retroperitoneal space, depriving the heart of any infusion from the lower extremities. A balanced salt solution such as Ringer's lactate solution is usually started until blood is available. Blood for typing and cross matching is drawn at the time the intravenous fluid is started, and the balanced salt solution is given in addition to the blood. Shock resulting from a blood loss of 500 to 750 ml can usually be corrected by rapid administration of 2 liters of Ringer's lactate solution over a 15- to 20-minute period. Blood loss in excess of 750 ml usually requires the administration of whole blood in addition to balanced salt solution. Often, 2 liters of balanced salt solution will replace the volume and correct hypotension so that no blood is necessary, reducing the possibility of blood transfusion reaction. When a patient initially responds to 1 to 2 liters of balanced salt solution, as evidenced by a normal blood pressure and decrease in pulse rate, but subsequently becomes hypotensive, whole blood usually is indicated. However, by this time, type-specific blood usually is available and often cross-matched, which reduces the chances for a transfusion reaction. Should a patient not respond to the rapid administration of 2 liters of balanced salt solution, un-cross-matched, type O, Rh-negative blood is administered without hesitation. The administration of blood from plastic bags markedly decreases the possibility of an air embolus when blood is being pumped.

External bleeding is best controlled by direct finger pressure on the bleeding wound or vessel. Tourniquets are of little benefit in the control of major arterial bleeding and often injurious if they occlude collateral circulation. A frequent mistake is the placement of a tourniquet on an extremity tight enough to obstruct venous return but loose enough not to inhibit arterial flow; this only increases the blood loss and edema. The danger of tissue loss from tourniquet use is always present.

Superficial vessels may be ligated if they are readily seen; however, wounds are not probed in a blind attempt to place a hemostat on a vessel. As soon as bleeding is controlled, the wound is covered with a sterile dressing, and the patient is taken to the operating room, where the wound is more adequately visualized and proper instruments are available. The needless probing of wounds in the emergency room may lead to severe infection, which can be avoided by proper exploration including adequate irrigation and sterile surgical technique in the operating room.

NEUROLOGIC EVALUATION. After an adequate airway has been obtained and hemorrhage has been controlled, a gross neurologic evaluation of the patient is undertaken. Motor function in the four extremities should be verified. A progressing neurologic deficit following injury to the spinal cord may indicate an emergency laminectomy. Decompression of a hematoma may result in return of function. Thoracoabdominal injuries usually take precedence over orthopedic or neurologic injury.

CHEST INJURIES. Airway obstruction may be due to mucus, fragments of bone from facial fractures, dirt and debris, and, commonly, broken teeth or dentures. If the patient does not ventilate normally after an endotracheal tube is inserted or a tracheostomy has been performed, several injuries should be considered. These include pneumothorax, hemothorax, cardiac tamponade, flail chest, and a ruptured bronchus.

Pneumothorax. If a pneumothorax is questionable, an 18-gauge needle may be inserted into the chest in the anterior axillary line and aspiration done to reveal the presence of air. A chest x-ray is preferable, but often severe respiratory distress precludes time for x-ray confirmation. Tension pneumothorax with mediastinal shift is suggested by displacement of the trachea to the opposite side. Auscultation of the chest may reveal decreased breath sounds.

The patient with a pneumothorax is treated with closed-chest drainage. As there is little danger from the insertion of a chest tube in the absence of a pneumothorax, an anterior chest tube should be inserted if there is doubt.

Hemothorax. Diagnosis of hemothorax is similar to that of pneumothorax. If the patient on the emergency-room cart is in distress, a needle may be inserted in the eighth interspace in the posterior axillary line and aspiration done to reveal a hemothorax. This is best drained with both anterior and posterior chest tubes. The anterior chest tube is placed in the second interspace in the midclavicular line, and the posterior chest tube is placed in the eighth interspace in the posterior axillary line in the region between the midaxillary and posterior axillary line. Chest tubes are of large caliber and soft rubber so that adequate drainage may be maintained. Thoracotomy may be indicated, depending on the rate of bleeding or the presence of intrathoracic clots.

Cardiac Tamponade. During initial observation, an unsuspected cardiac tamponade may develop secondary to blunt or penetrating trauma. This is often not present on arrival in the emergency room but may develop after 1 to 2 hours of observation. The clinical signs pathognomonic for cardiac tamponade are increased venous pressure, decreased pulse pressure, particularly with a paradoxical pulse and with or without cyanosis, and subsequent development of hypotension and decreased heart sounds. Emergency treatment includes aspiration of the pericardial sac with an 18-gauge needle through the xyphocostal angle. As little as 20 ml of aspirated blood may make a remarkable difference in the patient's vital signs. Depending on the cause of cardiac tamponade, immediate thoracotomy may be required to repair the cardiac wound, or the patient may be observed until a second aspiration is necessary. Following the development of the second cardiac tamponade, almost all patients will require an emergency thoracotomy. When a patient arrives at the emergency room in shock without evidence of blood loss, this diagnosis should be suspected.

Flail Chest. Unless patients sustaining blunt trauma to the thorax and abdomen are fully disrobed in the emergency room, a flail chest may not be recognized. Patients sustaining flail chest are best treated immediately with tracheostomy and intermittent positive-pressure breathing (IPPB). This promptly expands the lungs and provides adequate ventilation, often preventing the development of atelectasis and pneumonia. Some type of stabilizing apparatus such as towel clips may be beneficial. However, towel clips alone may not be effective, since the patient may not ventilate as well without intermittent positive-pressure breathing. Sandbags are of little value and may lead to the development of pulmonary complications such as atelectasis.

Ruptured Bronchus. After rupture of a bronchus, respiratory distress, hemoptysis, cyanosis, and a massive air leak with both mediastinal and subcutaneous emphysema and/or tension pneumothorax may be observed. Often the diagnosis is not obvious. There is a close relationship between fractures of the first and second ribs and rupture of a bronchus. If extrapleural hematoma is noted, special views of the first ribs are indicated. A ruptured bronchus is treated initially with closed-chest drainage. If this does not effectively keep the lung expanded, open thoracotomy with repair of the bronchus is indicated.

Open Chest Wounds. The patient with a chest injury resulting in a sucking chest wound is best managed by immediately covering the open wound with whatever material is available, such as a large gauze bandage. This prevents further shifting of the mediastinum and allows ventilation of the opposite lung. Chest tubes are usually inserted prior to operation, and immediate surgical intervention is indicated.

Ruptured Thoracic Aorta. The diagnosis may be suspected from chest x-ray showing a widened mediastinum and confirmed by arteriography. Immediate operation usually is indicated.

PENETRATING WOUNDS OF THE ABDOMINAL WALL. All penetrating injuries to the abdominal wall are explored locally in the emergency room to determine if the peritoneal cavity is penetrated. Exploration is usually accomplished by extending the stab wound and determining its depth. In the event that the extent of penetration cannot be determined or if the stab wound violates the posterior rectus abdominis sheath, the abdominal cavity is explored. The use of radiopaque material to determine abdominal cavity penetration has been reported, but until the accuracy of this method is better confirmed, questionable penetrating injuries of the abdominal cavity should be explored. The mortality and morbidity from a negative abdominal exploration is negligible, but failure to discover such injuries as colon or liver injury for several hours may allow peritonitis and other complications to develop. All gunshot wounds of the abdomen should be explored whether penetration is evident or not. Shock waves from nonpenetrating gunshot wounds of the abdominal wall often easily transect bowel or lacerate the liver or spleen without entering the abdominal cavity.

THE UNCONSCIOUS PATIENT. Patients with closed head injuries who are unconscious must have an airway established immediately. Hypotension rarely' results from a closed head injury but is almost always caused by blood loss, usually in the thorax or abdomen. The cause of the blood loss is most rapidly determined by using an 18-gauge needle for immediate abdominal and chest taps, which may reveal nonclotting blood. The absence of blood does not rule out an intraabdominal or thoracic injury. Extreme care should be used in moving unconscious patients until injuries of the spine have been ruled out, as repositioning the head may result in transection of the spinal cord.

Immediate Nonoperative Surgical Care

HEMATURIA. A Foley catheter is routinely inserted, particularly following blunt trauma to the abdomen, to determine the presence of hematuria as well as to follow the urinary output during and immediately following the surgical procedure. Gross hematuria is evidence of urinary tract injury resulting from contusion, laceration, or rupture.

If the patient's vital signs are stable and hematuria is present, a combined cystogram and intravenous pyelogram should be done. A single 15-minute film is usually adequate to determine kidney function as well as indicate extravasation from the bladder, ureter, or kidneys. Failure to demonstrate extravasation does not rule out the possibility of a ruptured bladder or kidney. Should a nephrectomy be required during a laparotomy, functioning of the kidney on the opposite side should be proved. It is useless to attempt to visualize the kidneys by intravenous pyelogram when the patient is hypotensive. X-rays are delayed until the patient has been resuscitated and bleeding has been controlled in the operating room. If time is not available preoperatively for an intravenous pyelogram, a cassette may be placed under the patient prior to the start of surgical procedures and a pyelogram obtained intraoperatively.

FRACTURES. Fractures of the extremities are best managed immediately with splints, such as a Thomas splint for the lower extremities and an arm board for the upper extremities. Immobilization may prevent additional nerve and blood vessel injury and conversion of a closed fracture to an open one. The presence or absence of pulses in the fractured extremities should be noted on initial examination. Intravenous infusions should not be started in an injured extremity. Massive thoracoabdominal bleeding takes precedence over fractures, unless there is an accompanying arterial injury of such magnitude that there is danger of loss of limb. In such instances, it is often necessary to have two surgical teams working simultaneously.

Pelvic fractures usually are managed conservatively with a pelvic binder, traction, or only bed rest. Inability to insert a Foley catheter into the urethra following a pelvic fracture may indicate a fractured urethra.

ARTERIAL INJURIES. Any penetrating injury in the region of a major blood vessel or nerve requires surgical exploration. On initial examination, 18 percent of subsequently proved arterial injuries are noted to have a normal pulse distal to the arterial injury, and one-third of the patients have a palpable but diminshed distal pulse. Arteriography is time-consuming and often will not demonstrate extravasation if the vessel injury is covered by a clot. If the platysma muscle in the neck has been violated, the neck is explored, and carotid and/or subclavian vessels also are explored. Vessel exploration in the region of the neck should be done under endotracheal anesthesia and may require resection of a portion of the clavicle for adequate visualization. Early recognition of an arterial injury is the most important factor in preserving a viable extremity or functioning distal organ.

Diagnosis and Management of Unapparent Injury

Blunt trauma to the abdomen may produce severe intraperitoneal or retroperitoneal injury with minimal physical findings. Bowel sounds may not be lost for several hours, and evidence of retroperitoneal or intraabdominal injury may not become apparent for as long as 18 hours.

An abdominal paracentesis may be performed early in the observation period in patients with injuries from blunt trauma to the abdomen. A 95 percent diagnostic accuracy is associated with the positive abdominal tap, and even a tap which yields only a few drops of nonclotting blood is indication for abdominal exploration. A negative abdominal tap does not rule out intraabdominal injury; if injury is still suspected, peritoneal lavage is indicated. Strong suspicion of intraabdominal injury in the female with a negative abdominal tap calls for culdocentesis. Patients with signs of peritoneal irritation require exploratory laparotomy even in the absence of a positive abdominal tap.

ROENTGENOGRAMS. These are taken when a patient's vital signs remain stable but are omitted for patients in severe shock. X-rays of the chest and abdomen are routinely performed to rule out foreign bodies such as knife blades within the depths of the wound. Patients sustaining gunshot wounds should have x-rays when possible in an attempt to trace the course of the missile. Patients sustaining blunt trauma often require multiple x-rays to rule out obscure fractures of the vertebral spine and retroperitoneal injuries. X-rays of extremities will be of value in determining whether or not the missile struck bone, fractured bone, or passed near vital structures.

NASOGASTRIC INTUBATION. A Levin tube is routinely inserted in the severely injured patient. Passage of the tube may provoke vomiting and empty the stomach of large particles, preventing subsequent aspiration during anesthesia. Stomach injury from penetrating or blunt trauma may be diagnosed by finding bright red blood in the Levin tube drainage. Gastric intubation prevents gastric dilatation during tracheal intubation and aids in the prevention of postoperative distension of the small bowel.

PROPHYLACTIC ANTIBIOTICS. Antibiotics are administered preoperatively to all patients sustaining penetrating wounds of the abdomen, beginning as soon as possible after the injured patient arrives in the emergency room. They may be discontinued if exploratory laparotomy is negative. Considerable experimental evidence indicates that prophylactic antibiotics in trauma are of benefit if administered within the first 3 hours following injury. A recent review of a group of patients at Parkland Memorial Hospital, Dallas, Texas, who sustained penetrating abdominal injuries showed that there was a statistically significant decrease in the incidence of wound infection in those patients who received antibiotics preoperatively or intraoperatively as opposed to those who received antibiotics in the immediate postoperative period or therapeutically. Following injury, immunized patients are administered a tetanus toxoid booster. In unimmunized patients the wound is debrided, and 250 units of tetanus human immune globulin is administered. Patients who were previously immunized but are now taking steroids, immunosuppressive therapy, or chemotherapy or who have had extensive irradiation should receive human immune globulin, since they may not have normal antibody response. Contaminated wounds should be left open or converted to open wounds when feasible.

METABOLIC RESPONSE TO TRAUMA

(by Malcolm O. Perry)

Trauma acutely and extensively alters the delicate integration of endocrine and metabolic systems in man (see Chap. 1). The wide range of response correlates with the magnitude of injury and the metabolic adjustments of which the patient is capable. Moore has divided the metabolic response into four phases: (1) the initial injury reaction, lasting 2 to 4 days; (2) the turning point, requiring 1 to 2 days; (3) an anabolic period, characterized by protein synthesis and lasting 2 to 5 weeks; (4) a period of several months of final adjustment in which "fat gain" is preponderant. These metabolic responses can be conveniently grouped into two categories: endocrine and catabolic.

Endocrine Response

Following injury, there is increased urinary excretion of epinephrine, norepinephrine, and their metabolic products. Although the measurement of blood levels of catecholamines does not always correlate well with the clinical findings, sympathicoadrenal activity is present. During the early stages the patient frequently exhibits tachycardia, sweating, and vasoconstriction, and is pale and apprehensive. Although the clinical signs may disappear relatively rapidly, elevated urinary levels of catecholamines and their metabolic products may persist for 1 or 2 days. If no complications follow the initial traumatic episode, the primary effects of sympathicoadrenal action are noted only during the early stages of the injury and pass rather rapidly.

Many of the metabolic changes noted following injury are similar to those induced by the administration of excessive amounts of cortisone or hydrocortisone. Urinary excretion of conjugated steroids is increased in the posttraumatic period. The normal excretion of 10 to 20 mg of 17-hydroxycorticosteroids may be tripled during the first 3 to 4 days following an injury of moderate severity. If shock or liver injury has not occurred, peak blood levels of 17-hydroxycorticosteroids are obtained about 6 hours after trauma. This reaction appears to be nonspecific and more closely related to the severity of the injury than to the specific type of injury. There is a less exact correlation between the negative nitrogen balance and the increasing levels of corticosteroid production. It has been observed that even in adrenalectomized rats urinary nitrogen excretion increases after injury if the animals are maintained on constant amounts of adrenocortical extracts, suggesting that the metabolic changes which follow injury are not directly related to the absolute level of corticosteroid production. This observation accords with the concept of the corticosteroids exerting a "permissive" or "conditioning" action.

The exact relationship between injury and the function of other endocrine glands remains unclear. The increase in oxygen consumption and carbon dioxide production following injury suggests that the thyroid gland may play an essential role, but similar effects can be produced by a variety of influences in the absence of trauma. Various measurements of thyroid function fail to correlate well with energy changes in the traumatized patient. The increased calcium excretion following injury can be related quite well to immobilization, and parathyroid function need not be invoked to explain calcium loss. Somatotropin, or growth hormone, has a profound effect on body metabolism, particularly skeletal growth and the synthesis of protein. Normal growth and development seem to be directly related to its presence, but there is no evidence that this hormone is necessary for normal convalescence. At the present time, the exact reaction of these other endocrine glands to injury is unclear.

Catabolic Response

Catabolism is increased following injury. Dissolution of body protein is reflected by increased urinary nitrogen excretion; after extensive trauma or with infection, levels of 15 to 20 Gm/day may be reached. The increased rate of excretion may persist for 3 to 5 days in the uncomplicated case. This can be reduced by the administration of exogenous protein and other compounds which supply calories, thus decreasing the effect of starvation. The inability to prevent these nitrogen losses completely indicates a definite catabolic effect in excess of that produced by starvation.

If water gain and loss are kept at minimal rates, careful weight measurements will reveal a loss of body tissue. A urinary loss of approximately 10 Gm of nitrogen represents about 62 Gm of protein loss, or about 300 Gm of wet lean muscle. The protein in bone and connective tissue and in plasma less readily reflect these changes. There can be, in fact, large losses or gains in protein without detectable changes in the concentrations of plasma proteins.

As initial responses to injury dissipate, a relatively abrupt change toward normal occurs in urinary nitrogen excretion. With sufficient caloric intake, protein balance is restored. If subsequent complications do not occur, net protein gain is prominent, and recovery proceeds rapidly. This gain, however, is usually much slower than the initial loss. It will often require three to six times as long to repair the protein deficit as it took to create it. If protein and caloric intake are satisfactory, the level eventually obtained is quite close to that prior to the loss.

Metabolic Requirements

ENERGY. The normal person at rest may require 2000 kcal/day, but a febrile, severely injured patient may use 4000 kcal in a single day. Variable periods of starvation almost inevitably follow severe trauma, and weight loss in excess of water loss may reach as high as 100 Gm daily as the energy demands are met by the consumption of body tissue.

Initial energy needs are supplied by the body stores of carbohydrate, 300 to 500 Gm being present as liver and muscle glycogen. The supply is exhausted within 14 to 18 hours after severe trauma, and subsequent energy requirements must be supplied by body tissues. In the postinjury period, 200 to 500 Gm of fat may be oxidized daily to yield 1800 to 4500 kcal. This is greatly in excess of the 1000 to 1300 kcal liberated by the oxidation of 100 to 150 Gm of fat/day in starvation.

Although the major contribution to energy needs comes from the oxidation of fat, protein catabolism yields a significant number of calories. Normal daily intake of 70 Gm of protein results in the urinary excretion of some 10 Gm of nitrogen daily. Following extensive injury, urinary nitrogen may reach levels as high as 20 Gm/day, representing the liberation of more than 500 kcal.

The production of energy is dependent upon the oxidation of metabolites via the tricarboxylic cycle. The two carbon fragments, active acetate or coenzyme A (CoA), assume a pivotal position in this important process. Acetyl CoA combines with oxaloacetic acid to form citric acid, which is subsequently degraded stepwise to yield eight hydrogen atoms, two molecules of carbon dioxide, and oxaloacetic acid. The eight electrons liberated by specific dehydrogenases then are introduced into the electron transport charge for transfer to oxygen. By oxidative phosphorylation the energy of foodstuffs is thus converted to adenosinetriphosphate (ATP), which is the ultimate driving force for most of the energy reactions within the cells (Fig. 6-1).

Intravenously administered carbohydrate solutions may supply a significant portion of the caloric needs for these energy processes. These solutions also may exert a protein-sparing effect, thus reducing the dissolution of lean body tissue. Approximately 100 Gm of carbohydrate appears to be adequate to obtain maximal protein sparing. As the first phase of injury passes, parenteral feeding is replaced by oral intake, and anabolic processes approach normal although the need for increased caloric supply often continues. Moore indicates that approximately 1 Gm of nitrogen and 20 kcal/kg of body weight/day are necessary to ensure restoration of body tissues during early convalescence.

CARBOHYDRATES. Although present in relatively small amounts, the monosaccharide glucose occupies a very important position because of its ready availability for energy. The two carbon fragments are intermediates in fatty acid metabolism and energy production. Via transamination reactions, glucose eventually may be converted to amino acids and proteins. Thus, glucose is an important precursor to fat and protein, as well as a supplier of oxidative energy.

Approximately 55 percent of absorbed carbohydrate is rapidly introduced into the Krebs cycle and converted into energy, carbon dioxide, and water. A portion of the remaining carbohydrate is converted to fat or protein, and about 5 percent is stored as liver and muscle glycogen. The carbohydrate in muscle is not readily available for use except by the muscle, but liver glycogen can easily be broken down and used elsewhere in the body. This glycogen is rapidly depleted in periods of starvation and in less

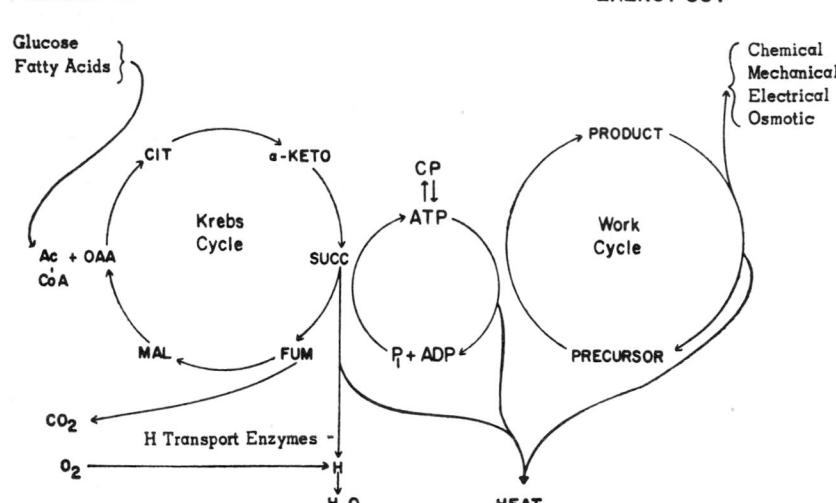

ENERGY IN

ENERGY OUT

Fig. 6-1. Schema of the mechanism of energy produced within the cell. OAA, oxalacetic acid; CIT, citric acid; α-KETO, α-ketoglutaric acid; SUCC, succinic acid; FUM, fumaric acid; MAL, malic acid; ADP, adenosinediphosphate; P_1, inorganic phosphate; ATP, adenosinetriphosphate; CP, creatine phosphate. (*From R. E. Olson, JAMA, 183:471, 1963.*)

than 5 hours may be exhausted if gluconeogenesis is interdicted. Without supplemental carbohydrate body tissues must be used to meet energy requirements.

FAT. Fat is rapidly oxidized to yield energy during starvation. From 75 to 100 Gm daily is mobilized under these conditions, but after extensive injury, as much as 500 Gm/day may be used. In addition to energy, free water is obtained. Although neutral fat contains little free water, the oxidation of 1 kg of fat liberates more than 1,000 ml of water.

VITAMINS. The suggested daily requirements of vitamins have been outlined by the National Research Council Committee on Nutrition. The exact vitamin requirements of the injured patient are not known, but it is probable that the vitamin C requirement is increased out of proportion to those of the other vitamins. There is a great individual variability in requirement for ascorbic acid in healthy adults, and it has been observed that blood level or buffy coat determinations for vitamin C do not necessarily reflect the magnitude of the deficit. It is widely held that the failure of wound healing and subsequent dehiscence is related more to the lack of vitamin C than to actual caloric starvation or protein depletion. It appears reasonable that the intake of vitamin C required to maintain normal body function in the posttraumatic patient is considerably higher than that customarily given for daily maintenance. If vitamin C is given intravenously in high levels, the renal threshold is soon exceeded, and a large portion of the administered dose is lost in the urine.

Most patients on parenteral therapy for short periods following surgical procedures for trauma will not require supplemental vitamins A and D. However, in addition to C, thiamine is certainly needed, as body stores of thiamine are rapidly depleted after the administration of large amounts of glucose. One of the important coenzymes in the tricarboxylic acid cycle necessary for oxidative decarboxylation of pyruvate to acetyl CoA is cocarboxylase, or thiamine pyrophosphate. The defect in oxidation of pyru-

vate therefore may be related to a preexisting thiamine deficiency in some patients.

Management

Most patients will reach the operating room in satisfactory nutritional status, but this desirable goal is not easily attained after extensive trauma. Preexisting nutritional and vitamin deficits may further complicate the severe metabolic response following trauma. Patients with hypoproteinemia may exhibit diminished tolerance to blood loss and reduced antibody production. There may be impaired wound healing and delayed union of fractures, and perhaps fatty infiltration of the liver in patients who are severely hypoproteinemic.

Although the normal patient at bed rest can be maintained easily on approximately 1 Gm of protein and 30 kcal/kg of body weight, after extensive trauma these requirements may be doubled or tripled. In the past it has been quite difficult to supply sufficient calories by the intravenous route.

Although protein may be supplied via administered blood plasma or albumin, these solutions are expensive, they require considerable metabolic work for their assimilation and caloric equilibrium for maximal use, and their caloric values are quite low. At one time there was widespread interest in the use of intravenous solutions containing protein hydrolysates and fat emulsions, which theoretically appeared to be more useful. However, this nutritional technique was not extensively employed because of doubtful effectiveness in preventing nitrogen losses and because of certain hazards attending their use. In 1968, Dudrick and associates reported that large quantities of protein hydrolysates and dextrose could be administered through a catheter inserted in the superior vena cava to consistently and safely achieve a positive nitrogen balance and weight gain. In over 300 patients, Dudrick and his colleagues induced weight gain and promoted healing of fistulas and wounds by this technique of *parenteral hyperalimentation*. Intravenous solutions containing adequate protein, essential amino acids, fat, carbohydrate, and vitamins to meet chronic nutritional requirements are now available. This important development in the pre- and postoperative care of patients is particularly useful when protein and caloric requirements are quite high and convalescence is prolonged.

Improvements in infusion technique are primarily responsible for the success of parenteral hyperalimentation, particularly the technique of catheterizing the subclavian vein to approach the superior vena cava for instillation of the concentrated solutions. As the subclavian vein is large, the catheter does not usually produce irritation of the vein wall and subsequent thrombosis, and the rapid blood flow prevents clotting and reduces bacterial growth. Placement of the catheter tip in the superior vena cava permits rapid dilution of the hypertonic solutions, thus decreasing the incidence of chemical phlebitis. Rigid sterile technique in placement and care of these catheters has allowed an acceptably low infection rate.

It is clear that with careful attention to strict asepsis and antisepsis in preparing and infusing these solutions (see Chap. 2) parenteral hyperalimentation may be considered a primary mode of both acute and long-term therapy, rather than a modified method of intravenous treatment, and can provide all essential nutrients without exceeding the daily fluid requirements. Initially, the solutions were prepared just prior to administration, but commercial products with a wide range of constituents now are available. Minor adjustments of essential amino acids, vitamins, and ion supplementation facilitate the preparation of individualized solutions.

ANESTHESIA

(by A. H. Giesecke, Jr., E. R. Johnson and James F. Lee)

Complicating Problems

Distinct problems differentiate the injured patient requiring emergency operation from the patient well prepared for elective operation (see Chap. 11). The major problems are possible airway difficulties, lack of comprehensive preoperative evaluation, multiple injuries, the full or nonemptied stomach, intoxication with alcohol or drugs, and shock.

AIRWAY OBSTRUCTION. Establishment and maintenance of the patient's airway may be the most important step in successful resuscitation. Some form of artificial airway is indicated for any patient with respiratory obstruction, inability to clear secretions, need for artificial ventilation, or unconsciousness. The type of airway must be individualized, but oropharyngeal or nasopharyngeal airways, orotracheal tubes, nasotracheal tubes, or tracheostomy should be considered.

Endotracheal intubation, if technically possible, is an effective method of rapidly clearing an airway obstruction to allow a more orderly, unhurried tracheostomy. Intubation should be performed under direct vision with a laryngoscope so that loose fragments of bone, teeth, or tissue will not be carried into the trachea by the advancing tube. The tube may be left in place for 48 hours or longer, if necessary, to support ventilation or maintain the airway until the patient can satisfactorily perform these functions. Meticulous care is as important for the indwelling endotracheal tube as for the tracheostomy. Inspired gases should be completely humidified. Periodic saline solution instillation followed by suctioning with a sterile catheter and hyperinflation of the lungs every other hour are prerequisites for proper management. Chest physiotherapy consisting of postural drainage, percussion, and vibration are beneficial in preventing and treating atelectasis.

The period of induction of anesthesia is probably the most hazardous time in the anesthetic period. During this time, hypotension, hypoxia, arrhythmias, and vomiting are likely to occur. The patient should be preoxygenated, allowing time for placement of intravenous infusions, further appraisal of the patient's status, and protection against hypoxia during induction. If general anesthesia is selected for the emergency repair of trauma, tracheal intubation is necessary. After consideration of the preanesthetic condition, the patient may be intubated while awake or following rapid induction. Awake intubation may avoid many dangers which may occur on induction of anesthesia, is generally easily performed, and is far less distressing to the patient than most physicians anticipate. Use of topical anesthesia will facilitate awake intubation in the more alert patient with a full stomach or hypotension. Awake intubation is contraindicated in patients with penetrating eye injuries and in patients with elevated intracranial pressure.

Intubation under general anesthesia will require consideration of other factors such as restoration of circulating volume and identification of associated injuries. Rapid intravenous induction is accomplished, and a cuffed endotracheal tube is inserted. The lungs must not be manually ventilated until the endotracheal tube is in place and the cuff inflated, except when intubation has been unsuccessful and hypoxia must be prevented or treated.

Many recent developments have improved a trauma patient's chances of survival with respiratory obstruction. The use of the esophageal airway by the EMTs (Emergency Medical Technicians) and evacuation of the unconscious injured in the lateral or prone position have saved many lives. In the desperate asphyxial emergency from supraglottic obstruction, oxygenation can be established by insufflating oxygen at a high flow through a 15-gauge needle inserted into the larynx via the cricothyroid membrane. Catheter-guided endotracheal intubation and fiberoptic intubation have made intubation possible in cases in which it was previously felt to be impossible.

For desperate asphyxia with supraglottic obstruction, a rapid flow of oxygen can be administered via a 15-gauge needle inserted through the cricothyroid membrane into the tracheal lumen. This will provide sufficient oxygenation for establishing an adequate airway by tracheal intubation or tracheostomy.

LACK OF COMPREHENSIVE PREOPERATIVE EVALUATION. Morbidity and mortality of trauma are inversely related to the preinjury state of health, but no patient should be assumed to have been healthy before injury. Evidence of prior diseases, allergies, or chronic drug therapy should be sought from the patient or an available informant. The main categories of drugs which create hazardous interactions with anesthetics are hormones (corticosteroids, insulin), psychopharmacologics, antihypertensives (including diuretics), cardiac drugs (including digitalis), and anticoagulants.

MULTIPLE INJURIES. When injuries involve many areas, problems arise in establishing priorities for operative intervention. In patients with head injuries, associated injuries may compel initial consideration. However, one must be alert to change in the patient's neurologic status during the anesthesia. Usually the pupils are the best indicators, and reduced requirement for anesthesia may indicate progression of the neurologic deterioration. Conversely, if the head injury is the primary surgical target, the anesthesiologist should be alert for progression of associated trauma, such as tension pneumothorax, hemoperitoneum, and cardiac tamponade. As shock rarely is directly caused by head injuries, its occurrence in the presence of head injury should engender suspicion of other injury. Unusual diagnostic skill may be needed to assess associated injuries with effects that become apparent only after an operation is progressing in another area. For example, hemorrhage from a torn spleen or liver may be minimal at the beginning of operation to correct extremity trauma but will require careful consideration if hypotension occurs. The diagnosis may be masked and delayed by the empiric administration of vasopressors for hypotension of uncertain cause.

THE FULL OR NONEMPTIED STOMACH. The chief hazard of the unprepared stomach is vomiting and aspiration of the vomitus. Peristalsis may cease at the time of the accident because of shock, anxiety, or abdominal or central nervous system trauma. For this reason all traumatized patients should be managed as if the stomach were full regardless of the interval since the last oral intake. Where appropriate, regional anesthesia should be selected for these patients, although aspiration remains a hazard. Regional analgesia is technically contraindicated for agitated, intoxicated patients and for those with significant hypovolemia.

Awake intubation with or without topical anesthesia has been shown to be safe for the emergency patient with a full stomach. An alternative choice for a vigorous patient is rapid induction with an intravenous thiobarbiturate followed by a paralyzing dose of succinylcholine to facilitate tracheal intubation. The hazard of anesthetic overdosage exists if, following intubation, volatile inhalation agents are pumped into the lungs by controlled ventilation. The stomach should be previously decompressed with a nasogastric tube. Following administration of the thiobarbiturate, an assistant should exert continuous pressure on the cricoid cartilage to occlude the esophagus. This should not be released until the tube is securely in the trachea and the cuff inflated. The endotracheal tube should not be removed until the patient is conscious postoperatively and has protective laryngeal reflexes to prevent aspiration during extubation.

Two clinical pictures of aspiration have been described: First is the aspiration of undigested food resulting in respiratory obstruction and distress. Depending on the amount of material aspirated, patients may have acute respiratory distress with cyanosis and cardiac arrest or may exhibit a milder, chronic course leading to lobar pneumonitis and lung abscess. A second form, Mendelson's syndrome, is caused by aspiration of liquid acid gastric secretions. This is equally hazardous in terms of morbidity and mortality and is manifest by generalized bronchospasm, dyspnea, tachypnea, and cyanosis. In severe cases cardiac arrest may develop. Immediate therapy includes oxygen, endotracheal suctioning, methylprednisolone given intravenously, and broad-spectrum antibiotics. Bronchoscopy is indicated if particulate material is found in the vomitus or if signs of obstructive atelectasis develop. Tracheobronchial lavage with large volumes of saline solution is no longer recommended.

ALCOHOL AND DRUG INTOXICATION. Based largely on animal studies, the statement has been repeatedly made that the manifestations of shock are more severe in the drunk patient than in the sober patient. However, mild to moderate intoxication (blood alcohol less than 250 mg/100 ml) is reported to have no effect on the incidence of hypotension, morbidity, or mortality of surgical treatment for trauma. Higher levels of blood alcohol are expected to increase intraoperative anesthetic complications. Regional anesthesia is not technically feasible for the agitated and intoxicated patient; intravenous induction is preferred. The airway should be protected by rapid endotracheal intubation.

Patients intoxicated with cannabis, LSD, and/or amphetamines may exhibit altered responses to anesthetics. Intoxication with barbiturates and methyl alcohol may result in delayed emergence from anesthesia.

SHOCK. The severely hypovolemic patient, unresponsive to pain or verbal stimulus, should receive no anesthetic drugs which may depress the cardiovascular system. Such a patient needs endotracheal intubation, ventilation with oxygen, and restoration of circulating volume. Satisfactory operating conditions should be provided, with muscle relaxants and analgesic concentrations of nitrous oxide.

Other aspects of care for the severely hypotensive, hypovolemic patient include (1) simultaneous infusion of large quantities of blood and electrolyte solutions, warmed to avoid myocardial hypothermia and irreversible cardiac arrhythmias; (2) administration of calcium as an antagonist to hyperkalemia, to prevent citrate intoxication and to strengthen myocardial force; (3) administration of sodium bicarbonate to correct the acidosis produced by anaerobic metabolism and infusion of acidotic blood; and (4) administration of large doses of steroids, although their efficacy is not firmly established.

Simultaneous infusions of type-specific whole blood and balanced salt solutions are used for the resuscitation of patients in hypovolemic shock. Balanced salt solutions are infused to correct the deficit in functional extracellular fluid volume which has been demonstrated to occur in hypovolemic shock and severe tissue trauma. The following guidelines are followed in the rational and moderate approach to the treatment of hypovolemic shock: (1) balanced salt solutions are not a substitute for whole blood; (2) blood should be given whenever losses approach 10 percent of blood volume; (3) balanced salt solutions are intended to replace deficits in functional extracellular fluid; (4) balanced salt solutions should be given to hypotensive, emergency room patients while type-specific whole blood is being obtained; (5) during surgery, blood loss is replaced with blood plus balanced salt solution at a rate of 7 to 10 ml/kg/hour; (6) patients with cardiac or renal disease deserve special consideration and care in fluid therapy; (7) intravenous infusions should be warmed; (8) microfiltration may be employed in transfusions of whole blood or packed cells; (9) packed cells should be reconstituted with normal saline solution prior to infusion.

Assessment of the Patient's Status

Blood pressure, pulse, skin color, capillary filling time, and pupil size should be monitored during all anesthesia. In addition, the central venous pressure of the severely traumatized patient should be monitored to detect early failure of the myocardium and overload with colloid solutions. The hourly urine output should be monitored to determine the efficacy of fluid therapy. Output should be at least 50 ml/hour if the extracellular fluid volume is being sufficiently replaced with a balanced salt solution.

Premedication

The emphasis in anesthesia for trauma is on resuscitation. An obligation exists to relieve suffering of a patient whose physical condition will tolerate the effects of analgesic drugs. However, hypoxic agitation must be differentiated from suffering. Barbiturates should not be used if the patient is in pain, as in this circumstance they tend to produce the paradoxic response of excitement or depressed agitation rather than sedation. Narcotics are contraindicated for patients with closed head injuries, because they deepen the depression, produce miosis, and mask the progression of intracranial injuries. For its drying effects and vagal depressant characteristics, an anticholinergic drug should be used for nearly all patients.

Choice of Anesthetic

The choice of agent varies from oxygen alone for the patient in hypovolemic shock to the full range of anesthetic agents for the patient with intact homeostatic mechanisms. Those agents and techniques should be chosen which tend to facilitate successful resuscitation. The patient who is hypoxic preoperatively should be managed with an anesthetic which can be given with the highest concentration of oxygen. Nitrous oxide is acceptable for obtunded or inebriated patients. Spinal anesthesia is useful for patients with injuries of the lower extremities if the central nervous system is not involved, if the blood volume has been replaced, and if the patient is not otherwise unmanageable.

A guiding principle in the choice of anesthetic agents and techniques is that complete supression of sensation is not necessary and may be harmful if achieved by deep anesthesia. Extensive surgical procedures can be performed in analgesic planes of nitrous oxide, ether, cyclopropane, or halothane, or by combining light general and local anesthesia. Severely traumatized and unconscious patients will require oxygen only and perhaps a muscle relaxant.

Postoperative Management

Not all the effects of massive trauma may be apparent at the same time. Following definitive correction of damage in one area, the patient must be closely observed for evidences of injury in other areas. The usual principles of recovery-room care must be applied. These include oxygen by mask, at least until the patient is awake and oriented; periodic use of intermittent positive-pressure breathing; frequent turning from side to side; and monitoring of the blood pressure, pulse rate, adequacy of ventilation, urine output, fluid infusion, gastric suction, emergence from anesthesia, and evidences of continued or recurring blood loss.

Delayed emergence from anesthesia may be caused by many factors, including possible head injury from the initial trauma or brain damage from prolonged shock or hypoxia. Progression of nervous system lesions should be watched for even if head injury was not suspected prior to operation. If the patient remains motionless except for breathing, anesthetic overdosage may be the cause, but the differential diagnosis should include spinal cord injury, brain damage, persistent partial curarization, overdosage with curare antagonists, hypothermia, and alcohol or drug intoxication. Bizarre causes for failure to awaken include myasthenia gravis, hypothyroidism, hypoglycemia, sickle cell crisis, intermittent porphyria, and nonketotic hyperosmotic coma.

Hypoventilation is a difficult problem to assess clinically in the postoperative patient. It can be caused by one condition or by a combination of several perplexing conditions. The list of reasons for hypoventilation includes most of those considered in delayed emergence from anesthesia, i.e., anesthetic overdosage or idiosyncrasy, relaxant overdosage or idiosyncrasy, overdosage with narcotics given for postoperative pain, endocrinopathies including myasthenia gravis and hypothyroidism, fluid overload, shock, neomycin or streptomycin administered intraperitoneally, upper and/or lower airway obstruction, respiratory restriction by dressings or casts, pneumothorax or hemothorax, abdominal distension, and pain.

An informed suspicion is required for the early diagnosis of hypoventilation, since the classic syndrome appears late and may be masked. Signs include restlessness, stridor or retractions, air hunger, disorientation or stupor, diminution of respiration (volume and/or frequency), hypertension which progresses to hypotension, tachycardia changing to bradycardia, and pallor or cyanosis. Chest roentgenograms may show atelectasis, pneumonitis, pneumothorax, or hemothorax. Spirometer measurements will confirm diminished tidal ventilation. Arterial blood-gas analysis will show hypercapnia, acidosis, and arterial unsaturation.

The proper treatment for hypoventilation is directed primarily at respiratory assistance or control with a breathing apparatus. Other measures may be indicated for specific causes: atropine and neostigmine to reverse residual paresis from curare; levallorphan or naloxone to antagonize narcotics; and analeptics. All are useful but are secondary to good ventilatory support.

PRINCIPLES IN THE MANAGEMENT OF WOUNDS

(by Ronald C. Jones and G. Tom Shires)

Primary Wound Management

The most important single factor in the management of contaminated wounds is adequate debridement. This old surgical principle frequently has been forgotten since the advent of antibiotics. All tissue which is dead, has a poor blood supply, or is heavily contaminated should be removed if at all possible. This is particularly true of subcutaneous fat and muscle. Skin with impaired blood supply should be removed initially because of its tendency to suppurate and become infected. Granulation tissue formation and later grafting procedures are preferable. Following sharp debridement and hemostasis, the wound is irrigated with copious quantities of saline solution, depending on the area and degree of soft tissue injury and contamination. That the incidence of wound infection is inversely proportional to the amount of irrigation and debridement at the time of injury has been demonstrated by Singleton et al. and by Peterson and confirmed clinically many times.

LOCAL CARE OF WOUNDS

Glass or sharp instruments usually carry a minimal amount of foreign material into a wound and cause a minimal amount of tissue trauma. X-rays should be taken of any area in which the depth of the wound cannot clearly be seen. It is not uncommon for the deep portion of a stab wound to contain the tip of a knife blade or other foreign body. Stab wounds of soft tissues are explored in the emergency room with the gloved finger or under local anesthesia by extending the length of the laceration to determine the direction and extent of the wound and to rule out any major vessel, nerve, or organ injury. The wound is then irrigated with copious amounts of saline solution. If the solution is found not to penetrate the peritoneal cavity, a small, soft-rubber Penrose drain is inserted, and the wound is left open for drainage. The drain is removed in 24 hours. Gunshot wounds are debrided externally and left open for drainage. Suturing these wounds leaves a closed contaminated space, and the infection can easily spread to surrounding soft tissue structures. Deep lacerations involving the extremity with damage to major vessels and tendons and massive muscle injury are managed by controlling major vessel bleeding and immediately wrapping the wound in sterile dressings. An x-ray is taken, if indicated, but a severe laceration is not explored until the patient is in the operating room. This procedure prevents undue contamination of the wound in the emergency room before the patient is adequately prepared. Minor lacerations can be managed in the emergency room.

Muscles usually can be approximated and, depending on the type of wound, the skin and subcutaneous tissue may or may not be closed initially. These wounds are often left open and have delayed primary closure in 3 to 5 days. Damaged muscle due to gunshot wounds is debrided, hemostasis is obtained, and the wound is irrigated as outlined above. The wounds are packed open and closed with delayed closure. All patients with such wounds receive antibiotics and tetanus toxoid.

Antibacterial soaps or detergent materials are not used to irrigate wounds when muscle, tendon, or blood vessels are visible. Severe chemical irritation to these structures may occur, with resultant structure impairment and delayed wound healing.

Many factors, such as the number and virulence of organisms, blood supply of tissue, host resistance, shock, adequacy of surgical debridement, tissue tension, dead space, hemostasis, age, and associated diseases, are responsible for infection. Condie demonstrated in dogs that obliterating dead space reduced the occurrence of wound infection in the presence of contamination. Viable bacteria can be demonstrated in many surgical wounds at the time of closure; however, few incisions become infected. Therefore, the number of bacteria encountered in clean operations is not, in itself, sufficient to produce sepsis.

Cosmetic appearance is a secondary consideration; the primary aim is to avoid infection and cover vital structures. No attempt at plastic repair is made at the initial closure of a potentially contaminated wound. Jagged edges of skin with poor blood supply are trimmed, and any resulting unpleasant scar can be cared for at a later date when no infection is present. Most lacerations, regardless of location, will never need revision if they meet the criteria previously outlined for the primary closure.

PUNCTURE WOUNDS. The most frequent puncture injury is that caused by a rusty nail in the foot. Initial treatment consists of ellipsing a small area of skin and subcutaneous tissue around the puncture site. A simple method of excising a portion of skin uses cuticle nippers. The wound is then irrigated with copious amounts of saline solution and left open for drainage. The patient is started on antibiotics both to prevent secondary infection and to aid in the prevention of tetanus, since this wound is not completely open to the air.

Puncture wounds elsewhere in the body are debrided more conservatively if they involve only the skin and subcutaneous tissue. Human tetanus immune globulin is given (250 mg) to the unimmunized patient. Debridement with conversion to an open wound and the administration of antibiotics and tetanus toxoid, whether or not the patient has been previously immunized, is also performed.

POWER MOWER INJURIES. Injuries resulting from the use of power mowers have increased in recent years. These include injuries from flying objects thrown from the power mower and from the mower itself to the hands and feet, particularly the fingers and toes. Treatment has consisted of covering exposed bones with muscle and leaving the entire wound open. These injuries almost uniformly become infected if an attempt is made to close the wound primarily. Patients are treated with systemic antibiotics and tetanus prophylaxis, and the wounds are packed with fine-mesh gauze. Skin grafting and reconstructive procedures should be delayed.

Emergency Laparotomy

INCISIONS. A longitudinal midline incision is regularly used for exploratory laparotomy in patients with abdominal trauma and does not endanger the abdominal muscle blood supply or nerve supply, or damage aponeuroses. Skin towels are routinely sewn into place, if time permits, to prevent skin contamination and drying of subcutaneous tissues. Minimal ligatures are used on bleeders which are contained in small bits of tissue, as each extra ligature is a foreign body and enhances the chance of a wound infection. Tissues should be kept moistened and gently handled. Surgical technique governs the development of wound infection as significantly as any single factor.

SUTURE. Number 30 stainless steel wire is the suture material of choice for closing the uncomplicated midline abdominal incision, particularly in operations for traumatic lesions. This has been shown to cause the least reaction and is of sufficient strength. It has not been the cause of draining sinuses following postoperative wound infections. Suture placement is probably the most important factor in the prevention of wound dehiscence. There is no longer need to overlap fascia, since new tissue comes from surrounding tissue, and if fascia is freed to allow overlapping, this surrounding tissue is damaged. Sutures should not be placed at equal distances from the edge of the fascia, as they will fall in the same group of fibers; should one suture tear the fascia longitudinally, the tear may extend from suture to suture until dehiscence occurs. Sutures should be staggered or placed at varying intervals from the edge of the fascia. With such a closure, there should be no fear in having a patient cough vigorously for adequate postoperative pulmonary care. No problem has occurred with wire sutures protruding through the skin. An occasional patient with minimal subcutaneous tissue will complain of pain in the incision when the wire is

under a pressure point such as a belt. These sutures are easily removed under local anesthesia.

Simple interrupted suture is used to close the fascia and peritoneum in a single layer. This is felt to be superior to the figure-of-eight suture, because less tissue is gathered and the suture can be placed faster, thus reducing anesthesia time. Interrupted sutures are used instead of running sutures, because a break in the suture material will not loosen the entire incision. Regardless of the type of suture or method of placement, the fascia should be loosely approximated and not strangulated. Tightening fascial sutures may lead to necrosis with the suture subsequently cutting through the tissue. Retention sutures have not been regularly used. Routine antibiotic irrigation of the wound for the prevention of infection has not been necessary. Fragmentation of wire sutures has been described as a complication, but this must be quite rare; we have seen no patients with fragmentation with erosion into a viscus such as the small bowel.

Through-and-Through Closure. Several local and systemic factors noted at the time of the original operation may make through-and-through closure the procedure of choice (Fig. 6-2). This uses plastic bridges and #4 stainless steel wire swaged on a large cutting needle. The bridges prevent cutting of skin by the wire and allow for swelling which occurs in the first 24 to 48 hours postoperatively. These sutures usually do not require postoperative adjustment. Wounds massively contaminated from shotgun wadding and fecal material, in patients on steroids, or associated with massive infection and peritonitis are best handled with through-and-through closure. Often a single patient may have several indications for this type of closure such as chronic pulmonary disease, obesity, and/or chronic debilitating disease. Occasionally through-and-through closure is used at the end of a lengthy operation with a long incision to shorten anesthesia time if the patient is not tolerating the procedure well. This type of closure is routinely used in the patient requiring reoperation in the early postoperative period because of gastrointestinal bleeding or intestinal obstruction. The wires are left in place for 3 weeks. This measure has proved to be sure, safe, timesaving, and often lifesaving.

INFECTION. Infection and severe abdominal distension are frequently mentioned as causative factors in dehiscence. Routine use of the Levin tube may prevent the latter. A severe wound infection may be prevented in the markedly contaminated abdomen by leaving the skin and subcutaneous tissue open down to the fascia for delayed primary closure. This method is frequently used in long operations or with excessive contamination such as from feces. Staphylococcus remains the number one organism causing wound infections in trauma patients. Abdominal wounds frequently harbor coliform organisms if bowel injury has been sustained. These wounds are packed open with fine-mesh gauze, changed daily for debridement, and either closed at 5 days or allowed to granulate until closure. This procedure will usually result in an excellent scar. Reoperation in the same area of a previous wound infection, even months later, will frequently result in a second wound infection.

Fig. 6-2. Through-and-through wire closure. (*From G. T. Shires, "Care of the Trauma Patient," p. 37, McGraw-Hill Book Company, New York, 1966.*)

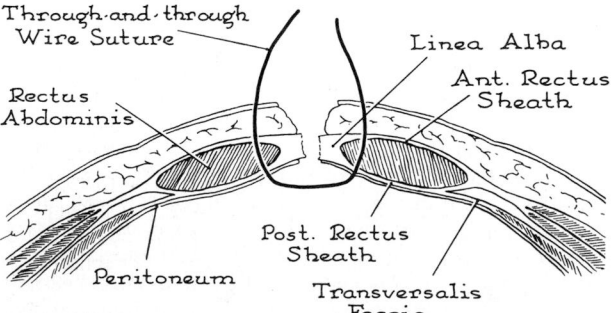

DRAINS. Subcutaneous drains will not substitute for good hemostasis. Failure to obtain hemostasis will give rise to a hematoma which is an excellent culture medium for an already contaminated wound. Drains from the abdominal cavity are usually brought out through a separate stab wound which will easily admit two fingers and by the most direct route, which occasionally may be through the midline incision. This is especially true for some liver and pancreatic injuries. Drainage of the free peritoneal cavity is not attempted unless drainage of a particular organ or a well-localized abscess is specifically indicated.

Antibiotics

Sepsis is related to the length of time which elapses between bacterial contamination of the traumatic wound or surgical incision and the start of treatment designed to prevent sepsis. The "golden period" for wound infection has been stated to be 6 hours, but the effectiveness of preventive antibiotics in surgical wounds has been shown to be no more than 3 hours. In fact, the shorter the time between contamination or surgical incision and the administration of antibiotics, the more effective are the antibiotics in preventing a bacterial infection.

Burke has demonstrated in animals injected with staphylococci that the steps which determine the size of a bacterial lesion take place very shortly after the bacteria reach the tissue. As the time interval between the injection of bacteria and the administration of an antibiotic increases, the antibiotic effect on the size of the lesion produced is decreased. Most of the antibiotic effect is over in 1 to 2 hours. As antibiotics injected more than 3 hours after staphylococci have been introduced have no effect on the size of the 24-hour lesion, it appears that there is little benefit from antibiotics administered 3 hours following the injection of staphylococci. This indicates that the antibiotic should be given early, so that it is in the tissue when the bacteria arrive. If given postoperatively, the antibiotic may reach the local dead tissue after the time period considered safe for traumatic injuries, and bacteria already may be beginning to multiply.

Viable bacteria can be demonstrated in many surgical wounds at the time of closure; however, only a minimal number later become infected. Therefore, the number of bacteria encountered in clean operations is not alone sufficient to produce sepsis. There is considerable evidence that other factors produce decreased host resistance.

Various regions of the body respond differently to wound contamination. Clinical experience has long shown an inverse relationship between the vascularity of an area and its susceptibility to infection. This probably is reflected in the low incidence of infection in head and neck operations, compared with the higher incidence with abdominal operations. Normal tissues have remarkable resistance to microorganisms, but devitalized tissues have limited resistance. Thus, the development of local wound infection depends greatly on the altered physiologic state of the wound. In addition, Ollodart and Mansberger have demonstrated in both animals and man that bacterial resistance is decreased following hypovolemic shock.

Surgical materials and technique are also important. Suture material enhances the virulence of staphylococci several-fold. Altemeier and Wulsin have shown that this occurs less with monofilament suture than with twisted or braided material. However, Condie and Ferguson have shown that dead space is more important in the production of wound infection than is increased amount of suture material.

Various regions of the body respond differently to wound contamination. Clinical experience has long shown an inverse relationship between the vascularity of an area and its susceptibility to infection. Normal tissues have remarkable resistance to microorganisms, but devitalized tissues have limited resistance. Thus, the development of local wound infection depends greatly on the altered physiologic state of the wound. Ollodart and Mansberger have demonstrated in both animals and human beings that bacterial resistance is decreased following hypovolemic shock. Routine antibiotic irrigation of the wound for the prevention of infection is not necessary if systemic antibiotics are being administered.

Approximately 80 percent of the organisms cultured from trauma patients with bacteremia are gram-negative. The mortality for polymicrobial bacteremia is almost twice that with single organisms. *Klebsiella pneumoniae, Bacteroides fragilis,* and *Pseudomonas aeruginosa* are the most frequent gram-negative organisms isolated. Enterococci remain the most common gram-positive organisms isolated from blood cultures on the trauma services, and are frequently associated with intraabdominal abscesses and wound infection. The treatment of choice for enterococcal infection is penicillin and an aminoglycoside such as gentamicin or tobramycin.

The systemic antibiotic treatment of choice for suppurative peritonitis in the absence of identification of organisms includes penicillin, Cleocin, and an aminoglycoside such as gentamicin or tobramycin. The combination of penicillin and an aminoglycoside is effective against the enterococci, and the aminoglycoside is effective against over 96 percent of gram-negative organisms. Clindamicin is effective against anaerobes, particularly *B. fragilis.* Two-drug combinations such as penicillin and an aminoglycoside or Cleocin and an aminoglycoside are also usually effective. If a single antibiotic is preferred, high-dose cephalothin, 12 Gm daily, is probably the drug of choice. Stone has demonstrated that cephalothin is as effective as clindamicin in the treatment of patients with peritonitis. The incidence of intraabdominal abscess formation appears to be common following the administration of penicillin and tetracycline since half the gram-negative organisms are resistant to tetracycline, and *Enterococcus* is a common pathogen. Penicillin and tetracycline appear to have little effect on the more resistant *E. coli* and *Klebsiella. Proteus mirabilis, Pseudomonas,* and *Providentia stuartii* are resistant to tetracycline, as are *B. fragilis* in most cases. After cultures are available, antibiotics can be stopped or changed, occasionally to a single antibiotic, although mixed gram-positive and gram-negative infections are common.

Following severe penetrating abdominal trauma, intraabdominal abscess formation is common, even with pro-phylactic antibiotic therapy. The organisms recovered from abscesses and peritonitis include *E. coli, Klebsiella,* and *B. fragilis.* Gram-positive organisms include enterococci, anaerobic streptococci, and *Clostridium.* Gorbach has demonstrated that *B. fragilis* is the most common anaerobe isolated following penetrating abdominal trauma, and these organisms were significantly altered by the adminis-tration of a combination of clindamycin and kanamycin. *B. fragilis* is the most significant anaerobic pathogen in infections below the diaphragm, and is the most common organism found in the colon, outnumbering gram-negative aerobes by a hundred times. Any abscess which fails to culture an organism is strongly suspected of containing anaerobes; this may be further supported by performing a Gram stain of the purulent material. Organisms present on Gram stain give some indication of which antibiotics are to be selected—i.e., antibiotics for gram-positive, gram-nega-tive, or a mixed infection.

A sinogram through any drain tract or wound is the simplest and most direct method of detecting an intraab-dominal collection. Unless the patient is producing large quantities of purulent material through a drain tract, rou-tine cultures of the drain tract are of limited benefit. How-ever, if large volumes of purulent material are produced, the organisms isolated in this instance frequently are those present in a deeper abscess. Occasionally a sump drain may be placed through this drain tract and the abscess aspirated without the necessity of a formal laparotomy; however, the majority of these cases require formal drain-age. Prompt drainage and identification of the continued source of sepsis are most important.

INTRAPERITONEAL ANTIBIOTICS. Since the advent of sulfa drugs, the administration of antibiotics intraperito-neally has been advocated. Artz demonstrated in dogs that antibiotics administered intravenously 2 hours after a fecal suspension had been injected intraperitoneally gave the same degree of protection as did intraperitoneal adminis-tration, without its complications. Because of the degrees of respiratory depression following intraperitoneal admin-istration of neomycin and kanamycin, the concentration should be no greater than $\frac{1}{2}$ %. Pittinger noted in 1959 the toxic responses that occur during anesthesia following administration of intraperitoneal antibiotics, and reported several instances of severe respiratory depression following intraperitoneal administration of neomycin. An effective antagonist of the respiratory and neuromuscular depres-sant actions of antibiotics is intravenous calcium gluconate and sodium bicarbonate. Intraperitoneal irrigations with-out systemic antibiotics reduce primary wound infection more than intraabdominal abscess formation. The question remains as to whether intraperitoneal antibiotics offer any value over systemic antibiotics.

Condon demonstrated, with the administration of 500 mg kanamycin intraperitoneally, that there was rapid absorption of the drug, producing serum levels comparable to those achieved with an intramuscular injection of kana-mycin. Rambo has demonstrated the rapid absorption of cephalothin by intraperitoneal irrigation, resulting in a serum level comparable to that obtained by systemic ad-

ministration and a high peritoneal fluid level following intravenous infusion of cephalothin. For single intraopera-tive instillation of cephalothin, 4 gm/liter may be used. Barnett has reported the effectiveness of cephalothin for established peritonitis; he believes it to be the drug of choice. The antibiotic used must be calculated into the total daily systemic dose unless rapidly removed.

Intraperitoneal antibiotic irrigation is not routine on a trauma service. Patients with significant intraperitoneal contamination are given systemic antibiotics, the abdomen is irrigated with saline solution, the fascia is closed, and the skin and subcutaneous tissue left open for delayed primary closure, usually within 3 to 4 days.

Singleton has shown that the incidence of infection in wounds already 4 hours old can be reduced by freshening with gauze sponges before irrigation, as opposed to irriga-tion without scrubbing the wound edges. Scrubbing the wound with a solution was significantly more effective than instillation of the solution intraperitoneally. Howes found that irrigation of a contaminated crushed wound in rabbits before 3 hours resulted in a significant reduction in infec-tions, but that infection was not prevented after 3 hours unless the wound was freshened with debridement.

A review of 400 patients sustaining gunshot and stab wounds to the abdomen indicated that the incidence of infection in patients with abdominal injuries who received prophylactic antibiotics penicillin and tetracycline in the emergency room or intraoperatively was lower (4.5 per-cent) than in patients who did not receive antibiotics until the immediate postoperative period or therapeutically (9 percent). Patients receiving gunshot wounds are at a four times greater risk of infection than stab wound victims. If no significant injury is found at laparotomy, antibiotics are discontinued in the recovery room or postoperatively dur-ing the first 24 hours. With severe contamination, antibiot-ics are administered for 3 to 5 days.

If the patient develops an infection following topical or intraperitoneal irrigation with antibiotics, the organisms isolated are usually resistant to the antibiotic used. This has been almost uniformly true in those patients receiving prophylactic antibiotics following penetrating abdominal trauma.

BITES AND STINGS OF ANIMALS AND INSECTS

(by Ronald C. Jones and G. Tom Shires)

Rabies

INCIDENCE. In the United States an estimated 2 million human beings are bitten by animals yearly, and $\frac{1}{2}$ million are bitten by dogs. Any mammalian animal may carry rabies. In 1975 there were 2,674 laboratory-confirmed cases of rabies. The animals most frequently reported infected and the percentage of the cases they accounted for were skunks (46 percent), foxes (15 percent), bats (11 percent), cattle (9 percent), dogs (5 percent), cats (5 percent), and raccoons (4 percent). In 1971, 80 percent of the rabies in this country was in wildlife species. Wildlife rabies was also reported in coyotes, opossum, otter, bobcats, bear, squirrel, deer, mink, woodchucks, coatis, and a badger. Domestic rabies was reported in cattle, dogs, cats, horses, mules, sheep, goats, swine, and guinea pigs in 1971. The Communicable Disease Center estimates that this represents less than 10 percent of the cases that actually exist. In the past 5 years, there has been an average of two cases of human rabies per year. Table 6-1 shows the incidence and frequency of reported rabies in the United States in various animals and in human beings by states or territory in 1975. Many of the few cases of human rabies reported in the past 10 years have resulted from exposure abroad.

EPIDEMIOLOGY. Saliva from a rabid animal contains large numbers of the rabies virus and is inoculated through a bite, any laceration, or break in the skin. Animal experiments and at least two human infections indicate that animals and man can become infected by bats, without being bitten, by inhalation of rabies virus. Girard examined bats and demonstrated rabies virus in the brain, kidney, urine, salivary gland, adrenal gland, and liver using the fluorescent antibody test. Most cases of racoon rabies are reported from Florida and Georgia, the only part of the United States where a cycle of transmission in raccoons has been established.

The maintenance of wild and exotic animals such as skunks, raccoons, ocelots, and bobcats as household pets is discouraged since many of these animals are infected with rabies. If people insist on maintaining wild and exotic animals as household pets, these animals should be quarantined for a minimum of 90 days after capture and vaccinated at least 30 days prior to being released to an owner. Annual vaccination is recommended.

Dogs and cats bitten by a known rabid animal should be destroyed immediately. If the animal has been vaccinated within the previous 3 years, it should be revaccinated immediately and confined for 90 days.

DIAGNOSIS. Circumstances of the Bite. Circumstances surrounding the attack frequently furnish vital information as to whether or not vaccine is indicated. Most domestic animal bites are provoked attacks; if this history is obtained, rabies vaccine can usually be withheld if the animal appears healthy. Children are frequently bitten while attempting to separate fighting animals or while teasing or accidentally hurting the animal. Bites during attempts to feed or handle an apparently healthy animal should generally be regarded as provoked. Frequently the patient has attempted to handle a sick animal.

Although vaccination of the animal does not totally rule out the possibility of transmitting rabies, it is over 90 percent effective. A small number of dog rabies have apparently involved vaccine failure.

Bites from rodents, including squirrels, chipmunks, rats, and mice, seldom require specific rabies prophylaxis. Each case of possible exposure must be studied individually before a conclusion can be reached as to whether antirabies therapy is indicated. An unprovoked attack is more likely to indicate that the animal is rabid.

Extent and Location of Bite Wound. The likelihood that rabies will result from a bite varies with its extent and location. For convenience in approaching management, two categories of exposure are widely accepted:

Severe: Multiple or deep puncture wounds, or any bites on the head, face, neck, hands, or fingers.
Mild: Scratches, lacerations, or single bites on areas of the body other than the head, face, neck, hands, or fingers. Open wounds, such as abrasions, suspected of being contaminated with saliva also belong in this category.

Laboratory Diagnosis. The fluorescent antibody test described by Goldwasser and his associates appears to be a more accurate test than the stain for Negri bodies. The intracerebral inoculation of mice combined with the microscopic examination of brain tissue for Negri bodies is still one of the most useful tests in the laboratory diagnosis of rabies and should be used whenever human beings have been bitten by suspect animals and the fluorescent antibody test is negative.

MANAGEMENT OF BITING ANIMALS. Most animal bites of human beings are caused by dogs and cats, and in most instances it is possible to observe the biting animal for the development of rabies. Domestic animals that bite a person should be captured and observed for symptoms of rabies for 10 days. If none develop, the animal may be assumed to be nonrabid. If the animal dies or is killed, the head should not be damaged but should be sent promptly to a public health laboratory for examination. The tissue requires refrigeration but not freezing, and transportation to the laboratory following death of the animal should be rapid. Clinical signs of rabies in wild animals cannot be interpreted reliably; therefore, any wild animal that bites or scratches a person should be killed at once (without unnecessary damage to the head) and the brain examined for evidence of rabies.

Information from the county health department regarding which animals, both domestic and wild, have been reported to be rabid within the past 10 years in the particular area may indicate a possible specific animal transmitting rabies.

EXPOSURE OF PERSONS PREVIOUSLY IMMUNIZED. For mild exposure of a person who has demonstrated an antibody response to antirabies vaccination received in the past, a single booster dose of vaccine is recommended. In the case of severe exposure, five daily doses of vaccine should be given followed by a booster dose 20 days later.

If it is not known whether an exposed person has had antibody, the complete postexposure antirabies treatment should be given. Because of variation in vaccine potency and individual response, immunization should not be considered complete until antibody is demonstrated in the serum. Farrar et al. have demonstrated that most persons receiving three or more injections of any rabies vaccine within 4 years will show antibody in the blood 30 days after a single booster injection of duck embryo vaccine (DEV), a killed virus.

PREEXPOSURE PROPHYLAXIS. The relatively low frequency of reactions to DEV has made it more practical to offer preexposure immunization to persons in high-risk groups, e.g., veterinarians, animal handlers, certain laboratory workers, and individuals, especially children, living in areas where rabies is a constant threat. Others whose vocations or avocations result in frequent contact with

Table 6-1. RABIES IN ANIMALS BY STATE AND BY TYPE OF ANIMAL, UNITED STATES, 1975

Area	Dog	Cattle	Other domestic	Fox	Skunk	Bat	Raccoon	Other wild	Total
United States	116	151	141	278	1,226	514	192	7	2,625
New England	2	7	2	36	5	26	..	..	78
Maine	2	7	2	36	4	1	..	..	52
New Hampshire	..	..	..	..	...	2	..	..	2
Vermont									
Massachusetts	..	..	..	..	1	11	..	..	12
Rhode Island	..	..	..	..	...	4	..	..	4
Connecticut	..	..	..	..	...	8	..	..	8
Middle Atlantic	2	5	2	21	25	64	1	..	120
New York	1	5	2	18	24	26	..	..	76
New Jersey	..	..	..	2	...	22	..	..	24
Pennsylvania	1	..	..	1	1	16	1	..	20
East North Central	20	8	12	5	87	41	2	..	175
Ohio	1	2	..	1	5	8	1	..	18
Indiana	1	..	1	1	1	6	..	..	10
Illinois	6	3	6	2	32	15	1	..	65
Michigan	..	..	3	..	2	5	..	..	10
Wisconsin	12	3	2	1	47	7	..	..	72
West North Central	27	66	52	3	402	24	4	1	579
Minnesota	10	12	7	..	143	10	1	..	183
Iowa	10	17	15	1	52	7	..	..	102
Missouri	4	2	4	1	24	6	1	..	42
North Dakota	1	16	11	..	74	..	1	..	103
South Dakota	..	12	11	1	60	..	..	1	85
Nebraska	..	2	1	..	...	1	..	..	4
Kansas	2	5	3	..	49	..	1	..	60
South Atlantic	7	6	8	113	6	54	175	1	370
Delaware	..	..	..	..	...	6	..	..	6
Maryland	..	..	..	..	...	15	..	..	15
District of Columbia									
Virginia	..	5	2	99	2	5	..	1	114
West Virginia	1	1	..	3	...	..	..	..	5
North Carolina	..	..	1	..	...	11	..	..	12
South Carolina	..	..	..	1	...	8	2	..	11
Georgia	4	..	3	10	3	7	143	..	170
Florida	2	..	2	..	1	2	30	..	37
East South Central	12	11	13	70	27	14	5	..	152
Kentucky	10	11	10	55	6	3	1	..	96
Tennessee	..	..	1	5	9	6	..	..	21
Alabama	2	..	2	10	12	4	4	..	34
Mississippi	..	..	..	..	...	1	..	..	1
West South Central	34	35	38	13	308	90	1	3	522
Arkansas	1	6	3	..	59	14	..	..	83
Louisiana	1	..	..	..	2	4	..	1	8
Oklahoma	8	15	8	..	70	4	..	..	105
Texas	24	14	27	13	177	68	1	2	326
Mountain	8	6	11	4	199	86	3	1	318
Montana	2	2	8	..	152	6	2	..	172
Idaho									
Wyoming	..	2	..	..	24	9	1	..	36
Colorado	..	..	..	1	5	26	..	..	32
New Mexico	5	2	3	1	13	18	..	..	42
Arizona	1	..	..	2	4	19	..	..	26
Utah	..	..	..	..	...	3	..	..	3
Nevada	..	..	..	..	1	5	..	1	7
Pacific	4	7	3	13	167	115	1	1	311
Washington	..	..	..	..	...	10	..	..	10
Oregon	..	..	..	..	...	6	..	..	6
California	4	7	3	7	167	99	1	1	289
Alaska	..	..	..	6	...	..	..	..	6
Hawaii	..	..	..	..	...	..	..	..	
Guam									
Puerto Rico	13	7	5	..	...	..	..	24	49
Virgin Islands	..	..	..						

SOURCE: Reported through the Rabies Surveillance Program, Center for Disease Control.

dogs, cats, foxes, skunks, or bats should also be considered for preexposure prophylaxis.

A significant number of citizens of the United States have been and, with increasing frequency, will continue to be exposed to rabies in other countries where rabies in dogs is a major problem. Because rabies in animals is widespread in large areas of Asia, Africa, and Latin America, the Foreign Quarantine Program of the United States Public Health Service has recently advised that preexposure immunization against rabies with DEV be suggested for Americans traveling in these areas.

Two 1-ml injections of DEV given subcutaneously in the deltoid area 1 month apart should be followed by a third dose 6 to 7 months after the second dose. This series of three injections can be expected to have produced neutralizing antibody in 80 to 90 percent of vaccinees by 1 month after the third dose. For more rapid immunization, three 1-ml injections of DEV should be given at weekly intervals with a fourth dose 3 months later. This schedule elicits an antibody response in about 80 percent of those vaccinated. All who receive the preexposure vaccination should have their serum tested for neutralizing antibody 3 to 4 weeks after the last injection. Tests for rabies antibody can be arranged with or through state health department laboratories. If no antibody is detected, booster doses should be given until a response is demonstrated. Persons with continuing exposure should receive 1-ml boosters every 2 to 3 years.

ACCIDENTAL INOCULATION WITH LIVE RABIES VIRUS VACCINE. Persons inadvertently inoculated with attenuated rabies vaccines for use in animals, such as the Flury strain vaccine, are not considered at risk, and antirabies prophylaxis is not indicated.

POSTEXPOSURE PROPHYLAXIS. Incubation Period. It is generally accepted that the incubation period for rabies in human beings ranges from 10 days to 1 year, most cases occurring within 4 months of the time of exposure. In cases of exposure of the head, neck, or upper extremities, the incubation period is potentially less than 30 days.

Immediate Local Care. Not all persons bitten by rabid animals contract the disease. Vigorous local treatment to remove possible rabies virus may be as important as specific antirabies therapy. Free bleeding from the wound is encouraged. Local care of an animal bite should consist of:

1. Thorough irrigation with copious amounts of saline solution.
2. Cleansing with a 20% soap solution.
3. Swabbing with a 1 or 2% solution of benzalkonium chloride (all soap should be removed before application of quaternary ammonium compounds, because soap neutralizes the activity of such compounds).
4. Debridement.
5. Administration of antibiotic when indicated to prevent bacterial infection.
6. Administration of tetanus toxoid.
7. Immediate suturing of the wound generally is not advised, since it may contribute to the development of rabies, but a severe laceration secondary to a dog bite may be sutured if exposure to rabies is unlikely.

Passive Immunization. RIG (rabies immune globulin) in combination with DEV is considered the best postexposure prophylaxis. RIG, 20 IU/kg body weight, is recommended

for most exposures classified as severe, for all bites by rabid animals or those suspected of having rabies, for unprovoked bites by wild carnivores and bats, and for nonbite exposure to animals suspected of being rabid. A portion of the RIG is used to infiltrate the wound, and the remainder administered intramuscularly. When indicated, RIG is used instead of equine serum and is used regardless of the interval between exposure and treatment. RIG is given only once, as early as possible following exposure. The use of human immune antirabies globulin is accompanied by 21 doses of vaccine over a 14-day period, with two doses given per day for the first 7 days (Table 6-2). If RIG is not available, the recommended dose of equine antibodies serum is 40 IU/kg body weight.

Active Immunization. *Primary Immunization.* At least 23 injections, including booster doses, of vaccine in the dose recommended by the manufacturer are administered. These are given subcutaneously in the abdomen, lower part of the back, or lateral aspect of the thighs; rotation of sites is recommended.

For severe exposure, 21 doses of vaccine are recommended. These 21 doses are administered as two doses per day for the first 7 days, followed by one dose per day for seven daily doses. This method is preferred to detect the slow responder. A shorter course of vaccine is not recommended, since passive immunity induced by serum may limit response to vaccine. The vaccine may be stopped if the animal is proved nonrabid.

Booster Doses. Two booster doses, one 10 days and the other 20 days after completion of the primary course, are administered. Two booster doses are particularly important if RIG or antirabies serum was used in the initial therapy. A serum antibody titer is drawn at the time of the second booster dose to detect the poor responder, and these poor responders are given additional boosters until an adequate titer is obtained. If two additional booster doses of vaccine do not result in demonstrable antibody, authorities at the state health department or Center for Disease Control should be consulted to determine if alternative procedures such as the use of experimental vaccine (human diploid rabies vaccine) should be used.

Factors that contribute to a poor antibody response include administration of steroid during postexposure prophylaxis and use of more than 55 IU/kg of equine antirabies serum.

Side Reaction to Vaccine and Antiserum. Rabies vaccine should not be given unless there is a definite indication for its use. Local reactions to DEV are frequent. These consist of erythema, pruritus, pain, and tenderness at the site of inoculation. Generalized reactions occasionally are observed, usually after five to eight doses.

Neurologic reactions following DEV are rare. Perhaps one death has been attributed to its use. Neurologic reactions to nerve tissue vaccine constitute the principal hazard to its use. They occur in three main types: peripheral neuritis, the spinal form, and the cerebral form with acute encephalitis. Dorsolumbar paralysis may be either flaccid or spastic. Peripheral neuritis may involve facial, oculomotor, glossopharyngeal, or vagal nerves.

Immediate reactions may occur in an individual sensi-

Table 6-2. POSTEXPOSURE ANTIRABIES TREATMENT GUIDE

The following recommendations are only a guide. They should be applied in conjunction with knowledge of the animal species involved, circumstances of the bite or other exposure, vaccination status of the animal, and presence of rabies in the region.

Species of animal	Condition of animal at time of attack	Treatment of exposed person
Skunk Fox Coyote Raccoon Bat	Regard as rabid	RIG + DEV*
Dog	Healthy Unknown (escaped) Rabid or suspected rabid	None† RIG + DEV RIG + DEV*
Cat		
Other	Consider individually—see Circumstances of the Bite	

*Discontinue vaccine if fluorescent antibody (FA) tests of animal killed at time of attack are negative.
†Begin RIG + DEV at first sign of rabies in biting dog or cat during holding period (10 days).
NOTE: RIG, rabies immune globulin, human; DEV, duck embryo vaccine.

tive to avian tissue. Epinephrine is helpful in anaphylactic reactions. Should a complication develop and if, in view of the severity of the exposure, the amount of immunization already obtained is considered adequate, the vaccine may be discontinued. If further immunization is indicated, steroids and antihistamines should be administered.

Antirabies serum is obtained from immunized horses and may be expected to produce side reactions in approximately 20 percent of persons. Serum sickness occurs in approximately 5 percent of persons.

Effectiveness of Vaccines in Human Beings. Over 30,000 people receive antirabies vaccine yearly. Comparative effectiveness of vaccines can be judged only by reported failures. During the years 1957 through 1968 when both nerve tissue vaccine and DEV were available, there were six rabies deaths among 125,000 individuals receiving the nerve tissue vaccine, or 1:20,800, and eight among the 225,000 treated with DEV, or 1:28,100. It is the opinion of the National Communicable Disease Center that the clinical effectiveness of the two vaccines has not been significantly different. Therefore, the lower frequency of central nervous system reactions with DEV makes it preferable to nerve tissue vaccine. Antibody tends to develop somewhat earlier following DEV than following nerve tissue vaccine, but the titers tend to be lower. Human beings may contract rabies even after 14 doses of DEV, particularly when the incubation period has been less than 30 days.

MANIFESTATIONS AND TREATMENT OF DISEASE. Rabid dogs are noted to have purposeless movements with snapping, drooling, and vocal cord paralysis. Death usually occurs in 2 to 5 days. Man dies essentially the same way. There are 2 to 4 days of prodromal symptoms before the patient reaches the excited stage. Paresthesia in the region of the bite is an important early symptom. Symptoms noted with the onset of clinical rabies include headaches, vertigo, stiff neck, malaise, lethargy, and severe pulmonary

symptoms including wheezing, hyperventilation, and dyspnea. The patient may have spasm of the throat muscles with dysphagia. The outstanding clinical symptom of rabies is related to swallowing. Drooling, maniacal behavior, and convulsions ensue and are followed by coma, paralysis, and death.

Instead of sedation and symptomatic treatment only, it is now recognized that intensive respiratory supportive care may be beneficial, in view of a case of human rabies in which the patient survived. Strict attention was given to the management of airway, pulmonary care, cardiac arrhythmias, and seizures. This included tracheostomy, vigorous suctioning, Dilantin for seizures, close monitoring of blood gases, electrocardiograms, electroencephalograms, and a ventricular shunt. Nursing care is extremely important. Probably many organs are involved, including brain, heart, and lungs.

Snakebites

INCIDENCE. In North America all the poisonous snakes of medical importance are members of the family Crotalidae, or pit vipers, with exception of the coral snake. Coral snakes are scattered from Florida to southern Arizona, are biologically related to the Indian cobra, and produce a different envenomation syndrome than the crotalids. The pit vipers include the rattlesnake, cottonmouth moccasin, and copperhead.

Approximately 8,000 persons are bitten each year by poisonous snakes. Over 98 percent of snakebites occur on the extremities. Thirty-five percent of snakebites occur in children less than ten years of age, usually in an area around their homes. Since 1960, an average of 14 victims have died annually as a result of snakebites. Seventy percent of all such deaths occur in five states: Texas, Georgia, Florida, Alabama, and Southern California. Rattlesnakes are responsible for approximately 70 percent of all deaths due to snakebite. Death from the bite of a copperhead snake is extremely rare, probably not exceeding an incidence of 0.01 percent.

POISONOUS VERSUS NONPOISONOUS SNAKES. Pit vipers are named for the characteristic pit, a heat-sensitive organ, that is located between the eye and the nostril on each side of the head. As a rule, these snakes may be identified by their elliptical pupils, as opposed to the round pupil of harmless snakes. Nonpoisonous snakes do not have pits. However, the coral snake does have a round pupil and lacks the facial pit. Pit vipers have two well-developed fangs that protrude from the maxillae, whereas nonpoisonous snakes have rows of teeth without fangs. Pit vipers also may be identified by turning the snake's belly upward and noting the single row of subcaudal plates. Nonpoisonous snakes have a double row of subcaudal plates (Fig. 6-3). The coral snake is a brightly colored small snake with red, yellow, and black rings. This color combination occurs also in nonpoisonous snakes, but the alternating colors are different. Only the coral snake has a red ring next to a yellow ring; when red touches yellow, it is a coral snake. The nose of the coral snake is black.

The venoms of poisonous snakes consist of enzymatic, complex proteins which affect all soft tissues. Venoms have been shown to have neurotoxic, hemorrhagic, thrombogenic, hemolytic, cytotoxic, antifibrin, and anticoagulant effects. Phospholipase A is probably responsible for hemolysis. Most venoms contain hyaluronidase, which enhances the rapid spread of venom by way of the superficial lymphatics. There may be considerable variation in the venom effect. Either neurotoxic features such as muscle cramping, fasciculation, weakness, and respiratory paralysis or hemolytic characteristics may predominate depending on the snake and the patient.

CLINICAL MANIFESTATIONS OF POISONOUS SNAKEBITES. Pain from the bite of a poisonous snake is excruciating and probably the symptom that most easily differentiates poisonous from nonpoisonous snakebites. Poisonous snakes characteristically produce one or two fang marks, whereas nonpoisonous snakes may produce rows of punctures. Swelling, tenderness, pain, and ecchymosis appear within minutes at the site of the venom injection. If no edema is present within 30 minutes following the injury, the pit viper probably did not inject any venom. Swelling may continue to increase for 24 hours. Hemorrhagic vesiculations and petechiae may appear in the first 24 hours, with thrombosis of superficial vessels and eventual sloughing of tissue.

Rattlesnake. Most rattlesnakes probably eject less than 50 percent of their venom during a single biting act. Following a rattlesnake bite ecchymosis, hemorrhagic vesiculations, swelling of the regional lymph nodes, weakness, fainting, and sweating commonly are reported. The venom produces deleterious changes in the blood cells, defects in blood coagulation, injuries to the intimal linings of vessels, damage to the heart muscles, alterations in respiration, and, to a lesser extent, changes in neuromuscular conduction. Pulmonary edema is common in severe poisoning, and hemorrhage into the lungs, kidneys, heart, and peritoneum may occur. Hematemesis, melena, changes in salivation, and muscle fasciculations may be seen. Urinalysis may reveal hematuria, glycosuria, and proteinuria. Red blood cells and platelets may decrease, and bleeding and clotting times are usually prolonged.

Coral Snakes. The coral snake contributes only 1.5 percent of all deaths from poisonous snakes. Bites by the coral snake occasionally provoke blurred vision, ptosis, drowsiness, increased salivation, and sweating. The patient may notice paresthesia about the mouth and throat, sometimes slurring of speech, and nausea and vomiting. Pain is not a constant complaint, nor is edema a constant finding. Thus coral snake venom causes more extensive changes in the nervous system, but death may occur from cardiovascular collapse.

CHARACTERISTICS OF SNAKES

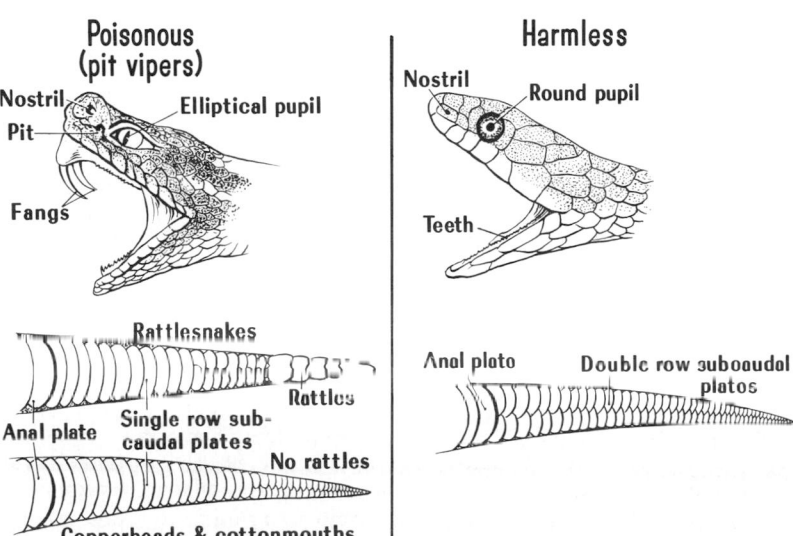

Fig. 6-3. Characteristics of poisonous and nonpoisonous snakes. (*From H. M. Parrish, Texas State J Med, 60:592, 1964.*)

LOCAL TREATMENT OF SNAKEBITES. The treatment of the bite of a poisonous snake varies considerably but is related to the length of time from the bite until treatment is instituted. The tourniquet, and incision and suction as well, are appropriate if employed within 1 hour from the time of the bite.

Immobilization. Patients are kept quiet, and the extremity is immobilized. Splinting the limb may inhibit the local diffusion of venom by stopping the movement of muscle bellies within their sheaths. Snyder and Knowles have shown in animals that exercise greatly enhances the absorption of venom, and as much as 30 percent may be absorbed within 30 minutes following vigorous exercise.

Tourniquet. The snake injects venom into the subcutaneous tissue, and this is absorbed by the lymphatics. As almost none of the venom is absorbed through the bloodstream, the tourniquet is applied loosely to obstruct only venous and lymphatic flow. The index finger should be easily inserted beneath the tourniquet after its application. The tourniquet is not released once applied and may be left in place during the 30 minutes that suction is being applied. Snyder and Knowles have injected ^{131}I-tagged venom into dogs and have demonstrated that if the tourniquet is applied promptly, less than 10 percent of the venom leaves the leg of the dog in 2 hours. The tourniquet may be removed as soon as an intravenous infusion is started and antivenin is ready for administration, if indicated.

Incision and Suction. Incision and suction should be accomplished as soon as possible after snakebite. Approximately 50 percent of subcutaneously injected venom can be removed when the suction is started within 3 minutes. Treatment in the first 5 minutes is important, since half the value of suction is lost after 15 minutes and almost all after 30 minutes. A 30-minute period of suction extracts about 90 percent of the venom which can be removed by this procedure. The incision should be $\frac{1}{4}$ in. long and $\frac{1}{8}$ to $\frac{1}{4}$ in. deep, longitudinal and not cruciate. When two fang marks are seen, the depth of the venom injection is generally considered to be one-third of the distance between the fang marks. A good rule of thumb has been to incise the skin and subcutaneous tissue the same distance between the fang marks to ensure adequate drainage. A superficial incision may be easily accomplished by raising the skin with a pinch between two fingers. This procedure rarely results in penetration of fascia or muscle. Incisions made proximal to the bite will usually recover venom insufficient to make the procedure worthwhile.

When a suction cup is not available after incisions have been made, mouth suction may be used if the mucosa of the mouth is intact. Snake venom is not absorbed through an intact oral mucosa but may be absorbed when there is any denuded area or minor laceration of the mucosa. The digestive juices neutralize poisonous snake venom if it is swallowed.

Russell has demonstrated that the serosanguinous fluid removed during suction contains substances which when injected into animals produced a fall in systemic blood pressure and changes in respiratory rates, and alterations in the electrocardiogram and electroencephalogram similar to those observed following injection of crude *Crotalus*

venom. If exudate removed during suction contains venom, its removal should increase the chances of survival.

Excision. Snyder and Knowles showed that wide excision of the entire area around the snakebite within 1 hour from the time of injection can remove most of the venom. Excision of the fang marks including skin and subcutaneous tissue should be considered in severe bites and in patients known to be allergic to horse serum who are seen within 1 hour following the bite.

Most fatalities from snakebites do not occur for 6 to 48 hours following the bite, giving time to institute these first-aid measures.

Cryotherapy. This form of therapy has been used but is not recommended, as it probably only increases the local area of necrosis. McCollough and Gennard analyzed cryotherapy in relation to amputation and noted that 75 percent of children requiring amputation following snakebite had received cryotherapy. In seven of nine snakebite cases requiring amputations in California, cryotherapy had been used. Cooling or refrigeration experimentally produces intense vasoconstriction and thus decreases the amount of antivenin getting into the area of the bite. Gill found that dogs developed edema and ecchymosis just as rapidly and extensively with cryotherapy as without it. There was no evidence to suggest inactivation of venom by tissue temperature of 15°C and below.

SYSTEMIC TREATMENT. The most important treatment for a snakebite is antivenin. Most snakebite fatalities in the United States during the past 20 years have involved either delay in obtaining treatment, no antivenin treatment, or inadequate dosage. Because antivenin contains horse serum, its administration requires prior skin testing.

Information concerning identification of a snake or proper antivenin frequently can be obtained from the nearest zoo herpetarium. A major problem with bites by exotic poisonous snakes is the choice and availability of suitable antiserum. Physicians confronted with this situation may obtain advice from the local poison control center or from the Antivenin Index Center of the American Association of Zoological Parks and Aquariums in Oklahoma City, Oklahoma (405-271-5454).

Because the rattlesnake, cottonmouth moccasin, and copperhead belong to the same biologic family, their bites can be treated by the same antivenin (antivenin Crotalidae polyvalent).

The coral snakebite is rare, and the antivenin is different from that for the pit vipers. A North American coral snake (*Micrurus fulvius*) antivenin has recently been developed and released. It effectively treats *Micrurus* coral snake bites but is not effective in treating bites of *Micruroides,* the genus native to Arizona and New Mexico. Coral snake antivenin can be obtained from many state public health departments. Also, a large supply has been stocked at the United States Public Health Service National Communicable Disease Center in Atlanta, Georgia.

The time of antivenin administration depends upon the snake involved. If the bite is from a snake with quick-acting venom, such as a king cobra or mamba, an initial dose of antivenin may be required as part of the first-aid treatment. However, for bites by most snakes, such as rattlesnakes and others with less virulent venom, antivenin should be withheld until a physician can determine if it is indicated. Approximately 30 percent of all poisonous snakebites in the United States result in no venenation.

The indication for antivenin is governed by the degree of venenation, as outlined by Wood et al. and modified by Parrish and by McCollough and Gennard:

Grade 0—no venenation: One or more fang marks; minimal pain; less than 1 in. of surrounding edema and erythema at 12 hours; no systemic involvement.

Grade I—minimal venenation: Fang marks; moderate to severe pain; 1 to 5 in. of surrounding edema and erythema in the first 12 hours after bite; systemic involvement usually not present.

Grade II—moderate venenation: Fang marks; severe pain; 6 to 12 in. of surrounding edema and erythema in the first 12 hours after bite; possible systemic involvement including nausea, vomiting giddiness, shock, or neurotoxic symptoms.

Grade III—severe venenation: Fang marks; severe pain; more than 12 in. of surrounding edema and erythema in first 12 hours after bite; grade II symptoms of systemic involvement usually present and may include generalized petechiae and ecchymoses.

Grade IV—very severe venenation: Systemic involvement is always present, and symptoms may include renal failure, blood-tinged secretions, coma, and death; local edema may extend beyond the involved extremity to the ipsilateral trunk.

Antivenin usually is not required for grades 0 or I venenation. Grade II may require three or four ampules, and grade III usually requires five ampules or more. If symptoms increase, several vials may be required during the first 2 hours. Because children are smaller, they receive relatively larger doses of venom, which places them in a higher-risk group. Thus, the smaller the patient, the relatively larger the required dose of antivenin. Proper dosage can be estimated by observing the clinical signs and symptoms. With frequent observations using this classification, the severity of the bite will be found to increase with time, and thus a change in grade is observed.

The injection of antivenin locally around the bite is not advised, as massive edema usually occurs in that area. Therefore, absorption from this area is poor, and additional antivenin fluid will further decrease perfusion and perhaps increase tissue anoxia.

Antivenin is given by intravenous drip in 250 ml of normal saline solution or 5% glucose solution. McCollough and Gennard have demonstrated in studies with radioisotopes that antivenin accumulates at the site of the bite more rapidly after *intravenous* than after *intramuscular* administration. The dose of intravenously administered antivenin can be more easily titrated with response to treatment. Antivenin is administered until severe local or systemic symptoms improve. When it is obvious that antivenin therapy will be instituted, the tourniquet should be left in place until antivenin is started intravenously.

Complications of Antivenin. If too much time has elapsed for excision to be effective and the patient is allergic to horse serum, a slow infusion of one vial of antivenin in 250 ml of 5% glucose solution may be given over a 90-minute period with constant monitoring of the blood pressure and electrocardiogram depending on the seriousness of the bite. If an immediate reaction occurs, the antivenin is stopped, and a vasopressor, epinephrine, and perhaps an antihistamine may be required, depending on the severity of the reaction.

The incidence of serum sickness is directly related to the volume of horse serum injected. Of patients receiving 100 to 200 ml of horse serum, 85 percent will have some degree of sensitivity in 8 to 12 days following injection. This complication will have to be dealt with at a later time since some patients may require from one to five vials of antiserum every 4 to 6 hours.

Steroids have been used but are of questionable benefit. Russell experimentally used doses of methlyprednisone up to 100 mg/kg in mice and noted that steroids neither affected survival nor prevented tissue damage and inflammation. When used in association with the antivenin, there is a decreased incidence of serum sickness. According to Parrish, cortisone and ACTH do not affect the survival rate of animals poisoned with pit viper venom. Antibiotics are started immediately to prevent secondary infection, and tetanus toxoid is administered. Tracheal intubation and prolonged ventilation may be required for respiratory failure. Acute renal failure may require renal dialysis.

Intravenous fluids are frequently required to replace the decreased extracellular fluid volume resulting from edema formation. Fascial planes may become very tense, with obstruction of venous and later arterial flow, requiring fasciotomy.

Blood should be immediately drawn for typing and cross matching, since hemolysis may later make this difficult. Since hemolysis and injury to kidneys and liver may occur, it is important to follow alterations in clotting mechanism and renal and liver function as well as electrolyte status. Bleeding and clotting time, platelet count, prothrombin time, fibrinogen level, and partial thromboplastin times are included in the base-line studies. These patients may need blood, since anemia can develop from the hematologic effects. As afibrinogenemia has been reported, fibrinogen may be required. Vitamin K may also be required, according to Stahnke. The patient is started on antibiotics immediately to prevent secondary infection, and tetanus toxoid is administered on arrival at the emergency ward. Prolonged artificial ventilation may be required for respiratory failure.

Stinging Insects and Animals

HYMENOPTERA

The most important insects that produce serious and possibly fatal anaphylactic reactions are the arthropods of the order Hymenoptera. This group includes the honeybee, bumblebee, wasp, yellow and black hornet, and fire ant. The venom of these stinging insects is just as potent as that of snakes and causes more deaths in the United States yearly than are caused by snakebites. Davidson states that, drop for drop, the venom of the bee is just as potent as that of the rattlesnake. Parrish noted that, of 460 deaths between 1950 and 1959, 50 percent were due to Hymenoptera, 30 percent due to poisonous snakes, and 14 percent due to spiders. Scorpions accounted for eight deaths. No other poisonous creature killed more than five persons.

Insects of the Hymenoptera group, except the bee, retain their sting and are in a position to sting repeatedly, each time injecting some portion of the venom sac contents. The worker honeybee sinks its barbed sting into the skin, and it cannot be withdrawn. As the bee attempts to escape, it is disemboweled. The stinger with the bowel, muscles, and venom sac attached are left behind. The muscles controlling the venom sac, although separated from the bee, rhythmically contract for as long as 20 minutes, driving the sting deeper and deeper into the skin, and continuing to inject venom.

Bee venoms contain histamine, serotonin, acelytcholine, formic acid, phospholipase A, hyaluronidase, and other proteins. Once the proteins of these insects are injected, the patient may become sensitized and be a candidate for anaphylactic response with the next sting.

CLINICAL MANIFESTATIONS. Symptoms consist of one or more of the following: localized pain, swelling, generalized erythema, a feeling of intense heat throughout the body, headache, blurred vision, injected conjunctiva, swollen and tender joints, itching, apprehension, urticaria, petechial hemorrhages of skin and mucous membranes, dizziness, weakness, sweating, severe nausea, abdominal cramps, dyspnea, constriction of the chest, asthma, angioneurotic edema, vascular collapse, and possible death from anaphylaxis. Fatal cases may manifest glottal and laryngeal edema, pulmonary and cerebral edema, visceral congestion, meningeal hyperemia, and interventricular hemorrhage. Death apparently results from a combination of shock, respiratory failure, and central nervous system changes.

The acute, allergic phase of the simple reaction is thought to be due to protein allergens rather than to toxicity of venom. These allergens may be found in dust from the wings, bodies, venom, saliva, or feces of the insect. Most deaths from insect stings occur within 15 to 30 minutes following the bite or sting.

TREATMENT. Early application of a tourniquet may prevent rapid spread of the venom. Affected persons should be taught to remove the venom sacs if present, being careful not to squeeze the sac. It may be necessary for some patients to carry an emergency kit, which is commercially available, supplied with a tourniquet, sublingual isoproterenol in 10-mg tablets, epinephrine hydrochloride aerosol for inhalation to reduce bronchospasm and laryngeal edema, and tweezers to remove the sting and venom sac until a physician is available. The patient should be taught to give himself an epinephrine injection. Patients having severe reactions should first receive 0.3 to 0.5 ml of a 1:1,000 solution of epinephrine intravenously. Antihistamines also may be intravenously administered, and oxygen may be given. If wheezing continues, aminophylline may be given slowly intravenously. Occasionally the patient may require a tracheostomy.

DESENSITIZATION. The Insect Allergy Committee of the American Academy of Allergy noted that 50 percent of people who had a severe generalized reaction to stings had no previous history of a severe reaction. A sharp rise was noted in the proportion of serious reactions after the age of thirty, suggesting increasing sensitivity as the total number of stings increase. Patients with a history of severe local or systemic involvement following insect stings should be desensitized.

The efficacy of desensitization to insect stings has been demonstrated. Of persons desensitized and stung again, 88 percent experienced milder reactions than they had previously, and only 3 percent suffered more severe reactions. By comparison, 63 percent of those patients stung again but not desensitized suffered more severe reactions. It has been suspected that a refractory period of 10 to 14 days persists following an insect sting during which skin tests may be negative. Therefore, skin tests should be delayed several weeks after stinging and be performed with extreme caution. Cross reactions to the wasp, bee, and yellow jacket may occur.

Because the antigens eliciting hypersensitive reactions are present in the insect's body as well as its venom, whole insect extract should be used for skin testing before hyposensitization therapy is begun. The initial dilution should be weak, since shocklike reactions have been reported after intradermal testing with a 1:1 million dilution. Immunotherapy consists of weekly subcutaneous injections of whole body extract, containing equal parts of bee, hornet, wasp, and yellow jacket whole body extracts, administered for at least 3 years, perhaps indefinitely.

STINGRAYS

Approximately 750 persons each year are stung by stingrays. However, during the past 60 years, only two deaths in this country have been attributed to the venom of the stingray.

As the spine, which is curved and has serrated edges, enters the flesh, the sheath surrounding the spine ruptures, and venom is released. As the spine is withdrawn, fragments of the sheath may remain in the wound. The wound edges are often jagged and bleed freely. Pain is usually immediate and severe, increasing to maximum intensity in 1 to 2 hours and lasting for 12 to 48 hours.

TREATMENT. This consists of copious irrigation with water to wash out any toxin and fragments of the spine's integumentary sheath. Russell noted that the venom is inactivated when exposed to heat. Therefore, the area of the bite should be placed in water as hot as the patient can stand without injury for 30 minutes to 1 hour. After soaking, the wound may be further debrided and treated appropriately. Patients treated in this manner were shown to have rapid and uncomplicated healing of the wound. Patients not treated with heat had tissue necrosis with prolonged drainage and chronically infected wounds.

PORTUGUESE MAN-OF-WAR

This coelenterate is commonly found along our southern Atlantic coast. Its tentacles are covered with thousands of stinging cells, the nematocytes, capable of emitting microscopic organelles, the nematocysts, each of which consists of a small sphere containing a coiled hollow thread. When activated by touch, the thread is uncoiled with such force that it can penetrate skin and even rubber gloves. On contact, venom in the cyst is injected into the victim through the thread. This sting produces extreme pain and often signs of clinical shock; however, no deaths have been reported due to this sting alone.

Following a severe sting there may be almost immediate severe nausea, gastric cramping, and constriction and tightness of throat and chest with severe muscle spasm. There is intense burning pain with weakness and perhaps cyanosis with respiratory distress.

TREATMENT. The most important emergency treatment is to inactivate the nematocysts immediately, to prevent their continuous firing of toxins. This is accomplished by application to the involved area of a substance of high alcohol content, such as rubbing alcohol. This is followed by application of a drying agent, such as flour, baking soda, talc, or shaving cream. The tentacles may then be removed by shaving. Alkaline agents, such as baking soda, are then applied to the involved area in order to neutralize the toxins, which are acetic. Antihistamines may be helpful in controlling the inflammatory response after these emergency treatments. Demerol and Benadryl may dramatically relieve the pain and symptoms. Aerosol corticosteroid-analgesic balm is helpful.

Spider Bites

BLACK WIDOW SPIDER

The most common biting spider in the United States is the black widow (*Latrodectus mactans*) (Fig. 6-4). This spider is black and globular, with a red hourglass mark on the abdomen. The bite of this species in the 10-year period 1950–1959 accounted for 63 deaths. *Latrodectus* venom is primarily neurotoxic in action and appears to center on the spinal cord. Following a bite by the black widow spider, the patient usually experiences sudden pain, and in a few minutes a small wheal with an area of erythema appears. The most prominent physical finding is generalized muscle spasm. Even if bitten on an extremity, the spasm may involve the abdomen and chest. Although the abdomen is rigid, it is nontender. The severe symptoms last from 24 to 48 hours.

TREATMENT. Treatment has consisted of narcotics for the relief of pain and a muscle relaxant for relief of spasm. Either methocarbamol (Robaxin) or 10 ml of a 10% solution of calcium gluconate relieves symptoms. Methocarbamol can be administered intravenously, 10 ml over a 5-minute period, with a second ampule started in a saline solution drip. Specific treatment involves the use of antivenin. This is administered intramuscularly, after appropriate skin tests, since it contains horse serum.

NORTH AMERICAN LOXOSCELISM

The distinguishing mark of the *Loxosceles reclusa* is the darker violin-shaped band over the dorsal cephalothorax (Fig. 6-5). The spider is native to the South Central United States and is found both indoors and outdoors and under cliffs and overhanging rocks. The first recognized and documented case in the United States of a bite by *Loxosceles reclusa* was not published until 1957.

CLINICAL MANIFESTATIONS. The bite may go unnoticed because pain may not occur until 6 to 8 hours afterward.

Fig. 6-4. Abdominal view of a female black widow spider showing the hourglass marking. (*From B. C. Paton, Surg Clin North Am, 43:537, 1963.*)

A generalized macular and erythematous rash may appear in 12 to 24 hours. Erythema develops, with bleb or blister formation surrounded by an irregular area of ischemia. A zone of hemorrhage with induration and a surrounding halo of erythema may develop peripherally. The central ischemia turns dark, an eschar forms by the seventh

Fig. 6-5. The distinguishing mark of the *Loxosceles reclusa* is the darker violin-shaped band over the dorsal cephalothorax. (*From C. J. Dillaha, G. T. Jansen, W. M. Honeycutt, and C. R. Hayden, JAMA, 188:33, 1964.*)

day, and by the fourteenth day the area sloughs, leaving an open ulcer. Approximately 3 weeks is required for the lesion to heal. Severe systemic manifestations may occur in 24 to 48 hours in small children, with fever, chills, malaise, weakness, nausea, vomiting, joint pain, and even petechial eruption. The two principal systemic effects, hemolysis and thrombocytopenia, have been responsible for two deaths. Hemoglobinemia, hemoglobinuria, leukocytosis, and proteinuria may also occur. *Loxosceles* venom is chiefly cytotoxic in action.

TREATMENT. Immediate excision with primary closure has been advocated as the treatment of choice. This usually is not possible since the patient rarely can be certain of what bit him or has failed to recognize the type of spider. Several writers immediately administered steroids. The dose has varied from 30 to 80 mg of methylprednisolone daily, tapered over a period of several days. This seems to be the preferred treatment. Excision of the necrotic area with skin grafting may be required at a later date.

PENETRATING WOUNDS OF THE NECK AND THORACIC INLET

(*by Robert F. Jones, G. Tom Shires, and William H. Snyder III*)

INCIDENCE. Although major wounds of the soft tissues of the neck are relatively uncommon in civilian surgical practice, the number of vital structures in the small volume of the neck makes it imperative that every penetrating neck wound be considered a serious surgical problem.

Prior to World War II, the treatment of penetrating wounds of the neck was largely nonsurgical unless major bleeding or deep injuries were obvious. Reported mortality rates were 18 percent of 188 cases in the Spanish-American War and 11 percent of 594 cases in World War I. During World War II the mortality rate fell to 7 percent, probably because of a variety of factors, including earlier tracheostomy, earlier and more frequent surgical exploration, antibiotics, and improvements in surgical and anesthetic techniques.

Since 1960, several civilian series have been reported with no further reduction in mortality rate, which seems to have leveled off at about 10 percent. In the three previous series, the total number of deaths was 57. Of these, 43 were a direct result of blood vessel injuries. The other 14 deaths were due principally to complications from wounds of the larynx, trachea, and esophagus. In the study of Shirkey et al. 6 of the 22 deaths occurred in the group in which exploration was delayed beyond 6 hours or omitted entirely. Fogelman and Stewart pointed out that the mortality rate for their cases which were promptly explored was 6 percent, whereas for those in which surgical intervention was omitted or postponed the mortality rate was 35 percent. Their overall mortality was 11 percent. Since the initial phase of the Fogelman and Stewart series, it has been the policy at Parkland Memorial Hospital to "treat the platysma like the peritoneum" and explore virtually all neck wounds that penetrate the platysma in the

operating room under general endotracheal anesthesia, regardless of preoperative opinion as to the extent and severity of the damage.

Recently, 274 penetrating wounds of the neck treated at Parkland Memorial Hospital have been reviewed. There were 11 deaths, for a mortality rate of 3.6 percent. Of the fatalities, four were due to complications from spinal cord injuries, three from massive hemorrhage, one from extensive aspiration of blood from a bleeding tracheal wound, one from blast injury to the brainstem, one from a cerebral embolus following repair of a common carotid artery injury, and one from blast injury to the trachea unrecognized at the original exploration and leading to laryngeal edema and obstruction in the absence of a tracheostomy.

Of the 274 cases, 103 explorations were negative, i.e., with no hematoma, no significant bleeding, and no damage to any named structure in the neck, although the tract of injury frequently was within millimeters of vital structures. Of these negative cases, there were no deaths and no complications except one superficial wound infection which cleared promptly with drainage. These patients usually were discharged within 72 hours to clinic follow-up if there were no associated injuries.

Table 6-3 summarizes the injuries found in 15 patients with clinically "negative" neck wounds, i.e., with no visible bleeding, no visible hematoma, no evidence of hemorrhagic shock. At some hospitals these wounds would not have been explored, and many probably would have healed uneventfully without surgical exploration. However, unexplored patients, apparently free of significant injury on examination in the emergency room, may bleed massively later when a blood clot is shaken loose, or a deep abscess may develop from a small perforation of the esophagus, or other complications may develop from unrecognized injuries. Even those less serious injuries associated only with damage to subcutaneous tissues and muscles will heal faster with less chance of infection if hemostasis, debridement, and adequate drainage are accomplished. It is a fundamental fact that bacteria thrive on extravasated blood and damaged tissue, and every penetrating wound is contaminated.

TREATMENT. The safest treatment for penetrating neck wounds appears to be prompt and thorough surgical exploration under local or general anesthesia.

Initial Treatment. On admission to the emergency room, all patients with neck injuries are immediately evaluated

Table 6-3. INJURIES IN 15 CLINICALLY "NEGATIVE"* NECK WOUNDS

Total series = 274 patients

Innominate vein	2
Subclavian vein	1
Internal jugular vein	5
Thyrocervical artery	3
Thoracic duct	2
Esophagus (blast injury)	2
Ascending pharyngeal artery	1

*No visible bleeding, no visible hematoma, no shock.

regarding their systemic condition, i.e., airway and adequacy of ventilation, blood pressure, pulse, mental state, and peripheral signs of shock such as sweating, cold skin, and collapsed veins. If there is external bleeding, some type of pressure is applied for temporary hemostasis. If there is upper airway obstruction, an endotracheal tube is passed immediately, or if there is sufficient time, a tracheostomy is performed. Meanwhile, one or two large-bore intravenous cannulas or needles are inserted in peripheral veins and Ringer's lactate solution is started while blood is drawn for typing and cross matching. If shock is present, the fluid is given rapidly, and if there is no evidence of significant blood loss, the intravenous infusions are kept going by slow drip. When indicated, whole blood is administered as soon as it is available. Usually the salt solution will temporarily reverse the shock state until cross-matched blood is available. If shock is severe and is not improved promptly by the Ringer's lactate solution, type O, Rh-negative low-titer unmatched blood is infused rapidly until the matched blood is available. Plasma has also been used, but there is little advantage over salt solutions; i.e., both are quite helpful temporarily, although neither is a substitute for whole blood.

If it is apparent that blood or air is free in a pleural cavity, closed-chest drainage is immediately instituted. If there is no clinical evidence or a pneumothorax or hemothorax and the missile or blade could have possibly reached the pleura, and if the patient's systemic condition is stable, an upright chest film is obtained with a physician in constant attendance. Special x-ray studies such as arteriograms have rarely been worthwhile.

If the depth of the injury is not apparent, the wound is very gently probed with a small hemostat only to the depth of the platysma muscle. If the platysma has been penetrated, the probing is discontinued. Nonbleeding neck wounds should not be deeply probed in an emergency room. The patient is then transferred to the operating room. No attempt is made to pass a nasogastric tube in the emergency room because of the danger of hemorrhage with coughing or gagging.

Anesthesia. Virtually all neck wounds are explored under general anesthesia, using an orotracheal airway with an inflatable cuff. The anesthetic agent varies considerably according to the specific problem, necessity for rapid induction, circulatory status, preexisting disease, etc. There are no specific contraindications in neck injuries per se to any of the commonly used anesthetic agents or relaxants.

The chest is again examined just prior to induction, since pneumothorax or hemothorax may develop slowly following a neck wound, appearing an hour or longer after an initially negative chest x-ray. Wounds at the root of the neck following a downward path may barely penetrate the pleura so that a pneumothorax is not apparent initially and may not be manifest until after the patient is intubated. This should be kept in mind as a cause for hypotension or hypoxia during anesthesia, especially if closed thoracotomy drainage has not been instituted.

Technique of Exploration. With adequate control of the ventilatory and cardiovascular systems, the surgeon can now safely and adequately explore the structures that are apparently or potentially injured. The incision is planned to allow full exposure of the tract of injury. Proximal and distal control of the major vessels must also be considered in the length and position of the incision. The sternocleidomastoid muscle and/or any other neck muscles are transected whenever necessary to provide adequate exposure. An oblique incision along the anterior border of the sternocleidomastoid muscle is often useful, or any transverse incision may be used if it gives adequate exposure. The tract of injury is followed to its depth, with systematic examination of each structure in or near the tract. It should also be pointed out that blast injury from gunshot wounds may not be immediately apparent in the tissues adjacent to the tract.

Specific Injuries

CERVICAL BLOOD VESSELS. If injuries to the major vessels are suspected, umbilical tapes are passed around the vessels proximal and distal to the point of suspected injury before local clots are removed if bleeding has previously occurred and stopped. This happens frequently with venous and occasionally with arterial injury. The vessels are then carefully inspected, all clots are removed, and repair is carried out.

When the injury involves the low anterior neck, it may be necessary to resect a portion of the clavicle or to split the sternum to obtain proximal control and prevent uncontrollable hemorrhage. The medial one-third or one-half of the clavicle is resected whenever necessary, disarticulating the sternoclavicular joint. There is no significant disability following this procedure, and if the periosteum is preserved, bony regeneration will usually occur. When this does not adequately expose the great vessels for repair or for proximal control, the entire clavicle is removed, or the sternum may be split with a Lebsche knife. The sternal incision may be carried off laterally into the second or third intercostal space to avoid opening the full mediastinum unnecessarily.

The internal carotid, common carotid, subclavian, and innominate arteries should be repaired if at all possible. An internal or external shunt may be utilized during carotid repair, as with carotid grafting or endarterectomy, or the vessel may be partially occluded with a curved vascular clamp to allow partial flow during repair. The vertebral artery is usually very difficult to repair in the bony canal but may be controlled by prolonged pressure, suture ligatures, and bone wax. The external carotid artery and/or its branches may be ligated except in patients with carotid arteriosclerosis with an occluded common or internal carotid vessel. In these cases, the external carotid may be a major source of collateral flow.

When the carotid arteries are to be handled or pressed upon in the region of the bifurcation, the adventitia of the carotid bulb is infiltrated with a local anesthetic to prevent hypotension from reflexes originating in pressor receptors of the carotid sinus. Atropine may be given at intervals during the procedure when hypotension results from such stimuli.

The internal jugular vein is repaired if feasible but may

be ligated unilaterally if necessary without adverse seque- lae. All other neck veins are routinely ligated if injured. Prompt pressure on an open vein and a slight head-down tilt to the table will prevent the occurrence of air em- bolism.

BLOOD VESSELS OF THORACIC INLET. Injuries to the major vascular structures in the base of the neck or tho- racic inlet are a significant challenge in management. Rapid resuscitation, liberal surgical exploration, and a thorough knowledge of the operative approach are the necessary ingredients of success. The vascular structures involved are the common carotid, subclavian, and innomi- nate arteries and their corresponding veins. A penetrating wound due to an act of violence is the usual cause. Indica- tions for early surgical exploration are listed in Table 6-4. Diagnostic errors and subsequent inappropriately con- servative management rarely occur with overt signs of major vascular injury. Unfortunately, a significant number of these injuries appear innocuous at the time of pres- entation, and a high index of suspicion is necessary. It is in this context that platysmal penetration and proximity of the wound to a major vascular structure must be re- garded as absolute indications for surgical exploration. This concept is emphasized by data from a recent Parkland Memorial Hospital series, to be presented later. Arteriog- raphy to modify the principle of proximity and penetration exploration remains controversial. It may prove useful if always immediately available. However, valuable time should not be wasted obtaining studies if objective evi- dence of major vascular injury exists.

Immediate formal exploration in the operating room generally is recommended. Massive bleeding progressing to exsanguination can occur rapidly from a wound that initially appears innocent if increased intrathoracic pres- sure dislodges a tamponading clot. For this reason, every effort is made to avoid vomiting, coughing, or agitation. Smooth anesthetic induction is most important. Endo- tracheal intubation of patients with wounds in the base of the neck is most safely accomplished following infusion of muscle relaxants, thus minimizing the danger of "buck- ing the endotracheal tube" with a sudden increase in intra- vascular pressure.

As preoperative prediction of the specific vessels injured

Table 6-4. FINDINGS SUGGESTING MAJOR VASCULAR INJURY

Obvious or direct evidence of injury:
  1. Circulatory instability
  2. Excessive external bleeding
  3. A large or progressing hematoma
  4. Distal pulse deficit
  5. Neurologic deficit involving nerves anatomically adjacent to major vascular structures
  6. Massive or continued intrathoracic bleeding

Indirect evidence indicating exploration:
  1. A wound above the clavicle or manubrium that penetrates the platysma muscle
  2. Thoracic wounds whose trajectory traverses the superior mediastinum or thoracic inlet
  3. Mediastinal widening demonstrated roentgenographically

often is inaccurate, a flexible operative approach is neces- sary. The entire neck, thorax, and proximal arms are in- cluded in the surgical field. The supine position with slight cervical extension provides the greatest flexibility for per- forming the primary incision and any necessary extensions. The major technical problem is to provide adequate ex- posure for establishing proximal and distal vascular control prior to dissecting the area of injury. Familiarity with several basic incisions and their extensions is necessary. These are demonstrated in Fig. 6-6. They include the oblique neck incision, the horizontal clavicular incision with resection of the medial portion of the clavicle, the median sternotomy, and the bilateral fourth intercostal space anterolateral thoracotomies.

The right oblique incision generally is adequate to ex- pose the entire right common carotid artery. The hori- zontal clavicular incision with subperiostial resection of the medial half of the clavicle adequately exposes the right subclavian vessels. Extension to a median sternotomy gen- erally is necessary to expose the innominate artery; the distal left common carotid artery is easily exposed through a left oblique neck incision. The proximal left common carotid and the distal left subclavian can be reached

Fig. 6-6. Incisions and extensions for base-of-the-neck vascular injuries.

INCISIONS AND EXTENSIONS FOR BASE OF THE NECK VASCULAR INJURIES

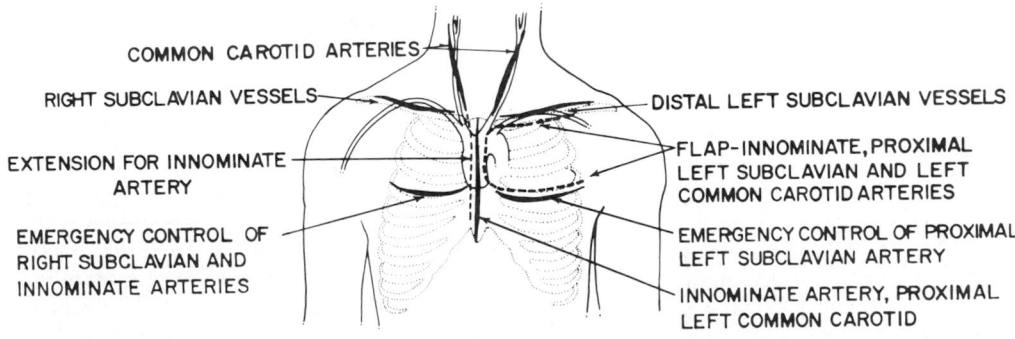

through a horizontal clavicular incision; further exposure can be gained by extension to a median sternotomy. However, the proximal portion of the left subclavian artery is best approached through a left anterolateral thoracotomy. The entire left subclavian artery is adequately exposed through a combined left clavicular and left anterolateral thoracotomy incision. The construction of a musculoskeletal flap, or "trapdoor," has been used by some to expose the innominate and subclavian vessels. This is formed by combining horizontal clavicular, superior median sternotomy, and anterolateral thoracotomy incisions. As a general rule, the majority of these injuries are exposed through the oblique neck or horizontal clavicular incisions. Major extensions should be made without hesitation when these incisions provide inadequate exposure. The vascular repair seldom is difficult and most often can be accomplished by lateral arteriorrhaphy or end-to-end anastomosis. When graft interposition is required, autogenous material is preferred.

Important factors in the management of these injuries are emphasized by a recent series from Parkland Memorial Hospital. During a 10-year period, 99 patients with 122 injuries of the major vascular structures at the base of the neck were seen. Arterial injuries accounted for 40 percent, including 23 injuries to the subclavian artery, 21 to the common carotid, and 3 to the innominate artery. Of 74 venous injuries, there were 35 to the subclavian vein, 31 to the internal jugular, and 8 to the innominate vein. Signs and symptoms of significant vascular injury were equivocal in many patients and totally absent in 32 patients. These patients were explored on the basis of platysmal penetration and the proximity of the wound to a major vascular structure. The overall mortality was 5.1 percent, generally related to the magnitude of associated injuries or the extent of blood loss prior to operation. Eleven percent of the patients with arterial trauma died, compared with 1.3 percent of those with venous injuries. Postoperative complications were related to vascular injury or repair in only 20 percent of patients. Essentially all injuries of the common carotid arteries or internal jugular veins were exposed through oblique neck incisions. Extension into a median sternotomy or horizontal clavicular incision was required only with associated vertebral or subclavian vessel injuries or when the proximal left common carotid artery was involved. Horizontal clavicular incisions with resection of the medial portion of the clavicle adequately exposed injuries of the subclavian vessels in most instances. An anterolateral thoracotomy was necessary only for immediate control of bleeding or when the proximal portion of the left subclavian artery was involved. The majority of the innominate vein injuries could be managed through horizontal clavicular incisions. However, median sternotomy was necessary to adequately expose innominate artery injuries. Early and liberal surgical exploration with emphasis on adequate exposure has resulted in the low mortality and morbidity rates in this large series.

LARYNX AND TRACHEA. Whenever laryngeal or tracheal injury is apparent in the emergency room, tracheostomy is performed promptly, prior to transfer of the patient to the main operating suite. If the injury is not apparent until the time of exploration, a tracheostomy is done during exploration. When the patient is hoarse or the wound is near the thyroid or larynx, indirect laryngoscopy is performed preoperatively when feasible to determine the integrity of the recurrent laryngeal nerve. Laryngeal blast injury may result from a bullet tract near the larynx; in such a case, a tracheostomy is also performed.

Subcutaneous air may be present with such injuries and may increase rapidly under observation. However, air may spread subcutaneously from outside via the entrance wound in the absence of tracheal, pharyngeal, or esophageal penetration. Cervical extension of mediastinal air from an injured bronchus or lung may also occur.

Clean lacerations of the trachea or larynx are closed using a nonabsorbable suture, usually cotton or silk. If the defect cannot be closed primarily, a fascial flap may be used as a patch. Synthetic patch grafts such as Marlex have been successful. The tracheostomy is maintained until healing is complete and laryngeal or tracheal edema has subsided, usually 4 to 8 days.

PHARYNX AND ESOPHAGUS. If a small esophageal injury is suspected but cannot be demonstrated during exploration, an anesthetic mask may be applied to the nose and mouth and positive pressure exerted while the wound is filled with saline solution. Bubbles may disclose the point of injury. The pharynx and esophagus may be repaired primarily using chromic catgut suture, following debridement as necessary. It is vital to drain all such wounds, since infection and/or a salivary leak is not an infrequent complication. If there is massive loss of tissue, as with a close-range shotgun blast, it may be necessary to perform a cutaneous esophagostomy for feeding purposes and cutaneous pharyngostomy for salivary drainage. A secondary plastic reconstruction will be required after initial healing is complete. A small plastic nasogastric tube is used for feeding for 8 to 10 days following all esophageal injuries, unless for some reason a gastrostomy is deemed preferable.

NERVES. A preoperative neurologic examination is performed whenever possible to identify an injured nerve. The brachial plexus, the deep cervical plexus, the phrenic nerve, and the cranial nerves are systematically tested. The vagus and recurrent laryngeal nerves can be checked by examination of the vocal cords. A hypoglossal or spinal accessory nerve injury is particularly easy to miss unless a preoperative neurologic examination is performed. An associated head injury or alcoholic intoxication will frequently complicate the neurologic evaluation.

Whenever possible, all severed or lacerated nerves are debrided and repaired primarily, using interrupted fine silk sutures on the perineurium. If a motor nerve deficit is apparent, an expendable sensory nerve such as the great auricular nerve may be interposed as a nerve autograft to allow anastomosis without tension.

THYROID. After debridement of devitalized tissue, hemostasis may be secured by suture ligature. Adequate drainage is particularly important.

THORACIC DUCT. Wounds near the inferior segment of the left internal jugular vein may sever the thoracic duct at or below the point of entry; the location is quite variable. Repair of the duct is not feasible because of its friability, but simple ligation is adequate. Since the duct may divide just before entering the vein or there may be tributaries for the head and arm, multiple ligatures may be required for lymphostasis. The area should be thoroughly dried and inspected before closing, since a large collection of lymph may occur postoperatively from even a small leak. If lymph does accumulate, incision and drainage with the application of a bulky pressure dressing will usually allow closure of the lymph fistula within a few days. Occasionally, an injured right lymphatic duct is encountered on the opposite side in the same location and is treated in like manner.

SALIVARY GLANDS. A sialogram may be used preoperatively to establish the diagnosis, or it may be determined during exploration. Injuries to the gland may be handled by debridement, hemostasis, and simple drainage. In the absence of ductal obstruction, a salivary fistula will rarely occur following injury to the gland substance. When the major duct is injured, it may be repaired with fine silk over a ureteral catheter stent. The catheter should be removed after repair is effected. When repair is not feasible because of the patient's condition or for some other compelling reason, the duct may be ligated and the gland allowed to atrophy, or the duct may be reimplanted in the mucosa at a later time.

When the parotid gland is involved, the major facial nerve branches should be identified and repaired if injured. Primary repair has a better prognosis for nerve function than does delayed repair, unless there is gross bacterial contamination or massive loss of tissue.

If a salivary fistula does occur postoperatively and fails to close spontaneously, irradiation is usually effective in arresting salivary flow but is not used for this purpose in children or young adults.

CLOSURE. Almost all soft tissue neck wounds are drained for 24 to 48 hours using soft Penrose drains to prevent the accumulation of blood and serum. If the pharynx or esophagus is injured, drainage is continued for 4 to 8 days. All muscles are repaired. In the case of massive gunshot wounds, such as a close-range shotgun injury, the wound is left open initially and a delayed primary closure performed 3 to 4 days later, if possible.

ABDOMINAL TRAUMA

(by Robert N. McClelland, Ronald C. Jones, Malcolm O. Perry, G. Tom Shires and Erwin R. Thal)

The incidence of abdominal trauma increases each year. About 5 million persons in the United States are injured yearly in automobile accidents, and many of these injuries are abdominal. Blunt abdominal trauma generally leads to higher mortality rates than penetrating wounds and presents greater problems in diagnosis. The spleen, liver, kidneys, and bowel are the most frequently injured abdominal viscera. In a review of several series of abdominal trauma by Griswold and Collier, the frequency of injury was determined (see Table 6-5).

Evaluation of Blunt Trauma

The greatest difficulty in the management of blunt abdominal trauma is in the diagnosis. This is largely due to masking of abdominal injury by associated injuries. The most frequently associated injuries are head trauma, chest trauma, and fractures. Often the patient is unconscious because of alcoholism, shock, or associated head injury. Another misleading factor in diagnosis, often not recognized, is that relatively trivial injuries may rupture abdominal viscera. The index of suspicion of abdominal trauma must be high, even in cases of supposedly minor abdominal trauma, if diagnostic errors are to be avoided.

CLINICAL MANIFESTATIONS. The evaluation of the patient with blunt abdominal trauma begins with a careful history and physical examination. The entire patient must be examined as well as the abdomen because of the high incidence of associated trauma. Fitzgerald et al. have reported extraabdominal injuries in 97 percent of patients with abdominal injuries who were dead on arrival at the hospital and in 70 percent of those admitted alive. When the diagnosis is doubtful, one must often depend on repeated physical examinations alone, done at frequent intervals by the same examiner to decide whether the patient requires laparotomy.

Abdominal pain and tenderness are the most frequent findings. Abdominal rigidity, or involuntary guarding, is the most helpful sign and even when present alone warrants exploratory laparotomy. Hinton, in 1929, recommended a period of watchful waiting before exploration because of fear of uncontrollable hemorrhage and infection, as well as the difficulty of performing the necessary surgical procedures under adverse conditions. There is no excuse for this course today, and a policy of watchful waiting frequently may be disastrous. Fitzgerald et al. reported no deaths of patients who had exploratory laparotomy without a finding of intraabdominal injury. However, three deaths in their series occurred from intraabdominal hemorrhage because abdominal injury was masked by associated head injuries. The absence of any mortality for negative abdominal exploration for suspected abdominal trauma has been reported from several trauma centers.

In patients with blunt abdominal trauma, determinations of alterations in blood pressure are often useful. In a series of patients with blunt trauma reviewed recently from this institution, approximately 65 percent had systolic

Table 6-5. FREQUENCY OF INJURY
IN ABDOMINAL TRAUMA

Viscera injured	Frequency, %
Spleen	26.2
Kidneys	24.2
Intestines	16.2
Liver	15.6
Abdominal wall	3.6
Retroperitoneal hematoma	2.7
Mesentery	2.5
Pancreas	1.4
Diaphragm	1.1

blood pressures below 80 mm Hg on admission to the emergency room. It was found that a valuable sign of continuing intraabdominal hemorrhage was transient elevation of the blood pressure to normal levels for a few minutes followed by return to hypotensive levels with rapid infusion of 500 to 1,000 ml of Ringer's lactate solution. Patients who are hypotensive from minimal blood loss or from neurogenic shock usually do not behave in this manner. The Ringer's lactate solution generally is infused over a period of 15 to 20 minutes while other measures, such as blood typing and cross matching, are being carried out. Postural hypotension, when the patient assumes the erect position, is another useful sign of continuing intraabdominal bleeding.

DIAGNOSTIC PROCEDURES. Berman et al. state that if the leukocyte count is greater than 15,000 following abdominal trauma, a ruptured solid viscus is likely, especially if other findings are compatible with that diagnosis. Knopp and Harkins and Williams and Zollinger, however, have not found the leukocyte count to be so helpful. Several studies of the hemoglobin and hematocrit done at intervals of 30 minutes to 1 hour in suspicious cases may be helpful, but they may be misleading if the findings are overinterpreted. Naffziger and McCorkle note that the serum amylase level is valuable in recognizing acute pancreatic trauma. Elevated amylase levels may also indicate injury to the upper small bowel and duodenum with leakage of amylase-containing fluid from the injured bowel into the peritoneal cavity, where the amylase is freely absorbed into the blood. Studies of urinary sediment are useful, since hematuria may indicate injury to the genitourinary tract. If the patient with abdominal injury cannot void, catheterization should be done to obtain urine for examination. Examination of vomitus or insertion of a nasogastric tube to obtain gastric contents to be checked for evidence of upper gastrointestinal tract bleeding is helpful.

Radiologic Findings. For patients who have sustained severe abdominal injury and in whom other clinical signs obviously point to such injury, roentgenography, for diagnosis, may dangerously delay surgical intervention. However, for about one-third of patients with stable vital signs and questionable diagnoses of intraabdominal injury, x-ray studies may be helpful. Roentgenography is of least aid in injury to solid viscera, notably the liver, spleen, and pancreas.

When a patient is suspected of having intraabdominal injuries, upright films of the chest should be made, in addition to supine films of the abdomen. Occasionally additional information may be obtained from lateral and left lateral decubitus films. In addition: (1) Skeletal parts are checked for fractures or dislocations. (2) Examination of the soft tissues may give information concerning alterations of size, shape, or position of many viscera. (3) Pneumoperitoneum may be diagnosed with the patient in the erect or lateral decubitus positions. (4) Indirect evidence of solid viscera rupture with secondary hemorrhage may be presumed by an increase in density in the region, by displacement of neighboring viscera, or by accumulation of fluid between the gas shadows of bowel loops. Also, if a gastric, duodenal, or upper jejunal rupture is possible, the frequency of pneumoperitoneum may be increased by injecting 750 to 1,000 ml of air into a nasogastric tube, after which the patient sits in a semierect position for 10 minutes before an upright chest film or left lateral decubitus film of the abdomen is made. Films should also be made prior to the air injection for purposes of comparison if the patient's condition permits.

Another study which may be useful is examination of the upper gastrointestinal tract by x-ray after ingestion of a water-soluble opaque medium, which may indicate injury of the stomach, duodenum, or upper small bowel. The use of barium mixtures for this is dangerous, since a severe peritoneal reaction is caused by barium if it leaks through a perforation in the gastrointestinal tract. This is especially true if there is fecal contamination in the peritoneal cavity from concomitant colon injury.

Intravenous or retrograde pyelograms should be done if feasible for patients with hematuria or other evidence of genitourinary injury, not only to establish the nature of the injury, but also to determine if both kidneys are functioning prior to surgical intervention in case an injured kidney must be removed. If necessary, intravenous pyelograms may be done during the surgical procedure to determine the presence of a functional kidney on one side before removing the other kidney.

Cystograms may also be useful for diagnosing bladder injury or perforation from blunt abdominal trauma, but normal cystograms do not rule out bladder injury.

Intravenous cholangiography has also been helpful at times in suspected trauma to the hepatobiliary system.

Levin Tubes. Levin tubes are inserted in all patients sustaining blunt abdominal trauma. The stomach contents are aspirated, and the aspirate is examined for the presence of blood. In addition, a Levin tube provides for decompression of the stomach, prevents gastric dilatation, and prevents aspiration with the induction of anesthesia.

Paracentesis. Needle abdominal paracentesis is a useful diagnostic aid only for those cases of abdominal trauma in which, after physical examination, the examiner continues to suspect intraabdominal hemorrhage. The abdominal tap has been particularly useful as a diagnostic adjunct for comatose patients with head injury in whom adequate physical examination of the abdomen is not possible. A recent review with this procedure shows a diagnostic accuracy of 95 percent with positive paracentesis. A negative tap is not definitive, particularly if other elements of the physical examination indicate other reasons for exploring the abdomen. In female patients with suspected intraabdominal hemorrhage, culdocentesis may be positive for blood when abdominal taps are negative.

The technique is well described by Drapanas and McDonald and illustrated in Fig. 6-7. The abdomen is surgically cleansed with pHisoHex or an iodophor compound. An 18 gauge short-bevel spinal needle is attached to a syringe and inserted through the abdominal wall after prior infiltration of the site of tap with a local anesthetic agent. Suction is applied to the syringe as the needle is slowly advanced into the abdomen at the sites illustrated. Return of a minimum of 0.1 ml of nonclotting blood constitutes a positive tap. Occasionally, an intraabdominal

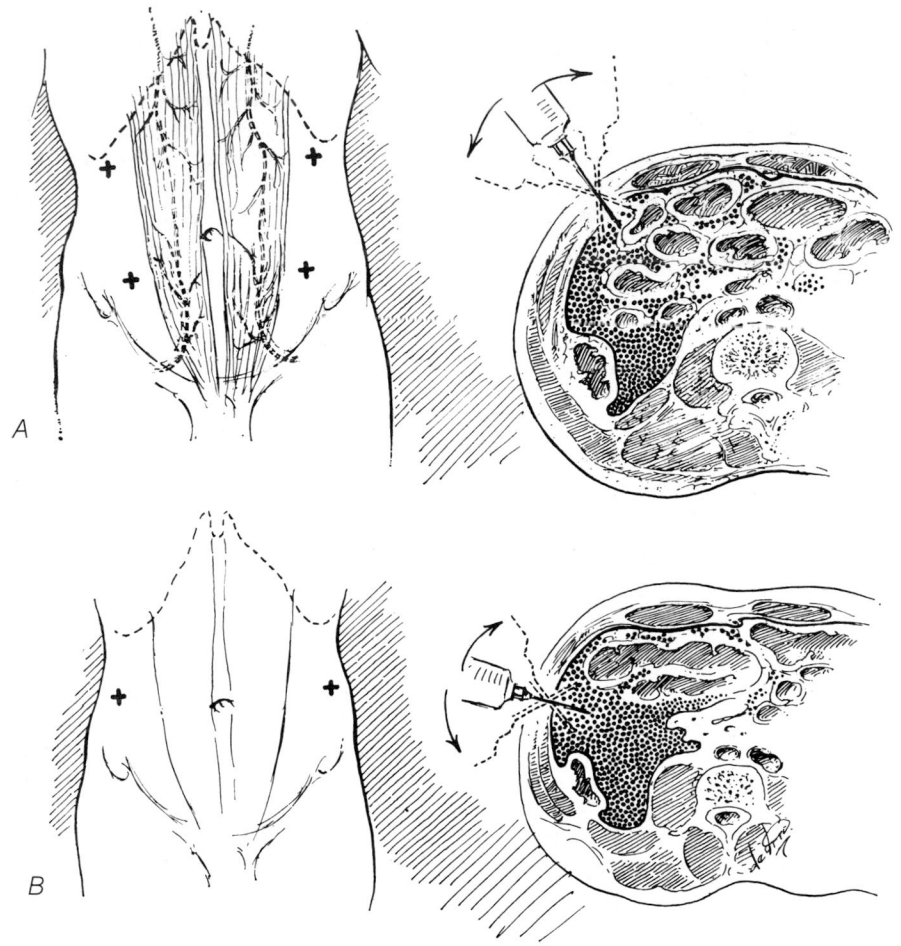

Fig. 6-7. *A.* Technique for four-quadrant peritoneal taps. Preferred location for aspiration of each quadrant is shown. Note that puncture through the rectus abdominis sheath is avoided. *B.* Technique for bilateral flank taps. Aspiration is performed in each flank midway between the costal margin and iliac spine. In our experience, bilateral flank taps are equally reliable as, and more easily performed than, four-quadrant taps in cases of abdominal trauma. (*From T. Drapanas and J. McDonald, Surgery, 50:742, 1961.*)

blood vessel may be entered, but this blood will clot and differentiate it from blood obtained from the free peritoneal cavity. Puncture of the rectus abdominis sheath anteriorly should be avoided to prevent a rectus abdominis sheath hematoma from injury to the epigastric vessels and to diminish the chance of the needle's penetrating the bowel, since gas-filled loops of bowel tend to float anteriorly in the abdomen containing fluid or blood. Actually, the danger of penetrating the intestine is slight; several studies have shown that penetration with an 18-gauge needle is harmless, as a hole in the bowel seals off quite rapidly with no leakage. Other technical considerations include the following:

1. Areas of abdominal scars or other points of possible bowel fixation to the abdominal wall should be avoided.
2. The direction of the needle inside the abdominal cavity should be changed only by withdrawing the point of the needle just superficially to the peritoneum, redirecting the needle, and reintroducing it into the peritoneal cavity.
3. Peritoneal taps should be avoided in the presence of markedly distended bowel, because abnormally elevated intraluminal pressure may cause continued leakage.

Paracentesis is simple and quick with relatively few complications. The major drawback is the high percentage of false-negative results.

Peritoneal Lavage. Because of the poor reliability of paracentesis, other procedures have been developed to detect intraabdominal injury. Canizaro et al. described in 1964 the use of intraperitoneal saline infusions in animals. Root et al. described in 1965 the technique of peritoneal lavage in human beings and subsequently reported a series of 304 patients with a 96 percent accuracy. A recent review of this procedure has proved peritoneal lavage to be a safe and reliable adjunctive procedure for evaluating patients with blunt abdominal trauma. The indications for this technique are closed head injuries, altered consciousness, spinal cord injuries, equivocal abdominal findings, and negative needle paracentesis. It is not recommended for patients with either gunshot or stab wounds to the abdomen, multiple abdominal procedures, dilated bowel, pregnancy, or positive needle paracentesis.

The technique used is similar to that described by Perry et al. A point is selected in the lower midline below the umbilicus approximately one-third of the distance between that and the pubic symphysis. After decompression of the urinary bladder, the skin is cleansed and prepared with an iodinated antiseptic solution. A wheal is raised with 1% lidocaine and the skin incised with a #11 scalpel. A standard peritoneal dialysis catheter (McGaw V-4900) is inserted, and the trocar is advanced carefully until it just penetrates the peritoneum (Fig. 6-8). Once the peritoneum is penetrated, the trocar is removed and the dialysis catheter advanced toward the pelvis. A syringe is then attached to the catheter and the peritoneal cavity aspirated.

Nonclotting blood often will be aspirated through the larger catheter even with a negative needle paracentesis. If no blood or fluid is aspirated, a liter of balanced saline solution (Ringer's lactate) is rapidly infused into the peritoneal cavity over 5 to 10 minutes, using 10 ml/kg for small adults and children. The patient is then turned from side to side in order to further mix the blood and fluid. If other injuries such as pelvic or long bone fractures are present, this step is eliminated.

The empty intravenous-fluid bottle is lowered and the fluid siphoned out of the peritoneal cavity. A sample is sent to the laboratory for quantitative analysis. In addition to obtaining red cell and white cell counts, it is important to determine the presence or absence of amylase, bile, or bacteria. Some have recommended colorimetric methods, but these do not appear to be as accurate as quantitative analysis of the fluid. The criteria for positive peritoneal lavage include the following determinations: gross blood in lavage fluid; greater than 100,000 RBC/mm^3; greater than 500 WBC/mm^3; elevated amylase level; bacteria or bile.

It must be emphasized that the lavage is very inaccurate in indicating retroperitoneal injuries. Unless the posterior peritoneum has been torn or considerable time has elapsed between the injury and lavage, most pancreatic injuries are not detected. The same is true for duodenal, urologic, and major vessel injuries which are retroperitoneal. Complications occur frequently enough that lavage is not recommended for every patient suspected of abdominal injury. However, a negative lavage may spare the patient exploratory laparotomy.

Arteriography. Selective arteriography is another available aid to the diagnosis of blunt abdominal trauma. This procedure, advocated by Freeark, employs percutaneous retrograde arteriography by the Seldinger method. Depending upon the skill of the technician, selective catheterization of celiac, mesenteric, or renal vessels may be performed. The arteriogram provides visualization of the arteries supplying the abdominal viscera and pelvis. A film taken several minutes after injection can be used as an excretory urogram.

The benefits of arteriography are directly related to the capabilities of the radiology department. Again, it must be emphasized that time should not be wasted on adjunctive procedures when surgical intervention is indicated.

Scintiscanning. Both liver and splenic scanning have been described in conjunction with blunt abdominal trauma. This technique primarily is limited to those patients whose diagnoses are uncertain and whose conditions remain stable. The radionuclide most frequently used is 99mTc sulfur colloid. Most series reporting results of this technique are small and emphasize the relative inaccuracy of the examination.

A filling defect representing a parenchymal hematoma frequently is seen with damage to the spleen or liver. In addition, displacement, increased size, and mottled ap-

pearance of the spleen may increase the suspicion of splenic trauma. Filling defects also may indicate cysts, abscesses, infarcts, or tumors secondary to trauma.

Other Procedures. Newer, noninvasive modalities, such as sonography and computerized tomography, may have a place in the diagnostic armamentarium, but their value is as yet unproved. Needleoscopy and laparoscopy provide a less than complete examination and cannot be recommended at this time for the multiply injured patient.

Penetrating Trauma

STAB WOUNDS

The diagnosis of penetrating injuries of the abdomen does not usually present the difficult problem often posed by blunt abdominal trauma. Three methods of managing stab wounds of the abdomen have evolved: (1) routine exploration of all abdominal stab wounds, (2) selective management, and (3) laparotomy following demonstration of peritoneal cavity penetration.

Abdominal stab wounds frequently were managed by routine exploration. Since the incidence of negative laparotomy results was as high as 60 percent in some series, a more conservative approach recommending selective management for those patients with abdominal stab wounds and no clinical evidence of intraabdominal injury has been advocated. The vital signs should be stable, with no evidence of upper or lower gastrointestinal bleeding, pneumoperitoneum, or signs and symptoms of peritoneal irritation if the patient is to be selectively managed. These patients are admitted to the hospital and reevaluated frequently, preferably by the same observer. If the patient's condition deteriorates or changes significantly, exploratory laparotomy is performed. Objections to selective management are that (1) minimal physical findings may be common in spite of significant visceral injury, (2) peritonitis may develop prior to laparotomy, and (3) the incidence of negative laparotomies may still run as high as 30 percent.

Instead of subjecting the patient to general anesthesia and exploratory laparotomy, it is often possible to deter-

Fig. 6-8. Insertion of catheter for peritoneal lavage in the lower midline below the umbilicus.

mine by other means whether the wound has penetrated the peritoneal cavity. Cornell et al. have described the diagnostic injection of radiopaque contrast material. Following aseptic preparation of the wound site, a small catheter is inserted into the wound and held tightly by a purse-string suture. Fifty to one hundred milliliters of contrast media is injected, and anteroposterior, lateral, and oblique films of the abdomen are obtained. Contrast media seen within the peritoneal cavity is an indication for surgery. Objections to this technique are the following: (1) Some patients are hypersensitive to the radiopaque material. (2) Injection of this material may be quite painful, thereby masking further evaluation. (3) The incidence of false-positive and false-negative results may be as high as 15 to 25 percent in some series. (4) The technique is impractical for multiple stab wounds.

Local exploration may provide useful information. The abdominal wall is prepared with an antiseptic agent, and, with local anesthesia, the abdominal wound is opened sufficiently to visualize the complete course and depth of the wound. Often with adequate light, instruments, assistance, and exposure it is obvious that a wound thought to have penetrated the peritoneal cavity is actually superficial and not damaging to viscera. These patients are managed by simple drainage and outpatient follow-up if other injuries do not require hospitalization. Usually, local wound exploration involves more than simple instrument probing to determine penetration. This blind probing may be misleading since a tortuous wound tract may allow passage of the probe for only a short distance, creating a false impression of nonpenetration. In this case, the course of penetration must be directly visualized. If the end of the tract cannot be visualized or if the peritoneum is penetrated, the patient is taken to surgery. This technique is equally useful for stab wounds of the back, although the thickness of the paraspinous muscles may prevent visualization of the end of the wound tract and exploration in the operating room may be necessary. Frequently, innocuous small stab wounds of the back significantly damage such

retroperitoneal structures as the inferior vena cava, ureter, pancreas, or duodenum.

Many wounds which appear to penetrate only the thorax also penetrate the abdomen, injuring abdominal viscera as well as intrathoracic organs. Figure 6-9 indicates the diaphragmatic excursion on maximal expiration and maximal inspiration; it is apparent that certain penetrating wounds of the lower thoracic region often involve the diaphragm and adjacent abdominal viscera. Consequently, an exploratory laparotomy is performed when penetrating injuries involve the lower thoracic region.

Prior to abdominal exploration of these thoracic wounds, anterior and posterior chest tubes are inserted to drain air and blood from the thorax and to prevent pulmonary complications during the operative procedure from concurrent thoracic injuries. Although a pneumothorax or hemothorax may not be indicated by x-ray or physical examination, prophylactic insertion of an anterior chest tube will decrease the danger of a tension pneumothorax developing during induction of anesthesia and subsequent abdominal exploration.

GUNSHOT WOUNDS

Any bullet passing in proximity to the peritoneal cavity requires laparotomy, since visceral injury from "blast effect" may occur whether or not the cavity is entered. In a report by Edwards and Gaspard, 14 percent of 35 patients sustaining gunshot wounds to the abdomen without penetration of the peritoneal cavity sustained at least one visceral injury. It is not possible to predict the path of a missile by merely observing the entrance and exit wounds or by connecting a line between an entrance wound and the appearance of a bullet on the x-ray film. Missiles may bounce, tumble, ricochet, and embolize. If the patient's condition permits, anteroposterior and lateral films of the abdomen should be made to locate the missile and determine its probable trajectory. Selective management, the use of radiopaque material, or local exploration is not recommended.

🎟 MAXIMUM EXPIRATION
▨ MAXIMUM INSPIRATION

Fig. 6-9. Maximum diaphragmatic respiratory excursion. (*From L. M. Shefts, Surg Clin North Am, 38:1577, 1958.*)

Once the diagnosis of intraabdominal injury is established and resuscitation instituted, the abdomen is explored. A long midline incision is preferred for the following reasons: (1) It may be made much more rapidly than other incisions—a matter of vital importance when attempting rapid control of exsanguinating hemorrhage; (2) it gives wide access to all parts of the abdomen, which transverse incisions do not; (3) it may be readily extended into either side of the thorax in case of combined thoracoabdominal injury or when better abdominal exposure is required; and (4) it may be rapidly closed, which is of great importance in decreasing the anesthesia and operative time for gravely injured patients.

MANAGEMENT OF PATIENTS WITH EXSANGUINATING ABDOMINAL HEMORRHAGE. With improvement of prehospital care, more patients are arriving at the hospital in extremis. Frequently this condition is due to massive intraabdominal hemorrhage that is refractory to standard resuscitative measures. Ledgerwood and associates have recently advocated performing preliminary left thoracotomy and temporary thoracic aortic occlusion prior to opening the abdomen in patients with massive hemoperitoneum, tense abdominal distension, and persistent hypotension. The descending thoracic aorta is quickly and bluntly dissected circumferentially and occluded by a straight vascular clamp just above the diaphragm.

Once the abdomen is opened, the aortic clamp can be slowly released following stabilization of the patient, and proximal control gained at a lower level. A medium or large Richardson retractor may be used to obtain rapid temporary occlusion of the abdominal aorta just below the diaphragm. The lesser curvature of the stomach is pulled inferiorly and the flat surface of the retractor blade is compressed firmly against the abdominal aorta, thus occluding it against the vertebra just beneath the diaphragm.

With effective control of massive hemorrhage, resuscitation can be successfully completed, ensuring continuous perfusion to the heart and brain and minimizing the possibility of sudden cardiac arrest.

Stomach

Injuries to the stomach from blunt trauma are not frequent, perhaps because of the relative lack of fixation of the stomach and its protected position. However, penetrating injuries of the stomach from gunshot wounds occur frequently.

DIAGNOSIS. The diagnosis is generally suspected from the course of the penetrating object, and, at times, additional suspicion of gastric injury arises from the presence of bloody fluid aspirated from the Levin tube. Generally, wounds of the anterior stomach wall are easily seen at laparotomy. Because of the possibility of missing posterior stomach wall wounds, it is important in all cases of proved or possible gastric injury to open the lesser sac through the gastrocolic omentum. This allows the entire posterior aspect of the stomach to be searched for injury. The points of insertion of the greater and lesser omentum into the greater and lesser curvature of the stomach, respectively, should also be carefully inspected. If a hematoma is noted

at the mesenteric attachment, it should be evacuated and the stomach wall at that site carefully inspected for injury of that part of the wall located between the leaves of the greater or lesser omentum.

TREATMENT. Gastric wounds are repaired by first placing a continuous locked 2-0 chromic catgut suture through all the layers of the gastric wall; a purse-string suture does not give adequate hemostasis. This hemostatic stitch is very important to control extensive bleeding which may occur from the rich submucosal network of blood vessels in the stomach. Following the first layer closure, an outer inverting row of interrupted nonabsorbable mattress sutures of the Lembert or Halsted type is placed. The outer row of sutures provides adequate serosal approximation of the stomach wall, seals off readily, and prevents leaks. These sutures in the outer layer should not be through-and-through, as is the first row of sutures, but should extend through the seromuscular coat and the submucosal layer of the stomach. Wounds of the stomach are not drained, since they are unlikely to break down and leak, as duodenal wounds sometimes do. However, it is very important to suction the peritoneal cavity, with particular attention to the subhepatic and subphrenic spaces and the lesser sac, so that all food particles and gastric juice spilled into these areas are removed.

After operation for a gastric wound, Levin tube suction should be maintained for several days until active peristalsis has resumed and the danger of postoperative gastric dilatation has passed. The gastric aspirate should be observed for inordinate bleeding, which may occur if the hemostatic suture line is inadequate. If bleeding is brisk or persists, the patient should be immediately reexplored for control of the gastric bleeding point. After peristalsis resumes, gastric aspiration is discontinued, and the patient is started on clear liquids in the usual fashion and advanced to a normal diet over the next few days.

COMPLICATIONS. Complications which may develop following stomach wounds are hemorrhage from, or leakage of, the suture line and development of subhepatic, subphrenic, or lesser sac abscesses secondary to spilling of contaminated gastric contents. The development of such abscesses is suspected following gastric wounds in patients who fail to do well postoperatively and who persist with unexplainable fever for more than a few days. If contamination seems heavy, the skin should be left open until the wound appears clean.

Duodenum

Injuries to the duodenum and small bowel comprise about 24 percent of blunt and penetrating abdominal trauma. Lauritzen reported the mortality rate for retroperitoneal duodenal perforation as approximately 60 percent and related it to the difficulty in establishing an early diagnosis. A mortality of 55.9 percent has been reported for abdominal wounds with all types of duodenal injury. Burrus et al. have reported a series of 86 duodenal injuries with a total mortality of 26 percent.

Mortality rates for duodenal injuries have steadily decreased and are directly proportional to the number and severity of associated injuries as well as the time interval between injury and treatment. Lucas reported a mortality rate of 40 percent in those patients who were not operated upon in the first 24 hours after injury, as contrasted to a mortality rate of only 11 percent among the patients operated upon within less than 24 hours. The average overall mortality rate is about 20 percent. The mortality rate for simple stab wounds involving only the duodenum should be significantly less than five percent, while the mortality rate for severe blunt trauma or shotgun wounds to the duodenum ranges from about 35 percent to more than 50 percent, especially when such trauma is combined with serious pancreatic injuries.

DIAGNOSIS. The diagnosis of blunt trauma to the duodenum and small bowel is considerably more difficult than that of penetrating trauma to these organs. With duodenal or small bowel trauma, all the characteristic signs of trauma to abdominal viscera may be minimal or absent, particularly in the early period following injury for several reasons: (1) The injury of the duodenum following blunt trauma is frequently retroperitoneal, so that duodenal contents leak into the retroperitoneal area, rather than into the free peritoneal cavity. (2) Duodenal and small bowel fluid is generally sterile and does not lead to early signs of bacterial peritonitis, as occurs following colon injury. (3) The pH of the small bowel contents if frequently nearly neutral and, thus, produces only slight chemical irritation of the peritoneum. This is not true of injuries to the duodenum, in which duodenal fluid freely flows into the peritoneal cavity. The highly alkaline pH of this fluid causes immediate chemical irritation of the peritoneum and physical signs of such irritation.

One should be suspicious of injuries to the duodenum or upper small bowel in any patients who have received a blow to the upper abdomen or lower chest, such as from a steering wheel. Testicular pain should raise suspicion of a retroperitoneal duodenal rupture. Also, pain referred to the shoulders, chest, and back is associated with perforation of the duodenum and small intestine.

Several diagnostic aids may be helpful in determining rupture of the duodenum or small bowel. First, needle paracentesis of the abdomen, particularly in the right gutter region or in the upper quadrants, may be helpful if blood, bile, or abnormal amounts of small bowel content are aspirated. Roentgenograms are helpful and may be diagnostic, but the absence of free intraperitoneal air does not rule out bowel perforation. Retroperitoneal rupture of the duodenum is not often diagnosed by x-ray. The diagnosis may be based on finding a large accumulation of air about the right kidney. It is also important to inspect the psoas muscle margins on the plain film of the abdomen for the presence of air, indicating retroperitoneal rupture of a viscus. After x-ray films of the abdomen and upright chest films are made to search for free air collections, it is valuable to inject air through the Levin tube in order to produce or enlarge these air collections. Such a maneuver frequently increases the diagnostic accuracy of x-ray films for free air. An additional aid is to give the patient a water-soluble radiopaque dye orally and then to make abdominal x-ray films to detect any dye leak from the duodenum or small bowel. Such diagnostic procedures are unnecessary if other clinical signs indicate the need for exploratory laparotomy.

When laparotomy is done for suspected intraabdominal injury, duodenal lesions are often missed, especially retroperitoneal lesions of the third and fourth portions of the duodenum. This is due to superficial observation, inadequate exposure, and lack of persistence on the part of the surgeon. Hinton has reported that duodenal perforations have been missed initially in 33 to 50 percent of the various reported series of retroperitoneal duodenal injuries. To avoid overlooking duodenal trauma and contributing to the high mortality from duodenal wounds, it is important to inspect the entire duodenum during abdominal exploration for trauma. This is particularly true if a retroperitoneal hematoma is noted near the duodenum or if there is crepitation or bile-stained fluid along the lateral margins of the duodenum retroperitoneally. If these signs are noted or if the duodenum is contused, it should be widely mobilized by the Kocher maneuver, incising the peritoneum along its lateral margins, so that it is completely mobilized along with the head of the pancreas. Thus, small areas of perforation in the retroperitoneal aspect of the duodenum may be seen. Often retroperitoneal wounds of the duodenum which have been missed are not recognized until several days later, when bile-stained fluid drains from the abdominal wound of a patient who has continued to do poorly postoperatively. As Cohn et al. state, the following signs, in addition to those mentioned previously, indicate careful exploration of the duodenum and the retroduodenal area: elevation of the posterior peritoneum with a glassy edema; petechiae or fat necrosis over the ascending and transverse colon or mesocolon; retroperitoneal phlegmon; hematoma over the head of the pancreas extending into the base of the mesocolon; fat necrosis of the retroperitoneal tissues; and/or discoloration of retroperitoneal tissues—dark from hemorrhage, grayish from suppuration, or yellowish from bile.

TREATMENT. The local treatment of the duodenal perforation itself will depend more on the size of the perforation than any other single factor. Generally, an attempt is made to close the duodenal perforation if this can be done without decreasing the lumen of the duodenum. This closure is done with a continuous locking 3-0 chromic catgut suture through all layers of the duodenal wall, followed by an outer layer of nonabsorbable interrupted mattress sutures in the seromuscular layer of the duodenum. After this, the duodenum should be carefully palpated to exclude stenosis. If the perforation is so large that closure will cause a stricture of the duodenum, consideration should be given to (1) complete division of the duodenum and an end-to-end anastomosis or (2) division of the duodenum, closure of both ends, and gastroenterostomy.

Kobold and Thal have reported another method of handling large duodenal defects, which previously might have necessitated one of the above techniques of duodenal division. This consists of using a retrocolic loop of proxi-

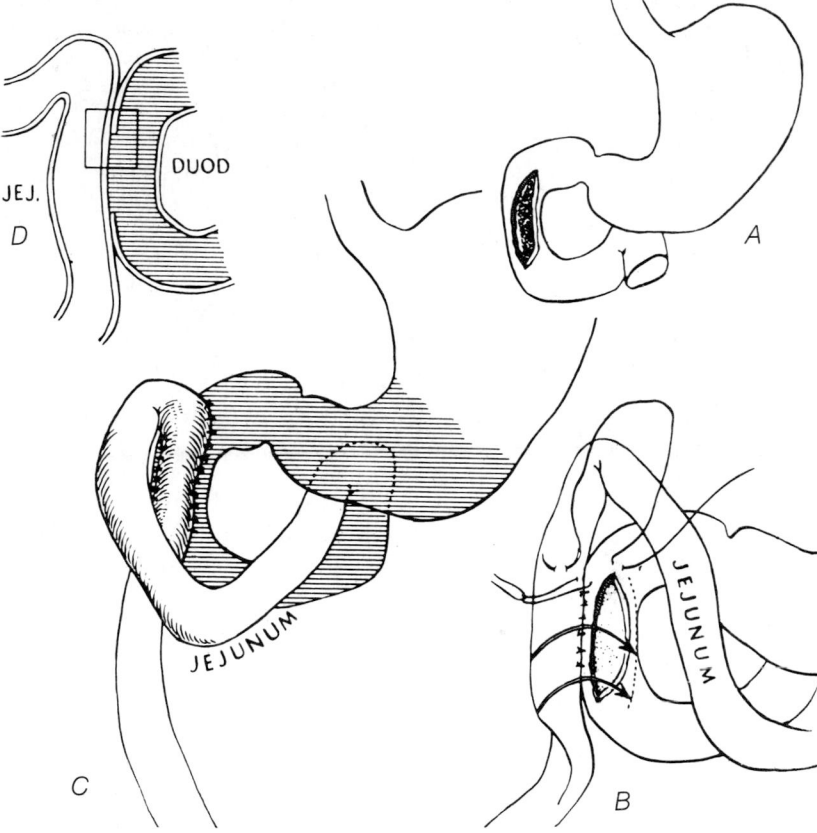

Fig. 6-10. *A.* Area of excision of duodenal wall. *B.* Technique of placement of intact jejunum over the wound to form a patch. *C.* The completed closure. *D.* Cross section of the completed closure showing the relationship of the intact jejunum to the duodenal perforation. The boxed area is the site from which tissue was subsequently removed for study. (*From E. E. Kobold and A. P. Thal, Surg Gynecol Obstet, 116:340, 1963.*)

mal jejunum with suture over the large defect in the duodenum, with an inner row of absorbable catgut sutures taken between the torn edge of the duodenum and the seromuscular layer of the jejunum and an outer layer of nonabsorbable mattress sutures taken between the seromuscular coats of the duodenum and the jejunum. Animal studies, as well as clinical usage, have demonstrated the feasibility of this "patching" technique in managing large duodenal defects (Fig. 6-10).

Large duodenal wounds and duodenal wounds which have dehisced also have been managed by anastomosing the open end of a defunctionalized Roux en Y loop of proximal jejunum over the duodenal defect.

The common bile duct should be identified with insertion of a T tube if the region of the ampulla is involved in a duodenal injury, since reimplantation of the common bile duct sometimes may be necessary. Approximately 75 to 80 percent of all duodenal injuries may be closed by debridement of the wound edges and simple suture. For the other 20 to 25 percent, however, one of the reparative procedures described above or recommended by Cleveland

and Waddell is used. Rarely, even a pancreatoduodenectomy may be necessary to manage large defects of the duodenum with extensive trauma to the duodenum and periampullary region (Fig. 6-11).

A recent report from the Lahey Clinic describes a technique for wide exposure of the third and fourth portions of the duodenum. This involves mobilizing the cecum, right colon, hepatic flexure of the colon, and mesenteries of these organs up to and including the ligament of Treitz, carrying the dissection of the mesocolon along the attachment at the root of the small bowel mesentery, as shown in Fig. 6-12.

It is also frequently important after duodenal injuries to establish adequate drainage. This is done by placing two or three Penrose drains near the injury, bringing them out of the abdomen by the most direct route possible. This reduced markedly the mortality from duodenal wounds in the several series in which drainage was evaluated. It is even more important to institute drainage if there appears to be associated pancreatic injury, as often occurs.

Fistulas. Fistula formation following duodenal injury occurs frequently because of poor blood supply, infection, excessive tension on suture lines, distal obstruction, and leads to approximately a 50 percent mortality. The occurrence of a fistula may be related to the lack of a serosal surface in which to sew the retroperitoneal portion of the duodenum, so that an insecure closure is obtained.

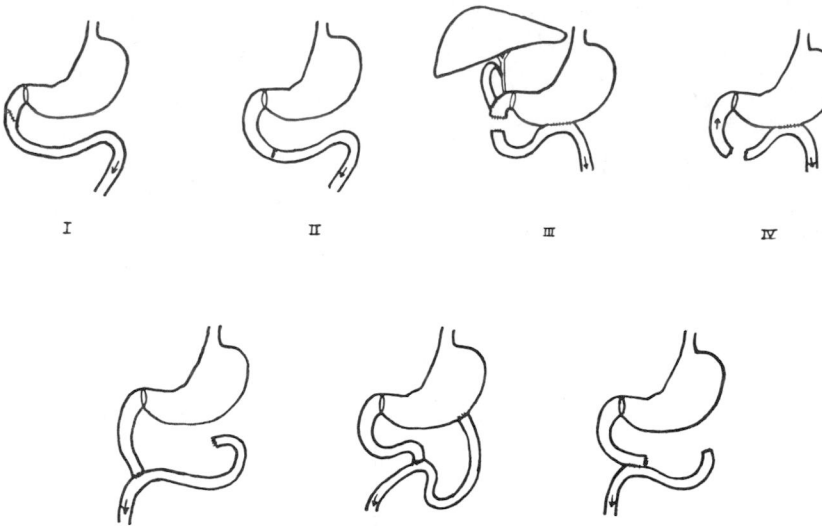

Fistulas may be prevented by prolonged decompression of the duodenum following closure of the wound. This is especially indicated in more severe injuries of the duodenum and is accomplished by several means:

1. A Levin tube may be threaded through the entire course of the duodenum with sufficient holes in the tube to allow simultaneous decompression of the duodenum and stomach. The tube may be brought through the anterior wall as a gastrostomy tube and placed on suction or may be inserted through the nasopharynx. A similar approach may be used via a retrograde jejunostomy (Witzel).

2. A # 10 Foley catheter may be placed through a small stab wound in the duodenum, adjacent to the area of duodenal injury, to serve as a vent. The tube is maintained on gentle suction until active bowel sounds return. At this time, suction is discontinued, and the tube is attached to a glass Y tube fixed to a stand at the level of the duodenum. This arrangement does not allow siphonage of

Fig. 6-11. Diagrammatic representation of various operative procedures in a series of cases. I, Simple closure; II, end-to-end duodenoduodenostomy; III and IV, closure of both ends of duodenum and gastroenterostomy; V, closure of distal duodenum and duodenojejunostomy; VI, duodenojejunostomy and gastroduodenostomy; VII, resection of fourth part of duodenum and duodenojejunostomy. (*From H. C. Cleveland and W. R. Waddell, Surg Clin North Am, 43:413, 1963.*)

Fig. 6-12. A technique for the exposure of the third and fourth portions of the duodenum. *A and B.* Initial dissection for mobilization of the right side of the colon, small intestine, and mesentery. *C.* Exposure obtained of the third and fourth portions of the duodenum. (*From R. B. Cattell and J. W. Braasch, Surg Gynecol Obstet, 111:379, 1960.*)

duodenal contents, as does gravity drainage, but does provide a decompressive vent if the pressure rises in the duodenum. After 9 or 10 days, at which time a fibrinous tract has formed about the small Foley catheter, the bag, which contains only 2 ml of water, is deflated. The Foley tube is again placed on gentle suction and is pulled just outside the duodenum, where it remains on suction for an additional 24 hours. At the end of the 24-hour period, the Foley catheter is removed if drainage is minimal. This small tube has been used for duodenal trauma at Parkland Memorial Hospital and also has been used to decompress the duodenum following gastric resection in which closure of the duodenal stump is insecure. In none of the approximately 75 cases in which the Foley tube was used following gastric resection and duodenal trauma has there been a significant complication, and no fistulas have occurred.

Postoperative Care. Postoperative care of these patients may be extremely difficult. Extracellular fluid volume deficits may be large, particularly if fistulas, retroperitoneal inflammation, or pancreatitis occur. It is very important to maintain the extracellular fluid volume with adequate infusions of balanced salt solution. In addition, these patients should be maintained on adequate doses of broad-spectrum intravenously administered antibiotics. Gastric and duodenal decompression should be continued for long periods of time in order to protect the suture lines. The average period of gastroduodenal decompression for duodenal wounds is about 5 to 7 days following exploration. If fistulas form, gastroduodenal decompression should be continued for longer periods, and a sump drain should be inserted into the drain site for continuous active suction of the fistular tract. This is instituted to prevent the collection of duodenal fluid with possible spread throughout the peritoneal cavity, to promote collapse and healing of the fistular tract, to prevent digestion of the skin by duodenal fluid draining onto the skin, and to aid calculation and replacement of fluid and electrolyte losses. Although several types of sump drains are now available commercially, recent experience with a simple sump drain made from two red rubber catheters has shown it to be more effective. A #18 French and a #14 French red rubber catheter are sewn together with nonabsorbable suture material at two or three points along the distal one-third of the catheters. Extra holes are cut in the sides of both tubes in their distal thirds. This sump drain is placed among several large Penrose drains through the abdominal drainage site. Postoperatively, suction is applied to the #18 catheter, and the smaller tube parallel to it serves as an effective air vent. This sump device was adapted from Waterman et al., although we have found it to be more effective when placed among several Penrose drains rather than through a single Penrose drain.

When a duodenal fistula develops, the patient should be placed on central intravenous hyperalimentation according to the principles of Dudrick and associates, which are discussed in Chap. 2. This regimen maintains excellent nutrition and may reduce the volume of gastrointestinal secretions.

With central intravenous hyperalimentation, it is now frequently unnecessary to perform feeding jejunostomies to provide nutritional support for patients with duodenal fistulas. If for some reason central intravenous feeding is not possible or if copious fistular drainage persists, a jejunostomy may become necessary. Two tubes are inserted through separate Witzel (serosal-lined) tunnels in the proximal jejunum and brought out through separate sites in the left upper quadrant of the abdomen. One jejunostomy tube is inserted in a retrograde direction so that its tip lies within the duodenum just below the duodenal fistula, and the other tube is inserted in an antegrade direction into the upper jejunum. Suction is applied to the retrograde tube lying within the duodenum; this usually greatly reduces the volume of drainage and promotes closure. Standard jejunostomy feedings are given through the antegrade tube in the proximal jejunum. Also, the duodenal fluid is slowly refed through this tube as it is removed by suction from the sump drain in the fistula and from the retrograde jejunostomy tube. This feeding is ideally done with constant slow infusions through a Barron pump.

If, after 5 to 7 days of Levin tube or gastrostomy decompression of the duodenum, the patient is doing well, shows no evidence of duodenal leak, and has adequate bowel activity, he is given 1 oz of water orally every hour for approximately 12 hours, after the Levin tube is removed or the gastrostomy tube clamped. If water is tolerated, the diet is increased in the usual fashion. Also, after feeding has been instituted for 1 to 2 days and there has been little or no drainage, the Penrose drains are advanced and removed over 3 days unless further drainage ensues. In the face of continued drainage, the drains should be left for at least 2 or 3 weeks, or as long as any significant drainage continues. After about 3 weeks, if drainage persists, the Penrose drains may be removed; the only drainage tube which should remain is the previously described sump drain, which is removed when drainage has dropped to a minimum.

Occasionally, the duodenal fistula does not close despite adequate nonoperative treatment described above. In such cases, when a reasonable trial of conservative treatment has been made and the patient is in optimal condition for reoperation, the abdomen is opened and completely explored to rule out distal bowel obstruction which may be causing the fistula to persist. The fistula is exposed at its origin from the duodenum, and a Roux en Y defunctionalized limb of proximal jejunum is brought up to the fistula and anastomosed to it. This anastomosis may use either the end or the side (after closing the end of the jejunal limb) of the defunctionalized jejunum. This procedure permanently diverts the fistular drainage internally and has been very effective in treating persistent duodenal fistulas.

INTRAMURAL HEMATOMA

Another interesting but infrequently reported lesion of the duodenum secondary to trauma is intramural hematoma of the duodenum.

This lesion is generally caused by blunt abdominal trauma which causes rupture of intramural duodenal blood vessels with formation of a dark, sausage-shaped mass in the submucosal layer of the duodenal wall. This hematoma causes partial or complete duodenal obstruction, usually partial. The patient shows signs of a high small bowel obstruction, with nausea and vomiting associated with upper abdominal pain and tenderness, and sometimes a suggestion of a right upper quandrant mass. Flat films of the abdomen may show an ill-defined right upper quadrant mass and obliteration of the right psoas shadow. An upper gastrointestinal tract series is almost diagnostic, showing dilatation of the duodenal lumen with the appearance of a "coiled spring" in the second and third portions of the duodenum due to the crowding of the valvulae conniventes by the hematoma, according to Felson and Levin. The serum amylase level may be elevated. The lesion has occurred spontaneously in patients on anticoagulants.

Treatment generally consists of celiotomy, evacuation of the duodenal hematoma, and closure of the defect in the seromuscular coat of the duodenum with interrupted nonabsorbable sutures after control of any bleeding points. Fullen has recently recommended conservative treatment of this injury. Eleven patients treated with restriction of oral intake, nasogastric suction, and intravenous fluids and electrolytes all survived without complication. Nonoperative treatment is considered only after satisfactorily excluding the possibility of duodenal perforation or other associated injuries requiring celiotomy. The prognosis is excellent.

Small Bowel

Injuries to the small bowel are more frequent than injuries to the duodenum or colon. Counseller and McCormack, in a review of 1,313 cases of intestinal trauma, found that 80 percent of bowel injuries occur between the duodenojejunal junction and the terminal ileum, with approximately 10 percent each in the duodenum and large intestine. The usual mechanism of small bowel injury from blunt trauma is the crushing of the small bowel against the vertebral column. Rupture of the small bowel is also caused by shearing and tearing forces applied to the abdomen, and rarely by sudden elevation of the intraluminal pressure of the bowel with bursting from such sudden high pressure. Work by Williams and Sargent has shown that rupture due to sudden elevation of pressure is quite unusual.

In exploring the abdomen for injuries to the small bowel, it is important to inspect minutely the entire circumference of the small bowel and its attached mesentery from the ligament of Treitz to the ileocecal valve. The bowel may be completely transected in one or more places by blunt trauma with or without severe injury to the mesentery and its blood supply; at times, the mesentery may be torn from a segment of bowel, thus depriving the bowel of its blood supply. Penetrating trauma to the small bowel from a gunshot wound or stab wound is frequent, although, surprisingly, it has been noted at times that in patients with a stab wound of the abdomen the small bowel has been spared. This is probably because the great mobility of the small bowel allows it to slide away from the knife, a much less likely occurrence with gunshot wounds than with stab wounds.

TREATMENT. Small, single perforations of the small bowel may be closed safely with a single layer of interrupted nonabsorbable mattress sutures which include and invert the seromuscular and submucosal coats of the bowel. A hemostatic stitch, as required for stomach wounds, is not necessary for small bowel wounds, because the small bowel does not tend to continue bleeding from the submucosal plexus, as does the stomach. Individual bleeders, however, should be ligated with fine suture material. An advantage of a single-layer closure is its rapidity of performance, which is important in patients in precarious condition following multiple trauma.

Two small perforations of the bowel which are very close together may often be repaired by converting the wounds into one and closing the resulting defect as a single linear wound. This type of repair does not constrict the lumen of the bowel as much as two separate lines of suture placed close together and is more secure. Multiple perforations of the small bowel may occur following injury from shotgun pellets. Each one of these injuries should be carefully sought out and closed with interrupted rows of nonabsorbable mattress sutures.

Long linear lacerations of the lumen also should be closed with a single row of nonabsorbable sutures after ligating any persistent bleeders with small nonabsorbable suture. Longitudinal lacerations may be closed in a longitudinal direction or transversely according to the Heineke-Mikulicz principle.

Small bowel injuries produced by high-velocity missiles cause severe contusions of tissue surrounding the actual perforation. Because the contusion is a site of potential tissue necrosis and bowel leakage caused by thrombosis of vessels in the area of blast injury, it should be debrided. The debridement should extend into viable bowel where active bleeding is obtained.

If the wound is too large or is long and longitudinal, the bowel may not be adequately closed without loss of lumen, and the damaged segment should be resected. Also, if there are multiple wounds in a short segment of bowel, it is much safer and easier to resect the injured segment than to attempt to suture each of the closely spaced wounds, with resulting impairment of the bowel lumen and blood supply and subsequent obstruction and/or necrosis and leakage. Perforations or lacerations to the mesenteric border, unless they are quite small, are difficult to repair and frequently are associated with vascular impairment. They also should be managed by resection of the involved bowel if an adequate closure cannot be obtained without interference with blood supply. Bowel transections should be reanastomosed after debriding contused and damaged bowel on either side of the wound back to normal bowel with good blood supply. Careful attention should be given to leaving uninjured mesentery adjacent to the suture line of the reanastomosis. Extensive segments of bowel may be avulsed from the mesentery, so that the bowel loses its blood supply. All the necrotic or potentially necrotic bowel and injured mesentery must be resected and an end-to-end anastomosis made between uninjured bowel attached to uninjured mesentery.

Contusions of the small bowel should be assumed to

be larger than is apparent. Such injuries are dangerous, since they may lead to necrosis and perforation. Contusions up to 1 cm in diameter may be turned in with a row of fine, nonabsorbable mattress sutures. Larger contusions should be resected.

Postoperative care of patients with wounds of the small bowel includes maintenance on nasogastric suction and no oral intake until adequate bowel activity has returned. Also, these patients are usually maintained on antibiotics, most frequently penicillin and tetracycline, which are given preoperatively and postoperatively. Usually, the antibiotic is discontinued at about the time that the nasogastric tube is removed, unless there is some other indication to continue antibiotic treatment. Leakage from suture lines and intestinal obstruction are rarely seen if the wounds are properly managed. In the report of Giddings and McDaniel concerning wounds of the jejunum and ileum during World War II, leakage from suture lines occurred in only 1 percent and intestinal obstruction in 1.7 percent, in a series of 1,168 patients with small bowel injuries, most of whom had multiple visceral injury. Again, extracellular fluid volume deficits should be replaced in patients with small bowel injury, with adequate amounts of balanced salt solution given during the surgical procedure and in the postoperative period to maintain sufficient urine volume and prevent extracellular fluid volume deficit.

Colon Injuries

The morbidity and mortality from acute injuries to the colon and rectum have been significantly reduced by an aggressive surgical approach. This has been largely influenced by the experiences of military surgeons during World War II and the Korean conflict. In the American Civil War, wounds of the abdomen carried a mortality rate of approximately 90 percent; it was not until the Boer War that the mortality rate of 80 percent of cases treated conservatively was thought to be excessive and active intervention was viewed more favorably. During this time, the fatalities from wounds of the colon eventually dropped to less than 60 percent. In World War II, an impressive improvement in the mortality from wounds of the colon was noted. This was due to several factors including improved methods of triage and transportation, effective replacement of blood and fluid, and early surgical intervention combined with ancillary use of antibiotics.

The mortality rate for wounds of the colon of 37 percent in World War II was reduced to approximately 15 percent during the action in Korea. The majority of military surgeons treating acute injuries of the colon tended to exteriorize the wound as an artificial anus to prevent further soilage of the peritoneal cavity. This approach to these particular wounds was duly carried over into civilian practice and reflected in the subsequent reduction in mortality and morbidity. In the later phase of the Korean conflict, however, some modification of the aggressive technique was noted in that small, primary wounds treated early were handled by primary closure without exteriorization.

Acute wounds of the colon which occur in a civilian environment exhibit features that may modify the indica-

tions for exteriorization of the wound. The types of injury usually noted in a military situation resulted from either high-velocity missiles or fragmentation missiles in which there was massive destruction of tissue and usually gross soilage of the peritoneal cavity. In the civilian environment, the wounds more often are caused by low-velocity missiles and usually are unassociated with massive destruction of surrounding organs and tissue. The time from wounding to initial treatment in the civilian situation is generally somewhat less than that noted during military conflict. Similarly, associated injuries occurring in civilian accidents do not tend to be so numerous nor so massive as those in a military environment, and this has a definite influence on morbidity and mortality.

ETIOLOGY. Acute injuries of the colon and rectum may be divided into penetrating wounds and wounds resulting from blunt trauma. In the former group, accidental colon injuries may be the result of industrial accidents involving explosions resulting in impalement, penetrating injuries from flying objects, or blast injuries. These injuries may be either the direct result of explosives or the result of accidents involving sources of greatly compressed air. External acts of violence constitute an important source of injuries to the colon, and these are generally penetrating injuries caused by guns or knives or, on rarer occasions, blunt abdominal trauma. Wounds of the rectum, particularly, may be the result of instrumentation during the process of sigmoidoscopy or the administration of enemas. There may also be perforations of the colorectum by foreign bodies which pass through the alimentary canal into the colon. Inadvertent penetration of the colon or rectum may occur during difficult operations; this is especially true of operations in the pelvis for severe neoplastic or inflammatory disease. Falls resulting in impalement upon sharp objects may produce wounds of the rectum. Automobile accidents and other forms of blunt trauma may produce acute injuries to the colon and rectum.

DIAGNOSIS. A systematic diagnostic approach to problems of abdominal trauma is necessary, but specific examinations of the colon and rectum may be necessary to delineate an injury. This is particularly pertinent in those instances in which instrumentation is the cause of suspected perforation of the rectum or colon. Rectal examination and sigmoidoscopy should occupy a prominent place in the examination of these patients. Diagnostic abdominal x-ray studies should be employed to determine if there is a perforated colon with leakage of air into the free peritoneal cavity. Anteroposterior and lateral decubitus views are particularly helpful in these instances. Contrast studies of the colon should be employed rarely and cautiously in view of the high morbidity and mortality associated with leakage of barium and feces into the free peritoneal cavity. Aqueous opaque media, such as Gastrografin, are preferable when penetration of the colon is suspected.

TREATMENT. The general principles of management of patients with abdominal trauma apply to those patients who have acute injuries of the colon. It is important that the time from wounding to definitive operation be as short as possible, and aggressive replacement of fluid and blood losses should be undertaken at once. Preoperatively, penicillin and tetracycline should be started in all patients suspected of having penetrating injuries of the colorectum. Two million units of aqueous penicillin and 0.5 Gm of tetracycline are added to the intravenous solution.

These patients are explored through a midline incision in order to allow access to all parts of the abdominal cavity. A thorough and complete exploration of all abdominal viscera is made, for the morbidity and mortality vary directly with the number of associated injuries. Bleeding should be controlled as rapidly as possible and immediate efforts made to reduce peritoneal soilage from any penetrating wound of an abdominal viscus. The specific care of the wound of the colon should be approached by noting the anatomic differences between the intraperitoneal and extraperitoneal large intestine. Particular attention must be paid to the type of wound, its location, the amount of tissue destruction, the presence of associated injuries, and the time from wounding to definitive care.

Wounds of the intraperitoneal colon may be divided into two groups: First, small, primary wounds located on the antimesenteric border which are seen quite early, in which there is minimal tissue destruction, and minimal or no peritoneal soiling. These wounds, especially of the left colon and in the absence of associated injuries of other abdominal viscera, may often be adequately managed by a primary two-layer closure. The mucosa is approximated with a running lock suture of 3-0 chromic catgut, and the seromuscular layers are closed with interrupted #50 cotton sutures, the Lembert technique. Second, wounds of the right colon, containing liquid feces, are less amenable to this type of primary closure, for often gross and extensive peritoneal soiling follows the colon penetration. High-velocity missile wounds should rarely, if ever, be closed primarily, for tissue destruction is often excessive and may not be readily apparent. The injured area should be extensively debrided.

Acute injuries of the intraperitoneal colon resulting from high-velocity missiles which are associated with extensive destruction of tissues or which are large and ragged in nature and are located near or involve the mesenteric border should not be closed primarily. If located in the ascending, transverse, or descending colon, the wound may be exteriorized as a colostomy. Similarly, if the time from wounding to definitive care is relatively long, allowing seeding of the peritoneal cavity with a large number of bacteria, some type of colostomy should be performed either as a wound exteriorization or as a proximal diverting colostomy. Primary closure of the distal wounds is then permissible. Although a loop colostomy may be done for expediency, a completely diverting double-barrel colostomy is favored. It is preferable to open the loop colostomy immediately, usually with the cautery, and secure early, complete fecal diversion. This is performed in the operating room after all the wounds are closed and dressed. When there are associated massive injuries to other viscera, although the colon wound itself might fulfill the indications for primary closure, a colostomy is indicated. In some instances, there may be massive injury of the cecum or of the ileocecal area, in which case it will be necessary

to resect the injured bowel and do an ileotransverse colostomy. This is preferable to an ileostomy and, with suitable antibiotic coverage and intraluminal antibiotics, is an adequate procedure.

Localized minor wounds of the right colon and cecum which do not produce extensive destruction of the large bowel and are not associated with massive soilage or serious injuries to other viscera may often be managed by primary closure and appendicostomy. In these instances, after debridement and careful closure of the laceration of the cecum, tube appendicostomy is performed to decompress this segment. Seromuscular sutures are placed about the base of the appendix and secured to the lateral parietal peritoneum in order to prevent intraperitoneal leakage about the area of tube insertion. By this technique, suitable decompression of the cecum and right colon may be obtained, and removal of the tube appendicostomy permits the vent to close spontaneously. This route may also be used for intraluminal installation of neomycin or kanamycin solutions, which may offer some protection from bacterial invasion of the suture line.

The extraperitoneal perforations of the rectum must be evaluated under the same principles employed for colon injuries within the peritoneal cavity. If clean lacerations with minimal spillage are seen early, primary bowel repair may be indicated if the wound is accessible. Presacral drains should then be inserted. Associated perineal wounds should be debrided and, if grossly contaminated, left open. If debridement is adequate and these wounds are clean, they may be closed with drainage. Any damage to the anal sphincter may be repaired at this time. When a perineal wound is present but not penetrating the colon, it should be debrided widely and if not grossly contaminated then may be closed with drainage. Where there is no perineal wound but there is significant tissue destruction about the extraperitoneal rectum, presacral drainage should be instituted.

For all injuries of the rectum, complete diversion of the fecal stream is mandatory and can be accomplished by constructing a proximal double-barrel colostomy. Even in those instances where the rectal wound has been closed and diverting colostomy performed, presacral drainage is necessary.

Drainage of the retrorectal area is extremely important. This can be established by making a curvilinear incision in the posterior perianal area, incising the anococcygeal ligament, and bluntly dissecting into the presacral space. Two Penrose drains will usually suffice, but with extensive injuries, it may be necessary to utilize sump drainage for a few days.

Lavenson and Cohen, on the basis of their experience in the Vietnam conflict, strongly recommend removal of all feces from the distal rectum. This is accomplished by irrigating copious amounts of saline solution through the defunctionalized segment until the return is clear. They report a significant decrease in mortality and complication rates when utilizing this technique. Military injuries are generally associated with higher-velocity missiles and cause more fecal contamination and blast injury to surrounding pelvic tissue. In civilian injuries, distal irrigation may not be as important, as evidenced by Trunkey and Shires, who report a lower morbidity and mortality rate in their series, in which distal irrigation was not employed but adequate drainage and diversion were used.

Serious perineal injuries are treated in a similar manner. Even in the absence of rectal injury, sepsis can be avoided by early fecal diversion. Failure to recognize this potential problem may lead to extensive soft tissue infections extending from the knee to the axilla, with potential involvement of the anterior and posterior abdominal wall.

Early closure of the colostomy is indicated in patients who have completely recovered and have no distal colon injury. It is desirable to close the simple colostomy in 2 or 3 weeks. Prior to closure, both limbs of the colon should be visualized radiographically to assure that no lesion persists. Mechanical and bacterial cleansing of the colon is effected preoperatively.

Adjunctive Measures. Aggressive replacement of fluid and blood loss should be undertaken immediately and general supportive measures instituted. Attention to possible injuries elsewhere is mandatory. The systemic antibiotics begun in the preoperative period are continued for 5 to 7 days postoperatively. The use of peritoneal and intraluminal instillation of antibiotics has been advocated by many. Certainly, removing all gross fecal material from the peritoneal cavity is indicated, but instillation of intraperitoneal antibiotics has been followed by some complications, notably respiratory depression. These have been most frequently seen in anesthetized patients who received intraperitoneal neomycin. Extensive lavage of the peritoneal cavity with saline solution may actually result in dissemination of fecal material and is not recommended. The use of an intraluminal catheter for postoperative instillation of antibiotics as advocated by Cohn may add further protection from late wound disruption. The antibiotics may be instilled through a small polyethylene catheter, which is inserted into the bowel proximal to the areas of injury. It is desirable to place the catheter through a taenia and secure it with a purse-string suture. The bowel is then sutured to the parietal peritoneum at the point of entrance of the catheter. A 1% solution of neomycin or 15 ml of sterile saline solution with 1 Gm of kanamycin may be instilled at 6-hour intervals for the first three or four postoperative days. The small polyethylene catheter may then be removed without difficulty. The use of antibiotics systemically and locally may reduce the incidence of septic complications, particularly septic shock.

Liver

Injury to the liver is suspected in all patients with penetrating or blunt trauma that involves the lower part of the chest and upper part of the abdomen. Among patients with penetrating abdominal trauma, the liver is second only to the small bowel as the structure most commonly injured; among those with blunt trauma, the liver is second only to the spleen as the most commonly injured organ. About 80 percent of liver injuries occur as a result of penetrating trauma from stab wounds or gunshot wounds; only 15 to 20 percent occur from blunt trauma. In the past decade, the incidence of stab wounds has diminished while the incidence of gunshot wounds, especially those caused by higher-velocity and larger-caliber missiles, and blunt trauma has increased. These changes in the types of liver injury, the more rapid transport of patients with hepatic trauma to treatment facilities, and better resuscitation methods have caused an increase in severity of liver injuries that are likely to confront the surgeon.

Early exploration, prompt replacement of blood and use of balanced electrolyte solution, use of antibiotics, proper choice of surgical treatment, and adequate drainage are all factors that have led to increased survival rates. The average overall mortality rate of patients with hepatic trauma is about 13 to 15 percent. However, this rate is directly related to the severity of the liver injury and the injury to other intraabdominal organs. The mortality rate of stab wounds to the liver without associated organ injury is only about 1 percent. When significant liver trauma is associated with injuries of more than five other intraabdominal organs, or when major hepatic resection is required to control bleeding, the mortality rate rises to about 45 to 50 percent.

TREATMENT. After initial resuscitation and diagnostic maneuvers, patients with suspected hepatic injuries are rapidly moved to the operating room. The entire abdomen and chest are "prepped" and draped, and a long upper midline incision is made. Sources of bleeding from the liver and the abdomen are quickly appraised, and temporary control of the bleeding is achieved by manual compression of packs placed over the bleeding sites and by temporary occlusion of appropriate major vessels. Digital compression of the hepatic artery and portal vein to occlude temporarily the blood flow to the liver (the Pringle maneuver) may control or slow hepatic hemorrhage in some patients, but more often it is necessary to combine the Pringle maneuver with compression packs placed over the liver injury to control hemorrhage effectively. There is general agreement that, in the normothermic liver, blood flow to the liver can be completely occluded for about 15 minutes without causing any hepatocellular damage. If it is necessary to occlude the hepatic blood supply for more than 15 minutes, the vascular occlusion can be briefly interrupted every 10 or 15 minutes to allow short periods of uninterrupted hepatic blood flow.

Definitive treatment may be accomplished by drainage alone, suture or hemostatic maneuvers and drainage, or variations of hepatic resection.

Drainage Alone. Hepatic hemorrhage will have ceased spontaneously by the time the abdomen is opened or stops soon after compression of the bleeding site in about 50 to 70 percent of patients with liver injuries. In such patients, the only treatment necessary is adequate drainage of the injury. Suturing of nonbleeding liver injuries is unnecessary. This is emphasized by Trunkey, Shires and McClelland, who reported no rebleeding among several hundred patients with liver injuries that stopped bleeding spontaneously or soon after temporary pack compression. Suturing of nonbleeding liver wounds may cause bleeding and needlessly traumatize hepatic tissue.

All liver injuries should be drained with large, 1-in. wide Penrose drains, and several drains should be used in patients with larger injuries. The drains are brought out posterolaterally, as dependently as possible, through an abdominal wall stab wound in order to achieve the best drainage by gravity. This greatly reduces the formation of infected collections of bile, blood, and tissue fluid in the subphrenic and subhepatic spaces. Also, dependent gravity drainage is more reliable than nondependent suction drainage. In most patients with liver injury it is unnecessary to resect the twelfth rib to achieve dependent drainage. Usually the drains can be brought through the stab wound at the tip of, or just below, the twelfth rib. However, in large patients with more extensive liver wounds, it may be preferable to resect the lateral half or two-thirds of the right twelfth rib, to achieve more effective drainage. An adequate opening, easily admitting two fingers, must be made in the abdominal wall to be certain that these injuries are effectively drained. The drains are left in place 5 to 10 days thereafter, being slowly removed over a 3-day period. Not until the end of this time is a firm, fibrinous tract formed about the drains which ensures adequate external drainage of any material that accumulates in the abdomen after the drain is removed.

Suture, Hemostatic Techniques, and Drainage. Bleeding persists despite temporary compression packing of the injury site in 30 to 50 percent of patients with liver injuries. Definitive hemostasis of persistently bleeding liver injuries usually can be achieved by liver sutures. Simple interrupted sutures are placed 2 cm from the wound margins, using 2-0 or 0 chromic suture swaged onto a 2-in. blunt-tipped "liver needle." This will allow gentle but firm approximation, thereby stopping most bleeding which originates from the outer 2 cm of the liver parenchyma immediately beneath the capsule of the liver. Larger wounds may require placement of figure-of-eight liver sutures to prevent cutting through the liver capsule. Passage of the liver suture through buttressing materials such as Surgicel, Gelfoam, or omentum is seldom needed if the sutures are placed 2 cm from the margin of the injury and tied gently. However, if a bolster is needed, it is preferable to use a vascularized pedicle of omentum instead of foreign material. Trunkey, Shires, and McClelland have abandoned the technique previously described using interlocking mattress sutures for hemostasis. These authors now recommend direct suture ligation of the bleeding vessel as an attempt to reduce the chance of strangulation and subsequent necrosis.

Recently, microcrystalline collagen powder (Avitene) has been reported to be successful in controlling bleeding from liver wounds. Unlike other material such as Gelfoam, Avitene can be left in liver wounds without inciting significant foreign body reaction. The use of other hemostatic agents as well as gauze packs to tamponade hemorrhage is not recommended.

The use of liver sutures to obtain hemostasis from both the entrance and exit sites of long gunshot tracts in the liver is controversial. However, Lucas and Ledgerwood state that this technique was successfully used in several of their patients who otherwise would have required extensive surgery. Placement of the liver sutures at both ends of the bullet tract stops bleeding arising from the subcapsular area, which is the usual source. During their 5-year prospective review, Lucas and Ledgerwood found that only one patient developed an intrahepatic abscess following this technique, and no patients developed hemobilia after closure of both ends of a long gunshot tract. Continued bleeding which persists after closure of both ends of the tract is usually identified at the initial operation by blood oozing between the liver sutures or by an increase in the size of the liver within 10 minutes after placement of the sutures. If the persistently bleeding tract is short and close to an accessible surface of the liver, hemostasis can be achieved by limited wedge resection or by resectional debridement incorporating the tract as part of the debridement. Persistently active bleeding from deep bilobar tracts that do not lend themselves to resectional debridement is best controlled either by ligation of an appropriate branch of the hepatic artery or by tractotomy and ligation of the intraparenchymal bleeding vessels. However, tractotomy may cause further bleeding, and for this reason, ligation of one of the main hepatic artery branches is preferable, since it usually stops arterial bleeding from deep tracts and is likely to cause less morbidity than tractotomy.

Ligation of an appropriate major branch of the hepatic artery (i.e., the right or left branch) is a safe and effective means for controlling liver bleeding in patients with active arterial bleeding from wounds that do not permit suture ligature or wedge resection and in whom bleeding stops with temporary hepatic artery occlusion. Mays reported achieving liver hemostasis in 15 of 16 patients who underwent ligation of hepatic artery branches. Lucas and Ledgerwood did not find ligation of major branches of the hepatic artery as effective in arresting hemorrhage as Mays did, possibly because some of these patients were bleeding from major venous injuries. It is suggested that the right or left hepatic artery should not be ligated if a simple temporary compression pack or suturing of a bleeding liver injury controls the hemorrhage. However, if compression or suturing does not control bleeding and temporary occlusion of the hepatic artery branch supplying the injured area of the liver does stop hemorrhage, then the appropriate major hepatic artery branch should be ligated, especially if the alternative treatment is a hepatic resection.

Resection. Resectional debridement or limited wedge resection is recommended for control of bleeding from the ragged liver injuries that may be caused by shotgun wounds, high-velocity rifle wounds, and severe blunt injuries. Limited resectional debridement of shattered liver tissue usually achieves hemostasis from such injuries effectively and safely. The margins of resectional debridement should be 2 or 3 cm beyond the point of injury, and bleeding during debridement is controlled by digital parenchymal constriction and/or temporary occlusion of the inflow of blood to the liver at the porta hepatis. The liver parenchyma is separated bluntly by finger fracture, a suction tip, or a scalpel handle. Vessels and bile ducts are secured by individual suture ligation or by metal clips as they are encountered. It is not necessary to oppose the margins of resection with interrupted liver sutures if bleeding from the resected surface is controlled. This suture technique may be undesirable, since it may create a potentially infected closed space within the liver.

Anatomic hepatic lobectomy for control of bleeding, especially from the right lobe, is best reserved for patients in whom (1) hepatic suturing is unsuccessful; (2) resectional debridement of hepatotomy with intraparenchymal hemostasis is precluded by the anatomic location of the injury; (3) occlusion of the hepatic artery is ineffective in controlling hemorrhage. Although resectional debridement or sublobar hepatic resection may be required in about 4 or 5 percent of all patients with liver injuries, no more than 2 or 3 percent require anatomic, lobar resection to control hemorrhage. Most of the few patients with liver injuries who require major hepatic lobectomies to control bleeding have massive, shattering injuries of the liver, injuries of the retrohepatic vena cava, or injuries to the major hepatic vein (Fig. 6-13). If it becomes apparent that major lobar resection is necessary, the hepatic bleeding is temporarily controlled by manual compression packing and a Pringle maneuver while the midline abdominal incision is extended by performing a median sternotomy.

A median sternotomy is much more quickly and easily made and closed than a right thoracoabdominal incision, causes considerably less diaphragmatic injury, provides much easier access to the vena cava and hepatic veins, permits easier insertion of a retrohepatic vena caval shunt if this is required, and causes less postoperative pain and pulmonary morbidity than a right thoracoabdominal incision.

After wide exposure is obtained by the median sternotomy extension of the midline abdominal incision, Rumel tourniquets are placed about the vena cava superior and inferior to the liver. The superior tape is placed about the vena cava superior to the central tendon of the dia-

phragm after this portion of the vena cava is exposed by opening the pericardium. These tapes permit temporary occlusion of the vena cava for insertion of a retrohepatic intracaval shunt if vascular isolation of the liver is required during hepatic lobectomy because of major retrohepatic vena cava or major hepatic vein injury. The hepatic artery, portal vein, and bile ducts supplying the lobe to be resected are then suture-ligated and divided. After this, hepatic resection can be carried out by dividing Glisson's capsule with a cautery along the line appropriate for the lobe being removed. The lobe is removed by fracturing through the liver substance along the line of resection with the thumb and forefinger or with the tip of an abdominal suction tube from which the guard has been removed. The back of a scalpel handle may also be used to fracture through the liver parenchyma. As the blood vessels and bile ducts are encountered within the liver, they are isolated by passing a right-angle clamp around them and are then sharply divided. After the larger vessels and ducts are suture-ligated, the smaller ones are secured with tantalum (Weck) clips. No attempt is made to secure the hepatic veins at their junction with the retrohepatic vena cava before beginning the resection; instead, it is much easier and safer to isolate and suture-ligate or oversew the appropriate major hepatic veins as they are encountered posteriorly during the liver resection. The resection begins anteriorly and progresses posteriorly toward the right or left side of the vena cava, keeping to the right or left of the middle hepatic vein (depending upon whether a right or left lobectomy is being done). The middle hepatic vein demarcates the right from the left lobe of the liver and passes in a line from the middle of the gallbladder bed posteriorly to the midportion of the retrohepatic vena cava. The hepatic veins and other large vascular structures must be oversewn, since simple ligatures on these large structures often slip off and cause catastrophic bleeding.

Fig. 6-13. Typical liver injury requiring hepatic resection.

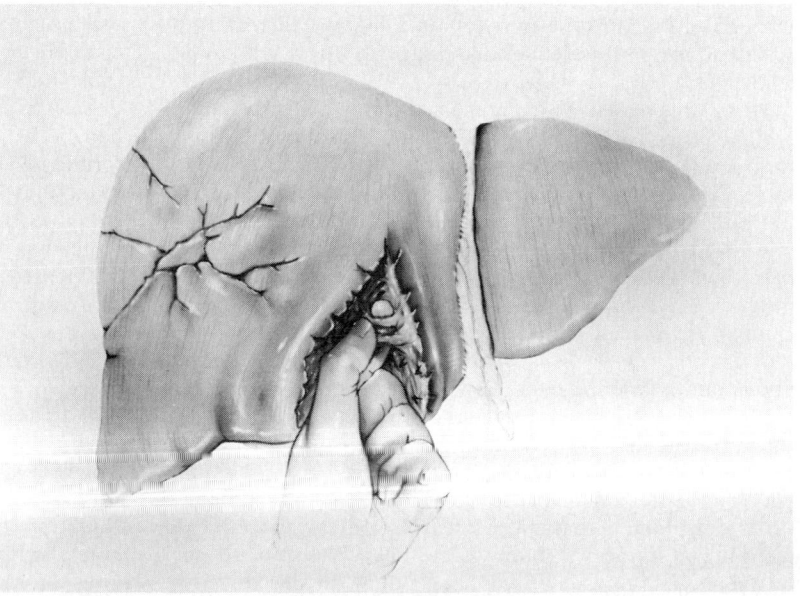

The recently described Lin liver clamp may be helpful in performing resections. There is considerable reduction in blood loss and operating time with the use of this clamp, but its availability should not cause a broadening of the indications for liver resection. The clamp can be used for resecting the liver only when the liver has been severely shattered and devitalized without injury to the retrohepatic vena cava or the major hepatic veins near the junction with the vena cava.

Although Merendino et al., Longmire and Marable, and Perry and LaFave suggest that T-tube drainage of the common bile duct should be carried out after hepatic resections, reports by Lucas and by Pinkerton et al., suggest that septic complications and bleeding from gastroduodenal stress ulcers are significantly increased by this practice. Although T-tube drainage may not lower pressures in the common bile duct and therefore probably does not prevent bile leakage from the liver and bile collections in the operative site, the T-tube does help identify the right and left hepatic ducts with certainty during liver resections, and thus aids in preventing operative injury to the remaining major bile duct. Also, the T-tube does provide a useful port through which such postoperative complications as hematobilia and biliary fistula formation can be recognized and the type of drainage observed. Cholangiography may also be done through the tube postoperatively, and this may be very useful in determining the cause of prolonged jaundice after hepatic resections. Lucas and Walt, in a well-controlled prospective study, support the position that effective biliary decompression is not achieved by the T-tube and that drainage of the common duct may, indeed, increase the incidence of complications in patients with hepatic trauma, especially those due to infection and bile duct obstruction (i.e., jaundice, cholangitis, and bile duct stricture). The increased likelihood of bleeding from gastroduodenal stress ulcers caused by T-tube drainage of the common bile duct after hepatic resection may be offset by frequently lavaging the stomach with antacid solution through the Levin tube to maintain a high gastric pH for several days postoperatively, as suggested by Curtis and associates.

Vascular Isolation. Vascular isolation may be required in a highly selected group of patients with liver injuries. This technique allows the surgeon to control bleeding from and to repair retrohepatic vena caval or major hepatic venous injuries. Vascular isolation of the liver is attained by using one of two techniques. The first technique was initially described and reported by Heaney in 1966; when this method of vascular isolation is used, occlusive vascular clamps are placed across the aorta just below the diaphragm, the porta hepatis, and the inferior vena cava above and below the liver. This technique may be associated with cardiac dysrhythmias and renal insufficiency. The second technique for obtaining vascular isolation of the liver was first described and reported by Shrock and associates in 1968. When this technique is used, retrohepatic vena caval and hepatic venous isolation is attained by inserting an intracaval shunt via the right atrial appendage of the heart; control of vascular inflow to the liver is obtained by placing a Rumel tourniquet or vascular clamp

on the porta hepatis. Defore and associates reported survival of 7 of 15 patients with major vena caval or hepatic vein injuries following vascular isolation and the introduction of intracaval shunts. The introduction of the intracaval shunt via the right atrial appendage is most expeditiously done via a median sternotomy. It is suggested that three equidistant "guy" sutures be placed in the right atrial wall somewhat outside the atrial purse-string suture before making the atrial opening in the center of the purse-string suture to insert the shunt. These "guy" sutures are then split apart and held up by assistants as the atrium is opened; this greatly facilitates the insertion of the shunt as the atrial wall is stabilized.

Another method for controlling hemorrhage from the retrohepatic vena cava or major hepatic veins has been described. If the major venous laceration is in such a position in the suprahepatic vena cava or the extrahepatic portion of the hepatic veins, a Foley catheter may be quickly inserted into the exposed laceration. The balloon of the Foley catheter is then inflated and pulled up against the wall of the vena cava or hepatic vein to occlude the laceration, arrest the hemorrhage, and thus permit repair of the venous laceration with relatively good exposure and little blood loss.

It is reemphasized that these methods should not be used except by a skillful and experienced surgeon in whose judgment exsanguination will occur unless vascular isolation is carried out.

SUBCAPSULAR HEMATOMA. The treatment of subcapsular hematomas is somewhat controversial. Left alone, these may (1) resolve spontaneously; (2) expand and burst with delayed intraperitoneal bleeding; (3) cause development of hepatic abscess; or (4) decompress into the biliary tree and cause hemobilia. The risk of inducing massive hemorrhage, at times uncontrollable, accompanies attempts at incision and evacuation.

Richie and Fonkalsrud reported on a series of patients treated nonoperatively. They emphasized that severe bleeding may result in some patients in whom hematomas of the liver are unroofed, and they further note that since some hematomas are centrally located within the liver, they often do not lend themselves to resection or control by hepatic artery ligation. These authors recommend performing an emergency liver scan on patients with probable blunt hepatic trauma who do not have evidence of persistent hemorrhage or shock and who do not have other indications for immediate celiotomy, such as positive needle paracentesis of the abdomen or positive peritoneal lavage. If the patient's condition remains stable, and a subcapsular hematoma is seen on liver scan, they recommend close observation of the patient in the hospital by means of frequent physical examinations, serial hematocrits, and performance of liver function studies. The status of the hematoma is appraised by serial liver scans to be certain it is resolving, not increasing in size.

Emergency hepatic arteriography for patients in stable condition with probable intrahepatic hematomas due to blunt trauma is probably preferable to emergency scanning. Arteriography more definitely delineates the size and location of a subcapsular or intrahepatic hematoma, indicates whether there is persistent intrahepatic or extrahepatic hemorrhage, and may show the source and severity of the bleeding.

Another notable advantage of hepatic arteriography, in some stable patients with intrahepatic hematomas, is that this technique may be used therapeutically as well as diagnostically. If a site of arterial hemorrhage is visualized arteriographically, the hemorrhage may be stopped nonoperatively and atraumatically by embolizing several 2-mm² pieces of Gelfoam through the hepatic catheter. These emboli obstruct the bleeding site and thus prevent further bleeding.

Hemobilia. Hemobilia is caused by arterial hemorrhage into the biliary tract after liver trauma; it classically presents with a triad of findings consisting of upper or lower gastrointestinal hemorrhage, obstructive jaundice, and colicky abdominal pain. In the past the standard treatment for this condition has consisted of hepatic resection or hepatotomy with direct exposure and suture ligation of the bleeding artery. Such treatment is often associated with considerable blood loss and high operative mortality and morbidity rates. There are now several reports of successful management of traumatic hemobilia by ligation of the hepatic arteries supplying the involved lobe of the liver. Recent experience with hepatic artery ligation in the management of hepatic trauma and hepatic tumors has proved this to be a safe technique.

COMPLICATIONS. Major nonfatal complications occur in approximately 20 percent of patients with liver injuries. Since the thorax is involved in a large number of hepatic injuries, there is a high incidence of pulmonary complications. A large number of patients develop intraabdominal abscesses, and approximately 50 percent of these are associated with injuries to the colon.

Patients with major lobar resections may be expected to have some degree of postoperative bilirubin elevation, secondary probably to transient biliary obstruction by blood clots and temporary hepatic insufficiency (due to shock, loss of hepatic mass, operative trauma, and on occasion, perhaps secondary to postoperative sepsis). Such hyperbilirubinemia usually disappears in about 3 weeks, with no further surgical treatment for the relief of jaundice required. Liver function studies generally demonstrate hepatic impairment but usually return to normal after several weeks. Glucose metabolism is altered following resection, and in the early postoperative period it may be necessary to give the patient supplemental glucose solutions. Studies indicate that survival is possible with only 20 percent of the normal hepatic mass and that within 1 to 2 years most of the resected hepatic tissue is replaced as a result of hepatic regeneration.

Gallbladder

Although perforations of the gallbladder due to blunt trauma are very unusual, penetrating abdominal trauma frequently causes gallbladder injury. Penetrating or avulsion injuries of the gallbladder are best managed by cholecystectomy, but in unstable patients with other severe injuries when, in the surgeon's judgment, cholecystectomy

is inadvisable, a tube cholecystostomy should be done, with placement of Penrose drains around the gallbladder in the subhepatic space. In general, simple suture of a gallbladder perforation is not recommended because of the probability of bile leakage. After about 4 weeks, if a patient who has had a tube cholecystostomy is doing well, a cholangiogram is performed through the cholecystostomy tube, and if this shows that the gallbladder and biliary ducts are normal, with free flow of contrast material into the duodenum, the cholecystostomy tube can be removed. Routine cholecystectomy after removal of the cholecystostomy tube in patients who have sustained gallbladder trauma is unnecessary, but it is probably advisable to perform an oral cholecystogram several months after injury to determine the status of the gallbladder.

Extrahepatic Biliary Tree

PENETRATING INJURIES

The diagnosis of penetrating injuries of the extrahepatic biliary tree generally presents no problem as compared with the diagnosis of blunt trauma of the biliary tree, which may be difficult unless intraabdominal hemorrhage occurs. When the hepatic artery and portal vein are involved, the mortality rate is inordinately high because of massive hemorrhage which may be virtually impossible to control before irreversible hypoxic damage occurs to the brain and myocardium. Probably most patients with injuries to the extrahepatic biliary tree and one of the major vessels in the hepatoduodenal ligament do not survive to come to surgical exploration. This is particularly true when the wounding agent is a large-caliber, high-velocity missile. In contrast, wounds of the gallbladder which are seen frequently following penetrating abdominal trauma have a low mortality rate and are not so frequently associated with injuries to the major vessels in the hepatoduodenal ligament.

On opening the abdomen, blood and bile seen issuing from the subhepatic region indicate possible injury to the biliary tree. At times, the amount of bile, blood, or contusion may be minimal, and the gallbladder, cystic duct, and hepatoduodenal structures must be carefully inspected to evaluate the significance of any subserosal hematoma or bile staining. If the patient has survived to be surgically explored, generally no massive bleeding from the subhepatic region will be noted initially. However, many times in obtaining exposure of the hepatoduodenal ligament structures, clots which have formed and caused tamponade of major bleeding sites may be dislodged, with recurrence of vigorous bleeding from the portal vein, hepatic artery, or their branches, which are so frequently injured when the bile ducts are injured.

Generally, the hemorrhage may be immediately arrested by placing the fingers in the foramen of Winslow and compressing the hepatoduodenal ligament. Following this, after removing the free blood and obtaining good exposure while maintaining finger tamponade as above, more definitive control of the hemorrhage may be obtained by placing vascular clamps or rubber-shod clamps across all structures in the hepatoduodenal ligament. One clamp should be placed as far distad as possible on the hepatoduodenal ligament, and this maneuver is aided by dividing the lateral serosal reflection of the duodenum and reflecting the duodenum and the head of the pancreas mediad. Another clamp is then placed on the hepatoduodenal ligament through the foramen of Winslow as near the liver hilus as possible.

After hemorrhage is controlled, the serosa of the hepatoduodenal ligament at the point of the hematoma formation is incised, and the disruption of the portal vein or hepatic artery is visualized by rapidly dissecting out these structures. When the defects in the major vessels are located, repair is done with 5-0 silk arterial sutures using the general principles and techniques of vascular surgery. The vascular repair should be done only after careful exposure of the defect but also with dispatch, since the safe occlusion period of hepatic vascular inflow is only 15 to 20 minutes unless the patient is under hypothermia.

After repair of any vascular injuries, the biliary tract is carefully dissected out along the course of the penetrating missile. Knife wounds of the bile ducts may be closed with interrupted 4-0 silk suture. The common duct should be decompressed with a T tube inserted through a separate incision in the ductal system a short distance above or below the injury, so that one arm of the T tube serves as a stent for the wounded portion of the bile duct. For injuries caused by bullets or other large penetrating objects which may produce destruction or avulsion of a segment of the biliary ductal system, the wound should be carefully debrided and all devitalized ductal tissue removed. This may require completing a partial transection of the bile ducts, so that an end-to-end anastomosis may be made between viable portions of the common duct. This anastomosis is again made with interrupted simple sutures of 4-0 silk, and the repair is stented with a rubber T tube placed through a separate incision in the duct, above or below the injury. Medial reflection of the duodenum relaxes tension and allows the ends of the divided ducts to come together more readily, particularly when duct tissue has been destroyed and the ducts are shortened.

If the loss of biliary ductal structure is extensive, end-to-end repair of the duct may not be possible, and a bypass procedure is necessary. Generally, the Roux en Y bypass is effective. This is done by bringing up a 30-cm Roux en Y limb of jejunum made by transecting the jejunum about 30 cm below the ligament of Treitz. The end of the defunctionalized limb of jejunum is closed with two layers of suture. Following this, the distal end of the common duct is doubly ligated with heavy nonabsorbable suture material, and the choledochojejunostomy is performed in the following manner: a small incision is made in the side of the defunctionalized limb of jejunum about 2 cm from the closed end, at a site where the free limb of jejunum comfortably opposes the divided proximal bile duct. The anastomosis is performed by placing a posterior row of 4-0 silk arterial sutures between the seromuscular coat of the jejunum and the common duct. Usually, it is possible to place only two or three silk sutures in the posterior layer of the anastomosis.

After this, the inner row of the anastomosis is made with 4-0 chromic gastrointestinal catgut sutures, placing the sutures so that the knots are tied within the lumen of the anastomosis. These catgut sutures are continued around from the posterior to the anterior row, and, again, it is usually possible with a small duct to place only about four of these catgut sutures. Following this, the anterior row of silk sutures is placed in the same manner as described above for the posterior row. It is best to perform this anastomosis over a T-tube stent to help prevent stenosis of the anastomosis and to reduce bile leakage from the anastomosis in the immediate postoperative period. The T tube should be placed in the bile duct, just above the anastomosis to the jejunum, so that one limb of the tube goes across the anastomosis. If the anastomosis is made so high in the hilus of the liver that it is impossible to place a T tube above it, then the T tube may be placed through a stab wound in the wall of the jejunal limb and one limb led through the anastomosis into the biliary ductal system. A purse-string suture should be placed in the jejunum about the T tube to secure it in position.

The abdomen should be closed with extensive drainage of the biliary-jejunal anastomosis. The T tube should be left in place for 3 or 4 weeks, following which cholangiography is performed to ensure adequate healing and patent anastomosis, and the T tube is removed. The drains are left in until all biliary drainage has ceased, or until a firm drainage tract has formed, which occurs about 3 weeks postoperatively.

If the gallbladder and cystic duct are intact, the bypass also may be done between the gallbladder and jejunum with ligation of the distal and proximal limbs of the damaged common duct. Also, it may be more expedient at times to use a simple loop of jejunum instead of a Roux en Y limb to perform the bypass procedure.

If the patient is in poor condition and cannot tolerate a prolonged procedure for definitive repair, then the defects of the biliary ductal structures may be repaired by simple bridging with a T tube fixed in place with a suture at either end of the ductal defect; secondary repair may be done later as soon as the patient can tolerate it. If possible, however, definitive repair should be done, since recurrent strictures are more likely to occur following the more difficult secondary repairs of the bile ducts.

Injuries to the gallbladder generally may be handled in one of two ways: (1) If the patient has other extensive injuries or is in poor condition from hemorrhagic shock and other complications, the most rapid means of dealing with the gallbladder injury is to suture the wound with a one-layer row of interrupted nonabsorbable mattress sutures and to decompress the gallbladder with a #28 to 30 French mushroom catheter, placed in the fundus of the gallbladder through a purse-string suture. The catheter is brought out through a separate stab wound in the right upper quadrant of the abdomen. This catheter remains for approximately 3 weeks, or until a good tract has formed around it in order to prevent bile leakage into the peritoneal cavity following removal of the tube. Before removing the tube, cholangiography should be done through it to demonstrate patent cystic and common ducts. (2) If the patient is in good condition, however, it is preferable to remove the gallbladder when it has been injured.

BLUNT TRAUMA

Blunt trauma to the biliary tree deserves separate discussion, not because the surgical management differs, but because of its relative rarity and difficulty of diagnosis. Barnes and Diamonon reported in 1963 that only 48 cases of traumatic rupture of the gallbladder due to blunt trauma to the abdomen had been reported up to that time. According to Rydell, complete division of the common duct by blunt trauma was reported in 25 cases up to 1970. The usual means of closed injury to the extrahepatic biliary tree is a shearing force applied to the common duct or impingement of the bile duct between the vertebral column and a crushing force applied to the abdominal wall.

When blunt trauma to the biliary tree is severe enough to result in a free flow of bile, the characteristic picture of bile peritonitis occurs. According to Sturmer and Wilt, the usual history reveals a crushing injury to the right upper quadrant, the epigastrium, or the lower part of the chest, which results in severe pain and is followed by shock. The shock usually is of relatively short duration, seldom more than a few hours. Generally during this period, the diagnosis of probable intraabdominal injury may be established by signs of peritoneal irritation, such as abdominal rigidity and guarding. Bile or nonclotting blood may be found on peritoneal tap or lavage. Shock is usually secondary to the marked outpouring of extracellular fluid into the peritoneal cavity due to the chemical irritation of the peritoneum by bile. The initial chemical peritonitis caused by bile may be followed shortly by a bacterial peritonitis. If biliary leakage is minimal, shock may be of relatively short duration or absent, and abdominal signs initially may be slight. This may be followed by the recovery and well-being of the patient, which lasts for periods up to 5 or 10 days. However, the onset of jaundice on about the third day is a fairly constant sign. The appearance of clay-colored stools and the presence of bile in the urine may be noticed from about the second to the fifth day after injury.

A considerable gradual increase in abdominal size occurs during the first 10 days that may be unattended by the usual signs of peritonitis. This condition is accompanied by progressive signs of extracellular fluid volume deficit and by evidence of infection, such as rising temperature and elevated white cell count. In the reported cases of complete transection of the common duct, the site of transection was uniformly in the retroduodenal area, thus again indicating the importance of extensive medial reflection of the duodenum to explore the retroperitoneal duodenum as well as the distal common duct and pancreas.

When blunt trauma to the extrahepatic biliary tract is diagnosed, the repair is generally the same as in the previous discussion of penetrating trauma. End to end repair of the ducts over a T tube should be done, if possible, or a bypass procedure between the ducts and the jejunum should be done by bringing up a Roux en Y limb or loop of jejunum to perform an anastomosis between the biliary tract and the jejunum as described in the discussion of penetrating trauma. The ducts should not be implanted in the duodenum, since anastomotic leaks occur more often with this than with the anastomosis to a defunctionalized limb of jejunum. Leak of a choledochoduodenal anastomosis produces not only a biliary fistula but a duodenal fistula as well, with all the grave consequences of such a fistula. If a biliary-jejunal anastomosis leaks, only a bile leak occurs, which is easier to manage generally and has a better prognosis than a biliary duodenal fistula.

The postoperative therapy of biliary tract injuries, in which bile peritonitis is an important complicating feature, should include adequate replacement of extracellular fluid volume deficits, which may require several liters of balanced salt solutions in 24 hours. These solutions should be given as soon as possible preoperatively and continued throughout the surgical procedure and postoperatively to avoid extracellular fluid volume deficit. Broad-spectrum antibiotics should be given prior to the surgical procedure and continued throughout the procedure and for several days after, until the chances of sepsis and infection have diminished.

Mortality from biliary tract injuries should be below 5 to 10 percent if they are discovered early and treated by adequate reconstruction, adequate drainage and decompression of the biliary tree, adequate coverage with antibiotics, and proper fluid replacement. Patients with more severe injuries probably do not survive to be diagnosed and treated.

Portal Vein

Approximately 90 percent of portal vein injuries occur because of penetrating trauma. They are frequently associated with other visceral injuries, most commonly to the inferior vena cava, liver, pancreas, and stomach. Mattox and associates recently reported a survival rate of 50 percent in their series of 22 patients.

Lateral venorrhaphy, if possible, is the preferred method of treatment. Mattox suggests performing a portacaval or mesocaval shunt as an alternate treatment of portal vein injury if suture repair is impossible and the patient's general condition is stable. Fish, on the other hand, reported that four of five patients who had portacaval shunts for portal vein reconstruction after trauma developed hepatic decompensation or encephalopathy, whereas these complications were not observed in patients undergoing portal vein ligation.

The insertion of an autogenous vein graft to bridge the defect in the portal vein (using the left common iliac vein, left renal vein, or a paneled saphenous vein graft) may be preferable to a portacaval shunt if the patient's condition is stable and the proximal and distal ends of the injured vein are suitable for the insertion of a graft. This procedure should prevent portal hypertension or hepatic deterioration that may occur if the vein is ligated. If, however, associated injuries are severe, then ligation of the portal vein may make it possible to save the patient. Even though portal vein ligation may cause portal hypertension, interruption of the vein is compatible with the patient's survival in about 80 percent of the cases. It should, of course, be emphasized that in those associated hepatic arterial injuries, a good repair of the hepatic artery must be achieved before accepting treatment of portal vein injuries by ligation.

Pancreas

Travers described the first pancreatic injury found in an intoxicated woman who was struck by a stage coach wheel in England in 1827. Although about two-thirds of pancreatic injuries are caused by penetrating trauma, recently there has been an increase in the incidence of blunt pancreatic trauma; most of this increase is caused by steering wheel injuries. Northrup and Simmons recently reviewed 734 cases of pancreatic trauma in the English literature. They describe three basic mechanisms of blunt pancreatic trauma: (1) when the blunt forces are concentrated to the right of the vertebral bodies, the head of the pancreas may be crushed, and, in addition, there may often be hepatic lacerations, avulsions of the common bile duct, and rupture of the duodenum; (2) when the blunt abdominal trauma is concentrated in the midline, where the pancreas normally crosses the vertebral bodies, the classic pancreatic transection injury is often produced, frequently without associated injuries; (3) if the impact forces are directed to the left of the vertebra, distal pancreatic contusions and lacerations, with associated splenic lacerations, may occur.

DIAGNOSIS. Diagnosis of pancreatic injuries is based upon a complete history, including the mechanism of injury, thorough physical examination, serum amylase level, and adequate visualization of the pancreas at surgical exploration. The history of trauma may be the only clue to the diagnosis of pancreatic injury. Signs and symptoms may initially be absent. In patients with isolated blunt pancreatic trauma, clinical manifestations of the injury typically appear slowly. Symptoms have been reported to be absent for as long as 5 days even after a complete pancreatic transection, and for up to 92 hours after avulsion of the pancreatic and biliary ductal systems from the duodenum. Moreover, symptoms following isolated blunt pancreatic trauma may even be delayed until a pseudocyst develops weeks, months, or years later. The delay in appearance of symptoms in patients with isolated pancreatic injuries may be caused either by an initial secretory inhibition of the pancreas after injury or by failure of pancreatic enzymes to be activated in the absence of other visceral injuries.

Not only are symptoms of isolated blunt pancreatic trauma often mild and delayed, but physical signs may also be absent or minimal. Usually, however, there is at least mild upper abdominal tenderness, but in the absence of a history of significant trauma or severe symptoms this sign may be overlooked. Injuries to retroperitoneal organs such as the pancreas may not produce clinical findings of loss of bowel sounds, tenderness, guarding, or spasm for several hours.

Serum Amylase Determination. Over 25 years ago Matthewson and Halter advocated routine serum amylase determinations in patients sustaining blunt trauma and emphasized that pancreatic injury was more common than

had been previously appreciated. Serum amylase elevation alone has not been considered an indication for exploratory celiotomy. If signs of peritonitis are present (such as spasm, tenderness, and absent bowel sounds), then a celiotomy is performed. Unrecognized severe pancreatic injury can be a fatal lesion, particularly when it is accompanied by disruption of pancreatic tissue and leakage of pancreatic juice.

Many patients have been found to have an elevated serum amylase level but negative abdominal findings. These patients are closely observed for evidence of peritonitis or until the amylase level returns to normal. An amylase determination is performed on peritoneal lavage fluid, but the elevation is more often due to small-bowel injury than to pancreatic injury.

Recent studies by Olsen, Moretz and associates, and White and Benfield have indicated that improper interpretation of elevated amylase determinations may be misleading. Olsen stated that 33 percent of patients with hyperamylasemia had no significant intraabdominal trauma, and no patient in his series with hyperamylasemia had significant intraabdominal injury without other evidence of such trauma. He reemphasized that hyperamylasemia alone without any other evidence of visceral injury is not an indication for exploratory celiotomy. White and Benfield found that only 26 percent of the patients in their series who had significant blunt or penetrating pancreatic trauma had preoperative hyperamylasemia.

Though these various reports show that it is unwise to perform exploratory celiotomy on the basis of elevated amylase levels alone, nevertheless, the detection of hyperamylasemia in asymptomatic patients who have sustained abdominal trauma cannot simply be dismissed. These patients are admitted to the hospital and closely observed. Plain abdominal x-ray films may show evidence of retroperitoneal trauma. This is suspected when there is obliteration of the psoas margin, retroperitoneal air along a psoas margin or around the upper pole of the right kidney, or displacement of the stomach. Upper gastrointestinal studies with water-soluble media may show leakage of contrast media from the retroperitoneal duodenal area. Serial sonographic studies of the upper part of the abdomen, when strongly positive, may also indicate pancreatic or other retroperitoneal injuries and thus give sufficient reason for performing exploratory celiotomy in patients with blunt abdominal trauma who have asymptomatic hyperamylasemia.

Visceral arteriography may be helpful in these diagnostically challenging patients. It may clearly show vascular injuries in the region of the pancreas that definitely indicate the wisdom of exploratory celiotomy. As more experience is gained with endoscopic retrograde pancreatography it is quite possible that this technique may have a role in the diagnosis of pancreatic injury.

Surgical Exploration. When preoperative diagnostic studies indicate a probability of pancreatic injury, it is very important to visualize the entire pancreas. The head of the pancreas and the duodenum are completely mobilized to the midline by performing a Kocher maneuver. The gastrocolic omentum is also divided in order to enter the lesser sac and view the entire body of the pancreas. The tail of the gland is mobilized by freeing the spleen and retracting it medially, along with the tail of the pancreas, thus allowing direct visualization and palpation of both sides of the distal part of the gland. Cattell and Braasch described a technique that provides easy access to the third and fourth portions of the duodenum, the head and part of the uncinate process of the pancreas, and the superior mesenteric vessels where they cross the duodenum. This technique entails mobilization of the right region of the colon and its mesentery along with the small bowel and its mesentery from the retroperitoneal attachments.

Any retroperitoneal hematoma in the upper part of the abdomen or a peripancreatic hematoma should be considered presumptive evidence of pancreatic injury and should be explored.

ASSOCIATED INJURIES. Isolated pancreatic injury is rare and occurs in less than 10 percent of all patients with pancreatic trauma. Associated injuries are usually more obvious indications for surgical exploration than suspected pancreatic injury. Death and serious complications are frequent in pancreatic trauma but are only rarely caused by the pancreatic injury. Massive hemorrhage from associated vascular, hepatic, or splenic injury is the main cause of death.

Although the pancreas is a vascular organ, it is not often responsible for uncontrollable hemorrhage. When profuse bleeding occurs from the pancreatic area, the pancreas is mobilized and the superior mesenteric and the splenic vessels, the aorta, and the vena cava are inspected, since they are often the source of severe hemorrhage. Because of the location of the pancreas, injuries to the liver and the stomach are frequent. In a series of 175 patients with pancreatic injuries reported by Jones and Shires, 58 percent had an associated retroperitoneal injury in addition to the pancreatic injury.

MANAGEMENT OF PANCREATIC INJURIES. It is essential to control all bleeding at the time of initial exploration of pancreatic injuries. Bleeding vessels in the pancreas are exposed by carefully debriding surrounding devitalized tissue sufficiently to gain secure hemostasis by precise placement of shallow mattress sutures of fine nonabsorbable material. Complete mobilization of the injured pancreas permits temporary control of bleeding by anterior and posterior compression of the bleeding site with the fingers of one hand while hemostatic stitches are placed with the other hand. Nonabsorbable sutures must be used, since absorbable material is quickly digested away by the proteolytic enzymes from the pancreas. Suturing of the bleeding points should be done without preliminary application of hemostatic clamps, since such clamps cause more damage to the viable pancreas and often cause tearing and further bleeding from the fragile pancreatic vessels. Control of bleeding from the pancreas should not be attempted by blind clamping, by mass ligatures, or by deep sutures which may injure or obstruct major pancreatic or biliary ducts or major mesenteric blood vessels and thus cause further serious complications.

After bleeding from the pancreas or from adjacent major blood vessels is controlled, the extent of the pancreatic injury is determined. In general, pancreatic injuries may be classified as follows: (1) simple pancreatic contusion without rupture of the pancreatic capsule or significant hemorrhage; (2) more severe contusion and disruption of the pancreatic parenchyma with rupture of the capsule but without major ductal injury; (3) severe pancreatic injury with major ductal disruption; and (4) combined pancreatic and duodenal injury.

Simple Contusions without Capsular or Ductal Disruption. Simple pancreatic contusions without capsular or ductal disruption and without persistent hemorrhage require no suturing or debridement. These injuries should be drained with a sump and several large Penrose drains placed directly at the site of the pancreatic contusion and brought out along a short, direct tract. A properly functioning sump drain allows air to enter the tract, preventing the occurrence of a vacuum. It also allows measurement of the amount of pancreatic juice being lost and helps prevent skin digestion. These drains should exit through a stab wound in the upper part of the flank which is placed as dependently as possible and made sufficiently large to admit two fingers easily. The drains are left in place for 10 days to 2 weeks, since moderate drainage may not occur during the first week following injury. Drainage from the pancreas might not be expected with a simple contusion and an apparently intact pancreatic capsule; however, minor capsular disruptions might be easily missed during exploration of the pancreas. Lack of drainage to such areas of unrecognized capsular injury may lead to complications associated with intraabdominal collections of pancreatic secretions such as pseudocysts, pancreatic abscesses, lesser-sac abscesses, and subphrenic abscesses.

Capsular Laceration without Ductal Injury. Most surgeons agree that simple pancreatic penetration or lacerations with capsular disruptions without loss of tissue or major ductal injury are best treated by simple suture of the capsule with nonabsorbable material and extensive drainage. Such injuries with significant loss of pancreatic tissue that precludes suture repair to the capsule obviously can be treated only by direct suture of any bleeding points and extensive drainage. Extensive drainage to control leakage from a pancreatic injury is more important than attempting to prevent a fistula by capsular repair.

Injury with Ductal Disruption. Disruption of the main pancreatic duct is a much more serious injury than capsular disruption and requires especially careful management. Major ductal injury almost always causes a pseudocyst or abscess if not recognized and drained. If treated by drainage alone, these injuries usually produce a troublesome and persistent fistula.

Distal Pancreatectomy. An effective method of treatment for pancreatic injuries with disruption of the pancreatic duct in the body or tail of the gland is distal pancreatectomy. This is performed at the point where the main duct is injured, and allows removal of the traumatized and devitalized tissue.

When performing a distal pancreatectomy, suture stick ties are placed in the superior and inferior borders of the pancreas approximately 1.5 to 2 cm from the edge. This, along with isolation of the splenic vessels during distal pancreatectomy, prevents unnecessary blood loss and provides better visualization. In resecting the distal pancreas, the cut edge is beveled in a fishmouth fashion. This enables a better closure of the proximal end of the pancreas. The transected duct of Wirsung in the remaining proximal gland is ligated with a transfixion suture of fine monofilament, nonabsorbable material such as Prolene, to discourage fistula formation. The cut surface of the transected proximal pancreas is oversewn with interrupted, interlocking mattress sutures, which facilitate hemostasis. The stump of the pancreas is extensively drained with a sump and large Penrose drains.

Yellin and associates reported excellent results with distal pancreatectomy in 60 patients. In eight of their patients, the injury was located considerably to the right of the superior mesenteric vessels and as much as 13 to 15 cm of distal pancreas was resected. (The average normal pancreas has a length of 15 cm, is 3 cm thick, and weighs 60 to 125 Gm.) Only one patient (1.6 percent) developed diabetes mellitus after distal pancreatectomy; this percentage is similar to the result in the series from Parkland Memorial Hospital in which Jones and Shires reported no incidence of pancreatic insufficiency or diabetes following distal pancreatectomy.

Distal Pancreatectomy with Roux-en-Y Anastomosis. This technique has been utilized in patients undergoing primary distal pancreatectomy for trauma when there is much contusion and edema of the remaining pancreatic head. In these cases the surgeon may anticipate that there will be significant obstruction in the proximal ductal system, leading to persistent leakage of pancreatic secretions from the end of the transected pancreas, if the pancreatic duct and stump are simply oversewn and drained instead of being implanted in a defunctionalized Roux-en-Y limb of jejunum. This procedure is time-consuming and is not recommended in patients whose condition is tenuous because of hemorrhage and severe injuries to structures adjacent to the pancreas.

Roux-en-Y Pancreaticojejunostomy. Several methods of treating pancreatic transection have been described. For the pancreas completely transected over the superior mesenteric vessels and to the right of these vessels, a Roux-en-Y anastomosis suturing both ends of the pancreas to the defunctionalized limb has proved satisfactory (Fig. 6-14). This treatment has been recommended by Jones and Shires

Fig. 6-14. Technique of Roux-en-Y anastomosis of both ends of transected pancreas.

for treatment of injuries which require removal of 75 percent or more of the pancreas. Transections of less magnitude are treated by simple distal pancreatectomy. A Roux-en-Y anastomosis to both ends of the severed pancreas has eliminated the need to find a severed duct or to reanastomose it. This method leaves all functioning pancreatic tissue, thereby avoiding the possibility of pancreatic insufficiency or diabetes. The risk of injury to the underlying superior mesenteric vessels seems less with this mode of treatment than with resection. The possibility of fistula and pseudocyst formation is also minimized.

The easiest method of accomplishing the Roux-en-Y anastomosis to both ends of the severed pancreas is an end-to-end anastomosis of one end of the pancreas to the jejunum and of the remaining end of the pancreas to the side of the jejunum. This is accomplished using permanent sutures placed approximately 1 cm apart in a single-layer anastomosis. Once this anastomosis is accomplished, drainage tract is established with Penrose and sump drains.

Jordan and associates advocate complete transection of the pancreas with a Roux-en-Y anastomosis to the pancreatic fragment with oversewing of the proximal pancreas. The Roux-en-Y limb should be at least 30 cm in length and is usually passed through the transverse mesocolon to the site of injury. As long as the duodenum is intact and viable, there is little justification for a pancreaticoduodenectomy for this type of injury.

Unless the completely severed pancreatic duct is managed with definitive surgery, a pseudocyst or fistula will almost always result. A Roux-en-Y anastomosis to one fragment of the severed pancreas is little more time-consuming than resection of the distal fragment, which requires a splenectomy.

If location of the pancreatic injury suggests the possibility of injury to the intrapancreatic portion of the common bile duct, the common bile duct is opened in its supraduodenal position and a cholangiogram obtained. If a partial tear of the distal common duct has occurred but some ductal continuity remains, a T tube is inserted for decompression.

Repair and Stent of Pancreatic Duct. It is difficult to locate the pancreatic duct with considerable bleeding and hematoma, and even more difficult to suture it after it is found. Nevertheless, several reports have appeared in which the pancreatic duct has been identified, found to be completely transected in the region of the neck of the pancreas, and successfully repaired by stenting and suture repair. The stent may be inserted into the duct at the area of injury and threaded through the ampulla into the duodenum. The second method by which this has been accomplished is by duodenotomy and catheter cannulation of the pancreatic duct through the ampulla, with or without a sphincterotomy, with passage into the distal pancreatic duct past the point of transection. The pancreatic duct is then reapproximated with 6-0 or 7-0 nonabsorbable suture. This is not a preferred but an alternate method, which might be of some benefit in selected cases in which the injury would require radical resection of the pancreas in the critically ill patient. Although fistula, late stricture formation at the site of injury, or recurrent pancreatitis secondary to partial obstruction of the pancreatic duct is possible, these complications have not been reported.

Anterior Roux-en-Y Pancreaticojejunostomy. A Roux-en-Y pancreaticojejunostomy may be placed to the anterior surface of the pancreas over the injury in selected cases. This method of treatment has been satisfactory only if the posterior pancreatic capsule is intact. If the posterior pancreatic capsule is broken, drainage will continue into the retroperitoneal space rather than into the Roux-en-Y limb and result in abscess, pseudocyst, or fistula formation.

The most severe form of pancreatic injury is extensive laceration and shattering of the head of the pancreas, which leaves virtually none of the proximal pancreas or its main ductal system intact. Extensive injuries of the pancreatic head not involving the duodenum are preferably treated by either a Child 95 percent pancreatectomy or a Jones-Shires double pancreaticojejunostomy. Only rarely should pancreaticoduodenectomy be done for injuries of the pancreatic head alone.

Combined Duodenum and Pancreatic Injuries

Northrup and Simmons reported an overall mortality of duodenal injuries alone of 20 percent, which is equal to the overall mortality of pancreatic injuries alone. Combined pancreatic and duodenal injuries, however, increase the mortality rate to an average of 44 percent, with some reports exceeding 60 to 70 percent. Some 30 percent of duodenal injuries are associated with pancreatic trauma, and approximately 20 percent of pancreatic injuries are associated with duodenal trauma. The high mortality rate among patients with combined injuries is related not only to the intensity and severity of forces that cause injury to the pancreas and duodenum but also to the frequent involvement of the adjacent major blood vessels, with resultant immediate or early death from hemorrhage. A large amount of devitalized tissue and complicated pancreaticoduodenal fistulas also contribute to the high mortality rate.

Combined injuries of the pancreas and duodenum are treated by either a Berne duodenal "diverticulization" procedure (Fig. 6-6), as previously described under Duodenum, for relatively less severe combined injuries or a Whipple procedure for very severe combined pancreaticoduodenal injuries.

Pancreaticoduodenectomy. Prior to performing a pancreaticoduodenectomy the presence of a pancreatic ductal injury should be verified. This may be accomplished by duodenotomy, cannulation of the pancreatic duct, and pancreatogram. The common duct is identified and proved to be intact by operative cholangiogram. An alternate method of determining ductal injury is by mobilizing the tail of the pancreas and performing a pancreatogram through the distal pancreatic duct. Hemostatic sutures are placed 1.5 to 2 cm into the superior and inferior portions of the pancreas prior to incising the tail. If the common bile duct and major duct system are intact and the duodenal injury can be closed, then a pancreaticoduodenectomy is usually not indicated.

Indications for pancreaticoduodenectomy include rupture of the duodenum and head of the pancreas, avulsion of the common duct from the duodenum with avascular duodenal wall, and stellate fracture with bleeding from a crushing injury of the head of the pancreas. This procedure also is indicated for combined injuries to the head of the pancreas and duodenum with destruction of both, to control hemorrhage, remove devitalized tissue, and restore ductal continuity. The overall condition of the patient and associated injuries must be considered prior to submitting the patient to several more hours of surgery. There are times when this procedure is necessary, but they are rare, particularly if the duodenum is intact. Complications following pancreaticoduodenectomy are common. Thus, mortality rate of this procedure must be low to justify its use if any other form of management can be employed.

In addition to fistula formation and abscesses, marginal ulceration with upper gastrointestinal bleeding has occurred following pancreaticoduodenectomy in which a vagotomy or subtotal gastric resection was not performed. Symptoms of dumping, diabetes, and weight loss with diarrhea and semiformed bowel movements have occurred following pancreaticoduodenectomy for trauma. Foley and associates have reported a postoperative complication following pancreaticoduodenectomy with bleeding into the intestinal tract from the site of the pancreaticojejunostomy which was demonstrated by arteriographic studies and required reoperation to suture the bleeding point.

The average mortality rate for patients treated with the Whipple procedure continues to be about 35 percent, with some series reporting as high as 50 to 60 percent. This high mortality rate is frequently due to associated injuries, and it is probable that some of these patients would have died if a pancreaticoduodenectomy had not been done. Despite a very justifiable concern about the inappropriate use of the Whipple procedure in the treatment of less serious pancreatic and duodenal injuries, Yellin and Rosoff conclude that pancreaticoduodenectomy is an effective procedure for removing severely devitalized pancreas and duodenum when these organs are irreparably injured.

COMPLICATIONS. Complications following pancreatic trauma include fistula, pancreatic abscesses, vascular necrosis with hemorrhage from the drain site, pseudocyst formation, and duodenal fistula secondary to suture line breakdown from pancreatic juice activation.

Pancreatic enzymes liberated in an inactive form do not digest living tissue. In extensive injuries, duodenal and biliary enzymes are often released and the proteolytic pancreatic enzymes activated. Trypsinogen activated by enterokinase and hydrolyzed to trypsin breaks down protein. Mixtures of bile, gastric, and pancreatic juice are capable of digesting soft tissues with which they come in contact. As a result of digestion of surrounding tissues, any attempt at delayed definitive operation in this area becomes hazardous.

Fistula. Jordan et al. have reported the occurrence of pancreatic fistula as the most common complication following operative therapy, occurring in 35 percent of the cases and usually following blunt trauma. Most pancreatic fistulas are minor and close within a period of one month. Major pancreatic fistulas have been arbitrarily defined as those which drain longer than 1 month. The serum amylase level is frequently elevated while the fistula is present, probably because of transperitoneal absorption.

Almost all pancreatic fistulas will eventually close spontaneously; therefore treatment is mainly conservative. Attention must be given to preventing autodigestion of the surrounding skin. Dressings should never be applied to any fistula, since skin irritation will result from the fistula fluid in the dressings even in the presence of relatively bland pancreatic juice.

The use of Stomahesive provides an excellent method for managing the drainage from pancreatic or other types of gastrointestinal fistulas. An opening is made in the Stomahesive sheet just large enough to permit drains from the fistula tract to pass through. Stomahesive securely adheres to the skin for several days before it must be replaced and is virtually nonreactive and nonallergenic. A gas-sterilized polyethylene bag with adherent backing and a "drainable stoma" at the bottom is applied so that it adheres to the Stomahesive sheet rather than to the patient's skin. The Penrose drains, if these are still in place, are completely contained within the bag, and the suction catheter in the fistula tract exits through the "drainable stoma" in the bag. Leakage is prevented by placing rubber bands around the suction catheter and the polyethylene bag in order to make a tight seal where the catheter passes through the stoma. This method protects the skin, isolates the drains from outside infection, and permits accurate measurement of fluid loss from the fistula.

Vigorous fluid replacement with balanced salt solution to prevent volume deficit is indicated: the volume may be equal to that lost through the fistula. In order to minimize fluid and electrolyte losses, the pancreatic fluid from a fistula may be returned to the alimentary tract by way of a nasogastric tube, a gastrostomy tube, or a jejunostomy. However, except with very large-volume fistulas, refeeding of this fluid usually is unnecessary.

Many patients with pancreatic fistulas can continue oral intake of food, especially if the fistula drains less than 500 to 600 ml each day and the volume does not increase significantly when the patient eats. In the presence of large-volume pancreatic fistulas, it is preferable to institute intravenous hyperalimentation. Intravenous hyperalimentation has two beneficial effects on such patients: (1) it maintains excellent nutrition and nitrogen balance without stimulating the pancreas, as do oral feedings, and (2) intravenous hyperalimentation can significantly reduce the volume of pancreatic exocrine secretion (by one-half or more).

Baker and associates have advocated the use of atropine or other anticholinergics to reduce pancreatic secretion and decrease fistula drainage. These agents may cause discomfort to the patient by inducing dryness of the mouth, blurring of vision, urinary retention, and inspissation of pulmonary secretions.

With good supportive care of the patients who develop pancreatic fistulas following pancreatic trauma, surgical repair should be necessary in less than 5 percent. Although there are no rigid criteria indicating when conservative treatment should be abandoned, Baker and associates suggest that closure probably should be carried out in most patients who have fistulas that have persisted for more than 60 days and continue draining more than 1,000 ml/day. Internal drainage of these fistulas via a Roux-en-Y defunctionalized limb of jejunum is a very satisfactory method of management.

Pseudocyst. A pancreatic pseudocyst is a cyst whose wall of inflammatory fibrous tissue does not contain epithelium but is made of those structures surrounding the region of the pancreas in the retroperitoneum. The most frequent symptoms associated with a pancreatic pseudocyst are an abdominal mass, pain, nausea, and vomiting. The serum amylase level is usually elevated for a prolonged period of time during this illness. The pseudocyst rarely resolves spontaneously. Pancreatic pseudocyst is now a rare complication following pancreatic trauma if the pancreas has been explored and managed appropriately, such management including adequate drainage with a sump and numerous drains. The preferred method of draining pancreatic pseudocysts is internally by either cyst gastrostomy or Roux-en-Y cyst jejunostomy.

Sepsis. Intraabdominal abscess is a common complication following multiple abdominal trauma. Although pancreatic fistulas rarely cause death, they occasionally give rise to pseudocyst formation and lesser-sac abscesses requiring reoperation for drainage. A lesser-sac abscess may contribute to either sepsis or retroperitoneal bleeding and death. Cultures of the abscess grow a predominance of mixed gram-negative organisms; however, staphylococci and enterococci may often be present. The serum amylase level is not consistently elevated in patients with a pancreatic or lesser-sac abscess.

The method of management of pancreatic abscesses consists of adequate debridement and drainage plus insertion of gastrostomy and feeding jejunostomy tubes. Complications are often associated with a duodenal fistula. If such a condition is present, a Roux-en-Y jejunostomy is placed over the duodenal fistula wall when possible. Antibiotics are instituted in all cases.

MORTALITY. The mortality rate caused by pancreatic injury is quite variable and is chiefly related to hemorrhage from adjacent major blood vessels. Northrup and Simmons, in a review of 734 patients, found that the wounding agent was directly related to the mortality rate as follows: stab wounds—8 percent; gunshot wounds—25 percent; steering wheel injuries and other severe blunt trauma—up to 50 percent; and shotgun wounds—60 percent. Whatever the wounding agent, the average mortality rate of pancreatic head injuries was 28 percent, in contrast to the mortality rate of 16 percent from all types of injuries to the body or tail. This result is similar to that in the series reported by Jones and Shires (Table 6-6).

Early surgical intervention in both blunt and penetrating abdominal trauma, meticulous abdominal examination of all organs, and an aggressive approach to pancreatic injuries, including resection when indicated, are essential if the mortality rate is to be lowered. Jones and Shires reported a decrease in mortality due to blunt trauma to the pancreas from 37 percent in 1965 to an overall 16 percent in 1970. The mortality for isolated pancreatic injury was less than 5 percent.

Table 6-6. MORTALITY AND TYPE OF TRAUMA

	No. of patients	Died	Mortality, %
Penetrating . .	143	27	19
Stab	30	2	6
Gunshot . .	95	14	15
Shotgun . .	18	11	61
Blunt	32	5	16
Total	175	32	18

Spleen

The spleen is the abdominal organ most frequently injured by blunt trauma; such injuries to the spleen represent approximately one-quarter of all blunt injuries of the abdominal viscera. The spleen also is often injured by penetrating abdominal trauma and is frequently associated with blunt and penetrating thoracoabdominal injuries.

DIAGNOSIS. The diagnosis of splenic injury is usually easily made with penetrating trauma but is often more difficult in patients sustaining blunt trauma. The clinical manifestations are the systemic symptoms and signs of hemorrhage and local evidence of peritoneal irritation in the region of the spleen. Only about 30 to 40 percent of patients with splenic injury present with a systolic blood pressure below 100 mm Hg. However, many patients with splenic trauma may develop hypotension and tachycardia when assuming the sitting position. A tender abdomen with guarding and distension is apparent in only about 50 to 60 percent of those patients with splenic rupture.

A history of injury, which may be seemingly slight, followed by abdominal pain, predominantly in the left upper quadrant, left shoulder pain, and syncope is very significant. Often the left shoulder pain, or Kehr's sign, occurs only when the patient is in a supine or head-down position. This is caused by irritation of the inferior surface of the left side of the diaphragm by free blood or blood clots. Elevation of the foot of the bed or pressure in the left subcostal region may occasionally reproduce pain at the top of the left shoulder. Ballance's sign, which refers to fixed dullness to percussion in the left flank and dullness in the right flank that disappears on change of position of the patient, thus indicating large quantities of clot in the perisplenic region and free blood in the remainder of the peritoneal cavity, may be helpful in establishing the diagnosis. Whereas a decreased or falling hematocrit, leukocytosis of more than 15,000, x-ray findings such as fractures of the left lower ribs, gastric displacement, loss of splenic outline, and splinting or elevation of the left diaphragm are useful diagnostic findings, they are frequently absent. Abdominal paracentesis and diagnostic peritoneal lavage are extremely helpful in establishing the diagnosis in doubtful cases, particularly in patients whose sensibility is obtunded by other injuries. In patients with splenic trauma the incidence of false-negative diagnostic peritoneal lavage is reported in repeated series to be less than 1 percent.

Delayed rupture of the spleen was first described by

Baudet in 1902, and the asymptomatic interval between abdominal injury and rupture of the spleen is known as the latent period of Baudet. It was postulated that bleeding appeared several days after injury because (1) a subcapsular splenic hematoma gradually increased in size until it caused a delayed rupture of the splenic capsule and intraperitoneal hemorrhage, or (2) there was initial bleeding from a splenic laceration which ceased spontaneously but began again in several days or weeks when the perisplenic hematoma became dislodged. This concept has recently been challenged by Olsen and Polley and by Benjamin and associates. These authors report a delayed rupture of the spleen of less than 1 percent in over 600 patients. They suggest that splenic rupture is an unusual occurrence and that the 15 percent incidence reported in older papers actually represents a delay in diagnosis rather than a delayed rupture in those patients.

TREATMENT. Splenectomy remains the only acceptable treatment for splenic injury. Even a slight nonbleeding tear of the splenic capsule may lead to recurrent fatal bleeding. Also, it is likely that a splenic hematoma will increase in size secondary to increasing osmotic pressure of the hematoma and imbibition of fluid, even though no further hemorrhage occurs. The splenic hematoma eventually reaches such size that the spleen ruptures, either spontaneously or following slight trauma, causing massive bleeding which may be rapidly fatal.

Nonoperative treatment was recognized very early to carry a high mortality rate; and when no operation is performed, the mortality rate is 90 to 95 percent. If an attempt is made to suture the spleen to stop bleeding or to tamponade it with omentum or other hemostatic agents, the estimated mortality rate ranges from 25 to 50 percent because of the high incidence of rebleeding.

Controversy surrounds the proper treatment of a minor nonbleeding splenic injury in the pediatric age group. Singer reported an incidence of fatal sepsis in children that was 58 times greater than that in the general population following splenectomies for trauma. Increasing experimental data and clinical evidence indicate that an intact spleen is required to produce important opsonic antibodies which are necessary for optimal function of the macrophage system in production of immunoglobulins.

Sepsis is a rather frequent occurrence following splenectomy for certain hematologic disorders, many of which have a diffuse reticuloendothelial abnormality. Many of these patients, however, receive various forms of therapy that alter immunity and response to infection.

There is no large series of carefully evaluated patients having had splenectomy for trauma in which overwhelming infection has developed. Without more proof that splenectomy in a patient with a normal reticuloendothelial system predisposes to infection, it is difficult to justify conservative management or partial splenectomy for splenic trauma, even in infants.

Another area of controversy is the issue of prophylactic antibiotics in the postsplenectomized patient, particularly in the pediatric age group. Most authors advocate prophylactic penicillin therapy until at least age five years, but it has been recommended that protection be extended into the teenage years, and isolated reports suggest indefinite protection. The use of long-term antibiotics is not without untoward effects, such as drug sensitivity, bacterial resistance, and suppression of natural immunologic defenses.

Operative Technique. Splenectomy is best performed through a long upper midline abdominal incision. The advantages of this incision are (1) it can be made very quickly; (2) it offers easy access not only to the spleen but also to other intraabdominal organs that may be injured; (3) it can be closed quickly and heals securely if closed with nonabsorbable, noninterrupted sutures of appropriate strength.

Good exposure can be obtained by downward retraction of the splenic flexure of the colon and the body of the stomach and by firm retraction on the left upper portion of the midline incision. The operator's right hand is then placed low and posterior to the spleen, and the spleen is grasped and delivered into the wound, either directly or after freeing the peritoneal reflection, which often attaches the lateral surface of the spleen to the diaphragm. Warm, moist sponges are packed into the splenic bed to aid in controlling bleeding from the bluntly divided ligaments and diaphragm and to maintain exposure of the spleen. Occasionally it is necessary to divide the splenorenal ligament by sharp dissection to obtain complete rotation of the spleen and optimum delivery through the incision. If there is considerable splenic hemorrhage, bleeding may be temporarily controlled by compressing the pedicle of the spleen between the index and middle fingers of the left hand or, if necessary, by placing a nontraumatic clamp such as a DeBakey vascular clamp or a Glassman clamp across the pedicle.

In some patients in whom the splenic pedicle cannot be quickly mobilized and compressed in order to control hemorrhage, the lesser sac can be rapidly entered by pulling the stomach inferiorly, opening the gastrohepatic omentum above the lesser curvature of the stomach, and then grasping and occluding the splenic artery and vein at the superior margin of the tail of the pancreas with the fingers of the left hand. This then permits rapid mobilization of the spleen and its pedicle by blunt dissection with the right hand, with much less blood loss during the mobilization.

Rotation of the spleen anteriorly and medially out through the midline abdominal incision in order to visualize the posterior aspect of the splenic pedicle is very important. This is necessary to avoid injury to the pancreas and to permit individual ligation of the hilar vessels of the spleen under direct vision. Whitesell in performing 50 anatomic dissections found the tail of the pancreas was either intimately applied to the spleen or within 1 cm of it in half the dissections, and in another 15 percent the tail approached to within 1.5 cm of the splenic hilum.

When the spleen is delivered, the pedicle is divided between long chest Péan clamps and ligated with heavy nonabsorbable suture. Suture ligatures should be used to control the portions of the pedicle containing the splenic artery and vein.

When delivering the spleen through the midline incision, care must be taken to avoid tearing the gastrosplenic vessels. These must be carefully ligated in order to avoid injuring the wall of the stomach by including it in a mass ligature. Such injuries may cause necrosis of the stomach at this point and subsequent formation of a gastric fistula. After the spleen has been removed, the proximal greater curvature of the stomach should be carefully inspected; if there is any question about its integrity or viability the questionable area should be buttressed by imbricating the fundus on itself with several interrupted Lembert sutures.

Although drainage of the splenic bed following elective splenectomy is controversial, there is little question that drainage should be employed when splenectomy is performed under emergency conditions. The incidence of drain tract infections and subphrenic abscesses has been reported to be as high as 25 to 50 percent when drains were used, in contrast to 5 to 12 percent when drains were not employed. Many of these infections, however, were related to the presence of associated injuries, usually in the gastrointestinal tract, or to the immunologic defects often present in patients requiring splenectomies for conditions other than trauma, and not to the drains per se. The routine use of drains following splenectomy for trauma is supported by the series reported by Naylor and Shires. These authors reported an incidence of subphrenic abscess of only 3.4 percent in 408 patients undergoing splenectomy for trauma. Among the 72 patients who had splenectomy for trauma involving the spleen alone, there were no subphrenic abscesses and an incidence of drain tract infection of only 1.3 percent.

Thus, while it cannot be proved that drainage of the splenic bed after splenectomy for trauma reduces the incidence of subphrenic collections, it is most probable that drainage in such cases does not increase the incidence of subphrenic abscess. Also in those instances of splenic injury in which there is any question of associated pancreatic or gastric trauma, drainage of the splenic bed may prevent complications that could arise if such unrecognized injuries were not drained. Even those authors who incriminate the usage of splenic bed drains report no higher incidences of subphrenic abscess or other infections if the drains are removed before the sixth postsplenectomy day.

MORTALITY. Factors contributing to mortality following splenic injury include (1) associated injury; (2) mechanism of injury; (3) presence of shock on admission to hospital; and (4) advanced age. Naylor and associates reported an overall mortality rate of 11.2 percent in their series of 408 patients, which compares favorably with that in other reports.

Retroperitoneal Hematoma

The management of traumatic retroperitoneal hematoma is a controversial problem. The most common cause of retroperitoneal hemorrhage, according to Baylis et al. and according to the experience at Parkland Memorial Hospital, is pelvic fracture, which accounts for about 60 percent of all traumatic retroperitoneal hematomas. The diagnosis of retroperitoneal hematoma is most difficult following blunt, nonpenetrating trauma to the abdomen, and should be suspected in any patient following trauma who has signs and symptoms of hemorrhagic shock but no obvious source of hemorrhage. Hemorrhage within the retroperitoneal area may be massive and may exceed 2,000 ml of blood. Experimental data have shown that as much as 4,000 ml of fluid can extravasate into the retroperitoneal space under pressure equal to that in the pelvic vessels.

DIAGNOSIS. Abdominal pain occurs in approximately 60 percent of patients, and back pain in about 25 percent. The abdominal pain is usually vague and generalized but is occasionally localized over the hematoma. Local or generalized tenderness is present in about two-thirds of the patients, and shock occurs in approximately 40 percent. Occasionally, a tender mass is palpable through the abdomen or in the flanks, and in some cases, rectal examination will reveal a boggy mass anterior or posterior to the rectum. Dullness to percussion over the flanks or the abdomen which does not vary with changing positions of the patient has been recorded in some instances. At times, discoloration of the flanks from retroperitoneal hemorrhage has been noted after the lapse of a few hours (Grey Turner's sign). Progressive decrease in the hemoglobin and hematocrit is a consistent finding, and hematuria is found in 80 percent of patients. Hematuria may represent the first clue to the development of a retroperitoneal hematoma.

Somewhat more than half the patients produce free, nonclotting blood on diagnostic paracentesis or lavage of the abdomen; this blood is generally related to the presence of both retroperitoneal and intraabdominal hemorrhage. However, if the retroperitoneal hematoma which occurs without intraperitoneal hemorrhage is large enough to yield a so-called "false-positive" peritoneal tap or lavage from retroperitoneal hemorrhage alone, then the hematoma itself may require abdominal exploration to search for the persistent source of the retroperitoneal bleeding.

Roentgenography, according to Baylis et al., has been valuable in several respects; approximately two-thirds of the patients with peritoneal hematoma have had fractures of the pelvis, and other x-ray findings have included obliteration of the psoas shadow in 30 percent, abdominal mass in 5 percent, and paralytic ileus in 8 percent. Also, displaced bowel-gas shadows and fractured vertebrae have been noted. Baylis et al. also noted that in one patient a pelvic phlebolith was displaced by an expanding retroperitoneal hematoma. Intravenous pyelograms and/or retrograde cystograms are routinely obtained in all patients with suspected retroperitoneal hematomas, if the patient's condition is stable enough to have these studies performed. Arteriography has also been helpful in establishing the diagnosis of retroperitoneal injury. In the patient whose condition is deteriorating, however, immediate exploration is performed without obtaining such studies, in order to attempt rapid control of progressive bleeding. Most retroperitoneal hematomas from pelvic fractures will tamponade themselves within a short time, and the patient's condition will remain stable and the hematocrit normal, perhaps after transfusion of several units of blood.

TREATMENT. It has been recommended by some that retroperitoneal hematomas not be explored at the time of operation. This nonexploration is considered poor practice, an opinion based on experience which indicates that nonoperative treatment of retroperitoneal hematomas (with the exception of retroperitoneal hematoma secondary to pelvic fracture) has led to an excessive mortality from continued or recurrent hemorrhage from injured retroperitoneal vessels such as the vena cava, aorta, lumbar veins, or renal veins. In addition, it is felt that nonexploration of retroperitoneal hematomas adjacent to partially extraperitoneal bowel is dangerous because of the possibility of missing a perforation in the bowel's extraperitoneal portion (e.g., duodenum). Consequently, it is recommended to explore all retroperitoneal hematomas discovered during celiotomy for the source of bleeding, as well as for associated injuries to the bowel, kidney, ureter, bladder, etc. This is done regardless of the size of the hematoma or whether or not it is increasing in size at the time of exploration. This policy has not been associated with any complications arising solely from such exploration.

Warnings have been made that if a small hematoma which is not enlarging is disturbed, uncontrollable bleeding may occur. However, it is felt that if such bleeding is to occur, it is best for it to take place at the time of the surgical procedure rather than postoperatively. If major vessels are not explored at the time that hematomas occur near them, major and sometimes fatal postoperative bleeding may occur. Present-day vascular surgical techniques obviate the fear of incurring massive hemorrhage as a contraindication to exploring retroperitoneal hematomas. This is with the sole exception of the treatment of large retroperitoneal hematomas due to pelvic fracture.

In massive retroperitoneal hematomas following pelvic fractures, it is often impossible adequately to control multiple small bleeding points. Consequently, it is advisable not to explore this type of massive pelvic hematoma (for fear of causing bleeding which may be very difficult to control) unless the hemorrhage from the fracture site fails spontaneously to tamponade itself and exsanguination threatens. However, spontaneous tamponade usually occurs. When not exploring these hematomas, it is important to be certain that there is no injury to the distal aorta, common iliac, or external iliac vessels.

Seavers et al. advise that the ligation in continuity of one or both hypogastric arteries may, at times, control persistent bleeding in the pelvic retroperitoneal space from pelvic fractures which cannot be controlled by any other means. This will often control the venous bleeding from this source, also. Certainly it is preferable to locate a single vessel which is bleeding and either ligate or repair it, than blindly to ligate the hypogastric arteries. Recent studies now indicate that infusion of vasospastic drugs or the embolization of autologous clots or hemostatic agents may be beneficial in controlling this type of hemorrhage. On rare occasions it may be necessary to pack the pelvis with large lap packs for 24 to 48 hours in order to achieve hemostasis.

Inferior Vena Cava

Inferior vena caval injuries associated with penetrating abdominal wounds are being seen with increasing frequency. It has been reported that one in every 50 gunshot wounds and one in every 300 knife wounds of the abdomen will injure the vena cava. These are serious injuries; one-third of the patients die before reaching the hospital, and up to half the remaining persons will die during hospitalization. Most deaths occur from bleeding because of the inherent difficulties in controlling injuries of large veins, but significant wounds of other structures, especially in the retroperitoneum, are common and often adversely affect therapeutic efforts.

ETIOLOGY AND DISTRIBUTION. Most injuries of the inferior vena cava are caused by gunshot wounds, but stab wounds or blunt trauma may also be involved (Table 6-7). Simple penetrating wounds produced by knives and low-velocity missiles are less lethal than those wounds caused by shotguns, high-velocity bullets, and especially blunt trauma. Widespread serious damage to other structures, particularly liver and major arteries and veins, are likely to result from shotgun wounds and blunt trauma to the abdomen and lower part of the chest.

The infrarenal vena cava is most susceptible and often injured (Table 6-8). The level of injury is a major determinant of survival, and injuries of the suprarenal, intrahepatic vena cava are extremely dangerous, especially when accompanied by wounds of hepatic and renal veins. Difficulties in exposure and control are invariably encountered, and adjunctive measures are often necessary.

DIAGNOSIS. Injuries of the inferior vena cava should be considered in all cases of penetrating wounds of the abdomen and lower part of the chest. Because of the vagaries of the trajectory of bullets, innocent-appearing small-caliber wounds may produce serious damage to retroperitoneal structures, without intraabdominal organ injury. Patients who have suffered stab wounds of the back or lower part of the chest may also harbor unsuspected caval injuries.

One of the major determinants of survival of these patients is the presence of hemorrhagic shock on admission. This is often a clue that despite the absence of identifying physical findings, major vascular injuries are present. Hemoperitoneum, hemothorax, subcutaneous blood staining from retroperitoneal bleeding, and evidence of distal vena caval obstruction may be helpful in diagnosis.

Except for direct venous studies with contrast media, radiographic examination is rarely specific. Routine x-ray studies, including anteroposterior and lateral films of the chest and abdomen, are useful and are recommended, but in a patient in unstable condition these should be obtained

Table 6-7. CAUSES OF INFERIOR VENA CAVAL INJURIES

	Total	Died	Mortality, %
Bullet	69	23	30
Shotgun	8	6	75
Stab	12	2	17
Blunt	12	11	84
Total	101	42	42

Table 6-8. LOCATION OF INFERIOR VENA CAVAL INJURY

	Total	Died	Mortality, %
Above renal veins	19	11	58
At renal vein level	21	13	62
Below renal veins	47	14	29
Bifurcation	14	4	27

in the operating room as preparations for surgery are in progress. It is usually best not to delay surgery for elaborate studies if firm indications for exploration exist.

TREATMENT. As alluded to in the discussion of other vascular injuries, associated injuries are common and are a major factor in survival of these patients (Table 6-9). Prior to exploration, resuscitation and attention to other problems often are important. An adequate airway must be obtained, volume and blood deficits repaired, and often fractures stabilized. Vena caval injuries may preclude the use of lower-extremity veins for fluid administration, and at least one large-bore catheter should be placed into the upper-extremity venous system. This line is best reserved for blood and fluid administration, and should not be used for primary anesthetic manipulations.

Thoracotomy may be required, especially in patients with suprarenal caval injuries. If transatrial intracaval shunts are needed, a median sternotomy offers good exposure for this maneuver as well as for control of associated hepatic injuries.

Abdominal exploration is performed through a midline incision which can be extended as required, and median sternotomy can be added if necessary. Rapid abdominal exploration will usually expose major injuries and establish priorities of repair. It is usually wise to control the bleeding, pause, and complete volume and blood restoration before definitive repairs are begun. Attempts to complete bowel repairs while bleeding persists from other injuries often extend the hypotensive episode and increase blood loss.

Centrally located retroperitoneal hematomas above the pelvis often harbor significant injuries, and usually are explored. Damage to other retroperitoneal structures is common (79 percent) and not always evident without formal exploration. The size or stability of the hematoma does not offer reliable evidence as to the presence or absence of significant injuries. Continued bleeding from the vena caval injury, however, is ominous. Patients actively bleeding at the time of operation have a very high mortality rate, especially if the vena caval injury is at or above the renal arteries and veins (Table 6-10).

Table 6-9. INJURIES ASSOCIATED WITH INFERIOR VENA CAVAL INJURY

Aorta, iliac artery 13	Kidney 21
Major splanchnic vessel . . . 26	Pancreas 18
Renal artery or vein 20	Spleen 10
Liver 46	Colon 27
Duodenum 27	Other 21

Table 6-10. RELATIONSHIP OF BLEEDING
AND MORTALITY FROM
INFERIOR VENA CAVAL INJURIES

	Total	Died	Mortality, %
Active bleeding	41	32	79
Tamponade	57	9	16
Not specified	3	0	0

Initial control of bleeding can usually be obtained with pressure and packs. Occasionally temporary occlusion of the abdominal aorta at the diaphragmatic hiatus is useful in reducing blood loss from high caval injuries. Exposure of the inferior vena cava is obtained by reflecting medially the right colon, duodenum, and pancreas. Direct tamponade, manually or with sponge sticks, is usually effective in controlling bleeding. Simple lacerations or punctures are most common, but transections, avulsion, or multiple lacerations may be encountered, and control may be very difficult in the last group.

Simple lacerations can be controlled with gentle digital pressure and sutured by simply passing the needle under the occluding finger. In some cases the edge of the wound can be held gently in apposition with vascular forceps or blunt Allis clamps while repair is effected. Balloon catheter tamponade has also been employed for control of these wounds. Partial occlusion with vascular clamps is a useful technique and can be instituted after the initial use of other maneuvers (Fig. 6-15). These simple tangential wounds usually can be repaired without injury to lumbar veins, but occasionally ligation of gonadal and lumbar tributaries is required (Fig. 6-16).

Transections may be repaired by end-to-end vascular surgical techniques after mobilizing the vena cava. If there are multiple caval wounds requiring complicated repairs, or if repair poses an undue risk in a patient with multiple injuries, infrarenal ligation is preferable. In most cases construction of venous grafts is not required, and the time and effort necessary to perform these repairs may increase the operative morbidity and mortality.

Wounds at or above the renal veins are difficult to expose and repair. If bleeding from behind the liver is encountered and is not easily identified as coming from a laceration of the anterior cava wall below the caudate lobe, an intracaval shunt may be needed. The liver can be rotated medially after division of supporting ligaments, and if intrahepatic vena cava or combined hepatic vein lacerations are present, the shunt can be inserted as described by Blaisdell. The transatrial approach is easier than inserting the shunt from the intrarenal vena cava, and is very useful in managing these extremely dangerous wounds. A large chest tube (34 to 38 Fr) with a proximal side hole is inserted through the atrial appendage, and the tip is placed near the orifices of the renal veins. Umbilical tapes encircling the inferior vena cava within the pericardium and above the renal veins secure the catheter. The side hole in the catheter is placed at a level to permit the return of blood via the tube into the right atrium. This shunt, occa-

Simple Anterior Repair

Fig. 6-15. Repair of anterior laceration of the inferior vena cava. Note the use of a partially occlusive clamp.

sionally combined with temporary occlusion of the portal triad, will usually allow sufficient control of bleeding to effect repairs.

Unlike injuries of the infrarenal cava, all wounds above the renal veins should be repaired. Ligation of the inferior vena cava at this level produces serious complications. Few survivors have been reported, and those were in elective operations uncomplicated by hypotension, shock, or other injuries.

Those vascular procedures used in other areas are effective in repairing the suprarenal vena cava. Simple venorrhaphy often may suffice, but patch graft angioplasty or anastomosis may be needed (Fig. 6-17). If graft interposition is required, autogenous venous grafts obtained from the infrarenal cava or iliac vein are preferred (Figs. 6-18,

Fig. 6-16. Repair of through-and-through injury to the inferior vena cava. *A.* Anterior laceration is enlarged to permit closure of the posterior wall from within the lumen. *B.* Rotation of the posteroinferior vena cava.

Anterior and Posterior Rotation Repair Repair

A

B

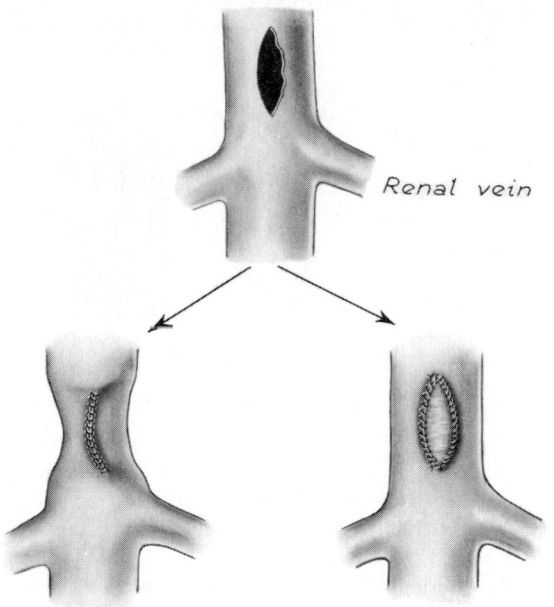

Fig. 6-17. Repair of the inferior vena cava using a patch graft to prevent stenosis.

6-19). Concomitant repair of hepatic vein injuries can be effected, but in some cases ligation may be preferable.

These repairs can usually be completed within 30 minutes, a period of ischemia well tolerated by the normothermic liver. Regional hypothermia may be induced with iced saline solution by irrigation techniques, thus conferring further protection of the liver during more prolonged ischemia.

Fig. 6-18. Construction of an inferior vena caval conduit from the saphenous vein.

COMPLICATIONS. In patients with isolated wounds of the inferior vena cava, repair is usually effective and complications are few. In these patients, two episodes of ileofemoral venous thrombosis have been encountered, and an additional patient had a pulmonary embolus. Pancreatitis has also been encountered, and recurrent retroperitoneal bleeding occurred in one patient.

The mortality in patients with isolated inferior vena caval injuries was 11 percent in the present series, but 67 percent of the patients with one or more major vessel injuries died. All the patients with inferior vena caval wounds at or above the renal veins had significant associated injuries, usually liver and bowel, occasionally pancreas, stomach, and lung. The mortality is high in this group of patients, especially if the inferior vena cava is actively bleeding at surgery.

Female Reproductive Organs

Injuries to the female reproductive organs are infrequently seen following either blunt or penetrating trauma to the abdomen. A series reported by Quast and Jordan revealed only 27 patients with gynecologic injuries in a 16-year period at their hospital. Two of those injuries resulted from blunt trauma with rupture of the uterus in patients who were in the immediate postpartum period. These are apparently the only cases recorded of rupture of the nonpregnant uterus. The remaining injuries were penetrating wounds. An enlarged uterus was present in 10 of their patients. Six patients were pregnant, two had large uterine myomas, and two were in the postpartum period. No cases of rupture of an unenlarged uterus by blunt trauma have been recorded, however. Rupture of the pregnant uterus due to blunt trauma is rare, but has occurred in a number of instances. Of blunt and penetrating wounds to the female reproductive tract, 90 percent involve the uterine corpus, and 10 percent involve the remaining adnexa.

TREATMENT. The signs and symptoms from a ruptured pregnant uterus are those of abrupt and massive intraperitoneal hemorrhage. Associated with these findings are generalized abdominal pain and tenderness, abdominal distension, ileus, and the absence of fetal heart sounds and movements. If the patient arrives at the hospital alive (which is not often the case), immediate blood volume and extracellular fluid replacement must be instituted through several large-bore intravenous cathethers, preferably placed in the upper extremities, since there may be an interference with venous return from lower extremities of these patients. Urgent celiotomy is necessary to control hemorrhage, even though the patient may still be in shock at the time, since the only means of controlling the shock is to stop the hemorrhage. Probably the only anesthesia which will be required is assisted respiration with 100 percent oxygen administered through an endotracheal tube. Other agents may be added if and when shock abates. The treatment of choice is evacuation of the uterus, closure of the disruption with large chromic catgut sutures, and thorough peritoneal toilet with removal of all blood and foreign tissue.

Wounds of the uterus and adnexa are repaired by fig-ure-of-eight chromic catgut sutures without drainage in most instances, although in occasional patients hysterec-tomy is indicated, as in injury of the lower uterine segment and major uterine vessels caused by high-velocity missiles. In these instances, hysterectomy is preferable to an at-tempted suture repair, since repair may cause stenosis of the cervical canal with resultant hematometra and dystocia. Also, hysterectomy for lower-uterine-segment injuries is indicated to obtain proper control of bleeding vessels and to help rule out urethral injury at the point where the ureter and uterine artery are in juxtaposition.

It is wise to leave the vaginal cuff partially open follow-ing hysterectomy for trauma, because of the likelihood of vaginal cuff or cul-de-sac abscess formation, especially if there is appreciable blast injury or concomitant colon injury. If abscesses occur and the vaginal cuff has been left open, it is usually a relatively simple matter to drain the abscess with a finger inserted through the vagina into the open cuff. If gross fecal contamination is present from colon injury, the cuff should be left open and a Penrose drain led out of the vagina from the cul-de-sac. This drain may be secured to the vaginal cuff by a single small chro-mic catgut suture.

If massive uncontrollable or recurrent bleeding occurs following trauma to the female pelvic organs, it may be rapidly and adequately controlled by bilateral in-continu-ity ligations of the hypogastric arteries with nonabsorbable suture material. This will not often be required, but should be borne in mind as a very helpful and possibly lifesaving procedure.

Following injury to the pregnant uterus, the loss of the fetus is quite high. Quast and Jordan reported a salvage of only 1 of 10 pregnancies. One patient who was pregnant at the time of a tangential knife injury of the uterus had a uterine repair for penetrating trauma and subsequently delivered the child uneventfully per vagina.

Other instances have been reported in which penetrating uterine injury during pregnancy has been repaired with ensuing normal delivery. Quast and Jordan found that 81 percent of their patients with uterine injuries during preg-nancy delivered subsequently per vagina with no difficulty. The cesarean section rate was 19 percent. Of the patients they followed after uterine injury, all who were in the childbearing age subsequently were able to conceive chil-dren. In this group, the abortion rate for these later preg-nancies was 16 percent, with no apparent cause found.

By far the majority of pregnant patients with uterine injuries will abort shortly after the injury, frequently re-quiring curettage to control bleeding after spontaneous abortion. Others will require elective emptying of the uterine contents at the time of celiotomy in order to secure adequate hemostasis and uterine repair. Intravenous oxy-tocin should be given in such instances to aid in uterine contraction and hemostasis after hysterotomy.

Abdominal Wall

Injury to the abdominal wall without peritoneal injury is often difficult to diagnose. Muscular guarding and rigidity

Fig. 6-19. Interposition of an excised segment of the infrarenal inferior vena cava to establish continuity of the suprarenal inferior vena cava.

are frequently present, and it may be impossible to rule out intraabdominal injury from a hematoma of the abdominal wall. Such hematomas are usually due to rupture of the rectus abdominis or the epigastric artery by direct trauma or severe muscular exertion. The epigastric artery may be injured also by penetrating trauma, so that a hemoperi-toneum results. The patient may become hypotensive from such an injury because of the severe intraperitoneal bleed-ing which sometimes occurs.

The mass from the rectus abdominis hematoma is below the umbilicus in over 80 percent of the cases. To distinguish this mass from intraperitoneal masses, the patient should be requested to raise his head against resistance; the mass should disappear if it is intraperitoneal and remain the same if it is in the abdominal wall. This sign is not com-pletely reliable, and if adjunctive diagnostic aids such as paracentesis and lavage are equivocal, then abdominal celiotomy should be performed.

References

General Considerations

Patman, R. D., Poulos, E., and Shires, G. T.: The Management of Civilian Arterial Injuries, *Surg Gynecol Obstet*, **118:**725, 1964.

Shires, G. T.: "Care of the Trauma Patient," McGraw-Hill Book Company, New York, 1966.

Metabolic Response to Trauma

Abbott, W. E., Krieger, H., Holden, W. D., Bradshaw, J., and Levey, S.: Effect of I.V. Administered Fat on Body Weight and Nitrogen Balance in Surgical Patients, *Metabolism*, **6:**691, 1957.

Cohn, I., Singleton, S., Hartwig, Q. L., and Atik, M.: New I.V. Fat Emulsion, *JAMA*, **183:**755, 1963.

Coon, W. W.: Ascorbic Acid Metabolism in Postoperative Patients, *Surg Gynecol Obstet*, **114:**522, 1962.

Doolas, A.: Planning Intravenous Alimentation of Surgical Pa-tients, *Surg Clin North Am*, **50:**103, 1970.

Elman, R.: Acute Starvation following Operation or Injury with

Special Reference to Caloric and Protein Needs, *Ann Surg,* **120:**350, 1944.

Hardy, J. D.: "Surgery and the Endocrine System: Physiologic Response to Surgical Trauma—Operative Management of Endocrine Dysfunction," W. B. Saunders Company, Philadelphia, 1952.

Krebs, H. A., and Lowenstein, J. M: "Tricarboxylic Acid Cycle: Metabolic Pathways," vol. 1, Academic Press, Inc., New York, 1960.

Lehr, H. B., Rhoads, J. E., Rosenthal, O., and Blakemore, W. S.: The Use of I.V. Fat Emulsion in Surgical Patients, *JAMA,* **181.**745, 1962.

Moore, F. D.: Hormones and Stress-Endocrine Changes after Anesthesia, Surgery, and Unanesthetized Trauma in Man, *Recent Prog Horm Res,* **13:**511, 1957.

———: Systemic Mediators of Surgical Injury, *Can Med Assoc J,* **78:**85, 1958.

———: "Metabolic Care of the Surgical Patient," W. B. Saunders Company, Philadelphia, 1959.

Olson, R. E.: The Two-Carbon Chain in Metabolism, *JAMA,* **183:**471, 1963.

Rea, W. J., Wyrick, W. J., Jr., McClelland, R. N., and Webb, W. R.: Intravenous Hyperosmolar Alimentation, *Arch Surg,* **100:**393, 1970.

Selye, H.: "Conditioning" vs. "Permissive" Actions of Hormones, *J Clin Endocrinol Metab,* **13:**122, 1954.

Shires, G. T., Williams, J., and Brown, F.: Acute Changes in Extracellular Fluids Associated with Major Surgical Procedures, *Ann Surg,* **154:**803, 1961.

Anesthesia

Bastron, R. D., and Hamilton, W. K.: Perils of Rapid Induction Techniques, *JAMA,* **201:**875, 1967.

Beck, G. P., and Neill, L. W.: Anesthesia for Associated Trauma in Patients with Head Injuries, *Anesth Anal (Cleve),* **42:**687, 1963.

Bowers, W. F.: Priority of Treatment in Multiple Injuries and Summation of Surgery for Acute Trauma, *Arch Surg,* **75:**743, 1957.

Clark, K.: The Incidence and Mechanisms of Shock in Head Injury, *South Med J,* **55:**513, 1962.

Crighton, H. C., and Giesecke, A. H.: One Year's Experience in the Anesthetic Management of Trauma—1964, *Anesth Anal (Cleve),* **45:**835, 1966.

Greene, N. M.: General Considerations in Anesthesia for Emergency Surgery, *Clin Anesth,* vol. 2, 1963.

Hamilton, W. K.: Atelectasis, Pneumothorax and Aspiration as Postoperative Complications, *Anesthesiology,* **22:**708, 1961.

Jacoby, J. J., Hamelberg, W., Ziegler, C., Flory, F. A., and Jones, J. R.: Transtracheal Resuscitation, *JAMA,* **162:**625, 1956.

Lee, J. F., Jenkins, M. D., and Giesecke, A. H.: The Anesthetic Management of Trauma: Influence of Alcohol Ingestion, *South Med J,* **60:**1240, 1967.

Nicholas, T. H., and Rumer, G. F.: Emergency Airway: A Plan of Action, *JAMA,* **174:**1930, 1960.

Sellick, B. A.: Cricoid Pressure to Control Regurgitation of Stomach Contents during Induction of Anesthesia, *Lancet,* **2:**404, 1961.

Walts, L. F.: Anesthesia of the Larynx in the Patient with a Full Stomach, *JAMA,* **192:**705, 1965.

Principles in the Management of Wounds

Alexander, J. W., Kaplan, J. Z., and Altemeier, W. A.: Role of Suture Materials in the Development of Wound Infection, *Ann Surg,* **165:**192, 1967.

Altemeier, W. A., and Wulsin, J. H.: Antimicrobial Therapy in Injured Patients, *JAMA,* **173:**527, 1960.

Artz, C. B., Barnett, W. O., and Grogan, J. B.: Further Studies concerning the Pathogenesis and Diagnosis of Peritonitis, *Ann Surg,* **155:**756, 1962.

Burke, J. F.: The Effective Period of Preventive Antibiotic Action in Experimental Incisions and Dermal Lesions, *Surgery,* **50:**161, 1961.

Cohn, I., Jr., and Kotler, A. N.: Intraperitoneal Kanamycin, *Ann Surg,* **155:**532, 1962.

Condie, J. P., and Ferguson, D. J.: Experimental Wound Infections: Contamination versus Surgical Technique, *Surgery,* **50:**367, 1961.

Crawford, D. T., and Ketcham, A. S.: Late Complications of Wire Sutures and Some Causative Factors, *Am J Surg,* **106:**898, 1963.

Douglas, D. M.: The Healing of Aponeurotic Incisions, *Br J Surg,* **40:**79, 1952.

Dunphy, J. E., and Jackson, D. S.: Practical Applications of Experimental Studies in the Care of the Primarily Closed Wounds, *Am J Surg,* **104:**273, 1962.

Elek, F. D., and Conen, P. E.: The Virulence of Staphylococcal Pyrogenes for Man: A Study of the Problems of Wound Infection, *Br J Exp Pathol,* **38:**573, 1957.

Houston, A. N., Roy, W. A., Faust, R. A., and Ewin, D. M.: Tetanus Prophylaxis in the Treatment of Puncture Wounds of Patients in the Deep South, *J Trauma,* **2:**439, 1962.

Jones, R. C.: "Care of the Trauma Patient," 2d ed., G. Thomas Shires (ed.), McGraw-Hill Book Company, New York, 1978.

Localio, S. A., Lowman, E. W., and Gibson, J.: Wound Healing in the Paraplegic Patient, *Surgery,* **44:**625, 1958.

Mann, L. S., and Levin, M. J.: Respiratory Depression with Intraperitoneal Neomycin, *Arch Surg,* **81:**690, 1960.

———, Spinazzola, A. J., Lindesmith, G. G., Levine, M. J., and Kuzerepa, W.: Disruption of Abdominal Wounds, *JAMA,* **180:**99, 1962.

McMullan, M. H., and Barnett, W. O.: Cephalothin—Effective Choice for Peritonitis, *Surgery,* **67:**432, 1970.

Ollodart, R., and Mansberger, A. R.: The Effect of Hypovolemic Shock and Bacterial Defense, *Am J Surg,* **110:**302, 1965.

Pissiotis, C. A., Nichols, R. L., and Condon, R. E.: Absorption and Excretion of Intraperitoneally Administered Kanamycin Sulfate, *Surg Gynecol Obstet,* **134:**995, 1972.

Pittinger, C. B., and Long, J. P.: Potential Dangers Associated with Antibiotic Administration during Anesthesia in Surgery, *Arch Surg,* **79:**207, 1959.

Rambo, W. M.: Irrigation of the Peritoneal Cavity with Cephalothin, *Am J Surg,* **123:**192, 1972.

Robertson, W. H.: Postoperative Wound Disruption, *Am Practitioner Dig Treat,* **9:**1615, 1958.

Rosen, R. G., and Enquist, I. F.: The Healing Wound in Experimental Diabetes, *Surgery,* **50:**525, 1961.

Singleton, A. O., and Julian, J.: An Experimental Evaluation of Methods Used to Prevent Infections in Wounds Which Have Been Contaminated with Feces, *Ann Surg,* **151:**912, 1960.

Sisson, R., Lang, S., Serkes, K., and Parevia, M. D.: Comparison of Wound Healing in Various Nutritional Deficiency States, *Surgery,* **44:**613, 1958.

Smith, P. S.: Management of Abdominal Incision: A Survey of Current Practices, *Arch Surg,* **88:**515, 1964.

Spencer, F. C., Sharp, E. H., and Jude, J. R.: Experiences with Wire Closure of Abdominal Incisions in 293 Selected Patients, *Surg Gynecol Obstet,* **117:**235, 1963.

Stanley, V. F., Giesecke, A. H., and Jenkins, M. T.: Neomycin-Curare Neuromuscular Block and Reversal in Cats, *Anesthesiology,* **31:**3, 1969.

Stone, H. H., Kolb, L. D., and Geheber, C. E.: Incidence and Significance of Intraperitoneal Anaerobic Bacteria, *Ann Surg,* **181:**705, 1975.

Thadepalli, H., Gorbach, S. L., Broido, P. W., Norsen, J., and Nyhus, L.: Abdominal Trauma, Anaerobes and Antibiotics, *Surg Gynecol Obstet,* **137:**270, 1973.

Thorngate, S., and Ferguson, D. J.: Effect of Tension on Healing of Aponeurotic Wounds, *Surgery,* **44:**619, 1958.

Wagner, D. H.: Errors in the Choice of Abdominal Wall Incisions and in Their Closure, *Surg Clin North Am,* **38:**175, 1958.

Bites and Stings of Animals and Insects

Auer, A. I., and Hershey, F. B.: Surgery for Necrotic Bites of the Brown Spider, *Arch Surg,* **108:**612, 1974.

Bitseff, E. L., Garoni, W. J., Hardison, C. D., and Thompson, J. M.: The Management of Stingray Injuries of the Extremities, *South Med J,* **63:**417, 1970.

Corey, L., Hattwick, M., Baer, G., and Smith, J.: Serum Neutralizing Antibody after Rabies Postexposure Prophylaxis, *Ann Int Med,* **85:**170, 1976.

Davidson, T.: Inside World of the Honeybee, *Natl Geograph,* **154:**188, 1959.

Dillaha, C. J., Jansen, G. T., Honeycutt, W. M., and Hayden, C. R.: North American Loxocelism, *JAMA,* **188:**33, 1964.

Fardon, D. W., Wingo, C. W., Robinson, D. W., and Masters, F. W.: The Treatment of Brown Spider Bites, *Plast Reconstr Surg,* **40:**482, 1967.

Farrar, W. E., Warner, A. R., and Vivona, S.: Pre-exposure Immunization against Rabies Using Duck-Embryo Vaccine, *Milit Med,* **129:**960, 1964.

Gill, K. A.: The Evaluation of Cryotherapy in the Treatment of Snake Envenomization, *South Med J,* **63:**552, 1970.

Girard, K. F., Hitchcock, H. B., Edsall, G., and MacCready, R. A.: Rabies in Bats in Southern New England, *N Engl J Med,* **272:**75, 1965.

Hattwick, M. A. W., Weis, T. T., Stechschulte, C. J., Baer, G. M., and Gregg, M. B.: Recovery from Rabies: A Case Report, *Ann Intern Med,* **76:**931, 1972.

Hershey, F. B., and Aulenbacher, C. E.: Surgical Treatment of Brown Spider Bites, *Ann Surg,* **170:**300, 1969.

Hildreth, E. A.: Review: Prevention of Rabies, *Ann Intern Med,* **58:**833, 1963.

Huang, T. T., Lynch, J. B., Larson, D. L., and Lewis, S. R.: The Use of Excisional Therapy in the Management of Snakebite, *Ann Surg,* **179:**598, 1974.

Langlois, C.: Allergic Reaction to Insect Stings, *Postgrad Med,* **45:**190, May, 1969.

Levine, M. I.: Insect Stings, *JAMA,* **217:**964, 1971.

McQueen, J. L., Lewis, A. L., and Schneider, N. J.: Rabies Diagnosis by Fluorescent Antibody, *Am J Public Health,* **50:**1743, 1960.

Marr, J. J.: Portuguese Man-of-War Envenomization, *JAMA,* **199:**115, 1967.

Parrish, H. M.: Fatalities from Venomous Animals, *Am J Med Sci,* **245:**129, 1963.

——: Intravenous Antivenin in Clinical Snake Venom Poisoning, *Mo Med,* **60:**240, 1963.

——: Texas Snakebite Statistics, *Tex State J Med,* **60:**592, 1964.

——: Incidence of Treated Snakebites in the United States, *Public Health Rept (US),* **81:**269, 1966.

—— and Carr, C. A.: Bites by Copperheads in the United States, *JAMA,* **201:**927, 1967.

—— and Schwichtenberg, A. E.: Treatment of Venomous Snakebites: Fiction versus Fact, *Med Times,* **97:**153, 1969.

Paton, B. C.: Bites: Human, Dog, Spider and Snake, *Surg Clin North Am,* **43:**537, 1963.

Portuguese Man-of-War, *JAMA,* **192:**994, 1965. (Editorial.)

Russell, F. E.: Pharmacology of Animal Venoms, *Clin Pharmacol Ther,* **8:**849, 1967.

——, Carlson, R. W., Wainschel, J., and Osborn, A. H.: Snake Venom Poisoning in the United States—Experiences with 550 Cases, *JAMA,* **233:**341, 1975.

Shaffer, J. H.: Stinging Insects: A Threat to Life, *JAMA,* **177:**473, 1961.

Sikes, R. K.: Guidelines for the Control of Rabies, *Am J Public Health,* **60:**1133, 1970.

Snakebite Symposium, *J Fla Med Assoc,* **55:**307, 1968.

Snyder, C. C., and Knowles, R. P.: Snake Bite! *Consultant (SKF),* **3:**44, 1963.

Sparger, C. F.: Problems in the Management of Rattlesnake Bites, *Arch Surg,* **98:**13, 1969.

Strauss, M. B., and Orris, W. L.: Injuries to Divers by Marine Animals: A Simplified Approach to Recognition and Management, *Milit Med,* February, 1974.

Wood, J. T., Hoback, W. W., and Gran, T. W.: Treatment of Snake Venom Poisoning with ACTH and Cortisone, *Va Med Mon,* **82:**130, 1955.

Penetrating Wounds of the Neck and Thoracic Inlet

Ashworth, C., Williams, L. F., and Byrne, J. J.: Penetrating Wounds of the Neck, *Am J Surg,* **121:**387, 1971.

Brawley, R. K., Murray, G. F., Crisler, C., and Cameron, J. L.: Management of Wounds of the Innominate, Subclavian and Axillary Blood Vessels, *Surg Gynecol Obstet,* **130:**1130, 1970.

Bricker, D. L., Noon, G. P., Beall, A. C., Jr., and DeBakey, M. E.: Vascular Injuries of the Thoracic Outlet, *J Trauma,* **10:**1, 1970.

Fitchett, V. H., Pomerantz, M., Butsch, D. W., Simon, R., and Eiseman, B.: Penetrating Wounds of the Neck, *Arch Surg,* **99:**307, 1969.

Fogelman, M. J., and Stewart, R. D.: Penetrating Wounds of the Neck, *Am J Surg,* **91:**581, 1956.

Huhay, C. A.: Soft Tissue Injuries of the Cervical Region, *Surg Gynecol Obstet,* **111:**511, 1960.

Hunt, T. K., Blaisdell, F. W., and Okimoto, J.: Vascular Injuries of the Base of the Neck, *Arch Surg,* **98:**586, 1969.

Imamoglu, K., Read, R. C., and Huebl, H. C.: Cervicomediastinal Vascular Injury, *Surgery,* **61:**274, 1967.

Jones, R. F., Terrell, J. C., and Salyer, K. E.: Penetrating Wounds of the Neck: An Analysis of 274 Cases, *J Trauma,* **7:**228, 1967.

Shirkey, A. L., Beall, A. C., and DeBakey, M. E.: Surgical Management of Penetrating Wounds of the Neck, *Arch Surg,* **86:**955, 1963.

Steenburg, R. W., and Ravitch, M. M.: Cervico-thoracic Approach for Subclavian Vessel Injury from Compound Fracture of the Clavicle: Considerations of Subclavian-Axillary Exposures, *Ann Surg,* **157:**839, 1963.

Stone, H. H., and Callahan, G. S.: Soft Tissue Injuries of the Neck, *Surg Gynecol Obstet,* **117:**745, 1963.

Abdominal Trauma

Ahmad, W., and Polk, H. C., Jr.: Blunt Abdominal Trauma. A Prospective Study with Selective Peritoneal Lavage, *Arch Surg,* **111:**489, 1976.

Allen, R. E., and Blaisdell, F. W.: Injuries to the Inferior Vena Cava, *Surg Clin North Am,* **52:**699, 1972.

Awe, W. C., and Eidemiller, L.: Selective Angiography in Splenic Trauma, *Am J Surg,* **126:**171, 1973.

Anane-Sefah, J., Norton, L. W., and Eiseman, B.: Operative Choice and Technique following Pancreatic Injury, *Arch Surg,* **110:**161, 1975.

Anderson, C. B., Connors, J. P., Mejia, D. C., and Wise, L.: Drainage Methods in the Treatment of Pancreatic Injuries, *Surg Gynecol Obstet,* **138:**587, 1974.

Backwinkel, K.: Rupture of the Rectus Abdominis Muscle, *Arch Surg,* **90:**35, 1965.

Baker, R. J., Bass, R. T., Zajtchuk, R., and Strohl, E. L.: External Pancreatic Fistula following Abdominal Injury, *Arch Surg,* **95:**556, 1967.

Barnes, J. P., and Diamonon, J. S.: Traumatic Rupture of the Gallbladder Due to Nonpenetrating Injury, *Tex State J Med,* **59:**785, 1963.

Bartizal, J. F., Boyd, D. R., Folk, F. A., Smith, D., Lescher, T. C., and Freeark, R. J.: A Critical Review of Management of 392 Colonic and Rectal Injuries, *Dis Colon Rectum,* **17(3):**313, 1974.

Bass, E. M., and Crosier, J. H.: Percutaneous Control of Post-traumatic Hepatic Hemorrhage by Gelfoam Embolization, *J Trauma,* **17(1):**61, 1977.

Baudet, quoted by J. H. Terry, M. M. Self, and J. M. Howard: A Discussion of Injuries of the Spleen, *Surgery,* **40:**615, 1956.

Baylis, S. M., Lansing, E. H., and Glas, W. W.: Traumatic Retroperitoneal Hematoma, *Am J Surg,* **103:**477, 1962.

Beall, A. C., Bricker, D. L., Alessi, F. J., Whisennand, H. H., and DeBakey, M. E.: Surgical Considerations in the Management of Civilian Colon Injuries, *Ann Surg,* **173:**971, 1971.

Benjamin, C. I., Engrav, L. H., and Perry, J. F., Jr.: Delayed Rupture or Delayed Diagnosis of Rupture of the Spleen, *Surg Gynecol Obstet,* **142:**171, 1976.

Berman, J. K., Habeller, E. D., Fields, D. C., and Kilmer, W. L.: Blood Studies as an Aid in Differential Diagnosis of Abdominal Trauma, *JAMA,* **165:**1537, 1957.

Berne, C. J., Donovan, A. J., White, E. J., and Yellin, A. E.: Duodenal "Diverticulization" for Duodenal and Pancreatic Injury, *Am J Surg,* **127:**503, 1974.

Bollinger, J. A., and Fowler, C. F.: Traumatic Rupture of the Spleen with Special Reference to Delayed Splenic Rupture, *Am J Surg,* **91:**952, 1956.

Brawley, R. K., Cameron, J. L., and Zuidema, G. D.: Severe Upper Abdominal Injuries Treated by Pancreaticoduodenectomy, *Surg Gynecol Obstet,* **126:**516, 1968.

Bricker, D. L., Morton, J. R., Okies, J. E., and Beall, A. C.: Surgical Management of Injuries to the Vena Cava: Changing Patterns of Injury and New Techniques of Repair, *J Trauma,* **11:**725, 1971.

Bull, J. C., Jr., and Mathewson, C., Jr.: Exploratory Laparotomy in Patients with Penetrating Wounds of the Abdomen, *Am J Surg,* **116:**223, 1968.

Burrington, J. D.: Surgical Repair of a Ruptured Spleen in Children: Report of Eight Cases, *Arch Surg,* **112:**417, 1977.

Burrus, G. R., Howell, J. F., and Jordan, G. L.: Traumatic Duodenal Injuries: An Analysis of 86 Cases, *J Trauma,* **1:**96, 1961.

Buscaglia, L. C., Blaisdell, W., and Lim, R. C.: Penetrating Abdominal Vascular Injuries, *Arch Surg* **99:**764, 1969.

Canizaro, P. C., Fitts, C. T., and Sawyer, R. B.: Diagnostic Abdominal Paracentesis: A Proposed Adjunctive Measure, *U.S. Army Surg Res Unit Annl Rept,* June, 1964.

Cassebaum, W. H., Bukanz, S. L., Baum, V., and Azzi, E.: Ligation of the Inferior Vena Cava above the Renal Vein of a Sole Kidney with Recovery, *Am J Surg,* **113:**667, 1967.

Cattell, R. B., and Braasch, J. W.: A Technique for the Exposure of the Third and Fourth Portions of the Duodenum, *Surg Gynecol Obstet,* **111:**379, 1960.

Cerise, E. J., and Scully, J. H., Jr.: Blunt Trauma to the Small Intestine, *J Trauma,* **10(1):**46, 1970.

Chunn, C. F.: Wounds of the Rectum, *Surg Clin,* 1960, p. 1649.

Cleveland, H. C., and Waddell, W. R.: Retroperitoneal Rupture of the Duodenum Due to Nonpenetrating Trauma, *Surg Clin North Am,* **43:**413, 1963.

Cohn, I., Jr., Hawthorne, H. R., and Frabese, A. S.: Retroperitoneal Rupture of the Duodenum in Nonpenetrating Abdominal Trauma, *Am J Surg,* **84:**293, 1952.

Cornell, W. P., Ebert, P. A., Greenfield, L. J., and Zuidema, G. D.: A New Nonoperative Technique for the Diagnosis of Penetrating Injuries to the Abdomen, *J Trauma,* **7:**307, 1967.

Curtis, L. E., Simonian, S., Buerk, L. A., Hirsch, E. F., and Soroff, H. S.: Evaluation of the Effectiveness of Controlled pH in Management of Massive Upper Gastrointestinal Bleeding, *Am J Surg,* **125:**474, 1973.

Defore, W. W., Jr., Mattox, K. L., Jordan, G. L., Jr., Beall, A. C., Jr.: Management of 1,590 Consecutive Cases of Liver Trauma, *Arch Surg,* **111:**493, 1976.

Dickerman, J. D.: Bacterial Infection and the Asplenic Host: A Review, *J Trauma,* **16(8):**662, 1976.

Drapanas, T., and McDonald, J.: Peritoneal Tap in Abdominal Trauma, *Surgery,* **100:**22, 1960.

Dudrick, S. J., Wilmore, D. W., Steiger, E., Mackie, J. A., and Fitts, W. T.: Spontaneous Closure of Traumatic Pancreato-duodenal Fistulas with Total Intravenous Nutrition, *J Trauma,* **10(7):**542, 1970.

Duke, J. H., Jones, R. C., and Shires, G. T.: Management of Injuries to the Inferior Vena Cava, *Am J Surg,* **110:**759, 1965.

Edwards, J., and Gaspard, D. J.: Visceral Injury Due to Extraperitoneal Gunshot Wounds, *Arch Surg,* **108:**865, 1974.

Felson, B., and Levin, E. J.: Intramural Hematoma of the Duodenum: Diagnostic Roentgen Sign, *Radiology,* **63:**828, 1954.

Fish, J. C.: Reconstruction of the Portal Vein: Case Reports and Literature Review, *Am Surg,* **32:**472, 1966.

Fitzgerald, J. B., Crawford, E., and DeBakey, M. E.: Surgical

Considerations of Abdominal Injuries: Analysis of 200 Cases, *Am J Surg*, **100:**22, 1960.

Fogelman, M. F., and Robison, L. J.: Wounds of the Pancreas, *Am J Surg*, **101:**698, 1961.

Foley, W. J., Gaines, R. D., and Fry, W. J.: Pancreaticoduodenectomy for Severe Trauma to the Head of the Pancreas and the Associated Structures: Report of Three Cases, *Ann Surg*, **170:**759, 1969.

Forde, K. A., and Ganepola, A. P.: Is Mandatory Exploration for Penetrating Abdominal Trauma Extinct? The Morbidity and Mortality of Negative Exploration in a Large Municipal Hospital, *J Trauma*, **14(9):**764, 1974.

Freeark, R. J.: Role of Angiography in the Management of Multiple Injuries, *Surg Gynecol Obstet*, **128:**761, 1969.

Fullen, W. D., McDonough, J. J., Popp, M. J., and Altemeier, W. A.: Sternal Splitting Approach for Major Hepatic or Retrohepatic Vena Cava Injury, *J Trauma*, **14(11):**903, 1974.

———, Selle, J. G., Whitely, D. H., Martin, L. W., and Altemeier, W. A.: Intramural Duodenal Hematoma, *Ann Surg*, **179:**549, 1974.

Giddings, W. P., and McDaniel, J. R.: Wounds of the Jejunum and Ileum, in "Surgery of World War II," chap. 19, Office of the Surgeon General, Washington, 1955.

——— and Wolff, L. H.: Penetrating Wounds of the Stomach, Duodenum, and Small Intestine, *Surg Clin North Am*, **38:**1605, 1958.

Graham, A. S.: Penetrating Wounds of the Colon, *Surg Clin*, 1960, p. 1639.

Haddad, G. H., Pizzi, W. F., Fleishmann, E. P., and Moynahan, J. M.: Abdominal Signs and Sinograms as Dependable Criteria for the Selective Management of Stabwounds of the Abdomen, *Ann Surg*, **172:**61, 1970.

Hinshaw, D. B., Turner, G. R., and Carter, R.: Transection of the Common Bile Duct Caused by Nonpenetrating Trauma, *Am J Surg*, **104:**104, 1962.

Jones, R. C., and Shires, G. T.: The Management of Pancreatic Injuries, *Arch Surg*, **90:**502, 1965.

———, McClelland, R. N., Zedlitz, W. H., and Shires, G. T.: Difficult Closures of the Duodenal Stump, *Arch Surg*, **94:**696, 1967.

——— and Shires, G. T.: Pancreatic Trauma, *Arch Surg*, **102:**424, 1971.

Jordan, G. L., Burns, G. R., and Howell, J. F.: Surgical Management of Pancreatic Injuries, *Am J Trauma*, **1:**32, 1940.

King, J. C.: Trauma to the Abdominal and Retroperitoneal Viscera As It Concerns the Radiologist, *Southern Med J*, **49:**109, 1956.

Kobold, E. E., and Thal, A. P.: A Simple Method for the Management of Experimental Wounds of the Duodenum, *Surg Gynecol Obstet*, **116:**340, 1963.

Lauritzen, G. K.: Subcutaneous Retroperitoneal Duodenal Rupture, *Acta Chir Scand*, **96:**97, 1947.

Lavenson, G. S., and Cohen, A.: Management of Rectal Injuries, *Am J Surg*, **122:**226, 1971.

Ledgerwood, A. M., Kazmers, M., and Lucas, C. E.: The Role of Thoracic Aortic Occlusion for Massive Hemoperitoneum, *J Trauma*, **16(8):**610, 1976.

Letton, A. H., and Wilson, J. P.: Traumatic Severance of Pancreas Treated by Roux-y Anastomosis, *Surg Gynecol Obstet*, **109:**473, 1959.

Lim, R. C., Glickman, M. G., and Hunt, T. K.: Angiography in Patients with Blunt Trauma to the Chest and Abdomen, *Surg Clin North Am*, **52(3):**551, 1972.

LoCicero, J., III, Tajima, T., and Drapanas, T.: A Half-Century of Experience in the Management of Colon Injuries: Changing Concepts, *J Trauma*, **15(7):**575, 1975.

Lucas, C. E.: What Is the Role of Biliary Drainage in Liver Trauma? *Am J Surg*, **120:**509, 1970.

——— and Ledgerwood, A. M.: Factors Influencing Outcome after Blunt Duodenal Injury, *J Trauma*, **15(10):**839, 1975.

——— and ———: Prospective Evaluation of Hemostatic Techniques for Liver Injuries, *J Trauma*, **16(6):**442, 1976.

——— and Walt, A. J.: Analysis of Randomized Biliary Drainage for Liver Trauma in 189 Patients, *J Trauma*, **12(11):**925, 1972.

———, Canizaro, P. C., and Shires, G. T.: Repair of Hepatic Venous Intrahepatic Vena Caval and Portal Venous Injuries, in Madding, G. F. and Kennedy, P. A., "Trauma to the Liver," 2d ed., Saunders, Philadelphia, 1971, chap. 10, pp. 146–153.

McClelland, R. N., and Shires, T.: Management of Liver Trauma in 259 Consecutive Patients, *Ann Surg*, **161:**248, 1965.

———, ———, and Poulos, E.: Hepatic Resection for Massive Trauma, *J Trauma*, **4:**282, 1964.

McInnis, W. D., Aust, J. B., Cruz, A. B., and Root, H. D.: Traumatic Injuries of the Duodenum: A Comparison of 1° Closure and the Jejunal Patch, *J Trauma*, **15(10):**847, 1975.

Madding, G. F., Lawrence, K. B., and Kennedy, P. A.: War Wounds of the Liver, *Tex J Med*, **42:**267, 1946.

Mattox, K. L., Espada, R., and Beall, A. C., Jr.: Traumatic Injury to the Portal Vein, *Ann Surg*, **181:**519, 1975.

Maynard, A. L., and Oropeza, G.: Mandatory Operation for Penetrating Wounds of the Abdomen, *Am J Surg*, **115:**307, 1968.

Mays, E. T.: Lobar Dearterialization for Exsanguinating Wounds of the Liver, *J Trauma*, **12(5):**397, 1972.

Merendino, K. A., Dillard, D. H., and Cammock, E. E.: The Concept of Surgical Biliary Decompression in the Management of Liver Trauma, *Surg Gynecol Obstet*, **117:**285, 1963.

Miller, D. R.: Median Sternotomy Extension of Abdominal Incision for Hepatic Lobectomy, *Ann Surg*, **175:**193, 1972.

Moretz, J. A., III, Campbell, D. P., Parker, D. E., and Williams, G. R.: Significance of Serum Amylase Level in Evaluating Pancreatic Trauma, *Am J Surg*, **130:**739, 1975.

Morgenstern, L.: Microcrystalline Collagen Used in Experimental Splenic Injury: A New Surface Hemostatic Agent, *Arch Surg*, **109:**44, 1974.

Morton, J. R., and Jordan, G. L.: Traumatic Duodenal Injuries: Review of 131 Cases, *J Trauma*, **8(2):**127, 1968.

Naffziger, H. C., and McCorkle, H. J.: Recognition and Management of Acute Trauma to Pancreas with Particular Reference to Use of Serum Amylase Test, *Ann Surg*, **118:**594, 1943.

Nance, F. C., and Cohn, I., Jr.: Surgical Judgment in the Management of Stab Wounds of the Abdomen: A Retrospective and Prospective Analysis Based on a Study of 600 Stabbed Patients, *Ann Surg*, **170:**569, 1969.

———, Wennar, M. H., Johnson, L. W., Ingram, J. C., and Cohn, I., Jr.: Surgical Judgment in the Management of Penetrating Wounds of the Abdomen: Experience with 2212 Patients, *Ann Surg*, **179:**639, 1974.

Naylor, R., Coln, D., Shire, G. T.: Morbidity and Mortality from Injuries to the Spleen, *J Trauma*, **14(9):**773, 1974.

Northrup, W. F., III, and Simmons, R. L.: Pancreatic Trauma: A Review, *Surgery,* **71(1):**27, 1972.

Ochsner, J. L.: Discussion of Buscaglia, L. C., Blaisdell, W., and Lim, R. C.: Penetrating Abdominal Vascular Injuries, *Arch Surg,* **99:**764, 1969.

———, Crawford, E. S., and DeBakey, M. E.: Injuries of the Vena Cava Caused by External Trauma, *Surgery,* **49:**397, 1961.

Olsen, W. R.: The Serum Amylase in Blunt Abdominal Trauma, *J Trauma,* **13(3):**200, 1973.

——— and Polley, T. Z., Jr.: A Second Look at Delayed Splenic Rupture, *Arch Surg,* **112:**422, 1977.

———, Redman, H. C., and Hildreth, D. H.: Quantitative Peritoneal Lavage in Blunt Abdominal Trauma, *Arch Surg,* **104:**536, 1972.

O'Mara, R. E., Hall, R. C., and Dombroski, D. L.: Scintiscanning in the Diagnosis of Rupture of the Spleen, *Surg Gynecol Obstet,* **131:**1077, 1970.

Parvin, S., Smith, D. E., Asher, W. M., and Virgilio, R. W.: Effectiveness of Peritoneal Lavage in Blunt Abdominal Trauma, *Ann Surg,* **181:**255, 1975.

Pellegrini, J. N., and Stein, I. J.: Complete Severance of the Pancreas and Its Treatment with Repair of the Main Pancreatic Duct of Wirsung, *Am J Surg,* **101:**707, 1961.

Perry, J. F., Jr., DeMeules, J. E., and Root, H. D.: Diagnostic Peritoneal Lavage in Blunt Abdominal Trauma, *Surg Gynecol Obstet,* **131:**742–743, 1970.

——— and LaFave, J. W.: Biliary Decompression without Other External Drainage in Treatment of Liver Injuries, *Surgery,* **55:**351, 1964.

Perry, M. O., Thal, E. R., and Shires, G. T.: Management of Arterial Injuries, *Ann Surg,* **173:**403, 1971.

Pinkerton, J. A., Sawyers, J. L., and Foster, J. H.: A Study of the Postoperative Course after Hepatic Lobectomy, *Ann Surg,* **173:**800, 1971.

Printen, K. J., Freeark, R. J., and Shoemaker, W. C.: Conservative Management of Penetrating Abdominal Wounds, *Arch Surg,* **96:**899, 1968.

Quast, D. C., and Jordan, G. L.: Traumatic Wounds of the Female Reproductive Organs, *J Trauma,* **4:**839, 1964.

———, Shirkey, A. L., Fitzgerald, J. B., Beall, A. C., and DeBakey, M. E.: Surgical Correction of Injuries of the Vena Cava: An Analysis of Sixty-one Cases, *J Trauma,* **5:**3, 1965.

Reich, W. J., and Nechtow, M. J.: Ligation of the Internal Iliac (Hypogastric Arteries): A Life-saving Procedure for Uncontrollable Gynecologic and Obstetric Hemorrhage, *J Intern Coll Surg,* **36:**167, 1961.

Reinhardt, G. F., and Hubay, C. A.: Surgical Management of Traumatic Hemobilia, *Am J. Surg,* **121:**328, 1971.

Resnicoff, S. A., Morton, J. H., and Bloch, A. L.: Retroperitoneal Rupture of the Duodenum Due to Blunt Trauma, *Surg Gynecol Obstet,* **125:**77, 1967.

Richie, J. P., and Fonkalsrud, E. W.: Subcapsular Hematoma of the Liver, *Arch Surg,* **104:**781, 1972.

Roof, W. R., Morris, G. C., and DeBakey, M. E.: Management of Perforating Injuries to the Colon in Civilian Practice, *Am J Surg,* **99:**641, 1960.

Root, H. D., Hauser, C. W., McKinley C. R., LaFave, J. W., and Mendiola, R. P., Jr.: Diagnostic Peritoneal Lavage, *Surgery,* **57:**633, 1965.

Rosoff, L., Cohen, J. L., Telfer, N., and Halpern, M.: Injuries of the Spleen, *Surg Clin North Am,* **52(3):**667, 1972.

Rydell, W. B., Jr.: Complete Transection of the Common Bile Duct Due to Blunt Abdominal Trauma, *Arch Surg,* **100:**724, 1970.

Ryzoff, R. I., Shaftan, G. W., and Herbsman, H.: Selective Conservatism in Abdominal Trauma, *Surgery,* **59:**650, 1966.

Salyer, K., and McClelland, R. N.: Pancreaticoduodenectomy for Trauma, *Arch Surg,* **95:**636, 1967.

Schrock, T., Blaisdell, F. W., and Mathewson, C.: Management of Blunt Trauma to the Liver and Hepatic Veins, *Arch Surg,* **96:**698, 1968.

——— and Christensen, N.: Management of Perforating Injuries of the Colon, *Surg Gynecol Obstet,* **135:**65, 1972.

Schwartz, S. I., Adams, J. T., Cockett, A. T. K., and Morton, J. H.: Blunt Trauma to the Upper Abdomen, *Surg Annu,* **3:**273, 1971.

Seavers, R., Lynch, J., Ballard, R., Jernigan, S., and Johnson, J.: Hypogastric Artery Ligation for Uncontrollable Hemorrhage in Acute Pelvic Trauma, *Surgery,* **55:**516, 1964.

Shaftan, G. W.: Indications for Operation in Abdominal Trauma, *Am J Surg,* **99:**657, 1960.

Sheldon, G. F., Cohn, L., and Blaisdell, W.: Surgical Treatment of Pancreatic Trauma, *J Trauma,* **10:**795, 1970.

Shires, G. T., Jackson, D., and Williams, J.: Temporary Duodenal Decompression as an Adjunct to Gastric Resection for Duodenal Ulcer, *Am Surg,* **28:**709, 1962.

Singer, D. B.: Postsplenectomy Sepsis, in H. S. Rosenberg and R. P. Bolande (eds.), "Perspectives in Pediatric Pathology," vol. 1, pp. 285–3111, Year Book Medical Publishers, Inc., Chicago, 1973.

Smiley, K., and Perry, M. O.: Balloon Catheter Tamponade of Major Vascular Wounds, *Am J Surg,* **121:**326, 1971.

Smith, A. D., Jr., Woolverton, W. C., Weichert, R. F., and Drapanas, T.: Operative Management of Pancreatic and Duodenal Injuries, *J Trauma,* **11:**570, 1971.

Smithwick, W., III, Gertner, H. R., Jr., and Zuidema, G. D.: Injection of Hypaque (Sodium Diatrizoate) in the Management of Abdominal Stab Wounds, *Surg Gynecol Obstet,* **127:**1215, 1968.

Sparkman, R. S.: Massive Hemobilia following Traumatic Rupture of the Liver, *Ann Surg,* **138:**899, 1953.

Sperling, L., and Rigler, L. G.: Traumatic Retroperitoneal Rupture of Duodenum: Description of Valuable Roentgen Observation in Its Recognition, *Radiology,* **29:**521, 1937.

Starzl, T. E., Kaupp, H. A., Beheler, E. M., and Freeark, R. J.: Penetrating Injuries of the Inferior Vena Cava, *Surg Clin North Am,* **43:**387, 1963.

Sturmer, F. C., and Wilt, K. E.: Complete Division of the Common Duct from External Blunt Trauma, *Am J Surg,* **105:**781, 1963.

Thal, E. R.: Evaluation of Peritoneal Lavage and Local Exploration in Lower Chest and Abdominal Stabwounds, *J Trauma,* **17:**642, 1977.

——— and Saretsky, N.: Negative Laparotomy, Morbidity, Mortality and Rationale. (In preparation.)

——— and Shires, G. T.: Peritoneal Lavage in Blunt Abdominal Trauma, *Am J Surg,* **125:**64, 1973.

Travers, B.: Rupture of Pancreas, *Lancet,* **12:**384, 1827.

Trunkey, D., Hays, R. J., and Shires, G. T.: Management of Rectal Trauma, *J Trauma,* **13(5):**411, 1973.

————, Shires, G. T., and McClelland, R. N.: Management of Liver Trauma in 811 Consecutive Patients, *Ann Surg,* **179(5):**522, 1974.

Turpin, I., State, D., and Schwartz, A.: Injuries to the Inferior Vena Cava and Their Management, *Am J Surg,* **134:**25, 1977.

Vannix, R. S., Carter, R., Hinshaw, D. B., and Joergensen, E. J.: Surgical Management of Colon Trauma in Civilian Practice, *Am J Surg,* **106:**364, 1963.

Weckerson, E. C., and Putman, T. C.: Perforating Injuries of the Rectum and Sigmoid Colon, *J Trauma,* **2:**474, 1962.

Weichert, R. F., III, Hewitt, R. L., and Drapanas, T.: Blunt Injuries to Intrahepatic Vena Cava and Hepatic Veins with Survival, *Am J Surg,* **121:**322, 1971.

Werschky, L. R., and Jordan, G. L.: Surgical Management of Traumatic Injuries to the Pancreas, *Am J Surg,* **116:**768, 1968.

White, P. H., and Benfield, J. R.: Amylase in the Management of Pancreatic Trauma, *Arch Surg,* **105:**158, 1972.

Whitesell, F. B.: A Clinical and Surgical Anatomic Study of Rupture of the Spleen Due to Blunt Trauma, *Surg Gynecol Obstet,* **110:**750, 1960.

Wilder, J. R., Habermann, E. T., and Schachner, S. J.: Selective Surgical Intervention for Stab Wounds of the Abdomen, *Surgery,* **61:**231, 1967.

————, Lotfi, M. W., and Jurani, P.: Comparative Study of Mandatory and Selective Surgical Intervention in Stab Wounds of the Abdomen, *Surgery,* **69:**546, 1971.

Williams, R. D., and Sargent, F. T.: The Mechanism of Intestinal Injury in Trauma, *J Trauma,* **3:**288, 1963.

———— and Zollinger, R. M.: Diagnostic and Prognostic Factors in Abdominal Trauma, *Am J Surg,* **97:**575, 1959.

Witek, J. T., Spencer, R. P., Pearson, H. A., and Touloukian, R. J.: Diagnostic Spleen Scans in Occult Splenic Injury, *J Trauma,* **14:**197, 1974.

Yajko, R. D., Seydel, F., and Trimble, C.: Rupture of the Stomach from Blunt Abdominal Trauma, *J Trauma,* **15(3):**177, 1975.

Yellin, A. E., Chaffee, C. B., and Donovan, A. J.: Vascular Isolation in Treatment of Juxtahepatic Venous Injuries, *Arch Surg,* **102:**566, 1971.

———— and Rosoff, L., Sr.: Pancreatoduodenectomy for Combined Pancreatoduodenal Injuries, *Arch Surg,* **110:**1177, 1975.

————, Vecchione, T. R., and Donovan, A. J.: Distal Pancreatectomy for Pancreatic Trauma, *Am J Surg,* **124:**135, 1972.

Burns

by P. William Curreri

The complex pathophysiologic alterations which accompany major thermal injury present the surgeon with an extraordinary therapeutic challenge. During the past two decades, few areas of medical science have experienced more rapid development of new treatment modalities. As a result, marked improvement in the care of patients with major burn injury has been noted. Comprehensive treatment centers now utilize sophisticated, multidisciplinary teams to aid in the diagnosis of rapidly changing physiologic responses to the injury and to assist in providing the vast array of specialized therapeutic services which are necessary to minimize morbidity and mortality.

Burn injury constitutes a major national health problem. More than 2,000,000 persons suffer thermal injury annually, of whom 70,000 must be hospitalized. As in other types of trauma, thermal injury frequently afflicts children and young adults. Prolonged morbidity, as well as temporary or permanent disability, associated with thermal injury results in a staggering economic drain on social resources. Financial support is often required to defray expenses associated with prolonged hospitalization, loss of family income sources, and replacement of lost manpower within the working force.

ETIOLOGY OF BURNS

Burns are caused by the application of heat to the body. The depth of the resulting burn injury will be dependent on the intensity and duration of heat application and the conductivity of the tissues involved. The most common heat sources are an open flame and hot liquid. In addition, thermal injury is frequently observed in patients who have been exposed to direct contact with hot metal, toxic chemicals, or high-voltage electric current. Damage as a result of heat rarely occurs below 45°C. Between 45 and 50°C, gradations of cell injury may occur; and above 50°C, denaturation of protein elements of the cell becomes apparent.

Laboratory accidents, civilian assaults, industrial mishaps, and inexpert application of agents used for medical purposes account for most of the chemical burns in the civilian population. A principal difference between thermal and chemical injury is the length of time during which tissue destruction continues, since the chemical agent causes progressive damage until inactivated by reaction with tissue, while thermal injury ceases shortly after removal of the heat source. Tissue destruction associated with exposure to chemicals may be limited by the application of neutralizing agents or by dilution with water. When compared to thermal injury, the severe, full-thickness chemical burn may appear deceptively superficial, with only mild bronze discoloration of intact skin during the first few postburn days.

In contrast to both thermal and chemical burns, electrical injury usually results in minimal destruction of skin. The magnitude of the injury is directly related to the amount of current passing through tissue between the point of contact with the electrical source and the exit site at which the patient is grounded. The magnitude of current passing through various organs is indirectly related to the resistance of the tissue. Nerve, blood, and muscle offer the least resistance to electric current and thus sustain the maximum amount of tissue damage. As a result, cutaneous injury may be apparent only at the entrance and exit sites, although considerable deep tissue destruction of upper and lower extremity musculature may be present. The electrical resistance of skin is markedly reduced by moisture. Thus small burns in the antecubital space or the axilla often are observed in the patient with severe electrical injury of the upper extremity. These burns result from the arcing of current across the joint through skin moistened with perspiration. When arc burns are present, they are nearly always accompanied by extensive, deep muscular destruction. Thermal injury to musculature is frequently associated with release of hemachromagens into the bloodstream which are subsequently excreted via the urinary tract. Thus "port wine"–colored urine containing myoglobin is not unusual following major electrical injury.

IMMEDIATE THERAPY

Initial therapy of the patient with a major burn should be directed toward restoration of normal physiologic parameters and prevention of life-threatening complications. With the exception of chemical burns, in which the toxic agent must be diluted with water and physically removed as rapidly as possible to prevent further tissue destruction, the burn wound is of secondary importance during the first few hours after the injury.

Maintenance of Airway

Immediate pulmonary complications may become manifest in the thermally injured patient. Excessive exposure to smoke may result in carbon monoxide poisoning. Patients exhibit the signs and symptoms of hypoxia, which may range from pronounced tachypnea and agitation to respiratory arrest and coma. The diagnosis may be quickly confirmed by analyzing the concentration of carboxyhemoglobin in the blood. Treatment includes the administration of 100% oxygen, with ventilatory support if necessary, in order to displace the tightly bound carbon monoxide from the hemoglobin molecule. Since carbon monoxide is not toxic to lungs per se, the syndrome is entirely reversible, provided anoxic damage to distant tissues (e.g., the central nervous system) has not occurred. Although several decades ago few patients with severe carbon monoxide poisoning survived long enough to reach the emergency room, the development of sophisticated paramedical teams trained to insert endotracheal tubes and administer ventilatory support in the field has allowed greater salvage of such patients in the last several years.

Upper airway obstruction in patients with burns of the head and neck may occur during the first 48 hours after injury. The obstruction is related to soft tissue edema of the oral pharynx and vocal cords following exposure to hot gases. Direct thermal injury to the lower respiratory tract is exceedingly unusual, since the nose and oral pharynx are extremely efficient heat exchangers, allowing cooling of inhaled hot gas prior to its entrance into the trachea. Since it is more difficult to extract heat from liquid, direct thermal injury of the lower respiratory tract is occasionally noted in patients injured by superheated steam.

Upper airway obstruction is usually heralded by an increase in the respiratory rate and progressive hoarseness. In addition, a patient may exhibit increased difficulty in clearing bronchial secretions as the vocal cords become more edematous. Confirmation of impending obstruction is made by direct visualization of the posterior oral pharynx and cords, utilizing either direct laryngoscopy or fiberoptic endoscopy. The latter is usually preferred, since at the same time, assessment of smoke inhalation may be accomplished by visualizing the lower respiratory tract.

Impending upper airway obstruction is treated by the immediate insertion of an endotracheal tube. Soft tissue edema is maximal at between 24 and 48 hours. Therefore the endotracheal tube is usually not removed until the third postburn day, since reintubation often is technically difficult to perform.

Intravenous Resuscitation

Cardiovascular alterations occur almost immediately following burn injury. There is a massive shift of fluid and electrolytes from the intravascular and extracellular fluid space into the cells. Reversion of water and sodium from the intracellular fluid back into the extracellular fluid begins between 24 and 48 hours but is not complete until the tenth postburn day. In general, these changes are directly proportional to the extent and depth of burn. Therefore any consideration of fluid resuscitation to prevent hypovolemic shock requires an accurate estimation of the magnitude of burn injury. The burned wound is three-dimensional, therefore not only the depth but the surface area involved must be estimated.

Burns are classified as first, second, or third degree (Table 7-1). First-degree burns are characterized by simple erythema of the skin, with only microscopic destruction of superficial layers of the epidermis. A mild sunburn is characteristic of a first-degree injury. The first-degree injury is of little clinical significance, since the water barrier of the skin is not disturbed. Systemic cardiovascular disturbances are rarely observed following first-degree burn injury. The burns rapidly heal if the patient avoids further exposure to a heat source. First-degree burns are *not* considered when estimating the magnitude of burn injury for purposes of planning intravenous fluid replacement.

Second- and third-degree burns are of equal physiologic significance and may be summated in the estimate of total body surface burn injury. Second-degree burns extend through the epidermis into the dermis. By definition, viable epithelial elements from which epithelial regeneration can occur are retained in second-degree burn injury; thus the burn is often described as *partial-thickness*. Even when most of the epithelium is destroyed, regeneration may occur from epithelial cells surrounding hair follicles or sweat glands. On the other hand, third-degree burns are characterized by total irreversible destruction of all the

Table 7-1. CLASSIFICATION OF BURNS

Classification	Morphology	Clinical appearance	Cause
First degree.	Only superficial layers of epidermis devitalized; dilatation and congestion of intradermal vessels.	Erythema only—blanches on pressure.	Ultraviolet exposure (ultraviolet light, sunburn), very short flash
Second degree	Destruction of varying depths of epidermis with coagulation necrosis; clefting of epidermis with fluid collection (blister formation); congestion and coagulation in subdermal plexus. Some skin elements remain viable (often only skin appendages), from which epithelial regeneration can occur.*	Erythematous, weeping, painful. Blisters and bullae often present. Superficial layers of skin can be readily wiped away. Remaining skin elements waxy white, soft, dry, insensitive.	Short flash, spill scald
Third degree	Destruction of all skin elements; coagulation of subdermal plexus.	Dry, hard, inelastic, translucent, with thrombosed vein visible.	Flame, immersion scald, chemical contact, electric current

*Initial injury may be partial-thickness, with only dermal appendages (hair follicles and glands) remaining, but these skin elements are readily destroyed by infection, with resulting conversion to full-thickness (third-degree) burn.

skin, dermal appendages, and epithelial elements. Spontaneous regeneration of epithelium is not possible, and the burns are described as *full-thickness.* Such burns require the application of skin grafts if the development of scar tissue is to be avoided.

Since skin varies in thickness in different parts of the body, application of the same intensity of heat for a given period of time will result in a burn which will vary in depth, depending on the thickness of the skin itself in the local area, as well as the existence and degree of development of the dermal appendages (sweat glands and hair follicles) and dermal papillae. In the very old person, in whom dermal papillae and appendages are atrophic, and in the very young, in whom they have not yet fully developed, deep burns result from the same heat intensity that produces a moderate second-degree burn in the middle-aged adult. Since the skin of the back is thicker than that on any other part of the body, full-thickness burns are less common in this area. On the other hand, skin covering the inner arm is extraordinarily thin, thus full-thickness injury is frequently observed in this area.

The length and width of the burn wound is expressed as a percentage of the total body surface area displaying either second- or third-degree burns. The extent of the body surface involved is most commonly estimated by the "rule of nines" (Table 7-2). The major anatomic portions of the adult may be divided into multiples of 9 percent of the body surface area. The proportion of each of these areas with second- or third degree burns is estimated, and the summation of these estimates represents the percentage of the total body surface area burn. Because the surface area of the head and neck in childhood is significantly larger than 9 percent of the total body surface area and the surface area associated with the lower extremities is

smaller, the rule of nines may not be used to estimate total body surface area burns in children. For example, a one-year-old child has 19 percent of the total body surface area associated with the head, as compared to only 7 percent in the adult patient. In contrast, each lower extremity represents only 13 percent of the total body surface area in the year-old infant. Thus the total body surface area burn in children is best estimated by the utilization of charts which relate regional body surface to age.

Over the past 20 years, many resuscitation formulas have been developed as guides to initial resuscitation in hypovolemic shock following thermal injury. Most utilize various combinations of crystalloid and colloid solutions but differ widely in the ratio of colloid to crystalloid, as well as the rate of fluid administration. The ideal resuscitation formula would rapidly restore normal hemodynamic stability. However, such a response is dependent on the rate at which fluid is lost from the extracellular fluid compartment, the composition of the fluid lost, and the ability of various solutions to restore an effective circulating extra-

Table 7-2. "RULE OF NINES" FOR ESTIMATING PERCENTAGE OF BODY SURFACE INVOLVED IN BURNS

Anatomic area	Percent of body surface
Head	9
Right upper extremity	9
Left upper extremity	9
Right lower extremity	18
Left lower extremity	18
Anterior trunk	18
Posterior trunk	18
Neck	1

cellular volume. Unfortunately, most formulas have been derived empirically from clinical experience, in which the amount of fluid required to restore renal function was accepted as optimal replacement therapy.

Although much controversy still remains over "the solution" for resuscitation in burn shock, scientific investigation supports the need for both crystalloid and colloid solutions. *It is of relatively little consequence which formula is utilized to begin such therapy, as long as this is modified according to the patient's changing requirements.* The formula shown in Table 7-3 has been popularized by Baxter and is known as the "Parkland formula." This formula has been adopted in most burn centers and is currently the standard against which new formulas must be compared. Data from numerous studies now suggest that both volume and the sodium ion are critical to providing adequate resuscitation in hypovolemic burn shock. Administration of crystalloid solution results in early expansion of depleted plasma and extracellular fluid volumes and return of the cardiac output toward normal. After 24 hours, colloid remains the most effective solution to maintain plasma volume without further increasing edema formation. The Parkland formula was derived to provide specific replacement of known deficits measured by simultaneous determinations of red cell volume, plasma volume, extracellular fluid volume, and cardiac output during burn shock. The formula calls for the administration of 4 ml of lactated Ringer's solution/kg of body weight/percent of body surface area burn during the first 24 hours postinjury. Fluid therapy during the second 24 hours, according to this formula, consists in the administration of free water (5% dextrose in water) in quantities sufficient to maintain the serum sodium concentration at 140 mEq/L (approximately 4 to 5 liters in a 70-kg patient with a 50 percent burn) and plasma sufficient to return the plasma volume to normal and sustain adequate perfusion of peripheral organs and tissues (approximately 250 ml for each 10 percent total body surface area burn over 20 percent). Potassium replacement is required to replace increased urinary losses associated with both the resuscitation and the subsequent catabolic state.

During the first 24 hours, the rate of fluid administration is adjusted to correspond as closely as possible with the rate of extracellular fluid loss. Baxter's studies have confirmed that extracellular deficits occur rapidly within the first 6 to

12 hours postinjury. Therefore one-half of the total calculated fluid volume is delivered during the first 8 hours *from the time of injury* and the remaining fluids more slowly over the next 16 hours.

The adequacy of resuscitation can best be judged by frequent measurements of vital signs, central venous pressure, hourly urine output, and observation of general mental and physical response. Urine output (normal, 30 to 100 ml/hour in the adult) still remains one of the most reliable guides to adequacy of fluid therapy. Acute tubular necrosis, with resultant renal failure, is extremely rare in an adequately resuscitated patient, with the possible exception of a patient in whom there is extensive muscle damage (electrical burns) resulting in hemachromogen release and intratubular protein precipitation. Therefore oliguria during the early postburn period is most often an indication of inadequate resuscitation, and increased fluid administration is the treatment of choice. Restriction of fluid is almost never indicated, and the administration of diuretics should be reserved for those cases in which tubular damage from circulating pigments appears likely, and then only after a sufficient amount of resuscitation fluids has been administered.

Urinary outputs of 30 to 100 ml/hour should be maintained during the first 24 hours in the adult patient. In the absence of hypoxia related to respiratory dysfunction, the patient's sensorium accurately reflects cerebral circulation. Well-resuscitated patients with major thermal injury rarely display hysteria, acute anxiety, or hostility.

Sedation

One of the most frequent therapeutic errors in the treatment of patients with major burns is the overuse of sedation. An insignificant burn of a minute area incurred during a common household mishap may be quite painful. Projection of such an experience by medical and paramedical personnel has resulted in marked overestimation of the pain associated with a major burn. If there is full-thickness skin destruction, the intrinsic sensory nerve endings have also been destroyed and the wound itself is painless. In contrast, the second-degree burn can be quite painful initially. Therefore the requirement for sedation is inversely proportional to the depth of the initial thermal injury.

Sedation should be kept at an *absolute minimum* to prevent depression of cardiopulmonary function and to allow evaluation of the sensorium, an important indicator of the adequacy of fluid resuscitation. Decreased peripheral circulation to muscle and skin is often associated with the hypovolemic state, so any narcotics administered intramuscularly or subcutaneously are subject to erratic uptake. Therefore narcotics should always be administered in small doses by the intravenous route during the first 4 to 5 days. Administration by this route assures rapid and predictable concentrations of the drug in the central nervous system and prevents the narcosis which may result following fluid resuscitation if repeated doses of narcotics have been administered by the intramuscular route. After 48 hours, the requirements for sedation are markedly reduced, except

Table 7-3. FLUID RESUSCITATION OF BURNED PATIENTS: PARKLAND FORMULA

First 24 Hours:
  Electrolyte solution (lactated Ringer's): 4 ml/kg body wt./% second- and third-degree burn
  Administration rate: $\frac{1}{2}$ first 8 hours, $\frac{1}{4}$ second 8 hours, $\frac{1}{4}$ third 8 hours
  Urine output: 30–70 ml/hr
Second 24 Hours:
  Glucose in water (D_5W): To replace evaporative water loss, maintaining serum sodium concentration of 140 mEq/L
  Colloid solution (plasma): To maintain plasma volume in patients with more than 40% second- and third-degree burns
  Urine output: 30–100 ml/hr

during times when the wound is actively debrided during the waking state.

Antibiotics

Subsequent to thermal injury, microorganisms contaminating the surface of the wound and persisting in the depth of the hair follicles and sweat glands begin to proliferate rapidly if topical chemotherapeutic agents are not applied. In the absence of topical chemotherapy, the superficial areas of the burn wound contain up to 100 million organisms per gram of tissue within 48 hours following injury.

Characteristically, gram-positive organisms are responsible for this initial proliferation and colonization of the burn wound. Therefore most experienced clinicians prophylactically administer penicillin to patients with major burn injuries for a period of 3 to 4 days. Antibiotic treatment with penicillin prevents overgrowth of the gram-positive organisms and has virtually eliminated streptococcal infections, one of the most common causes of death following burn injury 30 years ago. The systemic administration of antibiotics after the fourth postburn day has not resulted in decreased morbidity from infection. Since the full-thickness burn is relatively avascular after 48 hours, the concentration of antibiotic which reaches the burn wound from the bloodstream is inadequate to prevent subsequent gram-negative bacterial colonization. Therefore systemic antibiotics are not usually administered after the fourth postburn day unless a specific distant bacterial infection (e.g., pneumonia) has complicated the burn.

Tetanus Prophylaxis

All burn injuries must be considered contaminated, and tetanus prophylaxis is mandatory except in those patients actively immunized within the preceding 12 months. If a booster was received within the preceding 10 years, the intramuscular administration of 0.5 ml of absorbed tetanus toxoid will usually provide adequate prophylaxis. In the absence of active immunization within 10 years prior to the burn injury, 250 to 500 units of tetanus immunogobulin (human) should be simultaneously administered at another site, utilizing a different syringe and needle so as to prevent inactivation of the immune globulin by toxoid.

Escharotomy

A principal characteristic of human skin is a remarkable degree of elasticity, which allows the skin to stretch with only minimum applied force. The elasticity of skin allows considerable edema of underlying soft tissues without increasing central limb pressure, which might impede either venous outflow or arterial inflow. If the skin were unyielding, a patient with a severely sprained ankle might lose blood flow to the distal foot as soft tissue edema occurred. Skin with second-degree injury retains its elastic properties. However, full-thickness injury (third degree) is characterized by almost complete loss of elasticity. Thus circumferential third-degree burns are frequently associated with decreased peripheral blood flow as fluid resuscitation, ac-

companied by soft tissue edema, progresses. Failure to recognize this situation may result in unnecessary loss of distal extremities.

The usual clinical signs associated with poor peripheral blood flow in the nonburned patient, that is, diminished peripheral pulses and decreased skin temperature, are unreliable in patients with severe thermal injury. Hypovolemia with peripheral vasoconstriction usually results in decreased temperature of distal extremities in all patients with major second- and third-degree burns, and distal pulses often may not be felt as a result of overlying soft tissue edema preventing palpation of the underlying artery. More reliable signs of decreased peripheral flow in patients with circumferential third-degree burns are slow capillary refill (observed in the nail beds) and the onset of neurologic deficits. The most accurate monitoring device for assessing distal blood flow to extremities is the ultrasonic Doppler, which allows repetitive evaluation of both venous and arterial flow in the digital arteries and veins.

Patients with circumferential third-degree burns of the extremities should be encouraged to actively exercise those extremities in order to maintain patency of the small venules. In addition, the extremities should be elevated in order to promote venous and lymphatic drainage and minimize soft tissue edema. However, should vascular impairment become apparent, escharotomies should immediately be performed. An escharotomy is simply an incision through the full depth of the skin, allowing the eschar to separate, thus relieving underlying pressure on the central arteries and veins. These incisions may be performed without anesthesia, since third-degree burns are anesthetic. Blood loss is minimal because of the extensive intracapillary coagulation which has occurred as a result of the thermal injury. The escharotomies are usually performed on the lateral and medial aspects of the extremity and must be carried across the joints, since the skin is most tightly adherent to the underlying fascia at these points and vascular obstruction is most likely to occur in these areas. In the upper extremity, the escharotomy should extend through all areas of third-degree burn down to and including the thenar and hypothenar spaces, in order to preserve the intrinsic muscles of the hand. Similarly, in the lower extremities, escharotomies should extend to the base of the large and small toes if the foot exhibits extensive third-degree burns.

Fasciotomy, that is, linear excision of the deep fascia surrounding the muscles, is rarely indicated in patients with severe burns. In rare instances of extensive incineration when burns involve not only the skin but the underlying fat and muscle, fasciotomy becomes necessary as a result of swelling within the muscle compartments. More frequently, fasciotomy is required in the treatment of electrical burns where there has been extensive muscle injury which appears potentially reversible.

Gastric Decompression

Most patients with more than 20 percent total body surface area burns will develop a reflex paralytic ileus some time during the first 24 hours. Although bowel sounds are usually active for 6 to 10 hours following the injury, intestinal motility is gradually lost for a short period of time during the latter half of the first 24 hours. Unfortunately, the development of ileus frequently occurs at the time when medical and nursing surveillance has relaxed and the patient is asleep following sedation and restoration of fluid volume. Vomiting in such a patient carries a high risk of pulmonary aspiration, a complication which is associated with severe morbidity and high mortality. For this reason, patients with major burns require placement of a nasogastric tube, in order that the stomach may be effectively decompressed until normal gastrointestinal motility has been demonstrated.

The insertion of a nasogastric tube will also serve to allow inspection of the gastric contents at periodic intervals. Patients with major burns are at risk of hemorrhagic gastritis as a result of increased stress. For this reason, gastric aspirates should be monitored frequently for the presence of frank blood or guaiac-positive material, and antacid should be instilled through the nasogastric tube at hourly intervals to prevent superficial erosions of the gastric mucosa.

Medical Evacuation

Although most hospitals are equipped to provide emergency therapy of the patient with a major burn, the majority of community hospitals have neither the nursing nor the paramedical expertise to comfortably care for a patient with massive burn injury. Furthermore, because of the special physical requirements necessary for optimal treatment of such patients, it is not uncommon for personnel in community hospitals to transfer such patients to special facilities as soon as appropriate arrangements can be made.

Extensive experience with medical evacuation of severely burned soldiers during the Korean and Vietnam wars has yielded valuable information which may assist in assuring safe transfer of burned patients. In general, such patients tolerate evacuation best if they are moved within the first 24 to 48 hours. Prior to transfer, a fluid resuscitation program should be started. Patients with a larger than 20 percent burn should have a Foley catheter inserted into the bladder, so that urinary output can be monitored during the evacuation and fluid administration appropriately adjusted. Pulmonary function should be assessed, and if impending upper airway obstruction or severe smoke inhalation is suspected, an endotracheal tube should be inserted prior to transfer. Extensive debridement or treatment of the burn wounds is unnecessary and is generally to be avoided, since it interferes with evaluation of the burn wound by the receiving hospital. Rather, the wounds should be temporarily wrapped in sterile dressings to provide maximal comfort during the transfer. If air evacuation is to be utilized, it is especially important to insert a nasogastric tube, since air within the stomach will expand at increased altitude, often inducing acute gastric distension and vomiting. This, in turn, could result in aspiration pneumonitis, which would be particularly compromising in a patient with the smoke inhalation syndrome.

THERAPY OF THE BURN WOUND

Debridement and Excision

Second-degree wounds (partial-thickness burn injury) usually present as vesicular lesions. Unless very small, the overlying blister should be punctured and the nonviable skin removed. This permits the direct application of topical chemotherapeutic agents to the underlying viable dermal remnants. Failure to prevent secondary bacterial infection of deep second-degree burn wounds may result in conversion of the partial-thickness injury to a full-thickness injury. Debridement can usually be accomplished without anesthesia, utilizing careful surgical technique and modest amounts of sedation prior to removing the nonviable superficial epithelium.

The nonviable skin of the third-degree burn is referred to as the "eschar." Usually the eschar remains tightly adherent to the underlying subcutaneous tissues and cannot be sharply debrided without severe hemorrhage and significant pain. Therefore, except in special circumstances, only loose eschar, which may be debrided without anesthesia or excessive blood loss, is removed initially. The remaining eschar is left intact, and efforts are made to prevent bacterial colonization and invasion by the use of topical chemotherapeutic agents. Topical chemotherapeutic agents do not sterilize the third-degree burn eschar, and eventually bacterial growth will occur. The topical agents are employed to control the rate of proliferation of bacteria within the burn wound, so as to prevent invasion of underlying viable tissue, with entrance of bacteria into the bloodstream. At about 18 to 24 days following burn injury, the third-degree burn eschar will separate from the underlying viable tissue as a result of the liberation of bacterial proteases. At this time, it is extraordinarily important that the eschar be promptly debrided, in order to prevent systemic sepsis as a result of localized abscess formation beneath the eschar. Normally, the patients are taken to a hydrotherapy area once or twice a day during the first 3 weeks in order to cleanse the surface of the eschar and to inspect the wound. Each day, the physician debrides any loose areas of eschar and carefully inspects the wound and unroofs any localized abscess pockets.

Modern surgical principles dictate the surgical debridement of nonviable tissue in the treatment of major injury. However, in the case of burn injury, immediate total debridement of nonviable eschar has not proved to be a safe procedure because of the extensive hemorrhage associated with major excision of eschar. Some investigators have advocated the use of topical enzyme preparations to more rapidly remove the eschar. The advantages of such an approach include debridement without anesthesia and limitation of associated hemorrhage. However, the efficacy of currently available enzymes has not been conclusively demonstrated. Furthermore, most enzyme preparations require the use of overlying wet dressings to maintain the activity of the enzyme. Such dressings promote wound infection, since they provide a warm, moist environment. In addition, some of the enzyme preparations inhibit the effectiveness of topical chemotherapeutic agents in controlling the rate of proliferation of bacterial growth. Therefore other authors have condemned the use of enzymatic debridement, maintaining that the risks of sepsis far outweigh the benefits of early debridement. In addition, some enzyme preparations do not effectively differentiate nonviable eschar from underlying normal tissues, and erosion of vessels in viable tissue occasionally induces unexpected bleeding from the wound.

Other surgeons have advocated tangential excision to rapidly and safely remove full-thickness eschar. The eschar is tangentially excised, utilizing either a specially designed knife or an air-driven dermatome, to sequentially remove layers of the eschar in sheets of approximately 0.015 inches in thickness until viable tissue, as evidenced by capillary bleeding, is encountered. This procedure can usually be accomplished without anesthesia, since the third-degree burn is anesthetic. The procedure is technically rather difficult after full-thickness removal of skin is accomplished, since the underlying subcutaneous fat does not debride easily at uniform thickness, and viability of the relatively avascular fat is often difficult to appreciate. The exposed subcutaneous fat must be covered with either heterograft or homograft to preserve its integrity, and, unfortunately, adherence of the physiologic dressing is nonuniform.

Several investigators have utilized the carbon dioxide laser to excise third-degree burn eschar. The CO_2 laser allows removal of tissue with relatively little blood loss, and the level of excision can be readily selected by the surgeon. However, the procedure is very slow, because of the limited power which can be generated by the CO_2 laser with safety for both the patient and the operating room personnel. Thus the procedure results in prolonged operating time. Furthermore, the required equipment is expensive and somewhat cumbersome to use. Since the laser beam may cause serious damage to the retina following exposure, operating room personnel must wear protective glasses. Finally, the laser energy is partially dissipated in the underlying viable tissue (the graft recipient site), and the resulting injury to superficial cells may prevent acceptance of heterograft, homograft, and autograft.

When third-degree burns are relatively limited in size (less than 5 percent), as may occur following contact with a hot piece of metal, the full-thickness eschar may be excised primarily under anesthesia without excessive hemorrhage. The wound should be covered immediately with autograft. This approach markedly decreases postburn morbidity and often results in a better cosmetic appearance. Others have now suggested that patients with massive burn injury, that is, more than 70 percent total body surface burns, of which at least 60 percent is third-degree, should undergo early, deep burn wound excision in order to reduce the burn size to a total body surface area which is more compatible with survival. Such procedures should be attempted only in major centers, since this approach is still unproved and requires enormous medical, paramedical, and nursing support. Prior to excision, the burn wound must be sterile or contain only a relatively low concentration of bacteria (less than 10^4 organisms per gram of tissue). Some authors advocate the preoperative infusion of antibiotics by subeschar clysis into the eschar which is to be excised. In this manner, maximum antibiotic concentration is achieved in the relatively avascular eschar, and the chances of seeding the bloodstream during the procedure are presumably reduced. Both the eschar and the underlying subcutaneous fat are excised. The exposed deep fascia must be immediately covered with homograft. Failure to provide immediate physiologic coverage results in desiccation of the fascia and subsequent secondary infection. Thus an unlimited bank of homograft, obtained from cadavers, must be maintained. Furthermore, excision of 20 percent of the total body surface is frequently associated with loss of the patient's complete blood volume. Therefore centers evaluating this approach must have blood banks capable of providing significant quantities of both stored and fresh blood. In some cases, the blood loss has been reduced by utilizing deliberate hypotensive anesthesia during the procedure. Obviously, the operative procedure inflicts great stress on the patient, who already will have evidenced marked pathophysiologic alterations. Extraordinary intensive care support by both physicians and specialized nursing personnel is therefore required postoperatively in the intensive care area.

While most patients are gradually debrided of full-thickness injury over a period of 2 to 3 weeks, patients with electrical injury require more aggressive therapy. Since these patients often have injury to the muscle compartments of the extremities, early surgical exploration, fasciotomy, and removal of nonviable muscle should be performed when motor dysfunction or massive edema of the extremity occurs. If possible, hemodynamic stability should be obtained by the intravenous administration of lactated Ringer's solution prior to operative exploration.

Cutaneous burns resulting from contact with hot tar or asphalt are not infrequently encountered. By the time the physician sees the patient, the tar has solidified on the burn wound as it has cooled. It may be removed by applying generous quantities of Neopolycin ointment to the burn wound, over which a large occlusive dressing is applied. The dressing may be removed 18 to 24 hours later. At this time most or all of the tar will be dissolved, and a water-soluble topical chemotherapeutic agent may be applied.

Topical Chemotherapy

Modern antibacterial topical therapy was advocated by Monafo and Moyer in the early 1960s. These investigators utilized aqueous silver nitrate (0.5%) solution as a continuous wet soak, in combination with large, bulky dressings. The mode of action of silver nitrate is not specifically known but probably depends on the free silver ion, which is active at relatively low concentrations. Silver nitrate is effective against most gram-positive organisms and most strains of *Pseudomonas,* although it has limited effectiveness against other gram-negative bacteria such as *Enterobacter* and *Klebsiella.* The agent sterilizes the surface of the wound but has limited penetration of deeper tissues. Therefore the eschar must be removed rapidly when deep bacterial colonization occurs, in order to prevent invasion of underlying viable tissue. The major complication associated with the use of silver nitrate solution is severe electrolyte depletion (primarily sodium and chloride), necessitating frequent monitoring of serum electrolytes, since specific replacement therapy is required. Silver nitrate therapy has been acclaimed as the most economical topical agent. The drug itself is inexpensive and available in most hospital pharmacies. However, the large quantities of dressings required, the increased nursing personnel requirements to effect the dressing changes, and the major housekeeping problems associated with discoloration caused on contact by precipitation of silver salts, significantly increase the cost of this form of treatment. In addition, the necessity for bulky dressings inhibits the early active movement of extremities and therefore encourages less than optimum joint function.

In the mid-1960s, Lindberg, Moncrief, and Mason introduced mafenide acetate (Sulfamylon), a topically applied cream that allowed open treatment of burn wounds. Mafenide acetate has proved effective against a wide range of gram-positive and gram-negative organisms, as well as most anaerobes. This drug actively diffuses through the eschar, thus providing protection in the depth of the eschar at the interface between the viable and nonviable tissue. Since the burns remain exposed, wounds can be more readily examined. In addition, the treatment does not interfere with intensive physical therapy and allows uninhibited treatment of associated soft tissue injuries. Unfortunately, the drug is a potent inhibitor of carbonic anhydrase and therefore may induce acid-base derangements. Acidosis may develop rapidly in the presence of pulmonary dysfunction. The use of the drug is associated with a pronounced reduction of the buffering capacity of the blood, as a result of increased bicarbonate excretion by the kidney, and simultaneous hypocapnea secondary to hyperventilation. Other disadvantages associated with the use of this drug include pain on application, an occasional hypersensitivity reaction (5 to 7 percent), delayed eschar separation due to improved bacterial control, and the emergence of opportunistic infections, including *Providencia, Serratia,* fungal, yeast, and viral infections.

Silver sulfadiazine (Silvadene), developed by Fox in the late 1960s, has essentially the same bacterial spectrum as mafenide acetate but is associated with fewer disadvantages. The major side effects are hypersensitivity reaction to sulfa (5 to 7 percent), delayed eschar separation, and emergence of opportunistic infections. The agent appears to desiccate the wound less than other topical drugs and consequently keeps the eschar soft, allowing for greater joint mobility. It does not inhibit carbonic anhydrase activity, and its application is soothing rather than painful.

Betadine, a water-soluble topical antiseptic complex of polyvinylpyrrolidone (povidone) iodine, is effective against a wide range of gram-positive and gram-negative organisms, as well as some fungi. The drug is manufactured as an ointment and as an aerosol cream. The drug readily diffuses through the eschar and is absorbed and excreted rapidly. Systemic toxicity is apparently rare. One major disadvantage of this agent is its propensity to cause rapid desiccation of the eschar, resulting in interference with progressive active physical therapy programs. In addition, its application to partial-thickness burns may be associated with mild to moderate pain. This agent has only recently been extensively utilized for the topical therapy of burns and, as in the case of other topical agents, emergence of opportunistic infections may be expected after more extensive experience.

The properties of each of the currently utilized topical chemotherapeutic agents are summarized in Table 7-4. Newer and even more effective topical agents are currently in clinical trial and may be expected to be marketed in the near future. It is important to emphasize that burn wounds treated with these topical agents are not sterilized; rather, the bacterial population is effectively suppressed and remains at levels below that associated with the development of invasive burn wound sepsis. Furthermore, the agents are effective in preventing bacterial conversion of second-degree burns to full-thickness injury, thus reducing the amount of skin grafting which might be required had the agents not been employed.

Table 7-4. PROPERTIES OF TOPICAL CHEMOTHERAPEUTIC AGENTS

Agent	Antibacterial spectrum	Dressings required?	Disadvantages
Sodium mafenide (Sulfamylon)	Gram-positive and gram-negative organisms and most anaerobes	No	Pain on application; skin allergy; carbonic anhydrase inhibition; resistant organisms
Silver nitrate 0.5%	Most gram-positive organisms and some strains of *Pseudomonas*	Yes	Hyponatremia; hypochloremia; failure to penetrate eschar; methemoglobinemia
Silver sulfadiazine (Silvadene)	Gram-positive and gram-negative organisms and *Candida albicans*	No	Skin allergy; resistant organisms
Povidone-iodine (Betadine)	Gram-positive organisms and fungi; possibly less effective vs. some gram-negative organisms	Yes (cream) No (aerosol)	Pain on application; excessive drying of eschar

Bacteriologic Monitoring

Despite the use of topical chemotherapeutic agents, some patients, particularly those with burns of more than 60 percent of the total body surface, will evidence progressive colonization of the burn wound, with subsequent invasion of viable tissue and bloodstream dissemination of the bacteria. Therefore clinical bacteriologic monitoring of the burn wound is imperative in order to diagnose incipient burn wound sepsis and effect immediate treatment.

In general, cultures of the burn wound surface have failed to accurately predict progressive bacterial colonization or incipient burn wound sepsis. Qualitative and quantitative correlation is poor between flora on the surface of the burn wound and bacterial colonization of the deep layers of the eschar. Blood cultures, although helpful if bacterial growth is demonstrated, have not proved particularly useful, since life-threatening sepsis may occur in the absence of bacteremia, and the presence of bacteria in the bloodstream is a relatively late phenomenon, often just preceding death. Bacterial growth in burn wounds is best monitored by semiquantitative burn wound biopsy cultures. Multiple full-thickness wound biopsies are obtained serially from representative areas of the burn wound. The tissue is weighed, homogenized, serially diluted, and inoculated on blood agar and eosin–methylene blue plates. In this manner, the precise number of viable organisms per gram of tissue can be calculated. When wound biopsy cultures reveal more than 10^5 organisms per gram of tissue or a hundredfold increase in the concentration of organisms per gram of tissue is observed within a 48-hour period, it may be assumed that the organisms have escaped effective control by the topical chemotherapeutic agent and that burn wound sepsis is incipient.

Heterograft and Homograft

Immediately following eschar separation, the wound is seldom ready to accept a cutaneous autograft. However, all terrestrial mammals require an intact epithelial covering in order to maintain water, electrolyte, and thermal homeostasis. During the time interval between eschar separation and definitive cutaneous autograft, the open wound of granulation tissue can be temporarily covered with a physiologic dressing. Either porcine heterograft or homograft obtained from cadavers is most commonly utilized. The application of these materials, providing early temporary wound closure, can contribute to the prevention and control of infection, the preservation of healthy granulation tissue, and maintenance of joint function. Specifically, the physiologic dressings decrease evaporative water loss and diminish heat loss secondary to evaporation; they cover exposed sensory nerves and therefore decrease pain associated with the open wound, and they protect neurovascular tissue and tendons which would otherwise be exposed. When the physiologic dressing adheres to the underlying granulation tissue, bacterial proliferation is readily inhibited, since the heterograft or homograft provides an acceptable surface against which neutrophils may entrap

bacteria. Until the wound is ready for definitive autograft, the granulation tissue is protected from desiccation. The physiologic dressings prevent the development of hypermature granulation tissue and promote a well-nourished recipient bed; and they act as an excellent test material to determine the optimal time for subsequent autograft. When adherence is observed, the granulation tissue may be assumed to be in optimal condition for autograft and postoperative loss of split-thickness skin grafts (autografts) will rarely occur.

Heterograft and homograft are most commonly used for temporary coverage of granulation tissue, as described above. The grafts are removed within 5 days and replaced with new physiologic dressing until autografting has been accomplished. These physiologic dressings may also be utilized to debride untidy wounds immediately after eschar separation. The heterograft or homograft hastens separation of very tiny pieces of eschar left behind at the time of debridement. It should be emphasized, however, that physiologic dressings may be used for this purpose with safety only if more than 95 percent of the eschar has been mechanically removed in the course of daily debridement.

Either heterograft or homograft may be utilized electively over reepithelializing deep second-degree burns, once superficial necrotic debris has been entirely removed (usually 7 to 10 days postburn). Adherent physiologic dressings at this time will promote the rate of reepithelialization and decrease pain in the wound, allowing decreased hospitalization time. Some clinicians utilize heterograft or homograft to immediately cover superficial second-degree burns. The advantages of such treatment include marked decrease in pain, decreased hospitalization, earlier return of joint function, and more rapid reepithelialization of the burn. However, utilization of physiologic dressings in this manner must be undertaken with caution. One must be certain that the wound is indeed partial thickness, since coverage of a full-thickness wound essentially closes an open abscess and may precipitate burn wound sepsis. In addition, the homograft or heterograft must be applied within hours after the burn injury, at the time of the initial debridement. It is important that the physiologic dressing and burn wound be inspected within 24 hours to assure continued adherence to the dermal remnants. Should the physiologic dressing become dislodged or should fluid accumulate beneath it, the material should be removed immediately and the wound treated with topical chemotherapeutic agents in the conventional manner. If the heterograft or homograft remains adherent, it is important that it not be removed but rather be allowed to separate spontaneously as reepithelialization occurs. Frequent changing of physiologic dressings applied to second-degree burns results in sequential removal of epithelial cells at the time of removal and may convert them to full thickness burn wounds.

Autograft

Definitive closure of burn wounds as soon as possible after injury is the ultimate objective of all burn wound care. As soon as an area of full-thickness burn wound has been adequately prepared by the use of temporary physiologic dressings as described above, it should be covered with the patient's own skin. There are, however, priorities of coverage dictated by functional and cosmetic considerations. In general, the hands, feet, joints, and face should be covered prior to nonfunctional surfaces. Autografts may be applied as sheets of skin without the need of suture fixation or "pie-crusting" incisions to allow release of plasma, provided the wound has been preoperatively prepared by application of physiologic dressings. Fixation with bandaging is not required unless accidental dislodgement is likely, e.g., on circumferentially burned limbs or on burns of patients with uncontrollable motion. Exposure of the freshly applied autograft allows continuous graft inspection and early evacuation of any collections of blood or serum which may occur beneath the graft. When dressings are utilized, they should be removed 72 hours following grafting. If the grafts are adherent, active motion of the burned area may be begun.

Patients with extensive burns often present a serious disproportion between the area requiring autografting and available donor sites. Mesh or expanded grafts may be utilized to cover large areas from limited donor sites. After harvest of the skin grafts, the grafts are placed on plastic carriers and passed through a Tanner-Vanderput mesh dermatome. A series of parallel incisions is made in the sheet graft, allowing expansion of up to six times the area of the original donor site. The small interstices are rapidly filled by epithelialization (4 to 8 days), resulting in a somewhat thinner but physiologically functional skin cover. In general, mesh grafts are not used on the face, hands, feet, and flexion creases, since the healed grafts are not as cosmetically acceptable as intact autografts. In addition, mesh grafts are less able to withstand recurrent localized trauma.

GENERAL THERAPEUTIC CONSIDERATIONS

Metabolism and Nutrition

Hypermetabolism characterizes the human response to major injury. Several investigators have now shown a direct relationship between the magnitude and duration of the hypermetabolic response and the severity of the sustained trauma. Wilmore has demonstrated a curvilinear relationship between the resting metabolic expenditure and the magnitude of total body surface burn in human patients. Resting metabolic rate approached a maximum response of approximately twice normal in patients with burns of more than 60 percent of the total body surface. Both Reese and Wilmore have documented caloric expenditure in excess of 60 kcal/m^2/hour in patients with major thermal injury. Total daily energy consumption during the nonresting state in severely burned patients approached 40 kcal for each percent of body surface burned, plus 25 kcal/kg body weight.

Previously, the hypermetabolic response was attributed in part to obligatory energy losses in the form of heat associated with a marked increase in evaporative water loss. The increase in evaporative water loss results from destruction of the water barrier within the skin. However, if water evaporation is mechanically prevented, there is no significant decrease in the metabolic rate observed in the burn patient. Furthermore, one cannot reduce oxygen consumption in thermally injured patients to normal levels by manipulation of environmental temperature and humidity. This suggests that the hypermetabolic response is non-temperature-dependent. A close correlation has been demonstrated between oxygen consumption and urinary catecholamine excretion. In addition, hypermetabolic response has been partially blocked by the administration of alpha- and beta-adenergic blocking agents. The hypermetabolic response in human beings is associated with increased rectal and skin temperatures, and animal experiments have demonstrated that burn injury is associated with a true increase in critical temperature. These studies suggest that the hypermetabolic response to burn injury is mediated through the hypothalamic temperature center, which emits an efferent signal expressed via catecholamine excretion.

In addition to elevated energy requirements, a marked catabolic response accompanies severe burn injury. The postburn catabolism is associated with weight loss, retarded wound healing, and negative nitrogen, potassium, sulfur, and phosphorus balance. Again, the magnitude and duration of the catabolic response roughly parallels the severity of the burn injury. Up to 30 Gm of nitrogen/day may be recovered from the urine of severely burned patients. If extraordinary means to provide excessive dietary nitrogen are not pursued, negative nitrogen balance may be observed for up to 2 months following the thermal accident. However, protein catabolism does not proceed uniformly in all tissues. Structural and functional integrity of vital organs such as the heart and liver are maintained at the expense of muscle protein.

Posttraumatic negative nitrogen balance can be ameliorated if sufficient caloric and nitrogen intake is provided. More than 20 Gm of nitrogen/m^2 of body surface/day is required in patients with major burns during the first postburn month in order to maintain positive nitrogen balance. During the second postburn month, nitrogen intake of 13 to 16 Gm/m^2/day will maintain nitrogen equilibrium. The catabolic response in burn patients is associated with increased levels of glucagon and catecholamine (catabolic hormones) in the plasma and depressed levels of insulin (anabolic hormone).

Total oxidation of a normal 70-kg male would yield approximately 166,000 endogenous kcal. It is estimated that healthy persons can tolerate acute losses of up to one-third of lean body weight before death ensues. Thus an extensively burned adult, with energy requirements of 5,000 kcal/day, becomes a severe nutritional risk within 2 weeks, assuming no oral or parenteral caloric intake. Since most of the kinetic energy requirements of the supine, bedridden patient are associated with maintenance of normal respiratory function, the most common cause of death in these patients is pulmonary sepsis. An ineffective respiratory effort results in progressive atelectasis and subsequent lung infection by opportunistic pathogens.

The clinical consequences of inadequate nutritional replacement include profound weight loss, development of superior mesenteric artery syndrome, decreased immunologic response, diminished leukocyte function (host resistance), impaired wound healing, and severe inhibition of cellular active transport, resulting in cellular dysfunction.

Current knowledge of the hypermetabolic response following injury allows more rational therapy aimed at preventing morbid consequences of acute malnutrition. Control of the environment by maintaining an externally warm temperature (31°C) will alleviate patient discomfort and shivering associated with a cold environment and prevent further increases in the metabolic rate subsequent to cold stress. Furthermore, apprehension and pain may be treated appropriately with narcotics and tranquilizers, since both these stresses are known to potentiate the release of catecholamines.

Effective prophylaxis against infection and timely closure of the burn wound will ameliorate both the catabolic and the hypermetabolic response to burn injury. A progressive physical therapy program will also enhance the deposition of protein into lean muscle mass, which allows performance of kinetic work required for maintenance of normal function.

However, the cornerstone of nutritional management of the burn patient is the provision of adequate exogenous calories and nitrogen to prevent prolonged catabolism. Whenever possible, the gastrointestinal tract should be utilized for the various dietary regimens designed to supply the nutritional needs of the patient. Maintenance of adequate nutrition is best monitored by accurate daily measurements of body weight. Postburn weight loss of less than 10 percent is usually well tolerated, provided the patient was not nutritionally depleted prior to his burn injury. Weight loss which exceeds 10 percent of the preburn weight is often associated with an increased incidence of morbidity.

When the voluntary food intake of the burned patient is insufficient to provide for positive energy balance, the physician must intervene with forced feedings, by either the parenteral or the enteral route. Enteral feedings may be accomplished by insertion of a small silastic nasogastric feeding tube through which nutrients are delivered 24 hours a day via a constant delivery pump. Usually patients with major burns tolerate a complete homogenized diet. Partially digested or elemental diets are usually contraindicated, since the higher osmolality associated with these diets often results in gastric distension, profuse diarrhea, or dehydration when large caloric intakes are administered. When positive energy balance is unobtainable by utilization of the gastrointestinal route alone, intravenous hyperalimentation should be employed simultaneously in order to avoid prolonged periods of malnutrition. The intravenous administration of fat emulsions and amino acid solutions by peripheral vein may also be used to supplement enteral caloric intake, if necessary.

Physical Therapy, Splinting, and Rehabilitation

Contractures associated with serious loss of joint function may complicate severe thermal injury. It has now been documented that a progressive physical therapy program implemented immediately after hospital admission is associated with preservation of range of motion in joints with overlying burn injury. It should be emphasized that the program must begin on the day of admission and be continued until the burn wounds are healed and normal range of joint motion can be maintained by the patient. Major burn centers have found it necessary to employ full-time physical therapists to supervise active physical therapy at the bedside during waking hours. Repetitive exercises are conducted in the direction opposite that of any anticipated deformity.

Prolonged immobilization must be avoided, and early motion following skin grafting should be encouraged. In addition, proper positioning during bed rest must be monitored, and splints must be manufactured to maintain anticontracture positions during sleep. When a carefully supervised program of physical therapy is an integral part of burn wound care, 85 percent of the joints underlying surface burns should have a normal range of motion at the completion of therapy. The upper extremities are more susceptible to the deleterious effects of prolonged immobilization than the lower extremities. The ideal position for the lower extremities (knees extended, feet in neutral position) is comfortable to the patient and relatively easy to maintain in either the prone or supine position. However, the shoulders are difficult to position or splint in patients with extensive burns. Elevation and abduction of the arm at the shoulder joint are often uncomfortable, and a patient with burns at the shoulder invariably assumes and maintains a position of adduction and extension if not carefully monitored by nursing personnel and therapists.

Many factors influence the success of a physical therapy program, including patient motivation, but no factor is more deleterious to the preservation of motion than delay of treatment. Daily range-of-motion evaluation and appropriate daily exercises to achieve maximum potential range of motion in joints underlying both second- and third-degree surface burns are of paramount importance. Goals should be established during the early postburn period, which must be rapidly achieved and thereafter maintained. The patient should be encouraged to pursue daily self-care activities as soon as possible. By the time of discharge, the patient should be as independent as possible and should have mastered a home physical therapy program to maintain function.

The development of hypertrophic scars may occur after hospital discharge. The resultant scar overgrowth may inhibit function and often causes severe disfigurement. Larson and his associates have reported reduction of hypertrophic scar formation following the application of conforming isoprene splints and/or elastic dressings (Jobst stockings) during the convalescent period. These devices exert pressure on the scar, causing better alignment of collagen fibrils and reduction of local interstitial edema.

Such splints and elastic dressings should be used following hospital discharge for at least 6 months to discourage delayed development of hypertrophic scar.

COMPLICATIONS

Smoke Inhalation Syndrome

Smoke inhalation syndrome is an acute pulmonary dysfunction related to lower respiratory tract pathophysiology occurring within 72 hours after exposure to gaseous products of incomplete combustion (primarily aldehydes). The severity of this syndrome is a function of the type of smoke inhaled, its amount, and the magnitude of the accompanying thermal injury. Patients with smoke inhalation syndrome frequently exhibit *no* physical signs or symptoms of injury during the first 24 hours after sustaining a major burn. Smoke inhalation should be highly suspected in patients burned within an enclosed space, patients injured while under the influence of alcohol or drugs, and patients who lost consciousness at the time of the accident. Such patients are most likely to have inhaled large amounts of smoke prior to being evacuated from the scene of the fire.

Diagnosis is dependent on a high index of suspicion and careful physical and laboratory examination (Table 7-5). At the time of initial examination, sputum should be obtained from the lower respiratory tract and examined for the presence of carbon. When carbonaceous sputum is noted, the patient should be hospitalized and observed for the development of severe respiratory dysfunction within 18 to 36 hours. Carboxyhemoglobin concentration should be measured as soon as the patient reaches the hospital. Normal carboxyhemoglobin levels are of relatively little value, since the patient may have been exposed to smoke containing low concentrations of carbon monoxide or may have been treated effectively with oxygen by paramedical personnel prior to arrival at the hospital. However, the presence of increased concentrations of carboxyhemoglobin suggests the inhalation of a significant amount of smoke, and the patient should be retained in the hospital for observation, since most such patients will later develop a pathophysiologic condition of the lower respiratory tract

following recovery from carbon monoxide poisoning. Within 6 to 12 hours after injury, the hospitalized patient should be subjected to fiberoptic bronchoscopy to assess the lower respiratory tract. Direct visualization of the trachea and bronchus provides approximately 86 percent accuracy in indicating significant smoke inhalation. Objective findings include the extramucosal appearance of carbonaceous material, bronchorrhea, mucosal edema, vesicles, erythema, hemorrhage, and ulceration.

The Pa_{O_2} while the patient is breathing 100 percent oxygen may also be utilized to monitor for the development of smoke inhalation syndrome. Patients with an initial Pa_{O_2} of less than 300 should be suspected of significant smoke inhalation. This test also has an accuracy of approximately 86 percent.

Other authors have utilized a [133]xenon scan to diagnose lower respiratory tract injury. An abnormal scan following the injection of [133]xenon into a peripheral vein is indicated by incomplete washout from the lungs within 90 seconds or the presence of local radioisotopic trapping. The test is 87 percent accurate but has been infrequently utilized, since it requires the movement of severely ill patients to special radioactivity-counting facilities.

Between 24 and 48 hours after injury, the patient exhibits progressive bronchospasm with expiratory wheezes, rales, tachypnea, and progressive respiratory failure. The subsequent development of bronchopneumonia secondary to bacterial growth distal to occluding plugs (consisting of inspissated mucus and sloughed bronchial epithelium) is a fairly constant feature. Radiographic changes are usually not noted until 72 hours after the injury.

The treatment of smoke inhalation syndrome can be divided into nonspecific and specific therapy. Nonspecific modalities include rapid fluid resuscitation of burn shock, performance of escharotomies of the chest and the abdomen, the provision of external dry heat, and frequent monitoring of respiratory function. Prompt intravenous fluid resuscitation and restoration of normal intravascular volume prevents exacerbation of central nervous system hypoxia. When circumferential third-degree burns of the chest and abdomen are present, chest wall and diaphragmatic excursion are inhibited unless escharotomies are performed. The provision of an externally warm environ-

Table 7-5. SMOKE INHALATION SYNDROME

History: Enclosed space, alcohol/drugs, unconsciousness
Physical Exam: Altered mental status, carbon in sputum, delayed symptoms

Diagnostic tests	*Advantages*	*Disadvantages*
Carboxyhemoglobin	Simple, rapid	Nonspecific, rapid disappearance
Fiberoptic bronchoscopy	Simple, rapid objective	
[133]Xenon scan	Objective	Complicated, expensive
AaD_{O_2} gradient	Simple, rapid, ? objective	Unproved

ment minimizes oxygen demand associated with an increased metabolic rate. Most important, however, is the frequent assessment of respiratory function by repetitive physical examination, serial determinations of arterial P_{O_2}, and evaluation of the P_{O_2}/F_{IO_2} ratio, which often decreases prior to a significant fall in the arterial P_{O_2}.

Specific treatment includes the provision of humidified air and oxygen as required. If respiratory failure is incipient, endotracheal intubation should be performed and the patient supported with mechanical ventilation. Often it is necessary to institute positive end-expiratory pressure (PEEP) to prevent progressive respiratory failure. Intravenous administration of bronchodilators often alleviates the severe bronchospasm. When smoke inhalation syndrome is complicated by pneumonia, appropriate antibiotics should be administered by a parenteral route.

Burn Wound Sepsis

One of the principal causes of death following massive thermal injury is burn wound sepsis. Burn wound sepsis is characterized by the active invasion of microorganisms into viable subeschar tissue, with subsequent bacteremia. Third-degree burn wounds are essentially avascular, so systemic delivery of antibiotics via the bloodstream does not substantially affect microbiological growth within the burn wound. Moreover, host resistance to infection is now known to be markedly diminished in patients with major thermal injury. Complement abnormalities, hypogammagobulinemia, cell-mediated immunity, decreased neutrophil intracellular bacterial killing, and abnormalities in the inflammatory response within the burn wound have all been described. In addition, there is a marked decrease in neutrophil and monocyte chemotactic responsiveness. These two factors, markedly decreased perfusion of the eschar and severely compromised host resistance to infection, may result in rapid bacterial colonization if topical chemotherapeutic agents are not utilized. Although the topical agents have reduced the incidence of bacterial invasion of the viable subeschar tissue, bacterial proliferation may still escape the control of all currently used chemotherapeutic preparations. When bacterial escape is proved by quantitative wound biopsy, administration of antibiotics by needle clysis beneath the eschar has been employed with success. This therapy is most effective when initiated at the time wound colonization reaches 10^4 organisms per gram of tissue. Antibiotics administered by subeschar clysis should be selected after review of in vitro sensitivity of the offending organism. The entire daily "systemic" dose of the selected antibiotic should be dissolved in a solution of isotonic saline solution or half-strength saline solution of sufficient quantity to infuse each 44-cm^2 area of burn eschar with 25 ml of solution once daily.

Utilization of antibiotics administered by subeschar clysis has allowed recovery of children with documented *Pseudomonas* burn wound sepsis accompanied by ecthyma gangrenosum. Prior to the utilization of subeschar antibi-

otics, this complication of *Pseudomonas* septicemia was uniformly fatal in burn patients. Up to 50 percent survival was reported in such patients in 1974 by Loebl and his colleagues.

Distant Septic Complications

Because of decreased host resistance, distant septic complications are not unusual in patients with severe burn injury. Bronchopneumonia is the most common complicating infection. Sputum cultures from such patients usually reveal the same microorganism which has colonized the burn wound. Bacteria may be aerosolized from the burn wound and inhaled in large doses as the patient is manipulated during the course of daily wound care. In about one-third of burn patients with pneumonia the bacteria are seeded via the bloodstream (hematogenous pneumonia) as a complication of burn wound sepsis. Conventional treatment with systemic antibiotics and respiratory support is indicated when septic pulmonary infiltrates are diagnosed by physical examination or chest radiography.

Suppurative thrombophlebitis occurs more frequently in patients with massive thermal injury than in other hospitalized patients with severe illness. This complication follows prolonged venous cannulation with polyethylene catheters utilized for the delivery of intravenous fluid. In contrast to bland thrombophlebitis, this type often exhibits no abnormal physical signs. Calf tenderness and edema are only infrequently present. More commonly, the patient presents with bacteremia of unknown origin. Blood cultures often yield staphylococci. The diagnosis may be confirmed by surgical exploration of all peripheral veins which have been cannulated during hospitalization. The vein is opened and milked in a retrograde manner, and any effluent is observed. If pus can be identified, the diagnosis is confirmed. In the absence of liquefied suppurative material, the vein should be biopsied and subjected to frozen section. Bacterial colonization of the intima of the vein also strongly suggests the presence of suppurative thrombophlebitis. The incidence of suppurative thrombophlebitis may be markedly reduced in the burn population by limiting the duration of any single intravenous catheter to periods of 72 hours or less. Should the complication occur, the offending vein must be excised in its entirety. Failure to employ prompt surgical treatment usually results in fatal bacteremia.

Thermally injured cartilage is another common site of bacterial infection. Cartilage is relatively avascular, and local host resistance to established infection is diminished as a result. The cartilage of the external ear is covered only by cutaneous tissue and thus frequently is injured when full-thickness burns of the ear are sustained. The development of suppurative chondritis often may be prevented in patients with severe ear burns by minimizing external pressure upon the ear. Such patients should sleep without bed pillows and be prevented from assuming a lateral position with the burned ear down. When suppurative chondritis occurs, either in the cartilage of the external ear or in other cartilaginous structures, surgical excision of the involved cartilage is necessary to arrest progressive septic destruction.

Gastrointestinal Complications

Gastric and duodenal ulcers have been reported previously as a common complication of major thermal injury. These ulcers were first described by Curling in 1842 and have been reported to occur in as many as 25 percent of hospitalized burn cases. The incidence of Curling ulcers has been markedly reduced during recent years, and operative intervention for upper gastrointestinal bleeding following burn injury is only rarely necessary today. In the past, 85 percent of upper gastrointestinal hemorrhage was associated with bacteremia. The decreased incidence of Curling's ulcer is associated with the reduced frequency of major septic complications, the prophylactic introduction of antacids into the stomach via a gastrointestinal tube (maintenance of a neutral pH in gastric aspirates), and the improved provision of nutritional supplements, allowing more rapid healing of small acute mucosal erosions.

If major upper gastrointestinal hemorrhage should occur, the patient should be promptly treated with iced saline solution gavage and blood volume replacement begun. When hemorrhage cannot be controlled by conservative means, prompt surgical intervention is indicated, since these critically ill patients do not tolerate prolonged periods of hypovolemic shock. The abdominal cavity can be, and often must be, opened through the burn wound. At closure, the subcutaneous tissue and skin are left open to prevent soft tissue infection. Once the bleeding source is identified by gastrotomy or duodenotomy, hemostasis is obtained by oversewing the base of the ulcer. Blood volume replacement is continued until the patient's condition is stable, and then a vagotomy and hemigastrectomy should be performed. Lesser procedures are associated with an unacceptable incidence of rebleeding, and reoperation carries a prohibitive surgical risk.

SPECIAL PROBLEMS

Long Bone Fractures

Often physicians are confronted with a patient who has sustained a long bone fracture with overlying cutaneous burns. Such a patient cannot be treated with closed cylinder casts, since second-degree burns will rapidly convert to full-thickness injuries as a result of bacterial growth. Furthermore, bacterial growth will be unchecked in third-degree burns, resulting in subsequent burn wound sepsis. Open repair of the fracture is generally contraindicated in the presence of potentially infected soft tissue defects. The fracture should be immobilized by insertion of Steinman pins or Kirschner wires in order to effect suspension of the extremity in balanced skeletal traction. The burn wounds can then be left exposed and treatment with topical chemotherapeutic agents initiated. The wounds must be cleansed and inspected daily and the chemotherapeutic agent reapplied.

Following electrical burn, bone may be thermally injured at the entrance and exit sites. This is most likely to occur when the entrance or exit site is on the scalp, the sternum, or the anterior leg. In these locations the underlying bone is in close approximation to the overlying skin. The burn wound is debrided of nonviable soft tissue, and topical chemotherapeutic agents are applied to remaining soft tissue defects and the exposed nonviable bone. When granulation tissue has developed over the soft tissue, temporary coverage with physiologic dressings is instituted until the soft tissue is definitively grafted. After soft tissue wounds are closed, the devitalized bone is decorticated until bleeding bone is encountered. Granulation tissue will develop from the endothelium of the vessels and eventually cover the remaining viable bone. Split-thickness skin graft can then be successfully applied.

Burn Injury of Joints

Occasionally burn injury may extend down to and include the joint capsules. Such injuries are most likely to occur where the overlying skin and soft tissue are relatively thin. The interphalangeal joints of the dorsal surfaces of the fingers and toes are most commonly involved. When it is apparent that the joint capsule has been devitalized and the joint is open, the cartilage should be surgically removed and a formal arthrodesis performed to allow ankylosis of the joint in an optimal position. Interphalangeal joints should be fixed in the extended position or with just a few degrees of flexion. Crossed Kirschner wires are utilized to hold joint position until healing of adjacent bony surfaces has occurred at about 6 weeks. When arthrodesis of joints is necessary, it is particularly important to maintain maximal function of adjoining joints. Ankylosis of the interphalangeal joints results in little long-term disability as long as metacarpophalangeal and metatarsophalangeal joint function is maintained.

Occasionally patients with burns of the hand cannot be maintained in appropriate position by splints during the acute postburn period. This problem most frequently occurs in infants and young children, in whom the fingers are not long enough to allow application of appropriate pressure dressings to maintain optimal extremity position within the splint. In such patients the temporal insertion of a single axial wire through both interphalangeal joints of each finger prevents interphalangeal flexion contractures. The wires are removed at 3 weeks and aggressive active physical therapy is employed to regain finger flexion.

Burns of the Face

Because of its exposed position, the head, with its appendages and orifices, is an anatomic area frequently burned. The protective action of the lids and the constant moisture which surrounds the ocular structures prevents the eyes from being directly involved by thermal injury, except in cases of contact, chemical, or electrical burns.

Injury due to these agents often results in perforation of the cornea or opacification of the cornea, which may require later correction with a corneal graft. Moreover, third-degree burn injury of the lids may cause retraction of the lids, allowing the cornea to be constantly exposed to the drying action of air. Thus extreme care must be directed toward protecting the cornea of the eye. The instillation of artificial tears (methyl cellulose) and the use of antibiotic ointments are often required to prevent corneal desiccation. When such third-degree burn injuries are present, it is often beneficial to perform tarsorrhaphies shortly after the burn injury, limiting subsequent lid contraction deformity. The upper and lower tarsal plates are sewn together in such a fashion as to allow union of the two cartilaginous structures. The patient is able to see through a small peep-hole in the center of the eye, where the upper and lower lids are not joined. The tarsorrhaphies are not released until long after autografting has been accomplished and further lid contraction is not expected. Skin should be grafted over the lids as soon as eschar separation is complete. If subsequent lid retraction still occurs, reconstruction of the eyelids is accomplished by blepharorrhaphy.

Patients with second- or third-degree burn injury of the face may develop microstomia as a result of gradual fibrosis of the circumoral tissues. Prophylactic treatment to prevent this complication is particularly cumbersome and of only limited success. Surgical reconstruction of the mouth may be carried out one year after the burn injury.

Frequently patients become very self-conscious about major or minor postburn scarring on the face. Most scars should be treated initially by conservative management, utilizing elastic pressure masks for a period of 1 to 2 years. Attempts at early surgical reconstruction are often unsuccessful, since the tissue remains extraordinarily hyperactive for a year or more. Scar revision for cosmetic purposes should generally not be attempted for an interval of 1.5 to 2 years following the burn injury.

MORBIDITY AND MORTALITY

Whereas survival after burns of 30 percent of the total body surface area was infrequent 25 years ago, today very few patients with injuries of this magnitude die. In several series, 50 percent patient survival has been observed in patients between the ages of 8 and 45 with 75 percent total body surface burn. However, patients over the age of 65 with burns of more than 25 percent of the total body surface still have markedly reduced survival, and prognosis should be guarded. Chronic disease states in this group frequently interfere with appropriate physiologic response to major thermal injury.

More importantly, the development of multidisciplinary teams to provide total care of the burn patient has markedly reduced the morbidity associated with this severe injury. At several centers, more than 90 percent of surviving patients have been able to return to an occupation as remunerative as their preinjury employment. Self-respect and independence are preserved, and the quality of life experienced by the patient usually approaches, or in some cases exceeds, the preinjury level.

References

General

Artz, C. P., Moncrief, J. A., and Pruitt, B. A., Jr.: "Burns: A Team Approach," W. B. Saunders Company, Philadelphia, 1978.

Baxter, C. R.: Burns, in G. T. Shires (ed.), "Care of the Trauma Patient," p. 197, McGraw-Hill Book Company, New York, 1966.

Curreri, P. W., and Marvin, J. A.: Advances in Clinical Care of Burn Patients, West J Med, 123:275, 1975.

Krizek, T. J., Robson, M. C., and Wray, R. C., Jr.: Care of the Burned Patient, in W. F. Ballinger, R. B. Rutherford, and G. D. Zuidema (eds.), "The Management of Trauma," p. 650, W. B. Saunders Company, Philadelphia, 1973.

Monofo, W. W.: "The Treatment of Burns: Principles and Practice," W. A. Green, Inc., St. Louis, 1971.

Polk, H. S., and Stone, H. H.: "Contemporary Burn Management," Little, Brown and Company, Boston, 1971.

Shuck, J. M., and Moncrief, J. A.: The Management of Burns, Curr Probl Surg (Monograph), February, 1969.

Etiology of Burns

Baxter, C. R.: Present Concepts in the Management of Major Electrical Injury, Surg Clin North Am, 50:1401, 1970.

Curreri, P. W., Asch, M. J., and Pruitt, B. A., Jr.: The Treatment of Chemical Burns: Specialized Diagnostic, Therapeutic, and Prognostic Considerations, J Trauma, 10:634, 1970.

DiVincenti, F. C., Moncrief, J. A., and Pruitt, B. A., Jr.: Electrical Injuries: A Review of 65 Cases, J Trauma, 9:497, 1969.

Gruber, R. P., Laub, D. R., and Vistnes, L. M.: The Effect of Hydrotherapy on the Clinical Course and pH of Experimental Cutaneous Chemical Burns, Plast Reconstr Surg, 55:200, 1975.

Jelenko, C.: Chemicals That Burn, J Trauma, 14:65, 1974.

MacArthur, J. D., and Moore, F. D.: Epidemiology of Burns: The Burn-prone Patient, JAMA, 231:259, 1975.

Moncrief, J. A., and Pruitt, B. A., Jr.: Electrical Injury, Postgrad Med, 48:189, 1970.

Immediate Therapy

Baxter, C. R.: Crystalloid Resuscitation of Burn Shock, in H. C. Polk and H. H. Stone (eds.), "Contemporary Burn Management," p. 7, Little, Brown and Company, Boston, 1971.

——, Marvin, J. A., and Curreri, P. W.: Fluid and Electrolyte Therapy of Burn Shock, Heart and Lung, 2:707, 1973.

——, ——, and ——: Early Management of Thermal Burns, Postgrad Med, 55:131, 1974.

—— and Shires, G. T.: Early Resuscitation of Patients with Burns, in C. E. Welch (ed.), "Advances in Surgery, Vol. IV," p. 308, Year Book Medical Publishers, Chicago, 1970.

Curreri, P. W., and Marvin, J. A.: Advances in the Clinical Care of Burn Patients, West J Med, 123:275, 1975.

—— and Pruitt, B. A., Jr.: The Evaluation and Treatment of the Burn Patient, Am J Occup Ther, 24:475, 1970.

——, Rayfield, D. L., Vaught, M., and Baxter, C. R.: Extravascular Fibrinogen Degradation in Experimental Burn Wounds: A Source of Fibrin Split Products, *Surgery,* **77:**86, 1975.

Hummel, R. P., MacMillan, G. B., and Altemeier, W. A.: Topical and Systemic Antibacterial Agents in the Treatment of Burns, *Ann Surg,* **172:**370, 1970.

Loebl, E. C., Baxter, C. R., and Curreri, P. W.: The Mechanism of Erythrocyte Destruction in the Early Post-burn Period, *Ann Surg,* **178:**681, 1973.

———, Marvin, J. A., Curreri, P. W., and Baxter, C. R.: Erythrocyte Survival Following Thermal Injury, *J Surg Res,* **16:**96, 1974.

Salisbury, R. E., McKeel, D. W., and Mason, A. D., Jr.: Ischemic Necrosis of the Intrinsic Muscles of the Hand after Thermal Injury, *J Bone Joint Surg [Am],* **56-A:**1701, 1974.

Simon, T. L., Curreri, P. W., and Harker, L. A.: Kinetic Characterization of Hemostasis in Thermal Injury, *J Lab Clin Med,* **89:**702, 1977.

Zikria, B. A., Weston, G. C., Chodoff, M., and Ferrer, J. M.: Smoke and Carbon Monoxide Poisoning in Fire Victims, *J Trauma,* **12:**641, 1972.

Therapy of the Burn Wound

Baxter, C. R.: Topical Use of 1.0% Silver Sulfadiazine, in H. C. Polk and H. H. Stone (eds.), "Contemporary Burn Management," p. 217, Little, Brown and Company, Boston, 1971.

Burke, J. F., Bondoc, C. C., and Quinby, W. C.: Primary Burn Excision and Immediate Grafting: A Method Shortening Illness, *J Trauma,* **14:**389, 1974.

———, Quinby, W. C., Bondoc, C. C., Cosimi, A. B., Russell, P. S., and Szyfibein, S. K.: Immunosuppression and Temporary Skin Transplantation in the Treatment of Massive Third Degree Burns, *Ann Surg,* **182:**183, 1975.

Bromberg, B. E., Song, I. C., and Mohn, M. P.: The Use of Pig Skin as a Temporary Biological Dressing, *Plast Reconstr Surg,* **36:**80, 1965.

DiVincenti, F. C., Curreri, P. W., and Pruitt, B. A., Jr.: Use of Mesh Skin Autografts in the Burn Patient, *Plast Reconstr Surg,* **44:**464, 1969.

Fox, C. L., Roppole, B. W., and Stanford, W.: Control of *Pseudomonas* Infection in Burns by Silver Sulfadiazine, *Surg Gynecol Obstet,* **128:**1021, 1969.

Hummel, R. P., Kautz, P. D., MacMillan, G. B., and Altemeier, W. A.: The Continuing Problem of Sepsis Following Enzymatic Debridement of Burns, *J Trauma,* **14:**572, 1974.

Lindberg, R. B., Moncrief, J. A., and Mason, A. D., Jr.: Control of Experimental and Clinical Burn Wound Sepsis by Topical Application of Sulfamylon Compounds, *Ann NY Acad Sci,* **150:**950, 1968.

MacMillan, B. G.: Deep Excision and Early Grafting, in H. C. Polk and H. H. Stone (eds.), "Contemporary Burn Management," p. 357, Little, Brown and Company, Boston, 1971.

Monofo, W. W., Aulenbacher, C. E., and Pappalardo, E.: Early Tangential Excision of the Eschars of Major Burns, *Arch Surg,* **104:**503, 1972.

——— and Moyer, C. A.: Effectiveness of Dilute Aqueous Silver Nitrate in the Treatment of Major Burns, *Arch Surg,* **91:**200, 1965.

Polk, H. C.: Treatment of Severe Burns with Aqueous Silver Nitrate (0.5%), *Ann Surg,* **164:**753, 1966.

Pruitt, B. A., Jr., and Curreri, P. W.: The Burn Wound and Its Care, *Arch Surg,* **103:**461, 1971.

——— and ———: The Use of Homograft and Heterograft Skin, in H. C. Polk and H. H. Stone (eds.), "Contemporary Burn Management," p. 397, Little, Brown and Company, Boston, 1971.

Salisbury, R. E., Hunt, J. L., Warden, G. D., and Pruitt, B. A., Jr.: Management of Electrical Burns of the Upper Extremities, *Plast Reconstr Surg,* **51:**648, 1973.

Silverstein, P., Ruzicka, F. J., Helmkamp, G. M., Jr., Lincoln, R. A., Jr., and Mason, A. D., Jr.: In Vitro Evaluation of Enzymatic Debridement of Burn Wound Eschar, *Surgery,* **73:**15, 1973.

Snyder, W. H., Bowles, B. M., and MacMillan, G. B.: The Use of Expansion Meshed Grafts in the Acute and Reconstructive Management of Thermal Injury: A Clinical Evaluation, *J Trauma,* **10:**740, 1970.

Stone, H. H.: Mesh Grafting, in H. C. Polk and H. H. Stone (eds.), "Contemporary Burn Management," p. 383, Little, Brown and Company, Boston, 1971.

General Therapeutic Considerations

Curreri, P. W.: Long-term Supranormal Dietary Programs in Extensively Burned Patients, in W. L. Sheets and G. S. M. Cowan, Jr. (eds.), "Intravenous Hyperalimentation," p. 136, Lea & Febiger, Philadelphia, 1972.

———: Metabolic and Nutritional Aspects of Thermal Injury, *Burns,* **2:**16, 1975.

———, Hicks, J. E., Aronoff, R. J., and Baxter, C. R.: Inhibition of Active Sodium Transport in Erythrocytes from Burn Patients, *Surg Gynecol Obstet,* **139:**538, 1974.

———, Richmond, D., Marvin, J. A., and Baxter, C. R.: Dietary Requirements of Patients with Major Burns, *J Am Diet Assoc,* **65:**415, 1974.

———, Wilmore, D. W., Mason, A. D., Jr., Newsome, T. W., Asch, M. J., and Pruitt, B. A., Jr.: Intracellular Cation Alterations Following Major Trauma: Effect of Supranormal Caloric Intake, *J Trauma,* **11:**390, 1971.

Dobbs, E. R., and Curreri, P. W.: Burns: Analysis of Results of Physical Therapy in 681 Patients, *J Trauma,* **12:**242, 1972.

Larson, D. L., Abston, S., and Evans, E. B.: Splints and Traction, in H. C. Polk and H. H. Stone (eds.), "Contemporary Burn Management," p. 419, Little, Brown and Company, Boston, 1971.

———, ———, ———, Dobrkovsky, M., and Linares, H. A.: Techniques for Decreasing Scar Formation and Contractures in the Burn Patient, *J Trauma* **11:**807, 1971.

Linares, H. A., Kischer, C. W., Dobrkovsky, M., and Larson, D. L.: On the Origin of the Hypertrophic Scar, *J Trauma,* **13:**70, 1973.

Reiss, E., Pearson, E., and Artz, C. P.: The Metabolic Response to Burns, *J Clin Invest,* **35:**62, 1956.

Rickler, J. M., Bruck, H. M., Munster, A. M., Curreri, P. W., and Pruitt, B. A., Jr.: Superior Mesenteric Artery Syndrome as a Consequence of Burn Injury, *J Trauma,* **12:**979, 1972.

Salisbury, R. E., and Palm, L.: Dynamic Splinting for Dorsal Burns of the Hand, *Plast Reconstr Surg,* **51:**226, 1973.

Soroff, H. S., Pearson, E., and Artz, C. P.: An Estimation of the Nitrogen Requirements for Equilibrium in Burned Patients, *Surg Gynecol Obstet,* **112:**263, 1961.

Willis, B. A., Larson, D. L., and Abston, S.: Positioning in Splinting the Burned Patient, *Heart and Lung,* **2:**696, 1973.

Wilmore, D. W.: Hormonal Responses and Their Effect on Metabolism, *Surg Clin North Am,* **56:**999, 1976.

————, Curreri, P. W., Spitzer, K. W., Spitzer, M. E., and Pruitt, B. A., Jr.: Supranormal Dietary Intake in Thermally Injured Metabolic Patients, *Surg Gynecol Obstet,* **132**:881, 1971.

————, Mason, A. D., Jr., Johnson, D. W., and Pruitt, B. A., Jr.: Effect of Ambient Temperature on Heat Production and Heat Loss in Burn Patients, *J Appl Physiol,* **38**:593, 1975.

————, ————, and Pruitt, B. A., Jr.: Insulin Response to Glucose in Hypermetabolic Burn Patients. *Ann Surg,* **183**:314, 1976.

————, Orcutt, T. W., Mason, A. D., Jr., and Pruitt, B. A., Jr.: Alterations in Hypothalamic Function Following Thermal Injury, *J Trauma,* **15**:697, 1975.

Zawacki, B. C., Spitzer, K. W., Mason, A. D., Jr., and Johns, L. A.: Does Increased Evaporative Water Loss Cause Hypermetabolism in Burn Patients? *Ann Surg,* **171**:236, 1970.

Special Problems

Achauer, B. M., Allyn, P. A., Furnas, D. W., and Bartlett, R. H.: Pulmonary Complications of Burns: The Major Threat to the Burn Patient, *Ann Surg,* **177**:311, 1972.

————, Bartlett, R. H., Furnas, D. W., Allyn, P. A., and Wingerson, E.: Internal Fixation in the Management of the Burned Hand, *Arch Surg,* **108**:814, 1974.

Agee, R. N., Long, J. M., III, Hunt, J. L., Petroff, P. A., Lull, R. J., Mason, A. D., Jr., and Pruitt, B. A., Jr.: Use of ^{133}Xenon in Early Diagnosis of Inhalation Injury, *J Trauma,* **16**:218, 1976.

Alexander, J. W.: Emerging Concepts in the Control of Surgical Infections, *Surgery,* **75**:934, 1974.

————: Host Defense Mechanism against Infection, *Surg Clin North Am,* **52**:1367, 1972.

————: Immunologic Considerations and the Role of Vaccination in Burn Injury, in H. C. Polk and H. H. Stone (eds.), "Contemporary Burn Management," p. 265, Little, Brown and Company, Boston, 1971.

————, Dionigi, R., and Meakins, J. L.: Periodic Variation in the Antibacterial Function of Human Neutrophil and Its Relationship to Sepsis, *Ann Surg,* **173**:206, 1971.

Altman, L. C., Klebanoff, S. J., and Curreri, P. W.: Abnormalities of Monocyte Hemotaxis Following Thermal Injury, *J Surg Res,* **22**:616, 1977.

Asch, M. J., Curreri, P. W., and Pruitt, B. A., Jr.: Thermal Injury Involving Bone: A Report of 32 Cases, *J Trauma,* **12**:135, 1972.

————, Moylan, J. A., Jr., Bruck, H. M., and Pruitt, B. A., Jr.: Ocular Complications Associated with Burns: Review of a Five-year Experience Including 104 Patients, *J Trauma,* **11**:857, 1971.

Bartlett, R. H., and Allyn, P. A.: Pulmonary Management of the Burned Patient, *Heart and Lung,* **2**:714, 1973.

Baxter, C. R., Curreri, P. W., and Marvin, J. A.: The Control of Burn Wound Sepsis by the Use of Quantitative Bacteriologic Studies and Subeschar Clysis with Antibiotics, *Surg Clin North Am,* **53**:1509, 1973.

Bruck, H. M., and Pruitt, B. A., Jr.: Curling's Ulcer in Children: A 12-year Review of 63 Cases, *J Trauma,* **12**:490, 1972.

Curreri, P. W., Heck, H. M., Lindberg, R. B., Mason, A. D., Jr., and Pruitt, B. A., Jr.: *Providencia stuartii* Sepsis: A New Challenge in Treatment of Thermal Injury, *Ann Surg,* **177**:133, 1973.

————, Heck, E. L., Brown, L., and Baxter, C. R.: Stimulated Nitroblue Tetrazolium Test to Assess Neutrophil Antibacterial Function: Prediction of Wound Sepsis in Burned Patients, *Surgery,* **74**:6, 1973.

DiVincenti, F. C., Pruitt, B. A., Jr., and Reckler, J. M.: Inhalation Injuries, *J Trauma,* **11**:100, 1971.

Heck, E. L., Browne, L., Curreri, P. W., and Baxter, C. R.: Evaluation of Leukocyte Function in Burned Individuals by *in vitro* Oxygen Consumption, *J Trauma,* **15**:486, 1975.

Loebl, E. C., Marvin, J. A., Heck, E. L., Curreri, P. W., and Baxter, C. R.: The Method of Quantitative Burn-wound Biopsy Cultures and its Routine Use in the Care of the Burned Patient, *Am J Clin Pathol,* **61**:20, 1974.

————, ————, ————, ————, and ————: Survival with Ecthyma Gangrenosum, a Previously Fatal Complication of Burns, *J Trauma,* **14**:370, 1974.

————, ————, ————, ————, and ————: The Use of Quantitative Biopsy Cultures in Bacteriologic Monitoring of Burn Patients, *J Surg Res,* **16**:1, 1974.

Marvin, J. A., Heck, E. L., Loebl, E. C., Curreri, P. W., and Baxter, C. R.: Usefulness of Blood Cultures in Confirming Septic Complications in Burn Patients: Evaluation of a New Culture Method, *J Trauma,* **15**:657, 1975.

Moncrief, J. A.: Burns of Specific Areas, *J Trauma,* **5**:278, 1965.

Munster, A. M., and Artz, C. P.: A Neglected Aspect of Trauma Pathophysiology: The Immunologic Response to Injury, *South Med J,* **67**:935, 1974.

Petroff, P. A., Hander, E. W., Clayton, W. H., and Pruitt, B. A., Jr.: Pulmonary Function Studies after Smoke Inhalation, *Am J Surg,* **132**:346, 1976.

Pruitt, B. A., Jr., Erickson, D. R., and Morris, A.: Progressive Pulmonary Insufficiency and Other Pulmonary Complications of Thermal Injury, *J Trauma,* **15**:369, 1975.

———— and Foley, F. D.: The Use of Biopsies in Burn Patient Care, *Surgery,* **73**:887, 1973.

Reckler, J. M., Flemma, R. J., and Pruitt, B. A., Jr.: Costal Chondritis: An Unusual Complication in the Burned Patient, *J Trauma,* **13**:76, 1973.

Rosenthal, A., Czaja, A. J., and Pruitt, B. A., Jr.: Gastrin Levels and Gastric Acidity in the Pathogenesis of Acute Gastroduodenal Disease after Burns, *Surg Gynecol Obstet,* **144**:232, 1977.

Silverstein, P., and Peterson, H. D.: Treatment of Eyelid Deformities Due to Burns, *Plast Reconstr Surg,* **51**:38, 1973.

Teplitz, C., Davis, D., Mason, A. D., Jr., and Moncrief, J. A.: *Pseudomonas* Burn Wound Sepsis: I. Pathogenesis of Experimental *Pseudomonas* Burn Wound Sepsis, *J Surg Res,* **4**:200, 1964.

————, ————, Walker, H. L., Raulston, G. L., Mason, A. D., Jr., and Moncrief, J. A.: *Pseudomonas* Burn Wound Sepsis: II. Hematogenous Infection at the Junction of the Burn Wound and the Unburned Hypodermis, *J Surg Res,* **4**:217, 1964.

Voorhis, C. C., Law, E. J., and MacMillan, B. G.: Operative Treatment of Curling's Ulcer in Children: Report of 4 Cases with 3 Survivors, *J Trauma,* **14**:175, 1974.

Wanner, A., and Cutchavaree, A.: Early Recognition of Upper Airway Obstruction Following Smoke Inhalation, *Am Rev Respir Dis,* **180**:1421, 1973.

Warden, J. D., Mason, A. D., and Pruitt, B. A., Jr.: Suppression of Leukocyte Chemotaxis *in vitro* by Chemotherapeutic Agents Used in Management of Thermal Injuries, *Ann Surg,* **181**:363, 1975.

Chapter 8

Wound Healing and Wound Care

by **Erle E. Peacock, Jr.**

INTRODUCTION

During the course of man's evolution he lost a valuable defense mechanism—the ability to regenerate compound tissues—and accepted in its place a much less complicated and far less valuable process—the phenomenon of healing. Although the ability to heal has been of enormous importance in natural selection, restoration of physical integrity by synthesis of scar tissue can be regarded, at best, as only a method of preserving homeostasis and cannot be compared to the more pristine function of multi-germ-layer regeneration. Moreover, the fibrous tissue synthesis stage of healing can be detrimental even to the extent of destroying the organism which it sought to preserve. Examples are the potentially fatal deformity of valve leaflets incurred during healing of rheumatic fever valvulitis, development of posthepatic cirrhosis, and development of esophageal stenosis after swallowing a corrosive agent. The patient may survive the initial disease or injury only to succumb months or years later from complications of fibrous tissue synthesis during healing.

Posthepatitic cirrhosis is of special interest to students of the biology of wound healing, because the liver is probably the only example of a compound organ in human beings in which almost embryonic propensity for secondary regeneration appears to be retained. Under most circumstances, the liver can be counted upon to regenerate about four-fifths of its preinjury mass; in fact, the failure of regeneration to occur with normal rapidity in severe nodular cirrhosis gives the distinct impression that only overgrowth of fibrous tissue may have prevented hepatic regeneration. The significance of this hypothesis is based on the possibility that fibrous protein synthesis anywhere in the body chokes or overpowers cellular regeneration; from an evo-

lutionary standpoint, such a hypothesis has some factual basis. The hydrozoan *Tubularia* will sometimes regenerate an amputated hydranth without formation of a connective tissue scar; at other times the organism will merely heal the wound by formation of scar tissue. When scar tissue is found, only an abortive attempt at regeneration can be identified. There is a very critical time in the development of newts when the ability to regenerate is disappearing. If during this time connective tissue synthesis is blocked by pharmacologic methods, the power to regenerate a new limb will be slightly prolonged.

With the exception of the liver, regeneration in man is essentially limited to simple tissue such as epithelium; compound structures such as skin, deep organs, and nervous system can heal only by sealing the wound in a manner to be described. The sealing process varies, depending upon whether structural integrity is interrupted or tissue substance is removed. In both types of wounds, epithelization is the fundamental process which seals the wound, and fibrous tissue synthesis is the process which provides structural strength. When tissue is missing, an additional process—contraction—moves tissue edges into closer approximation so that epithelization and fibrous protein synthesis can accomplish their objectives. Simple as this description may sound, most of the mistakes made by physicians in treating wounds are attributable to failure to realize and understand the limitations and end results of each of these fundamental processes and how they differ from pristine regeneration. Thus optimal wound management requires detailed knowledge of epithelization, fibrous protein synthesis, and the biology of wound contraction. Study of these processes requires, in addition, some knowledge of the milieu in which they occur—the ground substance.

WOUND CONTRACTION

In 1793 John Hunter wrote, "In the amputation of the thick thigh (which is naturally 7, 8, or more inches in diameter) . . . the cicatrix shall be no broader than a crown piece." The essence of this quotation is that full-thickness wounds of organs (including skin) do not heal by synthesis of fibrous scar with the exact dimensions of the original defect. A crown piece in Hunter's time was $1\frac{1}{2}$ in. in diameter, thus over 90 percent of the amputation wound was closed by central movement of skin edges. This process is called *contraction*—a dynamic term denoting action, which should not be used interchangeably with "contracture," the term for the end result (Fig. 8-1*A* and *B*). Just as loss of

A

B

Fig. 8-1. *A.* Severe contracture produced by full-thickness skin loss in burn wound of neck and face. Note ectropion of lower lip. *B.* Release of contracture in same patient shown in Fig. 8-1*A.* Contracture was released by excising scar tissue and resurfacing the defect with several split-thickness skin grafts. Note absence of wrinkling of graft and restoration of cervical profile. Facial scars ultimately will be excised and resurfaced.

brain or stomach produces a permanent defect in man, loss of skin also is permanent, and when a defect in the integument occurs, restoration of integrity is largely dependent upon stretching surrounding skin to cover exposed subcutaneous tissue. Obviously, stretching skin will distort movable features such as lips, eyelids, breasts, or digits. The fundamental process in contraction can be illustrated perfectly and the end result predicted positively by simply grasping the edges of a gaping wound and manually coapting them. Such replication of the contraction process produces the exact deformity that will result from natural wound contraction over a longer period of time. If it is not physically possible to coapt the edges of a wound by reasonable external force, one can be certain that natural processes also will not be effective, as the amount of skin present is all that will be available to be stretched over the wound. The area which remains uncovered will either remain as an open granulating wound or, if it is small enough, be covered by epithelium, which is a poor substitute for normal skin and establishes a potentially dangerous area for the development of epidermoid carcinoma.

Thus the effectiveness of the contraction process in producing complete wound closure and the cosmetic and functional deformity which closure by contraction will produce are related to the amount of skin available in a given area of the body. Because the hands and face of a young person do not contain excess skin, closure of a defect by contraction will cause distortion of facial features or restriction of joint motion. In areas where there is redundancy of skin, such as the cervical region or face of old people, wound contraction can be extremely effective in closing defects without producing cosmetic or functional abnormalities. Where an excess of skin is not present but flexion or extension of a joint will move wound edges together, wound contraction inexorably results in movement of the joint into an extreme position. After healing has occurred, the joint will be fixed because of lack of a satisfactory envelope. When loss of skin occurs over an area such as the malleolar area of the lower leg and ankle, wound contraction simply cannot occur because there is not enough skin to stretch over the defect. In this instance the wound either becomes covered by a thin, almost gelatinous film of epithelium or remains open for an indefinite length of time.

Three questions immediately arise about the contraction process: What starts it? What stops it? What is the mechanism by which it occurs? On first consideration, the answer to the first question appears obvious, in that interruption of the integrity of skin always seems to be the initiating stimulus. Close examination of the series of events which occur following removal of a piece of full-thickness skin, however, reveals that wound contraction does not begin immediately and that about 4 days elapse before movement of the edges is measurable. The so-called "lag phase" of healing seems to include the contraction phenomenon, and it can only be surmised that a set of conditions must be established or an assembly of cells or energy source completed before the actual work of mobilizing skin edges begins. One might surmise also that reestablishment of physical integrity is the stimulus which stops contraction; but again, measurement of the timing of other events reveals that contraction of a wound does not stop immediately with closure; indeed, wounds which were not caused by a loss of tissue and which have their edges approximated immediately will sometimes undergo considerable contraction. Even closure of a wound by the application of a free split-thickness skin graft or pedicle graft does not stop the contracting process once movement of wound edges has begun (Fig. 8-2). An interesting observation is that the rate of wound contraction is not the same for all points on the circumference of a wound unless the wound is a perfect circle. The ultimate configuration of the scar produced by a contracting wound is the result of variations in the rate of movement of different segments as well as the firmness of attachment of different areas of the skin to both movable and immovable structures. From a practical standpoint, the surgeon may use such information to reduce the final extent of wound contraction. For example, a wound created by bringing ileum through the abdominal wall to form a permanent ileostomy can produce ileal obstruction if the skin opening undergoes contraction. One way to minimize skin wound contraction is to make the skin incision a perfect circle.

The first step in studying the mechanism of wound contraction is to try to define precisely where the fundamental process is located. In the crudest analysis it must be determined whether centripetal movement occurs because an energy or power source located outside the defect is pushing the skin edges in or whether a centrally located power source is pulling the skin edges to the center of the defect. Curiously, even after 15 years of intensive study, the answer is not entirely clear. There is good evidence that energy is being expended in both areas, and the question becomes whether both processes are effective or whether only one is effective and the other is either reacting to wound contraction or is insufficient to produce effective tissue movement.

Over the years most investigators have assumed either that central granulation tissue in a contracting wound was retracting and pulling the normal skin over the granulating base or that contents of the wound were being absorbed as the skin edges moved toward the center. In 1958, Grillo et al. awakened interest in this question by reporting some experiments designed to determine whether changes in the central mass of wound tissue were pulling the skin edges together or whether central wound tissue was merely adjusting to movement of wound edges propelled by peripheral force. The commonly held opinion that dehydration of wound tissue was responsible for contraction was destroyed by their measurements, which showed that water content of central wound tissue at the beginning of wound contraction had not changed significantly at the end of contrac-

Fig. 8-2. Appearance of split-thickness skin graft applied to granulating wound while it was undergoing contraction. Note wrinkled appearance of graft and effect of continued contraction on surrounding skin.

tion. The assumption that collagen synthesis and contraction might be responsible for drawing wound edges together also was disproved by direct measurements of the collagen content of wound tissue during the process of contraction. Although collagen content increases markedly between the fifth and eighth day of healing, total collagen in the wound falls significantly after this period and cannot be correlated with rate of wound contraction.

The result of these studies was that attention was focused upon living cells as the motor units in the contraction process. Wound contraction occurs only in living organisms, and the force producing migration of wound edges is generated by living cells. As might be expected, cytochrome poisons, such as potassium cyanide, can be shown to impair wound contraction although they do not abolish it completely. Migration of mesodermal cells in tissue culture also have been shown to be sharply restricted by cytochrome poisons. These observations are readily reversible, which suggests an inverse relationship between inhibition of aerobic respiration and cell migration.

In an attempt to see if the cells responsible for wound contraction were located in granulation tissue, Grillo excised all the central wound tissue from wounds in guinea pigs every day during the contracting process. Curiously, excision of central tissue did not affect rate of wound contraction. Such data are not conclusive in localizing the mechanism of wound contracture, however, because they cannot be correlated with results produced by other manipulations of the central mass of wound tissue. For instance, if a square of granulation tissue in the center of a healing wound is outlined by tattoo marks and then separated from the rest of the wound tissue by circumferential incision during wound contraction, two interesting observations can be made: The centrally migrating wound edge will retract peripherally, and the centrally circumcised area of granulation tissue will contract centrally. This finding leads one to the inescapable conclusion that granulation tissue between two wound edges was not being compressed by peripheral skin moving inward but was under considerable tension between the advancing wound edges. Moreover, in other experiments, wounds which were splinted for several days and then released did not show marked acceleration of wound contraction following removal of the splint if any central granulation tissue was incised. Additional evidence that tension in granulation tissue is causally related to wound contraction is found in the ingenious experiments of James and Newcombe, who measured the contraction force of granulation tissue and plotted it against the length of tissue elements and the cross-sectional area of granulation tissue. No significant correlation between wound tension and overall wound area could be shown, but a highly significant correlation was found between cross-sectional area of granulation tissue and the tension which was developed during wound contraction. Such studies suggest that granulation tissue under tension resembles stretched elastic tissue, in that the amount of tension produced is related to cross-sectional area and not to overall length or surface area. These data, plus the demonstration that granulation tissue contains cells of a type which can exert migratory force of a magnitude necessary to mobilize skin edges, strongly suggest that the machinery for wound contraction is located in the central granulating mass. A recent discovery by Majno et al. of highly specialized cells (which he termed *myofibroblasts*) with smooth-muscle-like contracting powers lends additional support to this concept. Because myofibroblasts have been found ubiquitously in human beings, many investigators are uncertain about their specific role in wound contraction. Demonstration that topical application of Trosinate, a smooth-muscle antagonist, inhibits wound contraction supports the notion that contractile protein in living cells provides the energy necessary for movement of wound edges.

Grillo found that although wound contraction was not inhibited by excising the entire central mass of granulation tissue, it could be stopped decisively by excising a very limited zone of tissue just beneath the advancing dermal edge. He coined the term "picture frame area" to describe the strategic location of cells which appeared to constitute the machinery for wound contraction. Histologic examination of the "picture frame area" reveals a collection of large, stellate, pale-staining cells which have been thought to be the cells responsible for moving the overlying dermis.

Presently it can be said only that recent investigations have eliminated changes in nonliving materials as the cause of wound contraction and have established that the movement of wound edges requires a high order of energy transfer which is performed by living cells. No unifying hypothesis exists by which all the available data can be explained or the exact site or mechanism of action of wound contraction identified. The apparently incompatible findings of Grillo and of Abercrombie and James concerning the importance of the central granulation tissue can be explained in one of three ways. The first involves the contribution of the panniculus carnosus muscle, which is well developed in some animals and not as well developed in others. The excision of central or peripheral tissue could have vastly different effects on wound contraction depending upon the presence or absence of this structure and whether it was cut in either the primary wound or the secondary excision. The second explanation is that although central granulation tissue can and obviously does contract to some extent during wound contraction it may be contracting as the result of peripheral wound-edge movement and not actually producing it. The third, and in the opinion of the author the most likely, explanation for the seemingly incompatible data of Grillo and Abercrombie is that the wound margin makes its way over the surface of the movable granulation tissue, and as it does so, it forces it by counteraction in a centrifugal direction, thus putting central granulation tissue under enough tension to cause retraction when it is excised or divided. Whatever the mechanism, however, the phenomenon of wound contraction is one of the most predictable and powerful of all biologic reactions and must be positively reckoned with in the management of wounds where tissue has been lost.

EPITHELIZATION

An attempt to cover by regenerating epidermis any area of the body denuded of skin is the first irrefutable sign of wound repair and occurs long before any evidence of connective tissue synthesis can be detected. Factors which control the movement of epidermal cells and the mechanism by which they cover a denuded area are important to students of wound healing for two reasons. The first is that epithelization is necessary in the repair of all types of wounds if a watertight seal is to occur. Protection from fluid and particulate-matter contamination and maintenance of an internal milieu are dependent upon the physical characteristics of keratin. It should be pointed out, however, that just as the plastic liner of a home swimming pool contributes only a watertight seal while structural stability is maintained by concrete blocks, the epidermis provides very little structural strength for the wound. It is the surrounding fibrous protein framework which gives strength to the scar (Fig. 8-3). Actually, no cellular structure or globular protein can impart much strength in the repair of a wound. When structural strength is needed, fibrous protein must be synthesized. Thus highly cellular organs, such as liver, spleen, kidney, or brain, have almost no structural strength and cannot be sutured as effectively as fibrous tissue organs, such as dura, dermis, fascia, or peritoneum. A wound healed only by epithelium will stop "weeping" and be safe from bacterial invasion as long as the epithelium is intact, but the slightest trauma will literally wipe off what is hardly more than a gelatinous film; thus no degree of permanent protection has been achieved.

Second, epithelization is of great importance in the study

of wound healing because when certain variations in the control of cell division and cell movement occur, normal epithelization becomes uncontrolled growth, with awesome invasive potential. The recognized propensity to development of cancer in certain types of wound scars (radiant-energy-induced wounds particularly) and in all wounds which are prevented from healing emphasizes the close similarity between cancer and the healing process (Fig. 8-4A and 4B). Actually, a histologic section from a 5-day-old healing wound can be interpreted easily as fibrosarcoma if none of the historical details are available. Healing is dependent upon what may be thought of as a return to embryonic status; at certain times in the healing process the overall picture—characterized by mitosis, pleomorphism, disorganization, and loss of polarity—resembles the uncontrolled growth of a malignant neoplasm. A major difference exists, however: the factor of control. In a healing wound, the embryonic state is temporary and some controlling influence brings order out of disorder, a resting state to rapidly multiplying cells, and a remodeling of recently synthesized fibrous tissue to produce purposeful structural patterns. In the neoplasm, however, one may consider the situation as a healing wound in which the factor of control never reappears, so that healing continues without purpose or control until the entire organism is consumed by direct extension or metastasis of the products of regeneration. Considered in this way, there may be only a very fine distinction between healing and malignant growth; it may be that when we understand all the factors which influence cells to return to embryonic activity during healing, and even more important, the factors which control their growth and movement after healing has been accomplished, an important step will have been taken in solving the riddle of cancer. For now, however, it is important to remember that the stimulus following injury to overcome entropy and develop embryonic kinetics is one of the most powerful and predictable phenomena in biology.

Apparently cell division and ameboid movement cease only when cells are surrounded by other cells of their own type, and this characteristic behavior of individual cells has something to do with determining the direction in which a mass of cells will move. Weiss observed that when epithelial and mesenchymal cells are mixed and suspended in a proper medium, random movement of cells will occur, causing numerous collisions. Collisions of dissimilar cells (i.e., epidermal and mesenchymal) result in repulsion, whereas collision of similar cells results in the two cells sticking together and later developing protoplasmic bridges and protofibrils. Thus random movements and collisions over a sufficient period of time invariably result in all the cells of one type becoming agglutinated on one side of the medium and the remainder of the cells becoming agglutinated in a similar manner on the other side. As increasing portions of the circumference of a cell membrane become satisfied by attaching to cells of similar lineage, the remaining unsatisfied sides become the exploring or searching surface; thus some degree of polarity for the whole mass may be established. Failure to achieve complete surface contact with other cells results in a con-

Fig. 8-3. Third-degree burn of lower leg following healing by epithelization. Absence of dermis accounts for shiny appearance and relative fragility of the surface.

tinued state of embryonic activity. One does not have to use much imagination to predict that as the cells continue to be driven by an insatiable desire to contact cells of their own types, the risk of loss of control over replication and locomotion increases with time. Until more is known about the factors involved in the control of cell growth and movement, however, one can only take cognizance of the fact that any wound which is prevented from healing is potentially a malignant neoplasm.

Wounds caused by certain agents such as radiant energy or specific chemicals have an unusual propensity for developing cancer in healed scars or unhealed wounds. In wounds induced by radiant energy, the length of time before cancer develops appears to be directly proportional to the wavelength of the damaging ray. Thus thermal burn wounds and scars may require 20 years for invasive cancer to develop, while in gamma- or x-ray wounds cancer may develop in a matter of a few months. Solar and cosmic radiation, a causative agent in most human skin cancer, is short-wavelength radiation, but because it is filtered by atmosphere and melanin, human development of epidermoid cancer from this source usually does not occur until late in life.

The development of cancer is more rare in surgical or traumatic wounds than in radiant-energy or chemical-induced wounds. No type of wound is exempt, however, when healing has been prevented by constant reinjury or inadequate skin replacement. Even in postphlebitic leg

A

B

Fig. 8-4. *A.* Epidermoid carcinoma in open third-degree burn wound of thigh. Burn is 15 years old. *B.* Microscopic appearance of carcinoma shown in Fig. 8-5. Carcinoma developing in burn wounds metastasizes by vascular routes more frequently than other carcinomas.

ulcer (a common chronic ulcer) cancer may develop over a long period of time.

The mechanism by which epithelium attempts to close a wound has caused considerable speculation. Previous descriptions of the process, based on the assumption that mitosis was not a prominent occurrence, are not correct. Although it is difficult to find mitotic figures in the advancing margin of epithelium, the works of Bullough and of Gillman and Penn have shown conclusively that mitosis does occur in several layers of epithelium and that it is an important part of epithelization. Theoretically, it should be possible for a wound of any size to be epithelized, although there is a practical limit to the size of the area which can be covered. Mitosis is not an unlimited opera-

tion which assures that enough cells will always be present to cover any area.

Two important gross and histologic differences between normal epithelization in a healing wound and abnormal epithelial growth in epidermoid cancer are the size and the shape of the peripheral cell mass. A striking feature in a normally healing wound is the diminishing thickness to monolayer proportions of the advancing cell front (Fig. 8-5*A* and *B*). In carcinoma, cells pile up and tumble over one another to produce a grossly umbilicated appearance (Fig. 8-6*A* and *B*). Thus in normal epithelial regeneration, even though mitosis does occur, the most fundamental process is dedifferentiation and cell movement by development of ruffled membranes and pseudopods. The process begins early (within hours) and results in flat, thin, resting cells at the margin of the wound. These cells develop ruffled membranes and move across the center of the wound. When this occurs, the cell seems to adopt the characteristics of a typical basal cell; if it comes to rest in a more superficial position, it becomes a typical prickle cell.

In incised and sutured wounds, epithelization produces a watertight seal in 24 hours even though there is a dip where the cells have migrated into the crevice. Although the area of regeneration thickens with the addition of more cells, the center of the wound remains somewhat inverted until underlying connective tissue synthesis pushes the epithelium into an everted position. Gillman and Penn have pointed out that the cutaneous tract of a skin suture on either side of the scar is also a wound of the epithelium, and that the inverted contour of the epithelium over the main wound also occurs along the path of a suture to the extent that a completely epithelized tract may be produced or a small cyst formed after a suture is removed.

Epithelization of a surface wound (whether partial thickness of skin such as an abrasion, or split-thickness skin-graft donor site, or full-thickness wound such as postphlebitic ulcer of the ankle) involves similar movement of epithelial cells but over a much more hazardous terrain and greater distance than incised and sutured wounds. The early escape of blood and serum in open wounds produces a scab, and the regenerating epithelium moves beneath the scab, literally detaching it from the underlying surface as it seals the wound. Actually, epithelium does not move along the interface between dermis or fat and the scab but seems to prefer to infiltrate or actually cut through the fibrous tissue substrate by elaborating an enzyme which renders collagen soluble. This mysterious behavior has been somewhat clarified recently by identification of a collagenolytic enzyme found at the interface between epithelium and mesenchymal tissue. Confirmation of the observation that epithelium literally cuts its own path through fibrous tissue may be extremely important in understanding the remodeling of deep fibrous tissue to produce a new dermis.

The protective influence of a scab or other cover (eschar, surgical dressing, etc.) to prevent physical trauma, drying, hemorrhage, contact with caustic materials, and the like is the basis for medical care of secondarily healing wounds. In the final analysis, successful epithelization occurs only if the cumulative effect of physical manipulation, drying, bacterial enzymes, wound area, etc., does not exceed the finite capacity of available cells to divide, dedifferentiate, and move across the surface. Considered in the simplest analysis, it may be that interruption of epidermis merely allows the epidermis to do what it normally would do if it had room, since cell movement and cell division are to a large extent prevented in the intact epidermis by the compression effect of surrounding cells; to interrupt the integrity of an epithelium-lined surface may merely allow the cells to do what they would naturally do if they were not orderly and compactly arranged.

GROUND SUBSTANCE

Even as late as 1952, some treatises on wound healing made no mention of the role of ground substance. The mystery surrounding ground substance is nowhere better exemplified than in the name itself, a mistranslation of the German *grundsubstance,* which referred to a mysterious matrix from which all the formed elements of connective tissue were believed to originate. A similar connotation was expressed by the French *substance fondamentale.* Modern definitions have done little to clarify the true nature of this amorphous material, and the best that can be said, even now, is that the term "ground substance" usually refers to a continuous nonfibrillar matrix including water and electrolytes through which metabolites diffuse between blood vessels and cells. Histologically, ground substance is identified by a remarkable propensity to absorb certain dyes such as toluidine blue and to undergo characteristic reactions with periodic acid. By such staining reactions it can be seen that ground substance is relatively organized in some areas, such as basement membrane, and undergoes, during inflammation and healing, characteristic changes in staining reaction called *metachromasia.* Such histochemical reactions seem to be due to reactions with mucopolysaccharides, many of which contain hexosamine. Because of the characteristic staining reactions which they produce, attention has been focused on the acid mucopolysaccharides, even though it must be remembered that they account for only a small portion of ground substance. As a result, errors have been made by measuring hexosamine in connective tissues and drawing conclusions about the relative amount and importance of the ground substance on the basis of change in one small sugar moiety.

Meyer's division of the acid mucopolysaccharides into two major groups has been useful in the study of wound healing. These groups are nonsulfated mucopolysaccharides, of which hyaluronic acid and chondroitin can be easily identified, and sulfated mucopolysaccharides, of which chondroitin sulfate A, chondroitin sulfate B, chondroitin sulfate C, heparitin sulfate and keratosulfate have been identified. Presently it seems that the nonsulfated group is the main component of the structureless gel fraction of ground substance and that the sulfated group is most closely associated with the fibrillar elements of connective tissue. Thus changes in sulfated acid mucopolysaccharides are most likely to be of significance during the healing process, and, indeed, such substances are

Fig. 8-5. *A.* Low-power view of epithelium advancing over granulating surface in a human wound. Note decreased thickness of advancing margin. *B.* High-power view of advancing epithelium in granulating human wound. Note dedifferentiation of cells, deep migratory activity suggesting subsurface enzyme activity at epithelial-mesenchymal tissue interface, and absence of mitotic activity.

found to be increased during early stages of wound healing. Determination of actual amounts of any of the components of ground substance may be misleading, however, as we are dealing with a very complex substance which involves polymerizing reactions and the formation of giant molecules with molecular weight varying between 10,000 and 10,000,000.

Because the healing process is characterized by polymerizing, cementing reactions, it is interesting to speculate upon the role of these complex substances. Discovery that acid-sulfated mucopolysaccharides accumulate during healing raises the question of whether linkages between fibrillar proteins and ground substance occur. The same question has been raised about normal tissues such as tendons, where chondroitin C is a prominent portion of

Fig. 8-6. *A.* Low-power view of epidermoid carcinoma of skin. Note accumulation of cells producing increased thickness of epithelium without purposeful migratory activity. *B.* High-power view of epidermoid carcinoma. Note numerous mitotic figures.

the ground substance; stabilization of tendon by cross linkages between collagen fibrils and chondroitin C has not been demonstrated conclusively. Chondroitin A protein complex seems important in stabilization of cartilage, and destruction of this complex by local injection of papain in a rabbit's ear will produce a lop-ear deformity which will return to normal as soon as the complex is reconstituted. It seems likely that ground substance is most important in the phenomenon of healing because of its relation to collagen synthesis and remodeling. Although chemical linkages between mucopolysaccharides and collagen have been extremely difficult to identify, chemical bonds are present which may be important in the development of strength or orientation of collagen fibers and fibrils. Certainly the assembly of collagen subunits into fibrils and fibers is dependent upon many environmental conditions, which ground substance provides. Variations in

the relative amounts of sulfated fractions are believed by many to be instrumental in determining the configurations of collagen fibrils, but how much this complicated substance actually participates in other aspects of the healing process awaits further investigation.

COLLAGEN

As far as the questions which patients ask their physicians following repair of wounds are concerned, fibrous protein synthesis is the essence of healing. Accurate answers to such questions as "When do the stitches come out?" "When can I go back to work?" "How bad will the scar be?" and others are dependent upon a thorough knowledge of collagen synthesis, collagen degradation, and the factors which influence the equilibrium between the two. Unfortunately, there are gaps in our knowledge about collagen metabolism; but enough is known so that the care of wounds does not have to be a mixture of craft and religion, as Paré expressed it, but can be, in most instances, a scientific exercise with a predictable outcome. Even such seeming trivia as the selection of a suture or dressing material can be the result of logical reasoning based upon factual knowledge.

Collagen is an extracellular secretion from specialized fibroblasts, and the monomeric particles or basic molecules which fibroblasts synthesize are frequently called *tropocollagen.* The tropocollagen molecule is one of the largest biologic macromolecules, with a molecular weight of about 300,000 and dimensions of 15 Å in width and 2800 Å in length. It is a stiff, elongated rod which can be visualized by an electron microscope and is soluble in cold salt solution. Thus tropocollagen is sometimes referred to as saline-extractable, or salt-soluble, collagen.

Recently it has become evident that genetic pleomorphism is expressed in subtypes of collagen molecules. Three types of collagens can be recognized by analyzing the composition of α1 and α2 chains. Type I collagen is the most prevalent type in the mature vertebrate organism. Type II collagen appears limited to cartilage and is found primarily in human articular and costal cartilages and in chick embryo bones. Type III collagen is found in association with Type I collagen and is most prevalent in tissue undergoing remodeling or fetal organogenesis. Type III collagen also appears to be an important component of tissues with an unusual degree of elasticity, such as those of the aorta, esophagus, and uterus.

The amino acids found only in collagen, and used to identify it in analytical procedures, are hydroxyproline and hydroxylysine. The amount of collagen in a specimen of tissue is determined by measuring the amount of hydroxyproline and multiplying the result by a factor of 7.8. Other fibrous tissues such as elastin do not contain significant amounts of hydroxyproline. Formerly it was believed that hydroxyproline in collagen had much to do with the formation of various intra- and intermolecular cross links which give collagen molecules, fibers, and fibrils their characteristic rigidity. The three-plane fixation of the triple helix structure results, teleologically speaking, in our being able to rely on collagen to transmit energy accurately in tendons or to support nonfibrous structures such as muscle. The supporting nonelastic properties of collagen can be destroyed by rupturing cross links within and between molecules, but fortunately, the destruction of cross links to this extent requires rather harsh treatment for mature collagen, such as temperatures over 70°C or exposure to strong acids or alkalies. Under these circumstances, what is produced is gelatin, which, of course, has no structural strength even though the essential amino acids are present. It seems evident now that hydroxylation of proline and lysine is most important in transport of the molecule across cell membranes.

Synthesis of collagen is an intracellular phenomenon which occurs on polysomes; a critical stage in construction of the molecule is the hydroxylation of proline to produce hydroxyproline. Externally administered hydroxyproline is rapidly excreted in the urine and apparently cannot be utilized by fibroblasts to synthesize collagen. Among other things, one of the metabolic defects which can be identified in collagen-deficiency diseases such as scurvy is the accumulation of proline-rich precursors and deficiency of hydroxyproline containing polypeptides. During active collagen synthesis the ergastoplasm of fibroblasts forms characteristic parallel lines, or canaliculi, and it appears that monomeric molecules are excreted into the extracellular milieu through these canaliculi. In ascorbic acid deficiency, the microsomes do not form parallel lines of canaliculi but are arranged, instead, in large cystic spaces. It is from these areas that proline-rich and hydroxyproline-poor amorphous material is found.

Before aggregation and normal assembly can occur, a specific enzyme, procollagen peptidase, is needed to remove nonhelical terminal extensions from both the N-terminal and C-terminal ends of the molecule. Recent evidence suggests that the terminal peptide extensions of the collagen molecule are registration peptides facilitating triple helix formation. They interfere with subsequent fibril aggregation, however, and failure to remove the registration peptides because of congenital absence of procollagen peptidase results in poorly assembled collagen with marked structural abnormalities. A type of Ehlers-Danlos syndrome has been found to be the result of persistent pro-αchains. A similar condition appears to be responsible for the structural malformations in a disease of Belgian cattle called dermatosparaxis.

Monomeric collagen particles exposed to proper pH, temperature, osmotic conditions, etc., in the intercellular milieu aggregate or polymerize rapidly by the formation of cross links of various types. The most important such cross links are covalent ester bonds such as a Schiff's base between an amino group of one molecule and an aldehyde group of another. Oxidative deamination of lysine by an important enzyme, lysyl oxidase, is a necessary first step to formation of covalent ester cross links. In addition, other types of cross links, such as oppositely charged electrostatic groups and Van der Waals interactions, are involved in assembling monomeric particles into polymerized aggregates.

The rodlike collagen molecules appear to lie in staggered, overlapping, parallel formation, with one-quarter-length overlap. It is this staggered one-quarter-overlap arrangement of tightly packed units which gives collagen its typical repeating axial periodicity of 640 Å. Whenever collagen molecules are assembled under physiologic conditions such as those provided by the extracellular ground substance, typical fibrils with 640 Å repeating periods are produced. In certain laboratory preparations, however, it is possible to alter the characteristic 640 Å periodicity by forcing the monomeric particles to line up exactly parallel or end-on. This can be accomplished by adding glycoprotein to the milieu or by charging the preparation with a high-energy system such as adenosine triphosphate. Under these conditions, fibrils with band widths of 2000 Å can be produced; such atypical fibers are called *segment long-spacing fibers,* or *fibrous long-spacing fibrils.* These preparations have been extremely valuable in the laboratory, as they have revealed much about the size and method of polymerization of collagen molecules; they are not of any physiologic importance, however, as far as is known.

Although the collagen molecule is basically a triple-helix molecule with a spiral configuration, heat-sensitive intramolecular cross links prevent it from having elastic or recoil properties. However, if a collagen fiber or fibril is placed in a water bath with a small weight suspended from one end and the temperature of the bath is elevated, a point will be reached when the heat-sensitive intramolecular cross links will be destroyed and recoil of the spiral polypeptide chain will occur. The temperature at which this phenomenon occurs is called the *thermal shrinkage temperature,* and the magnitude of this reaction is such that a fiber or fibril will shrink to one-third of its physiologic length. The thermal shrinkage temperature of collagen, therefore, is an excellent indicator of the strength and degree of inter- and intramolecular bonding. By measuring the thermal shrinkage temperature of various types of collagen, it has been possible to learn something about variations in bonding under physiologic conditions and, in some instances, to correlate the development of physical properties of collagen with the extent of cross linking. From such studies it has become clear that cross linking, among other factors, is a function of aging; the older a specimen of collagen becomes, the firmer and more numerous the cross links are. Thus, collagen gel which is only a few minutes old has relatively few cross links and a low thermal shrinkage temperature and is so flimsy that cold salt solution solubilizes it. If the gel is allowed to mature for 24 hours, the number and strength of the cross links increase to the extent that a weak acid may be needed to depolymerize even a portion of it and a higher temperature will be required to cause it to undergo thermal shrinkage. If the aggregate is allowed to polymerize for several weeks, the maximum number and firmness of cross links will be realized, with the result that a strong acid may be needed to get even a portion of the collagen into monomeric units and the thermal shrinkage temperature will be the highest yet. In summary, therefore, both solubility and thermal shrinkage temperatures can be used to measure the age of collagen as represented by the effectiveness of the cross-linking process.

In addition to naturally occurring cross links such as ester bonds, artificial cross links can be added to change the physical properties of collagen. Just as adding an agent which shares electrons easily, such as a sulfur molecule, will increase the stength of rubber (vulcanization) seven-fold, addition of a similar agent such as the methyl group in formaldehyde will increase the number and kinds of cross links in collagen. Just how much the addition and destruction of cross links has to do with the physical properties of wound-repair collagen in scar tissue is not known. It has been shown, however, that addition of methyl or amide cross links will increase the tensile strength of scar tissue in incised and sutured wounds in rats as much as threefold on the eighth postwound day. That variations in cross linking are partially responsible, however, for the final appearance, texture, or elasticity of human scars is becoming more certain for many investigators. Early studies suggested that apparent rapid acceleration of the rate of gain in tensile strength in dehisced and sutured wounds was the result of more efficient cross linking between collagen molecules. Recent data, however, strongly suggest that the phenomenon of secondary healing really is nothing more than briefly interrupted primary healing. Apparently brief physical disruption of coapted skin edges has little or no effect upon the fundamental biology and biochemistry involved in tensile strength gain of a healing wound.

At this point, other factors involved in tensile strength must be considered, for cross linking may have very little to do with tensile strength after fibrils and fibers have been formed. It is highly unlikely, in the opinion of the author, that fibrils and fibers are cross-linked very efficiently, because the average distance between fibrils is of the order of 1 μ. Chemical cross links are approximately 2.8 Å, which means that the distance is roughly 500 times too great for the usual types of cross links to span the distance between fibrils. However, because addition of cross links such as methyl or amide bonds definitely increases tensile strength in wet scar tissue, the inescapable conclusion seems to be that rupture of scar tissue must occur, to some extent, along inter- and intramolecular planes. There is not uniform agreement on this point, and the question of the importance of cross linking in the development of strength in scar tissue must be investigated further.

After a certain amount of collagen has been synthesized, the most important factor in gain of strength may be the physical weave of fibrils and fibers. Certainly it is possible to vary the physical properties of other fibrous materials by varying the weave of the small components exclusive of any chemical bonds. A good example of this principle is to be found in the physical weave of a nylon stocking. Nylon thread is nonelastic, yet a nylon stocking can be made elastic by properly weaving the fibers. Transposed to a biologic system, nonelastic tendon or fascia shows physical characteristics similar to nylon thread, while elasticity of the wall of the aorta is similar to that of a nylon stocking.

The old concept of collagen as a static, adynamic substance—the excelsior of the body—is erroneous. Actually, as will be shown later, collagen in wound scar is a relatively dynamic structure which, like other tissues, is undergoing constant remodeling and replacement. After the forty-second day of wound healing there is no measurable increase in the amount of collagen in a healing wound, yet the scar continues to gain strength for at least 2 years. Thus changes in collagen, such as increased cross linking and rearrangement of fibers and fibrils, must be occurring.

Before leaving the subject of remodeling, it is important to mention a disease, lathyrism, which has been useful in the study of collagen metabolism and which may have far-reaching implications for control of human scar tissue. The disease, recognized by Hippocrates, is caused by excessive ingestion of certain peas of the genus *Lathyrus*. Considerable differences exist between the human form of the disease, which is manifested by spastic paralysis, and the disease in laboratory animals, which is characterized by skeletal and cardiovascular abnormalities secondary to altered collagen metabolism. Curiously, attempts to produce neurolathyrism in rats have been unsuccessful; the *Lathyrus* species toxic to man and domestic animals are not toxic to rats, which thrive on them. The active and highly potent fraction which produces altered collagen metabolism is beta-aminopropionitrile. Considerable data are available on the effect of this substance on both developing and mature tissues. Most of these data support the hypothesis that the primary effect of beta-aminopropionitrile is to block the formation of inter- and intramolecular cross links during all stages of collagen aggregation. Thus beta-aminopropionitrile affects growing tissue more than adult tissue. Characteristically, beta-aminopropionitrile produces an enormous increase in the saline-extractable collagen, as it seems to block the assembly of monomeric collagen units into stable fibrils and fibers. There is some evidence to indicate that fibril formation is not stopped during lathyrism but that cross linking in fibrils is so unstable that cold saline will solubilize most of the collagen which was assembled during beta-aminopropionitrile poisoning. Growing embryos literally become saline-soluble under the effect of beta-aminopropionitrile, and mature animals will develop hernias or die suddenly of dissecting aneurysms. Wound healing, as might be predicted, is affected by beta-aminopropionitrile; there is a cessation of gain in tensile strength within hours after the agent is administered, while saline-extractable collagen increases approximately ten times. Clinical implications of the beta-aminopropionitrile effect are exciting, for it is a clear-cut demonstration that it is possible to alter the physical properties of collagen in dramatic fashion. Because some of the effects of fibrous tissue healing in specialized organs, such as the liver or heart, can be more ruinous to the health of the individual than the disease or injury which preceded healing, the demonstration that some control over deep scar formation is possible is an exciting one. If, in addition, mature recently synthesized collagen also could be solubilized selectively, a major breakthrough in many disease processes could evolve. Highly purified beta-aminopropionitrile has been administered to human beings with scleroderma, urethral stricture, and keloid. It can be given safely to human beings, and it is anticipated that clinical trials presently being performed will establish the effectiveness of induced controlled lathyrism as a therapeutic modality.

Several times in this chapter the term "remodeling" of scar tissue has been used. The thoughtful student is likely to be concerned over such a term, as it connotes not just synthesis of collagen but collagen breakdown as well. Because no enzyme able to lyse collagen had been identified in human beings until approximately 15 years ago, collagen turnover in either normal tissue or wound scar was suspect. Even though no such mechanism could be demonstrated, however, indirect evidence has been abundant that some enzyme or mechanism for solubilizing collagen must exist. There is always some extractable collagen in the skin of even the oldest and most depleted individuals. Obviously, if all tropocollagen were going into the skin, the dermis would soon be as thick as elephant hide. Some collagen must be coming out of the dermis, and the relatively constant thickness of skin only attests to an equilibrium which exists between collagen synthesis and degradation. Surface scars are raised above the surface 2 to 4 weeks after injury; yet they usually soften, become pliable, and decrease considerably in size with the passage of time. The loss of 50 percent of collagen from the gravid uterus 36 hours after parturition and the rapid disappearance of dermis when tetraplegic patients are allowed to lie unattended attest that man possesses an effective enzyme capable of degrading mature collagen. Search for such an enzyme previously has been unsuccessful because it was assumed that the enzyme could be extracted from tissues. In 1963, Gross, Lapiere, and Tanzer hypothesized that collagenolytic enzyme was the product of living cells and that contact with a living cell was necessary in order for collagenolysis to occur. In one of the most important experiments performed in the wound-healing field during the last decade, the hypothesis was tested by preparing culture plates of reconstituted collagen and amphibian Tyrode culture medium. Specimens of tissue from the rapidly absorbing tail of a metamorphosing tadpole (a structure containing mostly collagen which is absorbed and not broken off during metamorphosis) were placed on the collagen-Tyrode substrate, and the culture plates were incubated under suitable tissue culture conditions. After several days a clear zone appeared around each implant, and if the tissues were kept alive long enough, the entire substrate became lysed by collagenolytic activity. Failure of the cells to survive stops collagenolytic activity immediately; even after lysis has begun, it can be stopped by killing the cells. Thus Gross and Lapiere demonstrated that collagenolytic enzyme is a product of living cells and that cells which produce enzyme need to be in close contact with collagen fibers for lysis to occur. Grillo, using the same tissue-culture technique, cultured wound tissues from actively healing wounds in guinea pigs and found extremely active enzyme activity at the wound edge. Moreover, the most active lysis in a granulating healing wound appeared to be at the epidermis-dermis interface of an advancing wound margin. Riley and Peacock cultured a variety of normal and pathologic human tissues and found collagenolytic enzyme to be widely distributed, particularly in epithelium-containing structures.

The most uniformly positive tissue for collagenolytic enzyme in human beings is cutaneous scar. Scar tissue reveals positive lytic activity approximately 10 days after closure of a cutaneous laceration, and a high level of activity has been found in dermal scars as long as 30 years after injury. Granulation tissue is only slightly active; burn eschar does not show any activity for about 2 weeks. Between 2 and 3 weeks after a third-degree burn, however, cultures of separating dermal eschar are strongly positive for collagenolytic activity. These findings suggest that invasion of dead eschar by underlying connective tissue cells or undermining epidermal cells is necessary for contact between cells and heat-tanned collagen. Retarded wound healing may be the result of excessive collagenolysis. Serum, cysteine, and progesterone have been shown to inhibit tissue collagenase acting at neutral pH. Progesterone in ophthalmic concentrations may be the agent of choice in treating corneal injury, particularly alkali burns in which delayed tissue collagenase activity is the cause of rupture of the globe.

By measuring collagen synthesis and collagen breakdown, it is now possible to study healing from the standpoint of variations in metabolic equilibrium. Considered as such, scar tissue becomes a product of opposing forces of collagen synthesis and collagen destruction, and the result of such forces will vary according to the relative rate and effectiveness of each. The maximum amount of total collagen in a healing wound is found by the forty-second day. Although increased amounts of saline-extractable collagen (compared with nonwounded resting dermis) can be extracted from the scar for as long as 18 months, there is no further gain in insoluble (or mature) collagen. The conclusion would seem to be that, even though remodeling of the collagen continues, equilibrium has been established between collagen synthesis and collagen destruction. Recent demonstration by Cohen of accelerated collagen synthesis and deposition and collagenolytic activity in human keloids probably represents an abnormaility of such an equilibrium.

The concept that all collagen to some extent, and healing wound collagen particularly, is undergoing simultaneous construction and destruction can serve as a basis for speculation concerning some of the previously unexplainable findings in the healing process. One such enigma is the behavior of wounds during ascorbic acid depletion. In the classic descriptions of scurvy it is important to remember that sailors' wounds did not just fail to heal; they actually disrupted months after they had healed perfectly. This observation has been verified in animals and raises the question of whether collagen is dependent upon ascorbic acid for structural integrity. It is known that collagen can be repeatedly depolymerized and reconstituted in the laboratory without contact with ascorbic acid, and artificially reconstituted collagen does not lose tensile strength. Therefore, the notion that vitamin C has anything to do with strength of mature scar tissue is untenable. Because synthesis of new collagen is blocked during ascorbic acid deficiency, and because collagenolytic activity probably proceeds normally, a possible explanation for old scar dehiscence would seem to be that tissue previously in equilibrium becomes unbalanced by having synthesis knocked out and lysis continue. Inexorably, the scar will become weaker until a point is reached where normal tissue tension produces complete disruption.

Although to some extent hypothetical (actual quantitative measurements of lysis and synthesis are not sensitive enough now to prove or disprove the equilibrium hypothesis), the theory is important as it relates to the whole field of conditions erroneously referred to in the past as "collagen diseases." The collagen in these diseases is precipitated under physiologic conditions and, as might be predicted, is normal as far as can be determined by electron or light microscopy, x-ray defraction, or amino acid analysis. Thus all the evidence supports the idea that so-called "collagen diseases" represent abnormal amounts of collagen in abnormal places but are not specific diseases of the collagen molecule or fibril. Such an explanation is entirely logical, as one cannot have a disease of a nonliving structure. Collagen is a long-chain polymer in which the nearest thing that could be classified as a disease process is the abnormal construction of collagen during lathyrism. The collagen in such diseases as rheumatic fever, dermatomyositis, and scleroderma is probably much more accurately considered as the ash or scar from a burnt-out primary wound or inflammatory process. In the other direction, destruction of collagen in diseases such as rheumatoid arthritis is, at least partially, the result of excessive tissue collagenase activity. The concept of the collagen system as a dynamic, constantly remodeling one opens the door for investigation of a large number of diseases of unknown cause which are characterized by deficient or excessive collagen formation.

SEQUENCE OF EVENTS: SUMMARY

Once the basic processes in the healing phenomenon have been mastered, the student has only to relate them to one another in proper sequence to be ready to start the study of what physicians can do to aid healing. The most important concept in this regard is the understanding that healing is not a series of events but is a concert of simultaneously occurring processes, some of which continue for many years after physical integrity of wounded tissue has been reestablished. The most dramatic events, such as sealing the wound, regaining tensile strength sufficient to permit normal stress, and acquiring a scar which is cosmetically and functionally acceptable, occur in a relatively short period of time. Long-term processes, such as remodeling of collagen and development of cancer in scar tissue, fortunately are not processes which cause patients much concern. Although the basic processes are much the same in an incised and sutured wound properly coapted (healing by primary intention) and a wound in which tissue has been lost so that healing must occur by contraction and epithelization (secondary healing, or healing by secondary intention), the time required for secondary healing is so much longer and the area involved usually so much greater that it is convenient to study the secondary healing process

to see how the basic steps in wound healing relate to one another.

The first thing which happens after full-thickness skin loss is that normal elasticity of the skin and external tension produced in some areas by muscle pull enlarge the defect according to the amount of force exerted and the direction over which it acts. Thus the shape of a skin defect may have little relation to the size or shape of the fragment of tissue which was removed. If hemorrhage is not too severe, a clot forms quickly, then contracts and dehydrates to form a scab. Because a scab is essentially a dehydrated, fully contracted blood clot, it is less durable and effective in closing the wound than collagenous eschar. Nevertheless, a scab serves a useful purpose in providing limited protection from external contamination, satisfactory maintenance of internal hemostasis, and a surface beneath which cell migration and movement of the wound edges can occur. Classically, the beginning of wound healing is described as the "lag" phase—an inaccurate term which carries the connotation that there is a period when nothing of importance is happening. Actually, a great number of important things are happening even though they usually are not considered part of the healing process. One soon recognizes, however, that almost instantly following infliction of an injury the stage for healing is set, and the props and background for the events which are to follow are essentially those of controlled inflammation. Study of the biology of repair has emphasized that the most successful reparative processes occur against a background of inflammation and that, up to the point of necrosis, how well the wound heals is directly related to the amount of inflammation present. Specifically, the release of various amines from connective tissue mast cells, perfusion of capillaries surrounding the defect, change in permeability of capillary walls, release of enzymes, fluid, and protein into extracellular spaces, accumulation of white blood cells and connective tissue cells, and formation of thrombi in peripheral lymphatic channels are all well-known changes in general inflammation which are important in providing the best milieu for repair to proceed. It is only when bacteria, foreign bodies, medications, or accumulation of destructive enzymes cause necrosis of tissue that inflammation becomes a deterrent to healing. Therefore the author prefers to see the term "lag" phase replaced by strong emphasis on inflammation as an active part of the reparative process.

Approximately 12 hours after injury has occurred, and at a time when inflammation has been established, epithelial migration—the first clear-cut sign of rebuilding—occurs. In a primary wound, epithelization is complete in a few hours; in a secondary healing wound, migration of cells is rapid at first, but as the line of cells from the wound margin becomes extended and the epithelial probe dwindles to a monolayer, progress becomes slower, so that days or even weeks elapse before epithelization is complete. After 4 or 5 days, however, epithelization is assisted as the machinery of wound contraction begins, and the wound margins begin central movement.

A great amount of activity takes place in the center of the wound after a scar or eschar has been removed and before epithelium has covered the surface. Grossly, the surface which was once gray or yellow-brown and smooth becomes bright red and granular. The reason for this is an extravagant proliferation of richly perfused capillary loops. The knuckles or loops of blood vessels impart a granular appearance to the surface, and it is because of them that the wound is often described as granulating or showing granulation tissue. Granulation tissue provides a good defense against invasion by surface contaminants, but it is fragile and produces a difficult terrain for advancing epithelial cells. This is particularly true if surface infection, edema, or deep fibrous tissue interferes with return circulation. When this happens, the fiery red granular dots will change to a purple, soggy, gray-black cluster which may fill the entire wound cavity and spill over the wound edge, thus eliminating the possibility of epithelization.

Although no visible signs of collagen synthesis can be found until the fourth to sixth day, biochemical evidence of collagen synthesis can be found between the second and fourth days. The level of hydroxyproline in wound tissue rises rapidly, and the saline-extractable-collagen level becomes elevated shortly thereafter. Before signs of collagen synthesis occur, the ground substance changes, as evidenced by accumulation of sulfated mucopolysaccharides and development of metachromasia. On or about the seventh day wounds will show a delicate fine reticulum of young collagen fibrils. Actually, the gelation which is occurring at this time is so random that polymerization of new collagen fibrils is much like that of a new gel in a laboratory beaker—without purposeful orientation or polarity. There is a short period when young fibrils and fibers take silver stains selectively, and it is thought that this property reflects the presence of large numbers of unsatisfied bonding sites; mature collagen fibers do not stain selectively with silver. As fibrogenesis proceeds, purposefully oriented fibers seem to become thicker, presumably because they are accruing more collagen particles; nonpurposefully oriented fibers seem to disappear. The overall effect appears to be one of lacing the wound edges together by a three-dimensional weave. In secondary wounds the mass of scar tissue becomes dense, compact, and smaller in circumference but shows little in the way of purposeful organization. The overall direction is one of replacing granulation tissue, allowing the surface to become covered with epithelium, and filling in the remaining skin defect with scar tissue after contraction is complete. As far as filling the defect is concerned, contraction is the major influence; it exerts full potential before scar-tissue synthesis is complete. The central scar seems to remodel itself to fill the defect after contraction is over. Thus wounds surrounded by mobile and redundant skin will have a small central scar, while wounds surrounded with tight nonmovable skin will have relatively large central scars regardless of the size of the defect.

Development of tensile strength (strength per unit of scar tissue) and burst strength (strength of the entire wound) are the results initially of blood vessels growing across the wound, epithelization, and aggregation of globular protein. Later, collagen synthesis is important. The effect of vascularization and epithelization, although relatively small, is adequate on the fifth day to hold wound edges, if not under excessive tension, coapted without sutures. The really significant gain in tensile strength begins about the fifth day, however, when collagen synthesis becomes apparent; tensile strength measurements in laboratory animals usually are recorded from that day. Increase in strength is rapid for 17 days and slow for an additional 10 days; there is an almost imperceptible gain in tensile strength for at least 2 years. In spite of the measurable increase in tensile strength for such a long period, strength of scar in rat skin never quite reaches that of unwounded skin.

Collagen content of the wound tissue rises rapidly between the sixth and the seventeenth days but increases very little after the seventeenth day and none at all after the forty-second day. Gain in strength after the seventeenth day, therefore, is due primarily to remodeling of collagen and, hence, is not correlated with total collagen content except for a very short portion of the healing curve.

When a normally healing wound is disrupted mechanically after the fifth day and immediately resutured, the return of tensile strength is so rapid that within 2 days the burst strength is nearly what it would have been had the secondary wound not occurred. This phenomenon, commonly called the *secondary healing effect,* has been studied intensely to determine the exact mechanism of rapid gain of tensile strength following a secondary wound. Curiously, it is neither more rapid collagen synthesis nor more rapid assembly of collagen subunits; secondary wounds contain slightly less collagen than primary wounds of the same age. Because the thermal shrinkage temperature of secondary wound collagen is significantly higher than that of primary wounds of the same age, it has been suggested that more effective cross linking or better physical weave of collagen subunits is responsible for the rapid gain in strength of secondary wounds. The recent demonstration by Madden and Smith that secondary healing is really nothing more than continued primary healing (without a lag phase) invalidates previous cross-linking theories of secondary wound healing. Whatever the explanation, however, the machinery for producing rapid gain in tensile strength in secondary wounds is limited to an area of 7 mm around the first wound. Excision of skin edges more than 7 mm circumferential to the primary wound results in secondary wound healing at the same rate as in a primary wound.

WOUND CARE

From a treatment standpoint, there are essentially two types of wounds: those which are characterized by loss of tissue and those in which no tissue has been lost. Lacerations are an example of wounds without tissue loss, and avulsions or burns are examples of wounds which, in addition to interruption of surface continuity, result in destruction of tissue. A question which must be answered for both is whether immediate closure can be done safely.

Whether the wound can be closed by suturing the edges together or a graft of some sort is required, a decision must be reached about whether closure can be immediate or should be delayed until the danger of infection is past.

The history of wound surgery is, in large measure, the history of military surgery, and the decision of many surgeons about whether to close a wound primarily or to delay closure is based on principles and practices developed in military hospitals. The tendency of many surgeons to set a certain number of hours after a wound is sustained as the time during which primary closure can be performed safely probably dates back to World War I and a study of wound bacteriology made in French military hospitals. In an attempt to determine the number of hours within which immediate wound closure would be safe and beyond which closure should be delayed, many wounds were cultured and the growth of bacteria measured. It was determined that about 12 hours after wounding, the number of colonies on the wound surface doubled; this was interpreted as meaning that debridement and wound closure were safe before 12 hours had elapsed but likely to be dangerous after that time. It is interesting to follow the effect of this study through subsequent years and to note the difficulties that surgeons have encountered in performing primary wound closure in any predetermined length of time. As a result, the time set for closure has been shortened to the point where it is sometimes recommended that wounds should not be closed more than 2 hours after injury. Obviously, there is no fixed length of time within which primary closure is always safe and beyond which secondary closure must be done. The key to deciding when a wound should be closed is an understanding of the difference between contamination and infection; the trick to determining when one has become the other is the ability to recognize and interpret signs of inflammation. A contaminated wound can be converted by skillfully performed surgery into a clean wound which can then be closed safely; an infected wound cannot be surgically debrided without high risk of failure, including the potentially lethal complications of interfering with natural localizing processes. The history and physical examination contribute valuable information, because the length of time needed for contamination to become infection reflects, among other things, the strength of the bacterial inoculum and the ability of the substrate to combat invasion. A clean razor slice of highly vascular skin of the face might be closed safely 48 hours after injury, whereas a stable-floor-nail penetration of the foot of an elderly person might not be closed safely 1 minute after injury.

Once the decision has been made to close a laceration, the surrounding skin should be prepared with suitable antiseptic and local anesthetic injected. A guide to application of antiseptic is never to put anything in a wound that could not be tolerated comfortably in the conjunctival sac. Any caustic solution which is capable of sterilizing the surface of the skin will also destroy delicate cells on the surface of the wound. Therefore, harsh antiseptics should be applied only to the edge of a wound, never within it. Debridement of a wound can be done either hydrodynamically or mechanically. When the wound contains only surface contaminants not attached to wound tissues, a copious stream of saline solution will flush foreign bodies and undesirable organisms out of the wound cavity. When devitalized or contused tissue fragments are still attached to the wound tissues and external contaminants are partially driven into the tissues, however, surgical excision of affected tissues must be performed. When there is a redundancy of tissue and there are no important structures in the depth of the wound, such as nerve or tendon, the best type of debridement is excision of the entire wound to produce a new wound which is surgically clean. When there is a shortage of tissue or when a wound involves important structures which cannot be sacrificed without producing disability, damaged tissue must be carefully dissected until all dead tissue and extraneous material have been removed. In a wound of the hand involving numerous tendons and nerves, this type of debridement may be tedious and require several hours to perform.

After the wound has been debrided, proper suture materials must be selected for closure. There are two major types of sutures, absorbable and nonabsorbable, and selection of the proper suture should be based on what has been learned about the biology of the healing process. For the most part, absorbable sutures, which are made of sheep intestines or synthetic polymers, are used when infection is known to be present or when debridement has been difficult and thoroughness is in doubt.

Plain gut sutures will be solubilized by tissue collagenase in less than 10 days, while gut which has been tanned lightly with chromium salts will remain structurally intact for approximately 3 weeks. Absorbable sutures are usually not used when they can be avoided, because the reaction to a foreign animal protein is considerably greater than the reaction to such substances as cotton, silk, and nylon. Synthetic absorbable sutures may not be as locally irritating as animal proteins. Because the collagen-synthesis stage of wound healing is barely under way at 10 days and the scar tissue is far from mature even at 3 weeks, a more permanent material may be needed. Chromic gut sutures produce less soft tissue reaction than plain gut sutures, possibly because more available cross-linking sites have been satisfied by the tanning agent.

Nonabsorbable sutures are usually preferable because they produce less tissue reaction and can remain permanently below the surface of the integument. The major disadvantage of permanent sutures is that if they are placed in areas where infection develops, the suture material can harbor organisms; hence infection will not subside until the sutures are removed. A nonabsorbable suture of steel or some alloy may be mechanically irritating, and sometimes an inflammatory reaction develops around nonabsorbable sutures which resembles a local allergic phenomenon. Sutures are placed in different types of tissue for different reasons; before selecting and placing a suture in a wound, one should ask these questions: What is the suture being asked to do? and How long does it need to do it? Sutures which are placed in tissues to hold wound edges together under tension should be placed in fibrous tissue. Sutures placed in cellular tissues such as fat, epidermis, liver, or kidney provide little structural strength, as they tend to cut through the tissues, which have no appreciable strength. Sutures in weak tissues usually are used to obliterate a potential cavity (dead space), provide hemostasis, or act as a fine-adjustment leveling device on the surface of the skin. Objectives for such sutures are met in a few hours, thus absorbable sutures can be used satisfactorily if they are desirable.

A typical facial wound involving skin, subcutaneous fat, fascia, and superficial muscle might be repaired in the following way: After local anesthesia has been administered, the skin prepared, contaminants flushed out with saline solution, and any dead fragments of tissue excised, closure is performed. The muscle, being primarily cellular, would not support a suture, so the fibrous tissue surrounding it is closed with a permanent suture of silk or cotton. If hemorrhage has been significant in the muscle, a separate suture or ligature may be used to control it. If the skin is closed in a single layer, the retracted subcutaneous fat might not come together completely, thus producing a cavity which would become filled with blood and possibly infected. Another loosely tied stitch, which has no strength because it does not pass through fibrous tissue, may be utilized to obliterate a subcutaneous cavity and discourage hemorrhage. After the subcutaneous tissue has been closed, a decision should be made about the desired final appearance of the surface scar. The width of the wound following closure of the subcutaneous tissue will be a good indicator of how wide the final cutaneous scar will be if the next sutures merely approximate the skin edges and are tied on the outside. The reason is that, if suture marks are to be avoided, silk sutures should be removed in 6 to 8 days because of development of inflammatory reaction, epithelial lined tracts, or small stitch abscesses. Although the wound edges may be accurately coapted with only a hairline scar at the time that such sutures are removed, the wound is held together only by epithelium, blood vessels, and globular protein. Even though it usually will not dehisce before collagen production takes over, the scar will stretch and widen during the ensuing 21 days while collagen formation and remodeling are occurring. The result usually is that a 7-day-old 1-mm-wide scar may become a 1-cm-wide scar 3 weeks after the sutures have been removed. One way to reduce widening of a scar after skin sutures are removed is to place permanent sutures in the fibrous protein layers of the skin to bring the edges together. This is accomplished by a subcuticular or intradermal suture of fine silk or cotton. The overlying epidermis is gently retracted, and sutures are placed in the lower part of the dermis. The knot is sometimes placed deep in subcutaneous tissue but can be tied superficially provided that the ends of the suture are cut close and the knot and suture ends are covered by overlying epithelium. It is important to use a very fine suture that will not be palpable beneath the epithelium and a clear or light colored suture material that will not show through translucent epithelium. It has been shown recently that permanent subcuticular sutures will not eliminate completely secondary widening of a scar; such sutures will reduce the extent of transverse remodeling in many wounds, however.

After subcuticular sutures have been placed, the skin edges will be as close together as it is possible to bring them, yet the overlying epithelial edges may be vertically uneven. A final row of sutures of fine silk or nylon which serve as a fine adjustment or leveler of the epithelial edges is frequently utilized to produce an even surface. Because these sutures are in cellular tissue, they contribute little to the strength of the wound and should not be placed more than 1 mm away from the wound edge. They should be tied loosely and removed before any epithelial reaction develops. Actually, external sutures in a wound closed in this manner probably can be removed in a few hours or as soon as the plasma clot seals the epithelial edges. For practical purposes, however, they are not removed until the first dressing, whenever that may be. In recent years the use of external cutaneous sutures has been partially eliminated by the development of various types of adhesive strips which can be used to hold skin edges together without producing epithelial sinuses or reaction.

When do you remove stitches? is a question frequently asked of surgeons. The answer is simple: when they have done the job they were put in to do, namely, hold the wound edges together until adequate tensile strength has developed. To set a finite period of time for removal of sutures is to imply that wounds heal at a standard rate; but the rate of healing is variable even in different parts of the body and under different conditions in a single individual. Instead of counting days until sutures can be removed, the wound must be examined; sometimes one or two sutures must be removed to see if the skin edges are sufficiently adherent to permit removal of all sutures. In wounds where a narrow scar is important and where some tension is unavoidable, it is advisable to splint the immature scar with adhesive strips for 2 or 3 weeks or until new collagen has attained sufficient strength and reliability.

The appearance of a linear scar is frequently worse between the third and fifth weeks after wound closure than it is at the time sutures are removed. The irregular, raised, purplish appearance of immature scar tissue can be a cause of great concern to young patients. Resorption of excess collagen, development of pliability, and the fading of undesirable color are called *maturation* of the scar, and maturation occurs more rapidly in older people than in the young. Children and teen-age patients, particularly, may have a distressing amount of red color in scars for several years. This condition is temporary, however, and redness should not be an indication for secondary surgical revision.

Scars should be revised secondarily only after they have undergone maximum maturation. Beefy, red, hypertrophic, immature scars usually recur after excision, and it is often amazing how much natural improvement will occur if sufficient time is allowed. It is seldom wise to attempt surgical improvement of a scar in less than 6 months; often natural improvement will continue for as long as 12 months.

Secondary revision should not be performed with the idea of changing the color of a scar or with the idea that a scar can be eliminated completely. All that secondary revision can accomplish is to take out a scar which resulted from unskilled closure or closure under unsatisfactory conditions and to close the defect as skillfully as possible under optimal conditions. Leveling uneven edges, changing the direction so that the scar does not cross lines of changing dimensions, and supporting a wide scar by the use of meticulously placed subcuticular sutures are the main improvements which can be accomplished. If scar tissue is elevated slightly above the level of surrounding skin, abrasion of that area by sandpaper or rotating brush will produce a smooth denuded surface over which new epithelium will spread in a more even sheet.

Wounds characterized by a loss of skin can be allowed to heal by contraction and epithelization if there is sufficient skin to be stretched across the defect. This is usually permitted only when infection prevents primary closure and when contraction does not produce a contracture which would interfere with function or produce a cosmetically unacceptable scar. In all other wounds, a skin graft should be performed to replace the skin which has been lost.

At the moment, there is no known catalyst to speed up wound healing; about all that a physician can do to aid normal healing is to protect the wound from physical, chemical, or bacteriologic complications which retard or prevent healing. One useful exception to this statement is the utilization of topical vitamin A to correct inhibition of epithelization caused by cortisone therapy. Vitamin A does not accelerate epithelization over normal expectation, it only corrects inhibition of epithelization caused by a specific drug effect. Protection usually means the use of an artificial dressing unless a natural dressing material, such as an eschar or scab, can serve the same purpose. Once the scab or eschar deteriorates, however, it, like any other dressing material, must be changed (debrided), and either definitive coverage provided or an artificial dressing applied. As in the selection of suture materials, choosing dressing materials involves a clear understanding of the objectives of each component of the dressing and the fundamental biologic processes that the dressing is supposed to protect. The first layer of a dressing is usually made of fine-mesh gauze, so that granulation tissue will not penetrate the interstices and cause hemorrhage when the dressing is removed. A long search for a pharmacologic substance to incorporate in the gauze to stimulate epithelial growth has been unsuccessful so far. Because certain by-products of the azo dye industry are carcinogenic, it was hoped that related dyes such as scarlet red might offer epithelial stimulation without being carcinogenic. All such substances have been disappointing, however, although most surgeons do use a gauze impregnated with some bland substance such as petroleum jelly or topical antibiotic in a water-soluble base. The main value of such medicated dressings is that there is less adherence of epithelium and vascular tissue to the dressing, hence less interference with wound healing when the dressing is changed. Dry gauze is a perfectly satisfactory dressing for most wound surfaces, however, and when carefully applied and removed, it can be as atraumatic as any other material. The usual coarse 4 × 4 hospital gauze sponge with its cotton-filled center is not a good material to place against open wounds; the interstices permit permeation by vascular tissue, and the cotton lint which is included becomes embedded in the wound. Sponges, mechanics' waste, cotton, and the like are used to give bulk to a dressing after the fine-mesh gauze has been applied to make the dressing conform to a desired shape and immobilize the wounded part. Nonstretchable, firm, roller gauze bandage and adhesive tape are used to complete the dressing in a typical occlusive (erroneously called "pressure") type of dressing. The nonstretchable gauze and adhesive tape provide a compact and stable immobilizing influence. A clean wound has very little drainage and no odor, and does not have to be dressed very often.

Infected wounds have considerable drainage and odor and, therefore, must be dressed often to provide suitable drainage and tolerable appearance. It is common practice to use a wet dressing on infected wounds, which means that the inside layers of the dressing are intentionally moistened with saline solution or some other substance. The realization that there is no catalytic effect upon healing or any control of infection from water and that maceration of skin or eschar produces favorable conditions for bacterial or fungus growth throws doubt upon the beneficial effects to be obtained by applying a wet dressing. The usual answer is that drainage is increased by capillary action or that debridement is accomplished as detritus sticks to the dressing. Such reasoning has never seemed logical to the author; a dry dressing will absorb more wound drainage than a saturated one, and debridement can usually be accomplished more efficiently by mechanical means. It often appears that wounds become cleaner more quickly with the use of wet dressings, but in the author's experience this is partly because wet dressings are changed more often. Of course, less pain may be associated with wet-dressing changes than with dry-dressing changes. However, when dry dressings are changed frequently and skillfully, surface detritus may be removed more effectively by dry dressings than by wet ones. One sound reason for using a wet dressing, however, is that wet heat is more penetrating than dry heat, and when additional warmth is desirable to increase the local inflammatory response, a warm moist dressing is effective. Failure to keep a moist dressing warm by the addition of external heat, however, results in a cold soggy dressing which has no particular virtue and which is definitely inferior to a frequently changed dry one.

SKIN GRAFTS

Skin grafts are classified as free grafts (meaning that they are separated completely from their donor sites before being transferred to recipient areas) and pedicle grafts (which maintain a vascular connection with the general circulation). Free grafts are full-thickness (which means that the entire thickness of the skin, including epidermis and dermis, is transferred) and split-thickness (which means that the entire epidermis and only a portion of the dermis are transferred). The remainder of the dermis after split-thickness skin grafting remains at the donor site.

The "take" of a free graft refers to the pink appearance of a graft which occurs between the third and fifth days after transfer, signifying that vascular connections have developed between the recipient bed and the transplant. Before this time, free grafts are white, unless microvascular surgery has provided instantaneous restoration of circulation, and do not show any change in color when pressed upon and released. It is a matter of considerable conjecture whether there is any diffusion of gases and nutrients between cells of the graft and underlying capillaries prior to development of actual vascular connections, and it has been assumed in the past that diffusion was necessary to keep cells nourished during the first few days. When grafts which include more than full thickness of the skin do not survive as free transplants, or when split-thickness grafts with pus or blood interposed between graft and capillary bed do not survive, it has been considered that diffusion could not occur through fat, pus, blood, etc. It seems more likely now, however, that diffusion is not important in the take of a graft and that mechanical barriers such as pus, blood, or fat prevent the take of a free graft by preventing vascular connections from occurring. Whatever the reason, the thicker the graft, the more likely will be the failure of take if mechanical or inflammatory conditions at the graft-wound interface are less than optimal. For this reason, thin grafts are used to cover less than ideally prepared wounds; full-thickness grafts are reserved for surgically produced wounds under optimal conditions.

In taking a full-thickness skin graft the surgeon will produce a wound which will have to be closed by suturing the edges together or by applying a split-thickness skin graft from another donor site. If this is not done, closing of the wound in one area with the graft will leave a wound of the same size and shape at the donor site. Full-thickness grafts are usually small grafts which can be taken from a place where there is an excess of thin skin, such as the inframammary fold or the groin, where the donor site can be closed by suturing the skin edges together.

It was once thought that split-thickness skin grafts must be taken through the level of the dermal-epidermal undulating interface so that small islands of stratum germinativum cells would remain to reepithelize the denuded surface. Because of this notion, surgeons were careful to take grafts as thin as possible, and the taking of a split-thickness skin graft was relegated to only a few highly skilled individuals (Fig. 8-7). It seems obvious now that if it were possible to take a graft through only the epithelium, a satisfactory take would be unlikely. Most of the cells would be dead, and the covered wound would be resurfaced by cells which would provide no better coverage than that which would have occurred from normal epithelization. The qualities of skin other than waterproofing (strength, flexibility, appearance, etc.) which are desired in a graft are qualities provided by the dermis. The final appearance of both the recipient and donor sites, therefore, reflects the amount of dermis which has been transferred and the amount of dermis which is left behind. Epithelial cells migrate out of deeply located glands and hair follicles, and donor sites which do not extend through the entire depth of the dermis will be reepithelized from these sources. Dermis, being a complex organ and not a simple tissue, does not regenerate, however, and if all the prop-

Fig. 8-7. Removal of thick split-thickness skin graft with a free-hand knife. The largest possible grafts can be taken by this method.

erties of normal dermis are desired in the recipient area, full-thickness dermis must be transferred; if less than the full thickness is transferred, the resulting graft will be abnormal in appearance and function.

In choosing the thickness of a free skin graft, qualities which are desired in the recipient area must be balanced against cost incurred in the donor site. How such factors influence selection of graft thickness can be illustrated by comparing two extremes in wound and donor-site conditions. In a large thermal burn, the recipient area is not optimal in that it is usually infected and edematous and involves a large area. The take of a graft is therefore uncertain, and revascularization is problematic. From the standpoint of the donor site, it may be necessary to procure several grafts from the same area to obtain enough skin for the entire wound; thus rapid healing, with a remaining dermis thick enough for subsequent grafts to be taken, is mandatory. In this case, both donor-site and recipient conditions require thin grafts. In contrast, a 2-cm-diameter wound caused by loss of skin from the cheek of a young person presents an entirely different set of requirements for an optimal graft. The recipient bed should be optimal if excised immediately or prepared later in the operating room. The need for full-thickness dermis is mandatory so that normal texture, color, and thickness will produce the most cosmetically acceptable result. The graft is small, so a variety of areas with a 2-cm redundancy of skin can be found for a donor site. Thus all factors point to the selection of a full-thickness graft. In other wounds the choice may not be quite so clear, but the principles involved in these two cases are the factors which must be considered in selection of any free graft (Fig. 8-8A and B).

Split-thickness skin grafts have a tendency to develop deep pigmentation after transfer. The thinner the graft, the more pronounced is postoperative pigmentation for 6 to 9 months following transfer. It is important to warn patients who have recently had split-thickness skin grafts placed on exposed areas of the body that protection from

Fig. 8-8. *A.* Hypertrophic scar produced by deep second-degree burn. Although a significant amount of full-thickness skin has not been lost, overproduction of collagen has produced an unsightly scar. *B.* Patient shown in Fig. 8-8*A* following excision of facial portion of scar and application of a thick split-thickness skin graft. Cervical portion of scar will be resurfaced later. A single graft covering facial and cervical areas would obliterate submandibular groove. Note that scar at junction of graft and skin is most prominent near angle of mouth where motion and tension are unavoidable. Although different in texture, hue, and thickness from normal skin, the graft provides a smooth surface over which cosmetics can be applied more effectively than over previous scar.

solar radiation is mandatory for at least 6 months. Thick grafts have less tendency to develop undesirable pigment, and they will usually blend into their new surroundings more quickly than thin ones.

Finally, a word should be said about the concept of the "dressing graft." Split-thickness skin is the best possible dressing material for an open wound, and failure of many surgeons to take advantage of this fact in treating complicated wounds is usually based on the mistaken notion that placing a split-thickness skin graft on a wound is tantamount to closing the wound. Although the possibility that some portion or all of the graft may take and thus close the wound is the main advantage in using split-thickness skin grafts as a dressing material, placing the graft on a wound of questionable suitability for closure does not in itself produce a closed wound in the same manner as suturing two full-thickness skin edges together. Actually, a skin dressing does not close the wound any more than a petroleum jelly gauze dressing. If the wound has been inadequately debrided or infection is not yet controlled, the graft will slough in a few days and may disappear by the time of the first dressing. In such instances nothing will have been lost except a few square centimeters of split-thickness skin from the donor area. Dressing a questionable wound of relatively small size with split-thickness skin, therefore, is a sort of biologic test to determine suitability for closure, as well as providing some benefit if even a part of the graft survives. Xenografts of porcine skin and human allografts of split-thickness skin are useful also as biologic dressings and seem to improve various aspects of the healing process. Such grafts should be removed before take occurs and often are changed several times before optimum conditions for autograft application are obtained.

When more than the skin has been lost, and the skin plus some other tissue such as fat, tendon, muscle, or nerve must be replaced to restore function and appearance, transfer of skin by pedicle flap or direct vascular anastomosis is required (Fig. 8-9). As the name implies, pedicle transfers maintain vascular connection with the host, so that interruption of the capillary circulation never occurs. The vessels which are most important during transfer of tissue are the vessels in the subdermal plexus. These vessels are relatively large, frequently longitudinally oriented, and found on the undersurface of the dermis between it and the subcutaneous fat. One frequently hears that a pedicle flap has been made thicker than actually needed for cosmetic or functional purposes in order to provide a safe blood supply. Fat on the undersurface of a flap does not add any appreciable blood supply, and it may be removed safely to produce as thin a pedicle as needed, provided that surgical manipulation does not injure the important vessels lying on the undersurface of the dermis. The problem in transplanting tissue by the pedicle method is to design a pedicle so that the base is as narrow as possible in relation to the length needed to cover the deficient area. It becomes a matter of considerable judgment, therefore, to gauge the shape and dimensions of a flap so that blood supply through the intact pedicle will be adequate to nourish the distal end of the flap. A great deal depends upon the natural profuseness of vascular beds; thus it is possible to move a pedicle flap on the face or cervical region which is three times as long as it is wide, while it may not be possible (without performing preliminary procedures to increase the blood supply) to transfer a flap on the leg which is no longer than it is wide. The blood supply in the base of a contemplated flap can be improved by performing a procedure commonly referred to as delay of the flap. The principle of delay is to gradually reduce blood supply to small segments of the circumference of the flap and thus improve the remaining blood supply to the point where a pedicle which was of insufficient width before the flap was delayed becomes adequate to nourish the flap. The mechanism by which delay (gradual interruption of a portion of the blood supply to a flap) improves the circulation in the base is not completely clear. It seems doubtful that new blood vessels actually grow into the area, although casual observation of changes in the vessels at the base suggests that this is what may happen. The rapidity with which delay improves the circulation strongly suggests, however, that the release of various amines, probably in response to changes in pH secondary to increased anaerobic metabolism, causes a closure of normally open shunts that prevent perfusion of the entire capillary network. The effect is a substantial hyperemia at the base of the flap; over a period of several weeks and after several delaying procedures, the vessels in the pedicle base become racemose in appearance, and the amount of blood flow is increased to the extent that a relatively long flap can be transferred on a narrow pedicle. Following transfer of the flap, circulation must be observed carefully for the first 48 hours, as signs of impending circulatory embarrassment occur before irreversible thrombosis and cell death. It is not unusual for the distal end of a flap to be dusky following transfer; venous spasm secondary to the trauma of rotation may be all that is involved. Improvement usually occurs in a few hours, but during this time the danger of a venous thrombosis is increased; if there is any progression of cyanosis and edema, the possibility that tension on veins is interfering with return circulation must be investigated by removing a few sutures. Perhaps the most serious, but still reversible, sign of impending venous thrombosis is the development of a sharp line of color differentiation. A gradual change from normal pink to slight cyanosis is not so significant as a clear-cut line demarcating the area of circulatory deficiency from normal circulation. Even if all the sutures have to be removed and the flap returned to its original bed, the sign must be attended to, or an irreversible demarcation will soon develop, signifying complete thrombosis and certain distal necrosis. In sensibly planned and adequately prepared flaps, one does not have to be particularly concerned about arterial insufficiency; venous drainage is the function in which complications develop. Complications usually are the result of too much tension, poor dressing, hematoma, or infection. The use of heparin and low-molecular-weight dextran have seemed to be beneficial in dangerously compromised circulation. Hyperbaric oxygenation has been reported instrumental in saving flaps of laboratory animals, but is not practical for managing human flaps.

Fig. 8-9. Abdominal pedicle flap applied to dorsum of hand. Scar on hand has been turned back to resurface the raw side of pedicle and a portion of the donor site. Flap will be separated from the abdominal wall in 18 days.

Advancement flaps and rotation flaps are the simplest pedicle transfers. These are dependent upon a redundancy of soft tissue adjacent to a defect so that the donor defect can be closed by approximating the skin edges or applying split-thickness skin grafts. More complicated flaps require the use of an arm as a carrier to provide circulation during the period that skin is detached from the original donor site, such as abdominal wall, and transferred to a distant site, such as the lower leg. Because of similarity of tissue characteristics, safety in transfer, and expense and time involved, it is desirable to design flaps as close to the point where they are needed as possible. Widespread interest, perfecting of instruments and visual aids, and perfecting of technical procedures have made transfer of composite tissue grafts by direct small blood vessel anastomosis possible during recent years. As more experience is gained, microvascular anastomosis will circumvent the need for delays and carrier procedures in many patients.

One of the most sophisticated flaps is an island pedicle flap (Fig. 8-10), which combines the pedicle principle of intact blood and nerve supply with some of the advantages of a free graft. The principle of the island pedicle is that careful dissection of the artery and vein (and sometimes the nerve) to a piece of skin can be performed so that the skin is detached from surrounding skin and remains attached to the body only by essentials for survival—an artery, a vein, and sometimes a nerve. Depending on the length of these structures, it is possible to move a full-thickness skin and fat graft, or an intact finger, or a portion of a finger or toe, a surprising distance. Transfer of hair-bearing portions of the scalp on a temporal artery-and-vein supported flap to the supraorbital region for eyebrow reconstruction and transfer of a finger to replace a missing thumb are examples of island pedicle transfers which are useful.

Finally, it should be pointed out that, in the opinion

Fig. 8-10. Island pedicle flap developed during amputation of long finger. The flap is nourished by a single digital artery and nerve. Sensation is preserved by including a digital nerve in the vascular pedicle.

of many, maturity in restorative surgery can be measured, in part, by how often one thinks of a pedicle flap as the only means of rebuilding a damaged area and then devises a way to make a free graft do as well. Pedicles are dramatic, particularly as used by military surgeons to rebuild enormous tissue defects caused by high-explosive wounds; fortunately, however, civilian injuries are not often so devastating, and the practical points of expense, length of time away from work, shortage of hospital facilities, and the like have to be considered in each case where a pedicle could be used. In addition, although areas such as the face may appear in photographs to have been superbly restored by massive flaps, yet it must be remembered that flaps have no dynamic function; they are expressionless, and often look better in photographs than they do as part of the constantly moving facial features. When a pedicle flap is needed, nothing else will suffice, and pedicles are an extremely valuable part of restorative surgery. The high cost of donor-site mutilation, length of time required for transfer, and adynamic features, however, make the pedicle flap definitely second choice to a free graft if a free graft can be used as well.

References

General

Dunphy, J. E., and Van Winkle, W.: "Repair and Regeneration: The Scientific Basis for Surgical Practice," McGraw-Hill Book Company, New York, 1968.

Madden, J. W.: Wound Healing: Biologic and Clinical Features, in Sabiston, D. (ed.), "Textbook of Surgery," 10th ed., p. 249, W. B. Saunders Company, Philadelphia, 1972.

Montagna, W., and Billingham, R. E.: Advances in Biology of Skin, vol. V, "Wound Healing," *Proc Brown Univ Symp Biol Skin, 1963,* The Macmillan Company, New York, and Pergamon Press, New York, 1964.

Patterson, W. B.: Wound Healing and Tissue Repair, *Dev Biol Conf Ser Rept, 1956,* The University of Chicago Press, Chicago, 1959.

Peacock, E. E., Jr.: Wound Healing and Care of the Wound, in "Manual of Preoperative and Postoperative Care, A.C.S.," p. 3, W. B. Saunders Company, Philadelphia, 1971.

———, and Van Winkle, W.: "Wound Repair," 2d ed., W. B. Saunders Company, Philadelphia, 1976.

Wound Contraction

Abercrombie, M., Flint, M. H., and James, D. W.: Wound Contraction in Relation to Collagen Formation in Scorbutic Guinea-Pigs, *J Embryol Exp Morphol,* **4:**167, 1956.

———, James, D. W., and Newcombe, J. F.: Wound Contraction in Rabbit Skin, Studied by Splinting the Wound Margins, *J Anat,* **94:**170, 1960.

Billingham, R. E., and Russel, P. S.: Studies on Wound Healing with Special Reference to the Phenomenon of Contracture in Experimental Wounds in Rabbit's Skin, *Ann Surg,* **144:**961, 1956.

Danes, B., and Leinfelder, P. J.: Cytological and Respiratory Effects of Cyanide on Tissue Cultures, *J Cell Comp Physiol,* **37:**427, 1951.

Grillo, H. C., and Gross, J.: Studies in Wound Healing: III. Contraction in Vitamin C Deficiency, *Proc Soc Exp Biol Med,* **101:**268, 1959.

———, Watts, G. T., and Gross, J.: Studies in Wound Healing. I. Contraction and Wound Contents, *Ann Surg,* **148:**145, 1958.

James, D. W.: Intussusceptive Growth of Skin Islands within Wounds, *J Anat,* **93:**161, 1959.

———, and Newcombe, J. F.: Granulation Tissue Resorption during Free and Limited Contraction of Skin Wounds, *J Anat,* **95:**247, 1961.

Madden, J. W., Carlson, E. E., and Hines, J.: Presence of Modified Fibroblasts in Ischemic Contracture of the Intrinsic Musculature of the Hand, *Surg Gynecol Obstet,* **140:**509, 1975.

———, Morton, D., Jr., and Peacock, E. E., Jr.: Contraction of Experimental Wounds. I. Inhibiting Wound Contraction by Using a Topical Smoothe Muscle Antagonist, *Surgery,* **76:**18, 1974.

Majno, G., Babbiani, G., Hirschel, B. J., Ryan, G. B., and Statkov, P. R.: Contraction of Granulation Tissue *in vitro:* Similarity with Smooth Muscle, *Science,* **173:**548, 1971.

Phillips, J. L., and Peacock, E. E.: Importance of Horizontal Plane Cell Mass Integrity in Wound Contraction, *Proc Soc Exp Biol Med,* **117:**539, 1964.

Ryan, G. B., Cliff, W. J., Gabbiani, G., Iole, C., Montandon, D., Statkov, P. R., and Majno, G.: Myofibroblasts in Human Granulation Tissue, *Hum Pathol,* **5:**55, 1974.

Van den Brenk, H. A. S.: Studies in Restorative Growth Process in Mammalian Wound Healing, *Brit Surg,* **43:**525, 1956.

Watts, G. T., Grillo, H. C., and Gross, J.: Studies in Wound Healing: II. The Role of Granulation Tissue in Contraction, *Ann Surg,* **148:**153, 1958.

Epithelization

Abercrombie, M.: The Control of Growth and the Cell Surface, *Lect Sci Basis Med,* **8**(1958–1959):19, 1960.

Arey, L. B., and Covode, W. M.: The Method of Repair in Epithelial Wounds of the Cornea, *Anat Rec* **86:**75, 1943.

Brophy, D., and Lobitz, W. C.: Injury and Reinjury to Human Epidermis: II. Epidermal Basal Cell Response, *J Invest Dermatol,* **32:**495, 1959.

Bullough, W. S.: Mitotic and Functional Homeostasis, *Cancer Res,* **25:**1683, 1965.

—— and Lawrence, E. B.: The Control of Epidermal Mitotic Activity in the Mouse, *Proc R Soc Land [Biol],* **B151:**517, 1960.

Coman, D. R.: Decreased Mutual Adhesiveness: A Property of Cells from Squamous Cell Carcinomas, *Cancer Res,* **4:**625, 1944.

Gelfant, S.: Initiation of Mitosis in Relation to the Cell Division Cycle, *Exp Cell Res,* **26:**395, 1959.

Gillman, T., and Penn, J.: Studies on the Repair of Cutaneous Wounds, *Med Proc,* **2**(*Suppl.* 3):121, 1956.

Lobitz, W. C.: The Histochemical Response to Controlled Injury, *J Invest Dermatol,* **22:**189, 1954.

Medawar, P. B.: Biological Aspects of the Repair Process, *Br Med Bull,* **3:**70, 1945.

Meyer, K., Hoffman, P., and Linker, A.: Chemistry of Ground Substances, in I. Page (ed.), "Connective Tissue, Thrombosis and Atherosclerosis," p. 181, Academic Press, New York, 1959.

Needham, A. E.: "Regeneration and Wound Healing," Methuen & Co., Ltd, London, 1952.

Pace, D. M., and Layon, M. E.: Effect of Cell Density on Growth in HeLa Cells, *Growth,* **24:**355, 1960.

Sullivan, D. J., and Epstein, W. S.: Mitotic Activity of Wounded Human Epidermis, *J Invest Dermatol,* **41:**39, 1963.

Weiss, P.: The Biological Foundations of Wound Repair, *Harvey Lect,* (**55**)(1959–1960):**13,** 1961.

Winter, G. D.: Formation of the Scab and the Rate of Epithelialization of Superficial Wounds in the Skin of the Young Domestic Pig, *Nature* (*Lond*), **193:**293, 1962.

Collagen

Allgower, M., and Hulliger, L.: Origin of Fibroblasts from Mononuclear Blood Cells: A Study of *in vitro* Formation of the Collagen Precursor, Hydroxyproline, in Buffy Coat Cultures, *Surgery,* **47:**603, 1960.

Bornstein, P.: Disorders of Connective Tissue Function and the Aging Process: A Synthesis and Review of Current Concepts and Findings, *Mech Ageing Dev,* **5:**305, 1976.

Cohen, I. K., Keiser, H. R., and Sjoerdsma, A.: Collagen Synthesis in Human Keloid and Hypertrophic Scar, *Surg Forum,* 22:488, 1971.

Dayer, J., Russell, R. G., and Krane, S. M.: Collagenase Production by Rheumatoid Synovial Cells: Stimulation by a Human Lymphocyte Factor, *Science,* **195:**181, 1977.

Duskin, D., and Bornstein, P.: Impaired Conversion of Procollagen to Collagen by Fibroblasts and Bone Treated with Tunicamycin, an Inhibitor of Protein Glycosylation. *J Biol Chem,* **252:**955, 1977.

Gould, B. S.: Ascorbic Acid and Collagen Fiber Formation, *Vitam Horm,* **8:**89, 1960.

Grillo, H. C.: Origin of Fibroblasts in Wound Healing: An Autoradiographic Study of Inhibition of Cellular Proliferation by Local X-irradiation, *Ann Surg,* **157:**453, 1963.

Gross, J.: On the Significance of the Soluble Collagens, in I. H. Page (ed.), "Connective Tissue, Thrombosis and Atherosclerosis," pp. 77–95, Academic Press, Inc., New York, 1959.

——, Highberger, J. H., and Schmitt, F. O.: Extraction of Collagen from Connective Tissue by Neutral Salt Solutions, *Proc Natl Acad Sci USA,* **41:**1, 1955.

—— and Lapiere, C. M.: Collagenolytic Activity in Amphibian Tissues: A Tissue Culture Assay, *Proc Natl Acad Sci USA,* **48:**1014, 1962.

Hance, A. J., and Crystal, R. G.: The Connective Tissue of Lung, *Am Rev Respir Dis,* **112:**657, 1975.

Hoffmann, H., Olsen, B., Chen, H., and Prockop, D. J.: Segment-long-spacing Aggregates and Isolation of COOH-Terminal Peptides from Type I Procollagen, *Proc Natl Acad Sci USA,* **73:**4304, 1976.

Leven, C. I., and Gross, J.: Alterations in State of Molecular Aggregation of Collagen Induced in Chick Embryos by Aminopropionitrile (lathyrus factor), *J Exp Med,* **110:**771, 1959.

Madden, J. W., and Peacock, E. E.: Studies on the Biology of Collagen during Wound Healing: III. Dynamic Metabolism of Scar Collagen and Remodeling of Dermal Wounds, *Ann Surg,* **174:**511,1971.

——, and Smith, H. C.: Studies on the Biology of Collagen during Wound Healing: II. Rate of Collagen Synthesis and Deposition in Dehisced and Resutured Wounds, *Surg Gynecol Obstet,* **130:**487, 1970.

——: Some Aspects of Fibrogenesis during the Healing of Primary and Secondary Wounds, *Surg Gynecol Obstet,* **115:**408, 1962.

—— and Biggers, P. W.: Measurement and Significance of Heat-labile and Urea-sensitive Cross Linking Mechanisms in Collagen of Healing Wounds, *Surgery,* **54:**144, 1963.

Miller, E. S.: Biochemical Characteristics and Biological Significance of the Genetically-Distinct Collagens, *Mol Cell Biochem,* **13:**165, 1976.

Olsen, B., Hoffmann, H., and Prockop, D. J.: Interchain Disulfide Bonds at the COOH-Terminal End of Procollagen Synthesized by Matrix-free Cells from Chick Embryonic Tendon and Cartilage, *Arch Biochem Biophys,* **175:**341, 1976.

Prockop, D. J., Peterkofsky, B., and Udenfriend, S.: Studies on the Intracellular Localization of Collagen Synthesis in the Intact Chick Embryo, *J Biol Chem,* **237:**1581, 1962.

Raju, D. R., Jindrak, K., Weiner, M., and Enquist, I.: A Study of the Critical Bacterial Inoculum to Cause a Stimulus to Wound Healing, *Surg Gynecol Obstet,* 144:347, 1977.

Riley, W. B., Jr., and Peacock, E. E., Jr.: Identification, Distribution, and Significance of a Collagenolytic Enzyme in Human Tissue, *Proc Soc Biol Med,* **214:**207, 1967.

Ross, R., and Benditt, E. P.: Wound Healing and Collagen Formation: I. Sequential Changes in Components of Guinea Pig Wounds Observed in the Electron Microscope, *J Biophys Biochem Cytol,* **11:**677, 1961.

——— and ———: Wound Healing and Collagen Formation: III. A Quantitative Autoradiographic Study of the Utilization of Proline H³ in Wounds from Normal and Scorbutic Guinea Pigs, *J Cell Biol,* **15:**99, 1962.

Schiffman, E., and Martin, G. R.: Spontaneous Generation of Cross-Links in Aldehyde Containing Collagen, *Arch Biochem,* **138:**226, 1970.

Trelstad, R. L., Kimiko, H., and Gross, J.: Collagen Fibrillogenesis Intermediate Aggregates and Suprafibrillar Order, *Proc Natl Acad Sci USA,* **73:**4027, 1976.

Woessner, J. F.: Catabolism of Collagen and Non-collagen Protein in the Rat Uterus during Post-partum Involution, *Biochem J,* **83:**304, 1962.

Chapter 9

Oncology

by **Donald L. Morton, Frank C. Sparks, and Charles M. Haskell**

INTRODUCTION

Oncology (from the Greek *onkos,* mass, or tumor, and *logos,* study) is the study of neoplastic diseases. Neoplasms are an altered cell population characterized by an excessive, nonuseful proliferation of cells that have become unresponsive to normal control mechanisms and to the organizing influences of adjacent tissue. Malignant neoplasms are composed of cancer cells that exhibit uncontrolled proliferation and impair the function of normal organs by local tissue invasion and metastatic spread to distant anatomic sites. Benign neoplasms are composed of normal-appearing cells that are not locally invasive, or characterized by metastatic spread.

Cancer has plagued man since antiquity, and many of its clinical manifestations were described by Hippocrates (460–375 B.C.). Neoplasms have been identified in all species of animals including the lower vertebrates, such as amphibia and fish. The wide distribution of neoplasia in natural and human history suggests that cancer may be common to all multicellular organisms.

Neoplastic disease is the second most frequent cause of death in the United States. The magnitude of the cancer problem is exemplified by the fact that one of every four persons living today has or will develop cancer. An estimated 54 million Americans, one in four presently alive in the United States, will develop cancer sometime during their lifetime. Approximately one-third of those who get cancer will survive for at least 5 years after treatment. Until recently those facts caused many physicians and surgeons to approach the cancer patient with feelings of pessimism and despair that frequently interfered with adequate therapy. This aversion to the problems of cancer was reflected by the paucity of physicians willing to devote full time to its clinical studies. Furthermore, basic scientists were somewhat hesitant to investigate fundamental problems posed by the malignant state.

Fortunately, recent exciting developments in tumor immunology, viral oncology, and molecular biology and advances in the therapy of some neoplasms have led to a rebirth of interest in the basic biologic and clinical problems posed by cancer. The United States government has launched a massive Conquest of Cancer Program for cancer research. Specialty boards have been established in medical oncology and gynecologic oncology. A wide variety of scientists from many disciplines have been attracted to its study. As a result, it is probable that more advances will be made in cancer therapy during the next 10 years than in all previous times. This chapter is designed to introduce the student to general principles that can be used as the basis for acquiring further knowledge in this rapidly growing field.

EPIDEMIOLOGY

The changes in death rates caused by cancer by body site for males and females in the United States during the past 45 years are summarized in Figs. 9-1 and 9-2. Although there has been a decrease in mortality from certain neoplasms, the overall cancer death rates continue to show a slow, steady increase.

Age-Adjusted Cancer Death Rates* for Selected Sites, Males, United States 1930–1973

Sources: U.S. National Center for Health Statistics and U.S. Bureau of the Census.
*Standardized on the age distribution of the 1940 U.S. Census Population.

Fig. 9-1. Male cancer death rates by site, United States, 1930–1973 (standardized for age on the 1940 United States population). (*From National Vital Statistics Division and Bureau of the Census, United States.*)

The mortality rates from lung cancer have increased steadily and probably represent the most dramatic change for any cancer site. Compared with 40 years ago, the mortality is now eighteen times greater for men and six times greater for women. Lung cancer represents the leading cause of cancer death when both sexes are considered.

Pancreatic cancer death rates also have steadily increased through the years. Today, the rates are twice what they were in women and three times that in men when compared to 1930.

There has been a striking reduction during the past 40 years in death rates caused by cancers of the stomach and uterus. The stomach cancer death rate is now less than one-third the 1930 rate in men and less than one-fourth the 1930 rate in women, although there has been little improvement in the survival rates of stomach cancer. The

decreasing mortality is due to a decreased incidence of stomach cancer in both sexes. The reason for this declining incidence is unknown.

There has been a similar striking decline in death rates due to uterine cancer with mortality rates today only one-third what they were 40 years ago. In this case, the causes of the reduction are known to be earlier detection and improved treatment for cancer of the uterine cervix and corpus.

The incidences of cancer in different sites and the mortality rate in each sex are compared in Fig. 9-3. The sites most frequently causing cancer death in males, in order of decreasing frequency, are (1) lung, (2) colon and rectum, (3) prostate, (4) pancreas, and (5) stomach. The sites, in order of decreasing frequency in females, are (1) breast, (2) colon and rectum, (3) uterus, (4) lung, and (5) ovary.

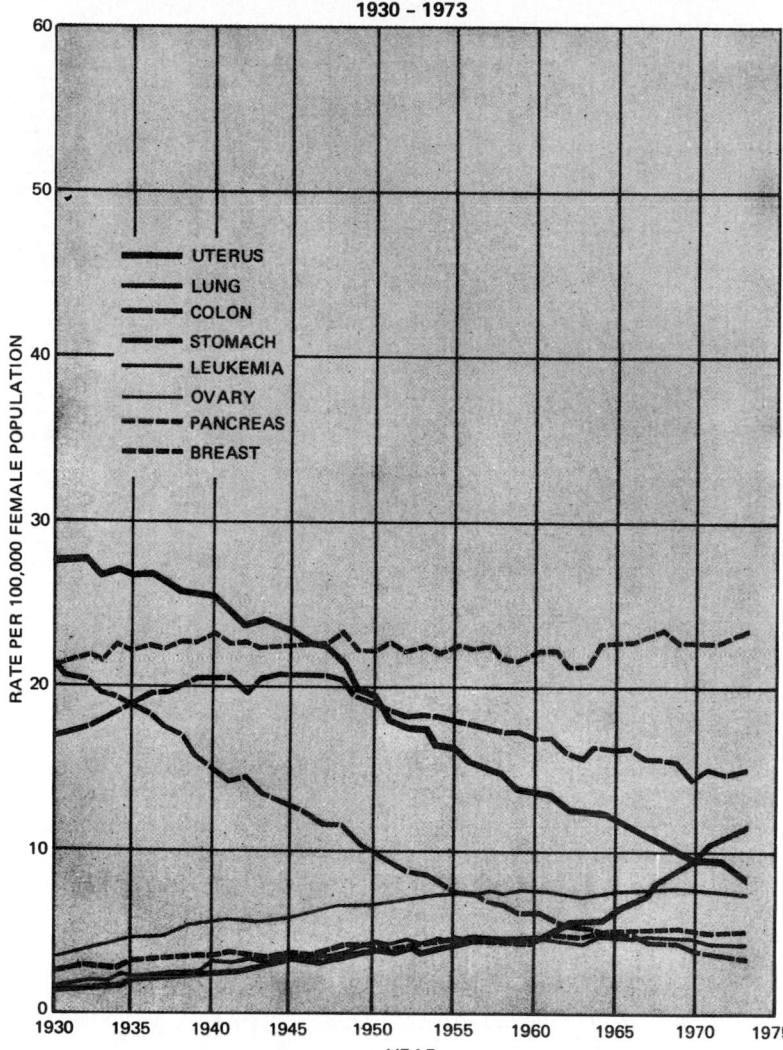

Age-Adjusted Cancer Death Rates* for Selected Sites, Females, United States 1930 – 1973

Fig. 9-2. Female cancer death rates by site, United States, 1930–1973 (standardized for age on the 1940 United States population). (*From National Vital Statistics Division and Bureau of the Census, United States.*)

Sources: U.S. National Center for Health Statistics and U.S. Bureau of the Census.
*Standardized on the age distribution of the 1940 U.S. Census Population.

It is obvious that there are differing incidences of kinds of cancer occurring in the male and female.

The incidence of various types of neoplasms differs from the death rates for the same neoplasms (Fig. 9-4) because different forms of cancer are not equally lethal. The most significant 5-year survival rates are achieved in patients with cancer of the skin (94 percent) and uterus (70 percent); the lowest survival occurs in patients with lung cancer (9 percent). Lung cancer is the leading cause of cancer death even though skin cancer occurs more commonly.

Females tend to have a greater number of 5-year survivals with cancers of any given primary site than males, although the reasons are unknown at this time. The overall 5-year survival for women with cancer is 50 percent, compared with only 31 percent for men. The overall 5-year

cancer survival rates for common malignant tumors of selected sites are shown in Fig. 9-5.

ETIOLOGY

The primary etiologic factors responsible for most neoplasms in man are still unknown. In experimental animals, a wide variety of causative agents have been identified. These agents may be classified as chemical and physical, viral and genetic. There is no reason to doubt that a similar variety of factors is responsible for causing human cancer. Although the primary mechanisms by which these agents cause neoplastic transformation is unknown, it seems relatively certain that the inciting agents represent but one link in the chain of factors that leads to the development of

1977 ESTIMATES

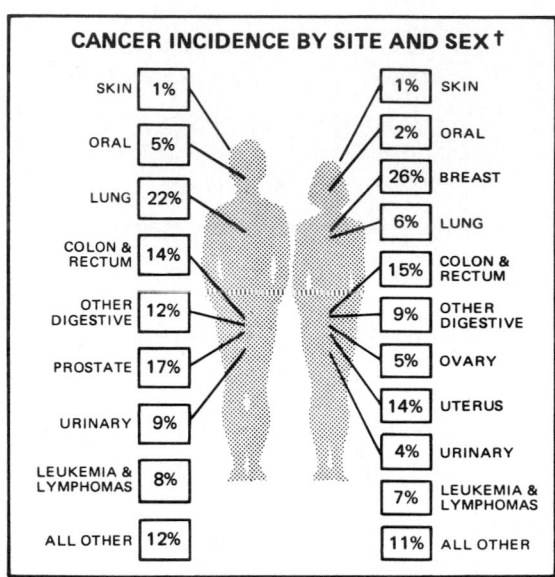

CANCER INCIDENCE BY SITE AND SEX †

SKIN	1%	1% SKIN
ORAL	5%	2% ORAL
		26% BREAST
LUNG	22%	6% LUNG
COLON & RECTUM	14%	15% COLON & RECTUM
OTHER DIGESTIVE	12%	9% OTHER DIGESTIVE
PROSTATE	17%	5% OVARY
		14% UTERUS
URINARY	9%	4% URINARY
LEUKEMIA & LYMPHOMAS	8%	7% LEUKEMIA & LYMPHOMAS
ALL OTHER	12%	11% ALL OTHER

† Excluding non-melanoma skin cancer and carcinoma in situ of uterine cervix.

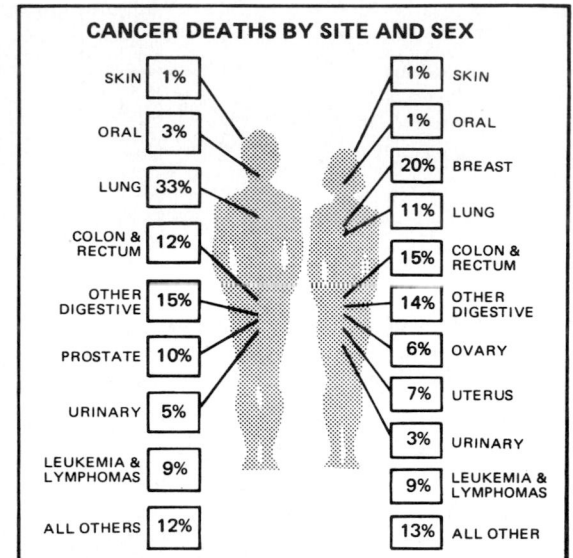

CANCER DEATHS BY SITE AND SEX

SKIN	1%	1% SKIN
ORAL	3%	1% ORAL
		20% BREAST
LUNG	33%	11% LUNG
COLON & RECTUM	12%	15% COLON & RECTUM
OTHER DIGESTIVE	15%	14% OTHER DIGESTIVE
PROSTATE	10%	6% OVARY
		7% UTERUS
URINARY	5%	3% URINARY
LEUKEMIA & LYMPHOMAS	9%	9% LEUKEMIA & LYMPHOMAS
ALL OTHERS	12%	13% ALL OTHER

Fig. 9-3. Estimated cancer incidence and resultant deaths by site and sex. Incidence for major sites = 391,000 and deaths = 213,000. If carcinoma in situ is included in cancer of the uterus, incidence = 87,000; if nonmelanoma is included, incidence for skin = 300,000. (*From National Cancer Institute, Third National Cancer Survey, 1969–71.*)

cancer. Therefore, the identification of carcinogenic agents, although their mechanisms of action are unknown, can be extremely important in cancer prevention.

CHEMICAL CARCINOGENS. The first cause-and-effect relation between a carcinogenic stimulus and the development of cancer in man was described by Percival Pott, an English surgeon, in 1775, when he described a cancer of the scrotum frequently occurring in the chimney sweeps. However, Yamagiwa and Ichikawa, working from 1915 to 1918, identified the carcinogen when they experimentally produced cancers by painting the ears of rabbits with coal tar. Kennaway and Cook in studies from 1924 to 1932, demonstrated that pure hydrocarbons, such as 1, 2-dibenz-anthracene and similar compounds isolated from coal tar,

were carcinogenic agents. Subsequently, a variety of chemical agents have been found that are capable of inducing neoplasms in experimental animals and in man. These chemicals are called *carcinogens*. There may be many years separating the time of exposure to a carcinogen and subse-

Fig. 9-4. *A.* Cancer death rates by sex, United States, 1900–1968 (standardized for age on the 1940 United States population). *B.* Forecast of cancer deaths based on present trends. (*From National Vital Statistics Division and Bureau of the Census, United States.*)

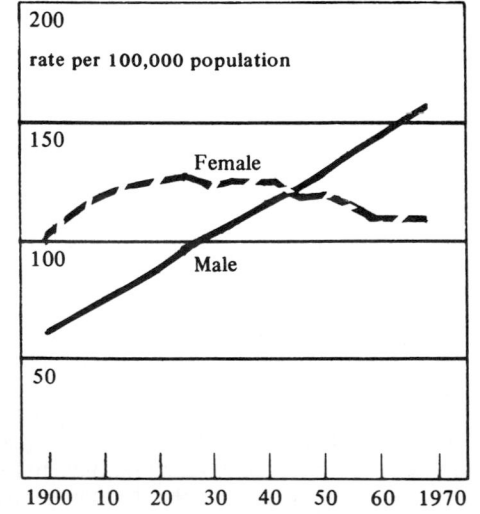

A — rate per 100,000 population. Female, Male. 1900 10 20 30 40 50 60 70

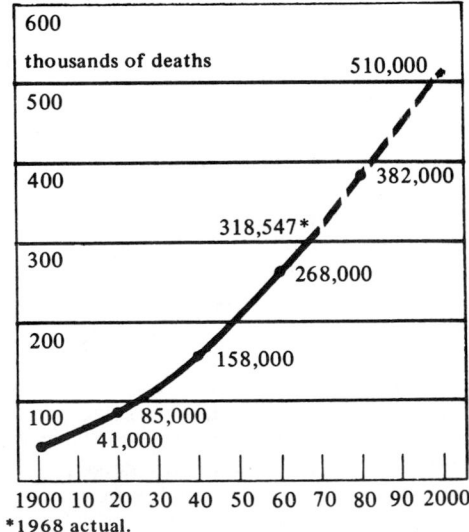

B — thousands of deaths. 510,000; 382,000; 318,547*; 268,000; 158,000; 85,000; 41,000. 1900 10 20 30 40 50 60 70 80 90 2000. *1968 actual.

quent development of a neoplasm. Consequently, the present-day evaluation of the safety of food additives or other products for human consumption that are chronically ingested over long periods of time is a most difficult task.

A variety of chemicals which have been associated with different types of human neoplasms are summarized in Table 9-1. Aromatic amines are known to cause tumors of the urinary tract; workers in the dye industry have a higher incidence of this type of cancer. Benzene has been associated with acute leukemia, in shoe repairmen in Italy, solvent manufacturers, painters, and printers who use it as a solvent. Coal tar, pitch, creosote, and anthracene have been associated with cancer of the skin, larynx, and bronchus. A variety of paraffin oils, waxes, and tars are associated with cancer of the skin. Isopropyl oil has been associated with cancer of the sinuses, larynx, and bronchus in workers exposed to it. Mesotheliomas occur very frequently in miners and ship workers who have been exposed to asbestos. Certain metals have been associated with tumors, including chromium, nickel, and arsenic.

PHYSICAL CARCINOGENS. Ionizing radiation was found in the 1920s to be carcinogenic when subcutaneous sarcomas were induced by radium implants in experimental animals. The carcinogenic effects of radiation in man was recognized when radium dial painters who commonly licked brushes containing radioactive materials developed bone cancers. Since then, many examples of the carcinogenic effects of radiation in man have been recognized. In physicians and dentists who experience multiple x-ray exposures recurrent skin cancer has developed. Cancer of the thyroid in adults is frequently associated with neck irradiation in early childhood. The survivors of the atomic bomb detonations show an increased incidence of leukemia. Ultraviolet light on exposed areas may foster the development of skin cancer. Farmers and sailors have an increased incidence of skin cancers from excessive exposure to sunlight, as do fair-skinned people living in tropical regions.

Mechanical Irritation. Chronic mechanical irritation may be associated with the development of cancer, although the exact mechanisms are unknown. Examples include the malignant degeneration in old burn scars (the chronic ulcer of Marjolin), and cancer of the liver and bladder subsequent to parasitic infestation by schistosomes.

VIRUSES. These are carcinogenic in several animal species, and it is likely that some cancers in man are caused by viruses. Many animal-oncogenic viruses have been described since 1911 when Rous discovered a filterable agent which caused sarcoma in chickens. At least two distinct classes of viruses can cause tumors. Ribonucleic acid (RNA) viruses have been associated with sarcomas, lymphomas, leukemias, and mammary cancer in chickens, mice, rats, cats, monkeys, and gibbons. Deoxyribonucleic acid (DNA) viruses also are oncogenic. The polyoma virus can cause multiple tumors in mice, rats, and hamsters. Simian virus (SV-40) can cause a sarcoma in hamsters; papilloma virus causes papillomas in a variety of animals; adenoviruses have caused sarcomas in rodents. Pox viruses have been associated with fibromas in the rabbit and

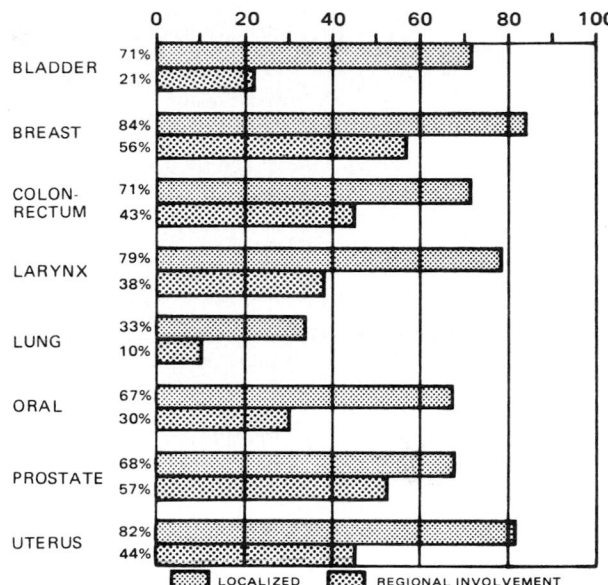

Fig. 9-5. Five-year cancer survival rates for selected sites.

squirrel, and a tumor in the monkey. Herpes viruses cause neoplasms in frogs, chickens, and monkeys.

Despite clear-cut evidence for a viral cause of a variety of animal tumors, there has been no proof that viruses can cause human neoplasms. Yet, it would be surprising if man were not susceptible to some form of viral carcinogenesis because it is so common in all other animal species, and basic biologic phenomena are generally quite similar throughout nature. In fact, there is increasing evidence linking viruses with certain types of human neoplasms and suggesting a prominent role in etiology. The Epstein-Barr (EB) virus, probably the cause of infectious mononucleosis in man, is linked to the occurrences of Burkitt's lymphoma in Africa and to nasopharyngeal cancer in the Orient. RNA viruses of a characteristic type (type C) similar to those agents known to cause leukemias, and sarcomas in mice, have been associated with leukemias, sarcomas, and papillary urinary neoplasms in man. RNA viruses resembling the mammary tumor virus of mice have been found in the breast cancers and milk from women with this malignant disease.

Two modes of oncogenic viral transmission, vertical and horizontal, have been described. Vertical transmission involves passage of virus from parent to offspring. For example, the mouse mammary tumor virus is transmitted to progeny in the mother's milk, and the Gross leukemia virus is transmitted in the gametes of the parents to the offspring. Horizontal transmission is passage of virus to close contacts in excreta and airborne particles, as with the polyoma virus.

Table 9-1. CHEMICAL AND PHYSICAL CARCINOGENS IN HUMAN BEINGS

Carcinogen	Site of neoplasm	Site exposed	Persons at risk
Chemical agents:			
Aromatic amines, especially β-naphthylamine	Urinary tract	Cutaneous and respiratory	Chemical workers producing dye stuffs, rodenticides, laboratory reagents
Benzol or benzene	Blood, lymphatic organs	Cutaneous and respiratory	Coal tar refiners, solvent manufacturers, painters, printers, mechanics
Coal tar, pitch, creosote, anthracene, tobacco	Skin, larynx, bronchus	Cutaneous and respiratory	Coke oven workers, coal tar distillers, lumber industry workers, chemical workers, smokers
Petroleum, shale and paraffin oils, waxes, tars	Skin	Cutaneous	Workers in oil refineries, wax and asphalt producers, mechanics
Isopropyl oils	Sinus, larynx, bronchus	Respiratory	Producers of isopropyl alcohol
Asbestos	Bronchus, mesothelioma of pleura	Respiratory, generally > 2 years	Asbestos miners, shippers, millers
Chromium	Bronchus	Respiratory and cutaneous	Workers engaged in chromate ore reduction
Nickel	Nasal cavity, sinus, bronchus	Respiratory	Nickel miners, shippers, and refiners
Arsenic	Skin, bronchus, bladder	Respiratory	Smelters, pesticide manufacturers
Physical agents:			
Ionizing radiation	Skin, thyroid, tongue, tonsil, sinus, bone, blood	Local or systemic, therapeutic (e.g., treatment of spondylitic polycythemia)	Radium dial workers
	Bronchus	Respiratory	Pitchblend miners
Ultraviolet radiation	Skin	Cutaneous	Farmers, other outdoor workers, sailors, fishermen, and fair-skinned people in tropical climates

Experimental animals must be infected as newborn offspring with almost all oncogenic viruses to produce neoplastic change in adulthood. The immunologic immaturity of the neonate allows viral infection and induction of neoplastic transformation. Adult animals are resistant to infection with oncogenic viruses unless they are immunosuppressed.

Studies of viral oncogenesis can become quite complex in situations where multiple factors may interact to produce a situation which ultimately causes cancer. The development of mouse mammary cancer depends upon the cooperation of (1) genetic susceptibility, (2) proper hormonal stimuli, and (3) infection with the virus in the first 6 weeks of life. When all these conditions have been met, the breast cancer still requires 1 to 2 years to develop.

HEREDITARY FACTORS. Genetic factors have been demonstrated to be of major importance in determining the effectiveness of chemical, physical and viral carcinogens in animals.

Clear-cut examples of genetic factors playing a role in human cancer development are demonstrated when the same type of cancer occurs in identical twins, when colon cancer develops in persons with familial polyposis, and with the familial patterns associated with breast cancer. Cancer of the breast is about three times more common

in the daughters of women with breast cancer and in women whose blood relatives have had at least two incidences of breast cancer. Furthermore, the daughters develop breast cancers at a younger age than did their mothers.

A more indirect genetic role was noted in certain families who seemed to have an increased incidence of neoplastic diseases. A clearly defined pattern of inheritance has been established for some of these tumors. It is often difficult to assess the importance of environmental factors in these cases. Substantiated examples include a pattern of dominant inheritance in some families for diseases such as retinoblastoma, lipomatosis, and colonic polyposis. In other families, there may be an association of multiple diseases that may include one or more neoplasms. An example of this is the association of pheochromocytoma with medullary (amyloid-producing) carcinoma of the thyroid, cerebellocortical hemangioblastoma, or neurofibromatosis. Other examples where tumors appear to be inherited in families as a dominant trait include some cases of polyendocrine adenomas (pituitary, parathyroid, pancreas), including the Zollinger-Ellison syndrome and hereditary adenocarcinomatosis (adenocarcinoma of the colon, stomach, uterus, and ovary occurring in different members of the same family). There are also several relatively rare heritable nonneoplastic diseases which have been associated with malignant tumors with great frequency. An example of this is the high incidence of skin cancer in patients with xeroderma pigmentosa. There also is an association between dermal inclusion cysts and multiple carcinomas of the colon, polyposis, multiple bony exostoses, and benign connective tissue tumors (Gardner's syndrome).

There are marked differences in the frequency of certain neoplastic diseases with respect to age, sex, and other constitutional factors suggesting that additional host determinants may be important. Acute lymphocytic leukemia is essentially a disease of childhood, whereas malignant melanoma is essentially a postpubertal disease. Testicular tumors and Hodgkin's disease are more frequent in young adults, and breast cancer is far more common in women than in men. In many other tumors, the frequency in both sexes increases markedly with increasing age.

GEOGRAPHIC FACTORS. Neoplasms may be found in all human populations, but there are some striking racial and regional differences in the occurrence of specific types of cancer. Although it is difficult to separate the genetic from the environmental factors, such as diet or habits, it is important to be aware of certain particularly strong differences. In a comparison study with the Caucasian population of the United States, Shimkin noted the following differences in cancer incidence:

1. High incidence of cancer of the stomach in Scandinavia, Iceland, and Japan
2. High incidence of primary cancer of the liver in South and West Africa
3. High incidence of cancer of the nasopharynx in China
4. High incidence of cancer of the urinary bladder in Egypt
5. Low incidence of cancer of the breast in Japan
6. Low incidence of cancer of the uterine cervix in Israel and in Jewish women in general
7. Low incidence of cancer of the skin in Negroes
8. Low incidence of cancer of the prostate in Japan and China

Custom and environment obviously play an important role in the development of cancer. It is almost certain that some of the geographic factors noted above are due more to environmental factors than to genetic ones. Migration of populations usually causes a shift toward the patterns of cancer incidence of the host country. For example, in Japan there is a very high incidence of stomach cancer and a relatively low incidence of lung cancer. However, a second generation Japanese-American has a low risk of stomach cancer, and if a heavy smoker, he has as high a risk of lung cancer as his smoking American counterpart.

For unknown reasons, socioeconomic factors may also influence cancer incidence. Cancer of the stomach and of the cervix are three to four times more frequent in lower economic groups than in middle and higher economic groups. On the other hand, cancer of the breast, leukemia, and multiple myeloma are more frequent in higher socioeconomic groups.

PRECANCEROUS CONDITIONS. Some clinical disorders are described as precancerous because they are so frequently followed by the development of cancer. It is particularly important that the physician be aware of these conditions in order to conduct careful follow-up of these patients. Some precancerous conditions are leukoplakia, actinic keratoses, polyps of the colon or rectum, neurofibromas, dysplasia of the cervix or bronchial mucosa, and chronic ulcerative colitis.

MULTIFACTORIAL ETIOLOGY. It is likely that in any given individual cancer is the result not of just one but of multiple factors. There may be an interaction of an oncogenic virus with a chemical or physical carcinogen. It is also possible that two chemical carcinogens may act synergistically to increase the incidence of cancer. A chemical may be a carcinogen only in those with a hereditary susceptibility. When condensations of smog or cigarette smoke are applied separately to the cheek pouch of the golden hamster, there is a low but definite incidence of tumor. However, a synergistic interaction is observed when they are applied together, with a markedly increased incidence of tumors. Similarly, viruses have enhanced the oncogenic effects of smog and cigarette smoke in tissue culture. It is very possible that such synergistic interactions also occur in man.

The possibility that multiple factors may be involved in the etiology of human neoplasia, although it makes the proof of any one factor as a causative agent more complex, may in itself increase the chances of ultimate cancer prevention by providing a larger number of factors to be manipulated. For example, in carcinoma of the lung, it may be that in addition to heavy cigarette smoking (perhaps only chronic irritation), one requires a specific genetic background (since not all heavy smokers develop cancer of the lung), suitable male hormonal factors (since males are more frequently affected), and a virus. In addition, the latent period between start of smoking and high incidence of lung cancer is roughly 35 years. Although cigarette smoking may not be the only cause of lung cancer, it is the only factor which is known at the present time that can be controlled. On the basis of present knowledge, lung cancer could be prevented by eliminating cigarette smoking altogether or by limiting cigarette smoking to a shorter period of time.

Custom and environment obviously play an important part in the etiology of cancer. Although cigarette smoking has been strongly implicated as a cause of squamous cell carcinoma of the lung, the habit is sufficiently ingrained in people in the United States to make its total elimination extremely difficult. Habits and customs in other parts of the world may be equally difficult to eliminate. The inhalation of snuff and the mastication of betel nuts have been associated with nasal and oral pharynx tumors, but the use of such materials continues despite their known carcinogenic effects. Nevertheless, efforts to identify the causative factors and to educate people regarding these factors must be continued.

BIOLOGY

Regardless of the etiologic agent, the cancer cell is a progeny of a normal cell that has lost its cellular mechanisms for controlling proliferation. The cancer cell differs from a normal cell in a variety of ways, but none of its new characteristics are absolutely indicative of malignancy. Cytogenetic studies of some cancer cells have revealed various abnormalities in chromosome number and appearance. However, these changes have not been shared by all cancer cells, and many cancer cells have normal chromosomal profiles.

Almost all malignant neoplasms seem to arise from a single cell that has undergone malignant transformation to form a malignant clone (group of cells); however, other human neoplasms such as the neurofibromas occurring in von Recklinghausen's disease may develop from multiple clones of cells. Simultaneously multifocal origins of carcinoma of the breast, oral pharynx, colon, and other organs also have been observed. Studies of breast carcinoma have demonstrated that at least 30 percent have other areas involved with in situ carcinoma. Nevertheless, the primary tumor mass which was the cause for clinical presentation arises from a single cell alone.

Although the proliferative rate of cancer cells is generally greater than the overall average of normal cells, the former do not divide more rapidly than some normal cells, such as leukocytes or cells of the intestinal mucosa. The proliferative rate of cancer cells generally decreases as the tumor mass grows. It has been shown that the proportion of cells undergoing mitosis is much greater when there are only a few cancer cells present than when there are many cells present in a large tumor mass. There are many rapid changes in the mitotic fraction of neoplasms during the initial growth phase, but after the tumor mass is 1 cm in diameter, the rate of division usually follows a predictable pattern.

After neoplastic transformation has occurred, the cancer cell differs from the normal cell not only in proliferative index but also in morphology, biochemistry, antigenetic expression, and many other aspects.

MORPHOLOGIC CHANGES. Malignant cells tend to revert to more primitive cell types, that is, to dedifferentiate. The normal orderly tissue patterns are lost or replaced by the random piling up of malignant cells without definite pattern. Other histologic changes may include cellular pleomorphism, a high index of mitoses, and hyperchromatism in the nucleus and nucleoli. Invasion of adjacent normal structures also may be seen microscopically. These morphologic changes are the basis for histopathologic or cytologic diagnoses of cancer and usually allow very accurate diagnosis of neoplastic diseases.

BIOCHEMICAL CHANGES. The biochemical activity of cancer cells is similar, though not identical, to that of normal cells. A great diversity exists in the biochemical characteristics of different tumor cells, usually correlating with rate of proliferation. Changes in DNA, RNA, and the chemical architecture of the cellular membrane of malignant cells are associated with the loss of contact inhibition to proliferation and intercellular adhesiveness. However, no single biochemical alteration has yet been defined that is absolutely characteristic of malignant transformation.

Reversion of the normal cellular biochemistry to that of the embryonal cells produces distinctive embryonal substances whose presence in the adult may be used to diagnose cancer. The carcinoembryonic antigen associated with gastrointestinal cancers, and α-fetoglobulin associated with hepatoma and embryonal cancers are thought to be examples of this type. The synthesis of these substances may be due to depression of fetal gene function that occurs during oncogenesis.

Malignant cells may also produce biologically active substances that are normally produced by the cells from which the neoplasm originated. The release of these substances may cause symptoms similar to hyperfunction of that particular organ, for example, hyperparathyroidism produced by parathyroid carcinomas. Neoplasms may also produce biologically active substances that are not normally produced by the cells of origin. Some bronchogenic carcinomas may produce parathyroidlike hormones, ACTH, antidiuretic hormones, and other hormones.

The mechanism of this ectopic hormone secretion is based upon the hypothesis of variable genetic activity or *selective derepression* of a specific gene. All cells contain the same genes; however, only about 10 percent of these genes are expressed in any one cell type; the remainder are repressed. Cancer cells are primitive cells; with the dedifferentiation, they acquire the ability to express some of these previously repressed genes. This new genetic expression is responsible for the production of a new specific-messenger RNA and the production of new polypeptides and hormones.

GROWTH RATES OF NEOPLASMS. Approximately two-thirds of the growth of human neoplasms occurs before they are clinically detectable. If one assumes that a cancer begins from a single cell, then it takes about 30 exponential divisions to produce a 1-cm nodule (1 billion cells). At 45 exponential divisions the patient is apt to be dead from the sheer bulk of the malignant tumor.

The growth rate of tumors can be expressed by the *tumor doubling time,* i.e., the time it takes for a tumor to double in volume. Tumor doubling times appear to be an accurate and precise method for comparing the biologic aggressiveness of neoplasms in different patients. This measurement is particularly applicable to metastatic pulmonary lesions, since these are usually peripheral in location and are discretely delineated on chest roentgenograms, so that accurate serial measurements are easily obtainable.

The method used in the measurement of the tumor doubling time is illustrated in Fig. 9-6. Briefly, the average of the greater and the lesser diameters of each metastatic nodule is determined from successive chest roentgenograms. The averages are plotted on semilogarithmic paper against the time in days between these points; the slope of this line represents the rate of tumor growth. Where this line crosses any two doubling lines, the horizontal distance between them represents the tumor doubling time in days. This measurement has been shown to be an accurate and reproducible method for the quantitation of the rate and pattern of tumor growth in individual patients.

The tumor doubling time of neoplasms varies from 8 to 600 days, most tumors doubling in 20 to 100 days. The measurement of tumor doubling times can be extremely helpful in determining prognosis, in evaluating response

Fig. 9-6. Method of plotting tumor doubling time, based upon the direct measurement of the changing diameters of metastatic pulmonary nodules. (*From W. L. Joseph et al., J Thorac Cardiovasc Surg, 61:23, 1971.*)

to chemotherapeutic agents, and in comparing responses to different therapeutic regimens.

In one study the tumor doubling times of a large series of patients with pulmonary metastases from tumors of different histologic types were measured. Wide variations within particular types of neoplasms were found. The tumor doubling time correlated closely with the length of survival in three distinct groups of patients. This is illustrated in Fig. 9-7. This correlation might be expected, because the tumor doubling time represents the balance between the intrinsic proliferative rate of the tumor cell and the patient's inhibiting defense mechanisms.

Based on growth dynamics, most human tumors have been present in the body for at least 1 year and many for as long as 10 to 15 years prior to their clinical detection. Thus, it appears that there is a long period of time between the inception of neoplastic transformation and the development of clinical cancer. During this time, detection may be possible and surgical treatment might result in cure. Tests must be perfected to detect cancer earlier, thus shorten this preclinical interval, and make surgical treatment more successful.

Immunobiology

The concept that cancer patients may develop an immune response against their neoplasms is not new. This view became very popular at the turn of the century when

it was found that strong immunity could be induced against transplantable neoplasms in randomly bred laboratory rodents. A period of intense laboratory and clinical investigation followed, in anticipation that tumor immunity might lead to control of malignant disease. However, it soon became evident that the immunity was not directed against tumor-specific antigens (TSA), but instead against normal tissue antigens in the neoplasm due to genetic differences between tumor donor and recipient. Thereafter, interest in tumor immunology declined because no antigens other than the transplantation antigens could be demonstrated in neoplasms.

Interest in the immunology of neoplastic diseases was reawakened in the 1950s when tumor-specific antigens were conclusively demonstrated in methylcholanthrene-induced sarcomas of mice. In order to eliminate any histocompatibility factors the investigators used inbred strains of rodents that, after many years of inbreeding, had the genetic homogeneity of monozygotic twins. Specific tumor transplantation resistance was induced by presensitization with a transplant of tumor tissue which was allowed to grow for a time and then was excised. The immunized rodents were then resistant to challenge with further transplants of the same neoplasm (Fig. 9-8). However, the limitations of tumor immunity were evident by the fact that the immunity induced in these animals was relative, not absolute. Whereas a challenge with 100,000 tumor cells produced a growing tumor in control mice, it did not in

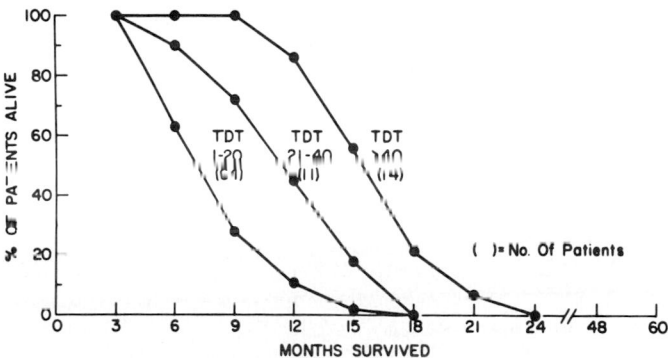

Fig. 9-7. Survival curves in 89 untreated patients following the onset of pulmonary metastases, showing three groups based upon tumor doubling time. (*From W. L. Joseph et al., J Thorac Cardiovasc Surg, 61:23, 1971.*)

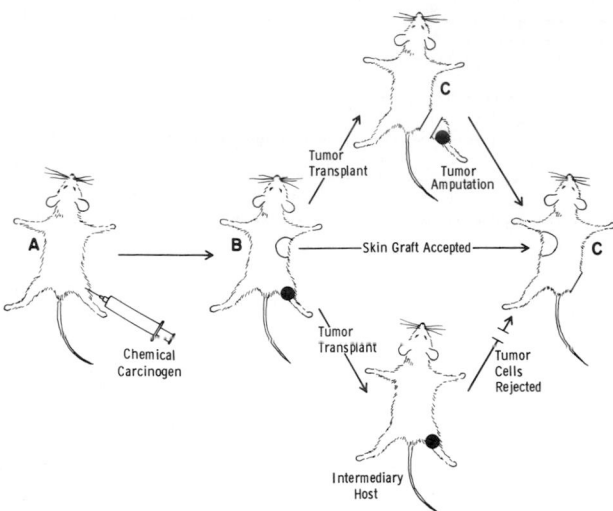

Fig. 9-8. Tumor induced with benzpyrene in mouse A is transplanted into mouse B. Mouse C, immunized by amputation of a tumor-bearing extremity, demonstrates tumor-specific immunity by rejecting tumor cells while accepting a normal skin graft from the same mouse.

Table 9-2. TUMOR-SPECIFIC ANTIGENS CAPABLE OF INDUCING REJECTION RESPONSES IN SYNGENEIC HOSTS

Inducing agent	*Antigenic specificity*
Chemical carcinogens:	
3-Methylcholanthrene	
1,2,5,6-Dibenzanthracene	
9,10-Dimethylbenzathracene	
3,4,9,10-Dibenzpyrene	Antigens distinct for
3,4-Benzpyrene-dimethylam-	each individual
inoazobenzene	neoplasm
Physical agents	
Films	
Millipore filter	
Cellophane film	
Radiation:	
Ultraviolet	
^{90}Sr	
Virus:	
DNA:	
Polyoma	
SV-40	
Adenovirus 12,18	
Shope papilloma	
RNA:	Common antigens in
Mammary tumor agent	each neoplasm in-
Leukemia	duced by the same
Gross	virus
Moloney	
Rauscher } Shared common	
Friend } antigens	
Graffi	
Rich	
Rous (Schmidt-Ruppin)	

the immune mice. Challenge with larger numbers of cells (1 to 10 million), however, usually overwhelmed the immunologic defense, and progressive tumor growth was observed.

During the past 15 years there has been tremendous progress in tumor immunology. Tumor-specific antigens have been demonstrated in most viral, chemical, and physical-carcinogen-induced neoplasms, as well as in many spontaneous tumors. These tumor-specific antigens can elicit tumor-specific immunity against tumor transplantation in syngeneic animals; thus, they are known as *tumor-specific transplantation antigens* (TSTA).

ANTIGENIC SPECIFICITY OF ANIMAL NEOPLASMS. The wide variety of viral, chemical, and physical-carcinogen-induced neoplasms for which tumor-specific transplantation antigens have been demonstrated are summarized in Table 9-2. The antigenic specificity of these major types of carcinogenic agents have been found to be quite different.

Tumor-specific Antigens of Neoplasms Induced by Chemical and Physical Carcinogens. These are individually distinct for each tumor, even if induced by the same carcinogen, in the same strain, and of the identical histologic type (Fig. 9-9). For example, injection of a chemical carcinogen such as benzpyrene in two inbred mice of the same strain will result in two antigenically different tumors, t_1 and t_2. If mouse *A* is immunized with irradiated tumor cells from t_1, it will subsequently reject tumor cells from the same tumor transplanted into an intermediate host. However, the same animal, immune to t_1, will develop a tumor when injected with the same number of tumor cells from t_2.

Tumor-specific Antigens of Neoplasms Induced by Viral Carcinogens. In contrast to the unique tumor-specific antigens of chemical-carcinogen-induced tumors, the tumor-specific antigens of viral-induced neoplasms are common to all neoplasms induced by the same virus, but differ from those induced by other viruses (Fig. 9-10). For example, with inbred mice of the same strain, mouse *A* is immunized with SV-40 virus alone, mouse *B* is immunized with *irradiated* tumor cells from a SV-40 virus–induced mouse tumor, and mouse *C* is immunized with tumor cells from an SV-40 virus–induced rat tumor. All will reject challenge of tumor cells from SV-40 virus–induced tumor t. However, challenge with the same tumor cells in mice *D* and *E,* immunized with either polyoma virus alone or polyoma virus–induced tumor cells, leads to progressive tumor growth and death.

Although the generalization that virus-induced neoplasms contain common antigens and chemical-carcinogen-induced neoplasms contain individually distinct antigens is usually correct, more recent studies have demonstrated that this distinction is not as absolute as originally believed. Common antigens related to leukemia viral antigens have been found in chemical-carcinogen-induced sarcomas, and some carcinogen-induced neoplasms arising in the bladder have contained common antigens. Furthermore, spontaneous mouse mammary carcinomas induced by the mammary tumor virus contain individually distinct antigens in addition to the common antigens of the mammary tumor virus.

MECHANISMS OF TUMOR-SPECIFIC IMMUNE REJEC-TION. The cellular immune response is thought to be more important in controlling tumor rejection than the humoral antibody response for several reasons: (1) tumor-specific immunity can be adoptively transferred by lymphocytes (Fig. 9-11) much more readily than by humoral antibody; (2) immune lymphocytes or macrophages that kill tumor cells in vitro can be demonstrated.

Many immune responses may be mediated by products of stimulated macrophages or lymphocytes. These products are collectively called *lymphokines* and may be important for the modification and development of the cellular immune response. For example, macrophage inhibition factor and chemotactic factor are both produced by lymphocytes after antigenic stimulation and may control the movement of macrophages or granulocytes in the development of delayed cutaneous hypersensitivity or inflammation. Many other such products have been described and probably contribute to the interaction between different cell types.

The lymphocyte may have a receptor site on its surface that is specific for the tumor-associated antigen on the tumor cell. Once contact is established, the lymphocyte could mediate a cytotoxic event (perhaps via a toxic protein such as lymphotoxin) that causes disruption of the tumor cell membrane and subsequent tumor cell death.

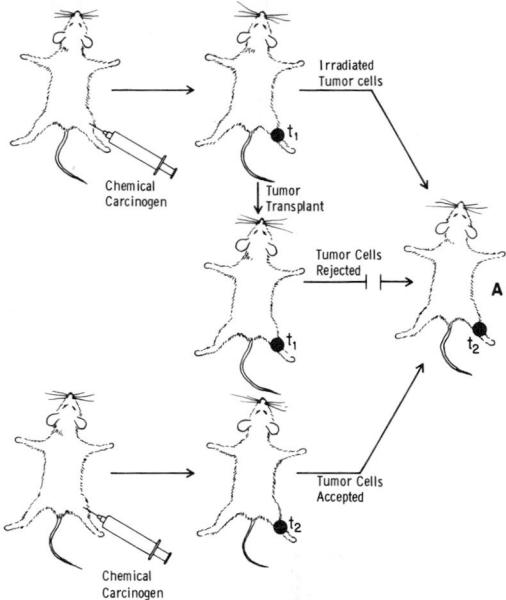

Fig. 9-9. Mouse A, immunized with benzpyrene-induced tumor t, resists subsequent challenge with t tumor cells. Challenge with cells from another benzpyrene-induced tumor, t_2, leads to progressive tumor growth and death of the mouse.

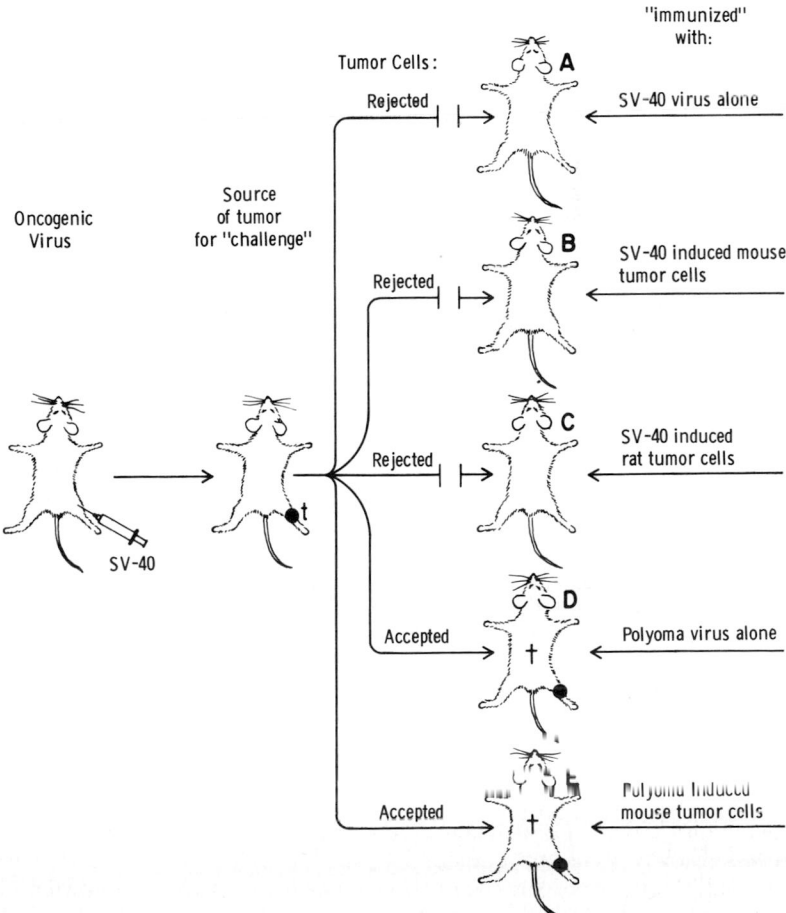

Fig. 9-10. Mice A, B, and C, immunized with SV-40 virus or SV-40 virus–induced tumor cells, reject challenge of tumor cells from SV-40 virus–induced tumor t. Challenge with the same tumor cells in mice D and E, immunized with polyoma virus or polyoma virus–induced tumor cells, leads to progressive tumor growth and death of the mouse.

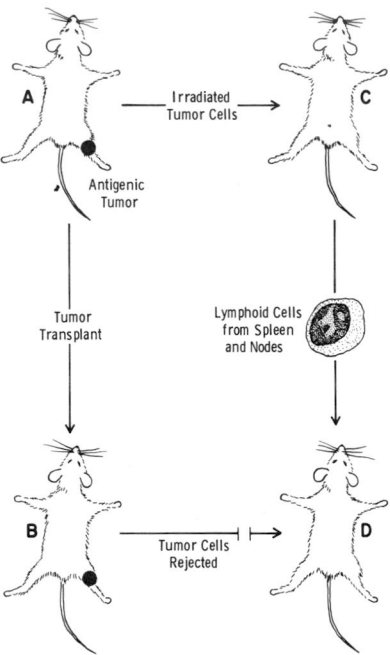

Fig. 9-11. Tumor induced in mouse A with benzpyrene is serially passed into another mouse, B, of the same strain. Mouse C is immunized with irradiated tumor cells of the same tumor. Immune lymphocytes transferred from mouse C to mouse D confer tumor-specific immunity to subsequent tumor challenge.

Thymus-derived lymphocytes have been credited as the main effector cells for tumor immunity. However, recent experiments have demonstrated the importance of macrophages and thymus-independent lymphocytes. Among the thymus-independent lymphocytes are cells known as *killer* or K cells. These K cells may or may not include B lymphocytes and are potentiated or armed by an antibody specific for antigens on the tumor cell in order to cause tumor cell destruction. This antibody-dependent cellular cytotoxicity (ADCC) is neither complement-dependent nor phagocytic, although monocytes can mediate ADCC. Antibody able to induce ADCC is usually of the IgG class.

Macrophages also play an important role in killing tumor cells. Two types of tumorocidal macrophages have been identified: the nonspecifically activated macrophage and the specifically armed macrophage. BCG and other microbes or microbial products can nonspecifically activate macrophages, which then are cytotoxic for tumor cells in vitro but not for normal cells. Sensitized lymphocytes specifically cytotoxic for a tumor or specific antisera can transmit their specificity to normal macrophages, which in turn become specifically cytotoxic to the sensitizing tumor.

Humoral antibodies can inhibit tumor growth in vivo and destroy tumor cells in vitro in the presence of complement. Usually, antibody must be given prior to or immediately after tumor transplantation in order to be effective. The sensitivity of various types of neoplasms to cytotoxic antibodies varies considerably. Leukemias and lymphomas are most sensitive, sarcomas and carcinomas more resist-

ant. There appears to be a correlation between the sensitivity of the tumor to cytotoxic antibodies in vitro and its response to antibodies in vivo. However, it is clear that the different classes of antibodies vary considerably in their ability to reduce tumor cell viability in vitro and inhibit tumor growth in vivo. Antibodies of the IgM class are generally more effective in inducing immunity by passive transfer.

In summary, T and B lymphocytes, K cells, macrophages, and antibody all have a role in controlling tumor growth. At best, they interreact to cause tumor cell destruction. At worst, they can lead to enhanced tumor growth both in vivo and in vitro. Much more research needs to be done before we can expect to understand how to manipulate the immune system for the maximum benefit of the patient.

IMMUNE SURVEILLANCE. The concept of immunologic surveillance is based upon the premise that carcinogenesis occurs frequently as a spontaneous mutation, from chemical carcinogens or from oncogenic viruses. Burnet postulated that the teleology of the immune system was to recognize the foreignness of tumor-specific antigens on the neoplastic cells and to mount an immune response capable of eliminating them. In this context, clinical cancer would represent a failure of the mechanisms for immunologic destruction, although it may be the exception rather than the rule.

Mechanisms for Evasion of Immune Surveillance. If neoplastic cells are capable of eliciting a host immune response that leads to their specific destruction, it is pertinent to ask why or how cancer develops. A variety of possible ways by which cancer cells evade the immune surveillance mechanisms have been described:

Insufficient antigenicity to evoke an immune response may account for the growth of some neoplasms. Tumor-specific antigens are usually weaker immunogens than transplantation antigens. Some neoplastic cells may have either an extremely weak tumor-specific antigen or an extremely low density of tumor-specific antigens on the cell surface. Thus, the tumor cell with the stronger tumor-specific antigen may be recognized and eliminated, whereas those cells with weak tumor-specific antigens may escape detection and destruction.

Antigenic modulation of a thymus leukemia (TL) antigen has been observed on a murine lymphoma cell. The TL antigen disappears when the cell is transplanted in immunized hosts or carried in tissue culture containing specific antibody, but it will reappear when the tumor cells are passed in tissue culture without antibody or transplanted in unimmunized hosts. Furthermore, antigenic shift may be another form of antigenic modulation whereby tumor cells escape control of immunologic surveillance. This phenomenon has been described with certain animal neoplasms in which the lung metastases are antigenically different from the primary tumor.

Immunologic indifference may explain the observation by Old and associates that small numbers of tumor cells having tumor-specific antigens develop into progressively growing tumors although larger numbers of cells are rejected. In this instance the small number of cells may not be immunogenic enough and can "sneak through" the host immune response.

Immunosuppression by irradiation, neonatal thymectomy, chemotherapy, or steroid or antilymphocyte globulin administration usually increases the frequency and growth rate, and shortens the latency period, for both virus- and carcinogen-induced neoplasms in experimental animals. The incidence of cancer in man increases significantly with advancing years as his immune response to a variety of antigens decreases. Furthermore, in human beings with congenital immunodeficiency diseases, the incidence of spontaneous cancer is 10,000 times that of the general age-matched population. In human organ transplant recipients on immunosuppressive drugs, the incidence of spontaneous cancer is more than seventy times that of the general age-matched population.

Immunologic tolerance that develops during the fetal or neonatal periods due to exposure to tumor-specific antigens or an oncogenic virus may account for tumor growth in some animals when the immunologic surveillance system would otherwise afford protection. Bittner discovered in 1936 that C3H female mice transmitted mammary tumor virus (MTV) through the milk to their nursing young which later induced mammary tumors in a high percentage of their adult female progeny. Morton demonstrated that mice infected as neonates subsequently became tolerant to the tumor-specific antigens of the MTV-induced neoplasms and consequently could not be immunized against them as adults. Newborn mice foster-nursed on non-MTV-carrying mothers from another strain were not tolerant to the virus and, when adult, could be effectively immunized against the MTV-induced mammary tumors. The incidence of mammary tumors in these foster-nursed mice was much lower than in those nursed on MTV infected mothers.

Low-dose immunologic tolerance similar to that seen with transplantation systems, but secondary to prolonged exposure to small amounts of weak tumor-specific antigens may account for the growth of some tumors. Low-dose tolerance may explain the development of metastases from breast cancer in immunocompetent patients many years after radical mastectomy.

Immunologic enhancement refers to the facilitated growth of some tumors in the presence of specific antibody against the tumor-specific antigen. The antibody may work on the afferent limb, the efferent limb, or the central portion of the immune response.

Afferent enhancement occurs when the antibody coats the antigen on the tumor cell and prevents processing of the tumor-specific antigen, either at the regional node or by a macrophage at the tumor cell. *Central enhancement* occurs when the antibody directly inhibits the reactivity of the immunocompetent cells. *Efferent enhancement* occurs when the antibody coats the antigenic site and prevents intimate contact between the immune cell and the tumor cell.

An important point to stress concerning the enhancement of tumor growth by specific antibody concerns the temporal relation between the transfer of antibody and tumor or organ allotransplantation. The antibody must be administered shortly before, at the same time as, or shortly after tumor or organ transplantation in order for enhancement to occur. If administration of the antibody is delayed for a week, the host cellular immune response has already been stimulated, and tumor rejection occurs in a normal fashion. Most animal and human neoplasms have a long latency period prior to clinical detection, and the host immune response is already sensitized to the tumor-specific antigens. Therefore, it is unlikely that immunologic enhancement by antibody is responsible for tumor enhancement or plays an important role in evasion of immunologic surveillance in naturally occurring neoplasms.

CLINICAL EVIDENCE FOR TUMOR IMMUNITY IN MAN

Until recently there was little evidence for the existence of tumor-specific antigens on human neoplasms. For obvious reasons the tumor transplantation techniques used to demonstrate these tumor-specific antigens of animal neoplasms were not applicable to the study of human tumors. Nevertheless, there are a number of well-documented clinical observations which suggest human host immune defenses against cancer. Although other physiologic, endocrinologic, and biologic explanations can be given for these observations, they are most easily explained on an immunologic basis:

1. Spontaneous regression of established tumors is a rare but well-documented phenomenon. Sometimes these regressions have followed a minor viral or bacterial infection. Although spontaneous regression has been observed in many different tumor types, it is most frequently seen in neuroblastomas of children, malignant melanoma, choriocarcinoma, adenocarcinoma of the kidney, and soft tissue sarcomas. However, spontaneous regression occurs less frequently than 0.5 percent in all types, except for neuroblastomas.

   Spontaneous regression of small pulmonary metastases following the surgical removal of the primary tumor has been observed and occurs most frequently in hypernephromas. Spontaneous regression also may account for the prolonged survival or cure of patients after incomplete surgical excision of the cancer.

2. Recurrence of tumor 10 years after successful treatment of the primary is often manifested by rapid tumor growth and death. Although endocrinologic changes may account for some of these observations in breast cancer, in other tumors this course suggests a host defense which inhibits the tumor growth during the disease-free interval.

3. Microscopic evidence of the histiocytic, plasmocytic, lymphocytic, and eosinophilic infiltration, which resembles that seen in an organ transplant or tumor transplant that is undergoing rejection in man, is associated with an improved prognosis. For example, in stomach cancer, these findings correlate better with survival than does adequate surgical removal of the tumor.

4. The presence of many tumor cells in the peripheral blood, lymphatics, pleural cavity, and operative wounds of patients who subsequently never develop metastases suggests host immune defense.

5. There is a low incidence of successful growth of tumor tissue, or autotransplants in patients with advanced disease. The resistance against tumor growth was relative rather than absolute, since challenge with greater numbers of cancer cells usually resulted in tumor growth. The immune nature of this resistance was suggested when autologous leukocytes or plasma was mixed with these tumor cells, and cancer growth decreased in approximately half the patients studied.

IMMUNOLOGIC EVIDENCE FOR TUMOR-SPECIFIC ANTI-GENS IN HUMAN NEOPLASMS. During the past decade, a variety of sensitive serologic techniques have demonstrated that every human neoplasm adequately studied contained specific antigens which elicited both cellular and humoral responses in cancer patients.

Humoral antibodies have been shown by the immuno-fluorescence, complement fixation, immunocytolysis, and immunodiffusion techniques. Cellular immunity has been demonstrated by lymphocyte-mediated cytotoxicity (the ability of lymphocytes to kill tumor cells in tissue culture), lymphocyte blastogenesis tests (the ability of lymphocytes to be stimulated to proliferate by tumor-specific antigens), and migration inhibition tests (macrophages or other blood leukocytes inhibited in their migration by tumor-specific antigens). Finally, it has been found that cancer patients develop delayed cutaneous hypersensitivity reactions to tumor-specific antigens. Thus, it has become increasingly apparent that tumor-specific antigens are capable of eliciting an immune response which can be monitored by the immunologic techniques used to study other types of immune reactions. The wide variety of human neoplasms in which tumor-specific antigens have been detected are listed in Table 9-3.

The antigenic pattern of most human neoplasms is similar. Neoplasms of the same histologic type contain common tumor-specific antigens which differ from tumor-specific antigens of other types of neoplasms. Thus, human sarcomas share a common antigen which is different from the antigens shared by bladder cancer.

In addition, some neoplasms such as malignant melanoma have additional antigens with a pattern of more limited specificity, as well as the common melanoma-specific antigen. This pattern of both individually distinct and common antigens may be characteristic of other types of human neoplasms as well, although studies undertaken thus far have not demonstrated it. The discovery of the common antigen in neoplasms of the same histologic type may allow precise immunotherapeutic and immunoprophylactic maneuvers based upon vaccines prepared for this common tumor antigen rather than from each patient's own tumor-specific antigens.

Carcinoembryonic, or Fetal, Antigens. Most of the tumor-associated antigens described above are located on the cell surface, where they are susceptible to immune attack by antibodies or lymphocytes. Thus, they are probably of

Table 9-3. HUMAN NEOPLASMS WITH DEMONSTRATED TUMOR-ASSOCIATED ANTIGENS

Burkitt's lymphoma
Malignant melanoma
Neuroblastoma
Osteosarcoma
Soft tissue sarcomas
Colon carcinoma
Breast carcinoma
Leukemia
Lung carcinoma
Bladder carcinoma
Renal carcinoma

considerable importance in the tumor-host relationship. However, there are other types of antigens which may not be located at the cell surface, although they are more or less specific for the neoplastic state. One such group is composed of the fetal, or carcinoembryonic, antigens.

Fetal antigens are produced by normal fetal organs during embryonic development. Their production is repressed shortly after birth, and they are not produced in significant quantities in normal adult organs. However, during neoplastic transformation, reversion of the cell to the embryonic state is accompanied by a renewed production of these fetal antigens. The fetal antigens are thought to represent the phenotypic expression of genes active during fetal life but not expressed during normal adult life. Their occurrence in tumors is thought to be secondary to alterations in the pattern of gene regulation as the result of the dedifferentiation and reversion of the cell to a primitive embryonic state.

The carcinoembryonic, or fetal, antigens may be a useful means of detecting malignant disease before other clinical evidence of disease is apparent or as a detector of recurrence following therapy to provide a basis for further treatment. Fetal antigens that are common to many different histologic types of human neoplasms have been described, as have those that are restricted to the organ of origin.

α-Fetoglobulin. The α-fetoglobulin circulating in approximately 70 percent of patients with primary hepatomas is found in normal human fetal serum up to 1 year after birth. The fetal antigen also has been found occasionally in patients with gastric cancer, prostatic cancer, and primitive testicular tumors such as teratomas, although it appears to be relatively specific for hepatomas. The specificity of the test was demonstrated when adult monkeys were given hepatic carcinogens; α-fetoglobulin appeared in the serum of a high percentage of these monkeys prior to any histologic evidence of neoplastic change.

The α-fetoglobulin test has been clinically evaluated and found to be useful in the diagnosis of hepatomas. It is not positive in patients with rapidly dividing cells due to hepatic regeneration following liver resection or in those with cirrhosis.

Carcinoembryonic Antigen. The carcinoembryonic antigen (CEA) reported in 1965 by Gold and Friedman is another tumor-associated antigen occurring in fetal gut, liver, and pancreas during the first two trimesters of gestation. This antigen was originally thought to be specific for adenocarcinomas arising in the gastrointestinal tract and pancreas, but more recently it has been found in a variety of carcinomas, sarcomas, and lymphomas of many different histologic types.

Since the CEA appears in the bloodstream, it was initially thought to be of great importance as a diagnostic tool for malignant disease prior to other clinical evidence of cancer. A radioimmunoassay capable of detecting nanogram quantities of CEA in the blood was developed. However, elevated CEA levels were found in patients with a variety of nonmalignant conditions including alcoholic cirrhosis, pancreatitis, cholecystitis, colonic diverticulitis, and ulcerative colitis. As a result, the incidence of elevated

CEA levels in mass screening of normal or hospitalized populations has been over 10 percent in some series. Therefore this test has not been useful as a serologic method for the diagnosis of malignant tumor.

The serum levels of CEA do appear to correlate with the extent of known carcinomas of the colon. Less than 20 percent of patients with early lesions (Dukes Stage A or B) have elevated CEA levels, whereas one-half of patients with Dukes C lesions and almost all patients with Dukes D lesions have elevated levels of CEA. Metastasis to the liver is frequently associated with the highest levels. These statistics suggest that CEA may have limited use in detecting early carcinoma of the bowel. It has been shown that the CEA level drops during the postoperative period in those patients who have successful resection of the tumor. Patients who develop tumor recurrence often show a rise in CEA titer to the preoperative levels. Thus, CEA may be extremely useful in following the clinical course of patients with known malignant disease in order to detect evidence of recurrence prior to its becoming clinically detectable.

GENERAL IMMUNE COMPETENCE OF CANCER PATIENTS. A number of studies have tested the general functional capacity of the cancer patient's immunologic system. Such studies can be grouped into two categories—those concerned with humoral antibody production and those dealing with cell-mediated immune reactions.

Formation of humoral antibody to known antigenic substances has been studied by many investigators, who have found most cancer patients have the ability to form humoral antibodies against a variety of antigenic substances, even in the presence of advanced disease. There is no evidence to implicate a defect in humoral antibody production in most cancer patients.

The cell-mediated immune reactions have been measured by the cancer patient's ability to manifest delayed cutaneous hypersensitivity to a variety of common skin test antigens to which most normal persons are reactive by virtue of previous exposure such as to mumps, tuberculin, streptokinase, or streptodornase. In addition, a primary immune response was tested against a new antigen by studying the survival of skin allografts and by sensitizing patients to an antigen, such as the contact sensitizer dinitrochlorobenzene (DNCB). DNCB reacts with proteins in the skin and forms a hapten which sensitizes the immunocompetent patient (Fig. 9-12). Cell-mediated immunity can

Fig. 9-12. Positive reaction to dintrochlorobenzene (DNCB), showing initial exposure and subsequent challenges.

be studied with an in vitro test which requires lymphocyte recognition and proliferation in response to foreign tissue antigens or mitogens such as phytohemagglutinin.

These immunologic studies revealed that cell-mediated immune reactions are significantly impaired in patients with lymphoreticular neoplasia. Since these diseases usually diffusely involve the immune effector system, this might be expected. However, a similar impediment in cell-mediated immune reactions was found in patients with localized or advanced solid neoplasms that did not involve the immune system. The explanation for this immunologic defect in cancer patients is unknown, but there does appear to be a strong correlation between an impaired cell-mediated response and the clinical course of the malignant disease.

This correlation becomes particularly evident when the postoperative course of cancer patients is compared with their ability to become sensitized to DNCB (Fig. 9-13). More than 95 percent of normal control volunteers, patients with benign neoplasms, patients free of disease 5 years or more following cancer surgery, and patients with a history of spontaneous regression of cancer could be sensitized to DNCB. On the other hand, only 65 percent of patients who presented for definitive cancer surgery could be sensitized to this chemical. Seventy-two percent of these immunocompetent patients had localized neo-

Patients	DNCB Positive		DNCB Negative	
Control	19/20	= 95%	1/20	= 5%
Benign	10/10	= 100%	0/0	= 0%
Longterm survival (>5 yrs) .	16/16	= 100%	0/16	= 0%
Spontaneous regression	8/8	= 100%	0/8	= 0%
All cancer patients	152/237	= 64%	85/237	= 35%
Free of disease (6 mo) . . .	110/152	= 72%	1/85	= 1%
Inoperable or early recurrence	42/152	= 28%	84/85	= 99%

Fig. 9-13. Correlation between delayed cutaneous hypersensitivity to DNCB and prognosis.

Fig. 9-14. Antisarcoma antibody titers determined by complement fixation against the HuSA-I liposarcoma antigen. Serial serum samples obtained from patients who remained free of disease up to 5 years after resection of the primary sarcoma. (*From D. L. Morton et al., Ann Intern Med, 74:587, 1971.*)

plasms that could be resected, and they subsequently remained free of disease for at least 6 months after surgery. However, those patients who were anergic had a poor prognosis following operation. Ninety-nine percent were inoperable because of local or metastatic spread of the disease or, when resected, had recurrence of disease within 6 months after surgery. Regardless of the histologic type of neoplasm, most patients who had severe impairment of their cell-mediated immune reactions apparent from cutaneous anergy to DNCB had a poor prognosis after operation.

There were considerable differences, however, in the pattern of DNCB reactivity in patients with different histologic types of solid neoplasms. Patients with epidermoid carcinoma of the cervix, mouth, pharynx, or larynx showed a very strong correlation between the positive DNCB response and a good prognosis after cancer surgery. Most of these patients who could be sensitized were operable and free of disease for at least 6 months, whereas those who were anergic had a poor prognosis. There was little correlation between a positive DNCB test and recurrence after surgery with the skeletal or soft tissue sarcomas and melanomas; many of these patients developed a recurrence even though they were immunologically competent. The explanation for the differences in cutaneous reactivity with various tumor types is unknown at the present time. It is possible that these patterns are indicative of some important variations in either the causes of or the response to the different types of human neoplasms. In some instances, it appears that the presence of a neoplasm is clearly related to the immunosuppression, because resection of the neoplasm results in return of immunologic competence. This is particularly true in patients with large, bulky skeletal and soft tissue sarcomas.

Some clarification of the immunosuppression that results

from malignant disease has come from recent studies. Patients who converted from anergic to positive during sequential skin testing with DNCB appeared to have gained control of their tumor just as often as those patients who were initially reactive to DNCB and who maintained their reactivity after surgical procedures. Conversely, those patients who converted from positive to an anergic response usually had progression of their disease. It would seem, therefore, that the defect in systemic immunity was the result of the neoplastic process and that the immunosuppression could be reversed by successful therapy. Other studies have shown that lymphocyte function is depressed in cancer patients when compared to normal controls and that this depression is directly related to the extent of tumor burden. Another investigation demonstrated serum factors in samples from cancer patients that inhibited function of lymphocytes from normal donors. These factors undoubtedly contribute to the immunosuppression observed in cancer patients.

Thus it appears that the immunosuppression seen in cancer patients could be the result of a humoral factor dispensed by the cancer cell or a complex physiologic response against the cancer cell that can depress normal cell-mediated immunity.

CORRELATIONS BETWEEN IMMUNE RESPONSE TO TUMOR-SPECIFIC ANTIGENS AND CLINICAL COURSE OF HUMAN CANCER. More sophisticated immunologic studies demonstrated a correlation between the cell-mediated and humoral immune responses and the clinical course of malignant disease. Such studies show that patients with a normal immune response to DNCB may have instead abnormalities in their response to the tumor-specific antigens of their neoplasms that can be detected by other immunologic techniques.

While the antibody role in controlling tumor growth is controversial at the present time, there is a marked correlation between the antibody titer detectable by immunofluorescence and complement fixation and the clinical course in patients with melanomas and sarcomas. This correlation was especially striking when sera from sarcoma patients were tested by complement fixation.

Analyses of sera from patients who enjoyed long-term survival from previous sarcomas showed a persistently elevated antisarcoma antibody titer (Fig. 9-14). Little variation was noted, and persistence of antibody was evident 3 to 4 years after removal of the primary tumor. When sequential antisera samples were obtained before and after surgery for primary sarcomas, it was found that all those patients who had primary surgery and continued to be free of disease had at least a fourfold rise in tumor antibody following removal of the tumor. These antibody titers remained elevated as long as those patients remained free of disease (Fig. 9-15). In contrast, most patients who had no antisarcoma antibody preoperatively with no increase in antibody titer following surgery developed recurrence within 6 months. Furthermore, of the several patients with low antibody titers preoperatively who had a transient rise in antibody titer following tumor removal, all who developed subsequent pulmonary metastases showed a progres-

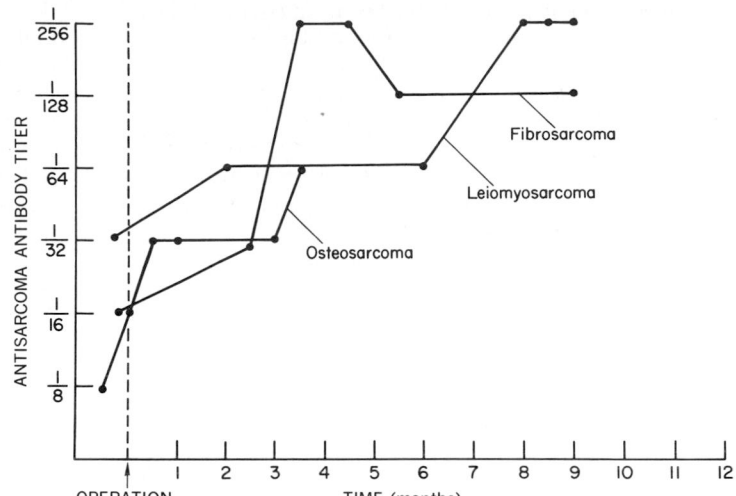

Fig. 9-15. Antisarcoma antibody titers determined by complement fixation against the HuSA-I liposarcoma antigen. Serial serum samples obtained following resection of the primary sarcoma in patients who remained free of disease. (*From D. L. Morton et al., Ann Surg, 172:740, 1970.*)

sive decline in antisarcoma antibody titers to nondetectable levels as the metastatic disease progressed (Fig. 9-16). In careful, frequent sampling of a few sarcoma patients, it appeared that the antibody titer fell 2 to 3 months prior to development of detectable pulmonary metastatic disease. Thus, careful monitoring of the sarcoma patient's complement fixing antibody titer in the postoperative period may be helpful in early detection of recurrence of disease.

The observation of Hellstrom and associates regarding the presence of blocking factors in the sera of sarcoma patients who have growing neoplasms or who subsequently will develop recurrent disease is probably of considerable importance in the tumor-host relationship. They found that lymphocytes specifically cytotoxic for tumor cells can be demonstrated throughout the course of malignant disease regardless of whether patients have been cured of their tumors or have growing neoplasms. However, the sera of those patients with growing tumors contained blocking factors that inhibited the cytotoxic action of the killer lymphocytes upon tumor cells in vitro. Further stud-

ies suggested that the blocking factors were probably circulating tumor antigen-antibody complexes or tumor antigen alone rather than simple enhancing antibodies. This blocking factor could be completely neutralized by admixture with serum that had the cytotoxic or deblocking antibodies from patients free of malignant disease. A most significant correlation to clinical course was found when these in vitro studies demonstrated the deblocking antibodies in patients free of disease but found the blocking serum factors in patients who had recurrence of the disease. Obviously such techniques can be useful in predicting in which patients the disease will recur. The day may come when the balance between antibody and cellular immunity may be manipulated to the patient's benefit through such studies as this.

In addition to the correlations of clinical course to specific humoral immunity, it does appear that delayed cutaneous hypersensitivity reactions to tumor-specific antigens extracted from various types of human neoplasms also correlate in a general way with clinical course. Patients with arrested melanomas, Burkitt's lymphoma, and leuke-

Fig. 9-16. Antisarcoma antibody titers determined by complement fixation against the HuSA-1 liposarcoma antigen. Serial serum samples obtained following resection of primary sarcoma in patients who developed recurrent disease with pulmonary metastases. The time at which pulmonary metastases were detected on the chest roentgenogram is indicated by an arrow. (*From D. L. Morton et al., Ann Intern Med, 74:587, 1971.*)

mia exhibit delayed skin reactions to antigens extracted from their tumor cells. These skin reactions become negative with relapse.

POSSIBLE APPLICATIONS OF IMMUNOBIOLOGY TO CANCER THERAPY. There are many possible applications of cancer immunobiology to cancer therapy besides those of the immunotherapy. Immunoprevention by vaccine prepared from the common tumor antigens or tumor viral antigens is theoretically possible. However, because of the long latency period of most human neoplasms, it would require several decades to evaluate such a vaccine even if it were already in hand.

Immunobiology has great potential as a guide to standard cancer therapy. Immunologic monitoring of cancer patients undergoing therapy for malignant disease could be extremely useful in determining choice of therapy, as well as determining the patient's response to the therapy. Immunologic testing also may be useful in following the patient's response to certain therapeutic modalities that are known to be immunosuppressive, such as chemotherapy or radiation therapy, so that therapeutic regimens that are nonimmunosuppressive may be devised. Furthermore, with multiphasic immune monitoring, it may become possible to carry out immunologic engineering in patients with defective immune responses. The deficiencies then might be corrected by appropriate adjunctive therapy once the site of the defect has been diagnosed.

PATHOLOGY

When confronted with a tumor mass, the clinician must first determine whether it is a neoplastic or inflammatory process and, if neoplastic, whether it is benign or malignant. This is usually accomplished by biopsy of the mass.

In general, biopsy of a neoplasm should always be obtained before therapy is instituted. The pathologist's interpretation of materials submitted for microscopic examination depends not only upon his experience and the quality of the material submitted but also upon the clinical history and findings on the patient and a review of any previous biopsy material. The features to which the pathologist must direct his attention are partly histologic, that is, the arrangement of the tumor cells and their relation to the surrounding tissue, and partly cytologic, namely, the nature of the tumor cells and, in particular, the appearance of the nucleus and nucleoli.

The characteristics of benign and malignant neoplasms are listed in Table 9-4. *Anaplasia* means lack of differentiation. *Polarity* is the normal orderly alignment of epithelial cells, which are arranged in sheets. One of the early signs of malignant change is the loss of this normal polarity, so that the cells may present as a disorderly arrangement in relation to the surface and to each other. *Nuclear changes* of the malignant cells are often seen as enlarged and hyperchromic nuclei. These three features may all be seen before invasion of the deeper tissues has occurred. This is known as *preinvasive carcinoma,* or *carcinoma in situ.*

One of the most characteristic features of malignant disease is *local infiltration of adjacent tissues,* i.e., malignant colonic epithelial cells invading the muscular or serosal layers of the colon. In contrast, a benign tumor grows by expansion, compressing the surrounding tissues to form a capsule.

Based upon these microscopic criteria, the pathologist usually has no difficulty in determining whether the neoplasm is malignant or benign. Sometimes the microscopic diagnosis is difficult and opinions are divided among the different pathologists examining the tissue. When this happens, several paths are open to the clinician: If the biopsy is not adequate, more material should be obtained. Special stains are sometimes helpful, such as oil red O, to show fat globules as in liposarcoma. Outside expert opinion may be useful, such as from the Armed Forces Institute of Pathology or the National Cancer Institute, which act as referral centers for patients with unusual malignant neoplasms.

The electron microscope has been helpful in diagnosing some undifferentiated tumors, such as malignant melanoma and soft tissue sarcomas. Tissue culture characteristics also may be useful in identifying some malignant

Table 9-4. GENERAL CHARACTERISTICS OF BENIGN AND MALIGNANT NEOPLASMS

Characteristic	Benign neoplasms	Malignant neoplasms
Nuclear structure	Normal size, staining and shape	Large, hyperchromatic with variation in size and shape
Mitotic figures	Usually rare	Frequent and perhaps atypical
Anaplasia	Absent	Varying degree
Polarity	Orderly arrangement	Disorderly arrangement
Local invasion or infiltration	Absent (except angioma)	Usually present
Capsule	Present	Absent or a pseudocapsule
Recurrence	Absent or rare	Frequent
Metastases	Absent	Frequent
Growth	Slow, self-limited	Often rapid
Systemic effects	Rare, except for neoplasms	Frequent

Table 9-5. SIMPLE CLASSIFICATION OF NEOPLASMS

Tissue of origin	Site of origin	Benign	Malignant
Epithelial origin (ectoderm or entoderm)	Skin, mouth, larynx, lung, esophagus, urinary tract, cervix	Papilloma	Squamous cell carcinoma
	Breast, stomach, colon pancreas, liver	Adenoma	Adenocarcinoma
Mesodermal origin	Fibrous tissue	Fibroma	Fibrosarcoma
	Muscular tissue	Leiomyoma, rhabdo-myoma	Leiomyosarcoma, rhabdo-myosarcoma
	Fatty tissue	Lipoma	Liposarcoma
	Vascular tissue	Angioma	Angiosarcoma
	Hemopoietic tissue		Leukemia, multiple myeloma, lymphoma
	Bone	Osteoma, chondroma	Osteogenic sarcoma, chondrosarcoma
Special types:			
Melanocytes	Skin, eye	Nevus	Malignant melanoma
Neural tissue	Brain, spinal cord nerve	Astrocytoma Ganglioneuroma	Glioblastoma multiforme Neuroblastoma
Trophoblast	Placenta testis	Chorioepithelioma	Choriocarcinoma
Notochord	Spine	Chordoma	Chordoma
Blastoderm	Mediastinum, ovary, testis	Teratoma	Teratoma

neoplasms. Hormonal assay may be helpful, as in diagnosing a glucagon-producing alpha cell cancer of the pancreas. However, it is well to remember that sometimes tumors produce biologic substances that are not normally produced by the tissue from which they originated.

It may not be possible, in certain situations, to differentiate histologically between a benign and a malignant neoplasm, as with the parathyroid carcinomas, giant cell sarcomas of bone, and thymomas. In these cases, clinical characteristics of the lesions in terms of the development of recurrence, metastases, and progressive growth may be the only differentiating criteria available to the clinician.

CLASSIFICATION OF NEOPLASMS. Many different classifications of tumors exist, but the most useful one is based upon the cell type of tissue of origin. When the neoplasm is undifferentiated, the special methods discussed above may help to classify it.

Neoplasms arising from epithelial cells regardless of whether in the ectoderm or the entoderm are known as carcinomas. Sarcomas arise from connective tissue and include tumors of fibrous, muscular, fatty, vascular, and skeletal origin. Teratoma signifies a neoplasm in which anaplastic, immature somatic cells, comparable to blastoderm, are usually dominant; it exhibits varying degrees of differentiation into mature somatic cells of ectodermal, mesodermal, and entodermal types. Teratomas occur in the testis, ovary, and mediastinum. A simplified classification of benign and malignant neoplasms arising from different sites is given in Table 9-5.

GRADING OF MALIGNANCY. Broders classified carcinomas into four grades according to their degree of differentiation, the appearance of cells, their nuclei, and the number of mitotic figures. On this basis, the least malignant are classified as grade 1, and the most malignant are grade 4. In general, the lower-grade, more differentiated neoplasms are less malignant and tend to metastasize less frequently than the higher-grade, more anaplastic ones.

Although the grading of neoplasms is sometimes useful, growth rate and presence of metastasis may be more important in determining prognosis.

CARCINOMA IN SITU AND OTHER PREMALIGNANT LESIONS. Carcinoma in situ is a lesion with the cytologic characteristics of malignant tumors but with no detectable invasion into the surrounding tissue. It seems to develop into invasive cancer after variable delay periods. The interval between the detection of carcinoma in situ of the cervix and invasive carcinoma may be 10 to 15 years. Carcinoma in situ also occurs in the skin, bronchus, stomach, and pharynx. When these lesions are adequately treated, a complete cure is assured.

ROUTES FOR SPREAD OF NEOPLASMS. There are few subjects of greater importance to the oncologist than the spread of cancer. Much is known about the routes of spread but little about the conditions which determine that spread. Some cancers are metastatic at the time of their clinical discovery, while others of the same type and in the same organ tissue may remain localized for years.

Metastases may entirely dominate the clinical picture, while the primary tumor remains latent and asymptomatic. For example, neoplasms of the brain secondary to silent cancers in the bronchus or the gastrointestinal tract are often mistaken for primary brain tumors.

Knowledge of the particular manner in which different types of cancer spread is important in planning therapy. In general, a malignant tumor may spread by four routes: directly by infiltrating surrounding tissue; via lymphatics; by vascular invasion; or by implantation in serous cavities (Fig. 9-17). Knowledge of the patterns of neoplastic spread in different types of cancer is important in planning definitive therapy. Metastatic patterns of various types of human tumors are summarized in Table 9-6.

Direct Extension. Cancer cells may spread by direct extension through tissue spaces. Some neoplasms, such as soft tissue sarcomas and adenocarcinomas of the stomach

Fig. 9-17. Four mechanisms of the dissemination of cancer cells. This is a diagrammatic illustration; the original tumor could be one of many organs with cells disseminating by the four mechanisms. (*From W. H. Cole, et al., "Dissemination of Cancer," Appleton-Century-Crofts, Inc., New York, 1961.*)

or esophagus, may extend for considerable distances (10 to 15 cm) along tissue planes beyond the palpable tumor mass. Other neoplasms, such as basal cell carcinoma of skin, rarely extend for more than a few millimeters beyond the visible margin.

Lymphatic Spread. Tumor cells can readily enter lymphatics and extend along these channels by permeation or embolism through the regional lymphatics to lymph nodes. Permeation is the growth of a colony of tumor cells along the course of the lymph vessel. This occurs commonly in the skin lymphatics in carcinoma of the breast and in the perineural lymphatics in carcinoma of the prostate.

Spread along the lymphatics by embolism to the regional nodes or distant lymph nodes is of much greater importance. Lymph node metastases are first confined to the subcapsular space; at this stage the node is not enlarged and may appear normal to the naked eye. Gradually the tumor cells permeate the sinusoids and replace the paren-

chyma. There is little direct spread from node to node, because the capsule is not penetrated until a late stage. The tumor cells travel by anastomosing lymphatics, and the spread occurs in other nodes by way of collateral lymph channels. When a lymph node containing tumor is more than 3.0 cm in diameter, tumor has usually extended beyond the capsule into the perinodal fat.

The lymph from the abdominal organs and lower extremities drains into the cisterna chyli and then into the thoracic duct, which finally opens into the left jugular vein. Tumor cells pass from the lymph to the bloodstream by this route. Spread along the thoracic duct explains those cases in which cancer of the gastrointestinal tract is associated with pulmonary metastasis while the liver remains clear. Involvement of the supraclavicular lymph nodes is usually related to entrapment of tumor emboli from the thoracic duct behind the valves near the termination of the duct, followed by extension of these cells along the lymphatics to the node. Thus, lymphatic spread may eventually become vascular dissemination.

Lymphatic spread is extremely common in epithelial neoplasms of all types, except basal cell carcinoma of the skin, which does not metastasize to regional lymphatics. Sarcomas metastasize to lymph nodes in only a minority of cases, usually less than 10 percent.

VASCULAR SPREAD. Cancer cells may reach the bloodstream either by the thoracic duct, as just described, or by invasion of blood vessels. The veins are invaded frequently, the arteries rarely. The chief reason for the striking differences in invasion characteristics between arteries and veins appears to be that lymphatics frequently penetrate the walls of the large veins from without and form a plexus reaching to the subendothelial region, thus providing a portal of entry for tumor cells through the vein wall. When the vascular endothelium is destroyed, a

Table 9-6. ESTIMATED FREQUENCY* OF PATTERNS OF NEOPLASTIC SPREAD FOR COMMON HUMAN NEOPLASMS

Neoplasm	Hematogenous	Lymphatic	Local infiltration (expressed as local recurrence)
Adenocarcinoma			
Breast	4	3	2
Colon	3	3	1
Stomach	4	4	3
Pancreas	4	4	3
Epidermoid carcinoma			
Lung	4	3	2
Oral pharynx	1	3	3
Larynx	1	3	2
Cutaneous neoplasm			
Squamous cell carcinoma	1	2	1
Melanomas	3	3	2
Basal cell carcinomas	0	0	1
Sarcomas			
Bones	4	1	1
Soft tissue	4	1	3
Brain neoplasms	0	0	4

*0—Does not occur, 1—1 to 15 percent, 2—15 to 30 percent, 3—>30 percent, and 4—>50 percent.

thrombus forms that is quickly invaded by tumor. It is this combination of thrombus and tumor which detaches to form the emboli that result in metastases. Vascular invasion is commonly seen in both carcinomas and sarcomas and is frequently associated with a poor prognosis. Some types of neoplasms have a remarkable tendency to grow as a solid column along the course of veins, for example, renal carcinomas and sarcomas. Renal carcinomas have been known to grow out of the renal vein into the inferior vena cava and up the inferior vena cava to the right atrium.

Spread through Serous Cavities. Tumor cells occasionally gain entrance to serous cavities via direct growth of tumor through the wall of certain organs, or by growth on the surface of such potential spaces. Many tumor cells are capable of growth in suspension without a supporting matrix. In either case, it is common for tumor cells to spread widely when they encounter a space lined with a serous surface. Thus, widespread peritoneal seeding is commonly seen with gastrointestinal neoplasms and tumors of ovarian origin. A similar mechanism appears to operate in the case of malignant gliomas, which may spread widely within the central nervous system via cerebral spinal fluid.

CLINICAL MANIFESTATIONS OF CANCER

The manner in which neoplastic disease presents itself clinically is varied and inconstant. Current ability to define, detect, and quantify the neoplastic state is limited. Cancer may present as an asymptomatic lesion too small to be seen without magnification, as an asymptomatic lump, or as symptomatic disease. Often, symptoms are nonspecific and resemble those of nonmalignant diseases. The clinical abnormalities produced by advancing neoplastic diseases may be grouped into two categories—those abnormalities which stem directly from the presence of a tumor mass and those physiologic derangements which are produced indirectly. By including the possibility of neoplastic disease in every differential diagnosis and by teaching patients those key symptoms which require medical evaluation, one may be able to achieve earlier diagnosis and treatment, thereby improving the survival of cancer patients.

The onset of the neoplastic state is difficult to date in human beings. As previously discussed, a prolonged latent or induction period is likely before clinically detectable disease evolves. Therefore, the use of the word "early" in describing a cancer may lead to confusion. To avoid this, we will use the terms "early" and "late" in relation to the clinical stage of a neoplasm rather than to indicate its duration in the body. When viewed in this manner, the curable cancer may have been present a long time prior to its diagnosis and therapy. The term *early* usually means a neoplasm that can be effectively treated. These neoplasms are small rather than large, do not extend into essential organs, and have not metastasized. Some lesions that have been present for years still may be early, whereas other lesions with more rapid growth rates may be *late* even if present for only a few months.

The "Seven Danger Signals of Cancer," as formulated

Table 9-7. CANCER'S SEVEN WARNING SIGNALS

Change in bowel or bladder habits
A sore that does not heal
Unusual bleeding or discharge
Thickening or lump in breast or elsewhere
Indigestion or difficulty in swallowing
Obvious change in wart or mole
Nagging cough or hoarseness

by the American Cancer Society, are listed in Table 9-7. These may be helpful in the ongoing effort to educate people and increase the frequency of early diagnosis for certain major tumors. The more common patterns of clinical presentation, and some of the more common syndromes related to cancer will be discussed in detail in the paragraphs which follow.

Carcinoma in situ and other premalignant lesions were discussed earlier under pathology and will not be discussed further here.

SIGNS OF EXPANSILE GROWTH. The signs attributable to the expansile growth of a tumor depend upon its location. When the neoplasm is either on or near the surface of the body, it may present simply as a visible or palpable mass. In the gastrointestinal, biliary, respiratory, and urinary tracts, signs are frequently related to obstruction. Examples are vomiting, jaundice, cough, or urinary retention. Within the central nervous system, expansile growth may cause pain and paralysis.

Expansile growth of a tumor may also result in destruction of host tissues. Examples are pathologic fractures, hepatic insufficiency, and Addison's disease.

SIGNS OF INFILTRATIVE GROWTH. Pain and paralysis may result when tumor infiltrates nerves. Frequently, signs of nerve invasion are also signs of incurability. Examples are lumbosacral plexus pain in cancer of the cervix and rectum, dorsal and lumbar spine pain in cancer of the pancreas, and the shoulder and arm pain and palsy when carcinoma of the lung infiltrates the brachial plexus. Other signs of infiltration generally denoting incurability are thickening of the uterine ligaments in cancer of the cervix and fixation to the chest wall in breast cancer.

SIGNS OF TUMOR NECROSIS: BLEEDING AND INFECTION. Tumors may become necrotic, ulcerate, and bleed. Fatigue and weakness may be the only symptoms or signs in cancer of the stomach or right colon, because the tumor ulceration and bleeding have resulted in anemia. If gastric or colonic cancer becomes ulcerated and infected, the signs of inflammation include edema, pain, tenderness, and fever. The inflammation caused by cecal cancer can mimic the clinical symptoms of acute appendicitis or cholecystitis. Therefore, response of such inflammation to antibiotics or the healing of an ulcer does *not* necessarily indicate a nonneoplastic lesion.

Tumor necrosis at any site may produce fever, leukocytosis, elevation of sedimentation rate, anorexia, and malaise. Such necrosis constitutes one of the causes of the "fever of unknown origin." Keller and Williams, in studies of 46 patients with unexplained fever, found that in 19 who underwent exploratory laparotomy the cause of the fever was intraabdominal malignant disease.

UNKNOWN PRIMARY TUMORS PRESENTING AS METAS-TASES. Although the primary neoplasm often grows to considerable size before metastatic lesions are seen, in other cases the primary neoplasms may be so small as to be undetectable. The initial presentation of a tumor may be at a distance from its origin. In fact, the primary neoplasm giving rise to the metastases may have regressed completely and may never be detected in some neoplasms, such as malignant melanoma and carcinomas of the oral pharynx.

The most frequent sites of presentation of metastatic neoplasms are the cervical and supraclavicular lymph nodes, lungs, liver, bones, and brain. The most common metastatic sites for unknown primary neoplasms are listed in Table 9-8.

SYSTEMIC MANIFESTATION OF MALIGNANT DISEASE. Tumors may have a variety of remote and systemic effects that contribute to morbidity. Cancer patients frequently develop unusual symptoms and physiologic derangements which cannot be attributed to the mechanical presence of primary or metastatic disease, or to physiologic changes resulting from hormones normally secreted by the tissue of origin.

Some symptoms, such as the cachexia of carcinomatosis, may result from competition between the tumor and the host for basic components of the same metabolic pool. However, the pathogenesis of many of these disorders is unknown. Some of these nonmetastatic, systemic manifestations of malignant tumors are thought to result from (1) the ectopic production of known hormones; (2) the secretion of unidentified, physiologically active substances which do not resemble known hormones; (3) autoimmune phenomena in which the host is sensitized to an antigen

Table 9-8. UNKNOWN PRIMARY TUMORS PRESENTING AS METASTASES

Site of metastasis	Primary neoplasm
Lymph nodes:	
Cervical nodes	Nasopharynx, pharynx, oral cavity, thyroid, larynx, lymphomas
Supraclavicular nodes	Bronchus, breast, stomach, esophagus, pancreas, colon, testis, ovary, cervix
Axillary nodes	Breast, melanoma, lymphoma
Inguinal nodes	Genitalia, anus, melanoma
Skin and subcutaneous tissues	Melanoma, breast, bronchus, stomach, kidney
Lung	Breast, colon, kidney, stomach, testis, melanoma, thyroid, sarcomas
Liver	Stomach, colon, breast, pancreas, bronchus
Ovary	Stomach, colon
Bones	Breast, bronchus, prostate, thyroid
Central nervous system	Breast, bronchus, kidney, colon
Serous cavities	Bronchus, breast, ovary, lymphoma

from the tumor; and/or (4) toxic substances secreted from the tumor.

The nonmetastatic clinical manifestations of malignant disease and the neoplasms with which they are associated are presented in Table 9-9. Sometimes palliative surgery is indicated to treat these systemic manifestations, for example, resection of metastases which are producing hormones that induce hypercalcemia, or of a pulmonary osteoarthropathy.

CANCER DIAGNOSIS AND STAGING EXTENT OF CANCER

Diagnosis

Diagnosis of cancer should proceed in an orderly fashion: careful history, thorough physical examination with examination of the blood and urine, and investigation of suspicious findings by appropriate radiologic examinations and radioisotope scans.

A history of any of the following is suspicious and should prompt a search for cancer: weight loss; loss of appetite; bleeding or a discharge from any body orifice or nipple; a sore that has not healed in 3 weeks; changing color or size of a mole; persistent cough or wheeze; change in voice; difficulty in swallowing; growing lump either in or under the skin, in the breast, in the abdomen, or in the muscles; and/or change of bowel habits.

Physical examination includes a thorough search of the entire skin surface for squamous cell and basal cell carcinomas, indurated lesions, ulcers, suspicious or irritated nevi, nodules, and other signs of malignant disease. Lymph nodes should be palpated for enlargement. Breasts should be palpated with the patient rotated to take the tension off the suspensory ligaments. All body orifices should be examined. A Papanicolaou smear from the cervix should be examined prior to a bimanual pelvic examination. Rectal examination should include proctoscopic examination of patients who have hemorrhoids or rectal symptoms. The oral pharynx should be examined with special attention to the floor of the mouth. Indirect laryngoscopy should be performed if the patient is hoarse or is suspected of having an intrathoracic neoplasm in cancer of the thyroid gland.

Laboratory examination should include complete blood cell count, urinalysis, examination of stool for occult blood, and chest roentgenogram. Other tests should be ordered where indicated by symptoms. Before operating on a patient for cure or palliation, a metastatic work-up should be done, directed by symptoms and the most likely site of metastases. Prior to extensive disfiguring or disabling procedures, tomograms of the lungs, bone marrow biopsy, scalene node biopsy, isotope scans, or arteriography may be useful in determining whether the neoplasm is still localized. Cytologic examination should be performed if a pleural effusion or ascites is present.

Diagnosis of solid tumors rests upon locating a space-occupying lesion and taking a portion of it for histologic

Table 9-9. SYSTEMIC MANIFESTATIONS OF
MALIGNANT DISEASE

Clinical manifestations	*Associated neoplasms*
Cutaneous	
Acanthosis nigricans	Cancer of stomach, lung, and breast
Dermatomyositis	Cancer of stomach, breast, lung, and ovary
Erythema multiforme, exfoliative dermatitis, bullous phemphigoid	Allergic response to a variety of neoplasms, lymphoma, myeloma
Peutz-Jeghers syndrome	Intestinal polyposis
Hematologic	
Abnormal red cell mass	
Erythrocytosis (increased erythropoietin)	Renal cell carcinoma, hepatoma, uterine myoma, cerebellar tumors, pheochromocytoma
Anemia:	
Myelophthisic	All tumors
Hypoproliferative	Thymoma, renal cell carcinoma
Hemolytic	Hematopoietic neoplasm
Miscellaneous causes (infection, bleeding, radiation effects, uremia, etc.)	
Abnormal leukocyte or platelet mass	
Leukemoid reactions	Miscellaneous neoplasms
Leukopenia	Hemopoietic neoplasms, lung, pancreas
Thrombocytosis	
Coagulation and bleeding disorder	
Disseminated intravascular coagulation (DIC)	Mucin-secreting adenocarcinoma
Vascular	
Thrombophlebitis	Cancer of lung, reproductive tract, pancreas, and breast
Fibrinogen deficiency (increased fibrinolysin)	Cancer of prostate and lung
Flushing, vasodilatation, violaceous skin, asthma	Carcinoid tumor
Hormonal and metabolic effects of nonendocrine tumors	
Hypoglycemia (mechanism unknown)	Retroperitoneal or mediastinal mesenchymal tumors, hepatic tumors
Cushing's syndrome (increased ACTH)	Cancer of the lung, malignant thymoma, pancreatic cancer
Hypercalcemia (increased PTH, vitamin D–like substances or bone destruction)	Cancer of lung, kidney, breast, uterus, sarcomas, hemopoietic neoplasms
Hyponatremia (increased ADH)	Cancer of lung, intracranial tumors
Hyperthyroidism (increased TSH)	Choriocarcinoma, testicular embryonal carcinoma
Precocious puberty and/or gynecomastia (increased gonadotropin)	Hepatoma, lung, adrenal cancer, testicular tumors
Zollinger-Ellison syndrome (increased gastrin) or secretion	Pancreatic nonbeta islet cell adenomas

Clinical manifestations	*Associated neoplasms*
Elevated liver enzymes	Renal cell carcinoma
Anorexia and weight loss	Most neoplasms
Hyperuricemia	Hemopoietic neoplasms
Atypical carcinoid syndrome	Pancreatic duct, islet cell, gastric, thyroid, and oat cell cancer of lung
Nonmetastatic neuromuscular	
Multifocal leukoencephalopathy	Hemopoietic neoplasms
Subacute cerebellar degeneration	Multiple neoplasms, especially of lung, ovary, and breast
Polyneuropathy and/or myopathy	Multiple neoplasms, especially of lung, ovary, and breast
Myasthenia gravis	Thymoma

SOURCE: Modified from A. H. Owens, Jr., Neoplastic Diseases, in A. M. Harvey, et al., "The Principles and Practice of Medicine." Appleton-Century-Crofts, New York, 1972.

examination. This goal is most easily fulfilled when the tumor is near the body surface or involves one of the orifices of the body that can be examined with appropriate visual instruments, such as a bronchoscope, proctoscope, or cystoscope. Carcinomas of the breast, tongue, or rectum can be seen or palpated, and a portion can be excised for definitive diagnosis.

The most difficult cancers to diagnose, and unfortunately the most lethal ones, occur in the internal organs. Space-occupying lesions in the internal organs may grow quite large before causing symptoms. Techniques which may be useful in localizing such lesions include barium examinations of the stomach and colon, examination of the bronchial tree with soluble contrast media, selective arteriography of major vessels supplying internal organs, and the use of radioisotopes and radiopaque dyes that concentrate in various organs such as the liver, gallbladder, kidney, and lymph nodes. Despite the use of such indirect means of examination, major surgery is often required to confirm the diagnosis.

CANCER DETECTION EXAMINATION. Both physicians and patients have been rather slow to adopt the habit of regular examinations to detect asymptomatic neoplasms. The lack of popularity of cancer detection examinations is in direct relation to the low yield of cancers diagnosed. Any given individual stands approximately 1 chance in 4 of developing cancer during his lifetime. Therefore, in screening 1,000 persons for an entire life span, we will find cancer in 250 of them. Since a person can harbor more than one primary cancer and a second lesion will develop with increasing frequency as the number of people who have survived the first one increases, we might count on a very crude estimate of 350 cancers in our population of 1,000. Since we expect people to live an average of 72 years, we must carry out 72,000 annual examinations to discover 350 cancers, or less than 5 cancers per 1,000 examinations. By directing our search to the middle and late adult years when the incidence is highest, we might conceivably double the yield to 10 per 1,000. Thus, the chances of detecting cancer in a given annual examination are no more than 1 in 100 even under the most optimal circumstances.

The problem of cancer detection is further complicated by the relative insensitivity of our methods for clinical cancer detection. The earliest neoplasms must be at least 1 cm in size before they are detectable by physical examination, and often tumor masses up to 10 cm in diameter will go undetected if in the liver, retroperitoneum, or other "silent" areas.

Therefore, the best chance for early diagnosis will depend upon the development of biochemical or serologic methods for cancer diagnosis rather than on routine cancer examinations in asymptomatic patients.

BIOPSY. It is imperative that microscopic proof of malignant disease be obtained prior to institution of treatment, since significant morbidity and mortality may result from all forms of cancer therapy. Significant errors have been made when biopsies were not obtained; examples are radical mastectomies for fat necrosis and radiation therapy for renal cysts.

Even when biopsy reports from another hospital are available, the slides of the previous biopsy must be obtained and reviewed prior to the institution of therapy. This is essential because, not infrequently and particularly in rare neoplasms, an erroneous interpretation may have been made. *Definitive therapy cannot be planned rationally without knowing the nature of the neoplastic lesion.*

Three methods for biopsy of suspicious tissue are commonly used. They are the *needle,* the *incisional,* and the *excisional,* or open, biopsy; each has its advantages and disadvantages. Regardless of method used, the pathologic interpretation of the tumor mass can be valid only if a representative section of tumor is obtained. A problem of "sampling error" can occur with the needle and the incisional biopsies when only a small portion of the total tumor mass is submitted for pathologic examination.

Needle biopsy is the simplest method and may be used for biopsy of subcutaneous masses, muscular masses, and some internal organs, such as liver and kidney. Further, this method is inexpensive and causes minimal disturbance of the surrounding tissue. There is less chance of disrupting lymphatics and spreading cancer cells along tissue planes. The danger of implanting tumor cells in a needle track during aspiration biopsy is extremely small and can be avoided if the location of the needle track is such that it can be excised easily at the time of the definitive surgical procedure. Needle biopsy may be disadvantageous when the specimen is quite small and not representative of the total tumor, or the needle may miss the space-occupying lesion within the liver or kidney. Hence, a needle or aspiration biopsy does require experience to interpret. A negative report for malignant disease is always viewed with skepticism and should be followed by incisional or excisional biopsy if there is any doubt.

Incisional biopsy involves removal of only a portion of a tumor mass for pathologic examination. It is best performed under circumstances where, if tumor cells are spilled at the time of biopsy, the incisional wound can be encompassed and totally excised at the time of the definitive surgical procedure. Incisional biopsy includes removal of portions of tumor with forceps during endoscopic examination of the bronchus, esophagus, rectum, and bladder. Incisional biopsy is indicated for deeper subcutaneous or muscular tumor masses when needle biopsy fails to establish a diagnosis.

The incisional biopsy is also used when a tumor is so large that total local excision would prejudice any subsequent adequate, wide, locally curative resection because of the wide tissue planes that are necessarily exposed by biopsy. Such biopsy should take a deep section of tumor, as well as a margin of normal tissue, if possible. Incisional biopsy does suffer from the same hazard as the needle biopsy in that the removed portion may not be representative of all the involved tissue; hence, a negative biopsy does not preclude the presence of cancer in the remaining mass. Another theoretic objection to the incisional method is the possibility that the surgeon may seed cancer cells into the operative wound or that exposed open lymphatics may transport the cells to distant sites. Despite these dangers, one must keep in mind that definitive surgical procedures cannot be planned rationally without knowing the nature of the neoplastic lesion.

Excisional biopsy is total local removal of the tumor mass. This is used for small, discrete masses, 2 to 3 cm in diameter, when local removal will not interfere with the wider excision required for permanent local control. A major advantage of an excisional biopsy is that it gives the entire lesion to the pathologist. However, this method is contraindicated in large tumor masses because, again, the biopsy procedure often scatters tumor cells throughout a large biopsy incision that must be widely and totally encompassed by subsequent definitive surgical procedures. Therefore, excisional biopsy is usually contraindicated for skeletal and soft tissue sarcomas, although it is ideally suitable for superficial squamous or basal cell carcinomas and malignant melanomas. The surgeon should always mark the excisional biopsy margins with sutures so that if removal is incomplete, he will know where tumor margin was positive should further excision be indicated.

Biopsy incisions should be closed with meticulous hemostasis, since it may be possible for a collecting hematoma to extend tumor cell contamination by widespread infiltration of tissue planes. Contaminated instruments, gloves, gowns, and drapes should be discarded and replaced with noncontaminated substitutes when the definitive procedure is to follow immediately after the biopsy procedure.

The excisional method is principally used for polypoid lesions of the colon, for thyroid and breast nodules, for small skin lesions, and when the pathologist cannot make a definitive diagnosis from tissue removed by incisional biopsy. An unbiopsied lump is surgically removed when the suspicious character of the lesion, the need for its removal whatever the diagnosis, and the nonmutilating nature of the operation make such an approach reasonably definitive. Examples of such procedures include hemithyroidectomy for thyroid nodules, partial colectomy for lesions at any point beyond the reach of the sigmoidoscope, or a right colectomy for a cecal mass that might be inflammatory or neoplastic.

Lymph nodes should be carefully selected for biopsy. Cervical lymph nodes should not be biopsied until a careful search for a primary tumor has been made. Indirect laryngoscopy, pharyngoscopy, esophagoscopy, and bronchoscopy are included in the work-up. Enlargement of the upper cervical nodes is usually due to metastases from laryngeal, oropharyngeal, and nasopharyngeal neoplasms. Supraclavicular nodes are more frequently enlarged from metastases originating in the thoracic or abdominal cavity.

The specimen may be prepared for pathologic examination by either frozen or permanent sections. Frozen sections are made immediately, and pathologic diagnosis can be obtained within 10 to 20 minutes. Although frozen sections may be as adequate as permanent sections for diagnosis of some neoplasms, most pathologists would prefer to make a definitive diagnosis in questionable cases on permanent sections. Unfortunately, such sections require 1 to 2 days for processing. Therefore, frozen sections are used when the diagnosis is required at the time of major surgery and when it is in the patient's best interests to have the definitive resectional surgery carried out at that time. Examples in which the therapeutic decision will be based upon the results of frozen section examination include (1) deciding between a local or radical operation in carcinoma of the breast, (2) limiting the extent of excision in carcinomas of the lip or face, (3) determining the adequacy of surgical margins, and (4) identifying small structures such as parathyroid glands.

Occasionally, an exploratory thoracotomy or laparotomy will be necessary to obtain tissue for microscopic examination and confirmation of diagnosis. As a general rule, regardless of the clinical picture, the neoplastic nature of the disease process must be confirmed by frozen section examination prior to closure of the wound. This is critical because the permanent sections may fail to confirm the neoplastic nature of the pathologic process.

Exfoliative cytology constitutes one possible method for the early diagnosis of certain types of neoplasms. This technique is based upon the fact that cancer cells are shed from the surfaces of neoplasms arising in epithelial-lined body cavities and orifices, such as the vagina, bronchus, and stomach. These cells can be collected, stained, and recognized as malignant because of their individual morphologic changes.

Staging Extent of Cancer

The extent of the patient's tumor at a given point in time is expressed as its *clinical stage*. In addition to making an exact histologic diagnosis of cancer, it is essential that the clinical stage of the disease be determined prior to making a decision regarding therapy. This is especially important when the patient initially presents for treatment, but also it is often desirable to repeat some of the diagnostic procedures periodically during the patient's course in order to assess his true status. The recognized impor-

tance of this staging has led to a variety of international and national attempts to standardize the staging of the patient with cancer. To date, no single system has been universally accepted. However, Stage I usually indicates a neoplasm confined to its primary site of origin, Stage II indicates metastases to the regional lymph nodes, and Stages III and IV indicate distant metastatic spread.

The Union Internationale Contre Cancer (UICC) has attempted to standardize one system for all nations. This has been called the TNM system because it relies on a statement of tumor extent in terms of the primary tumor (T), presence or absence of node metastases (N), and the presence or absence of distant metastases (M). The system was developed following careful analysis of the results of treatment in patients with various constellations of clinical findings. It was found that patients with larger tumors did less well than those with smaller tumors; hence, the separation of various stages on the basis of tumor size. For different tumors size criteria vary, but in this system decreasing prognosis is indicated by increasing numbers after the T, such as T1, T2, T3, or T4 for lesions of increasing sizes. The presence or absence of regional spread is usually indicated by variations in the secondary category, under N for nodes. The absence of nodal metastasis is designated as N_0; the presence of nodal metastasis is N_1; for more extensive nodal involvement, additional numbers may be used. Finally, distant metastases are indicated by adding a subscript 1 following M for metastases, or a subscript 0 for their absence. Thus, a small lesion that has neither spread to regional nodes nor metastasized would be designated as a $T_1N_0M_0$ lesion. A lesion which was larger and involved regional nodes but without distant metastases might be identified as a $T_2N_1M_0$ lesion. A larger neoplasm with both regional and distant metastases would be designated a $T_3N_1M_1$ lesion.

Specific staging systems have been developed for Hodgkin's disease and other lymphomas. A distinction is made between the clinical stage, as defined by clinical tests, and the pathologic stage, as defined by biopsy or major operation. Stage I relates to diseases localized to one lymph node–bearing area. Stage II would be disease into adjacent regional areas, but on one side of the diaphragm and restricted to lymph node–bearing areas including the spleen and Waldeyer's ring (tonsilar area). Stage IV represents widespread metastases in organs, such as bone, bone marrow, liver, or lung.

Hodgkin's disease, which spreads from a localized region directly into an organ, in this classification scheme is identified as the respective stage plus the subscript E, for extension. Thus, a patient with disease in the mediastinum and neck, with extension into the pulmonary parenchyma adjacent to the mediastinal lesion, would have Stage II_E disease. For lymphomas, the importance of symptoms in prognosis is further identified by adding a designation for the absence or presence of symptoms. Patients with symptoms of night sweats, weight loss, or fever are identified as having Stage B disease, whereas patients lacking these symptoms are identified as having Stage A disease (for example, Stage II_EA). The tremendous importance of accurate staging is underlined by the fact that for many lymphomas an accurate decision regarding therapy may require pathologic staging of the presence or absence of disease below the diaphragm. Thus, patients with disease clinically limited to extensive areas above the diaphragm are commonly subjected to an abdominal exploratory operation in order to remove the spleen, examine the liver, and biopsy lymph nodes. This allows a much more precise designation of the extent of disease, and the findings frequently lead to a change in decision regarding a choice of therapy. Specifically, Hodgkin's disease in Stages I and II is curable by radiation therapy, while Stages IIIB and IV are generally treated with chemotherapy.

The importance of accurate staging when designating a therapeutic program for a patient with cancer cannot be overemphasized. It is an important consideration when comparing the results of therapy in different centers, and as therapeutic methods for cancer improve, it is only by careful staging that new forms of therapy can be appropriately evaluated.

Unfortunately, one of the great difficulties in the present staging methods is their inability to detect subclinical microscopic metastatic lesions. Many patients who are treated for apparently localized cancers already have disseminated metastases. For example, about one-half of those patients who have cancer of the breast and who undergo mastectomy have subclinical distant metastasis at the time of operation.

THERAPY

General Considerations

At present, approximately 55 percent of all cancer patients are treated by surgical resection (40 percent by surgery alone); 34 percent by radiation therapy (16 percent by radiation therapy alone); and 22 percent by chemotherapy alone or in combination with the other modalities. As the use of chemotherapy as an adjuvant to surgery increases, it is likely that a much larger percentage of patients will have chemotherapy as part of their cancer treatment. Fifteen percent of cancer patients receive no treatment.

Surgery and radiation therapy today represent the most successful means of dealing with cancer as long as it remains localized to the primary site and regional lymph nodes. Neither can be considered curative once the disease has metastasized beyond the local region, although both methods of therapy may be useful as palliative treatment. Chemotherapy and immunotherapy, unlike surgery and radiation therapy, represent systemic forms of treatment effective against tumor cells already metastatic to distant organ sites. These systemic therapeutic modalities have a greater chance of curing patients with a minimum number of tumor cells than those with clinically evident disease. Thus, though surgery and radiation therapy cannot be curative unless the tumor is confined locally or regionally, they can decrease the patient's tumor burden so that chemotherapy or immunotherapy may become more effective. During the past several years, enough evidence has

accumulated to suggest that treatment combining surgery, radiation therapy, chemotherapy, and, possibly, immunotherapy will significantly improve cure rates above those achieved with any single therapeutic modality.

Future cancer treatment, therefore, will be approached in an interdisciplinary manner. Just as oncology should be approached as a unique field of study, so cancer should be regarded as a single but complex disease requiring a multidisciplinary approach. The practice of assigning certain types of neoplasms to surgery, radiation therapy, or medicine with a further division into various anatomically oriented specialties should be discontinued.

GOALS OF THERAPY—CURE OR PALLIATION. Once the diagnosis of malignant disease has been made and the extent of disease determined, a decision must be made about the specific therapy. *Is the patient curable?* This is the foremost question that must be answered before the physician recommends aggressive therapy with its attendant complications. The goals of therapy vary with the extent of the cancer. If the cancer is localized without evidence of spread, the goal is to irradicate the cancer and cure the patient. However, when the cancer is spread beyond local cure, the goal is to control the patient's symptoms and to maintain his maximum activity for the longest possible period of time. Palliation should be measured in terms of useful life. Diabetes is not cured, but the manifestations of the disease are controlled so that a patient has many years of activity and useful life. Goals for the palliation of patients living with cancer are similar.

Patients are generally judged as incurable if they have distant metastases or evidence of extensive local infiltration of adjacent organs or structures. The most common criterion for incurability is distant metastases. However, some patients are potentially curable even if they have distant metastases. For example, patients with solitary pulmonary metastases may be curable by resection, and even those with widespread metastases who have choriocarcinoma may be curable with chemotherapy. Histologic proof of distant metastases should be obtained before the patient is assessed as incurable. Occasionally, an exploratory celiotomy or thoracotomy may be necessary to determine the nature of equivocal lesions in the lungs or liver. In some situations, e.g., multiple pulmonary metastases, the clinical situation may point so overwhelmingly to distant metastases that the patient may safely be considered incurable without biopsy.

Local extension may be a criterion of incurability. For each anatomic site, there are certain local criteria which place the patient unequivocally in an incurable status, while others imply a poor prognosis but are not absolutely indicative of incurability. In equivocal situations after extensive studies have failed to demonstrate metastatic or incurable local extension, the patient deserves the benefit of doubt and should be treated for cure.

CHOICE OF THERAPY. Surgery, radiation therapy, and chemotherapy are the most frequently used therapeutic modalities in the fight against cancer. Each may play a role in both curative and palliative therapy. Immunotherapy is a new modality that has a limited role in cancer therapy at the present time, but one which should become increasingly useful in the future. In choosing therapy, a variety of factors must be considered regardless of whether the aim is cure or palliation. The natural history of the disease and the results obtained from each type of therapy must be known prior to choosing a modality or combination of modalities.

The patient's general medical condition and the presence of any coexisting disease must be considered in planning therapy. Surgery may be contraindicated in a patient who has recently experienced a myocardial infarction. A patient with preexisting diabetes will be much more susceptible to the toxic effects of hormonal therapy with corticosteroids. Renal disease may increase the toxicity of some of the chemotherapeutic drugs, such as methotrexate. In addition, any evidence of infection or bleeding in a patient may make any form of cancer therapy dangerous, requiring vigorous treatment prior to the initiation of definitive therapy.

The psychologic makeup of the patient and the patient's life situation must be considered. A patient who is unable to accept the realities of a given treatment should be offered an alternative approach when possible. This is particularly true of any surgical procedures that significantly alter appearance or that involve change of organ function requiring the patient's daily care, such as colostomy. Experimental forms of therapy, such as intraarterial infusion of drugs, should also be avoided by some patients. Obviously, a patient who is going to be unwilling to tolerate the inconvenience of an intraarterial catheter and who might remove it without medical approval should not undergo such treatment.

Surgical Therapy

Surgical treatment represents the most frequently used and the most successful single method of cancer therapy currently available. More patients are cured of cancer by surgery than by any other therapeutic modality. However, only about one-third of cancer patients are cured by surgery alone, since surgical therapy, with few exceptions, is curative only in those patients in whom the disease is localized in the primary site and regional nodes.

Cancer surgery is based upon the concept that cancer begins as a local disease and spreads in an orderly fashion from the primary site to adjacent tissues by direct extension, to the regional lymph nodes by lymphatics, and through the blood vessels. The surgical procedure is designed to remove the primary neoplasms and the usual contiguous routes of spread with the aim of removing *every* cancer cell from the body.

Advances in surgical techniques, anesthesia, and supportive care (blood transfusion, antibiotics, and fluid and electrolyte management) have permitted the development of more radical and extensive operative procedures. This has resulted in significant improvements in the cure rates for certain human neoplasms. Ultraradical cancer surgery has extended operations to their anatomic limits, permitting the surgical removal of nearly all organs. Unfortunately, these more radical procedures have often failed to significantly increase cure rates.

There have been few significant improvements in the management of most human neoplasms by surgery alone during the past two decades. Furthermore, advances in cancer surgery techniques beyond those presently practiced are unlikely to significantly change the cure rates of most human neoplasms. It would appear, then, that any therapeutic advances must come from the combination of other modalities with cancer surgery.

PREOPERATIVE PREPARATION. Often, the physical condition of cancer patients is relatively poor. Many malignant tumors seem to have a toxic effect on the host disproportionate to the size of the lesion. Patients may have a poor nutritional status because of interference with normal alimentary function as with cancers of the oral pharynx, esophagus, and intestinal tract. Pain may contribute to anorexia and severe electrolyte disorder. Anemia, vitamin deficiencies, and defects in the coagulation mechanisms must be corrected before an operation can be safely performed.

Every effort should be made to correct nutritional deficiencies, restore depleted blood volumes, and correct hypoproteinemia prior to extensive surgical procedures. Otherwise the operative morbidity and mortality following extensive cancer operations will be excessive.

CANCER SURGERY

Once the decision has been made to proceed with surgical therapy, the operative procedure should be planned carefully. It is essential to realize that the best, and often the only, opportunity for cure is at the time of the first operation. If the neoplasm is incompletely excised at that time, tissue planes, lymphatics, and blood vessels are violated and tumor cells seeded throughout the wound. Any recurrence that follows may be difficult to separate from the inflammatory reaction and scarring that can distort tissue planes to a point where tumor margins are indistinct. Therefore, enucleation or incomplete excision of tumor masses is *never* indicated as a therapeutic measure.

PREVENTION OF CANCER CELL IMPLANTATION DURING SURGERY. Local recurrence of cancer following surgery may be due to incomplete removal or spillage of cancer cells into the operative area (Fig. 9-18). The cancer surgeon constantly must be aware of the possible danger of transferring cancer cells by inoculation into the surrounding tissues during the course of an operation. As soon as the incision is made, all edges of the wound should be protected with a plastic drape to prevent tumor cell contamination. This precaution is exemplified best when laparotomy or thoracotomy is performed for malignant disease within the abdomen or thorax.

Tumor cells may be inadvertently transplanted from the primary site to other sites during the surgical procedure. When preliminary biopsy has been done, the entire operative field should be reprepared after the biopsy incision is closed. The instruments and gloves used during the biopsy are not used again, because they may have been contaminated. Even the basin of saline solution in which the surgeon dips his gloved hand may be contaminated with cancer cells. The importance of this is illustrated by a patient with breast cancer who had a skin graft taken

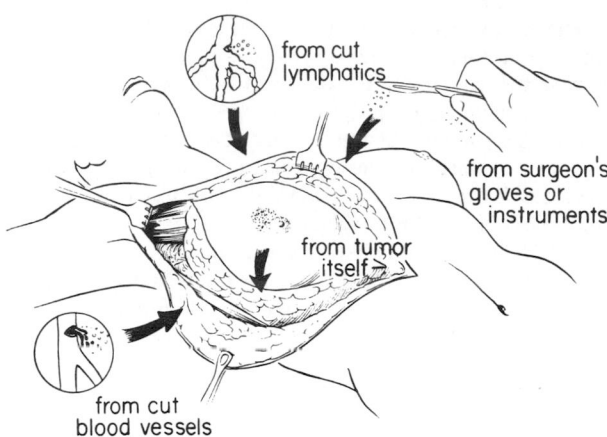

from cut lymphatics

from surgeon's gloves or instruments

from tumor itself →

from cut blood vessels

Fig. 9-18. During the operative procedure, cancer cells may be seeded in the wound by direct contact with the primary tumor, with lymph nodes containing metastatic tumor, or with contaminated gloves and instruments. Cancer cells may also enter the wound via cut lymphatics and divided blood vessels. (*From W. H. Cole et al., "Dissemination of Cancer," Appleton-Century-Crofts, Inc., New York, 1961.*)

from the thigh to close a skin defect after a mastectomy. Later, tumor nodules having the same histologic characteristics as the primary neoplasm developed on the thigh at the skin graft donor site.

If the tumor is entered during the operative procedure, the risk of implanting cancer cells into the wound is greatly increased. Should this happen, the operative field must be isolated; the cut surface of the tumor must be cauterized with the electrocautery and isolated from the remainder of the wound; and the contaminated knife, instruments, and gloves must be discarded. Then, and then only, can the operation continue through a new plane of dissection allowing a much wider margin around the tumor.

Many different cytotoxic solutions have been used to irrigate the wound following cancer surgery in an effort to sterilize the operative site. None have been very effective in decreasing the local recurrence rate, with the exception of 0.5% formaldehyde used to prevent local recurrence from carcinoma of the cervix. Sodium hypochlorite solution, nitrogen mustard, and thiotepa have all been tried, with little success.

The rate of local recurrence in the suture line following resection for carcinoma of the colon is about 10 percent. There has been some success with various techniques to prevent this local recurrence. Ligation of the bowel with umbilical tape proximal and distal to the tumor, or anastomosis, or irrigation of the cut ends of the colon with bichloride of mercury solution and then excision of the edge of each end of the bowel have been used and have decreased the recurrence rate to less than 2 percent. The use of closed anastomosis and iodized sutures has decreased the anastomotic recurrence rate in the laboratory.

PREVENTION OF VASCULAR DISSEMINATION AT SURGERY. Blood-borne metastases are a major factor in the death of patients with most tumors. Although cancer cells have been identified in the blood of many cancer patients, only a small number of these circulating cancer cells sur-

vive because of host resistance and other factors. Thus, tumor embolism and metastases are not synonymous. In fact, there appears to be little difference in the prognosis of patients with or without tumor cells in their blood preoperatively. However, there is a correlation between the presence of tumor cells seen in the blood during the operative procedure and prognosis. Furthermore, manipulation of the tumor at any time in the surgical procedure can greatly increase the number of cancer cells recovered from the blood.

Definite measures should be taken to prevent the dissemination of tumor cells during the operation. These can include (1) avoiding manipulation of the tumor ("no-touch" technique), (2) early ligation of the vascular pedicle, (3) the use of tourniquets on all extremity tumors.

Since any manipulation of the tumor mass may result in exfoliation of tumor cells into the lymphatics and blood, such manipulation must be kept to a minimum prior to the operative procedure, during preparation of the skin with antiseptic agents, as well as during the operative procedure. Furthermore, it is imperative to use an incision of proper size to minimize unnecessary manipulation of the tumor. One that is too small will not permit the necessary wide excision without excessive handling. Turnbull and associates have reported a significant higher survival in left colon cancer using the no-touch technique which combines minimal manipulation, early ligation of the vascular pedicle, and wide excision. However, the importance of early ligation of the vascular pedicle has been questioned by Stearns, who reported similar results without the early ligation.

TYPES OF CANCER OPERATIONS. Local Resection. Wide local resection in which an adequate margin of normal tissue is removed with the tumor mass may be adequate treatment for certain low-grade neoplasms that do not metastasize to regional nodes or widely infiltrate adjacent tissues. Basal cell carcinomas and the mixed tumors of the parotid gland are examples of such neoplasms.

Radical Local Resection. Some neoplasms may spread widely by infiltration into adjacent tissues. This is especially true for soft tissue sarcomas and esophageal and gastric carcinomas. For this reason, it is necessary to remove a wide margin of normal tissue with the neoplasm in these cases. The wide normal-tissue margin between the line of excision and the tumor mass also acts as a protective barrier against tumor cell spill into the severed lymphatics and vessels. The greater the thickness of normal tissue between the plane of dissection and the tumor, the greater likelihood of a complete local excision.

If the tumor was previously explored but not removed or if an incisional biopsy was performed, it is extremely important that a wide segment of skin and the underlying muscles, fat, and fascia be removed far beyond the limits of the original incision.

It must be constantly emphasized that malignant neoplasms are not well encapsulated. A pseudocapsule composed of a compression zone of neoplastic cells usually covers the tumor. This apparent encapsulation offers a great temptation for simple enucleation, because the tumor may be dislodged from its bed so easily. However, this temptation must be resisted. The surgeon must cut through normal tissue at all times and should never encounter the neoplasm during its removal. Dissection should proceed with meticulous care to avoid tumor cell spill. Retraction always should be away from, rather than toward, the tumor. It is important for the surgeon to remember that he must be as far as possible from the gross extent of the tumor on all sides including the deep aspect. He must be prepared to sacrifice important nerves, muscles, and blood vessels if necessary in order to encompass the tumor. Skin, subcutaneous fat and muscle usually can be sacrificed with impunity and little functional loss. However, involvement of major vessels, nerves, joints, or bones may require sacrifice of these structures and even amputation in order to obtain a curative result. During the surgical procedure, the extent of operation should be determined only by the concern for cure.

All deeply situated sarcomas lying between or within muscle groups require the removal of all muscle bundles from their origin to insertion within that particular fascial compartment; all surrounding or adjacent fascia, periosteum, vessels, nerves, and connective tissues; and all skin adjacent to the lesions. These procedures are imperative because sarcomas of the soft somatic tissues tend to infiltrate along fascial and muscle planes far beyond the palpable limits of the tumor. As the surgeon proceeds with the operation, he may be forced to alter his initial operative plan as he visualizes the extent of tumor and as the pathology reports of frozen section examinations of surgical margins are made available. These decisions as to extent of resection are difficult and require experienced judgment. In borderline situations, it is usually better to proceed with a potentially curative resection of the tumor mass unless there is histologic confirmation that the lesion has extended beyond the boundaries of possible surgical resection. Recent advances in the use of combined modality therapy for skeletal and soft tissue sarcomas have permitted the salvage of extremities rather than amputation in selected patients (see the section on Combined Modality Therapy).

Radical Resection with En Bloc Excision of Lymphatics. Since many neoplasms commonly metastasize by way of the lymphatics, operations have been designed to remove the primary neoplasms and the regional lymph nodes draining that area in continuity with all the tissues intervening between the primary neoplasm and regional nodes. Conditions are best for this type of operation when the collecting nodes of the lymphatic channels draining the neoplasm lie adjacent to the primary site or if there is a single avenue of lymphatic drainage which can be removed without sacrificing vital structures. The regional nodes farthest from the tumor should be dissected first, with dissection proceeding toward the tumor mass in order to prevent any confiltation of tumor cells from the primary tumor into the regional lymphatics of the venous system.

This principle was applied to breast cancer by Meyer and by Halsted at the turn of the century and has formed the foundation of cancer surgery for many years. At the present time, it is generally agreed that such en bloc regional lymph node dissections should be performed in patients having clinical involvement of nodes by metastatic tumor. However, in many such cases, the tumor has already spread beyond the regional nodes, and the cure rates following such procedures may be quite low.

The high rate of local cancer recurrence following surgical removal when lymph nodes are grossly involved and the high error rate when trying to ascertain by palpation those nodes involved by tumor have led to routine dissection of regional nodes close to the primary tumor even though they are not clinically involved. Microscopic examination of the excised lymph nodes in these patients who have no clinical evidence of palpable enlargement reveals evidence of tumor spread in 20 to 40 percent of carcinomas. This concept is supported by comparison of the higher 5-year survival rate of patients showing microscopic involvement of lymph nodes with that of patients in whom lymph node involvement was clinically recognizable.

Recently, some surgeons have challenged the concept of elective or prophylactic resection in cases where the regional nodes are not obviously involved, because of the possibility that such removal may interfere with the patient's immune response to the tumor. This concept originated from experiments in laboratory animals in which removal of the regional nodes within 1 to 2 weeks after implantation of tumor transplants in an extremity interfered with the development of tumor immunity. The validity of these experiments must be challenged, however, because it has been demonstrated with other animal tumors that regional lymphadenectomy has little influence upon host immunity if the removal of the regional nodes is delayed 4 to 6 weeks until the immune response is already underway. The differences between these two sets of experiments depends upon the well-established observation that early excision of regional nodes will interfere with a primary immune response.

It is possible that the immune response against cancer in man is similar. Most human neoplasms have been present in the body for many months or years prior to clinical detection. Hence, cancer patients already have an active systemic immune response to their malignant condition, best demonstrated by the presence of killer lymphocytes in the blood and circulating antitumor antibodies. Thus, the importance of the regional lymph nodes as an immune barrier controlling tumor dissemination in man probably should not be considered an adequate argument against regional lymphadenectomy. In addition, when metastatic cancer cells are found in 20 to 40 percent of operative specimens, it seems likely that the regional nodes obviously are not doing an effective job of controlling the dissemination of cancer.

Nevertheless, this is a very controversial issue at the present time, with sufficiently numerous conflicting reports concerning the effectiveness of elective regional lymphadenectomy that a definite conclusion regarding its use cannot be made. We advocate regional lymphadenectomy in selected patients with clinically negative nodes who have neoplasms which frequently metastasize to lymph nodes because of data supporting higher 5-year survival rates with this technique. Furthermore, most studies comparing identical stages of primary disease have shown slightly improved survival when lymphadenectomy was done. There has been little evidence that removal of the regional nodes adversely affects the survival figures.

An important benefit of lymphadenectomy is the provision of more accurate staging in order to identify those patients at high risk for disease recurrence. Now that we have presumptive evidence for the effectiveness of adjuvant chemotherapy and immunotherapy in a variety of malignant diseases, it is particularly important to identify those patients who will benefit most from these therapies.

This controversy can be settled by a controlled clinical trial to demonstrate the effectiveness of elective or prophylactic lymph node dissections. Such studies are currently underway for several different types of neoplasms. Until more data are available, en bloc resection of regional nodes should continue as standard therapy for carcinoma of the mouth, pharynx and larynx, colon and rectum, breast, uterus and cervix, malignant melanoma, and testicular neoplasms.

Extensive Surgical Procedures. Some slow-growing primary tumors may reach enormous size and may locally infiltrate widely without developing distant metastasis. Supraradical operative procedures can be undertaken in these extensive, nearly inoperable tumors, with cure of occasional patients. Although surgical care, anesthesia, blood replacement, and physiologic monitoring are much improved over the past, these procedures should not be undertaken except by experienced surgeons who can select those patients most likely to benefit from such procedures. Since these extensive surgical procedures sometimes offer a chance for a cure that is not possible by other means, they are justified in selected situations when extensive laboratory work-up shows no evidence of distant metastases. However, the surgeon must be willing to accept the responsibility for the postoperative emotional rehabilitation of the patient before undertaking such extensive procedures as the pelvic exenteration, hemipelvectomy, forequarter amputation, or mutilating operations for head and neck carcinomas.

Pelvic exenteration is a well-conceived operation capable of curing patients with radiation-treated recurrent cancer of the cervix and certain well-differentiated and locally extensive adenocarcinomas of the rectum. This operation removes the pelvic organs (bladder, uterus, and rectum) and all soft tissues within the pelvis. Bowel function is restored with colostomy. Urinary tract drainage is established by anastomosis of ureters into a segment of bowel (ileum or sigmoid colon). The 5-year survival cure rate from pelvic exenteration is 25 percent in this situation.

Hemipelvectomy (resection of the lower extremity and iliac bone) can sometimes be curative for skeletal sarcomas limited to the head of the femur or acetabulum or to one-half of the pelvic structures, and in some slowly growing soft tissue sarcomas of the upper thigh and buttock which recur locally but metastasize slowly. Forequarter amputation (resection of the upper extremity and scapula) can offer similar cure when the neoplasm is limited to the bones of the scapula and upper humerus or to the soft tissues of the shoulder girdle.

SURGERY OF RECURRENT CANCER. There is a definite role for surgical resection of localized recurrent neoplasms of low-grade malignancy and slow growth where further resection may produce a long period of remission. Additional surgical procedures are frequently successful in controlling recurrent soft tissue sarcomas, anastomotic recurrences of colon cancer, and certain basal and squamous carcinomas of skin.

Gilbertsen and Wangensteen advocated routine "second look" operations over a scheduled period, perhaps 6 months after the original procedure, whether or not symptomatic or objective evidence of recurrence was evident. The results of these operations have not been impressive, although a few patients experienced an unexpected long-term control of their disease. However, many of these patients might have been salvaged anyway if reoperation and excision had been delayed until a symptomatic recurrence developed, since this is not uncommon. Thus, it is difficult to prove the second-look theory; for this reason, second-look operations have not become common practice.

RESECTION OF METASTASES. Although logic would suggest that once a neoplasm has metastasized to a distant site it should no longer be curable by surgical resection, removal of metastatic lesions in the lung, liver, or brain has occasionally resulted in a clinical cure. Therefore, in selected patients with slowly growing neoplasms, resections of the metastatic lesions may be indicated especially if the metastasis is solitary. Prior to undertaking resection, an extensive laboratory work-up should rule out metastatic spread to other body areas.

Most patients with diffuse liver metastases are candidates for systemic or intraarterial chemotherapy. Most will not survive beyond 2 years, and few, if any, will survive for 5 years. Therefore, prior to embarking on such therapy, it is important to remember that significant palliation and an occasional cure can be achieved by resecting hepatic metastases in selected patients. Resection can be recommended when the primary tumor is controlled and no other metastases are present and when the patient's condition, the location of the tumor, and the capability of the surgical team allows safe resection.

In a survey involving 126 patients who had resection of metastases from carcinoma of the colon and rectum, Foster and Berman reported an 18 percent 5-year survival. These patients were obviously chosen from a large group of patients and do not represent statistics that can be applied across the board to all patients with hepatic metastases. Nonetheless, it is advisable to consider resection prior to beginning systemic chemotherapy, since an occasional 5-year cure can be achieved (Fig. 9-19).

The results of resection of pulmonary metastatic lesions have been much more satisfactory than those of resection of liver or brain metastases. In fact, resection of solitary pulmonary metastases has given a higher rate of 5-year survival than has resection of primary bronchogenic carcinoma of the lung. Resection of pulmonary metastases may be indicated even when more than one metastatic lesion is present. Many patients die with pulmonary metastases and no other evidence of tumor at autopsy; resection of the pulmonary metastases could have resulted in cure.

Fig. 9-19. Resected liver and smiling patient at 5-year anniversary of operation for hepatic metastases. (*From D. L. Morton, E. C. Holmes, and S. H. Golub, Chest, 71:640, 1977.*)

Our experience has shown measurement of the tumor doubling time to be useful in selecting those patients who will benefit most from resection of pulmonary metastases. Patients with tumor doubling times greater than 40 days received significant palliation from their pulmonary resections and remained free of disease for as long as 5 years. In contrast, patients with tumor doubling times of less than 20 days have not significantly benefited from resection of their metastatic lesions (Fig. 9-20).

Hepatic Dearterialization. Hepatic dearterialization has been advocated for the treatment of liver metastases, based upon the observation that metastases derive their blood supply predominantly from the hepatic artery whereas normal liver tissue receives blood from both the arterial and portal systems. In the absence of hypotension and sepsis, hepatic artery ligation is surprisingly well tolerated and results in selective necrosis of liver tumors. Because some tumor cells remain viable, postoperative chemotherapy is necessary to help control tumor growth. This procedure is not without risk and needs further evaluation to determine its role in managing patients with either primary hepatic carcinoma or hepatic metastases.

ADMINISTRATION OF CHEMOTHERAPY BY ARTERIAL INFUSION OR ISOLATED PERFUSION. The concentration of chemotherapeutic drugs can be greatly increased when the drug is administered directly into the artery supplying the neoplastic lesion. Continuous infusion of chemotherapeutic drugs over a period of weeks can be carried out with portable infusion pumps attached to a catheter placed in the artery. Some striking remissions using this technique have been observed, although they usually have been of short duration. It appears logical to assume that this manner of administering chemotherapeutic agents would increase their effectiveness because of the greater concentrations obtainable. Patients with hepatoma have responded well to the intraarterial infusion of 5-FU. Hepatic artery ligation and 5-FU infusion have been combined with some success in treating patients with metastatic colon carcinoma.

One ingenious method of administering increased concentrations of chemotherapeutic drugs involves the isolated perfusion technique. The artery and veins supplying the tumor-bearing extremity are cannulated and isolated from the systemic circulation by connection to a pump-oxygenator. The tumor is then perfused for up to 90 minutes with oxygenated blood containing cancerocidal drugs in amounts that would be prohibitively poisonous if infused through the general circulation.

Recently it has been found that heating the blood with a heat exchanger similar to that used for cardiopulmonary

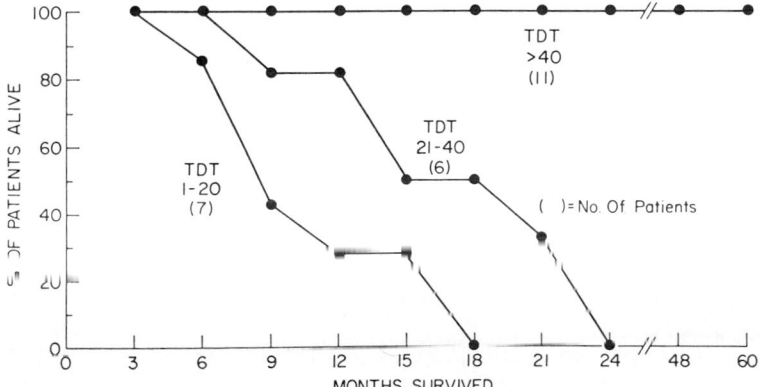

Fig. 9-20. Survival curves of 24 untreated patients following onset of pulmonary metastases. (*From W. L. Joseph et al., J Thorac Cardiovasc Surg, 61:23, 1971.*)

bypass appears to increase the effectiveness of the chemotherapeutic drugs. Hyperthermic perfusion with chemotherapeutic agents may be worthwhile in treating satellite or intransient metastasis from malignant melanoma and primary or recurrent sarcomas of the extremities. Some long-term survivors with malignant melanoma treated by this technique have been reported. Furthermore, Stehlin reports that hyperthermic perfusion of chemotherapeutic drugs, when combined with radiation therapy, may decrease the necessity of amputation in some primary or recurrent sarcomas which are bordering on vital structures of the extremity.

Despite a long experience with intraarterial infusion and regional perfusion for the administration of chemotherapeutic drugs, there is still no general agreement about their usefulness. Many chemotherapists believe systemic administration of drugs would be equally effective. However, we have observed more dramatic responses from the infusion/perfusion techniques than from systemic administration of chemotherapeutic drugs.

PALLIATIVE SURGERY. Surgical procedures are sometimes indicated to relieve symptoms, to reduce the severity of the patient's illness, or to prolong a useful comfortable life without attempting to cure the patient. Such an operation is justified to relieve pain, hemorrhage, obstruction, or infection when it can be done without great risk to the patient, and when it improves the quality of life even if it does not prolong it. Surgery that only prolongs a miserable existence certainly does not benefit the patient.

Some examples of palliative surgical procedures are (1) colostomy, enteroenterostomy, or gastrojejunostomy to relieve obstruction; (2) chordotomy to control pain; (3) cystectomy for infected, bleeding tumors of the bladder; (4) amputations for painful infected tumors in the extremities; (5) simple mastectomy for carcinoma of the breast, even in the presence of distant metastases, when the primary tumor is infected, large, ulcerated, and locally resectable; and (6) colon resection in the presence of hepatic metastases.

Radiation Therapy

Radiation therapy, like surgical therapy, can cure only localized cancer. The palliative effects of radiation therapy in treating symptoms of metastatic or recurrent cancer are well recognized. In fact, 40 percent of all cancer patients will receive radiation therapy at some time in the course of their disease. Irradiation can destroy neoplastic tissue with a minimum of damage to normal tissues surrounding the tumor and thus, when successful, leads to good functional and cosmetic results. Some neoplasms are best treated by this method, whereas other neoplasms can be managed equally well with surgery. Radiation therapy and surgery need not be competitive if specialists in each of the two areas understand the indications and limitations of each form of treatment. Often the two modalities can be used in combination to increase the cure rates for certain types of neoplasms.

MECHANISM OF ACTION. Regardless of the primary source of radiation energy, radiation penetrates and collides with the atoms in tissue, releasing energy that causes the ionization of water in cells. The hydroxy and peroxide radicals thus formed cause DNA and chromosome breaks in both tumor cells and normal cells. Thus, the mechanism of radiation damage relates to a direct effect on certain vital substrates within living cells. Although such effects occur in both normal and neoplastic cells, there are quantitative differences in toxicity, apparently related primarily to a more adequate mechanism for cellular repair in the normal cells, which can be translated into a useful therapeutic effect.

The cellular effects of radiation are both immediate and delayed. Changes in the appearance and behavior of individual cells are observed within a few minutes of exposure, whereas gross changes in irradiated tissue may not appear until weeks, months, or even years after exposure. Microscopic changes occur in both the cytoplasm and nucleus of the cell. Vacuoles often appear in the cytoplasm of the cell, which then becomes swollen. Nuclear chromatin may clump and shrink. The chromosomes may appear abnormal in the cell undergoing mitosis at the time of radiation exposure. Although the radiation may not cause immediate cell death, the cell may be unable to divide again.

The *rad* is the unit of measurement used to express the amount of radiation absorbed, whereas *roentgens* refer to the air dose. With unidirectional radiation therapy, the dose absorbed varies throughout the depth of the radiation field and is dependent upon the energy of the radiation source (Fig. 9-21). Since a tumor is three-dimensional, the dose varies across the tumor volume. There is a maximum and a minimum tumor dose. Without further qualification, a dose of 4,500 rads refers to the average tumor dose at the midpoint of the tumor.

By using various techniques such as multiple ports, rotational fields, lead shielding, and others, it is often possible to deliver larger doses of radiation to the tumor-bearing area than to the surrounding tissue.

Usually, patients tolerate radiation therapy much better when the total dose is fractionated over a number of days or when it is split into two treatment courses, allowing for a rest period between. The margin of safety between destruction of tumor and damage to surrounding tissue also is increased by these techniques.

Rets express the relation between the total dose delivered, the number of fractions, and the time it took to deliver the dose. The ret concept is a method of comparing dissimilar treatment schedules by reducing them to a similar unit of measurement.

There are three basic types of radiation: *alpha particles, beta, or electron, particles,* and *electromagnetic rays,* such as gamma rays and x-rays. Their qualitative effects upon tissue are similar. However, there is great variation in the distance to which these rays can penetrate tissues. Alpha particles penetrate only a few microns and are stopped by the epidermis. Beta particles penetrate tissue in proportion to their energy and in inverse proportion to the density of the tissue, but they do not usually penetrate tissues for more than a few millimeters. Gamma rays can penetrate several centimeters of metal, depending upon the energy and the distance from the target source. The penetration

Fig. 9-21. Typical isodose distributions for low-energy (200 kv), high-energy (^{60}Co), and very high energy (22 Mev) radiation. The average patient is 20 cm thick. When treating a tumor situated midway through the patient, or at 10 cm, each of the three sources would deliver a different percentage of the maximum dose at that point—25 percent with 200 kv, 52 percent with ^{60}Co, and 83 percent with 22 Mev.

of x-rays depends upon the voltage of the machine used to produce the radiation and the distance from the source. Supervoltage machines producing 1,000 to 50,000 kv of energy are available. Such radiation can penetrate to greater depth and will cause less ionization, hence less skin damage, as it passes through the skin than the 250-kv machines used routinely in the past.

The relative biologic effectiveness of x-rays, gamma rays, and beta rays are approximately equal, although neutrons and alpha rays are ten to twenty times as effective, respectively. Therefore, it is possible that new types of neutron radiation may eventually prove very useful in reaching those deep-seated tumors which are relatively insensitive to the present forms of radiation treatment.

RADIOSENSITIVITY VERSUS RADIOCURABILITY OF TUMORS. Radiosensitivity and radiocurability are *not* synonymous terms. A tumor may be radiosensitive but not radiocurable, because of recurrence developing either locally or at a distant site. For instance, very few patients with Ewing's sarcoma, a very radiosensitive tumor, can be cured with radiation therapy, because they develop distant metastases. Some tumors, such as undifferentiated soft tissue sarcomas, initially may respond very rapidly, only to recur locally several months later. Other tumors, such as epidermoid carcinoma of the cervix or adenocarcinoma of the uterus, do not disappear immediately, but hyster-

ectomy several months later may reveal no evidence of tumor, and the patient may be cured.

Radiocurability depends upon radiosensitivity; however, tumors differ in their response to radiation therapy, as shown in Table 9-10. In general, tumor cells which are undifferentiated or in active mitosis are more sensitive to radiation. Furthermore, radiosensitivity of malignant tumors usually parallels the radiosensitivity of their cell of

Table 9-10 RELATIVE RADIOSENSITIVITY OF MALIGNANT TUMORS

(Listed in order of decreasing radiosensitivity)

Malignant tumors arising from hemopoietic organs (lymphosarcoma, myeloma)
Hodgkin's disease
Seminomas and dysgerminomas
Ewing's sarcoma of the bone
Basal cell carcinomas of the skin
Epidermoid carcinomas arising by metaplasia from columnar epithelium
Epidermoid carcinomas of the mucous membranes, mucocutaneous junctions, and skin
Adenocarcinomas of the endometrium, breast, gastrointestinal system, and endocrine glands.
Soft tissue sarcomas
Chondrosarcomas
Neurogenic sarcomas
Osteosarcomas
Malignant melanomas

SOURCE: From L. V. Ackerman and J. A. del Regato, "Cancer: Diagnosis, Treatment, and Prognosis," 4th ed., The C. V. Mosby Company, St. Louis, 1970.

origin. Hemopoietic cells, epidermoid cells, lymphocytes, germ cells of the gonads, and the lining epithelium of the alimentary tract are most sensitive to radiation. Usually tumors derived from these cells are also radiosensitive. However, there are exceptions, such as adenocarcinoma of the stomach and gonads. Tumor volume, tumor oxygenation, and the histology of the tumor are of equal importance in determining radiosensitivity and radiocurability.

COMPLICATIONS OF RADIATION THERAPY. Although usually associated with no immediate mortality, the morbidity, complications, and long-term effects of radiation therapy may be considerable. The complications of radiation therapy may limit the dose and the rate of delivery. Both systemic and local complications of radiation therapy may be seen, as well as the less frequent genetic and carcinogenic effects. The acute and chronic local effects of radiation on different organs are outlined in Table 9-11. The acute changes are caused by edema and inflammation, while the chronic changes are caused by scarring and fibrosis. Megavoltage radiation has largely obviated the skin changes seen in the past with lower-voltage radiation.

Many patients undergoing radiation therapy temporarily develop systemic symptoms associated with malaise, nausea, vomiting, weakness, and weight loss. These symptoms are directly related to dose, volume, and rate of delivery, and to type of tissue treated. Radiation sickness usually can be prevented, and the nausea and vomiting can be successfully treated with antiemetics such as Compazine.

The genetic and carcinogenic effects of radiation therapy are seen less frequently as these problems have become better understood. The genetic effects of radiation expressed as mutations and congenital abnormalities have been demonstrated in lower animals, but not conclusively in human beings. The late carcinogenic effects of radiation are manifested by lung tumors in uranium miners, skin cancer in radiologists, bone tumors in clock dial painters, leukemia in radiologists and atomic bomb survivors, and thyroid cancer in patients who have had radiation in childhood for an enlarged thymus, tonsils, or adenoids.

INDICATIONS FOR RADIATION THERAPY. A variety of localized neoplasms can be cured with radiation therapy.

Curative radiation therapy usually requires doses of 4,500 to 6,000 rads, delivered over 4 to 6 weeks. As most patients are unable to work during this time, the total time the patient is incapacitated is similar for both radiation therapy and surgery. The doses and complications for curative radiation therapy are significantly higher than those for palliative radiation therapy. To avoid unnecessary complications, it is vital that the stage of the tumor be carefully established in order to assure that the disease is still localized and therefore curable by radiation therapy. The best example of this is Hodgkin's disease, which is treated by aggressive and curative radiation therapy for Stages I, II, and possibly III without organ involvement other than the spleen. If other organs are involved, then systemic chemotherapy is indicated.

When the cure rate for a particular tumor appears equal by either radiation therapy or surgery, a variety of other factors must be considered by the surgical oncologist before making a decision on treatment. These include age, operative risk, cosmetic and functional deformity, and logistical problems such as distance and time. Squamous cell and basal cell carcinomas of the skin are good examples. Many of these tumors can be cured with a simple and quick diagnostic biopsy as an outpatient procedure. However, if these tumors are located in areas where surgery would lead to extensive cosmetic deformity, such as the nose or eyelid, then radiation therapy is usually the treatment of choice.

Some useful generalizations regarding choice between radiation therapy and surgery can be made. Usually surgery, rather than radiation therapy, should be used to treat radiation-induced (actinic) skin cancer in people with prolonged exposure to the sun. Radiation therapy may be the preferred treatment for recurrent carcinomas when the primary therapy was surgery, and vice versa. However, surgery is more likely to salvage a cure after a radiation failure, especially in the head and neck area.

Neoplasms in which radiation therapy is preferred to surgical therapy are lymphomas, Ewing's sarcoma, some malignant thymomas, locally unresectable carcinoma of the breast, oat cell carcinoma of the lung, locally advanced carcinoma of the prostate, and carcinomas of the skin

Table 9-11. LOCAL EFFECTS OF RADIATION

Organ	Acute changes	Chronic changes
Skin	Wet or dry epidermitis Radiodermatitis Epilation	Running Ulceration
Gastrointestinal tract	Edema, ulceration, infection, diarrhea, hepatitis	Stricture, ulceration, and perforation
Kidney		Nephritis, renal insufficiency
Bladder	Dysuria	Ulceration
Gonads	Sterility	Atrophy, menopause
Hemopoietic tissue	Lymphopenia	Pancytopenia
Bone	Cessation of epiphyseal growth	Necrosis
Lung	Pneumonitis	Pulmonary fibrosis
Heart	Acute pericarditis, myocarditis	Chronic pericarditis, myocarditis
Eye	Conjunctivitis	Cataracts
Nervous system	Cerebral edema	Radiation myelitis

Table 9-12. COMPARISON OF RADIATION THERAPY AND SURGERY IN TREATMENT OF MALIGNANT TUMORS

A. Cure rate higher with radiation therapy
   1. Lymphomas and Hodgkin's disease
   2. Ewing's sarcoma
   3. Certain malignant thymomas
   4. Carcinoma of the breast (locally unresectable)
   5. Certain basal and epidermoid carcinoma of the skin where surgery would lead to extensive cosmetic deformity
   6. Oat cell carcinoma of the lung
   7. Carcinoma of prostate (locally advanced)
   8. Nasopharynx
B. Cure rate higher with surgery
   1. Carcinoma
      a. Gastrointestinal tract [esophagus (distal one-third), stomach, pancreas, liver and biliary ducts, colon and rectum]
      b. Lung
      c. Breast (localized to breast and axilla)
      d. Urinary tract [kidney, renal pelvis, ureter, bladder, and prostate (early)]
      e. Genital tract (ovary, testis, penis, vulva, vagina, uterus, in situ cervix)
      f. Thyroid and parathyroid glands
      g. Salivary glands
      h. Adrenal gland
      i. Paranasal sinuses
      j. Carcinoma from any site with lymph node metastases (not bulky or mixed)
   2. Neuroblastoma
   3. Sarcomas (skeletal and soft tissue)
   4. Melanoma
   5. Cancer of the brain and spinal cord
C. Cure rate of radiation therapy and surgery approximately equal (choice depends on stage, size of tumor, and other factors—see text)
   1. Epidermoid carcinoma
      a. Skin
      b. Cervix
      c. Anus
      d. Lip
      e. Oral pharynx (tongue, floor of mouth, tonsil, gingiva)
      f. Hypopharynx
      g. Larynx
      h. Esophagus, upper two-thirds (low cure rate)

(basal or epidermoid) where surgery would lead to extensive cosmetic deformity. Table 9-12 compares the effectiveness of radiation therapy to surgery in the treatment of various types of neoplasms.

Palliative Radiation Therapy. Radiation therapy can relieve symptoms such as pain, hemorrhage, intractable cough, inability to swallow, intestinal obstruction from tumor, edema such as that produced by lung carcinomas with an associated superior vena cava syndrome, pathologic fractures, spinal cord compression, and varying degrees of paralysis secondary to brain metastases from a number of different tumors. In the presence of diffuse metastases, aggressive radiation therapy should not be given except for specific indications, because patients may be made more uncomfortable by the side effects of the radiation itself. An exception would be palliative radiation of metastases in weight-bearing bones such as the neck of the femur; this can prevent pathologic fractures and unnecessary hospitalization.

Even when a tumor is considered to be radioresistant, a trial of radiation therapy will sometimes result in unexpected palliation with regression or stabilization of the tumor. For instance, soft tissue sarcomas are not considered by many to be very radiosensitive or radiocurable. Yet, radiation therapy for palliation of soft tissue sarcomas often produces an objective response and relief of symptoms. However, radiation therapy should not be used for radioresistant tumors such as melanoma and osteogenic sarcoma unless it is clearly the best form of therapy or other methods of therapy are no longer available.

Combined Radiation Therapy and Surgery. Radiation therapy is a logical adjunct to surgery for treating many *locally advanced neoplasms.* Table 9-13 lists the tumors for which preoperative or postoperative radiation therapy has improved the cure rate or decreased the local recurrence rate.

Preoperative Radiation Therapy. Radiation therapy can sometimes convert an inoperable tumor into an operable one by decreasing both the size of the tumor and its fixation to surrounding tissues. In this manner, radiation therapy is a logical adjunct to surgery, because it is known that the cells at the periphery of a tumor are more radiosensitive because of their more rapid rate of growth and the availability of adequate oxygen. In contrast, tumor cells in the center of the tumor are often hypoxic and more slowly dividing, which makes them less sensitive to radiation therapy.

Preoperative radiation therapy may increase the cure rate or decrease the rate of local recurrence from tumor cells disseminated into the wound, lymphatics, or body cavities during surgery, either by killing the cells or by

Table 9-13. RADIATION THERAPY AS AN ADJUNCT TO SURGERY (LOCALLY ADVANCED CANCERS)

Preoperative radiation therapy
   Cure rate increased with these locally advanced carcinomas:
      Larynx
      Laryngopharynx
      Esophagus
      Bladder
      Uterus
      Retinoblastoma
      Paranasal sinuses
      Superior pulmonary sulcus
      Soft tissue sarcomas (liposarcomas)
      Bulky cervical node metastases from epidermoid carcinoma of the head and neck
   Local recurrence decreased with these locally advanced carcinomas:
      Rectum
      Endometrium
      Head and neck (epidermoid) with clinically positive lymph nodes
Postoperative radiation therapy
   Carcinoma of the lung for mediastinal node metastases
   Seminoma (periaortic and iliac node areas)
   Medulloblastoma (after biopsy)
   Wilms' tumor
   Bladder
   Ovary (dysgerminoma, granulosa cell, and cystadenocarcinoma)

destroying their ability to multiply. In experienced hands, preoperative radiation therapy usually can be given with little increased morbidity or mortality. Its usefulness needs to be further evaluated for a number of neoplasms, such as carcinomas of the breast, pancreas, and stomach. In cancer of the rectum, preoperative radiation therapy can convert an inoperable tumor into an operable tumor, decrease the local recurrence rate, and decrease the incidence of metastases seen in the regional nodes. As survival is usually determined by spread of cancer beyond the pelvis and regional nodes, it does not follow that decreasing the incidence of histologically positive nodes will increase survival. Nonetheless, a slight increase in survival has been reported in some studies. However, none of the prospective randomized studies have clearly demonstrated an increase in survival. Furthermore, one randomized study failed to substantiate a prior optimistic report from the same institution. Several prospective randomized trials of pre- and postoperative radiation therapy using higher doses are currently under way. One may hope that the results will clearly show whether adjunctive radiation therapy will increase the survival for patients with cancer of the rectum.

Preoperative radiation is not justified when a cancer is small and freely movable, and can be removed with a wide margin of normal tissue. With these tumors there is both a high cure rate and a very small chance of local recurrence.

Postoperative Radiation Therapy. Postoperative radiation therapy has some advantages over preoperative treatment. Once the histopathologic findings are available, those patients at high risk for local recurrence can be identified and treated. This approach saves those patients at low risk from the discomfort, expense, and potential long-term complications of radiation therapy. When the "tumor margin" of normal tissue surrounding the tumor is inadequate or when further surgery is either impossible or unacceptably deforming, postoperative radiation therapy is indicated. However, it should not be given in place of proper (adequate) surgery or when further "curative" surgery can be performed.

Postoperative radiation therapy is given routinely for Wilms' tumor, medulloblastoma, seminoma (to treat periaortic and iliac node-bearing areas), and in Stage II cancer of the ovary. For carcinoma of the bladder, both preoperative and postoperative radiation therapy appears to have some benefit in selected cases, though the data are not totally convincing.

Recent evidence suggests that postoperative radiation therapy may be useful in carcinoma of the lung for treating residual mediastinal node metastases. For breast cancer, radiation therapy can be effective in treating local recurrences and bone metastases. However, the routine use of postoperative radiation therapy, even in patients with positive nodes, has not been found to be of value in increasing the cure rate.

Chemotherapy

The treatment of cancer with drugs was initiated in 1941 by Huggins and Hodges, with the discovery that estrogens palliated prostatic cancer. Polyfunctional alkylating agents were developed in the later 1940s, as a result of experimental work performed during World War II. Since then there has been a tremendous increase in the number of chemotherapeutic drugs available; at present at least five major classes of drugs, plus an additional group of miscellaneous drugs, are available (Table 9-14). Although full elucidation of this complex field is beyond the scope of this chapter, certain general principles will be described regarding the use of chemotherapy. This section will consider the mechanisms of action of the major classes of chemotherapeutic drugs, the biologic and pharmacologic factors which are important in understanding drug therapy, and guidelines for the use of chemotherapy in patients with nonhematologic malignant conditions.

MECHANISMS OF ACTION. The majority of antineoplastic drugs appear to affect either enzymes, directly, or substrates of enzyme systems. In most cases the effects on enzymes or substrates relate to DNA synthesis or function, apparently by inhibiting cells which are undergoing DNA synthesis. Drugs which act by inhibiting the enzymes of nucleic acid synthesis are called *antimetabolites,* or *structural analogs.* Methotrexate, a structural analog of folinic acid, appears to act as a nearly irreversible inhibitor of the active site of the enzyme dihydrofolate reductase, which is necessary for DNA synthesis. Another commonly used antimetabolite is 5-fluorouracil, which appears to act as a reversible inhibitor of the enzyme thymidylate synthetase, which is necessary for the synthesis of thymidine, which is then used in DNA synthesis. This class of compounds acts directly on enzymes as either reversible or irreversible inhibitors, leading to the synthesis of abnormal DNA due to the incorporation of an abnormal building block or to disruption of DNA synthesis due to the lack of an essential building block.

Other major drugs appear to work primarily by affecting substrates. The usual substrate affected is the DNA macromolecule, although some of these agents will interfere with other substrates, such as proteins, and may have other diverse effects. Three major chemical classes of drugs appear to act by affecting specific substrates. The alkylating agents are extremely reactive compounds which can substitute an alkyl group (for example, $R—CH_2—CH_2^+$) for the hydrogen atoms of many organic compounds. The primary compounds affected appear to be the nucleic acids, especially DNA. Such alkylation produces breaks in the DNA molecule and cross linking of the twin strands of DNA, thus interfering with DNA replication and the transcription of RNA. Since these effects are somewhat similar to that seen with ionizing radiation, alkylating agents are sometimes called "radiomimetic." Another group of compounds which appear to work primarily on substrates are the *antibiotics.* These are natural products derived from certain soil fungi. They produce their antineoplastic effect by forming relatively stable complexes with DNA, thereby inhibiting the synthesis of DNA and RNA. The final class of drugs acting primarily on substrates is the *vinca alkaloids.* Although their total mechanism of action may not be completely defined, it is apparent that they can bind to microtubular proteins necessary for cell division. These proteins form the spindle apparatus which allows the chromosomes to separate to either end of the dividing cell; the vinca alkaloids appear to be able to dissolve this protein, leading to death of the cell during mitosis.

Other than these two known major mechanisms of drug action, the mechanisms of action for many drugs useful in the treatment of cancer are unknown. In some cases there may be combinations of activities, particularly for those steroid hormones which are active in treating cancer.

Table 9-14 lists representative examples of each group along with selected characteristics of their clinical importance.

BIOLOGIC AND PHARMACOLOGIC FACTORS IN CANCER THERAPY. A major theme in pharmacology has been the study of variations in drug absorption, distribution, metab-

olism, and excretion as related to a stable, invariant biologic receptor. In cancer chemotherapy, however, the biologic receptor, the cancer cell, is a variable and fluctuating target. Thus, the kinetics of tumor growth must be given as much attention as the kinetics of drug absorption or metabolism when considering cancer chemotherapy. Specifically, four general principles of tumor biology relevant to treatment appear to be extremely important. These include an understanding of (1) antineoplastic drug action as a function of the cell cycle, (2) tumor cell population growth, (3) the log–cell kill hypothesis, and (4) the critical role of drug scheduling in optimizing therapy.

Drug Action and the Cell Cycle. The life cycle of all cells, both normal and neoplastic, starts with mitosis, or cell division. This is followed by either differentiation or a

Table 9-14. DRUGS USED IN TREATMENT OF NONHEMATOLOGIC NEOPLASMS

Drugs	Route of administration	Cell cycle phase specificity*	Acute toxicity†	Principle delayed or cumulative toxicity†
Alkylating agents:		Nonspecific	N & V§	BM§; cyclophosphamide may cause alopecia, hemorrhagic cystitis.
Nitrogen mustard	I.V.		N & V	
Chlorambucil	P.O.§		None	
Phenylalanine mustard	P.O., I.V.‡, I.A.‡		None	
Cyclophosphamide	P.O., I.V.		N & V	
Thiotepa	I.V.		None	
Antimetabolites:				
Methotrexate	P.O., I.M., I.V.	Specific	None	BM, stomatitis, hepatitis.
5-Fluorouracil	I.V.	Nonspecific	N & V	BM, stomatitis, diarrhea, nausea, alopecia.
Hydroxyurea	P.O., I.V.‡	Specific	None	BM.
Cytosine arabinoside*	I.V.	Specific	N & V	BM.
Antibiotics:				
Actinomycin D	I.V.		N & V	BM, alopecia, stomatitis.
Mithramycin	I.V.		None	BM & hemorrhagic diathesis.
Adriamycin	I.V.		N & V, fever	BM, cardiac toxicity, stomatitis, alopecia.
Bleomycin	I.V., S.C., I.M.		Fever	Skin changes, pulmonary fibrosis.
Vinca alkaloids:				
Vincristine	I.V.	Specific	N & V, rare	Constipation, BM, peripheral neuropathy, alopecia.
Vinblastine				
Steroid hormones				
Adrenal corticoids	P.O., I.V., I.M.	(?) Nonspecific	None	Hypertension, peptic ulcer, diabetes, increased susceptibility to infection.
Androgens	P.O., I.M.	Unknown	None	Fluid retention, masculinization; may cause hypercalcemia in breast cancer.
Estrogens	P.O.	Unknown	N & V, occasional	Fluid retention, uterine bleeding; may cause hypercalcemia in breast cancer.
Progestins	P.O., I.M.	Unknown	None	May cause hypercalcemia in breast cancer.
Miscellaneous				
Nitrosoureas‡	I.V., P.O	Nonspecific	N & V	BM (may be delayed 4–6 weeks), liver dysfunction.
BCNU				
CCNU	I.V., I.A.‡			
Imidazole carboxamide		Nonspecific	N & V	BM, hepatotoxicity, fever.
Mitotane (*o, p*-DDD)	P.O.	Unknown	N & V	Skin eruptions, mental depression, muscle tremors.

*The distinction between a phase-specific and non-phase-specific drug may not be absolute. Some authorities distinguish additional categories or use different names for these categories, but these are not considered in this chapter since their clinical relevance remains to be defined.

†See manufacturer's package inserts for usual doses and for additional toxicity data.

‡Experimental drug or route of administration; not yet approved by the Federal Drug Administration or Division of Biological Standards; it may be available from the Cancer Chemotherapy National Service Center, Bethesda, Maryland.

§N & V = nausea and vomiting; BM = bone marrow depression; P.O. = orally (per os); I.A. = intraarterial.

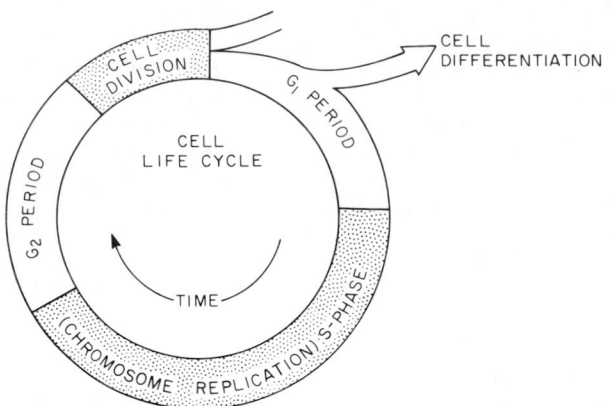

Fig. 9-22. Schematic diagram of the cell life cycle. G_1 is the first "gap" period, and G_2 is the second "gap" period. (*From R. Baserga (ed.), "The Cell Cycle and Cancer," Marcel Dekker, Inc., New York, 1971.*)

series of biochemically distinct phases known, in sequence, as G_1 (the first "gap" phase), S phase (DNA synthesis), G_2 (second "gap" phase), and mitosis (Fig. 9-22). Although these events are similar in neoplastic and normal cells, there appear to be some quantitative differences in the duration of the cycle and the sensitivity of cells to drugs during various phases of the cell cycle. Because of these differences, it has become apparent that one must differentiate between drugs which kill cells only during specific

phases of the cycle (*phase-specific*), and drugs which kill cells during all or most phases of the cell cycle (*phase-nonspecific*). The distinction between a phase-specific and phase-nonspecific drug may not be absolute. Some authorities distinguish additional categories or use different names for these categories. In particular, some workers separate the phase-nonspecific drugs into an additional two categories: *cycle-specific* and *non-cycle-specific*. For this discussion, drugs which can affect multiple phases of the cell cycle or which appear to be effective against nondividing cells are grouped together under the term *phase-nonspecific*, since the clinical usefulness of this group appears to be correlated with their lack of phase specificity.

Gompertz and Cell Population Growth. The human organism consists of communities of cells, many of which are capable of self-renewal through cell division. Generally these renewable populations grow rapidly when they are small in number and slowly when they are large. Thus, the fetus grows rapidly, but the adult organism remains constant in size, thanks to a balance between cell production and cell loss. This relation between size and growth rate may be expressed quantitatively in either of two ways: (1) as a function of volume doubling times (time for any given number of cells to double in number) or (2) as a function of the growth fraction (that fraction of cells undergoing division at any one time). Figure 9-23 presents a logarithmic plot of human fetal and childhood growth against time and includes specific data on the volume doubling times during growth. Growth in the early years

Fig. 9-23. Human fetal and childhood growth as a Gompertzian process, and the theoretic consequences of accumulation of leukemic cells at different rates over varying population ranges. (*From H. E. Skipper and S. Perry, Cancer Res, 30:1883, 1970.*)

is clearly exponential with a high growth fraction and very short volume doubling times. As time passes, the doubling time lengthens and the growth fraction decreases. The general slope of this curve can be expressed mathematically as an exponentially decreasing function. The specific equation describing this relationship was originally derived by the eighteenth-century mathematician Gompertz; therefore, biologic growth that conforms to this pattern is referred to as *Gompertzian growth*. Interestingly, evidence that not only normal cell growth but neoplastic cell growth follows a Gompertzian pattern is increasing. At least 18 different animal tumors conform to a Gompertzian growth curve, and Sullivan and Salmon have recent, preliminary evidence suggesting that human myeloma follows a Gompertzian growth pattern.

The Log–Cell Kill Hypothesis. Antineoplastic drugs are incapable of killing all cancer cells at any given exposure; rather, they will kill a variable fraction of cells from a very few up to a maximum of 99.99 percent. The fractional cell kill observed can usually be graphed as a line with a negative exponential slope, and so experimental chemotherapeutic data are usually expressed in logarithmic terms. Since the body burden of tumor cells in man with an advanced malignant tumor may be greater than 10^{12} cells, and since the best one can hope for with a single maximal exposure of tumor cells to a drug is 2 log cell kill, it is apparent that treatment must be repeated many times in order to achieve even partial control. Theoretically, this hypothesis also suggests that chemotherapeutic drugs may not be capable of totally eradicating any given population of tumor cells. There is good evidence that immunotherapy does not face this restriction, since it can completely eradicate small numbers of tumor cells; however, it may be totally ineffective against larger tumor cell masses (greater than 0.1 mg of tumor in most model systems).

DRUG SCHEDULING AND COMBINATION THERAPY. Studies with experimental animal tumors have conclusively demonstrated the critical importance of drug scheduling in therapy. Cytosine arabinoside, an antimetabolite which kills only cells in S phase, must be given frequently in order to assure contact with cancer cells during this critical period. When this drug is so employed, it is possible to "cure" some forms of murine leukemia, whereas maximally tolerated doses of the drug given at less frequent intervals fail to prolong survival. On the other hand, cyclophosphamide (Cytoxan), which is phase-nonspecific, achieves optimal suppression of most experimental neoplasms when given on an intermittent schedule.

A second factor related to drug scheduling is the growth status of any given tumor. In general, solid tumors with a large tumor mass will be growing slowly, and will have a small growth fraction (less than 10 percent) and a prolonged tumor volume doubling time. Since relatively few of these cells are dividing, these tumors are generally resistant to phase-specific drugs. Thus, the usual treatment for advanced nonhematologic tumors has been with phase-nonspecific drugs, such as the alkylating agents or 5-fluorouracil. However, successful treatment with such phase-nonspecific drugs may render the tumor more susceptible to phase-specific drugs, by converting the tumor

from one with a low growth fraction with few of the cells in S phase to one with a higher growth fraction with many cells in S phase. Good experimental data exist supporting this concept. Schabel has shown that a hamster plasmacytoma, which grows with Gompertzian kinetics, can be "cured" with cyclophosphamide therapy when followed by cytosine arabinoside therapy. When either drug is used alone or in the reverse sequence, "cures" were not seen. These results are consistent with tumor conversion, i.e., by changing an insensitive tumor with a low growth fraction and few cells in S phase to one with a higher growth fraction and many cells in S phase and therefore sensitive to the phase-specific drug cytosine arabinoside.

Theoretic Model for Combination Chemotherapy. The practical application of these concepts in man remains to be accomplished, but studies are in progress. One approach (Fig. 9-24) is proposed by Schabel. The vertical axis gives the number of viable tumor cells in a patient, on a log scale, versus arbitrary time units on the horizontal axis. At the initial tumor mass of 100 Gm, a likely growth fraction of less than 10 percent can be predicted. The class of drug to be used initially will be phase-nonspecific because of the low growth fraction. A 2 log cell kill with such drugs is possible in many types of tumors. During the recovery time only those viable tumor cells that are in the cell division cycle will repopulate the tumor. A phase-specific drug might be capable of suppressing this process by a selective effect on dividing cells, although doses and scheduling would have to be carefully chosen to minimize toxicity to the vital normal cells of the patient. Alternating courses of the phase-nonspecific and phase-specific agents, provided cellular resistance or excessive host toxicity does not intervene, would be expected to result in progressively more successful killing of tumor cells. This prediction (Fig. 9-24*E* and *G*) relates to the decreasing tumor cell mass and the associated increase in tumor cell growth fraction. Specifically, as the tumor cell mass becomes smaller, the percentage of cells in S phase or mitosis will be greater, leading to increased cell killing by drugs specific for such phases. Finally, "cure" may be possible with continued chemotherapy, or possibly by appropriate immunotherapy.

Schabel's model is attractive but difficult to evaluate in man. Nevertheless, it is clear that the optimal way to use chemotherapy against human cancer is by using combinations of drugs. Since cancer chemotherapy usually involves the use of toxic drugs, one must design programs of combination chemotherapy with care in order to minimize dangerous toxicity. In general, the successful programs of combination chemotherapy have been designed with the following criteria in mind: (1) only drugs active against the tumor in question are included; (2) drugs included have different mechanisms of action, in order to minimize the possibility of drug resistance; and (3) drugs chosen generally have different spectra of clinical toxicity, thus allowing the administration of full or nearly full doses of each of the active agents. A final factor relates to the preference of most investigators for utilizing intermittent courses of intensive combination chemotherapy rather than continuous programs of drug administration. This approach tends to

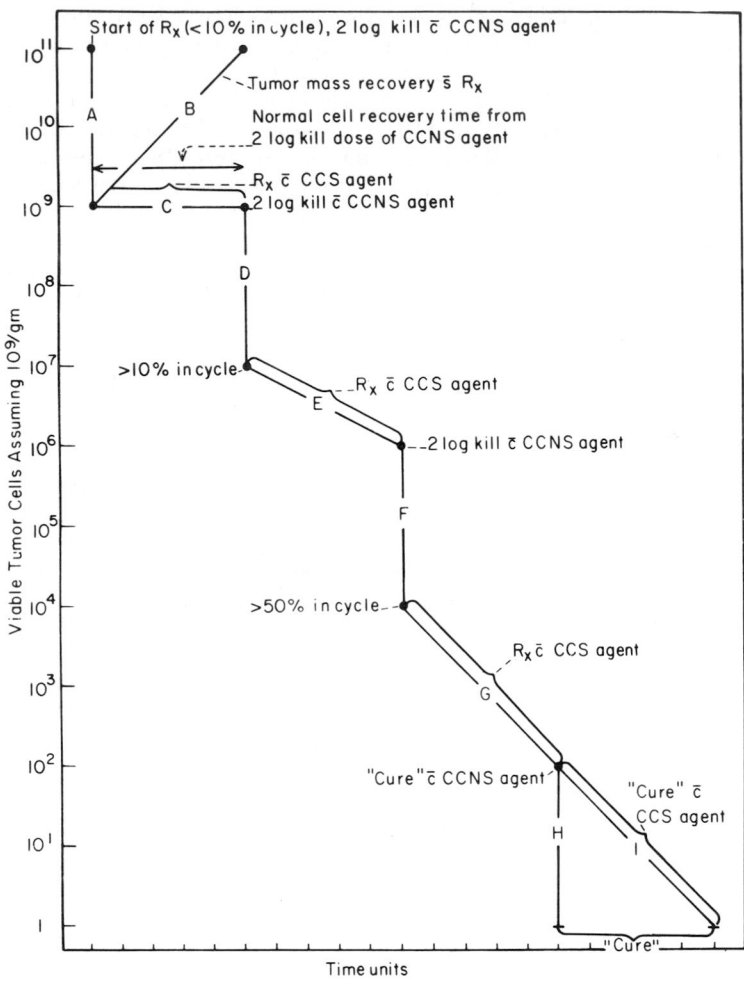

Fig. 9-24. Idealized approach to "curative" therapy of advanced tumors using a phase-nonspecific (CCNS) agent (for example, an alkylating agent) followed by a phase-specific (CCS) agent (for example, certain antimetabolites) in repeated courses. (*From F. M. Schabel, Jr., Cancer Res, 29:2384, 1969.*)

maximize tumor cell killing, is usually better tolerated by patients, and appears to cause less immunosuppression.

CHEMOTHERAPY AS AN ADJUVANT TO CANCER SURGERY. The proved ineffectiveness of surgical resection alone for many types of neoplasms has led many investigators to the use of cancer chemotherapeutic agents as adjunctive treatment. It was postulated that these agents might control microscopic foci of cancer already disseminated in the body. Controlled clinical trials have been carried out to determine the effectiveness of single chemotherapeutic agents when combined with surgical resection for carcinomas of the breast, lung, stomach, and colon. Very few significant benefits have been demonstrated thus far using single agents. However, the chemotherapeutic agents chosen for these studies, their dosage, and the duration of administration may not have been optimal for the desired result. It is likely that future applications of this concept using newer chemotherapeutic agents in combination for prolonged periods of time may well result in improved survival for these patients. This approach may be further enhanced by advances in immunotherapy and radiation therapy. An example of one approach to adjuvant chemotherapy as applied to breast cancer appears later in this chapter.

CLINICAL PHARMACOLOGY. In addition to the principles relating to tumor biology described above, numerous pharmacologic principles must be considered in cancer chemotherapy. The first such consideration relates to the route of administration of a drug or a combination of drugs. A variety of routes can be chosen, such as oral, intravenous, intramuscular, intraarterial, or local application. By using a carefully selected parenteral route of administration, difficulties related to absorption of drugs are avoided. It also may be possible to improve the antitumor effect of a given drug. Particularly promising in this regard has been the use of intraarterial administrative drugs, such as when the primary tumor is in the liver or on an extremity. Using a portable infusion pump, drugs can be continuously infused over weeks or months. An extension of this approach has been with isolation-perfusion of an extremity with high doses of chemotherapy. As newer drugs are developed, particularly drugs with very short half-life periods, it is likely that the choice of the route of administration will become increasingly important.

A second consideration relates to transport mechanisms for the drug in question. If the drug is transported on serum proteins, it is possible that other drugs may alter significantly the proportion of the bound and free anticancer drug. An example of this is the ability of salicylates to displace methotrexate from its binding site on albumin. In this setting, high doses of salicylates may result in augmented host toxicity from methotrexate.

Another consideration is the possible effect of drug interactions when drugs are given in combinations. One well-established drug interaction involves allopurinol, a xanthine oxidase inhibitor, when it is used with 6-mercaptopurine (6-MP). Since degradation of 6-MP is catalyzed by xanthine oxidase, the use of allopurinol along with full doses of 6-MP has been shown in the past to be dangerous. Normal function of organs important in drug metabolism or degradation may be critical to the biologic fate of a drug. For example, serious liver disease may increase the toxicity of drugs which are cleared by that route, such as vincristine or adriamycin. Severe neurotoxicity has been observed in patients with concomitant liver disease when given otherwise clinically well-tolerated doses of vincristine.

The route of excretion of a drug may be critical. Methotrexate is primarily excreted by the kidney, and even modest elevation of the BUN (blood urea nitrogen) may be associated with major hematologic toxicity from the use of relatively low doses of methotrexate. For this reason the status of the kidneys must be observed very closely in all patients receiving methotrexate therapy. In fact, it is wise to observe renal function in all patients receiving cancer chemotherapeutic drugs, since nearly all of them have some extent of excretion by the renal route. In addition, it is not unusual for a brisk response to chemotherapy to result in elaboration of large amounts of uric acid, from the breakdown of the nucleic acids of the destroyed cancer cells. Uric acid nephropathy may result. Pretreatment with allopurinol may prevent this complication.

A final factor relates to the ability of a given drug to enter the cancer cell: many drugs require direct access to a specific biochemical pathway within the cell, and failure to gain entry will be associated with drug resistance. To some extent this effect may be overcome by giving very large doses of the drug; however, this is usually associated with unacceptable drug toxicity. An exception to this limitation may be the experimental use of large doses of methotrexate and its antidote, citrovorum factor. Cancer cells appear to lack this transport system. When normal and cancer cells are exposed to massive doses of methotrexate, a high intracellular drug concentration results. When the antidote is subsequently given in lower doses, the normal cells are "rescued" by virtue of the cell membrane trans-port system. Further work with this treatment and with others that rely on the transport of drugs across cell membranes may result in further improvements in drug therapy.

Ultimately, all factors which might alter either the concentration of the critical drug at its primary site of action or the duration of time available for such activity should be considered in the use of drugs. This may be expressed as a function of concentration times time, and because of its importance it is commonly referred to as the $C \times T$ function.

GUIDELINES FOR THE USE OF CHEMOTHERAPY IN PATIENTS WITH NONHEMATOLOGIC MALIGNANT TUMORS. The initial major question a physician must ask himself when considering chemotherapy for any patient with a neoplasm is whether benefit will result with tolerable toxicity. The physician must have all the facts regarding the patient, including the type, extent, and grade of the malignant tumor, its expected natural history, the results of current therapy, and the psychologic makeup of the patient. In addition, he must consider the following three principles:

1. The patient should have a histologic diagnosis of a malignant disease that is known to respond in a reasonable percentage of cases in a manner beneficial to the patient. Table 9-15 outlines the current status of cancer chemotherapy for a variety of nonhematologic neoplasms. Brief comments on specific drug-sensitive neoplasms will be presented subsequently. In general, patients in whom disease usually or often responds to chemotherapy should receive drug treatment, unless there is a specific contraindication. In addition, patients suspected of having minimal residual disease (micrometastases) after local therapy also may be candidates for adjuvant chemotherapy. Such therapy would be questionable for those patients with a tumor known to be minimally inhibited by commercially available drugs. Experimental therapy may be warranted for these patients.

2. It is absolutely essential that there be adequate facilities to monitor the potential toxicity outlined in Table 9-14, and a physician should not initiate therapy unless he is adequately trained in the use of drugs and committed to monitoring the patient for drug therapy. Chemotherapy is generally contraindicated for patients with nonhematologic malignant conditions if they have major bleeding or infection, although patients with leukemia and, in some cases, lymphomas may require treatment even during such episodes in order to control life-threatening bleeding or infection. Patients with major dysfunction of an organ system particularly susceptible to the toxicity of a cancer chemotherapeutic drug must be followed carefully and may be more suitably treated with an alternative drug. An example of this latter situation would be a patient with a severe neuromyopathy, who might be better treated with drugs other than vinca alkaloids, as these may exacerbate the condition. Patients in whom a rapid response to therapy is possible or who have preexisting renal disease should be treated with allopurinol to prevent the complication of uric acid nephropathy. Finally, patients who are under active chemotherapy and develop severe toxicity may require aggressive support with platelets, red blood cells, antibiotics, or in some cases, white blood cells for control of infection.

3. Cancer chemotherapeutic drugs are toxic. In order to minimize unwarranted toxicity, the physician should conduct a diligent search for disease markers to assist in monitoring treatment. Ideally, several parameters of tumor response should be followed in order to objectively assess the response to therapy. Some factors which can be considered in assessing response to treatment are described in more detail in Table 9-16. As a general rule, tumor size is of particular importance. Most oncologists require a 50 percent reduction in the product of the greater and lesser diameters of any given tumor to accept the change as a "partial response."

The specific choice of a drug or drugs for a given patient with

Table 9-15. CURRENT STATUS OF CANCER CHEMOTHERAPY FOR NONHEMATOLOGIC NEOPLASMS

Disease	Agent	Benefit
Highly Responsive Neoplasms:		
Trophoblastic tumors	Methotrexate, actinomycin-D, alkylating agents, vinca alkaloids	>80% response with permanent regression
Carcinoma of prostate	Estrogens	80% response; prolonged survival
Wilms' tumor, neuroblastoma	Actinomycin-D, vincristine	80% 2-year survival with combined surgery, radiation, and chemotherapy
Ewing's sarcoma	Cyclophosphamide, vincristine, actinomycin-D, adriamycin	>50% response; prolonged survival when combined with radiation therapy
Testicular carcinoma, germinal cell tumors	Actinomycin-D, vinca alkaloids, methotrexate, alkylating agents, mithramycin, Bleomycin, cis-platinum (experimental)	Clinical improvement in approximately 80%
Carcinoma of breast	Estrogens, androgens, 5-fluorouracil, alkylating agents, combination chemotherapy	25–75% response; prolonged survival for responders
Moderately Responsive Neoplasms:		
Sarcomas of bone and soft tissue (adult)	Actinomycin-D, vinca alkaloids, alkylating agents, adriamycin	15–50% objective response
Carcinoma of ovary	Alkylating agents	Clinical improvement in 30–50%
Adrenal carcinoma	o,p'-DDD	Occasional clinical improvement, sometimes prolonged
Carcinoma of bowel and stomach	5-Fluorouracil	Clinical improvement in 15–25%
Carcinoma of endometrium	Progestins	Clinical improvement in 25%
Minimally Responsive Neoplasms:		
Head and neck tumors	Bleomycin, methotrexate, adriamycin	10–30% objective response, usually of short duration
Hepatic and pancreatic tumors	5-Fluorouracil	10% objective response
Carcinoma of cervix	Alkylating agents	5% objective response
Lung cancer	Alkylating agents, adriamycin, nitrosoureas, 5-fluorouracil	25% objective response, usually of short duration
Melanoma	Imidazole carboxamide	20% objective response, but duration of response usually short

SOURCE: Modified and updated from M. J. Cline and C. M. Haskell, "Cancer Chemotherapy," 2d ed., pp. 10–11, W. B. Saunders Company, Philadelphia, 1975.

cancer and the precise choice of a dose and schedule for such single agent or combination therapy are best decided in the light of current therapeutic research. To some extent such choices can be determined by referring to Table 9-16 and the following section. Other useful sources of information include the *Medical Letter on Drugs and Therapeutics,* which periodically publishes information on the choice of therapy in the treatment of cancer (Dec. 17, 1976); monographs on cancer chemotherapy (such as that by Cline and Haskell); and the specialty journals of cancer (*Cancer; Cancer Treatment Reports; Seminars in Oncology*).

ILLUSTRATIVE NEOPLASMS HIGHLY RESPONSIVE TO CHEMOTHERAPY. Trophoblastic Tumors of the Uterus. Metastatic gestational choriocarcinoma is curable in 80 to 90 percent of women using chemotherapeutic drugs alone. The discovery by Li et al. in 1956 that methotrexate could control metastatic disease in women with choriocarcinoma represents a landmark in the history of cancer chemotherapy. Subsequent systematic study of this disease has markedly increased our understanding about cancer and its treatment. Certain points are worthy of special mention.

1. Methotrexate must be started as soon as possible after the diagnosis has been made. This relates to the finding that the

best prognosis, with cure rates of 95 to 100 percent, is seen in patients whose disease is treated within 4 months of onset, in whom metastases do not include the brain or liver, and in whom 24-hour urine quantities of human chorionic gonadotropins (HCG) are less than 100,000 I.U.

2. Combination chemotherapy should be used if the initial response to chemotherapy is suboptimal or if the patient presents with high titers of HCG, with liver or brain involvement, or with symptoms present longer than 4 months. Second-line drugs for this disease include actinomycin D, vincristine, alkylating agents, and adriamycin.

3. Therapy should be continued for 6 months after the chorionic gonadotropin titer has returned to normal. This is even more important than eliminating radiographic evidence of disease, since residual pulmonary lesions may be present despite cure of clinical growths. This is analogous to the residual changes of many nonneoplastic diseases, such as tuberculosis.

Carcinoma of the Prostate. The mainstays of therapy for disseminated cancer of the prostate are orchiectomy and estrogen therapy. These modalities have increased survival of these patients two- to threefold. Many different doses of the most commonly used estrogenic hormone have been employed. However, data from the Veterans Administration Cooperative Research Group have shown up to a

Table 9-16. CRITERIA FOR RESPONSES IN
PATIENTS WITH SOLID TUMORS

Tumor size	Palpation and measurement with calipers. Radiologic measurement. Radioisotope scans. Ultrasound.
Tumor products	Quantitative level of chorionic gonadotropin (choriocarcinoma and certain testicular tumors). Quantitative level of carcinoembryonic antigen (CEA) in bowel cancer. Quantitative level of α-fetoprotein in hepatoma. Serum or urine paraproteins in myeloma. Urinary adrenal hormone (adrenal carcinoma treated with *o,p'*-DDD).
Improvement in symptoms or sign of tumor	Improvement in hypercalcemia (particularly with carcinoma involving bone). Improvement in obstruction due to tumor (such as bowel obstruction or obstructed ureter). Disappearance of effusions from tumors involving pleura, peritoneum, or obstructing lymphatics. Subjective symptoms are important to patient but are generally poor indicators of antitumor response.

25 percent increased mortality from cardiovascular diseases in a group of patients treated with moderately high doses (5 mg daily) of diethylstilbestrol. A prospective study has since proved that a low dose of 1 mg daily results in good antitumor effects without significant cardiovascular toxicity.

Wilms' Tumor. Improvements in survival for patients with Wilms' tumor have developed steadily in recent years. Whereas this was once considered a hopeless tumor to treat, it is now possible to control the disease for substantial periods of time in 80 percent of children with the disease. This improvement involves the sequential use of optimal surgery, radiation therapy, and chemotherapy with actinomycin D and/or vincristine. A national study group is currently trying to resolve the optimal combination of these modalities; however, it is clear that the addition of effective chemotherapy has substantially improved the care of these patients.

Carcinoma of the Breast. Recent developments as a result of combination chemotherapy, estradiol receptor protein, competitive inhibitors of estrogen, medical adrenalectomy, and adjuvant chemotherapy have made breast cancer one of the most interesting tumors to treat.

Most physicians are currently treating advanced breast cancer with multiple combinations of drugs. One such combination includes 5-fluorouracil, cyclophosphamide, vincristine, methotrexate, and sometimes prednisone (CMFVP). Another combination includes adriamycin and cyclophosphamide (AC) or 5-fluorouracil, adriamycin, and cyclophosphamide (FAC). Response rates for these combinations have been generally 50 percent or greater, compared to 20 to 35 percent for the same drugs used as single agents. The median duration of response with combination chemotherapy has been in the range of 9 months.

Changing concepts of the biology of breast cancer have stimulated a number of clinical trials of adjuvant chemotherapy using single or multiple agents given intermittently over prolonged periods after operation. Many such studies are currently in progress, and most have demonstrated a reduced early recurrence rate for patients treated with adjuvant chemotherapy. One study has also shown an improved 3-year survival rate for patients treated after operation with cyclophosphamide, methotrexate, and 5-fluorouracil (CMF). If these exciting preliminary results are confirmed, they will mark the first real impact on the natural history of breast cancer since the Halsted radical mastectomy.

A number of interesting therapeutic options in breast cancer are being evaluated by studies currently in progress. These include investigations to determine (1) the optimal combination and sequence of drugs and/or hormonal agents; (2) the efficacy of adjuvant chemoimmunotherapy, chemohormonal therapy, or hormonal manipulation used alone in women with estradiol receptor–positive tumors; (3) whether surgical adrenalectomy and medical adrenalectomy using aminogluethimide are comparable; and (4) the usefulness of the estrogen antagonist or competitive inhibitors.

COMBINED MODALITY THERAPY. Pediatric oncologists pioneered the use of combined modality therapy—radiation in combination with chemotherapy and surgical therapy—to overcome childhood neoplasms. The cure rate for localized retinoblastoma and other sarcomas in children has been increased with radiation therapy and chemotherapy with cyclophosphamide. Wilms' tumor can be cured 75 percent of the time if surgical therapy is followed by radiation and chemotherapy with actinomycin, an increase of 40 percent over operation alone. Embryonal rhabdomyosarcoma responds best to combinations of radiation, chemotherapy, and operation.

Until recently, the effectiveness of multimodality therapy had been demonstrated only occasionally for adult neoplasms. A recent example illustrates the complexity of such combined therapy for skeletal and soft tissue sarcomas.

Surgical therapy, the accepted method for management of most skeletal and soft tissue sarcomas of the extremity, has been associated with frequent treatment failure. Even with amputation, approximately 50 percent of patients with soft tissue sarcomas and 80 percent of those with sarcomas of bone eventually developed and died from their distant metastases. In an attempt to improve results of treatment for the sarcomas, a regimen of combined pre- and postoperative therapy was developed. Preoperative continuous intraarterial infusion of adriamycin, radiation therapy followed by surgical resection, and postoperative adriamycin were found to result in improved short-term recurrence-free survival and preservation of a functional extremity in most patients. This regimen dramatically reduced the incidence of pulmonary metastases from both the osteosarcomas and the soft tissue sarcomas.

The preoperative therapy with intraarterial adriamycin followed by radiation was found to produce extensive tumor cell necrosis as high as 88 percent (Table 9-17 and

Table 9-17. SKELETAL AND SOFT TISSUE SARCOMAS:
HISTOLOGIC EFFECTS OF TREATMENT

Treatment	No. of cases	Percent necrosis*	
		Pre-treatment	Post-treatment
Surgical resection	67	. . .	9*
I-A Adriamycin	6	5	63
I-A Adriamycin & x-radiation	11	12	88†

*Average of the percent necrosis of specimens examined.
†Four of the eleven had no identifiable tumor.

Fig. 9-25*a, b, c*). The effectiveness of this preoperative therapy permitted local resection of the sarcoma and salvage. Diseased bone, in this instance, was replaced by cadaver allografts obtained from the National Naval Medical Center. The donor grafts were matched to the diseased bone for intercondylar width and for intramedullary diameter to facilitate fixation (Fig. 9-26). After operation, patients with femur replacement were placed in non-weight-bearing long leg casts for up to 8 weeks and then wore weight-bearing long leg braces. Subsequently, some of the patients used only a routine hinged knee brace (Fig. 9-27). Patients with homograft replacements in the upper extremity were placed in full arm casts and then in a supporting splint. Function of the extremity in both sets of patients has been excellent, even though knee motion is limited in those with leg homografts.

Although it is too early to tell whether these results represent merely a delay in recurrence of disease or possible cure, certainly for those patients who would have had to sacrifice an arm or an entire leg, the functional results are far superior to any achieved by prosthetic replacement.

Immunotherapy

One of the basic problems associated with all forms of cancer therapy is caused by the similarities in the biochemical and subcellular constituents of the cancer and normal cells. Although some cancer cells may have a rapid rate of cell division when compared to normal cells of the same organ, there are other normal cells in the body (e.g., those in the bone marrow and intestinal epithelium) that may grow even more rapidly. Hence, any therapy designed to inhibit the proliferation rate of cancer cells may also inhibit the function of these normal cells. Herein lies the fundamental deficiency of both radiation and chemotherapy. Similarly, cancer surgery often requires the sacrifice of normal tissues and organs to ensure an adequate margin around the cancer cells. In contrast, immunotherapy depends upon basic antigenic differences between neoplastic and normal cells for its therapeutic effect. Because the immune attack is directed only at those cells possessing tumor antigens, while sparing normal cells from damage, this treatment method can achieve a specific tumor cell kill greater than any other known therapeutic modality. At the present time, however, immunotherapy has limited potency.

Immunity against cancer is relative rather than absolute. Host defenses are quite capable of destroying small numbers of tumor cells, 1 to 10 million, but 100 million tumor cells almost always result in progressive tumor growth. Since a neoplasm only 1 cm in diameter contains approximately 1 billion tumor cells, by the time most tumors are clinically detectable, they have already outgrown the patient's immune defenses. Therefore, it is unlikely that immunotherapy alone will ever bolster host offenses sufficiently to reverse tumor growth in patients with advanced disease.

In contrast, immunotherapy is a logical adjunct for the treatment of subclinical microscopic disease following definitive cancer surgery, radiation therapy, or chemotherapy, for the following reasons: (1) Patients who have only small foci of cancer cells remaining after destruction of the major tumor bulk are the most likely to benefit from immunotherapy, because the tumor mass that must be destroyed is smallest at that time. (2) The specificity of the immune response provides a possible therapeutic tool that has selectivity for small numbers of cancer cells not possible with any other therapeutic modality. (3) Patients with disease in earlier stages are more likely to respond to immunotherapeutic maneuvers, since the cancer patient's general immune competence is greatest when the disease is localized and is often impaired after metastasis. (4) Immunotherapy should complement rather than interfere with currently available methods of cancer therapy. However, since both irradiation and chemotherapy are immunosuppressive, the use of immunotherapy in combination with these therapeutic modalities must be carefully controlled. Because these treatment modalities can stimulate immune response when immunization is carried out under special conditions, the results of cancer therapy may improve when the influence of radiation therapy and chemotherapy upon the immune response is better understood.

Numerous attempts at immunotherapy of cancer have been undertaken since the turn of the century. Although an occasional striking regression was obtained, in most cases the results were neither impressive nor consistent, and interest in this treatment modality declined until re-

Fig. 9-25. *A.* Photomicrograph of pretreatment biopsy showing osteosarcoma with minimal necrosis. (×250.) *B.* Resected surgical specimen following preoperative treatment with intraarterial adriamycin and radiation therapy. Note gross tumor liquefaction and necrosis. *C.* Photomicrograph of posttreatment specimen showing 99 percent tumor necrosis with loss of nuclei. (×40.) (*From D. L. Morton et al., Ann Surg, 184:268, 1976.*)

cently. A rational basis for cancer immunotherapy was provided only during the past 10 years as compelling evidence accumulated indicating the participation of immune components in human cancer. It was found that cancer patients develop two types of immune response to the antigens of their neoplasms, *humoral antibodies* and *cell-mediated immune reactions.*

The relative importance of these two types of immune

responses and their influence upon the host's defense against cancer is somewhat controversial at the present time. Most approaches to immunotherapy do, in fact, stimulate both types of immune response. Three possible approaches to immunotherapy in man will be discussed—active; passive, or adoptive; and nonspecific.

ACTIVE IMMUNOTHERAPY

The greater effectiveness of active immunization over passive immunization in infectious diseases provided a

Fig. 9-26. Postoperative radiograph showing cadaver bone graft held in place by a Sampson rod and Stone staples used to reattach collateral ligaments. (*From D. L. Morton et al., Ann Surg, 184:268, 1976.*)

Fig. 9-27. Results 9 months after operation. Patient walks without crutches and can flex knee joint 20°. Brace is worn to assure stability of knee joint. (*From D. L. Morton et al., Ann Surg, 184:268, 1976.*)

treatment. Although such techniques have prevented progressive tumor growth, they may have inactivated the tumor-specific antigens as well. For example, the same freezing and thawing technique frequently used to prepare human tumor vaccines has often inactivated tumor-specific antigens of carcinogen-induced animal neoplasms.

Studies with animal neoplasms demonstrate that living tumor cells administered intradermally in numbers insufficient for progressive tumor growth generally are the most effective immunogens. The possibility that living tumor cells might result in tumor growth at the inoculation site has inhibited the use of such vaccines in man. However, it would seem that with certain tumors that share common tumor-specific antigens, such as skeletal and soft tissue sarcomas, one patient could be immunized with an allogenic vaccine of living tumor cells from another patient. An immune response could be induced against the foreign HLA transplantation antigens on the tumor cells, causing their rejection. Theoretically this immunization should induce a strong immune response against a common cross-reacting tumor-specific antigen as well.

Repeated attempts have been made to increase the antigenicity of tumor vaccines by modifying the tumor cells in a variety of ways. These have included coupling highly antigenic carrier proteins such as rabbit γ-globulin to the tumor cells, and chemical treatment by agents such as iodoacetate and, more recently, with neuraminidase and concanavalin A. Regression of established tumors has been observed in animals following active immunotherapy with such vaccines.

Many of these experiments have used immunological adjuvants as well, such as bacillus Calmette-Guérin (BCG) vaccine, *Corynebacterium parvum,* and Freund's adjuvant, in an attempt to enhance the host's immune response to the native or modified tumor antigens.

The ideal tumor vaccine in many respects, however, would be one composed of the isolated and purified tumor-specific transplantation antigens from the cell surface. Such vaccines would have the advantages of safety, stability, and ease of administration. Previous experience gained with guinea pig sarcomas from which isolated and partially purified tumor-specific antigen preparations induced good immunity to tumor challenge suggests that success can be anticipated for this approach. However, to date, there has been little progress along these lines with the human tumor-specific transplantation antigen.

In summary, active immunotherapy using vaccines prepared in a variety of ways combined with many different types of immunoadjuvants has been used in clinical trials. It can be demonstrated clearly that such autoimmunization procedures do enhance the patient's immune response to his own tumor (Fig. 9-29). Results to date, however, have not been impressive in patients with advanced disease where active immunization is used alone. Active immunotherapy has great potential when used in combination with other types of cancer therapy, such as surgery, chemotherapy, or radiation therapy. Preliminary experiences by Mathe with leukemia and Morton with melanomas and sarcomas would suggest that this potential will become increasingly evident in the future.

strong stimulus for studies of active immunotherapy against cancer. The rationale for this approach is based upon animal studies demonstrating that a growing tumor does not induce a maximum immune response in the host (Fig. 9-28). In this method of treatment, efforts are made to increase the patient's tumor immunity by altering the tumor-specific antigen in such a way that it becomes more antigenic, or by stimulating the patient's lymphoreticular system with immunologic adjuvants.

Most attempts at immunotherapy in man have involved vaccines composed of whole tumor cells inactivated by a variety of different methods to render the cells incapable of proliferation. These methods have included radiation, mitomycin C treatment, freezing and thawing, or heat

PASSIVE AND ADOPTIVE IMMUNOTHERAPY

Since patients with cancer develop two types of immune responses to their neoplasms—humoral antibodies and cell-mediated immune responses—passive immunotherapy is logically based upon the administration of either anti-tumor sera or lymphoid cells.

PASSIVE IMMUNOTHERAPY WITH ANTITUMOR SERA. In the past, antitumor sera produced in a foreign species proved to be very toxic to the recipient, because it contained antibodies against normal tissue antigens of the host. However, this problem may be resolved soon when successful isolation and purification of the tumor-specific transplantation antigens are achieved so that the antisera can be directed specifically against the tumor-specific transplantation antigens of the tumor cells. Another source of potential antisera may be from those patients cured of their malignant condition who demonstrate high titers of cytotoxic or deblocking antibodies.

An important concept of antisera therapy concerns the discovery of certain blocking factors that appear to inhibit the effectiveness of the lymphocytes. Thought to be circulating antigen or antibody-antigen complexes, these blocking factors may contribute to tumor growth by interfering with cellular immunity. In experiments using mouse and guinea pig sarcomas, as well as leukemias, tumor regression can be induced with antisera containing high titers of antitumor antibody. The mechanism for antitumor effectiveness is unclear. It could be due to a direct cytotoxic effect on tumor cells acting as cytophilic antibody that induces macrophages or lymphocytes to kill tumor cells or by neutralizing blocking factors. Nevertheless, these observations clearly indicate that antitumor sera can induce regression of established neoplasms and as such should receive serious consideration for immunotherapy of cancer.

Fig. 9-28. Immunotherapy experiments with a transplantable liposarcoma in syngeneic strain 2 guinea pigs: 1×10^5 liposarcoma tumor cells were inoculated intramuscularly into the leg, and immunotherapy was initiated intradermally in four sites on the back with 1×10^6 living or 1×10^7 irradiated tumor cells mixed with bacillus Calmette-Guérin (BCG). (*From D. L. Morton et al., Ann Surg, 172:740, 1970.*)

IMMUNOTHERAPY WITH LYMPHOID CELLS. Adoptive immunotherapy with lymphoid cells from an immunized donor was accomplished with ease between inbred laboratory animals of the same strain and suggested that antitumor immunity was primarily cell-mediated. However, these animal experiments indicated that the transferred lymphocytes must persist in the host to have a significant immunotherapeutic effect. As studies were done in human cancer, the primary difficulty was with rejection of the transferred lymphocytes due to HLA dif-

Fig. 9-29. Antisarcoma antibody titers determined by complement fixation against the HuSA-I liposarcoma antigen on serial serum samples from a sixteen year old boy with a primary osteosarcoma of the right femur in whom pulmonary metastases developed 10 months after resection of the primary, for which a left pneumonectomy was performed and immunotherapy initiated. (*From D. L. Morton et al., Ann Surg, 172:740, 1970.*)

ferences between host and donor. This problem was overcome when the lymphoid cells were obtained from family members who were identical by HLA matching or by bulk growth of the patient's own lymphocytes in tissue culture. The lymphocytes of the family members may be already sensitized to the tumor-specific antigens in certain neoplasms, such as human sarcomas, where our investigations have shown a high incidence of antibodies in close family members.

As with antisera, another source of lymphocytes may be those cancer patients who have been cured of their malignant disease. Sumner and Foraker reported one of the earliest successes by this means when they transfused a melanoma patient with whole blood from a second melanoma patient who had undergone complete remission. However, multiple attempts to repeat this transfer have been unsuccessful.

Moore and Gerner attempted to increase the lymphocyte ratio to tumor cells by growing a patient's lymphocytes in tissue culture and reinfusing them back to the patient. They reported significant regressions in two of three patients. However, the logistic problems of growing such large numbers of lymphocytes are considerable.

IMMUNOTHERAPY FOLLOWING IN VITRO ACTIVATION OF LYMPHOCYTES. Further studies of adoptive immunotherapy have concerned in vitro, nonspecific stimulation of lymphocytes with agents such as phytohemagglutinin. Some success has been reported when these treated autologous lymphocytes were reinfused into the patient or injected directly into tumor deposits. Another approach has involved specific sensitization of lymphocytes with tumor cells in vitro by incubation with mitomycin C-treated tissue culture tumor cells. The mitomycin C prevented replication of the tumor cells by eliminating their potential to form metastases. Though the results were not impressive in these human investigations, recent animal experiments suggest this means as a very effective way to induce an effective antitumor immunity. The ability to obtain large numbers of lymphocytes from any donor by continuous lymphophoresis using the NCI-IBM blood cell separator has considerably increased the feasibility of this approach.

IMMUNOTHERAPY WITH LYMPHOCYTES SENSITIZED BY TRANSPLANTATION OF TUMORS. Several investigators have attempted passive immunotherapy with cross immunization with tumor tissue followed by cross transfusions of lymphocytes or lymphocytes and serum. These studies have been undertaken in the following manner: Patients with incurable cancer were paired according to blood type and tumor types. Tumors from patients in group A were transplanted subcutaneously to patients in group B, and vice versa. Following sensitization to each other's tumors, the transfusions of lymphocytes from patients in group B to patients in group A, or vice versa, were begun and continued daily for variable periods of time. The response rate reported following this type of immunotherapy is from 15 to 20 percent. However, the criteria for therapeutic response have varied between investigators and in many cases have not met rigid specifications acceptable to many oncologists.

IMMUNOTHERAPY WITH EXTRACTS OF SENSITIZED LYMPHOID CELLS. One particularly appealing method of adoptive immunotherapy is the injection of informational molecules. These extracts of sensitized lymphoid cells are able to induce a specific immune response when injected into the host. Preliminary clinical investigations have been performed with two such substances, transfer factor and immune RNA.

Transfer factor, originally described by Lawrence, is of low molecular weight (4000 to 8000). Injections of this substance have induced immune reactions against fungal and bacterial antigens. Ongoing preliminary trials are using transfer factor in the immunotherapy of malignant tumors. There appears to be no toxicity, but therapeutic results are not definitive at this time.

Immune RNA, an RNA-rich extract of immune lymphoid cells, is the other means of transferring immunity by informational molecules. Immune RNA extracted from the lymphoid tissues of xenogeneic donors immunized with tumor tissue can induce immunity against that tumor in syngeneic recipients of the tumor transplants. The substance can stimulate normal human lymphocytes to react against human tumor cells in vitro. Ramming and deKernion recently reported a nonrandomized clinical trial of immune RNA in patients with metastatic renal cell carcinoma. There is a suggestion that such treatment may have clinical benefit, although these results must be subjected to a randomized, prospective clinical trial. Immune RNA is not antigenic, and there has been no toxicity associated with its use. Such a modality has significant theoretical advantages, since it is the only currently available system that uses the immunologic capacity of another species for the immunotherapy of humans.

NONSPECIFIC IMMUNOTHERAPY

The theoretic basis for nonspecific immunotherapy depends upon the observation that certain substances, such as mixed bacterial toxins and fractions of the tubercle bacillus, have the ability to nonspecifically enhance host resistance to most viral, fungal, and bacterial agents. Although the exact mechanism is unknown, these agents do appear to stimulate immune response to a wide variety of antigens, including tumor-specific antigens.

Historically, a type of nonspecific immunotherapy was described by Bradford Coley at the turn of the century in one of the first reports of a tumor regression possibly induced by immunologic means. Coley's interest in the possible value of such therapy was stimulated when he observed a recurrent inoperable sarcoma of the neck regress completely for 7 years after the patient had had attacks of erysipelas. This observation led to the development of Coley's toxins, a mixture of killed bacterial vaccines. Coley injected this admixture directly into tumor lesions or gave it intravenously. Some impressive regressions of tumors and long-term cures resulted from these agents. Because the responses were inconsistent, Coley's toxins never received widespread use, and interest in them died out. Recently a nonspecific immunotherapy of a similar type has been revived using attenuated bovine tuberculosis bacillus (BCG).

Our work with BCG began more than 10 years ago, when we injected BCG into metastatic nodules in the skin and subcutaneous tissues in patients with malignant melanoma. We observed that the intratumor injection of BCG caused 90 percent of the intradermal metastases to regress in patients who were immunologically competent as judged by their ability to develop delayed cutaneous hypersensitivity to DNCB and PPD. In addition, in about 20 percent of these patients, a few uninjected nodules were observed to regress. Satellite and in-transit metastases can be controlled in the extremity by this technique in two-thirds of patients. However, many of these patients still develop systemic metastases, as shown by our own experience in treating 24 patients with satellite and in-transit metastases in the leg. Ten of eighteen patients in whom local control was achieved later developed disseminated metastases, and seven of these ten patients have died. Although the intratumor injection of BCG may not control systemic disease, it is nonetheless a very useful method to control local disease that avoids the side effects of chemotherapy and can result in long-term survival.

There are several possible mechanisms to explain tumor regression following BCG injection; both specific and nonspecific immune reactions were probably involved. The tumor cells may be killed as "innocent bystanders" during the delayed cutaneous hypersensitivity reaction that occurs when lymphocytes and macrophages attack BCG dispersed throughout the tumor nodule. This is supported by the observation that the intratumor injection of BCG works only in patients who can be sensitized to BCG, as shown by their delayed cutaneous hypersensitivity reaction to PPD.

In addition to the nonspecific effect, a specific immune response to the melanoma tumor antigens also occurs in some patients because an associated rising titer of antimelanoma antibody is observed following BCG immunotherapy. Sequential biopsies of tumor nodules following BCG inoculation reveals that the regression of these nodules is associated with a granulomatous infiltration of lymphocytes, monocytes, and fibroblasts surrounding and infiltrating the melanoma cells. Furthermore, the regression of melanoma nodules not given injection with BCG is accompanied by the appearance of lymphocyte infiltrates within the regressing melanoma tumor nodules (Fig. 9-30). The specific antitumor effect may result from more lymphocytes and macrophages coming into contact with the tumor cells so that the afferent limb of the immune response is increased. Conversely, it may work via the effector limb of the immune response by bringing greater numbers of both stimulated and unstimulated lymphocytes to the tumor.

Our results have now been confirmed by a number of investigators. The observation that the intratumor injection of BCG occasionally led to the regression of uninjected nodules suggested that BCG might be useful as an adjuvant to operation to control micrometastatic disease in man. BCG has been shown to prevent the growth of spontaneous metastases in some animal tumor models where the variables of tumor load and time of BCG vaccination can be carefully controlled. In man, a number of preliminary reports have suggested that intradermal BCG delays

A

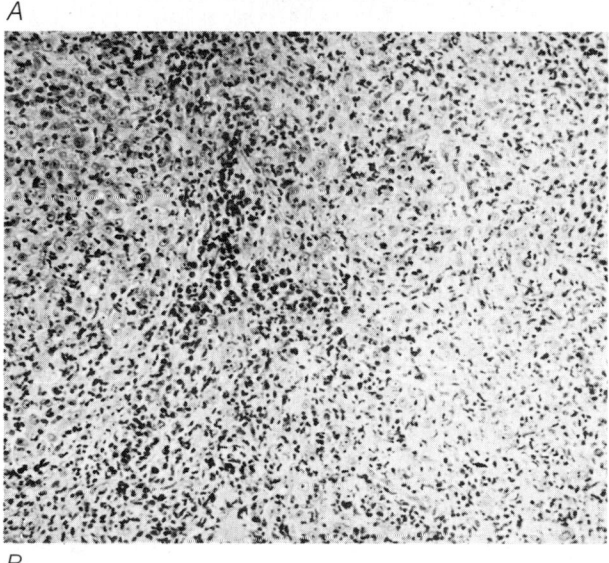

B

Fig. 9-30. *A.* Subcutaneous metastasis of malignant melanoma prior to immunotherapy with BCG. Note the absence of lymphocytic and monocytic infiltration among the tumor cells. *B.* Subcutaneous metastasis which had decreased in size from 10 to 5 mm during the 6-week period following immunotherapy with BCG injections into other melanoma nodules. BCG was *not* injected into this nodule. Note the marked lymphocytic and monocytic infiltration among the melanoma cells. (*From D. L. Morton, et al., Ann Surg, 172:740, 1970.*)

recurrence in patients with melanoma who are at high risk because of metastases to regional nodes (Fig. 9-31). However, the definitive answer on the usefulness of BCG in patients with melanoma will come from other prospective randomized controlled trials currently under way.

The most impressive results with BCG used as an adjuvant to operation for lung cancer have been reported by McKneally, who randomized patients to receive either BCG plus isoniazid or isoniazid alone administered as a single postoperative intrapleural dose following pulmonary resection. Patients with Stage I lung cancer who received

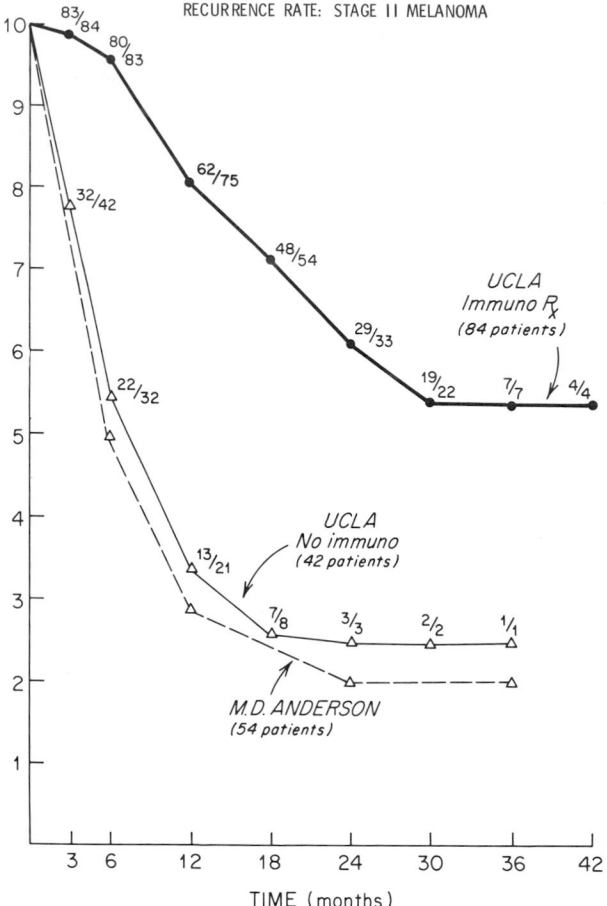

Fig. 9-31. Recurrence rate of Stage II melanoma showing the percentage of patients free of recurrent melanoma after regional lymphadenectomy alone or lymphadenectomy with postoperative immunotherapy. Numbers separated by a slash (/) indicate number of patients who remained free of disease over number of patients at risk of recurrence during that interval. $P < 0.01$ at each interval up to and including 30 months. Statistics on 54 patients from M. D. Anderson Hospital and Tumor Institute, University of Texas, Houston. (*From F. R. Eilber et al., N Engl J Med, 294:237, 1976.*)

Fig. 9-32. Schematic of cancer cell factory as it might function to enhance its growth by producing immunosuppression in the host. Theoretically, cancer surgery removes the cancer factory and its associated immunosuppressants, which allows the host immune responses to return to normal. (*From D. L. Morton et al., Chest, 71:640, 1977.*)

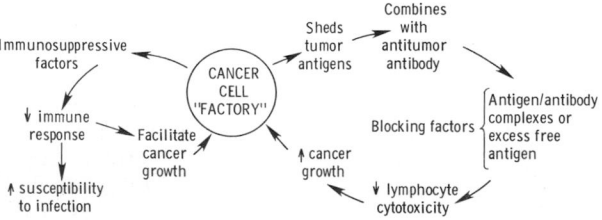

BCG had a significantly lower rate of recurrence and a correspondingly higher survival rate.

BCG is only one of a wide variety of agents that can nonspecifically stimulate the immune system's response to a variety of different types of antigens. Examples of other agents include *Corynebacterium parvum,* MER (methanol-extractable residue of BCG), bacterial antitoxins, and polynucleotides. We can anticipate that nonspecific immunotherapy will be tested in a wide variety of neoplasms and that new immunologic adjuvants will be developed.

Other impressive results with nonspecific immunotherapy come from the studies of Klein in patients with basal and squamous cell carcinomas of the skin. Here the induction of delayed hypersensitivity reactions to DNCB resulted in the resolution of more than 90 percent of superficial basal or squamous cell carcinomas. Klein observed that the mixture of multiple antigens such as PPD, mumps, and *Candida* increased the delayed hypersensitivity and effectiveness of this form of immunotherapy.

Another form of nonspecific immunotherapy involves the use of agents capable of restoring depressed immune responses. Several agents have been proposed in such a context, including thymic hormones such as thymosin and the antihelminthic drug levamisole, which is reported to increase host resistance to the benefit of patients with lung carcinoma.

The rational application of immunotherapy to human cancer will depend, to a large extent, on a better knowledge of tumor-associated antigens in human neoplasms and methods for increasing the immune response against these antigens. Specificity for cancer cells cannot be achieved by any other known therapeutic means; but the potency of immunotherapy is limited.

At the present time, the tumor immunologist is faced with a paradox in the clinical application of immunotherapy. Ideally, the patients who are most likely to respond to this therapeutic modality are those who are in the early stages of the disease and have minimal residual tumor burden following treatment with other therapeutic modalities. However, many of these patients may have been cured of their cancer by the primary treatment, so that immunotherapy can be evaluated only by controlled clinical trials of large numbers of patients. It should be emphasized, however, that the dosage indications, therapeutic results, and long-term toxicity of immunotherapy are largely unknown at the present time.

SURGERY AS IMMUNOTHERAPY

A tumor may promote its own growth by a number of immune mechanisms. The cancer cell may act as a "factory" that is constantly producing both immunosuppressive factors and tumor-associated antigens (Fig. 9-32). The specific and nonspecific immunosuppression decreases the patient's immune defenses and facilitates growth of the tumor.

The key to recovery of the balance in the host-tumor relationship depends on destruction or removal of the tumor cell "factory." Surgery appears to be the most efficient means of removing the factory. Once the mass of tumor is gone, the patient with cancer is more likely to be able to mount an immune response that may destroy any subclinical foci of tumor cells scattered through the body. However, if the recovery of the immune response is inadequate or if the number of tumor cells in any distant metastatic focus is too large, the patient may fail to regain control of the disease. Nonetheless, surgery for cancer becomes the first step in immunotherapy.

If this thesis is correct, it would follow that the approach to the surgical treatment for solid neoplasms must change dramatically. The future lies not in treating every patient with a solid neoplasm as one with localized disease but in assuming that the local disease is merely a manifestation of a systemic illness, whether or not the patient has overt metastatic disease. Not until we accept surgery as merely the first step in the treatment of cancer can we significantly improve our rates of cure. Therapeutic advances eventually must come from a multimethod combination of immunotherapy and chemotherapy with surgical therapy or radiotherapy. Unlike surgery and radiotherapy, both local treatments, the triple combinations represent a systemic treatment effective against tumor cells already metastatic to distant sites. However, at present, systemic therapeutic techniques have greater potential for curing those patients with a minimal number of tumor cells, rather than those with clinically evident disease. Thus, although surgery for cancer is not curative by itself, in most cases it can decrease the patient's burden of tumor cells and allow the immune response to normalize so that further chemoimmunotherapy has a chance to be more effective.

PROGNOSIS

Predicting the future course of a patient's malignant disease is one of the most difficult problems an oncologist faces. At the present time, it is impossible to predict the future course of a given patient except in general terms. However, a number of known factors are important in determining prognosis.

The *site of origin* of the primary tumor is one of the most important factors influencing prognosis. The propensity of a neoplasm to metastasize to distant sites varies according to its tissue of origin. Over 90 percent of carcinomas of the lung, pancreas, and esophagus spread beyond their primary site and cause death, whereas carcinomas of the skin, breast, and thyroid glands are frequently localized and curable, even when metastatic in some patients.

The *stage of disease* at the time of initial treatment is of considerable importance in determining survival for all types of neoplasms. The chance for cure is best when the neoplasm is confined to the organ of origin. The smaller the primary neoplasm, the better the prognosis, as well. Thus, in situ carcinoma of the cervix, carcinomas of the breast less than 1 cm in diameter, and small polypoid carcinomas of the colon are generally curable; larger neoplasms may not be curable. Direct extension into adjacent organs or metastases to regional nodes suggest a more

guarded prognosis, although many patients are still curable at this stage of the disease. The spread of cancer by the bloodstream with metastases to distant sites portends a grave prognosis, and few patients are curable at this stage. As a general rule, lymph node involvement sharply reduces survival probability by about one-half that of patients without involved nodes. If only one node is involved, the prognosis is better than if the majority of lymph nodes are involved.

The *histopathologic features* of the neoplasm correlate in a general way to prognosis. The more undifferentiated, highly malignant-appearing neoplasms with frequent mitosis are more likely to develop early distant spread and local recurrence. However, some very malignant neoplasms still can be cured with adequate treatment. Venous invasion is a grave prognostic factor in all types of neoplasia.

Host immune factors, as previously discussed, may be the most important single factor in determining prognosis. Immunologic methods for monitoring immune responses are currently under development. It is already apparent that those patients who have spontaneous depression of their immune responses have a uniformly poor prognosis following therapy.

The *age of the patient* may be an important factor affecting prognosis. Some oncologists believe that neoplasms in younger patients carry a poorer prognosis than the same tumors in middle-aged or elderly patients, although elderly patients may have associated medical problems that do not permit adequate treatment of the cancer. While there may be some validity in this concept, it should not be overemphasized, because many young patients have a good prognosis. In fact, some have a much better prognosis than adults with the same neoplasms. Those neoplasms which occur prior to one year of age generally have a better prognosis than those which occur later in childhood. This can be determined in the following manner: The child is usually cured of the neoplasm if he is free of disease for 9 months after treatment, plus double the age at the time treatment was begun. This concept is based upon the supposition that if the earliest cancer cell started with conception and if the cancer grew at a constant rate, then it would reach a certain size at the time treatment was initiated. If treatment was successful in eliminating all cancer cells except one, then in a period equal to 9 months plus double the age of the child, the cancer size would again be equivalent to the original tumor mass. Therefore, if there is no recurrence after this time span, it can be assumed that the patient is cured.

The *adequacy of treatment* is most relevant to prognosis for certain types of neoplasms. The cure rate for some neoplasms, such as soft tissue sarcomas and certain childhood neoplasms, may be twice as high in sophisticated cancer centers when compared to cure rates in small community hospitals. Furthermore, some patients with seemingly hopeless prognoses may be cured with aggressive therapy by an experienced oncologist, whereas they might not be by the physician who only occasionally treats cancer patients and might be unwilling to undertake the aggressive therapy.

PSYCHOLOGIC MANAGEMENT OF THE CANCER PATIENT

The cancer patient's great fear of his disease usually can be decreased by understanding derived from free and open communication with the physician. Psychologic support and education to deal with any disability that may result from therapy are important. Examples include training in the care of a stoma following curative surgery for colonic and rectal cancer or referral to lay groups associated with the American Cancer Society for counseling the anxious patient with an altered body image resulting from mastectomy.

Despite the prognostic factors discussed previously, it is still impossible to predict the exact course of any malignant tumor. Patients with the most grim prognoses are occasionally cured by aggressive therapy, and spontaneous regressions are sometimes observed even in patients with metastases. In contrast, some patients with apparently localized disease may be dead of disseminated cancer in a few months. This uncertainty about the future is one of the most difficult adjustments faced by the cancer patient and his family. Most reassuring in this regard is to emphasize that for each month that passes following successful treatment of the primary neoplasm, the chances for cure improve. This is particularly correct for tumors such as squamous cell carcinoma of the lung or oral pharynx. Although other, more slowly growing neoplasms, such as carcinoma of the breast and malignant melanoma, may recur after disease-free intervals of 10 or 20 years, the chances of recurrence also decrease with time. Recognition that cancer is a chronic disease is an important aspect of management. Long-term, consistent follow-up provides opportunities for reassurance and usually can ensure detection of recurrence at an early stage.

Some patients do not want to know about their illness for fear of having their suspicions verified. Never lie to a patient, if possible, even if requested by the family. In general, gentle and optimistic truth is best. Untruths often create barriers between the patient and his family which can lead to psychologic isolation of the patient who is unable to discuss his fears and anxieties with those he needs most.

With the patient for whom primary cancer therapy has failed, one of the most difficult problems faced by the physician is "What should the patient be told?" Most oncologists who deal exclusively with cancer patients agree that the incurable patient also must be told the truth as gently and optimistically as possible. Hope and reassurance as to the physician's continuing concern are best sustained by continuing active treatment until it is certain that the patient can no longer benefit. Realistic and consistent support is actually more important to the patient and the family at this stage of the disease than earlier. There is increasing evidence that patients tolerate the process of dying much better when cared for in this manner.

Some incurable patients are unable to accept the realities of the situation. In this case, it is essential that a responsible family member be informed. The life duration of the incurable patient is so uncertain that predictions should be avoided. If, as frequently happens, the relatives insist upon some estimate, a combined minimum-maximum prognosis, such as from 6 months to 2 years, will help the family accept this uncertainty.

The basic aim in caring for the patient with advanced cancer is to prolong useful life, but not useless suffering. The patient should be permitted to die with dignity when active therapy can no longer benefit him.

References

Etiology

Barratt, R. W., and Tatum, E. L.: Carcinogenic Mutagens, *Ann NY Acad Sci*, **71:**1072, 1958.

Blum, H. F.: Sunlight as a Causal Factor in Cancer of the Skin, *Cancer Res*, **5:**592, 1945; **9:**247, 1948.

Buell, P., and Dunn, J. E., Jr.: Cancer Mortality among Japanese Issei and Nisei of California, *Cancer*, **18:**656, 1965.

Burdett, W. J.: "Viruses Inducing Cancer," University of Utah Press, Salt Lake City, 1966.

Cutler, S. J.: A Review of the Statistical Evidence on Association between Smoking and Lung Cancer, *J Am Statis Assoc*, **50:**267, 1955.

Gallo, R. C., and Todaro, G. J.: Oncogenic RNA Viruses, *Semin Oncol*, **3:**81, 1976.

Green, M., and Wold, W. S. M.: Oncogenic RNA Viruses: Replication, Tumor Gene Expression, and Role in Human Cancer, *Semin Oncol*, **3:**65, 1976.

Haenszel, W.: Cancer Mortality among the Foreign Born in the United States, *J Natl Cancer Inst*, **26:**37, 1961.

Hammond, E. C., and Horn, D.: The Relationship between Human Smoking Habits and Death Rates, *JAMA*, **155:**1316, 1954.

Heuper, W. C.: Environmental Cancer, in F. Homburger (ed.), "The Physiopathology of Cancer," p. 919, Harper & Row, Publishers, Incorporated, New York, 1959.

Kennaway, E. C.: The Formation of a Cancer Producing Substance from Isoprene (2-Methyl-Butadiene), *J Pathol Bacteriol*, **27:**233, 1924.

Khanolkar, V. R.: Oral Cancer in Bombay, India: A Review of 1,000 Consecutive Cases, *Cancer Res*, **4:**313, 1944.

Lorenz, E.: Radioactivity and Lung Cancer: A Critical Review of Lung Cancer in the Miners of Schneeburg and Joachimstall, *Cancer Res*, **5:**1, 1944.

Martland, H. S.: Occupational Poisoning in Manufacture of Luminous Watch Dials: General Review of Hazard Caused by Ingestion of Luminous Paint with Special Reference to the New Jersey Cases, *JAMA*, **92:**466, 1929.

Mayo, C. W., DeWeerd, J. H., and Jackman, R. J.: Diffuse Familial Polyposes of the Colon, *Surg Gynecol Obstet*, **93:**87, 1951.

Pifer, J. W., Toyooka, E. T., Murray, R. W., Ames, W. R., Hempelmann, L. H., Crump, S. L., and Dutton, A. M.: Neoplasms in Children Treated with X-rays for Thymic Enlargement: I. Neoplasms and Mortality; II. Tumor Incidence as a Function of Radiation Factors; III. Clinical Description of Cases, *J Natl Cancer Inst*, **31:**1333, 1357, 1379, 1963.

Porter, C. D., and White, C. J.: Multiple Carcinomata following Chronic X-ray Dermatitis, *Ann Surg*, **46:**649, 1970.

Prehn, R. T.: Specific Isoantigenicities among Chemically Induced Tumors, *Ann NY Acad Sci*, **101:**107, 1962.

Rapp, R.: Viruses as Etiologic Factors in Cancer, *Semin Oncol,* **3:**49, 1976.

Rous, P.: Transmission of a Malignant New Growth by Means of a Cell-free Filtrate, *JAMA,* **56:**198, 1911.

Shimkin, M. B.: Cancer Research, in L. V. Ackerman and J. A. Del Regato (eds.), "Cancer," pp. 35–57, The C. V. Mosby Company, St. Louis, 1962.

Biology and Immunobiology

Black, M. M., Opler, S. R., and Speer, F. D.: Structural Representations of Tumor-Host Relationships in Gastric Carcinoma, *Surg Gynecol Obstet,* **102:**599, 1956.

Burnet, F. M.: "Immunological Surveillance," Pergamon Press, New York, 1970.

DeVries, J. E., Cornain, S., and Rumke, P.: Cytotoxicity of Non-T versus T-Lymphocytes from Melanoma Patients and Healthy Donors on Short and Long Term Cultured Melanoma Cells, *Int J Cancer,* **14:**427, 1974.

Dhar, P., Moore, T. L., Zamcheck, N., and Kupchick, H.: Carcinoembryonic Antigen (CEA) in Colonic Cancer: Use in Pre- and Postoperative Diagnosis and Prognosis, *JAMA,* **221:**31, 1972.

Eilber, F. R., and Morton, D. L.: Impaired Immunologic Reactivity and Recurrence following Cancer Surgery, *Cancer,* **25:**362, 1970.

——— ———, Nizze, A., and Morton, D. L.: Sequential Evaluation of General Immune Competence in Cancer Patients: Correlation with Clinical Course, *Cancer,* **35:**660, 1975.

Everson, T. C., and Cole, W. H.: "Spontaneous Regression of Cancer," W. B. Saunders Company, Philadelphia, 1966.

Fass, L., Ziegler, J. L., Heberman, R. B., and Kiryabwire, J. W. M.: Cutaneous Hypersensitivity Reactions to Autologous Extracts of Malignant Melanoma Cells, *Lancet,* **1:**116, 1970.

Fenyö, E. M., Klein, E., Klein, G., and Swiech, K.: Selection of an Immunoresistant Moloney Lymphoma Subline with Decreased Concentration of Tumor-specific Surface Antigens, *J Natl Cancer Inst,* **40:**69, 1968.

Foley, E. J.: Antigenic Properties of Methylcholanthrene-induced Tumors in Mice of the Strain or Origin, *Cancer Res,* **13:**835, 1953.

Gatti, R. A., and Good, R. A.: Occurrence of Malignancy in Immunodeficiency Diseases: A Literature Review, *Cancer,* **28:**89, 1971.

Gold, P., and Freedman, S. O.: Specific Carcinoembryonic Antigens of the Human Digestive System, *J Exp Med,* **122:**467, 1965.

Goodwin, W. E.: Regression of Hypernephromas, *JAMA,* **20:**609, 1968.

Griffiths, J. D., McKinna, J. A., Rawbotham, H. D., Tsolakidis, P., and Salsbury, A. J.: Carcinoma of the Colon and Rectum: Circulating Malignant Cells and 5-Year Survival, *Cancer,* **31:**226, 1973.

Haagensen, D. E., Jr., Mazoujian, G., Holder, W. D., Kister, S. J., and Wells, S. A., Jr.: Evaluation of a Breast Cyst Fluid Protein Detectable in the Plasma of Breast Carcinoma Patients, *Ann Surg,* **185:**279, 1977.

Hakala, T. R., and Lange, P. H.: Serum Induced Lymphoid Cell Mediated Cytotoxicity against Human Transitional Cell Carcinomas of the Urinary Tract, *Science,* **184:**795, 1974.

Hammond, W. G., Fisher, J. C., and Rolley, R. T.: Tumor Specific Transplantation Immunity to Spontaneous Mouse Tumors, *Surgery,* **62:**124, 1967.

Hellstrom, I., Sjogren, H. O., Warner, G., and Hellstrom, K. E.: Blocking of Cell Mediated Tumor Immunity by Sera from Patients with Growing Neoplasms, *Int J Cancer,* **7:**226, 1971.

Hellstrom, K. E., and Hellstrom, I.: Lymphocyte Mediated Cytotoxicity and Blocking Serum Activity to Tumor Antigens, *Adv Immunol,* **18:**209, 1974.

Hibbs, J. B., Lambert, L. J., and Remington, J. I.: Possible Role of Macrophage Mediated Nonspecific Cytotoxicity in Tumor Resistance, *Nature [New Biol],* **235:**48, 1972.

Klein, G.: Tumor Antigens, *Ann Rev Microbiol,* **20:**223, 1966.

Mach, J. P., Jaeger, P., Bertholet, M. M., Ruegsigger, C. H., Loosli, R. M., and Pettavel, J.: Detection of Recurrence of Large Bowel Carcinoma by Radioimmunoassay of Circulating Carcinoembryonic Antigen (CEA), *Lancet,* **2:**535, 1974.

Morton, D. L.: Acquired Immunological Tolerance and Carcinogenesis by the Mammary Tumor Virus. I. Influence of Neonatal Infection with the Mammary Tumor Virus on the Growth of Spontaneous Mammary Adencarcinomas, *J Natl Cancer Inst,* **42:**311, 1969.

———, Eilber, F. R., Joseph, W. L., Wood, W. C., Trahan, E., and Ketcham, A. S.: Immunological Factors in Human Sarcomas and Melanomas: A Rational Basis for Immunotherapy, *Ann Surg,* **172:**740, 1970.

———, Holmes, E. C., Eilber, F. R., and Wood, W. C.: Immunological Aspects of Neoplasia: A Rational Basis for Immunotherapy, *Ann Intern Med,* **74:**587, 1971.

Old, L. J., and Boyse, E. A.: Antigens of Tumors and Leukemias Induced by Virus, *Fed Proc,* **24:**1009, 1965.

———, ———, and Stockert, E.: Antigenic Properties of Experimental Leukemias: I. Serological Studies In Vitro with Spontaneous and Radiation-induced Leukemias, *J Natl Cancer Inst,* **31:**977, 1963.

———, Stockert, E., Boyse, E. A., and Kin, J. H.: Antigenic Modulation: Loss of TL Antigen from Cells Exposed to TL Antibody: Study of the Phenomenon In Vitro, *J Exp Med,* **127:**523, 1968.

O'Toole, C., Stejeka, V., Perlmann, P., Karlsson, M.: Lymphoid Cells Mediating Tumor-Specific Cytotoxicity to Carcinoma of the Urinary Bladder: Separation of the Effector Population Using a Surface Marker, *J Exp Med,* **139:**437, 1974.

Piessens, W. F.: Evidence of Human Cancer Immunity, *Cancer,* **26:**1212, 1970.

Pilch, Y. H., Meyers, G. H., Sparks, F. C., and Golub, S. H.: Prospects for the Immunotherapy of Cancer: Part I, Basic Concepts of Tumor Immunology, *Curr Probl Surg,* January 1975, p. 1.

Prehn, R. T., and Main, J. M.: Immunity to Methylcholanthrene-induced Sarcomas, *J Natl Cancer Inst,* **18:**769, 1957.

Shearer, W. T., and Parker, C. W.: Humoral Immunostimulation. V. Selection of Variant Cell Lines, *J Exp Med,* **110:**1133, 1975.

Sjogren, H. O.: Transplantation Methods as a Tool for Detection of Tumor-specific Antigens, *Prog Exp Tumor Res,* **6:**289, 1965.

Smith, R. T.: Tumor-specific Immune Mechanisms, *N Engl J Med,* **278:**1207, 1968.

Sophocles, A. M., and Nadler, S. H.: Immunologic Aspects of Cancer, *Surg Gynecol Obstet,* **133:**321, 1971.

Southam, C. M., Brunschwig, W., Levin, A. G., and Dixon, Q. S.:

The Effect of Leukocytes on Transplantability of Human Cancer, *Cancer,* **19:**1743, 1966.

Sparks, F. C., and Breeding, J. H.: Tumor Regression and Enhancement Resulting from Immunotherapy with Bacillus Calmette-Guérin and Neuraminidase, *Cancer Res,* **34:**3262, 1974.

——, O'Connell, T. X., Lee, Y-T., and Breeding, J. H.: BCG Therapy Given as an Adjuvant to Surgery: Prevention of Death from Metastases from Mammary Adenocarcinoma in Rats, *J Natl Cancer Inst,* **53:**1825, 1974.

Sugarbaker, E. V., and Cohen, A. M.: Altered Antigenicity in Spontaneous Pulmonary Metastases from an Antigenic Murine Sarcoma, *Surgery,* **72:**155, 1972.

Zamcheck, N. and Kupchic, H.: The Interdependence of Clinical Investigations and Methodological Development in Early Evaluation of Assays for Carcinoembryonic Antigen, *Cancer Res,* **34:**2131, 1974.

——, Moore, T. L., Dhar, P., and Kupchic, H.: Immunologic Diagnosis and Prognosis of Human Digestive Tract Cancer: Carcinoembryonic Antigens, *N Engl J Med,* **286:**83, 1972.

Pathology

Anderson, W.: The General Pathology of Tumors, in "Boyd's Pathology for the Surgeon," p. 92, W. B. Saunders Co., Philadelphia, 1967.

Bloom, H. J. G., Richardson, W. W., and Harries, E. J.: Natural History of Untreated Breast Cancer (1805–1933): Comparison of Untreated and Treated Cases according to Histological Grade of Malignancy, *Br Med J,* **2:**213, 1962.

Boyd, W.: "An Introduction to the Study of Disease," p. 210, Lea & Febiger, Philadelphia, 1971.

Cole, W. H., McDonald, G. O., Roberts, S. S., and Southwich, H. W.: "Dissemination of Cancer," Appleton-Century-Crofts, Inc., New York, 1961.

Collins, V. P., Leoffler, R. K., and Tivey, H.: Observations on Growth Rates of Human Tumors, *Am J Roentgenol Radium Ther Nucl Med,* **76:**988, 1956.

Cowan, D. R.: Mechanisms Responsible for the Origin and Distribution of Blood-borne Tumor Metastases, *Cancer Res,* **13:**397, 1953.

Everson, T. C.: Spontaneous Regression of Cancer, *Ann NY Acad Sci,* **114:**721, 1964.

Garland, L. H., Coulson, W., and Wollin, E.: The Rate of Growth and Apparent Duration of Untreated Primary Bronchial Carcinoma, *Cancer,* **16:**694, 1963.

Knox, L. C.: The Relationship of Massage to Metastases in Malignant Tumors, *Ann Surg,* **75:**129, 1922.

MacMahon, B., and Feng, M. A.: Prenatal Origin of Childhood Leukemia: Evidence from Twins, *N Engl J Med,* **270:**1082, 1964.

Moertel, C. G.: Incidence and Significance of Multiple Primary Malignant Neoplasms, *Ann NY Acad Sci,* **114:**886, 1964.

Pearson, H. A., Grello, F. W., and Cane, E. C., Jr.: Leukemia in Identical Twins, *N Engl J Med,* **268:**1151, 1963.

Pund, E. R., Nettles, T. B., Caldwell, T. D., and Nieburgs, H. E.: Preinvasive and Invasive Carcinoma of the Cervix Uteri: Pathogenesis, Detection, Differential Diagnosis, and Pathologic Basis for Management, *Am J Obstet Gynecol,* **55:**831, 1948.

Rigler, L. B.: Natural History of Untreated Lung Cancer, *Ann NY Acad Sci.* **114:**755, 1964.

Russell, W. O., Ibanex, M. L., Clark, R. L., and White, E. C.: Thyroid Carcinoma: Classification, Intraglandular Dissemination, and Clinicopathologic Study Based upon Whole Organ Sections of 80 Glands, *Cancer,* **16:**1425, 1963.

Slaughter, D. P.: Multicentric Origin of Intraoral Carcinoma, *Surgery,* **20:**133, 1946.

Clinical Manifestations

Barrie, J. G., Knapper, W. H., and Strong, E. W.: Cervical Nodal Metastases of Unknown Origin, *Am J Surg,* **120:**466, 1970.

Bhattacharya, S. K., and Sealy, W. C.: Paraneoplastic Syndromes Resulting from Elaboration of Ectopic Hormones, Antigens, and Bizarre Toxins, *Curr Probl Surg,* May, 1972.

Greenberg, B. E.: Cervical Lymph Node Metastases from Unknown Primary Sites, *Cancer,* **19:**1091, 1966.

Jesse, R. H., and Neff, L. F.: Metastatic Carcinoma in Cervical Nodes with an Unknown Primary Lesion, *Am J Surg,* **112:**547, 1966.

Keller, J. W., and Williams R. D.: Laparotomy for Unexplained Fever, *Arch Surg,* **90:**494, 1965.

Myers, W. P. L., Tashima, C. K., and Rothschild, E. O.: Endocrine Syndromes Associated with Non-endocrine Neoplasms, *Med Clin North Am,* **50:**763, 1966.

Owens, A. H., Jr.: Neoplastic Diseases, in A. M. Harvey, R. J. Johns, A. H. Owens, and R. S. Ross (eds.), "The Principles and Practice of Medicine," p. 641, Appleton-Century-Crofts, Inc., New York, 1972.

Smith, P. E., Krementz, E. T., and Chapman, W.: Metastatic Cancer without a Detectable Primary Site, *Am J Surg,* **113:**633, 1967.

Diagnosis and Staging

Commission on Clinical Oncology of the Union Internationale Contre Cancrum: "TNM Classification of Malignant Tumors," International Clinics against Cancer, Geneva, 1968.

Copeland, M. M.: American Joint Committee on Cancer Staging and End Results Reporting: Objectives and Progress, *Cancer,* **18:**1637, 1965.

Eilber, F. R., Holmes, E. C., and Morton, D. L.: Immunotherapy as an Adjunct to Surgery in Treatment of Cancer, *World J Surg,* **1:**547, 1977.

Glatstein, E., Guernsey, J. M., Rosenberg, S. A., and Kaplan, H. S.: The Value of Laparotomy and Splenectomy in the Staging of Hodgkin's Disease, *Cancer,* **24:**709, 1969.

Goldman, J. M.: Laparotomy for Staging of Hodgkin's Disease, *Lancet,* **1:**125, 1971.

Kennedy, W. B.: History and Physical Examination in the Diagnosis of Cancer, in T. F. Nealon, Jr. (ed.), "Management of the Patient with Cancer," p. 62, W. B. Saunders Co., Philadelphia, 1966.

Surgery

Ansfield, F. J., Ramirez, G., Skibba, J. L., Bryan, G. T., Davis, H. L. Jr., and Wirtanen, G. W.: Intrahepatic Arterial Infusion with 5-Fluorourocil, *Cancer,* **28:**1147, 1971.

Barnes, J. P.: Physiologic Resection of the Right Colon, *Surg Gynecol Obstet,* **94:**722, 1952.

Cole, W. H., Packard, D., and Southwich, H. W.: Carcinoma of the Colon with Special Reference to Prevention of Recurrence, *JAMA,* **155:**1549, 1954.

Deckers, P. J., Ketcham, A. S., Sugarbaker, E. V., Hoye, R. C., and Thomas, L. B.: Pelvic Exenteration for Primary Carcinoma of the Uterine Cervix, *Obstet Gynecol,* **37:**647, 1971.

Flanagan, L., and Foster, J. H.: Hepatic Resection for Metastatic Cancer, *Am J Surg,* **113:**551, 1967.

Foster, J. H., and Berman, M. M.: Solid Liver Tumors, Major Problems in Clinical Surgery, vol. 23, W. B. Saunders Company, Philadelphia, 1977.

Gilbertsen, V. A., and Wangensteen, O. H.: A Summary of Thirteen Years' Experience with the Second Look Program, *Surg Gynecol Obstet,* **114:**438, 1962.

Halsted, W. S.: The Results of Operations for the Cure of Cancer of the Breast Performed at the Johns Hopkins Hospital from June 1889 to January 1894, *Ann Surg,* **20:**297, 1894.

Huggins, C., and Bergenstal, D. M.: Inhibition of Human Mammary and Prostatic Cancer by Adrenalectomy, *Cancer Res,* **12:**134, 1952.

Kiselow, M., Butcher, H. R., and Bricker, E. M.: Results of the Radical Surgical Treatment of Advanced Pelvic Cancer: A Fifteen-Year Study, *Ann Surg,* **166:**436, 1967.

Krementz, E. T., and Ryan, R. E.: Chemotherapy of Melanoma of the Extremities by Perfusion: Fourteen Years Clinical Experience, *Ann Surg,* **175:**900, 1972.

Miles, W. E.: A Method of Performing Abdomino-perineal Excision for Carcinoma of the Rectum and the Terminal Portion of the Pelvic Colon, *Lancet,* **2:**1812, 1908.

Miller, D. R., and Albritten, F. F., Jr.: Principles of Surgery for Cancer, in T. F. Nealon Jr. (ed.), "Management of the Patient with Cancer," p. 154, W. B. Saunders Company, Philadelphia, 1966.

Mockman, S., Curreri, A. R., and Ansfield, F. J.: Second-Look Operation for Colon Carcinoma after Fluorouracil Therapy, *Arch Surg,* **100:**527, 1970.

Mueller, C. B., and Jeffries, W.: Cancer of the Breast: Its Outcome as Measured by the Rate of Dying and Causes of Death, *Ann Surg,* **182:**334, 1975.

Pierce, E. H., Clagett, O. T., McDonald, J. R., and Gage, R. P.: Biopsy of the Breast Followed by Delayed Radical Mastectomy, *Surg Gynecol Obstet,* **103:**559, 1956.

Ramming, K. P., Sparks, F. C., Eilber, F. R., Holmes, E. C., and Morton, D. L.: Hepatic Artery Ligation and 5-Fluorouracil Infusion for Metastatic Colon Carcinoma and Primary Hepatoma, *Am J Surg,* **132:**236, 1976.

———, ———, ———, and Morton, D. L.: Management of Hepatic Metastases, *Semin Oncol,* **4:**71, 1977.

Roberts, S. S., Hengesh, J. W., McGrath, R. G., Valaitis, J., McGrew, E. A., and Cole, W. H.: Prognostic Significance of Cancer Cells in the Circulating Blood: A Ten Year Evaluation, *Am J Surg,* **113:**757, 1967.

Sparks, F. C., Mosher, M. B., Hallauer, W. C., Silverstein, M. J., Rangel, D., Passaro, E., and Morton, D. L.: Hepatic Artery Ligation and Postoperative Chemotherapy for Hepatic Metastases: Clinical and Pathophysiological Results, *Cancer,* **35:**1074, 1975.

Stearns, M. W., and Schottenfeld, D.: Techniques for the Surgical Management of Colon Cancer, *Cancer,* **28:**165, 1971.

Stehlin, J. S.: Hyperthermic Perfusion with Chemotherapy for Cancer of the Extremities, *Surg Gynecol Obstet,* **129:**305, 1969.

Stehlin, J. S., Jr., Giovanella, B. C., Ipolyi, P. D., Muenz, L. R., and Anderson, R. F.: Results of Hyperthemic Perfusion for Melanoma of the Extremities, *Surg Gynecol Obstet,* **140:**339, 1975.

Turnbull, R. B., Kyle, K., Watson, F. R., and Spratt, J.: Cancer of the Colon: The Influence of the No-Touch Isolation Technic on Survival Rates, *Ann Surg,* **166:**420, 1967.

Watkins, E., Khazei, A. M., and Nabra, K. S.: Surgical Basis for Arterial Infusion Chemotherapy of Disseminated Carcinoma of the Liver, *Surg Gynecol Obstet,* **130:**581, 1970.

Wilkens, E. W., Jr.: The Surgical Management of Metastatic Neoplasms of the Lung, *J Thorac Cardiovasc Surg,* **42:**298, 1961.

Zike, W. L., Safaie-Sharazi, S., and Gulessarian, H. P.: Hepatic Artery Ligation and Cytotoxic Infusion for Treatment of Liver Neoplasms, *Arch Surg,* **110:**641, 1975.

Radiation Therapy

Higgins, G. S., Jr., Conn, J. H., Jordan, P. H., Jr., Humphrey, E. W., Roswit, B., and Keehn, R. J.: Preoperative Radiotherapy for Colo-Rectal Cancer, *Ann Surg,* **181:**624, 1974.

Johns, H. E., and Cunningham, J. R.: in "The Physics of Radiology," p. 345, Charles C Thomas, Publisher, Springfield, Ill., 1971.

Kligerman, M. M.: Radiotherapy and Rectal Cancer, *Cancer,* **39:**896, 1977.

Moss, W. T., and Brand, W. N.: "Therapeutic Radiology; Rationale, Technique, Results," 3d ed., The C. V. Mosby Company, St. Louis, 1969.

Paulson, D. L., Shaw, R. R., Kee, J. L., Mallams, J. T., and Collier, R. E.: Combined Preoperative Irradiation and Resection for Bronchogenic Carcinoma, *J Thorac Cardiovasc Surg,* **44:**281, 1962.

Powers, W. E., and Tolmach, L. J.: Preoperative Radiation Therapy: Biologic Basis and Experimental Investigation, *Nature,* **201:**272, 1964.

Stearns, M. W., Jr., Deddish, M. R., Quan, S. H. Q., and Leaming, R. H.: Preoperative Roentgen Therapy for Cancer of the Rectum and Rectosigmoid, *Surg Gynecol Obstet,* **138:**584, 1974.

Stevens, K. R., Jr., Allen, C. V., and Fletcher, W. S.: Preoperative Radiotherapy for Adenocarcinoma of the Rectosigmoid, *Cancer,* **37:**2866, 1976.

Chemotherapy

Bailor, J. C., and Byar, D. P.: Estrogen Treatment for Cancer of the Prostate, *Cancer,* **26:**257, 1970.

Baserga, R. (ed.): The Cell Cycle and Cancer, Marcel Dekker, Inc., New York, 1971.

Bonadonna, G., Brusamolino, E., Valagussa, B. S., Rossi, A., Brugnatelli, L., Brambilla, C., DeLena, M., Tancini, G., Bajetta, E., Musumeci, R., and Veronesi, U.: Combination Chemotherapy as an Adjuvant Treatment in Operable Breast Cancer, *N Engl J Med,* **294:**405, 1976.

Bruce, W. R.: The Action of Chemotherapeutic Agents at the Cellular Level and the Effects of These Agents on Hematopoietic and Lymphomatous Tissue, *Can Cancer Conf,* **7:**53, 1966.

Calabresi, P., and Parks, R. E., Jr.: Chemotherapy of Neoplastic Diseases, in L. S. Goodman and A. Gilman (eds.), "The Pharmacological Basis of Therapeutics," 5th ed., p. 1248, The MacMillan Company, New York, 1975.

Chabner, B. A., Myers, E. E., Coleman, C. N., and Johns, D. G.: The Clinical Pharmacology of Antineoplastic Agents, N Engl J Med, 292:1107, 1159, 1975.

Cline, M. J., and Haskell, C. M.: Cancer Chemotherapy, 2d ed., W. B. Saunders Company, Philadelphia, 1975.

D'Angio, G. J., Evans, A. E., Breslow, N., Beckwith, B., Bishop, H., Feigl, P., Goodwin, W., Deape, L. L., Sinks, L. F., Sutow, W., Tefft, M., and Wolff, J.: The Treatment of Wilms' Tumor, Cancer, 38:633, 1976.

Gilman, A.: The Initial Clinical Trial of Nitrogen Mustard, Am J Surg, 105:574, 1963.

Haskell, C. M.: Immunologic Aspects of Cancer Chemotherapy, Ann Rev Pharmacol Toxicol, 17:179, 1977.

———, Sparks, F. C., Graze, P. R., and Korenman, S. G.: Systemic Therapy for Metastatic Breast Cancer, Ann Int Med, 86:68, 1977.

Huggins, C., and Hodges, C. V.: Studies on Prostatic Cancer. I. The Effect of Castration, of Estrogen and Androgen Injection on Serum Phosphatases in Metastatic Carcinoma of the Prostate, Cancer Res, 1:293, 1941.

Laird, A. K.: Dynamics of Growth in Tumors and in Normal Organisms, Natl Cancer Inst Monogr, 30:15, 1969.

Lewis, J. L.: Chemotherapy of Gestational Choriocarcinoma, Cancer, 30:1517, 1972.

Li, M. C., Hertz, R., and Spencer, D. B.: Effect of Methotrexate Therapy upon Choriocarcinoma and Chorioadenoma, Proc Soc Exp Biol Med, 93:361, 1956.

Mathe, G.: Immunotherapy in the Treatment of Acute Lymphoid Leukemia, Hosp Prac, 6:43, 1971.

Schabel, F. M., Jr.: The Use of Tumor Growth Kinetics in Planning "Curative" Chemotherapy of Advanced Solid Tumors, Cancer Res, 29:2384, 1969.

Skipper, H. E.: Cancer Chemotherapy Is Many Things: GHA Clowes Memorial Lecture, Cancer Res, 31:1173, 1971.

——— and Perry, S.: Kinetics of Normal and Leukemic Leukocyte Populations and Relevance to Chemotherapy, Cancer Res, 30:1883, 1970.

Strawitz, J. G.: Cancer Chemotherapy Using Isolation Perfusion, in I. Brodsky, S. B. Kahn, and J. H. Moyer (eds.), "Cancer Chemotherapy II," p. 443, Grune & Stratton, New York, 1972.

Sullivan, P. W., and Salmon, S. E.: Kinetics of Tumor Growth and Regression in IgG Multiple Myeloma, J Clin Invest, 51:1697, 1972.

Sullivan, R. D., and Semel, C. J.: Arterial Infusion Cancer Chemotherapy for Solid Tumors, in I. Brodsky, S. B. Kahn, and J. H. Moyer (eds.), "Cancer Chemotherapy II," p. 453, Grune & Stratton, New York, 1972.

Combined Therapy

Ariel, I. M., and Briceno, M.: Rhabdomyosarcoma of the Extremities and Trunk: Analysis of 150 Patients Treated by Surgical Resection, J Surg Oncol, 7:269, 1975.

Cortes, E. P., Holland, J. F., Wang, J. J., and Sinks, L. F.: Doxorubicin in Disseminated Osteosarcoma, JAMA, 221:1132, 1972.

———, ———, ———, ———, Blom, J., Senn, H., Bank, A., and Glidewell, O.: Amputation and Adriamycin in Primary Osteosarcoma, N Engl J Med, 291:998, 1974.

DiPietro, S., DePalo, G., Gennari, L., Molinari, R., and Domascelli, B.: Cancer Chemotherapy by Intra-arterial Infusion with Adriamycin, J Surg Oncol 5:421, 1973.

Gerner, R. E., Moore, G. E., and Pickren, J. M.: Soft Tissue Sarcomas, Ann Surg, 181:803, 1975.

Gilbert, H. A., Kagan, R. A., and Winkley, J.: Soft Tissue Sarcomas of the Extremities: Their Natural History, Treatment and Radiation Sensitivity, J Surg Oncol, 7:303, 1975.

Haskell, C. M., Eilber, F. R., and Morton, D. L.: Adriamycin (NSC-12317) by Arterial Infusion, Cancer Chemother Rep, 6:187, 1974.

———, Silverstein, M. J., Rangel, D., Hunt, J. S., Sparks, F. C., and Morton, D. L.: Multimodality Cancer Therapy in Man: A Pilot Study of Adriamycin by Arterial Infusion. Cancer, 33:1485, 1974.

Jaffe, N., Frei, E., III, Traggis, D., and Bishop, Y.: Adjuvant Methotrexate and Citrovorum Factor Treatment of Osteogenic Sarcoma, N Engl J Med, 291:994, 1974.

Lindberg, R. D.: The Role of Radiation Therapy in the Treatment of Soft Tissue Sarcoma in Adults, in "Proc. 7th Natl. Cancer Congress," J. B. Lippincott Company, Philadelphia, 1972.

Martin, R. G., Butler, J. J., and Albores, S. S.: Soft Tissue Tumors: Surgical Treatment and Results, in "Tumors of Bone and Soft Tissue," p. 333, Year Book Medical Publishers, Chicago, 1965.

Morton, D. L.: Soft Tissue Sarcomas, in J. F. Holland (ed.), "Cancer Medicine," p. 1845, Lea & Febiger, Philadelphia, 1974.

———, Eilber, F. R., Townsend, C. M., Jr., Grant, T. T., Mirra, J., and Weisenburger, T. H.: Limb Salvage from a Multidisciplinary Treatment Approach for Skeletal and Soft Tissue Sarcomas of the Extremity, Ann Surg, 184:268, 1976.

McNeer, G. D., Cantin, J., Chu, F., and Nickson, J. T.: Effectiveness of Radiation Therapy in the Management of Sarcoma of the Soft Somatic Tissues, Cancer, 22:391, 1968.

Murphy, W. T.: The Role of Radiation Therapy in the Management of Soft Somatic Tissue Sarcoma, Proc. 6th Natl. Cancer Congress, p. 775, 1968.

Rosen, G., Murphy, M. L., Huvas, A. G., Guitierrez, M., and Marcove, R. C.: Chemotherapy, En Bloc Resection and Prosthetic Bone Replacement in the Treatment of Osteogenic Sarcoma, Cancer, 37:1, 1976.

———, Suwansirikal, S., Kwan, C., Tan, C., Wu, S. J., Beattie, E. J., and Murphy, M. L.: High Dose Methotrexate with Citrovorum Factor Rescue and Adriamycin in Childhood Osteosarcoma, Cancer, 33:1151, 1974.

Suit, H. D., and Russell, W. O.: Radiation Therapy of Soft Tissue Sarcomas, Cancer, 36:759, 1975.

———, ———, and Martin, R. G.: Sarcoma of Soft Tissue: Clinical and Histopathological Parameters and Response to Treatment, Cancer, 35:1478, 1974.

Townsend, C. M., Jr., Eilber, F. R., and Morton, D. L.: Skeletal and Soft Tissue Sarcomas: Results of Treatment with Adjuvant Immunotherapy, JAMA, 236:2187, 1976.

———, ———, and ———: Skeletal and Soft Tissue Sarcomas: Results of Surgical Adjuvant Chemotherapy, Proc Am Soc Clin Oncol, 17:265, 1976.

Immunotherapy

Deckers, P. J., and Pilch, Y. H.: RNA-Mediated Transfer of Tumor Immunity: A New Model for Immunotherapy of Cancer, *Cancer,* **28:**1219, 1971.

Eilber, F. R., Morton, D. L., Holmes, E. C., Sparks, F. C., and Ramming, K. P.: Adjuvant Immunotherapy with BCG in Treatment of Regional Lymph Node Metastases from Malignant Melanoma, *N Engl J Med,* **294:**237, 1976.

Gutterman, J. U., Mavligit, G. M., and Hersh, E. M.: Chemoimmunotherapy of Human Solid Tumors, *Med Clin North Am,* **60:**441, 1976.

Halpern, B. N., Biozzi, G., Stiffel, C., and Mouton, D.: Correlation entre l'activitie phagocytaire du système reticulo-endothelial et la production d'anticorps antibacteriens, *C R Soc Biol* (*Paris*), **152:**758, 1958.

Holland, J. F., and Bekesi, J. G.: Immunotherapy of Human Leukemia with Neuraminidase-modified Cells, *Med Clin North Am,* **60:**539, 1976.

Israel, L., and Edelstein, R. L.: "Nonspecific Immunostimulation with *Corynebacterium parvum* in Human Cancer," The Williams & Wilkins Company, Baltimore, 1974.

Klein, E.: Hypersensitivity Reactions at Tumor Site, *Cancer Res,* **29:**2351, 1969.

———, Holterman, O., Milgrom, H., Case, R. W., Klein, D., Rosner, D., and Djerassi, I.: Immunotherapy for Accessible Tumors Utilizing Delayed Hypersensitivity Reactions and Separated Components of the Immune System, *Med Clin North Am,* **60:**389, 1976.

Lawrence, H. S.: Transfer Factor, *Adv Immunol,* **11:**195, 1969.

LoBuglio, A. F., and Neidhart, J. A.: Transfer Factor: A Potential Agent for Cancer Therapy, *Med Clin North Am,* **60:**585, 1976.

McKhann, C. F.: Immunobiology of Cancer, in J. S. Najarian and R. L. Simmons (eds.), "Transplantation," p. 297, Lea & Febiger, Philadelphia, 1972.

McKneally, M. F., Maver, C., and Kausel, H.: Regional Immunotherapy of Lung Cancer with Intrapleural BCG, *Lancet,* **1:**377, 1976.

Mathe, G., Schwarzenberg, L., and Amiel, J. L.: Bone Marrow, in J. S. Najarian and R. L. Simmons (eds.), "Transplantation," p. 588, Lea & Febiger, Philadelphia, 1972.

Moertel, C. G., Ritts, R. E., Jr., Schutt, A. J., and Hahn, R. G.: Clinical Studies of Methanol Extraction Residue Fraction of Bacillus Calmette-Guérin as an Immunostimulant in Patients with Advanced Cancer, *Cancer Res,* **35:**3075, 1975.

Moore, G. E., and Gerner, R. E.: Cancer Immunity: Hypothesis and Clinical Trial of Lymphocytotherapy for Malignant Diseases, *Ann Surg,* **172:**733, 1970.

Morton, D. L.: Cancer Immunotherapy: An Overview, *Semin Oncol,* **1:**297, 1974.

———: Immunotherapy of Cancer: Present Status and Future Potential, *Cancer,* **30:**1647, 1972.

———, Eilber, F. R., Holmes, E. C., Hunt, J. S., Ketcham, A. S., Silverstein, M. J., and Sparks, F. C.: BCG Immunotherapy of Malignant Melanoma: Summary of a Seven-Year Experience, *Ann Surg,* **180:**635, 1974.

———, ———, Joseph, W. L., Wood, W. C., Trahan, E., and Ketcham, A. S.: Immunological Factors in Human Sarcomas and Melanomas: A Rational Basis for Immunotherapy, *Ann Surg,* **172:**740, 1970.

———, Haskell, C. M., Pilch, Y. H., Sparks, F. C., and Winters, W. D.: Recent Advances in Oncology, *Ann Intern Med,* **77:**431, 1972.

———, Holmes, E. C., and Golub, S. H.: Immunologic Aspects of Lung Cancer, *Chest,* **71:**640, 1977.

Nathanson, L.: Use of BCG in Treatment of Human Neoplasms: A Review, *Semin Oncol,* **1:**337, 1974.

Oettgen, H. F., Pinsky, C. M., and Delmonte, L.: Treatment of Cancer with Immunomodulators: *Corynebacterium parvum* and Levamisole, *Med Clin North Am,* **60:**463, 1976.

Old, L. J., Benacerraf, B., Clark, D. A., Carswell, E. A., and Stockert, E.: The Role of the Reticuloendothelial System in the Host Reaction to Neoplasia, *Cancer Res,* **21:**1281, 1961.

Powles, R.: Immunologic Maneuvers in Management of Acute Leukemia, *Med Clin North Am,* **60:**463, 1976.

Ramming, K. P., and deKernion, J. B.: Immune RNA Therapy for Renal Cell Carcinoma: Survival and Immunologic Monitoring, *Ann Surg,* **186:**459, 1977.

Rojas, A. F., Feierstein, J. M., Mickiewicz, E., Glait, H., and Olivari, A. J.: Levamisole in Advanced Human Breast Cancer, *Lancet,* **1:**211, 1976.

Sparks, F. C.: Hazards and Complications of BCG Immunotherapy, *Med Clin North Am,* **60:**499, 1976.

———, and Ramming, K. P.: Immunotherapy of Gastrointestinal Cancer: The Potential, *Clin Gastroenterol,* **5:**855, 1976.

Stockert, E.: The Role of the Reticuloendothelial System in the Host Reaction to Neoplasia, *Cancer Res,* **21:**1281, 1961.

Sumner, W. C., and Foraker, A. C.: Spontaneous Regression of Human Melanoma: Clinical and Experimental Study, *Cancer,* **13:**79, 1960.

Prognosis

Berkson, J., and Gage, R. P.: Specific Methods of Calculating Survival Rates of Patients with Cancer, in G. T. Pack and I. M. Ariel (eds.), "Treatment of Cancer and Allied Diseases," Harper & Row, Publishers, Incorporated, New York, 1958.

Dunphy, J. E.: On Caring for the Patient with Cancer, *N Engl J Med,* **295:**313, 1976.

Kelly, W. D., and Friesen, S. R.: Do Cancer Patients Want to be Told? *Surgery,* **27:**822, 1950.

Wangensteen, O. H.: Should Patients Be Told They Have Cancer? *Surgery,* **27:**944, 1950.

Psychologic Management

Sherman, C. D., Jr., and Feasel, W. P.: "General Aspects of Cancer," University of Rochester School of Medicine and Dentistry, Rochester, N.Y., 1969–1970. (Syllabus.)

Silverberg, E., and Holleb, A. I.: "Cancer Statistics 1972," American Cancer Society, Inc., New York. (Reprinted from CA, 22:1, 1972.)

Chapter 10

Transplantation

by Richard L. Simmons, John E. Foker, Richard R. Lower, and John S. Najarian

Man does not burst like a balloon—he falls apart, piece by piece. Clinical organ transplantation is designed to replace the exhausted parts as they fall. Because the immunologic barrier of allograft rejection stands in the way of attaining chimerism between host and graft, immunologists and surgeons have been working together since World War II to circumvent the rejection reaction. Unfortunately, the problems remain unsolved. Despite the clinical success of kidney transplantation, organs are still rejected, and attempts to prevent rejection can be fatal. The field of clinical transplantation, though no longer totally experimental, remains in flux, and many apparently well-founded principles are soon washed away. Much of the material presented in this chapter will not survive the decade.

 The first part of this chapter discusses the immunobiology of the allograft, the rejection reaction, and the means for achieving immunosuppression. The current and incipient clinical applications of these biologic principles and techniques to the human patient are discussed in the second section.

IMMUNOBIOLOGY OF THE ALLOGRAFT

Tissue or organ grafts between individuals of the same species (allografts, or homografts) are rejected with a vigor proportional to the degree of the genetic disparity between them. Grafts between individuals of different species (xenografts, or heterografts) are rejected even more rapidly. Grafts between identical twins (isografts, isogeneic grafts, or syngeneic grafts), or from an individual to himself (autografts, or autogenous grafts) survive indefinitely once vascular supply has been reestablished.

Allografts normally survive surgical manipulation as well as isografts. If the recipient has not previously encountered the antigens present on the donor graft, the allograft is not morphologically or physiologically distinguishable from the isograft in the early posttransplant period—the rejection process normally takes several days. Medawar, in his classic demonstration of the immunologic nature of the allograft response, noted that skin grafts between randomly selected adult rabbits appeared normal until the fourth or fifth day. At that time inflammation appeared within the graft bed in the form of a dense leukocyte infiltrate which led to necrosis of the entire graft by about the tenth day. Medawar further demonstrated that the rejection process is the result of immunologic mechanisms. Whereas the "first-set rejection" takes place in 10 or 11 days, a second graft from the same rabbit resulted in an accelerated "second-set rejection." This process of first-set and second-set rejection of allogeneic graft takes place whether or not the graft is orthotopic (a graft placed in the anatomic position normally occupied by such tissue) or heterotopic (those grafts placed in abnormal recipient locations). The reaction is immunologically specific for the antigens involved, and the second-set rejections occur only when the recipient has previously encountered the antigens of the first graft.

Transplantation (Histocompatibility) Antigens

Tissue transplanted from one individual to another will be rejected if the new host can recognize that tissue as foreign. Foreignness is equated with the presence of antigens on the donor cells which the host does not possess and thereby recognizes as nonself. Foreign antigens on a tissue or organ graft are considered histocompatibility antigens if they can be related to graft rejection. Any histocompatibility antigen will lead to graft rejection if the antigen is present on donor tissue but absent from the host. In fact, some histocompatibility differences are probably present in all donor-recipient combinations with the exception of identical twins in human beings, and inbred strains in other animal species. The "strength" of different antigenic in-

compatibilities varies, however, and a "strong" mismatch can lead to graft rejection within 8 days, while "weaker" differences will permit graft survival of well over 100 days. The strongest antigens are xenogeneic antigens, i.e., those which elicit the rejection of grafts from animals of a different species. Xenograft rejection is often accomplished within minutes. In contrast, one of the weakest histocompatibility antigens is linked to the Y chromosome of male mice, so that female mice gradually reject grafts from male mice of the same inbred strain.

THE NATURE OF HISTOCOMPATIBILITY ANTIGENS

Antigens which stimulate the rejection of grafts are predominantly located on the cell surface. A group of strong histocompatibility antigens has been found in several species, including human beings, which are the products of a single chromosomal region. Although they have been given different names in different species, they are the major histocompatibility antigens. Mismatch of these antigens inevitably leads to graft rejection. The ABO system leaves the more complex and elusive major histocompatibility antigens as the main determinants of graft survival. Because of the ease of typing the ABO antigens they will not be further considered in this discussion of major histocompatibility antigens.

Tissues vary in the amount of the histocompatibility antigens present. In the mouse, for example, the strong histocompatibility antigens are found in high concentration in the liver, spleen, and lymphoid tissue. Intermediate amounts of the antigens are found on cells of the kidney, lung, adrenal gland, and gastrointestinal tract, while heart, muscle, and brain cells contain very little. The histocompatibility antigens appear on the cell surface very early in the development of the individual—Simmons and Russell found evidence that they are expressed on the fertilized egg. Age of the donor is, therefore, not a consideration in the antigenic strength of a potential organ graft.

The biochemical nature and the cell membrane relationships of the histocompatibility antigens are slowly yielding to investigation. Most of the studies have centered on the major antigens, and although they have not been completely characterized, much is known about them. They are proteins of approximately 45,000 mol wt and associated noncovalently in the membrane with B_2 microglobulins. Peptide mapping and amino acid analyses of tryptic digests of highly purified antigens indicate that the variability occurs in small discrete regions of the molecule. A constant framework of amino acids characterizes the remainder of these molecules. The large number of antigens results from changes in the amino acids at only a few locations. This phenomenon is not unique and has many counterparts in the biological world. Mutations may be acceptable at only a few locations; otherwise the functional capabilities of the molecule are destroyed. With antigens, as with other molecules, variety with preservation of activity is gained by amino acid changes at these few sites.

The complexities of the cell membrane are only beginning to be unraveled, but the membrane appears to be a bilayer of lipid molecules interspersed with globular protein islands (Fig. 10-1). The bilayer has a fluid character, and consequently the proteins, which provide the many membrane functions, have considerable mobility within the lipid shell. This fluid mosaic model of membrane structure has several important consequences. Some of the proteins may traverse the entire membrane, as those making up the transport sites would be expected to do. Other proteins seem to be related only to the inner or outer surface of the membrane and may be useful in receiving or sending various signals and providing communication with the cytoplasm. The fluid nature of the membrane also means that the density of the active protein sites can be varied as the cell requires.

The histocompatibility antigens are among the protein islands of the cell surface. Their function is not yet understood, but obviously they have not evolved to thwart graft rejection. More likely, they are important in recognition phenomena and cell-to-cell interactions, but the mechanisms are unknown. Susceptibility to certain diseases, including ankylosing spondylitis, acute uveitis, celiac disease, psoriasis, Hodgkin's disease, and several immune-based maladies, has been linked to the major histocompatibility locus and associated with certain antigens. These seemingly unrelated conditions may prove to have obvious connections when cell membrane function is better understood.

THE IMMUNOGENETICS OF HISTOCOMPATIBILITY

The strongest of the transplantation antigens is the expression of a single chromosomal region called the *major histocompatibility complex* (MHC). In human beings the MHC is located on chromosome 6. Several species commonly used in immunological studies have a similar MHC which governs the major transplantation antigens. These antigens, however, were discovered and named before much was known about their genetic origins, and so the nomenclature varies among species. In human beings, transplantation antigens were first investigated on leukocytes and were named human leukocyte antigens (HLA). Naturally, the first-discovered antigens would be likely to be the major determinants. In mice, the strongest antigens are called H-2 antigens, in rats AgB antigens, etc. All seem to originate from an MHC, suggesting that considerable similarity exists between species.

The HLA locus has begun to be dissected through immunogenetic analysis. The presence of HLA antigens on a cell surface is detected in one of two ways. The serological method uses antigen-specific antisera which either agglutinates or lyses cells carrying the antigen. This has identified the serologically defined (SD) HLA antigens, which had been expected to encompass all the major antigens. When this proposition was tested in cell culture by measuring the reactivity of host lymphocytes to lymphocytes from potential graft donors, it was found that certain SD identical combinations still provided considerable stimulation. The lymphocytes were reacting to other cellular transplantation antigens. By screening hundreds of potential donors and recipients by these mixed leukocyte cultures (MLC) it was found that another transplantation locus existed. The lymphocyte-defined (LD) locus was

Fig. 10-1. Protein islands within the lipid bilayer of the cell membrane. Some proteins, such as those associated with transport, are thought to traverse the membrane; others are located only on the inner or outer surface. The transplantation antigens are complex proteins and are among the islands. Undoubtedly they are located on the outer portion of the membrane and perhaps extend to the inner surface as well. Their exposed position permits them to interact with immunocompetent cells and antibodies. (*From S. J. Singer and G. L. Nicolson, The Fluid Mosaic Model of the Structure of Cell Membranes, Science, 175:720, 1972.*)

found to be part also of the HLA complex but genetically distinct from the SD region. The two antigen testing methods, therefore, subdivided the HLA complex into SD and LD regions. Further genetic analysis has revealed the presence of additional components which do not code for cell antigens, and it is now clear that the human MHC consists of multiple genes—the number is not yet known but may be as large as several hundred.

At least three SD antigenic groups have now been found. The HLA-A and HLA-B antigens have formed the basis for transplantation tissue typing for many years, while HLA-C is a more recent discovery. Both the HLA-A and HLA-B loci have about 20 different alleles or antigens. Alleles are the alternative forms of a given gene locus, and, as noted, the allelic antigens may differ by only one or two amino acids. Less is known about the LD locus (now called HLA-D), but multiple alleles exist. Each individual inherits one chromosome and, hence, one set of HLA antigens from each parent. All the HLA antigens are expressed (codominant) on the cell surface, and thus, two A antigens, two B antigens, etc., are present.

The known loci of the HLA complex have been mapped on chromosome 6; their relative positions are shown in Fig. 10-2. The three SD loci (A, B, and C) are plotted, as is the LD locus (HLA-D). The site for complement factor C2 has also been found to be within the HLA complex. The relative positions of these five loci are known, but they are separated by a considerable amount of unidentified genetic material. Several other genes have been assigned to the HLA region, but their relative position is not known. The complement factors C4 and C8 are located somewhere within this region, and perhaps, as shown, a second LC locus is present. Recent evidence also suggests that the immune responsiveness of an individual is controlled by

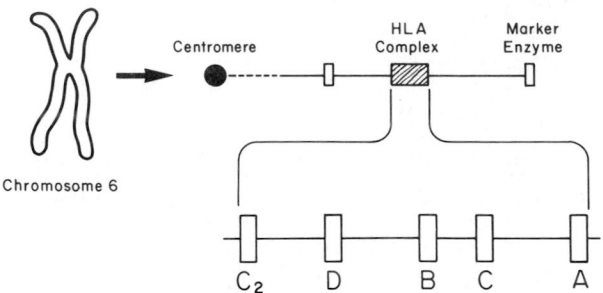

Fig. 10-2. Schematic representation of the HLA complex, the major histocompatibility determinants in human beings. The HLA complex is located on chromosome 6, although it is not known whether it is on the long or short arm. Many genes comprise the HLA complex; pictured are the relative positions of the HLA-A, -B, -C, and -D loci. Also shown is the location of the gene coding for the C2 component of the complement pathway. Many other genes, including that for the C4 component of complement, are probably found within the complex but are not yet well defined.

one or more genes within the HLA complex. How the products of these immune-response genes function is virtually unknown, but they may be of considerable importance in regulating the ability to react to antigens and thus to the immunological capabilities of the individual. Ultimately, the HLA region may be found to control a wide variety of membrane structures and functions.

The MHC loci have been found to be closely linked but

Fig. 10-3. Hypothetic examples of inheritance of serologically detectable HLA antigens of the A and B series. Four offspring of mating between parents with chromosomes labeled I-II and III-IV are shown, as well as one possible result of recombination within the HLA region and subsequent inheritance. The parental chromosomes are usually transmitted intact, and the offspring receive one chromosome containing an A and B pair from each parent. Occasionally, however, crossover occurs and the child receives a recombinant antigen pair from a parent. For simplicity, genes coding for the C and D series of antigens within the HLA complex are not shown. See Fig. 10-2 for the presumed location of the genes within the HLA complex.

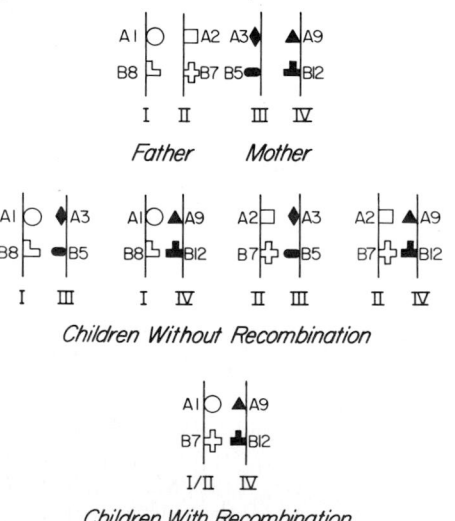

separable, and therefore genetic crossover between them, though rare, can occur. As shown in Fig. 10-3, the parental HLA-A and HLA-B pairs are usually inherited together, and the antigens originating from one chromosome are called an *HLA haplotype.* Almost always the haplotype the child receives from each parent corresponds to the haplotype of one of the parental chromosomes. When crossover occurs during meiosis, however, the child receives a recombinant haplotype from a parent. (In the example shown, recombination occurred between A and B antigens.)

Detection of the A and B alleles for tissue typing requires banks of monospecific sera. Typing is necessary because it seems clear that survival of transplanted organs correlates with the closeness of the A and B antigen match. The third SD locus, HLA-C, is presumably also a strong histocompatibility determinant, but the proof will come with greater use of HLA-C typing in transplantation studies. The role of the HLA-D sublocus (LD antigens) in transplantation is unclear. Lymphocytes in mixed leukocyte cultures respond to cells with different D antigens by proliferating. Even when the SD antigens are identical, lymphocytes with different LD antigens proliferate actively in MLC. The presence of proliferation in culture cannot be directly translated into antigraft activity, since the dividing lymphocytes acquire little cytotoxicity against the donor cells if only D differences are involved. Nevertheless, the proliferation induced by D antigens is essential for full development of cellular immunity against A and B antigens. Clinical tissue matching by mixed leukocyte culture to minimize HLA-D differences has proved to be valuable for bone marrow transplantation and may be valuable for kidney transplantation as well.

It is important to recognize that there are genes on other chromosomes outside the MHC which control weaker histocompatibility loci. In human beings, such antigens are not well understood, but a graft from a sibling identical at the HLA locus will be rejected if immunosuppressive drugs are not utilized. Such rejections are the natural consequence of these minor histocompatibility loci.

The Immune Apparatus

The presence of the histocompatibility antigens on the cells of transplanted organs triggers the rejection reaction. At birth, human beings are already immunologically competent and have undergone a complex developmental process. It is now agreed that there is a single hemopoietic stem cell, found in the extraembryonic yolk sac, which begins to proliferate. The resulting daughter stem cells migrate to various centers for further differentiation. Within these centers, progenitor cells for erythrocytes, eosinophils, basophils, neutrophils, and lymphoid cells arise, depending on the local microchemical environment. It is likely that further proliferation of these progenitor stem cells depends on the action of "poietins," which tend to expand the populations of specialized cells in the way that erythropoietin acts on the erythrocyte line (Fig. 10-4).

The lymphoid cell line first appears within two primary (or central) lymphoid tissues. The thymus governs the

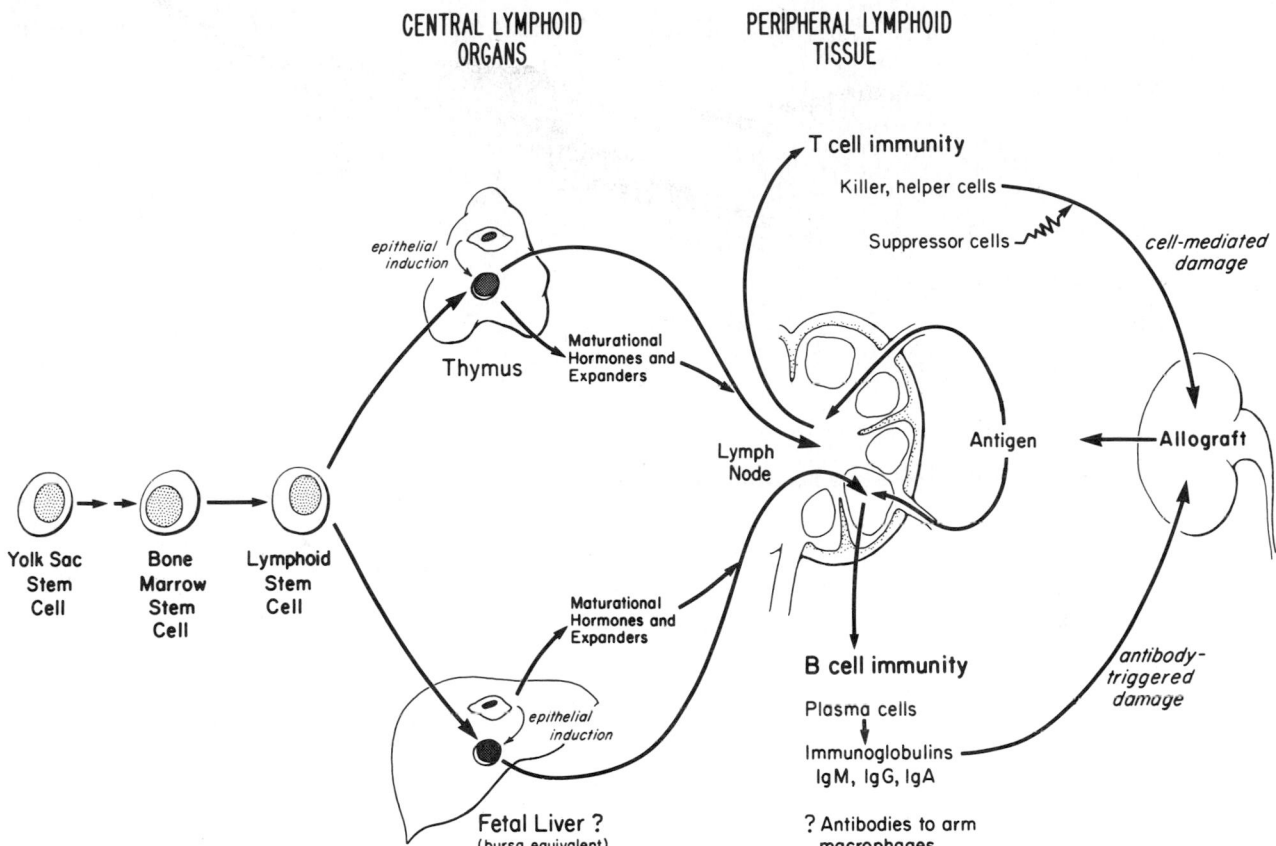

CENTRAL LYMPHOID ORGANS

PERIPHERAL LYMPHOID TISSUE

epithelial induction

Thymus

Maturational Hormones and Expanders

Lymph Node

Antigen

Allograft

T cell immunity

Killer, helper cells

Suppressor cells

cell-mediated damage

Yolk Sac Stem Cell

Bone Marrow Stem Cell

Lymphoid Stem Cell

Maturational Hormones and Expanders

epithelial induction

Fetal Liver ? (bursa equivalent)

B cell immunity

Plasma cells

Immunoglobulins IgM, IgG, IgA

? Antibodies to arm macrophages

antibody-triggered damage

Fig. 10-4. Encapsulation of the extraordinarily complex developmental sequences of the immune system. Certain of the known inducers, expanders, growth factors, and sites of maturation needed to establish the T and B cell lines are presented. Much of this takes place before birth, so transplant recipients are fully competent with established peripheral lymphoid populations in the lymph nodes, Peyer's patches, and spleen. Therefore, clinical immunosuppression consists principally of lymphocyte depletion and inhibition of the activation of antigen-stimulated lymphocytes. [*From J. E. Foker, R. L. Simmons, and J. S. Najarian, Principles of Immunosuppression, in D. C. Sabiston, Jr. (ed.), "Davis-Christopher Textbook of Surgery," p. 506, W. B. Saunders Company, Philadelphia, 1977.*]

development of cellular immunity. In birds, the bursa of Fabricius governs the development of humoral immunity. The bursa exists as a clearly defined central lymphoid structure only in birds. The equivalent of the bursa of Fabricius has not been defined in mammals, but there is evidence that it exists—perhaps within the fetal liver. In human beings the characteristics of sex-linked agammaglobulinemia of the Bruton type—very low levels of immunoglobulins, with normal cellular immunity and thymus-derived lymphocytes—suggest that the bursa equivalent has failed to develop.

Both the thymus and the bursa (or its equivalent) are responsible for the further development of the peripheral lymphoid tissues, i.e., spleen, lymph nodes, Peyer's patches. Certain areas of the lymph node can be shown to be dependent on the functional presence of the thymus and bursa (Fig. 10-5). The paracortical regions between the

cortical germinal centers and the medulla are dependent on the thymus, while the germinal centers themselves and the medullary cord lymphoid tissue are under the developmental control of the bursal equivalent. Therefore, thymectomy early in the neonatal period or congenital thymic deficiency results in failure of development of the paracortical regions of the lymph nodes. In chickens, bursectomy leads to failure of development of germinal centers and medullary cord lymphoid tissues.

During ontogeny, the thymus is the site of a vigorous cell proliferation. Many of these cells migrate to the paracortical areas of lymph nodes. All such cells which were once dependent on the thymus for their development are called T cells. Among their several functions T cells represent the immunocompetent cell population responsible for the development of cellular immunity, rather than humoral immunity. These reactions include delayed hypersensitivity reactions, as well as many of the early reactions responsible for allograft rejection.

Once these cells have migrated from the thymus, they seldom return. There is some evidence that the thymus produces a "hormone" (thymosin), perhaps a poietin, that is necessary for the maintenance of the full functional capacity of the T-cell system. The thymus increases in size until puberty, at which time it begins to atrophy. The function of the T-cell system is maintained by T cells established in the bone marrow and peripheral lymphoid tissue.

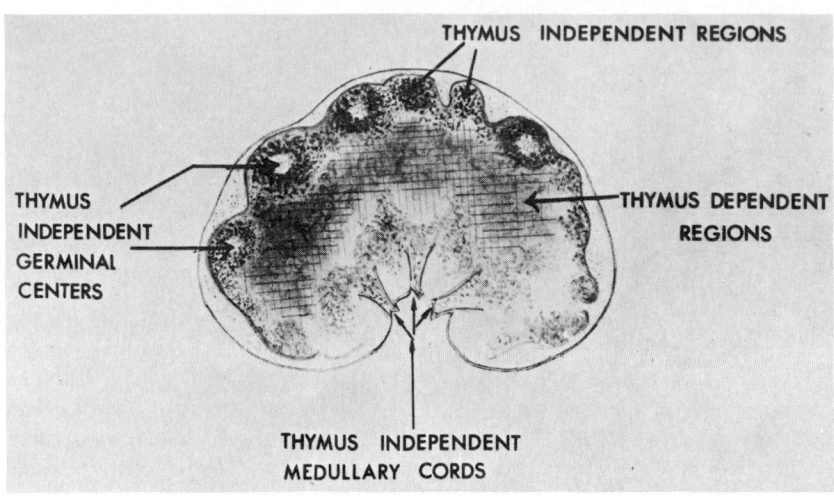

THYMUS INDEPENDENT REGIONS

THYMUS INDEPENDENT GERMINAL CENTERS

THYMUS DEPENDENT REGIONS

THYMUS INDEPENDENT MEDULLARY CORDS

Fig. 10-5. The thymus-dependent and thymus-independent areas are illustrated in this schematic representation of a lymph node. [*From R. A. Good and J. Finstad, Structure and Development of the Immune System, in J. S. Najarian and R. L. Simmons (eds.), "Transplantation," p. 26, Lea & Febiger, Philadelphia, 1972.*]

A humoral factor similar to that secreted by the thymus may also be at work here in maturing and maintaining the population of immunocompetent cells known as *B cells.* The B cells descend from stem cells in the bone marrow and become responsible for the manufacture of circulating immunoglobulins and thus for humoral immunity (Fig. 10-4).

It appears that the lymphoid system is the seat of the body's immunologic response and the small mature lymphocytes and the plasma cells are the immunocompetent cells. Once the lymphocytes (T or B cells) have migrated to the peripheral lymphoid tissue, they are fully immunocompetent. It is likely that Burnet's clonal selection theory holds true—i.e., a state of preparedness for a certain antigen or group of related antigens exists within a lymphoid cell so that it is capable of responding to only a narrow range of antigenic specificities. Whether this degree of specificity is "built in" or acquired during embryonic or early postnatal life is unknown. Nevertheless, only a small percentage of the lymphocytes in the body will respond to a specific antigen. Conversely, each cell can respond to only a narrow spectrum of antigens.

The B cells appear to be relatively sessile, but their end products, immunoglobulins and antibodies, can interact with foreign antigens at distant sites. The T cells responsible for cell-mediated immunity are of necessity more peripatetic and must migrate to the periphery in order to neutralize foreign antigens.

Immunologic Events in Allograft Rejection

INDUCTION OF IMMUNITY

ROLE OF THE SMALL LYMPHOCYTE. Mature lymphocytes appear to sit in a state of immunologic readiness. Whatever role other cells play in the development of immunity, there is little doubt that the small lymphocyte is the seat, and perhaps the only specific site, of immunologic recognition. The small lymphocyte has the capacity to recognize whether or not a molecule is foreign. Once

having reacted to an immunogen, the small lymphocyte, or its descendants, produces the molecules (antibodies or cellular receptor sites) that recognize and react with the antigenic determinants of the immunogen.

One of the major proofs in immunology was the demonstration of the ability of a virtually pure suspension of small lymphocytes from the thoracic duct of rats to cause a graft-versus-host (GVH) immune reaction in histoincompatible animals. Similarly, transfused small lymphocytes can bring about the adoptive destruction of long-tolerated skin allografts in rats. Gowans and associates observed that the small lymphocyte did not incorporate tritiated thymidine into deoxyribonucleic acid (DNA) until an appropriate immunogenic stimulus was encountered. When stimulated, the small lymphocyte transformed in the lymphoid tissue to large activated cells. This transformation heralds the onset of the lymphocyte response to an antigen.

Small lymphocytes not only initiate the immune response, they also carry immunologic memory. Gowans and Uhr showed that thoracic duct lymphocytes taken from rats immunized with phage particles would respond with high antibody titers after transfer to syngeneic irradiated recipients. These cells, or a portion thereof, have a life-span of many months in rats and many years in human beings. It is tempting to conclude that the small lymphocyte can carry out primary, secondary, and memory functions of the lymphoid system for allograft response, if not for all immunologic situations.

As stated above, the small lymphocyte recognizes the immunogenic determinants and translates that recognition into an immunologic response. The first phase of the immunologic response has been called the *afferent arc.* It involves the grafting process itself, the release of the immunogenic histocompatiblity antigens from the graft, the processing and recognition of the immunogens, and the stimulation of the responsive lymphoid cell population.

IMMUNOGEN RELEASE FROM THE GRAFT. The immunogens of a grafted organ, being surface components of the cell membrane, are readily available to the recipient's immune system. Most sensitization to allografts probably takes place within the peripheral lymphoid tissue of the host by antigens shed from the graft or on donor lymphocytes carried over in the transplanted organ. The remainder of the sensitization occurs in circulating host lymphocytes which migrate to the graft.

The route of administration of the immunogen is important in determining the onset of immunity, as well as its strength. The intravenous route will evoke the earliest response, but it is also the poorest immunogenic route and results in a less profound and less persistent state of immunity. The subcutaneous and the intraperitoneal avenues are more effective, and an intradermal route is the most efficient immunizing route. Thus permanent strong immunity follows intradermal injection of allogenic cells, and only weak immunity results from the intravenous infusion of dissociated cells. These findings may well account for the capacity of vascularized allografts (i.e., kidney, liver, heart) to withstand a graft rejection better than nonvascularized grafts (i.e., skin), which must develop a blood supply as they heal. Skin grafts appear to immunize primarily via the lymphatic system, whereas vascularized organ grafts immunize by the bloodstream, a far less immunogenic route.

PROCESSING OF THE IMMUNOGENS. The travels of microgram quantities of ^{125}I-labeled *Salmonella adelaide* flagella injected into rats were studied by Nossal and associates. Flagellar antigen was trapped in two locations in the lymph node. Antigen found in the medullary sinuses was overwhelmingly located inside macrophages. As will be discussed, the ingestion of antigen by macrophages may be the first step in the processing of antigens. In contrast to this, the immunogen in the follicular area of lymph nodes was retained in an extracellular location for as long as 3 weeks. It was most frequently found at or near the surface of fine processes of dendritic reticular cells, which in turn often interdigitated with the equally fine processes of lymphocytes (Fig. 10-6). Evidence for the development of immunity was the finding of transformed lymphocytes in the area that were identical morphologically to lymphocytes responding to antigens in vitro. When the rats had been previously sensitized to the flagellar antigen, the number of these responding cells greatly increased. The reticular cell may only facilitate contact between antigen and lymphocyte, or it may function in a more complex fashion as an inducer of lymphocyte transformation. Admittedly, these morphologic events are the response of an experimental animal to a bacterial flagellar immunogen, but nonetheless the events should be applicable to histocompatibility immunogens arriving at a lymph node (Fig. 10-7).

ROLE OF THE MACROPHAGE IN THE INDUCTION OF ALLOGRAFT IMMUNITY. The macrophage not only efficiently traps antigens but may also participate in the afferent arc as an antigen-processing cell. How the macrophage participates is not clear. It may simply partially digest the antigen to facilitate uptake by the lymphocyte. Others have proposed the macrophage processes the antigen more completely and transfers to the lymphocyte either an informative RNA (ribonucleic acid) molecule or an equally specific RNA-antigen complex (Fig. 10-7). The importance of the macrophage to transplantation immunity is not yet known. Considerable evidence obtained in cell culture indicates that the presence of macrophages is necessary to the development of immunity. Neither the subcellular mechanism, on one hand, nor the extension to the transplant patient, on the other, has been determined.

RECOGNITION OF THE IMMUNOGEN BY LYMPHOCYTES. The center of the immune response lies in the reaction of the lymphocyte to the immunogen. This most certainly requires direct interaction of the lymphocyte with the antigen or its products, since the most striking aspect of the immune response is its specificity. For each unique stimulus a distinctive population of antibodies or immune cells is elicited. The specificity of the immune response provides an important clue regarding the nature of the antigen receptors on the antigen recognition cells. The receptor

Fig. 10-6. An electron microscope radioautograph of a primary lymph node follicle which includes a reticular cell (*R*) and several lymphocytes (*L*). The labeled antigen (*A*) is located within or near surface invaginations of the reticular cell membrane and in close proximity to the lymphocytes. This relationship of lymphocytes, reticular cells, and antigens is appealing as a site of immunization. (From G. J. V. Nossal, A. Abbot, J. Mitchell, and Z. Lummus, Antigens in Immunity: XV. Ultrastructural Features of Antigen Capture in Primary and Secondary Lymphoid Follicles, J Exp Med, 127:277, 1968.)

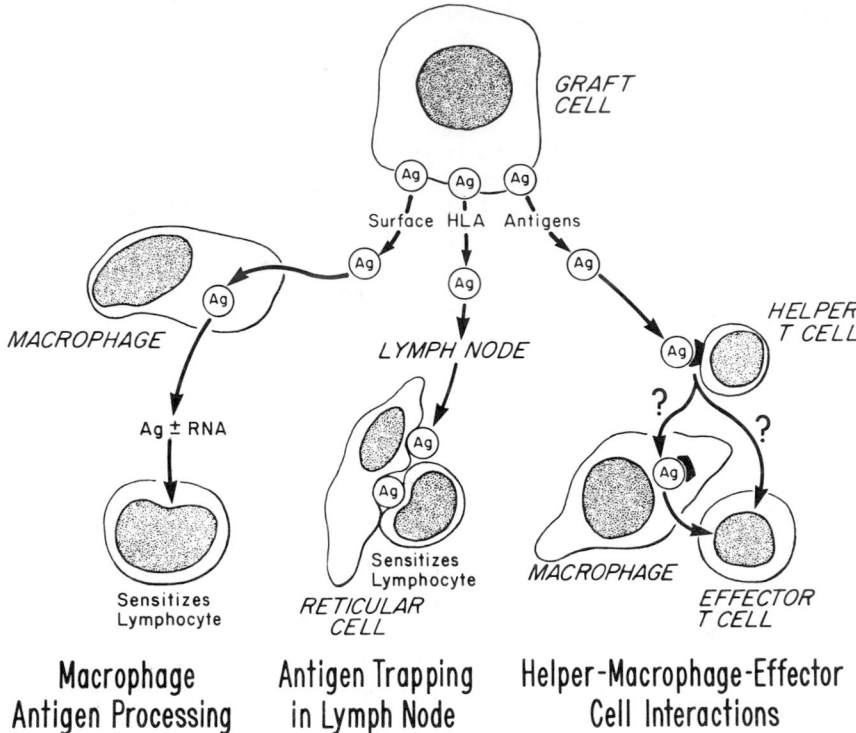

Macrophage Antigen Processing   **Antigen Trapping in Lymph Node**   **Helper-Macrophage-Effector Cell Interactions**

Fig. 10-7. Three possible mechanisms of antigen processing and presentation. Macrophages may first need to process the histocompatibility antigens and pass them in more immunogenic form to lymphocytes. The processing may or may not require the attachment of an RNA molecule. The antigen may not need to be internalized, however, and may need to be presented only on the surface of the lymph node reticular cells. This may facilitate sensitization of the lymphocytes. More recently, it has been found that maximum sensitization may require an even more complex interaction. In this scheme the antigen is first recognized by a helper T cell, which in turn may pass it to a macrophage for processing or directly to an effector T cell to produce sensitization. Some of these helper-macrophage–effector cell studies have utilized transplantation antigens, and these conclusions may be applicable to allograft immunity. It is clear, however, from the extensive experimental data that the cell-cell interactions involved are complex and not yet understood.

sites must be at least as discriminatory as the antibody-combining sites or the cellular recognition sites on hypersensitive cells. The presence of recognition molecules has been shown by (1) the ability of radioactive antigens to interfere with lymphocyte activation, (2) inhibition of hapten-sensitive cells by the haptens themselves, and (3) the removal of specific lymphocytes by passage through antigen-coated columns.

It is probable that the receptors on B lymphocytes are antibodies because immunoglobulins have been demonstrated on the cell surface. Furthermore, antisera to immunoglobulins will stimulate B cells, suggesting that the antibody combining with the recognition site immunoglobulin mimics the signal generated by antigen-antibody combination. The antigen-recognizing molecule on T cells has been more difficult to demonstrate. There is no question that T cells possess specific antigen receptors; it is their nature that is unclear. Several investigators have demonstrated evidence that at least portions of immunoglobulins are located on these surfaces and presumably they may contain the recognition sites.

How recognition molecules on either T or B cells are induced during lymphocyte development is unknown. Burnet's clonal selection theory proposes that clones of lymphocytes specifically reactive to an antigen arise, probably by somatic mutation, prior to any actual experience with the antigen itself. Thus, the lymphocytes are precommitted and equipped with recognition molecules to the antigen before the initial encounter with it. An alternative, and currently less favored, theory would have an instructional role for the antigen in the first exposure with the

individual's lymphocytes, with the recognition sites and sensitivity resulting from the encounter.

LYMPHOCYTE TRANSFORMATION. When lymphocytes encounter foreign alloantigens, the clones of cells precoded to these antigens respond in two essential ways—they proliferate and they differentiate into specifically sensitized cells either actively manufacturing antibody (B cells) or capable of inflicting damage directly to the foreign graft (T cells). The activation of resting small lymphocytes was first described by Scothorne and McGregor, who noted the cellular changes which occurred in the regional lymph nodes and spleen following the placement of skin allografts in the rabbit. In these nodes, large lymphoid cells appeared which stained heavily for ribonucleic acid. The supposition was that lymphoid cells had enlarged and transformed in response to allograft stimulation, and that the transformation involved RNA synthesis. Further investigation has uncovered a myriad of subcellular and molecular events that accompany this transformation. This is not surprising, for small lymphocytes are very inactive—as they await antigenic stimulation. Whatever the subgroup of T or B lymphocytes and whatever their response to the antigen, this transformation from resting to large, active cells seems necessary to further events.

CELL-CELL INTERACTIONS. The lymphocytes do not act individually in graft rejection. A great deal of cellular cooperation is required, and such cooperation is not confined to the enlistment of immunologically nonspecific cells such as macrophages, neutrophils, and platelets into the inflammatory response. It is becoming more certain that extensive lymphocyte-lymphocyte interaction is needed for the development of maximum lymphocyte proliferative and cytotoxic activity. The cooperation occurs both between subpopulations of T cells and between T and B cells. Many studies of cell-cell cooperation have used histocompatibility antigens to provide the immunological stimulus, indicating these mechanisms are operating in graft rejection.

The requirement for cooperation between T and B cells was established by showing that neither cell population alone could mount an immune response to certain antigens, whereas mixtures of the two cell types resulted in the production of high levels of antibody. Because B cells are the precursors of antibody-forming cells, and T cells do not synthesize readily detectable amounts of immunoglobulin, the T cells must serve as "helper cells" which assist B cells to differentiate into producers of antibody. Response to the major histocompatibility antigens requires this cooperation, and suspensions of B cells alone or lymphocytes from athymic mice in tissue culture will not effectively produce antibodies to these antigens unless T cells are added. Therefore, T-cell recognition of at least a portion of the antigen is necessary for the production of specific antibody by the B cell. Not all T cells can function in this role, only the subgroup of helper T cells (T_H). Production of IgG, IgE, and probably IgA also seems to require aid from T_H cells for full efficiency.

Just as T_H cells are necessary for B-cell antibody responses, other T_H cells are needed for the development of lymphocyte-mediated cytotoxicity. The lymphocytes that produce direct cytotoxicity are also T cells; effector (T_E) or killer cells. The T_H cell is required for the T_E cell to develop fully the capacity to inflict cell damage. Cell-associated histocompatibility antigens are prominent among the antigens that require T_H–T_E cell cooperation for induction of maximum cytotoxicity.

There is evidence that yet another T-cell subgroup can inhibit either the development of antibody-producing B cells or the generation of T_E cells. These regulatory lymphocytes have been called *suppressor T (T_S) cells.* The functional presence of suppressor cells has been demonstrated in a variety of in vitro experimental preparations but their role in modulating the immune response in general and allograft rejection in particular is incompletely understood. Nevertheless, suppressor cells offer considerable promise as a potential avenue to better immunosup-

pression. A schematic diagram of these several interactions is presented in Fig. 10-8.

The precise mechanisms by which cells interact are unknown but almost certainly quite complex. The collaboration could occur either (1) by direct contact and interaction of the involved cells in which the T_H cells focus and present antigen to either B cells or T_E cells of the appropriate specificity; or (2) by a mechanism in which the T_H cells release a molecule which can stimulate B cells or T_E cells. Among the uncertainties posed by these models are identifying which cells specifically recognize the antigen. Do the T_H, T_E, and B cells all precisely identify the same foreign antigen? Add to these interactions the apparent need for macrophages during the antigen-processing stage and the presence of one or more small molecules released by lymphocytes which either stimulate or suppress the reaction, and the complexity of the development of transplantation immunity is apparent.

One scheme for which there is good evidence has suggested that the T_H antigen receptors capture the antigens and both antigens and receptors are released for concentration on the surface of the macrophage. The concentrated antigen can then more efficiently stimulate either the B or T_E cells. In addition, soluble factors have been found released into the culture media which foster or hinder cellular cooperation and may serve as regulatory molecules. Much remains to be learned about these cell-cell interactions, and this scheme will certainly be heavily modified in the future. What is raised by this discussion are the roles of lymphocyte differentiation and proliferation in the development of allograft immunity.

LYMPHOCYTE DIFFERENTIATION AND PROLIFERATION. One of the most basic questions in cell biology is whether

Fig. 10-8. The development of specifically immune cells. The T-cell family is very active in these pathways, and helper T cells may be required to recognize the antigens for both B cells and other T cells. Following this recognition step and subsequent interaction with other lymphocytes, either cytotoxic killer T cells or antibody-producing B cells arise. The B-cell effect can be amplified by antibody attaching to other lymphocytes or macrophages. Specific immunity is thereby conferred on these antibody-directed cells. The development of immune cells is kept in check by either suppressor T cells or antibody providing feedback inhibition.

Allograft Rejection

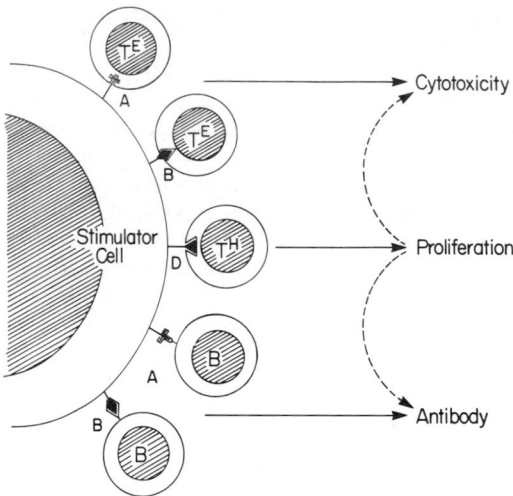

Fig. 10-9. The complexity of the antigen-cell relationships which occur during the development of allograft immunity. Helper T cells (T_H), which seem to be needed for maximal initial response to a foreign cell, respond to incompatible HLA-D antigens and begin to proliferate. The activated helper cells interact with other T cells or B cells to develop sensitized effector cells. Both the antibody-producing B cells or the cytotoxic T_E cells which result, however, develop their immunity against incompatible HLA-A or HLA-B antigens on the stimulator cell. Thus, lymphocytes proliferate in response to certain allogenic antigens and differentiate against other allogenic antigens on the graft cells. Effective immunity and graft rejection probably require both processes.

or not a cell must proliferate in order to differentiate further. Investigations into transplantation biology have not answered this question but have uncovered some surprising relationships between proliferation and differentiation in lymphocytes.

Dutton and Mishell have provided evidence that lymphoid differentiation to antibody-producing cells is accompanied by cellular proliferation. By combining assays indicative of DNA synthesis (uptake of tritiated thymidine) with an assay of antibody production by individual cells (Jerne plaque assay), they found virtually all the antibody-forming B cells had synthesized DNA. These results argue that production of antibodies, an example of cellular differentiation, also requires proliferation. At the end of the B-cell line is the plasma cell which has an abundance of rough endoplasmic reticulum engaged in the specialized production of antibody. Conversion from a transformed cell to a plasma cell is seen within a few days of grafting, in both organ allografts and the lymphoid tissues stimulated by these transplants. When the B cell proliferates, morphologic differentiation accompanies the proliferation, and the end result is a plasma cell busily engaged in making specific antibody.

The situation for T cells has proved to be a fascinating variation. The allogenic stimulation which occurs between two lymphocyte populations in MLC has become a standard model of the allo-immune response in vitro. The amount of immunogenic stimulation can be measured by the uptake of tritiated thymidine into DNA or by the

mitoses which soon follow. The ability of histocompatibility antigens on the surface of intact cells to stimulate lymphocyte proliferation is compelling evidence that similar cell activation occurs in vivo when an organ is allografted. Further investigation has yielded some surprising results, however. The T cell which proliferates most turns out to be the helper T cell (T_H), which recognizes the alloantigen but which develops little capacity to react against the foreign cells. The cell which differentiates and acquires the capability to inflict cytotoxic damage is the effector T cell (T_E), which undergoes relatively little proliferation. This has been best shown in mice, where the proliferating but noncytotoxic T_H cells bear one marker antigen (Ly 1) on their surface and the destructive but nondividing T_E cells have different (Ly 2,3) membrane antigens.

An analogous system almost certainly exists for human lymphocytes. Not only do the two cell types respond differently, but different antigens stimulate the T_H and T_E cells. The A and B loci of the HLA complex code for antigens which induce cytotoxicity, while the D antigens promote proliferation. It now appears that the precursor of the T_E cell has receptors for the A and B antigens, but when these antigens are mixed with a suspension of pure T_E cells proliferation of effector cells does not result. The helper T cell seems to be essential, but the T_H cell does not respond to A and B alloantigens; rather it requires a foreign D antigen to proliferate (Fig. 10-9). Thus T_E and T_H precursors respond to different alloantigens within the closely linked HLA complex, and different T-cell types appear to accomplish differentiation and proliferation. Differentiation requires proliferation, but quite unexpectedly they occur in different cells. In summary, lymphocyte differentiation and proliferation are complex subcellular events which are central to the development of transplantation immunity. Obviously, much remains to be learned about them, and the answers may be of considerable general biological importance.

EXPRESSION OF IMMUNITY: GRAFT DESTRUCTION

The recognition of antigens by sensitized cells or antibodies marks the beginning of the active effort of disposal of the foreign graft, but the reaction of an antibody, for example, with a graft antigen will not by itself destroy the graft. The recognition phase merely triggers the activation of several cascading enzyme systems, which include the complement, clotting, and probably the kinin pathways. In addition, a number of cellular mediators (macrophages, platelets, and polymorphonuclear leukocytes) are recruited, both as a consequence of the specific immunologic reaction itself and as a result of the subsequent enzymatic events. If the recognition molecule is on the surface of a cytotoxic T_E lymphocyte or an activated macrophage, destructive factors are released. Consequently, a variety of molecules and cells play an active role in disposing of the allograft. The efferent limb of the allograft reaction has both an immunologically specific (recognition) phase and an immunologically nonspecific (effector or amplification) phase.

ROLE OF SPECIFICALLY IMMUNIZED LYMPHOCYTES IN ALLOGRAFT REJECTION. The presence of inflammatory cells at the time and site of graft rejection has had a strong influence on immunobiologic thinking. The earliest and simplest explanation was that sensitized lymphocytes both recognized and destroyed the graft. Indeed, specifically sensitized T cells are present within most rejecting allografts and are capable of inflicting damage. It is only that their numbers do not seem capable of explaining the magnitude of the rejection reaction. It is more likely that a small number of specifically sensitized lymphoid cells initiate the rejection reaction but that the completion of the reaction requires many nonsensitized mononuclear cells, as well as PMNs, eosinophils, and plasma cells. Furthermore, there is convincing evidence that antibody can initiate graft destruction in the relative absence of a cellular reaction under appropriate circumstances.

In Vitro Lysis of Target Cells by Lymphocytes. The specifically sensitized lymphoid cells which collect at the site of an allograft have long been thought to damage the donor tissues directly. Recent in vitro studies support such a role for the specifically sensitized lymphocyte which can operate in the total absence of humoral antibody or complement. Direct contact between the sensitized lymphocyte and the target cell appears to be important. The ameboid lymphocyte contacts the target cells with its uropod and remains attached for 10 minutes. The lymphocyte then moves off, and 10 to 20 minutes later the target cells lyse.

Fig. 10-10. Activated (transformed) lymphocytes give off a variety of biologically active molecules (lymphokines). A number of properties have been ascribed to these lymphokines from cell culture experiments. These activities have obvious importance to allograft rejection. Chemotactic and migration inhibitory activity for macrophages and neutrophils, activating factors for lymphocytes, cytotoxicity for target cells, and vascular permeability factors all contribute to graft damage. What is not clear is how many kinds of molecules are involved; do a few have multiple properties?

The mechanism of cell membrane damage has not been identified, although several cytotoxic agents have been found which may be released by the lymphocytes. Such cytotoxic factors may well be the effector agents of cell-mediated immunity, but the specificity of the reaction in vitro favors the idea that interaction of cell surfaces is important to direct the damage of the target cell. The cytotoxic factors may be later released into the surroundings.

EFFECTOR MOLECULES (LYMPHOKINES) RELEASED BY ACTIVATED LYMPHOCYTES. The release of cytotoxic factors by lymphocytes infiltrating an allograft would be the most direct way to damage foreign cells, but probably not the most efficient since nonspecific cell killing would result. Several other kinds of molecules are released by specifically sensitized T cells, and these products or lymphokines serve to activate and enlist macrophages, polymorphonuclear leukocytes (PMNs), lymphocytes, etc., and thus amplify the initial cellular response. Several lymphokines have been identified, but it is not yet clear whether there is a small number of molecules with multiple functions or whether a different molecule is specific for each function. In Fig. 10-10 are depicted some of the best-studied lymphokines.

Macrophages seem to be very active participants in graft rejection; their role does not end with antigen processing. Two of the most investigated lymphokines, migration inhibitory factor (MIF) and chemotactic factor (CF), have similar properties and may be the same molecule. By attracting macrophages and then inhibiting their escape, the CF and MIF activities released by lymphocytes lead increased numbers of macrophages to the area. Another property of these factors, and perhaps of MIF itself, is macrophage activation. Macrophages resemble lymphocytes in that they have resting and activated states. In the later phase, the cytoplasm has the appearance of great activity, both morphologically and enzymatically. Phago-

UNSTIMULATED LYMPHOCYTES

Mitogenic, Transfer, and Antibody-producing Factors

Cytotoxic, Growth Inhibitory, and Vascular Permeability Factors

MACROPHAGES

Migration Inhibitory, Chemotactic, and Activating Factors

Chemotactic and Leukocyte Inhibitory Factors

TARGET CELLS

Transformed Lymphocyte *releases Lymphokines*

NEUTROPHILS

cytosis, pinocytosis, bacteriostatic, and tumoricidal activities are increased. Many enzymes, including the digestive enzymes found in lysosomes, are markedly elevated. Macrophages found at the site of graft rejection appear to be in the activated state and thus better able to participate (Fig. 10-11).

A host of other activities has been ascribed to the lymphokines. Neutrophils, basophils, and eosinophils are attracted by them. Growth inhibitory and cytotoxic activities against target cells have been described in vitro. Several apparent lymphokines affect lymphocytes themselves and can be shown under suitable experimental conditions to stimulate mitoses and increase antibody production. Transformed lymphocytes also release a vascular permeability factor in addition to the cytotoxic lymphokines. Little is known about the permeability factor(s) and its possible effect on an allograft rejection. Tissue edema is, however, a prominent feature of graft rejection, and it may join the vascular permeability factors released by complement activation and neutrophil and platelet participation in the efferent arc of rejection.

It is apparent that the lymphokines are only beginning to be understood. How many and by what mechanisms these factors operate are unknown. To date what little information is available has been gathered from in vitro systems, and their role in allograft rejection has yet to be determined—it seems that both the number and the activities will increase with further investigation.

RECRUITMENT OF SPECIFICALLY SENSITIZED CELLS. It is apparent that the few specifically sensitized cells which migrate to the site of the allograft cannot be totally responsible for graft death. Their effect is amplified both by the nonspecific lymphokines and by expansion of the specifically sensitized cells.

It is likely that the specifically immune cell, upon encountering the antigen which elicited its maturation, can recruit specifically sensitized cells from unsensitized lymphocytes in their environment. Among the antibody-producing population there is evidence that the number of active cells is expanded in this way. When the kinetics of plaque-forming (antibody-producing) cells were looked at in one experiment, more cells arose than could be accounted for by cell division. Recruitment of lymphocytes producing cellular hypersensitivity may be accomplished in several ways: A recognition molecule manufactured and released by the specifically sensitized cell could be attached to the cell surfaces of adjacent cells. Such factors would quickly convert lymphoid cells into specific cells which on encountering the antigen could transform and become metabolically active. The impressment of the cells in this manner would allow quick amplification of the number of sensitized cells.

One recognition molecule that could be transferred from lymphocyte to lymphocyte is specific antibody. Clark and Weiss showed that immunoglobulin synthesis of cultured and stimulated lymphocytes appeared simultaneously with their ability to inflict cellular damage. Cell-bound or cytophilic antibody released in the presence of unsensitized lymphocytes does adhere to those lymphocytes. It has not yet been established, however, that cytophilic antibody can enlarge the lymphocyte population specifically sensitized to an allograft.

A second recognition molecule which may expand the sensitized cell population is the transfer factor described by Lawrence. Transfer factor is dialyzable material of less than 10,000 molecular weight which can be extracted from specifically sensitized lymphocytes, and will convert previously unsensitized lymphocytes to a specific antigen-responsive state both in vitro and in vivo. When the converted lymphocytes are subsequently exposed to the specific

Fig. 10-11. Macrophages are stimulated by products of an immune reaction, which include lymphokines, to participate actively in graft rejection. A variety of macrophage functions and cellular parameters have been shown to be increased by activation. Clearly the ability of these cells to contribute to allograft rejection is enhanced by these stimulatory factors.

Lymphokines $\left\{\begin{array}{l}\text{CIF} \\ \text{MIF} \\ \text{AF}\end{array}\right\}$ CIRCULATING INACTIVE MACROPHAGE

Site of Rejection Reaction

ACTIVATED MACROPHAGE

Increased Functions	Increased Cell Components
Phagocytosis	Metabolic Enzymes
Pinocytosis	Membrane Synthesis
Adherence	Lysosomal Enzymes
Cytotoxicity	Adenylate Cyclase

antigen, they will transform and proliferate. Transfer factor itself appears not to be an immunoglobulin but has a polypeptide-polynucleotide composition, although it is resistant to pancreatic ribonuclease (RNase). Transfer factor may act as a transmitter of immunologic information. Much controversy revolves around its presence and nature, however, and some writers regard it as transferred antigen or question its importance in allograft rejection.

Another potential mechanism for recruitment of specifically sensitized cells would be by transfer of the information needed to produce recognition molecules. In addition to the possible role of RNA in the transfer of processed antigenic information from macrophage to lymphocyte, RNA from sensitized cells may enlist other lymphocytes into specific immunity. Mannick and Egdahl were the first to extract RNA from the nodes of rabbits immunized to skin allografts. This RNA fraction conferred the capacity to produce transfer reactions on normal lymphoid cells when they were injected into the skin of the graft donor. In later experiments, they demonstrated that rabbit spleen cells exposed in vitro to RNA extracted from the lymph nodes of immune rabbits would sensitize isogenic rabbits to subsequent grafts from the skin donor. These RNA extracts would confer sensitivity to the immunizing antigen on lymph node cells as measured by the ability to inhibit the migration of macrophages or the production of delayed skin hypersensitivity.

The obvious conclusion has been that the transfer and incorporation of a messenger RNA (mRNA) will establish immunity in lymphoid cells. Although these experiments suggest such a conclusion, more understanding of the development of immunity at the molecular level will be needed before it can be established. In addition, it has not been shown that the RNA comes from lymphocytes. The RNA could be from macrophages.

The recruitment, or horizontal expansion, of sensitized cells is an appealing concept, and certain evidence suggests it may be true; however, it has not been established for

immunity in general, and its role in the allograft reaction is unknown.

ROLE OF ANTIBODY IN ALLOGRAFT REJECTION. Any discussion of the role of humoral antibody in the rejection of allografted tissues should take into consideration two recognized facts: First, circulating antibody is not an obligatory participant in the rejection of solid tissue allografts. In fact, the inability to make an immunoglobulin of any recognizable type does not preclude graft rejection. Animals incapable of making antibody (neonatally bursectomized chickens or bursectomized irradiated chickens) can still reject allografts. Agammaglobulinemic fetal sheep were also found to be capable of rejecting skin allografts even in the presence of heterologous antisheep immunoglobulins.

Second, humoral antibody provides only the recognition portion of graft rejection and tends to be obscured by the effector mechanisms it activates. Unlike cell-mediated immunity, where the recognition system is intimately associated with the destruction of the target, humoral antibody must activate other systems in order to effect cell death.

Even during the early days of organ transplantation it was known that antibodies are formed in concert with allograft rejection. It was initially concluded, however, that antibodies were formed in association with rejection but were not of great functional significance. There is now no doubt that rejection can be mediated by alloantibodies—especially the rejection of vascularized organ allografts.

Effector Pathways and Their Amplification: Antibody-induced Molecular Cascade Systems. Although antibodies bind to allografts, such binding is of no consequence by itself, and the antibody would probably be cleared during the course of normal cell membrane repair. The combination of antibody with the antigen produces an active complex, which triggers a number of nonspecific effector pathways (Fig. 10-12). Each effector pathway typically consists of a sequential activation of enzymes which attract and hold active cells, produce vascular permeability, release enzymes capable of degrading cell surfaces and other pro-

ANTIBODY STRUCTURE

Fig. 10-12. Structure of the IgG antibody molecule. V_H and V_L are the variable portions of the heavy and light chains, respectively, and together they form the antigen-combining site. C_L is the constant portion of the light chain. CH_1, CH_2, and CH_3 are the subunits forming the invariable area of the heavy chain. The approximate positions of the inter- and intrachain disulfide bridges are shown. [From J. E. Foker, R. L. Simmons, and J. S. Najarian, Allograft Rejection: I. The Induction of Immunity: The Afferent Arc, in J. S. Najarian and R. L. Simmons (eds.), "Transplantation," p. 63, Lea & Febiger, Philadelphia, 1972.]

teins, release factors causing smooth muscle contraction, and precipitate the formation of fibrin clots.

The immunologic response can be therefore both efficient and discriminatory. Relatively few specifically differentiated cells can produce molecules that will perform the recognition function. Since few cells are committed to each antigen, many more antigens can be discriminated. The antibodies in turn initiate a relatively general effector mechanism which can destroy the graft.

THE COMPLEMENT SYSTEM. The combination of antibody (of IgG_1, IgG_2, IgG_3, or IgM classes) with antigen changes the conformation of the antibody molecule. Included in this change is the activation of a site on the constant (Fc) end of the antibody molecule, which then triggers the complement pathway, is initiated by antigen-antibody complexes, and is presumably of greatest importance in rejection reactions. The alternate (properdin) pathway can be set off by the immunologically nonspecific serum proteins of the properdin system reacting with sugar structures found on bacterial surfaces and conceivably mammalian cells, or perhaps by combining with certain antibodies; its role in graft rejection, however, is unknown. The components of both pathways are circulating protein molecules which, when activated, react in a sequential fashion. At present, the system is known to be made up of at least 15 (11 classical, 4 alternate) chemically and immunologically distinct molecules which are capable of interacting with one another, with antibody, and with cell membranes, for the C1 to C5 components acquire enzymatic activity after interaction with the previous factor. Once activated they can act enzymatically on the next molecule in the sequence which serves as the inactive substrate. Components C6 to C9 are nonenzymatic and bind to the previous components, resulting in conformational and activity changes.

Most of the biologically significant activities of the complement system arise during activation of the last six react-

ing complement components, C3 and C5 through C9 (Fig. 10-13). The two parallel but entirely independent initial pathways—the classical and the alternate pathways—converge at the C3 component, and the remainder of the reaction sequence, involving the reactions of C5 through C9, is common to both pathways. Both lead to activation of the terminal, biologically important portion of the sequence. The terminal portion of the complement sequence may also be directly activated by certain noncomplement serum and cellular enzymes without participation of the early reaction factors. For example, fibrinolytic enzymes in plasma and certain lysosomal enzymes will activate the C3 and C5 stages.

The classical complement pathway (Fig. 10-13) appears to be the most important for immune reactions. Three biologic consequences of complement activation are most important in transplantation rejection. (1) Complement has been shown to be capable of mediating lytic destruction of many kinds of cells to which antibodies have bound. The active components are in the C8 and C9 complexes, but the mechanism of lysis is not clear; perhaps enzymatic activity of the complex damages the membrane directly. (2) Many kinds of cells possess receptors for the C3b or C4b (activated) components, including B lympho-

Fig. 10-13. The complement pathways and the biological activity released at each step. The classical pathway begins with a specific antigen-antibody reaction. The properdin pathway is triggered by a more nonspecific interaction between cell surfaces and the molecules which comprise the properdin systems. Both pathways, however, converge at the C3 step, where most of the biological activity associated with complement activation begins. Amplification also occurs at several steps, but it is greatest at C3. The subsequent steps lead to the molecular condensation on the target cell surface, which ultimately results in membrane damage and lysis. There are several other important consequences of complement activation. The presence of these molecules on the target cell surface makes them adherent to other cells. Macrophages, platelets, polymorphonuclear leukocytes, and lymphocytes adhere and increase the damage to the graft cells. The steps through C5 are largely enzymatic in nature; the C3 and C5 components, for example, are split during activation, releasing chemotactic and vasoactive (anaphylatoxins) molecules. Attachment of the C5b molecule to the cell begins the condensation ending in membrane damage; this seems to occur away from the immune complex. Interaction of the C6,C7 components results, additionally, in the release of another chemotactic factor. The activation of the complement pathway, therefore, contributes to many of the features seen in allograft rejection; cellular infiltrates, adherent PMNs and platelets, thrombosed vessels, interstitial edema, and cellular damage.

Cell Ag + Ab ⟶ Active Immune Complex (I^*)

C1q + C1r + C1s ⟶ I^*C1 (Recognition of I^* by C1q)

C4 ⟶ I^*C14 (Adherence to target cell)

C2 ⟶ I^*C142 (Kinin-like activity)

C3 ⟶ I^*C1423b (Amplification, adherence to lymphocytes, PMNs, macrophages) + 3a (Anaphylatoxin)

Certain cell surfaces and antibodies

Properdin System

C5 ⟶ I^*C14235b (Begin membrane attack) + 5a (Anaphylatoxin, chemotaxis)

C67 ⟶ Cell-C567 (Chemotaxis)

C8 ⟶ Cell-C5-8 (Slow membrane damage)

C9 ⟶ Cell-C5-9 (Rapid cell lysis)

cytes, neutrophils, monocytes, and macrophages. If C3b or C4b attach to a damaged cell they may act as opsonins, bringing the target cells in contact with the phagocytic macrophages and monocytes or exposing the surface antigens of these cells to B lymphocytes. (3) Many of the complement cleavage products have biologic actions of their own. For example, C4a and C2b act as kinins. C3a has chemotactic activity for polymorphonuclear leukocytes, causes the release of histamine from mast cells (anaphylatoxin activity), has a kinin activity, and causes immune adherence. C5a is a very potent chemotactic factor, stimulates histamine release from mast cells, and liberates lysosomes from polymorphonuclear leukocytes. Therefore, the complement activation releases kinins which increase vascular permeability, leading to edema; attracts polymorphonuclear leukocytes which release other vasoactive compounds and lysosomal enzymes; encourages phagocytosis of damaged tissue; releases lysosomal enzymes from macrophages; opsonizes cells; binds cells to damaged cell surfaces (immune adherence); and leads to cell death.

An important biological characteristic of the complement system, as well as the other cascade systems discussed in this section, is that they are capable of self-amplification. Thus, in one study 450 C4 molecules were found fixed to each sensitized sheep red blood cell, but each erythrocyte had approximately 100,000 C3 components on its surface. In addition, the C3 components were distributed over the cell membrane surface, rather than confined to the site of the antigen-antibody combination, thus enlarging the area of effect. Although this step produces the greatest numerical amplification, other steps in the complement pathway also expand the number of active molecules.

THE CLOTTING SYSTEM. Theoretically the deposition of fibrin in the allografted organ may arise in two ways: The first, the so-called *extrinsic pathway* of thrombin formation, requires tissue thromboplastin to initiate the sequence of events. The release of this cellular substance may follow

damage to the endothelial cell membranes either by antibody and complement or through the direct cytotoxic effect of lymphocytes. The activation of complement through C_3 would also promote the adherence of platelets which, in turn, would stimulate platelet retraction and release of platelet phospholipids. These phospholipids have been shown to promote clotting.

The second method of inducing clot formation, the *intrinsic pathway,* has the potential to be activated directly by immunologic reaction. In the intrinsic pathway, Hageman factor (factor XII) begins a sequence which proceeds through factors XI, IX, VII, and V to the activation of prothrombin factor to form thrombin with the eventual polymerization of fibrin. Antigen-antibody complexes will activate Hageman factor to trigger this cascade and produce clotting in vitro in the absence of platelets. Thus, an entry into the intrinsic pathway is present within the interactions of antigens and antibodies (Fig. 10-14).

As the reaction proceeds and tissue damage is produced, tissue thromboplastin is released, collagen fibers are exposed, and clotting is facilitated. It is now generally hypothesized that the progressive obliterative vascular reaction of a chronically rejecting allograft is a by-product of fibrin laid down along endothelium that has been damaged by immune mechanisms.

THE KININ SYSTEM. The kinin or killikrein system is initiated by activation of coagulation factor XII, leading eventually to the formation of kallikrein, which acts on kininogen, an alpha-globulin substrate in the plasma, and results in bradykinin. Bradykinin is one of the kinins, a group of active peptides which are rather rapidly inactivated, after formation, by kininases present in plasma. The kinins possess a variety of biological activities, including chemotaxis of PMNs, smooth muscle contraction, dilatation of peripheral arterioles, and increase of capillary permeability. The involvement of the kinin system in graft rejection is likely but is as yet unproved.

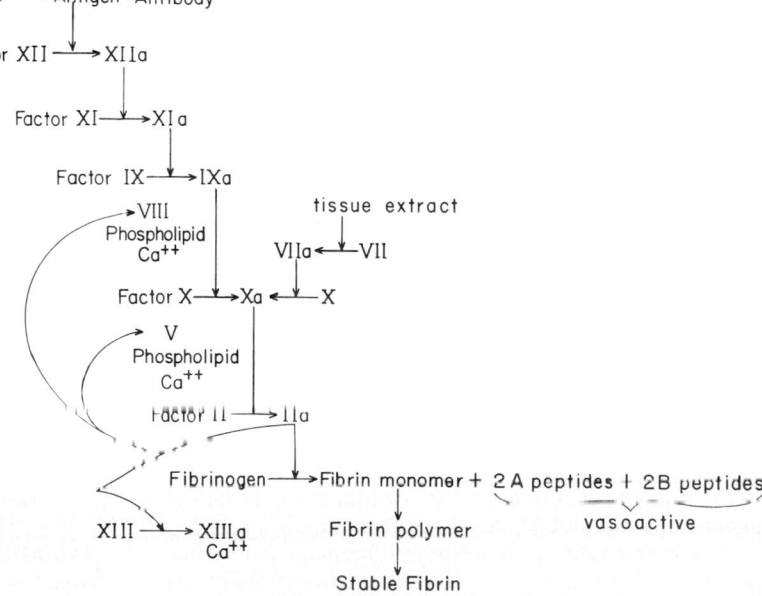

Fig. 10-14. The coagulation cascade system. Fibrin and two vasoactive peptides are the final products of the cascade. The two modes of activation of the system are diagrammed. Factor XII (Hageman factor) can be activated by immune complexes initiating the "intrinsic pathway." Tissue damage (presumably produced by immunologic damage) could precipitate the extrinsic system. In both systems, the factors shown, with the probable exceptions of V and VIII, are enzymes. Activation of the pathways involves the sequential conversions of these enzymes to active forms (reproduced by XIIa, XIa, etc). [From J. S. Najarian and J. E. Foker, Allograft Rejection: II. The Expression of Immunity: The Efferent Arc, in J. S. Najarian and R. L. Simmons (eds.), "Transplantation," p. 94, Lea & Febiger, Philadelphia, 1972.]

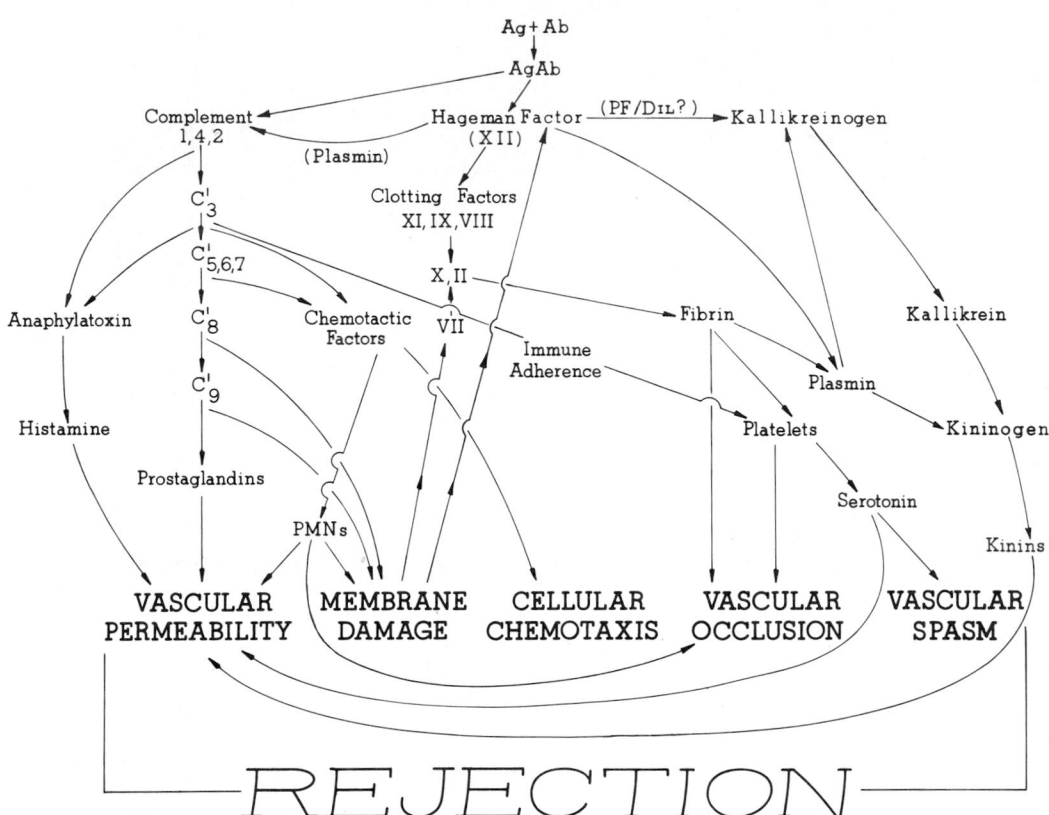

RECOGNITION

Ag + Ab

AgAb

Complement 1,4,2 ← AgAb — Hageman Factor (XII) —(PF/DIL?)→ Kallikreinogen

(Plasmin)

C'$_3$

Clotting Factors XI, IX, VIII

C'$_{5,6,7}$

X, II

Anaphylatoxin   C'$_8$ Chemotactic Factors   VII   Immune Adherence   Fibrin   Kallikrein

Histamine   C'$_9$ Plasmin

Platelets   Kininogen

Prostaglandins   Serotonin

PMNs   Kinins

VASCULAR PERMEABILITY   **MEMBRANE DAMAGE**   **CELLULAR CHEMOTAXIS**   **VASCULAR OCCLUSION**   **VASCULAR SPASM**

REJECTION

INTERRELATIONSHIPS OF THE MOLECULAR CASCADE SYSTEMS

(Fig. 10-15). Antigen-antibody complexes activate complement and Hageman factor. Hageman factor in turn produces clotting, activates plasmin, and perhaps directly activates complement. Plasmin in turn can activate C_3 to produce, among other effects, chemotactic factors, immune adherence, and opsonization. Activation of Hageman factor also leads to kinin production. Activation of the complement system produces aggregation of platelets and, consequently, initiation of the clotting mechanism. Thrombin formation, in turn, stimulates the production of plasmin from plasminogen. Prostaglandin activity is released following complement activation, and may contribute to vascular permeability, although the significance of this in allograft rejection remains unclear.

Not only are the activators of these systems interrelated, but also the inhibitors are intertwined. The C_1 esterase inhibitor also decreases the activity of the kinin and plasmin systems. Neither activation nor inhibition of one system can occur without affecting the other pathways.

The complexity of the allograft reaction is just beginning to be understood. Not only does it involve a variety of recognition molecules (antibodies) and presumably a similar variety of specifically sensitized cells; there is much recent evidence that unsensitized lymphocytes can be specifically directed and actively lyse target allogenic cells by a coating with antibody. In addition, the main force of the reaction may be produced by a bewildering array of am-

Fig. 10-15. Integration of the humoral amplification system in graft rejection. This diagram suggests the complexity of allograft rejection. The three main cascade pathways—complement, clotting, and kinin—generate many active molecules, including the kinins, chemotactic factors, anaphylatoxins, histamine, and serotonin. These molecules, together with platelets and polymorphonuclear leukocytes (PMNs), produce the destructive effects on the graft. The most prominent consequences include increased vascular permeability (edema), spasm, and occlusion as well as cell and basement membrane damage and cellular chemotaxis (infiltration). It is clear that these systems do not operate singly but tend to activate each other. Not shown are the many interlocking inhibitory factors that keep these systems in check once they are activated. [*From J. S. Najarian and J. E. Foker, Allograft Rejection: II. The Expression of Immunity: The Efferent Arc, in J. S. Najarian and R. L. Simmons (eds.), "Transplantation," p. 94, Lea & Febiger, Philadelphia, 1972.*]

plifying chain reactions which include both molecular amplification schemes and cellular amplifiers. The activation of complement, the clotting system, kinin formation, and the stimulation of PMN, macrophages, and platelet assault produce a variety of damage to the transplanted organ. Included are occlusive phenomena within the graft vessels, induced permeability of these same vessels with interstitial edema accumulation, disruption of cellular basement membranes, and the infiltration of the graft with a profusion of cell types (Fig. 10-15).

AN INTEGRATED VIEW OF THE REJECTION OF ORGAN ALLOGRAFTS.
Rejection morphology has two main components: The first component is the host response, and it is

Fig. 10-16. Canine renal allograft 48 hours after transplantation into unmodified recipient. Round cell infiltration, usually the first overt sign of host activity against the allograft, is apparent within 6 to 12 hours after transplantation. By 48 hours the number of invading cells is substantial. The original perivascular infiltrate has surrounded a glomerulus and adjacent tubules. [From J. E. Foker and J. S. Najarian, Allograft Rejection: III. The Pathobiology of Organ Rejection, in J. S. Najarian and R. L. Simmons (eds.), "Transplantation," p. 122, Lea & Febiger, Philadelphia, 1972.]

composed of effector cells and molecules, both immunologically specific and nonspecific. In rapid rejections these comprise most, if not all, of the pathologic picture so that the speed of the reaction virtually precludes response by the organ cells. The second component becomes prominent only with longer survival of the transplanted organ and encompasses the various morphologic alterations of the organs. In fact, the responses of these cells can form an important part of the pathologic picture.

A predictable series of events ensues when an unsensitized patient is allografted. The first visible change is a perivascular infiltration of round cells accomplished by migration through the cytoplasm of the endothelial cells (Fig. 10-16). The accumulation of cells is not significant for several hours after transplantation but can reach considerable numbers within 24 hours. This delay suggests that although the immunogenicity of the graft may be a sufficient stimulus to transmigration by the lymphoid cells, transformation of the host cells or other cellular events must transpire before migration occurs. The confrontation between graft and host immunocompetent cells may be important in the development of this infiltrate.

The temporal aspects have been best worked out for the kidney, but the sequence appears to be the same for most organs. During the first 48 hours following grafting the number of infiltrating cells continues to increase. The original enclaves around small vessels spread, and the interstitial space is further infiltrated. A potpourri of cells accumulates: cells resembling small lymphocytes are seen, as well as large transformed lymphocytes with basophilic cytoplasm. Large histiocytes or macrophages are just beginning to arrive in numbers. Plasma cells are still relatively scarce: as a terminal product of cellular differentiation, they may require several cell divisions before they appear in the organ (Fig. 10-17).

Antibody and complement are deposited in the area of the capillaries, and some of the infiltrating lymphoid cells are producing immunoglobulins by the third day. Recognition molecules (antibody) as well as sensitized cells are therefore present early in the allograft reaction.

Sensitized lymphoid cells, upon recognizing the foreign tissue, release several mediators of inflammation and cell damage. The release of cytotoxic factors directly injures membranes of adjacent cells. Mitogenic products stimulate division of lymphoid cells, perhaps expanding the immunocompetent population. Activated, phagocytic macrophages are effectively concentrated in the area by migration inhibitory factor and other chemotactic factors. In addition vascular permeability agents are released.

Meanwhile, complement is fixed, thereby producing chemotactic factors, anaphylatoxins, and finally cellular damage when the terminal components are activated. Capillary permeability is increased by anaphylatoxins from the complement chain and probably by kinins. Interstitial edema becomes prominent. At the same time there are several additional inducements to cellular infiltration. The complement cascade generates molecules which produce immune adherence and others which have chemotactic activity. Damaged cells release additional compounds which contribute to infiltration by PMNs as well as other cells. PMNs in turn release vasoactive amines (including histamine or serotonin, depending on the species) and

Fig. 10-17. Canine renal allograft 4 days after transplantation into an unmodified recipient. Invading cells all but obscure the architecture of the kidney. Numerous mitoses (circles) can be found, and this cellular proliferation may be producing immunologically competent cells within the graft. A plasma cell (arrow) is present, but most of the cells resemble lymphocytes and macrophages. [*From J. E. Foker and J. S. Najarian, Allograft Rejection: III. The Pathobiology of Organ Rejection, in J. S. Najarian and R. L. Simmons (eds.) "Transplantation," p. 122, Lea & Febiger, Philadelphia, 1972.*]

additional vascular permeability–promoting factors. The PMNs squeeze through the enlarged endothelial cell junctions and release proteolytic cathepsins D and E, causing basement membrane damage.

Fibrin, and α-macroglobulins, whose contribution is not understood, are deposited by 7 days. During this time, lymphoid cells have continued to accumulate and, joined by significant numbers of plasma cells and PMNs, obscure the normal architecture. The round cell population presumably contains many macrophages and other immunologic nonspecific cells at this point. Increasingly frequent mitoses may indicate the production of immunocompetent cells within the graft.

The small vessels become plugged with fibrin and platelets, diminishing the perfusion and preventing function. In this relatively rapid sequence of events the organ has little chance to respond, and the pathologic process is dominated by the host effector pathways.

Obviously, rejection modified by immunosuppressive agents is not a distinct morphologic classification but is only a continuation of the events comprising the rejection reaction. The morphologic features associated with this more chronic rejection become dominated by the response of the organ tissue itself. Here the normal response of tissue to injury predominates in the pathologic picture. A good deal of endothelial cell damage occurs in the allograft, and the responses of cellular repair, hypertrophy and hyperplasia, follow.

Endothelial cell damage also elicits repair processes. Aggregations of platelets within the intimal layer are resolved, and the dissolution of the thrombi is accompanied by the infiltration of macrophages and foam cells. The result is a thickened intimal layer with the loss of smooth endothelial lining and the presence of vacuolated cells. The lumen narrows as a result. Narrowing of the

vessel lumen is also a consequence of the medial thickening. Studies using nonimmunologic disease models have shown that most of the cells proliferating in response to the stimulus of injury are smooth muscle cells. A reasonable extrapolation is that hyperplasia of these cells produces much of the lumenal narrowing in the allograft (Fig. 10-18).

Although the exposed position of the endothelial cells and the striking proliferation of the smooth muscle cells argue for their being an important target of the immune reaction, there is evidence that the basement and elastic membranes of the vessel absorb a major portion of immune-mediated damage. Either immune complexes or antibodies to the vascular basement membrane activate complement and attract polymorphonuclear cells. These nonspecific effector cells release at least four protein factors which increase the permeability of the vessel and in addition produce cathepsins D and E, which digest basement membranes. The PMNs are active in reaching the basement membrane and will lift the endothelial cells to gain this access.

Platelets may be of greater significance than PMNs in mediating damage. Immune complexes (which activate complement) will result in platelet adherence and the release of vasoactive substances. Platelet aggregation leads to the release of histamine, serotonin, and other capillary permeability factors which expose more basement membrane; the exposed collagen fibers of the basement mem-

Fig. 10-18. A rejected human allograft removed 18 months post-transplant. The lumen of the arteriole has all but disappeared as a consequence of hyperplasia of the cells of the vessel. Most of the thickening of the wall is probably due to proliferation of smooth muscle cells, with spindle-shaped nuclei. Endothelial cells, with rounder nuclei, almost fill the lumen. [*From J. E. Foker and J. S. Najarian, Allograft Rejection: III. The Pathobiology of Organ Rejection, in J. S. Najarian and R. L. Simmons (eds.), "Transplantation," p. 122, Lea & Febiger, Philadelphia, 1972.*]

brane further enhance platelet aggregation. Platelets and PMNs drawn to these sites release cathepsins, elastases, and phosphatases which increase destruction and attract other nonspecific cellular effectors including macrophages.

The myocardial cell is the characteristic cell of the heart, the tubular cell of the kidney, the acinar and islet cell of the pancreas, etc. The differentiation and function of these cells demand an ample oxygen supply and if destroyed they cannot be replaced by further cellular division. Therefore, compromise of respiration by vascular endothelial and medial hypertrophy, intravascular aggregations of platelets, and interstitial accumulations of edema and mononuclear cells will have predictable consequences for these cells. They will atrophy, and death may be followed by replacement fibrosis (Fig. 10-19).

The interstitial area concomitantly increases in size. The interstitial area, however, has much activity in its own right. Repair of immunologic damage stimulates many fibroblastic cells to proliferate, and it attracts macrophages. The persisting immunogenic capacity of the allograft is indicated by the inevitable presence of infiltrating plasma cells and lymphoid cells.

It is impossible to determine what proportions of these effects result from ischemia produced by vascular occlusion, interstitial edema, or cellular infiltrates. Similarly, the contribution made by the direct cytotoxic action of specific and nonspecific effector cells and molecules is unknown.

CIRCUMVENTING REJECTION

Clinical Immunosuppression

Theoretically, there are nine methods by which the allograft rejection response can be suppressed: (1) destroying the immunocompetent cells prior to transplantation, (2) making the antigen unrecognizable or even toxic to the reactive lymphocyte clones, (3) interfering with antigen processing by the recipient cells, (4) inhibiting lymphocyte transformation and proliferation, (5) limiting lymphocyte differentiation into killer or antibody-synthesizing cells, (6) activating sufficient numbers of suppressor lymphocytes, (7) inhibiting destruction of graft cells by killer lymphocytes, (8) interfering with the combination of immunoglobulins with target antigens, or (9) preventing tissue damage by the nonspecific cells and molecules that are activated by sensitized cells or antigen-antibody complexes.

In practice, clinically useful immunosuppression largely depends on the destruction or elimination of the immunocompetent cells and on inhibiting the differentiation and proliferation of these cells. Methods of inducing specific immune tolerance by various antigen preparations prior to grafting, or by inhibiting sensitized cells and antibodies once they have been produced, have not been clinically successful. Furthermore, it is more difficult to inhibit the immune response after it is underway, and less clinical effect can be gained after sensitization has occurred. To be most effective, immunosuppression must be present at the time of transplantation, or even before. Nevertheless, some success can be achieved in reversing the exacerbations of the rejection reaction seen in clinical transplantation. Lesser, but still significant, benefits have also resulted from

Fig. 10-19. Extensive damage to this small artery in a human renal allograft removed 14 months posttransplant is apparent. The elastic membranes are badly frayed, and the elastica interna has been destroyed entirely along half the circumference of the vessel. The intimal layer shows extensive disruption and loss of cells. The cells remaining are often vacuolated. The lumen is narrowed by tissue from several origins: proliferation of smooth muscle cells in the media, endothelial cell swelling and hyperplasia, and the presence of an organized thrombus. The adventitial area shows damage and edema formation. Note also that severe tubular atrophy and interstitial fibrosis are present. [*From J. E. Foker and J. S. Najarian, Allograft Rejection: III. The Pathobiology of Organ Rejection, in J. S. Najarian and R. L. Simmons (eds.), "Transplantation," p. 122, Lea & Febiger, Philadelphia, 1972.*]

inhibiting such immunologically nonspecific cells as platelets.

The true complexity of immune rejection is only beginning to be revealed, but many potential points for inhibition have already been exposed. At this time, however, a similar complexity does not exist in clinical immunosuppression. Virtually all clinical transplantation immunosuppression regimens include azathioprine, steroids, radiation, and antilymphocyte antibodies. Agents which are occasionally used or are purely experimental will be presented more briefly.

ANTIPROLIFERATIVE AGENTS

Most of the commonly used immunosuppressive agents, including antimetabolites, alkylating agents, toxic antibiotics, and x-rays, have been borrowed from cancer chemotherapy for their antiproliferative activity. They inhibit the full expression of the immune response by preventing the differentiation and division of the immunocompetent lymphocyte after it encounters the antigen. The plethora of investigational immunosuppressive drugs has been reduced to a few for clinical use. All of them, however, fall into one of two broad mechanistic categories. Either they structurally resemble needed metabolites or they combine with certain cellular components, such as DNA, and thereby interfere with cell function.

The former group, the antimetabolites, have a structural similarity to cell metabolites and either inhibit enzymes of that metabolic pathway or are incorporated during synthesis to produce faulty molecules. The antimetabolites include purine, pyrimidine, and folic acid analogs, which are most effective against proliferating and differentiating cells. They are given at the time of transplantation when the immunocompetent cells are first stimulated, and then

for the life of the graft to interfere with the continuing stimulus to the immune system.

Alkylating agents and certain antibiotics include those compounds which combine with DNA and other cellular components. Although these agents would be useful in the pretransplant period to reduce the number of effective immunocompetent cells in the recipients, and thereafter to prevent proliferation, they are so toxic that their use has been limited to bone marrow transplantation and as occasional substitutes for azathioprine.

PURINE ANALOGUES. The purine analogue azathioprine (AZ) (Imuran) is the most widely used immunosuppressive drug in clinical organ transplantation. Azathioprine is 6-mercaptopurine (6-MP) plus a side chain to protect the labile sulfhydryl group. In the liver, the side chain is split off to form the active compound, 6-MP. The mechanism of action would seem to be similar for these two compounds; however, azathioprine seems to enjoy the advantage of slightly lower toxicity.

Full metabolic activity comes in the cell with the addition of ribose 5-phosphate from phosphoribosyl pyrophosphate to form 6-MP ribonucleotide. The structural resemblance of this molecule to inosine monophosphate is obvious, and 6-MP ribonucleotide inhibits the enzymes that begin to convert inosine nucleotide to adenosine and guanosine monophosphate (Fig. 10-20). In addition, the presence of 6-MP ribonucleotides slows the entire purine biosynthetic pathway by fraudulent feedback inhibition of an early step. The steric similarity to either adenosine or guanine nucleotides is not great enough to allow significant incorporation into DNA or RNA and synthesis of faulty molecules. The result of inhibiting these several enzymes, however, is to block the synthesis of cellular RNA, DNA, certain cofactors, and other active nucleotides.

Fig. 10-20. Mechanism of antimetabolite action. 6-Mercaptopurine (6-MP) ribonucleotide resembles inosine monophosphate in its steric configuration. It thereby competes with inosine in its transformation into adenosine monophosphate and guanosine monophosphate and their subsequent incorporation into RNA and DNA. In addition, 6-MP inhibits the purine biosynthetic pathway, since it resembles a product of that biosynthetic pathway (feedback inhibition). [From R. L. Simmons, J. E. Foker, and J. S. Najarian, Principles of Immunosuppression, in D. C. Sabiston, Jr. (ed.), "Davis-Christopher Textbook of Surgery," p. 471, W. B. Saunders Company, Philadelphia, 1972.]

The biologic activity of azathioprine and 6-MP is greatest when nucleic acid synthesis is most required. They will inhibit the development of both humoral and cellular primary immunity by interfering with the differentiation and proliferation of the responding lymphocytes. The inhibition of nucleic acid synthesis by azathioprine is most effective in these rapidly replicating cells. Once expansion of fully immunocompetent cells has been completed, nucleic acid synthesis is less important and the drug is less effective. The benefit of azathioprine may also result from a reduction of neutrophil production and macrophage activation. This effect would reduce the nonspecific inflammatory aspect of the immune reaction.

The toxicity of azathioprine results from the same mechanisms. The primary toxic effect of azathioprine is bone marrow suppression, leading to leukopenia. Again, it is the antiproliferative effect of inhibiting nucleic acid synthesis that affects this rapidly dividing cell population. Liver toxicity can also result, possibly because of the high rate of RNA synthesis by these cells, but because hepatic dysfunction does not seem to be dose-related, the mechanism is unclear.

PYRIMIDINE ANALOGUES. Although pyrimidine analogues have been studied extensively as immunosuppressants in the laboratory, they have had only limited clinical use. The structure of 5-bromodeoxyuridine resembles thymidine, and it is incorporated into DNA (Fig. 10-21). Once incorporated, however, it does not have the precision in base pairing that thymidine has, and subsequent synthesis of DNA and RNA is defective. Although 5-bromodeoxyuridine will prolong animal skin grafts and act in synergy with antilymphocyte globulin, its clinical use is untested.

Another pyrimidine analogue, cytosine arabinoside, also inhibits DNA synthesis and, therefore, the proliferative phase of the immune response. This molecule has an altered sugar moiety and is confused with cytosine riboside. Experimentally, the immunosuppressive effect of cytosine arabinoside has been more easily demonstrated in primary humoral antibody responses than in cell-mediated reactions. Clinically it is used to prepare leukemic recipients for eventual bone marrow transplantation. With more experience this agent may become more widely employed.

FOLIC ACID ANTAGONISTS. The immunosuppressive effect of a diet deficient in pteroylglutamic acid was originally noted by Little, and set the stage for the use of the folic acid antagonists, aminopterin and methotrexate. Both drugs inhibit the enzyme dihydrofolate reductase, and prevent the conversion of folic acid to tetrahydrofolic acid. This step is necessary for the synthesis of DNA, RNA, and certain coenzymes, Again, proliferating cell systems are most affected.

Some of the toxicity of aminopterin and methotrexate can be abrogated by the administration of folinic acid some hours or even days after the use of the antagonist. Nevertheless, the ratio of immunosuppression to toxicity has not justified their use in clinical kidney transplantation.

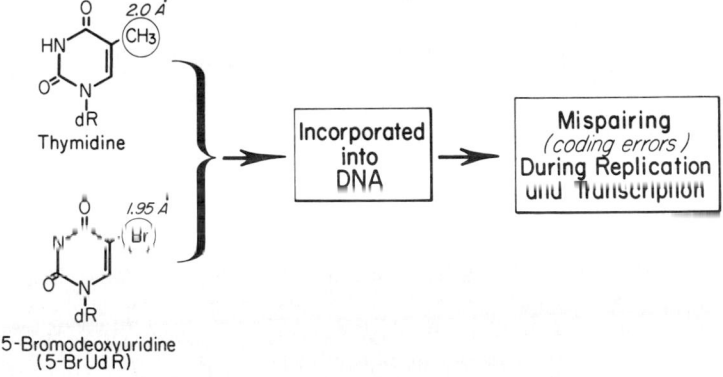

Fig. 10-21. Mechanism of antimetabolite action. 5-Bromodeoxyuridine (5BrUdR) strongly resembles thymidine in its steric configuration. Even the bromine molecule is similar in size to the methyl. 5-BrUdR thereby competes with thymidine incorporation into DNA. [From R. L. Simmons, J. E. Foker, and J. S. Najarian, Principles of Immunosuppression, in D. C. Sabiston, Jr. (ed.), "Davis-Christopher Textbook of Surgery," p. 471, W. B. Saunders Company, Philadelphia, 1972.]

The immune reactions that accompany bone marrow transplantation are more difficult to control, and methotrexate is used to both prevent and reverse the severe graft-versus-host reactions that occur. Since methotrexate is usually used with one or more other drugs, its toxic effects can be difficult to identify. Megaloblastic hemopoiesis, mucosal breakdown with severe gastrointestinal bleeding, and liver damage seem to be related to methotrexate therapy. These effects, even with high dosages of methotrexate, can usually be prevented by folinic acid (citrovorum rescue). Obviously, depression of the transplanted marrow may also result from the activity of methotrexate, although assigning the cause may be difficult in the complex clinical situation.

ALKYLATING AGENTS. The alkylating agents have highly reactive rings as part of the molecular structure. These unstable rings have electron-seeking points which combine with electron-rich nucleophilic groups such as the tertiary nitrogens in purines and pyrimidines, or with $-NH_2$, $-COOH$, $-SH$, and $-PO_3H_2$ groups on a variety of molecules. The high-energy rings of alkylating agents break and combine with these constituents to form stable covalent bonds. Obviously, many cell components have such groups, including DNA, RNA, and the enzymatic and structural proteins. Alkylation of DNA is probably the most detrimental. If the DNA strands are not repaired, chromosomal replication will be faulty in proliferating cells. Both DNA and RNA can be alkylated at several points, but a common site appears to be N-7 of the guanine ring (Fig. 10-22). Mispairing of DNA during replication may result from the presence of the alkylating agent itself, the clipping out of the alkylated guanine residue, or the cleavage of an alkylated guanine ring. Also chain breaks and cross-linkages frequently interfere with chain replication.

Since the damage to DNA can be repaired, these effects are apparently time-dependent. Consequently, the administration of alkylating agents just before and during stimulation by the antigen would most interfere with the ability of the immunocompetent cells to respond to that antigen. Continued use of the alkylating agents would also muffle the proliferative response of these cells in the face of a persistent stimulus. There are differences, however, in the response of T and B cells. The B cell seems to be more susceptible to cyclophosphamide than the T cell. This drug is a potent inhibitor of antibody formation, but its effect on skin or kidney rejection is much less spectacular. The reason for this apparent difference is unknown.

The usefulness of alkylating agents, which include nitrogen mustard, phenylalanine mustard, busulfan, and cyclophosphamide, is limited by their toxicity. Even so, cyclophosphamide has been used with good results in renal transplantation when liver toxicity prohibited the use of azathioprine. Cyclophosphamide is frequently used in clinical bone marrow transplantation, where it potentiates the effects of radiation and enhances the disruption of DNA. When cyclophosphamide is used, lower doses of radiation are required to deplete the recipient bone marrow population and provide space for donor cells. When leukemia is the indication for bone marrow transplantation, cyclophosphamide will aid in the destruction of these cells.

Toxicity is high, however, and predictable reactions occur, principally to rapidly replicating cell populations. Stomatitis, nausea, vomiting, diarrhea, skin rash, anemia, and alopecia are all common reactions. The more specific effects of cyclophosphamide administration are prompt fluid retention, occasionally severe hemorrhagic cystitis, and cardiac toxicity. The cardiac and edema problems suggest that even nonreplicating cell populations are adversely affected by this drug.

ANTIBIOTICS. The immunosuppressive antibiotics include the inhibitors of nucleic acid synthesis, and chloramphenicol and puromycin, which interfere with cellular protein synthesis. Actinomycin D binds to the guanine residue of DNA, thereby sterically interfering with RNA

Fig. 10-22. Mechanism of the action of the alkylating agent cyclophosphamide (CP). CP binds to the guanine molecule within the DNA chain. The guanine-CP complex leads to further damage to the DNA molecule. Four examples of the damage to DNA are shown. [From R. L. Simmons, J. E. Foker, and J. S. Najarian, Principles of Immunosuppression, in D. C. Sabiston, Jr. (ed.), "Davis-Christopher Textbook of Surgery," p. 471, W. B. Saunders Company, Philadelphia, 1972.]

polymerase and, consequently, with DNA-directed RNA synthesis. This potentially effective means of suppressing the development of immunity led to its use in reversing acute rejection of kidney grafts. The toxicity of actinomycin D has limited the overall clinical benefit, however, and it has been used less and less frequently. Mitomycin C combines with cellular DNA and hinders replication. This compound would also be useful in inhibiting allograft immunity, but its toxicity has precluded clinical use.

Both puromycin and chloramphenicol inhibit protein synthesis, and both can be immunosuppressive. Puromycin structurally resembles an amino acid–charged transfer RNA molecule and is accepted into the ribosome. There is no amino acid to be donated, however, and the peptide chain is prematurely terminated. Although protein synthesis is obviously central to immunological expression, it is so general a requirement for other cells that inhibition, and hence toxicity, will be widespread. Chloramphenicol has also been investigated experimentally. It is most potent in prokaryotic (bacterial) cell systems, and its effects on mammalian cells may be due to inhibiting mitochondrial synthesis. Unfortunately, it is only weakly immunosuppressive, and its potentially severe bone marrow toxicity precludes its use.

In general, only the antibiotic agents which primarily affect DNA synthesis can be expected to be clinically successful. Inhibition would be concentrated on dividing cell populations, and generalized toxicity would be less likely. This would potentially allow a favorable benefit/toxicity ratio.

IMMUNOSUPPRESSION BY LYMPHOCYTE DEPLETION

ADRENAL CORTICOSTEROIDS. Adrenal corticosteroids are the immunosuppressive agents most commonly used in clinical practice. They are effective in a variety of situations, from transplantation to the treatment of lupus erythematosus, childhood nephrotic syndrome, and asthma. Why steroids are beneficial for patients is not clear in most clinical situations. Experimentally, many effects have been described in a variety of cells from numerous species. Consequently, much of the uncertainty of mechanism of action stems from the difficulty in relating the many isolated in vitro effects to the patient. This is compounded by the variation in species susceptibility to steroids, which makes extrapolation difficult. In fact, direct evidence for immunosuppression by corticosteroids in human beings is lacking, and their benefit may be due primarily to inhibition of the inflammatory response. Despite this uncertainty about the mechanism of action, steroids are necessary for successful human transplantation and are commonly used to produce immunosuppression in other types of patients.

Many effects of steroids are known (Fig. 10-23). The problem is deciding which are primary and which are secondary actions. Steroids cross the cell membrane and bind to specific receptors in the cytoplasm of most cells,

Fig. 10-23. Adrenocortical steroids play an important role in clinical allograft immunosuppression. Many apparent sites of action have been located experimentally. These compounds bind to cytoplasmic receptors, and this complex combines with DNA. How this relates to the many functional consequences of steroids presented in this diagram is unclear. In the complex clinical transplantation setting it is not possible to determine if the primary suppression of lymphocytes is more important than the anti-inflammatory effects on neutrophils and macrophages in the suppression of allograft rejection reactions. Nevertheless, they produce a significant portion of the immunosuppressive effect of current clinical therapy.

lymphocytes included. Many experiments have shown a corollation between binding affinity and steroid potency, specifically between binding and lymphocyte resistance or susceptibility. The steroid-receptor complex then enters the nucleus and interacts with DNA in an unknown way. Subsequently in lymphocytes DNA, RNA, and protein synthesis are inhibited, as are glucose and amino acid transport. At a sufficient dosage, lymphocyte degeneration and lysis occur. Cytolysis can readily be produced in vivo, and T cells appear to be most susceptible. In some experiments the disintegration of nuclear membranes takes place within hours of exposure to steroids. Depletion of small T lymphocytes occurs both in the peripheral and central lymphoid tissues. Although it is unclear why the resting small lymphocyte should be so susceptible, it would seem that the primary antilymphocyte action of steroids may be to deplete small lymphocytes before they are activated by antigen.

The functional effects of steroids are predictable, and all T-cell responses are depressed. Paradoxically, the steroid-resistant thymocytes that remain after an injection of steroids have increased activity, but the net immunological capability of the treated animal is reduced.

Although B-cell activity and antibody production are relatively unaffected by steroids, many other cell types which participate in graft rejection are damaged. Neutrophil chemotaxis is inhibited, but whether or not suppression of phagocytosis occurs remains controversial. Similar results and controversies surround the effects on macrophages. It seems certain, however, that the accumulation of neutrophils, macrophages, and monocytes at sites of immune and inflammatory activity is reduced when steroids are given. Steroids also increase the membrane stability of digestive lysosomal particles in these cells, which reduces their inflammatory activity. These observations provide a basis for understanding the anti-inflammatory action activity of steroids. Inflammation is so intertwined with any substantial immune reaction that the various effects are inseparable. The variety of immunologic activities that steroids will suppress means that their effectiveness against the rejection reaction is probably the sum of many influences. When these effects are understood at the molecular level, however, there may prove to be a common discrete point of inhibition.

The effectiveness of cortisone in suppressing the allograft reaction was first recognized by its prolongation of skin graft survival in rabbits. Increased skin graft survival was subsequently shown in mice and guinea pigs, but the results were not as conclusive in pigs, dogs, monkeys, and human beings when cortisone was used alone. In experimental kidney allografts, steroids have not been convincingly effective by themselves, but they are valuable in combination with such agents as azathioprine, nitrogen mustard, and antilymphocyte globulin. Similarly, steroids alone cannot prevent clinical allograft rejection but, together with other compounds, are potent in both preventing and reversing rejection reactions.

Steroid toxicity of some degree is frequent and commonly includes a Cushinoid appearance. Other characteristic problems from steroid therapy are hypertension, weight gain, peptic ulcers and gastrointestinal bleeding, euphoric personality changes, cataract formation, hyperglycemia which may progress to steroid diabetes, and osteoporosis with avascular necrosis of bone. The appearance and severity of these complications vary considerably, but all too frequently they are life threatening. Clinical transplantation will be improved tremendously when more specific means of immunosuppression are developed and present steroid dosages can be reduced.

ANTILYMPHOCYTE GLOBULIN. The use of antilymphocyte antibodies to suppress the immune response is an interesting aspect of the transplantation story. In experimental studies, antilymphocyte globulin is a potent immunosuppressive agent, yet evidence for its value in clinical transplantation is controversial. This apparent contradiction results more from the difficulties which surround analyzing a complex clinical situation than from the ineffectiveness of antilymphocyte globulin. Evidence for the benefit of antilymphocyte globulin exists, but better-designed studies will be needed to measure the effects accurately.

The ability of an antiserum to destroy white cells was noted as early as 1899 by Metchnikoff. After guinea pigs were stimulated with lymph node or spleen cells from either rats or rabbits, their serum would agglutinate and kill polymorphonuclear leukocytes of the donor species. In the same year, Flexner found that lymphoid depletion occurred in animals treated with anti-lymph node serum. It was only during the last decade, however, that the functional consequences of heterologous sera made against lymphoid tissue were investigated. Certain immunologic reactions, e.g., tuberculin sensitivity and allograft rejection, were found to be depressed. Monaco and Russell induced potent antisera that were very effective in prolonging skin graft with strong histocompatibility differences, even including xenografts. Starzl was the first to use antilymphocyte serum in clinical kidney transplantation, and subsequently these preparations have been widely used.

Antilymphocyte globulins (ALG) are produced when thoracic duct, peripheral blood, lymph nodes, thymus, or spleen lymphocytes are injected into animals of a different species. Cell membranes or cultured lymphocytes serve equally well to provide the antigenic stimulation. The addition of adjuvants, usually Freund's complete adjuvant, is used to enhance the immunogenicity of the foreign lymphocytes and produce sera that are consistently more immunosuppressive. The rabbit, goat, and horse are commonly used to produce antisera for clinical transplantation.

Most of the relatively specific antibody against human lymphocytes resides in the IgG fraction. Further purification of the sera by separating the globulin fraction can be achieved by Cohn fractionation, column chromatography, or forced-flow electrophoresis. The purified material can be administered intravenously, intramuscularly, or subcutaneously. Unlike the immunosuppressive drugs used clinically, the course of ALG is short—usually the first few days or weeks after transplantation.

The action of ALG seems to be directed mainly against the T cell. The suppression produced by ALG can be at least partially reversed by T cells, but not by bone marrow cells. Thymectomy will enhance the effect of ALG, and ALG decreases the number of circulating T cells. Even in vitro, ALG will reduce the number of T cells. As would be expected, ALG administration interferes most with the cell-mediated reactions—skin or renal allograft rejection, tuberculin sensitivity, and the graft-versus-host reaction. ALG can abolish preexisting delayed hypersensitivity reactions, and larger doses will prolong the survival of some xenografts. ALG has a definite, but lesser, effect on humoral reactivity, and this, too, is concentrated on T cell–dependent antibody production.

The net effect of the relatively selective antilymphocyte activity of ALG is to enhance the activity of steroids, alkylating agents, and azathioprine against graft rejection. Most simply, the background of lymphocyte depression provided by ALG potentiates the effect of these agents without adding to the toxicity against other rapidly dividing cell systems. The fact that ALG and the other immunosuppressive drugs reinforce one another means that large doses of ALG can be used as a priming agent, followed by small doses of the more toxic immunosuppressants for a more effective and safer clinical regimen.

Many theories have been used to explain why ALG is a powerful (at present the most potent) inhibitor of cell-mediated immunity but only weakly affects antibody formation. Most of the explanations can be discarded because the anti-T-cell activity is more a function of the structure of the immune system than of the specificity of ALG itself. The spectrum of in vitro ALG activity can be easily shifted from anti-T to anti-B cell by changing the cells used to stimulate antibody production. Antithymus sera are richer in anti-T antibodies, anti-bone marrow sera have more anti-B-cell activity, while anti-spleen and lymph node sera contain large amounts of both types of antibodies. When ALG is given to the transplant patient, however, there is poor penetration of the antilymphocyte antibodies in the lymphoid regions where most of the relatively sessile B cells reside. The circulating long-lived lymphocytes, which are overwhelmingly T cell in origin, therefore absorb the bulk of the antibody. Lymphocytes coated with ALG share the fate of erythrocytes coated with antibody. They are either lysed or cleared from the blood by reticuloendothelial cells in the liver and spleen. More prolonged administration of ALG will deplete the paracortical regions of the lymph nodes where T cells reside, but high doses will also reduce the B cells in the medullary regions and follicles of the nodes.

Antilymphocyte globulin is widely used in clinical transplantation, with apparently beneficial results. Absolute proof of the effect of ALG is lacking, but the weight of the evidence suggests it is of value. What the many studies show is that it is difficult to analyze one factor, here ALG, in a complex clinical situation. Several studies have shown an increased percentage and length of survival, and renal function was increased among cadaver allografts when high doses of ALG were given (Fig. 10-24). The studies were not randomized, however, and the treatment groups not strictly comparable. Many considerations must be balanced in such a study, including (1) the length of time on dialysis, (2) the presence of presensitization, (3) the number of patients with depressed immune response, (4) the condition of the recipient, and (5) the condition of the graft, if it is from a cadaver donor.

The factors influencing the results are so numerous that a broad randomized study may not be able to equalize them all. Such an attempt has been made, however, by the Medical Research Council of Canada, with interesting results. There was no apparent effect of horse antithymocyte globulin on the 1-year survival of either living related or cadaver kidney allografts. But these patients did show a decrease in the average number of acute rejection episodes, an improvement in renal function, and a decrease in the amount of steroids given. These results could be interpreted to mean that the effect of ALG is greatest on the early, cell-mediated rejection reactions and less on later, antibody-produced graft damage. Unanswerable at this time is how much ALG adds to the risk of infection in the immunosuppressed patient. The benefit of ALG may be offset by an increased susceptibility to infection, and this may account for the lack of improved survival of patients in the clinical studies.

Fig. 10-24. The effect of ALG on kidney allograft function in transplant patients at the University of Minnesota. All kidneys were from cadavers; graft losses due to technical difficulties and hyperacute rejection were excluded. Although this is not a randomized study, improved function seems to occur in patients treated with ALG. The results with high doses (> 25 mg/kg/day) and medium doses (10 to 25 mg/kg/day) of ALG given for 14 days after transplantation do not seem to be significantly different. An accurate dose-response analysis is not possible, however, because of the lack of a satisfactory assay for the potency of individual batches of ALG. [*From J. E. Foker, R. L. Simmons, and J. S. Najarian, Principles of Immunosuppression, in D. C. Sabiston (ed.), "Davis-Christopher Textbook of Surgery," W. B. Saunders Company, Philadelphia, 1977.*]

The use of ALG is not confined clinically to kidney transplantation, and beneficial results have also been reported in bone marrow transplantation. These studies have suggested that ALG pretreatment of the recipient is of value in suppressing the response to the donor cells and for enlarging the marrow space. Also in this situation, a potentiating effect with certain drugs, such as procarbizine, has been described. Furthermore, it seems that ALG may be useful in the treatment of the graft-versus-host reactions which arise in these patients.

The toxicity of any heterologous serum preparation prepared against human tissue depends on two factors, (1) its cross-reactivity with other tissue antigens, and (2) the ability of the patient to make antibodies against the protein itself. When administered intramuscularly, ALG produces an area of erythematous induration accompanied by high fever. This probably results from the combination of antibodies with cellular antigens at the injection site. The combination of anemia and thrombocytopenia can also occur and presumably results from a reaction between ALG and host erythrocytes and platelets. Although prior absorption with human platelets and red cell stroma reduces the severity, some cross-reactivity to these cells persists in most ALG preparations. Cross-reactivity to renal glomerular basement membranes has occasionally been found, but no evidence for functionally significant nephrotoxic serum nephritis has been presented. These cross-

Fig. 10-25. X-ray-induced damage of DNA molecule. Irradiation frequently induces single breaks in the deoxyribotide backbone of the DNA double helix. More rarely, irradiation induces double breaks within the backbone. [*From R. L. Simmons, J. E. Foker, and J. S. Najarian, Principles of Immunosuppression, in D. C. Sabiston, Jr. (ed.), "Davis-Christopher Textbook of Surgery," p. 471, W. B. Saunders Company, Philadelphia, 1972.*]

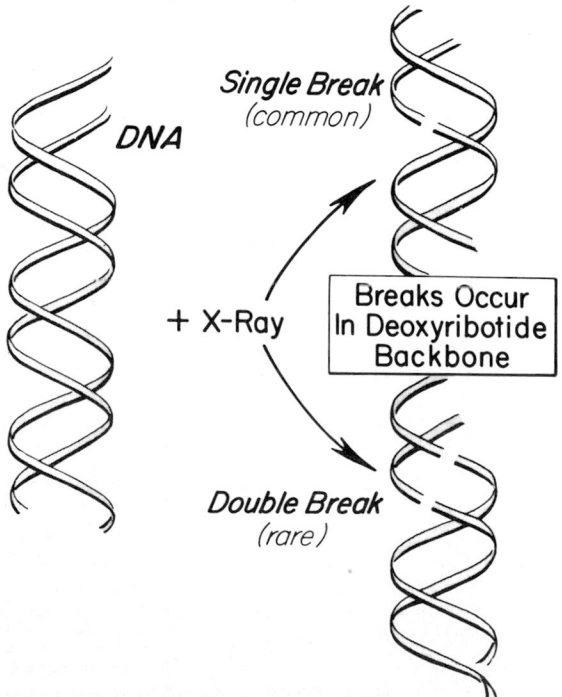

reactions can be reduced by using a purer lymphocyte suspension to stimulate ALG production. Either cultured lymphoblasts or thoracic duct lymphocytes will produce a more specific ALG than will the heterogeneous cell populations found in the spleen or bone marrow.

Allergic reactions to the antiserum itself were formerly the most common clinical problem associated with the use of ALG. Urticaria, anaphylactoid reactions, and serum sickness, including joint pain, fever, and malaise, all resulted from the patient developing immunity to the heterologous globulin. The incidence of these reactions has been reduced by inducing immunologic unresponsiveness to the foreign proteins in ALG by intravenous administration of a highly purified, deaggregated IgG fraction. This method has been used experimentally to produce tolerance to foreign proteins, and it is especially effective in the presence of the other immunosuppressive drugs used in renal transplantation.

The major problem in the production of a standardized antihuman ALG is the inability to develop a satisfactory method of assaying its in vitro immunosuppressive potency. Other immunosuppressive drugs are available in measurable quantities; therefore the response is more predictable. Unfortunately, individual laboratories make their own ALG preparations, and a standard method of assay has not been developed. Cytotoxic assays, the formation of cellular rosettes by antibody-coated cells, and animal assays for immunosuppressive activity have all been attempted, but their correlation with graft prolongation has been inconsistent. Standardization is important because two batches of ALG prepared by the same method will have varying degrees of immunosuppressive potency. A suitable assay is necessary to identify the better ALG preparations and make their use increasingly beneficial.

RADIATION. Radiation was probably the first agent used to produce immunosuppression. Ionizing radiation (x-rays, alpha rays, beta rays) affects both cellular proteins and nucleic acids. Despite the fact that relatively small doses of irradiation may disrupt the secondary protein structure formed by hydrogen bonding and the tertiary conformation that results, biologically significant alterations of protein function seem to require very high dosages. Consequently, most of the immunosuppressive effects of x-radiation are caused by changes produced in nucleic acids. DNA is particularly vulnerable, and therefore so is cellular replication. The most important of the several modes of damage is the production of scattered breaks in the deoxyribose-phosphate backbone of DNA (Fig. 10-25). Disruption of either the carbon-carbon bonds of the deoxyribotides or the bonds involving the phosphate groups produces breaks in one of the DNA strands. Occasionally both strands are broken at the same point. Other sites of damage, such as the bases themselves, are even less frequent.

Repair mechanisms exist to mend the breaks, but insufficient time may be available in the dividing cell. Therefore, the effectiveness of radiation is dependent upon the phase of the cell cycle in which the cell is found (Fig. 10-26). Cells in the M or G_2 phase are most sensitive to irradiation. Presumably, DNA breaks that occur during these phases cannot be repaired quickly enough, and the synthetic events and precise apportionment of cellular components which occur during mitosis may become scrambled. Conversely, the early G_1 phase and the latter part of the S phase are the most resistant portions of the cell cycle. Although irradiation is, in general, most effective just prior to or during mitosis, lymphocytes are a special case. For reasons that are not known, these cells are also sensitive in their resting, or G_0, phase.

Despite the complexity of the subcellular mechanisms, the effect of irradiation on the immune response is predictable and depends greatly on its timing with relation to antigen exposure. The possibilities are best seen when a relatively simple response, antibody production against a defined antigen, is measured. When the antigen is given soon after irradiation, the immune response will be inhibited because there is insufficient time for the immunocompetent cell population to recover before the antigen is encountered. If radiation is given during the time of maximal proliferation of the immunocompetent population to an antigen (soon after antigen administration), the response will be strongly inhibited. On the other hand, if antigenic stimulation is delayed long enough for the precursor cells to recover from the radiation, there will even be a slight augmentation of the response. Radiation is also ineffective if given long after the antigen, when a mature population of antibody-synthesizing cells has been formed. Fully differentiated plasma cells, and presumably cytotoxic lymphocytes, are radioresistant. Although radiation is relatively ineffective in blocking the secondary response of an immunized animal, paradoxically, an augmented antibody response may occur under certain circumstances. The timing of radiation must be carefully planned for the greatest immunosuppressive effect.

X-radiation has limited use in clinical transplantation. Effective suppression of the recipient's lymphoid tissues can be achieved, but the toxicity associated with the total body radiation is too great. Local irradiation of the graft, however, may provide some immunosuppressive effects. When given prior to transplantation, x-ray of the kidney may destroy the passenger leukocytes in the graft. These cells seem to be a potent source of antigen to the host, and thus the stimulus is somewhat diminished. After transplantation, radiation of the graft may damage invading cells, as well as produce nonspecific anti-inflammatory effects. Although proof of the benefit is lacking, some centers irradiate the kidney graft at the onset of a rejection reaction.

Other methods of using radiation have been tried. Selective irradiation of circulating lymphocytes has been done experimentally by diverting blood via a shunt through an extracorporeal radiation source. The circulating lymphocytes are depleted, and immunocompetence is reduced. Selective irradiation has the advantages that the neutrophils remain active in clearing infection, and protein loss is avoided. The inefficiencies of the system, however, and the need for nearly continuous irradiation make this technique impractical for clinical use.

Total body radiation does have one application at present in clinical transplantation. It is used to eliminate the immune reactivity of patients in preparation for bone

Lymphocyte Cell Cycle

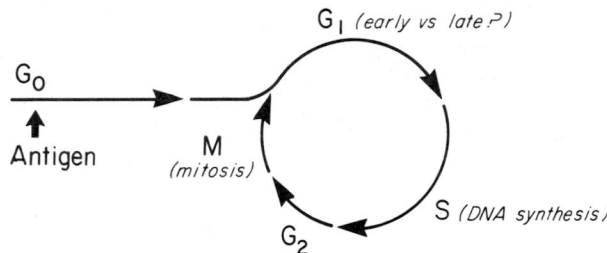

Fig. 10-26. The phases of the cell cycle. Following stimulation by an antigen, or other type of mitogen, small lymphocytes are activated. They are converted from the resting G_0 phase to the active G_1 phase. The G_1 phase lasts 10 hours or longer before DNA synthesis (S phase) begins. The S phase lasts about 10 hours and is followed by a short (2 to 4 hours) G_2 phase before mitosis (M phase). M phase is relatively brief, usually less than 2 to 3 hours, after which the cells are returned to the G_1 phase. The susceptibility of the cell to the immunosuppressive agents used in transplantation varies with the phase of the cycle. Periods of most intense nucleic acid synthesis, particularly S phase, are most vulnerable to the antimetabolites. As discussed in the text, the resting, G_0, lymphocyte is also susceptible to several of the clinically used immunosuppressive agents. [*From J. E. Foker, R. L. Simmons, and J. S. Najarian, Principles of Immunosuppression, in D. C. Sabiston, Jr. (ed.), "Davis-Christopher Textbook of Surgery," p. 509, W. B. Saunders Company, Philadelphia, 1977.*]

marrow transplantation. The toxicity is predictable. The rapidly replicating skin and gastrointestinal tract are universally affected, and nausea, vomiting, diarrhea, and skin changes occur. Late problems—growth retardation, vertebral deformities, sterility, cataracts, and a likely increased incidence of cancer—are also probably attributable to damage to the cellular genetic apparatus.

THYMECTOMY. There is some evidence that the adult mammalian thymus continues to play a role, albeit a diminished one, in maintaining the immunologic responsiveness of the animal. Its extirpation, therefore, may enhance the effects of immunosuppressive agents or irradiation. Unfortunately, although thymectomy can be performed rather simply through a cervical incision as well as by the classical transsternal route, it has not proved to be of use in clinical transplantation. In the early days of renal transplantation, Starzl tried thymectomy in a number of patients but had little improvement in results. It may be that a relatively small increment of benefit may be more apparent now when better results are regularly achieved. Perhaps thymectomy deserves another try. It must be conceded, however, that the thymus in an adult has largely completed its inductive functions and removal may have no measurable consequence. Furthermore, even if thymectomy could augment immunosuppression, it may not be desirable to produce greater general immunological incompetency in transplant recipients. In summary, it seems unlikely that the admittedly small potential gain will stimulate another clinical trial of thymectomy unless it is shown to be important to the production of tolerance.

LYMPHOID EXTIRPATION. Immunity becomes rapidly systemic. It is not confined for long to the regional lymph nodes or to a single major lymphoid organ like the spleen. Experimentally, the acquisition of immunity can be delayed for only brief periods by interrupting the lymphatic channels, by placing grafts in sites with poor lymphatic drainage, or by excising local lymphoid tissue. In one of the earliest clinical experiments, transplanted kidneys were placed in plastic bags after completion of the vascular anastomoses. This approach failed because vascularized organ grafts do not require lymphatic drainage to disseminate the antigen to awaiting lymphocytes. Excision of locally draining lymph nodes or the spleen is also ineffective as an immunosuppressive technique.

THORACIC DUCT DRAINAGE. Cannulation and drainage of the thoracic duct will successfully deplete the body of a large proportion of its circulating T lymphocytes. Such depletion will lead to prolongation of allograft survival, and to lesser, but real, decreases in the capacity for antibody synthesis. Thoracic duct cannulation and drainage have been used for clinical immunosuppression; although the technique seems to produce prolongation of allografts, it is cumbersome, the indwelling cannula can become plugged or infected, and protein depletion may result. There has been a recent resurgence of interest in this technique.

CONSEQUENCES OF CLINICAL IMMUNOSUPPRESSIVE THERAPY

The complications of immunosuppressive therapy in recipients of organ allografts are difficult to distinguish from the complications of recurrent rejection. Patients who do not have rejection episodes generally do not suffer major complications of immunosuppressive therapy. Conversely, the patient who requires repeated large doses of prednisone to avoid further rejection episodes or who suffer diminished renal function in the presence of high doses of azathioprine will have potentially lethal complications. The major complications all relate to a relative inability to respond effectively to a large variety of pathogenic, and even to normally saprophytic, organisms. There may be, moreover, a decrease in the normal capacity to destroy mutant, potentially neoplastic cells. This leads to a number of interesting and clinically important consequences of immunosuppression that must be considered.

PARAMETERS OF IMMUNOSUPPRESSION. Obviously the process of graft rejection can be prolonged, but are other parameters of immunocompetence concurrently depressed in the transplant patient? Can immunosuppression be measured in any other way than by the life of the graft? All methods of clinical immunological monitoring are restricted to measuring the specific or nonspecific responses in peripheral blood—the spleen, thymus, and lymph nodes not being readily available. With this restriction in mind, a number of studies have been performed. During the first two weeks after kidney transplantation an immunosuppressive effect can be detected. The response of the patient's circulating lymphocyte to either the mitogen phytohemagglutinin (PHA) or to foreign leukocytes is depressed. The loss of reactivity seems to be roughly proportional to the decrease in T cells among the peripheral lymphocytes and to the rise in null cells which occurs. The latter are

lymphocytes, coated with ALG and consequently inhibited.

Overall, the depressed lymphocyte reactivity probably results from a combination of acute destruction of T cells by ALG steroids, inactivation of other lymphocytes by masking with ALG, and inhibition of the lymphocyte proliferative response by azathioprine. Among these agents, ALG would seem to be the most responsible, because lymphocyte reactivity begins to return shortly after the ALG course is ended. Surprisingly, peripheral lymphocytes from kidney graft recipients show a normal response to PHA and foreign lymphocytes shortly thereafter. Because the kidney grafts continue to survive, an immunosuppressive effect which is not measured by these assays must persist. At the present time, there is no way to monitor the level of immunosuppression achieved after the effect of ALG has disappeared. Nor is it possible to predict incipient rejection accurately, although some success has been claimed for the detection of a rise in lymphocyte-dependent antibodies immediately prior to rejection. Because the degree of immunosuppression cannot yet be measured, the dosages of immunosuppressive agents are regulated instead by the toxicity produced.

BACTERIAL AND FUNGAL INFECTION. Immunosuppression understandably increases the risk of infection, but the consequences may offer some surprises. The routine post-transplant immunosuppression regimen does not necessarily result in a higher bacterial infection rate. With suitable precautions the postoperative wound infection incidence is very low. These patients seem to cope satisfactorily with inevitable contamination during the operation despite the increased immunosuppressive therapy used at the time. When there are no severe rejection reactions and the graft maintains good function, the day-to-day bacterial challenge to the recipient is handled. Although urinary tract infections are frequent, they are usually mild and easily controlled by antibiotics.

We do not mean to imply that bacterial infection is an insignificant problem for transplantation patients. On the contrary, infection is still the most common complication of immunosuppression, and overall it is the most common cause of death in transplant recipients. Even so, increasing experience has both lowered the incidence of serious infection and lengthened the time before it occurs.

The recent report of the American College of Surgeons/National Institute of Health Organ Transplant Registry stated that sepsis was the primary cause of death in 47 percent of all renal allografts recipients who died. Graft rejection not associated with sepsis accounted for less than 10 percent of deaths. Rejection of a kidney graft should not be fatal because the patient can be maintained on hemodialysis. The difficulties seem to arise with the treatment of rejection. Rejection causes decreased kidney function, which further potentiates the increased immunosuppression used to combat the rejection episode. The consequence is usually a severely immunodepressed patient, often with very few circulating polymorphonuclear leukocytes, who is highly susceptible to infection. In this setting, particularly if it is prolonged, severe bacterial infections and generalized sepsis can occur.

Most deaths, early in the history of kidney transplantation, occurred in the first few posttransplant months as a result of highly pathogenic bacterial infections. For example, pneumococcal pneumonia has been reported to be the most common type of pneumonia in kidney recipients. Since then, improved antibiotics and greater skill in immunosuppression therapy have shifted the spectrum of organisms. There has been a relative increase in lethal infection caused by organisms that are normally weakly pathogenic. Antibiotics will eradicate the more aggressive bacteria, but they leave opportunistic organisms free to colonize the susceptible transplant patient.

The opportunistic organisms, that are normally eliminated by cellular mechanisms, can now blossom in the face of the relative T-cell depression. Fungi are prominent opportunists, and they can cause urinary tract and pulmonary infections, skin lesions, and central nervous system involvement, as well as generalized sepsis. *Candida albicans* infections are probably the most common. The inevitable mucosal candidiasis can be satisfactorily prevented by oral mycostatin. Candida can become more deep-seated, and the pneumonia, usually part of a mixed infection, can be lethal. Characteristically, it produces soft, bulky, pulmonary infiltrates, although invasion of pulmonary arteries can lead to infarction and wedge-shaped peripheral infiltrates. Candida sepsis is most often associated with indwelling catheters, but it can take a more entrenched systemic form.

Aspergillus species are probably the second most common cause of fungal infection and typically produce upper lobe pulmonary cavities. *Rhizopus oryzae, Histoplasma capsulatum,* and *Cryptococcus neoformans* also invade the lung, and the latter occasionally causes meningitis. The indolent bacterium *Nocardia asteroides* occasionally infects, producing nodular pulmonary lesions. The protozoan *Pneumocystis carinii,* more commonly seen in patients undergoing cancer chemotherapy, usually causes an alveolar infiltrate with disproportionate dyspnea and cyanosis.

Standard patient isolation precautions are useless against these organisms, and prophylactic antibiotics are not available for most of them. Prevention is dependent upon avoiding excessive doses of immunosuppressive agents in a futile attempt to prolong the function of a rejected graft. An exception seems to be the protection against *P. carinii* provided by prophylactic trimethoprim and sulfamethoxazole.

VIRAL INFECTIONS. Viral infections seem to be almost ubiquitous among kidney transplant recipients. The herpes group of DNA viruses are most commonly present. Infection or antibody response to cytomegalovirus (CMV) is found in up to 90 percent of patients after renal transplantation. Herpes simplex infection occurs in about 25 percent and herpes zoster in 10 percent of graft recipients. Reports from England have shown that the Epstein-Barr virus commonly infects transplant patients, but the clinical significance of this is unclear. Antigenic evidence for hepatitis B virus infection can be detected in 15 percent of transplant patients. It seems almost certain that as detection methods improve, evidence will appear for other kinds of viral infections in these transplantation patients.

Several questions are raised by the recent appreciation of viral infections in kidney recipients. Are these infections of any consequence, or are they merely laboratory curiosities? The case of the hepatitis B virus is particularly interesting. Paradoxically, transplantation and hemodialysis patients who have circulating HB antigens usually have no symptoms of hepatitis. The intriguing question is why the disease is apparently much milder in these patients. It seems likely that liver cell damage results from an immune reaction against the viral antigens on the cell and that this may be reduced in these immunodepressed patients. The hepatitis virus does not seem directly cytotoxic for liver cells.

The situation with cytomegalovirus infection appears to be only slightly clearer and no less intriguing. Most evidence suggests that cytomegalovirus infection usually produces a clinical illness characterized by fever, neutropenia, and frequently a decrease in kidney function and apparent rejection. The virus may be newly acquired from blood transfusions or from foreign graft itself, but it is far more likely that apparently new infection is a reactivation of latent intracellular viruses. The finding that most normal adults have antibodies to CMV supports the latent virus hypothesis.

In transplant patients, does the infection cause the rejection or does the rejection encourage viral activation? Rejection reactions are accomplished by bursts of lymphocyte proliferation, cell division is known to activate latent viruses experimentally, and most immunosuppressive agents are mutagenic. Viral infections, on the other hand, can be associated with either an augmented or a depressed immune response. If the patient is able to produce antibody against virus, graft rejection is also enhanced. In preimmunized individuals, viruses seem to act as immunological adjuvants and enhance the response both to virus and to graft. When no antibody response accompanies the viral infection, a generalized immunodepression is usually present. At present it can be said only that viral infections and rejection reactions are clearly linked; which initiates and which follows is usually unknown.

A special case of CMV infection is worthy of note. The typical CMV infection is a mild febrile illness, followed by an antibody response and regression of viral symptoms. A rejection episode usually accompanies the viral infection and raises the controversy discussed in the previous paragraph. These patients remain asymptomatic but may continue to excrete CMV in urine or saliva despite the presence of antibodies to CMV. In certain patients, however, there is no antibody response or apparent rejection and the infection can be lethal. These severely immunodepressed patients are at the mercy of this usually trivial parasite. This would suggest that rejection is not essential for viral infection. Certainly the ability of the patient to respond to the virus is very important to his or her survival. Recently, surgical specimens taken from patients with bleeding gastric or cecal ulcers have shown heavy cellular infestation with CMV.

The other herpes viruses seem to behave in a similar manner. Transplant patients also have infections typical of herpes simplex and varicella zoster. The infections may be more severe than in normal patients, and although the lesions may be localized, the viruses are systemic and can be recovered in the urine. Fever, neutropenia, and allograft rejection may accompany the infection, and antibody response to the virus seems to be important for the patient.

We are not sure when the viral infections actually occur in relation to the clinical symptoms. With the exception of the hepatitis infection, these may represent activation of a normal intracellular viral flora, rather than recent infection. In transplant patients, studies suggest that cytomegalovirus "infection" takes place about the time of transplantation, when the mutagenic antirejection drugs are begun at high levels. This obviously may merely result from activation of latent intracellular viruses.

PREVENTION OF INFECTION. The incidence of severe, near-fatal infections can be reduced through a number of precautions: (1) The most important precaution is to eliminate all sources of infection prior to transplantation, especially those in the urinary tract and shunt site. Other sources of infection should be sought by routine preoperative cultures of nasopharynx, throat, sputum, urine, stool, and hemodialysis cannula sites. If any source is found, it should be eliminated by the appropriate use of surgical drainage or antibiotic therapy. (2) Technical problems clearly predispose to sepsis. Urinary extravasation frequently leads to wound infections. Abscesses deep to the transplant are difficult to drain, and mycotic aneurysms may develop at sites of anastomosis or in the iliac vessels. It is frequently necessary to remove the kidney to obtain control of the infection. (3) Organs from related and well-matched cadavers elicit less frequent and less vigorous rejection reactions. If repeated rejection can be avoided, the doses of immunosuppressive drugs can be minimized and the rate and severity of infection will diminish. (4) Many patients who die of infection develop leukopenia (especially neutropenia) at some time. Some bouts of leukopenia can be attributed to cytomegalovirus infections. Leukopenia can be prevented by careful reduction in azathioprine doses when the leukocyte count or platelet count falls and when renal function is lost for whatever reason. The use of other bone marrow depressants (chloramphenicol) should be scrupulously avoided in patients already on azathioprine therapy. (5) Gowns, masks, and gloves were formerly used to minimize infections in the initial postoperative care. Most transplant units have discontinued their use because they restrict access to the patients, impose psychologic stress, and are probably ineffective against viral, fungal, or endogenous bacteria.

MALIGNANCY. Cancer has been an unexpectedly frequent companion of clinical transplantation. The incidence of cancer is not high enough, however, to contraindicate the transplant procedure. Tumors in kidney recipients have come from two general sources. Some have been unfortunately transplanted from cadaver donors in whom the cancer was unsuspected. These tumors usually can be treated simply by halting immunosuppression therapy and allowing rejection of the tumor tissue, as well as the kidney, to occur. The more common cancers are the primary tumors which appear in the immunosuppressed recipient.

The data are still accumulating on these primary tumors, and precise frequencies are not yet available. It would seem, however, that the rate of development of malignancy in patients surviving renal transplantation may be as high as thirty times that of a similar, normal population.

Only certain tumors grow more readily in immunodepressed patients. Seventy-five percent of the spontaneous cancers are either lymphoid or epithelial in origin. Carcinoma in situ of the cervix, carcinoma of the lip, and squamous or basal cell carcinomas account for about half of this group, while lymphomas, predominantly reticulum cell carcinoma, make up the remainder. It has been estimated that the risks to the transplant recipient of developing skin cancer, lymphoma, or reticulum cell sarcoma are increased by 4, 40, and 350 times, respectively. The lymphomas are unusual both in their frequency and behavior. Almost 50 percent of the immunosuppressed patients with lymphomas have brain involvement, which occurs in only 1 percent of nontransplanted related cases of lymphoma. These lymphomas, moreover, are difficult to treat and have led to death in almost all cases.

Recent evidence suggests that the lymphomas are not true neoplasms. Immunological analysis has indicated that these tumors secrete several different types of immunoglobulins, i.e., they do not have the nomenclatural characteristics of cancer. Other evidence suggests that they may represent uncontrolled B cell proliferative responses to Epstein-Barr virus. The superficial malignant lesions of the lip, skin, and cervix are usually successfully treated by standard operative techniques. There is no need to jeopardize the allografts by reducing the immunosuppressive therapy.

We do not know why transplant patients have an increased risk for cancer in general and epithelial (and perhaps lymphoid) cancers in particular. It has been postulated that the surveillance and elimination of tumor cells as they arise by lymphocytes is an important natural defense of human beings against cancer. Certainly this function would be depressed in transplantation patients who are immunodepressed by antirejection therapy. Despite this, two observations argue that this explanation is incomplete: (1) only a few kinds of cancer are increased in these patients, and, perhaps more telling, (2) patients receiving hemodialysis have an increased risk of cancer, but tumors arise with the usual spectrum and frequency distribution. Dialysis patients have decreased immunological competence. Perhaps, the inhibition of a surveillance mechanism contributes to their increased risk.

Transplant patients, however, must have additional factors operating which contribute to the development of cancer. They are immunosuppressed, which may be important, but the presence of the mutagen azathioprine is a more certain factor. Azathioprine, theoretically, could either act as a primary mutagen on dividing lymphocytes and epithelial cells or contribute to the activation of viruses and their transformation of normal cells into tumors. It is unclear what consequences steroids and ALG have, but at least two reticulum cell sarcomas have sprung up at the site of ALG injections. It would seem possible that the most important effect the immunosuppressive agents have on tumor development is to encourage viral transformation of normal cells into cancer cells.

Cancers of the epithelium, for example, may be a consequence of herpes virus transformation. This group of viruses is carcinogenic in animals, and circumstantial evidence exists for a role in human cervical cancer. Herpes viruses are usually dormant, but the stress of transplantation or the action of antimetabolite may activate them. The viruses might then either proliferate and cause a clinical viral illness or produce cellular transformation into cancer cells. Similar possibilities exist for the lymphomas. Several animal lymphomas are produced by RNA viruses, and transformation by related viruses could be occurring in these patients. Perhaps a simpler explanation would do. Active lymphoid proliferation occurs after transplantation, and cell division in the presence of the mutagenic immunosuppressants may carry an increased risk of transformation of normal cells into cancer.

CUSHING'S DISEASE. Most transplant patients receiving steroid therapy undergo a series of changes that are referred to as iatrogenic Cushing's syndrome. The rate of its development is a result of the dose of steroid and number of rejection episodes. The appearance of the face is altered by rounding, puffiness, and plethora; fat tends to be redistributed from the extremities to the trunk and face. There is also an increased growth of fine hair over the thighs and trunk and sometimes over the face. Acne may increase or appear, and insomnia and increased appetite are noted; however, the underlying metabolic changes that accompany the obvious changes can be serious by the time the latter actually appear. The continuing breakdown of protein and diversion of amino acids to glucose increase the need for insulin and result in weight gain, fat deposition, muscle wasting, thinning of the skin with striae and bruising, hyperglycemia, growth suppression (in children), and sometimes the development of steroid diabetes, cataracts, and osteoporosis. In some patients a myopathy develops, the nature of which is unknown.

The cushingoid changes may on rare occasions represent such a psychologic problem that transplant nephrectomy will be necessary on that basis alone. Women and adolescents are more severely affected physically, and the psychologic problems are greater. These problems can be enormous in children, who grow less well, and most particularly in small girls on chronic steroid therapy, who seem to grow very little after age thirteen. The male psyche tolerates steroids better; the plethora and broad faces give many men a healthier look than they had while on dialysis.

STEROID DIABETES. Steroid diabetes is an occasional complication of chronic steroid administration, even when the steroid doses are not high. This may represent exacerbation of a prediabetic state. The diabetes is often mild, but its onset is frequently insidious, and the patient may have diabetic acidosis before the diabetic state is discovered.

GASTROINTESTINAL BLEEDING. Gastrointestinal bleeding due to reactivation of a preexisting ulcer or diffuse ulceration of the gastrointestinal tract is a frequently fatal complication. The relative contribution of progressive uremia and repeated massive steroid administration in the pathogenesis of gastrointestinal hemorrhage is unknown, but when bleeding appears, it is severe and difficult to control by nonoperative means. Occasionally the use of cimetidine or the intramesenteric arterial infusion of vasopressin is effective.

During moderate doses of steroid therapy, episodes of gastrointestinal bleeding can be almost totally prevented by the use of antacids between meals. Magaldrate (Riopan) is a useful antacid, since it is required in only small doses. In patients with recurrent rejection who require many episodes of high steroid dosage, antacid therapy must be intensified with each increase in steroid administration. Magnesium-containing antacids, however, are contraindicated in patients with poor renal function, since hypermagnesemia will result.

OTHER INTESTINAL COMPLICATIONS. A number of colonic complications, including diverticulitis, bleeding, and ulceration, is associated with immunosuppressive treatment. A syndrome of acute cecal ulceration with gastrointestinal bleeding has also been reported in transplant patients.

CATARACTS. Cataracts are common in patients who require steroids. The cataracts, which develop slowly, appear to be independent of the absolute prednisone dosage.

THROMBOSIS AND THROMBOEMBOLIC PHENOMENA. Thrombophlebitis may occur in the transplant recipient, particularly on the side of the graft where the venous anastomosis may become partially or completely thrombosed. This complication has occurred in patients who previously had steroid-resistant nephrotic syndrome, and it has been speculated that this is related to recurrence of the original kidney disease. No reason is known for this possible association.

When attention is focused on immunologic and infectious phenomena, thrombophlebitis and pulmonary embolism may be overlooked. Swelling of the leg on the side of the transplant site is a frequent sign of rejection, associated with increases in weight, pulmonary infiltrates, and slight increases in serum creatinine level. When the differential diagnosis is difficult, a femoral venogram is indicated. The diagnosis of pulmonary embolisms may also be difficult, and multiple pulmonary infiltrates should not be treated as fungal pneumonia on the basis of sputum cultures alone.

HYPERTENSION. Many of the patients who come to renal transplantation are already hypertensive. Hypertension can usually be controlled with dialysis or, if more refractory, with nephrectomy. Hypertension in most patients will develop soon after transplantation, but posttransplant hypertension is mild and easily controlled with dietary salt restriction and drugs. The hypertension seems to be due not only to prednisone but also to failure to regulate the normal salt and water balance in the early posttransplant period and secretion of renin by the kidney. Nevertheless, antihypertensive drugs can usually be stopped as maintenance levels of prednisone are reached. Hypertension returns with rejection and may be a sign of this problem. It should be remembered, however, that significant hypertension may be due to renal arterial stenosis, and arteriography may be necessary for the differentiation.

DISORDERS OF CALCIUM METABOLISM. Patients frequently come to transplantation with renal osteodystrophy. Alterations in vitamin D metabolism and secondary hyperparathyroidism are prominent factors in the pathogenesis of skeletal disease. Long-standing acidosis may likewise be contributory. The resulting osteoporesis, osteomalacia, and osteitis fibrosa cystica in the child can lead to growth restriction, epiphysiolysis, skeletal deformities, and pathologic fractures. The bone disease in some cases can be arrested with pharmacologic doses of vitamin D or aluminum hydroxide, or by total or subtotal parathyroidectomy.

Hemodialysis can correct the uremic state, but the bone disease may actually progress if the stimulus to parathyroid hormone secretion is not effectively eliminated. Great attention should be directed toward keeping the dialysate calcium concentration at a level (6 to 7 mg/100 ml) that does not promote calcium loss from the blood. Again, parathyroidectomy may be indicated if osteitis fibrosa cystica is progressive and cannot be reversed by maintaining the calcium concentration in the serum at normal or slightly elevated levels.

Parathyroidectomy performed in the patient with renal failure or on hemodialysis may help to arrest progressive bone disease. Frequently, however, the calcium levels will remain high and will fall only after renal transplantation. Conversely, if prompt transplantation from a related donor is planned or if the cadaver list is short, transplantation by itself will usually lead to the reversal of the hyperparathyroid state. The hypercalcemia of the immediate posttransplant period can be managed with a high-phosphate diet, low calcium intake, and furosemide diuretics. Even patients with flagrant osteitis fibrosa cystica with metastatic calcification will respond to transplantation alone without parathyroidectomy. Parathyroidectomy seems primarily indicated for patients on chronic hemodialysis in whom transplantation is not planned.

The role of persistent (tertiary) hyperparathyroidism after successful renal transplantation has been difficult to assess. At the present, parathyroidectomy is rarely indicated after transplant.

MUSCULOSKELETAL COMPLICATIONS. A most disturbing complication of successful renal transplantation is avascular necrosis of the femoral heads and other bones. Its occurrence is most closely correlated with the dosage of steroid used. Transient rheumatoid symptoms precede changes visible by radiography by several months. The bone changes apparently occur secondarily to steroid osteopenia or osteonecrosis with resulting microfractures. Alterations in lipid metabolism caused by fluctuating high levels of steroids likewise appear to be important in explaining the pathogenesis. The treatment is for the most part symptomatic. It is doubtful that bone lesions can revascularize sufficiently to restore normal architecture in the presence of maintenance steroids. Should symptoms increase in the hip and bone destruction progress, replacement arthroplasty may be indicated.

Migratory arthralgis, myalgia, and tendonitis are common, but persistent joint pain and swelling are most often signs of intraarticular infection. Occasionally, an unexplained septic arthritis crops up in these patients.

PANCREATITIS. Pancreatitis may appear suddenly and unexpectedly in renal allograft recipients; it may occasionally be fatal. Its cause is obscure; it has been attributed variously to corticosteroid therapy, azathioprine, cytomegalovirus, or hepatitis virus. The clinical course is sometimes accompanied by increases in serum creatinine, which may or may not be related to rejection. Most cases subside with conventional therapy and do not recur.

ERYTHREMIA AND ANEMIA. The transplanted kidney is apparently fully capable of manufacturing and secreting erythropoietin. During rejection, the serum level may be increased. Erythremia also may appear, but apparently it is not related to elevated erythropoietin levels.

Anemia usually is not present except in association with uremia or immunodepression secondary to azathioprine toxicity. A microangiopathic hemolytic anemia has also been thought to be induced by the vascular changes within the chronically rejecting organ.

GROWTH. The antiproliferative effects of immunosuppressive drugs would seem to make satisfactory growth in children unlikely after transplantation. Since chronic renal failure itself is inhibitory to development, these children are usually far behind their peers in size. After successful transplantation their growth response is highly variable and may depend on age, previous growth rate, renal function, and immunosuppressive drug regimen. Many children return to a normal growth rate; unfortunately the growth that was lost during their original illness is not made up, so these children will always be smaller than their peers.

Wound healing, a specific case in this category, is to all outward appearances normal. It is apparent clinically, however, that wound healing is severely affected when debilitation, chronic renal failure, and high steroid levels are present.

PREGNANCY. Many arguments can be raised against the likelihood of a successful pregnancy and a normal child being born when a patient has received a kidney graft. Excessive steroid levels, the antigrowth and mutagenic effects of the immunosuppressive agents, and viral activation and infection all should be detrimental to the fetus. As usual, however, the story is complicated.

By 1975 the Human Transplant Registry had reported on 132 graft recipients who had become parents. The experience at the University of Minnesota has been examined in detail and seems to be representative. Of these patients, 17 became pregnant after transplantation, and 12 children were born. Only one spontaneous abortion occurred. The children had a normal size distribution, and no congenital defects were found. There is no doubt, however, that azathioprine, and probably steroids, are mutagenic and that the risk of congenital abnormalities is real. Multiple defects have been reported in the child of a male transplant recipient. From the overall experience, it would appear that the risk is not high, but the incidence is still unknown. Steroids also cause their own peculiar problems, and a few cases of severe neonatal adrenocortical insufficiency, as well as lymphopenia, have been reported.

Transplant recipients who are pregnant are often beset with medical problems. Toxemia has occurred in over half the pregnancies, and bacterial and viral infections, particularly of the urinary tract, are common. Both these factors may contribute to the higher incidence of premature labor that has been reported. Another important medical concern is the effect of the pregnancy on renal functions. Although the data are insufficient to judge whether or not pregnancy is deleterious to kidney function, each series has apparent examples that show it may be. An indication for the termination of pregnancy is the compromise of graft function. The increased risk of cancer, in particular of the cervix, in transplant patients has already been discussed. The effect of pregnancy on this tendency is unknown. Another important problem that must be faced is the decreased life expectancy of the transplant recipient. Parenthood is a long-term obligation, and counseling of these patients should include a discussion of these considerations.

TOLERANCE. Many kidneys survive for years in their new host. That this represents an acquired tolerance, a specific nonreactivity to the graft antigens, has been suggested in the literature and is hoped for in immunosuppressive therapy. The question of tolerance has been raised earlier in this chapter, and the possible means of achieving it will be discussed under Experimental Immunosuppression, below. It has been found that even after long accommodation of graft and host, cessation of immunosuppressive therapy almost invariably leads to rejection. Some adaptation must occur, however, and long-term graft survival can be achieved at immunosuppressive dosages which do not immunologically cripple the recipient or produce other severe toxic consequences.

EXPERIMENTAL IMMUNOSUPPRESSION

The complexity of the immune response gives rise to the hope that many potential points of vulnerability exist. New approaches are constantly being tried and old ones refined to produce better immunosuppressive therapy.

ANTIGEN RECOGNITION AND PROCESSING. An obvious, if difficult, approach to immunosuppression would be to alter or mask graft antigens. Evidence exists that by perfusing the organ, before transplantation, with concanavalin A (Con A) the host response to it may be reduced. Although the mechanism is not known, presumably, Con A aggregates on graft cell surfaces and interferes in some way with host recognition. Subsequently, the cell membrane is cleared by normal repair processes, but may no longer be as antigenic as before.

Many agents have been tried to generally blockade the reticuloendothelial systems. Talc and gold, to name a few, can depress particle uptake and presumably antigen processing, by these cells. The effect of talc and gold on graft survival, however, has been negligible.

IMMUNOSUPPRESSION BY SPECIFIC ANTIGENS. The complications of immunosuppression constantly reinforce the importance of developing modes of immunosuppression that will be specific for the incompatible graft antigens. The immunosuppressive drugs and antilymphocyte globulin all act by suppressing the capacity of the immunocompetent cell to respond to any antigen. Thus, even ALG, with its predilection for cellular immunity, cannot select between T cells destined to reject an allograft and T cells necessary for immunity against viruses and tumors. The ability to produce a state of tolerance would obviously be of enormous benefit to the field of transplantation. Experimentally, a functional state of tolerance has been produced in two general ways—manipulation of the stimulating antigens, and infusion of specific antibodies; both have been successful.

A variety of conditions has been shown to predispose to the introduction of tolerance, rather than immunity, on exposure to antigen. The best example of antigen-directed immunologic unresponsiveness is the tolerance enjoyed by animals to their own body constituents. This apparently develops early, before or during maturation of the immune mechanism, and is usually maintained throughout life. Burnet, as part of his clonal selection hypothesis, considered this unresponsive state to result from direct contact between "self" antigens and the individual's own lymphocytes. The clones of lymphocytes reactive to "self" are eliminated, and tolerance ensues. He further predicted that specific unresponsiveness could be induced to foreign antigens if they were given very early in life. Experimental proof by Billingham, Brent, and Medawar followed and demonstrated tolerance to histocompatibility antigens after neonatal injection of replicating allogeneic cells.

Obviously this opportunity has passed for transplant patients, but under certain carefully controlled conditions, tolerance has been produced experimentally in adult animals. Thus, hope exists for future progress in this area, and several techniques have yielded limited but encouraging results. Repeated injection of small, subimmunogenic doses of antigen or the use of very large amounts of antigen preparations has produced unresponsiveness. When these preparations are cleared of aggregated material, the tendency to induced tolerance is greater. Certain antigens (e.g., serum proteins) are endowed with properties that are particularly favorable for the induction of immunologic unresponsiveness. These seem to be the ability to persist in the circulation and equilibrate within the extravascular spaces, thereby coming in contact with antigen-reactive cells in effective concentration. Whether or not this results in deletion of the antigen-reactive lymphocytes, however, is unknown. More likely suppressor cells are selectively or predominantly stimulated by such antigenic presentation.

Unfortunately, viral and bacterial antigens and transplantation antigens do not have these properties and, in addition, may possess multiple antigenic specificities. A diminished response to transplantation antigens can be induced in adult animals, but the antigen dose, physical state of the antigen, and route of injection all must be carefully chosen to avoid immunization. Tolerance is more easily produced to weak antigens; therefore, close histocompatibility matching is desirable. Irradiation, chemical immunosuppression, and antilymphocyte globulins have been used to inhibit the immune response and potentiate the emergence of a relatively unresponsive state. Although only modest successes have been achieved so far by these approaches, careful control of the conditions of antigen presentation may yet be important in the production of tolerance.

Recently, attempts to produce tolerance have utilized antigens tagged with radioactive compounds or alkylating agents. The purpose is to form a lethal combination with the specifically reactive lymphocyte clones and eliminate them. So far, only a hyporesponse state of short duration has been induced, but this approach may yet be fruitful.

In summary, the induction of tolerance by manipulating the presentation of the incompatible antigens is an attractive idea. So far, success for allografts has not been achieved, but it remains a promising pathway.

IMMUNOSUPPRESSION BY SPECIFIC ANTIBODIES. Tolerance can be easily defined. A conceptual understanding of tolerance is readily attained by considering the lack of reactivity toward self. Understanding the subcellular mechanisms involved is far more difficult, and they are unknown at this time. Tolerance may result from the absence of the reactive clone of lymphocytes or from the predominance of a suppressor clone. An alternative to these mechanisms is that tolerance is due to an antibody that interferes with the development of immunity. Certainly the immune system is regulated and subject to feedback control; the presence of an adequate level of antibody may block further activity. Experimentally, the immune response can be eliminated by the passive transfer of specific antibody prior to, or shortly after, giving the antigen.

Two general mechanisms for this phenomenon have been proposed. In the first the antibodies formed are inactive and do not trigger the effector mechanisms such as complement. These blocking antibodies have been best demonstrated in tumor immunology, where they have been shown to enhance the growth of transplanted tumors and prevent rejection. The second explanation is that these antibodies produce a negative feedback effect. The most striking example of this is the prevention of erythroblastosis fetalis in newborns by the administration of an Rh factor antiserum to the pregnant mother. The antiRh antibodies suppress the synthesis of antibodies in response to the foreign Rh antigens. Both these mechanisms for production of tolerance require the presence of antibody to the antigen. While the appropriate antibodies cannot always be detected in animals following the induction of "tolerance," they are often present. Furthermore, antibodies are frequently detected in patients with well-functioning, long-term kidney allografts. Graft function is thought to be prolonged by the presence of a specific antibody that inhibits the development of truly effective antigraft immunity. If immunosuppression is reduced, however, the balance is tipped and the common result of graft rejection is observed. Consequently, the apparently paradoxical hypothesis that tolerance to an antigen requires the presence of antibodies to that antigen may yet be valid.

When applied to transplantation, the application of this theory has yielded some success. The best results, however, for experimental kidney graft prolongation have been following the administration of both graft-specific antigens and antibodies against them. Therefore, the distinction between antigen and antibody-induced tolerance is blurred, and they may meet at virtually the same point in the subcellular response.

IMMUNOSUPPRESSION BY CELLULAR MECHANISMS. Even more theoretical than the preceding are two recent proposals for inducing immunological unresponsiveness. As previously mentioned, the ability to induce a sufficient number of suppressor T cells could effectively block graft rejection. A further requirement, of course, would be that the suppressor cells are antigen-specific or general immunosuppression would result.

Additional leverage on the immune response may be gained by manipulating the genes which govern the response to histocompatibility antigens. Not all individuals respond in the same way to different histocompatibility antigens, and part of this difference may be ascribable to a specific genetic locus. Matching the immune response governing loci in a similar way to aligning histocompatibility antigens may yield improved results.

INHIBITION OF LYMPHOCYTE METABOLISM. Normal cell metabolism results in turnover of adenine and other purines and pyrimidines. Several enzymes, including adenosine deaminase and purine nucleoside phosphorylase, are necessary for purine salvage and are present in all tissues. Lymphocytes may be unique in that absence of either enzyme cripples cell function and clinically is associated with a severe immunodeficiency state. This has stimulated investigation of experimental production of immunosuppression using adenine analogues to inhibit these enzymes selectively. It is possible that this approach may become clinically useful because other tissues do not seem to require this pathway and toxicity is low. Part of the immunosuppressive activity of azathioprine may be due to this mechanism.

INTERFERENCE WITH NONSPECIFIC EFFECTORS. The combination of sensitized cells or antibodies with the foreign antigens marks the beginning of the active effort to dispose of the graft. The complex of sensitized cells or antibodies with the antigens triggers the recruitment of a multitude of effector systems. We have mentioned the cascading enzyme systems, the complement, clotting, and kinin pathways, as well as the cellular mediators, lymphocytes, macrophages, platelets, and polymorphonuclear leukocytes. These are enlisted both by the specific immunological reaction itself and as a result of subsequent events. All play an active role in disposing of the allograft.

It is conceivable that one could reduce the effect of an immune response by (1) interfering with the complement, clotting, and kinin cascades that are activated by antigen-antibody complexes; (2) destroying factors secreted by activated cells (migration-inhibiting factor, chemotactic factor, cytophilic antibody, transfer factor, mitogenic factor); or (3) neutralizing the vascular permeability factors, lysosomal enzymes, or lymphotoxins.

A number of agents or combination of agents that interfere with the expression of immunity have been tested. For example, anticomplementary drugs (vitamin A, cobra venom factor) are either ineffective or, if potent, are short-acting and not clinically useful. Antimacrophage globulin, carrageenin, and silica all destroy macrophages but are weak transplant immunosuppressants. Antibodies to lymphotoxins or migration-inhibitory factors and other effector molecules are still in very early experimental states of evaluation. Antihistamines and antiserotonin agents are also relatively weak immunosuppressant drugs. Anticoagulants (heparin), agents that interfere with platelet aggregation (dipyridamole, aspirin), and fibrinolytic agents have been employed to interfere with the thrombosis of graft vessels. The antiplatelet agents have been found to improve long-term clinical function in both kidney and cardiac grafts and will undoubtedly be more widely used in the future. More information is needed on the role platelets play in the production of arterial narrowing, which seems often to limit graft survival.

The limited success with these agents reinforces the difficulty in attempting to interfere with the immune response after antibody has been synthesized and large numbers of immunologically committed effector cells have been mobilized. In fact, it is difficult to inhibit the secondary or anamnestic response of any immune reaction. Successful interference with the effector mechanism of graft rejection is prohibited by both the complexity and the interdependence of the reaction. Many pathways and cellular participants need to be blocked. In addition, there are points of cross activation between these pathways which make it difficult effectively to inhibit any or all of them. If true immunosuppression is to be achieved, with respect to a certain antigen, interference must take place during the early phases of the primary immune response.

PRIVILEGED SITES FOR ALLOGRAFTS. First-set grafts need to develop either vascular or lymphatic connections to sensitize the host. Certain sites within the recipient, therefore, may permit extended graft survival of first-set grafts. A presensitized recipient can usually reject a second-set allograft before these connections are made, however.

The anterior chamber of the eye has been the most frequently used privileged space for allografts and xenografts of both normal and malignant tissues. Grafts at this site were originally thought to survive because of their inability to sensitize the host, not because they are protected from immunologic mediators of rejection. Tissues in the anterior chamber are rejected if the host is sensitized by conventional means. Therefore, the anterior chamber of the eye has been considered an excellent site for the study of the afferent arc of immunity. It is one of the rare locations in which lymphatic vessels are completely lacking, and the prolonged survival of grafts provides further evidence for the importance of lymphatic connections in host sensitization.

Absence of lymphatic connections may not be the only explanation. Raju and Grogan have presented evidence that grafts within the anterior chamber become vascularized rapidly and sensitize the recipient only slightly less rapidly than other grafts. Despite such sensitization, however, the grafts continue to survive unless sensitization is induced by more conventional techniques. Implants in unsensitized recipients become infiltrated by small round cells which somehow are *not* associated with graft destruc-

tion. The extended survival of grafts in the anterior chamber may represent a combination of both afferent arc delay and efferent arc blockade.

Other sites provide a special environment for allografts. It has been known for almost 50 years that the meninges of the brain shelter grafts. The implants must be within the meninges and without encroachment on the ventricles. The extended survival is dependent on a lack of vascular connections to the host, which in turn prevents sensitization. The immunologic insulation of the testis may relate to its circuitous lymphatic supply. Presentation of the antigens to the host may be inefficient. Cartilage, too, can be successfully allografted without immunosuppression. The mucoprotein matrix seems to shield the graft cells from host lymphocytes.

The cheek pouch of the hamster has been used as a location for a variety of foreign grafts. Once again, graft survival is due to reduced ability to sensitize the host, since grafts will not survive in the cheek pouches of hamsters previously sensitized to donor antigens. Even well-established grafts will be rejected promptly if the host is sensitized through conventional means. The immunologic arc seems to be interrupted on the afferent side because the mucopolysaccharide-containing connective tissue of the pouch acts as an immunologic insulator.

HISTOCOMPATIBILITY MATCHING

It is obvious that, other things being equal, the less antigenic the graft, the less the host will react against the graft. In human transplantation, when the donor and recipient are identical twins, there is no antigenic difference of any significance, and the tissues will be readily accepted. When the donor and recipient are siblings or when a parent donor is used for offspring, there is a greater statistical likelihood of antigen sharing between donor and recipient than when a cadaver or other unrelated donor is used.

Several methods have been developed for the purpose of demonstrating antigenic similarities between donor and recipient prior to transplantation, so that donor and recipient pairs may be selected which are relatively histocompatible. This should lessen the need for large doses of immunosuppressive drugs and increase the likelihood of an ultimately successful outcome. Although many methods have been tried, the currently most promising are leukocyte typing and MLC (mixed lymphocyte culture).

LEUKOCYTE TYPING. The rationale for leukocyte typing is based upon two observations: The first is that leukocytes are capable of immunizing animals to a subsequent skin or kidney graft and thus must share many important antigens with these and other tissues of the body. The second rationale is that antisera from certain patients who have received multiple transfusions will react with cells from some patients but not from others. Investigators observed that antisera of this type were also found in certain multiparous women. Subsequently, many antisera obtained from multiply transfused patients or from women with multiple pregnancies (and occasionally from other sources) have been assembled and tested for their ability to detect leukocyte antigens. Some of the antisera seem to recognize groups of antigens, and others recognize single antigens (monospecific antisera). Using the patient's leukocytes and a group of standard antisera it is thus possible to characterize many, if not all, of the strong HLA-A and -B histocompatibility antigens on the human lymphocyte membrane. This is done for both donor and recipient, and the two patterns are then compared to determine whether the donor is likely to be compatible with the recipient or not.

Antigens found less frequently have been identified which appear not to be at this locus; it is likely that other antigenic loci may be defined in the future. The inheritance of HLA antigens was discussed above. Weaker histocompatibility antigens at other loci have not been detected by serologic techniques in human beings.

Currently antigens are detected by isolating lymphocytes from the peripheral blood of potential donors or recipients. The cells are incubated with antisera of various specificities and rabbit serum as a source of complement. Cells which react with antibodies in the serum die in the presence of complement and can be stained with vital dyes. Typing sera is becoming increasingly standardized. A typical set of results from the University of Minnesota typing laboratories is illustrated in Table 10-1.

Histocompatibility typing is useful in determining the best match between donor and recipient when family donors are utilized. Siblings who share all four HL-A antigens in common and who have inherited identical HL-A haplotypes from their parents are the best possible donor-recipient pair. But several points about histocompatibility matching deserve emphasis: (1) Recipients receiving grafts even from donors who are "perfect" matches with them will still reject the graft (although more slowly) unless immunosuppressive drugs are utilized. Only an identical twin is truly a perfect match. In the context used here "perfect" simply means that there are no detectable antigenic differences between donor and host with the antisera employed and that the degree of compatibility is suffi-

ciently high so that, with the judicial use of immunosuppressive drugs, the outcome is likely to be good. (2) Even with poor histocompatibility matches between relatives, the results are frequently good. Those results probably indicate that, with the current immunosuppressive drugs, it is sometimes possible to suppress even great degrees of antigenic incompatibility. (3) Even in the presence of a good histocompatibility match, the graft may fail if the host happens to have preformed antibodies against a donor's tissues. These antibodies can be recognized if recipient serum is allowed to react with donor lymphocytes in a cytotoxicity test. This test, called *cross matching*, should be performed with fresh serum as a final test of compatibility prior to transplant. Preformed cytotoxic antibodies to donor tissue cannot be detected by the usual typing procedure itself. (4) The presence of ABH antibodies will lead to the prompt rejection of tissue bearing incompatible blood group substances. Transplants in the face of such barriers should not be performed. (5) Despite the results of tissue typing, a related donor will generally yield better transplant results than an unrelated (cadaver) donor. This statement is controversial, but the results of kidney transplantation strongly support it. (6) Tissue typing for unrelated cadaver donors is not as successful as typing for related donors, but increasing evidence supports the correlation between graft success and HLA-A and -B locus matching (Fig. 10-27).

MIXED LYMPHOCYTE CULTURE (MLC). The other method of detecting degrees of histocompatibility between donor and recipient is the MLC test, which detects differences principally at the HLA-D locus. Lymphocytes of the recipient are mixed with lymphocytes of the donor in tissue culture. If significant antigenic differences exist between the two, they will respond by transformation into blast cells, DNA synthesis, and mitosis. The incorporation of tritiated thymidine into DNA can be quantified to assess the degree of stimulation. As the test was originally de-

Table 10-1. LYMPHOCYTE ANTIGEN TYPING REPORT OF THEORETIC FAMILY*

Family member	ABO	Genotype	HL-A locus (LA)								HL-A 2d locus (four)														
			HL-A1	HL-A2	HL-A3	HL-A9	HL-A10	HL-A11	W19	W28	HL-A5	HL-A7	HL-A8	HL-A12	HL-A13	W5	W10	W14	W15	W16	W17	W18	W21	W22	W27
Father AB	A	AO	+	+	−	−	−	−	−	−	−	+	+	−	−	−	−	−	−	−	−	−	−	−	−
Mother CD	A	AO	−	−	+	+	+	−	−	−	+	−	−	+	−	−	−	−	−	−	−	−	−	−	−
Son AC (patient)	O	OO	+	−	+	−	−	−	−	−	+	−	+	−	−	−	−	−	−	−	−	−	−	−	−
Son AD	A	?	+	−	−	+	+	−	−	−	−	−	+	+	−	−	−	−	−	−	−	−	−	−	−
Daughter BC	O	OO	−	+	+	−	−	−	−	−	+	+	−	−	−	−	−	−	−	−	−	−	−	−	−
Daughter BD	A	?	−	+	−	+	+	−	−	−	−	+	−	+	−	−	−	−	−	−	−	−	−	−	−
Daughter AC	O	OO	+	−	+	−	−	−	−	−	+	−	+	−	−	−	−	−	−	−	−	−	−	−	−

*The specificities for the first and second loci are those currently used at the University of Minnesota.

Son AC is the prospective transplant recipient. Daughter AC is a perfect match for all four antigens; she shares the inheritance of both HL-A haplotypes and is the ideal donor. Both parents, son AD, and daughter BC share only one haplotype with the potential recipient and are theoretically not as good donors. Daughter BD shares no HL-A haplotypes with the recipient and is the poorest donor in the family.

More important than the HL-A type are the ABO blood types. The father, mother, son AD, and daughter BD *cannot* donate, because they are all blood group A and the recipient is blood group O and possesses anti-A antibodies in his serum.

vised, it was a two-way test—cells of the donor were capable of reacting against cells of the recipient and vice versa. In order to isolate the response of the recipient cells to the donor antigens, the donor lymphocytes can be inactivated by irradiation or exposure to mitomycin C. More and more evidence supports the usefulness of this test in predicting success in organ and bone marrow transplantation.

CLINICAL TISSUE AND ORGAN TRANSPLANTATION

Clinical allotransplants may be of several types: (1) temporary free grafts, such as skin allografts and blood transfusions; (2) partially inert struts which provide a framework for the ingrowth of host tissue, such as bone, cartilage, nerve, tendon, and fascial grafts; (3) permanent, partially privileged, structurally free grafts, such as cornea, blood vessels, and heart valves; (4) partially privileged functional free grafts such as parathyroid, ovary, and testes; (5) whole organ grafts, such as pancreas, kidney, liver, lung, and heart; and (6) bone marrow which acts as a functional replacement of the entire hemopoietic and lymphopoietic systems. Immunosuppression is warranted only for grafts essential for life. Tooth bud and thyroid grafts, which would require immunosuppression for any success, are trivial grafts and are easily replaced by prostheses or medication.

Clinical autotransplants have been carried out with hair, skin, teeth, kidney, legs, arms, veins, arteries, pericardium, valves, bone, cartilage, fascia, fat, tendons, nerves, stomach, bowel, parathyroid, thyroid, ovary, testis, adrenal, and hemopoietic tissue. Allotransplants have been carried out employing cornea, teeth, thyroid, parathyroid, adrenal, ovary, testis, pituitary, spleen, lymph node, bone marrow, skin, bone, cartilage, fascia, tendons, nerves, arteries, valves, veins, hemopoietic tissue, pancreas, duodenum, kidney, liver, lung, and heart. Xenografts of skin, heart valves, heart, kidney, testis, bone, and cartilage have been tried in the past.

Skin

Autotransplants of skin containing hair are used to reconstruct eyebrows or to replace the scalp after traumatic avulsion. Autotransplants of individual hair roots are sometimes used as a treatment for baldness. Skin autotransplants have been used to reconstruct the esophagus, urinary tract, vagina, and hernial weaknesses as well as the usual surface defects. The main use of skin autografts is to cover and replace areas destroyed by trauma, burn, or operation.

Skin allotransplants are also used quite extensively in burned patients. They are commonly used in three different ways: In the first they are applied as a dressing to the burned area and are removed after 3 or 4 days. At this time additional allografts are reapplied if the area does not appear to be clean enough to accept autografts. If the area does appear to be clean, autografts are applied. The theory behind this is that the skin allograft provides a better

Fig. 10-27. The effect of tissue typing on the subsequent function of cadaver renal allografts at the University of Minnesota. If more (two to four) of the antigens are matched between graft and recipient, better kidney function is likely to result. If only zero to one of the four HLA-A and -B antigens on graft and recipient cells are the same, success is less likely. This difference is enhanced if diabetic recipients, technical kidney losses, and kidneys rejected by hyperacute reactions are excluded.

coverage than any other material, and during the period of time when it is taking, it prevents the continued spread of sepsis.

The second method is to place alternate thin strips of autografted and allografted skin side by side to cover large defects. As the allografted skin is gradually rejected, it is replaced by epithelial cells which grow in from the autografts.

In the last method the allograft is applied and allowed to take. When it begins to be rejected, it is removed, and autografts are applied. Prolongation up to 50 days of skin allograft survival can be achieved with immunosuppression. Massive burns can now be treated with excision and allografting within the first 10 days postburn. The allografts are then serially excised and replaced with autografts as the initially limited autograft donor sites regenerate. Bacterial complications of the burn and immunosuppression are minimized by temporarily housing the patient in protected "germ-free" environments.

Xenografts of skin are commonly used as temporary biologic dressings to be replaced at 2- to 4-day intervals. The commercial preparations of pig skin are nonviable and do not become vascularized. Similarly, chemically fixed grafts might be useful in the future as temporary covers to reduce burn mortality and morbidity.

Vascular Grafts

AUTOGRAFTS

Vein autografts have been used for over 50 years to replace segments of damaged arteries. This is still by far the best bypass graft for occluded vessels in the lower extremity below the level of the inguinal ligament. After a period of time in the arterial circuit the vein wall thickens, and the vein becomes somewhat arterialized. Although there are occasional instances in which vein grafts weaken and rupture, by and large they make very satisfactory arterial substitutes. The three most common usages at the present time are in femoro–popliteal artery–saphenous vein bypass grafts, aorto–renal artery–saphenous vein bypass grafts, and coronary artery bypass grafts. Pieces of autologous vein are also used as patch grafts either for small stenotic areas, such as the renal artery, or over long segments of endarterectomized artery. It is also possible to carry out successful autologous vein grafts to bridge defects in veins, although veins are less likely to stay open than arteries. Autologous vein grafts have also been used as tendon sheath and bile duct replacement without success.

Autografted arteries are also sometimes used as vascular replacements—most often the hypogastric artery is utilized. Pieces of pericardium are sometimes used to patch defects or divert flow in the repair of intracardiac defects.

ALLOGRAFTS

The use of allografted arteries had a considerable vogue a few years ago, but they are seldom used now. There are three reasons for this: (1) aneurysms sometimes occur, with rupture and a fatal outcome; (2) plastic prostheses have proved so suitable for the larger blood vessels; (3) for smaller blood vessels the use of the autologous saphenous vein has proved to be better than either prostheses or allografts. Arterial allografts, even if viable, do not survive but in part are replaced by host tissue and in part persist as semi-inert material.

When organs are transplanted, the artery supplying the organ becomes an arterial allograft. It has been shown that the epithelium of smaller blood vessels is antigenic and some degree of allograft rejection occurs.

Fresh, sterile aortic valve allografts have been used quite extensively. They appear to elicit a minimal antigenic response when compared with arterial allografts. Even so, gradual thickening, immobility, and calcification of these valves occur; their functional life expectancy in patients has not yet been determined.

Vein allografts have been used for a number of years in sporadic fashion, and umbilical vein allografts have become commercially available for arterial bypass. Allografts have always been, and will almost certainly continue to be, inferior to fresh autografts. There is, of course, no reason whatsoever for the inferiority of arterial and venous grafts to autografts of the same type *except* for the antigenicity of the allograft and the mild rejection reaction which these grafts elicit. For some reason there has been a great reluctance among surgeons and others to accept the fact that arterial and venous allografts are antigenic. It is true that the antigenicity is relatively mild and that the graft can provide structural function even in the face of the immunologic response, but it eventually limits the life of the graft.

Fascia

Fascial autografts, either free or attached at one end, are used as living sutures to repair inguinal hernias; for the repair of chest wall defects, torn ligaments and tendons, abdominal wall hernias, and defects in the pleura, dura, diaphragm, trachea, and esophagus; for wrapping aneurysms; in arthroplasty; for fascial slings to correct paralysis of the facial muscles; in the stabilization of fractures and joints; in the construction of flexor sheaths; and to correct urinary incontinence. Fascial autografts have been used most commonly because of their convenience and ready availability. Some freeze-dried, preserved (nonviable) allografts have been used, however, and these dead grafts have united with muscle nearly as quickly as living fascia. Such allografts lose much of their histoincompatibility and serve as strong lattice for the ingrowth of autologous tissue.

Tendon

Free tendon autografts are used every day in standard surgical procedures. By far the most common use is that of repairing severed flexor tendons to the fingers. Usually the palmaris longus or extensor tendons of the toes are used, and the graft is inserted from the level of the midpalm of the hand to the distal phalanx.

The only use of a tendon allograft is that suggested by Peacock and Madden, in which both flexor tendons and all surrounding tissue are removed from the hand and finger of a cadaver prior to transplantation into a recipient with loss of digital flexor mechanism. Under these circumstances, adhesions form only to the outer layer of the tissue, and the graft continues to glide against the inner surfaces which are normally against it. The advantage of this technique is to prevent adhesions from disrupting the function of the digital flexor mechanism. The cadaver allograft apparently works better and for longer periods of time than the more frequently utilized silastic rod to develop a nonadherent tunnel. The technique, however, is cumbersome, and cadavers are not readily available. Stored, freeze-dried, nonviable flexor tendons should serve as well, and the development of tissue banks may permit wider application of this technique.

Nerve

Nerve autotransplants are used to bridge defects in important motor nerves or sometimes to transfer the function of one nerve into the distal end of another, to repair a severed facial or recurrent laryngeal nerve, for instance. It has been nearly 100 years since it was demonstrated that a nerve autograft was capable of conducting impulses across a nerve defect. The autografts undergo wallerian degeneration with proliferation of Schwann cells and are penetrated by regenerating fibers of the host's nerve after a few weeks. When the nerve graft is thick, the center of the graft may develop a zone of avascular necrosis in which regeneration fails to occur, whereas this does not happen with thin grafts. As a consequence of this, some investigators have advocated the use of cable grafts consisting of several strands of smaller nerves to bridge defects in nerves of large caliber. Sensory recovery can occur as well as motor recovery.

When allografts are used, wallerian degeneration also

takes place but occurs a little more slowly than in autografts. The proliferation of Schwann cells is not as vigorous as in autografts, and after a few days the cells appear to become necrotic. Despite this fact, allografts are capable of penetration by the nerve fibers and have permitted return of nerve function across the defect. The rate and intensity of nerve fiber penetration is less in allografts than in autografts. The ultimate outcome of allografts is clearly far inferior to that obtained with autografts, and in general they should probably be used only when autografts cannot be obtained. Xenografts have been tried but appear to be of no value to man. It is likely that the inflammatory rejection response interferes with the passage of autologous nerve endings down the transplanted nerve sheath.

Cornea

Perhaps the most common clinical allotransplant is that of the cornea. The eye should be harvested from cadavers within at least 1 hour after death, although intervals up to 5 hours are permissible. Eyes removed more than 15 hours after death are unsuitable for corneal transplantation. The whole eye is generally preserved in sterile liquid paraffin at a temperature of 3 to 5°C, and the graft is cut from it at the time of use. The eye is suspended from a suture passed through the severed optic nerve to keep it from coming in contact with the sides of the vessel. Frozen corneas are not as good as those preserved this way, and freeze-dried corneas are completely unsatisfactory. Xenografts are useless.

Two types of corneal transplants are utilized; the full-thickness graft and the lamellar, or partial-thickness, graft. The full-thickness graft should give the best results, but complications such as secondary glaucoma, anterior synechiae, and a partial lifting off of the graft, causing astigmatism or opacification, are frequent. These complications are avoided in lamellar keratoplasty, which is the operation of choice when the corneal opacity does not involve the full thickness of the cornea. In order to achieve a successful graft there must be good apposition between the graft and the host, the graft must be in contact with healthy cornea at some point in the circumference if it is to remain transparent, and blood vessels must not invade the graft to any appreciable extent.

The best patients for grafting are those with central corneal scars and healthy surrounding cornea with no vascularization; keratoconus, especially if the apex of the cone is beginning to break down; corneal dystrophy; indolent corneal abscesses; and perforating ulcers of the cornea which have resulted in a descemetocele. The results are somewhat less good in acne rosacea and herpetic keratitis because of the danger of recurrence of the disease.

Corneal grafts are apparently so successful because they remain effectively isolated from the host's cells so long as the graft itself and the cornea directly around it remain avascular. Many corneal grafts remain clear indefinitely, although occasionally a graft which has remained clear for several weeks becomes opaque. Apparently the fibrous barrier which is formed at the junction between the host and the graft is almost impervious to blood vessels and helps to maintain the isolation of the graft even when vessels have entered the host's cornea. The clouding over of a previously clear graft is due to the allograft reaction, usually because of vascularization. It has been demonstrated experimentally that if a graft of skin from the donor of the cornea is put on 2 to 6 weeks after corneal transplantation, the graft becomes opaque, whereas if a skin homograft from another donor is applied, nothing happens. Skin from the original donor transplanted 6 weeks or more after the corneal transplantation is no longer capable of causing it to become opaque. This is presumably due to adaptation, the development of the scar tissue barrier between the host and the graft, or replacement of the cells of the graft by host's cells. Recently, short-term organ culture of corneas in order to reduce graft immunogenicity has been tried, but it is not yet known if this will improve the clinical results.

Bone

Bone implants are used for the following indications: (1) to hasten the healing of defects and cavities, e.g., the use of cancellous bone chips in the residual defect after curettage of a unicameral bone cyst; (2) to supplement the arthrodesis of joints, e.g., extraarticular arthrodesis of the tuberculous hip; (3) to achieve bony union in cases of delayed healing or pseudarthrosis arising after fracture, e.g., sliding or barrel stave grafts for nonunion of tibial shaft fractures; (4) to supplement the healing of certain fresh fractures for which open reduction and internal fixation are required, e.g., cancellous implants for fractures of both bones of the forearm in an adult; (5) to reconstruct major skeletal defects arising as a result of trauma, disease, or congenital malformation; (6) to reconstruct contour, e.g., replacement of calvarial defects after surgery for trauma by compact bone implants.

A variety of grafting techniques has been devised to meet the differing clinical requirements. The most frequent types of bone grafts are inlay grafts, onlay grafts and/or internal fixation, barrel stave grafts, sliding grafts, and application of cancellous chips. In addition, there are pedicled grafts of two types, those with a bony base and muscle pedicle grafts. The pedicle technique applies strictly to autografts and was devised to circumvent devitalization, thereby hastening healing.

Autografts are preferred for clinical use, since the cellular elements of bone allografts usually elicit a rejection response. Bone allografts do elicit new bone formation (osteoinduction) and serve as struts for the ingrowth of autologous bone (osteoconduction). As such, allografts are of great clinical use although they are always somewhat inferior to autografts.

For the most part stored or processed bone allografts are used in human beings. Preservation methods include (1) refrigeration, (2) freezing, (3) freeze drying, (4) boiling or autoclaving, (5) deproteinization, (6) decalcification, (7) any one of the above plus irradiation for sterilization, and (8) removal of marrow elements and replacement by autologous marrow. Such nonviable grafts mainly serve to stimulate and conduct new autologous bone formation.

Cartilage

It has been long known that cartilage can be successfully transferred between individuals of different genetic backgrounds without the need for immunosuppression therapy. This immunologic privilege is attributable to the presence of the mucoprotein matrix, which acts as an insulation to prevent host lymphocytes from reaching the graft chondrocytes. Cartilage cells can elicit allograft responses, but cartilage grafts will survive even in highly immunized hosts.

Free autografts of cartilage have been used most extensively in plastic reconstructive surgery (1) to rebuild the contours of the nose after congenital or posttraumatic deformity, (2) to reconstruct the pinna, and (3) to fill out defects in the facial bones and the skull.

The fresh cartilage autograft comes closest to fulfilling the description of an ideal cartilage graft: it should maintain its structure, have the potential for growth and repair, provoke no untoward reaction, and form a firm union with host tissues, persisting without loss of viability or absorption.

The fresh cartilage allograft, however, has been a reasonable substitute for the autograft, particularly because of its greater ease of procurement. The major drawback of such grafts is that despite the immunologic privilege of cartilage, the bulk of experimental and clinical evidence suggests that the tendency for late deterioration and absorption is somewhat greater than that of autografts.

The preserved cartilaginous allograft has been used as a substitute for the fresh implant primarily because of the convenience that storage of such implants in cartilage banks provides. Boiled, refrigerated, frozen, and chemically preserved sections of cartilage have all been used with success.

The cartilage xenograft should be mentioned since it enjoys a prolonged survival and relative exemption from transplantation rejection unrivaled by any other tissue. Even so, the exemption is not complete, and some xenografts elicit strong inflammatory responses and are absorbed.

COMPOSITE GRAFTS OF BONE AND CARTILAGE

Composite grafts involve the surgical transfer of entire functional units rather than the implantation of bits and pieces of cartilage or bone.

EPIPHYSEAL GROWTH PLATES. The object of the transplantation of epiphyseal growth plates is to restore longitudinal growth in hypoplastic limbs, whether congenital or acquired. This type of procedure has been used in efforts to improve the function of children with congenital deficiency of the radius. In these cases, autotransplantation of the proximal fibula has been used as a substitute for the radial deficiency. Although, in some cases, enlargement of the transplant could be demonstrated, this was always inferior to the natural growth potential and has not been sufficient to justify incorporation of this procedure into the surgical armamentarium.

OSTEOCHONDRAL GRAFTS. The diseases that destroy the articular cartilage are common. The osteochondral or osteoarticular graft might be a useful substitute. Transplants of articular cartilage, in conjunction with a very thin shell of subchondral supporting bone, are still in the experimental stage. Such operations will require allografting.

TRANSPLANT OF HEMIJOINTS OR WHOLE JOINTS. The experimental transplantation of joints was initiated by Judet in 1908. Autografts tend to heal their osteosynthesis sites, revascularize the bony component, and in general maintain the articular surfaces in a fair state of preservation. On the other hand, both fresh and preserved allogenic transplants give unpredictable results, sometimes healing well with good function, and other times showing progressive deterioration. These latter changes in the allogenic groups are associated with delayed revascularization of the bony component, subchondral fracture and collapse, and the late development of degenerative arthritic change. Artificial hemijoints or whole joints have superseded transplantation, at least for the present.

Extremity Replantation

Autotransplants or replantation of extremities have been carried out with increasing frequency in recent years. This has usually involved the upper extremity, because the chances for nerve regeneration are far greater in the arm than in the leg. Satisfactory prostheses exist for the lower extremity, but they are much more complex and unsatisfactory for the upper. Shortening of the reimplanted extremity usually is necessary, and this produces much more incapacity in the leg than in the arm. Replantation of the leg might be considered when the opposite leg has been extensively damaged or lost or when the amputation has been so high that good prostheses are not available. Advances in microsurgery have permitted replantation of digits to become almost routine if adequate experience and appropriate instrumentation, including an operating microscope, are available.

The technique of limb replantation initially requires a general evaluation of the patient to assess other associated injuries. This should include roentgenography of the proximal stump as well as the amputated extremity itself, and particularly of the spine to be certain that the spinal roots to the extremity have not been avulsed. After securing hemostasis and being certain that no serious injury has been overlooked, the replantation can begin. During this initial phase the severed limb should be packed in ice. It should not be frozen, however, and dry ice should be avoided. If the facilities are available, the artery of the limb should be perfused with cold Ringer's lactate solution to which albumin and heparin have been added. The limb may be replanted even though several hours have elapsed between its severance and the start of replantation. The exact critical period has not definitely been established, but it appears that at least 6 hours and sometimes even more can elapse with successful results after replantation. Satisfactory hypothermia of the extremity increases this period. The more distal the amputation, the better the preservation of the extremity, and the more prolonged is the tolerance to ischemia.

When perfusion is completed and replantation is about

to begin, a limited debridement of grossly devitalized tissue is carried out. Questionably viable tissue is not removed. Then the bone is fixed so that the limb will be stabilized before beginning the repairs of the vessels and nerve supply. Larger bones may require slight shortening to freshen up the ends and to gain additional length for relaxation of the arteries and nerves. Intramedullary fixation is used whenever possible.

After proper fixation of the bones the blood vessels are joined. The largest vein is joined first, so that there will be an outflow tract at the moment when the blood is ready to flow through the artery.

If the nerve injury has been a crushing one, nerve repair is delayed until healing is complete. If the nerve has been cleanly severed with a sharp instrument, particularly if the injury has been at the level of the wrist, immediate primary repair is carried out. While the results of nerve allografts are still highly problematic, an autograft or allograft should be used to bridge any large defect in the nerve. A better result is obtained in distal nerve transections than in proximal ones, and in young people as compared with older ones. Motor recovery in the median nerve is much more common than in the ulnar nerve.

After completing the arterial and venous anastomoses and after either joining the ends of the nerves or deciding to perform nerve suture as a secondary procedure, attention is turned to the soft tissues. With the blood supply restored, viability of tissues is easier to ascertain, and debridement can be completed. The shortening of the bone makes it possible to join several muscles together with a particular view to covering the blood vessels with living tissues. If soft tissue loss is minimal, the covering can be achieved with the skin of the extremity, and other defects can be covered with split-thickness skin grafts. If the soft tissue defect is great and no covering is available, the defect must be covered by a pedicle flap.

In the postoperative period the patient's arm must be kept in an elevated position to minimize edema. It is important to do a fasciotomy at the end of the replantation to avoid severe ischemia from swelling if damage to the arm was severe. Heparin and dextran are not generally used postoperatively. Some degree of hypotension may occur as a consequence of leakage of plasma into the replanted extremity. This is particularly true of a lower extremity. The hypotension is counteracted by the administration of plasma. There may be an acute period of acidosis as a consequence of absorption of metabolic products from the ischemic extremity, and this is counteracted by the administration of bicarbonate. Both bicarbonate and mannitol are administered to protect against renal damage, and prophylactic antibiotics are also administered. If early severe sepsis supervenes, the extremity may have to be amputated. Low-grade late infection, usually consisting of osteomyelitis, is treated by drainage and irrigation, and the fixation materials are left in place until the bone heals even in the face of sepsis—because fixation must be achieved if possible.

Passive movement of all joints is begun immediately and continued throughout the course of treatment. Galvanic stimulation of the intrinsic muscles of the hand is utilized to maintain the tone of the muscles. Extensive physical therapy is instituted. If primary nerve suture has not been carried out, the nerves are reexplored 6 weeks or more after the injury, and repair is carried out then. In subsequent months and years many reconstructive but functional results have been surprisingly good.

Hemopoietic and Lymphoid Tissues

BONE MARROW

Bone marrow is easily destroyed by whole-body ionizing irradiation, drugs, or chemicals. The erythrocyte stem cell compartment is the most sensitive site. Its final products, the mature peripheral blood cells, are in most instances not sensitive to injury by irradiation or by chemical substances, but these cells have a relatively short life-span, and a regular supply of new cells is needed. In leukemia, the bone marrow is replaced by tumor cells, a situation effectively the same as that existing when marrow is destroyed by other means.

Injury to bone marrow by drugs, chemicals, and disease poses several clinical problems. Bone marrow transplants between identical twins have been successfully carried out in many cases of irradiation exposure, aplastic anemia, and leukemia. Autologous marrow transplantation has also been found useful in a few patients after planned treatment with toxic levels of alkylating agents.

Marrow allotransplants are far less successful. Marrow is highly immunogenic and will be readily rejected by the immunologically normal host. If, however, the marrow is allotransplanted into an immunologically crippled (irradiated, immunosuppressed) host, a chimera is produced. The problem then becomes, not destruction of the marrow by the host, but the maturation of donor marrow stem cells to total immunological competence and rejection of the host by the graft. This graft-versus-host (GVH) phenomenon is not seen with skin, kidney, heart, liver, grafts, etc., but it is a major, unsolved problem in the transplantation of foreign bone marrow, white blood cells, and lymphoid tissues. Theory predicts, and practice shows, that GVH disease does not occur in bone marrow transplants between identical human twins. An important additional point is the finding of reduced severity of the GVH reaction when the donor and host, even though not genetically identical, have been closely matched at the HLA locus.

The major sites of injury in GVH reactions are the lymphatic tissues, the skin, the intestine, and the liver of the host. Dermatitis, diarrhea, loss of weight, poor liver function, and infection associated with immunoincompetence are intrinsic parts of the reaction. The GVH reactions in bone marrow transplantation in human beings have been of overwhelming importance and are the major problem in this new clinical area. Congdon has summarized some of the experimental and clinical approaches to the problem of the control of GVH disease (Table 10-2). A combination of tissue typing and immunologic suppression is now utilized to control the GVH reaction in human beings.

A long-range goal in marrow transplantation is the use

Table 10-2. SOME APPROACHES TO THE CONTROL OF GRAFT-VERSUS-HOST DISEASE

A. Immunologic compatibility: histocompatibility typing and matching of donor and recipient
B. Immunologic suppression
   1. Treatment of marrow recipient
      a. Methotrexate
      b. Cyclophosphamide
      c. Antilymphocyte serum
   2. Treatment of marrow donor: antilymphocyte serum
C. Removal of immunologically active cells
   1. Manipulation of the marrow in vitro
   2. Cell separation
D. Innate absence of immunocompetent cells: use of fetal and newborn blood-forming tissue as the donor source

of these grafts as a means of promoting acceptance of other organs, such as liver, heart, and kidney. Investigations in the mouse have shown that once the foreign marrow is established, a state of relative or complete specific nonreactivity against donor antigens is conferred, and other tissues taken from the same donor as the marrow can be successfully transplanted without further immunosuppression. The transplantation of foreign bone marrow in laboratory animals is an experiment in the production of tolerance and, as such, has potential wide application. The mechanism of adaptation by the graft to the host is not clear, but once such adaptation is accomplished, other grafts from the same donor will survive without immunosuppression.

In practice, human bone marrow allotransplantation has enjoyed increasing success. HLA identical marrow transplants (from matched siblings) are commonly used to treat aplastic anemias. Transplantation with HLA matched but nonidentical twin marrow usually produces a mild to moderate (but occasionally lethal) GVH reaction. Dramatic success has been achieved in the treatment of certain congenital immunodeficiency diseases, where no host-versus-graft reaction is possible, so that host immunosuppression is not required. In all other patients, marrow allotransplantation requires doses of immunosuppressive cytotoxic drugs much larger than those used to gain acceptance of kidney grafts, and the use of non-HLA matched donors has rarely been successful.

A few patients with leukemia have been helped by intensive chemotherapy followed by HLA matched marrow transplantation, but many die of GVH disease, recurrent leukemia, or infection. The hope, seldom realized thus far, is that the leukemia cells surviving chemotherapy will be killed by the GVH reaction.

THYMUS

The congenital absence of thymic tissue prevents the maturation of the entire T-cell system. Such patients are deficient in cell-mediated immune responses and those B-cell responses requiring T-cell interaction. Transplantation of an embryonic fresh or cultured thymus into such patients has resulted in considerable improvement in these normal defense mechanisms. The exact indications and

success rate have not been fully defined, but this is a promising field of investigation.

SPLEEN AND LYMPH NODE

Patients with agammaglobulinemia have been treated by free transplantation of lymph nodes or by transplantation of the spleen with vascular anastomoses. No success has been achieved, but, surprisingly, neither have any serious difficulties eventuated. If a patient with agammaglobulinemia were indeed able to accept allotransplants readily, it might be expected that the spleen or lymph node would react against the immunologically inadequate host.

Several splenic allografts have been carried out in human beings for a variety of indications. These include attempts (1) to transplant immunoglobulin-producing tissue for agammaglobulinemia, (2) to transplant enzyme-producing tissues to treat congenital enzymatic deficiencies (e.g., Gaucher's disease), and (3) to treat cancer with spleen immune to tumor antigens. None of these transplants were successful. Spleen transplants have also been proposed to treat hemophilia, since splenic tissue may be one source of antihemophilic globulin. Since the spleen and lymph nodes are highly antigenic tissues, their successful transplantation must require one of two circumstances: (1) either that the host have a severe type of congenital immunologic deficiency, thus permitting a successful allotransplant but subjecting the patient to the GVH disease, or (2) if the host has a somewhat greater degree of immunologic competence, that immunosuppressive drugs be administered, thus rendering the host even more vulnerable than before to serious infection. These transplants do not, therefore, hold out much hope of clinical success, and bone marrow transplantation may be a better solution which does not entail an operative procedure.

Endocrine Autografts

Most of the clinical experience with endocrine autografts is of only historical significance, because little scientific information has been acquired and there has been only doubtful benefit to the patient. At best such clinical attempts provided temporary indirect evidence of function. Claims of long-term success were never supported by histologic proof.

The placement of endocrine fragments as autografts into intramuscular pockets has proved successful in several clinical situations. For example, the indications for parathyroid autotransplantation have recently been listed by Wells et al. (Table 10-3). When it appears possible that a patient may have insufficient parathyroid tissue following removal of the thyroid gland, the implantation of small fragments into the exposed neck muscles has repeatedly proved worthwhile. Parathyroid glands excised during removal of thyroid mass should be diced and implanted into intramuscular pockets. When removal of the parathyroid tissue is planned, as in cases of secondary hyperparathyroidism, the volar forearm muscle is a useful site for autotransplantation. The parathyroids are readily available for subsequent excision if hyperparathyroidism recurs. Be-

Table 10-3. INDICATIONS FOR PARATHYROID
TRANSPLANTATION

A. Autotransplantation
  1. Severe secondary hyperparathyroidism
  2. Primary generalized parathyroid hyperplasia
  3. Inadvertent removal of parathyroid tissue
B. Allotransplantation
  1. Congenital absence of parathyroid glands—DiGeorge's syndrome
  2. Iatrogenic aparathyroidism which is not controllable with a medical regimen

cause secondary hyperparathyroidism is common in chronic renal failure, and hemodialysis is now possible for many years, the indications for total parathyroidectomy and autotransplantation may increase in the years ahead.

Similar indications may exist for other endocrine organs: in a child with lingual thyroid, the tissue from the lingual mass may be the only functional thyroid. Perhaps it should be autotransplanted. Woodruff has made a similar plea for the autotransplantation of ovarian fragments into the rectus muscle in selected cases. Testicular slices have been successfully autotransplanted (albeit without histologic or functional documentation) to prevent the need for replacement therapy in case of accidental castration. Such a procedure should always be attempted when uncontaminated tissue is available, with placement of the implants in a readily accessible muscle. The fragments must not exceed 1 mm in thickness if function is to be expected.

In adrenal hyperplasia with Cushing's syndrome, the accepted surgical therapy has changed from subtotal adrenalectomy to total adrenalectomy with indefinite steroid replacement therapy, because of high incidence of recurrent disease after subtotal adrenalectomy. Autotransplantation of hyperplastic slices with functional and histologic success has been reported, with placement of the grafts at a site accessible for secondary removal. It may represent a reasonable surgical alternative in selected cases of Cushing's syndrome.

Endocrine Allografts (Other than the Pancreas)

The prognosis for endocrine allotransplants as a useful surgical procedure is in doubt. Replacement therapy for endocrine deficiency (aside from insulin deficiencies, to be discussed below) is efficient and generally adequate, and there is seldom an indication for the use of systemic immunosuppressive drugs to eliminate the need for endocrine replacement therapy. In the case of parathyroid allotransplants, there has been an insistent and recurrently hopeful effort. Parathyroid deficiency is not treated with specific hormone replacement, but rather with calcium and vitamin D, which give inadequate results. Groth et al. have reported a successful parathyroid allotransplant in a patient with a functioning renal allograft already receiving immunosuppressive drugs. Most other reports of parathyroid allotransplant success have been based on indirect evidence of decreased replacement therapy, and none has

been substantiated by histologic or functional evidence. There is no evidence that parathyroid tissue is immunologically privileged in human beings, and effective immunosuppressive therapy is probably not worthwhile.

Although endocrine allografts are of little clinical usefulness at present, two important experiments used endocrine transplantation to advance the field of endocrinology. Harris and Jacobsohn first illustrated the control of pituitary secretion by releasing factors from the hypothalamus traveling through the portal-hypophyseal vessels. Pituitary transplants functioned normally when returned to that location but did not function when transplanted to an area vascularized by temporal lobe vessels. Parathyroid physiology was advanced by Barnicot, who found that glands transplanted onto the surface of parietal bone resorbed directly. This observation is the cornerstone of the accepted hypothesis that parathyroid hormone acts directly on bone to raise the calcium in the blood, rather than indirectly by the phosphaturic effect on the kidney.

Pancreas

The discovery of insulin in 1921 was hailed as the cure of diabetes; it prevented death from diabetic coma, controlled the overt symptoms of diabetes, and provided an increased life expectancy. As diabetic patients lived longer, however, previously unseen complications developed. Diabetes was responsible for at least 30,000 deaths in 1974, and it is the leading cause of new cases of blindness in adults. Diabetics are 17 times more liable to kidney disease, five times more liable to gangrene of the extremities, and twice as likely to develop heart disease. Obviously, new approaches to treatment are required. Pancreas and islet transplantation offer the possibility that the development and progression of diabetic lesions will be prevented by precise regulation of carbohydrate metabolism—control not achieved by injected insulin.

An unresolved question is whether juvenile-onset diabetics suffer only from a lack of insulin or whether the absence of insulin reflects other subcellular derangements. Whether normalization of carbohydrate metabolism in these patients will prevent the development of systemic lesions is still unanswered. Several observations, however, support the hypothesis that angiopathic lesions associated with diabetes are secondary to abnormal metabolism: (1) Nephropathy and retinopathy occur in patients who develop diabetes as a result of other disease states (e.g., hemochromatosis) or after total pancreatectomy. (2) Numerous longitudinal, clinical studies have shown a relationship between duration of the disease, control of plasma glucose, and development of lesions. (3) Nephropathy and retinopathy occur in animals with induced diabetes. (4) Studies in animals have demonstrated that reduction of hyperglycemia by insulin therapy or by transplantation of whole pancreas or islets prevents or minimizes formation of diabetic lesions in the eye, kidney, and nerve. (5) Kidneys transplanted from normal to diabetic rats develop histologic lesions characteristic of diabetes in the rat, whereas kidneys transplanted from diabetic to normal rats

Fig. 10-28. Technique used for pancreaticoduodenal allotransplantation in the first four patients. The distal end of the duodenum was brought out as a cutaneous duodenostomy. [*From R. C. Lillehei and J. O. Ruiz, Pancreas, in J. S. Najarian and R. L. Simmons* (eds.), *"Transplantation," p. 627, Lea & Febiger, Philadelphia, 1972.*]

Fig. 10-29. Present technique of grafting donor duodenum to recipient small intestine. Both renal and pancreaticoduodenal allografts are illustrated. [*From R. C. Lillehei and J. O. Ruiz, Pancreas, in J. S. Najarian and R. L. Simmons* (eds.), *"Transplantation," p. 626, Lea & Febiger, Philadelphia, 1972.*]

showed disappearance or lack of progression of these lesions. These observations suggest that it may be possible to prevent the systemic complications of diabetes by insulin released from transplanted pancreatic islets. Alternative methods to provide precise glucose homeostasis, such as an implantable glucose sensor coupled to an insulin pump are also possible, however.

EXPERIMENTAL TRANSPLANTATION OF THE WHOLE PANCREAS

The ability of pancreatic transplants to ameliorate diabetes has long been known. The major problems with the procedure include vascular thrombosis, difficulty in establishing drainage of the pancreatic duct, autodigestion of the pancreas, and graft rejection. Theoretically, ligation of the pancreatic duct results in atrophy of exocrine tissue without affecting endocrine tissue. But in practice a severe inflammatory reaction occurs and leads to a constricting fibrosis which damages even the islets. Therefore, transplantation of the duct-ligated pancreas has included attempts to decrease pancreatic exocrine activity by irradiation of the duct-ligated pancreas, administration of 5-fluorouracil, methylprednisolone, or glucagon. These measures have helped but not solved the problem.

The alternative approach, transplantation without ligation of the pancreatic duct, has many variations. Initial attempts used a combined pancreaticoduodenal approach, with the duodenum serving as a conduit for drainage of exocrine enzymes (Figs. 10-28 and 10-29). The transplanted duodenum, however, is particularly susceptible to rejection and to anastomotic leakage, bleeding, ulceration, or perforation, even when evidence of pancreatic graft rejection is minimal. These complications can be eliminated by direct anastomosis of the pancreatic duct to a drainage site. If a small rim of mucosa is left around the pancreatic papilla, a direct anastomosis of the duct to the jejunum can be made which maintains exocrine and endocrine function of the graft. The anastomosis of the main duct of a segmental pancreatic graft to the recipient ureter has also been reported in animals as well as several patients.

Successful whole-organ pancreatic transplants produce circulating insulin and normal plasma glucose levels. When the venous drainage of the pancreatic graft was hooked up to the systemic circulation, the circulating insulin levels were higher than when the venous anastomosis was made to the portal system, although the plasma glucose levels were similar. Animals given whole pancreas isogenic transplants soon after induction of diabetes do not develop the renal, eye, and neural lesions that develop in the nontransplanted diabetic animals. In allograft models, rejection is heralded by increasing serum amylase followed by return to the diabetic state.

CLINICAL TRANSPLANTATION OF THE WHOLE PANCREAS

Since 1966, 49 whole-pancreas transplants have been reported. Evidence from patients 10, 12, 22, and 47 months following transplantation have shown that a functioning vascularized pancreatic allograft will correct the metabolic deficiency in diabetes. The fact that only one of these recipients, however, is still alive with a functioning graft reflects the severe problems associated with pancreatic transplantation.

Of the first 20 pancreatic transplant procedures, 11 were pancreaticoduodenal grafts performed in conjunction with a kidney transplant. The eventual graft failure and subsequent death of the patient were frequently caused by sepsis as a consequence of duodenal rejection and associated complications. Duodenal rejection seemed to occur frequently while the pancreas was functioning, and gave the impression that pancreatic grafts were less immunogenic than duodenum or kidney grafts. This impression, however, has not been confirmed, and the pancreas seems to have an average amount of histocompatibility antigens on its surface.

Variations in clinical pancreatic transplantation have been tried in an attempt to improve the results. Staggering the pancreatic and kidney grafts for end-stage diabetic nephropathy has been done. One patient had a segmental pancreatic graft with anastomosis of the main pancreatic duct to the ureter so that exocrine pancreatic drainage was via the bladder, and then received a renal allograft 145 days later. This patient, the sole survivor with a long-term functioning pancreatic graft reported to the ACS/NIH Transplant Registry, had complete abolishment of insulin requirements, a normal insulin response to glucose, improvement in vision, and abatement of neuropathy 47 months later. Segmental pancreatic transplants have been tried with exocrine drainage into a retroperitoneal jejunal Roux-en-Y loop. In the two patients whose grafts functioned, an intravenous glucose load resulted in a rapid, although subnormal, rise in plasma proinsulin and insulin levels.

Clinical transplantation of the whole pancreas can produce normal glucose homeostasis and an excellent functional result. Unfortunately, technical problems are severe, rejection can be disastrous, and the morbidity and mortality rates are high at this time. The clinical results may improve, however, especially if the allograft rejection can be more effectively suppressed.

EXPERIMENTAL TRANSPLANTATION OF ISLET TISSUE

Immediate vascularization, in general, is not essential for endocrine tissue transplantation to be successful, and in the last several years it has been possible to cure experimental diabetes by transplantation of islet tissue. The transplantation of adult pancreatic fragments was unsuccessful because the associated exocrine enzymes autodigested the transplanted tissue or injured the host. When specific techniques to separate islets from the nonendocrine pancreas were developed, transplantation of isolated adult islets was successful. The current technique for isolation of adult islets from the pancreas involves mechanical disruption, enzymatic digestion, and density gradient separation. Isolated adult islets will produce long-lasting control of diabetes in rats. Transplantation via the portal vein is more effective than intraperitoneal transplantation, and more islets survive in the liver, either because of the immediate availability of the blood supply or because of a physiologic

advantage to this site. Furthermore, transplantation via the portal vein can be accomplished without deterioration of liver function.

The isolation of islets from the adult pancreas is a laborious process, and the yield is low. In contrast, the neonatal pancreas can be successfully transplanted without separation of the islets from exocrine components, since it possesses such an extraordinarily low exocrine enzyme content that damage to autologous islets or recipient tissues is minimal. The successful transplantation of dispersed neonatal pancreatic tissue suggested that the adult pancreas could be transplanted without islet isolation if the digestive enzyme content of the exocrine tissue could be reduced. New techniques designed to reduce the exocrine effect have included (1) the use of donors whose pancreatic duct had been previously ligated, (2) short-term tissue culture of pancreatic fragments, and (3) transplantation of fresh pancreatic fragments into the spleen, which is better able to tolerate the exocrine enzymes. The successful transplantation of adult pancreatic fragments by one of these methods may solve a major problem: the procurement of sufficient islet tissue from a single cadaver donor to cure one diabetic recipient, since an increased quantity of islet tissue is available when the islets are not separated.

An even more frustrating aspect of islet transplantation is the apparent increased susceptibility of islets to allograft rejection. Survival is difficult to achieve even when immunosuppression that will prolong skin, kidney, or heart allografts is used. The clinical application of islet transplantation will also require techniques such as cold storage or culture to preserve the cells.

Despite these formidable difficulties, the numerous experimental demonstrations that transplanted islet tissue can prevent, halt, and even improve the vascular and neurological lesions of diabetes provide a tremendous impetus to continue to attack these problems.

Gastrointestinal Transplants

Various segments of intestine have been experimentally and clinically autotransplanted by removal from the body and reimplantation. Stomach, small bowel, and colon can all be used to replace esophagus, with reimplantation of the vascular supply. Allotransplantation of the small bowel and stomach has been carried out experimentally (Fig. 10-30). These grafts are rejected in the usual fashion, and within the same general time period as those in kidneys and other organs. There is some evidence that the lymphoid tissue within the intestinal wall can initiate a graft-versus-host reaction.

Although there is little apparent clinical use for a gastric transplant, there is a definite need for transplantation of the small bowel. Infarction of the bowel sometimes requires excision of the entire small bowel, and this leads to a fatal nutritional deficiency. Patients with various nutritional and motility problems, as well as certain patients with Crohn's disease, might well benefit from safe and successful bowel transplantation. A few attempts in human beings have been successful for several months, but no long-term survival has been achieved.

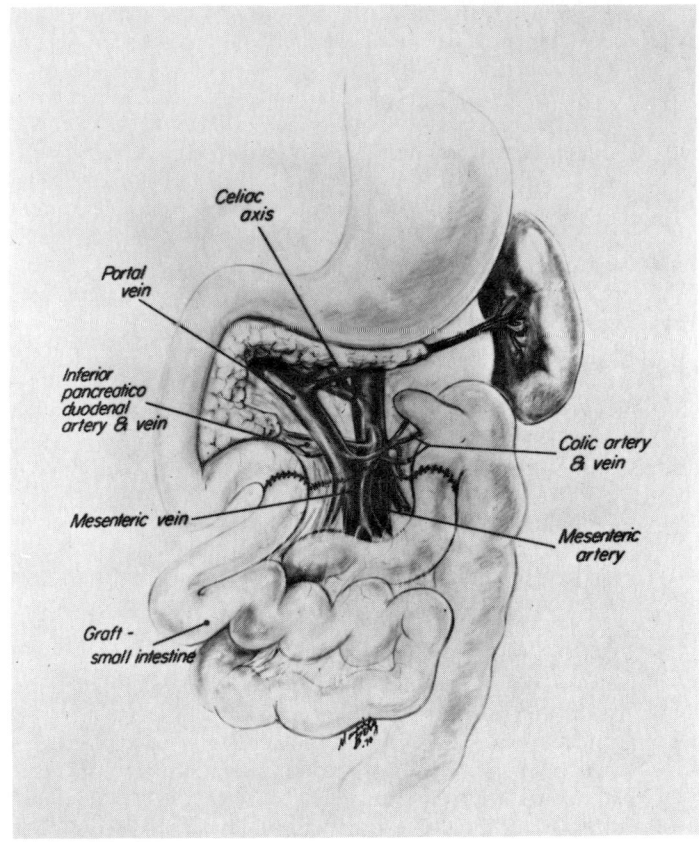

Fig. 10-30. Diagram showing the operative technique of orthotopic transplantation of the entire small intestine in a dog. [*From J. O. Ruiz, H. Uchida, and R. C. Lillehei, Intestine, in J. S. Najarian and R. L. Simmons (eds.), "Transplantation," p. 646, Lea & Febiger, Philadelphia, 1972.*]

Liver

EXPERIMENTAL TRANSPLANTATION IN ANIMALS

Two major surgical approaches to the transplantation of the liver are presently employed. The graft may be positioned in the normal anatomic location (orthotopic transplantation) following a recipient hepatectomy. Alternatively, the donor organ is placed in an ectopic site (heterotopic transplantation), generally with retention of the host's liver (auxiliary transplantation). Each of these techniques has unique inherent advantages, disadvantages, and requirements. The greatest success has been obtained with orthotopic transplantation, even though it is more technically difficult.

ORTHOTOPIC TRANSPLANTATION. The earliest studies evaluating orthotopic liver transplantation in the dog had an extremely high operative mortality rate. Initially, the inferior vena cava and portal vein of the anhepatic dog recipient were cross-clamped during total extirpation of the host's liver prior to receipt of the graft. Dogs subjected to this insult, without an adequate pathway for return of blood from the intestines and lower extremities, often died. To circumvent this dilemma, temporary shunts from the inferior vena cava and portal vein into the superior vena cava are necessary (Fig. 10-31). In human beings collateral venous networks usually develop as a consequence of existing liver disease, thereby eliminating the clinical need for shunts.

Experimentally, the graft is transplanted in its normal anatomical position by performing vena cava–to–vena cava and portal vein–to–portal vein anastomoses. An arterial anastomosis is created between the aorta of the graft and the aorta of the recipient. Biliary drainage is provided through construction of a cholecystoenterostomy (Fig. 10-32) after ligating the transected end of the graft's common duct.

With good surgical technique there is little early evidence of coagulation defects, severe acidosis, hypoglycemia, or biochemical derangements indicative of a significant hepatic injury pattern. But in the nonimmunosuppressed recipient, a pattern of rejection is almost invariably present by the fifth day. Elevations in the level of alkaline phosphatase, serum glutamic oxaloacetic transaminase (SGOT), and serum glutamic pyruvic transaminase (SGPT) develop at the same time as, or shortly prior to, the onset of jaundice. By the seventh day there are usually a progression of hyperbilirubinemia and other biochemical parameters reminiscent of biliary obstruction, as well as hepatic parenchymal cellular injury. A periportal mononuclear cell infiltrate, centrilobular necrosis, and intracanalicular bile stasis are present on microscopic examination. The recipient usually dies by the tenth postoperative day.

The pig appears to have inherent advantages as an experimental animal compared to the dog. In the pig there are fewer bacteria within the liver parenchyma and a greater

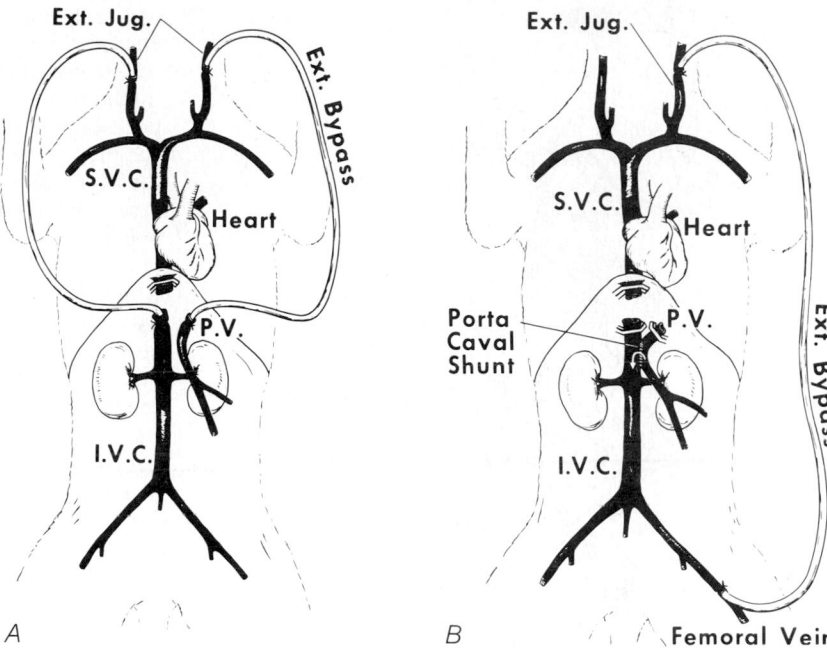

Fig. 10-31. Various splanchnic and systemic venous decompression techniques are employed during removal of the recipient liver in the healthy dog prior to revascularization of a hepatic graft. *A*. Two external shunts may provide for venous return from the inferior vena cava and portal vein into the jugular veins. *B*. Alternatively, a temporary side-to-side portacaval anastomosis establishing continuity between both venous systems permits the use of a single external bypass between the femoral and external jugular veins. [*From L. Brettschneider, Liver: I. Experimental (Transplantation), in J. S. Najarian, and R. L. Simmons (eds.), "Transplantation," p. 497, Lea & Febiger, Philadelphia, 1972.*]

resistance to problems caused by interrupting the portal circulation. Most remarkably, a number of liver transplant recipients have lived for many months, without much evidence of rejection. The cause of the absent or mild rejection pattern following transplantation of the pig liver is speculative. Most evidence supports the idea that the pig's reactions to vascularized organ grafts are less strong and the liver is a less immunogenic organ.

HETEROTOPIC TRANSPLANTATION. The theoretic advantages of auxiliary liver homotransplantation are great. The procedure is technically less arduous than orthotopic transplantation, retains the residual function of the host's liver, and avoids the necessity of removing the diseased organ from a critically ill recipient. These theoretic advantages have proved to be less useful in practice, however, because of complicating mechanical and physiologic factors.

The original technique (Fig. 10-33) placed the allograft outflow into the transected vena cava of the host below the renal vessels. The failure rate following auxiliary transplantation by this technique is extremely high. Even if survival can be obtained for several weeks in canine recipients of auxiliary grafts with immunosuppression (using azathioprine), the transplanted organ atrophies after 2 to 3 weeks.

The lack of hepatotrophic factors in splanchnic venous blood flow to the auxiliary transplant probably contributes to hepatic allograft atrophy. If splanchnic blood flow to the allograft is maintained, atrophy can be prevented. Splanchnic blood flow can be maintained by an anastomosis between the donor portal vein and recipient superior mesenteric vein, followed by ligation of the host's portal vein. This provides for retrograde flow of portal blood through the allograft, rather than through the host's own liver (Fig. 10-34).

Fig. 10-32. Orthotopic transplantation involves total substitution of the host's own liver with the donor organ placed in its normal location. The vena cava and portal vein are generally reestablished anatomically. In the earlier experiences, a segment of donor aorta in continuity with the celiac artery was sutured to the recipient's aorta. A cholecystoduodenostomy afforded biliary drainage. [*From L. Brettschneider, Liver: I. Experimental (Transplantation), in J. S. Najarian and R. L. Simmons (eds.), "Transplantation," p. 496, Lea & Febiger, Philadelphia, 1972.*]

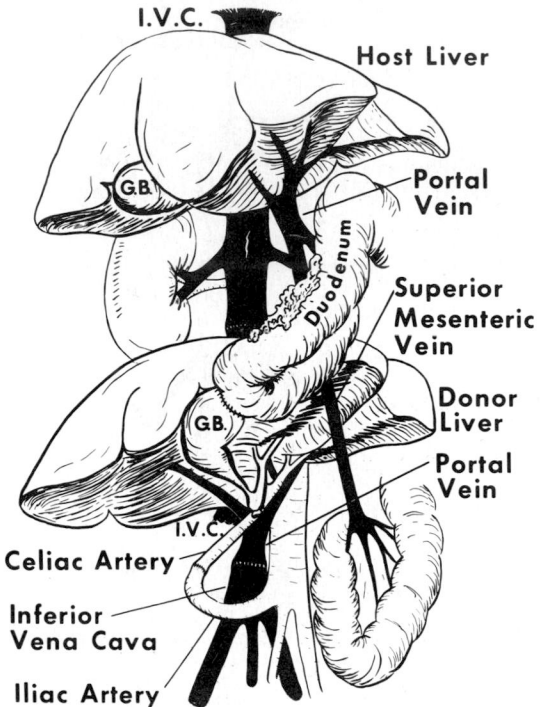

Fig. 10-33. Canine heterotopic transplantation as described by Welch. Anastomosis of the host's vena cava with the portal vein of the donor organ provides a systemic venous inflow. The hepatic artery is anastomosed to the transected iliac artery. Biliary drainage is afforded through a cholecystoduodenostomy. Graft atrophy is almost invariably noted following this procedure. [*From L. Brettschneider, Liver: I. Experimental (Transplantation), in J. S. Najarian and R. L. Simmons (eds.), "Transplantation," p. 496, Lea & Febiger, Philadelphia, 1972.*]

HEPATOCYTE TRANSPLANTATION. Over the past few years, orthotopic liver transplantation has been attempted in certain metabolic diseases with the hope that the grafted tissue would provide the enzyme or "factor" missing in the disease. An alternative approach has been proposed: viz., the transplantation of isolated hepatocytes. Several experimental investigations have demonstrated that intraportal and intramuscular transplantation of isolated hepatocytes in an enzyme-deficient animal can, at least partially, replace that enzyme. The advantages of such a rather simple surgical procedure compared with the more complex surgical procedures involved in whole-organ liver transplantation are obvious.

CLINICAL TRANSPLANTATION

Clinical hepatic transplantation is still experimental, and progress has been slow. Orthotopic transplants appear to be more successful than heterotopic grafts.

INDICATIONS. In the United States, approximately 15,000 persons, between the ages of five and sixty years, died in 1963 as a result of primary hepatic disease. Some patients with this disease will never be good candidates for liver transplantation, but others may benefit substantially.

Intrahepatic or extrahepatic congenital biliary atresia, if not surgically correctable, will generally lead to death before the age of two; few patients survive up to 5 years. Such a child is the ideal candidate for a liver transplant.

Patients with either primary hepatomas or cholangiocarcinomas are far less ideal candidates. If, however, it can be ascertained that the malignant condition is entirely confined to the liver, these patients should be considered for liver transplantation. Often the final diagnosis of disease confined to the liver may not be made until the operation.

The patient with cirrhosis raises additional problems. Rapid death is not as certain in these patients as in those with biliary atresia or primary malignant disease. On the other hand, the terminal stages of the cirrhosis make these patients extremely poor candidates for any operative procedure. Patients with postnecrotic cirrhosis without a history of alcoholism may be better risks, as will be the patient with primary biliary cirrhosis, Wilson's hepatolenticular degeneration, or hemochromatosis.

Acute liver failure may represent one of the best indications for liver transplantation, especially in those patients who have been exposed to hepatotoxins. Viral hepatitis, on the other hand, may or may not recur in the transplanted liver.

Each indication may require a different type of transplant. For example, acute liver failure may respond well to the temporary support of an auxiliary liver or the injection of isolated hepatocytes that will permit the host liver to recover. The child with biliary atresia will almost certainly require an orthotopic transplant with total hepatectomy, since the small child also has no abdominal space for an auxiliary liver. Patients with hepatic malignant disease will also require total hepatectomy and orthotopic transplantation.

In choosing a hepatic donor, the same guidelines should be followed as in choosing a donor for cadaver renal transplantation. Size is a more important criterion in liver transplantation than it is in renal transplantation, particularly when children with congenital biliary atresia are the potential recipients. Usually these children (weighing from 3 to 15 kg) cannot tolerate a liver larger than that from a child weighing 30 kg. Severe postoperative respiratory distress has occurred when donor livers from larger children were used.

PRECAUTIONS. The hepatic transplantation candidate is usually in severe preterminal hepatic failure. In addition, anemia, pulmonary insufficiency, myocardial fibrosis, inanition and protein depletion, and ascites may be present, singly or in combination. The anemia and hypoalbuminemia should be corrected with packed red blood cells and protein-containing solutions as soon as transplantation is contemplated.

Pulmonary insufficiency in hepatic failure can be traced to several causes: First, chronic abdominal ascites restricts the diaphragm and fosters compression atelectasis of the lower portions of the lungs. Also, extensive collateral circulation consequent to portal vein hypertension shunts blood from the portal system to the pulmonary veins via enlarged paraesophageal, mediastinal, and bronchial veins, resulting in venous admixture of systemic blood. Intrapulmonary shunts may also develop in cirrhotic patients, so that arterial hypoxemia is frequently encountered. These conditions make it more difficult for the anesthesiologist to provide adequate ventilation and oxygenation during surgery and require that he avoid techniques employing borderline oxygen concentration.

In cirrhotic patients, diffuse myocardial fibrosis frequently develops that reduces ventricular contractility, stroke volume, and work capacity.

The bedridden patient with hepatic failure invariably suffers from debilitation and poor nutrition, which make him vulnerable to hypotension following anesthesia, moderate hemorrhage, or positional change. Drugs which ordinarily produce mild vasodilation often evoke unusually severe and prolonged effects in the cirrhotic patient that are out of proportion to the dose administered. Most anesthetic drugs provoke such responses and must therefore be administered slowly in small increments. Sudden removal of ascitic fluid may also precipitate or exaggerate hypotension, but the mechanism of this response is obscure.

It is apparent from these considerations that in undertaking to provide anesthesia for the transplant patient, the anesthesiologist faces several difficult challenges. He must, on the one hand, provide conditions adequate for a massive intraperitoneal procedure; at the same time, he must keep in mind that his patient will probably not tolerate deep anesthesia and that the implanted liver may be slow to metabolize and detoxify anesthetic drugs. Most of all, intraoperative and postoperative respiratory distress must be anticipated and minimized. In addition, there is almost no time for proper preparation of the patient. Once a donor is available, the operation must commence promptly so that agonal ischemia of the donor organ may be as brief as possible. The recipient frequently comes to surgery unexpectedly, perhaps an hour or two after a meal. A full stomach is added to the already imposing list of preoperative problems.

The following preparatory procedures are carried out either before anesthesia is induced or immediately after: (1) A central venous pressure catheter is positioned in the right atrium or superior vena cava and a Swan-Ganz catheter for measurement of pulmonary wedge pressures is placed. (2) A second large-bore plastic needle is placed in an upper extremity vein for fluid and blood replacement; it is important to remember that intravenous input via the lower extremities is not adequate during the actual transplantation phase, since the inferior vena cava is clamped. (3) Another needle is placed in either the brachial or radial artery for direct blood pressure monitoring and arterial blood sampling. (4) A rubber warming blanket is placed under the patient and kept between 100 and 105°F. (5) An esophageal temperature probe is positioned so that its sensor lies directly behind the heart. (6) A catheter is placed in the urinary bladder and connected to a graduated collecting flask.

TECHNIQUE OF ORTHOTOPIC HEPATIC TRANSPLANTATION. A transverse abdominal incision with an extension into the thorax, if necessary, is the most common incision.

Recipient hepatectomy must be preceded by careful inspection to determine the feasibility of the procedure. This is particularly true of patients with primary hepatic

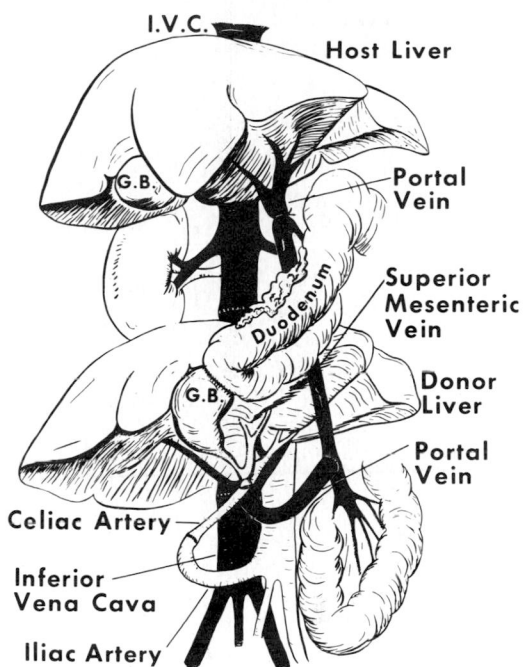

Fig. 10-34. Marchioro et al. modified the technique described in Fig. 10-33. By ligating the portal blood supply to the host's own liver and diverting the splanchnic blood to the homograft by creating an anastomosis between the graft's portal vein and the in situ superior mesenteric vein, homograft atrophy was prevented. [*From L. Brettschneider, Liver: I. Experimental (Transplantation), in J. S. Najarian and R. L. Simmons (eds.), "Transplantation," p. 496, Lea & Febiger, Philadelphia, 1972.*]

neoplasms to ensure that no extrahepatic spread of the tumor has occurred.

The allograft anastomoses are shown in Fig. 10-35. The suprahepatic caval anastomosis is the most difficult to perform. The second anastomosis is usually the hepatic artery but if visceral congestion is great, the portal vein anastomosis should be performed before the hepatic artery to relieve the venous congestion of the intestine. After the hepatic artery or portal vein anastomosis is completed, the inferior hepatic caval clamps should be briefly removed, leaving the suprahepatic vena cava clamped. The arterial or portal vein inflow should be opened to allow the liver to be perfused with warm blood. This sequence is useful to remove the cold perfusate from the liver and prevent systemic hypothermia and heparinization. As soon as the perfusate is washed from the liver and it becomes firm and pink, the intrahepatic vena cava is clamped, and the suprahepatic vena cava clamp is removed. The remaining vascular anastomoses can then be accomplished.

Following the vascular anastomoses, biliary drainage must be obtained. A Roux-en-Y cholecystojejunostomy is most often used, but occasionally a cholecystoduodenostomy is employed. No universally satisfactory technique has been devised, and obstruction, biliary leakage, and necrosis of the gallbladder are common complications. Biliary catastrophes may be the most common cause of death in these patients.

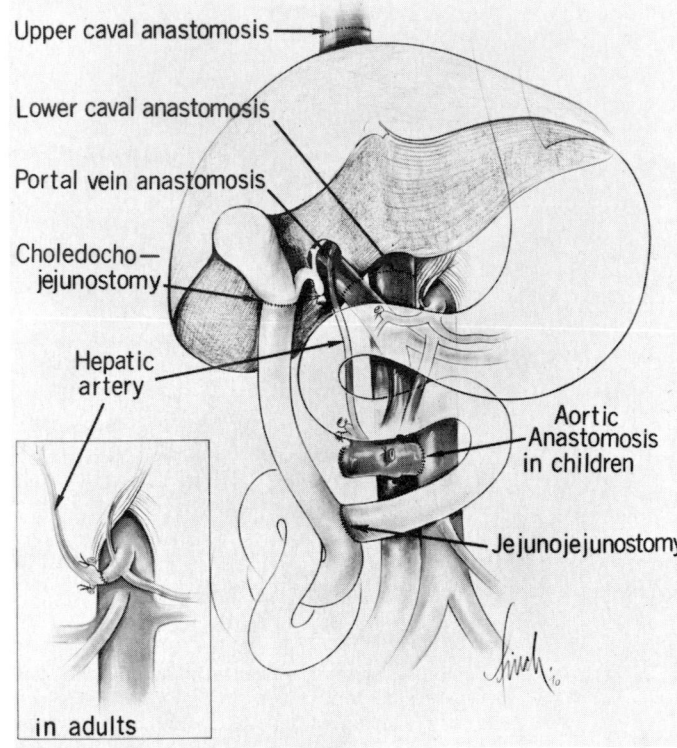

Upper caval anastomosis

Lower caval anastomosis

Portal vein anastomosis

Choledocho—
jejunostomy

Hepatic
artery

Aortic
Anastomosis
in children

Jejunojejunostomy

in adults

Fig. 10-35. Orthotopic liver transplantation in children and adults. In children an aortic cuff can be used for anastomosis; in adults (inset) a direct anastomosis of the hepatic artery and celiac axis can be used. [*From J. S. Najarian, Liver: III. Clinical (Transplantation), in J. S. Najarian and R. L. Simmons (eds.), "Transplantation," p. 522, Lea & Febiger, Philadelphia, 1972.*]

TECHNIQUE OF AUXILIARY LIVER TRANSPLANTATION. Auxiliary, or heterotopic, transplantation is the second alternative for patients with benign liver disease. The major disadvantage of this procedure is its requirement for abdominal volume in which to accommodate the second large organ. When auxiliary transplants are performed, the recipient's own liver is retained to offer some metabolic support during and after the operation. Thus, with the auxiliary liver transplant there is no urgent need for immediate function of the graft, and the operation is shorter and less traumatic.

As noted above, splanchnic blood should be supplied to the graft. This technique is illustrated in Fig. 10-36. The portal vein may be anastomosed to the side of the superior mesenteric vein or to the end of the splenic vein. The advantage of this technique is twofold. It allows for the decompression of the hypertensive recipient portal system, and it provides splanchnic blood flow through the auxiliary liver transplant.

OPERATIVE COMPLICATIONS. Technical Complications. Bleeding is the major technical problem during hepatic transplantation. Portal hypertension predisposes to an extensive collateral venous circulation, and laceration of any smaller vein precipitates extensive bleeding, especially during recipient hepatectomy. The failure of the diseased liver to produce a normal quota of coagulation factors compounds this problem.

It is important to remember that the cystic duct may not enter the common duct except in its terminal course. Therefore, during the donor operation one must be sure that the common duct is ligated distal to its anastomosis

with the cystic duct, if bile is to be expected to flow down the common duct and into the gallbladder. As noted above, biliary leakage due to primary anastomotic breakdown or thrombosis of the cystic artery is a common postoperative problem. Late complications of the biliary drainage procedure may include obstruction of the anastomosis by biliary sludge.

As many as 30 to 40 percent of patients have double hepatic arteries, and one of them may arise from the superior mesenteric artery. Care must be taken during the donor operation to preserve this arterial supply.

A common complication is paralysis of the right side of the diaphragm, which apparently results from crushing of the right phrenic nerve by the vascular clamp applied to the suprahepatic inferior vena cava. Enough length must be preserved during total hepatectomy for the clamp to be applied without impinging on the diaphragm.

Metabolic Complications. Because pulmonary insufficiency is common following hepatic transplantation, a sterile nasotracheal tube should be placed at the outset of anesthesia, with the intention of maintaining intubation and mechanical ventilation until respiratory competence is reestablished.

Because of increased tissue uptake of glucose and reduced glycogen conversion, hypoglycemia develops insidiously in response to hepatic ischemia, hypotension, and acidosis. Hyperglycemia is a hazard of hypertonic glucose infusion. The blood sugar should be regularly measured, and glucose infusion should be modified according to the values obtained.

Precise measurement of blood loss and fluid sequestration is not possible, and evaluation and correlation of suction loss, weight loss, arterial blood pressure, cardiac rate, venous pressure, acid-base status, and urine volume must be made frequently by the anesthetist. At this point of the operative procedure, central venous pressure measurement is useful as a guide to the adequacy of the filling pressure of the right side of the heart, but manipulation of the liver and its great vein attachments may produce high-pressure artifacts and make an estimation of left atrial pressure more useful.

Hypotension is a particular danger during the anhepatic period, its severity depending upon the adequacy with which collateral venous circulation maintains venous return to the heart. If blood pressure is seriously depressed, the transfusion rate is increased, but often the hypotension cannot be fully overcome until the caval clamps are removed. This disturbance of cardiac output is the major cause of the progressive metabolic acidosis that characterizes this portion of the transplant operation.

When the anastomoses are completed, further dangerous metabolic and hemodynamic changes occur. The great veins draining the intestines and lower half of the body now discharge blood containing a heavy load of acid metabolites. At the same time, the vascular space within the liver takes up a considerable volume of blood and discharges additional products of ischemia as it again becomes an integral part of the circulation. Thus the metabolic acidosis suddenly worsens and is accompanied by hypovolemia. Severe hypotension, cardiac arrhythmias, bradycardia, and other bizarre configurations of the ECG pattern appear abruptly at this point. Blood loss from leaks in the vascular anastomoses frequently compounds the hemodynamic problems. Whole blood must be rapidly administered at this phase of the operation until the systolic arterial blood pressure stabilizes at 100 mm Hg or better. Simultaneously, blood-gas analyses are made every 5 minutes to provide guidance in adjustment of acid-base balance at this critical juncture.

Hypothermia is a concomitant hazard as the donor liver is revascularized. The whole transplantation procedure, with its extensive visceral exposure and heavy blood loss, tends to produce hypothermia. Furthermore, the donor liver is flushed with iced saline solution prior to transplantation into the host's circulation to increase its tolerance of ischemia. The *coup de grâce,* therefore, is the sudden inclusion of this ice-cold organ directly upstream of the heart. Consequently the core temperature usually falls 3 to 4°C within 2 minutes of release of the clamps. Such abrupt cardiac cooling fosters arrhythmias and poor myocardial function. Perfusion of the liver through the infrahepatic vena cava prior to opening the suprahepatic vena cava will warm the liver and work out the cold perfusate. In addition, irrigation of the abdominal cavity with warm saline solution (40°C) and transfusion with warm blood can also compensate for this problem.

Potassium disturbances impose an additional hazard during revascularization. Several factors (hepatocellular ischemia, massive blood replacement, and metabolic acidosis) favor hyperkalemia when hepatic circulation is restored. There may be a concomitant decrease in serum

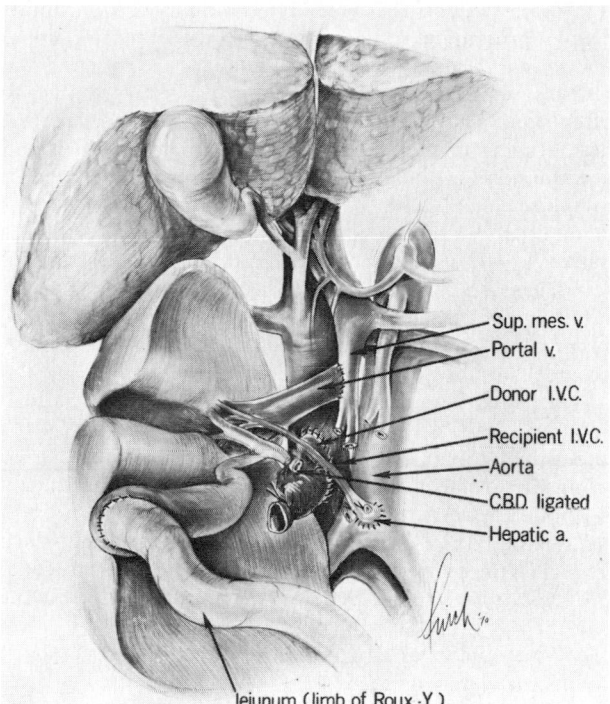

Fig. 10-36. The method of auxiliary liver transplantation utilizing splanchnic blood flow. The hepatic arterial supply comes directly from the aorta, and the portal vein supply to the liver is derived from the splanchnic circulation. The portal vein can be anastomosed either to the superior mesenteric vein, as shown, or to the portal vein, whichever is most convenient. The donor's inferior vena cava is anastomosed end to end to the inferior vena cava. In this method portal decompression is provided, as well as splanchnic circulation to the transplanted liver. [*From J. S. Najarian, Liver: III. Clinical (Transplantation), in J. S. Najarian, and R. L. Simmons (eds.), "Transplantation," p. 522, Lea & Febiger, Philadelphia, 1972.*]

Labels on figure: Sup. mes. v. / Portal v. / Donor I.V.C. / Recipient I.V.C. / Aorta / C.B.D. ligated / Hepatic a. / Jejunum (limb of Roux-Y)

calcium due to the heavy citrate load from the multiple transfusions and the impaired capacity of the new liver to metabolize that load. These cation shifts have not been systematically quantified, but the abrupt appearance of peaked T waves and conduction disturbances have been observed on the ECG as liver circulation is reestablished. Disturbance of the potassium/calcium ratio is known to depress myocardial function and cardiac output; when acidosis, hypothermia, and a sudden increase in the vascular bed add their own special depressant effects, severe hypotension and arrhythmias result. Prompt correction of hypovolemia and acidosis are the keys to success in negotiating this critical period. Then, if myocardial weakness still persists, one can assume that a potassium/calcium ratio disturbance is present and slowly inject 0.5 to 1.0 Gm of calcium chloride. The serum electrolyte determinations made every 15 minutes until the circulation stabilizes provide guidance in adjusting ionic balance. Hypokalemia is the most prominent electrolyte problem in the early postoperative period.

POSTOPERATIVE CARE. There is a high potential for postoperative respiratory insufficiency in most hepatic transplant patients, because (1) pulmonary dysfunction is always present in some degree, (2) the extensive upper abdominal incision causes abdominal muscle splinting and reduces vital capacity, and (3) the transplanted liver is often significantly larger than the organ it replaces, so that breathing is further compromised until abdominal wall accommodation takes place. The nasotracheal tube is therefore usually left in place after surgery. Mechanical ventilation is applied for at least 12 hours or until the patient's own respiratory competence is proved by normal blood gases. Strict adherence to sterile technique in respiratory care is essential because of the patient's immunosuppressed state. Sterile distilled water should be used to provide humidification of respiratory gases.

After operation, the transplant recipient is kept in a 30°-angle head-up position to reduce the pressure of the abdominal contents on the diaphragm. He is also turned from side to side each hour, and vibratory chest percussion is applied each time a positional change is made. Chest roentgenograms are made daily to detect atelectasis, which is dealt with by postural pummeling, directional tracheobronchial suction, and hyperinflation with a self-inflating bag.

Most of the remaining problems are related to metabolic changes that may be minimal if the quality of the new liver is good. If, however, the liver quality is impaired by prolonged ischemia or agonal changes in the donor, the liver will be unable to regulate blood sugar, and either hypoglycemia or hyperglycemic nonketotic coma may occur.

The coagulation changes that accompany the transplantation of the liver have been thoroughly discussed by the Denver group. Because most of the coagulation factors are hepatic in origin and the liver is involved in the clearing of substances active in coagulation and fibrinolysis, a damaged liver frequently fails to produce sufficient coagulation factors to prevent hemorrhage. The problem is compounded by the probability that intravascular coagulation accompanies the trauma and shock of the procedure, thereby consuming whatever factors are present. A rapid return of coagulation tests to normal in the early posttransplant period is a good indicator of satisfactory hepatic function.

Hepatic transplant recipients receive the same immunosuppressive drugs used in renal transplant recipients (azathioprine, prednisone, and ALG). The hepatotoxicity of azathioprine, however, requires that a reduced level be utilized (1 mg/kg), although the levels of prednisone and ALG remain the same. Cyclophosphamide has recently been used in place of azathioprine.

DIFFERENTIAL DIAGNOSIS OF HEPATIC MALFUNCTION. Many causes of hepatic malfunction other than rejection exist. Since there is evidence that rejection of the liver is less severe than that of other organs, technical complications should be ruled out prior to treating hepatic malfunction with more immunosuppression. The diagnosis may require surgical exploration.

While the milder rejection episodes may not be clinically apparent, severe rejection crises are accompanied by systemic signs that may mimic toxic hepatitis. Fever, malaise, anorexia, and hepatomegaly are present, and the patient generally appears quite ill. The laboratory findings reveal elevated serum bilirubin, alkaline phosphatase, and serum transaminase levels. The 99m technetium liver scan will reveal either a patchy or diffuse decrease in hepatic uptake and an increased uptake in the bone marrow and lungs. The serum bilirubin level is such a reliable indication that it should be tested two or three times weekly in the posttransplant period.

Septic infarcts within the liver are among the most severe problems encountered after liver transplants; they are usually fatal. This syndrome appears as a distinct clinical triad: (1) gram-negative septicemia, (2) evidence of massive liver necrosis with increased serum levels of liver enzymes, and (3) liver scans showing absence of isotope concentrations in one area of the liver allograft. Ischemic infarction then follows, and the liver can no longer deal with the enteric organisms normally traversing the portal venous system. The ischemic segment soon becomes abscessed. An increase in serum transaminase, a positive blood culture, and an area that fails to concentrate the isotope on liver scan are all positive indications of an abscessed ischemic segment. The cause is more likely to be technical problems of surgery than immunological rejection.

RESULTS. Of the 106 patients receiving orthotopic liver grafts in Denver prior to August, 1976, 27 were alive 1 year or more after grafting and 16 survived longer than 2 years. The longest survival period was 6.3 years. Of the 50 patients in the Cambridge/King series, 12 survived more than 6 months, four of these lived beyond a year, 10 were currently living, one was alive 2.5 years after transplantation. The longest survivor lived 5.2 years after orthotopic grafting. Younger patients seem to do better, and one-third of the recipients under age eighteen survived more than 1 year in the Denver series.

In all series, uncontrolled rejection reactions were the primary cause of death in about 10 percent of the patients. More commonly, the deaths were due to a wide variety of biliary tract problems and intraabdominal sepsis. The longest survivor of the Cambridge series lived for 5.2 years until calcified sludge blocked the anastomosis between the gallbladder and recipient common duct. Deaths were also caused by a variety of problems, including pneumonia, cerebrovascular accidents, and the recurrence of cancer in patients who had primary hepatomas or cholangiocarcinomas.

Heart

Cardiac transplantation is emerging as a truly therapeutic intervention for some patients with terminal or intractable heart disease for whom no alternative therapy is currently available. By July 1977, 346 cardiac transplants had been performed in human beings by 65 teams in various countries of the world. Though the overall survival rate has been disappointingly low, the potential for long-term survival has been established by 11 patients who are currently alive between 5 and 9 years after transplantation. Equally gratifying is their high degree of rehabilitation.

HISTORICAL BACKGROUND

Prior to the initiation of human trials, a number of fundamental areas required extensive laboratory investigation—development of a surgical technique, demonstration of adequate postoperative function of the acutely denervated heart, early detection and prevention of homograft rejection, and resuscitation and preservation of the cadaver heart. An encouraging degree of progress was made in each of these areas during the 10 years preceding the first clinical transplant in Cape Town, South Africa, in December of 1967.

Before the development of modern methods for cardiopulmonary bypass, studies of cardiac transplantation, of necessity, were confined to placement of the heart in an ectopic position, usually in the neck of a larger dog. As early as 1905, Carrel and Guthrie, using previously unknown suturing techniques, carried out heterotopic transplantation of the heart and of the heart and lungs and demonstrated the capacity of the transplanted heart to continue beating despite severance from its nerve supply. Subsequent studies by other investigators using various modifications of the original preparation added considerably to our knowledge of the transplanted heart. Much was learned about the susceptibility of the heart to the process of rejection; its vulnerability to hypoxia, thrombosis, and air embolism; and the protective effect of hypothermia against the metabolic abnormalities which occur with transplantation. In addition to these studies, the heterotopically transplanted heart has been investigated as a means of assisting circulation.

Subsequent to the development of techniques for generalized hypothermia and extracorporeal circulation, the possibility of complete cardiac replacement was investigated by several groups. Survival in the initial dog studies was limited to a few hours, but much was learned about the technical problems. In December of 1959, Lower and Shumway demonstrated that a dog could recover fully after orthotopic replacement of the heart with a homograft. In an initial series of 10 animals, 6 survived from 6 to 21 days without immunosuppression. Five days of survival was also achieved after orthotopic homotransplantation of the heart and both lungs as a unit.

Subsequent animal studies demonstrated that the ECG voltage was a useful means of monitoring the transplant in order to detect impending rejection episodes and that prolonged survival could be achieved in some animals by appropriate use of azathioprine and high doses of steroid to combat rejection crises. The feasibility of using cadaver hearts was also established, as was the successful hypothermic storage of the donor heart for several hours prior to transplantation.

Extensive physiologic studies of autotransplanted dog hearts confirmed the capacity of the denervated heart to function normally for several years under a variety of physiologic stresses and demonstrated that signs of autonomic reinnervation would frequently reappear within months to a year after transplantation. These laboratory investigations established the technical and physiologic feasibility of cardiac transplantation in man and set the stage for the clinical trials which were initiated in December of 1967 and carried out most extensively in 1968 in several centers. In subsequent years, because of the high rate of immunologic failure of the grafts, cardiac transplantation has been performed less frequently and only in a few centers as carefully studied clinical investigations.

SELECTION OF PATIENTS

Because of the relatively high risk of allograft failure from rejection or of death from complications of immunosuppression, patient selection for cardiac transplantation generally has been reserved for those under age fifty with terminal or intractable heart failure for whom no alternative therapy is available. The majority have had severe coronary disease with multiple infarctions and extensive or diffuse loss of left ventricular myocardium. Many of these patients have been failures of prior revascularization attempts, but these have proved to be an especially favorable group (see below). Another group for consideration includes patients with cardiomyopathy who do not respond satisfactorily to medical therapy. It has now been established in some long-term survivors that the cardiomyopathy is not likely to recur in the transplanted heart, and one such patient in our own series is alive after 4 years with normal cardiac function. Another group is composed of infants with the hypoplastic left-heart syndrome for whom transplantation from anencephalic donors might prove successful. Of particular interest is the high success rate reported by the Stanford University Medical Center group for patients who had prior cardiopulmonary bypass procedures, which suggest that, rather than the anticipated high rate of sensitization to donor antigens, some measure of graft enhancement may have occurred.

Up to the present time histocompatibility typing has provided no predictive value in matching donor and recipient, but to avoid the problem of accelerated rejection a lymphocyte cross match must establish that the recipient harbors no preformed antibodies against the potential donor. Otherwise, successful transplantation has required only the geographic and temporal proximity of recipient and donor with appropriate ABO compatibility. Cardiac donors have sustained brain death usually from trauma or from spontaneous intracerebral hemorrhage, and complete cessation of brain function has been certified by an independent team of neurologists and neurosurgeons.

TECHNIQUE

The operative approach (Fig. 10-37) for cardiac transplantation used by most groups follows with a few modifications the procedure which proved successful in the animal model. The recipient is prepared for cardiopulmonary bypass using a median sternotomy incision. Venous drainage catheters are placed through the right atrial wall in a posterior position, or they may be inserted through peripheral veins. Arterial cannulation is via the femoral artery or ascending aorta. The recipient's diseased heart is excised by appropriate incisions in the right and left atrial walls and atrial septum, retaining in the recipient the posterior portions of both atria. This residual atrial tissue not only facilitates anastomosis of the donor heart but

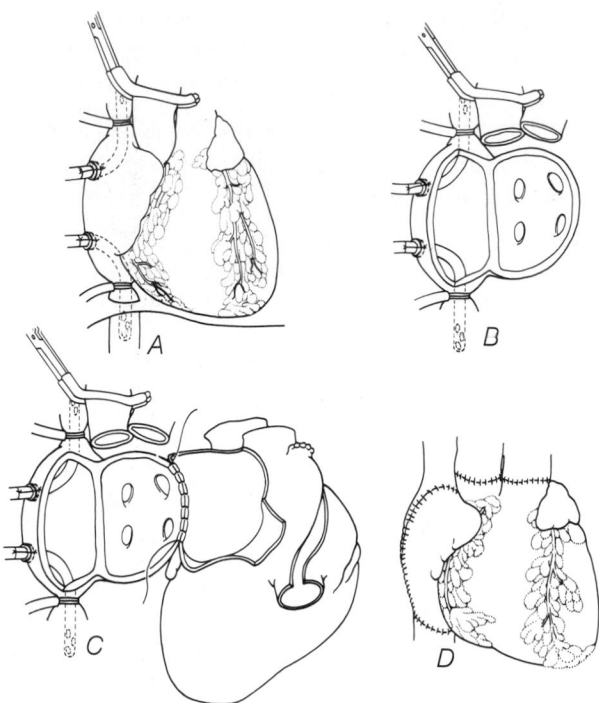

Fig. 10-37. *A*. The recipient has been prepared for cardiopulmonary bypass with insertion of caval catheters through the posterior portion of the right atrium. *B*. The recipient's heart has been excised leaving in place the posterior remnants of right and left atria. *C*. Suturing of the donor heart is begun with the left atrial wall, followed in sequence by the atrial septum, right atrium, pulmonary artery, and aorta. *D*. Suturing is complete, and coronary circulation is restored by removal of the aortic clamp. [*From R. R. Lower, Cardiac Transplantation, in J. C. Norman (ed.), "Cardiac Surgery," 2d ed., p. 599, Appleton Century Crofts, New York, 1972.*]

preserves some of the afferent innervation to the atria which may play a significant role in maintaining homeostatic fluid balance in the postoperative period. Blood supply to the retained atrial tissue is adequately provided by the bronchial circulation, but retention of excessive amounts, particularly the appendages, is avoided to minimize the risk of ischemia, stasis, and thrombosis. The aorta and pulmonary artery are transected at a convenient point distal to the semilunar valves.

Simultaneously, the donor is heparinized and the heart exposed by a second team. Removal of the donor heart is carried out by division of the venae cavae, the pulmonary veins, and the great arteries. The excised heart is then immersed in saline solution at 5 to 10°C to provide protective cooling of the myocardium during transport to the recipient, as well as during the remainder of the transplantation procedure. Further preparation of the donor heart includes suture ligation of the superior vena cava, incision of the lateral right atrial wall from the inferior vena cava to the atrial appendage avoiding the major internodal pathways, and preparation of the left atrium by incision between the pulmonary venous openings.

Implantation of the donor heart consists of suturing the left atrial wall, atrial septum, and right atrial wall in suc-

cession by continuous suture, followed by anastomosis of the pulmonary artery and ascending aorta. Prior to completing the final anastomosis, care is taken to evacuate all residual air from the cardiac chambers. With release of the aortic clamp and rewarming of the heart, cardiac rhythm often returns spontaneously, or ventricular fibrillation may require electrical cardioversion. In each of our cases, the transplanted heart has resumed vigorous contractions once coronary circulation has been restored, and cardiopulmonary bypass has been discontinued.

In 1977 we extended the procurement of donor hearts for urgent transplantation to include long-distance transportation of the hearts up to 900 miles by chartered jet. In four such cases ischemic times were from 1 hour 53 minutes to 3 hours 17 minutes, during which periods the hearts were protected by simple hypothermia. In each instance excellent cardiac function was restored in the recipient. Two patients later died, one of rejection, one of infection, and two recipients of the long-distance transplants remain alive.

POSTOPERATIVE CARE

The most immediate problem in the postoperative period is the capacity of the transplanted right ventricle to cope with the preexisting pulmonary hypertension which usually results from long-standing failure of the left side of the heart. Under these circumstances, the heart may temporarily require inotropic support for 1 or 2 days. The precise level of pulmonary hypertension which precludes a successful transplant has not yet been defined, but adequate cardiac function without prolonged pharmacologic support has been recovered in most instances despite the additional theoretic problems of acute denervation and interrupted cardiac lymphatics.

Once the posttransplant circulatory status is stable, the major emphasis in management shifts to the immunologic problem. The heart transplant recipient appears to be less immunologically depressed than a kidney transplant recipient with prolonged uremia and thus requires higher levels of immunosuppression in the early posttransplant weeks. Azathioprine is given in the maximally tolerated daily dose of 3 to 4 mg/kg, with careful observation for signs of hematologic toxicity. Prednisone is begun at a dose of 200 mg/day and tapered gradually to 60 mg/day by the end of 2 weeks. Further tapering of the dose is more gradual, reaching a level of 30 mg/day at 3 months, if the clinical condition permits. Antithymocyte globulin is administered over a 10-day period, although its importance and dosage are incompletely known at this time. To minimize the emergence of resistant microorganisms, antibiotics are administered only at the time of operation and for specific indications thereafter.

Monitoring for episodes of impending rejection depends almost entirely on daily or twice daily observation of the ECG. The majority of patients will have a rejection episode during the first 2 postoperative weeks, and the most significant ECG changes will include a stepwise decrease in voltage, rightward shift in the frontal plane axis, and the occasional occurrence of atrial arrhythmias or right bundle branch block (Fig. 10-38). An epicardial electrode implanted at operation serves to enhance the accuracy of voltage changes in the first few postoperative weeks.

Clinical signs of rejection may include the development of a protodiastolic gallop sound and the murmur of tricuspid insufficiency. Other signs and symptoms, such as pericardial friction rub, fever, and malaise, are rather nonspecific in the early postoperative period and therefore of little diagnostic value. Other confirmatory diagnostic maneuvers include fluoroscopy or ultrasound to demonstrate cardiac chamber enlargement, decreased amplitude of ventricular wall pulsations, and diminished ventricular compliance. A suspected rejection crisis may be further confirmed by transvenous endocardial muscle biopsy as described by the Stanford University Medical Center group (Fig. 10-39).

The treatment of a rejection episode requires a large intravenous dose of steroid, usually 1 Gm of methylprednisolone on the first day and 0.5 Gm on the second day, with subsequent return to maintenance levels if the clinical condition permits. The adjunctive value of graft irradiation and anticoagulant therapy is incompletely settled at the present time. Late postoperative management includes a vigorous exercise program to minimize the catabolic effects of steroid therapy. The likelihood of acute rejection diminishes after 4 months, and ECG studies are reduced to twice weekly.

The major late problem, aside from infectious complications, has been the development of vascular lesions characteristic of chronic rejection. Even small lesions may produce ischemic damage to the conduction system, and the occurrence of conduction defects may require transvenous pacing. The value of prolonged therapy with warfarin and dipyridamole is under investigation in the hope of minimizing the vascular complications. Control of hyperlipidemia is also carefully managed in the appropriate patients.

RESULTS

Survival data have been periodically compiled and published by the ACS/NIH Organ Transplant Registry. The majority of cardiac transplants from 1971 to 1977 were performed at the Stanford University Medical Center, and this group has also published several detailed analyses of their steadily improving results which currently indicate a 48 percent 1-year and 38 percent 2-year survival rate.

Seventy-seven patients are currently alive in the world experience, of whom 11 have survived more than 5 years, attesting to the therapeutic potential of this procedure. Late deaths occurring more than 3 months after operation have usually resulted from infectious complications or from the graft arteriosclerosis associated with chronic rejection (Fig. 10-40). Four patients have died of disseminated malignant disease.

The majority of patients surviving beyond 6 months have returned to an active and productive existence and have enjoyed an excellent exercise tolerance. Postoperative cardiac catheterization studies reported by the Stanford

CARDIAC TRANSPLANT   L.R.   ECG LEAD III

11-22-68

12-5-68

12-11-68

12-13-68

12-14-68

12-16-68

1-2-69

Fig. 10-38. ECG evidence of an acute rejection episode 3½ months after cardiac transplantation. The significant changes include a decrease in voltage and the development of right bundle branch block; these changes were reversed with a temporary increase in the steroid dose, and the patient remains the longest surviving transplant 5 years after operation. [*From R. R. Lower, Cardiac Transplantation, in J. C. Norman (ed.), "Cardiac Surgery," 2d ed., p. 599, Appleton Century Crofts, New York, 1972.*]

group on seven patients 12 to 14 months after operation revealed normal resting pressures in the right and left sides of the heart and a fall in pulmonary vascular resistance from a preoperative average of 5.8 units to an average of 2.4 units in the postoperative study. There was no evidence in any patient of autonomic reinnervation, but the cardiac index increased from 2.5 liters/min/m^2 at rest to 4.8 liters/min/m^2 during moderate exercise with a concomitant increase in left ventricular end-diastolic pressure to an average of 21 mm Hg. It is thus concluded from the patient and animal studies that the denervated transplanted heart increases cardiac output during exercise by two sequential mechanisms: in the initial phase of 2 to 3 minutes there is predominantly an increase in stroke volume due to the Starling mechanism with little change in rate, followed later by a gradual increase in heart rate in response to peripherally produced catecholamines.

Additional considerations include retransplantation as employed successfully by the Stanford group for uncontrolled acute rejection or severe chronic rejection. Also, Barnard's group in Capetown has employed the donor heart as a heterotopic transplant, placing it in tandem with the recipient's heart to avoid the lethality of a severe rejection episode. The exact role of these two approaches in improving the results of cardiac transplantation remains to be defined.

Fig. 10-39. Right atrial myocardium from a patient who died from acute rejection 7 days after cardiac transplantation. There are marked interstitial edema, hemorrhage, and an extensive mononuclear cell infiltration. [*From R. R. Lower, Cardiac Transplantation, in J. C. Norman (ed.), "Cardiac Surgery," 2d ed., p. 599, Appleton Century Crofts, New York, 1972.*]

Lung

Transplantation of the lung presents some rather unique problems: (1) for a long time it appeared that technical factors related to denervation of the transplanted lung would make it impossible to achieve normal or even adequate function of the transplant (this, however, no longer seems to be the case); (2) with the currently employed immunosuppressive agents, the lung is by far the most common site of infection in patients with kidney transplants. As an allotransplant, with the added hazard of immunosuppression, it is even more likely that the lung will become involved in bacterial, fungal, or viral infections which lead to its destruction and to the death of the host. Despite these formidable barriers to successful transplantation of the lung, some progress has been made in this field.

AUTOTRANSPLANTATION

EXPERIMENTAL STUDIES. Autotransplantation of the lung involves division of pulmonary and bronchial arteries, the pulmonary veins, the nerves, and the lymphatics. Each of these structures has a role in subsequent pulmonary events. Permanent division of the pulmonary artery results in fibrosis, but not necrosis, of the lung. Simple ligation of the bronchial arteries is without adverse effect upon the

function of the lung but probably contributes to the high incidence of disruption, leakage, and stenosis at the bronchial anastomosis after lung transplantation. Completion of the pulmonary venous anastomosis without residual stenosis has proved to be a common technical problem. If obstruction exists, pulmonary edema may result, especially if contralateral pneumonectomy or pulmonary artery ligation is carried out. Unilateral denervation of the lung by hilar stripping has sometimes been said to produce a decrease in ventilation, oxygen consumption, and compliance, while in other instances no alteration of pulmonary function has been observed. Bilateral denervation by hilar stripping reduces lung function but permits survival of the animal. In summary, the physiological effects of unilateral lung reimplantation are not life threatening in the absence of technical error.

The chief technical advance in transplantation of the lung has been the technique described by Metras and later by Neptune et al., in which a portion of the left atrium is removed along with the pulmonary veins. The venous anastomosis can be made using the wall of the left atrium instead of suturing the individual pulmonary veins (Fig. 10-41). This, in turn, reduces the likelihood of pulmonary venous obstruction. Bilateral autotransplantation has even been successfully carried out in dogs and baboons.

CLINICAL EXPERIENCE. Autotransplantation was once used in the treatment of severe bronchial asthma in human beings. A single lung was replaced in six patients, and in one additional patient bilateral staged autotransplantations were carried out. Two patients died ultimately of pulmonary hemorrhage from bronchovascular fistulae, while the other five patients, including the one with bilateral reimplantation, survived. The asthma was said to be improved. The procedure is not recommended.

ALLOTRANSPLANTATION

EXPERIMENTAL STUDIES. As with renal and hepatic transplantation, the function of the allotransplanted lung in the untreated recipient lasts for 6 to 8 days. Death of the recipient usually occurs within 2 weeks. A variety of drugs has been used in attempts to obtain prolonged survival of lung allotransplants. The function of the transplanted lung is often severely diminished even in those animals which survive for long periods of time. If the contralateral lung is removed or the contralateral pulmonary artery ligated in animals living for a long time with a lung allograft, only a few animals survive.

CLINICAL EXPERIENCE. More than 37 lung transplants have been performed in patients with end-stage pulmonary disease. Although one patient survived as long as 10 months, all efforts have ultimately failed. These failures have provided important information and have indicated areas for futher evaluation and study.

Certain technical considerations should be kept in mind. The transplanted lung must be capable of immediate function: there are no adequate artificial lungs available with which life can be maintained while waiting for the transplanted lung to function. Therefore, it is particularly important to perform a perfect venous anastomosis between the pulmonary veins and the left atrium. If this anastomosis is defective, thrombosis will occur in most cases, and even those patients with patency will demonstrate an increased vascular resistance and poor function. Other technical problems have frequently developed at the bronchial suture line because of the deficient blood supply of the transplanted bronchus, which must derive its blood supply from collaterals between the pulmonary and bronchial arteries. There is a high incidence of bronchial leakage and stenosis due to varying degrees of ischemic necrosis at the transplanted bronchus.

Lungs can be transplanted singly or along with the heart as a cardiopulmonary bilateral lung transplant. The latter procedure has been used on several patients and is preferred by some surgeons, since the anastomoses are rather simple. Bronchial anastomoses are eliminated, and a simpler tracheal anastomosis is substituted. In addition, cardiopulmonary transplantation circumvents the possibility that overexpansion of the emphysematous contralateral lung will compress the freshly transplanted lung causing immediate malfunction. This complication has been reported in several human unilateral transplants but has not proved to be a problem in most cases.

Lung transplantation in human beings has not been very successful and most patients have died within a few days. Veith has recently reviewed the difficulties which have led to this dismal state and found three groups of problems: First suitable donor lungs are extremely scarce. Even minimal ischemia of a donor lung produces transient malfunction after transplantation, and this cannot be tolerated by a recipient who is almost totally dependent on his transplanted lung. To minimize donor lung ischemia, donor and recipient must be located in the same institution, or new procedures for lung preservation must be developed. Infections other than pulmonary problems are common in prospective donors, most of whom have had long periods of tracheal intubation and controlled ventilation. Finally, the size of the donor lung, its hilar structures, and particularly its bronchus, must approximate those of the recipient to minimize technical problems.

The second major problem in lung transplantation consists of complications resulting from imperfect handling of the bronchial anastomosis, and include anastomotic disruption with air leakage, infection, bleeding, stenosis, or mucosal necrosis. The pathogenesis of these problems has been attributed to ischemia of the transplant bronchus, which must be nourished retrograde by collaterals from the pulmonary artery. Additional factors probably include rejection, high-dose corticosteroids, and size discrepancy between donor and recipient bronchi. A number of potential remedies have been suggested such as shortening the donor bronchial stump, reinforcing the anastomosis with surrounding vascularized tissue, or intussuscepting the donor bronchus within the recipient bronchus during anastomosis. Some investigators have also advocated revascularization of the transplant bronchial arteries by implanting a button of donor aorta containing their origin into the recipient aorta.

The final problem is lung allograft rejection, and Veith has postulated that this tends to take one of two forms. In one, an infiltrative rejection due to inflammatory cells

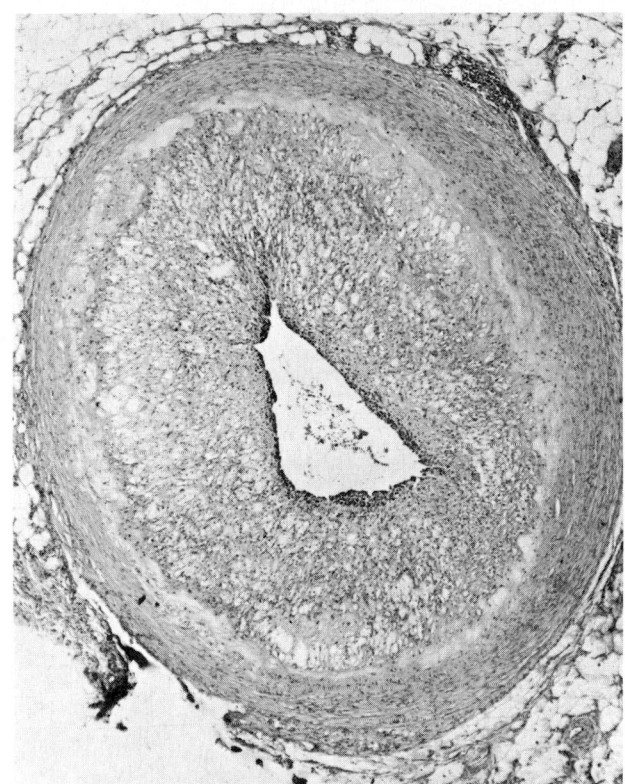

Fig. 10-40. An epicardial coronary artery from a patient dying 8 months after cardiac transplantation showing marked arteriosclerosis characteristic of chronic rejection. [*From R. R. Lower, Cardiac Transplantation, in J. C. Norman (ed.), "Cardiac Surgery," 2d ed., p. 599, Appleton Century Crofts, New York, 1972.*]

predominates; in the second, pulmonary edema is the major finding. Both are associated with opacification or infiltration of the transplanted lung on chest x-ray film and a decrease in arterial oxygen tension, fever, leukocytosis, and importantly, no change in sputum cultures. Obviously, better methods are needed for reliable differentiation of rejection from pneumonia; needle biopsy may prove helpful.

Kidney

The technical knowledge necessary to perform kidney transplants has been available since Carrel and Guthrie developed the techniques of vascular suture at the turn of the century.

Between the years 1951 and 1953 Hume performed nine cadaver kidney transplants. Function was adequate to maintain these patients for a limited period; one patient survived for 6 months. Steroids were used in some of these patients, but the doses were apparently inadequate. In 1954 Murray et al. successfully transplanted kidneys between identical twins, and the technical feasibility of routine human renal transplantation was confirmed. The discoveries by Schwartz and Dameshek that 6-mercaptopurine was immunosuppressive in rabbits, and the subsequent demonstrations by Calne and by Zukoski et al. that immuno-

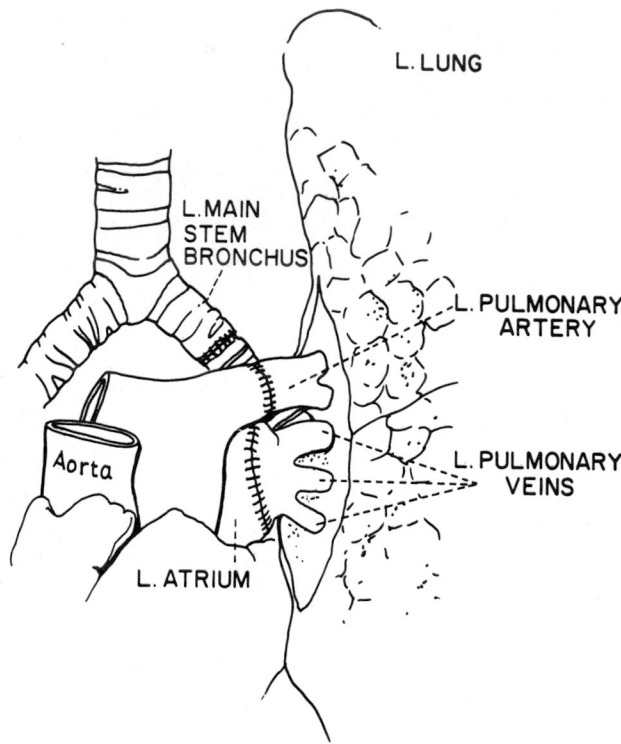

Fig. 10-41. Technique for lung transplantation (described by Metras). A portion of the left atrium is removed along with the pulmonary veins, so that the anastomosis can be made through the wall of the left atrium instead of through each individual pulmonary vein.

suppression would prolong renal allografts in dogs, led directly to the success of human renal allotransplantation. Renal transplantation is now the treatment of choice for most patients with renal failure, although hemodialysis can serve as an adequate substitute for certain patients.

RECIPIENT SELECTION AND INDICATIONS FOR TRANSPLANTATION

CRITERIA FOR SELECTION. Rigid criteria for the selection of recipients of renal allotransplants have never been defined. In general, irreversible renal failure in the patient less than sixty years of age with a normal urinary outflow tract, without active infection, severe malnutrition, disseminated malignancy, or incapacitating systemic disease should be considered for transplantation. We have found that most of the generally accepted contraindications to renal transplantation are unnecessarily exclusive. The only absolute contraindications are active infection or malignant disease that cannot be brought under control.

Renal transplantation has been carried out for almost every imaginable renal disease. Results of transplantation in most cases justify the indications, although certain precautions should be taken.

Congenital or hereditary diseases of the urinary tract are obvious indications without contraindication. Of particular note is the high degree of success with congenital obstruction and ureterovesical reflux and neurogenic bladders. It is possible to correct most such abnormalities or to substitute

intestinal conduits for bladders that cannot be repaired.

Among the acquired diseases, most transplants are carried out for either chronic glomerulonephritis or chronic pyelonephritis. In fact, many patients do not present a classic history of either disease, and the kidney disease is so far advanced by the time biopsy is performed that the pathogenesis is indeterminate. Rather than assign a definitive diagnosis suggesting a cause, it is best to regard such patients as having end-stage renal disease of unknown cause.

The more specific glomerulonephritides include Goodpasture's disease, in which antibodies to glomerular basement membrane can be detected by fluorescent techniques within the kidney. Such patients may or may not also have pulmonary hemorrhage, and they usually pursue a rather acute course of renal failure. It is generally agreed that serum titers of antiglomerular basement membranes should be performed and that the nephrectomy should precede transplantation in these patients. Transplantation should be delayed until the antiglomerular basement membrane antibody has reached a low level, and the patient should be maintained on dialysis for 6 months to 1 year following nephrectomy before transplantation.

The other glomerulonephritides are less well defined. One that is becoming increasingly well understood is related to low complement levels within the bloodstream and a proliferative membranoglomerulonephritis. Here, complement ($\beta\text{-}C_1$) can be detected in discrete fragments along the basement membrane without marked degrees of antibody deposition. Although the cause of this disease is not understood, it does not seem to be related to direct antikidney antibodies, so that delay in transplantation is not necessary. In the absence of well-defined disease, renal failure that follows an acute course complicated by a nonspecific glomerulonephritis should probably be treated by nephrectomy and delayed transplantation, although prompt transplants have been performed with success in such cases.

Most children with a nephrotic syndrome recover spontaneously or with steroid or immunosuppressive therapy. Other patients, however, develop the nephrotic syndrome and progress toward terminal renal failure despite the use of steroids. Following transplantation, some of these patients will develop recurrent nephrotic syndrome because of transmission of the disease to the fresh kidney—but most such patients will ultimately receive successful transplants.

Most patients with hypertensive nephrosclerosis present with gradual increase in hypertension and renal failure. A number of patients, however, have presented with sudden onset of malignant hypertension and renal failure. Emergency nephrectomy can occasionally be performed in such patients with resolution of the hypertension prior to transplantation.

Transplantation has been carried out in a number of patients with both benign and malignant tumors primarily arising within the kidney. Patients with benign tumors associated with tuberous sclerosis respond well to transplantation. If the tumor is malignant, it is best to maintain these patients on hemodialysis for several years prior to transplantation to avoid grafting patients with metastatic malignant disease. Diabetic end-stage renal disease was formally a contraindication to transplantation. Large series now confirm that more than half these patients will survive more than 5 years with transplants. Chronic hemodialysis is a poor second therapeutic choice.

Lupus erythematosus appears to produce an immune complex nephritis. Anti-DNA antibodies combine with systemic DNA and are filtered out in the kidney, leading to renal damage. There has not been much experience with transplantation for lupus erythematosus with renal disease, but is felt to be satisfactory if other manifestations of lupus erythematosus have been brought under control by immunosuppressive drugs.

A number of metabolic diseases (gout, oxalosis, cystinosis, hyperoxaluria, nephrocalcinosis, and amyloidosis) have very little in common except for the accumulation of abnormal deposits within the kidney leading to or associated with renal failure. Transplants in most of these diseases can be successful, although recurrence after oxalosis is common.

Patients with chronic obstructive pulmonary disease in addition to their renal disease require careful individual scrutiny. Such patients tolerate pulmonary infections poorly, and since pulmonary infections are a frequent cause of death in patients with renal transplantation, careful selection of these patients is required. Heavy smokers should be given a long period to discontinue smoking. Prolonged physical therapy for chronic pulmonary disease should also be done prior to transplantation. This is of particular importance in chronic granulomatous diseases, such as histoplasmosis, coccidioidomycosis, and tuberculosis. Such diseases may remain inactive prior to the institution of immunosuppression and be exacerbated in the presence of immunosuppressive drugs. Transplantation is not absolutely contraindicated—but the patient must be carefully followed for exacerbations.

The social and psychologic barriers to selection used by some groups seem capricious. It is extremely difficult to judge the psychologic and social stability of a patient who is dying of long-term renal disease. Similarly, one cannot exclude, out of hand, patients with coronary disease or cerebrovascular accidents. Patients with peptic ulceration do quite well if surgical correction of the peptic ulcer disease is carried out prior to transplantation. Patients with severe liver disease, however, may be more susceptible to azathioprine toxicity. Liver disease therefore remains a relative contraindication.

In short, all transplantation centers are now rapidly expanding their indications for transplantation and finding that the number of contraindications has greatly diminished.

CLINICAL EVALUATION OF POTENTIAL RECIPIENTS AND TIMING OF DIALYSIS. More important than the actual selection technique of the potential recipient is the choice of time for the institution of dialysis treatment. The conservative management of renal failure will not be discussed in detail here. In principle, homeostasis can be achieved by manipulation of the sodium, potassium, chloride, bicarbonate, water, and protein intake. An occasional dialysis may be necessary for exacerbations of renal failure secondary to infections in urinary tract or elsewhere. The protein-limited (high-quality) diets developed by Giodono and Giovanetti, and described by Anderson and associates, are essential. It is even possible to maintain patients in positive nitrogen balance over several months and even years on this diet. The main problem, however, has been motivation of the patient, and near-suicidal binges of eating are a constant problem over a long period.

Dialysis should always be instituted prior to the development of uremic complications. Once hypertension, pericarditis, cardiac failure, severe bone disease, bleeding, malnutrition, severe anemia, and neuropathy appear, management is markedly complicated and rehabilitation compromised. Ideally, the conservative management of patients treated for progressive renal functional deterioration should be carried out in conjunction with nephrologists associated with both dialysis and transplant centers. In this way, the complication of severe uremia can be rapidly prevented by dialysis without the delays inherent in the referral process.

The main indication for the institution of dialysis has been a serum creatinine level greater than 15 mg/100 ml or a creatinine clearance less than 3 ml/minute despite meticulous conservative care. It is obvious that there are exceptions to this rule. Some patients, particularly patients with polycystic kidney disease, with serum creatinine levels greater than 15 mg/100 ml can be maintained well for months on dietary management. In other patients, especially diabetic patients, severe complications of uremia will develop long before the serum creatinine level reaches that level. The most pernicious of these complications is peripheral neuropathy. If there are signs of motor involvement, the patient should have dialysis and transplantation without delay, since very rapid progression of the disease can make it impossible ever to rehabilitate such a patient. Another indication for early dialysis-transplantation is uncontrollable hypertension, or hypertension that can be controlled only at the expense of severe orthostatic hypotension and other side effects. Severe anemia with anemic symptoms (dyspnea at the mildest exertion), severe bone disease (especially in children), and the failure to maintain his diet or carry on his social and family obligations all should lead to early dialysis and transplantation. There is little to be gained by a delay of 3 to 6 months, and lives may be lost in futile attempts at conservative management.

Since some of the complications of uremia may appear suddenly during conservative management, it is extremely important that the patient be fully evaluated prior to the institution of dialysis, if possible. In addition to the medical evaluation, this preparation should include interviews with the patient and his family by the business office of the hospital, the rehabilitation clinic, and social service in order to ameliorate the financial and social difficulties that may accompany dialysis and transplantation. Rehabilitation of the patient can be actively pursued even prior to the institution of dialysis.

PREPARATION FOR HEMODIALYSIS AND TRANSPLANTATION. The pretransplantation studies are listed in Table 10-4. Most of these studies are used by many transplant

Table 10-4. WORK-UP OF POTENTIAL RECIPIENTS OF RENAL TRANSPLANTATION

1. General
   a. History and physical examination
   b. Chest x-ray
   c. ECG
   d. Electrophoresis
   e. Fasting blood sugar
2. Hematologic
   a. Hemoglobin
   b. Leukocyte count and differential count
   c. Platelet count
   d. Bleeding-clotting time
   e. Prothrombin time, partial thromboplastin time, thrombin time
3. "Allergic" potential for complications
   a. Serum electrophoresis
   b. LE test
   c. Antiglomerular basement antibodies
4. Renal
   a. Flat plate of abdomen (kidney size) (tomography)
   b. Creatinine clearance
   c. 24-hour protein excretion
   d. (Electrophoresis/urine, protein excretion selectivity)
   e. Electrolyte status in blood
   f. (Electrolyte status in urine)
   g. Urinalysis × 3
   h. Urine culture × 3
   i. (Renal biopsy)
5. Signs of hyperparathyroidism
   a. Bone x-ray (hands, skull, clavical, lamina dura)
   b. Ca, PO_4, Mg, alkaline phosphatase
6. Hypertensive work-up
   a. Chest x-ray (heart size)
   b. ECG
   c. Ophthalmic examination
   d. Serial blood pressure
7. Urologic evaluation
   a. Voiding cystogram
   b. (Retrograde pyelography)
   c. (Cystometrography)
   d. (Bladder biopsy)
   e. (Bladder stimulation)
8. Upper gastrointestinal x-ray
9. (Colon x-ray in older patients)
10. Typing
    a. ABO
    b. Blood pedigree
    c. Tissue typing including serial cytotoxic antibody determinations
11. (Pulmonary function studies)
12. Infectious work-up
    a. Chest x-ray
    b. Purified protein derivative (fungal skin tests)
    c. Urine culture
    d. Blood culture
    e. Skin-nose-throat culture
    f. Feces culture
    g. (Sinus-teeth x-ray-ear, nose, throat consultation)
13. Financial-social rehabilitation
    a. (Psychologic-psychiatric)

Note: The tests listed within parentheses are not administered routinely during the potential recipient work-up, but only when the circumstances so indicate.

groups and for patients on dialysis. A few deserve elaboration.

The urinary tract should be evaluated for patency of its outflow and absence of ureterovesical reflux. In general, a voiding cystogram suffices. That test makes it possible to determine that the urethra is unobstructed, that the bladder empties, that there are no abnormalities of the bladder wall, and that there is no ureteral reflux. Prostatic obstruction, urinary stricture, and bladder neck obstruction should be repaired prior to transplantation but only after the patient has been dialyzed for several weeks.

It is difficult or almost impossible to evaluate bladder emptying in the presence of ureterovesical reflux. Contraction of the bladder wall leads to reflux of the urine into the ureters, which then empty back into the bladder when the bladder wall is relaxed. It may be necessary to remove both ureters at the ureterovesical junction prior to evaluation of the bladder for competence.

The upper gastrointestinal tract should be evaluated for the possibility of a preexisting peptic ulceration. If significant disease is present, vagotomy and pyloroplasty or a comparable operation should be carried out at least several weeks prior to transplantation. Such precautions have almost completely eliminated upper gastrointestinal tract bleeding as a problem.

Electromyography may be useful for documenting the progress or improvement of peripheral neuropathy. Because so many patients with uremia also have hearing deficits, periodic audiograms should be carried out.

Obviously dialysis frequently must be instituted prior to the completion of these studies. Most of the studies listed are primarily designed to prepare for transplantation. Dialysis is both a definitive therapy and the most important part of the preparation for transplantation. It should not be delayed in order to complete other studies, the results of which no longer exclude the patient from treatment.

Tissue Typing and Cross Matching. The principles of transplantation immunogenetics have been presented in detail above. Prior to transplantation, tissue typing to match donor and recipient should be carried out—both for the selection of the most appropriate donor and for the determination of the prognostic implications of tissue matching. It is possible at present to type most patients completely at the HLA-A and HLA-B locus of the HLA major histocompatibility complex (Table 10-1). Typing at the HLA-D locus previously was thought to depend on mixed leukocyte reactivity of recipient against potential donor, but more recently antibodies have been developed which can detect antigenic differences at both C and D subloci of the HLA complex. What role matching at the C and D sublocus will have in prognosis is not yet known.

It is important to determine whether a putative recipient has antibodies against one or more A or B antigens by utilizing a panel of lymphocytes derived from persons bearing known HLA-A or -B specificities. Patients who have been presensitized by blood transfusion, pregnancy, or previous transplantation can then be identified; it may be possible actually to identify those A or B specificities to which the antibodies are directed. Some patients will have antibodies to the entire spectrum of A and B subloci. The detection of preformed antibodies against the C or D sublocus is far less advanced, but almost certainly such antibodies will be found.

There is strong evidence that typing for A and B sublocus antibodies and matching donor and recipient at those antigens will have beneficial consequences for the outcome of renal transplantation. Whether this is true for C and D subloci is as yet unknown.

Since patients who have preformed antibodies against the HLA-A and -B subloci might possibly have antibodies against a potential renal allograft donor, cross matching of the patient's serum to detect antibodies against donor leukocytes should be carried out immediately prior to the transplant. If these preformed antibody barriers are crossed, immediate (hyperacute) rejection almost always ensues. Varying cross-matching techniques have varying degrees of sensitivity, and the most sensitive method should be utilized, since organ preservation techniques currently permit prolonged storage of kidneys (up to 48 and frequently to 72 hours). Cross-matching techniques which take several hours should always precede transplantation.

Most transplant units draw serum samples monthly on all patients awaiting transplantation in order to detect the formation of anti-HLA-A and -B antibodies. The use of several of these sera for final cross matching should always be performed, since antibodies appear and disappear without apparent reason in recipients. Nevertheless, if a patient has previously made antibodies against the putative donor, it is likely that an accelerated rejection will occur and that that donor should not be utilized.

Principles of Hemodialysis

Dialysis removes toxic products of small molecular size from the blood and reinstitutes acid-base balance and electrolyte homeostasis. Although such treatment will not relieve all the complications of uremia, it will prevent death in a large percentage of cases. Blood is passed through a tubing composed of a semipermeable membrane, so that dialyzable substances within the blood pass into the dialysis bath and dialyzable materials within the bath pass into the blood. Fluid can be removed (ultrafiltration) (1) by increasing the osmolarity of the dialysate bath (by adding glucose), (2) by constricting the outflow of blood from the dialyzer, or (3) by running dialysate at negative pressure to raise the filtration pressure.

Transplant dialysis is not an end in itself. It merely maintains the patient while he awaits transplantation, prepares him for the operations required, and retrieves him if the transplant is temporarily or permanently unsuccessful. Three requirements are necessary to perform dialysis: (1) access to a flow of blood, (2) a semipermeable membrane tubing, and (3) a dialysate bath of appropriate composition.

Access to Blood Flow. Indwelling Cannulae The Quinton-Scribner silastic Teflon cannula was the instrument first widely used for access to blood in dialysis. The technique currently used for insertion is shown in Fig. 10-42A and B. A number of other devices similar in principle are also currently in use. Either upper or lower extremities can be used for cannulation, but the upper extremity is preferable in order not to immobilize the patient while the wounds are healing. The ideal vessels are the radial artery and the cephalic or basilic vein on the nondominant arm.

The persistence of the cannulae within the vessels and the subsequent passage through the skin have predictable consequences—the vessels may clot, the cutaneous fistulae may become infected, and the shunt is in danger of bleeding. The clotting problem looms especially large after major surgical procedures.

Infectious complications at the shunt site are particularly dangerous before transplantation. *Staphylococcus aureus* is the most common infecting agent. Long-term treatment with synthetic penicillinase-resistant penicillin plus intensive local treatment with heat and elevation can cure these infections in most instances. Systemic gram-negative infections have been rare when using disposable dialyzers. Infections are best prevented by handling all shunts with sterile technique. Mask and glove precautions should be enforced whenever the shunt is opened or manipulated. The shunt should be removed as soon as possible after function of the transplanted kidney has been established.

Arteriovenous Fistulae. Because the problems of shunt care increase with time, external shunts are most satisfactory when transplantation is scheduled within a few weeks or months. In patients being dialyzed for prolonged periods while awaiting a kidney from a cadaver, the subcutaneous arteriovenous fistula described by Brescia et al. and modified by many others has been a major advance. Here an arteriovenous anastomosis is performed, usually between the radial artery and the cephalic vein at the wrist (Fig. 10-43). The superficial veins become dilated, and blood can be obtained for passage through the dialyzer by the use of two large-bore needles inserted into the dilated venous system.

There are several advantages to this type of fistula: (1) no foreign bodies inviting infection pass through the skin except during dialysis; (2) the fistula has a lesser tendency to clot than does the Quinton-Scribner shunt; (3) the arteriovenous fistula can remain open in the posttransplant period, thereby facilitating dialysis if rejection occurs months or even years later; (4) the dilated veins are useful for the administration of any thrombogenic substance (e.g., antilymphoblast globulin) because of the rapid flow through the veins; and (5) it provides rapid access for the frequent blood samples required in the posttransplant period. Many modifications of these fistulas have been devised which utilize vascular or prosthetic grafts to bridge gaps between artery and vein; but all provide a dilated subcutaneous vessel for repeated puncture with large-bore needles.

SELECTION AND EVALUATION OF LIVING DONORS

The principles of histocompatibility typing and matching have been described above. From the recipient's point of view it is generally preferable that the donor be a biologic relative. It is still controversial whether or not histocompatibility typing can discern cadaver donors who will be more suitable than a relative. Even mismatched sibling and parent kidneys may survive with better function and for

① Artery is elevated by
ligation suture and
vessel loop →

② Arteriotomy accomplished
by scalpel puncture
medially, continuing
upward (Angle forceps
are used)

③ Arteriotomy
retracted by one of
2 methods:

OR

In
Children

In
Adults

④ Cannula
inserted thru
arteriotomy

⑤ Vessel loop and
ligation sutures tied
over cannula

⑥ Anchoring suture is
double looped and tied

⑦ Stab wound made
for exit of arterial
cannula

⑧ Cannula is pulled thru
stab wound, and positioned
subcutaneously

Anchoring suture is then run
along top of vessel and tied
over cannula and vessel

A

Fig. 10-42. Insertion of Scribner shunt (*A*) and connecting the two shunt limbs (*B*). [*From C. M. Kjellstrand, R. L. Simmons, T. J. Buselmeier, and J. S. Najarian, Kidney: I. Recipient Selection, Medical Management, and Dialysis, in J. S. Najarian and R. L. Simmons (eds.), "Transplantation," p. 418, Lea & Febiger, Philadelphia, 1972.*]

more prolonged periods than do closely matched cadaver kidneys. Before the advent of histocompatibility typing, it was shown that kidneys from sibling donors functioned better than kidneys from parental donors. Because the genes governing the expression of histocompatibility antigens are situated at one (complex) locus, there will always be one major allelic difference between the parent and the offspring, whereas one-fourth of siblings will be identical, one-half will have a one haplotype difference, and one-fourth will have both haplotypes different. Tissue typing can usually identify that sibling (if any) who shares all the serologically detectable antigens at the major histocompatibility complex (MHC). Such sibling grafts have a better than 90 percent chance for long-term success.

A living related donor offers other advantages to the recipient: the delay between renal failure and rehabilitation is shorter, posttransplant renal function is usually immediate, and there are fewer rejection episodes, so that smaller doses of immunosuppressive drugs are required.

The major blood group antigens (ABO) are strong transplantation antigens. Although a number of successful allotransplants have been carried out across isoantibody barriers, it is generally unwise to perform transplants into patients with known preformed isohemagglutinins against the donor blood type. The same rules apply to clinical transplantation that apply to transfusion: i.e., AB is the universal recipient and O the universal donor. When such blood type barriers are crossed, the most violent type of

⑨ Following venous anastomosis, both cannulae are prepared for connection

Arterial cannula

Teflon connector

Venous cannula

Silastic

⑩ 2 Plastic rings, and 2 metal crimp rings are placed over cannulae prior to connection

Arterial

Venous

⑪ The cannulae are connected and crimp rings tightened

Point of connection

⑫ Clamps released, flow established

B

Fig. 10-42. Continued.
See legend on facing page.

hyperacute rejection reaction may occur. While there is no convincing evidence to suggest that minor blood group factors (Rh, Duffy, Kell) act as histocompatibility antigens, the possibility exists that they may make a minor contribution to graft antigenicity.

The living related donor should be in perfect health to minimize any risks inherent in an operation of this magnitude. A death following renal donation from a healthy person has been reported, and the utmost caution must be exerted not to harm or diminish the renal reserve of a healthy volunteer. Table 10-5 lists the examinations routinely carried out on volunteer related donors.

ETHICAL PROBLEMS. Selection of a related donor is made on the basis of histocompatibility testing when possible; often, however, there is only one volunteer. The ethical and social problems of donor selection have been

extensively discussed elsewhere, but brief consideration is pertinent here.

In practice, the recipient is informed of the risks and benefits of receiving a kidney from a related donor. The recipient knows best which relatives he can approach and which he cannot. When a volunteer appears he is blood-typed and tissue-typed. If he is acceptable on these grounds, the risk of donor nephrectomy is explained to him. The risk to life in an otherwise perfectly healthy patient has been estimated to be 0.05 percent. The long-term risk has been estimated by actuarial statistics to that incurred by driving a car 16 miles every working day. Much evidence suggests that no long-term harm results from life with a single kidney. Although the risks are small, the pain, anxiety, and loss of work time are real.

It is difficult to conceive of a living related donor who is

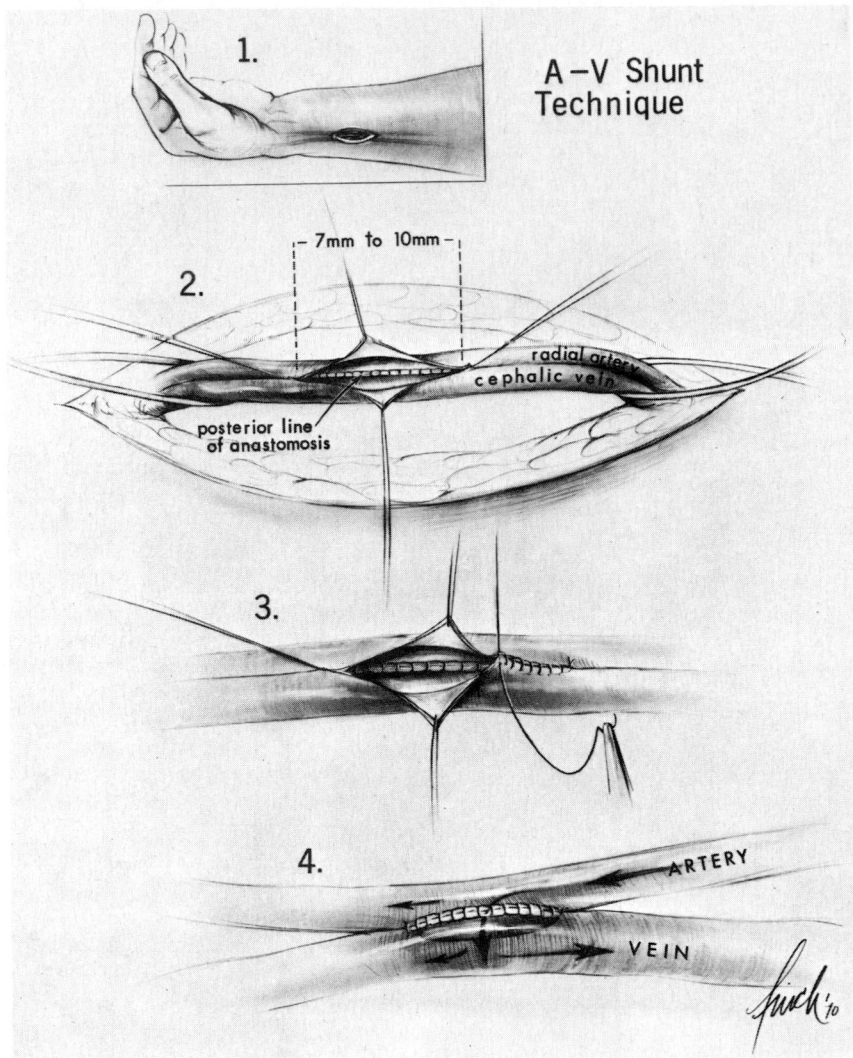

Fig. 10-43. Technique for constructing an arteriovenous anastomosis between radial artery and cephalic vein at the wrist. [*From C. M. Kjellstrand, R. L. Simmons, T. J. Buselmeier, and J. S. Najarian, Kidney: I. Recipient Selection, Medical Management, and Dialysis in J. S. Najarian and R. L. Simmons (eds.), "Transplantation," p. 418, Lea & Febiger, Philadelphia, 1972.*]

Table 10-5. PROTOCOL FOR LIVING RELATED DONOR WORK-UP

1. History and physical examination
2. Hematology: hematocrit, leukocyte count, differential count, platelet count
3. Coagulation: prothrombin time, partial thromboplastin time, thrombin time
4. Chemistry: serum Na^+, K^+, Cl^-, $CO^=$, SGOT, bilirubin, uric acid, Ca^{++}, P, BUN, creatinine, fasting blood sugar, glucose tolerance test
5. Urine: urinalysis, 24-hour urine for creatinine clearance
6. Microbiology: clean-catch urine culture $\times$ 2
7. Immunology: blood type (major and minor), tissue typing, leukocyte cross match for recipient antidonor and leukocyte antibodies; VDRL; Australian antigen
8. X-ray: chest x-ray, posteroanterior and lateral; intravenous pyelogram (IVP), renal arteriograms
9. Isotope: bilateral renogram
10. Electrocardiogram

not subject to some family pressure to donate. That such pressures exist, however, is evidence that people have feelings of family and role obligations within the society. When a person freely volunteers to donate, both the benefits to the recipient and the risks to the donor are explained. No pressure is exerted to persuade or dissuade the potential donor. He is not subjected to extensive psychologic interviews or testing. Careful studies of actual donors indicate a remarkably favorable psychologic response in most donors, but some ambivalence and conflict within the family occur in a minority. On occasion, when the potential donor expresses anxiety concerning his donation, it is necessary to fabricate a medical excuse not to donate that can be used by the otherwise medically and immunologically compatible donor.

Sometimes it is necessary or advisable to use donors under the age of eighteen. This has frequently been necessary for identical-twin transplants. The use of such donors, however, should be restricted to those circumstances in which other donors are not available. A court of law will also find it difficult to decide whether an adolescent should donate to his parents or siblings when family pressure may exist. Teen-aged donors have been used when they insisted on donation and the court has agreed to it.

Unrelated persons are not generally encouraged to donate, since the results are no better than that achieved with cadaver donors. It is possible that a pool of living unrelated donors may exist that could be typed and matched against a similar recipient pool in order to obtain ideal donors within unrelated populations. Such a system was tried at the University of California but with results no better than if cadaver donors were used. Prisoners, mental defectives, and psychiatric patients are not generally used as donors for the obvious reason that undue pressure might be exerted on these persons against their own best interests. The purchase of organs, with its inevitable consequences, the selling of living unrelated organs, or even the selling of a cadaver organ must be discouraged.

SELECTION OF A CADAVER DONOR

The ideal cadaver kidney donor (1) is young, (2) has remained normotensive until a short time before death, (3) is free of transmissible infection and malignant disease, and (4) has died in the hospital after observation for a number of hours, during which time blood group and tissue type have been determined and urinary function has been assessed. Under these ideal conditions the donor kidneys can be removed within minutes to minimize the warm ischemia time. It is often necessary, however, to compromise with these ideal principles. The age of the donor is not of crucial importance. A donated kidney can recover from long periods of shock and anuria that occur while it is still in the donor. But not more than 1 hour of warm ischemia time should elapse during harvesting.

CRITERIA OF BRAIN DEATH. The procurement of cadaver organs for transplantation has raised some serious moral, ethical, legal, and psychologic problems. The first problem is to establish when death occurs. Since the decision is a clinical one, made by the physician in the interest of the patient (potential donor), it should be based primarily on clinical criteria of irreversible brain damage—fixed dilated pupils, absent reflexes, unresponsiveness to external stimuli, and the inability to maintain vital functions such as respiration, heartbeat, and blood pressure without artificial means. The decision should be made by physicians who are not associated with the potential recipient in any way, either as the referring physician or as a member of the transplant team. The exact criteria vary among institutions and have been fully discussed by Schwab, Potts and Bonazzi, the Harvard Committee, and Juul-Jensen. An increasing number of states have passed laws which permit the absence of brain function to be used to define death.

Juul-Jenson established four criteria of brain death: (1) The type of cerebral lesions must be established; the donors must therefore be selected among neurosurgical

patients with severe trauma, vascular lesions, or tumors. Neuroradiologic studies, arteriography revealing the absence of cerebral blood flow, and surgical exploration assist in the diagnosis of irreversible brain damage. (2) The level of consciousness must be that of deep coma, in which the patient does not respond to any form of external stimulus. Neurologic examination must reveal dilated and reactionless pupils, absence of corneal and pharyngeal reflexes, no reaction to tracheal suction, absence of deep and plantar reflexes, and hypotonia. The patient must be without spontaneous respiration and must require controlled respiration. In this state, atropine will evidence no change in cardiac rhythm. These two criteria have generally been sufficient for most neurosurgeons to pronounce cerebral brain death after a period of observation and knowledge of the cerebral disease. A recent autopsy study confirmed that the brain damage in 24 consecutive cadaver donors was incompatible with recovery when these clinical criteria also were satisfied.

Despite this evidence, Juul-Jensen considers two more criteria, (3) a negative caloric test and (4) an isoelectric electroencephalogram (EEG), to be important. Juul-Jensen feels that the isoelectric EEG is essential, but points out that isoelectric EEGs have been described in anesthetized patients in hypothermia. He furthermore requires that the tests be repeated within a 24-hour interval where the EEG is recorded with normal amplification and double amplification with both a normal time constant and an increased time constant. These stringent EEG criteria are felt to be excessive by most physicians; vital signs will frequently fail before an isoelectric EEG will appear. A number of donors have been unnecessarily lost because of delay despite the presence of a destroyed brain.

In the past, a falling blood pressure has been used as a criterion of brain death, but it is frequently the result of dehydration due to diabetes insipidus. This is aggravated by loss of vasomotor tone, which produces hypotension. Almost all patients with total brain death can be maintained for prolonged periods with normal vital signs using plasma and vasopressors; cardiac stimulants are rarely required. Urinary output can likewise be maintained with hydration and diuretics. Even the head-injury patient who has been anuric and in shock for many hours can be restored to hemodynamic stability by restoration of a normal blood volume.

All decisions regarding the death of the potential donor must be made by physicians who understand the criteria of brain death and who have had no contact with the potential recipient. Various administrative techniques have been used; the best require the determination of brain death to be made by a team of neurologists and neurosurgeons.

The principles of organ preservation are described in a subsequent section. The advances in organ preservation have alleviated the urgency of cadaver transplantation. It is possible to harvest kidneys at the moment of death and preserve them in iced solutions for 24 hours until the transplant recipients are ready. Kidneys can now be routinely preserved by hypothermic perfusion for more than 48 hours (see subsequent section). The use of machines for this purpose has increased the availability of cadaver kidneys, because the kidneys can be transported for long distances. The development of preservation also allows for more careful typing, matching, shipping, and sharing of organs between various centers.

ORGAN HARVEST

RELATED LIVING DONOR. The actual technique of the donor operation is not as crucial as those factors that maintain urinary output in the donated kidney and in the remaining donor kidney. An active diuresis in the donor at the moment of renal artery occlusion favors prompt function in the recipient. Conversely, a soft cyanotic kidney in spasm after a difficult dissection frequently is slow to put out urine even if the period of ischemia has been short. For these reasons, the urine output is monitored throughout the donor operation and should not fall below 1 ml/minute/ kidney. The patient is hydrated during the night prior to operation, and both colloid (5 ml/kg/hour) and crystalloid solutions (5 ml/kg/hour) are administered during the operation, with constant attention to the central venous pressure and the urine output. Mannitol and furosemide

are given shortly before the kidney is removed. In addition, systemic heparinization is carried out 5 minutes before the renal artery is occluded. The heparin is then counteracted with protamine.

The technique of donor operation is described in Fig. 10-44. It is carried out through a flank incision. The peritoneum is retracted, the ureter identified, and a length of ureter is dissected free. The ureter is then transected (preserving its blood supply from the renal pelvis) so that the urinary output of the donor kidney can be observed throughout the operation. The remainder of the ureter is dissected free up to the renal vein. A large lumbar vein, the ovarian or testicular vein, and the adrenal branch of the renal vein are doubly ligated on the left side. There are no major branches of the renal vein on the right side. Dissection on the renal vein is carried down to the vena cava. The artery is not dissected free until the dissection of the renal

Fig. 10-44. Harvest of a kidney from a living related donor. [*From R. L. Simmons, C. M. Kjellstrand, and J. S. Najarian, Kidney: II. Technique, Complications, and Results, in J. S. Najarian and R. L. Simmons (eds.), "Transplantation," p. 445, Lea & Febiger, Philadelphia, 1972.*]

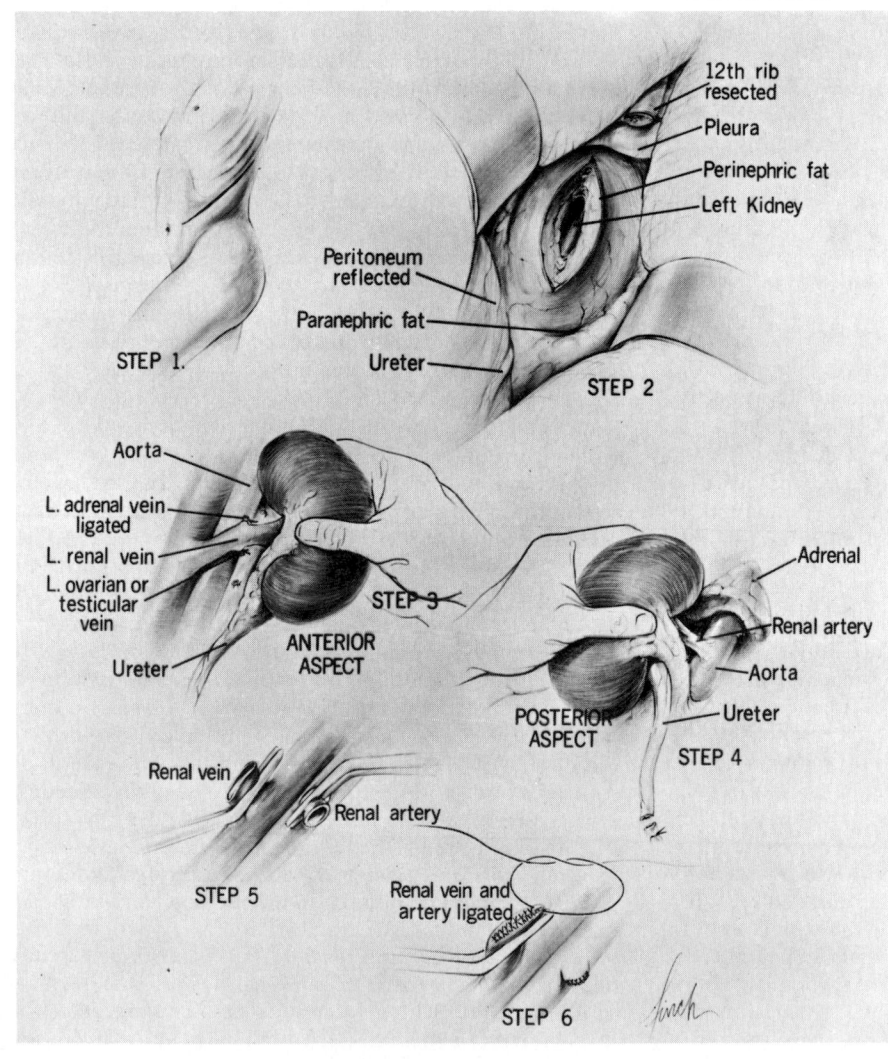

vein is complete. The kidney is not removed until urinary output from the donor kidney itself is excellent. At that time the renal artery and vein are sequentially clamped and divided.

Minor complications of nephrectomy in healthy related donors are common, but serious complications are quite rare. The function of the remaining kidney increases very quickly. Within the first hours after surgery, the renal clearance is 70 percent of the preoperative value. By 2 to 3 days cellular hypertrophy and hyperplasia have taken place and the kidney size has increased. Prolonged follow-ups indicate that the health and life expectancy of the donor are not adversely affected by donation.

CADAVER DONOR. The technique of kidney harvest from a cadaver donor depends to a large degree on the status of the donor's circulation. If the cadaver is brain-dead but with intact circulation and urine output, nephrectomy can be performed as in living donors, but by the transperitoneal route. The circulatory function of the cadaver can also be maintained by closed heart massage or artificial circulatory devices during the harvest procedure.

If the donor has a sudden irreversible circulatory collapse, the kidneys must be removed more rapidly to minimize ischemia time. The donor is heparinized, and both kidneys are removed together by clamping the aorta and vena cava above the origin of the renal arteries and veins and pulling the kidneys up together, prior to transection of the aorta and vena cava below the origin of the renal vessels and the ureters in the pelvis. Prompt cooling of the organs is required, and both kidneys can be perfused with iced crystalloid solution prior to storing them in the cold or perfusing them on preservation machines.

PREPARATION OF THE RECIPIENT
FOR TRANSPLANTATION

NEPHRECTOMY. It is probably not necessary to remove the kidneys from most patients, but the decision should be carefully considered for all. Removal of the patient's diseased kidney may be desirable to (1) control hypertension, (2) eliminate a potential or real source of infection, (3) remove ureters from patients with ureterovesical reflux, and (4) eliminate the patient's diseased kidneys as potential pathogenetic agents in the recurrence of the primary disease. The latter reason is of theoretic importance only, since the recurrence of the glomerulonephritis in the transplanted kidney is not known to be aggravated by the presence of the diseased kidneys.

When indicated, many transplantation centers perform bilateral nephrectomy at the time of the transplantation. Others feel that it is better to stage the operations and perform the nephrectomy sometime prior to transplantation in order (1) to minimize the surgical stress at transplantation; (2) to minimize the surgical shock incurred, which might interfere with the function of the transplanted kidney; (3) to apply the minimal surgical stress when immunosuppressant drugs are utilized; (4) to eliminate completely urinary tract infection before immunosuppression is begun; and (5) to control hypertension prior to transplantation.

When two-stage transplantation is carried out (i.e., ne-

phrectomy preceding the transplantation by a week or 10 days), the postnephrectomy management is simple. Hyperkalemia is a recurrent postnephrectomy problem, but it can usually be prevented if a 20% glucose solution is administered prophylactically (with insulin if the patient has diabetes). Rectal ion-exchange resins may be required to control hyperkalemia. Dialysis can usually be postponed 2 or 3 days with these techniques. Delay in reinstituting dialysis is preferred because heparinization is required and although it is regional, systemic effects may occur and invite postoperative hemorrhage.

Splenectomy and/or thymectomy have also been performed in kidney recipients prior to transplantation. Thymectomy has fallen into disuse since its performance was associated with a high rate of morbidity without improvement of renal function survival. Most groups still debate whether splenectomy contributes to the well-being of the recipient. There is no evidence that splenectomy increases the functional survival of the graft, although excision of a large portion of the bodies of lymphoid mass was the original indication for splenectomy.

During preparation for transplantation, sepsis from any source must be scrupulously removed. Frequent sources of sepsis are (1) the hemodialysis cannulae, if present, (2) the bladder in patients with preexisting urinary tract infections, and (3) the skin of patients with uremic dermatitis. The bladder of the nephrectomized patient frequently becomes infected, and the bladder should be irrigated with appropriate antimicrobial agents several times weekly, prior to grafting.

Dialysis should be frequent and intense in the immediate pretransplantation period. Recipients of cadaver kidneys will have little preparation time prior to transplantation. Many patients will be maintained on systemic anticoagulants because of clotting problems in hemodialysis shunts; the anticoagulants must be discontinued, and vitamin K must be administered.

TECHNIQUE OF RENAL TRANSPLANTATION

The operative technique of renal transplantation used at the University of Minnesota is described in Figs. 10-45 and 10-46.

OPERATIVE MANAGEMENT. There must be no deficit in blood volume following the vascular anastomoses. Hypovolemia interferes with the rapid resumption of renal function. Urine usually appears within a few minutes of completion of the vascular anastomoses in related living donor kidneys; mannitol and furosemide may be helpful in hastening the appearance of urine, a useful sign that there are no serious technical deficiencies.

Three methods are generally available for establishing urinary tract continuity. The preferred method involves ureteroneocystostomy. Pyeloureterostomy and ureteroureterostomy have also been recommended, but the incidence of urinary extravasation is far more common with the latter techniques.

Renal biopsy at the time of transplantation can be useful where hyperacute rejection is suspected, but it is rarely necessary in a primary transplant from a living related donor.

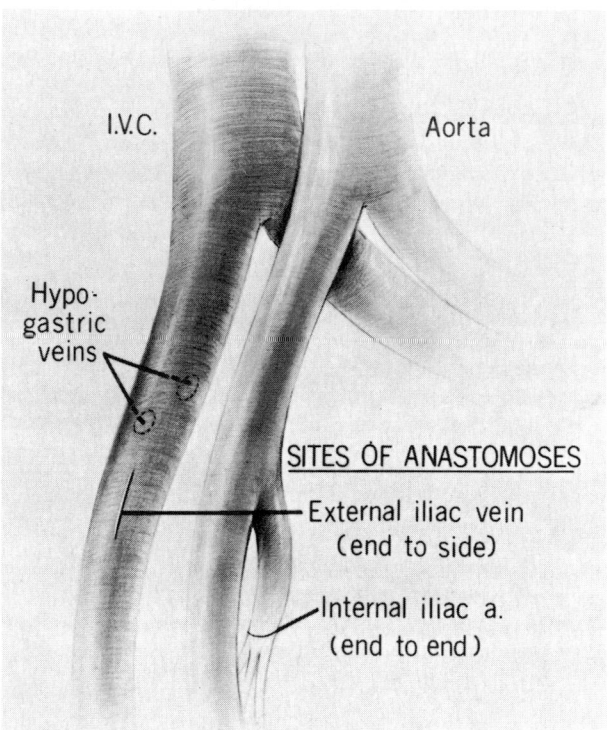

Fig. 10-45. Sites of anastomoses of renal vein to the side of the iliac vein. [*From R. L. Simmons, C. M. Kjellstrand, and J. S. Najarian, Kidney: II. Technique, Complications, and Results, in J. S. Najarian and R. L. Simmons (eds.), "Transplantation," p. 445, Lea & Febiger, Philadelphia, 1972.*]

Fig. 10-46. Anastomosis of hypogastric artery to renal artery. [*From R. L. Simmons, C. M. Kjellstrand, and J. S. Najarian, Kidney: II. Technique, Complications, and Results, in J. S. Najarian and R. L. Simmons (eds.), "Transplantation," p. 445, Lea & Febiger, Philadelphia, 1972.*]

ANESTHESIA IN THE ANEPHRIC PATIENT. Certain precautions are necessary during any operation on an anephric patient. In particular, certain anesthetics are excreted almost exclusively by the kidney and should not be used. These include the muscle relaxant gallamine triethiodide. Both curare and succinylcholine are metabolized by the liver, but both may also be accompanied by prolonged paralysis in the postoperative period. In the case of succinylcholine, a number of investigators have found that serum cholinesterase is broken down during hemodialysis. In such patients, succinylcholine would be expected to have prolonged action. Conduction anesthesia has been used, but most anethesiologists prefer general anesthesia.

In the administration of anesthetics and fluids, it should always be assumed that the kidney will not function immediately after transplantation, even if dialysis is rarely required after transplantation. Similar thinking should be employed with regard to hyperkalemia in the uremic patient. Other concerns of the anesthesiologist are the loss of the hypertensive state after induction of anesthesia to normal levels, and the low hematocrit in patients with chronic uremia. The hematocrit should be raised to 30 prior to transplantation, and hypovolemia due to excessive ultrafiltration during hemodialysis should be avoided.

ROUTINE POSTTRANSPLANT CARE

The management of kidney allograft patients in the early posttransplant period does not differ radically from the management of other postoperative patients. Vital signs are monitored frequently for the first day, and the central venous pressure is utilized as a guide to blood volume. A Foley catheter is left in the bladder, and it is not irrigated unless clots are thought to be occluding the catheter. The urine output is measured at least every hour. The volume of urine should be replaced with intravenous fluids. A convenient replacement solution consists of one-half normal saline solution with 5% dextrose and water and 10 mEq of sodium bicarbonate per liter. Potassium need not be added to the intravenous fluids except in small children, whose urinary electrolytes should be replaced milliequivalent for milliequivalent.

The urinary output in the early postoperative period may be enormous, partly because of tubular dysfunction but primarily because of the overhydrated state of even the best-dialyzed patient. A creatinine clearance obtained on the evening of transplantation will be helpful in assessing renal function. So called high-output renal failure has an associated obligatory diuresis, so urine output is not an infallible guide. If the clearance is satisfactory, however, acute renal failure is not present. The lower the clearance, the greater the degree of failure. When high-output ischemic damage has been ruled out, fluid restriction can be practiced to keep from "chasing" the urinary output with intravenous fluids. The use of 1% dextrose and water with half-normal saline solution (as an intravenous infusion when urinary outputs are greater than 500 ml/hour) will diminish the osmotic diuresis due to glycosuria.

The Foley catheter can be removed almost any time after the first day. The tip of the catheter should be cultured at that time. Prophylactic antibiotics are used during the perioperative period. Thereafter oral antibiotics which are concentrated in the urine are used to prevent urinary tract infections. Moderate hypertension is frequently seen in the early posttransplant period, and a low-sodium diet and low doses of antihypertensive medication (α-methyldopa, hydrochlorothiazide, or hydralazine) are useful to counteract this tendency. Antacids appear to be useful in preventing the appearance of gastrointestinal ulceration of patients on immunosuppressive drugs.

The patient is allowed out of bed and oral fluids are begun on the first postoperative day.

ROUTINE POSTTRANSPLANT LABORATORY DETERMINATIONS. The creatinine clearance is determined for two 2-hour periods. The first is during the second to fourth postoperative hours, and once more in the sixth to eighth postoperative hours. These determinations are extremely useful in interpreting early oliguria. The hematocrit should be followed at 4-hour intervals, since rebleeding is a rare but severe complication which can produce oliguria and the onset of acute tubular necrosis (ATN).

A ^{131}I Hippuran renogram is usually performed soon after transplantation. Intravenous pyelography (IVP) is rarely necessary. Determinations of blood urea nitrogen (BUN), serum creatinine, and creatinine clearance suffice to estimate daily renal function. Serum electrolyte determinations can usually be discontinued after good renal function is established. Periodic leukocyte and platelet counts are necessary to assay the state of the bone marrow during immunosuppression. Rarely, hyperglycemia and hypercalcemia are complications, and therefore blood sugar and calcium levels should be determined from time to time. The diabetic patient will require frequent blood sugar determinations and adjustments of insulin dosage.

Prophylactic Immunosuppression. The principles of immunosuppression have been described above. Standard immunosuppressive management at most clinical transplant centers consists of azathioprine with or without prednisone or ALG. A number of centers also use prophylactic irradiation of the graft. So many factors are involved in the success or failure of the transplant that the differences in immunosuppression methods used at different centers cannot easily be evaluated. The present regimen used at the University of Minnesota is typical. It is summarized in Table 10-6.

COMPLICATIONS OF RENAL TRANSPLANTATION

RENAL FAILURE. The most serious complication of renal transplantation is the failure of the graft to initiate or maintain function. Although the causes of failure can easily be defined, the differential diagnosis may, at the time, be impossible. The functional failure of the kidney is best examined in relation to the time after transplantation: The kidney may (1) never function, (2) have delayed onset of function, (3) fail to function after a brief or prolonged time, or (4) gradually lose its function over a period of months or years. In each phase, four general diagnoses should be considered: (1) ischemic damage to the kidney; (2) rejection of the kidney by reactions directed against

Table 10-6. PROPHYLACTIC IMMUNOSUPPRESSION FOR RENAL TRANSPLANTATION AT THE UNIVERSITY OF MINNESOTA

A. Antilymphoblast globulin (ALG)
  1. 30 mg/kg intravenously daily for cadaver and mismatched related organ recipients for 2 weeks
  2. 10 mg/kg intravenously daily for related organ recipients for 2 weeks
B. Azathioprine (evening dose after checking leukocyte count)
  1. Preoperative dose is 5 mg/kg/day for 2 days
  2. First and second postoperative days: 5 mg/kg
  3. Third through sixth postoperative days: 4 mg/kg
  4. Seventh postoperative day: 3 mg/kg; maintain at 2 to 3 mg/kg
  5. Adjust at all times with respect to WBC, platelet count, and renal function
  6. Caution: Reduce dosage to 1.5 mg/kg for severe renal functional impairment
C. Prednisone
  1. Related kidney
    a. 0.25 mg/kg every 6 hr beginning 36 hr prior to transplant
    b. First and second postoperative days: 1 mg/kg/day
    c. Third through sixth postoperative days: 0.75 mg/kg/day
    d. Seventh through ninth postoperative days: 0.5 mg/kg/day
    e. Reduce level slowly to achieve a maintenance dose of 0.15 to 0.25 mg/kg/day
  2. Cadaver kidney
    a. 0.5 mg/kg every 6 hr on first 3 postoperative days (total dose 20 mg/kg)
    b. 1.5 mg/kg/day for the next 3 days
    c. 1.0 mg/kg/day for 3 days
    d. 0.75 mg/kg/day for 3 days
    e. 0.5 mg/kg/day until discharge
    f. Reduce dose slowly to achieve a maintenance dose of 0.3 to 0.4 mg/kg
D. Methylprednisone
  1. 20 mg/kg/day intravenously on evening of transplantation and on first 2 postoperative days

histocompatibility antigens on the kidney, (3) technical complications; and (4) the development of renal disease, either a new disease or recurrence of the original.

The simplest and best assay for decreased renal function is the frequent determination of BUN, serum creatinine, and the determination of creatinine clearance. Occasional renograms or intravenous pyelograms are also useful. The differential diagnosis of renal malfunction, however, may require echography, retrograde pyelography, arteriography, and renal biopsy.

Early Anuria and Oliguria

Early anuria or oliguria is a major diagnostic problem. The possibilities include (1) hypovolemia, (2) thrombosis of the renal artery or renal vein, (3) hyperacute rejection of the kidney, (4) ischemic renal damage (ATN), (5) compression of the kidney (by hematoma, seroma, or lymph), and (6) obstruction of the urinary flow.

Differential Diagnosis of Early Oliguria. The investigation of early posttransplant anuria should be rapidly performed in a strict sequence. The Foley catheter should first be irrigated and/or changed to remove any question of catheter obstruction. Unfortunately, whatever the cause of anuria, a clot can be obtained by bladder irrigation in the first posttransplant day. The clot may not be the primary cause of anuria, however, because blood will clot within the bladder if the urine is not copious enough to wash it out prior to coagulation. Therefore, even if a clot is present within the urinary catheter, the urine output should be monitored for the first 10 to 15 minutes after emptying the bladder to determine urine output adequacy.

If the obstructed catheter has not caused the oliguria, one must rule out hemorrhage and hypovolemia combined with compression or displacement of the kidney by the hematoma. If hypotension and tachycardia are present and the central venous pressure is low, hypovolemia is very likely. A roentgenogram of the abdomen will reveal displacement of the intraperitoneal contents by a massive hematoma. Echography and repeated hematocrit determinations will confirm the diagnosis. The normal degree of ischemic damage to the transplanted kidney plus hypovolemia and compression of the kidney and vessels by a hematoma all conspire to impair renal function. If anuria or severe oliguria is present, restoration of the blood volume will seldom suffice to restore renal function, even if furosemide or other diuretics are used. Many patients will require reexploration to control the bleeding point. After exploration, if the period of hypovolemia and renal compression has been relatively brief and diuretics have been used during ischemia, prompt restoration of renal function usually occurs.

The diagnosis of bleeding is frequently apparent and obviates the need for the next step in the investigation sequence—an [131]I Hippuran renogram (Fig. 10-47A and B). The renogram permits assessment of the blood flow to the kidney and the ability of the kidney to concentrate and excrete the Hippuran. The results are never diagnostic. If the vascular phase and concentration are near normal, however, the renal arterial and venous anastomoses are

patent. If the Hippuran uptake by the kidney is severely depressed, a renal arteriogram should be done. Arteriography will assess the renal arterial anastomosis, and if it reveals the presence of intravascular thrombosis of the kidney the diagnosis of hyperacute rejection will be suggested.

Technical Complications Causing Early Oliguria. Thrombosis of the renal arterial anastomosis is rare. Partial obstruction due to torsion or kinking of the vessels is more common and should be promptly repaired. When the renogram demonstrates poor concentration of the [131]I Hippuran, an arteriogram should be performed to detect correctable technical complications (Fig. 10-48A and B). Thrombosis of the renal vein occurs even more rarely than thrombosis of the renal artery. When it does occur, thrombosis of the artery ensues because the collateral venous circulation of the kidney has been interrupted by the transplant procedure. Partial thrombosis of the renal and iliac veins has occurred. Usually, this is accompanied by swelling of the ipsilateral lower extremity, fever, and evidence of pulmonary embolism.

Formerly, one of the most common, and most frequently fatal, complications following renal transplantation was urinary extravasation due to distal ureteral necrosis. Rejection was seldom at fault. The problem can generally be avoided by (1) shortening the ureter as much as possible; (2) avoiding tension at the ureteroneocystostomy site; (3) avoiding hematomas within the wound, which put tension on the ureter and also interfere with the developing

Fig. 10-47. Function of a homotransplanted kidney. *A.* A radiorenogram showing a half-life of 6.3 minutes and a completely normal-appearing curve. *B.* A scan of the same transplant showing excellent uptake in the kidney and the appearance of the radioactive material in the bladder. This transplant continued to have excellent function 5½ years later. (*From D. M. Hume, "Advances in Surgery," vol. II, Year Book Medical Publishers, Inc., Chicago, 1966.*)

Fig. 10-48. Correctable arterial complications in the early post-transplant period. Oliguria was present in both patients. [131]I Hippuran revealed poor vascular phase. The arteriograms revealed (A) torsion distal to the renal arterial anastomosis, which was corrected by a reanastomosis, and (B) a suture that had caught the periadventitial tissues of the superior renal artery, kinking it. The defect was corrected by prompt lysis of the adventitial band. [From R. L. Simmons, C. M. Kjellstrand, and J. S. Najarian, Kidney: II. Technique, Complications, and Results, in J. S. Najarian and R. L. Simmons (eds.), "Transplantation," p. 445, Lea & Febiger, Philadelphia, 1972.]

collateral blood supply to the distal ureter; (4) avoiding transperitoneal "clotheslining" of the ureter by always placing the ureter in the retroperitoneal position where tension will be minimal and the collateral blood supply can develop. Urinary extravasation from ureteroureterostomies and from pyeloureterostomies occurs much more commonly than that from ureteroneocystostomies.

Urinary extravasation is a serious complication that leads to infection and frequently to death. It demands urgent reexploration with reimplantation of the ureter into the bladder, nephrostomy, or performance of a pyeloureterostomy to the host ureter. On occasion, the pelvis of the transplanted kidney may be involved, and nephrectomy may be required. Delay in definitive repair will frequently lead to infection, the development of mycotic aneurysms, loss of the kidney, and death.

Technical errors can become manifest long after the immediate posttransplant period. Arterial stenosis, venous thrombosis, and late ureteral leaks and strictures are frequently confused with rejection (see below). Prior to any antirejection treatment, technical problems should be ruled out by echography, arteriography, renography, or intravenous or retrograde pyelography.

Hyperacute Rejection Causing Early Oliguria. Hyperacute rejection of the kidney is almost always mediated by humoral antibody, with the subsequent participation of the complement, coagulation, and kinin cascade systems. Platelets, PMNs, and vasospasm may also play a role. Hyperacute rejection occurs most frequently in patients who have demonstrable cytotoxic antibody directed against donor histocompatibility antigens. A lesser number of patients will reject renal allografts in the absence of demonstrable cytotoxic antibody, but a degree of subliminal sensitization that cannot be detected with current techniques may be present. Indeed, detectable cytotoxic antibody will appear and disappear at intervals in patients awaiting transplantation. The classic hyperacute rejection appears in patients who have received multiple transfusions or who have rejected a previous transplant. In these patients, the kidney will fail to regain its normal turgor and healthy pink color after anastomoses are established, despite patent anastomoses. Biopsy and histologic study at this time may reveal leukocytes in the glomerular capillaries, and intravascular renal thrombosis follows (Fig. 10-49). On rare occasions, the intravascular coagulation will be so severe that a consumptive coagulopathy with a bleeding diathesis is produced. Definite evidence of a hyperacute rejection should be treated by immediate nephrectomy. A less acute rejection may occur, however, and renal function may not fail until a day or two following transplantation. Such rapid rejection has been differentiated by the term "accelerated rejection."

Since the advent and improvement of in vitro cytotoxic cross-match tests, antibodies against donor leukocytes can be detected prior to operation. Careful cross matching is therefore essential to any transplant program (see above).

Acute Tubular Necrosis Causing Early Oliguria. The diagnosis of ischemic renal injury is one of exclusion. If all other causes of renal functional failure in the early posttransplant period have been ruled out, one must assume that the diagnosis is ATN. "Acute tubular necrosis" in

Fig. 10-49. Hyperacute rejection. A biopsy of the kidney transplant taken 90 minutes after transplantation. The glomerulus may be seen to be filled with polymorphonuclear leukocytes. These cells fill the small vessels of the cortex and aid in the rapid destruction of the endothelium.

clinical parlance refers to kidneys whose function is impaired from ischemia or a variety of other causes. If kidneys from this clinical spectrum are biopsied, they most frequently show only hydropic changes. The more severe the insult, the more likely will be the presence of tubular necrosis. The correlation between tubule pathology and function, however, is not always good and suggests the interplay with other mechanisms, including prolonged vasoconstriction and vascular endothelial cell swelling. Most kidneys will recover, but disruption is so severe that cellular repair is not possible.

ATN occurs most commonly in cadaver recipients when the donor had undergone long periods of stress and hypotensive insult to the kidney to be transplanted. Another cause of recipient ATN is a long period of warm ischemia preceding transplantation. Kidneys with warm ischemic intervals greater than 1 hour should not be utilized for transplantation, because function will seldom return to normal. Cold ischemia is much better tolerated, and preservation up to 48 hours is now very satisfactory.

Almost all transplanted kidneys have undergone some degree of damage secondary to trauma and ischemia. A second trauma (hypovolemia, hypoxemia, renal compression, bacteremia, allergic reactions to ALG) that normally might not result in ATN in normal kidneys may cause oliguria in transplanted kidneys. One must not diagnose rejection and institute massive steroid therapy in the early posttransplant period without ruling out the possibility that an additional insult to an already damaged kidney has occurred and that the diagnosis is not acute rejection but ATN. Renal biopsy may be necessary to make this differentiation.

The management of the patient with ATN is simple. Urinary flow will resume in almost all cases within 2 or 3 weeks, but anuria for as long as 6 weeks with total recovery has been observed. [131]I Hippuran renograms are useful in following improvement prior to resumption of urinary flow. Dialysis is maintained intermittently during the period of oliguria. A number of studies have shown that the long-term function of renal transplants is independent of the presence or absence of oliguria in the early posttransplant period.

Rejection

Technical errors may not become evident for several weeks post grafting, and any trauma can aggravate the degree of ATN in a previously damaged kidney. Nevertheless most renal failure appearing after the first posttransplant week can be attributed to rejection.

With better immunosuppression, the acute rejection episodes that formerly appeared in the first month following transplantation are seen less and less frequently. The majority of patients, however, will sustain at least one acute rejection episode during the first 3 to 4 months following transplantation. Clinical rejection is rarely an all-or-nothing reaction, and the first episode seldom progresses to complete renal destruction. The functional changes induced by rejection appear to be in large part reversible; therefore, the recognition and treatment of the rejection episode prior to the development of severe renal damage is of extreme importance. Usually the rejection reaction responds to increased prednisone doses and local irradiation. Even with prompt treatment the creatinine clearance may be permanently impaired, however slightly, following each clinical rejection episode.

Differential Diagnosis of Renal Allograft Rejection. The clinical picture of a rejection reaction may be distressingly similar to several other problems: ureter leak or obstruction, hemorrhage with consequent ATN infection, or stenosis or twist in the renal artery or vein. Classic renal rejection is characterized by oliguria, enlargement and tenderness of the graft, malaise, fever, leukocytosis, hypertension, weight gain, and peripheral edema. Laboratory studies have shown lymphocyturia, red cell casts, proteinuria, immunoglobulin fragments, fibrin fragments in the urine, complementuria, lysozymuria, decreased urine sodium excretion, renal tubular acidosis, and increased lactic dehydrogenase in the urine. The level of the blood urea nitrogen increases, as does serum creatinine and lactic dehydrogenase, while the serum complement level is unstable. Creatinine clearance is obviously decreased; renograms will show slow uptake of the Hippuran and slow urinary excretion. An intravenous pyelogram is usually normal. The renal cortical blood flow is also decreased during rejection, and an arteriogram may show narrowing of the cortical vessels with irregularity of the distal vessels.

The most important parameter to follow is the serum creatinine level. Unlike the BUN, which is sensitive to a number of changes (steroid administration, fever, and high-protein diet), serum creatinine levels are relatively stable for each patient. The creatinine clearance is more sensitive, but it depends on a carefully timed collection of urine. The most reliable confirmatory test of renal functional deterioration (whatever the cause) is the radiorenogram. When compared with previous renograms, the early signs of rejection are a decreased excretory rate and a slight

Fig. 10-50. Human allografted kidney 11 months posttransplant. The flattened, atrophic-appearing tubules are the most striking feature. The narrowed arteriole in the lower left quadrant of the picture suggests that the basis for the atrophy may be ischemia. The paucity of infiltrating host immune cells reflects both the patchy nature of the rejection reaction and the indolent pace imposed by relatively effective immunosuppression. [*From J. E. Foker, and J. S. Najarian, Allograft Rejection: III. The Pathobiology of Organ Rejection, in J. S. Najarian and R. L. Simmons (eds.), "Transplantation," p. 122, Lea & Febiger, Philadelphia, 1972.*]

delay in the vascular phase. These changes are probably related to decreased cortical blood flow and may appear prior to changes in serum creatinine. More sophisticated modes of evaluating the disturbances in renal blood flow that always occur in transplant rejection have been described, but they have not yet achieved widespread clinical acceptance.

The most reliable clinical signs of renal functional deterioration are a slight decrease in urinary output, slow weight gain, small increases in diastolic blood pressure, and edema of the lower extremity on the side of the graft. A peripheral leukocyte count and a serum creatinine level should be determined to confirm renal functional deterioration. A renogram and intravenous pyelogram should be promptly performed and compared with those obtained at the peak of renal function (usually prior to discharge from the hospital). In the face of poor renal function, tomograms during intravenous pyelography may outline a normal ureter. If ureteral obstruction cannot be ruled out, retrograde pyelography can be carried out, although it may be difficult to cannulate the ureteral orifice. Finally, arteriography may reveal (1) characteristic changes of decreased concentration of dye flowing into the kidney, (2) decreased nephrogram effect, (3) an irregularity of the cortical vasculature and intralobar vasculature characteristic of rejection, and (4) normal renal artery and anastomosis, eliminating the possibility of a technical problem.

Renal biopsy should be a definitive diagnostic tool. Both open biopsy and needle biopsy techniques have been described, and the histologic changes of rejection are characteristic (Figs. 10-18, 10-19, 10-49 through 10-52). A normal kidney biopsy is diagnostic, but a biopsy that reveals renal damage may merely reflect acute rejection, a chronic ongoing process, exacerbation of the preexisting renal dis-

ease, or damage due to infection or radiation. Nevertheless, needle biopsy of transplanted kidneys is a safe procedure in experienced hands and gives very useful additional information.

Infection and Rejection. Many apparent allograft rejection episodes are preceded or accompanied by rather mild bacterial or viral infections (Fig. 10-53). The cause-effect relationship here is unclear. The infectious agent may act as a nonspecific adjuvant, upsetting the delicate immunologic balance that exists between donor organ and host and stimulating the rejection reaction. Alternatively, the antigens on the bacteria or virus may cross-react with the histocompatibility antigens and exacerbate the host immune response. Whatever the cause, appearance of mild infection in a renal transplant recipient often precedes renal functional deterioration. Conversely, the appearance of a rejection episode should prompt a search for underlying infection.

Treatment of Rejection. Most institutions have developed a standard rejection regimen for allografted kidneys (Table 10-7). This standard regimen can be repeated as many as three times within a 2-month period in patients for whom rejection appears to be unremitting. If it is repeated more often than that, infection may appear and be lethal. The decision to stop immunosuppression and sacrifice the transplant frequently depends on subtle factors and is difficult to make, particularly in patients who have deterioration of renal function over a period of months and years.

Renal Failure Due to Recurrent Disease

Renal grafts between identical twins have been performed in human beings for 20 years. Even though such transplants do not encounter the severe immunologic barriers to success that allografts do, they have not been

Fig. 10-51. Human renal allograft 27 months posttransplant. The interstitium dominates the morphologic features of this chronically rejected kidney. The area formerly occupied by tubule cells is largely replaced by ill-defined strands. The vacuolated appearance suggests the presence of edema. A modest round cell infiltrate, tubular atrophy, and occluded glomerular loops are also part of chronic rejection. [*From J. E. Foker, and J. S. Najarian, Allograft Rejection: III. The Pathobiology of Organ Rejection, in J. S. Najarian and R. L. Simmons (eds.), "Transplantation," p. 122, Lea & Febiger, Philadelphia, 1972.*]

uniformly successful. Recipients of renal isografts whose original disease was glomerulonephritis frequently develop a lesion in the graft identifiable as glomerulonephritis. An original disease of rapidly progressive glomerulonephritis is associated with the earlier and more frequent appearance of glomerular lesions on the isografts and subsequent progression to chronic renal failure. In contrast, a slowly

progressive glomerulonephritis is correlated with lower instances of glomerular lesions in isografts and a greater opportunity for survival. Glomerulonephritis of the isograft rarely appears in recipients whose primary disease was not categorized as glomerulonephritis.

The recurrent disease in the isografts in some respects resembles the late-onset glomerular lesion of the allo-

Fig. 10-52. Chronic rejection in a human renal allograft 11 months after transplantation. A small artery shows the result of endothelial cell damage and medial hypertrophy—a pinpoint lumen may be damaged endothelial cells. The bulk of the increase in vessel wall thickness, however, may be due to smooth muscle cell proliferation. The stimulus to cellular division among these cells may result from the immunologic activity on the elastic membranes of the vessel. [*From J. E. Foker and J. S. Najarian, Allograft Rejection: III. The Pathobiology of Organ Rejection, in J. S. Najarian and R. L. Simmons (eds.), "Transplantation" p. 122, Lea & Febiger, Philadelphia, 1972.*]

Fig. 10-53. The course of a patient whose "rejection episode" was preceded by an upper respiratory infection in both the patient and his wife. Despite prolonged and vigorous antirejection therapy, renal function returned to normal slowly. (*From R. L. Simmons, R. Weil III, M. B. Tallent, C. M. Kjellstrand, and J. S. Najarian, Do Mild Infections Stimulate Allograft Rejection? Transplant Proc, 2:419, 1970.*)

grafted kidney; the nephrotic syndrome may occur in either situation. The glomerulonephritis of isografts is associated with basement membrane and mesangial deposition of IgG, complement, and fibrinogen. The presence of preformed antiglomerular basement antibodies as well as immune complexes has been implicated in the pathogenesis of the recurrent disease. The high recurrence rate of glomerulonephritis in isografts and the apparent low rate in allografts is thought to be due to the relative universal use of immunosuppressive therapy in the latter group. Genetic predisposition to glomerulonephritis may also exist among the donor-recipient pairs in the isograft series.

Although experience is limited, prophylactic immunosuppression appears to have merit in the prevention and treatment of recurrent glomerulonephritis in isografts. Whether it is beneficial to remove the diseased host kidneys is not known. The general strategy is not to delay allotransplantation or isotransplantation after the nephrectomy of patients with proved glomerulonephritis unless the disease is of acute onset or there are high circulating titers of antiglomerular basement membrane (anti GBM) antibody present. If the disease is of recent onset with rapid progression to failure, nephrectomy is performed and the

titer of anti-GBM antibody follows until it falls to negligible quantities. At that time, transplantation should be carried out with immunosuppressive coverage in both isogeneic and allogeneic recipients.

Because so many of the changes that accompany chronic kidney disease are nonspecific, there is still active debate about the incidence of recurrent nephritis in renal allotransplants. In patients with complex nephritis, either of unknown cause or secondary to lupus erythematosus, it is possible that precipitation of complexes on the transplanted kidney GBM will reactivate the disease. It is also

Table 10-7. STANDARD ANTIREJECTION THERAPY AT THE UNIVERSITY OF MINNESOTA

1. Therapy
   a. Solumedrol: 20 mg/kg/day intravenously × 3.
   b. Prednisone: 2 mg/kg × 3 days; then 1.5 mg/kg × 3 days; then 1.0 mg/kg × 3 days; thereafter reduce prednisone slowly to a maintenance dose.
   c. Azathioprine: Regulate dose to prevent leukopenia; do not increase.
   d. Irradiate kidney transplant: 150 r every other day for three doses.
2. Adjuncts
   a. Reinstitute antacid therapy.
   b. Reinstitute oral nystatin (100,000 units twice daily) to prevent mucosal candidiasis.
   c. Reduce protein and fluid intake if renal function is significantly impaired.

possible that complexes of antibody will be filtered with streptococci, other bacteria, viruses, or ALG. Alternatively, direct binding of antibody with the GBM may take place, not only as a consequence of preexisting anti-GBM antibodies, but also secondary to GBM binding by ALG or by the development of Masugi nephritis. One or more mechanisms may be operating in a given patient, but, in general, most of the glomerular changes in allotransplants can be considered to be part of the rejection process.

RESULTS OF RENAL TRANSPLANTATION

TRANSPLANT REGISTRY RESULTS. The results presented here are the results of the "Thirteenth Report (1977) of the ACS/NIH Human Renal Transplant Registry" (Tables 10-8 and 10-9). All the data reported to the Registry are analyzed collectively. Although large numbers aid analysis, the reported results are neither as good as those of the most experienced centers nor as poor as those centers with the worst record. The report, therefore, should be thought of as an average of performance achieved by groups reported to the Registry.

The data for calculations in this report were derived from 19,631 transplants reported to the Registry. These include transplants performed in the United States, Europe, Australia, and Canada. It is clear from Tables 10-8 and 10-9, pooled from first transplants performed from around the world, that kidneys from living related donors survive much better than do those from cadaver donors. This has been a fairly consistent finding throughout all the years of renal transplantation. It is also clear that the improvements in results seen in the early days following transplantation have now leveled off and that the results of transplantation are not better than they were in 1968, although the mortality statistics continue to improve.

Other consistent findings from the Transplant Registry include the following: (1) Results of transplantation do not depend on the diagnosis of that disease which caused end-stage renal disease. There are several exceptions to this rule, i.e., patients with familial nephritis are usually children or adolescents and appear to have better survival, while poorer survival rates are seen in patients with malignant hypertension and cancer of the kidney. Similarly, diabetics have poorer survival, and patients with Fabry's disease and oxylosis have very poor results. (2) In general, when the results of transplantation in infants are excluded, the results of transplantation get worse with the age of the recipient. This is particularly striking after age forty or fifty. (3) The Registry has not been able to detect differences associated with splenectomy, although patients with splenectomy appear to do slightly better. (4) The Registry has not been able to detect differences associated with bilateral nephrectomy prior to transplantation.

Other registries and compilations of data from many centers have yielded slightly different data but have given indications that the following relations are also true: (1) Patients who receive blood transfusions prior to transplantation, i.e., transfusions at some time during their uremic anemia, appear to do better following transplantation than those who do not receive blood transfusions. This result is unexpected, since blood transfusions have been traditionally avoided by nephrologists for fear of sensitizing recipients to the HLA-A and -B antigens. Two factors may be at work here: (a) the patients who become sensitized, presumably from the blood transfusion, are excluded from transplantation, and this selects against the vigorous responders; and (b) patients who receive blood transfusions and who do not become sensitized may be a hypoimmunized group, i.e., have less immune capacity to respond against the graft as demonstrated by their failure to respond to the transfusion. (2) Certain registries have demonstrated poorer results in kidneys preserved by perfusion rather than ice-cold storage (see below). These results have not been confirmed by others, who show no difference in kidney survival regardless of the method of preservation. (3) Certain registries have found that patients who develop antibodies to the HLA-A and -B series of antigens reject donor kidneys more often than those who do not develop antibodies to the HLA-A and -B antigens prior to transplantation. Although sensitization is to be avoided at all costs, most investigators cannot confirm these findings and show only that if patients are transplanted with kidneys to which they have already developed cytotoxic antibodies, the results of transplantation are less favorable.

TRANSPLANTATION IN CHILDREN. Renal failure in children is a common cause of death. Traditionally, young children have not been considered ideal candidates for renal transplantation, although excellent results have been reported by a number of investigators. The small caliber of vessels and active social behavior of children make their management on hemodialysis extremely difficult. Long-term immunosuppressive therapy is also thought to interfere with normal growth with resultant social problems. Long-term hemodialysis is seldom satisfactory, and a parent is almost always willing to donate a kidney. The Human Renal Transplant Registry statistics reveal that patients above the age of five do extremely well posttransplant, confirming the impression of several large pediatric transplant groups. Several infants have had transplants, and at least one has survived for more than 1 year. The growth of children following transplantation has been the subject of several studies. Most children with allografts grow slightly slower than normal. The adolescent growth spurt is absent in children with transplants and adolescent growth is particularly depressed in girls.

This early cessation of growth causes the typical appearance of girls with transplants who are short and more cushingoid than the boys. Attempts to correlate the amount of first-year posttransplant growth with the kidney donor, renal function, or prednisone dosage have been unsuccessful. No such correlations can be made, even though it is generally felt that prednisone interferes with growth.

Sexual maturation in boys appears to be normal, although the period of observation has been short. Similarly, some girls have failed to menstruate at the usual age despite relatively normal renal function and only moderate doses of prednisone. Most girls have resumed menstruating if previously mature, or they undergo a normal menarche upon reaching age thirteen or fourteen.

MULTIPLE TRANSPLANTS. A number of studies have

Table 10-8. SURVIVAL OF PATIENTS: FIRST TRANSPLANT ONLY BY DONOR SOURCE AND YEAR OF TRANSPLANT

Donor source and year of transplant	Sample size	3 Months		6 Months		1 Year		2 Years		3 Years		4 Years		5 Years	
		Percent functioning	± SE	Percent functioning	± SE	Percent functioning	± SE	Percent functioning	± SE	Percent functioning	± SE	Percent functioning	± SE	Percent functioning	± SE
Sibling															
1968	207	94.0	1.7	90.4	2.1	87.7	2.3	82.4	2.7	79.7	2.9	76.2	3.1	73.6	3.3
1969	226	90.5	2.0	85.3	2.4	82.4	2.6	78.6	2.8	77.1	2.9	72.8	3.1	71.6	3.2
1970	280	91.6	1.7	88.6	1.9	85.8	2.1	83.8	2.3	80.6	2.5	78.2	2.6	78.2	2.6
1971	420	94.2	1.2	91.0	1.5	85.5	1.8	82.0	2.0	81.0	2.1	78.9	2.3		
1972	484	94.2	1.1	91.7	1.3	89.8	1.4	85.5	1.7	82.2	2.0				
1973	449	92.2	1.3	89.7	1.5	88.1	1.6	84.6	2.0						
1974	395	92.6	1.4	88.6	1.7	84.8	2.2								
Parent															
1968	210	86.7	2.4	83.2	2.6	79.6	2.8	75.4	3.1	70.4	3.3	66.1	3.5	64.0	3.6
1969	242	89.3	2.0	85.7	2.3	77.4	2.8	72.2	3.0	68.1	3.2	63.7	3.3	61.2	3.4
1970	274	94.7	1.4	90.0	1.9	85.9	2.2	81.6	2.5	78.4	2.6	75.3	2.8	74.5	2.9
1971	340	91.7	1.5	89.1	1.7	86.8	1.9	82.1	2.2	78.1	2.4	76.8	2.6		
1972	402	91.2	1.5	88.4	1.7	86.0	1.8	81.5	2.1	77.3	2.4				
1973	424	92.6	1.3	88.7	1.6	84.2	1.9	81.1	2.2						
1974	315	93.7	1.4	91.8	1.7	88.2	2.4								
Cadaver															
1968	655	73.4	1.8	64.3	2.0	58.5	2.1	51.5	2.1	46.4	2.2	44.3	2.2	42.0	2.2
1969	862	78.7	1.4	71.3	1.6	64.5	1.7	58.5	1.8	54.2	1.8	50.8	1.9	49.0	1.9
1970	1,183	81.0	1.2	74.9	1.3	68.5	1.4	62.5	1.5	57.6	1.6	54.0	1.7	51.0	1.8
1971	1,617	80.9	1.0	74.5	1.2	68.7	1.3	62.7	1.3	59.6	1.4	55.0	1.5		
1972	1,877	82.1	.9	75.7	1.1	69.8	1.2	63.7	1.3	61.4	1.3				
1973	2,110	82.4	.9	76.6	1.0	71.2	1.1	65.4	1.3						
1974	1,836	84.6	.9	79.3	1.1	72.3	1.4								

SOURCE: Data from the "Thirteenth Report of the ACS/NIH Human Renal Transplant Registry."

Table 10-9. FUNCTION OF TRANSPLANTED KIDNEYS: FIRST TRANSPLANT ONLY BY DONOR SOURCE AND YEAR OF TRANSPLANT

Donor source and year of transplant	Sample size	3 Months		6 Months		1 Year		2 Years		3 Years		4 Years		5 Years	
		Percent functioning	± SE	Percent functioning	± SE	Percent functioning	± SE	Percent functioning	± SE	Percent functioning	± SE	Percent functioning	± SE	Percent functioning	± SE
Sibling															
1968	207	88.4	2.2	83.6	2.6	80.2	2.8	74.4	3.0	71.4	3.1	65.8	3.3	61.9	3.4
1969	226	86.3	2.3	79.6	2.7	76.5	2.8	72.1	3.0	69.3	3.1	65.0	3.2	62.4	3.3
1970	280	87.1	2.0	83.6	2.2	80.3	2.4	77.2	2.5	72.7	2.7	68.8	2.9	65.9	3.1
1971	420	84.3	1.8	80.0	2.0	73.9	2.1	69.7	2.3	68.3	2.3	66.1	2.4		
1972	484	86.8	1.5	82.2	1.7	78.6	1.9	72.9	2.0	68.8	2.2				
1973	449	83.4	1.8	79.1	1.9	75.7	2.0	70.2	2.3						
1974	395	83.8	1.9	77.7	2.2	72.5	2.5								
Parent															
1968	210	83.3	2.6	78.1	2.9	72.4	3.1	67.1	3.2	59.9	3.4	53.2	3.5	50.5	3.5
1969	242	83.5	2.4	78.1	2.7	69.0	3.0	62.3	3.1	56.7	3.2	50.4	3.3	45.1	3.3
1970	274	87.6	2.0	82.8	2.3	75.2	2.6	69.6	2.8	62.4	2.9	58.0	3.0	54.7	3.2
1971	340	84.4	2.0	80.0	2.2	74.7	2.4	67.4	2.6	61.1	2.7	56.9	2.9		
1972	402	80.8	2.0	76.1	2.1	72.1	2.2	64.7	2.4	57.5	2.7				
1973	424	80.1	1.9	74.7	2.1	68.7	2.3	62.2	2.6						
1974	315	80.0	2.3	74.5	2.6	66.2	3.2								
Cadaver															
1968	655	63.0	1.9	53.1	2.0	46.4	2.0	38.8	1.9	33.8	1.9	31.1	1.8	28.6	1.8
1969	862	69.5	1.6	61.4	1.7	53.7	1.7	46.8	1.7	41.7	1.7	37.7	1.7	35.4	1.7
1970	1,183	69.4	1.3	61.9	1.4	55.4	1.4	47.1	1.5	42.3	1.5	38.4	1.5	34.6	1.5
1971	1,617	67.0	1.2	60.0	1.2	53.0	1.2	45.9	1.2	42.0	1.2	37.1	1.3		
1972	1,877	66.5	1.1	58.3	1.1	50.8	1.2	43.8	1.2	40.0	1.2				
1973	2,110	64.3	1.0	56.3	1.1	49.5	1.1	41.1	1.2						
1974	1,836	62.2	1.2	53.9	1.2	46.3	1.3								

SOURCE: Data from the "Thirteenth Report of the ACS/NIH Human Renal Transplant Registry."

shown that second and third transplants are less successful than the first, if the first was rejected soon after transplantation. The rejection of one transplant may sensitize the patient to a number of weaker histocompatibility antigens that cannot be easily detected by sensitive cross-match techniques. In addition, such patients may have less compromised immune systems which permitted the rejection of the first transplant. In contrast, patients who have maintained a successful first transplant for several years will, after losing the first transplant, accept the second transplant more readily.

XENOGRAFTS

Xenografts between related species are rejected by the same immune mechanisms as are allografts. Xenografts between distant species are rejected by an additional mechanism—the reaction of the xenograft with preformed antibodies which then trigger the efficient complement and clotting cascades. In short, xenografts across distant species barriers are rejected like hyperacute rejections.

There is not much information about clinical xenografts, because, in general, they have not proved to be useful. Xenografts of calf skin have sometimes been used for burn dressings and appear to offer some advantage over other dressing material, although they are not as useful as allografts. Some xenograft calf heart valves have been placed in patients, although it seems likely that these will not be as successful as are allografts, and they might be expected to calcify and become incompetent over a period of years. One xenograft chimpanzee heart has been placed in a patient, but this functioned for only about an hour. Since allografted hearts are invariably rejected experimentally, it would be expected that cardiac xenotransplants would suffer the same fate even more quickly. Renal xenografts using both chimpanzee and baboon donors have been done in a number of human beings, but this procedure has been abandoned. Surprisingly enough a few relatively long-term survivors were achieved with chimpanzee transplants which were considerably better tolerated than baboon transplants. Some testicular xenografts have been carried out in man in the past but have long since been abandoned. Bone and cartilage xenografts are still used from time to time but seem to offer no advantage over allografts. The use of organs from nonhuman species for extracorporeal perfusion, both kidneys and livers, has been tried but currently is of little value.

ORGAN PRESERVATION

The viable preservation of whole organs is one of the essential components of any transplantation program. Only cadaver donors can be used for some organs (heart and liver), and even when the organ is expendable (as in one of a pair of kidneys), the use of cadaver donors avoids the risks inherent in surgical removal of the organ from living persons. If tissue typing and matching ever achieve their true potential, it may be necessary to store the organ

until these matching procedures can be carried out. Even more time-consuming procedures, such as tolerance induction, may ultimately become available to pretreat the recipient and make him unresponsive to specific histocompatibility antigens. Table 10-10 lists some of those procedures which might be useful to carry out during organ preservation.

Methods of Viable Organ Preservation

The main problem associated with preservation of organs in a viable state seems to be hypoxia. When the organ is removed from its physiologic state, it is deprived of its normal oxygenation. The two major approaches to organ preservation have been what might be called metabolic inhibition and metabolic maintenance.

Metabolic inhibition seeks to prevent the normal catabolic processes from causing severe or irreversible damage to the tissues during the period of preservation. It is currently best achieved by hypothermia, which protects the organ by slowing metabolic activity and decreasing oxygen need. Two techniques of cooling are currently available: (1) simple cooling of a kidney by immersing it in, or flushing it with, a cold solution, which allows many hours of preservation and is almost always used for short periods of time, prior to transplantation of any organ, and (2) perfusion cooling, which allows longer periods of preservation.

Metabolic maintenance, the second approach to organ preservation, attempts to sustain a level of metabolic activity as close to physiologic normalcy as is feasible. Usually it implies perfusion of the organ in vitro with a carefully controlled fluid medium, although tissue oxygenation may be attempted. In practice metabolic maintenance is always best combined with perfusion cooling. The best system, at present, utilizes a pulsatile pump and pooled homologous plasma passed through a membrane oxygenator. Excellent transplantation results are obtained after perfusion as long as 72 hours. These moderately long preservation

Table 10-10. PROCEDURES DURING ORGAN STORAGE

A. Evaluation of the organ
   1. Typing and matching
     a. ABO typing
     b. Lymphocyte typing
     c. Organ cell typing
     d. Mixed lymphocyte culture with the recipient
   2. Diagnosis of disease in the donor or donor tissue
     a. Malignant tumors
     b. Infections
     c. Degenerative conditions
   3. Determination of functional state
     4. Restoration of normal function
B. Preparation of the recipient
   1. Induction of tolerance
   2. Immunosuppression
   3. Surgical procedures
C. Logistical procedures
   1. Stockpile various sizes and types
   2. Transport to a distant recipient
D. Modification of the immunogenicity of the organ

periods provide adequate time for accurate matching of donors and recipients.

Not all organs can be perfused equally well by the same approach. Certain precautions are necessary. It is necessary *to maintain optimal organ function* up to and beyond the moment of clinical death. For kidneys, adequate hydration and maintenance of systemic blood pressure are recommended. Manipulation of the organ also contributes to vasospasm, and so surgical dissection should be as rapid and efficient as possible. The *period of time* between the cessation of blood flow through the organ and the establishment of the organ in its new environment (warm ischemia time) is critical in preservation studies. *Temperature* is also important. Successful perfusion systems have incorporated hypothermia to reduce the need for oxygen and metabolic nutrients. *Oxygenation* is also critical. Oxygen dissolves in aqueous solution more readily at lower temperatures; a membrane oxygenator is incorporated into the system.

The *flow rate* necessary at 37°C can be substantially reduced when metabolic activity is lessened by hypothermia; flow rates of one-fifth to one-third of normal have been satisfactory. The *viscosity of the perfusion fluid* may have some influence on perfusion pressure and flow rate. The perfusion pressure is significant. If the flow rate is adequate to provide the nutrients and waste removal, then the absolute level of pressure is not critical, but excessive perfusion pressure invariably causes transudation of the perfusate, tissue edema, and, ultimately, obstruction to the flow. Another factor is *pulsation*. Perfusion results in less damage when the flow is pulsatile, particularly at normothermic temperatures. The necessity for pulsatile flow during hypothermic perfusion is less well documented. It is probably not necessary to maintain any *venous pressure gradient*. The *perfusate composition* has apparent significance. Whole plasma probably is the most physiologic perfusate and contains most of the nutrient ingredients, including fatty acids, which might be required for the metabolic activity of organs. Many other formulations have been successful, including dextran, albumin, other plasma expanders, tissue culture media, and balanced salt solutions. *Osmolarity* is important. Crystalloids are poor perfusates and lead to edema. The perfusate must be maintained at "normal" *pH* range of 7.35 to 7.45. CO_2 buffering may be necessary with the addition of 2.5 to 5 percent of this gas to the oxygenator. Extremes of alkalosis and acidosis can be prevented with the addition of HCl or $NaHCO_3$ as necessary. A number of *additives* to the perfusate have been tried. These include membrane stabilizers, vasodilators, and anticoagulants. *Hyperbaric oxygenation* has also been used to prolong the viability and storage time of organs in conjunction with hypothermia or a combination of hypothermia and perfusion. Hyperbaric oxygenations will probably play no significant role in organ preservation, or at least its effects may not prove to be additive to those of hypothermia and perfusion.

There is evidence that an adequate flow rate during perfusion is a good prognostic sign of the viability and transplantability of the organ. The most significant indica-

tion of inadequate flow rate is the swelling caused by fluid retention. This edema is usually the result of anoxia with subsequent lysosomal and cellular damage. Poor perfusion itself can produce anoxia, so that a vicious cycle of edema-anoxia-edema can be started. Other possible causes of interstitial edema are perfusate osmolarity and excessive perfusion pressure. Even hypothermia alone may cause cellular swelling. Another important factor in the obstruction of flow is simple blockage of the microvasculature. The many causes of this blockage have been described in detail and include bubbles in the perfusion system, fibrin, red cell agglutination, the adherence of platelets and leukocytes to endothelial cells, cell breakdown due to mechanically imperfect pumps, crystal formation, and even agglutination of bacteria. Some of this blockage can be prevented with adequate filtration, but even blood-derived perfusion media like whole plasma have been shown to contain aggregates that appear during hypothermic perfusion. This aggregated material has been identified as lipoprotein. Fortunately, these substances can be removed from plasma quite easily by freezing, which causes flocculation of the lipoprotein, and by subsequent filtration and/or ultracentrifugation to remove the aggregates.

When plasma or plasma products are used as perfusates, immunological damage is possible. This may be due to antibodies directed against organ antigens or to the precipitation of circulating antigen-antibody complexes within the organ. Although complement cannot be activated at hypothermic temperatures, bound antibody will activate complement within the recipient's body soon after transplantation. Although this has led to few recognized complications after renal transplantation, elimination of immunoglobulins from perfusates would be preferable.

One of the major problems in organ preservation research is the lack of methods to assay the functional state of organs in vitro and the consequent inability to measure the effectiveness of innovations in organ preservation techniques. Ultimately, of course, each preservation method must be tested by reimplantation of the organ. This is an all-or-none test which requires a large number of transplants in order to get statistically valid data. What is needed is an in vitro assay technique that can predict the transplantability of an organ and provide quantitative assessment of viability as the organ is subjected to the various preservation protocols. For practical purposes, such an assay should be utilized both before preservation (to determine whether postmortem changes have rendered the organ unfit for preservation) and immediately before transplantation (to determine whether the preservation efforts have been effective). As mentioned, the currently most popular technique involves the measurement of perfusate flow to the preserved kidney. Studies of enzymes or metabolites (like lactate) released from the graft appear promising.

Various pharmacologic agents have also been used as metabolic inhibitors. These include such drugs as magnesium sulfate, chlorpromazine, chloroquine, hydrocortisone, and diuretics such as mersalyl. Unfortunately, experiments utilizing such agents in addition to hypothermia show little additive effect. Most recently, however, allopurinol has been shown to protect against some of the anoxic damage to organs.

Organ Freezing

Since hypothermic storage is the mainstay of most preservation systems, it would seem logical to extend hypothermic to subfreezing temperatures in order to produce total inhibition of metabolic activity. It has long been possible successfully to store individual tissue cells bathed in cryoprotective agents and frozen at controlled rates. Bone marrow cells for transplantation and lymphocytes for immunologic typing and cross matching are stored by these techniques. Freeze preservation of intact solid organs presents several unique cryologic problems not present on homogeneous cell suspensions. (1) Solid organs are composed of a mixture of cell types that at least have the potential of having different optimal requirements for cryoprotective concentration and freezing and thawing rates. (2) The large volume-to-surface area ratio of solid organs leads to a lack of uniform heat distribution throughout the organ during freezing and thawing. Thus irregularity in both freezing and thawing are common. (3) Vascular patency is required for adequate perfusion of all organ parts, and the vascular integrity must be maintained for ultimate organ function. (4) An organ requires the integrated function of its many component tissues.

The best results utilizing frozen kidneys have required (1) gentle surgical technique harvested without warm ischemia while undergoing diuresis, (2) a quick, effective perfusion technique which will ensure the distribution of cryoprotectant uniformly throughout the kidney, (3) the proper choice of cryoprotective agent. Nondiffusible macromolecules or polymers are not satisfactory for solid organs since they have difficulty diffusing out of blood vessels to exert their cryoprotective effects on the cell membranes. The highly diffusible penetrating types of cryoprotectant, e.g., dimethylsulfoxide (DMSO), ethylene glycol, or glycerol, equilibrate rapidly (in 20 to 30 minutes) but exert a direct cellular toxicity and have a high osmotic effect. Therefore, the cryoprotectant must be added or removed in a gradual or stepwise fashion in order to prevent osmotic shock resulting in organ edema and vascular endothelial injury. Direct toxic effects of these agents are minimal in very cold temperatures. (4) The temperature of the kidney should be lowered to about 10°C/minute to minimize both cold shock and mechanical cellular fracturing due to differential freezing rates of the core and surface layers of the organ. These rates also minimize damage from intracellular ice formation or osmotic effect. (5) Long-term storage of freeze-preserved organs requires consideration of the fact that there is continual biodegradation through enzymatic activity even at subfreezing temperatures. Therefore storage at −70° to −100°C permits safe storage of bone marrow for weeks to months. The longest storage periods require temperatures of −196°C. Controlled freezing-cooling rates for these temperatures have not been thoroughly studied.

There seem to be two main components to the rewarming of frozen organs. The first aspect is rate of temperature increase and the second is the rate of thawing, i.e., the rate of solid to liquid phase transition. There is probably an optimal thaw rate, but the best rate for cells, tissues, and complex organs is not yet known. Some method for uniform thawing is necessary, and emersion will not work because of the difficulties in the large volume-to-surface areas of solid organs. Electromagnetic radiation appears promising, but this technique is not perfected yet. Finally, the reinstitution of hypothermic ex vivo perfusion is necessary to permit the gradual removal of cryoprotectant, which in turn reduces osmotic shock to the organ. Hypothermic perfusion also reduces the direct toxic effect of the cryoprotectant and permits evaluation of organ function. At this time, organ-freezing research is still in an empirical stage and even the general method is theoretical.

Storage of Nonviable Tissues by Freeze-Drying

Tissue grafts have been used in human reconstructive surgery for several decades. A majority of these grafts are from connective tissue and do not require that the graft be viable to function adequately. A major constituent of most of these tissues is collagen, which seems to maintain its integrity (or at least its strength) even after long-term storage by freezing or freeze-drying. Many thousands of patients each year receive bone, fascia, dura, tendon, heart valve, or skin grafts in treatment of traumatic or surgical defects. The architecture of these grafts is used as a framework for reconstruction as the host slowly replaces the tissue.

These tissues are probably best preserved by freeze-drying, which consists of rapid freezing of the tissue and the application of vacuum for removal of the water from the frozen state to the vapor state without permitting it to become liquid. Such a process usually results in maintenance of morphologic structure and therefore maintains the strength and structural integrity of the tissue. The rapidity of the initial freeze is important, as slow freezing can result in the formation of large ice crystals which can disrupt the tissue. This is apparently not a severe problem in tissues which consist largely of collagen. Other tissues, such as vascular grafts that contain elastic fibers, can show a disruption of these fibers due to crystal formation. In this instance, the most rapid freeze possible would be indicated to minimize crystal size. The graft is then dehydrated to a residual moisture of 5 percent. At this level it has been noted that tissues can subsequently be stored under vacuum at room temperature for years without further degradation or activation of metabolic processes. On reconstitution, it has been found preferable to inject water or saline solutions into a vacuum bottle containing tissue, so that the fluid can enter the tissue before it is exposed to air. Prior exposure to air apparently allows air molecules to enter the tissue and delays or prevents subsequent penetration of the water molecules necessary to rehydrate the tissue.

The usefulness of freeze-dried allografts is at least partly due to reduced antigenicity remaining in such grafts. The results of using freeze-dried allogeneic bone and autografting bone are not remarkably different. The dura has also been preserved by freeze-drying and functions extremely well when used to cover large cranial defects. Flexor tendon grafts of the hand have also been freeze-dried and used successfully, particularly when removed with their tendon sheaths intact. Many other freeze-dried tissues have been used with greater or lesser success. Cornea for nonpenetrating lamellar transplants, fascia, cartilage, heart valve, and nerve have all been tried.

Similarly, freeze-dried grafts have served as temporary biologic dressings to cover large burn wounds. In these instances the nonviable, freeze-dried graft "takes" and is even revascularized. It remains in place for several weeks or months, before it is finally sloughed. These grafts can be applied repeatedly without sensitization or acceleration of sloughing. Skin grafts have proved to be the best biologic dressing to prevent infection and to promote maximum granulation tissue formation in open skin wounds.

The usefulness of these techniques for the preservation of transplantable tissue has recently led to the organization of the American Association of Tissue Banks. The purpose of this organization will be to encourage research into and to standardize successful methods for the harvest, storage, and distribution of tissues and organs to needy patients.

References

General

Bloom, B. R., and David, J. R.: "In Vitro Methods in Cell-Mediated and Tumor Immunity," Academic Press, Inc., New York, 1976.

Calne, R. Y.: "Clinical Organ Transplantation," Blackwell Scientific Publications, Ltd., Oxford and Edinburgh, 1971.

Castro, J. E.: "Immunology for Surgeons," University Park Press, Baltimore, Md., 1976.

Fundenberg, H. H., Pink, J. R. L., Stites, D. P., and Wang, A. C.: "Basic Immunogenetics," Oxford University Press, New York, 1972.

Munster, A. M.: "Surgical Immunology," Grune & Stratton, Inc., New York, 1976.

Najarian, J. S., and Simmons, R. L.: "Transplantation," Lea & Febiger, Philadelphia, 1972.

Nelson, D. S.: "Immunobiology of the Macrophage," Academic Press, Inc., New York, 1976.

Peer, L. A.: "Transplantation of Tissues," The Williams & Wilkins Company, Baltimore, 1959.

Rapaport, F. T., and Dausset, J. (eds.): "Human Transplantation," Grune & Stratton, Inc., New York, 1968.

Russell, P. S., and Monaco, A. P.: "The Biology of Tissue Transplantation," Little, Brown and Company, Boston, 1965.

Snell, G. E., Dausset, J., and Nathenson, S.: "Histocompatibility," Academic Press, Inc., New York, 1976.

Starzl, T. E.: "Experience in Renal Transplantation," W. B. Saunders Company, Philadelphia, 1964.

——: "Experiences in Hepatic Transplantation," W. B. Saunders Company, Philadelphia, 1969.

Woodruff, M. F. A.: "The Transplantation of Tissues and Organs," Charles C Thomas, Publisher, Springfield, Ill., 1960.

Yunis, E. J., Gatti, R. A., and Amos, D. B. (eds.): "Tissue Typing and Organ Transplantation," Academic Press, Inc., New York, 1973.

Transplantation Immunology

Anderson, N. F., Delorme, E. J., and Woodruff, M. F. A.: Induction of Runt Disease in Rats by Injection of Thoracic Duct Lymphocytes at Birth, Transplant Bull, 7:93, 1960.

Anderson, R. E., and Warner, N. L.: Ionizing Radiation and the Immune Responses, Adv Immunol, 24:215, 1976.

Bach, F. H.: Genetic Control of Major Complex Histocompatibility Antigens, Genetics, 79:263, 1975.

—— and Carnaud, C.: Thymic Factors, Prog Allergy, 21:342, 1976.

—— and Kisken, W. A.: Predictive Value of Results of Mixed Leukocyte Cultures for Skin Allograft Survival in Man, Transplantation, 5:1046, 1967.

Becker, E. L., and Henson, P. M.: In Vitro Studies of Immunologically Induced Secretion of Mediators from Cells and Related Phenomena, Adv Immunol, 17:94, 1973.

Billingham, R. E., and Brent, L.: Further Attempts to Transfer Transplantation Immunity by Means of Serum, Br J Exp Pathol, 37:566, 1956.

—— and ——: Simple Method for Inducing Tolerance of Skin Homografts in Mice, Transplant Bull, 4:67, 1957.

——, ——, and Medawar, P. B.: "Actively Acquired Tolerance" of Foreign Cells, Nature (Lond), 172:603, 1953.

—— and Silvers, W. K.: Studies on Homografts of Foetal and Infant Skin and Further Observations on the Anomalous Properties of Pouch Skin Grafts in Hamsters, Proc R Soc Lond (Biol), 161:168, 1964.

Boak, J. L., Christie, G. H., Ford, W. L., and Howard, J. G.: Pathways in the Development of Liver Macrophages: Alternative Precursors Contained in Populations of Lymphocytes and Bone-Marrow Cells, Proc R Soc (Biol), 169:307, 1968.

Boyse, E. A., Old, L. J., and Thomas, G.: A Report on Some Observations with a Simplified Cytotoxic Test, Transplant Bull, 29:435, 1962.

Brent, L., Brown, J., and Medawar, P. B.: Skin Transplantation Immunity in Relation to Hypersensitivity, Lancet, 2:561, 1958.

—— and Medawar, P. B.: Quantitative Studies on Tissue Transplantation Immunity: V. Role of Antiserum in Enhancement and Desensitization, Proc R Soc Lond (Biol), 155:392, 1962.

Burnet, F. M.: "The Clonal Selection Theory of Acquired Immunity," Vanderbilt University Press, Nashville, Tenn., 1959.

—— and Fenner, F.: Genetics and Immunology, Heredity (Lond), 2:289, 1948.

Carpenter, C. B., d'Apice, A. J. F., and Abbas, A. K.: The Role of Antibodies in the Rejection and Enhancement of Organ Allografts, Adv Immunol, 22:1, 1976.

Cerottini, J.-C., and Brunner, K. T.: Cell-Mediated Cytotoxicity, Allograft Rejection, and Tumor Immunity, Adv Immunol, 18:67, 1974.

Claman, H. N., Chapman, E. A., and Triplett, R. F.: Thymus-Marrow Cell Combinations: Synergism in Antibody Production, Proc Soc Biol Exp Med, 122:1167, 1966.

—— and Mosier, D. E.: Cell-Cell Interactions and Antibody Production, Prog Allergy, 16:40, 1972.

Clark, D. S., Foker, J. E., Good, R. A., and Varco, R. L.: Humoral Factors in Canine Renal Allograft Rejection, Lancet, 1:8, 1968.

Cochrum, K. C., and Najarian, J. S.: Quantitation of Antigen Release from Renal Allografts, *Fed Proc,* **26:**572, 1967 (abstract).

David, J. R., and David, R. R.: Cellular Hypersensitivity and Immunity: Inhibition of Macrophage Migration and the Lymphocyte Mediators, *Prog Allergy,* **16:**300, 1972.

Dickler, H. B.: Lymphocyte Receptors for Immunoglobulin, *Adv Immunol,* **24:**167, 1976.

Diener, E., and Langman, R. E.: Antigen Recognition in Induction of Immunity, *Prog Allergy,* **18:**6, 1975.

Dupont, B., Hansen, J. A., and Yunis, E. J.: Human Mixed-Lymphocyte Culture Reaction: Genetics, Specificity, and Biological Implications, *Adv Immunol,* **23:**107, 1976.

Dutton, R. W., and Mishell, R. I.: Cellular Events in the Immune Response: The In Vitro Response of Normal Spleen Cells to Erythrocyte Antigens, in L. Frisch (ed.), "Cold Spring Harbor Symposia on Quantitative Biology (Vol. XXXII, Antibodies)," p. 407, Cold Spring Harbor Laboratory of Quantitative Biology, New York, 1967.

Egdahl, R. H., and Hume, D. M.: Immunologic Studies in Renal Homotransplantation, *Surg Gynecol Obstet,* **102:**450, 1956.

Feldman, J. D.: Ultrastructure of Immunologic Processes, *Adv Immunol,* **4:**175, 1964.

———: Immunological Enhancement: A Study of Blocking Antibodies, *Adv Immunol,* **15:**167, 1972.

Ferrone, S., Pellegrino, M. A., and Reisfeld, R. A.: The Major Histocompatibility Complex in Man: Biological and Molecular Approaches, *Prog Allergy,* **21:**114, 1976.

Fishman, M.: Induction of Antibodies In Vitro, *Annu Rev Microbiol,* **23:**199, 1969.

Foker, J. E., Clark, D. S., Pickering, R. J., Good, R. A., and Varco, R. L.: Mechanisms of Leukocyte Infiltration of Allografts: I. The Separation and Early Appearance of Two Components, *Surgery,* **66:**42, 1969.

George, M., and Vaughan, J. H.: In Vitro Cell Migration as a Model for Delayed Hypersensitivity, *Proc Soc Exp Biol Med,* **111:**415, 1962.

Globerson, A., and Auerbach, R.: Reactivation In Vitro of Immunocompetence in Irradiated Mouse Spleen, *J Exp Med,* **126:**223, 1967.

Goldstein, A. L., Asanuma, Y., Battisto, J. R., Hardy, M. A., Quint, J., and White, A.: Influence of Thymosin on Cell-Mediated and Humoral Immune Responses in Normal Immunologically Deficient Mice, *J Immunol,* **104:**359, 1970.

Gorer, P. A.: Some Recent Work on Tumor Immunity, *Cancer Res,* **4:**149, 1956.

Götze, O., and Müller-Eberhard, H. J. O.: The Alternative Pathway of Complement Activation, *Adv Immunol,* **24:**1, 1976.

Gowans, J. L.: The Fate of Parental Strain Small Lymphocytes in F1 Hybrid Rats, *Ann NY Acad Sci,* **99:**432, 1962.

———, McGregor, D. D., and Cown, D. M.: The Role of Small Lymphocytes in the Rejection of Homograft Skin, in G. E. Wolstenholme and J. Knight (eds.), "The Immunologically Competent Cell," p. 20, Little, Brown and Company, Boston, 1963.

——— and Uhr, J. W.: The Carriage of Immunological Memory by Small Lymphocytes in the Rat, *J Exp Med,* **124:**1017, 1966.

Grebe, S. C., and Streilein, J. W.: Graft-versus-host Reactions: A Review, *Adv Immunol,* **22:**119, 1976.

Greeves, M. F., Torrigiani, G., and Roitt, I. M.: Blocking of the Lymphocyte Receptors Site for Cell Mediated Hypersensitivity and Transplantation Reactions by Antilight Chain Sera, *Nature (Lond),* **222:**885, 1969.

Häyry, P.: Problems and Prospects in Surgical Immunology, *Med Biol,* **54:**1–38, 73–107, 1976.

Howard, J. G., and Mitchinson, N. A.: Immunological Tolerance, *Prog Allergy,* **18:**43, 1975.

Hume, D. M., and Egdahl, R. H.: Progressive Destruction of Renal Homografts Isolated from the Regional Lymphatics of the Host, *Surgery,* **38:**194, 1955.

Interbitzen, T.: Histamine in Allergic Responses of the Skin, in J. G. Shaffer, G. A. LoGrippo, and M. W. Chase (eds.), "Mechanisms of Hypersensitivity," p. 493, Little, Brown, and Company, Boston, 1958.

Jureziz, R. E., Thor, D. E., and Dray, S.: Transfer with RNA Extracts of the Cell Migration Inhibition Correlate of Delayed Hypersensitivity in the Guinea Pig, *J Immunol,* **101:**823, 1968.

———, ———, and ———: Transfer of the Delayed Hypersensitivity Skin Reaction in the Guinea Pig Using RNA-Treated Lymphoid Cells, *J Immunol,* **105:**1313, 1970.

Kaliss, N.: Immunological Enhancement of Tumor Homografts in Mice: Review, *Cancer Res,* **18:**992, 1958.

Katz, D. H., and Benacerraf, B.: The Regulatory Influence of Activated T Cells on B Cell Responses to Antigen, *Adv Immunol,* **15:**1, 1972.

Lawrence, H. S.: Transfer Factor, in F. J. Dixon, Jr., and H. G. Kunel (eds.), "Advances in Immunology," vol. II, p. 195, Academic Press, Inc., New York, 1969.

Liacopoulos, P., and Ben-Efraim, S.: Antigenic Competition, *Prog Allergy,* **18:**97, 1975.

McClusky, R. T., Benacerraf, B., and McClusky, J. W.: Studies on the Specificity of the Cellular Infiltrate in Delayed Hypersensitivity Reactions, *J Immunol,* **90:**466, 1963.

Mannick, J. A., and Egdahl, R. H.: Transformation of Nonimmune Lymph Node Cells to State of Transplantation Immunity by RNA, *Ann Surg,* **156:**356, 1962.

Medawar, P. B.: Second Study of Behavior and Fate of Skin Homografts in Rabbits: Report to War Wounds Committee of Medical Research Council, *J Anat,* **79:**157, 1945.

Miller, J. F. A. P.: Immunological Function of Thymus, *Lancet,* **2:**748, 1961.

——— and Mitchell, G. F.: The Thymus and the Precursors of Antigen Reactive Cells, *Nature (Lond),* **216:**659, 1967.

Mitchison, N. A.: Passive Transfer of Transplantation Immunity, *Proc R Soc Lond (Biol),* **142:**72, 1954.

Monaco, A. P., Wood, M. L., and Russell, P. S.: Some Effects of Purified Heterologous Antihuman Lymphocyte Serum in Man, *Transplantation,* **5:**1106, 1967.

Murphy, J. B.: "Lymphocyte in Resistance to Tissue Grafting, Malignant Disease and Tuberculous Infection," Rockefeller Institute for Medical Research Monograph 21, p. 168, 1926.

Najarian, J. S., and Feldman, J. D.: Passive Transfer of Tuberculin Sensitivity by Tritiated Thymidine-Labeled Lymphoid Cells, *J Exp Med,* **114:**779, 1962.

——— and Ferguson, R. M.: Transplantation Immunology, in J. R. Schmidtke and R. M. Ferguson (eds.), "Immunology for the Practicing Physician," p. 113, Plenum Press, New York, 1977.

Nelson, D. S., and Gatti, R. A.: Humoral Factors Influencing Lymphocyte Transformation, *Prog Allergy,* **21:**261, 1976.

Nossal, G. J. V., Abbot, A., and Mitchell, J.: Antigens in Immunity: XIV. Electron Microscopic Radioautographic Studies of Antigen Capture in the Lymph Node Medulla, *J Exp Med,* **127:**263, 1968.

Parker, C. W.: Control of Lymphocyte Function, *N Engl J Med,* **295:**1180, 1976.

Perey, D. Y., Cooper, M. D., and Good, R. A.: Normal Second Set Wattle Homograft Rejection in Agammaglobulinemic Chickens, *Transplantation,* **5:**615, 1967.

Raju, S., and Grogan, J. B.: Immunology of the Anterior Chamber of the Eye, *Transplant Proc,* **3:**605, 1971.

Rapaport, F. T., Dausset, J., Hamburger, J., Hume, D. M., Kaho, K., Williams, G. M., and Milgram, F.: Serologic Factors in Human Transplantation, *Ann Surg,* **166:**596, 1967.

Riesfeld, R. A., Pellegrino, M. A., Ferrone, S., and Kahan, B. D.: Chemical and Molecular Nature of HL-A Antigens, *Transplant Proc,* **5:**447, 1973.

Ritzmann, S. E.: HLA Patterns and Disease Association, *JAMA,* **236:**2305, 1976.

Scothorne, R. J., and McGregor, I. A.: Cellular Changes in Lymph Nodes and Spleen following Skin Homografting in the Rabbit, *J Anat,* **89:**283, 1955.

Sercarz, E., and Coons, A. H.: The Exhaustion of Specific Antibody Producing Capacity during a Secondary Response, in M. Hašek, A. Lengerová, and M. Vojtíšková (eds.), "Mechanisms of Immunological Tolerance," p. 73, Academic Press, Inc., New York, 1962.

Shreffler, D. C., and Chella, S. D.: The H-2 Major Histocompatibility Complex and the I Immune Response Region: Genetic Variation, Function, and Organization, *Adv Immunol,* **20:**125, 1975.

Simmons, R. L., and Russell, P. S.: The Histocompatibility Antigens of Fertilized Mouse Eggs and Trophoblast, *Ann NY Acad Sci,* **129:**35, 1966.

Singer, S. J.: Molecular Biology of Cellular Membranes with Applications to Immunology, *Adv Immunol,* **19:**1, 1974.

Snell, G. D.: Histocompatibility Genes of Mouse: II. Production and Analysis of Isogenic Resistant Lines, *J Natl Cancer Inst,* **21:**843, 1958.

Spitler, L. E., Levin, A. S., and Fudenberg, H. H.: Transfer Factor, *Clin Immunobiol,* **2:**153, 1974.

Stuart, F. P., Saitoh, T., Fitch, F. W., and Spargo, B. H.: Immunological Enhancement of Renal Allografts in the Rat, *Surgery,* **64:**17, 1968.

Terasaki, P. I., and McClelland, J. D.: Microdroplet Assay of Human Serum Cytotoxins, *Nature (Lond),* **204:**998, 1964.

Unanue, E. R.: The Regulatory Role of Macrophages in Antigenic Stimulation, *Adv Immunol,* **15:**95, 1972.

Ward, P. A.: Chemotaxis of Mononuclear Cells, *J Exp Med,* **128:**1201, 1968.

Warner, N. L.: Membrane Immunoglobulins in Antigen Receptors on B and T Lymphocytes, *Adv Immunol,* **19:**67, 1974.

Weaver, J. M., Algire, G. H., and Prehn, R. T.: Growth of Cells In Vivo in Diffusion Chambers: II. Role of Cells in Destruction of Homografts in Mice, *J Natl Cancer Inst,* **15:**1737, 1955.

Weigle, W. O.: Immunological Unresponsiveness, *Adv Immunol,* **16:**61, 1973.

Wilson, D. B.: The Reaction of Immunologically Activated Lymphoid Cells against Homologous Target Tissue Cells In Vitro, *J Cell Comp Physiol,* **62:**273, 1963.

Woodruff, M. F. A., and Anderson, N. A.: Effect of Lymphocyte Depletion by Thoracic Duct Fistula and Administration of Anti-lymphocyte Serum on Survival of Skin Homografts in Rats, *Nature (Lond),* **200:**702, 1963.

Liver Transplantation

Brettschneider, L.: Liver: I. Experimental, in J. S. Najarian and R. L. Simmons (eds.), "Transplantation," p. 496, Lea & Febiger, Philadelphia, 1972.

Calne, R. Y.: Clinical and Experimental Liver Grafting, *Guys Hosp Rep,* **123:**1, 1974.

———: The Present Status of Liver Transplantation, *Transplant Proc,* **9:**209, 1977.

———, White, H. J. O., Binns, R. M., Herbertson, B. M., Milard, P. R., Pena, D. R., Samuel, J. R., and Davis, D. R.: Immunosuppressive Effects of the Orthotopically Transplanted Porcine Liver, *Transplant Proc,* **1:**321, 1969.

Daloze, P., Fourtanier, G., Beaudouin, M., Corman, J., Smeesters, C., and Saric, J.: Biliary Function after Liver Transplantation, *Transplant Proc,* **9:**309, 1977.

DuBois, R. S., Rodgerson, D. O., Martineau, G., Schroter, G., Giles, G., Lilly, J., Halgrimson, C. G., and Starzl, T. E., with Sternlieb, I., and Scheinberg, I. H.: Orthotopic Liver Transplantation for Wilson's Disease, *Lancet,* **1:**505, 1971.

Fortner, J. G., Beattie, E. J., Jr., Shiu, M. H., Kawano, N., and Howland, W. S.: Orthotopic and Heterotopic Liver Homografts in Man, *Ann Surg,* **172:**23, 1970.

———, Kim, D. K., Shiu, M. H., Yeh, S. D. J., Howland, W. S., and Beattie, E. J., Jr.: Heterotopic (Auxiliary) Liver Transplantation in Man, *Transplant Proc,* **9:**217, 1977.

Groth, C. G., Arborgh, B., Björkén, C., Sundberg, B. and Lundgren, G.: Correction of Hyperbilirubinemia in the Glucoronyltransferase-Deficient Rat by Intraportal Hepatocyte Transplantation, *Transplant Proc,* **9:**313, 1977.

———, Porter, K. A., Otte, J. B., Daloze, P. M., Marchioro, T. L., Brettschneider, L., and Starzl, T. E.: Studies of Blood Flow and Ultrastructural Changes in Rejecting and Non-rejecting Canine Orthotopic Liver Homografts, *Surgery,* **63:**658, 1968.

Halgrimson, C. G., Marchioro, T. L., Faris, T. D., Porter, K. A., Peters, G. N., and Starzl, T. E.: Auxiliary Liver Homotransplantation: Effect of Host Portacaval Shunt, *Arch Surg,* **93:**107, 1966.

Jonasson, O., Reynolds, W. A., Snyder, G., and Hoversten, G.: Experimental and Clinical Therapy of Diabetes by Transplantation, *Transplant Proc,* **9:**223, 1977.

Lilly, J. R., and Starzl, T. E.: Liver Transplantation in Children with Biliary Atresia and Vascular Anomalies, *J Pediatr Surg,* **9:**707, 1974.

Machado, M. C. C., Monteiro da Cunha, J. E., Margarido, N. F., Bacchella, T., Gonçalves, E. L., and Raia, A. A.: Hyperosmolar Coma Associated with Clinical Liver Transplantation, *Int Surg,* **61:**368, 1976.

Marchioro, T. L., Porter, K. A., Kickinson, T. C., Faris, T. D., and Starzl, T. E.: Physiologic Requirements for Auxiliary Liver Homotransplantation, *Surg Gynecol Obstet,* **121:**17, 1965.

Martineau, G., Porter, K. A., Corman, J., Launois, B., Schroter, G. T., Palmer, W., Putnam, C. W., Groth, C. G., Halgrimson, C. G., Penn, I., and Starzl, T. E.: Delayed Biliary Duct Obstruction after Orthotopic Liver Transplantation, *Surgery,* **72:**604, 1972.

Najarian, J. S.: Liver: III. Clinical Transplantation, in J. S. Najarian and R. L. Simmons (eds.), "Transplantation," p. 522, Lea & Febiger, Philadelphia, 1972.

——, Sutherland, D. E. R., Matas, A. J., Steffes, M. W., Simmons, R. L., and Goetz, F. C.: Human Islet Transplantation: A Preliminary Report, *Transplant Proc,* **9**:233, 1977.

Portmann, B., Schindler, A.-M., Murray-Lyon, I. M., and Williams, R.: Histological Sexing of a Reticulum Cell Sarcoma Arising after Liver Transplantation, *Gastroenterology,* **70**:82, 1976.

Putnam, C. W., Bell, R. H., Jr., Beart, R. W., Jr., and Starzl, T. E.: Hepatic Transplantation, 1975, *Postgrad Med J,* **52** (suppl 5): 104, 1976.

——, Porter, K. A., Weill, R., III, Reid, H. A. S., and Starzl, T. E.: Liver Transplantation for Budd-Chiari Syndrome, *JAMA,* **236**:1142, 1976.

Roddy, H., Putnam, C. W., and Fennell, R. H., Jr.: Pathology of Liver Transplantation, *Transplantation,* **22**:625, 1976.

Schröter, G. P. J., Hoelscher, M., Putnam, C. W., Porter, K. A., Hansbrough, J. F., and Starzl, T. E.: Infections Complicating Orthotopic Liver Transplantation: A Study Emphasizing Graft-Related Septicemia, *Arch Surg,* **111**:1337, 1976.

Starzl, T. E.: "Experience in Hepatic Transplantation," W. B. Saunders Company, Philadelphia, 1969.

——, Porter, K. A., Putnam, C. W., Schroter, G. P. J., Halgrimson, C. G., Weil, R., III, Hoelscher, M., and Reid, H. A. S.: Orthotopic Liver Transplantation in Ninety-Three Patients, *Surg Gynecol Obstet,* **142**:487, 1976.

Stuart, F. P., Torres, E., Hester, W. J., Dammin, G. J., and Moore, F. D.: Orthotopic Autotransplantation and Allotransplantation of the Liver: Functional and Structural Patterns in the Dog, *Ann Surg,* **165**:325, 1967.

Sutherland, D. E. R., Matas, A. J., Steffes, M. W., Simmons, R. L., and Najarian, J. S.: Transplantation of Liver Cells in an Animal Model of Congenital Enzyme Deficiency Disease: The Gunn Rat, *Transplant Proc,* **9**:317, 1977.

Welch, C. S.: A Note on the Transplantation of the Whole Liver in Dogs, *Transplant Bull,* **2**:54, 1955.

Cardiac Transplantation

Barnard, C. N.: A Human Cardiac Transplant, *S Afri Med J,* **41**:1271, 1967.

Campeau, L., Pospisil, L., Grondin, P., Dyrda, I., and Lepage, G.: Cardiac Catheterization Findings at Rest and after Exercise in Patients following Cardiac Transplantation, *Am J Cardiol,* **25**:523, 1970.

Childs, J. W., and Lower, R. R.: Preservation of the Heart, *Prog Cardiovasc Dis,* **12**:149, 1969.

Cooley, D. A., Bloodwell, R. D., Hallman, G. L., and Nora, J. J.: Transplantation of the Heart: A Report of Four Cases. *JAMA,* **205**:479, 1968.

DeBakey, M. E., Diethrich, E. B., Glick, G., Noon, G. P., Butler, W. T., Rossen, R. D., Liddicoat, J. E., and Brooks, D. K.: Human Cardiac Transplantation: Clinical Experience, *J Thorac Cardiovasc Surg* **58**:303, 1969

Fish, R. J., Lillehei, C. W., and Zabriskie, J. B.: Detection of Circulating Heart-reactive antibody in Human Heart Transplants, *JAMA,* **211**:1505, 1970.

Griepp, R. B., Stinson, E. B., Bieber, C. P., Reitz, B. A., Copeland, J. G., Oyer, P. E., and Shumway, N. E.: Human Heart Transplantation: Current Status, *Ann Thorac Surg,* **22**:171, 1976.

Grinnan, G. L., Graham, W. H., Childs, J. W., and Lower, R. R.: Cardiopulmonary Homotransplantation, *J Thorac Cardiovasc Surg,* **60**:609, 1970.

Hardy, J. D., Chavez, C. M., Kurrus, F. D., Neely, W. A., Eraslan, S., Turner, M. D., Fabian, L. W., and Labeck, T. D.: Heart Transplantation in Man: Developmental Studies and Report of a Case, *JAMA,* **188**:1132, 1964.

Kahn, D. R., Reynolds, E. W., Jr., Walton, J. A., Kirsh, M. M., Vathayanon, S., and Sloan, H.: Human Heart Transplantation for Cardiomyopathy, *Surgery,* **67**:122, 1970.

Kosek, J. C., Bieber, C., and Lower, R. R.: Heart Graft Arteriosclerosis, *Transplant Proc,* **3**:512, 1971.

——, Hurley, E. J., and Lower, R. R.: Histopathology of Orthotopic Canine Cardiac Homografts, *Lab Invest,* **19**:97, 1968.

Lower, R. R.: Cardiac Transplantation without Complete Cardiac Denervation: The Role of the Afferent Receptors, *Am Heart J,* **72**:841, 1966.

——, Dong, E., Jr., and Shumway, N. E.: Long Term Survival of Cardiac Homografts, *Surgery,* **58**:100, 1965.

——, Stofer, R. C., and Shumway, N. E.: Homovital Transplantation of the Heart, *J Thorac Cardiovasc Surg,* **41**:196, 1961.

——, Szentpetery, S., Thomas, F. T., and Kemp, V. E.: Clinical Observation on Cardiac Transplantation, *Transplant Proc,* **8**:9, 1976.

Milan, J. D., Shipkey, F. H., Lind, C. J., Jr., Nora, J. J., Leachman, R. D., Rochelle, D. G., Bloodwell, R. D., Hallman, G. L., and Cooley, D. A.: Morphologic Findings in Human Cardiac Allografts, *Circulation,* **41**:519, 1970.

Schroeder, J. S., Popp, R. L., Stinson, E. B., Dong, E., Jr., Shumway, N. E., and Harrison, D. C.: Acute Rejection following Cardiac Transplantation: Phonocardiographic and Ultrasound Observations, *Circulation,* **40**:155, 1969.

Sewell, D. H., Kemp, V. E., and Lower, R. R.: The Epicardial ECG in Monitoring Cardiac Homograft Rejection, *Circulation,* **39** (*Suppl* 1):21, 1969.

Thomas, F., Kemp, V. E., Szentpetery, S., and Lower, R. R.: Monitoring and Modulation of Immune Reactivity in Cardiac Recipients, in J. Davila (ed.), "Second Henry Ford Hospital International Symposium on Cardiac Surgery," Appleton-Century-Crofts, Inc., New York, 1977.

Thomas, K. E., Linehan, J. D., and Lower, R. R.: Size Disparity in Dogs between Donor and Recipient in Cardiac Transplantation, *Surg Forum,* **21**:183, 1970.

Willman, V. L., Kaiser, G. C., Harades, Y., Cooper, T., and Hanlon, C. R.: Physiological Alterations following Transplantation of the Heart, *Adv Transplant Proc 1st Cong Transplant Soc,* 1968, p. 661.

Lung Transplantation

Arnar, O., Andersen, R. C., Hitchcock, C R., and Haglin, J. J.: Reimplantation of the Baboon Lung after Extended Ischemia, *Transplantation,* **5**:929, 1967.

Blumenstock, D. A., Transplantation of the Lung, *Transplantation,* **5**:917, 1967.

—— and Veith, F. J.: Lung (Clinical Transplantation), in J. S. Najarian and R. L. Simmons (eds.), "Transplantation," p. 569, Lea & Febiger, Philadelphia, 1972.

Haglin, J. J., and Arnar, O.: Physiologic Studies of the Baboon

Living on Only the Reimplanted Lung, *Surg Forum,* **15:**175, 1964.

Veith, F. J.: Lung Transplantation, *Transplant Proc,* **9:**203, 1977.

Kidney Transplantation

Advisory Committee to the Renal Transplant Registry (Barnes, B. A., Bergan, J. J., Braun, W. E., Fraumeni, J. F., Jr., Kountz, S. L., Mickey, M. R., Rubin, A. L., Simmons, R. L., Stavens, L. E., and Wilson, R. E.): Renal Transplantation in Congenital and Metabolic Diseases, *JAMA,* **232:**148, 1975.

Advisory Committee to the Renal Transplant Registry: Twelfth Report of the Human Renal Transplant Registry, *JAMA,* **233:**787, 1975.

Aldrete, J. S., Sterling, W. A., Hathaway, B. M., Morgan, J. M., and Diethelm, A. G.: Gastrointestinal and Hepatic Complications Affecting Patients with Renal Allografts, *Am J Surg,* **129:**115, 1975.

Alfrey, A. C., Jenkins, D., Groth, C. G., Schorr, W. S., Gecelter, L., and Ogden, D. A.: Resolution of Hyperparathyroidism, Renal Osteodystrophy and Metastatic Calcification after Renal Homotransplantation, *N Engl J Med,* **279:**1349, 1968.

Anderson, C. B., Codd, J. E., Graff, R. J., Gregory, J. G., Gorce, M. A., and Newton, W. T.: Serum Lactic Dehydrogenase and Human Renal Allograft Failure, *Surgery,* **77:**674, 1975.

Anderson, C. F., Nelson, R. A., Margie, J. D., Johnson, W. J., and Hunt, J. C.: Nutritional Therapy for Adults with Renal Disease, *JAMA* **223:**68, 1973.

Asbury, A. K.: Recovery from Uremic Neuropathy, *N Engl J Med,* **281:**1211, 1971.

Astle, J. N., and Ellis, P. P.: Ocular Complications in Renal Transplant Patients, *Ann Ophthalmol,* **6:**1269, 1974.

Balch, C. M., Morgan, J. M., Sterling, W. A., Bradley, E. L., and Diethelm, A. G.: Kidney Transplantation in Patients with End Stage Congenital Renal Disease: Report of Eighteen Cases and Review of the Organ Transplant Registry, *Am J Surg,* **130:**303, 1975.

Bartrum, R. J., Jr., Smith, E. H., D'Orsi, C. J., and Tilney, N. L.: Evaluation of Renal Transplants with Ultrasound, *Radiology,* **118:**405, 1976.

Baxby, K., Taylor, R. M. R., Anderson, M., Johnson, R. W. G., and Swinney, J.: Assessment of Cadaveric Kidneys for Transplantation, *Lancet,* **2:**977, 1974.

Beecher, H. K.: After the "Definition of Irreversible Coma," *N Engl J Med,* **281:**1070, 1968.

Belzer, F. O., Ashby, B. S., Gulyassy, P. F., and Powell, M.: Successful Seventeen-Hour Preservation and Transplantation of Human-Cadaver Kidney, *N Engl J Med,* **278:**608, 1968.

———, Perkins, H. A., Fortmann, J. L., Kountz, S. L., Salvatierra, O., Cochrum, K. C., and Payne, R.: Is HL-A Typing of Clinical Significance in Cadaver Renal Transplantation?, *Lancet,* **1:**774, 1974.

Bernstein, W. C., Nivatvongs, S., and Tallent, M. B.: Colonic and Rectal Complications of Kidney Transplantation in Man, *Dis Colon Rectum,* **16:**255, 1973.

Blaufox, M. D., Birbari, A. E., Hickler, T. B., and Merrill, J. P.: Peripheral Plasma Renin Activity in Renal-Homotransplant Recipients, *N Engl J Med,* **275:**1165, 1966.

Bolton, C. F., Baltzan, M. A., and Baltzan, R. B.: Effects of Renal

Transplantation on Uremic Neuropathy: A Clinical and Electrophysiologic Study, *N Engl J Med,* **284:**1170, 1971.

Braun, W. E., Banowsky, L. H., Straffon, R. A., Nakamoto, S., Kiser, W. S., Popowniak, K. L., Hewitt, C. B., Stewart, B. H., Zelch, J. V., Magalhaes, R. L., Lachance, J.-G., and Manning, R. F.: Lymphoceles Associated with Renal Transplantation: Report of 15 Cases and Review of the Literature, *Am J Med,* **57:**714, 1974.

Brescia, M. J., Cimino, J. E., Appel, K., and Hurwich, B. J.: Chronic Hemodialysis Using Venipuncture and Surgically Created Arteriovenous Fistula, *N Engl J Med,* **275:**1089, 1966.

Butt, K. M. H., Friedman, E. A., and Kountz, S. L.: Angioaccess, *Curr Probl Surg,* **8:**1, 1976.

Callender, C. O., Simmons, R. L., Yunis, E. J., Toledo-Pereyra, L. H., DeShazo, M. T. M., and Najarian, J. S.: Anti-HL-A Antibodies: Failure to Correlate with Renal Allograft Rejection, *Surgery,* **76:**573, 1974.

Calne, R. Y.: Cadaveric Kidneys for Transplantation, *Br Med J,* **2:**565, 1969.

Casali, R., Simmons, R. L., Ferguson, R. M., Mauer, S. M., Kjellstrand, C. M., Buselmeier, T. J., and Najarian, J. S.: Factors Related to Success or Failure of Second Renal Transplants, *Ann Surg,* **184:**145, 1976.

Cosimi, A. B., Wortis, H. H., Delmonico, F. L., and Russell, P. S.: Randomized Clinical Trial of Antithymocyte Globulin in Cadaver Renal Allograft Recipients: Importance of T Cell Monitoring, *Surgery,* **80:**155, 1976.

Dausset, J., Hors, J., Busson, M., Festenstein, H., Oliver, R. T. D., Paris, A. M. I., and Sachs, J. A.: Serologically Defined HL-A Antigens and Long-Term Survival of Cadaver Kidney Transplants: Joint Analysis of 918 Cases Performed by France-Transplant and the London Transplant Group, *N Engl J Med,* **290:**979, 1974.

David, D. S., Sakai, S., Brennan, B. L., Riggio, R. A., Cheigh, J., Stenzel, K. H., Rubin, A. L., and Sherwood, L. M.: Hypercalcemia after Renal Transplantation: Long-Term Follow-Up Data, *N Engl J Med,* **289:**398, 1973.

Demling, R. H., Salvatierra, O., Jr., and Belzer, F. O.: Intestinal Necrosis and Perforation after Renal Transplantation, *Arch Surg,* **110:**251, 1975.

Dietzman, R. H., Rebelo, A. E., Graham, E. F., Crabo, B. G., and Lillehei, R. C.: Long-Term Functional Success following Freezing of Canine Kidneys, *Surgery,* **74:**181, 1973.

Dossetor, J. B., Zqeig, S. M., Treves, S., and Ross, W. M.: The [131]I Ortho-iodohippurate Photoscan in Human Renal Allografts, *Can Med Assoc J,* **102:**1373, 1970.

DeShazo, C. V., Simmons, R. L., Bernstein, D. M., DeShazo, M. M., Willmert, J., Kjellstrand, C. M., and Najarian, J. S.: Results of Renal Transplantation in 100 Children, *Surgery,* **76:**461, 1974.

Ettenger, R. B., Terasaki, P. I., Ting, A., Malekzadeh, M. H., Pennisi, A. J., Uittenbogaart, C., Garrison, R., and Fine, R. N.: Anti-B Lymphocytotoxins in Renal-Allograft Rejection, *N Engl J Med,* **295:**305, 1976.

Evans, D. B., and Calne, R. Y.: Renal Transplantation in Patients with Carcinoma, *Br Med J,* **4:**134, 1974.

Fellner, C. H., and Schwartz, S. H.: Altruism in Disrepute: Medical versus Public Attitudes toward the Living Organ Donor, *N Engl J Med,* **284:**583, 1971.

Ferguson, R. M., Schmidtke, J. R., Simmons, R. L., and Najarian, J. S.: Functional and Anatomic Lymphocyte Subpopulation Redistribution following Transplantation, *Transplant Proc,* **9:**55, 1977.

———, Simmons, R. L., Noreen, H., Yunis, E. J., and Najarian, J. S.: Host Presensitization and Renal Allograft Success at a Single Institution: First Transplants, *Surgery,* **81:**139, 1977.

Festenstein, H., Oliver, R. T. D., Hyams, A., Moorhead, J. R., Pirrie, A. J., Pegrum, G. C., and Balfour, I. C.: A Collaborative Scheme for Tissue Typing and Matching in Renal Transplantation, *Lancet,* **2:**389, 1969.

Franksson, C., Lundgren, G., Mangnusson, G., and Ringden, O.: Drainage of Thoracic Duct Lymph in Renal Transplant Patients, *Transplantation,* **21:**133, 1976.

Frich, M. P., Loken, M. K., Goldberg, M. E., and Simmons, R. L.: The Use of 99-M Technetium Sulfurcolloid in the Evaluation of the Function of Renal Transplants, *J Nucl Med,* **17:**181, 1976.

Glassock, R. J., Feldman, D., Reynolds, E. S., Dammin, G. J., and Merrill, J. P.: Human Renal Isografts: A Clinical and Pathologic Analysis, *Medicine (Baltimore),* **47:**411, 1968.

Greene, J. A., Jr., Vander, A. J., and Kowalczyk, R. S.: Plasma Renin Activity and Aldosterone Excretion after Renal Homotransplantation, *J Lab Clin Med,* **71:**586, 1968.

Griffiths, H. J., Ennis, J. T., and Bailey, G.: Skeletal Changes following Renal Transplantation, *Radiology,* **113:**621, 1974.

Gustafsson, A., Groth, C. G., Halgrimson, C. G., Penn, I., and Starzl, T. E.: Fate of Failed renal Homografts Retained after Retransplantation, *Surg Gynecol Obstet,* **137:**40, 1973.

Hall, M. C., Elmore, S. M., Bright, R. W., Pierce, J. C., and Hume, D. M.: Skeletal Complications in a Series of Human Renal Allografts, *JAMA,* **208:**1825, 1969.

Hamburger, J., and Crosnier, J.: Moral and Ethical Problems in Transplantation, in F. T. Rapaport and J. Dausset (eds.), "Human Transplantation," p. 37, Grune & Stratton, Inc., New York, 1968.

Hansen, H. E., and Sell, A.: Isotope Renography Combined with Recording Isotype Cystogram in Patients with Renal Transplants, *Acta Med Scand,* **188:**205, 1970.

Harvard Medical School Committee: A Definition of Irreversible Coma: Report of the Ad Hoc Committee of the Harvard Medical School to Examine the Definition of Brain Death, *JAMA,* **205:**337, 1968.

Hattler, B. G., Jr., Rocklin, R. E., Ward, P. A., and Rickles, F. R.: Functional Features of Lymphocytes Recovered from a Human Renal Allograft, *Cell Immunol,* **9:**289, 1973.

Hinman, F., Jr., and Belzer, F. O.: Urinary Tract Infections and Renal Homotransplantation: I. Effect of Antibacterial Irrigations on Defenses of the Defunctionalized Bladder, *Trans Am Assoc Genitourin Surg,* **60:**46, 1968.

Ho, M., Suwansirikul, S., Dowling, J. N., Youngblood, L. A., and Armstrong, J. A.: Transplanted Kidney as a Source of Cytomegalovirus Infection, *N Engl J Med,* **293:**1109, 1975.

Hoover, R., and Fraumeni, J. F., Jr.: Risk of Cancer in Renal Transplant Recipients, *Lancet,* **2:**55, 1973.

Hume, D. M.: Homotransplantation of Kidneys and of Fetal Liver and Spleen after Total Body Irradiation, *Ann Surg,* **152:**354, 1960.

Husberg, B. S., and Starzl, T. E.: Outcome of Kidney Retransplantation, *Arch Surg,* **108:**584, 1974.

Irby, R., and Hume, D. M.: Joint Changes Observed following Renal Transplants, *Clin Orthop,* **57:**101, 1968.

Ireland, P., Rashid, A., Von Lichtenberg, F., Cavallo, T., and Merrill, J. P.: Liver Disease in Kidney Transplant Patients Receiving Azathioprine, *Arch Intern Med,* **132:**29, 1973.

Jeannet, M., DeWeck, A., Frei, P. C., Grob, P., and Thiel, G.: Cooperative Kidney Typing and Exchange Program, *Helv Med Acta,* **35:**239, 1969–1970.

Juul-Jensen, P.: "Criteria of Brain Death: Selection of Donors for Transplantation," Munksgaard, Copenhagen, 1970.

Kauffman, H. M., Swanson, M. K., McGregor, W. R., Rodgers, R. E., and Fox, P. S.: Splenectomy in Renal Transplantation, *Surg Gynecol Obstet,* **139:**33, 1974.

Kincaid-Smith, P.: Histological Diagnosis of Rejection of Renal Homografts in Man, *Lancet,* **2:**849, 1967.

Kjellstrand, C. M., Casali, R. E., Simmons, R. L., Shideman, J. R., Buselmeier, T. J., and Najarian, J. S.: Etiology and Prognosis in Acute Post-transplant Renal Failure, *Am J Med,* **61:**190, 1976.

———, Shideman, J. R., Lynch, R. E., Buselmeier, T. J., Simmons, R. L., and Najarian, J. S.: Kidney Transplants in Patients over 50, *Geriatrics,* **31:**65, 1976.

———, Simmons, R. L., Buselmeier, T. J., and Najarian, J. S.: Kidney: I. Recipient Selection, Medical Management and Dialysis, in J. S. Najarian and R. L. Simmons (eds.), "Transplantation," p. 418, Lea & Febiger, Philadelphia, 1972.

Kohler, B.: The Prognosis after Nephrectomy: A Clinical Study of Early and Late Results, *Acta Chir Scand,* **91** (suppl 94):1, 1944.

Koranda, F. C., Dehmel, E. M., Kahn, G., and Penn, I.: Cutaneous Complications in Immunosuppressed Renal Homograft Recipients, *JAMA,* **229:**419, 1974.

Ku, G., Varghese, Z., Fernando, O. N., Baillod, R., Hopewell, J. P., and Moorhead, J. F.: Serum IgG and Renal Transplantation, *Br Med J,* **4:**702, 1973.

Kyriakides, G. K., Simmons, R. L., and Najarian, J. S.: Wound Infections in Renal Transplant Wounds: Pathogenetic and Prognostic Factors, *Ann Surg,* **182:**770, 1975.

———, ———, and ———: Mycotic Aneurysms in Transplant Patients, *Arch Surg,* **111:**472, 1976.

Lacombe, M.: Arterial Stenosis Complicating Renal Allotransplantation in Man: Study of 38 Cases, *Ann Surg,* **181:**283, 1975.

Lazarus, J. M., Birtch, A. G., Hampers, C. L., and Merrill, J. P.: Hemodialysis Duration and Renal Transplant Survival, *Transplantation,* **15:**508, 1973.

Light, J. A., Annable, C., Perloff, L. J., Sulkin, M. D., Hill, G. S., Etheredge, E. E., and Spees, E. K., Jr.: Immune Injury from Organ Preservation: Potential Cause of Hyperacute Rejection in Human Cadaver Kidney Transplantation, *Transplantation,* **19:**511, 1975.

Linn, B. S., Portal, P., and Snyder, G. B.: Complementuria in Renal Transplantation, *Life Sci,* **6:**1945, 1967.

Lucas, Z. J., Palmer, J. M., Payne, R., Kountz, S. L., and Cohn, R. B.: Renal Allotransplantation in Humans: I. Systemic Immunosuppressive Therapy, *Arch Surg,* **100:**113, 1970.

McLean, R. H., Geiger, H., Burke, B., Simmons, R., Najarian, J.,

Vernier, R. L., and Michael, A. F.: Recurrence of Membranoproliferative Glomerulonephritis following Kidney Transplantation: Serum Complement Component Studies, *Amer J Med,* **60:**60, 1976.

Matas, A. J., Hertel, B. F., Rosai, J., Simmons, R. L., and Najarian, J. S.: Post-transplant Malignant Lymphoma: Distinctive Morphologic Features Related to Its Pathogenesis, *Am J Med,* **61:**716, 1976.

———, Simmons, R. L., Buselmeier, T. J., Kjellstrand, C. M., and Najarian, J. S.: Successful Renal Transplantation in Patients with Prior History of Malignancy, *Am J Med,* **59:**791, 1975.

———, ———, ———, ———, and ———: The Fate of Patients Surviving Three Years after Renal Transplantation, *Surgery,* **80:**390, 1976.

———, ———, Kjellstrand, C. M., Buselmeier, T. J., Johnson, T. L., and Najarian, J. S.: Increased Incidence of Malignancy in Uremic Patients and Its Significance to Transplantation, *Transplant Proc,* **9:**1137, 1977.

———, ———, and Najarian, J. S.: Chronic Antigenic Stimulation, Herpes-Virus Infection, and Cancer in Transplant Patients—Hypothesis, *Lancet,* **1:**1277, 1975.

Mauer, S. M., Barbosa, J., Vernier, R. L., Kjellstrand, C. M., Buselmeier, T. J., Simmons, R. L., Najarian, J. S., and Goetz, F. C.: Development of Diabetic Vascular Lesions in Normal Kidneys Transplanted into Patients with Diabetes Mellitus, *N Engl J Med,* **295:**916, 1976.

Miller, J., Kyriakides, G., Ma, W. K., Masler, D., and Brown, D. C.: Factors Influencing Morbidity and Mortality of Renal Transplantation in a High-Risk Population, *Surg Gynecol Obstet,* **140:**1, 1975.

Mills, S. A., Siegler, H. F., and Wolfe, W. G.: Incidence and Management of Pulmonary Mycosis in Renal Allograft Patients, *Ann Surg,* **182:**617, 1975.

Mohandas, A., and Chu, S. N.: Brain Death: A Clinical and Pathological Study, *J Neurosurg,* **35:**211, 1971.

Moore, T. C.: Effective Use of Isoniazid and an Antihistamine in Clinical Renal Transplantation, *Surg Gynecol Obstet,* **133:**75, 1971.

Murphy, G. P., Mirand, E. A., and Grace, J. T.: Erythropoietin Activity in Anephric or Renal Allotransplanted Man, *Ann Surg,* **170:**581, 1969.

Murray, J. E., Merrill, J. P., and Harrison, J. H.: Renal Homotransplantation in Identical Twins, *Surg Forum,* **6:**432, 1955.

Myburgh, J. A., Maier, G., Smit, J. A., Shapiro, M., Meyers, A. M., Rabkin, R., Van Blerk, P. J. P., and Jersky, J.: Presensitization and Clinical Kidney Transplantation: I. Favorable Course of a Substantial Number of Patients, *Transplantation,* **18:**206, 1974.

Najarian, J. S., Kjellstrand, C. M., Simmons, R. L., Buselmeier, T. J., Von Hartitzsch, B., and Goetz, F. C.: Renal Transplantation for Diabetic Glomerulosclerosis, *Ann Surg,* **178:**477, 1973.

———, Simmons, R. L., Condie, R. M., Thompson, E. J., Fryd, D. S., Howard, R. J., Matas, A. J., Sutherland, D. E. R., Ferguson, R. M., and Schmidtke, J. R.: Seven Years' Experience with Antilymphoblast Globulin for Renal Transplantation from Cadaver Donors, *Ann Surg,* **184:**352, 1976.

———, ———, Kjellstrand, C. M., Vernier, R., and Michaels, A.: Renal Transplantation in Infants and Children, *Ann Surg,* **174:**583, 1971.

Olsson, C. A., Mannick, J. A., Schmitt, G. W., Idelson, B. A., Williams, L. F., Lemann, J., Harrington, J. T., and Nabseth, D. C.: Nephrostomy in Renal Transplantation, *Am J Surg,* **121:**467, 1971.

Opelz, G., and Terasaki, P. I.: Prolongation Effect of Blood Transfusions on Kidney Graft Survival, *Lancet,* **2:**696, 1974.

Pasternack, A.: Fine Needle Aspiration Biopsy of Human Renal Homografts, *Lancet,* **2:**82, 1968.

Penn, I., Halgrimson, C. G., Ogden, D., and Starzl, T.: Use of Living Donors in Kidney Transplantation in Man, *Arch Surg,* **101:**226, 1970.

——— and Starzl, T. E.: Immunosuppression and Cancer, *Transplant Proc,* **5:**943, 1973.

Perkins, H. A., Howell, E., Gantan, Z., Mims, M. C., Dickerson, T., and Senecal, I.: Variation in Cytotoxic Antibody Response to Transfusion in Prospective Renal Allograft Recipients, *Transplantation,* **17:**216, 1974.

Pien, F. D., Smith, T. F., Anderson, C. F., Webel, M. L., and Taswell, H. F.: Herpesviruses in Renal Transplant Patients, *Transplantation,* **16:**489, 1973.

Pierce, J. C., and Hume, D. M.: The Effect of Splenectomy on the Survival of First and Second Renal Homotransplants in Man, *Surg Gynecol Obstet,* **127:**1300, 1968.

Quinton, W. E., Dillard, P. H., Cole, I. J., and Scribner, B. H.: Eight Months Experience with Silastic-Teflon Bypass Cannulas, *Trans Am Soc Artif Intern Organs,* **8:**236, 1962.

Rapaport, F. T., McCluskey, R. T., Hanaoka, T., and Shimada, T.: Induction of Renal Disease with Antisera to Group A Streptococcal Membranes, *Transplant Proc,* **1:**981, 1969.

Rattazzi, L. D., Simmons, R. L., Spanos, P. K., Bradford, D. S., and Najarian, J. S.: Successful Management of Miliary Tuberculosis after Renal Transplantation, *Am J Surg,* **130:**359, 1975.

Rosenberg, J. C., Azcarate, J., Fleischmann, L. E., McDonald, F. D., Menendez, M., Pierce, J. M., Jr., and Whang, C. W.: Indications for Pretransplant Nephrectomy, *Arch Surg,* **107:**233, 1973.

Salvatierra, O., Potter, D., Cochrum, K. C., Amend, W. J. C., Duca, R., Sachs, B. L., Johnson, R. W. J., and Belzer, F. O.: Improved Patient Survival in Renal Transplantation, *Surgery,* **79:**166, 1976.

Schwab, R. S., Potts, F., and Bonazzi, A.: EEG as an Aid in Determining Death in the Presence of Cardiac Activity (Ethical, Legal and Medical Aspects), *Electroencephalogr Clin Neurophysiol,* **15:**147, 1963.

Schwartz, R. S., and Dameshek, W.: Drug Induced Immunological Tolerance, *Nature (Lond),* **183:**1682, 1959.

Sciarra, J. J., Toledo-Pereyra, L. H., Bendel, R. P., and Simmons, R. L.: Pregnancy following Renal Transplantation, *Am J Obstet Gynecol,* **123:**411, 1975.

Scott, D. F., Whiteside, D., Redhead, J., and Atkins, R. C.: Ice Storage versus Perfusion for Preservation of Kidneys before Transplantation, *Br Med J,* **4:**76, 1974.

Sheil, A. G. R., Boulas, J., Drummond, J. M., May, J., Rogers, J. H., and Storey, B. G.: Controlled Clinical Trial of Machine Perfusion of Cadaveric Donor Renal Allografts, *Lancet,* **2:**287, 1975.

Shillito, J., Jr.: The Organ Donor's Doctor: A New Role for the Neurosurgeon, *N Engl J Med,* **281:**1071, 1969.

Simmons, R. L., Kjellstrand, C. M., Buselmeier, T. J., and

Najarian, J. S.: Renal Transplantation in High Risk Patients, *Arch Surg,* **103**:290, 1971.

——, ——, and Najarian, J. S.: Kidney: II. Technique, Complications, and Results, in J. S. Najarian and R. L. Simmons (eds.), "Transplantation," p. 445, Lea & Febiger, Philadelphia, 1972.

——, Lopez, C., Balfour, H., Jr., Kalis, J., Rattazzi, L. C., and Najarian, J. S.: Cytomegalovirus: Clinical Virologic Correlations in Transplant Recipients, *Ann Surg,* **180**:623, 1974.

——, Ozerkis, A. J., and Hoehn, R. J.: Antiserum to Lymphocytes: Interactions with Chemical Immunosuppressants, *Science,* **160**:1127, 1968.

——, Thompson, E. J., Yunis, E. J., Noreen, H., Kjellstrand, C. M., Fryd, D. S., Condie, R. M., Mauer, S. M., Buselmeier, T. J., and Najarian, J. S.: 115 Patients with First Cadaver Kidney Transplants Followed Two to Seven and a Half Years: A Multifactorial Analysis, *Am J Med,* **62**:234, 1977.

——, Van Hook, E. J., Yunis, E. J., Noreen, H., Kjellstrand, C. M., Condie, R. M., Mauer, S. M., Buselmeier, T. J., and Najarian, J. S.: 100 Sibling Kidney Transplants Followed 2 to 7½ Years: A Multifactorial Analysis, *Ann Surg,* **185**:196, 1977.

——, Yunis, E. J., Noreen, H., Thompson, E. J., Fryd, D. S., and Najarian, J. S.: Effect of HLA Matching on Cadaver Kidney Function: Experience at a Single Large Center, *Transplant Proc,* **9**:491, 1977.

Starzl, T. E.: "Experience in Renal Transplantation," W. B. Saunders Company, Philadelphia, 1964.

——, Groth, C. G., Terasaki, P. I., Putnam, C. W., Brettschneider, L., and Marchioro, T. L.: Heterologous Antilymphocyte Globulin Histoincompatibility Matching, and Human Renal Homotransplantation, *Surg Gynecol Obstet,* **126**:1023, 1968.

——, Halgrimson, C. G., Penn, L., Martineau, G., Schroter, G., Amemiya, H., Putnam, C. W., and Groth, C. G.: Cyclophosphamide and Human Organ Transplantation, *Lancet,* **2**:70, 1971.

Stenzel, K. H., Stubenbord, W. T., Whitsell, J. C., Lewy, J. E., Riggio, R. R., Cheigh, J. S., Marshall, V. F., and Rubin, A. L.: Kidney Transplantation: Use of Intestinal Conduits, *JAMA,* **229**:534, 1974.

Stewart, J. H., Johnson, J. R., Sharp, A. M., Sheil, A. G. R., Wyatt, K. M., and Johnston, J. M.: Successful Renal Allotransplantation in Presence of Lymphocytotoxic Antibodies: Importance of Preoperative Cross-Matching, *Lancet,* **1**:176, 1969.

Strauch, B., Andrews, L.-L., Siegel, N., and Miller, G.: Oropharyngeal Excretion of Epstein-Barr Virus by Renal Transplant Recipients and Other Patients Treated with Immunosuppressive Drugs, *Lancet,* **1**:234, 1974.

Swales, J. D., and Evans, D. B.: Erythraemia in Renal Transplantation, *Br Med J,* **2**:80, 1969.

Tallent, M. B., Simmons, R. L., and Najarian, J. S.: Birth Defects in a Child of a Male Kidney Transplant Recipient, *JAMA,* **211**:1854, 1970.

Terasaki, P. J., Kreisler, M., and Mickey, M. R.: Presensitization and Kidney Transplant Failures: I, *Postgrad Med,* **47**:89, 1971.

Thomas, F. T., and Lee, H. M.: Factors in the Differential Rate of Arteriosclerosis (AS) between Long Surviving Renal Transplant Recipients and Dialysis Patients, *Ann Surg,* **184**:342, 1976.

Toledo-Pereyra, L. H., Simmons, R. L., Moberg, A. W., Olson, L. C., and Najarian, J. S.: Organ Preservation in Success of Cadaver Transplants, *Arch Surg,* **110**:1031, 1975.

Tunner, W. S., Goldsmith, E. I., and Whitesell, J. C.: Human Homotransplantation of Normal and Neoplastic Tissue from the Same Organ, *J Urol,* **105**:18, 1971.

Weil, R., III, Simmons, R. L., Tallent, M. B., Lillehei, R. C., Kjellstrand, C. M., and Najarian, J. S.: Prevention of Urological Complications after Kidney Transplantation, *Ann Surg,* **174**:154, 1971.

West, T. H., Turcotte, J. G., and Vancer, A. J.: Plasma Renin Activity, Sodium Balance, and Hypertension in a Group of Renal Transplant Recipients, *J Lab Clin Med,* **73**:564, 1970.

Williams, G. M., dePlanque, B., Lower, R., and Hume, D. M.: Antibodies and Human Transplant Rejection, *Ann Surg,* **170**:603, 1969.

——, White, H. J., and Hume, D. M.: Factors Influencing the Long-Term Functional Success Rate of Human Renal Allografts, *Transplantation, Suppl.,* **51**:837, 1967.

Wilson, D. R., and Siddiqui, A. A.: Renal Tubular Acidosis after Kidney Transplantation: Natural History and Significance, *Ann Intern Med,* **79**:352, 1973.

Wood, R. F. M., Gray, A. C., Briggs, J. D., and Bell, P. R. F.: Prediction of Acute Rejection in Human Renal Transplantation Using Leukocyte Migration Test, *Transplantation,* **16**:41, 1973.

Zukoski, C. F., Lee, H. M., and Hume, D. M.: The Prolongation of Functional Survival of Canine Renal Homografts by 6-Mercaptopurine, *Surg Forum,* **11**:470, 1960.

Transplantation of Organs other than Kidney, Liver, Lung, and Heart

Advisory Committee of the Bone Marrow Transplant Registry: Bone Marrow Transplantation from Donors with Aplastic Anemia: A Report from the ACS/NIH Bone Marrow Transplant Registry, *JAMA,* **236**:1131, 1976.

Baird, R. N., and Abbott, W. M.: Vein Grafts: An Historical Perspective, *Am J Surg,* **134**:293, 1977.

Barnicot, N. A.: The Local Action of the Parathyroid and Other Tissues on Bone in Intracerebral Grafts, *J Anat,* **82**:233, 1948.

Bortin, M. M.: A Compendium of Reported Human Bone Marrow Transplants, *Transplantation,* **9**:571, 1970.

Burke, J. F., Quinby, W. C., Bondoc, C. C., Cosimi, A. B., Russell, P. S., and Szyfelbein, S. K.: Immunosuppression and Temporary Skin Transplantation in the Treatment of Massive Third Degree Burns, *Ann Surg,* **182**:183, 1975.

Burwell, R. G.: The Fate of Freeze-Dried Bone Allografts, *Transplant Proc,* **8**(suppl 1):77, 1976.

Calhoun, A. D., Bauer, G. M., Porter, J. M., Houghton, D. H., and Templeton, J. W.: Fresh and Cryopreserved Venous Allografts in Genetically Characterized Dogs, *J Surg Res,* **22**:687, 1977.

Cohen, Z., MacGregor, A. B., Moore, E. T. H., Falk, R. E., Langer, B., and Cullen, J. B.: Canine Small Bowel Transplantation, *Arch Surg,* **111**:248, 1976.

Congdon, C. C.: Bone Marrow Transplantation, *Science,* **171**:1116, 1971.

Corry, R. J., and Russell, P. S.: Replantation of Severed Fingers, *Ann Surg,* **179**:255, 1974.

Fefer, A., Einstein, A. B., Thomas, E. D., Buckner, C. D., Clift, R. A., Glucksberg, H., Neiman, P. E., and Storb, R.: Bone-

Marrow Transplantation for Hematologic Neoplasia in 16 Patients with Identical Twins, *N Engl J Med,* **290:**1389, 1974.

Flosdorf, E., and Hyatt, G. W.: The Preservation of Bone Grafts by Freeze Drying, *Surgery,* **31:**716, 1952.

Fortner, J. G., Sichuk, G., Litwin, S. D., and Bettie, E. J., Jr.: Immunological Responses to an Intestinal Allograft with HL-Al Identical Donor-Recipient, *Transplantation,* **14:**531, 1972.

Friedlaender, G. E.: The Antigenicity of Preserved Allografts, *Transplant Proc,* **8**(suppl)**1:**195, 1976.

Gittes, R. F.: Endocrine Tissues, in J. S. Najarian and R. L. Simmons (eds.), "Transplantation," p. 698, Lea & Febiger, Philadelphia, 1972.

Green, W. T., Sr.: Fascia Grafts, *Transplant Proc,* **8**(suppl)**1:**113, 1976.

Groth, C. G., Hammons, W. S., Iwatsuki, S., Popovtzer, M., Cascardo, S., Halgrimson, C. G., and Starzl, T. E.: Survival of a Homologous Parathyroid Implant in an Immunosuppressed Patient, *Lancet,* **1:**1082, 1973.

Hardy, J. D., and Langford, H. G.: Surgical Management of Cushing's Syndrome: Including Studies of Adrenal Autotransplants, Body Composition and Pseudotumor Cerebri, *Ann Surg,* **159:**711, 1964.

Harris, G. W., and Jacobsohn, D.: Functional Grafts of the Anterior Pituitary Glands, *Proc R Soc Lond* (*Biol*), **139:**263, 1952.

Harris, J. E., and Rathbun, W. B.: Ocular Tissues, in J. S. Najarian and R. L. Simmons (eds.), "Transplantation," p. 613, Lea & Febiger, Philadelphia, 1972.

Hickey, R. C., and Samaan, N. A.: Human Parathyroid Autotransplantation, *Arch Surg,* **110:**892, 1975.

Jaffe, S., Earle, A. S., Fleegler, E. J., and Husni, E. A.: Replantation of Amputated Extremities: Report of Five Cases, *Ohio State Med J,* **71:**381, 1975.

Kelly, W. D., Lillehei, R. C., Merkel, F. K., Idezuki, Y., and Goetz, F.: Renal and Pancreatic Allotransplantation in the Treatment of Diabetic Nephropathy in Man, in J. Dausset, J. Hamburger, and G. Mathé (eds.), "Advance in Transplantation," The Williams & Wilkins Company, Baltimore, 1968.

Koumans, R. K. J., and Burke, J. F.: Skin Allografts and Immunosuppression in the Treatment of Massive Thermal Injury, *Surgery,* **66:**89, 1969.

Lance, E. M.: Bone and Cartilage, in J. S. Najarian and R. L. Simmons (eds.), "Transplantation," p. 655, Lea & Febiger, Philadelphia, 1972.

Leapman, S. B., Deutsch, A. A., Grand, R. J., and Folkman, J.: Transplantation of Fetal Intestine: Survival and Function in a Subcutaneous Location in Adult Animals, *Ann Surg,* **179:**109, 1974.

Lillehei, R. C., and Ruiz, J. O.: Pancreas, in J. S. Najarian, and R. L. Simmons (eds.), "Transplantation," p. 627, Lea & Febiger, Philadelphia, 1972.

Lohrmann, H.-P., Niethammer, D., Kern, P., and Heimpel, H.: Identification of High-Risk Patients with Aplastic Anemia in Selection for Allogeneic Bone-Marrow Transplantation, *Lancet,* **2:**647, 1976.

Malt, R. A., and Harris, W. H.: Replantation of Limbs, in J. S. Najarian and R. L. Simmons (eds.), "Transplantation," p. 711, Lea & Febiger, Philadelphia, 1972.

———, Remensnyder, J. P., and Harris, W. H.: Long-Term Utility of Replanted Arms, *Ann Surg,* **176:**334, 1972.

Mankin, H. J., Fogelson, F. S., Thrasher, A. Z., and Jaffer, F.: Massive Resection and Allograft Transplantation in the Treatment of Malignant Bone Tumors, *N Engl J Med,* **294:**1247, 1976.

Matas, A. J., Sutherland, D. E. R., and Najarian, J. S.: Current Status of Islet and Pancreas Transplantation, *Diabetes,* **25:**785, 1976.

———, ———, Steffes, M. W., and Najarian, J. S.: Islet Transplantation, *Surg Gynecol Obstet,* **145:**757, 1977.

Mathe, G., Schwarzenberg, L., and Amiel, J. L.: Bone Marrow, in J. S. Najarian and R. L. Simmons (eds.), "Transplantation," p. 588, Lea & Febiger, Philadelphia, 1972.

Metras, H.: Note préliminaire sur la greffe totale du poumon chez le chien, *C R Acad Sci* [*D*] (*Paris*), **231:**1176, 1950.

Meuwissen, H. J., Rodey, G., McArthur, J., Pabst, H., Gattis, R., Childgren, R., Hong, R., Frommel, D., Coifman, R., and Good, R. A.: Bone Marrow Transplantation-Therapeutic Usefulness and Complications, *Am J Med,* **51:**513, 1971.

Nasseri, M., and Voss, H.: Late Results of Successful Replantation of Upper and Lower Extremities, *Ann Surg,* **177:**121, 1973.

Norman, J. C., Covelli, V. H., and Sise, H. S.: Transplantation of the Spleen: Experimental Cure of Hemophilia, *Surgery,* **66:**1, 1968.

Paloyan, E., Lawrence, A. M., Brooks, M. H., and Pickleman, J. R.: Total Thyroidectomy and Parathyroid Autotransplantation for Radiation-Associated Thyroid Cancer, *Surgery,* **80:**70, 1976.

Parrish, F. F.: Total and Partial Half-Joint Resection Followed by Allograft Replacement in Neoplasms Involving Ends of Long Bones, *Transplant Proc,* **8**(suppl 1):77, 1976.

Peacock, E. E., Jr.: A Review of Composite Tissue Allografts of the Digital Flexor Mechanism, *Transplant Proc,* **8**(suppl 1):119, 1976.

——— and Madden, J. W.: Human Composite Flexor Tendon Allografts, *Ann Surg,* **166:**624, 1967.

Rapaport, F. T., and Converse, J. M.: Skin Transplantation, in F. T. Rapaport and J. Dausset (eds.), "Human Transplantation," p. 304, Grune & Stratton, Inc., New York, 1968.

Rapaport, I., Pepino, A. T., and Dietrick, W.: Early Use of Xenografts as a Biologic Dressing in Burn Trauma, *Am J Surg,* **120:**144, 1970.

Ruiz, J. O., Uchida, H., and Lillehei, R. C.: Intestine (Clinical Transplantation), in J. S. Najarian and R. L. Simmons (eds.), "Transplantation," p. 646, Lea & Febiger, Philadelphia, 1972.

Schechter, I.: Prolonged Retention of Glutaraldehyde-Treated Skin Allografts and Xenografts: Immunological and Histological Studies, *Ann Surg,* **182:**699, 1975.

Schneider, J. R., and Bright, R. W.: Anterior Cervical Fusion Using Preserved Bone Allografts, *Transplant Proc,* **8**(suppl 1):73, 1976.

Slavin, R. E., and Santos, G. W.: The Graft Versus Host Reaction in Man after Bone Marrow Transplantation: Pathology, Pathogenesis, Clinical Features, and Implication, *Clin Immunol Immunopathol,* **1:**492, 1973.

Stamford, W. P., and Hardy, M. A.: Fatty Acid Absorption in Jejunal Autograft and Allograft, *Surgery,* **75:**496, 1974.

Sutherland, D. E. R., Matas, A. J., and Najarian, J. S.: Pancreas and Islet Transplantation, *World J Surg,* **1:**185, 1977.

Taylor, A. C.: Rates of Freezing, Drying and Rehydration of Nerves, *J Cell Comp Physiol,* **25:**161, 1945.

Thomas, E. D., Storb, R., Clift, R. A., Fefer, A., Johnson, F. L., Neiman, P. E., Lemer, K. G., Glucksberg, H., and Buckner, C. D.: Bone-Marrow Transplantation, Part 1, *N Engl J Med,* **292:**832, 1975; Part II, *N Engl J Med,* **292:**895, 1975.

Toledo-Pereyra, L. H., Raij, L., Simmons, R. L., and Najarian, J. S.: Role of Endotoxin and Bacteria in Long-Term Survival of Preserved Small-Bowel Allografts, *Surgery,* **73:**474, 1974.

———, Simmons, R. L., and Najarian, J. S.: Prolonged Survival of Canine Orthotopic Small Intestinal Allografts Preserved for 24 Hours by Hypothermic Bloodless Perfusion, *Surgery,* **75:**368, 1974.

Transplantation and Burns, *Lancet,* **1:**1017, 1975.

U.C.L.A.: Bone Marrow Transplant Team: Bone-Marrow Transplantation in Severe Aplastic Anaemia, *Lancet,* **2:**921, 1976.

Waksman, B. H., Arbouys, S., and Arnason, B. G.: The Use of Specific "Lymphocyte" Antisera to Inhibit Hypersensitive Reactions of the "Delayed" Type, *J Exp Med,* **114:**997, 1961.

Wells, S. A., Gunnells, J. C., Shelburne, J. D., Schneider, A. B., and Sherwood, L. M.: Transplantation of the Parathyroid Glands in Man: Clinical Indications and Results, *Surgery,* **78:**34, 1975.

White, R. J.: Experimental Transplantation of the Brain, in F. T. Rapaport and J. Dausset (eds.), "Human Transplantation," p. 692, Grune & Stratton, Inc., New York, 1968.

Organ Preservation

Filo, R. S., Bell, R. T., Small, A., and Sell, K. W.: Current Status of Kidney Freeze Preservation, *Transplant Proc,* **8**(suppl 1):215, 1976.

Sell, K. W., and Friedlaender, G. E. (eds.): Proceedings of the Tissue Bank Symposium, *Transplant Proc,* **8**(supplement 1): June, 1976.

Chapter 11

Anesthesia

by **Nicholas M. Greene**

GENERAL CONSIDERATIONS

Anesthesiology consists of two parts. One lies outside the operating (or delivery) room, the other within. The former centers about management of critically ill patients, especially their ventilatory care (Chaps. 12 and 13). It also involves diagnosis and treatment of chronic pain problems. The latter centers about operative anesthesia, that is, relief of pain, provision of operating conditions adequate for the surgery at hand, and supportive treatment with fluids, electrolytes, blood, and vasoactive drugs.

Surgical anesthesia inevitably entails risk. This is so because while each anesthetic has its advantages, each also has its disadvantages. But there is no anesthetic magic bullet that relieves pain without side effects. Each anesthetic, even the simplest, creates a state of physiologic trespass with attendant risk. The risk may be greater or smaller depending upon the circumstances, but it can never be eliminated.

Quantitation of anesthetic risk is difficult to achieve in terms of either morbidity or mortality. The problem lies in obtaining epidemiologically sound data. All deaths or complications associated with anesthesia are iatrogenic by definition. This immediately raises the specter of mediocolegal action if an anesthetic death is honestly recorded as such. Death certificates and discharge diagnoses become completely unreliable indices of anesthetic mortality rates under such circumstances. Added to this is the fact that many anesthetic deaths are so subtly related to the anesthetic and so cryptic in origin that the true relation between the fatal outcome and the anesthetic may be missed. Spectacular deaths due to anesthetic explosions or to cardiac arrest during induction of anesthesia are relatively easily identified. Less obvious, though considerably more frequent, are the "quiet" anesthetic deaths due to effects of anesthetics on pulmonary ventilation, hepatic function, cerebral blood flow, coronary blood flow, and metabolism—effects which may linger far into the postoperative period and prove particularly inimical to the poor-risk patient but may be extremely difficult to identify under clinical conditions. Finally, anesthetic deaths appear, especially to the casual observer, to occur only very infrequently. Their true incidence can be determined only when statistically accurate data are gathered from many thousands of patients over long periods of time. This is seldom done. The expense in terms of time, effort, and money usually aborts efforts to obtain such data long before statistical validity can be achieved. The vagaries of human memory and clinical impression further compound the problem. An average surgeon performing 400 operations per year may not encounter an anesthetic death for several years at a time. If the surgeon fails to recognize such a death for what it is when it does occur or fails to remember a previous anesthetic death, he or she soon comes to believe that no problems exist insofar as the safety of anesthetics is concerned; anesthetics are seen as a necessary but not particularly important accompaniment of surgery. The same thing can occur with the anesthesiologist caring for 800 patients a year, even though the time span between exposures to anesthetic death may be shorter.

Despite the problems inherent in quantitating anesthetic death rates, several studies in the past have addressed themselves to the matter using adequate statistical techniques. The results of these studies, while varying in detail, are remarkably consistent in finding that of approximately every 1,600 patients given an anesthetic, one patient dies primarily as a result of having received the anesthetic. The figure of 1 in 1,600 is based on all types of operative anesthesia, from the most "minor" to the most major. There is no evidence to suggest that contemporary anesthetic death rates are materially lower than those determined 15 years or more ago; indeed, the opposite may even be true.

The consideration of anesthetic death is not merely an

academic exercise. Approximately 18,000,000 anesthetics are said to be administered annually in hospitals in the United States, although it is hard to obtain figures and the number is probably higher. If the anesthetic death rate of 1 in 1,600 applies nationally—and there is every reason to believe it does—then the annual number of deaths associated with anesthesia in the United States is in excess of 10,000. Furthermore, antibiotics and blood banks have decreased death rates associated with certain so-called "minor" procedures such as tonsillectomy, inguinal herniorrhaphy, and hemorrhoidectomy to the vanishing point. There has, however, been no parallel decrease in deaths associated with anesthesia. The result is that anesthetic risk now exceeds surgical risk in many operations. Anesthetic death rates remain a major, if hidden, public health problem.

Because of the magnitude of the risk involved, the patient's safety must always be the first and most important consideration in any discussion of surgical anesthesia. True patient safety based upon sound physiologic and pharmacologic principles is not synonymous with the ability to "get away with" a calculated risk a certain number of times.

Bearing in mind the primacy of patient safety and the fact that no anesthetic agent or technique is without its disadvantages and dangers, it may be said that the selection of anesthetic agents and techniques in an individual clinical case depends upon five factors:

1. The condition of the patient. The presence of concurrent conditions such as obesity, a full stomach, coronary artery disease, or chronic pulmonary disease may contraindicate certain anesthetics.

2. The physiologic and pharmacologic effects of the various anesthetic agents. It is this aspect of anesthetic management which will be emphasized in the present chapter, noting that these effects are not necessarily the result of the anesthetic agent itself. A major portion of the physiologic trespass associated with anesthesia is due to factors such as mechanical effects of the apparatus used to administer the anesthetic, changes in blood-gas tensions, changes in fluid and electrolyte balance resulting from blood loss, creation of a surgical third space, and administration of intravenous fluids.

3. The site and type of surgical procedure to be performed. The anesthetic requirements for inguinal herniorrhaphy are different from those for pneumonectomy. Failure to recognize that the anesthetic should be tailored to the type of operation has led to inaccurate and dangerous generalizations as to anesthetic selection based solely upon the patient's condition and the pharmacologic effects of the anesthetic agent.

4. The experience, training, and background of the person who is to administer the anesthetic. Not all persons who can administer an anesthetic are necessarily equally qualified to administer all types of anesthetics. It is frequently advisable for an anesthetist to administer the type of anesthetic with which he has had the most experience, hence that in which he has the most confidence, rather than to administer on rare occasions an anesthetic which theoretically may have certain advantages but with which he has had little experience.

5. The skill, training, and requirements of the surgeon. The anesthetic requirements for an appendectomy by an experienced surgeon who will accomplish the entire operation in 20 minutes are markedly different from those for a surgeon who is less experienced and who may require an hour and a half of anesthesia.

Selection of anesthetic agent and technique based upon the preceding five factors will result in maximal patient safety. Convenience, surgical or anesthetic, should not play a significant role in selecting anesthetic agents, especially convenience measured in terms of minutes saved during induction of anesthesia. Similarly, what is most pleasant for the patient or what is acceptable to the patient should not be a primary consideration in selection of anesthetic agent or technique. Patient acceptability and surgical or anesthetic convenience may coincide with selection of the anesthetic which is also safest for the patient, but this should be regarded as fortuitous rather than the goal of selection of anesthetic agent and technique.

GENERAL ANESTHESIA

General anesthesia is produced either by anesthetics directly injected into the blood via the intravenous route or by anesthetics absorbed into the blood from the alveoli following inhalation. The advantages and disadvantages of inhalation general anesthesia as opposed to intravenous anesthesia and the physiologic and pharmacologic effects of the two techniques are such that it is best to discuss the two methods separately. These methods, however, do have two things in common, the risk of overdosage and the risk of inadequate ventilation. The vast majority of cardiac arrests, if not all cardiac arrests due to general anesthesia, result from one or both of these two factors. Avoidance of overdosage may prove difficult under clinical conditions, especially in the hands of a novice, for two reasons: First, individual variations of patients' responses to general anesthetics are so great that reliable dose/response relationships do not exist. General anesthetics cannot be administered in a predetermined dosage based on milligrams of anesthetic per kilogram of patient's body weight without running the risk of serious overdosage in some patients and inadequate depth of anesthesia in others. Second, evaluation of depth of anesthesia is neither easy nor precise but instead highly subjective, clinical signs varying not only with each general anesthetic but also with each patient. Even electroencephalography, a technique perhaps suitable for research purposes, is of no use in judging depth of anesthesia under clinical conditions. Signs such as pupillary size, eye motion, and character of respirations, as described by Guedel, apply only to ether and then only under select circumstances. The signs of depth of anesthesia with the more widely used present-day anesthetics are less well defined. Many anesthetics are such potent respiratory depressants, even in barely anesthetic concentrations, that respirations become an inadequate guide to depth of surgical anesthesia. Pragmatically, overdosage, whether absolute or relative, can be said to exist when arterial hypotension or (less frequently) cardiac arrhythmias are produced by a general anesthetic and is best avoided by repeated measurements of blood pressure and heart rate and by continuous electrocardiographic monitoring.

There are three principal causes of inadequate ventilation during general anesthesia: obstruction of the airway, pharmacologic interference with normal respiratory mechanisms, and anesthetically induced abnormalities of gas exchange between alveoli and pulmonary capillary blood. Obstruction may occur at any level in the airway, from pharynx to bronchi, and may be caused by anything from the tongue falling back into the pharynx to laryngospasm, bronchospasm, or aspiration of blood, gastric contents, secretions, or foreign bodies. Airway obstruction must immediately be treated by correction of the cause, whether by manipulation of the soft tissues of the upper airway (elevation of the chin or entire mandible), by insertion of artificial pharyngeal or endotracheal airways, or by endotracheal suctioning. If left untreated, obstruction results in hypoxia and hypercapnia, i.e., asphyxia. *General anesthesia is contraindicated unless a patent airway can be assured at all times.*

Pharmacologic causes of inadequate ventilation include interference with the normal neural or muscular mechanisms of respiration. These, together with anesthetically induced inadequacies of respiratory gas exchange secondary to abnormal alveolar ventilation/perfusion ratios, are included in the subsequent discussion of the individual anesthetic agents. It must be emphasized that pharmacologic derangements of respiration are often subtle and difficult to recognize although they are potentially as dangerous as, or more dangerous than, the more obvious forms of inadequate ventilation due to obstruction. They are especially insidious because the classic signs and symptoms of hypoxia and carbon dioxide retention are notoriously unreliable during clinical anesthesia. Respiratory rate, tidal volume, blood pressure, pulse rate, and color of the skin are all inaccurate indices of potentially dangerous levels of hypoxia or hypercapnia in a patient who is under general anesthesia. The only method by which abnormal blood levels of oxygen or carbon dioxide can be verified is measurement of the tensions (i.e., partial pressures) of these gases in *arterial* blood. Because of the difficulties inherent in estimating the adequacy of pulmonary ventilation and because of the dangers of inadequate ventilation compared with only minor and rather hypothetic disadvantages of hyperventilation, it is better to overventilate patients artificially during general anesthesia than to permit possible underventilation to occur. Hyperventilation is readily accomplished by intermittent manual compression of the anesthesia reservoir bag. Mechanical ventilators are not required. Neither is an endotracheal tube invariably required. Although this may prove necessary or desirable, endotracheal intubation does not guarantee adequate alveolar ventilation or even airway patency.

Inhalation Anesthesia

The principal advantage of inhalation anesthetics is controllable reversibility. As what enters via the lungs exits via the lungs, the rate at which the inhalation anesthetic exits can be as readily controlled as the rate at which it enters. Therefore, the administrator of an inhalation anesthetic can control its duration of action. This control does not exist following the intravenous administration of anesthetics and muscle relaxants, which require biotransformation or excretion for termination of action, processes over which the anesthetist has no control. Even specific antagonists to narcotics and muscle relaxants are not invariably reliable means for reversal of intravenous anesthetics. The half-life of the antagonist often differs significantly from the half-life of the agonist it is given to reverse, a situation which can lead to recurarization or reanesthetization of the patient after leaving the operating room.

Controlled reversibility and the ability to depress excitability of neuronal tissues are the only pharmacologic properties common to all inhalation anesthetics. Their pharmacologic effects and the physiologic responses they induce are otherwise too diverse to allow generalization. For one thing, inhalation anesthetics vary widely in their potency. Potency of inhalation anesthetics is commonly measured in terms of minimum alveolar anesthetic concentration (MAC), that is, the alveolar concentration of an anesthetic which prevents somatic response to painful stimuli in 50 percent of subjects. Alveolar concentration is emphasized in this definition because at equilibrium the partial pressure of an anesthetic in the alveoli is the same as it is in arterial blood, which, in turn, is the same as the partial pressure of the anesthetic in the central nervous system. Partial pressure of an anesthetic, not concentration in blood or brain, determines anesthetic effect. Differences in molecular weight and in air/blood and blood/lipid coefficients of distribution mean that equal partial pressures of different anesthetics are associated with quite different concentrations in blood, tissues, and cell membranes. MAC is widely used as a standard of reference for comparisons of different inhalation anesthetics. The side effects of anesthetics on, for example, respiration or cardiovascular function are meaningful only when equieffective concentrations of the anesthetics are compared. This is most conveniently done by comparing similar MAC values.

The concept of MAC represents an important advance both clinically and in understanding the mechanism of action of inhalation anesthesia. It has, however, limitations which must be understood if its value is to be appreciated. For example, the MAC of an anesthetic often shows substantial differences depending upon the species in which it is determined, thereby making difficult the application to man of MAC values derived in experimental animals. Furthermore, since MAC is defined as the alveolar concentration of anesthetic which prevents response to a painful stimulus in 50 percent of subjects, it follows that at MAC the other 50 percent of subjects are not anesthetized. More meaningful than MAC under clinical circumstances is the alveolar concentration which anesthetizes all subjects, the EC_{100} or AC_{100}. This is difficult to determine, however. An AC_{100} cannot be differentiated from an AC_{110}. Also important is the fact that MAC refers to alveolar, not inspired, concentration of anesthetic. The difference between inhaled and alveolar concentrations depends upon the level of total body equilibration with the anesthetic. This, in turn, is a function of duration of administration, as well as solubility of the anesthetic in various body fluids and tissues. Furthermore, although 1.0 MAC values of different anesthetics represent equal levels of anesthesia, multiples of MAC may not represent equianesthetic levels. Dose-response curves of inhalation anesthetics are not identical. They are not even parallel. In addition, since MAC refers to alveolar concentration, not tension, MAC values vary with atmospheric pressure, i.e., with altitude. Finally, although alveolar and arterial tensions of anesthetics are usually identical, alveolar-arterial pressure gradients may exist, especially with the more highly soluble anesthetics and in the presence of abnormalities of distribution of ventilation and perfusion within the lung.

All inhalation anesthetics have the potential for contaminating the air within operating rooms with subanesthetic trace amounts of anesthetic which have either escaped from the anesthesia circuit or been exhaled by the patient. The resulting pollution of air in operating rooms has been shown to produce demonstrable if subtle impairment of higher cerebral cortical functions, including judgment, among those exposed to such atmospheres. Data also suggest that contamination of operating-room air with trace concentrations of inhalation anesthetics may be associated with an increased incidence of spontaneous abortion and perhaps even increased frequency of congenital birth defects in children born to mothers repeatedly exposed to such an atmosphere in early pregnancy. It has also been suggested, though not proved, that hepatic and renal diseases as well as malignant diseases may be more frequent in those working in an atmosphere contaminated by trace concentrations of inhalation anesthetics. The danger involves not only those who administer anesthetics but surgeons, nurses, and others who work in operating rooms. Trace concentrations of anesthetics can be effectively controlled by scavenging systems attached to each anesthesia machine. All operating rooms should be equipped with such devices.

NITROUS OXIDE

Nitrous oxide (N_2O) is an inhalation analgesic. Nitrous oxide 20% provides analgesia equal to that produced by 10 mg of morphine sulfate. Increasing the concentration of nitrous oxide increases the degree of analgesia, but the MAC for nitrous oxide is over 100, so true anesthesia cannot be achieved (at 1 atmosphere) without decreasing inspired oxygen to the point where hypoxia occurs.

The analgesia produced by nitrous oxide differs substantially from the analgesia produced by narcotics. It is not associated with the profound respiratory and cardiovascular side effects characteristic of narcotics. And it is rapidly, almost immediately, reversible. These properties of nitrous oxide, combined with the fact that it is nonexplosive and odorless (and therefore enjoys high patient acceptance), make nitrous oxide the most widely used drug in surgical anesthesia. It is rarely used alone because of its lack of anesthetic potency. Instead it is employed in conjunction with other, more powerful, agents to decrease the amounts

of them that are needed and thus to diminish the magnitude of adverse side effects with which the more potent anesthetics are associated. Nitrous oxide 70%, for example, decreases the MAC of halothane by 60 percent. Nitrous oxide is also employed for the same reason during intravenous anesthesia: when nitrous oxide is used, fewer narcotics and barbiturates are needed. Because of the effectiveness of nitrous oxide as a nondepressant analgesic, it has been used in low concentrations for the relief not only of postoperative pain but also of the pain of myocardial infarction. The utility of nitrous oxide for this purpose is limited by the difficulty in maintaining its concentration at a level adequate to relieve pain yet not great enough to cause the delirium characteristic of the excitement state of light levels of general anesthesia.

Nitrous oxide is not, however, devoid of side effects. It increases sympathetic activity, probably by direct action on medullary vasomotor centers, and thereby increases peripheral vascular resistance, blood pressure, and heart rate. It also appears to have a slight stimulatory effect on respiration, shifting the CO_2-ventilation response curve to the left. These subtle effects are usually obscured under clinical conditions by the cardiovascular and respiratory effects of other more potent anesthetics simultaneously being administered. Chronic exposure to nitrous oxide also produces leukopenia.

Two clinical situations exist in which nitrous oxide may have unexpected and potentially undesirable effects not because of its pharmacologic action but because of its physical properties. Both situations are due to the fact that nitrous oxide is 30 times more soluble than nitrogen in blood. The first situation, diffusion hypoxia, may occur when a patient who is equilibrated with 80% nitrous oxide–20% oxygen spontaneously starts to breathe room air (80% nitrogen in 20% oxygen). The blood solubility differences between nitrous oxide and nitrogen being such that at equal partial pressures approximately thirty times more nitrous oxide than nitrogen is dissolved, when the patient starts to inhale room air there will be thirty times greater diffusion of nitrous oxide out of the bloodstream than of nitrogen into the bloodstream at the alveolar level. The net result is an increase in gas volume within the alveoli. Since intraalveolar pressure equals ambient pressure, the increased gas volume displaces oxygen molecules from the alveoli, with resulting transient hypoxemia. The phenomenon of diffusion hypoxia is transitory, lasting only moments, and involves at the most a 40-torr decrease in alveolar (and arterial) oxygen tension. It may be prevented by increasing alveolar oxygen tension to 150 to 200 torr at the conclusion of anesthesia. All nitrous oxide need not be eliminated to avoid diffusion hypoxia, nor should it be eliminated if analgesia is required during extubation of the trachea at the end of anesthesia.

The opposite of diffusion hypoxia, hyperoxia, occurs during induction when a patient starts breathing 80% nitrous oxide in oxygen instead of 80% nitrogen in oxygen (room air). The greater solubility of nitrous oxide means that uptake of nitrous oxide exceeds excretion of nitrogen, a concentrating effect which increases alveolar oxygen tension. The same concentrating effect also causes a transitory increase in alveolar carbon dioxide tension. Alveolar concentration of an inhalation anesthetic such as halothane is additionally accelerated, so induction of anesthesia is more rapid when nitrous oxide is used for induction of anesthesia, in part because of the concentrating effect of nitrous oxide.

The second situation in which solubility of nitrous oxide may cause difficulties occurs in patients with gas pockets containing room air, as in pneumothorax, intestinal obstruction, pneumoencephalography. When such patients are anesthetized with nitrous oxide, the anesthetic enters the air pocket at a faster rate than the nitrogen exits from it. The result is that the volume of the gas pocket increases. This can produce a shift in the mediastinum or collapse of adjacent aerated lung in the case of penumothorax or an increase in intraabdominal or intracranial pressure in the case of intestinal obstruction or pneumoencephalography.

During the administration of nitrous oxide–oxygen, the degree of oxygenation of the arterial blood cannot be accurately estimated merely by observing the flows of oxygen and nitrous oxide being delivered by the anesthesia machine. The reasons for this are twofold: First, when nitrous oxide–oxygen is administered at a time when respirations are controlled by intermittent positive pressure, a progressive and significant decrease in arterial oxygen tension can take place even though oxygen tension in the inspired air remains constant. Reasons for this are discussed in the section dealing with muscle relaxants. Second, following equilibration with the anesthetic gases, the concentration of oxygen in the inspired air during nitrous oxide–oxygen anesthesia on a semiclosed system is influenced by the amount of oxygen being metabolically consumed. For example, if a patient consumes 250 ml of oxygen per minute and is anesthetized on a semiclosed circuit into which 1 liter each of oxygen and nitrous oxide are flowing per minute, after equilibration the patient will not be inhaling 50% oxygen, because over the period of 1 minute he will consume 250 ml of the 1,000 ml of oxygen being delivered in that minute. He will therefore be inhaling approximately 42% oxygen. The importance of the metabolic requirements for oxygen as a determinant of the concentration of oxygen in the inspired mixture on semiclosed systems is a function of the total flow of anesthetic gases. The 250 ml of oxygen being metabolized per minute has little significant effect if the total flow rate into the anesthesia circuit is 8 liters per minute, but the same 250 ml will have a major effect if the total flow rate into the semiclosed system is only 1 liter per minute, e.g., 500 ml each of nitrous oxide and oxygen per minute. The concentration of oxygen in the inspired air when nitrous oxide is being administered is related not only to the percentage of oxygen delivered to the anesthesia circuit but also to the total flow rates at which these gases are being delivered.

HALOTHANE

Halothane ($CF_3CHBrCl$) is an extremely potent inhalation anesthetic. The MAC for halothane is 0.75. Surgical levels of anesthesia can usually be obtained with alveolar concentrations of about 1.0 vol %. The advantages of halo-

thane are that it is nonexplosive, that it is not unpleasant for the patient to breath, and that both onset of action and emergence are rapid. A potential advantage of halothane is that because it is so potent it can be administered with 98–99% oxygen. Such potency can also be a disadvantage. The difference between lethal and clinically effective concentrations of halothane in the inspired air is well below 1.0 vol %. Halothane should be administered only by experienced persons employing calibrated vaporizers, the accuracy of which must be independent of changes in temperature and changes in volume of gas flow through them. These specially designed vaporizers must be placed outside the anesthesia circuit to prevent accumulation of halothane within the circuit.

Cardiovascular depression is a frequent accompaniment of surgical levels of halothane anesthesia. It is the result of multiple actions of halothane on different parts of the cardiovascular system: direct depression of medullary vasomotor centers; inhibition of ganglionic transmission within sympathetic nerves innervating the heart and peripheral vasculature; alteration of threshold responses of baroreceptors within the carotid and aortic arch sinuses; and direct depression of both myocardial muscle fibers and peripheral vascular smooth muscle fibers. Hypotension and decreased cardiac output often occur during halothane anesthesia, especially in aged or hypovolemic patients and in patients with myocardial ischemia, valvular heart disease, or coronary artery insufficiency. Halothane also increases the sensitivity of ventricular pacemakers to arrhythmogenic stimuli, including epinephrine, probably because of anesthetically induced depression of conduction within the heart. It is for this reason that use of epinephrine must be restricted to less than 10 ml/70 kg body weight of a 1:100,000 solution every 10 minutes during halothane anesthesia.

Since the cardiovascular-depressant actions of halothane are dose-dependent (i.e., concentration-dependent), a frequent technique for decreasing the magnitude and frequency of such adverse side effects is to administer halothane with nitrous oxide. Nitrous oxide 70% decreases the anesthetic requirements of halothane by 60 percent. Since nitrous oxide has a slight stimulatory rather than a depressant effect on cardiovascular function, the combination of 70% nitrous oxide and 0.3% halothane produces less physiologic trespass against the cardiovascular system than does 0.7% halothane in 100% oxygen, yet depth of anesthesia is the same in each instance. Use of nitrous oxide to decrease halothane concentration diminishes the magnitude of the arterial hypotension and decreased cardiac output produced by the halothane, but it does so at the cost of decreasing arterial oxygen content below the level obtainable when 100% oxygen is given with the halothane. The increase in oxygen content of arterial blood associated with 100% oxygen is sufficient to maintain at normal levels the rate at which oxygen is delivered to peripheral tissues even if cardiac output decreases 15 percent. Decreasing the amount of halothane by using nitrous oxide and thus lowering inspired oxygen to 30% will be of little avail in terms of the rate at which oxygen is delivered to the periphery if the combination of N_2O and halothane is still associated with a 15 percent decrease in cardiac output. Addition of nitrous oxide in this situation may even be deleterious.

Halothane is a potent vasodilator. The vasodilation affects the circulation of almost all organs. Notable is the effect of halothane on the cerebral vasculature. Even when the respiratory-depressant effects of halothane are compensated for by artificial respiration to assure a normal arterial carbon dioxide tension of 40 torr, surgical levels of halothane anesthesia are associated with significant increases in cerebral blood flow due to the decrease in cerebrovascular resistance produced by the halothane. The resultant increase in intracranial pressure can be deleterious in patients with preexisting increase in pressure due to space-occupying lesions. This potential danger can be offset to a major extent by artificially hyperventilating the patient during halothane anesthesia to lower arterial carbon dioxide tension to 30 torr or less and thus restore cerebral blood flow and intracranial pressure to preanesthetic levels.

Halothane, like the majority of general anesthetics, decreases the sensitivity of the respiratory center to carbon dioxide. Spontaneous ventilation during surgical levels of halothane anesthesia is therefore inevitably associated with elevation of arterial carbon dioxide tension. The resultant respiratory acidosis can be only partially compensated for by assisting respirations. The increase in apneic threshold produced by halothane means that as long as any inspiratory effort remains, an inspiratory movement is needed to signal the exact moment when positive pressure must be applied to the anesthesia reservoir bag if inhalation is to be assisted, when carbon dioxide tension is above normal levels of 40 torr. When artificial ventilation succeeds in lowering carbon dioxide to 40 torr, apnea usually ensues and assisted ventilation becomes impossible. Eucapnia during halothane anesthesia can be assured only when respirations are controlled, not assisted.

Halothane, in common with other commonly used inhalation anesthetics, is metabolized by hepatic microsomal enzyme systems. The amount metabolized averages about 20 percent of that absorbed by the patient, but this varies from patient to patient and can be expected to be increased in patients in whom enzyme induction has been produced either by prior administration of drugs such as phenobarbital or by recent prior exposure (self-induction). The metabolism of halothane has no clinically significant effect on uptake, distribution, or MAC. The metabolites are pharmacologically largely inert. With prolonged exposure to high concentrations of halothane, however, enough inorganic bromine may be released to elevate serum bromine levels to the point where they may produce sedation. For this reason, prolonged (6 to 8 hours) administration of halothane may be inadvisable, especially in neurosurgical patients in whom rapid return of normal cerebral function postoperatively may be desirable. The possibility that the metabolites of halothane are toxic has been extensively studied. The consensus is that they are not, except possibly to the liver, as discussed below.

Because halothane is a highly halogenated hydrocarbon, the possibility that it might be a hepatotoxin has received considerable attention. Objective clinical data remain difficult to obtain, and the clinical significance of much of the data obtained from experimental animals remains obscure. Three things are, however, generally agreed upon. First, though rare and sporadic, instances of postoperative hepatic damage have been reported often enough in association with halothane to indicate that the matter deserves careful scrutiny and investigation. Second, halothane is not a true hepatotoxin in the sense that carbon tetrachloride is, for example. Halothane does not produce predictable dose/concentration–dependent hepatic damage in all species the way a true hepatotoxin does. And, third, the risk of an adverse hepatic response to halothane is not greater in the presence of preexisting liver disease. It may even be less in the case of cirrhosis. Halothane, furthermore, causes no greater exacerbation of preexisting liver disease than do other anesthetics. It is therefore not necessarily contraindicated in patients with liver disease.

Those who believe halothane is capable of producing hepatic damage describe a clinical picture in which a diffuse hepatitis develops 2 to 5 days following anesthesia. The onset of jaundice is preceded by high, unexplained fever for about 12 to 24 hours and is accompanied by eosinophilia. The syndrome is said to be more frequent in females than in males, more frequent following multiple exposures to halothane, and more frequent if a previous exposure to halothane was associated with unexplained fever. Biopsy specimens reveal a picture indistinguishable from that observed in infectious hepatitis. The damage to the liver may be mild and short-lived or it may progress to fatal liver failure.

"Halothane hepatitis" has been ascribed to an allergic or hypersensitivity reaction to halothane or its metabolites. This, it is said, agrees with its reported higher incidence among females and the associated eosinophilia and with the higher incidence of the syndrome following multiple exposures to halothane. Yet substantial series of cases have also been reported in patients who have been exposed on multiple occasions to halothane without adverse effects. The fact that "halothane hepatitis" has been reported in patients following a first exposure to halothane is explained on the basis of relatively nonspecific sensitization, comparable to the sensitivity of certain persons to horse serum even though they have not previously been exposed to it. The most compelling evidence that "halothane hepatitis" does indeed represent a sensitization phenomenon is a report of an anesthetist who developed hepatitis whenever he employed halothane as an anesthetic. When challenged with a trace concentration of halothane under controlled conditions at a time when the hepatitis had been quiescent for several months, there was prompt and immediate onset of fever and arthralgia and recrudescence of the hepatitis confirmed by biopsy.

The response of such a person to a challenge exposure to halothane is compatible with the hypothesis that the syndrome is a sensitization reaction. The response does not rule out, however, other possibilities. The trace concentrations of halothane or its metabolites may have been adequate to depress normal immune responses to a virus causing hepatitis and thereby cause a smoldering or incipient infection to become active enough to be clinically and histologically evident. The stress, both emotional and physical, of such a challenge test may also be sufficient to cause acute exacerbation of a previously quiescent condition. Finally, extensive in vitro immunologic tests have consistently failed to prove the existence of a sensitization reaction or an allergy to halothane in patients recovering from "halothane hepatitis."

Another explanation offered for "halothane hepatitis" is that certain persons are susceptible to halothane or its metabolites not on an immunologic or sensitivity basis but rather on the basis that they have an inherent abnormality of metabolism, either acquired or genetic in origin, which results in production of abnormal metabolites from halothane which are in themselves hepatotoxic. This view receives support from the demonstration that under the proper circumstances a small portion of the metabolites of halothane can produce damage to liver cells in vitro or in vivo in experimental animals. That this applies to man remains to be proved.

A major problem in determining the true incidence of "halothane hepatitis" lies in the fact that many other conditions encountered in surgical patients are capable of producing a similar picture. Chief amongst these is viral hepatitis. Making a differential diagnosis in an individual case between viral hepatitis and "halothane hepatitis" with absolute certainty is so difficult as to border on the impossible. Yet it is essential to do so. The natural incidence of viral hepatitis is such that the condition is bound to occur in a substantial number of the 18,000,000 persons anesthetized annually in this country, regardless of whether they had halothane or not. To complicate matters further, many drugs other than halothane administered to surgical patients are also capable of producing hepatic dysfunction; and shock, sepsis, and other complications of surgery can result in liver damage. Not all cases of hepatic damage following halothane are due to the halothane.

A fundamental question with regard to "halothane hepatitis" is the overall safety of halothane compared to other anesthetics. The massive National Halothane Study studied this insofar as deaths associated with postoperative liver failure are concerned. The results of this study conclusively demonstrated that the frequency of postoperative hepatic dysfunction not related to shock, sepsis, other forms of hepatitis, or the like is no greater following halothane than it is following any other anesthetic, and may even be less. The study also showed that otherwise inexplicable hepatic dysfunction was rare, occurring at most about once in 8,000 to 10,000 anesthesias, and not every case was fatal. But the safety of halothane as a clinical anesthetic cannot be judged solely by the incidence of associated hepatic damage. Substitution of another anesthetic for halothane in hope of avoiding a rare but perhaps possible case of "halothane hepatitis" may introduce risks greater than that of hepatitis. To replace halothane with an anesthetic associated with an incidence of ventricular fibrillation of 1 in 2,500 accomplishes little in terms of overall patient safety.

To summarize: Whether "halothane hepatitis" even exists as a clinical syndrome is debatable. If it does exist, the mechanism by which halothane causes hepatitis remains unproved. Even if it exists, the risk involved in the judicious use of halothane has not been proved to be greater than the risk of avoiding it in favor of other anesthetics; it may well be less. Halothane remains a safe and effective inhalation anesthetic when properly administered.

Finally, mention should be made of the fact that halothane is a potent depressant of uterine musculature. This property of halothane has been utilized for relaxing contraction rings and for performing internal versions. It is a property, however, which contraindicates use of halothane in most obstetric situations.

ENFLURANE

Enflurane (CHF_2OCF_2CHFCl) is representative of a group of recently synthesized compounds which combine an ether linkage (for anesthetic effect) with halogenation (F for nonflammability, Cl for anesthetic effect). About half as potent as halothane (the MAC of enflurane is 1.2), enflurane has nevertheless many of the properties of halothane. They are about equally rapid in onset of action. Recovery is also about equally rapid. Both depress respiration and the cardiovascular system to about the same extent when administered in equianesthetic concentrations.

Enflurane differs from halothane, however, in four respects. First, in a small percentage of normal patients it is associated with development of electroencephalographic patterns characteristic of epilepsy. This occurrence is markedly diminished in frequency and can perhaps even be eliminated if hyperventilation and hypocapnia are avoided. The clinical significance of these EEG patterns is dubious. Rarely are they associated with corresponding behavioral changes in the form of mild epileptiform movements. The appearance of these abnormal EEG patterns does not appear to be more frequent in epileptics.

Secondly, while enflurane does not protect against the arrythmogenic effects of epinephrine and similar compounds to the extent that a halogenated ether such as methoxyflurane does, it does not increase the irritability of ectopic ventricular pacemakers to the extent that halothane does. Enflurane is a particularly useful inhalation anesthetic when epinephrine is used by intravenous infusion for its inotropic effects or by injection for its vasoconstrictor effects to decrease operative blood loss. Enflurane is also useful in patients with pheochromocytomas when inhalation anesthesia is employed.

Thirdly, enflurane is metabolized, but the percentage of enflurane which undergoes biotransformation is but a fraction of that with other halogenated anesthetics, including halothane. This may be particularly advantageous during inhalation anesthesia of long duration. Enflurane avoids the problem of possible prolonged postoperative sedation due to increased bromine levels associated with lengthy halothane anesthetics.

Finally, cases of postoperative "hepatitis" have been reported following enflurane anesthesia, although less frequently than following halothane anesthesia. Since enflurane is metabolized less than halothane, this has been said to support the hypothesis that the metabolic products of halothane rather than halothane itself are responsible for sensitization reactions leading to "halothane hepatitis."

Equally possible is the alternative explanation, that enflurane and the few metabolites it produces are so immunologically inert that they are incapable of initiating a sensitization reaction. But whether "hepatitis" is in fact less frequent after enflurane than after halothane is in doubt. It has yet to be proved statistically. Perhaps the incidence of "hepatitis" associated with enflurane appears to be lower because enflurane has only recently been available for general clinical use, or perhaps there is a lower level of suspicion in regard to enflurane.

OTHER INHALATION ANESTHETICS

CYCLOPROPANE. Cyclopropane (C_3H_6) is a highly explosive, extremely rapidly acting inhalation anesthetic of intermediate potency (its MAC is 9.2). Anesthetic concentrations are associated with a pronounced centrally mediated increase in sympathetic activity. The blood pressure rises. The pulse slows, however, because of activation of baroreceptor reflexes the sensitivity of which is probably increased by the anesthetic. Blood levels of catecholamines, norepinephrine especially, rise as the rate of norepinephrine release from postganglionic sympathetic fibers exceeds the capacity for reuptake and local enzymatic breakdown. The elevated blood levels of catecholamines predispose to ventricular arrhythmias, including ventricular fibrillation, particularly if catecholamine levels are further increased by the exogenous administration of epinephrine or the endogenous release of still more catecholamines by hypoxia or carbon dioxide accumulation. Hypercapnia is particularly liable to occur in the absence of controlled ventilation because of the respiratory-depressant effects of cyclopropane. Because of the increase in sympathetic activity, cyclopropane is particularly advantageous in hypovolemic patients. Cyclopropane, however, is now infrequently used because of its explosiveness and the widespread use of electrocautery for surgical hemostasis.

DIETHYL ETHER. Ether ($CH_3CH_2OCH_2CH_3$) is an explosive, potent (its MAC is 1.9) inhalation anesthetic that differs from other general anesthetics in that respiration is not depressed by anesthetic concentrations. Like cyclopropane, it increases sympathetic activity, but to a somewhat lesser extent. Ether is rarely used today in the United States for three reasons: it is explosive; it is the most difficult of all general anesthetics to administer smoothly, principally because of its high solubility, especially in blood and other extracellular fluids; and finally, it is osmically offensive, an esthetic point—it smells bad. Ether remains, nevertheless, uniquely valuable in those rare instances in which surgical levels of anesthesia must be maintained with spontaneous respiration. Ether is also still widely employed in developing countries because it is the least expensive of all general anesthetics and because, being an easily handled and easily vaporized liquid that does not depress respiration, it can be administered with a minimum of equipment.

METHOXYFLURANE. Methoxyflurane ($CH_3OCF_2CHCl_2$) is another nonexplosive, halogenated ether. It is the most potent of all inhalation anesthetics, with a MAC of 0.16, and it has the lowest vapor pressure of all anesthetics, 20 torr at 18°C. Furthermore, it is the most highly soluble of all anesthetics in lipids: its oil/gas partition coefficient is

about 1,000. The physical properties of methoxyflurane mean that induction of anesthesia may be prolonged. Recovery may also be prolonged, often for hours. Its pharmacologic properties are much like those of other halogenated inhalation anesthetics. It depresses respiration and the cardiovascular system about as much as equieffective concentrations of halothane or enflurane. It protects against epinephrine-induced arrhythmias, however. The major distinguishing characteristic of methoxyflurane is that it is extensively metabolized with release of inorganic fluoride. Fluoride is nephrotoxic when serum levels exceed a level of about 50 μm/liter. These levels are apt to be equaled or exceeded under clinical conditions, especially when methoxyflurane is administered for more than an hour or two and especially in an obese patient. The danger of high-output renal failure in the postoperative period is so real that today methoxyflurane is infrequently used. When it is employed, it is most often used for brief periods in low concentrations, often intermittently, as an inhalation analgesic, especially in labor.

Intravenous Anesthesia

General anesthesia is also produced by the intravenous injection of one or, more commonly, a combination of two or more depressants. Intravenous anesthesia almost always also includes the simultaneous administration of nitrous oxide. When a single drug is used intravenously, it is most often a thiobarbiturate. When combinations of drugs are used, they are usually of different types, including narcotics, ketamine, hypnotics, or neuroleptics. "Balanced anesthesia" means different things to different people but most often refers to a combination of drugs used intravenously to obtain amnesia, analgesia, sedation, and muscular relaxation. A thiobarbiturate and a narcotic are almost always included (along with nitrous oxide). Neuroleptics and sedative-tranquilizers such as diazepam (Valium) may also be used, as well as a muscle relaxant.

An advantage of intravenous anesthesia is agreeableness for the patient. The rapid onset of unconsciousness without exposure to odorous vapors and without the claustrophobic feeling of a mask applied to the face makes intravenous anesthesia popular with patients. Another advantage is convenience for the anesthetist. Rapid induction of anesthesia without the problems inherent in the somewhat longer and certainly more exacting induction of anesthesia by inhalation techniques has appealing aspects.

Against these advantages must be weighed the disadvantages of intravenous anesthesia. Chief among these is the fact that although intravenous anesthetics produce immediate and profound depression, true anesthesia—that is, absence of response to painful stimuli—may not be complete. This can lead to a situation, for instance, in which depression is great enough to cause obstruction of the upper airway as the tongue and other soft tissues fall back into the pharynx, yet the patient is not deeply enough anesthetized to permit instrumentation in the airway by insertion of an artificial airway or an endotracheal tube to remove the obstruction. The result can be a patient unable to breathe adequately because of airway obstruction yet not deeply enough anesthetized to allow the situation to be corrected. The dilemma can be solved by paralyzing the patient with a muscle relaxant and then immediately performing a laryngoscopy and placing an endotracheal tube in place for artificial ventilation. This solution to the problem is based on the assumption that endotracheal intubation can *always*—in *all* patients—be immediately accomplished. If this assumption proves incorrect, as it occasionally may even in the most skilled hands, the obstructed, semianesthetized patient who is at least trying to breathe past an obstruction is converted to an obstructed, semianesthetized patient who is apneic, not trying to breathe, and cannot be ventilated artificially. The result can be disastrous. Even if endotracheal intubation is accomplished, the patient is still not anesthetized, although this will not be evident because the lack of anesthesia is covered up by paralysis. A corollary of this situation can arise during intravenous anesthesia in which a muscle relaxant is administered during maintenance of anesthesia. Redistribution of the intravenously administered neuronal depressants may cause blood levels and hence brain levels of narcotics and hypnotics to decrease to the point where awareness is regained. When the patient is paralyzed the anesthetist may be unable to recognize the fact that the patient is aware of his surroundings and may even be experiencing pain. Changes in blood pressure and pulse rate in response to surgical stimulation are sufficiently blunted under these circumstances by the intravenous anesthetics so that they are no longer reliable indications of the depth of anesthesia. The difficulty in maintaining constant and predictable levels of anesthesia with intravenous anesthetics is reflected by the fact that MAC values for intravenous anesthetics cannot be determined. The pharmacokinetics of uptake, distribution, metabolism, and excretion are too complex to allow establishment of a pharmacologic state steady enough for such a determination.

Another disadvantage of intravenous anesthesia, as already mentioned, is that the duration of action of the drugs used is determined by factors the anesthetist has no control over, namely biotransformation and renal or biliary excretion. Specific antagonists to narcotics and relaxants are available for use at the conclusion of intravenous anesthesia and are often helpful, but antagonists are often only a partial answer to the problem of controlled reversibility. There are no specific antagonists to barbiturates, neuroleptics, and other hypnotics which may be used during intravenous anesthesia. Furthermore, the duration of action of the antagonist may be less than the duration of action of the agonist.

Finally, the polypharmacy involved in intravenous anesthesia holds the potential for drug interactions of such complexity that they are difficult to unravel even under controlled experimental conditions in laboratory animals, let alone in human beings under clinical conditions. Intravenous anesthesia commonly involves use of at least ten drugs often more, including premedicants and antagonists in addition to the intravenous anesthetics. The theory behind such polypharmacy is that the desirable attributes of each drug in a combination of drugs supplement or potentiate one another. Less desirable attributes may also,

however, be supplemented or potentiated. A combination of neuronal depressants may produce a more satisfactory state of anesthesia, analgesia, and amnesia than would a single drug. At the same time, however, the adverse side effects of the drugs on cardiovascular function and on respiration may also be, and often are, greater.

Despite its disadvantages, intravenous anesthesia enjoys a well-deserved niche in the armamentarium of the anesthetist. Its apparent simplicity, however, belies the fact that intravenous anesthesia requires even more skill and experience than does inhalation anesthesia if it is to prove equally safe.

BARBITURATES

The intravenous agents most frequently used to produce surgical anesthesia are thiobarbiturates. Their popularity is based on the fact that they are "ultra-short-acting" barbiturates, i.e., rapid in onset and short in duration. Their pharmacologic actions, using thiopental (Pentothal) as a prototype, may be considered according to the cause of their "ultrashort action," with a brief comparison of their effects with those of inhalation anesthetics.

The rapid onset and apparently short duration of action of thiobarbiturates is a function primarily of increased lipoid solubility associated with the substitution of a sulfur atom for the oxygen atom in the barbituric acid ring. Thiopental is structurally similar to pentobarbital (Nembutal), except that a sulfur atom has been substituted for the oxygen atom in the latter. The increased lipoid solubility, plus a pK which makes thiopental only slightly dissociated at a pH of 7.40, cause the rapid onset of action. The rate at which drugs cross the so-called blood-brain barrier is directly related to their lipoid solubility and inversely related to their degree of ionization. These properties of thiopental combined with high cerebral blood flow result not only in an immediate onset of action (one circulation time) but also in an extremely short duration of action. Because the central nervous system has such a high flow compared to other areas of the body, more thiopental is delivered to it; this combined with high lipoid solubility produces a higher concentration in the central nervous system than elsewhere in the body immediately after administration of a single dose. With the passage of time other areas of the body with lesser blood flows gradually receive the barbiturate. In lean body mass, represented primarily by skeletal muscle, a concentration of thiopental develops after peak central nervous system concentrations have been achieved and in so doing produces a decrease in concentration of thiopental within the central nervous system. This hemodynamic redistribution of thiopental following a single intravenous injection is later followed by further redistribution to the areas of the body with the least blood flow, namely, adipose tissue. The buildup of thiopental in fatty depots throughout the body is relatively slow because of the low blood flow, but as time goes on the concentration in these areas becomes significant because of thiopental's high lipoid solubility in such tissues. As a result of this redistribution there is a relatively rapid reversal of the high central nervous system concentration following a single intravenous injection, and consciousness rapidly returns toward normal. This apparently ultrashort duration of action results not from a high rate of metabolism or excretion but from the dynamics of uptake and redistribution. The same sequence of events takes place, but to a less pronounced degree, following repeated intravenous injections of small amounts of the drug. The redistribution of thiopental within the body results in a regression of the state of central nervous system depression but does not result in its complete reversal until all the barbiturate has been metabolized or excreted.

The pharmacologic properties of thiopental are qualitatively comparable to those previously outlined for inhalation anesthetics, but with the additional disadvantage that when administered in equianesthetic doses thiopental is more depressant than true inhalation anesthetics. Thus thiopental is a cardiovascular and respiratory depressant. As a cardiovascular depressant, it acts directly on the myocardium to decrease the force of ventricular contraction. In addition it causes peripheral vasodilatation. The hypotension which may accompany thiopental administration may be extreme, especially in patients in or bordering on oligemic shock. But the hypotension of thiopental does not have the saving grace of being associated with a state of true surgical anesthesia, as is usual with an agent such as halothane. The respiratory depression of thiopental resulting in an elevated threshold response of the respiratory center to carbon dioxide is unassociated with the production of a truly anesthetic state and so is of completely different clinical significance from that produced by, for example, halothane.

Another major disadvantage of thiopental is that its depressant effects last longer than those observed with inhalation anesthetics. For example, the respiratory depression with enflurane is rapidly reversed moments after its administration has been terminated, while the effects of intravenous anesthetics such as thiopental may linger on for hours. The complete metabolism or excretion of thiopental occurs at an extremely slow rate. Thus, although the greater part of the thiopental-induced anesthesia may be reversed within moments following a single injection, a long-lasting and subclinical degree of central nervous system depression may persist for many hours until the barbiturate has been metabolized in the liver and removed not only from the brain but also from the lean body mass and the fatty depots. The prolonged but subtle central nervous system depression following thiopental anesthesia is exemplified by the electroencephalographic changes, which may be detected for 18 hours following a brief period of thiopental anesthesia.

Thiobarbiturates today are mainly used to supplement other relatively weak anesthetics such as nitrous oxide or other intravenous anesthetics or to induce general anesthesia prior to the administration of other more potent inhalation anesthetics. When employed as a means of inducing general anesthesia, thiobarbiturates are best administered in "sleep" or hypnotic doses of 150 to 200 mg/70 kg of body weight and not in anesthetic doses (500 to 600 mg). Thiopental is contraindicated (as is any general anesthetic) in the presence of a full stomach or in other situations in which the patency of the patient's airway cannot be assured at all times.

NARCOTICS

Narcotics are not anesthetics. Nevertheless they are employed frequently and advantageously enough as adjuncts to anesthesia to warrant discussion in this chapter. Narcotics are primarily used in two situations: during general anesthesia in combination with weak anesthetics such as nitrous oxide or intravenous anesthetics to provide more intense analgesia and during regional anesthesia to provide relief of pain or discomfort. In such instances narcotics should be administered only intravenously. Intramuscular and subcutaneous injections are so slowly and erratically absorbed and have such unpredictable onset and intensity of action that administration by such routes should be limited to premedication. When administered intravenously, narcotics must be given in repeated small doses rather than in a single therapeutic dose, to prevent development of transient dangerously high blood and brain levels.

The main disadvantage of narcotics as adjuvants to anesthesia is that some degree of respiratory depression is inevitably produced whenever narcotics are employed in therapeutic amounts. There is no significant difference in the degree of depression caused by the different narcotics *when administered in equianalgesic dosages.* Duration of action may, however, differ among the narcotics. Notable is the short duration of action of fentanyl (Sublimaze), the most potent narcotic presently available. With approximately fifty times the activity of morphine, fentanyl has a duration of action less than half that of morphine. Attempts to increase the usefulness of narcotics during anesthesia by administration of narcotic antagonists in the belief that respiratory depression will be alleviated without affecting analgesia have proved futile.

A completely different anesthetic use of narcotics involves their administration in amounts large enough to produce true anesthesia. Morphine is especially useful in this regard when given in doses of 2 to 3 mg/kg during cardiac surgery requiring cardiopulmonary bypass. Use of morphine in this manner is predicated on the assumption that respirations will be continuously controlled via an endotracheal tube in the immediate postoperative period, which is of considerable benefit to many cardiac patients.

Narcotics also are used during regional anesthesia, whether spinal, epidural, or nerve block, either to supplement inadequate sensory blocking or to relieve patient discomfort if the regional anesthesia wears off before the operation has been completed. The wisdom of using narcotics in either situation is often doubtful, because considerable depression is produced without real relief of pain. It is often wiser to give the patient a small amount of intravenous narcotic followed by a nondepressant, rapidly reversible analgesic such as nitrous oxide rather than try to provide true anesthesia with the narcotic alone. Intravenous narcotics in small amounts, however, are often of real value for patients undergoing lengthy procedures under regional anesthesia, as the immobile patient with spinal anesthesia on an uncomfortable operating table for 4 hours becomes restless because of the physical discomfort of the unanesthetized portions of the body.

OTHER INTRAVENOUS ANESTHETICS

Neuroleptic anesthesia (or analgesia) is an intravenous anesthetic technique in which a potent psychomotor sedative, the neuroleptic, is combined with a narcotic and a hypnotic. The most widely used neuroleptic is droperidol (Inapsine), which is supplied commercially either alone or in combination with the potent narcotic fentanyl in a ratio of 50:1 as Innovar. The combination of drugs in Innovar presupposes that when sedation is required a narcotic is required and vice versa, and furthermore that both are always needed in the same arbitrarily predetermined proportions. This may be true at times, but scarcely all the time. Innovar is best used in intravenous anesthesia to help establish a basic level of sedation and analgesia during induction of anesthesia. Subsequent analgesia is thereafter best maintained with nitrous oxide together with repeated injections of small amounts of fentanyl, while sedation is maintained either with further droperidol alone or with a thiobarbiturate.

Ketamine, although not a narcotic in the classic sense, produces profound analgesia combined with striking subjective dissociation from the environment. Administered intravenously or intramuscularly in the proper dosage, ketamine provides anesthesia adequate for superficial operations requiring no muscle relaxation without producing respiratory or cardiovascular depression. In fact, the arterial pressure frequently is elevated and the heart rate increased. Ketamine also has the important advantage of not relaxing muscles and soft tissue of the upper airway, as other narcotics and sedatives are prone to do. Therefore, airway obstruction is infrequent, though by no means impossible, during ketamine anesthesia. However, ketamine has the disadvantage of being occasionally associated with highly unpleasant hallucinations or subjective responses best described as nightmares. Since this adverse psychic response is particularly liable to occur in adults, ketamine is often restricted to children. As ketamine accentuates pharyngeal and laryngeal reflexes, it is usually contraindicated for operations on or about the mouth, lips, and nose because of the possibility of precipitating severe laryngospasm. It also rather sharply increases intracranial pressure and so is contraindicated in certain neurologic conditions.

RELAXANTS

Intravenously administered muscle relaxants allow profound muscular relaxation without deep levels of anesthesia. The avoidance of the adverse physiologic effects of deep general anesthesia by such means is not, however, without its disadvantages. These are related to the profound interference with normal respiration produced by all muscle relaxants when administered in amounts adequate to provide required degrees of muscular relaxation. The respiratory effects of muscle relaxants must be compensated for by artificial ventilation to maintain a normal arterial oxygenation and a normal carbon dioxide excretion. This is not always readily achieved under clinical circumstances, and the clinical signs of respiratory acidosis or hypoxia are unreliable in the anesthetized patient.

An additional problem associated with the use of muscle relaxants is that their duration of action may exceed the duration of surgical procedures, with the result that a patient is apneic or hypoventilated after the operation and anesthesia have been completed. Although prolonged apnea following the use of muscle relaxants is not always due solely to their prolonged action, the apnea cannot always be reversed at will.

A third difficulty associated with the use of muscle relaxants is that the intermittent positive-pressure ventilation which their use necessitates may be associated with arterial hypoxemia even though alveolar ventilation adequate for removal of carbon dioxide is provided. Arterial hypoxemia may supervene despite amounts of oxygen in the inspired air adequate to maintain normal arterial oxygenation in the unanesthetized patient. The reason is that intermittent positive-pressure ventilation often is associated with derangements of normal alveolar ventilation/perfusion ratios, and certain alveoli are perfused with blood when they are not ventilated. The uneven alveolar ventilation, which to some extent inevitably follows the institution of positive-pressure respirations, results in an increased gradient in oxygen tension between alveoli and pulmonary venous (i.e., peripheral arterial) blood because of the continued perfusion of unventilated or underventilated areas. For this reason it is necessary to provide at least 33% oxygen in the inspired air when artificial respiration is being carried on for long periods of time, as during nitrous oxide–oxygen anesthesia with muscle relaxants or halothane. The same events can occur in patients on controlled respiration for long periods of time in the postoperative recovery room and in intensive care units.

Muscle relaxants may be divided into two major categories depending on the method by which they produce muscle paralysis: those such as curare and pancuronium (Pavulon), which interfere with transmission of the nerve impulse at the myoneural junction by competing with acetylcholine for the motor end plate (nondepolarizing muscle relaxants), and those such as succinylcholine, which interfere with myoneural transmission by producing depolarization of the motor end plate, rendering it unresponsive. Agents such as curare are, by and large, longer acting than depolarizing agents. Curare, for example, shows significant regression from its peak action approximately 20 minutes after administration, the greater part of its action disappearing within approximately 40 minutes. Although curare is to a large extent ultimately excreted by renal mechanisms, its action is terminated after about 45 minutes primarily because of its redistribution throughout the body. Therefore, curare, like thiopental, may have a subtle subclinical effect persisting beyond its peak effect. Thus, curare has a cumulative effect, and a subsequent dose to produce muscular relaxation equal to that produced initially will be considerably lower than the first.

Unlike curare, the depolarizing agent succinylcholine

has a short duration of action, because it is metabolized by the enzyme pseudocholinesterase in approximately 8 minutes. However, after prolonged periods of administration the method by which succinylcholine produces neuromuscular block becomes more complex; it no longer resembles a depolarizing type of block so much as a nondepolarizing or curare type of block. This nondepolarizing phase of myoneural block is especially liable to be encountered after prolonged intravenous administration of dilute concentrations of succinylcholine.

The initial depolarization produced by single injections of large amounts of succinylcholine frequently results in onset of brief fasciculation of skeletal muscles and often in equally brief uncoordinated myoclonic contractions gross enough to resemble seizures. One result of the depolarization is an increase in intraocular pressure due to fasciculations of extrinsic muscles of the eye. This is of no consequence in normal patients, but in a patient with an open orbit or with preexisting increased intraocular pressure due, for example, to glaucoma, this side effect of succinylcholine can prove highly deleterious. Succinylcholine is often also associated with an increase in intraabdominal pressure due to fasciculation of muscles of the anterior abdominal wall and, perhaps, the diaphragm. This also is of little consequence in normal patients. In a patient suffering from disruption of an abdominal incision, however, the increased intraabdominal pressure can make the dehiscence worse. Intragastric pressure also increases when intraabdominal pressure is elevated during fasciculations. This is particularly dangerous in a patient with a full stomach because of the possibility of massive regurgitation of gastric contents into the upper airway and mouth, with subsequent aspiration into the trachea and bronchi.

Depolarization of skeletal muscles induced by succinylcholine is accompanied by efflux of potassium from skeletal muscles. In normal subjects this results in minor and quite transitory elevations of serum potassium levels of no clinical significance. In other patients, however, the hyperkalemia may be so pronounced as to result in ventricular fibrillation. This is particularly liable to occur in patients suffering from burns, from crush injuries involving skeletal muscles, and from injuries involving denervation of skeletal muscles.

Finally, the depolarization of succinylcholine can result in severe and distressing postoperative muscle pains. Clinical impression to the contrary, these pains are not related to gross jactitations of muscles which occur as muscle masses undergo depolarization at different rates. Muscle pains are due to the depolarization per se and can be observed postoperatively in patients who exhibited no gross movements of muscles following succinylcholine.

Increases in intraocular and intraabdominal pressures, hyperkalemia, and postoperative muscle pains associated with succinylcholine can all be prevented if a small amount of a nondepolarizing relaxant (e.g., 3 mg of d-tubocurarine/70 kg) is administered 5 to 8 minutes prior to injection of succinylcholine. When this is done, the amount of succinylcholine subsequently administered must be increased, because a nondepolarizing relaxant shifts the dose-response curve of a depolarizing relaxant to the right.

Succinylcholine, along with halothane and other inhalation anesthetics, has been shown to be capable of triggering, in certain rare individuals, a potentially lethal and rapidly progressing condition referred to as *malignant pyrexia*, often (though not invariably) characterized by muscular rigidity instead of relaxation following succinylcholine. The body temperature is rapidly elevated to levels as high as 107°F within 30 minutes or less. Once established, the pyrexia often proves fatal because of associated neurologic damage, cardiovascular collapse, and profound metabolic derangements. The biochemical events responsible for the massive increase in body heat remain to be fully elucidated, though they obviously involve skeletal muscles. The syndrome has, however, been shown to represent a genetically transmitted susceptibility to succinylcholine and many inhalation anesthetics which, when encountered, is most likely to be seen in young, muscular males who are otherwise quite healthy. There is no accurate method of diagnosing the condition in advance except for sophisticated and complex metabolic studies performed on muscle biopsies from those suspected of being at risk. Most valuable is a detailed family history in all patients to detect a familial history of adverse responses to anesthetics. Malignant pyrexia in a patient at risk because of a positive family history can be avoided by use of anesthetic techniques which do not rely on muscle relaxants or halogenated inhalation anesthetics. Management of the condition once it has been triggered depends on prompt recognition based on a high level of suspicion when patients respond atypically to succinylcholine, plus routine monitoring of body temperature, followed by immediate and aggressive physical measures to lower temperature as rapidly as possible. Pharmacologic treatment of malignant hyperpyrexia previously rested upon the uncertain benefits of intravenous procainamide. More promising is dantrolene, a drug currently under investigation but not yet commercially available for this purpose in an intravenous form.

The duration of action of muscle relaxants is altered by a number of clinically important conditions. In the case of succinylcholine, duration may be prolonged when, following continuous infusion of dilute solutions of succinylcholine to maintain surgical relaxation for long periods of time, the block has changed from depolarizing to nondepolarizing in character. Prolonged apnea is also observed in rare patients suffering from a genetically transmitted abnormal form of pseudocholinesterase incapable of metabolizing succinylcholine and other esterases as rapidly as normal. Prolonged apnea due to lack of pseudocholinesterase may be diagnosed by determination of plasma pseudocholinesterase levels. This is a test so difficult to perform as to preclude its routine use to screen for susceptible patients and to preclude most routine laboratory measurement of pseudocholinesterase activity in cases of prolonged apnea suspected as being of this origin. Treatment of prolonged apnea due to pseudocholinesterase insufficiency is mainly expectant. Artificial ventilation, together with monitoring of blood-gas tensions and twitch responses of muscles to indirect electrical stimulation, should be maintained for hours if necessary until such amounts of pseudocholinesterase as are present have been able to metabolize the succinylcholine. Transfusions of plasma or whole blood containing normal amounts of pseudocholinesterase should be reserved for rare instances in which little or no metabolism is effected after many hours.

In the case of nondepolarizing relaxants, prolongation of action can be observed in patients suffering from water intoxication or other abnormalities of electrolyte balance, especially calcium, and in patients given certain antibiotics, e.g., neomycin. The most frequent causes of prolonged apnea following muscle relaxants remain, however, not lack of pseudocholinesterase, electrolyte abnormalities, or antibiotics, but rather residual effects of inhalation anesthetics or narcotics, especially when combined with hyperventilation to the point where arterial carbon dioxide tensions have been reduced to below the apneic threshold.

Since the duration of action of muscle relaxants can and usually does exceed the duration of an operation, even in normal patients, the question is frequently raised whether the relaxants should be pharmacologically reversed at the conclusion of anesthesia. Only neuromuscular blocks of the nondepolarizing type seen after curare or pancuronium are susceptible to reversal. They can be safely and effectively reversed by the intravenous administration of an anticholinesterase such as neostigmine (Prostigmin). Neostigmine administration must always be accompanied by injection of atropine or a similar compound in amounts adequate to block the muscarinic stimulation and profound bradycardia otherwise produced by anticholinesterases. Atropine in doses of 1.5 to 2.0 mg intravenously is required for this purpose. Neostigmine should not, however, be routinely given to all patients at the conclusion of anesthesia during which nondepolarizing relaxants have been administered. The magnitude of neuromuscular blockade must first be measured to ascertain whether prolonged apnea or relaxation is due to residual effects of relaxants or to other factors. If the existence of significant impairment of neuromuscular transmission is established, the susceptibility of the blockade to anticholinesterases must then be established. Persisting depolarizing block from succinylcholine, for example, must be proved absent. This requires that tests be performed to obtain objective data on the function of the patient's muscle. One such test involves evaluation of the ability of the patient to lift the head and to maintain his head off the pillow for at least 30 seconds. This test requires a level of cooperation and motivation often lacking in a patient recovering from anesthesia while still on the operating table. The ability to lift the head may furthermore not always give an accurate indication of the status of the muscles of respiration. Different muscle groups not only have different sensitivities to muscle relaxants but also recover from their effects at different rates. The same limitations apply to hand grip as a measure of normal muscle function. More reliable are measurements of tidal volume and maximum inspiratory capacity, using a ventilation meter attached to an endotracheal tube. Equally useful is measurement of the patient's ability to generate at least 20 cm negative pressure during inhalation when ventilation is momentarily obstructed.

The most reliable means for determining the magnitude of neuromuscular blockade following muscle relaxants, as well as for defining the type of blockade, is electrical stimulation of a peripheral motor nerve (often the ulnar) while observing the response of peripheral muscle(s). This not only gives information of value in determining when muscle relaxants should be reversed at the conclusion of anesthesia but also provides an important means of monitoring the degree of paralysis during the course of anesthesia and operation and thus contributing to maintenance of constant intraoperative levels of surgical relaxation, while avoiding the dangers of relaxant overdosage. Three responses to electrical stimuli are evaluated: the magnitude of response to a single electrical stimulus; the ability to maintain contraction during tetanic stimulation; and the presence or absence of posttetanic facilitation. The resulting information defines whether a neuromuscular blockade is present and, if it is, whether it can be reversed by neostigmine. To be most accurate, these measurements should include recorded tracings of muscle responses. This technique of nerve stimulation cannot, however, quantitate percentage of recovery of normal neuromuscular transmission unless control data have been recorded prior to administration of relaxants. The problem of control observations can be solved by use of train-of-four stimuli, a technique also of value for monitoring intraoperative relaxant requirements. The ratio between the magnitude of response to the fourth of four stimuli and the magnitude of response to the first stimulus gives perhaps the most accurate appraisal of return to normal function of previously paralyzed muscles. The major disadvantages of the train-of-four technique are that it, too, gives information on function of hand muscles, not muscles of respiration; that it involves paper write-out of motor twitches to measure the ratios involved; and that it requires precise positioning of the wrist and hand.

REGIONAL ANESTHESIA

Regional anesthesia has the advantage of producing nonexplosive maximal sensory anesthesia and profound muscular relaxation without profound physiologic effects, *provided that the extent of anesthesia is limited*. The disadvantages of regional anesthesia include the fact that if it is extensive, the resultant physiologic trespass may be greater than during well-administered general anesthesia. For example, the regional anesthesia necessary for a gastrectomy is associated with physiologic changes more profound and potentially more dangerous than the changes accompanying a well-administered general anesthetic for the same operation. On the other hand, the physiologic disturbance associated with regional anesthesia for an operation such as hemorrhoidectomy is considerably less than that associated with general anesthesia for this procedure. The difference between the effects of extensive regional anesthesia and regional anesthesia limited in area is frequently unrecognized or forgotten but is one of the major considerations in evaluating the usefulness of this method. The inherent limitations of regional anesthesia relate both to the anesthetist and to the surgeon. For regional anesthesia to be smooth and successful, the anesthetist must have extensive experience and be highly skilled. Errors of omission or commission during regional anesthesia not only are dangerous but are immediately (and painfully) apparent to all. The surgeon operating with regional anesthesia must be gentle and silent to realize its full benefits.

Spinal Anesthesia

Spinal anesthesia consists of the injection of a local anesthetic into the subarachnoid space. The resulting anesthesia of somatic motor and sensory fibers is its raison d'être, but from a physiologic point of view the most important result of spinal anesthesia is the concurrent blocking of preganglionic sympathetic fibers. Almost all the profound physiologic changes which may be associated with spinal anesthesia are due to the effects of the sympathetic denervation. The sensory denervation produced by spinal anesthesia has little or no physiologic effect. The somatic motor denervation also has little physiologic effect, despite theories that somatic motor paralysis causes venous pooling, with a decrease in cardiac output. Succinylcholine is not associated with such changes, though the muscle relaxation is as profound as with spinal anesthesia. The physiologic effects of spinal anesthesia are also not due to any hypothetic ascent of the local anesthetic agent intracranially into the ventricular system to cause a direct depression of the vasomotor or respiratory centers.

Since the sympathetic nervous system block of spinal anesthesia is such an important determinant of the physiologic response to anesthesia, there are three aspects which deserve special emphasis. The first is that different types of nerve fibers are blocked by different concentrations of local anesthetic, smaller nerve fibers being blocked by lower concentrations of local anesthetic than larger fibers. The largest fibers in the human subarachnoid space being somatic motor fibers, these are the most resistant to local anesthetics. The next smaller fibers are somatic sensory fibers. The smallest fibers are the preganglionic fibers. These are blocked by concentrations of local anesthetic which have no effect on either sensory or motor nerve roots. Because the concentration of local anesthetic within the subarachnoid space decreases as the distance from the site of injection increases, a point is reached at which the concentration of local anesthetic in spinal fluid is no longer adequate to block somatic sensory fibers even though it is adequate to block sympathetic fibers. As a result, the sympathetic denervation of spinal anesthesia extends an average of two spinal segments beyond the level made anesthetic to pinprick. The physiologic response to spinal anesthesia may therefore be more profound than indicated by the extent of sensory denervation, especially if, as is sometimes the case, the zone of differential block extends beyond the usual two spinal segments to as much as six spinal segments. For the same reason, the level of somatic motor block during spinal anesthesia extends approximately two spinal segments below (i.e., caudal to) the level made anesthetic to pinprick. This is one reason why it is possible to have sensory anesthesia adequate for skin incision during appendectomy performed under spinal anesthesia without adequate muscular relaxation. The zone of differential anesthesia involving sympathetic, sensory, and

motor nerves also explains why phrenic paralysis rarely occurs even during high spinal anesthesias, including those with cervical sensory levels.

The second factor concerning the sympathetic denervation associated with spinal anesthesia is related to the fact that the highest (i.e., most cephalad) preganglionic sympathetic fiber arises at the T_1 level. Because sympathetic block extends approximately two spinal segments higher than sensory block, complete sympathetic denervation will be present in patients who have spinal anesthesia with a sensory level at approximately T_3. In other words, spinal anesthesia with high sensory levels is associated with the physiologic changes inherent in total sympathetic denervation. As a corollary, since the vast majority of the physiologic effects of spinal anesthesia are due to the concurrent sympathetic block and since the sympathetic block is complete with sensory levels to T_3, the physiologic response to cervical levels of anesthesia is no greater than to high thoracic levels. A patient with a sensory block to the T_3 level has essentially the same physiologic response as a patient with a sensory level at C_5 or C_6.

The third important aspect of sympathetic block produced by spinal anesthesia relates to the fact that each preganglionic sympathetic fiber, after penetrating the dura and entering the paravertebral sympathetic chain, ascends and descends in the chain, synapsing with a number of postganglionic fibers which are distributed to the periphery in a nonsegmental fashion. A single preganglionic fiber may synapse with as many as 18 postganglionic fibers. Stimulation (or block) of a single preganglionic fiber accordingly produces a diffuse peripheral response extending over a large number of peripheral segmental dermatomes, a response which is not limited to the peripheral segmental dermatome corresponding to the spinal segmental level at which the sympathetic fiber was stimulated (or blocked). Therefore, the sympathetic response to spinal anesthesia may be surprisingly extensive peripherally.

Just as the sympathetic blocking of spinal anesthesia is the most important determinant of the physiologic response, the cardiovascular changes resulting from the sympathetic blocking represent the most important physiologic alteration during this type of anesthesia.

The sympathetic denervation produces peripheral arterial and arteriolar vasodilatation. In the presence of a fixed cardiac output, the resulting decrease in peripheral vascular resistance produces a decrease in mean arterial pressure. The decrease in resistance is, however, relatively modest, amounting to 12 to 15 percent even in the presence of a total sympathetic denervation. It also is limited because peripheral vascular resistance is not eliminated by the denervation. The major site of resistance is merely shifted more peripherally, and there is still resistance to flow through the postarteriolar capillary circulation. In the normal individual, approximately 60 percent of the total peripheral vascular resistance arises at the arteriolar level, approximately 40 percent arising at the postarteriolar level. Following sympathetic denervation, approximately 40 percent of the resistance is at the arteriolar level, and 60 percent at the postarteriolar level. Even maximal vasodilatation on the arterial side of the circulation does not eliminate resistance to flow at the tissue level. Since total peripheral vascular resistance decreases so modestly during even high levels of spinal anesthesia, arterial and arteriolar vasodilatation cannot be accepted as the cause of severe arterial hypotension during spinal anesthesia. A 10 to 15 percent decrease in systolic pressure during spinal anesthesia can be ascribed to a decrease in peripheral resistance, but the severe degrees of hypotension must be ascribed to another cause, a decreased cardiac output.

From a cardiovascular point of view the most important result of the sympathetic denervation of spinal anesthesia is the effect on venous circulation. Because veins are innervated by the sympathetic nervous system, spinal anesthesia also results in venodilatation in the denervated areas. There is, however, a major difference between the sympathetic denervation produced on the venous side of the circulation and that produced on the arterial side. Although vasodilatation is not maximal following denervation on the arterial side of the circulation, it can be and often is maximal on the venous side. The smooth muscle in the arterial side of the circulation and in the postarteriolar bed maintains a considerable degree of autonomous tone after removal of its sympathetic nervous supply, with the result that sympathectomy is rarely associated with maximal vasodilatation. There is little or no autonomous tone in veins, however, after their sympathetic denervation. Whether or not a vein is dilated following sympathetic denervation depends primarily upon the effects of gravity. If the sympathectomized vein is below the level of the right atrium, gravity causes the blood to pool in the dependent vein and venodilatation becomes maximal. On the other hand, if the sympathectomized vein is above the level of the right atrium, gravity causes the blood to drain out, and essentially no venodilatation occurs.

If a significant degree of peripheral venodilatation occurs during spinal anesthesia because the patient is in a position in which the greater part of the denervated peripheral circulation is below the level of the right side of the heart (e.g., in the head-up position), there will be a pronounced decrease in venous return to the right side of the heart and resultant decrease in cardiac output. This in turn will cause a severe arterial hypotension. Decreases in cardiac output, including those great enough to lead to cardiac arrest, during spinal anesthesia are almost always consequent to significant decreases in venous return to the right side of the heart.

The most frequent cause of impaired venous return to the heart during spinal anesthesia is the head-up position. The second most frequent cause is administration of spinal anesthetic to a patient with decreased blood volume. Since the safety of spinal anesthesia is related to maintenance of an adequate arterial blood pressure and cardiac output and since these are related to maintenance of normal venous return to the right side of the heart, the head-up position should be employed only very cautiously during high levels of anesthesia. Of course, this position should be employed to regulate the level of anesthesia when hyperbaric spinal solutions are being used, but if severe hypotension ensues or if an inadvertently high level of anesthesia is obtained, there should be no hesitation about putting the patient in the head-down position in order to assure adequate venous return and cardiac output. The head-down position may result in a higher level of anesthesia, but it will not result in cardiac arrest. Injudicious use of the head-up position during spinal anesthesia, under the misapprehension that limiting the spread of the anesthetic is the primary consideration, constitutes the major cause of cardiac arrest during spinal anesthesia.

Respiratory function during spinal anesthesia remains normal even during high levels of sensory block. The intercostal paralysis accompanying a high spinal anesthetic is compensated for by the diaphragm, especially in the presence of a relaxed abdominal musculature so that arterial carbon dioxide and oxygen tensions remain within normal limits. This occurs even during cervical sensory levels of anesthesia, because the phrenic nerves are highly resistant to the effects of local anesthetics. Respiratory arrest can occur during spinal anesthesia, but the most frequent cause is not phrenic paralysis but a centrally induced apnea consequent to decreases in cardiac output great enough to result in ischemic medullary paralysis. The association between respiratory arrest and cardiac output is exemplified by the fact that the vast majority of respiratory arrests during spinal anesthesia immediately precede or follow cardiac arrest. Furthermore, once resuscitation has restored cardiac output, the patient usually exhibits spontaneous respiration. Respiratory arrest due to phrenic paralysis during spinal anesthesia undoubtedly can occur, but it is infrequent and only exceptionally the cause of apnea. Misguided attempts to avoid respiratory arrest by use of the head-up position lead to more cardiac and respiratory arrests than does judicious use of the head-down position. Even if apnea due to phrenic paralysis were to occur during spinal anesthesia, artificial means of ventilation are today such a standard part of every anesthetist's armamentarium that no harm will result. The same cannot be said for artificial means of maintaining cardiac output.

It is apparent from the above that the physiologic effects of high levels of spinal anesthesia are inevitably greater than with low levels of anesthesia. The difference in physiologic responses to high and low levels of spinal anesthesia is so great that from a practical and clinical point of view the two techniques should not be considered together. The advantage of low levels of spinal anesthesia is that profound sensory and muscular denervation can be achieved with relatively little other physiologic change. This is especially advantageous in patients with concurrent disease involving the cardiovascular or respiratory systems. The same cannot be said for high levels of anesthesia. The patient for whom a low spinal anesthesia is indicated during repair of an inguinal hernia because of concurrent disease, for example, is often the one for whom spinal anesthesia during cholecystectomy or gastrectomy is contraindicated because of concurrent disease. In modern practice there are few indications for the use of spinal anesthesia for surgical procedures above the level of the umbilicus, as the resulting total or near-total sympathetic denervation is too great a price to pay.

One potential drawback to spinal anesthesia is the association of the technique with postoperative headaches.

So-called "spinal headaches" are especially frequent in the younger age groups and in females, the highest incidence being in obstetric patients. Although all the etiologic factors producing headaches following spinal anesthesia have not yet been completely defined, it has been demonstrated that the incidence of headache is related to the size of the needle used to perform the lumbar puncture. The use of 18-gauge needles is associated with postspinal headaches in as many as 20 percent of patients. On the other hand, the routine use of 24- or 25-gauge spinal needles is associated with postspinal headaches in less than 2 percent of patients. If a spinal headache does occur, it should be treated conservatively with hydration (by intravenous routes if necessary) plus mild analgesics. If the headache is severe or if imminent discharge from the hospital indicates more radical therapy, injection of 8 to 10 ml of the patient's own blood (freshly and aseptically obtained) into the lumbar epidural space will usually produce prompt and permanent relief of the headache.

In modern practice the risk of possible neurologic complications from spinal anesthesia is more potential than actual. It is now apparent that the vast majority of neurologic complications associated with spinal anesthesia are the result of chemical contamination of the material being injected into the subarachnoid space. If the contaminating material is injected in a high concentration or if it is a strongly neurolytic substance such as alcohol or phenol, the resulting neurologic damage may be a chemical transverse myelitis which appears immediately and is irreversible. This is most frequently due to mistaken identification of ampules used to produce spinal anesthesia. On the other hand, if the contaminating material is injected in low concentrations or is only weakly neurolytic, the resultant neurologic deficit is more often a chronic adhesive arachnoiditis which may not become apparent for days or even weeks after the anesthesia but which, once it appears, progresses inexorably as the arachnoiditis spreads cephalad from the site of the injection. Since chemical contamination constitutes the most frequent single cause of neurologic complications associated with spinal anesthesia, the spinal set and drugs used should be not only bacteriologically sterile—a condition readily achieved by autoclaving—but also chemically sterile and free of all pyrogens and other contaminating substances, a condition achieved only by meticulously detailed preparation techniques. Not all neurologic deficits following spinal anesthesia are due to the anesthetic techniques. While the risk of neurologic or other complications with spinal anesthetics is negligible, it does exist. However, the risk of neurologic deficits following spinal anesthesia for operations on the lower extremities and perineum may well be less in the long run than that involved in the use of general anesthesia for such procedures.

Efficiency and safety in spinal anesthesia are best achieved by relying upon one or two local anesthetics (one of long, one of short duration) and regulating their spread in the subarachnoid space solely by changing the position of the patient, keeping constant the specific gravity of the solution injected. A satisfactory local anesthetic of proved safety for spinal anesthesia is 1% tetracaine (Pontocaine).

When mixed with equal volumes of 10% dextrose, a hyperbaric solution is achieved. The dosage of tetracaine will vary with the size of the patient and the extent and duration of anesthesia required but should not exceed 18 mg. The duration of tetracaine spinal anesthesia may safely be approximately doubled by the addition of 0.3 to 0.5 mg epinephrine.

Epidural Anesthesia

The physiologic response produced by the injection of local anesthetic agent into the epidural space is similar to that associated with spinal anesthesia in that sympathetic denervation is produced. But differences exist in the responses to the two techniques: First, the large amounts of local anesthetic agent used to produce epidural anesthesia may be absorbed and produce systemic effects on the cardiovascular system which add to the effects of the sympathetic block. The small amounts of local anesthetic employed in spinal anesthesia, on the other hand, produce no systemic effects. The physiologic response to epidural anesthesia also may be altered if epinephrine is injected with the anesthetic into the epidural space to prolong the duration of anesthesia. Epinephrine, even when administered in the pharmacologically ideal concentration of 1:200,000, can have peripheral systemic effects, whereas vasoconstrictors used intrathecally during spinal anesthesia are unassociated with such systemic responses.

The clinical advantage of epidural (i.e., peridural) as opposed to spinal anesthesia is to a large extent a function of the degree of apprehension on the part of the patient, anesthetist, or surgeon regarding spinal anesthesia. The pharmacologic and actuarial basis of a psychologic advantage is dubious, and epidural anesthesia, like spinal anesthesia, can on rare occasions also be associated with neurologic complications. Moreover, epidural injection of local anesthetic involves transfer of the local anesthetic across the dura into the subarachnoid space. Therefore, since epidural anesthesia is essentially spinal anesthesia, it is not clear why one is pharmacologically superior to the other with regard to the dangers of neurotoxic reactions. Properly performed epidural anesthesia does have the advantage of being associated with a lower incidence of spinal headache. But epidural anesthesia in clinical practice does not eliminate the danger of spinal headache, since the needle sometimes inadvertently may penetrate the dura instead of stopping in the epidural space during induction of this anesthesia. In large series of unselected cases, the incidence of spinal headache following routine use of 24-gauge needles for spinal anesthesia has been essentially the same as the incidence following epidural anesthesia complicated by occasional inadvertent perforation of the dura by the larger needles employed in epidural anesthesia.

There are two situations in which epidural anesthesia appears to have significant advantages over spinal anesthesia, the first being when rectal surgery is to be performed in the prone, jackknife position. In such a position it is clinically more convenient to produce caudal anesthesia with minimal patient manipulation and minimal physiologic effects from the anesthesia than to rely on spinal anesthesia, hypobaric or hyperbaric. Second, continuous epidural anesthesia with use of catheters has more to recommend it than does continuous spinal anesthesia when regional anesthesia is to be continued for long periods of time.

Nerve Block

Nerve block, infiltration, and topical anesthesia are advantageous techniques but present technical complexities beyond the scope of the present chapter. The disadvantages of infiltration anesthesia arise from two sources: First, too much is expected of the anesthesia. A laparotomy cannot be performed under infiltration anesthesia alone. Second, the systemic toxicity of local anesthetics is often ignored when infiltration anesthesia is used. Toxic reactions to local anesthetics are the result of inadvertently high blood levels of local anesthetics. They are not the result of allergic reactions or hypersensitivity. The high blood levels may be the result of using total dosages exceeding the recognized safe limits, injection of the local anesthetic into highly vascular areas, or accidental intravenous injection.

Toxic reactions to local anesthetics may involve either the central nervous system, in which case they are characterized by twitching progressing to convulsions, or the cardiovascular system, in which case they are characterized by sudden hypotension. Treatment and prevention of the former consists in the intravenous injection of small amounts of diazepam (Valium). Treatment of cardiovascular depression due to absorption of local anesthetics consists of placing the patient in the head-down position, followed by use of intravenous vasopressors. Oxygen should be administered in both cases. Safe dosage levels of local anesthetics depend upon the age, weight, and physical status of the patient and the speed and site of injection. A healthy 70-kg adult should not receive over 1.0 Gm of procaine or over 500 mg of lidocaine (Xylocaine) within 20 minutes. Tetracaime as a topical anesthetic for mucous membranes should not be administered in doses exceeding 40 mg.

Although nerve blocks and infiltration anesthesia have a definite role in surgery, the physiologic and pharmacologic effects of large amounts of local anesthetic injected into the operative area are often more adverse than the physiologic and pharmacologic effects of a well-administered general anesthetic. Present anesthesia techniques are such that *major* surgery is generally more safely and efficiently performed with techniques other than infiltration anesthesia. This is especially true in the poor-risk patient, in whom the systemic toxicity of a local anesthetic may be unusually difficult to handle. Major intraabdominal surgery under infiltration anesthesia is especially contraindicated if the surgical diagnosis is not definite. The initiation of an exploratory laparotomy in a poor-risk patient under infiltration anesthesia all too frequently results in the necessity of inducing general anesthesia under the most adverse circumstances possible: a poor-risk patient in pain, often with a full stomach, with the abdomen

open, and suffering from the adverse systemic effects of local anesthetics.

PREMEDICATION

The objectives of preanesthetic medication are, in order of decreasing importance, alleviation of anxiety, decreased reflex irritability, and decreased requirement for general anesthetic agents. Mental relaxation and detachment, not coma or unconsciousness, are the goals. The establishment of rapport between the anesthetist and the patient is more predictably able to produce the desired state of tranquility than is the use of drugs affecting the central nervous system. Nevertheless, drugs will continue to be used for psychic premedication. When pharmacologic agents are to be relied upon, those agents should be employed which produce the maximal desired effect with the greatest predictability and the fewest side effects. Evidence indicates that in the absence of pain, therapeutic amounts of barbiturates most frequently achieve the desired state of mental relaxation. Barbiturates, when employed for such purposes, also have the advantage of producing no respiratory depression. This is in contrast with the respiratory depression produced by narcotics in the absence of pain. Since maintenance of adequate ventilation during and after anesthesia is a frequent concern, it is often inadvisable to administer drugs preanesthetically which will further depress respiration. Barbiturates used in therapeutic amounts as premedicants also do not undermine the stability of the cardiovascular system to the same extent that narcotics do. Finally, normal persons without pain do not find the administration of a narcotic a pleasant experience; in fact, they show a high incidence of dysphoria rather than euphoria following narcotic administration. Barbiturates, on the other hand, do not have this effect.

The role of narcotics as premedicants is best limited to two major areas: First, narcotics should be administered preanesthetically to those patients who are in pain or who will experience pain prior to the induction of anesthesia. Second, narcotics are useful premedication for patients without pain but whose anesthetic management is to include balanced anesthesia. In such cases, the preoperative narcotic is essentially part of the anesthetic.

Tranquilizers have been used as premedicants with varying degrees of success. The disadvantage of routine preoperative tranquilizers is that many have diverse and frequent side effects in addition to their tranquilizing effects. This is particularly true of phenothiazine tranquilizers, which have adrenolytic, antihistaminic, parasympatholytic, and other actions. While nonphenothiazine tranquilizers such as diazepam (Valium) and hydroxyzine (Vistaril, Atarax) may not have such high incidences of undesirable side effects, their effectiveness in producing tranquility without physiologic response has not been demonstrated to be superior to barbiturates. The pharmacologic shotgun effect characteristic of many tranquilizers often represents a major disadvantage during subsequent general anesthesia. Tranquilizers have also been employed preoperatively to decrease the incidence of postoperative nausea and vomiting. The antiemetic effect of tranquilizers in such cases is unquestioned, but the incidence and severity of side actions such as arterial hypotension and prolongation of unconsciousness postoperatively detracts considerably from their usefulness. Since it has been demonstrated that any agent, including pentobarbital, which prolongs "sleep time" following general anesthesia will decrease the incidence of nausea and vomiting, the use of barbiturates as antiemetics is often more effective because of their lower incidence of side effects.

Finally, drugs may be administered preoperatively to decrease adverse reflex activity. Since the reflexes causing most concern are parasympathetic reflexes, in particular vagal cardiac and laryngeal reflexes, parasympatholytic agents are the most widely used. When they are employed in proper dosage, the incidence of bradycardia during anesthesia is lessened by the use of parasympatholytic agents. Whether the incidence of laryngospasm is significantly decreased by these agents is difficult to determine, since it is affected by so many factors, including the skill and training of the person administering the anesthetic.

Whether atropine, glycopyrrolate, or scopolamine is employed as the parasympatholytic agent is a matter of personal preference. The theoretic advantage of scopolamine in producing amnesia is offset in practice by the increased incidence of postoperative delirium in patients who have received the drug. When scopolamine is employed it should be administered in doses equal to two-thirds the atropine dose. Glycopyrrolate has the advantage of being unable to cross the blood-brain barrier and so is devoid of central nervous system actions. Of all the drugs used for premedication, parasympatholytic drugs are perhaps the most misused, in that they are either administered in doses incapable of producing the degree of parasympathetic block which is intended or they are administered when parasympathetic denervation is not required.

References

General

Beecher, H. K., and Todd, D. P.: A Study of Deaths Associated with Anesthesia, *Ann Surg,* **140**:2, 1954.

Bodlander, F. M. S.: Deaths Associated with Anaesthesia, *Br J Anaesthiol,* **47**:36, 1975.

Cullen, S. C., and Larson, C. P., Jr.: "Essentials of Anesthetic Practice," Year Book Medical Publishers, Chicago, 1974.

Eger, E. I.: "Anesthetic Uptake and Action," The Williams & Wilkins Company, Baltimore, 1974.

Kaufman, R. D.: Biophysical Mechanisms of Anesthetic Action, *Anesthesiology,* **46**:49, 1977.

Taylor, G., Larson, C. P., Jr., and Prestwich, R.: Unexpected Cardiac Arrest during Anesthesia and Surgery, *JAMA,* **236**:2758, 1976.

Inhalation Anesthetics

Bruce, D. L., Bach, M. J., and Arbit, J.: Trace Anesthetic Effects on Perceptual, Cognitive, and Motor Skills, *Anesthesiology,* **40**:453, 1974.

Cohen, E. N., Brown, B. W., Bruce, D. L., et al.: Occupational Disease among Operating Room Personnel: A National Study: Report of an Ad Hoc Committee on the Effects of Trace Concentrations on the Health of Operating Room Personnel, *Anesthesiology,* **41**:321, 1974.

———, and Van Dyke, R. A.: "Metabolism of Volatile Anesthetics: Implications for Toxicity," Addison-Wesley Publishing Company, Inc., Menlo Park, Calif., 1977.

Cousins, M. J., and Mazze, R. I.: Methoxyflurane Nephrotoxicity: A Study of Dose-Response in Man, *JAMA,* **225**:1611, 1973.

Dykes, M. H. M.: Is Halothane Hepatitis Chronic Active Hepatitis? *Anesthesiology,* **46**:233, 1977.

Eger, E. I., and Saidman, L. J.: Hazards of Nitrous Oxide Anesthesia in Bowel Obstruction and Pneumothorax, *Anesthesiology,* **26**:61, 1965.

———, ———, and Brandstater, B.: Minimum Alveolar Anesthetic Concentration: A Standard of Anesthetic Potency, *Anesthesiology,* **26**:756, 1965.

Fukunaga, A. F., and Epstein, R. M.: Sympathetic Excitation during Nitrous Oxide–Halothane Anesthesia in the Cat, *Anesthesiology,* **39**:23, 1973.

Hornbein, T. F., Martin, W. E., Bonica, J. J., et al.: Nitrous Oxide Effects on the Circulatory and Ventilatory Responses to Halothane, *Anesthesiology,* **31**:250, 1969.

Klatskin, G., and Kimberg, D. V.: Recurrent Hepatitis Attributable to Halothane Sensitization in an Anesthetist, *N Engl J Med,* **280**:515, 1969.

Merin, R. G.: Inhalation Anesthetics and Myocardial Metabolism: Possible Mechanisms of Functional Effects, *Anesthesiology,* **39**:216, 1973.

Saidman, L. J., and Eger, E. I.: Effects of Nitrous Oxide and of Narcotic Premedication on the Alveolar Concentration of Halothane Required for Anesthesia, *Anesthesiology,* **25**:302, 1964.

Tinker, J. H., Gandolfi, A. J., and Van Dyke, R. A.: Elevation of Plasma Bromide Levels in Patient following Halothane Anesthesia: Time Correlation with Total Halothane Dosage, *Anesthesiology,* **44**:194, 1976.

Intravenous Anesthesia

Ali, H. H., and Savarese, J. J.: Monitoring of Neuromuscular Function, *Anesthesiology,* **45**:216, 1976.

Bendixen, H. H., Hedley-Whyte, J., and Laver, M. B.: Impaired Oxygenation in Surgical Patients during General Anesthesia with Controlled Ventilation: A Concept of Atelectasis, *N Engl J Med,* **269**:991, 1963.

Britt, B. A., and Kalow, W.: Malignant Hyperthermia: A Statistical Review, *Can Anaesth Soc J,* **17**:293, 1970.

Graves, C. L., Downs, N. H., and Browne, A. B.: Cardiovascular Effects of Minimal Analgesic of Innovar, Fentanyl, and Droperidol, *Anesth Analg (Paris),* **54**:15, 1975.

Gronert, G. A., and Theye, R. A.: Pathophysiology of Hyperkalemia Induced by Succinylcholine, *Anesthesiology,* **43**:89, 1975.

Katz, R. L. (ed.), "Muscle Relaxants," Excerpta Medica, Amsterdam, 1975.

Lee, C., Barnes, A., and Katz, R. L.: Neuromuscular Sensitivity to Tubocurarine: A Comparison of 10 Paramaters, *Br J Anaesthiol,* **48**:1045, 1976.

Lowenstein, E.: Morphine "Anesthesia": A Perspective, *Anesthesiology,* **35**:563, 1971.

Pender, J. W.: Dissociative Anesthesia, *JAMA,* **215**:1126, 1971.

Rehder, K., Marsh, M., et al.: Airway Closure, *Anesthesiology*, **47:**40, 1977.

Traber, D. L., and Wilson, R. D.: Involvement of the Sympathetic Nervous System in the Pressor Response to Ketamine, *Anesth Analg (Paris)*, **48:**248, 1969.

Regional Anesthesia

Bonica, J. J., Akamatsu, T. J., Berges, P. U., et al.: Circulatory Effect of Peridural Block: Effects of Epinephrine, *Anesthesiology*, **34:**514, 1971.

Bromage, P. R.: Physiology and Pharmacology of Epidural Anesthesia, *Anesthesiology*, **28:**592, 1967.

Covino, B. G., and Fassallo, H. G.: "Local Anesthetics: Mechanisms of Action and Clinical Use," Grune & Stratton, Inc., New York, 1975.

Dripps, R. D., and Vandam, L. D.: Long-Term Follow-up of Patients Who Received 10,098 Spinal Anesthetics, *JAMA*, **156:**1486, 1954.

Greene, N. M.: "Physiology of Spinal Anesthesia," 2d ed., The Williams & Wilkins Company, Baltimore, 1969. (Reprinted by R. E. Knieger Co., Huntington, N.Y., 1976.)

Sivarajan, M., Armory, D. W., and Lindbloom, L. E.: Systemic and Regional Blood Flow during Epidural Anesthesia without Epinephrine in the Rhesus Monkey, *Anesthesiology*, **45:**300, 1976.

Strichartz, G.: Molecular Mechanisms of Nerve Block by Local Anesthetics, *Anesthesiology*, **45:**421, 1976.

Premedication

Beecher, H. K.: "Measurement of Subjective Responses," Oxford University Press, New York, 1959.

Frumin, M. J., Herekar, V. R., and Jarvik, M. E.: Amnesic Actions of Diazepam and Scopolamine in Man, *Anesthesiology*, **45:**406, 1975.

Leighton, K. M., and Sanders, H. D.: Anticholinergic Premedication, *Can Anaesth Soc J*, **23:**563, 1976.

Lo, J. N., and Cumming, J. F.: Interaction between Sedative Premedicants and Ketamine in Man and in Isolated Perfused Rat Livers, *Anesthesiology*, **43:**307, 1975.

Ramamurthy, S., Ylagan, L. B., and Winnie, A. P.: Glycopyrrolate as a Substitute for Atropine, *Anesth Analg (Paris)*, **50:**732, 1971.

Chapter 12

Complications

by **Seymour I. Schwartz**

GENERAL CONSIDERATIONS

Surgical care must encompass an appreciation and anticipation of postoperative complications which may result from the disease process per se, errors of omission, or errors of commission in technique. In regarding the patient postoperatively, any deviation from the anticipated norm for clinical evaluation and/or diagnostic findings should alert one to focus on complications of the disease and also to retrace the operative procedure. It is unusual, although certainly possible, that clinical and laboratory abnormalities may be caused by the chance occurrence of an unrelated disease during the postoperative period. Acute cholecystitis and appendicitis are two examples of diseases which may become manifest during the postoperative course of the patient. Routine care of a patient following surgical treatment includes repeated evaluation of the vital signs, i.e., temperature, pulse, blood pressure, and respiration. The extent of pain in the region of the incision and generalized discomfort are assessed, anticipating progressive improvement. The chest is auscultated for pleural rubs, bronchial breathing, and rales, while the abdomen is auscultated to determine the return of intestinal activity. The lower extremities are palpated in order to detect physical signs of deep venous thrombosis. The hematocrit and white blood cell count are measured at appropriate intervals to assess blood loss and continued infection, respectively. These determinations plus appropriate clinical chemistry determinations should be carried out when they are pertinent, not routinely.

TEMPORAL CONSIDERATIONS. Fever which presents shortly after surgical treatment in a patient who was previously afebrile is generally related to atelectasis or aspiration. Fever may also appear early in the postoperative course secondary to urinary tract infection, particularly if the patient has been catheterized. Fever of wound infection and leakage of an intestinal anastomosis or closure more frequently become evident on the fourth to seventh postoperative day. Hypotension in the early postoperative phase may be due to continued hemorrhage or the effects of depressive drugs which have been administered during the recovery period. Hypotension later in the postoperative course in a patient with sepsis should alert one to the possibility of endotoxin shock. The incidence of deep venous thrombosis and pulmonary embolism increases with duration of bed rest. Wound dehiscence usually does not become manifest until the fifth postoperative day.

WOUND COMPLICATIONS

Wound Dehiscence

Wound disruption, or dehiscence, generally refers to a separation of an abdominal wound, involving the anterior fascial sheath and deeper layers. The inaccuracy of computing the frequency of wound disruption is notorious; the incidence in the literature ranges from 0.5 to 3 percent, averaging 2.6 percent when all abdominal operations are considered collectively. The incidence is definitely related to age and is reported to be 1.3 percent for patients under forty-five years in contrast to 5.4 percent for those over forty-five years. There is a higher incidence in elderly, debilitated patients with poor nutrition and in the presence of significant ascites. Carcinoma is also associated with an increased incidence. In a collective review by Hartzell and Winfield, 22 percent of disruptions occurred when cancer was present, and 38 percent of dehiscences in Wolff's series were in cancer patients. Over 5 percent of laparotomies in patients in whom cancer was found are reported to have wound disruption in contrast to a 2 percent incidence when laparotomy demonstrates a benign condition. Other general factors which have been implicated include hypoproteinemia and atelectasis with its associated coughing, which, along with retching and hiccuping, increases the intraabdominal pressure and puts a strain on the incision. A lack of correlation between anemia and wound disruption has been reported. Obesity is definitely associated with an increased incidence.

Local factors involved in wound disruption include hemorrhage, infection, excessive suture material, and poor technique. Prompt wound healing is facilitated by a minimum of necrotic residue, bacterial contamination, and foreign material. Sutures should not be tied too tightly but should be positioned so that there is minimal peritoneal defect, since several theories suggest that wound disruptions start with a tiny wedge of omentum or bowel finding its way through such a defect, which is then enlarged.

Several series have suggested that the incidence of wound dehiscence is increased with vertical incisions. This has been related to the relative holding power of the fascia. The rectus abdominis sheath fascia runs horizontally, and therefore a transverse incision is in line with the fascial fibers, while a vertical paramedian incision transects the fascial fibers which act as a distracting force on the incision. It has been demonstrated that the pull on the fascial edges of a vertical incision is thirty times greater than that exerted on a transverse incision. A midline incision represents an exception, since there is marked decussation of the fibers with varying lines of forces. In reference to incisions for cholecystectomy, Pemberton and Manax noted no difference in incidences of dehiscence when vertical and transverse incisions were compared in a thoroughly randomized series. When an intestinal stoma or a drain is brought out through any incision, the incidence of wound dehiscence increases.

CLINICAL MANIFESTATIONS. Most disruptions are concealed in the deeper layers of the wound and do not manifest themselves until the fifth postoperative day, although the separation may, in fact, occur in the operating room or recovery room. The presenting sign is serosanguineous drainage from the wound, and if this occurs subsequent to the first 24 postoperative hours, it is virtually pathognomonic. Frequently, wound dehiscence becomes manifest when the skin sutures are removed and evisceration of intraperitoneal contents, either intestine or omentum, occurs. In some instances, wound disruptions remain concealed beneath an intact cutaneous closure and go unrecognized initially, only to become manifest later in the form of a postoperative ventral hernia.

TREATMENT. The management depends on the patient's condition. If the patient can tolerate the procedure, a secondary operative closure is indicated. The author prefers through-and-through horizontal mattress sutures placed superficial to the peritoneum or buried figure-of-eight monofilament stainless steel sutures to approximate the muscle and fascial layers. In some instances, it is preferable to treat the patient conservatively with an occlusive wound dressing and binder and to accept the complication of a postoperative hernia. If evisceration occurs, sterile moist towels should be applied to cover the extruded intestine or omentum, and the patient should be taken directly to the operating room. After general irrigation, the abdomen is closed with one of the two previously mentioned techniques.

The mortality associated with wound disruption depends on the patient's age and original pathologic condition; reported incidences range from 11 to 85 percent. The incidence of postoperative hernia in one large series was 31 percent.

Wound Infection

Postoperative wound infection results when bacteria within the wound multiply, exciting a local reaction and, frequently, a systemic response. Most wounds become infected in the operating room while they are open, but the presence of bacteria in the wound at the end of the surgical procedure does not usually result in a wound infection. The bacterium most frequently implicated is *Staphylococcus aureus*. Enteric organisms are the causative agents when bowel operation has been performed, and hemolytic streptococci account for about 3 percent of infections. Other common pathogens include enterococci, *Pseudomonas*, *Proteus*, and *Klebsiella*.

The reported incidence of wound infection has a wide range. In 1963, Howe and Mozden reported 350 major and 117 minor wound infections following 15,658 major operations. Barnes et al., in reporting "standardized operations," noted rates ranging from 1.7 to 9.4 percent for various procedures. The Public Health Laboratory Service of England and Wales reported an overall wound infection rate of 9.7 percent. In a combined study conducted by the Division of Medical Sciences, National Academy of Science-National Research Council, and reported in 1964, the overall incidence of infection in five participating hospitals varied from 3 to 11.1 percent. Clean atraumatic and uninfected operative wounds in which neither the bronchi, nor the gastrointestinal tract, nor the genitourinary tract was entered and which were elective, primarily closed, and undrained had an overall incidence of definite infection of 3.3 percent, while similar wounds which were either not elective, or not primarily closed, or drained mechanically through the incision or via a stab wound had a 7.4 percent incidence of wound infection. Operative wounds in which the bronchus, gastrointestinal tract, or oropharyngeal cavity were entered but without unusual contamination had an overall incidence of infection of 10.8 percent. Open, fresh traumatic wounds, operations with a major break in sterile technique, and incisions encountering acute non-purulent inflammation were associated with an incidence of wound infections of 16.3 percent. Old traumatic wounds and those involving abscesses of perforated viscera had the highest rate of infection (28.6 percent).

A variety of factors other than the nature of the wound also influences the incidence of infection. Age is a definite factor; the rate of wound infection rises steadily from 4.7 percent in the fifteen- to twenty-four-year-old group to 10.7 percent in the sixty-five to seventy-four-year-old group. There is virtually no difference in sex and race. The presence of diabetes is associated with an increase in infection rate, but when this is adjusted for age, there is no statistical significance to this figure. Steroid therapy affects the wound infection rate adversely. An incidence of 16 percent for patients receiving steroids has been contrasted with 7 percent for those not on such drugs. Patients who are extremely obese also have a more than doubled rate of wound infection when compared with control groups. In the combined study, patients with severe malnutrition also displayed a markedly increased rate of wound infection, but this was distorted by other factors, which, if corrected, cast doubt on the widely held belief that malnourished patients are intrinsically more susceptible. Patients who harbor infections remote from the operative incision have an increased infection rate. The duration of operation exerts a profound influence on wound infection, the incidence rising steadily from 3.6 percent for procedures lasting less than 30 minutes to 18 percent for those lasting over 6 hours.

The urgency of operation only indirectly influences the wound infection rate. The type of closure also influences the rate indirectly. Although 7 percent of wounds primarily closed became infected, 15 percent of those not closed or incompletely closed became infected. The difference appears to result from the greater proportion of nonclean operations in the group without primary closure. When adjusted for wound classification, the infection rate of the two groups was essentially the same. Secondary wound closure, however, was associated with a 28 percent infection rate and skin graft closure with a 17 percent rate. The use of a drain was associated with an 11 percent infection rate, whereas undrained wounds had a rate of 5 percent, but it could not be concluded that the drains themselves were responsible for the infection. Patients hospitalized for fewer than 2 days preoperatively had an infection rate of 6 percent, whereas those hospitalized for periods greater than 3 weeks preoperatively had a rate of 14 percent, and this relationship could not be explained on the basis of other associated factors. The prophylactic use of antibiotics was paradoxically associated with a much higher wound infection rate in the combined series, and similar findings were reported by Schonholtz et al. for orthopedic cases. In contrast, Ketcham et al., in a double-blind study, reported a reduction of wound infection in patients with extensive cancer who were placed on prophylactic antibiotics. In addition, Polk and Lopez-Mayor noted that preoperative and early postoperative cephaloridine reduced the incidence of wound infection in patients in whom segments of stomach or intestine were opened.

The two factors of importance in the genesis of infection are breaks in surgical technique and the host parasite relationship. Two potential sources of contamination are the patient himself, particularly the gastrointestinal tract, and the environment of the operating room including the operating team. Carriers of *S. aureus* in the hospital population have become an increasing source. It has been demonstrated that patients who are nasal carriers of *S. aureus* have a higher incidence of wound infection than noncarriers.

CLINICAL MANIFESTATIONS. In a typical situation about 3 to 4 days following operation, there is some increase in pulse rate, and about the fourth postoperative day, a low-grade, intermittent fever is noted. Usually there is edema and redness of the wound, but the most important early sign is undue pain. In some types, marked thrombosis of surrounding blood vessels is an important feature. Wound dehiscence is usually not caused by infection per se unless the infection is neglected. The diagnosis is usually made on the fifth to seventh day, but this interval may be extended if the patient has been on antibiotics. At that time, the wound is commonly seen as a suppurative process, essentially an abscess. Systemic features of septicemia may be present.

TREATMENT. The most important prophylactic measure is excellent technique. In human volunteers, Elek and Conen have shown that the presence of suture material enhances the infective power of *S. aureus* 1,000 to 10,000 times. Therefore, fine sutures and accurate hemostasis should reduce the incidence. It is generally felt that prophylactic antibiotics do not contribute to a reduction in the incidence of wound infection.

Once diagnosed, the treatment consists of surgical drainage. The skin sutures should be removed and the wound irrigated with saline solution and lightly packed. As a general principle, antimicrobial drugs are not required unless the offending organism is *S. pyogenes* or hemolytic streptococci, which should be treated with penicillin for a period of at least 1 week. Also, patients with wound infections around the central area of the face should receive antimicrobial therapy to prevent intracranial extension. Finally, if the wound sepsis is associated with bacteremia or spreading cellulitis, antimicrobial therapy is also indicated.

See Chap. 5 for a discussion of specific infections, i.e., staphylococcal infections, streptococcal infections, anaero-

bic clostridial cellulitis, clostridial myonecrosis, streptococcal myositis, and tetanus.

Wound Hemorrhage, Hematoma, and Seroma (Accumulation of Serum)

Wound hemorrhage is generally related to an error in
technique in which hemostasis is not accomplished. There
is a higher incidence in patients with polycythemia vera,
myeloproliferative disorders, or coagulation defects and in
patients receiving anticoagulant therapy (see Chap. 3).
Postoperative hemorrhage usually becomes manifest with
a sensation of pressure or pain within the wound shortly
after the patient awakes from anesthesia. There may be
leakage of sanguineous or serosanguineous material at that
time. To control bleeding from the wound edges, pressure
may be applied initially, but if the bleeding continues,
additional sutures or reexploration of the wound may be
required.

The placement of drains in areas of anticipated wound
bleeding is usually not indicated. If the bleeding is trivial,
the drain is unnecessary, while if the bleeding is severe,
it will not evacuate the material. Drains or catheters connected to closed suction are appropriately used to evacuate
serous fluid from underneath skin flaps, such as that associated with radical mastectomy, in order to prevent the
vicious cycle in which an expanding serous collection produces significant bleeding as it separates the wound. If a
large skin flap has been raised, it should be anticipated that
fluid will develop, and in order to facilitate apposition
between the subcutaneous tissue and deep fascia, the
drainage should be effected. This obviates formation of a
serous accumulation, a seroma.

Once a seroma develops, it should be aspirated initially;
if multiple aspirations are required, a polyethylene catheter may be inserted and attached to negative suction.
Prompt treatment is indicated, since the presence of contained serous fluid increases the incidence of subcutaneous
infection. The same situation pertains to a subcutaneous
hematoma, and drainage is required, since the blood
affords an excellent culture medium and also prevents
apposition between the two surfaces.

POSTOPERATIVE PAROTITIS

Postoperative parotitis is a serious complication and is
associated with a high mortality that is related to it and
to the primary disease with which it is associated. Recent
reviews indicate an incidence of 1:1,000 postoperative
cases, and there is a real recrudescence which is related
to the increasing age of the surgical population. The right
and left glands are involved equally, and in 10 to 15
percent of cases, the disease presents bilaterally. Seventy-
five percent of patients are seventy years or older, and the
overwhelming majority have associated diseases. Patients
having major abdominal surgical treatment, fractured hip,
debilitating diseases, and severe injury are among the most
commonly afflicted.

The factors which have been implicated in the etiology
include poor oral hygiene, dehydration, and the use of
anticholinergic drugs. In one large series, one-third of the
patients with acute suppurative parotitis had carcinoma,
and one-half had preexisting major infection elsewhere in
the body. In only one-third of the cases in this series the
acute suppurative process developed in the postoperative
period.

The pathogenesis is thought to be a transductal inoculation of the parotid, and the majority of infections are due
to staphylococci. The combination of poor oral hygiene
and lack of oral intake predisposes to bacterial invasion
of Stensen's duct. The inflammatory lesions of early parotitis are confined to an accumulation of cells within the
larger ducts. The parenchyma of the smaller ducts are
initially spared, but once penetration of the parenchyma
occurs, multiple abscesses form and later coalesce. If the
process continues, the purulent material penetrates the
capsule and invades the surrounding tissue along one of
three routes: downward into the deep fascial planes of the
neck, backward into the external auditory canal, or outward into the skin of the face.

CLINICAL MANIFESTATIONS. The interval between operation and the onset of parotitis varies from a few hours
to many weeks. The patient initially presents with pain
in the parotid region. The pain is usually unilateral but
may become bilateral in a short period of time. Initially,
inspection shows the gland to be slightly swollen, and
palpation demonstrates exquisite tenderness. The course
of postoperative parotitis is rapid and fulminating with
severe cellulitis developing on the affected side of the face
and neck. The temperature and leukocyte count may be
extremely high. Obstruction of the airway may necessitate
tracheostomy, and the abscess may rupture into adjacent
structures of the ear, mastoid, pharynx, or anterior and
posterior triangles of the neck. Parotitis is to be differentiated from benign postoperative swelling of the parotids,
which occurs more frequently in Negroes and may be
related to straining, belladonna, and neuromuscular depolarizing drugs.

TREATMENT. Prophylactic therapy consists of adequate
hydration and good oral hygiene which can be aided by
allowing the patient to take ice chips and stimulating
salivary flow. Prophylactic antibiotics are apparently of no
value.

Once the diagnosis is entertained, pus should be expressed from Stensen's duct and culture and sensitivity
tests performed. A broad-spectrum antibiotic which acts
against the staphylococci should be started while awaiting
results. In one series of 66 glands cultured, 64 contained
staphylococci. In some cases, these were combined with
streptococci, gram-negative bacilli, and pneumococci. If
there is considerable pain and the disease is less than 24
hours old, irradiation of the gland in small doses is indicated. Irradiation may provide symptomatic relief by reducing the secretions of the obstructed gland, but this type
of therapy does not affect the course of the disease as much
as antibiotics or surgical drainage.

Frequent observation of the patient is essential. If the

disease persists or progresses, drainage should be considered as early as the third day. If there is moderate improvement, drainage may be delayed for a day or two, but in no circumstance should it be delayed beyond the fifth day. An incision is made anterior to the ear, extending down to the angle of the mandible, and flaps are reflected, exposing the gland. A hemostat is inserted through the capsule and opened in the direction of the course of the branches of the facial nerve. Multiple drainage sites are thus established, and the wound is packed lightly open. Deferring drainage until fluctuation is apparent is unwise. Stimulation of the salivary flow by massage of the gland or other means is contraindicated, once the inflammatory process is established.

PROGNOSIS. In a recent series, the mortality rate approximated 20 percent, but this was frequently related to the patient's basic disease. However, 36 percent of the patients who died demonstrated active parotitis. In 80 percent of patients treated with incision and drainage the parotitis was palliated or cured.

POSTOPERATIVE RESPIRATORY COMPLICATIONS

Respiratory Failure

The availability of techniques to measure the arterial P_{O_2} (Pa_{O_2}) has focused attention on respiratory failure in the postoperative period. Neely and associates, Moore et al., and Pontoppidan et al. have indicated that respiratory failure is a major cause in 25 percent of postoperative deaths and a major contributory factor in another 25 percent. Acute respiratory failure has been defined as a situation in which the Pa_{O_2} is below the predicted normal for the patient's age or the Pa_{CO_2} is above 50 mm Hg in the absence of metabolic acidosis. A broad spectrum of patients fall in this category; well over two-thirds have experienced surgery or trauma.

PATHOPHYSIOLOGY. Physiologic causes of acute respiratory insufficiency following surgery include (1) hypoventilation, (2) diffusion defects, (3) abnormalities in the ventilation/perfusion ratio, (4) shunting which is either anatomic or related to atelectasis, (5) reduction in cardiac output with concomitant persistent shunt, and (6) alteration in the hemoglobin level and/or dissociation curve.

A variety of measurements of ventilation and oxygenation have been applied, with multiple refinements. Those which are relatively routinely performed will be considered in this discussion. Ventilatory mechanics are evaluated by routine monitoring of the respiratory rate and determination of the vital capacity and inspiratory force. Ventilation, itself, is assessed by consideration of respiratory rate, tidal volume, and, more particularly, Pa_{CO_2}. A frequently employed refinement to assess CO_2 elimination is VD/VT, where VD is the physiologic dead space and VT is the tidal volume. This ratio is defined as that portion of the tidal volume which is ineffective in the removal of CO_2 from the blood. The technique involves collection of expired gas over several respiratory cycles for about 2 minutes and simultaneous measurements of Pa_{CO_2}. VD/VT is influenced by cardiac output, tidal volume, and the pattern of respiration.

The adequacy of intrapulmonary blood-gas exchange is determined by measuring the Pa_{CO_2} and the Pa_{O_2} in relation to the inspired P_{O_2}. The efficacy of oxygen exchange within the lung is expressed as the alveolar-arterial oxygen tension difference ($A-aDO_2$). Factors which influence the $A-aDO_2$ include the difference between the arterial and venous oxygen content; the mixed venous oxygen content, itself, which may reflect oxygen consumption; the cardiac output; the inspired oxygen concentration (Fi_{O_2}); the position of the oxygen hemoglobin dissociation curve; and the position of the Pa_{O_2} on the curve. Abnormalities in the ventilation/perfusion ratio ($\dot{Q}_S/\dot{Q}_T$) express right-to-left physiologic shunt. This ratio can be determined precisely by measuring the oxygen content of the pulmonary end-capillary arterial and mixed venous blood, but more frequently a nomogram can be used to define $\dot{Q}_S/\dot{Q}_T$ based on the measurement of Pa_{O_2} and pulmonary alveolar oxygen tension (PA_{O_2}), as shown in Fig. 12-1. As can be seen, small changes in the $\dot{Q}_S/\dot{Q}_T$ are more readily detected when the patient is breathing 100% oxygen for 20 or 30 minutes. Determinations are affected by alterations in the cardiac output and pH.

Fig. 12-1. Analog-computed relationship between percent right-to-left shunt ($\dot{Q}_S/\dot{Q}_T \times 100$), arterial P_{O_2} and inspired oxygen or alveolar oxygen tension (PA_{O_2}). The alveolar-arterial oxygen tension gradient can be obtained by drawing a horizontal line from the ordinate (arterial P_{O_2}) to the appropriate PA_{O_2} line. For example, when $\dot{Q}_S/\dot{Q}_T \times 100 = 20$, and $PA_{O_2} \times 680$ mm Hg, then the arterial P_{O_2} is approximately 175 mm Hg and the $A-aDO_2 = 680 - 175 = 505$ mm Hg. Note that below a right-to-left shunt value of 30, small changes in $\dot{Q}_S/\dot{Q}_T \times 100$ can produce drastic alterations in arterial P_{O_2} particularly when the subject is breathing high concentrations of oxygen. The curves were drawn assuming a hemoglobin concentration of 15 Gm/100 ml, an arterial pH of 7.40, an $A-V_{O_2}$ difference of 6 ml/100 ml, and a standard oxyhemoglobin dissociation curve. (*From H. Pontoppidan et al., Adv Surg 4:163, 1970. Copyright 1970 by Year Book Medical Publishers, Inc., Chicago. Used by permission. Graphs kindly prepared by Dr. M. A. Duvelleroy.*)

PATHOGENESIS. The major etiologic and contributory factors are conveniently considered under the categories listed in pathophysiology. Hypoventilation may be related to thoracic trauma; muscle weakness; and deleterious changes in the respiratory mechanics, which have been shown to exist for several days following thoracotomy and laparotomy. Diffusion defects may exist in patients who are chronic long-term smokers with consequent intra-alveolar septal thickening. The defects also may be related to the aspiration of gastric content, which is now appreciated to occur more commonly; an incidence of 10 percent has been reported for intubated patients undergoing elective surgery, and a higher percentage for patients undergoing emergency surgery. There is no evidence that tracheostomy protects against such aspiration. Oxygen, itself, has intrinsic toxicity, and when Fi_{O_2} is over 60%, destruction of respiratory epithelium may occur. Therefore, it is preferable to maintain patients with congestive heart failure and emphysema at Pa_{O_2} of 70 mm Hg with Fi_{O_2} of 60% rather than expose the airway to 100% oxygen for a long period of time. If Pa_{O_2} remains low, mechanical measures such as positive end-expiratory pressure (PEEP) or constant positive airway pressure (CPAP) should be used in an intubated patient. Fluid overload with pulmonary edema initially decreases compliance and ultimately impairs gas exchange (see below). Other intrapulmonary lesions which may contribute to interference with diffusion include microemboli, fat emboli, and pulmonary infection. Abnormalities of the ventilation/perfusion ratio ($\dot{Q}_S/\dot{Q}_T$) result when areas which are well perfused with blood are underventilated. Maintaining the patient in a supine position accentuates this maldistribution, and the pathophysiologic consequence of atelectasis is a significant abnormality in $\dot{Q}_S/\dot{Q}_T$. Other factors which alter the ventilation/perfusion ratio are obesity and upper abdominal surgery with consequent collapse of the basal aveoli. Both atelectasis and reduced cardiac output result in intrapulmonary shunting. A shift in the oxygen-hemoglobin dissociation curve to the left decreases oxygen delivery to the tissues. This may be caused by respiratory alkalosis and also from deficiency in 2,3-diphosphoglycerate, which results from transfusion of banked blood more than 3 days old.

It is now felt that the term "shock lung" is inappropriate. Hemorrhagic shock unassociated with sepsis rarely causes acute pulmonary insufficiency. Davis and Pollack have shown that there is no distinct pathologic lung lesion in patients dying of hemorrhagic shock. $Na^+ - K^+$ transport and adenosine nucleotides in the lung are unchanged in hemorrhagic shock, indicating that cellular energy utilization or production in the lung is unchanged.

CLINICAL MANIFESTATIONS. Among the situations which should alert the observer to the development of the syndrome of postoperative pulmonary insufficiency are (1) congestive failure, (2) dyspnea, (3) cyanosis, (4) evidence of obstructive lung disease, and (5) pulmonary edema. Early in the evolution of the syndrome, the patient manifests hyperventilation associated with a reduction in Pa_{CO_2} below 35 mm Hg which precedes any significant reduction in Pa_{O_2}. Ultimately there is a reduction in Pa_{O_2} which becomes more significant when the patient does not respond to increases in Fi_{O_2}. Roentgenologic changes tend to occur late in the course of the condition and may represent the effects of therapy. These lesions are characteristically scattered, ill-defined, bilateral densities. A correlation exists between the extension of the densities and deterioration of pulmonary function.

TREATMENT. This should be mainly preventive and consists of ancillary measures and respiratory support. Antibiotics are indicated to treat established infections, and diuretics are useful in the management of pulmonary edema. Care is taken to avoid fluid overload of the patient, and the colloidal osmotic pressure of the plasma should be maintained at normal level. A difference of opinion regarding the use of albumin persists. There is concern as to whether administration of albumin will result in more substantial and longer-lasting interstitial pulmonary edema. Normal hemoglobin level is also important. Respiratory support includes physical therapy; the importance of moving the patient in order to avoid ventilation-perfusion abnormalities is emphasized.

The prophylactic use of artificial ventilation for respiratory support represents a major recent advance in the management of these patients. The indications for respiratory support have been categorized according to pathologic alterations (Table 12-1). Ventilatory support may be accomplished either through an endotracheal tube or a tracheostomy, since ventilation via a face mask or mouthpiece is rarely effective for more than short periods. Endotracheal intubation is considered the technique of choice when control of airway is urgently required.

The prolonged use of endotracheal intubation for ventilatory support is now gaining popularity as an alternative to tracheostomy. Although endotracheal tubes are not tolerated as well as tracheostomy tubes and it is appreciated that prolonged intubation is associated with laryngeal swelling, 6 days in adults and up to 3 weeks in children are regarded as reasonable periods of prolonged endotracheal intubation. In general, intubation via a nasotracheal route is tolerated better than via the orotracheal route, but insertion may be more difficult. The major advantage of endotracheal intubation is that the mortality is low, the complications are minimal, and the hazards associated with tracheostomy are avoided.

Tracheostomy is now generally reserved for the patient who requires prolonged ventilatory support and, as is pointed out in Chap. 19, may be associated with the complications of stenosis which are generally related to cuff pressure. The introduction of low-pressure cuffs may reduce the incidence of this complication.

In general, ventilatory support is first accomplished using intermittent positive-pressure breathing (IPPB) in which expiration is unobstructed and intrapulmonary pressure returns to atmospheric level. The patient's blood gases are monitored while on ventilatory support, and if necessary the Fi_{O_2} is increased up to 60% to maintain the Pa_{O_2} at normal levels. If IPPB is ineffectual, positive end-expiratory pressure ventilation (PEEP) is instituted. PEEP results in increased functional residual capacity, reduced normal negative intrathoracic pressure with, at times, conversion to positive values, increased venous pressure, and

Table 12-1. INDICATIONS FOR RESPIRATORY SUPPORT

		Acceptable range	*Chest physical therapy, oxygen, close monitoring*	*Intubation, tracheostomy, ventilation*
Mechanics	Respiratory rate	12–25	25–35	>35
	Vital capacity, ml/kg	70–30	30–15	<15
	Inspiratory force, cm H_2O	100–50	50–25	<25
Oxygenation ...	$A - aDO_2$, mm Hg*	50–200	200–350	>350
	Pa_{O_2}, mm Hg	100–75 (Air)	200–70 (On mask O_2)	<70 (On mask O_2)
Ventilation	VD/VT	0.3–0.4	0.4–0.6	>0.6
	Pa_{CO_2}, mm Hg	35–45	45 60	>60†

* After 15 minutes of 100% O_2.
† Except in chronic hypercapnia.

decreased venous return to the heart. PEEP ventilation is particularly effective in causing a rise in Pa_{O_2} and a fall in physiologic shunt, and the greater amount of shunting across the lung, the greater the effect of this modality. PEEP ventilation is preferred for patients with profound hypoxemia, significant physiologic shunting, atelectasis, and high cardiac output. It is particularly appropriate for patients with massive chest wall injuries. PEEP is contraindicated for conditions characterized by normal oxygenation, hyperexpansion of the lung, and low cardiac output. In general, it is felt that the end-expiratory pressure should be maintained at 5 cm H_2O and should rarely be increased above 10 cm H_2O because of the danger of producing pneumothorax.

Prolonged artificial ventilation has been characterized by the formation of edema and deterioration of blood-gas interchange, which is generally manageable by water restriction and the administration of diuretic agents such as furosemide or ethacrynic acid. When there is objective evidence that lung function is adequate to permit transfer from artificial to spontaneous ventilation, a gradual weaning process is required. The patient on PEEP is initially converted to IPPB. Difficulty in weaning can be attributed to abnormalities in blood-gas exchange, pulmonary mechanics, reduction in cardiac output, and general muscle weakness. A more gradual weaning, employing intermittent mandatory ventilation (IMV), may expedite the process. Weaning should be accomplished only with careful monitoring of blood gas and exchange; the pulmonary mechanics are indicated in Table 12-1.

Atelectasis

Atelectasis comprises 90 percent of all postoperative pulmonary complications, but a lack of definition and difficulty in diagnosis has resulted in a wide range of reported incidences varying between 1 and 80 percent depending on the type of operation and the reporting institution. The term "atelectasis" is derived from the Greek meaning "incomplete expansion" but is generally applied to the situation in which there are airless alveoli. Although collapse of alveoli may occur within definite anatomic units such as segments, lobes, or an entire lung, the most commonly encountered variety is platelike and subsegmental. Moersch reported atelectasis in 10 percent of operations on the thorax or upper abdomen and 4 percent of operations on the lower abdomen. Clendon and Pygott found 38 percent in patients undergoing abdominal surgical treatment and only 2.7 percent when operations were performed in areas other than the abdomen or thorax. Kurzweg indicated that atelectasis occurred in 3 percent of all operations, 10 to 20 percent of cases with abdominal surgery, and 20 to 30 percent of cases involving upper abdominal surgery. Becker et al., who took roentgenograms in a series of patients postoperatively, demonstrated that 51 percent of patients with upper abdominal surgical treatment had atelectasis. Three percent were lobar, fourteen percent segmental, and thirty-one percent platelike in distribution. When pulmonary function studies were used to determine the diagnosis, Beecher found evidence of collapse in 83 percent of laparotomies.

ETIOLOGY. The two major factors which have been implicated as causes of atelectasis are bronchial obstruction with distal gas absorption and hypoventilation or ineffectual respiration. The loss of chemical elements which stabilize the lung at low volumes by reducing alveolar surface tension, i.e., *surfactants,* has been implicated.

Obstruction of the tracheobronchial airway occurs secondary to changes in bronchial secretion, defect in the expulsion mechanism, and reduction in bronchial caliber. Subsequent to tracheobronchial obstruction by secretion, vomitus, blood, or tumor material, there is a period during which a change occurs in the composition of gases within the alveolus, following which the gas composition in the obstructed alveoli remains constant until absorption is complete. The rate of absorption is a function of the pressure difference between the gas in the alveoli and the gas in the blood, the absorption coefficient of the gas, and the rate and quantity of blood flow.

Obstruction of a large conductive airway certainly leads

to atelectasis of the distal lung segment. However, there are many observations which cast doubt on bronchial obstruction as the sole or major causative factor in postoperative atelectasis. It is common to find atelectasis at autopsy with no obstructive plug. Conversely, it is uncommon for atelectasis to be accompanied by a definite plug, the removal of which leads to recovery. The excessive secretions associated with atelectasis might be a secondary effect rather than a cause. For atelectasis to occur on an obstructive basis, the obstruction must be complete; it seems unlikely that postoperative secretions could establish an obstruction in so short a time. Also, the fact that atelectasis can be prevented or relieved by hyperventilation suggests that the obstructive origin is improbable. Finally, Van Allen and Adams found that, in dogs breathing normally, bronchial occlusion did not result in atelectasis, and they felt that this was due to sufficient collateral respiration or circulation of gas to prevent collapse of the alveoli. Perhaps the strongest case against the etiologic necessity of airway obstruction is the demonstration by Griffo and Roos that the time course of atelectatic changes does not vary with the varying solubility of inspired gases.

Currently, many feel that atelectasis usually consists of small and diffuse lesions which are nonobstructive in origin and are due to inspiratory insufficiency. The concept of inspiratory failure was first demonstrated by Mead and Collier and subsequently expanded by several writers, particularly Bendixen and his associates. It has been shown that spontaneous or artificial ventilation at constant tidal volumes usually will result in decreased compliance, decreased lung volume, and increased shunting (venous admixture). These signs all suggest a decrease in the number of functioning alveoli and occur more rapidly than could be explained by the absorption of gases due to an obstructing lesion. The changes are almost completely reversible with pulmonary inflation beyond the tidal volume range or with intermittent deep breathing. Thus, atelectasis is thought to occur without airway obstruction as a result of a constant volume ventilation with volumes approximating normal tidal volume, and the process is reversible by hyperinflation. The validity of this etiologic concept is also debatable as evidenced by the findings of Brattstrom, who noted that before and after operation in patients with and without lung complications, the course of ventilation was essentially similar. There was no evidence of decreased effectivity of ventilation in the functioning alveoli nor of impaired pulmonary mixing.

The third major cause of alveolar collapse is related to the surface forces acting at the gas-liquid interface within the alveolar units. Normally, there is a film, surfactant, which has the property of reducing surface tension when the alveolar volume is decreased. Increased surface tension of this film encourages collapse or decrease in the size of the alveolus and makes it more difficult to inflate. Regional changes in the pulmonary circulation may alter the characteristics of surfactant. Clements postulates that deep breathing mobilizes surfactant from within the alveolar cell to augment or replace the aging surfactant on the alveolar surface, maintaining stability and preventing atelectasis.

Many factors predispose to the development of post-

operative atelectasis. There is an increasing incidence in patients who smoke and those who suffer from bronchitis, asthma, emphysema, or other chronic lung diseases. Anesthesia and postoperative narcotics depress the cough reflex, while chest pain, immobilization, and splinting with bandages reduce the effective nature of the cough. The incidence of atelectasis is related to the duration and depth of anesthesia, and although higher incidences have been reported with general anesthesia than with regional anesthesia, when the same postoperative care was applied to the two groups, the difference disappeared. Nasogastric tubes have been implicated because of the increased secretions and predisposition toward aspiration. Bronchospasm is a predisposing factor, but severe bronchospasm is rarely encountered during clinical anesthesia. Congestion of the bronchial walls due to edema represents another source of decrease in the bronchial lumen. As mentioned previously, there is a definite increase in atelectasis associated with upper abdominal as opposed to lower abdominal or extraabdominal surgical procedures. Transverse incisions are associated with a lower incidence of atelectasis when compared to vertical incisions in the same area.

CLINICAL MANIFESTATIONS. Atelectasis usually becomes manifest in the first 24 hours after an operation and rarely appears after 48 hours. There is usually a sudden onset of fever and tachycardia. Frequently, the pulmonary manifestations are so minor that they are not recognized. Early findings include rales located posteriorly in the bases, diminished breath sounds, and bronchial breathing. With massive involvement, there may be a shift of the trachea, mediastinum, and heart to the involved side, but this is not present with the more common subsegmental lesions. Pronounced dyspnea and/or cyanosis are relatively uncommon. Roentgenograms may demonstrate areas of consolidation, but in early cases bronchial breathing is detected more frequently than roentgenographic changes. Determination of blood gases indicating intrapulmonary shunting of blood provides the diagnosis. Characteristically with atelectasis and significant shunting, the arterial Pa_{O_2} is decreased while the arterial Pa_{CO_2} may be normal or decreased. The ventilation is normal or increased.

If atelectasis persists, the clinical manifestations are those generally associated with pneumonia. The temperature increases to a greater extent, and there is increasing tachycardia, dyspnea, and cyanosis. It is felt that the great majority of postoperative pneumonias begin as atelectasis, since atelectatic areas are poorly drained and represent good sites for infection. In some instances, however, pneumonia may result from the aspiration of infected material. Another consequence of atelectasis is the development of lung abscess, which also may be initiated by the aspiration of foreign material, such as teeth or blood during tonsillectomy and purulent material from putrid abscesses in the mouth. Aspiration of gastric contents also represents a possible cause of lung abscess.

TREATMENT. Prophylaxis begins preoperatively by having the patient cease smoking, if possible, for at least 2 weeks prior to operation and instructing the patient in deep abdominal breathing and productive coughing. Postoperative prophylaxis includes the minimal use of depressant drugs, the prevention of pain which may limit respiration, frequent changes of body position, deep breathing and coughing exercises, and early ambulation. Sustained maximal inspiration, which can be accomplished with the aid of a variety of devices, is the most important factor in the prevention and treatment of atelectasis. The usual IPPB units do not have the mechanism for instituting sighing or deep breathing, but manual inflation using an Ambu bag may accomplish this end. Becker et al. reported that the routine use of IPPB with bronchodilator and bronchodetergent drugs did not prevent the occurrence of atelectasis or accelerate its disappearance, once it was established.

Three groups of medications have been applied to the prophylaxis and therapy of atelectasis. These are (1) expectorants to provide more liquid and less viscous secretions, (2) detergents and mucolytic solutions to alter the surface tension of secretions and render their elimination more likely, and (3) bronchodilators used primarily by inhalation to provide increased size of the tracheobronchial tree and elimination of bronchospasm. The mucolytic agents, such as Mucomist or Alevaire, are indicated because inhaled air with a relative humidity lower than 70% inhibits ciliary activity and tends to desiccate secretions.

Once atelectasis becomes clinically manifest, coughing, clearing of secretions, and increase in depth of respiration may be stimulated by endotracheal suction with a soft rubber catheter or the instillation of 1 to 2 ml of saline solution directly into the trachea via an intracatheter polyethylene tube. If these measures are not successful, bronchoscopy may be required, and if multiple bronchoscopic aspirations are necessary, tracheostomy should be performed to facilitate subsequent aspiration.

Atelectasis, pneumonia, aspiration pneumonia, and lung abscesses are also discussed in Chap. 17.

Pulmonary Edema

Pulmonary edema may occur during or immediately after an operation. The increased use of massive blood transfusions, plasma expanders, and other fluids during operative procedures has resulted in an increased incidence of this complication. Circulatory overload represents the most common cause of pulmonary edema. Other factors which have been implicated include incomplete cardiac emptying, shift of blood from the peripheral to pulmonary vascular bed, negative pressure on the airway which increases the gradient between the transmural capillary pressure and the alveolar pressure favoring transudation, and injury to the alveolar membrane by noxious substances.

Although circulatory overload is most frequently due to infusion of fluid during operative procedure, it may also result from the absorption of solutions during irrigation of hollow viscera, such as the bladder, and is frequently associated with subclinical heart failure in those patients in whom pulmonary edema becomes manifest.

Incomplete cardiac emptying may be attributed to any anesthetic, narcotic, or hypnotic agent, since all are capable of decreasing myocardial contractility. Incomplete cardiac emptying may also be due to gross irregularities in rhythm.

Pulmonary edema is rarely the result of this single factor, and there is usually elevated atrial and pulmonary blood pressure associated with incomplete cardiac emptying. Similarly, the etiologic mechanism of shift of blood to the pulmonary vascular bed is usually associated with other factors. Peripheral vascular beds may vasoconstrict, causing blood to shift centrally and result in pulmonary edema. A reflex mechanism of neurogenic origin which causes redistribution of blood from the periphery to the pulmonary bed has been reported to occur during manipulation of the brain and following head trauma.

Pulmonary edema caused by injury to the alveolar membrane is associated with the inhalation of noxious gases or vapors and the aspiration of gastric contents or chemicals, particularly kerosene, which are pulmonary irritants.

CLINICAL MANIFESTATIONS. The initial disturbance of pulmonary edema is thickening of the capillary and alveolar membranes. In the early stage, the principal effect is a reduction in diffusion, and unless increased oxygen tension is present, hypoxemia results. A reduction in lung compliance precedes evidence of carbon dioxide retention in the blood. Bronchospasm usually occurs and contributes further to reducing the compliance. As frank edema develops, a frothy pink-stained fluid appears in the alveoli, bronchi, and trachea, and at this time the problem is one of airway obstruction rather than diffusion. Clinically, bronchospasm and marked reduction in lung compliance in a patient being ventilated should provide premonitory evidence and anticipate the development of dyspnea and cough. A few scattered rales may appear early, but as the process intensifies, bubbling rales and rhonchi are heard all over the chest. The systemic blood pressure is usually raised initially but may be normal or reduced, and characteristically there is a marked tachycardia. Shock may appear with signs of peripheral circulatory failure, and death may occur from asphyxia.

TREATMENT. Therapy is directed at (1) providing oxygen, (2) allowing oxygen access to the alveoli by removing obstructive fluid, and (3) correcting the circulatory overload. Oxygen saturation can be restored by increasing the concentration of oxygen in inspired air. An increase in alveolar oxygen tension of 50 mm Hg, which can be achieved by a 7 percent increase in inspired oxygen, is sufficient to restore arterial oxygen tension to normal, even in the presence of the more severe diffusion defects. Hypoxemia, however, will persist even if pure oxygen is breathed unless the fluid is removed from the alveoli.

Measures to reduce the pulmonary capillary pressure include venous occlusion tourniquets, placing the patient in a head-up or sitting position to reduce the flow of venous blood to the heart, and phlebotomy. Since systemic vasoconstriction has been shown to be a precipitating cause, therapy may be indicated to reverse this mechanism. Spinal anesthesia has been applied successfully in the treatment of pulmonary edema, as has the ganglionic blocking agent Arfonad.

In the intubated patient, IPPB with PEEP or CPAP can rapidly reverse the process. However these modalities must be used with caution, since they may impair the efficiency of an already failing circulation. Drug therapy includes furosemide or ethacrynic acid for rapid diuresis and digitalis glycosides for situations where myocardial failure and lower output coexist (particularly in mitral stenosis) or where there is arrhythmia such as flutter or fibrillation. Morphine has been shown to be of value, though its mode of action remains unclear.

CARDIAC COMPLICATIONS

This section considers cardiac arrhythmias and myocardial ischemia and infarction related to surgery. A discussion of cardiac arrest and the postcardiotomy syndrome is presented in Chap. 19.

Arrhythmias

Although cardiac arrhythmias are frequently associated with operative repair of congenital and acquired lesions of the heart (see Chaps. 18 and 19), they represent a potential complication of any surgical procedure. As the age of the surgical population increases, one should encounter an increasing incidence of these disturbances.

INCIDENCE. The incidence varies and is somewhat determined by whether sinus tachycardia is included in the series. In a recent review, Reinikainen and Pontinen report that the incidence of cardiac arrhythmias occurring during extrathoracic operative procedures ranged between 30 and 100 percent. During thoracotomies carried out under general anesthesia, incidences as high as 77 percent have been recorded. Heart diseases increased the incidence; in one series, in 51 percent of cardiac patients as contrasted with 20 percent of other patients, arrhythmia developed during anesthesia. Kuner and associates, monitoring continuous electrocardiographic signals on magnetic tape for prolonged periods of time, found the incidence of cardiac arrhythmia during anesthesia to be 61 percent. The arrhythmias which they noted most frequently were wandering pacemaker, atrioventricular (AV) dissociation, and nodal rhythm and premature ventricular systoles. Relating intraoperative arrhythmias to type of anesthesia, Reinikainen and Pontinen recorded arrhythmias in 24 percent of patients in whom operations were carried out under local anesthesia. The majority of these were of vagal origin and caused by the occulocardiac reflex. There were also ventricular systoles related to anxiety or fear. Under epidural anesthesia, the incidence was 23.5 percent, and this was frequently related to blood pressure reduction. When general anesthesia was established with halothane, arrhythmias occurred during intubation in 29 percent and during maintenance of anesthesia in 13 percent of patients.

A study of over 3,000 noncardiac cases revealed 2.4 percent had abnormal postoperative electrocardiograms. The majority of patients were asymptomatic, and most of the abnormalities were conduction disturbances. Taylor reported postoperative arrhythmias in about 5 percent of cyclopropane administrations. Buckley and Jackson studied 100 patients immediately after surgical treatment and noted sinus tachycardia in 32 percent, sinus bradycardia in 2 percent, sinus arrhythmia in 3 percent, occasional ventricular contractions in 7 percent, and trigeminy in 1 percent. Arrhythmias occur much more frequently following thoracic surgical procedures, with paroxysmal fibrillation and atrial flutter or fibrillation representing the most common types. The time of onset is variable, 30 percent occurring on the first postoperative day and 60 percent with 72 hours of operation, though the onset has been noted as late as the eighteenth day. Wheat and Burford reported that 20 to 30 percent of patients recovering from thoracic operations exhibited cardiac arrhythmias. The site and extent of the procedure represented important factors. Arrhythmia occurred in 11 to 32 percent of cases following pneumonectomy and in only 5 percent following lobectomy or lesser resection procedures. When the thoracic lesions involved the vagus nerve, an increasing frequency was noted.

ETIOLOGY. Important predisposing factors include the patient's age and the presence of preexisting heart disease, arteriosclerosis, or hypertension. The highest incidence of arrhythmias occurs in patients over sixty, and it has been shown that the diseased heart is definitely more excitable. Other determining factors include the type of anesthetic, the duration of surgical procedures, the need for intubation, and hyperventilation. The anesthetic agents most frequently implicated are halothane and cyclopropane, though arrhythmias occur with all types of anesthesia. Halothane is usually associated with bradycardia and AV dissociation, and when vasopressors are used in combination with halothane, there is an increased incidence of paroxysmal arrhythmia. Atropine also has been noted to cause AV dissociation during anesthesia and in patients undergoing breast and perineal surgery. There is a high incidence of sinus bradycardia during Pentothal induction. Serum electrolyte abnormalities during the postoperative course are contributory factors, particularly acidosis and hypokalemia. Hypercalcemia following parathyroid manipulation or with inappropriate intravenous calcium therapy may precipitate rapid ectopic atrial arrhythmia. Thoracic surgery is associated with an increased incidence of arrhythmias. During the postoperative period, myocardial infarction and pulmonary complications are frequently associated with ventricular arrhythmias.

Postoperative cardiac arrhythmias frequently have their genesis in the preoperative period. Atrial arrhythmias are usually due to vagal stimulation. Other provoking factors are hypotension, hypoxia, and hypercapnia, all of which may cause inhibition of the sinus node and activation of a local pacemaker or reentrant atrial mechanisms. The most important reason for ventricular arrhythmia is increased excitability of the myocardium and specialized conduction pathways. This may be attributed to sympathomimetic drugs, such as epinephrine, and increase in blood pressure. It is generally held that some common anesthetic agents like halothane and cyclopropane produce sensitization of the myocardium, making it more responsive to the catecholamines, thus potentiating the development of arrhythmia. Muscle of the diseased heart is also more excitable, and hypercapnia provokes ectopic rhythm by decreasing pacemaker activity. Electrolyte disturbances, particularly alterations in potassium concentration, can cause ventricular arrhythmia. The vasovagal cardiac reflex has been implicated in arrhythmias which develop during intubation, surgical manipulation of the lung, and operations on the gallbladder and stomach. Positive-pressure breathing mechanisms may induce a high resistance in the pulmonary circulation, reduce venous return, and stimulate ventricular arrhythmia. Specific diseases which have been implicated as causes of arrhythmia during operative procedures are thyrotoxicosis and pheochromocytoma with its high catecholamine concentration in the plasma.

TREATMENT. In view of the high incidence of arrhythmia in elderly patients undergoing thoracic surgical procedures, some have suggested prophylactic digitalization, and others have employed quinidine and procaine amide therapy preoperatively. Digitalization is particularly applicable in patients with frequent atrial premature systoles, while withholding of digitalis is indicated in the presence of sustained or intermittent paroxysmal nodal rhythms. Many have advised discontinuing all myocardial depressant agents, including quinidine and procainamide preoperatively, and withholding all cardiac drugs in the operating room, unless an arrhythmia compromises cardiac output. A bipolar electrode may be inserted preoperatively into the apex of the right ventricle for emergency electronic pacing in patients with advanced second-degree heart block or third degree AV block.

Once an arrhythmia develops, if it is tolerated well by the patient, it may be simply observed, since a high percentage convert spontaneously. In general, therapy is directed at maintaining adequate cardiac output and coronary blood flow. Vasopressors may be administered to maintain the blood pressure while the definitive treatment is organized. If congestive failure threatens, digitalis is the treatment of choice. Digitalis is also the drug of choice in the presence of all supraventricular arrhythmias. For rapid digitalization, 1 mg of digoxin is administered in divided doses. However, paroxysmal and atrial tachycardia with block and nonparoxysmal nodal tachycardia may all be caused by inappropriate administration of digitalis. Although quinidine may convert atrial fibrillation to sinus rhythm, it does not represent the prime treatment in any real emergency. Cardioversion limits the applicability of quinidine to the prevention of arrhythmias. It is also unwise to administer calcium and depressant agents indiscriminately. If the arrhythmia is related to overdigitalization, potassium should be administered as 40 mEq of potassium chloride in 50 ml of solution, limiting the dose to 20 mEq/hour. Lidocaine, 1 mg/kg intravenously administered rapidly or as a continuous drip of 1 to 2 mg/minute, is preferred for ventricular arrhythmias. It has the advantage over procainamide that it is not associated with hypotension. Diphenylhydantoin (Dilantin) is effective as treatment for digitalis-induced supraventricular tachycardia and ventricular irritability. However, it may reduce myocardial contractility, increase AV block, and cause cardiac arrest. Propranolol, a beta-adrenergic blocker, is used for digitalis intoxication and for slowing ventricular rate in atrial flutter or fibrillation.

Sinus Tachycardia. By definition this disturbance in normal rhythm is not an arrhythmia. Sinus tachycardia is caused by increased sympathetic tone or decreased vagal tone frequently secondary to hypoxia, hypovolemia due to blood loss, and pain. Hypercapnia, dehydration, hyperthyroidism, and congestive heart failure are frequently associated with sinus tachycardia. A variety of drugs, including meperidine, atropine, and epinephrine, all increase the heart rate, as does digitalis intoxication. Treatment is directed at the cause.

Paroxysmal Supraventricular Tachycardia. This is usually characterized by the sudden onset of a regular heart rate ranging between 140 and 220 beats per minute. Rogers et al. reported an incidence of 0.2 percent during the postoperative period. The disturbance may be caused by digitalis or quinidine toxicity, myocardial infarction, congestive heart failure, thyrotoxicosis, and hypoxemia. The arrhythmia is more likely to occur in patients with a history of previous attacks.

The disturbance usually responds to carotid sinus stimulation, but immediate therapy is required only with extremely rapid ventricular rates. Depressive drugs may increase vagal tone via the carotid, and aortic sinus reflex stimulation associated with elevated blood pressure and phenylephrine hydrochloride is effective in about 80 percent of cases. Treatment includes cardioversion or rapid digitalization. Propanolol has also been effective in this situation.

Atrial Flutter. While the atrial rate resulting from ectopic stimuli ranges between 200 and 400 per minute, the ventricular rate is dependent upon the degree of heart block which characteristically occurs. The ventricular rate decreases with carotid sinus pressure only to increase again when the pressure is released, in contrast to the permanent conversion of an atrial nodal paroxysmal tachycardia to sinus rhythm. Atrial flutter occurs more frequently in elderly patients with cardiovascular disease and in patients undergoing intrathoracic surgical treatment. Vagal nerve stimulation, hypotension, and hypoxemia have all been considered as etiologic factors. Continued atrial flutter frequently causes congestive heart failure, particularly when the ventricular rate is rapid.

Digitalis is usually effective, and the flutter is usually converted to atrial fibrillation with a slower ventricular response. Quinidine also has been used therapeutically, but only after digitalization. However, cardioversion is now the treatment of choice.

Paroxysmal Ventricular Tachycardia. This is a rare disorder which has serious implications, since it is associated with a damaged myocardium. The pulse rate is usually between 140 and 180. There is no effect with carotid sinus pressure, and there may be some irregularities of rhythm. Ventricular tachycardia may represent one of the first findings in a patient with myocardial infarction. This disorder of rhythm has also been precipitated by hypercapnia and may progress rapidly to ventricular fibrillation.

Cardioversion or lidocaine given intravenously are the treatments of choice. If the disorder is related to digitalis intoxication, diphenylhydantoin and correction of hypokalemia may be therapeutic.

Sinus Bradycardia. This refers to irregular rhythm with

a rate less than 60 per minute. The low rate is normal in young athletic patients. The bradycardia may also be induced by drugs such as neostigmine, quinidine, procainamide, digitalis, methoxamine, and levarterenol. Arrhythmia usually does not require treatment unless there is evidence of reduced cardiac output, in which case atropine may be indicated.

AV Nodal Rhythm. This arrhythmia is usually a temporary disturbance caused by vagal inhibition of the sinus node and may be manifest only by a slow pulse, 40 to 50 per minute. Pronounced jugular venous cannon waves may be noted. The rhythm may be caused by carotid sinus pressure, endotracheal intubation, digitalis, and the vasopressor drugs. It usually corrects itself spontaneously, and no treatment is necessary.

AV Block. Incomplete block is an uncommon arrhythmia which is due to organic or surgically induced disturbance of the conduction pathway. Vagal stimulation, carotid sinus pressure, and vasovagal reflexes have also been implicated as have digitalis, quinidine, and morphine. The pulse is slow and regular, and the neck veins may demonstrate atrial pulsation. If the cause is reflex in origin, atropine is indicated, whereas if the condition is drug-induced, the drug should be withdrawn.

Complete AV block results in a ventricular rhythm of between 30 and 60 beats per minute and occasionally follows trauma to the conduction system during heart operation or intraoperative and postoperative septal infarction. Surgically induced blocks are best treated by a pacemaker.

Sinus Arrhythmia. This is more frequently noted in younger patients and children, and irregularity is characteristically associated with phases of respiration. It is occasionally seen in patients with digitalis toxicity. No treatment is required, though atropine will correct the abnormality, since it is related to vagal tone.

Sinoatrial Block. Either single beats drop out with regular sequence, or there are runs of two or three dropped beats. If the block is prolonged, nodal or ventricular escape occurs. The block is caused by increased vagal tone and depression of the sinus node impulse. It occurs during tracheobronchial suctioning, with carotid sinus pressure, and in hyperkalemia, and is associated with neostigmine administration. It may reverse itself spontaneously or with atropine administration.

Atrial Fibrillation. Atrial fibrillation with its characteristic irregular pulse most frequently appears postoperatively in arteriosclerotic patients subjected to thoracic surgical treatment. In early cases, the ventricular rate is usually rapid, but when digitalis has been given, a slow ventricular rate may be noted. In the absence of failure, no treatment is indicated, since spontaneous correction may occur. In the case of a paroxysmal atrial fibrillation, which may precipitate congesive heart failure, digitalis therapy is indicated. Quinidine or electric cardioversion may be used when there is no associated failure.

Premature Contractions. These represent the most common irregularities of the pulse, and they may originate from any portion of the conduction system. The premature beat characteristically occurs earlier than expected and is followed by a pause due to failure of the ventricle to respond to the next normal impulse. The abnormality occurs in 2 to 8 percent of postoperative patients. The occurrence has been associated with changes in posture, drug therapy with ephedrine and epinephrine, digitalis toxicity, and myocardial infarction. Usually premature contractions have no clinical significance and require no therapy, though if they occur with disturbing frequency, quinidine or lidocaine is recommended unless there is congestive failure, in which case digitalis is the drug of choice, provided it does not represent a possible cause.

Myocardial Infarction

The magnitude of the problem of postoperative coronary occlusion is evidenced by the fact that Master and associates, in 1938, reported that 5.6 percent of attacks of coronary occulsion in patients hospitalized during a given period of time occurred after an operative procedure. The majority of patients who died suddenly during the operative and immediate postoperative period demonstrated coronary artery thrombosis or myocardial infarction at autopsy in another series. The reported incidence for postoperative myocardial infarction ranges between 0.1 and 1.2 percent of all surgical patients, and between 0.9 and 4.4 percent of all surgical patients over the age of fifty. The incidence rose to 6 percent in a group of men over fifty with histories of previous coronary occlusion, and this relationship was more pronounced when the previous occlusion occurred within 2 years of surgical treatment. Eleven unsuspected acute myocardial infarctions were detected by routine postoperative electrocardiograms taken on 1,000 patients in the recovery room.

Tarhan et al. recently assessed the significance of operative procedures under general anesthesia performed in patients who had previous myocardial infarction; 6.6 percent had another infarct in the first week after operation, and 54 percent of these died. Reinfarction occurred most frequently after operations on the thorax or upper abdomen. In over one-third of patients operated on within 3 months of infarction, reinfarction occurred. This rate decreased to 16 percent in patients at 3 to 6 months postinfarction and to 4 to 5 percent when infarction occurred more than 6 months prior to surgery.

CLINICAL MANIFESTATIONS. The majority of cases occur on the operative day or during the first 3 postoperative days, and although infarction has been associated with all anesthetics, the incidence is higher after general anesthesia for abdominal or pelvic surgical treatment. The most important precipitating factor is shock, either during the operation or in the early postoperative phase. The more prolonged the shock, the greater the risk of coronary thrombosis and myocardial ischemia. The electrocardiogram may show ST depression and T-wave flattening with the loss of as little as 500 ml of blood in patients with previous coronary occlusion.

The diagnosis may be difficult, because chest pain is often absent or obscured by narcotics. It is appropriate to consider routinely monitoring patients with previous infarction in an intensive care unit. In the study of

Wroblewski and LaDue, chest pain occurred as a primary clinical manifestation in only 27 percent of patients, which is less than the 97 percent generally reported in patients in whom a coronary occlusion is not related to surgery. The sudden appearance of shock, dyspnea, cyanosis, tachycardia, arrhythmia, or congestive failure should alert one to the diagnosis. The triad of dyspnea, cyanosis, and arterial hypotension requires a differential diagnosis between cardiac and respiratory problems. The electrocardiogram may provide the diagnosis with a characteristic infarction pattern. However, this is not an unequivocal finding, since, in older patients, ST segment and T-wave changes may be associated with myocardial ischemia, and the same changes may be observed with postoperative shock. A study of arterial gases may provide a differential diagnosis in reference to respiratory problems. Left ventricular failure with pulmonary edema is not generally accompanied by carbon dioxide retention, and, in contrast to airway obstruction and alveolar hypoventilation, there is usually a reduction in arterial carbon dioxide tension (P_{CO_2}) and respiratory alkalosis when cardiac failure accompanies myocardial infarction. Increasing data indicate that the CPK-MB isoenzyme is the most precise method for detection of myocardial necrosis following operation. If myocardial infarction is suspected, serial studies, including ECG, SGOT, and CPK-MB, should be done daily.

TREATMENT (See Chap. 4). Preoperative preparation of patients with signs of cardiac insufficiency should include digitalization for patients with enlarged hearts or histories of previous cardiac failure. Anemia, if present, requires treatment, and attention should be directed toward the regulation of fluid and electrolyte balance and hypovolemia. Operation is contraindicated for a period of at least 6 weeks and preferably 6 months following myocardial ischemia or infarction, except in an emergency. During the operation, a broad spectrum of factors which precipitate myocardial infarction should be avoided. These include anoxia, hypotension, hemorrhage, dehydration, electrolyte disturbance, and arrhythmias. The regulation of blood pressure during anesthesia is probably the most important measure in the prevention of myocardial ischemia and infarction. When the blood pressure falls significantly, in the absence of blood loss, the prompt correction of anoxia by adequate ventilation with oxygen and the administration of vasopressors is indicated. Digitalization may be required when shock is combined with heart failure. The administration of blood or fluid is indicated to maintain blood volume.

Treatment of myocardial infarction itself consists of relief of pain and anxiety using morphine and sedation. Relief of anoxia is accomplished with 33 to 50 percent oxygen delivered via a BLB mask or nasal catheter. Suctioning of the tracheobronchial tree may be required to clear obstructing secretions. Shock is treated by vasopressor agents. Promptness in instituting vasopressor therapy will increase the chances of its being effective. Rapid digitalization is applicable in treatment of shock when the myocardial insufficiency may be responsible for the severe hypotension. Digitalization is also indicated for the treatment of heart failure, which is a frequent manifestation

of postoperative myocardial infarction. In addition to digitalization, parenteral diuretic therapy may be used in the treatment of cardiac failure. Some writers have advocated the use of anticoagulant therapy after the danger of excessive bleeding from an operative site ceases.

In 1952, Wroblewski and LaDue reported the mortality attributable to postoperative myocardial infarction to be 40 percent, which at the time was in keeping with the mortality rate for coronary occlusion unassociated with surgery. In contrast, Tarhan et al. and Mauney et al. reported that myocardial infarction after anesthesia and a major operation was more lethal than myocardial infarction alone.

DIABETES MELLITUS

Diabetes mellitus occurs in 2 to 3 percent of the general population with a higher rate among older people. In two series, the disease was discovered in the paraoperative period in 16 and 23 percent of patients. The most commonly associated operative procedures were complications of vascular disease, but in a high percentage of patients diabetes was discovered prior to an emergency procedure. Diabetic patients represent a special challenge during total surgical care, because the impairment of the homeostatic mechanism for glucose may result in ketoacidosis if untreated or hypoglycemia if overtreated and also because of the associated incidence of generalized vascular disease.

PATHOPHYSIOLOGY. Diabetes mellitus is characterized by hyperglycemia, usually accompanied by glycosuria. The basic defect is a lack of metabolically effective circulating insulin. The elevated blood sugar level is a result of deficient utilization on the part of peripheral tissues and an increased output of glucose by the liver. Excess glucose comes from dietary carbohydrates, liver glycogen, and glucose formed from protein and fat. In the course of metabolism, free fatty acids are released and metabolized in the liver to an end product of acetoacetate, which, by hydrogenation, is converted to β-hydroxybutyric acid or by decarboxylation to acetone. The three products are known collectively as *ketone bodies*. In diabetes, the breakdown of fatty acids is increased, and since the metabolism of the ketone bodies is limited, they accumulate in the bloodstream and are eliminated via the kidneys. Glycosuria itself produces an osmotic diuresis which is enhanced by the presence of ketone bodies and the associated loss of sodium and potassium. Evaluation of decompensated diabetes, therefore, includes not only measuring the blood glucose but also measuring acetone, electrolytes, and carbon dioxide–combining power of the serum.

The anesthetic agent may affect carbohydrate metabolism. Moderate elevation in blood glucose level occurs with cyclopropane and halothane; marked elevation occurs with ether, chloroform, and ethyl chloride; and only minor elevation is associated with nitrous oxide and trichloroethylene anesthesia. The hyperglycemia is related to an increased breakdown of liver glycogen and a concomitant catabolism of muscle glycogen with the formation of lactic acid. Also, the anesthetic agents affecting glucose catabolism cause an exaggerated hyperglycemic epinephrine response and an increased resistance to exogenously administered insulin. It has been suggested that these phenomena are related to activation of the sympathoadrenal system.

The stress of surgical treatment aggravates hyperglycemia because of the increased secretion of epinephrine and glucocorticoids. Increased epinephrine secretion results in an increased breakdown of liver glycogen to glucose, which is released into the general circulation. The glucocorticoids also increase hepatic glucose output via mobilized protein and exert an anti-insulin effect by stimulating a circulating insulin antagonist. The effects of both epinephrine and glucocorticoids are offset to some extent by an increased secretion of endogenous insulin in the normal person but may require the administration of larger doses of insulin in diabetic patients.

MANAGEMENT. In the diabetic patient, essential laboratory studies include hemoglobin determination, white cell count, urinalysis for sugar and acetone, fasting and timed postprandial blood glucose determination, blood urea nitrogen, and, in older patients, serum cholesterol determination and electrocardiography. Diabetic patients should have a preference for an early place on the operative schedule to minimize the effects of fasting and ketosis. Preoperative medication should be kept to a minimum, since diabetic patients, particularly elderly ones, are sensitive to narcotics and sedatives and there is a danger of hypercapnia and hypoxia. The choice of anesthesia should be determined by the operative procedure and the preference of the anesthesiologist. It should not be influenced by the presence of diabetes. It is true, however, that spinal anesthesia has little tendency to evoke hyperglycemia apart from the stress of the operation; among the inhalation anesthetics, nitrous oxide, trichloroethylene, and halothane have the least effect on carbohydrate metabolism. The degree of control is assessed by serial determination of the blood sugar and urinalysis for glycosuria and acetonuria. In general, it is safer to permit mild glycosuria and minimal elevation of the blood sugar level in the paraoperative periods, particularly in the elderly and cardiac patients. In the patient with postoperative hypotension, blood glucose determination should be obtained to rule out hypoglycemia as an etiologic factor.

Mild diabetics frequently do not require insulin, and dietary control is sufficient. The cornerstone of all diabetic management is the dietary or parenteral intake. The preoperative diabetic intake should contain 140 to 200 Gm of carbohydrates, 60 to 100 Gm of protein, and adequate vitamins and minerals, and should furnish 1200 to 2100 kcal daily. If parenteral fluids are required, there is a theoretical advantage to the use of fructose or sorbitol, which can be utilized in amounts up to 50 Gm daily in the diabetic patient. The goal of the dietary or parenteral fluid regimen is to keep the patient free of acetonuria and without excessive hyperglycemia. The patients in whom diabetes is well controlled with oral agents should continue the use of these drugs until the day prior to operation, particularly if the medication is tolbutamide or phenformin. With longer-acting agents, such as chlorpropamide, the drug should be discontinued 72 hours preopera-

tively if the administration of insulin is contemplated. Galloway and Shuman stated that patients who take tolbutamide preoperatively usually require insulin during and immediately after major surgical treatment whereas patients receiving chlorpropamide usually do not require insulin during the immediate paraoperative period.

Insulin Therapy. A variety of programs for the administration of insulin have been proposed. One of the popular methods of treatment employs a regimen in which the daily carbohydrate requirement is divided into four equal doses and given parenterally as 5 to 10% dextrose in water every 6 hours. This initiation of the parenteral glucose infusion is accompanied by the subcutaneous injection of unmodified regular insulin in doses equal to approximately one-fourth the dose of insulin which the patient required prior to operation. Urine is checked regularly, and supplementary doses of crystalline insulin are given as indicated. Based on the extent of glycosuria, 4 to 10 units of additional insulin is provided for each unit of positivity. Larger doses may be indicated when acetonuria, severe stress, infection, or marked hyperglycemia is present. The advantage of this method is that glucose and insulin are given at regular intervals permitting adjustment in the dose during the day. The major disadvantage is that inadvertent interruption of glucose infusion may result in hypoglycemia. With this regimen as with others, slight glycosuria is preferable provided there is no acetonuria.

For more labile diabetics and for patients in whom surgical treatment of great magnitude is anticipated, the use of short-term, unmodified insulin is preferable. In the case of the most labile patients, this regimen may be begun as early as 72 hours prior to operation and is sometimes continued well into the postoperative period. Although the caloric intake is generally less on the day of operation, the normal stress of anesthesia and the operative procedure usually more than compensate for the dietary deficiency. Some writers report having employed regular insulin directly in the intravenous glucose infusion, in doses ranging from 0.16 to 0.2 units/Gm of glucose, depending on the magnitude of the stress of surgical procedures and the fasting blood sugar level. Supplementary doses of 3 to 6 units of regular insulin are then given according to the glucose content of the urine. In general, however, the subcutaneous administration of insulin is preferred, since some of the insulin added to a solution may adhere to the walls of the bottle and tubing.

The second basic regimen is directed at patients who are under control with single-injection therapy employing long-acting insulin and in whom a complicated postoperative course is not anticipated. On the day of operation, the patient receives 50 Gm of glucose in 1,000 ml of solution, and at the time the intravenous solution is started, one-half the daily dose of insulin which previously was required is administered. Following operation and return to the recovery room or ward, the remainder of the usual daily dose of insulin is given subcutaneously. Thus, the amount of insulin given on the day of operation approximates that given the day before. On the day following operation, the usual dose of insulin is given in the morning prior to breakfast or at the time of starting an intravenous infusion. Modifications of this approach employ small doses of regular insulin subcutaneously during the postoperative period based on the extent of glycosuria. Supplementary doses of regular insulin are used if there is evidence of rapid deterioration of the metabolic status. In patients who have been treated with single daily injections and who are not under control prior to operation, conversion to a regimen of soluble insulin is indicated.

Management of Ketoacidosis. The preparation for surgical treatment of a patient with ketoacidosis is critical, and one should keep in mind that ketoacidosis itself may masquerade as a surgical emergency. The patient with frank diabetic coma is no candidate for surgical treatment regardless of the indication. Crystalline insulin should be used in all cases to establish control. Following the determination of the blood sugar level an appropriately large dose of crystalline insulin, occasionally higher than 200 units, is administered. A proportion of this may be given intravenously in an infusion of water and electrolytes. At this stage, the intravenous fluid should not contain glucose. Serial determinations of the blood glucose at 2-hour intervals are carried out, and additional doses of crystalline insulin are given as indicated. There is an associated deficiency of dehydration and electrolyte abnormality which must be corrected, and the ordinary patient with advanced coma will require an average of 2 to 4 or more liters of fluid to overcome the dehydration. The serum potassium should be determined at 6- to 8-hour intervals and potassium added to the fluid in quantities of 40 mEq/L administered at a rate of no greater than 25 mEq/hour. Usually the need for potassium does not exceed 80 mEq. There is generally no need to add glucose to intravenous fluid unless the blood glucose level falls below normal. Lactate solutions are contraindicated in acidosis with shock, since the excretion of lactate may be impaired and lactic acidosis may be potentiated. Gastric atony is a frequent accompaniment of diabetic ketoacidosis, and suction is frequently required to minimize pulmonary aspiration. It is usually possible to correct ketoacidosis in sufficient time so that the patient's surgical status is not compromised.

Nonketotic Hyperglycemic Hyperosmolar Coma. Hyperosmolar dehydration and coma is a relatively uncommon syndrome which usually occurs in elderly diabetic or nondiabetic obese patients and patients receiving total parenteral nutrition. The blood sugar level is frequently above 1,000 mg/100 ml, and ketone bodies are absent from the plasma and urine. Treatment consists of large amounts of hypotonic solutions plus insulin. Marked lowering of the blood sugar level may result with small doses of insulin, and it is recommended that a test dose of 10 units be given to determine responsiveness.

FAT EMBOLISM

Fat embolism is one of the important causes of increased morbidity and mortality in patients with fractures and extensive trauma. A distinction must be made between fat as a pathologically demonstrable phenomenon and fat embolism as a clinical entity. The presence of pulmonary fat embolism is a relatively common accompaniment of trauma, while the clinical entity is an infrequent occurrence. The pathologic entity of fat emboli in the pulmonary capillaries following trauma was described initially by Zenker in 1862. In World War I, Sutton estimated that 10 percent of the wounded suffered from fat embolism, and by 1931, 112 cases in which fat embolism was implicated as the cause of death had been reported. Mallory et al. reported that 65 percent of 60 patients who died of battle wounds in World War II had pulmonary fat embolism, and a similar finding was noted in 39 percent of 79 patients dying from war wounds in the Korean conflict. In 1962, Sevitt described 100 cases of fat embolism, 82 percent of which were related to long bone fractures.

There are two peaks of age distribution: the second and third decades, when fractures of the tibia and fibula are most frequent, and the sixth and seventh decades, at which time fractured hips are common. The occurrence of the pathologic entity of fat embolization is correlated with the degree of injury and survival time. In a study of 300 accident victims, 80 percent of those dying immediately had embolization of varying degrees. In those living up to 6 hours after accident, fat embolism was found in 96 percent of autopsies, and 12 hours after a fatal accident from mechanical trauma, there was not a single case without fat embolism. Massive fat embolism occurred in 26 percent of the cases with one fracture and 44 percent of those with multiple fractures.

In addition to fat embolization associated with extensive trauma, the clinical syndrome has been reported in blast concussion, with liver trauma, in burns, in severe infection (particularly that due to clostridia, which mediate alphatoxins that disintegrate fat), in closed-chest cardiac massage, with the use of extracorporeal circulation, and following renal transplantation and high-altitude flights.

PATHOGENESIS AND PATHOPHYSIOLOGY. There is disagreement as to whether the embolized fat originates from bone marrow and soft tissue or from circulating blood lipids. The most popular theory, which implicates mechanical causes, proposes that with trauma there is a liberation of liquid fat and intravasation of fat into the vascular channels. Bone, with its high fat content, vascularity, and rigidity, provides an ideal setting. It is theorized that the thin-walled intraosseous veins are prevented from collapsing by their adherence to the bony framework and permit the pressure generated by trauma to force fat into the general circulation. Supporting this theory is the fact that most of the cases of fat embolism occur after fracture of major long bones with high fat content and also the occasional finding that hemopoietic marrow fragments have been found within the lung as an accompaniment of fat embolization.

The second theory is based on physicochemical changes in the circulating blood lipids. It is proposed that the normal emulsion of fat within the plasma is altered to allow coalescence of the chylomicrons into larger fat droplets with subsequent embolization. This is supported by the fact that emboli may be found in nontraumatic conditions and that the chemical makeup of the embolic fat more closely resembles circulating lipids than marrow or depot fat. Several contributing factors are important in the pathogenesis. These include shock, disseminated intravascular coagulation, sepsis, local pressure, and release of kinins.

Circulating fat macroglobules larger than 20 μ in diameter are the offending elements. The lung usually acts as a very effective filter, as evidenced by the observation of Kuhne and Kremser that 95 percent of patients dying of injury had pulmonary involvement while only 23 percent demonstrated systemic fat embolism. Thus, in approximately three-fourths of the patients with fat embolism the lesion is confined to the lung. The first stage is hypoperfusion due to the mechanical effects of the macroglobules and adherent platelets, red cells, and fibrin plus the chemical effects of released serotonin and kinins. Local lipolysis leads to the second stage, chemical pneumonitis. Damage to the alveolar wall interferes with lung surfactant activity. Pathophysiologically, early hyperpnea leads to a transitory respiratory alkalosis, but combined respiratory and metabolic acidosis evolves rapidly. The cardiac effects are related primarily to the increased pulmonary vascular resistance and, to a lesser degree, to diffuse fat embolism within the myocardium itself. If the fat emboli pass through the pulmonary filter to reach the circulation, they may lodge in the cerebral vessels, accounting for central nervous system manifestations, and in the skin, producing the characteristic petechial changes. Although the kidneys are involved quite regularly when there is systemic fat embolism, they are usually not severely damaged.

CLINICAL MANIFESTATIONS. Although pathologic pulmonary fat embolization is a common occurrence, the clinical manifestations are rare. Symptoms characteristically occur within 12 to 48 hours but have been noted as late as 10 days following injury. The main manifestations relate to pulmonary pathology. Before symptoms become apparent, blood gas determinations may define significant hypoxemia. Tachypnea and tachycardia are characteristic. Pulmonary infection may ensue and lead to augmented respiratory symptoms plus manifestations of sepsis. Rarely, massive pulmonary embolization of fat will result in the sudden onset of right heart failure.

Cerebral fat embolism usually does not occur without evidence of pulmonary involvement. Symptoms which suggest cerebral involvement include changes in personality, drowsiness leading to coma, muscle weakness, spasticity, or rigidity, diplopia or blindness, and, rarely, extreme pyrexia. The cerebral manifestations must be differentiated from delirium tremens, cerebral contusion, and epidural hematoma. The lucid interval with cerebral contusion is usually absent, whereas it characteristically lasts 6 to 10 hours with epidural hematoma and 24 hours with fat embolism. Coma may be present immediately with cerebral contusion and evolves rapidly with fat embolism and slowly with an epidural hematoma. Decerebrate rigidity occurs early in fat embolism and is a terminal event with epidural hematoma. Tachypnea and tachycardia are characteristic of fat embolism, whereas the pulse and respiratory rate are slow with epidural hematoma.

The classic physical finding of fat embolism is the appearance of petechial hemorrhages in the capillary plexus of the dermis. They occur in a distinctive pattern over the shoulders, chest, axilla, and, rarely, the abdominal wall and extremities. They may also be noted in the subconjunctival region and on the palate. Petechiae occur as early as the second or third day and as late as the ninth day after injury and are present in 20 percent of patients found at autopsy to have fat embolism. A counterpart to the petechial hemorrhages is evident on funduscopic examination as emboli within the retinal vessels, and there may be streaks of hemorrhage throughout the retina and macular edema. Renal involvement usually does not produce severe damage, and both gross hematuria and impaired function are rare occurrences. Recently, an association with acute peptic ulceration has been noted.

DIAGNOSTIC STUDIES. A sudden and precipitous drop in the hematocrit is frequently noted and has been related to trapping of red cells and occasionally an associated D.I.C. within the pulmonary parenchyma. It may occur as early as the second or third day following injury, just prior to the onset of dyspnea, disorientation, and the appearance of petechial hemorrhages. Thrombocytopenia occurs less frequently. Roentgenographic pulmonary changes are noted in about 36 percent of the cases, and when roentgenograms are taken at intervals following injury, they are helpful in establishing the diagnosis. The characteristic pattern is that of unevenly distributed areas of radiodensity, congestive hilar shadows, and increased bronchovascular markings with dilation of the right side of the heart (Fig. 12-2). Serial measurements of Pa_{O_2} offer a better index of the degree of pulmonary involvement. The electrocardiogram may reveal changes which reflect myocardial ischemia and right ventricular strain. These are usually noted 24 to 48 hours after injury. The important findings are the sudden appearance of a prominent S wave in lead I and prominent Q waves in lead III. Inversion of the T wave indicates severe overloading of the right ventricle. Depression of the RS-T segments suggests subendothelial ischemia. There may be a right bundle branch block. Arrhythmias are frequent. The electroencephalogram may indicate a diffuse slow wave pattern.

Detection of Fat. Lipuria occurs in the first few days following injury and is usually associated with a serious degree of fat embolism. Free fat in the urine has been demonstrated in over 57 percent of cases in one series. Examination of the urine is simple but must be precise. The collecting apparatus must be free of fat, and the bladder must be emptied completely, since the fat floats and the majority of globules remain in the bladder residue. The patient should be catheterized using a non-oily lubricant and the fluid collected in a volumetric flask. The meniscus may be skimmed, or, after centrifugation, the supranatant is smeared and stained with Sudan III. Deep-orange-colored droplets represent fat globules. Another method of demonstrating fat in the urine is the Scuderi "sizzle" test, which involves placing a wire loop containing the supranatant fluid over a flame and listening for a pop or sizzle produced by burning fat. The fat can be detected in concentrations as small as 1:1,000. The demonstration of fat in the sputum has little diagnostic value, since it is a common phenomenon following trauma. Biopsy of petechiae may establish the diagnosis, and frozen section is mandatory to determine the presence of fat. Needle biopsy of the kidney also has been applied to demonstrate fat globules.

Serum Lipase. A serum lipase level elevation occurs in about 50 percent of the cases, the rise usually beginning on the third day and reaching a maximum on the seventh or eighth day after injury. An elevation greater than 1 ml is significant, and this determination is considered by Peltier to be the best laboratory test between the third and seventh day. The serum lipase level can be suppressed by the administration of ethyl alcohol and augmented by heparinization. Once elevated, the level is thought to reflect the prognosis, and elevations greater than 2 ml are associated with a higher incidence of favorable outcome. In a patient with extensive trauma, an elevated serum lipase level in the first 48 hours is more suggestive of pancreatitis.

TREATMENT. Prophylaxis against potentiating fat embolization includes careful handling of the patient and early splinting of fractures. Vigorous applications of resuscitative measures are indicated to correct oligemic shock, since it has been demonstrated that fewer emboli may be lethal in the hypotensive than in the normotensive patient. There is some suggestion that Trasylol, which inhibits the effect of kinins and antagonizes hypercoagulability, may prevent or reduce the extent of the fat embolism syndrome. High doses of corticosteroids (1.0 to 1.5 Gm hydrocortisone) administered during the first 2 days may inhibit the pneumonitis or expedite its resolution. Pulmonary manifestations are treated with oxygen therapy, rapid digitalization, and intensive endotracheal suction to minimize the accumulation of secretions. IPPB or PEEP are frequently indicated. Pa_{O_2} should be monitored and maintained between 80 and 100 mm Hg. Endotracheal intubation is preferred over tracheostomy, since the latter has been associated with a high mortality rate in these patients. Cerebral manifestations are treated with sedation and anticonvulsive therapy.

Trasylol has been beneficial in several instances. Heparin in doses which do not have an anticoagulant effect will clear lipemic plasma and stimulate lipase activity. A dose of 5,000 units may be administered intravenously every 6 hours. In the presence of acute systemic toxicity or a rapidly rising lipase level, the drug should be discontinued, since the release of fatty acids is undesirable. Low-molecular-weight dextran (40,000) has been administered intravenously to counteract intravascular thrombosis. One thousand milliliters is administered per 24 hours for two days. Ethyl alcohol, which may decrease the rate of hydrolysis of neutral fat and slow the release of toxic free fatty acids, has been used. Presently, this applicability of alcohol is debatable.

PROGNOSIS. Old age, preexisting lung disease, and reduced cardiac reserve have adverse effects. The early appearance of marked hypoxemia and the requirement of persistently high Fi_{O_2} are bad prognostic signs, as is hypocalcemia resulting from ion binding by FFA, while a persistently high serum lipase level is a favorable sign. At the Birmingham Accident Hospital, a fatality rate of 12 percent has been reported for 25 cases diagnosed according to strict criteria (all had petechial rash). While the "pure" cerebral form of the fat embolism syndrome generally has a better prognosis, the presence of coma is a poor sign. Acute respiratory disease usually is self-limiting.

Fig. 12-2. Pulmonary fat emboli. Note bilateral extensive ill-defined nodular densities situated primarily in peripheral lung fields. Patient was in an automobile accident and fractured his femur and two metatarsals. Twenty-four hours after admission fever developed, and 3 days later hemoptysis and mental confusion. Changes were seen roentgenographically on the fourth day after trauma. There were lipid bodies in the urine, and the serum lipase level was elevated. The patient was treated with antibiotics, heparin, and dextran, and the symptoms subsided 7 days after therapy.

PSYCHIATRIC COMPLICATIONS

Severe psychiatric disturbances may occur any time during an illness, but their appearance in the postoperative period is particularly significant. The first account of postoperative psychiatric disturbance presented by a surgeon was that of Dupuytren who, in 1834, wrote that "the brain itself may be overcome by pain, terror, or even joy and reason leaves the patient at the instant when it is most necessary to his welfare that he should remain calm and undisturbed." In 1910, Da Costa indicated that the anticipated frequency for such complications is as high as 1 in 250 laparotomies, while Lewis, more recently, suggested an incidence of 1 in 1,500. Scott described 11 cases in 2,000 surgical procedures. The validity of any of these figures, however, is open to question, since "postoperative psychosis" per se does not appear in the standard nomenclature and is frequently not coded on the patient's record, thus limiting the value of retrospective studies. Even more pertinent for surgical consideration is the study of Titchener et al., who evaluated 200 patients admitted to the surgical service of the Cincinnati General Hospital utilizing interview and the Minnesota Multiphasic Personality Inventory to substantiate a psychiatric diagnosis. Eighty-six percent of the sample had either distressing psychologic symptoms, disabling patterns of behavior, or both. The patients considered were in a municipal hospital and represented a lower socioeconomic group, but the figures of 21 percent having neuroses, 11 percent psychophysiologic reactions, 14 percent psychoses, 34 percent character behavior disorders, and 3 percent chronic brain syndrome are most impressive.

GENERAL CONSIDERATIONS. "Postoperative psychosis" cannot be considered as a distinct clinical entity. No single factor has been shown to be responsible, and the physical illness and operative procedure may merely bring to light a latent psychotic tendency. Both illness, particularly when prolonged, and surgical procedures represent threats to the integrity of the organism on somatic and psychologic grounds. In nearly every person informed of the need for a surgical procedure, some degree of anxiety arises. There may be fear of loss of life, of loss of body part, and of castration as with pelvic and hernia operations. The anxiety signal is assimilated and integrated by the patient in preparation for the surgical stress. Surgical intervention to cure, modify, or prevent illness is the beginning of a complicated and multifaceted process. The psychodynamic processes at work during the preoperative, postoperative, and convalescent periods may be classified as (1) psychophysiologic factors, (2) somatopsychic factors, and (3) psychosocial factors. Psychophysiologic factors represent processes originating from psychologic stress which act along neurogenic or humoral pathways to modify the healing process. A poorly functioning gastroenterostomy or marginal ulcer in a patient with emotional stress represents an example of this type. The somatopsychic factors have to do with the psychologic adaptation involved when the surgical procedure imposes a somatic defect, such as an ileostomy or colostomy. The psychosocial factors refer to the patient's concern with the effects of his physical illness or surgical procedure on his ultimate position in society. All these may interplay and contribute to anxiety, neurotic symptoms, severe depression, and frank psychosis.

CLINICAL MANIFESTATIONS. The time of occurrence of psychiatric derangement during illness is variable, and the duration of latent interval between surgical treatment and the psychologic disturbance may be days to weeks. Winkelstein and associates reported that, in the recovery room, patients who had been subjected to surgical procedures under general anesthesia exhibited a lack of concern about the operation and an absence of affective response, despite the fact that they were sufficiently oriented to be interviewed. After 24 hours the patients responded with these concerns and emotions which were so conspicuously absent in the immediate postoperative period. Both psychologic and pharmacologic factors are implicated in this response, since patients under spinal anesthesia exhibit immediate and overt emotional reaction.

The manifestations are extremely variable. Fear may be accompanied by depression or elation and overactivity. The clinical picture may be that of acute delirium with confusion and disorientation or merely a vague alteration in perception and mood. The manic type of reaction may incorporate psychomotor excitement, delirium, delusions, visual or auditory hallucinations, agitated depression, and feelings of persecution. The psychotic reactions which were observed in 44 of 200 patients in the Cincinnati series are indistinguishable from the range of psychoses observed under other circumstances. The acute brain syndrome, or delirium, was manifest in 20 patients.

Delirium may begin with an inappropriate remark or a dramatic agitated outburst and is frequently the first sign of continued mental deterioration leading to a chronic brain syndrome, particularly in an elderly patient. Therefore, delirium must be regarded as a potentially dangerous situation. It occurs most commonly in elderly patients who have lost closeness and support of family or friends and in patients who are immobilized for long periods of time.

Depressive reactions represented the second most important psychosis in surgical patients and occurred in 4.5 percent of patients in the Cincinnati series. The patient is characteristically uncooperative in an active way, or recovery may be impeded by listlessness, anorexia, and disinterest. The depressive reaction may be accompanied by physiologic changes; Moore et al. have demonstrated the effects of emotion on the pituitary-adrenal axis during the immediate and subsequent postoperative period. Suicide is a major risk in patients with depressive reaction.

Another category includes the paranoid psychotic disorder. Although it is not rare for schizophrenic reaction to have its onset in the surgical patient, no acute breaks of the schizophrenic type were noted among the 200 patients studied by Titchener et al. Generally, there is no contraindication to surgical treatment of patients with schizophrenia. Manic excitement is a particularly difficult problem in the management of surgical patients and requires the close cooperation of psychiatrist, surgeon, and anesthetist.

MANAGEMENT. The first step in the management of psychiatric disturbances occurring in the course of the surgical illness or following surgical procedures is that of anticipation. Although Knox has indicated that the incidence of postoperative psychosis was not related to the duration of preoperative hospital stay, the duration of illness, particularly when prolonged, does determine the patient's psychologic reaction to surgical experience. At the other end of the spectrum, sudden emergency operation often results in reactions marked by acute anxiety, nightmares, insomnia, irritability, and protective withdrawal from all stimuli. Age is an important factor, the highest incidence occurring in children under the age of two and in the elderly patients. In the latter group, this is particularly true of patients who have lost their proximity to and support of family and friends, and who have not developed a close relation with the hospital personnel. Knox has presented evidence of constitutional predisposition, and although 17 percent of his patients had had previous surgical treatment uncomplicated by psychiatric disturbances, 11 percent did have a previous psychiatric illness. Twenty-two percent of patients had a family history of mental illness of serious proportion. There is an increasing incidence of delirium in response to anesthesia and surgical treatment in patients who are alcoholic, while patients suffering from extensive trauma may have organic psychosis. Acidosis, acetonuria, hyperglycemia, and hepatic insufficiency may all cause postoperative mental aberrations, and cerebral hypoxia frequently results in behavioral changes. Medications, such as barbiturates, anticholinergics, and cortisone, also have been implicated.

There is an obvious need for integrating psychologic treatment with the management of surgical patients. As Titchener and Levine emphasize, it is not necessary, possible, or advisable for these needs to be turned over to psychiatrists, and it is frequently preferable that the measures be carried out by the surgeon in charge. Verbal communication between the surgeon and patient is the best means of overcoming emotional or mental difficulty. The anesthetist is regarded as an impersonal distant figure who carries out his task without emotional impact on the patient. The surgeon should become aware of the patient's feelings and attitudes and be appreciative of the effects of these factors on a patient's general well-being. Also, changes to increase the patient's positive adaptation to his illness should be constantly considered. The striking incidence of significant postoperative disturbance suggests the need for "mental check" to be incorporated into the usual postoperative surgical rounds. Efforts should be directed at removing toxic causes of the acute brain syndrome, removing undue stimuli without isolating the patient, and providing psychologic or pharmacologic tranquilization.

The physician's psychologic approach should include repeated reassurance of the patient. In some instances, specific counseling and directive treatment, which may require direct intervention in the patient's personal or family affairs and the assistance of the social service department, is indicated. The best prophylactic therapy, however, can be classified as supportive, in that the surgeon allows himself to be the object of dependency on the part of the patient. This relationship is fostered by interest on the part of the surgeon and trust on the part of the patient.

The provocative patient who emits anger or attempts to irritate others as a mechanism for covering fear or relieving guilt needs understanding of the emotional reason for the provocation and an attitude of firmness rather than anger from the physician. The attempt on the part of a patient to sign out against advice is a mechanism of expressing anger or fear and should be handled by the surgeon in such a way that the patient is allowed to change his mind without becoming embarrassed. In these and other situations, the patient may hide his real feeling behind an intellectual screen. For understanding himself, the patient must bring forth both the emotional and intellectual aspects of his personality.

Consultation with a psychiatrist is indicated in the case of any acute and severe emotional disturbance, and the referral should be candidly discussed between the surgeon and the patient. It is necessary for the patient to come to the conclusion that he requires expert help for his problems. Referral is also indicated for long-standing disturbances discovered during hospitalization and is frequently appropriate in patients with psychosomatic illness. Browning and Houseworth, in a study of patients with peptic ulcer, demonstrated that the removal of symptoms without altering the psychosomatic disorders led to the formation of a new spectrum of symptoms.

Special Surgical Situations

The very young and old patients are particularly vulnerable to the development of psychiatric complications following surgical treatment. Psychotic disturbances have been found in 2 to 3 percent of patients following cataract extraction. The combination of surgical procedure and the awareness of the implications of the illness is critical in the patient with cancer. Because of the high incidence of emotional disorders following surgical procedures, special consideration is indicated for mastectomy and gynecologic procedures, cardiac surgical treatment, dialysis and transplantation, and prolonged periods in an intensive care unit. The management of drug addicts is assuming greater importance.

PEDIATRIC SURGERY

In children, severe anxiety states may be precipitated by the shock of operation. Levy reported that of a group of 124 children who had operations, 20 percent showed residual emotional disturbances. This occurred most frequently in the one- to two-year-old group; after the age of three there was a sharp decrease with age. The age distribution was attributed to a greater dependence on home and mother, and Levy went so far as to suggest postponement of elective surgical treatment until the child could comprehend something about the situation. Postoperative reactions consisted of negativism, disobedience, tantrums, defiance, destructive behavior, and dependency, as manifested by clinging to the mother or attendant. The responses have been related to a feeling of betrayal and the consequent desire for revenge and rebellion. When a child is suffering from fears engendered by an operation, a second operation usually intensifies the earlier fears.

Prophylactic therapy is important. The maturity of the child's emotional adaptation is more a factor in the response than the operation per se. Parental absence is frequently associated with emotional difficulty. Prugh and associates compared two groups, one treated without organized consideration for emotional needs and another in which these needs were considered and ample opportunity for play was provided. Moderate or severe anxiety reactions, immediately after leaving the hospital, were observed in 92 percent of the control group and in 68 percent of the experimental group, with a peak incidence in children under three. Three months after discharge, the incidence of persisting anxiety had fallen to 58 percent for the control group and 44 percent for the experimental group. The youngest children reacted more severely with apprehension, feeding disturbances, and depression. The pattern for the four- to six-year-old group was a tendency toward obsessive worries, phobias, and accentuated aches and pains. The six- to ten-year-olds manifested conversion symptoms, compulsive behavior, and restlessness.

SURGERY IN THE AGED

Elderly patients are more prone to become emotionally disturbed when confronted with new situations, especially if they have inadequate comprehension and a generalized feeling of insecurity. The operative procedure also presents an obvious physical threat to the integrity of the nervous system. Titchener and associates reported a 25 percent incidence of significant and, at times, irreversible change in cerebral function in the patients in their group over the age of sixty-five. Some degree of depression was observed in 90 percent of the older patients, and this was of a disabling nature in about 50 percent. Indifference of the family, friends, and society contributed to the evolution of a paranoid cycle.

Attempts should be directed at limiting the physical insult to the brain, and postoperative mental evaluation is indicated on a routine basis in order to detect the early changes of the organic brain syndrome and delirium. Efforts should be made to familiarize the patients with the hospital and personnel, and visitors should be encouraged to maintain a human contact and prevent withdrawal. Collaboration with a social worker is frequently indicated for long-term rehabilitation.

GYNECOLOGIC SURGERY

Removal of the breast and a variety of gynecologic procedures are highly represented in most series of postoperative psychosis. Hysterectomy is associated with emotional disturbance more frequently than other gynecologic operations, and the more the procedure antedates the menopause, the more the likelihood of associated psychologic disturbance. The loss of menstrual function is perceived by the woman as a blow to normal feminine esteem. Hollender reported that of 203 women admitted to psychiatric hospital, 9 had pelvic surgical treatment as a precipitating event, and this was in contrast to a total of 5 women admitted following operations of all other kinds. Lindemann noted that the relative frequency of restlessness, insomnia, agitation, and preoccupation with depressive thoughts was greater after pelvic operations than after cholecystectomy.

CANCER PATIENTS

The cancer patient is exposed to two major threats, disease and extensive surgical treatment. He is concerned with death or injury during operation and disruption of his pattern of living as a result of the effects of cancer or the surgical procedure. Patients with emotional problems involving self-destruction are particularly vulnerable to preoperative anxiety concerning death and mutilation.

This may be manifest by anorexia, insomnia, tachycardia, fear, and panic. Acute depression with suicidal tendencies has been reported in anticipation of surgical procedures. Postoperatively, depression is related to an anticipated interference with valued activities. Sutherland and associates have demonstrated that colostomy imposed on almost all patients a new order of living, and the subjects were powerfully motivated to avoid social rejection. A rigid life arose from the fearful expectation of rejection because of the colostomy combined with the fear of death from cancer. There is a tendency toward seclusion, withdrawal, and nonparticipation. Spells of depression are frequent, and Sutherland and his associates are of the opinion that loss of an important bodily part or function is more depressing than the fear or expectation of death. The management of patients with carcinoma must be based on an appreciation that they frequently suffer a sense of isolation, guilt, and abandonment.

CARDIAC SURGERY

Serious psychiatric disturbances have been observed to occur with considerable frequency following mitral valvulotomy and open heart surgery. Fox and associates and Bliss et al. reported, respectively, a 19 and 16 percent incidence of serious emotional disturbance following mitral valve surgery. In contrast, Bolton and Bailey, in an evaluation of 1,500 consecutive patients, noted an incidence of psychosis of 3 percent with no relation to age, sex, severity of heart disease, duration of failure, or complications of surgical treatment. Egerton and Kay noted delirium in 25 of 60 adults following open heart surgery.

Manifestations generally occur after an initial lucid interval 3 to 5 days after operation and clear shortly after the patient is transferred from an intensive care unit to a standard hospital ward. Postoperative incapacitation and increased time on the heart-lung machine apparently are factors increasing the likelihood of delirium, while age and sex do not alter the incidence. Zaks has suggested that cardiac operation may produce organic brain damage, thus sensitizing patients and increasing the incidence of postoperative psychologic symptomatology. A prediction equation was successful in differentiating reactors from nonreactors. Using the ego strength variable of the Minnesota Multiphasic Personality Inventory, there is a significant inverse correlation between the reaction and the incidence of acute psychotic episodes following cardiac operation. The incidence of psychoses is greater in males, older patients, and those expressing minimal preoperative anxiety. A preoperative psychiatric interview reduces the incidence of postoperative psychosis by 50 percent.

Following operations on the heart, the patients with emotional disturbances manifest perceptual distortion, visual and auditory hallucinations, disorientation, and paranoia. Twenty-eight percent of adult patients subjected to open heart surgery, as reported by Egerton and Kay, had delirious states ranging in duration from several nights to several weeks, averaging 5 days. The delirious patients had no psychologic sequelae, and no relation could be established between the incidence of delirium and the duration of cardiac bypass, but open heart procedures were more likely to produce delirium than other intrathoracic operations. The writers felt that the precipitating factors for delirium included dehydration, hyponatremia, and the performance of a tracheostomy, while the predisposing factors included a familial history of psychosis, previous brain damage, overwhelming personal problems, and the presence of a rheumatic valvular lesion. Other psychiatric disturbances noted in patients following open heart surgery were disabling anxiety state, conversion hysteria, tension headaches, and, in a surprising 5 percent of the operative cases, exacerbation of peptic ulcer. The almost total absence of delirium and other emotional disorders in children is of particular interest and may be related to the fact that the concept of death as a permanent biologic process usually does not develop until the age of nine.

DIALYSIS AND TRANSPLANTATION

A variety of emotional disturbances has been observed in patients undergoing hemodialysis. The suicide rate is 300 times greater than for a comparable healthy population. Uremia, debilitating disease, and the repeated technical procedures which are performed all constitute etiologic factors. Wright et al. followed 11 patients on chronic dialysis and noted a number of stresses affecting them, such as unpredictability of well-being, tensions arising in the marital situation from guilt and anger, effects of separation on the families, and financial anxiety. Following each episode of dialysis, the main patient response was one of relief. Cramond and associates noted that their patients at first denied their illness and later realized that they had lost their health and independence and their futures were uncertain. This has been referred to as a "mourning reaction." From time to time the patients wished to be dead. They felt that life dependent on chronic dialysis was not worth living. Some patients passed from the mourning reaction to a state of active depression.

All patients undergoing dialysis become extremely dependent on the staff and emotionally attached to them. The patients often react emotionally to a sense of loss when any replacement of staff occurs. During the course of the dialysis program, regression occurs relatively frequently, and the patient becomes withdrawn and pretends to sleep. Insomnia and frightening dreams also occur, and the frequency with which emotional disturbances have been noted suggests that psychiatric assistance plays an important role in a dialysis program.

Two distinct groups of patients, the donors and recipients, must be considered in a renal homotransplantation program. Psychologic screening of the potential donors is indicated, and selection should be from individuals who are stable and who have mature judgment. Individuals with psychopathologic motives such as sacrifice or exhibitionism should be excluded, particularly when they are unrelated donors. It is to be emphasized that those who refuse to cooperate risk being rejected by the family and are frequently made to feel guilty. Therefore, when potential donors are rejected on psychiatric grounds, the rejection should be ascribed to a minor physical variation. In four of five cases, Cramond noted an ambivalent relationship between the donor and recipient. The donor experienced emotional and physical investment in the patient and, at times, sought to overprotect the patient. He felt that his sacrificial gift was in jeopardy if the patient behaved in a manner with which he did not approve.

The recipient has been shown to be aware of his obligation to the donor and resents the dependency relationship. At times feelings of shame and guilt must be considered. Kemph, in a follow-up of recipients of renal homotransplants, has noted periods of severe depression and concern with bodily damage and sexual damage. After the operation the donors also experience depression. Many expressed the feeling that they were not attentively supported by the hospital personnel.

Some recipients regard the operation as symbolic of rebirth and may undergo a religious conviction. In some recipients, a graft from a donor of an opposite sex is considered a threat to sexual identity. All recipients demonstrate anxiety in reference to injury of the grafted kidney. Although severe depressions and emotional reactions are uncommon, psychologic adjustment takes longer than a year to accomplish. When given a choice, patients who have rejected their kidney transplants have almost uniformly chosen a second transplant over return to dialysis.

INTENSIVE CARE DELIRIUM

Delirium manifested by a wide variety of behavior patterns, ranging from apathy to restlessness and combativeness, is a common occurrence in intensive care units. Both environmental and metabolic factors have been implicated. The former can be corrected by transferring the patient to a regular hospital ward or room as soon as possible. Katz et al. indicated a physiologic abnormality, such as hypoxemia or electrolyte or acid-base abnormality, as the cause in the great majority of patients.

DRUG ABUSE

Beebe and Keats have shown that not all narcotic addicts require detoxification associated with an operation. Methadone is the drug of choice for treating withdrawal. Haloxone may be preferable in an emergency situation. For patients on methadone maintenance, this drug can be stopped temporarily and frequent doses of conventional narcotics substituted during the early postoperative period. Withdrawal from barbiturates prior to elective operation may take 2 to 3 weeks. There is no physiologic addiction requiring maintenance of amphetamines or hallucinogens.

COMPLICATIONS OF GASTROINTESTINAL SURGERY

The gastrointestinal complications considered in this section are divided into (1) vascular complications, including hemorrhage and gangrene; (2) mechanical problems of gastroenterostomy and enteroenterostomy, including stomal obstruction, the afferent, or blind, loop syndrome, extrinsic obstruction and internal hernia, and inadvertent gastroileostomy; (3) leakage of an anastomosis, including the duodenal stump blowout; (4) external fistulas and stomal problems; and (5) damage to adjacent organs, including postoperative pancreatitis and jaundice.

Vascular Complications

HEMORRHAGE

Gastrointestinal hemorrhage which occurs subsequent to a gastrointestinal anastomosis may become manifest postoperatively by hematemesis, melena, hematochezia, or, most frequently, the passage of bright blood via a nasogastric tube positioned in the stomach. Bleeding from the suture line is most commonly associated with gastric surgery, occurring in approximately 1 percent of patients following gastric resection, with a higher incidence in those patients in whom operation is performed for a duodenal ulcer. Bleeding from the suture line is apt to occur either immediately after the operation or on the first postoperative day, but a second minor peak in incidence has been noted between the seventh and tenth postoperative days. Bleeding arising from the suture line on the first postoperative day is usually minimal or moderate and requires no specific therapy, but if it is continuous, the stomach should be aspirated and irrigated with ice-cold saline solution. Hemorrhage which does not stop following conservative measures constitutes an indication for laparotomy, at which time the suture line should be inspected. It may be preferable to enter the stomach above the line of anastomosis and ligate vessels from within. Bleeding later in the course of convalescence is usually due to sloughing from the suture line and generally responds to iced saline lavage. Significant hemorrhage from the suture line of small intestinal and large intestinal anastomoses is extremely rare. Upper gastrointestinal bleeding following a surgical procedure in a patient who is debilitated or in whom sepsis develops frequently indicates a stress ulcer (see Chap. 26).

GANGRENE

Gangrene is a rare complication of resection of a segment of gastrointestinal tract, since the intestine is supplied with a rich network of arteries. Necrosis of the gastric remnant has been reported following a high subtotal gastrectomy, particularly if the procedure incorporates ligation of the left gastric artery and concomitant splenectomy. Devascularization of the areas to be anastomosed should not occur following small intestinal surgical procedures if attention is directed toward the vascular supply. A precautionary measure is to slant the lines of incision so that more intestine is resected on the antimesenteric aspect. Small intestinal gangrene is more frequently due to mechanical strangulation, obstruction secondary to postoperative adhesions, volvulus, internal hernias, or vascular thrombosis. Gangrene of the segment of intestine may be apparent in the case of a colostomy in which an inadequate vascular supply has been provided.

In each instance, the recognition of gangrene requires resection of the gangrenous segment of intestine or stomach and reestablishment of intestinal continuity or a colostomy in bowel which is viable.

Mechanical Problems

STOMAL OBSTRUCTION

Although obstruction of the stoma may follow any intestinal anastomosis as a result of technical factors, postgastrectomy stomal obstruction represents the most common type and is frequently related to local edema. Factors which have been implicated in the etiology of edema include electrolyte depletion, hypochloremia, incomplete hemostasis, hypoproteinemia, leakage from the anastomosis, inadequate proximal decompression, and incorporation of too much tissue within the sutures. Other causes include rotation of the jejunum on its long axis, obstruction by the transverse mesocolon, particularly in an obese patient, obstruction by a fatty omentum, effect of vagotomy, and, rarely, jejunogastric intussusception, which has been reported as a complication in slightly over 100 cases of Billroth II procedures.

Postgastrectomy stomal obstruction is a most troublesome complication, and the reported incidence has ranged between 1 and 3 percent. Magnuson and associates indicated an almost identical incidence of 3 percent subsequent to gastrectomy for gastric ulcer as compared with gastrectomy for duodenal ulcer. Hibner and Richards, in a review of 648 partial gastrectomies, noted an incidence of 4.6 percent for patients requiring further operative therapy, 4.1 percent for Billroth II operations, and 3.5 percent for Billroth I types. In most instances in their series, the efferent loop was obstructed by the transverse mesocolon.

Symptoms usually occur on the third to fourth postoperative day, at which time there is abdominal fullness and increased return from the nasogastric suction. If the patient has been on oral intake, nausea followed by vomiting of large quantities of bile-colored gastric fluid occurs. Instillation of barium or Gastrografin via the nasogastric tube may reveal stomal obstruction or a patent stoma with distal loop obstruction. The symptoms usually persist for only short intervals and cause little disability, but occasionally they are prolonged and then have severe metabolic effects.

Prophylaxis is directed at avoiding the factors which have been implicated. Therapy of established stomal obstruction consists of adequate decompression and replacement of fluids and nutrients, while waiting for the obstruction to become relieved spontaneously. The course may be prolonged, extending over a period of several weeks. If there is not relief after extended conservative management or if the patient's condition is deteriorating, operative intervention is indicated. Rarely, a simple release of adhesions may be therapeutic, but more often the anastomotic site requires revision, a procedure which is frequently difficult in view of the extensive reaction around the stoma. It is generally preferable to transect the proximal and distal loops of intestine at their entrance to and exit from the indurated mass. These are then anastomosed to one another, and the short segment of intestine and a cuff of stomach are removed with the gastroenterostomy. Continuity is reestablished with a long antecolic gastrojejunostomy.

AFFERENT (BLIND) LOOP SYNDROME

The blind loop syndrome is a consequence of small intestinal surgical procedures and is presented in Chap. 27. The present discussion is concerned with the afferent loop syndrome which represents a complication of subtotal gastrectomy with Billroth II gastroenterostomy. The afferent loop consists of duodenum and a segment of jejunum of variable length. Acute or chronic obstruction can occur at any point proximal to the gastrojejunostomy. The incidence is difficult to estimate and is dependent upon the criteria for diagnosis. Quinn and Gifford reported five cases in 500 gastrectomies, while Blomstedt and Dahlgren reported an incidence of 18 percent with mild to moderate symptoms (type I and type II). The symptom complex of partial obstruction of the afferent loop was reported by Magnuson et al. to occur following gastrectomy in 4.2 percent of patients with gastric ulcer in contrast to 0.9 percent of patients with duodenal ulcer.

PATHOGENESIS. Normally after partial gastrectomy, biliary and pancreatic secretions enter the afferent loop, pass through the gastrojejunostomy to mix with gastric juice, and then pass through into the efferent loop. During a 24-hour period, approximately 1 to 1.5 liters of secretion enters the afferent loop. The afferent loop syndrome is caused by partial and, rarely, total obstruction of flow from the afferent loop. The pressure within the duodenum and segment of jejunum rises, and the loop becomes dilated by bile and pancreatic juice. After the ingestion of food, particularly a fatty meal, the duodenal contents increase rapidly, thus explaining the postcibal nature of the syndrome. With incomplete obstruction, pressure within the intestine eventually becomes sufficient to overcome resistance, and the contents are emptied into the stomach, causing variable amounts to be vomited. With total obstruction, the loop no longer has any communication with the stomach, and vomitus is free of bile.

CLINICAL MANIFESTATIONS. The symptoms of partial obstruction of the afferent loop occur most commonly in the early postoperative period. Two-thirds of the cases occur during the first week, but in some instances the syndrome becomes apparent months to years following gastrectomy. The symptoms vary in intensity and are characterized by postcibal vomiting. Mild symptoms consist of eructation of a mouthful of green biliary fluid within an hour and a half after a meal. Vomiting is generally preceded by the sensation of fullness and, at times, pain in the epigastrium. In some instances, the symptoms of chronic obstruction persist for several months, and the amount of biliary vomiting and antecedent epigastric pain are appreciable. With persistence of partial obstruction, the stools become bulky and gray, and contain much fat. Roentgenographic examination may show passage of contrast material into the efferent loop, while the afferent loop, as a rule, fails to fill. Chronic partial obstruction is associated with anemia, and the vitamin B_{12} absorption test may provide the diagnosis. Urinary excretion of B_{12} is reduced or absent and is unaffected by the administration of intrinsic factor, in contrast to pernicious anemia. However, following a course of 3 to 5 days of tetracycline, B_{12} urinary excretion returns to normal.

In the rare situation of the acute complete obstruction of the afferent loop, the patient becomes acutely ill with severe epigastric pain, and bile is characteristically absent from the vomitus. A mass may be felt in the upper abdomen. The patient's condition may deteriorate rapidly, and shock may occur as a result of compromise of the circulation of the duodenal wall and/or perforation with generalized peritonitis. Roentgenograms are of little diagnostic assistance. There may be delayed emptying of contrast material from the gastric remnant, and no barium enters the afferent loop. The amylase level may be markedly elevated.

TREATMENT. Incomplete obstruction generally subsides on a conservative regimen. Capper and Welbourn collected 44 cases requiring surgical intervention and reported that 36 of them had a good outcome. Surgical decompression of the afferent loop may be accomplished by anastomosis between the afferent and efferent loops, by employing a Roux en Y anastomosis or converting a gastrojejunostomy to a gastroduodenostomy. In the case of acute total obstruction, early operation with decompression of the afferent loop is mandatory.

INTESTINAL OBSTRUCTION

Intestinal obstruction in the immediate postoperative period is most frequently due to ileus or fibrinous adhesions; however, a variety of mechanical causes should be considered. Internal herniation represents a complication of subtotal gastrectomy, generally following a Billroth II antecolic anastomosis. Internal herniation of the small intestine may also take place through improperly closed mesenteric rents or when the mesentery of the ileum or colon is not tacked to the peritoneum in the course of an ileostomy or colostomy. Closed-loop obstruction generally results and may rapidly progress to compromise the vascular supply with ultimate perforation. Operative reduction and repair of an internal hernia are required. Adhesions and/or volvulus may occur in the postoperative hospitalization and require surgical intervention for relief of obstruction. The incidence is particularly high following resection for congenital atresia in infancy, especially when the proximal dilated bowel is not resected. Postoperative intussusception, generally involving the small intestine, is also to be considered in the pediatric age group.

INADVERTENT GASTROILEOSTOMY

The error of anastomosing the stomach to the ileum rather than the jejunum is fortunately uncommon. In 1949, Moretz indicated that 27 cases were recorded in the literature. The situation results in a malabsorption syndrome which begins as soon as the patient is allowed to eat solid food. Diarrhea, weight loss, and inanition in the absence of abdominal pain are characteristic. The stool contains a high percentage of undigested food and a large quantity of unabsorbed fat. Fecal vomiting and hemorrhage occasionally occur, and an ulcer may develop at the site of the ileum, in which case abdominal pain may be present. The diagnosis can be established roentgenographically by demonstrating a rapid transit and short distal intestine. The error should be avoided by using the ligament of Treitz as a landmark in establishing a gastroenterostomy; in the absence of a ligament of Treitz an anomaly of rotation should be suspected, and the loop of intestine for anastomosis should be selected by tracing the duodenum distad or the small bowel proximally from the cecum. The preoperative management of patients with gastroileostomy requires a vigorous preparation, and a preliminary feeding jejunostomy is of value in these cases. A block resection of the gastroileostomy is advocated for patients who have had subtotal gastric resection, while, in the absence of gastric resection, the ileostomy may be taken down directly. A gastrojejunostomy and reconstitution of intestinal continuity are then performed.

Anastomotic Leak

Suture line leakage represents a potential complication of any intestinal anastomosis. The three prime etiologic factors are (1) poor surgical technique, (2) distal obstruction, and (3) inadequate proximal decompression. Leak from an enteroenterostomy becomes manifest as localized or generalized peritonitis. Small leaks with localized response may be treated by proximal decompression and administration of appropriate antibiotics, while large leaks and diffuse peritonitis frequently require surgical intervention. Fistulization may develop as a tract becomes established between the point of leakage and the skin. A leak from the line of anastomosis is a relatively rare complication following gastroenterostomy. Such leakage occurs more frequently when there has been impairment of the blood supply of the residual gastric pouch and a concomitant splenectomy has been performed. A common point at which leaks develop has been referred to as the "angle du mort," where the residual gastric pouch of a Hofmeister closure meets the line of anastomosis of the small intestine.

Duodenal stump leakage (blowout) is a more frequent and critical complication of gastric resection. A review of gastrectomies performed at the Mayo Clinic in 1956 revealed that 4.5 percent of patients subjected to the procedure for gastric ulcer had some evidence of leak, while 5.6 percent of patients in whom the same procedure was carried out for duodenal ulcer revealed similar evidence. In that study, drains had been inserted into the stump region, and in many patients increased drainage represented the evidence of a leak. Edmunds et al. indicate that a review of gastrectomies performed at the Massachusetts General Hospital from 1946 to 1959 showed that an incidence of dehiscence of the stump was 1.1 percent and the mortality due to this cause was 0.6 percent.

Duodenal stump leakage occurs most commonly after operation for a duodenal ulcer and frequently when gastrectomy is performed as an emergency procedure to stop hemorrhage. In a great majority of cases, the leak arises as a result of a technical error and failure of the suture line. A scarred and edematous duodenum predisposes to the complication, as does obstruction of the afferent loop and local pancreatitis. Complications of duodenal leakage include peritonitis, subhepatic abscess, pancreatitis, sepsis, and establishment of an external fistula with fluid and electrolyte abnormalities.

Specific measures can be taken to avoid this complication. Before embarking on a gastric resection, the surgeon should be as sure as possible that the duodenal stump can be safely closed. In the face of marked inflammatory disease in the duodenal region, vagotomy and gastroenterostomy definitely represent safer procedures. When resection has been undertaken and duodenal closure is difficult, catheter duodenostomy may be used as an adjunct. Rodkey and Welch reported that in 51 cases with difficult duodenal stump closures in whom planned duodenostomy was carried out, there was only one death, and only five patients had drainage from the fistula that lasted more than 48 hours after the catheter was removed. As a compromise between primary closure and planned duodenostomy, some surgeons have advised drainage of the right upper quadrant with a Penrose drain placed in the region of the duodenal stump in the hope that if perforation occurs, the contents will discharge along the tract. However, this does not provide the safety factor of planned duodenostomy, since the drain tract may wall off from the stump before the perforation becomes established.

Duodenal blowout is a major catastrophe which is most likely to occur between the second and seventh postoperative day and becomes manifest by sudden pain, elevation in temperature and pulse rate, and general deterioration of the patient's condition. Adequate drainage must be instituted at once and is best accomplished by an incision below the right costal margin and insertion of a large sump catheter which is passed down to the duodenal stump area, with constant suction applied. Attention must be directed toward fluid and electrolyte therapy, and a high caloric and nitrogen intake should be maintained. Fistula closure can be anticipated within 2 to 3 weeks. Another area in which leaks are a major concern is low colon anastomoses; incidences of 5 to 51 percent have been reported. Recently Everett reported a randomized control trial in which it was shown that a single-layer technique is preferable for low colonic anastomoses. Pedicled omentum may be applied to seal the anastomosis. The mortality rate in patients with major colon leaks is extremely high, and this has led to a resurgence of enthusiasm for protective transverse colostomy if the anastomosis appears compromised.

External Fistulas and Stomal Complications

FISTULAS

External fistulas may arise from stomach, small intestine, or colon. In a review of the experiences at the Massachusetts General Hospital from 1946 to 1959, it was reported that in 157 patients with external fistulas, 55 fistulas originated from stomach, duodenum, or gastrojejunal anastomosis; 46 from jejunum or ileum, with drainage of over 100 ml of intestinal content daily; and 56 from the lower ileum and colon. Surgical complications were the direct cause of 67 percent of these fistulas.

Gastric and Duodenal Fistulas

The incidence of gastrojejunal or duodenal stump fistulas following subtotal gastrectomy has been reported to be 1 to 2 percent, approximately one-quarter of which originated from the gastrojejunostomy. Suture line failure accounted for 82 percent of all gastroduodenal fistulas. The causes of fistulas arising from the gastrojejunostomy may be related to the suture line containing tumor, ischemia of the gastric stump due to high ligation of the gastric artery and vasa brevia, stomal obstruction, and pancreatitis or tension on the suture line. The causes of duodenal stump fistula have been referred to in the previous section on stump leakage. The complications of an established gastric or duodenal fistula include electrolyte abnormalities and malnutrition, sepsis, intraperitoneal abscesses and wound infection, jaundice, and pancreatitis.

Treatment. Intensive fluid, electrolyte, and nutritional therapy is frequently required, and quantitative control of imbalance is critical. The amount of drainage should be measured and analyzed, and these determinations plus the base-line requirements should provide a formula for replacement therapy (see Chap. 2). Sump suction is the most efficient method of managing the drainage, and protection of the skin from autodigestion is usually required. The majority of fistulas which close spontaneously do so in less than 2 months. Surgical intervention may be indicated to drain abscesses or to establish a feeding jejunostomy. An established gastric fistula may require resection and correction of distal obstruction if the latter is present. Fistulas arising at the gastrojejunostomy stoma may require re-resection and establishment of a new gastroenterostomy. Fistulas arising from the duodenal stump are not generally amenable to direct closure. The literature reveals that definitive procedures rarely have been employed for fistulas in this segment of the gastrointestinal tract, and the mortality rate of 55 gastric and duodenal fistulas treated at the Massachusetts General Hospital was 65 percent. These fistulas are readily managed with parenteral hyperalimentation. In the report of MacFadyen et al., all duodenal fistulas closed spontaneously.

Small Bowel Fistulas (See Chap. 27)

Seventy-two percent of the 46 fistulas in this group reported by Edmunds et al. represented surgical complications secondary to dehiscence of anastomoses or inadvertent injury during dissection or closure of an abdominal incision. Although jejunal and proximal ileal fistulas are frequently characterized by profuse drainage, the fluid loss is generally less than that associated with duodenal fistulas, and therefore fluid and electrolyte abnormalities occur less frequently. Malnutrition develops in about three-quarters of these patients, and sepsis is a major complication. Twenty-two percent of the patients reported by Edmunds et al. died of generalized peritonitis, and a large number of intraperitoneal abscesses developed. Skin digestion is a frequent occurrence, and many of these patients eventually develop a ventral hernia due to wound complications.

Treatment. Supportive management of small bowel fistulas is similar to that outlined for gastroduodenal fistulas. This includes maintenance of fluid and electrolyte balance and nutrition. Hyperalimentation may be applicable. In the case of a proximal jejunal fistula, a distal feeding jejunostomy is frequently indicated to permit adequate fluid and nutritional intake. Oral feeding of low-residue diets is feasible with ileal fistulas. Control of fluid loss and diarrhea may be accomplished with the use of Lomotil, Kaopectate, and opiates plus nonabsorbable antibiotics when indicated. Drainage is best controlled by sump suction, and protection of the skin in the region of the fistula is indicated.

Of 46 patients reported by Edmunds et al., definitive procedures were carried out in 50 percent. The operative procedures include direct attack on a fistula with resection both of the fistula and the segment of intestine from which it arises or an indirect attack through a clean abdominal incision with a bypass operation or complete exclusion of the fistula by means of end-to-end anastomosis of the proximal and distal intestine. The excluded loop is then decompressed completely through a large fistula by exteriorizing the ends of the intestine to prevent later blowout. In general, and particularly in the face of peritonitis, early direct attack on the fistula is safer and more satisfactory than exclusion procedures, and most fistulas can be operated on within 3 weeks of onset. In the series reported by Edmunds et al., only 1 patient of 17 treated by resection died, while the mortality rate of patients treated conservatively was 80 percent. Using hyperalimentation, MacFadyen et al. reported that over 70 percent of small bowel fistulas closed spontaneously. An average of 40 days of hyperalimentation was required. By contrast, Aguirre et al. reported that gastrointestinal fistulas treated in part by total parenteral nutrition healed spontaneously in only 11 of 38 patients.

Colonic Fistulas (See Chaps. 27 and 28)

These are generally caused by anastomotic leaks or inadvertent trauma to the segment of intestine. Anastomosis in the region of tumor or inflammation and distal partial obstruction are predisposing factors. Fluid and electrolyte abnormalities are uncommon, while the incidence of infection is extremely high. This includes peritonitis, intraperitoneal abscesses, and wound infections. Significant skin digestion and irritation are rare.

Treatment. The patients can generally be managed on a low-residue diet, using enteric or parenteral antibiotics when indicated, and rarely require sump suction. Spontaneous healing of fistulas in these regions is the rule rather than the exception, but defunctionalizing colostomies for descending colon fistulas or ileal transverse colostomies for ascending colon and distal ileal fistulas may be indicated. Medical management is generally indicated for about 6 weeks to permit any active inflammation to subside. If the inflammation persists after this time, a defunctionalizing procedure is indicated. Definitive surgical treatment is indicated for fistulas which fail to progress satisfactorily after 6 weeks. If the fistula is accompanied by generalized peritonitis, early emergency resection is indicated and frequently should be accompanied by a proximal defunctionalizing procedure. Definitive operations include a turn-in procedure or resection which may be coupled with a temporary protective colostomy or bypass. Seventy-nine percent of the patients in the experience at the Massachusetts General Hospital were cured. Seventy-five percent of patients with no operation experienced spontaneous cure. Lichtman and McDonald reported that 74 percent of chronic fecal fistulas treated by turn-in or resection were cured.

EXTERNAL STOMAL COMPLICATIONS (See Chap. 28)

Ileostomy

Ileostomy performed for ulcerative colitis may be associated with complications related to technical factors, presence of disease, and the nature of the intestinal contents which are discharged. The location of ileostomy is critical to permit application of an effective collecting device, while the method of fixation of the ileal mesentery is important to prevent internal herniation. Formation of the ileostomy itself is important in reducing the incidence of complications. The technique of operative maturation by everting the mucosa reduces the incidence of serositis and peritonitis. Frozen section of the transected ileum is indicated, since ulcerative colitis may extend into the segment of ileum and result in improper function. The liquid nature of the ileostomy discharge requires that measures be taken to avoid excoriation of the skin, which is usually due to delayed application of the bag and a poor fit. When excoriation appears, it is generally wise to discontinue the use of cement and apply a soothing powder. The patient may be placed in a prone position on a frame so that the ileal contents are allowed to drain into a container and contact with the skin is avoided. The complication of prolapse, which requires revision, should be seen infrequently if the mesentery has been fixed. Fistulas which develop at or below the skin level are an indication for early revision of the ileostomy.

Cecostomy and Colostomy

Cecostomies generally demand more attention than colostomies, and frequent irrigation is indicated. Subsequent to removal of the cecostomy catheter, spontaneous closure is to be anticipated, but in unusual circumstances, surgical closure is required. Complications following colostomy include ischemia, gangrene, bleeding, wound abscesses, stenosis, or retraction of the stoma. In the case of a terminal colostomy, fixation during the operative procedure should prevent retraction. If either retraction or gangrene becomes evident, immediate operation is indicated to revise the colostomy using viable bowel of sufficient length.

References

General Considerations

Artz, C. P., and Hardy, J. D.: "Complications in Surgery and Their Management," W. B. Saunders Company, Philadelphia, 1967.

Wound Complications

Ad Hoc Committee of the Committee on Trauma, Division of Medical Sciences, National Academy of Sciences–National Research Council: Postoperative Wound Infections: The Influence of Ultraviolet Irradiation of the Operating Room and of Various Other Factors, *Ann Surg* [Suppl], vol. 160, 1964.

Alexander, H. C., and Prudden, J.: The Causes of Abdominal Wound Disruption, *Surg Gynecol Obstet*, **122**:1223, 1966.

Barnes, J., Pace, W. G., Trump, D. S., and Ellison, E. H.: Prophylactic Postoperative Antibiotics: A Controlled Study of 1,007 Cases, *Arch Surg*, **79**:190, 1959.

Dineen, P.: A Critical Study of 100 Consecutive Wound Infections, *Surg Gynecol Obstet*, **113**:91, 1961.

————: Major Infections in the Postoperative Period, *Surg Clin North Am*, **44**:553, 1964.

Elek, S. D., and Conen, P. E.: The Virulence of *Staphylococcus pyogenes* for Man: A Study of the Problems of Wound Infections, *Br J Exp Pathol*, **38**:573, 1957.

Glenn, F., and Moore, S. W.: The Disruption of Abdominal Wounds, *Surg Gynecol Obstet*, **72**:1041, 1941.

Halasz, N. A.: Dehiscence of Laparotomy Wounds, *Am J Surg*, **116**:210, 1968.

Hartzell, J. B., and Winfield, J. M.: Disruption of Abdominal Wounds: Collective Review, *Int Abstr Surg*, **68**:585, 1939.

Howe, C. W., and Mozden, P. J.: Postoperative Infections: Current Concepts, *Surg Clin North Am*, **43**:859, 1963.

Ketcham, A. S., Lieberman, J. E., and West, J. T.: Antibiotic Prophylaxis in Cancer Surgery and Its Value in Staphylococcal Carrier Patients, *Surg Gynecol Obstet*, **117**:1, 1963.

Pemberton, L. B., and Manax, W. G.: Complications after Vertical and Transverse Incisions for Cholecystectomy, *Surg Gynecol Obstet*, **132**:892, 1971.

Polk, H. C., Jr., and Lopez-Mayor, J. F.: Postoperative Wound Infection: A Prospective Study of Determinant Factors and Prevention, *Surgery*, **66**:97, 1969.

Rees, V. L., and Coller, F. A.: Anatomic and Clinical Study of Transverse Abdominal Incision, *Arch Surg*, **47**:136, 1943.

Schonholtz, G. J., Borgia, C. A., and Blair, J. D.: Wound Sepsis in Orthopedic Surgery, *J Bone Joint Surg* [Am], **44A**:1548, 1962.

Singleton, A. O., and Blocker, T. G., Jr.: The Problem of Disruption of Abdominal Wounds and Postoperative Hernia, *JAMA*, **112**:122, 1939.

Thompson, W. D., Ravdin, I. S., and Frank, I. L.: Effect of Hypoproteinemia on Wound Disruption, *Arch Surg*, **36**:500, 1938.

Thomsen, V. F., Larsen, S. O., and Jepsen, O. B.: Post-operative Wound Sepsis in General Surgery: IV. Sources and Routes of Infection, *Acta Chir Scand*, **136**:251, 1970.

Wolff, W. I.: Disruption of Abdominal Wounds, *Ann Surg*, **131**:534, 1950.

Postoperative Parotitis

Branson, B., Kugel, A. I., Stafford, C. E., and Morel, E. E.: The Re-emergence of Postoperative Parotitis, *Western J Surg Obstet Gynecol*, **67**:38, 1959.

Carlson, R. G., and Glas, W. W.: Acute Suppurative Parotitis, *Arch Surg*, **86**:659, 1963.

Hemenway, W. G., and English, G. M.: Surgical Treatment of Acute Bacterial Parotitis, *Postgrad Med*, **50**:114, 1971.

Krippaehne, W. W., Hunt, T. K., and Dunphy, J. E.: Acute Suppurative Parotitis: A Study of 161 Cases, *Ann Surg,* **156:**251, 1962.

Lary, B. G.: Postoperative Suppurative Parotitis, *Arch Surg,* **89:**653, 1964.

Petersdorf, R. G., Forsyth, B. B., and Bernake, D.: Staphylococcal Parotitis, *N Engl J Med,* **259:**1250, 1958.

Reilly, D. J.: Benign Transient Swelling of the Parotid Glands following General Anesthesia: "Anesthesia Mumps," *Anesth Anal (Cleve),* **49:**560, 1970.

Postoperative Respiratory Complications

Adriani, J., Zepernick, R., Harmon, W., and Hiern, B.: Iatrogenic Pulmonary Edema in Surgical Patients, *Surgery,* **61:**183, 1967.

Ashbaugh, D. G., and Petty, T. L.: Positive End-expiratory Pressure: Physiology, Indications, and Contraindications, *J Thorac Cardiovasc Surg,* **65:**165, 1973.

Becker, A., Barak, S., Braun, E., and Meyers, M. P.: The Treatment of Postoperative Pulmonary Atelectasis with Intermittent Positive Pressure Breathing, *Surg Gynecol Obstet,* **111:**517, 1960.

Beecher, H. K.: Measured Effect of Laparotomy on Respiration, *J Clin Invest,* **12:**639, 1933.

Bendixen, H. H., and Bunker, J. P.: "Ventilation and Postoperative Period," paper presented at The Second World Congress of Anaesthesiologists, Toronto, Sept. 6, 1960.

―――, Hedley-Shyte, J., and Laver, M. B.: Impaired Oxygenation in Surgical Patients during General Anesthesia with Controlled Ventilation: A Concept of Atelectasis, *N Engl J Med,* **269:**991, 1963.

―――, ―――, and ―――: Increased Physiologic Shunting during Anesthesia and Surgery, *Anesthesiology,* **24:**122, 1963.

Brattstrom, S.: Postoperative Pulmonary Ventilation with Reference to Postoperative Pulmonary Complications, *Acta Chir Scand Suppl* **195,** 1954.

Clements, J. A.: Surface Phenomena in Relation to Pulmonary Function (Sixth Bowditch Lecture), *Physiologist,* **5:**11, 1962.

Clendon, D. R. T., and Pygott, F.: Analysis of Pulmonary Complications Occurring after 579 Consecutive Operations, *Br J Anaesth,* **19:**62, 1944.

Collins, J. A.: The Causes of Progressive Pulmonary Insufficiency in Surgical Patients, *J Surg Res,* **9:**685, 1969.

Davis, H. A., and Pollak, E. W.: Adult Respiratory Distress Syndrome in Postoperative Patients: Study of Pulmonary Pathology in "Shock Lung" with Prophylactic and Therapeutic Implications, *Am Surg,* **41:**391, 1975.

Griffo, Z. J., and Roos, A.: Effect of O_2 Breathing on Pulmonary Compliance, *J Appl Physiol,* **17:**233, 1962.

Hamilton, W. K.: Postoperative Respiratory Complications, chap. 10 in "Clinical Anesthesia," 1/1965.

Joffe, N.: Roentgenologic Findings in Post-shock and Postoperative Pulmonary Insufficiency, *Radiology,* **94:**369, 1970.

Kurzweg, F. T.: Pulmonary Complications following Upper Abdominal Surgery, *Am Surg,* **19:**967, 1953.

Laver, M. B., and Bendixen, H. H.: Atelectasis in the Surgical Patient: Recent Conceptual Advances, *Prog Surg* **5:**1, 1966.

Masson, A. H. B.: Pulmonary Edema during or after Surgery, pt. I, *Anesth Anal Current Res,* **43:**440, 1964.

―――: Pulmonary Edema during or after Surgery, pt. II, *Anesth Anal Curr Res,* **43:**446, 1964.

Mead, J., and Collier, C.: Relation of Volume History of Lungs to Respiratory Mechanics in Anesthetized Dogs, *J Appl Physiol,* **14:**669, 1959.

Moersch, H. J.: Bronchoscopy in Treatment of Postoperative Atelectasis, *Surg Gynecol Obstet,* **77:**435, 1943.

Moore, F. D.: Postoperative Pulmonary Insufficiency: Anoxia, the Shunted Lung and Mechanical Assistance, in D. E. Harken (ed.), "Cardiac Surgery 2," *Cardiovasc Clin,* vol. 3, no. 3, F. A. Davis Company, Philadelphia, 1971.

―――, Lyons, J. H., Pierce, E. C., Jr., Morgan, A. P., Jr., Drinker, P. A., MacArthur, J. D., and Dammin, G. J.: "Post-traumatic Pulmonary Insufficiency," W. B. Saunders Company, Philadelphia, 1969.

Neely, W. A., Robinson, T. W., McMullan, M. H., Bobo, W. O., Meadows, D. L., and Hardy, J. D.: Post-operative Respiratory Insufficiency, *Ann Surg,* **171:**679, 1970.

Overfield, W., and Powers, S. R., Jr.: Arterial Oxygen Tension: Significance in the Surgical Patient, *Surgery,* **71:**1, 1972.

Peters, R. M., Hilberman, M., Hogan, J. S., and Crawford, D. A.: Objective Indications for Respiratory Therapy in Post-trauma and Postoperative Patients, *Am J Surg,* **124:**262, 1972.

Pontoppidan, H., Geffin, B., and Lowenstein, E.: Acute Respiratory Failure in the Adult: Trends in Treatment of Acute Respiratory Failure, *N Engl J Med,* **287:**690, 1972.

―――, ―――, and ―――: Acute Respiratory Failure in the Adult: Assessment of Respiratory Function, *N Engl J Med,* **287:**743, 1972.

―――, ―――, and ―――: Acute Respiratory Failure in the Adult: Effect of Mechanical Ventilation and Airway Pressures on Circulation and Blood Gas Exchange, *N Engl J Med,* **287:**799, 1972.

―――, Laver, M. B., and Geffin, B.: Acute Respiratory Failure in the Surgical Patient, *Adv Surg,* **4:**163, 1970.

Sayeed, M. M., Chaudry, I. H., and Baue, A. E.: Na^+–K^+ Transport and Adenosine Nucleotides in the Lung in Hemorrhagic Shock, *Surgery,* **77:**395, 1975.

Van Allen, C. M., and Adams, W. E.: The Mechanism of Obstructive Pulmonary Atelectasis, *Surg Gynecol Obstet,* **50:**385, 1930.

Cardiac Complications

Buckley J. J., and Jackson, J. A.: Postoperative Cardiac Arrhythmias, *Anesthesiology,* **22:**723, 1961.

Dack, S.: Postoperative Myocardial Infarction, *Am J Cardiol,* **12:**423, 1963.

Dixon, S. H., Jr., Limbird, L. E., Roe, C. R., Wagner, G. S., Oldham, H. N., Jr., and Sabiston, D. C., Jr.: Recognition of Postoperative Acute Myocardial Infarction: Application of Isoenzyme Technics, *Circulation* [Suppl], **47** & **48:**137, 1973.

Dreifus, L. S., Rabbino, M. D., Watanabe, Y., and Tabesh, E.: Arrhythmias in the Postoperative Period, *Am J Cardiol,* **12:**431, 1963.

Krosnick, A., and Wassermann, F.: Cardiac Arrhythmias in Older Age Group following Thoracic Surgery, *Am J Med Sci,* **230:**541, 1955.

Ikuner, J., Iliescu, V., Otsu, F., Boszormenyi, E., Bernstein, H., and Corday, E.: Cardiac Arrhythmias during Anesthesia, *Dis Chest,* **52:**580, 1967.

Master, A. M., Dack, S., and Jaffe, H. L.: Postoperative Coronary Artery Occlusion, *JAMA,* **110:**1415, 1938.

Mauney, F. M., Jr., Ebert, P. A., and Sabiston, D. C., Jr.: Postoperative Myocardial Infarction: A Study of Predisposing Factors, Diagnosis and Mortality in a High Risk Group of Surgical Patients, *Ann Surg,* 172:497, 1970.

Merideth, J.: Cardiac Arrhythmias in the Postoperative Patient, *Surg Clin North Am,* **49:**1083, 1969.

Reinikainen, M., and Pontinen, P.: On Cardiac Arrhythmias during Anaesthesia and Surgery, *Acta Med Scand Suppl* 457, 1966.

Rogers, W. R., Wroblewski, F., and LaDue, J. S.: Supraventricular Tachycardia Complicating Surgical Procedures: Study of Contributing Causes, Course, and Treatment of This Complication in Fifty Patients, *Circulation,* 7:192, 1953.

Sharnoff, J. G.: Postmortem Findings in 25 Cases of Sudden Heart Arrest in the Perioperative Period, *Lancet,* 2:876, 1966.

Stein, I., and Caginalp, N.: The Postoperative Electrocardiogram, *Angiology,* **17:**323, 1966.

Tarhan, S., Moffitt, E. A., Taylor, W. F., and Giuliani, E. R.: Myocardial Infarction after General Anesthesia, *JAMA,* **220:**1451, 1972.

Taylor, I. B.: Cyclopropane Anesthesia: With Report of Results in 41,690 Administrations, *Anesthesiology,* 2:641, 1941.

Wheat, M. W., Jr., and Burford, T. H.: Digitalis in Surgery: Extension of Classical Indications, *J Thorac Cardiovasc Surg,* 41:162, 1961.

Wroblewski, F., and LaDue, J. S.: Myocardial Infarction as a Postoperative Complication of Major Surgery, *JAMA,* **150:**1212, 1952.

Diabetes Mellitus

Black, K.: Diabetes and the Surgical Patient, *Br J Clin Pract,* **20:**555, 1966.

Canary, J. J., Stoffer, R., Delawter, D. D., and Moss, J. M.: The Response of Tolbutamide-treated Patients to the Stress of Surgery, *Med Ann DC,* **28:**614, 1959.

Forsham, P. H.: Management of Diabetes during Stress and Surgery, in R. H. Williams (ed.), "Diabetes," chap. 36, Hoeber Medical Division, Harper & Row, Publishers, Incorporated, New York, 1960.

Galloway, J. A., and Shuman, C. R.: Diabetes and Surgery: A Study of 667 Cases, *Am J Med,* **34:**177, 1963.

Gastineau, C. F., and Molnar, G. D.: The Care of the Diabetic Patient During Emergency Surgery, *Surg Clin N Am,* **49:**1171, 1969.

Greenstein, A. J., and Dreiling, D. A.: Nonketotic Hyperosmolar Coma in the Postoperative Patient, *Am J Surg,* 121:698, 1971.

Marble, A., and Steinke, J.: Physiology and Pharmacology in Diabetes Mellitus: Guiding the Diabetic Patient through the Surgical Period, *Anesthesiology,* 24:442, 1963.

Packovich, M. J., Molnar, G. D., and Leonard, P. F.: Management of Diabetic patients during Surgery, *Surg Clin North Am,* 45:975, 1965.

Weisenfeld, S., Podolsky, S., Goldsmith, L., and Ziff, L.: Adsorption of Insulin to Infusion Bottles and Tubing, *Diabetes,* **17:**766, 1968.

Fat Embolism

Ashbaugh, D. G., and Petty, T. L.: The Use of Corticosteroids in the Treatment of Respiratory Failure Associated with Massive Fat Embolism, *Surg Gynecol Obstet,* 123:495, 1966.

Benoit, P. R., Hampson, L. G., and Burgess, J. H.: Value of Arterial Hypoxemia in the Diagnosis of Pulmonary Fat Embolism, *Ann Surg,* **175:**128, 1972.

Collins, J. A., Hudson, T. L., Hamacher, W. R., Rokous, J., Williams, G., and Hardaway, R. M., III: Systemic Fat Embolism in Four Combat Casualties, *Ann Surg,* 167:493, 1968.

Evarts, C. M.: The Fat Embolism Syndrome: A Review, *Surg Clin North Am,* **50:**493, 1970.

Greendyke, R. M.: Fat Embolism in Fatal Automobile Accidents, *J Forensic Sci,* 9:201, 1964.

Henzel, J. H., Smith, J. L., Pories, W. J., and Burget, D. E.: Fat Embolism: Diagnostic Challenge of a Potentially Lethal Clinical Entity, *Am J Surg,* 113:525, 1967.

Jackson, C. T., and Greendyke, R. M.: Pulmonary and Cerebral Fat Embolism after Closed Chest Cardiac Massage, *Surg Gynecol Obstet,* 120:25, 1965.

Musselman, M. M., Glas, W. W., and Grekin, T. D.: Fat Embolism, *Arch Surg,* **65:**551, 1952.

Palmovic, V., and McCarroll, J. R.: Fat Embolism in Trauma, *Arch Pathol,* 80:630, 1965.

Pazell, J. A., and Peltier, L. F.: Experience with Sixty-three Patients with Fat Embolism, *Surg Gynecol Obstet,* **135:**77, 1972.

Peltier, L. F.: The Diagnosis of Fat Embolism, *Surg Gynecol Obstet,* 121:371, 1965.

Scuderi, C. S.: Fat Embolism: Clinical and Experimental Study, *Surg Gynecol Obstet,* **72:**732, 1941.

Sevitt, S.: "Fat Embolism," Butterworth Scientific Publications, London, 1962.

Sutton, G. E.: Pulmonary Fat Embolism, *Ann Surg,* **76:**581, 1922.

Weisz, G. M.: Fat Embolism, *Curr Probl Surg,* November 1974.

Psychiatric Complications

Altschule, M. D.: Postoperative Psychosis, *Surg Clin N Am,* **49:**677, 1969.

Bakwin, H.: Psychic Trauma of Operations, *J Pediatr,* 36:262, 1950.

Beebe, H. G., and Keats, N. M.: Surgical Patients and Drug Abuse Syndrome, *Am Surg,* 39:88, 1973.

Bliss, E. L., Rumel, W. R., and Branch, C. H.: Psychiatric Complications of Mitral Surgery: Report of a Death after Electroshock Therapy, *Arch Neurol,* 74:249, 1955.

Bolton, H. E., and Bailey, C. P.: Surgical Aspects in Psychosomatic Aspects of Cardiovascular Surgery, in A. J. Cantor and A. N. Foxe (eds.), "Psychosomatic Aspects of Surgery," chap. 3, Grune & Stratton, Inc., New York, 1955.

Browning, J., and Houseworth, J.: Development of New Symptoms following Medical and Surgical Treatment for Duodenal Ulcer, *Psychosom Med,* 15:328, 1953.

Cramond, W. A.: Renal Homotransplantation: Some Observations on Recipients and Donors, *Br J Psychiat,* 113:1223, 1967.

————, Court, J. H., Higgins, B. A., Knight, P. R., and Lawrence, J. R.: Psychological Screening of Potential Donors in a Renal Homotransplantation Programme, *Br J Psychiat,* 113:1213, 1967.

————, Knight, P. R., and Lawrence, J. R.: The psychiatric Contribution to a Renal Unit Undertaking Chronic Haemodialysis and Renal Homotransplantation, *Br J Psychiat,* 113:1201, 1967.

Da Costa, J. C.: The Diagnosis of Postoperative Insanity, *Surg Gynecol Obstet,* 11:577, 1910.

Deutsch, H.: Psychoanalytic Observations in Surgery, *Psychosom Med,* 4:105, 1942.

Donovan, J. C.: Some Psychosomatic Aspects of Obstetrics and Gynecology, *Am J Obstet Gynecol,* **75:**72, 1958.

Egerton, N., and Kay, J. H.: Psychological Disturbances Associated with Open Heart Surgery, *Br J Psychiat,* **110:**433, 1964.

Fox, H. M., Rizzo, N. D., and Gifford, S.: Psychological Observations of Patients Undergoing Mitral Surgery: Study of Stress, *Psychosom Med,* **16:**186, 1954.

Hackett, T. P., and Weisman, A. D.: Psychiatric Management of Operative Syndromes. I. The Therapeutic Consultation and the Effect of Noninterpretive Intervention, *Psychosom Med,* **22:**267, 1960.

——, and ——: Psychiatric Management of Operative Syndromes. II. Psychodynamic Factors in Formulation and Management, *Psychosom Med,* **22:**356, 1960.

Halper, I. S.: Psychiatric Observations in a Chronic Hemodialysis Program, *Med Clin North Am,* **55:**177, 1971.

Hollender, M. H.: A Study of Patients Admitted to a Psychiatric Hospital after Pelvic Operations, *Am J Obstet Gynecol,* **79:**498, 1960.

Katz, N. M., Agle, D. P., DePalma, R. G., and DeCosse, J. J.: Delirium in Surgical Patients under Intensive Care: Utility of Mental Status Examination, *Arch Surg,* **104:**310, 1972.

Kemph, J. P.: Renal Failure, Artificial Kidney and Kidney Transplant, *Am J Psychiat,* **122:**1270, 1966.

Knox, S. J.: Severe Psychiatric Disturbances in the Postoperative Period: A Five-Year Survey of Belfast Hospitals, *J Ment Sci,* **107:**1078, 1961.

Kornfeld, D. S., Zimberg, S., and Malm, J. R.: Psychiatric Complications of Open-Heart Surgery, *N Engl J Med,* **273:**287, 1965.

Layne, O. L., Jr., and Yudofsky, S. C.: Postoperative Psychosis in Cardiotomy Patients: The Role of Organic and Psychiatric Factors, *N Engl J Med,* **284:**518, 1971.

Levy, D.: Psychic Trauma of Operations in Children and a Note on Combat Neurosis, *Am J Dis Child,* **69:**7, 1945.

Lewis, A.: "The Relation between Operative Risk and the Patient's General Condition," Report 16, Congrès International de Chirurgie, Copenhague, 1955.

Lindemann, E.: Observations on Psychiatric Sequelae to Surgical Operations in Women, *Am J Psychiat,* **98:**132, 1941.

Meyer, B. C.: Some Psychiatric Aspects of Surgical Practice, *Psychosom Med,* **20:**203, 1958.

——, Brown, F., and Levine, A.: Observations on the House-Tree-Person Drawing Test Before and After Surgery, *Psychosom Med,* **17:**428, 1955.

Moore, F., Steinberg, R., Bull, M., Wilson, G., and Myrden, J.: Studies in Surgical Endocrinology: I, *Ann Surg,* **141:**145, 1955.

Prugh, D., Staub, E., Sands, H., Kirschbaum, R., and Lenihan, R.: A Study of the Emotional Reactions of Children and Families to Hospitalization and Illness, *Am J Orthopsychiatry,* **22:**70, 1953.

Sand, P., Livingston, G., and Wright, R. G.: Psychological Assessment of Candidates for a Haemodialysis Program, *Ann Intern Med,* **64:**602, 1966.

Scott, J.: Postoperative Psychosis in the Aged, *Am J Surg,* **10:**38, 1960.

Shea, E. J., Bogdan, D. F., Freeman, R. B., and Schreiner, G. E.: Haemodialysis for Chronic Renal Failure: IV. Psychological Considerations, *Ann Intern Med,* **62:**558, 1965.

Sutherland, A.: Psychological Impact of Postoperative Cancer, *Bull NY Acad Med,* **33:**428, 1957.

——, and Ohrbach, C.: Psychological Impact of Cancer and Cancer Surgery: II. Depressive Reactions Associated with Surgery for Cancer, *Cancer,* **6:**958, 1953.

——, ——, Dyk, R., and Bard, M.: The Psychological Impact of Cancer and Cancer Surgery: I. Adaptation to the Dry Colostomy: Preliminary Report and Summary of Findings, *Cancer,* **5:**857, 1952.

Titchener, J. L., and Levine, M.: "Surgery as a Human Experience: The Psychodynamics of Surgical Practice," Oxford University Press, Fair Lawn, N.J., 1960.

——, Zwerling, I., Gottschalk, L., Levine, M., Culbertson, W., Cohen, S., and Silver, H.: Psychosis in Surgical Patients, *Surg Gynecol Obstet,* **102:**59, 1956.

Weisman, A. D., and Hackett, T. P.: Psychosis after Eye Surgery: Establishment of a Specific Doctor-Patient Relation in the Prevention and Treatment of "Black-patch Delirium," *N Engl J Med,* **258:**1284, 1958.

Weiss, S. M.: Psychological Adjustment following Open-Heart Surgery, *J Nerv Ment Dis,* **143:**363, 1966.

Winkelstein, C., Blacher, R. S., and Meyer, B. C.: Psychiatric Observations on Surgical Patients in Recovery Room: Pilot Study, *NY J Med,* **65:**865, 1965.

Wright, R. G., Sand, P., and Livingston, G.: Psychological Stress during Haemodialysis for Chronic Renal Failure, *Ann Intern Med,* **64:**611, 1966.

Zaks, M. S.: Disturbances in Physiologic Functions and Neuropsychiatric Complications in Heart Surgery, in A. A. Luisada (ed.), "Cardiology: An Encyclopedia of the Cardiovascular System," vol. 3, McGraw-Hill Book Company, New York, 1959.

Complications of Gastrointestinal Surgery

Aguirre, A., Fischer, J. E., and Welch, C. E.: Role of Surgery and Hyperalimentation in Therapy of Gastrointestinal-Cutaneous Fistulas, *Ann Surg,* **180:**393, 1974.

Beal, J. M., and Moody, F. G.: Postoperative Complications of Duodenal Surgery, *Surg Clin North Am,* **44:**379, 1964.

Blomstedt, B., and Dahlgren, S.: The Afferent Loop Syndrome, *Acta Chir Scand,* **120:**347, 1961.

Burnett, W. E., Rosemond, G. P., Caswell, H. T., Beauchamp, E. W., Jr., Tyson, R. R., and Wright, W. C.: Studies on So-called Postgastrectomy Pancreatitis, *Ann Surg,* **149:**737, 1959.

Capper, W. M., and Welbourn, R. B.: Early Postcibal Symptoms following Gastrectomy, *Br J Surg,* **43:**24, 1955.

Colcock, B. P.: Leakage from the Duodenal Stump following Gastric Resection, *Lahey Clin Bull,* **13:**190, 1964.

Edmunds, L. H., Jr., Williams, G. M., and Welch, C. E.: External Fistulas Arising from the Gastro-intestinal Tract, *Ann Surg,* **152:**445, 1960.

Everett, E. G.: Comparison of One-Layer and Two-Layer Technique for Colorectal Anastomosis, *Br J Surg,* **62:**135, 1975.

Habif, D. V.: Immediate Complications of Surgery of the Small Intestine, *Surg Clin North Am,* **44:**387, 1964.

Hibner, R., and Richards, V.: Stomal or Small Bowel Obstruction following Partial Gastrectomy, *Am J Surg,* **96:**309, 1958.

Hoffman, W. A., and Spiro, H. M.: Afferent Loop Problems, *Gastroenterology,* **40:**201, 1961.

Johnson, C. L., and McIlrath, D. C.: Management of Patients with Enterocutaneous Fistulas, *Surg Clin North Am,* **49:**967, 1969.

Lichtman, A. L., and McDonald, J. R.: Fecal Fistula, *Surg Gynecol Obstet,* **78:**449, 1944.

MacFadyen, B. V., Dudrick, S. J., and Ruberg, R. L.: The Management of Gastrointestinal Fistulae with Parenteral Hyperalimentation, *Surgery,* 1973. (To be published.)

McLachlin, A. D., and Denton, D. W.: Omental Protection of Intestinal Anastomes, *Am J Surg,* **125:**134, 1973.

Magnuson, F. K., Judd, E. S., and Dearing, W. H.: Comparison of Postgastrectomy Complications in Gastric and Duodenal Ulcer Patients, *Am Surg,* **32:**375, 1966.

Moretz, W. H.: Inadvertent Gastro-ileostomy, *Ann Surg,* **130:**124, 1949.

Morgenstern, L., Yamakawa, T., Ben-Shoshan, M., and Lippman, H.: Anastomotic Leakage after Low Colonic Anastomosis. Clinical and Experimental Aspects, *Am J Surg,* **123:**104, 1972.

Pettersson, S., and Wallensten, S.: Leakage at Suture Lines after Partial Gastrectomy for Peptic Ulcer, *Acta Chir Scand,* **135:**229, 1969.

Quinn, W. F., and Gifford, J. H.: Syndrome of Proximal Jejunal Loop Obstruction following Anterior Gastric Resection, *Calif Med,* **72:**18, 1950.

Rodkey, G. V., and Welch, C. E.: Duodenal Decompression in Gastrectomy, *N Engl J Med,* **262:**498, 1960.

Rousselot, L. M., and Slattery, J. R.: Immediate Complications of Surgery of the Large Intestine, *Surg Clin North Am,* **44:**397, 1964.

Spencer, F. C.: Ischemic Necrosis of Remaining Stomach following Subtotal Gastrectomy, *Arch Surg,* **73:**844, 1956.

State, D.: Immediate Complications of Gastric Surgery, *Surg Clin North Am,* **44:**371, 1964.

Turner, F. P.: Postoperative Complications following Gastric Resection, *Am J Surg,* **101:**711, 1961.

Chapter 13

Physiologic Monitoring of the Surgical Patient

by **Louis R. M. Del Guercio**

Introduction

Physiologic Concepts and Monitoring

Instrumentation and Clinical Techniques

Physiologic Sensing
Respiratory Monitoring
Cardiovascular Monitoring
Cardiac Output Determinations
Monitoring of Tissue Metabolism

INTRODUCTION

Among the 14 definitions of the word "monitor" which appear in one dictionary, three appear applicable to medicine: "Something that serves to remind or give warning"; "A device or arrangement for observing or recording the operation of a machine or system, esp. an automatic control system"; and "To observe, record or detect an operation or condition with instruments that have no effect on the operation or condition."

This last definition offers the key to a basic problem of all patient monitoring, i.e., that the measuring system tends to change the measurements. The application of electrodes, cannulas, mouthpieces, and other paraphernalia definitely has psychologic and physiologic effects on the patient. From this it follows that the ideal monitoring system should be noninvasive and unobtrusive.

Another point to be stressed is that the most sophisticated and advanced electronic system can never substitute for close surveillance by an experienced and qualified health professional. Monitors in surgery are worthwhile only if they provide physiologic information about the patient which cannot be detected by the five senses of a physician or nurse. In addition, the transducers, signal processors, or readout devices should not so encumber the patient as to interfere with essential nursing care.

There is a tendency to think of monitoring in terms of complicated electronic devices and computers; in fact, the serial recordings of temperature, pulse, respiratory rate, and blood pressure are forms of clinical monitoring in common use for decades. This approach to monitoring had been observed by Harvey Cushing on a visit to Italy and, overcoming considerable resistance, he introduced routine blood pressure recording to the United States in 1903. These simple techniques served the surgeon fairly well until the advent of cardiopulmonary bypass and open heart surgery. At that point, it was recognized that optimum clinical care in the period following what could be considered at best a controlled physiologic insult, required a better assessment of the cardiovascular and respiratory status of the patient. Decisions regarding therapy had to be made rapidly on the basis of reasonably accurate measurements of physiologic variables.

This led in the early 1960s to the clinical use of central venous pressure and cardiac output determinations. The invention of the densitometer for the continuous recording of indicator dilution and of electrodes for the rapid determination of the partial pressures of oxygen and carbon dioxide in whole blood provided the technical impetus for the modern era of clinical monitoring.

Subsequently, many specialized diagnostic and treatment centers established within the hospital have included physiologic monitoring as an adjunct to patient care. Coronary care units, respiratory care centers, burn centers, neurosurgical intensive care units, pediatric and neonatal intensive care units, renal dialysis centers, and surgical intensive care units all utilize some forms of patient monitoring. Only in the coronary care unit, however, can it be statistically documented that lives are saved by monitoring. In this case, the electrocardiograph is an almost ideal monitor because it is safe, noninvasive, and specific for the physiologic aberration, cardiac arrhythmias, which kills most myocardial infarction victims.

The problem of monitoring for the surgical patient is much more complex, because there is as yet no known single physiologic variable which can be used to warn against impending disaster. And although there are many systems in daily operation which on the basis of cardiac output, arterial pressure, central venous pressure, and blood-gas tensions provide assessment of cardiorespiratory function and oxygen transport, these techniques are primarily used when it is already obvious that the patient is in serious trouble. Such systems at the present time are generally invasive and are used intermittently to assess the response of a desperately ill patient to specific modes of therapy. There are many models of these "shock carts" currently available commercially.

The second type of surgical monitoring involves the

continuous recording of one or two fundamental physiologic variables in order to show trends and changes which may warn of impending disaster. At the present time there is no system of this type in operation which has been proved to be practical for most surgical patients. Continuous rather than intermittent monitoring would be desirable for surgical patients if it could be performed inexpensively and noninvasively, because more information can be obtained from a variable which is measured in relation to time. Patterns and trends can be detected and compared with mathematical models obtained from studies of patients known to be in jeopardy. For example, it is believed by most experts that there is no such thing as cardiac arrest without antecedent events. Clinical studies have shown that long before cardiac standstill or ventricular fibrillation occurs, serious derangements of blood-gas tensions or hemodynamic variables can be demonstrated. Continuous monitoring of certain variables might reveal catastrophic trends.

But since cardiac arrest is a rare event, the need for surgical monitoring in the general population might be questioned, were it not for the National Halothane Study. That prospective statistical analysis of over 850,000 operations performed in 35 highly regarded hospitals revealed an overall 6-week mortality rate of 1.97 percent! This included ophthalmologic, plastic, and other low-death-rate operations. The overall need for surgical monitoring is mandated by that totally unacceptable mortality rate, which is higher than that for 1 year of combat service in World War II, Korea, or Vietnam!

PHYSIOLOGIC CONCEPTS AND MONITORING

One of the problems with patient monitoring today is that we tend to measure the variables which we *can* rather than the variables which we *should*. Thus far in the twentieth century, instruments have directed medicine rather than vice versa; we use the instruments which happen to be available. For example, the entire discipline of diagnostic cardiology developed around measurement of intracardiac pressure gradients and electric potentials rather than volume and flow relationships, because the strain gauge pressure transducer and electrocardiograph were the first instruments available. Monitoring to warn against surgical disaster or to record the proper operation of such a complex "automatic control system" as the human body must be based upon physiologic principles. Instruments and monitoring systems must be developed and designed to detect specific physiologic events known to be associated with surgical morbidity or mortality.

The overall physiology of oxygen transport, or the delivery of oxygen from the atmosphere to the mitochondria of the body cell mass, can be used as a model to assess the abilities of particular monitoring systems to detect critical events and trends. This process involves many organ systems and complicated feedback loops for regulation and compensation. It is imperative for the survival of the individual that the oxygen transport system continue in operation without interruption.

Even in the basal state, 4 ml of oxygen is required each minute for each kilogram of body weight. Human beings can store only a 4- or 5-minute supply in the lungs and blood cells. With cessation of oxygen transport anywhere along the line serious defects of oxygen tension gradient develop within 2 minutes. Even the highly trained pearl divers of Northern Australia dive for less than 2 minutes, and they still manifest markedly elevated blood lactate levels and frequent cardiac arrythmias. The best of the diving mammals, the whale, cannot store proportionately more than twice the amount of oxygen stored by nondiving mammals such as man.

The upper airways serve to humidify and warm or cool the air entering the tracheobronchial tree during spontaneous respiration. The difference in temperature between inspired and expired air provides a basis for monitoring the rate of respiration in patients. Simple thermistor probes have been developed which are fixed in front of the external nares to record the passage of warmed expired air. It is not possible by this means to evaluate the adequacy of ventilation, but a simple noninvasive means of monitoring the respiratory rate and signaling respiratory arrest could be of value. Respiratory rate is regulated by changes in arterial oxygen content through the carotid and aortic body reflexes, and by changes in pH and carbon dioxide tension through brainstem chemoreceptors. Hyperpnea can be a relatively nonspecific warning sign suggesting hypoxia, sepsis, increased metabolic demands, emotional excitement, or simply painful stimuli.

Table 13-1 traces the oxygen flow and partial pressure gradients from this point on. The critical importance of each stage is related to the oxygen stored beyond that point. For example, respiratory failure is tolerated far longer than circulatory arrest, because the circulatory system stores more than twice as much oxygen as the lungs. Cyanide kills quickly because it blocks the ability of the mitochondria to utilize oxygen. This is a point beyond which there is no oxygen reserve. Total body oxygen stores are about 1,500 ml. A monitoring system should detect a block of this most critical step, delivery of oxygen to the mitochondrion within the cell. At this point, oxygen stores are nil and the tension gradient is low.

The partial pressure of oxygen in the atmosphere is 159 mm Hg (20.84 percent of 760 mm Hg). As inspired air is rapidly humidified in the upper airways by the mucosa of the nasal turbinates, pharynx, and tracheobronchial tree, the partial pressure drops to 149 mm Hg due to the dilutional effect of the water vapor pressure at body temperature (47 mm Hg). As the alveoli are approached, the oxygen tension rapidly falls, because approximately 4 ml/kg of body mass of that gas is removed from the alveoli each minute. The 45 mm Hg fall in oxygen tension is replaced by a similar rise in carbon dioxide tension in the alveoli. It is the rapid removal of oxygen from the alveoli by the unsaturated blood entering the pulmonary capillary bed which establishes this gradient. This is why it is possible to maintain adequate oxygenation for several minutes by

Table 13-1. OXYGEN TRANSPORT AND MONITORING

Oxygen stores, ml	Oxygen tension gradient, mm Hg	Medium	Measurements
370	159 149 105	Atmosphere Airway Alveoli Interstitial fluid	Tidal volume, dead-space-to-tidal-volume ratio, lung compliance, work of breathing, functional residual capacity, end tidal CO_2, percent shunt, alveolar-arterial O_2 gradient, pulmonary transit time, blood gases
880	100 95 90	Pulmonary capillary Plasma Red cell membrane Hemoglobin Left side of heart Arteries Arteriole	Cardiac output, stroke volume, ejection fraction, ventricular function curves, systolic time intervals, central venous pressure, pulmonary wedge pressure, left ventricular end-diastolic pressure
	90–40	Capillary	Oxygen consumption, effective oxygen transport, mixed venous oxygen levels, P_{50}, blood lactate concentration, tissue oxygen tension, muscle surface pH
56	40 38 20 10	Endothelium Extracellular fluid Pericapillary tissue cylinder Cell membrane	
240	6	Myoglobin	
0	5	Mitochondrion	

*(left margin, vertical:* Oxygen flow *)*

$\rightarrow$ Oxygen + electrons +
            hydrogen ions $\longrightarrow$ water

Cytochromes $\longrightarrow$ 2 ATP
Ubiquinone
Flavoprotein $\longrightarrow$ 1 ATP
Diphosphopyridine nucleotide (DPN)
Acetyl coenzyme A
Pyruvate
Glucose

*(left margin, vertical:* Electron flow *)*

flushing oxygen into a bronchoscope without any ventilation. Of course, the blood carbon dioxide level rises markedly. The energy cost of ventilation may represent a serious problem to some postoperative patients. Many physiologic variables associated with ventilation and lung mechanics can be measured at the bedside if necessary; among these are tidal volume, minute ventilation, dead-space-to-tidal-volume ratios, compliance, and functional residual capacity. All these give an assessment of the efficiency of the lung, chest, and diaphragm in exchanging air in the alveoli.

The next stage in oxygen transport is truly remarkable. In 5 seconds, the entire output of the right side of the heart is spread out over an area the size of a tennis court and sucked back up into the left atrium. The blood pressure differential across this system is only 6 mm Hg, and all of the blood, during the brief time which the red cells spend in the pulmonary capillaries, normally reaches equilibrium with the oxygen in the alveoli. Only 90 ml of blood is in the capillaries at one time. Moreover, this remarkably efficient manifold system can dynamically expand within seconds to handle three times the normal blood flow without any sacrifice in oxygenation. Roughton has estimated that at normal flow rates each red cell takes 0.8 second

to squeeze through two or three alveolar capillaries in succession. At high flow rates, during exercise or in hyperdynamic shock, the time spent in the capillary bed is reduced. When it is reduced below 0.35 second, there is insufficient time for the four heme positions of the hemoglobin molecule to take up oxygen, and unsaturation results because of this so-called "speed shunt." This situation can also occur when the cross-sectional area of pulmonary bed is reduced, as in pulmonary embolism, since a more rapid flow is forced past the remaining capillaries. Arterial hypoxemia is well known in pulmonary embolism.

It can be seen from Table 13-1 that oxygen flow from the alveoli to the hemoglobin within the red cell encounters a number of resistances: alveolar membrane, interstitial fluid, capillary membrane, plasma, red cell membrane, and the paracrystalline structure within the red cell. But since all these together are normally only a few microns thick, diffusion is rapid. Many things can go wrong with this efficient system, however, and opportunities for monitoring at this level have been recognized. The red cells normally leave the pulmonary capillaries with an oxygen tension of 100 mm Hg. When they arrive in the left side of the heart, the partial pressure has dropped to about 95 mm Hg because of the mixing effect of unsaturated blood from the bronchial and coronary circulation which empties into the left side of the heart. This shunted blood normally is 3 percent of the output of the right side of the heart.

The difference in the partial pressure of oxygen from the alveoli to the arterial blood is an important monitoring variable. It is called the *alveolar-arterial oxygen gradient* (A-aDO$_2$). It is most useful in assessing the efficiency of gas exchange in the lung and is an early indicator of incipient respiratory failure due to a variety of causes in surgical patients. The normal A-aDO$_2$ is 25 to 65 mm Hg when the inspired oxygen concentration is 100 percent.

When the arterial oxygen tension falls below 60 mm Hg in a surgical patient without previous lung disease or intracardiac defects, the diagnosis of acute respiratory failure is made. An arterial oxygen tension below 30 mm Hg is generally incompatible with survival for more than a few hours. Several factors, singly or in combination, can produce this severe hypoxemia. Abnormal distribution of blood to sections of the lung containing closed or non-ventilated airways or alveoli will result in so-called physiologic shunting of unsaturated blood into the arterial circulation. Injury to the pulmonary capillary endothelium or pulmonary vascular congestion frequently leads to increased interstitial lung water, which not only increases the diffusion distance for oxygen but causes collapse of alveoli. Pulmonary surfactant, which normally prevents alveolar collapse by reducing surface tension at low lung volumes, may be depleted by hypoxemia and lack of metabolic substrates in acute disease. Thus the collapse of more alveoli creates a vicious cycle of increasing hypoxemia. The reduced lung volume and loss of compliance, or distensibility, are characteristic of a group of nonspecific respiratory distress syndromes associated with shock, trauma, and other clinical problems. They all result in serious venous admixture, so that as much as 50 percent of the output of the right side of the heart may bypass ventilated alveoli. In this circumstance, the alveolar-arterial oxygen gradient may be more than 600 mm Hg, resulting in an arterial oxygen tension of only 60 mm Hg. It is important to detect such a problem early, before irreversible damage is done. The use of a respirator with continuous positive-pressure breathing (PEEP) reduces the cost of respiratory work and decreases shunting by ventilating more alveoli.

Thus far, in dissecting the oxygen transport system as a guide to physiologic monitoring, only oxygen loading has been considered. Other problems can occur downstream related to bloodflow, hemoglobin deficiency, hemoglobin affinity, or cellular defects. These more or less reflect the classic forms of hypoxia described by Barcroft and later appended by Van Slyke: anoxic, stagnant, anemic, and histotoxic hypoxia.

In considering the physiology of body blood flow, two important points must be made: the cardiac output alone is not an indicator of myocardial contractility, and arterial blood pressure alone is not an indicator of blood flow. Myocardial contractility refers to the state of health of the heart muscle and the rate at which the muscle fibers can shorten circumferentially around the bolus of blood within the ventricles. As will be seen later, myocardial contrac-

tility is intimately involved with myocardial oxygen transport.

Cardiac output, the actual amount of blood ejected by the heart, is related to three other factors besides contractility: preload, afterload, and pulse rate. The preload is the degree of muscle fiber stretch imposed by filling of the ventricles during diastole. According to Starling's law of the heart, this varies directly with cardiac output. The afterload is the impedance to cardiac ejection during systole imposed by vascular resistance, blood pressure, and blood viscosity. The stroke output of the heart varies inversely with the afterload. The cardiac output varies directly with the pulse rate up to a level of 160, at which point there is insufficient time for complete ventricular filling. Any monitoring system designed to assess the state of the myocardium must include these factors. The Sarnoff ventricular function curve is a plot of stroke work (the product of stroke volume and mean aortic blood pressure) against ventricular end-diastolic pressure or end-diastolic volume. It provides a good evaluation of myocardial contractility because it includes consideration of afterload and preload.

One manifestation of the human body as an automatic control system is the fact that a major determinant of cardiac output is increased metabolic activity which produces peripheral vasodilation and a reduced cardiac afterload. Increased metabolic activity also increases the venous return and thus slightly increases cardiac preload. The peripheral arterioles under control of the autonomic nervous system largely control the systemic vascular resistance. The systemic blood pressure varies with the product of the total vascular resistance and the cardiac output. This is why it is impossible to evaluate blood flow on the basis of the blood pressure alone. One seldom used clue to the level of total peripheral resistance is the pulse pressure or the difference between systolic and diastolic blood pressure. As total peripheral resistance increases, the pulse pressure narrows because of increased outflow impedance from the arterial tree.

The varying distribution of the cardiac output to the different organs and body tissues is the body's most important defense in oxygen transport deficiency. During resuscitation from cardiac arrest, the cardiac index is slightly over 1 liter/minute with open-chest cardiac massage. Closed-chest massage produces half of that. The normal cardiac index is 3 liters/minute/m^2 of body surface area. Yet these low flows are frequently enough to keep the brain alive, because flow to all other tissues except the myocardium is drastically curtailed.

The brain is particularly sensitive to hypoxia. It has no oxygen reserves and constantly requires 15 percent of the resting cardiac output and 20 percent of the total basal oxygen consumption just to maintain its structural and physiologic integrity. The reasons for this will be discussed later. However, irreversible brain damage occurs in man when cerebral oxygen consumption is 50 percent reduced, while the kidneys can tolerate one-third the normal flow for over an hour without damage although they normally receive 25 percent of the cardiac output. In general, organs with low oxygen extraction ratios tolerate decreased blood flow fairly well. The kidneys normally extract only 10 percent of the oxygen available in their arterial blood supply, the heart extracts 70 percent, and the body as a whole extracts 25 percent. An arm or a leg can survive total tourniquet occlusion of its blood supply for over an hour without permanent damage, and the cornea of the eye survives several hours after death of the individual.

During acute hypoxia or circulatory crises, blood is preferentially sent to the heart and brain. Since flow is curtailed to tissues with a low priority such as the skin, skeletal muscles, and corneas as soon as hypoxia or low flow threatens, monitoring flow or oxygen tension in these tissues would provide an early warning.

Organs other than the heart, which normally extracts most of the oxygen from coronary artery blood, can compensate for low blood flow by extracting more oxygen from their venous oxygen reserves. Thus, the arteriovenous oxygen difference of the body or of an individual organ is a measure of the extent to which blood flow matches the metabolic demand for oxygen. In the normal resting state, the entire body consumes only 25 percent of the oxygen transported to it by the cardiac output. This is confirmed from all the organs after it has been mixed in the right side of the heart. Normal mixed venous blood is found to be 75 percent saturated with a partial pressure of 40 mm Hg. Levels lower than this indicate increased oxygen demands which cannot be met because of decreased available arterial oxygen or decreased cardiac output. Since most surgeons would like to be warned of either of these circumstances, monitoring of mixed venous oxygen levels is becoming popular. Mixed venous oxygen tension during anesthesia responds to a fall in cardiac output before any change is noted in blood pressure, pulse rate, or central venous pressure. It would be useful to assess the oxygen supply to individual organs as well, particularly the brain. Cerebrospinal fluid from the cisterna magna of the brain responds promptly to hypoxemia or ischemia with a drop in oxygen tension, but this can hardly be considered a noninvasive approach.

Having considered the lungs, the heart, and major blood vessels, we now approach the business end of the oxygen transport system, where the partial pressure of oxygen rapidly drops from 90 to 40 mm Hg. The capillary bed of an organ is a rapidly changing dynamic system with precapillary sphincters under the control of tissue hypoxic feedback mechanisms as well as sympathetic and hemodynamic reflexes. When increased work, fever, inflammation, catecholamine stimulation, or increased thyroxine levels intensify the metabolic demands of an organ, precapillary sphincters relax and the capillary bed enlarges. A working skeletal muscle has ten to twenty times the number of functioning capillaries as a resting muscle. The myocardium has the most active set of sphincters and the most profuse capillary network of any organ. In the basal state, less than half the capillaries are open, but with increased demands the myocardial oxygen consumption can increase sixfold. Not only does more blood flow through the enlarged capillary bed, but the distance between open capillaries is reduced from 20 to 14 μ, so that oxygen has a shorter diffusion distance to the cells. This

increased vascularity further reduces peripheral resistance and cardiac afterload in addition to that achieved by arteriolar dilatation. Up until this point, very little oxygen is lost from the arterial blood, but in the capillaries many factors combine to encourage oxygen unloading in the cylinder of tissue surrounding each capillary. The natural affinity of hemoglobin for oxygen is decreased by heat, hydrogen ions, carbon dioxide (Bohr effect), and red cell diphosphoglycerate (DPG). These agents act at a stereochemical level to help form a hemoglobin molecule which is more stable in its unsaturated state. The heat of working tissues, hypoxic acidosis, and carbon dioxide from cellular metabolism all tend to shift the oxyhemoglobin dissociation curve to the right where more oxygen is released at a higher tissue oxygen tension. The relative position of the oxyhemoglobin dissociation curve is identified by the P_{50} value, the partial pressure of oxygen at which the hemoglobin is half saturated at 37°C and pH 7.4. There is a biologic feedback mechanism which increases the red cell diphosphoglycerate in chronic hypoxic states, but like renal erythropoietin regulation, the mechanism is too slow to be of significance in clinical monitoring.

Red cell diphosphoglycerate may be of considerable clinical significance in patients requiring massive blood transfusions. Bank blood stored for more than 2 weeks is depleted of diphosphoglycerate, reducing the P_{50} value from 26 to 11 mm Hg. Adequate oxygen release in the capillary bed can occur only at lower oxygen tensions, thus reducing the oxygen diffusion gradient in the tissue cylinder surrounding the capillary. The cells at the venous end of the capillary, where the oxygen tension is normally lower, are the first to suffer. For this reason, the periphery of the pericapillary cylinder at the venous end is called the *todlische Ecke*, or "deadly corner." This effect is best seen in centrilobular necrosis of the liver, wherein hypoxic cell death first occurs near the central venule.

Another frequently overlooked problem of hemoglobin affinity is carbon monoxide poisoning. Patients who have been burned in closed spaces may have serious defects of oxygen transport caused by carbon monoxide displacing oxygen from hemoglobin and poisoning the mitochondrial cytochrome a_3 system. In addition, carbon monoxide lowers the P_{50}, which further reduces available oxygen (Fig. 13-7).

Since oxygen tension falls off with the square of the distance from the capillary, by the time oxygen diffuses through the pores of the cell membrane, the partial pressure of oxygen is about 6 mm Hg. Table 13-1 shows a value of 10 mm Hg outside the membrane. This does not mean that there is resistance to diffusion across the cell membrane but that, within the tissues, consumption of oxygen must occur in the cells in order to establish a gradient. Within the cell, myoglobin facilitates the passage of oxygen by serving as a sort of bucket brigade. As might be expected from what has been described in previous paragraphs, the cardiac muscle is richest in myoglobin. Myoglobin has a very high affinity for oxygen and releases it only at very low tensions, as needed. The actual utilization of oxygen occurs in complex intracellular organelles called *mitochondria*.

In the mitochondrion, an array of catalysts and cofactors comprising the Krebs cycle oxidize pyruvate produced by the anaerobic glycolysis of glucose. Anaerobic glycolysis of glucose yields only 50 kcal/mole, whereas the complete oxidation of glucose to carbon dioxide and water in the mitochondrion yields 686 kcal/mole of glucose. The higher animals cannot survive on the lower-energy-producing fermentative process alone. Some 1.2 billion years ago, organisms learned to protect themselves from the toxic oxygen molecules slowly building up in the primeval atmosphere by enzymatically catalyzing the reduction of oxygen to water while at the same time oxidizing the end products of cellular fermentation such as lactic acid. Trillions of generations later, the cells harnessed the extra energy thus released to the reconstitution of the high-energy phosphate bond of adenosine triphosphate (ATP). Vestiges of the earlier process are still found, even in human cells, in the form of other organelles called *peroxisomes*. Peroxisomes are believed to protect cells from excess oxygen by the enzymatic oxidation of amino acids and lactic acid. However, this oxidation is not coupled to energy storage.

Within the mitochondrion, the oxidation of pyruvate is carried out anaerobically by removal of electrons rather than the addition of oxygen. The electrons are passed along the respiratory chain, alternately oxidizing and reducing diphosphopyridine nucleotide (DPN), flavoproteins, ubiquinone, and cytochromes. At the final step cytochrome C passes two electrons to an oxygen atom, which combines with two hydrogen ions to form one molecule of water. An obligatory coupling of this process to the conversion of adenosine diphosphate (ADP) to ATP fulfills two functions. First, much of the high energy of the complete oxidation of glucose is stored for all forms of cellular work. Second, the rate of this oxidative phosphorylation is governed by the energy needs of the cell. The cell is protected from excess oxygen by the fact that only when ADP is present will oxygen be utilized to allow the establishment of an oxygen gradient across the cell membrane. As long as the intracellular oxygen tension is above 5 mm Hg, the rate-limiting factor of cellular respiration is the availability of ADP, not oxygen.

Certain agents, the best known of which is dinitrophenol, uncouple oxidation from phosphorylation permitting runaway oxidation without energy storage. This is a rapidly lethal process. Less well known is the uncoupling ability of certain bacterial endotoxins. Abnormally high oxygen consumption has been demonstrated just before death in patients with septic shock. Cyanide and carbon monoxide have the reverse effect on the cell; they block the transfer of electrons from cytochrome C to oxygen.

Britton Chance has defined three cellular respiratory states. First, in the resting state, oxidative phosphorylation is limited by low levels of ADP and phosphates. Second, in the working state, most of the ATP has been converted to ADP, establishing a relatively high oxygen gradient from the capillary to the mitochondrion. Third, ADP and phosphate are in excess; if oxygen is not available for diffusion from the capillary, critical pyridine nucleotide reduction (CPNR) rapidly occurs. Critical levels of reduced DPN occur when oxygen tension in the mitochondrion falls to 0.1 mm Hg. This corresponds to a capillary oxygen tension of 4 mm Hg. The cell is forced to obtain energy from anaerobic glycolysis alone, thus building up an oxygen debt and conversion of pyruvate to lactic acid. Acidosis and elevated lactate levels can be detected in the peripheral circulation, but only if capillary perfusion is present to wash the cellular products into the venous circulation. This is why, in shock states, peripheral arterial pH may not accurately reflect intracellular pH. The autolytic washout products of critically hypoxic and injured cells have been monitored for decades on the false assumption that venous blood always equilibrates with ischemic tissue. A better approach would be to detect molecular signals at the cellular level.

Voluntary muscle can build up an oxygen debt of 40 ml/kg of cell mass, compared to a resting oxygen requirement of 4 ml/kg/minute. The 10 billion neuron units of the human brain can tolerate no oxygen debt. When the cerebral arterial oxygen tension falls to 20 mm Hg, that within the neurons is only 0.2 mm Hg. At this level of hypoxia, half of the electron carrier, DPN, is in the reduced state. When 90 percent of DPN is in the reduced state, even the respiratory center ceases to function, and irreversible damage occurs. As long as some circulatory flow exists, even with severe hypoxemia, there is a chance to maintain the critical 0.1 mm Hg tension within the neuron. With complete circulatory arrest, however, the oxygen is quickly used up, and the neuron dies. The brain requires constant energy supplies just to maintain the unsteady state of polarization for the transmission of the network of impulses which is an integral part of the cerebral life process. This peculiar and critical requirement of the brain is related to modern information theory, which explains the energy requirements of complex information systems. Long before the critical state of cerebral hypoxia is reached, other symptoms and signs occur, such as restlessness, unconsciousness, Cheyne-Stokes respiration, and EEG abnormalities. There is recent evidence by Safar's group that massive doses of short-acting barbiturates, given shortly after complete cerebral ischemia, provide protection for the brain and normalize its metabolism.

As other cells reach critical hypoxic states, they no longer have the energy to maintain important internal cell structures. One of these is the phospholipid lysosomal membrane which protects the cell from the necessary but potentially destructive enzymes contained within the lysosomes. When released into the cell, the powerful proteases, esterases, and phosphatases destroy the cell.

Britton Chance has led the way in developing methods to study cellular hypoxia. His fluorometric instrument makes it possible to measure intracellular oxygen tensions between 0.03 and 2 mm Hg. This is accomplished by measuring the fluorescence emission of the reduced state of DPN when it is stimulated by ultraviolet light. Other techniques of detecting molecular signals at a distance for monitoring purposes are possible, among them stimulated emission of oxygen in the microwave range, far infrared emission spectroscopy (chemiluminescence), and surface reflectance spectroscopy. Though exciting, all these are a long way from validation and routine clinical use in man.

INSTRUMENTATION AND CLINICAL TECHNIQUES

Physiologic Sensing

Rushmer has classified the methods used to obtain information from the human body for monitoring purposes. The most obvious is the analysis of samples of tissue, blood, respiratory gases, urine, cerebrospinal fluid, or other body fluids. Here the assumption is that the sample in question is a representative aliquot of the state of the entire organ system.

In surgical monitoring, the most useful aspects of this approach include continuous or intermittent analysis of arterial or mixed venous pH, blood gases (P_{O_2}, P_{CO_2}), and lactate. As pointed out earlier, the blood lactate level can be considered an indicator of the adequacy of oxygen transport to the Krebs cycle in the mitochondria. Elevated blood lactate levels indicate anaerobic metabolism as long as there is enough tissue perfusion to "wash out" the acid metabolites. Blood lactate, increased from above 1.5 mEq/L to levels above 10 mEq/L, is a grave prognostic sign unless the trend is promptly reversed.

The disadvantage of the tissue and fluid sampling approach to monitoring is that it is invasive and therefore carries some risk of infection or blood loss. An invasive technique is always more expensive than a noninvasive one, because it requires more highly trained personnel for insertion, sterilization of parts, and surveillance to prevent accidents. A corollary to this rule is that the more invasive a device, the less likely is its use before it is too late.

Rushmer's two other monitoring categories are (1) techniques which utilize intrinsic energy sources within the body of the patient and (2) methods which direct extrinsic energy probes at or into the body, with analysis of the emerging energy. Many physiologic processes are characterized by the generation of dynamic potentials, tensions, pressures, and electromagnetic emissions which constitute the intrinsic energy sources available for surgical monitoring. Examples of this approach include electrocardiography, electroencephalography, thermography, infrared emission spectroscopy, and muscle surface pH metering.

The energy used for interrogating beams in extrinsic energy probe monitoring can be ultrasound, mechanical stimuli, or photons originating at any point along the electromagnetic spectrum from gamma rays to microwaves. Examples include ultrasonic echography, videodensitometry, nuclear magnetic resonance flow probes, and impedance plethysmography.

Shannon and Weaver's classic work on information theory can be used to show that, in general, the higher the frequency of the interrogating beam or intrinsic energy source, the more information capacity (bits per second) it has. For example, a gamma ray probe could be expected to detect more physiologic information than an ultrasonic probe. Other variables such as signal-to-noise ratio, of course, are important in determining the ultimate monitoring value of a particular system. A monitoring system employing extrinsic energy probes usually yields information with good spatial discrimination with regard to functional lesions, whereas devices which detect intrinsic energy usually provide an information-rich signal which often requires data processing for exploitation of its full information content.

The greatest need in the field of monitoring is for new sensors and transducers to detect critical states along the train of oxygen transport. Even very complicated occult signals from new sensing techniques can be made useful by modern spectral search systems. Computer programs are already available to examine and characterize more complex information in large amounts in order to analyze the fundamental properties of living systems.

Four guides to the development of new physiologic sensors are the following:

1. Detection of functional integrity of cells and cellular perfusion rather than the washout of autolytic products into the bloodstream.
2. A noninvasive mode; the device must not reduce the frequency of contact between the health professional and patient.
3. An information-rich signal originating from the desired organ system.
4. Extrinsic energy probes for spatial discrimination and intrinsic energy sources for a broader view of biologic activity.

A transducer is a device which converts energy from one form to another. A sensor is a device which detects an energy signal related to a particular state. In physiologic monitoring, a sensor is often a transducer, but not always. Electrocardiographic and electroencephalographic electrodes are sensors which do not convert energy from one form to another. The suitability of a sensing device for a particular clinical application is related to such factors as sensitivity, response time, linearity, and accuracy. The *sensitivity* is measured by the smallest change which is detectable by the device. The *response time* of an instrument is the period required to record a given change of input. *Linearity* refers to the constancy of the ratio of output signal to the measured variable. *Accuracy* is evaluated in terms of the ability to calibrate the instrument so that the output conforms precisely to the quantity of the measured variable. Accuracy is related to the error induced by unwanted variables such as temperature, pressure, and vibration.

Respiratory Monitoring

Respiratory monitoring can be very simple or extremely complex, depending on the trend or event to be warned against. The detection of a low-probability event such as respiratory arrest is easy compared to the on-line assessment of lung mechanics. Nevertheless, there is need for the former type of monitoring.

Next in complexity is the measurement of blood gases. The widespread use of pressure-cycled or volume-controlled respirators in the postoperative period would not be safe without blood-gas monitoring. In order to take over the work of breathing, when the patient's own respiratory reflexes and servo-control mechanisms are overridden or suppressed by respiratory depressants, it is essential to know if ventilation and gas exchange suit the patient's requirements. Were it not for the invention of the Clark polarographic oxygen electrode and the Severinghaus potentiometric carbon dioxide electrode in the 1950s, the task of monitoring blood gases by the classic manometric technique of Van Slyke and Neill would have imposed enormous difficulties. The Clark electrode depends on the diffusion of oxygen from the blood sample through a gas-permeable plastic membrane surrounding a platinum polarographic electrode. The electrode current is proportional to the number of oxygen molecules, but careful calibration with water of known oxygen concentration is necessary because of variations in membrane permeability and electrolyte characteristics. The Severinghaus potentiometric electrode is a glass pH electrode with bicarbonate buffer within the gas-permeable plastic membrane. Diffusion of carbon dioxide from the blood sample to the electrode produces a change in pH, which is recorded.

There are several commercial apparatus available which include thermostatically controlled water baths, calibration equipment, and digital readout. It is impossible to care properly for many surgical patients today without access to a blood-gas and pH analyzer of this sort. Unlike blood chemistries or electrolytes, these determinations require, for reliability, a rapid turnaround time and rigid quality control. For this reason, the blood-gas laboratory is often located in proximity to the intensive care unit, recovery room, and operating room.

Continuous methods of blood-gas monitoring have been developed for on-line applications, but problems of calibration, quality control, and expense reduce their utility over that of intermittent determinations. Mass spectrometry, which will be discussed later, shows promise as an accurate, rapid method for intermittent or continuous blood-gas monitoring.

Samples of arterial blood for these determinations can be obtained using an ordinary 20-gauge needle, by percutaneous puncture of the radial, brachial, or femoral arteries. The 5- or 10-ml glass or plastic syringe is first heparinized and then capped and placed in ice after the sample is drawn. Iced samples can be kept for 1 hour with a 1 percent drop in oxygen tension. Indwelling arterial and mixed venous lines can also be used as sampling sites, but the volume of blood contained in the catheter must first be discarded.

In assessing the process of gas exchange outlined in the upper part of Table 13-1, the decrement in oxygen tension from the alveolar level to the arterial blood is of considerable importance as a measure of the efficiency of oxygen exchange in the lungs. In normal man breathing room air, the alveolar-arterial oxygen tension gradient, abbreviated as $P(A-aDO_2)$, varies between 10 and 15 mm Hg. Half of this venoarterial admixture is caused by true shunting of desaturated blood into the left atrium, and the other half by ventilation-perfusion imbalance. When the patient with normal cardiorespiratory function breathes pure oxygen for 15 to 20 minutes, the alveolar-arterial gradient is between 25 and 65 mm Hg. Barometric pressure, less arterial carbon dioxide tension, less water vapor pressure, less the normal gradient yields a value of around 630 mm Hg for arterial oxygen tension while breathing pure oxygen. In this condition the gradient represents both anatomic shunting and perfusion of totally nonventilated alveoli. The effects of alveolar capillary diffusion barriers and ventilation-perfusion imbalance are eliminated by the high oxygen tension in all alveoli.

As mentioned earlier, an increased alveolar-arterial gradient on 100 percent oxygen is a very useful early warning sign for many postoperative pulmonary problems, among them atelectasis, pneumonia, interstitial pulmonary edema, septic shock lung, and posttraumatic pulmonary insufficiency. Although not very specific, it is very useful since an increase is easily determined at the bedside and occurs long before most radiologic changes are evident.

It is estimated that in normal resting man approximately 2 percent of total oxygen consumption is used to provide energy for breathing. In postoperative patients this may increase to 50 percent as a result of increased airway resistance and decreased compliance of the lung, chest wall, and diaphragm. Since much of this work can be taken over with proper use of a volume-cycled respirator, the clinical evaluation of respiratory resistance, compliance, and work has been the subject of much bioengineering research.

Patients with chronic obstructive lung disease, in whom the excess work of breathing is related primarily to expiratory rather than inspiratory effort, benefit little from respirator therapy alone. This situation generally should be detected in the preoperative state by standard pulmonary function testing, and the patient prepared for surgery by physiotherapy, bronchodilators, and antibiotics if infection is present.

Compliance is the change in pressure associated with each cubic centimeter increase in lung volume. When airway pressure is used, rather than the intrapleural pressure minus the intratracheal pressure, the compliance measurement includes that of the chest wall and diaphragm as well as the lungs. This is of little importance if the patient is entirely relaxed. However, in a postoperative patient, the difference between intraesophageal balloon or intrapleural pressure and aiway pressure must be used for meaningful results.

Volume is measured by integrating flow measured across a pneumotachograph at the airway. A *pneumotachograph* is a transducer which converts a pressure difference across a screen to an electric signal related to flow. Resistance is a function of the pressure necessary to overcome resistance at a given point in the respiratory cycle. Work per breath is the integral of the power expended during the respiratory cycle, where power is the transpulmonary pressure times flow.

The manual calculations for these variables of lung mechanics are much too tedious to be of clinical value, so a number of investigators have automated the procedures. Peters and coworkers have designed a mobile cart and digital computer programs for this purpose. Analog voltages are transmitted from an infrared carbon dioxide analyzer, a polarographic oxygen monitor, a Fleisch pneumotachograph, and a differential pressure transducer. The temperatures of inspired and mixed expired air are used for correction of gas volumes. The apparatus can be used with patients on respirators or breathing spontaneously.

The commercial version of this cardiopulmonary measurement cart also provides a channel for indicator-dilution determination of cardiac output. Measured variables include air flow, transpulmonary pressure, inspired oxygen concentration, and mean expired oxygen and carbon dioxide concentrations. From these a small, dedicated computer derives variables associated with respiratory mechanics and gas exchange. These include tidal volume, rate, compliance, resistance, work, oxygen consumption, carbon dioxide output, respiratory quotient, alveolar-arterial oxygen gradient, shunt fraction and dead-space ratio. The results can be viewed on a cathode ray tube or as teletype copy. The prototype device has been in clinical operation for several years. An analysis of patients studied thus far indicated that multiple variables of lung mechanics were better predictors of the need for a respirator than single tests. The commercial version permits telephone transmission of digitized data to a dedicated small computer or a larger time-shared system.

Osborn and associates have used a similar approach but with the transducers built in at the bedside and reliance on continuous monitoring with sophisticated trend analysis. The pneumotachygraph is specially modified with a warm air flush between sampling periods to minimize water condensation and base-line drift. The device can be left on line for as long as 48 hours. Continuous gas samples from a side tube at the expiratory end of the pneumotachygraph are analyzed with a special ceramic oxygen cell and an infrared carbon dioxide analyzer. A digital computer is used to calculate the derived variables and determine trends. Their studies of postoperative patients have revealed wide swings in the pH and blood gases related to the loss of respiratory control or changing ventilation requirements. Sudden fluctuations in carbon dioxide tensions often lead to cardiac arrhythmias or hypotension. The most useful variable in this regard is end-expiratory carbon dioxide tension. The gradient is usually less than 5 mm Hg from arterial blood to end-expiratory gas in patients, with relatively normal dead space. Such a system reduces the number of arterial blood-gas determinations necessary for the management of seriously ill patients. It has also been shown to reduce morbidity and mortality of postoperative patients requiring respirator support.

Kinney's group uses a different method for continuous spirometric determinations. A specially constructed clear plastic chamber covers the head with a snug fit at the neck. This permits the measurement of gas exchange and lung mechanics in spontaneously breathing patients with a minimum of cooperation. Several other centers employ custom-tailored computer-based respiratory monitoring systems, usually developed in cooperation with a major research-oriented corporation or an engineering school (Fig. 13-1). It is unlikely at the present time that the costs of such respiratory monitoring systems could be borne by even a large hospital on the basis of third-party payments. Nevertheless, the value of such systems for postoperative care of the high-risk patient has been proved.

Cardiovascular Monitoring

Most monitoring systems require access to arterial blood for sampling and direct pressure determinations. Monitoring, in many ways like politics, is the art of the possible. What is it possible to measure in the patient with consistent success and minimum risk? Maintaining an open arterial line without risk or discomfort requires skill and dedication to detail. The radial artery at the wrist is the site most frequently used because of safety and convenience. The presence of a functioning ulnar arterial arcade must be checked by pressure occlusion of both arteries at the wrist with subsequent release of the ulnar to produce a palmar flush (the Allen test). It is dangerous to perform even a radial arterial puncture unless such evidence of ulnar collateral flow is present. For percutaneous catheterization or a cutdown and cannulation of the radial artery, the wrist should be attached to an arm board and moderately extended. Strict glove, mask, and sterile drape technique should be used, as with all intravascular cannulations. The standards established by Dudrick and associates for indwelling central venous catheters should be followed for arterial catheters as well. Sterility should be maintained by removing the protective dressing every 3 days, rubbing off skin oil with acetone, and applying iodine tincture to the surrounding skin and antibiotic ointment to the catheter exit site. The occlusive dressing should be small and fixed carefully to the skin, using compound tincture of benzoin for better adherence. Unused stopcock sidearms should be capped with sterile rubber or plastic nipples to prevent contamination. Cannula sepsis is an iatrogenic disaster which can largely be avoided by good technique.

The type of cannula chosen is important. The long Becton-Dickenson Teflon cannula is easily inserted and can be plugged with a plastic stylet when not in use. Other polyvinyl or polyethylene cannulas are available commercially. Patency is best maintained with a constant slow infusion of 2 units of heparin diluted in 5 ml of saline solution delivered in 24 hours. This can be accomplished with either a Sage electrolytic (Fig. 13-2) or a disposable clockwork infusion pump. Both of these can be attached to the patient's arm to allow mobility.

Intermittent manual flushing to discharge clots is dangerous, since it has been demonstrated that as little as 3 ml may flush emboli back up into the cerebral circulation from a radial artery cannula. Other sites for indwelling arterial lines are the brachial or femoral artery, but these present the risk of distal ischemia and thrombophlebitis.

Catheterization of the central venous system or right side of the heart for manometry, injection of indicator, or mixed venous sampling is used as an integral part of many surgical monitoring systems. There are several routes of access to the central venous system (Fig. 13-3). In order of increasing risk these are the median basilic vein in the

Fig. 13-1. Cardiorespiratory monitoring system based upon a central digital computer for physiologic data processing and storage. This is the equipment used by Weil and associates at the Center for the Critically Ill and the Shock Research Unit, University of Southern California School of Medicine.

antecubital fossa, the external jugular vein, the internal jugular vein, and the subclavian vein. The femoral vein is seldom used because of contamination and thrombophlebitis. The median basilic vein directs the catheter directly into the subclavian vein and superior vena cava if the arm is extended laterally during the procedure, whereas the cephalic vein is difficult to negotiate at the shoulder. The external jugular vein is best approached with the neck extended, turned to the opposite side and lower than heart level (to fill the vein and prevent air embolism). The vein can also be steadied and distended by proximal pressure at the neck. As with the antecubital approach, venisection is best done before the vein is ruined with multiple puncture attempts. If there is difficulty passing the jugular-subclavian junction, the catheter may pass if the shoulder is depressed. The internal jugular vein can be cannulated percutaneously above the clavicle. The puncture is made immediately lateral to the pulsation of the common carotid artery through the lateral head of the sternocleidomastoid muscle. The distance to the proper position in the superior vena cava requires a catheter 20 cm long.

Puncture and catheter introduction into the subclavian

vein involves a slightly greater risk of pneumothorax, but its ease of access makes it popular in emergency situations. As with the other sites, local anesthesia should be used as well as complete sterile precautions. Skin puncture is done just inferior to the clavicle at the junction of the middle and inner thirds, with the needle aimed at a point behind the manubrium. The catheter should not be threaded through or over the needle until venous blood is easily aspirated. When threaded through the needle, the catheter should never be withdrawn separately because of the danger of shearing if off with the sharp edge of the needle. Some commercial sets have protective sleeves which can be extended beyond the needle point to prevent cutting the catheter. A chest roentgenogram should always be obtained following central venous catheterization to check for pneumothorax and ascertain the position of the catheter tip. If a nonradiopaque catheter is used, it can be filled with contrast medium during the exposure. There are a number of commercial intravenous catheter sets available which are ingeniously designed to facilitate advancement of the catheter without contamination or kinking (Fig. 13-4). The Abbott set employs a reel device which is easily manipulated with one hand. The Sorenson catheter is housed in a longitudinally slit semirigid conduit with a sliding sleeve on the outside attached to the catheter inside through the slit. As the sleeve is advanced over the conduit, the catheter is pushed through the needle into the vein. These sets can also be used for arterial cannulations.

The proper interpretation of central venous pressure or pulmonary artery wedge pressure for monitoring surgical patients requires an understanding of *all* the factors which may cause elevated readings. Artifacts such as inaccurate zero level, blockage, or kinking should be excluded by observation of 1 to 2 cm pressure fluctuations with the respiratory cycle and careful sighting of the zero level at the midaxillary line. The zero level should correspond to the point of projection of the posterior leaflet of the tricuspid valve on the right chest wall. Noncardiac factors which increase central venous pressure are hypervolemia, vasoconstrictor drugs (metaraminol and mephentermine constrict the veins as well as arterioles), positive-pressure ventilation, pneumothorax, hydrothorax, flail chest, and mediastinal compression. If none of these factors exists, normal readings vary between 0 and 9 cm of water for central venous pressure and 5 to 12 mm Hg pulmonary artery wedge pressure ($\overline{PAw}$). Elevated values suggest the inability of either ventricle to handle its venous return. Filling pressure alone is not a measure of ventricular function or myocardial contractility, because afterload and ventricular work are unknown quantities. A high central venous pressure does serve as a warning that volume infusion should be continued with extreme caution. However, there are situations such as pericardial tamponade or pulmonary embolism where a high central venous pressure is essential to maintain an adequate cardiac output until definitive therapy is used to relieve the obstruction. The most logical use of central venous pressure or $\overline{PAw}$ as a guide to fluid replacement in seriously ill patients is the observation of the response to challenge with 100-ml increments of volume infusion. Infusion is stopped when a sharp rise in pressure occurs.

Fig. 13-2. Radial artery cannula with patency maintained by Sage electrolytic infusion pump. Note the sterile rubber nipple on the sidearm of the stopcock. A central venous catheter protected with adhesive tape is shown alongside the arm.

The distinction between right and left ventricular failure is not possible without some indication of left atrial or left ventricular end-diastolic pressure. For this reason, various techniques have been developed for bedside monitoring of pressures in the left side of the heart. Cohn et al. have

Fig. 13-3. Four routes of access to the central venous system. The direct line from the median antecubital vein to the superior vena cava makes this a safe approach, particularly with the arm extended. The cephalic vein empties into the subclavian vein at an acute angle, making central venous catheterization difficult. The external jugular vein is the next safest route. The arm should be at the side and the shoulder depressed to straighten the angle at which the external jugular enters the subclavian vein. The internal jugular vein can be cannulated by inserting the needle through the clavicular head of the sternocleidomastoid muscle, just lateral to the pulsation of the carotid artery. The subclavian cannulation over the first rib is shown. The danger of pneumothorax or hemothorax is greatest with this approach.

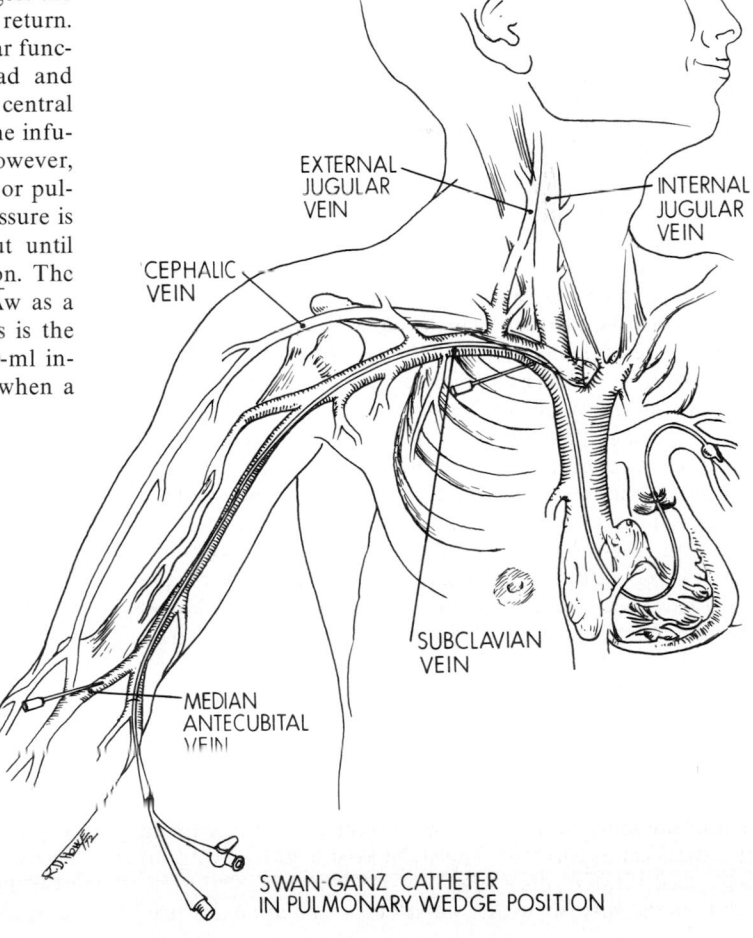

EXTERNAL JUGULAR VEIN

INTERNAL JUGULAR VEIN

CEPHALIC VEIN

SUBCLAVIAN VEIN

MEDIAN ANTECUBITAL VEIN

SWAN-GANZ CATHETER IN PULMONARY WEDGE POSITION

Fig. 13-4. Three popular types of monitoring catheters. The coiled Swan-Ganz balloon-tip catheter is designed to float into the pulmonary artery wedge position. The Sorenson catheter shown crossed in the photograph is contained in a conduit with a longitudinal slit to facilitate insertion into an artery or vein under sterile conditions. For similar purposes, the Abbott catheter is provided with a reellike device. The two halves of the sleeve which prevents shearing of the catheter are also shown.

used a precurved polyethylene catheter which is threaded over a wire guide from the femoral artery into the left ventricle. Fluoroscopic control is not used, but the electrocardiograph is observed for premature ventricular beats which signal entry into the ventricle and subside when the catheter is withdrawn a few centimeters. In shock associated with myocardial infarction, the left ventricular end-diastolic pressure is elevated in the 12 to 44 mm Hg range even though the central venous pressure may be normal. Such monitoring has permitted more precise fluid replacement and inotropic drug adjustment in patients with left ventricular failure.

The great majority of clinical physiologists prefer to approach the problem of bedside left ventricular dynamics from the right side of the heart. In 1959, Zohman and Williams described flow-guided pulmonary artery catheterization. The location of the catheter tip, as it floated along with the bloodstream through the right side of the heart, is determined by characteristic intracardiac electrocardiographic patterns conducted back through the soft catheter in a column of 7.5% sodium bicarbonate acting as a salt bridge. The pattern in the right atrium consists of a high, short inverted P wave, which becomes upright as the tricuspid valve is approached. The right ventricle pattern consists of a 7- to 9-mv downward QRS deflection. A standard low-voltage pattern is found in the pulmonary artery. The safety of flow-guided catheterization of the right side of the heart depends upon avoiding arrhythmias by careful observation of the intracardiac patterns. The hazard of ventricular fibrillation due to stray 60-cycle current should be minimized by careful appraisal of the electrocardiograph and the grounding capacity of its power supply. In 1966 Del Guercio et al. reported on a number of patients with suspected pulmonary embolism shock studied by a modification of this technique. Flow of the catheter was improved by a wind-sock effect created by heat curling the last 2 cm of catheter. The stylet kept it straight while it advanced through the veins.

More recently, a further advance of this approach was

the commercial development of the balloon-tipped Swan-Ganz catheter (Fig. 13-4). With the balloon inflated, the catheter sails through the right side of the heart into a wedge position in the pulmonary artery in less than 1 minute. In the absence of pulmonary vascular disease, pulmonary capillary wedge pressure ($\overline{PAw}$) is a reliable guide to left atrial and, in turn, left ventricular end-diastolic pressure. Without the wedge position, the pulmonary artery end-diastolic pressure is an acceptable indicator of mean left atrial pressure. Central venous pressure alone has been found to be an unreliable index of left ventricular function, since filling pressure in the left side of the heart may rise sharply and pulmonary edema occur without significant increases in right atrial pressures.

Right-sided catheterization with flow-guided catheters also can be monitored by intracardiac pressure changes or mobile radiologic image intensifiers. The catheter through the right side of the heart also can be used for obtaining mixed venous blood samples, injecting indicator, and infusion of medications. Extreme caution should be exercised when drugs are infused directly into the central circulation, because high myocardial concentrations are quickly achieved. These catheters also make it possible to obtain bedside pulmonary angiograms in cases of pulmonary embolism shock.

As pointed out earlier regarding physiologic concepts of monitoring, the mixed venous oxygen level reflects the extent to which the body must call upon the blood oxygen stores in states of cardiovascular stress. The value of right heart oxygen saturation monitoring during surgery has been demonstrated. Changes in cardiac output secondary to hemorrhage and other problems are reflected by early changes in right atrial oxygen saturations, usually before changes in arterial blood pressure, venous pressure, or heart rate. Changes in arterial oxygen content secondary to pulmonary shunting or decreased oxygen-carrying capacity also promptly affect mixed venous oxygen saturation. It was originally thought that pulmonary arterial samples would be necessary for this type of monitoring, but experience has shown that, in the stressed patient, right atrial or right ventricular samples correlate well with those from the pulmonary artery. Saturations below 50% from these sites are a bad prognostic sign and indicate either severe arterial hypoxemia or very significantly decreased cardiac output.

Border et al. originated a unique "no cost" bedside volumetric Van Slyke device for determining the volumes percent of unsaturation of mixed venous blood (Fig. 13-5). It is assembled from a heparinized 10-ml syringe, a stopcock, and the barrel of a 1-ml tuberculin syringe. Exactly 10 ml of mixed venous blood is drawn into the larger syringe followed by approximately 1 ml of pure oxygen. The smaller syringe, filled with saline solution, serves as a monometer to record the volume of the oxygen bubble used to saturate the blood. If the meniscus falls to the 0.5-ml mark, it indicates that the mixed venous blood required 5 vol % of oxygen for saturation. This is about normal. If the arterial blood is 100% saturated, this value would be equivalent to the arteriovenous oxygen difference. This device makes it possible for everyone to practice clinical physiology at the bedside, with little expense.

Cardiac Output Determinations

In spite of various questions regarding accuracy in high- or low-flow states, the description of indicator-dilution curves from central circulation remains the basic method for monitoring cardiac output. The technique, which goes back to 1897, involves the injection of an indicator into the right side of the heart and continuous determination of its concentration as it mixes with the cardiac output somewhere downstream. Any indicator can be used, as long as it does not affect hemodynamics or disappear from the blood before the concentration is measured. It can best be understood as a variation of the Fick principle, where the known amount of indicator is equivalent to a fixed amount of oxygen consumption, and the mean concentration of indicator after mixing is equivalent to the arteriovenous oxygen difference. It follows, then, that the faster the volume of blood flow, the lower the arteriovenous oxygen difference and mean concentration of indicator. All methods for the calculation of cardiac ouput from both continuous and single bolus injection of indicator use this principle in analyzing the time-concentration curves to obtain the mean concentration of indicator. The number of milligrams of indicator injected divided by the mean concentration of indicator gives the volume of flow during the time of the indicator-dilution curve. Thermal dilution curves are similar in principle, with use of cold saline solution as the indicator. They are popular because of their simplicity and the availability of bedside computers, but the required flow-directed balloon-tipped thermistor catheters are expensive. Since the cardiac output is usually expressed as flow per minute, the volume of flow during description of the curve is multiplied by 60 and divided by the number of seconds of duration of the curve.

It is convenient to mount the thermal dilution computer or the densitometer with its control box and motor-driven withdrawal syringe on a mobile cart, along with blood

Fig. 13-5. Border's volumetric Van Slyke device for bedside determination of mixed venous unsaturation. Each 0.1-ml fall in the meniscus indicates 1 vol % unsaturation of blood. Normal is 4 to 5 vol %. When the arterial blood is fully saturated, this device indicates the arteriovenous oxygen difference. (*From J. R. Border et al., J Trauma, 6:176, 1966.*)

pressure transducers, an electrocardiograph, and a multichannel recording device. As noted earlier, this mobile apparatus has been called a shock cart; it can be used to bring fairly complete cardiovascular assessment to the bedside, operating room, or emergency room, rather than transport a critically ill patient to a clinical laboratory (Fig. 13-6). Intracardiac and arterial blood pressure tracings, indicator-dilution curves, and electrocardiograph tracings combined with arterial and mixed venous blood-gas data permit calculation of a number of derived cardiorespiratory variables of physiologic significance. Practical considerations in the design of a shock cart require a sturdy chassis with large wheels for mobility through elevator doors. There should be a waterproof work surface on top, since dilutions for calibration purposes are best done immediately. The instrument panel should be recessed out of harm's way, and the power cord should be long and mounted on a reel of some sort. The multichannel recorder should be of the direct write-out type that does not require developing. It is also more convenient to have positioning arms for the support and alignment of the pressure strain gauges and the densitometer cuvette. Some of these units can be provided with built-in computers for calculation of the cardiac output and other derived cardiovascular variables. Others provide space for a programmable calculator to serve the same purpose (Fig. 13-7).

Several hand-held calculators with program cards specifically made up for shock-cart calculating are available. The primary data obtained from the recorder and blood gas machines are entered on the keyboard, and the derived values are immediately computed. Civetta's and Shoemaker's groups have made available magnetic card programs for the rapid automatic calculation of up to 27 derived cardiorespiratory variables, using Hewlett-Packard and Texas Instrument calculators, respectively.

Data become information only in the brain of the beholder. The average physician is "turned off" by a column of numbers representing cardiac index, stroke index, right and left ventricular stroke work, pulmonary and systemic vascular resistance, ventricular function indices, intracardiac and systemic pressures, arteriovenous oxygen differ-

Fig. 13-6. The bedside "shock cart" approach to monitoring is shown by this model which represents the advanced state-of-the-art. By means of a balloon flotation catheter in the pulmonary artery and a radial artery cannula, cardiac output, pressures and blood gas measurements are taken from the patient and fed into a microprocessor computer to calculate derived physiologic variables which are printed out on a graphic profile (Fig. 13-7). This system is essentially a mobile, computerized cardiac catheterization laboratory as distinct from the built-in, hard-wired monitoring systems based upon a central computer.

ence, venoarterial admixture, oxygen consumption, P_{50}, serum lactate and arterial base excess or deficit. In an attempt to make dull data attractive, Cohn and Del Guercio devised a system for displaying these derived variables on an easily scanned, logically organized, bar-chart format. Arterial and mixed venous blood gas and saturation values along with cardiac output, temperature, height, weight and inspired oxygen concentration are entered on the keyboard of a minicomputer, and within seconds the derived variables are drawn on a preprinted sheet (Fig. 13-7) by an X-Y alpha-numeric recorder. This system, called the *automated physiologic profile,* is a compromise between the hand-held calculator approach and the very expensive built-in digital computer monitors. The profile serves as a useful permanent record of cardiorespiratory status before and after therapeutic interventions.

The example shown in Fig. 13-7 demonstrates a number of points regarding monitoring of the critically ill patient.

This was a study, with Swan-Ganz thermistor catheter and radial artery cannula, of a young man who suffered a 30 percent burn and smoke inhalation. The physiologic assessment was done 24 hours after injury and showed a "normal" cardiac index and blood pressure with an increase in oxygen consumption resulting from a widened arteriovenous oxygen difference. Why, then, was there evidence of anaerobic metabolism and hypoxic acidosis with twice normal serum lactate levels and a base deficit of 6 mEq/L? Because the patient's oxygen needs were even greater, and had the state of increasing oxygen debt continued, the patient surely would have died. The ventricular function curve in the lower right quadrant shows why the patient could not increase his cardiac output enough to supply his increased oxygen needs. The plot, representing the Starling-Frank relationship, is significantly below the zone of normal ventricular function. The cause for this cardiac failure could have been circulating myocardial depressant factors, known to be associated with burns, early sepsis, or poisoning of myocardial mitochondrial cytochromes by the high level of carbon monoxide (SCO), which probably had been much higher on admission. The high right atrial and pulmonary artery wedge pressures indicate that both ventricles had more than adequate preload. Since total peripheral vascular resistance was normal, that determinant of cardiac output (afterload) also was not the limiting factor. It was obvious from this physiologic profile (but not from the ECG, $\overline{PAw}$, or systemic BP) that the patient would not survive unless inotropic therapy could stimulate the myocardium to at least normal contractility. This was accomplished with digitalis, dopamine, and GIK (glucose, insulin, potassium).

At the same time, the profile also illustrated the need for a volume cycled respirator with PEEP to reduce the severe pulmonary shunting (venoarterial admixture) caused by the smoke inhalation. The most appropriate setting of end-expiratory pressure (optimum PEEP) was determined by performing automated physiologic profiles sequentially at increased levels of PEEP. Beyond a certain level, reduced cardiac output, resulting from restricted preload, produced a net decrease in oxygen transport, even though arterial oxygen content continued to improve. Had it not been for the information provided by the monitoring of these derived cardiorespiratory variables, it is unlikely that lifesaving therapeutic decisions could have been made in time.

The effect of the 15 percent carboxyhemoglobin concentration on the position of the oxyhemoglobin dissociation curve is also shown. The P_{50} STD value of 30.2 excludes the effect of carbon monoxide, and the P_{50} STDX value of 24.9 indicates the shift to the left caused by carboxyhemoglobin. The lines with the Xs on the bar-charts for "A-V Diff," QO_2, and $\dot{Q}_A/\dot{Q}_T$ indicate those values at the patient's actual P_{50} compared with what they would have

Fig. 13-7. Graphic display of derived cardiorespiratory variables ▶ computed from arterial and mixed-venous blood gases, cardiac output, and other data obtained by means of a bedside "shock cart." For details of interpretation in this patient with 30 percent burns and smoke inhalation, see text.

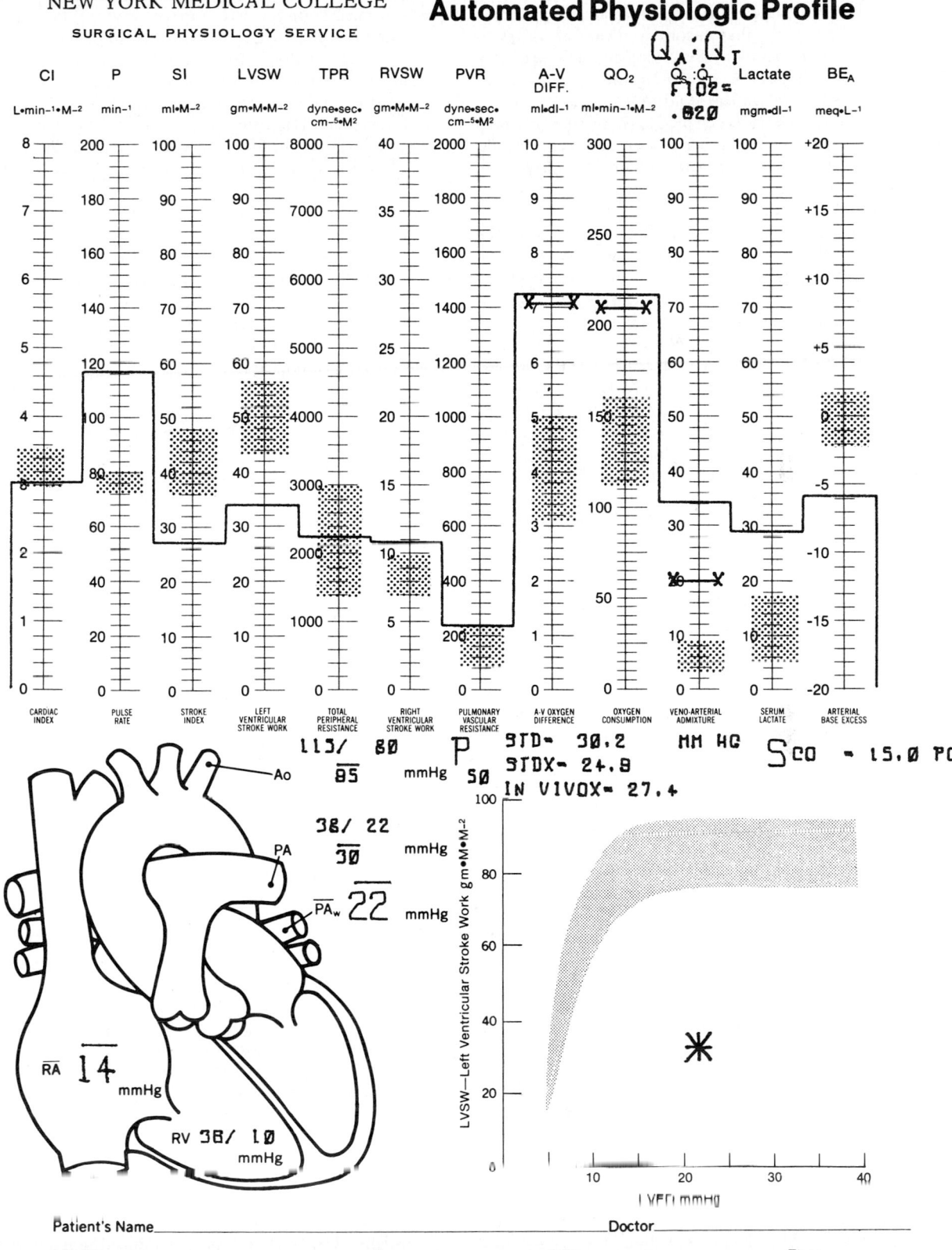

NEW YORK MEDICAL COLLEGE
SURGICAL PHYSIOLOGY SERVICE

Automated Physiologic Profile

$Q_A : Q_T$

$\frac{Q_S : Q_T}{FIO_2} =$

.020

CI	P	SI	LVSW	TPR	RVSW	PVR	A-V DIFF.	QO₂		Lactate	BE_A
L•min⁻¹•M⁻²	min⁻¹	ml•M⁻²	gm•M•M⁻²	dyne•sec• cm⁻⁵•M²	gm•M•M⁻²	dyne•sec• cm⁻⁵•M²	ml•dl⁻¹	ml•min⁻¹•M⁻²		mgm•dl⁻¹	meq•L⁻¹

CARDIAC INDEX — PULSE RATE — STROKE INDEX — LEFT VENTRICULAR STROKE WORK — TOTAL PERIPHERAL RESISTANCE — RIGHT VENTRICULAR STROKE WORK — PULMONARY VASCULAR RESISTANCE — A-V OXYGEN DIFFERENCE — OXYGEN CONSUMPTION — VENO-ARTERIAL ADMIXTURE — SERUM LACTATE — ARTERIAL BASE EXCESS

115/ 80   P STD= 30.2   MM HG   S CO = 15.0 PC
85 mmHg   STDX= 24.8
50   IN VIVOX= 27.4

Ao

38/ 22   PA
30 mmHg

$\overline{PA_w}$ 22 mmHg

$\overline{RA}$ 14 mmHg

RV 38/ 10 mmHg

LVSW—Left Ventricular Stroke Work gm•M•M⁻²

LVED mmHg

Patient's Name_____ Doctor_____

Lab. No._____ Rm._____ Date_____ Time_____

been had the P_{50} been normal (26 to 27 mm Hg). This type of calculation is of value clinically since it is possible to manipulate the P_{50} by pharmacologic means in order to improve oxygen transport. Harken's recent review of this aspect of monitoring emphasizes the importance of dissociation curve shifts in clinical syndromes.

The automated physiologic profile is in use in many institutions, including a number of community hospitals, where it has been proved cost-effective, particularly when used for preoperative assessment and physiologic fine tuning in the high-risk patient.

The technological goal in monitoring is to provide the maximum amount of cardiorespiratory and oxygen transport information with a minimum amount of blood sampling and trauma to the patient. In this regard thermal dilution techniques have become popular.

Another approach to this problem uses fiberoptic oximetry to record the concentration of green dye in the pulmonary artery after injection into the right atrium. A Swan-Ganz catheter was adapted with light-carrying glass fibers so that both oximetry for oxygen saturation measurement and densitometry for cardiac output determination could be carried out at the catheter tip. No arterial sampling is required when this technique is used.

There are other monitoring systems which involve the use of catheter-tip sensors. One measures pressure and electromagnetic flow velocity. When threaded retrograde into the left ventricle, this sensor permits the on-line recording of the left ventricular pressures, left ventricular pressure acceleration (dp/dt), intracardiac heart sounds, ascending aortic blood velocity, and ascending aortic blood acceleration. If the cross-sectional area of the aorta is known, total flow can be calculated. All these serve as very useful indices of left ventricular function, particularly following myocardial infarction. The problem of calibration of the electromagnetic flowmeter probe without a zero flow calibration point is a serious one, as it is for all clinical studies involving electromagnetic flowmeters.

A disposable, very thin polarographic oxygen-sensing electrode can be used for mixed venous oxygen tension monitoring. The miniature sensor is fabricated by dipcoating or painting the various insulators, diffusion membranes, and buffers directly onto the central wire electrode. Other similar devices are available complete with compact solid-state battery-powered recorders for use at the bedside.

The insertion of a long catheter from the radial artery up to the region of the aortic arch permits a detailed analysis of the aortic pulse contour. Warner has perfected this technique for clinical monitoring. Stroke volume is computed from the pulse contour on a beat-by-beat basis. This, combined with pressure variables, provides an almost instantaneous cardiovascular assessment. Unfortunately, McDonald et al. have pointed out, the method depends upon a stable vascular impedance, which is seldom the case in critically ill patients. For this reason, the technique is not in general use.

All the methods of estimating cardiac output described thus far are invasive to varying degrees and therefore present some risk and considerable expense because they require skilled personnel for their application. A number of promising noninvasive adaptations of the indicator-dilution principle are in clinical use. Included in this category are gamma densitometry (quantitative angiography), videodensitometry, isotope-dilution analysis, fluorescence excitation analysis, and magnetic fluid tracer dilution.

Information regarding flow rates, vascular volumes, distribution of pulmonary transit times, intracardiac and pulmonary shunting, and right or left ventricular ejection efficiency is theoretically contained in the shapes of indicator-dilution curves. With the conventional indocyanine green dye technique, sampling rates are too slow, and the injection and sampling sites are too far apart, for complete interpretation of the physiologic events that create the shape of the curve. Catheter lag between the sampling point and the densitometer cuvette also produces distortion of the curves and loss of potential information. Gamma densitometry, in which the indicator is a small bolus of radiopaque contrast medium and the blood vessels or cardiac chambers serve as the densitometer cuvettes, avoids these problems. Gamma rays or x-rays, projected through the cardiac silhouette, produce high-dynamic-response indicator time-concentration curves through the detection of changes in gamma photon density related, according to Beer's law, to the concentration of radiopaque indicator in the blood. In clinical practice, solid-state radiation detectors are placed behind the patient as in a portable x-ray unit. Five milliliters of Hypaque is then injected into the central venous catheter, and six simultaneous contrast dilution curves are recorded from the heart and great vessels. Analysis of these curves permits calculation of pulmonary circulation time, pulmonary blood volume, right and left ventricular ejection fraction, and other useful variables. More sophisticated interpretation requires electronic data processing for transfer function analysis.

Videodensitometry is similar in principle to gamma densitometry, except that an actual angiocardiogram is performed and recorded on magnetic tape. When played back on a television screen, the concentration of contrast medium is analyzed at any point in the heart and lungs by means of a movable electronic window. The advantages are that, at leisure, an infinite number of curves can be obtained from any point in the cardiac silhouette as the tape is played over and over. Disadvantages include great expense, lack of portability, and low signal-to-noise ratio requiring signal processing to obtain recognizable curves.

Isotope dilution analysis has made a great leap forward with the development of the Anger scintillation camera and other rapid-response isotope scanning devices. The ability to image and quantitate the distribution of a radioactive tracer second by second through the heart and lungs adds a new dimension of considerable value to surgical cardiovascular monitoring. High-photon-yield isotopes are injected intravenously and the gamma camera images recorded on magnetic tape. Later, specific areas can be analyzed to produce indicator-dilution curves which can be related to changes in size and position of the cardiac chambers. Jones et al. have produced good indicator-dilution curves for the right and left sides of the heart using an autofluoroscope. Spatial resolution and dynamic response, however, can never be as good as that obtained with the linear interrogating beams of radiation used in gamma densitometry. Furthermore, equipment for both isotope dilution and videodensitometry is expensive and bulky at present, and cannot be used for bedside studies.

Kaufman and associates have developed a highly innovative system for the bedside determination of cardiac output. Following the intravenous injection of a small amount of iodine containing radiographic contrast material, the iodine is caused to emit fluorescence in the gamma ray range by stimulation with an external gamma ray source. The stimulated emission of iodine is detected by a collimated silicon diode producing a characteristic indicator-dilution curve. The system is easily calibrated, and the radiation dose is low.

Another new method for the external noninvasive detection of indicator dilution has been described by Newbower. The indicator is a magnetic fluid tracer composed of fine ferromagnetic particles. The detection transducer is a simple set of air-core coils which easily measures the striking difference in magnetic susceptibility between the tracer and the background without the need for magnetic shielding. This novel approach has great potential because it does not involve ionizing radiation of any sort.

It is also possible to tag flowing blood in vivo by reversing the magnetic alignments of hydrogen nuclei in the water of the plasma by applying a powerful external magnetic field. These effects are detected further downstream by means of nuclear magnetic resonance. Nuclear magnetic resonance monitoring devices presently are under development. The technique is totally noninvasive.

It is obvious that noninvasive techniques for describing indicator-dilution curves will play a prominent role in surgical monitoring for years to come. Surgeons will be provided information regarding cardiac and circulatory function in their patients which will permit management of critical states on a firm physiologic basis.

The determination of systolic time intervals provides an external assessment of left ventricular function based entirely on intrinsic electrical and mechanical events. The methodology is gaining in popularity because it is physiologically sound and has been largely validated by extensive comparative clinical studies including catheterization of the left side of the heart.

Simultaneous recordings of the electrocardiogram, phonocardiogram, and external carotid pulse tracing are analyzed for the following time variables: total left ventricular systolic time (QRS complex to second heart sound), left ventricular ejection time (duration of carotid pulse upstroke), and preejection period (the difference between total left ventricular systolic and left ventricular ejection times). Although the calculations are straightforward, placement of the carotid pulse sensor and phonocardiogram microphone on the neck and chest is critical. With technical care in the performance of the recordings, remarkably good correlation with direct measures of the dynamics of the left side of the heart can be shown. Weissler et al. have found that the ratio of the preejection period to left ventricular ejection time (PEP/LVET) is relatively constant around 0.35 in patients with normal hearts. With failure of the left side of the heart, the PEP becomes longer and the LVET shorter, increasing the ratio. Serial studies reveal good correlation between the PEP/LVET ratio and left ventricular ejection fraction, end-diastolic volume, and end-diastolic pressure. This noninvasive approach, which requires inexpensive equipment, is useful for the continuous bedside monitoring of left ventricular function.

Alterations of left ventricular conduction, however, as in left bundle branch block, prolong the PEP selectively with no apparent change in LVET. Changes in peripheral impedance or vascular runoff, as occur in septic shock, may alter the relation between the PEP/LVET ratio and cardiac performance.

The application of ultrasound to clinical monitoring is undergoing a period of rapid growth. Both industrial and academic sectors are developing methods for cardiovascular assessment based on interrogating beams of high-frequency sound waves (less than 1 mm wavelength). Ultrasonic energy can penetrate all tissues except bone and air-filled structures and provide good spatial resolution for diagnostic studies. Thus far, at the levels of energy needed for clinical work, there has been no suggestion of injury to living tissue, not even the fetus. The lack of hazard and the reasonable cost of the equipment required has led to more clinical studies than with any other technique aside from electrocardiography.

There are two basic methods of operation of ultrasound for diagnostic purposes—the pulse-echo mode (sonar) and the backscatter frequency shift mode (Doppler effect). In the former, the distance between the emitter and any sound-reflecting interface deep within the body is measured in terms of the transit time of bursts of ultrasound to and from the tissue. An A-scan device is held stationary against the body and a recording of the depth of structures in the path of the beam made on the basis of the known speed of sound in tissue. The B scan is produced if the ultrasonic emitter is traversed across the body while echo-ranging, in order to produce a picture of the tissue cross section.

Not only is ultrasound less harmful than ionizing radiation, but it is capable of revealing internal surfaces which are invisible to roentgen rays. These include the internal structures of the heart and blood vessels. In addition, devices using the Doppler principle can detect rapid motions within the body. This makes them useful for studies of peripheral blood flow and cardiac valve function.

In echocardiography for ultrasonic determination of cardiac chamber size and stroke volume, a transducer is applied to the chest over the cardiac area. Sound in the 1- to 5-megacycle frequency is delivered through the chest in on-off bursts about 1,500 times per second. Echoes are detected during the off periods and recorded in terms of time lag (distance). The distances between the intraventricular septum and the posterior endocardial wall of the left ventricle are recorded at end diastole and end systole. The calculations of end-diastolic and end-systolic volumes are made on the assumption that the shape of the chamber is a prolate ellipse. The results from a number of investigators are remarkable. The left ventricular volumes measured by echocardiography and by biplane angiocardiography were very similar over a wide range of values (correlation coefficient .97). The problem with this technique for surgical monitoring is that the operator must be highly skilled and experienced in aiming the transducer and recognizing on the scan the exact structures he wishes to measure. The device cannot be simply strapped on and left alone for 24 hours to record left ventricular function. Some method will have to be devised for the ultrasonic beam to "lock on" to the left ventricular wall reflections. This will not be an easy task.

Fig. 13-8. Potentiometric electrode used to monitor muscle surface pH as an indicator of anaerobic metabolism related to inadequate perfusion. (*From N. P. Couch et al., Ann Surg, 173:173, 1971.*)

The Doppler flowmeter has achieved considerable sophistication as a clinical tool in the past few years. Readout varies from a simple audible signal related to pulse velocity to signals combining vessel cross section and velocity to provide actual flow measurements. These techniques cannot yet be applied to aortic flow determination, but the entire field of ultrasonics offers many possibilities for the evolution of the perfect cardiovascular monitor.

The concept of measuring pulse volume on the basis of the electric properties of blood goes back 40 years, but practical instruments for measuring electric impedance related to movement of electrolyte of the electromagnetic field have only recently been developed. In the instrument developed by Kubicek et al., two electrodes are placed around the neck and two around the abdomen just below the chest. The volume of blood between the electrodes decreases as the stroke volume flows up the carotids and down the aorta. This produces a decrease in electric impedance in the thorax. Since this cyclic change in impedance, compared to total chest impedance, is equivalent to less than one part in a thousand, considerable electronic sophistication is required for its detection. Alternating current is sent through the outer electrodes, and the change in voltage between the inner electrodes measured during cardiac systole indicates the impedance change due to left ventricular ejection. The problem, of course, is that venous inflow occurs more or less continuously, so that a net stroke volume during maximum ejection is measured. Great hopes were held for thoracic impedance plethysmography as a relatively inexpensive noninvasive means of monitoring cardiac output and ventricular function. Unfortunately, electrode motion artifacts and lack of correlation with other methods for the estimation of cardiac output in nonsteady states have dampened enthusiasm for this class of instruments.

There is no more consistently accurate method of measuring cardiac output than a properly calibrated electromagnetic flowmeter placed firmly around the ascending aorta. In fact, this approach is accepted as the standard against which other cardiac output monitoring equipment is evaluated for accuracy. Of course, electromagnetic flowmeters can be used only for assessing vascular operations.

Monitoring of Tissue Metabolism

It was pointed out early in the chapter that a systems approach to monitoring would direct most effort toward a study of tissue metabolism. Under certain conditions, such as hypoxemia or septic shock, a high cardiac output is no guarantee of adequate delivery of oxygen to the cells. Couch and colleagues have succeeded in developing a practical and simple solution to the problem of an early warning system for tissue hypoxia (Fig. 13-8). With an electrometer and right-angle pH electrode, skeletal muscle surface pH is continuously monitored. A 2-cm incision through skin, subcutaneous tissue, and fascia is required for placement of the electrode in gentle contact with the surface of the biceps muscle in adults and the quadriceps in children. Clinical monitoring by this technique has been continued for as long as 8 days.

The rationale for this approach is that with tissue deprivation of oxygen, oxidative phosphorylation ceases, and pyruvate is converted to lactic acid rather than carbon dioxide and water. Diffusion of the hydrogen ions and lactate across the cell membranes into the extracellular fluid is passive and rapid. Extracellular fluid acidosis related to anaerobic glycolysis precedes arterial pH depression because of a number of factors: in low flow states there is a delay of acid metabolite washout into the peripheral circulation; arterial pH will change only after the hemoglobin-, bicarbonate-, and phosphate-buffering capacity of the blood is exceeded; and metabolism of lactate by the heart and liver tend to reduce the peripheral lactate levels until late in shock. Skeletal muscle itself offers several advantages for surveillance of overall oxygen transport. Since it can tolerate hypoxia, its blood supply tends to get shut off early in critical states, and it tends to shift readily into anaerobic glycolysis and lactate production because of its high glycogen content. The surface of the muscle rather than the interior is monitored to avoid artifacts due to hematoma formation. Studies in man have shown that muscle surface pH is a sensitive indicator of muscle metabolism and as such is valuable as a practical monitoring instrument to alert against hypoxia of more vital tissues. The normal resting biceps pH is 7.38, slightly below arterial pH. When the normal oxygen gradient to the muscle cells is restored after the circulatory crisis is over, pH promptly returns to the normal resting level.

Couch's group has also done redox potential measurements of muscle as an indicator of balance between oxygen delivery and tissue needs. Redox potential of tissue reflects the overall balance of electron transfer which shifts toward the negative or reduced state with prolonged hypoxia. However, although the trends were found to be similar to the surface pH changes, absolute redox potential values were not as reliable indicators as pH changes. Muscle surface pH monitoring provides a good early warning of disaster during and after surgery. The small incision certainly can be justified in high-risk patients or those undergoing formidable operations.

Woldring et al. developed a mass spectrometer which accurately records partial pressures of oxygen, carbon dioxide, or other gases, sampled through plastic or rubber membranes mounted on a catheter tip. Using a mass spectrometer, Owens et al. measured intracerebral gas tensions continuously across a heparinized silastic membrane on a perforated cannula. Of course, the measurements represent the gas tensions in the extracellular fluid surrounding local tissue injury rather than intact cells. Other problems are related to changes in membrane permeability due to fibrin deposits and protein denaturation.

The quest for the perfect monitor of vital function is really just beginning, as investigators such as Chance learn about energy "spin-off" during bioenergetic exchange in the cells. More bioengineers are looking at the lower part of Table 13-1 to find noninvasive methods of scanning cellular bioenergetics. Huckabee has defined hypoxia as "the condition which exists when the supply of oxygen to the exterior of living cells is reduced to a rate insufficient for their current metabolic needs, with the result that

various cellular oxidation-reduction systems must shift toward a more reduced state." Detection of this state by a safe external sensor is the ultimate goal.

A number of attempts in this direction are in progress. One involves the stimulation of intracellular oxygen molecules with modulated soft x-rays. The stimulated emission of oxygen is in the microwave area of the 0.5-cm band and can be detected externally with a suitable waveguide and amplifier system. This approach would offer some degree of spatial discrimination of tissue hypoxia in specific organs. Another experimental method is a cross between Chance's fluorescence emission technique and thermography. Energy transfers within living cells emit specific wavelengths of electromagnetic radiation according to quantum bioenergetic laws. Energy dissipation associated with inefficient anaerobic metabolism or uncoupling of oxidative phosphorylation should be detectable by suitable instrumentation. Such a system has been developed to detect and identify narrow band and line spectra associated with abnormal tissue states. These signals in a physiologic situation are superimposed on the broad band (black body) radiation of the skin or organ surface along with the far infrared spectral pattern of cellular water and carbon dioxide. The desired signals are somewhat analogous to the Fraunhofer lines of the solar spectrum due to absorption in the sun's mantle. The approach differs from conventional infrared thermography in that the strategy is to analyze the spectral pattern rather than to determine the energy level within a specified wavelength. A Fourier interferometer, which is about the size of a bread box, is used to scan the patient at the bedside. The recorded interferogram is then transmitted by a time-shared system over telephone lines to a computer for Fourier transform and signature analysis. Emission power spectral density tracings have been obtained from human limbs as well as other tissues and superficial carcinomas. Cross-correlation techniques have been used to establish significant differences. Alterations in infrared emission spectra reflect changes in tissue metabolism from analysis of the frequencies of radiation corresponding to molecular vibrations and rotations. Although highly experimental, this is a good example of monitoring at the business end of the oxygen transport chain.

References

Physiologic Concepts and Monitoring

Barcroft, J.: "The Respiratory Functions of the Blood," Cambridge University Press, London, 1925.

Brown, J. H. U. and Dickson, J. F., III: Instrumentation and the Delivery of Health Services, *Science,* **166:**334, 1969.

Bunker, J. P., Forrest, W. H., Jr., Mosteller, F., and Vandam, L. D. (eds.): "The National Halothane Study," National Institute of General Medical Sciences, Bethesda, 1969.

Chance, B.: Regulation of Intracellular Oxygen, *Proc Int Union Physiol Sci,* **6:**13, 1968.

Clark, L. C., Jr. and Lyons, C.: Electrode Systems for Continuous Monitoring in Cardiovascular Surgery, *Ann NY Acad Sci,* **102:**19, 1962.

Cohn, J. D. and Del Guercio, L. R. M.: Cardiorespiratory Analysis of Cardiac Arrest and Resuscitation, *Surg Gynecol Obstet,* **123:**1066, 1966.

Cushing, H.: On Routine Determinations of Arterial Tension in Operating Room and Clinic, *Boston Med Surg J,* **148:**250, 1903.

Dammann, J. F.: Assessment of Continuous Monitoring in the Critically Ill Patient, *Dis Chest,* **55:**240, 1969.

Del Guercio, L. R. M., Feins, N. R., Cohn, J. D., Coomaraswamy, R. P., Wollman, S. B., and State, D.: A Comparison of Blood Flow during External and Internal Cardiac Massage in Man, *Circulation,* **32**(*Suppl* 1):171, 1965.

Dickens, F., and Neil, E.: "Oxygen in the Animal Organism," The Macmillan Company, New York, 1964.

Harken, A. H.: Lactic Acidosis, *Surg Gynecol Obstet,* **142:**593, 1976.

Hershey, S. G., Del Guercio, L. R. M., and McConn, R.: "Septic Shock in Man," Little, Brown and Company, Boston, 1971.

Huckabee, W. E.: Relationships of Pyruvate and Lactate during Anaerobic Metabolism: II. Exercise and Formation of O_2 Debt, *J Clin Invest,* **37:**255, 1958.

Irving, L.: Respiration in Diving Mammals, *Physiol Rev,* **19:**112, 1939.

Maloney, J. V., Jr.: The Trouble with Patient Monitoring, *Ann Surg,* **168:**605, 1968.

Pontoppidan, H., Geffin, B., and Lowenstein, E.: Acute Respiratory Failure in the Adult. *N Engl J Med,* **287:**690, 1972.

Roughton, F. J. W.: The Average Time Spent by the Blood in the Human Lung Capillary and Its Relation to the Rates of CO Uptake and Elimination in Man, *Am J Physiol,* **143:**621, 1945.

Safar, P., Myers, D., Snyder, J., et al.: Clinical Trial Protocols for Brain Resuscitation, *Intensive Care Med,* **3:**165, 1977.

Sarnoff, S. J., and Mitchell, J. H.: The Control of the Function of the Heart, in "Handbook of Physiology," vol. 1, The Williams & Wilkins Company, Baltimore, 1962.

Van Slyke, D. D.: The Carbon Dioxide Carriers of the Blood, *Physiol Rev,* **1:**141, 1921.

Weil, M. H., and Shubin, H.: "Critical Care Medicine, Current Principles and Practices," Harper & Row, Publishers, Incorporated, New York, 1976.

Physiologic Sensing

Collins, J. A., and Ballinger, W. F., II: "The Surgical Intensive Care Unit," *Surgery,* **66:**614, 1969.

Giles, A. F.: "Electronic Sensing Devices," William Clowes and Sons, London, 1966.

Johnson, H. A., Information Theory in Biology after 18 Years. *Science,* **168:**1545, 1970.

Rushmer, R. F. (ed.): "Medical Engineering: Projections for Health Care Delivery," Academic Press, Inc., New York, 1972.

Shannon, C. E., and Weaver, W.: "The Mathematical Theory of Communication," The University of Illinois Press, Urbana, 1959.

Respiratory Monitoring

Kinney, J. M., Morgan, A. P., Dominguous, F. G., and Gilder, K. J.: A Method for Continuous Measurement of Gas Exchange and Expired Radioactivity in Acutely Ill Patients, *Metabolism,* **13:**205, 1964.

Lewis, F. J., Shimizu, T., Scofield, A. L., and Rosi, P. S.: Analysis of Respiration by an On-Line Digital Computer System: Clinical Data following Thoraco Abdominal Surgery, *Ann Surg,* **164:**547, 1966.

————, Deller, S., Yokochi, H., Rosi, P. S., Quinn, M. L., Kite, M., and Rabin, S.: Automatic Monitoring in the Postoperative Recovery Room, *Surg Gynecol Obstet,* **130:**333, 1970.

Osborn, J. J., Badia, W., and Gerbode, F.: Respiratory or Cardiac Work and Other Analogue Computer Techniques, *J Thorac Surg,* **45:**500, 1963.

————, Beaumont, J. O., Raison, J. C. A., Russell, J., and Gerbode, F.: Measurement and Monitoring of Acutely Ill Patients by Digital Computer, *Surgery,* **64:**1057, 1968.

Peters, R. M.: Work of Breathing following Trauma, *J Trauma,* **8:**915, 1968.

———— and Hilberman, M.: Respiratory Insufficiency Diagnosis and Control of Therapy, *Surgery,* **70:**280, 1971.

———— and Stacy, R. W.: Automatized Clinical Measurement of Respiratory Parameters, *Surgery,* **56:**44, 1964.

Powers, S. R., et al.: Physiologic Consequences of Positive End-expiratory Pressure (PEEP) Ventilation, *Ann Surg,* **178:**265, 1973.

Rosi, P. S., Yokochi, H., Deller, S., Quinn, M., Greenberg, A. G., Rabin, S., Blatt, S., Lewis, F. J., and Jacobs, J. E.: Noninvasive Automatic Patient Monitoring, *Surg Forum,* **20:**234, 1969.

Cardiovascular Monitoring

Bondurant, S. (ed.): Research on Acute Myocardial Infarction, *Circulation,* vol. 40, Suppl 4, 1969.

Border, J. R., Gallo, E., and Shenk, W. G.: Alterations in Cardiovascular and Pulmonary Physiology in the Severely Stressed Patient: A Rational Plan for the Management of Hypotension, *J Trauma,* **6:**176, 1966.

Cohn, J. N., Khatri, I. M., and Hamosh, P.: Diagnostic and Therapeutic Value of Bedside Monitoring of Left Ventricular Pressure, *Am J Cardiol,* **23:**107, 1969.

Dalton, B., and Laver, M. B.: Vasospasm with an Indwelling Radial Artery Cannula, *Anesthesiology,* **34:**194, 1971.

Del Guercio, L. R. M.: Cardiogenic Shock, in J. D. Hardy (ed.), "Rhoads Textbook of Surgery," 5th ed., pp. 78–84, Lippincott Company, Philadelphia, 1977.

————, Cohn, J. D., Feins, N. R., Coomaraswamy, R. P., and Mantel, L.: Pulmonary Embolism Shock: The Physiologic Basis of a Bedside Screening Test, *JAMA,* **196:**751, 1966.

Dudrick, S. J., Wilmore, D. W., Vars, H. M., and Rhoads, J. E.: Can Intravenous Feeding as the Sole Means of Nutrition Support Growth in the Child and Restore Weight Loss in an Adult? An Affirmative Answer, *Ann Surg,* **169:**974, 1969.

Ganz, W., and Swan, H. J. C.: Measurement of Blood Flow by Thermodilution, *Am J Cardiol,* **29:**241, 1972.

Garcia, E., Michenfelder, J. D., and Theye, R. A.: Right Atrial Oxygen Saturation Levels during Anesthesia and Surgery, *J Can Anaesth Soc,* **15:**593, 1968.

Kazamias, T. M., Gander, M. P., Ross, J., Jr., and Braunwald, E.: Detection of Left-Ventricular-Wall Motion Disorders in Coronary Artery Disease by Radarkymography, *N Engl J Med,* **285:**63, 1971.

Krauss, X. H., Verdouw, P. D., Hugenholtz, P. G., Hagemijer, F., and Polanyi, M. L.: Continuous Monitoring of O_2 Saturation in the Intensive Care Unit, *Circulation,* **45**(*Suppl* 2):178, 1972.

Lee, J., Wright, F., Barber, R., and Stanley, L.: Central Venous Oxygen Saturation in Shock: A Study in Man, *Anesthesiology,* **36:**472, 1972.

Lowenstein, E., Little, J. W., III, and Lo, H. H.: Prevention of Cerebral Embolization from Flushing Radial-Artery Cannulas, *N Engl J Med.* **285:**1415, 1971.

Owens, G., Belmusto, L., and Woldring, S.: Experimental Intracerebral PO_2 and PCO_2 Monitoring by Mass Spectrography, *J Neurosurg,* **30:**110, 1969.

Sheppard, L. C., Kouchoukos, N. T., Kurtis, M., and Kirklin, J. W.: Automated Treatment of Critically Ill Patients, *Ann Surg,* **168:**596, 1968.

Shubin, H., and Weil, M. H.: Efficient Monitoring with a Digital Computer of Cardiovascular Function in Seriously Ill Patients, *Ann Intern Med,* **65:**453, 1966.

Weinberg, D. I., Artley, J. L., Whalen, R., and McIntosh, H. D.: Electric Shock Hazards in Cardiac Catheterization, *Circ Res,* **9:**1004, 1962.

Woldring, S., Owens, G., and Woolford, D.: Blood Gases: Continuous In Vivo Recording of Partial Pressure by Mass Spectroscopy, *Science,* **153:**887, 1967.

Zohman, L. R., and Williams, M. H., Jr.: Percutaneous Right Heart Catheterization Using Polyethylene Tubing, *Am J Cardiol,* **4:**373, 1959.

Cardiac Output Determinations

Ashburn, W., L., Moser, K. M., and Guisan, M.: Digital and Analog Processing of Anger Camera Data and a Dedicated Computer Controlled System, *J Nucl Med,* **11:**680, 1970.

Bender, M. A., and Blau, M.: The Autofluoroscope, *Nucleonics,* **21:**52, 1963.

Civetta, J. M.: Cardiopulmonary Calculations: A Rapid, Simple and Inexpensive Technique, *Intensive Care Med,* **3:**209, 1977.

Cohn, J. D.: A Pump System for Performing Indicator-Dilution Curves without Blood Loss, *J Appl Physiol,* **26:**841, 1969.

————, Engler, P. E., and Del Guercio, L. R. M.: The Automated Physiologic Profile, *Critical Care Med,* **3:**51, 1975.

Del Guercio, L. R. M.: Contrast Dilution Analysis, *Trans NY Acad Sci,* **33:**387, 1971.

————, and Cohn, J. D.: Monitoring: Methods and Significance, *Surg Clin North Am,* **56:**977, 1976.

Feigenbaum, H., Zaky, A., and Nasser, W. K.: Use of Ultrasound to Measure Left Ventricular Stroke Volume, *Circulation,* **35:**1092, 1967.

Franklin, D. L., Schlegel, W., and Rushmer, R. F.: Blood Flow Measured by Doppler Frequency Shift of Back-scattered Ultrasound, *Science,* **134:**564, 1961.

Ganz, W., and Swan, H. J. C.: Measurement of Blood Flow by Thermal Dilution, *Am J Cardiol,* **29:**241, 1972.

Harken, A. H.: The Surgical Significance of the Oxyhemoglobin Dissociation Curve, *Surg Gynecol Obstet,* **144:**935, 1977.

Hillenbrand, W. I.: Desk-top Computers and Electronic Calculators for Engineers, *Electronic Products,* June 1966, pp. 50–53.

Jones, R. H., Klaphaak, R. B., and Sabiston, D. C. Jr.: Anatomic Resolution in Dynamic Radionuclide Studies by Computer Identification of Radioactivity Fluctuation with Time, *Proc 2d Symp Sharing Computer Programs Technology Nucl Med* (*AEC Conf-720430*), 1972, p. 151.

Kaufman, L.: Clinical Applications of Silicon Lithium Radiation Detectors, *Proc IEEE Nucl Sci Symp,* December 1972.

Kubicek, W. G., Patterson, R. P., and Witsoe, D. A.: Impedance Cardiography as a Non-invasive Method of Monitoring Cardiac Function and Other Parameters of the Cardiovascular System, *Ann NY Acad Sci,* **170:**724, 1970.

McDonald, D. A., Kouchoukos, N. T., Shepard, L. C., and Kirklin, J. W.: Estimation of Stroke Volume and Cardiac Output from the Central Arterial Pulse Contour in Postoperative Patients, *Circulation,* **38**(*Suppl* 6):118, 1968.

Newbower, R. S.: Blood Flow Measurements with Magnetic Tracers, *Proc Conf Engineering Med Biol,* **14:**147, 1972.

Papp, R. L., and Harrison, D. C.: Ultrasonic Cardiac Echography for Determining Stroke Volume and Valvular Regurgitation, *Circulation,* **41:**493, 1970.

Pombo, J. F., Troy, B. L., and Russell, R. O., Jr.: Left Ventricular Volumes and Ejection Fraction by Echocardiography, *Circulation,* **43:**480, 1971.

Shabot, M. M., Shoemaker, W. C., and State, D.: Rapid Bedside Computation of Cardiorespiratory Variables with a Programmable Calculator, *Critical Care Med,* **5:**105, 1977.

Siegel, J. H., Fabian, M., Lankau, C., Levine, M., Cole, A., and Nahmad, M.: Clinical and Experimental Use of Thoracic Impedance Plethysmography in Quantifying Myocardial Contractility, *Surgery,* **67:**907, 1970.

————, Greenspan, M., Cohn, J. D., and Del Guercio, L. R. M.: A Bedside Computer and Physiologic Nomograms: Guides to the Management of the Patient in Shock, *Arch Surg,* **97:**480, 1968.

Warner, H.: The Role of Computers in Medical Research, *JAMA,* **196:**944, 1966.

Weissler, A. M., Harris, W. S., and Schoenfeld, C. D.: Bedside Techniques for the Evaluation of Ventricular Function in Man, *Am J Cardiol,* **23:**577, 1969.

Wood, E. H., Sturm, R. E., and Sanders, J. J.: Data Processing in Cardiovascular Physiology with Particular Reference to Roentgen Videodensitometry, *Mayo Clin Proc,* **39:**849, 1964.

Monitoring of Tissue Metabolism

Cohn, J. D., Del Guercio, L. R. M., Ito, K., Pan, C. H. T., and Moross, G.: Infrared Emission Spectroscopy from Human Limbs, *Proc 25th Conf Engineering Med Biol,* 1972, p. 55.

————, ————, ————, ————, and ————: Infrared Spectral Analysis of Metabolic Function, *Fed Proc,* **31:**350, 1972.

Del Guercio, L. R. M., Cohn, J. D., Ito, K., Moross, G. G., and Pan, C. H. T.: Non-invasive Assessment of Cellular Function and Organ Perfusion, in "Advances in Automated Analysis; Diagnostic Medicine, Biomedical Profiling," vol 2, Mediad Incorporated, Tarrytown, N.Y., 1973.

Laks, H., Dmochowski, J. R., and Couch, N. P.: The Relationship between Muscle Surface pH and Oxygen Transport, *Ann Surg,* **183:**193, 1976.

Owens, G., Belmusto, L., and Woldring, S.: Experimental Intracerebral PO_2 and PCO_2 Monitoring by Mass Spectroscopy, *J Neurosurg,* **30:**110, 1969.

Woldring, S., Owens, G., and Woolford, D. C.: Blood Gases: Continuous In Vivo Recording of Partial Pressures by Mass Spectroscopy, *Science,* **153:**885, 1966.

Chapter 14

Skin and Subcutaneous Tissue

by **Seymour I. Schwartz**

PHYSIOLOGY

The skin, which is the largest organ in the body, represents more than a structure covering vital organs and separating them from the environment. It is a complex organ that possesses unique physical properties and physiologic functions.

Physical Properties

Both *tension* and *elasticity* are physical properties which are related to elastic fibers within the skin. Tension is the characteristic which accounts for the fact that the skin resists stretching by weak forces; the maximal deforming force which is resisted by the skin, expressed in dynes per centimeter, is a measurement of tension. Tension varies in different areas and is most marked where the skin contains dense elastic fibers, particularly in regions where the skin is thin. The direction of the tension also varies anatomically and forms the basis of the line system described by Langer in 1861. The tension of skin is greater in young than in elderly patients. Elasticity refers to the skin's ability to resume its original shape after an external force has been applied to cause deformation. This also varies with age, being less in the elderly and also in patients with edema.

Quantification of the physical properties of the skin has been made by determining the *tensile strength,* or the resistance of skin to tearing under tension. The average tensile strength of the adult skin, without fat, is approximately 1.8 kg/m^2. This is significantly reduced in infants up to three months of age, and the lowest values are found in the Ehlers-Danlos syndrome, which is characterized by a reduction of elastic fibers. In patients with Cushing's syndrome or those taking high doses of cortisone for prolonged periods of time, the tensile strength of skin is significantly less than normal, and there is also a low modulus of elasticity.

The electrical behavior of skin has been the subject of much investigation. The skin generates polarization currents which provide great resistance to external electric forces. The intensity of imposed current passing through the skin is therefore very low. The skin also offers a resistance to alternating currents by its property of impedance.

Functions of Skin

Important physiologic functions of skin include (1) percutaneous absorption, (2) an important role in the circulatory system, (3) serving as an organ of senses, (4) secretion of sweat, (5) providing an avenue for the insensible loss of water, and (6) contributing to thermal regulation.

PERCUTANEOUS ABSORPTION. This refers to the penetration of substances through the skin, permitting them to enter the bloodstream. It has been shown that radioactive water, applied either as a vapor or as a solution, appears both in the circulation and the urine. If the skin is warmed after exposure, the concentration in the urine increases rapidly. Electrolytes applied to the skin in aqueous solution either do not penetrate or may enter in small amounts via the appendages. The skin is impermeable to sodium and calcium when these are applied to the skin in the form of a chloride solution. However, there is some evidence that the iodide ion may enter the skin either because it increases the negative electric charge of skin or because it penetrates via appendages. When radioactive electrolytes are rubbed onto the skin, they are absorbed, and the absorption is increased if the skin is abraded or has been shaved.

Lipid-soluble substances are fairly rapidly and completely absorbed through the skin, and absorption appears to be faster if the substances are also soluble in water to some degree. In the latter instance, the penetration is so rapid that the rate of absorption is comparable to gastrointestinal absorption and even absorption of the material injected subcutaneously. The percutaneous absorption of phenol has been recognized for many years, and fatal poisoning may be associated with the application of carbolic acid to large areas of skin. Salicylic acid also penetrates with great ease from alcoholic and aqueous solutions as well as from ointments. Estrogenic hormones, testosterone, progesterone, and desoxycorticosterone all penetrate the intact skin rapidly. Hydrocortisone may be therapeutically effective by percutaneous application, while cortisone acetate applied locally is poorly absorbed. Water-soluble hormones, such as insulin, are not absorbed. Lipid-soluble vitamins are absorbed with ease, while water-soluble vitamins do not penetrate the skin. Heavy metals may be absorbed to some extent, and their absorption is dependent upon the formation of compounds in combination with the fatty acid of the sebum. This is particularly true of mercury.

Substances in the gaseous form, with the exception of carbon monoxide, penetrate the skin easily. Oxygen, nitrogen, and carbon dioxide are examples of gases which perfuse readily. Carbon tetrachloride is also readily absorbed through the skin, as demonstrated by experiments with ^{14}C-labeled compound. Recently, the absorption of pharmaceutic agents through the skin has been employed by using dimethyl sulfoxide as a vehicle. The applicability of this technique has not been totally defined.

CIRCULATION AND VASCULAR REACTIONS. The cutaneous vascular system is extremely complex and contributes significantly to the general circulation and vascular reactions. Direct visualization of flow in minute vessels can be carried out by observing the capillary circulation of the base of the nail. The color of the skin is dependent upon the quantity of blood in the subpapillary plexus of vessels,

particularly in the Caucasian, while the skin temperature depends chiefly on the rate of flow through the whole skin. The range of pressure in human skin capillaries is between 12 and 45 mm Hg, and the average capillary pressure is equivalent to the colloid osmotic pressure of plasma proteins. Arteriovenous anastomoses of digital skin play an important role in temperature regulation and are implicated in the formation of the glomus tumor.

Local vascular responses may result from direct action on the vessel wall or its contractile elements. Local vasoconstriction follows gentle stroking. However, if the mechanical stimulus is of greater intensity than that which causes constriction, a red local reaction may develop secondary to dilatation of small vessels. Circumscribed superficial edema of the skin in areas responsive to stimuli is referred to as a "wheal" and is due to leakage of plasma from dilated blood vessels into the extracellular space. There are two distinct steps in the formation of the wheal: (1) local dilatation and (2) increased capillary permeability. Stimulation of the sympathetic fibers supplying the skin causes vasoconstriction of the cutaneous vessels, while interruption of these fibers results in dilatation of the small arteries and arterioles. The cutaneous circulatory system also responds to chemical agents. Acetylcholine causes vasodilatation, while norepinephrine and epinephrine are important vasoconstricting drugs. Vasopressin is also an active vasoconstrictor. Nicotinic acid and nitrites cause flushing and warmth, increased temperature, and increased blood flow. Ergot alkaloids act as vasodilators by their sympatholytic action, but the drugs also directly constrict the muscles of the peripheral arterioles, and the net effect is a decrease in blood flow.

SENSORY FUNCTION. The skin's sensory functions pertain to the modalities of pain (including itching), touch, and temperature. Skin consists of a mosaic of multiple sensitive spots, the relative density of which varies with the region of body. Cold sensitivity is probably mediated by Krause's end bulbs, whereas Ruffini's endings are probably receptors for warmth. Meissner's corpuscles and Merkel's discs are implicated in the tactile sensation, and the Pacinian corpuscles are involved in the sensation of pressure. Pain is mediated by free nonmyelinated endings, which are in a plexiform arrangement. Following injury to the skin, there is a widespread area of hyperalgesia which radiates from the point of injury. After traumatic injury of a peripheral nerve, causalgia, in which there is increased pain accompanied by cutaneous vasodilatation, may occur. Sympathectomy at the appropriate level in this case brings about almost complete relief.

SWEAT SECRETION. The skin contains two types of sweat glands, eccrine glands, which are small sweat glands, and apocrine, or large, sweat glands. The eccrine glands are distributed all over the body and are the true secretory glands which produce clear, aqueous sweat responsible for heat regulation. The apocrine glands in the human being are almost rudimentary structures. If the environmental temperature rises above 31 or 32°C (90°F), there is a sudden outbreak of visible sweating over the entire body. At lower environmental temperatures, the sweat glands secrete microscopically visible droplets in a periodic fashion. The insensible sweat secretion constitutes one part of the total insensible water loss.

The distribution of sweat glands is such that the highest number per square inch are located in the palms and soles and are also more dense on the dorsum of the hand, forehead, and trunk. There are fewer glands in the lower extremity than in the upper extremity. In most instances, sweating is almost exclusively the result of nervous impulses, but the glands are able to respond directly to application of heat if it is sufficiently intense. The nonnervous sweat response is strictly limited to the local area of stimulation. The nervous response is almost entirely mediated over sympathetic nerves and results from the pharmacologic action of parasympathetic substances. The nerve fibers to the sweat glands liberate acetylcholine at their endings upon stimulation. Atropine and other anticholinergics block the receptor sites so that they are unable to respond and thus interfere with secretion. Hyperhidrosis (increased sweating) may result from an abnormal increase in nerve impulses as in central nervous system lesions or emotional states. Increased tonicity of the sweat fibers may intensify the sweat response to normal nervous and nonnervous stimuli.

Primary hyperhidrosis usually presents as excessive sweating noted early in life. Mild cases can be managed with anticholinergic drugs and antiperspirant creams. Sympathectomy at T_2 to T_4 or T_5 abolishes eccrine sweating in the involved areas of the upper extremity. A modified Hurley-Shelley operation is used for axillary hyperhidrosis. The hair-bearing axillary skin is excised, and the ganglia at T_2 and T_3 are removed for accompanying hand sweating.

Eccrine sweat is a clear aqueous solution containing 99 percent water and 1 percent solids, half of which are inorganic salts and half organic compounds. Under normal circumstances, it is hypotonic, but at high rates of sweating it may approach isotonic concentration. Although the composition of sweat depends on material within the bloodstream, it is not a simple ultrafiltrate of plasma but represents an active secretion. The concentration of sodium and chloride is lower than that in plasma, while the concentration of potassium is somewhat higher. The concentration of chloride depends on many factors and is usually in the range of 15 to 60 mEq/L. The sodium concentration is almost always entirely equivalent to that of chloride and varies in a parallel fashion. Chloride and sodium concentrations rise with prolongation of sweating and with the rate of sweating and temperature of the skin. The chloride content of palmar sweat is greater than that from other parts of the body. The salt concentration of sweat also depends on the intake, and an adequate supply of drinking water depresses the concentration. The loss of potassium through the skin ranges between 2.7 and 3.1 mEq/L.

Nitrogen compounds are also lost transdermally, and the concentration of urea in sweat is twice as high as that in the blood. Creatinine is present in sweat in only a minute amount, and amino acids have also been noted. Ammonia is a primary constituent of sweat, and it can be concentrated by the sweat glands with nearly the same efficiency as the renal excreting unit. Large amounts of lactic acid and lactate have been demonstrated in sweat, particularly during heavy muscular exercise and in association with thermogenic sweat. The concentrations are ten to twenty times higher than that in the blood, and it is felt that the lactic acid originates from breakdown of glycogen within the sweat glands.

Sweat provides the skin with an "acid mantle." The average pH of freshly secreted sweat is 5.7 to 6.4. As the sweating progresses, the acidity decreases, but considerable amounts of acid are still lost with profuse thermal sweating. There is increasing acidity with evaporation of water from the sweat. The acidity retards the growth of many bacteria which reside in the keratin layer, glands, and hair follicles.

In contrast to the eccrine glands, which develop from the upper dermis, the apocrine glands are formed from follicular epithelium, as are sebaceous glands. Like sebaceous glands and hair follicles, the apocrine glands have major development during puberty. They are greater in number in females and respond to autonomic nervous stimulation rather than thermal stimulation. They function by producing a somewhat viscous milklike droplet.

INSENSIBLE WATER LOSS. Sweat secretion provides but one of two separate mechanisms contributing to insensible loss of water through continuous evaporation which occurs at all environmental temperatures. The other mechanism is that of loss through the epidermis which, unlike sweat secretion, is not affected by atropinization. Water loss through the epidermis is contrasted with sweat in that it does not contain salts or other solutes. The total insensible water loss through skin and lungs is constant under basal conditions and amounts to about 200 $Gm/m^2/24$ hours, 60 percent of which is cutaneous loss. Total cutaneous water loss in the adult man at rest without visible sweating is about 500 to 700 ml daily. The insensible loss from both the skin and the lungs shows a linear relationship to the basal metabolic rate. Water intake has no effect on cutaneous loss in the adult but does increase it in children. In hypothyroidism, the water loss is conspicuously low, whereas in thyrotoxicosis, total insensible perspiration is greatly increased.

THERMOREGULATION. The skin plays an important role in the regulation of body temperature. Heat is lost through the skin under the processes of radiation, convection, conduction, and evaporation. Sweating is a useful process only when the sweat can evaporate. It is therefore very efficient as a regulatory mechanism in a dry, hot environment, but with increased humidity the efficiency decreases markedly. Humidity begins to be of importance between 30 and 31°C (86 to 88°F) air temperature, at which point the difference between 50 and 100 percent relative humidity decides whether the person will be comfortable or hyperthermic. If heat production is raised or atmospheric temperature is raised, there is a shift of blood flow from the interior to the skin. The converse is also true, and this process is carried out reflexly.

Cold stimuli of a moderate degree result in the production of pallor. After the stimulus has ceased, there is reactive arterial vasodilatation. Cold stimuli of long duration are associated with livid discoloration as a result of paresis in the venous limbs of the capillaries. With extreme stimuli, there may be a reddish discoloration due to dilatation of the arterioles. The condition, however, is not associated with increased blood flow, and skin temperature does not rise. The reduction in temperature is also accompanied by interference with the utilization of oxyhemoglobin. Emersion foot, or "trench foot," occurs when the skin is exposed for long periods of time to cold water. There is vasoconstriction and capillary damage, and if the skin's temperature is returned to normal rapidly, reactive hyperemia and blistering result. Thrombosis may complicate the situation. It is therefore felt that exposure to the cold should be treated by gradual increase in temperature. The role of sympathectomy early in the course of frostbite has been debated, but there is some real evidence to indicate that it is applicable if carried out within 24 hours.

Heat exhaustion refers to a syndrome characterized by excessive loss of salt and water when people are exposed to high temperatures. A sweat retention syndrome has been recognized among troops in hot, humid climates, in which situation the personnel lose their ability to sweat and become moderately hyperthermic. Exhaustion, headache, palpitation, and dizziness are the characteristic manifestations.

PRESSURE SORES

Pressure on an area of skin for 2 or more hours, particularly in patients with impaired nutritional status, may result in sufficient ischemia to cause a decubitus ulcer. The ulceration usually occurs over bony prominences. Supportive therapy includes a nutritive diet, correction of anemia, and relief of pressure over the area. Routinely turning the patient and using special mattresses are effective. Surgical therapy requires sharp debridement to excise the ulcer and underlying fascia and necrotic material. The bony prominence frequently requires excision, with care to achieve hemostasis. The bone should be covered with muscle, and a large rotation flap of skin and fat provides the best skin coverage.

HIDRADENITIS SUPPURATIVA

This is a chronic acneform infection of the cutaneous apocrine glands, subcutaneous tissue, and fascia. It is generally confined to areas in which these glands are found, namely the axilla, areola of the nipple, groin, perineum, and circumanal and periumbilical regions. The disease was first described by Velpeau in 1839, and clinical manifestations vary with the duration of the lesion. At first, there is a slight subcutaneous induration, and as the tumor enlarges, the process advances to the skin, which becomes inflamed and adherent. Suppuration eventually develops, and cellulitis surrounds the abscess. At this stage, pain is often severe. Incision and drainage at this point result in a few drops of thick, viscous, purulent material. The proc-

ess may subside after 2 or 3 days, only to recur. In the chronic stage, the patient presents with multiple painful cutaneous nodules which coalesce and are surrounded by fibrous reaction. The pathologic picture is similar to that seen in any acute pyogenic infection of the skin, but involvement of the apocrine glands establishes the diagnosis. Culture of the pus yields a variety of saprophytic and pathogenic bacteria with a preponderance of staphylococci and streptococci.

Treatment consists of excision of the involved area or x-ray therapy for early cases. Cures can be achieved early in the course of the disease by improved hygiene and incision and drainage. In chronic cases, however, radical excision of all the pathologic tissue with split-thickness skin grafts for coverage affords the best opportunity for cure.

CYSTS

Epidermal Inclusion Cyst

When the epithelium of the skin is trapped subcutaneously, as a result of trauma or for other reasons, it may continue to grow and desquamate. This creates a cyst lined by epidermal cells and filled with keratin and desquamated cells. The lesions occur most frequently on the hand and are characterized by continued enlargement. Cure is effected by removal of the entire cyst and all its epithelial elements.

Ganglia

Ganglia are areas of mucoid degeneration of retinacular structures. They are tense, subcutaneous cystic masses occurring most commonly over the wrist and over tendon sheaths of the hands and feet. They grow very slowly and are usually associated with only minimal discomfort. The lesions consist of a wall of collagenous tissue which may or may not have synovial cells and contain thin clear collagenous material. They have been related to trauma, either accidental or occupational.

Treatment is by surgical excision which is usually performed after a tourniquet is applied to permit precise dissection. The ganglia which are closely adherent to a tendon sheath are relatively easy to remove, but those which communicate with the synovium of a joint require excision of the neck and base plate to protect against recurrence. Trauma to established ganglia usually results in rupture, but this is generally followed by recurrence.

Sebaceous Cyst

The ducts of ceruminous skin glands may be plugged or blocked for a variety of reasons. Sebaceous glands are most numerous on the face and in the midline of the trunk, and they are generally associated with hair follicles. They produce sebum, an oily material, which serves as a natural dressing for the hair and skin. If the exit of sebum is blocked, the material accumulates and a cyst is formed.

The lesions, which are lined with glandular epithelium and surrounded by an area of compression fibrosis, gradually increase in size. They are usually painless and nontender but may become secondarily infected.

If infection is present, incision and drainage should be performed followed by planned excision of the cyst as a second stage after the infection has totally disappeared. In the case of noninfected cysts, surgical excision of the entire cyst is indicated to prevent recurrence.

Dermoid Cyst

This is usually a congenital lesion which does not manifest itself until later in life. The dermoid cyst can be differentiated clinically from the sebaceous cyst in that it is cystic on palpation and does not exhibit a dimple or scar in the overlying skin. Dermoid cysts generally occur in the midline of the body, on the scalp over the occiput, on the nose, and in the abdominal and sacral regions. They are considered to be occlusion cysts, taking their origin from an embryonic process. Although it has been suggested that malignant degeneration may occur, Conway indicates that no authentic case has been reported. Surgical excision is the treatment of choice.

Pilonidal Cyst and Sinus

These are common malformations which occur over the sacrococcygeal region. Their origin is associated with the neurenteric canal, and it is thought that their development is related to blockage of a congenital coccygeal sinus which is a vestige of this canal. This is substantiated by evidence that some of the pilonidal cysts and sinuses result from penetration of local skin by growing hairs. The ingrowth of such hairs sets the stage for cyst formation and repeated infection. The lesions may often be present from birth but are usually not manifest until the late adolescent or early adult years. The disease has been referred to as "jeep-driver's disease," and it is thought that the bumpy driving merely aggravates a congenital condition. Histologically, both the cysts and sinuses are lined with the stratified squamous epithelium.

The clinical manifestations vary from a barely perceptible dimple at the superior end of the buttock crease to an obvious sinus tract or cyst at this site. The sinus may chronically drain or become infected. The cyst also gradually increases in size and is susceptible to secondary infection. There have been rare reports of escape of cerebrospinal fluid from the pilonidal sinuses and equally rare instances of meningitis resulting.

TREATMENT. If the cyst is acutely infected, tender, and erythematous, incision and drainage are indicated. Secondary removal of the cyst or sinus is then planned after the infection has subsided. Elective surgical removal must be complete, and methylene blue may be injected as a guide to determine the extent of arborization of the sinus tract. Following excision of the sinus, closure may be accomplished either primarily or by granulation. If there is any infection, it is preferable to leave the wound open, unroofing all the tracts and allowing it to heal by secondary

intention. Primary closure incorporates fascial flaps, and a great variety of techniques are directed at moving the scar from the midline. In some instances, a very thin split-thickness graft (0.005 to 0.008 in.) may be used to achieve early closure and still permit the desirable contracture of the wound which accompanies the open technique.

BENIGN TUMORS

Warts

The common wart, or verruca vulgaris, is caused by a filterable virus and is both contagious and autoinoculable. Lesions may occur on any part of the body but are most common on the hand and the soles of the feet. They appear as circumscribed intraepidermal tumors which may be elevated or flat. Verruca plantaris (plantar wart) is the most troublesome variety and is located on the soles of the feet in the region of the metatarsal heads or over the os calcis. These warts may become quite tender and painful.

Verruca vulgaris may be treated by a variety of simple methods including freezing with liquid nitrogen, caustic agents, and x-ray therapy. In general, however, electrodesiccation under local anesthesia is the best primary treatment. Surgical treatment has been somewhat disappointing in view of the infectious nature of the lesion and the incidence of recurrence. The symptoms of plantar warts may be relieved by using pads to remove direct weight bearing from the wart area. Chemotherapy and surgical paring have also been used, and injection of local anesthesia into the base of the wart has achieved some success. Hyfercation has been very effective. It is difficult to evaluate therapy of these lesions, since the clinical course is extremely variable and spontaneous disappearance, formation of daughter warts, and recurrence challenge conclusions.

Keratosis

This represents hypertrophy of the epidermis and is considered a precancerous lesion. Clinical classification includes senile keratosis, arsenical keratosis, and seborrheic keratosis.

Senile keratosis develops most commonly in individuals with fair complexion and characteristically presents as multiple lesions in the sixth, seventh, and eighth decades. Lesions suspected of being malignant should be treated by surgical excision, since other methods of therapy which may be applied, including trichloracetic acid, electrodesiccation, and x-ray, all deny microscopic evaluation.

Seborrheic keratosis (Fig. 14-1) develops in middle-aged or older people as multiple lesions occurring chiefly on the trunk. They appear as thickened areas and may be yellow, gray, brown, or black. They are often great in number and may be confluent. The darker lesions have been mistaken for melanotic tumors. Histologically, they may be differentiated from senile keratoses, and they generally remain benign, though occasionally they may de-

Fig. 14-1. Seborrheic keratosis: pigmented, greasy lesions which, when solitary, may be mistaken for melanotic tumors.

velop into basal cell carcinoma or, more rarely, squamous cell carcinoma. Treatment is usually conservative, employing electrocoagulation and curettage, but any rapid increase in size is indication for surgical excision.

Keloid

The term is derived from the Greek work meaning "crab's claw" and refers to a dense accumulation of fibrous tissue which extends above the surface of the skin and also circumferentially beyond areas which were originally traumatized or incised and sutured. The color may vary from red to pink to white, and the lesion is notorious for its recurrence following surgical excision. There is an increased incidence in Negroes and dark-haired Caucasians and a predilection for the lesions to occur on the face, neck, and skin over the sternum.

Treatment consists of excision with closure. In order to reduce the amount of foreign body reaction, sutures should not be left buried. Postoperative low-dose radiation has been applied with some success, and corticotropins also have been effective.

Vascular Tumors

CAPILLARY (PORT WINE) HEMANGIOMA

The lesion is made up of closely packed, dilated abnormal capillaries in the subpapillary, dermal, or subdermal region of the skin. Clinically, there is no elevation or contour change but rather a reddish or purplish patch of staining. Growth parallels that of the involved area. If the lesion is small, it may be treated by excision and closure with excellent results. Larger lesions, however, are most difficult to treat, since the entire dermis is involved and excision results in a contour defect and scar. The discoloration may be modified by tattooing, but repeated procedures are necessary, since the pigment is absorbed. Tattooing followed by the application of cosmetic preparations achieves the best approximation of normal skin color.

IMMATURE HEMANGIOMA (STRAWBERRY MARK) (Fig. 14-2)

This appears in infancy and undergoes a remarkable change with the growth of the child. The lesion generally enlarges, sometimes quite dramatically, during the first several months to 1 year, subsequent to which spontaneous regression usually occurs. Clinically, immature hemangiomas are raised and irregular, with some bright-red areas. They are compressible and may show superficial areas of opacity suggesting the beginning of regression. Regression takes the form of increasing opacity and whitening of the surface with progressive thickening and flattening. The hemangioma may become ulcerated if it is in an area subjected to trauma, but hemorrhage from these lesions is not common and is generally readily controlled by pressure. Such episodes of ulceration, minor hemorrhage, or superficial infection may actually hasten spontaneous resolution. Treatment in large part consists of reassuring the parents. Indications for surgical treatment, radiation, sclerosing agents, and local freezing are diminishing.

CAVERNOUS HEMANGIOMA

The lesions are full-sized in proportion to the child at birth and do not undergo changes with rapid growth or spontaneous regression. They consist of mature vessels and may include multiple arteriovenous communications. Cavernous hemangiomas frequently involve deep tissues, such as muscles and even the central nervous system. They may also be combined with lymphangiomatous elements. Rapidly growing tumors in childhood stop expanding or regress on a prednisone regimen. Treatment of established lesions is by wide surgical excision depending on the area of location.

SCLEROSING HEMANGIOMA

This is actually a subepidermal nodular fibrosis which occurs chiefly on the extremities and is related to trauma. It presents as a small nonpainful nodule, and the overlying epidermis may be pigmented in such a manner that the lesion is often mistaken for malignant melanoma. The treatment is surgical excision.

GLOMUS TUMOR

The glomus tumor is a benign, rare, and exquisitely painful small neoplasm of the skin and subcutaneous tissue occurring usually on the extremities and particularly in the nail beds of the hands and feet. The tumor is derived from the glomic end organ apparatus consisting of arteriovenous anastomoses which function normally to regulate the blood flow in the extremity. The organ contributes to the regulation of local and general body temperature through the dissipation or conservation of heat.

The tumors vary in structure but resemble the normal glomus unit and have often been referred to as *angiomyoneuroma*. The layers of circular muscle of the vessels may be separated from the endothelium by collagenous membrane, or the endothelium may be bordered directly by the so-called "glomus epithelioid" cells. In some tumors, the blood vessels are so enlarged that they resemble true angiomas. The glomus cells are supplied by nonmyelinated nerve fibers, which account for the painful nature of the lesion. Although the tumor per se is benign, a malignant counterpart exists and is referred to as a *hemangiopericytoma*.

The lesion is usually single, but multicentric origin has been reported. The color varies from deep red to purple or blue, and there is variation in color with changes in temperature. The patients usually present in the fifth decade, but the tumor has been reported at all ages. The pain associated with the lesion is the most prominent symptom and may occur either spontaneously, with pressure, or in association with trauma. The pain, which is described as stabbing, lancinating, and radiating from the tumor, may be intermittent in character or may occur only when the lesion is touched. The glomus tumor is radioresistant. Encapsulated tumors may be shelled out, but when an obvious capsule is not seen, wide excision is indicated.

LYMPHANGIOMA

Lymphangiomas, like hemangiomas, are congenital in origin. The most common type is deep and cavernous, consisting of lymph-filled spaces with thin-walled septums and some areas of fibrosis. A superficial variant presents as circumscribed lesions which appear as small blisters and slightly elevated skin patches. When deep lesions are present in the neck, mediastinum, and axilla, they are referred to as *cystic hygroma* (see Chap. 39). The treatment is surgical excision which, although frequently incomplete, is rarely associated with recurrence.

Fat Tumors

LIPOMA

This is an extremely common subcutaneous lesion which is composed of fat and is, at times, difficult to distinguish from the normal subcutaneous adipose tissue. Usually, however, there is a thin, fibrous capsule, and the lesion can be enucleated from surrounding normal fat. Benign lipomas occur more frequently over the back, between the shoulders, and on the back of the neck, and liposarcomatous transformation is extremely uncommon. Treatment is surgical excision.

WEBER-CHRISTIAN DISEASE

This is an uncommon inflammatory lesion of the subcutaneous fat characterized by painful reddened areas

Fig. 14-2. Immature hemangioma (strawberry mark). Note opacification in the center. Lesion is undergoing spontaneous resolution.

involving the panniculus. The diagnosis is made by biopsy and is based on the presence of inflammatory cells in the adipose tissue. Recently, it has been demonstrated that many of the lesions which were so classified represented facticial dermatitis or skin manifestations of fat necrosis associated with pancreatitis.

Neuromas

These benign tumors involving the nerve tissue may be classified as neurilemmomas when the lesion arises from the sheath cell of Schwann or neurofibroma in which there are subcutaneous masses of neurofibromatous tissue. Neurilemmomas frequently arise from relatively small nerves and do not produce much pain. Treatment is surgical excision. Neurofibromas may be multiple and may be associated with von Recklinghausen's disease, including café au lait spots and scoliosis. Patients with neurofibromatosis are prone to develop meningiomas, gliomas, and pheochromocytomas, and eventual sarcomatous degeneration occurs in approximately 10 percent.

MALIGNANT TUMORS

Carcinoma of the skin occurs predominantly in exposed areas, most frequently in the weather-beaten skin of the aging sailor or farmer. It is generally a low-grade malignant tumor which may metastasize late, in which case the metastasis is usually to regional lymph nodes, so that curability is high compared with that of other tumors.

Basal Cell Carcinoma

This is a localized malignancy which grows slowly, at times taking 1 or more years to double in area. Basal cell carcinoma is more common than the squamous cell tumor, accounting for at least three-fourths of all cases in most clinical series. Lesions may be found over most areas of the body and are waxy, grayish yellow, or pink, often with telangiectasia below the surface. There is a predilection for the head and neck. In some instances, the tumors are darkly pigmented and difficult to distinguish from melanoma (Fig. 14-3). The lesions are firm but not indurated, and there is little sign of inflammation. As growth progresses, the skin is stretched, and the center of the lesion tends to necrose, resulting eventually in a flat ulcer. Basal carcinoma may extend deeper subcutaneously than is initially apparent, and extensive ulceration into the deep tissue without marked induration or infiltration has been referred to as *rodent ulcer*. If the tumor is not treated, it may erode into the deep structures including the skull, orbit, or brain. Less commonly, basal cell carcinoma may appear fungoid and grow large externally.

Squamous Cell Carcinoma

Squamous cell carcinoma tends to be more clearly defined than basal cell carcinoma. It grows more rapidly and may achieve in weeks the same size that the basal cell carcinoma reaches in months or years. Differential diagnosis between basal cell and squamous cell carcinoma can usually be made on the basis of site, appearance, history, type of skin, and presence of scars. However, only biopsy provides an accurate diagnosis.

The primary lesion of the squamous cell carcinoma is frequently surrounded by satellite nodules, and central ulceration may occur. The degree of induration around the

Fig. 14-3. Pigmented basal cell carcinoma. Note characteristics of melanotic tumor.

lesion is significant. The center gradually deepens into a crater with an irregular base which is covered by crust. Small pearls may be expressed from the ulcer, and rolled margins surrounding the ulcer contribute to the lesion's resembling a small volcanic crater. Growth may be superficial, or the lesion may burrow into deeper tissue with minimal effect on the cutaneous surface. Squamous cell carcinoma is more malignant than the basal cell variety and will metastasize to regional glands more rapidly.

Squamous cell carcinoma is particularly common in the lip at the vermillion border and in the folds of the paranasal area or in the axilla. Lesions occur more frequently in blond individuals with thin dry skin which is subjected to frequent irritation by rubbing or shaving. Squamous cell carcinoma is also particularly likely to originate in papillomas, senile warts, or cutaneous horns and develops at the site of postradiation dermatitis and ulcerations in old burn scars (Marjolin's ulcer). The incidence is also higher in people exposed to arsenicals, nitrates, and hydrocarbons.

Sweat Gland Carcinoma

This rare tumor usually occurs in the sixth and seventh decades of life, but it has been reported in adolescents. Characteristically, a soft tissue mass has been present for many years. Therapy consists of wide local excision with consideration of lymphadenectomy, since regional lymph nodes are involved in about half the cases. Following treatment, the reported 5-year survival is 38 percent for all patients and 24 percent for those with lymph node involvement.

TREATMENT OF CARCINOMA. Both electrodesiccation and electrocoagulation have been used but are to be condemned, since they destroy more tissue than is needed, result in retardation of healing, and do not provide a diagnosis. Radiation therapy may afford good results in the treatment of basal cell carcinoma, whereas squamous cell carcinomas are generally more resistant. Resolution of superficial basal cell carcinomas has been achieved with topical dinitrochlorobenzene (DNCB).

Although there is wide disagreement, surgical excision generally shows rates of cure which are higher than those for radiation. The results of radiation are certainly not as good for basal cell carcinomas over 2 cm in diameter as those achieved with surgical excision. Radiation therapy is contraindicated for any lesion which has recurred following unsuccessful radiation or for lesions which have developed in tissue which has been scarred following burns, keratoses, or xeroderma pigmentosum.

Mohs has used an escharotic preparation which is applied to the surface of the skin; 24 hours later the area fixed by the preparation is removed and examined microscopically. From this evidence, decision is made as to the requirements for additional application. The procedure is repeated until marginal biopsy shows only healthy tissue. The advantage of this method is the possibility of eradicating small extensions of the central lesion with certainty, and the granulation tissue below the lesion heals rapidly. Mohs has achieved 93 percent cures for carcinoma of the skin in all locations on the surface of the body and 87.5 percent cures for carcinoma of the lip. Few surgeons have utilized this technique.

Surgical treatment for carcinoma of the skin should include complete excision of all malignant tissue and a sufficient margin of normal tissue. For smaller tumors, a margin of 0.5 cm laterally and in depth is usually sufficient, whereas for larger lesions, the margins must be significantly greater. Many of the larger lesions require planned reconstructive surgical procedures, frequently employing skin grafts. Prophylactic dissection of regional nodes is not practical and should be performed only if there is evidence of clinical involvement.

PROGNOSIS. This is difficult to evaluate, but recurrence rates are very low. Overall 5-year survival rates of 96 percent for basal cell carcinoma and 80 percent for squamous cell carcinoma have been reported. Sharp and Binkley reported on 983 cutaneous carcinomas of all types and found that a 14 percent recurrence rate followed surgical treatment, while 10 percent recurred following roentgen therapy and 17 percent following radium therapy. In contrast, Conway reported only one recurrence in 168 cases of basal cell carcinoma treated surgically as compared with a 7.2 percent recurrence rate following roentgen therapy.

Other Malignant Tumors

Since the skin has a mesodermal origin, it is logical that sarcomas should develop, and the skin represents the site of origin of 6 percent of all cases of sarcoma. Primary sarcomas vary in degree of malignancy and in histologic characteristics. Excision is associated with an overall incidence of recurrence of 61 percent.

FIBROSARCOMA

This occurs most commonly in women in the buttocks, thigh, and inguinal regions and particularly frequently in scars. The tumors are usually of relatively low-grade malignancy and are radioresistant. Wide surgical excision is the treatment of choice, but it is followed by a high incidence of recurrence. In one series, 56 percent survived 10 years without recurrence. Distant spread occurs in 25 percent.

HEMANGIOPERICYTOMA

This is a malignant tumor of angioplastic origin and is considered a malignant variant of the glomus tumor. The lesions are extremely malignant, and the prognosis is poor, with only 27 percent surviving 5 years without evidence of disease. Surgical excision has proved unsatisfactory for larger tumors, and x-ray therapy is considered the treatment of choice.

KAPOSI'S SARCOMA

The etiology and pathogenesis of this lesion have not been resolved. It occurs more commonly in men. In Western countries there is a predilection for Jews, Italians, and Prussians. The tumor is prevalent in equatorial Africa and constitutes 9 percent of malignant tumors in Uganda. The tumor usually starts in the hands or feet as multiple plaques which are reddish to purple and may be flat, ulcerated, or polypoid. The lymph nodes may be involved and obstruction of the lymph nodes may result in lymphedema.

X-ray may retard the growth of the lesion, but wide surgical excision and, at times, amputation offer more promise. Patients with florid lesions respond well to actinomycin D (dactinomycin). The prognosis is poor, although some cases have survived for prolonged periods of time. In the terminal stages, the tumor extends to the mucous membranes and portions of the gastrointestinal tract.

OTHER SARCOMAS

A wide variety of other tumors having origin in different cells have been described. Dermatrofibrosarcoma protuberans represents one tumor with relatively low-grade malignancy which generally occurs on the trunk. The tumors are radioresistant but respond to surgical excision, and 70 percent have been reported to be free of the disease for at least 5 years. Widespread dissemination is rare, but local recurrence may occur repeatedly.

Lymphangiosarcoma is almost always associated with chronic lymphedema. A recent review included 186 cases; 162 cases occurred postmastectomy an average of 10 years after surgery, with a range of 1 to 26 years. All patients had had radical mastectomy, and the overwhelming majority had received postoperative irradiation. Only 9 percent of the patients survived 5 or more years, and only 2 of 24 patients with nonpostmastectomy lymphangiosarcoma were alive at 5-year follow-up. Amputation gave significantly better results than radiation therapy.

MISCELLANEOUS LESIONS

Bowen's disease is a slowly growing cutaneous carcinoma in situ for which excision is recommended. *Adenoacanthoma*, which frequently develops on the face or ear, is characterized grossly by a verrucous appearance and microscopically by desquamated cells. Local excision is indicated, since it rarely metastasizes. *Keratoacanthoma* is an elevated, friable red lesion which may be of viral origin and is best managed by simple excision.

MELANOMA AND OTHER PIGMENTED LESIONS

General Considerations

Since melanoma is a relatively uncommon disease, occurring in 0.0018 percent of the general population, while the average Caucasian adult has 15 to 20 nevi, it is obvious that removal of all moles is not advisable. On the other hand, about 25 percent of patients who have malignant melanoma recall having had a "mole" at the site of origin of the malignant lesion. Therefore, in dealing with pigmented lesions, the surgeon must be aware of characteristics which should arouse suspicion of malignancy or premalignancy.

Several pertinent facts regarding the predilection for malignant melanoma aid in the evaluation of pigmented lesions of the skin. Melanoma is rare before puberty. Females and males are affected with equal frequency. The lesions tend to occur in people with fair skin. The type of mole is important in assessing the likelihood of development of melanoma. The junctional nevus, either alone or as part of a compound nevus, has been implicated more frequently than the pure intradermal nevus. The blue nevus is rarely the source of melanoma, and the development of malignancy in the small congenital hairy nevus is even more unusual. The incidence of malignant melanoma in giant pigmented nevi has been reported as 10 to 17.5 percent. Nevi of the palms, soles, nail beds, genitalia, and mucous membranes retain functional elements that are more prone to be the source of melanoma than moles at other sites. The ratio of the number of moles at this site to melanoma substantiates this notion. There is probably a genetic predilection for the development of melanoma as evidenced by the studies of Harnly, who has created a strain of flies in which melanotic tumors develop spontaneously. Kassel et al. have also induced melanotic cancer in *Drosophila,* using an extract of human tumors.

Many theories concerning pigmented lesions that enjoyed acceptance in the past have recently proved to be unfounded. MacDonald has shown that there is probably no difference in incidence among races. It is also untrue that melanoma occurs more frequently in areas of highest total sunlight. Although endocrine dysfunction is related to pigmentation in Addison's disease, Cushing's syndrome, thyrotoxicosis, and diabetes, there is no relationship to the development of malignant melanoma. Castration, adrenalectomy, hypophysectomy, and hormone therapy have all failed to alter the course of metastatic melanoma. White and George et al. have recently refuted the notion that pregnancy adversely affects survival in women with melanoma. Repeated trauma and its role in malignant transformation of moles remains theoretic and unproved.

Fig. 14-4. Typical malignant melanoma. Note central darkly pigmented elevation and surrounding halo of superficial satellite extensions. Sudden change in appearance and growth brought the patient to his physician.

Benign Pigmented Lesions

These include the intradermal nevus, or common mole, the junctional nevus, compound nevus, juvenile melanoma, and freckles. The *intradermal nevus* is characterized by nests of melanoblasts which are confined to the dermis. The lesions are smooth or papillary and rarely occur on the soles or palms. The presence of hair is strong presumptive evidence of the diagnosis. In the case of the *junctional nevus,* the proliferation of melanoblasts originates in the basal layer of the epidermis and extends down into the dermis. The lesions are smooth, flat, or slightly raised. They occur on the genitalia, soles, palms, nail beds, and mucous membranes. The *compound nevus* is formed from junctional and intradermal elements. It is smooth, elevated, occasionally papillary, and hairless. *Juvenile melanomas* are nevi which occur prior to puberty, and although the microscopic picture is similar to that of melanoma, the lesions are clinically benign. They may be purplish red, brown, or black; they are generally smooth and hairless with irregular edges. The majority occur on the face and enlarge slowly. *Freckles* occur most commonly in blond and red-headed people on exposed portions of their bodies and represent pigment in the basal layer and upper dermis. They are not of clinical significance.

DIFFERENTIAL DIAGNOSIS. Although the classic mole has a characteristic appearance, the differential between benign pigmented skin lesions and melanoma may be quite difficult. Other lesions which cause particular confusion are (1) seborrheic and senile keratoses (Fig. 14-1) and (2) pigmented basal cell tumors (Fig. 14-3). Small intradermal hematomas may have an appearance similar to melanomas, and subungual hematomas have been mistaken for melanomas. High-speed dental drills may force silver fillings into the buccal mucosa, and the appearance mimics that of melanoma.

TREATMENT. If the pigmented lesion is considered to be a junctional nevus, excision is advisable. Various characteristics of any pigmented lesions are indications for excision. These include change in color or pigment distribution; development of erythema; change in size or consistency; change in the surface characteristic, i.e., scaling, oozing, bleeding, crustings or erosion; subjective symptoms such as pain, numbness, burning, itching, diffusion of pigment into normal skin; satellite nodules; and regional lymphadenopathy.

The *Hutchinson freckle* (lentigo maligna) is worthy of special note. This is a circumscribed precancerous melanosis of the face, generally occurring in elderly people. There are two stages of disease: In the macular stage, the lesion is smooth and light brown with irregular borders and uneven color. About one-third of the lesions then evolve into a tumor stage characterized by induration and all the histologic features of melanoma, but the behavior is not like melanoma. The prognosis is excellent when the lesion is excised from the face, but it is guarded when the lesion is found in other body areas, in which case it should be treated as a melanoma.

Excision of any suspicious lesion should be complete and should include a margin of normal skin.

Fig. 14-5. Subungual melanoma. Lesion had been treated as an infection for nearly 1 year. Note pigmentation and replacement of nail. X-rays showed destruction of the distal phalanx. Axillary metastases were evident by this time.

Fig. 14-6. Clark's levels of invasion. Papillary and reticular dermis of normal skin of the right upper arm; hematoxylin and eosin stain. The tissue just below the epidermis is pale and delicate, without obvious collagen bundles. Deep to this, collagen is organized into bundles, and the upper part of this zone forms an almost straight line with the papillary dermis (small arrows). Piling up of cells at this interface constitutes level III invasion. The arrows and their respective roman numerals indicate invasion levels. Level V (not shown) is into fat. (*From Cancer Res., 29:725, 1969.*)

Melanoma

The term, by definition, refers to a malignant lesion originating in the melanoblast of the skin, and therefore "malignant melanoma" represents a redundancy. The tumor may develop in any area of the skin or in the pigmented region of the eye. There is an almost equal distribution between the head and neck, lower extremity, and trunk, each accounting for approximately 25 percent of the cases. About 11 percent occur in the upper extremity, and the remainder involve the genitalia or represent cases in which the primary lesion is never determined. The typical skin lesion (Fig. 14-4) is darkly pigmented, smooth, firm, and nonhairy. Subungual melanomas are more frequent than pigmented nevi in the nail beds and may present difficulty in reference to differentiation from subungual hematoma and chronic paronychial infection (Fig. 14-5). All melanomas originate from the melanoblast at the dermal-epidermal junction, but the cell does not contain melanin at all times; therefore some lesions may be amelanotic. The cells are characterized by a dopa-positive reaction.

Microstaging has been determined by direct measurement or according to Clark's levels of invasion (Fig. 14-6). Level I (in situ) applies when all tumor cells are above the basement membrane. Level II has tumor extension into the papillary but not the reticular dermis. Level III refers to tumor cells in the ill-defined interface between the papillary and reticular dermis. Level IV is characterized by tumor cells in the reticular dermis. Level V has invasion into the subcutaneous fat. Clinically, Stage I relates to isolated skin involvement, Stage II to involvement of regional lymph nodes, and Stage III to distant metastases.

TREATMENT. Incisional biopsy is performed only when the lesion is extremely large. Biopsy provides the definitive diagnosis and should indicate the depth of involvement.

When invasion does not extend beyond the papillary dermis, simple excision is generally sufficient. When the tumor extends below the papillary dermis, a 5-cm margin beyond the lesion is indicated. Inadequate excision has been associated with the development of satellite nodules (Fig. 14-7).

The major argument in therapy centers around removal of the regional lymph nodes. Some advocate removing these nodes only when they are involved clinically, since

Fig. 14-7. Recurrent satellite nodules. These followed inadequate excision of a malignant melanoma which was thought to be a simple nevus. Note the characteristic deep-black color and emergence of lesions from the subcutaneous tissues to and through the skin.

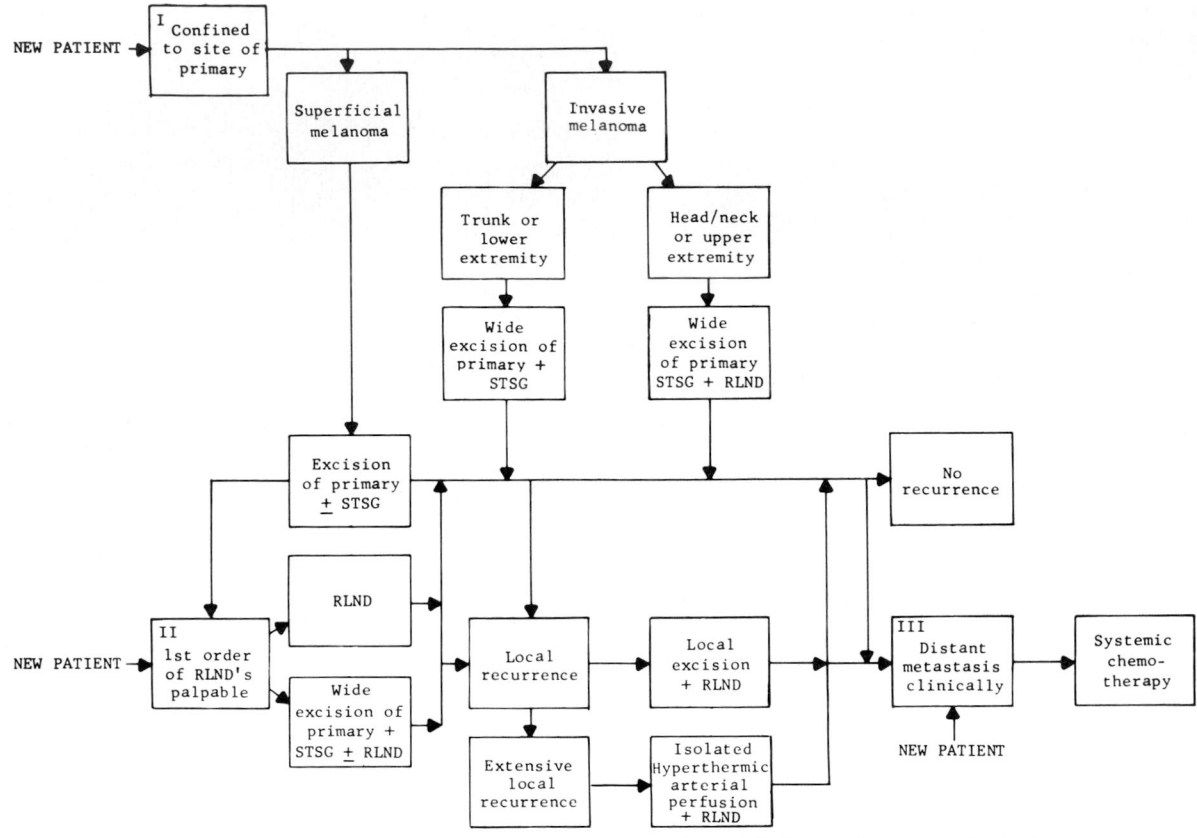

Fig. 14-8. Schematic diagram illustrating a treatment approach to melanoma patients. STSG, split-thickness skin graft; RLND, regional lymph node. (*From C. O. Knutson et al., Melanoma, Curr Probl Surg, The Year Book Medical Publishers, Inc., Chicago, December 1971.*)

there is significant morbidity associated with the procedure and statistical data do not demonstrate benefit. Others champion routine removal regardless of the clinical status in view of the accepted inaccuracy of clinical evaluation.

As a compromise, Knutson et al. recommend elective cervicofacial or axillary node dissection, in the absence of clinical involvement, for invasive lesions of the head and neck or upper extremity, since the consequent morbidity is minimal. Invasive melanomas of the trunk are treated with wide excision, and nodes are removed only if they are involved clinically, since lymphatic drainage is unpredictable. "Prophylactic" lymph node dissections generally are not advised for lower extremity lesions, since necrosis of skin flaps, delayed healing, infection, thrombophlebitis, edema, and satellitosis all contribute to a significant morbidity. Chronic lymphedema occurs in 6 percent of extremities following inguinal node dissection and 46 percent following ilioinguinal node dissection. The exception is a lesion which permits removal of the inguinal lymph nodes in continuity. Clinically palpable nodes should be excised (Fig. 14-8).

The appreciation of intermediate metastases between the primary tumor and regional nodes has led some writers to suggest aggressive amputation or, more recently, integumentectomy with removal of skin, subcutaneous tissue, and deep fascia from the foot to the inguinal ligament. In general, amputation is reserved for palliation of bulky, ulcerating, or painful lesions.

Groin Dissection (Fig. 14-9). The skin incision may be oblique and parallel to the inguinal ligament, vertical, or S-shaped with an oblique limb running parallel to the inguinal ligament and the vertical limbs running parallel to the lateral margin of the rectus femoris muscles craniad and to the medial portion of the femoral triangle caudad. If the primary lesion is close to the line of incision or if the proposed skin incision is overlying a large lymph node which might be attached to the subcutaneous tissue, a wide ellipse can be removed beginning medial to the anterior superior iliac spine and continuing over the femoral triangle. On the abdominal wall, the subcutaneous and fatty tissue is dissected cleanly from the aponeurosis of the external oblique down to the inguinal ligament. With genital primary melanomas, the presymphysial lymphatics and areolar tissue of the spermatic cord or round ligament must be included in the dissection. The lower flaps are retracted, the lateral margin is exposed first, and the superficial fascia and fascia lata are dissected off the bare sartorius muscle to the lateral margin of the femoral triangle. The femoral sheath is entered, and the femoral artery and vein are dissected clean of fatty tissue. The greater saphenous vein is transected at two levels, first at the medial inferior portion of the transected tissue and second where the vein enters the femoral vein. Since the deep inguinal

Fig. 14-9. Groin dissection. *A.* Dissection of upper thigh and sheath of femoral triangle. *B.* Dissection of inguinal region including excision of endopelvic fascia. Note exposure of iliac vessels. *C.* Dissection of obturator fossa containing medial chain of obturator lymph nodes. Note that external iliac vein is elevated and obturator nerve is isolated from the fascia. *(From J. S. Spratt, Jr., "Anatomy and Surgical Technique of Groin Dissection," The C. V. Mosby Company, St. Louis, 1965.)*

nodes lie in the areolar tissue about the femoral vessels, carrying the dissection down to the adventitial surface of the femoral artery and vein will include them in the dissected material. Mediad, the tissue is incised over the pectineus muscle, and eventually the specimen remains attached only by tissue passing into the femoral space medial to the femoral vein.

The iliac dissection represents a continuum of the inguinal dissection. The external oblique aponeurosis is incised, and a flap is established caudad down to the inguinal ligament. The fibers of the transversus abdominis and internal oblique muscles are separated from the inguinal ligament. The ligamentous attachment of the transversalis fascia to the inguinal ligament is divided, and the epigastric artery and vein are ligated and transected at the level of the inguinal ligament. Following the division of muscle and fascial fibers along the inguinal ligament to the anterior superior iliac spine, the peritoneum is exposed and reflected from the lateral pelvic wall by blunt dissection. This per-

mits visualization of the ureter and the iliac vessels. The endopelvic fascia is incised medial to the genitofemoral nerve from the inguinal ligament to above the bifurcation of the common iliac artery; the external iliac artery is rotated mediad, and the space between the artery and the muscle is dissected clear. The dissection then continues by reflecting the vascular sheath away from the external iliac artery and vein. The origin of the inferior epigastric arteries and veins will be exposed, and these are then transected. All the areolar tissue is swept down in a medial fashion. The medial chain of iliac lymph nodes is removed by dissection of the obturator fossa, retracting the external iliac vein laterally. In this dissection the bare muscle fibers of the internal obturator muscle are exposed, and the obturator veins must be transected. After the iliac dissection has been mobilized and freed from the margin of the inguinal-pectineal triangle, the inguinal ligament is elevated, and the iliac alveolar tissue and lymph nodes are delivered into the femoral triangle for completion of the en bloc dissection.

The lower abdominal wall is carefully reconstructed to avoid hernia formation, and the sartorius muscle transected and reflected mediad to cover the femoral artery and vein. Prior to closure of the subcutaneous tissue and skin, drainage is achieved with suction catheters.

Adjunctive Therapy. Systemic chemotherapy is used when there is recurrent or metastatic disease which precludes excision. Disseminated melanoma is one of the most chemoresistant cancers. Objective regression has been noted in about one-quarter of the patients receiving vinblastine or cyclophosphamide. Other effective agents include vincristine, hydroxyurea, and 1-phenylalanine mustard (melphalan), BCNU (1,3-bis[2-chloroethyl]-1-nitrosourea), and DTIC (dimethyl-triazeno-imidazole-carboxamine).

Isolated regional artery perfusion with L-phenylalanine mustard or a combination of drugs has had striking results as treatment for multiple local metastases or inoperable satellitosis of an extremity. Some writers have applied perfusion as an adjunct to patients without clinical subcutaneous or cutaneous metastases. Recurrence rates lower than those associated with conventional surgical treatment have been reported. However, the complications of arterial perfusion therapy are of such magnitude as to argue against this approach, with suggestion that perfusion be withheld until recurrences are noted.

Recent attention has been directed to the host immune response. A correlation between a patient's prognosis and his immune response to melanoma has been established. This response accounts for spontaneous regressions, which have been noted, and immunity to the tumor has been enhanced by active immunization with BCG (bacillus Calmette-Guérin) or autologous tumor cells. Dermal scarification has been associated with better results than intradermal vaccination. The best results have been noted for intradermal metastases, while subcutaneous and visceral metastases rarely respond. BCG therapy has toxic side effects, and deaths have been reported.

PROGNOSIS. In a recent review by Wanebo and associates, the 5-year cure rate was 100 percent for levels I and II, 88 percent for level III, 60 percent for level IV, and 15 percent for level V. In patients with level IV melanoma, the 5-year cure rate was 82 percent in those with negative nodes and 27 percent in those with nodal metastases after elective node dissection. In the same study the measured depth of invasion added significant clinical pathologic information. The incidence of nodal metastases at elective node dissection was 5 to 9 percent for melanomas showing 0.6 to 2.0 mm of invasion, 22 percent for melanomas measuring 2.1 to 3.0 mm, and 39 percent for melanomas

invading beyond 3 mm. The cure rate was 100 percent for melanomas measuring less than 1 mm, 83 percent for melanomas invading 1.1 to 2.0 mm, 58 percent for lesions measuring 2.1 to 3.0 mm, and 55 percent for melanomas invading over 3.0 mm. In another review, Cady et al. reported that the depth-of-invasion criteria of Clark were no more accurate in predicting survival than careful measurement of maximal diameter. Melanomas of the lower extremity offer a slightly better survival rate than those of the upper extremity and a markedly higher survival rate than lesions of the trunk.

References

Physiology

Allen, A. C.: "The Skin: A Clinicopathological Treatise," 2d ed., Grune & Stratton, Inc., New York, 1967.

Ellis, H., and Morgan, M. N.: Surgical Treatment of Severe Hyperidrosis, *Proc Roy Soc Med,* **64:**768, 1971.

Hartfall, W. G., and Jochimsen, P. R.: Hyperhidrosis of Upper Extremity and Its Treatment, *Surg Gynec Obst,* **135:**586, 1972.

Rothman, S.: "Physiology and Biochemistry of the Skin," The University of Chicago Press, Chicago, 1954.

Pressure Sores

Herceg, S. J., and Harding, R. L.: Surgical Treatment of Pressure Sores, *Pa Med,* **74:**45, 1971.

Hidradenitis Suppurativa

Conway, H., Stark, R. B., Climo, S., Weeter, J. C., and Garcia, F. A.: The Surgical Treatment of Chronic Hidradenitis Suppurativa, *Surg Gynecol Obstet,* **95:**455, 1952.

Knaysi, G. A., Jr., Cosman, B., and Crikelair, G. F.: Hidradenitis Suppurativa, *JAMA,* **203:**19, 1968.

Cysts and Benign Tumors

Brasfield, R. D., and Das Gupta, T. K.: Von Recklinghausen's Disease: A Clinicopathological Study, *Ann Surg,* **175:**86, 1972.

Brown, S. H., Jr., Neerhout, R. C., and Fonkalsrud, E. W.: Prednisone Therapy in Management of Large Hemangiomas in Infants and Children, *Surgery,* **71:**168, 1972.

Conway, H.: "Tumors of the Skin," Charles C Thomas, Publisher, Springfield, Ill., 1956.

Dwight, R. W., and Maloy, J. K.: Pilonidal Sinus: Experience with 449 Cases, *N Engl J Med,* **249:**926, 1953.

Hvid-Hansen, O.: Treatment of Ganglions, *Acta Chir Scand,* **136:** 471, 1970.

Mandel, S. R., and Thomas, C. C., Jr.: Management of Pilonidal Sinus by Excision and Primary Closure, *Surg Gynecol Obstet,* **134:**448, 1972.

Riveros, M., and Pack, G. T.: The Glomus Tumor: Report of Twenty Cases, *Ann Surg,* **133:**394, 1951.

Strahan, J., and Bailie, H. W. C.: Glomus Tumor: A Review of 15 Clinical Cases, *Br J Surg,* **59:**91, 1972.

Malignant Tumors

Ackerman, L. V.: "Surgical Pathology," The C. V. Mosby Company, St. Louis, 1964.

Castro, El B., Hajdu, S. I., and Fortner, J. G.: Surgical Therapy of

Fibrosarcoma of Extremities: A Reappraisal, *Arch Surg,* **107:**284, 1973.

Conway, H.: "Tumors of the Skin," Charles C Thomas, Publisher, Springfield, Ill., 1956.

De Cholnoky, T.: Cancer of the Face: A Clinical and Statistical Study of 1062 Cases, *Ann Surg,* **122:**88, 1945.

El-Domeiri, A. A., Brasfield, R. D., Huvos, A. G., and Strong, E. W.: Sweat Gland Carcinoma, *Ann Surg,* **173:**270, 1971.

Epstein, E.: Sarcoma Involving the Skin, *Arch Dermatol,* **60:**1130, 1949.

Futrell, J. W., Krueger, G. R., Morton, D. L., and Ketcham, A. S.: Carcinoma of Sweat Glands in Adolescents, *Am J Surg,* **123:**594, 1972.

Levis, W. R., Kraemer, K. H., Klingler, W. G., Peck, G. L., and Terry, W. D.: Topical Immunotherapy of Basal Cell Carcinomas with Dinitrochlorobenzene, *Cancer Res,* **33:**3036, 1973.

Mohs, F. E.: "Chemosurgery in Cancer, Gangrene and Infections," Charles C Thomas Publisher, Springfield, Ill., 1956.

Sharp, G. S., and Binkley, F. C.: The Treatment of Carcinoma of the Skin, *Am J Roentgenol Radium Ther Nucl Med,* **67:**606, 1952.

Vogel, C. L., Templeton, C. J., Templeton, A. C., Taylor, J. F., and Kyalwazi, S. K.: Treatment of Kaposi's Sarcoma with Actinomycin-D and Cyclophosphamide: Results of a Randomized Clinical Trial, *Int J Cancer,* **8:**136, 1971.

Woodward, A. H., Ivins, J. C., and Soule, E. H.: Lymphangiosarcoma Arising in Chronic Lymphedematous Extremities, *Cancer,* **30:**562, 1972.

Melanoma and Other Pigmented Lesions

Bluming, A. Z., Vogel, C. L., Ziegler, J. L., Mody, N., and Kamya, G.: Immunologic Effects of BCG in Malignant Melanoma: Two Modes of Administration Compared, *Ann Int Med,* **76:**405, 1972.

Cady, B., Legg, M. A., and Redfern, A. B.: Contemporary Treatment of Malignant Melanoma, *Am J Surg,* **129:**472, 1975.

Clark, W. J., Jr., From, L., Bernardino, E. A., and Mihm, M.C.: The Histogenesis and Biologic Behavior of Primary Human Malignant Melanomas of the Skin, *Cancer Res,* **29:**497, 1969.

Davis, N. C.: Cutaneous Melanoma: The Queensland Experience, *Curr Probl Surg,* vol. XII, No. 5, 1976.

George, P. A., Fortner, J. G., and Pack, G. T.: Melanoma with Pregnancy: A Report of 115 Cases, *Cancer,* **13:**854, 1960.

Goldsmith, H. S., Shah, J. P., Kim, D. H.: Prognostic Significance of Lymph Node Dissection in Treatment of Malignant Melanoma, *Cancer,* **26:**606, 1970.

Greeley, P. W., Middleton, A. G., and Curtin, J. W.: Incidence of Malignancy in Giant Pigmented Nevi, *Plastic Reconstr Surg,* **36:**26, 1965.

Harris, M. N., Gumport, S. L., and Maiwandi, H.: Axillary Lymph Node Dissection for Melanoma, *Surg Gynec Obst,* **135:**936, 1972.

Hueston, J. T.: Integumentectomy for Malignant Melanoma of the Limbs, *Aust NZ J Surg,* **40:**114, 1970.

Knutson, C. O., Hori, J. M., and Spratt, J. S., Jr.: Melanoma, *Curr Probl Surg,* December, 1971.

Krementz, E. T., Creech, O., Ryan, R., and Reemtsma, K.: An Appraisal of Cancer Chemotherapy by Regional Perfusion, *Ann Surg,* **156:**417, 1962.

McBride, C. M.: Advanced Melanoma of the Extremities, *Arch Surg,* **101:**122, 1970.

MacDonald, E. J.: Epidemiology of Melanoma, *Ann NY Acad Sci* **100:**4, 1963.

McKhann, C. F., Hendrickson, C. G., Spitler, L. E., Gunnarsson, A., Banerjee, D., and Nelson, W. R.: Immunotherapy of Melanoma with BCG: Two Fatalities Following Intralesion Injection, *Cancer,* **35:**514, 1975.

Morton, D. L., Eilber, F. R., Holmes, E. C., Hunt, J. S., Ketcham, A. S., Silverstein, M. J., and Sparks, F. C.: BCG Immunotherapy of Malignant Melanoma: Summary of 7-Year Experience, *Ann Surg,* **180:**635, 1974.

Polk, H. C., Cohn, J. D., and Clarkson, J. G.: An Appraisal of Elective Regional Lymphadenectomy for Melanoma, in G. D. Zuidema and D. B. Skinner (eds.), "Current Topics in Surgical Research," vol. 1, Academic Press, Inc., New York, 1969.

Raven, R. W.: The Clinicopathological Aspects of Malignant Melanoma, *Ann NY Acad Sci,* **100:**142, 1963.

Spratt, J. S., Jr., Shieber, W., and Dillard, B. M.: "Anatomy and Surgical Technique of Groin Dissection," The C. V. Mosby Company, St. Louis, 1965.

Wanebo, H. J., Woodruff, J., and Fortner, J. G.: Malignant Melanoma of the Extremities: A Clinicopathologic Study Using Levels of Invasion (Microstage), *Cancer,* **35:**666, 1975.

White, L. P.: The Role of Natural Resistance in the Prognosis of Human Melanoma, *Ann NY Acad Sci,* **100:**115, 1963.

Breast

by **Benjamin F. Rush, Jr.**

The breast is man's insignia of membership in the class Mammalia. It is somewhat humbling to reflect that this badge of status had its origin as a modified sweat gland. In the male the breast is, with few exceptions, a dormant structure. In the female, from puberty to death, the breast is subjected to a constant dynamic role of physical changes related to the menstrual cycle, pregnancy, lactation, and the menopause. Associated with this active role are numerous malformations and dysfunctions which make diseases of the breast common clinical problems.

EMBRYOLOGY

The human breast makes its first appearance in the sixth week of embryonic development as an ectodermal thickening extending from the axilla to the groin, a distinct linear elevation called the *mammary ridge,* or *milk line.* Lens-shaped thickenings appear along the milk line, presaging the sites of developing breasts. In man the caudal two-thirds of the line disappears rapidly, and the pectoral thickening progresses with the ultimate formation of a breast primordium. Man shares this pectoral location of the breasts with other primates and with the elephant and sea cow, in contrast to the multiple breasts of the dog and pig and the inguinal location in the cow, goat, and whale.

In the fifth month of embryonic development the human primordial breast develops 15 to 20 solid cords which fan out beneath the skin in the underlying connective tissue. These primary milk ducts branch, and the ends develop club-shaped dilatations. During the seventh or eighth month the ducts hollow to develop lumina. During this same period the point in the skin corresponding to the nipple develops a small depression. At birth the breast is represented by a slight pit pierced by 15 to 20 openings into the primary milk ducts. The areola is a slight thickening in the skin which contains a few glands (of Montgomery). Shortly after birth the nipples become everted, and the areola is distinguished by a slight increase in pigmentation.

A few days after birth, bilateral or unilateral enlargement of the breast occurs in 70 percent of infants. In half the infants the swelling is accompanied by the secretion of a cloudy fluid similar to colostrum, the "witch's milk" of folklore. Histologically, these changes are associated with hypertrophy of the duct system, the appearance of acini, and an increased vascularity of the stroma. These alterations are considered an indirect effect of the high level of maternal estrogens in the infant's circulating blood. Following birth the falling estrogen level stimulates the hypophysis to produce prolactin, resulting in the mammary changes. These changes occur equally in male and female infants and regress spontaneously by the second or third week of life. Attempts to strip the breasts of their milk, as advocated by some superstitions, provoke the breasts to remain in the secretory state. Hyperplasia of the infant breast persisting over many months with persistent secretions has resulted from such manipulations.

CLINICAL CORRELATIONS. A number of developmental errors of the breast are of clinical importance. Most often observed is the persistence of one or more of the additional nipples in the milk line. These are commonly mistaken for moles. A rare anomaly is the occurrence of extramammary breast tissue, usually seen in the axilla or over the upper abdomen (Fig. 15-1), often not appearing until the tissue is stimulated by pregnancy and lactation. Excision of these supernumerary structures is the treatment of choice. Absence of one or both nipples or of one or both breasts also occurs, though rarely. While these conditions are serious cosmetic and functional defects, a more important functional deficiency is the often associated absence of the underlying pectoralis muscles and chest wall.

Occasionally the nipple fails to evert following birth and remains retracted or inverted throughout life. This is a

Fig. 15-1. Supernumerary breast.

serious functional problem when the patient attempts to nurse a child.

In some infants the collecting ducts fail to open onto the apex of the nipple, opening onto the areola instead. In a few instances collecting ducts are observed to empty onto the skin of the breast, failing entirely to traverse the nipple. These nippleless collecting ducts recapitulate the normal anatomy of the nippleless breast of the duckbill platypus.

ANATOMY AND DEVELOPMENT

Except for the neonatal period of hypertrophy and a period of slight hypertrophy occurring at puberty, the male breast undergoes little change throughout life. The female breast shows little change through infancy and childhood, but in the prepubertal period and throughout the remainder of life the breasts undergo numerous gross and microscopic changes (Fig. 15-2).

ADOLESCENCE. During the prepubertal period (from eleven to fifteen years) growth of the breast begins with the development of the prepubertal "bud." The areola becomes elevated and forms with the nipple a small conical protuberance. Histologically, the rudimentary primary ducts begin a rapid process of elongation and terminal branching, pushing down through the subcutaneous tissue toward the pectoral fascia and carrying with them sheaths of periductal connective tissue. A firm plaque of fibrous breast tissue forms as the lobes of the breasts develop, crowding out the subcutaneous fat. Roentgenograms of the breast at this period show a featureless, fibrous mass without trabeculae. Lobules do not form, however, until ovulation begins. Following ovulation at age fourteen to fifteen the breasts mature into their normal nulliparous form.

THE YOUNG ADULT. Anatomic Limits. The breast is suspended from the anterior chest wall, extending from the second to the sixth rib. The medial boundary is at the lateral border of the sternum, and the lateral border stretches to the anterior axillary line (Fig. 15-3).

Areola and Nipple. The areola in the young female is convex and lens-shaped, surmounted at its center by the nipple. The areola gains a slight amount of pigmentation during adolescence, and although its surface is hairless, a few hairs may appear at the skin of the periphery. Both the subareolar area and the nipple contain much smooth muscle. The fibers of the areola are arranged in concentric rings as well as radially and are inserted into the base of the dermis. They function to contract the areola and to compress the base of the nipple. The bulk of the nipple is made up of smooth muscle fibers arranged both circularly and longitudinally. The nipple is made erect, smaller, and firmer by contraction of these fibers, and this involuntary action serves to aid in emptying the intrapapillary ducts. This response is evoked by suckling or by tactile stimuli. Sir Astley Cooper, a pioneer in describing the anatomy and diseases of the breast, first pointed out that the nipple lies to the lateral side of the center line of the breast and that its axis points upward and outward. The teleologic assumption is that this arrangement is for the convenience of the suckling child.

Glandular Tissue. The functional portion of the breast is a modified cutaneous gland, an appendage of the skin. It is enclosed between the superficial and deep layers of the superficial fascia. The glandular portion of the breast spreads out widely as a layer over the chest wall beneath the integument. It is roughly circular in outline except at the upper outer quadrant, where the axillary tail of Spence extends toward the axilla (Fig. 15-3). The tip of the axillary tail intrudes through an opening in the deep fascia of the axilla, Langer's foramen, to lie well up within the axilla. Neoplasms or deformities in this tail are sometimes mistaken for enlarged axillary nodes.

Portions of the fibrous tissue of the breast parenchyma extend from the surface of the glandular breast anteriorly to intermingle with the superficial layer of the superficial fascia. Similar processes arise from the deep surface of the gland to cross the retromammary space and fuse with the pectoral fascia. The anterior ligaments were described by Cooper, who noted, "The breast is slung upon the fore part of the chest, for [the ligaments] form a movable but very firm connection with the skin so that the breast has sufficient motion."

Blood Supply and Venous Drainage. Three major arteries generously supply the breast with blood. The perforating branches of the internal mammary artery pass through the first, second, third, and fourth intercostal spaces just lateral to the sternum to penetrate and pass through the origin of the pectoralis major muscle and enter the medial edge of the breast, supplying more than 50 percent of the blood to this organ. The lateral thoracic artery arises from the axillary artery and courses down along the lateral border of the pectoralis minor muscle. Its external mammary branches provide the second largest source of blood to the breast. The third artery of importance is the pectoral branch of the acromiothoracic artery, also a branch of the axillary artery. The pectoral artery is given off by the acromiothoracic at the medial edge of the pectoralis minor muscle. In its course between the pectoralis major and minor muscles, the pectoralis artery gives off branches to the posterior surface of the breast. The superior branch of the axillary artery, the lateral perforating branches of the intercostal arteries, and branches of the subscapular artery also contribute minor amounts to the blood supply.

The mammary glands have a rich, anastomosing network of superficial subcutaneous veins. These veins become markedly dilated during pregnancy and may sometimes become quite prominent over an area of underlying neoplasm. The majority of the superficial veins drain to the internal mammary vein. In some individuals these veins drain into the superficial veins of the lower neck.

The deep veins of the mammary gland drain along routes roughly corresponding to the arterial blood supply. Thus one major route is through the anterior intercostal perforating veins to the internal mammary veins. Another is by way of multiple branches to the axillary vein. A third route is by way of posterior branches anastomosing with the intercostal veins. This last route has special significance, since the intercostal veins communicate with the vertebral veins. This anastomosis with the vertebral veins is offered by Batson as the explanation for the often capricious metastasis of mammary cancer to the vertebral bodies or even the sacrum or pelvis without the presence of metastatic deposits in the lung. He holds that the wide variation in pressure within the thoracic cavity induced by straining or coughing may change the flow patterns within the valveless anastomosing veins so that blood from the breast draining through the lateral perforators to the intercostal vessels is forced down along the vertebral plexus.

The Lymphatics. A generous lymphatic plexus drains the skin and glandular tissues of the breast (Fig. 15-4). The lymphatic vessels empty into two main depots represented by the axillary and the internal mammary lymph nodes. There are an average of 53 lymph nodes in the axillary fossa, arranged along the course of the arteries and veins. Lymph from the lower outer quadrant of the breast drains to the lateral and inferior axillary nodes, while lymph from the areola, the upper outer quadrant of the breast, and the axillary tail drains to the medial superior axillary nodes. Within the axilla, lymph passes from the lateral inferior to the medial superior nodes at the apex of the axilla. Lymph then courses through lymphatic channels under the clavicle to the supraclavicular lymph nodes and by major lymphatic trunks to the junction of the subclavian and jugular veins. On the right, lymph enters the blood directly through these lymphatic trunks as they join the veins. On the left these trunks may first join with the thoracic duct, which shortly communicates with the venous system.

The internal mammary lymph nodes are much fewer in number than the axillary nodes, averaging but three or four nodes on each side lying along the internal mammary vessels, usually in the first, second, and third interspaces. Despite the scarcity and tiny size of these lymph nodes, most of the lymph from the upper and lower inner quadrants of the breast drains by this channel. Lymph from the nipple and areola may drain to both the internal mam-

Fig. 15-2. Gross and microscopic appearance of breast at different stages of development. Central pictures show three-dimensional projection of microscopic structure. A. Adolescence. B. Pregnancy. C. Lactation. D. Postmenopausal period.

mary and the axillary nodes. The internal mammary lymphatic trunks eventually empty into the great veins of the neck, usually by way of the thoracic duct or of the right lymphatic duct.

Histology of the Resting Mammary Gland. Each lobe of the mammary gland is an independent compound alveolar gland. The mammary gland is a conglomeration of a variable number of such independent glands, each with its own excretory duct which has its separate opening on the surface of the nipple. The excretory ducts measure from 0.4 to 0.7 mm in diameter at the nipple surface and run perpendicularly through the nipple to turn and radiate out toward the periphery of the breast. Beneath the areola they dilate into a short fusiform area called the *milk sinus*. Beyond the milk sinus the excretory ducts begin to subdivide into smaller and smaller branches forming the lobules of the lobe. Within the lobules the ducts subdivide further, forming terminal, elongated tubes, the alveolar ducts, which are studded by round evaginations, the alveolae. Lobules are peripheral and scanty in the nulliparous breast (Fig. 15-2A).

There is mild controversy as to whether alveolae are present in the resting mammary gland. Some claim that

Fig. 15-3. Normal distribution of mammary tissue of adult female breast. Note long tail of Spence extending into axilla.

Fig. 15-4. Lymphatic drainage of breast. Nipple drains both laterally and medially. Medial side of breast drains to small internal mammary lymph nodes.

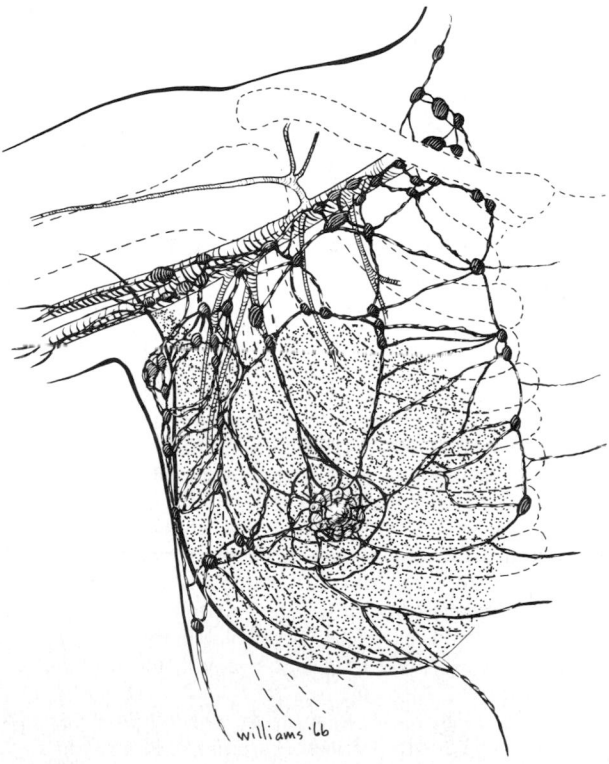

the resting gland is entirely a tubular structure and becomes tuboalveolar only during pregnancy. The majority opinion is that a few alveolae are scattered through the lobules in the resting state.

The walls of the alveolae and the alveolar ducts consist of a prominent basement membrane surrounding a layer of myoepithelial cells, which in turn lie beneath a layer of low columnar glandular cells. The myoepithelial layer is thin and difficult to identify in the acini and the alveolar ducts but becomes more prominent in the more major lobular ducts. These cells take a spiral course about the larger ducts and probably play a role in propelling milk from the acini to the nipple during lactation.

The collecting ducts are lined with a double layer of cuboidal to columnar epithelium until the milk sinus is reached. Here the lining changes to squamous epithelium. This continues through the milk sinus to the surface of the nipple.

Each lobule is surrounded by a coating of dense, firm, interlobular connective tissue, which is an intimate part of the breast parenchyma. The lobules are separated by a looser coating of less dense fibrous tissue, the interlobular connective tissue. This layer represents the supporting stroma of the breast. These layers are easily recognized histologically, but grossly the various lobules are intimately and firmly bound together and cannot be dissected apart.

Cyclic Changes of the Breast. Beginning about the eighth day of the menstrual cycle the female breast gradually increases in size, the volume often increasing by 50 percent by the immediate premenstrual period. At this point the breast is tense and may be somewhat tender. Part of the increase in size is due to interlobular edema and increasing congestion of the vasculature. Ingleby and Gershon-Cohen state that there is also a proliferation of the parenchyma, with the appearance of new lobules. These lobules then regress and fibrose during menstruation. Congestion and edema subside, and the breast again reaches its smallest size on about the eighth day after the onset of menstruation.

PREGNANCY AND LACTATION. Implantation of the ovum initiates a profound change in the gross and histologic structures of the breast. Grossly there is a pronounced enlargement of the breast, progressing throughout pregnancy. The normal size may be increased as much as two or three times. The nipple and areola become more prominent and more deeply pigmented. The openings of Montgomery's glands on the areola become prominent and are called *Montgomery's tubercles*. Pigmentation may spread beyond the areola onto the skin, forming a "secondary areola." The veins are engorged, and striae are frequently visible in the skin.

Histologically, the epithelium of the lobular ducts and alveolar ducts proliferates, and new ducts covered with multiple alveolar outpouchings are generated. The total number of lobules increases greatly. By the end of the sixth month the glandular cells of the acini produce small amounts of a secretion, colostrum, which increases toward the end of pregnancy (Fig. 15-2C).

Two or three days after delivery, globules appear in the supranuclear cytoplasm of the acinar cells. These push toward the cell lumen, increasing in size. The cell becomes tall and more columnar. Finally the globule is extruded into the lumen, and the cell shrinks to a cuboidal form, to begin the process again. The acini become distended with milk, which is propelled to the nipple during nursing. This process continues as long as suckling continues. When lactation ends, the extralobular tissue involutes, leaving small areas of fibrosis, and the breast gradually returns to the resting state. It never returns to the nulliparous form, however, but has the contour of maturity. The areola recedes into the breast tissue, with only the nipple projecting. Some of the darker pigmentation of the nipple and areola and residual skin striae persist.

MENOPAUSAL CHANGES. Following menopause the mammary gland gradually involutes (Fig. 15-2*D*). This change is slow and progressive, with gradual disappearance of lobules. Senile involution does not lead to complete extinction of mammary tissue; some lobules always remain, but they are scattered and small. In many areas only the larger lobular and collecting ducts may be found. The parenchyma and stromal fibrous tissue gradually blend together into a homogeneous mass, and the original lobular structure is almost completely lost. As the glandular tissues recede, there is a gradual invasion of fat, which aids in maintaining the breast outline, although in very thin women the breasts may become quite flabby as glandular tissue is lost.

CLINICAL CORRELATION. Both breasts of the adolescent girl usually develop at the same pace. Occasionally development is out of phase, and one breast will develop much more rapidly than the other, leading to distressing asymmetry (Fig. 15-5). The difference in size is usually repaired with time but occasionally persists. Patients complaining of asymmetric breasts during the adolescent period are advised to wait until maturation is complete. If asymmetry persists, a plastic surgical procedure may be required to adjust the difference.

A slight swelling of the breasts is often seen in adolescent boys. This is called *gynecomastia* and is a physiologic response to the change in the hormonal milieu in the pubertal male (Fig. 15-6). This slight hypertrophy normally subsides spontaneously but occasionally persists, either unilaterally or bilaterally. Persisting gynecomastia in young manhood requires an evaluation to exclude the possibility of abnormal endocrine secretion. If no abnormalities are found, the small button of hypertrophied breast tissue may be removed surgically to repair an embarrassing cosmetic defect in a young man.

Occasionally the growth of the female breast at puberty fails to cease and the breasts become huge—so-called virginal hypertrophy (Fig. 15-7). Breasts weighing 40 to 50 lb and descending to the level of the genitalia are described. Spontaneous regression does not occur, and the only solution is plastic surgical repair. This rare defect is seen in pregnant females as well and requires the same treatment.

EXAMINATION

INSPECTION. Physical examination of the breasts should begin with the patient erect, usually sitting on the edge

Fig. 15-5. Asymmetric breasts.

of the examining table. The breasts are observed for symmetry, dimpling of the skin, edema, deformity of outline, retraction of the nipple, or inflammation. Underlying masses will produce deformity or skin retraction, which is much more easily detected when the patient is erect and the breasts dependent. Haagensen suggests that the patient be allowed to lean forward to increase the breast dependency and further accentuate areas of deformity or dimpling.

PALPATION. Examination of the axillary and supraclavicular area is always part of a complete breast examination and is best done when the patient is erect. The axilla is examined with the humerus slightly abducted and the pectoralis muscle relaxed (Fig. 15-8*B*). The contents of the axilla are pressed gently against the rib cage, and the axilla is progressively palpated from apex to base. The apex of the axilla does not lie under the humeral head but anteriorly under the clavicle, where the axillary vein and artery

Fig. 15-6. Gynecomastia.

Fig. 15-7. Virginal hypertrophy. This growth occurred during 1 year in fifteen-year-old white girl and required plastic surgery for repair. (*Courtesy of Paul Weeks, M.D.*)

pass under the clavicle to become the subclavian vessels. Palpation of lymph nodes at this level is of great importance in predicting the prognosis in a patient with cancer.

The supraclavicular area is palpated with the tips of the fingers, making sure that the fingers are pressed down well behind the clavicle to roll the supraclavicular structures against the scalene muscles. In a thin neck the transverse fibers of the posterior belly of the omohyoid are sometimes mistaken for an enlarged lymph node. This can be differentiated by observing that a medial and lateral margin to

Fig. 15-8. Examination of breast. *A*. Observation with arms at side. *B*. Palpation of axilla. *C*. With arms raised. *D*. Palpation with patient supine.

the supposed node cannot be felt, although an upper and lower border are easily detected. Following palpation of the axilla and supraclavicular area, the breasts are also palpated, although masses in the breasts are best felt when the patient is supine.

After inspection and palpation with the patient erect, the entire mammary gland is palpated carefully with the tips of the fingers with the patient in the supine position, with the arm first over the head and then at the side (Fig. 15-8). This should be done systematically and in the same way in each examination so that the examiner follows a definite pattern. One may begin at the upper inner quadrant, gradually inspecting the breast tissue from above downward until the medial portion of the breast has been examined. The areolar area is then palpated. If the patient has complained of secretions or blood from the nipple, the areola should be stroked toward the nipple to see if this symptom can be reproduced. The lateral portion of the breast is palpated starting at the upper outer quadrant and completing the examination at the lower outer quadrant. The tail of the breast should also be examined as it extends into the axilla.

By self-examination a woman can usually detect a smaller mass in her own breasts than can a physician if she knows the proper methods to use. Since cancer of the breast is one of the major neoplasms in females, instruction in self-examination is a valuable addition to the physician's examination of the breast. A patient is instructed to emulate the physician's pattern of inspection and examination. She carries this out upon herself in both the erect and supine positions. Women thirty-five years of age and older should conduct such an examination at home once monthly.

MAMMOGRAPHY. Mammography is an x-ray examination of the breast. It requires special techniques and film, and a radiologist skilled in interpretation.

This technique is not a substitute for biopsy, which still provides definitive confirmation, but is a helpful adjunct in diagnosis. Mammography is especially useful in (1) follow-up examinations of the contralateral breast following radical mastectomy; (2) examination of an indeterminate mass which cannot be considered a dominant nodule, especially when there are multiple cysts or several vague masses and the indication for biopsy is uncertain; and (3) the large, fatty breast, when the patient has complaints but no nodules are palpated. Tumors cannot be easily felt in such breasts, but the mammogram is most accurate in the fatty breast.

A skilled radiologist can detect cancer of the breast with a false-positive rate of 11 percent and a false-negative rate of 6 percent. A fine stippling of calcium on the radiogram in the area of the lesion is very suggestive of cancer. There is also a characteristic infiltration of the surrounding tissues; a typical skin thickening may be seen, and the density of the lesion itself is often helpful in interpretation (Fig. 15-9).

Radiography of the breast can detect some cancers which cannot be found in any other way. It has been estimated that the lead time for treatment of lesions discovered at this small size is 1 or 2 years compared to

Fig. 15-9. Mammography of breast. *A.* Normal postmenopausal patient with atrophy of lobular tissue and ducts and predominance of fatty supporting tissue. *B.* Multiloculated cyst in menopausal patient. *C.* Scirrhous carcinoma in menopausal patient, demonstrating sunburst pattern; characteristic calcifications not present in this case.

cancers discovered by conventional palpation of the breast. Axillary nodal involvement is very rare in these early lesions, and preliminary results of follow-up indicate that 5-year survival rates for such tumors may exceed 90 percent. This data led to considerable activity in developing pilot mass screening programs for cancer of the breast which include mammography, careful physical examination, and thermography.

Recently increasing resistance has developed to the use of mammography for breast screening. If data obtained from women who had exposure of their breasts to 500 to 1500 rads is considered, the risk of breast cancer is increased markedly by radiation. Extrapolation of this data back to the low doses received from mammography indicates that the lifetime risk of breast cancer may be increased 1 percent for each rad absorbed, i.e., from 7.0 percent for the average American woman to 7.07 percent. Past studies of screening show that mammography in women over fifty years of age will save far more lives than might be threatened by the radiation used. Under fifty years of age there is no such evidence. Current guidelines of the National Institute of Health forbid screening women under fifty with mammography. The situation is very fluid, however, since much of the data being used to make these decisions are highly speculative. The situation is in flux, since the x-ray exposure produced by mammography has been decreased substantially to as low as 0.4 rads per examination, and newer techniques appear to be increasing the number of cancers found in younger women, so that the risk-benefit ratio may be shifting in this age group. It is likely that extended clinical trials will be necessary to solve this dilemma.

Xeroradiography of the breast is basically a radiographic technique which is carried out in exactly the same way as mammography, except that the image is recorded on a xerographic plate instead of the conventional x-ray transparency. The image is positive rather than negative and appears easier to read to the untrained eye. Unfortunately, a badly exposed xeroradiograph, too poor for proper interpretation, is harder to recognize than a poor radiomammograph and may fool the unwary physician.

THERMOGRAPHY. The skin over malignant tumors of the breast is usually warmer than the surrounding areas. Using special heat scanners it is possible to delineate these "hot spots" on film. This method may help to differentiate malignant and benign tumors. Infection may be associated with a false positive, and, conversely, not all cancers are "hot," so false negatives may occur. The method is still too new to have a definite place in the diagnostic armamentarium but may find a role in mass screening programs.

DISEASES OF THE BREAST

Neoplasms

From the standpoint of morbidity and mortality, cancer is by far the most important clinical problem that concerns the breast today. Most benign neoplasms of the breast would have little clinical importance if it were not for the difficulty in differentiating them from cancer. To emphasize this relationship, benign neoplasms are discussed in the section on differential diagnosis of cancer.

In recent years four major controversies have surfaced concerning breast cancer, concerning (1) the relation of treatment to the natural history of the disease; (2) the role of mammography in diagnosis, and especially in screening programs; (3) the appropriate operation for treatment; and (4) the use of postoperative chemotherapy as an adjuvant to primary therapy.

INCIDENCE

Cancer of the breast is the commonest form of cancer in females. Almost 6 percent of all women will develop cancer of the breast in their lifetime. The lifetime incidence of cancer of all types in females is 27 percent; thus one out of every four women with cancer will have cancer of the breast. In the United States, 50,000 to 70,000 new cases of breast cancer occur annually, and about 20,000 women die of the disease each year. According to the excellent cancer registry systems in Connecticut and upper New York State, the age-adjusted incidence of new cases has been increasing steadily since the middle 1940s.

Worldwide figures show that the Dutch have the highest national mortality of cancer of the breast, with 24.19 patients per 100,000 population. The United States ranks ninth, with 21.38 cases per 100,000 population. The Japanese rank lowest among all nations with reliable statistics, with an incidence of 3.76 per 100,000 population. The factors leading to this wide range of incidence are unknown, although studies seeking an answer are in progress.

ETIOLOGY

Sex is certainly an important contributing factor in this disease, since it is very rare in males. Maleness is not a complete protection, however; there is 1 carcinoma of the breast in men for every 100 carcinomas of the breast in women.

The age of the patient is also important (Fig. 15-10). Breast cancer is almost unknown in the prepubertal female and is very rare under the age of twenty. From the age of twenty onward there is a gradually increasing incidence, which reaches a plateau between the ages of forty-five and fifty-five at about 125 new cases each year for every 100,000 females of that age range. After fifty-five the incidence begins to rise again quite sharply, so that the annual risk of developing breast cancer for women eighty to eighty-five is twice as high as for women sixty to sixty-five (312 versus 153 new cases per 100,000 women per year). Some suggest that the plateau of incidence during the menopausal age period reflects the effects of a changing hormonal pattern in women at this time.

Genetic factors play a role in the development of this cancer, though the genetic effect does not seem to be strong and more than one allelic gene must be involved. When the mother has had a breast cancer, the chance of cancer of the breast developing in the daughter is two to three times greater than would be expected in the general population, but no specific pattern of inheritance is evident. Some hypothesize that there is a genotype which has a predisposition to the formation of cancer but which must interact with some nongenetic agent before cancer develops.

Patients in whom breast cancer develops and who have positive family histories for the disease are generally younger and have a higher frequency of bilaterality than breast cancer patients with negative family histories. Blood type O, benign breast disease, and ovarian cysts and tumors also tend to be more common in patients with early diagnoses of breast cancer. Blood type A, diabetes, hypertension, and uterine disorders are more common in those who are older at the time of diagnosis.

Interlinked with factors of age, sex, national origin, and inheritance in the development of breast cancer is the important role played by hormonal environment. Some breast cancers are highly susceptible to changes in the patient's hormonal pattern and will regress for a time when hormones of various types are given. Mammary cancer can be induced in the mouse and rat by repeated injections of estrogens and in the rat by a combination of estrogen and progesterone. There is a vast literature concerning both experimental and clinical induction and extinction of tumors with hormonal agents. The exact role of hormones in human cancer still remains elusive. It is not known whether hormonal maladjustment is responsible for human breast cancer or what predisposing causes may be required to produce a susceptibility to hormonal change.

Breast cancer may well be multifactorial. Other interesting correlations with breast cancer include the incidence of coronary artery disease, which has a positive correlation with breast cancer death rates in 24 parts of the world. Hems has concluded that "early" breast cancer (age group forty to forty-four) appears to be genetically influenced, while "late" breast cancer (age group sixty-five to sixtynine) is more closely associated with environmental factors, such as diet. Among younger women, higher risk is associated with late first pregnancy, while among women over fifty years of age the risk appears to increase with weight and the relation of weight to height. Zippin and Petrakis have reported an association between wet cerumen, or earwax, and breast cancer rates in diverse population groups, and breast cancer mortality is closely associated with wet cerumen. Such an association is plausible since the mammary and ceruminous glands are histologically of the apocrine type and have many similarities in their secretions. Cerumen exists in two phenotypic forms, wet and dry, which are controlled by a pair of genes in which the allele for the wet type is dominant over that of the dry type. The dry is homozygous recessive and is highly prevalent in the mongoloid population of Asia and in American Indians. The wet type predominates in Western Europeans, Caucasian Americans, and Negro Americans. These findings support the hypothesis that genetic variations in the apocrine system may influence susceptibility to breast cancer.

It has long been known that breast cancer in mice is related to a viral factor transmitted in the milk. Considerable excitement has attended the discovery of particles in human milk with the same morphologic characteristics as those found to be associated with breast cancer in mice. Antigens to these viral particles have been identified in human plasma. These particles have been found in the milk from the breasts of 60 percent of American women with family histories of breast cancer compared to 5 percent of women without positive family histories. The milk of thirty-nine percent of Parsi women in India also were found to contain these particles. The group of Parsi women is of particular interest because of their endogamous history over the centuries, resulting in an inbred population. Breast cancer accounts for approximately half of the cancers among Parsi women in contrast with Connecticut women, for example, in whom breast cancer represents one-fourth of all cancers.

NATURAL HISTORY

A typical carcinoma of the breast is a scirrhous adenocarcinoma beginning in the ducts and invading the parenchyma (80 percent). Beginning in the upper outer quadrant (40 to 50 percent), it grows slowly, doubling its volume every 2 to 9 months in 70 percent of patients. Starting from a single cell, it takes 30 doubling times for a tumor to attain a size of 1 cm—the smallest tumor of the breast normally found on physical diagnosis. Thus even the fastest-growing tumor of the more common type may require 5 years before it becomes clinically palpable. The use of doubling times to calculate the preclinical course of tumors of the breast is subject to many errors, the most obvious being that growth rates are not always constant, varying with areas of necrosis within the tumor and hormonal changes in the patient. Laboratory and clinical observations indicate, however, that growth rates are more consistent than is usually appreciated. The concept of the origin of these tumors in a single cell with increase in size by doubling is a useful model and suggests the long occult period which probably is present in many tumors before they are diagnosed and treated. Cancers of the breast are often multicentric (15 to 40 percent), but each tumor is assumed to have started from its own individual cell.

As the tumor increases in size and invades the surrounding glandular tissue, the accompanying fibrosis tends to shorten Cooper's ligaments, producing the characteristic dimpling in the skin (Fig. 15-11). Cords of tumor cells grow out along lymphatics, ultimately invading the skin itself. This invasion is preceded by localized edema of the skin as many lymphatic avenues are blocked and drainage of fluid from the skin is impeded. Eventually tumor cells replace the skin, which breaks down to form an ulcer. The tumor increases in size, and new areas of skin invasion may occur, indicated by small satellite nodules adjacent to the ulcer crater. As involvement and destruction of the skin progresses, blood vessels are invaded, and tumor cells seed into the circulation, passing into axillary or intercostal veins to be scattered through the pulmonary circuit into the lungs or by way of the vertebral veins up and down the vertebral column. When this seeding is early and small in amount, the majority if not all of these cells may fail to implant and are destroyed by an unknown mechanism, perhaps immunity. Eventually, perhaps as the number of

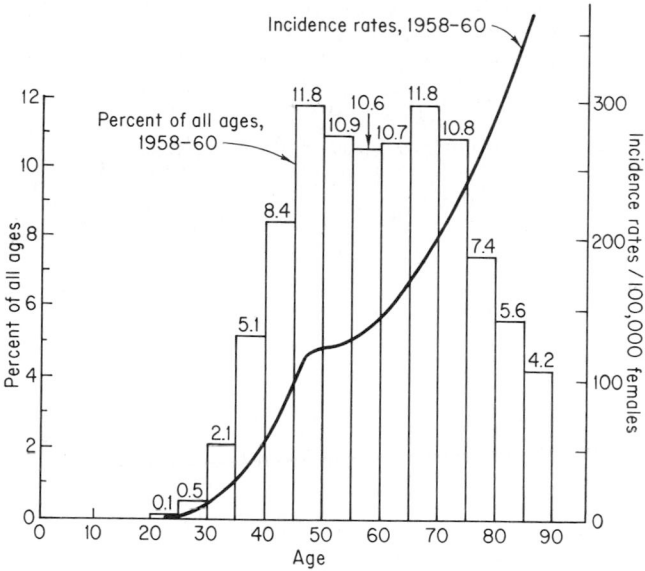

Fig. 15-10. Newly diagnosed breast cancer among women, 1958–1960: percentage distribution and incidence rates by age. Note plateau in incidence between ages forty-five and fifty-five.

cells seeded into the circulation begins to rise, they implant and grow in favorable locations. These implants may occur in the vertebral bodies, pelvis, lungs, liver, or brain.

As the breast tumor extends toward the skin, tumor cells simultaneously pass along the lymphatic vessels from the upper outer quadrant to the axillary nodes, where they implant and grow. As the axillary nodes enlarge, they are

Fig. 15-11. Dimpling of skin over primary carcinoma of breast in upper outer quadrant. Slowly growing lesion in seventy-year-old patient; dimpling had been present for 2 years.

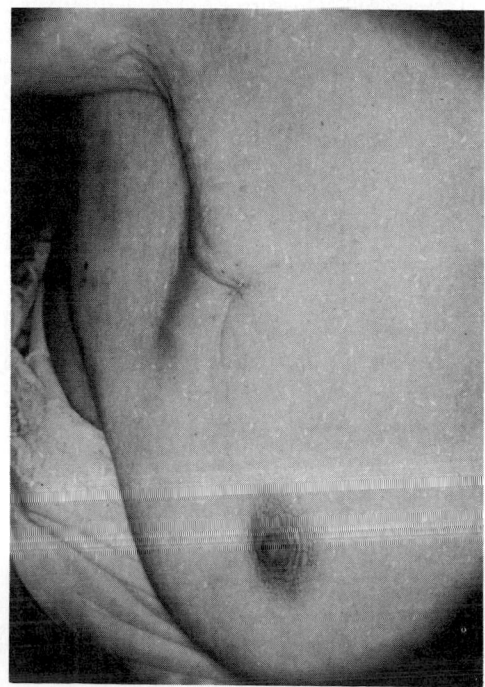

at first shotty and fairly soft, then firm and hard as they are increasingly replaced by tumor. Eventually the nodes adhere to one another in a large conglomerate mass, and as the tumor breaks out of the lymphatic capsule the mass of nodes become fixed to the medial wall of the axilla. As the axillary nodes become choked with tumor, cells are passed along the chain to the supraclavicular nodes, which also enlarge. Other cancer cells pass by way of the right lymphatic trunk or the thoracic duct into the bloodstream, heart, and lungs. Systemic spread is the rule, and 95 percent of patients who die of uncontrolled breast cancer have distant metastases. Lung (65 percent), liver (56 percent), and bones (56 percent) are the commonest sites for these deposits.

Patients today are rarely allowed to proceed through all stages of carcinoma without some therapeutic intervention. Data are available, however, from the latter half of the 1800s and the first few years of this century indicating the normal course of events in untreated tumors. The excellent report in 1962 by Bloom and associates summarizes much of the data. They cite the experience of the Middlesex Hospital in London, where in 1791 a cancer charity was founded to which patients were admitted to "remain an unlimited time, until either relieved by art or released by death." From the well-preserved records of this charity it was possible to collect a series of 250 advanced cases of untreated breast cancer seen between 1805 and 1933 (Fig. 15-12). All the patients reported died in the hospital, and in every case an autopsy was performed. In the last 86 cases, histologic sections were available. The mean survival in this series and for over 1,000 untreated cases collected from the literature was 38.7 months, with a range from 30.2 to 39.8 months. It must be noted that in all reports of untreated patients survival is calculated from the onset of the first symptom. Fifty percent of the patients died in 2.7 years (median survival); 18 percent survived 5 years,

3.6 percent 10 years, and 10.8 percent 15 years. The longest survivor in the group died in the nineteenth year after onset of symptoms. Histologic grading indicated that for 23 patients with grade 1 tumors the mean survival was 47 months. Autopsies indicated that 95 percent of the women died of their carcinoma, only 5 percent of intercurrent disease. Nearly three-fourths of the patients had ulceration of the breast at death, and in 21 percent this was very extensive, sometimes destroying the entire breast and excavating the chest wall. Bloom concluded that treatment of patients with breast cancer appeared to increase the length and improve the quality of survival.

DIAGNOSIS AND STAGING

The normal breast is a nodular structure by virtue of its lobular architecture, and this lobularity may be accentuated during the later portion of the menstrual cycle, pregnancy, or lactation. To the inexperienced examiner the normal nodularity may feel faintly suspicious throughout, although no obvious lesion can be felt. Palpation of the typical carcinoma of the breast normally leaves little doubt in the examiner's mind: the lesion is hard, almost cartilaginous; the edges are distinct, serrated, and irregular. This is true for the 75 to 80 percent of breast tumors associated with productive fibrosis. It is the remaining 20 to 25 percent of tumors, those associated with little fibrosis and those with a medullary or a colloid element or other less typical lesions, which form the spectrum of neoplasms most difficult to distinguish from benign lesions.

Physicians would prefer to have only the clues provided by the local mass to make the physical diagnosis of carcinoma, for it is only when the mass is localized to the breast that one can assume an "early" lesion and expect the best possible chance of long survival. Too often the later signs of breast cancer are present to confirm the diagnosis. As indicated previously, these are skin dimpling or nipple retraction, satellite skin lesions, edema or ulceration, and ipsilateral enlarged axillary or supraclavicular nodes. Signs of even wider spread may be present such as a history of back or leg pain, an enlarged and nodular liver, or perhaps a complaint of dyspnea associated with physical findings or fluid in the chest.

The physical examination of a patient with breast cancer should include an attempt on the part of the examiner to classify and record the stage of the patient's disease specifically. Only consistent classification can make possible clear conclusions concerning prognosis and type of treatment. The problem of comparing the results of treatment from institution to institution and among different operators has been impaired for years by a lack of adequate classification or by varying standards of classification. At present a strong effort is being made to promote the adoption of a standard system devised by the American Joint Committee on Cancer Staging and End Results Reporting, based on a system proposed by the International Union against Cancer in 1958. This system of classification is called the T.N.M. Classification, the T standing for "tumor," the N for "nodes," and the M for "metastasis." The general outline used in breast cancer is as follows:

Fig. 15-12. Survival of patients with untreated cancer of breast compared with natural survival. (*From H. J. G. Bloom, W. W. Richardson, and E. J. Harries, Br Med J, 5299:213, 1962, by permission.*)

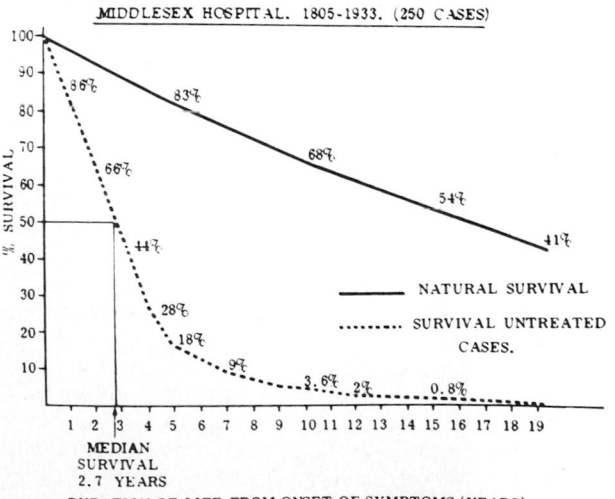

MIDDLESEX HOSPITAL. 1805-1933. (250 CASES)

T—Primary tumor

TX   Cannot classify (e.g., prior therapy)
T1S   Carcinoma in situ, lobular, ductal, Paget's (not a clinical classification)
T0   No tumor in breast (e.g., axillary mass; x-ray finding)
T1   Primary tumor freely movable, no fixation
T1a   Clinical classification not applicable (e.g., detected by mammography)
T1b   <1.9 cm
T1c   2–5 cm
T1d   >5 cm
T2a   Primary tumor <2 cm with fixation to skin, pectoral fascia, or muscle. *No* ulceration or edema (*peau d'orange*)
T2b   Primary tumor >2 cm with fixation to skin, pectoral fascia, or muscle. *No* ulceration or edema (*peau d'orange*)
T3   Primary tumor, any size, with skin edema (*peau d'orange*) and/or ulceration
T4   Primary tumor, any size, with fixation to chest wall (serratus, intercostals, ribs, or pectorals)
T5   Inflammatory carcinoma

N—Regional Axillary Nodes
(Infraclavicular are included as apical axillary)

NX   Cannot be evaluated (e.g., previous excision)
N0   Axillary nodes not involved by metastasis
N1   Clinical homolateral axillary nodes involved, 1–3 in number, less than 2 cm diameter; not fixed
N2   Clinical homolateral axillary nodes involved, >4 in number; any number fixed to one another but to no other structures, and/or any involved node >2 cm
N3   Homolateral axillary nodes involved fixed to neurovascular structures of axilla or chest wall (intercostals, serratus, ribs, *not* pectorals)
N4   Homolateral supraclavicular lymph node involved by metastasis

M—Distant metastasis

M0   No evidence of distant metastases
M1   Distant metastases, including skin beyond the breast area

Summary of clinical staging

In situ cancer (in situ lobular, pure intraductal, and Paget's disease of nipple without palpable mass):

Stage T1S   T1S, N0, M0

Invasive cancer:

Stage I   T1a, b, or c, N0, M0
Stage II   T0, N1, M0; T1d, N0, M0; T1a, b, c, or d, N1, M0; T2a, N0 or N1, M0
Stage III   T0, T1a, b, c, d, N2, M0; T2B, N0, M0; T3, N1 or N2, M0
Stage IV   T4, T5, and any N, M0; N3, 4, or 5 and any T, M0; M1 with any T and any N

DIFFERENTIAL DIAGNOSIS (BENIGN LESIONS)

CHRONIC CYSTIC MASTITIS. Chronic cystic mastitis was first described in the medical literature in the last two decades of the nineteenth century, by Reclus (1883), Brissaud (1884), Schimmelbusch (1890), and König (1893). For a time the disease was known as either Reclus' or Schimmelbusch's disease, but use of these eponyms dwindled following the introduction of the term *chronic cystic mastitis* by König. He chose this term to describe a group of pathologic lesions found in the breast because he thought

they were due to a "vicious cycle of secretion and irritation." While the disease is indeed chronic, it may not be cystic and is certainly not inflammatory, so this old name is at least two-thirds in error. Nonetheless, attempts to introduce more accurate or at least other nomenclatures have failed. Fibrocystic disease, fibroadenosis, mastopathy, nodular hyperplasia, cyclomastopathy, adenofibromatosis, mazoplasia, cystiphorous epithelial hyperplasia, adenocystic disease, and mammary dysplasia have all been offered, but chronic cystic mastitis is still the most widely used designation.

The term chronic cystic mastitis describes a family of lesions found in the breast. Pathologists disagree as to which lesions are legitimate family relations, so the morphology of the disease, like the terminology, appears rather fuzzy to the casual observer. Foote and Stewart have named 10 lesions often described as members of this group: cysts, papillomatosis, blunt duct adenosis, sclerosing adenosis, apocrine metaplasia, stasis and distension of ducts, periductal mastitis, fat necrosis, hyperplasia of duct epithelium, and fibroadenoma. These writers accept, however, only the first five of this group as being related lesions and forming part of chronic cystic mastitis; the others are held to represent different disease entities. They refer to the first five as the cystic and proliferative group, assuming that the proliferative lesions are responsible for the subsequent formation of cysts. A majority of pathologists accept this list, though some have argued for the inclusion of fibroadenoma. In addition, epithelial hyperplasia is usually accepted as part of the complex, with papillomas representing an advanced manifestation of hyperplasia.

The lesions of chronic cystic mastitis begin to appear in the breasts of a few women in their late twenties. The incidence is greater in the thirties and forties. Originally it was thought that the incidence of these lesions decreased after the menopause, but careful autopsy studies indicate that the lesions are common in the older age groups and may continue to increase in frequency with age. Frantz et al. found a 71 percent incidence of cystic and proliferative lesions in women over seventy years of age. Sandison noted epithelial hyperplasia of the ducts in 7 percent of women in their twenties and in 33 percent of women in their eighties. Rush and Kramer in 1963 reviewed step sections from the breasts of 20 women over seventy years of age. Approximately 100 sections were reviewed per patient, and with this close scrutiny two or more lesions of cystic mastitis were found in all the patients. Moderately severe epithelial hyperplasia was found in 14 of the 20 (Fig. 15-13). A case may be made for considering the lesions of cystic mastitis somewhat as one considers arteriosclerosis: a pathologic process which varies in degree and in time of onset but which is found to some degree in all adult females as they age.

Most of the lesions making up the complex of chronic cystic mastitis are proliferative, and almost from the first recognition of this disease there has been a suspicion that these lesions may represent a premalignant condition. Follow-up studies of patients shown by biopsy to have chronic cystic mastitis uniformly indicate that cancer sub-

Fig. 15-13. Benign marked intraductal hyperplasia in eighty-eight-year-old female. (Hematoxylin and eosin; ×32). (*From B. F. Rush, Jr., and W. M. Kramer, Surg Gynec Obstet, 117:425, 1963.*)

sequently occurs three to five times more often in these patients than in the general population.

If one assumes that all women eventually develop some degree of chronic cystic mastitis, how can one conclude that the finding of chronic cystic mastitis on biopsy is associated with an increase in the incidence of cancer of the female breast compared to patients in the general population? A reasonable hypothesis is that patients in whom this complex develops early enough or severely enough to warrant biopsy do indeed represent a special group with a greater hazard of eventual cancer.

The lesions of chronic cystic mastitis which are most likely to present a problem in differential diagnosis and to require biopsy are cysts, fibroadenoma, ductal papilloma, and sclerosing adenosis.

CYSTS. The cystic component of chronic cystic mastitis

Fig. 15-14. Cystic disease with apocrine metaplasia in seventy-three-year-old female. (Hematoxylin and eosin; ×32.) (*From B. F. Rush, Jr., and W. M. Kramer, Surg Gynec Obstet, 117:425, 1963.*)

is most prominent in patients in their thirties and forties. The cysts may vary in size from microcysts of 1 to 2 mm to large masses several centimeters in diameter (Fig. 15-14). They are felt in the breast substance as firm, round, fairly distinct masses, often with a rubbery feeling indicative of their cystic nature. Lesions in the anterior and dependent portions of the breast may be transilluminated. They are sometimes tender and, like many of the other lesions of this complex, may increase in size toward the end of the menstrual period.

If a lesion in a patient's breast is clearly suggestive of a cyst, aspiration is a good method for confirming the diagnosis. This technique should not be used unless the rules for its employment are clearly understood. The fluid obtained should be the characteristic clear, brown-green fluid of a cyst. When the cyst is aspirated dry, no underlying mass should be palpable. If a residual mass remains after aspiration or if the fluid is bloody, biopsy must be done. The patient should be followed at intervals for a month or two after aspiration; if the cyst reappears, biopsy is also indicated. Approximately half the cysts treated by aspiration will disappear, and fluid will not reaccumulate.

FIBROADENOMAS. These lesions are most common in the twenties and early thirties. They present as lobular but not serrated masses with a firm, rubbery consistency. Their edges are sharply defined. Most commonly solitary, they may occasionally be multiple. They are differentiated from cancer by the smooth rather than irregular lobulations and by the age group in which they occur. Although a skilled examiner can probably detect a fibroadenoma with an accuracy of 80 to 85 percent, biopsy is mandatory.

DUCTAL PAPILLOMA. The hallmark of the ductal papilloma is abnormal secretion from the nipple, which is often blood-stained. In 30 percent a small nodule, 3 or 4 mm in diameter, will be palpated in the major ducts underlying the areola. In the absence of a palpable nodule the papilloma's general position can often be detected by stroking the areola toward the nipple with the tips of the fingers, carefully working around the areola in a clockwise direction until an area is discovered which on pressure results in secretion from the nipple. A bloody nipple discharge may also be indicative of an intraductal carcinoma or even a deeper-lying infiltrating ductal carcinoma. The incidence of malignancy in the presence of this physical finding is 20 to 30 percent. Diagnosis is confirmed and treatment accomplished by excision of that portion of the collecting duct system shown on physical examination to be responsible for the secretion. Urban and Baker propose that the entire collecting duct system should be excised en bloc, since these lesions are often multiple and a partial excision of the duct system will often result in the retention of other lesions which will lead to further bloody secretions later.

SCLEROSING ADENOSIS. These lesions can sometimes result in an area of fibrosis within the mammary tissue which is firm and irregular and impossible to differentiate clinically from an ordinary scirrhous carcinoma. Biopsy is required to make the differential diagnosis.

OTHER BENIGN LESIONS. Fat necrosis, thrombophlebitis of the breast, and granular cell myoblastoma are three benign lesions of the breast which can be confused on physical examination with malignant growths. All three are uncommon. Fat necrosis is the most common of the group and is probably due to trauma, although only half the patients who have this lesion recall a trauma of the breast. The breasts are in an exposed position, however, and may be hurt at the time of a larger accident when the injury to the breast is overshadowed by more serious injuries. The lesions are always superficial and often near the areola. In 40 to 50 percent of patients with this lesion, accompanying ecchymoses are lingering stigmata of previous trauma. In one-third of the patients there is a history of pain or tenderness. Retraction of the skin over the lesion is seen in 50 to 60 percent. Retraction is due to the fibrosis and scarring in the fatty lobules which involve Cooper's ligaments. As the scarring progresses and matures, skin retraction, which may first be seen within two weeks of the original injury, becomes more prominent. The mass of subcutaneous scar tissue that forms is distinct, irregular, and often very firm. It is easy to understand how such a mass associated with skin retraction may be mistaken for carcinoma, and in every instance a biopsy specimen of the lesion must be examined histologically. In decades past, many unnecessary radical mastectomies were done in patients with fat necrosis. Today, the practice of routinely examining frozen sections of biopsy material prevents this tragedy.

Granular cell myoblastomas occur most commonly in the tongue but may also occur in the breast. The clinical importance of this rare tumor is that it can produce all the clinical signs of early cancer of the breast. The lesion is hard and relatively fixed to the breast tissue surrounding it. It sometimes causes dimpling of the overlying skin. Moreover, on gross examination of the specimen at operation the lesion looks and cuts like a scirrhous carcinoma of the breast. Only frozen sections can confirm that one is dealing with a benign rather than a malignant lesion.

Thrombophlebitis of a superficial vein of the breast, called *Mondor's disease,* may rarely be mistaken for a tumor because of the dimpling of the skin it produces. The tubular shape of the thrombosed vein and the accompanying tenderness usually indicate the diagnosis, but biopsy is often required for confirmation.

BREAST BIOPSY

Breast biopsy is a procedure with little risk and can be done under local anesthesia. It is still the general custom to do the biopsy under general anesthesia and proceed to a definitive cancer operation if the frozen section of the lesion indicates malignancy. However, there is an increasing trend to do the biopsy under local anesthesia, often in an outpatient setting, and to continue with the larger operation, if indicated, a few days later. This delay in definitive operation has no effect on the recurrence or survival rates. A curvilinear incision in the direction of the skin lines is made over the supicious mass. If the lesion is small, total excision is preferred, but if a large lesion is uncountered, a small excisional biopsy of the main mass is done.

Needle biopsy of breast masses is done in some institutions and is very satisfactory if the pathologist is familiar with this type of material. Negative needle biopsies have no significance, however, since an adequate sample may not be obtained.

HISTOPATHOLOGY

Malignant neoplasms of the breast, with few exceptions, are adenocarcinomas. The histologic features of these lesions vary considerably, and a number of classifications are available. The following was proposed by Foote and Stewart:

HISTOLOGIC CLASSIFICATION OF CANCER OF THE BREAST

A. Paget's disease of the nipple
B. Carcinomas of mammary ducts
  1. Noninfiltrating
  2. Infiltrating
    a. Papillary carcinoma
    b. Comedocarcinoma
    c. Carcinoma with productive fibrosis
    d. Medullary carcinoma with lymphoid infiltrate
    e. Colloid carcinoma
C. Carcinomas of mammary lobules
  1. Noninfiltrating
  2. Infiltrating
D. Relatively rare carcinomas
E. Sarcoma of the breast

PAGET'S DISEASE OF THE NIPPLE. This constitutes 1 percent of all breast carcinomas but has attracted an inordinate amount of attention and speculation, since for many years there was confusion as to whether this lesion arose primarily in the skin or in the mammary ducts. It is now generally accepted that this is a primary carcinoma of the mammary ducts of the nipple which has subsequently invaded the skin. The lesion presents as a scaling, eczematoid, and quite innocent-appearing lesion of the nipple (Fig. 15-15). In most instances it has a slow natural

Fig. 15-15. Typical scaling eczematoid lesion of Paget's disease; frequently misdiagnosed and treated by salves and ointments, with long delay in proper diagnosis.

history, and the skin lesion may be the only evidence of neoplasm for many years. Ultimately an underlying mass will develop if the lesion is untreated. Any eczematoid lesion of the nipple in a postmenopausal female which persists for more than a few weeks should be biopsied to exclude the possibility of Paget's disease. Adequate histologic studies of surgical specimens almost always reveal underlying carcinomas of the mammary ducts. Invasion of the skin by these cells produces the interesting Paget's cell, a large cell with clear cytoplasm and commonly with binucleation. This is associated with evidence of chronic inflammation and a surface crust. Robbins and Berg's study of 89 cases indicated that one-third of the patients showed noninfiltrating carcinoma, and in this group the survival rate was 100 percent at 5 years. The remaining patients had infiltrating carcinoma. The overall survival rate for the group was 64 percent, indicating a better prognosis for this lesion than for the average carcinoma of the breast.

NONINFILTRATING CARCINOMAS OF THE MAMMARY DUCTS. These constitute 1 percent of carcinomas of the breast. It is unfortunate that more cancers are not seen at the noninfiltrating stage, since these lesions are carcinomas in situ and operation should result in 100 percent 5-year survival. That this is not the case, 5-year survival being about 90 percent, reflects the fact that the breast is a large organ and that lesions which appear to be noninfiltrating may in fact be infiltrating at some area which the pathologist has not examined. Foote and Stewart report that they have traced progression of intraductal carcinoma from benign papillary hyperplasia through atypism to noninfiltrating intraductal carcinoma and ultimately to infiltrating carcinoma throughout a breast specimen. They state that while this may be one route for the development of cancer of the breast, cancer may arise from normal intraductal cells directly. The differentiation of a noninfiltrating intraductal carcinoma from a benign hyperplasia may be difficult; areas of atypism can blend gradually from one state into the other. Histologically, the duct

Fig. 15-16. Intraductal carcinoma with stromal invasion in eighty-three-year-old female. Field shows almost entire extent of this very early lesion. (Hematoxylin and eosin; ×32.)

epithelium is usually seen to be thrown up into papillae which show a loss of cohesiveness and disorientation of cells, with pleomorphism and occasionally mitotic figures but without evidence of invasion of the basement membrane. A more dramatic form is the noninfiltrating comedocarcinoma, in which hyperplasia is more extreme, choking the entire duct for long distances with masses of cells. These lesions commonly develop central necrosis of the cells. A gross section of such a lesion will extrude small cores of tissue from the ducts very much as the core is extruded from a comedo when it is squeezed, thus giving rise to the term comedocarcinoma.

INFILTRATING PAPILLARY CARCINOMA. Presumably a later stage or a more aggressive form of the noninfiltrating papillary lesion, these carcinomas still tend to evolve slowly and have a better 5-year survival rate than the average carcinoma of the breast. They produce a mass rather soft to palpation compared with the typical hard, fibrous lesion usually associated with breast cancer. They may reach large size before metastasizing to the axilla. Dimpling and skin edema are less commonly seen, another index of the late infiltration of the lymphatics and of the failure to stimulate a fibrous response. Noninfiltrating papillary carcinomas are often seen in association with the infiltrating form.

Infiltrating comedocarcinomas comprise approximately 5 percent of all breast cancers. They are often found in association with other forms of adenocarcinoma that result in productive fibrosis, and the presence of comedocarcinoma together with other elements of carcinoma of the breast does not significantly alter the prognosis from the average.

INFILTRATING DUCT CARCINOMA WITH PRODUCTIVE FIBROSIS. This is the commonest form of breast cancer, constituting 78 percent of the specimens seen. There is a tremendous variation in the amount of fibrosis. The lesion has been termed *scirrhous carcinoma, fibrocarcinoma,* and *sclerosing carcinoma.* The desmoplastic response to the invading cancer cells accounts for the remarkable hardness of the average breast cancer. Grossly the lesions have uneven serrated edges. They cut with great resistance and often with a rather gritty feeling as the knife edge passes through them. Histologically the lesions may vary from scattered, well-differentiated adenomatous clusters and a massive amount of fibrostroma to dense cellular aggregates with only minor amounts of fibroplasia (Fig. 15-16). Electron microscopic examination of these tumors indicates that they originate in the myoepithelial cells of the mammary duct.

MEDULLARY CARCINOMAS. Five percent of carcinomas of the breast assume this pattern, and the diagnosis indicates a favorable prognosis for the patient. Even in the presence of metastatic disease the prognosis remains favorable; the 5-year overall survival rate for the lesion is 85 to 90 percent. These lesions are soft, bulky, and often large. Necrotic areas of varying size are usually present. Occasionally one finds a lesion which is almost totally infarcted. On physical examination these tumors are freely movable, and smaller tumors are likely to be diagnosed clinically as cysts or fibroadenomas. Histologically the tumors are made up of large rounded or polygonal cells with an abundant cytoplasm arranged in broad or narrow plexiform masses anastomosing with one another. Electron microscopic and histochemical evidence suggests that these cells originate in the ductal epithelium. There is an abundant lymphoid infiltrate. Plasma cells are often seen and are sometimes very prominent. Axillary metastases occur less frequently than in the ordinary carcinoma of the breast but are not uncommon, occurring in about 40 percent. Metastasis frequently involves only a single node.

COLLOID CARCINOMA. This is an infrequent mammary cancer constituting about 1 percent of all breast cancers. The lesions contain a much greater amount of mucin than the usual adenocarcinoma and may be frankly gelatinous on cut section. Clinically these lesions are soft and ill defined and, like the medullary lesions, may be quite bulky before detection. Histologically the predominant picture is of large mucinous lakes in which epithelial aggregates float. Patients with these lesions have a better-than-average survival rate.

CARCINOMA OF THE MAMMARY LOBULES. This lesion arises in the mammary lobules from the cells of the acini and the terminal ducts. Most of the acini of a lobule are involved. Lobules may be of normal size or enlarged, with an unsystematic hyperplasia of the lining cells until the lumen is plugged. At the in situ stage of development these are the only changes, and simple mastectomy at this point should produce cure. The lesion subsequently becomes infiltrative and ultimately may give rise to regular scirrhous carcinoma.

Multicentricity and bilaterality are important features of lobular carcinoma. Eighty-eight percent of breast specimens removed for in situ lobular carcinoma show other in situ lesions scattered throughout the specimen. Examination of the contralateral breast has demonstrated in situ lesions in from 35 to 59 percent of specimens.

SARCOMA OF THE BREAST. Sarcomas of the breast are very rare. The commonest sarcoma seen is cystosarcoma phylloides, but only one in ten of these is truly malignant, the great majority being a benign variant of fibroadenoma. Great confusion is created because both the benign and malignant form are called "cystosarcoma." When Müller first described and named the lesion in 1838 he was aware of its predominantly benign nature. At that time "sarcoma" meant simply a fleshy tumor and did not carry the meaning of malignancy that it does today. Modern synonyms for the benign lesion are *giant intracanalicular or pericanalicular fibroadenoma* and *intracanalicular myxoma*. The malignant variant has been called *adenocarcinoma*.

Cystosarcoma phylloides occurs at an older average age (forty), is larger, and has a more cellular stroma than fibroadenoma. When first seen clinically these tumors average 5 to 10 cm, have a firm and rubbery consistency, and may have a bosselated surface. In cut section the tumors have a discrete capsule. Small lesions present leaflike intracanalicular protrusions, and larger lesions have cystic spaces into which project densely packed polypoid masses.

The malignant variant metastasizes most commonly to the lungs, bones, and subcutaneous tissues. Axillary metas-

tasis is so uncommon that simple mastectomy is an adequate procedure for both the benign and the malignant forms.

PRIMARY TREATMENT

The first historical reference to cancer of the breast appears in the Edwin Smith Surgical Papyrus (3000 to 2500 B.C.). The patient described is a man, but the description suggests most of the clinical features of breast cancer. The author concludes that "there is no treatment." References to cancer of the breast are scattered and brief over the following 2,500 years. Even in that large body of writings concerning Greek and Roman medicine, the Corpus Hippocraticum, direct reference to the treatment of breast cancer is absent, although it is clear that the condition was recognized.

Celsus, a Roman of the first century, spoke of operation and advised limiting it to early lesions: "None of these can be removed but the cacocthes [early lesion], the rest are irritated by every method of cure. The more violent the operations are, the more angry they grow." Galen, in the second century, inscribed one of the classic clinical observations:

We have often seen in the breast a tumor exactly resembling the animal the crab. Just as the crab has legs on both sides of his body, so in this disease the veins extending out from the unnatural growth take the shape of a crab's legs. We have often cured this disease in its early stages, but after it has reached a large size no one has cured it without operation. In all operations we attempt to excise a pathological tumor in a circle in the region where it borders on the healthy tissue.

Although Galen spoke of operations for tumors, his system of medicine ascribed the disease to an excess of black bile, and logically excision of a local outbreak could not cure the systemic imbalance. The Galenic theories dominated medicine until the Renaissance. Most established physicians looked down on attempts at operative treatment as misdirected and futile. Only when it was again established that a cancer could arise in a part as a local disorder quite separate from a systemic imbalance could excision of the tumor be recognized as rational therapy. Morgagni's definitive study of gross pathology, appropriately entitled *The Seats and Causes of Disease,* supplied this new rationale. Radical mastectomy until recently was the standard treatment for operable cancer of the breast in the United States. This operation involves the removal of the entire breast with a generous portion of overlying skin, all the underlying pectoralis major and minor muscles, and the entire lymphatic and fibrofatty contents of the axilla (Fig. 15-17).

This procedure evolved slowly from simple amputation of the breast. LeDran in the eighteenth century repudiated Galen's humoral theory and stated that cancer of the breast was a local disease which spread by way of the lymphatics to the regional nodes. He removed enlarged axillary nodes in his operations on patients with breast cancer. In the nineteenth century, Moore of Middlesex Hospital, England, emphasized wide removal of the breast and felt that when there was neoplasm in the axilla, the axillary con-

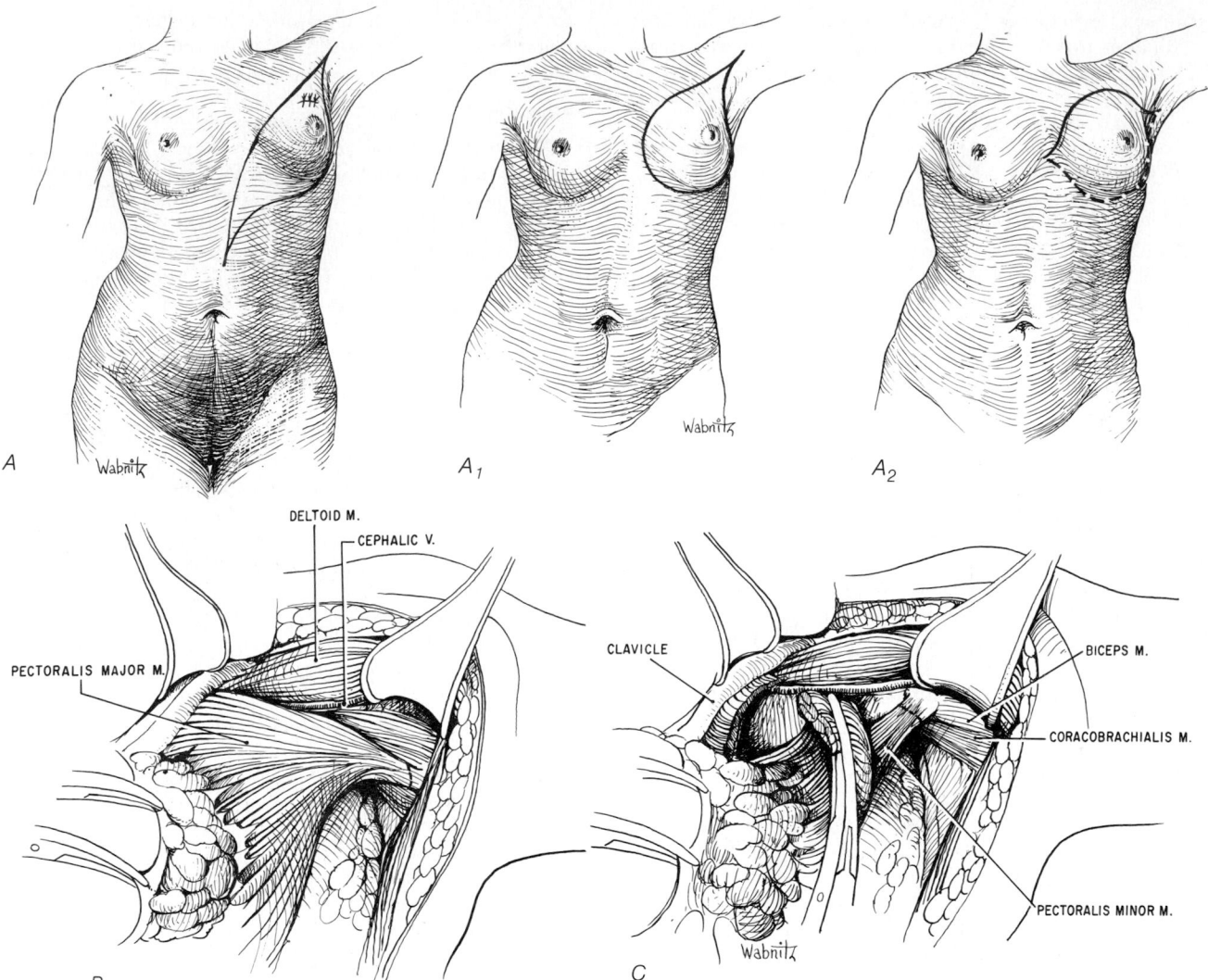

Fig. 15-17. Technique of radical mastectomy. *A.* Willy Meyer elliptical incision. *A₁* and *A₂.* Variations of mastectomy incision. *B.* Skin flaps developed and cephalic vein identified in order to delineate deltopectoral groove; tendinous insertion of pectoralis major muscle into humerus identified for transection. *C.* After transection of pectoralis major muscle, pectoralis minor insertion into coracoid process is defined. *D.* Pectoralis minor muscle transected and axilla being cleared of fatty tissue. *E.* Axillary vein cleared and all tributaries coursing caudad transected; long thoracic and thoracodorsal nerves identified and preserved; pectoralis major and minor muscle dissected with axillary fat and lymph nodes in medial direction. *F.* Dissection complete, showing chest wall including ribs and intercostal muscles cleared of pectoralis fascia, with sternum as medial limit of dissection. *G.* Incision closed and suction applied to obliterate dead space; with this technique, pressure dressing not needed.

tents should be removed in one block together with the breast. In a presentation before the British Medical Association in 1877, Banks supported Moore's concepts and advocated that axillary nodes should always be removed in one block with the breast tissue whether there were palpable nodes present or not, since occult involvement of the axillary nodes was so often present.

As Lewison notes, it remained for Halsted, the new professor of surgery at a young school called The Johns Hopkins Medical School, to "culminate the operation and germinate the present modern method." Halsted proposed a standard procedure, removing all the structures in one block. His first operation was performed about 1882, and he reported 13 cases in 1890. The procedure was almost exactly as it is today except that the pectoralis minor muscle was not removed. In 1894 he reported more than 50 cases over the preceding 12 years. In the same year Herbert Willy Meyer of New York reported six patients operated upon by a technique he had evolved independently. This procedure, almost a duplicate of the Hal-

sted mastectomy, added the removal of the pectoralis minor muscle. Halsted subsequently accepted this addition, and the modern radical mastectomy is often attributed to both these men. This procedure and the wide-block excision that it incorporated was soon adopted widely and for the following 50 years was the only operation used by the well-trained surgeon for treatment of breast cancer.

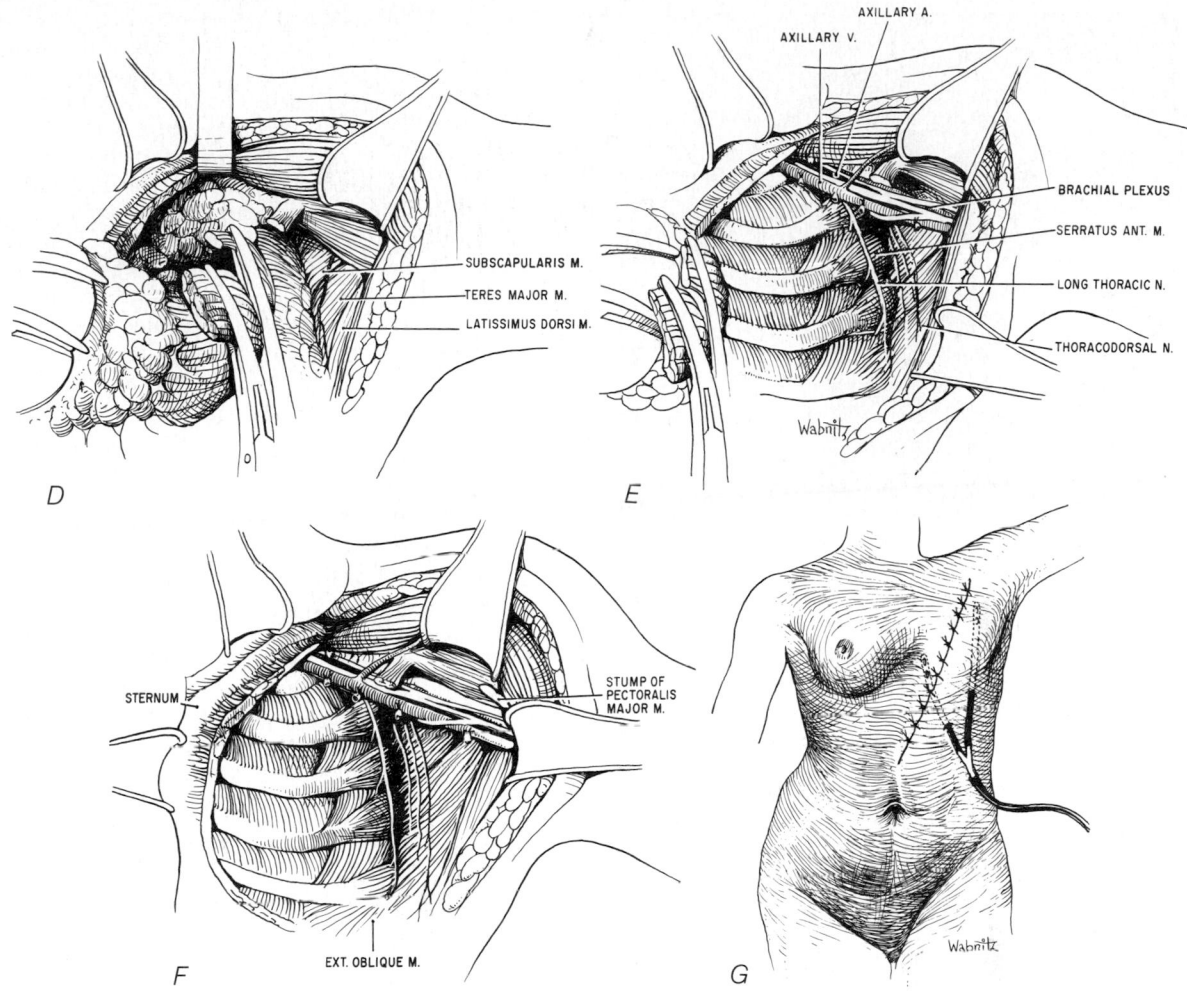

Fig. 15-17. See legend on facing page.

SELECTION OF PATIENTS. Operative treatment of breast cancer cannot be effective if disease has spread beyond the area removed by the operation. Distant spread to supraclavicular lymph nodes, lung, liver, or other sites is thus an absolute contraindication to the radical operation. Certain characteristics of the local lesion also indicate a high likelihood that operation would be futile. These generally accepted "criteria of inoperability" include fixation of the local breast lesion to the chest wall, fixation of the involved lymph nodes in the axilla, and inflammatory carcinoma of the breast. Haagensen compiled the following detailed list of criteria:

1. Extensive edema of the skin over the breast (Fig. 15-18)
2. Satellite nodules in the skin over the breast
3. Carcinoma of the inflammatory type (Fig. 15-19)
4. Parasternal tumor nodules
5. Proved supraclavicular metastases
6. Edema of the arm
7. Distant metastases
8. Any two or more of the following grave signs of locally advanced carcinoma
   a. Ulceration of the skin
   b. Edema of the skin of limited extent (less than one-third of breast skin involved)
   c. Solid fixation of tumor to the chest wall
   d. Axillary lymph nodes measuring 2.5 cm or more in transverse diameter
   e. Fixation of the axillary nodes to the skin or deep structures of the axilla

If these criteria are strictly applied, 75 percent of breast cancers seen will be operable. Figures from Connecticut indicate that from 1940 to 1959 ninety-five percent of all new patients there under sixty-five were treated by operation. This suggests that these clinical criteria are not observed in many institutions.

Haagensen has proposed an even stricter method of evaluation, called the *triple biopsy*. The object is "to exclude all patients who have no chance of cure." Patients who would otherwise be eligible for radical mastectomy are selected for triple biopsy if they have palpable axillary lymph nodes, primary lesions larger than 3 cm, or tumors in the center or the inner quadrants of the breast. Biopsy of the breast lesion, highest axillary nodes, and internal mammary nodes is done. If occult cancer is found in any of these areas, the patient is treated by radiation. This procedure reduces the number of patients eligible for operation to 50 percent of those seen.

Fig. 15-18. Large cancer of breast with retraction of nipple, skin edema, and several satellite skin nodules.

MacDonald introduced the term *biological determinism* into the consideration of cancer, meaning that the biologic nature of the tumor primarily determines the response to therapy. Concerning the breast he suggests that one-third of the lesions do not develop the propensity to metastasize, and while excision removes a disagreeable local growth, the procedure is not lifesaving since such a tumor would never be life-threatening. One-third of the lesions, he estimates, are incurable almost from inception, since they become generalized early, before they are clinically detectable, and no matter how early or how widely the tumor is excised, the procedure will not change the course of the disease. Finally, he assumes that in the remaining one-

Fig. 15-19. Inflammatory carcinoma of breast. Bright pink to red suffuses area of skin involvement, reflecting inflammatory response to extensive scattering of tumor cells in subcutaneous tissues. Large skin lesion above nipple is congenital pigmented nevus unrelated to the cancer.

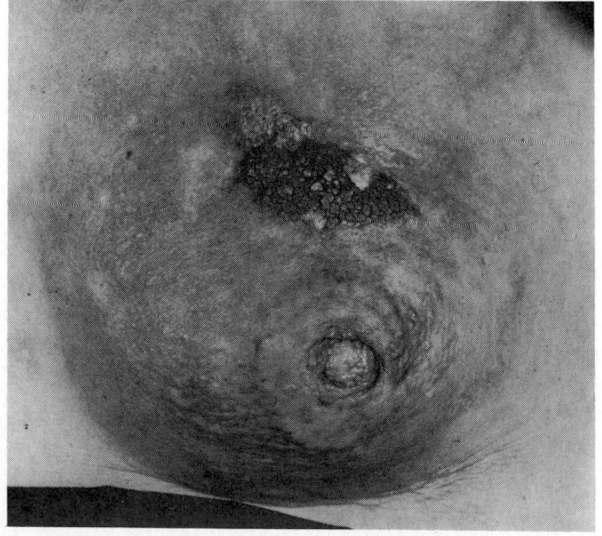

third of patients the systemic spread of the tumor is preceded by a long latent period in which the tumor reaches clinically detectable size before beginning to spread. In such patients early detection and excision of the tumor would be important, and treatment would have value in altering the course of the cancer. If this thesis is correct, a test to distinguish the different tumors, confining radical treatment to those of the last group only, would have great value. Such a test, as well as proof of this theory, remains to be provided.

The concept of biologic determinism would also explain much of the confusion that surrounds attempts to evaluate techniques of treatment by statistical methods. Butcher compares this effort to attempting to evaluate a remedy for snakebite in a series of patients who fell into a pit of vipers, some poisonous, some benign, and some moderately toxic, with no way of knowing which patients were bitten by which snakes.

Every effort should be made to identify patients with distant metastasis. Search for metastatic lesions preoperatively should include a chest film and liver and skeletal scintiscans. These tests, combined with urinary hydroxyproline, bone-derived alkaline phosphatase, and γ-glutamyl transpeptidase, have demonstrated a 40 to 45 percent incidence of distant metastasis in Stages I and II patients who were otherwise asymptomatic.

SELECTION OF THE OPERATION. For the past 20 years a controversy has been raging as to the appropriate operation for patients with operable breast cancer. Initially the debate was between radical mastectomy and total ("simple") mastectomy plus radiation therapy; then between radical mastectomy and total mastectomy alone; and finally between radical mastectomy alone and partial mastectomy with or without radiation therapy. While these have been the major themes, some minor variations of radical mastectomy have also appeared: either a little less than the radical mastectomy, sparing the pectoralis minor (Patey's operation) or both pectoral muscles (Madden's operation); or a little more than the radical mastectomy, taking the internal mammary lymph nodes and adjacent chest wall (Urban's operation).

The arguments for the various procedures have become remarkably bitter at times, with charges of bias, the citing of incomplete data, and irrationality being hurled not only in the scientific but in the lay press as well. Nonparticipants in this battle have been regarded darkly as agnostics who have failed to embrace either "true faith." American surgeons have remained reasonably level-headed during this period. At first they adhered to the traditional radical mastectomy. After all, the advantages of doing lesser operations were functional and cosmetic, while the penalty of being wrong was the life of a patient. A survey of New Jersey surgeons in 1971 showed that 75 percent would do a radical breast dissection and 15 percent a modified radical operation for a 2-cm lesion in the upper outer quadrant of a fifty-year old woman. Opinion is changing, however: in 1977, surgeons in the same state indicated that approximately 40 percent would do a radical mastectomy, 40 percent a modified radical mastectomy, 15 percent a total mastectomy, and 5 percent some other procedure.

My own rationale for selecting an operation involves the following considerations: Of the three major anatomic components in radical mastectomy—the breast, the axillary contents, and the muscles—current evidence strongly supports removal of at least the first two. Removal of all, rather than part, of the involved breast is required because of the high incidence of multicentricity of these malignant lesions. The risk of another tumor focus left in the remaining breast tissue following a segmental excision exceeds 50 percent.

The value of removing axillary contents has been defended in the past on the claim of improved survival. The results of controlled cooperative clinical trials indicate that treatment of the axilla does not change survival in patients with clinical Stage I tumors. Data from such trials are still accumulating concerning treatment of the axilla in clinical Stage II patients, and figures currently available are in conflict. On the other hand, the added information gained by knowing whether or not axillary nodes are histologically involved by malignancy is of enormous value to surgeons and patients, both in rendering an accurate prognosis and in influencing the trend of future therapy.

Hodgkin's disease, in which a major operation, exploratory laparotomy and splenectomy, is now felt justified for diagnostic and "staging" purposes, is an irresistible parallel. The addition of axillary dissection to breast resection adds very little in risk or morbidity, and the dividend in "staging" the extent of the disease is well worth the price whether survival is improved or not.

Should the muscles be removed as well, and if so, how much? In view of the enormous effort required to accumulate properly controlled series, this question may never be subject to scientific resolution. Pragmatically, muscle resection seems especially indicated for large or deep tumors which approach or invade fascia and muscle. This was the type of lesion most commonly seen in the late nineteenth century, for which the classic radical mastectomy was originally designed. Such large and often ulcerated tumors require the larger operations, often combined with radiation, to obtain proper local control of tumor. The object is to prevent recurrent uncontrollable local disease and improve the quality of survival, even though the eventual outcome will be death from distant metastasis.

Subcutaneous Mastectomy. The advent of mammography has led to an increasing diagnosis of in situ (T1S) and very small microinvasive cancers (T1a). This has coincided with the introduction of subcutaneous mastectomy, a technique in which most of the mammary tissue is removed but the skin of the breast is preserved. Contour is restored by inserting a silastic prosthesis into the subcutaneous pocket left by the excision of breast tissue. It is impossible to remove all breast tissue by this method, and 1 or 2 percent remains in the subcutaneous layer near the skin even if the nipple is sacrificed. Development of cancer in this residual mammary tissue has been reported, and in view of the multifocal nature of breast cancer, it is expected that some of the foci may be left behind. The risk/benefit ratio of this approach remains to be established and, while it is a very attractive alternative for women with in situ cancer of the breast, the accepted procedure for such lesions in the United States is still total mastectomy.

The Problem of Bilateral Mastectomy. Foote and Stewart have observed that "the most frequent precancerous lesion of the breast is a cancer of the opposite breast." Berg and Robbins noted that the incidence of occurrence of cancer in the contralateral breast following radical mastectomy was approximately 1 percent per year, so that the cumulative risk of cancer in the remaining breast among patients surviving radical mastectomy for 20 years was as high as 20 percent. As long ago as 1951, Pack published a plea for routine simple mastectomy of the remaining breast at the time of mastectomy for cancer. Presumably because of the psychologic blow to a woman who is asked to lose both her breasts, this approach has rarely been advocated by surgeons, and the usual routine after mastectomy has been to follow the contralateral breast with special care in the ensuing years. The recognition of the high risk of contralateral cancer in patients with in situ lobular carcinoma has caused a change in attitude toward this particular form of the disease. Currently recommended treatment for patients with either in situ or invasive lobular cancer of the breast is total mastectomy of the contralateral breast. Should this recommendation be refused, the patient is requested at least to permit a biopsy of the remaining breast in an area which represents a mirror image of the area of cancer in the involved breast. If this biopsy reveals in situ lobular cancer, a total mastectomy is carried out. If invasive lobular cancer is found, a radical or modified radical mastectomy is done. If the biopsy is negative, a very careful follow-up is recommended, with mammography and careful breast examination at least twice yearly.

A minority of physicians recommend a "watch" policy for in situ lobular carcinoma. They reason that only one-third of these lesions ultimately become invasive, and that even the invasive lesions of this tumor have a better prognosis than the usual invasive ductal lesion. Close follow-up would thus preserve a substantial number of women from what might be an unnecessary mastectomy. This view of therapy has not proved popular among patients and surgeons. Most women are uneasy about harboring a malignant breast lesion even if it is preinvasive, and most surgeons share this feeling. Moreover, the transition from preinvasive to invasive may go undetected for long periods, since it is not necessarily accompanied by any clinical signs.

ADJUVANT THERAPY FOLLOWING OPERATIONS FOR BREAST CANCER. Traditionally, patients who were discovered at operation for breast cancer to have metastatic tumor in the axillary nodes were subjected to radiation therapy given over the axilla and the parasternal and supraclavicular areas. This treatment was given in the hope of increasing the chance for survival in this high-risk group of patients. A number of cooperative clinical trials testing this hypothesis were launched in the 1950s and 1960s and have shown that such therapy has no effect on recurrence rate or survival. The National Surgical Adjuvant Breast Project (NSABP) conducted such a study starting in 1961 and found that at 5 years 50.6 percent of treated patients were disease-free, compared with 50.2 percent of patients who received no radiotherapy. Local recurrence of disease was affected, however, being twice as common (15.4 percent) when radiotherapy was not given as when it was (7.8 percent). Distant metastasis seemed to occur sooner in the radiated group. Current thinking is that adjuvant radiotherapy should be used only in breast cancer patients who are at very high risk of local recurrence.

It may be that cancer chemotherapy will provide an effective adjuvant to operative therapy where radiation has failed. In some of the early NSABP trials it was noted that a brief course of triethylene ethiophosphoramide (thiotepa), a nitrogen mustard analogue given at the time of operation, resulted in a decrease in recurrence rates in a special subset of the population treated. This special group comprised those premenopausal women with four or more axillary lymph nodes involved by tumor. This is a high-risk group with a recurrence rate of at least 90 percent in 5 years from operation. Long-term follow-up of these patients showed significantly improved survival at 5 and 10 years.

Subsequent cooperative clinical trials of adjuvant therapy with L-phenylalanine mustard (L-Pam, melphalan) were initiated. In the light of more modern concepts of cancer chemotherapy, the drug was given over a much longer period. Initial results again demonstrated significant improvement in the disease-free interval in the same subset of women up to 3 years after operation. More recent trials of a three-drug regimen suggest even more effective results in premenopausal women with four or more positive axillary lymph nodes (Fig. 15-20) and possible improvements in the disease-free period for women with similar advanced disease in the postmenopausal period as well. These are exciting results and seem to promise a real increase in survival in certain high-risk groups. However, another several years must elapse before final conclusions on these

Fig. 15-20. Early results of adjuvant therapy with a three-drug regimen (Cytoxan, methotrexate, and 5-fluorouracil) in women with four or more axillary lymph nodes involved by metastatic cancer. Major difference in recurrence rate is obvious. (*From U. Veronesi et al., World J Surg, 1:337, 1977, by permission.*)

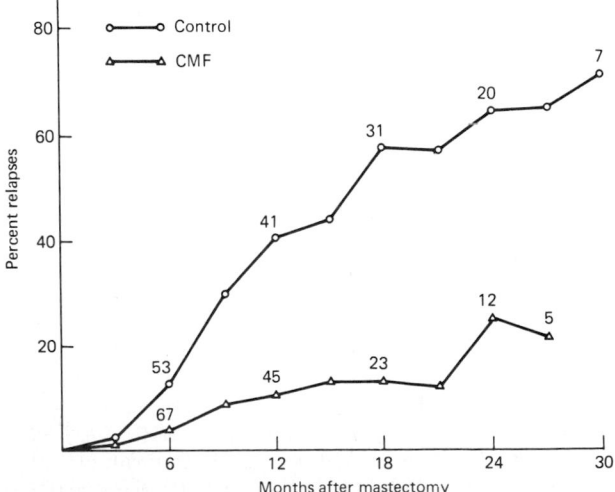

questions can be drawn. In the meantime, adjuvant chemotherapy of patients with Stage 1 lesions is not recommended, since the mortality due to cancer in this group is less than 15 percent at 5 and 10 years, and long-term hazards of chemotherapeutic drugs, especially the alkylating agents, have not been fully determined. There is some evidence that these are carcinogenic and may themselves induce some cancers.

Operative mortality is very low for all the various types of mastectomy. Kennedy and Miller reported no deaths following 212 simple mastectomies. Handley and Thackray reported no deaths following 143 modified radical mastectomies. Butcher reported 0.7 percent mortality in 425 radical mastectomies. Haagensen, Cooley, and their associates had no deaths in 556 radical mastectomies. In all the series cited above, any death of a patient up to 3 months after operation was considered an operative death. Even among patients with extended mastectomy, mortality is low: Sugarbaker reported 1 postoperative death in 250 patients with this procedure.

PROGNOSIS

The arguments for and against different forms of therapy in breast cancer are mainly statistical and are chiefly based on survival figures. Before an observer can appreciate this debate, a clear understanding of the data is required. The accurate comparison of results in different series demands that there be a common denominator. There is great variation in the base line of many published series, and astute investigation is often necessary to determine whether two sets of figures are truly comparable.

An older method of standard reporting required that all patients seen at an institution be reported in the final results, whether they were treated or not. This was called the "absolute," or "crude," survival figure. It had the advantage of indicating the effect of patient selection on the surgical, or "definitive," survival figures. Its disadvantage was that the total experience at different institutions varied greatly. Private hospitals and clinics have a much greater number of early and operable cases compared with cancer hospitals and charity institutions.

Favorable attention has been given to methods of clinical evaluation of the stage of the tumor. By this method the results in patients at an equal stage of disease can be compared among institutions. An advantage of this approach is that since the evaluation is based on pretreatment clinical findings, it is possible to compare the results in patients treated by radiation, radical mastectomy, simple mastectomy, or extended radical mastectomy even though microscopic evaluation of lymph node involvement is available with some forms of treatment and not with others. Disadvantages are that judgment of the extent of involvement is subjective and classification depends greatly on the skill and consistency of the examiner. The system of staging recommended by the American Joint Committee on Cancer Staging and End Results Reporting is most widely accepted; in addition there are the Columbia classification, the Manchester classification, and the Steinthal classification (Table 15-1).

Table 15-1. CLINICAL CLASSIFICATIONS OF CANCER OF THE BREAST

Manchester	*Steinthal*	*Columbia*
Stage I: Growth confined to breast, skin involvement over and in direct continuity with tumor and small in relation to breast	*Stage I:* Cancer limited to breast	*Stage A:* No skin edema, ulceration, or solid fixation of tumor to chest wall; axillary nodes not involved
Stage II: As Stage I but with palpable mobile axillary lymph nodes	*Stage II:* Limited to breast and axillary nodes	*Stage B:* As Stage A but axillary nodes present, not larger than 2.5 cm and without fixation to skin or deeper structures
Stage III: Growth extending beyond body of breast: *a.* Skin invaded or fixed over large area *b.* Tumor fixed to underlying muscle; nodes may be present but are mobile	*Stage III:* Adjacent structures involved, e.g., pectoral muscle skin (if ulcerated), opposite breast, cervical lymph nodes, viscera, skeletal tissue	*Stage C:* Any *one* of five grave signs present: 1. Edema of skin of limited extent (less than one-third) 2. Skin ulceration 3. Solid fixation to chest wall 4. Massive involvement of axillary nodes 5. Fixation of axillary nodes
Stage IV: Growth spread beyond breast: *a.* Fixation of axillary nodes *b.* Tumor fixed to chest wall (not just muscle) *c.* Supraclavicular nodes involved *d.* Satellite metastasis to skin beyond area of tumor *e.* Secondary deposits in opposite breast *f.* Distant metastasis		*Stage D:* All other more advanced cancer of breast

New diagnostic methods, especially mammography, have provided a new group of lesions not previously considered by any of the staging methods. Termed by some "minimal breast cancer," these are in situ and microinvasive lesions so small that they are not detectable by conventional palpation of the breast. Current data indicate that 5-year survivals in this group may exceed 90 percent.

The best way to evaluate methods of treatment is by cooperative programs among many institutions in which all factors are governed by the same rules and in which random selection of patients for the different methods of therapy is used. Even these trials are not an easy solution to the problem. Such trials tend to be biased toward false-negative results. Only in the largest of the cooperative trials is the chance of error in a negative result reduced to under 10 percent.

NO TREATMENT. In 1951 Park and Lees in a statistical analysis of 5-year survival figures for breast carcinoma tried to show that the course of the disease was not affected by operation. They regarded the improvement in 5-year survival seen following operation as an artifact introduced by operating upon patients earlier in the natural course of the disease. There are now available a number of studies of large groups of patients with untreated breast cancer. Survival computed from the onset of symptoms averages 19 percent at 5 years, 2.5 percent at 10 years. If one computes survival from onset of diagnosis, a figure more comparable to the situation in surgical series, the 5- and 10-year survivals average 8.6 percent and 1.2 percent, respectively. Bloom et al. found that untreated patients with histologically low grade (grade 1 of 4) neoplasms had survivals of 22 percent, 9 percent, and 0 at 5, 10, and 15 years, respectively. They compared these to survivals of 82, 56, and 37 percent at the same time intervals for lesions of comparable histologic grade in their own treated series (Fig. 15-12).

RADICAL MASTECTOMY. If survival data following radical mastectomy between 1915 and 1958 are examined, one may wonder why the procedure has received so much criticism. The absolute survival gradually increased from 30 to over 50 percent (Fig. 15-21). In California the incidence of patients with localized disease in different age groups has increased from 14–27 percent to 27–39 percent in county hospitals and from 39–44 percent to 43–48 percent in private hospitals. The end-result group of the National Cancer Institute and a number of state tumor registries have reported small but steady increases in 5-year survivals in patients with both regional and localized disease since about 1950. Epidemiologic reports from Connecticut and from Saskatchewan, Canada, establish a significant increase in the incidence of breast cancer in the last several decades accompanied by a decrease in mortality, thus implying an increase in survival (Fig. 15-22).

Survival for 5 years following radical mastectomy does not provide the same assurance against recurrence that it does for some other cancers. The risk of death continues higher than for the general population for at least 25 years after the operation, although this risk gradually diminishes with time (Fig. 15-23). According to Berg and Robbins, change in risk over the postoperative period follows a log-log curve. From this model it can be predicted that after operation the risk of recurrence and death will continue to decrease but will always be present, being about 1 percent in the decade from 30 to 40 years after operation and 0.5 percent from 40 to 50 years after operation. The 20-year survival rate after operation for patients without axillary lymph node involvement is 65 percent, and that for all patients with radical mastectomy is 41 percent [Berg

Fig. 15-21. Absolute survival figures in different series following treatment by radical mastectomy. Note improvement in survival from original observations to 1955. (*From H. Vermund, Trends in Radiotherapy in Breast Cancer, Proc 5th Natl Cancer Conf, Philadelphia, 1965, by permission.*)

Fig. 15-22. Contrary to past reports data from large population groups now indicate an increasing incidence and a decreasing mortality rate for breast cancer. (*From S. J. Cutler, B. Christine, and T. H. C. Barcley, Cancer, 28:1376, 1971.*)

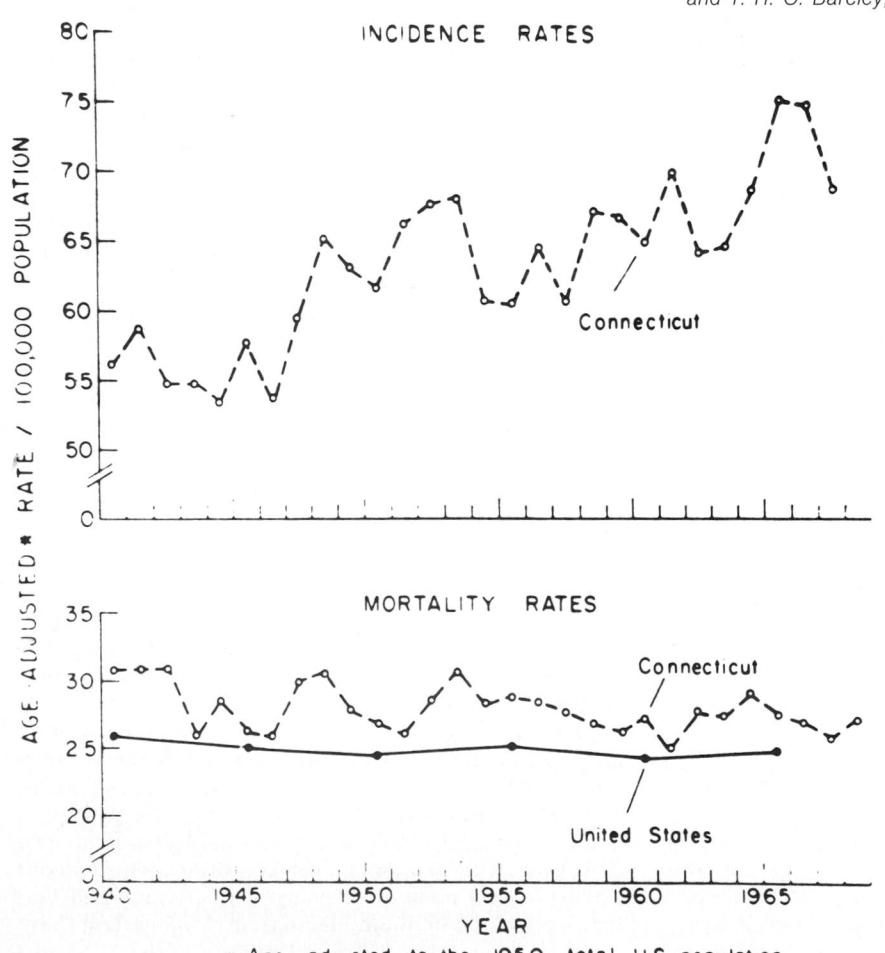

and Robbins]. If patients are considered who have node involvement at the apex of the axilla, the middle, and the lower portion, the 20-year survival is 11, 30, and 39 percent, respectively. These figures illustrate how important the absence or the extent of lymph node involvement is in determining patient survival. The increasing number of patients with primary lesions of the breast without lymph node involvement is the most important factor in the improving survival rates today compared with 25 years ago.

Our attitudes concerning survival and prognosis continue to be conditioned by our beliefs concerning the natural history of the disease. Mueller has reported data indicating that survival following treatment of breast cancer follows a log-normal curve, that is, that the annual risk of recurrence and death remains constant and if patients lived long enough all would eventually die of their tumor. If true, this would imply that all tumors have disseminated before clinical detection and treatment. In this circumstance treatment is effective only by altering the slope of the curve and delaying the ultimate death due to the cancer, long enough, it may be hoped, so that the patient dies of other "more natural" causes. This hypothesis is in conflict with the data of Berg and Robbins cited above and those of Blackwood and Rush, who indicated that the hazard function or risk of annual recurrence decreases significantly over time, following a well-known survival curve called the Wiebull distribution. Duncan and Kerr have examined a large series of patients treated in the 1940s with a follow-up of 20 or more years. Their data indicate that the "curability" of Stages I and II patients is 30.5 percent (Fig. 15-24).

Radical mastectomy is no longer the routine treatment for all patients with cancer of the breast, and even its stoutest defenders agree that there is a group of smaller cancers that can be treated by lesser procedures. It is still, however, the reference procedure, the operation with which we have the most experience over the greatest period of time. Defenders of radical mastectomy continue to be troubled by the fact that comparisons of survival with alternate procedures seem to favor the radical operation by 5 to 10 percent (Table 15-2). Such comparisons between institutional series have little or no statistical validity at this level of discrimination, and one must turn to the rapidly accumulating data from controlled cooperative clinical trials (Table 15-3).

RADICAL MASTECTOMY VS. OTHER SURGERY AND RADIATION THERAPY. There have been seven trials comparing total mastectomy plus immediate radiation therapy with radical mastectomy either with or without radiation since 1951 (Table 15-3). In every instance the results for survival and recurrence for Stage I tumors have been the same. For Stage II tumors the results were likewise similar except for the trial at Guy's, in which wide excision was done instead of total mastectomy. Stage II patients in this study had a significant increase in local recurrence and a significantly decreased survival at 5 years. Most such recurrences were in the axilla, and it has been noted that x-ray to the axilla in this series was considerably less than in other groups. By 10 years the survival rate in both groups was the same.

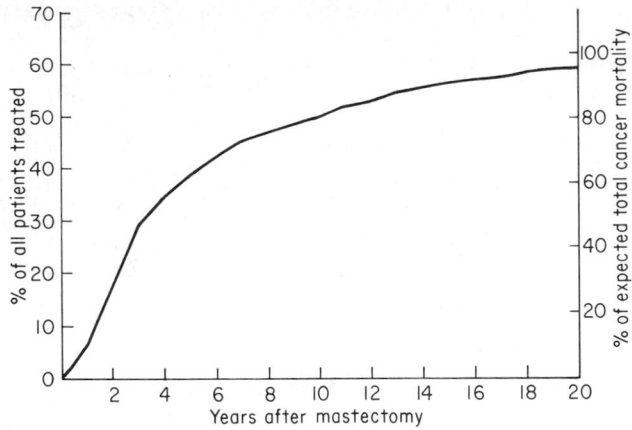

Fig. 15-23. Mortality 20 years after treatment by radical mastectomy; 95 percent of expected mortality has been realized, and over 40 percent of treated patients are still surviving. (*From J. W. Berg and G. F. Robbins, Surg Gynecol Obstet, 122:1311, 1966, by permission.*)

RADICAL MASTECTOMY VS. TOTAL MASTECTOMY. These trials are unique in that no radiation is used and that treatment to the axilla is omitted in one arm. Both the American and the Cardiff trials deal with Stage I disease. Early results in both trials show no difference in recurrence rate or survival. The Cape Town trial is the only one in this group in which axillary Stage II disease was observed and not treated. By the second year of the study, local recurrence rate (or continued growth of axillary nodes) was so great that the trial was stopped after entry of only 95 patients.

TOTAL MASTECTOMY AND RADIATION VS. TOTAL MASTECTOMY. Like the immediately previous trials, the effect of treating the axillary nodes versus watching them was being tested. In this case the primary treatment of the axilla was radiation. The three trials in this group differ in that the Edinburgh group and the NSABP-4 include only Stage I tumors—staged by histology in the former instance and clinically in the latter. In both groups early and thus

Fig. 15-24. "Curability" of breast cancer as determined in a group of patients treated 20 or more years. Survival rate in Stages I and II patients parallels the normal population at 20 years, and projection to the base line indicates that 30.5 percent of such patients are curable. (*From D. Brinkley and J. L. Haybittle, World J Surg, 1:287, 1977, by permission.*)

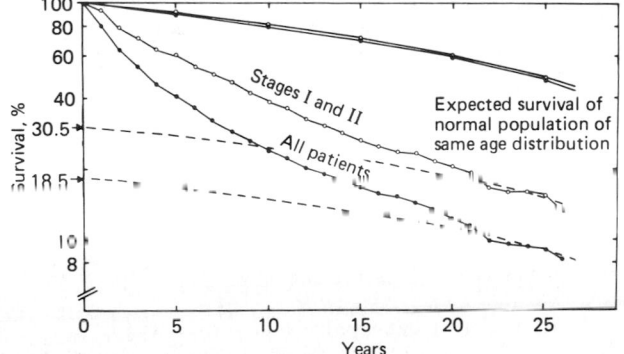

Table 15-2. METHODS OF TREATMENT COMPARED BY COLUMBIA CLASSIFICATION STAGES

Author	No. of patients		Method	5-yr survival, %	
	A	B		A	B
Kennedy and Miller	115	34	Simple mastectomy	62	41
Handley and Thackray	77	58	Limited radical mastectomy	75	57
Butcher	216	135	Classic radical mastectomy	76	48
Haagensen I	228	122	Classic radical mastectomy	82.5	59
Haagensen II	116	16	Classic radical mastectomy	87.9	62.5
Dahl-Iversen and Tobiassen	277	61	Extended radical mastectomy	77	48
Williams and Curwen	68	57	Limited radical mastectomy and radiation	72	60
Kaae and Johansen	159	28	Simple mastectomy and radiation	70	50
Baclesse	50	86	Radiation only	54	67

incomplete results show no differences. In the British Cancer Research Campaign trial, both clinical Stage I and Stage II lesions were included. In this trial, radiation significantly reduced the incidence of local recurrence or residual axillary disease. However, radiated patients with histologically positive axillary nodes had a 10 percent greater mortality in the first year of observation and a significantly higher incidence of distant metastasis.

RADICAL MASTECTOMY VS. EXTENDED RADICAL MASTECTOMY. A single cooperative trial has been conducted comparing these operative techniques. A total of 1,453 evaluable patients were admitted from 1963 to 1968 at several international hospitals. Five-year results indicate the same mortality and recurrence rate in both arms. But an interesting subset of patients, those with tumor in the axillary nodes with inner quadrant breast cancer, had a significantly better survival with the extended procedure, one of the rare reports in which removal of lymph nodes had any effect on prognosis.

SUMMARY. After a period of great confusion as to the proper treatment for breast cancer, during which surgeons continued to employ radical mastectomy because they were unsure what else to use, hard data are beginning to emerge from international cooperative clinical trials upon which we can base our future therapy: (1) Total mastectomy is as effective a treatment for clinical Stage I tumors as any other alternative tested, including radical mastectomy with or without radiation, total mastectomy with radiation, or extended radical mastectomy. (2) In Stage II breast cancer, the results of "watching" the axilla instead of treating it are still fairly early in controlled trials. On the basis of these early data, it appears that survival in the first 5 years of follow-up is unchanged. However, the local recurrence rate or continued growth of axillary nodes has proved unacceptable to one group of investigators and acceptable to another. Until such trials have matured further, physicians should continue to treat the axilla in Stage II patients by radiation or operation. (3) There is a

Table 15-3. SUMMARY OF INTERNATIONAL COOPERATIVE TRIALS

	Stage	Years	Patients
Radical and radiation vs. total and radiation			
Cambridge	II	1958–65	204
Cardiff/St. Mary's (part)	II	1967–73	139
Hammersmith			
Guy's (wide excision instead of total)	I,II	1961–71	370
Radical vs. total and radiation			
Denmark (superradical)	I,II,III	1951–57	400
Edinburgh I	I,II,III	1964–69	395
NSABP-4 (part)	I,II	1971–74	1226
Radical vs. total			
Cardiff/St. Mary's (part)	I	1967–73	154
Cape Town	I,II	1968–71	95
NSABP-4 (part)	I	1971–74	690
Total and radiation vs. total			
Cancer Research Campaign	I,II	1970–75	2268
NSABP-4 (part)	I	1971–74	689
Edinburgh II	I (histol.)	1974–	Still open

strong suspicion from several trials that radiation therapy increases the incidence of distant metastasis, and from one trial that early morbidity is significantly greater in patients with histologically positive axillary nodes. (4) No good data are available on the role of partial mastectomy in the treatment of breast cancer, and this procedure is contraindicated, used either alone or with radiation therapy, except as part of a controlled clinical trial.

As noted previously, this author believes that a prudent procedure for the treatment of Stages I and II breast cancer includes surgical removal of the breast and axillary contents. In more advanced malignant lesions of the breast, more extended operations such as radical mastectomy may be required, either with or without radiation therapy, to control local and regional disease and improve the quality if not the length of survival in such patients.

REHABILITATION. Most women require instruction in exercising the arm on the side of operation following radical mastectomy. Proper physical therapy in the immediate postoperative period should ensure complete return to normal function. Following operations which spare the pectoral muscles, full function of the arm usually returns promptly with little or no special help. Psychological support is also important in restoring the patient's self-image and her confidence that she is still desirable to a present or future husband. The Reach to Recovery program of the American Cancer Society has been most successful in providing advisors to the recent mastectomy patient from the ranks of women who have previously had the same operation.

Many women are interested in the possibility of subsequent reconstruction of the excised breast. If the previous operation was radical mastectomy, reconstruction is too complex a task to be worthwhile in most instances. In patients who have had a modified or total mastectomy, especially if the operation was performed through a transverse incision, reconstruction with a silastic implant is a relatively simple and feasible technique. The result is never a perfect match for the remaining breast, and decisions as to which patients will find these reconstructions worthwhile must be individualized.

TREATMENT OF RECURRENT CANCER

Prior to the 1950s recurrent cancer of the breast was treated either with radiation or operation or not at all. Radiation remains an extremely useful agent for painful osseous metastases and small subcutaneous lesions. Operation also may be useful for small local lesions. The basic problem in the patient with recurrent cancer is most often wide dissemination, and the new systemic agents of hormone therapy and chemotherapy are the treatments of choice.

Selection of hormonal therapy or chemotherapy as the initial treatment of recurrent disease depends on whether the patient's tumor is hormonally sensitive. For decades the only index of hormonal sensitivity was the patient's response to a trial of hormonal treatment. We now know that the response of breast cancers to hormones is dependent on the presence of hormone receptors in the substance of cancer cells. Hormonal receptors for estrogens, prolac-

tin, progesterone, and corticosteroids have been identified. Dependable clinical tests for estrogen receptors (ER) are now widely available, and all primary cancers should be submitted for testing when first removed; 50 percent of these tumors will prove to be ER-positive. Progesterone receptors (PR) also appear to have a predictive value. Eighty percent of patients with breast cancers which have both ER and PR will respond to hormonal manipulation. However, tests for PR are not widely available. A schema for treatment of patients tested for both ER and PR is shown in Fig. 15-25.

TREATMENT OF ESTROGEN RECEPTOR–POSITIVE RECURRENT TUMORS. Removal of estrogen-generating tissue in these patients will produce a remission in 60 percent. The major source of estrogens in the menstruating patient are the ovaries, and oophorectomy will result in an effective reduction in the estrogen level. In the postmenopausal patient some or most estrogen production has been assumed by the adrenals, thus bilateral adrenalectomy plus oophorectomy is required or, alternatively, hypophysectomy. Paradoxically, the postmenopausal woman also responds well to administration of estrogens in large doses, a far simpler procedure than the major operative procedures otherwise required.

Recently antiestrogen compounds have become available. These apparently block estrogen receptors at the cell. At best these may offer a useful substitute for ablative therapy, and at worst they offer a nonoperative test of which patients fall within the 60 percent who will respond to operative ablation.

TREATMENT OF ESTROGEN RECEPTOR–NEGATIVE RECURRENT TUMORS. Patients who have tumors which are estrogen receptor–negative rarely respond to estrogen ab-

Fig. 15-25. Schema for the treatment of patients with recurrent breast cancer when determinations for estrogen receptors and progesterone receptors are available. Patients who are estrogen receptor–positive (ERP) and progesterone receptor–positive (PRP) have an 80 percent response rate to surgical ablation. (*From G. A. Degenshein et al., Breast, 3:29, 1977, by permission.*)

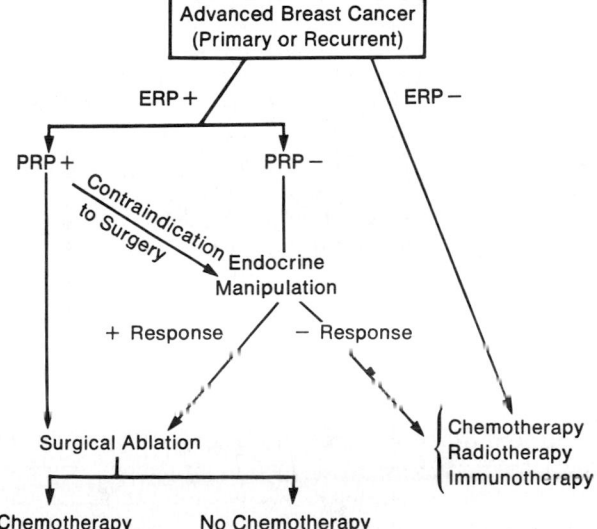

lative therapy (10 percent or less). Such patients, together with the 40 percent who fail to respond to a therapeutic trial of estrogen ablation or antiestrogens, are candidates for cancer chemotherapy. Multiple-drug regimens spaced at much longer intervals than the older single-drug programs are the current mode and have produced a doubling and even tripling of the improvement in the old results with single drugs. Arrest of tumor growth, partial remission, and even complete remissions can be expected in 65 percent of patients so treated. Because of the rapid improvement in the results of chemotherapy, there is now some controversy as to whether hormonal therapy should precede or follow chemotherapy. Wilson and Moore, among several clinicians, have combined total operative estrogen ablation with almost simultaneous cancer chemotherapy in patients with recurrent breast cancer. They suggest that the two forms of therapy work synergistically, with a better response for combination than for sequential use of these techniques when compared with historical controls. No controlled clinical trials are available to confirm this observation, and hormonal therapy remains the first treatment of recurrence at the present. Both therapies are palliative and not curative measures, and most patients will eventually receive most or all of the agents currently available. The aim of therapy is to improve the quality of life and the length of survival, but not as yet to provide cure.

Infection

ACUTE INFECTION

Bacterial infections almost always occur in the lactating breast in the first month or two following delivery. The portal of entry is an abrasion or fissure in the nipple. The best treatment is prevention, with the nursing mother carefully cleaning and drying her nipples after nursing. Because cleanliness is so important, infection more commonly occurs in patients from a lower socioeconomic stratum. It is also seasonal, being more common in the hot summer months.

The milk-containing ducts and acini of the lactating breast are a perfect culture medium, and infection, having gained access, often progresses rapidly through inflammation to suppuration. This is accompanied by extreme pain in the breast, and a good diagnostic sign of abscess is the patient's rapid withdrawal when the physician attempts to palpate the involved breast. The breast is red and the area of abscess indurated and firm. The tendency is to underestimate the size of the abscess on physical examination.

An abscess may be aborted by the use of systemic antibiotics given in the presuppurative period. Treatment of abscess, once it forms, is by surgical drainage. Antibiotics will suppress the process for a time, but it will flare up again when they are discontinued. A curvilinear transverse incision is made in the dependent portion of the breast and the gloved finger or a clamp used to break up the many septa which separate the cavity into loculations. A rubber drain is left in the wound. Culture of the pus usually demonstrates *Staphylococcus aureus*. Pain is relieved promptly by drainage, and the surrounding inflammation subsides rapidly.

CHRONIC INFECTION

Chronic infection of the breast is now rare. Tuberculosis is the major cause, and as the incidence of this disease has decreased, so have breast lesions caused by it. The genesis of breast tuberculosis is either pleural or, more commonly, the breaking down of a mediastinal node to involve one of the costal cartilages. Infection simmers in the cartilage for long periods, giving rise to lesions in the breast, which eventually form one or several fistulas to the skin. Antituberculosis drugs are now the primary treatment for this disease, but care of the breast lesion usually requires excision of the affected costal cartilage.

References

General

Geschickter, C. F.: "Diseases of the Breast," J. B. Lippincott Company, Philadelphia, 1943.
Haagensen, C. D.: "Diseases of the Breast," 2d ed., W. B. Saunders Company, Philadelphia, 1971.

Anatomy and Development

Batson, O. V.: The Function of the Vertebral Veins and Their Role in the Spread of Metastasis, *Ann Surg,* **112:**138, 1940.
Cooper, Sir A. P.: "The Anatomy and Diseases of the Breast," Lea and Blanchard, Philadelphia, 1845.
Ingleby, H., and Gershon-Cohen, J.: "Cooperative Anatomy: Pathology and Roentgenology of the Breast," University of Pennsylvania Press, Philadelphia, 1960.
Taylor, G. T.: Anatomy of the Breast with Particular Reference to Lymphatic Drainage, in W. H. Parson, "Cancer of the Breast," Charles C Thomas, Publisher, Springfield, Ill., 1959.

Examination of the Breast

Berger, S. M., and Gershon-Cohen, J.: Mammography of Breast Sarcoma, *Am J Roentgenol Radium Ther Nucl Med,* **87:**76, 1962.
Clark, R. L., Copeland, M. M., Egan, R. L., Gallagher, H. S., Geller, H., Lindsay, J. P., Robbins, L. C., and White, E. C.: Reproducibility of the Technic of Mammography (Egan) for Cancer of the Breast, *Am J Surg,* **109:**127, 1965.
Gershon-Cohen, J., and Berger, S. M.: Detection of Breast Cancer by Periodic X-ray Examinations: A Five-year Survey, *JAMA,* **176:**1114, 1961.
————, ————, and Klickstein, H. S.: Roentgenography of Breast Cancer Moderating Concept of "Biologic Predeterminism," *Cancer,* **16:**961, 1963.
———— and Ingleby, H.: Roentgenography of Unsuspected Carcinoma of Breast, *JAMA,* **166:**869, 1958.
Ingleby, H., Moore, L., and Gershon-Cohen, J.: A Roentgenographic Study of the Growth Rate of Six "Early" Cancers of the Breast, *Cancer,* **11:**726, 1958.
Snyder, R. E.: Mammography and Lobular Carcinoma In Situ, *Surg Gynecol Obstet,* **122:**255, 1966.
Treves, N., and Holleb, A. I.: Cancer of the Male Breast: A Report of 146 Cases, *Cancer,* **8:**1239, 1955.

Neoplasms

Abramson, D. J.: Delayed Mastectomy after Outpatient Breast Biopsy, *Am J Surg,* **132:**596, 1976.

Adair, F., Berg, J., Joubert, L. and Robbins, G. F.: Long-term Follow-up of Breast Cancer Patients: The 30-Year Report, *Cancer,* **33:**1145, 1974.

Anglem, T. J.: Management of Breast Cancer: Radical Mastectomy, *JAMA,* **230:**99, 1974.

Baclesse, F.: Five-year Results in 431 Breast Cancers Treated Solely by Roentgen Rays, *Ann Surg,* **161:**103, 1965.

Berg, J. W., and Robbins, G. F.: Factors Influencing Short and Long-Term Survival of Breast Cancer Patients, *Surg Gynecol Obstet,* **122:**1311, 1966.

———— and ————: Selection of Treatment Regimens for Women with Potentially Curable Breast Carcinoma, *Am Surg,* **43:**86, 1977.

Blackwood, J. M., Seelig, R. F., Hutter, R. V. P., and Rush, B. F., Jr.: Survival Distribution in Breast Cancer, *Surgery,* **82:**443, 1977.

Bloom, H. J. G., Richardson, W. W., and Harries, E. J.: Natural History of Untreated Breast Cancer (1805–1933): Comparison of Untreated and Treated Cases According to Histological Grade of Malignancy, *Br Med J,* **5299:**213, 1962.

Bonadonna, G., Brusamolino, E., Valagussa, P., Rossi, A., Brugnatelli, L., Brambilla, C., DeLena, M., Tancini, G., Bajetta, E., Musumeci, R., and Veronesi, U.: Combination Chemotherapy as an Adjuvant Treatment in Operable Breast Cancer, *N Engl J Med.,* **294:**405, 1976.

Branfield, J. R., Fingerhut, A. G., and Warner, N. E.: Lobular Carcinoma of the Breast—1969: A Therapeutic Proposal, *Arch Surg,* **99:**129, 1969.

Breslow, L.: Epidemiologic Considerations in Breast Cancer, *Proc 5th Natl Cancer Conf,* Philadelphia, 1965.

Brinkley, D., and Haybittle, J. L.: The Curability of Breast Cancer, *World J Surg,* **1:**287, 1977.

Butcher, H. R., Jr.: Effectiveness of Radical Mastectomy for Mammary Cancer: An Analysis of Mortalities by the Method of Probits, *Ann Surg,* **154:**383, 1961.

————: Radical Mastectomy for Mammary Carcinoma, *Ann Surg,* **157:**165, 1963.

Caceres, E., Lingan, M., and Delgado, P.: Evaluation of Dissection of the Axilla in Modified Radical Mastectomy, *Surg Gynecol Obstet,* **143:**395, 1976.

Cancer Research Campaign Trial: Management of Early Cancer of the Breast, *Br Med J,* **1:**1035, 1976.

Cant, E. L., Smith, A. F., Summerling, M. D., and Forrest, A. P. M.: "Superstaging" in Breast Cancer: A Correlation of Lymph Node Histology and Investigations Designed to Detect Occult Metastic Disease, *World J Surg,* **1:**303, 1977.

Crile, G., Jr.: Management of Breast Cancer: Limited Mastectomy, *JAMA,* **230:**95, 1974.

———— and Hoerr, S. O.: Results of Treatment of Carcinoma of the Breast by Local Excision, *Surg Gynecol Obstet,* **132:**780, 1971.

Cronin, T. D., Upton, J., and McDonough, J. M.: Reconstruction of the Breast after Mastectomy, *Plast Reconstr Surg,* **59:**1, 1977.

Cukier, D. S., Lopez, F. A., and Maravilla, R. B., Jr.: One-View Follow-Up Mammogram: Efficacy in Screening for Breast Cancer, *JAMA,* **237:**661, 1977.

Dahl-Iversen, E., and Tobiassen, T.: Radical Mastectomy with Parasternal and Supraclavicular Dissection for Mammary Carcinoma, *Ann Surg,* **157:**170, 1963.

Degenshein, G. A., Bloom, N., Ceccarelli, F., Daluvoy, R., and Tobin, E.: Estrogen and Progesterone Receptor Site Studies as Guides to the Management of Advanced Breast Cancer, *Breast,* **3:**29, 1977.

Duncan, W., Forrest, A. P. M., Gray, N., Hamilton, T., Langlands, A. O., Prescott, R. J., Shivas, A. A., and Stewart, H. J.: New Edinburgh Primary Breast Cancer Trials: Report By Co-ordinating Committee, *Br J Cancer,* **32:**628, 1975.

———— and Kerr, G. R.: The Curability of Breast Cancer, *Br Med J,* **2:**781, 1976.

Fisher, B.: Cooperative Clinical Trials in Primary Breast Cancer: A Critical Appraisal, *Cancer,* **31:**127, 1973.

————: United States Trials of Conservative Surgery, *World J Surg,* **1:**327, 1977.

————, Carbone, P., Economou, S. G., Frelick, R., Glass, A., Lerner, H., Redmond, C., Zelen, M., Band, P., Katrych, D. L., Wolmark, N., Fisher, E. R. (and Other Co-operating Investigators): 1-Phenylalanine Mustard (L-PAM) in The Management of Primary Breast Cancer: A Report of Early Findings, *N Engl J Med,* **292:**117, 1975.

———— and Fisher, B.: Lobular Carcinoma of the Breast: An Overview, *Ann Surg,* **185:**377, 1977.

————, Ravdin, R. G., Ausman, R. K., Slack, N. H., Moore, G. E., and Noer, R. J.: Surgical Adjuvant Chemotherapy in Cancer of the Breast: Results of a Decade of Cooperative Investigation, *Ann Surg,* **168:**337, 1968.

————, Slack, N. H., Cavanaugh, P. J., Gardner, B., and Ravdin, R. G.: Postoperative Radiotherapy in the Treatment of Breast Cancer: Results of the NSABP Clinical Trial, *Ann Surg,* **172:**711, 1970.

————, ————, ————, ————, and ————: Postoperative Radiotherapy in the Treatment of Breast Cancer: Results of the NSABP Clinical Trial, *Ann Surg,* **172:**711, 1970.

————, ————, Katrych, D. and Wolmark, N.: Ten Year Follow-Up Results of Patients with Carcinoma of the Breast in a Co-operative Clinical Trial Evaluating Surgical Adjuvant Chemotherapy, *Surg Gynecol Obstet,* **140:**528, 1975.

Fletcher, G. H., Montague, E., and White, E. C.: Evaluation of Preoperative Irradiation for Carcinoma for the Breast, *Proc 5th Natl Cancer Conf,* Philadelphia, 1964, 1965.

Foote, F. W., and Stewart, F. W.: Comparative Studies of Cancerous versus Noncancerous Breasts: I. Basic Morphology Characteristics, *Ann Surg,* **121:**6, 1945.

———— and ————: Comparative Studies of Cancerous versus Noncancerous Breasts: II. Mammary Carcinogenesis: Influence of Certain Hormones on Human Breast Structure, *Ann Surg,* **121:**197, 1945.

Forrest, A. P. M., Roberts, M. M., Cant, E., and Shivas, A. A.: Simple Mastectomy and Pectoral Node Biopsy, *Br J Surg,* **63:**569, 1976.

Gardner, B.: Cancer Revisited, *JAMA,* **231:**742, 1975. (Editorial.)

Gibson, E. W.: Reconstruction of the Breast after Mastectomy for Cancer, *Clin Plast Surg,* **3:**371, 1976.

Goldenberg, I. S.: Hormones and Breast Cancer: Historical Perspectives, *Surgery,* **53:**285, 1963.

Green, R. B., Sethi, R. S., and Lindner, H. H.: Treatment of Advanced Carcinoma of the Breast, *Am J Surg,* **108:**107, 1964.

Guttman, R.: Radiotherapy in the Treatment of Primary Operable Carcinoma of the Breast with Proved Lymph Node Metastases: Approach and Results, *Am J Roentgenol Radium Ther Nucl Med,* **89:**58, 1963.

Haagensen, C. D.: The Choice of Treatment for Operable Carcinoma of the Breast, *Surgery,* **76:**685, 1974.

———, Cooley, E., Kennedy, C. S., Miller, E., Handley, R. S., Thackray, A. C., Butcher, H. R., Jr., Dahl-Iversen, E., Tobiassen, T., Williams, I. G., Curwen, M. P., Kaae, S., and Johansen, H.: Treatment of Early Mammary Carcinoma: A Co-operative International Study, *Ann Surg,* **157:**157, 1963.

Handley, R. S.: The Conservative Radical Mastectomy of Patey: 10-Year Results in 425 Patients, *Breast,* **2:**16, 1976.

——— and Thackray, A. C.: The Internal Mammary Lymph Chain in Carcinoma of the Breast: Study of 50 Cases, *Lancet,* **257:**276, 1949.

——— and ———: Conservative Radical Mastectomy (Patey's Operation), *Ann Surg,* **157:**162, 1963.

Hayward, J. L.: The Guy's Trial of Treatments of "Early" Breast Cancer, *World J Surg,* **1:**314, 1977.

Hems, G.: Epidemiological Characteristics of Breast Cancer in Middle and Late Age, *Br J Cancer,* **24:**226, 1970.

Hoge, A. F., Bottomley, R. H., Shaw, M. T., and Asal, N. R.: Adrenalectomy and Oophorectomy plus Limited-Term Chemotherapy in the Treatment of Breast Cancer, *Cancer Treat Rep,* **60:**857, 1976.

Holleb, A. I., Montgomery, R., and Farrow, J. H.: The Hazard of Incomplete Simple Mastectomy, *Surg Gynecol Obstet,* **121:**819, 1965.

James, F., James, V. H. T., Carter, A. E., and Irvine, W. T.: A Comparison of in Vivo and in Vitro Uptake of Estradiol by Human Breast Tumors and the Relationship of Steroid Excretion, *Cancer Res,* **31:**1268, 1971.

Kaae, S., and Johansen, H.: Breast Cancer: A Comparison of Simple Mastectomy with Postoperative Roentgen Irradiation by the McWhirter Method with Those of Extended Radical Mastectomy, *Acta Radiol [Suppl] (Stockh),* **155:**185, 1959.

——— and ———: Simple Mastectomy plus Postoperative Irradiation by the Method of McWhirter for Mammary Carcinoma, *Ann Surg,* **157:**175, 1963.

Karpas, C. M., Leis, H. P., Oppenheim, A., and Mersheimer, W. L.: Relationship of Fibrocystic Disease to Carcinoma of the Breast, *Ann Surg,* **162:**1, 1965.

Kaufman, R. J.: Medical Management of Breast Cancer, *Clin Bull Mem Hosp,* **2:**21, 1972.

Kay, S., and Poulos, N.G.: Evaluation of the Criteria of Operability of Carcinoma of the Breast, *Surg Gynecol Obstet,* **113:**562, 1961.

Kennedy, B. J.: The Role of Castration in Breast Cancer, *Arch Surg,* **88:**743, 1964.

———, Meilke, P. W., Jr., and Fortuny, I. E.: Therapeutic Castration versus Prophylactic Castration in Breast Cancer, *Surg Gynecol Obstet,* **118:**524, 1964.

Kennedy, C. S., and Miller, E.: Simple Mastectomy for Mammary Carcinoma, *Ann Surg,* **157:**161, 1963.

Kleinfeld, G., Haagensen, C. D., and Cooley, E.: Age and Menstrual Status as Prognostic Factors in Carcinoma of the Breast, *Ann Surg,* **157:**600, 1963.

Kraft, R. O., and Block, G. E.: Mammary Carcinoma in the Aged Patient, *Ann Surg,* **156:**981, 1962.

Kramer, W. M., and Rush, B. F., Jr.: Mammary Duct Proliferation in the Elderly: A Histopathologic Study, *Cancer,* **31:**130, 1973.

Kusama, S., Spratt, J. S., Jr., Donegan, W. L., Watson, F. R., and Cunningham, C.: The Gross Rates of Growth of Human Mammary Carcinoma, *Cancer,* **30:**594, 1972.

Lacour, J., Bucalossi, P., Cacers, E., Jacobelli, G., Koszarowski, T., Le, M., Rumeau-Rouquette, C., and Veronesi, U.: Radical Mastectomy Versus Radical Mastectomy Plus Internal Mammary Dissection: Five-Year Results of an International Co-operative Study, *Cancer,* **37:**206, 1976.

Legha, S. S., and Carter, S. K.: Antiestrogens in the Treatment of Breast Cancer, *Cancer Treat Rev,* **3:**205, 1976.

Leung, B. S., Krippaehne, W. W., and Fletcher, W. S.: Prognostic Value of Estrogen Receptor to Endocrine Ablation in Cancer of the Breast, *Surg Gynecol Obstet,* **139:**525, 1974.

Levitt, S. H., and McHugh, R. B.: Radiotherapy in the Postoperative Treatment of Operable Cancer of the Breast: Part I. Critique of the Clinical and Biometric Aspects of the Trials, *Cancer,* **39:**924, 1977.

———, ———, and Song, C. W.: Radiotherapy in the Postoperative Treatment of Operable Cancer of the Breast: Part II. A Re-Examination of Stjernsward's Application of the Mantel-Haenszel Statistical Method: Evaluation of the Effect of the Radiation on Immune Response and Suggestions for Postoperative Radiotherapy, *Cancer,* **39:**933, 1976.

Lewison, E. F.: "Breast Cancer and Its Diagnosis and Treatment," The Williams & Wilkins Company, Baltimore, 1955.

———: The Problem of Prognosis in Cancer of the Breast, *Surgery,* **37:**479, 1955.

———: The Results of Treatment of Breast Cancer at the Johns Hopkins Hospital 1941–1945, with a Discussion, *Surg Gynecol Obstet,* **107:**313, 1958.

———: An Appraisal of Long-Term Results in Surgical Treatment of Breast Cancer, *JAMA,* **186:**975, 1963.

———, and Lyons, J. G., Jr.: Relationship between Benign Breast Disease and Cancer, *Arch Surg,* **66:**94, 1953.

——— and Neto, A. S.: Bilateral Breast Cancer at the Johns Hopkins Hospital: A Discussion of the Dilemma of Contralateral Breast Cancer, **28:**1297, 1971.

Linden, G., Cline, J. W., Wood, D. A., Guiss, L. W., and Breslow, L.: Validity of Pathological Diagnosis of Breast Cancer, *JAMA,* **173:**143, 1960.

MacDonald, I.: The Natural History of Mammary Carcinoma, *Am J Surg,* **111:**435, 1966.

Madden, J. L.: Modified Radical Mastectomy, *Surg Gynecol Obstet,* **121:**1221, 1965.

McWhirter, R.: Treatment of Cancer of the Breast by Simple Mastectomy and Roentgenotherapy, *Arch Surg,* **59:**830, 1949.

Missakian, M. M., Witten, D. M., and Harrison, E. G., Jr.: Mammography after Mastectomy: Usefulness in Search for Recurrent Carcinoma of the Breast, *JAMA,* **191:**1045, 1965.

Moore, D. H., Sarkar, N. H., Kramarsky, B., Lasfargues, E. Y., and Charney, J.: Some Aspects of the Search for a Human Mammary Tumor Virus, *Cancer,* **28:**1415, 1971.

Moore, F. D., Van Devanter, S. B., Boyden, C. M., Lokish, J., and Wilson, R. E.: Adrenalectomy with Chemotherapy in the Treatment of Advanced Breast Cancer: Objective and Subjective Response Rates; Duration and Quality of Life, *Surgery,* **76:**376, 1974.

———, Woodrow, S. I., Aliapoulios, M. A., and Wilson,

R. E.: Carcinoma of the Breast: A Decade of New Results with Old Concepts, *N Engl J Med,* **277:**293, 1967.

Moore, S. W., and Lewis, R. J.: Carcinoma of the Breast in Women 30 Years of Age and Under, *Surg Gynecol Obstet,* **119:**1253, 1964.

Mouridsen, H. T., Palshof, T., Brahm, M., and Rahbek, I.: Evaluation of Single-Drug Versus Multiple-Drug Chemotherapy in the Treatment of Advanced Breast Cancer, *Cancer Treat Rep,* **61:**47, 1977.

Mueller, C. B., and Jeffries, W.: Cancer of the Breast: Its Outcome as Measured by the Rate of Dying and Causes of Pain, *Ann Surg,* **182:**334, 1975.

Murad, T. M.: A Proposed Histochemical and Electron Microscopic Classification of Human Breast Cancer According to Cell of Origin, *Cancer,* **27:**288, 1971.

Murray, J. G., MacIntyre, J., Simpson, J. S., and McDonald, A. M.: Cancer Research Campaign Study of the Management of "Early" Breast Cancer, *World J Surg,* **1:**317, 1977.

Nissen-Myer, R., Kjellgren, K., and Mansson, B.: Preliminary Report from the Scandinavian Adjuvant Chemotherapy Study Group, *Cancer Chemother Rep,* **55:**561, 1971.

Norris, H. J., and Taylor, H. B.: Carcinoma of the Breast in Women Less than Thirty Years Old, *Cancer,* **26:**953, 1970.

Oberman, H. A.: Sarcomas of the Breast, *Cancer,* **18:**1233, 1965.

Owen, H. W., Dockerty, M. B., and Gray, H. K.: Occult Carcinoma of the Breast, *Surg Gynecol Obstet,* **98:**302, 1954.

Pack, G. T.: Argument for Bilateral Mastectomy, *Surgery,* **29:**929, 1951. (Editorial.)

Papaioannou, A. N., and Urban, J. A.: Scalene Node Biopsy in Locally Advanced Primary Breast Cancer of Questionable Operability, *Cancer,* **17:**1006, 1964.

Papdrianos, E., Cooley, E., and Haagensen, C. D.: Mammary Carcinoma in Old Age, *Ann Surg.,* **161:**189, 1965.

Park, W. W., and Lees, J. C.: Absolute Curability of Cancer of the Breast, *Surg Gynecol Obstet,* **93:**129, 1951.

Parson, W. H.: "Cancer of the Breast," Charles C Thomas, Publisher, Springfield, Ill., 1959.

Pennisi, V. R., Capozzi, A., and Perez, F. M.: Subcutaneous Mastectomy Data, *Plast Reconstr Surg,* **59:**53, 1977.

Pichon, M. F., and Milgrom, E.: Characterization and Assay of Progesterone Receptor in Human Mammary Carcinoma, *Cancer Res,* **37:**464, 1977.

Priestman, T., Baum, M., Jones, V., and Forbes, J.: Comparative Trial of Endocrine Versus Cytotoxic Treatment in Advanced Breast Cancer, *Br Med J,* **1:**1248, 1977.

Prohaska, J. V., Houttuin, E., and Kocandrle, V.: Mammary Carcinoma Metastes: Response to Bilateral Adrenalectomy and Oophorectomy, *Arch Surg,* **92:**530, 1966.

Prosnitz, L. R., Goldenberg, I. S., Packard, R. A., Levene, M. B., Harris, J., Hellman, S., Wallner, P. E., Brady, L. W., Mansfield, C. M., and Kramer, S.: Radiation Therapy as Initial Treatment for Early Stage Cancer of the Breast without Mastectomy, *Cancer,* **39:**917, 1977.

Richards, G. J., Jr., and Lewison, E. F.: Inflammatory Carcinoma of the Breast, *Surg Gynecol Obstet,* **113:**729, 1961.

Robbins, G. F., and Berg, J. W.: Bilateral Primary Breast Cancers, *Cancer,* **17:**1501, 1964.

—— and ——: Curability of Patients with Invasive Breast Carcinoma Based on a 30-Year Study, *World J Surg,* **1:**284, 1977.

——, Brothers, J. H., III, Eberhart, W. F., and Quan, S.: Is Aspiration Biopsy of Breast Cancer Dangerous to the Patient? *Cancer,* **7:**774, 1954.

Rosato, F. E., Fink, P. J., Horton, C. E., and Payne, R. L., Jr.: Immediate Postmastectomy Reconstruction, *J Surg Oncolol,* **8:**277, 1976.

Rosen, P. P., Fracchia, A. A., Urban, J. A., Schottenfeld, D., and Robbins, G. F.: "Residual" Mammary Carcinoma Following Simulated Partial Mastectomy, *Cancer,* **35:**739, 1975.

——, Snyder, R. E., Foote, F. W., and Wallace, T.: Detection of Occult Carcinoma in the Apparently Benign Breast Biopsy through Specimen Radiography, *Cancer,* **26:**944, 1970.

Rubin, P.: "Carcinoma of the Breast," American Cancer Society, New York, 1967.

Rush, B. F., Jr.: Axillary Dissection in Breast Cancer: A Staging Procedure, *Surgery,* **77:**478, 1975.

—— and Kramer, W. M.: Proliferative Histological Changes and Occult Carcinoma in the Breast of the Aging Female, *Surg Gynecol Obstet,* **117:**425, 1963.

Sandison, A. T.: An Autopsy Study of the Adult Human Breast, with Special Reference to Proliferative Epithelial Changes of Importance in the Pathology of the Breast, *Natl Cancer Inst Monogr* 8, June 1962.

Sanger, G.: An Aspect of Internal Mammary Metastases from Carcinoma of the Breast, *Ann Surg,* **157:**180, 1963.

Schmidt, M. L., Nemoto, T., and Bross, I. D. J.: Prognostic Factors Affecting Adrenalectomy in Patients with Metastatic Cancer of the Breast, *Cancer,* **27:**1106, 1971.

Schottenfeld, D., Nash, A. G., Robbins, G. F., and Beattie, E. J., Jr.: Ten-Year Results of the Treatment of Primary Operable Breast Carcinoma: A Summary of 304 Patients Evaluated by the TNM System, *Cancer,* **38:**1001, 1976.

Schwartz, H. M., and Reichling, B. A.: The Risks of Mammograms, *JAMA,* **237:**965, 1977.

Seidman, H.: Screening for Breast Cancer in Younger Women: Life Expectancy Gains and Losses: An Analysis According to Risk Indicator Groups, *Ca,* **27:**66, 1977.

Sherlock, P., and Hartmann, W. H.: Adrenal Steroids and the Pattern of Metastases of Breast Cancer, *JAMA,* **181:**103, 1962.

Shimkin, M. B.: Cancer of the Breast: Some Old Facts and New Perspectives, *JAMA,* **183:**358, 1963.

——, Koppel, M., Connelly, R. R., and Cutler, S. J.: Simple and Radical Mastectomy for Breast Cancer: A Re-analysis of Smith and Meyer's Report from Rockford, Illinois, *J Natl Cancer Inst,* **27:**1197, 1961.

Shingleton, W. W., Sedransk, N., and Johnson, R. O.: Systemic Chemotherapy for Mammary Carcinoma, *Ann Surg,* **173:**913, 1971.

Silverstrini, R., Sanfilippo, O., and Tedesco, G.: Kinetics of Human Mammary Carcinomas and Their Correlations with the Cancer and the Host Characteristics, *Cancer,* **34:**1252, 1974.

Strax, P.: New Techniques in Mass Screening for Breast Cancer, *Cancer,* **28:**1563, 1971.

Sugarbaker, E. D.: Extended Radical Mastectomy: Its Superiority in the Treatment of Breast Cancer, *JAMA,* **187:**95, 1964.

Surgical Adjuvant Chemotherapy Breast Group: Breast Adjuvant Chemotherapy: Effectiveness of Thio-tepa (Triethylenethiophosphoramide) as Adjuvant to Radical Mastectomy for Breast Cancer, *Ann Surg,* **154:**629, 1961.

Tellem, M., Prive, L., and Meranze, D. R.: Four-quadrant Study of Breast Removed for Carcinoma, *Cancer,* **15:**10, 1962.

Treves, N., and Holleb, A. I.: Cancer of the Male Breast: A Report of 46 Cases, *Cancer,* **8:**1239, 1955.

Urban, J. A.: Bilaterality of Cancer of the Breast: Biopsy of the Opposite Breast, *Cancer,* **20:**1867, 1971.

——— and Baker, H. W.: Radical Mastectomy in Continuity with En Bloc Resection of the Internal Mammary Lymph-Node Chain: A New Procedure for Primary Operable Cancer of the Breast, *Cancer,* **5:**992, 1952.

Veronesi, U., Rossi, A., and Bonadonna, G.: Adjuvant Combination Chemotherapy with CMF in Primary Mammary Carcinoma, *World J Surg,* **1:**337, 1977.

Wanebo, H. J., Huvos, A. G., and Urban, J. A.: Treatment of Minimal Breast Cancer, *Cancer,* **33:**349, 1974.

Watts, G. T.: Restorative Prosthetic Mammaplasty in Mastectomy for Carcinoma and Benign Lesions, *Clin Plast Surg,* **3:**177, 1976.

Williams, I. G., and Curwen, M. P.: Total Mastectomy with Axillary Dissection and Irradiation for Mammary Carcinoma, *Ann Surg,* **157:**174, 1963.

Willis, K. J., London, D. R., Ward, H. W. C., Butt, W. R., Lynch, S. S., and Rudd, B. T.: Recurrent Breast Cancer Treated with the Antiestrogen Tamoxifen: Correlation between Hormonal Changes and Clinical Course, *Br Med J,* **1:**425, 1977.

Zippin, C., and Petrakis, N. L.: Identification of High Risk Groups in Breast Cancer, *Cancer,* **28:**1381, 1971.

Benign Lesions

Davis, H. H., Simons, M., and Davis, J. B.: Cystic Disease of the Breast: Relationship to Carcinoma, *Cancer,* **17:**957, 1964.

Frantz, V. K., Pickren, J. W., Melcher, G. W., and Auchincloss, H., Jr.: Incidence of Chronic Cystic Disease in So-called "Normal Breasts": A Study Based on 225 Postmortem Examinations, *Cancer,* **4:**762, 1951.

Grow, J. L., and Lewison, E. F.: Superficial Thrombophlebitis of the Breast, *Surg Gynecol Obstet,* **116:**180, 1963.

Urban, J. A.: Excision of Major Ducts of the Breast, *Cancer,* **16:**516, 1963.

Chapter 16

Tumors of the Head and Neck

by Benjamin F. Rush, Jr.

HISTORICAL BACKGROUND

The head and neck are such public regions of the anatomy that one would expect ancient medical manuscripts to give considerable attention to tumors affecting these parts. Strangely, the ancient writers rarely mention such lesions. The Smith Papyrus (2300 B.C.) mentions wounds of the head frequently, but not a single tumor of the area is discussed. The Ebers Papyrus (1500 B.C.) contains references to "eating ulcer" of the gums and "illness of the tongue," but the descriptions are too brief to be adequately interpreted. Celsus (A.D. 178) is often credited with devising an operation for cancer of the lower lip. Martin notes that Celsus recognized and described cancer of the skin of the face, but his operation on the lower lip was for repair of a "mutilation," probably a war wound.

A perusal of *The Surgery of Theodoric* (A.D. 1267) in the translation of Campbell and Colton gives an interesting perspective of the personal experiences of a master surgeon of the era who had a profound knowledge of the writings of preceding centuries. Theodoric describes numerous lesions about the head and neck, mostly of minor significance, i.e., wens, "white pustules or spots which appear by the nose and over the cheeks," "lumps or swellings occurring on the head called horns," "nodes or wens which are formed on the eyelids," lipoma, pustules on the face, freckles, brown patches, wrinkles, and black and blue spots on the face. There is a lengthy section on "the scrofula." He had a much clearer concept of cancer than most of his contemporaries, but in his entire writing he does not mention the treatment of a single lesion of the lip or intraoral area.

This frequent failure to single out cancerous lesions in this area reflects the inability of our medical ancestors to differentiate grossly between chronic infections and cancer. Certainly some miraculous cures were achieved by ointments and spells applied to hard, round ulcers which, in fact, were chronic infections. An early, operable lesion was certain to be treated at length with salves and potions, and when it was evident beyond doubt that the treatment had failed, it was too late to do anything else.

Galen had established firmly the concept that cancer was a systemic disease, an oversupply of black bile. It made more sense by this concept to treat the systemic cause of the affliction by "proper balancing of the constitution" with bleeding or purging or hot and cold baths than it did to attack directly a symptom of the internal problem which happened to occur on the face or in the mouth. The beginnings of rational operations for cancer awaited the discovery of cancer's primary origin in the various organs and the ability to differentiate cancer grossly and microscopically from other confusingly similar diseases.

In addition to the problems of diagnosis, extensive cancer operations were impossible without anesthesia. Even minor operations about the head and neck were few when the patient had to be conscious to witness them. The gruesome habit of excising the tongue for torture and punishment is as old as man, but the first such excision for cancer is attributed to Marchette in 1664. Avicenna (980–1037) described excision of tumors of the lip, the wound being left open to heal by secondary intention, but the classic V excision for cancer of the lip was not described until the first part of the nineteenth century. Tracheotomy to relieve laryngeal obstruction was described by Galen and through the ages was occasionally used to prolong somewhat the lives of those with carcinoma of the larynx, but

laryngectomy was not accomplished until the late nineteenth century.

With the advent of anesthesia and microscopic pathology in the mid-1800s, operative attack upon cancer in all areas moved swiftly forward. This was especially true of tumors of the head and neck, since they involved easily seen structures and were so readily diagnosed and the suffering of the untreated patients was so apparent. Surgeons of the German school introduced an array of new techniques for operations upon the tongue, gingiva, mandible, maxilla, and larynx. Partial laryngectomy was introduced by Gurdon Buck in 1853, and total laryngectomy for cancer was first accomplished by Billroth in 1873.

In general, the results of these new procedures were more horrifying than gratifying. Operations in a septic field and without antibiotics produced a postoperative complication rate close to 100 percent with cellulitis, sepsis, abscess, pneumonia, and death the common results. Mortality rates exceeded 50 percent. Moreover, the results of many of the early and unsophisticated operations were not much better than if the cancer had not been treated. Billroth's famous first laryngectomy left the patient with an open pharyngostome and esophagostome, so that he constantly drooled saliva over his neck and had to feed himself with a rubber tube during the entire 8 months that he survived operation.

Operative excision was usually confined to the primary lesion, and in many of the patients fortunate enough to survive the initial operation metastatic disease subsequently developed in cervical nodes. Kocher and Butlin recognized this problem early and recommended excision of the lymphatic contents of the anterior triangle of the neck together with the removal of the primary lesion in the mouth.

At the turn of the century Crile devised radical neck dissection, removing all lymphatic tissue in both the anterior and posterior triangles of the neck together with the jugular vein and the sternocleidomastoid muscle. The basic elements of his classic procedure remain valid to the present.

Patients were willing to risk the high morbidity and mortality of operations in this region because the relentless progress of untreated disease offered a slow death by asphyxia, malnutrition, and eventual hemorrhage. Even the slimmest chance of avoiding this terrible triad seemed worthwhile.

As Crile was developing his operation for treating the cervical lymph nodes, radiation therapy for cancer was introduced. This, it was quickly apparent, offered a preferable alternative to operation, especially for primary lesions of the skin and oral cavity. Until the end of the 1930s most radical operations for cancers of the head and neck were abandoned, and the primary therapy was radiation. Techniques of radiation therapy became more refined and more successful. External radiation replaced radium as the treatment of choice, and fractionated therapy replaced the use of single applications of radium or a single dose of external therapy. With each refinement the percentage of patients who were cured increased. It was soon found that metastatic deposits in the neck did not respond as well to radiation as to operation, and radical neck dissection remained in use. Occasionally, patients who failed to respond to radiation or who had recurrent cancers were submitted to one or another of the old radical procedures. But when these operations were performed in a heavily irradiated fibrotic field, wound breakdown and complications often resembled the results of surgical treatment of the prior century.

In the 1940s, the introduction of endotracheal anesthesia, liberal use of blood transfusions, and antibiotics markedly changed the ability of surgeons to operate in and about the oral cavity. Postoperative morbidity and mortality dropped to a reasonable level. Radiation therapy, so long dominant in the treatment of oral lesions, seemed at a plateau with much dissatisfaction concerning the morbidity of overtreatment. These factors led to a reevaluation of operation. Grant Ward of The Johns Hopkins Hospital and Hayes Martin of the Memorial Center for Cancer led in devising combined operations whereby the primary lesions and the cervical contents were removed in a single block.

Application of this principle improved substantially the prognosis of patients with head and neck carcinomas, especially large lesions involving the oral cavity, hypopharynx, and larynx. In some institutions the pendulum swung from almost exclusive use of radiotherapy to almost exclusive use of operation. Increasing application of these combined operations during the 1950s made possible an evaluation of their mortality, morbidity, and effectiveness. By the end of the decade the place for surgical control of head and neck lesions was much more clearly defined and accepted.

Because of the late development of operative therapy after the long period of dormancy during the radiation era, this field of surgery is still something of a frontier with rapid developments of new techniques and the evolution of new ideas and approaches.

In the meantime, radiation therapy also acquired new techniques. Supervoltage radiation, originally with cobalt 60 and later with linear accelerators, delivered higher doses of therapy with a decreased morbidity, especially sparing the patient's skin and leaving a field more suitable for operation when this was required. Radiotherapists and surgeons who previously tended to disparage the results of each other's methods and to advance their own techniques as the primary treatment for tumors suddenly found that there was considerable common ground for the two methods and that there were patients who frequently could benefit from both operation and radiation as a planned course of integrated treatment.

Detection of most lesions of the head and neck is relatively easy, since the majority are readily available to the eye and the examining finger. Even so, it is tragic to find how often malignant lesions of this area are overlooked, not only lesions more difficult to diagnose, as in the maxillary sinuses and hypopharynx, but lesions readily visualized, such as tumors of the floor of the mouth, tongue, and tonsil.

DIAGNOSIS

Physical Examination

SKIN. The skin (see Chap. 14) of the face and neck should be closely scrutinized, keeping in mind that basal and squamous carcinomas of the skin are the most common of all cancers and that the most common site for such lesions is the area of the head and neck. Seborrheic keratosis, senile keratosis, and patches of atrophic skin often appear side by side with skin neoplasms. Differential diagnosis may be difficult, and biopsy is often required. Pigmented lesions must be examined closely to determine the presence of bleeding ulceration or satellitosis indicating melanoma. All lumps should be palpated to observe their firmness, whether they have a cystic or solid quality and whether they are fixed to the underlying tissues.

ORAL CAVITY. The oral cavity is often neglected in the course of a complete physical examination. It is said that the internist looks at the top of the tongue depressor, the otolaryngologist looks at the tonsils, and the general surgeon may not look at all. There is no excuse for this neglect, since the oral cavity is a rich source of pathologic processes, not only of local lesions, but often of lesions reflecting pathologic conditions elsewhere in the body.

Proper examination requires the use of a tongue depressor, finger cot or glove, and good lighting. If the examiner is skilled with the use of a head mirror, this will provide ideal illumination. However, there are numerous electric headlights which work equally well and which can be used at different points in the office or at the bedside without requiring an elaborate setup.

With the patient's mouth open, the light is directed into the oral cavity. If the patient has dentures of any sort, they should be removed. The examiner begins by looking at the anterior floor of the mouth and the openings of Wharton's ducts. Then the floor of the mouth is observed, progressing posteriorly along the gingivolingual gutter to the tonsillar pillars on either side. The undersurface of the anterior and lateral tongue can also be observed. This is a good place to detect early jaundice.

The lower gingiva and teeth are examined next. The condition of the teeth and the presence or absence of sepsis are considered. The gingivobuccal gutters are often the hiding place of small malignant lesions and should be inspected thoroughly.

The buccal mucosa can be examined next. Patches of hyperkeratosis are often seen here. The examiner looks for the nipple indicating the opening of Stensen's duct. Pressure on the parotid should express saliva from the orifice. The position and mobility of the tongue are observed. A deviated tongue may indicate injury to the hypoglossal nerve or a previous stroke. Numerous longitudinal fissures reflect previous syphilis, a condition now rarely seen. Malignant lesions are normally found on the edges or at the tip of the tongue.

Occasionally, a patch of dirty fibers will occupy the surface of the tongue. This condition, called "hairy tongue," often occurs in a dry mouth with impaired sali-

Fig. 16-1. Torus, a congenital lesion formed along the median raphe where the palatine processes of the maxilla join. These protuberances are normally smooth; the lobulation seen here is unusual.

vary secretion. Vitamin deficiencies are reflected by an atrophy of the taste buds with a flat, smooth, erythematous mucosa.

The tonsils and soft palate are considered next. The presence or absence of the tonsils or tonsillar tags should be noted. If the patient gags, the posterior tonsillar pillars rotate toward the midline, better exposing the tonsillar fossa itself. The anterior tonsillar pillar is a common site for patches of hyperkeratosis, or sometimes for very early carcinomas. Inappropriate hypertrophy of one tonsil may reflect a lymphoma. Paralysis of one side of the soft palate is often seen in patients who have had a cerebrovascular accident. Large tumors in the nasopharynx may push the soft palate forward and down.

The examiner can complete his observations with inspection of the hard palate. A smooth or occasionally lobular elevation running down the midline of the palate is usually a torus, a harmless, congenital deformity (Fig. 16-1). Tori of the mandible also occur, projecting into the mouth bilaterally at the level of the canine tooth. They have no particular importance except to the frightened patient who may notice them for the first time in adulthood and mistake them for new growths. Occasionally, patients with atrophied lower alveoli following total loss of the lower teeth will have a spur which projects backward from the midline into the floor of the mouth. This represents a prominence of the symphysis made detectable by the absorption of the surrounding bone.

Palpation is equal in importance to inspection. Many early lesions of the oral cavity cannot be detected except by the sense of touch. This is especially true of lesions buried within the substance of the tongue or in the salivary glands. The gloved finger is passed over the tongue, the floor of the mouth, and the gingivobuccal gutters. Any mass encountered can be made more prominent by bimanual or bidigital palpation, pressing the mass inward from the cheek or submental area toward the oral cavity. If the patient can tolerate it, palpation of the lateral pharyngeal wall may reveal masses in the deep lobe of the parotid. If the index of suspicion is high concerning lesions in the nasopharynx or base of tongue, these areas should be palpated as well.

NECK. Inspection and palpation of the cervical area are done methodically, keeping in mind a distinct list of structures to be felt. These should include the larynx, thyroid, trachea, sternocleidomastoid muscle, lymph node–bearing areas, and salivary glands. The submental area is examined for the presence of enlarged lymph nodes and the size and consistency of the submaxillary glands. In the older patient they may hang low in the anterior cervical triangle as the enveloping fascia becomes lax with age. In this location they often are mistaken initially for enlarged lymph nodes. The presence of any enlarged or firm lymph nodes incorporated within the substance of the submaxillary gland should be noted. Bimanual palpation through the floor of the mouth helps greatly.

The angle of the jaw is a common site for enlarged lymph nodes or not infrequently of a tumor in the tail of the parotid gland. The anterior border of the sternocleidomastoid may overlap a cystic mass representing a branchial cleft cyst. Cystic or fluctuant masses in the posterior cervical triangle may represent a lipoma or a cystic lymphangioma.

The most important consideration in the adult is the presence of enlarged lymph nodes. A number of structures in the neck deceive the novice and at first appear to be enlarged lymph nodes when in fact they are normal structures. The carotid bulb is commonly so mistaken, especially in older patients in whom arteriosclerosis has diminished or obliterated the pulse at the bulb. The tip of the hyoid bone adjacent to the carotid bulb sometimes fools the unwary, unless they are clever enough to palpate for this structure bilaterally. The posterior belly of the omohyoid muscle as it crosses the posterior triangle in the thin patient can mimic a fusiform node until the examiner realizes that the ends of the apparent node cannot be felt. Also in thin patients the tips of the transverse process of the second cervical vertebra are felt posterior to the ascending ramus of the mandible and may seem like a lymph node until it is realized that the structures are bony in consistency and bilateral.

Masses in the thyroid are best felt if the examiner stands behind the patient and palpates the lobes of the gland between thumb and forefinger. A midline mass just above the isthmus of the thyroid may represent an enlarged lymph node, a pyramidal lobe of thyroid, or a thyroglossal duct cyst.

PARANASAL SINUSES. The paranasal sinuses are relatively inaccessible to physical examination. Neoplastic lesions often hide within these recesses and are not manifest until quite late. Bulging, particularly asymmetric bulging of one maxillary sinus, can best be appreciated by observing the cheeks from above either by having the patient lean toward the examiner or by standing above the patient and looking down (Fig. 16-2). Palpation of the maxillary, ethmoid, or temporal areas may elicit tenderness or a sense of fullness. Transillumination of the sinuses by a bright light placed within the oral cavity of a patient in a dark room may reveal opacification of one or more of the sinuses. This is a relatively crude method of examination compared to x-ray examination.

INDIRECT LARYNGOSCOPY. There is a common misconception that indirect laryngoscopy is an examination to be performed only by specialists. Hoarseness and throat pain are such common symptoms and cancer of the pharynx and larynx so frequent that indirect laryngoscopy should be part of the armamentarium of any physician and part of the routine general physical examination.

The patient is seated in a chair slightly higher than the chair or stool of the examiner. The examiner sits opposite him with his right thigh and knee parallel and immediately adjacent to the right thigh and knee of the patient. The patient should extend his neck, thrusting his chin straight forward, as though he had just finished sneezing. The patient's tongue is wrapped in a gauze sponge, and the examiner, if he is right-handed, grasps the tip of the tongue between the thumb and second finger of the left hand, using the first finger to elevate the patient's upper lip. The tongue is drawn forward, and the patient is instructed to breathe rapidly in short, quick breaths, to "pant like a dog." As long as the patient continues to breathe in this fashion, gagging is inhibited. The examiner inserts a medium to large laryngeal mirror, previously flamed to keep it from fogging, into the oropharynx and shines his headlight on the mirror, reflecting a spot of light down into the hypopharynx (Fig. 16-3).

If one is a novice with the head mirror, an electric head lamp should be used. With the mirror in the oropharynx and directed downward, the posterior third of the tongue, the lateral pharyngeal wall, the posterior pharyngeal wall, the epiglottis, the valleculae, and the pyriform sinuses can all be examined thoroughly. The epiglottis will usually hide most of the glottic opening, and only the posterior portions of the arytenoids may be seen at first. The patient is told to breathe deeply several times. This often throws the uvula forward until more of the glottic opening and a little of the subglottic space is seen. The patient is asked to attempt to enunciate an "ee" sound. This throws the epiglottis even farther forward and usually brings the entire glottis, including the anterior commissure, into view.

The false cords, aryepiglottic folds, and posterior epiglottis can now be examined. The movement of the cords is considered, to determine whether both are moving adequately and whether they meet in the midline. Paralysis of one cord may indicate a malignant lesion in the mediastinum or cervical area or may be related to previous operation or cerebrovascular accident. If nodules in the pharynx or posterior tongue are noted, they should subsequently be palpated. As the examiner acquires skill in this procedure, most of these examinations can be accomplished without local anesthesia. Topical anesthesia with lidocaine 1% (preferably) or Pontocaine 1% should be used by the beginner.

In one or two patients out of every twenty, examination is incomplete or impossible because of a hypersensitive gag reflex or an acquired or congenital malformation of the

Fig. 16-2. Early swelling of the maxilla, seen best from above, as shown here. The patient had a space-occupying lesion within the sinus which was not as well appreciated in the frontal view.

epiglottis which makes visualization of the glottis impossible. In such instances, direct laryngoscopy must be used. While direct laryngoscopy is the more sophisticated and complex procedure, indirect laryngoscopy actually gives a

Fig. 16-3. Laryngeal mirror examination of the larynx. Cross section of the oral cavity illustrates the relation of the mirror to the larynx. Insert: View seen by the examiner. Note the epiglottis hiding the anterior portion of the cords.

BASE OF TONGUE

EPIGLOTTIS
VALLECULA

FALSE CORD

VOCAL CORD

ARYTENOID PROCESS

PYRIFORM
SINUS

better overall picture of the larynx and pharynx. The chief reason for resorting to direct laryngoscopy other than the above is the necessity of biopsy of lesions deep in the larynx. Direct laryngoscopy is sometimes performed using a *suspension laryngoscope,* which, once the cords are visualized, can be fixed in place so that the operator does not have to use his hands to hold the laryngoscope. This technique can be combined with the use of an optical device which greatly magnifies the cords so that small irregularities and tiny lesions may be examined. Occasionally in patients with unexplained hoarseness this approach will reveal very early any localized benign and malignant changes.

NASOPHARYNGOSCOPY. The mirror used for indirect laryngoscopy may be turned over and directed upward. The examiner, standing at the patient's shoulder and depressing the tongue with a tongue blade, may shine his headlight on the mirror and gain a fairly spacious view of the nasopharynx. In most instances the space between the soft palate and posterior pharyngeal wall is too small for the nasopharynx to be adequately visualized in this fashion. If physical findings or the history so indicate, complete examination of the nasopharynx is done by inserting a soft rubber #10 French catheter through either nasal passage, drawing its tip out through the mouth and retracting the soft palate forward, revealing the entire nasopharynx for indirect examination by the mirror (Fig. 16-4). The torus tubarius, the openings of the eustachian tubes, the posterior surface of the soft palate, the posterior aspect of the nasal septum arching back toward the sphe-

Fig. 16-4. Mirror view of the nasopharynx. Soft palate is drawn forward, and the mirror in the oropharynx is directed upward. Insert: View seen in the mirror.

MIDDLE
TURBINATE

INF. TURBINATE

SEPTUM

noid sinus, and the posterior tips of the turbinates are seen. The normal lymphatic tissue of the adenoids may lend a granular appearance to some of the posterior and superior mucosal surfaces.

The direct nasopharyngoscope is an instrument which can be used in the office. It is a small instrument like a miniature cystoscope and has a Foroblique or right-angled lens. The diameter of the tube is 5 to 8 mm, and the visual field is quite small and easily obscured by mucus or blood. Use of this instrument is a valuable adjunct to indirect inspection of the nasopharynx and is particularly helpful in searching for small neoplasms.

Diagnostic Studies

RADIOGRAPHY. Most of the bones of the face and neck are adjacent to air-filled cavities or are air-containing, creating an excellent situation for diagnostic roentgenograms. Lesions of the paranasal sinuses, nasal cavity, orbit, mandible, and larynx are readily revealed.

Arteriography. Injection of contrast medium into the vessels is a useful maneuver for evaluating tumors within the cranium or evaluating the arterial tree but has only rare indications for the evaluation of tumors in this region. The rare carotid body tumor can be nicely outlined by the use of radiopaque medium injected into the appropriate common carotid artery, and its appearance when examined in this fashion is pathognomonic. At times, arteriography is useful to outline the extent of a hemangioma of the face or oral cavity (Fig. 16-5).

Laminography. This technique is of great usefulness in examinations of the head and neck, especially for minute examination of the bony walls of the paranasal sinuses. Usually, the clouding of a paranasal sinus by tumor and by infection cannot be differentiated by x-ray unless obvious evidence of bone erosion is seen. Early detection of such erosions is best seen in laminographs. Tumors of the larynx are easily seen from above by indirect laryngoscopy, but their inferior extent is hidden from view unless the lesion is very small. Laminograms and lateral soft tissue views of the larynx play a useful role in revealing the extent of subglottic extension and often the degree of involvement of the pyriform sinuses, which may not otherwise be detectable (Fig. 16-6). Details of retropharyngeal and esophageal tumor spread can be seen on the lateral soft tissue view. Laryngograms are performed by the application of barium to the back of the tongue, cords, epiglottis, and all of the intrinsic larynx. A very clear examination of laryngeal structures can be obtained which offers excellent correlation with other diagnostic methods available.

BIOPSY. The vast majority of head and neck lesions can be easily biopsied in the office or clinic. The tools required are simple, and the procedure is short and uncomplicated. Lesions of the lip, skin, gingiva, floor of the mouth, tongue, and buccal mucosa can quickly be biopsied with a 4-mm dermatologist's skin punch. The area to be biopsied is cleansed with an antiseptic agent infiltrated with a small amount of local anesthesia, and the skin punch is pressed into the lesion to a depth of 4 to 6 mm, cutting a small disk of the tumor, and is withdrawn. The core of tissue which is still connected at its base is grasped with forceps, pulled up until the base is flush with the surface tissues, and cut off with a small pair of scissors. A silver nitrate stick thrust into the depth of the remaining cavity and mild pressure for a minute or two control bleeding in almost all instances. Lesions of the soft palate, tonsillar pillar, or posterior tongue which cannot be reached with a skin punch can often be biopsied easily and quickly with a cervical biopsy forcep; the techniques of anesthesia and hemostasis are essentially the same as described above.

If skill is obtained with indirect laryngoscopy, lesions of the lateral pharyngeal wall, pyriform sinus, epiglottis, and aryepiglottic folds can often be quickly biopsied in the office. While similar biopsies of the true and false cords sometimes can be achieved with skillful manipulation of the indirect mirror, such procedures are best carried out under direct laryngoscopy. Manipulation of biopsy forceps immediately above the cords is much more difficult for the patient to tolerate and may stimulate laryngeal spasm and bleeding at a site where aspiration of blood into the trachea is likely.

Biopsy of the primary lesion is always preferable, but sometimes although cervical nodes are enlarged, no primary tumor can be found. If so, needle biopsy of cervical nodes is indicated and is a rewarding procedure when the node contains metastatic squamous carcinoma. This neoplasm is easily diagnosed even with the smallest fragments of tissue. Nodes involved by lymphoma, on the other hand, are virtually impossible to diagnose by needle biopsy. Positive results of needle biopsy are useful and timesaving; the negative result of a needle biopsy has no significance and must be followed by open biopsy.

There has been much controversy concerning the tendency to spread tumor cells with the use of needle biopsies, and certainly it seems likely that tumor cells are spread into the needle tract by this manipulation. However, this is of greater theoretical than practical importance. Long experience with this technique at a number of major centers has not produced any gross difference in survival rates on long-term follow-up either in the head and neck or elsewhere. Open biopsy of a lymph node seems just as likely to scatter tumor cells, and even more widely.

VITAL DYES. Many cancers of the oral mucosa in their early stages are soft and superficial. They may have an erythematous appearance rather than a white color as usually thought and can easily escape detection even in a careful examination. If suspicion is aroused by a vaguely erythematous patch, the application of toluidine blue will aid in making the diagnosis. This technique will distinguish areas of dysplasia and carcinoma in situ as well as frank carcinoma of the mucosa. The method has its chief use in mapping out the full extent of dysplastic areas or areas of intraepithelial carcinoma.

CYTOLOGY. As used in the oral cavity exfoliative cytology is a superficial biopsy, since it does not reflect collection of fluid from the entire oral cavity but involves scraping a specific lesion with a spatula and spreading this scraping on a slide. Such cytologic examinations, therefore,

Fig. 16-5. Arteriographic demonstration of hemangioma of the oral cavity. On physical examination, only the cheek appeared involved. In the x-ray view, involvement of the lateral pharyngeal wall and oral cavity is noted. (*From B. F. Rush, Jr., Ann Surg, 164:921, 1966.*)

require a specific area of suspicion compared to sampling of an entire anatomic area such as in the cervix or bronchial tree. If a specific lesion is present, it is best evaluated by an actual biopsy. The chief virtue of oral cytology is that the physician who cannot bring himself to use office biopsy techniques or who feels they are beyond his competence can still have the opportunity to obtain a histologic specimen from the lesion in question. Unlike biopsy, cytology has no significance when it is negative. Thus, cytology will establish the presence of a lesion but cannot be relied on to rule that a questionable lesion is not malignant.

LIP

Squamous cell carcinomas of the lip are one of the common malignant tumors of the oral cavity, constituting 15 percent of all such lesions and 2.2 percent of all cancers. Basal cell carcinoma is much less frequent; only about 3 are seen for every 100 squamous cell carcinomas of the lip. Benign lesions which are occasionally seen in the lips include mucous cysts, tumors of the minor salivary glands, hemangiomas, lymphangiomas, venous lakes, fibromas, fissures, and hyperkeratosis.

ETIOLOGY. Like tumors of the skin, there is an important relationship between tumors of the lip and exposure to sunlight. About one-third of patients have a history of working outdoors, and the incidence of malignant squa-

Fig. 16-6. Laminogram of the pharynx. Indirect laryngoscopy would show only the supraglottic portion of the tumor. The laminographic view indicates the large transglottic and subglottic component of the lesion. [*From B. F. Rush and R. H. Greenlaw (eds)., "Integrated Radiation and Operation in Cancer Therapy: A Symposium," Charles C Thomas, Publisher, Springfield, Ill., 1968.*]

mous cancers of the lip increases progressively the farther south the latitude of the patient population being considered. Thus, in the United States the highest incidence is in Florida and Texas. Actinic rays are stronger at higher altitudes and in dryer air, and in areas having these features the incidence of lip (and skin) cancer is increased. Fishermen, sailors, and farmers are among the occupational groups with an increased incidence.

Complexion also plays a role. Susceptible types are fair-skinned, light, blond or ginger-haired, and blue-eyed, with the kind of complexion that freckles and burns rather than tans on exposure to the sun. Resistant people have the opposite characteristics: they are brunet and dark-skinned; blacks are rarely affected.

While there is a relation between lip cancer and tobacco, the exact cause for this is less apparent than in patients with lesions of the intraoral area, larynx, or lungs. The average cigarette smoker receives almost no carcinogen from his tobacco directly to the lips, since the smoke is drawn into the oral cavity and tracheobraonchial tree without passing over the mucosa of the lips themselves. Some feel that the inmates of nursing homes and institutions are more prone to have carcinoma of the lip from cigarette smoking. Smokers in this population usually treasure their cigarettes, smoking them down to the smallest possible butt. Macerated, moist tobacco and heat are directly applied to the lips.

Reports in the literature implicating pipe smoking as a cause of lip cancer have been appearing since 1795, and the Advisory Committee to the Surgeon General on Smoking and Health has accepted the causal relationship as established. Pipestems of wood and clay which soak up tobacco tars directly and apply a "tar poultice" to the lips have been viewed with special suspicion. In any case, such stems are little used now, and indeed the incidence of cancer of the lip in the United States has been gradually decreasing over the past 30 years. One may speculate whether this reflects the decrease in pipe smoking, outdoor work, use of wood and clay pipestems, or a combination of these and other factors.

Cancer of the lip in women is very rare, occurring in only 1 woman for every 20 to 30 men.

Benign Tumors

The mucosa of the inner surface of the upper and lower lips is subject to the same benign lesions as those throughout the mucosa of the oral cavity. These are discussed in greater detail in the following section, Oral Cavity, and include such lesions as mucous cysts, hemangiomas, tumors of the minor salivary glands, hyperkeratosis, and inflammatory hyperplasia. Specific benign lesions that involve the exposed borders of the lips include venous lakes, pigmented spots, hemangiomas, and very rarely neuromas. Venous lakes are a telangiectasis, usually of the lower lip, occurring in older individuals as a small bluish spot. They appear to have no pathologic significance. The other three lesions all have interesting systemic correlations. Multiple pigmented spots of the lips may be associated with Peutz-Jeghers syndrome and denote the presence of multiple small intestinal polyps, which sometimes lead to bleeding and intussusception but are rarely malignant. Scattered small hemangiomas of the lip may be associated with similar lesions elsewhere in the oral cavity and gastrointestinal tract, those of Rendu-Osler-Weber disease. Neuromas of the lips, particularly at the commissures, suggest a neuroendocrine dysplasia, a fascinating syndrome associated with pheochromocytomas, medullary carcinoma of the thyroid, hyperparathyroidism, and hypertrophy of the gastrointestinal myenteric plexus.

Hyperkeratosis

This is a premalignant condition of the lips, usually associated with long exposure to sunlight. It typically occurs in a fair-skinned individual in his sixties or seventies who has a long history of outdoor employment. The normal distinct line marking the mucocutaneous border becomes indistinct and gradually retreats, indicating a metaplasia of the outer portion of the mucosa to a keratosquamous epithelium. The mucosa of the lip becomes paler, thinner, and more fragile. There may be perpendicular cracks and fissures. On this base, a white film indicative of early hyperkeratosis appears. This may grow gradually thicker and more exophytic as the condition progresses (Fig. 16-7) or may remain stationary for many years. Gradually, a small area of scabbing and ulceration occurs. This breakdown within the hyperkeratotic tissue represents a failure of the less resistant areas of hyperkeratosis to tolerate normal wear and tear. When such areas of ulceration appear, they continue to break down and heal and often give rise to carcinoma in situ and eventually invasive carcinoma. Persistent hyperkeratosis is a distinct premalignant lesion, and 35 to 40 percent of all carcinomas of the lip are preceded by this condition. Cancers arising on such a base can be prevented by excising the entire exposed mucosa of the lip, elevating the protected mucosa of the inner lip, and advancing it over the bed of the excised mucosa to form a new lining for the lip. This procedure is called a *lip stripping and resurfacing*.

Carcinoma of the Lip

Most cancers of the lip are squamous carcinomas. When basal cell carcinomas appear, they usually involve the skin of the lip beyond the vermillion border and probably should be considered with the cancers of the skin of the face. Ninety-three percent of the squamous cancers occur on the lower lip. These are usually low-grade, well-differentiated lesions, 80 percent being grade 1 or grade 2. The lesions most frequently start on the outer edge of the mucosa at the vermillion border and seem to favor the middle two-thirds of the lip somewhat more frequently than the commissures (Fig. 16-8).

The natural history of these lesions is of slow but relentless growth. Some grow to great size, destroying the entire lip without ever metastasizing, but the incidence of metastasis gradually increases with the increasing size of the tumors (Fig. 16-9). About 5 to 10 percent of all patients with lip cancer have cervical lymph node metastasis, and in half of these patients only one lymph node is involved. The normal spread of cancer from the lower lip is by way of lymphatics to the submental node on the side of the lesion. Metastases do not involve the opposite submental node unless the primary lesion crosses the midline. Lesions of the upper lip drain to lymph nodes in the anterior portion of the submaxillary gland.

An ulcer of the lip which fails to heal is soon detected by the patient or his friends, and in most urban populations such lesions quickly come to the attention of physi-

Fig. 16-7. Hyperkeratosis of lower lip. This degree of hyperkeratosis merits serious concern. The entire lower lip is involved and should be treated by excision (lip stripping) and advancement of the mucosa of the inner lip to cover the defect.

cians. In rural populations it is surprising how long patients will carry these ulcerations before seeking medical aid.

Treatment for carcinoma of the lip has remained a topic of controversy between radiotherapists and surgeons for many decades. Recent controlled series comparing treatment by both modalities in randomly selected patients indicate that there is no statistical difference between the two methods in terms of cure rate. The choice for therapy must be made on other grounds. Small lesions of the lip can usually be excised under local anesthesia with little or no hospitalization time. Good radiation therapy producing maximal regression with minimal residual scarring requires 2 to 4 weeks of outpatient therapy. Medium-sized lesions require the use of flaps from the upper lip or elsewhere for closure, and for these lesions radiotherapy often requires the same or less time and less morbidity.

Fig. 16-8. Squamous carcinoma of lip. Any patient with a chronic ulcer of this sort should seek medical advice. The chance of cure at this early stage approaches 100 percent.

Fig. 16-9. Neglected carcinoma of the lip. A metastatic node is present along the line of the mandible. The chance of cure for this type of lesion is 50 percent or less.

For very large lesions which have destroyed most of the lip and are associated with metastasis to the neck, subsequent repair of the lip will be required under any circumstance as well as probable radical neck dissection for removal of cervical nodes; for these major lesions an integration of radiation and surgical therapy may be used to improve cure rates, which are relatively low for either radiation or operation alone. A final consideration is that most carcinomas of the lip are related to solar radiation. Since radiotherapy increases the sensitivity of tissues to such exposure, it is best to avoid radiotherapy in patients who expect to return to outdoor occupations.

Prognosis for lip cancers of 1 cm or less is excellent, ranging from an 87 to 95 percent 5-year survival rate without recurrence. Neglected lesions, especially with associated cervical metastasis, do much more poorly, with a 5-year survival of 50 percent.

ORAL CAVITY

The oral cavity includes the buccal mucosa, upper and lower gingivae, anterior two-thirds of the tongue (that portion anterior to the circumvallate papillae), floor of the mouth, and hard palate.

INCIDENCE. Eight percent of all malignant tumors occur in this area, 95 percent of such tumors being squamous carcinomas. The risk of carcinomas developing here in a male is approximately 1 percent in a lifetime. The risk in females is far less: oral cancer develops in about 1 woman for every 10 males. Benign tumors of the oral cavity are common in both sexes.

ETIOLOGY. Some benign lesions have a specific cause, which will be discussed with the descriptions of the lesions below. Contributing causes to squamous carcinoma are smoking, a heavy intake of alcohol, poor oral hygiene, and syphilis. While cancer often occurs without the presence

of any of these factors, they are associated with a majority of the lesions seen.

The *Report on Smoking and Health* by the Advisory Committee to the Surgeon General notes a suggestive relationship between smoking and oral carcinoma. This is especially true in pipe and cigar smokers, where oral cancer has the highest mortality ratio, 3.3,* of all causes of death compared with the nonsmoking population. There are a number of exotic cancers of the oral cavity which serve to indicate the relationship of tobacco to cancer. In Andhra Pradesh, a state in India, the habit of smoking a cigar (i.e., *chutta*) with the burning end inside the mouth is widespread. Carcinoma of the palate, called *chutta cancer,* is common. Presumably, repeated thermal trauma and/or tobacco smoke provide the carcinogenic agents.

In Uttar Pradesh and Bihar, a mixture of tobacco and slaked lime is habitually sucked by men of the districts. The quid is kept in the lower gingivolabial fornix for many hours during the day; a high incidence of carcinoma is found at this site. This has come to be called *khaini cancer,* from the name of the tobacco-lime mixture.

Betel-nut chewing is a common habit among the Indians, Javanese, and Malayans. The chew is made of a mixture of ground betel nut, slaked lime, and spices, such as ginger or pepper. These are wrapped in a betel leaf and chewed. The Indians add tobacco to their betel preparations and have a high incidence of oral cancer, whereas the incidence is low among the Javanese and Malayans, who consume their betel nut without benefit of the tobacco additive. Among betel nut–tobacco chewers, oral cancer comprises 36 percent of all cancers.

Alcoholism has a highly suggestive role in oral cancer. As many as 42 percent of all patients so afflicted have a history of alcoholism. As a corollary, cirrhosis of the liver is a common finding in patients with oral cancer, 20 percent having cirrhosis as compared to 9 percent in a control population. It has been proposed that alcohol acts as an adjuvant to the use of tobacco in producing oral cancer. This is a difficult point to prove, since finding a control population of patients who drink heavily but do not smoke is virtually impossible.

The roles of poor oral hygiene and oral sepsis, mentioned for decades as etiologic agents for oral cancers, are also difficult to evaluate. These conditions are seen most commonly in patients at the lower end of the social scale and in the ward population rather than in private practice. Oral hygiene is poor in this group, but it cannot be said whether poor hygiene or social level or other correlated factors are responsible.

Syphilis has a direct relation to cancer of one specific site in the oral cavity, the tongue. When syphilitic glossitis, a lesion of late syphilis, heals, it often leaves the tongue fibrotic and scarred with longitudinal fissures and thick hyperkeratotic plaques. It is on this base that lingual cancer develops (Fig. 16-10). In the days of Bloodgood (1921) 21

---

* That is, 3.3 times as many pipe and cigar smokers died of oral cancer as did nonsmokers in the same age group. The mortality ratio for cancer of the lung in pipe smokers was 1:1, no different from that of the nonsmokers.

percent of American men with lingual cancer had syphilis. Willis still calls this condition "the most clearly established causative factor in European males."

Benign Lesions

Common benign tumors of the oral cavity are inflammatory hyperplasias and cysts. Less commonly seen are giant cell granulomas, salivary tumors, granular cell myoblastomas, dermoids, and hemangiomas.

INFLAMMATORY HYPERPLASIA

The oral mucosa is subject to a number of irritating conditions producing tumorlike projections which are not true neoplasms. Patients develop the nervous habit of sucking a portion of mucosa from the cheek, tongue, or lip between the teeth or through an interdental or edentulous space. The traumatized mucosa becomes edematous and prominent, and the irritation may be compounded by the patient who bites as well as sucks on the offending mucosal fold. Initially, the overlying mucosa is swollen, and eventually this undergoes metaplasia to squamous epithelium. The tissue underlying the elevated mucosa changes from edematous connective tissue to a denser and more fibrotic collection of collagen. At this stage the lesion may be termed a *fibroepithelial polyp* (Fig. 16-11). Similar lesions are often seen in the gingivobuccal gutter and on the palate in patients with ill-fitting dentures. Those lesions which occur along the vestibular mucosa next to the gingiva in this relation are sometimes called *epulis fissurata*. Another appropriate term, more descriptive of the later stages of these lesions when the fibrosis and scarring has advanced, is *irritation fibroma*. In the early inflammatory phase of these lesions, the overlying mucosa is friable and bleeds easily.

The chief responsibility of the examiner who has recognized the lesion is to reassure the patient that it is not malignant. Although these lesions are usually not ulcerated and are easily recognized, diagnosis should be confirmed by biopsy. Treatment is by correction of the causative factor, either by the design of new dentures or by discouraging the patient from manipulating and traumatizing the area involved. Excision may be necessary, but if the basic problem is not abolished, recurrence is prompt.

CYSTS

Mucous cysts are a common oral lesion occurring on the posterior surface of the lip, floor of the mouth, tongue, and buccal mucosa. These cysts arise from the salivary gland–bearing areas of the oral mucosa and were thought to be due to obstruction of the excretory duct of minor salivary glands. It has been found, however, that these cysts have no epithelial lining and that they result from a rupture of the excretory duct. Saliva spills from the defect in the duct and begins to collect in the tissues. At first it forms a diffuse lesion, but soon a circumscribed cyst with a wall of granulation tissue develops. These mucoceles measure from 1 or 2 mm to 1 or 2 cm in diameter and appear as elevated, translucent, bluish lesions of the

Fig. 16-10. Syphilis of the tongue. The dense, white patches are sometimes mistaken for "geographic tongue." Cancers of the dorsal surface often follow this condition.

mucosa (Fig. 16-12). They frequently rupture, discharging sticky mucoid material, and then recur as the laceration in the overlying mucosa heals. Treatment consists of wide surgical unroofing of the lesion.

A somewhat larger and more dramatic mucocele may result from obstruction and rupture of the major excretory ducts in the floor of the mouth, ducts of the lingual or submaxillary glands. Except for size, these lesions resemble in every way the lesions which result from obstruction of the minor salivary glands but have received the special name of *ranula*.

Fig. 16-11. Irritation fibroma. The lesion seen here was caused by persistent sucking and irritation of mucosa through the edentulous space, which can be seen adjacent to this polyp. (*Courtesy of Sheldon Rovin, D.D.S.*)

Fig. 16-12. Mucous cyst of the lip, the most common location for this lesion. This mucocele has resulted from rupture of a minor salivary gland duct with spillage of mucus into the surrounding tissue.

Dermoids may develop in the floor of the mouth and the base of the tongue along the midline. If neglected, these lesions grow slowly as they accumulate the sloughed-off cells, secretion, and hair of the epidermal lining. They present both as a swelling in the submental triangle and an elevation of the floor of the mouth (Fig. 16-13). They will eventually elevate the floor of the mouth and tongue until it touches the palate and interferes with speech. Treatment consists of operative excision of the cyst, which may be done either intraorally or extraorally. The lesion has a definite, thick capsule and can be shelled out with ease from its relatively avascular midline location.

Fig. 16-13. Dermoid of the mouth. This huge dermoid has elevated the floor of the mouth until the tongue is forced against the hard palate and in this illustration is out of sight behind the cyst.

PERIPHERAL GIANT CELL REPARATIVE GRANULOMA

These benign tumors occur on the gingivae, affecting the maxillary or mandibular gingiva with equal frequency. Grossly, they appear as a slow-growing, reddish, smooth sessile tumor which bleeds easily. They often occur at an area of an interdental papilla (Fig. 16-14) but may also arise in edentulous patients. Histologically, the lesion is covered by stratified squamous epithelium. Endothelial and fibroplastic proliferations, multinucleated giant cells, and extracellular and intracellular hemosiderin are diagnostic microscopic criteria. Multinucleated giant cells are distributed unevenly throughout an area of rich fibroblastic proliferation. Some lesions show spicules of bone tissue. In general, the lesion closely resembles the giant cell tumor of bone seen in hyperparathyroidism. The descriptive term "peripheral" indicates that the lesion is of soft tissue, while the so-called "central" giant cell reparative granuloma is an intraosseous form found in the mandible or maxilla.

When these lesions arise in the mandible or maxilla, they may be confused with the giant cell tumors of long bones. The distinction between the two lesions must be made, since the oral lesions have no propensity for malignant transformation, as have the lesions seen elsewhere. Treatment of the soft tissue lesions is by complete excision. Inadequate removal may result in recurrence.

PERIPHERAL FIBROMA

These are also lesions of the gingiva and are in many respects similar grossly to the giant cell granuloma. They are usually firmer and under the microscope are made up of dense connective tissue. They may also contain bone spicules and may be calcified. One can speculate as to the relation of these lesions to the giant cell granuloma. They may represent a later stage of this lesion or may be a late stage of inflammatory hyperplasia. Excision is usually curative.

GRANULOMA PYOGENICUM

This is an elevated pedunculated or sessile lesion which may occur on the lips, tongue, buccal mucosa, or gingiva. It bleeds readily on being traumatized. Histologically it is made up of edematous, fibrous connective tissue with a prominent endothelial component arranged in lobules of varying sizes separated by bands of collagen. Numerous blood vessels are scattered throughout the tumor. No cause is known for the lesions of the lips, buccal mucosa, and tongue, but lesions of the gingiva are often associated with pregnancy. Thirty to forty percent of pregnant women show some degree of gingival enlargement. Of these, about 1 percent will have an isolated "tumor." These lesions in the pregnant female have been called "granuloma gravidarum." They appear about the third month of pregnancy and increase in size throughout the growth of the child in utero. They usually diminish in size and disappear following delivery, although with a subsequent pregnancy they may appear again in the same location. Lesions unassociated with pregnancy may be treated by excision. It is usually advisable to wait until the end of pregnancy to treat granuloma gravidarum.

SALIVARY TUMORS

Pleomorphic adenomas (mixed tumors) occasionally arise from any of the 400 to 700 minor salivary glands. Occurring most commonly on the lips, tongue, and palate, they can be found anywhere in the oral cavity where minor salivary glands are found. They are usually slow-growing, round masses of a rather rubbery consistency (Fig. 16-15). They have the potential of becoming malignant and if simply enucleated without adequate excision have a marked propensity for local recurrence. Treatment, therefore, is by wide local excision.

HEMANGIOMA

Capillary hemangiomas, not unlike the strawberry hemangioma of the skin, are sometimes seen in the mucous membranes of the oral cavity in infants. Like the lesions of the skin these lesions regress spontaneously, and unless they are so large that they interfere with function, they should be left to regress at their own pace. In most instances they will undergo involution by the end of the fifth year. Unlike the skin lesions they do not disappear completely and may still be seen as a small, dark lesion underneath the mucosa (Fig. 16-16). It is likely that the transparent nature of the mucosa reveals the sclerosed remnant in a manner that is not seen if the lesion is under the more opaque skin. The sclerosed hemangioma will remain visible throughout life but has no significance and does not require treatment. Rarely, large regional vascular malformations will involve the entire side of the mouth, including the tongue, gingiva, and buccal mucosa. Such lesions do not regress spontaneously. Their treatment is difficult, often requiring multiple plastic procedures to excise the hemangiomatous tissue and to return the contours of the mouth and oral cavity to normal.

GRANULAR CELL MYOBLASTOMA

This is a rare and interesting lesion which occurs most commonly within the muscle of the tongue, presenting as a small, firm spheroid mass detected best by manual palpation. These lesions have no malignant potential but may gradually increase in size with functional impairment. Treatment is by simple excision.

Hyperkeratosis

The gross finding of white patches on the oral mucosa elicits the diagnosis of leukoplakia from the clinician. "Leukoplakia" roughly translated means "white patches," so the physician need not feel too proud of his accomplishment; he has only managed to translate English into Latin. To some "leukoplakia" means a specific premalignant lesion. This meaning is not inherent in the original use of this term. Most pathologists adhere to a more rigid description of such lesions and describe the underlying microscopic changes: hyperplasia, keratosis, and dyskeratosis. White patches in the oral cavity may be associated with any of or all these basic changes (Fig. 16-17). Inflammation in this area often stimulates marked hyperplasia of cells, sometimes to the point where they resemble

Fig. 16-14. Peripheral giant cell tumor. These often arise in interdental spaces as seen in photograph.

epidermoid tumors and are spoken of as *pseudoepitheliomatous hyperplasia*. Keratosis is a common response of the buccal mucosa and may appear in the presence of lichen planus, chronic dyscoid lupus, and Darier's disease, as well as be a possible forerunner of malignant change.

Dyskeratosis, the loss of normal stratification or orientation of cells together with irregularity in the size and shape of cells and abnormal staining characteristics, is a much more treacherous lesion and much more likely to precede malignant disease.

Hyperkeratosis is announced by the gradual development of whitened patches of the mucosa which appear first as a thin, white, translucent or opalescent film in the normal mucous membrane. No malignant or premalignant changes will be found at this point but only evidences of

Fig. 16-15. Mixed tumor of palate. This is a benign lesion. Adequate removal to ensure prevention of recurrences includes resection of the underlying hard palate and gingiva.

Fig. 16-16. Fibrosing hemangioma. Lesions in the mucosal area remain visible under the buccal mucosa, whereas similar lesions may not be discernible under the skin.

hyperplasia or keratosis. Later these lesions can become thickened and rougher; the white patches are now quite opaque. Palpation will reveal a definite change in the consistency of the mucosa. Microscopic examination may still show advanced hyperkeratosis and hyperplasia, but now areas of mild to marked dyskeratosis may be present as well. Eventually, areas of distinct carcinoma in situ will appear, and this can be followed in rapid order by microinvasion or the frank invasion of a well-developed cancer.

Obviously, the early appearance of hyperplasia and hyperkeratosis may or may not foreshadow malignant disease. Since there is no way of telling which is the case, patients with such lesions should be warned to avoid smoking or heavy intake of alcohol and should embark on a campaign of improvement of oral hygiene. Cancer

Fig. 16-17. Hyperkeratosis of mucosa. The white mucosa in the gingivobuccal gutter of the patient is due to an ill-fitting denture causing hyperkeratosis, a normal response of the oral mucosa to irritation. (*Courtesy of Sheldon Rovin, D.D.S.*)

will ultimately develop in 5 percent of such patients, and it is significant that about 50 percent of all oral cancers develop in patients with associated areas of hyperkeratosis and dyskeratosis. The thin, early lesions require only a warning, and a biopsy is not necessary, but thickened lesions may already contain carcinoma in situ and should be biopsied in every instance and perhaps checked, as well, with vital dyes.

If a patch of dyskeratosis appears on biopsy to be particularly threatening and is limited in extent, local excision may be useful. More often, the extent of the lesion is so widespread that complete excision of the involved mucosa is impossible. Radiation therapy is contraindicated in these premalignant lesions. While the majority are associated with hyperkeratosis, which gives the whitish aspect to the surface, occasionally dyskeratosis and carcinoma in situ are the major elements. Such lesions may have a velvety erythematous appearance only slightly redder than the surrounding mucosa. These areas are difficult to detect, and toluidine blue may be very useful in mapping their true area.

Malignant Tumors

PATHOLOGY. Low-grade epidermoid carcinomas make up the overwhelming majority of all carcinomas of the oral cavity, varying from highly differentiated tumors, difficult to tell histologically from inflammatory hyperplasia, to less well-organized but still obvious epidermoid tumors usually with associated squamous pearls. Highly undifferentiated and anaplastic lesions are rare. The few adenocarcinomas found are derived from minor salivary glands. The occasional adenoid cystic carcinomas and mucoepidermoid carcinomas seen also arise from salivary tissues.

In the Southern United States a very low-grade cancer, verrucous carcinoma, is occasionally seen. This is an exophytic, shaggy white lesion usually found in the gingivobuccal gutter of patients who are tobacco chewers or "snuff dippers." Unless treated by radiation, the lesion never metastasizes, although it frequently invades surrounding tissues, including the mandible.

In general, lesions of the oral cavity are better differentiated and less malignant than lesions occurring in the oropharynx.

TONGUE

Carcinoma of the tongue commonly begins at the tip or along the free borders. It often starts in an area of hyperkeratosis and gradually develops as an ulcerated lesion with a moderately exophytic undermined border. The area of ulceration is related to the rest of the tumor as the tip of an iceberg is to its main mass, and palpation of the tongue may indicate that invasion has occurred deeply throughout underlying muscle (Fig. 16-18). Carcinomas beginning in an area of syphilitic glossitis are exceptions to the normal pattern and occur on the dorsal glossal surface.

Cancer of the tip of the tongue (Fig. 16-19) metastasizes to submental nodes, often bilaterally, while lesions along the borders of the tongue metastasize to ipsilateral submandibular nodes and occasionally to nodes at the angle of the mandible.

These lesions are quick to metastasize, and 40 percent of patients have nodes in the neck when first seen. In another 40 percent nodes develop at some point during therapy or during follow-up. For this reason therapy is designed to attack not only the primary lesion but also the nodes of the ipsilateral neck, as well. Combined operation including wide resection of the oral lesion together with radical neck dissection has been our treatment of choice in the past. More recently we have been inclined to treat all larger lesions of the oral cavity with radiation therapy, following this with radical neck dissection and in continuity excision of any residual cancer. The horizontal ramus of the mandible must be resected together with the tumor if the oral cancer has come in contact with the periosteum of the mandible at any point. Such contact seeds the periosteal lymphatics with tumor cells and makes resection of bone mandatory. The determinate 5-year survival for cancer of the tongue is 32 to 40 percent. If no palpable lymph nodes are present, the 5-year survival rate is 53 percent.

FLOOR OF THE MOUTH

The floor of the mouth is that portion of the oral cavity between the tongue and the inner surface of the mandible. This crescentic area of the mucosa lies over the sublingual and submaxillary salivary glands and contains their excretory ducts. It is divided into two halves by the frenulum, a fold of mucosa lying in the midline and extending to the tongue.

Squamous carcinomas developing in this area tend to develop a "run-around" extending anteriorly and posteriorly around the rim of the mandible, and if they are neglected long enough, the entire floor of the mouth becomes involved. This pattern of growth results in common bilateral involvement at the anterior floor of the mouth (Fig. 16-20) with frequent bilateral cervical metastases. These lesions tend to be less well differentiated than lesions of the tongue or gingiva and rapidly invade the surrounding structures, especially the periosteum of the adjacent mandible and the tissues of the submaxillary space. Metastases occur first to the submaxillary lymph nodes and are frequent. Taylor and Nathanson observed that 60 percent of these patients had palpable cervical metastases on admission, and in 90 percent cervical lymph node involvement had developed within a year of diagnosis.

The primary symptoms of these neoplasms are often neglected for some time, since they are quite minimal. Eventually the patient complains of pain, swelling of the tongue, and difficulty in eating and speaking. Early lesions are usually discovered by the patient himself while inspecting his mouth or have been noticed by an alert dentist or physician. Rarely, very early lesions may be seen involving only the superficial mucosa.

Large lesions of the floor of the mouth require wide excision in continuity with resection of a portion of the mandible and radical neck dissection. The neck dissection is done whether lymph nodes are palpable or not, in view

Fig. 16-18. Squamous carcinoma of the lateral border of the middle third of the tongue. The lesion is deeply invasive and much larger than the area of ulceration would indicate. The curled raised border is characteristic.

of the high incidence of positive cervical nodes. Operative therapy may be integrated with preoperative radiation in the larger lesions. The much less common superficial and in situ lesions can be treated by local excision only. The 5-year survival rates for cancers in this site are comparable with those for cancer of the tongue. James reports an average determinate survival of 37 percent, and the Tumor Registry of the Memorial Center for Cancer reports a 5-year survival rate of 39 percent.

GINGIVAE

Cancer of the gums is better differentiated and slower in its pattern of growth than lesions of the tongue and

Fig. 16-19. Squamous carcinoma of the tip of the tongue. An exophytic, fairly superficial lesion which histologically shows a well-differentiated structure. The prognosis for such a lesion is excellent.

Fig. 16-20. Squamous carcinoma of the floor of the mouth. This lesion is in a typical location in the midline with spread in both directions around the curve of the mandible. It has invaded deeply into underlying structures.

floor of the mouth. Patients first note a mass (Fig. 16-21) or slight tenderness of the gum, sometimes with loosening of teeth in the area of the tumor. This often leads them to consult their dentist, who, if he is not alert to the problem, may extract the teeth under the mistaken impression that the patient has an underlying abcess or cyst. As the lesion progresses, it ulcerates, bleeds, and interferes with mastication. As a neoplasm invades the underlying bone, it can involve the mandibular nerve with the appearance of numbness in the mental and submental areas. Extraction of a tooth often accelerates the invasion of the mandible.

Treatment of cancer of the lower gingiva requires resection of the involved mandible and overlying gum together with a radical neck dissection. Metastases from cancers at this site are usually to the submaxillary lymph nodes and are present in about half the patients at their first visit. Epidermoid cancers of the upper gingiva are less

Fig. 16-21. Carcinoma of the gingiva. The adjacent teeth are loose and easily removed. The underlying mandible is already invaded.

common and better differentiated than cancers of the lower gingiva. Metastases to cervical nodes are much less common. Therefore, treatment is restricted to local excision. Radical neck dissection is deferred until there is evidence of palpable cervical node involvement.

The definitive 5-year survival rate following treatment for carcinoma of the gingiva averages 45 percent.

HARD PALATE

The hard palate is the U-shaped area enclosed by the upper gingiva and bounded posteriorly by the attachments of the soft palate. It consists of the palatine processes of the maxillary bones in its anterior two-thirds and of the horizontal portions of the palatine bones in its posterior third.

The most common malignant lesions of the hard palate are tumors of the minor salivary glands. Adenoid cystic carcinomas (Fig. 16-22) and adenocarcinomas occur in almost equal number; malignant mixed tumors are somewhat less frequent. Epidermoid carcinomas primary in the hard palate are rare, although carcinomas primary in the maxillary sinus will occasionally invade the hard palate and perforate into the oral cavity.

The primary symptom is a mass usually noted first by the patient himself. There is no tenderness or other associated symptom until fairly late in the course of the tumor. As in most salivary malignant tumors, growth is very slow and metastases occur quite late, so that involved cervical lymph nodes are not found initially. Salivary neoplasms respond poorly to radiation therapy, and primary treatment is excision. The chief fault in treatment is underestimation of the extent and potential of these lesions. They are usually fixed to the underlying periosteum, and adequate excision must include resection of the hard palate together with the tumor mass. An attempt to enucleate the tumor from the underlying bone almost ensures a local recurrence. Excision with a wide margin including the bony palate leaves a substantial palatal defect requiring repair either by surgical reconstruction or the use of an upper plate constructed by a prosthodontist with an obturator which will plug the defect.

Despite the phlegmatic nature of these tumors, complete excision and complete eradication of the lesions are often elusive. The lesions tend to be of a higher grade than malignant lesions of the major salivary glands. Five-year survival rates between 30 and 40 percent are reported, but the incidence of new disease between the fifth and fifteenth year is frequent.

BUCCAL MUCOSA

The lateral walls of the oral cavity are formed by the cheeks, which consist of the buccinator muscle covered on its inner surface by a layer of mucosa extending from the upper to the lower gingivobuccal gutters and from the lateral commissure of the lips anteriorly to the ascending ramus of the mandible posteriorly. Lymphatics from this area pass through the buccinator muscle and follow the facial vein to end in the submaxillary and upper cervical lymph nodes.

The natural evolution of epidermoid carcinoma of the

buccal mucosa varies according to the grade of the tumor. About half of the lesions are rather undifferentiated and associated with ulceration, rapid invasion of the cheek, and sometimes even perforation of the skin and formation of an orocutaneous salivary fistula (Fig. 16-23). The majority of such lesions are accompanied by enlarged submaxillary lymph nodes when first seen.

A less aggressive form of buccal cancer is also encountered, especially in patients who are tobacco chewers and "snuff dippers." This is the so-called "verrucous carcinoma," which tends to occur in the gingivobuccal gutter and progresses very slowly, sometimes over a period of years. The tumor is locally invasive, but metastases have never been reported except in patients who have received previous irradiation. Verrucous lesions are easily recognized by their exophytic form and shaggy white appearance (Fig. 16-24). They may cover a wide area, sometimes the entire buccal surface, and have a propensity for bony invasion, often involving a large portion of the mandible or occasionally the maxilla.

Treatment of buccal carcinoma is dictated by the type of lesion encountered. External radiation therapy alone does not eradicate the less well-differentiated lesions, although it has been combined with interstitial therapy with some success. The highly differentiated verrucous carcinomas are fairly radiosensitive but have a marked tendency to recur following an early gratifying regression. In addition, the distressing propensity of these lesions for developing a higher grade of malignancy with metastases after being exposed to radiation is a unique characteristic which has discouraged many from using radiation in treatment. Therefore, the initial therapy for verrucous lesions is wide excision. Since cervical metastases are not ordinarily found, an accompanying radical neck dissection is not done.

For the high-grade lesions, block dissection of the cheek with radical neck resection is the operative treatment of choice. Additional benefit may be derived from combining this with preoperative radiotherapy; this type of combined treatment is still undergoing evaluation. James reported 5-year survival rates in 181 patients with carcinoma of the buccal mucosa of all types as 54.4 percent. The prognosis for the well-differentiated lesions, such as the verrucous carcinoma, should be much better than this.

OROPHARYNX

The oropharynx is the region of the mouth posterior to the anterior tonsillar pillars and the circumvallate papillae of the tongue (Fig. 16-25). It contains the soft palate, tonsil and tonsillar fossa, posterior third of the tongue, anterior surface of the epiglottis, and surrounding pharyngeal walls. The most common site for malignant tumors in this area is the tonsil.

TONSIL

The most common benign lesion of the tonsil is, as every layman knows, inflammatory swelling. This can lead to confusion in diagnosing nonulcerated tumors of these

Fig. 16-22. Adenoid cystic carcinoma of the hard palate. Although this lesion is much smaller than the mixed tumor in Fig. 16-15, it is malignant. Treatment is by wide excision, including the underlying bone.

organs. Common malignant lesions are high-grade epidermoid carcinomas (78 percent) and lymphosarcomas (16 percent). A large group of miscellaneous tumors are found, including hemangiomas, neurofibromas, and salivary gland tumors. High-grade epidermoid carcinomas in this area are often described as lymphoepitheliomas and transitional cell carcinomas. It is our feeling that these are simply microscopic variants of highly undifferentiated epidermoid carcinomas.

The frequent first symptom of carcinoma of the tonsil is a slight feeling of tenderness in the area, a typical sore throat. This is easily ignored by the patient for long periods until its persistence finally forces a consultation with the

Fig. 16-23. Carcinoma of buccal mucosa. A well-differentiated and slowly growing lesion which was neglected and mismanaged for many years. (*From B. F. Rush, Jr., Curr Probl Surg, May, 1967.*)

Fig. 16-24. Verrucous carcinoma. The shaggy white plaque along the gingivobuccal gutter is typical. The patient is seventy-five years old and has chewed tobacco for over 50 years.

physician. Even then the evidence of a growing tumor may be overlooked and the patient treated for some time with mouthwashes and antibiotics. The lesion will appear grossly as a swelling of the tonsil with a central ulcer. Palpation reveals firmness and induration spreading well beyond the area of ulceration. Trismus and pain in the ear are common complaints. The metastatic spread from this area is to the tonsillar node at the angle of the mandible, so often enlarged in children who have tonsillitis. The tonsil is a common site for very tiny "occult" carcinomas, which lead to large cervical masses and must be inspected minutely when one is searching for a primary

Fig. 16-25. Oropharynx. The shaded area delineates the oropharynx. The nasopharynx is located above, and the hypopharynx and larynx are located below.

OROPHARYNX

site for cervical metastases (Fig. 16-26). Lymphosarcomas of the tonsil usually present with a more bulky primary lesion and are not as inclined to ulceration. The primary lesions may be bilateral with involvement of both tonsils.

Treatment of tonsillar carcinoma either by radiation or operation has never been very satisfactory. Lymphosarcomas are quite radiosensitive and should be treated primarily by radiation. Carcinoma, on the other hand, yields poorly to either form of therapy. Still under evaluation, integrated therapy with preoperative radiation to the tonsil followed by resection in continuity with a radical neck dissection may prove to produce the best results. The definitive 5-year survival following treatment of cancer of the tonsil is 25 percent.

POSTERIOR THIRD OF THE TONGUE

Tumors in the posterior third of the tongue differ markedly in their natural history from those in the anterior two-thirds. Whereas the anterior lesions tend to be well differentiated, remain confined to the primary site, or involve only high cervical nodes for long periods, lesions in the posterior third are of much higher grade, often being classified as *lymphoepitheliomas,* or *transitional cell tumors.* They spread rapidly to the cervical nodes and often beyond to distant sites. A frequent initial symptom of carcinoma of the posterior third of the tongue is a large cervical lymph node accompanied by the complaint of pain on swallowing. Unfortunately, this is a fairly silent area, and lesions may attain considerable size before causing pain or dysfunction. Wide ulceration causes a malodorous breath and dysphasia. Weight loss is prominent. Treatment has been highly unsatisfactory in the past. Radiation therapy infrequently controls the primary lesion. Operation often results in total loss of the tongue, an overwhelming psychologic and functional deficit. Since these lesions are often across the midline, bilateral neck dissection must be combined with resection of the tongue. Initial experience with combined radiation and operation indicates that occasionally the lesions can be reduced in size sufficiently by preoperative radiation to permit a more conservative resection of the posterior tongue, leaving a functional anterior tongue behind.

SOFT PALATE

Malignant tumors of the soft palate are almost always epidermoid carcinomas. These tend to be well differentiated, slow-growing, and late to metastasize. They are generally superficial lesions spreading over the anterior surface of the soft palate and down the tonsillar pillars. Often it is difficult to determine whether the lesions arose in the tonsil or in the soft palate. Spread may be extensive, covering much of the soft palate, the tonsillar fossa, and the tongue. Pain and dysphagia are the usual first symptoms. Diagnosis by inspection and palpation is a simple matter, and biopsy is easily accomplished.

Response to radiation therapy is only fair. Resection is more likely to produce a cure but often leads to a difficult functional defect, since the patient is unable to close the nasopharynx and will tend to regurgitate food through the nose on swallowing. This is a situation where the clever prosthodontist can help greatly by installing an adequate extension on an upper plate which extends backward into the pharynx to seal the palatal defect. An even more convenient method of closing the palatal defect is to raise a flap from the posterior pharynx and swing it forward to close the defect at the time of the original operation. Prognosis is difficult to determine, since these tumors are usually classed in the literature with tumors of the tonsil or of the hard palate.

EPIGLOTTIS

Malignant tumors of the anterior surface of the epiglottis are usually exophytic and well differentiated and have a slow, natural evolution. Dysphagia and aspiration are early symptoms. Treatment by radiation therapy is quite successful. Hemilaryngectomy of the upper larynx above the cords has also produced good results. Patients who have had resection of the epiglottis must relearn swallowing, and this requires a reasonable level of intelligence. Senile patients or those with poor learning ability should be treated either by radiation or total laryngectomy.

LARYNX

When describing the site of tumors of the larynx, the terminology can be confusing and frustrating. According to current usage, the larynx is made up of those structures lying both above and below the true vocal cords. Thus, the mucosa of the larynx extends along the posterior surface of the epiglottis including its tip, along the aryepiglottic folds, and over the arytenoid cartilages posteriorly. It covers the inner surface of the aryepiglottic folds, the false vocal cords, and the ventricles. All of the larynx thus far described constitutes the supraglottic larynx, i.e., that which is above the true vocal cords. The glottic portion of the larynx is that portion made up of the true cords themselves. The mucosa lining the area underneath the true cords down to the lower border of the cricoid cartilage covers the infraglottic portion of the larynx.

In the past the area just described was called the "endolarynx," or the "intrinsic larynx," although the latter term gradually came to mean the true cords alone. Tumors taking their origin on the outside of the larynx for many years were designated as arising from the "extrinsic larynx." However, this term came to be used for supraglottic lesions as well, so this usage has now been abandoned. Lesions involving any portion of the exterior of the larynx are now spoken of as "hypopharyngeal" or, by some, "laryngopharyngeal."

INCIDENCE AND ETIOLOGY. Cancer of the larynx accounts for 1.62 percent of all cancers in men and only 0.14 percent of all cancers in woman; thus the ratio of incidence favors the male sex by over 11:1. The report of the Advisory Committee to the Surgeon General on Smoking and Health reviewed 10 retrospective studies and 7 prospective studies on the relationship of smoking to carcinoma of the larynx. There was a statistically positive relationship in every study. In the prospective studies the mortality ratios for smokers averaged 5.4 times greater for cigarette smok-

Fig. 16-26. Carcinoma of the anterior tonsillar pillar. These tiny lesions are invasive areas of carcinoma. Despite their size, the patient already had metastatic disease in the ipsilateral neck.

ers than for nonsmokers and 2.8 times greater for cigar and pipe smokers than for nonsmokers. Laryngeal cancer mortality has increased somewhat over the past three decades, but the increase has been much less than that for lung cancer. It appears that the induction of carcinoma of the larynx cannot occur solely as a result of tobacco tars but that a further agent, or cocarcinogen, is needed. One such agent may be alcohol, since a high percentage (30 to 40 percent) of patients with carcinoma of the larynx are alcoholics and come from population groups where the risk of alcoholism is great, such as bartenders and entertainers. Cirrhosis of the liver is a common complaint among patients with carcinoma of the larynx; this may be a secondary relationship due to the frequency of alcoholism in this group.

CLASSIFICATION. As it has for other cancers, the American Joint Committee on Cancer Staging and End Results Reporting has developed a "TNM system" for carcinomas of the larynx. Because of differences in prognosis at different sites the committee has divided the larynx into its three major areas: the supraglottic (posterior surface of the epiglottis, aryepiglottic folds, arytenoids, false cords, ventricles); the glottic (right and left vocal cords and anterior glottic commissure), and the subglottic (subglottic region exclusive of the undersurface of the true cords and down to the lower margin of the cricoid cartilage). About 56 percent of squamous epidermoid cancers of the larynx occur in the glottic region, 42 percent occur in the supraglottic region, and the remaining 2 percent are subglottic. The combination of topographic spread (T), nodal involvement (N), and distant metastasis (M) in a description of three separate anatomic sites results in a complex system, yet it is the most precise method whereby lesions can be classified and comparisons between institutions adequately made as to the results of treatment.

PATHOLOGY. Polyps, papillomas, granulomas, cysts, and areas of hyperkeratosis make up the common benign lesions of the cords. Rarely hemangiomas and chondromas of the laryngeal cartilages are seen. Ninety-nine percent of the malignant lesions of the larynx are epidermoid carcinomas, and most of these are of the ordinary cornifying (squamous cell) type. These lesions arise from the squamous epithelium of the cords themselves or from areas of metaplasia in the mucosa of the endolarynx. On the cord, carcinoma may be preceded by hyperkeratosis and stages of transition from hyperkeratosis to dyskeratosis, carcinoma in situ, and microinvasive carcinoma. Glottic cancers are usually very well differentiated, slow-growing, and late to metastasize. Supraglottic and infraglottic cancers are less well differentiated and more likely to have spread to lymph nodes when first seen.

DIAGNOSIS. Space-occupying lesions of the larynx produce initial symptoms through interference with phonation and respiration. Hoarseness, the usual first symptom, may be slight and intermittent but gradually becomes constant. What begins as a slight huskiness gradually progresses, until sounds are produced with difficulty. Respiratory obstruction is a later sign, although small lesions on the true cords will produce a greater degree of obstruction than somewhat larger lesions in supraglottic or infraglottic area. Obstruction progresses in severity until the patient may respire with visible effort, using his accessory muscles to force air through the cords, sometimes with audible stridor. At this point the patient's life is in jeopardy. At any moment the slightest additional swelling or edema can cut off breathing completely. The use of sedatives in patients at this phase of obstruction is fraught with danger. Under sedation the patient's tired muscles may fail, with a rapid shallowing of respiration, progressive anoxia, and cardiac arrest. The finding of a tumor on the cord associated with stridor, retraction, or the use of accessory muscles to breathe indicates immediate tracheostomy. It is far better to elect a tracheostomy done in the operating room than to be forced into an emergency tracheostomy on the ward or in the emergency room under much less favorable circumstances.

Late signs of malignant lesions of the larynx are a malodorous breath, pain on swallowing, weight loss, and hemoptysis.

Any patient who has persistent hoarseness for more than three or four weeks should have a careful inspection of his vocal cords by indirect laryngoscopy. If this reveals no pathologic conditions but hoarseness persists, then direct laryngoscopy should be used to examine the cords even more closely.

Benign Tumors

POLYPS

According to Holinger, 43 percent of all benign lesions of the larynx are simple polyps. These arise on the phonating edge of the cord at the junction between the anterior one-third and the posterior two-thirds (Fig. 16-27). Their cause is obscure. Treatment is by removal with a cupped forceps at direct laryngoscopy.

VOCAL NODULES

The second most common benign tumor of the larynx, these are usually bilateral and, like polyps, occur at the junction of the anterior one-third with the posterior two-thirds of the cords. They are often called "singer's nodules" but certainly are not confined to singers and can occur in any occupational group. Treatment is by removal with the biopsy forceps.

Fig. 16-27. Pedunculated polyp of the right vocal cord arising at the junction of the anterior and middle thirds. (*From P. H. Holinger et al., Ann Otol Rhinol Laryngol, 56:583, 1947.*)

Fig. 16-28. Carcinoma involving the left side of the larynx and anterior commissure. (*From P. H. Holinger et al., Ann Otol Rhinol Laryngol, 56:583, 1947.*)

RETENTION CYSTS

About half of these occur on the vocal cords, the remainder being found in the aryepiglottic folds, arytenoids, or epiglottis. They appear to occur as a result of the obstruction of small mucous glands. These lesions can reach considerable size and offer marked embarrassment to respiration.

HYPERKERATOSIS

Hyperkeratosis can affect the vocal cords as it does any of the mucosal areas of the lips, oral cavity, or pharynx. These lesions are evidence of a premalignant change and should be stripped off the cord with the use of the biopsy forceps. Patients who have developed hyperkeratosis should be followed at twice yearly intervals to guard against recurrence or the appearance of a frank carcinoma.

PAPILLOMAS

These multiple lesions are found most often on the true cords but may appear on any portion of the larynx or pharynx and even on the soft palate. While they are most commonly reported in children prior to adolescence, some adults are also affected. Like warts, these tumors appear to be caused by viruses. Frequently the growths cover the mucosa of the cords in great profusion, causing severe respiratory embarrassment and requiring tracheostomy. They can persist for many years; during this period the patient often must continue to wear a tracheostomy tube while papillomas are cleared from his airway by frequent excisions through the laryngoscope. Repeated excision is the only effective treatment to date. The large number of other forms of therapy attempted indicates the generally unsatisfactory state of therapy. Eventually, after a period of months or years of repeated excisions, the lesions gradually disappear.

Malignant Lesions

Carcinoma of the true cords (Fig. 16-28) is a lesion which should be easily detected. It gives warning of its presence at an early stage through hoarseness and grows slowly enough so that early therapy should be rewarded by a 90 percent or better 5-year survival rate. In many urban areas over half of the lesions of the true cords are stage 1 lesions confined entirely to the cord. In contrast, some rural areas report that in only 5 percent of patients reaching the physician the lesions are still in stage 1. As the tumor grows, it extends off the cord, either up into the supraglottic area or less commonly inferiorly into the infraglottic region. Invasion occurs slowly but relentlessly, eventually with perforation of the thyroid cartilage and direct invasion of the soft tissues of the thyroid gland and of the neck.

If cancer remains confined to the true cords, a high percentage of 5-year survivals can be obtained following treatment by radiotherapy alone. Holinger noted that in a series of 102 patients with cordal lesions treated with cobalt irradiation, only 9 patients had residual or recurrent cancer which required subsequent laryngectomy. None of the patients in this series died of carcinoma. Loss of the larynx is such a major functional and psychologic disability that if excellent results can be obtained by irradiation, this should be the treatment of choice.

Cancers which have invaded areas beyond the cord have a much different outlook. Involvement of cervical nodes becomes an important problem, and the ability to eradicate the disease by radiation alone is greatly decreased. For stage 2, 3, and 4 cancers, laryngectomy is mandatory. In addition, a radical neck dissection on the side of the lesion is usually performed, even though palpable nodes are not present. Using this approach, Norris has reported a 70 to 75 percent 5-year survival rate for stage 2 and 3 lesions of glottic and supraglottic origin. The very large stage 4 lesions do very poorly, with a 5-year survival rate of only 21 percent. Goldman et al. have combined radiation therapy and operation in treatment of advanced cancers of the larynx, and although the experience is still small, they feel that integration of the two modalities improves the long-term survival rate.

The major problem for the patient after laryngectomy is to regain a useful voice. About half of all such patients will learn to use effective esophageal speech, meaning they can communicate understandably with strangers and casual acquaintances. An additional 25 percent can make themselves understood to members of their family but find that their esophageal speech is too distorted to be useful in the general community. The remaining 25 percent of patients will be unable to conquer the technical problems of learning this method of conversation.

Esophageal speech is by far the most useful technique for speaking after laryngectomy, since it requires no additional paraphernalia and can be refined to the point where it very closely resembles the tone and expression of ordinary speech. It is produced by swallowing air and regurgitating it, creating a vibration in the pharynx—probably at the level of the cricothyroid muscle. The oral cavity modulates this tone just as it would a tone from the larynx.

For the 50 percent of patients who are partly or completely unable to learn esophageal speech, electric vibrating devices can be used to provide a tone in the oral cavity which is modulated by the patient's oral structures, giving a fairly reasonable method of communication.

HYPOPHARYNX

The hypopharynx is that area of the throat which surrounds the larynx. It is made up of the piriform sinuses on either side, the exterior portions of the aryepiglottic fold, and the lateral and posterior pharyngeal walls. It includes the mucosa overlying the posterior portions of the cricoid cartilage.

INCIDENCE. Cancer of the hypopharynx is three to four times as common as cancer of the larynx and constitutes 4.05 percent of all cancers in males. It is three times more common in men than in women. These tumors appear to be related to smoking. The correlation is stronger with pipe and cigar smoking than with cigarette smoking. Another etiologic factor is the Plummer-Vinson syndrome, found most commonly in Scandinavian women. This deficiency syndrome, now gradually disappearing, is clearly related to carcinoma of the hypopharynx and posterior tongue. At the Radiumhemmet in Stockholm carcinomas of the hypopharynx are seen more frequently in women than in men, and most of these cases are associated with a Plummer-Vinson syndrome.

PATHOLOGY. The great majority of these tumors are epidermoid carcinomas and compared with the oral cavity and endolarynx tend to be of a higher grade with a pre-

ponderance of grade 3 and 4 lesions. Better-differentiated forms are seen, however, most commonly on the exterior portions of the aryepiglottic folds and in the postcricoid area. Spread of the tumor occurs promptly and usually by way of the lymphatic channels which drain the hypopharynx, exiting between the lateral portion of the hyoid bone and the upper edge of the thyroid cartilage to travel with the superior thyroid artery to the midjugular chain of lymph nodes. Unlike most head and neck cancers, distant metastases are common with involvement of mediastinal nodes, lung, liver, and other distant viscera.

DIAGNOSIS. Since these lesions arise outside the endolarynx away from major paths of respiration and speech, hoarseness or dyspnea are uncommon findings until late in the growth of the tumor. Interference with swallowing, on the other hand, is the most common early symptom and is associated with choking and aspiration. Aspiration pneumonia may be the illness which first brings the patient to the physician. The lesions seem to have a long silent period and can grow to considerable size in the depths of the piriform sinus or on the pharyngeal walls before the first definite symptoms appear. Not uncommonly, the first sign is the appearance of a midjugular cervical node. The better-differentiated lesions invade and ulcerate widely, so that a malodorous breath is a common associated finding. Diagnosis is confirmed by indirect laryngoscopy and biopsy through a laryngoscope.

TREATMENT. Until recent years this was a highly lethal tumor with few cures either by operation or by irradiation. The introduction of wide radical excision with removal of the larynx and hypopharynx and en bloc radical neck dissection increased the cure rate perceptibly. This may be another area where judicious combination of irradiation and operation can improve the cure rate even more. Five-year survival rates with the older form of therapy were no more than 10 to 15 percent. With more aggressive operative approaches, cure rates in the vicinity of 30 percent have been reported.

NASOPHARYNX

The nasopharynx is at the top of the pharynx, just underneath the base of the skull. The body of the sphenoid bone forms a roof for this cavity, while its floor is formed by the soft palate. There is no anterior wall as such except for the posterior openings of the nasal passage together with the posterior aspects of the nasal septum and the turbinates. The roof of the cavity slopes into the posterior wall made up of the basiocciput and the atlas and the overlying covering of muscle and mucosa. Each lateral wall contains the opening of a eustachian tube guarded by a small prominence, the torus tubarius. The only structure lying within the nasopharynx is the lymphoid tissue of the adenoids scattered on the posterior and superior walls.

INCIDENCE. These tumors are uncommon but not rare, constituting about $\frac{1}{2}$ percent of all cancers. They are somewhat more common in males than in females (2.4:1). There is an interesting relation to race. This is a frequent tumor in the Near East, among the Filipinos, Malays, and

Dayaks, and especially among the Chinese. This cancer accounts for 30.4 percent of all cancers in males in Formosa. The incidence among the Chinese born in the Far East is more than thirty times greater than in this country, while the incidence among American-born Chinese is about six times as common as the incidence among the other racial groups here. This shift in pattern would suggest that both genetic and environmental causative factors are operating.

Benign Lesions

These include hypetrophied lymphatic tissue, juvenile nasopharyngeal hemangiofibroma, Rathke's pouch cyst, dermoids, and mixed tumors. Of these, hypertrophied adenoids occur commonly, and hemangiofibroma and Rathke's pouch cyst have a special predilection for this site.

Any enlarging, space-occupying lesion of the nasopharynx calls attention to itself by respiratory obstruction and nasal stuffiness. Obstruction to the eustachian tubes provokes earaches and often chronic ear infection. As the lesion encroaches on the soft palate, deglutition is disturbed with pain on swallowing or regurgitation of food and fluids into the nasopharynx and out of the nose.

HYPERTROPHIED ADENOIDS

The adenoids represent a portion of the large circle of lymphatic tissue surrounding the oral respiratory passageway at the level of the posterior tongue and tonsils. Chronic upper respiratory tract infections in infants and children often cause marked and persistent hypertrophy of some of this rim of tissue. In past decades resection of the adenoids and tonsils was one of the most common of operations in children. With the advent of the antibiotics the need for these procedures has diminished markedly. Nonetheless, in an occasional child a persistent hypertrophy of the adenoids will develop which disturbs his breathing pattern, causing mouth breathing, or more importantly will obstruct the eustachian tubes, leading to chronic ear infections with a threat to the child's hearing. These symptoms are adequate indication for operative excision.

JUVENILE NASOPHARYNGEAL HEMANGIOFIBROMA

Made up of a hard stroma of fibrous tissue, richly interlaced with capillaries and cavernous sinuses, this rare and interesting tumor appears to originate on the roof of the nasopharynx perhaps from the periosteum of the sphenoid bone (Fig. 16-29). It increases in size slowly but relentlessly and eventually begins to erode the anterior structures, obstruct the nasal passages and enter the maxillary sinus on one or both sides. The first symptom may be nasal obstruction but is usually epistaxis, which can be very profuse and even life-threatening.

This lesion is found exclusively in males, usually in the preadolescent or adolescent age groups. In some instances as the boy matures, the lesion appears to regress spontaneously. Just as often it persists, and hemangiofibromas of the nasopharynx have been described in males in their

Fig. 16-29. Juvenile nasopharyngeal hemangiofibroma. A fibrous, highly vascular lesion on the posterior wall of the nasopharynx. This was first noted because of epistaxis. Exposure was obtained by an incision between the hard and soft palate with retraction of the soft palate downward.

twenties and thirties, either persisting from childhood or appearing for the first time.

The progressive destruction of surrounding bone by pressure and the continuing threat of major hemorrhage require prompt treatment, preferably before the lesions grow too large. Radiation therapy is ineffective, and operative excision appears the only mode of treatment. There is a tendency toward local recurrence following excision, and these patients must be followed carefully for some years after operation.

Malignant Lesions

These are epidermoid carcinoma, lymphosarcoma, adenoid cystic carcinoma, cervical chordoma, sarcoma, and myeloma. The only lesions occurring with any frequency are epidermoid carcinoma and lymphosarcoma.

EPIDERMOID CARCINOMA

These develop from areas of metaplasia in the respiratory epithelium of the nasopharynx and are moderately to highly undifferentiated. There is a liberal amount of lymphoid tissue in the nasopharynx, and frequently malignant epithelial cells are seen mixed with a prominent lymphoid stroma. This mixture of epidermoid and lymphoid cells gave rise to the term "lymphoepithelioma" introduced by Regaud and Schmincke. Many pathologists feel there is no place for this special term, since these tumors are probably highly anaplastic epidermoid carcinomas and the lymphoid element may not constitute an actual malignant part of the growth. Some feel that a large percentage of lymphoid intermixing indicates a more radiosensitive and more radiocurable tumor.

Fig. 16-30. Metastatic lymph nodes in the neck from lympho-sarcoma of the nasopharynx. Note the characteristic location behind and inferior to the ear.

In addition to the obstructive symptoms described for benign tumors, the invasive qualities of malignant lesions produce a number of characteristic signs and symptoms. These lesions invade the roof of the nasopharynx entering the cavernous sinus with paralysis of the IIId, IVth, Vth, and VIth cranial nerves. The VIth nerve is usually para-lyzed first; this is frequently accompanied by pain in the distribution of the supraorbital and infraorbital branches of the Vth nerve. The tumor reaches these nerves by spreading along the eustachian tube into the space between the pharynx and the maxilla, then extending upward through the suture line between the petrous portion of the temporal bone and the lateral wing of the sphenoid. Thus, the symptom complex is called the *petrosphenoidal syn-drome*. Metastatic nodes in the retropharyngeal space tend to spread into the area along the base of the skull medial to the parotid gland, where they compress the IXth, Xth, XIth, and XIIth cranial nerves. This causes difficulties with deglutition from hemiparesis of the superior constrictor muscle, a perversion of the sense of taste in the posterior third of the tongue, and hypesthesia of the mucous mem-branes of the soft palate, pharynx, and larynx. Paralysis of the trapezius muscle, the sternocleidomastoid, the soft palate, and one side of the tongue may also occur. These signs may be associated with Horner's syndrome from compression of the cervical sympathetic chain. Invasion of the orbit and displacement of the globe will cause double vision and proptosis.

Unfortunately, the nasopharynx is a silent area, and tumors here can reach considerable size before any symp-toms are evident. The early signs of nasal obstruction or brief episodes of epistaxis are easily ignored. In two-thirds of the patients, by the time diagnosis is made, invasion of the sphenoid bone and base of the skull or nerve paral-ysis is present. Not infrequently, the primary growth will remain small, even microscopic, and is announced by its cervical metastases. These occur in a characteristic loca-tion, high in the neck behind the lower portion of the ear with additional involved nodes scattered along the path of the spinal accessory nerve as it courses down the trape-zius muscle (Fig. 16-30). Cervical metastases are found in 50 percent of patients when first seen and are the present-ing symptom in one-third.

There is no acceptable way of obtaining an adequate margin of resection when operating upon lesions of the nasopharynx, and the only operative procedure used is biopsy. Treatment of the primary lesion and usually of the metastases is by radiation therapy. Considering the ad-vanced state of most of these lesions when first seen, the 5-year survival rate as a result of therapy is remarkably good, with an overall absolute survival of 28 percent. For the occasional patient who does not have evidence of cervical node metastasis at the beginning of treatment the 5-year survival rate is 55 percent.

LYMPHOSARCOMA

Lymphosarcomas of the nasopharynx tend to occur at the extremes of age in childhood and in the seventh and eighth decades. The majority of these lesions announce their presence by the occurrence of cervical node metas-tases, which are usually bulky with a rubbery consistency; the nodes mat together but are less inclined to be invasive and fixed than nodes involved by carcinoma. While lym-phosarcoma may mimic all the symptoms produced by epidermoid carcinomas, they invade bone infrequently, and paralysis of nerves is much less common. If there is no evidence of spread beyond the area of the head and neck, the radiotherapist usually administers a high level of therapy in the vicinity of 6,000 rads of cobalt to both the nasopharynx and the cervical lymphatic tissues bilater-ally. Five-year survival in these highly radiosensitive tu-mors is slightly better than for epidermoid carcinoma, averaging 35 to 40 percent.

NASAL CAVITY AND PARANASAL SINUSES

The position of the eight nasal sinuses surrounding the nasal cavity is often poorly appreciated. The maxillary sinuses lateral to the nasal cavities and beneath the orbits are the largest and most important of the sinus structures. The ethmoid air cells occupying the space between the orbit and the upper nasal cavity are much smaller and are less commonly involved by tumors. The frontal sinuses bilaterally above the orbits are the second largest set of sinuses. The paired sphenoid sinuses divided by a thin septum just below the pituitary and over the roof of the nasopharynx are the most remote of the sinuses. The frontal and sphenoid sinuses are rare primary sites for tumors.

INCIDENCE. Tumors of the nasal cavity and paranasal

sinuses represent about 1 percent of all cancer seen. Malignant lesions are found here three times as commonly in men as in women. With the exception of the esthesioneuroblastoma no specific cause is known for lesions arising here.

Benign Tumors

Polyps of the nasal cavity and maxillary sinus are the most common growths seen. These are usually associated with chronic inflammation or, occasionally, allergy. Sometimes the underlying infection may be due to a tumor, so that the discovery of polyps should not be considered an adequate diagnosis until the possibility of an underlying tumor has been ruled out. While polyps can be eradicated by simple excision, they will usually re-form unless the basic pathologic condition leading to their growth has been determined and corrected. This may be allergy, septal deviation, or other factors which obstruct adequate drainage and promote infection.

Malignant Tumors

Of 293 patients with neoplasms of the nasal cavity and paranasal sinus examined at the Mayo Clinic approximately 50 percent had epidermoid carcinomas, 10 percent had lymphomas, and 20 percent had tumors which probably arose from minor salivary tissue. The remaining 20 percent had various soft tissue sarcomas such as fibrosarcoma, chondrosarcoma, neurofibrosarcoma, and osteogenic sarcoma. Among 648 patients seen in Sweden with epidermoid carcinomas arising from the paranasal sinuses, the average age ranged from fifty to seventy years, and the vast majority of the lesions arose in the maxillary sinus (Fig. 16-31). None of these tumors occurred in the sphenoid sinus and only one in the frontal sinus.

Tumors, whether benign or malignant, are announced by pain, nasal obstruction, and persistent nasal secretion. Fifty percent of the patients present with one or more of these three symptoms. Unfortunately, these are also the presenting symptoms of sinusitis; patients may be treated with antibiotics and other measures for long periods before the more serious nature of the disease is realized. Repeated epistaxis is more likely to suggest the presence of tumor but occurs in only 10 percent as a presenting symptom. Swelling or ulceration of the hard palate or gingiva, swelling of the cheek, or ocular symptoms are evidences of a much more advanced stage of tumor growth yet constitute the presenting symptom in 25 to 30 percent of patients (Fig. 16-32). Bone destruction seen on roentgenographic examination is almost certain evidence of a tumor and unfortunately is also a late sign. Absence of bone destruction does not rule out a malignant tumor. All tissue removed when polyps of the nose or maxillary sinus are treated or when the maxillary sinus is drained should be submitted for histologic examination. Not infrequently this is the first evidence of the presence of an underlying carcinoma and may be the only opportunity for diagnosis of such lesions at an early state.

TREATMENT. Electrosurgical therapy, radiation therapy,

Fig. 16-31. Squamous carcinoma of the maxilla. The lesion had its origin in the upper portion of the maxillary sinus and invaded the floor of the orbit.

Fig. 16-32. Squamous carcinoma of the ethmoid sinuses. This lesion began in the left ethmoid and invaded the nasal cavity and right ethmoid sinus.

and operative excision have all been used to treat these tumors. Lymphomas are ordinarily treated by radiation alone. Epidermoid carcinomas of this site are refractory to either irradiation or operation. Integration of irradiation preoperatively with operative excision has been used for many years and has gained wide acceptance. This approach yields a 5-year survival rate of 30 to 35 percent for lesions of the maxillary sinuses. Cervical lymph nodes are involved late, and radical neck dissections are not done unless palpable nodes are present.

MANDIBLE

Tumors of the mandible arise from two main sources, from the tooth-forming (odontogenic) tissue and from bone.

Odontogenic Tumors

These neoplasms arise from ectodermal odontogenic tissue, mesodermal odontogenic tissue, or a mixture of both. They are invariably benign. The lesions most commonly seen are ectodermal odontogenic cysts: the follicular and radicular cysts. A rare and intriguing tumor is the ameloblastoma. Other odontogenic tumors are too rare to merit consideration here.

FOLLICULAR CYST

Some cysts are derived from the dental lamina and outer enamel epithelium of developing teeth. Remnants of this tissue sequestered during development may undergo proliferation and cystic change. Microscopically, they have fibrous walls usually lined by squamous epithelium. Occasionally remnants of odontogenic epithelium are present from which ameloblastomas may develop. Often the cyst

Fig. 16-33. Roentgenogram of a radicular cyst. Note the root of the tooth from which the cyst took origin. (*Courtesy of Sheldon Rovin, D.D.S.*)

envelops an unerupted tooth. A pathognomonic x-ray finding is the appearance of a smooth symmetric cyst in the mandible containing an unerupted tooth in its cavity. Clinically the tumor is found as a mass causing enlargement of the ramus of the mandible or the rim of the gingiva. Treatment is by intraoral excision, removing the top of the cyst and excising its entire lining membrane.

RADICULAR CYST

Infection of the dental pulp is the most common cause of this frequent cyst. A dental granuloma forms when epithelial remnants of the sheath about the tooth root are entrapped. Nests of epithelial tissue proliferate to line a central lumen usually at the apex of the infected tooth (Fig. 16-33). Cysts may vary in size from 1 to several centimeters. Microscopically, there is a dense, fibrous connective tissue lining covered internally by squamous epithelium. Frequently, a generalized inflammatory reaction in the cyst wall is seen. Treatment is by extraction of the tooth involved and excision of the cyst with its lining.

AMELOBLASTOMA

Although very uncommon, this is the most frequent solid tumor of the mandible. It usually appears in the body of the mandible at its junction with the ramus. Growth is slow, and the lesion is relatively asymptomatic, although it may expand the bone about it and eventually attain enormous size, encroaching on soft tissues of the face and neck (Fig. 16-34). Microscopically, the tumor presents interlacing strands and nests of odontogenic epithelium enmeshed in a connective tissue stroma with numerous areas of cystic degeneration. Treatment is by segmental resection of the portion of the mandible affected by the tumor including a centimeter or two of normal bone on either side. Unless the wide excision is accomplished, recurrence is common. The adjacent soft tissues need not be resected, and a good bed is usually left for reconstruction of the mandible.

Osteogenic Tumors

The mandible is affected by the same group of benign and malignant tumors which affect other bones in the body. Benign lesions include exostosis (torus mandibularis), fibrous dysplasia, Paget's disease, and giant cell tumor. Primary malignant lesions are multiple myeloma, Ewing's sarcoma, osteogenic sarcoma, chondrosarcoma (Fig. 16-35), and periosteal fibrosarcoma.

Giant cell tumors of the mandible are often referred to as *central* reparative giant cell tumors and are equivalent to the peripheral giant cell tumors of the gingiva. Although this lesion grows slowly and expands the surrounding bone, it never appears to have the malignant potential of giant cell tumors seen elsewhere in the skeleton and may have a different histogenesis. Microscopically, no distinction can be made between mandibular giant cell tumors and giant cell lesions of other bones. Treatment is usually by unroofing the tumor and curetting its tissue from the bony cavity.

SALIVARY GLANDS

Salivary tissue is found in the parotid gland, the submaxillary gland, the lingual gland, and the numerous salivary glands. The parotid gland is a unilobular structure which is bent in a U shape about the posterior portion of the mandible in such a way that the larger external portion of the gland is often called the *superficial lobe* and the smaller internal portion lying on the internal surface of the ascending ramus is called the *deep lobe*. The VIIth nerve exiting from the skull by way of the stylohyoid foramen crosses the space between the mastoid and the ascending ramus of the mandible and plunges into the parotid gland at the point where it turns the corner around the posterior edge of the ascending ramus. The VIIth nerve usually bifurcates within the substance of the parotid. Each bifurcation further subdivides, and the branches eventually lie between the parotid gland and the underlying masseter muscle. The relationship of the VIIth nerve to the parotid gland is of clinical importance, since tumors of the parotid lie most commonly in the external portion of the gland; on excising such tumors great care must be taken not to cut the branches or the main trunk of this nerve.

The submaxillary gland is an ovoid structure lying in the submaxillary fossa beneath the horizontal ramus of the mandible. It is bounded by the anterior and posterior portions of the digastric muscle, thus occupying most of the digastric triangle in the neck. The important relationships of this gland are to the ramus mandibularis, the lowest branch of the VIIth nerve which courses over the upper portion of the gland. Injury to this nerve blocks innervation of the inferior quarter of the orbicularis oris on the side of the nerve and deprives the patient of the ability to pucker his lips normally. The lingual nerve, deep to the upper inferior surface of the submaxillary gland, provides the gland with some small branches. In addition, the lingual nerve parallels the course of Wharton's duct, which conducts saliva from the submaxillary gland to the mouth. When the gland is removed, injury to the lingual nerve can occur either when Wharton's duct is clamped or when the gland is pulled down into the neck dragging the lingual nerve along by its nerve attachments.

The lingual gland is the smallest of the three major salivary glands. It lies beneath the mucosa of the anterior floor of the mouth.

The minor salivary glands are small deposits of salivary tissue which are scattered throughout the mucosa of the oral cavity, maxilla, and nasopharynx. The term "ectopic salivary tissue" is sometimes used but carries an incorrect connotation, since this salivary tissue is a normal finding in all individuals and is not the result of an error in development.

INCIDENCE. About ⅓ percent of all malignant tumors occurs in the salivary tissues. These tumors are equally common in men and women. About 60 percent of these lesions occur in the parotid glands, which is not surprising, since this is the largest single collection of salivary tissues. The second largest concentration of tumors is found in the submaxillary gland and the third largest in the minor

Fig. 16-34. Ameloblastoma. These lesions can grow to fantastic size, as shown here. Aside from the mass and functional disability, they are painless and never become malignant. (*Courtesy of Sheldon Rovin, D.D.S.*)

salivary glands. Tumors of the lingual glands are rare. No specific cause is known for any of the benign or malignant tumors of the salivary glands other than the occasional congenital or obstructive cyst. Women with malignant tumors of the salivary glands are known to have a higher incidence of cancer of the breast.

Benign Lesions. A variety of lesions may arise in salivary tissue.

Fig. 16-35. Chondrosarcoma of the mandible. This is a slowly developing lesion and was present in this patient for 9 years before medical aid was sought. The pressure of the upper gingiva has caused the groove which is seen in the dorsal surface of the tumor. Even at this late date, the tumor had not metastasized, and the patient was still alive and well 5 years after resection. (*From B. F. Rush, Jr., and K. Trinkle, South Med J, 60:714, 1967.*)

Mixed Tumors. The most common lesion of the salivary glands is the mixed tumor (pleomorphic adenoma). Fifty percent of all tumors of the salivary glands and over eighty percent of all benign tumors are mixed tumors. These probably originate from adult glandular epithelium and, as their name implies, have an extremely diverse structural pattern. In 90 percent of the tumors one finds areas where the tumor grows in a network of strands made up of spindle and stellate cells not always connecting and sometimes lying entirely detached. In about a third of all cases this loose myxoid pattern predominates but is by no means the sole structural component. Half the tumors have pseudocartilaginous structures. Twenty percent show tissue closely resembling hyaline cartilage. Well-formed tubular structures are common and present a wide variety of patterns. The lining epithelium may be single-layered, conspicuously double-layered, stratified, or pseudostratified. Some areas of metaplasia into squamous epithelium may be seen, and well-differentiated squamous epithelium can be found in about a fourth of the cases.

Papillary Cystadenoma Lymphomatosum (Warthin's Tumor). These curious lesions occur only in parotid salivary tissue and almost exclusively (95 percent) in males. About 10 percent of them are bilateral. Characteristically they are made up of a papillary epithelial component intermingled with well-developed lymphoid tissue commonly containing germinal centers. Their histogenesis is uncertain, but many feel they represent parotid duct tissue sequestered in lymph nodes within the parotid gland. They represent the second most common benign tumor of salivary tissue but are a poor second to mixed tumors, which are at least eight times more common.

Mikulicz's Disease. This disease is characterized by a dense infiltration of lymphocytes occasionally arranged in follicles throughout the salivary tissue. This is accompanied by atrophy and disappearance of acinar tissue. Scattered throughout the lymphoid tissue are foci of epithelial and myoepithelial cells in close relationship to distal structures. The more popular modern term for this lesion is *benign lymphoepithelial lesion,* and many feel it represents a phase of the larger disease complex *Sjögren's syndrome.* The diffuse lymphocytic infiltrate, much as one sees in lymphomatous thyroiditis, suggests the possibility of an autoimmune disease. While several of or all the major salivary glands may be involved, a single parotid gland is the most frequent site (80 percent). The highest incidence of the disease is in patients between thirty-one and forty years of age.

Asymptomatic Enlargement of Salivary Tissue. This affection is usually observed in both parotid glands but may involve all the major salivary glands. The characteristic microscopic findings are an increase in size of the glandular acini due to swelling of the individual acinar cells. There is an increase of the secretory granules, a fatty infiltration, and a moderate fibrosis. These changes seem associated with nutritional deficiencies and have been found in patients suffering from cirrhosis of the liver, kwashiorkor, and diabetes mellitus. It also has been found in whole populations suffering from malnutrition in India, in Greece during the occupation of World War II, and in the inmates of German concentration camps. Katsilambros believes that this is a fundamental response to a deficiency of vitamin A and has duplicated his findings in vitamin A–deficient rats.

Other Lesions. Cysts of the parotid glands are seen quite rarely and in some instances may represent cysts of the first branchial cleft. Hemangiomas in children have a predilection for the area of the parotid gland and sometimes persist into adulthood. Neurofibromas and lipomas of the parotid gland have been described.

Malignant Lesions. About 75 percent of all malignant salivary tumors arise from the parotid gland, and 25 percent of all parotid tumors are malignant. Ten percent of malignant salivary lesions arise in the submaxillary gland and an additional twelve percent in the minor salivary glands. The incidence of malignant lesions in the submaxillary and minor salivary glands compared to benign lesions is somewhat higher than in the parotid gland, averaging one-third to one-half of all lesions seen. Roughly one-third of the malignant lesions of salivary tissue arise from the acinar epithelium and are adenocarcinomas. Another third arise from the ductal epithelium as various forms of epidermoid carcinomas. The remaining third appear either as highly anaplastic and unclassified lesions or as malignant mixed tumors.

Epidermoid Carcinoma. The most frequent of these are the mucoepidermoid carcinomas originally identified as a special group by Stewart et al. in 1945. These interesting tumors are made up, as the name indicates, of epidermoid cells and mucus-containing cells. The name falls short of being completely descriptive, since there is a third cell called an "intermediate" cell, smaller than either of the other two, which closely resembles certain cells of the salivary gland duct. They are commonly seen in stratifications lining dilated ductlike structures. Stewart et al. suggest that this intermediate cell is capable of differentiation into mucinous cells or into epidermoid and even squamous cells.

Mucoepidermoid carcinomas are usually divided on the basis of the microscopic appearance into low-grade and high-grade tumors. Low-grade tumors contain a large portion of mucus-secreting cells, often with the presence of microcysts and large amounts of mucoid material which may leak diffusely through the tissues, generating variable degrees of inflammatory reaction. In the highly malignant tumors epidermoid and intermediate cells dominate the picture. Pseudoglandular formation is fairly frequent, and the growth pattern is commonly sheetlike or in coarse plugs.

Squamous cell carcinomas like mucoepidermoid carcinomas must certainly originate in the ductal epithelium, and the ability of salivary duct epithelium to undergo squamous metaplasia is well known. Stewart et al. suggest that most squamous cell carcinomas represent diffuse squamous cell overgrowth of tumors that were fundamentally mucoepidermoid. Microscopically, these lesions share the usual features of squamous cell carcinomas seen in the skin, oral cavity, and elsewhere. In this location, however, they are usually more malignant, and local and regional metastases are common.

Adenocarcinoma. *Adenoid Cystic Carcinoma (Cylindroma).* The chief histologic feature of these lesions is the arrangement of rather small, darkly staining cells with relatively low cytoplasm in anastomosing cords between which are acellular areas which may contain mucous, hyaline, or mucohyaline material. The cystic components of an adenoid cystic carcinoma usually stain positively with mucicarmine, indicating the presence of mucin. While the lesions are of sluggish evolution, metastases to cervical lymph nodes develop in 30 percent of the cases.

Acinar Cell Adenocarcinoma. These histologically distinct tumors are of low-grade clinical malignancy and fairly rare. They appear to arise from the acinar cells of salivary tissue and to be limited to the parotid gland. In the usual microscopic arrangement rounded or polygonal cells with a dark eccentric nucleus and a finely granular basophilic cytoplasm are packed closely together, sometimes in crude, acinar groups. While low-grade, these lesions are capable of metastasis both regionally and to distant locations.

Miscellaneous Adenocarcinomas. Adenocarcinomas may have a trabecular pattern and may be anaplastic or resemble adenocarcinomas of the gastrointestinal tract. These are usually highly malignant with a high degree of local invasiveness and regional and distant metastases.

Malignant Mixed Tumors. It is usually assumed that malignant mixed tumors arise from a neoplastic transformation of a previously benign mixed tumor. Patients who demonstrate these lesions are generally older than those with benign mixed tumors and have had a mass in the parotid for a longer period. Moreover, the malignant lesions are usually larger than the benign. In general, the microscopic picture is of a definite mixed tumor which contains within it malignant elements which may be adenocarcinomas, squamous cell carcinomas, or a malignant spindle cell alteration. The malignant component of a mixed tumor may so greatly overgrow the area of origin that it is extremely difficult to identify the previous benign mixed tumor.

NATURAL HISTORY. With the exception of the mixed tumor the common benign lesions of salivary tissue have no malignant potential. While the mixed tumor may have a very long history without malignant transformation and may grow for 20 to 30 years at a slow pace (Fig. 16-36), a rapidly growing and even anaplastic component can suddenly develop which markedly changes its course. On rare occasions mixed tumors have been found which have metastasized to local nodes without apparent histologic change and in their new location have pursued a slow course of growth. The most common pattern, however, is the development of a squamous cell carcinoma, adenocarcinoma, or other tumor which rapidly overgrows the original mixed tumor. Some very slowly evolving "chronic" carcinomas are known to develop from salivary tissue. Notable among these are the adenoid cystic carcinomas, which may develop their metastases 10, 15, and even 20 years after treatment of the primary tumor.

Many such tumors have been reported in which metastatic nodules in the lungs have been observed growing very slowly, at times appearing almost stationary for 10 and 15 years. The mucoepidermoid carcinoma, while not as

Fig. 16-36. Giant mixed tumor of the parotid. This lesion had been present for 29 years. It was still benign and was excised without evidence of recurrence in a 5-year follow-up. (*From B. F. Rush, Jr., and K. Trinkle, South Med J, 60:714, 1967.*)

slow-growing as the adenoid cystic carcinoma, is rather slowly progressive; however, this trait is offset by its great degree of local invasiveness, especially by perineural invasion. The chances for local recurrence are great even after wide local excision. Squamous cell carcinomas and adenocarcinomas of the salivary glands are almost always highly malignant, quick to invade and metastasize, and fatal in a high percentage of the patients affected.

DIFFERENTIAL DIAGNOSIS. Most tumors of the salivary glands appear as painless, slowly growing nodules (Fig. 16-37). Lesions of the parotid are bound by the heavy

Fig. 16-37. Multilobulated mixed tumor of the parotid. The lesion presents in the upper pole of the superficial portion of the gland.

cervical fascia which splits on either side of the gland and invests it with a strong capsule. This dense covering obscures the actual size of the underlying tumor, and the surgeon may be surprised by the size and extent of a lesion at operation. Paralysis of the VIIth nerve is indicative of a malignant tumor and usually of a highly malignant lesion such as squamous carcinoma or adenocarcinoma. Mucoepidermoid carcinomas of the low-grade type or adenoid cystic carcinomas frequently spare the nerve until quite late in their course. Fixation of the gland to underlying structures and palpable nodes in the neck are also more commonly seen with the tumors of higher grade. Since there is nothing that can distinguish the benign mass in the salivary gland from an early malignant tumor, excision of the mass and histologic examination are indicated in every case.

TREATMENT. Benign mixed tumors, the most common solid tumors of salivary gland origin, are so easily disseminated that incisional biopsy is never indicated. In earlier decades the technique of choice for removal was enucleation. Follow-up of patients so treated indicated that local recurrence was late and slow to develop and occurred in as many as 50 percent. Attempt at excision of these lesions with a cuff of surrounding normal tissue was accompanied by a high rate of injury to one or more branches of the VIIth nerve.

Through these painful experiences the present method of therapy was developed. After isolation of the VIIth nerve, the superficial portion of the parotid gland is dissected from the underlying tissues and removed with the tumor contained within it, assuring against injury of branches of the facial nerve and against dissemination and local recurrence of the tumor.

Frozen section of the lesion should be done at operation. If a low-grade malignant lesion such as an acinar cell adenocarcinoma, a low-grade mucoepidermoid carcinoma, or an adenoid cystic carcinoma is identified, the remainder of the gland and probably the VIIth nerve should be removed. If a high-grade lesion such as an anaplastic adenocarcinoma or squamous carcinoma is identified, a radical neck dissection should accompany the procedure. Aside from the problem of dealing with the VIIth nerve, the same general rules apply for lesions in the submaxillary gland.

Most of the tumors of salivary glands have a reputation for being poorly radiosensitive; however, the more malignant the lesion, the less likely this is to be true. Many high-grade mucoepidermoid carcinomas, squamous carcinomas, and even an occasional adenocarcinoma will demonstrate considerable sensitivity to x-ray therapy.

PROGNOSIS. Benign mixed tumors will recur in 40 to 50 percent of patients if improperly excised. If excision is by superficial lobectomy, the recurrence rate should be 5 percent or less. Five-year survival rates tend to be misleading, particularly in the chronic, slow-growing tumors. Adenoid cystic carcinoma has an 86 percent 5-year survival rate but a 57 percent 10-year survival. Malignant mixed tumor may have a 5-year survival of 87 to 90 percent and a 10-year survival of 60 to 70 percent.

TUMORS OF THE NECK

Palpable or visible cervical swellings are a common complaint. Two to three percent of all admissions to hospital surgical services are for this condition. About half of these lesions occur in the thyroid gland; the remainder are due to a wide range of malignant, congenital, or inflammatory swellings.

Inflammation

Inflammatory swelling in the adult neck is now a rare hospital problem. Skandalakis and coworkers, in reviewing 1,616 nonthyroid masses of the neck, found that only 3.2 percent were inflammatory, whereas 84 percent were neoplastic and 12 percent congenital or miscellaneous. The inflammatory lesions requiring hospitalization of adults are largely acute, often resulting from drainage from infection elsewhere. A common source is an infected tooth draining to the nodes in the submandibular area and causing an abscess. Only two patients in Skandalakis' entire series had tuberculous adenitis (scrofula). This was once the most common cause of neck masses, but with the tuberculin testing of cows and the pasteurization of milk, bovine tuberculosis has virtually disappeared in this country.

Malignant Tumors

The vast majority of cervical masses in adults are due to neoplasms. About 80 percent of these are metastatic from some other site, while the remainder occur from primary lesions in the neck. Primary cervical neoplasms occur either in the major salivary glands (40 percent) or are lymphomas primary in the cervical lymph nodes (60 percent). At one time it was proposed the squamous carcinomas arose primarily in the neck from the lining of branchial cleft cysts. This diagnosis was often made only to discover at a later date that the lesion was actually a metastasis from the oral cavity, nasopharynx, or laryngeal area. While there is some evidence that branchiogenic cysts become malignant, the reported, provable cases number only a handful.

A knowledge of the statistics quickly indicates that a clinician's first suspicion concerning any nonthyroid, cervical mass in adults is of a malignant tumor. He may also suspect that it is metastatic and from a site at some point above the clavicle, since 85 percent of all metastatic cervical lesions come from a supraclavicular site.

When a firm to hard cervical node which suggests malignancy is found, the first responsibility of clinicians is a thorough exploration of possible sites of origin. Cervical tumors appearing below and behind the ear and along the cervical chain are more likely to come from the nasopharynx or lateral pharyngeal walls. Swollen lymph nodes at the angle of the mandible or in the area of the submaxillary gland are most commonly from lesions in the tonsillar area, buccal mucosa, floor of the mouth, and gingiva. Swelling of the lymph nodes in the submental area should provoke a thorough examination of the tip of the tongue, lower lip, and anterior gingivobuccal gutter. Lymph nodes involved by neoplasm which appear in the middle third of the neck should cast suspicion first on the hypopharynx, piriform sinus, larynx, or thyroid.

Only when enlarged lymph nodes appear in the supraclavicular area does metastasis from below the clavicle become a major possibility. These may stem from carcinoma of the upper lobes of the lung or mediastinum or, in women, from carcinoma of the breast. The left supraclavicular nodes are frequently involved by malignant tumors metastatic from the abdomen (Virchow's node). Advanced adenocarcinoma of the stomach, pancreas, biliary tree, and even large bowel metastasize to this site.

If a thorough search of all sites reveals no possible source of a primary lesion, biopsy of the cervical node is usually carried out. If this confirms the clinical impression of malignancy, further attempts to find the primary lesion are indicated. This can include surgical exploration of the maxillary sinuses. If all avenues have been searched thoroughly and no primary lesion has been found, the problem of local treatment still remains. The best course is to treat the lesion to achieve cure. If operation is chosen, it should be a radical neck dissection; if radiation therapy is used, it should be a full course of therapy. Since lymph nodes involved by metastatic disease respond poorly to radiation, the treatment of choice is normally operation. In the presence of advanced lesions a combination of radiation and operation may be used.

If a group of these patients treated without a known primary lesion is followed for 5 years, 80 percent of the patients will ultimately manifest the primary lesion. In some instances this may subsequently be resected for cure. A few patients may die over this period without ever demonstrating the source for the metastatic lesion, and even at postmortem examination it may not be found. Even more interesting, about 20 percent of the patients survive 5 or more years with apparent "cure" of their metastatic lesion even though the presumed primary lesion has not been found or treated. In those patients who received radiation therapy, either together with operation or alone, it may be that the port included the primary lesion as well. In those patients who are treated by operation alone, the fate of the primary lesion remains a mystery. A few of these patients may represent true branchiogenic carcinoma, or possibly the primary lesion regresses spontaneously.

Other Lesions

A host of other tumors, found infrequently in the area of the neck, present problems in differential diagnosis. Dermoids occur in the midline, most commonly in the submental area and sometimes along the line of the clavicle. Sebaceous cysts are common, especially in men, and probably are related to the trauma of shaving.

Carotid body tumors (chemodectomas) are rare tumors of the paraganglionic tissue found at the carotid bifurcation. Another lesion with a slow evolution, it gradually increases in size over many years, enveloping the bifurca-

tion and slowly compressing the adjacent nerves including the hypoglossal, vagus, and sympathetic chain. For many periods, the only symptom is the mass in the neck. Eventually nerve paralysis, dysphagia, and pain appear. Malignant transformation is rare, but early removal is indicated to avoid the late symptoms. Small lesions can be removed easily (Fig. 16-38), but advanced large tumors require resection of the carotid artery with the risk of subsequent hemiparesis.

TUMORS OF THE NECK IN CHILDREN

The order of frequency of masses in the neck in children differs markedly from that found in adults. Inflammatory lesions are by far the most common, often coming from related infections of the tonsils. The most common malignant lesion is the lymphoma, and the second most common is carcinoma of the thyroid. Congenital lesions, of course, are much more common in children than in adults.

CHEMOTHERAPY AND IMMUNOTHERAPY

In the past decade it has been discovered that certain types of neoplasms commonly found in the head and neck area can be cured by chemotherapy. Burkitt's lymphoma, a rare neoplasm in the United States but common in some parts of Africa, was the first such cancer. It became apparent that a predictable and consistent percentage of patients with this disease could be cured by the use of *systemic* chemotherapy alone. Recently we have also learned that squamous cancer of facial skin and of the lips, while in the in situ or microinvasive and superficial stages, can be

Fig. 16-38. Carotid body tumor of moderate size. The lesion lies between the internal and external branches of the carotid arteries; the adventitial layer binding it to the carotid bulb has been removed. (*From B. F. Rush, Jr., Ann Surg, 157:633, 1963.*)

cured by the topical application of 5-fluorouracil used as a cream or paste. These lesions are multiple and often tedious to eradicate by operation or radiation. A third head and neck lesion in which chemotherapy has become important is embryonal rhabdomyosarcoma, an uncommon lesion found in infants and children. Cure of this lesion occasionally has been obtained by combining radiation, chemotherapy, and operation.

Epidermoid cancers of the head and neck respond transiently to a number of single agents. Methotrexate has been the most extensively used. Response rates range from 15 to 57 percent. Bleomycin has also been found to have significant activity, comparable to methotrexate, with reported responses ranging from 15 to 50 percent. Other, less effective, single agents are cyclophosphomide (36 percent), vinblastine (29 percent), hydroxyurea (39 percent), 5-fluorouracil (15 percent) and procarbazine (10 percent). Reports of many of these latter drugs are based on small series and represent, at best, rough estimates. The most recent drug to excite interest in treatment of these tumors is cis-dichlorodiammine platinum (II) (DDP or cis-platinum), which appears to match or exceed methotrexate and bleomycin in activity, especially when used in high doses with mannitol-induced diuresis to avoid renal injury.

Arterial infusion for the treatment of cancer in the head and neck area has received much attention. This involves the introduction of chemotherapy, usually methotrexate or 5-fluorouracil, into the external carotid artery via a catheter. The agents are administered either continuously or intermittently over 1 to several weeks. At present, this technique is known to produce a substantial to complete regression of the lesions in a large percentage of patients—as high as 50 percent in some series. Unfortunately, the response is usually transient, and the cancers return to continued growth within 2 to 3 months after treatment is discontinued. Long-term regression is uncommonly seen, and the period of regression obtained is rarely worth the morbidity and complications of the treatment itself. Nonetheless, these observations continue to tantalize clinical investigators seeking a clue which will lead to longer or even permanent remissions.

The growing body of knowledge concerning the interrelationships between cancer and the body's immune system has touched the field of head and neck cancer through the work of Chretian and others. At least half the patients with epidermoid cancer of the oral cavity, hypopharynx, and larynx show some degree of immune incompetence. Moreover, this incompetence is correlated with treatment failure following either radiation or operation. Immune competence can be restored in a number of these patients by improving nutrition, by the use of immunostimulant agents such as BCG or c-Parvum, and by "reconstitution" agents such as Levamisole, thymosin, and transfer factor. Trials to determine the effectiveness of manipulations of the immune system in the immune-incompetent patient are being developed.

Combined forms of treatment for head and neck cancers, which include chemotherapy and immunotherapy as well as radiation and operation, have enjoyed marked clinical and investigative interest in the past several years. The more our knowledge of the natural history of tumor growth develops, the more rational and logical it appears to combine available treatment methods. In the next decade clinical research will be devoted to determining the best dose schedules and the best combinations of drugs and techniques.

OPERATIONS OF THE HEAD AND NECK

The most commonly performed major operation for cancer of the head and neck is radical neck dissection. This procedure was originally designed by Crile to eradicate the cervical lymphatic network, thereby eliminating sites of metastasis from cancer of the oral cavity, pharynx, paranasal sinuses, or other areas of the head and neck. In the early days of head and neck surgery radical neck dissections were usually performed after the primary lesion had been controlled through the use of radiation therapy. Today, we are more inclined to combine radical neck dissection with a simultaneous resection of the primary lesion. This is sometimes preceded by a course of radiation therapy to the primary area as part of a planned program of tumor treatment. Combined operations have been called by a number of terms including *composite resections* and *commando operations*. Other common operations in this area are superficial resection of the parotid gland, V excision of carcinoma of the lip, and resection of the maxillary antrum.

Fig. 16-39. Common operative incisions for radical neck dissections. (*From B. F. Rush, Jr., Curr Probl Surg, May, 1966.*)

CRILE (T-INCISION)

MARTIN (DOUBLE-Y INCISION)

WARD (Y-INCISION)

MACFEE (LADDER INCISION)

Radical Neck Dissection

Incisions for radical neck dissection are numerous and include a T-shaped incision originally used by Crile, a Y incision described by Ward, and a double Y incision described by Martin (Fig. 16-39). We prefer a hockey-stick-shaped incision with the ascending limb along the posterior border of the sternocleidomastoid muscle and the horizontal portion crossing the neck about 2 or 3 cm above the clavicle (Fig. 16-40). This last approach has the advantage of being outside areas of radiation when the neck has had previous exposure to radiation therapy and of being a simple linear incision avoiding small triangular-shaped flaps, which have a tendency to slough. The skin flap is reflected mediad, including the underlying platysma muscle, and dissection of neck structures begins in the posterior triangle, dissecting the fibroareolar tissue of this space away from the trapezius muscle and the underlying brachial plexus and scalene fibers. This portion of the dissection is carried mediad until the phrenic nerve lying on the anterior scalene muscle is identified.

The lower end of the sternocleidomastoid muscle is transected and the jugular vein identified and ligated. The accompanying vagus nerve next to the jugular vein in the carotid sheath is identified and spared. Dissection is then carried up the neck, gradually dissecting the lymph node chain free from underlying fascia and beneath the carotid artery. Just above the level of the carotid bulb the hypoglossal nerve is identified. In the upper portion of the neck the sternocleidomastoid muscle is again transected at the level of the mastoid together with the tip of the parotid gland. The submaxillary gland is dissected free from the digastric fossa and included with the specimen. The lingual nerve and artery in the depths of the submaxillary fossa are visualized and left intact. Care is taken to identify the ramus mandibularis, the tiny fiber of the VIIth nerve which innervates the lower lip, and to reflect this above the submaxillary gland so that its continuity is maintained. The spinal accessory nerve is usually sacrificed, being cut in the lower neck where it enters the trapezius muscle and in the upper neck where it enters the sternocleidomastoid muscle. The operation is completed with the transection of the jugular vein at the point where it leaves the base of the skull (Fig. 16-41). If a radical neck dissection alone is performed, the operation is ended at this point by closing the skin flaps. Multiperforated catheters are left underneath the flaps and are connected to suction. This helps to draw the flap firmly to the structures of the neck and eliminates the problem of fluid collecting under the flap.

COMBINED OPERATION

If a radical neck dissection is to be combined with the removal of structures within the oral cavity or tonsillar area, the contents of the neck dissection are left attached to the horizontal ramus of the mandible. The mandible is frequently divided. If the lesion is in the floor of the mouth or tongue, the horizontal ramus of the mandible may be resected. If the lesion is in the tonsillar fossa, the ascending ramus of the mandible is removed. If the lesion in the oral cavity is quite large, total removal of the hemi-

Fig. 16-40. Radical neck dissection through a hockey-stick incision (shown in insert) combined with an exposure of the mandible. The tumor has grown through the mandible and presented on the cheek so that a portion of the skin of the cheek has been left on the specimen. Structures of the neck are shown exposed and intact prior to the start of radical neck dissection. (*From B. F. Rush, Jr., Surg Gynecol Obstet, 121:353, 1965.*)

mandible on the side of the lesion may be necessary. Resection of the mandible is done to remove bone involved by tumor and sometimes to obtain a closure of the oral cavity which would not be feasible without removing a portion of the bony framework. Mandibular resection can be done with the acceptable cosmetic and functional result, especially when the anterior portion of the mandible is preserved (Fig. 16-42). The more anteriorly the mandible is resected, the more likely there is to be facial deformity. If the primary site of the tumor is in the larynx or thyroid, then these structures may also be removed with the radical neck dissection. The mortality for radical neck dissection alone is less than 1 percent. If neck dissection is combined with en bloc excision of a primary lesion, then mortality rates range from 2 to 3 percent.

BILATERAL RADICAL NECK DISSECTION

Lesions that are in the midline of the oral cavity often spread bilaterally, and it is necessary to remove lymph

Fig. 16-41. Radical neck dissection completed, combined with excision of the horizontal ramus of the mandible. The jugular vein and sternocledomastoid muscle have been removed. The phrenic nerve and the common carotid artery are seen coursing across the operative field. The closure of the neck incision is seen in the insert. (*From B. F. Rush, Jr., Surg Gynecol Obstet, 121:353, 1965.*)

nodes on both sides of the neck. Simultaneous bilateral neck dissections are feasible with an acceptable mortality; however, the postoperative course is likely to be prolonged, since there is a period of marked facial edema following this extensive resection which can persist for several weeks. Some operators will spare the jugular vein on one side when a bilateral neck dissection is done in order to decrease the amount of postoperative edema. Others stage the dissection, allowing a delay of several weeks before operating on the second side.

Parotidectomy

Most lesions in the superficial lobe of the parotid gland are removed by superficial parotidectomy. This operation is designed to give maximal safety in operating about the branches of the VIIth nerve (Fig. 16-43). The VIIth nerve pierces the parotid gland at its posterior margin and lies underneath the gland on the muscles of the face. A Y-shaped incision is made with the lower limb lying behind the angle of the mandible and the arms of the Y on either side of the lobe of the ear. Dissection is carried down to identify the main trunk of the VIIth nerve, which lies in the space between the mandible and the mastoid bone approximately one fingerbreadth below the external auditory meatus. Once the main trunk is identified, dissection is carried along the external surface of the nerve and its branches, gradually separating away the overlying portion of the parotid gland. Stensen's duct is identified at the most medial portion of the midpoint of the parotid gland and is ligated. This technique sometimes causes temporary weakness in the fibers of the VIIth nerve but prevents transecting any of the major trunks of the nerve. Recovery of function in all branches is ensured by the knowledge that they are intact and usually occurs within a week or two following completion of the operation.

V Excision of the Lip

Most cancers of the lower lip are removed with the use of V excision (see Chap. 51). Between one-fourth and one-third of the lower lip can be easily resected by simple excision without resulting in residual deformity or interference with function. While we refer to this excision as a V, a much better cosmetic result is obtained if the outline of the incision resembles that of a shield. A true V excision results in some flattening of the lower lip with a loss of normal eversion. If a shield-shaped incision is used, the lip will evert normally.

If the tumor involves more area than can be excised with a V excision, a flap is migrated from the upper lip. This involves outlining a V-shaped flap in the upper lip which is left attached at its lower medial corner and is then rotated into the defect in the lower lip. Using this type of closure excision of up to two-thirds of the lower lip can be accomplished without difficulty.

Maxillectomy

Cancer of the hard palate or the lower maxilla requires subtotal excision of the maxillary sinus. Cancer in the upper maxilla involving the orbital plate requires total excision of the maxillary sinus together with an exenteration of the orbital contents. While these excisions are basically mutilating, they can be accomplished with little visible external deformity. The Weber-Fergusson incision is used. This begins at the midpoint of the upper lip, extends to the columella of the nose, and is carried around the edge of the nose and up to the corner of the eye. A horizontal portion continues laterally from the inner canthus to a point just beyond the outer canthus and about 2 or 3 mm below the palpebral fissure. The skin and muscles of the cheek are undermined laterally, so that the entire cheek is turned outward, opening a door to the maxillary sinus. The bony attachments of the maxillary sinus are divided, including the midline of the hard palate, the zygoma, the pterygoid plates; if the orbital plate is to be removed, the bony walls of the medial and lateral orbit are also transected. When this is accomplished, the entire maxillary sinus can be lifted like a small box from its normal position. The inner surface of the Weber-Fergusson flap is covered with a split-thickness skin graft, and the incision is closed. Because it falls in the normal skin lines and about the normal structures of the face, this incision is often difficult to detect after it has healed as long as the structures have been replaced precisely and in good apposition. This operation leaves a large defect in the hard palate on the side of the procedure. This is occasionally closed by subsequent operations, but more commonly a

Fig. 16-42. Mandibular resection, 8 days after bilateral neck dissection and partial mandibulectomy on the left, with resection of a portion of the floor of the mouth and the anterior half of the tongue for carcinoma of the tongue. The portion of the jaw was replaced with a Steinmann pin. At 3 years postoperatively there still was no recurrence. Note that it is difficult to determine on which side the mandible was resected. (*From B. F. Rush, Jr., Curr Probl Surg, May, 1966.*)

Fig. 16-43. Superficial parotidectomy. *A.* Incision. *B.* Skin flaps established and fascia incised; greater auricular nerve transected and external jugular vein identified. *C.* External jugular vein transected; superficial lobe is being reflected anteriorly, and facial nerve with its mandibular and cervical branches are shown. *D.* Dissection continued anteriorly, demonstrating temporal, zygomatic, and buccal branches. *E.* Superficial lobe removed; if excision of the deep lobe is indicated, the facial nerve can be retracted craniad and the remaining parotid removed. *F.* Relationship of facial nerve and parotid gland. The nerve branches lie between the deep and superficial lobes of the parotid. (*Courtesy of Robert Chase, M.D.*)

dental prosthesis with a large obturator which fits into the defect is constructed by the prosthodontist. This restores normal speech and relatively normal mastication for the patient.

Total Laryngectomy

Total laryngectomy is traditionally accomplished through a midline longitudinal incision. We have found definite advantages in accomplishing this procedure through a transverse incision in the lower neck very much like the typical thyroidectomy incision. The incision is made 4 cm above the clavicles and approximately 4 cm beyond the edge of the sternocleidomastoid muscles on either side; it is carried down through the platysma muscle, and the upper flap is then developed. The upper limit of dissection is approximately 1 cm above the hyoid, and at this point the entire group of strap muscles and the midportion of the hyoid are exposed. In cancer operations for glottic tumors of any size, all the anterior strap muscles are removed. Occasionally at the election of the operator in the presence of somewhat smaller lesions, the strap muscles on the side contralateral to the lesion may be preserved, or, rarely, the larynx is skeletonized with the preservation of strap muscles on both sides. In the ordinary instance, however, the sternothyroid and sternohyoid muscles are transected at the level of the cricoid, the digastric and mylohyoid muscles are separated from the hyoid above, and the body of the hyoid bone is cut at the junction of the attachments to the lateral wings on either side. The larynx is rocked laterally exposing the pharyngeal constrictors, which are cut at the lateral edge of the thyroid cartilages bilaterally. One can now enter the pharynx laterally, usually on the side opposite the tumor, so that proper visualization of the area can be obtained, and an adequate margin of excision of pharyngeal mucosa will be developed around the tumor. Once the pharynx is entered, it is possible for the surgeon to operate both outside and inside the pharynx. The remaining muscles of the tongue are severed from the hyoid, and the larynx is pulled forward. The vascular pedicles containing the laryngeal arteries and the superior laryngeal nerves are ligated bilaterally. An incision is made in the pharyngeal mucosa just posterior to the arytenoids, entirely circumscribing the point at which the larynx projects into the pharynx. As all pharyngeal mucosa is now separated from the larynx, the larynx is pulled forward, and a plane of dissection is developed between the larynx and the anterior esophageal wall. This dissection is carried inferiorly until the only remaining structure holding the larynx in place is the trachea. This is then divided obliquely around the site of the tracheostomy (if one has been done previous to the operation), or if an endotracheal tube has been used in anesthesia, this is now removed, and a tube is placed in the severed trachea so that anesthesia can be continued. After the larynx has been removed, the defect in the pharynx is closed transversely with an inverting Connell stitch. This is reinforced by interrupted sutures of 4-0 silk which are used to imbricate the constrictor muscles up and around the pharyngeal closure. This closure may further be reinforced by stitches which catch the platysma muscle and draw it down snugly along with the overlying skin. A generous circular portion of skin is removed in the lower midline; this measures about 3 to 4 cm in diameter with three-quarters of the circle lying above the transverse skin incision and one-quarter of the circle lying below. The beveled end of the trachea is then drawn up to the skin by interrupted sutures of nylon. Every attempt is made to obtain a delicate mucosa to skin closure, since the smaller the size of the scar at the junction between mucosa and skin, the less likely there is to be subsequent stenosis of the tracheal opening. The generous amount of skin excised tends to evert the trachea in a slightly "trumpet-like" manner, and this too ensures against subsequent stenosis. This type of trachea skin closure can be maintained without the use of an indwelling tracheostomy tube except for the first 24 hours or so postoperatively. The remainder of the wound is closed with interrupted sutures to the platysma muscle and skin. Two suction catheters are left in place on either side of the neck and are usually removed in 24 to 36 hours. The patient is maintained on postoperative feedings through a nasal tube made up of a #18 whistle-tip red rubber catheter inserted at the time of operation through the nose and into the esophagus before the pharyngeal defect is closed. This tube is sutured to the nasal columella. The patient is maintained on nasal tube feedings for about 10 days. A liquid diet is usually begun on the fifth or sixth day, and the patient may take solid food on the ninth or tenth day. The nasal tube is removed as soon as it is apparent that the patient can well maintain his own nutrition.

Partial Laryngectomy and the Neolarynx

In the past all lesions extending beyond the true cords have been treated by total laryngectomy. The functional importance of the voice and the great benefit of preserving it for the patient has led to an evaluation of cancer operations which do not remove the entire larynx. Ogura and Biller have led this effort and have proposed a number of new operations which involve removal of most or all of the larynx above the cords (supraglottic laryngectomy) or excision of most of one side of the larynx (hemilaryngectomy) for lesions which are confined enough in their growth to be suitable for this technique. This approach requires careful selection of patients who are young and flexible enough to overcome some of the swallowing and aspiration difficulties that often arise postoperatively. Since the resected margin around the tumor may be very limited, careful diagnostic techniques must be used to identify the outer margins. This technique is almost always combined with preoperative radiation therapy to ensure a lesser threat from residual cells at the periphery of the tumor which may be left by the surgeon. Using these techniques in patients with tumors advanced enough to cause fixation of the cord, Ogura and Biller have reported a 77 percent 3-year survival.

An alternative method for preserving the voice, especially in patients with lesions not amenable to partial laryngectomy, is creation of a pseudolarynx. This is done by suturing the trachea, usually after preserving the lower cricoid, to the hyoid bone. The tracheal stoma is covered by a flap of mucosa and a new glottis is formed by a small incision in the mucosal flap. Following this procedure patients usually must wear a tracheostomy tube and speak by occluding the tube, diverting air through the new glottis. Aspiration of swallowed fluids is often an early problem, but patients usually learn to avoid this in time. This procedure was introduced by Serafini in Italy in 1970 and further refined by Vega of Spain. It has only recently been introduced in the United States and is still undergoing refinement. It may offer a good method of preserving the voice in patients with larger lesions.

POSTOPERATIVE CARE FOLLOWING HEAD AND NECK OPERATIONS

Tracheostomy is performed at the time of operation in any patient in whom a portion of the mandible is removed or when there is extensive removal of oral structures. Postoperative edema plus the tendency for the larynx to shift position following sacrifice of many of its suspensory muscles predispose to aspiration and obstruction. Catastrophic anoxia may supervene rapidly, with little apparent warning. The tracheostomy tube must be aspirated frequently. This requires the presence of well-trained nursing personnel. If a patient appears to be accumulating unusual amounts of tracheal secretions, it is probable that saliva is being aspirated through an incompetent larynx. This can be controlled by diligent suctioning. In extreme instances, a cuffed tracheostomy may be required temporarily.

The patient with a tracheostomy has lost the usual humidifying effects of the nasal and pharyngeal passageways. The best way to provide humidity for the patient's trachea is to tie an umbilical tape about the neck above the tracheostomy and to hang a moistened 4 by 4 sponge over this tape very much in the manner that a towel is hung over a rail. The sponge must frequently be moistened, and after the first day or two the patient can be taught to moisten his own sponge and arrange it for himself.

There is no need to leave the tracheostomy in place for prolonged periods. As soon as the patient is found to be maintaining a dry, unobstructed airway and the skin flaps are sealed, the tracheostomy tube is covered with a piece of adhesive tape. This is done about 5 days postoperatively. If the patient tolerates the covering of the tracheostomy tube for 24 hours, it can be removed. This tube should always be removed in the morning, so that the patient can be observed during the daylight hours following removal.

Patients who have undergone combined resections have had extensive superficial operation, but the body cavities have been undisturbed, and the normal function of the gastrointestinal tract resumes almost immediately. A nasoesophageal tube consisting of a #16 French urethral catheter is left in place at the end of the operative procedure. The tip of the standard urethral catheter reaches to the lower third of the esophagus but does not traverse the esophagocardiac junction. Such tubes can be left in place for long periods without the risk of acid regurgitation and

peptic esophagitis. The patient receives fluids intravenously on the day of operation, but on the first postoperative day nasal feedings of half-strength milk are given. On the second postoperative day a nasal formula consisting of a blenderized regular diet diluted with milk is begun. This is continued until the fifth or sixth postoperative day or until the patient shows evidence that he can tolerate an adequate diet by mouth.

Except for the different flora encountered, there is little difference in the principles of operating on the mouth and other areas in the gastrointestinal tract. This is a contaminated area, and numerous tissue planes are open to this contamination. All patients should be placed on appropriate antibiotics postoperatively. Ketcham et al. demonstrated in a controlled study the advantages of prophylactic antibiotics in these patients.

The mental stress in a patient undergoing an oral operation of any magnitude is considerable. He awakens unable to speak because of his tracheostomy. He is unable to control his saliva and finds that he is constantly aspirating small amounts of mucus. His neck and shoulder are completely numb and boardlike because of the section of all cervical sensory nerves on the side of the lesion, and while he has little or no sharp pain, he has a pounding and persistent headache due to the ligation of the jugular vein and concomitant rise of spinal fluid pressure. In a day or two he looks into the mirror and may not recognize the swollen, edematous, and possibly deformed face which stares back at him. It would be abnormal if he were not

Fig. 16-44. Construction of a pseudolarynx by covering the tracheal stoma left after laryngectomy with a flap of mucosa and constructing a new glottis by an incision in the mucosa as shown here is another attempt to obtain immediate functional reconstruction in the head and neck patient. (*From A. Swaminathan, K. Jefferies, and B. F. Rush, Jr., Am J Surg, in press.*)

Fig. 16-45. *A.* Resection of the entire anterior mandible is one of the most devastating procedures for patients both cosmetically and functionally. Attempts at immediate reconstruction include use of a tantalum tray as shown here filled with cancellous bone chips. *B.* The tray is concorporated in a flap of cervical skin from the anterior neck, which also is used to line the residual tongue and floor of the mouth. The remaining mandible is immobilized with external pins. Immediate appearance and function are very acceptable.

depressed under these circumstances. Support for the patient depends on good preoperative preparation. The patient must understand clearly what to expect in the postoperative period. Patients do not panic if they understand their problems and realize that most of their deficiencies are reversible as edema subsides and the tracheostomy tube is removed.

REHABILITATION

As Shedd has pointed out, progress in medicine often brings new problems. In head and neck oncology the successful control of major cancers may leave a considerable number of patients whose posttreatment life involves a significant degree of disability. Major impairment in appearance, swallowing, taste, and speech all reduce the quality of life and the effectiveness of treatment. While the field of rehabilitation of these patients is too broad to detail here, the major thrust of recent years has been to accomplish as much of the rehabilitation as possible on the

operating table at the primary procedure. Techniques such as the construction of a pseudolarynx (Fig. 16-44) or primary implantation of a new mandible at the initial procedure (Fig. 16-45*A* and *B*) produce immediate cosmetic and functional results much more gratifying to the patient and the surgeon than multistaged reconstructions done secondarily, which often take months to accomplish. If primary reconstruction is still unobtainable, then the surgeon must be certain to guide his patient to the appropriate speech therapy, prosthetic substitution, or secondary reconstruction required.

References

General

Advisory Committee to the Surgeon General on Smoking and Health, "Report on Smoking and Health," *Public Health Serv Publ,* 1103, 1964.

Arons, M. S., and Smith, R. R.: Distant Metastases and Local Recurrence in Head and Neck Cancer, *Ann Surg,* **154:**235, 1961.

Baker, H.: Oral Cancer: A Six Part Series, *CA,* pt. I: January–February, 1972; pt. II: March–April, 1972; pt. III: May–June, 1972; pt. IV: July–August, 1972; pt. V: September–October, 1972; pt. VI: January–February, 1973.

Conley, J. (ed.),: "Cancer of the Head and Neck," Butterworth Inc., Washington, 1967.

Gowen, G. F., and deSuto-Nagy, G.: The Incidence and Sites of Distant Metastases in Head and Neck Carcinoma, *Surg Gynecol Obstet,* **116:**603, 1963.

James, A. G.: "Cancer Prognosis Manual," American Cancer Society, Inc., New York, 1967.

Kark, W.: "A Synopsis of Cancer: Genesis and Biology," The Williams & Wilkins Company, Baltimore, 1966.

MacComb, W. S.: Treatment of Head and Neck Cancer, Janeway Lecture, 1960, *Am J Roentgenol Radium Ther Nucl Med,* **84:**589, 1960.

Moore, C.: Smoking and Cancer of the Mouth, Pharynx and Larynx, *JAMA,* **191:**107, 1965.

Rubin, P.: Current Concepts in Cancer: Cancer of the Head and Neck, *JAMA,* **221:**68, 1972. (First of a continuing series of articles.)

Rush, B. F., Jr., Chambers, R. G., and Ravitch, M. M.: Cancer of the Head and Neck in Children, *Surgery,* **53:**270, 1963.

———, Horie, N., and Klein, N. W.: Intra-arterial Infusion of the Head and Neck: Anatomical and Distributional Problems, *Am J Surg,* **110:**510, 1965.

——— and Trinkle, K.: The Management of Low-Grade, Neglected Neoplasms, *South Med J,* **60:**714, 1967.

Schottenfield, D.: Cancer of the Buccal Cavity and Pharynx: A Review of End Results of Primary Treatment in 2877 Cases 1949–1964, *Clin Bull Memorial Hosp,* **2:**51, 1972.

Serafini, I.: Larengectomia totale con mantenimento della respirazione per via naturale (resoconto sul primo case recentemente operato con technica personale), *Min Otorinolarin,* **20:**73, 1970.

Shedd, D. P.: Rehabilitation Problems in Head and Neck Patients, *J Surg Oncology,* **8:**11, 1976.

Taylor, G. W., and Nathanson, I. T.: "Lymph Node Metastases:

Incidence and Surgical Treatment in Neoplastic Disease," Oxford University Press, London, 1942.

Vega, M. F.: Larynx Reconstruction Surgery. A Study of Three-Year Findings: A Modified Surgical Technique, *Laryngoscope,* **85:**866, 1975.

Willis, R. A.: "Pathology of Tumors," Butterworth & Co. (Publishers), Ltd., London, 1960.

Historical Background

Absolon, K. B., Rogers, W., and Aust, J. B.: Some Historical Developments of the Surgical Therapy of Tongue Cancer from the Seventeenth to the Nineteenth Century, *Am J Surg,* **104:**686, 1962.

Campbell, E., and Colton, J.: "The Surgery of Theodoric," Appleton-Century Crofts, Inc., New York, 1955.

Fletcher, G. H., and Jesse, R. H., Jr.: The Contribution of Super-voltage Roentgenotherapy to the Integration of Radiation and Surgery in Head and Neck Squamous Cell Carcinomas, *Cancer,* **15:**566, 1962.

Lip

Ashley, F. L., McConnell, D. V., Machida, R., Sterling, H. E., Galloway, D., and Grazer, F.: Carcinoma of the Lip: A Comparison of Five Year Results after Irradiation and Surgical Therapy, *Am J Surg,* **110:**549, 1965.

Blackerby, J. N., and Hamilton, J. E.: Carcinoma of the Lip, *Surgery,* **51:**591, 1962.

Ward, G. E.: Carcinoma of the Lips, *Md Med J,* **5:**23, 1956.

Oral Cavity

Fayos, J. V. and Lampe, I.: Treatment of Squamous Cell Carcinoma of the Oral Cavity, *Am J Surg,* **124:**493, 1972.

Helfrich, G. B., Nickels, M. E., El-Doomeiri, A., and DasGupta, T.: Management of Cancer of the Floor of the Mouth, *Am J Surg,* **124:**559, 1972.

Kraus, F. T., and Perez-Mesa, C.: Verrucous Carcinoma: Clinical and Pathologic Study of 105 Cases Involving Oral Cavity, Larynx, and Genitalia, *Cancer,* **19:**26, 1966.

Lash, H., Erich, J. B., and Dockerty, M. B.: Pathologic Study of 217 Cases of Epithelioma of the Tongue, *Am J Surg,* **102:**620, 1961.

Marchetta, F. C., Sako, K., and Murph, J. B.: The Periosteum of the Mandible and Intraoral Carcinoma, *Am J Surg,* **122:**711, 1971.

Martin, H. E.: The History of Lingual Cancer, *Am J Surg,* **48:**703, 1940.

Niebel, H. H., and Chomet, B.: In Vivo Staining Test for Delineation of Oral Intraepithelial Neoplastic Change: Preliminary Report, *J Am Dent Assoc,* **68:**801, 1964.

O'Brien, P. H., and Catlin, D.: Cancer of the Cheek (Mucosa), *Cancer,* **18:**1392, 1965.

Rush, B. F., Jr.: Combined Procedures in the Treatment of Oral Carcinoma, *Curr Prob Surg,* May, 1966.

———— and Humphrey, L.: Primary Repair of Full Thickness Excision of the Cheek, *Am J Surg,* **114:**592, 1967.

Sandler, H. C.: Oral Cytology, *CA,* **16:**97, 1966.

Shedd, D. P., Hukill, P. B., Bahn, S., and Ferraro, R. H.: Further Appraisal of In Vivo Staining Properties of Oral Cancer, *Arch Surg,* **95:**16, 1967.

————, Von Essen, C. F., Bevin, A. G., and Greenberg, R. A.:

Ten Year Survey of Oral Cancer in a General Hospital, *Am J Surg,* **114:**844, 1967.

Southwick, H. W., Slaughter, D. P., and Trevino, E. T.: Elective Neck Dissection for Intraoral Cancer, *Arch Surg,* **80:**905, 1960.

Stecker, R. H., Devine, K. D., and Harrison, E. G., Jr.: Verrucose "Snuff Dipper's" Carcinoma of the Oral Cavity: A Case of Self-induced Carcinogenesis, *JAMA,* **189:**144, 1964.

Thoma, K. H.: "Oral Surgery," The C. V. Mosby Company, St. Louis, 1963.

Yonemoto, R. H., Ching, P. T., Bryon, R. L., and Riihimaki, D. U.: The Composite Operation in Cancer of the Head and Neck (Commando Procedure), *Arch Surg,* **104:**809, 1972.

Oropharynx

Baker, R. R., and Weiner, S.: The Clinical Management of Tonsillar Carcinoma, *Surg Gynecol Obstet,* **121:**1035, 1965.

Barkley, H. T., Fletcher, G. H., Jesse, R. H., and Lindberg, R. D.: Management of Cervical Lymph Node Metastasis in Squamous Cell Carcinoma of the Tonsillar Fossa, Base of Tongue, Supraglottic Larynx and Hypopharynx, *Am J Surg,* **124:**464, 1972.

Keller, A. Z.: Cirrhosis of the Liver, Alcoholism and Heavy Smoking Associated with Cancer of the Mouth and Pharynx, *Cancer,* **20:**1015, 1967.

McIlrath, D. C., ReMine, W. H., Devine, K. D., and Dockerty, M. B.: Tumors of the Parapharyngeal Region, *Surg Gynecol Obstet,* **116:**88, 1963.

Perez, C. A., Ackerman, L. V., and Mill, W. B.: Malignant Tumors of the Tonsil: Analysis of Failures and Factors affecting Prognosis, *Am J Roentgenol, Radium Ther Nucl Med,* **114:**43, 1972.

Rush, B. F., Jr., Reynolds, G., and Greenlaw, R.: Integrated Irradiation and Operation in Treatment of Cancer of the Larynx and Hypopharynx: A Preliminary Report, *Am J Roentgenol Radium Ther Nucl Med,* **102:**129, 1968.

Larynx

Baker, R. R., and Cherry, J.: Carcinoma of the Larynx: Results of Therapy in 209 Cases, *Arch Surg,* **90:**449, 1965.

Carveth, S. W., Devine, K. D., and ReMine, W. H.: Laryngectomy with Radical Neck Dissection in Extensive Cancer of the Larynx, *Am J Surg,* **104:**705, 1962.

Clinical Staging System for Cancer of the Larynx, American Joint Committee on Cancer Staging and End Results Reporting, June, 1962.

Donegan, W. L.: An Early History of Total Laryngectomy, *Surgery,* **57:**902, 1965.

Flynn, M. B., Jesse, R. H., and Lindberg, R. D.: Surgery and Irradiation in the Treatment of Squamous Cell Cancer of the Supraglottic Larynx, *Am J Surg,* **124:**477, 1972.

Goldman, J. L., Cheren, R. V., Silverstone, S. M., and Zak, F. G.: Combined Irradiation and Surgery for Cancer of the Larynx and Laryngopharynx, in J. Conley (ed.), "Cancer of the Head and Neck," Butterworth Inc., Washington, 1967.

Holinger, P. H.: Cancer of the Larynx: Classification and Partial Laryngectomy, in J. Conley (ed.), "Cancer of the Head and Neck," Butterworth Inc., Washington, 1967.

Krause, L. G.: Clinical Review of Carcinoma of the Larynx: Experience of a Large Cancer Hospital, *Am J Surg,* **111:**206, 1966.

Norris, C. M.: Treatment of Cancer of the Larynx and the Hypopharynx, *Proc Natl Cancer Conf,* **5**:265, 1964.

Ogura, J. W., and Biller, H. F.: Preoperative Irradiation for Laryngeal and Laryngopharyngeal Cancer, *Laryngoscope,* **80**:802, 1970.

Ono, J., and Shigejo, S.: Endoscopic Microsurgery of the Larynx, *Ann Otol Rhinol Laryngol,* **80**:479, 1971.

Powell, R. W., Redd, B. L., and Wilkins, S. A., Jr.: An Evaluation of Treatment of Cancer of the Larynx, *Am J Surg,* **110**:635, 1965.

Shahrokh, D. K., Devine, K. D., and Harrison, E. G., Jr.: Statistical Evaluation of 115 Cases of Carcinoma of the Epiglottis (1943 to 1952), *Am J Surg,* **102**:781, 1961.

Shedd, D. P.: Role of Surgical Measures in Voice Restoration after Laryngectomy, "Symposium on Malignancies of The Head and Neck," The C. V. Mosby Company, St. Louis, Mo., 1975.

Smith, R. R., Caulk, R. M., Russell, W. O., and Jackson, C. L.: End Results in 600 Laryngeal Cancers Using the American Joint Committee's Proposed Method of Stage Classification and End Results Reporting, *Surg Gynecol Obstet,* **113,** 435, 1961.

Spalt, L., Greenlaw, R., and Rush, B. F., Jr.: Integrated Therapy for Carcinoma of the Larynx, in B. F. Rush, Jr. and R. H. Greenlaw (eds.), "Integrated Radiation and Operation in Cancer Therapy: A Symposium," Charles C Thomas, Publisher, Springfield, Ill., 1968.

Nasopharynx

Jesse, R. H.: Preoperative versus Postoperative Radiation in the Treatment of Squamous Carcinoma of the Paranasal Sinuses, *Am J Surg,* **110**:552, 1965.

Moench, H. C. and Phillips, T. L.: Carcinoma of the Nasopharynx: Review of 146 Patients with Emphasis on Radiation Dose and Time Factors, *Am J Surg,* **124**:515, 1971.

Thomas, J. E., and Waltz, A. G.: Neurological Manifestations of Nasopharyngeal Malignant Tumors, *JAMA,* **192**:103, 1965.

Nasal Cavity and Paranasal Sinuses

Kurohara, S. S., Ellis, F., Fitzgerald, J. P., Webster, J. H., Shedd, D. P., and Badib, A. O.: Role of Radiation Therapy and of Surgery in the Management of Localized Epidermoid Carcinoma of the Maxillary Sinus, *Am J Roentgenol Radium Ther Nucl Med,* **114**:35, 1972.

Rush, B. F., Jr., Knightly, J. J., and Jewell, W.: Transoral and Transverse Incision for Excision of the Maxillary Sinus, *J Surg Oncol,* **3**:53, 1971.

Tabah, E. J.: Cancer of the Paranasal Sinuses: A Study of the Results of Various Methods of Treatment in Fifty-four Patients, *Am J Surg,* **104**:741, 1962.

Mandible

Bernier, J. L.: "Tumors of the Odontogenic Apparatus and Jaws," Armed Forces Institute of Pathology, Washington, 1960.

Cramer, L. M., Culf, N. K., Hulnick, S. J., and Kodsi, M. S.: Reconstruction Management of the Mandible in the Treatment of Head and Neck, "Symposium on Malignancies of The Head and Neck," The C. V. Mosby Company, St. Louis, Mo., 1975.

Salivary Glands

Beahrs, O. H., Woolner, L. B., Caveth, S. W., and Devine, K. D.: Surgical Management of Parotid Lesions, *Arch Surg,* **80**:890, 1960.

Bhaskar, S. N., and Bernier, J. L.: Mikulicz's Disease, *Oral Surg,* **13**:1387, 1960.

Connell, H. C. and Evans, J. C.: Mucoepidermoid Carcinoma of the Salivary Glands, *Am J Surg,* **124**:519, 1972.

Foote, F. W., and Frazell, E. L.: "Tumors of the Major Salivary Glands," Armed Forces Institute of Pathology, Washington, 1954.

Grage, T. B., and Lober, P. H.: Benign Lymphoepithelial Lesion of the Salivary Glands, *Am J Surg,* **108**:495, 1964.

——, ——, and Shahon, D. B.: Benign Tumors of the Major Salivary Glands, *Surgery,* **50**:625, 1961.

Katsilambros, L.: Asymptomatic Enlargement of the Parotid Glands, *JAMA,* **178**:513, 1961.

Reynolds, C. T., McAuley, R. L., and Rogers, W. P., Jr.: Experience with Tumors of Minor Salivary Glands, *Am J Surg,* **111**:168, 1966.

Rosenfeld, L., Sessions, D. G., McSwain, B., and Graves, H., Jr.: Malignant Tumors of Salivary Gland Origin: 37-year Review of 184 Cases, *Ann Surg,* **163**:726, 1966.

Stewart, F. W., Foote, F. W., and Becker, W. F.: Mucoepidermoid Tumors of Salivary Glands, *Ann Surg,* **122**:820, 1945.

Stuteville, O. H., and Corley, R. D.: Surgical Management of Tumors of Intraoral Minor Salivary Glands: Report of Eighty Cases, *Cancer,* **20**:1578, 1967.

Winsten, J., and Ward, G. E.: The Parotid Gland: An Anatomic Study, *Surgery,* **40**:585, 1956.

Tumors of the Neck

Albers, G. D.: Branchial Anomalies, *JAMA,* **183**:399, 1963.

Hoffman, E.: Branchial Cysts within the Parotid Gland, *Ann Surg,* **152**:290, 1960.

Jesse, R. H., and Neff, L. E.: Metastatic Carcinoma in Cervical Nodes with an Unknown Primary Lesion, *Am J Surg,* **112**:547, 1966.

MacComb, W. S.: Diagnosis and Treatment of Metastatic Cervical Cancerous Nodes from an Unknown Primary Site, *Am J Surg,* **124**:441, 1972.

Marchetta, F. C., Murphy, W. T., and Kovaric, J. J.: Carcinoma of the Neck, *Am J Surg,* **106**:974, 1963.

Mooney, C. S., Jewell, W., Greenlaw, R., and Rush, B. F., Jr.: Simultaneous Bilateral Radical Neck Dissection following High Level Radiation Therapy, *J Surg Oncol,* **1**:335, 1969.

Rush, B. F., Jr.: Current Concepts in the Treatment of Carotid Body Tumors, *Surgery,* **52**:679, 1962.

——: Familial Bilateral Carotid Body Tumors, *Ann Surg,* **157**:633, 1963.

Skandalakis, J. E., Gray, S. W., Takakis, N. C., Godwin, J. T., and Poer, D. H.: Tumors of the Neck, *Surgery,* **48**:375, 1960.

Chemotherapy and Immunotherapy

Adams, G. L., Berlinger, N. T., Good, R. A., Pollak, K., Tsakraklides, V., and Yang, M.: Immunologic Assessment of Regional Lymph Node Histology in Relation to Survival in Head and Neck Carcinoma, *Cancer,* **37**:697, 1976.

Alexander, J. C., Jr., Chretien, P. B., Henson, D. E., Silverman,

N. A., and Smith, H. G.: Viral-Specific Humoral Immunity to Herpes Simplex-Induced Antigens in Patients with Squamous Carcinoma of the Head and Neck, *Am J Surg,* **132:**541, 1976.

Couture, J., and Deschenes, L.: Intra-arterial Infusion: An Adjuvant to the Treatment of Oral Carcinoma, *Cancer,* **29:**1632, 1972.

Cvitkovic, E., Gerold, F. P., Shah, J., Strong, E. W., and Wittes, R. E.: cis-Dichlorodiammineplatinum (II) in the Treatment of Epidermoid Carcinoma of the Head and Neck, *Cancer Treat Rep,* **61:**359, 1977.

Donaldson, R. C.: Methotrexate plus Bacillus Calmette-Guerin and Isoniazid in the Treatment of Cancer of the Head and Neck, *Am J Surg,* **124:**527, 1972.

Freckman, H. A.: Results in 169 Patients with Cancer of the Head and Neck Treated by Intra-arterial Infusion Therapy, *Am J Surg,* **124:**501, 1972.

Ohnuma, T., Selawry, O. S., Holland, J. F., DeVita, V. T., Shedd, D. P., Hansen, H. H., and Muggia, F. M.: Clinical Study with Bleomycin: Tolerance to Twice Weekly Dosage, *Cancer,* **30:**914, 1972.

Williams, A. C.: Topical 5 FU: A New Approach to Skin Cancer, *Ann Surg,* **173:**864, 1971.

Woods, J. E.: Current Status of Chemotherapy in the Treatment of Head and Neck Cancer, *Arch Surg,* **111:**1055, 1976.

————: The Influence of Immunologic Responsiveness on Head and Neck Cancer, *Plast Reconstr Surg,* **56:**77, 1975.

Operations of the Head and Neck

Frazell, E. L., and Moore, O. S.: Bilateral Radical Neck Dissection Performed in Stages: Experience with 467 Patients, *Am J Surg,* **102:**809, 1961.

Ketcham, A. S., Liebermann, J. E., and West, J. T.: Antibiotic Prophylaxis in Cancer Surgery and Its Value in Staphylococcal Carrier Patients, *Surg Gynecol Obstet,* **117:**1, 1963.

Lore, J. M.: "An Atlas of Head and Neck Surgery," W. B. Saunders Company, Philadelphia, 1962.

Madan, S. C., Rosenthal, S. P. and Bochetto, J. F.: Pneumomediastinum and Pneumothorax following Lower Neck Surgery, *Arch Surg,* **98:**153, 1969.

Martin, H., Del Valle, B., Ehrlich, H., and Cahan, W. G.: Neck Dissection, *Cancer,* **4:**441, 1951.

Moore, O. S., and Frazell, E. L.: Simultaneous Bilateral Neck Dissection: Experience with 151 Patients, *Am J Surg,* **107:**565, 1964.

Norris, C. M.: Composite Resections of Laryngeal and Supralaryngeal Cancer, in J. Conley (ed.), "Cancer of the Head and Neck," Butterworth Inc., Washington, 1967.

Royster, H. P., Noone, R. B., Graham, W. P., and Theogaraj, S. D.: Cervical Pharyngostomy for Feeding after Maxillofacial Surgery, *Am J Surg,* **116:**610, 1968.

Rush, B. F., Jr.: A Standard Technique for In-Continuity Incisions of the Head and Neck, *Surg Gynecol Obstet,* **121:**353, 1965.

————, Swaminathan, A. P., and Jefferies, K.: The Use of Cervical Flaps from Radiated Necks in Immediate Reconstruction, *Am J Surg.* (in press.)

Swaminathan, A. P., Jefferies, K. R., and Rush, B. F., Jr.: Construction of a Pseudolarynx following Laryngectomy and Radical Neck Dissection: A Preliminary Report, *Am J Surg.* (in press.)

Ward, G. E., Edgerton, M. T., Chambers, R. G., and McKee, D. M.: Cancer of the Oral Cavity and Pharynx and Results of Treatment by Means of the Composite Operation (in Continuity with Radical Neck Dissection), *Ann Surg,* **150:**202, 1959.

Wise, R. A., and Baker, H. W.: "Surgery of the Head and Neck," The Year Book Medical Publishers, Inc., Chicago, 1962.

Chapter 17

Chest Wall, Pleura, Lung, and Mediastinum

by **Lester R. Bryant and Calvin Morgan**

INTRODUCTION

The existence of life from moment to moment depends primarily on adequate function of the heart and lungs. Surgical procedures for the treatment of thoracic diseases or injury must be performed under circumstances which can guarantee continuing cardiopulmonary function during operative manipulations. Preexisting impairment of pulmonary function, operative removal of tissue from the chest wall or lungs, and postoperative pain are routine hazards to the patient's ability to continue adequate respiratory exchange following operation. From these considerations it is apparent that the development of thoracic surgery has necessarily followed the development of techniques for tracheal intubation with positive-pressure ventilation. This is not to imply that surgeons were unable to operate on the thorax until recent times. Attempts to manage chest wounds received in battle were recorded in very ancient writings, including the Iliad (about 950 B.C.). Galen described a patient who recovered after partial excision of the sternum and pericardium for recurrent abscess due to an injury. Writing about chest wounds in the thirteenth century, Theodoric noted that "the stitches should be placed in accordance with the size of the wound so that the natural heat cannot escape in any way nor the air outside be able to enter."

The introduction of firearms in the fourteenth century complicated the management of chest wounds because of uncertainty about the extent of damage inside the thorax and whether or not wounds should be closed when an open pneumothorax had been produced. Many surgeons held the view that the wound must be kept open to allow the drainage of blood. In recording the opposite view, Napoleon's surgeon, Baron Larrey, confirmed the sporadic observations of other surgeons about the lifesaving value of closing an open wound of the thorax. His description of the cardiopulmonary effects of an open chest wound can hardly be improved upon:

A soldier was brought to the hospital of the Fortress of Ibrahyn Bey, immediately after a wound penetrated the thorax, between the fifth and sixth true ribs. It was about 8 cm in extent. A large quantity of frothy and vermilion blood escaped from it with a hissing noise at each inspiration. His extremities were cold, pulse scarcely perceptible, countenance discolored, and respiration short and laborious; in short, he was every moment threatened with a fatal suffocation. After having examined the wound, the divided edges of the part, I immediately approximated the two lips of the wound, and retained them by means of adhesive plaster and a suitable bandage around the body. In adopting this plan, I intended only to hide from the sight of the patient and his comrades, the distressing spectacle of a hemorrhage, which would soon prove fatal; and I, therefore, thought that the effusion of blood into the cavity of the thorax, could not increase the danger. But the wound was scarcely closed, when he breathed more freely, and felt easier. The heat of the body soon returned, and the pulse rose. In a few hours he became quite calm, and to my great surprise grew better. He was cured in a very few days, and without difficulty.

Drainage of lung abscesses and amputation of lung which has herniated through traumatic wounds in the chest wall have been performed for centuries. In the late 1800s successful transthoracic pulmonary resections were performed in animals, and methods for the control of respiration during operation were evaluated. On the basis of experiments that suggested a superiority of negative pressure over positive airway pressure, Sauerbruch developed a negative pressure chamber in 1904 in which the operating team and the patient could be housed during operation. Under these conditions, the lung would not collapse when the chest was open. The animal experiments gave some success, but the operations on patients were not so rewarding. Techniques of tracheal intubation and anesthesia were developing in parallel with the increasing desire to make surgery of the thorax an achievable reality at the close of the nineteenth century. Orotracheal intubation with metal tubes for the treatment of croup and for the prevention of aspiration during oral surgical procedures provided the early experience that led to endotracheal anesthesia for thoracic surgery. An artificial respiration device consisting of a hand bellows and a tracheostomy tube were introduced by Fell in 1893, and modified by O'Dywer in 1896. The latter substituted an orotracheal tube and a foot bellows with a greater volume capacity. Rudolph Matas in New Orleans advocated the use of the Fell-O'Dywer apparatus to allow a more general availability of thoracic surgical techniques, and he introduced his own modification of the equipment in 1900. The use of these early techniques to prevent lung collapse and ineffectual ventilation during thoracotomy were associated with hazards of their own. It is not surprising then to find that surgeons were still devising makeshift techniques to control the open pneumothorax associated with chest-wall resections as late as the first several decades of this century. These included various packing techniques, preoperative pneumothorax for "conditioning," and suturing the lung to the parietal pleura. It

Fig. 17-1. The relationship of the thoracic cage to the upper abdominal viscera must be remembered to avoid overlooking concomitant abdominal injuries in patients with thoracic trauma.

Anterior

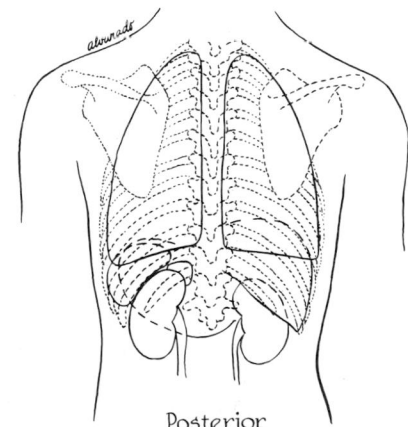

Posterior

was inevitable that refinements in laryngotracheal intubation, in design and materials of tracheal tubes, and in techniques of anesthesia would displace the local improvisations of a handful of surgeons. During the 1930s and the 1940s the majority of thoracic surgical techniques in use today for noncardiac disease were either developed or refined for widespread use.

Although the developments in cardiac surgery have overshadowed the progress being made in other areas of thoracic disease, the practice of thoracic surgery has nonetheless become more exciting as advances in technology are brought into clinical use. Though the flexible fiberscopes have transferred a major responsibility for endoscopic diagnosis to internists, these instruments have allowed the recognition of bronchopulmonary and esophageal neoplasms at an early stage. Surgical resection of the tumors in the "occult" stage has yielded cure rates previously considered to be unobtainable. Isotope methodology and computerized tomography for detection of systemic metastases have supplemented mediastinal exploration techniques, sharply reducing the percentage of unproductive thoracotomies in patients with incurable bronchogenic cancer. The early results of several methods to enhance immunocompetence in patients with pulmonary neoplasms strengthen the concept that surgical treatment of most neoplasms should be combined with continuing postoperative systemic therapy.

The current management of thoracic injuries has become more sophisticated, partly through the improvements and understanding of trauma pathophysiology and support techniques that can be attributed to the research-funded trauma centers. Lung transplantation remains out of reach for the present, but it seems inevitable that some limited success will be achieved in the near future.

ANATOMY OF THE THORAX AND PLEURA

Because of the palpable bony structures of the thoracic cage and the transmission of cardiac and breath sounds through the chest wall, the physician is aided in relating thoracic anatomy to principles of diagnosis. On the other hand, the overlap of the upper part of the abdomen by the lower ribs and the extension of the lung apices above the level of the clavicles can lead to serious errors, especially in patients with blunt trauma (Fig. 17-1). The lower ribs and costal margin overlap the liver, spleen, stomach, the upper pole of both kidneys, and the distal part of the pancreas. By providing support for the upper extremity, the thorax acquires the additional anatomic elements of the shoulder girdle. Because the skeletal and muscular components of the shoulder participate in several functions and diseases of the thorax, it is necessary to review the relations of these structures in any detailed study of thoracic anatomy.

The framework of the thoracic cage consists of the sternum, twelve thoracic vertebrae, ten pairs of ribs that end anteriorly in segments of cartilage, and two pairs of floating ribs (Fig. 17-2). The thoracic inlet is characterized by having a rigid structural ring formed by the sternal manubrium, the short, semicircular first ribs, and the vertebral column. As a result of its articulation with the manubrium and the attachment of the costoclavicular ligament, the clavicle participates in providing protection for the underlying vascular and neural structures which traverse the thoracic inlet. The same rigidity that provides protection from trauma, however, leaves little room for pathologic swelling, enlarging masses, or postural adjustments with age.

The cartilages of the first six ribs have separate articulations with the sternum; the cartilages of the seventh through the tenth ribs fuse to form the costal margin before attaching to the lower margin of the sternum. In children, significant flexibility is made possible by the vertebral joints and the elasticity of the costal cartilages. Although flexibility of the chest wall decreases progressively with age, serious trauma can be transmitted to the intrathoracic structures with little injury to the bony framework, even in adults.

The pectoralis major and minor muscles constitute the principal muscular covering of the anterior thorax, and the lower margin of the pectoralis major forms the *anterior axillary fold.* Auscultation of the chest in the axilla often allows the best determination of breath sounds, because the thoracic cage is covered only by the origins of the serratus anterior muscle in that location. The long thoracic nerve passes vertically on the axillary surface of that muscle—a point to be remembered when doing a thoracentesis or tube thoracostomy. A convergence of the latissimus dorsi and teres major muscles forms the *posterior axillary fold* on each side. The triangle of auscultation can often be palpated near the inferior medial border of the scapula, but the latissimus, trapezius, rhomboid, and other shoulder girdle muscles form a strong muscular coat for the posterior thorax. A disadvantage of the heavy muscle coat is the difficulty in accurately identifying specific ribs by palpation of the posterior chest wall.

Fig. 17-2. The radiolucent costal cartilages and the poor projection of the sternum on anteroposterior chest x-rays make it difficult to demonstrate major injuries or abnormalities of the anterior part of the chest wall.

The sternal angle is almost always palpable, and this allows quick identification of the second rib because of its articulation with the sternum at this location. A plane that is parallel to the floor and passes through the sternal angle of an upright patient will also pass through the fourth or fifth thoracic vertebra. The tracheal bifurcation lies in this same plane, while the apex of the aortic arch is located slightly higher. There is a gradual increase in the length of ribs from the first to the seventh and a progressive lateral displacement of the rib-costal cartilage junctions. Because of the radiolucency of the cartilages, standard anteroposterior chest x-rays may fail to document injury to the thoracic cage even though a severe blunt injury to the chest has disarticulated and fractured multiple costal cartilages.

The *pleura* is a serous membrane of flat mesothelial cells overlying a thin layer of connective tissue in which a vascular and lymphatic network is distributed. That part covering the lungs is referred to as the *visceral* pleura, and it is continuous over the pulmonary hilum and the mediastinum with the *parietal* pleura, which covers the inside of the chest wall and the diaphragm. The pleura thereby forms a closed sac around the pleural cavity. With normal lung expansion the pleural cavity is completely filled and only a potential space exists. As shown in Fig. 17-3, the line of pleural reflection extends slightly beyond the lung border in each direction. This is expected because of the dynamic process of respiration and the need for the pleural sac to accommodate maximum lung expansion with deep inspiration. Conversely, with acute decreases in lung volume, such as that with lobar atelectasis, there is a limit to

Fig. 17-3. The relation of the pulmonary lobes and pleural sinuses to the chest wall.

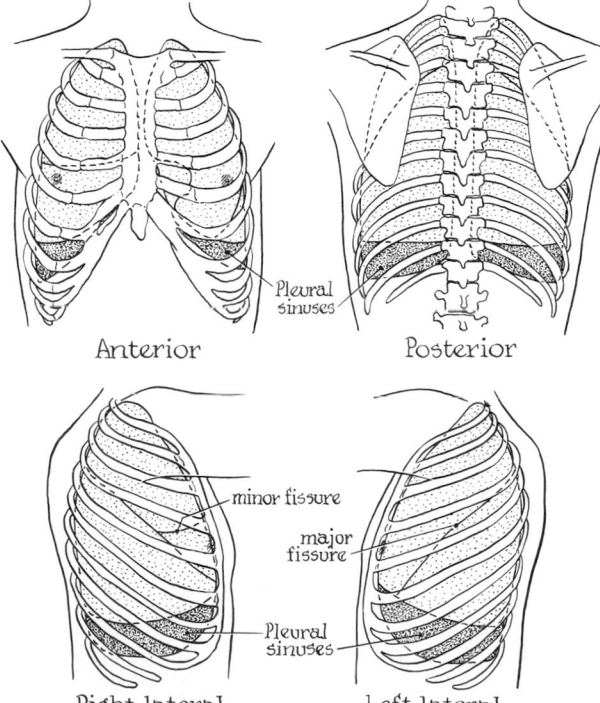

the pleural accommodation and fluid may be drawn into the pleural cavity to replace partially the lost lung volume.

There is no communication between the pleural cavity of each hemithorax, but the anteromedial borders of the two pleural sacs come nearly into apposition behind the sternum. A lateral divergence of the left pleural border between the fourth and sixth costal cartilages forms a cardiac notch which makes it possible to perform transthoracic aspiration of fluid from the pericardial cavity without entering the pleural cavity. The possibility of lacerating the internal thoracic artery as it descends just beyond the lateral sternal border must be remembered; aspiration through this approach should be attempted only when there is almost a certainty that significant pericardial fluid or blood is present. The inferior border of each pleural cavity is located at the ninth rib in the midaxillary line, and the borders continue posteriorly in the eleventh intercostal space. Occasionally the pleural sac extends as low as the twelfth rib. Posteriorly, the margins of the two pleural sacs lie on the anterolateral surfaces of the vertebrae, separated by the esophagus. A retroesophageal recess is occasionally formed when the pleural margins are in near-apposition. At the inferior margin of the lung hilum on each side, a double layer of mediastinal pleura is formed, the *inferior pulmonary ligament*.

The structures which occupy the *intercostal spaces* have considerable significance in relation to thoracic function, disease, and diagnostic procedures. The parietal pleura, for example, is well supplied with nerve endings for pain, while the visceral pleura is insensitive. Only when pulmonary disease extends to involve the parietal pleura or chest wall is pain produced. Figure 17-4 shows the structures in an intercostal space and emphasizes the layering effect of the muscles and fascia. Three layers of intercostal muscles are present in a major part of the thoracic wall, but some anatomists consider the innermost and the internal intercostals to be a single muscle entity. With quiet respiration the ribs are elevated by synchronous contraction of the intercostal muscles. Because the ribs of each side move as a unit in respiration, a localized painful lesion may eliminate effective function of the entire side. During quiet respiration, however, movements of the diaphragm provide approximately 75 percent of pulmonary ventilation and temporary loss of unilateral intercostal muscle function is not a threat to breathing. With labored breathing, the muscles of the upper extremity and those cervical muscles that attach to the chest wall assist in elevation and expansion of the thorax.

The *endothoracic fascia* is a layer of light areolar tissue subjacent to the parietal pleura. At the apex of each hemithorax it is thickened into a more substantial layer referred to as *Sibson's fascia.*

The vein, artery, and nerve of each interspace are located deep to the external and internal intercostal muscles and lie just behind the lower margin of the rib. For most interspaces a smaller collateral artery runs along the top border of the rib below. There is significant overlap of neural supply by adjacent nerves, and complete anesthesia in an interspace will generally not occur unless the intercostal nerve of the adjacent space above and below and the space in question are anesthetized. To minimize the risk of lacerating the intercostal artery, a thoracentesis needle or a clamp used to perforate the pleura for insertion of a catheter should be passed across the top of the lower rib of the selected interspace.

The lymphatic drainage of the chest wall extends in both anterior and posterior directions. Lymph draining from the anterior region of the first four or five intercostal spaces passes to lymph nodes along the internal thoracic arteries. These nodes may be connected by cross anastomoses before draining into a single or double trunk that joins the thoracic duct, a right lymphatic duct, or a bronchomediastinal trunk. Lymphatics that drain the posterior and lateral regions of the intercostal spaces are tributary to lymph nodes that lie near the vertebral ends of each interspace. In the lower part of the thorax these nodes join the drainage from the posterior mediastinum to contribute to the *cisterna chyli.* The posterior lymph nodes of the upper thorax drain into the thoracic duct or a right lymphatic duct.

A musculofibrous floor is provided for the thorax by the *diaphragm.* The peripheral muscular portions of the diaphragm arise from the lower six ribs and costal cartilages, from the lumbar vertebrae (right and left crus), and from the lumbocostal arches. Additional fibers arise from the xiphoid cartilage, and all the muscular elements converge into the central tendon. The central part of the tendon underlies the pericardium, while the right and left divisions extend posteriorly. Some of the lower intercostal nerves are thought to contribute to the sensory innervation of the diaphragm, but motor innervation is supplied by the phrenic nerve on each side.

Of the three major openings in the diaphragm the aortic hiatus is most posterior. The aorta, azygos vein, and thoracic duct pass through this opening. The esophageal hiatus transmits the esophagus and vagus nerves, and only the inferior vena cava goes through the foramen of that name.

Thoracic Incisions

A basic knowledge of the incisions used to perform thoracic operations is helpful in understanding the postoperative course of patients and the management of complications. Because of the rigidity of the thoracic cage, the incisions for major procedures must be relatively large and must disrupt the integrity of muscles and bone, or cartilage. The extensive division of tissues and the distortion or stretching associated with the use of strong mechanical retractors often result in severe postoperative pain.

There are two principal incisions: (1) *lateral thoracotomy,* performed either as an anterolateral or posterolateral incision, and (2) *median sternotomy,* performed as a vertical, sternal splitting incision. Other incisions are infrequently used, either because experience has shown them to be inferior, or because they are used in unusual circumstances. The *thoracoabdominal incision* combines an upper abdominal incision with an incision in a lower intercostal space (sixth, seventh, or eighth) that may be carried as far posteriorly as the posterior axillary line. The costal margin and diaphragm are divided to provide an extensive exposure of the upper part of the abdomen and the retroperitoneal and posterior thoracic structures. Prolonged pain associated with incomplete healing of the costal margin, as well as complicated wound management involving two body cavities if infection occurs, has reduced the enthusiasm for this incision. It still finds usefulness for certain operations involving retroperitoneal structures (kidney, thoracoabdominal aorta), and it may be the best incision to use for hepatic or thoracoabdominal trauma under emergency conditions.

A *bilateral transverse thoracotomy incision* with transection of the sternum is rarely used at present but was employed for routine operative approach to the heart and mediastinum before confidence was gained in the median sternotomy incision. The incision generally extends from

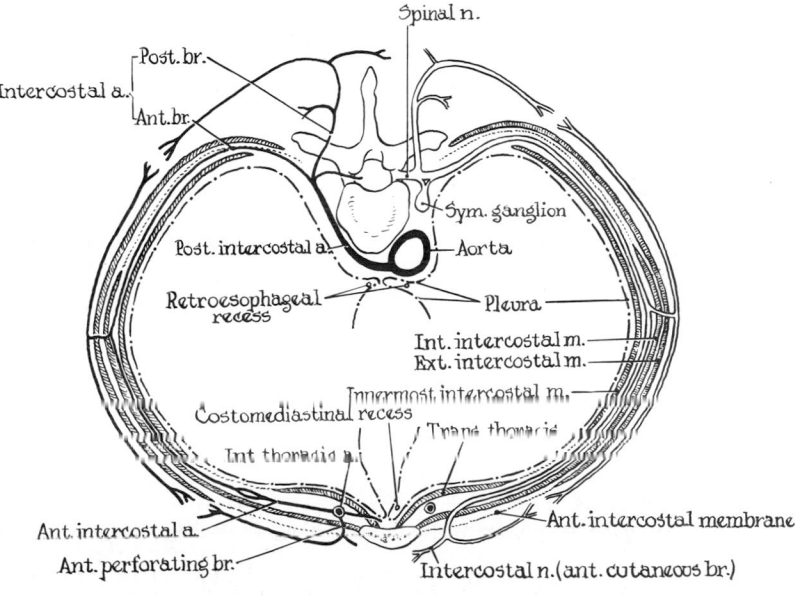

Fig. 17-4. An illustration of the structures within an intercostal space. [*Modified from C. E. Blevins, Anatomy of the Thorax and Pleura, in T. W. Shields (ed.), "General Thoracic Surgery," Lea & Febiger, Philadelphia, 1972, by permission of the author and publisher.*]

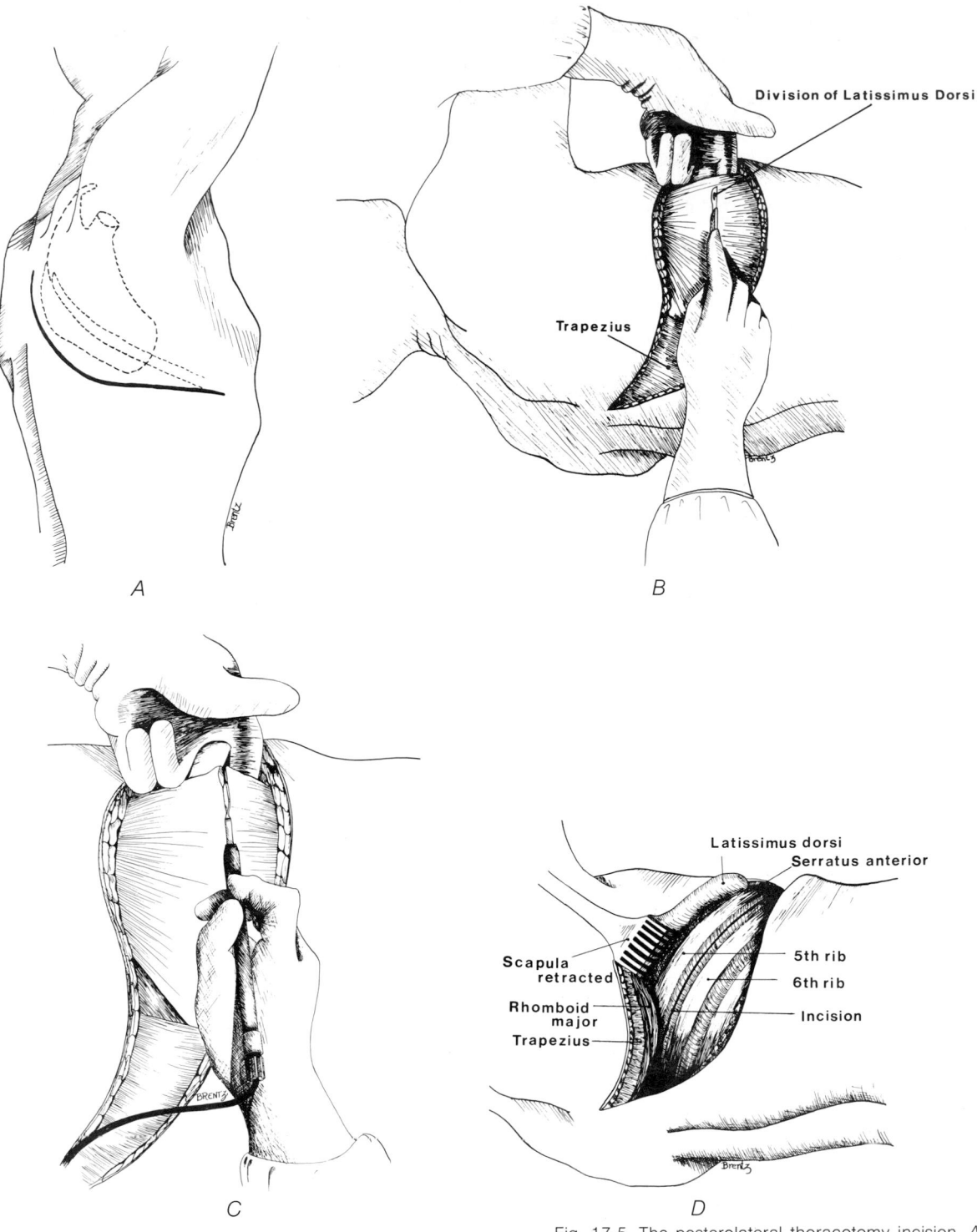

Fig. 17-5. The posterolateral thoracotomy incision. *A.* The skin incision begins near the anterior axillary line and curves posteriorly around the vertebral border of the scapula. *B.* The skin and muscle incisions are located in approximately the same position, whether the pleural cavity is entered in the fourth, fifth, or sixth intercostal space. *C.* Division of the shoulder-girdle muscles with the electrocautery may reduce blood loss and operating time. *D.* The pleural cavity is entered by dividing the intercostal muscles along the lower margin of the interspace.

one anterior axillary line to the other, either in the third or the fourth intercostal space. For reduced exposure needs the incision may be started on the side where the principal dissection will be done and extended only a short distance into the opposite hemithorax after transection of the sternum. The disadvantages of this incision include the longer time required to make the incision and to close the chest, compared to the median sternotomy incision. Both pleural cavities are usually entered with the transverse incision, but this may be avoided with the median sternotomy approach. In unusual circumstances, where the instruments necessary to perform median sternotomy are not available and there is urgent need to have access to both sides of the mediastinum, this incision may still be quite useful.

The *anterolateral and posterolateral* thoracotomy incisions are used most frequently for general thoracic operations. Each one requires division of one or more major shoulder girdle muscles, and this results in voluntary restriction of shoulder motion in the early postoperative period. Because they function as accessory muscles of respiration, it is possible that the selection and placement of the incision to minimize muscle injury could be important in an occasional patient with need for maximal muscle preservation. All patients must be encouraged to begin active shoulder and arm motion after operation, but elderly patients are especially likely to develop a restricted range of shoulder motion if not supervised carefully. The distal parts of the transected muscles lose their nerve supply and atrophy to a significant degree postoperatively. Commonly, patients note a zone of reduced sensation in the skin on the caudal side of the incision for months after operation.

The *posterolateral thoracotomy* is used for the majority of pulmonary resections (except lung biopsy), for esophageal operations, and for the approach to the posterior mediastinum and the vertebral column (Fig. 17-5). When the intent is to enter the pleural cavity in the fifth intercostal space, the most common selection, the skin incision is begun at the anterior axillary line just below the nipple level in the male, and at the corresponding position in the female. The incision extends posteriorly below the tip of the scapula and ascends midway between the vertebral border of the scapula and the spinous processes of the vertebrae. To expose the thoracic cage it is necessary to divide part of the serratus anterior, latissimus dorsi, trapezius, and rhomboid major muscles. The pleural cavity may be entered by dividing the intercostal muscles in the chosen interspace, or by resecting the posterior two-thirds of the corresponding rib. Only in circumstances where the rib is needed for bone grafting or when broad exposure is needed in a patient with a rigid thoracic cage is it necessary to resect the rib. The division of the rib posteriorly before the mechanical rib spreader is put in place may avoid accidental fracture of one or more ribs, or a costochondral separation by the instrument. The injury to the rib or cartilage may increase postoperative incisional pain and prolong the restricted motion of the chest cage.

Two advantages of the *anterolateral thoracotomy* may be important in trauma victims and in patients with an unstable cardiovascular system. The incision can allow rapid entry into the chest, and the patient may be placed in the supine position on the operating table. This is tolerated better than the lateral decubitus position, and it gives the anesthesiologist the maximum control over the patient's cardiorespiratory system. The incision may be used for mediastinal operations, for some cardiac procedures, and for wedge resections of the upper and middle lobes of the lung. It is preferable to make a submammary skin incision starting at the sternal border overlying the fourth intercostal space and extending to the midaxillary line. The pectoralis major muscle and part of the pectoralis minor are divided at the level of the fourth or fifth intercostal space, and the incision is extended into the serratus anterior. By extending the chosen intercostal muscle incision posteriorly along the top of the subjacent rib it is possible to obtain a wider opening in the chest than the length of the skin incision would suggest. Still further exposure may be obtained by transecting the sternum.

An *axillary thoracotomy incision* may be used in selected circumstances where only limited exposure of the upper hemithorax is needed. It is satisfactory for biopsy of an upper lobe, for resection of small apical pulmonary blebs and pleural abrasion in patients with recurrent pneumothorax, for upper thoracic sympathectomy, and for biopsy of upper mediastinal lymph nodes or masses. The skin incision parallels the course of the third rib in the axilla and extends from the anterior to the posterior axillary folds (Fig. 17-6). Retraction of the pectoralis major or latissimus dorsi muscles often makes it possible to enter the pleural cavity by dividing only the second or third intercostal muscles.

A hazard that is common to all the lateral thoracotomy incisions is the potential for injury to the brachial plexus and the axillary neurovascular structures from excessive displacement of the shoulder in positioning the patient on the operating table after anesthesia has been induced. By preventing posterior displacement of the shoulder this complication can be minimized.

The *median sternotomy incision* provides optimum exposure for anterior mediastinal lesions, and it is the principal incision used for cardiac operations. Either pleural cavity may be entered, or incision into the pleural cavities may be avoided if it is unnecessary. Disadvantages of the incision include an increased risk of infection if it is necessary to do a tracheostomy within a few days after operation, and the protracted course that occurs with infection because of involvement of the sternal fragments. An occasional patient who develops an acute wound infection also develops a severe mediastinitis associated with dehiscence of the sternal wound. The mortality rate for this complication is high but has decreased with the evolution of effective treatment.

The skin incision extends from just below the suprasternal notch to a point several centimeters below the xiphoid process (Fig. 17-7). Either an oscillating saw or a Lebsche knife and mallet may be used to split the sternum. A mechanical retractor is used to spread the incision, but the retractor blades may fracture the sternal halves with excessive pressure. After operation, patients who have had a sternotomy have less pain and less interference with pul-

A

B

Fig. 17-6. *A.* An axillary thoracotomy incision requires minimal muscle division for entrance into the pleural cavity. *B.* The exposure is limited to the upper hemithorax, but postoperative recovery is more rapid than after a standard thoracotomy.

monary function than those who have had a lateral thoracotomy.

The pleural cavity is usually drained with one or two chest tubes connected to an underwater seal system at the conclusion of the intrathoracic portion of the operation. Each chest tube should be brought through a separate stab wound in the chest wall at least two interspaces away from the incision. If the pleural cavity is not entered in operations through a median sternotomy, it is advisable to drain the retrosternal space for 24 hours with an intercostal tube that is brought out through a stab wound in the epigastrium.

EVALUATION OF THE THORACIC SURGICAL PATIENT

At the same time that specific diagnostic procedures are being completed in the patient with a thoracic lesion, it is

pertinent to assess the ability of the patient to undergo operative treatment. In the first instance, the surgical lesion should be evaluated with all possible techniques that will allow the soundest and most effective operative procedure. For many patients the effective operation may require a removal or alteration of tissues with immediate loss of function. This consideration is the tie that binds the thoracic lesion to the several components of the patient's overall state of health.

An experienced surgeon will make a preliminary decision that incorporates his evaluation of the patient's health, the operation that would be required, the patient's age, and the complications or disability that may occur postoperatively. Obviously the potential benefit from operation must be weighed against the involved risk. Increasingly, it has become possible to evaluate patients in terms of the morphologic and functional effects of their thoracic disease, and to control the intraoperative and postoperative events that could threaten the desired result.

The history and physical examination, done with the consideration of a thoracotomy in mind, constitute the

Fig. 17-7. *A.* The median sternotomy incision is outlined. *B.* Exposure of the anterior mediastinum is optimum with the use of a mechanical retractor.

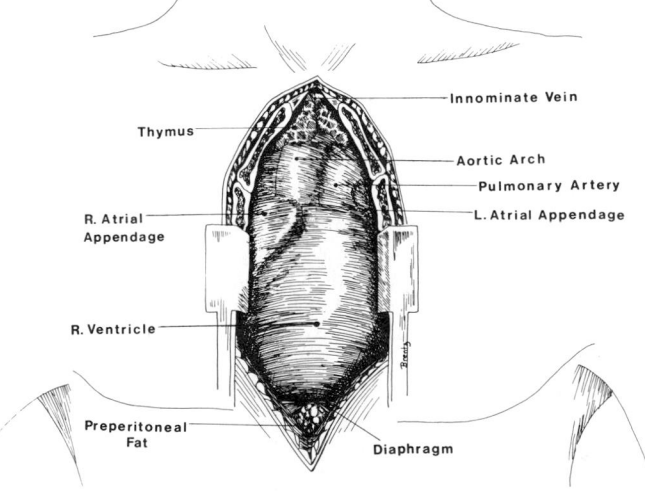

A

B

foundation of each patient's evaluation. If the patient is found to be in good health, is young, and has normal values for the hospital admission blood tests and urinalysis, no further evaluation may be necessary in some instances. Excision of a benign tumor of a rib, transthoracic sympathectomy for hyperhydrosis or causalgia, and resection of small apical pulmonary blebs are examples of operative procedures that may be performed with nothing more than clinical assessment of the patient's health.

More often the candidate for operation has a pulmonary or esophageal neoplasm or is a cigarette smoker with symptoms of chronic bronchitis and is at least middle-aged. If the person proves to be a satisfactory candidate for operation, a major procedure will be required that will almost certainly interfere with cardiopulmonary function. During an operation in one side of the thorax the corresponding lung will be either retracted or displaced in such a way that it can contribute little, if any, to respiratory gas exchange. Further, it may be necessary to retract intermittently against the pericardium in a way that either interferes with venous return to the atria or precipitates brief arrhythmias. Therefore, the functional status of the contralateral lung and the presence of preexisting cardiac disease are major determinants of the safety of the operation.

Following operation, the pain of a thoracotomy incision, whether or not the chest wall or pulmonary tissue has been resected, restricts the patient's ventilatory ability. A normally functioning lung on the side operated upon does not guarantee that the patient will recover without pulmonary complications, but there is a greater likelihood of recovery without major difficulty. If preexisting pulmonary disease is present, a significant effort will be necessary to prevent or reduce pulmonary complications. The additional factors of obesity, advanced age, abdominal distension, or infection can add to the risk of morbidity or mortality.

An assessment of the patient's nutritional state is always warranted, since thoracic operations result in severe degrees of surgical stress. A catabolic state is the expected result, and it may be important to plan for intensive preoperative and postoperative nutritional support. Though the relationship between infection and nutritional status is not objectively defined, there is a significant body of opinion that a catabolic state increases susceptibility to infection.

The need for preoperative cardiac evaluation is based on the expected postoperative demand for increased cardiac output, the frequency of coincidental cardiac disease, and the known frequency of cardiopulmonary complications. Any evidence of preexisting cardiac disease in a patient who is being prepared for a thoracic operation demands an adequate diagnosis, including cardiac catheterization if necessary. The development of even mild pulmonary edema can result in critical hypoxemia during or after operation. It is important to evaluate renal function as well, since fluid accumulation in the lungs or fluid and electrolyte imbalance may occur on the basis of renal insufficiency. The primary symptoms of the thoracic lesion may obscure any evidence of cardiorenal dysfunction, but the latter must be sought by screening examination.

A major consideration in recommending surgical treatment for a thoracic disease is whether the patient has adequate pulmonary function to tolerate the operation and the handicaps of the postoperative period. When the planned operation will result in a loss of functioning pulmonary tissue (lobectomy, pneumonectomy) there is a significant hazard of postoperative respiratory failure if the patient's preoperative pulmonary function is already compromised. Despite the common use of last-minute estimates of pulmonary function (such as the patient's ability to walk rapidly up two flights of stairs), it is better to measure function by objective techniques. This allows the most accurate interpretation of data and provides a permanent record for comparison with subsequent measurements.

No single test is yet available which provides an overall evaluation of lung function that would be adequate for surgical patients. The specific measurements that are of greatest value include lung volumes, mechanics of breathing, and arterial blood gases. Carefully performed spirometry forms the basis of the pulmonary function data most used in the evaluation of patients with thoracic lesions. Although most patients undergo pulmonary function testing in the hospital, the recent development of accurate electronic spirometers for office use makes it possible to perform satisfactory screening tests during an initial office visit. For the patient with compromised function, it is possible to institute a plan of management before hospitalization.

Figure 17-8 illustrates the subdivisions of lung volume in relation to a spirograph tracing. Functional residual capacity (FRC) and residual volume (RV) may be measured either by gas dilution techniques or by body plethysmography. FRC and RV are not routinely determined for surgical patients, but a broader use of these tests would be helpful. Body plethysmography has the additional advantage of permitting measurements of airway resistance and compliance.

Vital capacity, the amount of air that can be forcefully expelled from a maximally inflated lung position, can be a

Fig. 17-8. The lung volumes and their subdivisions related to a spirograph tracing. Functional residual capacity and residual volume must be measured by other techniques.

useful determination if its limitations are accepted. The predicted value decreases with age, and its measurement requires understanding as well as full cooperation from the patient.

The *mechanics of breathing* permits dynamic measurements of a patient's ability to move volumes of air during units of time. Individual laboratories vary in the panel of function tests that are performed, sometimes on the basis of an interest in a specific part of the expiratory flow curve of the spirogram. The *forced expiratory volume* in 1 second (FEV_1) is the commonest flow measurement, and it seems unlikely that measurements of an earlier portion of the curve, i.e., $FEV_{0.5}$, offer any advantage over FEV_1. Petty believes that the FEV_3 may be useful for detecting abnormalities in airflow that are not detected by the FEV_1. For example, small-airway disease is not generally detected at high lung volume flow, which is that part specifically measured by the FEV_1. In practice the FEV_1 is usually reported as a percentage of the VC (FEV_1/VC) as well as an actual volume. It is important to note its value both ways. If the VC is significantly reduced, the ratio FEV_1/VC may be satisfactory while the actual volume exhaled is markedly abnormal.

The *maximal midexpiratory flow* (MMEF) is derived from the midportion of the spirogram curve and is considered to be relatively *effort-independent*. It is not included in the report from many laboratories, but for surgical patients any flow rates below 1 liter/second suggest caution in advising a thoracotomy without an effort to improve pulmonary function.

Fig. 17-9. A fixed obstruction in the trachea markedly alters the maximum expiratory flow-volume curve (MEFV). The normal MEFV is shown by the interrupted line. (*Reproduced from R. E. Hyatt, Evaluation of Major Airway Lesions Using the Flow-Volume Loop, Ann Otol Rhinol Laryngol, 84:635, 1975, by permission of the author and publisher.*)

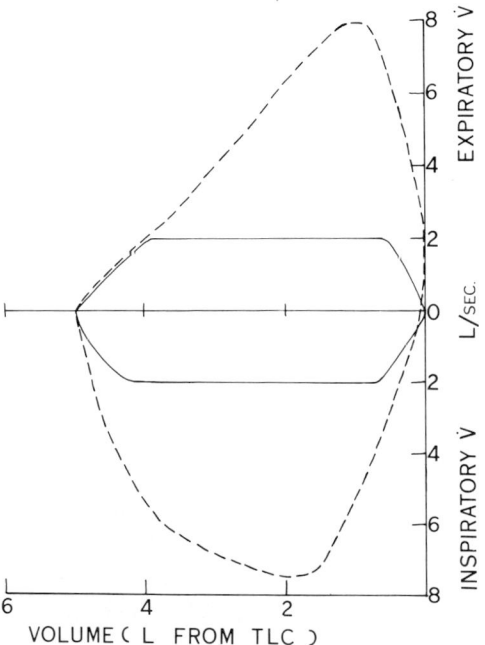

A test which is *effort-dependent* is the *maximal voluntary ventilation* (MVV—previously called the maximal breathing capacity), performed by having the patient inhale as deeply and rapidly as possible for 15 seconds. The MVV usually correlates well with the FEV_1, and in Petty's laboratory the expected relationship is $FEV_1 \times 34$ for males, $FEV_1 \times 40$ for females. If the actual measured value fails to correlate with the calculated value it suggests a poor effort or a fatigued patient. In most laboratories the patient is given an aerosol of a sympathomimetic amine bronchodilator and the spirometry is repeated. An improvement, sometimes significant, in flow rates and in VC may occur. A failure of severely decreased function values to improve does not mean that the patient has irreversible pulmonary disease. Aggressive therapy with the patient's cooperation can often improve pulmonary function, a benefit both to the patient's comfort and to the operative procedure.

The significance of early small-airway disease that is not demonstrated by standard spirometry has not been defined for thoracic surgical patients. Nevertheless, there is increasing interest in two tests of recent development that deserve evaluation. The *maximal expiratory flow-volume* curve (MEFV) is inscribed from a plot of airflow against the volume of vital capacity. This relationship of the data may provide information not given by a spirogram. Major airway lesions may distort the MEFV curve; Fig. 17-9 shows the abnormality seen with a fixed obstruction of the trachea. The *closing volume* (CV) depends on the fact that gravity results in a greater negative pressure at the apex of the lung than at the base in an upright person. That lung volume at which lung units in the dependent regions of the lung cease to ventilate, presumably because of airway closure, is referred to as the CV. The measurement can be made by monitoring the concentration of nitrogen in the exhaled gas during a vital-capacity maneuver after inspiration of a bolus of 100% oxygen. [133]Xenon or another gas may be used as the marker. An abrupt increase in the marker concentration in the terminal portion of the vital-capacity curve is the CV, and the value is expressed as a percentage of the vital capacity.

A measurement of the arterial blood gases and pH should be routine in the preoperative evaluation of a candidate for thoracic surgery. It would be an unusual situation in which the decision to advise operation depended solely on a single measurement of arterial oxygen or carbon dioxide tension. Even so, an occasional patient is discovered to have hypoxemia or CO_2 retention that was not suspected on the basis of clinical examination or spirometry. A measurement of the Pa_{CO_2} provides an immediate indication of the patient's alveolar ventilation; any value above 46 torr means that there is hypoventilation. There are multiple causes for this, and the specific reason should be sought in each patient. The ability of the lungs to excrete CO_2 is remarkable, and any persistent elevation of Pa_{CO_2} in a patient who might otherwise be considered a candidate for a major thoracotomy suggests serious abnormalities in distribution of ventilation and perfusion. Most operations will temporarily increase the ventilation-perfusion abnormality. A mild elevation of the Pa_{CO_2} in a patient with chronic lung disease may be treated aggressively to improve pulmonary function and allow the patient to be considered for operation. If pulmonary resection is contemplated in such an individual, the risk of postoperative respiratory failure is high and the decision to operate may depend on whether functioning pulmonary tissue would be removed.

The measurement of arterial P_{O_2} is valuable in the preoperative assessment of pulmonary function, but the number reported must be viewed with a consideration of the possibilities for error in its measurement. At sea level the normal Pa_{O_2} is above 85 torr. It is remarkable, however, how seldom one sees a patient with even minimal pulmonary disease who has an arterial oxygen tension in the normal range. The majority of patients considered by a thoracic surgeon have a Pa_{O_2} of 80 torr or below, and values in the range of 70 to 80 torr do not suggest unusual risk in the absence of other signals of caution. If the Pa_{O_2} is below 70 torr, an attempt should be made to determine the cause and to improve the patient's respiratory exchange. The possibilities include right-to-left shunting as a result of the thoracic disease for which the patient is being considered, uneven distribution of ventilation and perfusion, or diffusion barrier. More sophisticated pulmonary function tests may be indicated, including determination of alveolar-arterial oxygen difference, calculation of right-to-left shunt fraction, and split pulmonary function.

The pulmonary-function values obtained with spirometry in the individual patient must be compared with those obtained from other individuals of the same sex, age, and height who are known to be free of pulmonary disease. Data obtained from the spirometric studies in hundreds of normal males and females form the basis for *prediction nomograms* which facilitate that comparison. Figure 17-10 shows a prediction nomogram developed from studies of 422 normal adult males in a Veterans Administration–Army Cooperative Study of Pulmonary Function. To demonstrate the considerable information that may be accumulated about the individual patient's pulmonary function, Table 17-1 lists the values for a healthy young male breathing air at sea level. The panel of studies shown is adequate for most surgical patients, but it is possible that measurements of inspired gas distribution, diffusing capacity, pulmonary capillary blood volume, and the work of breathing could be determinants in the decision to operate on a patient with marginal pulmonary function.

Of the standard function tests, surgeons have come to place the greatest reliance on the expiratory flow rates and MVV as the critical determinants of operability for the patient with reduced function from respiratory disease, advanced age, or chronic illness. Mittman reported a 9 percent cardiopulmonary mortality rate in patients with a maximum breathing capacity (MBC) greater than 50 percent of the predicted value. By contrast, those patients whose MBC was less than 50 percent had a 45 percent cardiopulmonary mortality rate following thoracotomy. Similar results were reported by Miller for patients who underwent pneumonectomy, with a slightly lower mortality for those who had a lobectomy. Other studies have failed to support a precise correlation between a given level of reduced pulmonary function and an expected mortality

risk. In the last decade improvements in the facilities and tools (respiratory care units, arterial blood-gas measurements, volume-controlled respirators) for postoperative care have influenced many surgeons to become more aggressive in advising thoracotomy for patients with compromised pulmonary function. For example, a patient with a suspected bronchogenic carcinoma would be considered a high risk for pulmonary resection if the routine pulmonary function tests showed the VC, FEV_1, and MVV to be less than 50 percent of the predicted values. If operation would require right pneumonectomy, many surgeons would advise against surgical treatment. Others would insist on attempting to determine the contribution to pulmonary function of each lung.

Table 17-1. TYPICAL VALUES IN PULMONARY FUNCTION TESTS*

Lung volumes

Inspiratory capacity, ml	3,600
Expiratory reserve volume, ml	1,200
Vital capacity, ml	4,800
Residual volume (RV), ml	1,200
Functional residual capacity, ml	2,400
Thoracic gas volume, ml	2,400
Total lung capacity (TLC), ml	6,000
RV/TLC $\times$ 100, %	20

Ventilation

Tidal volume, ml	500
Respiratory dead space, ml	150
Respirations/min	12
Minute volume, ml/min	6,000
Alveolar ventilation, ml	4,200

Mechanics of breathing

Maximal voluntary ventilation, L/min	125–170
Forced expiratory volume, % in 1 sec	83
Forced expiratory volume, % in 3 sec	97
Maximal expiratory flow rate (for 1 L), L/min	400
Maximal inspiration flow rate (for 1 L), L/min	300
Compliance of lungs and thoracic cage, L/cm H_2O	0.1
Compliance of lungs, L/cm H_2O	0.2
Airway resistance, cm H_2O/L/sec	1.6

Alveolar ventilation/pulmonary capillary blood flow

Alveolar ventilation, L/min/blood flow, L/min	0.8
Physiologic shunt/cardiac output $\times$ 100, %	<7
Physiologic dead space/tidal volume $\times$ 100, %	<30

Arterial blood

Oxygen tension, torr	100
Carbon dioxide tension, torr	40
Oxygen tension (100% inhaled oxygen), torr	640
Alveolar-arterial P_{O_2} difference (100% inhaled oxygen), torr	33
Oxygen saturation (% saturation of hemoglobin)	97.1
pH	7.4

*The values shown are those of a resting young male, 1.7 m² body surface area, breathing room air at sea level, except where specified otherwise.
SOURCE: Modified from J. H. Comroe, Jr., "The Lung," 2d ed., Yearbook Medical Publishers, Inc., Chicago, 1962, with permission of the author and publisher.

It has been established that a centrally located neoplasm may sharply reduce the function of the ipsilateral lung even though the routine chest x-ray does not suggest this. Split lung function may be determined by bronchospirometry, but the difficulty in accurate placement of the double endotracheal tube (Carlen) has discouraged use of that technique. Radioisotope lung scintiscanning can be used more simply to suggest the relative contribution of each lung to total pulmonary function. Olsen has refined the radioisotope split-function test by measuring pulmonary artery pressure and calculating the predicted postpneumonectomy FEV_1 in a prospective study of patients considered at high risk for pulmonary resection. Although the cardiorespiratory mortality rate of nearly 18 percent for pneumonectomy in that series is impressive, it is likely that some of the surviving lung cancer patients would have been excluded from operation by standard function studies.

The interest in providing a satisfactory evaluation of the patient before thoracic operation must not obscure the ultimate purpose of the evaluation—to provide the patient with whatever physical and mental preparation is needed. Many patients are smokers, and every effort should be made to persuade them to stop smoking before operation, preferably for 2 weeks or more. The etiology of pulmonary infection should be identified and treated intensively, using respiratory therapy, physical therapy, or appropriate techniques. Thoracic operations often are associated with prolonged stays in intensive care units, with multiple chest tubes, with invasive catheters of several types, and with considerable pain. All patients deserve a full explanation of what to expect from the operation, presented in a way that assures them of excellence in their medical care and concern for their well-being.

THORACIC INJURIES

General Considerations

Increasing crime rates with deliberate attempts to kill the victims and a highly mobile population that rushes from one form of violent recreation to another provide a continuing high incidence of thoracic injuries. The spectrum of injury is especially broad and varies from a simple rib fracture or costochondral separation to fatal rupture of the heart from a crushing deceleration against an automobile steering wheel. When one realizes that chest trauma is the cause of approximately 25 percent of all accidental deaths, the need for accurate diagnosis and prompt treatment becomes obvious. Fundamental to the approach to any patient who has suffered a thoracic injury is a consideration of the preinjury cardiopulmonary functional status. The rib fracture or modest pneumothorax that is well tolerated without hospitalization in a healthy young man may lead to pneumonia, empyema, and even death in an older patient with chronic airways disease. Similarly, the patient with preexisting cardiac disease is particularly vulnerable to the development of pulmonary edema and hypoxia that may occur with the rapid administration of salt-containing intravenous fluids typically used for resuscitation of injured patients.

A rapid but perceptive overall evaluation of the patient is always indicated, whether the injury is thought to be serious or not. Chest trauma is often accompanied by other injuries, and the overlap of the upper part of the abdomen by the thoracic cage provides a border zone that is often the site of combination injuries. The young man who is complaining only of chest-wall pain because of one or two rib fractures received in a street fight may have a rapid pulse rate and vasoconstriction that are out of proportion to a broken rib. A consideration of the general region where the rib fracture is located may lead to a correct complete diagnosis that includes a rupture of the spleen or liver. Particularly challenging are those patients who cannot describe their chest pain, or their difficulty in breathing, because of associated head injuries or profound shock. From extensive experience Naclerio has recommended that patients with chest injuries should be approached on the basis of (1) physiologic, (2) etiologic, and (3) anatomic considerations. Since the primary aim of treatment is the prompt restoration of normal cardiopulmonary function, first consideration is given to the patient's physiologic status. Fundamental to this approach is an ability to detect physical abnormalities and relate them to the pathologic processes that are frequently associated with chest injuries. The classification of pathologic processes derived by Naclerio for clinical use is the following:

Group I	*Those peculiar to the outer region of the chest* 1. Subcutaneous emphysema 2. Paradoxical respiration (flail chest) 3. Open pneumothorax
Group II	*Those peculiar to the inner region of the chest* 1. Closed pneumothorax 2. Hemothorax 3. Secretional obstruction of lower airways (pulmonary contusion, "wet lung," aspiration pneumonitis)
Group III	*Those peculiar to the innermost region of the chest* 1. Mediastinal emphysema 2. Cardiac tamponade 3. Compression atelectasis (traumatic diaphragmatic hernia)

Fig. 17-10. A prediction nomogram for pulmonary function in men. *FRC*, functional residual capacity; *TLC*, total lung capacity; *RV*, residual volume; $FEV_{0.5}$, 0.5-second forced expiratory volume; MVV_F, maximal voluntary ventilation (free); FEV_1, 1-second forced expiratory volume; *FVC*, forced vital capacity. The predicted values for *FRC* and *TLC* can be read directly from the left-hand scale, based on the patient's height. The scale at the bottom is for convenience in converting centimeters to inches. *RV/TLC* (%) may be read directly from the age scale. For the other predicted values, lay a straight edge between the patient's height and his age. Predicted normal values can be read directly from the points where the straight edge crosses the *RV*, $FEV_{0.5}$, MVV_F, FEV_1, and *FVC* scales. (*Reproduced from H. C. Dorcn, R. C. Kory, and J. C. Syner, The Veterans Administration–Army Cooperative Study of Pulmonary Function: II. The Lung Volume and Its Subdivisions in Normal Men, Am J Med, 41:96, 1966, by permission of the authors and publishers.*)

Regardless of whether a classification of pathologic processes is used as a reference, the physician who manages thoracic trauma must know what specific injuries are possible (Fig. 17-11). It is traditional to classify thoracic injuries on the basis of whether the thoracic cage was penetrated by the wounding object. *Nonpenetrating* or *blunt* injuries result from application of force to the chest wall or from sudden deceleration of the chest against a relatively unyielding structure, such as a steering wheel.

Fig. 17-11. The approach to diagnosis and emergency treatment of patients with major thoracic trauma is facilitated by a sound knowledge of the specific injuries that can occur. (*Reproduced from E. A. Naclerio, "Chest Injuries," Grune & Stratton, Inc., New York, 1971, with permission of the author and publishers.*)

Minor impacts on the chest wall allow the dissipation of applied force with simple contusion of the soft tissues or the bony cage. With a blunt force of greater energy the chest wall transmits some of the wounding force to the intrathoracic structures. Because the lungs and heart present their surfaces to the inner chest wall, it can be expected that those organs are most likely to be injured by transmitted force. In some instances more complex relationships have to be considered to explain a laceration of the esophagus, a tear in the wall of a major bronchus, or a disruption of the thoracic aorta. For many such injuries the explanation is thought to lie in a difference of deceleration rates for adjacent regions of the same organ or structure, related to the degree of fixation of the adjacent regions.

The mortality rate of major blunt injuries has been reduced steadily during the past quarter century, but complications and death associated with pulmonary contusion, posttraumatic pulmonary insufficiency, and trauma to the heart and great vessels are still impressive. It is especially characteristic of blunt injuries that the maximal extent of cardiopulmonary functional loss and often the complete diagnosis require several days for development.

Penetrating injuries are those in which the wounding agent has at least entered the chest wall and generally has penetrated interior structures. In some classifications of wounds an additional category of perforating injuries is used to designate those penetrating wounds in which the wounding object passes through the body region and produces a wound of exit. The latter wound may be more ragged and larger than the wound of entrance. It is often possible to predict which tissue or organs have been damaged by estimating the direction from which the wounding object came and its apparent course. However, the bony structures of the thoracic cage can so markedly alter the course of a knife or small-caliber bullet that relatively little damage may be associated with an entrance wound that appears ominous because of its proximity to the mediastinum (Fig. 17-12). In general, the management of penetrating wounds depends on the same techniques for assessment and diagnosis that are applied in patients with nonpenetrating injuries. A greater utilization of emergency thoracotomy is required in those hospitals where the bulk of thoracic trauma consists of patients with penetrating injuries.

The penetrating injuries that produce a major disruption of the chest wall may result in an open wound—free communication between the pleural cavity and the outside. Because of the noise that is made by passage of air in and out of the wound with respiratory efforts, the open wounds are often referred to as "sucking wounds" of the chest. Shotgun blasts at close range, industrial accidents in which the victim's chest wall is impaled by motorized equipment, and high-speed car wrecks are examples of situations in which open chest wounds may be produced.

Naclerio's *anatomic* approach to chest injuries is especially useful for considering the management of knife wounds. When a stab wound has been made in the *upper part of the thorax* and there is no subcutaneous emphysema, it can be assumed that there is no injury to the trachea. If examination of the chest suggests only a minimal hemothorax, it sharply reduces the possibility that a major artery has been injured, either in the thoracic inlet or the superior mediastinum. But if a major hemothorax is present, injury to a large vessel is likely, and a decision must be made either to do an exploratory operation or to obtain immediate angiography. A patient whose esophagus has been penetrated by the stab wound may have some slight discomfort with swallowing, accompanied by mediastinal and subcutaneous emphysema. A contrast esophagogram is necessary to determine the level of an esophageal penetration and to help with the choice of procedure for its management.

If a patient has been stabbed in the *midthoracic region* the primary concern is whether the heart has been penetrated. When the entrance wound overlies the large central area occupied by the heart, and the patient is in shock, an immediate pericardiocentesis should be done to relieve any possible tamponade while preparations are made for emergency thoracotomy. A parasternal stab wound with evidence of hemothorax often requires operation for ligation of severed internal thoracic vessels, sometimes accompanied by cardiac injury. Stab wounds of the lung generally stop bleeding spontaneously, and the majority of patients who are stabbed in the lateral and posterior regions of the chest do not require thoracotomy. A moderate hemothorax resulting from penetration of the lung parenchyma may be managed by tube thoracostomy. However, if bleeding continues after the chest tube is put in, it is more likely to be due to an injured intercostal artery, and an exploratory thoracotomy will be required.

For stab wounds in the *lower thoracic region* the type of management is dominated by a consideration that the diaphragm may have been penetrated. Therefore, some surgeons believe that a stab wound of the left lower part of the chest mandates early abdominal exploration on the basis that the knife may have gone through the diaphragm to injure the spleen, stomach, or colon. An alternate approach, and the one generally used for patients with stab wounds of the right lower part of the chest, is to observe the patient carefully for evidence of peritoneal irritation, free air, or signs of bleeding in excess of the amount of blood drained by an intercostal catheter. Contrast radiologic studies of the stomach and colon may be done early if the patient's condition is good, or following the initial period of observation. Because the liver is generally the only abdominal structure injured by right-sided stab wounds that penetrate the diaphragm, it is reasonable to observe such patients for a period of some hours. Abdominal exploration is indicated if there is evidence of continuing blood loss, and additional thought must be given to possible late complications of delayed hemorrhage, bile peritonitis, or subphrenic abscess.

Rib Fractures

The most common injury of the chest is a fracture of one or more ribs, including fracture at the costochondral junction ("separation"). Children seem less liable to rib fractures, but chest x-rays are made less frequently in those young age groups with minor trauma. Fractures occur most

Fig. 17-12. This chest x-ray was taken less than 1 hour after the patient was shot in the left side of the chest with a .44-caliber pistol. The film shows mediastinal widening, greater on the right, with deviation of the trachea to the left (*upper arrows*). Coughing and pain were the only symptoms, but the patient underwent emergency mediastinal exploration with an expectation of finding major vascular injury. A hematoma was found in the mediastinum, but no major vascular structures were damaged. The bullet was lying free in the right pleural cavity in the location where it is seen on the x-ray.

commonly in the middle and lower ribs with blunt trauma, but the distribution with penetrating wounds varies with the distribution of the penetrating objects. The first rib is rarely fractured unless one or more upper ribs are also broken. There is inconclusive evidence that a direct relationship exists between first and second rib fractures and trauma to major vessels at the apex of the hemithorax (Fig. 17-13).

An inward displacement of the fracture fragments at the time of injury may lacerate the lung parenchyma and produce a pneumothorax with bleeding into the pleural cavity. With a single rib fracture the incidence of pneumothorax is not high, but there is an increasing likelihood of this complication as the number of fractured ribs increases. The occurrence of pneumothorax may be delayed for some hours or even days after the injury has occurred. Hemothorax of a significant degree occurring with rib fractures is usually due to laceration of an intercostal artery rather than to bleeding from the lung. Again, bleeding may be delayed in onset or it may recur after an interval of several days. Especially in the patient who has multiple rib fractures with segmental fractures of one or more ribs, a de-

A

B

Fig. 17-13. *A.* The first chest x-ray of a twenty-five-year-old man who was injured in a motorcycle accident shows a fracture of the right first rib (*upper arrow*) and a small extrapleural hematoma at the right apex (*lower arrow*). *B.* A subclavian arteriogram and venogram were done 3 days after admission because of the sudden development of a massive hemothorax (2,000 ml blood) on the right side. Bleeding stopped spontaneously, and the venogram shows a tear in the subclavian vein at the rib fracture site.

layed pneumothorax or hemothorax may coincide with some shift of the rib fragments demonstrated in serial chest x-rays. In elderly or chronically ill patients rib fractures may occur with severe coughing or hard straining. The occurrence of a spontaneous fracture in any patient should alert the physician to the possibility of a bone abnormality such as metastatic neoplasm or hyperparathyroidism. Pneumothorax and hemothorax are infrequent with rib fractures that do not result from external trauma.

The diagnosis of a rib fracture may be implied from the pleuritic type of pain and marked tenderness over the fracture area. A sharply localized contusion of the chest-wall structures may mimic the findings, including shallow respirations with chest-wall splinting. Green-stick fractures are those not associated with separation of the fragments, and they may not be demonstrated by the initial chest x-ray examination. Several weeks may elapse before a suspected fracture is confirmed. However, when the patient has two or more adjacent fractured ribs, especially if the ribs are broken in more than one place (segmental fractures), the diagnosis is made with greater certainty by examination alone. Cartilage fractures and separation from either the rib or sternum are not demonstrated by chest x-rays.

The acute complications of rib fracture are pneumothorax, hemothorax, and interstitial emphysema. These will be discussed as separate items because of their frequent association with multiple types of chest trauma. Atelectasis and pneumonia may develop as complications because of re-

stricted chest-wall motion, bed rest, and preexisting respiratory disease.

The principal goal of treatment for patients without serious injury is relief of pain. If this is accomplished, patients may resume their normal activities except those that require a vigorous work effort. Adhesive strapping of the chest or chest binders to splint the fracture area may be used to diminish pain in young or middle-aged persons. These techniques are not good for the elderly and for patients with chronic lung disease. The adhesive strapping must be done carefully to avoid blistering and excessive skin traction. A disadvantage that many patients find inconvenient is the inability to shower or to bathe adequately while the adhesive tape is in place. For the majority of patients an adequate oral analgesic or an intercostal nerve block plus oral analgesics provides reasonable pain relief with minimal risk of side effects (Fig. 17-14). The nerve block may need to be repeated once daily for several days, but a single injection may suffice for individuals whose injury does not require hospitalization. A patient whose rib fracture is accompanied by minimal pneumothorax (less than 1.5-cm separation between the lung and the inner

Fig. 17-14. Intercostal nerve blocks may be very effective in relieving the pain of rib fractures. The nerves above and below the fractured ribs must be blocked, in addition to those corresponding to the ribs fractured.

chest wall by x-ray), may be treated as an outpatient under ideal conditions of observation and follow-up. The management of more significant complications will be described below.

Sternal Fractures

Fractures of the sternum are generally the result of slamming against the steering wheel in car accidents. A fracture may occur with any type of blunt trauma to the anterior part of the chest, or occasionally may be produced by a penetrating missile. The fractures are usually transverse and most often occur in the body of the sternum at or near the junction with the manubrium (Fig. 17-15). Displacement of the fragments is not unusual, and when it occurs the upper fragment is behind the lower segment. There may be comminution of the sternal fracture as well as associated fractures of the costal cartilages and separation from the sternal borders. The term *crushed chest* refers to a constellation of blunt chest injuries in which there is extensive disruption of chest-wall structures, including sternal and rib fractures, associated with pulmonary and/or cardiac contusion. The instability of the chest wall is referred to as "flail chest," but fractures of the sternum are not a necessary component of all flail-chest injuries.

Sternal fractures should always signal the possibility of myocardial injury, rupture of the aorta or brachiocephalic vessels, or major tracheobronchial laceration. The pain of a sternal fracture may persist for a long time; when this occurs a nonunion should be suspected. This is usually the result of persistent displacement of the proximal fragment, and a closed reduction may be attempted under general anesthesia by hyperextension of the spine with the arms above the head. Occasionally, open reduction and wiring of the fragments are required.

Traumatic Pneumothorax

Pneumothorax due to penetrating or nonpenetrating trauma is usually the result of injury to the lung or the tracheobronchial tree. An occasional instance of esophageal perforation may be followed by a pneumomediastinum

Fig. 17-15. A lateral chest x-ray demonstrates the type of sternal fracture that occurs when the driver of a car is thrown against the steering wheel.

A

B

C

Fig. 17-16. *A*. In a tension pneumothorax there is compression of the contralateral lung and a displacement of the mediastinum that may sharply reduce venous return to the atria. *B*. If the diagnosis is strongly suspected, needle aspiration of the pleural space should be done without waiting for the chest x-ray. In this patient, the tension pneumothorax developed slowly and became symptomatic shortly after this film was taken. The lower arrow points to the displacement of the right heart border, and the lung is completely collapsed (*upper arrow*). *C*. Following needle aspiration a large intercostal tube was put in place, but a major air leak continued for several days and eventually required insertion of an additional chest catheter. The arrow points to the visceral pleura, showing incomplete expansion of the lung.

that ruptures into the pleural cavity. In addition, it is possible for a sucking wound of the chest to produce pneumothorax without pulmonary parenchymal injury. The term *closed pneumothorax* is sometimes used to distinguish a pneumothorax that is not in direct communication with the outside air from the type associated with sucking wounds of the chest. Whether the pneumothorax is associated with blunt injury and fractured ribs or is due to a penetrating wound, there is a variable amount of bleeding into the pleural cavity. The decision to use the term *hemopneumothorax* depends on the amount of blood in the pleural cavity and the likely consequences. If sufficient blood is present to require a concerted effort to assure its removal, or if its loss from the circulating volume requires transfusion replacement, it seems proper to use the double term.

Pneumothorax varies from that which is so slight that it may be missed on the initial x-ray examination to a massive, continuing air leak that displaces the mediastinum, depresses the diaphragm, and compresses the opposite lung—*tension pneumothorax* (Fig. 17-16). A pneumothorax due to a parenchymal lung injury tends to be self-limited because the developing lung collapse combines with blood clotting in the wound for a sealing effect. For some patients extensive adhesions already present between the visceral and parietal pleura may localize the pleural air and prevent a collapse of the lung (Fig. 17-17).

The mechanics of a developing tension pneumothorax may not be obvious when the patient is first seen. Pain may be the primary complaint, with no evidence of respiratory distress. But if the lung wound is behaving as a check valve, some air will escape into the pleural cavity with each inspiration or with each cough. Gradually, intrapleural pressure will build up, the lung collapses, and a tension pneumothorax may develop. A shift of the mediastinum and compression of the large veins result in a decreased cardiac output that may lead to sudden death.

With any chest injury it is wisest to presume that a pneumothorax is present until proved otherwise. Because of pain and limited chest motion on the injured side,

physical examination may be inadequate for diagnosis of a minimal pneumothorax. When there is no respiratory distress it is proper to base the diagnosis on the results of an upright or lateral decubitus chest x-ray. With tension pneumothorax of rapid development the patient's life depends on rapid decompression of the pleural space, without waiting to confirm the suspected diagnosis by chest x-ray. In addition to dyspnea, with or without cyanosis, the patient may show distended neck veins, a hyperresonant percussion note over the injured hemithorax, absent or distant breath sounds, and a shift of the heart sounds and trachea toward the opposite side. To accomplish rapid decompression, a large-gauge needle with a stopcock and syringe may be passed into the pleural cavity through the second intercostal space in the midclavicular line. After initial decompression the needle should be replaced with an intercostal catheter attached to an underwater seal. Subsequent treatment depends on whether the lung reexpands and whether the air leak is associated with a parenchymal injury versus a major bronchial disruption.

Treatment of the more usual pneumothorax depends on symptoms of respiratory insufficiency, the extent of the pneumothorax, and the presence of significant hemothorax. There is a tendency to think of pneumothorax in terms of a two-dimensional concept that is conveyed by the anteroposterior chest x-ray. Instead, the hemithorax must

Fig. 17-17. A free pleural space will allow the development of a complete pneumothorax or a massive hemothorax. These potentially fatal complications cannot occur in patients with an obliterated pleural space. (*Reproduced from E. A. Naclerio, "Chest Injuries," Grune & Stratton, Inc., New York, 1971, with permission of the author and publisher.*)

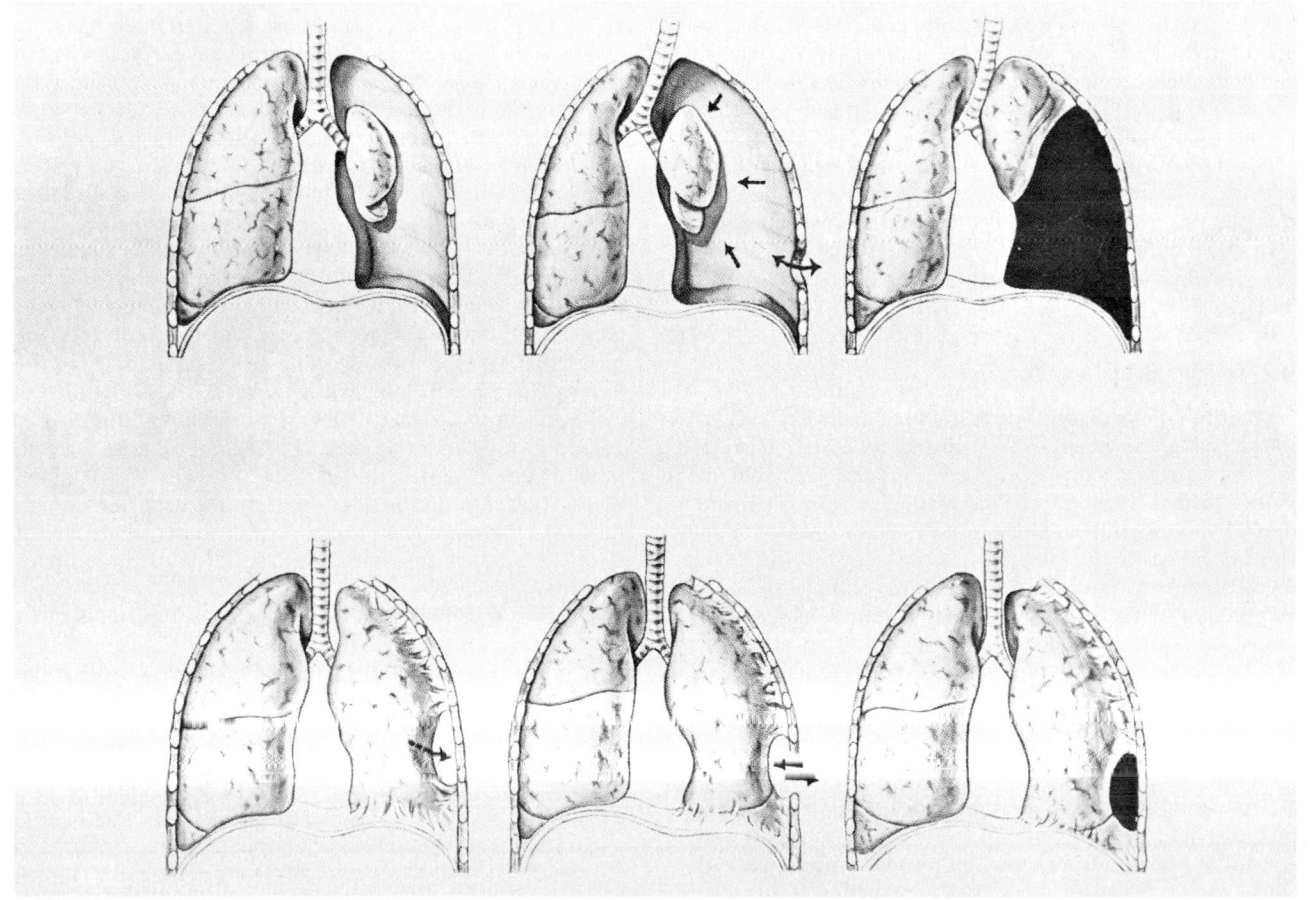

be considered a modified cylinder, and when the lung surface is separated from the chest wall by 3 cm or more the patient may have a 50 percent lung collapse (by volume) rather than the 25 or 30 percent collapse that the chest x-ray suggests. With a pneumothorax that is less than this amount, due to a nonpenetrating injury (theoretically, no contamination of the pleural space) and not accompanied by significant blood or fluid in the pleural cavity, no treatment may be required. A decision not to remove the pleural air implies that the patient has had a simple injury and that conditions for observation are ideal. Approximately 1.25 percent of the air will be absorbed each day, with full expansion expected in 3 to 6 weeks.

Aspiration of the air with a needle and insertion of an intercostal catheter only if lung collapse recurs is a reasonable method of treatment advocated by some physicians when the pneumothorax amounts to as much as 50 percent. In all cases with greater than 50 percent collapse, in those with hemopneumothorax, and in patients whose pneumothorax is the result of penetrating trauma, an intercostal catheter should be inserted and attached to a water seal with 10 to 25 cm H_2O negative pressure. In the majority of patients, lung reexpansion and cessation of the air leak will occur within a few hours or a few days. If not, a major bronchial injury may be present, and a thoracotomy may be required after appropriate diagnostic procedures.

There are three essential steps in the management of the open pneumothorax associated with sucking wounds. A watertight dressing should be used to cover the wound, and an intercostal catheter should be inserted in the pleural cavity. As soon as the patient's condition permits, debridement of the wound should be done, followed by wound closure if possible.

The use of prophylactic systemic antibiotics in patients with chest trauma is a subject of current debate, but their use in cases of nonpenetrating trauma seems unjustified. Certainly, the simple insertion of an intercostal catheter cannot be used as the justification for prescribing an antibiotic.

Interstitial Emphysema

Disruption of the respiratory tract at any level will result in the passage of air into the surrounding tissues. *Mediastinal emphysema* occurs when air enters the areolar tissue planes from a tracheobronchial wound or from a perforation of the esophagus. Occasionally, blunt injuries to the chest may disrupt the integrity of a group of bronchioles or alveolar units without disrupting the visceral pleura. As air escapes into the pulmonary interstitium it dissects centrally along the bronchi and pulmonary vessels to reach the mediastinum. When the mediastinal pleura remains intact, progressive loss of air into the tissue carries the dissection into the neck, where the air escapes the deep-tissue planes and spreads in the subcutaneous tissue (Fig. 17-18).

Subcutaneous emphysema may also be produced by penetrating or blunt injuries that disrupt the lung and parietal pleura so that air is forced into the tissues of the chest wall. An initial pneumothorax may be present, but the patients who develop the most massive subcutaneous emphysema

often have delayed onset of pneumothorax. The progressive development of subcutaneous emphysema causes marked distortion of the patient's appearance and significant discomfort. However, there is seldom any reason to "treat" the condition by making a cervical incision to provide a point of air escape. Instead, attention should be directed at confirming the presumed source of the air leak so that an esophageal perforation or major bronchial injury is not delayed in its recognition.

Traumatic Hemothorax

Intrathoracic bleeding occurs with any form of chest injury that disrupts the tissues. In most instances of either penetrating or nonpenetrating trauma the blood is shed into the pleural cavity, often with some degree of pneumothorax. Although hemothorax develops at the time of injury in most patients, the bleeding may be delayed for several days. Occasionally an extrapleural hematoma will break into the pleural cavity and give the impression of delayed hemorrhage.

Bleeding from the lung as the result of rib fractures or small-missile wounds will generally stop before a sufficient volume has been lost to mandate an emergency thoracotomy. From accumulated military and civilian experience it can be estimated that slightly more than 10 percent of patients with traumatic hemothorax will require thoracotomy for control of bleeding or determination of the extent of injury. A progressive hemothorax or continued bleeding at the rate of more than 100 ml/hour beyond a few hours after placement of an intercostal catheter suggests bleeding from an intercostal artery, the internal thoracic artery, or a source that will require operative control. In particular, a major pulmonary laceration due to blunt trauma is generally characterized by continued major blood loss and a large air leak.

Movement of the diaphragm and thoracic structures causes partial defibrination of blood that is shed into the pleural cavity, and clotting is usually incomplete. Sufficient coagulation does occur to interfere with efficient drainage of the pleural blood through intercostal catheters, and the latter often become plugged with blood clot. Pleural enzymes begin to produce clot lysis within a few hours after bleeding stops, and the process of hemolysis with protein breakdown increases the osmotic pressure. Unless the pleural space is drained adequately the transudation of fluid into the space can produce significant compression of the lung and a shift of the mediastinum toward the opposite hemithorax.

The diagnosis of hemothorax with chest injuries is not a matter of determining whether it is present. The question is how much is present, and whether bleeding is still going on. A consideration of the type and extent of injury, gen-

Fig. 17-18. *A* and *B*. A patient with extensive subcutaneous emphysema due to a laceration of the right lung from a rib fracture. *C*. There is massive involvement of the face, trunk, and scrotum. A tracheostomy was done for harassing cough due to chronic bronchitis. *D*. Note the face of the patient 10 days later.

A

B

C

D

A

B

Fig. 17-19. *A.* A major hemothorax resulted from a gunshot wound in the right side of the chest of the fifty-year-old man whose chest x-ray is shown here. *B.* This film was taken several weeks later with injection of contrast material through the chest tube. The contrast material outlines a large, irregular cavity in the pleural space, representing an empyema cavity that had developed because of inadequate drainage of the hemothorax by chest catheters. *C.* After decortication there is complete expansion of the right lung, but considerable exudate and fluid are still present in the costophrenic sulcus.

C

eral signs of blood loss, physical signs of fluid in the pleural cavity, and chest x-ray findings may all be needed to assess the extent of hemothorax. It should be remembered that as much as 400 to 500 ml of blood may be hidden by the dome of the diaphragm on the upright chest x-ray, and only the liquid part will be demonstrated by the lateral decubitus film.

A small hemothorax that produces little more than

blunting of the costophrenic angle on the chest x-ray does not require initial treatment. Instead, follow-up x-rays should be made at intervals of a few days to assist with the decision to drain the pleural cavity if there is a progressive accumulation. When the hemothorax exceeds an amount that fills the costophrenic sulcus, or when there is associated pneumothorax, one or more large catheters should be placed in the pleural cavity through the seventh, eighth, or ninth intercostal space in the posterior axillary line. Underwater drainage alone may be sufficient, but low suction applied to the catheters is often helpful when combined with active efforts at stripping the tubes of blood clot. If the initial drainage of blood is followed by continued bleeding in the absence of a clotting defect, a decision to operate must be made, with a broad consideration of the possible sources of the bleeding.

With a major hemothorax the success of tube drainage is often frustrated by extensive clot that obstructs the tubes (Fig. 17-19). An attitude should be adopted that a nonfunctioning chest tube represents a *liability* to the patient because of discomfort and the risk of carrying infection from the skin wound into the pleural clot. Patency of the intercostal tubes may be assured by careful irrigation with normal saline solution and by daily instillations of topical Varidase for lysis and drainage of remaining clotted blood.

Especially with penetrating trauma, a hemothorax that fails to drain adequately through intercostal catheters may develop into empyema. An additional hazard is the organization of residual clot to form a fibrothorax. Although the incidence of these complications is not high, the consequences are severe, and it is wiser to proceed with thoracotomy and evacuation of the hemothorax before an extensive decortication becomes necessary.

Pulmonary Injury

The lungs have a remarkable ability to tolerate penetrating injuries and blunt trauma without long-term residual effects. Civilian gunshot wounds of the chest penetrate a lung more frequently than any other structure, but the majority of patients with no other significant injury can be treated without a thoracotomy. Any penetrating object produces an air leak with a variable degree of pneumothorax. The disruption of tissue along the missile track causes bleeding, which usually ceases as the damaged parenchyma becomes swollen and filled with blood clot. With small-calibre and low-velocity bullet wounds that pass through the lung periphery, the amount of tissue damage produced may be sufficiently small that late follow-up chest x-rays fail to demonstrate the area of injury. With high-velocity bullets, the tissue destruction extends more widely, and even a peripheral bullet pathway may result in irreversible damage to a lobar or lung hilus. The occurrence of arterial air embolism as a cause of morbidity or death in patients with penetrating lung trauma has recently been emphasized by Thomas. The symptoms are related to involvement of either the cerebral or coronary circulation. A failure to produce systemic air embolism under experimental conditions and lack of clinical experience with the condition on a large trauma service have caused others to challenge the occurrence of this complication.

The immediate management of the patient with a penetrating injury is the insertion of at least one intercostal catheter for evacuation of the associated hemopneumothorax. Serial arterial blood gases and frequent evaluation of the patient's ventilatory ability allow an overall estimate of the effect of the injury on respiratory exchange. Civilian penetrating wounds do not require ventilatory assistance very frequently, but the effect of the injury may be underestimated. In some patients, the likelihood of injury to the heart or great vessels, a likely penetration of the diaphragm, or major bleeding may mandate immediate thoracotomy or abdominal exploration. More often, the need for thoracotomy to control bleeding or to perform pulmonary resection for an irreversibly injured lung becomes apparent only over a period of hours, or several days. A massive continuous air leak through the chest tube suggests a major bronchial laceration, but a similar air leak can occur with a peripheral lung wound that transects a number of small airways. A point of differentiation that can be helpful is the difficulty in achieving complete lung expansion and maintaining the expansion in the presence of a major bronchial injury.

Pulmonary contusion is the contemporary term used to indicate the consequences of blunt trauma to the lung. The frequent causes of contusion include rapid deceleration of the chest against an automobile steering wheel, falls from a height, and blast injuries. Particularly in young persons, severe pulmonary contusion can occur by transmission of force through the chest wall with minimal fractures of the ribs or sternum. In middle-aged or elderly persons significant pulmonary contusion is usually accompanied by multiple fractures of the thoracic cage.

The contused lung is characterized by capillary disruption that results in intraalveolar and interstitial hemorrhage, edema, protein and fluid obstruction of small airways, and leukocyte infiltration. Serial chest x-rays begun right after injury show a fluffy infiltrate that progresses in extent and in density over a period of 24 to 48 hours. Although the maximum lung injury is directly related to that region of the chest wall that receives the trauma, a "contrecoup" effect may be responsible for a wider distribution of the pulmonary damage. Unless the contusion involves only a small region of one lung, it may result in serious loss of respiratory function. The associated injury to the chest wall is aggravated by the loss of pulmonary compliance, increasing the work of breathing. Small areas of atelectasis become confluent, and progressive hypoxia further diminishes the patient's ability to compensate for the loss of function.

Pulmonary contusion is often part of a major chest injury that includes one or more fractures of the thoracic cage, pneumothorax, and hemothorax. If not present initially, a pneumothorax may subsequently develop from actual disruption of the contused pulmonary parenchyma. Although it is infrequent in patients who survive to reach the hospital, a major pulmonary laceration may represent the maximum extent of pulmonary contusion. In some instances the tissue disruption is the result of extensive penetration by rib fragments, but in others the causative factor is probably a severe shearing force. The clinical and x-ray findings suggest a serious chest injury but do not differentiate the patient with a major lung laceration from those with pulmonary contusion and associated hemopneumothorax. Continued or uncontrolled hemorrhage and massive air leak generally mandate an early thoracotomy. A major pulmonary resection is often necessary, and the mortality rate is high.

Treatment of pulmonary contusion must include an accurate clinical assessment of the patient's respiratory exchange and careful monitoring by serial measurements of the arterial blood gases. Unfortunately, the techniques of large-volume intravenous fluid administration commonly used to resuscitate patients with multiple injuries may worsen the pulmonary edema that accompanies pulmonary contusion. To reduce this likelihood, the rate of intravenous fluid administration should not exceed 50 to 75 ml/hour if this is at all possible. In addition, 20- to 40-mg doses of intravenous furosemide at intervals of 4 to 6 hours should aid the mobilization of edema fluid from the lung.

A high percentage of patients require temporary assisted ventilation, and it may be evident at the time of admission that endotracheal or nasatracheal intubation should be performed. Without question, aggressive respiratory therapy, including ventilatory support, should be initiated before cardiopulmonary decompensation requires treatment measures that add additional risks. Criteria for insti-

Table 17-2. CRITERIA FOR ASSISTED VENTILATION

Function	Normal values	Ventilate
Pulmonary mechanics		
Respiratory rate...........................	12–20	>35
Vital capacity, ml/kg.....................	65–75	<15
Maximum inspiratory force, cm H_2O		
(negative values).......................	75–100	<25–35
Gas exchange		
Pa_{O_2}, torr.................................	76–100 (room air)	<65–70 (added oxygen)
Alveolar-arterial oxygen difference, torr		
(100% oxygen)	30–70	>350
Pa_{CO_2}, torr	35–45	>50
Dead space/tidal volume ratio..........	0.25–0.40	>0.6

tuting assisted ventilation are shown in Table 17-2. For most patients the need for assisted ventilation does not extend beyond 48 to 72 hours unless there is major injury to the chest wall or to other body regions.

Tracheobronchial Injury

Penetrating wounds of the thoracic trachea and the stem bronchi are especially serious because of concomitant damage to the major intrathoracic vascular structures. Rapid assessment of the likely course taken by a bullet or knife that entered the patient's mediastinum and prompt evaluation of respiratory distress, hemoptysis, and interstitial emphysema may allow successful treatment. The patients often have an associated pneumothorax, which may rapidly develop into a tension pneumothorax. Shock is not uncommon because of associated bleeding into the mediastinum and one or both pleural cavities. The alert patient often has coughing, and this causes the subcutaneous emphysema to develop more rapidly. Chest x-rays generally show mediastinal emphysema, and if bilateral pneumothorax is also present, it suggests a lacerated trachea.

Early insertion of a large intercostal catheter for pneumothorax may fail to result in expansion of the lung despite a large air flow produced by high-suction drainage. As soon as the patient's respiratory exchange is under control, bronchoscopy should be done to confirm a suspected tracheal or bronchial injury. At the same time, esophagoscopy should be done because of the frequency of associated esophageal injury.

For small penetrating injuries of the intrathoracic trachea and major bronchi, tracheostomy and effective pleural decompression may provide satisfactory definitive treatment. Those injuries which are associated with an actual defect in the tracheobronchial wall, including partial disruption, require operative exploration and repair. Tracheostomy will frequently be necessary to prevent high intratracheal pressures and to allow tracheal care postoperatively.

Penetrating injuries of lobar or segmental bronchi may produce a similar clinical picture to proximal tracheobronchial injuries. Bilateral pneumothorax is rare, and the principal immediate problem is to begin management of the major air leak and confirm the presence of a major

bronchial injury. Hemoptysis may not be detected, and the bronchial air leak may stop soon after an intercostal catheter is put in place. The definitive diagnosis may be delayed if the bronchus becomes obstructed by blood clot or mucus and the air leak ceases. Under these conditions the pulmonary lobe or segment becomes atelectatic and resists conservative methods to produce reexpansion. If infection does not occur, the injured bronchus may heal with significant distortion and obstruction, or the atelectasis may persist and lead subsequently to a correct diagnosis. Operative repair of the disrupted bronchus can be achieved even years after injury. If infection occurs at the site of the bronchial injury the patient may develop pneumonia, distal bronchiectasis, and empyema. Resection of the bronchus and the involved pulmonary lobe is then required.

Severe blunt chest trauma may result in tracheobronchial tears or complete disruption. The most common intrathoracic location is in a main-stem bronchus, the left being more frequently injured than the right. Respiratory distress is generally present, and death may occur from progressive obstruction of the respiratory tract by secretions and blood. Again, an injury may seal itself off, fail to be recognized, and heal with severe stenosis.

The diagnosis and successful management of tracheobronchial injuries depend on a high index of suspicion. Unfortunately, a significant number of tracheal injuries in trauma patients are the result of faulty techniques of endotracheal intubation or tracheostomy when these are performed under emergency circumstances, particularly with head and neck injuries. Improved tracheostomy tubes and better tracheostomy care based on an understanding of the pathophysiology of tube-related tracheal damage have reduced the incidence of tracheal stenosis. Nevertheless, tracheal damage due to overinflated balloon cuffs still occurs, and the patient whose chest x-ray is shown in Fig. 17-20 developed a tracheoesophageal fistula.

Flail Chest

The terms *crushed chest* and *flail chest* have often been used interchangeably, although they are not synonymous. A crushed-chest injury indicates the general cause and implies a disruption of tissue integrity that would be likely to result in flail-like motion of a chest-wall region and a varying degree of crushing (contusion) of any or all underlying structures. It is better to restrict the use of *crushed chest* to indicate the mechanism of injury, rather than trying to have the term imply the several possible consequences of pulmonary contusion, myocardial injury, pneumothorax, hemothorax, and so on. Similarly, a diagnosis of flail chest should be accompanied by the tabulation of the specific associated injuries.

The diagnosis of flail chest is based on the presence of paradoxical respiratory movement in a segment of the chest wall. This generally requires at least two segmental fractures in each of three adjacent ribs or costal cartilages. Multiple combinations of rib or sternal fractures with costochondral or chondrosternal separations can result in the paradoxical respiratory motion that characterizes a flail chest. Figure 17-21 demonstrates the three major types of flail chest based on the location of the flail segment. The posterior type is rare, and in the absence of disrupted intrathoracic structures is the easiest to manage because of the strong muscular and scapular support, and because of the patient's natural tendency to lie with his back against the mattress.

Theoretically, the paradoxical motion markedly reduces respiratory efficiency and allows a back-and-forth movement of dead-space air across the carina between the two lungs during each respiratory cycle. This has been referred to as *Pendulluft* (pendulum-like movement of air), but it has been discounted experimentally.

Mediastinal motion away from the injured side with inspiration and toward the flail segment during expiration may reduce venous return and cardiac output if the flail area is large and if the patient's respiratory efforts are labored.

Emphasis on the chest-wall injury in patients with a flail chest may divert the physician's attention from the underlying pulmonary and/or myocardial injury. Pulmonary contusion is an important feature of the great majority of flail-chest injuries, and early treatment should be directed toward minimizing the evolution of that lesion. In some patients, the paradoxical motion of the injured chest wall

Fig. 17-20. This chest film shows a markedly overinflated tracheostomy balloon cuff in a patient who required assisted ventilation for multiple injuries. The cuff was one of the current "low-pressure" types, but the patient developed a tracheoesophageal fistula.

may become apparent only after the associated lung injury has produced a sharp reduction in pulmonary compliance and a corresponding increase in respiratory effort. Pneumothorax or hemothorax is often present with severe flail injuries, and rapid placement of an intercostal catheter may partially relieve the respiratory distress. Especially with anterior chest injuries that include sternal fractures or disruption of costal cartilages, the probability of myocardial contusion must be considered. Serial electrocardiograms, cardiac isoenzyme determinations, and radioisotope delineation of injured myocardium may be appropriate for correlation with clinical evidence of cardiac failure or pericardial friction rubs.

Chest-wall stabilization and reduction of respiratory dead space are major goals of treatment. For many years early tracheostomy has been considered routine in the management of patients with flail chest, because it allows

Fig. 17-21. The three major types of flail chest. (*Reproduced from E. A. Naclerio, "Chest Injuries," Grune & Stratton, Inc., New York, 1971, with permission of the author and publisher.*)

TYPES OF FLAIL CHEST

Lateral type   Anterior type   Posterior type

easy access for tracheobronchial suctioning, it reduces dead space, and it facilitates internal stabilization of the chest wall through mechanical ventilation. Other techniques for stabilizing the flail segment, such as the use of external compression dressings or the application of traction by encircling the fractured ribs with towel clips or wire, have largely been displaced by mechanical ventilation. For some patients with a small flail area and minimal pulmonary injury an intubation followed by tracheostomy may allow satisfactory recovery without the use of assisted ventilation. The improvements in respiratory therapy, including bedside measurements of pulmonary mechanics and the widespread availability of arterial blood-gas determinations, have allowed greater individualization in the treatment of patients with flail-chest injuries (Fig. 17-22).

Tracheostomy and mechanical ventilation are associated with significant complications, the incidence of which varies directly with the duration of ventilatory assistance. These modalities are still the basis of management for those patients with the more severe forms of flail chest and for those with associated head injuries or multiple trauma. In those patients with a minimal or moderate chest-wall injury treatment should be directed at the respiratory dysfunction rather than at stabilizing the area of paradoxical motion. If respiratory support is required it should be initiated with nasotracheal intubation and discontinued when the patient can maintain satisfactory gas exchange. A rare patient presents with localized chest-wall fractures that can be stabilized by direct operative approach. Surgical stabilization of the fractures considerably shortens the convalescence of these individuals.

Traumatic Rupture of the Diaphragm

The diaphragm may be ruptured either by blunt thoracoabdominal trauma or by penetrating injuries. Auto-mobile accidents are the most frequent cause of blunt trauma, and the left hemidiaphragm is ruptured more frequently than the right, in a ratio of about 9:1. Bilateral rupture is rare, but the actual incidence may be higher than the present reports indicate. The right hemidiaphragm is said to be protected from rupture by the liver, and when rupture of the right side does occur the liver is usually the only abdominal structure that herniates into the chest. With lacerations of the left hemidiaphragm, the stomach, spleen, left transverse colon, and omentum in any combination may enter the left pleural cavity. When the diagnosis is delayed for several days or longer, there is often a progressive displacement of the abdominal viscera into the chest, or a progressive gaseous distension of the herniated stomach. The latter may occur despite an indwelling nasogastric tube, and it may precipitate respiratory distress (Fig. 17-23).

This does not imply a casual approach to the diagnosis. Many patients with diaphragmatic rupture due to blunt trauma have associated injuries that demand first attention and prevent a detailed initial evaluation. The first chest x-ray after rupture of either hemidiaphragm may show nothing more than a blurring of the diaphragm with or without evidence of a small hemothorax. In some patients the diagnosis is made very early because the nasogastric tube is seen to lie within the confines of the left pleural cavity. Injection of air through the nasogastric tube during auscultation of the left side of the chest may add support to the diagnosis.

An occasional patient has minimal herniation and no symptoms to suggest the diagnosis. After several months or years, gastrointestinal obstruction may develop and lead to strangulation of herniated viscera. Penetrating diaphragmatic injuries rarely produce symptoms except those related to the other structures that are injured. The hole in the diaphragm is small, and herniation occurs slowly. At

Fig. 17-22. This chest x-ray demonstrates extensive subcutaneous emphysema and multiple segmental rib fractures on the right side. The patient had a severe flail chest and a left pneumothorax, requiring nasotracheal intubation for 6 days and assisted ventilation for 5 days. Tracheostomy was not required.

the time of injury an effort should be made to confirm the diagnosis by contrast studies, by the use of pneumoperitoneum, and by radioisotope liver and spleen scans. Early transabdominal operation is indicated when the diagnosis is confirmed, and associated intraabdominal injuries may be repaired at the same time. The wound in the hemidiaphragm may vary from a simple radial tear to an extensive and complex laceration. Repair can usually be accomplished by direct suture, but a prosthetic patch is occasionally required. If the diagnosis is delayed for months or years a transthoracic approach is more appropriate.

Posttraumatic Pulmonary Insufficiency

The development of acute respiratory failure can be expected in a high percentage of patients who suffer major thoracic trauma. Preexisting pulmonary status will influence the severity of respiratory insufficiency, and the extent of actual pulmonary damage will determine whether the patient survives. An initial evaluation of respiratory exchange and ventilatory ability, confirmed by measurement of pulmonary mechanics and arterial blood gases, should be followed by serial reevaluations.

Especially in patients who have suffered multiple trauma, a respiratory distress syndrome may develop that is out of proportion to the extent of thoracic injury. A series of terms has evolved over the years to designate several forms of respiratory insufficiency that follow trauma and may be associated with a constellation of causative factors. Such terms as "wet lung," "shock lung," "congestive atelectasis," and "adult respiratory-distress syndrome" reflect some principal features that seemed to be characteristic of the cases that came to the attention of those who coined the terms. There is certainly some overlap in the causation of the several forms of respiratory failure that follow major trauma, and it is important to determine the specific causes in individual patients. Blaisdell and Lewis have presented a thorough discussion of posttraumatic pulmonary insufficiency, choosing the term *respiratory-distress syndrome of shock and trauma* for those cases not due to a specific cause. They suggest that eight different explanations for respiratory failure other than the respiratory-distress syndrome occur with reasonable frequency in patients who suffer major injury. These include aspiration, simple atelectasis, lung contusion, fat embolism, pneumonia, pneumothorax, pulmonary edema, and pulmonary embolism.

On the basis of their experience with a large number of cases, Blaisdell and Lewis have concluded that the respiratory-distress syndrome (RDS) is one and the same as the fat-embolism syndrome. Originally thought to result from fat embolism from fracture of long bones, the syndrome consists of pulmonary, neurologic, and systemic manifestations. The pulmonary manifestations appear first, generally within 24 to 36 hours after injury, and consist of dyspnea, tachycardia, fever, and cyanosis. Documentation that much of the fat which appears in the blood following injury represents a mobilization of free fatty acids from body neutral fat as a result of shock and increased levels of catecholamines has helped in understanding the mecha-

Fig. 17-23. Bilateral traumatic rupture of the diaphragm occurred in this eighteen-year-old student when he was thrown from the passenger's seat in a car wreck. The arrow points to the top of the distended intrathoracic stomach. Subsequent staged repairs of the diaphragm allowed him to return to college.

nism of this condition. Because some degree of intravascular coagulation can be demonstrated in all cases, this is almost certainly a factor in development of the syndrome.

For patients who suffer major chest injury it may be impossible to define what part of their respiratory failure is a result of direct trauma and how much is a consequence of the RDS. Treatment must be based on correction of the direct results of injury and on the anticipation or early recognition of respiratory insufficiency. The radiologic changes of RDS, consisting of diffuse lung infiltrates that progress to become confluent, may be superimposed on the effects of pulmonary contusion and atelectasis. Changes observed on serial chest x-rays lag behind the changes in pulmonary function, and a patient may be in critical respiratory failure before the films suggest a progressive pulmonary lesion.

Management of the RDS requires maintenance of good cardiovascular function and prompt institution of ventilatory support. An adequate volume replacement for external fluid and blood losses is complicated by the internal fluid losses due to increased capillary permeability in the lung, in all areas of direct tissue trauma, and to a varying degree throughout the body. Monitoring central venous pressure is the minimum for guidance of fluid and diuretic therapy in these patients, but placement of a Swan-Ganz catheter to allow left atrial and pulmonary artery pressures is superior. The need for inotropic myocardial support can be detected earlier by this access to left-sided heart pressures.

Ventilatory support techniques have advanced to allow a wider selection of ventilators and methods of assisted respiration. Attention to detail can offer the patient a maximum chance of survival with a minimum risk of complications. An unanswered question is the place of steroid therapy. The experience with these agents has been variable, and their employment is generally delayed until the patient appears to be nearing an irreversible state of progressive respiratory failure. This is probably too late for a reasonable drug effect, and on the basis of accumulating data it seems appropriate to advocate a broad trial of repeated pharmacologic doses of methylprednisolone as described by Sladen. By using a regimen of 30 mg/kg of that agent, given intravenously every 6 hours for 48 hours in combination with ventilatory support, Sladen demonstrated a significant reduction in mortality rate.

CHEST WALL

Congenital Deformities

Developmental abnormalities of the thoracic wall have become more important in the recent era because of widespread participation in competitive school athletics and because of the evolution in clothing styles that uncover more of the individual's chest. Because no obvious handicap appears to accompany the more common abnormalities, the subjects are expected to participate in sports, in physical education classes, and in other activities that require some exposure of their deformity to public view. The chest deformities seem not to evoke the sympathy engendered by limb or head and neck anomalies, and the child with a thoracic deformity is often viewed as a curiosity by his classmates. Fortunately, the abnormality is mild is many instances, and the children without an actual functional limitation often learn to cope with the stares or teasing remarks until growth and maturity of their peers make it unnecessary to consider operation.

Except for the more severe sternal deformities, it is generally not possible to predict whether a given deformity will progress during early childhood. Therefore, children who have mild abnormalities can be observed during the first 2 to 5 years and be considered for operative correction on the basis of the cosmetic and physiologic effects which evolve.

Vertebral abnormalities such as scoliosis may result in secondary deformities of the thoracic cage, with significant physiologic effects. The primary approach to treatment involves the vertebral column, and attempts at surgical improvement of the chest-wall deformity are seldom performed.

PECTUS EXCAVATUM

The most common deformity of clinical importance is the sternal depression called *pectus excavatum* (Fig. 17-24). Additional terms that have been used include *schusterbrust, funnel chest,* and *thorax en embudo.* The body of the sternum is displaced posteriorly from its expected position, resulting in a concavity from above downward and from side to side. The costal cartilages participate in the deformity, and their configuration determines whether the concavity is deep and central or broad and shallow. Though the sternal depression most commonly begins at a variable point below the angle of Louis, the posterior displacement can involve the manubrium in the most severe cases. Whether or not the depression begins at the

sternal angle, the lower end of the sternum may approximate the vertebra or project laterally into the vertebral gutter in the extreme deformities.

Mild asymmetry is not uncommon, and it always is associated with greater depression of the right costal cartilages as well as rotation of the sternum to the right. Breast asymmetry is relatively frequent and results in a less well developed right breast in girls. In infants and young children the deep deformities are often accentuated by a potbelly. As growth occurs the older children often present a characteristic posture, with rounded and forward-thrust shoulders. The neck may also project forward, and there is often a dorsal kyphos of the spine.

The deformity results in a variable displacement of the heart to the left, sometimes associated with significant rotation in that direction. Associated systolic murmurs at the cardiac base are not uncommon, but the chest x-ray appearance of the heart has limited diagnostic value because of the displacement. Operative correction of the deformity usually is followed by disappearance of the murmurs, but angiocardiography and cardiac catheterization are occasionally required to decide whether an intracardiac defect is responsible for the murmur.

Pectus excavatum is present at birth, but the milder forms may not be recognized for some months. The cause of the condition is a matter for speculation, and the factors which determine whether the sternal depression deepens in relation to the development of the thoracic cage as the child grows have not been identified. A familial tendency has been noted, but this seems to be expressed by its occurrence in two or more siblings of the same generation more often than in parent and child. This anomaly occurs frequently in patients with Marfan's syndrome, and it is one of several chest-wall deformities that show an increased frequency in children with congenital heart disease.

There is strong difference of opinion about the physiologic effects of pectus excavatum with relatively little evidence of cardiopulmonary dysfunction. Some physicians have contended that no physiologic defect is associated with the deformity and that a corrective operation is indicated only for psychologic or cosmetic reasons. This is strongly disputed by the majority of surgeons who have had extensive experience with this anomaly. The latter contend that exercise tolerance and maximal physical activity are sharply limited in patients with a severe deformity and that operative correction allows the patient to develop toward a normal capacity for cardiopulmonary function. Many individual patients have been reported with specific cardiac problems that were relieved by correction of the depressed sternum. This includes individuals with supraventricular tachycardias and recurrent heart failure.

Fig. 17-24. A two-year-old child with moderate pectus excavatum. *A.* The posterior displacement of the sternum appears to start at the level of the third chondrosternal junction. *B.* The potbelly that accompanies pectus excavatum in the young child is accentuated in the sitting position. *C.* The postoperative photograph shows an excellent cosmetic result. (*Photographs courtesy of Dr. Harold A. Albert.*)

A

C

B

The spectrum of depression deformities is wide, and the remarkable ability of individuals to develop physiologic compensation for mild deviations from normal structure should not be surprising. Most studies of cardiac and respiratory function have shown either normal values or results that were in the lower range of normal. The short-coming in attempts to provide objective corroboration of the clinical improvement experienced by patients who have operative correction has probably been due to inadequate testing methods. More recently, Weg has demonstrated a decrease in maximum voluntary ventilation and forced expiratory flow in a group of Air Force trainees who complained of exercise intolerance associated with pectus excavatum. An especially significant study was done by Beiser in which cardiac output response to exercise was measured in both supine and upright positions, before and after correction of the deformity. The results indicated that a mild to moderate deformity interfered significantly with cardiac function, primarily when exercise was performed in the upright position. The effects on the heart were

Fig. 17-25. Operative correction of pectus excavatum. The distorted medial portions of the costal cartilages have been resected and a steel bar has been placed behind the lower end of the sternum to decrease the possibility of late posterior sagging of the bone. From 9 to 12 months after operation the steel bar is removed through a small incision at the lateral ends. (*From G. W. Holcomb, Jr., Surgical Correction of Pectus Excavatum, J Pediatr Surg, 12:295, 1977, with permission of author and publisher.*)

considered due to diminished space in the lower part of the thorax which interfered with optimal filling of the right side of the heart. In a completely asymptomatic patient, however, there is no reason to assume that such studies will show impairment of cardiac performance.

OPERATIVE TREATMENT. Though operation is rarely indicated in infants with pectus excavatum, Ravitch has noted an occasional infant with stridor who was relieved by early operation. Most surgeons prefer to observe children with this deformity until they are beyond two years of age. Because of the detrimental effect of the deformity on posture, however, operation should be performed between two and five years of age. There is no cause to wait until the child with a significant defect has developed a regressive personality or become a nonparticipator because of fear of exposing his chest. Although several operations have been described for correction of pectus excavatum; the procedure developed by Ravitch has been increasingly accepted. This includes excision of all the deformed costal cartilages, disarticulation of the xiphisternal joint, division of the intercostal muscle bundles from the sternum, and transverse posterior osteotomy of the sternum above the point of depression. The osteotomy is combined with a forward fracture of the sternum and insertion of a wedge of bone in the osteotomy site to provide an overcorrection of the deformity. Internal fixation of the sternum with metal pins or struts is usually not required, but in some instances the likelihood of recurrence can be minimized by use of temporary retrosternal support (Fig. 17-25).

At the end of the operation the loss in rigid support of the anterior part of the chest usually results in mild paradoxical motion of the sternum with respiration. Respiratory difficulty is rare, however, and the chest wall begins to be firm by 10 to 14 days postoperatively. Whether the indication for operation was exercise intolerance or to provide a more normal appearance of the chest, the results are so satisfying to the patient and his family that it is difficult to understand the opposition to treatment that is still seen with significant frequency.

PECTUS CARINATUM

The protrusion deformities of the sternum are much less frequent in occurrence than pectus excavatum. There is significant variation in the features of pectus carinatum from patient to patient, but Ravitch has pointed out that two principal types can be identified. In the chicken-breast type, a deep depression of the costal cartilages along each side of the sternum accentuates a mild protrusion of the sternum and creates an illusion of greater anterior projection. The deformity is usually developed maximally below the nipple level, involving the fourth through the seventh or eighth costal cartilages. There may be an asymmetry of the deformity with mild rotation of the sternum, most often to the right. Symptoms of exertional dyspnea or exercise intolerance may occur, but this is difficult to predict, and a teenage athlete with a severe deformity may have no symptoms.

In the second form of sternal protrusion, called "pouter-pigeon" variety by Ravitch, a double angle is formed in the sternum. The manubrium and upper costal cartilages project forward while the body of the sternum first angulates posteriorly for a variable distance and then sharply reverses to project anteriorly. This has the effect of creating a depression in the lower part of the sternum.

As with pectus excavatum, there is a range of severity in the deformity, and patients may be referred for operative treatment as infants or at any age. Operation may be performed at a time of convenience, but it should be done by five years of age to reduce secondary effects of the deformity on posture, thoracic development, and the child's personality. Operative correction of the chicken-breast deformity is done through a curved submammary incision that allows broad exposure of the deformed costal cartilages and costochondral junctions (Fig. 17-26). Sub-perichondral and subperiosteal resection of all the deformed cartilages and ribs is performed throughout the extent of their deformity. Reefing sutures are used to obliterate the excessive length of each perichondral bed, and a transverse osteotomy is used to adjust the contour of the distal sternum if it still projects forward. Correction of the pouter-pigeon deformity does not require a wide lateral dissection, but a cuneiform osteotomy of the sternum must be done at each of the two angulations in the bone.

The results of operative repair of pectus carinatum are usually excellent, with little likelihood of recurrence when the deformity is properly corrected.

STERNAL DEFECTS

The sternum is formed in embryologic life by the midline fusion of two lateral bars. Formation of the manubrium is contributed to from the developing ventral ends of the clavicles, and the process is generally complete by the tenth week. While the specific cause is yet unexplained, a partial or complete failure of fusion is responsible for the three types of congenital sternal defects that occur. Cardiac pulsations are quite prominent with each type of cleft sternum, giving rise to the visible suggestion that the heart is partially outside the chest wall (ectopia cordis). Fortunately, this is generally not the case, but in true examples of anterior ectopia cordis the sternum is partially cleft and the heart projects well beyond the chest wall. Associated cardiac defects and multiple anomalies in other body regions usually preclude survival.

Superior Sternal Cleft

In this type of sternal defect the cleft commonly extends inferiorly to the level of the fourth costal cartilage. The external appearance is that of a complete absence of the upper part of the sternum even though the unfused lateral halves are present. Because of the prominent pulsations of the heart, which is covered only by thoracic fascia and skin, there is an illusion that partial cardiac displacement into the neck accompanies the bony defect. Therefore, cervicothoracic ectopia cordis is occasionally used in reference to superior sternal cleft.

The anatomic defect may be either U shaped or V shaped, and some patients have been reported in whom the sternal cleft extended down to the xiphoid. If operative repair is done in early infancy it may be possible to suture the two sternal halves together without extensive relaxing incisions in either the costal cartilages or the intact part of the sternum. Repair may be done at any age, but there are obvious disadvantages to leaving the heart unprotected from external trauma. As the child grows, the heart may shift forward and direct repair may become impossible because of intolerance of the heart for the reduced space available for it. At that stage the defect must be closed with use of a prosthetic graft such as Marlex mesh or Teflon felt. Autogenous bone or cartilage grafts can supplement the prosthetic material for additional firmness.

Distal Sternal Cleft

A defect in distal closure of the sternum is usually part of a syndrome of cardiac and parietal anomalies. Commonly, the syndrome is referred to as a pentalogy with the following components: (1) a cleft distal sternum, (2) a ventral abdominal defect that may be a true omphalocele, (3) an inferior pericardial defect with pericardiopleural communication, (4) a deficiency of the anterior diaphragm, and (5) congenital heart disease, commonly in the form of tetralogy of Fallot and sometimes with a left ventricular diverticulum. The sternal cleft may occur without the full syndrome, but the reported cases include several types of midline lesions that have the appearance of keloids or surgical scars.

Operative correction of the cleft sternum and the associated defects may require a staged approach, depending on the priority of the several defects. The presence of an omphalocele would most likely mandate primary attention to that anomaly, with delay of treatment for the cardiac defect. Early repair offers the best opportunity for direct closure of the sternal defect with attachment of the diaphragm.

Complete Sternal Cleft

A cleft of the entire sternum is the rarest of the three forms of failed fusion of the sternal halves. The external appearance of the anterior part of the chest and abdomen is striking, whether or not there is an associated defect in the anterior abdominal wall. When a defect of the musculofascial structures of the abdominal wall is present, there may be communication between the pericardium and the peritoneal cavity, with herniation of bowel into the pericardial cavity. The reported cases have shown variations in the defects involving the diaphragm as well as the pericardium and heart. Operative repair in early infancy is highly desirable, and it may be possible to close the sternum directly if no other defects are present. In other instances a prosthetic graft may be required to bridge over the gap in the anterior part of the chest wall.

ABNORMALITIES OF RIBS AND COSTAL CARTILAGES

Even though the costal cartilages and ribs are involved in the pectus deformities, it is the sternal deformity that forms the basis for the pectus classification. A complete classification of rib and cartilage anomalies is not yet available, although Ravitch has suggested a grouping of costal abnormalities that are associated with soft tissue defects. In the simplest form of abnormality a patient may have a

A

B

C

D

deformed, deficient, or enlarged cartilage or rib that is asymptomatic. With more complex anomalies there may be absence of one or more lower ribs, sometimes associated with hemivertebra, fused bony paravertebral bars, and progressive scoliosis. An absence of ribs or a costal deformity associated with divergence of adjacent ribs may result in regional paradoxical respiratory motion of the chest wall with a lung hernia through the bony defect. Bridging of bone between adjacent ribs posteriorly may be seen as part of the Klippel-Feil type of syndromes as well as of more bizarre abnormalities. In most instances the vertebral anomaly, rather than the costal defect, requires treatment, but the surgeon may need to apply individual innovation in providing the best possible correction.

Absence of the pectoralis major, absence or hypoplasia of the pectoralis minor, hypoplasia of the breast, and partial absence of the upper costal cartilages on one side of the chest constitute an unusual syndrome that may be recognized at birth. Depending on the extent of cartilage deficiency there may be an impressive lung hernia, paradoxical respiratory motion, or simple flattening of the anterolateral part of the chest wall. The breast and nipple are underdeveloped, and the deficiency in subcutaneous tissue accentuates the absence of the costosternal portions of the pectoral muscles.

When the anomaly is left-sided there is significant vulnerability of the underlying lung and heart, since only the skin, fascia, and pleura form a protective covering for these structures. Regardless of which side the defect is on, the concavity becomes relatively more severe as the child grows. Operative repair is indicated for cosmetic reasons, to eliminate paradoxical motion, and to provide protection for the intrathoracic structures. Split rib grafts to bridge the cartilage defect may be combined with Teflon felt to cover the area of muscular deficiency. The repair does not correct the soft tissue defect, but plastic surgery techniques may be utilized later to improve the cosmetic result.

Poland's syndrome is a spectrum of chest-wall defects like that just described along with a complex of hand anomalies including syndactylism, brachydactyly, or ectrodactyly. Those patients least affected have a unilateral absence of the costosternal portion of the pectoral muscles, hypoplasia of the breast, and intact costal cartilages. Severe involvement includes an absence of the second, third, and fourth, or fifth costal cartilages, the deficiency of the pectoral muscles and breast, and the hand anomalies. Surgical treatment is based on the desired correction of the chest-wall defects and the need for reconstruction of the digital anomalies.

Fig. 17-26. A fourteen-year-old boy with pectus carinatum. A. The preoperative lateral chest x-ray shows remarkable anterior projection of the sternum. B. A line drawing demonstrates the forward projection of the sternum that is accentuated by the prominence of the knoblike costal cartilages. C. The postoperative photograph of the patient demonstrates a very satisfactory result. D. The postoperative lateral chest x-ray contrasts sharply with the preoperative film.

Cervical Ribs and Thoracic-outlet Syndrome

Cervical ribs are present in approximately 1 percent of the population, but symptoms attributable to the extra ribs are said to occur in only 10 percent of those who have the anomaly. The ribs are bilateral in 80 percent of cases, and they are characterized by their significant anatomic variation, including variation between the two sides in the same person (Fig. 17-27). In the simplest form, the rib is a short bar of bone that extends a few millimeters beyond the transverse process of C_7 vertebra and is completely enveloped in cervical and scalene muscles. Rarely, a complete rib is formed that articulates by a costal cartilage with the sternum. Between these two extremes are the majority that produce symptoms, and they vary in length, with occasional articulation with the superior surface of the first rib by a synchondrosis. The incompletely developed ribs often have a fascial condensation that extends as a ligament from the anterior tip to the superior surface of the first rib.

The lowest trunk of the brachial plexus (C_8 and T_1 nerve roots), the subclavian artery, and occasionally the subclavian vein course over the superior surface of the cervical rib, or over the ligament from the tip of the rib to the first thoracic rib. In symptomatic individuals it is most often the pressure on the lowest trunk of the plexus, particularly those fibers giving rise to the ulnar nerve, that causes progressive discomfort. Symptoms vary from vague and minor aching in the upper arm or shoulder to severe paresthesias down the medial side of the arm, forearm, and

Fig. 17-27. This patient's x-rays show a greater asymmetry in the cervical ribs than is usually seen. The right cervical rib is well developed (*arrows*), but the left one is represented only by a short bar of bone.

hand. Intermittent weakness in grip may cause the patient to drop things or to develop hand and forearm fatigue quickly when doing manual work. Neurologic symptoms are far more frequent than vascular symptoms, but the majority of patients demonstrate little objective evidence of nerve compression on physical examination. If compression of the brachial plexus has been progressive, the patient will begin to demonstrate atrophy and weakness of the intrinsic muscles of the hand, and eventually weakness of the forearm. Symptoms of arterial compression include numbness of the hand, pallor, fatigue, ischemic diffuse discomfort, coolness, occasionally a sensitivity to cold, and aggravation by postural elevation of the extremity. When venous compression occurs the patient notices intermittent swelling and a bluish discoloration of the extremity.

It has long been recognized that the symptoms of neurovascular compression at the thoracic outlet may occur whether or not a cervical rib is present. The compression is due to the small space between the first thoracic rib and the clavicle (Fig. 17-28). When a cervical rib is present it may be responsible for precipitating the symptoms by further reducing the space. Over the years several terms have been applied to the complex of symptoms that is now generally referred to as the *thoracic-outlet syndrome*. This includes hyperabduction syndrome, costoclavicular compression, and scalenus anticus syndrome. Symptoms are much more frequent in women, and the onset is rarely before the early adult years.

Many individuals with intermittent symptoms of shoulder or arm discomfort may consult a physician for relief. In the absence of other explanations for their symptoms a cervical rib that is discovered by x-ray examination is usually assigned the causative role. Whether or not the extra ribs are present, however, it is often difficult or impossible to distinguish symptoms representing brachial plexus compression from those caused by cervical nerve

root pressure or a herniated cervical disc. For that reason the work-up of the patient should include cervical spine films and a neurosurgical evaluation if there is suspicion of an abnormality affecting the cervical nerve roots or spinal canal.

A lack of conclusive evidence by physical examination that neurovascular compression at the thoracic outlet is responsible for a patient's symptoms has been characteristic. In slender patients a large cervical rib may be palpable and there may be distinct supraclavicular tenderness. A vascular bruit is occasionally heard over the subclavian artery, but this may be affected by the position of the arm. Rarely, a subclavian aneurysm may be suspected from the presence of a pulsating mass, or the patient may have serious ischemia of the arm and hand because of distal embolism or thrombosis of the aneurysm itself. Arterial compression tests, such as the Adson maneuver, have been found to be unreliable for diagnosis, since many asymptomatic persons show a positive response and the majority of symptomatic patients have intermittent neural compression rather than vascular obstruction. Selective subclavian arteriography or venography may be helpful by demonstrating vascular compression or by showing poststenotic dilatation of the subclavian artery (Fig. 17-29). Importantly, symptomatic neural compression can exist without a positive arteriogram, and many surgeons do not recommend arteriography in the absence of vascular symptoms.

Ulnar nerve conduction velocity has been proposed as an objective test to confirm a clinical diagnosis of thoracic-outlet syndrome with primary neural compression. An average normal value of 72 m/second across the thoracic

Fig. 17-28. The chest x-ray shows fusion of multiple cervical and thoracic vertebrae as well as posterior bridging of several upper ribs in this patient with Klippel-Feil syndrome. She had severe neurovascular compression at the right thoracic outlet because of encroachment on the space between the clavicle and the first rib.

A

B

Fig. 17-29. This patient had recurrence of arm pain and numbness and tingling in her right hand several years after a transaxillary resection of the right first rib. *A.* The x-ray shows a right cervical rib that was incompletely removed through the axillary incision. *B.* A right subclavian arteriogram shows kinking of the artery as it courses over the cervical rib and poststenotic dilatation. Removal of the cervical rib and neurolysis of the brachial plexus through a parascapular approach relieved her symptoms.

outlet has been reported by Urschel, with an average of 53 m/second in the patients with outlet compression. Other groups have not found the nerve conduction velocity to be an accurate discriminator because some patients with a normal conduction velocity have received an excellent result from surgical treatment. A difference in techniques of electromyography may be partly responsible for the differing results.

The treatment of thoracic-outlet syndrome depends on the severity of symptoms, the apparent cause, and the presence of complications such as subclavian artery aneurysm. Even in the presence of a small cervical rib, patients who have nothing more than mild symptoms of numbness and tingling or fatigue in the arm may require no treatment. Instruction in posture improvement may be adequate, but professional physiotherapy may give better relief. Urschel suggests that nerve conduction velocity may be used as a guide for treatment with operation not advised unless the velocity is below 60 m/second. For persistent or

progressive symptoms a resection of the first rib along with any cervical rib or abnormal congenital bands gives the best result in the experience of many surgeons. An axillary incision can be used to resect the first rib in most patients, but considerable skill is required to do an adequate resection of a cervical rib through this approach. An alternate surgical approach is provided by a posterior parascapular incision which allows a better exposure of the brachial plexus and is especially helpful for reoperation. The presence of a significant aneurysm requires an anterior incision, often with partial resection of the clavicle.

Approximately 90 percent of patients have excellent relief of symptoms following operation, although they may have occasional discomfort at the time of increased work activity.

Tumors

Primary neoplasms of the chest wall are uncommon; even large medical centers require long periods of time to acquire useful experience with their treatment. Metastatic tumors, especially to the ribs, and direct invasion of the chest wall from primary lung and breast carcinomas easily outnumber the tumors arising from the chest wall. Soft tissue tumors that occur in other body areas such as cavernous hemangiomas, hemangiopericytoma, rhabdomyosarcoma, and so on have a special significance when they develop in the chest wall, because treatment may require extensive resection of the thoracic cage. A classification of chest-wall tumors would be convenient for study, but the number of cases is sufficiently small that anything other than a division into benign and malignant and by tissue of origin is not practical. Table 17-3 shows the types of primary tumors and their relative frequency in Adkins' experience during the years 1954–1970. It is apparent that the majority of patients in his practice were in younger age groups. This should not mislead, however, since there is a wide age spread in other reports, and in this author's experience the majority of patients have been older than 30 years.

The clinical manifestation of a chest-wall neoplasm is most often either pain, a palpable mass, or an abnormality detected on a chest x-ray. Surprisingly, with either benign or malignant lesions the discomfort is relatively mild, and patients often present with tumors that have been enlarging for months or years. Many patients will attribute the tumor origin to some episode of localized trauma, or they will state that they discovered the mass while rubbing their chest after a minor injury. A differential diagnosis will include the less frequent pulmonary infections that invade the chest wall, such as actinomycosis and nocardiosis, tuberculous chondritis, costochondral separation, and Tietze's syndrome (nonspecific chondritis). A suspicion of fluctuation in the mass and a corresponding pulmonary lesion may suggest that a diagnostic aspiration should be done in instances of probable infection. A true history of trauma and the ability to reproduce a clicking sensation with local pressure may reinforce the diagnosis of a suspected costochondral separation.

The most important aspect of diagnosis is the correlation of physical findings with adequate radiographic examination. The latter often requires the help of the radiologist by having him examine the lesion and determine what special views or techniques will allow maximum information about the extent of the lesion, its possible relationship to

Table 17-3. PRIMARY CHEST-WALL TUMORS

Benign (average age of patients, 21 years)
Fibrous dysplasia 8
Chondroma 4
Osteochondroma. 4
Eosinophilic granuloma. 2
Hemangioma 3
    Total   21
Malignant (average age of patients, 25 years)
Chondrosarcoma 9
Osteogenic sarcoma 3
Myeloma 3
Ewing's tumor 2
Fibrosarcoma 3
Reticulum cell sarcoma. 2
Liposarcoma 1
Undifferentiated 2
    Total   25

SOURCE: Reproduced with permission from T. W. Shields, "General Thoracic Surgery," p. 445, Lea & Febiger, Philadelphia, 1972.

intrathoracic structures, and the presence of characteristics that may suggest malignancy. Radioisotope studies may be indicated to look for other areas of neoplastic involvement, and pulmonary function tests should be performed as a screening examination to determine the likelihood that chest-wall resection would be tolerated. Because the majority of tumors involving the costal cartilages and the sternum are malignant, the anterior location of a neoplasm will often suggest the need to plan for resection and extensive reconstruction.

BENIGN TUMORS

Fibrous Dysplasia

The ribs are the most common site of solitary fibrous dysplasia (osteofibroma, bone cyst), and this lesion constitutes 20 to 35 percent of the benign tumors of the thoracic cage. Located most frequently in the posterior or lateral portion of a rib, it usually presents as a slowly enlarging nonpainful mass. Diagnostic radiographs show expansion and thinning of the bony cortex, with a central trabeculated appearance. Histologic examination often shows fine calcification in a matrix of fibrous tissue, osteoid tissue, and occasional cysts. There may be involvement of more than one rib, suggesting metastatic malignancy. Fibrous dysplasia in ribs as well as other bones forms part of Albright's syndrome, a condition that includes skin pigmentation and precocious puberty in girls.

The lesion should be excised to establish the diagnosis and to prevent progressive enlargement that would eventually encroach on other structures.

Chondroma

According to Adkins, chondromas constitute 15 to 20 percent of benign tumors in the ribs. They occur at the costochondral junction, primarily in children or young people, and may be difficult to differentiate from chondritis or the sequela of a traumatic costochondral separation. Chest and rib x-rays show an expansion of bone with thinned but intact cortex. It is not possible to distinguish between a chondroma and chondrosarcoma by clinical examination, but the onset of pain and rapid growth in a preexisting lesion suggest a malignant change.

Chondromas slowly expand into the surrounding tissues without fixation, but adequate removal requires resection of a block of the chest wall to achieve an adequate margin. If the patient is operated upon when the lesion is small, no special techniques are required to close the defect that results from resection.

Osteochondroma

Osteochondromas generally arise from the cortex of a rib and slowly expand over a long period of time. They occur more frequently in men, but they are also seen in children. Pain is infrequent, but once the lesion has become palpable the patient is likely to complain of intermittent discomfort. As with other neoplasms, the occurrence of pain may signal accelerated growth, which produces concern over the possibility of malignant change.

Fig. 17-30. This operating-room photograph of a resected segment of rib and attached tumor shows the typical appearance of an osteochondroma.

The roentgenographic appearance is often that of a distorted rib cortex with an overlying mass that has a thin rim of calcification (Fig. 17-30).

The lesion should be removed by a block resection with a margin of normal tissue.

Eosinophilic Granuloma

The lesions of eosinophilic granuloma are sometimes part of a disease that includes pulmonary lesions called *histiocytosis X* or *eosinophilic granuloma of the lung*. When it occurs in a rib, the granuloma is a solitary destructive process, often associated with pain and localized tenderness. Roentgenograms reveal a punched-out osteolytic lesion, which, when subjected to excision and microscopic examination, is found to consist of a chronic granuloma. Healing may occur spontaneously, or a pathologic fracture may develop through the area of osteolysis. Resection is primarily advised for the purpose of diagnosis. If only a biopsy is done the granuloma may be observed and attention diverted to a survey for additional lesions in the lung, the reticuloendothelial system, and the other bones.

Other less frequent benign tumors may occur in the chest wall, including soft tissue neoplasms that arise in the muscular, fibrous, vascular, or other tissues that are normally there (Fig. 17-31). Because of the frequency of malignancy in soft tissue neoplasms, these tumors must be approached bearing in mind the possibility that extensive resection may be required.

MALIGNANT TUMORS

Chondrosarcoma

Chondroma and chondrosarcoma are the most frequently occurring primary tumors of the chest wall, with the question of whether chondromas undergo malignant transformation still unanswered. Some investigators believe that all chondrosarcomas arise as malignant lesions. Either way, chondrosarcomas comprise between 45 and 60 percent of all malignant tumors of the bony thorax. The tumors occur most commonly in the anterior part of the thorax, and the incidence is greatest between the ages of twenty and forty years. Growth is often relatively slow, and the neoplasm may extend either internally or outwardly into the soft tissue of the chest wall. The overwhelming majority of sternal tumors are malignant, with chondrosarcoma and osteogenic sarcoma comprising the greatest percentage.

The chest x-ray generally shows a lobulated mass that appears to destroy cortical bone, with or without fine calcification. Because of a varied histologic picture that often fails to provide proof of malignancy, a simple biopsy of a chondrosarcoma may not be used to guide treatment. Though the decision to do so may be difficult, the performance of a wide excision of the tumor with a block of surrounding tissue is the proper treatment for chondrosarcoma.

Osteogenic Sarcoma

Osteogenic sarcoma is more malignant than chondrosarcoma but less frequent in occurrence. A pleural effusion tends to develop early, and the tumor may have rapid growth, particularly in young people (Fig. 17-32). Pain is mild at first but may become severe when the tumor has reached a stage where resection is unlikely. The predominant component may be cartilaginous, bony, or fibrous and the lesion may result in both bone destruction and bone production.

There is often an early development of pulmonary metastases in osteogenic sarcoma, and in occasional instances it may be proper to resect the metastases at the same time

A

B

Fig. 17-31. An aneurysmal bone cyst. *A.* The posteroanterior chest x-ray shows a mass extending into the thoracic cavity and elevating the pleura on the posterolateral chest wall. *B.* A film for rib detail demonstrates the origin of the tumor from the left fifth rib. (*X-rays furnished by Dr. Arthur Lieber.*)

Fig. 17-32. An osteogenic sarcoma arising from the right tenth rib in this middle-aged man resulted in early pleural invasion with massive pleural effusion. Chemotherapy failed to affect rapid tumor growth, and he died with widespread metastases.

that the primary tumor is treated. For patients with a well-localized neoplasm the only form of adequate treatment is wide excision of the adjacent bony structures and soft tissue. When the sternum is involved, a complete resection must be done although 5-year survivals are unusual.

Ewing's Sarcoma

Occurrence during the first two decades of life, with a much reduced incidence beyond twenty years of age, characterizes Ewing's tumor. The tumor occurs more frequently in boys than in girls and is generally manifested by a painful mass that enlarges rapidly. Fever and malaise are common systemic symptoms.

Roentgenograms often show a characteristic onion-skin appearance that is due to elevation of the periosteum as the tumor enlarges. Spread to other bones occurs early in a high percentage of patients, but the tumor is generally radiosensitive. If the diagnosis is made by biopsy, the choice of treatment may be irradiation alone or radical excision combined with the irradiation. Unfortunately, the prognosis is poor regardless of the treatment chosen.

Myeloma

Plasma cell myeloma is more frequently a generalized disease than a solitary tumor affecting a single rib. When a solitary plasmacytoma does occur in the thoracic cage, the serum proteins are generally normal and Bence-Jones proteins are not found in the urine. Chest x-rays show the solitary lesion as a punched-out defect in the rib, with expansion and thinning of the cortex.

The clinical course of patients with a solitary myeloma is markedly different from that of patients who first appear with multiple lesions. The latter are almost always dead within 2 years after the diagnosis is made, but those who have a solitary lesion initially may live for many years without evidence of other disease. A careful survey for other sites of disease should be made in patients who present with a solitary lesion, and if none is found the involved rib should be resected.

SURGICAL TREATMENT OF MALIGNANT CHEST-WALL TUMORS. Particularly with the cartilaginous tumors, an excisional biopsy may not be adequate to determine whether a lesion is malignant (Fig. 17-33). The surgeon must often make a judgment on the basis of the history, the roentgenograms, and the gross appearance of the neoplasm. Because most chest-wall tumors are not radiosensitive the best chance for cure is related to the adequacy of the initial resection. When malignancy is suspected, preliminary plans must be made for chest-wall reconstruction that will allow resection of a generous margin of normal

Fig. 17-33. A giant-cell tumor of the right clavicle. A. The preoperative photograph of the upper part of the chest and neck shows a tumor at the right sternoclavicular junction in this elderly man. A biopsy suggested the diagnosis but did not indicate the degree of malignancy. B. A chest x-ray indicates the origin of the tumor from the medial end of the clavicle, and the arrows suggest the extent of the mass. C. An operating-room photograph shows the completely resected clavicle with an en-bloc resection of the upper sternum and the anterior end of the first rib. The rounded tumor mass which projects toward the knife handle is covered with intact pleura.

A

B

C

A

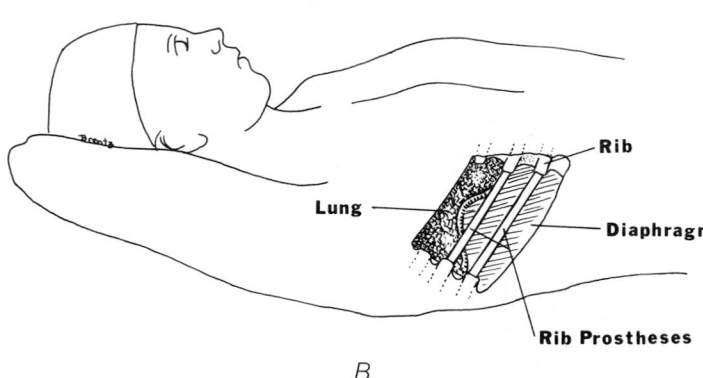

B

Fig. 17-34. A reoperation for chondrosarcoma. *A*. Two years earlier the patient had a localized resection of one rib for an apparent chondroma. The recurrence of a mass suggested the likelihood that chondrosarcoma was the correct diagnosis, and this operative photograph shows the extensive chest-wall resection that was done in continuity with a large wedge of the right lower pulmonary lobe. Two metal rib struts were used to provide stability to the anterolateral chest wall. *B*. The line drawing is intended to clarify the structures in the photograph.

tissue around the neoplasm. The resection should include at least one adjacent normal rib above and below the tumor, with all intervening intercostal muscles and pleura. When the lung periphery is involved in the neoplasm, it is proper to resect the adjacent part of the pulmonary lobe in continuity (Fig. 17-34). Presently available techniques for respiratory support are sufficiently good that a resection should not be compromised by a concern that the patient will not be able to ventilate satisfactorily during the immediate postoperative period.

Because the anatomy of the thorax appears to offer few, if any, natural limits to the spread of a neoplasm, and because of the sharply limited long-term survival with surgical treatment, there is a reasonable debate over the value of chest-wall resection. There is little to recommend radical treatment once a neoplasm has reached an advanced stage of musculoskeletal destruction with invasion of the pleural cavity. With selection of patients who have either slowly growing tumors or limited chest-wall involvement, extensive resection can provide excellent relief of pain and prolonged survival. In a series of 68 patients

who had chest-wall resections for malignant disease at the Memorial Sloan-Kettering Cancer Center, the cumulative 5-year survival rate was 34 percent. Table 17-4 shows that primary lung carcinoma with chest-wall invasion was slightly more frequent than thoracic sarcomas in that series. Of the 68 patients, 43 had a concomitant pulmonary resection, including 20 wedge resections and 20 lobectomies.

Reconstruction of a large defect in the chest wall requires the use of some type of material to avoid lung herniation or paradoxical respiratory motion. Marlex or prolene mesh, fascia lata, and metal struts are among the most frequently used materials for this purpose. When a loss of skin and subcutaneous tissue accompanies the musculoskeletal defect, reconstruction becomes more complicated because of the need to use skin flaps or a transposition flap of the omentum, covered by a skin graft.

Table 17-4. ORIGIN OF MALIGNANT TUMORS RESECTED FROM CHEST WALL

Type of tumor	No. of patients	
Primary chest-wall sarcoma..........	25	
Sarcoma metastatic to chest wall ...	7	
Carcinoma of lung...................	30	
Epidermoid carcinoma		17
Adenocarcinoma		7
Bronchiolar carcinoma		3
Miscellaneous.....................		3
Metastatic carcinoma................	6	
Kidney...........................		4
Miscellaneous.....................		2

PLEURA

Because primary diseases of the pleura are infrequent, it is easy to think of this tissue as a "membrane highway" for transport of infectious agents or neoplastic cells throughout the hemithorax, or as a reservoir for containing air, blood, or transudative fluids. A completely passive role for the pleura like that implied by the previous statement is obviously not correct. But from the surgeon's viewpoint it is a close description of pleural function as it affects surgical procedures. With few exceptions, most notably, the pleural tumors, the pathologic processes involving the pleura take origin from other sources. Symptoms and signs of pleural disturbance, therefore, may be first evidence of a disease process that has been developing in a relatively silent area such as the mediastinum or lung periphery.

The anatomy of the pleural space is altered by the disease processes that affect the space and the structures that form its boundaries. An injury to the phrenic nerve, for example, with paralysis of the diaphragm results in a reduced volume of the hemithorax. This could be significant if a thoracentesis were planned with an attempt to place the needle in the lowest part of the pleural cavity. Inflammation, trauma with hemothorax, or thoracic operative procedures often produce partial obliteration of the pleural space. A subsequent collection of pleural fluid, for whatever cause, may take an unusual appearance, including an isolated location in a fissure between pulmonary lobes, or confinement between the diaphragmatic surface of a lower lobe and the diaphragm. A more significant result of fibrosis in the pleural cavity is the occasional development of *fibrothorax,* in which the lung becomes encased in a layer of fibrous tissue. This generally results from incompletely treated hemothorax or empyema, and the lung is said to be "trapped." In addition to its restrictive effect on ventilation, fibrothorax may result in a mild scoliosis of the thoracic region of the spine. An age difference in the capability of the pleura to remove massive exudates without excessive fibrosis is suggested by the fact that decortication is required much less frequently in small children than in adults.

Pleural Effusion

The presence of fluid within the pleural space can have a variety of causes, a partial list of which is shown in Table 17-5. Additional rare causes have been reported, and in a few patients no cause is ever identified. The so-called "idiopathic effusions" are thought to have a viral causation in many instances, but careful skin testing for tuberculosis is always indicated, along with follow-up examination for at least a year.

Traditionally, effusions are classified as either transudates or exudates. Transudates have a specific gravity of less than 1.015 and a protein content of less than 3 Gm/100 ml. Most often a transudate is clear with a faint yellow tinge and no odor. Among the more common causes of transudates are the conditions associated with salt and water retention (e.g., congestive heart failure, nephrotic syndrome), ascites, and atelectasis. Pleural exudates vary greatly depending on the cause, but pleural inflammation is usually present. Infectious diseases, pulmonary infarction, and tumors are the common causes of pleural exudates. A hemorrhagic effusion is not easily classified as a transudate or exudate but may have properties of either. Neoplastic invasion of the pleura is the most frequent cause of bloody effusions, but pulmonary infarction, tuberculosis, and unrevealed trauma are additional causes that must be considered for individual patients.

A compromise of lung volume by fluid within the pleu-

Table 17-5. CAUSES OF PLEURAL EFFUSION

Relative frequency	Cause
Frequent	Congestive heart failure
	Infection: bacterial pneumonia, tuberculosis
	Neoplasm: bronchogenic carcinoma, pleural metastases, lymphoma
Common	Trauma
	Pulmonary infarction
	Cirrhosis
Occasional	Viral pulmonary and pericardial infections
	Atelectasis
	Pneumothorax
Rare	Meigs's syndrome
	Intraabdominal infection: pancreatitis, subphrenic abscess: mycotic infection; systemic bacterial infection; rheumatoid arthritis
	Fluid retention: nephrotic syndrome

ral space is usually manifested by dyspnea and tachycardia. If the effusion is massive, the mediastinum can be shifted to the contralateral side, causing compression of the opposite lung (Fig. 17-35). Severe cardiorespiratory embarrassment with cyanosis may result, and if unrelieved, may precipitate a fatal cardiac arrhythmia.

A diagnostic thoracentesis is indicated in most patients with a pleural effusion unless the cause is either without question or of no relevance in the patient's management. The technique of thoracentesis and the method for insertion of an intercostal tube are shown in Fig. 17-36. In many circumstances, even if the patient is suffering mild respiratory embarrassment from a large pleural effusion, the first step is a simple needle or needle-catheter aspiration of the fluid. This may relieve the patient's symptoms temporarily and allow a diagnosis to be made from examination of the fluid. The decision to insert an intercostal tube for continuous drainage depends on the rapidity of its reaccumulation and the cause. Because the placement of an intercostal tube results in continuous discomfort for the patient and a restriction of activities, it is not indicated unless the fluid is associated with empyema or requires aspiration as often as every other day.

Thorough examination of the aspirated fluid includes determination of specific gravity and total protein content, and chemical measurement of sugar, fat, lactic acid dehydrogenase, and, occasionally, amylase content. In addition, cultures for bacteria, fungi, and mycobacteria may be indicated, along with cytologic examination for malignant cells. If a diagnosis is not obtained from fluid examination, a pleural biopsy by needle technique is often indicated. Satisfactory tissue for examination can be obtained in 60 to 80 percent of patients for whom a closed biopsy appears

A

B

Fig. 17-35. A massive pleural effusion due to metastases from carcinoma of the left breast (previously excised by mastectomy). *A.* The arrow shows the tracheal displacement to the opposite side. *B.* After drainage of the malignant effusion by insertion of an intercostal tube, the trachea and mediastinum have shifted back toward a normal position. Paralysis of the left side of the diaphragm, presumably due to phrenic nerve involvement by the pleural metastases, was confirmed by fluoroscopy.

warranted. Open pleural biopsy is rarely done unless a concomitant lung biopsy has been suggested. However, there are patients who should have a definitive diagnosis made, and the technique of thoracoscopy described in the following section deserves wider application for this purpose.

THORACOSCOPY. In the past, visual inspection of the pleural surfaces by thoracoscopy was done primarily in association with induced pneumothorax therapy for patients with pulmonary tuberculosis. The technique has enjoyed somewhat of a revival in the United States and has been in constant use in Europe for many years. It has been reported highly successful in patients with pleural disease in whom a diagnosis could not be made by bronchoscopy, thoracentesis with closed pleural needle biopsy, or mediastinoscopy.

The one prerequisite for successful thoracoscopy is a reasonably free, nonadherent pleural space to permit adequate visualization of the pleura as well as manipulation of the thoracoscope and the biopsy forceps. Instruments such as the mediastinoscope and the flexible bronchoscope have been used for the examination in addition to the rigid thoracoscope.

If recurrent pleural effusion has been a problem and malignant pleuritis has been diagnosed, cytotoxic or pleurodytic agents can be introduced at the time of thoracoscopy. This has also been helpful in patients who are too ill for open thoracotomy, in children, and in cases of suspected traumatic rupture of the diaphragm.

Empyema

Empyema thoracis is the term generally applied to pyogenic infections of the pleural cavity, associated with purulent effusions. Bacterial pneumonia is the most frequent

cause of empyema, but trauma, pulmonary infarction, septic pulmonary emboli, and spread of infection from intraabdominal sepsis are additional major causes. Empyema may develop as a complication of thoracic surgical procedures, with or without infection of the incision.

When the pleura is invaded by infection there is an outpouring of pleural exudates that may have a localized or generalized distribution. If infection continues, the effects of gravity lead to a volume concentration of the effusion in the posterior and inferior areas of the pleural cavity. As the leukocyte and fibrin content increase, the pleurae may become fused around the margins of the fluid accumulation. This localization may be thought of as an abscess, but it is generally referred to as a loculated empyema (Fig. 17-37).

The management of a pyogenic empyema depends on the stage at which the diagnosis is made. If the condition is diagnosed early, when the fluid is still thin, intensive treatment by needle aspiration and appropriate antibiotics may suffice. In a well-established empyema, a continuous form of drainage by one or more large intercostal catheters is necessary to keep the pleura free of an accumulation that would promote pulmonary collapse. With empyema not accompanied by an air leak from the lung (bronchopleural fistula), the volume of drainage seems to be unaffected by the addition of negative pressure to the underwater seal. In the presence of a bronchopleural fistula, every effort

A

B

C

Fig. 17-36. The techniques for aspirating and draining a pleural effusion. *A*. From a consideration of the position of the pleural effusion on chest x-rays and by examination the proper interspace is selected for needle aspiration. The procedure should be explained to the patient and a comfortable position should be obtained, such as that shown in the drawing. After thorough preparation of the skin with surgical soap, the intended tract of the aspirating needle is anesthetized with 2 percent lidocaine. If a tube is to be inserted, the primary purpose of the aspiration is to confirm the locations and character of the effusion. *B*. For insertion of an intercostal catheter a short skin incision is made and the wound deepened by knife or scissors down to the rib level. After puncture of the intercostal muscles and pleura with a hemostat, the gloved finger is used to enlarge the intercostal opening and assess the character of the pleural lining. If loculations can be easily separated, this should be done. A large intercostal catheter (32 to 36F) should be inserted in the direction and distance suggested by the chest x-ray. *C*. Whether a simple underwater seal is adequate for drainage depends on the presence or absence of a bronchopleural fistula. If the patient has a continuous or an intermittent air leak, negative pressure should be utilized in the range of −10 to 50 cm of water.

should be made to keep the pulmonary lobes expanded. This requires the use of 10 to 50 cm of water negative pressure; if it is successful the need for open thoracotomy with decortication of the pleura may be avoided.

Unfortunately, patients are often referred to the surgeon for empyema management after the acute phase has been treated by antibiotics but without adequate drainage. Tube drainage may show that the lung is partially collapsed with no significant reexpansion after 48 to 96 hours of high-suction drainage. Although an excessive delay in the decision to perform decortication is frequent in these cases, Bryant showed that the need for operation could generally be determined within a few days after the drainage was initiated. Previous antibiotic treatment results in negative cultures of the aspirated fluid in more than half the patients who are seen at this stage, but the management is primarily a mechanical problem of draining the empyema

cavity or excising the inflammatory membrane that has trapped the lung and lines the chest wall.

Several complications of empyema thoracis may occur. Chronicity or persistence of a localized pleural infection with continuous or intermittent purulent drainage is not uncommon. This may be caused by premature removal of a drainage tube or failure to establish drainage at the dependent position of the empyema cavity. Inadequate drainage, particularly of a localized empyema, may be handled by converting to open drainage by rib resection (Fig. 17-38). When chronicity is the result of lung disease, especially in the presence of a bronchopleural fistula, decortication must be combined with pulmonary resection to effect a cure. When this is not possible, either because of the extent of lung disease or the failure of other methods, the pleural space may be obliterated by collapsing the chest wall down to meet the lung through performance of a thoracoplasty. Under special circumstances, such as chronic empyema following a pneumonectomy, techniques for long-term drainage by creating a defect in the chest wall (Eloesser flap) may be indicated.

Another complication of chronic empyema is *empyema necessitans*. In this condition a neglected or unrecognized pleural abscess may provide its own drainage by breaking through either the visceral or parietal wall. Perforation into the lung and communication with a bronchus is indicated by the sudden expectoration of large amounts of purulent material. Prompt evacuation of the pleura and intensive bronchopulmonary toilet are urgent. Proper treatment of

A

B

C

Fig. 17-37. A loculated pyogenic empyema. *A*. The posteroanterior chest x-ray shows a large opacity in the right hemithorax of a patient who was not recovering satisfactorily despite antibiotic treatment for an apparent pneumonia. *B*. The lateral x-ray shows that the opacity extends far posteriorly. The smooth, rounded borders suggested that the mass was fluid, and an empyema was confirmed by thoracentesis. *C*. Following aspiration the chest x-ray suggests significant pleural reaction and persistence of fibrinopurulent exudate in the costophrenic sulcus. A tube thoracostomy would probably need to be done to provide continuing drainage.

the empyema will often permit closure of the bronchial fistula. Penetration of the chest wall is less dramatic and usually presents as an enlarging local abscess. Appropriate treatment includes drainage of the abscess, including the underlying chronic pleural infection.

Tuberculosis

It is generally considered that pleural tuberculosis is the result of extension of tuberculosis to the pleura from a subjacent pulmonary lesion. The most common form is fibrinous pleurisy that causes localized pleural adhesions. Serofibrinous pleurisy develops in approximately 5 percent of all cases of pulmonary tuberculosis. In some patients the parenchymal lesion may be obscured by the overlying pleural involvement. Malaise and fever may be the presenting symptoms, and if the effusion is large the patient may have dyspnea.

It is important to recognize tuberculous empyema because the treatment differs from that for pyogenic empyema. Therefore, there is an increasing tendency to obtain a pleural biopsy to provide greater accuracy in diagnosis. Open drainage is necessary only when there is a bronchopleural fistula. Prior to the advent of effective chemotherapy for tuberculosis, a high mortality rate was associated with open drainage of tuberculous empyema. In selected instances pleural decortication is indicated, along with intensive chemotherapy, as an attempt to produce pulmonary reexpansion.

Pleural Calcification

Pleural calcification is occasionally seen in patients with chronic pleuritis. In most instances, there is considerable thickening of the parietal pleura, with plaques of calcium deeply embedded. Calcification of the pleura per se is usually not the cause of symptoms, and it rarely requires treatment even though the appearance of the chest x-ray may be impressive. The chief clinical importance lies in the association with a chronic empyema, of either tuberculous or nontuberculous origin. Almost certainly, the presence of the calcification makes the empyema more intractable.

Chylothorax

An accumulation of chyle in the pleural space may occur after trauma, or it may be spontaneous. Spontaneous chylothorax is frequently caused by a primary malignancy such as lymphosarcoma or a metastatic carcinoma which invades or compresses the thoracic duct. Rarely, a benign cystic lesion of the duct or its tributaries may be an etiologic factor. There is a low incidence of chylothorax after operative procedures such as thoracic sympathectomy, esophagectomy, aneurysmectomy, and cardiac procedures. Rupture of a normal duct has been seen as a result of blunt trauma, especially when accompanied by hyperextension of the spine.

The first indication of an injury to the thoracic duct may be a rapidly accumulating pleural effusion associated with tightness in the chest, dyspnea, and tachycardia. A specific diagnosis is made only when thoracentesis yields an opalescent or milky fluid which shows fat globules by microscopic examination. Chyle has a specific gravity which ranges between 1.010 and 1.020. The total lipid content varies from 1 to 4 percent, and the total protein content averages 3.5 to 4.5 Gm/100 ml. Normal chyle is sterile. The erythrocyte count may vary, and the lymphocyte count may be 6,000 per cubic millimeter or higher. After trauma, there is frequently an admixture of blood that can obscure the true nature of the effusion. Patients with large leaks can drain as much as 2,500 ml in 24 hours, and a prolonged loss of chyle can lead to dehydration, depletion of electrolytes and serum proteins, lymphocytopenia, low levels of blood lipids, and deficiencies of fat-soluble vitamins.

If an injury to the thoracic duct is recognized during an operative procedure, the structure should be mobilized only enough to permit double ligation. Reconstruction or repair of the injured duct is unnecessary. When a chylothorax is diagnosed several days after the causative event, the initial treatment should consist of repeated thoracentesis or tube drainage. Healing frequently occurs, especially if the patient is given a low-fat or elemental diet. Total parenteral alimentation is also helpful. If the chyle drainage does not respond in 7 to 10 days, operative exploration will frequently be necessary, especially if the injury involves the major thoracic duct on the right side.

Tumors

PRIMARY TUMORS

Primary pleural tumors are uncommon, and because of their origin in the thorax they are usually mistaken for pulmonary neoplasms on the initial chest x-ray. Since

Fig. 17-38. Open drainage of a localized chronic empyema by rib resection. This technique is good for relatively small empyema cavities where a 5- to 10-cm length of rib can be resected over the dependent area of the cavity. An incision is made through the bed of the rib to unroof the cavity partially. A plastic tube is maintained in the cavity to prevent closure of the skin opening as the cavity gradually heals.

tumors of mesothelial origin may closely resemble adenocarcinomas, there may be difficulty in establishing the correct diagnosis even with biopsy material. The most widely used classification of primary pleural tumors is an anatomic one which divides them into localized and diffuse types. Almost all diffuse mesotheliomas are malignant, but so are a significant number of the localized tumors.

Evidence of a relationship between asbestos exposure and malignant pleural tumors now seems as convincing as the relationship between the mineral and carcinoma of the lung. The great majority of patients with asbestos exposure who develop a mesothelioma (asbestos miners, insulation workers) are also cigarette smokers, and their asbestos exposure has taken place over a long period of time.

Localized mesotheliomas most frequently arise from the visceral pleura, and the chest x-ray may simply show a solitary pulmonary nodule (Fig. 17-39). This lesion is often referred to as "benign fibrous mesothelioma" because of its excellent prognosis if resected with a margin of normal tissue. On occasion the tumor may arise from the parietal, mediastinal, or diaphragmatic pleura, and it may grow to become a very large solitary mass. These tumors are generally asymptomatic unless they reach a size that is sufficient to produce pulmonary compression and dyspnea. Chest pain, fever, and painful osteoarthropathy have been reported with the larger localized mesotheliomas, and the symptoms disappear after the tumor is removed. A pleural effusion may accompany the larger fibrous lesions, and the presence of significant red blood cells in the fluid does not

Fig. 17-39. A localized benign mesothelioma. This operative photograph shows a fibrous mesothelioma arising from the visceral pleura just at the juncture of the patient's lower and upper lobes of the right lung. The tumor was removed with a margin of normal tissue by wedge resection.

necessarily indicate a malignant state or inoperability. Hypoglycemia with convulsions has been reported; it is presumably due to the production of an insulin-like substance by the tumor.

A less frequent form of the localized mesothelioma is one that involves the subjacent lung without seeding the pleural cavity or producing metastases (Fig. 17-40). It must be considered a malignant tumor, but its slow growth and the fact that it is curable by pneumonectomy put it in sharp distinction to the diffuse form of mesothelioma.

A *diffuse mesothelioma* may arise from any region of the pleura and may spread along the pleural surface to encase the ipsilateral lung completely. Direct extension over the pericardial surface to the pleural cavity on the opposite side occasionally occurs. The histologic appearance is often that of erratic spindle cells resembling sarcoma in combination with elements that appear to have epithelial origin. There is often some uncertainty about the true origin of a diffuse malignant lesion that is considered to be a mesothelioma. This is because it may be impossible to say that such a lesion, examined either at operation or autopsy, actually arose from the pleura rather than from the lung or chest wall. In true mesotheliomas, metastases to regional lymph nodes or distant sites are said to be unusual.

A serous or serosanguineous pleural effusion accompanies a diffuse mesothelioma, and the tumor is associated with significant chest pain. Cytologic study of the aspirated fluid is often negative for cells that a pathologist can associate with malignant mesothelioma. Chest x-rays generally show an effusion with pleural thickening and a contracted or fibrotic lung. A closed-needle biopsy may yield satisfac-

tory tissue for diagnosis, and the identification of hyaluronic acid in the pleural fluid may be used as presumptive evidence for mesothelioma.

The treatment for a diffuse mesothelioma must be considered palliative. Even extensive resection involving the chest wall with pneumonectomy has generally failed to produce long-term survival. Radiation therapy, with systemic chemotherapy, may reduce the patient's chest pain. The prognosis is bad; the majority of patients live less than 1 year after the diagnosis is made.

METASTATIC TUMORS

The pleura may be the site of metastases from neoplasms in other body regions. There is often concomitant involvement of the lungs, but it is the pleural effusion that produces symptoms by lung compression. In addition to metastatic involvement of the pleural surface, obstruction of the lymphatic channels by neoplastic cells may result in massive accumulation of pleural fluid. An occasional patient first presents because of pleural and respiratory symptoms before the primary tumor is known. Pleural needle biopsy may need to be combined with examination of the aspirated fluid to develop an accurate diagnosis.

The treatment of a malignant pleural effusion depends on the symptoms produced and the sensitivity of the primary tumor to radiation therapy or chemotherapy. If respiratory symptoms are significant, it is satisfactory to insert an intercostal tube and drain the effusion. If the pleural cavity is kept drained for several days the lung is given a chance to reexpand and radiation or chemotherapy may be started (Fig.. 17-41). A direct instillation of nitrogen mustard (0.2 to 0.4 mg/kg in 100 ml sterile water) through the intercostal catheter is very effective in reducing the reaccumulation of pleural fluid.

LUNG

Anatomy

The respiratory system arises as an outpouching from the primitive gut during the third week of embryonic life and undergoes a bifurcation of the distal end of the pouch into right and left primitive bronchial buds. Growth and secondary outpouching of each primary bud provides an early indication of the lobar development of each lung by the fourth week. Progressive branching then accompanies histologic differentiation from the cuboidal epithelium that lines the terminal buds during the first four fetal months to the flattened epithelium present at birth. Whether the lungs grow by additional branching of respiratory units after birth has been debated. On the basis of studies earlier in this century it was stated that the newborn infant's lung had 18 generations of branching. Comparison of this number with a reported 25 branchings in the adult middle lobe suggested that maturation continued by additional branching at least through early childhood. More recently, Boyden and Tomsett identified 23 to 27 branching generations in infants, adolescents, and adults, to support the concept that the lungs are completely developed at birth.

A

C

B

Fig. 17-40. A localized malignant mesothelioma. *A*. A chest x-ray in 1975 showed a small left hilar mass (*arrow*) in a twenty-six-year-old white male with pleuritic-type chest pain. He declined a recommended thoracotomy. *B*. By April 1977, the mass had become very large and was associated with pleural changes above the diaphragm. *C*. The lateral chest x-ray shows the posterior extent of the mass. Because of continued chest pain the patient accepted operation, and a left pneumonectomy was done. He has recovered satisfactorily without evidence of recurrence. (*Chest x-ray and case history courtesy of Jacqueline Coalson, Ph.D.*)

Although the number of respiratory units may not increase after birth, it does seem apparent that the newborn's lung is structurally immature. In place of alveoli, the lungs are made up of primitive air sacs that differentiate into alveolar ducts and sacs. Alveoli develop by outpouching and compartmentalization, so that by eight years of age the adult number of approximately 300 million alveoli is at-tained. The fully developed alveoli give a surface area of 70 to 80 m² at three-fourths maximal inflation of the adult lung.

The segmental anatomy of the lungs and bronchial tree is illustrated in Fig. 17-42. Although there is continuity of the pulmonary parenchyma between adjacent segments of each lobe, the separation of the bronchial and vascular stalks allows subsegmental and segmental resections rather than lobectomy for certain localized lesions. The object of performing lesser resections is to preserve the maximum amount of pulmonary tissue. Inflammatory diseases such as tuberculosis and bronchiectasis characteristically involve segmental units of the upper and lower lobes, respectively, but often do so in a way that leaves one or more segments of the same lobe unaffected. Both these diseases, as well as metastatic pulmonary neoplasms, may involve more than one pulmonary lobe, either synchronously or metachronously. The advantages of a segmental concept of surgical

A

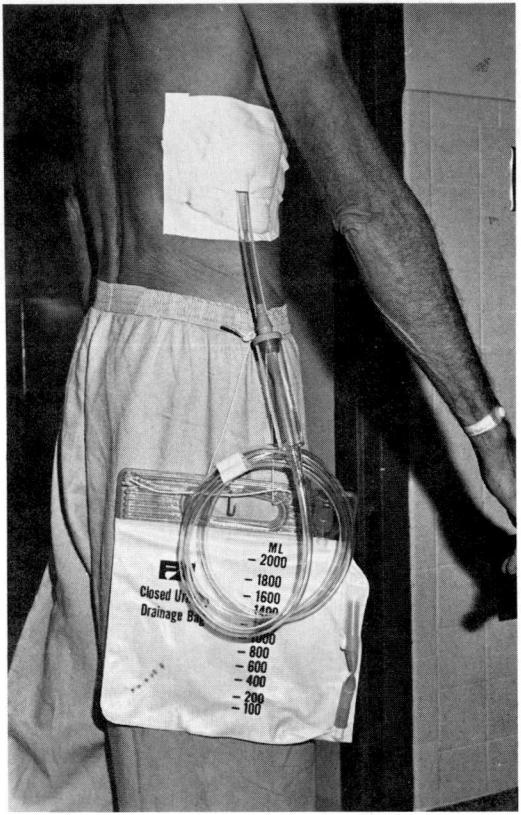

B

Fig. 17-41. Use of a one-way drainage valve to permit mobility of patients with a chest tube. *A.* The Heimlich one-way valve can be attached to an intercostal tube and eliminates the need for an underwater seal in some patients with either an air leak or drainage from the pleural cavity. *B.* By attaching the one-way valve to a collection bag the patient with a continuously draining pleural effusion can be completely ambulatory.

treatment are most apparent under these circumstances.

Abundant lymphatic vessels are located beneath the visceral pleura of each lung, in the interlobular septums, in the submucosa of the bronchi, and in the perivascular and peribronchial connective tissue. The lymph nodes which drain the lungs are divided into two large groups, the *pulmonary lymph nodes* and the *mediastinal nodes.* In turn, the pulmonary lymph nodes consist of (1) the intrapulmonary nodes, which lie at points of division of segmental bronchi or in the bifurcations of the pulmonary artery; (2) hilar nodes located along the main bronchi; and (3) interlobar nodes, situated in the angles formed by the bifurcation of the main bronchi into lobar bronchi.

The interlobar lymph nodes lie in the depths of the interlobar fissure on each side and have special surgical significance because they constitute a lymphatic sump for each lung. This designation results from the fact that all the pulmonary lobes of the corresponding lung drain into that group of nodes. On the right side the nodes of the lymphatic sump lie around the bronchus intermedius, bounded above by the right-upper-lobe bronchus, and below by the middle lobe and superior segmental bronchi. The lymphatic sump on the left side is confined to the interlobar fissure, with the lymph nodes disposed in the angle between the lingular and lower-lobe bronchi, and in apposition to the pulmonary artery branches.

The mediastinal lymph nodes consist of four principal groups: (1) anterior mediastinal, (2) posterior mediastinal, (3) tracheobronchial, and (4) paratracheal. The anterior mediastinal nodes are located in association with the upper surface of the pericardium, the phrenic nerves, the ligamentum arteriosum, and the left innominate vein. Within the inferior pulmonary ligament on each side are found the paraesophageal lymph nodes that constitute a major part of the posterior mediastinal group. Additional paraesophageal nodes may be located more superiorly between the esophagus and trachea in the region of the arch of the azygos vein.

The tracheobronchial lymph nodes are made up of three subgroups that are located about the bifurcation of the trachea. Included are the subcarinal nodes, the lymph nodes lying in the obtuse angle between the trachea and each main-stem bronchus, and a few nodes that lie anterior to the lower end of the trachea. The paratracheal lymph nodes are located in proximity to the trachea in the superior mediastinum. Those on the right side form a chain with the tracheobronchial nodes inferiorly and with some of the deep cervical nodes above. A few of the latter are referred to as the *scalene lymph nodes* because they lie on the anterior scalene muscle.

The high incidence of bronchial carcinoma is partly responsible for a continuing interest in identifying the precise patterns of lymphatic drainage of the lungs to the mediastinum. Previous studies suggested that drainage from the left lung was mainly contralateral and that from the right lung was ipsilateral. The development of mediastinoscopy and its extensive use in patients with bronchogenic carcinoma has allowed a slight modification of this concept. Lymphatic drainage of the right lung is ipsilateral except for an occasional incidence in which drainage to the

RIGHT LUNG AND BRONCHI

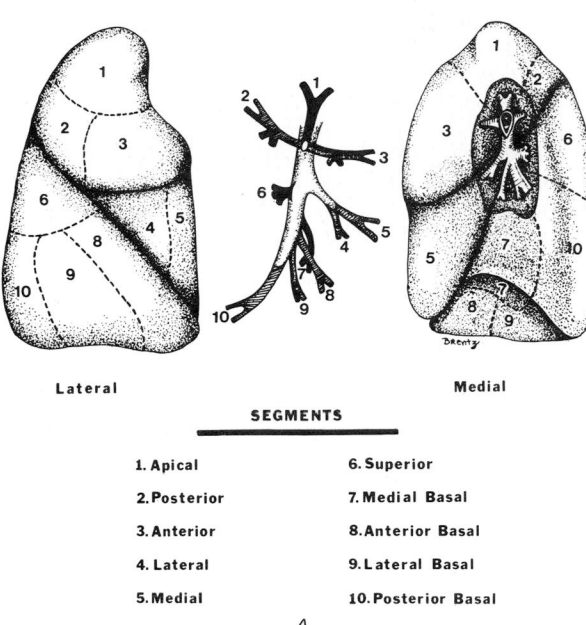

Lateral   Medial

SEGMENTS

1. Apical	6. Superior
2. Posterior	7. Medial Basal
3. Anterior	8. Anterior Basal
4. Lateral	9. Lateral Basal
5. Medial	10. Posterior Basal

A

LEFT LUNG AND BRONCHI

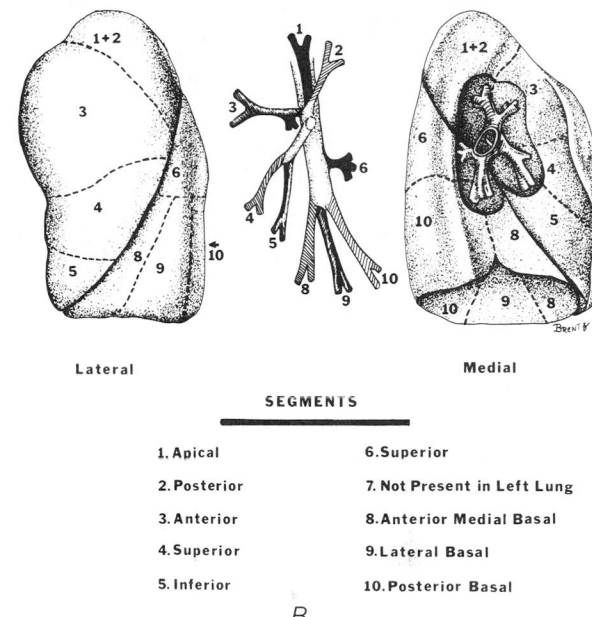

Lateral   Medial

SEGMENTS

1. Apical	6. Superior
2. Posterior	7. Not Present in Left Lung
3. Anterior	8. Anterior Medial Basal
4. Superior	9. Lateral Basal
5. Inferior	10. Posterior Basal

B

Fig. 17-42. *A* and *B*. The segmental anatomy of the lungs. An appreciation of these anatomic divisions often makes it possible to preserve pulmonary tissue by performing segmental resections for localized disease.

superior mediastinum is bilateral. Drainage from the left lung to the superior mediastinum is as frequently ipsilateral as it is to the opposite side.

Diagnostic Techniques

Despite their great variety, respiratory diseases, including congenital anomalies, have only a limited group of signs and symptoms, and there is considerable overlap in their clinical presentation. Notwithstanding the remarkable advances in roentgenographic techniques, it is often impossible to differentiate pulmonary inflammatory disorders from primary or secondary neoplastic diseases on the basis of chest x-rays. In addition, pulmonary lesions are sometimes found on a standard screening chest x-ray with a complete absence of symptoms. At least two factors may be considered conducive to continuing developments in pulmonary diagnostic techniques. The first is the free communication of the interior of the respiratory system with the oropharynx. This facilitates collection of secretions, infectious agents, and desquamated cells that may provide a definitive diagnosis. Second, roentgenograms and fluoroscopic techniques provide a "window" into the thoracic cavity for serial observations and for precise guidance of biopsy needles and forceps. Pulmonary angiography has been disappointing as a general diagnostic technique, but it can be important in defining congenital abnormalities.

In most acquired pulmonary diseases sputum collection and examination is indicated as an initial diagnostic procedure. The specific etiologic agent of infections is sought by examination of smears and by culture techniques. The flora of the upper part of the respiratory tract stops abruptly at the level of the larynx, and the tracheobronchial tree is normally sterile. Not infrequently, either the patient's sputum is scant or, because it is mixed with saliva and an oral bacterial flora, its diagnostic usefulness is reduced. To bypass these problems, percutaneous transtracheal aspiration may be performed through the cricothyroid membrane. A 16-gauge or 14-gauge intracatheter needle is used for the procedure after preparation of the skin with soap or iodine solution and local infiltration anesthesia with lidocaine. Coughing may be induced by injecting 5 to 10 ml sterile saline solution without preservative into the trachea. Aspiration of the diluted secretions into a 10- or 20-ml syringe should be followed by immediate delivery of the material to the laboratory.

This same technique may be used to collect material for cytologic examination in patients with a suspected pulmonary neoplasm, but because bronchoscopy is always indicated in these patients, it may suffice to collect secretions and saline irrigations (bronchial washings) through the bronchoscope. The sputum coughed up immediately after bronchoscopy is especially valuable for cytologic examinations. Chest physical therapy and intermittent positive-pressure breathing with saline solution and bronchodilators are additional techniques to facilitate the collection of sputum. Unfortunately, too little effort is spent in obtaining adequate samples of sputum in many hospitals, and the patient's diagnosis is often delayed while additional and more complicated procedures are done.

BRONCHOSCOPY. The visual examination of the tracheobronchial tree can be both diagnostic and therapeutic. Information can be gained from this procedure that is available from no other source: cell type of bronchial neoplasms by direct biopsy, mobility of surrounding structures, extent of endobronchial involvement in neoplasms and inflammatory disease, and on occasion, source of bleeding. In addition, the therapeutic aspects of bronchoscopy should not be overlooked. The removal of thick, inspissated secretions from the postoperative patient can be lifesaving. The benefit of foreign body extraction by endoscopic means is obvious.

The introduction of the flexible bronchoscope in 1967 by Ikeda greatly extended the benefits of this procedure. With this instrument examination of the tracheobronchial tree to the subsegmental level became possible. Brush biopsy and transbronchial lung biopsy also became practical.

Bronchoscopy may be performed under general or topical anesthesia, on conscious or unconscious patients, and under circumstances of spontaneous ventilation or with respirator support. Topical anesthesia is the preferred method under most circumstances.

BRONCHIAL BRUSHING. Bronchial-brush biopsy of pulmonary endobronchial lesions may be performed through the flexible fiberoptic bronchoscope, or it may be done as an independent procedure under fluoroscopic control. With the latter technique the patient is studied in the x-ray department and a catheter is guided into the appropriate segmental bronchus under topical anesthesia. After withdrawal of the guide wire, the special nylon brush is inserted through the catheter and advanced into the lesion. As the brush is passed back and forth through the lesion, the bristles entrap material that is scraped from its surface. As soon as the brush is removed from the catheter it is smeared on glass slides and the latter are placed in fixative solution according to the Papanicolaou technique. The brush may be cut off the guide wire and placed in any desired type of culture media.

Bronchial brushing has been very effective in the diagnosis of bronchogenic carcinoma, but less so with meta-

Fig. 17-43. This chest x-ray of a twenty-four-year-old black woman shows bilateral hilar masses that could be lymphoma or sarcoidosis. Mediastinoscopy was performed to obtain tissue that confirmed the diagnosis of sarcoidosis.

static pulmonary neoplasms. Tuberculosis and fungal diseases have been diagnosed by this method, but the increasing performance of fiberoptic bronchoscopy by physicians in pulmonary medicine seems to have stopped the development of brush biopsy as an independent procedure.

MEDIASTINOSCOPY-MEDIASTINOTOMY. Since its introduction in 1959 mediastinoscopy has gained increasing use as a technique for exploring the routes of mediastinal spread of pulmonary neoplasms. The procedure is usually performed under general endotracheal anesthesia and utilizes a small transverse incision in the suprasternal notch. Digital exploration is carried inferiorly in the plane between the anterior surface of the trachea and the posterior surface of the innominate artery and the aorta. The paratracheal, tracheobronchial, and subcarinal lymph nodes are accessible to visualization and biopsy through the mediastinoscope, and tumor masses such as thymomas or thyroid lesions may be biopsied directly. The decision to perform thoracotomy in a patient with proved or suspected bronchogenic carcinoma may be supported when mediastinoscopy fails to show evidence of mediastinal spread. In some circumstances, the procedure is used as a means of obtaining tissue for confirmation of a suspected diagnosis of bronchial neoplasm when other methods such as bronchoscopy have failed. The technique provides a positive diagnosis in almost all patients with lymphoma who have radiographic evidence of enlarged mediastinal lymph nodes, and the yield is similarly very high for patients with infectious granulomatous disease. Mediastinoscopy is considered the procedure of choice for diagnosis of sarcoidosis in most institutions, and it has largely replaced scalene lymph-node and fat-pad biopsy for both benign and malignant lesions (Fig. 17-43).

Unfortunately, a metastasis to lymph nodes between the trachea and esophagus and to posterior mediastinal lymph nodes cannot be determined by mediastinoscopy. In addition, direct mediastinal extension to an extent that makes it impossible to perform curative resection is not detectable by this procedure. Additional methods for exploring the mediastinum have been developed, and the procedure referred to as anterior mediastinotomy has been used most frequently. Through either a transverse or vertical parasternal incision the second costal cartilage is removed on the side of the lesion. An effort is made to avoid opening the pleural cavity as the mediastinal pleura is freed from the undersurface of the sternum and dissected away from the mediastinum. By additional removal of the third costal cartilage a wider exploration can be performed, the object being to sample mediastinal lymph nodes and determine the extent of mediastinal spread of a centrally located bronchial neoplasm. If it is pertinent to the confirmation of the diagnosis, the mediastinal pleura can be opened to allow direct lung or pleural biopsy. The pleura may be opened also during a mediastinoscopy for the same purposes, but most surgeons are reluctant to use this technique with the sharply limited exposure of the mediastinoscopy incision.

On the right side, mediastinotomy allows exploration along the superior vena cava and the trachea. The left pulmonary hilum may be evaluated, and the possibility of neoplastic extension to involve the aorta may be partly determined by left mediastinotomy.

More recently, Arom and his colleagues have described a subxiphoid approach for anterior mediastinal exploration in which a short incision over the xiphoid process is used to allow entrance into the inferior aspect of the anterior mediastinum. Digital exploration is combined with the use of a mediastinoscope to provide an access to the entire anterior mediastinal compartment (Fig. 17-44). Biopsy of tumor masses or lymph nodes may be performed through this approach in the same fashion as with conventional mediastinoscopy.

LUNG BIOPSY. An accurate diagnosis is fundamental in the management of pulmonary and bronchial disease, whether localized or diffuse. Bronchial lesions may be biopsied during bronchoscopy or by bronchial brushing. It is also possible to perform lung biopsy via the bronchoscope, but the number of individuals using the transbronchial technique was limited until development of the flexible fiberscope. An increasing number of endoscoptists are utilizing transbronchoscopic lung biopsy for obtaining sufficient tissue samples to allow diagnosis of diffuse pulmonary diseases such as sarcoidosis, pulmonary alveolar proteinosis, and *Pneumocystis carinii* pneumonia. It is also possible to obtain tissue for diagnosis of localized lung disease by the transbronchial technique, but this requires good cooperation from the x-ray department to provide bi-plane image intensification. The morbidity rate of transbronchial lung biopsy has been low, with pneumothorax as the principal complication. Though the incidence of pneumothorax has varied from 5 to 20 percent, few patients require active treatment.

Percutaneous needle biopsy and open lung biopsy through a limited anterolateral or transaxillary thoracotomy are the more established methods for obtaining a tissue diagnosis in those patients who are not candidates for primary surgical treatment. Whether the patient has a diffuse lung disease or a presumed bronchial cancer that is inoperable, needle biopsy is preferable to open thoracotomy. Both aspirating and cutting needles are available, but the disposable Tru-Cut needles have gained in popularity during the past few years. Contraindications to needle biopsy include (1) pulmonary hypertension, (2) suspected or proved bleeding diathesis, (3) an uncooperative patient, (4) a patient receiving continuous or frequent positive-pressure breathing, and (5) respiratory failure.

An occasional patient is encountered for whom thoracotomy represents a high risk, but operation would be recommended if the localized lesion were known to be malignant. Some surgeons would argue against needle biopsy on the basis of the rare but documented occurrence of seeding the needle tract with malignant cells. In this special circumstance needle biopsy does appear warranted.

Needle biopsy is performed under local anesthesia, preferably with fluoroscopic control. Aspirated material must be immediately smeared or cultured, but pathology departments vary somewhat in their preference for the handling of tissue removed with cutting needles. The complications include hemoptysis, pneumothorax, and rarely

Fig. 17-44. A modification of mediastinoscopy is the technique of subxiphoid anterior mediastinal exploration recently described by Arom and colleagues. (*Courtesy of Kit V. Arom, M.D.*)

hemothorax. Although an incidence of pneumothorax as high as 30 percent has been reported, only an occasional patient requires tube thoracotomy for treatment. A special form of trephine needle biopsy using a high-speed turbine drill has been used in a few medical centers, but the method has not gained widespread interest.

The chief indications for open lung biopsy are failure of closed methods for diagnosis, including needle biopsy, and presence of a small localized lesion that should be totally removed by the biopsy. An example of the latter circumstance is presented by the patient with a solitary pulmonary nodule and a previously controlled malignancy in another body region. Occasionally there is a need to remove a larger amount of tissue than can be obtained by needle biopsy in patients with either diffuse or localized disease.

Open lung biopsy is performed as a formal operation under general anesthesia, and the patient should be made to understand that it is not a minor procedure. One or more wedges of pulmonary tissue are removed with an automatic stapler or a careful suture technique to reduce the likelihood of postoperative air leak from the lung (Fig. 17-45). Since a leak does occur in a few patients, an intercostal tube is placed at the time of operation and removed the next day if possible. The morbidity of open lung biopsy is minimal, and patients can often be discharged from the hospital in 48 to 72 hours if they require no further in-hospital procedures. The need for close follow-up must be emphasized to the patient when early discharge is allowed.

Congenital Disorders

Abnormalities in development of the lung and tracheobronchial tree may occur at any stage of intrauterine life, with clinical manifestations immediately after birth or at any subsequent age. Under normal circumstances the lungs are considered immature at the time of birth, but immaturity to even a greater degree is associated with respiratory-

Fig. 17-45. Open lung biopsy is performed by delivering a margin of a pulmonary lobe through the small thoracic incision and applying the automatic stapler across the parenchyma, as shown here. The first line of staples has been applied, and the stapler is in place for the second line. A wedge of pulmonary parenchyma can then be amputated for appropriate studies.

distress syndromes, including hyaline membrane disease.

The most fundamental abnormality is bilateral *pulmonary agenesis,* in which there is failure of the primitive respiratory outpouching to develop. Unilateral pulmonary agenesis represents a failure of development of the right or left primary bronchial bud; its occurrence is twice as often on the left side. Unilateral agenesis is compatible with relatively normal physical growth and development if the child has no other major abnormalities. The lung that is present fills both hemithoraces. Lobar agenesis is probably more frequent than reported, because it produces no characteristic clinical picture and is most often found during examination for other conditions.

Congenital *tracheoesophageal fistulas* of several types are among the more serious abnormalities of pulmonary development. Esophageal atresia is present in the great majority of cases; these conditions are considered in detail in the chapter on diseases of the esophagus.

Small *diverticula* of the trachea or bronchi with a predilection for the distal trachea are occasionally seen. They are usually in free communication with the airway lumen, and symptoms are absent. Aberrant origin of a normal major bronchus is seen infrequently, but it can have major significance when pulmonary resection is indicated for another reason. The commonest example is origin of the right-upper-lobe bronchus or the apical segmental bronchus from the lateral wall of the trachea. In the *scimitar syndrome,* anomalous drainage of the right pulmonary veins into the inferior vena cava is associated with underdevelopment of the right lung, several bronchovascular abnormalities, and aberrant systemic arterialization of the right lung. A principal concern of management is redirection of the pulmonary venous flow into the left atrium and simultaneous repair of any intracardiac defects.

A *bronchocele* is a localized cystic structure filled with mucus and located immediately distal to an area of stenosis or atresia in the bronchial tree. Presumably, the lesion can be produced either by a congenital obstruction in the bronchial tree or subsequent to an acquired stenosis. It is generally asymptomatic in the absence of infection and presents as a density several centimeters in length on a routine chest x-ray. Most often, diagnosis is made by examination of the specimen following a segmental or subsegmental resection.

An interesting and rare pulmonary abnormality that may require urgent resection is the *cystic adenomatoid malformation.* Prematurity and stillbirth are frequent characteristics of this condition, and infants that survive may develop respiratory distress soon after birth. Mediastinal shift toward the normal side is common, and the chest x-ray shows a large mass in the lower part of the chest with depression of the hemidiaphragm. Emergency thoracotomy reveals replacement of the lower lobe by a greatly enlarged mass that may be studded with cysts. Some evidence of partial aeration may be present, but there is no suggestion of ventilatory function. A systemic arterial supply such as that which occurs with pulmonary sequestration is usually absent. A lobectomy is generally required, but pneumonectomy has been necessary in a few instances. If survival occurs without early operation, subsequent infection of the malformed lobe is likely to result in a diagnosis of congenital cystic bronchiectasis.

Microscopic examination of the resected tissue shows tubules lined with cuboidal or columnar epithelium, bronchial mucous glands, and occasionally bits of cartilage or smooth muscle. The presence of the multiple components of respiratory tissue has caused some authors to refer to this abnormality as a diffuse hamartoma.

An *accessory lung* or *lobe* occasionally develops in association with a supernumerary bronchus that communicates with the trachea or a major bronchial branch. Left-sided occurrence is more frequent, and the blood supply may come from either the pulmonary or systemic circuits. This lesion is distinguished from *pulmonary sequestration* by the lack of a bronchial communication in the latter condition. In addition, a pulmonary sequestration receives its blood

A

B

C

Fig. 17-46. An extrapulmonary sequestration discovered on a routine chest x-ray in a twenty-year-old male. *A.* The posteroanterior chest x-ray shows a triangular density adjacent to the right heart border and based on the diaphragm. *B.* An oblique view shows the density to be a large mass with sharp borders. *C.* An aortogram shows several arteries passing retrograde from the infradiaphragmatic aorta to supply the sequestration.

supply from an ectopic systemic artery, often arising from the aorta at a point below the diaphragm (Fig. 17-46). The sequestration may be located in a lower lobe of the lung (intrapulmonary) or as a cystic mass in the inferior mediastinum (extrapulmonary). Rarely, a sequestration may be intraperitoneal, or it may develop a fistulous communication with the distal esophagus.

Intrapulmonary sequestration is the commonest type, and it may remain without symptoms for years. The development of symptoms is usually the result of infection, even though no apparent communication exists between the lower-lobe bronchi and the cystic lumina of the sequestration (Fig. 17-47). Treatment requires surgical resection of the involved lower lobe for the intrapulmonary forms, and excision of the mass for the extrapulmonary lesions.

Several forms of *congenital cystic abnormalities* may occur in the lung. Unilateral absence of a pulmonary artery may be associated with hypoplastic development of the lung and a cystic transformation. Intrapulmonary bronchogenic cysts may occur that are thought to represent a pinching off of the developing bronchial buds well beyond the subsegmental level. They may be single or multiple, confined to a segment or a lobe, and histologically similar to the large bronchogenic cysts that are located in the mediastinum alongside the major bronchi. The cysts are typically lined with ciliated, pseudostratified epithelium, and they contain a viscid opaque fluid. Small communications with the bronchial tree can develop, and the cysts become partially air-filled. If infection occurs and resection is required, it may be difficult to distinguish a congenital cyst from a chronic pulmonary abscess or cystic bronchiec-

A

B

Fig. 17-47. An example of an intrapulmonary sequestration. The chest x-rays show consolidation and an air-fluid level in the posterior part of the right lower lobe. A lobectomy showed a cystic sequestration with infection.

tasis. Other organs such as the kidney, liver, and pancreas may be the site of cystic changes in these patients.

Pulmonary arteriovenous aneurysms consist of fistulas between the branches of the pulmonary arteries and veins (Fig. 17-48). They vary in size from 1 or 2 mm up to lesions that may occupy a major portion of a pulmonary lobe. The occurrence of a single fistula is less common than the presence of multiple fistulas involving more than one lobe, especially in those patients with hereditary hemorrhagic telangiectasia (Osler-Rendu-Weber disease). More than one arterial branch and more than one vein are generally involved in a single aneurysm. The aneurysms are often subpleural in location, and spontaneous hemothorax occasionally occurs. Even when their individual size is small, a sufficient number of aneurysms may be present to produce

massive right-to-left shunting, cyanosis, clubbing, polycythemia, and congestive heart failure in the first few years of life. In other patients the development of cyanosis may not occur until adult life, but cerebral symptoms may result from cerebral thrombosis or subacute bacterial endarteritis. Hemoptysis is unusual in young patients, but it may be life-threatening in the adult. Fluoroscopic examination

Fig. 17-48. *A.* The plain chest x-ray in this eight-year-old boy shows three lesions thought to be compatible with pulmonary arteriovenous aneurysms. *B.* The pulmonary arteriogram confirms the aneurysms, which were subsequently removed by staged bilateral thoracotomies.

A

B

during the Valsalva and Müller maneuvers may show changes in the size of lesions that are suspected to be arteriovenous fistulas on plain chest x-rays. Pulmonary angiography is necessary to confirm the diagnosis and allow proper planning for surgical treatment. Ordinarily, the confirmation of the presence of one or more fistulas is adequate indication for operation, because of the risk of eventual serious complications. Conservative segmental and subsegmental resections rather than lobectomy are the procedures of choice.

Multiple chest-wall *systemic-to-pulmonary arterial fistulas* may present as a localized lesion associated with hemic murmurs and changes such as unilateral rib notching on the chest x-ray. The internal thoracic or several intercostal arteries may give origin to the systemic arterial components, and the fistulous connections may be formed with branches of the pulmonary arteries rather than with the veins. Angiography is required to determine the extent of the lesion, and the decision for resection must be carefully planned because of the danger of intraoperative hemorrhage.

INFANTILE LOBAR EMPHYSEMA

Michelson has stressed the need to use the term *infantile* lobar emphysema rather than *congenital* because the condition is not necessarily congenital in origin. There is characteristically a mild to marked overdistension of an upper or middle lobe, with compression of the remaining ipsilateral pulmonary tissue and mediastinal shift to the opposite side. Progressive distension results in herniation across the anterior mediastinum and atelectasis of the contralateral upper lobe (Fig. 17-49).

Lobar emphysema affects newborn as well as older infants and produces varying degrees of respiratory distress. Those with limited experience often think of it as an acute irreversible condition, but chronic forms as well as acute reversible emphysema may occur. It is especially important to understand that deficiency of the bronchial cartilage with resulting obstruction to expiratory air flow is only one of several causes of the disease. For example, lobar emphysema may develop as a result of acute bronchial infection with obstruction due to inflammatory secretions and mucosal edema. Proper management under these circumstances requires intensive treatment of the infection and close observation of the overdistended lobe or lobes. Evidence that the emphysema is reversible is provided by stabilization of the infant's respiratory distress and beginning reversal of the radiographic evidence of pulmonary overdistension.

In a significant number of the studied cases there has been dissatisfaction with the attempt to explain lobar emphysema on the basis of bronchial obstruction. An interesting mechanism that may produce upper-lobe overdistension in any age group is related to the concept that there is a relatively positive intrapleural pressure at the lung base compared to a relatively negative pressure at the apex. In the supine position the anterior portion of the lung is better ventilated than the posterior portion. Since the infant has a pliable chest wall and a spacious anterior mediastinum, it seems possible that increased ventilation would promote an overexpansion of the anterior segment, especially in the presence of any resistance to expiratory air flow.

Asymptomatic lobar emphysema may be found by chest x-rays in the newborn. Clearing of the emphysema within a day or two and failure to develop symptoms have suggested that bronchial obstruction was due to aspiration of amniotic fluid or mucus. Lobar emphysema resulting from extrabronchial compression due to bronchogenic or mediastinal neuroenteric cysts may be especially difficult to diagnose. The structure responsible for compression may not be seen on the chest x-rays, and a confusing clinical picture may result. An esophagogram will generally suggest the presence of a mediastinal mass, and this procedure should be performed when the infant's condition permits it. The presence of thoracic hemivertebrae may suggest the likelihood that a neuroenteric cyst can be present. Anomalous location of vascular structures such as the left pulmonary artery and the ductus arteriosus has been reported as an extrinsic cause of lobar emphysema.

Typical irreversible lobar emphysema is a disease of the newborn. Approximately 50 percent of the reported cases have occurred during the first 4 weeks of life, and symptoms of respiratory distress may begin shortly after birth. Chest x-ray evidence of overdistension of an upper or middle lobe may be subtle at first, but progressive symptoms are accompanied by mediastinal shift and compression of the opposite lung. Overinflation is often confined to the anterior segment of either upper lobe or the middle lobe, but the lower lobes are rarely involved.

The treatment of severe, acutely symptomatic lobar emphysema is immediate operation if the likelihood that primary bronchial infection is not the cause. Nonoperative treatment may result in a mortality rate as high as 50 percent. Congenital heart disease is associated with approximately 15 percent of infants with lobar emphysema, and occasionally it is appropriate to treat both conditions at the same time. Exploration of the emphysematous lobe and the mediastinum is done through a standard posterolateral thoracotomy incision. If a clear-cut cause of extrinsic bronchial compression is found, this is dealt with and a decision is made about removal of the distended lobe. Generally, a lobectomy will be required, and satisfactory expansion of the remaining lung can be expected.

EMPHYSEMATOUS BLEBS AND BULLAE

Infrequent air-containing spaces that are located in apparently normal lung parenchyma may represent a form of congenital blebs. These spaces may also be referred to as congenital air cysts, and they are characterized by an epithelial lining of the respiratory type. The incidence is unknown and the relationship between the very occasional infant or child with pulmonary blebs and the more frequently seen teenager or young adult with recurrent spontaneous pneumothorax is unclear. Similarly, the occurrence of giant bullae in the lungs of young adults who have no evidence of obstructive airway disease suggests a congenital defect in the integrity of the pulmonary parenchyma (Fig. 17-50).

The congenital air cyst may enlarge to produce pressure on adjacent lung, and such cysts may become infected.

A

B

Fig. 17-49. Infantile lobar emphysema. *A.* The anteroposterior chest x-ray shows marked overinflation of the left upper lobe, with mediastinal shift to the right and compression of the right upper lobe. *B.* The lateral x-ray shows that most of the hyperinflation is anterior. *C.* Histologic examination of the resected left upper lobe bronchus shows incomplete cartilage development. (*From E. Michelson, Clinical Spectrum of Infantile Lobar Emphysema, Ann Thorac Surg, 24:182, 1977.*)

C

With infection, purulent fluid develops in the cyst (pyocyst), and treatment similar to that for lung abscess is required. The preferred treatment is surgical resection before infection occurs.

Emphysematous blebs and bullae are so much a part of the overall condition of pulmonary emphysema that it is difficult or impossible to consider their surgical significance without a consideration of the pathogenesis of emphysema. From the strict anatomic definition, pulmonary emphysema means enlargement of distal air spaces, often accompanied by destruction of septums. At least four processes are operative in the production of emphysema, but the relative role of each and the precise combinations that may be determinative in the individual patient are often uncertain. The processes are (1) traction, (2) airway obstruction, (3) destruction of interalveolar septums, and (4) loss of elasticity.

In the process of traction, overdistension of focal groups of alveoli occurs as an attempt to compensate for volume

Fig. 17-50. An operative photograph showing a giant bulla arising from the upper lobe of an eighteen-year-old man with no symptoms of obstructive airway disease.

loss due to multiple areas of microatelectasis or pulmonary fibrosis. The obstructive processes vary in location from the lobar bronchi to the bronchioles, with a varied etiologic picture that encompasses both extrinsic and intrinsic causes of bronchial obstruction. With focal obstructive emphysema, air trapping occurs in isolated alveolar units, and

Fig. 17-51. A. Multiple pulmonary bullae are shown arising in the right upper lobe of a thirty-one-year-old salesman who had three episodes of spontaneous pneumothorax over a 2-year period. B. The bullae have been opened to show the netlike interior resulting from progressive parenchymal destruction as the bullae evolved.

overexpansion leads to the formation of bullae. Diffuse obstructive emphysema involves all the air spaces to a limited degree, but there may be an intermix with focal areas of greater distension and resulting bullae. In the presence of bullous emphysema a self-perpetuating cycle may be established. An enlarging bulla can produce partial obstruction of adjacent bronchioles with further air trapping and progressive distension of the bulla.

A process of tissue destruction almost certainly plays a key role in the development of bullae, because the interalveolar septums must give way as recruitment of increasing volume occurs (Fig. 17-51). Through this process the

A

B

relatively simple air chamber of the bulla is formed from the complex of respiratory units that originally existed. The bulla communicates with a progressive number of bronchioles or bronchi as it enlarges. A loss of elasticity in the parenchymal structure accompanies the destruction of septums.

The surgical significance of pulmonary blebs and bullae is related to the complications that they may produce and to the implications of their presence when a patient is being considered for surgical treatment of another pulmonary lesion. Radiographic demonstration of bullae indicates the presence of emphysema and suggests (1) caution in the decision to offer a thoracic operation for treatment of the patient's primary problems, and (2) conservative resection when pulmonary tissue must be excised. Among the usual complications are (1) recurrent pneumothorax, often with prolonged air leak, (2) infection (pyocysts), and (3) occasional bleeding, (4) compression of adjacent parenchyma, and (5) respiratory insufficiency.

Giant bullae may be seen in all age groups, but decisions regarding surgical management seem to gather more attention and controversy in young adults and middle-aged persons. There are often minimal symptoms in the former, and any debate over surgical excision revolves around the question of whether the removal of the bullae will allow improved pulmonary function through reexpansion of the compressed parenchyma. Middle-aged and older patients with giant bullae often have symptoms of obstructive airway disease and evidence of generalized emphysema. The advocates of a nonoperative approach insist that data are lacking to support a significant improvement in pulmonary function due to removal of the bullae.

The apical region of the upper lobes and the superior segment of the lower lobes give rise to the greatest number of bullae (Fig. 17-52). While the walls of bullae may be

Fig. 17-52. This operative photograph shows multiple thick-walled blebs arising from the left upper lobe. Numerous adhesions were probably the result of many episodes of pneumothorax treated by tube thoracostomy.

extremely thin, it is surprising how often they may be opaque and collagenous in consistency. Microscopically, there is often smooth muscle that is said to derive from the walls of bronchioles, bronchial vessels, and lymphatics.

Dyspnea with exercise is characteristic in patients with giant bullae, but the results of pulmonary-function testing will depend on the stage of the disease and associated pulmonary abnormalities. The residual volume and the functional residual capacity are generally increased while the maximum voluntary ventilation is decreased. Arterial oxygen tension is usually normal at rest, but graded exercise often produces desaturation. Routine chest x-rays and laminograms may be supplemented by radioisotope lung scans and pulmonary angiography in completing the evaluation of a patient to be considered for excision of bullae. These tests show the distribution of functioning lung tissue and indicate the degree of compression of the adjacent pulmonary parenchyma.

For the young patient without evidence of generalized respiratory disease, the bullae are simply resected either through a lateral thoracotomy, or in some cases with bilateral giant bullae, through a median sternotomy incision. The older patient with chronic bronchitis and evidence of airways obstruction requires careful preparation for operation. All measures are taken to improve pulmonary function and eliminate chronic bronchial infection. At operation the guiding principle is that of conserving the maximum functional pulmonary tissue. Only if a lobe is largely replaced by bullae should lobectomy be performed. Otherwise the bullae should be resected individually and attention devoted to closing all possible communicating bronchi.

SPONTANEOUS PNEUMOTHORAX

Pneumothorax is one of the common complications, or manifestations, of pulmonary diseases and injuries. In addition, however, there are many patients who have episodes of pneumothorax in which there appears to be no apparent cause for the leak of air from the lung parenchyma into the pleural space. These episodes of "spontaneous" pneumothorax are almost always the result of rupture of subpleural blebs that are located at the apex of the upper lobe or in the superior segment of the lower lobe. The cause of the blebs continues to be unknown, and the patients do not have obstructive airway disease. Since typically the episodes occur in young men of college age, the condition is common at universities and military bases. Spontaneous pneumothorax occurs much less frequently in women, but a rare woman will have episodes that seem to coincide with her menses (catamenial pneumothorax).

The peak age incidence is between twenty and forty years, but episodes can occur at the extremes of age. Patients who have had several episodes commonly indicate that symptoms have occurred on both sides, but rarely at the same time. Tension pneumothorax can occur and, less frequently, hemopneumothorax. There is no consistent history of exertion preceding the onset of pneumothorax, and many patients relate symptoms that suggest very mild episodes that did not cause them to seek medical attention. In other instances, the onset of pneumothorax may be

A

B

Fig. 17-53. Spontaneous pneumothorax. *A.* The arrows point to the lung margin. Occasionally a partial pneumothorax is missed during a rapid examination of an emergency chest x-ray. *B.* The right lung was easily reexpanded by placement of a large intercostal tube and initiation of pleural suction. *C.* Another patient who had multiple episodes of pneumothorax underwent right thoracotomy and obliteration of apical blebs with a row of metal staples (*arrow*).

R

C

associated with significant chest or shoulder pain and dyspnea. The findings on examination may suggest a major collapse of the lung with tracheal shift, or there may be nothing more than reduced breath sounds.

The chest x-ray usually confirms the suspected diagnosis and shows the extent of pneumothorax. Occasionally, when only a small pneumothorax is present, it is possible to misread the roentgenogram and conclude that a pneumothorax is not present (Fig. 17-53). From the x-ray, an estimate of lung collapse should be made, remembering that the lung is a modified cylinder. The x-ray badly underindicates the degree (percent) of collapse because it is only two-dimensional.

When there is minimal pneumothorax in a patient without significant symptoms, it is reasonable simply to observe the course of the pneumothorax without attempting to aspirate air from the pleural cavity. This conservative approach applies only when the patient can be observed and when sufficient hours have passed from the occurrence of symptoms to the time when the x-ray was made to presume that the air leak has stopped. When the pneumothorax exceeds 25 percent, or when the patient is symptomatic, placement of a tube thoracostomy in the second intercostal space anteriorly or in the fifth, sixth, or seventh intercostal space laterally will ordinarily allow prompt reexpansion of the lung when pleural suction is applied. Prophylactic antibiotics are not needed simply because a tube thoracostomy has been performed.

For the majority of patients, 24 to 72 hours of pleural suction is adequate to ensure reexpansion and sealing of the air leak. An occasional patient continues to leak air for many days, and it may be necessary to adjust or replace the thoracotomy tube. A persistent air leak beyond 7 to 10 days requires open thoracotomy for excision of the blebs or adhesions that are responsible for the continued leak. At the same procedure pleural abrasion should be performed with sterile gauze pads to encourage obliteration of the pleural space by adhesions.

Patients who have had a single episode of pneumothorax stand about a 30 percent chance of having a second episode. After a second episode the chances are 50-50 that a third and further episodes will occur. Therefore, it is prudent to recommend open thoracotomy after the second episode, and certainly after the third pneumothorax, regardless of whether the episodes have occurred on one side or the other. Operation can generally be performed through a transaxillary third interspace incision, with wedge resection, oversewing, or stapling of any blebs. Pleural abrasion should be done at the same time.

Pulmonary Infections

Though thoracic surgeons must still concern themselves with active participation in the treatment of patients with serious pulmonary infections, it is strikingly apparent that their role has progressively decreased. As recently as the early 1960s thousands of patients in the United States required pulmonary resection for lung abscess, bronchiectasis, and chronic granulomatous disease each year. In some areas of the world where adequate diagnostic techniques and chemotherapy are still far below regional needs these diseases continue to progress to those stages that can yield only to surgical management. Effective antibiotics, aggressive methods for accurate diagnosis, an increased standard of living, and public health programs are among the factors that have reduced the need to remove chronically infected or destroyed pulmonary tissue.

LUNG ABSCESS

Necrosis of pulmonary tissue with associated infection is the principal distinction between a lung abscess and an infected bulla (pyocyst) or an infected bronchogenic cyst. Table 17-6 shows a classification of pulmonary abscesses based on the precipitating event.

Although it is uncommon, primary pneumonias with bacterial species that are noted for their necrotizing ability may proceed to abscess formation. Postpneumonic abscesses of this type are frequently located in the upper lobes and may simulate tuberculous cavities in a chronic phase. In infants and young children the *Staphylococcus aureus* is most frequently associated with an acute course that rapidly proceeds to abscess formation and pleural empyema. Aspiration of gastric contents followed by

Table 17-6. CLASSIFICATION OF LUNG ABSCESSES

A. Infection by specific necrotizing organisms
   1. Aerobic infection
      a. *Staphylococcus aureus*
      b. *Klebsiella pneumoniae*
      c. *Mycobacterium tuberculosis*
   2. Anaerobic infection
      a. *Bacteroides fragilis*
      b. *Bacteroides melaninogenicus*
      c. *Fusobacterium fusiformis*
      d. *Actinomyces*
B. Abscess following aspiration pneumonia
C. Abscess following pulmonary embolism
   1. Septic pulmonary emboli
   2. Infection of pulmonary infarct
D. Abscess following pulmonary trauma
   1. Infected hematoma
   2. Contaminated foreign body
E. Abscess due to bronchial obstruction
   1. Neoplasm
   2. Foreign body
F. Abscess due to extension from hepatic, subphrenic, or mediastinal abscess

pneumonia is probably the commonest mechanism of lung abscess at present, and the association with alcoholism is well-known (Fig. 17-54). An overdosage of drugs, general anesthesia, and vomiting associated with trauma are alternate items that may be significant in the patient's history. Abscesses that follow aspiration are usually located posteriorly and in the lower lobes. Retained foreign material (undigested food) is infrequent, but occasionally the endoscopist or the pathologist examining a resected lobe is surprised to find material that seemingly could have been expelled by coughing.

Lung abscesses due to septic emboli do not have a characteristic location but are distinguished by their association with septic pelvic, peritoneal, or musculoskeletal disorders. These abscesses are typically small, multiple, and bilateral. Infection developing in a pulmonary infarct is likely to lead to empyema as often as it produces a pulmonary abscess.

Rarely a pulmonary abscess will develop about a retained metallic fragment or other foreign material carried into the lung by a penetrating injury. The presence of foreign material is not necessary, however, if a parenchymal hematoma has been produced by the trauma, either penetrating or nonpenetrating.

Partial or complete bronchial obstruction is associated with pulmonary abscess frequently enough to make it mandatory that patients have bronchoscopy soon after management has begun. The cause of obstruction may be a bronchial neoplasm, bronchial stenosis from previous inflammatory disease, or trauma, and rarely, a foreign body. A question of the relationship between infected gums and teeth and the occasional development of an otherwise unexplained lung abscess remains unanswered. Such patients are usually found to have a generally accepted cause of their pulmonary infection if the history is sufficiently detailed.

A lung abscess usually forms communications with multiple bronchi as it develops, and the necrotic, purulent

A

C

B

Fig. 17-54. Lung abscess due to vomiting and aspiration after an alcoholic binge. *A.* The posteroanterior chest x-ray shows an abscess cavity in the superior segment of the left lower lobe. *B.* A tomogram confirms the thin wall of the abscess and reduces the likelihood that the lesion could be a cavitated carcinoma. *C.* After 4 weeks of antibiotic therapy the abscess appears to be healing.

contents are intermittently discharged in the sputum. A zone of inflammatory consolidation continues to surround the abscess cavity as it passes to a chronic stage. Unfortunately, an abscess ignores the vague segmental boundaries within a lobe, and slow parenchymal destruction can necessitate complete lobectomy if operative resection is required. The diagnosis is usually made on the basis of clinical manifestations of pulmonary infection, foul or putrid sputum, and the roentgenographic demonstration of a lesion with an air-fluid level. If the latter is absent and the patient is a smoker beyond thirty-five years of age the pressure may mount to differentiate the lesion from a bronchogenic tumor. Even when an air-fluid level is shown on the chest x-ray, the abscess can be difficult to distinguish from a cavitated epidermoid carcinoma. Occasionally, a cavitated pulmonary mycosis can mimic lung abscess, as can infected congenital lesions such as bronchogenic cysts and intralobar sequestration.

The treatment of lung abscess is based on intense antibiotic therapy combined with techniques to promote bronchial drainage of the abscess cavity. As mentioned, diagnostic bronchoscopy should be done early. Formerly, repeated bronchoscopy at intervals of several days to a week was advocated to promote bronchial drainage. Postural drainage, chest physical therapy, appropriate use of bronchodilators, and, occasionally, special procedures such as the endotracheal placement of an aspirating catheter in children should be adequate for 80 to 90 percent of patients. Occasionally a surgical emergency is created when a patient's abscess ruptures into the pleural cavity to form a pyopneumothorax. Tube thoracostomy for drainage of the pleural cavity is required initially, but the formation of a chronic bronchopleural fistula may necessitate pulmonary resection.

Failure of the patient to respond to medical management by loss of systemic signs of infection, and lack of beginning resolution of the abscess are the principal indications for surgical intervention. If the patient is not critically ill, several weeks may be allowed for a determination of the response. Surgical treatment may consist either of *pneumonotomy,* for drainage of the abscess, or *pulmonary resection.* Pneumonotomy is a technique of direct drainage of the abscess through the chest wall after subperiosteal resection of a short rib segment overlying the abscess. Although performed infrequently, pneumonotomy is especially valuable for debilitated or elderly patients for whom lobectomy would seem to have a high risk. The result may be excellent, with subsequent rapid reduction in the ab-

Fig. 17-55. An oblique view of a left-sided bronchogram shows bronchiectasis of the basal segmental bronchi.

scess cavity. Healing of the track through the chest wall generally requires several months as the drainage tubes are gradually shortened.

Resection of a pulmonary abscess generally requires lobectomy, and care must be taken with the induction of anesthesia or positioning of the patient to prevent a spill of the abscess contents into the contralateral lung. Because an abscess can extend across an interlobar fissure to involve the adjacent lobe, it is important to recognize the need for surgical treatment before a more extensive resection might be required.

BRONCHIECTASIS

Bronchiectasis is a complex of pulmonary and bronchial infection characterized by bronchial dilatation. It encompasses a spectrum of disease with involvement of bronchi at several levels, primarily the segmental and subsegmental bronchi and their branches (Fig. 17-55). The basal segments of the lower lobes, the lingula, and the right middle lobe are the principal areas of involvement. Upper-lobe involvement (other than the lingula) is unusual except as a complication of preceding conditions such as tuberculosis. Bronchiectasis may follow partial obstruction of any bronchus due to a variety of causes, i.e., foreign body, neoplasm, extrinsic pressure. An example of this variation is the so-called *middle-lobe syndrome,* in which compression of the middle-lobe bronchus by enlarged peribronchial lymph nodes leads to destructive infection of the segmental bronchi. Lobar atelectasis and peribronchial fibrosis accompany the chronic infection, with resultant destruction of the lobe if the process is not reversed by early reexpansion (Fig. 17-56).

There has been a wealth of literature on the pathogenesis of bronchiectasis, but the singular fact remains that the cause of the average case is unknown. For each patient who presents with the disease it is pertinent to look for features that may signal the likelihood of a special variation such as bronchial obstruction or Kartagener's syndrome (situs inversus, pansinusitis, and bronchiectasis).

The bronchial changes may vary in severity from a mild tubular or cylindrical dilatation to cystic or saccular structures that are no longer recognizable as bronchi. The cystic dilatations almost always contain residual mucus with varying amounts of debris or purulent material, depending on the infection status. Broncholiths are occasionally found in the destroyed bronchi, and they may be associated with active ulceration. Fibrosis surrounding the diseased bronchi along with retained secretions may lead to a progressive loss of volume in the involved pulmonary segment.

Bronchiectasis is diagnosed in both sexes throughout the entire age spectrum from infancy to old age. Its highest incidence seems to range from late childhood through the fourth decade in varying regions of the world. The complications of recurrent pneumonia, hemoptysis, and metastatic infection such as cerebral abscess often precipitate an effort to confirm the suspected diagnosis. Retarded physical development, digital clubbing, and voluminous sputum production are sometimes allowed to progress for remarkable periods before medical attention is sought.

Although the diagnosis may be strongly suspected on the

basis of the clinical history and changes seen in the standard posteroanterior and lateral chest x-ray, bronchography is the definitive diagnostic procedure. Bronchoscopy should precede the contrast study to determine the presence of bronchial obstruction or foreign bodies and to obtain material for cultures. If the patient has a large sputum production it is appropriate to gain control of the infection and reduce the volume of secretions before attempting bronchography. Excessive secretions will interfere with an accurate mapping of the bronchial tree, the most critical feature of the diagnostic work-up.

The initial treatment of bronchiectasis consists of medical management with a goal of assessing the severity of the disease, the extent of pulmonary involvement, and the response to antibiotic therapy combined with postural drainage (Fig. 17-57). Especially in children there are often a generalized bronchitis and an evolving development of the bronchiectasis which are best handled by avoiding a premature decision for operation. An ideal candidate for surgical resection is the older child or adult whose disease is localized to one lobe or to one lobe on each side. Patients with simple cylindrical bronchiectasis can often be managed satisfactorily without surgical treatment. With advanced bronchial destruction to the stages of saccular or cystic disease, the involved pulmonary segments cannot function normally and represent greater liabilities than assets to the patient (Fig. 17-58). If the disease is sufficiently localized, these anatomic changes alone are adequate indications for operation. Recurrent pneumonia, hemoptysis, sputum production that interferes with the patient's ability to enjoy normal activities, and the general debilitating effects of chronic infection are the principal indications for pulmonary resection.

A maximum effort should be made to reduce sputum volume and infection prior to operation. Segmental resections are the procedures of choice, especially when more than one lobe is involved and bilateral disease is present. Postoperative care must be meticulous to reduce problems of atelectasis, pneumonia, and empyema. The results of a well-planned medical and surgical program should be satisfactory in more than 75 percent of patients.

TUBERCULOSIS

The development of effective chemotherapy and its influence on the course of pulmonary tuberculosis have to be

Fig. 17-56. This lateral chest x-ray shows a wedge-shaped density overlying the cardiac shadow and corresponding to a collapsed middle lobe. Resection of the fibrotic lobe showed marked bronchiectasis of the segmental bronchi (middle-lobe syndrome).

counted among the remarkable accomplishments of the past quarter-century. As evidence that the disease is still with us is the fact that more than 30,000 new cases of active tuberculosis were reported in 1975. The surgical significance of this new case rate is a great deal different, however, than it would have been in 1955. During that era the

Fig. 17-57. Postural drainage combined with chest physical therapy is important in the medical management of bronchiectasis and in the preoperative care of patients who require pulmonary resection.

Fig. 17-58. The cut section of this right lower lobe shows one of several cystic bronchiectatic cavities with surrounding localized pneumonia.

surgical treatment of pulmonary tuberculosis required a significant amount of the available thoracic surgical manpower. In fact, the development of thoracic surgery was inseparably linked with the development of effective surgical techniques for the management of tuberculosis. Presently, the relatively few patients that are considered for operative treatment are insufficient to assure adequate experience with the disease for many thoracic surgery training programs.

Surgical techniques are rarely required in the treatment of first-infection ("childhood") tuberculosis. When there is a need, it is generally directed at complications such as massive pleural effusion or compression of mediastinal structures by enlarged lymph nodes (i.e., middle-lobe syndrome). Among patients with reinfection tuberculosis it is estimated that pulmonary resection will be indicated in about 1 percent of those undergoing first treatment with drug therapy, and in 5 percent of individuals receiving retreatment.

Fig. 17-59. Pulmonary tuberculosis, active. A. The posteroanterior chest x-ray shows an infiltrative lesion with pleural thickening at the left apex. B. A tomogram suggests cavitation in the lesion.

A

B

The typical lesion of reinfection tuberculosis begins as a bronchopneumonia in the apical or posterior segments of an upper lobe, less frequently in the superior segment of a lower lobe. Caseous necrosis occurs to a variable extent, along with an exudative reaction. A successful response by the patient, with or without drug therapy, may lead to resolution with predominant scar formation and some communication with bronchi (Fig. 17-59). If caseation is extensive, fibrous tissue is formed at the periphery and in multiple locules, producing a cavity in communication with the bronchi that provide its drainage. According to the patient's resistance to the continued growth of the *Mycobacterium tuberculosis* and the antibiotic effect of the chemotherapy regimen, the cavity may stabilize or continue to enlarge. Occasionally, a cavity undergoes rapid expansion as the result of air entrapment by stenotic bronchi (tension cavity).

With control of the organism and stabilization of the cavity an ingrowth of epithelium may occur. Thickening of the fibrous tissue follows, with eventual contraction and partial or complete obliteration of the cavity. In some patients, however, little contraction occurs and the cavity remains open—the so-called "open-negative" cavity that formerly was the subject of much debate over its validity as an indication for pulmonary resection.

Though bronchial artery branches in the walls of a cavity

may be the source of significant hemoptysis, the life-threatening hemorrhages of tuberculosis are more often from the pulmonary arteries. The latter may become involved by the necrotizing process in the formation and expansion of tuberculous cavities, and fistulas may develop between bronchi and major pulmonary arterial branches. A dilated pulmonary artery branch which protrudes into the lumen of a cavity is referred to as a Rasmussen aneurysm.

In some patients a tuberculous bronchitis develops in the bronchi draining an active parenchymal lesion. The response to chemotherapy is usually good, but the destruction of tissue may result in bronchial stenosis. Another bronchial sequela, tuberculous bronchiectasis, is thought by many to be the result of traction on the bronchial wall during the healing of extensive parenchymal lesions. In these circumstances it is not necessary that the wall of the bronchus be involved by the actual tuberculous process.

It is important to remember that pulmonary tuberculosis can produce a variety of lesions in the lungs and that the lesions may vary in their location (Fig. 17-60). In the absence of cavitation, and without acid-fast bacilli in the sputum smears, a parenchymal lesion may be indistinguishable from bronchogenic carcinoma by x-ray studies. This is particularly the case with tuberculomas, and the latter are often removed because they present as solitary undiagnosed lesions. Improvements in diagnosis by bronchial brushing, flexible bronchoscopy, and percutaneous needle biopsy have reduced the number of patients who undergo thoracotomy and resection for diagnostic pur-

Fig. 17-60. Pulmonary tuberculosis, active. *A* and *B*. A large mass in the left upper lobe that was associated with marked atypia of cells obtained by bronchoscopy, and negative sputum smears for acid-fast bacilli. The resected lobe showed active tuberculosis without cavitation.

A   *B*

poses. Skin testing for tuberculosis can be helpful in the diagnosis, but only if the patient's previous status is known. A high percentage of patients with bronchogenic carcinoma have a positive tuberculin skin test, but no more than 5 percent of individuals with active pulmonary tuberculosis have a negative test if the procedure is done properly.

The deliberate, planned surgical treatment of tuberculosis is based on pulmonary resection after a period of drug therapy. In most instances lobectomy or segmentectomy is the procedure of choice. Pulmonary destruction is so extensive in an occasional patient that only pneumonectomy will suffice. The principal indications for resection are (1) extensive pulmonary destruction with bronchopleural fistula and empyema, (2) persistently active disease with drug-resistant organisms, (3) open-negative cavitary disease in selected irresponsible patients, (4) posttuberculous bronchostenosis with recurrent nontuberculous infections, (5) pulmonary hemorrhage, and (6) suspected (or proved) concomitant bronchogenic carcinoma.

Collapse therapy, consisting either of thoracoplasty or pneumonolysis, preceded pulmonary resection as a practical surgical approach to the treatment of tuberculosis. These techniques are inferior to resection, but an occasional patient with significant loss of pulmonary function and persistently positive sputum may not be a proper risk for removal of pulmonary tissue. In these circumstances thoracoplasty may be appropriate. An extrapleural removal of the necessary number of ribs may be done in two stages.

Pulmonary disease produced by acid-fast bacilli that are referred to as *atypical mycobacteria* has gained relative prominence in recent years. The two groups that are primarily responsible for pulmonary lesions are listed in Table 17-7, along with two additional groups that are principally associated with nonthoracic disease. Although the atypical mycobacteria are easily confused with *M. tuberculosis* in smears, they can be differentiated by their specific cultural and biological characteristics. *Mycobacterium kansasii* infections are seen predominantly in the Middle West, the Southwest, and California, while patients with disease due to the Battey bacillus are mostly located in the Southeast.

The pulmonary lesions caused by the atypical mycobacteria may be clinically and radiographically indistinguishable from those due to *M. tuberculosis.* Histologic studies of resected tissue may show characteristics suggesting the atypical causation, or the lesions may resemble straightforward tuberculosis.

The important difference is due to the resistance of the atypical mycobacteria to antituberculous drugs, and to their different skin test characteristics. Chemotherapy must be based on the results of sensitivity studies of the cultured mycobacteria, and three or four drugs are commonly used for initial treatment. Prolonged therapy of 2 to 4 years is generally anticipated. The indications for surgical treatment are approximately the same as for patients with infection due to *M. tuberculosis,* but a higher percentage will require resection because of drug failure.

ACTINOMYCOSIS AND NOCARDIOSIS

Clinical infection due to the actinomycetes occurs infrequently despite the wide and abundant distribution of the organisms. The *Actinomyces* are anaerobic or microaerophilic organisms; the *Nocardia* are obligate aerobes that show an acid-fast characteristic in sputum or tissue smears.

Actinomycosis is characterized by seemingly indolent, burrowing tissue invasion that leads to the formation of sinus tracts, abscesses, and fistulas. Considerable care may be required to identify the *Actinomyces israelii* by anaerobic cultures, and there is presently no serologic or skin test to allow confirmation of a suspected diagnosis. The often-mentioned "sulfur granules" consist of colonies of the organism in which the filaments are coated with proteinaceous material.

The bulk of cases involve the craniofacial tissues or the abdomen, and only 15 percent of patients have pulmonary actinomycosis. Because the organism is so often found in the tonsillar crypts or other areas of the mouth it is assumed that the usual portal of entry is by bronchial aspiration. Embolic spread from other areas is also possible, as well as direct extension into the thorax. From an initial lesion of pneumonic consolidation the disease can extend to involve the pleura, mediastinum, and chest wall, with eventual discharge of an abscess through a cutaneous sinus if not treated. The chest x-ray generally shows a nonspecific pulmonary consolidation, sometimes with cavitation (Fig. 17-61).

Penicillin in doses in 6 to 12 million units daily forms the basis of treatment, but erythromycin may be used for those patients who cannot take penicillin. Pulmonary resection is not usually required, although an occasional patient undergoes operation because the lesion is an undiagnosed infiltrate compatible with neoplasm. Drainage of empyema or chest-wall abscesses may be needed, and sinus tracts may be biopsied to establish the diagnosis.

Nocardiosis occurs predominantly in males, and the majority have thoracic involvement. A pulmonary infiltrate or consolidation is the usual beginning lesion. *Nocardia aster-*

Table 17-7. CLASSIFICATION OF ATYPICAL MYCOBACTERIA

Group	Example	Principal lesion
I. Photochromogens.....	*Mycobacterium kansasii*	Pulmonary disease
II. Scotochromogens.....	*Mycobacterium scrofulaceum*	Cervical lymphadenitis
III. Nonchromogenic	*Mycobacterium intracellulare* (Battey bacillus)	Pulmonary disease
IV. Rapid growers........	*Mycobacterium marinum*	Swimming pool skin granuloma

oides may gain a foothold after prolonged steroid therapy for other conditions, or following vigorous chemotherapy for infections or neoplasms. Characteristically, the *Nocardia* produces a more acute infection than the *Actinomyces*, with necrosis and abscess formation. Hemoptysis occurs in a quarter of the patients, and metastatic involvement of the central nervous system is common. The patient can present with a mass in the chest wall from the progressive extension of the pulmonary lesion. Again, the chest x-ray is nonspecific and the infection may resemble either neoplasm or tuberculosis.

Surgical resection is rarely required, and when it has been performed the underlying reason has generally been that of providing a diagnosis for an individual at risk for lung cancer. Either sulfadiazine or sulfamerazine is the drug of choice, and the majority of lesions respond satisfactorily to a prolonged course of the drug.

FUNGOUS INFECTIONS

Pulmonary infections due to fungi are generally in the form of chronic granulomatous lesions that resemble tuberculosis. Their roentgenographic appearance often raises the possibility of a neoplasm and makes it necessary to follow an aggressive course for diagnosis. An increased use of steroid therapy and antibiotics has been blamed for a greater incidence of generalized fungous infections in recent years.

Histoplasmosis must be considered the most frequent pulmonary mycotic infection in this country because of the estimated millions of persons who are said to have a positive skin test. The disease has a high incidence of subclinical infection in the Mississippi and Ohio River Valleys, as reflected by the pulmonary and hilar lymph node calcifications that represent healed or arrested disease. Erosion of a calcified lymph node into a bronchus may occur rarely, with the production of hemoptysis. A *broncholith* produced by this mechanism can obstruct the bronchial lumen and result in segmental or lobar suppuration. The *Histoplasma capsulatum* may produce a rounded solitary granuloma with a necrotic center that grossly resembles a tuberculoma. Figure 17-62 shows a histoplasmoma that was resected from a forty-two-year-old construction engineer who moved to the Ohio Valley a year earlier. An attempt at diagnosis by percutaneous needle biopsy had failed. His skin test and the complement-fixation titer both were positive, but he was a heavy smoker with a family history of lung cancer. Drug therapy is generally not required for localized lesions, whether or not they are resected.

A rare patient develops a progressive granulomatous and cavitary form of histoplasmosis that resembles tuberculosis in many respects. The lesions are predominant in the upper lobes and frequently bilateral. Sputum smears may show the organisms, and the diagnosis is supported by a rising complement-fixation titer. Untreated, this form of the disease can progress to a fatal outcome. However, amphotericin B is effective in the great majority of cases, and slow healing may follow a prolonged course of therapy to maximum dosage. For the patient whose sputum remains positive, and for those who develop bronchiectasis or major hemoptysis, pulmonary resection is indicated.

Fig 17-61. The chest x-ray in this patient with proved pulmonary actinomycosis shows an infiltrate in the anterior segment of the left upper lobe.

North American blastomycosis is seen principally in the Central and Southeastern United States as a mycotic disease with pulmonary involvement alone, with cutaneous lesions, or with any combination of pulmonary, skin, and systemic disease. The *Blastomyces dermatitidis* can be demonstrated in the sputum and in pus or scrapings from skin lesions. Granulomatous lesions in the lungs may become confluent with cavitation. On the chest x-ray the findings may be an infiltrate, a perihilar consolidation, or a lesion with multiple cavities that can resemble tuberculosis. The pulmonary lesion may be mistaken for a bronchogenic neoplasm (Fig. 17-63), and it can extend into the mediastinal structures.

The diagnosis is often made because of modest respiratory symptoms and chest x-ray findings that prompt a complete work-up. A complement-fixation test is available that shows increasing titers with a pulmonary lesion. The blastomycin skin test is of limited value because patients with well-developed lesions often fail to react to the antigen. Chemotherapy with either 2-hydroxystilbamidine or amphotericin B is effective in almost all patients. Resection is occasionally indicated if there is a strong suspicion of malignancy or if there is no response to drug therapy.

Coccidioidomycosis is another fungal disease with principal pulmonary involvement and a strong geographical association. *Coccidioides immitis* is distributed in the Southwest, including California, and the fungus may produce a subclinical infection sufficient to convert the skin test to positive. An acute bronchopulmonary disease ("valley fever") and granulomatous lesions that have considerable resemblance to tuberculosis are additional forms of the disease. The diagnosis is suggested by residence or even

A

B

Fig. 17-62. Histoplasmosis. *A*. The posteroanterior chest x-ray shows a faint round lesion in the right lower lobe. *B*. Tomograms demonstrate the lesion clearly and show its sharp borders. *C*. The lesion was removed by wedge resection; the cut surface shows a histoplasmoma.

C

a brief visit in the endemic area coupled with a rising complement-fixation titer, a positive skin test, and the presence of the organisms in the sputum.

The mainstay of treatment for progressive coccidioidomycosis is amphotericin B. Pulmonary resection is required when the probability of neoplasm cannot be excluded, and for the management of recurrent hemoptysis, pneumothorax, or progressive cavitation.

The surgical significance of *aspergillosis* is related to the propensity of the *Aspergillus fumigatus* (and a few other species) to invade preexisting pulmonary cavities due to tuberculosis, histoplasmosis, chronic lung abscess, or even neoplasm. An accumulation of mycelia and exudate progressively fills the cavity to form a mycetoma, or "fungus ball," which can be recognized radiographically by a thin rim of air surrounding the mass (Fig. 17-64). Recurrent hemoptysis is often associated with this form of aspergillosis, and it may necessitate pulmonary resection. For those

patients with compromised pulmonary function the significance of the blood spitting must be carefully judged. If pulmonary resection seems formidable, a trial of amphotericin B may be warranted. An alternate or subsequent treatment is the performance of cavernostomy by which the cavity can be evacuated through the chest wall and a portal established for dressings and topical chemotherapy. While management of this type is time-consuming it may give excellent results.

Cryptococcosis is best known for the serious central nervous system infections that are its hallmark. The lungs are the usual route of infection with the *Cryptococcus neoformans*, and occasionally an infiltrative or solitary nodular lesion is removed because of a suspicion of malignancy. Other organisms, including *Candida albicans, Sporotrichum schenkii*, and *Geotrichum candidum*, are occasionally responsible for pulmonary infections that may proceed to cavitation or to other complications that require consideration for operative treatment. In a high percentage of cases factors such as prolonged steroid therapy, immunosuppression, or diabetes mellitus seem to have an effect on the initiation and course of the disease.

SOLITARY PULMONARY NODULES

A perplexing yet intriguing problem in pulmonary disease is presented by the patient with an asymptomatic solitary pulmonary nodule on the chest x-ray. Also referred to as a "coin lesion," the solitary pulmonary nodule (SPN) is an abnormal density up to 4 cm in diameter and rounded or ovoid in appearance (Fig. 17-65). The lesion may be located in any region of the lung, and to qualify as an SPN it should have delineated margins that need not be pencil sharp. Further, the density should be free of cavitation or associated lung infiltrates. Eccentric flecks of calcium may be present, but lesions that are largely calcified or that have concentric calcium rings are not considered.

The stimulus for a high interest in the patient with an SPN has come from the superior cure rate for bronchogenic carcinoma when pulmonary resection is performed at that stage of its growth. Therefore, when a chest x-ray shows a nodular density not present on previous films, a possibility of neoplasm must be given early consideration. Demonstrating that the lesion is of recent development depends upon the availability of previous chest x-rays, or the official report at the least. Occasionally, the review of an earlier film will show a faint, small lesion that was overlooked originally but now provides an indication of growth rate. When previous x-rays document radiologic stability of a solitary nodule for 2 years or more, this is a strong indication that the lesion is benign.

Unfortunately, the differential diagnosis of an SPN includes many entities, among which are pulmonary hamartoma, granuloma, pulmonary arteriovenous fistula, pulmonary infarct, and benign and malignant tumors. It would be desirable to have a correct diagnosis for every patient, but it is critical only for those with a malignant lesion. Extensive experience with this problem has allowed some basic information to be accumulated: (1) a significant percentage of the nodules will prove to be malignant tumors, either primary or metastatic. In the Veterans Administration–Armed Forces Cooperative Study, 51 percent of the resected lesions were primary bronchogenic carcinoma in patients older than fifty years. The subjects were all males,

and most of them were moderate to heavy cigarette smokers. (2) For patients under the age of thirty-five years the likelihood that a nodule is malignant is only 1 to 2 percent. (3) The great majority of benign nodules are granulomas, some of which prove to be histoplasmosis, tuberculosis, or fungal lesions. (4) Roentgenologic differentiation of benign from malignant lesions is usually not possible. (5) A 5-year cure rate greater than 50 percent can be expected for those peripheral bronchogenic carcinomas that are less than 2 cm in diameter when resected. (6) Resection of solitary metastatic neoplasms may be associated with a significant survival rate. Some difference of opinion exists about the approach to management of patients with an SPN that either was not present on previous x-rays or has increased in size during an interval of several months. With an enthusiasm to improve the cure rate of lung cancer some groups have advocated an early thoracotomy with resection of the lesion for all patients above thirty to thirty-five years of age. Because an aggressive surgical policy results in the removal of a high percentage of benign lesions, others have proposed a conservative approach with greater emphasis on diagnostic techniques and observation. Sputum cytology may yield a diagnosis in fewer than 50 percent of those patients with a primary malignant SPN if an aggressive program is followed. Failure to demonstrate malignant cells does not exclude a neoplasm, however, and bronchial brushing is a more productive technique if the method is available. The increasing skill with flexible fiberoptic bronchoscopy has allowed more widespread use of brush

Fig. 17-63. North American blastomycosis. *A.* The posteroanterior chest x-ray shows a mass in the right field adjacent to the heart border. *B.* The tomogram is consistent with a neoplasm, but pulmonary resection showed active blastomycosis in the middle lobe.

A   *B*

A

B

C

Fig. 17-64. A "fungus ball" due to *Aspergillus fumigatus. A.* The lordotic-view chest x-ray shows a probable fungus ball in a patient with recurrent hemoptysis. *B.* A cut section of the resected upper lobe confirms the presence of a fungus ball in an old fibrotic cavity. *C.* The microscopic section of the cavity wall stained for fungi shows the mycelia infiltrating the tissue. (×580).

A

B

C

Fig. 17-65. A solitary pulmonary nodule. *A* and *B*. The postero-anterior and lateral chest x-rays show a round density in the lingula that had not been present on the patient's previous x-rays. *C*. The lesion is homogeneous, with smooth borders, on tomo-grams. A wedge resection showed the lesion to be a resolving pulmonary infarct.

biopsy, with a corresponding decrease in the need for diagnostic thoracotomy. Percutaneous needle-aspiration biopsy under fluoroscopic guidance is appropriate for lesions with a diameter of nearly 2 cm or more. If the biopsy material is suggestive, clearly shows a malignant lesion, or is nonspecific, resection is warranted. Only if the aspirated material shows a specific benign process is a plan of ob-

servation warranted in the older patient who smoked cigarettes.

Another approach to the patient with an undiagnosed coin lesion is based on observation of the growth rate of the lesion and calculation of the time necessary for doubling its volume. Serial roentgenograms provide the data for calculation of growth rate, and it is generally possible to detect that a lesion is growing within a few weeks. It has been demonstrated that the doubling time of a malignant nodule is usually between 37 and 465 days. Therefore, if the lesion under review is growing more slowly or more rapidly than this, the evidence is in favor of benignancy. Advocates of a conservative approach insist that present knowledge supports the concept that a pulmonary nodule can be watched safely for a period of time to determine whether it is growing. There has not been widespread acceptance of this method of watchful waiting.

Presently, a reasonable approach includes the concept that if there is a significant chance of malignancy (older patient, large lesion, long smoking history), early thoracotomy is appropriate. If the chance of malignancy is small, then needle biopsy and bronchial brush biopsy are appropriate, with watchful waiting and observation under limited circumstances.

Neoplasms

PRIMARY CARCINOMA OF THE LUNG

From a position of infrequent occurrence before 1900, bronchogenic carcinoma has become the leading cause of death due to cancer in this country. It is estimated that more than 85,000 persons died of lung cancer in 1976. Until the present decade, the disease was infrequent in women, but it now accounts for approximately 5 percent of all female cancer. In addition to the concern caused by its steady increase in frequency, bronchogenic carcinoma has also been disheartening because of its low cure rate. Only 5 to 8 percent of patients survive for 5 years after the diagnosis is confirmed. The remarkable aspect of lung cancer is its clear relationship to cigarette smoking, together with the fact that knowledge of this association has had so little effect on the frequency of tobacco use.

Though it seems certain that 90 percent or more of bronchogenic carcinomas are due to tobacco smoking, it is not so clear why a long period of exposure is generally required. The great majority of patients have smoked cigarettes for more than 20 years when the diagnosis of bronchogenic carcinoma is first made. Equally puzzling is the fact that most smokers do not develop clinical bronchogenic carcinoma, even if they have evidence of severe bronchitis or emphysema. Hundreds of separate organic compounds have been identified in cigarette smoke, and many have been shown to have carcinogenic potential. Since there has been little success in discouraging the smoking habit, considerable research is now directed at altering the composition of cigarette tobacco and the inhaled smoke.

Other studies have implicated chromium, nickel, asbestos, arsenic, radioactive minerals, and hydrocarbon distillates of coal and petroleum in the causation of bronchogenic carcinoma. Individuals working in the mining or processing of these materials may increase their hazard even further by heavy cigarette smoking. A co-carcinogen concept of respiratory viruses working in concert with tobacco smoke to produce bronchial neoplasia has been partly supported by experimental work in the recent past.

PATHOLOGY. Most primary lung carcinomas arise from the surface epithelium of the bronchial tree (bronchogenic). Table 17-8 shows a histopathologic classification of lung tumors developed as a working guide by a panel of the World Health Organization. Noteworthy is the fact that the term *bronchial adenoma,* which formerly referred to bronchial carcinoid, cylindroma, and mucoepidermoid tumors, has been eliminated. The latter two neoplasms are considered to be of bronchial-gland origin.

Several forms of atypical epithelial proliferation are thought to precede pulmonary neoplasms, and the identification of these processes in a patient may heighten the suspicion that a tumor is present. Carcinoma in situ is probably the fully developed expression of squamous metaplasia and dysplasia. These processes have been considered to be a frequent precursor of squamous bronchogenic carcinoma. A type of atypical epithelial proliferation of

Table 17-8. HISTOPATHOLOGIC CLASSIFICATION OF LUNG TUMORS (WHO CLASSIFICATION)

1. Epidermoid carcinoma
2. Small-cell anaplastic carcinoma
3. Adenocarcinoma
4. Large-cell carcinoma
   a. Solid tumors with mucinlike content
   b. Solid tumors without mucinlike content
   c. Giant-cell carcinoma
   d. "Clear"-cell carcinoma
5. Combined epidermoid and adenocarcinoma
6. Carcinoid tumor
7. Bronchial gland tumors
   a. Cylindroma
   b. Mucoepidermoid tumor
   c. Others
8. Papillary tumors of the surface epithelium
9. "Mixed" tumors and carcinosarcomas
10. Sarcoma
11. Unclassified
12. Mesotheliomas
    a. Localized
    b. Diffuse
13. Melanoma

cuboidal or columnar cells is referred to as acinar proliferation. Interstitial fibrosis and honeycombing of the lung are especially associated with this process, and the atypical proliferation develops as a regenerative process lining the remodeled air spaces. Finally, an atypical proliferation of Kultschitzsky cells is associated with development of the carcinoid tumors.

Bronchogenic carcinomas develop twice as frequently in the upper lobes as in the lower lobes, and the neoplasms may be present for several years before symptoms occur. In fact, it has been estimated that a tumor nodule must go through approximately 30 doublings to become 1 cm in diameter, a size that is large enough to be seen on the routine chest x-ray. If true, this could mean that many pulmonary tumors may have been present for as long as 8 years before discovery. Slow growth of this type is most often a characteristic of *epidermoid* (squamous) carcinoma. The epidermoid type of bronchial tumor resembles squamous epithelium and is therefore considered to arise after a preliminary squamous metaplasia has replaced the normal respiratory pseudostratified epithelium. The degree of differentiation in epidermoid neoplasms varies widely, and an occasional lesion is so highly anaplastic that its designation as an epidermoid tumor is speculative. Squamous cell carcinoma has been the most prevalent type of lung cancer in the United States, even though the criteria for classification used by individual pathologists has influenced its incidence at different institutions. Reports from several large medical centers, however, have documented a progressive increase in the incidence of adenocarcinoma, suggesting that it may replace the epidermoid tumor as the leading pulmonary neoplasm.

An epidermoid tumor has a tendency to present either as a central bulky neoplasm associated with bronchial obstruction or as an expanding peripheral lesion that develops cavitation. When centrally located, the tumor may involve the peribronchial and hilar lymph nodes by direct extension rather than by lymphatic permeation. Central necrosis and cavitation may also occur in the tumors that arise near the pulmonary hilum, and evidence of metastases may be absent even with tumors of very large size. When the tumor is located in the periphery, the slow growth rate and late metastasis characteristic of squamous cell carcinoma may allow selected patients to have operative removal for cure even with localized chest-wall invasion. The Pancoast syndrome represents a specific example of this circumstance wherein a tumor in the superior pulmonary sulcus may invade the brachial plexus, the upper two ribs or transverse processes, and the vascular structures at the thoracic apex.

Adenocarcinoma of the lung generally arises in the subsegmental bronchi away from the pulmonary hilum. These tumors are often acinar in structure, with or without mucin production. In the absence of a smoking history or occupational exposure to known bronchogenic carcinogens, a malignant bronchial neoplasm has a high likelihood of this classification. Pulmonary adenocarcinoma is especially prevalent in women, and the age distribution is purportedly greater than that of epidermoid tumors. Growth may be rapid, and early metastasis by the vascular route is common. Occasionally an adenocarcinoma may undergo symmetrical expansion in the lung periphery to reach a size and configuration that led to its designation as a "cannonball" tumor in earlier days. When an adenocarcinoma is anaplastic in appearance the pathologist may be hardpressed to determine the classification with light microscopy alone. This is also true with other types of bronchogenic carcinoma, and multiple sections taken from separate areas of the same neoplasm may suggest a different classification for each area.

The pulmonary neoplasms that are designated as *bronchioloalveolar* tumors are considered by many to be variants of adenocarcinoma. For years, bronchioloalveolar cell carcinoma has been described as occurring in two forms, localized and diffuse, without a completely satisfactory explanation of the relationship between them. The localized tumor develops as a slowly growing peripheral neoplasm that is highly differentiated. Electron microscopy has been reported to show cellular features suggestive of alveolar origin in some instances, while other tumors have contained atypical Clara cells suggestive of an origin in bronchioles. Resection of the solitary or localized tumor has given a 5-year cure rate of approximately 50 percent. This contrasts remarkably with the diffuse form of bronchioloalveolar cell carcinoma, in which there is rapid dissemination of the neoplasm in one or both lungs, with no possible consideration of operative treatment. While the two forms of this neoplasm may be similar by microscopic appearance, the behavior necessarily raises the issue of whether they are two separate pulmonary tumors. Speculation that the diffuse form could represent uncontrolled metastases from an original single lesion developing after an unknown interval of time has not been corroborated to general satisfaction. Either multicentric origin or some other variant of biologic behavior that sets the diffuse neoplasm apart from the localized tumor seems more plausible.

The *small-cell anaplastic* carcinoma, sometimes referred to as "oat cell carcinoma," is a highly malignant, rapidly growing neoplasm that is most often central in location because of origin from a proximal bronchus. In addition to early spread by hilar and mediastinal lymph-node involvement, this tumor aggressively invades local structures and is disseminated by early vascular invasion. Because of its rapid growth and spread, many consider the oat cell carcinoma to have no place among the bronchogenic tumors that are treated by surgical resection.

Large-cell anaplastic bronchogenic carcinomas may have either a central or a peripheral location similar to epidermoid tumors. Mucin-producing cells are not uncommon, but this is not sufficient to classify these tumors as a variant of adenocarcinoma. Grouped with the large-cell neoplasms are the less common "giant-cell" bronchogenic tumors. The name for these highly malignant cancers is derived from the giant, multinucleated cells that characterize their microscopic appearance.

The term "scar carcinoma" has been used increasingly in recent years to refer to the concept that lung cancer occasionally arises at the site of previous pulmonary disease. This might be considered analogous to the circumstance of skin cancer arising in a burn scar. Therefore, when a patient with previous pulmonary tuberculosis develops a neoplasm in the same area that was scarred by the tuberculous process, there is generally a speculation about the cause-and-effect relationship. The majority of such lesions have been adenocarcinoma or bronchiolar cell carcinoma, but there is not yet convincing proof that the concept is valid.

CLINICAL MANIFESTATIONS. Bronchogenic carcinoma is seen predominantly in men of forty-five to sixty-five years of age with a peak incidence at fifty-five to sixty years. It is not rare in men less than forty-five years old, and the diagnosis is being made with increasing frequency in women who are in their fifth decade. The disease is discovered incidentally in a patient without symptoms in about 5 percent of cases. Such discovery is by means of chest x-ray for the greatest number of patients, but sputum cytology occasionally leads to the eventual identification of an otherwise occult tumor.

Because intermittent or chronic cough is so common among long-term smokers it may be difficult to establish an onset of symptoms. Nevertheless, about three-fourths of patients with bronchogenic carcinoma must be said to have coughing as a principal symptom. Hemoptysis in the form of blood streaking of sputum occurs in about half of all patients, but massive hemoptysis or spitting of blood clots is unusual. Chest pain of a dull, nonspecific type is described by some patients whose tumor is subsequently found to be free of chest-wall involvement. When there is invasion of the parietal pleura or chest wall the patient may have mild to severe pain that is either localized or radicular in form. Fever and purulent sputum may mark an increase of symptoms in the patient whose tumor is producing major bronchial obstruction, and wheezing or stridor may also be present.

Involvement of the left recurrent laryngeal nerve (rarely the right nerve), either by direct tumor invasion or by

A

B

C

extension from a metastatic lymph node, may result in hoarseness that is often minimized by the patient. Direct tumor extension into the superior vena cava or its compression by the expanding neoplasm produces early symptoms of edema of the eyes and prominence or distension of the superficial veins over the upper part of the body. Dyspnea occurring as a symptom of bronchogenic carcinoma is usually associated with a large pleural effusion, paralysis of a hemidiaphragm due to phrenic nerve invasion, or major bronchial obstruction.

A loss of appetite accompanied by weight loss of more than a few pounds is an ominous sign in the patient with a bronchial neoplasm; such patients usually have either an unresectable tumor or systemic metastases. A deliberate

D

Fig. 17-66. Pulmonary hypertrophic osteoarthropathy associated with oat cell carcinoma. *A.* The chest x-ray in a thirty-nine-year-old man shows a left hilar mass that proved to be oat cell carcinoma on bronchial biopsy. *B.* Painful clubbing of the fingers and toes developed during an interval of approximately 3 months. *C.* A close-up of the patient's foot demonstrates clubbing of the toes. *D.* The arrow points to the new bone formation on the femur.

search should be made for evidence of spread by isotope scanning and computed tomography. Because the metastatic spectrum of these tumors is so wide, almost any imaginable symptom can be produced. A rare patient may develop pulmonary hypertrophic osteoarthropathy with clubbing of the digits (Fig. 17-66). Evidence of metastases may be absent, and the process may be partially reversed if the tumor is resected.

A small percentage of patients with bronchogenic carcinoma present with *extrapulmonary nonmetastatic* manifestations that are considered due to elaboration of hormone-like substances by the neoplastic cells (Fig. 17-67). The occurrence of these signs and symptoms does not imply systemic spread of the bronchogenic tumor, and resection of the lesion is generally associated with a regression of the symptoms. Ultrastructural studies have demonstrated the presence of neurosecretory-type granules in the cells of many anaplastic tumors, and the more striking clinical symptoms are associated with oat cell carcinomas. An example is a Cushing-like syndrome which differs from the classic Cushing's syndrome by an older age incidence, a greater frequency in males, and a more rapid clinical course. The ectopic adrenocorticotropic hormone that has been demonstrated in the oat cell tumors appears indistinguishable from the normal hormone. An inappropriate antidiuresis associated with the anaplastic small-cell carcinoma occasionally results in the symptoms of water intoxication with hyponatremia and increasing cerebral symptoms. The carcinoid syndrome has been reported in a few patients with oat cell carcinoma, and either 5-hydroxytryptamine or 5-hydroxytryptophan may be secreted.

Hypercalcemia caused by a parathormone-like polypeptide has most often been associated with squamous bronchogenic carcinoma. Tender gynecomastia and ectopic gonadotropin secretion have been identified with large-cell anaplastic carcinoma. Satisfactory resection of the squamous neoplasm reverses the hypercalcemia, but it may return if the tumor recurs. A group of carcinomatous neuromyopathies is included in the nonmetastatic manifestations of lung cancer, and their incidence is thought to be as high as 15 percent. The symptoms may be subtle or somewhat overshadowed by the pulmonary complaints. Thus, the patient with bronchogenic carcinoma who mentions weakness along with his cough and chest pain is usually not questioned in detail about the characteristics of the weakness. This is the principal symptom, however, of a myasthenia-like syndrome that is probably due to a defect in neuromuscular conduction. Peripheral and central neuropathies also occur, and their differentiation from the symptoms of metastatic lesions can be important. With the former, pulmonary resection may be possible and result in disappearance of the symptoms.

DIAGNOSIS. In recent years the trend has been toward a maximal effort at obtaining a cytologic or tissue diagnosis of lung carcinoma before subjecting the patient with a suspected tumor to thoracotomy. Even further, mediastinoscopy and mediastinotomy have found increasing use to determine the presence of hilar and mediastinal spread of tumor, with a corresponding decrease in frequency of fruitless exploratory thoracotomy. Unfortunately, bron-

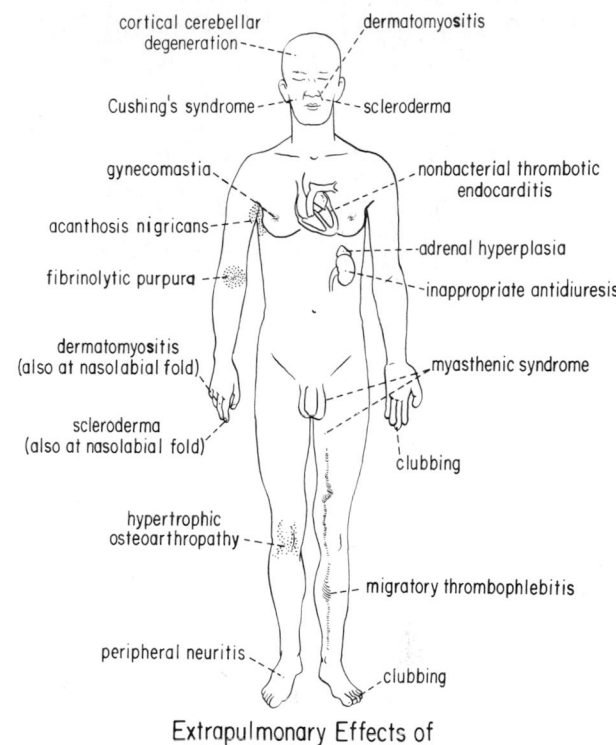

Extrapulmonary Effects of Pulmonary Neoplasms

Fig. 17-67. Various extrathoracic nonmetastatic manifestations of bronchogenic carcinoma occur, but their frequency varies and they are often overlooked. (*From J. H. Kennedy, Extrapulmonary Effects of Cancer of the Lung and Pleura, J Thorac Cardiovasc Surg, 61:514, 1971, with permission of the author and publisher.*)

chogenic carcinoma has no characteristic or unique radiographic appearance. Therefore, thought must be given to the possibility of carcinoma with almost any type of pulmonary infiltrate, nodule, mass, or atelectasis. A pyogenic lung abscess secondary to aspiration may closely mimic the appearance of cavitated epidermoid carcinoma, even with tomography (Fig. 17-68). Some help with differentiation is obtained when the wall of the cavitated lesion is irregularly thickened with projections of tumor into the cavity. In those incidences when attempts to obtain cytologic evidence of neoplasm have failed, and factors such as young age or alcoholism increase the likelihood of a true abscess, it may be proper to treat the patient for a short interval with antibiotics. Some modest improvement in the appearance of the chest x-ray and the patient's condition does not exclude carcinoma. Close observation must be continued, along with serial studies of sputum cytology.

The cytologic examination of properly obtained and preserved sputum specimens may yield a high percentage of positive diagnoses in patients with bronchial carcinoma. By examining serial daily specimens, often combined with chest physiotherapy to increase the yield of sputum, a cytologic diagnosis may be made in as many as two-thirds of patients. Bronchoscopy is the fundamental diagnostic technique for patients with suspected carcinoma, and the development of the flexible fiberscope has increased the

A

B

Fig. 17-68. Lung abscess masquerading as bronchogenic cancer. *A*. The posteroanterior chest x-ray shows a mass with a small cavity in the right apex, mediastinal lymph nodes (*arrow*). Several healed rib fractures are seen (*arrow*), and the patient was known to be a "social drinker." *B*. A tomogram confirms the presence of a cavity and suggests that the walls are thick. *C*. A chest x-ray 7 months later shows that the abscess has healed with antibiotic therapy. The decision to treat for abscess rather than for lung cancer hinged on the history of alcoholism.

C

positive diagnosis yield to better than 70 percent in some hands. These results include bronchial brushing and cytologic studies of bronchial washings that may be obtained at the same time. The endoscopist must determine the proximal extent of a visualized neoplasm because the patient's operability may be governed by the closeness of the tumor to the tracheal carina.

Small peripheral lesions often present a problem in diagnosis; this was discussed in the preceding section on solitary pulmonary nodules. An infrequent dilemma occurs when a patient is found to have persistently positive sputum cytology without a visible lesion on the chest x-rays. Other sources of the malignant cells, such as the nasophar-

ynx or piriform sinuses, have to be eliminated, and careful flexible bronchoscopic examination may need to be performed at intervals of 4 to 8 weeks. Selective bronchial brushing or selective washing may localize the lesion, but exfoliated cells can become displaced into a bronchus other than the one of origin. This suggests caution in planning a major resection on the basis of these techniques alone.

Percutaneous transthoracic needle biopsy as a technique for obtaining a tissue diagnosis is increasingly accepted for patients who are not considered operable because of tumor extent, evidence of metastases, or general factors such as age. For patients who are considered to be candidates for resection there is widespread resistance to needle biopsy among surgeons. This is based on the possibility of tumor seeding in the pleural cavity or the needle track through the chest wall. Though this rarely happens, many thoracic surgeons are influenced by recollection of a single occurrence. Pneumothorax is the most frequent problem following needle biopsy, but less than half of the patients with this complication require treatment. In a series of 5,300 percutaneous biopsies performed in 2,726 patients, Sinner reported a definitive diagnosis in 90.7 percent, with pneumothorax occurring in 27.2 percent. Two percent of the patients had hemoptysis, and one subcutaneous tumor implant occurred in the more than 1,200 patients with malignant lesions.

A pleural effusion in the presence of a suspected or confirmed pulmonary cancer is generally an indication of extensive tumor that is producing pleural or mediastinal invasion. However, an effusion can occur as a consequence of bronchial obstruction with atelectasis or infection. The fluid should be examined for the presence of blood and malignant cells with a simultaneous pleural needle biopsy if feasible. A demonstration of malignant cells in the effusion occurs in approximately half the patients with visceral or parietal pleural invasion by the neoplasm.

It is unfortunate that approximately 50 percent of all patients with bronchogenic cancer are beyond consideration for operative treatment when the opportunity for definitive diagnosis is first presented. For this reason diagnosis includes a conscientious effort to determine whether localized or metastatic spread has occurred. This is based on a careful history, a meticulous examination for suggestive lymph nodes, and a consideration of how detailed the work-up should be. Some physicians recommend a routine roentgenographic bone survey for all patients who might be considered for operative treatment. This is based on the known incidence of 21 percent skeletal involvement in autopsy series and the frequency of bone metastases in patients who are followed after pulmonary resection. In the absence of skeletal symptoms this has not been sufficiently productive to justify the cost. The same principle applies to the routine use of brain and liver scans. Scanning with radioactive gallium has been disappointing for revealing unsuspected metastases, but some groups use gallium scans to help in the decision to perform mediastinoscopy or mediastinotomy. There should be no hesitancy to utilize any or all of these techniques to survey for metastatic spread in the presence of suggestive symptoms, or if the patient's general condition suggests systemic spread. With any question of a metastasis an attempt at biopsy should be considered before treatment for the primary neoplasm is planned.

TREATMENT. Bronchogenic carcinoma can be cured by pulmonary resection. Though the preceding statement is true, many qualifiers must be added. In general, the factors that determine the likelihood of cure are (1) the cell type, (2) tumor size, (3) lymph-node metastases, (4) direct extension of tumor to adjacent structures, and (5) distant metastases. These factors are the same for malignant neoplasms arising in any region of the body and are listed here to indicate that the approach to treatment depends on an assessment of individual factors as well as the constellation of factors. For example, if bronchoscopic biopsy of the neoplasm shows that it is a small-cell anaplastic carcinoma (oat cell), the majority of surgeons would consider the patient not a candidate for surgery.

Unfortunately, any consideration of operative treatment for cure is impossible in about half of all patients with bronchogenic carcinoma at the time of hospital admission. These patients have centrally located neoplasms with evidence of mediastinal extension, symptoms of distant metastases, or compromised cardiopulmonary function that precludes a major pulmonary resection. A primary goal of the patient's work-up is to confirm the suspected diagnosis of carcinoma by means other than exploratory thoracotomy. Mediastinotomy and mediastinoscopy are occasionally used to obtain a tissue diagnosis in the patient with a pulmonary lesion whose sputum cytology and bronchoscopic procedures have failed to give a positive yield. Thus, there is an overlap of the diagnostic procedures with the techniques for establishing the patient's suitability for operation. Despite a proper application of all reasonable diagnostic procedures, 10 to 20 percent of patients will undergo thoracotomy without a proved diagnosis before operation.

Factors such as the patient's age and tumor extension outside the lung vary in their influence on the decision of individual surgeons to attempt pulmonary resection. Though there is increasing risk of morbidity and mortality for those who undergo major pulmonary resection after sixty years of age, it has been demonstrated that patients of seventy years and beyond tolerate lobectomy with an acceptable mortality rate. Invasion of either the phrenic or the recurrent laryngeal nerve is considered a contraindication to thoracotomy by the majority of surgeons. This is not totally accepted, and because the phrenic nerve involvement is most often along its course over the pericardium, the latter can be resected en bloc with the lung in selected patients.

Direct extension of tumor into the chest wall may be considered a contraindication to attempted resection in the presence of other risk factors. When the tumor is a well-differentiated squamous carcinoma, however, cure is occasionally achieved by localized chest-wall resection, thus justifying an aggressive approach for selected patients.

Though total pneumonectomy would seem to be the ideal operation for bronchogenic carcinoma, it carries a significantly higher mortality rate than lobectomy (Fig. 17-69). For this reason, and because the survivors have a greater ventilatory handicap after the removal of an entire lung, most surgeons have come to accept lobectomy as the procedure of choice for bronchial cancer. This applies only to those patients whose tumor can be adequately removed by lobectomy. Brock has emphasized that a routine adherence to the concept of lobectomy can compromise the chance for cure of some patients. Lobectomy sharply limits the extent of en bloc lymph-node removal that can be performed, and it is clear that hilar and mediastinal nodal metastases have a marked effect on 5-year survival. Radical pneumonectomy, as described by Brock, provides for removal of anterior and posterior mediastinal lymph nodes along with excision of the ipsilateral tracheobronchial nodes. This represents an extensive resection of the lymphatic field, but there is no agreement among surgeons about the selection of patients for the radical procedure. Table 17-9 from a recent report by Lord Brock shows the results in an extensive personal series of patients who underwent lobectomy, simple pneumonectomy, or radical pneumonectomy. The 5-year survival rates are impressive, but the patients who underwent resection represented only a small fraction of all those seen with lung cancer during the study period.

PERIOSTEUM

A 1

A 2

B

PARIETAL
PLEURA

LUNG

RIBS

SACROSPINALIS

A 3

C 1

C 2

D 1

D 2

E

INF. PULMONARY V.

F 1

BRONCHUS

F 2

G

PLEURAL
GRAFT

Table 17-9. COMPARATIVE RESULTS
IN 293 PATIENTS OPERATED ON
FOR BRONCHOGENIC CARCINOMA

Operation	Total no. of patients	Mortality, %	5-year survival, %	Still alive
Lobectomy..........	86	3.5	41	10
Simple pneumonectomy.	89	30.00	30	2
Radical pneumonectomy.	118	15.25	39	11
Total	293	13.00	32	23

SOURCE: Reproduced from Lord R. Brock, Long Survival after Operation for Cancer of the Lung, *Br J Surg,* **62**:1, 1975, by permission of the author and publisher.

Not infrequently, the surgeon is confronted with a circumstance in which the patient's neoplasm is relatively small but its growth has obviated the likelihood of cure with less than pneumonectomy. If the patient is young there is usually little hesitancy about removing the entire lung, especially if the pulmonary function studies are satisfactory. For an elderly patient, however, there is greater caution, and the decision may have to be supported by a combination of experience and objective data. Figure 17-70 shows the preoperative chest x-rays of a seventy-one-year-old obese man whose pulmonary function values were as follows:

	Predicted, L	Observed, L	% Predicted
Vital capacity	4.2	3.5	83
FEV$_1$ second	2.8	2.6	93
Maximal voluntary ventilation	123	149	121
Peak flow	510(L/min.)	560(L/min.)	110

Fig. 17-69. Resection of lung. *A.* Opening into pleural cavity: (1) periosteum incised over the rib; (2) subperiosteal resection being performed; (3) pleura opened through bed of resected rib. *B.* Freeing of pulmonary artery from adjacent structures. *C.* Ligation and division of pulmonary artery: (1) artery doubly ligated with an adequate distance between the two ligatures; (2) artery transected between two ligatures. *D.* Peripheral dissection of pulmonary artery to increase safety factor: (1) branches of pulmonary artery and main pulmonary artery identified; (2) branches individually double-ligated and transected. *E.* Division of pulmonary vein. Double ligatures are on inferior pulmonary vein which is to be transected. *F.* Transection of bronchus. This is performed after ligation of pulmonary arteries and veins. Diagram indicates bronchial transection during a left pneumonectomy. (1) Clamp is applied to bronchus distad, and on the bronchus is transected, the proximal end is closed with interrupted sutures in order to avoid a widely open bronchus with its associated ventilatory disturbance; alternately, the bronchus may be closed with an automatic stapler. (2) Progression of bronchial transection. *G.* Pleural flap placed over sutured bronchial stump.

At operation the upper-lobe tumor had extended across the major fissure to invade the lower lobe. Despite his age and obesity, his excellent pulmonary function and vigorous life-style suggested that he would tolerate pneumonectomy satisfactorily. More than 2 years following removal of his left lung with the epidermoid carcinoma he plays golf three times weekly and has shown no sign of recurrence.

For purposes of contrast, Fig. 17-71 shows the preoperative chest x-rays of a fifty-five-year-old man with a suspected carcinoma in the right pulmonary apex. He was smoking two packages of cigarettes daily and had clinical manifestations of significant chronic airways disease. After 2 weeks of sharply reduced smoking, chest physical therapy, and antibiotic treatment for his bronchitis, the following pulmonary function values were obtained:

	Predicted, L	Observed, L	% Predicted
Vital capacity.......	4.1	4.1	100
FEV$_1$ second........	3.1	2.0	65
Maximal voluntary ventilation.........	135	70	52

The marked reductions in his expiratory flow rates indicated that pneumonectomy would carry a prohibitive risk if the neoplasm had spread to the hilum. Therefore, a preliminary mediastinotomy was done, and no evidence of tumor was found in the pulmonary hilum or the right mediastinal lymph nodes. A subsequent right upper lobectomy was well tolerated, and the neoplasm was found to be a bronchioloalveolar cell carcinoma without lymph-node involvement.

Paulson has emphasized the great importance of selectivity in the surgical treatment of lung cancer. This requires a maximum use of preoperative evaluation through tomography, mediastinotomy, or mediastinoscopy, occasional pulmonary angiography, and acknowledgment of the differing biologic behavior of the different histologic types. The goal is to avoid exploratory thoracotomy in those patients whose tumor cannot be resected for cure. Figure 17-72 shows a comparison of survival for two 10-year time periods according to the stage of lymph-node involvement. For patients without lymph-node metastases (stage 0) the 5-year survival increased from 31 percent during the first period to 45 percent during the second 10-year era. For those with hilar node involvement (stage 1-2) the 5-year survival rate increased from 22 to 30 percent during the same time frames. Patients with mediastinal nodal involvement (stage 3) had very low survival rates in both decades.

Figure 17-73, also from Paulson's extensive experience, shows a survival comparison according to central or peripheral location of the patient's neoplasm, with relation to the extent of resection. The ability to perform lobectomy for a centrally located neoplasm generally implies a small tumor and a favorable cell type (epidermoid, most frequently). None of the 45 patients who underwent resection for small-cell undifferentiated carcinoma survived for 5 years. Interestingly, in a recent report by Shields, if oat cell

A

B

Fig. 17-70. *A*. The posteroanterior chest x-ray shows a mass in the left upper lobe that is compatible with pulmonary carcinoma. *B*. A tomogram indicates cavitation in the lesion compatible with epidermoid carcinoma. The diagnosis was confirmed by examination of the resected left lung.

cancer is discounted, the cell type per se had little or no significant influence on survival when curative resection was performed and lymph-node involvement was absent. A barely significant difference was noted in favor of squamous carcinoma when lymph nodes were involved.

A uniform method for staging lung cancer, based on the full definition of the extent of disease, is fundamental to the evaluation of treatment methods. Table 17-10 shows the definitions for tumor size and for lymph-node and distant metastases described by the American Joint Committee for Cancer Staging. From these definitions the extent of the neoplasm in any individual patient may be described as Stage I, II, or III as shown in Table 17-11. General adoption of this system should improve the meaning of reports on treatment results from differing medical centers. The place of radiation therapy in bronchogenic carcinoma is not easily defined. A hope for improved survival by combining preoperative radiation with resection has not been realized for the usual lung cancer patient. A generally recognized exception to this conclusion is the patient with Pancoast's syndrome, in whom preoperative radiation often relieves pain and allows a subsequent resection with a modest chance for long-term survival. Some surgeons also feel that preoperative radiotherapy is of benefit for the patient with chest-wall involvement in any location. Although firm data to prove its efficacy are still lacking, most surgeons request postoperative radiation therapy for those patients whose resection specimens show metastases to the hilar or mediastinal lymph nodes. The most extensive use of radiation therapy in lung cancer is for attempted palliation in those patients with extensive disease that precludes operation, or for those whose neoplasms are unresectable when thoracotomy is performed. In the occasional patient whose disease is still localized in the thorax, prolonged palliation may be achieved. Investigative work on therapy using particles with high linear energy transfer and interstitial implanta-

tion of radioactive ^{125}I is currently under assessment for local control of lung cancer.

Until very recently chemotherapy had little to offer for the patient with bronchogenic carcinoma. Now, the application of multiple-agent therapy has shown success in palliation of the condition of some patients with small-cell anaplastic carcinoma and disseminated epidermoid cancer. The successful chemotherapeutic programs have featured two characteristics: (1) a combination of agents that have shown some activity singly in at least one histologic type of lung carcinoma, but have different pharmacologic actions, and (2) the use of drugs that are active at different points within the cycle of cell division, and which are administered in a fashion to potentiate their cytotoxic activity. The combination of vincristine and bleomycin has proved to be effective for epidermoid carcinoma with use of a drug-scheduling technique that provides sequential administration of vincristine followed by the bleomycin. Other multiple-drug programs that include Adriamycin (doxorubicin HCL), bleomycin, nitrosureas, vincristine, and nitrogen mustard may show effective activity against epidermoid carcinoma as well as small-cell anaplastic cancer in at least 50 percent of patients. Significant palliation is often limited to 15 to 25 percent of patients, but chemotherapy is often used only in the far-advanced cases. At present, effective drug therapy for primary adenocarcinoma and large-cell undifferentiated carcinoma is lacking.

Concepts of adjuvant therapy are not new, and it is very disappointing that an effective systemic control of bronchogenic carcinoma is not available for routine use in those

A

B

C

D

Fig. 17-71. *A*. The posteroanterior chest x-ray shows an indeterminate lesion in the right apex of this fifty-five-year-old man with compromised pulmonary function. *B*. A lateral chest x-ray suggests a posterior location of the lesion and radiographic features of chronic lung disease. *C*. A tomogram indicates that the lesion is a solid mass with features of malignancy. *D*. Microscopic examination of the tumor in the lobectomy specimen showed a bronchioloalveolar cell carcinoma. (×250.)

Table 17-10. DEFINITIONS OF T, N, AND M CATEGORIES FOR CARCINOMA OF THE LUNG

Type	Definition
T—primary tumors:	
T0	No evidence of primary tumor
TX	Tumor proved by presence of malignant cells in bronchopulmonary secretions but not visualized roentgenographically or bronchoscopically, or any tumor that cannot be assessed
TIS	Carcinoma in situ
T1	A tumor 3 cm or less in diameter, surrounded by lung or visceral pleura and without invasion proximal to a lobar bronchus at bronchoscopy
T2	A tumor more than 3 cm in diameter, or any size with visceral pleural invasion or associated atelectasis or obstructive pneumonitis that extends to the hilar region but involves less than the entire lung; at bronchoscopy the proximal extent of tumor must be within a lobar bronchus or at least 2 cm distal to the carina
T3	A tumor of any size with extension into an adjacent structure such as the parietal pleura, chest wall, diaphragm, or mediastinum and its contents; or demonstrated bronchoscopically to involve a main bronchus less than 2 cm distal to the carina; any tumor associated with atelectasis or obstructive pneumonitis of an entire lung or with pleural effusion
N—regional lymph nodes:	
N0	No demonstrable metastasis to regional lymph nodes
N1	Metastasis to lymph nodes in the peribronchial or ipsilateral hilar region, or both, including direct extension
N2	Metastasis to mediastinal lymph nodes
M—distant metastasis:	
M0	No distant metastasis
M1	Distant metastasis such as supraclavicular, or contralateral hilar lymph nodes, lung, brain, etc.

patients who undergo pulmonary resection. Whether systemic therapy will take the form of antitumor agents or enhancement of the patient's innumocompetence is only speculated.

IMMUNOLOGY OF PULMONARY CARCINOMA. Recent studies have emphasized the important but not clearly defined role of immunodeficiency in the prognosis of patients with many forms of cancer. An impaired reaction to delayed cutaneous hypersensitivity testing with 2-4-dinitrochlorobenzene has been demonstrated in many lung cancer patients, and those who are unable to become sensitized to this antigen often have unresectable neoplasms. Impaired lymphocyte transformation with in vitro stimulation by several antigens and mitogens has also

demonstrated a marked decrease in immunocompetence in patients with pulmonary carcinoma. One of the mechanisms of immune deficiency is thought to be the presence of circulating immunosuppressive factors in the serum of the lung cancer patient. Whether such factors might be produced by the neoplasm is only speculative. The observation some years ago of improved survival in patients who develop pleural empyema after pulmonary resection for bronchogenic cancer seems to coincide with current concepts. Presumably the mechanism that increased the cure rate in those patients with postoperative empyema was an immunostimulation.

On the basis of the observations just described, clinical trials are under way to evaluate the usefulness of immunostimulation as adjuvant therapy in patients who undergo pulmonary resection for carcinoma. McKneally has utilized intrapleural BCG and shown a significant improvement in the 1-year recurrence rate of tumor. Two other nonspecific immunopotentiators, formalized *Corynebacterium parvum,* and L-tetramisole (levamisole) are being used in clinical trials. The early results are encouraging, and it is possible that combinations of both immunotherapy and chemotherapy may be appropriate to supplement the surgical treatment of bronchial cancer.

BRONCHIAL CARCINOID TUMOR

Carcinoid neoplasms of the bronchus arise from Kultschitzsky-type cells and histologically resemble the carci-

Table 17-11. STAGE GROUPING IN CANCER OF THE LUNG

Type	Definition
Occult carcinoma:	
TX N0 M0	An occult carcinoma with bronchopulmonary secretions containing malignant cells but without other evidence of the primary tumor or evidence of metastasis to the regional lymph nodes or distant metastis
Stage I:	
TIS N0 M0	Carcinoma in situ
T1 N0 M0	A tumor that can be classified T1
T1 N1 M0	without any metastasis or with
T2 N0 M0	metastasis to the lymph nodes in the ipsilateral hilar region only, or a tumor that can be classified T2 without any metastasis to nodes or distant metastasis
Stage II:	
T2 N1 M0	A tumor classified as T2 with metastasis to the lymph nodes in the ipsilateral hilar region only
Stage III:	
T3 with any N or M	Any tumor more extensive than T2,
N2 with any T or M	or any tumor with metastasis to
M1 with any T or N	the lymph nodes in the mediastinum, or with distant metastasis

SURVIVAL BY STAGE OF DISEASE (1950-1959)

SURVIVAL BY STAGE OF DISEASE (1960-1969)

Fig. 17-72. A comparison of survival after operation for patients with lung cancer during two consecutive decades. The staging is based on lymph-node involvement, and for patients with positive hilar nodes the 5-year survival increased from 22 to 30 percent. (*From D. L. Paulson and J. S. Reisch: Long Term Survival after Resection for Bronchogenic Carcinoma, Ann Surg, 184:324, 1976, with permission of author and publisher.*)

noid tumors of the small intestine. Along with cylindroma and mucoepidermoid tumors, the bronchial carcinoid was formerly referred to as a bronchial adenoma. This designation was awkward because the term *adenoma* implied a fundamental quality of benignancy that was not in keeping with the high incidence of malignant behavior shown by cylindroma and mucoepidermoid tumors. Further, a small number of bronchial carcinoids has shown metastases to regional lymph nodes, with the result that reference was occasionally made to "metastasizing bronchial adenomas." The recent classification of lung tumors (Table 17-8) eliminates the designation of adenomas, but many years may be required to discard the term from common usage.

More than 80 percent of carcinoids arise in the major proximal bronchi, but peripheral origin beyond cartilage containing bronchi does occur. The tumors grow slowly and protrude into the bronchial lumen to a degree that makes symptoms and signs of bronchial obstruction the principal form of clinical presentation. Unusual vascularity often is associated with significant hemoptysis as a presenting complaint. In addition, the vascularity gives the tumor a deep pink or red color when visualized through a bronchoscope, and biopsy can result in substantial bleeding (Fig. 17-74).

The extent of bronchial-wall involvement is variable, but there is usually some invasion of the underlying cartilages by the neoplasm. Rarely, a direct extension of tumor through the bronchial wall can result in invasion of adjacent mediastinal structures. Regional lymph-node deposits are found in approximately 10 percent of patients, but liver metastases have been reported in only a few percent. Because bronchial carcinoids and oat cell cancer both are thought to arise from Kultschitzky-type cells, there has

been speculation about their relationship. In their usual form these two neoplasms are widely separated in character. Nevertheless, a few carcinoids have been reported in which some part of the tumor had an anaplastic appearance. Further, a few patients with a bronchial carcinoid have had a Cushing-like syndrome that seemed attributable to the tumor.

Although the average age of patients with a carcinoid tumor is approximately forty years, the neoplasm does occur in children. Commonly, the clinical presentation is a result of bronchial obstruction with infection and pulmonary atelectasis. Sputum cytology is negative, but more

Fig. 17-73. A comparison of survival after operation for lung cancer based on location of the tumor. (*From D. L. Paulson and J. S. Reisch, Long Term Survival after Resection for Bronchogenic Carcinoma, Ann Surg, 184:324, 1976, with permission of author and publisher.*)

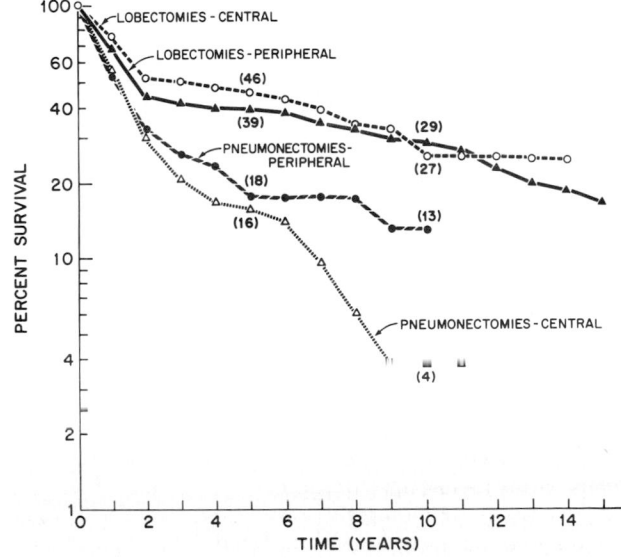

ACTUAL SURVIVAL RATES BY LOCATION AND EXTENT OF RESECTION (1960-1969)

A

B

C

Fig. 17-74. A forty-two-year-old woman with a bronchial carcinoid tumor. *A.* The chest x-ray shows collapse of the left lower lobe and shift of the mediastinum to that side. *B.* Bronchotomy of the left stem bronchus confirmed an obstruction of the lower-lobe bronchus by the vascular tumor projecting from the bronchus between the Allis clamps. *C.* Histologic examination of the neoplasm showed it to be a benign carcinoid tumor. ($\times$400.)

than 80 percent of the lesions can be visualized by bronchoscopy. The carcinoid syndrome is produced in a rare patient, but this can occur without extrathoracic metastases. It is wise to measure daily urinary 5-HIAA excretion and blood serotonin level, but these can be clearly elevated without corresponding symptoms.

The only treatment for bronchial carcinoid tumor is surgical resection. Neither the primary neoplasm nor lymph-node metastases are sensitive to radiation therapy. Lobectomy is an acceptable operation, but Jensik has correctly emphasized the low potential for malignancy of

the carcinoid neoplasm. He has advocated the use of conservative procedures such as sleeve resection or local bronchial excision with bronchoplasty whenever feasible (Fig. 17-75). Occasionally, a critical location of the neoplasm makes pneumonectomy unavoidable. The mortality rate for operation is low, and the expected long-term survival rate is close to 90 percent.

TUMORS OF BRONCHIAL GLAND ORIGIN

Cylindroma, or adenocystic carcinoma, and mucoepidermoid tumors are the commonest neoplasms arising from the bronchial glands. Their location is predominantly central, and they are said to take origin only from bronchi containing cartilage. Both neoplasms may show a spectrum of behavior from benign to malignant, with regional and distant metastases. The treatment is surgical resection, including en bloc removal of regional lymph nodes when possible. Though the long-term cure rate is considerably higher than that of primary carcinoma of the lung, it does not equal the results in bronchial carcinoid.

Other rare tumors of bronchial gland origin are occasionally reported; the majority seem to be forms of adenocarcinoma.

CARCINOSARCOMA

An interesting but very infrequent group of pulmonary neoplasms are designated as carcinosarcomas because of their mixed components. Both epithelial and mesenchymal types of tissue comprise the neoplasms, and electron microscopy has confirmed that the sarcomatous elements are not simply transformed components of epithelial origin. The term *blastoma* has recently been used for some tumors

that show histologic evidence of association with embryonal tissue.

Carcinosarcomas may be located in the lung periphery or in proximal bronchi, and they have been reported in a wide age range, including children. The treatment is surgical resection, and a cure rate generally exceeding that for bronchogenic carcinoma can be expected.

SARCOMA

A variety of mesodermal sarcomas and tumors of reticuloendothelial origin may occur in the lungs. As a group these tumors represent approximately 1 percent of all primary neoplasms removed at operation. The age range of presentation is considerably wider than that for bronchogenic carcinoma, and the tumors may arise anywhere in the lung or bronchial tree. Difficulty with true histologic identification of the neoplasms is not rare, and they may be mistaken for highly undifferentiated carcinomas or metastatic neoplasms.

In general, the symptoms may be the same as those expected with primary carcinomas, but there is no distinct association with cigarette smoking. When the tumors develop as intrabronchial polypoid neoplasms, the symptoms of bronchial obstruction lead to earlier diagnosis and, therefore, a relatively higher cure rate after resection. Leiomyosarcomas, for example, had a 5-year cure rate of approximately 40 percent in McNamara's report.

Lymphosarcoma and *reticulum cell sarcoma* may rarely develop in the lung without evidence of tumor elsewhere.

Fig. 17-75. Operative procedures to conserve pulmonary tissue in patients with bronchial carcinoid. *A.* Sleeve resection of tumor from left main bronchus. *B.* Superior segmentectomy and middle lobectomy with bronchial anastomosis. (*From R. J. Jensik, L. P. Faber, C. M. Brown, and C. F. Kittle, Bronchoplastic and Conservative Resectional Procedures for Bronchial Adenoma, J Thorac Cardiovasc Surg, 68:556, 1974, with permission of the author and publisher.*)

LEFT BRONCHIAL TREE

RIGHT BRONCHIAL TREE

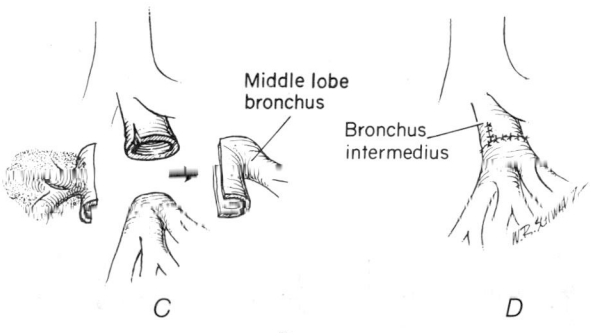

Routine chest x-rays discover an asymptomatic pulmonary lesion in a number of patients; other lesions become symptomatic because of pressure of the growing tumor or lymph nodes on adjacent structures. There is no characteristic roentgenographic appearance, and the diagnosis is rarely suspected from sputum cytology or bronchoscopy. Percutaneous needle biopsy may give the diagnosis with either neoplasm.

A sufficient number of lymphosarcomas are localized to make the prognosis good after pulmonary resection. A 5-year survival exceeding 50 percent may be anticipated, but the results with reticulum cell sarcoma are not as good because the neoplasm is less often resectable.

Hodgkin's disease frequently involves the lung, and a rare patient is seen in whom a solitary pulmonary lesion is unassociated with other evidence of tumor. If resection has been performed, the patient should have complete staging of the disease so that decisions regarding additional therapy can be made.

Fibrosarcoma, rhabdomyosarcoma, neurofibrosarcoma, and other tumors of mesodermal origin may occur rarely in the lung but without specific clinical presentation. The treatment is surgical resection, and the prognosis depends on the stage at which the neoplasm was discovered.

BENIGN TUMORS

The *hamartoma* (chondroadenoma), among the commonest benign pulmonary tumors, has a characteristic peripheral location (Fig. 17-76). Very slow growth and striking male preponderance are additional features. Although they have been reported in children, hamartomas have their greatest age incidence between forty and sixty years. An absence of symptoms is the rule, and the great

Fig. 17-76. This posteroanterior chest x-ray shows a smooth round density in the midlung field that proved to be a hamartoma when removed by wedge resection.

majority are discovered on chest x-rays taken for another purpose.

The major component of the hamartoma is cartilage, and it is often possible to shell the tumor out of the lung parenchyma. Epithelial elements are generally present, and there may be fat, muscular, or fibrous tissue interspersed. Removal by wedge resection is generally performed as the diagnostic procedure.

Neurofibromas may occur in the lung parenchyma, particularly in patients with neurofibromatosis. *Sclerosing hemangiomas, plasma cell granulomas, lipomas,* and rare examples of a few other neoplasms complete the list of benign tumors that may arise in the parenchyma. Many of the same neoplasms may develop in a major bronchus and present as a polypoid lesion. The *granular cell myoblastoma* is an example of this type of development in which the clinical presentation is that of bronchial obstruction. Lobar resection is often necessary because of the effects of chronic infection.

METASTATIC TUMORS

Metastases to the lungs are common during the clinical course of many uncontrolled primary neoplasms of extrathoracic origin. In some patients death occurs with pulmonary metastases in the absence of any other foci of recurrent tumor. Further, it has now been demonstrated that surgical resection of one or more pulmonary metastases can result in a significant 5-year survival rate for patients with several types of carcinomas or sarcomas. Unfortunately, in many communities there does not appear to be a general appreciation of the potential for cure that may result from an application of this knowledge.

The initial experience with surgical treatment of pulmonary metastases was based on the principle that resection was indicated only in those patients with a solitary metastasis, in whom a year or more had passed between control of the primary tumor and appearance of the metastasis. Occasionally, patients with an apparent solitary metastasis were observed for prolonged intervals so that any subclinical metastases could become apparent. Though a conservative approach of this type has most likely avoided fruitless thoracotomy for some patients who did have additional metastases, it also may have allowed additional metastases to develop from the lesion that was being observed. The occurrence of secondary metastases from a primary metastasis has been demonstrated to the satisfaction of most observers. Therefore, this phenomenon must now be considered in the decision about treatment for individual patients.

The original recommendation to consider for resection only those patients whose metastasis appeared approximately one year or more after control of the primary tumor has been challenged by more recent results. Five-year survivors have been reported who had their pulmonary metastasis resected within several months after resection of the primary neoplasm. It seems likely that the origin of the primary tumor and the biologic behavior of the individual neoplasm are the major factors in the prognosis for survival. Morton has shown that the measurement of the tumor doubling time (TDT) provides an accurate method for judging the biologic behavior of a neoplasm in the individual patient. From an experience with 60 patients who underwent resection for multiple pulmonary metastases, it was concluded that aggressive surgical resection is indicated when TDT is greater than 40 days. In that series, the estimated 5-year survival was approximately 60 percent for patients whose TDT exceeded 40 days.

Differing results in the literature have not allowed firm conclusions to be drawn regarding the tumors that offer the best change for cure with resection of metastases. In children the likelihood of 5-year survival after resection of single or multiple metastases from extremity sarcomas has seemingly been enhanced by effective chemotherapy. Breast carcinoma has not given favorable results in the experience of most surgeons, and the prognosis after resection of metastases from renal and colon neoplasms has varied widely.

The problem to be considered in a patient who presents with a solitary pulmonary nodule, either synchronous or metachronous with an extrathoracic cancer, is whether it is a metastasis, a primary pulmonary tumor, or a nonneoplastic lesion (Fig. 17-77). In a report on 54 colon cancer patients who had a solitary lung shadow at the Sloan-Kettering Cancer Center, 25 patients had colon cancer metastases and 29 had primary lung carcinoma. Resection of the metastases resulted in a 35 percent 5-year survival. In the absence of strong evidence to support a conclusion that the pulmonary lesion is nonneoplastic, an aggressive surgical approach is warranted under these circumstances.

In the evaluation of patients to be considered for resection of pulmonary metastases, the exclusion of metastases to other sites should be as thorough as possible. Besides the standard roentgenographic and radioisotopic surveys for metastatic disease, bone marrow biopsy, lymphangiography, and other special procedures may be indicated, depending on the known biologic behavior of the primary neoplasm. Metastatic neoplasms result in positive sputum cytology or positive bronchial washings much less frequently than primary lung cancers. If preoperative confirmation of the diagnosis is imperative, percutaneous needle biopsy may offer the greatest chance for success.

In all events it is important to assess the extent of the pulmonary lesions before operation. Standard x-ray tomography is rapidly being supplanted by computed tomography for this purpose. Although the survival rate for individuals who had bilateral metastases was not found to be significantly different (statistically) from those with unilateral metastases by Takita, other factors become operative (Fig. 17-78). Previously, the recommended approach for patients with bilateral lesions was that of staged thoracotomies and an interval of several weeks or months. The results achieved by Takita and his associates with a series of patients having simultaneous resection of bilateral metastases through a median sternotomy provides strong support for the single-stage operation.

McCormack has recently reported on 188 patients who underwent single or multiple thoracotomies for metastatic carcinoma from multiple sites of origin (Fig. 17-79). Only 26 patients had one or more metastases in each lung at the time of the first thoracotomy. The overall 5-year survival

Fig. 17-77. This chest x-ray shows a large round density in the right lung of a patient who had undergone abdominoperineal resection for anal carcinoma 2 years earlier. The arrow points to a small density in the upper lobe area that was not detected before his right thoracotomy. Both lesions were removed by wedge resection and proved to be metastases from the anal neoplasm. There has been no further evidence of neoplasm in 18 months.

Fig. 17-78. Even though the survival rate after resection of unilateral metastases was not significantly different from that of patients with bilateral metastases, the data of Takita do show a trend that coincides with the experience of other surgeons. (From H. Takita et al., The Surgical Management of Multiple Lung Metastases, Ann Thorac Surg, 24:359, 1977, with permission of the author and publisher.)

Multiple Lung Metastases: Survival by Unilateral vs. Bilateral Disease

Extent of Pulmonary Metastases at Initial Thoracotomy

Primary Site	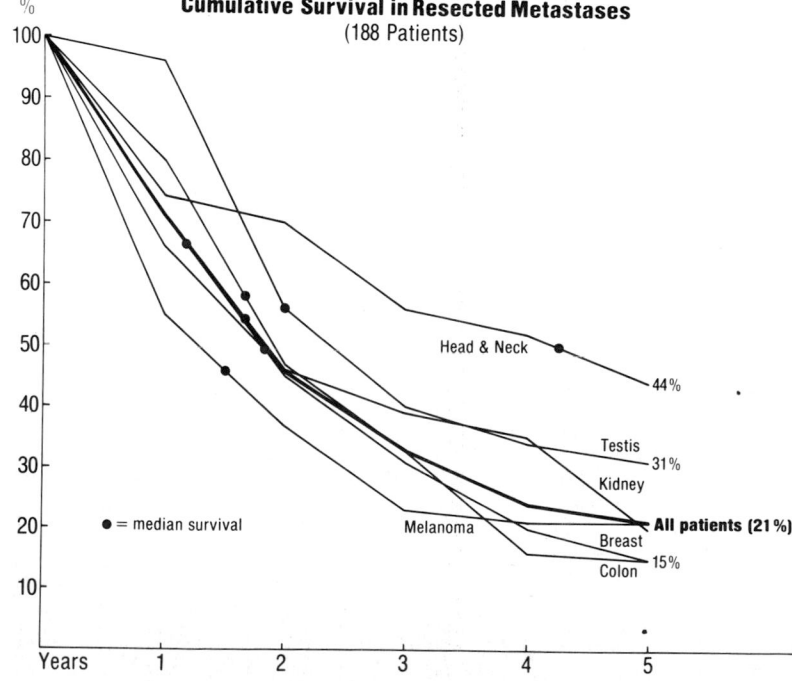				Number of Patients
Colon and Rectum	23	1	10	6	40
Melanoma	23	0	5	1	29
Breast	24	0	3	1	28
Testis	8	0	14	3	25
Head and Neck	10	0	12	1	23
Kidney	6	1	4	5	16
Bladder	2	0	4	2	8
Other	8	0	6	5	19
TOTAL	104	2	58	24	188

Fig. 17-79. The origin of the primary tumors and the unilateral or bilateral extent of pulmonary metastases at the time of the initial thoracotomy in 188 patients reported from the Sloan-Kettering Cancer Center. (*Reproduced from P. M. McCormack et al., Pulmonary Resection in Metastic Carcinoma, Chest, 73:163, 1978, with permission of the author and publisher.*)

Cumulative Survival in Resected Metastases
(188 Patients)

• = median survival

Head & Neck — 44%

Testis — 31%
Kidney

All patients (21%)

Melanoma
Breast — 15%
Colon

Years   1   2   3   4   5

Fig. 17-80. The overall 5-year survival in 188 patients who underwent resection of pulmonary metastases was 21 percent, but those who had primary tumors in the head and neck had a 44 percent survival. (*Reproduced from P. M. McCormack et al., Pulmonary Resection in Metastatic Carcinoma, Chest, 73:163, 1978, with permission of the author and publisher.*)

with resected solitary metastases was 21 percent, and that for multiple metastasis was 15 percent. As shown in Fig. 17-80, the overall rate of survival for all groups in her series was also 21 percent, but there was a significant difference between the groups according to tumor origin.

The extent of pulmonary resection for metastatic lesions is determined by the location of the lesions, the patient's pulmonary function, and the number of metastases. For a solitary lesion it may be necessary to do a lobectomy to distinguish between metastatic and primary carcinoma. Pneumonectomy is rarely indicated. For the majority of patients with multiple lesions, wedge resections must be done to conserve pulmonary tissue (Fig. 17-81).

Most recently a concept of "debulking" the lungs has developed in which the goal is to remove as much tumor volume as possible in the patient with extensive pulmonary metastases. Operation is then followed by intense chemotherapy with the hope of controlling tumor growth and prolonging survival. The preliminary results from this approach have been inconclusive to date except for isolated cases. Nevertheless, the concept seems valid and experience will lead to the proper selection of patients.

TRACHEA

Because of its singular importance to life and its relatively vulnerable position in the neck, the trachea must be considered among the few really vital structures in the body. Considering these facts one would have to say that it has been a relatively silent organ when compared to the attention demanded by the heart, the liver, etc. Research effort and money devoted to solution of the diseases or disorders affecting the trachea have been minuscule in comparison to that expended for other organs that are no more critical to human survival.

The adult trachea varies in length from approximately 10 to 13 cm, with an internal diameter of 2.3 cm laterally and 1.8 cm anteroposteriorly. There are generally 18 to 22 cartilaginous rings, but some degree of lateral fusion between adjacent rings, or lateral division of single rings is not infrequent. The flexible character of the trachea is complemented by its ability to maintain an adequate lumen during the extremes of neck motion and externally applied pressure. Loss of the cartilaginous support takes away the property of lumen integrity and is the principal threat to adequate tracheal function after injuries or benign disease.

The blood supply of the trachea is not generous, and this must be given major attention in operations involving repair or reconstruction. The cervical trachea receives its major blood supply from the inferior thyroid artery; the lower part of the trachea is supplied by bronchial arteries.

The most common significant congenital disorders of the trachea are the *tracheoesophageal fistulas* associated with esophageal atresia. Management of the tracheal part of these abnormalities consists essentially of interrupting the fistula and closing the posterior membranous wall of the trachea. It is the management of the esophagus that constitutes the long-term problem; that is discussed elsewhere.

Fig. 17-81. Two small metastases that were wedged from the left lung in a thirty-four-year-old woman who previously had amputation of her left leg for an alveolar cell sarcoma.

Several forms of *congenital tracheal stenosis* may occur, often associated with other congenital anomalies. Congenital webs in the form of diaphragms may produce acute or chronic obstruction in newborns as well as older children. In addition, three types of stenosis involving the tracheal wall have been described: (1) funnel stenosis in which the distal trachea tapers to a very small lumen above the carina; (2) segmental stenosis, which may occur at any level; and (3) hypoplasia of the entire tracheal length. Obstruction of the trachea can occur in association with anomalous origin of the left pulmonary artery from the right pulmonary artery (pulmonary artery sling) and passage of the left artery behind the trachea. Several types of vascular ring malformations may produce partial tracheal obstruction.

Diagnosis of tracheal abnormalities depends on a suspicion of the anomalies and the use of air tracheograms, fluoroscopy, and careful bronchoscopy. Obviously there is a danger that the attempts at diagnosis can convert a partial obstruction to near-total obstruction and a critical emergency. Corrective operative procedures must be highly selective in infants, and reconstruction of the trachea is seldom attempted in small children. Tracheostomy or careful dilatations are the usual procedures done for intrinsic tracheal obstruction, and they must be done with the concept of subsequent reconstruction in mind.

Penetrating or blunt trauma to the neck or thorax may produce tracheal injuries that vary from localized contusion with submucosal hematoma to penetrating defects and complete interruption. An alertness to the significance of dyspnea, coughing, blood spitting, wheezing, or stridor should lead to emergency bronchoscopy or exploration of the trachea in patients with trauma. Simple penetrating injuries may require tracheostomy, or occasionally with small wounds of minor consequence, only the placement of a drain to the point of injury. Rarely, a complete division of the trachea allows the patient to survive for a period of hours to weeks before the diagnosis is made. Reanastomosis with appropriate tracheoplasty is the goal of management. A complementary tracheostomy may be required.

The complications of tracheostomy have constituted the principal need for tracheal reconstruction since the era of mechanical ventilation started. Table 17-12 lists the complications of tracheostomy according to the time period in which they are usually seen. Improved tracheostomy tubes and tracheostomy care have reduced the frequency of many of these complications. Unfortunately, acquired tracheoesophageal fistula, tracheo-innominate artery fistula, and tracheal stenosis have not been eliminated. The development of a tracheoesophageal fistula rarely occurs before the second or third week after tracheostomy has been performed. Pressure from an overinflated tracheostomy balloon cuff, trauma to the posterior tracheal wall from the tube and from suction catheters, and an indwelling nasogastric tube are factors in the development of the fistula. Repeated aspiration through the fistula produces severe pulmonary infection, while the positive-pressure ventilation forces excessive amounts of air into the gastrointestinal tract. Confirmation of the suspected diagnosis is usually accomplished with endoscopy, and treatment most often requires urgent division of the fistula with repair of both structures.

Massive hemorrhage resulting from a tracheo-innominate artery fistula may be preceded by one or more minor bleeding episodes. This is a highly lethal complication, but survivors with emergency operation are being reported with increasing frequency. A fistula is most likely to occur if tracheostomy is performed below the fourth tracheal ring. Direct erosion of the inner curve of the tube into the innominate artery is the usual mechanism of the fistula. Control of bleeding should be attempted by adjustment of the tube position and reinflation of the cuff. If this is unsuccessful, it is necessary to insert a finger into the pretracheal space and compress the artery against the

Table 17-12. COMPLICATIONS OF TRACHEOSTOMY

1. Complications of the operative procedure
   a. Cardiac arrhythmias and arrest
   b. Hemorrhage
   c. Injury to adjacent structures
   d. Incorrect tracheal incision
   e. Pneumothorax
2. Early postoperative complications
   a. Tube obstruction
   b. Displaced tube
   c. Aspiration
   d. Tracheobronchial infection
   e. Tracheoesophageal fistula
   f. Tracheo-innominate artery fistula
3. Late complications
   a. Persistent stoma
   b. Tracheal stenosis
   c. Tracheomalacia
   d. Granuloma

sternum while preparations are made for median sternotomy and direct operative control of the innominate artery.

Tracheal obstruction becomes apparent only after decannulation, and it may occur immediately or gradually over a period of days or weeks. While the development of large-volume, low-pressure balloon cuffs has sharply reduced the frequency of posttracheostomy obstruction, the complication has not been eliminated. The location of the site of obstruction in the majority of patients has changed from the area of balloon cuff–tracheal wall contact to the site of the tracheal stoma. Even so, examples of tracheal stenosis at the cuff site are still seen because of circumferential fibrous stricture or tracheomalacia resulting from overinflation of so-called "soft cuffs." The ready availability of pressure manometers to allow frequent monitoring of intracuff pressure has not completely prevented a misconception that the first approach to unsatisfactory ventilation in a respirator patient is the addition of air to the balloon cuff. Development of the foam-cuff tracheostomy tubes may help reduce even further the incidence of tracheal injury at the site of contact of the cuff with the tracheal wall.

Obstruction at the stomal site may be due to excessive granulation tissue, tracheomalacia, or fibrous stricture (Fig. 17-82). Factors that have been implicated in producing stomal stenosis are related to the type of incision made in the trachea, severity of infection at the tracheostomy site, possible protrusion of the balloon cuff through the stoma, and duration of the indwelling tube. There are no clear data to define the specific role of any of these factors, and different investigations support different types of tracheal incisions.

Recognition or suspicion of tracheal stenosis before a critical obstruction forces emergency tracheostomy can significantly reduce the complexity of tracheal resection and repair. Dilatation is usually not successful for management of severe stenosis, but recent experience with local steroid administration, dilatation, and intraluminal stenting has given encouraging results. Two other techniques currently being evaluated for treatment of localized strictures are endotracheal cryotherapy and endoscopic laser treatment. Both methods have shown promise for correctly selected patients. In addition, laser therapy may have application for management of benign and malignant tracheal tumors.

The usual management for acquired tracheal stenosis with a lumen diameter of 1.5 cm or less is resection of the stenotic area with end-to-end reanastomosis. This can generally be done through a cervical incision that incorporates the tracheostomy scar. Approximately 4.5 to 5 cm of trachea can be resected and still allow primary anastomosis, but a partial sternotomy may be required for adequate mobilization. In a rare patient the extent of tracheal stenosis, including its length, may block the attempt to do a reanastomosis. This has usually resulted in multiple operations utilizing several techniques for attempted tracheal reconstruction. The results have often been poor, and the patient was left with a permanent tracheostomy. A tracheal prosthesis of silicone rubber recently developed by Neville has shown promise for relief of this problem and for

A

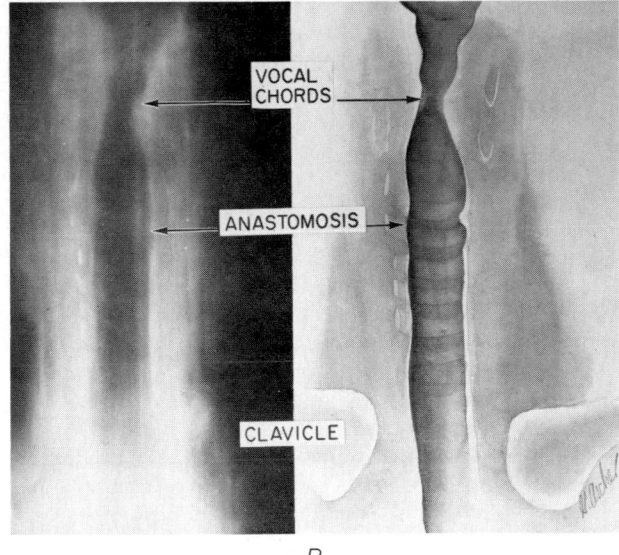

B

Fig. 17-82. Resection and the anastomosis of the trachea for tracheostomy stomal stenosis. *A*. A tomogram of the cervical trachea demonstrates the area of stenosis. *B*. A postoperative tomogram shows restoration of a normal tracheal lumen after resection and end-to-end anastomosis.

tracheal replacement in patients with carcinoma involving that structure (Fig. 17-83). Neville has been successful in achieving a "take" of the prosthesis in a modest group of patients; this represents significant progress in the area of tracheal surgery.

Fig. 17-83. *A*. An operative photograph furnished by Dr. William Neville shows a tracheal prosthesis that has been used to replace a length of the cervicomediastinal trachea. *B*. The drawing shows the relationship of the tracheal prosthesis to the aorta and innominate artery. (*From W. E. Neville et al., Prosthetic Reconstruction of the Trachea and Carina, J Thorac Cardiovasc Surg, 72:525, 1976, with permission of the author and publisher.*)

A

Tumors

Primary tracheal tumors are uncommon. The trachea is more frequently involved secondarily by direct extension of neoplasms arising in the bronchi, the esophagus, the larynx, or the thyroid gland. Of the primary tumors that do arise in the trachea more than 80 percent are malignant, with squamous cell carcinoma and cylindroma (adenocystic carcinoma) constituting the great majority. The commonest benign primary tumors are squamous papillomas and fibromas. Included among the other benign and malignant neoplasms are carcinoid tumor, chondroma, adenocarcinoma, mucoepidermoid tumor, giant-cell myoblastoma, chondrosarcoma, plasmacytoma, hemangioma, squamous papillomatosis, and fibrosarcoma.

The clinical manifestations of primary tracheal neo-

B

plasms are essentially the signs and symptoms of airway obstruction. Dyspnea on exertion may be the first evidence of developing obstruction, but cough, wheezing, and inspiratory stridor are frequently the complaints that cause the patient to seek help. Occasionally hemoptysis is the precipitating event, or it may be respiratory infection due to major obstruction of a mainstem bronchus. The chest x-rays are frequently of no help unless one requests laminagrams of the trachea because of the wheezing or stridor. Sputum cytology should be requested in the diagnostic work-up, but bronchoscopy should not be unduly delayed while numerous indirect techniques for diagnosis are performed. Because bronchoscopy can precipitate critical tracheal obstruction, however, the procedure should be carefully planned, with preparations made to proceed to definitive operation if indicated.

Pulmonary-function studies may have little meaning in the patient with high-grade tracheal obstruction, but they should be obtained if the patient's condition is satisfactory. With performance of flow-volume loops, significant obstruction will be indicated by plateaus of inspiration and expiration and flattening of the peak flow.

The goal of surgical treatment is complete resection of the neoplasm and restoration of tracheal continuity. From the bronchoscopic examination and biopsy the tumor should be identified sufficiently to plan the operative approach. Occasionally, tantalum bronchograms and tracheograms assist in the planning. Upper tracheal neoplasms are usually approached through a cervical incision, combined with median sternotomy as necessary. Lower tracheal tumors are generally operated upon through a right lateral thoracotomy. If possible a sleeve resection is done with end-to-end reanastomosis. When a more extensive resection is required, the technique of Moghissi for tracheal reconstruction with a Marlex mesh–pericardial graft may be employed (Fig. 17-84). The success reported by this author for reconstruction after major tracheal resection with both primary and secondary tumors is impressive. With a total experience of 27 patients, some of whom are alive and well from 3 to 7 years after resection for carcinoma, Moghissi suggests that an aggressive approach to tracheal resection is well justified.

For squamous carcinoma of the trachea, radiation may give temporary tumor control. At present, there is consid-

erable hope that the chemotherapy programs that are showing improved results in bronchogenic carcinoma will also be helpful in tracheal neoplasms.

MEDIASTINUM

The mediastinum is the extrapleural space between the two pleural cavities, bordered on each side by parietal pleura and containing the heart and great vessels, trachea, esophagus, vagus nerves and sympathetic chains, the thymus gland, and a lymphatic network consisting of several groups of lymph nodes and the thoracic duct. In this complex area between the thoracic inlet and diaphragm, the heart and great vessels develop, the pulmonary diverticulum arises from the primitive foregut, and the caudal branchial arches develop. It is not surprising that many congenital anomalies are found within the mediastinum.

For purposes of classification, it is customary to divide the mediastinum into several areas. Traditional anatomists have considered the mediastinum to have superior, anterior, posterior, and middle segments. It has become obvious that this classification relies upon criteria that do not coincide with clinical behavior. For this reason, Burkell and his associates have suggested that the mediastinum be subdivided into the three major areas illustrated in Fig. 17-85. With this modification, the anterior part of the superior mediastinum is incorporated into the anterior mediastinum, and the boundary of the posterior mediastinum is extended cephalad. This is more in keeping with the actual distribution of the clinical lesions and allows the three regions to be described as follows:

1. The anterior mediastinum—bounded by the posterior surface of the sternum anteriorly, the anterior border of the upper dorsal vertebrae posteriorly, and an oblique line running along the

Fig. 17-84. Tracheal reconstruction after major resection for carcinoma. *A.* The drawings show the technique used by Moghissi for reconstruction of the trachea with a composite Marlex mesh–pericardial graft after resection of a primary tracheal neoplasm. *B.* Resection of the lateral tracheal wall en bloc with a right upper-lobe carcinoma may be repaired with the Marlex mesh–pericardial graft. (*From W. E. Neville et al., Prosthetic Reconstruction of the Trachea and Carina, J Thorac Cardiovasc Surg, 72:525, 1976, with permission of the author and publisher.*)

A   *B*

A

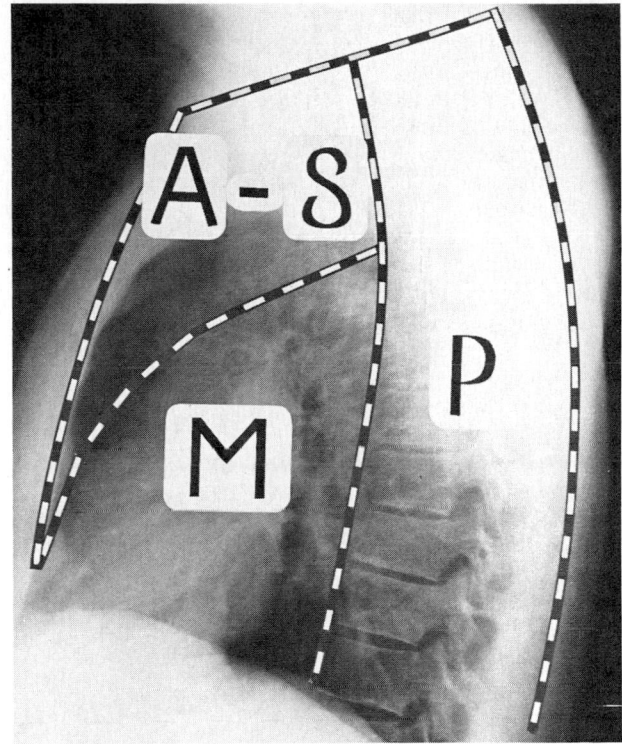

B

Fig. 17-85. The anatomic divisions of the mediastinum. *A*. The traditional consideration of the mediastinum provides for its division into superior (*S*), anterior (*A*), middle (*M*), and posterior (*P*) compartments. *B*. The anatomic divisions that Burkell and associates have suggested are shown as a cephalad extension of the posterior compartment, and a combination of the anterior and superior compartments (*A-S*). [*From C. C. Burkell, J. M. Cross, H. P. Kent, and E. N. Nanson, Mass Lesions of the Mediastinum, in M. M. Ravitch (ed.), "Current Problems in Surgery," Yearbook Medical Publishers, Inc., Chicago, June 1969, by permission of author and publisher.*]

anterior border of the heart with continuation upwards and posteriorly until it reaches the border of the dorsal vertebrae.

2. The posterior mediastinum—bounded posteriorly by the anterior surface of the curve of the ribs, anteriorly by a line drawn along the anterior border of the bodies of the dorsal vertebrae, and inferiorly by the diaphragm.

3. The middle mediastinum—a roughly triangular area with its base on the diaphragm and bounded front and back by the anterior and posterior compartments.

In addition to mass lesions, the principal concern for the surgeon, the mediastinum may be the site of acute and chronic infections, congenital malformations, and aneurysms.

Mass Lesions

The clinical presentation of primary mediastinal tumors and cysts varies from the asymptomatic and nonspecific systemic complaints to symptoms that are nearly pathognomonic for syndromes specifically associated with mediastinal lesions. Roughly 50 percent of mediastinal tumors and cysts are symptomatic in adults, with the figure being

closer to two-thirds in children. Malignant tumors are more often symptomatic than benign ones, and the most common symptoms are related to compression of adjacent mediastinal structures. Chest pain is common, and many patients have respiratory symptoms caused by displacement or erosion of the tracheobronchial tree. In infants and children symptoms of cough, stridor, and dyspnea are prominent because even a small mass may readily encroach on their compressible airways. Other frequent manifestations include dysphagia, due to displacement of the esophagus, superior vena caval obstruction, recurrent nerve palsy, and Horner's syndrome. Less frequently a mediastinal neoplasm is discovered because of systemic symptoms such as hypertension due to a pheochromocytoma, hypoglycemia resulting from secretion of an insulin-like substance, or a Pel-Ebstein fever due to Hodgkin's disease.

In most cases, the definitive diagnosis of a mediastinal mass has to await histologic examination. However, every effort should be made to localize the lesion, assess its site of origin, and evaluate its relationship to surrounding structures. The diagnostic evaluation of a patient with a mediastinal mass lesion begins with a complete history and physical examination. Further investigation of these patients should follow a logical sequence proceeding from simpler to more complicated techniques.

The routine chest x-rays in anteroposterior and lateral projections are usually the most useful diagnostic procedures. The localization is of diagnostic value since certain tumors or cysts have a predilection for arising in specific regions of the mediastinum (Fig. 17-86). Not infrequently

A

B

Fig. 17-86. *A.* Mediastinal lesions have a tendency to occur in specific areas; this figure indicates the expected location of the most frequently occurring lesions. *B.* The numbers shown in the mediastinal compartments indicate the distribution of lesions in 102 patients reported by Burkell and associates. [*From C. C. Burkell, J. M. Cross, H. P. Kent, and E. N. Nanson, Mass Lesions of the Mediastinum, in M. M. Ravitch (ed.), "Current Problems in Surgery," Yearbook Medical Publishers, Inc., Chicago, June 1969, by permission of author and publisher.*]

the precise localization is obscured because of overlying or adjacent structures, thus making it necessary to obtain further radiologic studies. Tomography may be useful in delineating middle mediastinal masses from normal hilar structures and in clarifying the presence of rib erosion or vertebral deformity in association with posterior neurogenic lesions. A barium swallow may show invasion, compression, or displacement of the esophagus resulting from either intrinsic or extrinsic lesions (Fig. 17-87). Fluoroscopy can be helpful for distinguishing mediastinal from pulmonary lesions in that a primary lung lesion will move with respiration in association with the adjoining lung parenchyma. Recently, computerized axial tomography has been helpful in certain cases because relative densities can be measured and vascular attachments can be assessed. Of further aid in assessing vascularity are angiocardiography and thoracic aortography. Pneumomediastinum has found application as a means of differentiating a true mediastinal mass from a normally enlarged thymus in infants. For patients with posterior mediastinal lesions, especially those with neurologic symptoms, myelography may be indicated in the diagnostic work-up.

Radioisotope scanning may be important in evaluating some patients, especially those with superior mediastinal lesions that may be substernal thyroid abnormalities. A recent development is the use of radioactive gallium to evaluate lymphadenopathy.

Ultrasonography is a noninvasive way to evaluate the density of a mediastinal lesion, such as differentiating a pericardial cyst from a primary tumor, but it has been shown that the technique is imperfect.

As noted previously, the above diagnostic procedures must be supplemented by tissue biopsy for precise diagnosis. Several techniques have been described for obtaining tissue, including needle biopsy, needle aspiration, anterior mediastinal exploration, and mediastinoscopy. Each method has specific advantages and disadvantages but the overall value of each probably depends most on the experience and expertise of the individual performing the procedure. The important role of exploratory thoracotomy as a diagnostic test should be emphasized, and the demonstration of a mediastinal mass may be sufficient indication for operative intervention. In modern practice there is no rationale for serial chest x-rays or the trial use of irradiation as a diagnostic technique.

ANTERIOR MEDIASTINAL LESIONS

Figure 17-86 shows those lesions which are most common in this area.

Thymoma

Thymomas are the most common neoplasms arising in the anterior mediastinum and comprise approximately 20 percent of all primary mediastinal tumors and cysts. There is an equal frequency of occurrence in males and females, with a peak incidence between ages forty and sixty years. These tumors do not have a characteristic radiologic appearance (Fig. 17-88), and the clinical presentations can be numerous and varied. Less than one-third are asympto-

matic at the time of diagnosis. Some patients present with compression effects such as chest pain, cough, dyspnea, or superior vena caval obstruction, but the majority have symptoms referable to one of the several systemic syndromes associated with thymoma. The most common of these is myasthenia gravis, the incidence being reported to vary from 10 to 50 percent. Conversely, the reported incidence of thymomas in patients with myasthenia gravis ranges from 8 to 15 percent. It is of interest that a thymoma can occur prior to, concomitant with, or subsequent to the onset of symptoms of myasthenia gravis. Unfortunately, myasthenic patients with thymoma derive less symptomatic benefit from thymectomy than patients without tumors.

The histologic classification of thymomas remains a

Fig. 17-87. Mediastinal bronchogenic cyst. *A.* The anteroposterior view of this barium esophagogram shows lateral displacement of the distal esophagus in an eighteen-year-old man who had slowly progressive dysphagia. *B.* The lateral view demonstrates mild dilatation of the esophagus and a rapid tapering at the site of obstruction just above the diaphragm. *C.* A tomogram shows an egg-shaped mass overlying the vertebral column. *D.* The cystic lesion removed through a left thoracotomy was filled with mucoid material and was lined by typical pseudostratified respiratory epithelium.

A

B

C

D

A

B

C

D

Fig. 17-88. A benign thymoma in a thirty-two-year-old man. *A.* The posteroanterior chest x-ray, taken because of persistent cough, showed a large smooth mass contiguous with the right heart border. *B.* An oblique projection again suggests that the mass is closely attached to the pericardium. *C.* The tumor was removed, along with the remnants of the thymus, through a high right thoracotomy. This photograph of the open neoplasm shows that it was a well-encapsulated fleshy neoplasm. *D.* Histologic examination of the tumor shows a predominance of lymphocytic elements that justifies its classification as a lymphocytic type of thymoma.

controversial problem. A categorization of thymomas into as many as 13 different types has been proposed; however, the prevalent opinion is to classify thymic neoplasms simply on the basis of the predominance of epithelial or lymphocytic cells. Thus, they may be typed as predominantly epithelial, lymphocytic, or mixed. Furthermore, there is no confirmed association between histologic appearance and biologic behavior. The important clinical classification of thymomas is that of benign or malignant, but the microscopic appearance is unreliable for this purpose. Benign tumors comprise 50 to 65 percent of all thymomas, they are well encapsulated, and they do not invade adjacent mediastinal structures. Tumors are designated as malignant when they locally infiltrate the pericardium, pleura, great vessels, heart, or chest wall.

The presence of a thymoma is sufficient indication for exploration regardless of whether or not the patient has an associated syndrome. A median sternotomy is the preferred approach because the extent of resection can be deter-

mined only at the time of operation. Encapsulated tumors should be completely resected, along with the entire thymus and the adjacent adipose tissue of the anterosuperior mediastinum. If the thymoma is invasive, complete resection should be attempted by excising all nonvital structures involved by contiguous spread. Radiation therapy in doses of 4,000 to 6,500 r is usually given postoperatively to patients with invasive tumors.

Lymphomas

Mediastinal lymph-node involvement is a frequent manifestation of disseminated lymphoma. In 50 percent of patients with Hodgkin's disease, there is evidence of mediastinal involvement; however, with the advent of accurate clinical staging, the mediastinum has been shown to be the sole site of involvement in only 5 percent of patients. Lymphomas are usually located in the anterior mediastinum but may present as hilar masses in the middle mediastinum, or even less frequently in the posterior compartment. Mediastinal lymphomas can occur at any age but most commonly are seen in the third or fourth decades of life with associated symptoms of cough, chest pain, fever, or weight loss. The diagnosis of mediastinal involvement by disseminated lymphoma is often inferred from the chest x-rays along with cervical lymph-node biopsy, bone marrow aspiration, or liver biopsy. When the tumor is confined to the mediastinum, thoracotomy or mediastinal exploration by anterior mediastinotomy or mediastinoscopy is required to obtain tissue for diagnosis.

Teratodermoid Tumors

A teratoma is a neoplasm composed of multiple tissues foreign to the area in which the teratoma is found. Mediastinal teratomas are believed to arise from cells originating from the branchial cleft and pouch in association with the thymus gland. The mediastinum is second to the gonads as the most frequent location of teratomas in adults, and to the sacrococcygeal area in children (Fig. 17-89). These tumors are most frequently found in the anterior mediastinum at the level of the pericardial reflection, but a rare teratoma is located intrapericardially in the posterior mediastinum. The term *dermoid cyst* is used to describe those lesions that are primarily cystic with a composition that varies in relative amounts of epidermis and dermal glands, hair, and sebaceous material. Careful histologic examination will often reveal that ectodermal elements predominate, but remnants of mesodermal and endodermal tissue are also present. Predominantly solid teratomas have a more complex structure and may contain well-differentiated elements of teeth, bone, cartilage, mucus or salivary glands, muscle, fibrous and lipoid tissue, nerve, thymus, pancreas, and lung.

Teratodermoid tumors occur most frequently in adolescents or young adults and with equal incidence in both sexes. Approximately 80 percent are benign. There is no correlation between the age of the patient or the size of the tumor and malignancy. Although not specific for teratocarcinomas, the most reliable diagnostic tests for suggesting malignancy preoperatively are the serum levels of alpha-fetoprotein and carcinoembryonic antigen. Elevated levels of these glycoproteins are due to their secretion by the malignant components of the tumor, most often adenocarcinoma.

Radiographically, the cystic lesions are well circumscribed, with a smooth outline that projects to either side of the sternum in the posteroanterior view. The solid lesions may be smooth and lobulated, or they may appear irregular.

Fig. 17-89. A mediastinal teratoma in a twenty-five-year-old woman. Chest x-rays taken for nonspecific respiratory symptoms showed a smooth mass overlying the pulmonary artery. Pulmonary arteriography was normal, and the lesion was removed through a median sternotomy.

Operative resection is the definitive treatment for all teratodermoid tumors. Even if benign, the tumors often are attached to the pericardium or thymus, and portions of these structures must be removed with the specimen. Malignant teratomas often invade the pericardium, heart, or superior vena cava, making curative resection impossible. The prognosis for all malignant teratomas is poor because the tumors tend to recur locally and to metastasize early.

Germ Cell Tumors

The entire spectrum of germ cell tumors may arise in extragonadal sites, and when they occur in the thorax, they are located in the anterior mediastinum. Though the histogenesis of such extragonadal germ cell tumors is unknown, most authorities agree that the lesions do not represent metastases from a primary gonadal site.

Seminoma is the most common germinal tumor, usually affecting young men between the ages of twenty to thirty years. Most patients are symptomatic at the time of diagnosis, with retrosternal chest pain, weight loss, hoarseness, or evidence of superior vena caval obstruction. The chest x-ray may show a large anterior mediastinal mass, but there are no pathognomonic features. Clinically and roentgenographically these tumors must be differentiated from thymic neoplasms and lymphomas. They commonly metastasize to the pleura, chest wall, lymph nodes, liver, bone, and retroperitoneum. Most often, only partial excision can be accomplished because of regional and distant spread. Seminomas are highly radiosensitive, and even if complete excision is done postoperative radiation therapy is mandatory.

Choriocarcinoma and embryonal carcinoma are highly malignant neoplasms that also have a predilection for young males. Almost all patients present with symptoms of cough, chest pain, shortness of breath, or hemoptysis. More than half the male patients have gynecomastia and widespread metastases at the time of diagnosis. Choriocarcinomas always produce human chorionic gonadotropin, while the embryonal carcinomas often release alpha-fetoprotein or carcinoembryonic antigen. These tumors are rarely sensitive to irradiation or chemotherapy, and they usually lead to a rapidly fatal course.

Mesenchymal Tumors

A variety of mesenchymal tumors arise in the mediastinum, and as a group they comprise approximately 7 percent of all primary mediastinal tumors and cysts. Lipomas are the most frequently encountered, with three out of four occurring in the anterior mediastinum. Because of soft consistency and lack of fixation to adjacent structures, they may reach enormous size before causing symptoms. When symptoms do occur they are nonspecific in type, such as chest pain and dyspnea. Operative resection of these lesions is curative.

Other mesenchymal tumors which have been reported in the mediastinum include liposarcoma, fibroma, fibrosarcoma, mesothelioma, myxoma, xanthogranuloma, leiomyosarcoma, and rhabdomyosarcoma.

Tumors of blood-vascular and lymph-vascular origin are included among the mesenchymal neoplasms of the anterior mediastinum. The several types of hemangiomas—capillary, cavernous, and venous—are differentiated by the size of the vascular spaces and the presence or absence of smooth muscle cells in the vessel walls. Operative excision is the treatment of choice for both benign hemangiomas and the rare malignant hemangiopericytoma.

The tumors of lymph-vascular origin may be thin-walled, unilocular cysts or multilocular tumors intimately related to surrounding structures. They usually present as a rounded or lobulated mass of homogeneous density on the chest x-ray. The most common variety is the benign lymphangioma, also known as cystic hygroma.

Endocrine Tumors

The two types of endocrine tumors most frequently found in the anterior mediastinum are those of thyroid and parathyroid origin. Perhaps 10 percent of parathyroid adenomas are located in the mediastinum, although many of these may be approached by a cervical incision. They are usually in close association with the upper pole of the thymus gland, a result of their common embryologic origin from the third branchial cleft. It is rare for a parathyroid tumor to present as a mediastinal mass. Instead, a patient with signs and symptoms of hyperparathyroidism will be found to have an adenoma located in the mediastinum after a negative cervical exploration.

Thyroid tumors found in the mediastinum are usually substernal extensions of the cervical gland. True aberrant thyroid tissue is found in the mediastinum only infrequently, and the blood supply in this location is derived from the great vessels. Theoretically, the mediastinal thyroid could represent all of the thyroid tissue that a patient has, but this can easily be determined by means of a radionuclide scan. The latter test should be a routine part of the work-up in any patient who presents with an otherwise undiagnosed mass high in the anterior mediastinum.

MIDDLE MEDIASTINAL LESIONS

Some of the lesions that have been described as occurring in the anterior mediastinum may also develop in the middle mediastinum (Fig. 17-86). Pericardial cysts, esophageal lesions, and Morgagni hernias are unique to the middle compartment.

Cysts

Collectively, congenital cysts comprise approximately 20 percent of primary mediastinal mass lesions. Included in this group are cysts of pericardial, bronchogenic, enteric, and nonspecific origin. *Pericardial cysts* are the most common. Whatever the developmental defect may be, the result is usually a solitary cyst adjacent to the pericardium with a diameter of 3 to 6 cm. Such cysts usually contain a clear fluid and occasionally communicate with the pericardium. Histologically, the cyst wall is composed of a single layer of mesothelial cells. Pericardial cysts, despite their congenital origin, are usually first detected in adult life as an incidental finding on a routine chest x-ray. The most frequent location is at the right cardiophrenic angle. Operative removal is indicated primarily for diagnosis. Accumulated experience with more recent technologies for diagnosis, computed tomography, and ultrasound, for example, may allow confident observation in the future.

Bronchogenic cysts may arise in any location in the mediastinum or lung parenchyma, but they are usually located posterior or inferior to the carina. Rarely, there is communication with the tracheobronchial tree. Bronchogenic cysts are recognized most often in young adults, and symptoms are usually the result of compression by the cyst, with cough, wheezing, dyspnea, or even dysphagia. The cysts are uncommon in infancy, but lesions in a critical position may cause life-threatening respiratory embarrassment. Infection of the cyst may develop and make distinction from a lung abscess very difficult. All bronchogenic cysts should be removed. If the cyst has been infected, dense adhesions in the hilar area can make dissection difficult and require pulmonary resection.

Hernias through the foramen of Morgagni are most often discovered as incidental retrosternal masses on chest x-rays taken for other purposes. Alternately, a herniation of omentum or retroperitoneal fat may be found during a thoracotomy. Even less frequently the transverse colon becomes displaced into the right or left side of the chest through the foramen of Morgagni, and it may then appear as an anterior mediastinal mass on the plain films. Retrosternal pain is sometimes produced and requires operative treatment. When the diagnosis is made preoperatively, an abdominal approach is recommended.

Esophageal lesions and aneurysms are discussed in other chapters.

POSTERIOR MEDIASTINAL LESIONS

Neurogenic Tumors

The several types of neurogenic tumors are the most common neoplasms arising in the mediastinum, accounting for approximately 21 percent of all primary mediastinal tumors and cysts. Classically, neurogenic tumors arise from either the intercostal nerves or the sympathetic ganglia, and they are usually located in the paravertebral gutter (Fig. 17-90). Though the peak incidence is in adult life, the tumors may be seen in children and older persons. An incidence of malignancy between 10 and 20 percent can be estimated from analysis of several reports, with the greater likelihood of malignancy in children. In adults, it is more common for neurogenic tumors to be discovered as an incidental finding. When symptoms are present, the most common complaint is chest pain due to compression of an intercostal nerve or erosion of adjacent bone. Pleural effusion may be found with both benign and malignant lesions, but a bloody effusion is usually a sign of malignancy. The intraspinal component of a "dumbbell" tumor can compress the cord, causing paresthesias and weakness.

Neurogenic tumors may produce systemic syndromes secondary to the endocrine functions of the tumor; e.g., the production of catecholamine by a pheochromocytoma, vanillylmandelic acid by gangliosarcomas and neuroblastomas, and immunoreactive insulin by neurosarcomas.

Neurilemomas are the most common neurogenic tumors, occurring usually in the third to fifth decades of life. They arise from Schwann cells of the nerve sheath and are also called *schwannomas.* The neurilemomas are well encapsulated and are seen on chest films as dense, homogeneous, circumscribed masses in the posterior mediastinum.

Neurofibromas contain nerve elements as well as nerve-sheath cells. They are poorly encapsulated, but radiographically resemble neurilemomas. Neurofibromas of the mediastinum may be one manifestation of generalized neurofibromatosis; however, if a patient with known von Recklinghausen's disease is found to have a posterior mediastinal mass, this more likely represents a *meningocele*, not a neurofibroma. Because of the infiltrating growth of these tumors, complete operative excision is often difficult.

When a neurofibroma or neurilemoma undergoes malignant degeneration, it becomes a *neurosarcoma.* The frequency of malignant change varies from 25 to 30 percent. There is an increased incidence of neurosarcoma associated with generalized neurofibromatosis, and a malignant neoplasm is more often found in older patients. Patients with neurosarcoma have a poor survival rate because of rapid tumor growth and invasion of adjacent mediastinal structures.

Ganglioneuromas originate from a sympathetic ganglion and are composed of mature ganglion cells and nerve fibers. They occur in patients of a younger age group than tumors of nerve-sheath origin and may become very large before causing symptoms. Roentgenographically, a ganglioneuroma often has a triangular configuration, with the broad base toward the mediastinum. In the lateral projection, they are poorly defined because of the radiographic density of the vertebrae. There is no association between endocrine function and malignancy.

Neuroblastomas are the most poorly differentiated malignant tumors arising from the sympathetic nervous system, and approximately 10 percent occur as a primary

Fig. 17-90. A neurilemoma of the posterior mediastinum. *A.* The posteroanterior chest x-ray suggests a dense mass behind the heart. *B.* A tomogram shows the somewhat lobulated appearance of the tumor in the paravertebral gutter.

A

B

lesion in the mediastinum. More than 75 percent occur in children less than four years of age, often with symptoms of fever, vomiting, diarrhea, and cough. Metastases to bone, brain, liver, and regional lymph nodes may be present at the time of diagnosis, and direct invasion of the spinal cord with resultant neurologic deficit is not uncommon. Evidence of catecholamine excretion by the tumor is manifested by systemic hypertension.

Mediastinal neuroblastomas are often unresectable at the time of diagnosis, because of either local invasion or distant metastases. However, the tumors are usually radiosensitive, and long-term survival may follow postoperative radiation therapy. Interestingly, mediastinal neuroblastomas have a more favorable prognosis than neuroblastomas originating at other sites.

Less than 1 percent of all *pheochromocytomas* occur in the mediastinum, but the tumors are most often situated in the posterior region. Clinically, these tumors are no different from the intraabdominal lesions.

The therapy of benign neurogenic tumors is complete excision through a standard posterolateral thoracotomy. The preoperative evaluation should include careful radiographic visualization of the thoracic spine so that any enlargement of the interspinal foramina adjacent to the neoplasm may be detected. If there is an intraspinal component, this portion should be excised prior to thoracotomy, because manipulation of the intrathoracic tumor may cause swelling or bleeding in the spinal canal and precipitate cord compression.

Enteric Cysts

In addition to neurogenic lesions, the posterior mediastinum is the usual location of enteric cysts. These cysts can be located at any level of the posterior mediastinum adjacent to the esophagus, but only rarely is there a communication with that structure. Approximately 60 percent occur in infants less than one year of age, and symptoms of tracheal or esophageal obstruction are common. The cysts usually contain a clear, colorless mucoid fluid. Occasionally, a lining of aberrant gastric mucosa leads to peptic ulceration and perforation of the adjacent bronchial or esophageal lumen, with resulting hemoptysis or hematemesis. Erosion into adjacent lung parenchyma can result in a lung abscess.

Operative removal of the cysts is always indicated, and the surgical approach depends on the level of the lesion as well as its projection toward either hemithorax. Previous episodes of inflammation may result in fibrous tissue proliferation that interferes with dissection of the lesion away from adjacent structures.

Acute Mediastinitis

Acute suppurative mediastinitis is a serious and potentially fatal infection that is generally distributed in the superior or posterior mediastinum. The areolar tissues of the mediastinum have little ability to deal with infection, but the mediastinal pleura on each side serves as a temporary barrier to the spread of the infection into one or both pleural cavities. The mechanism of infection is usually from contamination of the mediastinum due to (1) perforation of the cervical or thoracic esophagus during instrumentation; (2) esophageal perforation by foreign body; (3) leakage of an esophageal suture line following operative procedures; (4) inferior extension of a cervical suppuration; (5) spread of infection into the soft tissues from an infection involving the ribs, sternum, or vertebra; (6) mediastinal extension of pleural or pulmonary infection; (7) external trauma; and (8) spontaneous esophageal rupture (Boerhaave's syndrome).

Chills and fever, shock, tachycardia, dull or severe chest pain, and soft tissue crepitus in the suprasternal notch may progress rapidly in the patient with continuing contamination from esophageal perforation. The chest x-ray will usually show widening of the superior mediastinum as well as air in the tissue planes. As the infection spreads, pleuritic pain often occurs, associated with effusion. Thoracentesis or tube thoracostomy may become necessary to relieve both the pleural sepsis and respiratory distress.

Acute infections which involve the lower mediastinum, as seen with perforation of the distal esophagus, produce less definite signs and symptoms. The pain may be subxiphoid or epigastric, and the tenderness and muscle rigidity of the upper part of the abdomen may suggest an acute intraabdominal process. Crepitus is often absent or late in appearance, and gastric contents escaping through the esophageal laceration may not penetrate the pleura for 24 hours or longer.

Acute infections of the mediastinum require immediate and vigorous management if prolonged and complicated convalescence or death is to be avoided. Without continued contamination, localized acute mediastinitis may resolve completely with massive broad-spectrum antibiotic coverage. Most surgeons, however, recommend immediate exploration for mediastinitis associated with esophageal injury. A more detailed discussion of the management of esophageal perforation is given in Chap. 25.

Chronic Mediastinitis

Chronic inflammation and fibrosis in the mediastinum is most often the result of a specific granulomatous infection such as tuberculosis, histoplasmosis, or other mycotic infections. *Sclerosing mediastinitis* and *fibrosing mediastinitis* are terms that have developed common usage with continuing mediastinal inflammation because of the clinical effects of the process. Analysis of cases suggests that the mediastinitis begins as an extension of infection from involved mediastinal, tracheobronchial, or hilar lymph nodes. Though histoplasmosis and tuberculosis are thought to be the most frequent initiators of the process, it has been unusual to prove the relationship in individual patients by demonstration of the organisms.

The more notable clinical presentations are usually the result of progressive fibrosis with obstruction of the superior vena cava, the esophagus, or the pulmonary veins. Symptoms of chest pain, fever, exercise intolerance, and dysphasia may occur to correlate with mediastinal widening on standard chest x-rays. A clinical picture of superior vena caval obstruction may occur, however, in the absence of significant changes on the x-rays. Angiography and tomography are usually helpful in demonstrating the underlying process, but operative exploration may be required to define the morphologic and etiologic diagnosis.

The treatment depends on the determination of the cause of the mediastinitis, its degree of activity, and the functional effects. Obstruction of the superior vena cava or esophagus may require operative relief, or rarely, pericardiectomy may be necessary to relieve constrictive pericarditis.

Superior Vena Caval Obstruction

In this country the great majority of patients who develop obstruction of their superior vena cava have bronchogenic cancer. It is estimated that 10 to 15 percent of those with lung cancer will develop caval obstruction before death. Primary neoplasms of the right upper lobe are the most frequent tumors that involve the vena cava, but metastatic tumor and lymphomas account for a larger number than do benign lesions. Thoracic aortic aneurysms, including dissecting aneurysms, occasionally compress the vena cava, and rarely a benign tumor is responsible for the obstruction. The mechanism of obstruction varies from simple compression to malignant invasion and thrombosis. Rarely, thrombosis may accompany a septic thrombophlebitis due to drug injections in an addict or a contaminated central venous catheter. Fibrosing mediastinitis may lead to thrombotic occlusion, and this complication can apparently occur in the presence of polycythemia without an associated obstruction.

Headache, confusion, discomfort on bending over, swelling of facial structures, and distended veins in the upper half of the body are common clinical presentations of superior caval obstruction. Sudden occlusion can lead to rapid development of cerebral edema, intracranial thrombosis, and death. A suspected diagnosis of caval obstruction should be confirmed by venography regardless of cause.

For patients with proved malignant neoplasms the aggressiveness of therapy for relief of caval obstruction depends on the stage of their disease. Most of those with bronchogenic carcinoma will receive only temporary relief from radiation therapy combined with nitrogen mustard or other adjuvants. A rare patient with a controlled or slowly growing malignancy can benefit from a combination of radiation therapy and a vascular graft that bypasses the superior vena cava. For patients with nonmalignant caval obstruction it is reasonable to consider treatment with diuretics, salt restriction, and a Fowler's position in bed while collateral venous channels have an opportunity to develop. Failing this, operative reconstruction of the superior vena cava or a bypass graft may be done.

References

Introduction

Meade, R. H.: "A History of Thoracic Surgery," Charles C Thomas, Publisher, Springfield, Ill., 1961.

Anatomy of the Thorax and Pleura

Blevins, C. E.: Anatomy of the Thorax and Pleura, in T. W. Shields, (ed.), "General Thoracic Surgery," Lea & Febiger, Philadelphia, 1972.

Grant, J. C. B. and Basmajian, J. V.: "Grant's Method of Anatomy," 7th ed., The Williams & Wilkins Company, Baltimore, 1965.

Thoracic Incisions

Thurer, R. J., Bognolo, D., Vargus, A., Isch, J. H. and Kaiser, G. A.: The Management of Mediastinal Infection following Cardiac Surgery, *J Thorac Cardiovasc Surg*, **68:**962, 1974.

Evaluation of the Thoracic Surgical Patient

Boren, H. G., Kory, R. C. and Syner, J. C.: The Veterans Administration–Army Cooperative Study of Pulmonary Function: II. The Lung Volume and Its Subdivisions in Normal Men, *Am J Med*, **41:**96, 1966.

Miller, R. N.: Evaluation of Pulmonary Impairment in the Surgical Candidate, *Med Clin North Am*, **46:**885, 1962.

Mittman, C.: Assessment of Operative Risk in Thoracic Surgery, *Am Rev Resp Dis*, **84:**197, 1961.

Olsen, G. N., Block, A. J., Swenson, E. W., Castle, J. R., and Wynne, J. W.: Pulmonary Function Evaluation of the Lung Resection Candidate: A Prospective Study, *Am Rev Resp Dis*, **111:**379, 1975.

Petty, T. L.: "Pulmonary Diagnostic Techniques," Lea & Febiger, Philadelphia, 1975.

Thoracic Injuries

Blaisdell, F. W., and Lewis, F. R., Jr.: "Respiratory Distress Syndrome of Shock and Trauma," W. B. Saunders Company, Philadelphia, 1977.

Bryant, L. R., Spencer, F. C., Boyd, A. D., and Daly, J. F.: Tracheostomy and Assisted Ventilation, in D. L. Sabiston, Jr. and F. C. Spencer (eds.), "Gibbon's Surgery of the Chest," W. B. Saunders Company, Philadelphia, 1976.

Grover, F. L., Richardson, J. D., Fervel, J. G., Arom, K. V., Webb, G. E., and Trinkle, J. K.: Prophylactic Antibiotics in the Treatment of Penetrating Chest Wounds, *J Thorac Cardiovasc Surg*, **74:**528, 1977.

Hankins, J. R., McAslan, T. C., Ayella, R., Cowley, R. A., and McLaughlin, J. S.: Extensive Pulmonary Laceration Caused by Blunt Trauma, *J Thorac Cardiovasc Surg*, **55:**16, 1968.

Naclerio, E. A.: "Chest Injuries," Grune & Stratton, Inc., New York, 1971.

Neugebauer, M. K., Fasburg, R. G., and Trummer, M. J.: Routine Antibiotic Therapy following Pleural Space Intubation, *J Thorac Cardiovasc Surg*, **61:**882, 1971.

Patterson, L. T., Schmitt, H. J., Jr., and Armstrong, R. G.: Intermediate Care of War Wounds of the Chest, *J Thorac Cardiovasc Surg*, **61:**882, 1971.

Ruckley, C. V., and McCormack, R. J. M.: The Management of Spontaneous Pneumothorax, *Thorax*, **21:**139, 1966.

Shackford, S. R., Smith, D. L., Zarins, C. K., Rice, C. L. and Virgilio, R. W.: The Management of Flail Chest. A Comparison of Ventilatory and Non-ventilatory Treatment, *Am J Surg*, **132:**759, 1976.

Sladen, A.: Methylprednisolone: Pharmacologic Doses in Shock Lung Syndrome, *J Thorac Cardiovasc Surg*, **71:**300, 1976.

Thomas, A. N., and Stephens, B. G.: Air Embolism: A Cause of Morbidity and Death after Penetrating Chest Trauma, *J Trauma,* **14:**633, 1974.

Waldo, W. J., Harlaftis, N. N. and Symbas, P. N.: Systemic Air Embolism: Does It Occur after Experimental Penetrating Lung Injury? *J Thorac Cardiovasc Surg,* **71:**96, 1976.

Wise, L., Connors, J., Hwang, Y. H., and Anderson, C.: Traumatic Injuries to the Diaphragm, *J Trauma,* **13:**946, 1973.

Chest Wall

Congenital Deformities of the Chest Wall

Beiser, G. C., Epstein, S. E., Stempter, M. D., Goldstern, R. E., Noland, S. P., and Levitsky, S.: Impairment of Cardiac Function with Pectus Excavatum with Improvement after Operative Correction, *N Engl J Med,* **287:**267, 1972.

Haller, J. A., Jr., Peters, G. N., Mazur, D., and White, J. J.: Pectus Excavatum, *J Thorac Cardiovasc Surg,* **60:**375, 1970.

Ravitch, M. M.: Disorders of the Sternum and the Thoracic Wall, in D. L. Sabiston, Jr., and F. C. Spencer (eds.), "Gibbon's Surgery of the Chest," 3d ed., W. B. Saunders Company, Philadelphia, 1976.

Stallworth, J. M., Quinn, G. J., and Aiken, A. F.: Is Rib Resection Necessary for Relief of Thoracic Outlet Syndrome? *Ann Surg,* **185:**581, 1977.

Urschel, H. C., Jr., Razzuk, M. A., Wood, R. E., Parekh, M., and Paulson, D. L.: Objective Diagnosis (Ulnar Nerve Conduction Velocity) and Current Therapy of the Thoracic Outlet Syndrome, *Ann Thorac Surg,* **12:**608, 1971.

Weg, J. G., Krumholz, R. A., and Harkleroad, L. E.: Pulmonary Dysfunction in Pectus Excavatum, *Am Rev Resp Dis,* **96:**936, 1967.

Chest-Wall Tumors

Adkins, P. C.: Tumors of the Chest Wall, in T. W. Shields (ed.), "General Thoracic Surgery," Lea & Febiger, Philadelphia 1972.

Burnard, R. J., Martini, N., and Beattie, E. J., Jr.: The Value of Resection in Tumors Involving the Chest Wall, *J Thorac Cardiovasc Surg,* **68:**530, 1974.

Martini, N., Huvos, A. G., Smith, J., and Beattie, E. J., Jr.: Primary Malignant Tumors of the Sternum, *Surg Gynecol Obstet,* **138:**391, 1974.

Pleura

Bryant, L. R., Chicklo, J. M., Crutcher, R. R., et al.: Management of Thoracic Empyema, *J Thorac Cardiovasc Surg,* **55:**850, 1968.

Craenen, J. M., Williams, T. E., Jr., and Kilman, J. W.: Simplified Management of Chylothorax in Neonates and Infants, *Ann Thorac Surg,* **24:**275, 1977.

Green, R. A., and Johnson, R. F.: Diseases of the Pleura, in G. L. Baum (ed.), "Textbook of Pulmonary Diseases," 2d ed., Little, Brown and Company, Boston, 1974.

Sahn, S. A.: Evaluation of Pleural Effusions and Pleural Biopsy, in T. L. Petty (ed.), "Pulmonary Diagnostic Techniques," Lea & Febiger, Philadelphia, 1975.

Shearin, J. C., Jr., and Jackson, D.: Malignant Pleural Mesothelioma: Report of 19 Cases, *J Thorac Cardiovasc Surg,* **71:**621, 1976.

Lungs and Trachea

Anatomy and Diagnostic Techniques

Arom, K. V., Franz, J. L., Grover, F. L., and Trinkle, J. K.: Subxiphoid Anterior Mediastinal Exploration, *Ann Thorac Surg,* **24:**289, 1977.

Bartlett, J. G., Rosenblatt, J. D., and Finegold, S. M.: Percutaneous Transtracheal Aspiration in the Diagnosis of Anaerobic Pulmonary Infection, *Ann Intern Med,* **79:**535, 1973.

Boyden, E. A., and Tomsett, D. H.: Congenital Absence of the Medial Basal Bronchus in a Child: With Preliminary Observations on Postnatal Growth of the Lungs, *J Thorac Cardiovasc Surg,* **43:**517, 1962.

Neff, T. A.: Needle Lung Biopsy, in T. L. Petty (ed.), "Pulmonary Diagnostic Techniques," Lea & Febiger, Philadelphia, 1975.

Nohl, H. C.: "The Spread of Carcinoma of the Bronchus," Lloyd Luke, London, 1962.

Nohl-Oser, H. C.: The Lymphatic Spread of Carcinoma of the Bronchus, in "International Symposium of Mediastinoscopy," Odense University Press, Odense, Denmark, 1970.

Sinner, W. N.: Wert und Bedeutung der perkutanen transthorakalen Nadelbiopsie, *Fortschr Geb Roentgenstr Nuklearmed,* **123:**197, 1975.

Stanford, W., Steele, S., Armstrong, R. G., and Larsen, G. L.: Mediastinoscopy: Its Application in Central versus Peripheral Thoracic Lesions, *Ann Thorac Surg,* **19:**121, 1975.

Congenital Disorders

Glenn, W. L., Liebow, A. A., and Lindskog, G. E.: "Thoracic and Cardiovascular Surgery with Related Pathology," 3d ed., Appleton-Century-Crofts, Inc., New York, 1975.

Michelson, E.: Clinical Spectrum of Infantile Lobar Emphysema, *Ann Thorac Surg,* **24:**182, 1977.

Pulmonary Infections

Baum, G. L.: "Textbook of Pulmonary Diseases," 2d ed., Little, Brown and Company, Boston, 1974.

Elkadi, A., Salas, R., and Almond, C. H.: Surgical Treatment of Atypical Pulmonary Tuberculosis, *J Thorac Cardiovasc Surg,* **72:**435, 1976.

Fosburg, R. G., Baisch, B. F., and Trumner, M. J.: Limited Pulmonary Resection for Coccidioidomycosis, *Ann Thorac Surg,* **7:**420, 1969.

Glenn, W. L., Liebow, A. A., and Lindskog, G. E.: "Thoracic and Cardiovascular Surgery with Related Pathology," 3d ed., Appleton-Century-Crofts, Inc., New York, 1975.

Groff, D. B., and Marquis, J.: Transtracheal Drainage of Lung Abscesses in Children, *J Pediatr Surg,* **12:**303, 1977.

Larsen, R. E., Bernatz, P. E., and Gerasi, J. E.: Results of Surgical and Nonoperative Treatment for Pulmonary North American Blastomycosis, *J Thorac Cardiovasc Surg,* **51:**714, 1966.

Prather, J. R., Eastridge, C. E., Hughes, F. H., Jr., et al.: Actinomycosis of the Thorax: Diagnosis and Treatment, *Ann Thorac Surg,* **9:**307, 1970.

Sealy, W. C., Bradham, R. R., and Young, W. G., Jr.: The Surgical Treatment of Multisegmental and Localized Bronchiectasis, *Surg Gyncol Obstet,* **123:**80, 1966.

Solit, R. W., McKeown, J., Jr., Smullens, S., et al.: The Surgical Implications of Intracavity Mycetoma (Fungus Balls), *J Thorac Cardiovasc Surg,* **62:**411, 1971.

Sutaria, M. K., Polk, J. W., Reddy, P., et al.: Surgical Aspects of

Pulmonary Histoplasmosis: A Series of 110 Cases, *Thorax,* **25:**31, 1970.

Takaro, T.: Mycotic Infections of Interest to Thoracic Surgeons: Collective Review, *Ann Thorac Surg,* **3:**71, 1967.

Tunell, W. P., Koh, Y. C., and Adkins, P. C.: The Dilemma of Coincident Active Pulmonary Tuberculosis and Carcinoma of the Lung, *J Thorac Cardiovasc Surg,* **62:**563, 1971.

Solitary Pulmonary Nodules

Higgins, G. A., Shields, T. W., and Keehn, R. J.: The Solitary Pulmonary Nodule: Ten-Year Follow-up of Veterans Administration–Armed Forces Cooperative Study, *Arch Surg,* **110:**570, 1975.

Lillington, G. A., and Stevens, G. M.: The Solitary Nodule: The Other Side of the Coin, *Chest,* **70:**322, 1976.

Nathan, M. H.: Management of Solitary Pulmonary Nodules: An Organized Approach Based on Growth Rate and Statistics, *JAMA,* **227:**1141, 1974.

Primary Carcinoma of the Lung

Armentrout, S. A.: Chemotherapy in Carcinoma of the Lung, *Chest,* **71:**638, 1977.

Bates, M.: Results of Surgery for Bronchial Carcinoma in Patients Aged 70 and Over, *Thorax,* **25:**77, 1970.

Bell, J. W.: Positive Sputum Cytology and Negative Chest Roentgenograms: A Surgeon's Dilemma, *Ann Thorac Surg,* **9:**149, 1970.

Brock, Lord: Long Survival after Operation for Cancer of the Lung, *Br J Surg,* **62:**1, 1975.

Holmes, E. C.: Immunology of Lung Cancer, *Chest,* **71:**643, 1977.

Kennedy, J. H.: Extrapulmonary Effects of Cancer of the Lung and Pleura, *J Thorac Surg,* **61:**514, 1971.

McKneally, M. F., Maver, C., and Kausal, H. W.: Regional Immunotherapy with Intrapleural BCG for Lung Cancer: Surgical Considerations, *J Thorac Cardiovasc Surg,* **72:**333, 1976.

Mountain, C. F.: Assessment of the Role of Surgery for Control of Lung Cancer, *Ann Thorac Surg,* **24:**365, 1977.

Paulson, D. L., and Reisch, J. S.: Long Term Survival after Resection for Bronchogenic Carcinoma, *Ann Surg,* **184:**324, 1976.

—— and Urschel, H. C., Jr.: Selectivity in the Surgical Treatment of Bronchogenic Carcinoma, *J Thorac Cardiovasc Surg,* **62:**554, 1971.

Pearson, F. G., Thompson, D. W., and Delarne, N. C.: Experience with the Cytologic Detection, Localization and Treatment of Radiographically Undemonstrable Bronchial Carcinoma, *J Thorac Cardiovasc Surg,* **54:**371, 1967.

Shields, T. W., Yee, J., Conn, J. H., and Robinette, C. D.: Relationship of Cell Type and Lymph Node Metastasis to Survival after Resection of Bronchial Carcinoma, *Ann Thorac Surg,* **20:**501, 1975.

Bronchial Carcinoid and Tumors of Bronchial-Gland Origin

Axelsson, C., Burcharth, F., and Johansen, A.: Mucoepidermoid Lung Tumors, *J Thorac Cardiovasc Surg,* **65:**902, 1973.

Heilbrunn, A., and Crosby, I. K.: Adenocystic Carcinoma and Mucoepidermoid Carcinoma of the Tracheobronchial Tree, *Chest,* **61:**145, 1972.

McConaghie, R. J.: The Malignant Carcinoid Syndrome Associated with a Metastasizing Bronchial Adenoma: Report of a Case, *J Thorac Cardiovasc Surg,* **43:**303, 1962.

Meffert, W. G., and Lindskog, G. E.: Bronchial Adenoma, *J Thorac Cardiovasc Surg,* **59:**588, 1970.

Turnbull, A. D., Huvos, A. G., Goodner, J. T., et al.: The Malignant Potential of Bronchial Adenoma, *Ann Thorac Surg,* **14:**453, 1972.

Miscellaneous Lung Tumors

Arrigoni, M. G., Woolner, L. B., Bernatz, P. E., et al.: Benign Tumors of the Lung: A Ten-Year Surgical Experience, *J Thorac Cardiovasc Surg,* **60:**589, 1970.

Davis, P. W., Briggs, J. C., Seal, R. M. E., et al.: Benign and Malignant Mixed Tumours of the Lung, *Thorax,* **27:**657, 1972.

Guccion, J. G., and Rosen, S. H.: Bronchopulmonary Leiomyosarcoma and Fibrosarcoma: A Study of 32 Cases and Review of the Literature, *Cancer,* **30:**836, 1972.

Iverson, R. E., and Straehley, C. J.: Pulmonary Blastoma: Longterm Survival of Juvenile Patient, *Chest,* **63:**436, 1973.

Kakos, G. S., Williams, T. E., Jr., Assor, D., et al.: Pulmonary Carcinosarcoma: Etiologic Therapeutic and Prognostic Considerations, *J Thorac Cardiovasc Surg,* **61:**777, 1971.

Koutras, P., Urschel, H. C., Jr., and Paulson, D. L.: Hamartoma of the Lung, *J Thorac Cardiovasc Surg,* **61:**768, 1971.

McNamara, J. J., Paulson, D. L., Kingsley, W. B., et al.: Primary Leiomyosarcoma of the Lung, *J Thorac Cardiovasc Surg,* **57:**635, 1969.

Martini, N., Hajdu, S. I., and Beattie, E. J., Jr.: Primary Sarcoma of the Lung, *J Thorac Cardiovasc Surg,* **61:**33, 1971.

Ostermiller, W. E., Comer, T. P., and Barker, W. L.: Endobronchial Granular Cell Myoblastoma: A Report of Three Cases and Review of the Literature, *Ann Thorac Surg,* **9:**143, 1970.

Metastatic Pulmonary Neoplasms

Beattie, E. J., Martini, N., and Rosen, G.: The Management of Pulmonary Metastases in Children with Osteogenic Sarcoma with Surgical Resection Combined with Chemotherapy, *Cancer,* **34:**618, 1975.

Cahan, W. G., Castro, E. B., and Hajdu, S. I.: The Significance of a Solitary Lung Shadow in Patients with Colon Carcinoma, *Cancer,* **33:**414, 1974.

McCormack, P. M., Bains, M. S., Beattie, E. J., and Martini, N.: Pulmonary Resection in Metastatic Carcinoma, *Chest,* **73:**163, 1978.

Morton, D. L., Joseph, W. L., Ketcham, A. S., Geelhoed, G. W., and Adkins, P. C.: Surgical Resection and Adjunctive Immunotherapy for Selected Patients with Multiple Pulmonary Metastasis, *Ann Surg,* **178:**360, 1973.

Ochsner, A., and DeBakey, M.: Significance of Metastasis in Primary Carcinoma of the Lungs, *J Thorac Surg,* **11:**357, 1942.

Roth, J. A., Silverstein, M. J., and Morton, D. L.: Metastatic Potential of Metastases, *Surgery,* **79:**669, 1976.

Takita, H., Merrin, C., Didalkar, M. S., Douglass, H. O., and Edgerton, F.: The Surgical Management of Multiple Lung Metastases, *Ann Thorac Surg,* **24:**359, 1977.

Trachea

Bryant, L. R., Trinkle, J. K., and Dubilier, L.: Reappraisal of Tracheal Injury from Cuffed Tracheostomy Tubes, *JAMA,* **215:**625, 1971.

Grillo, H. C.: Congenital Lesions, Neoplasms and Injuries of the Trachea, in Gibbon, J. H., Jr., Sabiston, D. C., Jr., and Spencer, F. C. (eds.): "Surgery of the Chest," 3d ed., W. B. Saunders Company, Philadelphia, 1976.

Hajdu, S. K., Huvos, A. G., Goodner, J. T., Foote, F. W., Jr., and

Beattie, E. J., Jr.: Carcinoma of the Trachea: Clinicopathologic Study of 41 Cases, *Cancer,* **25:**1448, 1970.

Moghissi, K.: Personal communication.

————: Tracheal Reconstruction with a Prosthesis of Marlex Mesh and Pericardium, *J Thorac Cardiovasc Surg,* **69:**499, 1975.

Neville, W. E., Bolanowski, P. J., and Soltanzadeh, H.: Prosthetic Reconstruction of the Trachea and Carina, *J Thorac Cardiovasc Surg,* **72:**525, 1976.

Pearson, F. G., Thompson, D. W., Weissbert, D., Simpson, W. J. K., and Kergin, F. G.: Adenoid Cystic Carcinoma of Trachea: Experience with 16 Patients Managed by Tracheal Resection, *Ann Thorac Surg,* **18:**16, 1974.

Rodgers, B. M., Rosenfeld, M., and Talbert, J. L.: Endobronchial Cryotherapy in the Treatment of Tracheal Strictures, *J Pediatr Surg,* **12:**443, 1977.

Webb, W. R., Ozdemir, I. A., Ikins, P. M., and Parker, F., Jr.: Surgical Management of Tracheal Stenosis, *Ann Surg,* **179:**819, 1974.

Mediastinum

Burkell, C. C., Cross, J. M., Kent, H. P., and Nanson, E. N.: Mass Lesions of the Mediastinum, in M. M. Ravitch (ed.), "Current Problems in Surgery," Yearbook Medical Publishers, Inc., Chicago, June 1969.

Effler, D. B., and Groves, L. K.: Superior Vena Caval Obstruction, *J Thorac Cardiovasc Surg,* **43:**574, 1962.

Filler, R. M., Troggis, D. G., Jaffe, W., and Vawter, G. F.: Favorable Outlook for Children with Mediastinal Neuroblastoma, *J Pediatr Surg,* **7:**136, 1972.

Gomes, M. N., and Hufnagel, C. A.: Superior Vena Cava Obstruction, *Ann Thorac Surg,* **20:**344, 1975.

Grimes, O. F.: Infections of the Mediastinum and the Superior Vena Caval Syndrome, in T. W. Shields (ed.), "General Thoracic Surgery," Lea & Febiger, Philadelphia, 1972.

Kirwan, W. O., Walbaum, P. R., and McCormack, R. J.: Cystic Intrathoracic Derivatives of the Foregut and Their Complications, *Thorax,* **28:**424, 1973.

Sakulsky, S. B., Harrison, E. G., Jr., Dinea, D. E., and Payne, W. S.: Mediastinal Granuloma, *J Thorac Cardiovasc Surg,* **54:**279, 1967.

Wychulis, A. R., Payne, W. S., Clagett, O. T., and Woolner, L. B.: Surgical Treatment of Mediastinal Tumors: A 40-Year Experience, *J Thorac Cardiovasc Surg,* **62:**379, 1971.

Chapter 18

Congenital Heart Disease

by **Frank C. Spencer**

INTRODUCTION

With the declining incidence of rheumatic fever, congenital heart disease has become the most common form of heart disease seen in children. In several studies the frequency has been found to be about 3 cases of congenital heart disease occurring in every 1,000 live births. The frequency is about ten times greater in members of the same family than in the normal population, and a convenient approximation of risk of occurrence in younger siblings of a child with congenital heart disease is about 2 percent. In most patients the etiologic factor is unknown.

Rubella occurring in the first trimester of pregnancy is one of the few infectious diseases known to cause congenital heart disease. It produces the well-recognized syndrome of mental deficiency, deafness, cataracts, and congenital heart disease, usually a patent ductus arteriosus. Mongolism is another congenital abnormality associated with a high incidence of congenital heart disease. Usually congenital heart disease occurs as an isolated malformation resulting from defective embryonic development without known cause.

The surprisingly short period of time during which cardiac development occurs in uterine life should be emphasized, for virtually all the fetal heart structures are formed between the third and eighth week of pregnancy, a time interval of only 5 weeks. Atrial or ventricular septal defects result from incomplete formation of the respective septa, while transposition and other anomalies of the aorta result from abnormalities in the spiral division of the primitive bulbus cordis. Although there are six branchial aortic arches, all atrophy with the exception of the fourth left arch, remaining as the aorta, and the sixth left arch, remaining as the ductus arteriosus. Malformations with vascular rings arise from different remnants of these embryonic branchial arches.

The fetal circulation has several distinctive features, which may persist in association with congenital heart disease in adults. In embryonic life the lungs are collapsed, with a high vascular resistance, and pulmonary blood flow is small. Most of the blood returning through the inferior vena cava to the right atrium goes through the foramen ovale into the left atrium and thence to the left ventricle. Also, most of the blood expelled from the right ventricle into the pulmonary artery is shunted through the ductus arteriosus into the descending thoracic aorta. At birth, with expansion of the lungs, there is a fall in pulmonary vascular resistance, although the vascular resistance does not decrease to that normally found in older individuals for the first 1 to 3 years of life. There is a corresponding persistence during this time of the fetal histologic structure of the pulmonary arteries, characterized principally by an abundance of smooth muscle in the media of the arterial wall. Persistence of the fetal histologic structure of the pulmonary arterioles has been associated with pulmonary hypertension in small children.

With expansion of the lungs, the ductus arteriosus normally closes in the first few days after birth. It remains patent in only a small percentage of individuals, but this is one of the most common forms of congenital heart disease. The foramen ovale is a slitlike channel which is automatically sealed when left atrial pressure becomes higher than right atrial pressure and normally permits the flow of blood only from the right atrium to the left atrium, not in the reverse direction. Patency of the foramen ovale, usually an innocuous defect, remains throughout adult life in at least 10 to 20 percent of patients. With elevation of right atrial pressure above left atrial pressure from any cause, the foramen ovale may be stretched open and create a right-to-left shunt from the right atrium to the left atrium, resulting in cyanosis from shunting of unoxygenated blood. This characteristically occurs in patients with pulmonic valvular stenosis when right ventricular failure develops and right atrial pressure rises above left atrial pressure.

Although a large number of congenital heart defects have been recognized and classified, in a large pediatric cardiac clinic seven malformations will be found to comprise the majority of abnormalities seen. Ventricular septal defect, with or without pulmonic stenosis, is by far the most common, representing 20 percent or more of all patients. The other six malformations, each occurring in 10 to 15 percent of patients, are atrial septal defect, pulmonic valvular stenosis, aortic valvular stenosis, patent ductus arteriosus, coarctation of the aorta, and transposition of the great vessels. The frequency of different defects varies somewhat with the age of the patient studied; transposition of the great vessels is a much more common disease in the newborn, as many do not survive beyond six months of age.

Classification

Congenital heart disease may be conveniently classified by the type of anatomic abnormality present, which in turn produces a distinct physiologic disturbance, as follows: (1) obstructive lesions predominantly restrict the flow of blood, with corresponding increased work loads on the obstructed ventricular chamber; (2) left-to-right shunts occur through uncomplicated septal defects; (3) right-to-left shunts result from combination of a septal defect with obstruction to ventricular emptying; (4) complex malformations, as the name indicates, are more extensive disturbances of the structure of the heart from gross errors in development. These include abnormal origin or atresia of the aorta or pulmonary artery and hypoplasia or atresia of the right or left ventricle and the corresponding tricuspid and mitral valves.

Pathophysiology

Four stages in the severity of congenital heart disease often can be recognized. Initially, there may be only abnormal physical findings. In milder forms of congenital heart disease, such as trivial pulmonic valvular stenosis, there may never be any sign of heart disease except the characteristic systolic murmur. In the second stage of severity, physiologic disturbances can be measured by cardiac catheterization, such as pressure gradients across stenotic pulmonic or aortic valves, increased blood flow through shunts occurring through atrial or ventricular septal defects, or elevation in pulmonary artery pressure as pulmonary hypertension evolves. Sooner or later, these physiologic abnormalities produce corresponding anatomic changes (the third stage in severity) manifested principally by cardiac enlargement with hypertrophy of the right or left ventricle, best measured by the electrocardiogram and roentgenogram. With the development of pulmonary hypertension, histologic changes occur in the media and intima of the pulmonary arterioles. Only in the fourth stage do symptoms of cardiac failure appear.

This late appearance of symptoms is an important consideration in evaluating children with congenital heart disease, for parents are normally apprehensive about consenting to complex diagnostic studies or operative procedures on a child who seems, to the inexperienced eye, to have little disability. Postponing therapy until a child is disabled to a point that is clinically obvious may result in irreversible changes in ventricular muscle, for severe hypertrophy of the right or left ventricle does not always regress completely following surgical correction of the basic cause, such as pulmonic or aortic stenosis. Even more serious is an increase in pulmonary vascular resistance, which, with present therapy, is often irreversible.

The three main physiologic disturbances resulting from congenital heart disease are (1) obstruction to emptying of the ventricles, (2) left-to-right shunts with increase in pulmonary blood flow and corresponding decrease in systemic blood flow, and (3) right-to-left shunts producing oxygen unsaturation of the arterial blood. Each of these physiologic disturbances is considered in detail in subsequent sections. Also, with all forms of congenital heart disease there is an increased susceptibility to bacterial endocarditis, because the anatomic malformation creates a localized turbulent flow of blood predisposing to local deposition of bacteria during a transient bacteremia.

OBSTRUCTIVE LESIONS. The most common disorders are pulmonic valvular stenosis, aortic valvular stenosis, and coarctation of the aorta. These impede emptying of the involved ventricular chamber, resulting in what has been termed "systolic" overloading and corresponding concentric hypertrophy of the ventricle. As the ventricular response is predominantly concentric hypertrophy, cardiac enlargement cannot be detected by clinical means, and often the chest roentgenogram is only slightly abnormal. The electrocardiogram is a most useful guide, however, indicating the degree of ventricular hypertrophy which has occurred. With progressive left ventricular hypertrophy angina pectoris may occur, with susceptibility to arrhythmias and even sudden death. Cardiac failure is a late and often preterminal manifestation.

LEFT-TO-RIGHT SHUNTS. As pressures in the left atrium and left ventricle are normally greater than those in the right atrium and right ventricle, a defect in either the atrial or ventricular septum results in a shunt of oxygenated blood from the left side of the heart to the right side. This causes pulmonary congestion from an increase in pulmonary blood flow and often a corresponding decrease in systemic blood flow. Cyanosis, of course, does not occur. With the increase in pulmonary blood flow there is a tendency to develop pulmonary hypertension, varying both with the type of defect and with the individual patient. The most common defects producing left-to-right shunts are atrial septal defects, with or without anomalous pulmonary veins, ventricular septal defects, and patent ductus arteriosus.

Pulmonary Congestion. A shunt becomes physiologically significant when the pulmonary blood flow is 1.5 to 2.0 times as great as the systemic blood flow. Large shunts may produce a pulmonary blood flow three to four times greater than systemic blood flow, with a calculated pulmonary blood flow of even 10 to 15 liters/minute/square meter of body surface. The resulting pulmonary congestion produces a susceptibility to bacterial infection; recurrent bouts of pneumonia may occur in the first few years of life. Beyond early childhood, however, high pulmonary blood flows may be associated with surprisingly little disability for a period of time. With the increase in pulmonary blood flow there is a corresponding enlargement of the involved ventricle (right ventricle with atrial septal defect, left ventricle with patent ductus arteriosus, both ventricles with ventricular septal defect), resulting in so-called "diastolic" overloading of the ventricle, with cardiac dilatation rather than hypertrophy. The dilatation can be more easily recognized on clinical examination and on the chest roentgenogram than its counterpart, concentric hypertrophy. The changes in the electrocardiogram are often less prominent than those seen with concentric hypertrophy. Cardiac failure tends to occur somewhat earlier in the course of the disease than with concentric hypertrophy, and the prognosis with medical therapy is somewhat better than that for predominantly obstructive lesions.

Pulmonary Hypertension. With the increase in pulmonary blood flow there is a tendency to develop pulmonary hypertension. Although the mode of development has been a subject of intense study for over two decades, many factors remain unknown. An excellent analysis of the functional pathology of the pulmonary vascular bed was published by Edwards in 1957. Pulmonary hypertension may result from at least three factors: (1) an increase in pulmonary blood flow, (2) histologic changes in the pulmonary vascular bed with corresponding anatomic restriction of distensibility of the pulmonary vessels, or (3) pulmonary venous obstruction. It should be emphasized that the most important consideration in evaluating the pulmonary circulation is the pulmonary vascular resistance, not the systolic pulmonary arterial pressure per se. Pulmonary hypertension resulting from an increase in pulmonary blood flow subsides as soon as the cardiac defect producing the increase in

blood flow is corrected. Pulmonary hypertension due to increased pulmonary vascular resistance from a decrease in distensibility of the pulmonary vascular bed is often irreversible, however. When severe, surgical therapy may be of limited value or even contraindicated. Hence, in evaluating pulmonary hypertension, the significant physiologic measurement is the degree of change in the pulmonary vascular resistance, as calculated from the relation between flow and pressure, and not the absolute level of the pulmonary artery pressure per se.

Normally pulmonary arterioles are very distensible and can accommodate an increase in pulmonary blood flow up to three times normal values without any increase in pressure. Further distensibility is limited by the fibrous tissue in the adventitial sheath surrounding the arterioles. In infants and young children with pulmonary hypertension the prominent histologic change in the pulmonary arterioles is hypertrophy of the smooth muscle of the media of the arteriolar wall, which is similar to that normally found in embryonic life. Some feel that these histologic changes represent merely a failure of involution of the normal fetal pattern. In older children and adults, thickening of the intima occurs also, with associated fibrosis, and has a more serious prognosis, for such histologic changes are often irreversible and may not improve even after the underlying cause has been corrected.

More significant than the increase in pulmonary blood flow, however, is the pressure under which blood is expelled into the pulmonary artery, for pulmonary hypertension is much more frequent with ventricular septal defects than with atrial septal defects which produce a similar increase in pulmonary blood flow. In general, the incidence of hypertension with secundum atrial septal defects in children is about 5 percent, with atrioventricular canal defects about 10 percent, and with ventricular septal defects about 25 percent, as reported by Nadas.

In addition, there is an individual variation in susceptibility to development of pulmonary hypertension, for some children with a large ventricular septal defect and a large increase in pulmonary blood flow will not develop any change in pulmonary vascular resistance, while others with a smaller septal defect will develop significant pulmonary hypertension at an early age. Finally, there are unexplained variations in pulmonary hypertension for which no known cause can at present be discerned. In some children pulmonary hypertension is apparently present from birth and remains for several years without any change. In others pulmonary hypertension found at birth may be found to have regressed spontaneously when the patient is studied at repeat cardiac catheterization some years later. In most patients, however, pulmonary hypertension gradually but progressively increases in severity, eventually becoming incurable.

The earliest age at which pulmonary vascular changes become irreversible is both variable and uncertain, but certain defects such as truncus arteriosus or transposition apparently may produce permanent changes in some patients by the age of one year. With advances in surgical therapy, most lesions producing an increase in pulmonary vascular resistance, such as ventricular septal defect, patent ductus arteriosus, or aortopulmonary window, should be surgically corrected in the first two years of life. With simple atrial secundum defect, however, operation at such an early age is virtually never necessary, illustrating the unknown etiologic factors in the development of increase in pulmonary vascular resistance.

Restriction in Systemic Blood Flow. With large left-to-right shunts there is often a decrease in systemic blood flow, frequently associated with a retardation in normal growth and development. This is more prominently seen in children with a patent ductus arteriosus or an atrial septal defect. The appearance of frail, underweight children with atrial septal defect has been termed the *gracile* habitus. Although mental retardation is slightly more common in children with congenital heart disease, beyond this association there is no evidence that congenital heart disease retards mental development. Unfortunately, correction of the cardiac defect does not result in any improvement in mental function. There is, however, often a substantial increase in growth and weight once the cardiac defect has been corrected.

RIGHT-TO-LEFT SHUNTS. Right-to-left shunts of venous blood directly into the systemic circulation, producing arterial hypoxemia and cyanosis, result from the combination of an intracardiac septal defect with obstruction to normal flow of blood into the pulmonary artery. The classic example is the tetralogy of Fallot, a combination of ventricular septal defect and pulmonic stenosis. Other cyanotic disorders include the more complex malformations, such as transposition of the great vessels, tricuspid atresia, truncus arteriosus, and total anomalous drainage of the pulmonary veins. Right-to-left shunts produce a large number of physiologic disturbances because of the anoxia resulting from chronic hypoxemia in the arterial blood. These are considered in detail in the following paragraphs. It should be emphasized that all these disturbances result from deficient oxygen transport to tissues of the body. With right-to-left shunts there is no increase in cardiac output, and often the pulmonary blood flow is less than normal. Hence cardiac failure is rare with an uncomplicated right-to-left shunt, in contrast to its inevitable eventual occurrence with left-to-right shunts.

Cyanosis. This is the most prominent feature of a right-to-left shunt. The degree of cyanosis depends upon both the degree of anoxia and the blood hemoglobin concentration, for the visible intensity of cyanosis is determined by the number of grams of reduced hemoglobin in the circulation. It has been estimated that about 5 Gm of reduced hemoglobin is required to produce visible cyanosis. Normally in the capillaries about 2.25 Gm of reduced hemoglobin is present, so with an average hemoglobin concentration of 15 Gm/100 ml of blood, a decrease in arterial oxygen from the normal range of nearly 95% to 75% is needed to produce visible cyanosis. In the presence of anemia, however, a more severe degree of anoxia is required to produce visible cyanosis, while with polycythemia and hemoglobin concentrations of 20 Gm/100 ml of blood or more, severe cyanosis may represent less serious anoxia.

Cyanosis has been conveniently grouped into "central"
and "peripheral" types. *Peripheral* cyanosis results simply from a decrease in cardiac output with sluggish regional flow of blood through the capillary circulation, as a result of which more oxygen is extracted and a greater amount of reduced hemoglobin is present. This type of cyanosis occurs with conditions producing a low cardiac output, such as mitral stenosis, and varies with the condition of the patient. It is usually more prominent in certain regions of the body, such as the tips of the fingers, the lips, or the lobes of the ears.

Central cyanosis results either from a defect in oxygenation of blood in the lungs or from an intracardiac shunt. Cyanosis resulting from pulmonary insufficiency can usually be recognized from its prompt improvement when the patient breathes 100% oxygen, increasing the efficiency of pulmonary ventilation. In the catheterization laboratory it can be recognized from the finding that oxygen saturation of blood in the left atrium is less than 95%. Pulmonary insufficiency from cardiac disease occurs only with severe pulmonary congestion from cardiac failure or far advanced pulmonary vascular disease.

An intracardiac shunt, permitting direct entry of venous blood into the systemic circulation, is the cause of central cyanosis in most patients. The intensity of the cyanosis is related to the volume of pulmonary blood flow, for ultimately cyanosis depends upon the relative proportions of unoxygenated and oxygenated blood in the arterial circulation. Even though a large intracardiac shunt is present, an increase in pulmonary blood flow to produce a larger amount of oxygenated blood can substantially reduce cyanosis and improve oxygen transport. This was dramatically demonstrated by Blalock with the systemic-pulmonary artery anastomosis for tetralogy of Fallot.

Two distinctive changes which inevitably result with chronic cyanosis are clubbing of the digits and polycythemia. The triad of cyanosis, clubbing, and polycythemia is a familiar one in children with congenital heart disease. Clubbing of the digits, or hypertrophic osteoarthropathy, is an unusual change in the appearance and structure of the digits, consisting of a rounding of the tips of the fingers and toes, as well as a thickening of the ends, associated with deposition of fibrous tissue. In addition, there may be a pronounced convexity of the fingernails. Histologically, the fingers have increased numbers of capillaries, with a large number of tiny arteriovenous aneurysms. Clubbing is usually not prominent until a cyanotic child is one to two years of age, but in some instances of severe anoxia it may evolve within several weeks. It usually gradually subsides following correction of the intracardiac defect.

Polycythemia is a fortunate physiologic response of the bone marrow to chronic anoxia, as an increase in red cell and hemoglobin concentration increases the ability of the blood to transport oxygen. Hematocrit readings of 60 to 70 percent are frequent with chronic cyanosis, and readings exceeding 80 percent are found in extreme cases. There is a parallel rise in viscosity of the blood, with restriction to the flow of blood as the hematocrit reading increases. Once the hematocrit reading exceeds 75 to 80 percent, the increased viscosity constitutes a significant hazard, for transitory dehydration in an infant with a hematocrit reading above 80 percent may precipitate cerebral venous thrombosis and permanent neurologic injury, apparently from formation of thrombi in the viscous blood.

Limitation of Exercise Tolerance. A decrease in exercise tolerance, with dyspnea on exertion, is characteristic of cyanotic heart disease, for the circulation is unable to increase oxygen transport with exercise. The severity of the disability, or its progression, can be conveniently measured in terms of the patient's ability to walk a measured distance. Associated with exertional dyspnea is squatting, a phenomenon first emphasized by Taussig. The cyanotic child quickly learns that dyspnea on walking can be lessened by assuming a squatting position. Physiologic studies indicate that squatting produces an increase in peripheral vascular resistance, with a corresponding increase in pulmonary blood flow. Squatting is most commonly seen in tetralogy of Fallot, less frequently in other cyanotic conditions.

Neurologic Damage. Periodic episodes of unconsciousness, termed *cyanotic spells,* are grave signs of cerebral anoxia. They often appear in the third to fourth month of life in severely cyanotic children, even in the first few weeks of life with extreme anoxia, but are rare after the fifth to sixth year of life. They characteristically occur at different times, not always associated with exertion, and evolve as episodes of crying, deepening cyanosis, and coma, lasting a few minutes to a few hours. Such episodes are extremely grave, for although recovery may ensue promptly, the spells are recurrent, and any spell may either terminate fatally or result in permanent neurologic injury. Emergency surgical treatment to improve the oxygen content of the arterial blood is strongly indicated.

Another cause of neurologic injury in cyanotic children is brain abscess, for which there is increased susceptibility especially in children with tetralogy of Fallot. The increased susceptibility is partly related to direct access of bacteria in the venous circulation to the arterial circulation through the right-to-left shunt. This is probably not the entire explanation, however, for a similar increased frequency does not occur in other cyanotic conditions. A localized infarct with subsequent bacterial infection may explain the evolution in some patients.

Another rare cause of cerebral injury is paradoxic embolism through an intracardiac defect, in which a thrombus migrating in the venous circulation, which would normally produce a pulmonary embolus, traverses an intracardiac defect and lodges in the cerebral circulation. Hence permanent neurologic injury, most often seen as hemiplegia, is not uncommon in children with chronic severe cyanosis, constituting a strong indication for early surgical therapy when possible.

Other Changes. In older children with severe cyanosis there is a striking increase in bronchial circulation, apparently a compensatory response to the chronic decrease in pulmonary blood flow. The myriads of collateral vessels, often constituting a mass of varicosities in the mediastinum, are principally of surgical significance because of the risk of bleeding during operation. They may be associated with epistaxis in some children, but hemoptysis is rare because the pulmonary blood flow is usually less than

normal, even though the bronchial circulation is greatly increased.

Finally, with chronic polycythemia in children older than ten to fifteen years of age, multiple defects in blood coagulation occur, with abnormalities in several aspects of the blood-clotting mechanism. Clinically this may result in mild gastrointestinal bleeding, but the major significance is the increased susceptibility to hemorrhage following surgical procedures.

Clinical Examination

HISTORY. In obtaining the history of a patient with congenital heart disease, the presence of abnormal factors during pregnancy, especially during the first trimester, should be noted. Rubella in the first trimester has been emphasized because of the high incidence of cardiac and other defects. In some disorders, notably hypertrophic muscular aortic stenosis, there is a definite familial history of the disorder. Also, with the majority of patients with congenital heart disease there is about a 2 percent associated occurrence of congenital heart disease in other members of the same family. In most patients, however, no etiologic factors can be found.

The age at which a cardiac murmur was detected for the first time should be carefully noted, and the reliability of this observation should be estimated. Similarly the time of appearance of cyanosis is of significance, whether at birth or subsequently during infancy. Variations in the appearance of cyanosis, as well as its location, are also important. In some patients cyanosis may be recognized at birth, then disappear for months or years, and finally appear again.

A decrease in exercise tolerance manifested by dyspnea on exertion, is a common symptom and a convenient indication of the severity of the disorder in patients with right-to-left shunts. Squatting can be readily identified by the parents. Symptoms of lesser degrees of restriction in physical capacity, such as undue fatigability or inability to participate in exercise, should be noted, although the ability of many children with large left-to-right shunts to participate vigorously in athletics is impressive. Feeding habits and the pattern of weight are also important features.

Previous neurologic episodes such as cyanotic spells, cerebral embolism, brain abscess, or other signs of cerebral injury should be noted.

Finally, episodes of infection occurring as pneumonia, bacterial endocarditis, or rheumatic fever should be ascertained.

PHYSICAL EXAMINATION. Abnormalities in growth and development should be particularly assessed, because these are among the most common signs of cardiac disease. Cyanosis, with clubbing or polycythemia, may be obvious or may require close scrutiny for detection. On examination of the heart, any deformity of the left costal cartilages, indicating long-standing cardiac enlargement, should be noted. Palpation for a thrill is particularly important, for its presence almost uniformly indicates significant underlying cardiac disease. Cardiac size should be estimated, although this is difficult in small children and infants and is best determined by the roentgenogram. Systolic murmurs are commonly found but often are of little diagnostic significance. Basal systolic murmurs occur with pulmonic stenosis, aortic stenosis, patent ductus in infants, and coarctation of the aorta. A murmur along the left sternal border is particularly prominent with ventricular septal defect. With systolic murmurs the type of murmur, location, and transmission are of particular importance. Diastolic murmurs are infrequent in infants but when present are especially significant. They may occur from aortic insufficiency with prolapse of an aortic cusp, with pulmonic insufficiency from long-standing pulmonary hypertension, or in association with a systolic murmur as the continuous murmur of a patent ductus arteriosus. The cardiac sounds, especially the second sound at the base, may be of importance in certain conditions. The pulmonic second sound is increased with pulmonary hypertension, decreased or absent with pulmonic stenosis or atresia. Variation in splitting of the second sound may be recognized by experienced observers and is of diagnostic importance, especially with atrial septal defect. Disturbances of rhythm are infrequent. The gallop rhythm with its ominous prognosis is seen in terminal forms of cardiac disease.

Examination of the lungs may detect rales from cardiac failure in large left-to-right shunts, but characteristically no abnormalities are found in the lungs with right-to-left shunts producing cyanosis. The hallmark of congestive failure in children is hepatic enlargement, occurring with

Fig. 18-1. Chest roentgenogram of child with tetralogy of Fallot, showing typical cardiac silhouette (sabot-shaped heart). Features include heart of normal size with prominent apex from right ventricular hypertrophy. There is increased concavity at base of heart because pulmonic stenosis produces decrease in size or absence of shadow normally seen from pulmonary artery. Vascularity of lung fields may be normal or decreased. (*Courtesy of Dr. Raymond M. Abrams, Department of Radiology, New York University Medical Center.*)

surprising rapidity and regressing rapidly as failure improves. Hence estimation of the presence and extent of hepatic enlargement is of particular importance. Often hepatic enlargement precedes the detection of audible rales, in contrast to adult forms of cardiac disease. Similarly, edema is usually less prominent clinically than hepatic enlargement.

In the extremities, the presence and quality of the radial, femoral, and pedal pulses should be noted. Faint pulses are characteristic of aortic stenosis. With coarctation, radial pulses are prominent while femoral pulses are weak or absent. Easily palpable, bounding pulses are characteristic of defects producing an abnormal exit of blood from the aorta during diastole, such as patent ductus arteriosus, aortic insufficiency, or a ruptured aneurysm of the sinus of Valsalva. These are associated with an increase in pulse pressure, usually due to a decrease in diastolic pressure. Normally the systolic blood pressure in infants is in the range of 70 to 90 mm Hg, rising to about 100 mm Hg in the first five years of life and subsequently to the normal adult level of 120 mm Hg in the next few years. Diastolic pressures are usually in the range of 55 to 60 mm Hg.

Examination of the digits is particularly useful with cyanosis, because clubbing is inevitable with chronic severe cyanosis.

LABORATORY STUDIES. A noninvasive diagnostic tripod for congenital heart disease consists of the clinical examination, the chest roentgenogram, and the electrocardiogram. These three modalities are all important in arriving at the correct diagnosis. In the roentgenogram, contour of the heart, cardiac size, and vascularity should be particularly noted. Infrequent abnormalities include pleural effusion and notching of the ribs in coarctation of the aorta. Cardiac size is best estimated from the cardiothoracic ratio; a ratio greater than 0.5 indicates cardiac enlargement. In infants a cardiac shadow with a transverse diameter greater than 5.5 cm indicates cardiac enlargement. In oblique views with fluoroscopy, cardiac enlargement involving the atria, right ventricle, left ventricle, or both ventricles may be estimated. Enlargement of the left atrium occurs with mitral insufficiency, ventricular septal defect, patent ductus arteriosus, or any form of left ventricular failure. Left ventricular enlargement is characteristic of aortic disease, mitral insufficiency, coarctation of the aorta, patent ductus arteriosus, ventricular septal defect, or tricuspid atresia. Right atrial enlargement is especially prominent in Ebstein's malformation and also occurs in tricuspid atresia, atrial septal defect, and pulmonic stenosis. Selective enlargement of the right ventricle is frequent with pulmonic stenosis, pulmonary hypertension from any cause, atrial septal defect, and ventricular septal defect.

Changes in cardiac contour may be characteristic in certain conditions. The sabot-shaped heart of tetralogy of Fallot results from hypertrophy of the right ventricle in association with a small pulmonary conus (Fig. 18-1). The egg-shaped heart of transposition of the great vessels (Fig. 18-2) is caused by enlargement of the right ventricle and right atrium, with a narrow shadow at the base from the anteroposterior relation between the aorta and the pulmonary arteries. With total anomalous drainage of the pulmonary venous return, a figure-of-eight abnormality (Fig. 18-3), composed of a large left superior vena cava in the upper mediastinum separate from the cardiac shadow, is characteristic.

The size of the pulmonary vessels and the pulmonary vascularity are also important. This can be estimated by fluoroscopy, where the vigor of the pulsations can be observed. Defects with an increased pulmonary blood flow and pulmonary hypertension can be easily differentiated from conditions associated with a normal or a decreased pulmonary blood flow.

The electrocardiogram is the best guide to the presence of ventricular hypertrophy. Selective hypertrophy of the left ventricle, as in aortic valvular stenosis, or selective hypertrophy of the right ventricle, as in pulmonic valvular stenosis, can be recognized and also correlated with the degree of stenosis. Bundle branch block, typically seen as a right bundle branch block with an atrial septal defect, also occurs in certain conditions.

Cardiac catheterization with cineangiography is essential for a complete evaluation. With cardiac catheterization, intracardiac pressures can be determined; abnormal shunts of blood can be recognized, and the ratio between pulmonary and systemic blood flow determined. Direct passage of the catheter into an abnormal chamber, such as a patent ductus arteriosus, may provide visual confirmation of the diagnosis. Mitral or aortic insufficiency are best evaluated

Fig. 18-2. Chest roentgenogram of child with transposition of great vessels, showing egg-shaped heart with large ventricular silhouette and small "waist," which results from abnormal location of aorta directly anterior to pulmonary artery. (*Courtesy of Dr. Raymond M. Abrams, Department of Radiology, New York University Medical Center.*)

Fig. 18-3. *A.* Chest roentgenogram of child with total anomalous drainage of pulmonary veins through left superior vena cava. Shadow in left upper mediastinum is due to dilated left superior vena cava. *B.* Angiogram demonstrates left superior vena cava emptying into greatly dilated left innominate vein. This x-ray appearance is pathognomonic of total anomalous drainage of pulmonary veins into left superior vena cava. (*Courtesy of Dr. Raymond M. Abrams, Department of Radiology, New York University Medical Center.*)

by cineangiography. Dye-dilution curves, once widely used, are now seldom done, as simpler and more precise diagnostic methods have evolved.

In the normal heart the right atrial systolic pressure does not exceed 5 mm Hg, while left atrial pressure is in the

A

B

range of 5 to 10 mm Hg. In the normal right ventricle systolic pressure ranges from 15 to 30 mm Hg, while in the left ventricle pressures average 80 to 130 mm Hg systolic and 5 to 10 mm Hg diastolic. Continuous pressure recordings as a catheter is withdrawn from one cardiac chamber to another can readily detect the presence of stenosis; pulmonic stenosis can be measured as a catheter is withdrawn from the pulmonary artery to the right ventricle, and aortic stenosis as a catheter is withdrawn from the left ventricle into the aorta. Combined right- and left-heart catheterization is usually done with the introduction of a catheter through a systemic vein into the right side of the heart, combined with introduction of another catheter from a peripheral artery into the aorta and across the aortic valve into the left ventricle to obtain information from both the right and left sides of the heart simultaneously.

All variations from the normal pulmonary and systemic flow of 3 liters/minute/square meter of body surface may occur with intracardiac shunts. A rise in oxygen saturation of 1 vol % between cardiac chambers is usually sufficient evidence to diagnose an intracardiac left-to-right shunt. Smaller shunts may be detected with a hydrogen electrode. A pulmonary blood flow one and one-half to two times greater than systemic blood flow is associated with mild physiologic disturbances and is on the borderline of indications for surgical correction. Defects producing greater pulmonary blood flows are uniformly recommended for operation. From the combination of pulmonary blood flow and pulmonary pressure, pulmonary vascular resistance can be calculated, which with pulmonary hypertension is one of the most significant physiologic measurements influencing prognosis.

The most precise physiologic evaluation of the degree of valvular stenosis is obtained by calculation of the functional cross-sectional area of the stenotic valve orifice, as elucidated by Gorlin and Gorlin in 1951. A normal mitral valve has a functional cross-sectional area of about 5 cm²; mitral stenosis with an area of less than 1.5 cm² is functionally significant. In the aortic valve, normally with a cross-sectional area of 3 to 4 cm², a stenosis producing an opening of less than 0.8 cm² is functionally significant. Similarly, in the pulmonic valve, with a normal cross-sectional area of 2 to 4 cm², a stenosis producing an opening of less than 0.8 cm² is functionally significant.

Principles of Operative and Postoperative Care of Infants

Certain principles of management specifically pertain to infants undergoing cardiovascular surgery. For general principles of operative monitoring, extracorporeal circulation, cardiac massage, and defibrillation, Chap. 19 on acquired heart disease should be consulted.

OPERATIVE MANAGEMENT. Four important aspects of operative care are temperature control, fluid administration, prevention of air emboli, and serial blood-gas monitoring. Temperature control is essential in infants, especially in air-conditioned operating rooms, because body temperature will quickly decrease to 32 to 34°C when the

infant is anesthetized and shivering mechanisms abolished. Constant recording of the temperature with an electric esophageal or rectal probe is mandatory, and some method of warming the infant, preferably a water mattress, should routinely be employed.

Fluids must be administered with unusual precision; a 3-kg infant in cardiac failure should have no more than 20 to 40 ml of fluid in excess of measured losses during an operative procedure.

The danger of air embolism is frequently overlooked in cyanotic infants with right-to-left shunts, in whom air emboli can bypass the heart and lungs to enter the cerebral or the coronary circulation. With intravenous therapy, much care is required to prevent small air emboli, which almost routinely occur with the usual intravenous therapy during an operation. Only a few small bubbles, if lodged in a coronary artery, can precipitate ventricular fibrillation.

Serial measurement of the pH and the oxygen and carbon dioxide tensions of central venous blood, usually at 20- to 30-minute intervals during an operation, is perhaps the most essential part of monitoring. Metabolic and respiratory acidosis are extremely frequent in seriously ill infants and may quickly become intensified with compression of the lung, ineffective cardiac contraction, or hypovolemia. A pH of central venous blood below 7.30 should be promptly corrected by appropriate ventilation, bicarbonate infusion, cessation of anesthesia, or other measures to increase cardiac output. In the author's experience, changes in pH always well antedate cardiac arrest or ventricular fibrillation. With serial monitoring of blood-gas tensions during operation, desperately ill anoxic children may tolerate procedures which ordinarily would terminate in cardiac arrest or fibrillation.

POSTOPERATIVE CARE. Four important principles are constant observation, monitoring of the electrocardiogram, routine measurement of blood-gas tensions, and respiratory therapy.

Constant observation of the seriously ill infant by experienced staff on a 24-hour basis is mandatory. This includes observation of adequacy of ventilation, blood-gas tensions, fluid therapy, and arrhythmias appearing on the electrocardiogram. Ventricular fibrillation can appear virtually without warning but can be corrected, usually with electric cardioversion, if therapy can be started within 1 to 3 minutes. With a policy of constant observation, fibrillation has often been corrected with subsequent recovery in infants who otherwise would surely have succumbed to transitory ventricular arrhythmias following operation.

Serial measurement of blood-gas tensions by analysis of blood samples withdrawn through a central venous catheter, usually introduced through the saphenous vein and the inferior vena cava, is the best measurement of adequacy of ventilation and circulation. Venous carbon dioxide tensions above 45 mm Hg promptly develop with inefficient ventilation, and pH values below 7.30 quickly occur with either metabolic or respiratory acidosis. These changes far antedate any obvious clinical alteration in pulse or blood pressure and accordingly permit more effective therapy. Whether changes in pH and gas tensions are due to metabolic or respiratory causes can be determined by clinical evaluation and by gas analysis of peripheral arterial blood.

Proper ventilation is perhaps the most difficult postoperative problem in the infant following a thoracotomy. Secretions are difficult to remove, the tracheobronchial passages are so small that instrumental manipulation is difficult and can precipitate occlusive edema, and infants quickly develop cardiac arrest with transient anoxia or respiratory acidosis. Many advances in respiratory therapy of infants have been made in the past 5 to 7 years. These include mechanical respirators specifically designed for infants, the continuous positive-pressure breathing system developed by Gregory, and intermittent mandatory ventilation.

The following methods of management have been found useful, but the mode of application varies widely with individual patients. Adequate humidity, with the infant kept in a dense mist right from the time of operation, is essential. An endotracheal tube may be left in place for an indeterminate length of time following operation to assist ventilation and removal of secretions. Some have left endotracheal tubes in position for days or weeks, but the author prefers a much shorter period, usually less than 24 to 48 hours. When an endotracheal tube is left in position, it may require changing every 6 to 12 hours if inspissated secretions occlude the tip of the tube.

Translaryngeal aspiration of the trachea, accomplished with a laryngoscope to permit direct introduction of a soft catheter between the vocal cords into the trachea, is a valuable technique. It must be done by experienced personnel; otherwise trauma and edema of the vocal cords will quickly develop. It is simpler than bronchoscopy, less traumatic, and can be repeated frequently.

Tracheostomy should be avoided if possible but should be done if secretion cannot be adequately removed otherwise. With a precise technique avoiding excision of any tracheal cartilage, complications are far less frequent than in the past. At the University of South Africa in Cape Town, an extensive experience with tracheostomy and mechanical ventilation for several weeks in the treatment of neonatal tetanus has clearly demonstrated the safety of a properly performed tracheostomy.

OBSTRUCTIVE LESIONS

Pulmonic Stenosis

HISTORICAL DATA. In 1948 Brock and Sellors independently performed the first successful valvulotomies for pulmonic valvular stenosis, using a valvulotome through a transventricular approach. In 1954 Swan and Zeavin used hypothermia and venous inflow occlusion. These facts are of historical interest only, for operation with extracorporeal circulation is almost always the best approach. Rarely, a moribund infant may be best treated with one of the simpler methods.

INCIDENCE AND ETIOLOGY. Pulmonic stenosis is a common disease, representing about 10 percent of all patients with congenital heart disease. However, it was once considered a very rare disease. Taussig, in her monograph in

1947, wrote that she had not had an opportunity to study a proved case herself. The now well-established frequency of the disease indicates how interest in and recognition of a disorder is influenced by the diagnostic methods available.

There are no known significant etiologic factors.

PATHOLOGIC ANATOMY. Pulmonic stenosis was once considered to be a simple pathologic disorder due to stenosis of the pulmonary valve in most patients. From clinical experience, combined with the development of excellent angiography in recent years, it is now apparent that this simplistic concept was often erroneous and that pulmonic stenosis is a wide spectrum of disorders involving the pulmonary artery, pulmonary valve complex, and right ventricular muscle. For effective therapy these areas must be evaluated both with angiography and also at operation.

The most common variety is stenosis from fusion of the pulmonary valve cusp (Fig. 18-4). Frequently there is some hypoplasia of the main pulmonary artery, which normally should be larger than the aorta. Stenosis of the distal pulmonary artery is fortunately uncommon and is described subsequently.

Hypoplasia of a pulmonic annulus, in addition to stenosis of the valve leaflets, is important to recognize, and Kirklin and associates have recently reported a mathematical guideline of normal and abnormal cross-sectional areas of the pulmonic valve for different body weights. In the ventricle there may be a discrete infundibular stenosis (Fig. 18-5), obstruction from severe hypertrophy of ventricular muscle or combined with fibrosis, or, rarely, an anomalous papillary muscle. Hence at operation, all potential areas of stenosis should be carefully examined.

Pulmonary valvular stenosis results from fusion of the three semilunar cusps of the pulmonic valve to form a

Fig. 18-4. Pulmonic valvular stenosis with fused valve cusps creating central stenotic opening. Annulus of pulmonic valve ring is normal. (*Adapted from W. H. Cole and R. M. Zollinger, "Textbook of Surgery," Appleton-Century-Crofts, Inc., New York, 1963, 8th ed., p. 935.*)

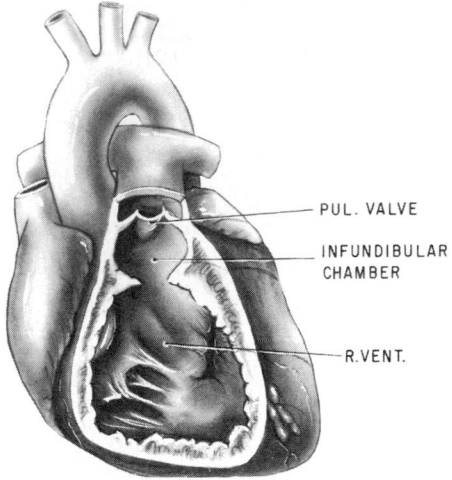

Fig. 18-5. Types of subvalvular or infundibular pulmonic stenosis. Infundibular stenosis may result in a discrete chamber between stenotic area and pulmonic valve. (*Adapted from W. H. Cole and R. M. Zollinger, "Textbook of Surgery," Appleton-Century-Crofts, Inc., New York, 1963, 8th ed., p. 936.*)

dome with a central opening usually 1 to 3 mm in diameter. In infants with severe obstruction only a pinpoint orifice may be present, while in milder forms the orifice may be 7 to 10 mm in diameter (Fig. 18-6). It has been estimated that the pulmonary valve orifice must be reduced to about one-third of normal size before significant physiologic obstruction results. Normally the three valve cusps are well formed, although variation in size is frequent. Variants include a bicuspid valve or, rarely, a fused dome-like structure with a central opening and only vestigial

Fig. 18-6. Pulmonic valvular stenosis exposed at operation following incision of pulmonary artery. Dome-shaped structure produced by fusion of valve cusps, with small central opening, is clearly shown. Suction tip has been placed in distal pulmonary artery.

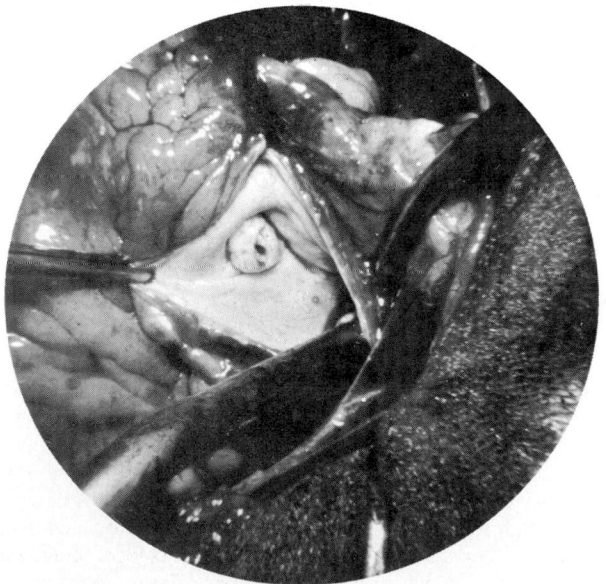

commissures. Some patients develop varying degrees of poststenotic dilatation of the main pulmonary artery. The mechanism of poststenotic dilatation was well elucidated by Holman in 1954, being related to increased lateral pressure resulting from deceleration of high velocity of flow through a small orifice. Other factors, however, must be present, for the degree of dilatation does not correspond to the severity of stenosis. Occasionally an asymptomatic patient in the fourth or fifth decade is seen following the detection of a mediastinal mass on a chest roentgenogram, who on later study will be found to have mild pulmonic stenosis with extensive poststenotic dilatation.

Compensatory hypertrophy of the right ventricle to eject blood through the stenotic orifice occurs regularly. In severe, chronic stenosis the massive ventricular hypertrophy (1 to 2 cm), may significantly reduce the lumen of the right ventricular cavity, constituting an additional element of obstruction to the flow of blood.

Isolated infundibular stenosis occurs in 5 to 10 percent of patients with pulmonic stenosis. It consists of a discrete fibrous diaphragm with a 3- to 6-mm central opening in the outflow tract of the right ventricle located 2 to 5 cm proximal to the pulmonic valve. The most frequent location is at the site of the crista supraventricularis. With infundibular stenosis, an "infundibular chamber" exists in the right ventricle between the site of stenosis and the pulmonic valve (Fig. 18-7). Detection of this chamber on cardiac catheterization or angiography readily confirms the diagnosis.

A patent foramen ovale is present in at least 50 percent of patients. This often is a slitlike opening apparently stretched open from the increased right ventricular pressure and dilatation of the right atrium. Rarely, a larger typical atrial septal defect, 1 to 3 cm in diameter, is present, Other associated abnormalities such as patent ductus arteriosus are rare.

PATHOPHYSIOLOGY. The physiologic disturbance is obstruction to flow of blood from the right ventricle with resulting hypertrophy of the right ventricle. Initially the severity of the obstruction is related to the diameter of the stenotic orifice. Right ventricular pressures of 75 to 100 mm Hg are found with moderate pulmonic stenosis, while severe obstruction results in right ventricular pressures of 100 to 200 mm Hg, and levels as high as 270 mm Hg have been recorded. With growth of the patient, two additional elements of obstruction occur. One of these is progressive hypertrophy of the right ventricle, until subsequently the contraction of the hypertrophied muscle of the right ventricular outflow tract also constitutes an obstruction to the flow of blood. The other factor is a relative one related to the growth of the child with corresponding increase in the flow of blood. Hence a 3- to 4-mm opening tolerated by an infant may produce serious symptoms in a child of twelve to fourteen years.

With the obstruction to the flow of blood, over one-half the patients have a patent foramen ovale with a right-to-left shunt producing unsaturation of the arterial blood. When the shunt through the foramen ovale is large, visible cyanosis develops, followed by polycythemia and clubbing. The usual clinical story is a progressive increase in cyanosis over a period of years, insidiously appearing in early child-hood and gradually increasing in severity.

Overt cardiac failure seldom occurs in children except in infancy. In infants with a pinpoint opening in the pulmonary valve, severe failure may constitute an emergency indication for pulmonic valvulotomy to prevent immediate death. Cardiac failure gradually becomes more common in older children and young adults, as cardiac reserve is progressively decreased.

CLINICAL MANIFESTATIONS. Symptoms. Dyspnea on exertion is the dominant symptom, increasing in severity as the cardiac reserve fails. Easy fatigability is common but less precise. Dizziness and/or syncope are occasionally seen; chest pain is infrequent. The history of the development of cyanosis may be characteristic. Cyanosis may have been noted in infancy, due to a right-to-left shunt through a foramen ovale, which subsequently disappeared as the foramen ovale closed. In later years, as right ventricular pressure increases and atrial dilatation occurs, the foramen ovale is gradually stretched open, resulting in the insidious appearance and progression of cyanosis as the right-to-left shunt progressively increases in magnitude. With chronic cyanosis, clubbing and polycythemia appear.

Sudden death in childhood has been reported but fortunately is rare. Symptoms of overt cardiac failure are rarely seen in children except in infancy but may be present in adults with severe stenosis.

Physical Examination. The characteristic finding is a harsh, loud systolic murmur heard best in the second left intercostal space and widely transmitted to the neck and adjacent areas. The murmur is of the ejection type, the peak intensity varying with the severity of the stenosis. Usually in infancy it can be clearly detected, although in advanced failure it may be faint. The pulmonic second sound is characteristically weak or absent. Diastolic murmurs are almost never heard. With increasing cardiac hypertrophy, the forceful contractions of the right ventricle can be palpated along the left sternal border. Cyanosis is present in varying degrees in patients with a patent foramen ovale and in the neglected chronic case is associated with polycythemia and clubbing.

Signs of cardiac failure, with hepatomegaly and edema, are usually found only in adults with severe obstruction.

LABORATORY FINDINGS. The chest roentgenogram characteristically shows cardiac enlargement confined to the right ventricle, although this is not marked until cardiac reserve fails. In older patients the poststenotic dilatation of the pulmonary artery, often unusually prominent in the left pulmonary artery, may be seen in association with normal or decreased vascularity of the peripheral lung fields. Changes in cardiac size are of particular importance, because cardiac enlargement precedes the onset of symptoms. In infants, marked cardiac enlargement may occur within only a few months.

The electrocardiogram is of great value in assessing the severity of the obstruction for signs of right ventricular hypertrophy are regularly present. With severe disease a right ventricular strain pattern with changes in the ST segment and T waves becomes apparent.

Cardiac catheterization and angiography are, of course,

Fig. 18-7. Heart with infundibular stenosis. Site of infundibular stenosis is visible as area of constriction in outflow tract of right ventricle. Infundibular chamber, consisting of dilated right ventricular muscle, is located between infundibular stenosis proximally and pulmonary vein distad.

necessary to define precisely the severity of the condition and the associated abnormalities. With moderate disease, a right ventricular systolic pressure of 100 mm Hg or more, associated with a systolic gradient across the stenotic pulmonary valve of 80 to 90 mm Hg, is frequent. With severe disease, systolic ventricular pressures may even exceed 200 mm Hg. The presence of a foramen ovale can be detected by noting oxygen unsaturation in the arterial blood. A right ventricular pressure exceeding systemic pressure almost always indicates an intact ventricular septum, although unusual exceptions have been recorded.

On angiography, as mentioned earlier, several structures should be carefully noted. These include the degree of stenosis of the right ventricular outflow tract by the hypertrophied muscle, especially noting any signs of a focal infundibular stenosis. The size of the pulmonary valve ring, the main pulmonary artery, and the distal pulmonary artery should also be carefully analyzed. The recognition of the frequency of multiple sites of obstruction constitutes a significant advance in effective therapy in recent years.

DIAGNOSIS. The diagnosis can usually be made with certainty in the presence of a loud systolic murmur with a weak pulmonic second sound, combined with roentgenographic evidence of enlargement of the right ventricle and electrocardiographic signs of right ventricular hypertrophy. An atrial septal defect or pulmonary hypertension may be confused with pulmonic stenosis, but the quality of the pulmonic second sound is a helpful guide. Ebstein's anomaly of the tricuspid valve is a rare malformation which can simulate pulmonic stenosis; catheterization and angiography are required to establish the correct diagnosis.

Differentiating pulmonic stenosis from tetralogy of

Fallot is a common problem when right-to-left shunting of blood through a foramen ovale has produced cyanosis. Cyanosis is usually a more prominent feature of the history with tetralogy of Fallot; cardiac enlargement and failure also are unusual with the latter. Cardiac angiography readily establishes the diagnosis.

TREATMENT. Indications for Operation. With mild pulmonic stenosis associated with a heart of normal size and no signs of hypertrophy of the right ventricle on the electrocardiogram, no treatment has been found necessary. Johnson and associates described the benign course of trivial pulmonic stenosis in a significant group of patients followed over many years. If there are electrocardiographic signs of significant right ventricular hypertrophy, cardiac catheterization should be done. Operation is usually recommended if the systolic pressure gradient across the stenotic pulmonary valve is greater than 50 mm Hg. It should be emphasized that the severity of the obstruction often increases with growth of the child, so a physiologically insignificant stenosis in a young child may become more significant in later childhood.

Operative Technique. Except for the rare emergency operation in an infant, all operations are done with extracorporeal circulation through a median sternotomy. The closed technique with the valvulotome developed by Potts (Fig. 18-8) is rarely used.

Our operative approach at New York University has undergone considerable modifications in the last few years following unsatisfactory results in unusual patients with severe obstruction in whom, although angiography indicated an isolated stenosis, multiple points of obstruction were found at operation. The approach currently used is briefly described in the following paragraphs.

With cardiopulmonary bypass established and body temperature lowered to 30°C, a small left ventricular vent is inserted to facilitate both decompression of the left ventricle and removal of any intracardiac air which might lodge in the left ventricle if a small unrecognized septal defect is present.

Initially, the atrial septum is palpated through a small stab wound in the right atrium to detect a foramen ovale. If present, this is sutured.

The size of the pulmonary artery in comparison to the aorta is carefully noted. If it is smaller than normal, a longitudinal arteriotomy is made and subsequently closed with a patch of pericardium or Dacron to produce a pulmonary artery of normal diameter. The size of the distal pulmonary artery is carefully measured with graduated Hegar dilators, and any stenoses found are corrected.

The external appearance of the pulmonary valve ring is carefully noted, as a hypoplastic annulus will require division of the ring and insertion of a patch. This is especially emphasized because occasionally excellent angiograms have been found to be misleading in this regard.

Contrary to our previous technique of either avoiding a ventriculotomy or using a transverse ventriculotomy, our preferred approach now is to make a short longitudinal ventriculotomy, beginning near the pulmonic annulus and extending proximally to the right ventricle for no more than 4 to 5 cm. Division of any significant coronary arteries is carefully avoided. Limiting the ventriculotomy to a short one in the outflow tract results in less impairment of ventricular function. Its use, however, usually requires closure of the ventriculotomy with a small woven Dacron patch. Through the vertical ventriculotomy, the pulmonic valve can often be adequately visualized and the commissures incised without opening the pulmonary artery. In addition, any areas of subcommissural fusion can be divided. If the valve ring is found to be hypoplastic according to the diameter guidelines recently published by Pacifico, Kirklin, and Blackstone, the ventriculotomy can be extended across the pulmonic annulus.

The short vertical ventriculotomy not only maintains ventricular function better but also, when combined with a patch, permits relief of the stenosis without radical excision of right ventricular muscle.

During the procedure, the aorta is intermittently occluded for periods of 10 to 15 minutes, venting the aorta through a small stab wound with a catheter when the aortic clamp is released, while compressing the coronary arteries to avoid air embolism and then defibrillating the heart and allowing it to beat for a few minutes before proceeding. Defibrillating the heart and allowing it to beat at 15- to 20-minute intervals for a few minutes seemingly has resulted in far less right ventricular failure than seen in the past, for subendocardial coronary blood flow is probably significantly impaired in a severely hypertrophied right ventricle with prolonged fibrillation. Care is taken to be certain that no air is present in the left ventricle before the heart is defibrillated.

With this approach, making certain that obstruction has been appropriately corrected in all areas, i.e., the right ventricle, the pulmonic annulus, the pulmonic valve, the main pulmonary artery, and its branches, even the most severe forms of pulmonic stenosis with right ventricular pressures exceeding 200 mm Hg can be promptly corrected with little cardiac failure afterward. Pressures are routinely checked, with the goal of obtaining a residual gradient between the right ventricle and pulmonary artery of less than 40 mm Hg.

Fig. 18-8. Dilator and valvulotome developed by Potts for pulmonic valvulotomy. Calibrated swivel mechanism permits precise opening or closing of instruments.

Postoperative Course. With the exception of emergency operations in infants, the operative risk is very low, approaching 1 to 2 percent, and most patients have an uneventful convalescence.

After recovery from operation, symptomatic improvement is usually prompt. A systolic murmur almost always remains audible, and a faint diastolic murmur of no known physiologic significance frequently can be heard. The electrocardiogram will show signs of gradual regression of right ventricular hypertrophy, although such changes may require 1 to 3 years to evolve completely. Often there is little change in the heart size as seen on the chest roentgenogram, unless cardiac dilatation from failure was present before operation. If significant right ventricular hypertension remains after valvulotomy, cardiac catheterization should be performed after 6 months to 1 year to evaluate the degree of residual hypertension. In the majority of patients the systolic pressure in the right ventricle will subsequently be found to be less than 50 mm Hg.

A study of a group of 108 patients reported by Tandon and associates included only 10 percent with significant residual abnormalities on the electrocardiogram or roentgenogram. Postoperative catheterization studies performed upon 22 patients demonstrated only 1 with significant hypertension in the right ventricle.

STENOSIS OF THE PULMONARY ARTERY

Focal stenosis of the pulmonary artery or its peripheral branches, either single or multiple, has been recognized as an unusual condition since the development of selective angiocardiography. An early review by Franch and Gay in 1963 reported experiences with 11 patients and found 90 previously reported cases.

The physiologic disability depends upon the severity of the stenosis and the artery involved. Usually no limitation is present unless multiple stenoses involving both pulmonary arteries are present.

Although plastic reconstruction of multiple stenoses can be done, long-term results are yet uncertain. The operative technique is not complicated, and one of the first such operations was reported by McGoon and Kincaid in 1964. However, recurrence of the stenosis at the site of patch grafting has been described in several reports, so the indications and the best method of patch grafting remain uncertain at this time.

Congenital Aortic Stenosis

HISTORICAL DATA. Adequate surgical treatment of congenital aortic stenosis was not possible until the development of extracorporeal circulation. In 1955 Swan and associates and Lewis independently performed valvulotomy under hypothermia, but this approach was quickly discarded in favor of the more precise approach possible with cardiopulmonary bypass. By 1958 Spencer et al. had reported successful operation upon 12 children without any mortality.

INCIDENCE AND ETIOLOGY. Congenital aortic stenosis is a common congenital cardiac anomaly, representing 8 to 10 percent of all patients with congenital heart disease.

For unknown reasons it is three to four times more frequent in males than in females. By contrast, congenital aortic regurgitation is an extremely rare lesion. The four patients with isolated congenital aortic regurgitation reported by Frahm and associates in 1961 were the first reported in whom the diagnosis was firmly established during life.

There are no known causative factors associated with valvular or subvalvular aortic stenosis. Only in the unusual forms of supravalvular or diffuse muscular stenosis are there associated factors suggesting a genetic basis for the disease. Rheumatic fever is rarely a cause of isolated aortic stenosis; it usually causes associated disease of the mitral valve.

PATHOLOGIC ANATOMY. In valvular stenosis the valve cusps are often well formed but are fused along the commissures to produce an opening varying from 2 to 6 mm in diameter. The pattern of fusion of the commissures is similar in many patients. The commissure between the right and left coronary cusps is often the least developed, the valve functioning as a bicuspid valve. Commissural fusion between the right and noncoronary cusps is usually moderate, and fusion between the left and noncoronary cusps is usually the least extensive. The valve cusps are usually thicker than normal cusps but have adequate mobility. Calcification is common in adults but is almost never seen before seventeen to eighteen years of age. In most patients the aortic annulus is of normal diameter, but mild poststenotic dilatation of the ascending aorta is common (42 percent of 100 patients reported by Braunwald et al.). Fortunately, only in a minority of patients are the more bizarre, extreme forms of valvular stenosis seen, with a hypoplastic annulus, unusual valve cusps with absence of commissures, and associated hypoplasia of the left ventricle.

Subvalvular stenosis usually occurs as a narrow ring of fibrous tissue, varying in length from a "ring" to a short "tunnel," 1 to 2 cm proximal to the aortic valve cusps. The orifice varies from 4 to 8 mm. The aortic outflow tract is usually of normal diameter proximal and distal to the stenotic ring, although muscular hypertrophy may be prominent in older patients. In some patients the base of the aortic cusps is immediately adjacent to the stenotic ring and must be protected from injury during surgical excision of the stenosis. Two other anatomic relations are of particular importance during surgical excision. Beneath the noncoronary cusp where the stenotic ring is attached to the ventricular septum, the conduction bundle is present and may easily be injured. Beneath the left coronary cusp the ring is attached to the base of the aortic leaflet of the mitral valve, which is also susceptible to injury.

Associated cardiac malformations are found in 15 to 20 percent of patients, being more frequent with valvular stenosis than with subvalvular stenosis. The most frequent associated conditions are patent ductus, coarctation, ventricular septal defect, and pulmonic stenosis.

PATHOPHYSIOLOGY. The physiologic limitations from aortic stenosis are directly related to the severity of obstruction. Mild stenosis of little physiologic significance can occur with "typical" findings on examination. At the other extreme, severe obstruction can cause death from congestive heart failure in infants or sudden death in older children. The severity of the stenosis can be quantitated only by left heart catheterization; it is usually expressed in terms of the peak systolic gradient between the left ventricle and the ascending aorta. A gradient of less than 40 mm Hg is usually associated with such mild disability that operation is not recommended. In such patients cardiac output should be measured as well as the pressure gradient in order to calculate the functional cross-sectional area of the aortic valve. A functional cross-sectional area less than $0.5 \text{ cm}^2/\text{m}^2$ of body surface should usually be surgically corrected. Systolic pressure gradients of 50 to 75 mm Hg are usual with aortic stenosis of moderate severity, while gradients exceeding 100 mm Hg may be found with severe stenosis.

Depending upon the degree of stenosis, there is resulting hypertrophy of the left ventricle. Cardiac failure may occur in infants and is often fatal: 19 of 25 infants with cardiac failure reported by Peckham et al. died from their illness. Operation is urgently indicated in these severely ill infants. The stenosis in infants is almost always valvular, not subvalvular, and is often associated with additional cardiac malformations.

Between the ages of two and ten there are usually few or no signs of impairment of function of the left ventricle. In older children symptoms representing limited cardiac reserve and a restriction in coronary or cerebral blood flow become increasingly common, although overt congestive heart failure is rare. Sudden death may occur in children, apparently from ventricular fibrillation. The frequency of sudden death varies with different reports. Braverman and Gibson reported 6 deaths in 73 patients, an 8.2 percent mortality rate. Nadas estimated the incidence of sudden death in his group of 250 patients as 7.5 percent. The lowest incidence of sudden death was reported by Peckham et al., who observed only 4 deaths in a group of 300 patients, approximately 1 percent. The occurrence of sudden death has not always correlated with clinical signs of severity of obstruction, so the risk of this tragedy cannot be predicted with certainty.

In young adults calcification of the fused valve cusps occurs with increasing frequency and probably approaches 100 percent in the third and fourth decades. Calcification adds the element of rigidity to the obstruction formerly originating only from the small size of the orifice. Consequently patients in the third or fourth decades may be seen with severe symptoms who have a history of a cardiac murmur during childhood without symptoms. It is now recognized that with the declining frequency of rheumatic fever, most adults with isolated calcific aortic stenosis represent calcification of a congenitally deformed valve. In the past year, the author has operated upon one patient over seventy-five years of age who had calcific aortic stenosis with the classic commissural abnormalities of a congenital deformity, well illustrating the long period of time that may elapse before rigidity from progressive calcification produces significant stenosis.

CLINICAL MANIFESTATIONS. Symptoms. Many young children with significant aortic stenosis are asymptomatic.

The most common symptoms are fatigue, dyspnea, angina pectoris, and syncope. These were found in 30 to 50 percent of a group of 100 patients studied by Braunwald et al. In most of these patients the systolic gradient was greater than 50 to 70 mm Hg.

Physical Examination. The four principal physical findings are a basal systolic murmur, palpable thrill, forceful left ventricular impulse, and narrow pulse pressure. The systolic murmur is a harsh, ejection-type murmur usually heard best in the second right interspace and is widely transmitted to the neck and arms. In infants and young children it may be loudest to the left of the sternum. A thrill can be felt in over 80 percent of patients. The left ventricular impulse is usually forceful and heaving. The pulse pressure was found to be decreased from the normal value of 30 mm Hg in 38 percent of 300 patients studied by Peckham and associates but was considered normal in 54 of 67 patients studied by Nadas.

An early diastolic murmur can be heard in about 20 percent of patients but is usually of no physiologic significance. For unknown reasons, it is considerably more frequent with subvalvular stenosis than with valvular stenosis.

LABORATORY FINDINGS. The electrocardiogram is the most sensitive guide to the severity of aortic stenosis but has distinct limitations. The usual abnormalities are signs of left ventricular hypertrophy, subsequently followed by depression of the ST segment and inversion of T waves. In about 75 percent of patients in whom the gradient exceeded 50 mm Hg, a left ventricular strain pattern was present. The limitations of electrocardiography have been emphasized by Braunwald and associates, for in some patients with severe obstruction the electrocardiogram may show few abnormalities.

The chest roentgenogram is frequently normal. In about one-half the patients slight enlargement of the left ventricle can be recognized, with a cardiothoracic ratio greater than 50 percent. Mild dilatation of the ascending aorta may be detected in 30 to 40 percent of patients. Calcification of the stenotic valve is rarely found except in adults.

Cardiac catheterization is necessary to determine whether operation is indicated. The critical determination is measurement of the systolic gradient between the left ventricle and the ascending aorta. With gradients of less than 50 mm Hg, cardiac output should be determined to permit calculation of the functional cross-sectional area of the aortic valve. It may be possible to differentiate valvular from subvalvular stenosis by noting changes in pressure as a catheter is withdrawn from the apex of the left ventricle into the aorta, but this information is of little value to the surgeon, as the two areas are immediately adjacent to each other and can be easily identified at operation. Usually on catheterization the pulmonary artery pressure, left atrial pressure, and cardiac output are normal. The left ventricular pressure is elevated when severe stenosis with early cardiac failure is present.

DIAGNOSIS. The diagnosis can be made with confidence in the presence of the characteristic murmur, thrill, left ventricular impulse, and narrow pulse pressure. Confirmation can be obtained from the chest roentgenogram and electrocardiogram, reserving cardiac catheterization to assess the severity of the obstruction. In infants, when the murmur is loudest to the left of the sternum, catheterization may be required to differentiate from ventricular septal defect or pulmonic valvular stenosis.

TREATMENT. Infants in congestive heart failure should usually be operated upon with a pump-oxygenator once the diagnosis has been established. The mortality from nonoperative therapy is extremely high, 19 of 25 patients having died in a series reported by Peckham et al. Before operation, catheterization is required to differentiate the condition from coarctation of the aorta or the hypoplastic left heart syndrome.

In most children operation is considered because of mild symptoms or the presence of changes in the electrocardiogram. A final decision can be made after left heart catheterization; operation is usually performed if the peak systolic gradients are greater than 40 to 50 mm Hg.

Operative Technique. Operation is performed with cardiopulmonary bypass, using a median sternotomy incision. After bypass is established, the temperature is lowered to about 25°C and a vent is inserted into the apex of the left ventricle to aspirate blood from the operative field. Subsequently the ascending aorta is clamped and opened with a curved incision, which is extended down into the noncoronary sinus but does not go to the base of the sinus. Extending the incision into the depth of the noncoronary sinus may increase exposure but theoretically may result in prolapse of the noncoronary cusp when the aortic circumference is narrowed by suture of the aortotomy.

Coronary perfusion was occasionally used in the past but has now been abandoned in favor of the potassium cardioplegia technique, injecting the cold (4°C) potassium cardioplegic mixture into the coronary ostia to stop the heart and lower the myocardial temperature below 20°C. With this technique, periods of ischemia for as long as 45 to 60 minutes seem completely safe.

Calibrated Hegar dilators are useful for measuring the diameter of the stenotic orifice both before and after commissurotomy. If an orifice admitting a #16 or #18 Hegar dilator can be obtained by commissurotomy, corresponding to a cross-sectional area nearly 2 cm², the obstruction will have been adequately relieved. (This, of course, varies with body size.) Even a larger opening is preferable, of course, if this can be obtained without risking the production of aortic insufficiency. Measuring the stenotic orifice before commissurotomy provides a good guide to the length of commissural incision necessary to obtain the desired opening.

With valvular stenosis, the fused commissures are gradually incised with a small (#15) knife blade, the fused commissure being incised exactly along the center of the fibrous raphe in order to have a thick margin on each of the two cusps which are thus separated (Fig. 18-9). Attempted division of the fused commissures with scissors will often result in division of the area to one side of the area of fusion and increase the likelihood of insufficiency. As far as possible, the incision of the commissures should be limited to areas where the commissures are well formed. When necessary, the commissural incisions may be carried

Fig. 18-9. *A.* Operative exposure of congenital aortic stenosis. Stenotic aortic valve has been exposed through longitudinal aortotomy. Fused commissures between three aortic cusps are clearly seen, with small central opening. *B* and *C.* Commissurotomy performed with knife, with center of fused commissures carefully incised and incision avoided in areas where commissures are not well developed. *(Reprinted by permission of The C. V. Mosby Company, St. Louis, from F. C. Spencer, C. A. Neill, and H. T. Bahnson, The Treatment of Congenital Aortic Stenosis with Valvulotomy during Cardiopulmonary Bypass, Surgery, 44:116, 1958.)*

completely to the aortic wall or, if not necessary, can be stopped 1 to 3 mm away. With the classic bicuspid valve, the commissure between the right and left coronary cusps is not well developed, and only a 2- to 4-mm incision, or no incision at all, may be made in this area, leaving the valve as a bicuspid valve. It is better to relieve the stenosis incompletely than to produce severe aortic insufficiency. Starr and associates have reported disappointing long-term results if significant insufficiency is produced at operation, with patients often requiring aortic valve replacement within a few years because of progressive cardiac enlargement and failure. In most patients, however, a stenosis can be adequately relieved by selective incision of the fused commissures without producing significant insufficiency. In one group of 23 patients studied, limited incision of the commissures was performed in 15 and obtained a satisfactory reduction in pressure gradient. The technique of commissurotomy is emphasized in some detail, for most difficulties with aortic insufficiency following aortic valvulotomy have resulted from inept valvulotomies rather than from the pathologic anatomy.

With subvalvular stenosis the valve cusps can be carefully retracted and the fibrotic ring incised. The tissue between the base of the valve cusps and the fibrotic ring must be clearly visualized to avoid injury of the base of the aortic valve cusps. The ring may consist of thin fibrous tissue, easily removed, or it may be a thick fibrotic structure requiring excision with a knife and rongeur. The surgical anatomy is of crucial importance in this area, for

A

B

C

Fig. 18-10. *A*. Operative exposure of congenital subaortic stenosis. Valve cusps are normal. Insert shows membranelike subaortic stenosis exposed by retraction of valve cusps. (*From Am Surg, 26:210, 1960.*) *B*. Diagram of pertinent surgical anatomy with subaortic stenosis. Beneath noncoronary cusps and part of left coronary cusp is aortic leaflet of mitral valve. Beneath part of right coronary cusp is membranous septum. Only in area beneath commissure between right and left coronary cusps is limited zone where underlying ventricular muscle can be safely excised. Failure to observe these landmarks can result in injury to mitral valve or to membranous septum with conduction bundle. *C*. Subaortic stenosis exposed at operation. Aorta has been opened with longitudinal aortotomy and retractor inserted to retract normal aortic cusps. Diaphragmlike subaortic stenosis can be clearly seen with small pinpoint central opening. (*Reprinted by permission of C. V. Mosby Co. from F. C. Spencer, C. A. Neill, and H. T. Bahnson, The Treatment of Congenital Aortic Stenosis with Valvulotomy during Cardiopulmonary Bypass, Surgery, 44: 117, 1958.*)

only in a narrow zone constituting less than 20 percent of the circumference of the stenotic ring can excision be safely carried into the underlying ventricular wall. This corresponds to the area beneath the commissure between the right and left coronary cusps (Fig. 18-10). Radical excision of the fibrotic ring beneath the left coronary cusp will perforate the aortic leaflet of the mitral valve, producing severe or fatal mitral insufficiency. Radical excision beneath the noncoronary cusp and part of the right coronary cusp will injure the ventricular septum, creating either a complete heart block or ventricular septal defect. The most useful instrument for excising the stenotic ring is a right-angled rongeur with a swivel for rotating the instrument to an appropriate angle (Fig. 18-11). With good exposure, an unhurried approach, and appropriate instru-

ments, a stenotic area can be regularly excised satisfactorily. Optical magnification and focal illumination with a headlight are excellent adjuncts in small children.

The aortotomy is sutured with a continuous Prolene suture. A small opening is left for removal of air. Following closure of the aortotomy, induced electrical ventricular fibrillation is carefully maintained with electrodes on the heart. The heart is then allowed to fill with blood by stopping the suction on the left ventricular vent, after which it is gently massaged to expel air from the ventricle and the aorta through the small opening remaining in the aortotomy. While compressing the right coronary artery digitally, the aortic clamp is cautiously removed and any remaining air expelled through the aortic vent site, which can later be sutured.

Following removal of the aortic clamp and meticulous removal of air from the heart, the heart can be defibrillated. Subsequently the left ventricular vent is removed and bypass slowed and stopped.

Following bypass, with a systemic pressure over 100 mm Hg, the residual gradient across the aortic valve can be measured by needle puncture of the left ventricle and the aorta. The residual gradient should be less than 40 mm Hg, and is often very small.

Postoperative care is little different from that for thoracotomy for other conditions. Arrhythmias or mild congestive failure may occur, but are infrequent.

The risks of operation are small and the results good. Nadas reported that only 2 of 54 patients with uncomplicated aortic stenosis died following operation. Some have expressed pessimism and dissatisfaction with operations for aortic stenosis, but the experience of the author has been most favorable. In a series exceeding 75 patients over the past several years, there have been no deaths among those with valvular stenosis, a satisfactory reduction in systolic gradient was achieved in almost all, and only a few have some aortic insufficiency. With subvalvular stenosis, there have been no operative deaths in several years. Earlier, deaths occurred in isolated patients from injury to adjacent anatomic structures, such as the mitral valve or attached aortic cusp, but with the present technique such injuries can be avoided.

Postoperative Course. Electrocardiographic changes may show improvement in some patients after recovery from operation, but in others little change may occur. The failure to show electrocardiographic improvement may indicate that operation should have been performed earlier than is customary. Changes in heart size on the chest roentgenogram are usually negligible. Usually a systolic murmur is audible, and a faint diastolic murmur without any signs of significant aortic insufficiency may be heard.

The long-term prognosis for these patients is yet unknown, although some patients have now survived for over 15 years after operation and recurrence of the stenosis has not been observed. A more probable complication is the eventual development of progressive aortic insufficiency from fibrosis and contraction of the thickened aortic cusp, ultimately requiring valvular replacement. To date, this has not occurred in a significant number of patients. Similarly, the persistence of abnormal changes in the electrocardiogram following operation has not been associated with any serious long-term complications.

Fig. 18-11. Right-angled sharp rongeur used for excision of subaortic stenosis. Swivel mechanism permits rotation of instrument to obtain proper exposure.

SUPRAVALVULAR AORTIC STENOSIS

Supravalvular aortic stenosis is the rarest form of aortic stenosis, although it has been recognized with increasing frequency in recent years. The first successfully treated patient was reported by McGoon and Kirklin in 1956, and 10 years later Rastelli et al. reported surgical experience with 16 patients. At that time a total of 88 cases were found in the medical literature, 51 of which had been treated surgically. In most patients there are no known etiologic factors. Both sexes are equally involved. In about 20 percent of patients there is a peculiar facies consisting of a broad forehead, heavy cheeks, protuberant lips, and pointed chin. This facies is similar to that found with idiopathic hypercalcemia of infancy, and experimental induction of hypercalcemia in rats may produce a vascular lesion resembling supravalvular aortic stenosis. Most but not all patients with the characteristic facies are mentally deficient.

There is considerable variation in the type of aortic obstruction in different patients. In a review of 68 cases, Peterson et al. found three types: membranous, 9 cases; diffuse hypoplastic, 14 cases; hourglass, 45 cases (Fig. 18-12). Surgical results with the diffuse hypoplastic type to date have not been very good. The left ventricular-aortic valve conduit has been used for some forms of severe

Fig. 18-12. Different types of supravalvular aortic stenosis, obstruction varying from localized constriction near aortic valve to diffuse hypoplasia of ascending aorta. (*Adapted from G. C. Rastelli et al., J Thorac Cardiovasc Surg, 51:878, 1966.*)

LOCALIZED   DIFFUSE

Fig. 18-13. *A.* Drawing of left ventricular aortic prosthesis coupled to valved Dacron conduit. (1) Inflow tube to be inserted through left ventricular apex to body of ventricle. (2) Curved part of prosthesis with movable outflow connection. (3) Clamp used to fix Dacron graft in place. (4) Dacron graft containing xenograft valve. *B.* Operative photograph showing left ventricular aortic prosthesis in place during cardiopulmonary bypass. Catheter used to decompress left ventricle can be seen entering lateral wall (on right). Vascular clamp placed beneath aortic anastomosis is visible at bottom of photograph. (*From W. F. Bernhard et al., J Thorac Cardiovasc Surg, 69:223, 1975.*)

obstruction to left ventricular outflow in the past two or three years by several investigators, including Weldon and Cooley and Bernhard and associates, and may be used for such patients in the future (Figs. 18-13, 18-14).

A new technique for insertion of a prosthetic aortic valve in patients with a hypoplastic aortic valve ring was reported by Konno in 1975. He described an ingenious method of extending the aortotomy down into the upper ventricular septum by a complex approach in which the anterior wall of the right ventricular outflow tract is also incised (Fig. 18-15). Favorable experiences have also been described by others, so initial experience with this technique seems sound. Most successful operations have been with the hourglass type, in which constriction of the aorta is found as a shelflike thickening and hypertrophy of the plica at the upper margin of the sinuses of Valsalva. The

Fig. 18-14. Technique for modifying a commercially available valve-bearing arterial prosthesis for use as an apical-aortic shunt. (1) A metal cylinder is drawn over a cloth cylinder. (2) The cloth is doubled over the metal cylinder in porous polyester cloth. (3) The cloth-covered cylinder is sewn to the prosthesis and a ring of felt is used to cover the junction. (*From W. P. Dembitsky et al., Ann Surg, 184:317, 1976.*)

outer diameter of the aorta may be normal or reduced. The stenotic ridge has thickened intima and hypertrophy of the media, with an increase in fibrous and elastic tissue.

Associated abnormalities are frequent. In about one-third of the patients abnormalities of the aortic valve cusps are present, frequently consisting of adherence of part of one of the free margins of the cusps to the aortic wall, which, when extensive, can result in aortic regurgitation. The coronary arteries are abnormal in over one-half the patients. Often the right coronary artery is markedly dilated and tortuous, with hypertrophy of the media and intima which produce narrowing of the lumen. Focal stenotic lesions of the branches of the aortic arch and of the peripheral branches of the pulmonary arteries have also been found.

The usual symptoms are either angina or syncope, as with other forms of aortic stenosis. Death usually either has been sudden, suggesting an arrhythmia, or has resulted from congestive heart failure. Physical examination provides no clues to the diagnosis except when the typical facies, first described by Williams and associates in 1961, is present. A precise diagnosis can be established only by aortography.

A satisfactory operation can be accomplished in the localized type of stenosis by widening the stenotic area by the insertion of a patch of Dacron or pericardium. Complete excision of the stenotic ridge is not possible because of the attachment of the aortic valve cusps (Fig. 18-16). Although some have reported sudden death of patients after such an operation, a report by Rastelli et al. in 1966 stated that 15 of 16 patients survived operation, and in subsequent follow-up evaluation 13 of the 15 were consid-

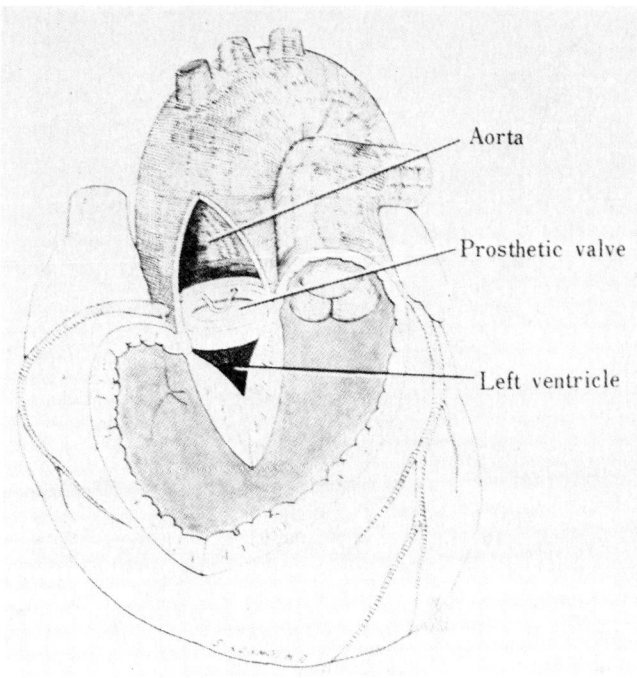

Fig. 18-15. Prosthetic valve is placed in subcoronary position. (*From S. Konno et al., J Thorac Cardiovasc Surg, 70:909, 1975.*)

ered to have had a good result (Fig. 18-17). In 1977 Doty described a more complex form of reconstruction of the aorta for severe supravalvular stenosis. This may be applicable for some of the more complex forms of obstruction.

IDIOPATHIC HYPERTROPHIC SUBAORTIC STENOSIS

This disease is basically a myopathy involving the left ventricle, with secondary obstruction of the left ventricular outflow tract. The hypertrophy is not uniform but may be most extensive in the septum, in some patients producing obstruction of the right ventricular outflow tract as well.

There is a familial history, in 30 to 40 percent of patients, of puzzling forms of heart disease in other members of the family, often terminated by sudden death at an early age. In one group of 27 patients reported by Braunwald et al., a positive familial history was found in 10. Often there is no sign of heart disease in childhood, with symptoms and physical findings appearing in later years, apparently as the hypertrophy of the left ventricle progresses. Pathologically, the heart shows massive ventricular hypertrophy with virtual obliteration of the lumen. The histologic structure of the hypertrophied muscle fibers is not distinctive. Although little is known of the natural history of the disease, the

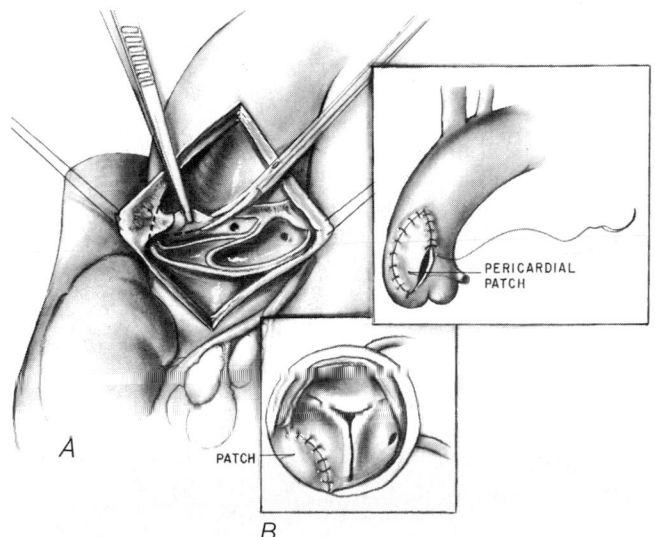

Fig. 18-16. Operation for localized supravalvular aortic stenosis. Stenotic area is widened by making longitudinal aortotomy and inserting pericardial patch. Partial excision of stenotic membrane is also shown. (*Adapted from G. C. Rastelli et al., J Thorac Cardiovasc Surg, 51:875, 1966.*)

A

B

Fig. 18-17. *A.* Operative photograph of the unusual lesion of supravalvular aortic stenosis. The waistlike narrowing of the ascending aorta just above the aortic valve can be clearly seen. *B.* Operative photograph of correction of supravalvular aortic stenosis by insertion of a Dacron patch to widen the area. The aortic valve gradient was reduced from 80 to near 30 mm Hg.

usual course has not been a favorable one, with death occurring at an early age.

The symptoms differ little from those of patients with the usual form of aortic stenosis, including syncope, angina, and dyspnea. On physical examination a systolic murmur, of medium intensity near the apex but not prominent at the base of the heart in the aortic area, may first arouse suspicion that a valvular stenosis is present. The chest roentgenogram will usually show some enlargement of the left ventricle, while the electrocardiogram shows left ventricular hypertrophy with depression of the ST segment and inversion of the T waves.

Diagnosis is best established by cardiac catheterization and angiography. On catheterization a gradient can usually be demonstrated over an area in the proximal outflow tract of the left ventricle. The systolic gradient may vary from 50 to 150 mm Hg, the average value being 80 to 90 mm Hg. An increase in the pressure gradient can characteristically be produced by the infusion of isoproterenol, apparently resulting from a more forceful contraction of the left ventricle. Cardiac angiography will show striking hypertrophy of the left ventricle, with a small lumen.

Operation is indicated in the presence of symptoms when there is a systolic gradient of more than 50 mm Hg. Although operation can relieve the left ventricular obstruction, it of course does not alter the basic disease of diffuse progressive ventricular hypertrophy.

The best operative results have been obtained with the technique developed by Morrow and associates. Their experience has been extensive, and catheterization studies 2 to 3 years after operation have demonstrated that recurrence of the obstruction is rare. At operation a trough of ventricular muscle is excised, going from the base of the aortic cusp into the ventricular cavity (Fig. 18-18). This procedure has been found to be superior to a variety of others attempted, including simple myotomy through the aorta, myotomy performed through a radical ventriculotomy, and even mitral valve replacement.

Coarctation of the Aorta

HISTORICAL DATA. In 1928 the characteristic features of coarctation of the aorta were outlined by Abbott in her classic analysis of 200 cases, including postmortem examinations. In 1944 and 1945 Blalock and Park, Gross, and Crafoord and Nylin all independently contributed to the first successful surgical treatment of coarctation by excision and direct anastomosis. Subsequently Gross provided a strong impetus to the study of vascular grafts by successfully using aortic homografts for patients with coarctation in whom direct anastomosis could not be performed.

INCIDENCE AND ETIOLOGY. Coarctation is one of the most common congenital abnormalities, occurring in 10 to 15 percent of patients with congenital heart disease. It is approximately twice as frequent in males as in females.

The exact cause of coarctation is unknown, but proximity of the coarctation to the ligamentum arteriosum has supported the most popular theory, that coarctation is an aberrant extension of the same fibrotic process that converts a patent ductus into a ligamentum arteriosum. Some observations indicate that a coarctation may increase in severity with time as a result of progressive thickening of the intima.

PATHOLOGIC ANATOMY. In most patients the coarctation is located as a diaphragmlike constriction in the first 2 to 4 cm of thoracic aorta distal to the left subclavian artery. Usually there is a 1- to 3-mm lumen, although complete occlusion may be present. On histologic examination the intima and media are both found to be markedly thickened. In older patients fibrosis and calcification may be found in the adjacent aortic wall. Usually the ligamentum arteriosum is attached to the medial surface of the aorta at the site of coarctation, although it may be inserted slightly above or below. The ligamentum clearly anchors the coarctation in this area, for when surgically divided, the two ends retract sharply, indicating the degree of tension previously exerted.

The aorta distal to the coarctation is usually dilated, more so in older patients; rarely it develops into an aneurysm. A striking feature of coarctation, becoming more prominent in older patients, is the large, dilated intercostal arteries which enter the distal aorta. As these vessels dilate, there is progressive thinning of the arterial wall, frequently resulting in the development of small aneurysms in adult patients.

The proximal aorta between the coarctation and the left subclavian artery is usually smaller than the distal aorta and may be hypoplastic, requiring excision along with the coarctation to relieve the obstruction completely.

The striking clinical characteristics of coarctation of the aorta are related to the growth of collateral circulation around the site of obstruction. These tributaries predominantly arise from the subclavian arteries and anastomose with the intercostal and epigastric vessels to enter the distal aorta. The development of collateral circulation through the intercostal arteries results in the characteristic "notching" of the ribs seen on the chest roentgenogram in patients over eight to ten years of age, virtually pathognomonic of coarctation.

A variety of unusual forms of coarctation are occasionally seen. A coarctation may extend proximally to involve the left subclavian artery or even left carotid and innominate artery, constituting an *interruption of the aortic arch*. In 1976 the different forms of this severe type of obstruction were well classified in the report by Fishman and associates.

A separate severe anomaly, often fatal in the first few months of life unless recognized and treated, is the so-called "preductal" coarctation, in which a number of severe anomalies are present. A large patent ductus supplies the distal aorta, with the coarctation proximal to this. Often additional severe cardiac defects are present. The syndrome, though rare, is well described in the textbook by Taussig. In the few patients surviving infancy, cyanosis may be recognized as localized in the lower half of the body.

PATHOPHYSIOLOGY. In infants, left ventricular failure may result from the obstruction to emptying of the left ventricle created by the coarctation. This is often fatal if untreated. Subsequently, enlarging collateral circulation partly relieves the obstruction; thus congestive failure is rare after the first year of life until late childhood or early adult life.

In infants with a preductal coarctation, severe symptoms are present, with pulmonary congestion, cardiac failure, and cyanosis. These disabilities cause death in the majority of infants unless effective surgical therapy can be performed. The disabilities result from the coarctation, the large patent ductus entering the distal aorta, and the other

Fig. 18-18. *A.* Second myotomy is made about 1 cm to right (clockwise) of first. Incisions are then deepened if necessary by digital splitting of muscle fibers. Myotomies are usually 12 to 15 mm in depth at most prominent aspect of septum. Transverse incision is then made at base of valve leaflet connecting proximal portions of the two myotomies. *B.* Bar of muscle isolated between incisions is held by traction suture as shown or by suitable clamp. Muscle is freed with rectangular knife (devised by Stinson) or with special angled rongeur. *C.* As traction is made on muscle bar, rectangular knife is pushed toward apex, freeing muscle bar from its anterior attachments to septum. Apical portion of resection is often more easily accomplished with rongeur, which may be introduced via aorta or via apical stab wound. In latter case, rongeur is positioned and directed by left index finger passed through valve ring. (*From A. G. Morrow et al., Circulation, 52:88, 1975.*)

Fig. 18-19. Chest roentgenogram in patient with coarctation of aorta, demonstrating classic notching of ribs from enlarged intercostal arteries. This roentgen appearance is virtually pathognomonic of coarctation of aorta, as it is rarely produced by any other condition. (*Courtesy of Dr. Raymond M. Abrams, Department of Radiology, New York University Medical Center.*)

associated cardiac malformations so frequently present, such as ventricular septal defect, fibroelastosis, or even transposition of the great vessels.

The hypertension from the coarctation causes rapid degenerative changes in the proximal aorta at such a rate that children in their early teens may have severe fibrosis that complicates surgical repair. Although some patients may live until the fifth or sixth decade, the average life expectancy is between 30 or 40 years. Before surgical therapy was possible, approximately 25 percent of untreated patients died from rupture of the aorta, 25 percent from cardiac failure, 25 percent from rupture of intracranial aneurysms, and 25 percent from superimposed bacterial endocarditis.

CLINICAL MANIFESTATIONS. Symptoms. Many children are asymptomatic for long periods of time despite severe hypertension and the progressive degenerative changes occurring in the aorta. When symptoms are present, headache, dizziness, and epistaxis are the most common. Dyspnea on exertion or occasionally chest pain may be mentioned. Claudication in the lower extremities is infrequent despite the restriction of peripheral blood flow.

Physical Findings. The combination of hypertension in the upper extremities and absence or decrease of pulses in the lower extremities in a child immediately suggest the

diagnosis of coarctation. In less severe forms measurements of the blood pressure in the upper and lower extremities may be required to confirm the diagnosis. Normally the blood pressure in the lower extremities is slightly higher than in the upper. Prominent pulsations are usually visible in the neck, and examination of the muscles of the shoulder girdle, especially the latissimus dorsi and supra-scapular muscles, will often reveal visible and palpable pulsations. Auscultation over these sites may detect a bruit. A systolic murmur, the origin of which is often obscure, is usually widely audible over the left hemithorax. It may result from the coarctation, an associated abnormality of the aortic valve, or dilated, tortuous arteries.

LABORATORY STUDIES. The chest roentgenogram in older patients may automatically establish the diagnosis by demonstrating bilateral notching of the ribs (Fig. 18-19). Notching of the ribs from other causes is extremely rare. Left ventricular hypertrophy also may be evident. The electrocardiogram shows signs of left ventricular hypertrophy or strain.

In most patients the diagnosis can be made from the clinical findings in combination with the roentgenogram and the electrocardiogram. Cardiac catheterization and aortography should be done routinely to detect additional anomalies and to outline the location and extent of the obstruction.

TREATMENT. The ideal age for operation is between five and seven years, preferably before the child begins to attend school. There is little reason and some risk in postponing operation beyond this time.

In adults, operation is complicated by the extensive degenerative changes of calcification and fibrosis. If these are so extensive that direct anastomosis is not feasible, a bypass graft with Dacron is preferable to attempting excision of the coarctation and insertion of a direct graft.

In the majority of infants with congestive failure, operation should be performed unless response to medical therapy is prompt. This may require operation within the first few weeks of life. Often there is an associated ventricular septal defect with a large increase in pulmonary blood flow; so banding of the pulmonary artery may be necessary at the time the coarctation is resected. When operation is performed in infants, there may be a recurrence as the child grows older, even though interrupted sutures are used to perform the anastomosis.

Operative Technique. A left posterolateral thoracotomy in the fourth intercostal space is used, usually dividing the fourth rib posteriorly in older patients (Fig. 18-20). After the lung is retracted inferiorly, the coarctation is usually obvious, with the indentation mediad at the site of insertion of the ligamentum arteriosum, and large, tortuous intercostal arteries entering the distal aorta (Fig. 18-21). After incision of the mediastinal pleura, the vagus nerve is retracted mediad; the aorta proximal to the left subclavian artery, the left subclavian artery, the ligamentum arteriosum, and the distal aorta are serially mobilized and encircled with tapes. The recurrent nerve coursing around the ligamentum arteriosum is usually not seen if dissection is kept close to the aorta but should be identified and protected if more extensive dissection is performed. Injury of

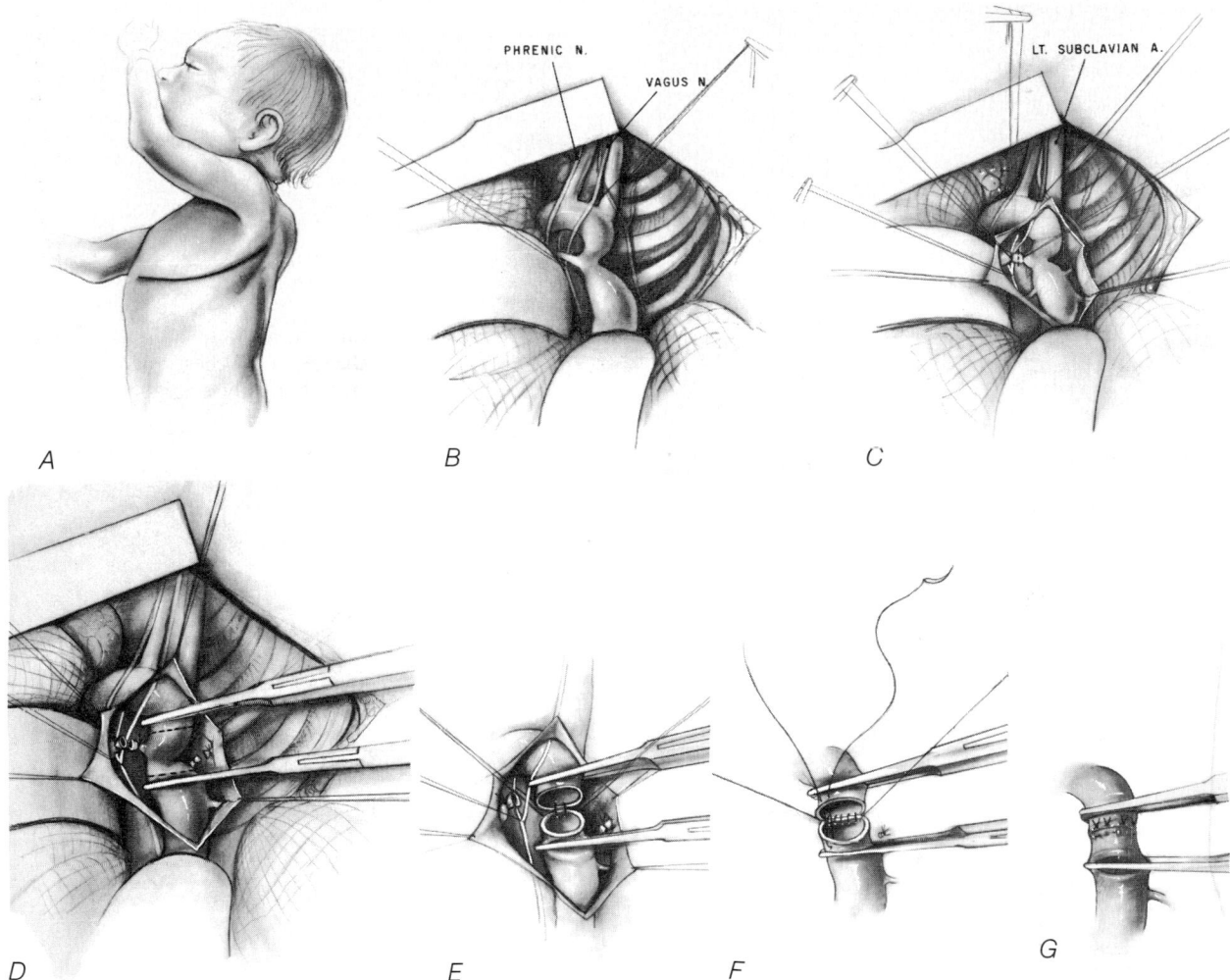

Fig. 18-20. Excision of coarction of aorta. *A*, Chest is opened with posterolateral incision in fourth intercostal space. *B*. Once chest has been opened and lung retracted, site of coarctation is often visible where aorta is angulated inward toward mediastinum just distal to left subclavian artery. This is site where ligamentum arteriosum is inserted. *C*. After incision of mediastinal pleura overlying coarctation, vessels are isolated proximal and distal to coarctation and ligamentum arteriosum is mobilized and divided. Recurrent laryngeal nerve, often not seen during operative procedure, is displaced mediad with vagus nerve. *D*. After division of ligamentum arteriosum, vascular occlusion clamps are applied to aorta proximal and distal to site of coarctation. Often it is necessary to apply proximal clamp to aorta between left carotid and left subclavian arteries, separately occluding left subclavian artery, in order to excise widely the narrowed segment of aorta. *E*. End-to-end anastomosis is constructed with continuous or interrupted sutures of silk. *F*. After completion of posterior row of anastomosis, interrupted sutures are often used in anterior row in young children to permit growth of anastomosis. *G*. Final view of completed anastomosis.

the thoracic duct may also occur if dissection is not kept next to the aorta. The proper plane for dissection of the aorta is between the adventitia and the media. This will avoid injury to the thoracic duct in the majority of patients. If the aorta is sharply angulated, division of the ligamentum will provide sufficient mobility. This may be done

before the aorta is occluded; otherwise the ligamentum may be divided at the same time that the coarctation is excised. Dissection of the distal aorta is the greatest hazard in the operation because of friable intercostal arteries. In older patients, intercostal aneurysms occur. Such aneurysms were found in 45 of 487 patients operated upon by Gross and associates. Usually the aorta can be mobilized sufficiently beyond the intercostal arteries. The intercostals are then individually isolated and can be separately occluded during performance of the anastomosis. Division of the intercostal arteries can be done but is seldom necessary.

One of the most feared hazards with operation for coarctation is paraplegia, fortunately rare. In a survey of published reports by Brewer et al., paraplegia has been reported to occur in approximately 0.5 percent of patients following operation (1 patient in 200). Although the author has personally never had a postoperative neurologic complication for several years the pressure in the aorta has been routinely monitored during excision of the coarctation by inserting a small catheter in the distal aorta before it is occluded. Though significant data are not available, it seems probable that there is little risk of neurologic injury if the distal aortic pressure remains above 60 mm, although

A

B

C

Fig. 18-21. *A.* Typical coarctation of aorta in child. Dilated sub-clavian artery is visible at top of field. At area of coarctation, aorta is angulated into mediastinum, where ligamentum arteriosum is inserted. *B.* Aortic anastomosis performed after excision of co-arctation. Anastomosis is made at point of origin of left subclavian artery. *C.* Resected coarctation of aorta, showing narrow lumen which was present.

the pressure has been found to vary widely, from as low as 30 mm to levels greater than 60 mm. Another safeguard is the fact that neurologic injury is virtually unknown if the aorta is occluded for less than 20 minutes. Hence it would seem wise to limit periods of aortic occlusion to less than 20 minutes if the distal pressure is less than 50 to 60 mm, or otherwise to employ a temporary shunt, as recommended by Hughes and Reemtsma.

With these precautions regarding paraplegia, once the vessels have been adequately mobilized, occluding vascular clamps are applied to the left subclavian artery, the proximal aorta, and the distal aorta, after which the coarctation is excised. The objective with excision, of course, is to obtain an anastomotic lumen as large as the proximal

aorta. Often this can be done in children by excising as much as 5 cm of the proximal aorta up to the level of the left subclavian artery and performing a primary anastomosis (Fig. 18-22). In older children, with fibrosis and decreased elasticity of the aorta, only 2.5 to 3.0 cm of aorta may be excised.

An end-to-end anastomosis is usually done with continuous and interrupted sutures of polypropylene (Prolene), using interrupted sutures especially in small children to provide the best opportunity for subsequent growth of the anastomosis.

Following completion of the anastomosis and removal of vascular clamps, the blood pressure is measured proximal and distal to the anastomosis to confirm that no significant gradient remains. In addition, the circumference of the anastomosis is measured and compared to that of the proximal aorta. If a gradient of more than 5 to 10 mm Hg is present and the circumference is smaller than the proximal aorta, clamps are reapplied after a short period of time, one or two sutures are removed from the anterior suture line, and a short anterior arteriotomy is made. This permits insertion of an appropriate patch of Dacron, widening the lumen sufficiently to construct an anastomosis equal to the proximal aorta. The combination of anastomosis and selective patch grafting is a valuable technique that permits complete correction of the obstruction without the insertion of a vascular graft. Less than 10 percent of children have an obstruction so diffuse that primary insertion of a graft is necessary. Schuster and Gross inserted grafts in 70 patients, 14 percent of their series, with excellent results over periods of observation as long as 12 years. Crafoord and Nylin employed grafts in only 1.0 percent of patients, while Brom reported the use of grafts in 5.0 percent.

A useful guideline for criteria of inadequate anastomosis in children was reported in 1965 by Brom, who observed from experience with over 1,000 operations for coarctation that recurrence was unlikely if the anastomosis had a circumference greater than 40 mm.

Postoperative Course. Antibiotics are given routinely during operation and for 3 to 4 days afterward. Patients usually recover rapidly and are discharged from the hospital in 10 to 12 days.

Fig. 18-22. *A.* Preductal coarctation exposed at emergency operation on thirteen-day-old infant. Large patent ductus equal in diameter to descending aorta is present. Proximal to patent ductus is coarctation of aorta with narrow proximal aortic segment and narrow subclavian artery. *B.* Appearance after excision of coarctation and suture of patent ductus arteriosus. Anastomosis was constructed proximally at point of origin of left subclavian artery from aorta.

Often there is a "paradoxical" hypertension to some extent in the first 48 to 72 hours after operation. This was first recognized by Sealy. Apparently it is related to a sudden perfusion of visceral arteries, previously functioning with a lower perfusion pressure. If this is untreated, a number of complications can occur, including intermittent abdominal pain or even intestinal necrosis in its extreme form, probably due to a mesenteric arteritis. With recognition of the syndrome and prompt treatment with appropriate antihypertensive medications, usually reserpine, serious complications are virtually unknown. Brom reported the abdominal pain syndrome in 16 of 548 patients, none of whom required laparotomy. With the liberal use of antihypertensive medications, the author has not seen any significant abdominal problems in the past 10 years.

With present techniques, the risk of operation is small and long-term results are excellent. In the series of 487 resections reported by Schuster and Gross, operative mortality was 4 percent. On long-term follow-up, 4 percent of the patients had systolic pressures above 150 mm Hg, 36 percent had values between 130 and 150 mm Hg, and 60 percent had pressures below 130 mm Hg. Crafoord and Nylin reported experiences with 249 patients, with a 4.5 percent mortality, and Brom reported experiences with 530 patients and a mortality of slightly greater than 3 percent. In a long-term evaluation of 350 patients, Brom found only 42 with some residual hypertension. At New York University, of patients operated upon beyond the first year of life, there has been no mortality and no significant complications since 1963.

Vascular Rings

HISTORICAL DATA. Although the clinical significance of vascular rings was recognized by Abbott in her classic survey of congenital heart disease in 1932, surgical therapy

A   *B*

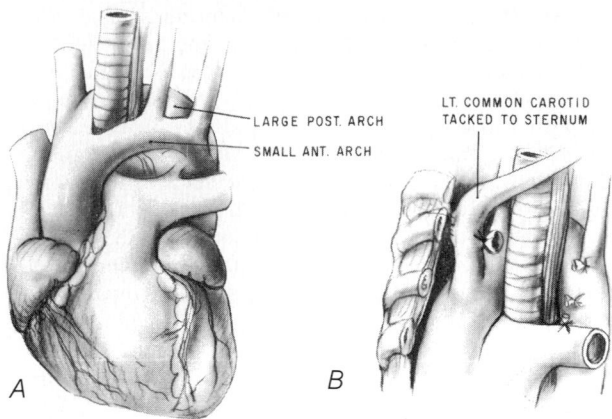

Fig. 18-23. Double aortic arch with small anterior and large posterior limb. *A.* Anterior view of double aortic arch with small anterior limb. *B.* Exposure after division of small anterior arch between left carotid and left subclavian artery, followed by displacement of carotid artery anteriorly toward sternum. (*Adapted from R. E. Gross, "The Surgery of Infancy and Childhood," W. B. Saunders Company, Philadelphia, 1953, p. 917.*)

was first successfully used with the division of a double aortic arch by Gross in 1945. Gross subsequently made many contributions to diagnosis and therapy of vascular rings, classifying and illustrating with clarity and precision the various anomalies found.

INCIDENCE AND ETIOLOGY. Vascular rings are fairly common among patients with congenital heart disease. Nadas reported seeing over 50 such patients during a

period of 10 years. Embryologically, the vascular rings result from variation in the formation of the aorta and pulmonary artery from the six embryonic aortic arches. In view of the fact that six aortic arches exist in the embryo, it is surprising that such abnormalities are not even more frequent. In embryonic life six pairs of aortic arches appear and disappear as the heart migrates caudad. The first two arches disappear before the fifth and sixth have developed, and the fifth never fully develops. Only the third, fourth, and sixth are significant in normal development. Ultimately the right common carotid artery arises from the third arch and the innominate from the right fourth. The left fourth contributes to the transverse aortic arch, while the ductus arteriosus originates from the sixth aortic arch.

PATHOLOGIC ANATOMY. Five types of vascular anomalies of clinical significance have been recognized: (1) double aortic arch; (2) right aortic arch with left ligamentum arteriosum; (3) retroesophageal subclavian artery; (4) anomalous origin of innominate artery; and (5) anomalous origin of left common carotid artery. The last two conditions, anomalous origin of the innominate or of the left common carotid artery, are rare malformations in which the origin of the artery from the aortic arch is such that the trachea is compressed. Briefly, surgical correction can be achieved by mobilizing the vessel and suturing it in

Fig. 18-24. *A.* Double aortic arch with large anterior arch. *B.* Small posterior arch, compressing esophagus. *C.* Appearance after division of small posterior arch. (*Adapted from R. E. Gross, "The Surgery of Infancy and Childhood," W. B. Saunders Company, Philadelphia, 1953, p. 918.*)

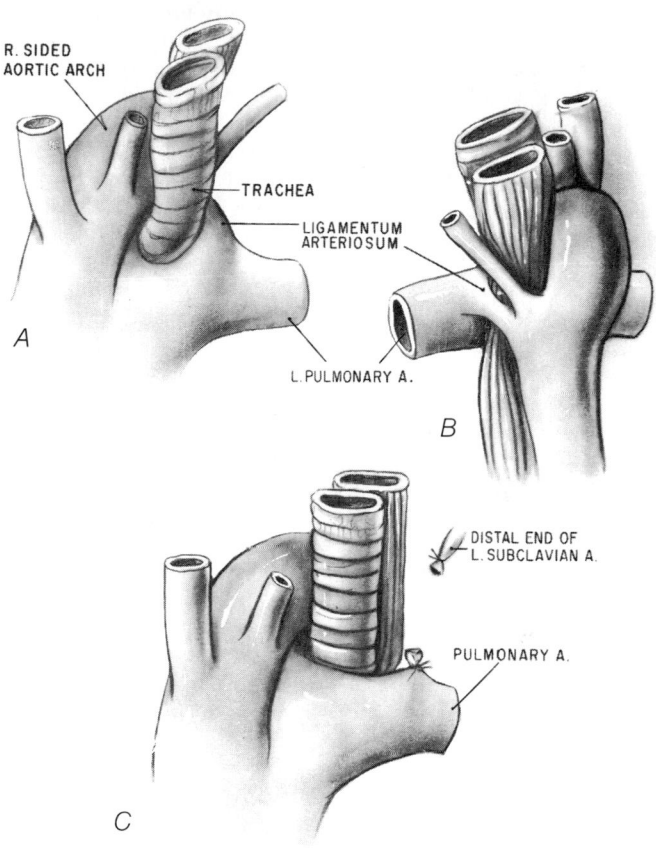

Fig. 18-25. *A.* Right aortic arch with left posterior ligamentum arteriosum. *B.* Posterior view of ligamentum arteriosum extending from right aortic arch to left pulmonary artery, compressing esophagus. Small left subclavian artery arising close to ligamentum arteriosum is also present. *C.* Appearance after division of ligamentum arteriosum and subclavian artery. (*Adapted from R. E. Gross, "The Surgery of Infancy and Childhood," W. B. Saunders Company, Philadelphia, 1953, p. 923.*)

a more normal position. The other three conditions are considered here in more detail.

A double aortic arch, with one limb anterior to the trachea and the other limb posterior to the esophagus (Figs. 18-23 and 18-24), is usually the most severe malformation, producing symptoms in early infancy. Usually one limb is smaller than the other. Often the thoracic aorta descends on the right rather than on the left.

A right aortic arch with a retroesophageal ligamentum arteriosum is an important anomaly, often producing symptoms in later childhood (Fig. 18-25). A retroesopha-

geal subclavian artery, usually consisting of a right subclavian artery originating beyond the left subclavian artery and coursing posterior to the esophagus to the right arm, is a common anomaly but usually does not cause symptoms (Fig. 18-26).

CLINICAL MANIFESTATIONS. Symptoms from vascular rings are usually due to respiratory obstruction from compression of the trachea. Less frequently, there is difficulty in swallowing from compression of the esophagus.

Symptoms. Infants with a double aortic arch often develop respiratory difficulty in the first few months of life

Fig. 18-26. *A.* Retroesophageal right subclavian artery, anomalous vessel arising from aortic arch distal to left subclavian artery. *B.* Appearance after division of anomalous vessel with retraction of distal stump to right of trachea. (*Adapted from R. E. Gross, "The Surgery of Infancy and Childhood," W. B. Saunders Company, Philadelphia, 1953, p. 932.*)

and become seriously ill. Episodes of serious respiratory distress, with "crowing" respirations, are common. During these attacks the infant prefers to lie in hyperextension, and there is visible retraction of the intercostal and supraclavicular spaces with inspiration. Feeding may precipitate such episodes, perhaps from flexing of the neck, and attempts at feeding may be interrupted by vomiting, and cyanosis, probably from aspiration. Because of the feeding difficulties, infants soon become underweight and malnourished.

Symptoms developing after infancy are more gradual in onset, with intermittent episodes of respiratory compression, at times precipitated by a respiratory infection. Mild difficulty in swallowing may be present, but this is seldom prominent. Recurrent pneumonic infections occur, perhaps from aspiration. The mildest clinical picture is seen with the retroesophageal subclavian artery, which may cause only mild or intermittent dysphagia for long periods of time. Some patients may be symptomatic in infancy and spontaneously recover with growth.

Physical Examination. The physical examination is within normal limits unless respiratory distress is present. During such episodes, the infant remains with the back arched and the neck extended. Attempts to flex the neck may precipitate severe dyspnea and cyanosis. Stridor is usually obvious. There are no abnormalities in the heart or peripheral circulation.

LABORATORY STUDIES. The chest roentgenogram is normal unless aspiration pneumonia is present, and the electrocardiogram is normal. Examination of the esophagus with a barium swallow usually establishes the diagnosis by demonstrating a typical area of compression from the retroesophageal vessel, usually at the level of the third or fourth thoracic vertebra. Such a finding is virtually all that is needed to establish the diagnosis of a vascular ring. To determine whether the ring is responsible for the symptoms may require further study. Tracheal compression may be defined with a tracheogram. In the anterior view, compression may be noted laterally, but the lateral tracheogram provides the best evidence for the vascular ring, demonstrating anterior compression of the trachea a short distance above the carina. The demonstration of anterior compression of the trachea combined with posterior compression of the esophagus firmly establishes the diagnosis of a vascular ring. Aortography can then precisely delineate the abnormal vessels.

TREATMENT. Since a vascular ring has no physiologic significance, no treatment is needed in the absence of symptoms. If symptoms are mild, their origin may be uncertain, and an observation period is required to be sure that other difficulties are not responsible. If obvious respiratory compression is present, operation should be performed promptly, however, because death from aspiration can occur.

Operative Technique. The preferred operative approach is through a left lateral thoracotomy, usually the fourth intercostal space. An important feature of the operation is to dissect the aortic arch completely and identify the innominate artery, the left common carotid artery, and both subclavian arteries. Opening the pericardium will facilitate identification of these vessels. The vagus nerve should be traced to the recurrent laryngeal nerve and, usually, the ligamentum arteriosum divided. Removal of part of the thymus gland will facilitate exposure. It should be emphasized that operative correction is more than simple division of an abnormal ring, because fibrosis surrounding the adventitia of the abnormal vessel may cause continued compression unless the vessels are widely mobilized and all possible compression relieved.

With a double aortic arch, the smaller of the two arches should be divided. Usually, with a left descending aorta, the anterior arch is smaller and should be divided between the left common carotid and left subclavian artery, after which the mobilized anterior arch can be sutured to the posterior surface of the anterior chest wall to prevent compression of the trachea. If the posterior arch is smaller, it can be divided behind the esophagus. With a right descending thoracic aorta, almost always the posterior arch is the smaller of the two.

With a right aortic arch and a retroesophageal ligamentum arteriosum, division of the ligamentum arteriosum, combined with mobilization of the abnormal vessels, may be all that is necessary. In some patients the left subclavian artery may be in a retroesophageal location and should also be divided. A nubbin of aorta, constituting an aortic diverticulum, has been found in a retroesophageal location in some patients and may require amputation to relieve compression.

With a retroesophageal subclavian artery as an isolated anomaly, simple division of the artery is all that is necessary. Division of this artery through a cervical incision, followed by reimplantation into the right carotid artery, has been reported.

Postoperative Course. Postoperative care consists primarily of careful attention to respiration, with the infant kept in a highly humidified atmosphere and tracheal secretions aspirated. Tracheostomy should be avoided if at all possible. If serious tracheal compression was present before operation, serious difficulties may develop after operation if extensive dissection around the trachea was necessary, creating postoperative edema. In such cases the patient may require unusually vigilant care for 24 to 72 hours because of edema of the trachea. After recovery from operation, symptoms promptly disappear without further disability. The risk of operation is primarily related to the age of the patient and the severity of compression of the trachea. Excellent results in a group of 70 patients have been reported by Gross, who had only 5 postoperative deaths, all of which occurred in a group of 26 infants with double aortic arches.

LEFT-TO-RIGHT SHUNTS (ACYANOTIC GROUP)

Atrial Septal Defects

A variety of malformations involve the atrial septum or the pulmonary veins and result in a left-to-right shunt of blood from the systemic to the pulmonary circulation.

These include atrial septal defects of the secundum type, anomalous drainage of the pulmonary veins, ostium primum defects, and atrioventricular canal malformations. These defects are serially considered below. The physiologic disturbance is identical with secundum-type atrial defects and with anomalous pulmonary veins, consisting simply in a left-to-right shunt. With ostium primum defects and atrioventricular canals, mitral and tricuspid insufficiency are present in addition to the left-to-right shunt.

SECUNDUM DEFECTS

HISTORICAL DATA. Several ingenious attempts were made to close atrial septal defects by closed techniques from 1947 to 1953, but only following the successful closure of an atrial septal defect by Lewis in 1953 under direct vision with inflow occlusion and hypothermia did a method of surgical closure become firmly established. In the same year Gibbon employed the pump-oxygenator successfully for the first time in man to suture an atrial septal defect. In subsequent years a large number of patients were successfully operated upon by using hypothermia to permit interruption of the circulation for 5 to 10 minutes, but extracorporeal circulation quickly became the preferred technique because of the additional time available to close the septal defect and also to correct any additional malformations which may be encountered.

INCIDENCE AND ETIOLOGY. Atrial septal defects are among the most common cardiac malformations, representing 10 to 15 percent of all cases of congenital heart disease. They are approximately twice as frequent in females as in males. Embryologically, the secundum defects result from failure of the septum secundum to develop completely.

PATHOLOGIC ANATOMY. Atrial septal defects vary widely in size and location. A "high" defect near the entrance of the superior vena cava is commonly referred to as a sinus venosus type of defect and is usually associated with anomalous entry of the superior pulmonary veins into the vena cava. The majority of secundum defects are located in the midportion of the atrial septum. "Low" defects are near the point of entry of the inferior vena cava, and caution must be taken in closing such defects to avoid compromising the entry of the inferior vena cava into the right atrium. Defects vary from as small as 1 cm in diameter to virtual absence of the atrial septum, but most are 2 to 3 cm. A foramen ovale should not be considered an atrial septal defect, for it is a normal opening in 15 to 25 percent of adult hearts. Because of its slitlike construction, a normal foramen ovale allows shunting of blood only from right to left. In some patients the atrial septum is fenestrated with multiple defects.

Anomalous pulmonary veins entering the right atrium are frequent, occurring in 10 to 15 percent of patients with atrial septal defects. An unusual variant of atrial septal defect is seen when a secundum defect occurs in association with mitral stenosis, the so-called Lutembacher's syndrome. The mitral stenosis retards flow of blood from the left atrium to the left ventricle and results in an enormous shunt of blood through the septal defect, with massive dilatation of the pulmonary arteries. With present diagnostic techniques, this syndrome has become rare.

PATHOPHYSIOLOGY. An atrial septal defect results in a left-to-right shunt of blood from the left atrium to the right atrium because of the pressure-volume characteristics of the left and right ventricles. The thick-walled left ventricle is less distensible than the right ventricle; with a closed atrial septum, left atrial pressure is normally 8 to 10 mm Hg, while right atrial pressure is 4 to 5 mm Hg. This difference in distensibility of the two ventricles results in a left-to-right shunt when an atrial septal defect is present. However, during infancy and the first few years of life the structure of the right ventricle more closely resembles the left ventricle, and usually only a small shunt is present. For this reason atrial septal defects are commonly not recognized during the first few years of life.

Depending upon the size of the atrial defect, as well as the difference in distensibility of the two ventricles, the size of the left-to-right shunt may vary from as little as 1 liter to as high as 20 liters/minute. Most septal defects have a pulmonary blood flow two to four times greater than the systemic blood flow. The great reduction in systemic blood flow may result in retardation of normal growth and development, with the so-called gracile habitus seen in some children with a large atrial septal defect. The increase in pulmonary blood flow increases susceptibility to pneumonia and also causes dyspnea on exertion. For unknown reasons patients are susceptible to rheumatic fever, but fortunately bacterial endocarditis is rare. Arrhythmias of different types are also frequently seen.

With the increased pulmonary blood flow, pulmonary vascular resistance in children is usually less than normal, but it gradually increases. Pulmonary hypertension is found in less than 5 percent of children with this condition but occurs in 20 to 25 percent of adult patients as fibrotic changes develop in the pulmonary vessels. Cardiac failure is similarly unusual in children but becomes more frequent in the second and third decades. It has been estimated that the average life span of an untreated patient with an atrial septal defect is about 40 years.

Some patients are seen in the fourth, fifth, or sixth decades for the first time with a previously unrecognized atrial septal defect. In these older patients, arrhythmias are especially common, a result of long-standing hypertrophy of the right atrium. Even in patients in the sixth decade a good result may be obtained following operation if increase in pulmonary vascular resistance has not occurred. However, arrhythmias may continue.

CLINICAL MANIFESTATIONS. Symptoms. Symptoms are uncommon in the first few years of life because the shunt may be small until the right ventricular hypertrophy of embryonic life has subsided. Frequently children with large shunts are physically active and completely free of symptoms. In a report of 275 surgically treated patients with hemodynamically significant atrial defects, Sellers et al found 113 asymptomatic. The most frequent symptoms are fatigue, palpitations, and exertional dyspnea. Slow growth and development may also be noted by the parents. In adults overt signs of congestive heart failure gradually appear, often with the first pregnancy.

Physical Examination. A soft systolic murmur is usually audible in the second or third left intercostal space. In the first few years of life this murmur may be scarcely detectable or may be diagnosed as a functional murmur. The murmur arises at the pulmonary valve from the increased flow of blood through the valve. The second pulmonic sound is characteristically widely split, and "fixed" splitting (not varying with respiration) is characteristic of the disorder. Slight to moderate cardiac enlargement is present with large defects. With large defects the cardiac enlargement may produce a distinct prominence of the left costal cartilages. The physical habitus of such patients is often thin, with long, narrow bones and limited muscular development—the gracile habitus.

LABORATORY FINDINGS. The chest roentgenogram shows mild to moderate cardiac enlargement limited to the right ventricle. The pulmonary artery is prominent, with increased vascularity in the lung fields. The electrocardiogram typically shows a right axis deviation with a right bundle branch block. Mild but not severe right ventricular hypertrophy is usually evident.

On cardiac catheterization the diagnosis can be confirmed by finding a rise in oxygen saturation of 1.5 to 2.0 vol % between the superior vena cava and right atrium. During catheterization the presence of anomalous veins should be noted, although the diagnosis cannot always be established with certainty. The right ventricular systolic pressure in children is usually 30 to 40 mm Hg. With large shunts there may be a 20 to 40 mm Hg gradient across a normal pulmonary valve as a result of the large flow of blood. Selective angiography with injection of dye into the pulmonary artery may disclose opacification of the right atrium as dye flows from the left atrium through the defect.

DIAGNOSIS. Diagnosis in infancy is virtually impossible on clinical grounds, because the systolic murmur is not distinctive. In older children the diagnosis can be made with reasonable certainty from the combination of a soft systolic murmur with fixed splitting of the pulmonic second

sound. These physical findings, combined with the chest roentgenogram and electrocardiogram, provide firm support for the diagnosis. A left axis deviation on the electrocardiogram immediately suggests that an ostium primum malformation is present.

TREATMENT. Indications. Since many children are asymptomatic, operation is frequently recommended on the basis of clinical findings and laboratory determination of the size of shunt present. Operation is usually performed if the pulmonary blood flow is one and one-half to two times greater than the systemic blood flow. The only contraindication to operation is the presence of severe pulmonary hypertension with an elevated pulmonary vascular resistance, fortunately almost unknown in children. In adults, if the pulmonary vascular resistance has increased to where pulmonary blood flow is only slightly greater than systemic flow, operation is hazardous, and patients who survive often show little benefit. However, if pulmonary blood flow is still significantly increased despite the presence of pulmonary hypertension, operation may be beneficial, although the operative risk is considerably greater than with uncomplicated atrial septal defect and improvement does not occur to an equal degree in all patients.

Operative Technique. All patients are operated on with extracorporeal circulation. A sternotomy or a right thoracotomy in the fourth intercostal space is used. Once bypass has been established, a finger is introduced into the right atrium through a stab wound to identify the pathologic anatomy, noting the atrial septal defect, the coronary sinus, the location of the pulmonary veins, the mitral and tricuspid valves, and the ventricular septum. Palpation beforehand minimizes the need for exploration of the heart once it has been opened and similarly lessens the hazards of air embolism.

At a perfusion temperature of 30°C, the heart is fibrillated, the aorta clamped, and the atrium opened widely to identify the margins of the defect (Fig. 18-27). In at least 90 percent of patients, closure can be done with a simple continuous suture, preferably polypropylene (Prolene). If

Atrial septal defect as seen thru incision in r. atrium

Fig. 18-27. Atrial septal defect of secundum type exposed at operation. Operation illustrated was performed under hypothermia several years ago with perfusion of aorta with oxygenated blood. Such operations are now performed with cardiopulmonary bypass. Large oval opening in atrial septum superior to coronary sinus is type usually found with secundum-type defects.

direct suture is not possible, a prosthetic patch of knitted Dacron or pericardium can be inserted.

Care is taken during operation to avoid aspiration of blood from the left atrium. As the suture line is completed, the lungs are ventilated and the aorta unclamped to expel blood from the left atrium into the right atrium and provide an additional protection against trapping air in the left atrium. With these safeguards, no problems with air embolism have occurred in several years.

Subsequently, after bypass has been stopped, correction of the left-to-right shunt can be confirmed by aspirating blood from the superior vena cava and pulmonary artery and demonstrating similar oxygen concentration in the two samples. Left atrial pressure should be measured afterward and serially monitored if elevated.

Postoperative Course. Postoperative convalescence is uncomplicated and recovery from any signs of cardiac disability is prompt in the usual patient with uncomplicated atrial septal defect.

The risk of operation with extracorporeal circulation is surprisingly small. Several groups have reported series of more than 100 patients operated upon with a mortality of 1 to 3 percent. Gerbode et al. reported one death in 77 patients, and Sellers et al. a 1.8 percent mortality in uncomplicated atrial defects in a group of 275 patients. In the author's experience with more than 100 secundum defects, no deaths have occurred in the past decade.

ANOMALOUS DRAINAGE OF PULMONARY VEINS

Partial and total anomalous drainage of the pulmonary veins are distinct clinical entities and are presented separately in the following sections. The physiologic handicap from partial drainage of the pulmonary veins resembles atrial septal defect, while total anomalous drainage is a much more serious physiologic derangement, often fatal in the first few months of life.

Partial anomalous drainage is frequent, occurring in 10 to 15 percent of patients with atrial septal defect. Total anomalous drainage, however, is much less common.

HISTORICAL DATA. Although anomalous pulmonary veins have been recognized at postmortem examinations for decades, emphasis was focused on clinical features by the analysis by Brody of 106 cases in 1942. Before open cardiac surgery was possible, only a few cases of successful surgical correction were reported. One of the first of these was reported in 1951 by Muller, who successfully implanted an anomalous left pulmonary vein into the left atrium. Subsequently, with operations performed under hypothermia, partial anomalous drainage of pulmonary veins, usually into the right atrium or superior vena cava, could be corrected by changing the position of the atrial septum. Successful correction of total anomalous pulmonary venous drainage, however, was accomplished only with extracorporeal circulation. A modification of the technique reported by Cooley and Ochsner in 1957 has subsequently proved to be the most useful.

PARTIAL ANOMALOUS DRAINAGE OF PULMONARY VEINS. Pathologic Anatomy. Anomalous drainage of the right pulmonary veins occurs approximately twice as frequently as that involving the left. Anomalous right pulmo-

nary veins usually enter the superior vena cava inferior to the point of entry of the azygos vein, the right atrium, or the inferior vena cava. Anomalous left pulmonary veins commonly enter a persistent left superior vena cava or innominate vein or, more rarely, the coronary sinus. Partial anomalous drainage usually involves only the veins from one lung, but a few unusual examples of partial drainage of pulmonary veins from both lungs have been described. One of the most detailed reports of the pathologic anatomy of anomalous pulmonary veins was published by Blake et al. in an analysis of data from the Armed Forces Institute of Pathology. In a group of 113 patients with anomalous pulmonary venous return, a total of 27 different variations were found, emphasizing the wide variation in physiologic derangement which occur.

Anomalous right pulmonary veins entering the superior vena cava are almost always associated with a characteristic high atrial septal defect at the point of entry of the superior vena cava, which has been termed a sinus venosus defect because of its embryologic origin. Pulmonary veins entering the right atrium are also usually associated with an atrial septal defect of the secundum type. Only rarely are anomalous pulmonary veins found with an intact atrial septum. Pulmonary veins entering the inferior vena cava usually communicate through a single channel with the inferior vena cava near the diaphragm.

An unusual variant of anomalous right pulmonary veins entering the inferior vena cava, in association with other anomalies, has been described as a "scimitar" syndrome, a term emphasizing a characteristic radiologic appearance resulting from the shadow of the anomalous vein parallel to the right border of the heart. Although this roentgenographic appearance is suggestive, other abnormalities may have a similar appearance. The malformation is often associated with defective development of the right lung and anomalous origin of the pulmonary arteries from the aorta. The physiologic disturbance is not severe, because the amount of blood shunted through the hypoplastic lung is small.

Pathophysiology. With partial anomalous drainage of the pulmonary veins, the volume of blood shunted is usually less than 50 percent of normal pulmonary blood flow, because less than one-half the pulmonary veins are involved. Hence the abnormal physiology is a left-to-right shunt identical to that of an atrial septal defect.

Clinical Manifestations. The symptoms and signs are identical to those of an atrial septal defect, and clinical separation of the two entities is not possible. Cardiac catheterization is the only method for establishing a precise diagnosis. Direct entry of an anomalous vein by the cardiac catheter may be diagnostic, especially if the vein is entered from the superior vena cava. In the right atrium, one often cannot be certain whether or not the catheter has traversed an atrial septal defect before entering the pulmonary vein. Selective angiography may confirm the diagnosis in some patients.

Treatment. A single anomalous pulmonary vein, usually from the right upper lobe entering the superior vena cava, is physiologically harmless and does not require treatment. More extensive malformations are usually operated upon in conjunction with closure of an atrial septal defect. Anomalous veins entering the right atrium can be corrected by insertion of a prosthetic patch so that the defect is closed and the pulmonary veins enter the left atrium. Pulmonary veins entering the superior vena cava in association with a sinus venosus defect can be corrected by the application of a prosthetic patch, preferably of pericardium, to shunt blood into the left atrium (Fig. 18-28). Anomalous veins entering the inferior vena cava are usually treated by division of the aberrant channel and direct implantation into the left atrium.

TOTAL ANOMALOUS DRAINAGE OF PULMONARY VEINS.

Pathologic Anatomy. Darling et al. have classified anatomically the types of total anomalous drainage of pulmonary veins according to location. Supracardiac drainage occurs in 55 percent of cases, paracardiac in 30 percent, and infracardiac in 12 percent. Multiple sites of entry are found in 3 percent.

With the supracardiac type of drainage, the most common point of entry of the anomalous veins is into a left vertical vein which in turn enters the left innominate vein. Rarely, the common anomalous venous trunk may drain directly into the posterior aspect of a right superior vena cava. With paracardiac drainage, the anomalous veins may enter the right atrium directly or, more rarely, may drain into the coronary sinus. With infracardiac drainage the pulmonary venous blood usually enters the inferior vena cava through a common channel traversing the diaphragm to connect with a hepatic vein or the portal vein.

Pathophysiology. Life is possible with total anomalous pulmonary venous drainage only as long as an atrial septal defect, often only a foramen ovale, is present. In addition, pulmonary venous hypertension often exists because of constriction of the point of entry of the anomalous pulmonary veins into the systemic venous system, which in turn results in pulmonary hypertension. With adequate communication between the anomalous pulmonary veins and the systemic venous circulation and a large atrial septal defect, patients may do surprisingly well for a period of time, the disability resembling that from a large atrial septal defect. This fortunate situation occurs in about 20

percent of patients. In the majority (80 percent) severe pulmonary hypertension is present; half these patients die in the first 3 months of life, and most within the first year. Cardiac failure develops with great rapidity, and cyanosis, varying with the degree of pulmonary blood flow, is frequent.

Clinical Manifestations. The dominant findings are a seriously ill infant with congestive failure, cyanosis, and rapidly progressive cardiac enlargement. In infants a murmur may not be audible. Hepatic enlargement is frequent.

The chest roentgenogram may be diagnostic when there is significant dilatation of the left vertebral and left innominate veins, creating a characteristic double contour on the x-ray termed a "snowman" appearance (Fig. 18-3).

Occasionally, with severe pulmonary venous obstruction, pulmonary congestion may be so severe in the infant as to suggest miliary tuberculosis. Diagnosis can be confirmed by cardiac catheterization. The hallmark of the physiologic disturbance in total anomalous pulmonary venous drainage is an almost identical oxygen content of the right atrium, pulmonary artery, and femoral artery because of complete mixing of oxygenated and unoxygenated blood in the right atrium before entering the left atrium through an atrial septal defect. Pulmonary hypertension is common. Also, the right atrial pressure is usually greater than the left atrial pressure.

Treatment. Infants with total anomalous pulmonary venous drainage may not survive more than the first few days or weeks of life without operation, so operation is often performed under emergency or desperate circumstances. Enlarging the atrial septal defect by the balloon septos-

Fig. 18-28. *A.* Sinus venosus type of atrial septal defect located near junction of superior vena cava with right atrium. Defect is partly obscured by crescentic lower margin. Anomalous pulmonary veins from right upper lobe enter superior vena cava near its juncture with right atrium. *B.* Prosthetic patch can be applied to encompass both atrial septal defect and ostia of anomalous pulmonary veins, avoiding undue constriction of point of entry of superior vena cava into right atrium. *C.* Final view of prosthetic patch which excludes anomalous veins and atrial septal defect from right atrium. (*Adapted from C. D. Benson et al., "Pediatric Surgery," vol. I, Year Book Medical Publishers, Inc., Chicago, 1962, p. 439.*)

A   *B*   *C*

tomy technique of Rashkind may provide valuable pallia-tion but unfortunately is not always successful. When surgical correction is done in infants, the deep hypother-mia–circulatory arrest technique, well developed by Barratt-Boyes and his colleagues, is the preferred ap-proach, for extracorporeal circulation is often not well tolerated in infants.

When the pulmonary veins drain into a left vertical vein, surgical correction includes creation of a long (2.5 to 3.0 cm) side-to-side anastomosis between the anomalous pulmonary veins and the left atrium (Fig. 18-29), followed by closure of the atrial septal defect and ligation of the left vertical vein. A similar procedure is followed with the unusual condition of drainage of the pulmonary veins into a single vein that courses beneath the diaphragm to join the portal venous system. If anomalous veins enter the right atrium or the coronary sinus, surgical reconstruction can be more simply performed (Fig. 18-30).

In infants, operative mortality has remained high, in the range of 30 to 50 percent. Most deaths are associated with pulmonary congestion and insufficiency. Beyond the first year of life, operative risk is small, approaching that of atrial septal defect if there is not a great increase in pulmo-nary vascular resistance. In 1975 Wukasch, Cooley, and associates reported experiences with 125 patients with an operative mortality in the first year of life remaining near 50 percent. By contrast, several groups have reported rea-sonable mortality rates in infants requiring operation be-fore the age of 6 months, often employing the technique of deep hypothermia and circulatory arrest. Kirklin stated in 1976 that he and his associates had not had a death in patients over 6 months of age since 1967.

OSTIUM PRIMUM DEFECT

Primum defects are relatively infrequent, occurring in 4 to 5 percent of patients with defects in the atrial septum. One of the first papers to emphasize clinical differentiation of ostium primum from secundum defects was published in 1956 by Blount and associates.

Ostium primum defects are often found in children with mongolism, occurring in 20 to 30 percent. Except for this unusual association, no etiologic factors are known.

A primum defect results from incomplete formation of the mitral and tricuspid valves and the atrial and ventricu-lar septa from the embryonic endocardial cushions. In embryonic life the endocardial cushions develop as dorsal and ventral partitions to separate the single atrium and ventricle of the embryo and join with the ventricular and atrial septa to form the normal four cardiac chambers. A synonym for ostium primum defects and the more severe associated malformation, atrioventricular canal, is *endo-cardial cushion defect,* partial (ostium primum) or complete (atrioventricular canal).

PATHOLOGIC ANATOMY. The two significant defects are a cleft in the anterior leaflet of the mitral valve and a low, crescent-shaped defect in the atrial septum (Fig. 18-31A). The sickle-like superior border of an ostium primum defect can be easily recognized on palpation at the time of surgi-cal correction. The cleft in the anterior leaflet of the mitral valve may be partial, extending for a short distance from

Fig. 18-29. *A.* Abnormal physiology with anomalous drainage of pulmonary veins into left superior vena cava. All pulmonary ve-nous blood flows through left innominate vein into large right superior vena cava and can enter systemic circulation only through atrial septal defect, usually foramen ovale. *B.* At opera-tion, wide opening is made between posteriorly located common pulmonary venous trunk and left atrium, after which opening in atrial septum is closed and left superior vena cava divided. *(Adapted from C. D. Benson et al., "Pediatric Surgery," vol. I, Year Book Medical Publishers, Inc., Chicago, 1962, p. 446.)*

the ventricular septum, or complete, separating the mitral valve leaflet into anterior and posterior halves.

Chordae tendineae are usually attached to the margins of the cleft and in some fortunate patients may prevent significant mitral insufficiency. In other patients, usually those with more severe malformations, abnormal chordae tendineae are present.

An associated partial or complete cleft in the tricuspid valve is also frequently seen. Conduction abnormalities from fibrosis or distortion of the conduction bundle, char-acteristically located along the posterior rim of the septal defect, are common.

Primum defects are anatomically distinguished from the more severe atrioventricular canal malformation by the

A

B

Fig. 18-30. *A.* Total anomalous drainage of pulmonary veins into coronary sinus. With this anomaly, atrial septal defect, usually foramen ovale, must be present to maintain life. It is possible to correct anomaly by excision of septum between foramen ovale and dilated coronary sinus. *B.* After excision of septum between foramen ovale and coronary sinus, resulting opening can be closed by suture of atrial septum, thus diverting all pulmonary venous blood, as well as blood draining from coronary sinus, into left atrium.

presence of distinct, separate mitral and tricuspid valve rings and an intact ventricular septum. With an atrioventricular canal malformation there is an additional defect in the ventricular septum, as well as extensive abnormalities of the mitral and tricuspid valve leaflets.

PATHOPHYSIOLOGY. The physiologic abnormalities are a left-to-right shunt combined with mitral insufficiency. When mitral insufficiency is minimal, the malformation is identical with that of atrial septal defect of the secundum type. When mitral insufficiency is severe, left ventricular failure and pulmonary hypertension appear early in life and produce a much more severe impairment of cardiac function than is seen in secundum-type septal defects. Increase in pulmonary vascular resistance with pulmonary hypertension may develop but is more frequent with atrioventricular canals.

CLINICAL MANIFESTATIONS. Symptoms. A variety of clinical profiles occur, varying with the degree of mitral insufficiency. When mitral insufficiency is minimal, the clinical picture is similar to that of atrial septal defect of the secundum type. Before the advent of precise diagnostic

techniques, ostium primum defects were often first recognized at operation. With significant mitral insufficiency, cardiac failure with pulmonary congestion, dyspnea, recurrent bouts of pneumonia, and retardation of growth may be prominent in the first years of life.

Physical Examination. On physical examination moderate cardiac enlargement is often found, with a thrill near the apex. A harsh apical systolic murmur from mitral insufficiency is usually present and should arouse suspicion of an ostium primum defect. An additional systolic murmur may be heard along the left sternal border. The intensity of the pulmonic second sound is often increased. With cardiac failure, signs of pulmonary congestion and hepatic enlargement are found. Growth is frequently retarded.

LABORATORY FINDINGS. The chest roentgenogram usually shows moderate cardiac enlargement, involving both the right and the left ventricle. Increased pulmonary vascularity is also common. The most useful diagnostic guide is provided by the electrocardiogram, which shows both right and left ventricular hypertrophy, with a left axis deviation. In the vectorcardiogram the inscription in the

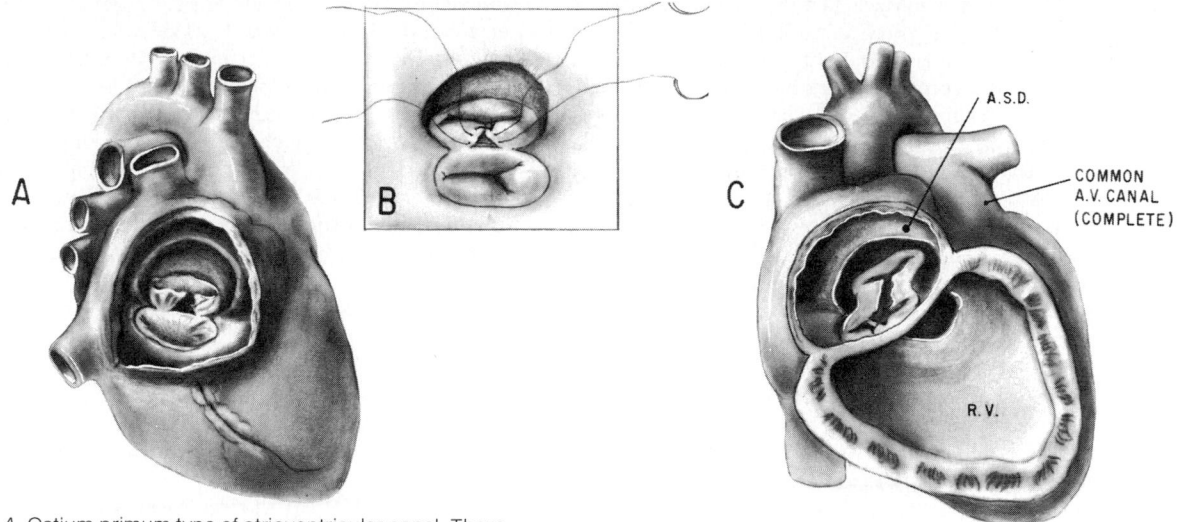

Fig. 18-31. *A.* Ostium primum type of atrioventricular canal. There is a cleft in anterior mitral leaflet, but ventricular septum is intact. *B.* Method of repair of cleft valve with interrupted sutures to produce competent mitral valve. Classic crescent-shaped atrial septal defect superior to valve ring is shown. *C.* Appearance of complete atrioventricular canal, showing complete division of mitral and tricuspid valves in association with atrial septal defect and ventricular septal defect. (*Adapted from D. C. McGoon et al., Am J Cardiol, 6:598, 1960.*)

frontal plane is in a counterclockwise loop, a finding almost pathognomonic of ostium primum defect. Conduction defects with prolongation of the P-R interval are frequent. These electrocardiographic abnormalities are due primarily to the conduction defect and not to the associated left ventricular hypertrophy.

On cardiac catheterization a left-to-right shunt is found at the atrial level; frequently the catheter will enter the left atrium or left ventricle. The pulmonary blood flow is frequently two to three times greater than systemic flow. Mitral insufficiency, suggested by prominent V waves in the left atrial pressure tracing, is best confirmed by injection of contrast media into the left ventricle.

DIAGNOSIS. The diagnosis usually can be made with reasonable certainty from the clinical picture of a child with cardiac enlargement, a left-to-right shunt with an apical systolic murmur, and an electrocardiogram showing left axis deviation with a frontal-plane counterclockwise loop in the vectorcardiogram. Differential diagnosis should exclude ventricular septal defect and atrial septal defect of the secundum type.

TREATMENT. In most patients operative correction of the defect should be performed between the ages of four and six years. Rarely, an adult is seen in the third or fourth decade with a history of little disability from a primum defect, but such patients are those in whom mitral insufficiency has been minimal and the clinical course has been more similar to the benign secundum-type defect. In most patients the combination of a left-to-right shunt with mitral insufficiency results in progressive cardiac enlargement and failure in childhood.

Operative Technique. Operation is performed with extra-

corporeal circulation, using a median sternotomy incision. The three principal objectives are correction of the mitral insufficiency, closure of the septal defect, and avoidance of the production of heart block from injury to the conduction bundle along the posterior margin of the septal defect. Incomplete correction of the mitral insufficiency can be disastrous. Closure of the septal defect with residual severe mitral insufficiency may produce severe or fatal pulmonary edema, because decompression of the left atrium into the right atrium has been abolished by closure of the defect.

Usually, operation is performed with intermittent aortic occlusion for 10 to 15 minutes at 30°C, alternating with periods of aortic unclamping and cardiac contraction. Appropriate measures are taken to avoid an air embolism. The right atrium is widely opened, and the septal defect, cleft in the mitral valve, associated cleft in the tricuspid valve, and ventricular septum are carefully examined. Initially the cleft in the mitral valve is closed with interrupted sutures placed from the ventricular septum out to the free margin of the mitral orifice (Fig. 18-31*B*), the points of insertion of the chordae tendineae being carefully noted. Usually a left ventricular vent is inserted through the apex of the left ventricle to avoid production of air embolism once the mitral valve has been rendered competent by closure of the cleft. After repair of the cleft mitral valve, the septal defect is repaired with a patch of pericardium inserted with interrupted sutures. Along the posterior rim near the conduction bundle the sutures are inserted superficially to the left of the rim of the defect along the annulus of the mitral valve, the electrocardiogram being checked after the sutures are inserted to avoid producing a conduction injury. A defect in the tricuspid valve is frequent but usually is not amenable to repair by direct suture. Air should be completely evacuated from the left atrium as closure of the septal defect is completed.

Postoperative Course. If adequate correction of the mitral insufficiency is accomplished and production of heart block avoided, postoperative recovery is usually uneventful and similar to that for closure of other septal defects. A conduction injury is a grave complication, but rare. It should be treated at operation by the temporary insertion of a pacemaker. If a complete heart block should persist, a permanent pacemaker should be inserted. Some patients have a residual systolic murmur, and some of these will be found on subsequent study to have significant mitral regurgitation. A small percentage of such patients require mitral valve replacement in the next 5 to 10 years. The functional results in the majority of patients, however, are satisfactory. At the Mayo Clinic, McGoon and associates in 1973 reported long-term results in 232 patients, the majority of whom had maintained an excellent result following operation. The operative mortality is less than 5 percent. At New York University since 1963, there have been no deaths or complete heart blocks following operation.

In early experiences with surgical repair, an unusual syndrome of severe hemolytic anemia was recognized in a small percentage of patients following repair of an ostium primum defect. This striking clinical picture resulted from residual mitral insufficiency accidentally oriented so that the regurgitant jet of blood struck the prosthetic patch closing the septal defect and intermittently dislodged fibrin from the surface of the patch with each systolic jet. Although rare, such a syndrome should be recognized, for reoperation and closure of the residual insufficiency is curative.

PERSISTENT ATRIOVENTRICULAR CANAL

This malformation is a more extensive error in development of the endocardial cushions, consisting of a large common defect involving both the atrial and ventricular septa, and extensive defects in the mitral and tricuspid valves (Fig. 18-31C). These are often connected across the incomplete septa to form large common valve leaflets in the anterior and posterior portions of the heart. The great variation in valve deformities in these patients was well described by Rastelli et al. in an analysis of 30 postmortem specimens. The physiologic defect is a left-to-right shunt at both the atrial and ventricular levels, resulting in cardiac failure in early life as well as pulmonary vascular obstruction and pulmonary hypertension. The severity of the malformation depends upon the extent of the mitral insufficiency and the size of the ventricular septal defect. In infants with severe deformities the course is a severe one, with death in the first few months of life, while patients with less severe lesions do reasonably well for the first few years of life.

An atrioventricular canal, rather than an ostium primum defect, may be suspected from the malignant clinical course of severe cardiac failure and cardiac enlargement in the first one or two years of life. Diagnosis is established principally by cardiac catheterization and angiography, demonstrating both a ventricular septal defect and mitral insufficiency.

Several years ago results of operative correction were very poor, the mortality exceeding 75 percent in infants. Prosthetic valves were employed in a few infants but with similarly unimpressive results. Great advances have been made in surgical therapy in recent years, due principally to the techniques of surgical correction developed by Rastelli et al. and McGoon, which have reduced mortality to a range of 10 to 15 percent in patients over 2 years of age.

Similar results have been reported by Mills in a smaller series. The original publication should be consulted for details of operative techniques. The essential steps include insertion of a large prosthetic patch, which is attached to the underlying ventricular septum, following which the valve is reconstructed and attached to the patch at an appropriate level, with subsequent closure of the atrial septal defect.

In 1976 Kirklin stated that the policy of his department for a long time had been that of primary repair of the complete atrioventricular canal at whatever age operation was required and elective repair in all patients by age 2. Results in a small series of infants have been quite good since 1974, in striking contrast to experiences before that time.

Ventricular Septal Defect

HISTORICAL DATA. A description by Roger in 1879 of two patients with ventricular septal defect led to the eponymic designation *Roger's disease* and emphasized the asymptomatic nature of the disease when the ventricular septal defect is small. Further contributions to clinical characterization of the syndrome were made by Abbott in 1932, by Taussig in 1947, and later by Selzer and by Wood. Surgical closure became possible with the development of the pump-oxygenator in 1955. In recent years the frequency of spontaneous closure of ventricular septal defects has been well delineated. It is now clear that spontaneous closure of septal defects, once thought to be a rare phenomenon, may occur in the first few years of life in a significant percentage of patients, so patients with few symptoms and without pulmonary hypertension may be safely observed for 3 to 4 years for signs of spontaneous closure.

INCIDENCE AND ETIOLOGY. There are no known significant etiologic factors, although ventricular septal defect is a common form of congenital heart disease, constituting 20 to 30 percent of all cases in various cardiac clinics.

PATHOLOGIC ANATOMY. Five types of ventricular septal defect have been recognized, depending upon the location in the ventricular septum: membranous septum defect; defect anterior to the crista supraventricularis near the pulmonic valve; posterior ventricular septum defect; low muscular defect; and left ventricular–right atrial defect. Defects in the membranous septum are by far the most frequent (85 to 90 percent of patients), the other types being seen only infrequently.

Defects in the membranous septum (Fig. 18-32, type B) are located posterior to the crista supraventricularis. With small defects a rim exists superiorly, while large defects are extremely close to the base of the septal leaflet of the tricuspid valve on the right and the mitral valve on the left. The bundle of His, of critical importance to the surgeon, is located at the posterior and superior rim of the defect, where it bifurcates into the right and left conduction bundles. The septal defects are located beneath the right aortic cusp or beneath the junction of the right aortic and septal cusps. Often these cusps are easily visible through the defect and must be protected from injury during surgical repair. The degree of dextroposition of the aorta varies widely. With some defects the aortic valve is not visible at all. At the other extreme are those defects in which the aorta partly arises from the right ventricle. This type is common with tetralogy of Fallot.

Anterior ventricular septal defects (Fig. 18-32, type A) occur anterior to the crista supraventricularis near the pulmonic valve. Surgical closure is simple because the defect is a safe distance from the conduction bundle. Posterior ventricular septal defects (Fig. 18-32, type C) are posterior to the papillary muscle of the conus and beneath the tricuspid valve. Often the rim is partly or completely muscular. Exposure is awkward but can be accomplished with appropriate retraction. Muscular ventricular septal defects (Fig. 18-32, type D) are located inferiorly in the ventricular septum and are often multiple. In the most extreme form, the "Swiss cheese" type of septum, there are multiple tiny serpentine communications which make complete surgical closure difficult or perhaps impossible. Left ventricular–right atrial defects are the rarest of all, consisting of a communication between the left ventricle and the right atrium through the membranous septum superior to the annulus of the tricuspid valve. Such defects are small but are associated with a large shunt because of the great difference in pressure between the left ventricle and right atrium. Once these defects are recognized, closure by direct suture is simple.

The size of ventricular septal defects varies from as small as 0.3 cm to greater than 3 cm. A diameter of 0.8 to 1 cm is a convenient one for separating "small" and "large" septal defects, for those smaller than 1 cm are often associated with a pulmonary blood flow less than twice systemic blood flow and few cardiac abnormalities. "Small" defects are seen in about 25 percent of patients. Defects larger than 1 cm, corresponding to about one-half the diameter of the aortic valve orifice, are regularly associated with more severe physiologic disturbances.

Histologic changes in the pulmonary vasculature are an important part of the pathologic anatomy, for these are related to the evolution of pulmonary hypertension. Young children with pulmonary hypertension have prominent smooth muscle in the media of the pulmonary arterioles, resembling that found in the pulmonary vasculature during fetal life. In subsequent years, with continued pulmonary hypertension, proliferative changes appear in the intima, becoming more prominent in late childhood and early adult life. The intimal proliferative changes apparently represent a permanent increase in pulmonary vascular resistance, with irreversible pulmonary hypertension. Though the pathogenesis of pulmonary hypertension has been studied intensely, the sporadic appearance and erratic course among different patients with similar defects remains a mystery.

Associated anomalies with ventricular defects are common. These include patent ductus arteriosus, coarctation of the aorta, atrial septal defect, mild infundibular stenosis of the right ventricle, and aortic insufficiency from prolapse

Fig. 18-32. Common types of ventricular septal defect. Most common is type B, with defect lying just proximal to crista supraventricularis. Type A defects are located immediately proximal to pulmonic valve. Type C defects are located beneath septal leaflet of tricuspid valve. Type D defects are in muscular part of ventricular septum and are often multiple. (*Adapted from J. W. Kirklin et al., J Thorac Surg, 33:45, 1957.*)

of an aortic valve cusp into the ventricular septal defect. Recognition of the additional anomalies is an obviously important part of preoperative diagnosis and planning prior to surgical correction.

PATHOPHYSIOLOGY. Since normally the systolic left ventricular pressure is about four times greater than the systolic right ventricular pressure, a ventricular septal defect results in a left-to-right shunt of blood from the left ventricle into the pulmonary circulation, producing a pulmonary blood flow greater than systemic blood flow. The size of the left-to-right shunt varies with both the size of the defect and the pulmonary vascular resistance. With a septal defect less than 1 cm in diameter, the pulmonary blood flow may be only about $1\frac{1}{2}$ times systemic blood flow, and few physiologic changes result. With septal defects greater than 1 cm in diameter and a pulmonary blood flow more than twice systemic flow, a strain on cardiac function becomes obvious. With huge septal defects, pulmonary blood flow may be four to five times greater than systemic flow, producing severe pulmonary congestion and heart failure.

The two major changes from a ventricular septal defect are cardiac failure and pulmonary hypertension. In infancy severe cardiac failure develops if a large defect is present. This may be fatal in some unless surgical therapy, either closure of the defect or banding of the pulmonary artery, is performed. Surgical closure of ventricular septal defects in severely symptomatic infants has been safely accomplished in recent years, using the technique of deep hypothermia and partial or complete circulatory arrest. A considerable experience with this technique has been reported by Barratt-Boyes and also by Kirklin, clearly indicating that in the majority of patients such defects may be safely closed in the first 1 to 2 years of life, rather than banding the pulmonary artery. After the first year of life, chronic pulmonary congestion may persist with large defects, resulting in recurrent pulmonary infections and limitation of growth and development. Death from congestive heart failure is unusual in children after the first year of life. In adults, however, congestive heart failure is frequent.

Pulmonary hypertension from progressive sclerosis of the pulmonary vascular bed is the other major pathologic change. As mentioned earlier, the principal histologic changes are in the pulmonary arterioles, with hypertrophy of the smooth muscle of the media and proliferation of the intima. These evolve slowly during childhood, becoming more prominent in the late teens and early adult life. Rarely, such changes may progress to an "irreversible" degree in the first few years of life. The cause of this great variability is unknown.

As pulmonary vascular resistance increases to approach systemic vascular resistance, definite changes in blood flow result, for right-to-left shunting through the defect appears in association with the predominant left-to-right shunt. This right-to-left shunt produces unsaturation of the peripheral arterial blood. When the pulmonary vascular resistance and the systemic vascular resistance are nearly equal, a *balanced shunt* results. Ultimately, when pulmonary vascular resistance has risen to exceed systemic vascular resistance, the right-to-left shunt is predominant, resulting in cyanosis, clubbing, and polycythemia. This advanced inoperable disease, formerly termed the Eisenmenger syndrome, is now recognized as simply the end stage of progressive pulmonary hypertension from a large left-to-right shunt. It usually results from a ventricular septal defect but can also occur from a neglected patent ductus arteriosus, atrial septal defect, or other malformations. With severe pulmonary hypertension, death usually occurs at about forty years of age from cardiac failure, respiratory infection, or hemoptysis. The natural course of disease in these patients has been well documented by Wood.

An increased susceptibility to bacterial endocarditis has been long recognized with ventricular defects and is the only known physiologic handicap from a small one. The susceptibility results from the jet of blood through the defect striking the right ventricular wall; bacterial fungations form here. The estimated frequency of the disease varies widely, from 15 to 30 percent, but the risk emphasizes the importance of prophylactic chemotherapy.

Patients with mild infundibular stenosis and a ventricular septal defect are in the midportion of the spectrum of malformations extending from ventricular septal defect at one end to tetralogy of Fallot at the other. The clinical picture varies with severity of the infundibular stenosis. As long as the infundibular stenosis is mild, pulmonary blood flow exceeds systemic blood flow, and the patient is acyanotic. However, if infundibular stenosis is more severe, with a systemic blood flow greater than pulmonary blood flow, cyanosis develops. Cases in this intermediate zone are often termed *acyanotic* tetralogies of Fallot.

The ultimate life expectancy of patients with a ventricular septal defect is unknown, but it appears that average life expectancy of patients with a pulmonary blood flow more than twice the systemic blood flow is near forty years of age. Death is from pulmonary hypertension, cardiac failure, or endocarditis.

CLINICAL MANIFESTATIONS. Symptoms. Patients with a small ventricular septal defect (0.3 to 0.8 cm in diameter) are often asymptomatic and enjoy unrestricted physical activity. Those with larger defects are usually symptomatic. Dyspnea on exertion with easy fatigability is most common, often accompanied by frequent pulmonary infections. Severe cardiac failure is usually seen only in infants or in adults, although chronic pulmonary congestion may occur throughout early childhood. Hemoptysis occurs only in older children or adults with severe pulmonary hypertension. In these unfortunate patients it is a frequent cause of death in the third and fourth decades.

Physical Findings. A loud, harsh, pansystolic murmur is typically present along the left sternal border in the third and fourth intercostal spaces. Frequently a thrill is palpable. The pulmonic second sound varies with pulmonary vascular resistance and may even be palpable when pulmonary vascular resistance is markedly elevated. Intensity of the systolic murmur also varies with the pulmonary vascular resistance, diminishing in many patients as the pulmonary vascular resistance increases. In some patients there is a paradoxic variation between signs and symptoms: pronounced physical findings with a loud murmur and thrill in an asymptomatic child, but a murmur of less intensity without a thrill with severe pulmonary hypertension.

Retardation of growth may be obvious, accompanied by rales from chronic pulmonary congestion and hepatic enlargement. Some cardiac enlargement is regularly present. When severe, it may produce a visible deformity of the left costal cartilages. Basal diastolic murmurs are infrequent but can originate from two sources: A murmur of aortic insufficiency can develop from prolapse of an aortic cusp into the underlying ventricular septal defect. Alternately, a murmur resulting from pulmonic insufficiency may appear with far advanced pulmonary hypertension.

LABORATORY FINDINGS. The chest roentgenogram with a small ventricular septal defect is usually normal. With larger defects, enlargement of both ventricles becomes visible, especially as pulmonary vascular resistance increases. When the pulmonary blood flow is significantly increased, there is visible enlargement of the pulmonary artery and its tributaries, pulmonary congestion, and enlargement of the left atrium.

The electrocardiogram varies with both the pulmonary blood flow and the pulmonary vascular resistance. With a small defect it is normal. A large pulmonary blood flow produces left ventricular hypertrophy, while an increase in pulmonary vascular resistance induces right ventricular hypertrophy. Often hypertrophy of both ventricles is evident, and the axis of the electrocardiogram varies with the relative degree of ventricular hypertrophy. Predominant right ventricular hypertrophy and a right axis deviation appear with severe pulmonary hypertension.

Cardiac catheterization confirms the diagnosis and assesses the extent of the left-to-right shunt and the pulmonary vascular resistance. A rise in oxygen saturation of more than 1 vol % between the right atrium and the right ventricle establishes the diagnosis, and calculation of the ratio between the pulmonary blood flow and the systemic blood flow will indicate both the size of the shunt and the pulmonary vascular resistance. At times the catheter may actually traverse the septal defect. Selective angiography, usually by injection of dye directly into the left ventricle from a catheter advanced from the aorta across the aortic valve, can opacify the defect.

DIAGNOSIS. The diagnosis is suggested by the loud systolic murmur along the left sternal border, often with a thrill. Similar physical findings may be present with aortic stenosis in infancy, infundibular pulmonic stenosis, or an ostium primum defect. An atrial septal defect usually has a softer systolic murmur near the base of the heart. Confirmation of the diagnosis requires cardiac catheterization, although the changes in the chest roentgenogram and electrocardiogram are helpful.

TREATMENT. Indications for Operation. Operation should be performed in the first 1 to 2 years of life for infants with either severe congestive failure or an increase in pulmonary vascular resistance. There are good data to indicate that an increase in pulmonary vascular resistance will regress if surgical correction is performed before 2 years of age, but there may be irreversible injury to the pulmonary vascular bed if operation is postponed beyond 2 years.

If symptoms are not disabling and pulmonary vascular resistance is not increased, the preferred time for operation is between 4 and 6 years of age. Often a period of observation is indicated to determine whether the defect will close spontaneously. Once observation has demonstrated that the defect is a persistent one, operation is usually done if the pulmonary blood flow is more than one and one-half to two times greater than normal. With smaller defects, operation is usually not recommended unless there is a demonstrated susceptibility to endocarditis, the only known hazard of a small ventricular septal defect.

In the unfortunate patients with marked elevation of pulmonary vascular resistance, the hazard of operation is increased and the benefit decreased. Criteria of inoperability vary among different institutions, but generally patients with a pulmonary vascular resistance greater than one-half the systemic resistance have a high operative mortality and little benefit from operation. With the increasing awareness of the problem and the ready availability of excellent diagnostic facilities, such unfortunate children are becoming increasingly rare, as most cases are detected and the patients successfully operated on within the first few years of life.

Technique of Operation. The operation is performed through a median sternotomy with extracorporeal circulation. If a patent ductus arteriosus, a commonly associated defect in infants, has been found by preoperative catheterization and angiography, this must be closed at the start of bypass before the ventricle is opened.

In selecting the site of ventriculotomy, the most important consideration is to avoid division of any underlying significant coronary arteries for anomalous coronary arteries are frequent. The most common anomaly is the origin of the left anterior descending from the right coronary artery, division of which is often fatal. With these considerations, a transverse, longitudinal, or oblique ventriculotomy can be made. If the coronary anatomy is satisfactory, the author prefers a short transverse incision. If a longitudinal ventriculotomy is performed, it should be in the infundibular part of the right ventricle and near the anterior descending coronary.

An alternate approach is closure of the ventricular septal defect through the right atrium. This is strongly indicated when pulmonary vascular resistance is significantly increased, to avoid any transitory injury to the right ventricle. In some institutions this technique is almost routinely employed, although it is more awkward than operation through a ventriculotomy.

A left ventricular vent is routinely used to aspirate blood from the operative field and facilitate removal of intracardiac air. A variety of surgical techniques have been employed successfully. The author's preference is for intermittent cardiac ischemia, intermittently occluding the aorta 10 to 15 minutes at a temperature of 30°C. This has the advantage of having the heart intermittently contract, with monitoring of the electrocardiogram to protect against heart block. Excellent results have been obtained by several groups with techniques of hypothermia and prolonged cardiac arrest, carefully placing the sutures to the right of the ventricular septum posteriorly to avoid heart block. In the author's personal experience there have been no complete heart blocks in the past decade.

Once the septal defect, usually located in the membranous septum posterior to the crista supraventricularis, has been identified, an oval patch of knitted Dacron is inserted with mattress sutures posteriorly and a continuous suture anteriorly, preferably polypropylene (Prolene) (Fig. 18-33).

Posteriorly, the sutures are inserted through the base of the septal leaflet of the tricuspid valve to the right of the posterior margin of the defect, avoiding the posterior superior angle where the conduction bundle is located. A useful surgical guide for avoiding the conduction bundle, described by Barratt-Boyes, is to identify the fibrous trigone located at the bottom of the noncoronary aortic sinus, inspecting this area through the ventricular septal defect with a dry, still operative field. The conduction bundle passes through this fibrous trigone and then along the area where the membranous ventricular septum joins the muscular septum posteriorly. Projecting an imaginary line between the fibrous trigone and the papillary muscle of the conus and subsequently inserting sutures to the right of this imaginary line avoids injury to the conduction bundle. This can be confirmed by observing the electrocardiogram after the posterior sutures are inserted but before the prosthetic patch is tied in position. The anterior portion of the closure can be simply done with a continuous suture. After the patch is inserted, adequacy of closure, as well as the presence of additional defects, can be checked by temporarily occluding the aorta, aspirating air through the left ventricular vent, and then forcefully injecting saline solution retrograde through the left ventricular vent into the left ventricle to distend the ventricular septum. This technique, used for several years, has been a valuable adjunct and has identified additional defects in several patients.

Subsequently, after closing the ventriculotomy and stopping the bypass, adequacy of closure can be confirmed by

Fig. 18-33. *A.* Ventricular septal defect exposed through longitudinal ventriculotomy. Cusps of aortic valve are clearly visible through large defect. Closure is carried out with prosthetic patch of Teflon felt. First sutures are inserted in posterosuperior margin where conduction bundle is located. Often sutures are placed to right of margin of defect, through base of septal leaflet of tricuspid valve. Heart is beating while sutures are inserted, in order to observe conduction disturbances on electrocardiogram. *B.* Subsequent sutures around margins of defect may be interrupted or continuous sutures. In aortic valve area, care is taken to insert sutures directly into aortic annulus, avoiding injury to valve cusps. *C.* Final position of prosthetic patch.

demonstrating a similar oxygen content of blood samples withdrawn simultaneously from the right atrium and the pulmonary artery.

The combination of ventricular septal defect with aortic insufficiency from prolapse of an aortic valve cusp is fortunately rare. The lesion is often a progressive one due to continued herniation of an aortic valve cusp, usually the right coronary cusp, into the underlying ventricular septal defect. Surgical correction can usually be done without insertion of a prosthetic aortic valve, even though some aortic insufficiency remains. A detailed report of the experience of the author, Bahnson, and Weldon with this condition was published in 1973 (Fig. 18-34). In the subsequent years, continued experience has been satisfactory.

Postoperative Course. A temporary pacemaker wire is routinely left in the ventricle before the thoracotomy incision is closed. If bradycardia appears, with a rate lower than 70 to 80 per minute, pacing is done for 1 to 2 days, as necessary. Transitory conduction disturbances often subside within 24 to 48 hours. A report years ago by Lillehei et al. indicated the grim prognosis with complete heart block. If a complete heart block persists for as long as 3 weeks after operation, a permanent pacemaker should be inserted before the patient is discharged from the hospital,

for the risk of sudden death is great even though the patient is asymptomatic.

Digitalis is usually given after operation, as some degree of right ventricular failure is common, especially if significant pulmonary hypertension was present. In most patients convalescence is uneventful.

The risk of operation increases if pulmonary vascular resistance is increased, but with earlier diagnosis and treatment such complicated problems are fortunately becoming rare. With normal pulmonary vascular resistance, postoperative mortalities as low as 1 to 2 percent have been reported. Similar results have been obtained at New York University. However, when the pulmonary vascular resistance is significantly elevated, the risk of operation rises, approaching 15 to 30 percent if pulmonary vascular resistance is as much as one-half systemic resistance.

Following recovery from operation, patients without an increase in pulmonary vascular resistance have a dramatic regression of all signs of cardiac disease. Heart size and the vascularity of the lung fields both return to normal. A right bundle branch block usually persists on the electrocardiogram as a consequence of insertion of sutures to the right of the margin of the septal defect. Life expectancy is probably that of a normal person. In patients with increased pulmonary vascular resistance, there may be regression in some. In general, the pulmonary vascular resistance decreases in about one-third of the patients, remains stationary in about one-third, and actually increases in the remainder, probably representing an inherent disease in the pulmonary vasculature separate from that due to the previous left-to-right shunt.

Patent Ductus Arteriosus

HISTORICAL DATA. Gibson, in Edinburgh, first reported in 1900 the classic clinical findings of a patent ductus arteriosus, but it was not until 1937 that Strieder first attempted ligation of the ductus in a patient with bacterial endocarditis. This patient died on the fourth postoperative day, but the following year Gross successfully ligated the patent ductus of a seven-year-old girl.

INCIDENCE AND ETIOLOGY. Patent ductus arteriosus is one of the most common forms of congenital heart disease, occurring once in about every 4,000 births and constituting about 15 percent of all cases of congenital heart disease. For unknown reasons it is two to three times more frequent in females than in males.

The patent ductus arteriosus, which develops as an embryologic remnant of the sixth left aortic arch, is an important normal fetal pathway connecting the pulmonary artery at its bifurcation to the aorta just beyond the origin of the left subclavian artery. Through this channel in embryonic life blood bypasses the collapsed lungs, flowing directly from the pulmonary artery into the aorta. With the expansion of the lungs at birth, the ductus normally closes within a few days, becoming fibrotic ligamentum arteriosum. The physiologic stimuli responsible for closure of the ductus have been studied in detail. Apparently changes in oxygen tension of the arterial blood exert a

D. A plicating suture draws up the excess to the commissural margin. No tissue is excised.

E. The leaflet is now normally proportioned and accurately suspended.

A

Fig. 18-34. *A*. Diagram of concept of one method of repair of the prolapsed valve cusp, developed by Weldon at Washington University in St. Louis. *B*. Operative view of the prolapsed aortic cusp through a right ventriculotomy, showing the cusp prolapsing into the ventricular septal defect. Partial occlusion of the ventricular septal defect by the prolapsing cusp is one reason that the left-to-right shunt is not large. *C*. Pre- and postoperative aortograms showing massive aortic insufficiency before operation and no insufficiency whatever several months later.

B

C

profound stimulus on the closure. The most important cause of closure, however, is probably related to the distinctive histologic structure of the wall of the ductus, which is different from that of either the pulmonary artery or the aorta. As the ductus closes, the wall of the ductus contracts, the internal elastic membrane fragments, and smooth muscle projects into the lumen as progressive fibrosis obliterates the patent channel.

If rubella occurs during the first trimester of pregnancy, a well-recognized syndrome of congenital defects can occur, including mental retardation, cataracts, and a patent ductus. For the majority of patients, however, the cause of persistent patency is unknown.

PATHOLOGIC ANATOMY. The diameter of a ductus ranges from as small as 2 to 3 mm to greater than 1 cm. Usually it is 5 to 7 mm. The length is usually slightly greater than the width, although in some cases the ductus is unusually short, creating some technical hazard at the time of surgical correction (Fig. 18-35).

Associated anomalies occur in approximately 15 percent of cases; the most common are ventricular septal defect and coarctation of the aorta.

PATHOPHYSIOLOGY. Depending upon the diameter of the ductus, a varying amount of blood is shunted from the aorta to the pulmonary artery, constituting a left-to-right shunt. In a large ductus, the shunt may constitute 50 to 70 percent of the output from the left ventricle, with resulting decrease of blood flow to other tissues and retardation of development. With such large shunts, the pulmonary blood flow may reach levels as high as 10 to 15 liters/minute. The symptomatology is directly proportional to the size of the shunt.

A large patent ductus in infants may result in serious or even lethal heart failure. However, after the age of two years heart failure is rare until adult life, although symptoms of limited cardiac reserve may occur.

In infancy the high pulmonary vascular resistance of fetal life subsides gradually in the first 1 to 2 years after birth. During this time only a systolic murmur may be audible. In some infants the increased pulmonary blood flow from the ductus causes the pulmonary vascular resistance to remain elevated and even increase, with resulting pulmonary hypertension. Usually the pulmonary vascular resistance will decrease to normal levels following surgical division of the ductus, but in older patients only a partial regression toward normal levels may occur. With a long-neglected patent ductus pulmonary resistance may, rarely, increase to exceed systemic vascular resistance, resulting in a "reversed" ductus, with blood flowing from the pulmonary artery to the descending thoracic aorta to produce cyanosis in the lower half of the body. Fortunately this is now almost unknown, for diagnosis and treatment are carried out at an early age.

An unusual feature of a patent ductus is susceptibility to development of bacterial endocarditis from viridans streptococci. Although this is most common in the second or third decade, it may occur rarely in children. It has been estimated that in untreated cases such an infection would ultimately develop in 20 to 25 percent of patients. The localization of the infection apparently is related to turbulent blood flow where blood forcefully ejected from the aorta through the ductus strikes the wall of the pulmonary artery. The fungations of bacterial endocarditis usually begin in this location, with septicemia initially limited to the lungs until systemic spread occurs. Fortunately such infections can usually be promptly controlled with antibiotic therapy.

With the dual tendency to develop either heart failure or bacterial endocarditis, it has been estimated that the life expectancy of a seventeen-year-old patient with a patent ductus is approximately one-half that of a normal individual.

CLINICAL MANIFESTATIONS. Symptoms. In infants a large patent ductus may cause serious heart failure, but many older children are asymptomatic. When symptoms are present, the most common are palpitations, fatigue, and dyspnea. More definite symptoms of congestive heart failure are usually seen only in adult patients. In the female these often appear during the first pregnancy. The author has successfully operated on one patient over sixty years of age who first developed signs of congestive failure after age sixty. Fortunately, though advanced cardiac failure was present, full recovery ensued after closure of the ductus.

Physical Examination. The hallmark of a patent ductus is the continuous murmur. This murmur is one of the most distinctive signs in clinical medicine, and usually a patent ductus can be diagnosed with confidence simply on this basis. Because of the continuous quality of the murmur it is often described as a "machinery" murmur. It is a

Fig. 18-35. Patent ductus arteriosus as regularly found just distal to left subclavian artery between aorta and pulmonary artery. It is encircled by recurrent laryngeal nerve, a useful surgical landmark in isolating patent ductus in mediastinal tissues. (*Adapted from R. E. Gross, "The Surgery of Infancy and Childhood," W. B. Saunders Company, Philadelphia, 1953, p. 807.*)

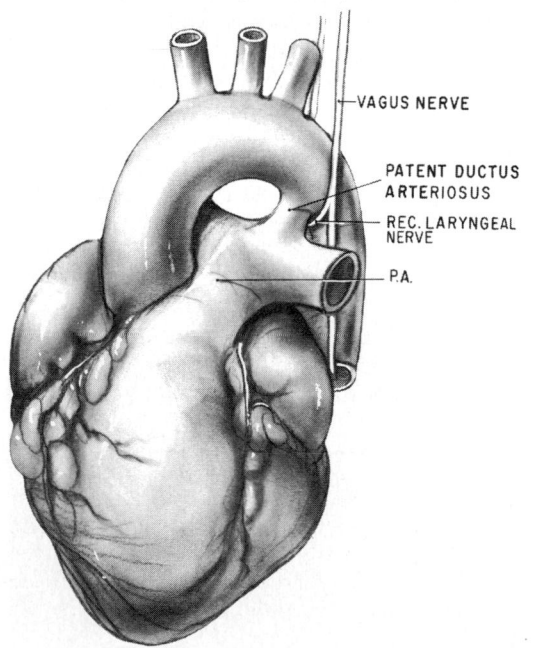

VAGUS NERVE

PATENT DUCTUS ARTERIOSUS

REC. LARYNGEAL NERVE

P.A.

harsh, rasping sound, accentuated in systole and diminishing in diastole. It is best heard in the second left intercostal space but is normally widely transmitted over the chest and into the neck. In many patients the murmur is so loud that it is associated with a palpable thrill. Often in infants either no murmur or only a systolic murmur can be heard until the age of one or two years, after which a continuous murmur may be detected for the first time. The absence of the diastolic component of the murmur during infancy is due to persistent elevation of the pulmonary vascular resistance, which limits flow of blood through the ductus during diastole.

A wide pulse pressure is usually found with a large ductus, resulting from a decrease in diastolic pressure. In the extremely large ductus the diastolic pressure may approach very low levels and be associated with peripheral vascular findings similar to those of severe aortic insufficiency.

Cyanosis is never present with an uncomplicated patent ductus. The presence of cyanosis indicates either an associated cardiac anomaly, such as tetralogy of Fallot, or a marked increase in pulmonary vascular resistance, either from progressive sclerosis of the pulmonary arteriolar bed or from congestive heart failure. The severity of the arterial hypoxia which can result from heart failure in infants often has not been recognized. Arterial oxygen saturations as low as 75% may occur with the severe pulmonary congestion of heart failure.

LABORATORY FINDINGS. With a small patent ductus the chest roentgenogram may be normal. With a larger ductus the pulmonary conus is prominent, the left ventricle is enlarged, and the pulmonary vascular markings are increased, all indicating a large left-to-right shunt. On fluoroscopy a "hilar dance" may be observed. The electrocardiogram is often normal with a small ductus but will show left ventricular hypertrophy with a larger one. Cardiac catheterization can readily localize the left-to-right shunt to the pulmonary artery and differentiate the condition from a ventricular septal defect or an atrial septal defect. Often with appropriate manipulation the cardiac catheter can be passed through the patent ductus, visually confirming the diagnosis. Aortography is the most definitive diagnostic measure, visually demonstrating the flow of dye from the aorta through the ductus into the pulmonary arteries (Fig. 18-36). It is of particular value with severe pulmonary hypertension, when only a systolic murmur may be audible.

DIAGNOSIS. In most patients the diagnosis can be made with confidence from the clinical findings combined with the chest roentgenogram and the electrocardiogram. Cardiac catheterization with aortography should then be done both for confirmation and for detection of additional anomalies.

There are several rare conditions which may produce a continuous murmur simulating a patent ductus arteriosus and requiring cardiac catheterization and angiography for differentiation from a patent ductus. These include an aortic-pulmonary window, a ventricular septal defect with a prolapsed cusp causing aortic insufficiency, a ruptured aneurysm of the sinus of Valsalva, and a coronary arterio-

Fig. 18-36. Aortogram performed by injection of dye into aorta demonstrates patent ductus arteriosus, as indicated by arrows, with opacification of pulmonary artery. (*Courtesy of Dr. Raymond M. Abrams, Department of Radiology, New York University Medical Center.*)

venous fistula. Most of these conditions create a physiologic left-to-right shunt and hence a continuous murmur simulating a patent ductus.

TREATMENT. In most patients over two to three years of age, a patent ductus should be surgically corrected as soon as convenient after the diagnosis has been made. The operative risk is low and the results are excellent. In infants, operation should be performed if serious heart failure is present.

The only contraindication to operation, rarely seen, is cyanosis. Cyanosis may be due to an associated cardiac anomaly such as tetralogy of Fallot, in which case the patent ductus is an important ancillary source of blood flow to the lungs. Cyanosis can also develop with a reversed ductus when pulmonary vascular resistance has increased to exceed systemic vascular resistance, as a result of which blood flows from the pulmonary artery to the aorta and creates cyanosis in the lower half of the body. A reversed ductus cannot be safely closed, for the patent ductus partly decreases the pulmonary hypertension, shunting blood from the pulmonary artery to the aorta. Attempted surgical closure usually results in immediate death. Fortunately, with early operations for patent ductus, such advanced pulmonary vascular disease is almost unknown. The author has not seen such a patient in the past 15 years.

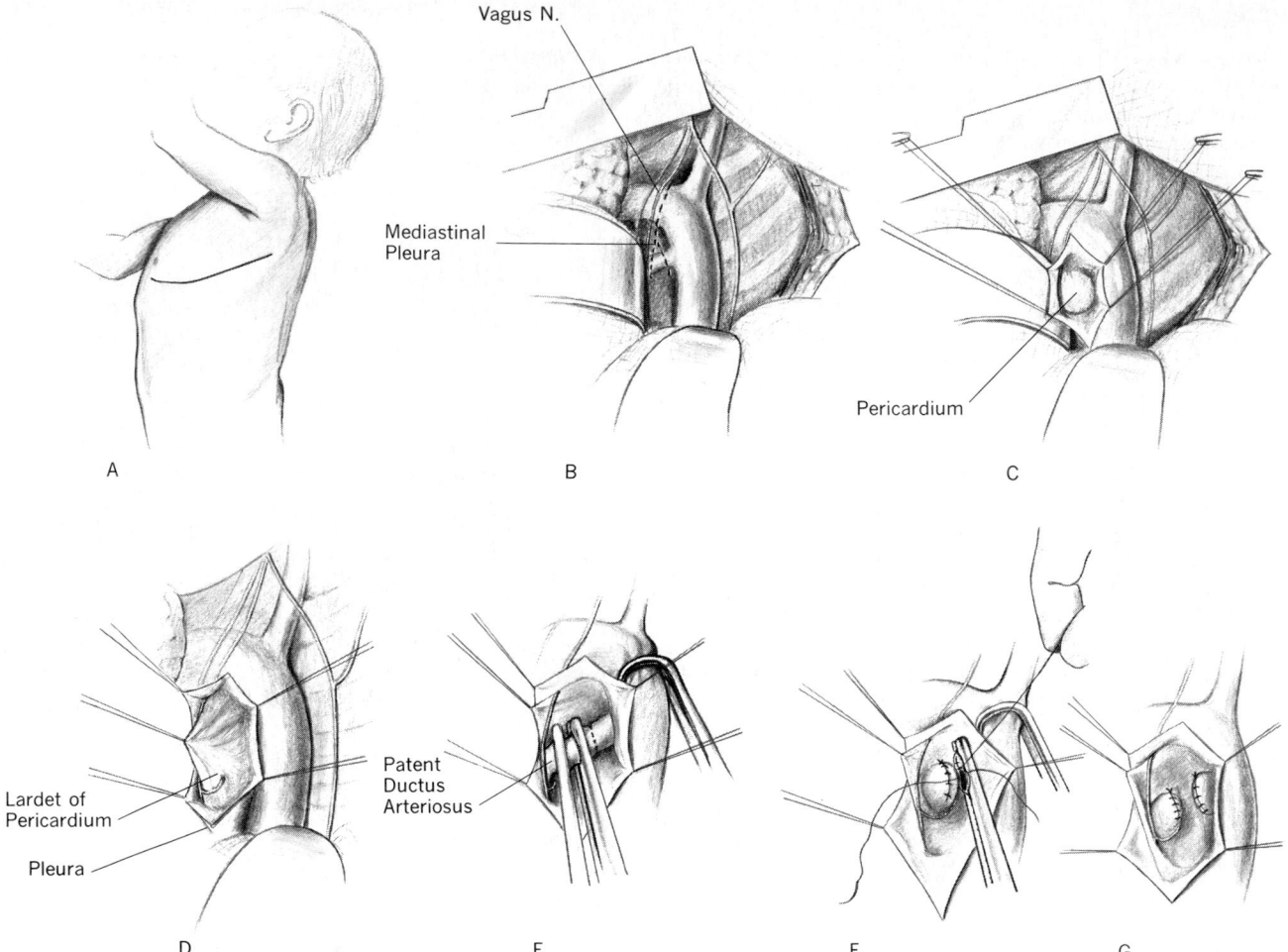

Fig. 18-37. Division of patent ductus arteriosus. *A*. Chest is opened with left posterolateral incision in fourth intercostal space. *B*. Once lung has been retracted, mediastinal pleura is incised longitudinally parallel to vagus nerve. *C*. Initial dissection is along vagus nerve to expose widely the recurrent laryngeal nerve originating from vagus and passing beneath ductus. Wide exposure of recurrent laryngeal nerve is essential part of operative procedure. *D*. After dissection of recurrent laryngeal nerve, lappet of pericardium overlying ductus is freed by sharp dissection proximally to expose pulmonary artery. *E*. Subsequently ductus is encircled, and vascular occlusion clamps are applied. *F*. Ductus is gradually divided and sutured, employing two rows of sutures. *G*. Final view of divided ends of ductus with recurrent laryngeal nerve well exposed.

With bacterial endocarditis, intensive antibiotic therapy will effect cure in most patients; operation can then be more safely performed several weeks later. If the endocarditis cannot be controlled with antibiotic therapy, operation should be undertaken as a last resort, although operations upon a friable, infected ductus have a high mortality rate from hemorrhage or subsequent infection.

Operative Technique. The operation is preferably done through a posterolateral thoracotomy in the fourth intercostal space, although a left anteriolateral thoracotomy in the third intercostal space has been satisfactorily used in previous years. The author's preferred operative technique is shown in detail in Fig. 18-37.

Patients in the third and fourth decade with pulmonary hypertension and sclerosis or calcification of the ductus constitute a difficult and dangerous technical problem because of friability of the ductus, especially at its junction with the pulmonary artery. Lacerations in this artery may quickly result in fatal hemorrhage. A temporary aortic shunt, either a left atrial–femoral artery bypass or the Gott aortic shunt, can be employed to permit temporary occlusion of the aorta above and below the ductus, which can be safely occluded with a single clamp placed near its junction with the aorta. The ductus can then be divided at its point of origin from the aorta, or alternately, the aorta can be incised and the orifice of the ductus obliterated with a patch applied from within the aorta.

Ligation of a patent ductus with multiple ligatures, well developed by Blalock, is now rarely used but is an effective technique in most patients. The original technique included four separate ligatures, with two purse-string sutures at the aortic and pulmonary artery ends of the ductus, followed by two transfixion ligatures on the remaining portions of the ductus.

In 1971 the author treated a sixty-five-year-old patient with congestive failure and extensive calcification of both the aorta and a large patent ductus. Even simple application of vascular clamps to the calcified vessels seemed unusually hazardous. Accordingly, the ductus was effectively obliterated with multiple mattress sutures placed through Teflon felt surrounding the ductus. The patient has subsequently remained well.

As illustrated in Fig. 18-37, a valuable technical point for safe division of any patent ductus is the application of a vascular clamp tangentially onto the aorta a few millimeters from the ductus, rather than on the ductus itself. This method of application of the clamp avoids the problem of a short ductus.

Postoperative Course. With an uncomplicated ductus, the operative risk is surprisingly small. As early as 1953 Gross reported experience with 611 patients, with a mortality rate of less than 0.5 percent in those with neither cardiac failure nor infection before operation. Similar figures were described by Jones in a total series of 909 patients. When patent ductus is associated with other abnormalities, a condition encountered in infants with cardiac failure, operative mortality is higher. At New York University there has been no mortality or serious complications following division of an uncomplicated patent ductus in several years.

Convalescence following operation is usually uneventful, most patients leaving the hospital within 7 to 10 days. A functional systolic murmur may remain audible in a few patients. This may be related to a localized irregularity in the wall of the pulmonary artery where the ductus was present. The electrocardiogram usually returns to normal within a few months. From data now available from over 30 years' experience, it appears that cardiac function becomes normal once the ductus has been surgically obliterated.

RIGHT-TO-LEFT SHUNTS (CYANOTIC GROUP)

Tetralogy of Fallot

HISTORICAL DATA. Tetralogy of Fallot was described as long ago as 1671 by Stensen, but it was not until 1888 that the combination of abnormalities regularly present was emphasized by Fallot. Effective therapy first became possible in 1944, when Blalock dramatically demonstrated that much benefit could be obtained by anastomosis of the subclavian artery and pulmonary artery to create an artificial ductus arteriosus. This operation was developed following the suggestion of Taussig, who had noted an increase in symptoms in infants when a patent ductus arteriosus spontaneously closed. Thereafter the operation was referred to as the *Blalock-Taussig procedure.* It constitutes one of the milestones in cardiac surgery. Subsequently over 1,500 such procedures were performed at the Johns Hopkins Hospital, and experience with these operations led to the development of many other aspects of cardiac surgery. Subsequent contributions were made by Potts et al., who developed an aortic pulmonary side-to-side anastomosis, especially applicable to infants, and by Brock who introduced partial excision of the infundibular obstruction. With the development of extracorporeal circulation, correction of the tetralogy first became possible in 1954–1955 and is now the preferred operation.

INCIDENCE AND ETIOLOGY. Tetralogy of Fallot is one of the most common cyanotic malformations, constituting over 50 percent of all cases of cyanotic heart disease. In cyanotic children who survive beyond the first 2 years of life, a tetralogy of Fallot is present in 70 to 75 percent. There are no known etiologic factors.

PATHOLOGIC ANATOMY. The four features of the tetralogy from which the name originates are obstruction of the outflow tract of the right ventricle, a ventricular septal defect, dextroposition of the aorta, and hypertrophy of the right ventricle. The right ventricular obstruction is severe enough to increase right ventricular systolic pressure to equal left ventricular systolic pressure. The ventricular septal defect is large (2 to 3 cm), approximately equaling the diameter of the orifice of the aortic valve. Right ventricular hypertrophy is the natural consequence of the severe obstruction to emptying of the right ventricle; dextroposition of the aorta is an anatomic variant of probably little physiologic significance.

The right ventricular obstruction may be an infundibular stenosis, a valvular stenosis, or a combined lesion (Fig. 18-38). Often it is a localized obstruction, although less frequently a diffuse stenosis of the entire right ventricular outflow tract is present. In one series of patients, Brock found a localized infundibular stenosis in slightly less than 50 percent of patients, a valvular stenosis in 35 percent, and a combined lesion in 22 percent. The pulmonary artery is often smaller than normal, while the diameter of the aorta is larger than normal. When a localized infundibular stenosis is present, an "infundibular chamber" exists between the right ventricle proximal to the stenosis and the pulmonary valve distad.

The ventricular septal defect is almost always located proximal to the crista supraventricularis and is usually 2 to 3 cm in diameter. The aortic cusps are readily seen through the defect, varying with the degree of dextroposition which is present.

With the decrease in pulmonary blood flow, there is striking enlargement of the bronchial arteries and other routes of collateral circulation to the lungs, creating extensive varicosities throughout the mediastinum and chest wall. In some older children with severe cyanosis, a progressive occlusive disease also develops in the peripheral pulmonary arteries. Absence of the left pulmonary artery has been found in a small number of patients, and in others one or more focal stenoses may be found in either one or both the pulmonary arteries.

Anomalous coronary arteries are also frequent, especially in the outflow tract of the right ventricle, where they are of particular surgical significance. A right aortic arch, for unknown reasons, occurs in about 25 percent of patients. An atrial septal defect is also frequent, at times referred to as part of a pentalogy of Fallot, although the malformation differs little physiologically from the tetralogy. It is noteworthy that although a patent ductus arteriosus may be essential to life, it gradually closes in almost all patients during the first few months of life, often with a disastrous increase in the severity of anoxia.

PATHOPHYSIOLOGY. Physiologically, a tetralogy of Fallot is a combination of a large ventricular septal defect

Fig. 18-38. Different types of right ventricular obstruction in tetralogy of Fallot. *A.* Combined obstruction from hypoplasia of pulmonic annulus in association with diffuse stenosis of outflow tract of right ventricle. This type of diffuse stenosis is commonly found and often requires insertion of prosthetic patch to widen annulus. *B.* Localized stenosis of infundibulum of right ventricle, with "infundibular chamber" distal to this which is proximal to normal pulmonic valve. *C.* Pulmonic stenosis of valvular type in association with normal right ventricular outflow tract. (*Adapted from C. D. Benson et al., "Pediatric Surgery," vol I, Year Book Medical Publishers, Inc., Chicago, 1962, p. 463.*)

with an obstruction in the right ventricular outflow tract of sufficient severity to elevate right ventricular systolic pressure to equal left ventricular systolic pressure. Venous blood entering the right ventricle then is shunted directly into the aorta to produce cyanosis. In addition to cyanosis, the malformation decreases pulmonary blood flow and hence limits the ability of the lungs to absorb oxygen. The inability to increase pulmonary blood flow constitutes the basis for the severe intolerance of exercise. The large ventricular septal defect has a separate influence, in that right ventricular pressure almost never exceeds left ventricular pressure, in contrast to isolated pulmonic valvular stenosis. Hence cardiac enlargement and cardiac failure are rare. Only a few unusual patients have been reported in whom the malformation was such that right ventricular pressure exceeded left ventricular pressure.

The severity of the anoxia varies with the degree of reduction in pulmonary blood flow. Arterial oxygen saturations of 70 to 85% are seen in older children, but in younger children, who may not survive through infancy without operation, astonishingly low arterial oxygen saturations are encountered. Saturations of 30 to 35% may be seen in patients who can walk only a short distance, and levels of 20 to 25% are found in some infants who are unable to walk. Saturations as low as 10% have been recorded, usually associated with loss of consciousness from cerebral anoxia. With exercise, there is often a precipitous fall in arterial oxygen saturation, decreasing from a resting level of 70% to 20 to 25%, which clearly indicates the physiologic basis for exertional dyspnea.

Chronic anoxia produces compensatory polycythemia and, subsequently, clubbing of the extremities. Polycythemia is seldom apparent until after two years of age, but later hematocrit readings varying from 60 to 75 percent are common. Wide variations in hematocrit readings are found, ranging from normal with mild tetralogies to readings as high as 85 to 90 percent in the most severe forms.

The degree of cyanosis increases significantly in the first few years of life, for visible cyanosis is proportional to the number of grams of unsaturated hemoglobin in the pe-

ripheral circulation and not to the actual oxygen concentration. Hence severe cyanosis is visible only after polycythemia has developed. The time of appearance has been used by Nadas for a convenient grouping of the clinical course of the disease. About one-third of patients are cyanotic at birth, another one-third become cyanotic in the first year of life, and one-third develop cyanosis only subsequently in childhood. Patients who are cyanotic at birth have severe anoxia and often do not survive infancy unless operation is performed. Patients who become cyanotic in the first year of life have a milder course but are seriously disabled, while those who develop cyanosis in later years may have little incapacity and little polycythemia—a so-called "pink" tetralogy. These patients, of course, have only moderate reduction in pulmonary blood flow.

The main threat to life in the first years of life is a cerebral vascular accident, either from cerebral thrombosis or from a localized infarct from anoxia. In severe cases, cyanotic "spells" are seen in which the infant becomes deeply cyanotic and comatose. Spontaneous recovery usually occurs, but death or hemiplegia may ensue.

Brain abscess is another serious, often lethal, complication to which patients are peculiarly susceptible. The right-to-left shunt, bypassing the lungs and providing direct access for bacteria into the venous blood to the arterial circulation, is the most convenient explanation of the high incidence of brain abscess, although localized cerebral infarcts may also play a role in etiology.

Cardiac failure is extremely rare with tetralogy, and

its presence always brings into question the accuracy of the diagnosis. It is seen in a few adults in the second or third decade but is virtually unknown in children. There is also a susceptibility to bacterial endocarditis, as with other cardiac malformations.

Life expectancy without treatment is relatively short. Infants cyanotic at birth formerly seldom lived beyond the first decade. Those becoming cyanotic in the first year of life might survive to early adult life, while those becoming cyanotic in later years would occasionally survive into the third or fourth decade or, rarely, beyond. In older, chronically cyanotic patients, other physiologic signs of chronic anoxia appear, with disturbances in the blood-clotting mechanism and secondary hemorrhage in the gastrointestinal tract.

CLINICAL MANIFESTATIONS. Symptoms. Almost all patients are symptomatic. Dyspnea and cyanosis, markedly aggravated by exertion, are the outstanding features. Two additional characteristics are cyanotic spells and squatting. Cyanotic spells are episodes of sudden increase in intensity of cyanosis, followed by unconsciousness, usually with spontaneous recovery within a few minutes or hours. Such episodes, representing acute cerebral anoxia, may be fatal or may result in hemiplegia. They are frequent in infants but seldom occur in older children, probably because symptomatic infants seldom survive without treatment. Squatting is an impressive characteristic, for children learn quickly to relieve dyspnea by assuming a squatting position. The physiologic benefit from squatting, apparently a redistribution of blood flow, is not clear. Walking for short distances, interrupted by squatting, is a well-recognized hallmark of the tetralogy. Hemoptysis is a rare symptom, occurring usually in older children with marked varicosities of the bronchial circulation.

Physical Examination. On physical examination the obvious features are cyanosis of varying severity and clubbing of the digits. The heart usually has a normal size, rate, and rhythm. A systolic murmur of grade II to III intensity is commonly present along the left sternal border at the third or fourth intercostal spaces, and a thrill is present in about one-half the patients. With severe pulmonic stenosis or pulmonary atresia, the murmur may be faint or even absent because of absence of flow through the pulmonic orifice. The second pulmonic sound is weak or absent, while the aortic second sound is increased above normal intensity.

LABORATORY FINDINGS. The chest roentgenogram shows a heart of normal size with an unusual contour, termed the *coeur en sabot*, or sabot-shaped heart (Fig. 18-1). This indicates the characteristic enlargement due to selective hypertrophy of the right ventricle, combined with a concavity in the area where the pulmonary artery is normally located. The lung fields often show decreased vascularity.

The electrocardiogram is always abnormal, showing right ventricular hypertrophy of varying severity with right axis deviation.

Cardiac catheterization demonstrates several characteristic features. A slight left to right shunt may be detected at the ventricular level in mild cases, but often no left-to-right intracardiac shunt is present. A large right-to-left shunt is indicated by arterial unsaturation. The right ventricular systolic pressure is usually identical with the left ventricular systolic pressure, while pulmonary artery pressure is decreased below normal levels, resulting in a large systolic pressure gradient between the right ventricle and pulmonary artery. The pulmonary blood flow is decreased, varying with the severity of the disorder. The degree of decrease in pulmonary blood flow will be found to parallel the severity of the arterial oxygen saturation. The hematocrit is usually between 60 and 75 percent, with a range from 45 to 90 percent.

Selective angiocardiography is of great importance in planning surgical correction, for the location of the right ventricular obstruction, either infundibular, valvular, or diffuse, can be outlined. The presence of associated abnormalities in the pulmonary arteries should be particularly noted. Simultaneous opacification of the aorta and pulmonary arteries when dye is injected into the right ventricle is typical of tetralogy of Fallot (Fig. 18-39).

DIAGNOSIS. The diagnosis can usually be made with certainty from clinical examination combined with roentgenogram and electrocardiogram. The important clinical features are cyanosis with severe exertional dyspnea and squatting. The important physical findings are a heart of normal size with a systolic murmur. Roentgenographic

Fig. 18-39. Cardiac angiogram in patient with tetralogy of Fallot, demonstrating large ventricular septal defect. Dye has been injected through catheter in right ventricle. Dye flows through large ventricular septal defect into left ventricle. Pulmonic stenosis which was present is not visible on this angiogram. (*Courtesy of Dr. Raymond M. Abrams, Department of Radiology, New York University Medical Center.*)

findings demonstrate a heart of normal size with decreased vascularity of the lung fields, while the electrocardiogram shows right ventricular hypertrophy. Cardiac catheterization and angiography should be done routinely to confirm the diagnosis and precisely define the pathologic anatomy.

Other cyanotic conditions to be distinguished from the tetralogy include tricuspid atresia, transposition of the great vessels, and pulmonic valvular stenosis with a patent foramen ovale. Tricuspid atresia can be suspected from the electrocardiogram, which characteristically shows a left axis deviation. Transposition often has cardiac enlargement and vascular lung fields, although cardiac catheterization is required for precise evaluation. Pulmonic valvular stenosis with a patent foramen ovale is suggested by the presence of cardiac enlargement with signs of cardiac failure. The most important feature in differentiating the tetralogy from other cyanotic malformations is the fact that the heart with a tetralogy is of normal size.

TREATMENT. Indications for Operation. Infants with cyanotic spells from anoxia require emergency operation to prevent death or hemiplegia. At present some type of shunt procedure is preferable, although a few groups have explored corrective operations even in the first few months of life. The best type of shunt in these critically ill infants, usually under four months of age, remains uncertain. The side-to-side anastomosis between the ascending aorta and the right pulmonary artery, developed by Waterston, is almost always possible but fraught with serious complications because the margin of safety between an adequate shunt and an excessively large shunt, producing serious or

lethal cardiac failure, is small (Fig. 18-40). Despite a number of variations, almost all groups report a mortality above 20 percent with the Waterston procedure in the first few months of life, so this has been virtually abandoned at New York University.

The Potts operation of aortic–pulmonary side-to-side anastomosis is also rarely used because of both the technical difficulties of construction and subsequent problems of dismantling such a shunt at the time of corrective surgery (Fig. 18-41).

The subclavian–pulmonary anastomosis of Blalock has been used more and more in infants (Fig. 18-42) but is not always technically feasible with small subclavian arteries.

At New York University for the past few years a homograft vein has been successfully used in several patients to establish a shunt between the ascending aorta and the pulmonary artery. This approach has several attractive features and may well become the procedure of choice.

Beyond six months of age, the increasing tendency is for primary corrective operation rather than performance of a shunt. Excellent data have been reported from several centers supporting this approach.

At New York University, the Blalock shunt is still employed in some children between six and twenty-four months of age with complex tetralogies, although the tendency is increasingly in favor of primary correction. Certainly beyond two years of age primary correction is considered the procedure of choice by most groups, although Chiariello in 1975, reviewing a 5-year experience with 403 patients operated on in Houston, Tex., still considered the

Fig. 18-40. Side-to-side anastomosis between ascending aorta and right pulmonary artery. *A.* Tangential clamp has been applied to ascending aorta, which is then incised for 4 to 5 mm. Corresponding incision is then made in right pulmonary artery, which has been occluded with proximal and distal ligatures. *B.* Posterior row of anastomosis is constructed with continuous suture of 5-0 silk. *C.* Anterior anastomosis may be done with interrupted or continuous sutures. *D.* Diagram of final anastomosis, depicting flow of blood from aorta into pulmonary artery. (*Adapted from D. A. Cooley and G. L. Hallman, "Surgical Treatment of Congenital Heart Disease," Lea & Febiger, Philadelphia, 1966, p. 128.*)

optimal age for elective correction to be between six and ten years.

Technique of Corrective Operation. A median sternotomy incision is preferred. If a previous shunt operation has been performed, the anastomosis is isolated before extracorporeal circulation is begun and subsequently occluded during bypass before the heart is opened. Once the pericardium has been opened, the outflow tract of the right ventricle is carefully examined for anomalous coronary arteries, selecting an incision in the right ventricle to avoid dividing any such arteries. Only rarely is the anatomy of the coronary circulation such that a ventriculotomy cannot be safely performed. In such instances the approach may be through the right atrium. Edmunds reported, in 1976, successful experiences with 15 patients using the transatrial approach.

Five potential zones of obstruction to flow of blood to the lungs should be considered for surgical correction, the location, the severity, and number varying with each patient. These include fusion of the pulmonary valve leaflets; a hypoplastic pulmonic annulus; varying degrees of infundibular stenosis in the right ventricle, either fibrous or muscular; hypoplastic main pulmonary artery; or hypoplastic distal pulmonary arteries. Precise selective angiocardiograms are of great value before operation in identifying these zones of obstruction.

For several years a high transverse ventriculotomy was employed but has been abandoned in favor of a short (4 to 5 cm) high vertical ventriculotomy stopping near the pulmonic annulus and being limited almost to the infundibular portion of the right ventricle. This incision is routinely closed with an appropriate Dacron patch. This approach of a short high vertical ventriculotomy combined with insertion of a prosthetic patch requires a less radical excision of the hypertrophied right ventricular musculature and better preserves ventricular function. Large muscle bundles of the hypertrophied crista supraventricularis are excised, but the infundibulectomy is considerably less radical than working through a transverse ventriculotomy.

If the pulmonic valve ring is of adequate size, the fused commissures of the pulmonic valve may be divided through the ventriculotomy without opening the pulmonary artery. Otherwise a separate incision is made in the pulmonary artery to facilitate appropriate commissurotomies.

A crucial part of the operation is deciding whether the diameter of the pulmonic valve ring is adequate. Sizing of the diameter of the pulmonic ring with graduated Hegar dilators has been used by our group for several years and has been similarly endorsed by several others. Kirklin and associates in 1976 precisely described the relationships between body weight and a pulmonic annulus of adequate size. These measurements are particularly useful for smaller children. In larger children, a pulmonic valve ring that will accommodate a No. 16 Hegar dilator, representing a cross-sectional area of slightly less than 2 cm², is satisfactory.

If the pulmonic annulus is hypoplastic, the ventriculotomy is extended accordingly across the annulus into the pulmonary artery and an appropriate patch applied.

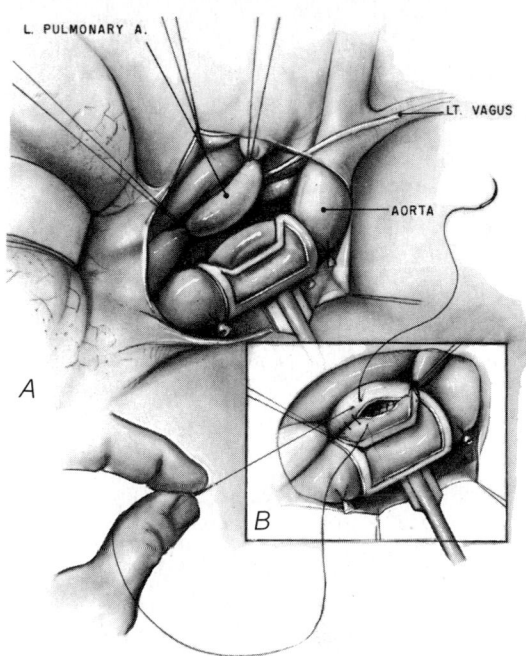

Fig. 18-41. Potts type of aortic-pulmonary anastomosis. *A.* Partial-occlusion clamp has been applied to aorta, and segment of pulmonary artery has been occluded by traction on ligatures. *B.* After approximation of two vessels, side-to-side anastomosis is constructed. Size of anastomosis is critical, an aortic incision 4 mm long being used in infants and one 6 mm in older children. This type of anastomosis is avoided whenever possible because of difficulties in dividing it during subsequent corrective surgery with cardiopulmonary bypass.

Following correction of the infundibular obstruction, the ventricular septal defect is closed in a manner identical to that described previously for ventricular septal defect. Adequacy of closure is confirmed by retrograde injection of saline solution through a left ventricular vent while the aorta is temporarily clamped. With the technique of closure of the septal defect as described, there has been no permanent heart block in any patient in the author's experience in the past decade.

If the diameter of the main pulmonary artery is less than 2 cm, it is also widened to an appropriate degree with a patch which may be extended when necessary beyond the bifurcation of the artery onto the left pulmonary artery.

Our preference for the prosthetic patch is a section of woven tubular Dacron graft, popularized by Kirklin. Pericardium is also a satisfactory material in most patients but has been associated with the subsequent formation of aneurysms in a small number of patients, usually with residual pulmonary hypertension.

Following closure of the ventriculotomy and removal of air from all cardiac chambers, extracorporeal circulation is stopped and intracardiac pressure is measured to confirm that right ventricular obstruction has been corrected. The right ventricular systolic pressure should be reduced to less than 60 to 70 percent of left ventricular systolic pressure. If right ventricular pressure is still elevated above this level, more adequate correction of the ventricular obstruction is

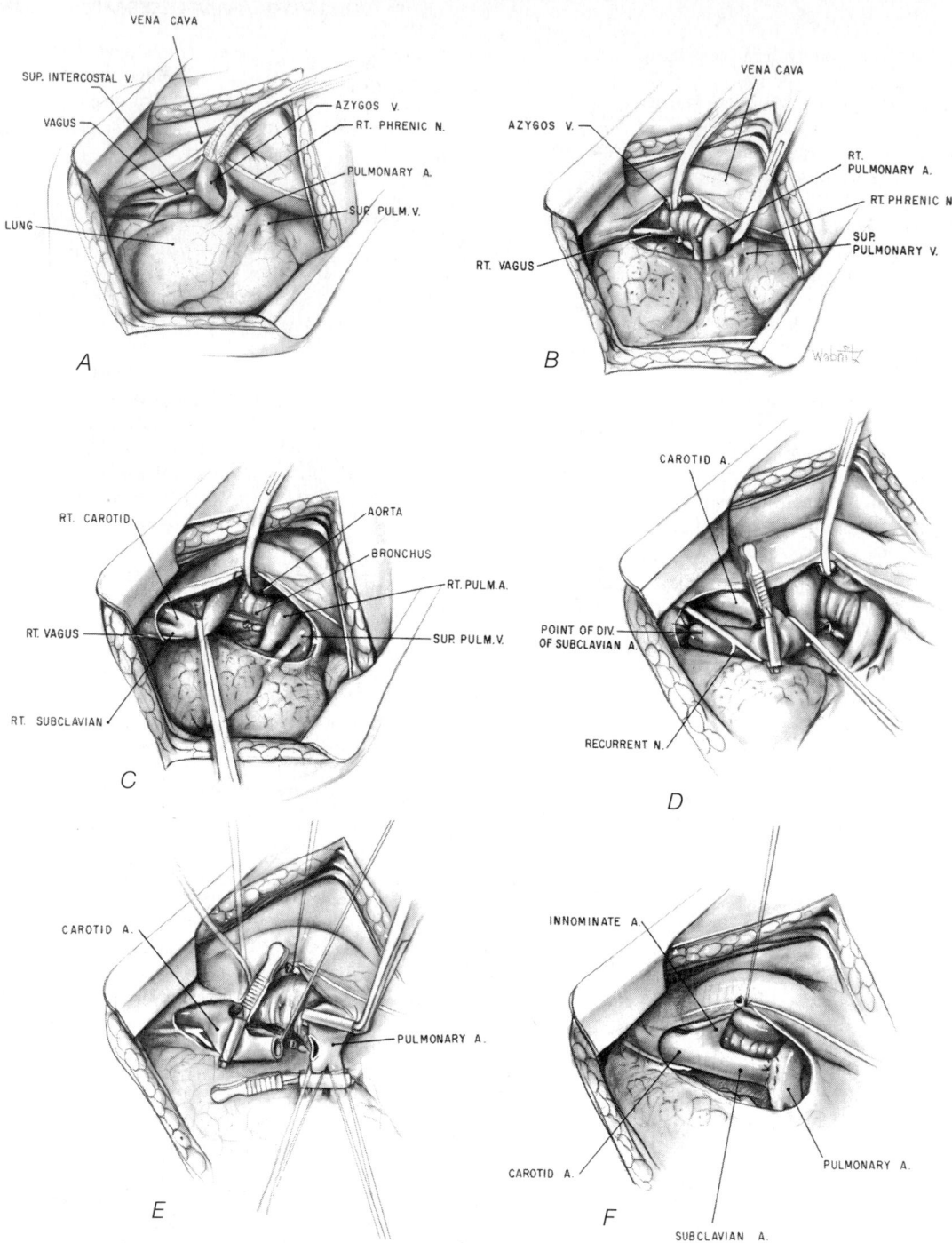

Fig. 18-42. Blalock procedure. *A*. Dissection is begun by isolation of azygos vein, followed by incision of mediastinal pleura in front of pulmonary artery. *B*. Pulmonary artery is isolated in hilum, dissecting artery distally to beyond point of origin of upper lobe branch. Medially, artery is freed well into mediastinum in order to permit displacement of artery superiorly during construction of anastomosis. Traction on stump of divided azygos vein retracts superior vena cava to expose pulmonary artery in mediastinum. *C*. Subclavian artery is mobilized at apex of thorax, mobilizing carotid artery and subclavian artery down into mediastinum. Wide mobilization of carotid artery greatly facilitates subsequent performance of anastomosis. Vagus and recurrent nerves are protected during this dissection. *D*. After mobilization of carotid and

subclavian arteries, tributaries of subclavian arteries are ligated, vertebral artery being ligated separately to avoid retrograde flow of blood from vertebral artery distad into arm, producing subclavian "steal" abnormality. *E*. After division of subclavian artery, longitudinal arteriotomy is made in pulmonary artery. Adventitia is carefully cleared from subclavian artery before performance of anastomosis. *F*. Appearance of completed anastomosis. Anterior row of anastomosis is usually made with interrupted sutures of 5-0 silk to permit growth of anastomosis. With wide mobilization of carotid artery superiorly and pulmonary artery inferiorly, satisfactory anastomosis can be accomplished with sublcavian artery as short as 1 to 1.5 cm in length. Vein graft is rarely necessary.

necessary. Otherwise fatal depression of cardiac output from right ventricular failure may occur in the early postoperative course. In most patients following bypass a satisfactory result is obtained, with a systolic pressure near 100 mm, a right ventricular systolic pressure between 35 and 50 mm, and a pulmonary artery systolic pressure of 20 to 25 mm.

Postoperative Course. Following operation, particular attention is required in the first 24 hours to intrathoracic bleeding, because older cyanotic patients have an increased hemorrhagic tendency from the long-standing polycythemia. Transfusion of fresh frozen plasma, often combined with platelet transfusions, is the best therapy. Close observation is necessary to avoid intrathoracic accumulation of blood with cardiac tamponade.

Adequacy of cardiac output is monitored by observing blood pressure, blood-gas concentrations in mixed venous blood, and urine output. Blood is transfused in sufficient amounts to keep central venous pressure near 12 to 15 mm Hg if necessary, possibly at higher levels. If cardiac output is inadequate despite these measures, small amounts of isoproterenol or epinephrine are infused (1 to 2 μg/minute). Acidosis is not a significant problem if cardiac output remains adequate. Assisted ventilation may be required for a few hours but seldom for longer.

Some degree of right ventricular failure is commonly encountered. Hence, digitalis is routinely given, combined with bedrest and restriction of sodium intake.

The risk of operation varies with the age of the patient and the degree of cyanosis, reflecting the severity of the right ventricular obstruction. The risk is only 3 to 5 percent in older children but larger in smaller ones with severe cyanosis. The excellent monograph by Kirklin et al. contains much data regarding experiences with tetralogy of Fallot. Large clinical series showing low operative mortality have also been published by Kirklin et al., Malm et al., Shumway et al., and McGoon et al.

Following recovery from operation, dramatic improvement is obvious. Cyanosis is, of course, absent, and exercise tolerance within a few months approaches that of a normal individual. If cardiac failure is significant following operation, convalescence may be slow for several weeks. Some cardiac enlargement may remain, but long-term studies show that most patients have excellent cardiac function. The tolerance for pulmonic insufficiency which results if the pulmonic annulus is incised and a prosthetic patch inserted is surprisingly good. Ultimate prognosis in such patients is uncertain, though some have now survived for over 20 years with continuing good results. Some groups have inserted homograft valves at the time of operation to avoid pulmonic insufficiency, but there is not sufficient evidence to warrant this as a routine procedure.

COMPLEX MALFORMATIONS

Transposition of the Great Vessels

HISTORICAL DATA. The clinical syndrome of transposition of the great vessels was clearly described by Taussig in 1938. The first surgical procedure to achieve significant benefit, creation of an atrial septal defect, was reported by Blalock and Hanlon. Another palliative surgical procedure, no longer used, was developed by Baffes, who transposed the inferior vena cava and the right pulmonary veins. Senning, in 1957, first completely corrected transposition of the great vessels by repositioning the atrial septum, but mortality was prohibitively high. Further experience with a modification of the technique was reported by Senning in 1975. Mustard, in 1964, developed a method of reconstructing the atrial cavity which has produced the best clinical results to date.

INCIDENCE AND ETIOLOGY. Transposition of the great vessels is one of the most frequent causes of cyanotic heart disease in the newborn, constituting 30 to 40 percent of all cases. It is the most common cause of cardiac failure in the newborn. As many patients die in infancy, it is much less common after the first two years of life.

Transposition of the aorta and pulmonary arteries results from abnormal division of the bulbar trunk in embryologic development, occurring between the fifth and seventh uterine week. Etiologic factors are unknown. It is about four times more frequent in males than in females.

PATHOLOGIC ANATOMY. With transposition of the arteries, the aorta originates from the right ventricle and the pulmonary artery from the left ventricle (Fig. 18-43). As a result of these abnormal locations, venous blood returning through the venae cavae to the right atrium enters the right ventricle and is then propelled directly into the aorta. Oxygenated blood returning from the lungs through the pulmonary veins to the left atrium enters the left ventricle and is then expelled through the pulmonary artery again to the lungs. This dual, parallel circulatory arrangement is obviously incompatible with life without communication between the pulmonary and systemic circulations. Three possible communications exist, a patent ductus arteriosus, an atrial septal defect or foramen ovale, or a ventricular septal defect. One or more of these, of course, must exist for the infant to survive even a few hours after birth. Normally a patent ductus is present for a few weeks after birth in over one-half the patients. A foramen ovale is frequently found, and a ventricular septal defect occurs in 50 to 70 percent of patients, varying with the group of patients studied.

Associated anomalies are common. One of the most frequent of these, pulmonic stenosis, occurs so commonly as to constitute a well-defined variant of the syndrome, because the prognosis is unusually favorable in such patients. A wide variety of other anomalies may occur, including coarctation of the aorta, pulmonary atresia, and dextrocardia.

PATHOPHYSIOLOGY. The two basic physiologic handicaps with transposition are severe anoxia from inability to transport oxygen from the lungs to the tissues of the body and progressive cardiac failure. The severe and rapidly progressive cardiac failure results partly from a high cardiac output and partly from the fact that the coronary arteries are filled with unoxygenated blood with resulting myocardial anoxia. The relative severity of the anoxia and the cardiac failure varies with the nature of the intracardiac

R. ATRIUM

AORTA

PUL. A.

L. ATRIUM

INTERVENT.
SEPTAL
DEFECT

R. VENT.

L. VENT.

Fig. 18-43. Transposition of great vessels, with aorta arising from right ventricle and pulmonary artery from left ventricle. Ventricular septal defect permits communication between pulmonic and systemic circulations; otherwise condition would be incompatible with life after birth. (*Adapted from H. B. Taussig, "Congenital Malformations of the Heart," 3d ed., Harvard University Press, Cambridge, 1960, p. 149.*)

communications and valvular stenoses. Nadas has found in his group of patients that cardiac failure was present at birth in 80 percent. Because of the severe cardiac failure and anoxia, physical development is severely retarded.

Transposition is a lethal condition, and a high percentage of patients die within the first 1 to 3 months of life. Mustard et al. estimated that 90 percent of their patients died within 7 months. A survey by Hanlon and Blalock in 1948 found only six patients reported in the literature at that time who had lived beyond ten years of age.

Nadas has conveniently grouped patients into four clinical categories related to prognosis. Those with an intact ventricular septum do poorly because of inadequate mixing of the pulmonary and systemic circulations. Similarly, those with a large ventricular septal defect do badly because of excessive pulmonary blood flow. Pulmonary hypertension in this group of patients is also associated with a poor prognosis. The most favorable prognosis is associated with a ventricular septal defect combined with pulmonic stenosis. This combination permits mixing of the pulmonary and systemic circulations through the ventricular septal defect, while the pulmonic stenosis prevents excessive pulmonary blood flow with pulmonary congestion and secondary pulmonary hypertension.

CLINICAL MANIFESTATIONS. Symptoms. A high percentage of infants are cyanotic at birth (80 percent in Nadas' series), and cardiac failure is similarly frequent. Cyanosis appears in most other patients in the first year of life. There is a corresponding severe retardation of growth and development, and anoxic spells of unconsciousness are frequent. Mental development, however, is not impaired. The most prominent symptoms are cyanosis and dyspnea. In children who survive beyond the first two years of life, clubbing and polycythemia appear.

Physical Findings. Cyanosis is frequently obvious on inspection and is often severe. In older children clubbing and polycythemia are similarly evident. Signs of congestive failure are almost always found, with cardiac enlargement, hepatomegaly, and pulmonary congestion. A systolic murmur is usually present but is variable and not diagnostic.

It can result from any of the different intracardiac communications which may be present. Severe retardation of physical development is obvious in older infants.

Absence of a murmur, often indicating absence of an intracardiac communication, indicates a particularly unfavorable prognosis because of inadequate communication between the pulmonary and systemic circulations.

LABORATORY FINDINGS. The chest roentgenogram shows cardiac enlargement, often with a distinctive silhouette, and pulmonary congestion. The contour of the heart has been described as "egg-shaped" and results from the prominent right ventricle projecting into the left side of the chest and the dilated right atrium bulging into the right side. The base of the cardiac shadow, termed the "waist," may be unusually narrow because of the location of the aorta directly in front of the pulmonary artery, rather than the conventional side-to-side relationship seen in the normal cardiac shadow (Fig. 18-2).

The electrocardiogram consistently shows severe right ventricular hypertrophy. Left ventricular hypertrophy varies with the pulmonary blood flow or with the presence of pulmonary valvular stenosis.

Cardiac catheterization reveals several distinctive features. It may not be possible to enter all four cardiac chambers because of the malformations. The systolic pressure in the right ventricle is the same as in the aorta, while that in the left ventricle varies with the size of the ventricular septal defect and the presence of pulmonic stenosis. The oxygen saturation in the pulmonary artery is increased, and a hallmark of the condition is the fact that oxygen saturation in the pulmonary artery is greater than that in the femoral artery. Varying degrees of arterial oxygen unsaturation are regularly found, ranging from as low as 12% to as high as 85%. Angiocardiography provides the best means for confirming the diagnosis, for it classically demonstrates the anterior origin of the aorta from the right ventricle, with the more faintly visualized pulmonary artery lying posterior to the aorta.

DIAGNOSIS. The diagnosis of transposition can be immediately considered in a seriously ill, cyanotic infant with cardiac enlargement and congestive heart failure. In older children the retardation of physical development is striking. It must be differentiated from tetralogy of Fallot, tricuspid atresia, and total anomaly of venous return. Tetralogy of Fallot is readily identified in many patients by the normal cardiac size and the absence of cardiac failure. Tricuspid atresia is easily recognized by the characteristic left axis deviation on the electrocardiogram. Total anomalous drainage of the pulmonary veins may require cardiac catheterization to establish the diagnosis with certainty.

TREATMENT. Indications for Operation. For several reasons transposition may be classified into four broad groups, as follows: (1) Intact ventricular septum, patent foramen ovale; (2) ventricular septal defect; (3) ventricular septal defect and pulmonic stenosis; and (4) complex transposition, one of the previous three forms in association with other severe defects such as coarctation of the aorta.

The most urgent problems are seen with an intact ventricular septum, for the only communication between the pulmonary and systemic circulations is through the foramen ovale. In these patients, balloon septostomy provides dramatic, though not permanent, improvement. In the other groups, balloon septostomy is of considerably less value.

Because of the high fatality rate in the first month of life, some type of surgical procedure must be done to increase communication between the pulmonary and systemic circulations at the time the diagnosis is established in the catheterization laboratory. The simplest procedure is the balloon septostomy, enlarging the foramen ovale or atrial septal defect present by passing a deflated balloon catheter through the defect into the left atrium, inflating the balloon, and forcefully pulling the inflated balloon across the septum to enlarge the opening. This ingenious technique was developed by Rashkind and has greatly helped in the initial treatment of these seriously ill infants. In most instances, balloon septostomy probably should be routinely done at the time of cardiac catheterization to establish the diagnosis.

When balloon septostomy is ineffective, an atrial septal defect may be created by the Blalock-Hanlon technique. With the attractive simplicity of balloon septostomy, this procedure is now performed much less frequently than in the past. The operative procedure is illustrated in Fig. 18-44. A right thoracotomy is performed, after which the pericardium is opened and the superior and inferior pulmonary veins are isolated. The atrial septum is identified at the point of entry of the right pulmonary veins and a vascular clamp applied to isolate a segment of both the right and left atria at this point. Parallel incisions are then made in the right atrium and pulmonary vein through the septum, after which the two incisions are connected and a portion of the septum is incised, creating a defect 1 to 2 cm in diameter. Although this procedure has provided dramatic palliation in many patients for 6 to 12 months, results are often not sustained. Hence the present trend is to consider total surgical correction if balloon septostomy is inadequate.

In patients with a large ventricular septal defect resulting

PARALLEL INCISIONS IN BOTH ATRIA

SEPTUM

SEPTUM

R.A.

L.A.

Fig. 18-44. Creation of atrial septal defect (Blalock-Hanlon Technique). Right pulmonary veins are mobilized and occluded by traction on ligatures. Pulmonary artery and right main bronchus are also occluded to avoid congestion of lungs during occlusion of pulmonary veins. Tangential occlusion clamp is applied to right and left atria, enclosing atrial septum. Separate incisions are then made in right atrium and left atrium. Exposed atrial septum is then removed, temporarily releasing clamp in order to withdraw more septum from between its jaws and create larger defect. After excision of this septum, incision is sutured, creating large atrial septal defect. (*Adapted from D. A. Cooley et al., Arch Surg, 93:704, 1966.*)

in flooding of the lung fields from excessive pulmonary blood flow, total correction may be considered or banding of the pulmonary artery may be done as a palliative procedure. Conversely, if pulmonic stenosis is present with severe reduction in pulmonary blood flow, a palliative subclavian-pulmonary anastomosis may be done.

Corrective Operations. All the previously described procedures are palliative only. If the ventricular septum is intact, many patients do reasonably well with a large atrial septal defect up to two to three years of age, and then total correction may be undertaken. In patients with ventricular septal defects, however, operation must be employed at an earlier age unless banding of the pulmonary artery is performed. Otherwise irreversible changes in the pulmonary vascular bed may develop before two years of age.

Dramatic advances have been made in recent years with the total correction of transposition in the first 1 to 2 years of life. In some instances operation has been successfully performed in the first 2 to 3 months of life, although operative mortality is higher. Performance of these complex procedures in small infants has been greatly facilitated by the deep hypothermia–circulatory arrest technique, developed extensively by Barratt-Boyes and his colleagues.

Data from several sources, including Barratt-Boyes, Kirklin, and Stark, now indicate that excellent results can be obtained by operation in the first 2 years of life. A more conservative approach is to perform palliative procedures described in earlier paragraphs, delaying the corrective procedure until the child is older. The strongest factor in support of early operation is the development of irreversible changes in the pulmonary vascular bed within the first 1 to 2 years of life in some patients. At New York University we have increasingly favored total surgical correction performed within the first 2 years of life.

A second important concept is that the durability of the Mustard baffle procedure, first reported in 1964, seems well established. In 1976 Mustard reported catheterization studies on 14 patients 4 to 10 years after the baffle operation, with continuing good results. Several technical modifications of the method of insertion of the baffle for the Mustard procedure are beyond the scope of this report, but complications from obstruction of either the pulmonary veins or the vena cavae have been described by several groups.

In 1975 Jatene, in South America, reported a successful surgical correction in an infant by switching the aorta and pulmonary arteries, with transposition of the abnormal coronary arteries. To date, attempts by others with this technique have had a prohibitive mortality; however, this method of total correction remains an attractive goal for the future.

Tricuspid Atresia

PATHOLOGIC ANATOMY. Tricuspid atresia is a rare form of congenital heart disease (Fig. 18-45) affecting 3 to 8 percent of children with cyanotic heart disease. However, series of 100 to 150 cases have been analyzed and reported from different cardiac centers. The basic abnormality is atresia of the tricuspid valve. Often only a dimple is found in the right atrial cavity where the tricuspid valve orifice is normally located. Several other cardiac malformations are associated with tricuspid atresia, and the severity of the disease varies with the associated malformations. The right ventricle is always underdeveloped, even absent, its place being taken by a solid mass of hypoplastic muscle. In other patients it exists as a small chamber, either a blind sac or one communicating with the left ventricle through a ventricular septal defect. The pulmonary artery and pulmonary valve are atretic with severe right ventricular hypoplasia, the pulmonary circulation being maintained through the ductus arteriosus. When a small right ventricular cavity is present, a normal pulmonary valve may be found. The ventricular septum is intact with right ventricular hypoplasia, but with a rudimentary ventricular chamber a septal defect is usually present. There is often an associated transposition of the great vessels. Edwards and Bargeron have described four anatomic variants of tricuspid atresia, differing in the presence of a ventricular septal defect, pulmonic stenosis, or transposition of the great vessels. An atrial septal defect must, of necessity, be present to maintain life. This may consist of a foramen ovale stretched open by a high right atrial pressure, a small atrial septal defect, or virtual absence of the atrial septum.

PATHOPHYSIOLOGY. The basic physiologic disturbance results from complete mixing of systemic venous blood and pulmonary venous blood in the left atrium, as blood returning to the right atrium is diverted by the hypoplastic tricuspid orifice through the atrial septal defect into the left atrium. The severity of the resulting cyanosis varies with the pulmonary blood flow. Cyanosis and anoxia are severe with pulmonary atresia, while they may be minimal with an adequate pulmonary blood flow. The hypoplastic right ventricle which is uniformly present is the most valuable clue to the diagnosis. An additional significant physiologic disturbance is the elevated right atrial pressure resulting from flow of systemic venous blood through the atrial septal defect and into the left ventricle. The right atrial pressure may be elevated 5 to 10 mm Hg if only a foramen ovale is present, resulting in hepatic enlargement and other signs of right-sided heart failure.

CLINICAL MANIFESTATIONS. Symptoms. The disease is a severe one, and most infants die in the first few months of life as the patent ductus arteriosus closes, unless an operation is performed. The severity of the malformation varies with the degree of reduction in pulmonary blood flow, which in turn is related to the degree of hypoplasia of the right ventricle. The patients are usually cyanotic at birth and have exercise intolerance, retarded development, and frequent anoxic spells of unconsciousness. Hemiplegia may develop after a severe anoxic spell. Death occurs during an anoxic episode or results from congestive heart failure. In older children endocarditis may occur.

The prominent symptoms are cyanosis and dyspnea with intolerance to exercise, squatting, and limited growth and development.

Physical Examination. On physical examination there is slight to moderate cardiac enlargement. A moderate systolic murmur along the left sternal border is present in about one-half the patients but is of no diagnostic significance. It presumably arises either from flow through the atrial septal defect or possibly from flow through a stenotic pulmonic valve. Absence of a murmur often indicates an unusually poor prognosis. The second heart sound is unusually "pure" because the pulmonic second sound is weak or absent. A particularly significant diagnostic finding is hepatic enlargement and other signs of right-sided failure, especially in association with absence of any signs of pulmonary congestion or left-sided failure.

LABORATORY FINDINGS. The chest roentgenogram regularly shows cardiac enlargement, and on fluoroscopy it may be possible to detect that the enlargement is predominantly in the left ventricle. There is decreased vascularity in the lung fields. The electrocardiogram is the most important diagnostic tool, for left ventricular hypertrophy and left axis deviation are uniformly present, in contrast to the classic right ventricular hypertrophy of most forms of cyanotic heart disease. There are often unusually tall, peaked P waves, indicating right atrial hypertrophy in association with a small atrial septal defect or foramen ovale. On cardiac catheterization there is a right-to-left

Fig. 18-45. A. Tricuspid atresia with rudimentary right ventricle, pulmonary atresia, and vestigial pulmonary artery which does not communicate with hypoplastic right ventricular cavity. B. Tricuspid atresia in which pulmonary artery is normally formed and arises from rudimentary right ventricular cavity. Small ventricular septal defect is present, permitting flow of blood from normal left ventricular cavity through rudimentary right ventricular cavity into pulmonary artery. C. Tricuspid atresia with rudimentary right ventricle in which normal pulmonary artery with normal pulmonic valves arises from rudimentary right ventricle. Right atrial cavity is dilated, with absence of tricuspid valve. (*Adapted from H. B. Taussig, "Congenital Malformations of the Heart," 2d ed., Harvard University Press, Cambridge, 1960, pp. 77–79.*)

shunt at the atrial level, with some elevation of the right atrial pressure. The right atrial pressure is higher than the left atrial pressure if only a foramen ovale is present. Characteristically it is impossible to advance the catheter into the right ventricle because of the tricuspid atresia. Selective angiocardiography establishes the diagnosis by demonstrating flow of blood from the right atrium to the left atrium and into the left ventricle.

DIAGNOSIS. Diagnosis can be reasonably well estab-

lished from the combination of clinical cyanosis with left ventricular hypertrophy shown on the electrocardiogram. The usual differential diagnosis is from tetralogy of Fallot or from transposition of the great vessels, with the electrocardiogram and other clinical features providing the best diagnostic clues. Confirmation can be obtained by catheterization and angiography.

TREATMENT. As the malformation is often incompatible with life once the ductus arteriosus closes, emergency operations in infants undergoing cyanotic spells are often necessary. In the rare patient who survives the first year of life without operation, the presence of cyanosis and severe retardation of growth are the usual indications for operation.

Operative Procedures. With this severe malformation, most operative efforts have been to provide effective palliation for a few years. The long-term results have been uncertain. Some encouragement, however, came from the initial report by Fontan in 1971 of a more effective corrective procedure, inserting a valve conduit between the right atrium and pulmonary artery in older children. The importance of palliative procedures has been enhanced, as, if successful, these procedures may support the patient for several years until the child is large enough for a Fontan-type operation or some other more effective corrective procedure.

In infants and small children, the Potts type of aortopulmonary shunt seems to provide the best results over several years, probably because of the gradual enlargement in size of the Potts anastomosis. These data were well demonstrated in an analysis of Williams et al., in 1975, of experiences with 104 patients in Toronto with different types of shunts. The results seem superior to those obtained from either the subclavian–pulmonary anastomosis or the aortopulmonary anastomosis. A similar preference for the Potts anastomosis was reported by Kyger and associates in 1975 in a series of 105 patients operated on.

The cable-pulmonary shunt developed by Glenn provides excellent palliation for 5 to 7 years and is most effective in older children (Fig. 18-46). Its future after this time, as collateral circulation enlarges, is uncertain. It has the distinct advantage of not increasing cardiac work. Hence, if there are signs of cardiac failure, this should be considered the procedure of choice.

Postoperative Course. The risk of operation in infants is significant because of the severity of the malformation; an operative mortality of 10 to 20 percent is common. Long-term evaluation of patients surviving operation has shown substantial improvement in 60 to 70 percent. In the next

few years more effective and sustained results may be obtained with valve-conduit procedures of the Fontan type.

RARE MALFORMATIONS

Cor Triatriatum

Cor triatriatum is a rare malformation. In 1960 a review by Niwayama found only 36 cases, and in 1965 McGuire et al. stated that only about 10 cases had been recognized in adult patients.

PATHOLOGIC ANATOMY. The anomaly results from incomplete absorption of the embryonic common pulmonary vein into the left atrium, so that it remains as an additional cardiac chamber superior and posterior to the normal left atrium. The pulmonary veins enter this accessory chamber, which communicates with the left atrium through a tiny opening, often only 3 to 4 mm in diameter. The mitral valve and atrial appendage are normal. The foramen ovale almost always opens into the left atrium and not into the accessory chamber.

CLINICAL MANIFESTATIONS. The disease is a severe one, with rapid progression of pulmonary congestion, pulmonary hypertension, and heart failure. Over 50 percent of affected infants do not survive the first year of life. Symptoms are identical to those of mitral stenosis, although in the few older patients who have been studied, hemoptysis has been an unusually prominent feature. On physical

Fig. 18-46. Anastomosis between superior vena cava and right pulmonary artery. *A.* Tangential clamp has been applied to superior vena cava to include origin of azygos vein. Right pulmonary artery has been divided, and end-to-end anastomosis will be constructed. *B.* Posterior row of anastomosis is constructed with continuous 5-0 silk suture. *C.* Completed posterior row of anastomosis. *D.* Anterior row of anastomosis is constructed with interrupted sutures to permit growth of anastomosis. After removal of occluding clamps, superior vena cava is doubly ligated at point of juncture with right atrium. (*Adapted from W. W. L. Glenn, N Engl J Med, 259:117, 1958.*)

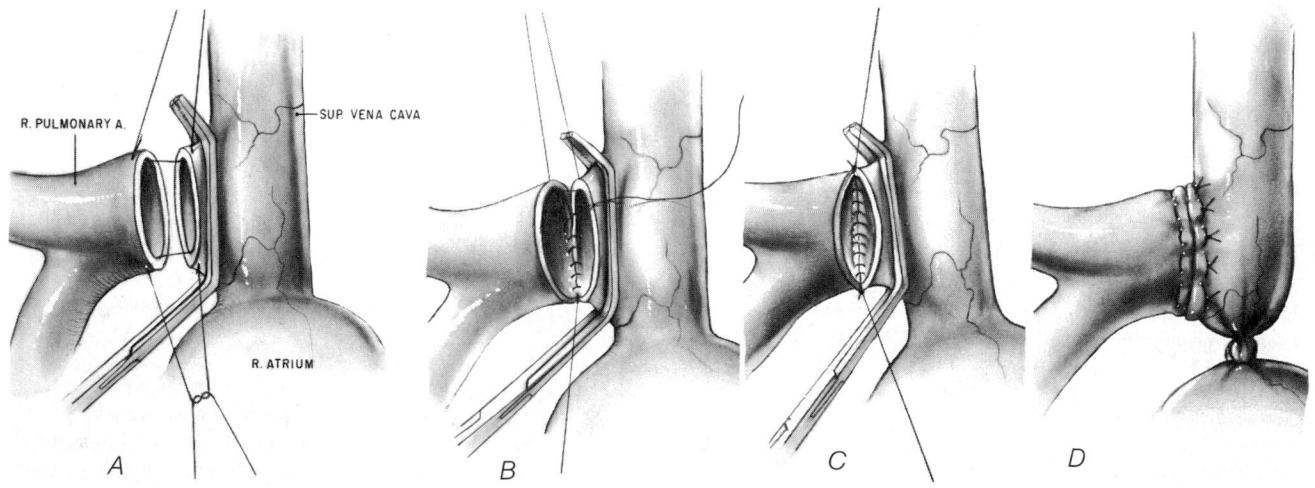

R. PULMONARY A.

SUP. VENA CAVA

R. ATRIUM

A   *B*   *C*   *D*

examination a typical diastolic rumbling murmur of mitral stenosis is usually not present, although a systolic murmur is audible. The absence of a typical murmur, combined with the presence of a sinus rhythm, should raise the suspicion that something other than mitral stenosis is present. A forceful impulse may be palpable in the left parasternal area because of marked right ventricular hypertrophy.

LABORATORY FINDINGS. The roentgenogram shows pulmonary congestion with enlargement of the right ventricle, and the electrocardiogram shows right ventricular hypertrophy. The diagnosis can be established at catheterization by the finding of elevated pulmonary artery pressure as well as an increased wedge pressure (often 25 to 30 mm Hg), *combined with a normal pressure in the left atrium.* Selective angiocardiography will disclose the accessory chamber superior and posterior to the normal left atrium.

DIAGNOSTIC CONSIDERATIONS. By far the most common condition that obstructs flow of blood from the pulmonary veins into the left ventricle is mitral stenosis. In the differential diagnosis, however, three rare conditions should be considered: stenosis of the pulmonary veins, cor triatriatum and supravalvular stenosing ring of the left atrium. Although all these are rare, if they are recognized, surgical treatment is relatively simple. With the precise diagnostic catheterization and angiographic methods now available, it may be hoped that earlier diagnosis and successful treatment will be reported more frequently in the next few years than it has in the past.

TREATMENT. Operation should be performed as soon as the diagnosis is established, because most patients succumb to cardiac failure at an early age. Although a successful operation was performed by Lewis and one by Vineberg in 1956, the collective review published in 1960 by Niwayama found a total of only five successful operations at that time. In 1964 Grondin et al. reported experiences with six cases, four of whom had been operated upon, with three survivors.

The operative procedure is theoretically a simple one, consisting of enlarging the small opening between the accessory atrium and the normal left atrium. It should ideally be performed with cardiopulmonary bypass, to permit extensive excision of the obstructing membrane. The few reported survivors have been asymptomatic.

Congenital Mitral Stenosis

Congenital mitral stenosis is a rare lesion which frequently results in congestive heart failure and death in the first year of life. Ferencz et al., in 1954, found 34 patients previously reported and described nine additional cases. Nadas has studied five cases, and Daoud and associates in 1963 described experiences with seven. In 1967 Tsuji et al. stated that 131 cases had been reported. Two additional patients who had been successfully operated upon were described, making a total of 41 patients operated upon with 21 known survivors.

In 1975 Khalil reported operative experiences with nine patients at the Ohio State University Hospital, with five

survivors, and in 1976, Carpentier reported an extensive experience with 47 children with congenital mitral lesions, in 14 of whom mitral stenosis was the dominant finding.

PATHOLOGIC ANATOMY. The wide spectrum of abnormalities which may be found is well described in the excellent report by Carpentier, probably the most extensive experience in the world with congenital mitral valve abnormalities. The abnormalities present include commissural fusion, abnormalities in the development of the leaflets (such as a parachute valve), and defects in the chordae tendinae and papillary muscles.

If the leaflets are well developed, commissurotomy and a reconstructive procedure may be feasible. With severe abnormalities, valve replacement may be necessary. In the extensive experience reported by Carpentier, valve reconstruction was possible in 38 patients, while valve replacement was necessary in 9. In most reports, valve replacement has been required much more frequently.

CLINICAL MANIFESTATIONS. Symptoms often appear in infancy, with dyspnea, pulmonary congestion, and repeated pneumonic infections. In milder forms of stenosis, symptoms may appear only in later childhood. On physical examination an apical diastolic rumbling murmur is almost always found and provides the best clue to the diagnosis. A thrill is also frequent. An associated systolic murmur, probably from concomitant mitral insufficiency, is common. Sinus rhythm is usually present.

LABORATORY FINDINGS. The main abnormality on the chest roentgenogram is enlargement of the left atrium, with some associated enlargement of the right ventricle. The electrocardiogram will demonstrate right ventricular hypertrophy and right axis deviation. On cardiac catheterization the diagnosis can be confirmed by the finding of an elevated pulmonary artery pressure and pulmonary capillary pressure. Selective angiography may outline the dilated left atrium.

TREATMENT. Operation should be avoided in infancy or early childhood because of the complexity of prosthetic valve replacement, which may be required in the young child. However, severe symptoms may necessitate operation at an early age. The excellent article by Carpentier should be consulted for the techniques of mitral valve reconstruction which he has employed. If a prosthetic valve is inserted, replacement with a larger prosthesis will almost certainly be necessary within a few years.

Aortic-Pulmonary Window

Several terms have been applied to this rare anomaly, including *aortopulmonary fenestration, aorticopulmonary fistula,* and *aortic septal defect.* It is an unusual lesion and has been recognized only with the development of diagnostic and surgical techniques for patent ductus arteriosus. In a group of 100 patients with a diagnosis of patent ductus arteriosus, 1 will usually be found to have an aortic-pulmonary window. A comprehensive report by Skall-Jensen in 1958 found 62 cases in the medical literature. One case was successfully treated by ligation by Gross in 1948, and another was treated by division and suture by Scott and

Sabiston in 1951 (Fig. 18-47), but correction with extracorporeal circulation is now the preferred procedure. Three such patients were reported by Cooley et al. in 1957. In 1962, Morrow and associates found 71 reported cases, 27 of whom had been operated upon. In 1976 Clark reported experiences with seven patients, all surviving operation. In five, the defect was closed with a Dacron patch through a transaortic approach, which was considered to be the best surgical technique.

PATHOLOGIC ANATOMY. Embryologically, the defect results from incomplete development of the spiral septum dividing the primitive truncus arteriosus into the aorta and the pulmonary artery. Persistent truncus arteriosus is a more severe malformation of similar cause but represents incomplete development of both the spiral septum in the truncus arteriosus and the bulbar septum in the bulbus cordis. In persistent truncus arteriosus there is both a ventricular septal defect and a failure of formation of the separate aortic and pulmonic valves, while in aortic-pulmonary window the aortic and pulmonic valves are normally formed, although a separate ventricular septal defect has been found in some patients.

The opening, or "window," between the aorta and the pulmonary artery may vary in diameter from 5 to 30 mm. It may be located proximally near the ostia of the coronary arteries and the pulmonic valve, or it may be as much as 2 cm distal to these structures.

PATHOPHYSIOLOGY. The defect produces a large left-to-right shunt similar to that of a patent ductus arteriosus. The course is a more malignant one, however, because the shunt is usually larger than that seen in the usual patent ductus, resulting in the rapid development of pulmonary hypertension, increase in pulmonary vascular resistance, and cardiac failure.

CLINICAL MANIFESTATIONS. The clinical findings may be identical to those found in patent ductus arteriosus, with a continuous murmur, wide pulse pressure, left ventricular enlargement, and pulmonary congestion. Often only a systolic murmur is present, however, because of severe pulmonary hypertension. Usually the condition is diagnosed as patent ductus arteriosus until cardiac catheterization, angiography, or surgical exploration discloses the correct diagnosis.

LABORATORY FINDINGS. At catheterization the findings are identical to those with a patent ductus arteriosus unless the cardiac catheter can be manipulated through the defect into the aorta, in which case the catheter takes a characteristic course to enter either the ascending aorta or the innominate artery; in patent ductus arteriosus, the catheter enters the aorta distal to the left subclavian artery and usually goes into the descending thoracic aorta. This observation of the course of the catheter can visually establish the diagnosis.

Angiography can also confirm the diagnosis, demonstrating dye flowing from the aorta into the pulmonary artery near the aortic valve rather than in the usual location distal to the left subclavian artery.

DIAGNOSIS. Differential diagnosis must exclude persistent truncus arteriosus, ventricular septal defect with a prolapsed aortic cusp, and patent ductus arteriosus. The exact diagnosis can be made only upon cardiac catheterization and angiography.

TREATMENT. Usually operation should be performed as soon as the diagnosis has been established, because irreversible changes in pulmonary vascular resistance develop rapidly. There is a paucity of data about the natural history of the disease because of its rarity and recent recognition, but irreversible changes in the pulmonary arterioles have been seen as early as three or four years of age. The author has had one three-year-old patient who died within a few hours from elevated pulmonary vascular resistance following an uncomplicated division and suture of a large aortic-pulmonary window with extracorporeal circulation, and Gross has reported similar experiences with two patients.

Operation should be performed with extracorporeal circulation because of the unpredictable variation in friability of the vascular structures. Once cardiopulmonary

Fig. 18-47. Aortic-pulmonary fistula, showing large communication between aorta and pulmonary artery near base of heart. (*Adapted from H. W. Scott and D. C. Sabiston, J Thorac Surg, 25:26, 1953.*)

AORTA

AORTIC-PUL. FISTULA

PUL. A.

R. VENT.

L. VENT.

bypass has been established, the aorta can be occluded distal to the window, lowering the pressure in the pulmonary artery.

The window may then be divided and the aortic and pulmonary openings sutured. If possible, tangential vascular clamps may be applied to the aorta and pulmonary artery at the site of the window before it is divided, but simple division is usually preferable. The main precaution is evacuation of air from the aorta before circulation is reestablished. Shumway has reported an alternate technique of opening the pulmonary artery and suturing the opening without dividing it. The alternate approach of opening the aorta and applying a patch to the opening, suggested by Wright in 1968 and endorsed by Clark, as mentioned earlier, seems to be reasonable.

The risk of operation is proportional to the increase in pulmonary vascular resistance and is probably in the range of 15 to 20 percent. Gross has operated upon seven patients with two fatalities, both in patients who had an elevated pulmonary vascular resistance. Following recovery from operation, prognosis is apparently as favorable as that found with patent ductus arteriosus.

Ruptured Aneurysm of Sinus of Valsalva

This unusual entity produces a distinct syndrome which can be readily diagnosed and effectively treated. Before the advent of extracorporeal circulation it usually caused death from cardiac failure within 1 to 2 years after onset. An aneurysm of the sinus of Valsalva can result from syphilis or other infections; at present most are congenital in origin.

A detailed review by Sawyer et al. in 1957 found 47 patients with congenital aneurysms, but the natural increased interest in diagnosis and therapy which followed the first successful surgical closure in 1956 has led to more widespread recognition. Paton and associates stated in 1965 that since the first operation performed, there had been reports of 91 additional patients operated upon and at least 60 other cases had been described.

PATHOLOGIC ANATOMY. The normal sinus of Valsalva is composed of an aortic valve cusp medially and the aortic wall laterally, which joins the annulus fibrosus of the aortic valve ring inferiorly. In embryonic development the developing ventricular septum inferiorly meets the spiral septum superiorly which separates the aorta and the pulmonary arteries. Incomplete merger of these two structures results in a ventricular septal defect in the membranous septum. An aneurysm of the sinus of Valsalva results from a less severe malformation of the same type, for the media of the aortic wall does not extend down to the annulus of the aortic valve ring. As might be expected, however, an associated ventricular septal defect is often found.

The right coronary sinus is involved in about 70 percent of patients, and rupture occurs into the right ventricle. The noncoronary sinus is involved in about 20 percent of patients, with rupture occurring into the right atrium. Involvement of the left coronary sinus is rare, and rupture into the left atrium or left ventricle is very unusual.

CLINICAL MANIFESTATIONS. Until rupture occurs, an aneurysm of the sinus of Valsalva does not cause any disability, and diagnosis can be made only accidentally during aortography performed for other reasons. The average age at rupture is thirty-one years, although a few such instances have been reported in childhood. Rupture usually occurs without known cause and is soon followed by cardiac failure. Once cardiac failure develops, life expectancy without surgical correction is about 1 year.

At the time of rupture there may be transitory pain in the chest, subsequently followed by dyspnea and palpitation, although in some patients the first symptom is dyspnea. Subsequently other symptoms of congestive heart failure appear. On physical examination, the important abnormality is the characteristic parasternal murmur, often accompanied by a palpable thrill. The murmur may be continuous or may be a to-and-fro murmur with a somewhat louder component in diastole. It is often located somewhat lower than the usual murmur of a ductus arteriosus, being heard in the third, fourth, or fifth parasternal spaces to the right or left of the sternum, depending upon the point of rupture of the aneurysm. The murmur is unusually superficial in location and is widely transmitted. These unusual qualities may lead to the suspicion that it is not arising from the usual patent ductus arteriosus. Other physical findings, including a wide pulse pressure, cardiac enlargement, and pulmonary congestion, resemble those of a patent ductus arteriosus.

LABORATORY FINDINGS. Cardiac enlargement and pulmonary congestion are noted on the roentgenogram, and cardiac hypertrophy on the electrocardiogram. On cardiac catheterization, a left-to-right shunt can be identified at the atrial or ventricular level. Diagnosis is best established by selective aortography, demonstrating the leakage of dye from the aorta into the involved cardiac chamber (Fig. 18-48). The differential diagnosis must exclude patent ductus arteriosus and aortic-pulmonary window.

Fig. 18-48. Aortogram confirms diagnosis of ruptured aneurysm of sinus of Valsalva by demonstrating flow of dye from region of aortic sinuses to right atrium. (*Courtesy of Dr. Raymond M. Abrams, Department of Radiology, New York University Medical Center.*)

Fig. 18-49. Diagram of unusual type of ruptured aneurysm of sinus of Valsalva. Aneurysm arose from left coronary cusp and developed fistulous tract before rupture into right atrium. Operative closure was performed by opening aorta and closing opening directly. (*From Ann Surg, 152:965, 1960.*)

TREATMENT. Operative correction should be performed as soon as the diagnosis has been established. This is done with extracorporeal circulation through a median sternotomy incision. The basic objective at operation is to close the defect in the aortic wall at the mouth of the aneurysm by attaching the aortic media superiorly to the aortic ring below (Fig. 18-49). Although initially operations were usually performed by approaching the lesion through the right atrium or right ventricle, excising the fistulous sac and suturing the opening, a transaortic approach, as suggested by Shumacker et al., permits a more precise closure, assuring adequate repair of the aortic wall without any risk of injury to the aortic valve cusps. The author has seen recurrence of the lesion in one young woman, occurring a few months after the aortic opening was closed by direct suture. With a large opening, transaortic closure with a Dacron patch may be preferable to direct suture. A concomitant ventricular septal defect may frequently be found and repaired at the same operation. The operative risk is small and the results have been excellent.

Truncus Arteriosus

Truncus arteriosus is a rare malformation resulting from failure of division of the fetal arterial channel into the aorta and pulmonary arteries and the left and right ventricles. Therapy of this condition is a good example of the rapid changes in cardiac surgery. When the first edition of this book was written in 1969, only palliative therapy was possible. Since that time McGoon and associates have developed a technique of surgical correction with an aortic homograft which has been successfully applied to a significant number of patients.

PATHOLOGIC ANATOMY. In this condition the entire circulation, including the coronary arteries, the pulmonary arteries, and the systemic arteries, arises from a common arterial trunk. There is always a ventricular septal defect, and a single ventricle occurs in 15 to 20 percent of patients. Only one semilunar valve is present, usually with four cusps, although the number may vary from two to six. Four anatomic types of truncus have been described, according to how the pulmonary arteries arise from the aorta. These are well illustrated in the publication by Poirier in 1975 (Fig. 18-50).

"Pseudotruncus" has been used by some to describe a condition in which a single large artery originates from the base of the heart, but the pulmonary arteries are absent and pulmonary blood flows through enlarged bronchial vessels. Others consider the condition as pulmonary atresia or a variant of severe tetralogy of Fallot.

PATHOPHYSIOLOGY. The disability with this condition is a severe one, with 70 to 80 percent of infants dying within the first year of life, usually from congestive heart failure. Incompetence of the truncal valve contributes to death in many of this group.

As blood entering the aorta is a mixture of blood from the systemic circulation and the pulmonary circulation, arterial oxygen unsaturation is always present, the degree varying with the volume of pulmonary blood flow. If large pulmonary arteries originate from the aorta, initially there is a large pulmonary blood flow with minimal cyanosis. Subsequently there is a progressive rise in pulmonary vascular resistance with diminution of pulmonary blood flow and increase in cyanosis. Hence the degree of cyanosis is directly related to the volume of pulmonary blood flow. Severe pulmonary vascular disease develops rapidly in

Fig. 18-50. Four anatomic types of truncus arteriosus. (*From R. A. Poirier et al., J Thorac Cardiovasc Surg, 69:169, 1975.*)

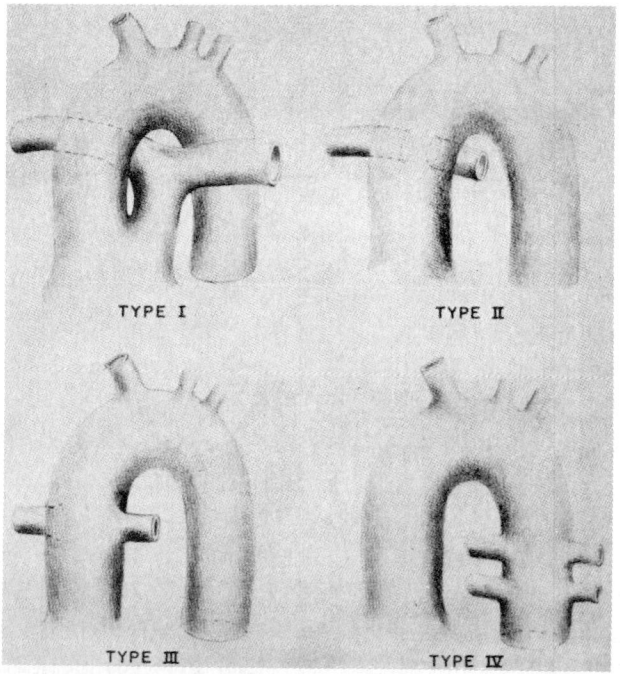

many patients, some of whom probably become inoperable before 2 to 3 years of age.

CLINICAL MANIFESTATIONS. Disability is evident in infancy, with cyanosis and dyspnea on exertion and retardation of growth and development. On physical examination, loud systolic and diastolic murmurs are audible over the base of the heart, often as a to-and-fro murmur rather than a true continuous murmur. In older children, continuous murmurs may be best heard over one or both lungs, originating from collateral circulation to the lungs; as emphasized by Taussig, this is virtually diagnostic of the malformation. The second heart sound is "pure" and increased in intensity.

LABORATORY FINDINGS. The chest roentgenogram and electrocardiogram show both right and left ventricular enlargement. Cardiac catheterization will demonstrate a left-to-right shunt in the ventricle with a systolic pulmonary artery pressure equal to aortic systolic pressure. The abnormal vessels can be outlined with selective angiography, but precise studies are required to demonstrate with certainty the exact point of origin of the pulmonary arteries.

In acyanotic children the condition must be differentiated from patent ductus arteriosus or an aortic-pulmonary window. With severe cyanosis, pulmonary atresia, tricuspid atresia, and transposition of the great vessels must be considered.

TREATMENT. The operation developed by McGoon et al. consists of construction of a new pulmonary artery with a valved conduit, preferably a Dacron tube with a glutaraldehyde preserved porcine heterograft (Hancock prosthesis). Employing extracorporeal circulation, the pulmonary arteries are detached from the aorta. The right ventricle is then opened in the outflow tract. The ventricular septal defect is then closed so that the aorta originates only from the left ventricle. The homograft with the aortic valve is then attached to the opening in the right ventricle, and distally is connected to the right and left pulmonary arteries, creating a new pulmonary artery.

Operative mortality has been low in the selective group of patients operated upon between five and ten years of age, in whom the pulmonary vascular resistance is less than 0.6 percent of systemic vascular resistance. However, this is a selective group of patients because, as indicated earlier, there is both a high mortality in infancy and also rapid development of irreversible pulmonary vascular disease in many. These considerations were well reviewed in the reports by Poirier in 1975 and by Applebaum in 1976.

Banding of the pulmonary arteries in infancy to protect the pulmonary vascular bed has a surprisingly high mortality, nearly 50 percent from different reports according to Applebaum, and also a significant mortality at the time of attempted correction at a later date. Hence the increasing tendency is to perform corrective surgery with a valve conduit at an earlier age, probably between two and three years, or in the first years of life if symptoms are severe. This has been accomplished in several patients described by Ebert in 1976.

When a conduit is inserted in such small children, it will have to be replaced as the child grows older; however,

Marcelletti and McGoon reported in 1976 that 22 aortic homograft conduits had been successfully replaced with a Dacron conduit.

Single Ventricle

A single ventricle is a rare, severe malformation for which corrective surgery has only recently become possible with the construction of a new ventricular septum [Malm]. Nadas found only 10 cases in a group of 577 patients.

PATHOLOGIC ANATOMY. The anomaly consists of a single functioning ventricular chamber into which both atrioventricular valves enter. Connected to the functioning ventricle is a rudimentary outlet chamber located in the position normally occupied by the outflow tract of the right ventricle. From this rudimentary chamber one or both of the great vessels may arise. Transposition of the aorta and pulmonary artery occurs in over one-half the patients. The clinical profile varies widely, depending upon whether or not the arteries are transposed and whether the artery arising from the rudimentary outlet chamber is of normal diameter or hypoplastic.

PATHOPHYSIOLOGY. The two physiologic characteristics are admixture of oxygenated and unoxygenated blood in the common ventricle before entering the aorta, and pulmonary hypertension resulting from origin of the pulmonary artery and the aorta from the same ventricle. The degree of cyanosis depends upon the pulmonary blood flow.

CLINICAL MANIFESTATIONS. Infants with an increased pulmonary blood flow, occurring when the aorta arises from the rudimentary outlet chamber and the pulmonary artery from the functioning ventricle, may be acyanotic but disabled from pulmonary congestion and cardiac failure. Conversely, with a decreased pulmonary blood flow from a hypoplastic pulmonary artery, cyanosis may be severe and the clinical picture dominated by signs of anoxia. Much variation between these two extremes is seen because of other anomalies frequently present. A single ventricle per se is most unusual, for concomitant cardiac malformations are frequent.

The disability is severe and associated with cardiac failure or cyanosis. In a group of 85 patients reviewed by Campbell and associates, over one-half died in the first year of life, although 18 lived to be twenty years of age. On physical examination variable systolic murmurs and cardiac enlargement are found, but variation in the murmurs precludes any diagnostic significance.

LABORATORY FINDINGS. The roentgenogram demonstrates cardiac enlargement, and the electrocardiogram shows left or right ventricular hypertrophy. Great variation is present, depending upon the relation of the aorta and pulmonary artery to the common ventricle and the rudimentary outlet chamber. The best diagnostic information is obtained on cardiac catheterization, with a rise in oxygen concentration of 4 to 5 vol % noted when a catheter is advanced from the atrium into the common ventricle. Similar pressures may be found in the aorta and pulmonary artery. Selective angiography may demonstrate the rudimentary outlet chamber.

TREATMENT. In the past few years, single ventricle has been successfully corrected in a few selected cases by construction of a new ventricular septum. To avoid complete heart block, the course of the conduction bundle should be electrically mapped at the time of operation as noted by Malm. Though experience thus far is limited, it indicates the ever-widening horizon of possibilities of correction of anomalies which in the past could only be treated by palliative methods.

Ebstein's Anomaly

This peculiar and unusual anomaly was described by Wilhelm Ebstein in 1866 following postmortem examination of a nineteen-year-old cyanotic youth who had died with signs of tricuspid insufficiency. Although the anomaly is uncommon, with improvement in cardiac diagnostic techniques it has been recognized with increased frequency. Vacca and associates in 1958 found the total number of cases reported to be 108. The cause is unknown.

PATHOLOGIC ANATOMY. The anomaly consists of a downward displacement of part of the tricuspid valve, creating a third chamber in the right side of the heart. Usually the anterior leaflet of the tricuspid valve arises normally from the tricuspid annulus and may be abnormally large and prominent. It has been described as saillike. The septal and posterior leaflets, however, are not attached to the normal tricuspid annulus but arise from the wall of the right ventricle at a varying distance from the true annulus. These two cusps may be small and adherent to the wall of the ventricle, with little functional ability (Fig. 18-51). The segment of right ventricular wall between the true annulus of the tricuspid valve and the origin of the displaced leaflets is then functionally a part of the right atrium and has been termed the *atrialized* ventricle. The wall of this part of the ventricle may be unusually thin. The foramen ovale is usually patent, and often an atrial septal defect is also present.

The malformation varies widely in severity, depending upon the relative size of the atrialized ventricle above the tricuspid valve and the functioning right ventricle below the abnormal valve. The anatomic spectrum of malforma-

tions which may be seen has been well illustrated by Taussig.

PATHOPHYSIOLOGY. The main physiologic disturbance is inadequate cardiac output from the right ventricle. This is probably due to both the tricuspid insufficiency and the paradoxic contraction of the atrialized segment of the right ventricle. Less significant causes are the small size of the functioning right ventricle and the frequent arrhythmias. With the low cardiac output and tricuspid insufficiency, the right atrium becomes massively dilated, and cyanosis of moderate degree is usually present because of a right-to-left shunt through the foramen ovale. The cyanosis tends to become more severe in later years of life, probably because of progressive right ventricular failure.

CLINICAL MANIFESTATIONS. The clinical course is often a severe one, although some adults survive for many years. Analysis of reported cases has found that about 40 percent of patients die in the first decade and 30 percent in the next. Death occurs from congestive failure in about one-third of patients, and at least another third may die suddenly from an arrhythmia.

The predominant symptoms are fatigue, with gradual increase in exertional dyspnea and cyanosis over the years. Symptoms may be present in some patients during early childhood, while in others they appear only after the first decade. Signs of right-sided failure gradually become more evident. Physical examination discloses soft, blurred systolic and diastolic murmurs along the left sternal border,

Fig. 18-51. *A.* Normal heart showing septal and posterior leaflets of tricuspid valve. *B.* Pathologic anatomy in Ebstein's malformation, with displacement of diminutive septal and posterior leaflets down into normal right ventricular cavity. Large anterior leaflet is not shown. *C.* Abnormal pathologic anatomy in Ebstein's malformation. There is large "saillike" anterior leaflet with hypoplastic septal and posterior leaflets, which are often displaced downward into ventricle, creating third cardiac chamber interposed between right atrium and functioning right ventricle. (*Adapted from K. L. Hardy et al., J Thorac Cardiovasc Surg, 48:931, 1964.*)

A   *B*   *C*

with muffled heart sounds and signs of feeble, ineffective cardiac contractions. The cardiac size is usually increased. The findings have been appropriately compared to those with a large pericardial effusion. Cyanosis and clubbing may be found but are usually not severe.

Nadas has stated that the auscultatory findings are pathognomonic of the condition. He emphasizes three findings: a slow cardiac rate with a triple or quadruple rhythm, a systolic murmur of tricuspid regurgitation, and frequently a low-pitched diastolic murmur.

LABORATORY FINDINGS. The roentgenogram may be remarkable for the great enlargement of the right side of the heart, including a huge right atrium and the atrialized part of the right ventricle. The pulmonary artery segment is often small, and the vascularity in the lung fields is less than normal. On fluoroscopy, feeble cardiac contractions are frequently seen. The electrocardiographic findings are also considered to be typical. Conduction disturbances with prolonged P-R interval and partial right bundle branch block are common. Right ventricular hypertrophy is absent after infancy, but the left chest leads show average potentials.

Cardiac catheterization may be hazardous; deaths from arrhythmias have occurred in several laboratories. Alertness to the possibility, however, in combination with use of electric defibrillators, has greatly decreased the risk of catheterization. With catheterization, a right-to-left shunt at the atrial level, with resulting arterial hypoxemia, is found in 25 to 50 percent of patients. Interestingly enough, the contour of the right atrial pressure wave may not be strikingly abnormal, perhaps because of the damping effect of the large cavity of the right atrium on the blood regurgitating through the incompetent tricuspid orifice. The abnormal course of the cardiac catheter in the atrialized part of the right ventricle can be of diagnostic significance, and with selective angiography, the huge right atrium can be outlined. Diagnosis can usually be made with certainty on the basis of the typical physical findings, combined with the abnormalities observed on the roentgenogram and electrocardiogram and those found at cardiac catheterization.

TREATMENT. A suggestion made by Hunter and Lillihei in 1958 to exclude the atrialized ventricle from the circulation seemingly remains sound, but there is a disappointing lack of data demonstrating good surgical results. Hardy and associates reported one successful operation in 1964 and Bahnson and associates two additional operations in 1965. Hardy subsequently operated on a few additional patients. Replacement of the abnormal valve with a prosthetic valve was performed by Barnard, and Timmis and associates combined prosthetic replacement with elimination of the atrialized ventricle in one patient.

Surprisingly little progress has been made in the surgical treatment of Ebstein's disease since the previous edition of this textbook. The report by MacPaul from the Mayo Clinic in 1976, summarizing experiences with 16 patients, expresses the continuing uncertainty about indications for operation as well as the best method of approach. Five patients had valve replacement performed, but only one survived, while much better results were obtained with

tricuspid annuloplasty and plication of the atrialized segment. However, two of seven patients who survived operation died suddenly with arrhythmias at a later date.

The four basic problems with Ebstein's anomaly are the insufficiency of the right ventricle from the atrialized segment, tricuspid insufficiency, arrhythmias, and the atrial septal defect. The atrial septal defect is surely the least important, except for the occasional instance of paradoxical embolization, although this is the mechanism of cyanosis in these patients, permitting right-to-left shunting if the right ventricle fails.

It seems clear that there is wide variation in the pathologic anatomy, making individualization of different patients necessary, as emphasized by Bahnson. A second therapeutic point is that the atrialized segment of the right ventricle must be appropriately treated if it is enwalled and moves paradoxically, treating this either by excision or by plication. On the other hand, if the segment is thick-walled with little paradoxical motion, treatment may not be necessary. This variation in the severity of the atrialized segment may explain the finding in some patients that valve replacement alone is sufficient, while in others it has promptly resulted in a fatality, perhaps because the incompetent right ventricle could no longer decompress through the insufficient tricuspid valve.

An additional therapeutic point is the malignant nature of the arrhythmias of some patients. Possibly earlier operation before right atrial hypertrophy becomes severe might be helpful, but this is only a hypothesis. Helpful advances in electrical mapping of the abnormal pathways are another possibility. A third possibility is that prostheses used in the past may have contributed to subsequent arrhythmias as the right ventricle decreases in size, as has been seen with other complications with ball-valve prostheses in the tricuspid position. Hence the tricuspid prosthesis of choice at present would seem to be a heterograft. An alternative approach is a form of annuloplasty, perhaps employing the Carpentier ring in severe cases.

Anomalies of the Coronary Arteries

ANOMALOUS ORIGIN OF LEFT CORONARY ARTERY FROM PULMONARY ARTERY

The first case of this unusual malformation was described by Abrikosov in 1911, but little clinical interest evolved until Bland et al. in 1933 described the clinical features of the syndrome and emphasized its similarity to myocardial infarction in adults. Over 50 cases were reviewed by Keith in 1959. A significant advance was made by Sabiston et al. in 1959 when they conclusively demonstrated retrograde flow of blood from the anomalous left coronary artery into the pulmonary artery, a theoretical possibility previously mentioned by several investigators. Subsequently, in two older children, four and five years of age, the ideal operation was accomplished by Cooley and associates, who detached the coronary artery from the pulmonary artery and connected it to the aorta by means of an interposed graft (Fig. 18-52).

PATHOLOGIC ANATOMY AND PHYSIOLOGY. The disease

Fig. 18-52. *A.* Anomalous left coronary artery arising from pulmonary artery. *B.* Vein graft is used to anastomose coronary artery to aorta. This theoretically ideal operation has rarely been accomplished as yet. (*Adapted from D. A. Cooley et al., J Thorac Cardiovasc Surg, 52:805, 1966.*)

is a severe one, and the majority of affected children die in the first year of life. The left ventricle is usually grossly dilated, with a thin fibrotic wall showing multiple areas of infarction. Other abnormalities are secondary to chronic congestive failure. Apparently the serious physiologic handicap from origin of the left coronary artery from the pulmonary artery is the low perfusion pressure and not the low oxygen content of blood in the coronary artery, because even more severe degrees of oxygen unsaturation in severely cyanotic children do not produce gross injury to the muscle of the left ventricle. The demonstration that the flow of blood may be retrograde through the coronary artery into the pulmonary artery indicates that the anomaly actually siphons oxygenated blood away from the ischemic myocardium. Retrograde flow is proved by finding a higher oxygen content in blood in the coronary artery than in the pulmonary artery, and also by demonstrating a *rise* in pressure in the coronary artery when its origin from the pulmonary artery is occluded. Survival of a few patients beyond infancy apparently results from an abundant collateral circulation with the right coronary artery, so that the left ventricle is supplied with blood first entering the right coronary artery and then flowing through collateral

channels into tributaries of the left coronary artery. Anomalous origin of the *right* coronary artery from the pulmonary artery is apparently an innocuous condition and compatible with normal longevity.

CLINICAL MANIFESTATIONS. Dyspnea and other symptoms often appear in the first 3 months of life. Characteristically, acute episodes may occur with feeding, between which the infant is completely normal. During these episodes there may be colicky pain, tachypnea, cyanosis, pallor, and sweating, apparently a syndrome resembling angina pectoris. Subsequently, with chronic congestive failure, tachypnea becomes a chronic symptom. On examination, obvious cardiac enlargement is found, with muffled heart sounds. Frequently no murmurs are audible.

LABORATORY FINDINGS. The chest roentgenogram will confirm the extensive enlargement of the ventricle. The electrocardiogram may be diagnostic, demonstrating inversion of the T waves and prominent Q waves in certain precordial leads. The diagnosis can be confirmed by catheterization and coronary arteriography, demonstrating the abnormal origin of the left coronary artery, a small left-to-right shunt at the level of the pulmonary artery, and dilatation of the left ventricle, often with a thin wall from multiple infarctions. On angiography the right coronary artery in older children will be dilated and tortuous, with dye filling the right coronary artery and subsequently opacifying the left coronary artery.

TREATMENT. Patients should obviously be operated on as soon as the condition is recognized, for it is frequently lethal in the first year of life. Ligation of the anomalous coronary artery can be done if reconstruction is not feasible. One study by Likar and associates of 27 patients who underwent ligation of anomalous artery included 20 infants, 11 of whom died after operation; but this report, published in 1966, is surely not representative of what might be achieved with present techniques.

With present techniques of microsurgery it would seem that reconstruction should be possible in the majority of infants, using the "button" concept of detaching the anomalous left coronary artery from the pulmonary artery with a button of wall of the pulmonary artery to facilitate reconstruction. This is well discussed in the 1976 report by Doty of reconstruction in a ten-month-old child.

Cooley first demonstrated possibilities with vein-graft reconstruction of the coronary artery and in 1975 summarized his experiences with 15 patients. Though initial results have been good, long-term results with the saphenous vein graft are disappointing, probably because of the disproportion in size.

The subclavian artery would seem far preferable and at present would seem to be the ideal graft. As discussed in the report by Doty, this has been used in a variety of methods, mobilizing either the left subclavian or the right subclavian artery as in the classic subclavian–pulmonary anastomosis.

The author has successfully used a free graft of subclavian artery in one patient, placing the free arterial graft *behind* the pulmonary artery, rather than in front, which makes it possible to use a much smaller graft. A similar technique has been reported by Bahnson. Hence, at present, although few data are available, the ideal form of reconstruction would seem to be detachment of the anomalous coronary with a button of arterial wall, followed by anastomosis to the subclavian artery, either directly to the mobilized subclavian artery or as a free graft of subclavian artery, placing the subclavian graft behind the pulmonary artery, if the graft is too short to reach the aorta otherwise.

CORONARY ARTERIOVENOUS FISTULA

Information concerning this unusual anomaly was crystallized in 1960 by Gasul and associates in their collective review of 52 cases.

PATHOLOGIC ANATOMY AND PHYSIOLOGY. The abnormality consists of a direct communication between a coronary artery and a cardiac chamber through one or more abnormal openings. Usually the coronary fistula opens into the right atrium or right ventricle, constituting a left-to-right shunt. Rarely it enters the left atrium or left ventricle, causing signs of mild aortic insufficiency. With the increased blood flow through the arteriovenous fistula there is dilatation of the coronary arteries, which become progressively elongated and tortuous (Fig. 18-53). Astonishing degrees of dilatation, with vessels 1 to 2 cm in diameter, have been reported.

When the fistula opens into the right side of the heart, the resulting left-to-right shunt is small, but with subsequent dilatation of the parent artery the shunt may eventually become large enough to cause significant cardiac enlargement.

CLINICAL MANIFESTATIONS. Although the arteriovenous fistula may cause myocardial ischemia from blood preferentially flowing through the fistula rather than through the myocardial capillaries, this is uncommon. Several patients with minor hemodynamic disability have been reported living normal lives without symptoms. When the fistula is large, however, significant cardiac symptoms appear, both from the left-to-right shunt and from the myocardial ischemia.

The most common symptoms are fatigue and dyspnea. On physical examination the significant finding is a continuous murmur that seems unusually loud and superficial, especially in combination with absence of symptoms and minimal signs of cardiac disability. The location of maximal intensity of the murmur varies with the site of the fistula; it usually is at a lower level than that of the typical patent ductus arteriosus.

LABORATORY FINDINGS. The chest roentgenogram may be normal or may show only slight cardiac enlargement. Similarly, the electrocardiogram may be normal or may show minimal signs of ventricular hypertrophy. Cardiac catheterization can detect the site of the left-to-right shunt and thereby identify the chamber into which the fistula empties. The most definitive study is coronary arteriography, outlining both the site of the fistula and the course of the abnormal vessels. The degree of dilatation and tortuosity in some patients is most impressive.

TREATMENT. If a patient is asymptomatic with no signs of cardiac disability, operation is not urgent. Some have been managed simply by continued observation. However, as the usual course is continued enlargement of the fistula,

Fig. 18-53. Arteriovenous fistula of right coronary artery. Enlarged, tortuous right coronary artery is clearly visible over surface of right ventricle. Fistulous communication directly into right ventricle was found, as illustrated by ligatures, and ligated.

with progressive hemodynamic disability, elective repair is preferable in most instances (Fig. 18-54).

A 1971 review by Oldham et al. well summarized clinical experiences. In a review of over 200 reported cases, including their own personal experiences with 12 cases, 183 of the fistulas entered the right side of the heart, and only 17 entered one of the chambers of the left side. A significant point facilitating surgical treatment is the fact that almost all fistulas had a single, rather than multiple, point of entry into the heart. The shunt was seldom large, with the pulmonary blood flow usually increased to about twice normal. Congestive heart failure appeared in two age groups, either in infancy or after forty years of age. The latter group probably resulted from progressive enlargement of the fistula. However, in the overall series there was a history of congestive heart failure in only 14 percent of the patients, and angina in 7 percent.

Precise coronary angiography has greatly facilitated treatment. The single point of entry of the fistula can be identified by angiography. Surgical dissection in this area can often locate the abnormal vessel and occlude it but preserve continuity of the involved coronary artery. Of 116 reported cases undergoing operation, only four deaths have occurred.

Little change in the status of the treatment of coronary arteriovenous fistula has occurred since 1974. The author has treated one patient over fifty years of age with congestive heart failure who has subsequently remained asymptomatic in the three years since occlusion of the fistula. A few other patients have been treated at New York University with an uneventful course. In all instances it has been possible to isolate the fistula and occlude it by the combination of precise angiography and appropriate dissection at operation, maintaining continuity of the involved coronary

A

B

Fig. 18-54. *A.* Operative photograph of the tortuous coronary vessels with a coronary arteriovenous fistula in a woman in the fifth decade who was virtually asymptomatic. *B.* Operative photograph of the site of entry of the fistula into the right ventricle near the apex of the heart. This was eliminated by simple ligature.

artery. Sudden death has been reported months following closure of a fistula in a patient with large dilated coronary arteries, presumably a case of arrhythmia. This may constitute an additional indication for early operation in these patients, once the diagnosis has been made, as the risk of operation is small and the results excellent.

Corrected Transposition

This unusual anomaly has been studied in detail in recent years, principally because of the influence of its unusual anatomic features on the surgical treatment of associated cardiovascular malformations. The clinical features of the syndrome were well summarized by Anderson et al. in their report of 14 patients in 1957. An additional group of 33 cases was reported by Schiebler and associates in 1961.

PATHOLOGIC ANATOMY AND PHYSIOLOGY. In this malformation the aorta and pulmonary artery are transposed to lie in a relation exactly the opposite of that normally occurring. The aorta arises from the anterior left border of the heart and the pulmonary artery from the right and posterior area of the heart (Fig. 18-55). The ventricle from which the aorta arises has the anatomic characteristics of a normal trabeculated right ventricle, and that from which the pulmonary artery arises resembles a left ventricle. The atrioventricular valves are similarly reversed, with the tricuspid valve opening into the aortic ventricle and the mitral valve opening into the pulmonary ventricle. Venous drainage into the atria, however, is normal; so despite the abnormal anatomic relations, the circulation is normal. Venous blood returns to the right atrium, flows through the mitral valve into an anatomic "left" ventricle, and is expelled into the pulmonary artery. From the lungs blood returns through the pulmonary veins to the left atrium, flows across a tricuspid valve into an anatomic "right" ventricle, and is expelled into the aorta. The anatomic

relations of the coronary arteries are also reversed, the right coronary artery arising anteriorly and the left coronary artery posteriorly and the noncoronary sinus being located at the anterior left border of the heart.

The significance of the malformation is primarily in the high incidence of associated abnormalities, for some additional malformation is almost always present. Nadas has stated that at least 50 percent of patients with this condition have mitral insufficiency, perhaps as a result of the tricuspid valve being poorly designed to withstand systemic ventricular pressures. A ventricular septal defect is common, and a wide variety of other malformations may be seen. Conduction defects are frequent. Approximately one-third of the patients have a first- to third-degree heart block, and another third have different types of arrhythmias, such as paroxysmal atrial tachycardia.

CLINICAL MANIFESTATIONS. The symptoms are principally determined by the associated malformations. In the unusual case of "pure" corrected transposition, there are no symptoms except for those resulting from the cardiac arrhythmias. Physical examination similarly discloses no abnormalities, except that the cardiac second sound to the left of the sternum is unusually loud because it originates from closure of the aortic valve.

LABORATORY FINDINGS. On the roentgenogram there is an unusual contour at the base of the heart from the unusual relation of the great vessels, but often this is not distinctive enough to be diagnostic. The electrocardiogram is almost always abnormal and is one of the best diagnostic guides. Conduction disturbances, arrhythmias, and unusual

Fig. 18-55. *A.* Normal cardiac anatomy with pulmonary artery arising from right ventricle and aorta from left ventricle. Comparison with *B* shows that in corrected transposition, relative positions of aorta and pulmonary artery are reversed. *B.* In corrected transposition of great vessels, aorta arises anteriorly from ventricle that has anatomic characteristics of right ventricle. Pulmonary artery arises posteriorly and to right of aorta—reverse of normal anatomic arrangement. Insert depicts origin of coronary arteries in corrected transposition. (*Adapted from A. S. Nadas, "Pediatric Cardiology," W. B. Saunders Company, Philadelphia, 1964, p. 714.*)

Fig. 18-56. Diagram of anomalous origin of left pulmonary artery from right pulmonary artery. Anatomic relationship of left pulmonary artery to trachea and esophagus is also shown. (*From F. L. Grover et al., J Thorac Cardiovasc Surg, 69:295, 1975.*)

patterns of ventricular hypertrophy in the precordial leads may all suggest the diagnosis. Diagnosis can be firmly established by angiography, which will demonstrate the aorta to the left of the pulmonary artery.

TREATMENT. The importance of this condition is predominantly related to the other anatomic defects often present. With ventricular septal defect, there is a high frequency of complete heart block, which occurs spontaneously during the course of the disease in some patients but is especially hazardous surgically because of the abnormal location of the conduction bundle. A significant contribution was reported by Waldo et al. in 1975, using electrophysiologic studies to map the course of the conduction bundle and finding the conduction system in the anterior rim of the defect. Clearly, mapping of the conduction bundle should be an important part of surgical operations performed for closure of a septal defect in patients with corrected transposition.

Kirklin and associates have had one of the most exten-

Fig. 18-57. Diagram of anatomy at completion of operation. Note that proximal stump of left pulmonary artery is to right of trachea after having been dissected free. Distal left pulmonary artery has been anastomosed to side of main pulmonary artery. (*From F. L. Grover et al., J Thorac Cardiovasc Surg, 69:295, 1975.*)

sive experiences with operations with corrected transposition, reporting 17 patients in 1976. With tetralogy of Fallot in the presence of corrected transposition, the location of the coronary vessels may preclude use of the usual operative approach, but the insertion of a valve conduit may make surgical correction possible.

In the absence of other anatomic defects, many patients with corrected transposition do well for some decades but subsequently develop mitral insufficiency and may require prosthetic valve replacement at that time.

Double Outlet Right Ventricle

Double outlet right ventricle was not included in the previous edition of this book, but significant advances have been made in the recognition of this anomaly. The classification developed by Van Praagh has been especially useful in recognizing the different variants of this syndrome, with appropriate modifications for effective surgical treatment. The reader is referred to the excellent recent article by Stewart in 1976, a collective review with 68 references, which provides an up-to-date summary of the present status of knowledge of this unusual but surgically significant lesion.

Pulmonary Artery Sling

This unusual anomaly, not included in the previous edition, is briefly mentioned here because of the facility of

its recognition with modern angiography and the simplicity of surgical correction.

The condition is essentially an aberrant origin of the left pulmonary artery, arising from the right pulmonary artery and passing between the trachea and esophagus to the left lung, forming a "sling" around the distal trachea and producing respiratory distress. The anomaly is usually fatal in the first year of life if not corrected then. In 1975, Grover and associates reported data on the eighteenth survivor of correction of this anomaly (Figs. 18-56 and 18-57). In their report they mention that 63 patients with the anomaly have been reported, one-half of whom had additional anomalies. Twenty of twenty-three unoperated patients died. Twenty-six had definite anatomic correction, with eight hospital deaths and one late death.

References

General

Abbott, M. E.: "Atlas of Congenital Cardiac Disease," The American Heart Association, New York, 1936.

Benson, C. D., Mustard, W. T., Ravitch, M. M., Snyder, W. H., and Welch, K. J. (eds.): "Pediatric Surgery," 2d ed., Year Book Medical Publishers, Inc., Chicago, 1971.

Breckenridge, I. M., Oelert, H., Graham, G. R., Stark, J., Waterston, D. J., and Bonham-Carter, R. E.: Open Heart Surgery in the First Year of Life, *J Thorac Cardiovasc Surg,* **65:**58, 1973.

Cooley, D. A., and Hallman, G. L.: "Surgical Treatment of Congenital Heart Disease," Lea & Febiger, Philadelphia, 1966.

Dammann, J. F., Jr.: Pulmonary Hypertension in C. D. Benson et al. (eds.), "Pediatric Surgery," 2d ed., vol. 1, Year Book Medical Publishers, Inc., Chicago, 1971.

Edwards, J. E.: Functional Pathology of the Pulmonary Vascular Tree in Congenital Cardiac Disease, *Circulation,* **15:**164, 1957.

Gorlin, R., and Gorlin, S. G.: Hydraulic Formula for Calculation of the Area of the Stenotic Mitral Valve, Other Cardiac Valves, and Central Circulatory Shunts: I, *Am Heart J,* **41:**1, 1951.

Gross, R. E.: "The Surgery of Infancy and Childhood," W. B. Saunders Company, Philadelphia, 1953.

Keith, J. D., Rowe, R. D., and Vlad, P.: "Heart Disease in Infancy and Childhood," 2d ed., The Macmillan Company, New York, 1967.

Nadas, A. S.: "Pediatric Cardiology," 2d ed., W. B. Saunders Company, Philadelphia, 1963.

Stewart, S., III, Edmunds, L. H., Jr., Kirklin, J. W., and Allarde, R. R.: Spontaneous Breathing with Continuous Positive Airway Pressure after Open Intracardiac Operations in Infants, *J Thorac Cardiovasc Surg,* **65:**37, 1973.

Taussig, H. B.: "Congenital Malformations of the Heart," 2d ed., Harvard University Press, Cambridge, Mass., 1960.

Pulmonic Stenosis

Brock, R. C.: Pulmonary Valvulotomy for the Relief of Congenital Stenosis: Report of Three Cases, *Br Med J,* **1:**112, 1948.

Engle, M. A., Holswade, G. R., Goldberg, H. P., Lukas, D. S., and Glenn, F.: Regression after Open Valvotomy of Infundibular Stenosis Accompanying Severe Valvular Pulmonic Stenosis, *Circulation,* **17:**862, 1958.

Gilbert, J. W., Morrow, A. G., and Talbert, J. L.: The Surgical Significance of Hypertrophic Infundibular Obstruction Accompanying Valvular Pulmonic Stenosis, *J Thorac Cardiovasc Surg,* **46:**457, 1963.

Holman, E.: On Circumscribed Dilation of an Artery Immediately Distal to a Partially Occluding Band: Poststenotic Dilatation, *Surgery,* **36:**3, 1954.

Johnson, L. W., Grossman, W., Dalen, J. E., and Dexter, L.: Pulmonic Stenosis in the Adult: Longterm Followup Results, *N Engl J Med,* **287:**1159, 1972.

Nadas, A. S.: Pulmonic Stenosis: Indications for Surgery in Children and Adults, *N Engl J Med,* **287:**1196, 1972.

Pacifico, A. D., Kirklin, J. W., and Blackstone, E. H.: Primary Patch Enlargement of the Pulmonary Valve Ring in the Repair of the Tetralogy of Fallot. Paper presented at the American Association for Thoracic Surgery, Ontario, Canada, April 1977.

Sellors, T. H.: Surgery of Pulmonic Stenosis, *Lancet,* **1:**988, 1948.

Spencer, F. C., and Bahnson, H. T.: Intracardiac Surgery Employing Hypothermia and Coronary Perfusion Performed on 100 Patients, *Surgery,* **46:**987, 1959.

Swan, H., and Zeavin, I.: Cessation of Circulation in General Hypothermia, *Ann Surg,* **139:**385, 1954.

Tandon, R., Nadas, A. S., and Gross, R. E.: Results of Open Heart Surgery in Patients with Pulmonic Stenosis and Intact Ventricular Septum: A Report of 108 Cases, *Circulation,* **31:**190, 1965.

Stenosis of the Pulmonary Artery

Franch, R. H., and Gay, B. B.: Congenital Stenosis of the Pulmonary Artery Branches, *Am J Med,* **35:**512, 1963.

McGoon, D. C., and Kincaid, O. W.: Stenosis of Branches of the Pulmonary Artery: Surgical Repair, *Med Clin North Am,* **48:**1083, 1964.

Wallsh, E., Reppert, E. H., Doyle, E. F., and Spencer, F. C.: "Absent" Left Pulmonary Artery with Tetralogy of Fallot, *J Thorac Cardiovasc Surg,* **55:**333, 1968.

Congenital Aortic Stenosis

Braunwald, E., Goldblatt, A., Aygen, M. M., Rockoff, S. D., and Morrow, A. G.: Congenital Aortic Stenosis: Clinical and Hemodynamic Findings in 100 patients, *Circulation,* **27:**426, 1963.

Braverman, I. B., and Gibson, S.: The Outlook for Children with Congenital Aortic Stenosis, *Am Heart J,* **53:**487, 1957.

Frahm, C. J., Braunwald, E., and Morrow, A. G.: Congenital Aortic Regurgitation: Findings in Four Patients, *Am J Med,* **31:**63, 1961.

Lawson, R. M., Bonchek, L. I., Menashe, V., and Starr, A.: Late Results of Surgery for Left Ventricular Outflow Tract Obstruction in Children, *J Thorac Cardiovasc Surg,* **71:**334, 1976.

Peckham, G. B., Keith, J. D., and Evans, J. R.: Congenital Aortic Stenosis: Some Observations on the Natural History and Clinical Assessment, *J Can Med Assoc* **90:**639, 1964.

———, ———, ———, and Bahnson, H. T.: The Treatment of Congenital Aortic Stenosis with Valvulotomy during Cardiopulmonary Bypass, *Surgery,* **44:**109, 1958.

———, ———, Sank, L., and Bahnson, H. T.: Anatomical Varia-

tions in 46 Patients with Congenital Aortic Stenosis, *Am Surg,* **26:**204, 1960.

Supravalvular Aortic Stenosis

Bernhard W. F., Poirier, V., and LaFarge, C. G.: Relief of Congenital Obstruction to Left Ventricular Outflow with Ventricular-Aortic Prosthesis, *J Thorac Cardiovasc Surg,* **20:**136, 1975.

Dembitsky, W. P., and Weldon, C. S.: Clinical Experience with the Use of a Valve-bearing Conduit to Construct a Second Left Ventricular Outflow Tract in Cases of Unresectable Intraventricular Obstruction, *Ann Surg,* **184:**317, 1976.

Doty, D. B., Polansky, D. B., and Jensen, C. B.: Supravalvular Aortic Stenosis: Repair by Extended Aortoplasty. Paper presented at the American Association for Thoracic Surgery, Ontario, Canada, April 1977.

Keane, J. F., Fellows, K. E., LaFarge, C. G., Nadas, A. S., and Bernhard, W. F.: The Surgical Management of Discrete and Diffuse Supravalvar Aortic Stenosis, *Circulation,* **54:**112, 1976.

Morrow, A. G., Waldhausen, J. A., Peters, R. L., Bloodwell, R. D., and Braunwald, E.: Supravalvular Aortic Stenosis, *Circulation,* **20:**1003, 1959.

Peterson, T. A., Todd, D. C., and Edwards, J. E.: Supravalvular Aortic Stenosis, *J Thorac Cardiovasc Surg,* **50:**734, 1965.

Rastelli, G. C., McGoon, D. C., Ongley, P. A., Mankin, H. T., and Kirklin, J. W.: Surgical Treatment of Supravalvular Aortic Stenosis: Report of 16 Cases and Review of Literature, *J Thorac Cardiovasc Surg,* **51:**873, 1966.

Williams, J. C. P., Barratt-Boyes, B. G., and Lowe, J. B.: Supravalvular Aortic Stenosis, *Circulation,* **24:**1311, 1961.

Idiopathic Hypertrophic Subaortic Stenosis

Barratt-Boyes, B. G., Neutze, J. M., and Harris, E. A. (eds.): "Heart Disease in Infancy," The Williams and Wilkins Company, Baltimore, 1973.

Bigelow, W. G., Trimble, A. S., Auger, P., Marquis, Y., and Wigle, E. D.: The Ventriculomyotomy Operation for Muscular Subaortic Stenosis: A Reappraisal, *J Thorac Cardiovasc Surg,* **52:**514, 1966.

Braunwald, E., Brockenbrough, E. C., and Morrow, A. G.: Hypertrophic Subaortic Stenosis: A Broadened Concept, *Circulation,* **26:**161, 1962. (Editorial.)

Frye, R. L., Kincaid, O. W., Swan, H. J. C., and Kirklin, J. W.: Results of Surgical Treatment of Patients with Diffuse Subvalvular Aortic Stenosis, *Circulation,* **32:**52, 1965.

Kelly, D. T., Barratt-Boyes, B. G., and Lowe, J. B.: Results of Surgery and Hemodynamic Observations in Muscular Subaortic Stenosis, *J Thorac Cardiovasc Surg,* **51:**353, 1966.

Kirklin, J. W., in B. G. Barratt-Boyes, J. M. Neutze, and E. A. Harris (eds.): "Heart Disease in Infancy," The Williams and Wilkins Company, Baltimore, 1973.

Konno, S., Imai, Y., Iada, Y., Nakajima, M., and Tatsuno, K.: New Method for Prosthetic Valve Replacement in Congenital Aortic Stenosis Associated with Hypoplasia of the Aortic Valve Ring, *J Thorac Cardiovasc Surg,* **70:**909, 1975.

Morrow, A. G., Reis, R. A., Epstein, S. E., Henry, W. L., Conkin, D. M., Itscoitz, S. B., and Redwood, D. R.: Operative Treatment in Hypertrophic Subaortic Stenosis: Technics and Results of Pre- and Postoperative Assessments in 83 Patients, *Circulation,* **52:**88, 1975.

Coarctation of the Aorta

Abbott, M. E.: Coarctation of the Aorta of the Adult Type: II. A Statistical Study and Historical Retrospect of 200 Recorded Cases, with Autopsy, of Stenosis or Obliteration of the Descending Arch in Subjects above the Age of Two Years, *Am Heart J,* **3:**392, 1928.

Allard, J. R., Williams, R. L., and Dobell, A. R. C.: Interrupted Aortic Arch: Factors Influencing Prognosis, *Ann Thorac Surg,* **21:**243, 1976.

Blalock, A., and Park, E. A.: The Surgical Treatment of Experimental Coarctation (Atresia) of the Aorta, *Ann Surg,* **119:**445, 1944.

Brewer, L. A., III, Fosburg, R. G., Mulder, A. G., and Verska, J. J.: Spinal Cord Complications following Surgery for Coarctation of the Aorta: A Study of 66 Cases, *J Thorac Cardiovasc Surg,* **64:**368, 1972.

Brom, A. G.: Narrowing of the Aortic Isthmus and Enlargement of the Mind, *J Thorac Cardiovasc Surg,* **50:**166, 1965.

Craafoord, C., and Nylin, G.: Congenital Coarctation of the Aorta and Its Surgical Treatment, *J Thorac Surg,* **14:**347, 1945.

DeBakey, M. E., Garrett, H. E., Howell, J. F., and Morris, G. C.: Coarctation of the Abdominal Aorta with Renal Arterial Stenosis: Surgical Considerations, *Ann Surg,* **165:**830, 1967.

Fishman, N. H., Bronstein, M. H., Berman, W., Roe, B. B., et al.: Surgical Management of Severe Aortic Coarctation and Interrupted Aortic Arch in Neonates, *J Thorac Cardiovasc Surg,* **71:**35, 1976.

Gross, R. E.: Coarctation of the Aorta: Surgical Treatment of One Hundred Cases, *Circulation,* **1:**41, 1950.

Hughes, R. K., and Reemtsma, K.: Correction of Coarctation of the Aorta: Manometric Determination of Safety during Test Occlusion, *J Thorac Cardiovasc Surg,* **62:**31, 1971.

Schuster, S. R., and Gross, R. E.: Surgery for Coarctation of the Aorta: A Review of 500 Cases, *J Thor Cardiovasc Surg,* **43:**54, 1962.

Sealy, W. C., Harris, J. S., Young, W. G., and Callaway, H. A.: Paradoxical Hypertension following Resection of Coarctation of the Aorta, *Surgery,* **42:**135, 1957.

Vascular Rings

Gross, R. E.: Arterial Malformations Which Cause Compression of the Trachea or Esophagus, *Circulation,* **11:**124, 1955.

Mahoney, E. B., and Manning, J. A.: Congenital Abnormalities of the Aortic Arch, *Surgery,* **55:**1, 1964.

Shumacker, H. B., Jr., and Burford, T. H.: Unusual Sequel to Operative Intervention for Vascular Ring, *J Thorac Cardiovasc Surg,* **65:**124, 1973.

Atrial Septal Defects: Secundum Defects

Gerbode, F., Harkins, G. A., Ross, J. K., and Osborn, J. J.: Experience with Atrial Septal Defects Repaired with the Aid of Cardiopulmonary Bypass, *Arch Surg,* **80:**846, 1960.

Gibbon, J. H., Jr.: Application of a Mechanical Heart and Lung Apparatus to Cardiac Surgery, *Minn Med,* **37:**171, 1954.

Sellers, R. D., Ferlic, R. M., Sterns, L. P., and Lillehei, C. W.: Secundum Type Atrial Septal Defects: Results with 275 Patients, *Surgery,* **59:**155, 1966.

Spencer, F. C., and Bahnson, H. T.: Intracardiac Surgery Employing Hypothermia and Coronary Perfusion Performed on 100 Patients, *Surgery,* **46:**987, 1959.

Anomalous Drainage of Pulmonary Veins

Bahnson, H. T., Spencer, F. C., and Neill, C. A.: Surgical Treatment of 35 Cases of Drainage of Pulmonary Veins to the Right Side of the Heart, *J Thorac Cardiovasc Surg,* **36:**777, 1958.

Blake, H. A., Hall, R. C., and Manion, W. C.: Anomalous Pulmonary Venous Return, *Circulation,* **32:**406, 1965.

Brody, H.: Drainage of the Pulmonary Veins into the Right Side of the Heart, *Arch Pathol,* **33:**221, 1942.

Cooley, D. A., Hallman, G. L., and Leachman, R. D.: Total Anomalous Pulmonary Venous Drainage, *J Thorac Cardiovasc Surg,* **51:**88, 1966.

———, and Ochsner, A., Jr.: Correction of Total Anomalous Pulmonary Venous Drainage: Technical Considerations, *Surgery,* **42:**1014, 1957.

Darling, R. C., Rothney, W. B., and Craig, J. M.: Total Pulmonary Venous Drainage into the Right Side of the Heart: Report of 17 Autopsied Cases Not Associated with Other Major Cardiovascular Anomalies, *Lab Invest,* **6:**44, 1957.

El-Said, G., Mullins, C. E., and McNamara, J. J.: Management of Total Anomalous Pulmonary Venous Return, *Circulation,* **45:**1240, 1972.

Gott, V. L., Lester, R. G., Lillehei, C. W., and Varco, R. L.: Total Anomalous Pulmonary Venous Return: An Analysis of 30 Cases, *Circulation,* **13:**543, 1956.

Muller, W. H.: Surgical Treatment of Transposition of Pulmonary Veins, *Ann Surg,* **134:**683, 1951.

Wukasch, D. C., Deutsch, M., Reul, G. J., Hallman, G. L., and Cooley, D. A.: Total Anomalous Pulmonary Venous Return, *Ann Thorac Surg,* **19:**622, 1975.

Ostium Primum Defect and Persistent Atrioventricular Canal

Alfieri, O., and Subramanian, S.: Successful Repair of Complete Atrioventricular Canal with Undivided Anterior Common Leaflet in a Six-month-old Infant, *Ann Thorac Surg,* **19:**92, 1975.

Blount, S. G., Jr., Balchum, O. J., and Gensini, G.: Persistent Ostium Primum Atrial Septal Defect, *Circulation,* **13:**499, 1956.

Braunwald, N. S., and Morrow, A. G.: Incomplete Persistent Atrioventricular Canal, *J Thorac Cardiovasc Surg,* **51:**71, 1966.

Castaneda, A. R., Nicoloff, D. M., Moller, J. H., and Lucas, R. V., Jr.: Surgical Correction of Complete Atrioventricular Canal Utilizing Ball-Valve Replacement of the Mitral Valve: Technical Considerations, *J Thorac Cardiovasc Surg,* **62:**926, 1971.

Cooley, D. A., and Hallman, G. L.: "Surgical Treatment of Congenital Heart Disease," Lea & Febiger, Philadelphia, 1966.

Gerbode, F., Sanchez, P. A., Arguero, R., Kerth, W. J., Hill, J. D., and deVries, P. A.: Endocardial Cushion Defects, *Ann Surg,* **167:**486, 1967.

Levy, M. J., Cuello, L., Tuna, N., and Lillehei, C. W.: Atrioventricularis Communis, *Am J Cardiol,* **14:**587, 1964.

McGoon, D. C.: Atrioventricular Canal, in D. C. Sabiston and F. C. Spencer (eds.), "Gibbon's Surgery of the Chest," W. B. Saunders Company, Philadelphia, 1976.

McMullan, M. H., McGoon, D. C., Wallace, R. B., Danielson, G. K., and Weidman, W. H.: Surgical Treatment of Partial Atrioventricular Canal, *Arch Surg,* **107:**705, 1973.

Mills, N. L., Ochsner, J. L., and King, K. D.: Correction of Type C Complete Atrioventricular Canal: Surgical Considerations, *J Thorac Cardiovasc Surg,* **71:**20, 1976.

Neill, C. A.: Postoperative Hemolytic Anemia in Endocardial Cushion Defects, *Circulation,* **30:**801, 1964.

Rastelli, G. C., Kirklin, J. W., and Titus, J. L.: Anatomic Observations on Complete Form of Persistent Common Atrioventricular Canal with Special Reference to Atrioventricular Valves, *Mayo Clin Proc,* **41:**296, 1966.

——, Weidman, W. H., and Kirklin, J. W.: Surgical Repair of the Partial Form of Persistent Common Atrioventricular Canal, with Special Reference to the Problem of Mitral Valve Incompetence, *Circulation,* **31:**31, 1965.

Ventricular Septal Defect

Barratt-Boyes, B. G., Neutze, J. M., Clarkson, P. M., Shardey, G. C., and Brandt, P. W. T.: Repair of Ventricular Septal Defect in the First Two Years of Life Using Profound Hypothermia–Circulatory Arrest Technics, *Ann Surg,* **184:**376, 1976.

Bloomfield, D. K.: The Natural History of Ventricular Septal Defect in Patients Surviving Infancy, *Circulation,* **29:**914, 1964.

Cartmill, T. B., DuShane, J. W., McGoon, D. C., and Kirklin, J. W.: Results of Repair of Ventricular Septal Defect, *J Thorac Cardiovasc Surg,* **52:**486, 1966.

Cooley, D. A., and Hallman, G. L.: "Surgical Treatment of Congenital Heart Disease," Lea & Febiger, Philadelphia, 1966.

Hallman, G. L., Cooley, D. A., and Bloodwell, R. D.: Two-stage Surgical Treatment of Ventricular Septal Defect: Results of Pulmonary Artery Banding in Infants and Subsequent Open-Heart Repair, *J Thorac Cardiovasc Surg,* **52:**476, 1966.

——, ——, Wolff, R. R., and McNamara, D. G.: Surgical Treatment of Ventricular Septal Defect Associated with Pulmonary Hypertension, *J Thorac Cardiovasc Surg,* **48:**588, 1964.

Lillehei, C. W., Anderson, R. C., Eliot, R. S., Wang, Y., and Ferlic, R. M.: Pre- and Postoperative Cardiac Catheterization in 200 Patients Undergoing Closure of Ventricular Septal Defects, *Surgery,* **63:**69, 1968.

——, Sellers, R. D., Bonnabeau, R. C., Jr., and Eliot, R. S.: Chronic Postsurgical Complete Heart Block: With Particular Reference to Prognosis, Management, and a New P-Wave Pacemaker, *J Thorac Cardiovasc Surg,* **46:**436, 1963.

McGoon, D. C.: Closure of Patent Ductus during Open-Heart Surgery, *J Thorac Cardiovasc Surg,* **48:**456, 1964.

Spencer, F. C., Doyle, E. F., Danilowicz, D. A., Bahnson, H. T., and Weldon, C. S.: Longterm Evaluation of Aortic Valvuloplasty for Aortic Insufficiency and Ventricular Septal Defect, *J Thorac Cardiovasc Surg,* **65:**15, 1973.

Walker, W. J., Garcia-Gonzalez, E., Hall, R. J., Czarnecki, S. W., Franklin, R. B., Das, S. K., and Cheitlin, M. D.: Interventricular Septal Defect: Analysis of 415 Catheterized Cases, *Circulation,* **31:**54, 1965.

Wood, P.: The Eisenmenger Syndrome, *Br Med J,* **2:**701, 1958.

Patent Ductus Arteriosus

Blalock, A.: Operative Closure of the Patent Ductus Arteriosus, *Surg Gynecol Obstet,* **82:**113, 1946.

Dammann, J. F., Jr.: Berthrong, M., and Bing, R. J.: Reverse Ductus, *Bull Johns Hopkins Hosp,* **92:**128, 1953.

Gross, R. E.: "The Surgery of Infancy and Childhood: Its Principles and Techniques," W. B. Saunders Company, Philadelphia, 1953.

—— and Hubbard, J. P.: Surgical Ligation of a Patent Ductus Arteriosus: Report of First Successful Case, *JAMA,* **112:**729, 1939.

Jones, J. C.: Twenty-five Years Experience with the Surgery of Patent Ductus Arteriosus, *J Thorac Cardiovasc Surg,* **50:**149, 1965.

Touroff, A. S. W., and Vesell, H.: Subacute Streptococcus Viridans Endarteritis Complicating Patent Ductus Arteriosus: Recovery following Surgical Treatment, *JAMA,* **115:**1270, 1940.

Tetralogy of Fallot

Bahnson, H. T., Spencer, F. C., and Neill, C. A.: Surgical Treatment and Follow-up of 147 Cases of Tetralogy of Fallot Treated by Correction, *J Thorac Cardiovasc Surg,* **44:**419, 1962.

Blalock, A.: Surgical Procedures Employed and Anatomical Variations Encountered in the Treatment of Congenital Pulmonic Stenosis, *Surg Gynecol Obstet,* **87:**385, 1948.

—— and Taussig, H. B.: The Surgical Treatment of Malformations of the Heart in Which There Is Pulmonary Stenosis or Pulmonary Atresia, *JAMA,* **128:**189, 1945.

Brock, R. C.: Pulmonary Valvulotomy for the Relief of Congenital Pulmonary Stenosis: Report of Three Cases, *Br Med J,* **1:**1121, 1948.

Chiariello, L., Meyer, J., Wukasch, D. C., Hallman, G. L., and Cooley, D. A.: Intracardiac Repair of Tetralogy of Fallot, *J Thorac Cardiovasc Surg,* **70:**529, 1975.

Cooley, D. A., and Hallman, G. L.: "Surgical Treatment of Congenital Heart Disease," Lea & Febiger, Philadelphia, 1966.

Ebert, P. A., and Sabiston, D. C.: Surgical Management of the Tetralogy of Fallot: Influence of a Previous Systemic-Pulmonary Anastomosis on the Results of Open Correction, *Ann Surg,* **165:**806, 1967.

Edmunds, L. H., Saxena, N. C., Friedman, S., Rashkind, W. J., and Dodd, P. F.: Transatrial Resection of the Obstructed Right Ventricular Infundibulum, *Circulation,* **54:**117, 1976.

Kirklin, J. W.: "Tetralogy of Fallot," W. B. Saunders Company, Philadelphia, 1971.

——, Wallace, R. B., McGoon, D. C., and DuShane, J. W.: Early and Late Results after Intracardiac Repair of Tetralogy of Fallot, *Ann Surg,* **162:**578, 1965.

Lillehei, C. W., Levy, M. J., Adams, P., and Anderson, R. C.: Corrective Surgery of Tetralogy of Fallot: Longterm Follow-up by Postoperative Recatheterization in 69 Cases and Certain Surgical Considerations, *J Thorac Cardiovasc Surg,* **48:**556, 1964.

Malm, J. R., Blumenthal, S., Bowman, F. O., Jr., Ellis, K., Jameson, A. G., Jesse, M. J., and Yeoh, C. B.: Factors That Modify Hemodynamic Results in Total Correction of Tetralogy of Fallot, *J Thorac Cardiovasc Surg,* **52:**502, 1966.

Potts, W. J., Smith, S., and Gibson, S.: Anastomosis of the Aorta to a Pulmonary Artery: Certain Types in Congenital Heart Disease, *JAMA,* **132:**627, 1946.

Shumway, N. E., Lower, R. R., Hurley, E. J., and Pillsbury, R. C.: Results of Total Surgical Correction of Fallot's Tetralogy, *Circulation,* **31:**I-57, 1965.

Wolf, M. D., Landtman, B., Neill, C. A., and Taussig, H. B.: Total

Correction of Tetralogy of Fallot: Follow-up Study of 104 Cases, *Circulation,* **31**:385, 1965.

Transposition of the Great Vessels

Baffes, T. G., Riker, W. L., Boer, A. D., and Potts, W. J.: Surgical Correction of Transposition of the Aorta and the Pulmonary Artery, *J Thorac Cardiovasc Surg,* **34**:469, 1957.

Barratt-Boyes, B. G., Neutze, J. M., and Harris, E. A.: "Heart Disease in Infancy," The Williams and Wilkins Company, Baltimore, 1973.

Blalock, A., and Hanlon, C. R.: The Surgical Treatment of Complete Transposition of the Aorta and the Pulmonary Artery, *Surg Gynecol Obstet,* **90**:1, 1950.

Cooley, D. A., Hallman, G. L., Bloodwell, R. D., and Leachman, R. D.: Two Stage Surgical Treatment of Complete Transposition of the Great Vessels, *Arch Surg,* **93**:704, 1966.

Cornell, W. P., Maxwell, R. E., Haller, J. A., and Sabiston, D. C.: Results of the Blalock-Hanlon Operation in 90 Patients with Transposition of the Great Vessels, *J Thor Cardiovasc Surg,* **52**:525, 1966.

Edwards, W. S., Bargeron, L. M., and Lyons, C.: Reposition of Right Pulmonary Veins in Transposition of Great Vessels, *JAMA,* **188**:522, 1964.

Glenn, W. W. L., Ordway, N. K., Talner, N. S., and Call, E. P.: Circulatory Bypass of the Right Side of the Heart, *Circulation,* **31**:172, 1965.

Godman, M. J., Friedli, B., Pasternac, A., Kidd, B. S. L., Trusler, G. A., and Mustard, W. T.: Hemodynamic Studies in Children Four to Ten Years after the Mustard Operation for Transposition of the Great Arteries, *Circulation,* **53**:532, 1976.

Hanlon, C. R., and Blalock, A.: Complete Transposition of Aorta and Pulmonary Artery: Experimental Observations on Venous Shunts as Corrective Procedures, *Ann Surg,* **127**:385, 1948.

Hermann, V., Laks, H., Kaiser, G. C., Barner, H. B., and Willman, V. L.: The Blalock-Hanlon Procedure: Simple Transposition of the Great Arteries, *Arch Surg,* **110**:1387, 1975.

Jatene, A. D., Fontes, V. F., Paulista, P. P., et al.: Successful Anatomic Correction of Transposition of the Great Vessels: A Preliminary Report, *Arq Bras Cardiol,* **28**:461, 1975.

McGoon, D. C.: Intraventricular Repair of Transposition of the Great Arteries, *J Thorac Cardiovasc Surg,* **64**:430, 1972.

Merendino, K. H., Jesseph, J. E., Herron, P. W., Thomas, G. I., and Vetto, R. R.: Interatrial Venous Transposition, *Surgery,* **42**:898, 1957.

Moss, A. J., Maloney, J. V., Jr., and Adams, F. H.: Transposition of the Great Vessels, *Ann Surg,* **153**:183, 1961.

Mustard, W. T.: Progress in the Total Correction of Complete Transposition of the Great Vessels, *Vasc Dis,* **3**:177, 1966.

———, Keith, J. D., Trusler, G. A., Fowler, R., and Kidd, L.: The Surgical Management of Transposition of the Great Vessels, *J Thorac Cardiovasc Surg,* **48**:953, 1964.

Senning, A.: Surgical Correction of Transposition of the Great Vessels, *Surgery,* **45**:966, 1959.

———: Surgical Correction of Transposition of the Great Vessels, *Surgery,* **59**:334, 1966.

Stark, J., de Leval, M. R., Waterston, D. J., Graham, G. R., and Bonham-Carter, R. E.: Corrective Surgery of Transposition of the Great Arteries in the First Year of Life, *J Thorac Cardiovasc Surg,* **67**:673, 1974.

Tricuspid Atresia

Fontan, F., and Baudet, E.: Surgical Repair of Tricuspid Atresia, *Thorax,* **26**:240, 1971.

Glenn, W. W. L., Ordway, N. K., Talner, N. S., and Capp, E. P.: Circulatory Bypass of the Right Side of the Heart: Shunt between Superior Vena Cava and Distal Right Pulmonary Artery; Report of Clinical Application in 38 Cases, *Circulation,* **31**:172, 1965.

Kyger, E. R., Reul, G. J., Sandiford, F. M., Wukasch, D. C., Hallman, G. L., and Cooley, D. A.: Surgical Palliation of Tricuspid Atresia, *Circulation,* **52**:685, 1975.

Williams, W. G., Rubis, L., Trusler, G. A., and Mustard, W. T.: Palliation of Tricuspid Atresia, *Arch Surg,* **110**:1383, 1975.

Cor Triatriatum

Grondin, C., Leonard, A. S., Anderson, R. C., Amplatz, K. A., Edwards, J. E., and Varco, R. L.: Cor Triatriatum: A Diagnostic Surgical Enigma, *J Thorac Cardiovasc Surg,* **48**:527, 1964.

McGuire, L. B., Nolan, T. B., Reede, R., and Dammann, J. F.: Cor Triatriatum as a Problem of Adult Heart Disease, *Circulation,* **31**:263, 1965.

Niwayama, G.: Cor Triatriatum, *Am Heart J,* **59**:291, 1960.

Oglietti, J., Reul, G. J., Leachman, R. D., and Cooley, D. A.: Supravalvular Stenosing Ring of the Left Atrium, *Am Thorac Surg,* **21**:421, 1976.

Congenital Mitral Stenosis

Carpentier, A., Branchini, B., Cour, J. C., Asfaou, E., et al.: Congenital Malformations of the Miral Valve in Children, *J Thorac Cardiovasc Surg,* **72**:854, 1976.

Daoud, G., Kaplan, S., Perrin, E. V., Dorst, J. P., and Edwards, F. K.: Congenital Mitral Stenosis, *Circulation,* **27**:185, 1963.

Ferencz, C., Johnson, A. L., and Wiglesworth, F. W.: Congenital Mitral Stenosis, *Circulation,* **9**:161, 1954.

Khalil, K. G., Shapiro, I., and Kilman, J. W.: Congenital Mitral Stenosis, *J Thorac Cardiovasc Surg,* **70**:40, 1975.

Tsuji, H. K., Shapiro, M., Redington, J. V., and Kay, J. H.: Congenital Mitral Stenosis: Report of Two Cases and Review of the Literature, *J Thorac Cardiovasc Surg,* **53**:850, 1967.

Aortic-Pulmonary Window

Clarke, C. P., and Richardson, J. P.: The Management of Aorto-pulmonary Window, *J Thorac Cardiovasc Surg,* **72**:48, 1976.

Cooley, D. A., McNamara, D. G., and Latson, J. R.: Aorticopulmonary Septal Defect, *Surgery,* **42**:101, 1957.

Gross, R. E.: Surgical Closure of an Aortic Septal Defect, *Circulation,* **5**:858, 1952.

Morrow, A. G., Greenfield, L. J., and Braunwald, E.: Congenital Aortopulmonary Septal Defect: Clinical and Hemodynamic Findings, Surgical Technique, and Results of Operative Correction, *Circulation,* **25**:463, 1962.

Putnam, T. C., and Gross, R. E.: Surgical Management of Aorto-pulmonary Fenestration, *Surgery,* **59**:727, 1966.

Scott, H. W., and Sabiston, D. C.: Surgical Treatment for Congenital Aortico-pulmonary Fistula, *J Thorac Cardiovasc Surg,* **25**:26, 1953.

Skall-Jensen, J.: Congenital Aortico-pulmonary Fistula: A Review of the Literature and Report of Two Cases, *Acta Med Scand,* **160**:221, 1958.

Ruptured Aneurysm of Sinus of Valsalva

Gerbode, F., Osborn, J. J., Johnston, J. B., and Kerth, W. J.: Transaortic Approach for the Repair of Ruptured Aneurysms of the Sinus of Valsalva, *Ann Surg,* 161:946, 1965.

Lillehei, C. W., Stanley, P., and Varco, R. L.: Surgical Treatment of Ruptured Aneurysms of the Sinus of Valsalva, *Ann Surg,* 146:459, 1957.

Paton, B. C., MacMahon, R. A., Swan, H., and Blount, S. G.: Ruptured Sinus of Valsalva, *Arch Surg,* 90:209, 1965.

Sawyer, J. L., Adams, J. E., and Scott, H. W.: Surgical Treatment for Aneurysms of Aortic Sinuses with Aorticoatrial Fistula, *Surgery,* 41:126, 1957.

Shumacker, H. B., King, H., and Waldhausen, J. A.: Transaortic Approach for the Repair of Ruptured Aneurysms of the Sinus of Valsalva, *Ann Surg,* 161:946, 1965.

Spencer, F. C., Blake, H. A., and Bahnson, H. T.: Surgical Repair of Ruptured Aneurysm of Sinus of Valsalva in Two Patients, *Ann Surg,* 162:963, 1960.

Truncus Arteriosus

Applebaum, A., Bargeron, L. M., Pacifico, A. D., and Kirklin, J. W.: Surgical Treatment of Truncus Arteriosus with Emphasis on Infants and Small Children, *J Thorac Cardiovasc Surg,* 71:436, 1976.

Ebert, P. A., Robinson, S. J., Stanger, P., and Engle, M. A.: Pulmonary Artery Conduits in Infants Younger than Six Months of Age, *J Thorac Cardiovasc Surg,* 72:351, 1976.

Marcelletti, C., McGoon, D. C., and Mair, D. D.: The Natural History of Truncus Arteriosus, *Circulation,* 54:108, 1976.

McGoon, D. C., Wallace, R. B., and Danielson, G. K.: The Rastelli Operation: Its Indications and Results, *J Thorac Cardiovasc Surg,* 65:65, 1973.

Poirier, R. A., Berman, M. A., and Stansel, H. C.: Current Status of the Surgical Treatment of Truncus Arteriosus, *J Thorac Cardiovasc Surg,* 69:169, 1975.

Single Ventricle

Campbell, M. G., Reynolds, G., and Trounce, J. R.: Six Cases of Single Ventricle with Pulmonary Stenosis, *Guys Hosp Rep,* 102:99, 1953.

Edie, R. N., and Malm, J. R.: Surgical Repair of Single Ventricle, *J Thorac Cardiovasc Surg,* 66:350, 1973.

——— and ———: Surgical Repair of Single Ventricle, in B. S. L. Kidd and R. D. Rowe (eds.): "The Child with Congenital Heart Disease after Surgery," Futura Publishing Co., Mount Kisco, N.Y., 1976.

McGoon, D. C., Danielson, G. K., Ritter, D. G., Wallace, R. B., Maloney, J. D., and Marcelletti, C.: Correction of the Univentricular Heart Having Two Atrioventricular Valves, *J Thorac Cardiovasc Surg,* 74:218, 1977.

Ebstein's Anomaly

Bahnson, H. T., Bauersfeld, S. R., and Smith, J. W.: Pathological Anatomy and Surgical Correction of Ebstein's Anomaly, *Circulation,* 31(Suppl 1):3, 1965.

Barnard, C. N., and Schrire, V.: Surgical Correction of Ebstein's Malformation with Prosthetic Tricuspid Valve, *Surgery,* 54:302, 1963.

Hardy, K. L., May, I. A., Webster, C. A., and Kimball, K. G.:

Ebstein's Anomaly: A Functional Concept and Successful Definitive Repair, *J Thorac Cardiovasc Surg,* 48:927, 1964.

Hunter, S. W., and Lillehei, C. W.: Ebstein's Malformation of the Tricuspid Valve, *Dis Chest,* 33:297, 1958.

Timmis, H. H., Hardy, J. D., and Watson, D. G.: The Surgical Management of Ebstein's Anomaly, *J Thorac Cardiovasc Surg,* 53:385, 1967.

Vacca, J. B., Bussmann, D. W., and Mudd, J. G.: Ebstein's Anomaly: Complete Review of 108 Cases, *Am J Cardiol,* 2:210, 1958.

Anomalous Origin of Left Coronary Artery from Pulmonary Artery

Bland, E. F., White, P. D., and Garland, J.: Congenital Anomalies of Coronary Arteries: Report of an Unusual Case Associated with Cardiac Hypertrophy, *Am Heart J,* 8:787, 1933.

Chiarello, L., Meyer, J., Reul, G. J., Hallman, G. I., and Cooley, D. A.: Surgical Treatment for Anomalous Origin of Left Coronary Artery from Pulmonary Artery, *Am Thorac Surg,* 19:443, 1975.

Cooley, D. A., Hallman, G. L., and Bloodwell, R. D.: Definitive Surgical Treatment of Anomalous Origin of Left Coronary Artery from Pulmonary Artery, *J Thorac Cardiovasc Surg,* 52:798, 1966.

Doty, D. B., Chandramouli, B., Schieken, Lauer, R. M., and Ehrenhaft, J. L.: Anomalous Origin of the Left Coronary Artery from the Right Pulmonary Artery, *J Thorac Cardiovasc Surg,* 71:787, 1976.

Likar, I., Criley, J. M., and Lewis, K. B.: Anomalous Left Coronary Artery Arising from the Pulmonary Artery in Adults: A Review of the Therapeutic Problems, *Circulation,* 33:727, 1966.

Neches, W. H., Matthews, R. A., Park, S. C., Lenox, C. C. et al.: Anomalous Origin of the Left Coronary Artery from the Pulmonary Artery: A New Method of Surgical Repair, *Circulation,* 50:582, 1974.

Sabiston, D. C., Neill, C. A., and Taussig, H. B.: The Direction of Blood Flow in Anomalous Left Coronary Artery Arising from the Pulmonary Artery, *Circulation,* 22:591, 1960.

Coronary Arteriovenous Fistula

Effler, D. B., Sheldon, W. C., Turner, J. J., and Groves, L. K.: Coronary Arteriovenous Fistulas: Diagnosis and Surgical Management; Report of Fifteen Cases, *Surgery,* 61:41, 1967.

Gasul, B. M., Arcilla, R. A., Fell, E. H., Lynfield, J., Bicoff, J. P., and Luan, L. L.: Congenital Coronary Arteriovenous Fistula: Clinical, Phonocardiographic, Angiocardiographic, and Hemodynamic Studies in Five Patients, *Pediatrics,* 25:531, 1960.

Hallman, G. L., Cooley, D. A., and Singer, D. B.: Congenital Anomalies of the Coronary Arteries: Anatomy, Pathology, and Surgical Treatment, *Surgery,* 59:133, 1966.

Oldham, H. N., Jr., Ebert, P. A., Young, W. G., and Sabiston, D. C., Jr.: Surgical Management of Congenital Coronary Arteriovenous Fistula, *Ann Thorac Surg,* 12:503, 1971.

Corrected Transposition

Anderson, R. C., Lillehei, C. W., and Lester, R. G.: Corrected Transposition of the Great Vessels of the Heart: A Review of 17 Cases, *Pediatrics,* 20:626, 1957.

Fox, L. S., Kirklin, J. W., Pacifico, A. D., Waldo, A. L., and Bargeron, L. M.: Intracardiac Repair of Cardiac Malformations with Atrioventricular Discordance, *Circulation,* **54:**123, 1976.

Schiebler, G. L., Edwards, J. E., Burchell, H. B., DuShane, J. W., Ongley, P. A., and Wood, E. H.: Congenital Corrected Transposition of the Great Vessels: A Study of 33 Cases, *Pediatrics,* **27:**851, 1961.

Waldo, A. L., Pacifico, A. D., Bargeron, L. M., James, T. N., and Kirklin, J. W.: Electrophysiological Delineation of the Specialized A-V Conduction System in Patients with Corrected Transposition of the Great Vessels and Ventricular Septal Defect, *Circulation,* **52:**435, 1975.

Double Outlet Right Ventricle

Stewart, S.: Double Outlet Right Ventricle, *J Thorac Cardiovasc Surg,* **71:**355, 1976.

Van Praagh, R., Perez-Trevino, C., Reynolds, J. L., et al.: Double Outlet Right Ventricle with Subaortic Ventricular Septal Defect and Pulmonary Stenosis, *Am J Cardiol,* **35:**42, 1975.

Pulmonary Artery Sling

Grover, F. L., Norton, J. B., Webb, G. E., and Trinkle, J. K.: Pulmonary Sling: Case Report and Collective Review, *J Thorac Cardiovasc Surg,* **69:**295, 1975.

Chapter 19

Acquired Heart Disease

by Frank C. Spencer

INTRODUCTION: CLINICAL MANIFESTATIONS

With the development of prosthetic cardiac valves, the scope of surgical therapy for heart disease was greatly enlarged. An additional major advance was the development of bypass grafting for coronary artery disease, starting in the year 1967–1968 and now widely employed.

Present frontiers include corrective operations for severe cardiac malformations in infancy, cardiac transplantation, and the development of an artificial heart. This steadily expanding scope of cardiac surgery requires that the surgeon become familiar with features of cardiac disease that have traditionally been the province of the cardiologist. Accordingly, basic clinical features of cardiac disease, which classically are found only in a textbook of cardiology, are briefly presented in this section. The objective is not to train a surgeon as an amateur cardiologist but to enable the surgeon to be familiar enough with the clinical manifestations of cardiac disease to recognize gross abnormalities and to appreciate further the great importance of having a cardiologist as an integral part of a cardiac surgical team. Unless a cardiologist works closely with a cardiac surgeon, many surgical mishaps can occur which otherwise might be prevented or promptly treated, such as arrhythmias or myocardial infarction.

The five major methods of evaluating a patient with heart disease can be conveniently grouped as history, physical examination, electrocardiogram, radiologic studies, and special diagnostic tests, especially cardiac catheterization and cineangiography. In this introductory section the major characteristics of cardiac disease, as elicited by the history, physical examination, and laboratory studies, will be briefly described. For additional details, a textbook of cardiology should be consulted.

HISTORY. It is particularly important to determine the degree of disability present and its rate of progression. These considerations are especially pertinent to a decision as to the advisability of surgical intervention, especially if the contemplated operative procedure would require insertion of a prosthetic mitral or aortic valve. The hazard of thromboembolism with prosthetic valves, though decreased to the range of 2 to 4 percent since about 1970, still limits their use to patients seriously disabled or to those developing marked cardiac enlargement. The relative freedom from thromboembolism of the glutaldehyde-preserved porcine heterograft prosthesis, used with increasing frequency in the past 5 years, has further expanded the indications for valve replacement.

Dyspnea, *fatigue*, *edema*, and *cyanosis* are all usually manifestations of decreased cardiac output and congestive heart failure. *Pain* is an especially prominent feature with coronary artery disease. *Palpitation* and *syncope* occur with many forms of heart disease, especially with disturbances of rhythm. *Hemoptysis* can result from either cardiac or pulmonary causes. Each of these disorders will be briefly discussed.

Dyspnea on exertion is an extremely common symptom with heart disease, resulting from pulmonary congestion from elevation of left atrial pressure with increased physical activity. The degree of exertion required to cause dyspnea, especially with any changes in recent months, should be carefully noted. Other clinical manifestations of pulmonary congestion include cough, orthopnea, paroxysmal nocturnal dyspnea, or frank pulmonary edema. In considering the possible causes of dyspnea, it should be remembered that probably the most common cause is an anxiety syndrome, not heart disease. This can usually be determined by careful examination. *Fatigue,* probably a reflection of decrease in cardiac output, is a more subtle sign of limited cardiac function than dyspnea and may be the only complaint when the patient has subtly restricted his physical activities to avoid dyspnea. Patients following a sedentary existence can tolerate serious cardiac disease for long periods of time without having any other symptoms from a significant underlying hemodynamic disturbance.

Cyanosis may appear with acute pulmonary congestion but is usually variable and not a reliable guide to the type or severity of cardiac disease. It is a more reliable and significant finding in patients with congenital heart disease. *Edema* is a late symptom of congestive heart failure, for it can be detected clinically only after 10 lb or more of extracellular fluid have accumulated. Few symptoms may result from the presence of edema except for generalized aching and discomfort from the increased weight of the legs.

Chest pain is a particularly significant symptom which must be closely analyzed. Angina pectoris is one of the most frequent causes and, in perhaps 75 percent of patients, can be readily diagnosed from the characteristic symptoms. It usually occurs as a substernal pain or constriction provoked by exercise, eating, emotion, or exposure to cold. The discomfort commonly lasts 1 to 4 minutes and may be immediately relieved by sublingual administration of nitroglycerin. In perhaps 20 to 25 percent of patients a bizarre discomfort develops with radiation of pain to numerous unusual locations, such as the ear, the right hand, or the epigastrium. In such patients establishing the correct diagnosis may challenge the most experienced cardiologist and require laboratory evaluation with exercise electrocardiography or coronary arteriography.

Other frequent causes of chest pain include myocardial infarction, dissecting aneurysm, pericarditis, or pulmonary infarction. As with dyspnea, anxiety is a frequent cause for a precordial discomfort described as pain or "tightness," and its frequency must be appreciated in considering the differential diagnosis. Other noncardiac conditions which may be easily confused with angina pectoris are diseases of the esophagus or, less frequently, biliary disease.

Palpitation is a generalized term for the patient's becoming aware of cardiac contractions. Rarely this occurs in a thin-chested individual without cardiac disease. Usually it results from increased force of left ventricular contraction as a result of underlying heart disease or from a cardiac arrhythmia, such as an extrasystole. Its significance is re-

lated to the underlying disease or disturbance which produces the discomfort. *Syncope* may result from several cardiac diseases, the most important of which are aortic stenosis, heart block, mitral stenosis, tetralogy of Fallot, or rarely pulmonary hypertension. It is a particularly ominous symptom in patients with aortic stenosis, for the life expectancy of such patients is brief unless surgical therapy is performed. In evaluating the significance of syncope, the possibility of epilepsy or cerebrovascular disease must be considered.

Hemoptysis, an alarming symptom, often results from pulmonary disease. The four most frequent disorders are tuberculosis, bronchogenic carcinoma, bronchiectasis, and pneumonia. The two cardiac conditions most commonly associated with hemoptysis are mitral stenosis and pulmonary infarction. Patients with fulminating pulmonary edema may expectorate a pink, frothy sputum as a result of rupture of pulmonary capillaries into the alveoli, but the frothy sputum of pulmonary edema can be easily distinguished from the blood clots expectorated with frank hemoptysis.

PHYSICAL EXAMINATION. The general body habitus of the patient should be carefully noted. A number of unusual genetic syndromes are associated with cardiac disease. Most of these are described in recent textbooks of cardiology. The Marfan syndrome is a familiar example of a disorder of connective tissue which may cause either a dissecting aneurysm or aortic insufficiency.

The prominence of the neck veins is a guide to venous pressure. With a normal venous pressure of 2 to 10 mm Hg, the internal jugular vein is visible for only 2 to 3 cm above the level of the clavicle. With obviously distended veins, measurement of central venous pressure should be considered. In patients with tricuspid valvular disease, the experienced cardiologist can detect prominent *a* waves in the jugular pulse generated from forceful contractions of the right atrium. Peripheral edema can be best noted in the legs, but in patients confined to bed edema may be more prominent in the flanks or buttocks.

Much information can be obtained from a careful examination of the peripheral pulse and the blood pressure. A disturbance of cardiac rhythm, such as atrial fibrillation, can be recognized from the pulse and then investigated more thoroughly by auscultation of the heart and study of the electrocardiogram. Pulsus alternans, a rhythmic alternation between a forceful pulse and a weak one, is a significant sign of serious left ventricular failure. A small, weak pulse is found with cardiac disease associated with a low cardiac output, increased peripheral vascular resistance, and a narrow pulse pressure. This may occur with myocardial failure, aortic stenosis, mitral stenosis, or cardiac tamponade. A forceful, bounding pulse results when there is an increased cardiac output with a wide pulse pressure and decreased peripheral vascular resistance. This is classically seen with aortic insufficiency but is also a prominent feature in any disease associated with a decreased peripheral vascular resistance, such as patent ductus arteriosus, peripheral arteriovenous fistula, hyperthyroidism, or pregnancy.

Inspection and palpation of the precordium is another

important part of the cardiac examination. Some cardiologists have almost discarded percussion of the cardiac shadow because of the wide range of normal findings among persons of different habitus and have found more significant information by careful inspection and palpation. Cardiac pulsations should be observed for their location, timing, amplitude, and distribution. Normally, the apical impulse is near the midclavicular line and can be detected as a moderately forceful tapping sensation in early systole over an area 2 to 3 cm in diameter. With left ventricular hypertrophy, as with aortic stenosis or insufficiency, both the size and vigor of the left ventricular impulse are increased. With right ventricular hypertrophy, a prominent parasternal impulse, which some cardiologists consider a better index of right ventricular hypertrophy than the electrocardiogram, can be felt. In the presence of marked dilatation of the heart from congestive heart failure, palpation becomes less reliable because of the diffuse nature of the cardiac impulse.

Characteristic thrills develop with certain types of valvular disease. The more common of these are the thrill in the aortic area from aortic stenosis, a similar one in the pulmonic area with pulmonic stenosis, and less frequently a diastolic thrill at the apex with mitral stenosis.

Auscultation is a very important part of the cardiac examination, because some serious disorders, such as mitral stenosis or aortic insufficiency, can be firmly diagnosed best by detection of the characteristic murmur. In auscultation the cardiac sounds should be carefully analyzed and any murmurs identified. A convenient method for beginning the examination is to identify the first and second sounds by auscultation at the base of the heart. Normally the second sound, produced by closure of the aortic and pulmonic valves, is of a higher pitch and shorter duration than the first sound, produced by seating of the mitral and tricuspid valves. If uncertainty exists, simultaneous palpation of the carotid pulse will identify the two sounds. Splitting of the pulmonic second sound is a familiar characteristic of conditions which increase pulmonary blood flow, especially atrial septal defect.

In defining the characteristics of a murmur, the timing, duration, intensity, and location are of particular significance. Aortic and pulmonic stenosis each produce so-called "diamond-shaped" murmurs, representing an early rise and late decline in intensity. Mitral insufficiency, by contrast, produces a loud apical systolic murmur without the characteristic sharp decrease heard in aortic stenosis. The diastolic murmur of aortic insufficiency is usually best heard along the left sternal border, while the typical diastolic murmur of mitral stenosis may be sharply localized at the cardiac apex. Murmurs of tricuspid stenosis and insufficiency often are similar to the more frequently encountered murmurs of mitral stenosis or insufficiency, except that they also may be audible near the lower end of the sternum and can be accentuated during inspiration. Confirmation of the diagnosis usually requires cardiac catheterization. A murmur of ventricular septal defect is usually a harsh holosystolic murmur near the lower border of the sternum, while the murmur of an atrial septal defect creased pulmonary blood flow. The classic murmur of

patent ductus arteriosus is a continuous murmur best heard in the left second or third intercostal space.

Functional murmurs are especially common in conditions with an increase in cardiac output, such as hyperthyroidism, anemia, or pregnancy. In general these are short systolic murmurs which may be audible at the apex or in the pulmonic area. Their differential diagnosis, which may necessitate cardiac catheterization, is beyond the scope of this presentation.

Two infrequent findings on auscultation are a pericardial friction rub or a gallop rhythm. A friction rub is particularly common after cardiac operations and may be unassociated with any other clinical signs, originating from resorption of fluid in the pericardium. In other patients it may indicate the so-called "pericardiotomy syndrome," which frequently occurs following cardiac surgical procedures. A gallop rhythm is of particular importance, because its presence usually indicates serious disease of the myocardium, such as myocardial infarction or impending cardiac failure.

ELECTROCARDIOGRAPHY. The electrocardiogram will be mentioned only briefly, for its proper interpretation requires the careful analysis of an experienced cardiologist. Disorders of cardiac rhythm are extremely common following cardiac surgical procedures, and a wide variety of rhythms can occur in a patient over a period of several hours. In analysis of the electrocardiogram, the cardiac rate, rhythm, and electrical axis should be noted. It is particularly useful for detection of hypertrophy of either the right or left ventricle. Conduction defects, such as right or left bundle branch block, can be diagnosed only by electrocardiography. With serious coronary artery disease, either as chronic coronary artery disease or with acute myocardial infarction, the electrocardiogram may provide the only positive laboratory findings.

RADIOLOGY. The chest roentgenogram provides many valuable guides in evaluation of cardiac disease. Determination of heart size is of basic importance, for cardiac enlargement immediately establishes the presence of cardiac disease. Alterations in cardiac contour occur with different diseases. Normally the right border of the heart is formed by the superior vena cava and the right atrium, and the left border by the aorta, pulmonary artery, and left ventricle. Selective enlargement of any of the four cardiac chambers is best recognized by oblique or lateral views. In the left anterior oblique position, enlargement of the left ventricle can be recognized as a posterior shadow against the spine, while an enlarged right ventricle can be seen bulging anteriorly into the retrosternal space. Enlargement of the left atrium is best recognized in the lateral view, by simultaneous opacification of the esophagus with barium, as it produces a characteristic concave indentation of the esophagus. Enlargement of the right atrium, bulging into the right hemithorax, can be easily seen in the usual posteroanterior view.

In analysis of the cardiac shadow, detection of calcification is of particular importance. Calcification of the aortic or mitral valves is very common with long-standing rheumatic disease. With constrictive pericarditis most patients will have visible areas of calcification.

Analysis of the pulmonary circulation provides many valuable guides to the status of the circulation. Pulmonary venous congestion develops when left atrial pressure is chronically elevated above the upper limit of normal of 12 mm Hg. With severe mitral stenosis, a typical picture of engorged pulmonary veins may be readily recognized. When severe left atrial hypertension is present, edema forms in the lungs in both the alveoli and the interstitial tissues. Edema accumulating in the interlobar planes forms transverse linear opacities on the chest roentgenogram which are perpendicular to the surface of the pleura, the so-called "Kerley lines." Their presence usually indicates a left atrial pressure exceeding 20 mm Hg.

The prominenence of the pulmonary arteries is also of particular significance. Marked enlargement of the pulmonary arteries may occur with either an increase in pulmonary blood flow or an increase in pulmonary vascular resistance with pulmonary hypertension. Normally, the central pulmonary arteries are three to five times larger than the peripheral arteries. With an increase in pulmonary blood flow, as with an atrial septal defect, both the central and peripheral pulmonary arteries are symmetrically enlarged. With an increase in pulmonary vascular resistance and pulmonary hypertension, the central pulmonary arteries may become strikingly enlarged, while the peripheral pulmonary arteries do not distend, producing a striking disproportion in the size of the two vessels. An estimation of the pulmonary blood flow by fluoroscopy is of particular importance in the presence of congenital heart disease. Wide variations are seen, ranging from the avascular lung fields with tetralogy of Fallot to the plethoric lung fields of ventricular or atrial septal defect.

CARDIAC CATHETERIZATION AND CINEANGIOGRAPHY. These two techniques have greatly advanced the precision of diagnosis of cardiac disease. Only by these studies can many cardiac disorders be properly diagnosed and quantitatively analyzed. It is our practice to perform cardiac catheterization and angiography upon virtually every patient undergoing cardiac surgical treatment to assess the hemodynamic disturbance, confirm the diagnosis, and detect any associated cardiac disease. This liberal policy has provided numerous dividends in the care of patients both during and following operation.

Cardiac catheterization, by obtaining oxygen concentration and pressure in different cardiac chambers, can establish the diagnosis of an intracardiac shunt, such as an atrial or ventricular septal defect, or the presence of a valvular stenosis, such as pulmonic stenosis, mitral stenosis, or aortic stenosis. The presence of cardiac failure, as indicated by an elevation of left atrial pressure, or pulmonary hypertension can also be measured. It is not of great value for analysis of aortic or mitral insufficiency, except to detect the development of cardiac failure.

Cineangiography, however, provides the best method for analysis of aortic or mitral insufficiency, visually demonstrating the amount of dye refluxing through the incompetent valve. In patients over forty years of age, simultaneous coronary arteriography is routinely done to evaluate the presence of associated coronary atherosclerosis.

The combination of cardiac catheterization and cineangiography in a well-equipped cardiac catheterization laboratory is an essential component of any cardiac surgical unit.

PATHOPHYSIOLOGY

A detailed analysis of the pathophysiology of mitral and aortic disease is presented in those respective sections. Accordingly, only a brief discussion of certain broad principles of pathophysiology of acquired heart disease is presented here.

As stated earlier, the degree of incapacity of a patient with cardiac disease should be carefully evaluated in deciding that an operation should be performed. Many patients with aortic or mitral disease can function well for years and should be treated by nonoperative methods until the disease has progressed to an incapacitating stage. The reason for this conservatism, which may change in the future, is the significant frequency of thromboemboli with prosthetic cardiac valves. Hence, an operation which entails insertion of a prosthetic cardiac valve should be postponed as long as a patient can carry out his normal activities with appropriate medical therapy. One exception to this policy is the presence of progressive cardiac enlargement. As very large hearts of 750 to 1,000 Gm may not decrease after operation, surgery is being performed earlier in some patients with only moderate symptoms but with progressive cardiac enlargement.

Conversely, it is important to realize that with present surgical techniques an operation almost always can be performed, even though advanced, severe cardiac failure is present. The immediate risk of operation is increased, but possibilities for rehabilitating a patient are fairly good, even though he is bedridden with severe edema from far advanced congestive failure. Our most extreme example of this is a patient who lost 80 pounds of edema fluid during prolonged preoperative treatment before undergoing an uneventful mitral valve replacement. The most important principle in operating upon such patients is to be certain that all existing valvular pathologic conditions are corrected, for multivalvular disease is common with intractable congestive failure. In some patients replacement of three cardiac valves, the mitral, aortic, and tricuspid, is necessary.

With mitral stenosis, different considerations apply, because many such patients can be effectively treated by commissurotomy. Accordingly, operation should be planned whenever the diagnosis is made if any symptoms are present. Surgical therapy should be especially considered once atrial fibrillation has occurred because of the risk of thromboembolism. Before either anticoagulant or surgical therapy was available, approximately 25 percent of patients with mitral stenosis ultimately died from cerebral embolism.

With aortic stenosis or insufficiency, once symptoms such as dyspnea, syncope, or chest pain have appeared, operation should be performed quickly, because sudden death is a real possibility. This is particularly true with aortic stenosis. Sudden death of patients with aortic stenosis either contemplating or scheduled for operation still occurs with distressing frequency.

Pulmonary hypertension is of considerably different significance with acquired heart disease than with congenital heart disease. With ventricular septal defect an elevated pulmonary vascular resistance may or may not decrease following closure of the defect. With pulmonary hypertension from mitral stenosis, however, even in its more severe forms with a pulmonary artery systolic pressure exceeding 100 mm Hg, improvement almost invariably occurs following adequate correction of the stenosis.

The heart size and presence of congestive failure are important indices of long-term rehabilitation following successful cardiac valvular surgical treatment. Unfortunately in most patients disabled by the disease significant cardiac enlargement has developed. A small percentage of patients with mitral disease following valvular replacement will have permanent cardiac disability, requiring careful limitation of physical activities and administration of diuretics. Whether this permanent disability reflects a rheumatic myocarditis or a permanent injury to the myocardium from long-standing valvular disease is unknown. Similarly, with aortic valvular disease and severe cardiac enlargement, sometimes to weights of 700 to 900 Gm, sudden death remains an ominous possibility following operation, especially in the first year. Death is probably due to a disturbance of rhythm from the severely hypertrophied left ventricle. As mentioned earlier, the probable solution for this group of patients is performance of operation at an earlier date, which will surely be done when cardiac valvular prostheses are completely free from the risk of thromboembolism.

PHYSIOLOGY
OF EXTRACORPOREAL CIRCULATION

HISTORICAL DATA. The pioneering imagination and efforts of Gibbon were largely responsible for the development of extracorporeal circulation. In 1932, Gibbon initiated laboratory investigations which continued for over 20 years until the first successful open heart operation in man was performed by him in 1953. Subsequent developments were rapid, with the brief use of cross circulation by Lillehei and associates at the University of Minnesota in 1954, followed a short time later by the development of the bubble oxygenator by DeWall, who was working in the group with Lillehei. Kirklin and associates at the Mayo Clinic first began routine, successful use of the Gibbon oxygenator in 1955. The disc oxygenator was developed in Sweden by Bjork and Crafoord and introduced to the United States by Kay and Cross. Since 1970, disposable bubble oxygenators have been adopted almost universally.

PUMPS. The majority of heart-lung machines utilize a simple roller pump, originally developed by DeBakey. The resulting flow is almost nonpulsatile, with a pulse pressure of about 15 mm Hg. A variety of other pumps have been employed, with no clear demonstration of any advantages over the simple roller pump. A recurrent physiologic question has been the importance of a pulsatile flow in the normal circulation. Available experimental data indicate that over long periods of time a pulsatile flow may be of importance, but for periods of 1 to 4 hours a nonpulsatile flow seems adequate. The gradual increase in vasomotor tone which occurs during extracorporeal circulation may be a physiologic response to nonpulsatile perfusion.

OXYGENATORS. Since 1970 the disposable bubble oxygenator has become the most widely used type (Fig. 19-1). Technical improvements in the removal of bubbles from blood following oxygenation have made it possible to perfuse with surprisingly little difficulty for as long as 4 to 6 hours. Disposable membrane oxygenators have also been developed and are used frequently in some centers, particularly for infants, but are somewhat more cumbersome than disposable oxygenators.

PRIMING SOLUTIONS. Originally heart-lung machines were primed with heparinized blood collected within 24 hours before the time of operation, adding 20 mg heparin for each 500 ml blood used. Citrated blood (first demonstrated by Maloney and associates) is now used almost routinely, except in small infants. Some degree of hemodilution is now used routinely during perfusion by most groups. A variety of substances, such as dextrose-water, Ringer's lactate, and other solutions have been used. Our preference is for modified Ringer's lactate solution (Plasmalyte), which closely approximates the electrolyte composition of blood. Serum albumin is also added; so the priming mixture closely resembles plasma. Our preferred technique is to prime the pump-oxygenator with the electrolyte solution up to 40 ml/kg, which is adequate for adult patients but not adequate to fill the oxygenator in smaller children. Once bypass has started, blood is added as needed, but blood is not placed in the oxygenator until the time for initiation of bypass, to avoid prolonged contact of blood with the plastic surfaces of the oxygenator. Blood or packed red cells are added as necessary to keep the hematocrit reading between 20 and 25 percent. If there is significant hypotension, blood or albumin may be added to increase the oncotic pressure of the perfusate.

TECHNIQUE OF PERFUSION. Heparin, 3 mg/kg body weight, is given before the venous and arterial cannulae are inserted. Venous blood is aspirated by gravity or pump drainage through large cannulae inserted into the right atrium, except in some children and young adults, and advanced into the venae cavae. Oxygenated blood is returned to the arterial circulation, usually through a cannula directly inserted into the ascending aorta. Once widely popular, femoral artery cannulation has been almost abandoned to avoid the rare but dangerous complication of retrograde dissection of the aorta. Perfusion is done at a flow rate of about 2,500 ml/m²/minute, providing a flow rate between 4 and 5 liters/minute for adults of normal size. Oxygen flow rates through the oxygenator are adjusted to produce an arterial oxygen tension near 100 mm Hg. Temperature is controlled with a heat exchanger in the circuit and is often lowered to 30 to 32°C. This moderate

Fig. 19-1. Photograph of heart-lung machine, showing the Bentley bubble oxygenator with DeBakey roller pumps. The filters in the coronary suction return are also visible.

hypothermia increases the tolerance of the heart to ischemia produced by temporary occlusion of the ascending aorta in order to permit better visualization of intracardiac structures. Intracardiac blood is aspirated with a suction apparatus, filtered, and returned to the oxygenator.

During perfusion a number of modalities are monitored. Arterial pressure is monitored with a catheter previously inserted into a peripheral artery. Venous pressure in the superior vena cava is carefully observed to be certain that there is no obstruction to return of blood from the brain. The electrocardiogram and electroencephalogram are also monitored. Mean arterial pressure usually decreases sharply with the onset of perfusion, apparently from vasodilatation, and then subsequently rises to levels varying between 50 and 80 mm Hg. The importance of the actual level of mean arterial pressure, as long as flow rate is adequate, is debated. For several years we have preferred to maintain a mean perfusion pressure near that existing before bypass, achieving this by increasing the flow rate, increasing the volume of fluid in the patient, or infusing small amounts of vasopressor agents. This seems especially important in older patients with a history of hypertension or stroke and is of less importance in younger patients and children. There is a wide variability in the blood pressure

response to perfusion. Within a short period of time the blood pressure may stabilize. Some patients develop signs of progressive vasoconstriction after 1 to 2 hours. An occasional patient has a puzzling hypotension which requires rigorous therapy.

Oxygen and carbon dioxide tensions are periodically measured in the venous blood returned to the oxygenator and the oxygenated blood returned to the patient. Preferably the arterial oxygen tension should be near 100 mm Hg and the carbon dioxide tension 30 to 35 mm Hg. Venous blood returning to the heart-lung machine with the described flow rate will usually have an oxygen saturation greater than 50 percent. With flow rates and oxygen saturations in this range, metabolic acidosis of significant degree does not occur.

Heparin is gradually metabolized by the body; so, additional heparin is given each hour of perfusion in a dose of 1 mg/kg body weight. During perfusion the lungs are kept stationary in a partially inflated position with intermittent periods of inflation.

Termination of Perfusion. As perfusion is stopped, left atrial pressure is measured and blood transfused from the heart-lung machine until a left atrial pressure adequate to maintain cardiac output is obtained. The left atrial pressure needed will vary according to that existing before bypass. This technique has been found a better guide to adjustment of blood volume than either blood volume measurement or careful, balanced measurements of blood withdrawn versus blood transfused. Heparin is then neutralized with protamine. Initially 3 mg of protamine/kg is given, regardless of the total amount of heparin administered, assuming that the rate of heparin metabolism approximately equals the rate at which additional heparin is given. A protamine titration is then carried out and additional small amounts of protamine given as indicated. Several reports have emphasized the wide variations in response of patients to both heparin and protamine; so flexibility in management of the individual patient is necessary.

TRAUMA FROM PERFUSION. Extracorporeal circulation produces trauma to the blood, primarily from the exposure of blood to gas in the oxygenator and from the use of suction to aspirate intracardiac blood. At present tolerance for extracorporeal circulation is in the range of 6 to 8 hours; some patients undergo a very long perfusion with surprisingly few metabolic defects, but others show definite signs of physiologic injury after 6 hours of perfusion. Experimental studies of the capillary microcirculation during perfusion have found a progressive sludging of the blood elements, producing stasis and obstruction to capillary blood flow. The concentration of hemoglobin in the plasma is an index of hemolysis occurring during perfusion and may rise 40 to 50 mg/hour perfusion, the amount varying with the volume of urine secreted during perfusion. Some derangement of the clotting mechanisms invariably occurs and is reflected by an increased bleeding tendency afterward even though heparin activity has been neutralized. The coagulation defects, usually from multiple sources, subside within 6 to 12 hours. Bleeding problems are far less frequent than in previous years because of an appreciation of the vulnerability of platelets to injury from a wide variety of medications, especially aspirin, combined with availability of platelets and frozen plasma for correction of coagulation disorders. Fat embolism also has been demonstrated, although the significance is uncertain. Denaturation of plasma proteins occurs from the trauma at the gas-blood interphase and is probably responsible for some of the subtle physiologic changes with long perfusions.

In the past few years several studies have demonstrated microaggregates in the blood in the oxygenator, which can be partly removed with special filters in the pump circuit. Filters of different porosity are now widely used clinically, but their importance is yet uncertain. Our preference is for the Dacron wool (Swank) filter in the coronary suction line, but filters are not used in the venous or arterial lines.

The clinical counterparts of trauma with long perfusions have manifestations in different organs. A bleeding tendency develops, the degree varying with the duration of perfusion and the degree of trauma. This subsides within

12 to 18 hours. A mild degree of renal insufficiency is common after long perfusions, varying with flow rate during perfusion, blood trauma, and acidosis. Fortunately this is usually reversible. Varying degrees of respiratory insufficiency can develop with long perfusions. The cause is not completely clear and is probably related to multiple factors. Postoperatively, some patients require mechanical ventilation for a few hours but seldom for more than 8 to 12 hours. The central nervous system also becomes injured with long perfusions, as a result of which a variety of generalized neurolgic signs may appear. One of the most interesting of these is a psychosis, appearing unpredictably in a few patients, with all the symptoms of a severe toxic psychosis; fortunately this subsides within 2 weeks after operation.

RISK OF PERFUSION. At present the risk from extracorporeal circulation for 1 to 2 hours is extremely small, in the range of less than 1 percent. This low risk represents an astonishing achievement, especially when compared with the fact that as late as 1950 to 1952 the entire concept of extracorporeal circulation was purely hypothetic. Perhaps the most common complication is the development of serum hepatitis, related to the amount of blood used to prime the oxygenator and perform the operation. With longer periods of perfusion, the risk of perfusion per se gradually increases, though perfusion for as long as 6 hours is well tolerated in some patients. In some patients with severe respiratory insufficiency, partial perfusion with extrathoracic cannulation and a membrane oxygenator has been performed for as long as 7 to 8 days.

POSTOPERATIVE CARE AND COMPLICATIONS FOLLOWING EXTRACORPOREAL CIRCULATION

Postoperative care following extracorporeal circulation involves problems which are not encountered following other surgical procedures. Part of the complications arise from the use of extracorporeal circulation, involving several units of blood and moderate trauma to the blood, the degree varying with the duration of extracorporeal circulation as well as with the type of oxygenator. In general, extracorporeal circulation for 2 to 4 hours is well tolerated; periods of 4 to 6 hours may have moderate but reversible complications, while periods for 6 to 9 hours approach the physiologic limits compatible with survival with present pump-oxygenators. The complications are also related to the type of disease which is treated by open cardiotomy and often occur in patients with chronic congestive failure with the attendant impaired function of many organ systems.

GENERAL PROCEDURES. Following these operations, as with most major surgical procedures, temperature, pulse, blood pressure, and respirations are frequently measured. Intraarterial pressure recording is often used for 24 to 48 hours, because residual vasoconstriction following extracorporeal circulation may make auscultatory methods for blood pressure measurement difficult and unreliable. Central venous pressure is routinely measured. In addition, since 1958 or 1960, small polyvinyl catheters frequently have been left in the left atrium and pulmonary artery for 24 to 48 hours to measure oxygen and carbon dioxide tensions in left atrial and mixed venous blood, as well as to measure pulmonary artery and left atrial pressures. The oxygen saturation of mixed venous blood, representing the ability of the respiratory and circulatory systems to supply oxygen requirements, is a particularly useful guide, especially in seriously ill patients. Left atrial pressure is of more value than central venous pressure, especially with isolated left ventricular failure. Pulmonary artery diastolic pressure in most patients parallels left atrial pressure and may be substituted for direct measurement of left atrial pressure in many patients, but this relationship should be checked while the heart is exposed.

Chest roentgenograms are frequently made to evaluate hemothorax, pleural effusion, or atelectasis. The electrocardiogram is regularly monitored on an oscilloscope for varying periods of time because of the frequency of cardiac arrhythmias. Hematocrit, serum electrolyte concentrations (sodium, potassium, carbon dioxide, and chloride), and blood urea nitrogen (BUN) levels are serially measured.

Antibiotics are regularly given in large amounts during the operative procedure and for different lengths of time after operation. Although routines for antibiotic therapy vary widely among different institutions, we have preferred to administer oxacillin, 4 to 8 Gm daily, and more recently cephalothin, 2 Gm daily, for approximately 2 to 4 days following insertion of valvular prostheses. Digitalis is given routinely to patients who previously have been in congestive failure. Anticoagulant therapy is regularly used with valvular prostheses and continued for varying periods of time. It is usually begun 2 to 4 days after operation.

SPECIFIC COMPLICATIONS. Bleeding Syndromes. Although heparin is routinely neutralized with protamine following extracorporeal circulation, it is important to realize that blood-clotting mechanisms are abnormal for 8 to 12 hours following bypass. Unusually diligent care is required following extracorporeal circulation to obtain hemostasis before incisions are sutured, necessitating much more attention than after usual operations. The exact basis for the deficient clotting mechanisms is not certain, since detailed studies of the different components of the blood responsible for normal clotting show some derangement of several components, without any specific correctible factor. Residual heparin activity, the so-called "heparin rebound phenomenon," probably occurs in some patients. When serious defects of blood coagulation persist after operation, transfusion with fresh frozen plasma or platelets is the most effective therapy. Fortunately, the clotting derangements are transitory and will disappear in the majority of patients within a few hours.

Because of the bleeding tendency, unusual care is required to measure blood loss serially and transfuse appropriate amounts of blood. Soft plastic sump tubes are now used regularly in the mediastinum and pericardium after operation and seem superior to previous drainage techniques.

With the extensive bleeding, the possibility of cardiac tamponade from blood clots accumulating in the peri-cardium should be considered. The usual findings with cardiac tamponade include hypotension, elevated venous pressure, and a wide mediastinal shadow on the chest roentgenogram. In doubtful cases reoperation may be required to confirm or exclude the diagnosis. In most patients the right or left pleural cavity is opened at operation to lessen the subsequent risk of cardiac tamponade. Closure of the pericardium may be accomplished in many patients without undue constriction of the heart and has been found by Cunningham and others to lessen the frequency of tamponade.

The usual blood loss following operation is in the range of 400 to 800 ml, although this varies widely among individual patients. A blood loss exceeding 1 liter usually indicates active intrathoracic hemorrhage requiring reoperation. With improvements in pump-oxygenators and surgical technique, the frequency of reoperation for postoperative hemorrhage has greatly decreased.

Cardiac Failure. *Low-Cardiac-Output Syndrome.* In the early period of open heart surgery, a low-cardiac-output syndrome frequently developed. With increasing experience, however, the syndrome has progressively decreased in frequency and is now rarely encountered except in association with specific causes, most of which can be prevented. The normal cardiac output is near 3 liters/m^2/minute. Following cardiac surgical procedures, there may be a decrease to 2 liters/m^2/minute with moderate cardiac failure or to as low as 1 to 1.5 liters/m^2/minute with severe depression of cardiac function. With low cardiac output and deficient perfusion of different organs, a number of metabolic disturbances appear. There is hypotension, vasoconstriction, oliguria, and metabolic acidosis. After varying periods of time, ranging from a few hours to 1 to 2 days, death may result from either progressive hypotension or cardiac arrest.

Although a number of complex hypotheses were developed to explain the low-output syndrome, it is now realized that most of the causative factors are preventable. In the past 2 or 3 years, significant advances in myocardial preservation have been made. Undoubtedly, the most frequent cause of the low-output syndrome is some form of myocardial injury occurring insidiously at operation. Even with advanced cardiac failure, the majority of patients will maintain an adequate cardiac output following operation if the entire underlying valvular pathologic condition is corrected and significant injury to the heart does not occur during operation. Failure to correct the valvular pathologic condition completely, especially before the advent of satisfactory prosthetic cardiac valves, was a frequent cause of cardiac failure. Another frequent cause was hypovolemia.

Although a number of methods to adjust blood volume have been used following extracorporeal circulation, including blood volume determinations and careful fluid balance measurements, the most reliable technique has been transfusion of fluid to elevate the central venous pressure or left atrial pressure to normal or moderately high levels. Preoperatively, many patients with aortic or mitral valvular disease may have a mean left atrial pressure of 15 to 20 mm Hg, and at times even higher levels (20 to 40 mm Hg). As this pressure represents the pressure distending the left ventricle in diastole and hence determining stroke volume and cardiac output, transfusion to similar levels may be required following operation to maintain a satisfactory cardiac output. In retrospect, failure to transfuse adequate fluid was a frequent unrecognized cause of the low-output syndrome.

Coronary air emboli, transection of coronary arteries during a ventriculotomy, or prolonged cardiac ischemia from temporary aortic occlusion are all insults which can depress cardiac function but can be avoided in carefully executed operative procedures. With congenital heart disease, a greatly increased pulmonary vascular resistance, as with a ventricular septal defect and pulmonary hypertension, can severely impair cardiac function after operation and in some patients can result in death. Fortunately, with acquired valvular disease an irreversible increase in pulmonary vascular resistance almost never occurs.

An inadequate cardiac output can be suspected if hypotension, oliguria, or acidosis develops. Acidosis following operation is virtually unknown in the presence of an adequate cardiac ouput, for the acidosis results from production of lactate, pyruvate, and similar anions by anaerobic metabolism. A more precise method for evaluating the low-cardiac-output syndrome is either by direct measurement of cardiac output or by measurement of oxygen saturation of mixed venous blood obtained from the pulmonary artery through an indwelling catheter implanted at operation. The oxygen saturation of mixed venous blood, normally greater than 60 percent, is only an approximation of cardiac output, for it varies with the adequacy of ventilation, the blood volume, the hematocrit, and temperature. However, the oxygen saturation is an extremely useful guide, because it reflects how well the circulation is supplying the oxygen requirements of the body tissues. An oxygen saturation in the range of 50 to 80 percent (P_{O_2} 25 to 30 mm) indicates a moderate deficiency in oxygen transport, while a saturation in the range of 40 to 50 percent (P_{O_2} less than 25 mm) represents a serious deficiency and may be associated with a fatal outcome unless corrected.

Therapy of the low-cardiac-output syndrome includes transfusion of fluid to elevate the central venous pressure to an appropriate level, usually 10 to 12 mm Hg, or the left atrial pressure to 15 to 20 mm Hg. Acidosis which has developed can be corrected by infusion of sodium bicarbonate (50 to 200 mEq). If a low cardiac output remains despite transfusion of appropriate fluid, cardiac inotropic drugs, such as epinephrine or isoproterenol, may be cautiously administered, usually in the range of 1 to 3 μg/minute in adult patients. Premature use of inotropic drugs and vasopressors, such as norepinephrine or metaraminol, in the past perhaps accentuated the severity of the low-cardiac-output syndrome because hypovolemia was not recognized and was further masked by elevation of the blood pressure.

If respiratory insufficiency is present, as manifested by dyspnea or abnormalities in the oxygen and carbon dioxide tensions of arterial blood, artificial ventilation may be required. This is usually done initially by insertion of an endotracheal tube following appropriate sedation of the patient. Tracheostomy is rarely necessary. Digitalis, usually digoxin, should be administered to full therapeutic doses, although the immediate effect on cardiac output is often not significant.

The intraaortic balloon pump has been adopted widely in the last 3 or 4 years to provide an effective method of circulatory support by increasing cardiac index 0.5 to 0.7 liters/minute. Such support may be used for several days or longer and is undoubtedly lifesaving in certain critically ill patients.

Cardiac Arrhythmias. Minor arrhythmias, such as atrial fibrillation or a nodal rhythm, are very common after open heart surgical procedures. An important feature of postoperative care is constant, 24-hour-a-day, visual monitoring of the cardiac rhythm on an oscilloscope for 2 to 3 days following operation. Only by constant visual observation can serious arrhythmias be promptly detected, because such arrhythmias may develop in the presence of a normal cardiac output and without any other signs of circulatory failure.

Tachycardia, either as a sinus rhythm or rapid atrial fibrillation, may result from inadequate amounts of digitalis. Ventricular extrasystoles are the most common serious arrhythmias, because their appearance may herald the developing of more serious arrhythmias, such as bigeminy, ventricular tachycardia, or ventricular fibrillation. Digitalis toxicity is probably the most frequent cause of ventricular arrhythmias, resulting from varying sensitivity to digitalis after operation in relation to changes in plasma potassium concentration. Hypokalemia is particularly frequent, because patients in cardiac failure preoperatively may have significant depletion of body stores of potassium from chronic diuretic therapy.

Mild disturbance of cardiac rhythm from digitalis toxicity will subside following restriction of digitalis and administration of supplemental potassium. Intravenous lidocaine, 1 to 3 mg/minute, is a valuable form of therapy for temporary control of arrhythmias, although the drug is quickly metabolized. In selected arrhythmias the beta-blocking drug propranolol is of great value. Procainamide, in doses varying from 2 to 6 Gm/day, is also useful for more lasting control. In serious circumstances with ventricular tachycardia or other rhythms refractory to other forms of therapy, electrical cardioversion is invaluable.

Chronic Cardiac Failure. When the patient becomes ambulatory a few days after operation, fluid retention commonly becomes evident, especially if sodium intake is not carefully restricted. This can be easily detected by noting the appearance of edema in the flanks, hips, and legs. Weighing the patient daily is an important part of routine postoperative care. The edema usually responds promptly to diuretic therapy and restriction of sodium, but some patients with severe chronic cardiac failure before operation may require long periods of care before edema no longer develops.

Respiratory Insufficiency. Some disturbance of pulmonary function is very common following extracorporeal circulation. The frequency varies widely with different groups and also at different periods of time. The simplest numerical expression of the pulmonary dysfunction is indicated by the alveolar-arterial oxygen gradient, representing impaired diffusion of oxygen from the alveoli into the pulmonary venous blood. There are undoubtedly many causes of the pulmonary dysfunction, some of which are not well understood. Overtransfusion with resulting elevation of left atrial pressure and pulmonary congestion is one of the most frequent causes. Inadequate removal of pulmonary secretions, with resulting atelectasis and infection, is another. Microemboli or fat emboli are less well understood possible causative factors.

Ventilation through an indwelling endotracheal tube for 24 to 48 hours has much decreased the need for tracheostomy. The most effective measures for avoiding pulmonary congestion following operation are the familiar ones of humidification of inspired gas, usually with an oxygen mask, and diligent removal of tracheobronchial secretions, including frequent turning of the patient with coughing and deep breathing. Nasotracheal aspiration with a catheter may be done if necessary. Bronchoscopy is rarely necessary.

Postoperative Fluids. Fluids are restricted moderately during the first 48 hours following operation, though less stringently than in the past. An average intake would be about 30 to 35 ml/kg/24 hours, although wide variation exists. Oral intake is minimized for the first 24 hours after operation because of the risk of gastric dilatation with vomiting and aspiration.

Renal Function. Hourly urine output is carefully measured for 1 to 2 days after operation, preferably keeping the average urine output greater than 30 ml/hour. A transitory elevation of BUN level to 25 to 35 mg/100 ml is commonly seen after complex operative procedures, although the frequency has much decreased with the use of hemodilution priming of the pump-oxygenator. The renal injury may be produced by deficient perfusion, excessive hemolysis, or a transfusion incompatibility. Significant renal failure often presents a high-output renal failure, with daily secretion of 1 to 2 liters of dilute urine, associated with progressive elevation in BUN level. The degree of renal insufficiency in such circumstances can be most simply evaluated by performance of a simple urea clearance test, comparing the simultaneous urea concentration in the blood and the urine. Normally, urea concentration should be at least fifteen to twenty times greater in the urine than in the blood; a urea concentration less than ten times greater in the urine than in the blood usually represents a severe degree of renal insufficiency.

If serious renal insufficiency evolves, peritoneal dialysis is employed at an early stage, often within 2 to 3 days after operation with BUN levels of 75 to 90 mg/100 ml. Postponement of peritoneal dialysis, with progressive increase of BUN concentration above 100 mg/100 ml, may be associated with serious or even fatal cardiac arrhythmias. As the risk of arrhythmias cannot be predicted for an individual patient, the routine use of early dialysis has been of significant benefit. With frequent dialysis, recovery from the renal injury almost always takes place.

Oliguric renal failure of severe degree has a much more ominous prognosis, with a mortality rate exceeding 50 to 70

percent. Fortunately, this is rare. In some instances the etiology remains uncertain.

Fever. There is almost always some fever following extracorporeal circulation, temperatures of 38 to 39°C being very common in the first 1 to 3 days after operation. In some patients, unexplained fevers of 39 to 40°C may develop, probably as a result of minute areas of atelectasis. Contamination of the heart-lung machine with pyrogens was a frequent cause of fever in the early experiences with open heart operations but with disposable oxygenators now occurs rarely. Significant fever, with its detrimental effects on metabolic requirements, can be most simply controlled by the use of a hypothermia mattress beneath the patient through which cold fluid can be circulated at appropriate intervals.

Fever persisting beyond a few days after operation is commonly found to be due to atelectasis or a pleural effusion. Another frequent cause of fever is the so-called "pericardiotomy syndrome," which may develop in any patient in whom the pericardium has been opened at operation, even if extracorporeal circulation has not been employed. This puzzling syndrome, the cause of which still remains unknown despite numerous investigations, may be associated with sustained fever, a pericardial friction rub, and pericardial and pleural effusions. The white blood cell count may be increased in some patients, while in others it is normal or decreased to 5,000 to 7,000 white blood cells per cubic millimeter. In a minority of patients abnormal lymphocytes appear, the recognition of which greatly facilitates the diagnosis. Most patients respond promptly to administration of 50 to 60 mg prednisone daily, which is frequently employed for both a diagnostic and therapeutic test. Prednisone is given for 3 to 4 days and then stopped to see if fever recurs. Recurrences are not uncommon and may require administration of smaller amounts of prednisone, 10 to 20 mg daily, for several days.

Urinary tract infection is another frequent cause of postoperative fever and can be easily recognized by microscopic examination of the urine and appropriate bacterial cultures. With fever continuing more than a few days after operation, the dread question of bacterial endocarditis must always be considered. The diagnosis can be established or excluded only by serial blood cultures, which should routinely be done with persistent unexplained fever. Fortunately in recent years bacterial endocarditis has become extremely rare. With routine use of large amounts of antibiotics both during and following cardiac operations, staphylococcal endocarditis has almost disappeared. Rarely a fungal endocarditis, usually organisms of the *Candida* group, appears and is often lethal. Since our unit adopted the practice of stopping prophylactic antibiotics within 3 to 4 days after operation, as opposed to 7 to 14 days, fungal endocarditis has virtually disappeared.

Central Nervous System. Probably the most common cause of injury to the central nervous system following extracorporeal circulation is air embolism associated with incomplete evacuation of air from the cardiac chambers. It is extraordinarily difficult to remove all intracardiac air, because air pockets may be loculated in pulmonary veins, the left atrium, or the left ventricle. Rarely air accumulating in the right side of the heart with a functioning right ventricle may be propelled through the pulmonary vascular bed into the left side of the heart. Prevention of air embolism is more difficult when previous operations have been performed, producing adhesions which fix the heart in the pericardial cavity and limit manipulation and massage of the heart at the end of perfusion to displace air pockets. Use of both a left ventricular vent and an aortic vent, which function while the heart is beating, is a valuable method of protection from air emboli, since in some patients all air is not completely removed until the heart begins to beat.

Another cause of focal neurologic injury is calcium emboli, especially in patients with calcific aortic stenosis in whom extensive fragmentation of the calcific valve may occur as it is removed, often piecemeal, with rongeurs. Thrombi in the left atrium, usually in patients with chronic mitral stenosis, are another cause of emboli unless they are carefully removed. Fortunately, all these forms of cerebral injury are avoidable with a carefully planned and executed procedure.

With extracorporeal circulation for 5 to 6 hours or longer, especially when associated with significant trauma to the blood from extensive use of intracardiac suction, a diffuse depression of cerebral function may occur, almost always subsiding without residual neurologic injury in a few days. The exact cause of this difficulty is unknown but is probably sludging of blood elements in cerebral capillaries with focal areas of circulatory stasis. Fat emboli have been long considered as a possible cause, but their significance remains uncertain.

A curious postperfusion psychosis may develop in some patients, with all the emotional symptoms of a psychotic syndrome. Intensive therapy with appropriate sedation and physical restraints to avoid bodily harm is necessary. Fortunately such emotional disturbances almost always subside within 2 weeks after operation. They probably also result from diffuse disturbances in cerebral microcirculation.

With focal injuries to the central nervous system, convulsions are frequent and should be anticipated in therapy. With severe injuries, a tracheostomy is usually performed to facilitate removal of bronchial secretions and assist ventilation. In a seriously ill, comatose patient, a sustained convulsion with anoxia can precipitate a serious or fatal cardiac arrhythmia. This can be avoided if a tracheostomy with mechanical ventilation is performed prophylactically. Convulsions usually can be controlled satisfactorily with appropriate amounts of diphenylhydantoin (Dilantin) or phenobarbital. With neurologic injuries fever of 39 to 40°C is common but can be controlled simply by the use of a hypothermia mattress. A massive neurologic injury may be fatal, but less severe ones are seldom permanent. Although intensive care may be necessary for 3 to 4 weeks, virtually complete recovery usually results. If a neurologic deficit persists more than a month after operation, full recovery seldom occurs.

Gastrointestinal Disturbances. A mild paralytic ileus is frequent for the first 24 hours after operation, and for this reason patients are usually not allowed fluids by mouth for this period of time. Otherwise, gastric dilatation with the risk of vomiting and aspiration can occur. After this period of time, gastrointestinal disturbances are infrequent. Rarely, in seriously ill patients, a stress ulcer with serious gastrointestinal hemorrhage can develop. However, the routine use of a bland (antiulcer) diet, combined with antacid medications for the first few days after operation, has greatly decreased the frequency of this ulcer. Perforation of a stress ulcer, a rare and often fatal complication, has not been seen in our unit for several years.

Anemia. Often following operation there is a daily decrease in hematocrit to levels of 28 to 32 percent. Blood transfusion in appropriate amounts is usually given for severe anemia, while oral therapy with iron is sufficient for most patients. Although anemia can result from many causes, it is usually due to an accelerated rate of blood cell destruction, probably from trauma to the red blood cells during extracorporeal circulation.

Anticoagulant Therapy. Although policies vary at different cardiac centers, most patients with prosthetic valves are routinely started on anticoagulants in the 2 to 4 days following operation. Since 1971, with the use of cloth-covered valves, anticoagulant programs have varied widely among different centers, and the overall frequency of major thromboembolism is only 1 to 3 percent. At New York University, sodium warfarin is continued permanently for patients with prosthetic valves; when porcine heterografts are employed, the drug is prescribed for about 3 months following operation. Dosage levels are adjusted to maintain the prothrombin time at about two to two-and-a-half times normal. Once the dosage requirement for warfarin has stabilized, usually within 4 to 6 weeks after operation, aspirin, 0.6 Gm twice daily, is begun and continued daily for 2 years to minimize the hazard of platelet emboli.

CARDIAC ARREST AND VENTRICULAR FIBRILLATION

Cardiac arrest and ventricular fibrillation are considered together in this section because either of these catastrophes produces immediate cessation of the circulation. An injury causing generalized cardiac depression, such as anoxia, is more likely to lead to cardiac arrest, while agents increasing myocardial irritability, such as digitalis intoxication, are more likely to produce ventricular fibrillation. Diagnosis and treatment for the two conditions are, however, very similar.

HISTORICAL DATA. The first successful cardiac resuscitation was performed in 1901 by Igelsrud in Norway, but for many years this remained an isolated therapeutic triumph. The first successful case of electrical defibrillation was reported by Beck in 1947. In 1960 a dramatic advance in cardiac resuscitation occurred when Kouwenhoven, Jude, and Knickerbocker, working as a group at the Johns Hopkins Hospital, first introduced the concept of closed-chest massage. The same group also contributed greatly to the simultaneous development of methods of closed-chest defibrillation. The applicability of closed-chest cardiac massage and defibrillation has greatly enlarged the feasibility of cardiac resuscitation and has made it a responsibility of every physician to become familiar with these techniques. Resuscitative techniques have been successfully taught to large numbers of nonmedical personnel and have been applied effectively in many instances.

PATHOGENESIS. Etiology. A great many agents may cause cardiac arrest. The more frequent of these will be briefly mentioned.

Coronary Thrombosis. Coronary thrombosis, with or without myocardial infarction, may induce either cardiac arrest or ventricular fibrillation and is a frequent cause of cardiac arrest refractory to all forms of therapy.

Anoxia. The depressant effect of anoxia on the myocardium is a frequent major underlying factor in producing cardiac arrest. This can occur from many causes, including depression of respiration, airway obstruction, and aspiration of gastric contents.

Drugs. Several drugs may produce either ventricular fibrillation or cardiac arrest when excessive amounts are used or when an abnormal sensitivity to the drug is present. Digitalis is one of the most prominent of this group, for the sensitivity of the myocardium to digitalis varies with the serum electrolyte concentrations, especially potassium.

Serum Electrolyte Abnormalities. Either deficiency or excess of potassium can cause cardiac arrest. The effects of the abnormal potassium concentration are significantly influenced by the existing concentration of calcium ions, and also by the presence of acidosis or alkalosis.

Anesthesia. Almost any anesthetic agent in excessive amounts will depress the myocardium and precipitate cardiac arrest. Statistical surveys have disclosed that cardiac arrest occurs in approximately 1 in every 1,500 operations.

Bradycardia. A profound bradycardia, with a heart rate below 60 beats per minute, may result in ventricular extrasystoles, subsequently followed by ventricular tachycardia or fibrillation. This is frequently seen in patients with a complete heart block unless the heart rate is increased by electrical or chemical stimulation.

Cardiac Catheterization. Ventricular fibrillation is an infrequent but well-recognized complication of cardiac catheterization or angiocardiography, usually developing during manipulation of the cardiac catheter into different cardiac chambers.

Reflex Mechanisms. On many occasions cardiac arrest has developed in association with some event which stimulated the vagus nerve. Such episodes include endotracheal suctioning, insertion of a gastric tube, or vomiting. It is doubtful that a vagal reflex per se can ever arrest a normal heart. In the laboratory, normal hearts can be arrested for only a few seconds even with continuous electrical stimulation of the vagus nerve. It is probable in clinical circumstances that only a myocardium seriously injured from other causes will be arrested or fibrillated during some event which stimulates the vagus nerve.

Aberrant Electric Currents. When implanted pacemaker wires traverse the chest wall, faulty electrical mechanisms associated with monitoring, electrocardiography, or electrocautery can be responsible for fibrillating the heart. Malfunction of an implanted pacemaker is yet another cause.

Pathophysiology. The cerebral anoxia resulting from cessation of circulation produces significant brain injury within 3 to 4 minutes, depending upon the temperature. Periods of anoxia for 6 to 8 minutes may produce extensive but reversible brain damage, whereas longer periods regularly cause irreversible brain injury. Myocardial anoxia is, of course, also present but is of little clinical significance as compared to the central nervous system injury.

DIAGNOSIS. Since brain injury will develop following 3 to 4 minutes of cardiac arrest, it is imperative that a diagnosis be made rapidly and therapy begun. The physician considering a diagnosis of cardiac arrest should either confirm or exclude it within 30 to 60 seconds and act accordingly. In most patients the diagnosis can be simply made. There is an abrupt disappearance of peripheral pulses, most easily confirmed by palpation of the femoral or carotid arteries. Loss of consciousness quickly occurs, as well as absence of respiratory activity except for a few agonal gasps. Auscultation of the chest readily demonstrates that no cardiac sounds are audible. Complex diagnostic maneuvers which require larger amounts of time should be avoided. It should be emphasized that the *electrocardiogram is of little value for the diagnosis of cardiac arrest,* for electrical activity can continue on the electrocardiogram for some minutes after effective cardiac contractions have ceased. The main value of the electrocardiogram is to demonstrate the presence of ventricular fibrillation, because cardiac arrest can be differentiated from ventricular fibrillation only by the electrocardiogram or by direct inspection of the myocardium.

The most common differential diagnosis from cardiac arrest is the presence of extreme bradycardia with hypotension, as in someone who has fainted or developed anaphylactic shock from a hypersensitivity syndrome. Usually differentiation is not difficult, for although profound peripheral vascular collapse is present, there is some respiratory activity and not a total loss of consciousness.

TREATMENT. Ventilation. The most urgent first step in treatment of cardiac arrest is to provide adequate oxygenation (Fig. 19-2). It is futile to begin cardiac massage without ventilation of the lungs, although under the pressures of extreme circumstances, this obvious fact is often overlooked. Ventilation is most readily accomplished by mouth-to-mouth insufflation of the lungs. This can be begun immediately and continued until less laborious methods can be arranged. Most cardiac resuscitation kits include a laryngoscope and an endotracheal tube which can be inserted by any physician with moderate experience. Until an endotracheal tube can be inserted, however, mouth-to-mouth ventilation should be continued. Attempts to perform a hurried tracheostomy should not be made unless there is an obstruction at the larynx. Tracheostomy under emergency circumstances can be surprisingly difficult and quickly waste the precious few minutes available for preserving cerebral function. If an endotracheal tube cannot be inserted, a cricothyroidotomy, rather than an emergency tracheostomy, is probably preferable, as evidenced by the report of Brantigan and Grow.

Cardiac Massage. Closed-chest massage should be used in the majority of patients. Its efficacy depends upon intermittent compression of the heart between the sternum and the vertebral column, with lateral motion of the heart limited by the pericardium. For performing cardiac massage, the patient must be on a firm surface, such as the floor or a board under his shoulders. Certain points of technique are essential. The heel of the hand should be applied over the lower third of the sternum with the other hand above it to depress the sternum intermittently for 3 to 4 cm (Fig. 19-3). Sternal compression should be brisk, depressing the sternum sharply and then releasing it to permit cardiac filling. Compression of the sternum at a lower level near the xyphoid process may injure the liver, while compression more superiorly or laterally over the chest will result in multiple fractures of the ribs. Massage should be at a rate of about 60 per minute; more than one person is usually required, since the person performing massage will fatigue quickly. The amount of force applied should be gauged by palpation of a peripheral pulse, usually the femoral. Some caution is required to be certain that a regurgitant pulse in the femoral vein is not confused with a pulse in the femoral artery, because a strong retrograde pulse wave can be propagated down the vena cava during massage. Massage should be continued for as long as cardiac resuscitation remains feasible, especially if cerebral function is intact. A definite time limit cannot be given beyond which cardiac massage should be abandoned, although most successful cardiac resuscitations are accomplished within a few minutes. On one occasion we partici-

Fig. 19-2. Technique of mouth-to-mouth ventilation. The chin of the patient must be held forward with one hand to prevent obstruction of the nasopharynx by backward displacement of the tongue. The nostrils need to be occluded with the other hand. The head should be extended on the cervical spine to avoid obstruction in the nasopharynx.

pated in a successful cardiac resuscitation which required 2 hours and 20 minutes of direct massage before a fibrillating heart could be successfully defibrillated. The patient was still well 20 years later.

Open cardiac massage, performed through a lateral thoracotomy in the left fourth or fifth intercostal space, is seldom needed. It should, however, be used if there is an open pericardium, cardiac tamponade, or massive intrathoracic hemorrhage.

Drugs and Fluids. Epinephrine, sodium bicarbonate, and calcium are the most useful agents. Epinephrine, 1 to 2 ml of 1:10,000 dilution, may be injected directly into the heart or into a peripheral vein. Calcium, 3 to 4 ml of a 10% solution, is a similarly powerful stimulant of myocardial contraction. Acidosis is especially common with

Fig. 19-3. A. Closed-chest massage. The heel of the hand should be used to compress intermittently the lower portion of the sternum toward the vertebral column. The effectiveness of the compression should be monitored by palpation of a peripheral pulse by another member of the team. Artificial ventilation must be performed at the same time. B. Cross section of chest showing the anatomic basis for closed-chest massage. The heart is seen suspended in the midthorax between the sternum anteriorly and the vertebral column posteriorly. The pericardium must be intact for closed-chest massage to be effective. C. Compression of the heart as the sternum is depressed downward toward the vertebral column.

A   B   C

cardiac arrest and may require vigorous therapy to restore a normal pH before effective cardiac contractions can be obtained. Sodium bicarbonate, in amounts as large as 200 to 300 mEq, may be required if severe acidosis is present. Rapid intravenous infusion of fluids, up to 1 liter or more, is usually of value, especially if hypovolemia was present before cardiac arrest occurred. An intravenous infusion of vasopressors, usually 1 to 4 μg/minute of norepinephrine or epinephrine, is frequently of value. Other drugs, such as atropine or digitalis, are usually of little benefit.

Defibrillation. In the presence of ventricular fibrillation, which can be confirmed only by the electrocardiogram or by direct inspection of the myocardium, electrical defibrillation is required. This can be accomplished in the closed chest by applying electrodes over the base and apex of the heart or by applying one large electrode posteriorly near the vertebral column and a smaller electrode anteriorly near the cardiac apex (Fig. 19-4). Defibrillation can be done with either alternating or direct current, although studies in recent years have indicated that direct current defibrillation is preferable (approximately 400 joules). With an open chest, direct defibrillation can be easily accomplished by application of electrodes to the heart and administration of an appropriate electric impulse, usually 110 to 120 volts for 0.1 second. The usual cause of failure to defibrillate is either an anoxic or an acidotic myocardium. Vigorous massage before application of the electric shock may be required to oxgenate the myocardium sufficiently. Acidosis can be corrected with bicarbonate. Injection of epinephrine may also stimulate myocardial tone and enhance subsequent defibrillation. Unless a coronary thrombosis has occurred, it should be possible to defibrillate almost all fibrillating hearts, although the ensuing

Fig. 19-4. Technique of closed-chest defibrillation. One electrode paddle is applied at the apex of the heart and the other at the base. The most common errors are inadequate electrical contact between the electrodes and the skin or inadequate amounts of current.

cardiac arrest may be refractory to therapy. Inability to defibrillate is usually due to one or more correctible causes, such as inadequate electric stimulus, inadequate application of electrodes, anoxic myocardium, or acidosis. The heart should be observed closely when the electric shock is applied. If adequate current is transmitted through the myocardium, the fibrillations will cease almost immediately, though they may recur. If the fibrillations are not stopped completely for a short period, enough current has not been transmitted, and the stimulus should be adjusted accordingly. Causes of inadequate current include the voltage applied, the electrodes, and the manner in which the electrodes are applied to the heart.

Therapy following Cardiac Resuscitation. Following restoration of an adequate heartbeat, careful note should be made of the presence of injury to the central nervous system. This is usually indicated by continuing coma. Patients with significant brain injury are best treated by mild hypothermia, lowering the body temperature to 33 to 34°C and maintaining this temperature for 3 to 4 days. There are abundant experimental data indicating that this mild degree of hypothermia will significantly enhance recovery from cerebral injury. Hypothermia should be begun soon, because hyperthermia to 39 to 40°C often develops within 2 to 4 hours. Massive doses of a steroid, e.g., 2 to 3 Gm of prednisone, should be given every 6 to 8 hours for 24 to 48 hours to minimize cerebral edema. The efficacy is difficult to measure, although steroids have been shown to be beneficial in experimental cerebral edema.

Continuous visual monitoring of the cardiac rhythm with an oscilloscope is essential, because arrhythmias are frequent and some can progress to ventricular fibrillation unless promptly treated. Intravenously administered lidocaine, 1 mg/minute, and procainamide are both very useful drugs for suppressing cardiac arrhythmias. Adequacy of cardiac output and ventilation can be monitored by periodic measurment of arterial and central venous blood-gas concentrations (P_{O_2}, P_{CO_2}, and pH).

Fluid therapy should be carefully regulated, depending upon the blood volume and the renal function. Excessive fluids may intensify cerebral edema. Adequacy of ventilation should be carefully assessed, because anoxia can readily precipitate another episode of cardiac arrest. In comatose patients, a tracheostomy is usually performed, and frequent assisted ventilation with a mechanical respirator is performed for 2 to 3 days.

PROGNOSIS. Unless a myocardial thrombosis or some other irreversible injury is present, the majority of patients in whom cardiac arrest has developed may be effectively treated if the correct diagnosis is made promptly.

When a reversible cardiac injury is present, as with overdose of an anesthetic agent, cardiac resuscitation is almost uniformly possible if begun quickly. Similarly, ventricular fibrillation from a variety of mechanisms can be promptly and effectively treated by external defibrillation if defibrillation is done before severe myocardial anoxia has developed. The usual cause of failure of defibrillation is the presence of an underlying myocardial thrombosis.

MITRAL STENOSIS

HISTORICAL DATA. A valiant effort to treat mitral stenosis by excising a portion of the valve with a valvulotome was made by Cutler and Levine in 1923, but the resulting mitral insufficiency caused a prohibitive operative mortality. Souttar, in 1925, performed a digital commissurotomy in one patient. Thereafter surgical efforts virtually ceased for over 20 years until 1948–1949 when Harken et al. and Bailey independently demonstrated the value of digital commissurotomy. These early commissurotomies, often limited in extent, frequently produced striking clinical improvement, even though mitral stenosis frequently recurred within 5 years. A transventricular mitral dilator developed around 1957 produced a more extensive commissurotomy and was widely adopted. Subsequently the increasing safety of cardiopulmonary bypass made commissurotomy under direct vision the procedure of choice in most centers, though some groups still obtain excellent results with a closed commissurotomy. When a closed commissurotomy is undertaken, the heart-lung machine is usually kept on a standby basis to permit use of cardiopulmonary bypass if closed commissurotomy becomes hazardous or is unsuccessful. When the mitral valve has been virtually destroyed by fibrosis and calcification, effective commissurotomy is not possible, and replacement with a prosthetic valve is necessary.

ETIOLOGY. All evidence indicates that mitral stenosis is almost always due to rheumatic fever, even though a definite history of rheumatic fever can be obtained in only about 50 percent of patients. Congenital mitral stenosis is very rare, less than 300 cases having been reported. After the initial episode of rheumatic fever, symptoms of mitral stenosis may not appear for 10 or more years but may develop as soon as 3 years in some patients and as late as 25 years in others. Selzer and Cohn, in an excellent review of clinical characteristics of mitral stenosis, have suggested that scarring of the mitral valve from rheumatic fever may cause turbulent flow of blood which in turn causes progressive scarring and contraction over many years; this would explain the appearance of severe mitral stenosis 20 to 30 years after the last known bout of rheumatic fever.

PATHOLOGY. Although rheumatic fever produces a pancarditis, involving pericardium, myocardium, and endocardium, the most serious permanent injury results from the endocarditis. Permanent myocardial injury following recovery from acute myocarditis is ill defined and apparently seldom of clinical significance. Endocarditis produces ulceration of the endocardium along the edges of the valve leaflets where they normally appose in systole. Tiny, 1- to 2-mm nodules of fibrin and platelets accumulate and may progress to fusion of the leaflets at the commissures. A more serious injury evolves from extensive valvulitis with fibrosis and contraction of the body of the leaflets, compounded in subsequent years with calcification and decreasing leaflet mobility. Inflammation of the chordae tendineae similarly leads to fibrosis with contraction, thickening, and fusion. With severe disease the chordae contract to such an extent that the valve leaflets are pulled down to appose the tips of the underlying papillary muscles.

In many patients mitral stenosis gradually increases in severity over many years, at times more than 20. Previously these progressive changes were considered due to clinically silent episodes of rheumatic fever. A more plausible current hypothesis is that the changes are hemodynamic in origin, resulting from turbulent flow of blood originally produced by the initial inflammation and scarring.

The possibilities of surgical correction of mitral stenosis vary greatly with the nature of the valve injury. When simple fusion of the commissures is the only lesion, mitral commissurotomy is highly successful. With concomitant fibrosis and rigidity of the leaflets, commissurotomy is less effective. If the chordae tendineae have contracted and fused to make the leaflets immobile, commissurotomy may be impossible. With such advanced pathology replacement of the diseases valve with a prosthesis is necessary. How often this is required varies with the type of patient operated on. When operation is performed fairly "early" in the course of the disease, valvular reconstruction, rather than replacement, should be possible in the majority of patients, i.e., 85 to 90 percent.

PATHOPHYSIOLOGY. A normal mitral valve has a cross-sectional area between 4 and 6 cm^2. Reduction of the cross-sectional area to 2 to 2.5 cm^2 constitutes the mildest form of mitral stenosis. Typical auscultatory findings are present, but the patient is often asymptomatic (Class I). Further reduction to the range of 1.5 to 2.0 cm^2 produces some symptoms (Class II disability); these are more severe with a cross-sectional area in the range of 1 to 1.5 cm^2. Patients with a cross-sectional area of less than 1 cm^2 are usually seriously disabled (Class IV). A valve area near 0.6 cm^2 is said to be the minimal size compatible with life.

Three significant physiologic events result from mitral stenosis—increase in left atrial pressure, decrease in cardiac output, and increase in pulmonary vascular resistance. Increase in left atrial pressure (normally less than 10 to 12 mm Hg) is the immediate consequence of mitral stenosis. The degree of elevation of left atrial pressure varies with three factors: (1) the cross-sectional area of the mitral orifice, (2) cardiac output, and (3) cardiac rate. These three factors represent physical laws determining pressure-flow relations through a stenotic orifice, namely, cross-sectional area of orifice, total volume of flow, and duration of time during which flow occurs. When left atrial pressure rises to exceed oncotic pressure of plasma (25 to 30 mm Hg), transudation of fluid across the pulmonary capillaries will occur. The result of this transudation depends upon the capacity of the pulmonary lymphatics to transport the additional fluid. When the fluid load exceeds the capacity of the lymphatic circulation, pulmonary edema results. Clinically, therefore, left atrial pressure and concomitant pulmonary symptoms vary with the degree of mitral stenosis, the cardiac output as influenced by exercise or emotion, and the length of diastole determined by cardiac rate.

As the oncotic pressure of plasma is 25 to 30 mm Hg,

about that of a column of blood 12 to 14 in. high, pulmonary congestion in the upright position may be much greater in the lower lobes of the lung than in the upper, for the average thorax is about 20 in. high. A patient with only basilar rales in the upright position may develop extensive pulmonary congestion when supine, with cough, dyspnea, or frank pulmonary edema. Hence, the pathogenesis of paroxysmal nocturnal dyspnea.

The cardiac output is fixed at a low level by the rigid stenotic orifice. With exercise, cardiac output cannot be increased significantly, and dyspnea results. The general fatigue and limitation of physical activity with mitral stenosis is a clinical reflection of this physiologic inability to increase cardiac output.

The degree to which pulmonary vascular resistance increases with mitral stenosis varies greatly among different patients. The cause for the variation is unknown. Some, with severe mitral stenosis, have little change, while in others vascular resistance increases to levels fifteen to twenty times greater than normal. This increased resistance is primarily a result of vasoconstriction in the pulmonary arterioles, ultimately intensified by hypertrophy of the media and intima. In far advanced cases recurrent pulmonary emboli may create additional obstruction, but this is uncommon. Fortunately, in the vast majority of patients, the increased vascular resistance either decreases greatly or disappears following surgical correction.

Two other serious disabilities which appear with chronic mitral stenosis are atrial fibrillation and systemic embolization. Atrial fibrillation is the usual ultimate consequence of the atrial hypertrophy produced by chronic left atrial hypertension. Fibrillation produces some decrease in cardiac output and also is often a prelude to more serious arrhythmias. The most serious consequence, however, is the development of thrombi, usually in the ineffectively contracting left atrial appendage. The frequency of thrombi varies both with the duration of mitral stenosis and the presence of atrial fibrillation. Utlimately thrombi develop in 15 to 20 percent of patients, after which episodes of arterial embolism appear with increasing frequency. Before either anticoagulant therapy or operation was possible, cerebral embolism caused death in 20 to 25 percent of patients dying from mitral stenosis.

CLINICAL MANIFESTATIONS. Symptoms. The most important symptom is *dyspnea.* This appears whenever mean left atrial pressure exceeds 30 mm Hg long enough to produce significant transudation of fluid into the pulmonary capillaries. Characteristically, it first appears with extreme exertion and subsequently, with more severe stenosis, occurs with lesser degrees of exertion. It may also appear with emotion or other circumstances which increase cardiac output.

Several other symptoms subsequently appear, all developing as a result of recurrent pulmonary congestion. A chronic *cough,* worse in the evenings in the recumbent position, is frequent, reflecting basilar congestion. *Orthopnea* and *paroxysmal nocturnal dyspnea* similarly reflect the influence of the upright position on the localization of pulmonary congestion. In the upright position, congestion may be limited to the lower lobes but becomes more diffuse in the supine position. Mobilization of peripheral edema from the lower extremities when the patient is supine intensifies the degree of pulmonary congestion. *Hemoptysis* is a frequent symptom, varying from expectoration of blood-tinged sputum to massive amounts of bright red blood, in unusual circumstances exceeding 1 liter. Fortunately such severe hemoptysis, although an alarming symptom, usually subsides spontaneously. Rarely, an emergency mitral valvotomy is required. Episodes of *pulmonary edema* occur when pulmonary congestion greatly exceeds the capacity of the pulmonary lymphatics. In contrast to hemoptysis, pulmonary edema may be fatal unless quickly and effectively treated.

When pulmonary vascular resistance rises to produce pulmonary hypertension, failure of the right side of the heart appears, manifested by venous distension, hepatic enlargement, and peripheral edema.

As mentioned earlier, atrial fibrillation develops eventually in most patients. Initially it may be transient, but ultimately in most patients chronic atrial fibrillation is the most common rhythm.

Arterial embolism is a constant threat, especially with atrial fibrillation, although emboli can occur with a sinus rhythm. Emboli evolve from stasis in the dilated left atrium, especially in the atrial appendage. Rarely, huge thrombi 5 to 10 cm in diameter may fill much of the left atrium and partly obstruct the ostia of the pulmonary veins.

Angina pectoris develops in about 10 percent of patients. The basic cause is unclear, for it is usually not due to associated coronary atherosclerosis. Possible mechanisms include a low cardiac output, impaired blood flow during diastole because of tachycardia, and recurrent small emboli to the coronary arteries.

Physical Examination. A patient with chronic, severe mitral stenosis may be thin and frail, with the muscular wasting characteristic of a chronic illness. Dilated neck veins are visible if congestive failure is present. Rubor and/or cyanosis are often seen over the fingers or lips. These signs reflect a chronic severe restriction in cardiac output, resulting in blood flowing slowly through peripheral capillary beds. Rales are frequently audible over the lung bases.

On examination of the heart, the cardiac size and the quality of the apical impulse are of particular importance. Often with pure mitral stenosis, the cardiac size is normal, and the apical impulse is normal or decreased in intensity. A forceful, heaving left ventricular impulse immediately suggests that associated disease, such as mitral insufficiency or aortic valvular disease with resulting ventricular hypertrophy, is present. With increased pulmonary vascular resistance, palpation of the left parasternal area may find a "lift," resulting from contraction of a hypertrophied right ventricle. The pulse rhythm may be regular but is usually atrial fibrillation.

The three significant auscultatory findings with mitral stenosis are the diastolic rumble, an opening snap, and an increased first sound. The apical diastolic rumble, at times sharply localized to an area at the apex only 2 to 3 cm in diameter, is the hallmark of mitral stenosis. It may be of grade I or II intensity in some patients, while in others it is unusually loud with a palpable thrill. The intensity of the murmur, however, does not correlate with the severity of the stenosis. Rarely "silent" mitral stenosis is present without an audible murmur. This results from a calcified, fibrosed valve with little mobility. The increased first sound, the origin of which is not certain, is another distinctive feature and is often the first auscultatory abnormality detected. The opening snap, closely following the second sound, is the third distinctive feature. In many patients careful auscultation can immediately establish the diagnosis of mitral stenosis by finding the triad of an opening snap, followed by a diastolic rumble, and an accentuated first sound.

A short apical systolic murmur may be heard in patients with pure mitral stenosis without any associated mitral insufficiency. Loud pansystolic murmurs, however, which are transmitted to the axilla usually indicate associated mitral insufficiency. A systolic murmur from tricuspid insufficiency may be confused with one arising from mitral insufficiency. The systolic murmur of tricuspid insufficiency, although audible at the apex with hypertrophy of the right ventricle, is usually heard equally well near the sternum and may be accentuated with deep inspiration.

Laboratory Studies. The initial change in mitral stenosis is dilatation of the left atrium (Fig. 19-5). Hence, detection of slight degrees of enlargement of the left atrium is of particular importance in establishing the diagnosis. Once it has been determined that the left atrium is enlarged, however, there is little correlation between the actual size of the left atrium and the severity of the mitral stenosis. Left atrial enlargement is best detected with a lateral chest roentgenogram exposed during oral administration of barium to outline the esophagus. Characteristically, the middle third of the esophagus is displaced backward to form a slight concave curve. With additional degrees of enlargement, the dilated left atrium may be visible as a double shadow in the posteroanterior roentgenogram, forming a separate dense shadow behind the normal shadow of the right atrium. The left border of the cardiac shadow also shows characteristic changes with mitral stenosis, for the normal concavity between the shadow of the aortic knob and the left ventricle becomes obliterated as both the left atrium and the pulmonary artery enlarge to produce a "straight" left heart border. The overall cardiac size may be normal, but lateral views can demonstrate enlargement of the right ventricle when pulmonary vascular resistance has increased. Calcification of the mitral valve is visible with chronic disease in older patients.

Careful roentgenographic scrutiny of the lung fields is of particular importance, for several abnormalities occur. Engorged pulmonary veins can be unusually prominent, often with a greater degree of dilatation in the veins to the upper lobes. With pulmonary hypertension the pulmonary arteries are also enlarged. With chronic, severe left atrial hypertension, dilated pulmonary lymphatics become visible as transverse lines across the lower lung fields, "Kerley lines," indicating significant left atrial hypertension.

The electrocardiogram is normal in some patients. The earliest change is an increased P wave from hypertrophy of the left atrium. Unfortunately, this is not consistent, and different studies have reported variation in the frequency of P-wave abnormalities from as low as 20 to 30 percent to as high as 70 to 80 percent. Only with increase in pulmonary vascular resistance does right ventricular hypertrophy produce distinct electrocardiographic changes, with the development of a right axis deviation. Hence, the electrocardiogram often is an inaccurate guide to the severity of the mitral stenosis. It is of particular value, however, in differential diagnosis, for signs of left ventricular hypertrophy immediately suggest some disease in addition to mitral stenosis, usually mitral insufficiency or aortic valvular disease.

Cardiac catheterization is required to evaluate mitral stenosis precisely, as well as for detecting the presence of additional valvular disease, such as mitral insufficiency or aortic valvular disease. Left atrial pressure is usually estimated from the pulmonary capillary "wedge" pressure, although alternatively the left atrium can be entered directly with a catheter, usually by puncture of the atrial septum. The left atrial pressure in isolated mitral stenosis is increased from the normal range of 5 to 10 mm Hg to levels of 20 to 30 mm Hg with severe stenosis, producing a diastolic pressure gradient between the left atrium and left ventricle of 10 to 20 mm Hg. It is important to realize that the left atrial pressure varies not only with the severity of the stenosis, but also with the cardiac output and the cardiac rate. Hence, evaluation of an isolated determination must include assessment of these additional factors. The most precise measurement is mathematical calculation of the cross-sectional area of the mitral valve, determined by the pressure gradient and the cardiac output. Angiography may demonstrate rigidity and limited mobility of the valve leaflets but is not of great diagnostic value. It is of particular value, however, in determining the presence of mitral insufficiency by noting the reflux of dye after injection into the left ventricle. Coronary arteriography is an important part of the evaluation of cardiac catheterization, especially in patients over forty years of age in whom coronary atherosclerosis may be present.

DIAGNOSIS. A diagnosis of mitral stenosis can usually be made with certainty on physical examination, with the finding of the triad of an opening snap, an apical diastolic rumble, and an increased first sound. These abnormalities often occur in association with a normal left ventricle, an enlarged left atrium, signs of pulmonary congestion, pulmonary hypertension, and right ventricular hypertrophy. The differential diagnosis should include associated mitral insufficiency, tricuspid insufficiency, or aortic valvular disease.

TREATMENT. Indications for Operation. Operation is usually recommended for any patient with symptoms, because the risk is small (1 to 2 percent) and the slight but definite hazard of cerebral embolism is always present. If peripheral embolism has occurred, operation should be performed as soon as the patient has recovered from the embolic episode, for sooner or later emboli almost always recur. Until operation is performed, continuous anticoagulant therapy should be employed.

Fortunately, mitral stenosis almost always can be successfully operated upon, no matter how far advanced the disease or how severe the pulmonary hypertension. The immediate risk of operation is increased with far advanced disease, but surviving patients nearly always show remarkable improvement, with a significant decrease in, or complete disappearance of, pulmonary hypertension.

General Considerations. Since 1971 at New York University almost all mitral valve operations have been performed with cardiopulmonary bypass. The "closed" commissurotomy, performed blindly with the index finger introduced through the left atrial appendage, has been virtually abandoned. For some years mitral operations were performed with the heart-lung machine on a "standby" basis: a closed commissurotomy was attempted first, but if it was unsatisfactory, cardiopulmonary bypass was employed. For several reasons, an open operation with cardiopulmonary bypass is now preferred. The risk of bypass is very small, approaching less than 1 percent. The hazard of emboli from thrombi in the atrium or calcium in the mitral valve is much less than with blind, digital commissurotomy. Of even greater importance, perhaps, is that a more effective commissurotomy can be performed as the commissures can be clearly separated, underlying fused

chordae separated, and a wide mitral orifice obtained without producing mitral insufficiency. Not all cardiac centers agree with this policy, however, and some continue to report excellent short-term results with the classic digital commissurotomy.

Technique of Open Mitral Commissurotomy. A median sternotomy incision is employed in almost all cases unless a previous sternotomy incision has been made, in which case a left thoracotomy is used. A sternotomy is preferred because of ready access to the heart, including palpation of the mitral and tricuspid valves, cannulation of the aorta and venae cavae, as well as access to the aortic valve if needed. Once cardiopulmonary bypass is established, body temperature is lowered to 30°C and the heart fibrillated. The left atrium is opened with a longitudinal incision in the interatrial groove, anterior to the point of entry of the right pulmonary veins. By extending the atriotomy beneath the superior vena cava above and the inferior vena cava below, adequate exposure of the mitral valve can be obtained. Usually the aorta is intermittently occluded for periods of 10 to 15 minutes to attain a dry, quiet heart. Before the aortic occlusion clamp is intermittently released, a small catheter vent is placed in the ascending aorta through a stab wound to remove accumulated air.

A

Fig. 19-5. *A.* Chest roentgenogram of a patient with mitral stenosis showing a heart of normal size. The prominent pulmonary artery along the left cardiac border is characteristic of this condition. The enlarged left atrium can be seen as a double density behind the shadow normally formed by the right atrium.

Periodically the heart is defibrillated and allowed to beat for 3 to 4 minutes, to permit adequate distribution of coronary blood flow.

Any thrombi in the atrium or atrial appendage are carefully removed before the mitral valve is approached. The atrial appendage, a potential source of postoperative emboli, is routinely excluded from the atrial cavity, either by closure of the orifice from within the atrium or by amputating the appendage outside the heart (Fig. 19-6).

The fused commissures of the mitral valve are best exposed by inserting sutures into both the aortic and mural leaflets for traction. By applying *horizontal,* not vertical, traction on the two leaflets, the fused commissures can be clearly visualized. The commissure is then carefully separated with a knife, often with a right-angled clamp held open below the commissure to identify chordae arising from the underlying papillary muscle and inserting on the adjacent leaflets. Division of any chordae is scrupulously avoided. A technical problem encountered in 25 to 30 percent of patients is fusion and contraction of the chordae beneath the commissures, often with the fused commissures virtually attached to the papillary muscle. In such instances the papillary muscle is carefully split with a knife for as much as 1 cm, carefully preserving the chordae to each leaflet. This, of course, greatly increases the efficacy of

the commissurotomy and is one of the attractive features of routine open operation.

The question of having produced mitral insufficiency following commissurotomy can be assessed by selective induction of aortic insufficiency, using a small plastic catheter (#10 French) with multiple side perforations over a length of 6 to 7 cm. The catheter is introduced into the ascending aorta through a stab wound and manipulated across the aortic valve into the left ventricle, occluding the aorta momentarily to permit collapse of the valve leaflets. With the catheter in its proper position, some perforations are in the aorta while the remainder are in the ventricle (Figs. 19-7 to 19-9). Then, when the aortic clamp is released, removing intraaortic air, blood refluxes through the catheter into the ventricle, ballooning the aortic leaflets of the mitral valve and seating it firmly against the mural leaflet. Areas of regurgitation can be readily identified and corrected, usually with direct sutures, although a few patients may require an annuloplasty.

As originally reported by Mullin in 1974, this method has been used for about 5 years and has greatly simplified valvuloplasty, permitting a bolder approach. Hence a wider opening can be safely produced. This, in turn, should minimize the likelihood of turbulent flow and recurrence in the future. For a long time the reliability of the method

Fig. 19-5. *B.* Lateral roentgenogram of the same patient shows enlargement of the left atrium, producing a concave displacement of the esophagus, which has been filled with barium.

Fig. 19-6. Open mitral commissurotomy. *A.* The left atrium has been incised and the edges retracted. A small thrombus is present in the midportion of the field, demonstrating the pathologic condition which frequently causes cerebral embolism with mitral stenosis. *B.* Large clot found within the left atrium. With cardiopulmonary bypass functioning, the left atrium has been opened widely. The laminated clot is being removed with a large spoon. A clamp occluding the ascending aorta to avoid embolization of clot is visible at the top of the illustration. *C.* Large laminated clot removed at operation from a patient with mitral stenosis. The inability to detect the presence of such a clot before operation is the most cogent reason that all mitral commissurotomies should be performed with a pump-oxygenator as a "standby," to be employed if such a clot is found.

was routinely checked by subsequent digital palpation of the mitral valve with the heart beating and the systolic pressure near the preoperative level, but this now seems superfluous.

After discontinuing bypass, adequate correction of the mitral stenosis is confirmed by measuring left atrial and ventricular pressure by needle puncture and demonstrating elimination of the end-diastolic pressure gradient. This is an important check, surprisingly neglected in many reports, because with fibrosis and stiff mitral leaflets an opening that seems adequate may be restrictive because of the impaired mobility of the leaflets.

Following operation convalescence is usually benign, and the patient is discharged in 10 to 12 days. If atrial fibrillation is present, an attempt is made to convert it to a sinus rhythm. This is usually successful if chronic atrial fibrillation, with hypertrophy of left atrial musculature, has not been present.

Technique of Mitral Valve Replacement. An approach with a sternotomy incision similar to that for open commissurotomy is used. Mitral replacement, rather than commissurotomy, is almost always necessary if both insufficiency and stenosis are present. It is frequently needed for mitral stenosis with extensive calcification in the valve if the calcification is in the commissures, while calcification in the leaflets does not preclude effective commissurotomy. When replacement is done, the valve is excised by incising it a few millimeters from the annulus with a circumferential incision, which often removes the entire valve intact (Fig. 19-10). Underlying papillary muscles are divided near their apexes. A ball-valve prosthesis is used almost routinely, though excellent results also have been reported with a disc prosthesis. The ball-valve prosthesis has the advantages of longer experience in its use and less likelihood of prosthetic failure, which has been more frequent with a disc prosthesis. The problem of a small left ventricle with mitral stenosis has been avoided by careful selection of a valve of appropriate size. Rarely an obstructing collar of muscle in the wall of the left ventricle has been excised to avoid possible protrusion of muscle into the cage of the prosthesis. With these precautions a ball-valve prosthesis has functioned well. Some have proposed that ventricular function is better with a disc than with a ball-valve prosthesis, but data demonstrating a significant difference are meager (Figs. 19-11 and 19-12).

The prosthesis is inserted with a series of 12 to 18 mattress sutures of Dacron, with a pledget in each mattress suture to avoid the suture's cutting through a friable annulus (Fig. 19-13). Before pledgeted mattress sutures were routinely employed, significant postoperative insufficiency from suture leaks continued to occur, but the routine use of pledgets has virtually eliminated this complication. An alternative technique, widely and effectively used by others, is to insert 25 to 30 simple interrupted sutures. Care is taken to insert the sutures in the annulus, but no deeper, to avoid injury to the coronary sinus, the circumflex coronary artery, or the conduction bundle. Once the prosthesis has been tied in position, the motion of the ball in the cage is carefully checked to be certain that no muscle bundles in the ventricular cavity protrude into the cage

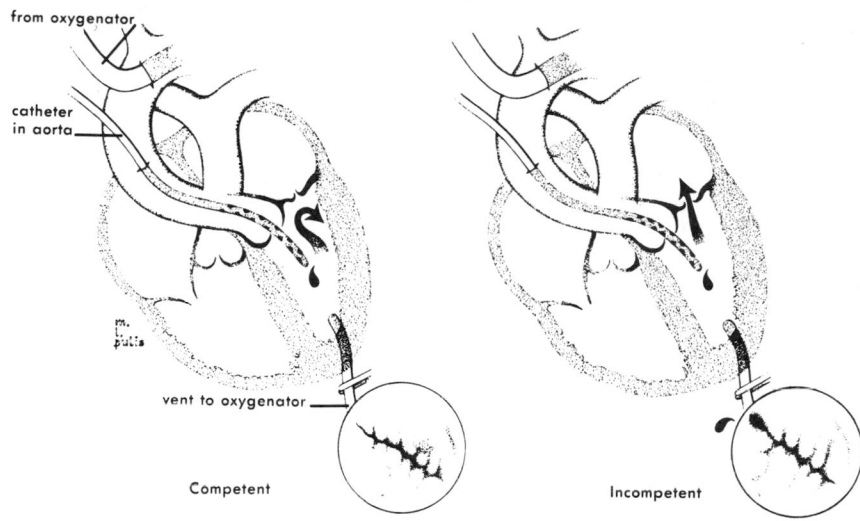

Fig. 19-7. Assessment of mitral regurgitation utilizing controlled aortic insufficiency to close mitral valve.

and restrict motion of the ball. With this important precaution, so-called postoperative thrombosis of a prosthetic valve has not been seen.

As the atriotomy is closed, air is removed from the heart with the conventional Foley catheter left across the mitral valve, but in addition the apexes of both the left ventricle and the ascending aorta are vented to remove air, as the simple use of the Foley catheter is not completely effective in removing air emboli. A catheter vent in the ascending aorta, rather than the needle vent previously used, has been found far more effective for prevention of air embolism.

Fig. 19-8. A. Closure of left atrial appendage. B. Exposure of mitral valve with horizontal traction on sutures. C. Right-angle clamp guides incision.

Convalescence is usually benign except in patients with long-standing congestive failure where the cardiac output may be low for 1 to 2 days and require careful supportive care. Antibiotics are given for 3 to 5 days. Anticoagulation with sodium warfarin is begun about 4 days after operation and maintained with a prothrombin time near 20 seconds, a significantly lesser degree of anticoagulation than the former prothrombin levels near 30 seconds. This more conservative approach has less risk of anticoagulant hemorrhage but has not been associated with an increase in frequency of thromboembolism. Anticoagulation is continued permanently. Acetylsalicylic acid, 0.6 Gm twice daily, is also given for 1 to 2 years for possible inhibition of platelet aggregation. The frequency of thromboembolism has been small, in a range of 2 to 4 percent.

Most patients improve promptly after operation, obtaining the full therapeutic benefit within 3 to 6 months. Dur-

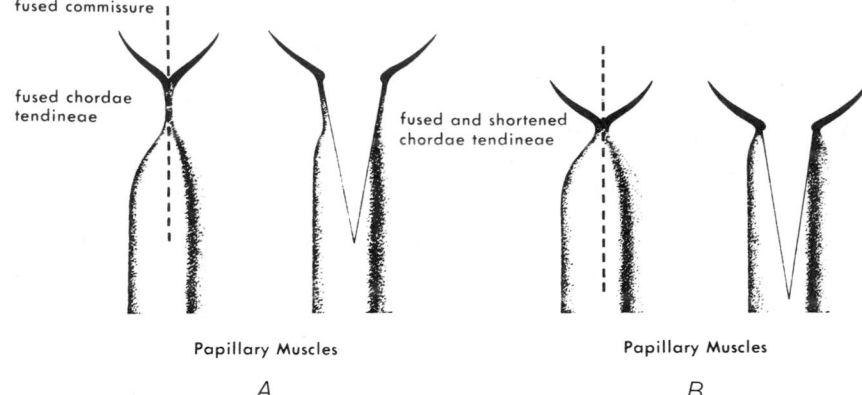

A   *B*

Fig. 19-9. *A.* Separation of fused chordae tendinae with incision into papillary muscle. *B.* Deeper incision into papillary muscle when valve leaflets are fused to underlying papillary muscle.

ing this time careful attention to salt intake and body weight is necessary, for renal excretion of sodium remains impaired for several weeks.

Within 6 months after operation most patients have little physical restriction of activity. However, a few, with chronic congestive failure and cardiac enlargement beforehand, continue to have some permanent limitation, apparently from irreversible myocardial injury before operation.

Different types of tissue valve have been used, including aortic homografts, fascia lata, dura mater, and most recently gluteraldehyde-preserved porcine heterografts.

Fig. 19-10. *A.* Excised mitral valve with severe calcification. When such calcification is present, satisfactory function can rarely be restored to the valve. *B.* Calcified mitral valve removed from another patient in whom prosthetic replacement of the mitral valve was necessary.

These are discussed in more detail in the following section on mitral insufficiency.

PROGNOSIS. Following an adequate mitral commissurotomy that does not produce insufficiency, long-term prognosis is very good. As the valve is not normal, long-term function will probably be determined by the degree of fibrosis in the leaflets and the chordae. If these fibrotic changes are extensive enough to produce significant turbulent flow of blood, eventual stiffening and calcification of the leaflets are likely. However, if disease is predominantly in the commissures, excellent long-term function may be expected. Formerly a recurrence rate of mitral stenosis as high as 30 to 40 percent within 5 years after operation was reported, but this group included a significant percentage of patients in whom commissurotomy was initially ineffective, either because of technique or because calcification and fibrosis prevented effective reconstruction, for which prosthetic replacement is now done.

With commissurotomy as now performed, recurrence at 5 years is probably near 10 percent, far less than that estimated in the past. In a group of patients operated upon by the author at the University of Kentucky between 1961 and 1966, reported in a larger series by Bryant and Trinkle in 1971, the recurrence rate was well under 10 percent. Similarly, Higgs and associates in 1970 and Morrow and Braunwald in a careful study of 45 patients from a series of 226 undergoing mitral commissurotomy found that true restenosis occurred in only 5 patients. As stated earlier, the frequent "restenosis" reported previously was often simply an ineffective commissurotomy. Valve complications which do occur at a later date, either restenosis or insufficiency, are probably due to fibrosis of the valve leaflets from turbulent flow of blood, much like that seen in a congenitally bicuspid aortic valve, and are not a result of recurrent rheumatic fever. Since 1966, the author has not had a single patient who developed recurrent stenosis of the mitral valve due to an inadequate commissurotomy.

Following prosthetic replacement of the mitral valve, the risk of endocarditis is small but permanent. Hence, prophylactic antibiotics should be routinely employed when episodes of transient bacteremia can be anticipated, as with

Fig. 19-11. *A.* Starr-Edwards mitral prosthesis. This prosthesis is completely covered with cloth and uses a steel ball. It is hoped that the complete covering of the prosthesis with cloth will decrease the incidence of thromboembolism. *B.* Mitral valve prosthesis with a Silastic ball used prior to 1967. In contrast to the prosthesis in *A,* the Teflon cloth does not cover the metallic ring and struts. *C.* Disc prosthesis. The disc prosthesis has a wider opening than a ball-valve prosthesis, and the cage does not protrude as far into the ventricle.

dental extraction or cystoscopy. Thromboembolism remains a small but definite hazard. For this reason anticoagulants are used permanently, as described in the earlier paragraphs. A detailed report by Starr in 1971 of all experiences with mitral valve replacement, beginning with the first model prosthetic valve in 1961, confirms the durability of prosthetic mitral replacement (Figs. 19-14 and 19-15).

In 1977, Isom et al. reported the long-term follow-up of 1,375 cloth-covered ball-valve replacements. The 5-year survival following mitral valve replacement was 71 percent.

MITRAL INSUFFICIENCY

HISTORICAL DATA. A number of ingenious attempts to treat mitral insufficiency surgically by a closed approach were made before cardiopulmonary bypass became clinically feasible in 1955. Since that time an open approach with cardiopulmonary bypass has been uniformly used. Prosthetic replacement of the insufficient valve is usually necessary, especially if calcification of the valve has occurred. In some patients with mobile valve leaflets it may be possible to correct the insufficiency with an annuloplasty. Long-term results following annuloplasty in selected cases have been reported by Merendino and by Reed et al. The Carpentier annuloplasty has provided another method of reconstruction rather than replacement.

ETIOLOGY. Mitral insufficiency is usually rheumatic in origin, although a definite history of rheumatic fever can be obtained in only somewhat over one-half of the patients. Other causes of mitral insufficiency include prolapse of the mitral valve, bacterial endocarditis, rupture of chordae tendineae, and papillary muscle dysfunction from extensive occlusive disease of the coronary arteries. Bacterial endocarditis can be suspected when protracted fever is

associated with the development and persistence of the systolic murmur of mitral insufficiency, but the diagnosis can be proved only by identification of the bacterial organism in serial blood cultures. Rupture of chordae tendineae is an unusual but important cause of mitral insufficiency in older patients. Clinically it simulates rheumatic mitral insufficiency closely, but the acute onset in an older patient without previous signs of cardiac disease should suggest the diagnosis. Papillary muscle dysfunction is usually associated with obvious extensive disease of the coronary arteries, causing either cardiac dilatation and failure or myocardial infarction.

In the past decade the surprising frequency of some degree of prolapse of the mitral valve has become widely recognized. It occurs to a slight degree in as many as 5 to 10 percent of the normal population. Fortunately, in the majority of patients the hemodynamic disturbance is minimal. In older patients, however, it has become an increasingly common cause of severe insufficiency requiring valve replacement.

PATHOLOGIC ANATOMY. The basic changes with rheumatic fever have been described under Pathology in the preceding section, Mitral Stenosis. Several alterations in the normal mitral valve, either singly or in combination, may produce mitral insufficiency. These include fibrosis and retraction of the valve leaflets, extensive calcification limiting mobility of the valve leaflets, fibrosis and contraction of the chordae tendineae, rupture of the chordae tendineae, or dysfunction of the papillary muscles. Although seldom a primary cause, dilatation of the mitral annulus develops with mitral insufficiency and accordingly intensifies the insufficiency over a period of time as progressive dilatation of the annulus occurs. The reason that rheumatic endocarditis produces mitral stenosis in one patient and mitral insufficiency in another is unknown and is probably fortuitous.

PATHOPHYSIOLOGY. The basic physiologic change is systolic elevation of left atrial pressure as blood regurgitates through the incompetent mitral valve during ventricular systole. The ventricular pressure spike is commonly to levels of 30 to 40 mm Hg, but levels as high as 80 to 90 mm Hg have been recorded. In diastole the left atrial pressure drops sharply to approach the left ventricular

Fig. 19-12. Insertion of mitral valve prosthesis. *A.* A median sternotomy is the preferred incision, providing ready access to all
areas of the heart. *B.* Cannulae are introduced through the atrial
wall into the venae cavae. Normally these are not snared with
encircling tapes unless a patent foramen ovale is encountered
which causes aspiration of air from the opened left atrium into
the right atrium. *C.* The mitral valve is exposed with an incision
in the left atrium anterior to the point of entry of the right pulmonary veins. Exposure is facilitated by intermittent occlusion of the
aorta, which will arrest and stop the heart, and also decrease
the amount of blood in the operative field. *D.* The mitral valve
with the papillary muscles is completely excised, leaving a small
rim of annulus. The cavity of the left ventricle is carefully inspected and a prosthesis of appropriate size chosen, making
certain that the cage of the prosthesis can be readily accommodated in the ventricular cavity. *E.* A Starr-Edwards ball-valve
prosthesis, cloth-covered and with a steel ball, is preferred. It is
inserted with 12 to 15 mattress sutures of #0 Dacron. Often
the mattress sutures are buttressed with Teflon felt on the ventricular surface (not shown). *F.* Following insertion of the valve,
a Foley catheter is placed across the valve to keep the valve
incompetent and avoid air embolism. *G.* Final view of the valve
in position before closure of the atriotomy. *H.* The atriotomy
incision is closed around the Foley catheter, after which the heart
is allowed to fill with blood and displace air. Subsequently the
Foley catheter is removed, which permits the left ventricle to
contract normally. (Figure continued on next page.)

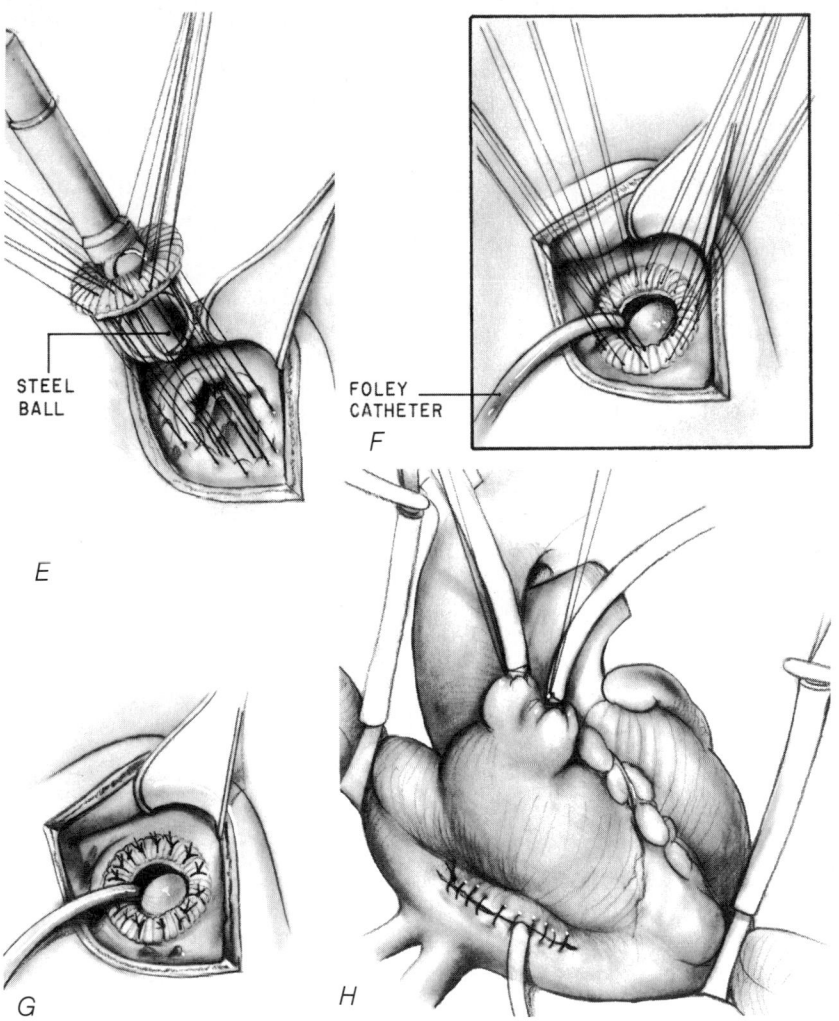

STEEL
BALL

FOLEY
CATHETER

F

E

G   H

Fig. 19-12. Continued.

diastolic pressure, although a small gradient usually remains because of the large blood flow through the mitral valve during diastole. Mean left atrial pressure is usually 15 to 25 mm Hg. The mitral regurgitation produces enlargement of the left atrium, although for unknown reasons the degree of left atrial enlargement varies greatly among different patients and is not proportional to the degree of regurgitation. In some patients with significant regurgitation only slight left atrial enlargement is present, while in others giant left atria evolve, enlarging to contact the right chest wall. In contrast to mitral stenosis, pulmonary vascular changes appear rather late in the course of the disease, perhaps as a result of a large left atrium absorbing much of the kinetic energy of the regurgitating blood without sustained elevation of left atrial pressure. Fortunately, the dilated left ventricle with mitral insufficiency may function adequately for surprisingly long periods of time, maintaining the left ventricular diastolic pressure near the normal range of 8 to 12 mm Hg until eventually left ventricular failure appears.

As there is little stasis of blood in the left atrium, in contrast to mitral stenosis, left atrial thrombosis and arterial embolism are much less frequent than with mitral stenosis.

CLINICAL MANIFESTATIONS. Symptoms. In some patients mild mitral insufficiency may be present without significant disability. This results from minimal rheumatic injury to the mitral leaflets, producing a systolic murmur but few other hemodynamic alterations. In a number of patients, mitral valve prolapse may have been misdiagnosed as rheumatic in origin. With developments in echocardiography, the differential diagnosis can be made readily. Such patients have an increased susceptibility to bacterial endocarditis, but in the absence of symptoms or cardiac enlargement additional therapy is not needed. With more significant mitral insufficiency, the most common symptoms are fatigue, dyspnea on exertion, and palpitation. Often these symptoms remain mild for long periods of time, despite impressive physical signs of mitral insufficiency and cardiac enlargement. Eventually left ventricular failure and increase in pulmonary vascular resistance both develop and intensify the cardiac disability. Respiratory symptoms then become prominent, with increasing dyspnea, cough, and paroxysmal nocturnal dysp-

Fig. 19-13. Technique for suturing a mitral valve prosthesis with Dacron pledgets seated below the mitral annulus.

nea, all of which are essentially similar to those occurring with mitral stenosis and are described in more detail in that section.

Physical Examination. The two characteristic features of mitral insufficiency are the apical systolic murmur and the increased force of the apical impulse. The systolic murmur is heard best at the apex, which is often displaced downward and to the left from enlargement of the left ventricle. It is well transmitted to the axilla. The quality is of a harsh, blowing type. With severe insufficiency, the murmur is pansystolic, appearing immediately after the first sound and continuing until the second sound. The intensity of the murmur does not correlate with the severity of the regurgitation, but the pansystolic characteristic does. Murmurs not extending completely through systole are seen with less serious degrees of regurgitation. The systolic murmur is a highly characteristic feature of mitral insufficiency and is absent only in most unusual circumstances. A diastolic murmur is usually present in addition, resulting from increased flow across the mitral valve as a result of blood regurgitated into the atrium during systole. The absence of an opening snap and the normal quality of the first heart sound both suggest that the diastolic murmur is due to increased flow of blood rather than anatomic mitral stenosis.

The apical impulse is typically forceful, prolonged, and

Fig. 19-14. A. Autopsy photograph of a Starr-Edwards valve prosthesis inserted before 1966, showing the tendency for original model of the prosthetic valve to develop extensive thromboembolism. Surprisingly enough the patient had had no clinical signs of emboli although myriads of scars were found in the kidneys at autopsy. Death occurred 7 years after operation, following a pulmonary infection. Thrombi extending from the ring of the prosthesis down the struts to the apex are clearly seen. B. Atrial view of valve, showing thrombi over approximately two-thirds of the metallic ring. Development of such thrombi was the principle reason for the development of cloth-covered prosthetic valves.

A   B

diffuse, occupying an area 3 to 4 cm². The first heart sound is usually normal, although it has been reported as decreased or absent, usually from confusion with the early onset of the systolic murmur. Atrial fibrillation is frequent with chronic disease.

Laboratory Examinations. The chest roentgenogram will show enlargement of both the left ventricle and the left atrium (Fig. 19-16). As mentioned earlier, in some patients for unknown reasons a giant enlargement of the left atrium occurs, with an atrial chamber extending to the right chest wall and producing a grotesque deformity of the cardiac shadow. Calcification of the regurgitant valve is infrequent, although with combined lesions of stenosis and insufficiency, calcification is common. Visible changes in the pulmonary vasculature are often minimal except with advanced disease.

The electrocardiogram is unfortunately variable and may not contribute greatly to assessment of the severity of the disease. In about 50 percent of patients there is definite left ventricular hypertrophy. Significant insufficiency may be present, however, with a normal electrocardiogram, or in some patients a right axis may develop as a result of pulmonary vascular changes. Atrial fibrillation is frequent.

Mitral insufficiency is best quantified by cardiac catheterization with cineangiography. Only by injection of dye into the left ventricle, with evaluation of the degree of reflux into the atrium, can the degree of insufficiency be best estimated. This is far superior to complex studies with indicator dilution dye curves. The left atrial pressure tracing with mitral insufficiency is greatly altered, usually with a prominent V wave developing from regurgitation of blood during systole. During diastole the left atrial pressure decreases sharply to approach left ventricular diastolic pressure, but usually some gradient remains throughout diastole because of increased flow of blood across the mitral valve.

DIAGNOSIS. The diagnosis of mitral insufficiency can be made with reasonable certainty from the characteristic systolic murmur radiating to the axilla in association with evidence of left ventricular hypertrophy obtained by palpation, the chest roentgenogram, or the electrocardiogram. The degree of severity of the insufficiency is best quantitated with cineangiography. When multivalvular disease is present, cardiac catheterization and angiography are needed to delineate the relative severity of the different valvular lesions.

TREATMENT. Indications for Operation. An acceptable operation for mitral insufficiency was not routinely available until the pioneering work of Starr and Edwards first developed a mitral valve prosthesis in 1961. With the mitral prostheses available between 1961 and 1966, the 5-year survival was only about 50 percent.

Over the past 5 to 7 years, the cloth-covered valve has been modified several times, the most recent modification being a "track" valve (Fig. 19-17). A tilting disc valve, the Bjork-Shiley, which is the most popular, is an excellent prosthesis and provides a wider orifice than is available with most ball valves (Fig. 19-18). The gluteraldehyde-preserved porcine heterograft has become increasingly

Fig. 19-15. Operative photograph of a Kay-Shiley disc prosthesis removed over 2 years after insertion because of recurrent emboli. Extensive thrombi, easily detached from the metallic surface of the prosthesis, are present. Development of these thrombi, intermittently dislodging into the circulation, is the principal reason for the development of cloth-covered prostheses.

Fig. 19-16. Chest roentgenogram of a patient with mitral insufficiency. The distinctive features include an enlarged cardiac shadow with a prominent pulmonary artery. The shadow of the left atrium is visible in the right border of the cardiac shadow behind the shadow of the right atrium. The pulmonary vascular markings are prominent.

Fig. 19-17. Starr-Edwards composite track valve available since 1972. Cloth covers the exterior portion of the valve cage and a metallic track is provided on the inner surface of each cage strut.

popular in the last 5 years and is now used at many centers as the valve of choice, because all other types of prosthetic valve require anticoagulation (Fig. 19-19).

Most patients at New York University have received cloth-covered steel ball valves (Fig. 19-20). The cloth usually becomes covered with a translucent layer of compacted fibrin less than 1 mm thick. This surface is very resistant to thromboembolism. Problems with cloth wear, hemolysis, and endocarditis have occurred in a minority of patients and there is limited enthusiasm for the prosthesis. Because of the limitations of all prostheses and the limited data about their 5- to 10-year durability, operation is usually recommended only for progressive disability resistant to customary medical therapy.

Fig. 19-18. Bjork-Shiley tilting disc valve.

Medical therapy includes appropriate use of digitalis, diuretics, and restriction of sodium intake in the presence of heart failure. Arrhythmias, usually atrial fibrillation, require frequent therapy, both to control tachycardia and to attempt conversion of the arrhythmia to a sinus mechanism.

Technique of Operation. The technique for mitral valve replacement was described under Mitral Stenosis and will not be repeated in detail here. In general, operation is performed through a median sternotomy, occasionally a right thoracotomy. The main precautions during mitral replacement are to anchor the prosthetic valve adequately in position to prevent subsequent partial dislodgment with recurrent mitral insufficiency and to avoid air embolism. Until recent years the prevalence of the two complications cited resulted in an operative mortality of 15 to 20 percent; now it is near 5 percent. Following operation anticoagulant therapy is begun on the fourth or fifth postoperative day and continued indefinitely.

In 10 to 15 percent of patients a mitral annuloplasty may be employed, rather than prosthetic replacement of the valve. Such patients are usually younger, with a dilated mitral annulus and mobile valve leaflets with little or no calcification. Several techniques of annuloplasty have been described, with the objective of producing a small, competent mitral orifice. In general, heavy sutures are used, often including more of the annulus of the mural leaflet rather than the aortic leaflet, because the aortic leaflet often has more mobility than the smaller mural leaflet. When annuloplasty can be satisfactorily performed, excellent long-term results may be obtained. Unfortunately, in many patients the insufficiency cannot be completely corrected at the first operation; also, it may recur at a later date. The Carpentier ring annuloplasty, developed in France, has not to date been widely used in this country.

Ruptured chordae tendineae causing mitral insufficiency create a special surgical problem, varying with the number and location of the chordae ruptured (Fig. 19-21). McGoon has described a technique of plication of the flail mitral leaflet which is applicable in some patients. Kay and Egerton have described other methods of repair, including suture of the flail leaflet directly to the underlying papillary muscle. In some patients excision of the valve with prosthetic replacement is necessary. Long-term results are usually excellent.

PROGNOSIS. Recovery from operation is usually followed by excellent rehabilitation. There is subsidence of pulmonary vascular changes and of signs of cardiac failure. For unknown reasons, however, cardiac function does not return to completely normal values, perhaps because of the rigid ring of the prosthesis in the mitral annulus or because of irreversible myocardial injury from longstanding mitral insufficiency. Most patients have few, if any, restrictions on physical activity. (For specific data following prosthetic valve replacement, see Prognosis, under Mitral Stenosis.)

Careful long-term management is required to supervise anticoagulant therapy, to detect any signs of malfunction of the prosthesis, and to protect from endocarditis during episodes of transient bacteremia by using prophylactic antibiotics.

Five-year survival following mitral valve replacement varies widely with the stage of the disease at which operation is performed. With Class II patients it is about 90 percent; with Class III, nearly 70 percent; and with Class IV, only about 50 percent.

AORTIC STENOSIS

HISTORICAL DATA. Effective treatment of aortic valve disease first became acceptable in 1961 with the development of satisfactory prosthetic valves by Starr and Edwards and by Harken and associates. Earlier attempts to correct aortic valvular disease by cusp replacement with prosthetic cusps of Teflon cloth or by extensive debridement of calcific material from calcified valve cusps initially gave satisfactory results in many patients, but a high failure rate within 1 to 2 years following operation led to abandonment of these techniques as soon as a satisfactory prosthetic valve became available.

With all prosthetic valves, the major limitation is thromboembolism. With the improvements in prosthetic valves in the past few years, especially with the use of cloth covering, thromboembolism has decreased to a range of 1 to 3 percent. Endocarditis following transient bacteremia remains a small but definite risk.

The most exciting data in recent years are those on the continuing excellent results obtained with the gluteraldehyde-preserved porcine heterograft, developed especially by the Hancock Laboratories. Aortic homograft valves have been discarded by many groups but are still preferred by Barratt-Boyes.

ETIOLOGY. A definite history of rheumatic fever can be obtained in only 30 to 50 percent of all patients, but the fact that associated mitral valve disease also is found in 30 to 50 percent of patients with aortic disease supports the relative frequency of rheumatic infection.

In the majority of other patients, calcification superimposed on a mild congenital aortic stenosis is probably the most frequent cause, rather than unrecognized rheumatic fever. In almost all untreated patients with congenital aortic stenosis, calcification in the aortic leaflets develops after thirty years of age. This adds an element of valve cusp rigidity to the obstruction already present because of congenital fusion. It is now clear that this calcification may gradually increase over several decades. Several patients in the sixth and seventh decades of life have been followed with a heart murmur since childhood but without symptoms until 2 or 3 years before operation, at which time a calcified bicuspid valve was found.

In patients in the seventh and eighth decades, an aortic systolic murmur, resulting from mild fibrosis and calcification of the valve leaflets, is extremely common. Only rarely, however, does this form of atherosclerosis in the elderly produce significant obstruction.

PATHOLOGY. The basic pathology of rheumatic fever has been detailed under Mitral Stenosis. The pathologic process with aortic valvulitis is similar, with ulceration of the endocardium developing over the valve leaflets where the margins normally appose in diastole. Tiny, beadlike

Fig. 19-19. Hancock gluteraldehyde-preserved porcine xenograft, now the valve of choice in many centers.

vegetations form and produce fusion of the commissures as healing takes place. Fibrosis and stiffening of the leaflets may develop as well as fusion of the commissures, both features producing obstruction to the flow of blood. In subsequent years superimposed calcification of the diseased leaflets, probably from turbulent flow of blood, regularly occurs and creates further rigidity of the valve cusps.

Mitral valve disease, either stenosis or insufficiency, is found in a high percentage of patients with aortic disease, indicating the underlying rheumatic cause. In older patients coronary atherosclerosis may be present, although the incidence is no greater than that in the normal population. When extensive coronary atherosclerosis is present in association with aortic stenosis of only moderate severity,

Fig. 19-20. Starr-Edwards cloth-covered steel ball aortic prostheses. *A.* The Starr-Edwards aortic ball-valve prosthesis developed in the latter part of 1967. The prosthesis is completely covered with Teflon cloth. A metal ball is used. *B.* The Starr-Edwards ball-valve prosthesis used prior to 1967. The ball is composed of silastic. The Teflon cloth, in contrast to the valve shown in *A*, only partially covers the metal surfaces of the prosthesis.

Fig. 19-21. Operative photograph of mitral valve showing rupture of a major chordae, creating severe mitral insufficiency. In some such patients, plication of the mitral leaflet will obviate mitral replacement.

it may be difficult to determine which of the two lesions is responsible for the symptoms.

PATHOPHYSIOLOGY. The normal aortic valve has a cross-sectional area of 2.5 to 3.5 cm². Moderately severe aortic stenosis is present when the valve orifice has been narrowed to a cross-sectional area of 0.8 to 1 cm², which is associated with a systolic gradient of about 50 mm Hg at a moderate cardiac output. Severe aortic stenosis exists if the cross-sectional area has been reduced to 0.5 to 0.7 cm², which requires a systolic pressure gradient near 150 mm Hg to produce a moderate cardiac output. When stenosis of such severity is present, increases in ventricular systolic pressure are very ineffective in producing further increases in cardiac output. A left ventricular systolic pressure of 250 mm Hg is near the maximum that a left ventricle can sustain for any period of time.

With the increased cardiac work imposed by the stenosis, there is progressive concentric ventricular hypertrophy but little cardiac dilatation, as a result of which the heart size may be near normal on the conventional chest roentgenogram. The cardiac output is often normal, though the left ventricular diastolic pressure is frequently elevated above the normal of 12 mm Hg, especially during exercise, because of the extensive muscular hypertrophy. Left atrial pressure may be temporarily elevated, but sustained elevation of left atrial pressure with production of pulmonary edema is a late and often a preterminal manifestation. Similarly, pulmonary vascular disease is infrequent. In contrast to mitral stenosis, a patient with aortic stenosis may have relatively few symptoms for a long period of time, but when cardiac decompensation with pulmonary congestion appears, a fatal outcome often ensues within a few months.

The quality of the pulse is frequently altered with aortic stenosis because of the restriction to ventricular ejection. The typical changes include a pulse wave of low amplitude, a slow rate of rise, and a rounded peak.

Myocardial ischemia, manifested as angina pectoris, is frequent in aortic stenosis from a combination of factors. These include increase in left ventricular work, myocardial hypertrophy with resulting fewer capillaries per gram of myocardium, decreased aortic pressure in diastole, during which the majority of coronary blood flow usually occurs, and in some patients superimposed atherosclerosis. Because of the myocardial ischemia, aortic stenosis is a most treacherous lesion, for sudden death is *always* a possibility. The risk varies with the severity of the disease but is always present, even with mild aortic stenosis. It is much more frequent with aortic stenosis than with any other form of acquired valvular heart disease.

CLINICAL MANIFESTATIONS. Symptoms. Characteristically there is a prolonged latent period in the development of aortic stenosis. For perhaps 10 to 20 years classic physical findings may be present with slight dyspnea on exertion as the only symptom. The turning point in the illness is heralded by the appearance of one or more of three symptoms: angina pectoris, syncope, or left ventricular failure. Sudden death, which accounts for about 20 percent of fatalities from aortic stenosis, becomes much more of a threat once these symptoms are present, although sudden death is an ever-present hazard in any patient with aortic stenosis. Once angina or syncope appears, the average life expectancy for the untreated patient is 3 to 4 years. Left ventricular failure is an even more serious symptom, death usually occurring within 1 to 2 years, although great variations are seen among different patients, ranging from periods as short as 1 week to as long as 10 years.

Syncope develops in about one-third of the patients. In a minority of patients syncope may result from a conduction abnormality, arising from involvement of the atrioventricular node by calcium spicules deposited on the stenotic valve. Usually syncope develops with effort, and it is commonly associated with angina pectoris. Once left ventricular failure has developed, syncopal attacks may be precipitated by very little effort and are of the gravest significance.

Angina pectoris develops in about two-thirds of the patients, representing myocardial ischemia from an inadequate cardiac output. With protracted angina, small areas of muscle necrosis may evolve, ultimately represented as myocardial fibrosis; infrequently large areas of silent infarction occur.

Left ventricular failure is a grave development and demands immediate therapy. Many patients do not survive long enough to develop associated right ventricular failure. Atrial fibrillation, developing as a consequence of prolonged elevation of left atrial pressure, is similarly a grave event, as it indicates an advanced stage of left ventricular failure.

Physical Examination. The classic physical finding with aortic stenosis is the systolic diamond-shaped ejection murmur produced by blood forced through the stenotic orifice. The murmur is usually heard best in the aortic area to the right of the sternum but in some patients is loudest at the cardiac apex. The intensity of the murmur varies from grade II to grade IV but has no correlation with the severity of the stenosis. Loud murmurs are associated with a palpable thrill and are readily transmitted to the carotid arteries. The aortic second sound is soft but can be detected in 70 to 80 percent of patients. A grade I to II diastolic murmur of aortic insufficiency can often be heard along the left sternal border.

The apical impulse has distinctive features. It is usually in a normal position, for cardiac size is not increased. Palpation of the apical contraction detects a prolonged heave but not a forceful thrust such as is found with ventricular dilatation from aortic or mitral insufficiency. In many patients the blood pressure is normal. Only with advanced stenosis is the pulse pressure significantly narrowed to less than 30 mm Hg.

Laboratory Studies. The chest roentgenogram often demonstrates a heart of normal size. Gross cardiac enlargement, resulting from ventricular dilatation and failure, is associated with an ominous prognosis. Mild degrees of left atrial enlargement are often found. Calcification of the aortic valve should be almost routinely visible in patients over thirty-five years of age. If calcification is not found, the validity of the diagnosis should be seriously questioned.

With advanced disease the electrocardiogram will show signs of left ventricular hypertrophy, including increased voltage of the QRS complex, in association with ST-segment and T-wave abnormalities. With less advanced stenosis, however, the changes may be much less specific, and in some dangerously ill patients the electrocardiogram is virtually normal. In older patients the prevalence of ST-segment and T-wave abnormalities from coronary artery disease makes correlation of the electrocardiogram with the severity of the aortic stenosis difficult. A left bundle branch block is occasionally seen in some patients with advanced stenosis.

Cardiac catheterization to determine the pressure gradient between the left ventricle and the aorta is required to estimate the severity of the stenosis. With mild aortic stenosis, a systolic pressure gradient of only 30 to 40 mm Hg is found, while severe stenosis may have a pressure gradient exceeding 100 mm Hg. Actually, the severity is best correlated with the cross-sectional area of the valve, calculated from simultaneous measurement of pressure gradient and cardiac output. In most patients simple determination of the gradient is sufficient if the patient is in a resting, basal state. At the time of catheterization the presence of mitral disease can also be determined, as well as associated aortic insufficiency. When feasible, coronary arteriography should be done in association with aortogra-

phy to detect associated coronary vascular disease.

DIAGNOSIS. A diagnosis of aortic stenosis can usually be made with certainty from detection of the characteristic ejection-type systolic murmur in the aortic area, associated with findings of left ventricular hypertrophy. Supportive evidence can be obtained from the chest roentgenogram, demonstrating calcification of the aortic valve and often a heart of normal size. The electrocardiogram will usually show variable degrees of left ventricular hypertrophy.

The diagnosis can be confirmed by cardiac catheterization, which also provides the only precise method of measuring the severity of the stenosis. In some patients with aortic systolic murmurs, especially those in the seventh and eighth decades, catheterization will demonstrate that significant obstruction is not present.

TREATMENT. Indications for Operation. Once a clinical diagnosis of aortic stenosis has been made, usually cardiac catheterization should be performed to measure the severity of the obstruction. Subsequent management of the patient depends upon the symptoms, the severity of the obstruction, and the degree of cardiac hypertrophy. Operation is recommended with a gradient exceeding 50 mm Hg, though some such patients are virtually asymptomatic.

Once syncope, angina, or congestive heart failure has appeared, operation should be performed promptly because of the high incidence of sudden death.

Technique of Operation. Detailed preoperative care is not often necessary. If diuretic therapy has been employed, supplemental potassium is usually given before operation to avoid postoperative hypokalemia and arrhythmias. Patients are usually hospitalized 2 to 3 days in advance of the scheduled operation.

A median sternotomy incision is usually employed, with cannulation of the venae cavae for withdrawal of venous blood from the patient to the pump-oxygenator and cannulation of the ascending aorta for return of arterial blood from the pump-oxygenator to the patient (Fig. 19-22). Before bypass is instituted, left atrial pressure is measured to indicate the degree of left ventricular failure. The preoperative left atrial pressure is a convenient guide to postoperative infusion of fluids, because left atrial pressure reflects the diastolic filling pressure of the left ventricle. With severe cardiac failure a mean left atrial pressure of 20 to 30 mm Hg may be present, and following operation elevation of left atrial pressure to similar levels by infusion of fluids may be required for a short time to maintain an adequate cardiac output.

Once cardiopulmonary bypass has been instituted, a vent is placed in the apex of the left ventricle to aspirate blood. The ascending aorta is then occluded distad and incised with an oblique incision which extends proximally into the noncoronary sinus. Perfusion of the left and right coronary arteries is then instituted following cannulation with Silastic coronary cannulae of appropriate size. Perfusions at 100 to 150 ml/minute are used in each artery, depending upon the size of the left ventricle (Fig 19-23)

In recent years the technique of topical hypothermia, long used by Shumway and associates, has become in-

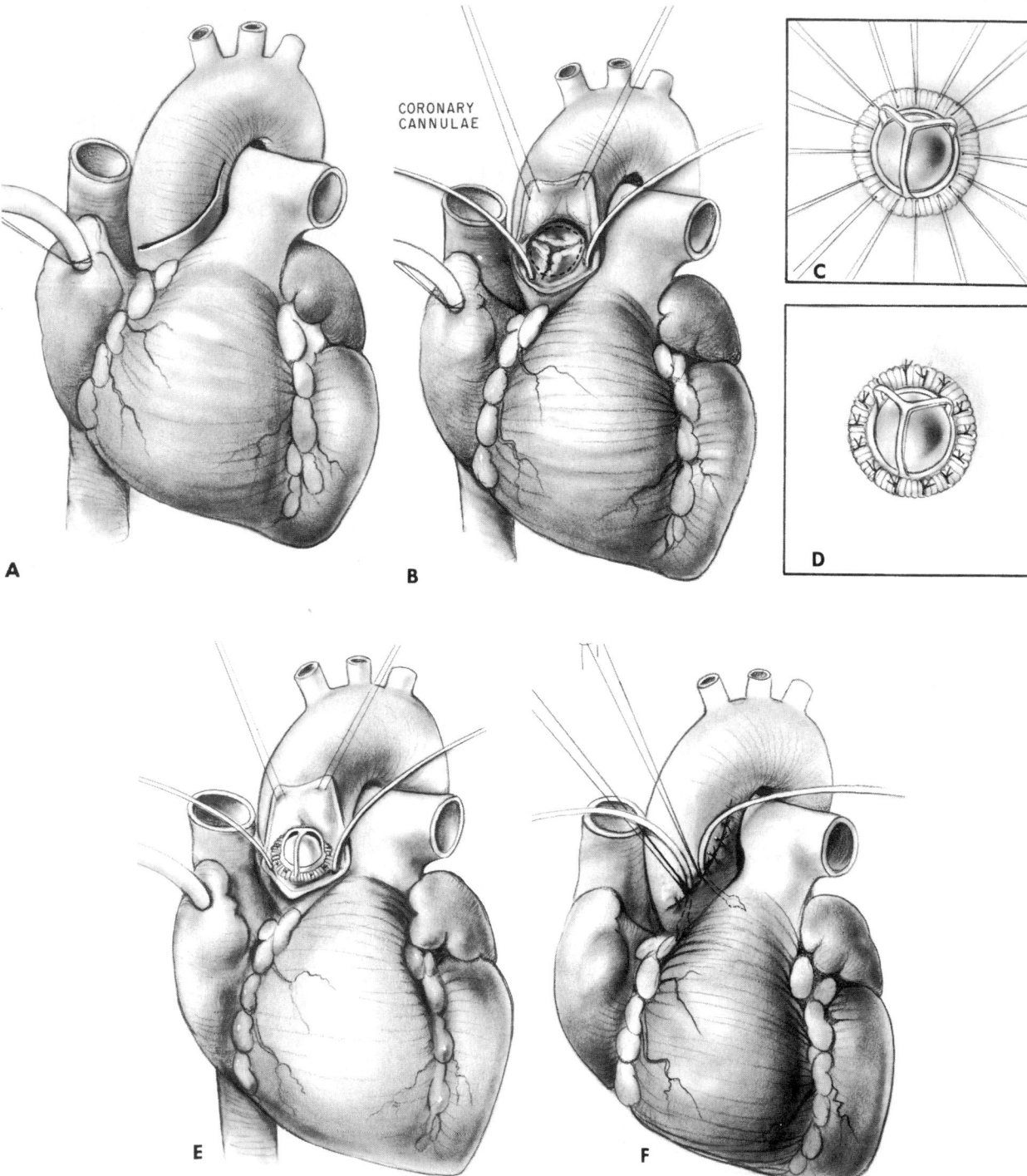

Fig. 19-22. Insertion of aortic valve prosthesis. *A.* Cardiopulmonary bypass is instituted following cannulation of the right atrium with a single large cannula. Usually the ascending aorta is cannulated for arterial return (not shown). The aorta is opened with an oblique incision, initially begun about a centimeter above the right coronary artery. *B.* The right and left coronary arteries are cannulated with Silastic coronary cannulae, held in position with purse-string sutures about the coronary ostia. Coronary perfusion is then begun at a rate of 200 to 250 ml/minute in each coronary artery. The aortic valve is then excised, with care to avoid the loss of any calcific fragments into the ventricle which might subsequently embolize. *C.* The Starr-Edwards ball valve which is normally used. *D.* Valve sutured in position. *E.* Final position of the valve. Care is taken, as the valve is tied in position, to seat the valve well below the coronary ostia, actually farther below than is shown here. *F.* The aortotomy is closed around the coronary cannulae, encircling each one with a mattress suture. Subsequently the contracting heart is allowed to fill with blood and expel air from the heart before the cannulae are removed.

creasingly popular. Hypothermic cardiac arrest, often combined with potassium cardioplegia, has become the most popular method of myocardial preservation, though the author and McGoon, among others, prefer coronary perfusion in routine cases unless significant coronary disease or coronary anomalies are present. There are seemingly valid data from several sources to indicate that myocardial ischemia for 1 hour is well tolerated if the myocardial temperature, as measured by an indwelling thermistor, is kept below 20 to 25°C.

The stenotic aortic valve is then completely removed (Fig. 19-24). Only in a small percentage of cases is simple fusion of the valve commissures found which can be treated by commissurotomy. In most patients there is extensive destruction of the valve cusps with superimposed calcification; complete removal has been found the only satisfactory therapy (Fig. 19-25). Removal of the calcified valve requires great care to avoid losing fragments of calcium into the left ventricle which could subsequently be embolized into the peripheral circulation. A gauze pack is routinely placed in the ventricle before removal of the valve is begun. Subsequent removal of the pack often reveals several fragments of calcium which have been dislodged during removal of the valve and would otherwise have been lost in the left ventricle.

Following removal of the diseased valve, a prosthetic ball valve of appropriate size is selected. It is important that the valve fit easily into the aortic lumen, choosing one that is neither too large nor too small. Once the appropriate valve has been chosen, 12 to 15 mattress sutures of 2-0 Dacron are placed in the valve annulus and inserted into the prosthetic valve. Each mattress suture is buttressed with a small pledget of Dacron cloth to avoid tearing of the

Fig. 19-24. A. Stenotic aortic valve exposed during cardiopulmonary bypass through a transverse aortotomy. The valve orifice has been almost obliterated by calcification and apposition of the cusps. B. Calcified aortic valve in another patient exposed through a transverse aortotomy. Fusion has produced a small eccentric rigid ostium which is both stenotic and insufficient.

Fig. 19-23. Silastic coronary cannulae used to cannulate the coronary arteries at operation for coronary perfusion. Once the cannulae are inserted, slight tension is applied through the snare shown here to a purse-string suture of 4-0 silk which has been sutured about the coronary ostium. If a short left coronary artery is present, the tip of the cannula is amputated back to the ball to avoid inadvertent perfusion of only one tributary of the left coronary artery.

sutures through the annulus (Fig. 19-26). During seating of the valve, care is taken to seat the valve well below the coronary ostia and to avoid any tilting of the valve in its final position. Following closure of the aortotomy, air is displaced from the left ventricle, the coronary cannulae are removed, effective cardiac contraction is restored, and bypass gradually is slowed and stopped (Fig. 19-27).

Coronary perfusion is maintained throughout operation at a flow rate of 250 to 300 ml/minute and a temperature of 32 to 34°C, interrupting perfusion for 5 to 10 minutes when necessary for adequate exposure. In the past three to four years, abundant data have demonstrated that subendocardial coronary blood flow is seriously impaired in fibrillating hypertrophied hearts. Accordingly, the author and many others have abandoned the use of ventricular fibrillation and keep the heart beating throughout the

Fig. 19-25. Calcified fragments removed with rongeurs from a patient with severe aortic stenosis. The multiplicity of such fragments emphasizes the grave risk of embolization of calcified material during aortic valve replacement with reduction of severe or fatal neurologic injury. Careful packing of the ventricle with gauze before removal of the calcified valve is essential.

entire procedure. In the rare instance when this cannot be done, coronary perfusion is abandoned and the potassium cardioplegia technique substituted.

Following bypass, blood is transfused to elevate left atrial pressure to a level adequate to maintain a satisfactory cardiac output. The actual mean left atrial pressure required varies with that existing before bypass but is usually between 10 and 20 mm Hg. The left atrial pressure has been found a more valuable guide for postoperative fluid infusion than measurement of blood volume or blood loss.

Postoperative Care. After initial adjustment of blood volume following operation, convalescence may be uneventful. Arrhythmias are among the more frequent complications. Because they are serious and can be fatal if untreated, early detection by 24-hour monitoring of the cardiac rhythm with an oscilloscope in a cardiac intensive care unit is necessary. Arrhythmias are often related to changes in electrolyte concentration, such as decreased potassium concentration and varying sensitivities to digitalis. The most frequently employed therapeutic measures include supplemental potassium, intravenously administered lidocaine for short-term therapy, procainamide, or propranolol.

Anticoagulant therapy is begun with sodium warfarin 4 days after operation, keeping the prothrombin time in the conservative range of 20 to 25 seconds, and continued permanently. Elevation of the prothrombin time to 25 to 30 seconds has resulted in serious hemorrhage in a few patients, especially in the early postoperative course. Acetylsalicylic acid, 0.6 Gm twice a day, is given for 1 to 2 years to inhibit platelet aggregation, for such aggregates

Fig. 19-26. Schematic representation of technique for suturing the aortic valve with Dacron pledgets seated below the aortic annulus.

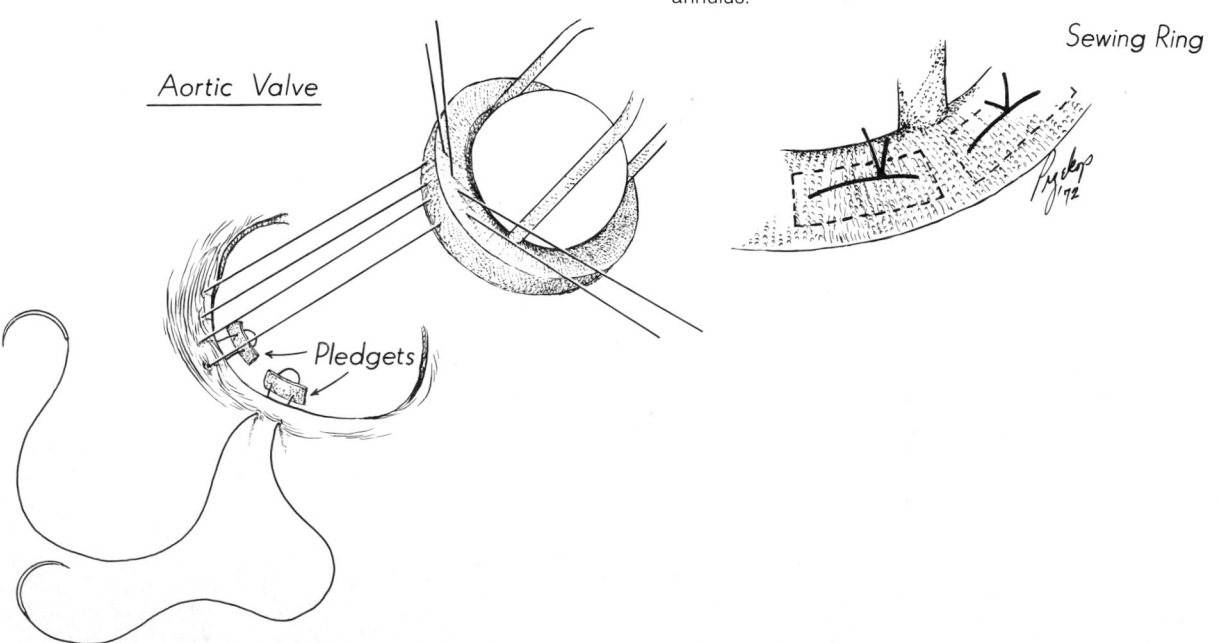

rather than fibrin appear to be the most frequent cause of thromboembolism with cloth-covered prostheses.

Within 3 to 4 months after operation the majority of patients are asymptomatic, with a normal range of physical activities. Careful long-term medical supervision is essential, however, especially in patients with marked cardiac hypertrophy. Actually there is a greater risk of death during the first year after leaving the hospital than from the operation itself. With severely hypertrophied hearts, arrhythmias remain a constant problem for months or longer and may be fatal if not treated. A mild degree of salt restriction and diuretic therapy may also be required if cardiac enlargement was severe beforehand. The rate of increase of physical activity should be determined from the patient's symptoms, heart size, and signs of left ventricular hypertrophy on the electrocardiogram.

PROGNOSIS. The average operative mortality for aortic valve replacement is in the range of 5 to 8 percent. It may be much higher in patients with far advanced disease from cardiac failure or less than 5 percent in good-risk patients. Probably the major factor influencing operative mortality is the ability to avoid serious myocardial ischemia. In 1965, McGoon et al. reported an impressive series of 100 consecutive aortic replacements without *any* operative mortality.

Most patients show a surprising degree of recovery following operation, and many subsequently have virtually no limitation of physical activity. With severe cardiac enlargement, however, there remains a risk of sudden death, even beyond 1 year after operation. This is probably due to arrhythmias, for the cause is often not found at postmortem examination.

AORTIC INSUFFICIENCY

ETIOLOGY. The most common cause of aortic insufficiency is rheumatic fever. A definite history of this illness can be obtained from 60 to 70 percent of patients. In the past, syphilis was a frequent cause, but it is now rare. Bacterial endocarditis produces insufficiency from destruction and perforation of valve cusps. Though formerly operation was strenuously avoided until the bacterial infection had been controlled, operation is now being performed much earlier, at times within the first 7 to 10 days of the illness in patients with life-threatening insufficiency. This is only possible, of course, if effective antibiotic therapy is used.

A dissecting aneurysm produces insufficiency by dissection of the aortic wall with detachment and prolapse of the valve cusps. Usually the noncoronary cusp is involved most. Diseases producing dilatation of the aortic annulus create insufficiency by preventing effective coaptation of the valve cusps in diastole. This is typically seen in the Marfan syndrome and also in less well defined diseases in which there is an isolated unexplained dilatation of the aortic annulus and ascending aorta. A similar pathologic process develops in a small percentage of patients with rheumatoid arthritis. Not infrequently a patient is seen with a "floppy valve," a connective tissue degeneration of the valve cusps resulting in elongation and prolapse without any signs of infection or fibrosis. Congenital aortic insufficiency is very rare.

Fig. 19-27. *A.* A Starr-Edwards ball valve being inserted in the operation shown in Fig. 18-17*B* following excision of the calcified valve. The operation was performed in 1963. The patient has done well since that time. *B.* The aortic ball valve in position.

PATHOLOGY. Normal function of the aortic valve depends upon sufficient mobility and length of the cusps so that the centers of the three cusps appose in diastole. With fibrosis and retraction of the cusps, varying degrees of distortion produce an incompetent valve (Fig. 19-28). It is probable that the turbulent blood flow produced by the initial distortion of the cusps results in progressive fibrosis stiffening, and eventual calcification, all of which result in a gradual increase in the degree of insufficiency. In the Marfan syndrome and other diseases associated with dilatation of the aortic annulus, the basic disturbance is stretching of the aortic valve ring, as a result of which the valve cusps can no longer meet centrally (Fig. 19-29).

Fig. 19-28. Three aortic valve cusps removed from an eighteen-year-old boy with rheumatic aortic insufficiency. The contracted free margins of each cusp are clearly shown, illustrating the mechanism of production of aortic insufficiency from contracture and retraction of the free margins of the aortic valve cusps.

The cardiac response to blood regurgitating into the left ventricle in diastole is an increase in left ventricular stroke volume, accomplished by dilatation of the heart. Progressive dilatation of the left ventricle gradually evolves. This response is quite different from that occurring with aortic stenosis, where there is concentric muscular hypertrophy but little increase in ventricular diastolic volume.

PATHOPHYSIOLOGY. Surprisingly large volumes of blood can regurgitate through an incompetent orifice of less than 1 cm² because of the large differential in diastolic pressure between the aorta and the left ventricle. The actual amount of blood regurgitating with each cardiac cycle can be only approximated by existing techniques, such as dye-dilution measurements, or experimentally with flow meters. The initial adjustment of the heart is an increase in diastolic fiber length and a corresponding increase in stroke volume. There is little elevation in left ventricular diastolic pressure until cardiac failure begins to develop. In the absence of elevation of left ventricular diastolic pressure, there is accordingly no increase in left atrial pressure or pulmonary congestion. Hence, in contrast to mitral disease, symptoms of pulmonary congestion appear only in the terminal stages, once left ventricular failure has occurred.

The amount of blood regurgitating during diastole varies not only with the size of the incompetent orifice but also with the degree of peripheral vasodilatation and the heart rate. Tachycardia has a somewhat beneficial effect, for diastole is shortened and less time is available for blood to regurgitate into the ventricle. Peripheral vasodilation apparently is a compensatory mechanism by which peripheral resistance and the amount of blood regurgitating

into the ventricle are decreased. It is often a prominent clinical finding.

With advanced aortic insufficiency and marked dilatation of the left ventricle, some mitral insufficiency may develop from dilation of the annulus of the mitral valve. When severe cardiac failure is present, with elevation of left ventricular end-diastolic pressure above 20 mm Hg, clinical findings of aortic insufficiency may actually decrease, for the total volume of blood regurgitating during diastole decreases as the left ventricular diastolic pressure rises.

CLINICAL MANIFESTATIONS. Symptoms. Although there is considerable variability among different patients, in general the symptom-free period after the appearance of aortic insufficiency averages about 10 years. With the onset of symptoms, death occurs in about 5 years, but the variability is great. Although in a large group, about 40 percent of patients will be dead within 10 years and over 50 percent within 20 years, another 25 percent may live for 20 years with very few symptoms. The terminal illness is usually a progressive downhill course from increasing cardiac failure, but sudden death occurs in about 5 percent.

The earliest symptom is palpitations because of the forceful contractions of the dilated left ventricle. Dyspnea on exertion is another early symptom, gradually increasing as the disease progresses. Angina pectoris is common in the later stages from myocardial ischemia, developing from the decreased coronary blood flow during diastole as well as the large size of the left ventricle. Peripheral vasomotor phenomena, including episodes of severe sweating and intolerance to heat, are common.

Physical Examination. The cardiac rhythm is usually normal. With significant aortic insufficiency palpation readily discloses a prominent cardiac impulse, located downward and to the left of the normal location because of dilatation of the left ventricle. The hallmark of aortic insufficiency is the high-pitched, decrescendo diastolic murmur along the left sternal border. The murmur starts immediately after the second sound and may be confused with it. The length of the murmur correlates approximately with the severity of the insufficiency; those lasting only through early diastole represent less severe degrees of regurgitation. Having the patient lean forward while listening along the left sternal border makes the murmur more audible. With faint high-pitched murmurs, having the patient stop breathing momentarily is helpful. If the murmur is loudest to the right of the sternum, dilatation of the aortic ring, as in the Marfan syndrome, is likely. As mentioned earlier, with advanced cardiac failure and increase in the left ventricular diastolic pressure, the intensity of the diastolic murmur may decrease to actually become inaudible in terminal stages. A systolic murmur of the ejection type, moderate in intensity, is frequently heard, arising from increased volume of blood expelled from the left ventricle, not from anatomic aortic stenosis.

Examination of the peripheral arterial circulation reveals many positive findings. The pulse pressure is increased, partly from an increase in systolic pressure, but principally from a decrease in diastolic pressure from the normal range near 80 mm Hg. The diastolic pressure may

Fig. 19-29. *A.* Aneurysm in the ascending aorta in a patient with the Marfan syndrome. Marked dilatation of the proximal ascending aorta has developed, stretching the aortic annulus and producing aortic insufficiency. The distal ascending aorta, proximal to the innominate artery, is nearly normal in diameter and has been encircled with an umbilical tape. The left innominate vein is retracted at the top of the field. *B.* With the patient on cardiopulmonary bypass, the aorta has been clamped and the aneurysm opened. The aortic annulus is shown with the stretched leaflets producing total insufficiency. Silastic coronary cannulae have been inserted into each coronary ostium for coronary perfusion while reconstruction is performed. *C.* A Starr-Edwards ball valve in position which has been inserted following excision of the insufficient valve leaflets. The coronary perfusion cannulae are still in position. *D.* Following insertion of the aortic valve, the ascending aorta was reconstructed with a short prosthesis of Dacron cloth. The distal suture line is just proximal to the origin of the innominate artery.

be as low as 40 mm Hg, but true diastolic pressure is never less than 30 to 35 mm Hg, as measured by direct arterial puncture. Auscultatory findings of a diastolic pressure of zero results from dilatation of peripheral arteries. The exact level of diastolic pressure does not correlate closely with the severity of the aortic insufficiency. For example, a blood pressure of 130/65 mm Hg may be present with either moderate or severe insufficiency. This lack of correlation is due to the influence of peripheral resistance. With vasodilatation, diastolic pressure may be low without marked regurgitation, while with severe vasoconstriction diastolic pressure may be higher but with severe regurgitation.

With significant insufficiency, peripheral pulses are easily visible, forceful, and bounding. "Pistol shot" sounds are readily heard with the bell of the stethoscope over peripheral arteries. A wide variety of other auscultatory phenomena have been described, all of which indicate vasodilatation and a hyperactive peripheral circulation.

Laboratory Studies. The chest roentgenogram usually shows enlargement of the left ventricle, with the apex displaced downward and to the left. Serial chest roentgenograms over months or years is the best method for evaluating progression of the disease. Lateral views are required to appreciate fully the degree of enlargement of the left ventricle because of its posterior location. The electrocardiogram may be normal with early aortic insufficiency, but with more advanced disease and the appearance of symptoms there are signs of left ventricular hypertrophy with abnormalities in the ST-T segments. The cardiac rhythm is usually sinus. Atrial fibrillation is rare. Its presence suggests either terminal aortic insufficiency or concomitant mitral valve disease.

Cardiac catheterization may show no abnormalities in

Fig. 19-30. Operative photograph of a Silastic ball removed from an aortic valve prosthesis, inserted before 1966. Development of a diastolic murmur fortunately led to reoperation before fatal embolization of the fragmented Silastic ball occurred. With improvement in Silastic ball prostheses this complication has been virtually unknown since 1966.

the early stages of the disease when left ventricular diastolic pressure is normal. With cardiac failure and elevation of the left ventricular diastolic pressure to 15 to 20 mm Hg, there is corresponding elevation of left atrial pressure. The best method for quantitating the degree of insufficiency is aortography, injecting dye into the ascending aorta and visually estimating the degree of reflux into the ventricle. Though subjective, this method is quite satisfactory for most clinical decisions.

DIAGNOSIS. A diagnosis can be readily made when the characteristic diastolic murmur is heard along the left sternal border. Quantitation of the degree of insufficiency, however, is more difficult. Mild insufficiency exists when only a murmur is audible without any changes in pulse pressure. Such patients may be treated optimistically, as their only serious risk is that of developing bacterial endocarditis. With more significant insufficiency, a diastolic murmur extending throughout diastole is audible in association with a decrease in diastolic blood pressure and prominent peripheral pulses. Cardiac enlargement as well as changes in the electrocardiogram of left ventricular hypertrophy are usually present. The degree of enlargement of the left ventricle is probably the most reliable indicator of the severity of the disease.

A significant surgical problem exists regarding the degree of aortic insufficiency when concomitant mitral valve disease requires operation. In such patients a decision needs to be made whether or not to replace the diseased aortic valve as well as the diseased mitral valve. Aortography is the best method for estimating the degree of insufficiency but is not totally accurate. A final decision must be made at operation, approaching the heart through a median sternotomy incision and noting the amount of blood regurgitating through the aortic valve after the mitral valve has been removed.

TREATMENT. Surgical treatment is recommended ordinarily only when symptoms become significant. In some patients progressive enlargement of the left ventricle develops with surprisingly few symptoms. Probably these patients should be operated upon to avoid extreme degrees of left ventricular hypertrophy, with heart weights approaching 900 to 1,000 Gm. Once symptoms become significant, surgical therapy should be prompt because of the rapid downhill course of the disease in most symptomatic patients.

When operation is performed, we prefer prosthetic replacement with a cloth-covered ball valve of the Starr-Edwards variety (Fig. 19-30). With small aortic roots, the disc valve of the Bjork-Shiley type is useful. Tissue prostheses, such as homografts and porcine heterografts, are described in the preceding section, Aortic Stenosis. They have been widely and effectively used by several groups.

TRICUSPID STENOSIS AND INSUFFICIENCY

ETIOLOGY. Organic disease of the tricuspid valve is almost always due to rheumatic fever. With the exception of septic endocarditis, usually in drug addicts, it virtually never occurs as an isolated lesion, but only in association with extensive disease of the mitral valve. With mitral disease the frequency of associated tricuspid disease is near 10 to 15 percent, although an incidence as high as 30 percent has been reported.

Tricuspid insufficiency is the more common lesion encountered, while pure stenosis is infrequent. Rarely, both stenosis and insufficiency are present.

Functional tricuspid insufficiency is actually more common than insufficiency from organic disease. It develops from dilatation of the tricuspid annulus and right ventricle as a result of pulmonary hypertension and right ventricular failure. The hypertension is usually a consequence of mitral valve disease with elevated left atrial pressure.

A more recent etiologic factor in isolated tricuspid disease is bacterial endocarditis among heroin addicts. This presents many very special problems because of the repeated infections which such patients tend to sustain.

PATHOLOGY. With tricuspid stenosis the pathologic changes are similar to those found with the more familiar mitral stenosis. There is fusion of the commissures to form a small central opening 1 to 1.5 cm in diameter. As right atrial pressure is normally only 4 to 5 mm Hg, significant tricuspid stenosis may be present with a valve orifice considerably larger than that seen with mitral stenosis.

Tricuspid insufficiency results from fibrosis and contraction of the valve leaflets, often in association with shortening and fusion of chordae tendineae. Calcification is rare. With dilation of the tricuspid annulus the valve leaflets appear stretched, but otherwise are pliable and seemingly normal even though serious regurgitation is present. An unexplained fact, however, is that such valves may not regain competence after correction of mitral valve disease and restoration of pulmonary artery systolic pressure to normal.

PATHOPHYSIOLOGY. With tricuspid stenosis the mean right atrial pressure is elevated to 10 to 20 mm Hg. The higher pressures are found with a tricuspid valve orifice smaller than 1.5 cm^2 and a mean diastolic gradient between the atrium and ventricle of 5 to 15 mm Hg. When mean right atrial pressure remains above 10 mm Hg, edema and ascites usually appear.

Moderate degrees of tricuspid insufficiency may be tolerated surprisingly well because the regurgitant blood is dissipated into the systemic veins with little adverse influence on circulation except for a decrease in cardiac output. This is in striking contrast to mitral insufficiency, where the regurgitating blood produces pulmonary congestion. The significance of tricuspid insufficiency alone is difficult to evaluate because it is almost always seen in association with the more serious mitral valve disease. However, rarely tricuspid insufficiency results from an isolated traumatic injury. Such patients may tolerate the disease well for many years, the only physiologic disturbance being elevation of venous pressure and a decrease in cardiac output.

CLINICAL MANIFESTATIONS. Symptoms. The symptoms of tricuspid valve disease are similar to those of failure of the right side of the heart resulting from the associated mitral valve disease. Prominent features include elevation of venous pressure with edema, ascites, and hepatomegaly.

As similar findings occur from failure of the right side of the heart without disease of the tricuspid valve, the concomitant presence of tricuspid disease may be easily overlooked. The general effects of tricuspid disease are to increase the severity of failure of the right side of the heart. Otherwise the clinical course is similar to that seen with isolated mitral stenosis or insufficiency.

Physical Examination. The characteristic murmur of tricuspid stenosis is best heard as a diastolic murmur at the lower end of the sternum. It is a low-pitched murmur of medium intensity and can easily be overlooked as it is well localized at the lower end of the sternum. During inspiration the intensity of the murmur increases as the volume of blood returning to the heart is temporarily increased by an increase in intrathoracic negative pressure. Tricuspid insufficiency produces a prominent systolic murmur at the lower end of the sternum and also at the cardiac apex, where it may be confused with the systolic murmur of mitral insufficiency. The murmur is often seen in association with an enlarged pulsating liver and prominent engorged peripheral veins. A prominent jugular pulse, especially when the cardiac rhythm is sinus, may be the best clue to unsuspected tricuspid disease.

Laboratory Studies. The chest roentgenogram and electrocardiogram may show enlargement of the right side of the heart, but this does not differentiate tricuspid disease from cardiac enlargement caused by pulmonary hypertension secondary to mitral disease. Cardiac catheterization and cineangiography are the most precise ways of establishing the diagnosis. At catheterization the presence of tricuspid stenosis can be established by measuring the diastolic gradient between the atrium and the ventricle. As the gradient may be quite small (5 to 7 mm Hg), careful measurements are necessary.

With serious tricuspid insufficiency, the contour of the right atrial pressure tracing is altered by the regurgitating of blood during systole. If the right atrium is large, however, significant regurgitation may be present with little alteration in contour of the right atrial pressure tracing; so a normal pressure tracing does not exclude significant insufficiency. Cineangiography is the best method for detecting insufficiency, noting the degree of reflux of dye into the atrium when dye is injected into the ventricle.

DIAGNOSIS. The diagnosis can be made with reasonable certainty if the characteristic systolic or diastolic murmurs are audible at the lower end of the sternum, especially in association with an enlarged, pulsating liver. Confirmatory studies are best obtained by catheterization and angiography. A good surgical routine at the time of mitral valve operation is to palpate the tricuspid valve through the right atrium before bypass is started to confirm or exclude the presence of tricuspid disease.

TREATMENT. Tricuspid disease is surgically treated at the time of correction of more serious mitral disease. Rarely the aortic valve is also involved; so replacement of three cardiac valves is necessary. There is not a uniform opinion about the necessity for treating minor to moderate degrees of tricuspid insufficiency secondary to pulmonary hypertension from mitral disease. Some have felt that correction of mitral valve disease, followed by regression of the pulmonary hypertension, would decrease the degree of tricuspid insufficiency to clinically unimportant levels. Braunwald and associates reported results with operation upon 23 patients with tricuspid disease, 4 of whom had an annuloplasty while 19 had no therapy other than correction of the mitral disease. Fairly good clinical results were obtained. With extensive tricuspid insufficiency, however, almost all surgeons have concluded that tricuspid replacement or annuloplasty, should be performed at operation because a significant impairment of cardiac output from untreated tricuspid insufficiency jeopardizes the patient's opportunity for recovery following mitral replacement.

Tricuspid stenosis may be treated by simple commissurotomy, usually opening the commissure between the anterior and septal leaflets and the commissure between the posterior and septal leaflets, but leaving the fused commissure between the anterior and posterior leaflets. Opening of this commissure usually produces insufficiency. Hence, following commissurotomy the valve functions as a bicuspid one.

With organic disease of the tricuspid valve producing tricuspid insufficiency, surgical correction has usually been ineffective except with prosthetic replacement. For a long time the ball-valve prosthesis seemed satisfactory in the tricuspid position, much as in the mitral position. However, late thrombosis of the tricuspid ball-valve prosthesis months or years after operation has been reported by several groups. This is presumably caused by decrease in size of the right ventricle with resulting impairment of motion of the ball within the cage of the prosthesis (Fig. 19-31). For this reason most groups have abandoned the use of the ball-valve prosthesis.

A disc prosthesis may be used but carries an increased risk of thrombosis because of the low pressures in the right side of the heart. For this reason, the prosthesis of choice at present is the gluteraldehyde-preserved porcine heterograft. This does not require anticoagulants, and a durability of up to 5 or 6 years is well established.

During insertion of the prosthetic valve, along the septal leaflet where the conduction bundle is located between the coronary sinus and the ventricular septum, sutures are placed through the base of the septal leaflet rather than through the annulus to avoid injury of the conduction bundle and production of heart block (Fig. 19-32). As arrhythmias are frequent after operation, two pacemaker wires are routinely left in the ventricle.

When moderate tricuspid insufficiency with pulmonary hypertension is present and the leaflets of the tricuspid valve appear normal but the annulus is dilated, an annuloplasty is preferable. Our results with posterior leaflet annuloplasty, as reported by Boyd et al., have been consistently good. Others have preferred the more complex annuloplasty techniques, using either the Carpentier ring or the method of annuloplasty developed by DeVega. Considerable pessimism had been expressed about the durability of annuloplasty, but enough long-term data are now available to indicate that annuloplasty is a sound procedure of permanent benefit.

An astonishing observation of some physiologic importance concerning tricuspid function is the finding reported by Arbulu and associates that total excision of the tricuspid

Fig. 19-31. A. Chest roentgenogram of a patient following prosthetic replacement of the mitral and tricuspid valves. The mitral valve has been replaced with a Starr-Edwards ball-valve prosthesis. A Kay-Shiley disc prosthesis was used for the tricuspid valve. B. Lateral-roentgenogram showing the mitral and tricuspid valves in position.

Tricuspid Valve

Autogenous Pledget

*Partially Resected Septal
Leaflet*

Fig. 19-32. Technique for suturing the tricuspid valve prosthesis with Dacron pledgets seated below the tricuspid annulus. The pledgets are used in all areas except the area of the partially resected septal leaflet, which is used as an autogenous pledget to avoid the conduction bundle and the production of heart block.

valve *without replacement* could be tolerated for at least short periods of time. These observations were made in treating the difficult problem of tricuspid valve endocarditis in heroin addicts, where repeated septic injections had resulted in endocarditis of the tricuspid valve. Chemotherapy in such instances has often been futile, and prosthetic replacement frequently resulted in reinfection. These writers made the significant observation that the value could simply be excised with fair cardiac function for at least several months. They reported one survivor who was without a tricuspid valve for 10 months. However, there is definite disability, therefore a two-stage procedure for the treatment of endocarditis seems to be the method of choice. Initially, all diseased valvular tissue is excised to eradicate the endocarditis, and an elective prosthetic replacement is done a few weeks later.

MULTIVALVULAR HEART DISEASE

With rheumatic heart disease, more than one cardiac valve is frequently involved. The physician must remain alert to this possibility, for prominent signs of disease of one valve can readily mask disease of additional valves. For this reason, cardiac catheterization and cineangiography are used to evaluate the function of all four cardiac valves to determine stenosis or insufficiency. In addition, at the time of operation other valves can be inspected or palpated. This is one of the great advantages of the sternotomy incision, which provides ready access to all cardiac chambers. The precise recognition of multivalvular disease is of considerable therapeutic importance, for widespread clinical experience has demonstrated that failure to correct all significant valvular disease at the time of operation significantly increases the surgical mortality.

A variety of clinical syndromes can be produced by

different combinations of valvular disease. Often the clinical diagnosis can be only suspected and must be decided either by cardiac catheterization and angiography or operative exploration. The more common types of multivalvular disease will be briefly mentioned.

AORTIC DISEASE WITH FUNCTIONAL MITRAL INSUFFICIENCY. With dilatation of the left ventricle from cardiac failure due to aortic insufficiency, rarely from aortic stenosis, dilatation of the mitral annulus can produce a functional mitral insufficiency without intrinsic disease of the mitral valve. Such insufficiency may regress following repair of the aortic lesion, or it may be corrected by annuloplasty at operation, narrowing the annulus to normal dimensions by placing sutures at the stretched commissures. Replacement of the stretched but normal mitral valve is not often necessary. Usually the procedure can be decided by palpation of the mitral valve in the functioning, beating heart by introducing a finger into the left atrium through a stab wound in the intraatrial groove, just before cardiopulmonary bypass is started.

A convenient approach for assessing the magnitude of functional mitral insufficiency is to palpate the mitral valve in the beating heart by introducing a finger into the left atrium through a stab wound in the intraatrial groove just before bypass is started. There is some danger of hemorrhage with this maneuver, and preparations for initiating bypass should be complete before the finger is introduced. If uncertainty remains, the mitral valve can be palpated in a similar manner after the aortic valve has been replaced and bypass stopped. In recent years we have found that annuloplasty is seldom necessary in the absence of organic disease of the mitral valve.

AORTIC STENOSIS AND MITRAL STENOSIS. When these two stenotic lesions coexist, the clinical signs of mitral stenosis often overshadow those of aortic stenosis, for the volume of blood entering the left ventricle is restricted by the stenotic mitral valve. Hence, functionally severe aortic stenosis may be present with minimal physical findings and a systolic pressure gradient between the left ventricle and aorta or only 20 to 40 mm Hg. Calculation of the cross-sectional area of the aortic valve by simultaneous measurement of cardiac output will quantitate the degree of aortic stenosis present. In uncertain instances, at the end of operative correction of the mitral stenosis, the aortic valve should be examined, either by pressure measurements or by inspection. Overlooking significant aortic stenosis at the time of correction of mitral stenosis can easily result in death early in the postoperative period.

AORTIC INSUFFICIENCY AND MITRAL STENOSIS. With prominent aortic disease, an underlying mitral stenosis can easily be masked because the classic diastolic rumble of mitral stenosis is overshadowed by the prominent aortic murmurs. Cardiac catheterization will usually detect significant mitral stenosis beforehand. If uncertainty remains, however, the mitral valve may be readily palpated or inspected through a short incision in the left atrium at the time of surgical correction of aortic valve disease.

MITRAL STENOSIS WITH TRICUSPID DISEASE. When signs of mitral disease are prominent, tricuspid disease can be easily overlooked. As mentioned earlier, the most significant clinical signs of tricuspid disease are a systolic or diastolic murmur at the lower end of the sternum, especially one accentuated during inspiration. Often the jugular veins are prominent with systolic pulsations, in combination with an enlarged, pulsating liver. These clinical signs, however, are not precise. Catheterization and angiography may establish the diagnosis, but again the technique is not totally reliable. The pressure gradient with significant tricuspid stenosis may be small, and tricuspid insufficiency can be assessed by angiography only by introducing a catheter across the triscupid valve to inject dye into the

right ventricle, a procedure which in itself may produce some tricuspid insufficiency. For these reasons, routine palpation of the tricuspid valve at the time of operation on the mitral valve is preferred. This is technically simple and quickly confirms or excludes the presence of tricuspid disease.

TRIVALVULAR DISEASE. In some unfortunate patients, significant disease of the mitral, aortic, and tricuspid valves is present. Such patients are usually in far advanced cardiac failure with generalized cardiomegaly. Hence, detection and surgical correction of all three valvular lesions is of critical importance if the patient is to survive operation. Attempting to shorten and simplify the operative procedure by not correcting all three diseased valves is usually unsatisfactory. Triple valve replacement, however, is an operative procedure of significant complexity and magnitude and has a mortality in the range of 15 to 20 percent, primarily because patients requiring triple valve replacement are usually critically ill with far advanced chronic congestive failure and extensive cardiomegaly. In such patients cardiac function often improves slowly over weeks or even months after operation (Fig. 19-33).

CARDIAC TRAUMA

HISTORICAL DATA. In 1896 Rehn first successfully sutured a stab wound of the heart, but for over 20 years this remained principally an isolated historic achievement until developments in anesthesia, blood transfusion, and

Fig. 19-33. Lateral roentgenogram in a patient with prosthetic replacement of the mitral, tricuspid, and aortic valves. The mitral and tricuspid valves were replaced with Kay-Shiley disc prostheses, while the aortic valve was replaced with a Starr-Edwards ball-valve prosthesis.

other surgical advances made thoracotomy progressively safer, especially after 1940. In 1943 Blalock and Ravitch recognized that many patients survived a penetrating injury of the heart because pericardial tamponade developed and prevented exsanguination. Their introduction of pericardial aspiration as a form of definitive treatment greatly lowered mortality from penetrating cardiac injuries. Asfaw et al., in 1975, reported experiences with 12 cases of traumatic intraventricular defects and reviewed previous published reports. Improvements in diagnosis, resuscitative therapy for shock, anesthesia, and operative technique have all contributed to lower mortality from cardiac injuries in recent years. At present, pericardial aspiration is used primarily in resuscitation before operating on the patient. It is used much less frequently as definitive therapy. The risks from a negative exploratory thoracotomy are small and outweigh the hazards of recurrent tamponade or of overlooking multiple injuries if nonoperative therapy is employed.

ETIOLOGY. Patients with penetrating cardiac injuries who are still alive when first seen by a physician usually have stab wounds from a small instrument such as an ice pick or small knife. Less common are similar injuries from low-velocity bullets, but injuries from high-velocity bullets or large knives often cause immediate death from exsanguination. Nonpenetrating cardiac injuries result from blunt trauma to the chest wall, the most frequent of which is the "steering wheel" injury from contusion of the chest wall by impact against the steering wheel in an automobile accident.

PATHOLOGY. Because of its anterior position, the right ventricle is the cardiac chamber most frequently injured with penetrating wounds. In surviving patients most wounds are penetrating rather than perforating wounds. Nonpenetrating crushing injuries usually cause diffuse contusion of the myocardium. With nonpenetrating injuries of severe force, however, actual cardiac lacerations occur, usually fatal. Rarely, a surviving patient is seen with a laceration of the tricuspid valve, the right atrium, or even the ventricular septum.

PATHOPHYSIOLOGY. The three principal physiologic disturbances following a cardiac injury are intrathoracic hemorrhage, pericardial tamponade, and cardiac failure. Hemorrhage of varying degree, of course, is present with every cardiac injury. The clinical signs are usually obvious with profound shock; death often occurs before definitive treatment can be started. Cardiac tamponade is frequently the dominant physiologic injury in surviving patients because patients surviving long enough for therapy often do so because tamponade has delayed or stopped the bleeding from the cardiac laceration. Tamponade quickly occurs because the normal pericardium can accommodate only 100 to 250 ml of blood. As the intrapericardial pressure rises with continuing tamponade, there is a progressive fall in cardiac output. Careful experimental studies by Isaacs found that elevation of intrapericardial pressure to 17 cm saline solution virtually stopped cardiac output unless venous pressure was elevated by infusion of fluid. This restriction of cardiac output results from prevention of

diastolic filling of the ventricles, not from impaired venous flow into atria from the venae cavae.

Impaired cardiac function from the penetrating injury per se is unusual. It is seen only with the rare instance of injury of specific structures, such as a major coronary artery, a heart valve, or the cardiac conduction bundle.

CLINICAL MANIFESTATIONS. Symptoms. Patients with a cardiac injury may collapse immediately in profound shock or develop shock more gradually over a period of 1 to 2 hours. The clinical appearance of some patients with tamponade is initially deceptive, for they may appear only moderately ill and then collapse suddenly with an imperceptible blood pressure. This rapid change is due to the fact that once the pericardial cavity becomes distended, only 5 to 10 ml additional fluid is sufficient to raise the intrapericardial pressure to the critical zone of 17 to 18 cm saline solution, where cardiac output falls to very low levels.

The most frequent symptoms are the familiar ones of shock, including weakness, thirst, and restlessness. Chest pain is seldom severe. An unusual degree of restlessness, at times with the patient wildly rolling about, in contrast to the usual quiet, apathetic state of patients in hemorrhagic shock, perhaps results from cerebral anoxia produced by both arterial hypotension and venous hypertension.

Physical Examination. If tamponade is not present, the findings are those of hemorrhagic shock, hypotension with collapsed peripheral veins, and intense vasoconstriction. Tamponade is immediately suggested by finding hypotension combined with venous hypertension, indicated by visible, dilated neck and arm veins. The chest roentgenogram often shows little cardiac enlargement with tamponade, because the pericardium does not distend easily. A hemothorax is common, especially if there is concomitant injury of the lung or if the laceration is large enough for blood to drain from the pericardium into the pleural space. Particular care should be taken in examining the film for the presence of a small foreign body. The electrocardiogram is often normal, except for the rare patient with injury of a coronary artery or the conduction bundle. Fluoroscopy, once a popular technique for evaluating tamponade, has been virtually abandoned because of the time required and the lack of precision. Accurate measurement of central venous pressure, an important early measurement in the treatment of any patient with hemorrhagic shock, may quickly establish or exclude tamponade. A venous pressure above 10 cm saline solution suggests the diagnosis, while one above 15 cm is virtually diagnostic.

DIAGNOSIS. With the combination of arterial hypotension and venous hypertension, combined with other clinical findings, cardiac tamponade can be diagnosed with considerable accuracy. The differential diagnosis includes venous hypertension from overtransfusion, cardiac failure, or pulmonary embolism. If tamponade is a possibility, the pericardium should be aspirated promptly, at times within 5 to 10 minutes after the patient is first seen in the emergency department. Aspiration both confirms the diagnosis and partially relieves the tamponade.

In urgent instances where death is imminent and the presence of tamponade uncertain, a subxiphoid incision can be made in the linea alba and the pericardial cavity entered by making a small opening in the diaphragm immediately behind the xiphoid process. This can be quickly done and the pericardial cavity digitally explored. This is particularly helpful when large clots in the pericardium make needle aspiration ineffective.

The diagnosis of chronic or subacute cardiac tamponade is difficult. The question may arise several days after a penetrating thoracic injury which initially was not thought to have entered the pericardium. It more commonly arises after cardiac surgery, usually several days after operation when the question of intrathoracic bleeding no longer exists. As with acute tamponade, the clinical findings are a decreased cardiac output with hypotension and elevation of venous pressure. The usual condition to be differentiated from chronic tamponade is cardiac failure, more rarely pulmonary embolism. Several years of experience have indicated the great variation in clinical signs with chronic tamponade and the unreliability of such findings as a paradoxic pulse, changes in intensity of cardiac sounds, or size of the cardiac silhouette on the chest roentgenogram. The safest approach seems to be the realization that in the presence of decreased cardiac output and elevated venous pressure tamponade cannot be excluded with 100 percent certainty except by thoractomy. Simply being aware of these diagnostic limitations is particularly important in treating a patient for supposedly congestive failure who does not respond to the usual therapy of digitalis and diuretics. In uncertain instances the pericardial cavity must be explored, either by needle aspiration, subxiphoid digital aspiration, or formal thoracotomy.

TREATMENT. With shock from penetrating cardiac injuries, therapy includes intravenous infusion of fluids, administration of catecholamines to stimulate myocardial contractility, pericardial aspiration, and thoracotomy. Appropriate amounts of fluid, 1 to 3 liters of electrolyte or blood, should be infused rapidly to elevate venous pressure and thus enhance cardiac filling, despite the elevated intrapericardial pressure. Cardiac filling results from the difference between venous pressure and intrapericardial pressure; hence, elevation of venous pressure by intravenously infused fluids will partly correct the impaired myocardial filling from the elevated pericardial pressures. For patients in extremis with bradycardia and impending cardiac arrest, probably from impaired coronary blood flow, catecholamines such as epinephrine or isoproterenol may be useful for short periods of time.

When a moribund patient with possible tamponade is first seen, pericardial aspiration should be done immediately. One of the most dramatic experiences in surgery is to aspirate as little as 10 to 15 ml blood from the pericardium of a moribund patient with an imperceptible blood pressure and see a prompt rise in blood pressure to 70 to 80 mm Hg and a return of consciousness. Aspiration is best done through a subxiphoid approach, inserting a 16- or 18-gauge needle slowly upward in the angle between the xiphoid process and the left costal margin. Ideally, the electrocardiogram should be monitored for an arrhythmia during the procedure. As the needle is angled upward, a sense of resistance can be noted as the diaphragm and pericardium are traversed. Varying amounts of blood may be obtained, ranging from as little as 10 ml to as much as 300 to 400 ml. The blood obtained from the pericardium may not clot, while blood obtained from inadvertent puncture of the heart, usually the right ventricle, does.

As mentioned earlier, when tamponade is likely but aspiration is ineffective, a prompt subxiphoid digital exploration should be done, making a short incision in the linea alba, separating the diaphragm behind the xiphoid process, and digitally entering the pericardium. The technique is well described by Berger et al.

Immediate thoracotomy should be considered and the operating room notified as soon as a patient is seen with a penetrating cardiac injury, because of the unpredictability of either continued hemorrhage or tamponade. Final decision about thoracotomy can be made after initial response to intravenously administered fluids.

Some patients with massive hemorrhage from cardiac wounds are near death on arrival in an emergency department and are often seen alive only because they were injured not far from the hospital. In such patients immediate thoracotomy in the emergency room, often with minimal aseptic technique, may be lifesaving. Once hemorrhage has been controlled by digital pressure or temporary suture, resuscitation can proceed in a more orderly fashion, usually followed by closure of the incision in the operating room. Since 1970, at Bellevue Hospital, several such patients have recovered uneventfully after immediate thoracotomy who clearly would not have survived otherwise.

Separate from the necessity of immediate thoracotomy for massive hemorrhage is the question of elective thoracotomy for penetrating cardiac injuries with tamponade. Data clearly indicate that 60 to 70 percent of the patients with tamponade can be safely treated by serial aspiration. In 1959 Isaacs reported that in a group of 60 patients with cardiac injuries treated at The Johns Hopkins Hospital, 40 had symptoms of tamponade for which aspiration was successful treatment in 75 percent; there was only one death in this group. However, there has been a gradual trend in recent years to perform thoracotomy upon virtually all patients with penetrating injuries and tamponade. The risk of thoracotomy is very small, probably no more than 1 to 2 percent, and the likelihood of delayed bleeding and recurrent tamponade small.

Sugg et al. in 1968 presented convincing data that routine thoracotomy gave overall better results in most institutions than selective thoracotomy for patients judged to have continuing hemorrhage or recurrent tamponade. In 1971 Beall et al. described a similar trend at Baylor University, where thoracotomy is now done almost routinely, rather than repeated pericardiocentesis.

Myocardial contusion from blunt thoracic trauma should be treated much as an acute myocardial infarction, with bed rest and serial observations with blood-enzyme measurements and the electrocardiogram. Complete recovery after a period of weeks can be expected in most patients. Rarely blunt injury may be associated with signs of intrapericardial bleeding from a laceration. Such instances are unusual, but because of the unpredictable nature of the laceration a pump-oxygenator should be available, and attachment of the pump-oxygenator to the femoral vessels in the thigh before the chest is opened should be considered. Without the pump-oxygenator, fatal hemorrhage may occur when the pericardium is opened if the laceration is too extensive to be promptly controlled by digital pressure. A recent report by Drapanas dramatically illustrates the utility of the pump-oxygenator in such injuries.

COMPLICATIONS. In the absence of injury of a discrete cardiac structure, recovery in most patients following suture of a cardiac laceration is uneventful. Formerly in those treated by serial aspiration alone, 15 to 20 percent developed a pericardiotomy syndrome with fever and effusion, lasting for several days to a few weeks but eventually resulting in complete recovery. Septic pericarditis from bacterial infection is very rare, and constrictive pericarditis has occurred as a late complication in only a few patients.

Foreign Bodies

Foreign bodies remaining in the heart after injury have naturally attracted much interest because of the unusual circumstances and the profound psychologic influences of having a missile embedded in the heart. Following World War II, Harken published a careful analysis of extensive experiences with foreign bodies, defining the complications and the indications for removal at that time. A reevaluation of the problem was published by Holdeger et al. in 1966. Data clearly indicate that symptomatic foreign bodies smaller than 1 cm are innocuous and can be safely left alone. Larger foreign bodies or those associated with a pericardial effusion or signs of pericarditis are best removed. Occasionally foreign bodies migrate in the circulation, moving from a large vein to the right ventricle or to a pulmonary artery.

In 1966 Bland and Beebe published a significant report of the 20-year course of 40 patients with foreign bodies remaining in the heart after World War II. All patients survived. A major complication occurred in only 1 patient, in whom a shell fragment in the left pulmonary artery moved to the right pulmonary artery and eroded the bronchus. The electrocardiogram became normal in all but 2 patients. Only 1 patient, who had a distinct injury of the aortic valve, had persistent cardiac enlargement. However, the emotional disability was impressive, apparently related to the strain of living with a condition of uncertain prognosis. Almost all patients were seriously concerned, and 5 were incapacitated with anxiety neuroses. Because of this significant emotional disability and the safety of current cardiac surgical procedures, most foreign bodies of significant size should be electively removed.

CARDIAC TUMORS

Metastatic neoplasms are the most common cardiac neoplasms, occurring in 4 to 12 percent of the autopsies performed on patients with neoplastic disease. The most frequent primary cardiac tumor is *myxoma,* comprising 50 to 60 percent of all primary cardiac neoplasms. *Sarcomas* are found in 20 to 25 percent of cases, and *rhabdomyomas* in 10 to 15 percent. Benign but extremely rare neoplasms include fibromas, angiomas, lipomas, teratomas, and cysts.

The clinical significance of cardiac tumors is similar to that of many other cardiac lesions in that accurate diagnosis and successful treatment first became possible with the development of extracorporeal circulation. Before 1950 cardiac tumors were usually first diagnosed at autopsy. Several excellent reviews have previously summarized the pathologic findings and clinical features. A classic analysis was published by Yater in 1931, and a detailed French monograph was published by Mahaim in 1945. In 1949 Whorton described the clinical findings in 100 sarcomas of the heart, and in 1951 Prichard reviewed 150 lesions, most of which were metastatic in origin.

In 1953 Steinberg et al. reported the diagnosis of an atrial myxoma in three patients by angiocardiography. An unsuccessful attempt was made to remove the myxoma in one of the patients studied by Steinberg et al., and in 1952 another unsuccessful attempt was made by Bahnson. Both these efforts preceded the development of open heart surgery. The first successful removal of an atrial myxoma was performed by Crafoord in 1954, using extracorporeal circulation. Other successful reports quickly followed, and in 1967 Thomas et al. stated that there had been 126 attempted excisions of atrial myxomas, either planned or inadvertent, 85 of which had been successful.

With the safety of extracorporeal circulation and the refinement of diagnostic techniques, including selective angiocardiography and more recently echocardiography, diagnosis and surgical excision have been greatly simplified. Typical of several reports is one by Symbas et al. in 1976, describing experiences with 13 patients.

Myxoma

Sixty to seventy-five percent of cardiac myxomas develop in the left atrium, almost always from the atrial septum near the fossa ovalis. Most other myxomas develop in the right atrium. Less than 20 have been found in either the right or left ventricle. The curious predilection for a myxoma to develop from the rim of the fossa ovalis in the left atrium has been studied by several observers, but a satisfactory explanation has not been found.

Myxomas are apparently true neoplasms, although their similarity to an organized atrial thrombus led to considerable debate at one time about whether they represented a true neoplasm or not. Their occurrence in the absence of other organic heart disease, histochemical studies demonstrating mucopolysaccharide and glycoprotein, and a distinct histologic appearance all indicate that myxomas are true neoplasms. In 1976 Dang and Hurley reported 19 recurrences of a myxoma following surgical excision in 16 patients, conclusively establishing the low-grade malignant potential of the tumor.

PATHOLOGY. The tumors are usually polypoid, projecting into the atrial cavity from a 1- to 2-cm stalk attached to the atrial septum. The maximal diameter varies from 0.5 to 10 cm. Careful histologic study of the point of origin of the myxoma from the atrial septum has demonstrated that only the superficial layer of the septum is involved, and invasion of the septum does not occur. Frequently myxomas grow slowly, some patients having symptoms for 10 to 20 years. There is no tendency to invade other areas of the heart, and metastases have not occurred. The consistency of a myxoma is of surgical significance, for extreme friability has been found in some tumors, resulting in fatal embolization when the tumor was digitally manipulated.

Histologically, a myxoma is covered with endothelium and composed of a myxomatous stroma with large stellate cells mixed with fusiform or multinucleated cells. Mitoses are infrequent. Lymphocytes and plasmacytes are regularly found. Hemosiderin, a result of hemorrhage into the tumor, is also common.

PATHOPHYSIOLOGY. A myxoma may cause no difficulty until it grows large enough to obstruct the flow of blood through either the mitral or tricuspid valve, or fragments to produce peripheral emboli. The rarity of embolization is surprising, for an astonishing degree of to-and-fro motion of a myxoma swinging on a small pedicle with each cardiac contraction may occur. This has been vividly demonstrated by angiographic and fluoroscopic studies.

Because of its rarity, myxoma is almost always confused with a more frequent cardiac condition. Left atrial myxomas simulate mitral stenosis or insufficiency or idiopathic pulmonary hypertension. Right atrial myxomas are confused with tricuspid valvular disease or constrictive pericarditis. Because of the polypoid nature of the myxoma, intermittent obstruction of the mitral or tricuspid valve may occur, with resulting variation in symptoms, but this has not been observed frequently enough to be of much diagnostic significance.

CLINICAL MANIFESTATIONS. The clinical course of the patient with a myxoma may be protracted, with a variety of erroneous clinical diagnoses. The rate of development and variation in symptoms depend upon the growth of the tumor with the associated obstruction to cardiac filling and obstruction at the valve orifice. There are no characteristic symptoms or signs from which a precise diagnosis can be made. The usual findings are those of mitral valvular disease, with progressive dyspnea, cough, and subsequent cardiac failure with hepatic enlargement and edema.

In a few patients unusual signs of a generalized systemic disease have developed, with recurrent fever, weight loss, malaise, and abnormalities in serum proteins gradually evolving over 1 to 3 years. Why these symptoms should occur with a myxoma is not known.

Peripheral emboli occur in a minority of patients and in some are the first sign of a myxoma. A few instances have been described in which the diagnosis was first made as a result of histologic examination of a surgically removed embolus recognizing the characteristic myxomatous structure. Such a patient was recently treated in our unit.

On physical examination patients with a left atrial myxoma may have either a diastolic murmur suggesting mitral stenosis or a systolic murmur simulating mitral insufficiency. With a right atrial myxoma, hepatic enlargement and edema characteristic of constrictive pericarditis are frequent.

The electrocardiogram is often normal unless pulmonary hypertension from long-standing mitral valve obstruction has produced right ventricular hypertrophy. The chest roentgenogram may show enlargement of the left atrium with pulmonary congestion. Rarely on fluoroscopy calcification is visible. Echocardiography has been a significant advance in diagnosis, since most myxomas can be readily identified by this simple, noninvasive technique. Selective angiography may graphically confirm the diagnosis if the left atrium can be opacified satisfactorily, but unfortunately this cannot always be accomplished.

Differential diagnosis includes more frequent cardiac lesions, such as mitral stenosis or insufficiency, pulmonary hypertension, constrictive pericarditis, rheumatic fever, and bacterial endocarditis.

TREATMENT. Operation should be performed upon all patients once the diagnosis has been established. Extracorporeal circulation is routinely employed because of the grave risk of dislodging emboli into the arterial circulation.

A sternotomy or a right lateral thoracotomy is preferred. Once extracorporeal circulation has been established, ventricular fibrillation may be induced and the aorta clamped to avoid the risk of embolism of tumor fragments. Palpation of the lesion is avoided. In recent years we have adopted the operative approach described by Cooley in 1973. With bypass functioning, the right atrium is opened and the fossa ovalis incised to expose the stalk of the myxoma. The left atrium is opened in the interatrial groove. With the myxoma visualized, the segment of fossa ovalis from which the tumor arises is excised, after which the myxoma is removed through the incision in the left atrium. The defect in the atrial septum is closed with a small patch. This technique is simple, avoids manipulation of the tumor, and should prevent the rare recurrences which have been described.

Following operation the prognosis is excellent for complete recovery. Complete regression of severe pulmonary hypertension has been reported in several patients. One of the earliest cases, a fifty-seven-year-old patient operated upon in 1956, was well and asymptomatic 8 years later (Fig. 19-34).

Metastatic Neoplasms

Cardiac metastases have been found in 4 to 12 percent of autopsies performed for neoplastic disease. Although they have occurred from primary neoplasms developing in almost every known site of the body, the most frequent have been carcinoma of the lung or breast, melanoma, and lymphoma. Cardiac metastases involving only the heart are very unusual. Similarly, a solitary cardiac metastasis is infrequent; usually there are multiple areas of involvement. Cardiac involvement is particularly common with leukemia or lymphoma, developing in 25 to 40 percent of patients. All areas of the heart are involved with equal frequency except the cardiac valves, perhaps as a result of the absence of lymphatics in the valves.

Most patients have no symptoms of heart disease, even though large areas of myocardium are involved by an infiltrating neoplasm. A pericardial effusion, which is hemorrhagic in about 15 percent of patients, is the most frequent abnormality. This was found in 45 of 217 patients studied by Gassman and associates, but only 3 of these had cardiac tamponade. Symptoms from cardiac failure are the most common disability, but these developed in only 17 of the 217 patients in Gassman's series. Recurrent arrhythmias are infrequent. The electrocardiogram is similarly nonspecific, usually showing T-wave changes, although a wide variety of conduction abnormalities have been reported.

The diagnosis can be suspected in a patient with malignant disease in whom a hemorrhagic pericardial effusion develops. Identification of malignant cells in fluid aspirated from the pericardium can establish the diagnosis. Thoracotomy should be avoided if possible, because no effective treatment is available and death usually occurs from generalized metastatic disease within a few months. The cardiac involvement per se is seldom a significant factor in the terminal illness.

Sarcoma

Sarcomas of the heart constitute about 25 percent of all primary cardiac neoplasms. In 1962 Dong et al. reported that 178 cases had been described. Spindle cell and round cell sarcomas are the most frequent, but the entire range of mesenchymal tumors has been reported, including leiomyosarcoma and fibrosarcoma. The right atrium and right ventricle are the most frequent sites of involvement, usually with a diffuse infiltrating tumor that does not involve the cardiac valves. Valvular obstruction or embolization, in contrast to atrial myxoma, is infrequent. Metastatic spread to the mediastinum is frequent, with death occurring 1 month to 3 years after onset of symptoms. Symptoms usually evolve from obstruction of the venae cavae, pericardial effusion, or arrhythmias from invasion of the conduction system.

Sarcomas developing in the pericardium, usually mesotheliomas, are rare lesions that grow rapidly and cause symptoms from obstruction of the venae cavae. Invasion of the myocardium develops in the late stages of the tumor.

The diagnosis of a primary cardiac malignant tumor can be suspected in a patient in whom an unexplained hemorrhagic pericardial effusion develops, especially in association with a bizarre cardiac shadow on the roentgenogram. Thoracotomy is usually required to establish the diagnosis. Only rarely is effective therapy possible. Scannell and Grillo, in 1958, reported one fortunate experience in a child in whom exploration for pericardial effusion found a localized fibrosarcoma in the right atrial wall which was successfully excised. In 1966, we removed an angiosarcoma of the right side of the heart, invading the tricuspid valve, along with a large segment of right atrial wall. Reconstruc-

Fig. 19-34. Pedunculated atrial myxoma removed at operation in 1957. The patient has remained free of cardiac symptoms since that time. (*Reprinted from H. T. Bahnson, F. C. Spencer, and E. C. Andrus, Diagnosis and Treatment of Intracavitary Myxomas of the Heart, Ann Surg, 145:915, 1957, by permission of J. B. Lippincott Company, Philadelphia.*)

tion was with a pericardial patch graft, reattaching the tricuspid valve to the reconstructed annulus. Postoperative radiotherapy was given, following which the patient lived for 18 months before dying of widespread metastatic disease.

Rhabdomyoma

A cardiac rhabdomyoma is a rare lesion which is not a true tumor but is probably a focal arrest in maturation of cardiac muscle. Seventy such patients were reviewed by Prichard in 1951. The nodules have been termed *nodular glycogenic degeneration,* being interpreted as an example of localized glycogen storage disease. It is uncertain whether they are hamartomas or merely localized manifestations of glycogen storage disease.

The cardiac lesions may be solitary or multiple nodules, or may present as diffuse infiltration of the cardiac muscle. The nodules are not encapsulated but merge imperceptibly with the surrounding healthy myocardium. The lesions do not grow, and metastases do not occur.

On histologic examination, the nodules are composed of tubular muscle cells with large vacuoles in which the nuclei appear suspended by threads of cytoplasm, like spiders in a web, giving origin to the term "spider cell." About one-half of the patients have tuberous sclerosis of the brain. The clinical significance of the cardiac lesions is uncertain, for disability is usually due to the associated tuberous sclerosis. Sudden death has been reported in some patients who, at postmortem examination, were found to have a rhabdomyoma. Isolated instances of obstruction of the outflow tract of the right ventricle from a large rhabdomyoma requiring surgical excision have been reported.

Miscellaneous Tumors

Unusual benign lesions of the heart include fibromas, lipomas, angiomas, teratomas, and cysts. Fewer than 50 examples of each of these types of lesions have been reported. Fibromas have been found most frequently in the left ventricle, often as 2- to 5-cm nodules within the muscle. Sudden death, probably from a cardiac arrhythmia, has been reported with such tumors and may be the reason that only 18 percent of the reported tumors have been found in adults.

Lipomas are usually asymptomatic tumors found projecting from the epicardial or endocardial surface of the heart in older patients. Only about 30 such cases have been reported. Angiomas are commonly small, focal vascular malformations of no clinical significance, except four that have been found associated with a heart block. Pericardial teratomas and bronchogenic cysts are rare lesions that may cause symptoms from compression of the right atrium and obstruction of venous return. About 30 such patients have been reported in the surgical literature, most of them children. Some of the larger cysts, up to 10 cm in diameter, may produce grotesque deformities from extensive invagination of the right atrial wall.

CORONARY ARTERY DISEASE

HISTORICAL DATA. Since the late 1930s, different investigators have attempted to increase the blood supply of a heart ischemic from coronary atherosclerosis. Beck pioneered these efforts by attempting to develop vascular adhesions around the heart to introduce additional blood supply and to redistribute blood flowing through patent coronary vessels. Many unusual, imaginative, and sometimes bizarre procedures were tried. These included abrasion of the epicardium, painting the epicardium with phenol, insertion of talc or asbestos into the pericardial cavity, and wrapping omentum around the heart. Unfortunately, consistent benefit could not be demonstrated from any of these procedures, and virtually all have been abandoned. Perhaps the fundamental biologic reason for failure is the natural tendency for vascular adhesions to progressively fibrose and become more avascular with time.

In 1946, Vineberg developed a new concept for revascularizing the heart when he found that an internal mammary artery implanted in a tunnel in the myocardium of a dog would remain patent in a high percentage of cases. The operation of implantation of the internal mammary artery into the wall of the left ventricle in man was begun by Vineberg in 1950 and has been consistently employed by him since that time. Objective analysis of the results of arterial implantation was not possible until the development of coronary arteriography by Sones in the year 1958–1959. Demonstration by Sones that the implanted artery remained patent in the majority of patients and in some patients connected with regional coronary arteries provided a stimulus to further investigation of methods of arterial implantation. Subsequently between 1960 and 1967 different arterial implants were extensively tried in several centers, but with the introduction of the bypass operation the procedure has greatly decreased in popularity and has been virtually abandoned in most institutions, including ours. The limited, often negligible, physiologic improvement in most patients is related to the fact that even though the artery remains patent in over 90 percent of patients, it often carries only a small amount of blood, as little as 5 to 10 ml/minute, to the myocardium. An occasional patient develops significant collateral circulation following implantation, and isolated instances have been reported in which the implanted artery clearly was of substantial benefit, carrying as much as 50 ml of blood per minute and causing obvious severe myocardial ischemia when temporarily interrupted. The reason for the wide variation in the development of collateral circulation after implantation has never been satisfactorily determined.

From 1956 to 1959 initial attempts were made with coronary endarterectomy to remove directly localized areas of obstruction caused by atherosclerotic plaques. Longmire and Cannon, Bailey, and others attempted such procedures, but results were discouraging because of a high operative mortality and a high rate of subsequent occlusion. Subsequent performance of such procedures with cardiopulmonary bypass, often combined with a pericardial roof patch, was satisfactory in a small percentage of patients but disappointing in many.

The development of the bypass operation for coronary occlusive disease from 1967 to 1968 was a dramatic achievement, for this represented the first such operation in which it was possible to immediately increase the blood flow to the myocardium. Most of the basic clinical investigations of the technique of bypass grafting evolved from studies in three centers in the United States during this period. Favaloro, discouraged with the limited application of endarterectomy and pericardial patch grafting, began using longer and longer segments of saphenous vein to bypass occlusive disease in the right coronary artery, eventually demonstrating that grafts could be effectively interposed between the aorta proximally and the termination of the right coronary artery at the posterior descending coronary artery distad. Johnson first showed that similar grafts could be effectively used for the left coronary artery, a most significant achievement, for previously all direct operative procedures upon the left coronary artery had had a prohibitive operative mortality well over 50 percent. At New York University, Green et al., following extensive experimental studies, first began direct anastomoses between the left internal mammary artery and the anterior descending coronary artery, using an end-to-side anastomosis. This procedure was not widely used by others for 2 to 3 years but subsequently greatly increased in popularity. The dramatic, virtually instantaneous relief of angina with bypass techniques led to performance of the procedure in thousands of patients in the past several years.

However, despite this widespread popularity, much remains unknown about the long-term results. For this reason considerable debate continues about indications and contraindications for bypass grafting, a question that will require several years' accumulation of data to answer.

ETIOLOGY AND PATHOGENESIS. Atherosclerosis is the cause of coronary occlusive disease in almost all patients. It is extremely common in the American male; autopsy studies of men killed in the Korean conflict who were between twenty and thirty years of age found some coronary atherosclerosis in 30 to 40 percent. The frequency gradually rises in men to approach 70 to 80 percent by seventy years of age. For a detailed analysis of the different theories concerning the cause of coronary disease, as well as its widely varying incidence according to race, sex, and other factors, recent monographs on epidemiology of atherosclerosis should be consulted.

The basic lesion is a segmental atherosclerotic plaque, often localized within the first 5 cm of the origin of the coronary arteries from the aorta. Involvement of the tributaries of the major coronary arteries, as well as the arterioles, is often minimal. This segmental localization makes bypass procedures possible. The atherosclerotic plaque is composed of focal deposits of lipid alternating with areas of fibrosis, perhaps a histologic reaction to the deposition of lipids. In older lesions spotty areas of calcification develop. Areas of intramural hemorrhage are visible in some lesions and often seem to precipitate thrombosis of the stenosed vessel.

The myocardial ischemia produced by coronary atherosclerosis results in a number of grave complications: sudden death, angina pectoris, myocardial infarction (with or without coronary thrombosis), and congestive heart failure. Any one or all of these events may occur unpredictably in a patient with coronary atherosclerosis.

Of these four, angina pectoris occurs most frequently. Patients experience a periodic discomfort, usually substernal, appearing typically with exertion, after eating, or with extreme emotion. Characteristically these symptoms subside within 3 to 5 minutes or may be dramatically relieved by sublingual nitroglycerin. In about 25 percent of patients, the symptoms are less typical and may have unusual areas of radiation to such remote areas as the teeth, the shoulder, the hand, or the epigastrium. Establishing a diagnosis of angina in such patients is difficult, perhaps impossible, without angiography, for results of the physical examination are usually normal. Differential diagnosis includes anxiety states, musculoskeletal disorders, and reflux esophagitis.

There is a constant risk of sudden death with angina pectoris: the risk varies both with the extent of disease and the degree of impairment of ventricular function, ranging from 2 percent to 10 to 15 percent per year. Often postmortem examination does not show any acute cause of death, such as myocardial infarction or coronary thrombosis. In such instances death is probably due to an acute disturbance of rhythm with terminal ventricular fibrillation.

Myocardial infarction, with or without thrombosis of a diseased coronary artery, is another frequent and often fatal complication. For a detailed discussion of myocardial infarction, a textbook of cardiology should be consulted.

Surgical procedures for acute myocardial infarction have been tried in a few instances, but thus far the procedures remain experimental. Results with bypass grafting seem best if it is performed within 6 hours after onset of infarction. Berg in 1976 reported operating on almost 100 such patients.

In some patients congestive heart failure develops and may become the principle disability, eventually causing death. Congestive failure may or may not be preceded by angina or a myocardial infarction. Probably congestive failure is a result of myriads of tiny myocardial infarctions, eventually destroying over one-third of left ventricular muscle mass. What determines angina as the dominant symptom in one patient and congestive failure in another is unknown. Repeated tiny emboli from an ulcerated atherosclerotic plaque have been suggested as one possible mechanism. Once congestive failure has developed, revascularization of the heart with bypass operations has been disappointing, for objective signs of improved cardiac function have been small in a few and negligible in most. Probably this unfortunate group of patients may be best treated by cardiac transplantation when advances in immunology make organ transplantation more feasible. At present congestive failure is significantly helped by operation only in patients with large left ventricular aneurysms.

DIAGNOSIS OF ANGINA PECTORIS. The history is the most important method for making the diagnosis, for usually there are no abnormal physical findings. With unusual symptoms, especially the absence of pain induced by exertion and relieved by nitroglycerin, laboratory studies are needed.

The electrocardiogram is normal at rest in about 70 percent of patients. Evaluation of changes in the electrocardiogram with graded exercise is a useful and widely used test, noting signs of ischemia in the cardiogram with increasing exercise, but the changes are difficult to quantitate. By far the most exact method for determining the presence and severity of coronary artery disease is selective coronary arteriography (Fig. 19-35). Coronary arteriography provided the first method for accurately determining the extent and severity of coronary disease in individual patients. Not only the presence of disease but progression and response to therapy over months or years can be evaluated by serial arteriograms. Since the introduction of arteriography, around 1958 or 1959, thousands of such procedures have been performed.

OPERATIVE PROCEDURES FOR CORONARY ARTERY DISEASE. Coronary Bypass Operations. *Indications and Contraindications.* There is some disagreement at present about indications for bypass grafting for angina. It is well established that operation can be performed in good-risk patients with a mortality of less than 3 percent and is followed by almost immediate and complete relief of angina in the majority of patients. Fifteen to twenty percent of vein grafts may occlude in the first year after operation but thereafter the rate of occlusion is reduced. Although the 5-year patency data are meager, it appears that the patency rate approximates 60 percent.

Bypass grafting is widely used for patients with disabling angina unresponsive to conventional medical therapy, and

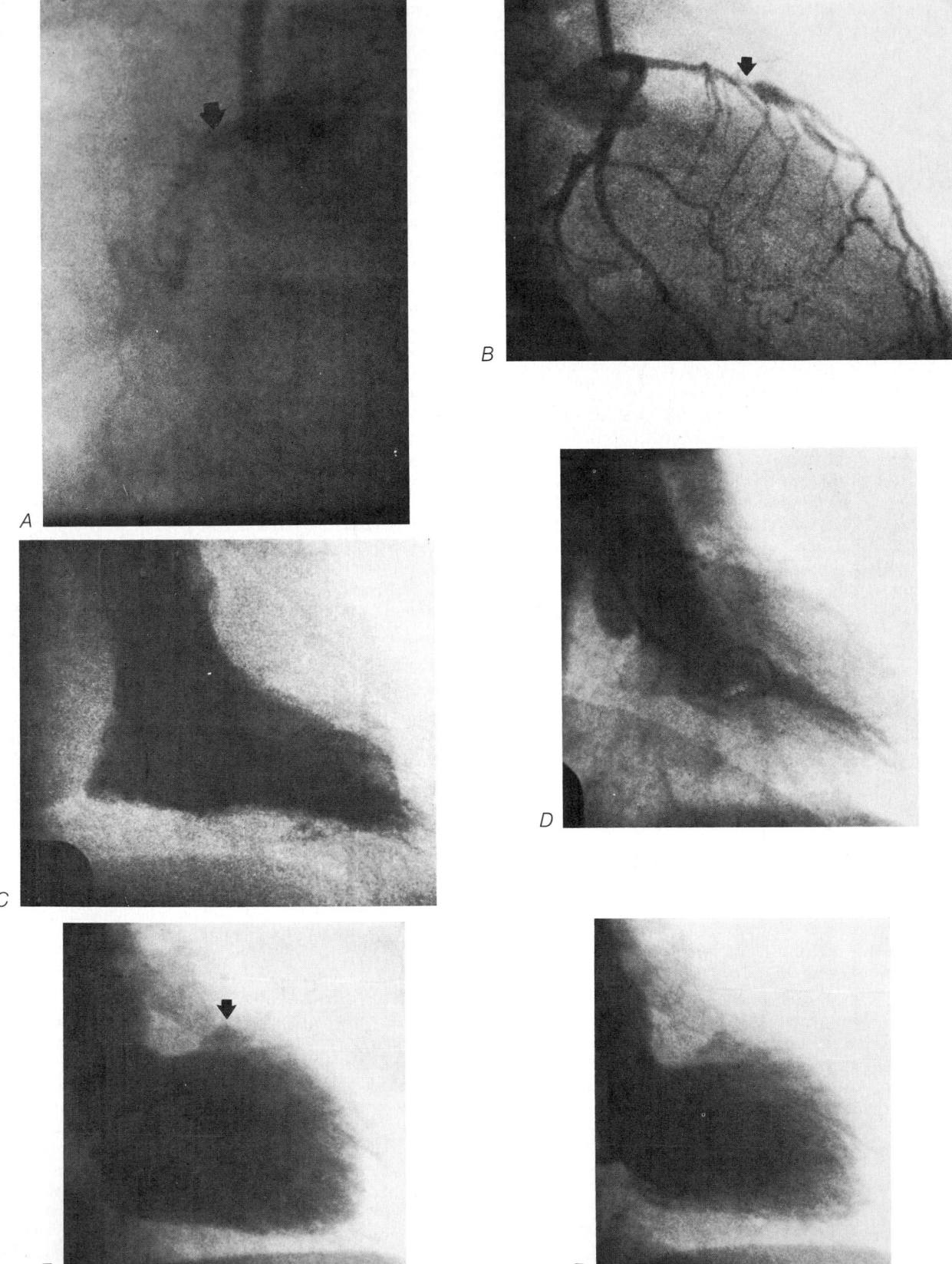

also for angina of increasing intensity, so-called preinfarction angina, for this is often a forerunner of acute myocardial infarction. At New York University most operations have been performed for patients in these two categories.

More uncertain is the use of bypass grafts for patients with mild, nonincapacitating angina or on a prophylactic basis in patients with few or no symptoms but with previous myocardial infarction and extensive occlusive disease seen on subsequent coronary arteriography. Some experienced groups routinely recommend operation for triple occlusive disease with few or no symptoms, while others, equally experienced, do not. In such patients the operation would provide protection from future myocardial infarctions, a very plausible hypothesis if the grafts remain patent for several years but one that has not yet been proved.

Severe congestive failure is a definite contraindication to operation, for the mortality is high and improvement small in surviving patients.

When a patient is considered for operation, coronary arteriography must be performed to determine the areas of obstruction, the size and patency of vessels beyond the area of obstruction, and the function of the left ventricle. Atherosclerotic obstruction is physiologically significant if the diameter of the vessel is narrowed more than 50 percent, corresponding to a reduction in cross-sectional area greater than 75 percent. The size and patency of vessels beyond the area of obstruction is also of importance, for patency rates after bypass grafting have been better with larger arteries in the range of 2 to 3 mm, as compared to 1 to 2 mm. However, ability to visualize vessels beyond an area of obstruction is a function of collateral circulation; so the angiographic evaluation is not precise. In some patients dissection at operation will find an adequate vessel beyond an area of obstruction not visualized by angiography because the flow of the injected dye was limited by sparse collateral circulation.

Multiple areas of obstruction are common. Nearly 50 percent of patients with severe angina have involvement of all three major coronary arteries, the anterior descending, the circumflex, and the right coronary.

Ventricular function, judged by contractility of the left ventricle during ventriculography, is a crucial part of preoperative evaluation, as it indicates the degree of previous muscle injury. In patients with normal ventricular function,

operative risk is less than 3 percent and the likelihood of improvement great. At the other extreme, severe impairment of ventricular function with congestive failure, representing infarction of areas of myocardium and replacement by scar, indicates an operative risk as high as 20 to 25 percent and far less likelihood of improvement.

Attempts have been made to quantitate the degree of impairment of ventricular function by measurement of ejection fractions, angiographically estimating the percentage of blood in the ventricle which is ejected during systole. Although this is an imprecise measurement, reduction of ventricular function to a point at which the ejection fraction is less than 0.15 to 0.20 indicates a serious operative risk. The degree of angina as compared with the degree of congestive failure is significant in deciding on operation.

Left ventricular end-diastolic pressure in patients with normal ventricular function is normal, less than 10 to 12 mm Hg. Some increase occurs with moderate failure, but the level of elevation varies so much with the medical management of congestive failure preceding catheterization that the actual value found at catheterization is not of precise prognostic value. Elevation beyond 20 to 25 mm Hg, however, indicates a poor prognosis. Nevertheless, over 100 such patients have been operated on at NYU with an operative risk near 10 percent and a 5-year survival of 83 percent.

Operative Technique. Coronary bypass operations are usually performed during extracorporeal circulation with the heart stilled either by inducing ventricular fibrillation or by ischemic arrest produced by temporary occlusion of the ascending aorta. Before bypass is started, a long segment of saphenous vein is removed from the thigh or leg, taking 15 to 20 cm of vein for each graft to be performed. It is reversed before insertion because of venous valves, attaching the distal end to the aorta. During bypass with the heart fibrillating, the left ventricle is decompressed with a vent to avoid overdistension. Either the aortic or the coronary anastomosis may be done first; our preference is to do the aortic first. The patent coronary artery beyond the area of obstruction is then dissected, and an arteriotomy about 1 cm long made. Care is taken to avoid dissecting the coronary artery from its bed, for inclusion of the surrounding soft tissue in the subsequent anastomotic suture line greatly aids hemostasis. The vein-coronary artery anastomoses are performed end-to-side with interrupted and continuous sutures of 6-0 or 7-0 synthetic suture material, usually Prolene. Three- to four-power optical magnification is routinely employed and greatly facilitates the performance of these small anastomoses. Following completion of the distal anastomosis, the vein graft is attached in gentle curves to the epicardium over the surface of the heart.

One theoretic objection to the use of vein grafts is the discrepancy in size between the vein and the artery, which results in turbulent flow. For example, if a 6-mm vein is anastomosed to a 2-mm artery, the rate of blood flow in the vein will be only one-ninth of that in the artery because of the difference in cross-sectional area. For this reason there has been an increased tendency to use veins from

Fig. 19-35. *A.* Right coronary artery, left anterior oblique projection. There is total obstruction of the vessel immediately distal to its aortic origin (arrow). A network of collateral vessels on the anterior surface of the right atrium and the right ventricle is apparent. *B.* Left coronary artery, right anterior oblique projection. There is severe narrowing of the left anterior descending coronary artery (arrow) distal to the origin of the second septal branch. *C.* Left ventricle in right anterior oblique projection in diastole. There is a normal contour of the chamber. *D.* Same ventricle in systole showing inadequate contraction of all areas of the ventricle. *E.* Left ventricle in diastole, right anterior oblique projection. There is increased rounding of the ventricle and bulging of the anterolateral wall. A localized bulge on the superior portion of the anterolateral wall is evident (arrow). *F.* The same ventricle in systole. The degree of left ventricular contraction is generally markedly impaired.

the leg, with a diameter near 4 mm, rather than larger veins from the thigh. However, significant data regarding influence of the size of veins on long-term patency rates are not available.

Because of the frequency of multiple areas of occlusion, double or triple bypass grafts are used in most patients, usually attaching each graft separately to the aorta. At New York University in the past 5 years, during the performance of over 1,000 bypass procedures, nearly 50 percent of patients have had a triple bypass. With the techniques described, a graft can be attached to a vessel on almost any surface of the heart, the most difficult being the posterior wall of the left ventricle near the termination of the circumflex coronary artery. With optical magnification, grafts can be attached to vessels as small as 1 mm internal diameter. This fact, combined with the ability to attach grafts to any area of the heart, makes it possible to perform bypass grafts in the majority of patients with angina, over 95 percent of patients seen. The artery is technically inoperable when there are multiple areas of occlusion throughout the length of the artery, fortunately an unusual pattern of involvement.

Once the bypass grafts have been constructed, rate of blood flow is measured with a flowmeter. Though accuracy in the operating room is sometimes questionable, these measurements are of particular prognostic value, for there is good correlation between rate of flow and long-term patency. A mean flow rate of less than 20 ml/minute is associated with a high rate of subsequent occlusion, while high mean flow rates, greater than 70 to 80 ml/minute, have a much better prognosis. The flow rate, of course, varies with the size of the distal artery and the patency of the distal vascular bed. Patency rates have not been good with grafts attached to vessels as small as 1 mm in diameter, probably because of the small rate of flow.

Following operation careful observation in a cardiac intensive care unit is necessary to maintain adequate ventilation and cardiac output and to detect arrhythmias. Arrhythmias are quite frequent following operation but can be controlled by appropriate measures. These include infusion of lidocaine, procainamide, digitalis, propranolol, and electrical cardioversion. In most patients convalescence is comparatively uneventful, with the patient leaving the hospital in 10 to 14 days. A pericardiotomy syndrome, with fever, pleural effusion, and pleural or pericardial friction rubs, occurs in a small percentage of patients but responds well to administration of prednisone in small amounts for several days.

Angiographic studies performed within 1 to 2 weeks after operation have found a patency rate well above 90 percent. However, angiograms performed 6 to 12 months later have found occlusion of 20 to 25 percent of vein grafts. Though extensive data are not yet available, with periods of observation now between 4 and 5 years in small numbers of patients, the rate of occlusion beyond the first year after operation apparently is small. Several factors may cause early or late thrombosis in a vein graft. These include technical factors at the time of operation in the construction of the anastomoses and ischemic injury to the vein during removal from its bed, such as excessive removal of adventitia or other mechanical trauma. As mentioned earlier, the size of the coronary artery grafted and the rate of flow through the vein graft both correlate reasonably well with late patency. A progressive fibrosis has been seen in some vein grafts, usually segmental in location, which progresses to complete obliteration within a few months. This curious histologic response at times is observed in one vein graft but not in others in the same patient. It probably represents segmental ischemic or mechanical injury to the vein at the time of operation. With appropriate care in removal of the vein graft, dissecting the vein gently and gradually distending it with cold heparinized blood, segmental stenosis has virtually disappeared in our unit over the past 3 to 4 years. Other factors influencing thrombosis of vein grafts include turbulent blood flow producing intimal proliferation at the anastomotic sites, pericardial adhesions, and theoretically progressive coronary atherosclerosis. The last factor, to date, has been rare.

With the natural concern about the significant rate of thrombosis of vein grafts, arterial grafts have been used with increasing frequency. The left internal mammary-anterior descending coronary anastomosis was first developed at New York University by Green and Tice and has been used consistently by Green since (Fig. 19-36). Since 1970 there has been increasing use of the internal mammary artery by several groups because of the long-term patency rates above 90 percent, a much more favorable finding than that with vein grafts. Unfortunately the internal mammary artery is small, and the rate of flow of blood is not as great as with vein grafts. However, the size of the internal mammary closely approximates that of the coronary artery in many patients. Another objection is the fact that use of the internal mammary is much more restrictive than that with free vein grafts. It is possible to attach the right internal mammary artery to the anterior descending, and the left internal mammary artery to the circumflex, but the right internal mammary will not reach to the termination of the right coronary on the posterior surface of the heart. For this reason, pedicled splenic arterial grafts have

Fig. 19-36. Angiogram performed several months after left internal mammary–left anterior descending coronary bypass, showing a good flow from the internal mammary artery into the anterior descending coronary and its branches.

been tried, but the rate of occlusion within one year was prohibitive (40 to 50 percent). A search for other arterial grafts continues, and at this time a few experiences with the radial artery have been verbally reported but not published. At present the feasibility of bypass grafting has been thoroughly established, but undoubtedly the best technique for grafting will require long periods of comparison of data with different methods.

The critical question with coronary bypass grafting is, of course, the long-term protection from myocardial infarction and death. This will require several years of careful study. A cooperative study among several universities is currently being coordinated by the National Institutes of Health.

The total experience with elective coronary bypass at New York University between February 1968 and December 1975 included 1,172 patients; 98 percent of the cases were reassessed in 1976. Overall operative mortality over this $7\frac{1}{2}$-year period was 5 percent, decreasing to about 2 percent for the last few years. Hence a total of 1,111 patients left the hospital. Only 48 cardiac-related deaths subsequently occurred. Thus the long-term survival, calculated by the actuarial method and including operative deaths, was 88 percent at 5 years and 80 percent at 7 years. To further emphasize the surprisingly low late mortality, of each 95 patients discharged from the hospital, only 7 died from cardiac causes in the next 5 years, an annual mortality of 1.5 percent, closely paralleling the normal population. Although the study was not randomized, most patients were operated on for angina refractory to available medical therapy, and multiple coronary grafts were performed in over 80 percent of the group, indicating the extent and severity of disease. These data strongly indicate that coronary bypass does indeed prolong life. Similar data were recently reported by Jones et al. and by Mills and Ochsner.

When significant obstruction of the left main coronary artery is present, which fortunately occurs in only 5 to 10 percent of patients, virtually all published data agree that a bypass procedure should be done promptly, regardless of symptoms, because complete occlusion of the left main coronary is almost always fatal.

Other Operative Procedures. It is significant that when the previous edition of this textbook was published, most of the discussion of surgical procedures concerned implantation of a systemic artery into the myocardium, the Vineberg procedure. In the intervening years, with the dramatic results obtained with the bypass operation, the popularity of arterial implants has waned sharply. Almost none have been performed at New York University since 1970, primarily because bypass grafts can be used in the majority of patients. The implanted artery remains patent in the majority of patients, a range of 80 to 90 percent, but the amount of blood flowing through the implanted artery seems to be small in most. Hence, the degree of improvement in myocardial ischemia is disappointingly small. A few unusual exceptions have been cited where at repeat operation months or years later when disease developed in other areas, direct flow measurements of an implanted artery found blood flow as high as 50 ml/minute.

Endarterectomy, either with carbon dioxide gas or with mechanical strippers, is employed particularly on the right coronary artery but in selected instances on the left. The procedure now is done almost always in conjunction with bypass grafting to improve flow rates through the graft.

Operative procedures for acute myocardial infarction, performing bypass grafting within hours after the vessel has become occluded, are under evaluation. Experimentally, total ischemia to an area of myocardium produces irreversible necrosis within less than 1 hour; so the potential value of bypass grafting is to improve blood flow to critically ischemic areas which have not yet undergone necrosis. Excision of myocardial infarcts has been studied experimentally and in a few instances clinically, but results have usually been poor.

Intestinal bypass procedures to decrease absorption of cholesterol and to stop or even reverse the coronary atherosclerotic process have been cautiously but hopefully evaluated primarily by Buchwald and Varco and by others. Results are somewhat encouraging, but significant data are not yet available. Such observations require several years.

VENTRICULAR ANEURYSM

HISTORICAL DATA. A few early attempts to excise ventricular aneurysms by a closed technique were made before the development of pump-oxygenators, but a precise, safe surgical technique with a pump-oxygenator was first employed by Cooley et al. in 1958. Initially the operation was rarely done; by 1962 a total of only 28 cases operated upon had been reported. By 1965 Effler et al. reported that 61 patients with such aneurysms had been operated upon at the Cleveland Clinic. With coronary bypass, excision of such aneurysms has become commonplace, usually combined with bypass grafting. By 1971 the Cleveland Clinic group alone had performed over 300 such procedures.

ETIOLOGY. Almost all aneurysms develop as a complication of myocardial infarction (Fig. 19-37). The reported frequency with which an aneurysm develops after an infarction varies from 10 to 15 percent.

PATHOLOGY AND PATHOPHYSIOLOGY. Most of the aneurysms which have been surgically treated have been located in the anterior portion of the left ventricle in the area supplied by the anterior descending coronary artery. Aneurysms of the posterior portion of the ventricle, an area supplied by the circumflex artery, are much less frequent. It has been suggested that large aneurysms seldom arise in the posterior part of the left ventricle because of the attachments of the papillary muscles in this area, for a large infarction involving the attachments of the papillary muscles is usually fatal. Calcification may develop in the wall of a chronic aneurysm, but is not common. Lower recently described several uncommon types of ventricular aneurysms.

An aneurysm with an expansile wall can impair function of the left ventricle, since energy developed during contraction of the left ventricle is dissipated into expanding the wall of the aneurysm. This may be recognized by fluoroscopy. The resulting decrease in cardiac function can increase the severity of congestive heart failure. Mural

Fig. 19-37. Ventricular aneurysm. *A.* Chest roentgenogram showing a heart of normal size 2 days following an acute myocardial infarction. *B.* Chest roentgenogram showing cardiac enlargement from a large left ventricular aneurysm which progressively enlarged before a fatal episode of cardiac arrhythmia.

thrombi often develop in the aneurysm and may be a source of systemic embolization, although this is not frequent. Also, the aneurysm may enlarge and rupture, fortunately an uncommon complication. Rupture occurred in only 2 of 65 cases studied at autopsy by Abrams et al. Death in most patients with a left ventricular aneurysm is from further complications of the underlying coronary atherosclerosis, usually a subsequent myocardial infarction.

Prognosis of patients with an untreated left ventricular aneurysm was found by Schlichter et al. to be grim; 75 percent of the patients died within 3 years after the myocardial infarction. In contrast, a study of 65 patients by

Abrams et al. found a much more favorable prognosis; the 5-year survival rate following myocardial infarction was 69 percent, and in only 14 percent of the patients was death considered to be a complication of the aneurysm. The patients studied by Abrams et al., however, had small aneurysms in the posterior portion of the left ventricle, with an average diameter of 4 cm, which may explain the discrepancy in the two reports.

CLINICAL MANIFESTATIONS. Clinical findings are meager, often absent. A diffuse forceful apical impulse is seen in some. The chest roentgenogram may show a suspicious bulge in the area of the left ventricle, but with small aneurysms the roentgenogram may appear normal. The electrocardiogram shows only the changes of coronary artery disease with a previous myocardial infarction. Small aneurysms are probably often not recognized, and in only 4 of the 65 cases studied by Abrams et al. was the diagnosis made before autopsy. The size of the aneurysm ranged up to 8 cm, with an average diameter of 4 cm, and all were located in the posterior portion of the ventricle.

Diagnosis can be made principally by cineangiography, outlining the size, location, and expansile nature of the aneurysm. Simultaneous coronary arteriography is of significant value, indicating the extent of the coronary artery disease and the consequent risk of operation. Preferably the cardiac output should be measured at the time of cardiac catheterization, in order to evaluate subsequent improvement of the patient following operation. In equivocal cases evaluation by cineangiography and catheterization should form the basis for a decision to excise the aneurysm. It seems probable that small left ventricular aneurysms are of negligible physiologic significance, while larger ones significantly impair cardiac function. Operation should usually be postponed for a minimum of 3 months after the preceding myocardial infarction because of the friability of the ventricular muscle.

TREATMENT. Technique of Operation. A sternotomy incision is preferred. Dissection of adherent pericardium over the aneurysm, usually obliterating the major portion of the pericardial cavity overlying the left ventricle, is postponed until cardiopulmonary bypass is started. Once bypass is established, the heart is fibrillated and the left atrium opened to decompress the left heart (Fig. 19-38). Adhesions over the ventricle and aneurysm are divided to mobilize the heart. The aneurysm is then incised in its central portion and widely opened, carefully removing any laminated clot. If pericardial adhesions are extensive, the wall of the aneurysm is simply divided a short distance from the pericardial adhesions, leaving this part of the aneurysmal wall in situ and thus avoiding troublesome bleeding. Similarly, the wall of the aneurysm is divided about 2 cm from its junction with left ventricular muscle. When the opening of the aneurysm is sutured, most of the suture line includes the scar at the point of junction, and there is little compromise of the adjacent left ventricular muscle and no reduction in size of the left ventricular cavity (Fig. 19-39).

At New York University the frequency with which the wall of the aneurysm includes the area of the anterior descending coronary artery has been significant, for the scar may extend over into the ventricular septum. Preservation of the anterior descending coronary artery, often occluded proximally, may not be significant in some patients because the ventricular muscle supplied by the anterior descending coronary artery has been previously infarcted, but in other patients significant tributaries arise from this artery, especially to the ventricular septum. For this reason, before the aneurysm is excised, the anterior descending coronary artery is identified to avoid injury during excision of the aneurysm. Later, a bypass graft is attached if the artery is of adequate size. Following excision, the wall of the aneurysm is closed with two or three rows of continuous sutures, placing these through Teflon felt to reinforce the closure. Air is removed subsequently from the heart and the ventricle defibrillated.

This technique avoids several hazards associated with excision of an aneurysm. Extensive bleeding is avoided by cautiously dissecting adhesions without tearing the epicardium. There is no danger of reduction in size of the ventricular cavity or loss of functioning ventricular muscle from incorporation in the suture line to close the aneurysm, and the anterior descending coronary artery is revascularized. With these guidelines and precautions, operative excision has a very low mortality, and convalescence is usually uneventful. If the other coronary vessels, the right and the circumflex, are involved, bypass grafts are also inserted to these vessels.

The impressive advances made in the therapy of complications of myocardial infarction and ventricular aneurysms were well illustrated with a recent patient at New York University. The patient, seventy-seven years of age but previously in good health, sustained a massive myocardial infarction complicated by refractory congestive failure, a large ventricular aneurysm, multiple interventricular septal defects, left ventricular end-diastolic pressure of 30, cardiac index 1.2 liters/minute, and a pulmonary blood flow three times normal. At operation the aneurysm was excised, the ventricular septal defects closed with application of a large patch, and two bypass grafts done. Recovery was strikingly uneventful, and the patient remains in excellent health 4 months later.

PROGNOSIS. Substantial improvement has been reported following excision of large ventricular aneurysms. Actually this is the only cardiac operation in which preoperative congestive failure has been greatly improved by the surgical procedure. Disruption of the suture line with recurrence of the aneurysm has not been reported. In 1964 Cooley et al. reported experiences with 37 patients, with eight hospital deaths and five subsequent deaths. Thirteen patients at that time were living more than 3 years after operation, and substantial improvement had occurred in most of these. Catheterization studies before and after operation in seven patients showed an increase in cardiac output and regression of pulmonary hypertension, confirming the physiologic benefit following excision of large aneurysms.

In the past few years excision of aneurysms has become commonplace. Most patients undergoing excision of a left ventricular aneurysm now often have concomitant bypass grafting; so the benefit from excision of the aneurysm per se cannot be easily determined.

A

B

Fig. 19-38. *A.* Operative photograph of left ventricle, showing advanced destruction of the left ventricle from multiple myocardial infarcts. The heart has been turned upward so that the posterior surface of the left ventricle is exposed. *B.* During cardiopulmonary bypass, when suction was applied to the left ventricle, the ventricle collapsed readily, demonstrating that most of the ventricular muscle had been replaced by scar. The patient did not survive operation, and in retrospect it appears that the condition was probably inoperable because of extensive destruction of left ventricular muscle.

PERICARDITIS

Acute Pyogenic Pericarditis

A purulent infection of the pericardium has been reported for many centuries, and some of the earliest operations in thoracic surgery involved resection of costal cartilages to drain a purulent pericarditis. In recent years, with the widespread availability of antibiotics, purulent pericarditis has become a rare disease, and few institutions have experiences with more than a few cases. In 1961 Boyle and associates reviewed 414 cases reported in the literature and added 11 of their own. At that time their group of 11 patients constituted one of the largest single series ever reported.

Formerly pneumococcal pericarditis was one of the most common types and developed in association with a pneumonic infection in the lungs. Such infections are now infrequent. Staphylococcal infection, by contrast, usually occurs as a complication of generalized septicemia from a septic focus in another area of the body. Less frequent forms of pericarditis include a streptococcal pericarditis, now rarely seen, and infection with such unusual organisms as *Hemophilus influenzae* or *Salmonella*.

An unrecognized, untreated purulent pericarditis usually terminates fatally. The clinical picture is that of an acute septic course, which soon includes signs of a pericardial effusion and may progress to cardiac tamponade. Simply considering the possibility of the disease is probably the main factor in making a correct diagnosis. Once the diagnosis has been considered, needle aspiration of the pericardial cavity can confirm or exclude it. If uncertainty remains, a subxyphoid exploration can easily be done.

Both the rarity and the lethal nature of purulent pericarditis are well illustrated in the report by Rubin et al. of 18 cases, with only six patients surviving. The rarity was clearly indicated by the fact that only 14 patients were seen over a 14-year period. In eight of the patients the pericarditis developed as a complication after thoracic surgery; in others it developed from primary pleural mediastinal or pulmonary foci; in six it was a result of systemic bacteremia, probably the most difficult diagnosis of all. In these patients, resistance to infection was decreased because of other diseases, such as extensive burns or immunosuppressive therapy.

Treatment is with parenteral administration of appropriate antibiotics, combined with serial pericardial aspiration and instillation of antibiotics directly into the peri-

Fig. 19-39. *A.* Photograph of left ventricular aneurysm involving the posterior part of the left ventricle, an unusual location. *B.* The aneurysm has been excised, and the interior of the left ventricle is being inspected. The suction tip is within the ostium of the mitral valve, showing the proximity of the aneurysm to the mitral valve. The unusual occurrence of these aneurysms may be related to the fact that myocardial infarction in this area is often fatal because of concomitant mitral insufficiency. *C.* Completed repair of the aneurysm with a long suture line buttressed with Teflon felt. A coronary bypass graft is visible at the top of the field which was inserted into a branch of the circumflex coronary artery.

cardial cavity. In patients not responding to therapy, surgical drainage may be required, but this has not always been necessary.

Chronic Constrictive Pericarditis

HISTORICAL DATA. The first successful pericardiectomy was performed by Rehn in 1913, although the theoretical basis for the operation had been suggested some years before. Subsequently, the first pericardiectomy in the United States was performed by Churchill in 1929. Initial operations were limited in scope, partly because of differences in philosophy as to what part and how much of the constricted pericardium should be removed. In the 1960s routine performance of a radical pericardiectomy became widely accepted with considerable improvement in results.

ETIOLOGY. In most patients the cause is unknown. Possibly the disease represents the end stages of an undiagnosed viral pericarditis. Tuberculosis was formerly thought to be the most frequent cause, but in recent years it has been responsible for less than 20 percent of cases in most series. The author has personally never seen a proved case. Rarely, a traumatic hemopericardium can evolve to a constrictive pericarditis.

PATHOLOGY AND PATHOPHYSIOLOGY. The pericardial cavity is obliterated by dense scar tissue which encases and constricts the heart. In chronic cases areas of calcification develop in the fibrous tissue, resulting in an additional element of constriction.

The physiologic handicap from pericardial constriction is limitation of diastolic filling of the ventricles. Several sequelae result: Stroke volume is decreased with a resulting decrease in cardiac output, despite a compensatory tachycardia. Right ventricular diastolic pressure increases, with a corresponding increase in right atrial and central venous pressure, ranging from 15 to 40 cm water, the average elevation being 25 to 30 cm water. The venous hypertension produces hepatic enlargement, ascites, peripheral edema, and venous distension, accompanied by a gradual increase in blood volume.

CLINICAL MANIFESTATIONS. Symptoms. The disease is most common in patients in their second or third decade, but patients ranging from two to seventy-eight years have been reported. The youngest patient in our personal series of cases was three years old. The disease is a slowly progressive one with increasing ascites and edema. Fatigability and dyspnea on exertion are common complaints, but dyspnea is rare at rest. Ascites may be unusually severe. The diagnosis is easily confused with cirrhosis.

Physical Findings. Several unusual physical findings are commonly present. There may be striking enlargement of the liver with ascites, often in association with only moderate peripheral edema. Dilatation of peripheral veins is also prominent. Although these findings are the familiar ones of advanced congestive failure from heart disease, with constrictive pericarditis the usual cardiac findings are a heart of normal size without murmurs or abnormal sounds. Atrial fibrillation is present in about one-third of patients, and a pleural effusion in about one-half. The pulse pressure is normally decreased to a variable degree, and a paradoxic pulse, with obliteration of the pulse during deep inspiration, is found in a small percentage of patients.

Laboratory Findings. The venous pressure is regularly elevated to levels between 20 and 40 cm water. The electrocardiogram is not diagnostic but is almost always abnormal, with a low voltage and inversion of T waves. A chest roentgenogram often shows a heart of normal size, but calcification in the pericardium can be seen, often as a linear sheet, in about 50 percent of patients. Fluoroscopy may demonstrate decreased cardiac pulsations.

On cardiac catheterization several characteristic abnormalities are usually detected, although rarely these can also result from diffuse myocardial fibrosis from other causes. There is elevation of the right ventricular diastolic pressure to levels greater than one-third of right ventricular systolic pressure, and a corresponding increase in right atrial pressure. The contour of the right ventricular pressure pulse is characteristically altered, showing an early "dip" in diastole. A similarity of pressures in different cardiac chambers is frequently found, the right atrial pressure, the right ventricular diastolic pressure, the pulmonary artery diastolic pressure, and the pulmonary wedge pressure often being almost identical.

DIAGNOSIS. Once the diagnosis has been suspected from the clinical picture, it can usually be confirmed with findings from the electrocardiogram, chest roentgenogram, and catheterization data. Most diagnostic errors arise from failure to consider constrictive pericarditis, for it is a comparatively rare disease. The most frequent erroneous diagnoses are cirrhosis of the liver and congestive heart failure from other causes.

TREATMENT. Once the diagnosis has been established in a symptomatic patient, pericardiectomy should be performed. The incision may be a sternotomy or a bilateral thoracotomy in the left fifth and right fourth intercostal spaces with oblique division of the sternum. Bilateral thoracotomy provides ready exposure to all areas of the heart, but in recent years we have found sternotomy simpler and adequate. The objective is extensive removal of the constricting pericardium from both ventricles, extending from the right to the left pulmonary veins. Recently the adherent pericardium over the posterior (diaphragmatic) part of the ventricle also has been excised, thus removing the pericardium from the entire surface of both ventricles. Removal of the pericardium from the atria and the venae cavae is physiologically less important, although we remove most of this pericardium as well. Dissection over the thin-walled atria involves some hazard of perforation and hemorrhage and must be done with caution. Particular care is required over the coronary vessels, leaving a small segment of thickened pericardium if it cannot be satisfactorily mobilized from the underlying coronary arteries.

In performing pericardiectomy, where possible the plane of dissection should be external to the epicardium, which greatly decreases operative hemorrhage.

It is helpful to measure intracardiac pressures by direct needle puncture before and following pericardiectomy. With an extensive pericardiectomy, the characteristic pressure changes present before operation are either eliminated or greatly improved.

Following operation many patients improve immediately with a massive diuresis of edema fluid, but others recover more slowly and require careful restriction of sodium intake with appropriate diuretic therapy for several months before recovery. Atrophy of myocardial muscle fibers compressed by scar tissue has been considered a probable cause of the prolonged convalescence. In the past, inadequate removal of the scarred pericardium was undoubtedly the most frequent cause of a poor result. Some groups have used bypass to facilitate pericardiectomy, but to date we have not found this necessary. Copeland et al., reporting experiences in 1975, described the use of bypass to perform pericardiectomy in 11 patients with an excellent short-term result in all.

PROGNOSIS. The risk of operation varies with the age of the patient and the severity of the disease, but it is in the range of 10 to 12 percent. A good result can be anticipated in 80 to 85 percent of patients, although there is considerable discrepancy in the reports in the literature. In a series of 26 patients reported by Effler, 15 of the 26 obtained substantial improvement from operation while there was a total of nine early and late deaths. Schumacker and Roshe, however, have reported a total of 19 patients with 18 good results. In a long-term follow-up of 78 cases reported by Dalton et al., sustained improvement continuing over many years was found in patients initially obtaining a good result. A group of 40 cases has been reported from Vanderbilt University by Collins et al., including patients originally studied by Blalock and Burwell in 1941. Only 53 percent of 32 patients subjected to operation obtained an excellent result, but this series includes the early operations which are now considered inadequate. At New York University an excellent short-term result has been obtained in most patients, but detailed long-term data are not available.

HEART BLOCK AND PACEMAKERS

by Joseph N. Cunningham

HISTORICAL DATA. Surgical therapy of complete heart block with an electric pacemaker has evolved with astonishing rapidity in the past 20 years. In 1951 Callaghan and Bigelow developed a transvenous pacemaker which could be used to stimulate the sinoatrial node, and the following year Zoll first described successful treatment of ventricular standstill by external electrical stimulation of the heart through the intact chest wall. In 1958 Lillehei and associates demonstrated that direct cardiac pacing could be performed with an electrode implanted in the left ventricle, but long-term electrical stimulation with such electrodes traversing the chest wall ultimately resulted in infection. Between 1958 and the present, many investigators contributed to the development of implantable, battery-powered pacemakers, including Chardack, Zoll, Frank, Senning, Kantrowitz, Furman, Escher, and Parsonnet. Glenn has intensively studied radiofrequency stimulation of the heart with a transmitter through the intact chest wall, while Nathan and Center have evaluated pacemakers activated

from impulses arising in the atrium, which are subsequently transmitted to the ventricle. Furman and Schwedel, in 1959, described permanent pacing of the heart with a transvenous catheter wedged into the endocardial surface of the right ventricle. Since 1962 modifications of this technique have made it the procedure of choice, with the catheter implanted under local anesthesia and subsequently connected to an implanted pacemaker in a subcutaneous pocket.

In 1957 the first implantable pacemakers were being used. As of 1972, 120,000 implantations had been made in the United States alone, with a 15-year survival rate for that population of about 75 percent and an average age of approximately 70 years. Since 1972 an astronomical number of implantations have been performed. This appears to be a function not only of increased awareness on the part of the physician but also of new developments in pacemaker hardware, with increased battery longevity and improved electrode design the major factors in the increasing success and popularity of these procedures.

ETIOLOGY. Congenital heart block is extremely rare, less than 200 patients having been reported in the literature. Heart block from surgical trauma during repair of intracardiac defects has decreased in frequency but still remains a serious postoperative complication, usually resulting from direct injury to the bundle of His associated with repair of ventricular septal defects and occasionally with aortic valve replacement in the severely calcified aortic annulus. Heart block following myocardial infarction is usually transitory in surviving patients and requires no permanent pacing. Temporary pacing through a transvenous route is often indicated and can be performed with low morbidity. Infection or tumors have been reported in rare cases to cause heart block.

The most common cause of complete heart block in the elderly patient is degenerative fibrosis of the conduction system (75 to 80 percent of cases). The most common indication for implantation of pacemakers continues to be the occurrence of Stokes-Adams attacks; these have been the indication in 80 to 90 percent of patients requiring pacemakers.

PATHOLOGY AND PATHOPHYSIOLOGY. In normal cardiac conduction the cardiac impulse arises in the sinoatrial node located near the junction of the superior vena cava with the wall of the right atrium. The impulse is propagated through the wall of the right atrium to the atrioventricular (AV) node, lying medial to the ostium of the coronary sinus. From this node it travels along the bundle of His near the annulus of the tricuspid valve to pass through the central fibrous body of the ventricular septum near the junction of the muscular and membranous components. In this area the conduction bundle divides into the right and left bundles, which in turn travel to different areas of the respective ventricles. The most common surgical trauma producing complete heart block occurs during repair of a ventricular septal defect or an ostium primum defect. More rarely it occurs during prosthetic replacement of the aortic valve, mitral valve, or tricuspid valve, as there are areas along the annulus of each of these three valves where the bundle of His can be injured. Surgical injuries of either the right or the left conduction bundle are usually not of clinical significance.

Heart block, of whatever degree, may seriously impair cardiac output by any of a number of mechanisms. With complete heart block the resulting bradycardia, varying from 25 to as high as 60 beats per minute, depending on the idioventricular response, may decrease coronary and cerebral circulation. There may be progressive refractory congestive heart failure even with rates as high as 45, marked intolerance to exercise, and even symptoms of cerebrovascular insufficiency with syncope and convulsions. With complete AV dissociation there may be periods of transient ventricular asystole with cessation of cardiac output, syncope, convulsions, and death. In some patients, rather than standstill, there may be equally disastrous bouts of ventricular tachycardia or ventricular fibrillation, as ventricular "escape" mechanisms result from absence of normal AV conduction. In others there may be only periodic marked accentuation of the bradycardia. With lesser degrees of heart block, although the cardiac rate is usually normal, abrupt transition to complete AV dissociation with any of its complications can occur. Any one episode may be followed by complete recovery with resumption of the preattack rhythm or may result in death.

Attacks of syncope and convulsions due to sudden alterations of cardiac output from heart block have long been designated the *Stokes-Adams syndrome*. Some patients with low cardiac output from severe bradycardia become disabled with progressive cardiac failure but never develop Stokes-Adams syndrome.

It is a curious and as yet unexplained phenomenon that with ventricular standstill from heart block, mechanical or electrical energy delivered to the heart will result in intermittent ventricular contractions. Thus, even rhythmic thumping of the chest wall may result in 1:1 ventricular responses until the ventricles resume their intrinsic rhythmic contractions.

CLINICAL MANIFESTATIONS. Although some patients may be asymptomatic with a rate as low as 30 to 35 beats per minute, most patients have symptoms with a rate less than 45 per minute. Episodic Stokes-Adams attacks are the most frequent disability; between attacks the patient feels entirely well. During such episodes there is the sudden onset of syncope, often followed by convulsions. Examination reveals severe bradycardia or cardiac standstill. Recovery depends on the spontaneous return of cardiac contractions. In milder forms, recurrent syncope for a short period may be the only symptom. Then the differential diagnosis must consider heart block, aortic stenosis, simple syncope, carotid sinus syndrome, epilepsy, and occlusive arterial disease of the cerebral circulation. When complete heart block is present, the diagnosis can be quickly established by the electrocardiogram. When intermittent heart block or the presence of a "sick-sinus syndrome" (tachy-brady arrhythmia) is etiologic in the production of symptomatology, a 24-hour recording by Holter monitor may be necessary to determine the diagnosis. This test is performed by having the patient carry a portable ECG which produces a 24-hour recording of the intrinsic cardiac rhythm. The tape recording of the patient's rhythm can be quickly analyzed with a computer to determine what arrhythmia is present.

With intermittent heart block there may be no definite findings between syncopal attacks. However, certain electrocardiographic findings are suggestive. Trifascicular block, degrees of block less than complete AV dissociation, and the Mobius II type usually signify impending or intermittent AV dissociation. Attempts have been made to induce heart block under controlled conditions to confirm the diagnosis. One method reported by the author involved atrial pacing to rates of 120 or less, which ordinarily does not affect normal conduction.

Some patients become disabled from progressive heart failure simply as a result of inadequate cardiac output, while other patients tolerate rates of 40 to 50 beats per minute with no apparent symptoms. Dramatic improvement, with prompt diuresis of many liters of fluid, may follow insertion of a pacemaker.

TREATMENT. Physiology of Cardiac Pacemakers. The electrical resistance of the normal heart is 300 to 350 ohms, and the fibrillating threshold to electrical stimulation is at least ten times greater. The efficacy of cardiac pacemakers depends on the ability of the heart in ventricular standstill to respond to short bursts (2 milliseconds) of electric current, ideally less than $1\frac{1}{2}$ to 2 milliamperes. This amount of current is effective if delivered directly to the heart, but much larger currents are necessary to pace the ventricle directly through the chest wall, a method of pacing generally not employed at present.

Ventricular pacing may be accomplished by one of two methods, bipolar or unipolar. In the bipolar system both the positive and the negative pole of the electrode are in contact with the endocardium of the heart. In epicardial implantation, two separate electrodes (positive and negative) must be implanted. If unipolar pacing is desired, the tip of the endo- or epicardial electrode acts as the stimulating pole, while the cathode or indifferent pole is usually the ground plate on the generator implanted in the subcutaneous tissue. The choice of unipolar or bipolar pacing modes is purely a personal preference. Most cardiologists feel that use of a bipolar system allows more accurate reading of the patient's intrinsic underlying electrocardiogram, since the stimulus artifact when this system is used is much less than when a unipolar system is employed. Bipolar electrodes can be converted to unipolar systems at any point where indicated by simply capping off the lead which has the highest threshold and connecting the remaining lead to a unipolar generator, which is then implanted in the subcutaneous tissue.

Ventricular stimulation by current generator and electrode systems generally results in ventricular rates of 72 beats per minute. Such rates not only effectively override and suppress spontaneous ventricular activity of hearts in complete AV dissociation with rates of 45 or less but also prevent Stokes-Adams attacks due to complete ventricular standstill. Resultant improvement in cardiac output on the basis of rate increase alone may be as much as 50 to 80 percent. Frequently an impressive improvement in exercise tolerance, with regression of any overt signs of cardiac failure and even with diuresis, occurs. Despite the fixed rates of stimulation, variations in cardiac output are usually effectively achieved by variations in cardiac stroke volume in most patients. In some instances, however, variations in pacemaker rate and amplitude are necessary. The present availability of pacemakers with variable rate and amplitude settings now allows effective control of such syndromes as the tachy-brady arrhythmia type and syndromes characterized by refractory ventricular arrhythmias. In such patients, not only the rate but also the amplitude of the pacemaker generator may be increased to permit chronic "overdriving" of the arrhythmia. In the "sick-sinus syndrome," where the patient's rate often varies from 40 to 120 beats per minute, it is possible to control the bradycardia by use of a pacemaker which has been surgically implanted, while Inderal is given to control the intermittent bouts of tachycardia which these patients experience. An occasional patient with angina who is not a surgical candidate may be extremely sensitive to digitalis or propranolol. Such patients may require instillation of pacemakers with variable rate settings so that rates as low as 60 can be achieved by the pacemaker while the patient receives adequate doses of digitalis and propranolol for heart failure and/or angina.

Variations of the fixed-rate mode of delivery of the stimulus were sought to correct certain problems which became evident during early pacemaker experience. The most significant of these was a markedly decreased fibrillatory threshold to electric currents under certain conditions such as hypokalemia and acute myocardial infarction. In patients who either did not have complete AV dissociation at the time of pacemaker implant or had return of intermittent AV conduction after periods of electrical pacing, the coincidence of the fixed-rate stimulus with the "supernormal phase" of the cardiac cycle could precipitate ventricular fibrillation if the patient sustained an acute myocardial infarct or became hypokalemic. This led to the so-called "demand" pacemaker, which may be of the R-wave-suppressed or R-wave-triggered type. In both, the electrode acts as an element which senses beginning ventricular depolarization. In one, the pacemaker output is suppressed and no artifact appears on the electrocardiogram, while in the other the pacemaker discharge occurs during the refractory period of the heart and the artifact is seen on the electrocardiogram within the QR segment. This seems to have effectively eliminated the problem of pacemaker-induced arrhythmias in postinfarction patients or those with severe electrolyte abnormalities. Suppressing pacemaker discharge does not appear to significantly increase the life expectancy of the pacemaker generator.

Many currently used pacemaker generators are programmed to produce a fixed output and impulse at 72 beats per minute irrespective of ventricular response or activity. The generated impulse is either received or suppressed by the cardiac muscle in relation to the refractory period of the QRS complex. Fixed-rate pacemakers should only be used in patients who have not had documented evidence of competitive rhythms. This should be established by exercise testing, which will often reveal the presence of competitive arrhythmias in patients who had been presumed to have complete heart block. When using fixed-rate units,

efforts should be made to use low-output pacemakers to prolong the life of the generator. Demand pacemakers, on the other hand, are always indicated for patients with intermittent AV dissociation or block and for those who occasionally have competitive intrinsic rhythms of their own.

Asynchrony between atrial and ventricular contractions, which impairs cardiac output and limits the rate imposed by ventricular pacemakers, led to the development by Nathan and associates of the P-wave-activated pacemaker. This pacemaker senses atrial depolarization and delivers a subsequent synchronized stimulus to the ventricle which follows atrial activity in a timely electrical fashion, thereby resulting in optimal cardiac output. This system is more "physiologic." However, it requires more complex circuitry and implantation of electrodes in the atrium as well as the ventricle. Previously such implantation was possible only via thoracotomy. More recently, advances in technology have resulted in production of generator and electrode systems which may be adapted to either transthoracic or pervenous implantation. By either modality, a pair of electrodes (one in the atrium and one in the ventricle) is utilized to sense and stimulate in a synchronous fashion both atrial and ventricular contractions. This clever and extremely physiologic pacemaker system is most indicated in the patient whose cardiac output would otherwise be inadequate without the "atrial kick" prior to ventricular systole, most commonly the patient with severe chronic failure and heart block, or the younger person with heart block who is athletic. In the latter instance, exercise-induced increase in atrial activity is sensed by one electrode and transmitted in a similar fashion to the ventricular electrode. This allows for atrioventricular rates of 100 to 120 beats per minute with exercise.

Selection of Patients for Operation. Medical therapy of symptomatic complete heart block with myocardial stimulants such as isoproterenol has been associated with a high mortality. In one group of 100 patients treated before pacemakers were developed, 30 percent were dead in 6 months and 75 percent within 5 years. Heart block resulting from acute myocardial infarction usually can be treated by temporarily pacing the heart with an electrode catheter introduced through a peripheral vein and advanced into the right ventricle. The block usually disappears as the patient recovers from the infarction, and implantation of a permanent pacemaker is rarely indicated.

Heart block following intracardiac operations is a grave complication, requiring a pacemaker if the block is permanent. Most such problems develop at operation and can be prophylactically treated by leaving a temporary electrode wire in the ventricle before the thoracotomy or sternotomy incision is sutured. Stimulation can be given through the wire for several days, but prolonged use of the unit is inadvisable because of the risk of infection. It was found by Lillehei and associates, reporting experiences with 40 patients with complete heart block in 1963, that heart block lasting more than 1 month after operation is almost always permanent; until 1 month, some hope remains that complete block is temporary and may subside with healing of the intracardiac wound. Low-dose steroids (Dexamethasone 1 mg/hour) may be useful for reduction of edema of the conduction system and improvement in AV conduction during the first 24 hours postoperatively.

In some unfortunate patients complete block may develop several months after a cardiac operation, probably from progressive fibrosis near the conduction bundle. With a cardiac rate less than 50 beats per minute, it is probably wise to implant a permanent pacemaker before the patient leaves the hospital, especially if the block has persisted longer than 1 month after operation. A study of 20 patients discharged without pacemakers found an appalling mortality of 80 percent in subsequent years. Because of the complications of pacemaker use in a small child, some investigators have cautiously managed a few asymptomatic children without pacemaker implantation with better long-term results than those reported earlier by Lillehei and associates. However, ultrasmall units weighing 40 to 100 Gm are now available for implantation into small children. It is imperative to use epicardial electrodes with sufficient length to ensure that growth patterns do not result in need for electrode replacement. While pacemaker implantation in the small infant generally requires a minithoracotomy, the long-term results can be gratifying if sufficient electrode length is left to accommodate the child's growth. This, coupled with use of the previously mentioned small pacemaker generators, makes management of heart block in the infant or young child more promising than it was 5 years ago.

Technique of Endocardiac Catheter Pacing. Fluoroscopic placement of a transvenous endocardial electrode in the anterior wall of the right ventricle is the preferred method of pacemaker implantation at this time. The procedure can be performed with minimal risk (0.5 percent in large series). It is generally done under local anesthesia and, for reasons of sterility, should generally be done in the operating room or cardiac catheterization laboratory under totally aseptic techniques. Most large centers currently employ a C-arm fluoroscopic unit which enables a surgeon to place the electrode in proper position in the operating room or cardiac catheterization laboratory. Numerous reports by Lagergren, Furman, Parsonnet, Escher, and others have described experiences with large numbers of patients who underwent successful transvenous electrode placement with low mortality and morbidity rates.

The operative approach involves a semilunar incision, preferably made on the right side below the clavicle in the deltopectoral groove. A single incision is utilized to expose the right cephalic vein and at the same time fashion a subcutaneous tissue pocket inferiorly to implant the generator. If the cephalic vein is inadequate for electrode advancement, a separate incision can be made in the neck in the area of the external jugular vein to permit introduction of the pacemaker electrode and proper placement in the right anterior ventricular wall under fluoroscopy. Once the electrode is introduced into the right side of the heart through a pervenous route, it is necessary to position the tip of the electrode properly in the anterior and apical portion of the right ventricle. Care must be taken to ensure that the tip of the electrode is properly wedged into the right ventricle and does not move significantly with cardiac pulsations or when the patient coughs or breathes deeply. Diaphragmatic contractions at the rate of 72 per minute, observed under fluoroscopy, should alert the surgeon to the possibility of perforation of the right ventricle. In this case the electrode should be withdrawn and replaced, as perforation generally does not occur. Once the electrode is wedged properly into a motionless area of the right ventricle, thresholds should be checked. With current equipment, thresholds for complete and consistent capture of less than 2 milliamperes should be obtained if electrode positioning and placement are correct. Care should be taken to ensure that the electrode not only paces but also adequately senses the intrinsic rhythm of the ventricle.

Once the electrode is properly placed, it is securely tied to the cephalic vein by suture ligature and then connected to the appropriate generator. The generator, in turn, is implanted in the subcutaneous pocket previously fashioned from the original semilunar incision in the deltopectoral area. It is generally advisable to seal the connections between the electrode and generator with silastic adhesive. Antibiotic lavage of the incisions and the subcutaneous pocket is carried out, and a simple mound closure follows. All patients should be placed on preoperative antibiotics for 12 to 24 hours and kept on antistaphylococcal drugs for at least 2 to 3 days following implantation. A closed, airtight occlusive dressing should be applied to the deltopectoral incision and not removed for 72 hours, since retrograde contamination by bacteria through the skin is a possibility. Many pacemaker-generator pockets collect serous fluid. Despite the appearance of fluid or hemotomas in the area, the cardinal rule is "never aspirate a pacemaker generator pocket." The hazards of introducing bacteria by aspiration of fluid from a pacemaker-generator pocket are obvious, and infection often ensues.

Technique of Direct Myocardial Implantation. In certain instances, endocardial electrode placement is not possible. Patients with pulmonary hypertension, extremely dilated right ventricles and right atria, or tricuspid regurgitation are usually poor candidates for endocardial electrode placement in the right ventricle, for there is a high frequency of electrode displacement in the first few days following operation. Also, a rare patient with endocardial fibrosis will prove to be an unsatisfactory candidate for endocardial pacing. In these instances, direct approach to ventricular pacing by implantation of epicardial electrodes is indicated. Small, coiled platinum-iridium electrodes of a fragile nature, often used in the past, have proved unsatisfactory after lengthy analysis; fracture of the electrode coils resulted at varying lengths of time after implantation. More recently, sutureless myocardial electrodes of the screw-in variety have been perfected (Medtronics), which allow for extremely fast implantation of epicardial electrodes through a minimal surgical approach. Generally, a subxiphoid approach through the "space of Larrey," where the rectus abdominus muscles attach to the underside of the rib cage, is utilized. A transverse or diagonal incision in the left upper quadrant anterior to the left side of the rectus muscle is made just below the left costal arch. The rectus sheath is entered and the muscle retracted. With blunt dissection in a cephalad fashion, the free space anterior to the pericardium can be reached through the insertion of the rectus sheath and muscles on the costal arch. The pericardium can be opened in a T-shaped incision and the inferior wall of the right or left ventricle visualized. The screw-in electrode is mounted on a 12- to 15-inch applicator which allows placement of the electrode in the inferior wall of the ventricular muscle. Generally, three turns of the electrode are necessary to implant the corkscrew apparatus deeply into the ventricular muscle. Placement of the electrode in the left ventricle is preferable, as perforation of the corkscrew apparatus into the right ventricle may result in increased pacemaker thresholds. Three- to five-year follow-up on this type of epicardial electrode implantation would suggest that it is superior to the previously employed small coil electrodes implanted through a thoracotomy incision. There is no evidence of late electrode breakage, and the only negative aspect of such implantation is that late threshold rise after implantation may occur.

Implantation of epicardial electrodes by direct approach should be reserved for patients in whom endocardial electrode placement is inadvisable, as mentioned above. It is also ill-advised to use such an approach in the elderly patient, in whom chronic lung disease or other cardiac problems may exist. Implantation of electrodes by this approach usually requires general anesthesia for a brief period of 15 to 20 minutes and is best employed in the young, healthy patient who cannot tolerate endocardial pacing.

Temporary Cardiac Pacing. After an acute myocardial infarction associated with heart block, temporary cardiac pacing is preferably done by insertion of a transvenous electrode catheter under fluoroscopy through an internal jugular or subclavian vein approach. If transvenous catheter placement cannot be quickly achieved, direct insertion of an electrode via a transthoracic route through the third or fourth left intercostal space into the left ventricle is now routinely carried out. As a last resort, the heart can be stimulated directly through needles implanted subcutaneously over the anterior chest wall; this requires generators which produce considerable milliamperage output for pacing.

Postoperative Care. Following operation, electrocardiograms should be obtained promptly to determine that the pacemaker is functioning properly, and a chest x-ray should be obtained to confirm that the pacemaker electrode is correctly placed in the anterior portion of the right ventricle.

To protect from infection, antibiotics should be started before operation and continued for 3 or 4 days after operation, using the antistaphylococcal antibiotics. Dressings over the generator should be carefully sealed for about 72 hours because of the hazard of infection.

Subsequently, after recovery and discharge from the hospital, the patient should enroll in a pacemaker clinic for long-term follow-up. An alternate approach is for the patient to enroll in a telephonic pacemaker program, now being routinely offered by Intermedics, Medtronics, and others.

Complications of Pacemaker Implantation. Mortality rates for transvenous pacemaker implantation in most institutions are about 0.5 percent and for epicardial implantation between 1 and 2 percent. Morbidity likewise is quite low, ranging from 10 to 30 percent, depending on the series involved. The most common pacemaker complication is early electrode displacement when the transvenous approach is used, generally within the first 24 hours and infrequently at a later time. Electrode perforation may occur after transvenous implantation and often is indicated by diaphragmatic twitching or pacing and, more ominously, by signs of cardiac tamponade. Immediate electrode removal, with preparations if necessary for emergency thoracotomy, is indicated.

Rise in thresholds for endocardial electrodes usually occurs 1 to 2 months after implantation, with subsequent return of thresholds to preoperative levels. Since most generators put out 9 to 10 milliamperes of current, the early rise in threshold appears to be no problem. Late rise in thresholds of epicardial screw-in electrodes has been reported but does not appear to be a serious problem.

Erosion of the pacemaker generator or electrode in a thin person with sparse subcutaneous tissue has occurred, and implantation of the unit below the pectoralis muscle may be indicated in such persons. Infection is an inevitable consequence of erosion, and removal or replacement of the generator and electrode generally follows. Subclavian vein thombosis due to electrode implantation through the pervenous route has been reported and generally is of no consequence. Infectious complications of transvenous pacemaker insertion have been reported in about 5 percent of patients, usually involving the generator pocket. Occasionally bacteremia exists without subsequent evidence of clinical infection. Most cases can be treated effectively with adequate antibiotics. Pericarditis following implantation of epicardial pacemakers is frequent and probably occurs in 10 to 15 percent of the patients in the form of a postcardiotomy syndrome secondary to incision of the pericardium for electrode implantation.

Equipment malfunction continues to be the commonest cause of pacemaker failure. Fortunately, federal regulations (FDA) now require all companies to register their pacemakers, and failures of the generators are reported with regularity. All companies are about equal in terms of their failure or success rate.

Finally, an unusual cause of electrode displacement should be mentioned, the "pacemaker twiddler's syndrome." This occurs when the patient inadvertently turns the pulse generator over and over in its subcutaneous pocket in a manner that dislodges the endocardial or epicardial electrode.

PROGNOSIS. The long-term outlook following pacemaker implantation has progressively improved and now approaches that of patients with cardiac disease without conduction problems. There has been progressive improvement in the durability of pacemaker generators worn with the standard nickel-mercury-cadmium batteries, with a life span approaching 5 to 6 years. Recently lithium-powered units have been developed by most pacemaker companies which are guaranteed to last 6 years and will probably last 8 to 10 years. These units are more expensive, costing approximately $2,000, but are not only longer-lasting but also much smaller than other units, weighing 100 to 200 Gm. An additional significant development, principally at the research level at the present time, is the atomic energy–powered pacemaker, using plutonium 238 or promethium 137, which will last for 20 years or more. The units cost about $10,000 and are under careful federal regulation at present. They are tiny, weighing less than 100 Gm, and are particularly applicable for young patients who may require a generator for decades.

Two other recent developments in this rapidly changing field are also of significance. Programmable pacemakers have been developed which permit the physician to change the rate and amplitude of the pacemaker's generator externally by a radiofrequency beam. Hence the patient may use a rate of 65 to 70 beats per minute while sleeping and increase it to 80 to 90 beats per minute while playing tennis. Rechargeable generators are also now available in which a unit can be recharged once a month by a radiofrequency console, which can be kept at the patient's bedside at home. It is predicted that such rechargeable pacemakers will last for 8 to 10 years.

It is obvious that the entire field has not only developed rapidly but is making progress in several areas and will certainly constitute an important segment of cardiac surgery in the future.

ASSISTED CIRCULATION, AND ARTIFICIAL HEARTS

For certain forms of advanced heart disease, cure seems possible only with cardiac transplantation or the implantation of an artificial heart. This is true in some complex congenital anomalies, but most commonly in advanced coronary artery disease in which more than 40 percent of the left ventricular muscle mass has been destroyed. Significant experimental progress has been made with both forms of treatment, but ultimate solution remains unclear at this time. Both are active fields of laboratory investigation. Subsequent paragraphs briefly describe the status of these areas as of mid-1977.

THEORETIC CONSIDERATIONS. The concept of assisting the failing heart by pumping part or all of the circulation through a heart-lung machine as a parallel circuit is, on first glance, a simple and attractive one. One of the first observations of the possible beneficial effects of assisted circulation was made by Senning, who noted that an injured left ventricle incapable of supporting the circulation after an intracardiac operation might recover if extracorporeal circulation was continued for 30 to 60 minutes. Apparently the injury of the left ventricle was reversible.

Subsequent investigation of this seemingly simple hypothesis encountered many problems. First, attempting to "rest" a contracting left ventricle is a complex undertaking. Unless the left ventricle is decompressed during cardiopulmonary bypass, which requires the insertion of a can-

nula into the left atrium and left ventricle, blood will continue to accumulate in the left ventricle, which in turn will contract as a closed chamber against closed mitral and aortic valves. Left ventricular systolic pressure must then exceed that produced in the aorta by the extracorporeal pump, as a result of which oxygen requirements of the contracting left ventricle remain near those levels existing before the extracorporeal pump was used. Hence, although most of the circulation may be supplied from an extracorporeal pump, a contracting left ventricle intermittently ejecting a small amount of blood may metabolize a large amount of oxygen, and thus not be significantly "rested."

If a peripheral circulatory bypass is employed, as with a venoarterial circuit, the left ventricle can actually be harmed. Blood pumped into a peripheral artery from the extracorporeal pump may increase work requirements of the ventricle as it contracts and attempts to propel blood through the aortic valve, which is being maintained in a closed position by the pressure generated from the "assist" circulatory device. Electronic synchronization of the natural heart and the artificial heart so that the artificial heart infuses blood during diastole is physiologically of greater benefit.

A second hypothesis—that recovery of a failing heart would be aided by "resting" the heart with assisted circulation—has also been difficult to demonstrate. The most encouraging data are from experiments in which an acute, reversible injury has occurred, such as transient anoxia, where extracorporeal circulation for 30 minutes to 1 hour may permit recovery. With an extensive injury, such as a myocardial infarction, how long extracorporeal circulation would be required is unknown. It seems likely that bypass for several days may be necessary, during which time collateral circulation could develop around the acutely occluded coronary artery.

TECHNIQUES OF ASSISTED CIRCULATION. Intraaortic Balloon Pumping. In the past 5 or 6 years the most effective technique for assisted circulation has been intraaortic balloon pumping. A balloon catheter is inserted into a peripheral artery, usually the femoral, and advanced into the thoracic aorta. With electronic synchronization, the balloon is alternately inflated during diastole and deflated during systole. This intermittent inflation is of significant benefit to the peripheral circulation, but careful synchronization is essential. Inflation of the balloon during systole actually may harm the left ventricle as it attempts to open the aortic valve against the pressure generated by the inflating balloon. Early experimental and clinical studies with balloon pumping were reported by several investigators. In the past few years balloon pumping has been widely employed, as morbidity is small and the benefit, though limited, is critical to some patients. It seems to increase cardiac index about 0.5 to 0.7 liters and can be used for several days. We use the balloon pump often in our unit and firmly believe several patients would not have survived without it.

Left Heart Bypass. A decade ago Dennis demonstrated the benefits of assisted circulation with left heart bypass, withdrawing blood from the atrium and infusing it into a peripheral artery. Difficulties with closed chest cannulation of the left atrium, however, have thus far greatly limited application of the procedure. Several years ago the author and associates applied left heart bypass in a small group of patients by direct cannulation of the left atrium through a thoracotomy incision and employing perfusion for periods of 3 to 4 hours, but longer periods of perfusion were impractical because of the necessity for thoracotomy. At New York University, a special transvenous cannula has been developed by Glassman and associates which permits closed-chest cannulation of the left atrium through a modification of the transseptal puncture technique. First a standard transseptal left atrial puncture is done, introducing the needle and catheter through the femoral vein. A guide wire is subsequently introduced, after which the special large bore (28 F) catheter is advanced over the guide wire into the left atrium. With this large catheter bypass flow rates as great as 4 liters/minute have been obtained. This technical advance may increase the applicability of left heart bypass, especially as the circulatory support feasible is far greater than that attainable with intraaortic balloon pumping. At this time, it has had limited clinical application.

Litwak and associates in 1976 reported a new type of left heart bypass, used in patients who could not be weaned from the heart-lung machine at the time of operation. Especially designed silastic cannulae were left in the left atrium and femoral artery and brought through the chest wall, which was then closed. Pumping was done with a roller pump with silastic tubing, infusing enough heparin to keep the activated clotting time near 150 seconds and to prevent clotting in the pump, but not enough to cause serious bleeding. There is significant platelet destruction, however, requiring serial infusion of platelets. In their report they describe using the device in 14 patients, in some for 1 week or longer. Of the 14, nine could be weaned from the device, six left the hospital, and four remained alive at the time of the report, one 22 months after operation. We have unsuccessfully used the technique at New York University in three or four moribund patients and believe that, with some modification to lessen the destruction of platelets, it may have significant possibilities.

Peripheral Bypass. A peripheral bypass may be a venoarterial bypass in which venous blood is withdrawn, oxygenated, and returned into a peripheral artery. As indicated earlier, such perfusion should be synchronized to return blood during diastole. Alternatively, a venovenous bypass can be used, returning the blood from the oxygenator into a peripheral vein. Hill and associates have reported on extensive use of this technique for the treatment of acute pulmonary insufficiency, employing a membrane oxygenator and continuing perfusion for several days. In 1977 Hill and associates were still employing the technique, but to date ultimate survival has been poor, primarily because of lack of reversibility of the primary disease causing the acute respiratory insufficiency.

A number of other techniques have been attempted for assisted circulation, such as counterpulsation or synchronized application of external pressure to the extremities, but none have found widespread clinical use. The main limitation of all techniques is that short periods of assisted circulation seem of little value unless the underlying cardiac injury can be corrected.

ARTIFICIAL HEARTS. The ideal solution of many difficult cardiac problems would be a satisfactory mechanical heart, but this seems to be far on the horizon. The National Heart and Lung Institute for several years coordinated a large interdisciplinary program, studying many of the engineering, physical, chemical, and hematologic problems involved. Results were meager, however, primarily because of lack of basic knowledge that would make an artificial heart feasible at this time. One major obstacle, among many, is the inability to pump blood without the use of heparin. Continuous heparinization results in intractable bleeding, while pumping without heparin results in thromboembolism.

Experiences in an attempt to develop a nuclear-fuel support system were summarized by Norman and Huffman in 1972. Bernhard has precisely studied left ventricular bypass pumps in calves for several years and summarized his experience in 1975. The pump functioned successfully in 20 consecutive calves for at least 2 weeks, with an average flow rate of 5 liters/minute. One calf was maintained for over a year. The technique has subsequently been applied successfully to two or three patients.

Weldon and Cooley, as well as others, have successfully implanted conduits between the left ventricle and the aorta for severe forms of obstruction to left ventricular outflow, usually a hypoplastic aortic annulus. The conduit consists of a Dacron tube with a porcine heterograft. Long-term results are not yet available.

Studies of total replacement of the heart, rather than simple left heart bypass, have continued. Kolff and associates have periodically reported the status of their investigations, obtaining survivals for a few weeks, with death ultimately occurring either from thromboembolism or from infection. Excellent work has been done by Pierce and associates with left heart bypass pumps functioning in calves for several weeks, and significant progress is being made toward total heart replacement.

At present the most realistic immediate goal for artificial hearts is their use for bypassing the left heart for a few days or 1 or 2 weeks until the heart recovers from either operative injury or an acute infarction. If recovery is not possible, such a device would simply postpone inevitable death, so its use would require considerable judgment and caution.

References

Introduction; Clinical Manifestations

Gibbon, J. H., Jr., Sabiston, D. C., Jr., and Spencer, F. C.: "Surgery of the Chest," 2d ed., W. B. Saunders Company, Philadelphia, 1969.

Hurst, J. W., and Logue, R. B.: "The Heart, Arteries, and Veins," 2d ed., McGraw-Hill Book Company, New York, 1970.

Extracorporeal Circulation

Allen, J. G. (ed.): "Extracorporeal Circulation," Charles C Thomas, Publisher, Springfield, Ill., 1958.

Bahnson, H. T., and Spencer, F. C.: Extracorporeal Circulation, in C. D. Benson et al. (eds.), "Pediatric Surgery," vol. I, Year Book Medical Publishers, Inc., Chicago, 1962.

Boyd, A. D., Tremblay, R. E., Spencer, F. C., and Bahnson, H. T.: Estimation of Cardiac Output Soon after Intracardiac Surgery with Cardiopulmonary Bypass, *Ann Surg,* **150:**613, 1959.

Brantigan, C. O., and Grow, J. B.: Cricothyroidotomy: Elective Use in Respiratory Problems Requiring Tracheostomy, *J Thorac Cardiovasc Surg,* **71:**72, 1976.

Clowes, G. H. A., Jr.: Extracorporeal Maintenance of Circulation and Respiration, *Physiol Rev,* **40:**826, 1960.

DeWall, R. A., Warden, H. E., Varco, R. L., and Lillehei, C. W.: The Helix Reservoir Pump-Oxygenator, *Surg Gynecol Obstet,* **104:**699, 1957.

Ellison, L. T., Duke, J. F., III, and Ellison, R. G.: Pulmonary Compliance following Open-Heart Surgery and Its Relationship to Ventilation and Gas Exchange, *Circulation,* **35**(*Suppl 1*):217, 1967.

Gibbon, J. H., Jr.: Application of a Mechanical Heart and Lung Apparatus to Cardiac Surgery, *Minn Med,* **37:**171, 1954.

Jones, R. E., Donald, D. E., Swan, H. J. C., Harshbarger, H. G., Kirklin, J. W., and Wood, E. H.: Apparatus of the Gibbon Type for Mechanical Bypass of the Heart and Lungs: Preliminary Report, *Proc Staff Meetings Mayo Clin,* **30:**105, 1955.

McGoon, D. C., Moffitt, E. A., Theye, R. A., and Kirklin, J. W.: Physiologic Studies during High Flow, Normothermic, Whole Body Perfusion, *J Thorac Cardiovasc Surg,* **39:**275, 1960.

Porter, G. A., Kloster, F. E., Herr, R. H., Starr, A., Griswold, H. E., and Kimsey, J. A.: Renal Complications Associated with Valve Replacement Surgery, *J Thorac Cardiovasc Surg,* **53:**145, 1967.

———, Starr, A., Kimsey, J., and Lenertz, H.: Mannitol Hemodilution-Perfusion: The Kinetics of Mannitol Distribution and Excretion during Cardiopulmonary Bypass, *J Surg Res,* **10:**447, 1967.

Sachdev, N. S., Carter, C. C., Swank, R. L., and Blachly, P. H.: Relationship between Post-Cardiotomy Delirium, Clinical Neurological Changes, and EEG Abnormalities, *J Thorac Cardiovasc Surg,* **54:**557, 1967.

Spencer, F. C., Benson, D. W., Liu, W. C., and Bahnson, H. T.: Use of a Mechanical Respirator in the Management of Respiratory Insufficiency following Trauma or Operation for Cardiac or Pulmonary Disease, *J Thorac Cardiovasc Surg,* **38:**758, 1959.

Cardiac Arrest and Ventricular Fibrillation

Cunningham, J. N., Spencer, F. C., Zeff, R., Williams, C. D., Cukingnam, R., and Mullin, M.: Influence of Primary Closure of Pericardium after Open Heart Surgery on Frequency of Tamponade, Postcardiotomy Syndrome and Pulmonary Complications, *J Thorac Cardiovasc Surg,* **70:**119, 1975.

Joseph, W. L., and Maloney, J. V., Jr.: Extracorporeal Circulation as an Adjunct to Resuscitation of the Heart, *JAMA,* **193:**600, 1965.

Jude, J. R., and Elam, J. O.: "Fundamentals of Cardiopulmonary Resuscitation," F. A. Davis Company, Philadelphia, 1965.

Kouwenhoven, W. B., Jude, J. R., and Knickerbocker, G. G.: Closed Chest Cardiac Massage, *JAMA,* **137:**1064, 1960.

———, Milnor, W. R., Knickerbocker, G. G., and Chestnut,

W. R.: Closed Chest Defibrillation of the Heart, *Surgery,* **42:**550, 1957.

Spencer, F. C., and Bahnson, H. T.: Treatment of Cardiac Arrest, in C. D. Benson et al. (eds.), "Pediatric Surgery," vol. I, p. 522, Year Book Medical Publishers, Inc., Chicago, 1962.

Williams, G. R., and Spencer, F. C.: The Clinical Use of Hypothermia following Cardiac Arrest, *Ann Surg,* **148:**462, 1958.

Zimmerman, J. M., and Spencer, F. C.: The Influence of Hypothermia on Cerebral Injury Resulting from Circulatory Occlusion, *Surg Forum,* **9:**216, 1958.

Mitral Stenosis

Bailey, C. P.: The Surgical Treatment of Mitral Stenosis (Mitral Commissurotomy), *Dis Chest,* **15:**377, 1949.

Bryant, L. R., and Trinkle, J. K.: Mitral Valvotomy in the Valve Replacement Era, *Ann Surg,* **173:**1024, 1971.

Cutler, E. C., and Levine, S. A.: Cardiotomy and Valvulotomy for Mitral Stenosis, *N Engl J Med,* **188:**1023, 1923.

Ellis, L. B., Harken, D. E., and Black, H.: A Clinical Study of 1000 Consecutive Cases of Mitral Stenosis Two to Nine Years after Mitral Valvuloplasty, *Circulation,* **19:**803, 1959.

Gerbode, F.: Transventricular Mitral Valvulotomy, *Circulation,* **21:**563, 1960.

Higgs, L. M., Glancy, D. L., O'Brien, K. P., Epstein, S. E., and Morrow, A. G.: Mitral Restenosis: An Uncommon Cause of Recurrent Symptoms following Mitral Commissurotomy, *Am J Cardiol,* **26:**34, 1970.

Kiser, I. O., Hoeksema, T. D., Connolly, D. C., and Ellis, F. H., Jr.: Long-Term Results of Closed Mitral Commissurotomy, *J Cardiovasc Surg,* **8:**263, 1967.

Logan, A., and Turner, R.: Surgical Treatment of Mitral Stenosis with Particular Reference to the Transventricular Approach with a Mechanical Dilator, *Lancet,* **2:**874, 1959.

Mullin, M. J., Engelman, R. M., Isom, O. W., Boyd, A. D., Glassman, E., and Spencer, F. C.: Experience with Open Mitral Commissurotomy in 100 Consecutive Patients, *Surgery,* **76:**974, 1974.

Nathaniels, E. K., Moncure, A. C., and Scannell, J. G.: A Fifteen-Year Follow-up Study of Closed Mitral Valvuloplasty, *Ann Thorac Surg,* **10:**27, 1970.

Nichols, H. T., Blanco, G., Morse, D. P., Adam, A., and Baltazar, N.: Open Mitral Commissurotomy: Experience with 200 Consecutive Cases, *JAMA,* **182:**268, 1962.

Olinger, G. N., Rio, F. W., and Maloney, J. V., Jr.: Closed Valvulotomy for Calcific Mitral Stenosis, *J Thorac Cardiovasc Surg,* **62:**357, 1971.

Roe, B. B., Edmunds, L. H., Jr., Fishman, N. H., and Hutchinson, J. C.: Open Mitral Valvulotomy, *Ann Thorac Surg,* **12:**483, 1971.

Selzer, A., and Cohn, K. E.: Natural History of Mitral Stenosis: A Review, *Circulation,* **45:**878, 1972.

Souttar, P. W.: The Surgical Treatment of Mitral Stenosis, *Br Med J,* **2:**603, 1925.

Spencer, F. C., Cortes, L., Marcarenhas, G., Ifuku, M., and Hoopke, J.: The Mechanism of Thrombus Formation upon the Starr Edwards Prosthetic Mitral Valve, *Ann Surg,* **165:**814, 1967.

Starr, A.: Mitral Valve Replacement with Ball Valve Prostheses, *J Thorac Cardiovasc Surg,* **64:**354, 1972.

——— and Edwards, M. L.: Mitral Replacement: Clinical Experience with a Ball Valve Prosthesis, *Ann Surg,* **154:**726, 1961.

————, Herr, R. H., and Wood, J. A.: Mitral Replacement: Review of Six Years' Experience, *J Thorac Cardiovasc Surg,* **54:**333, 1967.

Mitral Insufficiency

Anderson, A. M., Cobb, L. A., Bruce, R. A., and Merendino, K. A.: Evaluation of Mitral Annuloplasty for Mitral Regurgitation: Clinical and Hemodynamic Status Four to 41 Months after Surgery, *Circulation,* **26:**26, 1962.

Barnhorst, D. A., Oxman, H. A., Connolly, D. C., Pluth, J. R., Danielson, G. K., Wallace, R. B., and McGoon, D. W.: Long-term Follow-up of Isolated Replacement of Aortic or Mitral Valve with the Starr-Edwards Prosthesis, *Am J Cardiol,* **35:**228, 1975.

Bjork, V. O., Book, K., And Holmgren, A.: The Bjork-Shiley Mitral Valve Prosthesis, *Ann Thorac Surg,* **18:**379, 1974.

Bonchek, L. I., Anderson, K. P., and Starr, A.: Mitral Valve Replacement with Cloth-Covered Composite-Seat Prostheses, *J Thorac Cardiovasc Surg,* **67:**93, 1974.

Braunwald, N. S., and Bonchek, L. I.: Prevention of Thrombus Formation on Rigid Prosthetic Heart Valves by the Ingrowth of Autogenous Tissue, *J Thorac Cardiovasc Surg,* **54:**630, 1967.

Isom, O. W., Williams, C. D., Falk, E. A., Glassman, E., and Spencer, F. C.: Long-Term Evaluation of Cloth-covered Metallic Ball Prostheses, *J Thorac Cardiovasc Surg,* **64:**354, 1972.

————, Spencer, F. C., Glassman, E., Teiko, P., Boyd, A. D., Cunningham, J. N., and Reed, G. E.: Long-Term Results in 1375 Patients Undergoing Valve Replacement with the Starr-Edwards Cloth-Covered Steel Ball Valve Prosthesis, *Ann Surg,* **186:**310, 1977.

Kay, J. H., and Egerton, W. S.: The Repair of Mitral Insufficiency Associated with Ruptured Chordae Tendineae, *Ann Surg,* **157:**351, 1963.

McGoon, D. C.: Repair of Mitral Insufficiency Due to Ruptured Chordae Tendineae, *J Thorac Cardiovasc Surg,* **39:**357, 1960.

Pakrashi, B. C., Mary, D. A., Elmufti, M. E., Wooler, G. H., and Ionescu, M. I.: Clinical and Hemodynamic Results of Mitral Annuloplasty, *Br Heart J,* **36:**768, 1974.

Reed, G. E.: Repair of Mitral Regurgitation, *Am J Cardiol,* **31:**494, 1973.

————, Tice, D. A., and Clauss, R. H.: Asymmetric Exaggerated Mitral Annuloplasty: Repair of Mitral Insufficiency with Hemodynamic Predictability, *J Thorac Cardiovasc Surg,* **49:**752, 1965.

Starr, A.: Mitral Valve Replacement with Ball Valve Prostheses, *Br Heart J Suppl,* **33:**47, 1971.

———— and Edwards, M. L.: Mitral Replacement: Clinical Experience with a Ball Valve Prosthesis, *Ann Surg,* **154:**726, 1961.

Stinson, E. B., Griepp, R. B., and Shumway, N. E.: Clinical Experience with a Porcine Aortic Valve Xenograft for Mitral Valve Replacement, *Ann Thorac Surg,* (In press.)

Zerbini, E. J.: Results of Replacement of Cardiac Valves by Homologous Dura Mater Valves, *Chest,* **67:**706, 1975.

Aortic Stenosis

Angell, W. W., Shumway, N. E., and Kosek, J. C.: A Five Year Study of Viable Aortic Valve Homografts, *J Thorac Cardiovasc Surg,* **64:**329, 1972.

Bahnson, H. T., Spencer, F. C., Busse, E. F. G., and Davis, F. W., Jr.: Cusp Replacement and Coronary Artery Perfusion in Open Operations on the Aortic Valve, *Ann Surg,* **152:**494, 1960.

Barnhorst, D. A., Oxman, H. A., Connolly, D. C., Pluth, J. R., Danielson, G. K., Wallace, R. B., and McGoon, D. W.: Long-Term Follow-up of Isolated Replacement of Aortic or Mitral Valve with the Starr-Edwards Prosthesis, *Am J Cardiol,* **35:**228, 1975.

Isom, O. W., Spencer, F. C., Glassman, E., Teiko, P., Boyd, A. D., Cunningham, J. N., and Reed, G. E.: Long-Term Results in 1375 Patients Undergoing Valve Replacement with the Starr-Edwards Cloth-Covered Steel Ball Valve Prosthesis, *Ann Surg,* **186:**310, 1977.

Magovern, G. J., Kent, E. J., Cromie, H. W., Cushing, W. B., and Scott, S.: Sutureless Aortic and Mitral Prosthetic Valves: Clinical Results and Operative Technique on 60 Patients, *J Thorac Cardiovasc Surg,* **48:**346, 1964.

McGoon, D. C., Ellis, F. H., and Kirklin, J. W.: Late Results of Operations for Acquired Aortic Valvular Disease, *Circulation,* **31:**108, 1965.

————, Pestana, C., and Moffitt, E. A.: Decreased Risk of Aortic Valve Surgery, *Arch Surg,* **91:**779, 1965.

Pacifico, A. D., Karp, R. B., and Kirklin, J. W.: Homografts for Replacement of the Aortic Valve, *Circulation,* **45:**I-36, 1972.

Senning, A.: Fascia Lata Replacement of Aortic Valves, *J Thorac Cardiovasc Surg,* **54:**465, 1967.

Starr, A., Edwards, M. L., McCord, C. W., and Griswold, H. E.: Aortic Replacement: Clinical Experience with a Semi-rigid Ball-Valve Prosthesis, *Circulation,* **27:**779, 1963.

————, Bonchek, L. I., Anderson, R. P., Wood, J. A., and Chapman, R. D.: Late Complications of Aortic Valve Replacement with Cloth-Covered, Composite-Seat Prostheses, *Ann Thorac Surg,* **19:**289, 1975.

Stinson, E. B., Griepp, R. B., Oyer, P. E., and Shumway, N. E.: Long-Term Experience with Porcine Aortic Valve Xenografts, *J Thorac Cardiovasc Surg,* **73:**54, 1977.

Zerbini, E. J.: Results of Replacement of Cardiac Valves by Homologous Dura Mater Valves, *Chest,* **67:**706, 1975.

Tricuspid Stenosis and Insufficiency

Arbulu, A., Thoms, N. W., and Wilson, R. F.: Valvulectomy without Prosthetic Replacement: A Lifesaving Operation for Tricuspid *Pseudomonas* Endocarditis, *J Thorac Cardiovasc Surg,* **64:**103, 1972.

Boyd, A. D., Engelman, R. H., Isom, O. W., Reed, G. E., and Spencer, F. C.: Tricuspid Annuloplasty, *J Thorac Cardiovasc Surg,* **68:**344, 1974.

Breyer, R. H., McClenathan, J. H., Michaelis, L. L., McIntosh, C. L., and Morrow, A. G.: Tricuspid Regurgitation, *J Thorac Cardiovasc Surg,* **72:**867, 1976.

Grondin, P., Lepage, G., Castonguay, Y., and Meere, C.: The Tricuspid Valve: A Surgical Challenge, *J Thorac Cardiovasc Surg* **53:**7, 1967.

————, Meere, C., Limet, R., Lopez-Bescos, L., Delcan, J. L., and Rivera, R.: Carpentier's Annulus and DeVega's Annuloplasty: End of the Tricuspid Challenge, *J Thorac Cardiovasc Surg,* **70:**852, 1975.

Isom, O. W., Spencer, F. C., Glassman, E., Teiko, P., Boyd, A. D.,

Cunningham, J. N., and Reed, G. E.: Long-Term Results in 1375 Patients Undergoing Valve Replacement with the Starr-Edwards Cloth-Covered Steel Ball Valve Prosthesis, *Ann Surg,* **186:**310, 1977.

Kay, J. H., Maselli-Campagna, G., and Tsuji, H. K.: Surgical Treatment of Tricuspid Insufficiency, *Ann Surg,* **162:**53, 1965.

Spencer, F., C., Shabetai, R., and Adolph, R.: Successful Replacement of the Tricuspid Valve 10 Years after Traumatic Incompetence, *Am J Cardiol,* **18:**916, 1966.

Starr, A., Herr, R., and Wood, J.: Tricuspid Replacement for Acquired Valve Disease, *Surg Gynecol Obstet,* **122:**1295, 1966.

Multivalvular Heart Disease

Bonchek, L. I., and Starr, A.: Ball Valve Prostheses: Current Appraisal of Late Results, *Am J Cardiol,* **35:**843, 1975.

Starr, A., McCord, C. W., Wood, J., Herr, R., and Edwards, M. L.: Surgery for Multiple Valve Disease, *Ann Surg.* **160:**596, 1964.

Cardiac Trauma

Asfaw, I., Thoms, N. W., and Arbulu, A.: Interventricular Septal Defects from Penetrating Injuries of the Heart, *J Thorac Cardiovasc Surg,* **69:**450, 1975.

Bahnson, H. T., and Spencer, F. C.: Pericardial Aspiration and the Treatment of Acute Cardiac Tamponade from Penetrating Wounds in the Heart, in J. H. Mulholland, E. H. Ellison, and S. R. Freisen (eds.), "Current Surgical Management," W. B. Saunders Company, Philadelphia, 1957.

Beall, A. C., Jr., Gasior, R. M., and Bricker, D. L.: Gunshot Wounds of the Heart: Changing Patterns of Surgical Management, *Ann Thorac Surg,* **11:**523, 1971.

——, Ochsner, J. L., Morris, G. C., Jr., Cooley, D. A., and DeBakey, M. E.: Penetrating Wounds to the Heart, *J Trauma,* **1:**195, 1961.

Berger, R. L., Loveless, G., and Warner, O.: Delayed and Latent Postcardiotomy Tamponade: Recognition and Nonoperative Treatment, *Ann Thorac Surg,* **12:**22, 1971.

Blalock, A., and Ravitch, M. M.: A Consideration of the Nonoperative Treatment of Cardiac Tamponade Resulting from Wounds to the Heart, *Surgery,* **14:**157, 1943.

Bland, E. F., and Beebe, G. W.: Missiles in the Heart: A 20-Year Follow-up Report of World War II Cases, *N Engl J Med,* **274:**1039, 1966.

Boyd, T. F., and Strieder, J. W.: Immediate Surgery for Traumatic Heart Disease, *J Thorac Cardiovasc Surg,* **50:**305, 1965.

Harken, D. E.: Foreign Bodies in and in Relation to the Heart and Thoracic Vessels, *Surg Gynecol Obstet,* **83:**117, 1946.

Holdeger, W. F., Lyons, C., and Edwards, W. S.: Indications for Removal of Intracardiac Foreign Bodies, *Ann Surg,* **163:**249, 1966.

Isaacs, J. P.: Sixty Penetrating Wounds to the Heart: Clinical and Experimental Observations, *Surgery,* **45:**696, 1959.

Spencer, F. C.: Treatment of Chest Injuries, *Curr Probl Surg,* January, 1964

—— and Kennedy, J. H.: War Wounds of the Heart, *J Thorac Cardiovasc Surg,* **33:**361, 1957.

Sugg, W. L., Ecker, R. R., Webb, W. R., Rose, E. F., and Shaw, R. R.: Penetrating Wounds of the Heart: An Analysis of 459 Cases, *J Thorac Cardiovasc Surg,* **56:**531, 1968.

Symbas, P. N., Harlaftis, N., and Waldo, W. J.: Penetrating Cardiac Wounds: A Comparison of Different Therapeutic Methods, *Ann Surg,* **183:**377, 1976.

Tabatznik, B., and Isaacs, J. P.: Post-Pericardiotomy Syndrome following Traumatic Hemopericardium, *Am J Cardiol,* **7:**83, 1961.

Cardiac Tumors

Bahnson, H. T., Spencer, F. C., and Andrus, E. C.: Diagnosis and Treatment of Intracavitary Myxomas of the Heart, *Ann Surg,* **145:**915, 1957.

Crafoord, C.: Case Report, *Int Symp Cardiovasc Surg Henry Ford Hosp,* p. 202, 1955.

Dang, C. R., and Hurley, E. J.: Contralateral Recurrent Myxoma of the Heart, *Ann Thorac Surg,* **21:**59, 1976.

Gassman, H. S., Meadows, R., and Baker, L. A.: Metastatic Tumors of the Heart, *Am J Med,* **19:**357, 1955.

Geha, A. S., Weidman, W. H., Soule, E. H., and McGoon, D. C.: Intramural Ventricular Cardiac Fibroma: Successful Removal in Two Cases and Review of the Literature, *Circulation,* **36:**427, 1967.

Gerbode, F., Keith, J. W., and Hill, J. D.: Surgical Management of Tumors of the Heart, *Surgery,* **61:**94, 1967.

Hanfling, S.: Metastatic Cancer to the Heart, *Circulation,* **22:**474, 1960.

Mahaim, I.: "Les Tumors et les polypes du coeur: Étude anatomo-clinique," Masson et Cie, Paris, 1945.

Prichard, R. W.: Tumors of the Heart, *Arch Pathol,* **21:**98, 1951.

Scannell, J. G., and Grillo, H. E.: Primary Tumors of the Heart, *J Thorac Cardiovasc Surg,* **35:**23, 1958.

Spencer, F. C.: The Heart, in T. F. Nealon (ed.), "Management of the Patient with Cancer," p. 537, W. B. Saunders Company, Philadelphia, 1965.

Steinberg, I., Dotter, C. T., and Glenn, F.: Myxoma of the Heart: Roentgen Diagnosis during Life in Three Cases, *Dis Chest,* **24:**509, 1953.

Symbas, P. N., Hatcher, C. R., Jr., and Gravanis, M. B.: Myxoma of the Heart: Clinical and Experimental Observations, *Ann Surg,* **183:**470, 1976.

Thomas, K. E., Winchell, C. P., and Varco, R. L.: Diagnostic and Surgical Aspects of Left Atrial Tumors, *J Thorac Cardiovasc Surg,* **53:**535, 1967.

Whorton, C. M.: Primary Malignant Tumors of the Heart, *Cancer,* **2:**245, 1949.

Yater, W. M.: Tumors of the Heart and Pericardium, *Arch Intern Med,* **48:**627, 1931.

Coronary Artery Disease

Berg, R., Kendall, R. W., Duvoisin, G. E., Ganji, J. H., Rudy, L. W., and Everhart, F. J.: Acute Myocardial Infarction: Surgical Emergency, *J Thorac Cardiovasc Surg,* **70:**432, 1975.

Buchwald, H., and Varco, R. L.: A Bypass Operation for Obese Hyperlipedemic Patients, *Surgery,* **70:**62, 1971.

Cheanvechai, C., Groves, L. K., Reyes, L. A., Sility, E. K., and Soner, E. M., Jr.: Manual Coronary Endarterectomy Clinical Experience in 315 Patients, *J Thorac Cardiovasc Surg,* **70:**524, 1975.

Dilley, R. B., Cannon, J. A., Kattus, A. A., MacAlpin, R. N., and Longmire, W. P.: The Treatment of Coronary Occlusive Disease by Endarterectomy, *J Thorac Cardiovasc Surg,* **50**:511, 1965.

Favaloro, R., Effler, D. B., Groves, L. K., Sones, F. M., Jr., and Fergusson, B. J. G.: Myocardial Revascularization by Internal Mammary Artery Implant Procedures, *J Thorac Cardiovasc Surg,* **54**:359, 1967.

Green, G. E., Stertzer, S. H., and Reppert, E. H.: Coronary Arterial Bypass Grafts, *Ann Thorac Surg,* **5**:443, 1968.

Grondin, C. M., Lesperance, J., Bourassa, M. G., and Campeau, L.: Coronary Artery Grafting with the Saphenous Vein or Internal Mammary Artery, *Ann Thorac Surg,* **20**:605, 1975.

Isom, O. W., Spencer, F. C., Glassman, E., Cunningham, J. N., Teiko, P., Reed, G. E., and Boyd, A. D.: Does Coronary Bypass Increase Longevity? *J Thorac Cardiovasc Surg,* **75**(1):28, 1978.

————, ————, Dembrow, J. M., and Pasternack, B. S.: Long-Term Survival Following Coronary Bypass Surgery in Patients with Significant Impairment of Left Ventricular Function, *Circulation,* **51–52**(*Suppl 1*):141, 1975.

Jones, J. W., Ochsner, J. L., Mills, N. L., and Hughes, L.: Impact of Multiple Variables on Operative and Extended Survival Following Coronary Artery Surgery, *Surgery,* **83**(1):20, 1978.

Kouchoukos, N. T., and Kirklin, J. W.: Coronary Bypass Operations for Ischemic Heart Disease, *Mod Concepts Cardiovasc Dis,* **41**:47, 1972.

McNeer, J. F., Starmer, C. F., Bartel, A. G., Behar, V. S., Kong, Y., Peter, R. H., and Rosati, R. A.: The Nature of Treatment Selection in Coronary Artery Disease, *Circulation,* **49**:606, 1974.

Mills, N. L., and Ochsner, J. L.: Coronary Artery Bypass Surgery: 322 Consecutive Patients with No Hospital Mortality, *J La State Med Soc,* **128**:1, 1976.

Mundth, E. D., and Austen, W. G.: Surgical Measures for Coronary Heart Disease: Part I, *N Engl J Med,* **293**:13, 1975.

————, and Austen, W. G.: Surgical Measures for Coronary Heart Disease: Part II, *N Engl J Med,* **293**:75, 1975.

————, and Austen, W. G.: Surgical Measures for Coronary Heart Disease: Part III, *N Engl J Med,* **293**:124, 1975.

Oglietti, J., Angelini, P., Leachman, R. D., and Cooley, D. A.: Myocardial Revascularization, *J Thorac Cardiovasc Surg,* **71**:736, 1976.

Olinger, G. N., Po, J., Maloney, J. V., Jr., Mulder, D. G., and Buckberg, G. D.: Coronary Revascularization in "High-" versus "Low-Risk" Patients: Role of Myocardial Protection, *Ann Surg,* **182**:293, 1975.

Reul, G. J., Cooley, D. A., Sandiford, F. M., Kyger, E. R., III, Wukasch, D. C., and Hallman, G. L.: Aortocoronary Artery Bypass, *Arch Surg,* **111**:414, 1976.

Schimert, G., Vidne, B. A. and Lee, A. B., Jr.: Free Internal Mammary Artery Graft: Improved Surgical Technic, *Ann Thorac Surg,* **19**:474, 1975.

Slater, S. D., Sallam, A., Bain, W. H., Turner, M. A., and Lawrie, T. D. V.: Hemolysis with Bjork-Shiley and Starr-Edwards Prosthetic Heart Valves: Comparative Study, *Thorax,* **29**:624, 1974.

Spencer, F. C.: Bypass Grafting for Preinfarction Angina, *Circulation,* **40**:274, 1972.

————: Surgical Procedures for Coronary Atherosclerosis, *Prog Cardiovasc Dis,* **14**:399, 1972.

————, Green, G. E., Tice, D. A., and Glassman, E.: Surgical Therapy for Coronary Artery Disease, *Curr Probl Surg,* September, 1970.

————, ————, ————, Wallsh, E., Mills, N. L., and Glassman, E.: Coronary Artery Bypass Grafts for Congestive Heart Failure, *J Thorac Cardiovasc Surg,* **62**:529, 1971.

————, Isom, O. W., Glassman, E., Boyd, A. D., et al.: The Long-Term Influence of Coronary Bypass Grafts on Myocardial Infarction and Survival, *Ann Surg,* **180**:439, 1974.

Stiles, Q. R., Lindesmith, G. G., Tucker, B. L., Hughes, R. K., and Meyer, B. W.: Long-Term Follow-Up of Patients with Coronary Bypass Grafts, *Circulation,* **54**(*Suppl 3*):32, 1976.

Tecklenberg, P. L., Alderman, E. L., Miller, D. C., Shumway, N. E., and Harrison, D. C.: Changes in Survival and Symptom Relief in a Longitudinal Study of Patients after Bypass Surgery, *Circulation,* **51–52**(*Suppl. 1*):98, 1975.

Vineberg, A. M.: Technical Considerations for the Combined Operation of Left Internal Mammary Artery or Right and Left Internal Mammary Implantations with Epicardiectomy and Free Omental Graft, *J Thorac Cardiovasc Surg,* **53**:837, 1967.

Ventricular Aneurysm

Abrams, D. L., Edelist, A., Leuria, M. H., and Miller, A. J.: Ventricular Aneurysm: A Re-appraisal Based on a Study of 65 Consecutive Autopsy Cases, *Circulation,* **27**:164, 1963.

Cooley, D. A., Hallman, G. L., and Henly, W. S.: Left Ventricular Aneurysm Due to Myocardial Infarction: Experience with 37 Patients, *Arch Surg,* **88**:114, 1964.

Effler, D. B., Groves, L. K., and Favaloro, R.: Surgical Repair of Ventricular Aneurysm, *Dis Chest,* **48**:37, 1965.

Schlichter, J., Hellerstein, H. K., and Katz, L. N.: Aneurysm of the Heart: A Correlative Study of 102 Proved Cases, *Medicine,* **33**:43, 1954.

Pericarditis

Berger, R. L., Loveless, G., and Warner, O.: Delayed and Latent Postcardiotomy Tamponade: Recognition and Nonoperative Treatment, *Ann Thorac Surg,* **12**:22, 1971.

Boyle, J. D., Pearce, M. L., and Guze, L. B.: Purulent Pericarditis: Review of Literature and Report of 11 Cases, *Medicine,* **40**:119, 1961.

Collins, H. A., Woods, L. P., and Daniel, R. A.: Late Results of Pericardectomy, *Arch Surg,* **89**:921, 1964.

Copeland, J. G., Stinson, E. B., Griepp, R. B., and Shumway, N. E.: Surgical Treatment of Chronic Constrictive Pericarditis Using Cardiopulmonary Bypass, *J Thorac Cardiovasc Surg,* **69**:236, 1975.

Dalton, J. C., Pearson, R. J., and White, P. D.: Constrictive Pericarditis: A Review and Long-Term Follow-up of 78 Cases, *Ann Intern Med,* **45**:445, 1956.

Effler, D. B.: Chronic Constrictive Pericarditis Treated with Pericardectomy, *Am J Cardiol,* **7**:62, 1961.

Holman, E.: The Pericardium, in J. H. Gibbon (ed.), "Surgery of the Chest," chap. 24, 1st ed., W. B. Saunders Company, Philadelphia, 1962.

Rubin, R. H., and Moellering, R. C., Jr.: Clinical Microbiologic and Therapeutic Aspects of Purulent Pericarditis, *Am J Med,* **59**:68, 1975.

Heart Block and Pacemakers

Chardack, W. M., Gage, A. A., Federico, A. J., Schimert, G., and Greatbatch, W.: The Long-Term Treatment of Heart Block, *Prog Cardiovasc Dis,* **9:**105, 1966.

Corman, L. C., and Levison, M. E.: Sustained Bacteremia in Transvenous Cardiac Pacemakers, *JAMA,* **233:**264, 1975.

Furman, S., Escher, D. J., Solomon, S., and Schwedel, J. B.: Implanted Transvenous Pacemakers: Equipment, Technic and Clinical Experience, *Ann Surg,* **164:**465, 1966.

Glenn, W. W. L.: Cardiac Pacemakers and Heart Block, in J. H. Gibbon (ed.), "Surgery of the Chest," 1st ed., W. B. Saunders Company, Philadelphia, 1962.

Imparato, A. M. and Kim., G. E.: Electrode Complications in Patients with Permanent Cardiac Pacemakers, *Arch Surg,* **105:**705, 1972.

———, Reppert, E., and Spencer, F. S.: Rapid Atrial Pacing to Produce Heart Block, *Surgery,* **63(1):**198, 1968.

Johnson, R. A., Hutter, A. M., Desanctis, R. W., Yurchak, P. M., Leinbach, R. C., and Hartone, J. W.: Chronic Overdrive Pacing and Control of Refractory Ventricular Arrhythmias, *Ann Intern Med,* **80:**380, 1974.

Lagergren, H., et al.: Three-hundred-five Cases of Permanent Intravenous Pacemaker Treatment for Adams-Stokes Syndrome, *Surgery,* **59:**494, 1966.

Lillehei, C. W., Sellers, R. D., Bonnabeau, R. C. and Eliot, R. S.: Chronic Postsurgical Complete Heart Block: With Particular Reference to Prognosis, Management, and a New P-wave Pacemaker, *J Thorac Cardiovasc Surg,* **46:**436, 1963.

Nathan, D. A., Center, S., Wu, C., and Keller, W.: An Implantable Synchronous Pacemaker for the Long Term Correction of Complete Heart Block, *Am J Cardiol,* **11:**362, 1963.

Parsonnet, J.: Power Sources for Implantable Cardiac Pacemakers, *Chest,* **61:**165, 1972.

Parsonnet, V., Feldman, S., Parsonnet, J., and Rothfeld, E.: Arrhythmias Induced by Exercise in Paced Patients, *Am Heart J,* **86:**76, 1974.

———, Furman, S., and Smyth, N.: Implantable Cardiac Pacemakers: Status Report and Resource Guideline, *Circulation,* **50:**A21, 1974.

Sowton, E., Hendrix, G., and Row, P.: Treatment with Implantable Cardiac Pacemakers, *Br Med J,* **3:**155, 1974.

Zoll, P. M.: Historical Development of Cardiac Pacemakers, *Prog Cardiovasc Dis,* **14:**421, 1972.

———, Frank, H. A., and Linenthal, A. J.: Four Year Experience with an Implanted Cardiac Pacemaker, *Ann Surg,* **160:**351, 1964.

Assisted Circulation and Artificial Hearts

Bergman, D., and Goetz, R. H.: Clinical Experience with a New Cardiac Assist Device: The Dual-Chambered Intra-aortic Balloon Assist, *J Thorac Cardiovasc Surg,* **62:**577, 1971.

Bernhard, W. F., Poirier, V., LaFarge, C. C., et al.: A New Method for Temporary Left Ventricle Bypass: Preclinical Appraisal, *J Thorac Cardiovasc Surg,* **70:**880, 1975.

———, Griepp, R. B., Stinson, E. B., and Shumway, N. E.: Clinical Transplantation of the Heart, *Ann Surg,* **176:**503, 1972.

Dembitsky, W. P., and Weldon, C. S.: Clinical Experience with the Use of a Valve-Bearing Conduit To Construct a Second Left Ventricular Outflow Tract in Cases of Unresectable Intraventricular Obstruction, *Ann Surg,* **184:**317, 1976.

Glassman, E., Engelman, R. M., Boyd, A. D., Lipson, D., Ackerman, B., and Spencer, F. C.: Method of Closed-Chest Cannulation of Left Atrium for Left Atrial-Femoral Artery Bypass, *J Thorac Cardiovasc Surg,* **69:**283, 1975.

Gold, H. K., Leinbach, R. C., Mundth, E. D., Sanders, C. A., and Buckley, M. J.: Reversal of Myocardial Ischemia Complicating Acute Infarction by Intra-aortic Balloon Pumping (IABP), *Circulation,* 1973.

Griepp, R. B., Stinson, E. B., Biever, C. P., Reitz, B. A., Copeland, J. G., Oyer, P. E., and Shumway, N. E.: Human Heart Transplant, *Ann Thorac Surg,* **22:**171, 1976.

Hall, D. P., Moreno, J. R., Dennis, C., and Senning, A.: An Experimental Study of Prolonged Left Heart Bypass without Thoracotomy, *Ann Surg,* **156:**190, 1962.

Hill, J. D., deLeval, M. R., Fallat, R. J., Bramson, M. L., Eberhart, R. C., Schulte, H. D., Osborn, J. J., Barber, R., and Gerbode, F.: Acute Respiratory Insufficiency: Treatment with Prolonged Extracorporeal Oxygenation, *J Thorac Cardiovasc Surg,* **64:**551, 1972.

Kaiser, G. C., Marco, J. D., Barner, H. B., Codd, J. E., Laks, H., and Willman, V. L.: Intraaortic Balloon Assistance, *Ann Thorac Surg,* **21:**487, 1976.

Liotta, D., Maness, J., Bourland, H., Rodwell, D., Hall, W. C., and DeBakey, M. E.: Recent Modifications in the Implantable Left Ventricle By-pass, *Trans Am Soc Artif Intern Organs,* **11:**284, 1965.

Litwak, R. S., Koffsky, R. M., Jurado, R. A., Lukban, S. B., et al.: Use of a Left Heart Assist Device after Intracardiac Surgery: Technique and Clinical Experience, *Ann Thorac Surg,* **21:**191, 1976.

Norman, J. C., Molokhia, F. A., Harmison, L. T., Whalen, R. L., and Huffman, F.: An Implantable Nuclear-fueled Circulatory Support System: I. Systems Analysis of Conception, Design, Fabrication, and Initial *In Vivo* Testing, *Ann Surg,* **176:**492, 1972.

Okura, T., Tjonneland, S., Fred, P. S., and Kantrowtiz, A.: U-shaped Mechanical Auxiliary Ventricle, *Arch Surg,* **95:**821, 1967.

Skinner, D. B., Anstadt, G. L., and Camp, T. F., Jr.: Applications of Mechanical Ventricular Assistance, *Ann Surg,* **166:**500, 1967.

Spencer, F. C., Eiseman, B., Trinkle, J. K., and Rossi, N. P.: Assisted Circulation for Cardiac Failure following Intracardiac Surgery with Cardiopulmonary Bypass, *J Thorac Cardiovasc Surg,* **49:**56, 1964.

Chapter 20

Diseases of Great Vessels

by **Frank C. Spencer**

ANEURYSMS OF THE THORACIC AORTA

Aneurysms of the thoracic aorta may be classified in five groups, varying with the anatomic location: (1) ascending aorta; (2) transverse aortic arch; (3) traumatic thoracic aorta, uniformly occurring distal to the left subclavian artery; (4) descending thoracic aorta; and (5) thoraco-abdominal. The etiology, disability, and surgical approach all vary with these different types. Hence, each one is discussed separately.

Aneurysms of the Ascending Aorta

Aneurysms localized to the ascending aorta are often due to a degenerative connective tissue disease of the aortic media. This is seen typically as cystic medial necrosis, one manifestation of a generalized disorder in the Marfan syndrome, or as an isolated disease in Erdheim's cystic medial necrosis. Syphilitic destruction of the media of the aorta was formerly a frequent cause of such aneurysms but is now uncommon. Atherosclerotic aneurysms are seldom limited to the ascending aorta, usually evolving as diffuse fusiform lesions involving both the ascending aorta and the transverse arch.

PATHOLOGY. As an aneurysm develops in the proximal ascending aorta, dilatation of the annulus of the aortic valve often develops, stretching the cusps of the aortic valve apart and producing aortic insufficiency (Fig 20-1). Often cardiac failure from aortic insufficiency is the significant disability, rather than enlargement of the aneurysm with rupture or compression of adjacent structures. Large saccular syphilitic aneurysms can enlarge and erode through the sternum (Fig. 20-2), but these are now rare.

Once aortic insufficiency has resulted from an aneurysm, progression of disability is fairly rapid with death from cardiac failure in 1 to 2 years in many patients unless operation is performed. In the Marfan syndrome, the degenerated wall of the aorta may also rupture and form a dissecting aneurysm. Before surgical therapy was available, most patients with the Marfan syndrome died from one of two complications—either dissecting aneurysm or aortic insufficiency.

CLINICAL MANIFESTATIONS. Patients are often asymptomatic when the diagnosis is made following detection of a mass on a chest roentgenogram performed for other purposes. Expanding saccular aneurysms may cause symptoms from compression of the superior vena cava or the trachea, but compression rarely occurs from fusiform aneurysms. Frequently, the first symptom is due to congestive heart failure from aortic insufficiency. Physical examination usually demonstrates no abnormalities except the aortic diastolic murmur and wide pulse pressure of aortic insufficiency.

DIAGNOSTIC FINDINGS. The diagnosis can be suspected from the chest roentgenogram, disclosing enlargement of the ascending aorta, but aortography is required to establish the exact diagnosis. The aortographic finding of a fusiform aneurysm in the proximal ascending aorta, tapering to an aorta of near-normal diameter at the level of the innominate artery, is virtually diagnostic of cystic medial necrosis (Fig. 20-3).

TREATMENT. Because of the progressive nature of the aortic insufficiency, operation should be performed as soon as possible after the diagnosis is made. The operative procedure must include both correction of the aortic insufficiency and excision of the aneurysm. This, of necessity, involves the use of extracorporeal circulation. If aortic insufficiency is minimal, simple excision of the aneurysm may be adequate.

At operation, once cardiopulmonary bypass has been started, the aorta can be occluded and the aneurysm excised. A critical point is whether the aorta proximally can be divided distal to the coronary ostia or whether excision should extend proximal to the ostia. Usually this decision can be made based on preoperative angiography.

If excision distal to the coronary ostia, which is preferable, can be done, the aorta is divided at this level. The author's preference is for cannulation of both coronary arteries and perfusion during the operative procedure. Others prefer a hypothermic cardioplegic technique, often with potassium.

Fig. 20-1. Operative photograph of a patient with a large aneurysm of the ascending aorta. *A.* The aneurysm in the proximal aorta has been isolated and the aorta elevated by encircling umbilical tapes. *B.* Once the aorta has been incised, the incompetent aortic valve is exposed. The aortic insufficiency was produced by dilatation of the aortic annulus.

If aortic valve replacement is required, this is done initially, inserting the prosthetic valve of choice. Our preference is for the Starr-Edwards cloth-covered steel ball prosthesis. With a narrow aortic root, the tilting disc prosthesis of the Björk-Shiley type is preferred.

Subsequently, a preclotted, short, woven Dacron graft, usually about 10 cm long, is inserted to reestablish aortic continuity. Because the aortic wall is thinned by the disease in the media, care must be taken in performing the anastomosis to avoid serious or even fatal hemorrhage. Buttressing the suture lines with pledgets of Teflon felt (Fig. 20-4) is valuable. Other techniques are either preserving the wall of the aneurysm and wrapping it about the graft afterward or constructing a tube of pericardium and sewing this about the graft if there is serious hemorrhage.

Liddicott et al., in 1975, described excision of 100 ascending aortic aneurysms (including 45 dissecting aneurysms) over a period of 10 years. Concomitant replacement of the aortic valve was necessary in 63 patients. Of the 100 aneurysms, 69 were considered to be due to atherosclerosis, 22 to cystic medial necrosis, and 9 to syphilitic aortitis. The average follow-up of 82 surviving patients was 4.7 years, with an actuarial survival rate of 83 percent at 2 years and 70 percent at 8 years.

If the aneurysm extends proximal to the ostia of the coronary arteries, the complex composite operation developed by Dentall in 1968 and later described by Edwards in 1970 seems to be quite satisfactory. In this procedure an aortic prosthetic valve is placed inside a Dacron tube and the composite graft sutured to the aortic annulus. The distal anastomosis is to the distal aorta, and the ostia of the coronary artery are reimplanted into windows made in the side of the graft. The wall of the aneurysm is then closed around the graft. Zubiate and Kay, in 1976, reported experiences with six patients, and recently Kouchoukos et al. described operations on 25 patients with no operative

Fig. 20-2. Patient with a large syphilitic aneurysm eroding through the sternum and projecting beneath the skin. Fortunately such lesions are now rare. An attempt at operative extirpation of the lesion was unsuccessful because of hemorrhage.

mortality. We have used the procedure several times and have found it quite satisfactory.

In 1975 Griepp et al. reported the use of deep hypothermia and circulatory arrest for simplifying the procedure in four patients, three of whom survived. His technique is shown in Fig. 20-5. Further experience with this method, which could simplify the operative approach, will be significant.

Aneurysms of the Transverse Aortic Arch

Aneurysms of the transverse aortic arch are almost always due to atherosclerosis, rarely syphilis. The diagnosis is usually established by aortography, differentiating the aneurysm from a malignant mediastinal tumor. The degree of involvement of the great vessels arising from the aortic arch also can be determined.

Detailed consideration of the technical management of these aneurysms is beyond the scope of this textbook, but limited pertinent references are listed in the bibliography at the end of the chapter. Because of the complexity of the operative procedure and the high mortality, excision should be attempted only for expanding aneurysms with an obviously impending fatal outcome, usually from tracheal obstruction, unless operation is performed. Surgical excision is a complex undertaking, requiring perfusion of the distal aorta, the great arch vessels, and often the coronary arteries. Hemorrhage and neurologic complications from perfusion of the innominate and carotid arteries have been responsible for an operative mortality often exceeding 60 to 70 percent (Fig. 20-6). Retrograde perfusion of the right brachial artery has been the most satisfactory method of perfusing the right vertebral and right carotid arteries arising from the innominate artery, while perfusion of the left carotid artery has been through direct cannulation. Pressure in the carotid artery should be monitored during perfusion to avoid the extremes of inadequate or excessive perfusion. Surgical techniques have gradually improved and undoubtedly will continue to do so. One remarkable example was published in 1972 by Lefrak et al., who described excision of a massive aneurysm of the aortic arch in a seventy-six-year-old patient which had virtually occluded the trachea. One year later the patient remained well and free of symptoms.

Traumatic Thoracic Aneurysms

ETIOLOGY AND PATHOLOGY. Traumatic aneurysms almost invariably arise from transection of the thoracic aorta associated with closed chest trauma. The section on traumatic rupture of the aorta in this chapter should be read in conjunction with this one, as traumatic rupture and traumatic thoracic aneurysms have a common etiology but a different clinical course. In those few patients fortunate enough not to succumb from exsanguinating hemorrhage an aneurysm will subsequently develop. If a patient survives longer than 6 to 8 weeks following injury, the risk of acute rupture is small. In a review of the English and French literature between 1950 and 1965, Bennett and Cherry found rupture occurring nine times in a total of 105

Fig. 20-3. *A.* Posteroanterior view of a thoracic aortogram demonstrating a large aneurysm in the ascending aorta, stopping near the innominate artery. Resection of the aneurysm was successfully performed. The patient was well 5 years following operation. *B.* Lateral view of a thoracic aortogram in the same patient.

aneurysms. The usual course is one of progressive enlargement with compression of adjacent structures.

The aneurysm virtually always arises just distal to the left subclavian artery, opposite the point of insertion of the ligamentum arteriosum. Although a huge aneurysm filling most of the hemithorax may be found, at operation the point of origin is almost invariably found in this area. This localization is a significant one in planning operative therapy, for little disease of the adjacent segments of aorta exists. Reconstruction can usually be done with a short prosthetic graft; occasionally direct anastomosis is possible.

Fig. 20-4. Procedure for excision of dissecting aneurysm of the ascending aorta. *A.* A dissecting aneurysm of the ascending aorta in a patient with the Marfan syndrome. The lesion had produced acute aortic insufficiency. *B.* Initially at operation the aneurysm was excised, and the coronary arteries were perfused to support coronary circulation. Distad the dissected wall of the aorta was approximated with interrupted sutures. *C.* The mechanism of production of aortic insufficiency by an aortic dissection. The area of dissection proceeds proximally to detach the aortic cusps from the aortic wall, permitting them to prolapse into the lumen and cause aortic insufficiency. Prolapse of the right and left coronary cusps is minimized by the location of the coronary artery; hence, dissection of the noncoronary cusp is the most extensive. Reapproximation of the aortic wall may correct the insufficiency. *D.* Aortic reconstruction is performed with a woven Dacron graft, performing the anastomosis with continuous silk sutures. The disease in the aortic wall results in unusual friability, which may make adequate hemostasis difficult. *E.* The proximal anastomosis is completed, leaving the coronary cannulae in position. The distal anastomosis is then similarly performed, after which the coronary catheters are withdrawn and aortic circulation reestablished.

CLINICAL MANIFESTATIONS. Unlike most aneurysms from other causes, traumatic thoracic aneurysms enlarge slowly and in some patients have apparently remained stationary for 10 to 20 years, the diagnosis being made in retrospect after finding an asymptomatic aneurysm with a history of closed-chest trauma 10 to 20 years before. A detailed study of the natural "life history" of such aneurysms was reported by Bennett and Cherry in 1967. As the aneurysm enlarges, compression of the left main bron-

Fig. 20-5. Operative procedure for aortic arch replacement. (*Griepp et al., Thorac Cardiovasc Surg, 70:1051, 1975.*)

Fig. 20-6. Operative photograph of a patient with aneurysm of the aortic arch. The procedure is a complicated one requiring multiple bypass grafts, temporarily diverting blood through bypass channels to the carotid arteries and distal aorta while the aneurysm is excised and the aortic arch reconstructed.

chus with pain, dyspnea, cough, and atelectasis are the predominant complications. Hoarseness from compression and distortion of the left recurrent laryngeal nerve may appear. These symptoms usually well precede enlargement of the aneurysm to such a degree that rupture occurs. This course of events is emphasized because of the small risk of rupture, which is in direct contrast to factors governing the surgical policy with the majority of aneurysms from atherosclerosis or syphilis, where the threat of rupture constitutes a major reason for recommending elective excision as soon as possible.

Frequently there are no abnormalities on physical examination unless compression of the main bronchus has produced atelectasis of the left lung. A murmur is usually not heard, and there is no abnormality of peripheral pulses.

DIAGNOSTIC FINDINGS. The chest roentgenogram usually discloses an ovoid density near the left subclavian artery. If an aneurysm has been present for several years, calcification is often visible in the wall. The diagnosis can be established by aortography, which is required to delineate the extent of the aneurysm and to differentiate it from other mediastinal tumors (Fig. 20-7).

TREATMENT. The problem of management of acute rupture of the thoracic aorta, with the risk of exsanguinating hemorrhage, is presented in the section on Wounds of the Great Vessels. Elective excision is recommended for the majority of patients, although probably 20 to 30 per-

Fig. 20-7. *A.* Chest roentgenogram following an automobile accident, demonstrating widening of the mediastinum with subcutaneous emphysema. Traumatic rupture of the aorta was not recognized at this time. *B.* Chest roentgenogram 5 months after the injury demonstrated a left upper mediastinal mass. *C.* Posteroanterior view of an aortogram demonstrating a localized thoracic aneurysm. This lesion was excised successfully. *D.* Lateral view of an aortogram in the same patient. *E.* Chest roentgenogram in a different patient 2 years after an automobile accident demonstrated an asymptomatic mass in the upper mediastinum. *F.* Aortography demonstrated a saccular thoracic aneurysm, which was subsequently resected successfully. *G.* Aortogram in the same patient as in *F.* This film demonstrated the size and extent of the aneurysm as additional contrast material flowed freely within the lesion.

cent of aneurysms remain stationary and asymptomatic for many years. Apparently most aneurysms, despite long latent periods of stability, eventually progressively enlarge. When serious associated disease, such as coronary atherosclerosis, is present, observation with serial chest roentgenograms may be safely employed.

Technique of Operation. A left posterolateral thoracotomy through the fourth or fifth intercostal space is used. Initially the aorta is mobilized and encircled proximal and distal to the aneurysm. Proximal involvement of the left subclavian artery often requires encirclement of the aorta between the left carotid and the left subclavian arteries. This is facilitated by opening the pericardium and dissecting the intrapericardial portion of the aortic arch. The vagus nerve with the recurrent laryngeal nerve should also be mobilized and protected, for the recurrent laryngeal is often adherent to the wall of the aneurysm.

Once the aorta has been encircled proximally and distad and the recurrent laryngeal nerve mobilized as much as possible, further dissection is unnecessary. Some form of

aortic bypass should then be established to maintain flow to the distal aorta during aortic occlusion and prevent ischemic injury of the spinal cord and kidneys. Without an aortic bypass, paraplegia has been reported to develop within as short a time as 20 to 25 minutes of aortic occlusion.

The first effective technique of aortic bypass was the left

Fig. 20-7 E-G. (See legend on facing page.)

shunts was greatly aided by the work by Gott, who developed a method of temporarily binding heparin to the surface of polyvinyl tubes. Different techniques for temporary shunts without any heparin have been reported, but there seems to be little reason not to use the temporary heparin tubes.

In 1972 Krauss and associates described experiences with the Gott shunt in 8 patients. Several reports from that time have described good results with the shunt. A recent report by Donahoo et al. described a ten-year experience.

As described in the following section, Crawford and associates have utilized the interesting approach of not employing any type of shunt at all, simply minimizing the period of ischemia of the aorta. They have properly emphasized that many factors besides the use of a shunt influence paraplegia, such as vessels arising from the aneurysm which may supply the spinal cord and blood pressure before and after excision of the aneurysm, which in turn would influence the rate of flow of blood through the impaired collateral circulation. Although this technique is not one the author would prefer, the Crawford observations are quite significant.

After the type of shunt has been selected and the aorta appropriately localized and occluded proximal and distal to the aneurysm, it is incised, after which the point of origin can be identified as a transverse laceration or transection near the point of insertion of the ligamentum arteriosum. The aorta proximal and distal is usually normal; therefore it is unnecessary to excise any significant length of aorta. The inner lining of the aneurysmal sac may be removed, but it is unnecessary and unwise to attempt complete excision, partly because of vascular adhesions surrounding the wall of the aneurysm. In most patients a 5- to 8-cm segment of woven Dacron graft is sufficient to restore arterial continuity.

Convalescence following operation is usually uneventful, and long-term results are excellent. The risk of operation is probably less than 5 percent. One of the largest groups of patients has been reported by Cooley et al., operating on over 86 such lesions without any operative mortality. The low mortality is due to both the young age and the localized nature of the aneurysm.

Aneurysms of the Descending Thoracic Aorta

ETIOLOGY AND INCIDENCE. Aneurysms in the descending thoracic aorta may result from atherosclerosis, syphilis, trauma, or a dissection of the aortic wall. Most are due to atherosclerosis and are exceeded only by abdominal aneurysms in frequency of occurrence. They are most frequently found in men in the fifth to the seventh decades. Formerly, saccular aneurysms from syphilis were common, but these are now rare. Dissecting aneurysms and traumatic aneurysms are considered in the accompanying sections.

The majority of atherosclerotic aneurysms are located in the proximal part of the descending thoracic aorta, beginning distal to the left subclavian artery. They extend for varying distances and in some instances can involve the entire descending thoracic aorta. They are generally

atrial-femoral bypass, withdrawing blood through a cannula inserted into the left atrium, which in turn is pumped to the distal arterial tree, usually the left iliac, occasionally the distal aorta. Flow rates of 2 to 2.5 liters/minute are required to maintain the base-line pressure in the proximal aorta as well as to maintain distal aortic pressure between 60 and 75 mm Hg. This technique has been widely used but has the disadvantage of increased bleeding associated with systemic heparinization.

If access to the left atrium is awkward, a femoral artery–femoral vein cannulation can be carried out and a pump oxygenator used in the circuit to perfuse the lower half of the body while the aorta is clamped, letting the heart and lungs perfuse the upper half normally.

To avoid the need for heparin, there has been increasing use of different types of temporary shunt inserted between the proximal and distal aorta. This technique has become the one of choice at New York University. The safety of

Fig. 20-8. *A.* Chest roentgenogram of a forty-five-year-old patient with a large diffuse aneurysm of the thoracic aorta from atherosclerosis. The aneurysm was excised and the aorta reconstructed with a Teflon graft. *B.* Chest roentgenogram 6 months after operation shows the area of insertion of the Teflon graft. *C.* Operative photograph of atherosclerotic aneurysm demonstrated in the chest roentgenogram seen in *A.*

fusiform (Fig. 20-8), in contrast to syphilitic saccular aneurysms. Their rate of growth is significantly slower than that of abdominal aneurysms, with a less malignant tendency toward rapid enlargement and rupture, but eventual rupture is the outcome in most cases unless other complications of atherosclerosis appear. Syphilitic saccular aneurysms, by contrast, usually rapidly enlarge and rupture, a high percentage rupturing within 2 years after the diagnosis is made. Erosion of bone, commonly seen with saccular syphilitic aneurysms, is unusual with fusiform atherosclerotic aneurysms.

CLINICAL MANIFESTATIONS. In many patients a thoracic aneurysm is found as an asymptomatic mass on a chest roentgenogram made for other reasons. Probably the most common symptoms from enlargement result from compression or erosion of the lung, or compression and obstruction of the left main bronchus with resulting dyspnea and atelectasis. Erosion into the bronchus will produce hemoptysis. Involvement of the left recurrent laryngeal nerve where it encircles the ligamentum arteriosum may lead to paralysis of the vocal cord with hoarseness. In contrast to abdominal aneurysms, where acute rupture may be the first indication of a previously unsuspected aneurysm, such a sequence of events is unusual with a thoracic aneurysm.

Physical examination often yields entirely normal findings. Infrequently, a bruit may be heard over the left chest, loudest in the left paravertebral area. Peripheral pulses are frequently normal, unless involvement of the left subclavian artery produces hypotension in the left arm.

DIAGNOSTIC FINDINGS. The diagnosis can usually be suspected from the appearance of the mass in the region of the aorta on the chest roentgenogram. The differential diagnosis includes other conditions producing an opacity on the chest roentgenogram, such as bronchogenic carcinoma, metastatic carcinoma, or rarely esophageal tumors. Laminar calcification may be visible in the wall of the aorta. Aortography is used both to confirm the diagnosis and to delineate the precise extent of the aneurysm. An electrocardiogram and a blood urea nitrogen determination should be routinely obtained, because atherosclerotic disease in other organs, especially the heart and kidney, is frequent.

Fig. 20-9. Procedure for excision of an aneurysm of the thoracic aorta. *A.* An aneurysm of the thoracic aorta. Initial dissection is limited to isolation of the aorta proximal and distal to the aneurysm. Left atriofemoral bypass is then instituted at a flow rate near 2 liters/minute. Pressures should be monitored in the aorta and also in the femoral artery to ensure adequacy of perfusion of the arterial circulation proximal and distal to the aneurysm. *B.* Aneurysm is widely opened, excising the anterior wall but removing only the inner lining posteriorly to avoid excessive bleeding where the aneurysm may be adherent to the vertebral column and lung. *C.* Bleeding intercostal arteries may be oversewed from within the lumen of the aneurysm. *D.* A woven Dacron prosthesis is used for reconstruction of the aorta, employing a continuous suture for the anastomosis. *E.* Following completion of the anastomosis the adventitial sac remaining from the aneurysm can be used to partly surround the graft.

TREATMENT. In most patients once the diagnosis of a discrete aneurysm has been made, excision should be recommended. With small aneurysms, associated with significant coronary or cerebrovascular disease, observation with frequent chest roentgenograms to evaluate the rate of enlargement may be safely employed. Serial observations also may be preferable in some patients with a diffuse fusiform dilatation of the entire thoracic aorta.

The technique of operation is detailed in Fig. 20-9. As mentioned in the section on Traumatic Thoracic Aneurysms, the major hazards are operative hemorrhage and ischemic injury to the spinal cord and kidneys while the aorta is clamped and the aneurysm excised. The different methods for perfusing the distal aorta to protect the spinal cord and kidneys are discussed in that section. Either the conventional left atriofemoral bypass, which has the advantage of simplicity but the disadvantage of systemic heparinization, should be used, or some type of temporary shunt without heparin should be employed. Our preference for the last 3 or 4 years has been the Gott shunt, inserted proximally into the ascending aorta and distally into the femoral vessels. In the unusual case where this does not function satisfactorily, one of the forms of bypass with heparin can be employed. Whatever method of perfusion is employed, it is important to monitor pressure in the distal aorta, keeping mean pressure above 60 mm Hg. Pressure in the proximal aorta is similarly monitored to avoid excessive hypertension which may precipitate left ventricular failure, especially in the presence of preexisting coronary disease.

As with aneurysms elsewhere, an important principal in minimizing operative hemorrhage is to avoid an attempt to completely excise the aneurysm, especially when the wall is adherent to the lung or vertebral column. Initial dissection should be limited to encircling the aorta proximally and distad. Once aortic bypass has been instituted, the aorta can be occluded with clamps and the aneurysm opened widely. The inner wall then can be removed, suturing the ostia of any patent intercostal vessels but leaving the outer adventitial layers to avoid bleeding. Following excision of the aneurysm, aortic continuity is reestablished with a vascular prosthesis (Fig. 20-10). Our preference is for woven Dacron prostheses, carefully preclotted, inserted with continuous synthetic sutures. The remaining adventitial wall of the aneurysm then can be wrapped around the prosthesis to further minimize bleeding.

The most serious complication is paraplegia. Fortunately this is rare with adequate aortic bypass. In some instances, however, some degree of spinal cord injury has occurred despite seemingly adequate bypass, probably as a consequence of ligation of intercostal arteries during excision of the aneurysm. As the blood supply to the spinal cord is highly variable, it is impossible to know which, if any, intercostal arteries are vital to spinal cord circulation. Fortunately, with many thoracic aneurysms intercostal arteries arising from the aneurysm have become occluded beforehand by thrombus. Although some patients have tolerated excision of the entire thoracic aorta uneventfully, it is probably wise to limit the degree of excision of adjacent thoracic aorta, even though moderate disease and dilatation are present, especially if large patent intercostal arteries are seen arising from this segment.

Following recovery from operation, the prognosis is favorable and related chiefly to the extent of atherosclerotic disease in other organs. Complications from the prosthetic graft or the adjacent diseased aorta are unusual. With experienced surgical groups, the operative mortality is in the range of 10 to 15 percent. This varies both with

Fig. 20-10. *A.* Operative photograph of saccular syphilitic aneurysm of distal thoracic aorta. *B.* Teflon graft used to restore continuity following excision of a syphilitic aneurysm of the lower thoracic aorta. This graft was used in the patient seen in *A.*

the size of the aneurysm and with the age of the patient; for larger aneurysms there is a greater operative risk from hemorrhage. Actually there is only a limited amount of data in the surgical literature concerning excision. It is probable that infrequently performed operations for thoracic aneurysm have a much higher mortality rate. In a report of 237 aneurysms treated at The Johns Hopkins Hospital between 1952 and 1959 by Vasko and associates, there were only eight patients with thoracic aneurysms due to syphilis or atherosclerosis. All survived operation, but three died within 2 years from further vascular complications. In 1966 Bloodwell and associates described experiences with nearly 400 thoracic aneurysms, but detailed analysis of these cases was not presented. The low mortality reported by Krauss et al. in 1972 in the series of eight patients with seven survivors in whom the temporary heparinized shunt was used indicates the progressive improvement in surgical mortality with improved techniques.

Thoracoabdominal Aneurysms

These aneurysms fortunately are rare, because their excision is a complicated surgical procedure, involving restoration of blood flow to the celiac, superior mesenteric, and renal arteries. Such procedures have usually been performed with multiple bypass techniques to minimize duration of ischemia to different organs, but operative mortality has remained high. More recently some procedures have been performed with a simple left atriofemoral bypass, opening the aneurysm widely and attempting to reestablish flow to different organs with a relatively short period of ischemia.

INCIDENCE AND ETIOLOGY. The rarity of such aneurysms is indicated in the report by DeBakey and associates of experiences with treating over 2,000 aneurysms of the abdominal aorta below the renal arteries, during which less than 50 of these aneurysms above the renal arteries were treated. They are usually due to atherosclerosis, rarely to cystic medial necrosis as in the Marfan syndrome. In the group of 42 patients reported by DeBakey et al., 62 percent resulted from atherosclerosis, and 26 percent were due to syphilis.

CLINICAL MANIFESTATIONS. The rate of enlargement is slow, and excision should be attempted only for expanding aneurysms causing symptoms from compression and displacement of adjacent structures. Often the aneurysm cannot be palpated, because it is concealed in the upper abdomen by the stomach and pancreas. The diagnosis may be suspected from the chest roentgenogram disclosing enlargement of the thoracic aorta near the diaphragm, but aortography is required to confirm the diagnosis.

TREATMENT. Most of the earlier operations have been performed with a multiple bypass technique, inserting an initial bypass graft from the thoracic aorta above the aneurysm to the abdominal aorta below the origin of the renal arteries. From this initial graft, branch grafts are then serially inserted to the celiac artery, superior mesenteric artery, and both renal arteries. Once the grafts have been inserted, avoiding prolonged ischemia of any individual organ, the aneurysm can be opened widely and the inner lining removed. Anastomosis to the right renal artery may be more conveniently performed at this time.

These procedures have been performed through a variety of thoracic and abdominal incisions. A thoracoabdominal incision from a left lateral position has been employed, or a separate midline abdominal incision combined with a left thoracotomy incision.

In recent years Cooley and others have reported the use of left atriofemoral bypass for excision of the aneurysm, establishing bypass and then opening the aneurysm widely, followed by direct anastomoses to the involved visceral arteries with a long straight graft. This technique must be accomplished in a short period of time, however, to avoid significant ischemic injury.

Patients surviving this complex operative procedure have had a fairly good prognosis. In the group of 42 surgically treated patients reported by DeBakey in 1965, 11 died within 1 month of operation, a mortality of 26 percent. There were four deaths subsequently, but the remaining 27 patients were alive without significant disability at the time of the report. The longest individual follow-up was about 10 years (Fig. 20-11).

Fig. 20-11. Angiogram of Dacron graft 1 year after excision of thoracoabdominal aneurysm. The graft was inserted between the thoracic aorta, as an end-to-side anastomosis, and the abdominal aorta, not shown in this illustration. Side branches to the superior mesenteric artery, celiac artery, and right and left renal arteries are individually visible.

A most significant report came from Crawford and associates in 1973, reporting experiences with 84 patients, 38 in whom some type of bypass was used and 45 more recent cases in which shunting was avoided. The significance of this paper is that with a simplified technique mortality was 8.8 percent versus 21 percent when a shunt was employed. It may be hoped that others can duplicate this impressive record. Basically, their technique avoided heparin or shunting but opened the aneurysm widely and used the "button" technique to anastomose the ostia of the distal vessel to appropriate windows in the side of the aneurysm, minimizing the ischemia time.

DISSECTING ANEURYSMS

ETIOLOGY AND INCIDENCE. Dissecting aneurysms are related to degenerative disease of the media of the aorta, the cause of which is unknown. The disease is about three times as common in males as in females and is most frequently seen in patients in the fifth and sixth decades. However, it can occur in almost any age group, one of the youngest patients being only 14 months of age. The most frequently associated factor is hypertension, present in 75 to 85 percent of patients, although the reported incidence has varied widely.

Conditions associated with abnormalities of connective tissue have a greater frequency with dissecting aneurysm. The most common of these is the Marfan syndrome. Before surgical therapy was available, most patients with the Marfan syndrome succumbed either from a dissecting aneurysm or from aortic insufficiency as a result of dilatation of the aortic annulus. Other conditions occasionally associated with dissecting aneurysm include coarctation of the aorta, pregnancy, and kyphoscoliosis. Atherosclerosis is not a definite causative factor. The segment of aorta most frequently involved is different in the two diseases, since dissecting aneurysm usually involves the proximal thoracic aorta while atherosclerosis is most severe near the bifurcation of the abdominal aorta. There is also no known relationship to trauma or syphilis.

Experimentally, dissecting aneurysm can be produced in young rats with a diet containing 50 percent sweet peas, which causes a distinct abnormality of connective tissue, known as *lathyrism*. The abnormal chemical agent that weakens the cross-linking of collagen is a β-amino nitrite.

PATHOLOGY. The term "dissecting aneurysm" is actually a misnomer, for the pathologic lesion is more accurately described as a "dissecting hematoma," consisting of a hemorrhagic separation of the layers of the aortic wall (Fig. 20-12). The basic lesion is degeneration of the aortic media, often associated with rupture of the vasa vasorum. Most patients also have a tear in the intima of the aorta, establishing a communication between the lumen of the aorta and the hematoma in the aortic wall. Whether the tear in the intima is a primary or secondary event is uncertain. If it is the primary event, superimposed upon underlying disease of the aortic media, the progressive dissection of the aortic wall which follows may result from establishing a communication between the lumen of the aorta and the aortic wall. The alternative hypothesis is that

Fig. 20-12. *A.* Photograph of dissecting aneurysm of the thoracic aorta operated upon a few days after onset of the dissection. The lung is being separated from the aneurysm. Hematoma in the wall of the dissected aorta is visible. *B.* With a left atriofemoral bypass functioning and the aorta occluded, the aneurysm has been incised. The lacerated edges of the aortic wall from the dissection can be seen. Clot is visible in the wall of the aorta superior to the tip of the metal aspirator.

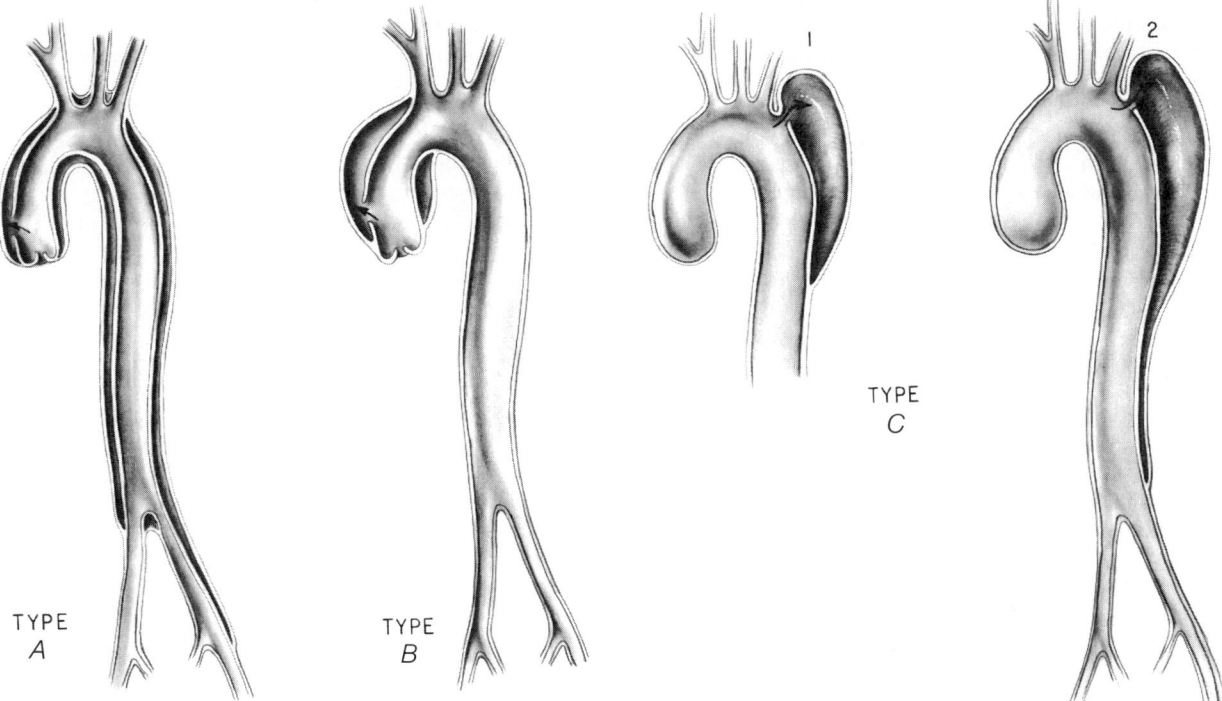

Fig. 20-13. Different types of aortic dissection. A. Dissecting aneurysm which begins in the ascending aorta near the aortic valve and extends throughout the aorta down to the external iliac arteries. Unfortunately, this is a common type of dissecting aneurysm. B. Dissecting aneurysm limited to the ascending aorta. This is commonly seen in the Marfan syndrome. C1. Dissecting aneurysm beginning distal to the left subclavian artery. The localized nature of this aneurysm makes it readily accessible to surgical excision. 2. Dissecting aneurysm arising distal to the left subclavian artery but extending into the abdominal aorta. Only partial excision of the area of dissection is possible.

rupture of the vasa vasorum is the primary event, creating an intramural hemorrhage, which secondarily ruptures through the intima to establish communication with the aortic lumen. Rarely no intimal laceration can be found at autopsy, which indicates that rupture of the vasa vasorum was the primary event. The frequency with which tears of the intima are localized either to the ascending aorta or near the ligamentum arteriosum, however, suggests that laceration of the intima is probably the initial event in the majority of patients.

Two clinical observations indicate that in the majority of patients the tear of the intima is the significant event. First, at operation often not all of the diseased aorta is excised but simply the area in which the intima is torn in the major area of disruption of the aorta. With dissection starting near the left subclavian, the origin is excised and perhaps one-half of the distal thoracic aorta with the remaining dissected aorta is left, approximating the intima to obliterate the false lumen. In these patients the dissection process often extends below the diaphragm. The fact that "recurrent" dissecting aneurysms have not been reported, although corrective operations have now been performed for several years, reinforces the fact that if the tear in the

intima is excised and the hypertension controlled, recurrence is rare. This is particularly noteworthy with Marfan's syndrome, where the primary connective tissue defect cannot be corrected. In such patients, recurrence following successful excision of a dissecting aneurysm is thus far virtually unknown.

In 60 to 70 percent of patients the dissection originates in the ascending aorta, while in about 25 percent it originates beyond the left subclavian artery near the ligamentum arteriosum (Fig. 20-13). Infrequently it may originate in the aortic arch or at more distal locations in the aorta.

Once a dissection has begun, it may extend progressively to involve all of the thoracic and abdominal aorta as well as many of the arterial tributaries. This occurs in a high percentage of patients. As dissection progresses, branch vessels are sheared off, either becoming obliterated or establishing a communication with the false lumen created by the dissection. Proximally, the coronary arteries may be involved, and frequently one or more aortic valve cusps are detached and prolapse into the lumen, creating aortic insufficiency. More distad the vessels involved may include any tributary of the aorta. Involvement of the carotid arteries may produce neurologic injury. Obstruction of the subclavian arteries produces differences in blood pressure between the two arms. Dissection of intercostal arteries may cause spinal cord injury with paraplegia. Dissection of renal arteries may produce fatal renal insufficiency. In the extremities acute obstruction of the iliac or femoral arteries can result in either claudication or gangrene.

The dissection may terminate fatally at any time by rupture of the false lumen. The usual mode of death is rupture into the pericardial cavity from proximal dissection or rupture into the left pleural cavity. In the extensive review of 425 cases by Hirst et al., 21 percent of the patients died within 24 hours and 74 percent within 2 weeks. Ninety-one percent had succumbed within 6 months. In a group of 50 patients reported from the Massachusetts General Hospital by Austen et al., 45 percent died in the first week, 75 percent in the first month, and 86 percent within the first year. In evaluating mortality statistics, it is important to differentiate dissections arising in the ascending aorta from dissections arising distal to the left subclavian artery. The former have a much higher mortality rate. In a group of 62 patients reported by Lindsay and Hurst, almost all 40 patients with dissection involving the ascending aorta succumbed within 3 weeks, while in the group of 19 patients in whom the disease began distal to the aortic arch the survival was greater than 50 percent.

In patients who survive with a dissecting aneurysm an endothelial lining of the false lumen, termed a *healed dissecting aneurysm,* may develop and establish a so-called "double-barreled" aorta. A wide variety of bizarre circulatory patterns may be found in such patients. For example, one renal artery may arise from the "false" lumen and the other from the true lumen (Fig. 20-14), or alternatively both renal arteries can arise from the false lumen. In other patients, one iliac artery may originate from the false lumen, and the other from the true lumen.

In the few patients surviving an aortic dissection, rupture of the false lumen back into the true aortic lumen has often been found at the termination of the dissection. This spontaneous "reentry" into the aortic lumen suggested that establishing a communication between the false lumen and the true lumen might terminate the dissecting process. These observations led to the development of the aortic fenestration operation, originally attempted by Gurin and by Shaw, and later extensively used by DeBakey and associates. At the time of introduction of this operation, little else could be offered such patients. Significant benefit

from fenestration operations has been meager, however, and the operation has now been almost completely abandoned as more effective methods of therapy have been developed. The failure of development of a reentry area to protect against external rupture was noted by McCloy and associates. In a group of 22 patients who died from external rupture of a dissecting aneurysm, 11 had developed a point of reentry of the dissection into the aortic lumen, but this had not prevented fatal rupture.

CLINICAL MANIFESTATIONS. The abrupt onset of excruciating pain, almost immediately reaching its peak intensity, is very characteristic of a dissecting aneurysm. A myocardial infarction, by contrast, may gradually develop pain of increasing severity over several minutes. Usually anterior chest pain develops with dissection of the ascending aorta, while back pain is more common with dissection beginning distal to the aortic arch. Pain may be in both the front and back of the chest with dissection of either type, but usually predominant back pain suggests dissection beyond the left subclavian artery. Another significant characteristic of the pain is its tendency to migrate into different areas as dissection extends distad. As might be predicted from the wide variation in the extent of the dissection process, many pain syndromes may occur. Pain

Fig. 20-14. *A.* Aortogram showing an unusual pattern of aortic dissection in which dissection extended from the thoracic aorta into the abdominal aorta, creating two lumens, with the right renal artery arising from one and the left renal artery from the other. Focal stenosis of the right common iliac artery is seen at the lower part of the field producing intermittent claudication, which was the presenting complaint of the patient. *B.* Aortogram performed by a different root opacifies the left kidney and the left common iliac artery. The condition of the dissected aorta is illustrated in the accompanying drawing. Circulation was reestablished by excising the septum between the two channels at the aortic bifurcation. (*Adapted from W. Gryboski and F. C. Spencer, Intermittent Claudication Caused by a Dissecting Aneurysm of the Aorta, South Med J, 58:593, 1965.*)

A

B

TRUE LUMEN

FALSE LUMEN

PARTIAL OBSTRUCTION

may radiate to the neck, the arm, the epigastrium, or the leg. Seldom is pain completely absent, probably in no more than 10 percent of patients.

Syncope occurs in 10 to 20 percent of patients, and some neurologic symptoms are present in 20 to 40 percent. These may result from ischemia of the brain, spinal cord, or a peripheral nerve, depending upon whether a carotid artery, an intercostal artery, or a peripheral artery has been compromised.

Hypertension, often of severe degree, is present in 75 to 85 percent of patients. Often the hypertension with severe vasoconstriction contrasts with the clinical picture of an acutely ill patient, pale, sweating, and in acute distress. An aortic diastolic murmur appears in 20 to 30 percent of patients and is of great diagnostic significance, usually originating from detachment of an aortic valve cusp. Less frequently a pericardial friction rub may be audible due to leakage of blood into the pericardial cavity. Inequality of the carotid or subclavian pulses may be found, caused by unequal compression of these vessels. A variety of neurologic abnormalities may be detected, the most common being either a monoplegia or paraplegia.

DIAGNOSTIC FINDINGS. On the chest roentgenogram a widened mediastinum or a left pleural effusion from extravasation of blood is frequently seen. In some patients, however, the roentgenogram may be completely normal. The electrocardiogram is of particular value in distinguishing dissecting aneurysm from myocardial infarction, but there are no characteristic features of aortic dissection. The most common abnormality is left ventricular hypertrophy from the antecedent hypertension.

Aortography to demonstrate the double lumen created by the dissection is the most definitive diagnostic procedure. In some patients a diagnosis cannot be established by any other technique, especially if there are no abnormal physical findings and the only abnormality is a history of severe back pain.

The importance of aortography in any patient with unexplained sustained severe pain cannot be overemphasized. The history of pain may be the *only* abnormality found on subsequent examination. Occasionally a patient is seen a few days or weeks after an acute dissection with no symptoms and no abnormality on physical examination, electrocardiogram, or chest x-ray. Only aortography provides the diagnosis. Similarly, severe pain without abnormal findings in patients in whom aortography was not done has been followed by exsanguination within a few hours or days.

TREATMENT. The most effective treatment for acute dissecting aneurysm has not yet been determined. The ideal form of therapy, drug or surgical, is still uncertain, but with improvement in surgical techniques, the trend is toward the emergency use of drug therapy until the patient is stabilized, followed by prompt operation. How promptly operation should be performed varies among different centers, with Najafi et al. operating on some such patients with the same urgency as for a ruptured abdominal aneurysm, while others may wait for 2 to 7 days.

There is no question that emergency institution of antihypertensive therapy is the top priority in treatment, for this may arrest the dissection process and lessen the risk of fatal hemorrhage. Unfortunately, fatal hemorrhage has occurred in some patients who were asymptomatic and seemingly stable with drug therapy. Hence the prevailing trend is for operation at an appropriate time, probably the sooner the better, once the patient's condition has stabilized, perhaps earlier if drug therapy is not satisfactory and signs of rupture persist such as continued pain, hemothorax, or other signs of leakage of blood into the body cavities. As mentioned earlier, the appearance of a diastolic murmur, indicating detachment of an aortic cusp, is a particularly ominous finding. In 1976 Kirklin reported experiences from the University of Alabama, a total of 108 cases, and concluded that operation was the therapy of choice. The urgency of treatment is well emphasized by the grim mortality statistics, with 40 to 50 percent of patients dying within 2 weeks and the majority of those surviving the first 2 weeks succumbing within 1 year. Only about 10 percent of untreated patients survive beyond this time.

It is important in evaluating different forms of therapy to separate patients with dissections of the ascending aorta from patients in whom the dissection is distal to the aortic arch. The prognosis is much worse with dissections in the ascending aorta, with an acute mortality exceeding 90 percent in some series.

A significant addition to the therapy of dissecting aneurysms was made by Wheat and associates in 1965 when they reported the successful treatment of six patients with antihypertensive drugs. These studies were partly stimulated by observations from the poultry industry that certain flocks of turkeys had a high fatality rate from spontaneous dissecting aneurysm which could be reduced dramatically by adding to the food a small amount of reserpine (0.1 part to 1 million). Wheat et al. noted that their patients often lived a few hours to a few days following onset of the aortic dissection, only to succumb from continued dissection with eventual rupture. Because of the high frequency of hypertension in this group of patients, antihypertensive drugs were utilized to ameliorate the dissecting process. The therapeutic program included the immediate lowering of blood pressure by an intravenous infusion of Arfonad (trimethaphan), combined with the simultaneous administration of reserpine, chlorothiazide (Diuril), and guanethidine (Ismelin). Other investigators employing this form of therapy have substituted methyldopa (Aldomet) for guanethidine. Harris et al. stated that 19 of 21 patients had survived treatment with induced hypotension, 18 of whom were living and well with no progression of the disease. Austen and associates, in contrast, had a 60 percent mortality in patients with acute dissection.

At this time the ultimate role of drug therapy remains uncertain. Although Wheat and associates have obtained an impressively low mortality in their series of patients, others have been unable to duplicate these findings. With improved surgical techniques there has been an increasing tendency to perform early operation, within either a few hours or a few days after onset of symptoms. Data supporting an early operative approach were published in 1970 by Daily et al. and in 1972 by Liotta et al., by Shumacker, and by Najafi and associates.

Fig. 20-15. *Opposite.* Thoracic aortogram, performed with a catheter introduced retrograde through the femoral artery, showing a dissecting aneurysm arising distal to the left subclavian artery. The outer channel is faintly visualized as a double density beyond the left subclavian artery. *Lower left.* Operative photograph of dissecting aneurysm arising distal to the left subclavian artery. A clamp is visible on the aorta proximal to the left subclavian artery, which has been encircled with an umbilical tape. The vagus nerve is visible proximally. Laminated clot was found in the lumen of the aneurysm. *Lower right.* Dacron graft inserted to restore aortic continuity following excision of the aneurysm.

Although the final role of antihypertensive therapy is uncertain, its value is obvious as emergency therapy in the presence of severe hypertension to slow or reduce the dissecting process. Once the patient's condition is stabilized, emergency aortography can be performed to identify the area of dissection. From the location of the dissection, a decision can be made whether to perform emergency operation or not. Operation is simpler if dissection is located distal to the left subclavian artery. At New York University most patients in this category have been operated upon promptly, excising the area of dissection and restoring arterial continuity with a woven Dacron prosthesis (Figs. 20-15 and 20-16). If the dissection extends throughout the thoracic aorta, only the major area of involvement is removed, and the layers of the dissected aorta are sewed together distad before insertion of the prosthetic graft.

When operation is performed upon patients with dissection of the ascending aorta, the preferred treatment is excision of the ascending aorta and reconstruction with a Dacron prosthetic graft. Concomitant aortic insufficiency may be treated by reattachment of the prolapsed aortic valve cusps, occasionally by prosthetic valve replacement (Fig. 20-4). If the dissection has extended into the transverse arch and involves the origin of the great vessels, excision is probably best limited to the ascending aorta, sewing the layers of the dissected aorta together before the prosthetic graft is inserted. The long-term prognosis for these dissected aortas is yet unknown, but data thus far available indicate that prognosis is reasonably good if hypertension is controlled. More than 10 years have now elapsed since some surviving patients underwent excision of dissecting aneurysms.

Several years ago DeBakey and associates reported an extensive series of 142 patients with a mortality of 20 percent. Austen and associates had a similar mortality of 22 percent in 23 patients, while Harris et al. reported a mortality near 50 percent in 22 patients. In 1975, Reul et al. described experiences with 91 patients over a period of 10 years. Those operated on for acute dissection had an operative mortality of 25 percent; with chronic dissection the mortality was 17 percent. Only 1 of 31 patients with simple aneurysms above the diaphragm, operated on electively, died. According to recent reports, with improved techniques mortality rates have been significantly improved.

WOUNDS OF THE GREAT VESSELS

Penetrating Injuries

Penetrating injuries of the aorta or venae cavae are a frequent cause of death with penetrating chest injuries. Fatal hemorrhage occurs so quickly that only a few patients survive long enough for treatment. Patients alive with such injuries when first seen are usually in profound shock with signs of massive intrathoracic bleeding. Immediate thoracotomy offers the only chance for survival. In some instances this must be employed in the emergency department, often with conditions less than ideal. Once hemorrhage has been stopped, the patient is often transferred to the operating room for more definitive surgical exploration and subsequent closure of the incision. Depending upon the location of the injury, a variety of thoracic incisions have been used, including thoracotomy, median sternotomy, resection of the clavicle to expose the subclavian artery, or a cervicothoracic approach. In all likelihood a median sternotomy should be employed far more frequently than in the past, as was emphasized by Brawley et al. in 1970. Injuries involving the origin of the innominate or left common carotid artery, with cerebral ischemia, may be most safely managed with a temporary shunt. Experiences with shunts for injuries of this type were described recently by Ecker et al.

A number of recent case reports have described successful repair of unusual injuries of the aortic arch or its branches from either penetrating or nonpenetrating trauma. These successful experiences result from the avail-

Fig. 20-16. *Left.* Operative photograph of dissecting aneurysm of upper thoracic aorta, starting a few days before operation. The hematoma in the aortic wall is visible. *Center.* With a functioning left atrial bypass, the aorta has been occluded and the aneurysm incised. A tape encircles the left subclavian artery. The vagus nerve with the recurrent nerve encircling the aorta is visible. The aneurysm began in the classic location, just beyond the left subclavian artery. A large thrombus is present in the aortic wall. *Right.* Aortic reconstruction was accomplished with a short woven Dacron graft. The proximal anastomosis is immediately beyond the left subclavian artery.

ability of excellent angiography and the increasing trend to prompt thoracotomy with a sternotomy which provides excellent exposure of the vessels of the aortic arch. Undoubtedly in the next few years such injuries will be treated even more successfully than they have been in the past.

An unusual type of penetrating injury is one involving the intrapericardial portion of the ascending aorta; development of cardiac tamponade may temporarily control bleeding and allow more time for operation. In 1961 Dively et al. reported successful treatment of three patients with this type of unusual injury and described published experiences with others. Rarely a small penetrating injury may produce a fistula between the aorta and right ventricle, between the aorta and vena cava, or between the aorta and pulmonary artery.

Fig. 20-17. *A.* Transected aorta found at autopsy when the patient was exsanguinated 24 hours following injury. The patient had only minor chest pain before the terminal event. The sharp, transverse laceration of the aorta is the usual finding, resulting from the deceleration forces at the time of injury. *B.* Partial transection of the aorta found at autopsy when the patient was suddenly exsanguinated 3 weeks following an automobile accident. An aortic lesion had not been previously suspected.

Nonpenetrating Injuries

Traumatic injury of the aorta following blunt trauma is important to recognize, because effective surgical therapy is possible in many patients. Unfortunately the diagnosis is often not considered because of the unusual nature of the lesion. It is a frequent finding at autopsy following a fatal injury, but careful analysis of 171 cases by Parmley et al. emphasized that surgical therapy was often possible because 20 percent of the patients lived longer than 30 minutes after injury and several survived for several days before fatal hemorrhage occurred. Only in the past decade has increasing familiarity with the lesion occasionally resulted in early diagnosis and successful therapy.

ETIOLOGY AND PATHOLOGY. A rupture of the aorta is usually produced from a deceleration-type injury, typically in an automobile accident. In 70 to 75 percent of patients the aortic laceration occurs just distal to the left subclavian artery. Apparently the descending thoracic aorta and the aortic arch decelerate at different rates because of differences in anatomic structure, and a transverse tear of the aorta is produced near the site of insertion of the ligamentum arteriosum. The tear may involve part or all of the layers of the aortic wall, varying from laceration of the intima to transection of the aorta with retraction of the two ends. Part or all of the circumference of the aortic wall may be involved (Fig. 20-17). Fatal hemorrhage is prevented in some patients by the adventitia, which has been reported to constitute 60 percent of the tensile strength of the aortic wall.

The next most frequent site of injury is in the ascending aorta near its origin from the left ventricle. Other sites are very unusual and may be produced by various forms of injury, such as direct trauma or vertical deceleration injuries as in a fall from a building. A dissecting aneurysm following trauma is extremely rare.

In patients who do not exsanguinate soon after injury, a hematoma forms in the mediastinum and produces a characteristic roentgenographic appearance due to enlargement of the mediastinum. Disturbances in blood flow through the aorta usually do not occur. Only a few instances of paraplegia appearing after aortic injury from acute interruption of blood flow have been described. Following the acute injury, a latent period is often present before the mediastinal hematoma surrounding the aortic laceration suddenly ruptures into the pleural cavity and causes fatal hemorrhage. The fatal rupture almost always occurs within 4 weeks after injury. Spencer et al. described a few examples of rupture 30 to 90 days after injury.

In patients who survive longer than 2 months after injury a false aneurysm of the aorta gradually develops and may pursue an unusually benign course. Unlike the more common atherosclerotic or syphilitic aneurysms, traumatic aneurysms may remain as asymptomatic mediastinal masses for many years, or even decades, until enlargement occurs. Calcification develops in most such lesions after varying periods of time and may provide the first clue to the diagnosis when first recognized on a chest roentgenogram made for other reasons. Only a moderate amount of data is available about the long-term course of traumatic aneurysms, probably because many have been misdiagnosed as calcified atherosclerotic or syphilitic aneurysms. In 1961, in a detailed review of reported experiences with traumatic aneurysms Spencer et al. found only about 60 reported cases. Apparently most such lesions tend to enlarge after months or years, producing compression of the left main bronchus and the recurrent laryngeal nerve. With such enlargement, symptoms from obstruction of the left bronchus appear and require therapy. Usually enlargement of traumatic aneurysms proceeds slowly for a long period of time before rupture occurs, providing ample time for diagnosis and therapy.

Associated injuries are common. Most patients have fractures of the ribs, and fractures of the extremities occur in about 50 percent of patients, reflecting the severity of trauma producing the aortic injury.

CLINICAL MANIFESTATIONS. Following injury to the thorax, there are usually no symptoms or signs to indicate that an aortic injury has occurred. Dyspnea and chest pain are usually present, but these commonly result from the almost universally present rib fractures and do not aid in recognizing rupture of the aorta. A hemothorax, with varying degrees of shock, is also frequent, but again such findings frequently arise from rib fractures and pulmonary lacerations which do not involve the aorta. A murmur has been present in only a few patients. Rarely, signs of acute obstruction of the aorta, apparently from prolapse of a segment of intima with obstruction of the lumen, have occurred, with weak or absent femoral pulses and even acute paraplegia.

Patients with a traumatic aortic aneurysm who are first seen months or years following injury are often asymptomatic and are evaluated because of the accidental discovery of a mediastinal mass on a chest roentgenogram. Symptoms, if present, are usually due to compression of the left main bronchus from an expanding aneurysm, causing cough, wheeze, dyspnea, and pneumonia. Compression and paralysis of the left recurrent laryngeal nerve may produce hoarseness. (See the section on Traumatic Thoracic Aneurysms.)

DIAGNOSTIC FINDINGS. The chest roentgenogram provides the best clue to the diagnosis. In acutely injured patients with rupture of the aorta, widening of the mediastinum (Fig. 20-18) is almost invariably present. It is important to realize, however, that this may result from a hematoma arising from some cause other than rupture of the aorta. When widening of the mediastinum is recognized on the chest roentgenogram, an aortogram should be performed immediately, for only with an aortogram can the diagnosis be firmly established (Fig. 20-19). In 1976 Marsh and Sturn described six radiologic abnormalities which

Fig. 20-18. Chest roentgenogram of a patient with traumatic rupture of the thoracic aorta, illustrating the characteristic widening of the mediastinum. When this is observed following a chest injury, emergency aortography should be performed to establish the diagnosis of rupture of the thoracic aorta.

Fig. 20-19. Aortogram demonstrating traumatic rupture of the thoracic aorta distal to the left subclavian artery. The point of rupture can be seen as an irregular border of the thoracic aorta, in association with localized bulging. This angiogram represents the first instance in which emergency aortography was employed to establish firmly the diagnosis of traumatic rupture of the aorta.

were indications for the prompt performance of thoracic aortography following chest trauma. These observations were obtained from a study of 100 patients without trauma and 47 consecutive patients who underwent aortography following blunt trauma. Postponing aortography may be fatal, for the mediastinal hematoma surrounding the lacerated aorta often ruptures without any warning symptoms. In asymptomatic patients who are seen because of an undiagnosed mediastinal mass, aortography also provides the most definitive means of establishing the diagnosis.

TREATMENT. Thoracotomy should be performed as soon as possible after the diagnosis has been established. A 1961 review of all reported experiences found only one patient who had survived repair of an aortic laceration. In the subsequent 16 years, fortunately, many patients have been sucessfully treated, a result of increasing familiarity with the clinical picture combined with the availability of emergency aortography and thoracotomy.

As with thoracic aneurysms, the surgical approach is through a left posterolateral thoracotomy in the fourth intercostal space. The preference in our unit is some form of aortic bypass, usually the Gott intraaortic shunt, to minimize the risk of paraplegia during occlusion of the aorta (Fig. 20-9). An alternate approach was recently reported by Applebaum et al., describing experiences with 25 patients. In 18 treated by some method of perfusing the distal aorta, two developed paraplegia, while seven treated with simple aortic cross-clamping recovered satisfactorily. Their conclusion was that simple aortic cross-clamping might be preferable to attempts to insert a shunt. The author would disagree with this conclusion, but our data clearly indicate that a shunt per se may not prevent paraplegia. The operation was initially performed with the conventional left atriofemoral bypass, but more recently systemic heparinization has been avoided by the use of aortic shunts. A report by Kirsh et al. in 1976 described experiences with 43 patients treated over a period of 10 years. Overall survival was 70 percent with five patients dying without undergoing operation. Twenty-eight patients underwent operation within 12 hours, with the remaining nine patients undergoing operation from 24 hours to more than 5 days after hospital admission. Most repairs were completed using an external shunt. Successful repair was accomplished in 30 of the 37 patients operated on.

OBSTRUCTION OF THE SUPERIOR VENA CAVA

Obstruction of the superior vena cava produces an unusual but distinctive clinical syndrome which can be easily recognized once the diagnosis is considered. Diagnostic errors are surprisingly common, however, partly because of the infrequent occurrence and partly because of a lack of familiarity with the distinctive clinical features.

ETIOLOGY. In 70 to 80 percent of patients superior vena cava obstruction is due to a malignant neoplasm. This was true in 48 of 64 patients described by Effler and Groves and in 90 percent of 60 cases reported by Hanlon and Danis. Usually the neoplasm is a bronchogenic carcinoma

of the right upper lobe which is invading the mediastinum. Less frequently seen are primary mediastinal tumors, such as thymoma or lymphoma. Metastatic neoplasms from a distant source are unusual.

In the past, saccular aneurysms were found in about 30 percent of patients with vena cava obstruction, but with the marked decrease in frequency of syphilitic aneurysms, these are now infrequently seen. If superior vena cava obstruction is not due to a malignant tumor, a chronic fibrosing mediastinitis, usually of unknown origin, is the most common cause. Probably many of the cases undiagnosed in the past were due to histoplasmosis. Obstruction from a benign tumor, such as a substernal thyroid, is unusual.

PATHOPHYSIOLOGY. With obstruction of the superior vena cava there is an increase in venous pressure in its tributaries in the arms and head to levels ranging between 200 and 500 cm of water. The degree of increase in venous pressure varies with the rate of development and the site of the obstruction. Obstruction proximal to the site of entry of the azygos vein is more disabling than more distal sites of obstruction in which a patent azygos vein can function as a collateral pathway. Acute obstruction of the vena cava, as during a thoracic operation, can produce fatal cerebral edema within a few minutes. At the opposite extreme are instances where superior vena cava obstruction develops slowly, permitting time for the development of collateral circulation, as a result of which symptoms are mild.

CLINICAL MANIFESTATIONS. With mild obstruction, frequent symptoms are headache, swelling of the eyelids, puffiness of the face, or enlargement of the neck. In males there may be a noticeable increase in collar size. The severity of symptoms is closely related to posture, for the patient quickly notes that his symptoms increase if he bends over or lies down. If obstruction of the vena cava develops rapidly, as with hemorrhage into a rapidly growing neoplasm, more serious symptoms of cerebral congestion are present, including drowsiness and blurring of vision. Edema of the vocal cords may produce hoarseness or dyspnea. As the majority of cases are due to a rapidly growing bronchogenic carcinoma, pulmonary symptoms such as cough and hemoptysis are also frequently present. In most patients death results in a few months.

In the minority of patients in whom obstruction is due to a benign process, collateral circulation may enlarge sufficiently to where little disability is present. Prominent features include dilated veins with edema and cyanosis, the degree varying with the degree of stasis. Venous hypertension is manifested by prominence and distension of the veins. Effler and Groves have reported 16 patients with obstruction from a benign process, all of whom eventually developed sufficient collateral circulation to have minimal symptoms; there were no fatalities as a direct result of the chronic venous obstruction. We have observed one patient over a period of 20 years in whom the superior vena cava was obstructed following an intracardiac operation for correction of anomalous pulmonary veins entering the superior vena cava. Initially there was serious venous hypertension to levels of 350 cm of water, producing a bilateral chylothorax ultimately controlled by ligation of the thoracic duct. Within a few months, however, all symptoms subsided, and the patient, now a young married woman with children, has no limitation of physical activities.

DIAGNOSTIC STUDIES. Although the clinical picture is characteristic when fully developed, early manifestations of the disease, such as swelling of the eyes or headache, may be confused with angioneurotic edema, congestive heart failure, or constrictive pericarditis. The diagnosis can be confirmed by measuring the venous pressure, which is usually in the range of 200 to 500 cm of water. The location and extent of the obstruction can be best outlined by venography. In some patients the underlying disease process is uncertain, although usually signs of a bronchogenic carcinoma are visible on a chest roentgenogram. Bronchoscopy and biopsy may be helpful in confirming the diagnosis. Aortography can be used if necessary to exclude the presence of an aneurysm.

TREATMENT. With a malignant process, involvement of the superior vena cava almost precludes surgical resection, although isolated exceptions have been reported. Thoracotomy is a serious undertaking, encountering serious bleeding from the venous hypertension. If a diagnosis can be established without thoracotomy—e.g., by bronchoscopy, mediastinoscopy, or biopsy of a peripheral node—it may be preferable to proceed directly to radiation rather than perform a thoracotomy.

Significant palliation can be obtained by intensive radiation therapy, often in combination with diuretics and chemotherapy. Improvement in symptoms soon occurs, probably from diminution in edema associated with a growing neoplasm. Death from the neoplasm, however, usually occurs within a few months.

With benign obstructions, the report of Effler and Groves clearly indicates that there is no urgency in performing an operation if symptoms are mild. In all likelihood symptoms will improve or subside completely as collateral circulation develops. A number of ingenious attempts have been made to reconstruct an obstructed superior vena cava. Prosthetic grafts have been almost uniformly unsuccessful, with the possible exception of a crimped Teflon graft, which experimentally has given the best results. The most favorable graft is a composite one of autogenous veins, prepared by combining both superficial femoral veins into a graft of larger diameter. Good results lasting for several years have been reported by Hanlon and Danis in three patients in whom such grafts were used.

A good collective review was published by Gomes and Hufnagel in 1975, describing experiences with two patients and reviewing previous reports by others. Methods of constructing a large composite vein graft from the saphenous vein were described by Doty and Baker in 1976. The experimental studies with Gore-Tex, a type of polyethylene, may eventually find applicability in treatment of this unusual condition.

Rarely a localized granuloma may compress and thrombose the vena cava; patency can be restored by opening the vein and removing the clot. Three such cases have been reported by Pate and Hammon and one such patient by Hanlon and Danis. Other ingenious attempts to bypass the obstructed vena cava, applicable in certain specific in-

stances, have been reported. Cooley and Hallman rotated the azygos vein to provide a bypass route for draining blood directly into the atrium, while Schramel and Olinde reversed the saphenous vein in a subcutaneous tunnel to drain blood from the superior vena cava system to the common femoral vein.

References

Aneurysms of the Ascending Aorta

Bahnson, H. T., and Spencer, F. C.: Excision of Aneurysm of the Ascending Aorta with Prosthetic Replacement during Cardiopulmonary Bypass, *Ann Surg,* **151:**879, 1960.

Bloodwell, R. D., Hallman, G. L., and Cooley, D. A.: Aneurysm of the Ascending Aorta with Aortic Valvular Insufficiency, *Arch Surg,* **92:**588, 1966.

Connors, J. P., Ferguson, T. B., Weldon, C. S., and Roper, C. L.: The Use of the TDMAC Heparin Shunt in Replacement of Descending Thoracic Aorta, *Ann Surg,* **181:**735, 1975.

Griepp, R. B., Stinson, E. B., Hollingsworth, J. F., and Buehler, D.: Prosthetic Replacement of the Aortic Arch, *J Thorac Cardiovasc Surg,* **70:**1051, 1975.

Kidd, J. N., Reul, G. J., Cooley, D. A., Sandeford, F. M., Kyger, E. R., III, and Wukasch, D. C.: Surgical Treatment of Aneurysms of the Ascending Aorta, *Circulation,* **54**(Suppl. III):118, 1976.

Kouchoukos, N. T., Karp, R. B., and Lell, W. A.: Replacement of the Ascending Aorta and Aortic Valve with a Composite Graft: Results in 25 Patients, *Ann Thorac Surg,* **24:**140, 1977.

Liddicott, J. E., Bekassy, S. M., Rubio, P. A., Noon, G. P., and DeBakey, M. E.: Ascending Aortic Aneurysms: Review of 100 Consecutive Cases, *Circulation,* **51–52**(Suppl. 1):202, 1975.

Liotta, D., Hallman, G. L., Milam, J. D., and Cooley, D. A.: Surgical Treatment of Acute Dissecting Aneurysm of the Ascending Aorta, *Ann Thorac Surg,* **12:**582, 1971.

Shumacker, H. B., Jr.: Operative Treatment of Aneurysms of the Thoracic Aorta Due to Cystic Medial Necrosis, *J Thorac Cardiovasc Surg,* **63:**1, 1972.

Spencer, F. C., and Blake, H. A.: A Report of the Successful Surgical Treatment of Aortic Regurgitation from a Dissecting Aortic Aneurysm in a Patient with the Marfan Syndrome, *J Thorac Cardiovasc Surg,* **44:**238, 1962.

Weldon, C. S., Ferguson, T. B., Ludbrook, P. A., and Mcknight, R. C.: A New Operation for Far-Advanced Cystic Medial Necrosis of the Aortic Root, *Ann Thorac Surg,* **23:**499, 1977.

Zubiate, P., and Kay, J. H.: Surgical Treatment of Aneurysm of the Ascending Aorta with Aortic Insufficiency and Marked Displacement of the Coronary Ostia, *J Thorac Cardiovasc Surg,* **71:**415, 1976.

Aneurysms of the Transverse Aortic Arch

Allard, J. R., Williams, R. L., and Dobell, A. R. C.: Interrupted Aortic Arch: Factors Influencing Prognosis *Ann Thorac Surg* **21:**243, 1976.

Bloodwell, R. D., Hallman, G. L., and Cooley, D. A.: Total Replacement of the Aortic Arch and the "Subclavian Steal" Phenomenon, *Ann Thorac Surg,* **5:**236, 1968.

DeBakey, M. E., Beall, A. C., Jr., Cooley, D. A., Crawford, E. S., Morris, G. C., Jr., and Garrett, H. E.: Resection and Graft

Replacement of Aneurysms Involving the Transverse Arch of the Aorta, *Surg Clin North Am,* **46:**1057, 1966.

Griepp, R. B., Stinson, E. B., Hollingsworth, J. F., and Buehler, D.: Prosthetic Replacement of the Aortic Arch, *J Thorac Cardiovasc Surg,* **70:**1051, 1975.

Lefrak, E. A., Stevens, P. M., and Howell, J. F.: Respiratory Insufficiency Due to Tracheal Compression by an Aneurysm of the Ascending, Transverse, and Descending Thoracic Aorta: Successful Surgical Management, *J Thorac Cardiovasc Surg,* **63:**956, 1972.

Traumatic Thoracic Aneurysms

Bennett, D. E., and Cherry, J. K.: The Natural History of Traumatic Aneurysms of the Aorta, *Surgery,* **61:**516, 1967.

Connors, J. P., Ferguson, T. B., Weldon, C. S., and Roper, C. L.: The Use of the TDMAC Heparin Shunt in Replacement of Descending Thoracic Aorta, *Ann Surg,* **181:**735, 1975.

Cooley, D. A.: Discussion of R. J. Stoney, B. B. Roe, and J. V. Redington, Rupture of Thoracic Aorta Due to Closed-Chest Trauma, *Arch Surg,* **89:**840, 1964.

Donahoo, J. S., Brawley, R. K., and Gott, V. L.: The Heparin-Coated Vascular Shunt for Thoracic Aortic and Great Vessel Procedures: A Ten Year Experience, *Ann Thorac Surg,* **23:**507, 1977.

Kirsh, M. M., Behrendt, D. M., Orringer, M. B., Gago, O., Gray, L. A., Jr., Milts, L. J., Walter, J. F., and Sloan, H.: The Treatment of Acute Traumatic Rupture of the Aorta: A 10 Year Experience, *Ann Surg,* **184:**308, 1976.

Marsh, D. G., and Sturm, J. T.: Traumatic Aortic Rupture: Roentgenographic Indications for Angiography, *Ann Thorac Surg,* **21:**337, 1976.

Spencer, F. C., Guerin, P. F., Blake, H. A., and Bahnson, H. T.: A Report of Fifteen Patients with Traumatic Rupture of the Thoracic Aorta, *J Thorac Cardiovasc Surg,* **41:**1, 1961.

Aneurysms of the Descending Thoracic Aorta

Bahnson, H. T.: Definitive Treatment of Saccular Aneurysms of the Aorta with Excision of the Sac and Aortic Suture, *Surg Gynecol Obstet,* **96:**382, 1953.

Bloodwell, R. D., Hallman, G. L., Beall, A. C., Jr., Cooley, D. A., and DeBakey, M. E.: Aneurysms of the Descending Thoracic Aorta: Surgical Considerations, *Surg Clin North Am,* **46:**901, 1966.

Connolly, J. E., Kountz, S. L., and Boyd, R. J.: Left Heart Bypass: Experimental and Clinical Observations on its Regulation with Particular Reference to Maintenance of Maximal Renal Blood Flow, *J Thorac Cardiovasc Surg,* **44:**577, 1962.

Crawford, E. S., and Rubio, P. A.: Reappraisal of Adjuncts To Avoid Ischemia in the Treatment of Aneurysms of Descending Thoracic Aorta, *J Thorac Cardiovasc Surg,* **66:**693, 1973.

DeBakey, M. E., Cooley, D. A., Crawford, E. S., and Morris, G. C., Jr.: Aneurysms of the Thoracic Aorta. Analysis of 179 Patients Treated by Resection, *J Thorac Surg,* **36:**393, 1958.

Donahoo, J. S., Brawley, R. K., and Gott, V. L.: The Heparin-Coated Vascular Shunt for Thoracic Aortic and Great Vessel Procedures: A Ten Year Experience, *Ann Thorac Surg,* **23:**507, 1977.

Gerbode, F., Braimbridge, M., Osborn, J. J., Hood, J., and French, S.: Traumatic Thoracic Aneurysms: Treatment by Resection and Grafting with the Use of Extracorporeal Bypass, *Surgery,* **42:**975, 1957.

Kahn, D. R., Vathayanon, S., and Sloan, H.: Resection of Descending Thoracic Aneurysms without Left Heart Bypass, *Arch Surg,* **97:**336, 1968.

Krauss, A. H., Ferguson, T. V., and Weldon, C. S.: Thoracic Aneurysmectomy Using the Tedmac Heparin Shunt, *Ann Thorac Surg,* **14:**123, 1972.

Reul, G. J., Jr., Cooley, D. A., Hallman, G. L., Reddy, S. B., Kyger, E. R., III, and Wukasch, D. C.: Dissecting Aneurysm of Descending Aorta: Improved Surgical Results in 91 Patients, *Arch Surg,* **110:**632, 1975.

Vasko, J. S., Spencer, F. C., and Bahnson, H. T.: Aneurysm of the Aorta Treated by Excision: Review of 237 Cases Followed Up to Seven Years, *Am J Surg,* **105:**793, 1963.

Wechsler, A. S., and Wolfe, W. G.: Heparinless Shunting during Cross-clamping of the Thoracic Aorta, *Ann Thorac Surg,* **23:**497, 1977.

Thoracoabdominal Aneurysms

Crawford, E. S., and Rubio, P. A.: Reappraisal of Adjuncts to Avoid Ischemia in the Treatment of Aneurysms of Descending Thoracic Aorta, *J Thorac Cardiovasc Surg,* **66:**693, 1973.

DeBakey, M. E., Crawford, E. S., Garrett, H. E., Beall, A. C., Jr., and Howell, J. F.: Surgical Considerations in the Treatment of Aneurysms of the Thoraco-abdominal Aorta, *Ann Surg,* **162:**650, 1965.

Garrett, H. E., Crawford, E. S., Beall, A. C., Jr., Howell, J. F., and DeBakey, M. E.: Surgical Treatment of Aneurysm of the Thoracoabdominal Aorta, *Surg Clin North Am,* **46:**913, 1966.

Dissecting Aneurysms

Appelbaum, A., Karp, R. B., and Kirklin, J. W.: Ascending versus Descending Aortic Dissection, *Ann Surg,* **183:**296, 1976.

Austen, W. G., Buckley, M. J., McFarland, J., DeSanctis, R. W., and Sanders, C. A.: Therapy of Dissecting Aneurysms, *Arch Surg,* **95:**835, 1967.

Daily, P. O., Trueblood, H. W., Stinson, E. B., Wuerflein, R. D., and Shumway, N. E.: Management of Acute Aortic Dissections, *Ann Thorac Surg,* **10:**337, 1970.

DeBakey, M. E., Henly, W. S., Cooley, D. A., Morris, G. C., Crawford, E. S., and Beall, A. C.: Surgical Management of Dissecting Aneurysms of the Aorta, *J Thorac Cardiovasc Surg,* **49:**130, 1965.

Gryboski, W., and Spencer, F. C.: Intermittent Claudication Caused by a Dissecting Aneurysm of the Aorta, *South Med J,* **58:**593, 1965.

Harris, P. D., Malm, J. R., Bigger, J. T., and Bowman, F. O.: Follow-up Studies of Acute Dissecting Aortic Aneurysms Managed with Antihypertensive Agents, *Circulation,* **35** (*Suppl* 1): I-183, 1967.

Hirst, A. E., Johns, V. J., and Kime, S. W.: Dissecting Aneurysm of the Aorta: A Review of 505 Cases, *Medicine (Baltimore),* **37:**217, 1958.

Lindsay, J., and Hurst, J. W.: Clinical Features and Prognosis in Dissecting Aneurysm of the Aorta, *Circulation,* **35:**880, 1967.

Liotta, D., Hallman, G. L., Milam, J. D., and Cooley, D. A.: Surgical Treatment of Acute Dissecting Aneurysm of the Ascending Aorta, *Ann Thorac Surg,* **12:**582, 1971.

McCloy, R. M., Spittell, J. A., and McGoon, D. C.: The Prognosis of Aortic Dissection (Dissecting Aortic Hematoma or Aneurysm), *Circulation,* **31:**665, 1965.

Najafi, H., Dye, W. S., Javid, H., Hunter, J. A., Goldin, M. D., and Julian, O. C.: Acute Aortic Regurgitation Secondary to Aortic Dissection: Surgical Management without Valve Replacement, *Ann Thorac Surg,* **14:**474, 1972.

Schumacker, H. B., Jr.: Operative Treatment of Aneurysms of the Thoracic Aorta Due to Cystic Medial Necrosis, *J Thorac Cardiovasc Surg,* **63:**1, 1972.

Spencer, F. C., and Blake, H. A.: A Report of the Successful Surgical Treatment of Aortic Regurgitation from a Dissecting Aortic Aneurysm in a Patient with the Marfan Syndrome, *J Thorac Cardiovasc Surg,* **44:**238, 1962.

Wheat, M. W., Jr., and Palmer, R. F.: Dissecting Aneurysms of the Aorta, *Curr Probl Surg,* July 1971.

———, ———, Bartley, T. D., and Seelman, R. C.: Treatment of Dissecting Aneurysms of the Aorta without Surgery, *J Thorac Cardiovasc Surg,* **50:**364, 1965.

Wounds of the Great Vessels

Applebaum, A., Karp, R. B., and Kirklin, J. W.: Surgical Treatment for Closed Thoracic Aortic Injuries, *J Thorac Cardiovasc Surg,* **71** (3): 458, 1976.

Bennett, D. E., and Cherry, D. K.: The Natural History of Traumatic Aneurysms of the Aorta, *Surgery,* **61:**516, 1967.

Blake, H. A., Inmon, T. W., and Spencer, F. C.: Emergency Use of Antegrade Aortography in Diagnosis of Acute Aortic Rupture, *Ann Surg,* **152:**954, 1960.

Brawley, R. K., Murray, G. F., Crisler, C., and Cameron, J. L.: Management of Wounds of the Innominate, Subclavian, and Axillary Blood Vessels, *Surg Gynecol Obstet,* **131:**1130, 1970.

Castagna, J., and Nelson, R. J.: Blunt Injuries to Branches of Aortic Arch, *J Thorac Cardiovasc Surg,* **69:**521, 1975.

Clarke, C. P., Brandt, P. W. T., Cole, D. S., and Barratt-Boyes, B. G.: Traumatic Rupture of the Thoracic Aorta: Diagnosis and Treatment, *Br J Surg,* **54:**353, 1967.

DeMuth, W. E., Jr., Roe, H., and Hobbie, W.: Immediate Repair of Traumatic Rupture of Thoracic Aorta, *Arch Surg,* **91:**602, 1965.

Dively, W. L., Daniel, R. A., and Scott, H. W.: Surgical Management of Penetrating Injuries of the Ascending Aorta and Aortic Arch, *J Thorac Cardiovasc Surg,* **41:**23, 1961.

Ecker, R. R., Dickinson, W. E., Sugg, W. L., and Rea, W. J.: Management of Injuries of the Innominate and Proximal Left Common Carotid Artery, *J Thorac Cardiovasc Surg,* **64:**618, 1972.

Gerbode, F., Braimbridge, M., Osborn, J. J., Hood, M., and French, S.: Traumatic Thoracic Aneurysm: Treatment by Resection and Grafting with the Use of Extracorporeal Bypass, *Surgery,* **42:**975, 1957.

Jahnke, E. J., Jr., Fisher, G. W., and Jones, R. C.: Acute Traumatic Rupture of the Thoracic Aorta: Report of Six Consecutive Cases of Successful Early Repair, *J Thorac Cardiovasc Surg,* **48:**63, 1964.

Kahn, A. M., Joseph, W. L., and Hughes, R. K.: Traumatic Aneurysms of the Thoracic Aorta: Excision and Repair without Graft, *Ann Thorac Surg,* **4:**175, 1967.

Kirsh, M. M., Behrendt, D. M., Orringer, M. B., Gago, O., Gray, L. A., Jr., Mills, L. J., Walter, J. F., and Sloan, H.: The Treatment of Acute Traumatic Rupture of the Aorta: A 10 Year Experience, *Ann Surg,* **184:**308, 1976.

Marsh, D. G., and Sturm, J. T.: Traumatic Aortic Rupture: Roentgenographic Indications for Angiography, *Ann Thorac Surg,* **21** (4): 337, 1976.

Parmley, L. F., Mattingly, T. W., and Manion, W. C.: Penetrating Wounds to the Heart and Aorta, *Circulation,* **17:**953, 1958.

———, ———, ———, and Jahnke, E. J., Jr.: Non-penetrating Traumatic Injury of the Aorta, *Circulation,* **17:**1086, 1958.

Spencer, F. C., Guerin, P. F., Blake, H. A., and Bahnson, H. T.: A Report of 15 Patients with Traumatic Rupture of the Thoracic Aorta, *J Thorac Cardiovasc Surg,* **41:**1, 1961.

Steenburg, R. W., and Ravitch, M. M.: Cervico-thoracic Approach for Subclavian Vessel Injury from Compound Fracture of the Clavicle: Considerations of Subclavian Axillary Exposures, *Ann Surg,* **157:**839, 1963.

Symbas, P. N., Tyras, D. H., Ware, R. E., and Hatcher, C. R., Jr.: Rupture of the Aorta: A Diagnostic Triad, *Ann Thorac Surg,* **15:**405, 1973.

Obstruction of the Superior Vena Cava

Cooley, D. A., and Hallman, G. L.: Superior Vena Caval Syndrome Treated by Azygos Vein–Inferior Vena Cava Anastomosis: Report of Successful Case, *J Thorac Cardiovasc Surg,* **47:**325, 1964.

Doty, D. B., and Baker, W. H.: Bypass of Superior Cava with Spiral Vein Graft, *Ann Thorac Surg,* **22:**490, 1976.

Effler, D. B., and Groves, L. K.: Superior Vena Caval Obstruction, *J Thorac Cardiovasc Surg,* **43:**574, 1962.

Gomes, M. N., and Hufnagel, C. A.: Superior Vena Cava Obstruction: Review of Literature and Report of Two Cases Due to Benign Intrathoracic Tumors, *Ann Thorac Surg,* **20:**344, 1975.

Hanlon, C. R., and Danis, R. K.: Superior Vena Caval Obstruction: Indications for Diagnostic Thoracotomy, *Ann Surg,* **161:**771, 1965.

Heydorn, W. H., Zajtchuk, R., Miller, F., and Schuchmann, G. F.: Gore-Tex Grafts for Replacement of the Superior Vena Cava, *Ann Thorac Surg,* **23:**539, 1977.

Pate, J. W., and Hammon, J.: Superior Vena Cava Syndrome Due to Histoplasmosis in Children, *Ann Surg,* **161:**778, 1965.

Schramel, R., and Olinde, H. D. H.: A New Method of Bypassing the Obstructed Vena Cava, *J Thorac Cardiovasc Surg,* **41:**375, 1961.

Chapter 21

Peripheral Arterial Disease

by Anthony M. Imparato and Frank C. Spencer

INTRODUCTION

Progress in vascular surgery has been so rapid since 1950 that it is difficult for a student of medicine at this time to realize that most of the vascular operations commonly performed today scarcely had been considered 30 years ago. For perspective, an historical review is worthwhile.

Prior to 1900, progress was greatly hampered by the lack of anesthesia and asepsis. Nevertheless in 1888 Matas reported his successful operation upon a patient with a traumatic aneurysm of the brachial artery upon whom he performed the first endoaneurysmorrhaphy. Nine years later (1897) Murphy performed the first end-to-end arterial anastomosis in man following excision of an arteriovenous fistula in the thigh. He performed a total of 34 experiments in dogs, sheep, and calves to evaluate methods of vascular suture prior to performing this first procedure in man. By 1906, Carrel and Guthrie developed many of the techniques of vascular surgery which are still in use today. Soon thereafter autogenous vein grafts were successfully used following excision of aneurysms. In 1915 Bernheim used a vein graft in man for the first time in the United States in treating a patient with a syphilitic popliteal aneurysm.

After World War I a curious lag occurred in vascular surgery until the 1940s, when the epochal work of Blalock, Gross, and Crafoord with tetralogy of Fallot, patent ductus arteriosus, and coarctation of the aorta launched the modern era of vascular surgery. The development of atraumatic vascular clamps by Potts, in conjunction with fine arterial sutures with swaged needles, greatly facilitated the techniques of vascular operations. The introduction of aortic homografts for repair of coarctation of the aorta by Gross stimulated intensive investigation of vascular prostheses. The successful excision of an abdominal aneurysm with replacement by an aortic homograft was reported by Dubost et al. in 1952, and in the same year Voorhees et al. reported the first use of a cloth material, Vinyon N, as a vascular prosthesis. Within the next 5 years this stimulated the development of the presently used vascular prostheses of Dacron and Teflon, with many contributions made by DeBakey, Cooley, Bahnson, Wesolowski, and others. The increasing use of arteriography, along with the development of safer radiopaque media, greatly enhanced further development of reconstructive surgery. Between 1955 and 1960 operations for carotid artery stenosis and renal artery stenosis were first done. With these many advances in both diagnostic and therapeutic surgical techniques the scope of vascular surgery has increased to the stage where it has become an increasingly large segment of surgical practice.

Since peripheral arterial diseases lend themselves to broad classification as occlusive, aneurysmal, and vasospastic the topics in this chapter are grouped in a sequence representing these three broad categories.

OCCLUSIVE DISEASE OF THE LOWER EXTREMITIES

Clinical Manifestations

HISTORY. The ischemic basis for symptoms can be strongly suspected from the history, which varies markedly depending upon whether ischemia develops acutely, as in embolic occlusion of arteries, or slowly, which is more characteristic of thrombotic occlusions. The key symptom which requires elaboration is *pain*. The characteristics of pain are related to the abruptness of the onset of arterial occlusion and the severity of the ischemia. When arterial interruption occurs abruptly, pain is usually sudden in onset and severe, and involves the entire portion of the extremity supplied by that artery. Characteristically, acute popliteal occlusion results in excruciating pain of the entire extremity below the knee, while common femoral occlusion produces a painful foot, calf, and thigh. Aortoiliac occlusions may result in pain in the lower half of the body. The pain, often associated with numbness, persists until one of three events occurs: (1) the ischemia is relieved by reopening the artery surgically, (2) the opening of the collateral channels over periods of days or weeks, (3) persistence of ischemia, resulting in nerves which are destroyed and consequent anesthesia of the affected limb. When arterial occlusion develops over longer periods of time ischemia may be subtle and may not become manifest until there are demands for blood beyond basal requirements, such as with exercise. Pain is experienced during exertion and gradually disappears within minutes upon cessation of activity. This represents the characteristic symptom of *intermittent claudication,* the most common complaint produced by limb ischemia. The areas which are felt to be painful are usually those requiring the largest amount of blood during exertion, viz., muscle groups.

With acute arterial occlusions, the level of arterial obstruction can often be diagnosed from the history, since exertional muscle pain occurs approximately one joint distal to the site of occlusion. Characteristically, superficial femoral occlusion causes pain in the calf, while external iliac occlusion results in thigh pain, and aortic occlusion is manifest by buttock pain. A characteristic finding in the diabetic who may have only tibial arterial occlusion is that of tightening of the ankle and foot on exertion.

Chronic arterial occlusion may progress, and intermit-

tent pain involving muscle groups may be supplanted by continuous *pain at rest* referred to the sites most distal to the arterial occlusion, viz., toes, feet, fingers, hands. The large muscle groups which are the first to express the ischemic state are almost never the site of rest pain in chronic arterial occlusions. Even rest pain is distinguishable by history from other types of foot or hand pain. Rest pain is worsened by elevation of the extremity, even to the supine position, and is relieved by placing the extremity in the dependent position. Patients with pain related to diabetic neuropathy report no such positional dependence.

Other aspects of history which are critically important include smoking, diabetes, cardiac disorders, trauma, familial disease, and occupational history, as well as drug therapy.

PHYSICAL EXAMINATION. Physical examination is of paramount importance in assessing the presence and severity of vascular disease. In this regard physical examination is relatively of greater importance than with abdominal or thoracic problems, where laboratory investigations play a more dominant role. Particular attention to the color, temperature, and pulse pattern of the extremities involved is required and usually permits estimation of the level of arterial occlusion, the severity of ischemia, and the abruptness of the onset. Acute arterial occlusion characteristically produces marked color and temperature differences; chronic occlusion may produce no visible changes but only a difference in palpable pulses early in the course of disease. When acute occlusion progresses to gangrene it is manifest frequently as "wet" gangrene, with blebs, bullae, and violaceous discoloration. When chronic occlusion progresses gradually to severe ischemia, characteristic changes associated with atrophy appear and progress to localized tissue necrosis, manifested by ulceration. The final stage is usually the mummification characteristic of dry gangrene, which starts peripherally in the toes and extends proximally to involve the entire foot and leg. Palpation of the peripheral pulses is the most important feature of the examination. In the lower extremity, the femoral, popliteal, posterior tibial, and dorsalis pedis pulses should be noted. It is important to remember that the common femoral artery extends only about 5 cm below the inguinal ligament before bifurcating into the profunda femoris and superficial femoral arteries. In the upper extremity the brachial, radial, and ulnar pulses should be noted. In many patients it is possible to feel the digital pulses at the bases of the phalanges. The integrity of the palmar arterial arches can be tested by the performance of the Allen test. This is done by having the patient make a tight fist, then occluding the radial and ulnar arteries at the wrist and having the patient slowly open the hand. With the hand in a relaxed position, the integrity of the radial artery in the hand is determined by releasing radial compression and noting the return of color. The maneuver is repeated releasing the ulnar artery while the radial remains compressed. The ability to determine definitely the presence or absence of a peripheral pulse is one of the most essential features of an adequate evaluation of the peripheral circulation.

With chronic ischemia, characteristic nutritional changes

develop in the feet. These include the loss of hair from the toes, the development of brittle, opaque nails, the appearance of atrophy and rubor in the skin, and atrophy of muscles of the feet with increasing prominence of the interosseous spaces. Hence, a simple glance at a foot can determine the presence or absence of serious vascular disease. The importance of this evaluation is emphasized by the fact that gangrene seldom appears in an extremity with chronic vascular disease until these stigmata of chronic ischemia have appeared.

Characteristic color changes also appear with advanced arterial insufficiency, consisting of a purplish rubor in dependency, changing to pallor when the extremity is elevated. The colors are quite different from the chronic congested extremity with venous insufficiency.

The location of ulcerations offers a major clue to cause, for ulceration from venous insufficiency is virtually unknown below the level of the malleolus. By contrast, most ulcers from arterial insufficiency begin over the toes, corresponding to the most distal parts of the arterial tree. Rarely ischemic ulcers develop on the leg or about the ankle without involvement of the toes, perhaps as a result of local tissue infarction, especially after localized trauma, or from arterioarterial embolization.

Palpation of the extremity for temperature and moisture may provide useful information, especially with vasospastic conditions with increased sympathetic tone, where the cool, sweaty extremity affords an important clue to the diagnosis.

Auscultation is of value for certain disorders, particularly arteriovenous fistulas, where detection of the classic continuous murmur quickly establishes the diagnosis. With localized stenotic lesions in peripheral arteries, usually from atherosclerotic plaques, a systolic bruit may be heard, promptly confirming the presence of arterial stenosis.

Estimation of venous filling time is of some value in the diagnosis of arterial insufficiency, but the test is of no value where incompetent valves are present in the venous system. In the absence of varicosities, the test is performed by elevation of the extremities until collapse of the veins has occurred. The extremities are then quickly lowered, and the time required for the veins to fill, usually on the dorsum of the foot or hand, is noted. Normally venous filling will occur within 10 to 15 seconds. Prolonged filling frequently denotes arterial insufficiency. Venous filling times of longer than 1 minute denote a very high degree of arterial compromise.

An oscillometer may be of some value in extremities with edema where peripheral pulses may be difficult to palpate. This instrument consists of a blood pressure cuff attached to a manometer and provides a method for evaluating pulsatile oscillations when the cuff is inflated to just above diastolic pressure. It is of value for specific problems such as determining that a palpable pulse is distal to a markedly stenotic or occluded artery. Other special instruments which can be used in the office or at the bedside to quantify the degree of ischemia and determine prognosis have limited usefulness. Doppler instruments, as well as other types of pulse recorders, may give information regarding the patency of particular distal arteries such as the dorsalis pedis or the posterior tibial. Pressures in these arteries may be determined by the use of a standard blood pressure cuff applied to the calf or ankle, inflated to above arterial systolic pressure, and released as one listens with the Doppler instrument over the vessel. As with the oscillometer, these determinations are most useful for defining arterial occlusions or stenoses proximal to palpable distal pulses.

The general physical examination is important to determine whether there are any underlying or associated disorders and whether there are additional areas of arterial involvement detectable by finding absent pulses elsewhere or bruits over arteries such as the carotids. It is vital to know about the presence of aneurysms in the abdomen, groins, or thorax. Examination of the heart is essential to determine whether there are valvular lesions, rhythm disorders, or congenital lesions which might serve as the nidus for thromboemboli.

LABORATORY EXAMINATION. The most important laboratory examination by far is selective arteriography to outline the location and extent of arterial obstruction. Selection of the appropriate method of examination varies with the disease present, for virtually every artery in the body can now be successfully outlined by appropriate catheter angiography. Percutaneous introduction of the arterial catheter is the most frequently employed technique. Arteriography may not be essential to confirm the diagnosis but is important to evaluate the possibilities of successful therapy. Illustrative angiograms are shown in specific disease sections in this chapter.

Other techniques for evaluating peripheral circulation are of little clinical value and are utilized mostly for investigative studies. These include precise measurements of skin temperature, sweating, plethysmography, radioactive isotope clearing rates, and various Doppler studies.

Manifestations of Acute Arterial Occlusion

Recognition of acute arterial occlusion is vital, since it may progress to ischemic necrosis within hours. A thrombus propagates distally as well as proximally to the point where it lodges, occluding collateral channels, thereby worsening the ischemia. Thrombosis may occlude the venous system as well, making restoration of flow impossible.

Acute occlusion usually appears without specific warning symptoms. Prompt diagnosis can be made only if the clinical picture is quickly recognized. This is essential for successful therapy, because within 4 to 8 hours after acute occlusion ischemic necrosis in the involved muscles may become irreversible. An additional feature in the pathogenesis of acute arterial occlusion that emphasizes the time factor is the tendency for thrombi to develop in the arteries distal to the point of occlusion where the flow of blood is either decreased or stagnant. This development superimposed upon the acute obstruction, makes surgical therapy to restore circulation much more difficult. With persisting ischemia, thrombosis finally develops in the venous system as well, making surgical therapy impossible.

The usual causes of acute arterial occlusion are embolism, trauma, or thrombosis. Thrombosis of a previously undiagnosed aneurysm, such as a popliteal aneurysm, is a less frequent cause. Each of these is discussed in subsequent sections. Embolism is noteworthy in that it often appears without any previous signs of underlying disease as an acute catastrophe involving an extremity. In many it is the first symptom of serious underlying heart disease: mitral stenosis, atrial fibrillation, or myocardial infarction. Arterial trauma, when occurring as an isolated injury, may be easily recognized. When complicated with associated fractures or head injuries, the diagnosis may be difficult.

FIVE P's. For emphasis the five prominent features of acute arterial occlusion may be summarized as five p's: *p*ain, *p*aralysis, *p*aresthesia, *p*allor, and absence of *p*ulses.

Pain is present in 75 to 80 percent of patients with acute arterial occlusion, representing the onset of ischemia in the involved tissues. It is absent in some patients, apparently from the prompt onset of complete anesthesia and paralysis. In others, when collateral circulation minimizes the degree of ischemia produced, pain may also be minimal.

Paralysis and paresthesias (or anesthesia) are the most important symptoms in evaluating the severity of arterial occlusion. The importance of these features is based on the fact that the peripheral nerve endings are the most sensitive tissues to anoxia in an extremity. A familiar illustration of the sensitivity of sensory nerve endings to anoxia is the common experience of one's foot "going to sleep" while one sits with the extremity flexed in an unusual position. The sensitivity of striated muscles to anoxia is almost as great as that of nerve endings. Hence, an extremity with paralysis and paresthesia will almost surely develop gangrene, while, conversely, if motor and sensory function are intact even though signs of ischemia are present, gangrene probably will not occur. The neurologic findings then are an important clue both to the urgency of prompt therapy and in the evaluation of the effectiveness of therapy in restoring circulation. Recognition that a paralysed anesthetic extremity will develop gangrene in most patients within 6 to 8 hours after onset emphasizes the urgency of immediate treatment.

Pallor is a less important sign, representing varying degrees of decreased circulation. Associated with visible pallor may be the sensation of coldness.

Absence of pulses confirms the diagnosis and localizes the point of occlusion. With uncertainty, as in an edematous extremity, an oscillometer may be of some value in confirming the absence of pulses. When palpation is indeterminate, the presence of neurologic symptoms indicates the urgency of deciding whether arterial occlusion is present. A frequent example is seen in a patient with a swollen extremity with a fracture of the femur in whom swelling of the extremity may make palpation of the pulses difficult. To determine whether or not an associated injury of the femoral artery is present may require arteriography. If neurologic symptoms are present, angiography should be performed on an emergency basis.

Manifestations of Chronic Arterial Occlusion

The picture of chronic progressive arterial ischemia is typically seen with atherosclerosis involving the abdominal aorta and its branches to the lower extremities, including the iliac, femoral, and popliteal arteries. The course of the disease may be a gradual, progressive one, or it may be interrupted with acute episodes of segmental arterial thrombosis or minor traumatic injuries to the toes resulting in gangrene. The disease almost always is due to atherosclerosis with its protean variations. Diabetic patients in general tend to have more distal arterial involvement of the popliteal and tibial arteries. Their clinical syndromes are further modified by the not infrequent presence of diabetic neuropathy and by characteristic susceptibility to necrotizing infections. This is more fully discussed in a subsequent section, The Diabetic Foot. In the upper extremities Buerger's disease, Raynaud's disease, and cervical rib are unusual causes of chronic ischemia.

The hallmark of chronic arterial insufficiency is claudication, the pathophysiology of which was discussed earlier. This is a highly specific symptom, virtually diagnostic of chronic arterial insufficiency. Hence, a carefully taken history to establish the presence of claudication is essential to establishing the diagnosis. For a long period of time the only measure of progression of arterial insufficiency is the appearance of claudication with progressively smaller amounts of exercise, usually measured in terms of walking two blocks, one block, or even shorter distances.

An important subsequent feature of progressive arterial insufficiency is the appearance of trophic changes in the feet, including loss of hair from the toes, the appearance of brittle, opaque nails, and atrophy of the skin with the development of rubor in dependency. These objective changes are associated with few symptoms except for an increasing susceptibility to cold. However, their presence in association with claudication indicates a much more advanced state of arterial insufficiency.

The importance of recognizing these changes in management of chronic ischemic disease is the fact that gangrene will readily occur in a foot or hand with advanced trophic changes following trivial trauma, such as trimming of a callus or corn, a blister from improper shoes, or minor exposures to extremes of heat or cold. Thirty to forty percent of patients with gangrene of the extremities ultimately requiring amputation may date the onset of gangrene in a toe to such trivial trauma. Apparently local trauma results in increased metabolic demands and perhaps in regional thrombosis of collateral circulation. The latter may be progressive despite all therapy unless immediate surgical revascularization can be carried out.

The end stages of chronic arterial insufficiency are represented by ischemic rest pain, usually in association with ulceration. Rest pain is due to ischemic neuritis and may be associated with tissue necrosis, often with superficial ulceration. It is seen in its most severe forms in patients with Buerger's disease, probably with superimposed ischemic neuritis. The recognition of ischemic rest pain and its ominous prognosis is of great significance, because unless ulceration or gangrene are already present, they will develop shortly if arterial circulation cannot be improved. Hence, surgical therapy if feasible should be done as soon as possible. Prolonged nonsurgical measures, consisting principally of rest to avoid trauma, vasodilators, and avoidance of tobacco, may be successful in a limited number of patients over a period of many weeks, probably because of the development of additional collateral circulation. In many patients, however, rest pain inevitably progresses to gangrene and amputation unless the occluded vascular bed can be reconstructed.

Fortunately, in the upper extremity, in contrast to the lower extremity, atherosclerosis which progresses to rest pain and gangrene is unusual. Claudication of the arm with exercise may be moderately disabling, but more serious symptoms are uncommon. Rest pain and tissue necrosis when present usually denote digital vessel occlusion either due to embolization from proximal atherosclerotic plaques or end-stage Raynaud's phenomenon.

Atherosclerotic Disease of the Lower Extremities

Atherosclerotic disease of the arteries to the lower extremities may be divided into three large groups, dependent upon the level of involvement. These are aortoiliac, femoropopliteal, and tibioperoneal. There are distinctive clinical features about each of the categories; more than one area is involved in at least one-third of patients seen. Aortoiliac disease in the fifth and sixth decades is characterized by relatively mild atherosclerosis with aortic occlusion from superimposed thrombosis, but in the seventh and eighth decades atherosclerosis is severe and thrombosis is relatively mild. Isolated femoropopliteal disease is especially frequent in cigarette smokers, while tibioperoneal disease occurs predominantly in diabetics. No matter where the obstruction is located, the physiologic deficit is decreased blood flow to the lower extremities, with symptoms ranging from intermittent claudication to gangrene. Tissue necrosis is more prone to occur with distal arterial disease and occlusive disease which progresses rapidly without time for collateral circulation to develop.

The choice of surgical therapy for the three different types depends upon several variables. These include the natural history of the arterial disease and the severity of the ischemic symptoms; the age and responsibilities of the patient; and the reliability of arterial reconstructive procedures, which varies greatly from one area to another.

AORTOILIAC DISEASE

HISTORICAL DATA. The ischemic syndrome produced by atherosclerotic disease of the bifurcation of the abdominal aorta has been recognized with increasing frequency over the past 30 years. Leriche is credited with emphasizing in the early 1940s the clinical characteristics of occlusion of the abdominal aorta, i.e., claudication, impotence, and absence of gangrene. The development of angiography, pioneered by dos Santos, greatly facilitated diagnosis.

ETIOLOGY AND PATHOLOGY. Some degree of atherosclerosis is almost universally seen at autopsy in the abdominal aortas of patients over sixty years of age, but symptoms from decrease in blood flow do not occur unless the diameter of the aorta has been greatly narrowed by as much as 90 percent. The process may simply be athero-

sclerosis with intimal thickening and fibrosis, or it may be complicated by ulceration of atherosclerotic plaques with superimposed thrombosis or embolization of portions of atherosclerotic plaques. As in other arteries, the disease often begins at bifurcations where flow patterns conducive to intimal thickening occur. Hence, involvement is often greatest at the aortic, the iliac, and the common femoral bifurcations. It may extend proximally in the abdominal aorta up to the level of the renal arteries, but fortunately occlusion proximal to the renal arteries is rare.

Patients are frequently seen in the fifth and sixth decades with thrombosis of the abdominal aorta but only mild atherosclerosis of the common iliac arteries. The thrombus often propagates up to the level of the renal arteries, rarely occluding one renal artery, and extending up to near the superior mesenteric artery. These patients contrast to a curious degree with patients in the seventh and eighth decades who may have unusually severe atherosclerosis but without thrombosis and total occlusion despite advanced stenosis. This variation with age suggests that some unrecognized factor in the younger group may precipitate the thrombotic process.

Fortunately clinically significant atherosclerosis of the abdominal aorta is virtually always segmental. Proximally it stops at the level of the renal arteries; distad the profunda femoris artery is almost always patent, though not infrequently involved with correctible stenotic lesions even in the presence of a totally occluded superficial femoral artery. Hence, reconstruction can be done in over 95 percent of patients, directing flow distad into the patent profunda femoris artery, which, however, may require either bypass or endarterectomy to serve as a suitable outflow tract. If the superficial femoral artery is also occluded, additional reconstruction is usually not required unless tissue necrosis is present. Otherwise simple aortoiliac or aorto-profunda femoris will suffice.

A separate therapeutic consideration is the 10 percent of persons with aortoiliac occlusive disease who have small aneurysms as well. This group must be treated by aortic graft replacement of the aneurysmal segment, for aneurysmal dilatation may develop following endarterectomy.

Concomitant coronary or cerebral atherosclerosis occurs frequently, probably in 30 to 50 percent of patients with symptomatic aortoiliac disease. Coronary disease is by far the principal cause of death in the 5-year period following surgical aortoiliac reconstruction. This has led to an increased interest in overcoming the effects of aortoiliac occlusions without invading the abdominal cavity, through the performance of so-called extraanatomical bypass grafts, popularized by Blaisdell et al. In these procedures one or both axillary arteries serve as the takeoff vessels for grafts leading to the groin. To overcome unilateral iliac arterial occlusions, cross-femoral grafts also have been used successfully.

In addition, patients with detectable involvement of cerebral or coronary arteries are evaluated for possible angiographic studies of those arteries and for possible cerebrovascular or coronary arterial reconstructive procedures.

PATHOPHYSIOLOGY. Aortoiliac disease decreases blood

flow to the pelvic viscera and lower extremities. Collateral circulation develops to an extensive degree when the aorta becomes completely occluded. The principal collaterals are through the lumbar arteries, anastomosing distad with the branches of the gluteal arteries and the profunda femoris arteries. Fortunately this collateral circulation is sufficient to prevent ischemia at rest, so symptoms appear only with exercise. In men impotence is frequent because of decreased blood flow through the hypogastric arteries. Claudication is present in the lower extremities, but as blood flow is adequate at rest, the extremity remains well nourished. Only with additional occlusions in the superficial femoral, profunda femoris, or popliteal and tibial arteries do nutritional changes with ulceration and gangrene appear. Rarely a few patients develop occlusion of the aorta at a rapid rate, before collateral circulation develops; these may show severe ischemic changes in the legs, even though no additional disease is present distad. Necrotic toe and foot lesions secondary to embolization of minute particles (atheroemboli) from the aorta or iliac arteries are being recognized with increasing frequency. These may occur in the presence of nonoccluding or even nonstenosing atherosclerotic plaques which give rise to emboli which occlude pedal or digital arteries, resulting in so-called "blue or purple toe" syndromes.

CLINICAL MANIFESTATIONS. The classic symptoms are intermittent claudication and impotence of varying severity in males. Claudication may be symmetric or asymmetric, depending upon the pattern of involvement of the iliac arteries. Characteristically with walking, discomfort is felt in the calf, thigh, and buttock muscles. The symptoms vary in severity from difficulty after walking three to four blocks to inability to walk even indoors. Rest pain, ulceration, or gangrene almost always indicate additional distal disease. This is particularly true in diabetics, where disease of the tibial arteries is common.

Symptoms may remain stable for years and progress only with progression of distal atherosclerosis. In some patients the symptoms improve with exercise as collateral vessels enlarge. Conversely, symptoms may worsen, sometimes dramatically, with hypotension secondary to myocardial infarction or cardiac arrhythmias. Impotence is a complex syndrome which may arise from multiple causes. Its presence or absence cannot be relied upon to diagnose aortoiliac disease. Although it may improve after successful arterial reconstruction, the likelihood in any particular patient is unpredictable.

Physical Examination. The principal finding is diminution or absence of the femoral pulses, combined with absence of popliteal and pedal pulses. Pulsations in the abdominal aorta may be palpable if occlusion is limited to near the aortic bifurcation, but these are absent if the abdominal aorta is occluded up to the renal arteries. A systolic bruit is often audible over the aorta or iliac arteries, confirming the presence of atherosclerosis. However, it does not correlate with the degree of stenosis. Nutrition in the extremities is usually normal. With signs of chronic ischemia, such as absence of hair, brittle nails, or rubor, additional atherosclerotic disease in the femoral or popliteal arteries is probably present.

Occasionally patients are seen with aortoiliac disease with acute episodes of severe ischemia of the toes or feet, often with cyanosis and rest pain. The diagnosis may be especially puzzling if the aortoiliac obstruction is not severe. Occasionally pedal pulses are palpable. The syndrome probably arises from arterioarterial embolization of fragments of atherosclerotic plaques or thrombi dislodged from the surface of such plaques. The diagnosis may be suspected if a localized bruit in the abdomen or groin is found.

As multiple areas of atherosclerosis are frequent, particular care should be taken to search for bruits over the carotid or subclavian arteries, as well as to note the adequacy of pulses in the upper extremities.

LABORATORY STUDIES. With the exception of patients experiencing arterioarterial embolization, the diagnosis usually can be established by the history and physical examination. Roentgenograms often show calcification in the wall of the aorta, but as the calcification is in the media, it does not correlate with the degree of flow obstruction. An unsuspected abdominal aortic aneurysm, however, may be outlined by the calcification within its wall. Aortography is performed if surgical reconstruction is being considered. It delineates the proximal extent of the occlusion and may outline the patent arteries beyond the obstruction, especially the profunda femoris vessels.

TREATMENT. Nonsurgical. The need for surgical reconstruction depends upon the severity of the symptoms and the age of the patient. Intermittent claudication in most instances denotes mild ischemia even in the presence of extensive arterial occlusions and, of itself, is a relative indication for surgical intervention. In 80 percent of patients affected, the course is relatively benign, the claudication either improving or disappearing over a period of months or remaining stable. Two-thirds of all patients affected can be managed successfully without operative intervention; 14 percent require an operation for "social" reasons. For example, mild claudication in a forty-five-year-old patient whose occupation necessitates frequent walking is a strong indication for operation. By contrast, a retired patient of seventy with angina pectoris and claudication does not require operation. The presence of trophic changes in the feet, rubor, absence of hair, and brittle nails is a useful guide to the risk of gangrene, for gangrene is rare except with acute arterial occlusion as long as trophic changes are absent. Only 2.5 percent of claudicators develop gangrene. These usually are the patients with the most severe claudication and the most marked involvement of the tibial arteries, in whom surgical reconstructions either cannot be done or, if done at higher levels, do not result in control of the necrotizing ischemia. Thus, prophylactic intervention in claudicators probably does not avert the appearance of gangrene at a later date (see Table 21-1).

If operation is not recommended, daily exercise to the point of claudication should be encouraged, for this may enhance collateral circulation, as manifested by gradual increase in walking tolerance. If walking is not feasible, a similar exercise can be performed indoors by having the patient raise himself on his toes and then rock back on his heels, repeating the sequence rapidly until calf cramps

Table 21-1. FATE OF 104 CLAUDICATORS*

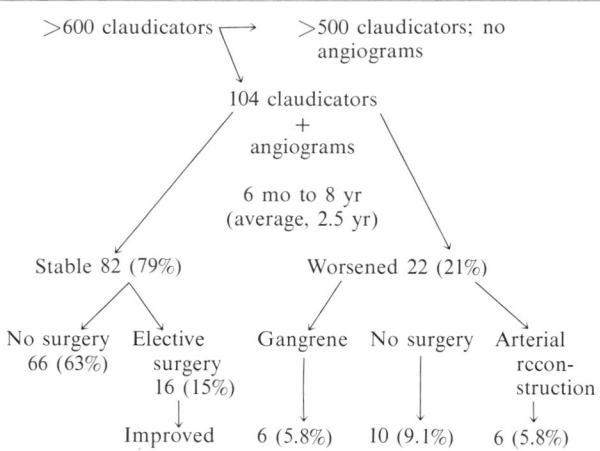

*These patients had arteriograms and were followed for 6 months to 8 years (average, 2.5 years) in an attempt at nonsurgical management.
SOURCE: From A. M. Imparato, G. E. Kim, and J. G. Crowley, Intermittent Claudication: Its Natural Course, *Surgery,* **78:**795, 1975, Table II, p. 796.

occur. Following a rest period the exercise is repeated, as often as twenty or more times daily.

Abstinence from tobacco in any form is mandatory. There is reasonable statistical evidence that claudication improves when smoking is stopped and that the risk of gangrene is greater in patients who smoke. The precise mechanism is unknown, but tobacco is a potent vasoconstrictor. Robichek et al. have reported that continued smoking after arterial reconstructions results in premature failures. Drug therapy with vasodilators may be tried, but unfortunately few patients have had any improvement in the claudication. Alcohol, orally administered, is employed for its peripheral vasodilator effect.

With severe ischemia, one of the most crucial points in management is educating the patient to protect the feet from any form of trauma. This includes extremes of heat or cold, improperly fitting shoes, or vigorous trimming of calluses, corns, or toenails. A familiar tragedy is that a trauma that would be minor in a foot with normal circulation will produce gangrene of a toe in a severely ischemic foot which not only fails to heal but may gradually progress upward to result in a low thigh amputation. Infection associated with unguis incarnatus or dermatophytosis similarly may cause decompensation of the circulation with gangrene, probably from an increase in local tissue metabolism.

Therapy directed toward lowering blood lipid concentrations by diet, drugs, or even surgical procedures remains of uncertain benefit. Anticoagulant therapy with heparin or warfarin sodium has not been helpful. The recent exciting discovery that acetylsalicylic acid in small doses critically alters platelet aggregation and may thereby prevent intravascular thrombosis is now undergoing clinical evaluation and holds considerable therapeutic promise.

Lumbar Sympathectomy. In patients with trophic changes in the feet not amenable to direct arterial reconstruction, lumbar sympathectomy may be of benefit both in improving symptoms and in protecting from gangrene. Unfortunately, the benefits of sympathectomy are variable and unpredictable although on occasion dramatic. In several reports objective signs of improvement were demonstrated in only 20 to 30 percent of patients, usually consisting of increased circulation in the skin which provides some protection from ulceration. Increased blood flow to the leg muscles, associated with improvement in claudication, is unfortunately rare.

Due to the great variability of the morphologic features of the lumbar sympathetic chain, lumbar sympathectomies should involve near-total denervation, removing the sympathetic chain from the level of the crus of the diaphragm superiorly down to the level of the common iliac inferiorly. Bilateral excisions of the uppermost lumbar ganglia may cause impairment of sexual function, usually disturbances in ejaculation, and must be considered in deciding the extent of bilateral sympathectomy in young men.

Aortic Reconstruction. The most frequently performed surgical procedures are thromboendarterectomy and a bypass graft, usually with Dacron or Teflon. As mentioned earlier, the almost uniform patency of the profunda femoris vessels makes reconstruction feasible in the vast majority of patients. The risk of operation is between 5 and 10 percent, determined principally by the degree of associated coronary or cerebral atherosclerosis. The superiority of one operative procedure over the other has not been demonstrated conclusively, although the late complications associated with each procedure differ considerably. Long-term patency rates after either procedure range from 65 to 90 percent. Though tedious, endarterectomies have been successfully performed from the level of the renal arteries proximally to the mid-profunda femoris vessels distad. Concomitant aneurysmal disease of the aorta is a definite contraindication to endarterectomy. In some instances the procedures are combined, performing an aortofemoral bypass in combination with localized endarterectomy of the common femoral and profunda femoris arteries.

The most frequent late complications after bypass procedures are false aneurysms developing at the suture lines, which have continued to occur since the introduction of synthetic suture material, and graft infection, which may occur years after implant. The most frequent complication after endarterectomy is a recurrent stenosis from progressive fibrosis and narrowing of the arterial lumen.

Extraanatomical Bypass Grafts. A number of factors have led to a growing interest in the use of extraanatomical bypass grafts to overcome the effects of aortoiliac occlusions. The magnitude of the direct aortic operation makes it less suitable for aged, debilitated patients, and has led to the development of the axillofemoral and femorofemoral bypass grafts. The high success rate of these grafts and the long-term course of the patients have made extraanatomical grafts attractive for use in this group of patients, in whom early death from coronary or other vascular disease is quite high. In many series these operations are being performed preferentially in patients with advanced arterial disease and severe ischemia.

Preoperative Considerations. An aortogram is usually performed to determine the extent of disease in the external iliac and femoral arteries. As it is not needed to confirm the diagnosis, which is readily made on physical examination, the aortogram is of little value unless the distal circulation is visualized. In some instances the authors perform operative angiograms of the common femoral artery to delineate the extent of disease in the proximal profunda femoris artery, for endarterectomies may be successfully

Fig. 21-1. Angiogram illustrating that the profunda femoris artery is usually patent in the presence of aortoiliac occlusive disease. Advanced lesions may be present, however, requiring surgical correction to render the profunda femoris suitable for an outflow tract. Arrow points to patent mid-profunda femoris artery.

performed down to the midportion of this artery (Fig. 21-1).

Operative Technique. A midline abdominal incision, usually extending from the xiphoid process to the pubis symphysis, is preferred. The intestines are retracted onto the right abdominal wall and placed in a plastic bag, after which the retroperitoneal tissues are incised to expose the aorta proximally up to the level of the left renal vein. Once the proximal and distal extent of arterial disease has been defined, a choice is made between a bypass graft or an endarterectomy.

As mentioned earlier, the presence of small aneurysms in the aorta or common iliac artery are absolute contraindications to endarterectomy. A small external iliac artery or severe atherosclerosis in the external iliac artery has influenced many surgeons to perform a bypass procedure to the common femoral artery because of the technical difficulties with endarterectomy of a small diseased external iliac artery. The availability of arterial strippers, as well as the eversion endarterectomy popularized by Conley, however, has extended the scope of endarterectomy and made the operation more satisfactory in these circumstances.

Thromboendarterectomy. A typical pattern of atherosclerotic involvement is extension of disease proximally to within 2 to 3 cm of the renal arteries and distad into the common iliac arteries, stopping in about 50 percent of patients just beyond the bifurcation of the common iliac arteries. Initially the aorta proximally and the external and hypogastric arteries distad are encircled with plastic tapes. The lumbar and inferior mesenteric arteries are similarly exposed. Fifty milligrams of heparin is then given by intravenous injection before occlusive clamps are applied to avoid thrombus formation during the periods of stasis. External iliac clamps are applied before clamping the abdominal aorta to protect from distal embolization. Incisions are made over the distal common iliac arteries, and cleavage planes between the plaques and media are developed. A longitudinal incision is made into the aorta above the level of the inferior mesenteric artery and an appropriate cleavage plane near the junction of the arterial intima and media identified. Using various techniques, including arterial strippers, the core of atherosclerotic material is freed proximally. Usually by blunt dissection the aortic and iliac cores can be mobilized and removed in one piece. A critical aspect of the operative procedure distad is careful inspection of the intima of the proximal external iliac artery to eliminate ledges of thickened intima by suturing. The caliber of the external iliac arteries may be measured with catheters. A diameter smaller than a #16 F catheter often indicates the necessity of extending the endarterectomy to the common femoral arteries. In the hypogastric arteries, endarterectomy is limited to removal of the occluding material near the ostia, for distal dissection of this artery is usually technically unsatisfactory.

The aortotomy incision is closed with a simple continuous suture of 4-0 or 5-0 Tevdek. The iliac arteriotomies may be closed similarly or with a patch graft of either autologous saphenous vein or a prosthetic patch of knitted Dacron. The choice depends upon both the diameter of the artery and the rigidity of the wall. After the incisions are sutured, the occluding clamps are sequentially removed to permit flushing initially into the hypogastric arteries and subsequently into the external iliacs. Strong pulses should be palpable immediately. Weak or absent pulsations indicate obstruction from either retained plaques or stenotic suture lines, in which case the arteriotomy should be promptly reopened and the obstruction corrected. Occasionally in such circumstances operative angiography is needed.

Once blood flow is restored, heparin may be neutralized with protamine, giving 1 to 1.5 mg for each mg heparin used. Often, unless bleeding appears to be excessive, heparin is not neutralized by protamine administration. The posterior peritoneum is sutured over the reconstructed aorta (Fig. 21-2). A concomitant bilateral lumbar sympathectomy is a simple adjunct to the reconstructive procedure but not clearly beneficial. Many uncontrolled data, including higher patency rates, are available regarding the beneficial effects of sympathectomy performed with arterial reconstruction. In our own series, sympathectomy has been performed on rare occasions in association with arterial reconstruction, with no apparent detrimental effect on patency. When it is performed, the sympathetic chain can be identified by palpation as cordlike nodular structures parallel to the aorta on the left and just under the lateral border of the vena cava on the right.

Bypass Grafting. When a bypass procedure is chosen, a knitted rather than a woven Dacron prosthesis is preferred, because of firmer adherence of the neointima which forms subsequently to the wall of the graft. In some tightly woven prostheses, the neointima remains loose, gelatinous, and relatively nonadherent.

After initial determination of where the occlusive disease stops distad, the femoral arteries are exposed if disease extends to the inguinal ligament. The aorta is then isolated proximally and incised longitudinally for 4 to 5 cm. The anastomosis is simpler if a short segment of aorta is identified and clamped, rather than employing a tangential clamp on the anterior wall, which is particularly awkward if the aorta is small and stiff.

The anastomosis is constructed end to side with a continuous suture of 3-0 or 4-0 Tevdek. The graft then can be clamped adjacent to the anastomosis and flow restored to the iliac vessels. Soft tissue tunnels are then developed by blunt dissection anterior and parallel to the iliac vessels, after which the limbs of the prosthesis are brought through the tunnels, lying parallel to the iliac arteries. If the distal anastomosis is performed to the common femoral artery, the graft is brought beneath the inguinal ligament, and the common femoral is incised near the origin of the profunda femoris artery to be certain that there is no obstruction of flow into either the deep or the superficial femoral artery. A continuous suture of 4-0 or 5-0 Tevdek is used. The graft is placed under slight tension at the time of performing the anastomosis to avoid buckling of the graft when it is distended with arterial pressure after the clamps are removed (Figs. 21-3 and 21-4).

A major technical hazard in bypass grafting is the formation of thrombi in the proximal or distal arterial tree with subsequent embolization into the extremity when blood flow is restored. This can be avoided by carefully flushing the graft and routinely inserting a balloon catheter down the distal arterial tree before the distal anastomosis is completed. As the knitted prostheses are porous, they should be preclotted with blood before insertion.

Antibiotics in large amounts are routinely begun at the start of the operation to have circulating blood levels at bactericidal concentrations during the operation. Antibiotics are repeated at appropriate intervals during long procedures.

In performing the axillofemoral bypass graft procedures, the outflow tract is the femoral artery, usually in the groin. This vessel must be made ready to accept a 10- to 12-mm Dacron graft, as for direct aortofemoral grafting. After suitable outflow tracts have been prepared, either unilaterally or bilaterally as the degree of ischemia of the extremities dictates, the axillary artery is exposed in the infraclavicular region. Care must be taken to select axillary arteries which are fully patent. Comparisons of bilateral upper extremity blood pressures are mandatory, since the relatively high incidence of subclavian arterial lesions, usually on the left side, may lead to graft failure. If a blood pressure differential exists or if supraclavicular bruits are heard, arch aortography is indicated. We now favor the right axillary artery, since the innominate, right subclavian complex seems to be involved less often by advanced atherosclerosis. An incision is made over the coracoid process parallel to the clavicle, exposing the pectoralis major muscle, which is divided in the direction of its fibers, exposing the tendon of the pectoralis minor muscle. This is severed from its attachment to the coracoid process, exposing the axillary artery surrounded by the brachial plexus. The artery is dissected free of these nerves, sometimes producing transient and seemingly inevitable brachial plexus neuropathies. The subscapular artery serves as a useful landmark, which is usually though not invariably preserved. A curved tunneler is used to create a subcutaneous tunnel between the infraclavicular incision and the groin incision. When indicated, a suprapubic tunnel is made to connect groin incisions, thereby permitting an additional femorofemoral bypass graft. This latter addition to unilateral axillofemoral grafts is said by some to have a higher late patency rate than the unilateral axillofemoral alone or than bilateral separate axillofemoral grafts.

It is advisable to check the condition of the entire system with operative angiograms, since there are many pitfalls to the procedure. These include not only the usual problems with operations upon atherosclerotic arteries but also accumulations of clot within the prosthesis caused by leakage of tissue thromboplastins from the subcutaneous tunnel into the prosthesis.

Postoperative Care. Peripheral pulses should be closely monitored, for sudden disappearance of a previously palpable pulse usually indicates thrombosis of the graft or an embolus, either of which should be treated by prompt reoperation. Ileus, the most frequent postoperative complication of the intraabdominal procedures, is simply managed by nasogastric suction until adequate peristalsis returns. Antibiotics are given for about 3 to 5 days.

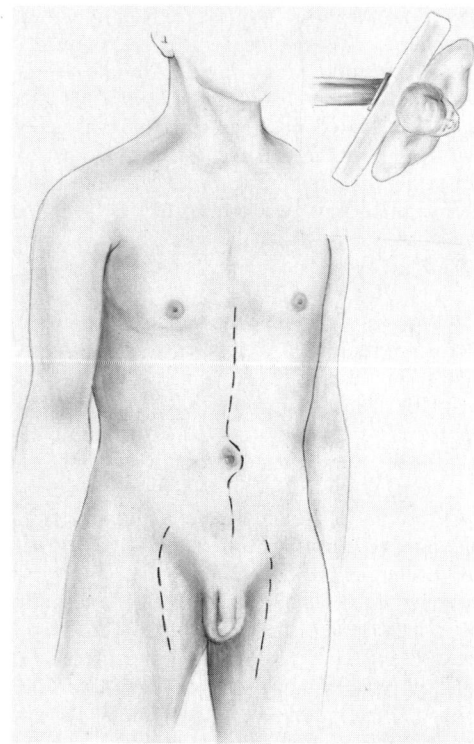

A

Fig. 21-2. Endarterectomy for atherosclerotic obstruction of the aortoiliac segments. *A.* A midline incision from xiphoid process to pubis symphysis is employed. Rotation of the operating table 30 to 40° to the right side facilitates retraction of the intestines. The thighs should be included in the operative field to permit exposure of the bifurcation of the common femoral arteries. *B.* The intestines are either encased in a plastic bag or covered with moist pads. The retroperitoneal tissues are incised exposing the aorta up to the left renal vein. *C.* The arteriotomy incisions are shown placed according to the distribution of the disease. *D.* Endarterectomy strippers may be used to separate the atherosclerotic cores in the iliac arteries. *E.* Following endarterectomy the distal intima is carefully attached to the arterial wall with vertically oriented interrupted sutures to prevent its dissection when circulation is reestablished. *F.* The multiple arteriotomies are either closed by direct suture or with roof patches of autologous vein or Dacron if the vessels are narrow.

B

Fig. 21-2 *C, D, E, F* Continued.

The most catastrophic postoperative complication, fortunately extremely rare, is infection developing around the prosthetic graft. In such circumstances the graft usually must be removed to prevent fatal hemorrhage. This can result in unilateral or bilateral amputation of the extremities unless another graft can be inserted. Probably the best form of management is the temporary insertion of axillary-femoral bypass grafts through long subcutaneous tunnels, followed by removal of the infected retroperitoneal prosthesis. Although a single axillary artery has been employed successfully to maintain circulation to the lower half of the body through axillofemoral, femorofemoral grafts, the end-type aortic closures following removal of aortic grafts have frequently ruptured as late as 1 year postoperatively.

Results and Prognosis. Immediate results of aortoiliac reconstructions are excellent. A nearly 100 percent patency rate can be achieved by meticulous technique and proper selection of operative procedures. The immediate functional results are predictable from the angiographic patterns of arterial involvement and the functional status of patients (Fig. 21-5). Claudication is almost always relieved. If tissue loss with gangrene is present, however, additional reconstructive procedures in the distal arterial tree are needed in about 50 percent of the patients.

Numerous data have been published about the long-term results following endarterectomy or bypass grafting. In general, good to excellent results have been sustained in the majority of patients for at least 5 years after operation. If reconstruction is limited to the aorta and common iliac arteries, the 5-year results are similar for endarterectomy and bypass grafts. In a study of 420 patients, Wylie reported that 108 patients with aortoiliac endarterectomy had a 10-year patency of 90 percent. Kouchoukos et al. reported a series of 206 patients treated either by endarterectomy or bypass grafting, after which the 5-year patency rates were virtually identical, 62 and 63 percent. Szilagyi et al. reported similar results 5 years after operation with patency rates of 89 and 85 percent, respectively, when comparing bypass grafting and endarterectomy. Gomes et al. described good results in 84 percent of 401 patients 5 years after operation, and Garrett et al. reported that in over 3,000 operations performed for aortoiliac disease using bypass grafts in the majority of patients good results approached 90 percent 5 years after operation. The results of axillofemoral grafts are not as well documented because of their more recent introduction and failure to receive

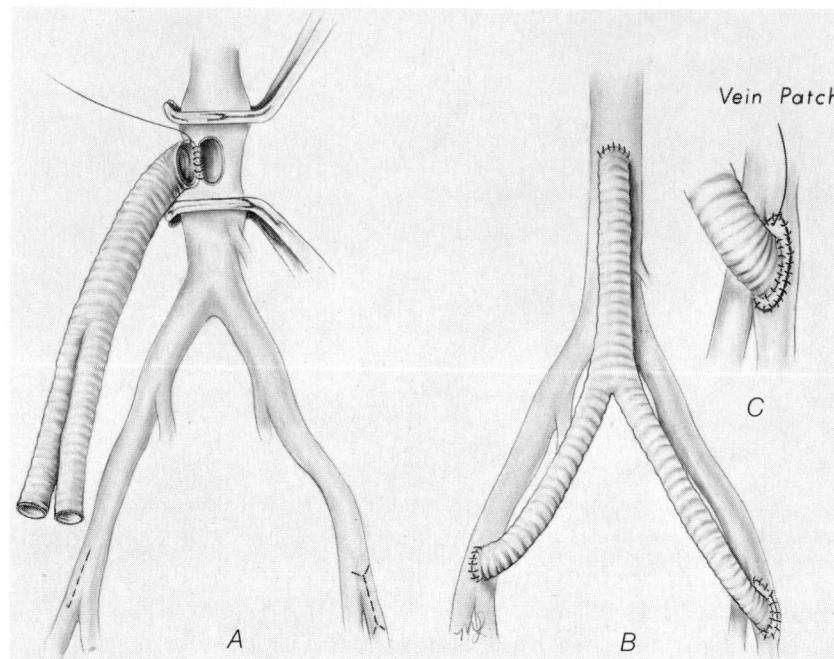

Fig. 21-3. Bypass graft of abdominal aorta. Dissection and exposure are similar to that for endarterectomy procedures. *A.* The proximal anastomosis is performed end to side to the aorta proximal to the point of obstruction. End-to-end aortic anastomosis is preferred by many to lessen the risk of distal embolization. Knitted Dacron is preferred. *B.* The distal anastomoses are performed as end-to-side anastomoses either to the iliac artery proximal to the inguinal ligament or to the common femoral artery at the point of origin of the profunda femoris artery depending upon the degree of atherosclerotic involvement of the external iliac artery. Anastomoses distal to the inguinal ligament are avoided whenever possible to avoid trauma to the prosthesis passing under the inguinal ligament and to lessen the risk of infection posed by having a plastic prosthesis in the groin. *C.* A vein roof patch may be employed to facilitate suture of the prosthesis to small arteries.

immediate universal acceptance. There are now series from Blaisdell, Mannick, and Parsonett which suggest that the immediate and long-term patency rates are comparable to those for aortofemoral grafts, while operative mortality is lower. They are subject to the same complications as other prostheses anastomosed in the groin, viz., false aneurysms and infection.

Hence, it is clear from the data available that the procedure chosen for an individual patient must vary with the disease present and the experience of the surgeon. Whichever technique is used, immediate patency rates should approach 100 percent. False aneurysms following the use of bypass grafts have greatly decreased in frequency with the use of synthetic sutures and the avoidance of excessive tension on the suture lines, although they still occur too frequently. False aneurysms generally do not occur following endarterectomy, and infection with endarterectomy in which autologous tissue only is used is rare.

The principal cause of late deaths after operation is coronary arterial disease, approximately 12 percent within 2 years at New York University. It is hoped that recent advances with coronary bypass operations will improve this poor prognosis.

FEMOROPOPLITEAL OCCLUSIVE DISEASE

PATHOLOGY. The most common site for atherosclerotic occlusion in the lower extremities is the distal superficial femoral artery within the adductor canal. The reason for this characteristic localization is unknown but may be related to the anatomic relationship between the distal femoral artery and the adductor magnus tendon as the artery traverses the adductor foramen to enter the popliteal fossa. The usual sequence of atherosclerotic occlusion is to extend gradually proximally in the superficial femoral artery until the artery is occluded at its origin from the common femoral. Fortunately, involvement of the profunda femoris artery is infrequent, a complete contrast to the frequency of involvement of the superficial femoral. For this reason atherosclerotic occlusion of the superficial femoral artery alone usually produces claudication but no more serious circulatory impairment.

The importance of the profunda femoris artery in arterial reconstructions of the aortoiliac system has been realized for many years, and correction of ostial stenoses, incident to femoral popliteal reconstructions, has been routinely performed by some. Recently Martin emphasized its importance as a valuable contributor of blood to the extremity in the presence of superficial femoral arterial occlusions, suggesting that the profunda femoris ostium be enlarged even in the absence of high-grade stenosis. Few direct measurements of flow have been made before and after this reconstruction.

When more extensive occlusive disease develops, usually from occlusion of the popliteal artery or its branches, the anterior and posterior tibial arteries, more serious circulatory insufficiency appears. With occlusion of this extent, ulceration and gangrene are common. Such diffuse patterns of atherosclerosis are particularly common in diabetic patients.

CLINICAL MANIFESTATIONS. Segmental occlusion of the superficial femoral artery produces claudication in the leg with moderate exercise, but no symptoms at rest. Physical examination finds a normal femoral pulse but absent popliteal and pedal pulses. Rarely pedal pulses are present at rest but disappear with exercise. The nutrition of the foot is normal. If additional occlusive disease is present beyond the femoral artery, claudication is more severe, perhaps associated with rest pain and trophic changes in the foot, and ulceration and gangrene ultimately ensue. Fortunately, the rate of progression of atherosclerotic occlusion is slow in many patients, and the risk of gangrene developing within 5 years in an extremity with claudication as the only symptom is only about 5 percent.

LABORATORY STUDIES. Arteriography is required to determine the segmental nature of the occlusive disease and the consequent possibilities of arterial reconstruction. Adequate visualization of the popliteal artery and its branches is essential (Fig. 21-6). Fortunately, with current techniques, revascularization procedures extended to the popliteal artery are quite satisfactory if the anterior or posterior tibial branches are patent. The peroneal artery, which does not directly contribute to the formation of the pedal arch, is less satisfactory. If all three branches are occluded, under special circumstances reconstructive procedures may be extended down to the pedal arches of the foot. This is discussed under Tibioperoneal Occlusive Disease.

TREATMENT. If claudication is the only symptom, operation is an elective decision, determined from the age and occupation of the patient. As the risk of gangrene with claudication alone is small, this alone does not constitute an indication for operation. Only when trophic changes appear in the feet is operation indicated because of the risk of gangrene. Care to avoid trauma to the foot, described in the section on aortoiliac occlusive disease, is similarly applicable, avoiding even minor trauma or exposure to extremes of heat or cold. Recommendations regarding tobacco, alcohol, exercise, and vasodilator drugs similar to those made for aortic occlusive disease are applicable. In patients able to walk at least one city block, or 300 feet, a vigorous exercise program of walking at least 1 mile daily has resulted in marked improvement in claudication in at least 50 percent of patients within 6 to 12 months.

Sympathectomy. Unfortunately, when claudication is the only symptom, sympathectomy is of little value. It may enhance the development of collateral circulation and thereby lessen the hazard of more serious insufficiency, but this is primarily theoretic. When trophic changes are pres-

Fig. 21-4. Interposition of vein roof patches over the profunda femoris and superficial femoral arteries facilitates suture of plastic prostheses to the common femoral artery in aortofemoral bypass procedures.

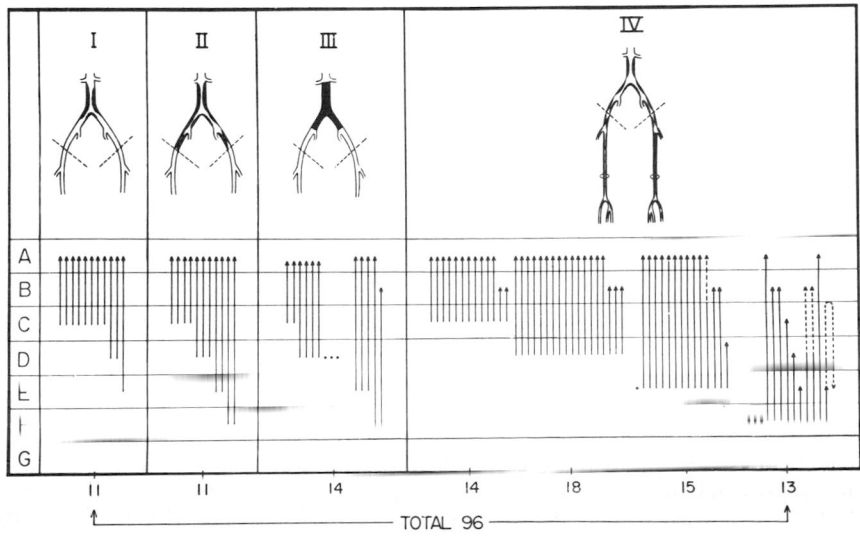

Fig. 21-5. Preoperative angiographic studies provide an excellent index of functional results which can be achieved by aorto-iliacfemoral reconstructions. Functional categories *A* to *D* are increasing severities of claudication, while *E* and *F* represent rest pain and gangrene respectively. Even in the presence of disseminated distal occlusive lesions and ischemic lesions aorto-iliac reconstructions to the profunda femoris artery resulted in marked improvement. (*From A. M. Imparato et al., Results in 96 Aorto-iliac Reconstructive Procedures, Surgery, 60:610, 1970.*)

Fig. 21-6. Representative angiographic study required to evaluate patients for arterial reconstruction for claudication. Only in this manner can the inflow and outflow tracts be critically evaluated and arterial reconstructions planned.

ent, however, and direct arterial reconstruction is not possible because of diffuse occlusive disease, a sympathectomy should be performed. The vasodilating effect of sympathectomy on the vessels of the skin provides some protection from ulceration of the ischemic foot. Statistically the results are disappointing, however, for objective improvement can be demonstrated in little more than 20 percent of patients receiving operation.

Direct Arterial Reconstruction. *Bypass Grafting; Endarterectomy.* The basic principle of arterial reconstruction is that there must be both adequate inflow and adequate outflow of blood from the area of reconstruction. Early operative failures are almost always due either to obvious technical faults or to inadequate inflow or outflow. Most groups have become dissatisfied with bypass prosthetic grafts. Although Crawford and associates reported in 1966 that crimped Dacron prostheses, 8 mm or more in diameter, employed in over 2,500 cases gave adequate long-term function, up to 10 years, in about 75 percent of patients, most others have had less satisfactory results. Szilagyi et al. reported a patency rate of only 40 percent in 193 cases 4 years after operation, and Linton achieved only a 6 percent patency 5 years after operation. These poor results contrast markedly to the excellent results following aorto-iliac reconstruction.

The bypass operation with the autologous saphenous

vein is used most commonly though not by all groups. Wylie described similar 5-year results following either endarterectomy or vein bypass. At New York University, three different techniques—venous bypass, long endarterectomy procedures with a venous roof patch, and endarterectomy performed through multiple arteriotomies with multiple vein roof patches—had almost identical results 5 to 7 years later. Analysis of the cause of late failures after reconstruction found that about one-third were due to progressive distal atherosclerosis and one-third to intimal proliferation in the areas of arterial reconstruction. Tissue specimens were not obtained to determine the cause of failure in the other one-third of the cases.

With prosthetic grafts, failure is due to stiffening of the prosthesis from the ingrowth of fibrous tissue, especially when the graft crosses a joint, as well as extensive scarring about the graft which results in poor adherence of the neointima. Venous bypass is favored if a saphenous or cephalic vein can be dilated to an internal diameter greater than 4 mm. If a suitable vein is not available, endarterectomy with wire strippers and multiple vein roof patches has given comparable results, even in diabetic patients. If, for some reason, this is not possible, usually due to a previous operative procedure, then a long endarterectomy with a long vein roof patch, originally described by Edwards et al., is favored. The least satisfactory choices are either a prosthetic graft, usually Dacron, or a homologous vein (Fig. 21-7).

Other techniques have been proposed but lack substantial experience. This includes carbon dioxide ("gas") endarterectomy, developed by Sawyer et al., bovine heterografts, or autologous tissue tubes prepared with a silicone mandril.

Bypass Grafting. The technique of bypass grafting is illustrated in Fig. 21-8. It is particularly attractive because of its simplicity and ease of performance. The precision required for obtaining nearly 100 percent immediate patency can best be evaluated by operative angiography. Relatively small imperfections in the anastomotic suture lines or within the body of the graft can lead to deposition of platelet-fibrin aggregates with occlusion within a few hours.

The saphenous vein is carefully removed from the inguinal ligament to the knee, reversed to permit blood to flow in the direction of the venous valves, and then attached with end-to-side anastomoses to the femoral and popliteal arteries proximal and distal to the obstruction. As mentioned earlier, the vein should be at least 4 to 5 mm in diameter. In 15 to 25 percent of patients a satisfactory vein is not available, because of either previous surgical removal or anatomic variations. A suitable cephalic vein is an acceptable substitute, though a lot of data are not yet available. Otherwise one of the techniques previously described is used.

Endarterectomy. Since its introduction over 20 years ago, between 1951 and 1953, endarterectomy has been modified several times. A completely open technique, incising the artery throughout its length, removing the atherosclerotic core, and suturing the long arteriotomy, had a very high failure rate. Similarly, closed techniques with mechanical

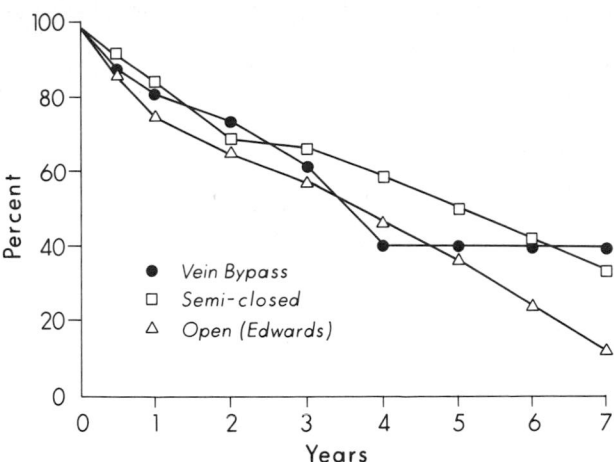

Fig. 21-7. Cumulative patencies of femoropopliteal arterial reconstructions performed by one of three techniques employing only autologous tissue are nearly statistically identical. The three groups are otherwise comparable for indications for operation and grading of severity of involvement of the outflow tracts. Inserts show the three basic techniques employed in reconstructions. (*From A. M. Imparato et al., Comparisons of Three Technics for Femoral-Popliteal Arterial Reconstructions, Ann Surg, 177(3):375, 1973.*)

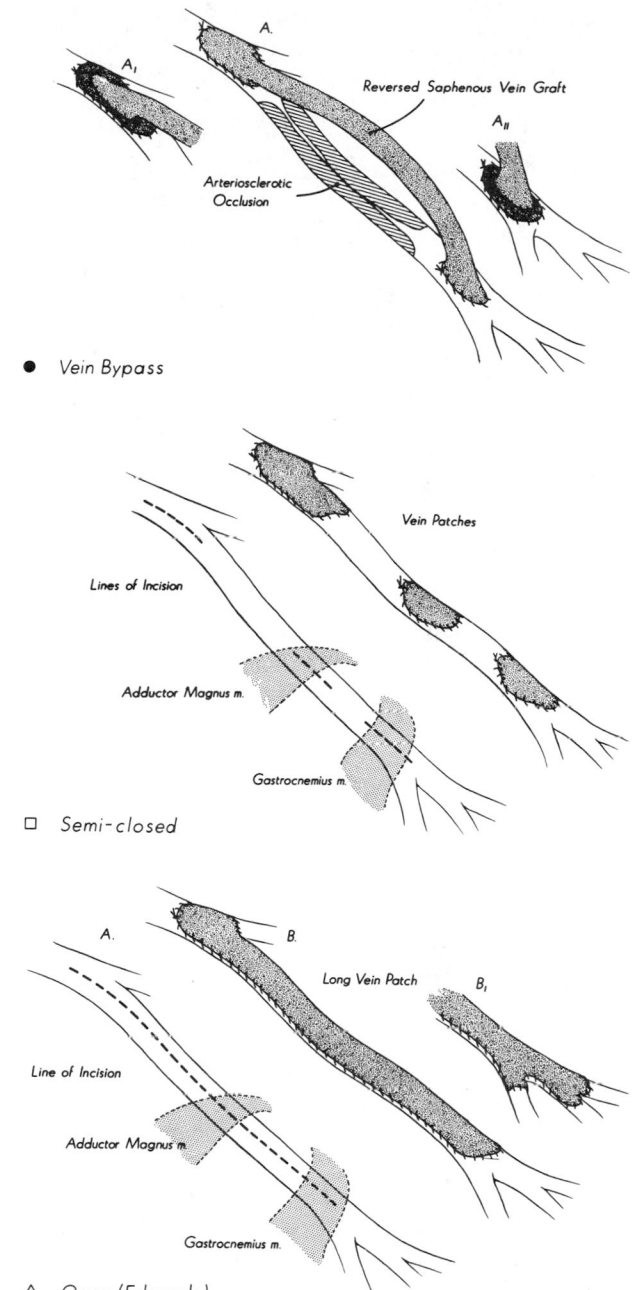

strippers often failed, usually from leaving loose fragments of intima or atherosclerotic plaque in the lumen. Closure of the long arteriotomy with a vein roof patch, developed by Edwards et al., gave significantly better results. A subsequent modification was the use of multiple vein roof patches to close multiple arteriotomies used for semiclosed endarterectomy. This technique is illustrated in Fig. 21-9. Operative angiography is essential to be certain that atherosclerotic debris has been entirely removed from the lumen.

A technique utilized in some patients is the so-called "in situ" vein graft, in which the saphenous vein is not removed from its bed but is mobilized proximally and distad to be anastomosed end to side to the femoral artery proximally and the popliteal artery or its branches distad. Before the anastomoses are performed, however, the valves in the vein are disrupted by passage of a mechanical instrument along the course of the vein. One limitation of the technique is the production of small arteriovenous fistulas from tributaries of the saphenous vein. Another objection is incomplete disruption of the venous valves with the production of turbulent flow. Some such grafts have been successfully inserted from the common femoral artery proximally to the posterior tibial artery near the ankle, but in general long-term results with the technique have been found unsatisfactory by most groups.

TIBIOPERONEAL ARTERIAL DISEASE

PATHOLOGY. Occlusive disease of the tibial arteries occurs most commonly in patients with diabetes mellitus. It is also seen in patients with Buerger's disease. Some instances of intra-arterial embolism are almost surely incorrectly diagnosed initially and considered as primary occlusive disease of the tibial arteries.

In the diabetic patient there are different patterns of disease which can be recognized, though the reason for development of such patterns is unclear. All tibial arteries may be involved, as well as occlusion of the pedal arches formed by branches of the anterior and posterior tibial vessels. In such instances surgical reconstruction is impossible. In other patients one or more of the tibial arteries may be entirely patent, or there may be proximal occlusion with patent vessels starting at the level of the midcalf. With this pattern of involvement, arterial reconstruction is possible if grafts are extended to the ankles. Unfortunately, in some diabetic patients there is additional disease in the aortoiliac or femoral areas.

Valves in Reversed Saphenous Vein

Fig. 21-8. Bypass graft procedure for occlusion of the superficial femoral artery. *A.* Incisions employed for exposure of the major vessels. A proximal incision is made over the saphenous vein from just below the inguinal ligament to the apex of Scarpa's triangle, avoiding undermining of adjacent skin flaps which might result in ischemic necrosis. The distal incision is made on the medial aspect of the popliteal fossa to expose the popliteal artery. The adductor magnus tendon, the site often of most severe superficial femoral arterial involvement, is shown. It is frequently cut to facilitate passing the vein graft from adductor canal to popliteal fossa. *B.* Completed bypass graft of the reversed saphenous vein. The anastomoses are performed end to side to the common femoral and popliteal arteries. The vein is brought either subcutaneously or through the subsartorial canal. Inserts show details of the bevel created in the vein bypass and reversal of the valves. An alternative technique is to leave the saphenous vein in its usual location, without reversal, destroying the valves, accomplishing an in situ nonreversed bypass graft.

CLINICAL MANIFESTATIONS. Occasionally occlusive disease of the tibial arteries merely produces claudication of the foot. Usually, however, there are signs of advanced ischemia. With diabetes there is the additional problem of diabetic neuropathy, difficult to differentiate from ischemic rest pain. Characteristically, ischemic pain is relieved by placing the foot in a dependent position, while that of diabetic neuropathy is not. A frequent problem in the diabetic patient is ulceration on the plantar surface of the foot, secondary to pressure associated with diabetic neuropathy. A more serious problem is a spreading necrotizing infection, with absent pedal pulses. Because of associated ischemia the infection is often refractory to both antibiotic therapy and surgical debridement unless revascularization can be done. This type of progressive, refractory infection may lead to amputation before tissue ischemia per se has caused widespread necrosis. Infection undoubtedly increases the metabolic requirements of the tissue and thereby accentuates the degree of ischemia. A third type of terminal event in the ischemic diabetic foot is soft tissue atrophy to a severe degree, terminating with progressive ischemic dry gangrene of the toes and foot.

LABORATORY STUDIES. Precise angiography is essential to determine the adequacy of the proximal circulation in the aorta and iliac arteries, as well as in the distal arterial tree, especially the small arteries of the ankle and foot. Significant advances in the technique of angiography have permitted excellent delineation of small arterial branches in these areas. Such studies may be done by direct needle puncture of the femoral artery, followed by injection of a large bolus (50 ml) of contrast medium with serial films made over a long period of time (Fig. 21-10). An alternative technique is to produce ischemic vasodilation by temporary arterial occlusion with an inflated blood pressure cuff for 5 minutes or longer, injecting the dye immediately after deflation of the cuff. This almost invariably produces excellent opacification of distal vessels.

TREATMENT. Unless the extremity is in jeopardy, arterial reconstructions into the tibial arteries are avoided because of the unpredictable outcome in any particular patient. When a reconstruction fails, amputation is usually necessary because the trauma of surgical dissection usually impairs collateral circulation to a significant degree. If operation is not considered indicated, treatment is primarily directed at careful avoidance of foot trauma, as emphasized in the preceding sections.

Surgical reconstruction may be undertaken if only a single tibial artery remains patent or if the pedal arch is found patent on angiogram, usually seen at the ankle as a communication between the anterior and posterior tibial arteries across the dorsum of the foot.

When a necrotizing infection is present, characteristically extending as a necrotic phlegmon rather than an abscess and requiring debridement as opposed to drainage, therapy is almost hopeless without arterial reconstruction. A combined approach of revascularization into the distal tibial and malleolar vessels, followed soon thereafter by debridement of all infected tissue, has been successful. As a practical guideline, if more than one-half of the sole of the foot has been destroyed, the limb will never be suitable for weight bearing, despite effective arterial reconstruction; so amputation is the primary choice. In all such difficult problems intensive antibiotic therapy for the specific organism involved is essential.

Direct Arterial Reconstruction. Bypass venous grafts, usually the greater saphenous vein, have been effective in some patients when connected distad to the anterior or posterior tibial arteries at the level of the malleolus. Tyson and Reichle recently described a substantial experience with the technique performed over the last 4 years. In our experience endarterectomy procedures are not feasible in the small vessels beyond midcalf, although they are quite satisfactory up to that level. However, they have succeeded in the proximal portion in the anterior tibial down to where it passes through the tibiofibular interosseous membrane and down the posterior tibial and peroneal arteries for about 2 in. beyond their origins, removing the overlying soleus muscle to expose the vessels in this area.

These procedures are performed by widely exposing the bifurcation of the popliteal artery through a long medial incision over the calf and lower thigh, a surgical approach described by Imparato and Kim. The endarterectomy is performed with a longitudinal arteriotomy, followed by endarterectomy and closure of the vessels with venous roof patches up to the level of the distal popliteal artery. If arterial reconstruction proximal to this level is required,

Fig. 21-9. *A*. Femoral popliteal endarterectomy performed by exposing the femoral artery proximally and the popliteal artery distad. *B*. An endarterectomy stripper is used to detach atherosclerotic material via a plane in the media or between media and adventitia. Cutting the adductor magnus tendon facilitates passage of the arterial stripper. The distal intima in the popliteal artery is carefully sutured to prevent detachment and dissection of this free edge when circulation is restored. Arteriotomies are closed with autologous vein roof patches. Angiographic studies are performed to ensure that all debris has been removed, since even minute fragments left behind may result in immediate rethrombosis. Alternative techniques are exposing the entire femoral artery, opening it longitudinally in its entirety and suturing a long roof patch for closure, or utilizing CO_2 intramural injection to accomplish endarterectomy.

a bypass procedure or an endarterectomy can be combined with a distal endarterectomy. Similarly if reconstruction is required distad down to the ankle, the reversed autologous vein bypass technique is employed. Although the arteries at the malleolus are small, with an internal diameter of 1 to 2 mm, the anastomoses can be performed with fine suture material (7-0) and optical magnification. Operative angiography is quite useful when such small anastomoses are performed (Fig. 21-11).

Prognosis. As mentioned earlier, arterial reconstructions in this area are performed only when ulceration and gangrene threaten amputation. Arterial reconstruction is initially successful in about 75 percent of patients, both with reconstruction at the proximal tibioperoneal level and with reconstruction extending down to the malleolus. Immediate failures are almost always due to inadequate outflow tracts. Failures occur invariably if the dorsal arch at the ankle is not complete. When the reconstruction is initially successful, limb salvage is excellent, for the necrotic tissue

can be debrided and the wound subsequently closed by skin grafting. If the arterial reconstruction fails before complete healing is obtained, however, amputation is usually required.

If healing is complete and the arterial reconstruction subsequently becomes occluded, a significant percentage of patients remain with a viable functional extremity. Some reconstructions into the proximal tibial arteries so far have remained patent for as long as 5 to 7 years. Fewer data are available for bypass grafts extending down to the ankle, but the failure rate within 2 years after operation seems to exceed 50 percent.

Lumbar Sympathectomy. Lumbar sympathectomy is often tried in desperation as an alternative to amputation when arterial reconstruction cannot be performed. It also may be combined with reconstruction, although its value in this case cannot be determined. As an isolated procedure, improvement can be significant in more than 50 percent of patients in this group. Occasionally a brilliant result occurs,

A   *B*

Fig. 21-10. Preoperative angiographic studies in the presence of tibial disease. *A.* Angiographic studies routinely performed showing poor visualization of tibial arteries. *B.* Angiograms in the same patient obtained 6 weeks later, when an ischemic lesion developed in the foot, showing patency of the anterior tibial artery. This degree of opacification was obtained using the ischemic hyperemia technique described in the text.

consisting of relief of rest pain and marked increase in temperature of the foot. Unfortunately it has not been possible to predict which patients with impending limb loss would respond favorably. Therefore, in our series all patients, whether diabetic or not, whose conditions were considered inoperable from the point of view of arterial reconstruction on the basis of angiographic studies had lumbar sympathectomies. Some 60 percent responded favorably for longer than 6 months, while 40 percent came to early amputation within 2 months.

Infected Prosthesis. The large number of patients now alive with artificial, plastic blood vessel replacements has introduced a numerically significant new pathologic entity, viz., the infected plastic prosthesis. Plastic blood vessel substitutes, especially if placed in the groins, are subject to infection, which usually cannot be eradicated unless the plastic material is removed from the infected area. Axillofemoral bypass grafts have been employed to permit removal of infected intraabdominal grafts. Infections in the

groin, in the presence of noninfected intraabdominal arteries, have been treated by performing iliac to superficial femoral or popliteal bypass grafts, avoiding the infected groins by leading the grafts through the obturator foramen to the posteromedial aspect of the thigh or to the medial aspect of the popliteal fossa, thus permitting the radical debridement of infected tissue and grafts from the groins. These have been highly successful when properly planned in association with prolonged antibiotic therapy. These procedures are indicated at a stage when infection may appear relatively innocuous. Injection of a radiopaque contrast medium into the sinuses has been helpful in delineating the true nature and extent of the problem. Aggressive and extensive surgical procedures are required to prevent exsanguinating hemorrhage from breakdown of suture lines secondary to the local infection. Although obturator bypass grafts have been successful in dealing with infections in the groins, removal of aortic prosthesis with end closure of the infrarenal aorta has resulted frequently in subsequent rupture of the aorta.

Amputation. Some important guidelines should be emphasized when amputation threatens because of progressive ulceration of the foot: First, an arterial reconstructive procedure may be successful if only one major arterial tributary is patent, a branch of the popliteal artery, the anterior tibial, the posterior tibial, or even the peroneal artery. Second, a foot will remain useful for weight bearing as long as the posterior half, including the heel, is intact. If more than 50 percent of the sole has been lost, however, the foot is probably useless for weight bearing even if arterial reconstruction is successful. With these two guidelines, angiograms should be seriously considered for virtually all patients in whom amputation is being considered. Data published by Dale in 1967 are quite significant in this regard. Of 100 patients threatened by amputation, either because of rest pain (38 percent) or ulceration with gangrene (62 percent), arterial reconstructive procedures were performed in 73 and lumbar sympathectomy in 13. The leg was salvaged in 64, and a minor amputation was possible in 10 others.

Both morbidity and mortality are surprisingly high in patients requiring amputation for peripheral vascular disease. Mortality is related to the advanced age in many and to a rate of severe coronary occlusive disease exceeding 50 percent. Morbidity is primarily related to failure of wound healing from improper selection of the site of amputation. In general, as long as gangrene is limited to a toe, the amputation should be delayed and the ischemic toe permitted to mummify and undergo virtual autoamputation. Delay permits growth of collateral circulation in the more proximal tissues so that wound healing may occur if the toe is allowed to gradually separate over a period of weeks; a definitive amputation often results in failure and extension of the wound onto the foot. A transmetatarsal amputation may be effective in some diabetic patients when infection superimposed upon a gangrenous toe requires operation. This is successful if pedal pulses are palpable but ineffective if gangrene has extended into the forefoot. Foot amputations proximal to the transmetatarsal level are generally unsatisfactory for weight bearing except for the Syme amputation, which is almost never successful in the presence of peripheral vascular disease.

A fortunate and surprising development in the past few years has been the demonstration by several groups that below-knee amputations can be successfully performed in a high percentage of patients, even in the absence of a popliteal pulse. Preservation of the knee joint greatly facilitates the wearing of a prosthesis. Guidelines are still being sought to determine the likelihood of wound healing if a below-knee amputation is performed in the absence of a popliteal pulse. The degree of skin bleeding is one of the most useful guidelines, though not infallible, that has yet appeared. An attempted below-knee amputation is a

reversed autologous femoral-dorsal pedal bypass graft. *A.* Posterior tibial artery forming pedal arch. *B.* Bypass graft in place.

significant benefit to the patient if successful but is detrimental if the wound fails to heal and a subsequent above-knee amputation must be performed.

THE DIABETIC FOOT

The foot of the diabetic patient has distinct problems, characteristic of the diabetic state, which can quickly progress to conditions that threaten limb and life. Three distinct characteristics can be delineated:

First, the diabetic has an extraordinary susceptibility to infection. This can develop after minor trauma to the toe, the sole of the foot, or the heel. After a seemingly trivial injury, within hours or days a virulent necrotizing infection can appear which rapidly spreads along musculofascial planes. It characteristically begins in an interdigital space, spreads along the plantar fascia, and may continue along tendon sheaths into the muscles of the leg. Frequently the infecting organism is gas-producing and may be of the clostridial group. A life-threatening infection quickly evolves. This same susceptibility to infection manifests itself in the development of carbuncles in the neck and in different types of necrotizing infections of the abdominal wall after elective abdominal operations. These infections often occur with patent major arteries and seemingly are not closely related to local ischemia.

A second peculiarity of the diabetic is diabetic neuropathy. Characteristically this appears as hypalgesia or true anesthesia of some portion of the sole of the foot, subsequently complicated by trophic ulcers. These also are unrelated to ischemia and often develop with strongly palpable pedal pulses. The trophic ulcer, anesthetic and painless initially, then becomes a portal of entry for necrotizing infection.

The third peculiarity of the diabetic foot is the type of arterial occlusive disease which typically involves the popliteal artery and its branches down to the pedal arches. The process may be diffuse, or one or more arteries may be spared. Arteries proximal to the popliteal may be normal or may show a typical "nondiabetic" pattern of atherosclerosis.

CLINICAL MANAGEMENT. Infection. In some unfortunate instances a rampant uncontrolled infection with clostridia may necessitate immediate open amputation through the midcalf or midthigh to prevent death from septic shock. If patients are seen earlier, immediate widespread incision and drainage with debridement of infected tissue may prevent amputation. At an earlier stage, when infection is the dominant process without extensive tissue necrosis, localized debridement combined with intensive antibiotic therapy may be successful. A basic guideline is that all necrotic tissue must be extensively debrided, for simple drainage is hopelessly inadequate in the presence of extensive tissue necrosis, as is radical debridement alone because of the underlying tissue ischemia. In such instances the combination of radical debridement with arterial reconstruction down to the ankle may permit salvage of the extremity. These considerations were discussed in the preceding section on tibioperoneal arterial reconstruction.

Gangrene. If gangrene of a toe is present and not complicated by infection, a much more leisurely approach is indicated, quite in contrast to the urgency of therapy if spreading infection is present. As discussed earlier, localized dry gangrene of a toe is best treated by postponing operation, often permitting autoamputation over a period of weeks, during which time the development of collateral circulation may permit wound healing to occur. In all likelihood such instances of gangrene of a digit represent occlusion of a critical digital vessel. This may be followed by the development of enough collateral circulation to salvage the foot, but such circulation requires time to develop.

Trophic Ulcers. A trophic ulcer can be readily recognized by several characteristics. It is usually a sharply demarcated, punched out area on the sole of the foot overlying a pressure point, usually the metatarsal heads. A location over the first or third metatarsal head is particularly common. Often the ulcers are completely anesthetic and hence relatively free of pain until secondary infection develops. Similarly, the pedal pulses may be entirely normal.

Treatment in the majority of patients consists of local cleansing, protection from trauma, and most important of all, avoidance of weight bearing. Reconstruction of shoes to distribute weight differently is often effective. Special types of shoes, such as those lined with lamb's wool, are useful. Effective therapy requires long-term careful periodic observation to readjust the weight-bearing characteristics of the foot so that pressure on the area of ulceration is avoided. Any superimposed infection requires antibiotics and local debridement. As most patients fortunately do not have any vascular occlusion, arterial reconstruction is not needed.

SUMMARY OF THERAPEUTIC CONCEPTS FOR ARTERIAL OCCLUSIVE DISEASE OF THE LOWER EXTREMITIES

Intermittent claudication with normal nutrition in the extremity is a comparatively benign disease in many patients. The risk of gangrene within 5 years is no more than 5 percent. If a patient stops smoking and exercises regularly, claudication may improve to a significant degree within months or years. This, combined with the fact that arterial reconstructions are not curative, indicates that a conservative approach can be applied to many patients with claudication, depending upon the patient's age and occupation.

A quite different approach is indicated when the nutrition of the foot is impaired from chronic ischemia, for the likelihood of ulceration and gangrene within 1 to 2 years is great. In these patients, the possibilities of arterial reconstruction should be carefully investigated by detailed angiography, examining the arterial tree from the abdominal aorta to the pedal arches at the ankle. This has been especially productive when ulceration and gangrene already have appeared and amputation appears imminent.

ARTERIAL EMBOLISM

It has been long recognized that the majority of arterial emboli originate in the heart. The embolus originated from the heart in 86 percent of 426 emboli reported by Darling and associates and in 91 percent of 214 emboli reported by Cranley et al. In the past few years there has been increasing recognition of emboli which originate in atherosclerotic arteries, either fragments of a plaque or thrombi adherent to the surface of an ulcerated plaque which subsequently dislodge. For simplicity in presentation, emboli arising from the heart, constituting the majority of emboli seen, are referred to as *cardioarterial embolization*. As a separate entity, the frequency of which is yet unknown, emboli arising from an atherosclerotic artery and lodging in the distal branches are referred to as *arterioarterial emboli*.

Cardioarterial Embolization

HISTORICAL CONSIDERATIONS. Emboli have been long recognized as a cause of acute arterial occlusion resulting in gangrene. Several unsuccessful embolectomies were attempted near the end of the nineteenth century, but the first successful embolectomy is credited to Lahey in 1911. For many years embolectomies performed within 4 to 6 hours after lodging of the embolus were successful, while those performed later had a progressively higher failure rate. Less than 15 years ago a serious proposal was made that emboli which had lodged more than 12 hours earlier should not be operated upon. It is now well established that such a viewpoint is erroneous. The difficulties with late operation have been found due to inadequate removal of distal thrombi. With the combination of operative angiography and the balloon catheter developed by Fogarty et al. in 1963, viability can be preserved in well over 90 percent of patients operated upon if operation is performed before the muscles become necrotic, regardless of whether the embolus lodged 3 hours or 3 days beforehand.

INCIDENCE AND ETIOLOGY. In about 90 percent of patients with emboli, the embolus originates in the heart from one of three causes: mitral stenosis, atrial fibrillation, or myocardial infarction. In some patients it is the first sign of previously unrecognized heart disease. Hence, an embolus, though a serious or catastrophic event, is best regarded as a symptom of serious heart disease which must be treated separately.

With mitral stenosis emboli originate from thrombi which have formed in the left atrium because of restriction of blood flow through the stenotic mitral valve. Most such patients also have atrial fibrillation with impaired contractility of the atrium. Atrial fibrillation from atherosclerosis without mitral stenosis can occur and becomes increasingly frequent in older patients. Emboli have been recognized to occur following the spontaneous or induced conversion of fibrillation to sinus rhythm, probably because the contractions of the atrial appendage expel thrombi which have accumulated during the impaired contractility from fibrillation. Emboli following a myocardial infarction originate from mural thrombi forming over the endocardial surfaces of the infarcts. Their frequency is greatest in the first 2 to 3 weeks following infarction, and in some patients they are the first sign that an infarction has occurred.

Unusual causes of peripheral emboli include a paradoxic embolus in which a thrombus arising in the venous circulation passes through a congenital atrial or ventricular septal defect and lodges in a peripheral artery. Other unusual causes include bacterial endocarditis, mural thrombi in subclavian or popliteal aneurysms, and atrial myxoma. In 4 to 5 percent of patients, despite the most diligent search, the source is never found.

PATHOLOGY. Most emboli ejected from the heart, 70 percent of the 426 emboli reported by Darling, lodge in the arteries of the lower extremities. Unfortunately 20 to 25 percent lodge in the cerebral circulation, usually intracranially, and are surgically inaccessible. Five to ten percent lodge in visceral arteries, the superior mesenteric or renal, and an unknown number lodge in silent areas of the circulation, such as the spleen, for which clinical signs are obscure.

Emboli usually lodge at bifurcations of major arteries where the diameter abruptly narrows. Common sites are the bifurcation of the abdominal aorta, the common iliac artery, the common femoral artery, and the popliteal arteries (Fig. 21-12). In the upper extremities similar patterns are found, including the distal subclavian artery and the bifurcation of the common brachial. The severity of the ischemia produced is due both to the abrupt occlusion and the fact that the site of occlusion involves two major arteries whereas an occlusion either immediately proximal or distal to a site of bifurcation would permit collateral circulation through the bifurcation.

PATHOPHYSIOLOGY. The physiologic consequences of an arterial embolus are the immediate onset of severe ischemia of the tissues normally supplied by the occluded artery. Depending upon the artery involved, if untreated, an embolus results in gangrene in about 50 percent of patients. The prominent early symptoms of pain, paralysis, and paresthesia all result from the great sensitivity of peripheral nerves to oxygen deprivation. Striated muscle is secondary only to peripheral nerves in susceptibility to anoxia. Necrosis may appear within 4 to 6 hours after onset of ischemia but varies with a number of factors. These include the size of the artery occluded, the collateral circulation around the site of occlusion, blood pressure, and temperature. If collateral circulation is well developed, necrosis may not appear for 8 to 12 hours; occasionally moderate ischemia is present but necrosis does not develop. The fact that muscle necrosis often begins within 4 to 6 hours is the reason that surgical embolectomy is uniformly successful within 4 to 6 hours but considerably less effective after longer periods of time.

Sluggish flow of blood in arteries distal to the embolus results in secondary thrombosis within the distal arterial tree. This may be a thrombus in continuity with the original embolus, or separate thrombi may develop in areas of severe stasis, varying with the degree of blood flow through collateral circulation. Secondary thrombi further occlude major collateral channels and intensify the ischemia. Effective therapy becomes more difficult because not only the primary embolus but also the secondary thrombus must be removed. Eventually the progressive circulatory stasis is further complicated by extensive venous thrombosis.

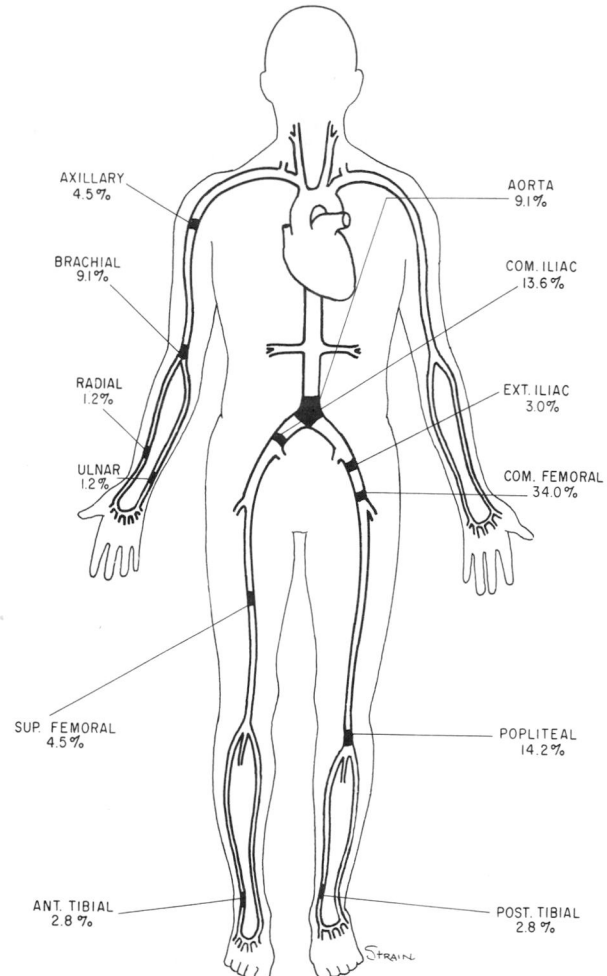

AXILLARY
4.5%

BRACHIAL
9.1%

RADIAL
1.2%

ULNAR
1.2%

AORTA
9.1%

COM. ILIAC
13.6%

EXT. ILIAC
3.0%

COM. FEMORAL
34.0%

SUP. FEMORAL
4.5%

POPLITEAL
14.2%

ANT. TIBIAL
2.8%

POST. TIBIAL
2.8%

Fig. 21-12. Frequency of involvement of different peripheral arteries by arterial emboli. In the majority of patients arteries in the lower extremity are involved. (*Redrawn from H. Haimovici, Peripheral Arterial Embolism, Angiology, 1:20, 1950.*)

CLINICAL MANIFESTATIONS. The five p's discussed earlier under manifestations of acute arterial occlusion, pain, paralysis, paresthesia, absent pulses, and pallor, describe the principal clinical features of arterial embolism. The onset is abrupt in most cases, gradual in a few. In 75 to 80 percent of patients there is severe and unremitting pain, usually referred to the most peripheral portions of the limb. The color may be extreme pallor or mottling from alternate areas of pallor and cyanosis. Sensory disturbances vary from anesthesia to paresthesia. Paralysis may be the most prominent feature; complete paralysis and anesthesia mask the true nature of the disorder, diverting the physician into investigations for neurologic disease while muscle necrosis is occurring.

The neurologic symptoms are the crucial prognostic signs for muscle necrosis usually appearing within 6 to 8 hours after onset unless therapy is effective. Conversely, if motor and sensory function is intact, the extremity will survive even though chronic ischemia may persist.

Physical Examination. The extremity is often pale and cold with collapsed peripheral veins. With less severe degrees of ischemia there may be cyanosis instead of pallor. A temperature level may be detected which coincides with the level at which the color changes. The arterial pulse is absent at the site of occlusion, frequently with accentuation of the pulse immediately proximal to this point. Sensory impairment varies from hypesthesia to anesthesia, and motor disturbances from weakness to paralysis.

The level of occlusion can often be estimated from the color, temperature level, and pulse findings. Ordinarily acute ischemia develops one joint below the site of occlusion. An iliac embolus produces ischemia at the level of the hip joint, while a common femoral embolus produces ischemia distal to the knee. These, of course, vary with the effectiveness of collateral circulation. Muscle turgor in the ischemic limb is most important. Shortly after the onset of ischemia, the muscles are soft. With continuing ischemia, edema appears, progresses to necrosis, and finally to rigor mortis. Early ischemic edema creates a "doughy" sensation on palpation, termed by some "football calf." The importance of this physical finding is the fact that as long as the muscles are soft to palpation, the extremity can be salvaged with effective embolectomy and thrombectomy, regardless of how long the embolus has been present. Conversely, the presence of stiff muscles warns that necrosis has occurred. This is most clearly apparent in the leg where the muscle tone of the gastrocnemius and soleus group can be easily evaluated. Some limbs with early muscle necrosis can be salvaged by embolectomy and thrombectomy, combined with extensive fasciotomy and later debridement of localized muscle necrosis, but failure is frequent.

An additional important aspect of physical examination is the cardiac examination for underlying heart disease. The cardiac rhythm, murmurs, or friction rubs may provide clues to atrial fibrillation, mitral stenosis, or acute myocardial infarction. Examination of other peripheral arteries for pulses and bruits provides additional clues to underlying cardiac or arterial disease.

LABORATORY STUDIES. A critical decision to be made when the patient is first encountered is whether an angiogram should be performed or not. The diagnosis of acute arterial occlusion can be readily made from the history and physical findings. An electrocardiogram and a chest roentgenogram should both be done to evaluate the presence of heart disease. If performance of angiography delays surgical therapy beyond the 4- to 6-hour "golden period" of therapy, it should be omitted. Intraoperative angiography is one alternative. Angiography is particularly useful where the site of the embolus is uncertain or in distinguishing between arterial embolism and arterial thrombosis superimposed upon an atherosclerotic plaque.

DIAGNOSIS. The condition most easily confused with an arterial embolus is acute thrombosis of an artery previously diseased with atherosclerosis. The importance of differentiating the two conditions is to determine the method of surgical therapy, for a more extensive operative procedure is required with thrombosis. Certain clinical findings suggest thrombosis rather than embolism. Atherosclerosis is usually seen in an older age group, and often symptoms of chronic ischemia, such as claudication, have been present for some time. The involved extremity may show signs of chronic ischemia such as loss of hair from the toes and atrophy of the skin and nails. The absence of heart disease which could cause an arterial embolus further supports the diagnosis of thrombosis. At times differential diagnosis is difficult or even impossible, because an embolus may occur in an older patient with atrial fibrillation who also has claudication from femoral atherosclerosis. Then, an arteriogram is of great value. With atherosclerosis and secondary arterial thrombosis, diffuse changes of atherosclerosis can be seen throughout the peripheral arteries, often with the development of prominent collateral circulation. By contrast, with embolism, the distal arteries are usually normal except at the site of occlusion.

Rarely, acute extensive thrombophlebitis may be confused with an embolus. Thrombophlebitis may be associated with extensive vasospasm, causing pain and peripheral vasoconstriction with diminished pulses. A bluish extremity, termed *phlegmasia cerulea dolens,* is also characteristic of venous thrombosis. With arterial embolism edema appears only after extensive gangrene has developed.

Even more rarely, acute dissecting aneurysm of the thoracic aorta with obliteration of peripheral pulses may suggest multiple peripheral emboli. A dissecting aneurysm can be suspected because of pain in the chest or back, often with a left pleural effusion.

TREATMENT. Indications for Operation. Because patients with arterial emboli usually have serious heart disease, the operative procedure must be planned with regard to the influence of anesthesia and operation on the heart disease. This is particularly critical when the embolus has resulted from a myocardial infarction. With modern vascular techniques, however, embolectomy can be performed in most patients with minimal trauma, often with local anesthesia. Hence, a decision not to operate because of heart disease should be made only if death is imminent. The reason for this is that failure to remove a peripheral embolus, which subsequently produces gangrene, of necessity requires a major amputation, a much greater surgical stress than simple embolectomy.

As repeated frequently in this chapter for emphasis, the urgency for performing arterial embolectomy can be simply estimated from the presence of paralysis and anesthesia. When these are present, muscle necrosis often occurs within 4 to 6 hours. If they are absent, a more conservative approach may be undertaken. However, their absence does not guarantee that claudication will not subsequently develop in the extremity with resumption of normal physical activity.

An unusual indication for nonsurgical therapy occurs with a migrating embolus. An embolus may lodge in a proximal artery, such as the common femoral, then fragment proximally within a few hours and migrate distad. Rarely such patients may recover completely, but most remain with significant residual occlusion of peripheral arteries. Peripheral pulses should be unequivocally present before simple observation is continued for a long period of time.

Preoperative Therapy. The prompt intravenous administration of heparin to inhibit the development of thrombi distal to the embolus is the most important therapeutic measure in the treatment of an arterial embolus. Heparin, 5,000 to 10,000 units, is given intravenously by continuous drip or repeated at 3- to 6-hour intervals, depending upon the clotting time, if embolectomy is delayed. Lumbar sympathetic blocks are of dubious value and cannot be safely performed in the presence of systemic anticoagulation. Other measures to influence collateral circulation, such as orally administered vasodilator drugs, are of little value. Intraarterial administration of drugs such as reserpine and priscoline sometimes dramatically improves the appearance of acutely ischemic extremities by eliminating functional arterial resistance to flow.

Operative Technique. For operations on the extremities, local anesthesia can be used in seriously ill patients. Frequently the operative incisions are short, for the location of the embolus can be accurately predicted from the clinical picture. The Fogarty balloon catheter has permitted removal of propagated clot both distal and proximal to emboli, making possible performance of the entire operative procedure through limited surgical incisions. Frequently, it is possible to perform the entire embolectomy and thrombectomy through incision in the upper thigh over the common femoral artery. Emboli and thrombi can be removed from the aorta and both iliac arteries by a retrograde approach. With emboli at the common femoral bifurcation, it is possible to remove thrombi from the arterial tree down to the ankle through the same incision. Rarely is it necessary to enter the peritoneal cavity for aortoiliac embolectomy and thrombectomy. This should be avoided when possible, for these patients are usually quite ill from their cardiac disease. Many have had a large myocardial infarction which in turn produced an embolus large enough to occlude the abdominal aorta. On other occasions, because of difficulty in passing Fogarty balloon catheters from the common femoral artery into the anterior tibial artery, a separate incision is made at the level of the knee joint to expose the origin of the anterior tibial from the popliteal artery.

In general, surgical incisions are placed directly over the uppermost level of arterial occlusion unless the aortoiliac system is involved, in which case incisions are placed over both common femoral arteries. Once the artery has been isolated proximal and distal to the embolus, 5,000 units heparin should be given intravenously. A transverse or a longitudinal arteriotomy is then made in the artery immediately proximal to its bifurcation, where the embolus is usually lodged. The embolus characteristically "pops" out as soon as the lumen is entered and can be recognized by its gray appearance and nonadherence to the arterial wall. Hence, removal is a simple procedure, but removal of thrombi which have formed distad or even proximally may be unusually complex. Fogarty balloon catheters have virtually eliminated the need to make multiple incisions along the course of the arterial tree for the laborious retrograde washing out of thrombi. The preferred technique is to pass the catheter into the distal artery as far as possible, inflate the balloon, and withdraw it in its inflated state. Comparison of the length of the catheter inserted with the length of the extremity indicates how far the catheter has been advanced. Passage of catheters into the aorta for the removal of aortoiliac thrombi is similarly performed. Occasionally it is impossible to pass the balloon catheter into various distal tributaries, either the anterior and posterior tibial in the calf or the radial and ulnar in the forearm. In such instances separate distal incisions are made over these vessels, followed by separate introduction of the catheter into each branch. Dale has used polyethylene catheters to aspirate clot. With these techniques, retrograde flushing of the artery through a distal incision is rarely necessary.

As indicated, the most crucial aspect of the operation is determining the completeness of removal of propagated thrombus. Back-bleeding is a notoriously unreliable indicator. Obviously if there is no back-bleeding, thrombus is still present. Back-bleeding can occur, however, through the nearest arterial branch, while the major artery distad is still occluded. Failure to remove all residual thrombus usually results in reocclusion (Fig. 21-13). The operative procedure should be continued until, by an appropriate combination of techniques, all pulses are restored at the ankle or wrist, or an operative arteriogram has demon-

strated that the arteries are patent. On occasion, restoration of a pulse can be misleading, and bounding pulses may be felt in an artery partly reopened but with persisting distal obstruction. For this reason operative angiography is often critical to success.

If severe ischemic injury has been present beforehand, wide fasciotomy of the fascial envelop containing the major muscles may help preserve limb viability. This should be particularly considered if embolectomy has been delayed beyond the golden first 4 to 6 hours and definite change in muscle turgor was palpable before operation.

Postoperative Care. The most important aspect of postoperative care is to be certain that peripheral circulation is adequate. A palpable pulse is the best clinical sign. This should be identified immediately after operation and its presence periodically confirmed by palpation. Pulses which

Fig. 21-13. Embolic material and secondary clot. The embolic material which was deposited in the heart chambers during active blood flow is gray to salmon-colored, of firm consistency, and unattached to the arterial wall. It is composed mainly of fibrin and degenerated platelets. The gelatinous clot which appears homogeneous is a secondary stasis clot and was formed when blood flow ceased. It contains all the blood elements, and is dark red in color.

are difficult to feel can be checked with the Doppler instrument, which permits not only auscultation over pedal arteries but also measurement of pressures within those vessels. Disappearance of a previously palpable pulse or a change in Doppler measurements associated with unsatisfactory appearance of the extremity is an indication for either arteriography or immediate reoperation.

The persistence of paralysis and anesthesia following operation is ominous; gangrene is almost a certainty. Conversely, restoration of normal neurologic function indicates adequate circulation for muscle viability. This is particularly reassuring either when pulses cannot be restored or palpation is inconclusive because of edema and swelling.

The mode of heparin administration in the postoperative period is critical, since fresh surgical wounds are subject to hemorrhage, while delay of anticoagulation may predispose to further embolization. Some surgeons give no heparin for 6 hours postoperatively and then administer it by intermittent intravenous injection in doses of 5,000 units every 4 to 6 hours. Oral therapy with Coumadin derivatives is begun after 3 to 4 days and continued as long as the patients are at risk. Salzman et al. have reported that continuously administered intravenous heparin, avoiding peak effects which reach infinity during the intermittent administration, is associated with a lesser incidence of hemorrhage. Thrombolysis may accompany heparin administration, especially when porous knitted vascular prostheses are employed. The importance of prompt and continuous anticoagulant therapy cannot be overemphasized, for the arterial embolus is only a symptom of serious heart disease. Recurrence of embolization, each incident associated with a 25 to 30 percent likelihood of lodging in the brain, is distressingly common unless the heart disease is effectively treated. Patients with intractable atrial fibrillation should be maintained on permanent anticoagulant therapy. Those with mitral stenosis should have a mitral valvulotomy performed soon. Those with myocardial infarction should receive anticoagulants for several weeks, by which time the endocardial surface of the infarct will have healed and the likelihood of embolism is small.

Antibiotic therapy, usually penicillin or methicillin, generally is started at the time of operation and continued for 2 to 4 days.

PROGNOSIS. The most important feature influencing survival of the extremity following embolectomy is the time elapsing between the occurrence of embolization and successful restoration of flow at operation. As mentioned repeatedly, removal within 4 to 6 hours after onset is almost always associated with an excellent prognosis, having the two great advantages of avoiding muscle necrosis and limiting the secondary thrombus formation beyond the site of embolism. In both of the large series reported by Darling et al. and by Cranley et al. excellent results were obtained in 85 to 95 percent of patients. When more than 6 hours elapsed between embolization and embolectomy, unsuccessful results were more common. These particularly occur with inexperienced vascular surgeons and limited facilities. The crucial concept is that as long as the calf muscles are "soft" before operation, indicating that muscle necrosis has not occurred, salvage of the extremity should

approach 95 percent or higher, regardless of the duration of ischemia. However, in delayed cases achieving this goal taxes the resources, skills, and ingenuity of the vascular surgeon to the utmost, for thrombi may have accumulated from the aortic bifurcation to the posterior tibial artery at the ankle and complete removal requires a combination of careful surgical exploration, frequently multiple incisions, and serial operative angiography. If muscle necrosis is present before operation, indicated by a rigid calf muscle, possibilities of limb salvage are small, though these findings are seldom clear enough to warrant primary amputation. Rarely, a functional extremity may be salvaged in which virtually all the calf muscles are lost from necrosis but a viable foot is preserved.

The crucial long-term feature determining prognosis is the ability to prevent further emboli. Without adequate prophylactic anticoagulation recurrence is dismally inevitable, eventually terminating with fatal or crippling cerebral thrombosis. Vigilance to prevent emboli can be relaxed only when a myocardial infarction has healed or mitral stenosis has been treated by valvulotomy.

In any large series of patients with arterial embolism, death occurs in 25 to 30 percent of patients during that hospitalization. This is almost always due to the underlying heart disease causing the embolus, indicating the gravity of the basic illness. In some instances death is due to either inadequate management of the embolic episode, with the complications of sepsis from gangrene, or to recurrent embolism to the brain or viscera, a result of inadequate anticoagulant therapy.

Arterioarterial Embolization

HISTORICAL CONSIDERATIONS. In the past decade there has been increasing awareness of the entity of arterioarterial embolism to produce ischemic syndromes previously unexplained. With cerebrovascular insufficiency, the ophthalmologic visualization of minute particles of atherosclerotic plaque or platelet fibrin emboli in the retina in association with an ulcerated atherosclerotic plaque at the bifurcation of the carotid artery indicated the genesis of minute emboli. In the lower extremities, sudden onset of toe and foot ischemia, the "blue toe" syndrome, with little or no impairment of peripheral pulses led to the finding that minute emboli were the mechanism, having originated in aortic or iliac atherosclerotic plaques. The occasional finding of peripheral emboli beyond aneurysms has been described periodically. Miles et al. have cited observations suggesting that small emboli in the coronary circulation could come from ulcerated plaques, producing diffuse myocardial scarring from myriads of tiny emboli.

PATHOGENESIS. The basic process seems to be ulceration of an atherosclerotic plaque with discharge of minute fragments of atherosclerotic debris into the circulation. The ulcerated surface may become covered by platelets and fibrin which in turn are intermittently dislodged. How often these are subsequently resorbed is unknown. The emboli may arise from an atherosclerotic artery near the end organ where the emboli lodge or may originate some distance away, occasionally seen when emboli in the toes

B

A

Fig. 21-14. Arterioarterial embolization, also known as athero-embolization, in a patient in whom marked ischemia of the toes developed in the presence of palpable pedal pulses. Several attacks occurred with progressive ischemia. *A.* Angiograms showing infrarenal abdominal aortic plaques. Occlusion of small calf arteries without involvement of renal arteries suggested that this infrarenal plaque was the source of emboli. *B.* Aortic plaque removed by endarterectomy. There has been no recurrence of embolization since operation 7 years ago.

apparently originate from plaques in the abdominal or thoracic aorta. Repeated embolic episodes are frequent, at times with almost complete recovery from ischemia between each episode; in other patients progressively greater degrees of ischemia occur, ultimately terminating in necrosis.

CLINICAL FINDINGS. A most striking syndrome occurs with emboli from the distal thoracic aorta, the "blue toe" syndrome. There is severe ischemia of the toes and feet, bilaterally, in association with renal failure. Before the pathogenesis was understood, the diagnosis remained an enigma, for pulses often remained palpable even while distal ischemia progressed to gangrene. There is a wide range in severity, from complete clearing of ischemia to progressive occlusion and gangrene.

Similar episodes occur in the cerebrovascular circulation with any combination of neurologic symptoms from the most transient, fleeting symptoms to complete stroke with cerebral infarction. In the upper extremity the subclavian artery is most frequently involved, with repeated attacks simulating Raynaud's phenomenon.

DIAGNOSIS. The diagnosis can be suspected from the combined findings of severe ischemia of a digit with palpable pulses. Determining the source of the emboli is crucial, for many can be corrected surgically, often by simple endarterectomy. Hence, detailed angiographic studies are necessary. The source of the embolus can be estimated by noting the peripheral circulation in other areas, where previous emboli may have lodged. For example, involvement of branches of the profunda femoris artery indicate emboli arising proximal to this level. Concomitant involvement of renal artery branches suggests that the emboli originated in the thoracic aorta. Similarly in the upper extremity emboli may arise from the subclavian artery or alternatively from lesions located far distad, such as small aneurysms in the palm of the hand. These diagnostic possibilities can be resolved only by precise, extensive angiography.

TREATMENT. When the atherosclerotic plaque can be related to the pattern of distal embolization (Fig. 21-14), arterial reconstruction of the atherosclerotic segment either by endarterectomy or replacement with a prosthetic graft has prevented further embolism. In the carotid system, there is now extensive experience with arterial reconstruction to prevent recurrent ischemic episodes, so-called transient ischemic attacks (TIA). The operation is effective and durable. Similar procedures have been performed in the subclavian artery to prevent TIA in the upper extremity. In the lower extremity experience is still limited, but good results in a series of 10 cases operated upon at New York University have confirmed both the validity of the concept and the surgical approach.

Theoretically emboli from platelet or fibrin aggregates should be inhibited or prevented by anticoagulants, but their effectiveness is yet uncertain. Paradoxically, anticoagulant therapy might prevent healing of an ulcerated plaque and thereby increase the tendency for embolization. This may explain the infrequent clinical puzzle of an embolus developing *after* heparin therapy has been started.

ACUTE ARTERIAL THROMBOSIS

ETIOLOGY AND PATHOLOGY. Acute arterial thrombosis usually occurs in an artery previously narrowed by atherosclerosis. In some patients the process of occlusion is gradual; no acute symptoms appear, but chronic arterial insufficiency slowly becomes more severe. In others, however, sudden thrombosis precipitates acute symptoms, closely mimicking an arterial embolus.

Unusual causes of arterial thrombosis are a cervical rib or repeated occupational trauma, such as operation of a pneumatic tool, the vibrations of which locally injure the arterial wall and produce thrombosis. Very rarely arterial thrombosis develops within a normal artery. This can happen with debilitating infections, especially in infants, usually with diarrhea and dehydration. It may also occur with primary hematologic disorders, such as polycythemia vera.

Iatrogenic thrombosis has become much more common from percutaneous introduction of catheters for cardiac catheterization or selective angiography. Thrombosis develops from detachment of a flap of intima from the arterial wall with subsequent formation of an occluding thrombus. Acute lower extremity arterial thrombosis also has been seen following long periods of immobilization such as in long automobile or plane trips, similar to acute venous thrombosis, which occurs more commonly.

CLINICAL MANIFESTATIONS. When thrombosis occurs suddenly, the findings are similar to those occurring with arterial trauma or embolism: pain, absence of pulses, paresthesias, and paralysis.

The usual question in differential diagnosis is the distinction between an arterial embolus and an arterial thrombosis. Such a distinction cannot always be made with accuracy, but several clues are helpful. A history of claudication in the involved extremity indicates chronic arterial disease. Similarly, examination of the extremity may show the stigmata of chronic arterial insufficiency, including ab-

sence of hair and trophic changes in the skin and nails. Significant findings may also be present in the contralateral, asymptomatic extremity. The absence of heart disease commonly associated with an arterial embolus is indirect evidence that thrombosis is the most likely cause.

Before successful techniques of arterial reconstruction were developed, the distinction between arterial thrombosis and arterial embolism in a patient in whom acute arterial occlusion suddenly developed was an important one. Surgical exploration of patients with arterial thrombosis usually was futile, because the underlying cause of the thrombosis, atherosclerotic stenosis of the artery, could not be treated. Futile surgical exploration often made the condition worse through interruption of collateral circulation. With present surgical techniques, differentiation between the two conditions is much less important, because operation is necessary with either if circulation is impaired to such an extent that gangrene is imminent. The main reason for recognizing which condition is present before operation is to anticipate the degree of vascular reconstruction which will be required. Restoration of blood flow in an extremity with chronic occlusive disease, with an arterial thrombosis superimposed upon an artery previously narrowed by atherosclerosis, is much more difficult than the performance of simple embolectomy upon an artery with no intrinsic vascular disease. Patients with arterial thrombosis should have an arteriogram before operation to assess the extent of occlusive disease and to evaluate the patency of the vascular bed beyond the point of occlusion in order to determine where a bypass graft can be inserted distad.

TREATMENT. Operative correction of the arterial occlusion requires both removal of the thrombus and correction of the atherosclerotic stenosis. The operative techniques are described in detail in the section on chronic arterial disease. Usually either the atherosclerotic narrowing is removed directly with an endarterectomy, or a bypass graft is inserted around the area of obstruction.

BUERGER'S DISEASE

HISTORICAL DATA. The entity referred to as Buerger's disease was first described by Winiwarter in 1879 and elaborated upon by Buerger in 1908 and again in 1924. The descriptive term *thromboangiitis obliterans* (TAO) emphasizes the inflammatory reaction in the arterial wall, with involvement of the neighboring vein and nerve, terminating in thrombosis of the artery. In 1960 doubt was cast upon the specificity of the pathologic findings when Wessler et al. pointed out that arterial occlusion from any cause, be it atherosclerosis or even embolic occlusion, may result in a similar type of angiitis, indistinguishable from what is usually considered to be specific for TAO. The relatively widespread use of arteriography has shown that many cases of so-called Buerger's disease probably represented presenile atherosclerosis occurring in the third, fourth, and fifth decades of life.

INCIDENCE AND ETIOLOGY. In our experience, we have made the diagnosis in fewer than 0.25 percent of all the patients with occlusive arterial disease of the extremities. The disease is found most frequently in men between twenty and forty years of age. In a Mayo Clinic series exceeding 500 patients, the youngest patient seen was seventeen years of age. The disease is uncommon in women, only 5 to 10 percent of patients with Buerger's disease being women. It is also rare in Negroes; of 936 cases found in the Armed Forces and analyzed by DeBakey and Cohen, only 2 percent were in Negroes. Initially it was felt that the disease was much more common in the Jewish race; subsequent statistical studies have shown that this frequency has been greatly exaggerated and the incidence is only slightly greater if at all.

Heavy tobacco smoking, usually 20 or more cigarettes per day, has been almost universally associated with this disease. The Mayo Clinic group found only three nonsmokers in a 30-year period. The tobacco habit is so entrenched in these individuals that very few successfully forego smoking although often warned of the dire consequences and in spite of obvious remissions which occur upon cessation. DeBakey and Cohen analyzed 936 patients and found that only 10 percent successfully stopped smoking over a 10-year period.

Although the correlation between Buerger's disease and smoking is strong, the mechanisms involved are not clear. There is either a particular response to tobacco (since there are so many more smokers than patients with Buerger's disease) or, as in the Orient, particular brands of cigarettes are associated with the disease. This has never been noted in the West.

PATHOLOGY. The gross features of Buerger's disease are characteristic of an inflammatory process. The diseased artery is usually surrounded by a dense fibrotic reaction, often incorporating the adjacent vein, less often the neighboring nerve. Although this is usually considered to be characteristic of thromboangiitis obliterans, it also occurs occasionally with atherosclerosis obliterans and very frequently in association with aneurysmal disease.

The distribution of arterial involvement is different from that of atherosclerosis in that smaller, more peripheral arteries, usually in segmental distribution, are involved. In the lower extremities the disease generally occurs beyond the popliteal arteries, starting in tibial vessels extending into the vessels of the foot, similar to the typical arterial involvement in the diabetic. In the upper extremities, where atherosclerotic and diabetic involvement are extremely rare, TAO is manifested by arterial involvement usually distal to the forearm in about 30 percent of these patients. The visceral and cardiac circulations can be involved but this occurs rarely.

Early in the course of Buerger's disease there is involvement of superficial veins, producing the characteristic migratory, recurrent superficial phlebitis, while the larger and deeper veins (such as femoral and iliac) are affected rarely.

Although some doubt has been raised about the specificity of the histologic findings, most observers consider them to be characteristic. Precise retrospective diagnoses have been made on the bases of histologic examination of amputated extremities.

Microscopic examination of small thrombosed arteries shows extensive proliferation of intimal cells and fibroblasts throughout all segments of the arterial wall, with preservation of the basic architecture of the artery. Lipid deposition and calcification, frequently seen in atherosclerosis, are absent. Inflammatory cells, usually lymphocytes, are observed, while giant cells, whose presence was noted originally by Buerger, generally are absent. Necrosis of the arterial wall is very unusual, as is abscess formation. The thrombus in the arterial wall shows an unusual degree of fibroblastic activity with endothelial proliferation, suggesting the presence of a primary antigen in the blood, though none has been found. Spaces within the thrombus, interpreted as partial though functionally ineffectual recanalization, are common but not particularly characteristic of Buerger's disease, since this is seen with all thrombotic occlusions.

Involvement of the neighboring vein and nerve by the inflammatory and fibrotic reactions completes the histologic appearance of the lesions.

Periods of exacerbation of the acute process may be manifested by acute superficial phlebitis, with eventual progression of arterial occlusions and ischemia counterbalanced by remissions, during which collateral circulation becomes effective in the younger patients. The ultimate severity and extent of the extremity ischemia are determined by the frequency and duration of the acute attacks and the length of the quiescent periods. The cycles can usually be broken by cessation of smoking.

DeBakey and Cohen studied this progression in a group of 936 patients followed during a 10-year period after the diagnosis had been made and noted a three times higher mortality rate (10 percent), predominantly from cardiovascular disease, than in a control population. Postmortem examination revealed the familiar pattern of atherosclerotic disease in coronary and cerebral vessels, rather than the characteristic histologic pattern of thromboangiitis obliterans found in upper and lower extremity vessels. The limb amputation rate was 20 to 30 percent in 10 years, with an additional 40 percent showing some progression of ischemia but not requiring amputation. The Mayo Clinic series showed a somewhat better prognosis in that the amputation rate in a 10-year follow-up period was only 20 percent, while the overall survival was similar to that in the control group.

CLINICAL MANIFESTATIONS. There may be a phase of recurrent migratory superficial phlebitis involving superficial veins of the feet, which may occur over a period of years before there is any suspicion of arterial involvement. Invariably the patient is a cigarette smoker, and with continued smoking intermittent claudication appears as the first manifestation of ischemia. Reflecting the peripheral involvement of pedal arteries, pain while walking is usually referred to the arch of the foot, somewhat less often to the calf of the leg, but almost never to the thigh or buttock unless there is associated atherosclerosis obliterans. Upper extremity claudication is rare, probably a reflection of the distribution of arterial involvement, which is usually distal to the wrist. Progression of ischemia is similar to that in all chronic progressive arterial occlusions, in which the initial pain induced by exercise progresses to rest pain, postural color changes, trophic changes, and eventually ulceration and gangrene of one or more digits and finally of an entire foot or hand, necessitating major amputations. Patients with Buerger's disease may eventually require quadruple extremity amputations.

One variant of the typical syndrome is first manifest by painful vesicles of the pulp of fingers with surrounding intensive hyperemia and hypersensitivity, recurring as acute attacks over 2- to 4-year intervals, associated with progressive claudication of the feet and calves. The prognosis appeared to be worsened not only by continued smoking but by smoking certain types of cigarettes.

Pain in Buerger's disease, as in other ischemic conditions of the extremities, is common and may result from phlebitis, ischemia neuritis, or progressive skin and muscle ischemia manifested by the typical ischemic rest pain. This is unremitting and prevents patients from sleeping but is somewhat ameliorated by placing the affected limb in the dependent position. There may be blanching on elevation and rubor on dependence, as well as marked blanching on exposure to cold.

Physical Examination. The most frequent finding is absence of the posterior tibial and dorsalis pedis pulses in the feet. Often the popliteal pulse is palpable, especially in the early stages of the disease. Absence of the posterior tibial pulse is highly suggestive of the diagnosis, especially when bilateral. In the upper extremity, the radial pulse may be congenitally absent in 5 to 10 percent of patients, but absence of both pulses again is very suggestive of the disease. Signs of chronic tissue ischemia include loss of hair from the digits, atrophy of the skin, brittle nails, and rubor on dependency. In more advanced cases there may be ulceration or gangrene in the digits, often beginning near the nail and involving only the distal portion of the digit. With more extensive disease, gangrene extends into the foot. In the upper extremity, fortunately, extension of gangrene beyond the fingers is rare, and amputation of the hand is almost never necessary.

Edema is also frequently seen with advanced ischemia. It may result from keeping the extremity in a dependent position for many hours in an attempt to relieve rest pain. Other mechanisms causing edema include abnormal dilatation of the capillaries, producing rubor, and, rarely, significant venous obstruction. Superficial phlebitis involving segments of superficial veins is frequent, but rarely is phlebitis found in the large veins, such as the femoral or iliac. Accordingly, edema on the basis of phlebitis is unusual.

Another helpful distinction from atherosclerosis is the fact that a bruit is virtually never heard over the involved arteries, whereas such a bruit is frequently audible over the iliac or femoral arteries when atherosclerotic plaques are present.

Laboratory Studies. The most significant laboratory examination is arteriography. Plain roentgenograms of the extremity are helpful only if calcification can be demonstrated in the diseased arteries. This virtually excludes the diagnosis of Buerger's disease. The arteriographic findings, as emphasized by McKusick et al., are frequently characteristic. Typically, the intimal lining of the large arteries

is smooth, without the characteristic irregularities seen from cholesterol plaques in atherosclerosis. In the small arteries, there are abrupt areas of occlusion, frequently surrounded by extensive collateral circulation. The collateral circulation, which evolves over many years, is unusually tortuous and has been termed "tree root" or "spiderlike." A "corkscrew" deformity also has been noted in peripheral arteries, probably representing partial recanalization of an artery previously occluded by a thrombus. The combination of extensive occlusive disease in small arteries with large vessels which remain smooth and normal in appearance, especially in association with extensive collateral circulation, is highly characteristic of Buerger's disease and is most useful in differentiating it from atherosclerosis (Fig. 21-15).

DIAGNOSIS. Buerger's disease can be differentiated from atherosclerosis without undue difficulty. Other entities with occlusive disease of small arteries, however, closely resemble Buerger's disease. These include diabetes mellitus or popliteal aneurysms, repeated episodes of arterioarterial embolization from proximal atherosclerotic plaques, and different collagen disorders. Patients with any of these may have palpable popliteal pulses, absent pedal pulses, and severe ischemia in the digits. In most of these, however, the upper extremities are not involved. Positive factors supporting the diagnosis of Buerger's disease are its onset in men between the ages of twenty and forty years, a history of migratory phlebitis, strong dependence upon tobacco, usually cigarettes, and frequent involvement of the upper extremities.

Factors suggesting that the disease is not Buerger's disease include diabetes mellitus, palpable popliteal or abdominal aneurysms, audible bruit over a major artery, high blood cholesterol, calcification of peripheral arteries, and onset after forty years of age.

Usually the diagnosis can be made from the history and physical examination. Angiographic studies are needed for confirmation and to define the possibilities of arterial reconstruction. Final proof of the diagnosis may require gross and microscopic examination of the diseased arteries.

TREATMENT. The most important aspect of treatment is to have the patient forego the use of tobacco in any form. Simply decreasing the frequency of cigarette smoking is ineffective. The great difficulty in getting the patient to stop smoking cannot be overemphasized, for the pernicious addiction to smoking in this disease closely resembles the tenacity of a heroin addict. In most teaching institutions there are one or more pathetic individuals who have undergone amputation of both legs and most of the fingers of each hand but who are trying to get someone to light a cigarette for them! The statistical facts cited by DeBakey and Cohen that a 10-year follow-up demonstrated that only 10 percent of patients had stopped smoking completely further indicates the magnitude of the problem. In the experience of one of the authors with a few patients with histologically proved Buerger's disease, almost none stopped smoking completely for a significant period of time.

A sympathectomy should be performed routinely in the involved extremity to limit the degree of vasospasm which,

A

B

Fig. 21-15. *A*. Femoral arteriogram in a patient with Buerger's disease, demonstrating extensive tortuous collateral circulation in the lower thigh which has developed over a period of years as a result of occlusion of the superficial femoral and popliteal arteries. *B*. Angiogram of vessels below the knee, demonstrating the usual tortuosity of small arterial tributaries and illustrating the extensive collateral circulation which may develop with Buerger's disease or any other long-standing arterial occlusion.

when superimposed on ischemia from organic occlusion, may precipitate tissue necrosis. The benefit from sympathectomy is difficult to measure because of the episodic characteristics of Buerger's disease, but at least 50 percent of patients significantly benefit from the procedure. Vasodilating drugs, such as alcohol or Arlidin, may be tried but are of less benefit than sympathectomy.

Exposure to extremes of cold or heat should be avoided. Education regarding foot care similar to that described for

the atherosclerotic patient is very important. Often gangrene is precipitated by minor trauma to the foot, such as unwise trimming of a callus or wearing tight shoes, which a foot with normal circulation can tolerate uneventfully. The patient must recognize that his foot has to be carefully protected from all forms of even minor trauma permanently if ulceration and gangrene are to be avoided.

Arteriography should be performed to confirm the diagnosis and exclude other forms of smaller arterial occlusions which may require surgical therapy. If a popliteal pulse is absent, it may indicate the possibility of performing local direct arterial reconstruction.

Occasionally patients with Buerger's disease develop atherosclerotic obstruction of major arteries which are surgically accessible to reconstruction. Such a combination of arterial disease is suggested if the popliteal pulse is absent. In these patients arterial reconstruction may be successfully done upon the atherosclerotic disease, with marked circulatory improvement. Direct surgical approach to the vessels primarily involved by Buerger's disease, however, is not possible.

A conservative procedure is indicated when amputation is required. Often the patients are among the younger of the twenty-to-forty age group, and the episodic nature of the disease indicates that conservatism may be rewarded by subsidence of the acute episodes with subsequent partial revascularization by the growth of collateral circulation. As long as gangrene is confined to a toe, amputation should be postponed as long as possible unless rest pain or infection cannot be controlled otherwise. Delaying amputation of a gangrenous digit can permit sufficient development of collateral circulation to allow healing following amputation, whereas amputation soon after gangrene has appeared is often followed by failure of wound healing and the necessity for a more extensive amputation.

Once gangrene has involved the foot extensively, there is little point in delaying amputation, because a functional foot can rarely be obtained if the point of amputation is more proximal than the base of the metatarsal bones. Often a below-knee amputation can be performed, rather than an above-knee, because the popliteal artery is frequently patent.

Long-term anticoagulant therapy has not been of measurable benefit. Therapy with adrenal steroids, so effective for many inflammatory conditions, has similarly not been of consistent value and may aggravate the intimal changes in the tibial arteries.

PROGNOSIS. As stated earlier, 10-year follow-up studies have not agreed upon the prognosis. The Mayo Clinic group have found the survival similar to that of the general population, whereas the group studied by DeBakey and Cohen had a 10-year mortality about three times greater than the normal population. The risk of amputation within 10 years after onset of symptoms is probably near 20 percent, although this varies with the continued use of tobacco as well as the degree to which the ischemic foot is carefully protected. In the few patients who stop smoking completely, progression of the disease may be greatly restricted. A marked advance in therapy would be the discovery of a method by which abstinence from tobacco could be achieved uniformly in this unfortunate group of individuals.

ARTERIAL TRAUMA

HISTORICAL DATA. The feasibility of routinely repairing injured arteries in military casualties was first demonstrated in the Korean conflict in 1952. Earlier attempts in World War II were generally unsuccessful, and rather pessimistic conclusions were reached concerning the possibilities. Following the Korean conflict experiences, injured arteries have been repaired almost routinely, for ligation of major arteries has an overall incidence of subsequent gangrene of about 50 percent. The advances in therapy in the Korean conflict were due to several factors. The most significant was the almost routine prevention of infection in traumatic wounds by extensive debridement, followed by antibiotics and secondary wound closure 4 to 10 days later. Familiarity with techniques of vascular surgical treatment, in combination with the availability of vascular instruments, was also important. The prompt evacuation of wounded men by helicopter, often bringing a wounded patient to the hospital within 2 to 4 hours after injury, also was a significant factor.

ETIOLOGY. Most arterial injuries result from penetrating wounds which partly or completely disrupt the wall of the artery. Nonpenetrating injuries, usually associated with a fracture in an adjacent bone, are less frequent but often have a more serious prognosis, partly related to extensive crushing injury to the wall of the artery and partly due to delay in diagnosis.

PATHOLOGY. Most injuries are either lacerations or transections of the arterial wall. Uncommon injuries include arterial spasm, arterial contusion with thrombosis, and arteriovenous fistula. With lacerations or transections, the extent of injury varies with the type of trauma, which is an important consideration in subsequent debridement and surgical therapy. With clean incised wounds, such as those made by a knife or an icepick, injury to the arterial wall is minimal. In contrast, trauma from a high-velocity missile will disrupt the intima and media for a short distance away from the actual laceration in the arterial wall and requires a wider debridement at the time of surgical repair.

Contusion or spasm often occurs in association with fractures and extensive soft tissue injuries from blunt trauma. The presence of multiple injuries obscures recognition of the arterial injury, especially with extensive comminuted fractures. With such problems arteriography has been found of increasing value. Arterial spasm is an infrequent response to injury in which sustained contraction of the smooth muscle in the wall of the artery may obstruct blood flow and precipitate thrombosis. The cause is obscure. The spasm results from direct muscular contraction rather than a neurogenic stimulus. It occurs most frequently in the brachial artery associated with fracture of the humerus.

Arterial contusion from a blunt injury may be characterized by multiple areas of fragmentation of the arterial wall with intramural hemorrhage. The intima may become detached and prolapse into the lumen, creating an intraluminal obstruction which can be detected only by performing an arteriotomy and inspecting the intima. A serious error occurs when a contusion is misdiagnosed as "spasm." The delay in treatment as a consequence of this diagnostic error can result in gangrene. The well-known Volkmann ischemic contracture of the muscles of the forearm is due to an untreated spasm or contusion of the brachial artery in association with a supracondylar fracture of the humerus.

PATHOPHYSIOLOGY. The severity of the ischemic response following an arterial injury varies with the tolerance of different tissues for anoxia. In the extremity the peripheral nerves are the most sensitive to anoxia; hence, paralysis and anesthesia quickly develop when arterial blood flow is seriously decreased. Striated muscle is almost equally sensitive to anoxia and will usually become necrotic if arterial blood flow is decreased to such a degree that anesthesia and paralysis are present. Skin, tendon, and bone all have a greater tolerance for anoxia and may survive an ischemic injury which has produced irreversible extensive muscle necrosis. This is seen in an extremity in which an arterial repair is performed several hours after injury. The skin may appear viable, but the extremity is anesthetic and paralyzed, and after a period of time will be found to have widespread necrosis of the muscles.

The period of tolerance of striated muscle for ischemia is in the range of 6 to 8 hours. Experimental studies by Miller and Welch found arterial repair successful in about 90 percent of experiments when performed within 6 hours after injury, but the success rate decreased to 50 percent when repair was delayed for 12 hours. Therefore, every effort should be made to complete arterial repair within 6 hours after injury if anesthesia or paralysis are present, indicating a severe degree of anoxia. A definite time limit does not exist, however, beyond which arterial repair is futile, for the importance of the time interval varies with the collateral circulation. The collateral circulation, in turn, varies with the artery injured, with the degree of soft tissue injury which has interrupted collateral circulation, with associated shock, and with ambient temperature. In some patients with little disturbance of collateral circulation, arterial repair may be successfully performed 12 to 15 hours after injury, but in general successful repairs are obtained much more frequently when accomplished within 6 hours after injury.

CLINICAL MANIFESTATIONS. Shock, from loss of blood, is present in over 50 percent of patients with an arterial injury, either as a result of hemorrhage from the injured artery or because of associated injuries. The degree of shock varies with the severity of the blood loss or the severity of other injuries. When profound shock is present, the severe peripheral vasoconstriction may conceal the presence of an arterial injury until blood pressure has been restored to near-normal levels.

With blunt trauma, multiple organ injuries are commonly present. These include skull fractures, rib fractures, or blunt abdominal injuries. Careful assessment of each injury, with subsequent assignment of priorities in therapy, is a critical part of initial evaluation of the patient.

In the injured extremity, fractures and nerve injuries are commonly present with either penetrating wounds or following blunt trauma. The presence of a fracture or extensive soft tissue injury greatly influences the prognosis of an arterial injury. For example, in one series of arterial injuries the presence of a fracture of a femur in association with an injury of the femoral artery raised the incidence of gangrene from 11 to 55 percent.

In the extremity, the arterial injury frequently produces four abnormal findings, conveniently remembered as four p's: *p*aralysis, *p*aresthesia or anesthesia, loss of *p*ulses, and *p*allor. Of these four, the neurologic findings, paralysis and paresthesia, are the most important, because, as previously stated, loss of neurologic function indicates a degree of tissue ischemia which will progress to gangrene unless arterial blood flow is improved. Absence of a pulse in the presence of a normal pulse in the contralateral extremity immediately suggests an arterial injury. If serious vasoconstriction is ascribed to hypotension, evaluation of peripheral pulses may be difficult until blood volume is restored. It is important to emphasize, however, that the presence of a peripheral pulse does not exclude an arterial injury. This is frequently seen with a tangential laceration of the wall of an artery which is sealed by a blood clot with preservation of some flow through the arterial lumen.

With penetrating wounds, bright red bleeding, even in small amounts, immediately suggests an arterial injury. In the absence of hemorrhage, a tense hematoma may be palpated around the wound, evolving from extravasation of blood under significant pressure beneath the fascia. Occasionally a systolic bruit may be audible over the wound, or rarely a continuous bruit if an acute arteriovenous fistula has been produced.

It should be emphasized that an arterial injury can be present with virtually no abnormalities in the extremity. Hence, the presence of a penetrating injury near a major artery should alert the physician to the possibility of an arterial injury. In a series of 85 arterial injuries reported by Dillard and associates, the correct diagnosis was delayed in 15 of the patients. Usually the diagnosis is missed if serious hemorrhage is not present or if a peripheral pulse can be felt. In unrecognized cases a secondary hemorrhage from the wound may subsequently develop a false aneurysm, or an arteriovenous fistula may form in the area where the hematoma has formed around the lacerated artery.

With uncertain cases, an arteriogram should be performed. This is of particular value with blunt trauma producing a fracture of the extremity. A critical question in such patients is whether a decreased or absent pulse is due to an arterial injury or to angulation of the artery from the fractured bone.

TREATMENT. Preoperative Considerations. Control of bleeding is the most urgent immediate problem. This can usually be accomplished by tightly packing the wound with gauze and applying a pressure dressing. A large amount of packing may be required, for the efficacy of the packing depends upon compression of the artery between the overlying skin and the underlying bone. Tourniquets are best avoided for most injuries. When used they must be carefully padded to avoid the risk of permanent injury to a peripheral nerve.

Shock, which is present in 50 to 60 percent of patients, should be treated by the rapid infusion of fluids (500 ml every 5 to 10 minutes) until the systolic blood pressure rises to 80 mm Hg, after which additional fluids can be infused more gradually. Usually 1,000 to 2,000 ml of fluid will be required. Blood is preferable, but until the necessary cross matching has been done, Ringer's lactate solution, plasma, or dextran may be used.

Antibiotic therapy should be started promptly and appropriate prophylactic therapy for tetanus begun. Sympathetic blocks and anticoagulant therapy have no significant role in preoperative care.

Operative Technique. An important basic attitude regarding arterial trauma is that almost all injuries can be repaired successfully with available surgical techniques. The prognosis then becomes a question of whether or not the repair was performed before irreversible muscle necrosis developed. The only special instruments required are atraumatic vascular clamps and arterial sutures, usually of synthetic fiber (Dacron, polypropylene) fashioned to be monofilamentous, sizes 4-0 to 5-0, with swaged needles. The surgical incision should be placed to expose the artery proximal and distal to the site of injury in order to avoid hemorrhage when clots are evacuated from the wound. Once proximal and distal control of the artery has been obtained, the hematoma surrounding the injury can be widely opened and the site of injury mobilized. Most injuries are best treated by excision of the injured area followed by end-to-end anastomosis. With injuries from high-velocity missiles, 2 to 4 mm of adjacent arterial wall should be excised. Tangential repairs of lacerations are deceptive in that the suture of the laceration often results in constriction and subsequent thrombosis. Usually excision followed by direct anastomosis is preferable.

With transection of an artery, elastic recoil will separate the two ends of the vessel for 1 cm or more, giving the erroneous impression that a segment of artery has been destroyed. In most instances application of gentle traction on the ends of the artery with vascular clamps will demonstrate that direct anastomosis can be performed. Normally 1 to 2 cm of a peripheral artery can be excised and the vessel ends still approximated after limited mobilization of the two ends. For example, in 180 arterial reconstructions for civilian injuries reported by Patman and associates, grafts were necessary in only 20 patients. Similarly, in a series of 190 arterial reconstructions reported by Morris et al., primary repair was done in 167 patients and vascular grafts in 23. Before the anastomosis is performed, the degree of back-bleeding from the distal artery should be noted and any blood clots removed with a catheter. The anastomosis should be performed with 4-0 or 5-0 arterial sutures, using a continuous suture interrupted in two or three areas to avoid a purse-string effect. Individual sutures should be 1 to 1.5 mm in depth and a similar distance apart. With small arteries, interrupted or horizontal mattress sutures may be employed. Either a continuous over-and-over suture or an everting suture is satisfactory (Fig. 21-16).

A vascular graft is needed only when direct anastomosis cannot be performed because of loss of 2 cm or more of artery, this occurs in about 10 to 15 percent of injuries. An autogenous vein is the preferable graft, reversing the ends of the vein which is employed, usually the saphenous. If for some reason a vein cannot be utilized, a graft of knitted Dacron is preferable. If a prosthetic graft is used, the diameter rarely should be less than 8 mm, for throm-

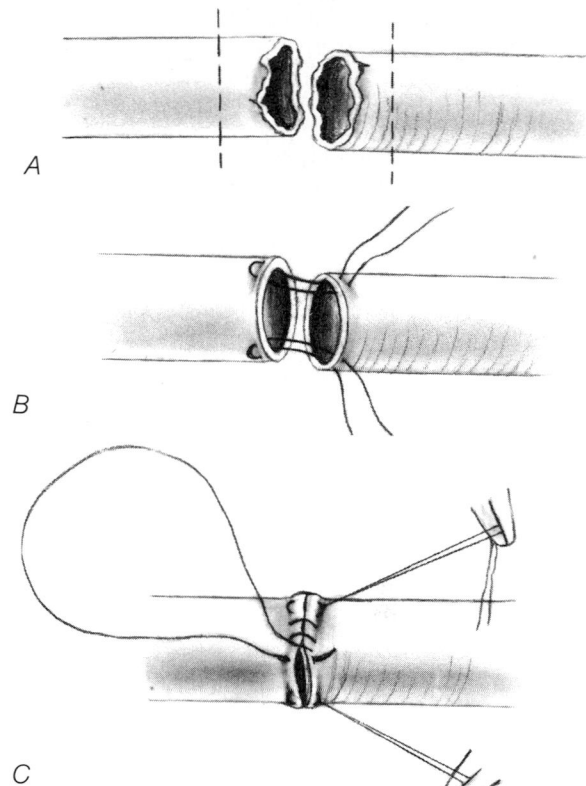

Fig. 21-16. *A.* Repair of traumatic transection of a peripheral artery. Initially the edges of the injured artery are debrided, removing 1 to 2 mm of normal arterial wall, especially if the injury was from a high-velocity missile which would traumatize adjacent segments of arterial wall. *B.* Initially the two ends of the artery are aligned with mattress sutures of 4-0 or 5-0 synthetic, monofilament material placed about 180° apart. *C.* Anastomosis is then performed with a continuous suture of the same material, usually as a simple over-and-over suture. Alternatively, an everting suture can be employed. With small vessels, simple interrupted or horizontal mattress sutures can be used to lessen the risk of constriction of the lumen.

bosis occurs much more frequently with smaller grafts.

With contaminated wounds, the best protection from infection following adequate debridement and arterial reconstruction is approximation of the adjacent soft tissues over the arterial repair and leaving the remaining wound open, to be closed by secondary suture 4 to 7 days later. This technique will almost routinely prevent the development of infection.

Ligation of an injured artery should be performed only for minor arteries, such as a radial or an ulnar artery which is not essential to survival of the limb. Back-bleeding is an inadequate guide to ligation of major arteries, indicating that some collateral circulation is present but not guaranteeing that collateral flow will be large enough to prevent gangrene. In the Korean conflict "good" or "fair" back-bleeding was recorded in 9 of 20 arterial ligations performed in one group of patients, all of which resulted in gangrene.

Arterial spasm, an unusual injury, may be treated by the topical application of 2 to 5% papaverine. Another technique, reported by Mustard and Bull, is the forceful dilatation of the area of spasm by the injection of saline solution into the lumen of the artery. The importance of differentiating spasm from contusion with disruption of the wall of the artery has been mentioned previously. Unless the area of constriction can be satisfactorily corrected, it should be excised and continuity reestablished by direct anastomosis or a vascular graft.

Postoperative Care. Anticoagulant therapy is not recommended after arterial repair, for it provides little protection from thrombosis but does increase the risk of bleeding into the wound. Sympathetic blocks are similarly of little value. The most important consideration following operation is to detect peripheral pulses, which indicate satisfactory restoration of arterial flow. If pulses cannot be detected or if previously palpable pulses disappear, an arteriogram should be performed, or alternatively the site of anastomosis should be reexplored. The important principle to reemphasize is that with modern vascular techniques a traumatic injury of a normal artery can almost always be successfully repaired.

When a femoral artery is repaired hours after injury, ischemic swelling may occur in the leg muscles in the anterior and posterior tibial compartments. The swelling can progress to such an extent that ischemic necrosis results. Prompt fasciotomies over the muscle compartments, decompressing the edematous, turgid muscles, may be of great value.

When an arterial repair is performed several hours after an injury, a peripheral pulse may be restored, but the extremity remains paralyzed and anesthetic. In such patients the skin may be viable, but the status of the underlying muscles is uncertain. Such patients must be carefully observed, because extensive muscle necrosis will result in serious toxic manifestations, with high fever and occasionally renal insufficiency. A decision to amputate such extremities, as opposed to widespread debridement of the necrotic muscles, is a difficult one to make, and each individual case must be evaluated carefully. In some patients the extremity may be salvaged following extensive debridement of necrotic calf muscles, with preservation of a limited but useful foot.

The development of a postoperative infection around the site of arterial repair is a grave complication, because frequently the anastomosis will disrupt with life-threatening hemorrhage. The infection should be treated promptly by widespread drainage, for there is usually inadequate removal of necrotic tissue. If infection involves the arterial reconstruction, ligation of the artery is usually required to prevent fatal hemorrhage or sepsis. Occasionally bypass grafts may be inserted through channels circumventing the area of infection, an anastomosis being performed between the artery proximal and distal to the point of injury. As mentioned earlier, the Korean conflict experiences well emphasized that despite massive contamination, the policy of widespread debridement, followed by secondary wound closure, almost always prevented postoperative wound infections.

PROGNOSIS. With present vascular techniques, arterial reconstruction almost always can be performed success-fully if undertaken within 6 hours after injury. In 209 patients with arterial injuries reported by Patman and associates, the amputation rate was 3.8 percent. In another series of 67 arterial reconstructions reported by Dillard et al., only two amputations were necessary. If a vein graft is needed for arterial reconstruction, the long-term patency is probably in the range of 80 to 85 percent, varying with the experience of the surgeon and the circumstances of the injury. If subsequent occlusion of a vein graft does occur, viability of the extremity is rarely jeopardized, although claudication may develop. In such patients a subsequent vascular reconstruction may be performed electively.

Popliteal Artery Entrapment Syndrome

Popliteal artery entrapment syndrome consists of intermittent claudication caused by an abnormal relation of that artery to the muscles, usually the medial head of the gastrocnemius, resulting in ischemia of the leg at an unusually early age.

HISTORICAL DATA. In 1879, a medical student named Stuart recognized an anatomical abnormality associated with a thrombosed aneurysm of the popliteal artery which led to amputation of the extremity. A number of reports, beginning with Hamming in 1959, documented approximately 60 cases. Inshua in 1970 was able to classify the anatomic abnormalities of the structures in the popliteal fossa which led to the development of the syndrome.

ETIOLOGY AND PATHOLOGY. Normally the popliteal artery enters the popliteal fossa through the arch of the adductor magnus muscle and passes along a longitudinal place accompanied by the popliteal vein and tibial vein. The artery exits dorsal to the popliteus muscle, having passed approximately midway between the lateral and medial heads of the gastrocnemius muscle, and divides into its branches at the terminal portion of the popliteal fossa. As a consequence of developmental abnormalities, the popliteal artery may be severely compressed by portions of the medial head of the gastrocnemius muscle, at times continuously and at other times only during tensing of that muscle. As repeated trauma to the vessel ensues, typical arteriosclerotic changes appear, with irreversible stenosis and thrombosis. On occasion, poststenotic dilatation and aneurysm formation may be seen.

CLINICAL MANIFESTATIONS. Almost all patients experience either gradual or sudden onset of progressive intermittent claudication of the leg and sometimes of the foot; the remaining few present with acute ischemia of the leg. Ischemic gangrene has been encountered very rarely. The symptoms are usually unilateral but may be bilateral.

On physical examination there are the usual findings of popliteal arterial stenosis or occlusion with diminished or absent popliteal, dorsalis pedis, and posterior tibial pulses. On occasion all pulses appear to be normal but can be made to disappear on dorsiflexion of the foot, and a pulsatile mass may be noted in the fossa.

DIAGNOSIS. It is essential to establish the diagnosis early, since correction of the abnormality may present irreversible changes which may require more complex arterial reconstructions. Any individual in the preatherosclerotic age group who presents with typical ischemic intermittent claudication or who is found to have a pulsatile popliteal mass should be suspected of having a popliteal artery entrapment syndrome. The physical findings may be minimal or nil; therefore angiographic studies are essential to making the diagnosis. Angiography may demonstrate stenosis, occlusion, or poststenotic dilatation of that artery. Occasionally there may be no visible abnormalities on the angiographic study until the foot is passively dorsiflexed, after which stenosis of the popliteal artery may be seen.

The differential diagnosis requires exclusion of all other causes of popliteal artery occlusion, including thromboangiitis obliterans, embolic occlusion, cystic degeneration of the popliteal artery, atherosclerosis obliterans, as well as other trauma to the vessel.

TREATMENT. Surgical correction is required. The type of surgical procedure which should be performed depends entirely upon the condition of the popliteal artery. When the popliteal artery has had no permanent structural changes, various types of myotomy procedures which can be determined only at the operating table may prove to be curative. In instances in which structural changes have already occurred, in addition to the correction of the anatomic abnormalities, replacement of the artery with vein or thromboendarterectomy angioplasty may be required to restore flow. The results in these young people, who ordinarily have normal arteries above and below the site of compression, are excellent. In most instances the reported case histories indicate that unilateral correction is sufficient, but it is essential that both limbs be studied, since bilateral corrections may be necessary.

PROGNOSIS. The prognosis for immediate restoration of flow to the extremity is excellent in these young people. The long-term prognosis will depend upon the material employed to reconstruct occluded arteries. It would appear desirable to avoid the use of plastic prostheses and employ autologous tissue for the arterial reconstruction.

Anterior Compartment Syndrome

The anterior tibial compartment syndrome is a progressive neuromuscular disability related to pressure from tissue fluid within the closed anterior tibial compartment.

ETIOLOGY. Any condition which increases the presence of fluid or compromises the outflow of fluid from this closed space may result in augmented pressure and clinical consequences. The swelling continues until the intracompartmental pressure exceeds arterial pressure. The critical structures coursing through the closed compartment and subjected to the effects of the intracompartmental pressure include the tibial artery, the anterior tibial nerve, and the anterior tibial, extensor digitorum longus, peroneus tertius, and extensor hallucis longus muscles. The unyielding walls of the compartment are composed of the tibia, the interosseous membrane, and the anterior crural fascia.

In some cases, there is a readily demonstrable arterial lesion; the syndrome has been associated with arterial trauma, arterial embolism, and acute arterial thrombosis; and it has been a complication of femoropopliteal bypass procedures and also of cardiopulmonary bypass. In a second group of patients, the syndrome is caused by severe exertion, and there is no proved anatomic lesion.

CLINICAL MANIFESTATIONS. In young patients with idiopathic anterior tibial syndrome, a history of marked exertion should be investigated. Characteristically, in most cases, the pain is the first and dominant symptom. Initially, it begins as a dull ache which soon becomes severe and is primarily located over the anterior compartment, where palpation may elicit tenderness. Motion of the leg or foot increases the severity of pain. Subsequently, erythema of the skin over the anterior compartment becomes apparent, and there is measurable increase in the size of the calf. As the syndrome progresses, these signs become more apparent. The dorsalis pedis pulse may be normal, diminished, or absent. Actually, its absence is a late sign and occasionally follows the loss of motor power of the muscles of the anterior compartment. The anterior tibial muscle and the extensor hallucis longus usually become paralyzed first, whereas the extensor digitorum longus loses its function later and is usually the first to return after release of pressure. Loss of the extensor digitorum brevis is an ominous sign. Loss of sensation is confined to the area served by the deep peroneal nerve.

The syndrome must be differentiated from a common condition known as "shin splints." The pain in the latter condition is usually over bone and can be relieved by rest, elevation, and application of cold. There is no associated marked swelling and muscle paresis with shin splints. Other conditions to be differentiated include cellulitis, thrombophlebitis, and stress fractures of the tibia.

TREATMENT. This is directed at decompressing the anterior tibial compartment and should be performed early to avoid anoxic necrosis of the muscle mass. Treatment can be effected with fasciotomy. The skin is incised lateral to the tibial crest over the midportion of the anterior tibial muscle, and the incision is carried through subcutaneous tissue and the fascia. Muscle bellies are then allowed to bulge. The skin may be closed over the bulging muscle or can be left open for secondary closure. A variation of the procedure employs two small incisions, one in the craniad and the other in the caudad portion of the anterior compartment. The fascia is then incised blindly between these two small incisions.

PROGNOSIS. If decompression is performed before muscle necrosis is present, return of function is complete. Thus, in many instances, fasciotomy is indicated prior to total disappearance of the pedal pulse. If fasciotomy is delayed until muscle necrosis occurs or neurologic findings are advanced, total recovery of function is not to be anticipated, and rehabilitation is required.

Traumatic Arteriovenous Fistulas

HISTORICAL DATA. The true nature of an arteriovenous fistula was first recognized by William Hunter in 1764. Previously the lesion had not been distinguished from a traumatic aneurysm. In a careful description of two patients in whom fistulas developed following phlebotomy, he described the typical clinical findings of a thrill, continuous murmur, dilated artery proximal to the fistula, and dilated pulsating veins. He first recognized that the lesion was basically a communication between an artery and a vein. Attempted therapy by proximal ligation of the involved artery, which was frequently effective for traumatic aneurysms, was often disastrous for arteriovenous fistulas, because gangrene resulted. The gangrene developed because blood flowing through collateral circulation around the ligated artery would flow through the fistula instead of into the distal extremity.

Matas in 1888 established effective therapy with his

Fig. 21-17. *A.* Immediately following the development of an arteriovenous fistula there is shunting of blood from the artery through the fistula into the vein, from which it returns to the heart. This results in a decrease in peripheral vascular resistance, a fall in diastolic blood pressure, and an increase in heart rate. The venous pressure rises in the involved vein. Peripheral blood flow is decreased in the involved artery. *B.* After several weeks, collateral circulation enlarges around the fistula because of the decreased vascular resistance at the site of the fistula. As the collateral circulation develops, the involved artery and vein also dilate, increasing the amount of blood flowing through the fistula. *C.* After several years, extensive dilatation may develop about a fistula with marked enlargement of collateral circulation. In addition there is enlargement of the artery immediately distal to the fistula, through which blood flows in a retrograde fashion through the fistula toward the heart. The vein may enlarge to marked proportions, creating varicosities in the extremity. Ultimately such progressive dilatation after a period of years may result in congestive heart failure from the increased cardiac output.

technique of endoaneurysmorraphy. Directly incising the fistulous sac, followed by suture of the communication between the artery and the vein, was more effective than indirect therapy of proximal and distal ligation of the involved artery and vein. The abnormal physiology of an arteriovenous fistula was carefully analyzed in a scholarly monograph published by Holman in 1937.

Although the collateral circulation which develops with an arteriovenous fistula made it possible to treat such fistulas by excision without gangrene resulting, intermittent claudication was frequently permanent. Consequently, after World War II, reconstruction of the injured artery became the preferable form of treatment.

ETIOLOGY AND PATHOLOGY. An arteriovenous fistula usually results from a penetrating injury which simultaneously injures an artery and an adjacent vein, permitting blood to flow directly from the injured artery into the vein. A fistula may be established immediately, in which case there is little external loss of blood, or the fistula may become apparent days or weeks following injury as clot surrounding the lacerated artery and vein is liquefied.

Unusual forms of arteriovenous fistulas have been reported following different surgical operations. Injury of the iliac artery and vein is a well-recognized, fortunately rare complication of removal of an intervertebral disc. Arteriovenous fistulas have been reported following thyroidectomy, nephrectomy, or even thoracentesis, in all instances representing a concomitant injury of an artery and a vein, sometimes due to simultaneous ligation of artery and vein by the same ligature.

PATHOPHYSIOLOGY. A series of anatomic and physiologic changes begin to evolve when an arteriovenous fistula is produced (Fig. 21-17). The immediate effects are a decrease in blood flow to tissues distal to the lesion and an increase in venous pressure. The peripheral vascular resistance is lowered as a result of blood flowing directly through the newly created arteriovenous shunt. This results in a decrease in systolic and diastolic blood pressure, an increase in heart rate, and an increase in cardiac output.

In the ensuing days, several compensatory events occur as a result of the decrease in peripheral vascular resistance: The blood volume is increased, systolic blood pressure increases with a corresponding increase in pulse pressure, and a decrease in pulse rate occurs. Locally there is the progressive development of extensive collateral circulation around the fistula, because the decreased vascular resistance at the site of the fistula is a very potent stimulus to development of collateral circulation. Within a few weeks the blood flow to the distal extremity may approach normal limits. There is a progressive dilatation of the "fistulous circuit," including the heart, the arteries leading to the fistula, the fistula itself, and the venous channels leading from the fistula to the heart.

In subsequent months or years, additional changes evolve. The artery both proximal and distal to the fistula may dilate in response to blood flowing through the fistula. The involved veins progressively dilate with marked tortuosity; external rupture with hemorrhage, however, is very rare. Chronic venous congestion may develop in the extremity, causing skin ulcerations resembling those from varicose veins. In growing children, there may be hypertrophy of the involved limb from increased growth of the bones and soft tissues. With large fistulas, involving vessels as large as the iliac artery and vein, continued dilatation of the heart eventually terminates in heart failure. This, however, is an unusual complication with the majority of arteriovenous fistulas, because the volume of blood shunted is not enough to produce heart failure. Only with large arteries and veins do cardiac symptoms appear.

Two rare complications with arteriovenous fistulas are bacterial endarteritis in the fistula and spontaneous closure. Bacterial endarteritis has been reported in only a few patients and is similar to bacterial endocarditis. Usually with intensive chemotherapy the infection can be controlled or eliminated, after which surgical excision of the fistula should be promptly carried out. A fistula may close spontaneously, occasionally after it has been present for several months. Shumacker reported eight such experiences in 245 patients.

CLINICAL MANIFESTATIONS. A penetrating injury producing an arteriovenous fistula often causes surprisingly few symptoms. External loss of blood can be small, and few disturbances of peripheral circulation develop. Subsequently the patient may be entirely asymptomatic. He is usually aware of a soft mass in the area of the fistula, which transmits a buzzing sensation when the fingers are placed over it. Rarely the patient is totally unaware of the presence of a fistula. In the experience of one of the authors, a fifty-five-year-old patient was admitted for congestive heart failure, presumably due to atherosclerotic heart disease, and was found on physical examination to have a popliteal arteriovenous fistula resulting from trauma many years before. Surgical correction of the fistula promptly eliminated the signs of congestive failure.

In some patients the venous hypertension produces varices with peripheral pigmentation and ulceration from venous insufficiency. Surgical mishaps have resulted from unwise attempts to remove such varices without recognizing their origin.

On physical examination, a soft, diffuse mass is usually palpable and often visible. Dilated veins may surround the area. On palpation a thrill is usually felt, maximal in systole. Auscultation reveals a continuous murmur, loudest in systole, which has been described as a "machinery" murmur, emphasizing the rhythmic rise and fall in intensity and pitch during systole and diastole. It is similar to the murmur of a patent ductus arteriosus. Detection of this classic finding establishes the diagnosis and differentiates the lesion from an arterial aneurysm.

Another significant finding is the demonstration of slowing of the pulse when the fistula is obliterated by digital compression, as evidenced by disappearance of the murmur. This phenomenon, generally known as Branham's sign, was first described by Nicoladoni in 1875. The slowing of the pulse results from the increase in peripheral vascular resistance when the fistula is digitally occluded causing the blood pressure to rise with reflex slowing of the heart rate. The bradycardia results from a neurogenic reflex mediated through pressure-sensitive receptors in the great vessels and carotid sinuses; it can be blocked by atropine.

Usually there are no signs of arterial insufficiency in the extremity. With large fistulas, the pulse pressure is increased, both from an elevation of systolic pressure and a decrease in diastolic pressure. If cardiac enlargement has occurred, a systolic murmur may be audible at the apex of the heart. Usually cardiac failure is found only with fistulas between large vessels, such as the aorta and the vena cava, or when the fistula has been present for many years, allowing time for progressive enlargement of the fistulous opening. In World War II cardiac failure was rarely seen in a collected series of 593 patients treated surgically.

The physical findings are usually sufficient to establish the diagnosis, but if uncertainty exists, an arteriogram readily demonstrates the rapid opacification of adjacent veins and the greatly increased collateral circulation. As the veins fill rapidly, the exact site of the fistula may be obscured unless serial angiograms are obtained. A common problem in differential diagnosis in the cervical area is with a venous "hum," an auscultatory curiosity resulting from flow of blood in the jugular veins. The murmur of a venous hum promptly disappears when intrathoracic pressure is raised by forced expiration against a closed glottis, which will differentiate it from the murmur of an arteriovenous fistula.

TREATMENT. Formerly treatment was delayed for 2 to 4 months to permit the development of collateral circulation in order for the extremity to survive following ligation of the involved artery. Although gangrene virtually never occurred following ligation, claudication frequently resulted, often in as many as 50 percent of patients, despite the abundant collateral circulation. Presently, the majority of patients are treated by division of the fistula and reconstruction of the involved artery, and preferably the injured vein. Excision is performed only for fistulas involving small vessels not essential to normal circulation of the extremity, such as the radial or ulnar arteries. Most fistulas are treated at the time of the arterial injury if the proper diagnosis is made. Otherwise operation is performed within 2 or 3 weeks, after the immediate effects of the injury on the soft tissues have subsided.

Operative Technique. The incision should be placed so as to permit exposure of the artery and vein proximal and distal to the fistula before the fistula is dissected. Once these vessels are isolated and temporarily occluded, the fistulous sac can be incised and the opening directly isolated. Although a large aneurysmal sac may be present, the basic lesion is usually an incomplete laceration of the arterial wall, involving only a short length of artery. A long segment of artery may be incorporated in the wall of the aneurysmal sac, however, which must be freed and mobilized to perform arterial repair. Once the involved vessels have been mobilized, most of the remaining sac may be left, for complete excision is difficult and of little benefit.

In many patients the artery can be repaired by direct anastomosis. In a group of 29 aneurysms and arteriovenous fistulas resulting from civilian injuries reported by Crawford et al., all were treated by end-to-end arterial anastomosis. In 134 fistulas treated by Hughes and Jahnke, an anastomosis was performed in 61, a vessel graft in 23, a lateral repair in 4, and simple division of the fistula in 10.

Repair of the involved vein is indicated if the vein is a large one, such as an iliac or common femoral vein. Permanent edema has been frequent following ligation of such large veins. Repair can often be done by lateral suture.

PROGNOSIS. Convalescence following operation is usually uneventful, and long-term results are excellent if arterial continuity is preserved. Hughes and Jahnke published a 5-year follow-up of 148 such lesions treated during the Korean conflict with satisfactory results in the majority of patients.

CONGENITAL ARTERIOVENOUS FISTULAS

Congenital arteriovenous fistulas are very uncommon lesions. In 1963 Tice et al. estimated that only about 200 cases had been reported in the American surgical literature. In 1956 Coursley and associates reported experiences with 69 patients, and Robertson in a Hunterian Lecture referred to 40 patients.

ETIOLOGY AND PATHOLOGY. As the name indicates, the basic lesion is a congenital abnormality of multiple communications between arteries and veins. A single communication is unfortunately very rare, for the multiplicity of lesions precludes surgical cure in most patients. The extent of the lesion varies from an angiomatous mass localized in a foot or a finger to diffuse involvement of an entire arm or leg. In addition to the presence of multiple lesions, the almost uniform recurrence suggests that a basic defect exists in the peripheral vascular tree as a result of which additional arteriovenous fistulas develop throughout the life of the patient.

The extremities are a common site for such fistulas. When present in childhood, there is increased growth of the affected extremity. Hemihypertrophy of moderate degree was found in over one-half of patients reported by Coursley and associates and also by Robertson. Fortunately, cardiac difficulties from the arteriovenous shunting are uncommon; an increase in heart size has been recorded in only about 15 percent of the patients. The dilated veins associated with the lesions tend to enlarge gradually, causing difficulty from periodic external rupture and bleeding. With involvement of the digits, ischemic pain may occur with gangrene of the tips of the fingers because of shunting of blood proximally through the fistulas.

CLINICAL MANIFESTATIONS. The finding of multiple dilated veins or small angiomas may suggest simple varicosities, but the location of the dilated veins in unusual areas should raise suspicion of congenital arteriovenous fistulas. Detection of a continuous bruit over the lesion establishes the diagnosis, but with some diffuse multiple fistulas involving an entire extremity a bruit may not be audible. In contrast to traumatic single arteriovenous fistulas, it is impossible to obliterate the bruit completely by

digital compression. Often a bruit is audible in several widely separated areas, indicating the presence of multiple fistulas.

Occasionally a patient first becomes aware of his condition following an injury, and an error can easily be made by concluding that a traumatic fistula with a single communication is present. Careful inquiry concerning earlier dilatation of the regional veins may give a clue to the correct diagnosis and prevent a long, futile surgical exploration for a single fistula. The finding of multiple bruits which cannot be eliminated by digital compression also suggests a congenital origin. Arteriography is needed to confirm the diagnosis, demonstrating many tortuous arteries with rapid opacification of numerous dilated veins (Fig. 21-18).

TREATMENT. The keynote to therapy is conservatism. Operation should be undertaken only when the lesion is of sufficient size to threaten with ulceration or bleeding, because surgical excision must be considered as palliative in the majority of patients. Only when the lesion is localized sufficiently to permit complete excision of adjacent soft tissue is a curative procedure possible. With most lesions, thorough understanding should be reached with the patient beforehand regarding the palliative nature of the surgical procedure.

On the other hand, amputation merely to remove the lesion is unwarranted, for excellent palliation can be obtained for many years by serial surgical procedures to excise all accessible varicosities. Cross et al. has reported eight patients successfully managed with such measures.

At operation, in contrast to traumatic arteriovenous fistulas, a widespread en bloc excision of the soft tissue should be planned, because excision of an isolated fistula is seldom possible. Amputation of one or more digits may be required. Precise arterial control is often impossible; so, a pneumatic tourniquet should be applied proximal to the lesion if possible. In some patients serious bleeding has been encountered which could be controlled only by resection of adjacent bone.

Some of the most difficult lesions to treat are those involving the head and neck. Ravitch and Gaertner described a remarkable patient treated for an extensive recurrence 48 years after the patient was originally operated upon by Halsted. Rosenfeld has described experiences with seven patients which well emphasize the value of conservative therapy. By prolonged, painstaking dissection, the facial nerve was preserved in most of these patients, but resection of the mandible was frequently required (Fig. 21-19).

A lesion operated upon by one of the authors, after several previous surgical procedures had been ineffective, required amputation of an ear to prevent hemorrhage. When the cartilage of the ear was divided adjacent to the skull, numerous large arteries closely adherent to the cartilage were transected. Within a year additional bruits were audible over the head and neck, but fortunately no symptoms were present.

Another area in which lesions generally are not resectable is in the pelvis and flank. One of the authors operated upon one such patient at the Walter Reed Army Hospital

Fig. 21-18. Series of angiograms demonstrating congenital arteriovenous fistulas. *A.* This series of three views shows a popliteal arteriogram in the same patient. The first view is a posteroanterior view which demonstrates the great degree of enlargement of the calf. The next two views are early and late exposures in the arterial phase in a lateral projection. The extensive staining in the late arterial phase is highly suggestive of congenital arteriovenous fistulas. *B.* Arteriogram in the thigh area of a second patient. Note the diffuse staining produced by injection into the profunda femoris vessel. *C.* These two views demonstrate early and late arteriograms in the shoulder area. In this patient the fistulas originate from the circumflex humeral vessels.

in 1958. Previous operation several years before with division of the iliac artery had resulted in only temporary improvement. During a surgical procedure which lasted several hours, numerous large vessels, including the internal iliac artery and vein, were excised and ligated, but it was obvious that a definitive procedure could not be accomplished. Within a week following operation a loud continuous murmur was again audible. Six years later the murmur persisted, but fortunately there was little disability. Such a course emphasizes the value of conservatism with these lesions.

A   *B*

C

Fig. 21-19. *A.* The usually extensive nature of these lesions is illustrated by the following case history. Large recurrent congenital arteriovenous fistula operated upon by Ravitch 48 years after the lesion had been removed by Halsted. Extensive collateral vessels were found in the neck around tributaries of the external carotid artery. *B.* Operative field following completion of the dissection, indicating the numerous unnamed collateral vessels which had developed over many years, causing recurrence of the lesion. (*Reprinted from M. M. Ravitch and R. A. Gaertner, Congenital Arteriovenous Fistula in the Neck: 48 Year Follow-up on a Patient Operated upon by Dr. Halsted in 1911, Bull Johns Hopkins Hosp, 107:31, 1960.*)

Increasingly favorable experiences with intraarterial embolization have been reported. Combinations of Gelfoam, pellets, and autologous muscle have been injected by the Seldinger technique. Inoperable lesions may be treated by embolization alone, while extensive lesions may be managed by embolization followed by excision.

THORACIC OUTLET SYNDROMES

A variety of physical abnormalities have been recognized which constrict or compress the brachial plexus, the subclavian artery, or the subclavian vein near the first rib and clavicle. Several descriptive terms have been employed, indicating the causative mechanism thought to be present. These include cervical rib, scalenus anticus syndrome, costoclavicular syndrome, and hyperabduction syndrome. The disability is dependent upon which of the major neural or vascular structures is compressed. Regardless of the specific mechanism involved, all such abnormalities may be conveniently grouped together as neurovascular compression syndromes occurring near the thoracic outlet.

HISTORICAL DATA. Cervical ribs have been reported as anatomic curiosities for hundreds of years. They occur in about 0.5 percent of the normal population. Murphy in 1905 described a successful operation upon a patient whose subclavian artery was compressed by a cervical rib. By 1916 Halsted was able to find reports of more than 500 cases of symptoms from a cervical rib. Attention was focused on the scalenus anticus muscle in 1927 when Adson and Coffey observed constriction of the subclavian artery by a scalenus anticus muscle and subsequently pro-

posed that compression by an abnormal scalenus anticus muscle created a syndrome identical to that caused by cervical rib. They also emphasized the role of the scalenus anticus muscle in producing symptoms from a cervical rib, the two structures jointly compressing the brachial plexus between them.

Subsequently the frequency of compression between the clavicle and first rib was recognized and the mechanisms well defined in 1943 by the report of Falconer and Weddel, who named this type of compression the *costoclavicular syndrome.* A short time later, in 1945, Wright observed patients in whom vascular symptoms resulted from hyperabduction and introduced the term *hyperabduction syndrome.*

Some degree of compression of the subclavian artery may be demonstrated in a high percentage of normal individuals in whom no symptoms whatever are present, but it formerly was thought that compression syndromes producing significant disability were rare. Recently, however, since the publication of Roos of a simplified approach to relieve compression syndromes at the thoracic outlet and since the introduction of peripheral nerve conduction velocity determinations, the conditions have been recognized with increasing frequency. It has even been suggested that for certain patients who have thoracic outlet syndromes a diagnosis of angina pectoris is erroneously made. Further experience will be needed to determine the exact frequency of these disorders, for the nerve conduction velocity studies have only recently been developed. The aforementioned transaxillary approach to resection of the first rib, first emphasized by Clagett in 1962, may help define the frequency of the condition more exactly, as removal of the first rib effectively decompresses the thoracic outlet.

REGIONAL ANATOMY. The subclavian artery leaves the thorax by passing over the first rib between the scalenus anticus muscle anteriorly and the brachial plexus and scalenus medius posteriorly. It then passes under the clavicle and subclavius muscle to enter the axilla beneath the pectoralis minor muscle. The subclavian vein has an almost identical course except that it passes anterior to the scalenus anticus muscle. The route of the brachial plexus nearly parallels that of the subclavian artery in the neck, lying posterolaterally between it and the scalenus medius muscle.

A potential area of compression exists in the interscalene triangle between the scalenus anticus anteriorly, the scalenus medius posteriorly, and the first rib inferiorly. Only slightly distal to this area, in the narrow space between the clavicle and the first rib, is another potential site of compression. Finally, in the axilla, where the pectoralis minor tendon attaches to the coracoid process, an area of potential obstruction of the axillary artery exists where it travels around the coracoid process. Lord and Rosati have emphasized that during hyperabduction the axillary vessels and brachial plexus are bent at an angle of approximately 90° in this area.

When a cervical rib persists, there may be in addition either a bony or a ligamentous structure, originating on the lowermost cervical vertebra, coursing between the anterior and medial scalene muscles, passing under the brachial plexus and subclavian artery, and attaching to the first rib.

ETIOLOGY. Although cervical ribs are found in about 0.5 percent of the normal population, only about 10 percent of these produce symptoms. Asymptomatic anomalies of the first rib are also frequently seen. Thus, additional factors other than the presence of a cervical rib or anomalous first rib must contribute to the compression syndrome. Symptoms are very rare in children and most frequently are seen in thin women in the third and fourth decades. An unusually well-developed musculature seems also to predispose to compression. A congenital variation in the anatomy of the head and neck has been suggested by Adson as a predisposing factor, a familiar type of patient being a thin woman with a long, narrow neck. The onset of symptoms in the second and third decade could be due to gradual descent of the shoulder girdle perhaps from atrophy of the regional musculature.

Local anatomic variations are probably of particular significance. The width of the first rib in individuals in whom we have resected this structure has appeared to be unusually great. The width of the scalene anticus muscle at its insertion into the first rib varies greatly. A wide scalenus anticus muscle, which narrows the space in the interscalene triangle, has often been found at operation in symptomatic patients. Cervical ribs vary from short and rudimentary to completely formed and articulating anteriorly with the first rib. Some incomplete ribs are connected by fascial bands to the first rib which compress the brachial plexus.

Fractures of the clavicle or first rib may subsequently produce a large bony callus, especially if there is poor alignment of the ends of the fractured bone. One patient treated by one of the authors for severe ischemia of the hand was found to have peripheral emboli from a small subclavian aneurysm, produced by fracture of the first rib in an automobile accident.

PATHOLOGY. Disability from compression may be produced in several ways and depends upon which portions of the neurovascular bundle are involved. Compression of the brachial plexus usually causes pain, paresthesias, and a feeling of numbness. Often these symptoms are greatest in the C_8–T_1 distribution, because the ulnar nerve is derived from this most caudad portion of the plexus which rides over the first rib. Muscular weakness, paralysis, or atrophy of muscles are less frequent and appear only in far advanced cases. Vascular symptoms may be intermittent from compression or temporary occlusion of the subclavian artery, producing claudication with exercise, pallor, or a sensation of coldness, numbness, or paresthesia. In chronic cases, a different and more serious mechanism evolves, for intermittent compression and trauma of the subclavian arteries produce atheromatous changes in the artery and, rarely, a poststenotic aneurysm. From either arterial abnormality, emboli may be dislodged into the peripheral circulation and produce ischemia in the hand, even with focal areas of gangrene requiring amputation of digits. Thrombosis of the subclavian artery may eventually result. On occasion Raynaud's phenomenon may occur. Schein and associates found a total of 29 cases of subclavian arterial involvement previously reported. Eleven of these lost part or all of one digit from gangrene, while two required more extensive amputation. Restoration of continuity of the subclavian artery following thrombosis was reported for the first time in a case cited by Schein and associates.

A third group of vascular symptoms are intermittent episodes of vasoconstriction, similar to those seen in Raynaud's disease. The unilateral appearance of the Raynaud's phenomenon, however, almost always suggests a focal disturbance in the blood supply to the involved extremity. Such vasomotor phenomena are uncommon. A possible explanation for this infrequent occurrence has been proposed by Telford and Mottershead, who, on anatomic dissection, found that in 10 to 15 percent of patients the sympathetic innervation of the extremity traveled in a separate cord not incorporated in the main trunks of the brachial plexus. This isolated filament of fibers presumably would be more prone to direct compression and irritation. Finally, intermittent compression of the subclavian vein may cause signs of venous hypertension in the upper extremity with edema and the development of varicosities.

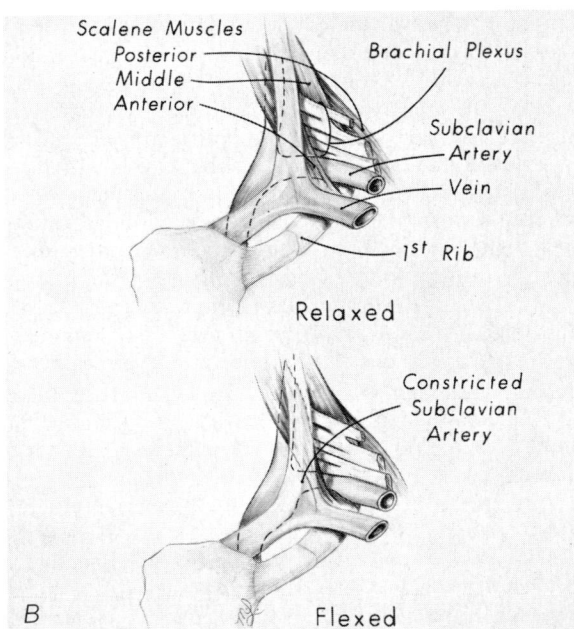

Fig. 21-20. Technique of performance of the Adson test for obstruction of the subclavian artery by the scalenus anticus muscle. *A.* The patient should be seated with his elbows at his sides and his neck extended. During deep inspiration his chin is turned to the affected side, while the intensity of the radial pulse is palpated. All these positions increase the tension on the scalenus anticus muscle. *B.* Course of the brachial plexus and subclavian artery between the scalenus anticus and medius muscles. A localized dilatation of the subclavian artery distal to the scalenus anticus is illustrated. Immediately distal to the scalenus anticus and medius muscles is another potential area of constriction, between the clavicle and the first rib. When the scalenus

The so-called "effort thrombosis," a condition of acute thrombosis of the subclavian vein, may be a result of a neurovascular compression syndrome, but the pathologic mechanisms have not been clearly identified.

CLINICAL MANIFESTATIONS. The symptomatology of the thoracic outlet syndrome depends on whether nerves, blood vessels, or both are compressed. Usually compression of one of these dominates the clinical picture. As reported in a paper by Urschel et al., symptoms of nerve compression manifested by pain and paresthesia were present in all but 6 of 138 patients, the pain usually being of insidious onset, commonly involving the neck, shoulder, arm, and hand with occasional radiation to the anterior chest or parascapular area. Paresthesias in specific nerve distribution occurred in 102 of their patients, the ulnar nerve being involved in 90 percent.

Symptoms of arterial compression were observed less frequently, in about one-quarter of their patients. Thirteen had symptoms of venous compression, including edema, venous distension, and discoloration; only three had the classic effort thrombosis, or Paget-Schroetter syndrome. Raynaud's phenomenon was present in 17 patients, all of whom were women.

Chronic ischemic pain has been observed in three of our patients following embolic occlusion of the radial or ulnar arteries with localized gangrene of one finger in one patient.

Physical Examination. Objective physical signs are more common in patients with vascular compression than in those with neural disorders. In only about 20 percent of patients with nerve compression are objective signs of decreased sensation found; some of these show additional muscle weakness or even atrophy. In the presence of neurologic symptoms at least one of the vascular compression signs can be expected, consisting essentially of loss of radial pulse with either Adson's maneuver, hyperabduction, or hyperextension. In the Adson maneuver, the patient sits with his hands on his knees, inspires deeply, extends his head backward, and turns his chin toward the affected side. Deep inspiration, extension of the neck, and turning of the head all tense the scalene anticus muscle and may decrease or obliterate the radial pulse (Fig. 21-20). Simultaneous auscultation of the supraclavicular space for bruit should be performed. In certain patients, a bruit will appear as the head is turned, reach a peak intensity, and cease as compression is increased to the point of obliterating the radial pulse. In other patients turning the head to the opposite side may demonstrate compression more effectively. The possibility of compression of the neurovascular bundle between the first rib and the clavicle also may be tested by displacing the shoulders backward and downward. The test is considered positive

anticus muscle is relaxed, there is minimal compression of the subclavian artery. With tension on the scalenus anticus muscle, compression of the subclavian artery results in decrease in the radial pulse, in some patients resulting in disappearance of the pulse. A bruit may become audible in the supraclavicular area as the scalenus anticus muscle is progressively stretched to compress the subclavian artery.

if the radial pulse is obliterated. The hyperabduction maneuver is performed by fully abducting the arm above the head and noting the effect upon the radial pulse.

The signs of arterial compression may be evident by direct physical examination. There may be differences in the qualities of the pulses between the two arms when the subclavian, brachial, radial, and ulnar arteries are compared. A localized supraclavicular bruit may be present. On occasion a particularly wide pulse, denoting a subclavian or axillary aneurysm, is palpable. With mild forms of ischemia there may be only pallor on elevation while in the more severe forms, especially with embolization, there may be atrophy of the skin, brittle nails, or even focal ulceration. In approximately 5 percent of patients frank Raynaud's phenomenon can be induced by application of cold to the extremity. In the approximately 10 percent of patients who have signs of venous obstruction, edema and venous distension are apparent.

In evaluating the maneuvers to detect neurovascular compression, it is important to remember that they are positive in a high percentage of normal individuals. This is particularly true of the costoclavicular compression or the hyperabduction test. A positive result, therefore, does not in itself establish a thoracic outlet syndrome; absence of any positive findings, however, suggests some other diagnosis.

LABORATORY STUDIES. Chest and cervical spine roentgenograms may demonstrate bony abnormalities in as many as one-third of the patients, either as cervical ribs, bifid first ribs, fusion of the first and second ribs, or clavicular deformities either congenital or traumatic.

For diagnosing arterial abnormalities, arteriography may be especially useful in demonstrating intimal irregularities, stenoses, or aneurysms of the subclavian artery. The arteriographic studies are of no value where there is no evidence of arterial compression or occlusion. Venographic studies are useful in patients with signs of venous compression, especially in establishing a differential diagnosis between thoracic outlet compression and other entities which mimic the condition.

The determination of nerve conduction velocities through the thoracic outlet as well as electromyographic determinations have been used to attempt to establish objective criteria for diagnosing neural compression. By applying electrical stimulation to various of the distal components of the brachial plexus and measuring conduction velocities to pinpoint areas of abnormal conduction, it is possible to evaluate sites of involvement of various neural structures. This technique used in conjunction with the specific determination of the ulnar nerve conduction velocity has been employed by Urschel to make diagnoses of thoracic outlet syndromes as well as to establish the differential diagnosis. Where atypical thoracic outlet neural compression syndromes are present, other nerves such as the median and the musculocutaneous can be similarly studied. Differential diagnoses between compression at the thoracic outlet, at the carpal tunnel at the wrist, and at the pronator level are possible. When this is combined with carefully performed electromyographic studies, very specific diagnoses are possible. With increasing experience, correlating the results of electrical studies with postoperative results may permit more precise selection of patients for different types of therapy available.

DIAGNOSIS. Formerly, thoracic outlet syndromes have been erroneously diagnosed on purely clinical criteria, frequently in the presence of neural compression occurring at sites other than the thoracic outlet. Cervical disc disease, arthritis of the cervical spine, and nerve and spinal cord tumors, especially of the extramedullary type, can produce similar symptoms. The most easily diagnosed of the neurologic syndromes is that involving the lowermost portion of the brachial plexus. In this, there are subjective symptoms along the course of the ulnar nerve; relief obtained frequently on moderate abduction at the shoulder joint and a positive vascular compression test confirm the diagnosis. Electrical studies of ulnar nerve conduction velocity, with or without electromyographic studies, can firmly establish the diagnosis. With atypical neural compression syndromes the diagnosis is more difficult in the absence of positive physical signs except for signs of vascular compression during one of the compression maneuvers. An extensive investigation may be required, looking for bony abnormalities in the region of the thoracic outlet and performing nerve conduction and electromyographic studies to establish the probable site of the neural disorder. In many, the diagnosis will be a combination of exclusion of other diagnostic entities associated with positive findings on the specific electrical studies.

Diagnosis of the occlusive vascular disorders is less difficult. Physical findings suggesting arterial or venous compression are usually present. Appropriate angiographic studies may be required to delineate the nature, the specific mechanism, and the indicated therapy.

Diagnosis of the vasospastic disorders (Raynaud's) is clear-cut, but other conditions associated with it must also be considered.

TREATMENT. The treatment can be divided into that for the arterial, venous, and neurologic compressions. Treatment of the arterial compression depends upon the specific entity produced: embolization, stenosis and thrombosis, aneurysm formation, or intermittent vasospasm (Raynaud's). Occlusion of the subclavian artery, if not associated with severe ischemia, may require no therapy except an exercise program to promote development of collateral circulation. With atherosclerotic plaques or aneurysms of the subclavian artery, frequently associated with embolic episodes, therapy should correct the underlying compression mechanism. This usually involves resection of the first rib, preferably by the transaxillary approach, as well as removing the source of emboli. The presence of a thrombus in an aneurysm or ulceration in an atherosclerotic plaque requires resection of the involved artery and replacement, preferably with autologous tissue: composite grafts of saphenous veins have been useful. On occasion direct exposure of the arteries in the arm or forearm is necessary to remove emboli.

The venous occlusions are more difficult to treat, for the compressing mechanism may not be apparent from either physical examination or laboratory studies. It appears clear from results of transaxillary resection of the first rib that the most proximal part of the vein can be decompressed by this procedure, but the roles of the clavicle, the pectoralis minor, and clavipectoral fascia in producing compression cannot be evaluated by this approach. Those patients with effort thrombosis seen within the first day or two of its occurrence should be considered for combined surgical procedures of venous thrombectomy and relief of the compressing mechanism. Anticoagulation therapy then should be used, perhaps for as long as 1 year.

The management of the neural compression syndromes generally involves a conservative, nonsurgical approach. An exercise program designed to strengthen the muscles of the shoulder girdle and lessen the tendency of the shoulder to droop has been of value in some patients with mild to moderate symptoms. A series of such exercises are carefully described by Allen et al. As an example of this approach, fewer than half of a group of 300 patients with thoracic outlet syndromes required surgical intervention. The selection of patients for operation should depend upon the severity of the symptoms, failure to respond to a nonsurgical program, and the specificity of the diagnosis.

Operative Technique. It is important to include the entire extremity in the sterile operative field, permitting manipulation of the extremity in order to define the most likely area of compression. Whether or not a cervical rib is present, the transaxillary approach is favored for its simplicity, the clarity with which the compression mechanisms can be diagnosed, the excellent cosmetic result, and the ease with which cervical ribs together with the first rib can be excised. If vasomotor symptoms are prominent, sympathectomy can be performed through the same transaxillary approach, exposing the third and second thoracic ganglia as well as the lower third of the stellate ganglion; this includes the first thoracic ganglion but avoids the production of Horner's syndrome. If removal of the second and third intercostal nerves with their ganglia is thought necessary, since the demonstration by Skoog that 10 to 15 percent of the sympathetic ganglia to the upper extremity is contained in these nerves, it can be similarly carried out.

The transaxillary approach is performed by making an incision in the lowermost portion of the axilla from the pectoralis major anteriorly to the latissimus dorsi posteriorly (Fig. 21-21). The incision is deepened to the muscles of the chest wall, the serratus anterior and the intercostal muscles coming into view. The dissection is continued upward, avoiding the intercostobrachial nerve, with the arm hyperabducted to raise the neurovascular bundle off the first rib. By gentle dissection, it is possible to outline the scalene muscles and identify the attachment of the cervical rib to the first rib if one is present. The scalene muscles are transected and permitted to retract, and the muscles along the inferior border of the first rib are similarly incised. The first rib and cervical rib usually can be removed in their entirety, including periosteum, from the costochondral junction anteriorly to the posterior angle of the rib. The parietal pleura lies deep to the dissection; care must be taken to avoid puncturing it. If the pleura is punctured, the wound is closed around a catheter in the axilla while the anesthetist expands the lung. This usually suffices to correct the pneumothorax. On occasion it has been necessary to aspirate air from the pleural cavity in the early postoperative period.

If a sympathectomy is indicated, the parietal pleura is stripped from the chest wall attachments and the sympathetic chain exposed, dissected free, and excised.

The postoperative course is usually benign, with the patient ready for discharge by the third postoperative day.

Other approaches have been described for excising the first rib. The posterior approach has been advocated by many but is an operation of greater magnitude. The anterior transthoracic approach has been proposed by others for more extensive exposure. However, most agree that the supraclavicular approach is probably archaic, since it does not permit thorough exploration of the area and easy excision of the first rib, which has become of paramount importance in treatment.

PROGNOSIS. The prognosis is dependent upon the specific syndrome present. The arterial compression syndromes can be quite satisfactorily relieved and arterial reconstructions performed with a high degree of precision, although a large series of patients treated with arterial compression has not been reported. In our experience it has been possible to stop embolic episodes and restore circulation to the upper extremity by standard arterial reconstructive procedures. However, patients with Raynaud's phenomena and cervical rib in whom associated sympathectomies have been performed have had variable results. Although immediate effects of sympathectomy have been excellent, relapses have occurred quite abruptly as early as 6 months following operation.

The venous compression disorders also have given variable results. It is not clear at present whether thrombectomy, with or without relief of the venous compression mechanism, is any better than prolonged anticoagulant therapy. Those patients with chronic venous occlusions of the subclavian and axillary veins who have been followed for years have shown remarkable recovery, with subsidence of edema coincident with the appearance of a prominent venous pattern on the chest wall and little or no resulting disability.

The surgical approach has often changed through the years. Other procedures include scalenotomy performed through the supraclavicular approach, then resection of the clavicle proposed by Lord and Rosati, and now resection of the first rib. Adson, predominantly performing scalenotomy through the supraclavicular approach, reported in 1947 that over a period of 22 years 142 patients had been operated upon with excellent results in about 50 percent and improvement in another 20 to 30 percent. In another series from the Mayo Clinic, Love reported that of 700 patients seen over a 5-year period with a wide variety of thoracic outlet syndromes, only about 3 percent underwent operation. Roos has reported from a wide experience with transaxillary resection of the first rib that 80 to 90 percent of those with predominantly neurologic symptoms obtained complete relief, while approximately 50 percent of those with predominantly vascular symptoms became free of symptoms.

The recent development of electrical conduction studies provides an objective method not only for making the

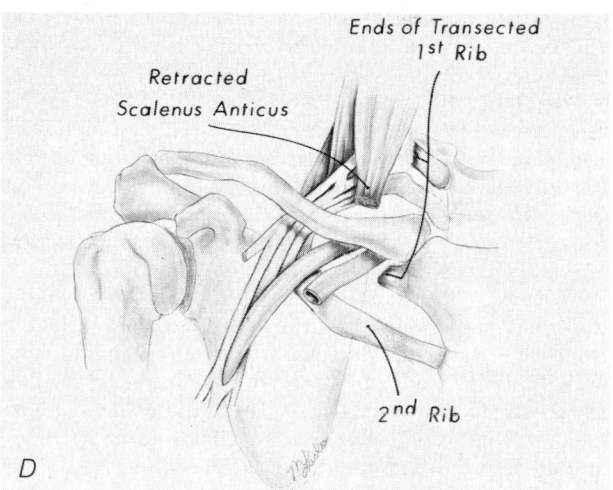

Fig. 21-21. Technique of transaxillary resection of the first rib.
A. The critical relations of the first rib, clavicle, scalene muscles
and neurovascular structures are shown. The lowermost portion
of the brachial plexus which gives rise to the ulnar nerve is in
contact with the first rib and explains the most characteristic
neurologic symptoms usually involving the ulnar aspect of the
forearm and fourth and fifth fingers. *B.* Operative incision below
the axillary hairline with hyperabduction of the arm which raises
the neurovascular bundle out of the operative field. *C.* Effect of
hyperabduction in exposing the first rib and scalene muscles,
retracting the neurovascular bundle. *D.* Effect of first rib resection, which requires cutting all three scalene muscles, in relieving
the compression of artery, vein, and brachial plexus.

diagnosis but for evaluating the results of therapy. The
wide variation in frequency of diagnosis and results with
operation from different groups is perhaps due to variation
in diagnostic criteria. Urschel emphasized the usefulness
of electrical conduction studies; in a series of 300 patients
seen between 1946 and 1970, only 138 were operated upon.
Seventeen of these had bilateral operations. Employing the
electrical conduction studies, 96 percent of patients im-

proved after resection of the first rib. There were only five
cases of failure, in two of which a cervical disc subsequently was removed. The most favorable group were
those with pain and paresthesia in the distribution of the
ulnar nerve, diminution of the pulse by one of the various
compression tests, and slowing of ulnar nerve conduction
velocity below 60 m/second. Failures following operation
were more common in those with atypical pain distributions, often with associated cervical syndromes secondary
to whiplash or trauma. Usually, pulse changes with the
compression tests were minimal or absent, and there was
less slowing of ulnar nerve conduction velocity.

EXTRACRANIAL OCCLUSIVE
CEREBROVASCULAR DISEASE

HISTORICAL CONSIDERATIONS. One of the most astonishing historical medical facts of the twentieth century
relates to the belated recognition 25 years ago that the

majority of ischemic strokes are due to occlusive atherosclerotic disease of the extracranial arteries in the neck, not to intravascular arterial occlusions. The earliest recorded recognition of this possible relationship was made by Savory in 1856. This concept was rediscovered in 1914 by Hunt, who described the postmortem findings of infarction of a cerebral hemisphere in a patient with patent territorial (middle cerebral) arteries but a thrombosed extracranial internal carotid artery. This fact was considered to be a curiosity for almost four more decades, because of both the unavailability of techniques for studying afflicted patients in vivo and the practice of performing incomplete postmortem examinations in order to preserve the cervical carotid arteries for the injection of embalming fluid. The intracranial arteries were examined, as were the origins of the great vessels from the aortic arch, but the critical carotid bifurcation in the neck was left untouched.

The development of safe techniques for cerebral angiography, combined with careful clinical pathologic studies of the type of vascular disease in large numbers of patients with strokes, led to recognition of the frequency with which stroke syndromes were due to extracranial vascular disease. Classic studies were reported by Fischer between 1951 and 1954 and by Hutchinson and Yates in 1956.

The report of Eastcott, Pickering, and Rob documenting the successful operation for carotid bifurcation disease stimulated wide interest in the surgical management of this condition, although three groups, including Carre et al, Stuly et al, and DeBakey, claimed priority in having performed earlier operations. The first significant series in the United States was reported by Lyons and Galbraith in 1957. It was soon established that the operation of endarterectomy for carotid bifurcation atherosclerotic lesions could be performed in large numbers of afflicted individuals with a high degree of safety, in spite of the unmatched sensitivity of the brain to ischemia, and that long-term patency could be expected. The effects of the surgical approach on the natural history of stroke syndromes, which were many and varied, however, had not been evaluated. Therefore, a "Joint Study of Extracranial Arterial Occlusion as a Cause of Stroke" was begun in 1961. Many universities throughout the country participated in a patient-informed prospective randomized study of the effects of surgical reconstructive procedures upon the natural history of the disease. In the ensuing 10 years, on the basis of the carefully collected protocols of 11,000 patients and frequent workshop meetings among the members, understanding of the natural history of the disease, the indications, contraindications, and hazards of diagnostic and surgical procedures were developed. The randomized nature of the study was fully justified by the rapidity with which understanding developed, permitting the elimination, as surgical candidates, of those patients in whom the surgical procedure was detrimental, and vastly improving the management of those in whom the surgical procedure was beneficial.

ETIOLOGY AND PATHOLOGY. Although the term *stroke* encompasses a variety of clinical situations in which major neurologic deficits occur because of involvement of the brain, the term *ischemic stroke* refers to cerebral infarction occurring as a result of impairment of regional blood flow. Atherosclerosis is the basis for this in the vast majority of patients. Smaller percentages are (1) secondary to cerebral embolization of thrombi which originate in the heart, (2) due to fibromuscular hyperplasia, (3) associated with obliterative arteritis of the great vessels as they originate from the aortic arch (see Aortic Arch Occlusive Disease, in Chap. 20), (4) due to blunt or penetrating trauma, (5) secondary to forceful hyperextension of the neck resulting in dissection and tearing of the carotid intima, and (6) due to dissecting thoracic aortic aneurysms which involve the carotid arteries.

A clinical pathologic correlation between the appearance of surgically removed plaques and the specific syndromes presented by patients operated on at New York University confirmed the early findings of Millard Fisher, showing that patients with generalized symptoms of cerebral ischemia had major stenotic fibrotic lesions which had smooth surfaces, while those with focal symptoms were found to have plaques with either frank ulcerations or cul de sacs which could have been the source of emboli. Intramural hemorrhage was the most common single, pathologic finding and could be responsible for fragmentation of plaques, development of sudden stenosis, breakdown of the plaque, and subsequent thrombosis. If patients with stroke syndromes are studied with four-vessel angiography, opacifying both carotid and both vertebral arteries from their origins to their point of entry into the skull, significant extracranial occlusive disease will be found in about 75 percent of the group (Fig. 21-22). The segmental localization is impressive. In the carotid artery, almost all plaques are found at the carotid bifurcation, starting in the distal centimeter of the common carotid and involving the proximal external carotid and the proximal 1 to 2 cm of the internal carotid. Fortunately for surgical reconstruction, and also a striking example of segmental localization of atherosclerosis, the internal carotid beyond the first 1 to 2 cm is usually uninvolved to beyond its point of entry into the skull, the area of the so-called carotid siphon. Because of the freedom of involvement of this portion, arterial reconstruction almost always can be done if the internal carotid is not thrombosed. Disease in the middle cerebral artery is rare. In the basilar-vertebral system, plaques are usually at the origin of the vertebrals from the subclavian, but disease of the vertebral beyond its origin is unusual. In the basilar artery localized atherosclerosis is more common. Within the thorax, the great vessels are infrequently diseased. The lesions are multiple in more than 50 percent of patients.

Soon after the recognition of the frequency of extracranial vascular disease, it became apparent that simple reduction in cerebral blood flow was not an adequate explanation for many of the neurologic syndromes encountered. As a result of several years of investigation by the National Cooperative Stroke Study, it now seems clear that arterioarterial embolization of fragments of plaque or platelet-fibrin aggregates is probably the most frequent mechanism of neurologic injury (Fig. 21-23). These plaques form on the irregular surface of atherosclerotic plaques, usually at the carotid bifurcation, and subse-

Fig. 21-22. Carotid plaque dynamics in the pathogenesis of stroke syndromes are suggested by the variations in the appearances of lesions surgically removed. *A.* Smooth fibrous plaque producing marked stenosis and decreased blood flow. *B.* Ulcerated plaque giving rise to embolization. *C.* Hemorrhage into the wall of a plaque which can result in sudden stenosis or ulceration and subsequent ulceration and embolization. *D.* Total occlusion of an internal carotid artery secondary to thrombosis.

quently embolize. Ophthalmologic visualization of these plaques suddenly appearing in the retina during transient ischemic attacks was one of the first clues to the mechanism of the syndrome. The second method for production of symptoms is the obvious one of simple decrease in flow from marked stenosis or occlusion. Because of abundant collateral circulation in the brain, major arteries may be-

come narrowed or occluded without any symptoms whatever unless multiple areas are diseased. As with stenotic lesions in the vascular system elsewhere there is little decrease in blood flow until the cross sectional area of the vessel is narrowed by more than 75 percent. If collateral circulation is adequate, even complete occlusion may be harmless. Routine postmortem studies by Martin and associates of a large group of patients dying from different causes at the Mayo Clinic found that in as many as 40 percent of the patients at least one of the four major extracranial arteries significantly was narrowed or oc-

STENOSIS   OCCLUSION

A   B

Fig. 21-23. Frequency distribution of lesions according to anatomic locations and stenosis versus occlusion. The predominance of stenotic lesions over occlusions favors embolization as a common mechanism for the production of cerebral ischemia. The predominance of extracranial lesions renders surgical intervention feasible.

cluded, even though there were no neurologic symptoms before death.

The atherosclerotic plaques removed from the vessels of symptomatic patients have varied greatly in composition and appearance. Some were principally fibrotic, with smooth internal surfaces; others showed advanced degenerative changes, with intramural hemorrhage and little stenosis, but with ulceration of the intimal surface. Plaques with a smooth intimal surface are probably harmless until the cross-sectional area of the artery is reduced to a marked degree. An ulcerated plaque, however, even though the lumen is compromised little, may cause serious or even catastrophic injury from repeated embolization.

CLINICAL MANIFESTATIONS. A great variety of clinical syndromes result from the different patterns of occlusive disease in the carotid, vertebral, and subclavian arteries. These will be only briefly summarized here, for they are described in considerable detail in standard texts of neurology. The classic stroke from unilateral carotid disease is ipsilateral blindness and contralateral hemiplegia. The presence of aphasia depends upon the dominant cerebral hemisphere. The other extreme is the most fleeting focal neurologic defect such as a transient monoplegia, transient hemiplegia, or transient ipsilateral blindness. These episodes, clearing within minutes to hours after an abrupt onset, are termed *transient ischemic attacks*. Between such

episodes the patient may be completely well, but unfortunately such attacks often precede a catastrophic stroke. One retrospective study of patients with severe strokes found that almost 75 percent had such premonitory symptoms in the weeks or months before the stroke appeared.

Between the transient ischemic attack on the one hand and the massive stroke on the other, a wide variety of motor and sensory syndromes are seen. Their unilateral localization is strongly suggestive of carotid artery disease. They may be precipitated by hypotension, hypoxia, or changes in position or posture, or they may be unrelated to any known cause.

With disease of the vertebral-basilar system, a number of brainstem symptoms occur. In contrast to carotid disease, the symptoms are often bilateral, involving either both arms or both legs, but may alternate in severity from one side of the body to the other. Tinnitus, dizziness, vertigo, diplopia, and dysarthria are also common. One type of characteristic syndrome is the so-called "drop attack," in which the patient may literally fall to the ground with little or no warning, with or without loss of consciousness, and recover equally rapidly with only residual dizziness or mild ataxia.

Disease of the subclavian artery proximal to the origin of one of the vertebral arteries, more commonly the left, produces the so-called "subclavian steal" syndrome. The proximal obstruction in the subclavian artery decreases the pressure in that artery at the point of origin of the vertebral artery; this results in an actual reversal of flow in the vertebral artery, with blood draining out of the basilar artery into the arm. Although this phenomenon is seen frequently on angiographic studies, production of symptoms from ischemia of the brainstem by exercising the arm is uncommon.

Physical Examination. Examination is directed primarily at determining the presence of any neurologic deficit as well as the pattern of arterial involvement. Palpation of the carotid pulses is useful only for the rare instance of intrathoracic occlusion of the common carotid artery. Palpation for the internal carotid pulse in the pharynx posterior to the tonsillar pillars is no longer advised. Separate palpation of the external and internal carotid arteries is impossible because of their location next to one another. Hence, the carotid pulses are normal on palpation in almost all patients with occlusive disease at the carotid bifurcation. However, auscultation over the carotid bifurcation for a bruit is essential. With high-grade stenoses at the bifurcation, a bruit is audible just anterior to the sternocleidomastoid muscle near the level of the angle of the mandible in at least 50 percent of patients with stenosis. Auscultation in the supraclavicular fossae may find bruits from subclavian-vertebral disease. When bruits are detected, they must be differentiated from cardiac valvular lesions, such as aortic stenosis, which produce murmurs transmitted along the great vessels. If occlusive disease of a subclavian artery is present, the blood pressure will be significantly different in the two arms.

Ophthalmodynomometry is a useful screening procedure when there is high-grade stenosis or total occlusion of one of the internal carotid arteries. The technique is simple comparison of the pressure in the retinal arteries of the two eyes; though not quantitative, it is a useful screening technique.

DIAGNOSIS. The differential diagnosis of cerebrovascular insufficiency syndromes is extremely complex and involves exclusion of a variety of intracranial lesions in addition to generalized conditions which can effect cerebral hypoxia. The latter include myocardial infarction, cardiac arrhythmias, Stokes-Adams syndrome, Ménière's syndrome, and a number of metabolic disorders such as diabetic ketosis and hypoglycemia.

The diagnosis of ischemic stroke syndromes ultimately depends upon angiographic delineation of the intra- and extracranial cerebral arteries. The risks related to angiography generally are assumed by the patients most seriously afflicted with arterial disease, particularly those who have already developed serious neurologic deficits. The overall risk of stroke or death incident to cerebral angiography is about 0.5 to 1 percent. Less serious complications, such as hematomas and temporary or permanent loss of arterial pulses distal to puncture sites, occur with greater frequency.

The presence of amaurosis fugax, transient paralysis or weakness of the extremity, weakness of facial muscles, and transient disorders of speech all require more extensive investigation, which should include skull x-rays, lumbar puncture, computed axial tomography of the head, and electroencephalograms. Electrocardiography with prolonged cardiac monitoring may be appropriate to rule out transient cardiac arrhythmias. The ultimate study in these patients is cerebral angiography.

The major questions related to cerebral angiography concern patients with massive and persistent neurologic deficits and those with asymptomatic bruits. Both cerebral angiographic studies and carotid-vertebral reconstructive procedures assume grave risks in patients who have had full-blown ischemic stroke within the week.

On the other side of the spectrum, the finding of neck bruits in asymptomatic patients during routine examination increasingly poses a problem. Doppler examination of the supraorbital arteries or ultrasound scanning of the cervical carotid arteries may permit detection of hemodynamically significant carotid lesions. However, it is clear that many carotid lesions which produce stroke manifest no local hemodynamic disturbances and act rather as a source of emboli. Thus, there are difficult decisions regarding performance of cerebral angiography in these patients.

The study by Thompson, in which patients with asymptomatic bruits were shown to have "significant" lesions by angiography and appeared to be protected from future stroke by operative intervention, suggests a more aggressive attitude. However, Gaspar and Movius, among others, report that patients who had neck bruits and underwent major abdominal procedures did not develop an increased incidence of postoperative strokes.

The attitude of the authors of this chapter toward asymptomatic bruits, in the face of conflicting data, is to study angiographically those patients with "loud, high-pitched" carotid bruits who are physiologically fit and

therefore thought to have long life expectancies. Operations are offered to patients who have 70 percent stenosis or lesions with irregular contour. Any patient with an asymptomatic carotid bruit discovered prior to a major intraabdominal or intrathoracic procedure is studied in a similar manner.

TREATMENT. General Considerations. Data accumulated from several years of study by the National Cooperative Stroke Study clearly show that effective surgical treatment must be performed before major neurologic deficits are produced from cerebral infarction. Hence, surgical therapy must be basically prophylactic. Operations are generally performed on patients who have had transient ischemic attacks. Operation upon patients with acute strokes is associated with a high mortality, considerably higher than that for patients treated medically. If operation for acute stroke is for an ulcerated plaque which does not narrow the artery, there is little benefit at all to the patient except prevention of subsequent episodes. If a totally obstructed internal carotid artery is reopened, the patient's condition may be exacerbated from edema or hemorrhage developing in the infarct as a result of restoring perfusion pressure. The question of operating on patients with asymptomatic bruits has not been resolved.

Recently, as the prevalence of arterioarterial embolization in the production of stroke syndromes has become clear, there has been renewed interest in altering the coagulability of the blood. The striking finding of the influence of acetylsalicylic acid on platelet aggregation may be of considerable therapeutic significance. Clinical trials are now in progress to determine the possible value of aspirin in preventing stroke syndromes.

Treatment of Atherosclerotic Disease of the Internal Carotid Artery. Atherosclerosis of the origin of the internal carotid artery is the most common form of extracranial vascular disease. As stated earlier, the disease fortunately is limited only to the first 1 to 2 cm of the origin of the internal carotid and hence is ideal for surgical correction (Fig. 21-24).

When complete occlusion develops in the carotid artery, however, an organized thrombus develops above the atherosclerotic plaque which extends superiorly into the intracranial internal carotid, making successful operation impossible. In approximately 10 percent of patients with complete occlusion, however, the thrombus has not propagated more than 2 to 3 cm, and surgical removal is still possible.

As stated earlier, the ideal patient for operation is one with transient ischemic attacks without any permanent neurologic abnormality. In such patients operation can be performed under regional cervical block with little risk. Mortality and major neurologic complications are in the range of 1 to 4 percent. Details of the operation are shown in Fig. 21-25.

The hazards of operation are greater and the likelihood of benefit much less when a stroke has occurred. If the internal carotid has become totally occluded, producing a major neurologic deficit, operation performed within 6 hours after onset of symptoms may produce dramatic recovery. The operative mortality, however, especially with altered states of consciousness, is considerably higher than with elective operations. If operation is delayed much beyond 6 hours after the onset of symptoms, reopening a totally obstructed carotid artery may be followed first by transient improvement, then worsening of symptoms and even death from hemorrhage into the area of infarction precipitated by the restoration of arterial perfusion pressure. It has been suggested by Warren and Triedman that this catastrophe might be prevented by careful avoidance of blood pressure elevation during operation and for some weeks afterward.

If the acute stroke has resulted from embolization of atheromatous debris or platelet aggregates, with occlusion of small intracerebral vessels, emergency operation upon the nonstenosing ulcerated plaque at the carotid bifurcation is neither helpful nor harmful. At a later time such patients perhaps should be considered for operation to prevent future embolization if the permanent neurologic deficit is not severe.

In patients with chronic strokes in whom acute injury weeks or months earlier produced a permanent neurologic deficit indicative of total hemispheric infarction, operation is of little value. A challenging group consists of asymptomatic patients with loud bruits. Thompson et al. have reported a lowered stroke incidence in such patients if angiographic studies revealed significant carotid lesions.

Following endarterectomy of the stenotic carotid artery, the likelihood of long-term patency of the reconstructed artery is excellent. In a group of 100 patients reported by

Blaisdell et al., 21 were evaluated by angiography more than 5 years later. There was only one late occlusion, an asymptomatic one found at autopsy. In 1968 Edwards and associates studied 75 patients operated upon 5 to 9 years earlier. Only five of the 75 had subsequently had a stroke. Three of the group had developed recurrent stenosis at the site of endarterectomy, but all experienced successful reoperation.

The effect of prophylactic carotid endarterectomy in altering the incidence of mortality in future stroke has been analyzed in detail by the National Cooperative Stroke Study. Although the results of the study were not completely definitive, certain facts emerged. The natural history of the disease definitely can be changed if the operative mortality and stroke rate can be kept at low levels (1 to 5 percent). Those patients with the most severe and extensive involvement, viz., those with bilateral carotid

Fig. 21-24. Angiographic studies of the cerebral circulation for stroke syndromes should outline the major extracranial as well as the intracranial arteries. This facilitates planning operative procedures and aids in making differential diagnoses of the various causes of stroke syndromes. Cervical carotid and vertebral arteries are outlined by retrograde right brachial arterial injection. *A.* Arrow points to significant lesion in the internal and external carotids. *B.* Arrow points to typical stenotic lesion at the origin of the vertebral with an associated kink.

A

B

Sternocleidomastoid
Muscle   *A*

C

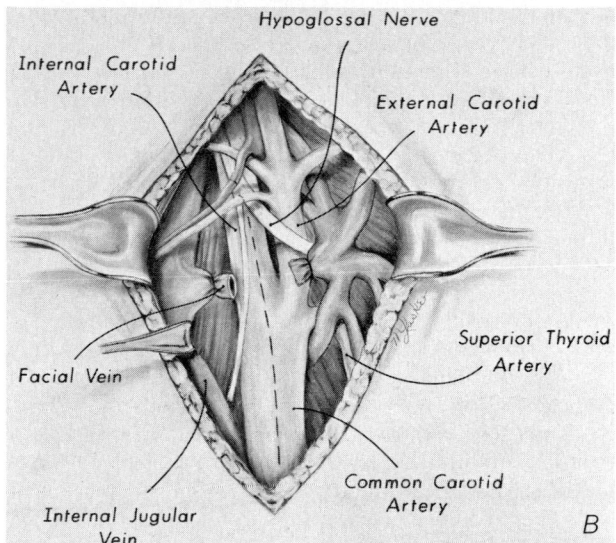

Hypoglossal Nerve

Internal Carotid
Artery

External Carotid
Artery

Facial Vein

Superior Thyroid
Artery

Internal Jugular
Vein

Common Carotid
Artery   *B*

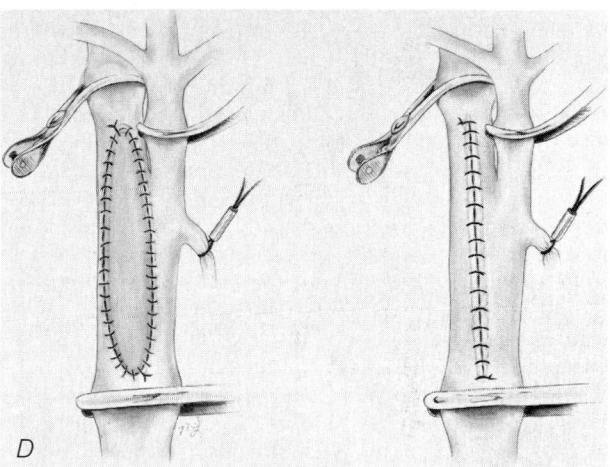

D

Fig. 21-25. Technique of carotid endarterectomy. *A.* A skin incision is made anterior to the sternocleidomastoid muscle. *B.* The carotid artery branches are widely mobilized. The internal carotid artery is clamped before widely mobilizing the frequently thrombus-containing bulb, thereby protecting the brain from embolization, which may occur during the dissection. The vagus and hypoglossal nerves are carefully protected. Mobilization of the hypoglossal is facilitated by dividing the sternocleidomastoid artery and vein. A longitudinal arteriotomy is made extending above and below the plaque at the carotid bifurcation. *C.* After division of the intima above the plaque, the plaque can be easily dissected from the underlying media or from the adventitia. The distal intima is carefully inspected and sutured if necessary. *D.* The arteriotomy is either closed primarily with 5-0 Tevdek, or a vein roof patch fashioned from autologous saphenous vein is used to avoid producing stenosis. The technique for restoring flow after completion of the closure is crucial to avoid embolization to the brain. The internal carotid clamp is temporarily removed and reapplied. The common and external carotid clamps are removed, and after 1 or 2 minutes of flushing of the carotid bulb the internal carotid clamp is removed.

lesions or with stenosis opposite complete occlusion, who survive operations enjoy the greatest protection from future stroke and from death from stroke. Strokes in the neurologic area corresponding to the surgically repaired artery are virtually eliminated.

In a series of 800 carotid and vertebral operations performed at our institution during a 15-year period, 70 had unilateral and 20 had bilateral carotid operations, 3 percent in conjunction with vertebral arterial reconstructions.

The combined death and stroke rate was 4 percent, being highest for patients with acute strokes (40 percent), 11 percent for strokes in evolution, and 0 for 106 patients who were neurologically intact and asymptomatic at the time of operation. Although patients with multiple extracranial arterial lesions have the highest operative risks, they enjoy the greatest long-term benefits from carotid surgery. Late mortality is primarily due to coronary artery disease.

Treatment of Subclavian-Vertebral Disease. Stenosis involving only the vertebral artery is infrequent. It is physiologically significant only when bilateral or if one vertebral is congenitally hypoplastic or absent. The disease is frequently limited to the site of origin of the vertebral from the subclavian. The atherosclerotic plaques in this area usually have a smooth intimal surface, contrasting to the frequency of ulcerated plaques in the carotid artery. In addition, there are frequently tortuous kinks in the first few centimeters of the vertebral artery, which can be shown to result in total occlusion when the head is turned to one side. Symptoms are probably due to decreased flow through the basivertebral system, although embolization cannot be entirely excluded. Concomitant disease in the basilar artery is frequent.

Atherosclerotic stenosis or occlusion of the subclavian artery proximal to the site of origin of the vertebral artery produces the clinical picture termed the subclavian steal syndrome. This abnormality was well defined by Reivich et al. in 1961, following an angiographic description in 1960 by Contorni of retrograde flow in the involved vertebral artery. The reduction in pressure in the subclavian artery beyond the stenosis results in retrograde flow from the brainstem down the vertebral artery to the arm; hence the term "subclavian steal." The clinical picture is that of ischemic neurologic symptoms in association with mild ischemia in the involved arm. Diagnosis can be easily made by finding a decreased pulse and blood pressure in the symptomatic arm, often in association with a localized bruit in the supraclavicular space. Serial angiograms after injection of contrast media into the opposite brachial artery or the ascending aorta will demonstrate reversal of flow in the involved vertebral artery by initially opacifying the opposite vertebral artery in a normal fashion, followed by retrograde opacification of the involved vertebral. Although this phenomenon is not infrequent on angiographic examination, clinical symptoms are not common, perhaps because collateral circulation in the brain can readily compensate for the amount of blood diverted away from the brain by the retrograde vertebral flow.

Operations upon the vertebral artery usually can be performed without thoracotomy. Surgical exposure of the subclavian-vertebral junction is obtained through a transverse supraclavicular incision which divides the clavicular head of the sternocleidomastoid muscle and the underlying scalenus anticus muscle. If the stenosing plaque has a smooth intimal surface, endarterectomy may not be necessary. The artery can be simply widened with a patch angioplasty with autologous saphenous vein. If the vertebral artery is significantly tortuous and redundant, predisposing to kinking, plication can be performed. In approximately 50 arterial reconstructions of the vertebral artery performed at New York University, there has been no neurologic deficit and no evidence of cerebral ischemia during the period of reconstruction.

Operations for the subclavian steal syndrome are seldom necessary. When done, a transthoracic approach to the subclavian artery can be avoided by employing a bypass graft from the ipsilateral common carotid artery to the distal subclavian artery. This is physiologically possible because the common carotid is large enough to deliver sufficient blood to supply both the brain and the upper extremity. On occasion, when the common carotid or in-nominate arteries are markedly stenotic and not suitable, axilloaxillary bypass grafting has been useful.

Treatment of Aortic Arch Occlusive Disease. In 1962 a report by Crawford et al. stated that during a period of 100 years since the first clinical description of the aortic arch syndrome by Savory in 1854, only about 90 patients were reported. In the report by Crawford et al., operative experiences with 67 patients in the 4-year period between 1957 and 1961 well indicated the increased recognition of the disease through the widespread use of angiography. Atherosclerosis was the most frequent cause. Formerly syphilitic arteritis was common, but this is now unusual. In the Orient a peculiar arteritis of unknown cause occurs, especially in young women. One eponym referring to this disease, Takayasu's disease, originated from an early description of the clinical syndrome by a Japanese ophthalmologist. An arteritis of this type is rarely seen in the United States.

For several years the occlusive lesions were approached directly with a transthoracic exposure. As the atherosclerotic process was often multiple and diffuse, endarterectomy was seldom possible. Bypass grafts were employed from the ascending aorta proximally to the carotid or subclavian arteries distad. This operative approach is extensive, requiring a thoracotomy incision and separate cervical or supraclavicular incisions.

In more recent years short bypass procedures in the neck establishing grafts from the normal artery to the obstructed artery have become increasingly popular. In a report of 125 patients, Dietrich and his associates expressed a preference for cervical carotid-subclavian bypass rather than the thoracic approach. A left carotid subclavian bypass was employed in 91 patients and a right carotid subclavian bypass in 20. The operative mortality was 5 percent, with good results in the majority of patients. This operative technique avoids an intrathoracic procedure but has the theoretic disadvantage of siphoning blood from a normal artery to a diseased artery. Apparently this theoretic objection is of limited clinical significance, for significant neurologic syndromes have not been produced from the shunting procedure.

ABDOMINAL ANEURYSMS

HISTORICAL DATA. The modern era of treatment of abdominal aneurysms began with the first successful excision of an abdominal aneurysm and replacement with an aortic homograft by Dubost in 1951. Previous therapeutic efforts, such as wiring to promote clotting, wrapping or coating with plastics, and other techniques to induce thrombosis, are now of historic interest only. Following the report of Dubost et al., advances in operative therapy came rapidly, especially those achieved by Cooley, DeBakey and his associates, and Bahnson. Late complications of aortic homografts soon appeared, following which replacement of the aorta with a prosthetic graft was developed. Although nylon was used briefly, Dacron or Teflon has been the preferred reconstruction material since 1957 (Fig. 21–26).

A   B   C   D

Fig. 21-26. Replacement of abdominal aorta. *A.* Aortic homograft inserted following excision of aneurysm of abdominal aorta by Bahnson in 1953. Homografts were among the earliest materials used for arterial grafts but were subsequently discontinued because of late degeneration of the homograft. *B.* Nylon graft used following excision of an abdominal aneurysm in 1954. Nylon was subsequently discontinued because experience found a marked loss in tensile strength 1 year after implantation. (*Courtesy of Dr. Henry T. Bahnson, Department of Surgery, University of Pittsburgh.*) *C.* Operative photograph of knitted Dacron graft inserted following excision of abdominal aneurysm. Dacron has been satisfactorily used since 1967 with excellent long-term results. *D.* Operative photograph of Teflon graft inserted following excision of abdominal aneurysm. Teflon, like Dacron, has given excellent long-term results with large vessels, but with small vessels, such as the femoral artery, results have been less satisfactory.

INCIDENCE. Abdominal aneurysms are the most common of the arteriosclerotic aneurysms. With the increasing age of the population, abdominal aneurysms are increasing in frequency, for most patients are in the sixth or seventh decade. Men are affected more frequently than women, in a ratio approximating 10:1.

ETIOLOGY AND PATHOLOGY. The vast majority of abdominal aneurysms are arteriosclerotic in origin. This is probably related to the frequency of involvement of the abdominal aorta by atherosclerosis, and perhaps to mechanical factors creating turbulent flow at the bifurcation of the abdominal aorta. The authors have never seen an abdominal aneurysm arising below the renal arteries from any cause except arteriosclerosis, although they have been reported from syphilis, trauma, the Marfan syndrome, or bacterial endocarditis.

The aneurysms characteristically originate just below the renal arteries and extend beyond the aortic bifurcation into the common iliacs. Fortunately, they seldom involve the external iliac arteries. Small aneurysms may be limited just to the abdominal aorta. The anatomic location of abdominal aneurysms, therefore, makes them accessible to surgical therapy, for a graft can be inserted proximally from the abdominal aorta below the renal arteries to the common iliac arteries distad. The size of abdominal aneurysms varies greatly, small ones 2 to 3 cm in diameter being

detected accidentally by aortography while others may enlarge to a diameter of 10 to 15 cm before being discovered accidentally by palpation. The usual course of untreated aneurysms was well documented in the classic report by Estes in 1950. Without treatment there is a 20 percent chance of rupture within 1 year after diagnosis and a 50 percent chance within 4 or 5 years. Complications seldom arise from expanding aneurysms until rupture occurs. Erosion of bone, so common in syphilitic aneurysms, virtually never occurs with abdominal aneurysms. There is usually no impairment of peripheral circulation, although larger aneurysms commonly are composed principally of laminated clot with a small central lumen. Emboli from the shaggy laminated clot lining abdominal aneurysms occur but rarely.

Although aneurysms frequently originate within 1 to 2 cm of the origin of the renal arteries, actual involvement of the origin of the renal arteries in the aneurysm, necessitating reconstruction of the renal arteries during surgical excision, is rare. In a series of over 170 abdominal aneurysms at the Johns Hopkins Hospital, only 3 aneurysms involving the renal arteries were found.

An abdominal aneurysm is often associated with generalized atherosclerosis. In a series of 1,400 patients operated upon by DeBakey and associates, some signs of coronary artery disease were present in 30 percent of the patients, and 40 percent of the patients had some increase in systolic blood pressure. Associated occlusive disease of the carotid arteries was found in 7 percent, of the renal arteries in 2 percent, and of the iliac arteries in 16 percent of the patients. Concomitant clinically significant aneurysms were found in the thoracic aorta in 4 percent, in the femoral artery in 3 percent, and in the popliteal artery in 2 percent of the group.

CLINICAL MANIFESTATIONS. Symptoms. Most patients are unaware of their abdominal aneurysms until a mass is accidentally discovered by the patient or his physician. The importance of careful deep palpation of the abdomen on routine physical examination, outlining the abdominal aorta when possible, is obvious. Occasionally, low back pain caused by an abdominal aneurysm may be diagnosed erroneously as due to an orthopedic condition. The pain apparently arises from tension on retroperitoneal tissues from the aneurysm; erosion of bone almost never happens. Virtually any intraabdominal condition may be simulated by an abdominal aortic aneurysm, such as renal colic, acute appendicitis, diverticulitis, peptic ulcer, pancreatitis, or cholecystitis. Rarely, there is gastrointestinal bleeding. With beginning leakage of the aneurysm or frank rupture momentarily contained retroperitoneally, acute abdominal conditions such as perforated ulcer, hemorrhagic pancreatitis, or generalized peritonitis may be simulated.

Sometimes, sudden vascular collapse with shock is the first indication. Most patients, however, have some premonitory symptoms. The absence of signs preceding fatal rupture is a strong reason for removing most abdominal aneurysms as soon as the diagnosis is made, even though the condition is asymptomatic. Symptoms from an aneurysm are an urgent indication for operation and are sometimes called a *syndrome of impending rupture.*

Physical Examination. On physical examination an abdominal aneurysm larger than 5 cm in diameter can be diagnosed with reasonable certainty. Once the patient has relaxed the muscles of the abdominal wall, careful deep palpation can usually outline the abdominal aorta near the bifurcation, generally slightly inferior to the umbilicus. The aorta may be traced proximally into the upper abdomen, where it is concealed beneath the pancreas and transverse colon. A normal aorta is seldom over an inch in

diameter. Careful palpation can usually distinguish the lateral walls of the aorta and hence provide an estimate of the width. Finding a pulsating mass greater than an inch in diameter usually establishes the diagnosis of aneurysm.

Confusion may arise in thin females with diastasis of the rectus muscles in whom the aortic pulsations are abnormally prominent. This is particularly true if an increased pulse pressure is present. Such patients may come to the physician because of concern over the prominent pulsations, and vague tenderness may be elicited in palpating the aorta. Formerly the unwary surgeon was led to perform a laparotomy on such patients because of the prominent pulse. Almost always careful palpation will demonstrate that the aorta is of normal diameter. When palpation is uncertain, an echogram or an aortogram may be required to exclude the presence of a small aneurysm. In the majority of patients palpation either establishes or excludes the diagnosis; confirmation by laboratory studies is often superfluous.

During the physical examination, peripheral pulses should be carefully examined, for associated occlusive vascular disease may be present. The presence of a bruit over the bifurcation of the carotid arteries is particularly

Fig. 21-27. X-ray films of the abdomen with the gastrointestinal tract opacified often reveal the calcific rim of abdominal aortic aneurysms quite clearly. The lateral film is most helpful since the thin shadow of the calcification is separated from the shadows of the spinal column. *A.* Anteroposterior view. *B.* Lateral view.

A

B

significant, because an asymptomatic stenosis of a carotid artery can significantly increase the risk of hypotension occurring during operation.

Laboratory Studies. A roentgenogram of the abdomen, including anteroposterior and lateral views, will establish the diagnosis in many patients by demonstrating calcification in the wall of the aneurysm. The lateral view is particularly helpful, since it permits visualization of the usually thin calcific rim of the aneurysm wall, which may be obscured by the shadows of the vertebral bodies in the frontal projections (Fig. 21-27). An accurate estimate of the size of the aneurysm is obtainable by measuring the distance from the anterior border of the vertebral bodies to the calcium in the anterior wall of the aneurysm and making the appropriate correction for the usual 20 percent magnification produced by the diverging x-rays. The uppermost extent of the aneurysm can be determined from this view. If combined with left lateral views of the chest it permits recognition of upper abdominal and thoracoabdominal aneurysms. A rapid-sequence excretory urogram may also be useful in detecting renal involvement. The use of ultrasound and CAT scan (computed axial tomography) also helps to delineate aneurysms, assisting in differentiation from other abdominal masses.

Aortography is now used infrequently by most vascular surgeons because of the small but definite risk it entails and because the diagnosis can usually be established by these other means. In addition, a laminated thrombus within the aneurysm may mask the true size of the lesion. Formerly, it was thought that in order to establish the relationship of the renal arteries to the aneurysm aortography was essential, but accumulated experiences have found renal artery involvement in only about 1 percent of patients. Nevertheless, some highly experienced vascular groups insist upon performing angiographic studies on all abdominal aortic aneurysm patients to delineate associated vascular lesions. It has not been shown that this has resulted in either increased survival or decreased morbidity.

Our own preference is to perform aortography only for specific indications, avoiding it in the majority of patients. These indications include uncertainty of diagnosis in the presence of small aneurysms (Fig. 21-28), the suspicion of an extensive lesion involving the upper abdominal and thoracic aorta as well, and the presence of lower extremity arterial occlusions manifested by absent pulses. Markedly depressed renal function, or controlled hypertension, though somewhat increasing the risk of aortography, are additional indications for this diagnostic procedure.

TREATMENT. Indications for Operation. Aneurysms smaller than 5 cm in diameter can be relatively safely observed unless they expand or become symptomatic. An asymptomatic aneurysm, measuring at least 5 to 6 cm in diameter, constitutes an indication for operation unless there are other conditions which either markedly increase the operative risk or promise to markedly shorten life expectancy. Asymptomatic aneurysms smaller than 5 to 6 cm are usually considered to carry a very small risk of rupture, while those 5 to 6 cm and larger carry at least a 20 percent yearly risk of rupture. There is very little correla-

tion between the size of the asymptomatic aneurysms beyond 5 to 6 cm, the absence of symptoms, and the tendency to rupture. Operative mortality with a ruptured aneurysm is nearly ten times greater than that for elective excision.

On the other hand, when the aneurysm becomes painful, operation ceases to be elective, for pain often denotes either rupture or impending rupture. The pain may be located in the back, the flank, or the abdominal region and may vary in both intensity and character, simulating many other intraabdominal and musculoskeletal conditions. Abdominal tenderness should increase the suspicion of impending or frank rupture. In such situations the indications for operation are extended to include conditions which might otherwise preclude an elective operation.

Preoperative evaluation should include, in addition to the studies already mentioned, an electrocardiogram, renal clearance studies, coagulation studies including platelet counts and, if indicated, platelet function studies. If carotid bruits are heard, cerebral angiograms may be indicated, and severe carotid stenotic lesions may have to be corrected first. If severe angina pectoris is present, coronary angiograms may be indicated, and coronary arterial surgery may be necessary as the initial procedure.

Technique of Operation for Abdominal Aneurysms. The operative procedure for excision of abdominal aneurysms is illustrated in Fig. 21-29. Separate from the obvious risk of hemorrhage, avoidable with careful technique, there are several common hazards. These include infection, renal failure, declamping shock, peripheral embolization, and ischemic necrosis of the colon. Infection of a plastic prosthesis is an ever-present and serious complication. It may be prevented by meticulous aseptic technique and by the administration of large doses of antibiotics, preoperatively, during the operation, and for about 5 days postoperatively. Renal insufficiency has virtually been eliminated (except in the presence of ruptured aneurysm) by careful attention to renal function during the entire operative procedure, especially during the phase of aortic clamping. Normal quarter-hourly urine output is achieved by carefully maintaining normal cardiodynamics and state of hydration, replacing lost blood promptly, and administering electrolyte solutions to compensate for the known fluid shifts which occur intraoperatively. Diuretics are not administered routinely but only to evaluate the function of the kidneys if anuria is encountered, or to expand circulating volume rapidly. An intrapulmonary catheter of the Swan-Ganz type is an invaluable aid to determine normal cardiodynamics and states of hydration.

Declamping hypotension varies with several factors, such as duration of aortic occlusion, adequacy of blood volume, and degree of collateral circulation to the lower extremities. While the aorta is occluded, the lower extremities are relatively ischemic as a result of which there is pooling of blood in dilated vessels and accumulation of ischemic products of metabolism. If the aorta is unclamped suddenly when ischemia has been severe, profound hypotension, cardiac arrhythmias, and even cardiac arrest can occur. Such problems can be almost completely avoided by different techniques. Hypotension is uncommon if the

A

B

C

D

aorta is occluded for less than 1 hour. With longer periods gradual restoration of the circulation is useful. An effective approach has been as follows: Once the proximal aortic anastomosis and one iliac anastomosis have been completed, flow is restored to that hypogastric artery, permitting gradual reopening of the circulation. When adjustment has occurred, the ipsilateral iliac artery is similarly unclamped while anastomoses are performed on the contralateral side, and the same sequence is repeated. In a series of 202 aortic operations reported by Imparato et al., declamping shock did not occur with this technique, vasopressors were not needed, and sodium bicarbonate was not required.

Distal embolization of atherosclerotic or thrombotic debris can be particularly hazardous, varying with the friability of the contents of the aneurysm. The following guidelines have been useful: The external and internal iliac arteries are mobilized and occluded before the aorta is clamped proximally. At this time 10 to 20 mg heparin is injected into the distal iliac vessels, or 50 mg heparin is given intravenously. Subsequently, as the individual iliac anastomoses are completed, retrograde flushing of the iliac arteries is allowed to occur. If this cannot be accomplished, a rubber catheter is passed into the external iliac arteries in order gently to pry apart the walls which may have been deformed by application of arterial clamps. Fogarty catheters are not routinely passed into the distal arteries because if aneurysmal disease is present in the femoral and popliteal arteries or if there is atherosclerosis, a thrombus or plaque may be dislodged. The selective iliac "flush" technique described above has been very effective. Finally, at the conclusion of the operation, the peripheral pulses are examined to be certain that they are the same as before operation.

Ischemic injury of the colon can be avoided by dissecting within the wall of the aneurysm rather than outside it and ligating the inferior mesenteric artery at its origin, carefully avoiding injury to any collateral vessels in the mesentery of the left colon. The technique of removing only the inner portion of the aneurysm, leaving the adventitial sheath, facilitates dissection, avoids injury to adjacent structures such as the vena cava, and provides a soft tissue covering of the prosthesis to prevent erosion of the duodenum or other structures subsequently. As the inferior mesenteric artery has been ligated, at least one hypogastric artery must be preserved to maintain collateral circulation to the colon through the middle hemorrhoidal arteries. If one or both

Fig. 21-28. *A.* Aortogram showing abdominal aneurysm in the distal aorta. Superimposed on the film is a photograph of a lesion excised at operation, indicating the large laminated clot filling the aneurysm. (*Courtesy of Dr. Henry T. Bahnson, Department of Surgery, University of Pittsburgh.*) *B.* Anteroposterior lumbar aortogram performed by percutaneous introduction of an arterial catheter, illustrating a large abdominal aneurysm arising in the lower abdominal aorta. Linear calcification of the lower thoracic and upper abdominal aorta is also visible. *C.* Lateral view in same patient. *D.* Abdominal aortogram in a patient with atherosclerotic occlusion of the abdominal aorta which has extended up to the level of the renal arteries. The superior mesenteric artery is visible as well as the right renal artery. Extensive collateral circulation has developed, particularly in the left flank.

hypogastric arteries have been ligated, either transplanting to the aortic prosthesis a button of aneurysm wall containing the inferior mesenteric artery or bypassing from the prosthesis to the inferior mesenteric artery should be performed. With these guidelines, significant ischemic injury of the colon is very rare, occurring probably only when atherosclerosis has compromised the collateral circulation. If ischemic injury is suspected, however, then a "second-look" laparotomy procedure is indicated to detect irreversible colon ischemia before bowel perforation and peritonitis occur.

An alternative technique to abdominal aortic aneurysm operation has been a retroperitoneal approach which avoids manipulation of the abdominal viscera. Postoperative recovery is said to be smoother by avoiding the problems of prolonged intestinal atony.

Postoperative Complications. The operative mortality for excision of an abdominal aneurysm is now 5 to 10 percent, varying with the age of the patient and the degree of associated atherosclerosis. Paralytic ileus for 2 to 4 days following operation is the most frequent complication. It is best treated by gastric decompression through a nasogastric tube until bowel function returns. Antibiotic therapy, usually with large amounts of penicillin or methicillin, is begun during operation and continued for 4 to 6 days. In uncomplicated aneurysms, convalescence is usually uneventful once postoperative ileus has subsided.

Following operation particular attention should be given to pedal pulses which were palpable before operation. Absence of a pedal pulse is usually an indication for prompt reoperation, for this is commonly due to embolization of atherosclerotic or thrombotic material during removal of the aneurysm. Renal insufficiency is now infrequent following uncomplicated operations. An unusual but often lethal cause of renal insufficiency is embolic occlusion and infarction of the kidneys from atherosclerotic material dislodged during manipulation of the proximal aorta during operation.

PROGNOSIS. The reported 5-year survival following resection of an abdominal aneurysm has varied from 30 to 60 percent. Fatalities are usually due to cardiac or cerebral complications of atherosclerosis. Complications from the prosthetic graft are unusual. The most frequent of these is development of a false aneurysm, often at the proximal suture line, with subsequent rupture or erosion into the duodenum. This can be minimized by limiting dissection of the proximal aorta at the time that the aneurysm is resected, covering the graft with the adventitia of the aneurysm, and subsequently carefully separating the prosthetic graft from the intestine.

Ruptured Abdominal Aneurysm

CLINICAL MANIFESTATIONS. A ruptured abdominal aneurysm constitutes a grave surgical emergency, for irreversible renal injury develops with great rapidity. The onset is characterized by acute vascular collapse, usually with abdominal or flank pain. With severe collapse, the diagnosis initially may be uncertain, because a stuporous or comatose patient cannot describe pain. Until a pul-

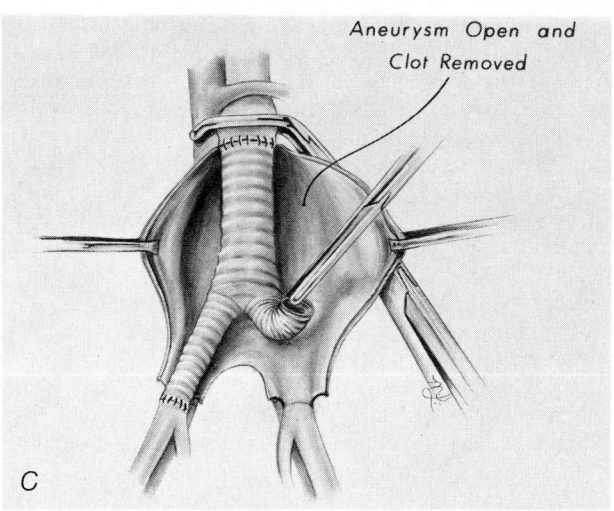

Aneurysm Open and
Clot Removed

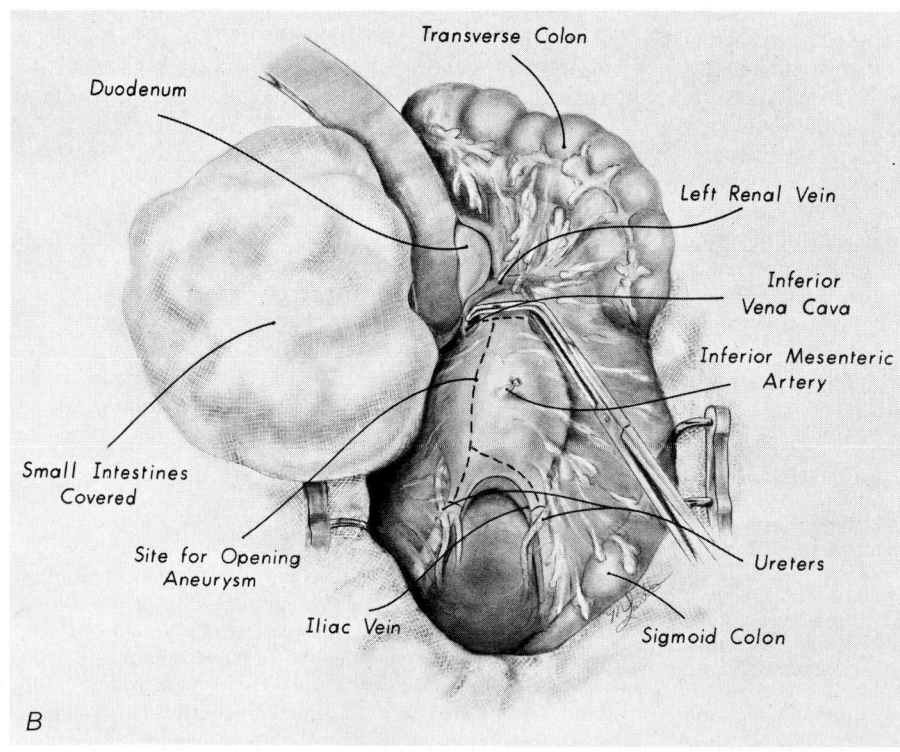

Transverse Colon

Duodenum

Left Renal Vein

Inferior
Vena Cava

Inferior Mesenteric
Artery

Small Intestines
Covered

Site for Opening
Aneurysm

Ureters

Iliac Vein

Sigmoid Colon

Clamp Opened Intermittently to Flush Aorta

Clamp Partially Opened

Clamp Opened

D   Aortic Flush

Flow Restored to Hypogastric

Flow Restored to Right Side

Fig. 21-29. Procedure for substituting aortoiliac bifurcation prosthesis for abdominal aortic aneurysm. *A.* A midline incision extending from xiphoid process to pubis symphysis is usually employed. Insert shows rotation of the table to the patient's right
side, which facilitates retraction of the small bowel. *B.* Surgical
exposure of vital structures and lines of incision of the aneurysm
are shown. *C.* Endarterectomy of the aneurysm wall is performed;
the lumbar arteries transfixed with sutures and the prosthesis in
place are shown. *D.* Technique for preventing embolization of
atherosclerotic debris to the lower extremities and gradually
restoring lower extremity circulation to avoid declamping shock.
(1) Aorta is flushed through one open limb of the prosthesis. (2)
Flow gradually restored to one hypogastric artery and, when the
blood pressure has been stabilized, to the ipsilateral external iliac
artery. (3) The sequence is repeated on the opposite side. *E.*
The remains of the aneurysm wall and the base of the left colon
mesentery are carefully sutured over the prosthesis and suture
lines to prevent adherence of the bowel and to bolster the suture
lines to prevent aorticointestinal fistulas. (*From A. M. Imparato et
al., Avoidance of Shock and Peripheral Embolism during Surgery
of the Abdominal Aorta, Surgery, 73(1):68, 1973.*)

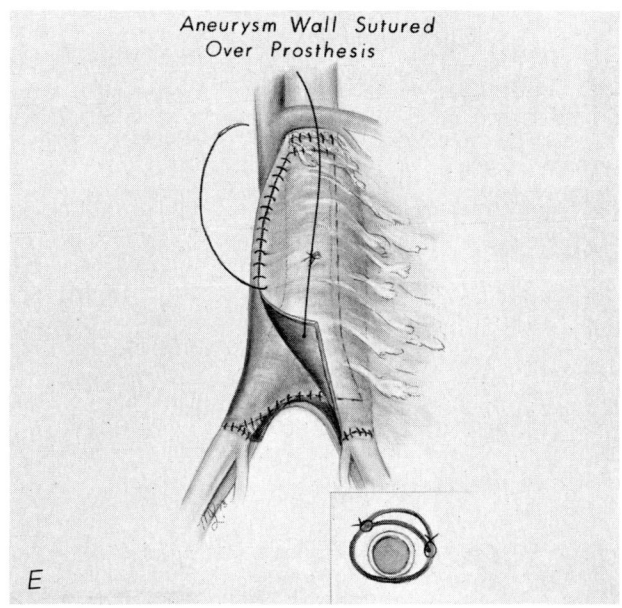

Aneurysm Wall Sutured Over Prosthesis

E

sating mass is palpated, a frequent erroneous diagnosis is
renal colic from a ureteral stone or massive myocardial or
pulmonary infarction. The diagnosis usually can be established by careful, deep palpation of the abdomen, which
should outline a pulsating, ill-defined mass in the epigastrium or flank.

TREATMENT. Operation should be performed as quickly
as possible, infusing 500 to 1000 ml of fluid every few
minutes until serious hypotension has been corrected. A
midline incision is preferred. Proximal control of the aorta
generally can be obtained by isolating the aorta above the
stomach just below the diaphragm. This should be done
initially, because once the posterior peritoneum is incised
and the hematoma surrounding the ruptured aneurysm
evacuated, massive hemorrhage can occur with exsanguination. The aorta can be safely clamped below the diaphragm for 20 to 30 minutes without serious ischemic
injury to the intestines or liver. Once it has been clamped,

the ruptured aneurysm can be widely incised, intraabdominal clots evacuated, and the proximal aorta below the renal
arteries isolated, after which a clamp can be applied to
the infrarenal aorta and the previously applied clamp
below the diaphragm released. Reconstruction is then similar to that with elective excision of an abdominal aneurysm, although excision of the wall of the aneurysm should
be limited because of the serious condition of the patient.
On occasion, the intradiaphragmatic portion of the aorta
cannot be clamped, because of either the massive amount
of retroperitoneal hematoma or free rupture into the peritoneal cavity. In this case, left thoracotomy is required to
achieve control. Consequently, in preparing the patient for

emergency operation for abdominal aneurysm, the chest as well as the abdomen must be made surgically accessible. Unfortunately, despite successful removal of the aneurysm, death results from renal insufficiency in 30 to 50 percent of patients.

The value of prompt excision of ruptured abdominal aneurysms is reflected by high survival rates if operation is performed within 1 to 2 hours of rupture. If operation is performed 8 to 10 hours after rupture, there is a very high fatality rate from renal insufficiency. The unheralded rupture of asymptomatic aneurysms, with resulting high fatality rates, is the most urgent reason for recommending routine excision of abdominal aneurysms as soon as the diagnosis is made.

PERIPHERAL ANEURYSMS

Aneurysms outside the major body cavities, the skull, thorax, and abdomen, are rare. If traumatic and congenital malformations, considered in different chapters, are excluded, almost all such aneurysms result from arteriosclerosis, for syphilitic aneurysms now are seldom seen. Similarly, mycotic aneurysms associated with bacterial

Fig. 21-30. Femoral angiogram indicating the presence of a popliteal aneurysm. Characteristic tortuosity of the involved artery is present. Such tortuosity often makes it possible to establish continuity by direct anastomosis following excision of the aneurysm.

endocarditis are infrequent with present methods of antibiotic therapy. The majority of peripheral arteriosclerotic aneurysms are in the popliteal artery. Infrequent sites include the femoral, carotid, or subclavian arteries. Each of these is considered separately.

The aneurysms in different locations are similar in that they usually occur in men in the fifth to seventh decades, often with hypertension and signs of atherosclerosis in other organs. Multiple aneurysms are frequent. In contrast to abdominal or thoracic aneurysms, where rupture is the greatest threat, peripheral aneurysms infrequently rupture but cause disability due to distal embolization or thrombosis with subsequent ischemia and gangrene of the extremity.

Because of their superficial location, peripheral aneurysms are readily amenable to successful therapy if operated upon electively before embolization and acute ischemia develop in the extremity. Tortuosity of the involved artery often makes it possible to mobilize the artery proximal and distal to the aneurysm and reestablish continuity following excision by end-to-end anastomosis. Continuity also can be established with a short graft, preferably of the saphenous vein. If this is not possible, a knitted Dacron prosthesis is preferred. In 1966 Howell and associates stated that over 400 such aneurysms had been treated at Baylor University during the previous 14 years with serious complications in only 3 percent of the patients. In patients with a distal pulse before operation, distal circulation was restored in all but one.

Popliteal Aneurysms

Almost all popliteal aneurysms originate from arteriosclerosis, usually in men in the sixth or seventh decade. As with other peripheral arteriosclerotic aneurysms, complications of arteriosclerosis in other organs are frequent. Bilateral popliteal aneurysms occur in at least 25 percent of patients. Aneurysms at other sites such as the abdominal aorta also are common. Hypertension is present in 40 to 50 percent of patients.

The aneurysms are often small, 3 by 4 cm, and asymptomatic. Nonetheless they pursue a malignant course of peripheral embolization with subsequent gangrene of the extremity. The marked tendency to progress rapidly to embolization and gangrene may be related to intermittent compression of the aneurysm by flexion of the knee. In one group of 29 aneurysms reported by Hara and Thompson, 18 progressed to acute ischemic occlusion despite their small size and lack of symptoms preceding acute vascular occlusion. In an extensive study of 100 popliteal aneurysms, Gifford et al. found that only about 20 percent remained free of symptoms within 5 years following diagnosis. In some patients, the tendency for silent aneurysms to embolize is demonstrated by the unheralded development of acute ischemic symptoms from occlusion of the popliteal artery; on subsequent physical examination the aneurysm is discovered.

CLINICAL MANIFESTATIONS. The clinical findings in most patients are characteristic enough to permit an accurate diagnosis. Some patients are unaware of the aneurysm, while others note a vigorous pulse behind the knee joint in a small mass which is otherwise asymptomatic. Rarely, the aneurysm may enlarge sufficiently to cause local pain and tenderness. Actual rupture is unusual.

A pulsating mass is usually found. If the aneurysm is thrombosed, pulsation may be absent, and a mass may or may not be felt. Differential diagnosis must include other cystic tumors about the knee joint, such as Baker's cyst, as well as other causes of tibial arterial occlusion, such as emboli, Buerger's disease, and diabetes mellitus. The presence or absence of pedal pulses should be carefully noted.

Calcification in the wall of the aneurysm is often visible on a roentgenogram. The diagnosis can be confirmed by arteriography, although much of the cavity of the aneurysm may be filled with thrombus (Fig. 21-30).

When a patient is seen with symptoms of acute ischemia in an extremity, such as pain, paralysis, or discoloration, the presence of pedal pulses is of particular importance, because the ischemic symptoms usually result from embolization of thrombotic material from the aneurysm distad into the posterior and anterior tibial arteries.

TREATMENT. Because of the hazard of thrombosis, embolization, and gangrene, operation should be performed as soon as possible after the diagnosis is made even though the aneurysm is small, asymptomatic, and seemingly stable. A retrospective study of gangrene and amputation from popliteal aneurysms which have embolized found no warning signs that such a catastrophe was imminent.

Operative Technique. With the patient in a prone position, an incision across the popliteal crease readily exposes the artery proximal and distal to the aneurysm. An alternative exposure, particularly useful when the femoral artery needs to be exposed for some distance from the popliteal, has been described by Imparato and Kim. An incision is made on the medial aspect of the lower thigh and extended across the knee joint into the upper calf, transecting the muscles inserting into the upper medial tibial plateau as well as the head of the gastrocnemius tendon. Transection of these muscles provides unusually wide exposure and has not resulted in any late impairment of function of the extremity.

Once the artery has been isolated distal to the aneurysm, vascular clamps are applied and the aneurysm widely opened. Any laminated thrombus is removed, as well as the inner lining of the wall of the aneurysm, preserving the adventitial sheath. The origins of the geniculate branches of the popliteal artery are sutured from within the lumen. This technique preserves branches of the popliteal vein which are usually stretched over the wall of the aneurysm, and also the collateral circulation is less disturbed. A small amount of heparin should be given either systemically or into the distal artery at the time that the clamps are applied.

If the aneurysm is small and the popliteal artery tortuous, an end-to-end anastomosis is sometimes possible. Most patients, however, require a short graft, preferably a reversed autologous saphenous vein (Fig. 21-31). Short grafts of knitted Dacron also have been satisfactory. As the anastomoses are completed, the distal popliteal artery

Fig. 21-31. Operative photograph of saphenous vein graft used to restore continuity of the popliteal artery following excision of a popliteal aneurysm. Long-term results of saphenous vein grafts following excision of such aneurysms have been excellent. At present, since most aneurysms of the popliteal artery are small, excision is no longer required and bypass with exclusion is practiced most often.

is cleared with a Fogarty balloon catheter to remove any laminated thrombus.

In a series of 48 popliteal aneurysms reported by Crichlow and Roberts, a vein graft was used in 21 and a Teflon graft in 14. The 21 saphenous vein grafts remained free of complications. Similar experiences were described by Hunter et al. for 27 patients with a total of 31 aneurysms.

Acute Ischemia. When operation is required because thrombosis has produced severe ischemia with impending gangrene, a different approach is needed. Simple excision of the aneurysm, of course, is futile with the obstructed distal circulation. The major consideration is removal of these distal thrombi followed by restoration of arterial continuity across the occluded aneurysm as in elective procedures. Operative incision and exposure should be planned to permit precise cannulation of the anterior and posterior tibial arteries with balloon-tipped catheters to remove propagated thrombus. Retrograde flushing with saline solution from the posterior and anterior tibial arteries is far less satisfactory than the Fogarty catheter technique. Operative angiography should be available to be certain that all thrombi have been removed. In some patients the distal thrombi have become adherent to the arterial wall and require repeated efforts for removal. If thrombi are not completely removed, as confirmed by angiography, rethrombosis terminating in gangrene and amputation is almost a certainty (Fig. 21-32).

Femoral Aneurysms

INCIDENCE AND PATHOLOGY. Femoral aneurysms are virtually all due to arteriosclerosis, with frequent signs of

Fig. 21-32. Angiographic study of tibial arteries after surgical repair of popliteal aneurysm showing persistent thrombi in the tibial arteries subsequently removed with Fogarty catheters. Such thrombi almost inevitably lead to occlusion of the tibial arterial outflow tract and may involve the arterial reconstruction itself.

atherosclerosis in other organs. In one series of 89 patients with 115 aneurysms, 86 of the 89 were men with an average age of sixty-four years. In this large series, 36 percent of the aneurysms were bilateral. At least one other aneurysm was present besides a single femoral aneurysm in 69 percent of the patients. Twenty-eight percent of the group had abdominal aneurysms, and 54 percent had hypertension.

In the femoral artery, the aneurysm was limited to the common femoral in 27 percent and to the superficial femoral in 26 percent, and involved both areas in the remainder. In only 1 percent of the entire group was the aneurysm limited to the profunda femoris artery.

As with popliteal aneurysms, the usual course is that of thrombosis, embolization, and ischemia. Rupture is rare. Of the two events producing ischemia, thrombosis is more common than embolization, in contrast to the usual course of popliteal aneurysms. This occurred in 26 percent of the 89 patients reported by Papas and associates, while rupture occurred only five times. Similar experiences were reported in a smaller series of 12 patients by Tolstedt et al. Eight of the twelve thrombosed, resulting in amputation in each patient.

CLINICAL MANIFESTATIONS. Symptoms usually consist of an awareness of a pulsating mass in the upper thigh until thrombosis or embolization produces ischemic symptoms in the extremity. The diagnosis can often be easily made on physical examination, outlining the pulsating mass in the femoral artery. A roentgenogram may show calcification in the wall of the aneurysm. Arteriography is useful to delineate the relationship of the aneurysm to the profunda femoris artery, as well as to define the patency of the distal circulation.

TREATMENT. Surgical correction should be performed promptly, unless coexisting cerebral or coronary artery disease makes the risk of operation prohibitive. If operation is postponed because of concomitant disease, such decisions should be made with the full realization that a subsequent amputation because of gangrene may entail an even greater operative risk to the patient.

At operation the arteries can be mobilized proximal and distal to the point of aneurysm and the aneurysm excised. Vascular continuity may be restored with either a saphenous vein graft or an 8- or 10-mm knitted Dacron prosthesis. Patency of the profunda femoris artery should be maintained by using a Y-bifurcation graft if necessary. Complications following operation are unusual unless peripheral arterial occlusion has already produced severe ischemic signs. In most patients following operation the prognosis is determined by the coexisting atherosclerotic disease, rather than the femoral aneurysm.

Carotid Artery Aneurysms

INCIDENCE AND PATHOLOGY. The infrequent occurrence of carotid aneurysms has been documented by several reports. Reid found only 12 cases in a 30-year survey at the Johns Hopkins Hospital ending in 1922. At the University of Pennsylvania in a 20-year period ending in 1947, five cases were encountered. Raphael and associates reported six patients seen at the Mayo Clinic in a 25-year period, and Beall et al. in 1962 stated that seven carotid aneurysms had been seen at Baylor University over a period of time during which 2,300 operations for aneurysms had been performed.

Most carotid aneurysms result from arteriosclerosis. As in other arteries, syphilis once was the most common cause but is now rare. Unusual causes include trauma, bacterial infection, or cystic medial necrosis. The most frequent location is in the common carotid artery near its bifurcation into the internal and external carotid arteries. Less frequently aneurysms are localized to the internal carotid. The main hazard from an aneurysm is embolization of thrombotic material into the cerebral circulation with production of cerebral infarcts. Infrequently such aneurysms may enlarge and rupture, but treatment is usually undertaken before this has occurred.

CLINICAL MANIFESTATIONS. Patients are usually seen because of a mass in the neck. Pulsations are often prominent and provide an easy clue to the diagnosis. A more difficult problem arises if pulsations are absent, because of laminated thrombus occupying most of the cavity of the aneurysm. Arteriography is the most definitive laboratory technique, establishing the diagnosis and also defining the relationship of the common and internal carotid arteries to the aneurysm (Fig. 21-33). The differential diagnosis should include prominent pulsations from buckling of the carotid artery, a condition seen in hypertensive women, and other solid tumors of the neck, such as a lymph node or a carotid body tumor.

TREATMENT. Because of the constant risk from cerebral infarction, the aneurysm should be excised as soon as possible. The major consideration in planning operation is protection of the brain from ischemic injury while the carotid artery is occluded during excision. In a review of reported experiences by Raphael and associates, 12 patients were described in whom the aneurysm was excised without any protection of the brain from ischemia. Six of the twelve had a transient neurologic injury, while four developed a permanent neurologic deficit.

The safest surgical technique is excision of the aneurysm under local or regional block anesthesia, keeping the patient awake to assess constantly the tolerance of the brain for temporary occlusion of the carotid artery. If ischemic symptoms develop, an internal shunt may be utilized to maintain cerebral blood flow. Even with a large aneurysm, regional block anesthesia is adequate.

The limited surgical experiences with carotid aneurysms was indicated by the report by Kianouri in 1967, who found a total of 28 patients in whom the aneurysm had been excised and arterial continuity reestablished. The first such report of successful excision of a carotid aneurysm, followed by end-to-end anastomosis, was published by Shea in 1955. Experiences at present indicate that in over one-half of the patients there is sufficient tortuosity and elongation of the carotid artery proximal and distal to the site of involvement of the aneurysm to permit mobilization of the ends of the carotid artery and direct anastomosis (Fig. 21-34). Following excision of the aneurysm with reconstruction of the carotid artery, convalescence has usually been uncomplicated, and long-term results are excellent.

Fig. 21-33. Carotid arteriogram illustrating saccular aneurysm of the internal carotid artery. The internal carotid proximal and distal to the aneurysm is opacified.

Subclavian Aneurysms

The majority of subclavian aneurysms develop as secondary complications of a cervical rib and are discussed in the section on Thoracic Outlet Syndromes. The extremely rare subclavian aneurysm which results from atherosclerosis is similar to other peripheral atherosclerotic aneurysms, occurring in older men, often with atherosclerotic aneurysms elsewhere. The diagnosis is usually readily made from physical examination. The most important differential diagnosis is from the frequently seen tortuosity of the innominate and subclavian arteries which occurs in hypertensive patients. Careful examination of the bulge will differentiate a true aneurysm from a tortuous vessel. If aneurysm cannot be excluded, an arteriogram should be done. Excision with reconstruction of the involved artery can be easily performed.

Visceral Aneurysms

SPLENIC ARTERY ANEURYSMS

Significant aneurysms of the splenic artery are uncommon. Because of their rarity and unusual manifestations, several detailed reviews have been published. In 1953 Owens and Coffey reported six patients and found a total of 198 cases in previous reports. Of historical interest is the fact that President Garfield in 1881 died from a traumatic aneurysm of the splenic artery 2 months after being shot by an assassin.

INCIDENCE AND PATHOLOGY. A report of unusual interest is that of Bedford and Lodge in 1960 who published findings from 250 consecutive postmortem examinations in older patients. Routine dissection of the splenic artery

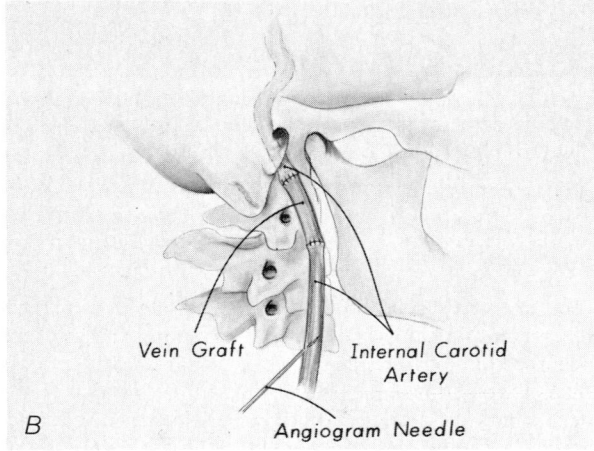

Fig. 21-34. Carotid aneurysmectomy is possible even when the internal carotid artery is involved in its upper extracranial portion, since the artery can be exposed through lateral neck incisions to the base of the skull. *A.* Internal carotid aneurysm. *B.* Replacement with vein graft. (*From G. M. Sanoudos et al., Internal Carotid Aneurysm, Am Surg, 39:118, 1973.*)

found 26 aneurysms, an incidence of nearly 10 percent. All had been asymptomatic. Their size was small, ranging from a few millimeters to as large as 2.5 cm; most were near 1 cm in diameter. In the 204 cases reviewed by Owens and Coffey, the average diameter was 3 cm. This great discrepancy between the high autopsy incidence and the rarity of clinically symptomatic aneurysms indicates that small aneurysms are probably of no clinical significance and are usually overlooked.

These aneurysms, like other atherosclerotic aneurysms, occur in older patients with an average age near fifty. Atherosclerosis is present in the splenic artery in over 95 percent of patients. Surprisingly, though, the aneurysms are more frequent in women, in contrast to the overwhelming predominance of the usual atherosclerotic aneurysm in men. In the Owens and Coffey series, 127 patients were women and 63 were men. Bedford and Lodge noted that the aneurysms tended to develop at bifurcations of the splenic artery and suggested that degeneration of the

media as well as atherosclerosis might be a predisposing factor.

The aneurysms are usually single and in the main trunk of the splenic artery. Rupture is more likely to occur during pregnancy. The actual risk of rupture is uncertain, for many are recognized only after rupture. Rupture is obviously a grave event, for of 131 symptomatic patients reported by Owens and Coffey 94 died from rupture and only 7 from other causes. In 37 female patients, rupture occurred during late pregnancy.

CLINICAL MANIFESTATIONS. Pain in the epigastrium or left flank is the most frequent symptom, occurring in 93 of 131 symptomatic patients in the Owens series. Other symptoms are nonspecific gastrointestinal symptoms, usually interpreted as due to peptic ulcer. These include nausea, vomiting, dyspepsia, and constipation or diarrhea. Gastrointestinal hemorrhage has occurred in about one-third of patients. For unknown reasons gastrointestinal symptoms may exist for months or years before the diagnosis is made. Perhaps this is fortuitous.

In one patient treated by one of the authors several years ago, acute gastrointestinal bleeding led to the erroneous performance of a subtotal gastrectomy a few days earlier, though an ill-defined mass suggesting an aneurysm was noted. When bleeding returned several days later, reoperation was performed. Recovery eventually ensued after a long and difficult convalescence.

Often rupture is the first sign of the aneurysm, in 46 percent of the patients in one series. A "double" rupture is a significant clinical sequence, recognized in about one-half of patients. The first rupture is hemorrhage into the lesser omental sac; this ceases temporarily but is followed in 1 to 2 days by secondary hemorrhage and exsanguination.

With the small size of the splenic aneurysms, physical abnormalities are usually not found. For unknown reasons, moderate splenomegaly has been reported in 40 to 50 percent of patients. However, a mass has been palpated in only 20 percent, and pulsations or a bruit in 10 percent. Roentgenographic identification of a mass with calcium in the walls suggestive of an aneurysm has been reported in 15 percent of the group.

TREATMENT. Obviously symptomatic aneurysms should be excised as soon as the diagnosis is made, usually with concomitant splenectomy. The widespread use of aortography for investigating many abdominal conditions has disclosed aneurysms smaller than 1 cm which are asymptomatic. Their treatment is uncertain because of the rarity of rupture. On the other hand, it is disquieting to note that rupture without preceding symptoms is the first event in one-half of the patients with splenic aneurysms. From data available, surgical treatment does not seem indicated for asymptomatic aneurysms smaller than 1 cm, but those greater than 3 cm should be excised. Further data are needed to be certain of these guidelines.

RENAL ARTERY ANEURYSMS

INCIDENCE AND PATHOLOGY. Aneurysms of the renal artery are similar to aneurysms of the splenic artery in that recognition has greatly increased with the use of vascular angiography. A collective review in 1957 by Garritano found only 180 patients. Nine years later, Cerny et al. found a total of 345 reported cases and described 25 patients from the University of Michigan alone. In discussing this report, Smith described 17 aneurysms at the Henry Ford Hospital, and Morris described operative experience with 58 patients at Baylor Medical Center. The widespread use of renal angiography to investigate patients with hypertension has been chiefly responsible for the increasing recognition of renal aneurysms. Apparently, about 1 percent of hypertensive patients will be found on angiography to have a small aneurysm of one renal artery.

These aneurysms are equally common in males and females, usually in the fifth and sixth decades, but they have been found in all age groups, even in patients as young as nine months. Anatomically they may be saccular or fusiform. Unusual varieties include a false aneurysm from trauma, a dissecting aneurysm, or an arteriovenous fistula. The saccular aneurysm is apparently congenital, arising from a defect in elastic tissue of the wall of the artery, often near a bifurcation. It varies from 1 to 3 cm in size and often develops extensive eccentric calcification, a so-called "signet ring" on the roentgenogram. It is infrequently associated with hypertension and rarely ruptures. The fusiform aneurysm develops distal to an area of constriction of the renal artery and is basically a poststenotic aneurysm similar to that seen in other parts of the arterial circulation. Because of the proximal stenosis, it is frequently seen with hypertension.

The aneurysms occur with equal frequency in either renal artery, usually in the main renal artery or one of its branches. An intrarenal location is uncommon. In one report, 92 aneurysms were in the main renal artery, 44 were in an extrarenal branch, and 15 were intrarenal.

Rupture has been reported in at least 24 patients with

a fatal outcome in 20. Eight of these episodes occurred during pregnancy. Rupture has been recognized only three times in a calcified aneurysm.

CLINICAL MANIFESTATIONS. Abdominal or flank pain has occurred in about 50 percent of the patients but is probably unrelated to the aneurysm. Investigation of the symptom subsequently led to finding the aneurysm. Hematuria, gross or microscopic, has also been reported in 30 to 40 percent of patients. As expected, hypertension has been frequently seen with poststenotic aneurysms and has been improved or cured in over one-half of these after operation. By contrast, hypertension in one series was present in only 7 of 12 with a saccular aneurysm and improved after operation in only 1 of the 7. A mechanism by which a saccular aneurysm can produce hypertension is not clear except for the rather nebulous possibility of compression or distortion of the renal artery. The association may simply be fortuitous.

There are usually no abnormalities on physical examination. Occasionally a localized bruit is audible. Roentgenographic examination may show signet ring calcification which must be differentiated from calcification of mesenteric lymph nodes or calcification of other visceral arteries. The intravenous pyelogram is abnormal in about one-half of the patients because of ischemia, infarction, or localized pressure defects. Aortography is essential to establish the diagnosis and define the precise location (Fig. 21-35). As mentioned earlier, most aneurysms have been found during aortography performed for other purposes.

TREATMENT. Prompt operation is indicated whenever an aneurysm is found during investigation of a patient for hypertension. With poststenotic aneurysms the aneurysm can be excised and the renal artery reconstructed, with an excellent likelihood of improving the hypertension. With a saccular aneurysm and hypertension, operation is probably indicated to reconstruct the renal artery, although the prognosis for improving the hypertension is less favorable. Of the 25 patients reported by Cerny et al., 20 were oper-

Fig. 21-35. Renal artery aneurysms are frequently saccular, as shown in the angiographic study, and may be associated with arterial hypertension.

ated upon. Unfortunately 9 required a nephrectomy, but there was no operative mortality. In the 17 patients reported by Smith, 5 had successful operations, while 12 with small aneurysms of questionable significance had been followed for an average of 3 years without complications. Morris stated that reconstructive operations had been performed on 58 patients with renal artery aneurysms, representing about 5 percent of all reconstructive operations upon the renal artery for patients with hypertension. In this group of 58 patients, 8 had previously lost the contralateral kidney, perhaps from complications of an aneurysm in that kidney. The "bench" technique, in which the kidney is removed from its bed by transecting the main arteries and veins and leaving the ureter intact, performing microsurgical arterial repair on branch arteries, and then reattaching the main vessels to the iliac vessels, has permitted removal of branch artery aneurysms without sacrifice of kidneys. In a patient with a small calcified aneurysm without symptoms or hypertension, there probably is little indication for operation, for the risk of rupture is almost negligible. With larger aneurysms, certainly with symptoms present, operation should be performed.

Traumatic Aneurysms

Several milestones in vascular surgery evolved from treatment of traumatic aneurysms produced in military combat. In the second century Antyllus treated an arterial aneurysm by ligature immediately above and below the lesion, followed by incision of the aneurysm, evacuation of the clot, and exteriorization of the cavity. John Hunter, in 1786, electively ligated a femoral artery proximal to a popliteal aneurysm to minimize blood loss during subsequent attempts at extirpation. The anatomic term *Hunter's canal,* referring to the distal third of the superficial femoral artery in the thigh, originated from this surgical episode. In 1888 Rudolf Matas described his operation of endo-aneurysmorraphy, in which the aneurysm was widely opened and the communications into the artery were sutured. This imaginative approach promptly became the standard treatment and was modified little during the next 55 years; even during World War II it was the operation performed for most traumatic aneurysms. Subsequently, as techniques of vascular reconstruction developed, the policy of restoring arterial continuity became preferred.

ETIOLOGY AND PATHOLOGY. A traumatic aneurysm is produced from a tangential laceration of the wall of an artery. Usually continuity of flow through the lacerated artery is maintained. By contrast, injuries that transect an artery often require immediate treatment because of hemorrhage or ischemia in the affected limb and consequently seldom evolve into an aneurysm.

Following the laceration, blood extravasates into adjacent soft tissues to form a hematoma that compresses and seals the point of injury. If the artery is confined within a small space surrounded by fascia, the hematoma may be small enough to escape recognition. Both the patient and the physician are unaware that an arterial injury has occurred. After days or weeks, the blood clot gradually liquefies; then the firm, immobile mass surrounding the

artery begins to pulsate. A descriptive term for these lesions was "pulsating hematoma." With the appearance of pulsation, the aneurysm begins to enlarge. This is ominous, for enlargement is progressive and relentless, destroying nerves, even eroding bone, and eventually terminating in rupture and death.

Traumatic aneurysms are often termed *false* aneurysms, as distinguished from *true* aneurysms, for the wall is composed of fibrous tissue rather than components of normal arterial wall, as with arteriosclerotic or syphilitic aneurysms.

As the hematoma enlarges in a recent wound, the tissues are firm, tender, perhaps warm. These findings of redness, tenderness, and heat are, of course, the usual characteristics of an abscess. Occasional vivid reports appear in the surgical literature in which an unsuspecting physician widely incised such a red, tender mass to drain an abscess, with resultant violent hemorrhage.

A similar therapeutic catastrophe occasionally occurs when a traumatic aneurysm stabilizes for years and is subsequently confused with a neoplasm. If the previous history of trauma is not available, the differential diagnosis is difficult, for the aneurysm is partly filled with clot and closely resembles a solid tumor. Attempted biopsy of such lesions, with frightening consequences, has been reported.

Usually there is no disability from a traumatic aneurysm except for the local mass until it enlarges to compress adjacent nerves, causing pain, paresthesias, and eventually paralysis. The peripheral arterial circulation is usually normal. Peripheral embolization of thrombi from the aneurysm is unusual except for the rare aneurysm of the subclavian artery following trauma. Here, intermittent compression by the clavicle may dislodge emboli. One of the authors treated such a patient in whom ischemic symptoms in the arm dominated the clinical picture. Arteriography disclosed a small traumatic aneurysm of the subclavian artery which had developed following an automobile accident some months before.

CLINICAL MANIFESTATIONS. A localized mass is often the only finding. As it enlarges, there is pain or paralysis from compression of nerves. On physical examination the borders of the mass are ill defined because the hematoma surrounding the aneurysm is beneath the deep fascia. Pulsations may or may not be present, depending upon the amount of thrombus in the lumen. A systolic bruit is frequently audible. Peripheral pulsations are normal.

If the mass pulsates, the diagnosis is reasonably certain from the physical findings. Otherwise arteriography is required to differentiate it from a neoplasm or a cyst. On arteriography the full size is not disclosed, as much of the cavity is filled with thrombus.

TREATMENT. Operation should be performed as soon as the diagnosis has been established because of the inevitable outcome of enlargement and rupture. If neurologic symptoms are present, operation should be done urgently, within hours, to prevent irreversible pressure injury of crucial nerves. At operation the incision should be placed to permit exposure of the uninvolved artery proximal and distal to the aneurysm. With these vessels temporarily occluded, the aneurysm can be widely incised, clots evacuated, and the point of origin from the artery identified. Dissection around the aneurysm before it is opened should be avoided; it is unnecessary, complicated, and often dangerous.

With unusually large aneurysms, it is important to remember that there is only one small opening in the wall of the aneurysm, the tangential laceration of the arterial wall from which the aneurysm began. Hence, if the aneurysm is inadvertently entered, this small opening can be digitally occluded to control bleeding while further exposure is obtained. This approach was once employed in desperation during emergency treatment of a badly neglected traumatic aneurysm of the proximal subclavian artery which had involved the brachial plexus and compressed the trachea to a near fatal degree.

Once the aneurysm has been opened and the inner contents removed, the site of communication with the parent artery can be mobilized and the injured area excised. Complete excision of the wall of the aneurysm is unnecessary and should be avoided because of the surrounding dense fibrotic reaction. Once the involved artery has been mobilized, arterial continuity can usually be restored by end-to-end anastomosis or by insertion of a short graft, preferably autologous vein. Ligation should be performed only for small arteries, such as the radial, not essential to normal circulation.

PROGNOSIS. Convalescence after operation is usually uneventful and long-term results excellent. Crawford et al. described experiences with a group of 29 patients with aneurysms or arteriovenous fistulas, all of whom were treated by excision and end-to-end anastomosis with a uniformly good result. Hughes and Jahnke similarly reported continuing good results 5 years after surgical treatment of 67 traumatic aneurysms during the Korean conflict.

VASOSPASTIC DISORDERS

Raynaud's Disease

A syndrome of intermittent vasospasm in the upper extremities without permanent vascular obstruction was described by Maurice Raynaud in 1862. The initial description included several disorders which subsequent observation found were not primary Raynaud's disease, but attention was focused on the disorder by this report. The syndrome described by Raynaud, now termed *Raynaud's phenomenon,* consists of recurrent episodes of vasoconstriction in the upper extremities, initiated by exposure to cold or emotional stress. Three sequential phases classically occur: pallor, cyanosis, and rubor. It is now recognized that Raynaud's phenomenon may exist as a primary disorder, termed *Raynaud's disease,* or may be a secondary manifestation of a more serious vascular disease, often not evident for 1 or 2 years after the initial appearance of the recurrent color changes. The more common disorders associated with Raynaud's phenomenon include Buerger's disease (thromboangiitis obliterans), scleroderma, cervical rib or other thoracic outlet syndrome, and atherosclerosis.

It occasionally results from recurrent minor trauma, such as the use of mechanical vibrating tools. Rarely, other collagen diseases, such as periarteritis nodosa or disseminated lupus erythematosus are found. Hence, in the evaluation of a patient the critical decision is to determine whether the disease is primary Raynaud's disease or a secondary manifestation of a more serious disorder. Some suspect that it is always secondary to some other underlying disorder.

ETIOLOGY. The cause of primary Raynaud's disease is unknown. It is much more frequent in women, with a ratio of about 5:1, and appears in over 90 percent of patients before forty years of age. In men, it is usually much less severe in intensity. DeTakats and Fowler observed abnormal electroencephalograms in some patients, suggesting a primary disease in the midbrain, but the existence of a primary neurologic disease has not been established.

PATHOLOGY. The clinical picture of Raynaud's phenomenon is related to the anatomy and physiology of the arteriolar circulation in the dermis. The arterioles penetrate the dermis at right angles with an irregular reticulate pattern and arborize into a capillary network. Some fluctuation in vasomotor tone, as with pallor or blushing, is a normal physiologic variation. In Raynaud's disease, vasospasm occurs with such severity that dermal circulation momentarily ceases, with the production of severe pallor. If the vasospasm is less severe, with slowing but not cessation of the dermal circulation, cyanosis appears, a result of sluggish flow of blood with an increase in the percentage of reduced hemoglobin in the capillaries. When the vasospasm subsides, a reactive hyperemia with vasodilatation develops, probably from the accumulation of tissue metabolites during the anoxic period, producing an unusual redness or rubor.

The basis for the increased tendency of the dermal arterioles to vasoconstriction is unknown. It may be a sensitivity in the arterioles themselves, or possibly may result from hyperactivity of the sympathetic nervous system. Initially the arterioles are normal on histologic examination. With chronic disease, there is progressive hypertrophy of the arteriolar walls and ultimate occlusion. Detailed histologic observation of early phases of Raynaud's disease are not available, because tissue biopsies are seldom performed at this time.

In the majority of patients the episodes of vasoconstriction are precipitated by exposure to cold. In about 25 percent of patients intense emotion, as well as cold, may be the initiating factor. Only rarely is emotion alone the significant stimulus without an abnormal sensitivity to cold.

In most patients the upper extremities are symmetrically involved. Unilateral involvement by Raynaud's phenomenon almost always denotes a proximal mechanical cause, either occlusion of one of the major proximal arteries, recurrent embolization, or neurovascular compression. In 10 to 15 percent of patients the legs are involved as well as the arms. This was found in 51 of 474 patients seen over a period of years at the Mayo Clinic.

With repeated episodes of vasoconstriction and ischemia, trophic changes gradually appear. These include atrophy of the skin with loss of elasticity and hair. The term *sclerodactylia* has been applied to this appearance, since it resembles the changes found in scleroderma in other organs. However, long-term studies by Gifford et al. have demonstrated conclusively that the presence of sclerodactylia in the fingers does not indicate that generalized scleroderma will appear in the future. Focal areas of ulceration develop and leave characteristic scars with healing. Recurrent superficial infections, such as paronychia, may occur. In the more extreme forms of ischemia, gangrene may require amputation of one or more digits, but fortunately gangrene almost never progresses to involve the hands.

CLINICAL MANIFESTATIONS. The patient is usually a young woman who has noted that episodes of cold precipitate vasoconstriction with a repetitive sequence of pallor, cyanosis, and rubor. Several variations in the color phenomena may occur with less severe disease. For example, there may be only cyanosis followed by rubor or only episodes of mild cyanosis.

In addition to the color changes, the patient may have paresthesias and localized pain in the digits. If infection or ulceration is present, pain is more severe. Except for the discomfort in the hands, the patients usually have no other symptoms.

Physical Examination. In the early phases of the disease, the extremities may be entirely normal with peripheral pulses of equal volume. The best index to the severity of the disease is the extent of trophic changes in the fingers, such as atrophy of the skin and nails with loss of hair over the terminal phalanges. In more advanced disease, signs of chronic ischemia are obvious, with punctate scars from healed ulcerations, chronic rubor, and absence of a radial or ulnar pulse.

Arteriography is of value in establishing the diagnosis by revealing the absence of occlusive arterial disease. The most critical examination is demonstration of the vasoconstrictor response to cold. Induction of the characteristic pallor-cyanosis-rubor sequence in both hands following exposure to cold establishes the diagnosis, although it does not differentiate between primary and secondary Raynaud's phenomenon. An electroencephalogram should be obtained to pursue the observation made by DeTakats that abnormal electroencephalographic tracings are present in some patients.

Once the presence of Raynaud's phenomenon has been confirmed, the principal question is whether the vasomotor changes are primary or secondary to some other vascular disease. The possibility of early scleroderma can be evaluated by study of the motility of the esophagus and small bowel. Other blood tests to screen for collagen disorders, such as lupus, should be done. The presence of cervical ribs can be easily determined by roentgenograms of the cervical spine and thorax. Other compression syndromes of the subclavian artery can be detected by performing the maneuvers described under Thoracic Outlet Syndromes. Complete angiographic studies to opacify the arterial circulation from the aortic arch to the small arteries of the hand should be done to exclude the possibility of proximal atherosclerotic plaques producing distal emboli. Occasionally skin and lymph node biopsies are useful.

An important principle in diagnosis is continued observation of the patient over a period of several years. Even after a thorough examination has failed to detect any underlying vascular disease, such a disease may appear in the next 2 to 3 years. In the Mayo Clinic series the diagnosis of Raynaud's disease is simply considered a tentative one for as long as 2 years.

TREATMENT. In the majority of patients the disability is mild. Avoiding cold or other stimuli which precipitate vasoconstriction is adequate. Moving to a warm climate may be considered, but this does not eliminate the attacks. Tobacco certainly should be avoided because of its potent vasoconstrictor action, but this alone does not abolish the syndrome. Various vasodilator drugs have been repeatedly tried, but none have been of consistent benefit. The most recent medications are orally administered methyldopa, employed for patients with ulceration of the fingers and severe pain, and intraarterially administered reserpine. Significant long-term data are not yet available, but one of the authors has used this therapy in some patients, with occasional dramatic and prolonged relief. Therapy for several weeks is required in increasing doses to be effective.

The most effective therapy is cervicodorsal sympathectomy. This is accomplished by removing the first, second, and third thoracic ganglia, preserving the cervical portion of the stellate ganglion to avoid a Horner's syndrome.

The immediate results after sympathectomy in patients with severe vasospasm is quite encouraging, but relapses are common. For this reason, sympathectomy is usually employed only when symptoms are severe and other therapy ineffective. In Gifford's series of 474 patients, only 77 were operated upon; about one-half of these had excellent to good results. DeTakats and Fowler tabulated reports from different groups, including 40 cases of their own, and found an average of 55 percent good results in 424 sympathectomies performed. More radical sympathectomies have not given any better results. Proximally all of the stellate ganglion has been removed, producing Horner's syndrome; distad the fourth thoracic ganglion has been included. Another technical modification has been to include the second and third intercostal nerves with the third ganglion because of the demonstration by Skoog that 10 to 15 percent of sympathetic ganglia to the upper extremity are contained in these two intercostal ganglia. Also there has been considerable discussion about differences in preganglionic and postganglionic sympathectomy. None of these variations have been found significant, however, and the conservative sympathectomy involving the first, second, and third thoracic ganglia is usually performed. Severe trophic changes before operation are unfortunately often associated with a poor result. Patients with scleroderma also obtain little benefit.

Operative Technique. At least four different surgical techniques have been employed at different times for sympathectomy. Originally most were done through a posterior approach, with the patient in a prone position and an incision similar to that for a thoracoplasty. The sympathetic chain was exposed by resecting a short segment of the second or third rib, followed by an extrapleural dissection to isolate the sympathetic chain. In large muscular individuals this approach is quite difficult and provides only limited exposure. It has been virtually abandoned.

A second technique, a supraclavicular approach, provides excellent exposure in patients of small stature with long thin necks. However, in those with short, thick necks, significant trauma to the brachial plexus, resulting in a painful neuritis, may complicate the postoperative course. An excellent description of the technique was published by Nanson.

Ideal exposure can be obtained by an anterior transthoracic incision, opening the hemithorax in the third or fourth intercostal space. This, of necessity, involves a major thoracotomy, though a simple one. It has been favored by Palumbo, who also emphasized that removal of the lower one-third of the stellate ganglion would adequately sympathectomize the extremity without producing a Horner's syndrome.

In recent years the transaxillary approach has become preferred. This is done through a short incision in the axilla, followed by resection of a short segment of the second or third rib and exposure of the sympathetic chain. Good technical descriptions have been published by Roos and by Kirtley et al. The thoracotomy is of much less magnitude than that through the anterior approach, and the incision is in an inconspicuous location.

PROGNOSIS. The prognosis in most patients with primary Raynaud's disease is good with the exception of the discomfort associated with the abnormal sensitivity to cold. Even in the more advanced forms, tissue loss seldom exceeds the loss of one or more digits. More serious systemic vascular disease does not develop, and although symptoms may continue for many years, there is no known impairment of longevity or health.

Uncommon Vasomotor Diseases

Rare, unusual vasomotor diseases include livedo reticularis and acrocyanosis, which primarily result from vasoconstriction, and erythromelalgia, apparently a result of vasodilatation. The disability with these disorders is usually episodic and mild. Their clinical significance is primarily in differentiating them from more serious underlying disease, such as Buerger's disease, scleroderma, or disseminated lupus erythematosus. Only salient clinical features of these bizarre diseases will be presented here.

LIVEDO RETICULARIS

This unusual vasomotor condition is characterized by a persistent mottled reddish blue discoloration of the skin of the extremities. It is more prominent in the legs and feet than in the hands or arms and only infrequently involves the trunk. Although the severity varies with temperature, becoming worse on exposure to cold it never entirely disappears spontaneously.

ETIOLOGY AND PATHOLOGY. The cause is unknown, although miscellaneous associated vascular diseases such as hypertension or emotional disorders have been found in different patients.

The pathophysiologic feature apparently is a stenosis of the arterioles which pierce the cutis at right angles and arborize into the peripheral capillaries of the skin. The obstruction of the arterioles, either spastic or organic, therefore affects the peripheral capillary arborizations and accounts for the peculiar reticular nature of the discoloration.

The pathologic change in the arterioles varies from no visible abnormality to proliferation of the intima, in some patients progressing to complete occlusion. With severe organic obstruction, focal ulceration of the skin, usually over the lower legs, may occur.

CLINICAL MANIFESTATIONS. Patients with livedo reticularis complain of the persistent reddish blue mottling over the legs and feet, varying somewhat with temperature. Often the cosmetic appearance is the only concern of the patient. In some there are localized symptoms of coldness, numbness, dull aching, and paresthesias. With severe forms and localized tissue ischemia, there may be pain from local ulceration. These symptoms are more prone to appear during the winter in association with cold temperatures.

The diagnosis is usually made from physical examination, with observation of the persistent blotchy discoloration, and a history of prolonged persistence in association with some variation with environmental temperature. Peripheral pulsations are normal, and trophic changes are not present in the digits. Only with more extreme forms are ischemic ulcers present over the lower legs. These usually heal after a short period of time.

TREATMENT. In most patients no treatment is necessary except reassurance regarding the benign nature of the condition. Only one patient is described in the Mayo Clinic series in whom gangrene developed in the legs. Avoiding extremes of cold is beneficial in some patients. Vasodilating agents may be tried, but none has been found of consistent benefit. Sympathectomy should be employed if the disability is severe enough to produce local ulceration. After sympathectomy the discoloration may decrease in extent and remain pink rather than blue. In most patients the disorder is a permanent one, remaining as a moderate cosmetic disturbance, but fortunately with no other disability.

ACROCYANOSIS

Acrocyanosis is a disorder characterized by persistent but painless cold and cyanosis of the hands and feet. The cause and the pathologic and pathophysiologic features are virtually unknown, for the disease consists primarily of persistent color changes. Usually it is confused with Raynaud's syndrome because of the prominent localized cyanosis. Detailed investigation of the pathophysiologic features by Lewis and Landis concluded that the fundamental disorder was a localized abnormality in vasomotor tone in the circulation of the hands and feet. Apparently the basic physiologic condition is a slow rate of blood flow through the skin, the result of chronic arteriolar constriction, which results in a high percentage of reduced hemoglobin in the blood in the capillaries and production of the cyanotic color. Endocrine dysfunction has been found in some patients, but no consistent pattern has been established.

Usually the disorder is found in a young woman who has noted persistent coldness and blueness of the fingers and hands for many years, often with symptoms of less severity in the toes and feet. The abnormalities are more prominent in cold weather, but the extremities are never completely normal. With heat the color may change from deep purple to red, but there are no episodes of blanching, such as occurs with Raynaud's disorder. The peripheral pulses are normal, and there are no trophic changes indicative of chronic tissue ischemia, such as atrophy of the skin, sclerosis, or ulceration.

The principal differential diagnosis is from Raynaud's disease because of the prominent color changes in both disorders. The absence of pallor, as well as the absence of signs of chronic ischemia, are the most useful features. Similarly, the constant presence of the color changes in acrocyanosis, as opposed to the intermittent episodic occurrence in Raynaud's disease, is characteristic.

Usually reassurance is the only treatment needed, with the avoidance of cold temperatures when possible. Sympathectomy can be employed with reasonably good results if the disability is more serious. Prognosis is excellent, with tissue loss virtually never occurring. Usually the color changes remain for many years or permanently.

ERYTHROMELALGIA

This rare disorder is characterized by red, warm, painful extremities. The clinical characteristics were described by S. Weir Mitchell in 1872 and the disorder named by him in 1878. The cause of the primary disease is unknown. Similar phenomena, so-called "secondary erythromelalgia," can occur as a result of hypertension or polycythemia vera.

The basic abnormality is an unusual sensitivity to warmth, for skin temperatures of 32 to 36°C, which produce no effects in normal individuals, will regularly induce the painful burning sensation. The exact temperature at which the distress can be produced varies with different patients but may be a precise one for any individual patient. It was termed by Lewis a "critical point." The increase in temperature is usually a result of vasodilatation with increase in blood flow. The exact basis for the spontaneous vasodilatation with the rise in temperature and the burning sensation is not known.

The disease is equally prevalent in men and women, usually of middle age. The distress may be greater in the summer months, but only a general relationship to extremes of heat or cold may be present. The patient soon learns that exposing the extremities to cold, such as by immersing them in ice water, may abort an attack.

Physical examination usually reveals no abnormalities of the peripheral arteries. The diagnosis is usually established by demonstration of a close relationship between the symptoms and skin temperature. This may be induced by direct application of heat, noting the skin temperature at which distress appears. Erythromelalgia should be differentiated from the painful red but cold extremities which occur with Buerger's disease and also with peripheral neuritis.

Aside from the troublesome symptoms, the disorder is a benign one. Avoiding extremes of heat is one of the most useful therapeutic measures. Acetylsalicylic acid, 0.65 Gm, has been found beneficial in many patients, although the mode of action is uncertain. A trial of therapy with vasoconstrictor drugs, such as ephedrine, should be employed, but consistent value from one drug has not been found. The disorder is usually a permanent one, but no permanent disability results.

FROSTBITE

Several forms of cold injury have been described, usually varying with the environmental conditions under which exposure occurs. These different syndromes include acute pernio (chilblains), chronic pernio, trench foot, immersion foot, and frostbite. Acute and chronic pernio are focal injuries of the skin and subcutaneous tissue resulting from exposure to cold of moderate intensity, representing an increased susceptibility to cold injury in a particular individual. The disorder is seldom a surgical problem, because the lesions are focal, superficial ones which heal readily. Trench foot and immersion foot are primarily military injuries produced by prolonged exposure to cold in damp surroundings, often with temperatures well above freezing, but in circumstances where there is an element of prolonged immobility. Immersion foot is probably simply the seagoing counterpart of trench foot. Such injuries are rarely seen in civilian practice. For practical purposes frostbite is the type of injury usually encountered and will be discussed in detail. The tissue response in the other disorders mentioned, however, is a similar type of response to cold, modified somewhat with the environmental conditions.

ETIOLOGY. Frostbite results when tissues are exposed to cold for varying periods of time. The severity varies both with the temperature and the duration of exposure. Experimentally, it has been demonstrated that freezing begins in mammalian tissues when the temperature in the deeper parts reaches 10°C and that −5°C is the lowest temperature to which cells may be slowly frozen and still survive. Frostbite injury usually results from exposure over a period of several hours. In the Korean conflict, 90 percent of the cases occurred at temperatures near −7°C after exposure for 7 to 18 hours. A different form of frostbite is produced by acute exposures to below zero temperatures, commonly occurring in airplanes at high altitudes and hence termed "high altitude" frostbite. In such injuries the exposed part is acutely frozen with deposition of ice crystals in the tissues. This unusual form of injury is different from the usual case of frostbite, where a "slow freeze" results.

Several factors influence the injurious effect of cold. Two of the most significant ones are humidity and the presence of wind, both of which accelerate the withdrawal of heat from body tissues. Immobility or occlusive vascular disease also are significant factors, both influencing the rate of peripheral blood flow. Acclimatization has been demonstrated in some persons repeatedly exposed to cold, such as those who live in northern latitudes, and probably is a localized vasomotor adaptation. By contrast, extremities previously injured by cold may remain permanently susceptible to future cold injury, perhaps from an intensified vasoconstrictor response.

PATHOLOGY. The degrees of severity of a frostbite injury have been conventionally grouped into four clinical types: a first-degree injury consists of edema and redness of the affected part without necrosis; formation of blisters represents a second-degree injury; necrosis of the skin constitutes a third-degree injury; in a fourth-degree injury gangrene of the extremity develops, requiring amputation.

As frostbite occurs, the injured tissue becomes numb and moderately stiff without extensive discomfort. Often the patient is unaware that frostbite is occurring. With subsequent rewarming the tissues become reddened, hot, and edematous. At this time blisters erupt and gangrene gradually appears in the more seriously injured tissues. Edema increases to a maximum within 24 to 48 hours and then gradually is resorbed as gangrenous tissue begins to demarcate. The extent of gangrene is difficult to estimate initially and requires observations for as long as 30 days or more. Fortunately the degree of gangrene is often much less than that initially feared, because the skin may be gangrenous but the underlying tissue viable. For this reason amputation is delayed until the extent of gangrene is definitely known.

Following recovery of the extremity, there is frequently a permanent increase in vasoconstrictor tone resulting in hyperhidrosis, and an abnormal sensitivity to cold. Pain and paresthesias are also common, perhaps as residuals from ischemic neuritis.

It is uncertain whether the fundamental injury from cold results from direct freezing with disruption of cell membranes or whether the injury is primarily an ischemic necrosis from widespread thrombosis of arterioles and capillaries. Certainly vascular occlusion is a prominent feature, whether it is a primary or a secondary event. With exposure to cold, there is severe vasoconstriction, decreasing the rate of blood flow in the chilled extremity, with resulting stasis, sludging of blood, and eventual widespread thrombosis. In clinical experiments, immersion of the arm for 2 hours in water at 13°C decreases blood flow to about 3 percent of normal, while immersion of a finger in water at 7°C stops blood flow altogether. In addition to sludging and capillary thrombosis, there is an increase in capillary permeability, resulting in the formation of edema when blood flow is increased after rewarming.

On histologic examination of the injured tissues, edema, infiltration of inflammatory cells, and deposition of fibrin are prominent findings. Widespread thrombosis of small vessels is frequently seen. In addition focal areas of necrosis may be evident in skin, muscle, and other tissues.

CLINICAL MANIFESTATIONS. Frequently, the patient is unaware that frostbite is occurring. The usual injury occurs with exposure to near freezing temperatures for several hours, often combined with wind, high humidity, damp or wet shoes, or immobility from tightly constricting shoes or confinement in a cramped position. All these factors influence the rate of heat transfer between the extremity and the environment. Initially there may be mild discomfort, but as the extremity becomes numb and somewhat stiff, frequently discomfort is minimal.

When rewarmed, the extremity quickly becomes red, edematous, hot, and painful. This is due to vasodilatation and widespread extravasation of fluid through the walls of capillaries whose permeability has been increased from injury. Edema reaches its peak intensity within 48 hours and then gradually subsides over several days. As described under Pathology, gangrene gradually becomes evident and slowly demarcates over a period of many days. An ominous sign, indicating that gangrene will develop, is the persistence of coldness and numbness in an area while surrounding tissues become edematous, hot, and painful. The persistent coldness and numbness indicate cessation of all circulation with the certain outcome of ischemic necrosis.

Following recovery from frostbite, a high percentage of extremities remain with an increased vasoconstrictor tone, manifested by increased susceptibility to cold, hyperhidrosis, paresthesias, and localized pain.

TREATMENT. Frostbite seldom occurs during exposure to cold if proper precautions are taken. This includes the wearing of dry, insulated, loosely fitting clothing and carefully avoiding long periods of immobility of the exposed extremities. Most cases of clinical frostbite occur in circumstances where exposure to cold inadvertently occurs for long periods of time because of coma from injury, alcohol, or other factors.

Rapid warming of the injured tissue is the most important aspect of treatment. Several studies have clearly demonstrated the advantages of the rapid-rewarming method over any other. The frozen tissue should be placed in warm water, with a temperature in the range of 40 to 44°C. Complete rewarming usually requires about 20 minutes. Higher temperatures are more injurious than beneficial. A frostbitten part should never be exposed to hot water, an open fire, or excessive dry heat, as in an oven, for the loss of sensitivity in the frozen area makes it especially vulnerable to injury. Warming in water is much more rapid than application of warm blankets, which require three or four times as long as the immersion method.

Following rewarming, the injured extremity should be elevated to minimize formation of edema and carefully protected in a sterile environment. Usually it is left exposed but surrounded by a protective cradle. Blisters are opened only when necessary to remove necrotic skin. Antibiotic therapy and tetanus antiserum are routinely given to lessen the risk of infection. Demarcation of gangrenous areas should be carefully observed, often for several weeks, before amputation is performed. Often a gangrenous area which initially appears to involve the foot will gradually regress with the separation of superficial areas of gangrenous skin, ultimately with the loss of one or more digits but preservation of the foot.

Dramatic reversal of the vasospasm has been achieved by the use of intraarterial reserpine, the effects being monitored angiographically. Angiography of the frostbite patient can define the extent of organic vascular stenosis and the degree of functional vasospasm, thus aiding the choice of therapy. The use of other fast-acting vasodilators such as papaverine might also be appropriate.

The role of sympathectomy has been studied by Shumacker and Kilman and by Golding et al. Both experimental and clinical experiences indicate a beneficial effect from sympathectomy, especially when employed in the first few days after frostbite has occurred. Shumacker and Kilman reported 66 sympathectomies in 38 patients, 24 of which were performed soon after injury. Their experience indicated that sympathectomy should be performed for injuries severe enough to produce necrosis of tissue, both to minimize the extent of necrosis and to prevent the usual late vasomotor sequelae. Golding et al. found in experimental and clinical studies (68 patients) that the proper time for sympathectomy was between 36 and 72 hours after injury. Earlier sympathectomies accelerated the rate of edema formation, while sympathectomies performed following the peak intensity of edema seemed to hasten absorption of edema and minimize eventual tissue necrosis. Sympathectomy is also beneficial in alleviating the late sequelae from cold injury, i.e., paresthesias, coldness, and hyperhidrosis.

If vascular injury is the primary event, therapeutic measures to decrease vasoconstriction or blood clotting, such as sympathectomy or the administration of heparin, should be of routine benefit. The theoretic benefit from sympathectomy is the release of vasospasm, which may precipitate thrombosis in injured capillaries and arterioles. Heparin and dextran have also been given in attempts to lessen the degree of small vessel thrombosis which is such a prominent feature on histologic examination of the injured tissues. Although theoretically plausible, consistent benefit has not been demonstrated from the routine use of either heparin or dextran.

PROGNOSIS. Following recovery from injury, all studies have found a significant percentage of residual disability in the extremity. Simeone evaluated 1,061 limbs 4 months after frostbite while the patients were still in the hospital and found painful feet and hyperhidrosis the most common complaints. Ervasti described similar sequelae in 812 cases of frostbite 5 to 18 years after injury. Orr and Fainer reported that gangrene occurred in only 6 percent of 1,880 cases from the Korean conflict, but some disability remained in 10 to 20 percent of patients.

References

Occlusive Disease: General

Barker, W. F.: Peripheral Vascular Disease in Diabetes: Diagnosis and Management, *Med Clin North Am,* **55**(4):1045, 1971.

Baumann, F. G., Imparato, A. M., and Kim, G. E.: The Evolution of Early Fibromuscular Lesions Hemodynamically Induced in the Dog Renal Artery: 1. Light and Transmission Electron Microscopy, *Circ Res,* **39**:809, 1976.

Beebe, H. G., Clark, W. F., and DeWeese, J. A.: Atherosclerotic Change Occurring in an Autogenous Venous Arterial Graft, *Arch Surg,* **101**:85, 1970.

Berardi, R. S., and Siroospour, D.: Lumbar Sympathectomy in the Treatment of Peripheral Vascular Occlusive Disease: Ten Year Study, *Am J Surg,* **130**:309, 1975.

Boyd, A. M.: The Natural Course of Arteriosclerosis of the Lower Extremities, *Angiology,* **11**:10, 1960.

Brewster, D. C., Retana, A., Waltman, A. C., and Darling, C.: Angiography in the Management of Aneurysms of the Abdominal Aorta: Its Value and Safety, *N Engl J Med,* **292**(16):822, 1975.

Cohen, S. I., Goldman, L. D., Salzman, E. W., and Glotzer, D. J.: The Deleterious Effect of Immediate Postoperative Prosthesis in Below-Knee Amputation for Ischemic Disease, *Surgery,* **76**(6):992, 1974.

Dale, W. A.: The Beginnings of Vascular Surgery, *Surgery,* **76**(6):849, 1974.

Friedman, S. A., Freiberg, P., and Colton, J.: Vasomotor Tone in Diabetic Neuropathy, *Ann Intern Med,* **77**:353, 1972.

Goldenfarb, P. B., Cathey, M. H., and Cooper, G. R.: The Determination of ADP Induced Platelet Aggregation in Normal Men, *Atherosclerosis,* **12**:335, 1970.

Greenhalgh, R. M., Rosengarten, D. S., and Mervart, I.: Serum Lipids and Lipo Proteins in Peripheral Vascular Disease, *Lancet,* **2**:947, 1971.

Hamaker, W. R., Doyle, W. F., O'Connel, T. J., Jr., and Gomez, A. C.: Subintimal Obliterative Proliferation in Saphenous Vein Grafts. A Cause of Early Failure of Aorta to Coronary Artery By-pass Grafts, *Ann Thorac Surg,* **13**:488, 1972.

Hardy, J. D., Conn, J. H., and Fain, W. R.: Nonatherosclerotic Occlusive Lesions of Small Arteries, *Surgery,* **57**(1):1, 1965.

Hill, G. L.: A Rational Basis for Management of Patients with the Buerger Syndrome, *Br J Surg,* **61**:476, 1974.

Honour, A. J., Pickering, G. W., and Sheppard, B. L.: Ultrastructure and Behavior of Platelet Thrombi in Injured Arteries, *Br J Exp Pathol,* **52**:482, 1971.

Imparato, A. M., Baumann, F. G., Pearson, J., Kim, G. E., Davidson, T., and Ibrahim, I.: Electron Microscopic Studies of Experimentally Produced Fibromuscular Arterial Lesions, *Surg Gynecol Obstet,* **68**:683, 1976.

———, Bracco, A., Hammond, R., Kaufman, B., Kim, G. E., Migrassi, P., Pearson, W., Baumann, G., and Nathan, I.: The Effect of Intimal and Neo-Intimal Fibromuscular Fibroplasia on Arterial Reconstructions, *J Cardiovasc Surg., (Torino),* Special Issue, **488**, 1975.

———, Kim, G. E., Davidson, T., and Crowley, J. G.: Intermittent Claudication: Its Natural Course, *Surgery,* **78**(6):795, 1975.

Jamieson, C. W., and Hill, D.: Amputation for Vascular Disease, *Br J Surg,* **63**:683, 1976.

Karayannacos, P. E., Yahson, D., and Vasko, J. S.: Narrow Lumbar Spinal Canal with Vascular Syndromes, *Arch Surg,* **111**:803, 1976.

Kelly, J. P., and James, J. M.: Criteria for Determining the Proper Level of Amputation in Occlusive Vascular Disease: A Review of 323 Amputations, *J Bone Joint Surg [AM],* **39A**:883, 1957.

Kim, G. E., Ibrahim, I. M., and Imparato, A. M.: Lumbar Sympathectomy in End Stage Arterial Occlusive Disease, *Ann Surg,* **183**(2):157, 1976.

————, Imparato, A. M., Chu, D. S., and David, S. W.: Lower Limb Amputation for Occlusive Vascular Disease, *Am Surg,* **42:**598, 1976.

Lassen, N. A., and Holstein, P.: Use of Radioisotopes in Assessment of Distal Blood Flow and Distal Blood Pressure in Arterial Insufficiency, *Surg Clin North Am,* **54**(1):39, 1974.

Otteman, M. E., and Stahlgren, L. H.: Evaluation of Factors Which Influence Mortality and Morbidity following Major Lower Extremity Amputations for Arteriosclerosis, *Surg Gynecol Obstet,* **120:**1217, 1965.

Raskin, N. H., Levinson, S. A., Hoffman, P. M., Pickett, J. B., and Fields, H. L.: Postsympathectomy Neuralgia: Amelioration with Diphenylhydantoin and Carbamazepine, *Am J Surg,* **128:**75, 1974.

Rich, N. M., Hobson, R. W., and Fedde, W.: Vascular Trauma Secondary to Diagnostic and Therapeutic Procedures, *Am J Surg,* **128:**715, 1974.

Robinson, K.: Long-Posterior-Flap Myoplastic Below-Knee Amputation in Ischemic Disease, *Lancet,* **1:**183, 1972.

Salzman, E. W.: The Limitations of Heparin Therapy after Arterial Reconstructions, *Surgery,* **57:**131, 1965.

Schatz, I. J.: Classification of Primary Hyperlipidemia, *JAMA,* **210:**701, 1969.

Schnetzer, G. W.: Platelets and Thrombogenesis: Current Concepts, *Am Heart J,* **83:**552, 1972.

Scott, H. W., Jr.: Metabolic Surgery for Hyperlipidemia and Atherosclerosis, *Am J Surg,* **123:**3, 1972.

Sethi, G. K., Scott, S. M., Takaro, T.: Multiple-Plane Angiography for More Precise Evaluation of Aortoiliac Disease, *Surgery,* **78**(2):154, 1975.

Stanley, J. C., Gewertz, B. L., Bove, E. L., Scottiurai, V., and Fry, W. J.: Arterial Fibrodysplasia: Histopathologic Character and Current Etiologic Concepts, *Arch Surg,* **110:**561, 1975.

Strandness, D. E.: Evaluation of the Patient for Vascular Surgery, *Surg Clin North Am,* **54**(1):13, 1974.

Tomatis, L. A., Fierens, E. E., and Verbrugge, G. P.: Evaluation of Surgical Risk in Peripheral Vascular Disease by Coronary Arteriography: A Series of 100 Cases, *Surgery,* **71**(3):429, 1972.

Vlodaver, Z., and Edwards, J. E.: Pathologic Changes in Aortic Coronary Arterial Saphenous Vein Grafts, *Circulation,* **44:**719, 1971.

Wray, C. H., Still, J. M., and Moretz, W. N.: Present Management of Amputations for Peripheral Vascular Disease, *Am Surg,* **38:**87, 1972.

Wright, C. J., and Cousins, M. J.: Blood Flow Distribution in the Human Leg following Epidural Sympathetic Blockade, *Arch Surg,* **105:**334, 1972.

Yao, J. S. T., and Bergan, J. J.: Application of Ultrasound to Arterial and Venous Diagnosis, *Surg Clin North Am,* **54**(1):25, 1974.

Aortoiliac Occlusive Disease

Cohn, L. W., Moore, W. S., and Hall, A. D.: Extra-abdominal Management of Late Aortofemoral Graft Thrombosis, *Surgery,* **67**(5):755, 1970.

Garrett, H. E., Crawford, E. S., Howell, J. F., and DeBakey, M. E.: Surgical Considerations in the Treatment of Aorto-iliac Occlusive Disease, *Surg Clin North Am,* **46:**949, 1966.

Guida, P. M., and Moore, S. W.: Obturator Bypass Techniques, *Surg Gynecol Obstet,* **128:**1307, 1969.

Imparato, A. M., Sanoudos, G., Epstein, H. Y., Abrams, R. M., and Beranbaum, E. R.: Results in 96 Aortoiliac Reconstructive Procedures: Pre Operative Angiographic and Functional Classifications Used as Prognostic Guides, *Surgery,* **68:**610, 1970.

Inihara, T.: Endarterectomy for Occlusive Disease of the Aorto-iliac and Common Femoral Arteries: Evaluation of Results of the Eversion Technique Endarterectomy, *Am J Surg,* **124:**235, 1972.

Kwaan, J. H. M., Molen, R. V., Stemmer, E. A., and Connolly, J. E.: Peripheral Embolism Resulting from Unsuspected Atheromatous Aortic Plaques, *Surgery,* **78**(5):583, 1975.

LoGerfo, F. W., Johnson, W. C., Corson, J. D., Vollman, R. W., Wasel, R. D., Davis, R. C., Nabseth, D. C., and Mannick, J. A.: Comparison of the Late Patency Rates of Axillobilateral Femoral and Axillounilateral Femoral Grafts, *Surgery,* **81:**33, 1977.

Lorentsen, E., Hael, B. L., and Hal, R.: Evaluation of the Functional Importance of Atherosclerotic Obliterations in the Aorto-iliac Artery by Pressure-Flow Measurements, *Acta Med Scand,* **191:**399, 1972.

Mannick, J. A., Williams, L. E., and Nabseth, D. C.: The Late Results of Axillofemoral Grafts, *Surgery,* **68**(6):1038, 1970.

May, A. G., Van de Berg, L., DeWeese, J. A., and Rob, C. G.: Critical Arterial Stenosis, *Surgery,* **54:**250, 1963.

Szilagyi, D. E., Smith, R. F., Elliott, J. P., and Varndecic, M. P.: Infection in Arterial Reconstruction with Synthetic Grafts, *Ann Surg,* **176**(3):321, 1972.

————, Smith, R. F., Elmquist, J. G., Gonzalez, A., and Elliott, J. P.: Angioplasty in the Treatment of Peripheral Occlusive Arteriopathy: A Summary of 12 Years' Experience, *Arch Surg,* **90:**617, 1965.

Femoropopliteal Occlusive Disease

Allan, J. S., and Taylor, G. W.: The Relationship between Blood Flow and Failure of Femoropopliteal Reconstructive Arterial Surgery, *Br J Surg,* **59:**549, 1972.

Brief, D. K., Brener, B. J., Alpert, J., and Parsonnet, V.: Crossover Femoropopliteal Grafts Followed up Five Years or More. An Analysis, *Arch Surg,* **110:**1294, 1975.

Crawford, E. S., Garrett, H. E., DeBakey, M. E., and Howell, J. F.: Occlusive Disease of the Femoral Artery and Its Branches, *Surg Clin North Am,* **46:**991, 1966.

Cutler, B. S., Thompson, J. E., Kleinsasser, L. J., and Hempel, G. K.: Autologous Saphenous Vein Femoropopliteal Bypass: Analysis of 298 Cases, *Surgery,* **79**(3):324, 1976.

Dale, W. A.: Autogenous Vein Grafts for Femoropopliteal Arterial Repair, *Surg Gynecol Obstet,* **123:**1282, 1966.

————: Salvage of Arteriosclerotic Legs by Vascular Repair, *Ann Surg,* **165:**844, 1967.

DeWeese, J. A., and Rob, C. G.: Autogenous Venous Bypass Grafts Five Years Later, *Ann Surg,* **174**(3):346, 1971.

Imparato, A. M., Bracco, A., and Kim, G. E.: Comparisons of Three Techniques for Femoral-Popliteal Arterial Reconstructions, *Ann Surg,* **177**(3):375, 1973.

Koontz, T. J., and Stausel, H. C., Jr.: Factors Influencing Patency of the Autogenous Vein Femoropopliteal By-pass Graft: An Analysis of 74 Cases, *Surgery,* **71:**753, 1972.

Linton, R. R., LeRoy, S., and Wirthlin, M. D.: Femoropopliteal Composite Dacron and Autogenous Vein Bypass Grafts: A Preliminary Report, *Arch Surg,* **107:**748, 1973.

Martin, P., and Jamieson, C.: The Rationale for and Measurement after Profundaplasty, *Surg Clin North Am,* **54**(1):95, 1974.

Plecha, F. R., and Pories, W. J.: Intraoperative Angiography in the Immediate Assessment of Arterial Reconstruction, *Arch Surg,* **105:**902, 1972.

Poliwoda, H.: Treatment of Acute and Chronic Arterial Occlusions with Streptokinase, *Aust Ann Med,* **19**(Suppl 1):25, 1970.

Rosenberg, N., Thompson, J. E., Keshishian, J. M., and Vander-Werf, B. A.: The Modified Bovine Arterial Graft, *Arch Surg,* **111:**222, 1976.

Sawyer, P. N., Kaplitt, M. J., Sobel, S., Golding, M. R., and Dennis, C.: Analysis of Peripheral Gas Endarterectomy in 127 Patients, *Arch Surg,* **97:**859, 1968.

Skinner, J. S., and Strandness, D. E., Jr.: Exercise and Intermittent Claudication: Effects of Physical Training, *Circulation,* **36:**23, 1967.

Szilagyi, D. E., Smith, R. F., Elliott, J. P., and Allen, H. M.: Long-Term Behavior of a Dacron Arterial Substitute: Clinical, Roentgenologic and Histologic Correlations, *Ann Surg,* **162:**453, 1965.

Vollmar, J., Frede, M., and Laubach, K.: Principles of Reconstructive Procedures for Chronic Femoro-popliteal Occlusions: A Report of 546 Operations, *Ann Surg,* **168:**215, 1968.

Tibioperoneal Occlusive Disease

Imparato, A. M., Kim, G. E., and Chu, D. S.: Surgical Exposure for Reconstruction of the Proximal Part of the Tibial Artery, *Surg Gynecol Obstet,* **136:**453, 1973.

———, ———, Madayag, M., and Haveson, S.: Angiographic Criteria for Successful Tibial Arterial Reconstructions, *Surgery,* **74**(6):830, 1973.

———, ———, ———, and ———: The Results of Tibial Artery Reconstruction Procedures, *Surg Gynecol Obstet,* **138:**33, 1974.

Kahn, S. P., Lindenauer, M., Dent, T. L., Kraft, R. O., and Fry, W. J.: Femorotibial Vein Bypass, *Arch Surg,* **107:**309, 1973.

Reichle, F. A., and Tyson, R. R.: Comparison of Long-Term Results of 364 Femoropopliteal or Femorotibial Bypasses for Revascularization of Severely Ischemic Lower Extremities, *Ann Surg,* **182**(4):449, 1975.

Arterial Embolism

Billig, D. M., Hallman, G. L., and Cooley, D. A.: Arterial Embolism, *Arch Surg,* **95:**1, 1967.

Cranley, J. J., Krause, R. J., Strasser, E. S., Hafner, C. D., and Fogarty, T. J.: Peripheral Arterial Embolism: Changing Concepts, *Surgery,* **55:**57, 1964.

Crawford, E. S., and DeBakey, M. E.: The Retrograde Flush Procedure in Embolectomy and Thrombectomy, *Surgery,* **40:**737, 1956.

Darling, R. C., Austen, W. G., and Linton, R. R.: Arterial Embolism, *Surg Gynecol Obstet,* **124:**106, 1967.

Fisher, E. R., Hellstrom, H. R., and Myers, J. D.: Disseminated Atheromatous Emboli, *Am J Med,* **29:**176, 1960.

Flory, C. M.: Arterial Occlusions Produced by Emboli from Eroded Aortic Atheromatous Plaques, *Am J Pathol,* **21:**549, 1945.

Fogarty, T. J., Cranley, J. J., Krause, R. J., Strasser, E. S., and

Hafner, C. D.: A Method for Extraction of Arterial Emboli and Thrombi, *Surg Gynecol Obstet,* **116:**241, 1963.

Haimovici, H.: Peripheral Arterial Embolism, *Angiology,* **1:**20, 1950.

Kassirer, J. P.: Atheroembolic Renal Disease, *N Engl J Med,* **280:**817, 1969.

Miles, R. M., Dale, D., and Booth, J. L.: The Dynamics of Peripheral Arterial Embolism, *Ann Surg,* **167:**801, 1968.

Spencer, F. C., and Eiseman, B.: Delayed Arterial Embolectomy: A New Concept, *Surgery,* **55:**64, 1964.

Buerger's Disease

Kjeldsen, K., and Mozes, M.: Buerger's Disease in Israel: Investigations on Carboxyhemoglobin and Serum Cholesterol Levels after Smoking, *Acta Chir Scand,* **135:**495, 1969.

McKusick, V. A., Harris, W. S., and Ottesen, O. E.: The Buerger Syndrome in the United States: Arteriographic Observations, with Special Reference to Involvement of the Upper Extremities and the Differentiation from Atherosclerosis and Embolism, *Bull Johns Hopkins Hosp,* **110:**145, 1962.

———, ———, ———, Goodman, R. M., Shelley, W. M., and Bloodwell, R. D.: Buerger's Disease: A Distinct Clinical and Pathologic Entity, *JAMA,* **181:**5, 1962.

McPherson, J. R., Guergels, J. L., and Gifford, R. W., Jr.: Thromboangiitis Obliterans and Arteriosclerosis Obliterans: Clinical and Prognostic Differences, *Ann Intern Med,* **59:**288, 1963.

Silbert, S.: The Etiology of Thromboangiitis Obliterans, *JAMA,* **129:**5, 1945.

Wessler, S.: Buerger's Disease Revisited, *Surg Clin North Am,* **49:**703, 1969.

———, Si-Chun, M., Gurewich, V., and Freiman, D. G.: Critical Evaluation of Thromboangiitis Obliterans: Case against Buerger's Disease, *N Engl J Med,* **262:**1149, 1960.

Arterial Trauma

Hughes, C. W., and Cohen, A.: The Repair of Injured Blood Vessels, *Surg Clin North Am,* **38:**1529, 1958.

Miller, H. H., and Welch, C. S.: Quantitative Studies on Time Factor in Arterial Injuries, *Ann Surg,* **130:**428, 1949.

Morris, G. C., Jr., Beall, A. C., Jr., Roof, W. R., and DeBakey, M. E.: Surgical Experience with 220 Acute Arterial Injuries in Civilian Practice, *Am J Surg,* **99:**775, 1960.

Mustard, W. T., and Bull, C. A.: A Reliable Method for Relief of Traumatic Vascular Spasm, *Ann Surg,* **155:**339, 1962.

Patman, R. D., Poulos, E., and Shires, G. T.: The Management of Civilian Arterial Injuries, *Surg Gynecol Obstet,* **118:**725, 1964.

Spencer, F. C.: Vascular Injury and Arteriovenous Fistula, in "Lewis-Walters Practice of Surgery," vol. XI, chap. 8, W. F. Prior Co., Inc., Hagerstown, Md., 1965.

——— and Grewe, R. V.: The Management of Arterial Injuries in Battle Casualties, *Ann Surg,* **141:**304, 1955.

Popliteal Artery Entrapment Syndrome

Albertazzi, V. J., Elliott, T. E., and Kennedy, J. A.: Popliteal Artery Entrapment, *Angiology,* **20:**119, 1969.

Brightmore, T. G. J., and Smellie, W. A. B.: Popliteal Artery Entrapment, *Br J Surg,* **58:**481, 1971.

Hamming, J. J.: Intermittent Claudication at an Early Age, due to an Anomalous Course of the Popliteal Artery, *Angiology,* **10:**369, 1959.

Harris, J. D., and Jepson, R. P.: Entrapment of the Popliteal Artery, *Surgery,* **69:**246, 1971.

Inshua, J. A., Young, J. R., and Humphries, A. W.: Popliteal Artery Entrapment Syndrome, *Arch Surg,* **101:**771, 1970.

Stuart, A. T. P.: Note on Variation in the Course of the Popliteal Artery, *J Anat Physiol,* **XIII:**162, 1879.

Anterior Compartment Syndrome

Carter, A. B., Richards, R. L., and Zachary, R. B.: The Anterior Tibial Syndrome, *Lancet,* **2:**928, 1949.

Getzen, L. C., and Carr, J. E., III: Etiology of Anterior Tibial Compartment Syndrome, *Surg Gynecol Obstet,* **125:**347, 1967.

Mavor, G. E.: The Anterior Tibial Syndrome, *J Bone Joint Surg* [*Br*], **38B:**513, 1956.

Moretz, W. H.: The Anterior Compartment (Anterior Tibial) Ischemia Syndrome, *Am Surg,* **19:**728, 1953.

Traumatic Arteriovenous Fistulas

Creech, O., Jr., Gantt, J., and Wren, H.: Traumatic Arteriovenous Fistula at Unusual Sites, *Ann Surg,* **161:**908, 1965.

Hughes, C. W., and Jahnke, E. J., Jr.: The Surgery of Traumatic Arteriovenous Fistulas and Aneurysms: A Five-Year Follow Up Study of 215 Lesions, *Ann Surg,* **148:**790, 1958.

Shumacker, H. B., Jr.: Arterial Aneurysms and Arteriovenous Fistulas: Report on Spontaneous Cures, in D. C. Elkin, and M. E. DeBakey (eds.), "Vascular Surgery," Office of the Surgeon General, U.S. Public Health Service, 1955.

Spencer, F. C.: Vascular Injury and Arteriovenous Fistula, in "Lewis-Walters Practice of Surgery," vol. XI, chap. 8, W. F. Prior Co., Inc., Hagerstown, Md., 1965.

Congenital Arteriovenous Fistulas

Cross, F. S., Glover, D. M., Simeone, F. A., and Oldenburg, F. A.: Congenital Arteriovenous Aneurysms, *Ann Surg,* **148:**649, 1958.

Fry, W. J.: Surgical Considerations in Congenital Arteriovenous Fistula, *Surg Clin North Am,* **54**(1):165, 1974.

Olcott, C., Newton, T. H., Stoney, R. J., and Ehrenfeld, W. K.: Intra-arterial Embolization in the Management of Arteriovenous Malformations, *Surgery,* **79**(1):3, 1976.

Robertson, D. J.: Congenital Arteriovenous Fistulae of the Extremities: Hunterian Lecture, *Ann R Coll Surg Engl,* **18:**73, 1956.

Rosenfeld, L.: Experiences with Vascular Abnormalities about the Parotid Gland and Upper Neck, *Arch Surg,* **79:**553, 1959.

Spencer, F. C.: Vascular Injury and Arteriovenous Fistula, in "Lewis-Walters Practice of Surgery," vol. XI, chap. 8, W. F. Prior Co., Inc., Hagerstown, Md., 1965.

Szilagyi, E. D., Smith, R. F., Elliott, J. P., and Hageman, J. H.; Congenital Arteriovenous Anomalies of the Limbs, *Arch Surg,* **111:**423, 1976.

Tice, D. A., Clauss, R. H., Kierle, A. M., and Reed, G. E.: Congenital Arteriovenous Fistulae of the Extremities: Observations Concerning Treatment, *Arch Surg,* **86:**460, 1963.

Thoracic Outlet Syndromes

Adams, J. T., and DeWeese, J. A.: Effort Thrombosis of the Axillary and Subclavian Veins, *J Trauma,* **11:**923, 1971.

Adson, A. W.: Surgical Treatment for Symptoms Produced by Cervical Ribs and the Scalenus Anticus Muscle, *Surg Gynecol Obstet,* **85:**687, 1947.

Beyer, J. A., and Wright, I. S.: The Hyperabduction Syndrome: With Special Reference to Its Relationship to Raynaud's Syndrome, *Circulation,* **4:**161, 1951.

Dale, W. A.: Thoracic Outlet Syndrome, *J Tenn Med Assoc,* **64:**941, 1971.

Falconer, M. A., and Weddell, G.: Costoclavicular Compression of the Subclavian Artery and Vein: Relation to the Scalenus Anticus Syndrome, *Lancet,* **2:**539, 1943.

Jochamisen, P. R., and Hartfall, W. G.: Per Axillary Upper Extremity Sympathectomy: Technique Reviewed and Clinical Experience, *Surgery,* **71**(5):686, 1972.

Kirtley, J. A., Riddell, D. H., Stoney, W. S., and Wright, J. K.: Cervico-sympathectomy in Neurovascular Abnormalities of the Upper Extremities: Experiences in 76 Patients with 104 Sympathectomies, *Ann Surg,* **165:**869, 1967.

Lord, J. W., Jr., and Rosati, L. M.: Neurovascular Compression Syndromes of the Upper Extremity, *Ciba Found Clin Symp.* **10:**35, 1958.

Nanson, E. M.: The Anterior Approach to Upper Dorsal Sympathectomy, *Surg Gynecol Obstet,* **104:**118, 1957.

Patman, R. D., Thompson, J. E., and Persson, A.: Management of Post-traumatic Pain Syndromes: Report of 113 Cases, *Ann Surg,* **177**(6):780, 1973.

Roos, D. B.: Transaxillary Approach for First Rib Resection to Relieve Thoracic Outlet Syndrome, *Ann Surg,* **163:**354, 1966.

——— and Owens, J. C.: Thoracic Outlet Syndrome, *Arch Surg,* **93:**71, 1966.

Ross, J. P.: The Vascular Complications of Cervical Rib, *Ann Surg,* **150:**340, 1959.

Schein, C. J., Haimovici, H., and Young, H.: Arterial Thrombosis Associated with Cervical Ribs: Surgical Considerations: Report of a Case and Review of the Literature, *Surgery,* **40:**428, 1956.

Telford, E. D., and Mottershead, S.: Pressure at the Cervicobrachial Junction: An Operative and Anatomical Study, *J Bone Joint Surg* [*Br*], **30B:**249, 1948.

Urschel, H. D., Paulson, D. L., and McNamara, J. J.: Thoracic Outlet Syndrome, *Ann Thorac Surg,* **6:**1, 1968.

Extracranial Occlusive Cerebrovascular Disease

Bahnson, H. T., Spencer, F. C., and Quattlebaum, J. K., Jr.: Surgical Treatment of Occlusive Disease of the Carotid Artery, *Ann Surg,* **149:**711, 1959.

Baker, Dennis J., Gluecklich, B., Watson, W., Marcus, E., and Vijaylakshmi, K.: An Evaluation of Electroencephalographic Monitoring for Carotid Study, *Surgery,* **78**(6):787, 1975.

Barner, H. B., Kaiser, G. C., and Willman, V. L.: Hemodynamics of Carotid-Subclavian Bypass, *Arch Surg,* **103:**248, 1971.

Barnes, R. W., Bone, G. E., Reinertson, J., Slaymaker, E. E., Hokanson, E., and Strandness, E.: Noninvasive Ultrasonic Carotid Angiography: Prospective Validation by Contrast Arteriography, *Surgery,* **80**(3):328, 1976.

Bornhard, W. M., Johnson, W. D., and Peterson, J. J.: Carotid Artery Stenosis, *Arch Surg,* **105:**837, 1972.

Blaisdell, F. W., Lim, R., and Hall, A. D.: Technical Result of Carotid Endarterectomy: Arteriographic Assessment, *Am J Surg,* **114:**239, 1967.

Bone, G. E., and Barnes, R. W.: Limitations of the Doppler

Cerebrovascular Examination in Hemispheric Cerebral Ischemia, *Surgery,* **79**(5):577, 1976.

Capistrant, T. D.: Thermographic Facial Patterns in Carotid Occlusive Disease, *Radiology,* **100**:85, 1971.

Cervantes, F. D., and Schneiderman, L. J.: Anticoagulants in Cerebrovascular Disease. A Critical Review of Studies, *Arch Intern Med,* **135**:875, 1975.

Cohen, A., Manion, W. C., Spencer, F. C., Czarnecki, S. W., and DeBakey, M. E.: Occlusive Lesions of the Great Vessels of the Aortic Arch, *Arch Surg,* **84**:628, 1962.

Crawford, E. S., DeBakey, M. E., Garrett, H. E., and Howell, J.: Surgical Treatment of Occlusive Cerebrovascular Disease, *Surg Clin North Am,* **46**:873, 1966.

———, ———, Morris, G. C., Jr., and Cooley, D. A.: Thrombo-obliterative Disease of the Great Vessels Arising from the Aortic Arch, *J Thorac Cardiovasc Surg,* **43**:38, 1962.

Dent, T. L., Thompson, N. W., and Fry, W. J.: Carotid Body Tumors, *Surgery,* **80**(3):365, 1976.

Fields, W. M.: Selection of Stroke Patients for Arterial Reconstructions, *Am J Surg,* **125**:527, 1973.

Ford, J. J., Baker, W. H., and Ehrenhaft, J. L.: Carotid Endarterectomy for Nonhemispheric Transient Ischemic Attacks, *Arch Surg,* **110**:1314, 1975.

Gresham, G. E., Fitzpatrick, T. E., Wolf, P. A., McNamara P. M., and Dawber, T. R.: Residual Disability of Survivors of Stroke—the Framingham Study, *N Engl J Med,* **293**(19):954, 1975.

Hachinski, V. C., Lassen, N. A., and Marshall, J.: Multi-Infarct Dementia, a Cause of Mental Deterioration in the Elderly, *Lancet,* **2**:207, 1974.

Hays, R. J., Levinson, S. A., and Wylie, E. J.: Intraoperative Measurement of Carotid Back Pressure as a Guide to Operative Management for Carotid Endarterectomy, *Surgery,* **72**(6):953, 1972.

Higgs, W. A., and Bullington, S. J.: Correlation between Opthalmodynamometry and Arteriography in Diagnosing Carotid Arterial Occlusive Disease, *Eye Ear Nose Throat Mon,* **49**:369, 1970.

Humphries, A. W., Young, J. R., Beven, E. D., LeFevre, F. A., and deWolfe, V. G.: Relief of vertebrobasilar symptoms by carotid endarterectomy, *Surgery,* **57**(1):48, 1965.

Imparato, A. M.: Bracco, A., Kim, G. E., and Bergmann, L.: The Hypoglossal Nerve in Carotid Arterial Reconstructions, *Stroke,* **3**:576, 1972.

———, Kricheff, I., Capetillo, A., and Post, K.: Circulatory Dynamics of the Cerebrovascular System in Surgery for Stroke, *Circulation,* **42**(Suppl 3):94, 1970.

——— and Lin, J. P. T.: Vertebral Arterial Reconstruction, Internal Plication and Patch Vein Angioplasty, *Ann Surg,* **166**:213, 1967.

Jacobson, J. H., Mozersky, D. J., Mitty, H. A., and Brothers, M. J.: Axillary-Axillary Bypass for the Subclavian Steal Syndrome, *Arch Surg,* **106**:24, 1973.

Joint Study of Extracranial Arterial Occlusion as a Cause of Stroke:

I. Fields, W. S., North, R. R., Hass, W. K., Galbraith, J. G., Wylie, E. J., Ratinov, G., Burns, M. H., MacDonald, M. C., and Meyer, J. S.: Organization of Study and Survey of Patient Population, *JAMA,* **203**:955, 1968.

II. Hass, W. K., Fields, W. S., North, R. R., Kricheff, I. I.,

Chase, N. E., and Bauer, R. B.: Arteriography, Techniques, Sites and Complications, *JAMA,* **203**:961, 1968.

III. Bauer, R. B., Meyer, J. S., Fields, W. S., Remington, R., MacDonald, M. C., and Callen, P.: Progress Report of Controlled Long Term Survival in Patients With and Without Operation, *JAMA,* **208**:509, 1969.

IV. Blaisdell, W. F., Clauss, R. H., Galbraith, J. G., Imparato, A. M., and Wylie, E. J.: A Review of Surgical Considerations, *JAMA,* **209**:1889, 1969.

V. Fields, W. S., Maslenikov, V., Meyer, J. S., Hass, W. K., Remington, R. D., and MacDonald, M.: Progress Report of Prognosis Following Surgery or Non Surgical Treatment for Transient Cerebral Ischemic Attacks and Cervical Carotid Lesions, *JAMA,* **211**:1993, 1970.

Killen, D. A., Foster, J. H., Gobbel, W. G., Jr., Stephenson, S. E., Jr., Collins, H. A., Billings, F. T., and Scott, H. W., Jr.: The Subclavian Steal Syndrome, *J Thorac Cardiovasc Surg,* **51**:539, 1966.

Kollarits, C. R., Lubow, M., and Hissong, S. L.: Retinal Strokes: I. Incidence of Carotid Atheromata, *JAMA,* **222**(10):1275, 1972.

Lazar, M. L., and Clark, K.: Microsurgical Cerebral Revascularization: Concepts and Practice, *Surg Neurol,* **1**(6):355, 1973.

Lyons, C., and Galbraith, G.: Surgical Treatment of Atherosclerotic Occlusion of the Internal Carotid Artery, *Ann Surg,* **146**:487, 1957.

Millikan, C. H.: The Pathogenesis of Transient Focal Cerebral Ischemia, *Circulation,* **32**:438, 1965.

Najafi, H., Javid, H., Dye, W. S., Hunter, J. A., Wideman, F. E., and Julian, O. C.: Emergency Carotid Thromboendarterectomy: Surgical Indication and Results, *Arch Surg,* **103**:610, 1971.

Ranson, J. H. C., Imparato, A. M., Clauss, R. H., Reed, G., and Hass, W. K.: Factors in Mortality and Morbidity Associated with Surgical Treatment of Cerebrovascular Insufficiency, *Circulation,* **39**(Suppl 1):269, 1969.

Reivich, M., Holling, E., Roberts, B., and Toole, J. F.: Reversal of Blood Flow through the Vertebral Artery and Its Effect on Cerebral Circulation, *N Engl J Med,* **265**:878, 1961.

Rhodes, L. E., Stanley, J. C., Hoffman, G. L., Cronenwett, J. L., and Fry, W. J.: Aneurysms of Extracranial Carotid Arteries, *Arch Surg,* **111**:339, 1976.

Rosenberg, J. C., and Spencer, F. C.: Subclavian Steal Syndrome: Surgical Treatment of Three Patients, *Am Surg,* **31**:307, 1965.

Rosenthal, J. J., Gaspar, M. R., and Movius, H. R.: Intraoperative Arteriography in Carotid Thromboendarterectomy, *Arch Surg,* **106**:806, 1973.

Ross, R. S., and McKusick, V. A.: Aortic Arch Syndrome, *Arch Intern Med,* **92**:701, 1953.

Sand, B. J., Barker, W. F., Freeman, W. L., and Hummell, S.: Ophthalmic Arterial Blood Pressures Measured by Oclular Plethysmodynamography, *Arch Surg,* **110**:813, 1975.

Santschi, D. R., Frahm, C. J., Pascale, L. R., and Dumanian, A. V.: The Subclavian Steal Syndrome: Clinical and Angiographic Considerations in 74 Cases in Adults, *J Thorac Cardiovasc Surg,* **51**:103, 1966.

Spencer, F. C., and Eiseman, B.: Technique of Carotid Endarterectomy, *Surg Gynecol Obstet,* **115**:114, 1962.

Thompson, J. E., Austin, D. J., and Patman, R. D.: Carotid Endarterectomy for Cerebrovascular Insufficiency: Long-Term

Results in 592 Patients Followed up to Thirteen Years, *Ann Surg,* **172**(4):663, 1970.

——, Kartchner, M. M., Austin, D. J., Wheeler, C. G., and Patman, R. D.: Carotid Endarterectomy for Cerebrovascular Insufficiency (Stroke): Follow Up of 359 Cases, *Ann Surg,* **163**:751, 1966.

—— and Patman, R. D.: Endarterectomy for Asymptomatic Carotid Bruits, *Heart Bull,* **19**:116, 1970.

——, Patman, R. D., and Persson, A. V.: Management of Asymptomatic Carotid Bruits, *Am Surg,* **42**(2):77, 1976.

Thompson, N. W., Olsen, W., Schmidt, C. M., and Kraft, R. O.: Occlusive Disease of the Subclavian Artery and the Subclavian Steal Syndrome, *Univ Mich Med Cent J,* **33**:8, 1967.

Warren, R., and Triedman, L. J.; Pulseless Disease and Carotid-Artery Thrombosis: Surgical Considerations, *N Engl J Med,* **257**:685, 1957.

Wylie, E. J., Hein, M. F., and Adams, J. E.: Intracranial Hemorrhage following Surgical Revascularization for Treatment of Acute Strokes, *J Neurosurg,* **21**:212, 1964.

Abdominal Aneurysms

Bahnson, H. T.: Surgical Treatment of Abdominal Arteriosclerotic Aneurysms, *Surg Clin North Am,* **36**:983, 1956.

DeBakey, M. R., Crawford, E. S., Cooley, D. A., Morris, G. C., Royster, T. S., and Abbott, W. P.: Aneurysm of Abdominal Aorta: Analysis of Results of Graft Replacement Therapy One to Eleven Years after Operation, *Ann Surg,* **160**(4):622, 1964.

Dent, T. L., Lindenauer, M., Ernst, C. B., and Fry, W. J.: Multiple Arteriosclerotic Arterial Aneurysms, *Arch Surg,* **105**:338, 1972.

Estes, J. E., Jr.: Abdominal Aortic Aneurysm: A Study of One Hundred and Two Cases, *Circulation,* **2**:258, 1950.

Hardy, J. D., and Timmis, H. H.: Abdominal Aortic Aneurysms: Special Problems, *Ann Surg,* **173**(6):945, 1971.

Imparato, A. M., Berman, I. R., Bracco, A., Kim, G. E., and Beaudet, R.: Avoidance of Shock and Peripheral Embolism during Surgery of the Abdominal Aorta, *Surgery,* **73**(1):68, 1973.

Jarrett, F., Darling, C. R., Mundth, E. D., and Austen, G.: Experience with Infected Aneurysms of the Abdominal Aorta, *Arch Surg,* **110**:1381, 1975.

Lawrence, R. J., Ferguson, M. D., Bergan, J. J., Conn, J., Jr., and Yao, J. S. T.: Spinal Ischemia following Abdominal Aortic Surgery, *Ann Surg,* **181**(3):267, 1975.

Mehrez, I. O., Nabseth, D. C., Hogan, E. L., and Deterling, R. A., Jr.: Paraplegia following Resection of Abdominal Aortic Aneurysm, *Ann Surg,* **156**:890, 1962.

Porter, J. M., McGregor, F., Acinapura, A. J., and Silver, D.: Renal Function following Abdominal Aortic Aneurysmectomy, *Surg Gynecol Obstet,* **123**(4):819, 1966.

Sethi, G. K., Hughes, R. K., and Takaro, T.: Dissecting Aortic Aneurysms, *Ann Thorac Surg,* **18**(2):301, 1974.

Shumacker, H. B., Barnes, D. L., and King, H.: Ruptured Abdominal Aortic Aneurysms, *Ann Surg,* **177**(6):772, 1973.

Smith, R. F., and Szilagyi, D. E.: Ischemia of the Colon as a Complication in Surgery of the Abdominal Aorta, *Arch Surg,* **80**:806, 1960.

Stanley, J. C., and Fry, W. J.: Pathogenesis and Clinical Significance of Splenic Artery Aneurysms, *Surgery,* **76**(6):898, 1974.

Szilagyi, D. E., Elliot, J. P., and Smith, R. F.: Clinical Fate of the Patient with Asymptomatic Abdominal Aortic Aneurysm and Unfit for Surgical Therapy, *Arch Surg,* **104**:600, 1972.

Szilagyi, D. E., Smith, R. F., De Russo, F. J., Elliott, J. P., and Sherrin, F. W.: Contribution of Abdominal Aortic Aneurysmectomy to Prolongation of Life, *Ann Surg,* **164**(4):678, 1966.

Thompson, J. E., Hollier, L. H., Patman, R. D., and Persson, A. V.: Surgical Management of Abdominal Aortic Aneurysms: Factors Influencing Mortality and Morbidity—a 20 Year Experience, *Ann Surg,* **181**(5):654, 1975.

Vasko, J. S., Spencer, F. C., and Bahnson, H. T.: Aneurysm of the Aorta Treated by Excision: Review of 237 Cases Followed Up to Seven Years, *Am J Surg,* **105**:793, 1963.

Peripheral Aneurysms: General

Howell, J. F., Crawford, E. S., Morris, G. C., Jr., Garrett, H. E., and DeBakey, M. E.: Surgical Treatment of Peripheral Arteriosclerotic Aneurysm, *Surg Clin North Am,* **46**:979, 1966.

Popliteal Aneurysms

Alpert, J.: Aneurysms of the Popliteal Artery, *J Med Soc NJ,* **67**:791, 1970.

Edmunds, L. H., Darling, R. C., and Linton, R. R.: Surgical Management of Popliteal Aneurysm, *Circulation,* **32**:517, 1965.

Gifford, R. W., Jr., Hines, E. A., Jr., and Janes, J. M.: Analysis and Follow-up Study of 100 Popliteal Aneurysms, *Surgery,* **33**:284, 1953.

Hunter, J. A., Julian, O. C., Javid, H., and Dye, W. S.: Arteriosclerotic Aneurysms of the Popliteal Artery, *J Cardiovasc Surg,* **2**:404, 1961.

Femoral Aneurysms

Crawford, E. S., Edwards, W. H., DeBakey, M. E., Cooley, D. A., and Morris, G. C., Jr.: Peripheral Arteriosclerotic Aneurysm, *J Am Geriatr Soc,* **9**:1, 1961.

Papas, G., Janes, J. M., Bernatz, P. E., and Schirger, A.: Femoral Aneurysms: Review of Surgical Management, *JAMA,* **190**:489, 1964.

Stoney, R. J., Albo, R. J., and Wylie, E. J.: False Aneurysms Occurring after Arterial Grafting Operations, *Am J Surg,* **110**:153, 1965.

Tolstedt, G. E., Radke, H. N., and Bell, J. W.: Late Sequela of Arteriosclerotic Femoral Aneurysms, *Angiology,* **12**:601, 1961.

Carotid Artery Aneurysms

Beall, A. C., Jr., Crawford, E. S., Cooley, D. A., and DeBakey, M. E.: Extracranial Aneurysms of the Carotid Artery: Report of Seven Cases, *Postgrad Med,* **32**:93, 1962.

Kianouri, M.: Extracranial Carotid Aneurysms, *Ann Surg,* **165**:152, 1967.

Sanoudos, G. M., Ramp, J., and Imparato, A. M.: Internal Carotid Aneurysm, *Am Surg,* **39**:118, 1973.

Spencer, F. C.: Aneurysm of the Common Carotid Artery Treated by Excision and Primary Anastomosis, *Ann Surg,* **145**:254, 1957.

Subclavian Aneurysms

Howell, J. F., Crawford, E. S., Morris, G. C., Jr., Garrett, H. E., and DeBakey, M. E.: Surgical Treatment of Peripheral Arteriosclerotic Aneurysm, *Surg Clin North Am,* **46**:979, 1966.

Splenic Artery Aneurysms

Bedford, P. D., and Lodge, B.: Aneurysm of the Splenic Artery, *Gut,* **1:**312, 1960.

Owens, J. C., and Coffey, R. J.: Aneurysm of the Splenic Artery, Including a Report of 6 Additional Cases, *Int Abstr Surg,* **97:**313, 1953.

Renal Artery Aneurysms

Cerny, J. C., Chang, C., and Fry, W. J.: Renal Artery Aneurysms, *Arch Surg,* **96:**653, 1968.

Garritano, A. P.: Aneurysm of the Renal Artery, *Am J Surg,* **94:**638, 1957.

Poutasse, E. F.: Renal Artery Aneurysm: Report of 12 Cases, Two Treated by Excision of the Aneurysm and Repair of Renal Artery, *J Urol,* **77:**697, 1957.

Traumatic Aneurysms

Crawford, E. S., DeBakey, M. E., and Cooley, D. A.: Surgical Considerations of Peripheral Arterial Aneurysms, *Arch Surg,* **78:**226, 1959.

Dickinson, E. H., Hood, R. H., and Spencer, F. C.: Traumatic Aneurysm of the Innominate Artery, *U.S. Armed Forces Med J,* **3:**1871, 1952.

Hughes, C. W., and Jahnke, E. J., Jr.: The Surgery of Traumatic Arteriovenous Fistulas and Aneurysms: A Five Year Follow-up Study of Lesions, *Ann Surg,* **148:**790, 1958.

Raynaud's Disease

Burton, E. E., Jr., et al.: Raynaud's Phenomenon: Treatment with Intraarterial Reserpine, *Cutis (N.Y.),* **9:**464, 1972.

DeTakats, G., and Fowler, E. F.: The Neurogenic Factor in Raynaud's Phenomenon, *Surgery,* **51:**9, 1962.

Farmer, R. G., Gifford, R. W., Jr., and Hines, E. A., Jr.: Raynaud's Disease with Sclerodactylia: A Follow-up Study of Seventy-one Patients, *Circulation,* **23:**13, 1961.

Gifford, R. W., Jr., Hines, E. A., Jr., and Craig, W. McK.: Sympathectomy for Raynaud's Phenomenon: Follow-up Study of 70 Women with Raynaud's Disease and 54 Women with Secondary Raynaud's Phenomenon, *Circulation,* **17:**5, 1958.

Kirtley, J. A., Riddell, D. H., Stoney, W. S., and Wright, J. K.: Cervicothoracic Sympathectomy in Neurovascular Abnormalities of the Upper Extremities: Experiences in 76 Patients with 104 Sympathectomies, *Ann Surg,* **165:**869, 1967.

Palumbo, L. T.: Anterior Transthoracic Approach for Upper Thoracic Sympathectomy, *Arch Surg,* **72:**659, 1956.

Varadi, D. P., and Lawrence, A. M.: Suppression of Raynaud's Phenomenon by Methyldopa, *Arch Intern Med,* **124:**13, 1969.

Willerson, J. T., and Decker, J. L.: Raynaud's Disease and Phenomenon, a Medical Approach, Am Heart J, **82:**572, 1971.

Uncommon Vasomotor Diseases

Estes, J. E.: Vasoconstrictive and Vasodilative Syndromes of the Extremities, *Mod Concepts Cardiovasc Dis,* **25:**355, 1956.

Lewis, T., and Landis, E. M.: Observations upon the Vascular Mechanism in Acrocyanosis, *Heart,* **15:**229, 1930.

Frostbite

Ervasti, E.: Frostbites of the Extremities and Their Sequelae: A Clinical Study, *Acta Chir Scand Suppl,* **299,** 1962.

Couch, N. P., Sullivan, J., and Crane, C.: Predictive Accuracy of Renal Vein Renin Activity in Surgery of Renovascular Hypertension, *Surgery,* **79:**70, 1976.

Golding, M. R., Martinez, A., deJong, P., Mendosa, M., Fries, C. C., Sawyer, P. N., Hennigar, G. R., and Wesolowski, S. A.: The Role of Sympathectomy in Frostbite, with a Review of 68 Cases, *Surgery,* **57:**774, 1965.

Mundth, E. D., Long, D. M., and Brown, R. B.: Treatment of Experimental Frostbite with Low Molecular Weight Dextran, *J Trauma,* **4:**246, 1964.

Penn, I., and Schwartz, S. I.: Evaluation of Low Molecular Weight Dextran in the Treatment of Frostbite, *J Trauma,* **4:**784, 1964.

Shumacker, H. B., Jr., and Kilman, J. W.: Sympathectomy in the Treatment of Frostbite, *Arch Surg,* **89:**575, 1964.

Simeone, F. A.: A Preliminary Follow-up Report on Cases of Cold Injury from World War II, in M. I. Ferrer, Cold Injury, *Trans 4th Conf Josiah Macy Jr. Found NY,* 1956, pp. 197-223.

Snider, R. L., and Porter, J. M.: Treatment of Experimental Frostbite with Intra-arterial Sympathetic Blocking Drugs, *Surgery,* **77(4):**557, 1975.

Chapter 22

Venous and Lymphatic Disease

by **James A. DeWeese**

VENOUS THROMBOSIS AND PULMONARY EMBOLISM

Venous thrombosis is a common direct and indirect cause of morbidity and mortality. During its acute phase, pain and swelling may be incapacitating. The threat of embolization of the thrombus to the pulmonary artery constantly exists. Postthrombotic scarring of the veins may lead to venous insufficiency with chronic discomfort and ulceration. The relatively frequent occurrence of venous thrombosis following operations or trauma arouses the surgeon's interest in the problem. In addition, operative intervention may be indicated to prevent or treat the complications of the thrombosis.

Etiology

Virchow, in the mid 1800s, first recognized three general causes of vascular thrombosis: stasis; injury to the vessel wall; and increased coagulability of the blood. Much more detailed information is now available regarding each of these general causes. Identification of the specific cause for a venous thrombosis seen in a given patient, however, may be very difficult. For example, a patient may present with a deep venous thrombosis following a long car ride, with-

out any history of trauma and without measurable abnormalities of coagulation factors. It is currently popular to incriminate stasis of blood as the etiologic agent. However, thousands of people may be in similar positions for equally long periods without developing thrombi. In other words, at the present time the reasons for thrombotic tendencies in certain patients are not known. The situations (as recorded by DeBakey and by Coon and Coller) in which thrombosis is more likely to occur, however, can be identified: following major injuries, following operations, during pregnancy, after previous thrombosis, with cancer, following long periods of sitting or bed rest, with infection, with varicose veins, and in obese females.

The incidences of at least minor thrombosis in these high-risk states have recently been emphasized in the studies of Kakkar. Using a radioiodinated fibrinogen test, venous thrombi were identified in the legs of 27.8 percent of elective surgery patients, in 54 percent of patients with hip fractures, in 3 percent of postpartum women, and in 19 percent of patients with myocardial infarction.

Pathophysiology

Venous thrombosis may be associated with an acute inflammatory response causing pain, local swelling, redness, tenderness, and tachycardia; the syndrome may then be labeled *thrombophlebitis*. Although acute inflammatory changes are present in the vein wall, bacteria are rarely present. The thrombus, on the other hand, may produce no local signs or symptoms and may be loosely attached to a vein wall which microscopically contains only a few chronic inflammatory cells; the condition may then be labeled *phlebothrombosis*. The differentiation of the two types of venous thrombosis, however, is only of academic interest. From a practical viewpoint it is the thrombus which is responsible for the early and late pathologic and physiologic changes, and it is the thrombus which may become a pulmonary embolus.

The thrombus initially causes obstruction of the vein; if the vein is a major one or if many veins are involved, there may be an increase in distal venous pressure. If the pressure in the venous capillaries becomes sufficiently high, water and solutes are not resorbed, and edema occurs. If the pressure becomes higher than local arterial pressures, blood flow ceases and venous gangrene occurs.

Some veins may remain obstructed following thrombosis; others may recanalize. In either case the venous valves are destroyed, leading to chronic venous valvular insufficiency. Thrombi which break loose in the moving venous bloodstream may be swept through the right heart and lodge in the pulmonary arteries as pulmonary emboli.

Although it is not important to differentiate thrombophlebitis and phlebothrombosis, it is important to differentiate superficial and deep venous thrombosis. Thrombi in the superficial veins rarely, if ever, embolize to the lung and can be treated symptomatically unless they propagate into a deep vein. Thrombi in the deep veins frequently embolize, cause permanent damage to the vein, and should be diagnosed early and treated aggressively.

Types of Venous Thrombosis

SUPERFICIAL VENOUS THROMBOSIS

SYMPTOMS. Patients usually complain of aching and swelling localized to a "knot" or "bump" on the leg or arm.

PHYSICAL FINDINGS. The diagnosis can usually be made by palpation of a firm mass or cord along the known course of a superficial vein. In the leg it is helpful to examine the patient in a standing position, since a distended or varicose vein may be palpated above and below the thrombus. In addition, redness, tenderness and *local* induration frequently are present (Fig. 22-1).

DIFFERENTIAL DIAGNOSIS. Insect bites may mimic superficial phlebitis but usually can be differentiated by the history of exposure, the presence of itching, and their lack of relation to the usual anatomic course of the significant superficial veins. Cellulitis or abscesses may at times be difficult to differentiate from thrombophlebitis, but in general, the more marked erythema, tenderness, and finally fluctuance define the diagnosis. The presence of a

Fig. 22-1. Superficial venous thrombosis. There is usually redness, tenderness, and swelling surrounding a palpable thrombosed superficial vein.

red lymphatic streak or tender lymphadenopathy may also make the diagnosis of infection more obvious. It may be difficult to differentiate a subcutaneous hematoma from a bland thrombus unless a clear-cut history of trauma is present or the site of injury is away from the course of a major vein.

TREATMENT. Nonoperative management is the method of choice in patients with localized disease, since embolization almost never occurs and late morbidity is insignificant. However, superficial venous thrombosis may be present in patients with deep venous thrombosis. The presence of significant distal swelling or of tenderness over the deep veins should make one suspect deep venous thrombosis. A phlebogram may be helpful in ruling out deep-vein involvement.

Nonoperative Management. In general the acute discomfort of the process is over within a few days and symptomatic therapy is adequate. Bed rest is rarely indicated. Hot baths or compresses may be helpful in relieving discomfort. Propagation of the thrombus can usually be prevented by preventing venous stasis. The patient is advised to be either walking with elastic support or lying down with the legs elevated above the level of the heart. Sitting and standing are discouraged. Anticoagulants are not needed. The various enzymatic "clot dissolvers" have little if any effect on the outcome. Expensive and potentially dangerous "anti-inflammatory" drugs do not appear any more effective than aspirin. Antibiotics are not indicated, despite the presence of redness and tenderness, unless a septic cause is obvious.

Operative Treatment. *Ligation.* Thrombi in the greater saphenous system above the level of the knee may propagate into the common femoral vein, and any evidence of the ascension of such thrombi should be treated by ligation of the vein at the saphenofemoral junction, using local anesthesia. Similarly, the lesser saphenous vein may be ligated in the popliteal fossa.

Excision or Stripping. Veins which are the site of recurrent phlebitis and are stubbornly symptomatic can be ligated at their junctions with the deep system and then excised or in some instances "stripped," as suggested by Herrmann.

DEEP VENOUS THROMBOSIS

The deep veins are hidden within their muscular compartments, and the diagnosis of thrombosis, particularly of the bland type, may be difficult. DeBakey, as well as Barner and DeWeese, have reported that venous thrombosis is recognized prior to death in less than 55 percent of patients with fatal pulmonary emboli. This poor record exists despite the fact that the sources of approximately 85 percent of pulmonary emboli are the veins of the lower extremity, according to the experiences of Byrne and O'Neil, Ravdin and Kirby, and Short.

CLINICAL MANIFESTATIONS. Symptoms. There may be an aching pain, which is aggravated by muscular activity, at the site of a deep venous thrombus. In the presence of a massive thrombosis, there may be an extremely severe aching or cramping pain in the calf and thigh. At other times, however, only a feeling of "heaviness," accentuated by standing, will be noticed. Depending on the site of thrombosis, noticeable swelling may be absent, minimal, or marked. Few, if any, symptoms may be noticed by a patient confined to bed.

Physical Findings. The three signs most frequently described as being useful in the diagnosis of deep venous thrombosis include swelling, tenderness, and Homans' sign. Swelling must be searched for with the aid of a measuring tape; the eye cannot be trusted to tell small or even moderate differences in the size of two extremities. When properly looked for, this sign appears to be the most reliable in making a positive diagnosis of deep venous thrombosis. Tenderness over the thrombosed vein is also usually present if carefully looked for by palpation of the calf, popliteal space, adductor canal, and groin.

Homans was one of the first physicians to emphasize the importance of venous thrombosis in the legs as a source of pulmonary emboli. He popularized a simple test for detecting early thrombosis which is now known as Homans' sign. It is performed by dorsiflexing the foot and is considered positive if the patient complains of calf pain. It is thought that passive elongation of the gastrocnemius and soleus muscles causes irritative pain in the calf when the veins of the calf contain thrombi. Although this test is the easiest to perform, it is unfortunately the least reliable, according to the author's personal experience and to McLachlin et al.

The presence of superficial venous dilatation due to deep vein obstruction is considered by some to be a useful observation, but deep venous obstruction can be more objectively determined by measurement of the venous pressure.

Relation to Site of Involvement. The most frequent site of thrombosis is probably in the veins of the calf, particularly in the venous sinuses of the soleus muscle. Untreated, the thrombi may propagate to involve the femoral vein or even the iliac vein. Actually, however, thrombi that involve the iliac and femoral veins most frequently begin in the valve pockets of those veins and propagate distally, according to Gibbs and to McLachlin and Paterson. The signs and symptoms differ according to the veins involved, and it is worthwhile to consider each of the more common sites individually.

Calf Vein Thrombosis (Fig. 22-2*A*). Although the calf is the most frequent site of thrombosis, diagnosis in this location is probably the one most frequently missed. Calf pain and calf tenderness are usually present, but swelling is present in only 70 percent of cases. If present, the swelling is almost always minimal, the circumference of the involved calf and ankle being less than 1.5 cm greater than the normal limb. Homans' sign may or may not be present. The venous pressure is usually normal, which explains why there is little if any edema.

Femoral Vein Thrombosis (Fig. 22-2*B*). Although combined thrombosis of the calf veins and femoral veins is frequently seen, in some instances the thrombus is localized to the femoral vein. There is usually tenderness in the calf, popliteal region, or adductor canal. Swelling is usually present at the ankle and calf level, as might be predicted from the fact that the venous pressure is usually

two to five times normal. Homans' sign may or may not be present.

Iliofemoral Venous Thrombosis (Fig. 22-2*C*). Thrombosis which involves the iliac and femoral veins may also involve the calf veins, but it is frequently sharply localized to the iliofemoral or even iliac level. The left leg is involved two or three times more frequently than the right leg, apparently due to the longer course of the vein, its constriction by the right iliac artery, and the occasional presence of congenital webs at its junction with the vena cava. Iliofemoral venous thrombosis is the most dramatic of the thromboses, since pain, tenderness, and marked swelling of the entire leg are usually present. The venous pressure is considerably elevated, which explains the marked edema and also the bluish discoloration frequently observed during the early course of the process. When pain and cyanosis are present, the process may be termed *phlegmasia cerulea dolens*. This syndrome may progress to venous gangrene secondary to massive thrombosis of all the venous drainage of the part involved. Arterial spasm may also be present in some instances.

Pelvic Vein Thrombosis. Thrombosis of the pelvic veins, including the branches of the internal iliac veins, may be seen in women with pelvic inflammatory disease or in men with involvement of the prostatic plexus. The diagnosis is best made by pelvic or rectal examination plus a high degree of suspicion. Leg signs are not present unless the external and common iliac veins are also involved.

Primary Deep Venous Thrombosis of the Upper Extremity. Although this process of deep thrombosis may be seen in patients with congestive heart failure or with terminal carcinomas, it is more dramatic when it appears in otherwise normal individuals. It has been termed "Paget-Schroetter syndrome," "axillary vein thrombosis," or "effort thrombosis," since it most frequently occurs after some unusual muscular activity of the arm. In otherwise healthy patients, the thrombosis apparently originates in the subclavian vein at the point where the vein can be compressed between the first rib and clavicle. The diagnosis is usually made from swelling of the arm and the presence of tenderness over the axillary vein. Phlebography can confirm the diagnosis and determine the site of the obstruction.

SPECIAL TESTS. Special tests which are helpful in the diagnosis of deep venous thrombosis include (1) phlebography, (2) venous pressure measurements, and (3) non-invasive techniques.

Phlebography. Phlebography provides a means of visualizing the deep veins of the extremities (Fig. 22-3*A*,*B*,*C*). It is particularly useful in the patient with equivocal signs or symptoms, since it can provide ancillary evidence for or against the diagnosis of venous thrombosis. It is also helpful in determining the source of pulmonary emboli in patients without significant signs of venous thrombosis. It is helpful in determining the extent of thrombosis in patients who will undergo operative treatment, and it offers an objective means of evaluating any form of therapy.

Since the technique of phlebography was first described by Dos Santos and popularized by Bauer, there have been continued improvements in methods. The following tech-

CALF   FEMORAL   ILIO-FEMORAL

A   B   C

nique has been used in over 400 patients with suspected deep venous thrombosis and has been found safe, reliable, and relatively simple to perform.

1. A #21 scalp-vein needle is inserted into a superficial vein on the dorsum of the foot and a slow infusion of saline solution begun to maintain patency of the needle. With experience, a cut-down to expose a vein is rarely necessary.
2. The patient is placed in a semierect position 15 to 45° from the horizontal on a tilt table.
3. A snug rubber tourniquet is placed around the ankle.
4. Over a 1- to 2-minute period, 50 to 100 ml of an angiographic contrast material is injected.
5. Two sets of 14- by 34-in. radiographs are exposed about 30 seconds apart. If the patient was ambulatory prior to the test, he is asked to stand on his toes five times between exposures.

Thrombi are identified as globular or serpentine defects in well-opacified veins. Lack of filling of a vein is considered evidence of venous thrombosis, but only if clots are also seen in the vein, or if the lack of filling of a major vein is associated with visualization of numerous collateral veins at the same level.

Venous Pressure Measurements. Venous pressure is easily measured by inserting a needle into a superficial vein of the foot or ankle and connecting it to a saline solution manometer. The pressure should be compared with those in the other leg and the arm; the test will be positive in the presence of significant venous obstruction only early in the course of the disease before sufficient collaterals have developed.

Fig. 22-2. *A.* Calf vein thrombosis. Thrombosis is localized to veins of calf and popliteal vein. There is minimal, if any, swelling at level of ankle. Calf pain and tenderness are usually present. Homans' sign may or may not be present. *B.* Femoral vein thrombosis. There is thrombosis of femoral vein and usually associated thrombosis of calf vein. Swelling is usually present and extends to just above level of knee. Popliteal tenderness and calf tenderness may be present. Homans' sign may or may not be present. *C.* Iliofemoral venous thrombosis. There is thrombosis of iliac and proximal femoral vein, and frequently calf veins also are involved. Edema is present from foot to level of inguinal ligament. There is usually tenderness in groin and sometimes popliteal and calf tenderness. Homans' sign may or may not be present.

Noninvasive Technique. During the past few years, progress has been made in developing noninvasive methods for diagnosing venous thrombosis, i.e., those which require neither incision nor the introduction of needles into the involved extremity. These methods include isotope studies, the Doppler ultrasound technique, and an electrical impedance test, and presently are most valuable in screening patients. The ^{125}I-labeled fibrinogen test is particularly helpful in identifying small areas of thrombosis in the calf, while the Doppler technique is best for identifying significant venous occlusion in the femoral region. However, phlebography may still be necessary in cases where equivocal results are obtained by noninvasive methods, and it is still recognized as the most definitive test for the diagnosis of deep venous thrombosis.

Fig. 22-3. *A.* Phlebogram demonstrating calf thrombi. Note areas of relative radiolucency in opaque-filled veins. *B.* Phlebogram demonstrating femoral and calf thrombosis. *C.* Phlebogram demonstrating iliofemoral thrombosis without involvement of calf vein. Note extensive formation of collaterals in upper thigh. (*From J. A. DeWeese and S. M. Rogoff, Surgery, 53:99, 1963.*)

Isotope Studies. Gomez et al. and Schwartz described methods for the scanning detection of venous thrombi in which radioactive elements are attached to thrombi by either tagged fibrinolytic enzymes or fibrinogen antibodies (Fig. 22-4). Kakkar and Browse more recently reported extensive clinical experience with the use of ^{125}I-labeled fibrinogen to detect venous thrombi.

Human fibrinogen is fractionated from the plasma of a restricted pool of accredited donors to minimize the risk of transmitting viral hepatitis. The fibrinogen is labeled with ^{125}I under sterile conditions and stored at $-20°$C. The patient is given 100 mg of sodium iodide 24 hours before the test to prevent excessive accumulation of the radioactive iodine in the thyroid gland. The test is performed by injecting 100 μCi of the labeled fibrinogen into a femoral vein, and the radioactivity over the legs is measured 2 hours later. Portable bedside equipment is available for this measurement.

The test cannot differentiate thrombi from an inflammatory fibrinous exudate and, therefore, is of no value for patients with superficial thrombophlebitis, recent operative incisions, traumatic wounds, hematomas, cellulitis, active arthritis, or primary lymphedema. In addition, thrombi cannot be accurately diagnosed in the upper thigh and pelvis because of high background counts.

The test is positive only during the active formation or propagation of a thrombus. It is most valuable in detecting the onset of thrombosis in patients at risk, such as during the postoperative period when the test is performed daily with corroborated accuracy in the range of 90 percent. Test accuracy falls to the 80 percent range when it is used for patients with suspected established deep venous thrombosis.

Doppler Ultrasound Technique. The Doppler ultrasound blood velocity detector emits a sound beam which alters frequency when moving blood cells are encountered. When reflected and detected, the altered frequencies are amplified to drive a loudspeaker or for display on a recorder. Manual compression of the leg augments flow through the veins, producing characteristic "A" sounds for Doppler detection which are hampered or obliterated when venous thrombosis significantly occludes the deep veins.

Sigel et al. have had extensive experience with this technique. The ultrasound method recognized 78.1 percent of new thrombotic venous occlusion corroborated by phlebography. However, the technique cannot differentiate new occlusion from old, and small areas of thrombosis which do not significantly occlude major venous channels cannot be diagnosed.

Impedance Tests. Significant venous obstruction and replacement of blood by thrombi decreases the venous volume changes occurring with respiration. Liquid blood conducts electric currents, and instruments capable of measuring small changes in the electrical resistance of the leg can indirectly assess changes in venous volume. Wheeler et al. have devised an electrical impedance test which uses these principles to detect venous thrombosis indirectly. Cranley et al. use a modified plethysmographic technique for measurement of these venous volume changes.

Unfortunately, several factors other than patency of the major veins may influence venous volume changes. These include venous tone, extravascular compression which may vary with leg position, and adequacy of the collateral circulation, plus the ventilatory excursion. Dmochowski et al. were able to demonstrate only 53.5 percent test accu-

Fig. 22-4. Isotope scan following injection of ^{131}I-labeled anti-fibrinogen. Right leg normal; left leg shows femoral and popliteal thrombus confirmed by phlebography. (*From I. L. Spar, M. I. Varon, R. L. Goodland, and S. I. Schwartz, Arch Surg, 92:752, 1966.*)

racy, and for the present the test must be considered experimental.

DIFFERENTIAL DIAGNOSIS. Superficial venous thrombosis may be associated with deep venous thrombosis. This should be suspected if there is edema other than at the site of thrombosis; if there is calf, popliteal, or groin tenderness; and if Homans' sign is positive. A superficial thrombosis extending to the popliteal space or groin should also arouse suspicion.

A tear of the gastrocnemius, soleus, or plantaris muscles may mimic a calf vein thrombosis and cause edema, calf tenderness, and a positive Homans' sign. A history of a sharp stinging pain in the calf associated with walking or running and the appearance of ecchymosis over the calf and below the malleoli will usually make the diagnosis of muscle tear obvious. An effusion of the knee joint may produce distal edema and popliteal tenderness but can be differentiated from venous thrombosis by detection of a ballotable patella. A cellulitis in a lymphedematous limb may cause edema of the entire limb and tenderness, but the presence of erythema, high fever, and leukocytosis usually differentiates this condition from an iliofemoral or subclavian vein thrombosis. Phlebography is helpful in differentiating deep venous thrombosis from all these conditions.

PREVENTION. Attempts to prevent venous thrombosis have been aimed at avoidance of venous intimal injury, minimization of venous stasis, and use of anticoagulants. Venous intimal injury can occur with rough handling of vessels during operations. This should be avoided. Hypertonic or irritating intravenous solutions should not be introduced into the veins of the lower extremity and are best given by an indwelling catheter in the high-flow superior vena cava.

Elevation of legs above heart level during operations and in the postoperative period can decrease venous stasis. Although the value of elastic stockings has been questioned, recent studies, including phlebographic studies of Lewis et al., confirm that properly fitting compression stockings can increase flow and clear stagnant blood from behind venous valves. In addition, Flanc and Tsapogas, in separate studies, have demonstrated significant decreases in thrombosis as diagnosed by phlebography or ^{125}I-labeled fibrinogen scanning techniques when elevation, elastic stockings, and bed exercises were used following major operations. Cotton and Roberts have demonstrated that either pedaling of the foot or the intermittent compression of the leg during an operation decreases the incidence of isotopically detectable deep venous thrombosis postoperatively.

Dextran, Coumadin, and heparin have been used in operative patients in hopes of preventing venous thrombosis. The occasional occurrence of pulmonary edema following a dextran fluid load and increased incidence of bleeding and hematomas following the use of dextran or anticoagulants has hampered their routine use. The use of small doses of heparin—5,000 units of concentrated aqueous heparin (25,000 units/ml) subcutaneously 2 hours prior to operation and every 8 hours thereafter for 7 days—was evaluated by Kakkar et al. in a prospective randomized trial. The miniheparin regimen significantly decreased the incidence of deep venous thrombosis as diagnosed by the ^{125}I-labeled fibrinogen test. Many surgeons are now using prophylactic heparin, 5,000 units twice or three times a day, and others are awaiting reports of larger clinical trials before committing their patients to the regimen.

TREATMENT. This generally relies on a medical regimen but occasionally requires an aggressive surgical approach.

Nonoperative Treatment. The primary aims of nonoperative therapy are to prevent thrombi which have already formed from embolizing and to prevent new thrombi from forming.

Bed Rest and Elevation. It is generally agreed that bed rest is indicated for approximately 7 days after onset or progression of symptoms to allow thrombi which are present to become firmly adherent to the vein wall. Bed rest prevents the fluctuations of pressure in the deep venous system that occur with walking. Unfortunately, it does not prevent the more marked fluctuations that may occur with straining during defecation, which all too commonly precipitates a fatal pulmonary embolus. Elevation of the legs above the level of the heart to a height equal to the venous pressure in a superficial vein of the foot, if possible, decreases the pressure in the veins and relieves the edema and pain. In addition, the increased rate of flow in the nondistended veins prevents venous stasis and formation of new thrombi. Elastic support is not required with adequate elevation. When ambulation begins, it is limited to walking with elastic support. The elastic support compresses the superficial veins, and, with walking, the rate of flow in the veins is increased and the venous pressure is kept at a minimum, which impedes the development of edema. Standing and sitting are initially forbidden, since the additional hydrostatic ·pressure in the veins would increase edema and discomfort. Limitation of the amount of standing and sitting may be necessary for periods of 3 to 6 months in patients with extensive iliofemoral venous thrombosis. In this way edema can be reduced until recanalization of the major veins and/or dilation of collaterals has occurred.

Anticoagulation. The propagation of established thrombi may be prevented with anticoagulants such as heparin or one of the coumarin derivatives.

Heparin. Heparin is believed to prevent thrombus formation by inhibiting the formation of thromboplastin and acting as an antithrombin to inactivate thrombin. Its effect can be determined by measuring the whole blood clotting time and partial thromboplastin time (PTT). Propagation of thrombi can be prevented if the clotting time or the PTT is at least twice normal. Such times can be achieved by the administration of aqueous heparin intravenously, either continuously or every 4 hours in 5,000- to 10,000-unit amounts. Similar results can be obtained by administering 15,000 to 20,000 units of concentrated aqueous heparin (20,000 units/ml) into the deep fat of the abdominal wall every 12 hours. Continuous intravenous administration is the preferred method if a reliable infuser is available. Heparin therapy is advised for varying lengths of time, but it seems reasonable to use it for a period of 7 days, until the thrombi have become firmly adherent to the vein; the amounts given are then tapered off over a 3- to 5-day period. If the drug is discontinued abruptly, new thrombosis is frequently observed within the next few days. This is described as "heparin rebound" by some but may merely be a return of a pretreatment thrombotic tendency. It is advisable to continue anticoagulant therapy with the coumarin derivatives after discontinuing heparin. Possible complications of heparin therapy are bleeding and arterial emboli. Bleeding is most apt to occur in fresh surgical wounds. If necessary the heparin effect can be reversed by injecting protamine sulfate intravenously in 50- to 100-mg amounts. Platelet emboli have been observed by Roberts et al. in patients receiving heparin, but at this time the mechanism is unknown.

Controlled and comparative studies indicate that heparin therapy is superior to no anticoagulation but that pulmonary emboli may still occur. The incidence of pulmonary emboli in patients with venous thrombosis during treatment with heparin is variously reported as 0.9 to 7.7 percent.

Coumarin Derivatives. The coumarin derivatives may interfere with four factors in the clotting mechanism, but the effect of clinical importance is its reduction of the plasma concentration of prothrombin. Its effect can therefore be determined by measuring the prothrombin time, which must be less than 10 percent of normal to inhibit the propagation of thrombi as effectively as heparin does. This, unfortunately, is the level at which bleeding complications are most likely to occur. However, somewhat higher prothrombin times are apparently able to prevent formation of new thrombi. Coumarin derivatives can be administered orally and at the present time are the drugs of choice for prophylactic therapy or long-term therapy following initial heparin therapy. It appears logical to continue anticoagulation with the coumarin derivatives for approximately 4 weeks after an acute venous thrombosis or pulmonary embolism, since recurrence is most likely within that period. Patients with iliofemoral venous thrombosis may be maintained on therapy for 6 months after the onset, since recurrence is most likely during this period when venous stasis is still being decreased by the enlargement of collaterals.

Other Medications. The administration of fibrinolytic drugs or dextran for the treatment of venous thrombosis shows some promise. At present, however, it would seem best to consider their use experimental until further clinical studies are available.

Operative Treatment. Thrombi can be successfully removed from major veins such as the subclavian, iliac, or femoral. Iliofemoral venous thrombectomy is performed through an incision in the groin, using a local anesthetic (Fig. 22-5), via a femoral venotomy. The iliac system is cleared with forceps and suction applied to polyethylene tubing or long fine catheters with an inflatable balloon on

Fig. 22-5. Venous thrombectomy. (*Courtesy of C. Rob and R. Smith.*)

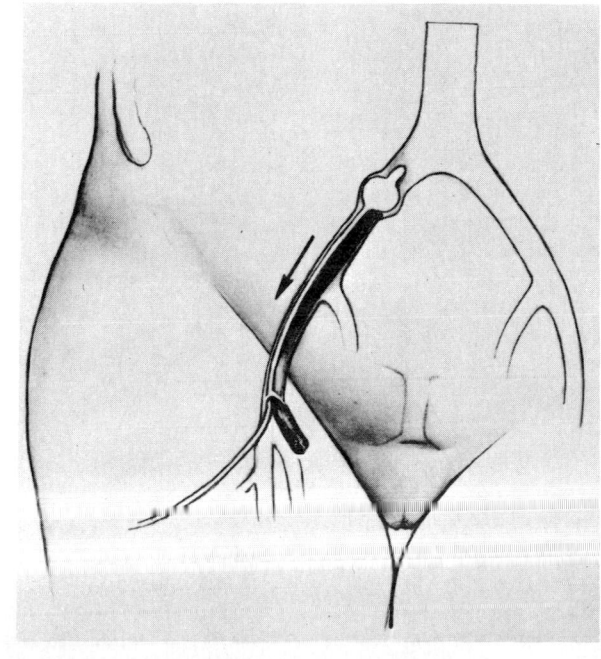

the end. Thrombi can be removed from the femoral vein by the same method plus tight wrapping of the leg with an elastic bandage. The venotomy is then closed with fine arterial suture. In general, venous interruptions are not necessary. Heparin is administered after the operation. The best results are obtained in patients operated on within 1 week of onset and in those in whom the thrombus is segmental in nature as determined by an ascending phlebogram. Care must be taken not to push thrombi into the moving flow of blood in the common iliac vein or inferior vena cava, but pulmonary embolization has rarely if ever occurred during the operation. Despite the use of heparin, thrombosis occasionally recurs, probably secondarily to the mechanical or inflammatory processes which initiated the thrombosis originally. In general, thrombectomy has successfully decreased the early and late morbidity of massive venous thrombosis, and phlebograms have demonstrated restoration of patent veins with normal valves in at least one-third of patients. Mavor et al. demonstrated 85 percent of 42 iliac veins to be patent 14 days after successful venous thrombectomy.

Subclavian Venous Thrombosis. Primary subclavian venous thrombosis is probably secondary to localized thrombosis of the vein at the site where the vein passes between the clavicle and first rib. This theory is supported by the facts that patients may be seen with intermittent venous obstruction at this site and that this obstruction may be relieved by removal of the first rib or clavicle. This theory

Fig. 22-6. Chest x-ray demonstrating peripheral wedge-shaped area of infarction.

is further supported by observations at the time of subclavian venous thrombectomy that the older thrombi and venous scarring are also found at the point where the vein passes between the clavicle and first rib. Thrombectomy with removal of the clavicle or first rib may provide definitive therapy. Patients who have had a subclavian venous thrombosis develop large collaterals between the axillary vein and the internal jugular venous system, which also passes between the clavicle and first rib. These collaterals may be obstructed by hyperextension of the arm or hyperabduction of the shoulder, and this condition may also be relieved by removal of the clavicle or first rib.

Pulmonary Emboli

INCIDENCE. Complete autopsy studies by Hunter et al. indicate that deep venous thrombi may be found in approximately 50 percent of patients who die in a hospital. Approximately 1 in 5 of these patients demonstrated nonfatal emboli, while 1 in 10 had fatal emboli.

PATHOPHYSIOLOGY. Thrombi, which break loose from their point of origin, pass through the right atrium and ventricle and lodge in the pulmonary arteries. Large thrombi which lodge in major pulmonary arteries may cause immediate death secondary to vasovagal shock, right ventricular failure, and inadequate transfer of oxygen and carbon dioxide in the pulmonary circulation. It is debatable whether small emboli lodging in a lobar or segmental artery can cause death, and if so, by what mechanisms. It is postulated, and supported by some laboratory data, that intense bronchoconstriction and vasoconstriction might explain such an occurrence. Such single small emboli may also result in infarctions. Infection and even abscesses and empyema may ensue. Multiple small emboli may eventually produce enough arterial obstruction to cause pulmonary hypertension and right ventricular failure.

Various autopsy series indicate that the lower extremity (including the iliac veins) is the source of pulmonary emboli in approximately 85 percent of patients. Approximately 10 percent of emboli arise from the right atrium. The remaining 5 percent come from the pelvic veins, vena cava, or upper extremities.

SYMPTOMS. Classically, patients with pulmonary emboli complain of dyspnea, pain, and hemoptysis. The dyspnea is usually the first and may be the only symptom. There may be crushing substernal pain in the presence of a massive embolus lodged in the main pulmonary artery. The pain may be sharp, localized, and stabbing, occurring with breathing, in the presence of a peripheral infarct. This is referred to as *pleuritic* pain. Epigastric pain is occasionally described. Hemoptysis, with coughing up of small flecks or even massive amounts of blood, may occur in the presence of infarction of segments of the lung.

PHYSICAL FINDINGS. Tachycardia is frequently observed, and tachypnea is common. Shock is an ominous sign of a massive embolus. Cyanosis may be present if there is a massive embolus. Splinting of the chest and pleural friction rubs are observed in the presence of peripheral infarcts. Râles may be heard in the region of infiltrates or may be bilateral and bubbling with secondary pulmonary edema. Small pleural effusions are frequently present and sometimes large enough to be recognized on examination.

Less than 50 percent of all pulmonary embolisms found at autopsy had been suspected before death. A retrospective study by Coon and Coller of patients later shown at autopsy to have pulmonary emboli indicates the following frequency of certain signs and symptoms: dyspnea, 58 percent; chest pain, 22 percent; hemoptysis, 11 percent; shock, 28 percent; friction rub, 16 percent. Epigastric pain, cough, fever, and cyanosis are less frequently seen. The classic triad of dyspnea, pain, and hemoptysis was observed in only 3 percent of the patients, and 27 percent appeared to have had no signs or symptoms.

SPECIAL TESTS. Chest X-rays. Since pulmonary emboli do not always cause infarction, the wedge-shaped infiltrate may not be seen (Fig. 22-6). Other signs such as areas of decreased vascularity, dilated pulmonary arteries, or pleural fluid may be found. Stein et al. state that the diagnosis can be suspected from x-rays in approximately 50 percent of patients with pulmonary emboli.

Electrocardiogram. The classic finding of right heart strain is usually not present. However, Henderson reports some significant abnormality concomitant with the acute event in over 60 percent of patients.

Chemical Tests. The triad of elevated serum lactic dehydrogenase (LDH) and serum bilirubin in the presence of normal serum glutamic oxalacetic transaminase (SGOT) level is no longer considered reliable in the diagnosis of pulmonary embolism. Szucs et al. found the triad to be positive in only 18 percent of pulmonary emboli proved by pulmonary arteriogram.

Pulmonary Angiograms. Pulmonary angiography provides the most effective means of diagnosing pulmonary emboli. It is indicated in patients with unexplained pulmonary infiltrates and in those with recurrent symptoms suggestive of pulmonary emboli. It is most helpful in diagnosing the presence and extent of a massive pulmonary embolus. The procedure may be performed by rapidly injecting a radiopaque material into the right atrium or main pulmonary artery through a catheter threaded into position through a peripheral vein. It can also be performed by the simultaneous rapid injection of a bolus of radiopaque material through needles placed in superficial veins in both arms. Visualization of the significant pulmonary arteries can be obtained by either technique, and occlusion of the arteries can be identified by the lack of filling (Fig. 22-7).

Gas Analysis. Pulmonary arterial obstruction with decreased perfusion of the lung results in a decrease in the alveolar carbon dioxide tension (P_{CO_2}). Therefore, the gradient between the brachial arterial P_{CO_2} and the end-tidal ("alveolar") P_{CO_2}, which is usually minimal, is increased in the presence of significant pulmonary emboli.

Radioisotope Scanning. The rapid intravenous injection of radioactive substances such as [131]I- tagged macroaggregated albumin accompanied by scintillation scanning of the chest may be used to diagnose areas of decreased vascularity in the lung field. Obstruction of the pulmonary

Fig. 22-7. Pulmonary angiogram demonstrating absence of filling of left pulmonary arterial branches, indicative of large embolus obstructing left main pulmonary artery.

arteries by emboli usually results in the appearance of crescent-shaped defects along the lateral borders of the lung (Fig. 22-8). A normal ventilation scan can provide confirmatory evidence that the perfusion scan is demonstrating pulmonary emboli.

DIFFERENTIAL DIAGNOSIS. Inflammatory infiltrates of the lung may mimic recurrent pulmonary emboli, particularly on the chest roentgenogram. Significant fever, leukocytosis, and positive sputum cultures usually differentiate the inflammatory from the embolic lesions. Pulmonary edema may result from pulmonary emboli as well as heart disease. The differentiation is easy only in the absence of heart disease or murmurs. It is frequently difficult to differentiate a massive pulmonary embolism from acute myocardial infarction, and in this situation it may be necessary to perform pulmonary angiography to make an accurate diagnosis.

TREATMENT. Venous Interruption. It is generally agreed that interruption of the veins of the lower extremity is indicated if a pulmonary embolus occurs in a patient receiving adequate anticoagulant therapy or in one for whom anticoagulant therapy is contraindicated. In some centers, venous interruptions are even performed prophylactically or instead of administering anticoagulants. The interruption, which can be performed at the femoral vein level if the thrombi are localized in the distal veins, would be the procedure of choice in the desperately ill patient. Phlebography is routinely used in the author's clinic to assist in localizing the thrombi. The interruption should always be performed at the vena cava level in the presence of pelvic vein or iliac vein thrombosis.

Ligation or Division. Ligation or division of the femoral

Fig. 22-8. Radioisotope scans following intravenous injection of macroaggregated albumin tagged with [131]I. *A*. Massive pulmonary embolus to right lung. *B*. Small bilateral emboli evidenced by crescent-shaped defects.

vein is variously performed below the entrance of the deep femoral vein or below the entrance of the greater saphenous vein. The postligation sequelae are less severe if only the superficial femoral vein is ligated. However, the deep femoral vein is also frequently the site of thrombosis, and in such instances ligation of the superficial femoral vein would offer no protection. Donaldson et al. report that approximately 4 percent of patients treated by femoral vein interruption alone develop pulmonary emboli. This is an incidence approximately equal to that following anticoagulation therapy alone.

Ligation or division of the vena cava should be performed just distal to the right renal vein to prevent forming a pocket in which thrombi might develop. The operation requires a general or spinal anesthetic, as opposed to femoral vein ligation, which can be performed under local anesthesia. The incidence of pulmonary embolism following this procedure is generally lower than the reported incidence following femoral vein ligation. Its routine use

in desperately ill patients, however, can result in an increased mortality rate which may equal that from pulmonary embolism following femoral vein ligation.

The ligation of a vein in which there is distal venous thrombosis usually results in propagation of the thrombus to the site of the ligature. Recurrent phlebitis, pain, edema, and ulceration may ensue. Adams and DeWeese report a 30 to 35 percent incidence of these distressing postligation sequelae.

Partial Vein Interruption. In the hope of preventing postligation sequelae, partial interruptions of the femoral vein or inferior vena cava have been performed to allow normal venous flow and yet trap potential pulmonary emboli (Figs. 22-9, 22-10). The methods described include creation of a grid filter of silk sutures [DeWeese], compartmentalization of the vein with sutures [Spencer et al.], constriction of the vein with a plastic clip [Moretz], and compartmentalization of the vein with a plastic clip having serrated edges [Miles et al.]. Although thrombosis may occur at the site of the partial interruption or the vein may be occluded by a trapped embolus, the results of such an occurrence would be no worse than if the vein were ligated. Mobin-Uddin et al. devised a filter which can be introduced under local anesthesia through a small incision into the jugular vein. Under fluoroscopic control, the collapsed filter is passed to the lower vena cava on the tip of a catheter. As the catheter is withdrawn, the filter is dislodged, opens like an umbrella, and is impinged against the wall of the vena cava distal to the renal vein. However, the umbrella can be misplaced or subsequently dislodged, and at present it appears to be ideally suited for the desperately ill patient who requires interruption at the vena cava level. Greenfield has described the use of an intraluminal steel wire filter that can be introduced through the femoral vein and positioned in the inferior vena cava.

Fig. 22-9. Partial interruption of inferior vena cava: grid and compartmentalization.

DE WEESE
1958

SPENCER
1959

Table 22-1. VENA CAVA INTERRUPTIONS:
COMPARISON OF LIGATIONS AND
PARTIAL INTERRUPTIONS*

	Ligation	Partial interruptions
Operations	1,159	569
Operative mortality	14.0%	10.3%
Fatal emboli	1.3%	0.7%
Fatal shock	2.9%	0
Nonfatal emboli	4.1%	6.7%
Patent vena cava	0†	72.0%†
Disabling symptoms	23.0%‡	7.0%‡

*A summary of 30 reports.
†In patients who had postoperative vena cavagrams.
‡When late follow-up information was available.

Comparison of the reported results of all types of vena cava interruption indicates a slightly higher incidence of nonfatal pulmonary emboli following partial interruption than following ligation (6.7 versus 4.1 percent) (Table 22-1). The incidence of fatal emboli following both procedures is about 1 percent. However, fatal shock secondary to ligation of the vena cava with sudden decrease in venous return or massive distal venous thrombosis occurred in 2.9 percent of cases, compared to no observed occurrence following partial interruption.

When postoperative vena cavagrams are performed following partial interruptions, at least 70 percent are patent, and the incidence of significant late postphlebitic sequelae is only 7 percent following partial interruption compared to 23 percent following ligation. In addition, the large collaterals observed by Parrish et al. following vena cava ligation are capable of transmitting fatal pulmonary emboli from the lower extremities within a few weeks after operation.

Partial interruption of the femoral veins was also found by Adams et al. to be at least as effective as ligation in preventing pulmonary embolism and associated with less late extremity morbidity.

Urokinase Therapy. Urokinase activates the available plasminogen which causes lysis of thrombi. Treatment of pulmonary embolism with materials of high specific activity which are much less toxic and pyrogenic than previously available plasminogen activators was evaluated in a cooperative study. Twelve-hour urokinase infusion followed by at least 5 days of heparin was more effective than heparin alone in lysing thrombi, as seen by significantly greater improvement in pulmonary arteriograms, lung scans, and right heart pressure measurements. Unfortunately, bleeding complications were sufficiently frequent and severe that Sautter et al. felt urokinase therapy to be contraindicated within 10 days of childbirth or any operation within the major body cavity. Severe systemic hypertension, a recent cerebrovascular accident, active gastrointestinal bleeding, renal or hepatic insufficiency, active rheumatic disease, bacterial endocarditis, a history of nephritis, or pregnancy at any stage were also considered contraindications. No significant differences in the rate of pulmonary embolism recurrence or in the 2-week mortality rate were observed. The report concluded that further evaluation of urokinase in the treatment of pulmonary thromboembolism is indicated before specific therapeutic recommendations can be made.

Pulmonary Embolectomy. Approximately 95 percent of patients with a pulmonary embolism massive enough to cause hypotension die. Although most of them die within a few minutes, at least 25 percent live longer than 1 hour. In 1908 Trendelenburg first advocated the emergency removal of large emboli from the pulmonary artery. From 1908 to 1962 only 17 survivors of such a procedure were reported. Since the development of cardiopulmonary bypass, however, pulmonary embolectomies are performed much more frequently. With this technique the main pulmonary arteries can be opened leisurely and emboli removed. Peripheral emboli can also be evacuated by massaging the lung and by the use of catheters to which suction is applied. It may be possible to use a portable temporary

Fig. 22-10. Partial interruption of inferior vena cava using serrated clip. *A.* Transperitoneal approach is preferred to permit high interruption of vena cava and concomitant ligation of the left spermatic or ovarian veins. *B.* Kocher maneuver. *C.* Vena cava cleared immediately below renal veins. *D.* Clip applied. *E.* Clip closed. *F.* Final position of clip in the immediate infrarenal region to prevent cul-de-sac. (*From J. T. Adams and J. A. DeWeese, Surg Gynecol Obstet, 123:1087, 1966.*)

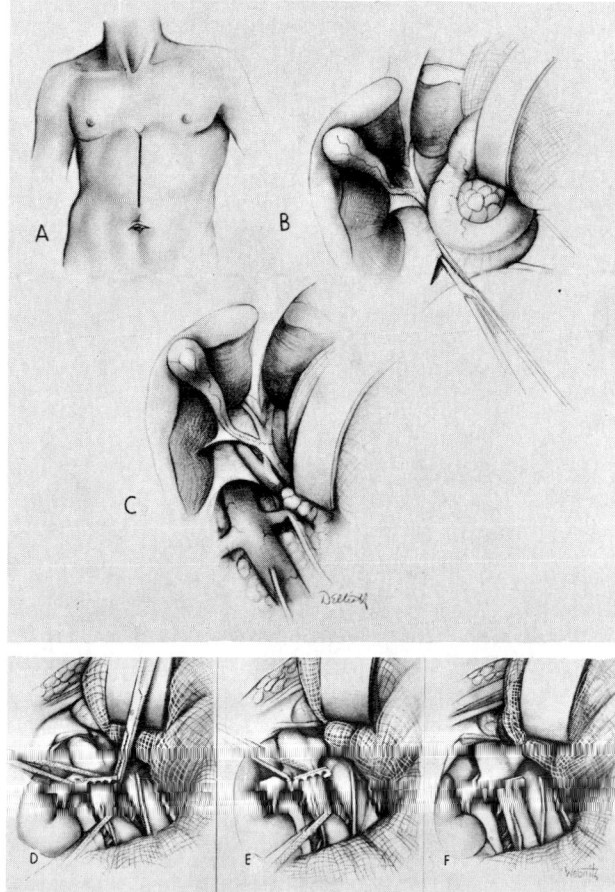

cardiopulmonary bypass to sustain desperately ill patients until they can be transported to the operating room. The studies of Sautter et al. suggest that urokinase therapy is preferable to pulmonary embolectomy for patients recovering from shock. Patients with cardiac arrest or unresponsive shock are still candidates for emergency cardiopulmonary bypass and pulmonary embolectomy.

VENOUS INSUFFICIENCY AND VENOUS ULCERS

There are three conditions of the veins of the lower extremities associated with venous ulcers. These are varicose veins, incompetent perforators, and deep venous abnormalities. Venous ulcers usually appear in the presence of one, two or all three of these conditions, and they are therefore best discussed together. The abnormality common to all is reflux of blood from the deficiency or absence of competent valves.

Hippocrates (460–377 B.C.) is credited with first noting the association between varicose veins and ulcers of the leg and recommending the use of compression bandages in their treatment. However, many centuries elapsed before the role of deep venous abnormalities in the etiology of venous ulcers was appreciated. Gay and Homans demonstrated the relation between postthrombotic changes including the destruction of venous valves, and venous ulcers. More recently Linton and also Dodd and Cockett have emphasized the role of the incompetent perforator in causing ankle ulceration.

Anatomy and Physiology

The veins of the lower extremity consist of superficial veins, deep veins, and perforating veins which join the superficial and deep systems. The superficial veins consist of the greater saphenous and lesser saphenous veins. The greater saphenous vein begins on the dorsum of the foot, passes *anterior* to the medial malleolus, ascends the medial calf and thigh lying close to the deep fascia, and enters the common femoral vein in the groin through the fossa ovalis. Several smaller veins join the greater saphenous vein along its course. The important branches, clinically, include the anterior and posterior branches of the lower leg, which enter the major vein in the upper medial calf region, and the lateral and medial branches of the upper leg, which join the saphenous in the upper thigh (Fig. 22-11A). The lesser saphenous vein begins posterior to the lateral malleolus, ascends the posterior calf, where it pierces the deep fascia, usually near the popliteal fossa, and enters the popliteal vein (Fig. 22-11B).

The deep veins, in general, follow the course of the major arteries and carry the same names. In the lower leg, however, the veins are routinely paired. The paired anterior tibial, posterior tibial, and peroneal veins join to form the popliteal vein in the region of the knee. The popliteal vein passes beneath the adductor tendon, where it becomes the superficial femoral vein and is joined by the deep femoral vein in the upper thigh to become the common femoral vein. The common femoral veins become the external iliac veins as they pass beneath the inguinal ligament and are joined in the pelvis by the internal iliac

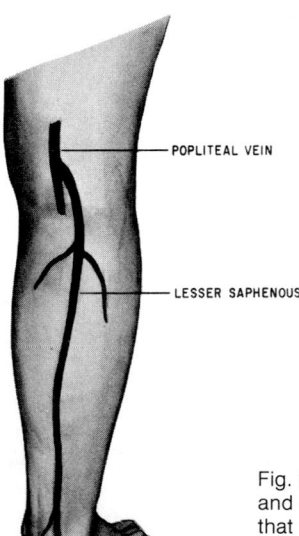

Fig. 22-11. A. Usual course of greater saphenous vein and its major branches in lower leg, emphasizing fact that branch varicosities are the ones usually seen. Perforating veins, posterior and superior to medial malleoli, are indicated. B. Usual course of lesser saphenous vein in lower leg.

veins to become the common iliac veins; these veins join to become the inferior vena cava.

There are numerous veins perforating the deep fascia connecting the superficial and deep veins. The most constant and clinically important of these perforators are those posterior and superior to the medial malleoli. These perforators, which usually are three in number, connect the posterior branch of the greater saphenous vein to the paired posterior tibial veins. One perforator usually lies posterior to the medial malleolus, the second is 5 to 10 cm superior to the first, and the third is 5 to 10 cm higher (Fig. 22-11*A*). A similar perforator connects the lesser saphenous and peroneal veins posterior and superior to the lateral malleolus.

Normal veins contain bicuspid valves, which, although sometimes found in other areas, are almost always just distal to major branches. In the upper leg only a few valves are found, whereas in the lower leg they are numerous in both the superficial and deep systems. The valves are oriented to permit flow of blood superiorly in the superficial and deep veins. More important is the fact that the valves in the perforators normally allow flow only from the superficial to the deep veins (Fig. 22-12).

There is normally a progressive decrease in mean pressure in the bloodstream beginning in the left ventricle and ending in the right atrium. It is this force from behind, or vis a tergo, that guarantees the continued flow of blood in the venous system. The actual pressure in any one vessel, however, is also dependent on the effect of gravity. In the standing resting position, therefore, the actual pressure in any vein includes a hydrostatic pressure approximately equivalent to the distance between the vein and the heart. The actual pressures in the arteries are also increased by hydrostatic pressure, and venous flow continues.

In addition to vis a tergo, venous return is aided by muscular action and possibly by respiration. Contraction of the calf muscles, for example, squeezes blood from the intramuscular veins into the deep veins. In addition, the veins which pass through the relatively rigid fascial compartment about the muscle are also compressed by the muscle. The combined result is an increase in pressure and flow in the popliteal vein and increased venous return with muscular contraction. During relaxation of the muscles the popliteal venous pressure falls below the resting pressure, and increased emptying of the superficial veins into the deep veins occurs, so that with repeated muscular activity the quantity of blood in the superficial veins decreases and superficial venous pressure decreases to below normal resting pressures. It must be emphasized that these normal variations in venous pressure and flow are dependent upon normal valves. Valves in the calf veins prevent reflux of blood distad when the venous pressure is increased by muscle contraction. Valves in the perforators prevent reflux of blood from the deep into the superficial veins during muscular contraction. The negative intrathoracic pressure which is accentuated by inspiration is believed by some to increase venous return. This positive effect is probably offset by the increased abdominal pressure secondary to descent of the diaphragm, which slows venous return.

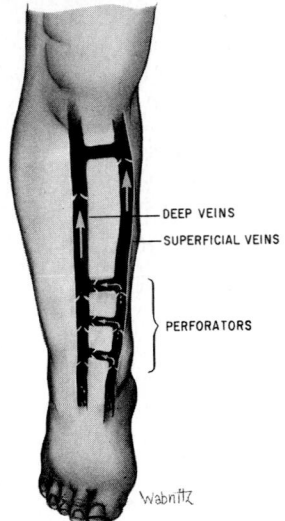

Fig. 22-12. Orientation of valves and flow of blood in superficial, deep, and perforating veins of lower leg.

Etiology of Venous Insufficiency

The causes of venous insufficiency are varicose veins, incompetent perforators, and deep vein abnormalities.

VARICOSE VEINS. The term *varicose veins* is usually applied to dilated, tortuous, elongated branches of the greater and lesser saphenous veins. These branches are quite superficial and are, therefore, most easily seen. The same changes occur to a much lesser extent in the greater and lesser saphenous veins themselves. The important abnormality in both the branches and the major superficial veins is the incompetency of their valves.

It is not known whether the valvular incompetency is the cause of the dilatation of the veins in varicosities or whether the dilatation of the valvular ring occurs first and causes secondary valvular incompetence. There are probably several causes of varicose veins. The rare presence of varicose veins in very small children without other visible arterial and venous malformations indicates that they may be congenital. The occurrence of severe varicosities in several members of a family suggests that heredity may be important in some cases. The frequent appearance of varicosities during pregnancy is well known, but it is not known whether hormonal influence, increased pelvic venous blood flow, or the mechanical effect of the enlarged uterus is the primary cause of these varicosities. The appearance of varicose veins in patients with congenital or acquired arteriovenous shunts implicates these as causative factors. The appearance of branch varicosities following superficial venous thrombosis indicates that trapping and fragmentation of the valves by the thrombus as it retracts to the wall and becomes organized is of importance in some instances. The predilection of varicose veins for the lower extremities in human beings, as opposed to quadrupeds, and for people in professions requiring long periods of standing indicates that the hydrostatic pressure in the veins of the lower extremities in the standing resting position aggravates and may actually cause varicosities.

INCOMPETENT PERFORATORS. There are numerous perforators between the superficial and deep veins. The largest and most constant are those posterior and superior to the medial and lateral malleoli. Normally these perforators cannot be demonstrated clinically. When their valves are incompetent, however, they become dilated and may form rather large localized dilatations at their junctions with the superficial vein. Defects in the deep fascia of the leg at the site where the dilated perforators pierce the fascia may be palpated. The frequent occurrence of incompetent perforators following deep venous thrombosis suggests that the valvular damage in these instances is secondary to recanalization of the perforators. Incompetent perforators, however, may be found in patients without known previous venous thrombosis but with varicose veins. It is likely, therefore, that the factors which cause venous dilatation and valvular incompetency in the valves of other veins may also cause incompetency of the valves of the perforating veins.

DEEP VEIN ABNORMALITIES. The most common abnormalities of the deep veins result from thrombosis of the veins. Following thrombosis, the major deep veins may become patent by gross recanalization, or they may remain functionally occluded, with only microscopic recanalization. With gross recanalization, the veins have the phlebographic appearance of irregular walled valveless tubes. If the veins remain occluded, numerous dilated collaterals *without apparent valves* are visualized. Examination of the occluded major veins demonstrates only microscopic recanalization. The deficiency or absence of valves and the dilatation of the deep veins is observed also in many patients with complicated varicose vein problems. This suggests that the congenital or familial causes of varicosities may also cause deep vein abnormalities.

Symptoms of Venous Insufficiency

The symptoms most frequently attributed to venous insufficiency of the lower extremities include aching, swelling, and night cramps.

An "aching" discomfort in the lower legs is frequently described by patients with severe venous insufficiency. With lesser degrees of insufficiency, "tenderness" of the legs or a "heaviness" may be described. The discomfort may occur soon after arising in the morning but usually begins after a period of relatively inactive standing or sitting. In many women the symptoms are worse just before and during the first part of the menstrual period. The symptoms are relieved by elevation of the legs.

Edema of the lower leg may also occur in venous insufficiency. Although it may occur with varicose veins alone, it is almost always seen in patients with deep venous abnormalities and incompetent perforators. It usually appears during the course of the day and is aggravated by prolonged standing or sitting. It usually disappears or is markedly decreased during a night's sleep.

The explanation for the heaviness, tiredness, and aching is the increase in the weight of the lower extremities sec-

ondary to an increase in volume of blood and edema fluid. In a normal individual the erect position is associated with an increased volume of blood in the legs. This volume is increased in venous insufficiency, where dilated veins increase the potential storage space and incompetent valves hinder venous return. Normally the erect position is also associated with an increased amount of interstitial fluid, transferred across the capillary membrane. This fluid is normally resorbed by the capillaries or lymphatics. Resorption by the veins is primarily due to the osmotic force exerted by the intravascular protein, but an increase in venous pressure can overcome the osmotic force and prevent resorption. The venous pressure at the ankle in the normal erect individual is sufficient to prevent resorption, and an increase in interstitial fluid is observed. In normal individuals, however, the venous pressure is markedly decreased by the frequent muscular contractions occurring with daily living. The same exercise in patients with venous insufficiency causes lesser decreases in the pressure and hence more significant increases in interstitial fluid (or edema). Lymphatic abnormalities can also decrease the resorption of the interstitial fluid. Such abnormalities may be observed in patients following venous thrombosis.

Night cramps are due to sustained contractions of muscles and most frequently occur in the muscles of the calf and feet. They usually appear after a few hours of sleep. They are relieved by massage or by standing and walking. Night cramps may be associated with a number of other abnormalities besides venous insufficiency. Night cramps secondary to venous insufficiency, however, can be relieved by proper management. The underlying cause of the increased muscular irritability or increased muscular stimulation is unknown.

Physical Findings

The changes which may be observed in patients with venous insufficiency include edema, brawny induration, brownish discoloration, dermatitis, and ulceration.

Edema may not be observed in patients with varicose veins, but it is almost always present to some degree in patients with deep vein pathologic conditions and incompetent perforators. It may be soft and pitting initially and may completely disappear overnight. In the presence of long-standing venous insufficiency, however, the edema becomes more firm and may decrease slowly and minimally with elevation. It then acquires a "woody" feeling, termed *brawny induration,* due to increased connective tissue in the subcutaneous tissue. This scarring may be secondary to excess protein in the interstitial tissue (see section below on lymphedema) or to repeated trauma, infection, and phlebitis.

Brown pigmentation of the lower leg is frequently observed in long-standing venous insufficiency, particularly about healed ulcers. It is known to be secondary to hemosiderin in the subcutaneous tissue, presumably derived from the breakdown of extravasated blood.

Various types of dermatitis may be seen in patients with venous insufficiency. Dryness and scaling with some pruritis may be seen over prominent varices, particularly at the ankle level. Although the cause is unknown, this condition is apparently related to the underlying venous abnormalities, since it will disappear with treatment of the venous insufficiency alone. Skin infections secondary to dermatophytosis (athlete's foot) may be seen. The most frequent dermatitis, however, is secondary to local medications. The allergic dermatitis may be particularly difficult to control.

Venous ulcers are almost always found in the lower third of the lower leg and are particularly common posterior and superior to the medial and lateral malleoli (Fig. 22-13). Characteristically they are shallow ulcerations with surrounding rims of bluish discoloration and erythema. They may penetrate to the level of the deep fascia or tendons, but not through them. They can, however, erode veins or even arteries. They may on occasion encircle the leg.

The ulcers may appear spontaneously or follow trivial trauma. The underlying problem, however, is venous insufficiency, a point frequently forgotten by the patient and ignored by the physician treating him. Their occurrence in the ankle region incriminates the high venous pressure of the superficial veins in that region as a prime cause. Further support for this hypothesis is the fact that ulcerations are more common in patients with deep vein abnormalities and incompetent perforators than in patients with varicose veins alone. The high venous pressure results in localized varicosities and edema, with consequent increased deposition of fibrous tissue. A localized area of redness, tenderness, and brawny induration frequently precedes an ulcer. Dodd and Cockett present interesting pathologic material to support the thesis that this preulcer state is due to thrombosis of small end veins in the subcutaneous tissue resulting in fat necrosis. A contusion, laceration, or necrosis of the skin over this area results in a deep ulceration because of the underlying fat necrosis.

Although the above chain of events may occur rapidly after the onset of venous insufficiency, it more commonly occurs several years later. Bauer followed a group of patients with known deep venous thrombosis for several years: ulcers appeared in 20 percent of the patients within 5 years, in 52 percent within 10 years, and in 79 percent at a later date.

Tests for Venous Insufficiency

There are a number of tests for diagnosing of venous insufficiency which are also helpful in understanding the pathophysiology of the condition and differentiating the various causes.

PERCUSSION TEST. This test was originally described as a means of determining the incompetency of valves in superficial veins. The saphenous vein is tapped near the saphenofemoral junction and the opposite hand placed over the knee to feel the impulse transmitted through an unbroken column of blood if the valves are incompetent. The percussion of veins may actually be more helpful in other ways. The greater saphenous vein in the thigh usually lies quite close to the deep fascia and is neither visible nor palpable, particularly in obese individuals. Percussion of a varix in the region of the knee, with the opposite hand

Fig. 22-13. Venous ulcers of lower leg.

following the expected course of the greater saphenous vein, can confirm the association of the varix with the greater saphenous vein. In addition, once the varicose saphenous vein is found by percussion, its size can be estimated. In a similar fashion the size, position, and importance of the lesser saphenous vein in the popliteal space can be determined by tapping varicosities on the posterior calf.

COMPRESSION TESTS. These tests are usually associated with the name of Trendelenburg. The patient lies down and elevates the involved leg until the superficial veins are collapsed. The saphenous vein is then compressed high in the thigh with the fingers of the hand or with a *tight* tourniquet (part 1). With the hand or tourniquet in place, the patient stands up. The sites of previously noted varicosities are carefully observed for 20 to 30 seconds (part 2). The tourniquet is then removed and the veins again carefully observed. There are four possible results of the test:

1. Negative-negative (Fig. 22-14*A*). In the presence of normal veins there is gradual ascending filling of the superficial veins when the patient stands up; part 1 is negative. With release of compression the gradual filling continues; part 2 is negative.
2. Negative-positive (Fig. 22-14*B*). In the presence of incompetent valves in the greater saphenous vein without incompetent valves in the perforators, part 1 is negative. With release of compression, however, there is rapid reflux of blood from the femoral vein into and down the greater saphenous vein, with rapid distension of the varicosities; part 2 is positive.
3. Positive-negative (Fig. 22-14*C*). In the presence of incompetent valves in the perforators, there is reflux of blood from the deep to the superficial system when the patient stands up. The varices in the region of the perforator becomes rapidly filled, and part 1 is positive. If the saphenofemoral valve is competent, there is no further rapid distension of the veins when the compression is released, and part 2 is negative.
4. Positive-positive (Fig. 22-14*D*). In the presence of incompetent valves in the perforators and also in the greater saphenous vein, filling of the varices occurs on standing, and further rapid filling occurs after the compression is released. Both part 1 and part 2 are positive.

Thus the test can detect the presence of an incompetent saphenous vein and determine the site of incompetent perforators.

VENOUS PRESSURE. The normal standing resting pressure in the saphenous vein at the level of the ankle is

NEGATIVE   **A**   NEGATIVE   NEGATIVE   **B**   POSITIVE

Fig. 22-14. Four possible results of Trendelenburg compression test. Patient has been lying down with leg elevated; he then stands up with compression over saphenofemoral junction. *A.* Negative-negative response, in which there is gradual filling of veins from below over a 30-second period and there is continued slow filling after release of hand. *B.* Negative-positive response. On standing, there is gradual filling of distal veins; on release of compression there is rapid retrograde filling of saphenous vein. *C.* Positive-negative response. With hand in place, filling of superficial varicosities through incompetent perforators occurs; with release of compression there is further slow filling of the veins. *D.* Positive-positive response. On standing with hand in place, there is filling of varices through incompetent perforators. On release of compression there is additional rapid filling of saphenous vein.

slightly higher than the hydrostatic pressure of a column of blood reaching from the tip of the catheter to the level of the right midatrium. There are no significant differences in the standing resting pressures for normal extremities and for extremities with varicose veins, incompetent perforators, or abnormal deep vein valves. With walking or rhythmic contraction of the calf muscles, different venous pressure responses are noted (Fig. 22-15). Normally there is a marked decrease in the saphenous vein pressure with exercise, indicating that the muscular action has increased the flow of blood in the deep veins and allowed increased drainage of blood from the superficial to the deep veins during muscular relaxation. When exercise stops, there is a gradual return of venous pressure to normal levels, indicating that the valves in the deep and the superficial systems are competent, preventing rapid reflux of blood. Extremities with varicose veins demonstrate lesser decreases in venous pressure with exercise and more rapid return to normal levels when walking ceases; that is, some of the effect of the rapid emptying of the superficial veins with exercise is counteracted by reflux of blood from the femoral vein into the saphenous vein with its incompetent valves. When exercise stops, there is rapid reflux of blood down the saphenous vein. In the presence of uncomplicated varicose veins, pressure on the saphenofemoral junction or operative removal of the varicosity can result in a normal venous pressure response. Extremities with postthrombotic veins demonstrate little if any decrease in pressure with exercise. After cessation of exercise the venous pressure rapidly returns to normal. The normal decrease in pressure with exercise is prevented by the reflux of blood

back down the abnormal valveless deep veins during muscular relaxation and the propulsion of blood through incompetent perforators during muscular contraction. Ligation of the femoral vein in these patients does not significantly improve the venous pressure response. In the presence of significant obstruction of the deep veins, such as may be seen following a major venous thrombosis or during some pregnancies, the venous pressure actually increases with exercise. Following exercise, the pressure slowly decreases to normal.

FUNCTIONAL PHLEBOGRAPHY. Phlebograms performed with the patient in the semierect position before and immediately after a standard active exercise may demonstrate important pathologic and physiologic abnormalities:

1. The patient lies on a table tilted 60° from the horizontal.
2. A #21 needle is inserted into any superficial vein on the dorsum of the foot and a tourniquet applied snugly to the ankle.

POSITIVE   **C**   NEGATIVE

Fig. 22-14 (continued)

3. Over a 1-minute period, 50 ml of any suitable angiographic contrast material is injected.
4. Radiographs of the entire lower extremity are taken before and after the patient stands on his toes ten times.

Normally, slender veins with prominent valves are visualized, and after exercise little radiopaque material is seen except in the cusps of the valves. In the presence of varicose veins alone, the appearance of the deep veins before and after exercise is usually the same as with normal veins. If the superficial veins are visualized, tortuosity and dilatation of the veins may be seen. Following deep venous thrombosis, the veins may be completely recanalized but valveless. They may also remain obstructed, in which case numerous dilated valveless collaterals are visualized. Following exercise there is poor emptying of the radiopaque material from the deep veins, and increased filling of collateral veins, perforating veins, and superficial veins may be seen. Similar changes and responses to exercise may be seen in patients with dilated valveless deep veins presumably of congenital or familial origin. The poor emptying of the radiopaque dye from the veins and dye reflux through perforators into the superficial veins is another demonstration of the abnormal valvular function seen in patients with venous insufficiency.

Differential Diagnosis

Lymphedema may be confused with the edema of venous insufficiency in the early postthrombotic phase

POSITIVE   **D**   POSITIVE

Fig. 22-15. Responses in venous pressure of superficial veins at ankle with exercise. In standing position, venous pressure is slightly higher than hydrostatic pressure in column extending from ankle to heart. This pressure is approximately the same for normal persons and for those with venous insufficiency or chronically obstructed veins in which collaterals have formed. With walking, however, normal persons demonstrate rapid decrease in venous pressure and slow return to normal when exercise stops; patients with varicose veins show lesser decrease in pressure with walking but more prompt return to normal following cessation of exercise; patients with postthrombotic veins demonstrate little if any decrease in venous pressure with walking and rapid return to normal; patients with obstructed veins show increase in pressure with walking and slow return to normal.

AMBULATORY VENOUS PRESSURE CHANGES

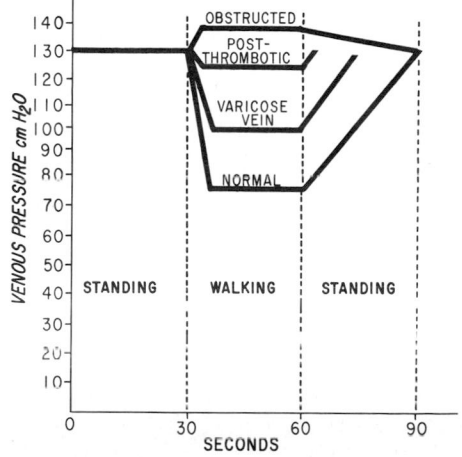

before brawny induration, brownish discoloration, and ulceration occur. Lymphedema, however, generally is of a rubbery consistency and is nonpitting. The edema of congestive heart failure and renal failure is usually bilateral and should also be differentiated by the history and physical examination. Phlebography is particularly helpful in ruling out deep venous thrombosis as a cause of edema.

Venous ulcers almost always occur behind the medial and lateral malleoli. Their positions and associated brawny induration and brownish discoloration generally differentiate them from arterial ulcers, which may occur anywhere on the lower leg, usually have a surrounding blue and then erythematous ring, and are much more painful than venous ulcers. It should also be noted that venous ulcers do not penetrate fascia as arterial ulcers commonly do. A malignant tumor should be suspected in ulcerations of long duration, particularly if they do not respond to proper management.

Treatment

The management of these patients is demanding but rewarding. A single operative procedure is rarely curative except in the mildest cases. Careful education of the patient in the nonoperative management is of utmost importance. In addition, the patients must be seen periodically in order to be sure that they are continuing proper elastic support and periodic elevation.

NONOPERATIVE MANAGEMENT. The nonoperative management of patients with venous insufficiency is based on decreasing the amount of blood sequestration in the veins of the lower extremities and decreasing the venous pressure in the superficial veins.

Elevation of the legs overcomes the hydrostatic pressure in the veins and thereby decreases the pressure and the amount of blood in the dilated valveless veins. It should be emphasized that this is accomplished ideally only when the legs are elevated above the level of the heart, which is facilitated by having the patient sleep with the foot of the bed or the foot of the mattress elevated. During the day, the patient should lie on a couch with the feet elevated on pillows. A sitting posture in a chair with the legs outstretched does not provide adequate elevation.

Active exercise, except in the presence of obstruction, also decreases the volume and pressure in the veins of the lower extremities. Walking is excellent exercise. Standing, without muscular contraction, and sitting increase the volume and pressure of the peripheral venous blood.

Compression of the superficial veins also decreases the volume of the venous pool and if strong enough overcomes the venous pressure transmitted through the superficial veins via incompetent perforators. Means of providing compression vary in strength and, in order of increasing effectiveness, include nylon support hose, ordinary cotton elastic stockings, snugly applied Ace bandages, heavy-duty cotton elastic stockings (Truform), specially constructed pressure-gradient stockings (Jobst), Gelucast, Unna's paste, or Elastoplast boots, and canvas boots containing an inflatable rubber bladder (Aeropulse). The goals of any compression therapy are the relief of symptoms and the prevention of measurable evening swelling of the legs. The importance of proper elastic support in accomplishing this goal cannot be overemphasized. Nylon support hose and ordinary cotton elastic stockings are effective only in the management of patients with very mild venous insufficiency. Ace bandages are only as good as the care with which they are applied. The management of patients with moderate to severe insufficiency and particularly those with ulceration demands the use of one of the stronger means of support.

The severity of the venous insufficiency governs the type of therapy prescribed. A patient with mild symptomatic varicosities might find relief of symptoms and edema with ordinary cotton elastic stockings and elevation of the legs whenever there is a choice between lying down and sitting down. A patient with severe venous insufficiency would need more aggressive treatment similar to the "new way of life" described by Luke. The patient may require overnight elevation of the legs, planned periodic elevation of the legs during the day, and strong elastic support. The nonoperative management of patients with venous ulcers is primarily an aggressive management of the venous insufficiency as outlined above. The use of local medications should be avoided unless a definite secondary infection is present. Increasing the local pressure over the ulcer by means of a sponge rubber pad beneath a strong elastic support can usually heal ulcers of silver-dollar size and sometimes larger.

OPERATIVE MANAGEMENT. Surgical treatment may in some instances be curative, but in most instances is merely helpful as an adjunct to the conservative management of venous insufficiency.

Ligation and Stripping of Greater or Lesser Saphenous Veins. The ligation and stripping of the saphenous veins should not be performed unless incompetency of the vein is demonstrated by the Trendelenburg test. The indications for the procedure are (1) moderate to severe symptomatic varicosities, (2) severe varicosities, even though the patient does not admit to symptoms, (3) severe venous insufficiency with recurrent ulcerations, in association with aggressive nonoperative management. Patients with mild varicosities and significant symptoms usually do not benefit from the procedure, and it is usually found that the symptoms are due to some unrelated cause or to deep venous abnormalities. Significant edema rarely accompanies greater saphenous varicosities alone and is not appreciably helped by vein stripping. Treatment of other underlying conditions or the aggressive nonoperative management of deep venous abnormalities is necessary.

The operative procedure (Fig. 22-16) consists of ligation of the greater saphenous vein at its junction with the femoral vein and ligation of its four major branches at the margin of the transverse groin incision. The entire vein is then stripped from its bed by making a separate incision at the ankle, passing a wire within the lumen in a craniad direction the length of the vein, transecting the vein in the ankle, and avulsing the entire vein by pulling on the wire from the groin incision. The branches of the veins break off near their junctions with the saphenous vein, but bleeding is minimal, particularly if the feet are markedly ele-

Fig. 22-16. Ligation and stripping of saphenous vein. *A,* Groin incision, showing junction of greater saphenous and femoral veins. Note four major branches of saphenous vein which required ligation and division. *B,* counterincision at knee or ankle to permit stripping of saphenous vein. Additional incisions to permit removal of branch varicose veins.

vated during the operation. As noted before, however, the visible varicosities are usually found in the branches of the vein, and attention must also be directed toward them. Some surgeons prefer to remove the veins through separate incisions at the time of the original operation, others prefer to inject the remaining branches with sclerosing solutions at a later date. These solutions produce a localized phlebitis and thrombosis of the veins. The veins will remain obstructed unless complete recanalization of the lumen occurs.

Fegan has advocated the injection of veins, followed by 6 weeks of continuous elastic compression, for the treatment of varicosities. Doran and White, in a randomized study, concluded that patients who were treated by Fegan's method required significantly less additional treatment at 1 year than those who underwent operation. Long-term results were not available, however, and it is still generally agreed that an operation followed by injection, if necessary, is the treatment of choice.

Following operation, snug elastic stockings are applied, and the foot of the bed is elevated above the level of the heart. During the first week after operation patients are allowed up to walk or allowed to lie in bed with the feet elevated. Sitting is prohibited except for bathroom privileges. During the second week patients find it necessary to elevate the legs during a portion of the day to avoid discomfort. During the third or fourth week after operation they gradually increase their activities to their preoperative level.

Ligation of Incompetent Perforators. Incompetent perforators rarely occur without other types of venous insufficiency. Their ligation, however, may be a valuable adjunct to the nonoperative management of patients with venous insufficiency. It is particularly effective if performed before the patient develops an ulcer. This preulcer state may be recognized by the presence of telangiectasia, brownish pigmentation, or mild brawny induration behind the medial or lateral malleoli. The operation is also indicated

after the nonoperative healing of recurrent ulcers. It should not be performed in the presence of an active infected ulcer.

Various techniques for ligation of the perforators in the lower leg have been described by Linton, Felder and associates, and Dodd and Cockett. Dodd and Cockett point out that the perforators most frequently associated with ulcers are those posterior and superior to the medial and lateral malleoli. Longitudinal incisions are made posterior and superior to the malleoli; then the perforators are interrupted above or below the fascia near their communication with the deep veins (Fig. 22-17). Extensive undermining of the tissue should be avoided, since there is a risk of sloughing of the overlying skin. Ligation of perforators is only an adjunctive measure, and aggressive nonoperative treatment of the underlying deep venous abnormalities is still indicated.

Ligation of the Superficial Femoral or Popliteal Veins. Some surgeons advocate the ligation of the superficial femoral or popliteal veins in the presence of deep venous abnormalities. The procedure was originally advocated to prevent reflux of blood down valveless normal deep veins. However, postoperative phlebograms in patients who have had this type of operation indicate that the obstructed deep veins are only replaced by dilated valveless collaterals. In addition, venous pressure measurements indicate that after such ligations increased venous hypertension occurs.

LYMPHATICS AND LYMPHEDEMA

Anatomy and Physiology of Lymphatic Return

The lymphatic system provides a means of returning certain extravascular materials in the interstitial space to the bloodstream. Normally there is a constant leakage of fluid and protein through the arterial capillary membrane into the interstitial space. The water and solutes can be resorbed by the vascular capillaries; the protein cannot. Proteins, however, can readily enter the lymphatic capillaries. Other materials, including red blood cells, bacteria, and small particulate matter, can also pass through the lymphatic capillary membrane.

The lymphatic capillaries form a superficial plexus within the dermis which covers the whole body surface.

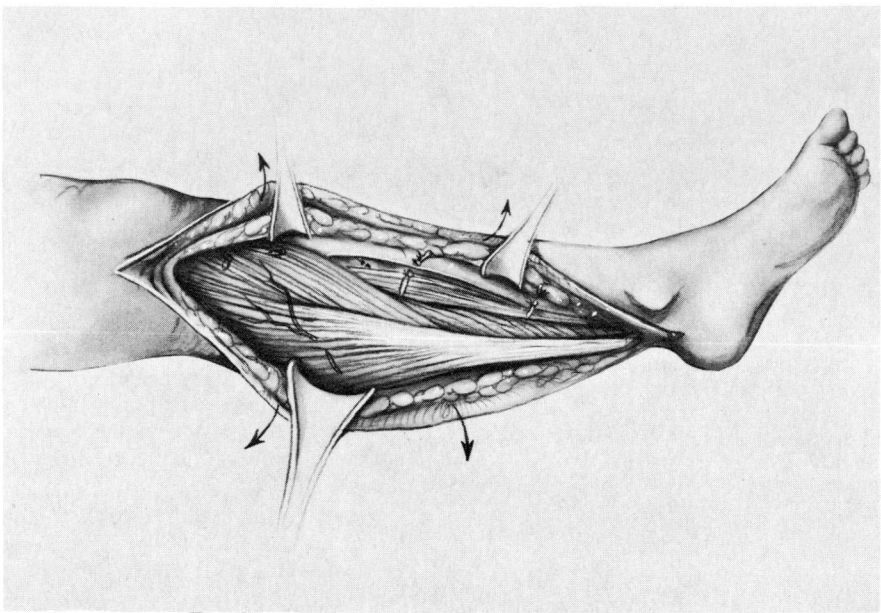

Fig. 22-17. Perforating veins interrupted subfascially. Skin flaps are carefully developed, and the great and small saphenous veins and the subcutaneous tissue, with many communicating veins, are excised. (*After D. Silver, J. J. Gleysteen, G. R. Rhodes, N. G. Georgiade, and W. G. Anlyan, Surgical Treatment of the Refractory Postphlebitic Ulcer, Arch Surg, 103:554, 1971. Copyright 1971, American Medical Association.*)

Another similar plexus lies in the deep dermis or subdermal region. These join other deeper lymphatics to form larger vessels which, in general, follow the course of the major blood vessels to the neck, where they empty into the bloodstream at the junction of the internal jugular and the subclavian vein. The continuity of the larger lymphatics is interrupted by lymph nodes, which acts as filters and also contribute lymphocytes to the lymph. The lymph vessels contain valves which direct the flow of lymph toward the neck. The movement of the lymph is aided by extrinsic factors such as muscle contraction, arterial pulsations, respiratory movement, and massage.

Information regarding the normal or altered anatomy and physiology of the lymphatics can be obtained from special examinations, including (1) dye injections of the superficial dermal lymphatics, (2) lymphangiography, and (3) analysis of the protein content of edema fluid.

DYE INJECTIONS. Hudack and McMaster introduced patent blue dye, and Butcher and Hoover used 4% direct sky blue dye for the intradermal injection of the human superficial dermal lymphatics; 0.2 ml is inserted via a 30-gauge needle, and in normal skin a network of very fine intradermal lymphatic capillaries is demonstrated within 30 to 60 seconds after injection (Fig. 22-18).

LYMPHANGIOGRAPHY. Kinmonth demonstrated the feasibility of obtaining radiographs of the lymphatics. Patent blue dye or direct sky blue dye is injected into the subcutaneous tissue of the foot. The dye rapidly enters the lymphatics. Massage of the foot and muscular contractions increase the lymph flow. An incision is then made on the dorsum of the foot and a cannula inserted into a blue-dye-filled lymphatic; 10 ml of radiopaque dye is injected, and x-rays of the entire extremity are made.

Normally the slender lymphatics, unlike veins, appear of uniform caliber throughout their course. Unlike veins, they bifurcate as they proceed proximally. As with veins,

slight dilatations at the level of the valves are visualized (Fig. 22-18).

ANALYSIS OF THE PROTEIN CONTENT OF EDEMA FLUID. Edema fluid can be collected by the insertion of a special Southey tube into the subcutaneous tissue. The protein content of peripheral edema fluid secondary to venous, heart, or renal disease is less than 1.5 Gm/100 ml. Since the lymphatics are responsible for removal of protein from the interstitial space, abnormally high levels of protein would reflect abnormal lymphatic function.

Lymphedema

Congenital or acquired abnormalities of the lymphatics may hinder the lymphatic capillaries from absorbing materials such as proteins or prevent the main channels from carrying sufficient quantities of tissue fluid from a limb. The result is an accumulation of plasma protein in the tissue spaces. This protein concentration is of high osmotic pressure, causing absorption of fluid into the extravascular space. Edema, or in other words lymphedema, is the result.

ETIOLOGY. The various types of lymphedema have been outlined by Taylor as follows:

1. Primary lymphedema
   a. Congenital
   b. Lymphedema precox
2. Secondary lymphedema
   a. Neoplastic invasion
   b. Surgical excision

Fig. 22-18. Diagnostic procedures for lymphedema: dye injections, lymphangiograms, and protein analysis.

c. Radiotherapy
d. Inflammation or parasitic invasion
e. Motor paralysis

Primary Lymphedema. Primary lymphedema of the lower extremities is caused by abnormal development of the lymph vessels. The edema may be present at birth and is then called *congenital lymphedema*. More frequently the edema appears during the teens and is then termed *lymphedema precox*. It may appear insidiously or may follow minor trauma or infection. Primary lymphedema is about three times more common in females than in males. It involves both legs in about 50 percent of patients.

Secondary Lymphedema. Secondary lymphedema is usually due to obstruction or destruction of normal lymphatic channels. It may, therefore, follow obstruction of the lymphatics by tumor, repeated infection, or parasitic infestation. It may also follow the excision of lymph nodes, as during a radical mastectomy or radical groin dissection. Irradiation therapy, particularly for malignant disease, may similarly destroy the lymphatics.

PATHOPHYSIOLOGY. Primary Lymphedema. Kinmonth et al. performed lymphangiograms on 87 patients with pri-

mary lymphedema. Aplasia, or the absence of any significant lymphatic trunks in the subcutaneous tissue, was observed in 14 percent of the extremities. Dye injected beneath the skin, however, would travel great distances through dilated dermal vessels. Hypoplasia, a deficiency in size or number of lymphatic vessels, was seen in 55 percent of the extremities. Dye injected subcutaneously in the interdigital webs would frequently appear in the dermal plexus of the dorsum of the foot. Varicose lymphatics which were broader and more tortuous than normal were observed in 24 percent of the patients. Dye injected subcutaneously would frequently appear in dermal lymphatics some distance from the site of the injection. This "dermal backflow" in the lymphatics is assumed to be secondary to incompetency of valves in the lymphatics. It can be demonstrated also by the intradermal injection of dye, when "skip areas" in the filling of the dermal lymphatics is observed. The protein content of the edema fluid of patients with primary lymphedema, studied by Crockett and by Taylor et al., was found to be greater than 2 Gm/100 ml in 41 of 48 patients. It would appear, therefore, that the underlying cause of the edema is the inability of the lymphatic system to remove protein from the interstitial fluid at a normal rate. In primary lymphedema this lymphatic insufficiency may be due to aplasia, hypoplasia, or varicosities of the lymphatic vessels (Fig. 22-18).

Secondary Lymphedema. Lymphangiograms of patients with acquired lymphedema demonstrate the point of obstruction of the lymphatics. The remaining vessels appear normal, but there is considerable dermal backflow of the radiopaque material. Intradermal dye injections demonstrate dilatations and prominence of the dermal lymphatics. The inability of the lymphatics to effectively remove protein from the interstitial fluid can be demonstrated by measurements of the protein content of the edema fluid (Fig. 22-18).

CLINICAL MANIFESTATIONS. Symptoms. The usual symptoms of primary and secondary lymphedema are the same. Edema increases during the course of the day and decreases overnight, but the limb always remains larger. There is gradual increase in the degree of swelling over a period of years. The edema may cause some fatigue and be cosmetically objectionable but in most instances causes no real concern. In others the disability is significant, particularly in those with elephantiasis secondary to filariasis.

Physical Findings. Lymphedema is characteristically a firm, rubbery, nonpitting edema. Early in the course of the disease the edema is somewhat softer, and much of it will disappear overnight with elevation of the legs. With the passage of time the edema may become woody in character. This is a result of an increase of fibrous tissue within the subcutaneous tissue, which is believed to be secondary to the increase in protein-rich edema fluid. Repeated infections will hasten growth of fibrous tissue. Some patients develop small blisters containing edema fluid of high protein content. These blisters may occur on the lower abdomen and upper thigh and contain a milky white fluid with the characteristics of chyle; they are believed to be secondary to reflux from the retroperitoneal lymphatics. Hyperkeratosis of the skin is common in long-standing lymphedema.

COMPLICATIONS. Recurrent Cellulitis and Lymphangitis. The major complication of lymphedema is recurrent attacks of cellulitis and lymphangitis. These attacks may occur without warning or may follow minor injuries or infections in the extremity. They are characterized by an elevated temperature, constitutional symptoms of malaise, nausea and vomiting, and local symptoms of redness, pain, and increased swelling of the involved limb. Beta-hemolytic streptococci are the offending organisms and, if carefully looked for, may be found at the site of minor injuries, in the nose and throat, in blood cultures, or in edema fluid. The protein-rich edema fluid is apparently an excellent culture medium, since the lymphedematous limb is very susceptible to repeated infections. Once the infection starts it spreads rapidly.

Lymphangiosarcoma. A rare but serious complication of lymphedema is the appearance of lymphangiosarcoma. This malignant tumor is most frequently described in patients with lymphedema following a radical mastectomy for breast cancer but is also seen in long-standing lymphedema due to other causes. It is usually first recognized as a bruiselike blue or reddish purple nodule in the skin of the lymphedematous extremity. As the primary lesion enlarges, satellite tumors appear about it. Metastases appear early in the course of the disease, particularly to the lung.

Protein-losing Enteropathy. Very rarely patients with primary lymphedema of their legs may also develop a protein-losing enteropathy. Using mesenteric lymphangiography, Kinmonth and Cox have been able to demonstrate localized lymphatic obstructions of bowel wall treatable by resection of a segment of bowel.

DIFFERENTIAL DIAGNOSIS. The firm, rubbery, non-pitting character of unilateral lymphedema usually differentiates it from the soft, pitting, bilateral edema secondary to heart failure, renal failure, hypothyroidism, or aldosteronism. Some deep cavernous hemangiomas may be confused with lymphedema, but the presence of overlying birthmarks, the sponginess of the hemangiomas, and their decrease in size on elevation usually indicate the correct diagnosis. The edema of an acute postoperative or infectious lymphedema may be confused with deep venous thrombosis, and a phlebogram may be most helpful in establishing the correct diagnosis. The edema of chronic venous insufficiency can usually be differentiated from lymphedema because of its brawniness, overlying brownish discoloration, and telangiectasia. However, lymphedema is commonly a complication of acute thrombophlebitis, and venous insufficiency and lymphedema may coexist. Streptococcal infection should be carefully searched for in the patient with a postphlebitic extremity who is repeatedly admitted to the hospital with high fever and redness, tenderness, and marked swelling of the leg. In the author's experience these cases are usually labeled "recurrent phlebitis" but in actuality are recurrent cellulitis and lymphangitis secondary to lymphedema.

Whenever there is a question of deep venous disease versus lymphedema, a phlebogram may be helpful in establishing the diagnosis of deep venous disease, and the author has found dye injections of the superficial dermal lymphatics helpful in confirming the diagnosis of lymphedema. Lymphangiograms and, in confusing cases, analysis of the protein content of the edema fluid may be necessary to establish the diagnosis.

TREATMENT. Nonoperative Management. The conservative management of lymphedema is directed toward control of the edema and prevention of recurrent infection. Elevation of the involved extremity above the level of the heart will increase lymph drainage by reducing the hydrostatic pressure within the lymph vessels. Patients are therefore instructed to elevate the foot of the bed; they are also instructed to lie down and elevate the extremity whenever they have the opportunity. Massage is also known to increase lymph flow. Special apparatuses are available to accomplish this: one is a cloth sleeve containing a plastic bladder that can be alternately inflated and deflated to produce a rhythmic pneumatic compression of the entire extremity; another is a series of bladders that can be sequentially inflated and deflated to give a massaging effect beginning at the hand or foot and extending to the shoulder or thigh. When the maximal decrease in edema is achieved by these methods, very tight elastic stockings or canvas boots containing an inflatable rubber bladder can be applied. These supports can prevent reaccumulation of edema fluid. In addition they provide a semirigid encasement of the extremity so that muscular action, which causes alterations in the volume of the leg, can produce a massaging effect on the lymphatics. Diuretics may be helpful in reducing the size of the limb temporarily. However, none of the procedures mentioned can completely return the limb to its normal size, particularly in long-standing cases; they can only delay or prevent progression of the process.

The control of the recurrent bouts of infection associated with lymphedema is important. Ideally it should be possible to prevent these by control of edema, local hygiene, avoidance of trauma, and prevention of athlete's foot. These procedures alone are usually not sufficient, however, and the use of prophylactic antibiotics may be indicated. Since the offending organism is almost always the streptococcus, oral penicillin is the drug of choice.

Surgical Treatment. Surgical treatment is indicated for a very small percentage of patients with lymphedema. The indications include excessive edema, when the weight and size of the limb interfere with normal activities, and recurrent bouts of cellulitis. Surgery for cosmetic reasons alone is rarely indicated, since after an effective operation a disproportion in the size of the two limbs will still usually remain, and in addition the scars resulting from the operation may still call attention to the limb.

Numerous surgical approaches to the problem are described, including (1) insertion of silk threads, Teflon wicks, or polyethylene tubing into the subcutaneous tissue in the hope of draining the edema fluid into normal tissue; (2) removal of long strips of fascia in the hope that new anastomoses will form between the superficial and deep lymphatics, as advocated by Thompson; (3) construction of pedicle grafts from the involved limb to the trunk in the hope of bypassing obstructed lymphatics; (4) excision of long strips of subcutaneous tissue and deep fascia to reduce the size of the limb; (5) complete excision of all the skin, subcutaneous tissue, and deep fascia from the limb, followed by application of split-thickness skin grafts to the exposed muscle and periosteum, as originally described by Charles.

The Charles procedure is, in the author's opinion, the most effective of the surgical procedures. The size and weight of the limb are effectively reduced, and there is lower incidence of recurrent cellulitis and lymphangitis after removal of the edematous subcutaneous tissue. It should be reemphasized, however, that this, like other treatments for lymphedema, cannot return the limb to a normal appearance.

References

Venous Thrombosis and Pulmonary Embolism

Adams, J. T., and DeWeese, J. A.: Experimental and Clinical Evaluation of Partial Vein Interruption in the Prevention of Pulmonary Emboli, *Surgery*, **57:**82, 1965.

——— and ———: Comparative Evaluation of Ligation and Partial Interruption of the Femoral Vein in the Treatment of Thromboembolic Disease, *Ann Surg*, **172:**795, 1970.

——— and ———: "Effort" Thrombosis of the Axillary and Subclavian Veins, *J Trauma*, **11:**923, 1971.

———, Feingold, B. E., and DeWeese, J. A.: Comparative Evaluation of Ligation and Partial Interruption of the Inferior Vena Cava, *Arch Surg*, **103:**272, 1971.

Allen, E. V., Hines, E. A., Jr., Kvale, W. F., and Barker, N. W.: The Use of Dicumarol as an Anticoagulant: Experience in 2,307 Cases, *Ann Intern Med*, **27:**371, 1947.

Artz, C. P., and Amspacher, W. H.: Evaluation of Various Methods of Administration of Heparin, *Surg Forum*, **3:**530, 1952.

Barner, H. B., and DeWeese, J. A.: An Evaluation of the Sphygmomanometer Cuff Pain Test in Venous Thrombosis, *Surgery*, **48:**915, 1960.

Barritt, D. W., and Jordan, S. C.: Anticoagulant Drugs in the Treatment of Pulmonary Embolism: A Controlled Trial, *Lancet*, **1:**1309, 1960.

Bauer, G. A.: Roentgenological and Clinical Study of the Sequels of Thrombosis, *Acta Chir Scand* [*Suppl*], **86:**74, 1942.

Bauer, G.: Clinical Experiences of a Surgeon in the Use of Heparin, *Am J Cardiol*, **14:**29, 1964.

Berger, R. L.: Pulmonary Embolectomy with Preoperative Circulatory Support, *Ann Thorac Surg*, **16:**217, 1973.

Brockman, S. K., and Vasko, J. S.: Phlegmasia Cerulea Dolens, *Surg Gynecol Obstet*, **121:**1347, 1965.

Browse, N. L.: The ^{125}I Fibrinogen Uptake Test, *Arch Surg*, **104:**160, 1972.

Byrne, J. J., and O'Neil, E. E.: Fatal Pulmonary Emboli: A Study of 130 Autopsy-proven Fatal Emboli, *Am J Surg*, **83:**47, 1952.

Carey, L. C., and Williams, R. D.: Comparative Effects of Dicumarol, Tromexan, and Heparin on Thrombus Propagation, *Ann Surg*, **152:**919, 1960.

Cegelski, F. C., DeWeese, J. A., and Lund, C. J.: Deep Iliofemoral Venous Thrombosis during Pregnancy, *Am J Obstet Gynecol*, **89:**510, 1964.

Cooley, D. A., and Beall, A. C., Jr.: A Technic of Pulmonary Embolectomy Using Temporary Cardio-pulmonary Bypass, *J Cardiovasc Surg (Torino)*, **2:**469, 1961.

Coon, W. W.: The Spectrum of Pulmonary Embolism: Twenty Years Later, *Arch Surg*, **111:**398, 1976.

——— and Coller, F. A.: Clinicopathologic Correlation in Thromboembolism, *Surg Gynecol Obstet*, **109:**259, 1959.

——— and ———: Some Epidemiologic Considerations of Thromboembolism, *Surg Gynecol Obstet*, **109:**487, 1959.

———, Mackenzie, J. W., and Hodgson, P. E.: A Critical Evaluation of Anticoagulant Therapy in Peripheral Venous Thrombosis and Pulmonary Embolism, *Surg Gynecol Obstet*, **106:**129, 1958.

Cosgriff, S. W.: Thromboembolism, *Am J Med*, **3:**758, 1947.

Cotton, L. T., and Roberts, V. C.: The Prevention of Deep Vein Thrombosis, with Particular Reference to Mechanical Methods of Prevention, *Surgery*, **81:**228, 1977.

Crane, C.: Deep Venous Thrombosis and Pulmonary Embolism, *N Engl J Med*, **257:**147, 1957.

——— : Femoral vs. Caval Interruption for Venous Thromboembolism, *N Engl J Med*, **270:**819, 1964.

Cranley, J. J., Gay, A. Y., Grass, A. M., and Simeone, F. A.: Plethysmographic Technique for the Diagnosis of Deep Venous Thrombosis of the Lower Extremities, *Surg Gynec Obstet*, **136:**385, 1973.

Dale, W. A.: Inferior Vena Caval Ligation for Venous Thrombo-embolism, *Rev Surg,* **19:**1, 1962.

Deaton, H. L., Anlyan, W. G., Silver, D., and Webster, J.: Thrombosis: Prevention and Treatment, *Surgery,* **49:**130, 1961.

DeBakey, M. E.: A Critical Evaluation of the Problem of Thromboembolism, *Surg Gynecol Obstet,* **98:**1, 1954.

DeWeese, J. A.: Current Status of Plastic Procedures on the Venous System, *NJ Acad Med Bull,* **7:**1, 1961.

———: The Role of Pulmonary Embolectomy in Venous Thromboembolism, *J Cardiovasc Surg (Torino),* **17:**348, 1976.

———: Thrombectomy for Acute Iliofemoral Venous Thrombosis, *J Cardiovasc Surg (Torino),* **5:**703, 1964.

———, Adams, J. T., and Gaiser, D. L.: Subclavian Venous Thrombectomy, *Circulation,* **41, 42** (*Suppl* II):158, 1970.

———, Kraft, R. O., Nichols, W. K., Six, H. H., and Thompson, N. W.: Fifteen-Year Clinical Experience with the Vena Cava Filter, *Ann Surg,* **178:**247, 1973.

——— and Rogoff, S. M.: Phlebographic Patterns of Acute Deep Venous Thrombosis of the Leg, *Surgery,* **53:**99, 1963.

———, ———, Phillips, C. E., Jr., and Pories, W. J.: Deep Venous Thrombosis, *Postgrad Med,* **29:**614, 1961.

DeWeese, M. S., and Hunter, D. C.: A Vena Cava Filter for the Prevention of Pulmonary Embolism, *Arch Surg,* **86:**852, 1963.

Dmochowski, J. R., Adams, D. F., and Couch, N. P.: Impedance Measurement in the Diagnosis of Deep Venous Thrombosis, *Arch Surg,* **104:**170, 1972.

Donaldson, G. A., Linton, R. R., and Rodkey, G. V.: A Twenty-Year Survey of Thromboembolism at the Massachusetts General Hospital, 1939–1959, *N Engl J Med,* **265:**208, 1961.

Edwards, W. H., Sawyers, J. L., and Foster, J. H.: Iliofemoral Venous Thrombosis: Reappraisal of Thrombectomy, *Ann Surg,* **171:**961, 1970.

Engelberg, H., and Berk, M. Z.: Prolonged Anticoagulant Therapy with Subcutaneously Administered Concentrated Aqueous Heparin, *Surgery,* **36:**762, 1954.

Flanc, C., Kakkar, V. V., and Clarke, M. B.: Postoperative Deep-Vein Thrombosis: Effect of Intensive Prophylaxis, *Lancet,* **1:**477, 1969.

Fogarty, T. J., and Krippaehne, W. W.: Catheter Technique for Venous Thrombectomy, *Surg Gynecol Obstet,* **121:**362, 1965.

Fontaine, R., and Tuchmann, L.: The Role of Thrombectomy in Deep Venous Thromboses, *J Cardiovasc Surg (Torino),* **5:**298, 1964.

Gibbs, N. M.: Venous Thrombosis of the Lower Limbs with Particular Reference to Bed-Rest, *Br J Surg,* **45:**15, 1957.

Gomez, R. L., Wheeler, H. B., Belko, J. S., and Warren, R.: Observations on the Uptake of a Radioactive Fibrinolytic Enzyme by Intravascular Clots, *Ann Surg,* **158:**905, 1963.

Greenfield, L. J., Peyton, M. D., Brown, P. P., and Elkins, R. C.: Transvenous Management of Pulmonary Embolic Disease, *Ann Surg,* **180:**461, 1974.

Hafner, C. D., Cranley, J. J., Krause, R. J., and Strasser, E. S.: A Method of Managing Superficial Thrombophlebitis, *Surgery,* **55:**201, 1964.

Haller, J. A., and Abrams, B. L.: Use of Thrombectomy in the Treatment of Acute Iliofemoral Venous Thrombosis in Forty-five Patients, *Ann Surg,* **158:**561, 1963.

Henderson, R. R.: Pulmonary Embolism and Infarction, *Med Clin North Am,* **48:**1425, 1964.

Herrmann, L. G.: Superficial Venous Thrombosis (Saphenous Thrombophlebitis): Should Treatment be Empirical or Definitive? *J Cardiovasc Surg (Torino),* **5:**239, 1964.

Hughes, E. S. R.: Venous Obstruction in the Upper Extremity (Paget-Schroetter's Syndrome): A Review of 320 Cases, *Int Abstr Surg,* **88:**89, 1949.

Hume, M.: The Relation of "Hypercoagulability" to Thrombosis, *Monogr Surg Sci,* **2:**133, 1965.

Hunter, W. C., Sneeden, V. D., Robertson, T. D., and Snyder, G. A. C.: Thrombosis of the Deep Veins of the Leg, *Arch Intern Med,* **68:**1, 1941.

Jorpes, J. E.: Heparin: Its Chemistry, Pharmacology and Clinical Use, *Am J Med,* **33:**692, 1962.

Kakkar, V.: The Diagnosis of Deep Vein Thrombosis Using the ^{125}I Fibrinogen Test, *Arch Surg,* **104:**152, 1972.

———: Prevention of Fatal Postoperative Pulmonary Embolism by Low Doses of Heparin, *Lancet,* **2:**45, 1975.

Lawen, A.: Weitere Erfahrungen über operative Thrombenentfernung bei Venenthrombose, *Arch Klin Chir,* **193:**723, 1938.

Lewis, C. E., Jr., Antoine, J., Mueller, C., Talbot, W. A., Swaroop, R., and Edwards, W. S.: Elastic Compression in the Prevention of Venous Stasis, *Am J Surg,* **132:**739, 1976.

Mahorner, H., Castleberry, J. W., and Coleman, W. O.: Attempts to Restore Function in Major Veins Which Are the Site of Massive Thrombosis, *Ann Surg,* **146:**510, 1957.

Mavor, G. E.: Deep Vein Thrombosis, *Postgrad Med J,* **47:**311, 1971.

McLachlin, J., and Paterson, J. C.: Some Basic Observations on Venous Thrombosis and Pulmonary Embolism, *Surg Gynecol Obstet,* **93:**1, 1951.

———, Richards, T., and Paterson, J. C.: An Evaluation of Clinical Signs in the Diagnosis of Venous Thrombosis, *Arch Surg,* **85:**738, 1962.

Miles, R. M., Chappell, F., and Renner, O.: A Partially Occluding Vena Caval Clip for Prevention of Pulmonary Embolism, *Am Surg,* **30:**40, 1964.

Mobin-Uddin, K., McLean, R., Bolooki, H., and Jude, J. R.: Caval Interruption for Prevention of Pulmonary Embolism: Long Term Results of a New Method, *Arch Surg,* **99:**711, 1969.

———, Trinkle, J. K., and Bryant, L. R.: Present Status of the Inferior Vena Cava Umbrella Filter, *Surgery,* **70:**914, 1971.

Moretz, W. H., Rhode, C. M., and Shepherd, M. H.: Prevention of Pulmonary Emboli by Partial Occlusion of the Inferior Vena Cava, *Am Surg,* **25:**617, 1959.

Moser, K. M., Guisan, M., Cuomo, A., and Ashburn, W. L.: Differentiation of Pulmonary Vascular from Parenchymal Diseases by Ventilation/Perfusion Scintiphotography. *Ann Int Med,* **75:**597, 1971.

———, Houk, V. N., Jones, R. C., and Hufnagel, C. C.: Chronic, Massive Thrombotic Obstruction of the Pulmonary Arteries: Analysis of Four Operated Cases, *Circulation,* **32:**377, 1965.

Murray, G.: Anticoagulants, in Venous Thrombosis and the Prevention of Pulmonary Embolism, *Surg Gynecol Obstet,* **84:**665, 1947.

Nabseth, D. C., and Moran, J. M.: Reassessment of the Role of Inferior-Vena-Cava Ligation in Venous Thromboembolism, *N Engl J Med,* **273:**1250, 1965.

Parrish, E. H., Adams, J. T., Pories, W. J., Burget, D. E., and DeWeese, J. A.: Pulmonary Emboli Following Vena Caval Ligation, *Arch Surg,* **97:**899, 1968.

Ravdin, I. S., and Kirby, C. K.: Experiences with Ligation and Heparin in Thromboembolic Disease, *Surgery,* **29:**334, 1951.

Robb, G. P., and Steinberg, I.: Visualization of the Chambers of the Heart, the Pulmonary Circulation, and the Great Blood Vessels in Man, *Am J Roentgenol Radium Ther Nucl Med,* **41:**1, 1939.

Roberts, B., Rosato, F. E., and Rosato, E. F.: Heparin—A Cause of Arterial Emboli? *Surgery,* **55:**803, 1964.

Robin, E. D., Julian, D. G., Travis, D. M., and Crump, C. H.: A Physiologic Approach to the Diagnosis of Acute Pulmonary Embolism, *N Engl J Med,* **260:**586, 1959.

Sautter, R. D., Myers, W. O., Ray, J. F., III, and Wentzel, F. J.: Pulmonary Embolectomy: Review and Current Status, *Prog Cardiovasc Dis,* **17:**371, 1975.

———, ———, and Wenzel, F. J.: Implications of the Urokinase Study Concerning the Surgical Treatment of Pulmonary Embolism, *J Thorac Cardiovasc Surg,* **63:**54, 1972.

Sawyer, R. B., Moncrief, J. A., and Canizaro, P. C.: Dextran Therapy in Thrombophlebitis, *JAMA,* **191:**740, 1965.

Schwartz, S. I.: Diagnosis of Thromboembolic Disease, *J Cardiovasc Surg (Torino),* suppl. issue, VII Congress of International Cardiovascular Society, Philadelphia, Sept. 5–18, 1965.

Sharp, E. H.: Pulmonary Embolectomy: Successful Removal of Massive Pulmonary Embolus with Support of Cardiopulmonary Bypass: Case Report, *Ann Surg,* **156:**1, 1962.

Short, D. S.: A Survey of Pulmonary Embolism in a General Hospital, *Br Med J,* **1:**790, 1952.

Sigel, B., Felix, W. R., Jr., Popky, G. L., and Ipsen, J.: Diagnosis of Lower Limb Venous Thrombosis by Doppler Ultrasound Technique, *Arch Surg,* **104:**174, 1972.

Spencer, F. C., Quattlebaum, J. K., Quattlebaum, J. K., Jr., Sharp, E. H., and Jude, J. R.: Plication of the Inferior Vena Cava for Pulmonary Embolism: A Report of 20 Cases, *Ann Surg,* **155:**827, 1962.

Stein, G. N., Chen, J. T., Goldstein, F., Israel, H. L., and Finkelstein, A.: The Importance of Chest Roentgenography in the Diagnosis of Pulmonary Embolism, *Am J Roentgenol Radium Ther Nucl Med,* **81:**255, 1959.

Szucs, M. M., Jr., Brooks, H. L., Grossman, W., Banas, J. S., Jr., Meister, S. G., Dexter, L., and Dalen, J. E.: Diagnostic Sensitivity of Laboratory Findings in Acute Pulmonary Embolism, *Ann Int Med,* **74:**161, 1971.

Templeton, J. Y.: Endvenectomy for the Relief of Obstruction of the Superior Vena Cava, *Am J Surg,* **104:**70, 1962.

Trenwith, B. J., and Dooss, T. W.: Soleus Rupture: Differential Diagnosis of Calf Thrombosis, *NZ Med J,* **82:**18, 1975.

Tsapogas, M. J., Goussous, H., Peabody, R. A., Karmody, A. M., and Eckert, C.: Postoperative Venous Thrombosis and the Effectiveness of Prophylactic Measures, *Arch Surg,* **105:**561, 1971.

Urokinase-Streptokinase Embolism Trail, Phase 2 Results, *JAMA,* **229:**1606, 1974.

Wagner, H. N., Sabiston, D. C., Jr., McAfee, J. G., Tow, D., and Stern, H. S.: Diagnosis of Massive Pulmonary Embolism in Man by Radioisotope Scanning, *N Engl J Med,* **271:**377, 1964.

Wessler, S., and Morris, L. E.: Studies in Intravascular Coagulation: IV. The Effect of Heparin and Dicumarol on Serum-induced Venous Thrombosis, *Circulation,* **12:**553, 1955.

Wheeler, H. B., Pearson, D., O'Connel, D., and Mullick, S. C.: Impedance Phlebography: Technique, Interpretation, and Results, *Arch Surg,* **104:**164, 1972.

Williams, J. R., Wilcox, W. C., Andrews, G. J., and Burns, R. R.: Angiography in Pulmonary Embolism, *JAMA,* **184:**473, 1963.

Williams, R. D., and Zollinger, R. W.: Surgical Treatment of Superficial Thrombophlebitis, *Surg Gynecol Obstet,* **118:**745, 1964.

Zilliacus, H.: On the Specific Treatment of Thrombosis and Pulmonary Embolism with Anticoagulants, with Particular Reference to the Post-thrombotic Sequelae, *Acta Med Scand [Suppl],* **171:**13, 1946.

Venous Insufficiency and Ulcers

Bauer, G.: A Roentgenological and Clinical Study of the Sequels of Thrombosis, *Acta Chir Scand,* **86**(Suppl 74):1, 1942.

DeCamp, P. T., Schramel, R. J., Ray, C. J., Feibleman, N. D., Ward, J. A., and Ochsner, A.: Ambulatory Venous Pressure Determinations in Postphlebitic and Related Syndromes, *Surgery,* **29:**44, 1951.

DeWeese, J. A.: Functional Popliteal Phlebography in the Patient with a Complicated Varicose Vein Problem, *Surgery,* **44:**390, 1958.

———, and Rogoff, S. M.: Clinical Uses of Functional Ascending Phlebography of the Lower Extremity, *Angiology,* **9:**268, 1958.

——— and ———: Functional Ascending Phlebography of the Lower Extremity by Serial Long Film Technique: Evaluation of Anatomic and Functional Detail in 62 Extremities, *Am J Roentgenol Radium Ther Nucl Med,* :841, 1959.

Dodd, H., and Cockett, F. B.: "The Pathology and Surgery to the Veins of the Lower Limb," E. & S. Livingstone Ltd., Edinburgh and London, 1956.

Doran, F. S. A., and White, M.: Clinical Trial Designed to Discover if Primary Treatment of Varicose Veins Should be by Fegan's Method or by Operation, *Br J Surg,* **62:**72, 1975.

Edwards, E. A., and Edwards, J. E.: The Effect of Thrombophlebitis on the Venous Valve, *Surg Gynecol Obstet,* **65:**310, 1937.

Felder, D. A., Murphy, T. O., and Ring, D. M.: A Posterior Subfascial Approach to the Communicating Veins of the Leg, *Surg Gynecol Obstet,* **100:**730, 1955.

Fell, S. C., McIntosh, H. D., Hornsby, A. T., Horton, C. E., Warren, J. V., and Pickrell, K.: The Syndrome of the Chronic Leg Ulcer: The Phlebodynamics of the Lower Extremity; Physiology of the Venous Valves, *Surgery,* **38:**771, 1955.

Gay, J.: On Varicose Diseases of the Lower Extremities, in "The Lettsomian Lectures of 1867," J. & A. Churchill Ltd., London.

Homans, J.: The Etiology and Treatment of Varicose Ulcer of the Leg, *Surg Gynecol Obstet,* **24:**300, 1917.

Linton, R. R.: The Post-thrombotic Ulceration of the Lower Extremity: Its Etiology and Surgical Treatment, *Ann Surg,* **138:**415, 1953.

Luke, J. C.: The Deep Vein Valves, *Surgery,* **29:**381, 1951.

Myers, T. T.: Results and Technique of Stripping Operation for Varicose Veins, *JAMA,* **163:**87, 1957.

Pollack, A. A., Taylor, B. E., Myers, T. T., and Wood, E. H.: The Effect of Exercise and Body Position on the Venous Pressure at the Ankle in Patients Having Venous Valvular Defects, *J Clin Invest,* **28:**559, 1949.

Schneewind, J. H.: The Walking Venous Pressure Test and Its Use in Peripheral Vascular Disease, *Ann Surg,* **140:**137, 1954.

Scott, W. J. M., and Radakovich, M.: Venous and Lymphatic Stasis in the Lower Extremities: I. A. Test for Incompetence in the Perforating Veins; II. A Simple Method of Adequate Control, *Surgery,* **26:**970, 1949.

Staffon, R. A., and Buxton, R. W.: Deep Vein Ligation in the Postphlebitic Extremity, *Surgery,* **41:**471, 1957.

Veal, J. R., and Hussey, H. H.: The Venous Circulation in the Lower Extremities during Pregnancy, *Surg Gynecol Obstet,* **72:**841, 1941.

Warren, R., White, E. A., and Belcher, C. D.: Venous Pressures in the Saphenous System in Normal Varicose and Postphlebitic Extremities: Alterations following Femoral Vein Ligation, *Surgery,* **26:**435, 1949.

Lymphatics and Lymphedema

Brush, B. E., Wylie, J. H., Jr., and Beninson, J.: Some Devices for the Management of Lymphedema of the Extremities, *Surg Clin North Am,* **392:**1493, 1959.

Butcher, H. R. Jr., and Hoover, A. L.: Abnormalities of Human Superficial Cutaneous Lymphatics Associated with Stasis Ulcers, Lymphedema, Scars, and Cutaneous Autografts, *Ann Surg,* **142:**633, 1955.

Charles, R. H.: In A. Latham and T. C. English (eds.), "A System of Treatment," vol. 3, p. 516, J. & A. Churchill, Ltd., London, 1912.

Crockett, D. J.: The Protein Levels of Oedema Fluids, *Lancet,* **2:**1179, 1956.

Gibson, T., and Tough, J. S.: The Surgical Correction of Chronic Lymphoedema of the Legs, *Brit J Plast Surg,* **7:**195, 1954.

Hudack, S. S., and McMaster, P. D.: The Lymphatic Participation in Human Cutaneous Phenomena: A Study of the Minute Lymphatics of the Living Skin, *J Exp Med,* **572:**751, 1933.

Jantet, G. H., Taylor, G. W., and Kinmonth, J. B.: Operations for Primary Lymphedema of the Lower Limbs: Results after 1–9 Years, *J Cardiovasc Surg (Torino),* **2:**27, 1961.

Khodadadeh, M., and Johnson, R.: Lymphangiosarcoma Arising from Postmastectomy Lymphedema, *JAMA,* **186:**1097, 1963.

Kinmonth, J. B.: Lymphangiography in Man: A Method of Outlining Lymphatic Trunks at Operation, *Clin Sci,* **11:**13, 1952.

——— and Cox, S. J.: Protein-Losing Enteropathy in Primary Lymphoedema: Mesenteric Lymphography and Gut Resection, *Br J Surg,* **61:**589, 1974.

———, Taylor, G. W., Tracy, G. D., and Marsh, J. D.: Primary Lymphoedema: Clinical and Lymphangiographic Studies of a Series of 107 Patients in Which the Lower Limbs Were Affected, *Br J Surg,* **45:**1, 1957.

Scott, W. J. M., and Radkovich, M.: Venous and Lymphatic Stasis in the Lower Extremities: I. A Test for Incompetence in the Perforating Veins; II. A Simple Method of Adequate Control, *Surgery,* **26:**970, 1949.

Taylor, G. W.: Lymphoedema, *Postgrad Med J,* **35:**2, 1959.

———, Kinmonth, J. B., and Dangerfield, W. G.: Protein Content of Oedema Fluid in Lymphoedema, *Br Med J,* **1:**1159, 1958.

Wakim, K. G., Martin, G. M., and Krusen, F. H.: Influence of Centripetal Rhythmic Compression on Localized Edema of an Extremity, *Arch Phys Med Rehabil,* **36:**98, 1955.

Yoffey, J. M., and Courtice, F. C.: "Lymphatics, Lymph and Lymphoid Tissue," Harvard University Press, Cambridge, Mass., 1956.

Chapter 23

Surgically Correctible Hypertension

by **John H. Foster**

Systemic hypertension and its associated cerebrovascular, renal, and cardiovascular sequelae are among the most common causes of crippling illness and death in the world today. Gordon and Devine estimated in the early 1960s that there were 17 million people with hypertension in the United States; current estimates are that 30 million people have hypertension. Although the vast majority of hypertensive patients have essential hypertension, an increasingly significant percentage, estimated to be between 5 and 10 percent of all hypertensive patients, are being found to have a specific underlying lesion which is surgically correctible.

PHYSIOLOGY AND PATHOPHYSIOLOGY

Blood flows through a series of elastic arterial tubes. The peak pressure within arteries, a reflection of ventricular contraction, is referred to as systolic pressure. Residual resting pressure during ventricular diastole accounts for the diastolic pressure. The accepted upper limit of normal blood pressure in the adult is 140/90 mm Hg. The so-called "normal" varies with age as follows. Infants, 70/45 mm Hg, early childhood 85/55 mm Hg, and adolescence 100/75 mm Hg.

The factors influencing arterial blood pressure include (1) viscosity of blood, (2) blood volume, (3) cardiac output, (4) elasticity of arterial wall, and (5) peripheral resistance.

An increase in viscosity results in an increase in resistance to blood flow and may give rise to hypertension, as in polycythemia. An increase in the amount of blood or fluid circulating in the vascular system may also result in hypertension, just as a reduction in the blood volume is manifest by hypotension. The cardiac output, which refers to the volume of blood pumped into the vascular system per unit of time, is an important determinant. An increase in output, as in thyrotoxicosis, may cause hypertension, whereas the decrease which accompanies myocardial disease and cardiomyopathies is attended by hypotension. The arterial wall normally relaxes in systole and contracts in diastole; loss of this function, as in rigid arteriosclerotic vessels, results in increased systolic and decreased diastolic pressure. Perhaps the most important determinant in the development of systemic hypertension is the peripheral resistance within the arteriolar segments of the vascular system. Small changes in arterial caliber result in marked changes in resistance and pressure, chiefly the diastolic pressure.

Although each of these factors may influence the blood pressure, the effect depends largely on the modifying influence of the autonomic nervous system and on renal and hormonal contributions. Reflex arcs within the nervous system control the vasomotor tone, cardiac rate, and cardiac output. Proprioceptors or baroreceptors in the aortic wall and carotid sinus participate in the reflex arcs and play an important role in the regulation of blood pressure.

In most cases of hypertension, little is known about the factors which alter the arteriolar tone and caliber. Age, race, and environment are significant but ill-defined factors in essential hypertension. A more precise role has been determined for certain humoral agents in a small percentage of patients. Excessive production of catecholamines such as epinephrine and norepinephrine by the adrenal medulla in cases of pheochromocytoma has been shown to increase small-vessel tone and consequently increase peripheral resistance. Adrenal cortical hormones have also been implicated in clinical hypertension. Aldosterone, the sodium-retaining hormone of the cortex, has been shown to potentiate the rise in blood pressure caused by pressor agents. Excessive secretion of aldosterone is accompanied by retention of sodium and water, with consequent expansion of the blood volume and resultant hypertension. Although sodium seems to have an unquestioned role in human hypertension, the mechanism or locus of its effect is unclear. The volume-expansion effects of sodium are the most obvious. In addition, an increased sodium content of the vascular wall appears to make the blood vessels more responsive to vasoconstrictor agents. Production or accentuation of experimental hypertension by salt feeding is well documented and carries over into the clinical management of hypertensive patients, where salt restriction is commonly advised. However, the relation between aldosterone and hypertension does not seem to be limited to salt retention and volume expansion. In many cases of malignant hypertension of renovascular origin there is an associated hyperplasia of the cortex and increase in aldosterone secretion, and in such cases the urinary excretion of sodium may be high and the blood volume normal.

The role of other adrenocortical hormones in human hypertension is even more obscure. Hypertension is a manifestation of Cushing's syndrome which is associated with excessive production of cortisol. The effects of this hormone on hypertension have not been defined. In Cushing's syndrome, an increase in aldosterone is inconstant, and hyperresponsiveness of blood vessels to pressor amines, which has been related to an increase in glucocorticoids, has not been observed. Androgenic adrenal tumors are also occasionally associated with hypertension, but the mechanism is obscure.

Humoral mechanisms are also involved in the role of the kidney in the production of hypertension, an area of intense interest and controversy for over half a century. In response to the compromising of the arterial blood supply, the kidney releases renin, which by interaction with a serum globulin produces angiotensin I. A plasma enzyme acts to convert angiotensin I to angiotensin II, which is a powerful vasoconstrictor. Angiotensin also stimulates aldosterone production, which, with its resultant sodium and water retention and expansion of blood volume, plays an important role in the production of hypertension. More obscure renal mechanisms which may play a role in the formation of systemic hypertension include the production of antirenins and vasoexciter material (VEM), which may potentiate arteriolar response to epinephrine, and the excretion or metabolism of circulatory pressor substances.

CLINICAL MANIFESTATIONS

The signs and symptoms of hypertension are rarely to be attributed to the elevated blood pressure per se but rather to the effects of the elevated pressure on a given organ system. Early in the course of hypertension there are usually no signs or symptoms. Headache, weakness, palpitation, and dizziness are among the early symptoms. Epistaxis occurs more frequently in older patients with established hypertension. A history of flushing, sweating, paroxysmal headaches, and episodic hypertension suggests pheochromocytoma. The combination of paresthesia, muscular weakness, transient paralysis, polyuria, and polydipsia is associated with aldosteronism. Urinary tract infection may suggest renal parenchymal disease, and the presence of peripheral vascular disease intensifies suspicion of renal vascular hypertension.

The duration of hypertension and the presence or ab-

sence of visual disturbances, angina, stroke, and myocardial infarction should all be documented, since these provide an index of the severity of hypertension and have prognostic implications.

On physical examination, the finding of a persistently elevated diastolic pressure establishes the diagnosis of systemic hypertension. Vascular changes in the optic fundi, graded on the Keith-Wagener-Barker scale from 0 to 4 for increasing severity, are indicative of general systemic changes and of the degree of hypertension. With all types of hypertension, signs of specific organ involvement may be apparent. These include congestive failure, renal failure, hypertensive encephalopathy, and manifestations of cerebrovascular accident. Certain causes of surgically correctible hypertension are associated with specific findings. Coarctation of the aorta is suggested by decreased femoral pulses and decreased blood pressures in the leg. A loud systolic bruit may be heard over the precordium and posterior chest wall. After the first decade of life, patients have well-developed shoulders and arms, and enlarged collateral arteries are palpable in the musculature of the thorax posteriorly. The finding most suggestive of renovascular hypertension is the presence of a bruit in the upper abdomen. This is most frequently encountered in young females with fibromuscular hyperplasia of the renal artery. Evidence of arteriosclerotic disease of the aorta or of the iliac, femoral, or carotid arteries in hypertensive patients increases the likelihood of similar lesions in the renal arteries.

Cushing's syndrome is associated with the physical findings of central obesity, "buffalo hump," moon face, abdominal striae, ecchymoses, hirsutism, and evidence of osteoporosis. Pheochromocytoma is characterized by sweating, blanching or flushing, syncope, tachycardia, or angina associated with extreme fluctuations in blood pressure. These paroxysms may be induced by painful stimulus, exercise, or palpation of the tumor. The physical manifestations of primary aldosteronism are nonspecific except for those associated with advanced hypokalemic alkalosis, in which a positive Chvostek's sign may be present and carpal spasm may occur when the blood pressure cuff is inflated. Muscle weakness or paralysis also may be noted.

LABORATORY STUDIES

The chest x-ray and electrocardiogram serve as indices for the extent of cardiomegaly and left ventricular hypertrophy. The x-ray may provide the diagnosis in cases of coarctation of the aorta, in which rib notching and the silhouette of a coarcted segment of aorta may be seen. In hyperaldosteronism, the electrocardiogram demonstrates the typical findings of hypokalemia.

Abnormalities demonstrated in routine urine examination such as bacterial growth and proteinuria, accompanied by an elevation of the blood urea nitrogen (BUN) and impaired creatinine clearance, suggest bilateral parenchymal disease. However, these findings do not rule out the possibility of renovascular hypertension. If the urine culture shows bacterial growth, split renal function studies should be delayed until the infection is brought under control.

In pheochromocytoma, a 24-hour urinary output of catecholamines in excess of 200 μg/day and an excretion of the catecholamine metabolite VMA (3-methoxy-4-hydroxymandelic acid) in excess of 7 mg/day are key diagnostic findings. However, certain drugs and foods give false-positive results. The fasting blood sugar level and basal metabolic rate are often elevated. In Cushing's syndrome, the critical determination is an elevated 24-hour urinary output of 17-hydroxysteroids in relation to the daily excretion of creatinine; the fasting blood sugar and glucose tolerance tests often show a diabetic-type response.

In primary aldosteronism, serum electrolyte determinations reveal the potassium to be less than 3 mEq/L and the carbon dioxide more than 30 mEq/L, while the sodium is normal or only slightly increased. The daily urinary potassium excretion exceeds 40 mEq/L, while sodium excretion is normal. The urinary specific gravity is low and there is an alkaline pH. The changes of hypokalemic alkalosis may also occur with secondary aldosteronism related to renovascular hypertension.

CLASSIFICATION

In general, surgically correctible hypertension involves the consideration of diastolic hypertension. Systolic hypertension with normal or decreased diastolic pressure is usually dependent upon cardiac output, and changes in the elasticity of the aortic wall are not commonly associated with pathologic sequelae in the small vessels or target organ systems. Examples of systolic hypertension include arteriovenous fistulas, thyrotoxicosis, and atherosclerosis of the aorta in the elderly patient. Elevation of diastolic pressure is primarily the result of a chronically increased residual resistance in the peripheral vascular bed.

Table 23-1 lists the more important surgically correctible causes of hypertension. Although several entries might be added, those which are included have the greatest practical importance, because of their relative frequency and the lasting benefits which may result from their recognition and treatment. Correction of any of these disease processes may save a patient from a lifetime of antihypertensive drug therapy.

The first three causes listed in the table, i.e., pheochromocytoma, primary aldosteronism, and Cushing's syndrome, are related to abnormalities in the adrenal glands and are discussed in detail in Chap. 37; coarctation of the

Table 23-1. SURGICALLY CORRECTIBLE
CAUSES OF HYPERTENSION

Pheochromocytoma
Primary aldosteronism
Cushing's syndrome
Coarctation of the aorta
Renovascular hypertension
Unilateral renal parenchymal disease

Table 23-2. STUDY OF THE HYPERTENSIVE
PATIENT FOR EVIDENCE OF A
SURGICALLY CORRECTIBLE
LESION

History
Physical examination
Roentgenogram of the chest
Electrocardiogram
Laboratory studies:
  Urinalysis, urine culture, and 24-hour urine protein
  Hemogram
  Serum: BUN, creatinine, and cholesterol
  Serum*: CO_2, K, Cl, Na
  Fasting blood sugar and glucose tolerance test
  24-hour urinary excretion of catecholamines†, VMA†, and 17-hydroxy steroids
  24-hour urinary excretion of K and Na
  Creatinine clearance
Special tests:
  Rapid-sequence excretory urogram
  Radioisotope renogram
  Renal arteriography, via aortic injection and selective injection if indicated

If the above studies show or suggest one of the following correctible causes, further procedure is as indicated:

Renal artery stenosis: Split renal function study and renal vein renin assay.
Aldosteronism: Plasma renin activity and aldosterone secretion rates.
Cushing's syndrome: Adrenopituitary function studies.
Pheochromocytoma: Reconfirm results and proceed with operation.
Coarctation of the aorta: Thoracic aortogram.
Unilateral renal parenchymal disease: Split renal function study and renal vein renin assay.

  *Patient should not be receiving diuretic therapy.
  †A number of drugs or foods may cause false-positive results.

aorta is considered in Chap. 18. These causes are briefly summarized in this chapter, with special emphasis on their relation to the diagnostic study of a patient with hypertension.

In September of 1963, at Vanderbilt University Hospital, a careful search was initiated for patients with surgically correctible hypertension. As of July 1, 1972, a total of 1,070 patients with diastolic hypertension had been investigated. In this study, the history, physical examination, and laboratory and special diagnostic studies (Table 23-2) were designed to detect the causes listed in Table 23-1. The results of this study are referred to throughout the chapter. The very low incidence of patients with hypertension secondary to adrenal causes or coarctation of the aorta in this study may be somewhat misleading. In most patients with hypertension secondary to an adrenal pathologic condition the diagnosis of a pheochromocytoma, Cushing's syndrome, or primary aldosteronism is established or strongly suspected before they are referred. Ordinarily such patients are not included in our general study of patients with hypertension; the same is true of most patients with coarctation of the aorta. Therefore the incidence of this condition will be very small, which indeed it is, but not so small as may be indicated.

PHEOCHROMOCYTOMA

Pheochromocytoma is undoubtedly the most dramatic and treacherous of the surgically correctible causes of hypertension. Unfortunately, many reported cases to date have been undiagnosed during the patient's life or have been suspected only at the last minute during a lethal paroxysmal hypertensive crisis and confirmed at autopsy. The incidence of pheochromocytoma even in the hypertensive population is very low. It has been estimated by Barbeau et al. and Kvale et al. that 0.4 to 2 percent of patients with hypertension have a pheochromocytoma. In the 9-year study of 1,070 consecutive hypertensive patients investigated for evidence of a surgically correctible cause, only 3 patients with pheochromocytoma were found at Vanderbilt University Hospital. During that time, approximately 150 patients presented with a clinical picture suggestive of pheochromocytoma which subsequent study failed to confirm.

CLINICAL MANIFESTATIONS AND LABORATORY STUDIES. The clinical manifestations of these neoplasms are related to their secretion of norepinephrine and epinephrine, and the resultant hypertension may be paroxysmal or sustained. It occurs in all age groups, although 80 percent of the reported cases have been in adults. Although pheochromocytoma is rare, the lethal propensities of the tumor in the untreated case and the extremely good result attending well-planned surgical treatment make it important to screen all patients with hypertension for the lesion. From a practical point of view, this can be done by determining the 24-hour urinary excretion of catecholamines (normally less than 100 $\mu g/24$ hours) and of the catecholamine metabolite VMA (usually excreted in the urine in excess of 7 mg/24 hours in patients with pheochromocytoma). This latter test is especially useful in patients taking an antihypertensive drug such as alpha-methyldopa, which interferes with the measurement of catecholamine excretion but does not alter the validity of the VMA determination. Other pharmacologic tests useful in the study of patients suspected of having pheochromocytoma are discussed in Chap. 37.

Pheochromocytoma should be strongly suspected in all patients who have hypertensive or hypotensive reactions associated with anesthesia, pregnancy, or antihypertensive drug therapy, and in patients with family histories of pheochromocytoma, von Hippel-Lindau syndrome, von Recklinghausen's disease, or Sipple's syndrome. When performing any diagnostic study which may involve painful stimuli or provoke catecholamine release in a patient suspected of having a pheochromocytoma, adequate means of supporting or lowering the patient's blood pressure should be instantly available. Although aortography may demonstrate the location of a pheochromocytoma, the powerful stimulation attending this procedure can precipitate a paroxysmal crisis, and deaths have resulted. It is for this reason that, in the Vanderbilt University Hospital study protocol for hypertensive patients, the catecholamine and VMA levels are routinely determined before aortography if there is any suggestion of a pheochromocytoma in the history or physical examination. Although we formerly believed that aortography should not be done in the patient with a pheochromocytoma, we now believe that with certain precautions it can be done safely and will provide important localizing information. In general the tumor is very vascular, and an intense tumor stain is demonstrated. Obviously if a palpable adrenal mass is present or is demonstrated on an intravenous pyelogram (IVP), aortography assumes less importance. However, many of the tumors are small, 10 percent occur in extraadrenal locations, and 7 to 11 percent are multiple or bilateral.

TREATMENT. Once the diagnosis of pheochromocytoma has been established, the preoperative preparation becomes very important. The use of alpha- and beta-adrenergic blockage in preparing these patients for operation as well as during and after the operation is presented in Chap. 37. These advances have contributed significantly to the greatly lessened operative mortality noted below. Anesthesia for these operations is critical. There is a paramount need for smooth, nonstressful induction, atraumatic tracheal intubation, and avoidance of anesthetics which stimulate catecholamine release or enhance responsiveness to these amines. The operative approach is shown in Fig. 23-1.

During the last decade, reports by Greer et al., by Hume, and by Scott et al. indicate that better understanding of the pharmacologic problems engendered by pheochromocytoma and adherence to a careful plan of treatment have resulted in a reduction of operative mortality from 25 percent to less than 5 percent. Following removal of the tumor, the majority of patients (70 to 75 percent) become normotensive and remain so. About 25 percent of the patients have persistent mild to moderate hypertension, which is thought to be due to hypertensive vascular changes in the kidney.

PRIMARY ALDOSTERONISM

Primary aldosteronism refers to a syndrome caused by autonomous hypersecretion of aldosterone by hyperplastic

Fig. 23-1. Abdominothoracic approach to the adrenal glands. This approach is preferred in cases of pheochromocytoma and in Cushing's syndrome due to adrenal carcinoma; it allows radical nonmanipulative removal of the adrenal tumor.

ABDOMINO-THORACIC APPROACH
TO THE ADRENAL

ADRENAL TUMOR

RETRACTED STOMACH and SPLEEN

EXTENDED INCISION

LEFT KIDNEY

adrenal, or by an adrenal adenoma or (rarely) carcinoma. Aldosterone, a mineral corticoid discovered in 1952, regulates extracellular fluid volume by controlling the excretion and resorption of sodium and water by the kidney. It is the most potent sodium-retaining hormone naturally occurring in man. In 1955, Conn described a syndrome of hypertension, hypokalemia, and alkalosis due to overproduction of aldosterone by an adrenal adenoma. Since that time several hundred cases have been reported.

In the vast majority of reported cases of primary aldosteronism, the cause is an adrenal adenoma. Less frequently, bilateral adrenal hyperplasia with or without nodularity has been reported as causing primary aldosteronism. Adrenal carcinoma is rare as a cause of aldosteronism.

CLINICAL MANIFESTATIONS AND LABORATORY FINDINGS. Conn collected 145 cases and found females predominated 3 to 1. Patients have ranged in age from fifteen to seventy-five years, but most have been in the fourth and fifth decades of life. Hypertension is usually present but is rarely severe. However, it may be associated with headache, cardiomegaly, and retinopathy. In the juvenile cases, severe and even malignant hypertension may occur. Symptoms related to the hypokalemia and alkalosis include muscle weakness, often episodic, which sometimes progresses to paralysis. Paresthesias of the hands and feet are common. Frank tetany may occur, with positive Chvostek's and Trousseau's signs. Polyuria and polydipsia are often prominent. Edema is usually absent.

Laboratory findings include hypokalemia (usually below 3 mEq/L), increased serum bicarbonate, normal or increased serum sodium, and elevated serum pH. Urinary potassium exceeds 40 mEq/24 hours, while urinary sodium is normal. Conn has recently stressed the opinion that hypokalemia may be a late manifestation of the disease and has reported cases of primary aldosteronism with persistent normokalemia. In primary aldosteronism, the plasma renin activity is low and the daily aldosterone secretion rates are high. The reasons for these pathophysiologic changes are discussed in detail in Chap. 37.

Primary aldosteronism is to be suspected in any hypertensive patient with the signs and symptoms listed above, especially the patient with hypertension, lack of edema, low serum potassium level, and increased serum sodium and carbon dioxide. Hypokalemia has proved to be the most valuable simple laboratory test. Plasma renin activity is low, usually 100 m μg/100 ml (nanograms) or less. The definitive diagnosis depends on the finding of a low serum renin with an increased urinary aldosterone excretion. The normal range for the latter study is 3 to 17 μg/24 hours, while in patients with primary aldosteronism the excretion rate may be elevated to levels as high as 160 μg/24 hours.

A number of factors influence the serum potassium, aldosterone, and renin levels, two of the most important being salt restriction and diuretic therapy. Thiazide diuretics cause potassium depletion and hypokalemia. A low-salt diet may prevent the hypokalemia and alkalosis of primary aldosteronism. Finally, a low-salt diet may cause a considerable rise in aldosterone and renin secretion. Patients being screened for evidence of primary aldosteronism should therefore be off diuretic therapy and on a liberal-salt diet (200 mEq sodium for 4 to 5 days) if meaningful serum potassium, aldosterone, and renin levels are to be obtained.

Secondary aldosteronism occurs in renovascular hypertension, congestive heart failure, nephrosis, cirrhosis of the liver, and other edematous states. In all these, the urinary sodium level is low as contrasted to normal or high levels in primary aldosteronism, and plasma renin activity is usually high.

At one point in the initial Vanderbilt University Hospital series of 341 patients with diastolic hypertension, 90 consecutive patients were studied for evidence of primary aldosteronism. After the patients had received a high-salt diet for 4 to 5 days, peripheral venous renin activity and aldosterone secretion rates were determined. Any patient with a suggestive elevation of aldosterone secretion or depression of plasma renin activity was readmitted to the hospital and again studied. Of these 90 patients, none proved to have primary aldosteronism due to an adrenal adenoma; one had a marked decrease in aldosterone secretion following removal of the left adrenal gland and 50 percent of the right adrenal. An initial serum potassium of less than 3.5 mEq/L was encountered in 42 of 341 patients. Many of these patients actually turned out to have a syndrome of hypokalemia, suppressed renin levels even with stimulation, normal aldosterone levels, and hypertension which was controlled by aldactone.

Conn's early estimate that 15 to 20 percent of patients designated as having essential hypertension have primary aldosteronism was excessive. Simpler and better methods of renin and aldosterone assays for widespread use will provide the means of answering many of the troublesome questions about this form of surgically correctible hypertension. Treatment and results are discussed in Chap. 37.

CUSHING'S SYNDROME

In 1932, Harvey Cushing described a syndrome consisting of central obesity ("buffalo hump" and moon face), osteoporosis, amenorrhea, hirsutism, abdominal striae, hypertension, and weakness. Cushing's syndrome is presently defined as a constellation of clinical and metabolic disorders which result from a chronic excess of cortisol (hydrocortisone). The source of the excess cortisol may be an adrenocortical tumor or, more commonly, bilateral adrenocortical hyperplasia under the stimulation of ACTH from the pituitary or a nonendocrine ACTH-secreting tumor of the lung, pancreas, or other organ. Untreated Cushing's syndrome is a highly incapacitating and lethal disorder. With early recognition and treatment a favorable outcome may be expected.

PATHOLOGY. The underlying adrenal pathologic condition in Cushing's syndrome is bilateral adrenocortical hyperplasia in 60 to 70 percent of cases. The remainder have adrenocortical tumors, of which two-thirds are adenomas and one-third carcinomas. The incidence of Cushing's syndrome due to nonendocrine ACTH-secreting tumors (ectopic ACTH syndrome) is unknown, but this type probably accounts for fewer cases than do adrenocortical tumors. In cases due to adrenal hyperplasia under the influence of pituitary ACTH, the pituitary may or may not contain an adenoma.

Normal adults excrete 3 to 12 mg of 17-hydroxycorticosteroids (17-OHCS) in 24 hours, while adults with Cushing's syndrome usually excrete in excess of 12 mg/day. However, it is more accurate to relate the daily urinary output of 17-OHCS to the quantity of creatinine excreted per 24-hour period. In this way variation due to body size and to the collection of less than the 24-hour output can be averted. Normal persons usually excrete 3 to 7 mg of 17-OHCS/Gm of creatinine; with Cushing's syndrome more than 7 mg of 17-OHCS/Gm of creatinine is usually excreted.

CLINICAL MANIFESTATIONS AND LABORATORY FINDINGS. Cushing's syndrome is three times as frequent in females as in males. It is found at all ages but is most common in the third and fourth decades. In children it almost always is due to an adrenocortical tumor, usually a carcinoma. The frequency of the various clinical and metabolic manifestations of the syndrome is shown in Table 23-3.

The florid case of Cushing's syndrome may be recognized by the clinical picture alone. However, many patients present only a few of the classic findings. The basic diagnostic study is the measurement of 24-hour urinary excretion of 17-OHCS. If the 17-OHCS output is abnormally elevated, special adrenopituitary function studies as described by Liddle are performed to confirm the diagnosis and to determine the underlying pathologic condition. These are discussed in detail in Chap. 37.

In the Vanderbilt University Hospital study of 1,070 consecutive hypertensive patients one patient with Cushing's syndrome was encountered. Interestingly enough, the initial determination of 17-OHCS had been in the normal range. Aortography revealed a tumor of the right adrenal gland. Subsequent 17-OHCS determinations and the other tests of adrenopituitary function indicated that the lesion was an adrenal adenoma, and this was confirmed when the tumor was removed.

TREATMENT. Diagnostic precision is important because appropriate therapy depends on recognition of the under-

lying pathologic condition. Before surgical treatment is undertaken, severe metabolic derangements, infections, and complications related to hypertension should be brought under control. The views on treatment expressed here primarily reflect the experience of Liddle's Division of Endocrinology at Vanderbilt University Hospital.

Cushing's Syndrome Due to Adrenal Tumors. The only satisfactory treatment of Cushing's syndrome due to adrenocortical neoplasm is complete surgical removal of the tumor. In cases due to an adenoma, the posterior approach (Fig. 23-2) through the bed of the twelfth rib provides satisfactory exposure. Hayes has advocated bilateral adrenal exploration, because bilateral adenomas are found in about 10 percent of the cases. The most practical approach is perhaps the use of two surgical teams carrying out simultaneous posterior exposure of the two adrenal glands. This approach is less difficult, especially in the obese patient, and is associated with a lower postoperative morbidity than is the transperitoneal approach (Fig. 23-3). Following surgical excision of the adenoma, prompt and permanent regression of the syndrome is to be expected in the overwhelming majority of cases, although the hypertension may take some time to subside completely. An important consequence of "autonomous" production of cortisol by an adrenal tumor is the supression of ACTH production by the pituitary with resultant atrophy of the remaining adrenal tissue. A careful regimen of adrenal substitution therapy (usually hydrocortisone) must be initiated during the operation and continued until it has been demonstrated (by ACTH stimulation tests and 17-OHCS urinary levels) that the remaining adrenal tissue is functionally adequate.

In cases of Cushing's syndrome known or suspected to be due to an adrenocortical carcinoma, a thoracoabdominal incision is preferred so that a radical, nonmanipulative resection can be performed (Fig. 23-1). If preoperative roentgen studies have failed to localize the tumor, the abdominal component of the incision is made first and then extended into the appropriate hemithorax after the tumor has been identified. If the carcinoma can be completely removed, the results are the same as described above for an adenoma; the remarks regarding adrenal substitution therapy also apply. Obviously, if the tumor has metastasized beyond the limits of the resection or if the carcinoma is so extensive as to defy complete excision, the ultimate result is usually poor.

Cushing's Syndrome Due to Ectopic ACTH Syndrome. The only satisfactory treatment of an ACTH-secreting tumor (usually of the lung or the pancreas) is complete surgical removal. This has been accomplished in few cases to date; widespread metastases are usually present by the time the diagnosis is established. Irradiation or chemotherapy has been of little if any benefit in these cases. Bilateral adrenalectomy or therapy with adrenal-inhibiting agents may offer substantial benefit in selected cases, even though it has no influence on the tumor or on ectopic ACTH production.

Cushing's Syndrome Due to Bilateral Adrenocortical Hyperplasia. Treatment is dependent on the severity of the syndrome. If the patient has severe hypertension, osteo-

Table 23-3. FREQUENCY OF THE
MANIFESTATIONS OF CUSHING'S SYNDROME
(61 Cases, Vanderbilt University
Hospital, 1954–1964)

Manifestation	Frequency, percent
Central obesity	100
Hypertension	83
Impaired glucose tolerance	83
Protein wasting	77
Osteoporosis	70
Hirsutism	70
Weakness	60
Menstrual aberrations	50
Ecchymoses	47
Edema	33
Striae	27

porosis, or psychosis, bilateral total adrenalectomy should be performed. The bilateral posterior approach is preferred for the reasons indicated earlier. Patients so treated usually have complete regression of the syndrome. Lifelong adrenal replacement therapy is required. Mild to moderate hypertension persists in about 10 percent of the cases.

If Cushing's syndrome is only mild to moderate and not associated with the severe manifestations listed above, irradiation of the pituitary with 4,000 to 5,000 r should be the initial treatment. Approximately 30 percent of the patients so treated with irradiation will obtain complete and lasting remission of the syndrome. Patients who fail to respond to this form of therapy should have bilateral adrenalectomy.

Patients with sellar enlargement or neurologic deficits attributable to a pituitary tumor should have the tumor removed. Transsphenoidal hypophysectomy employing magnification technique is being used with increasing frequency and success.

In patients treated by bilateral adrenalectomy as the initial therapy evidence of pituitary tumors may develop subsequently. Thorn has reported the incidence as 15 to 20 percent in his experience; in the Vanderbilt University Hospital experience, as reported by Liddle, it had occurred in three of seven cases. Of 11 patients treated by irradiation and then bilateral adrenalectomy, none had developed evidence of a pituitary tumor; of 18 patients treated with irradiation alone, none had developed evidence of a pituitary tumor. This experience would support the belief that pituitary irradiation lessens the incidence of pituitary tumor in patients who have bilateral adrenalectomy.

Finally, mention must be made of subtotal adrenalectomy in the treatment of Cushing's syndrome with bilateral adrenocortical hyperplasia. Subtotal adrenalectomy refers to complete removal of one adrenal and 80 to 90 percent of the other. This procedure had its origin at the time when adrenal steroid substitution therapy was not available. Persistent severe hypertension has been common in patients with hyperplasia who were treated by subtotal adrenalectomy. As Orth has reported, in our experience every patient treated by subtotal adrenalectomy was a treatment failure.

COARCTATION OF THE AORTA

Coarctation of the aorta is to be suspected in all infants, children, and adults with hypertension. The coarctation can occur anywhere in the aorta from the midpoint of the aortic arch down to the aortic bifurcation; however, 98 percent of coarctations are located in the first part of the descending thoracic aorta. The association of coarctation and systemic hypertension has long been known. It was not until 1945, however, that both Crafoord and Gross performed successful surgical correction of the coarctation and demonstrated that this form of hypertension was surgically correctible.

The mechanism of hypertension in coarctation remains debatable. The explanation that it is caused by mechanical

Fig. 23-2. Posterior approach to the adrenal glands. This approach is recommended in cases of Cushing's syndrome due to an adrenal adenoma or bilateral adrenocortical hyperplasia and in primary aldosteronism.

obstruction of the aorta causing increase in resistance to blood flow, with resultant hypertension in the circulation of the arms and head, has never seemed valid, since obstruction of the lower abdominal aorta does not produce hypertension. The experimental studies of Scott and associates have suggested that the coarctation results in reduced renal blood flow and activation of the renal pressor system. Convincing corroborative evidence in patients with coarctation has not yet been presented. Sealy performed angiotensin assays in five patients with coarctation of the aorta and found elevated levels in only two of them.

CLINICAL MANIFESTATIONS AND LABORATORY FINDINGS. The presence of vigorous pulses in the upper extremities and absence or profound decrease in the pulses of the lower extremities provide the basis for prompt recognition of this important cause of hypertension. Decreased blood pressure in the legs, normally 20 to 40 mm Hg higher than in the arms, and a precordial systolic murmur are valuable confirmatory findings. In infants and young children, the blood pressure in the arms may be normal or only mildly elevated. In older children and

Fig. 23-3. Anterior transperitoneal approach to the adrenals for removal of adrenal adenoma or hyperplastic adrenal glands.

adults, hypertension is the rule. After the first decade of life, the shoulders and arms of a patient with coarctation are often extremely well developed and collateral arterial pulsation can be palpated in the musculature of the posterior thorax. The chest roentgenogram frequently reveals a silhouette of the coarcted segment in the descending thoracic aorta and notching of the ribs due to compensatory changes in the collateral circulation. The electrocardiogram usually shows left axis deviation.

A detailed consideration of coarctation of the aorta is presented in Chap. 18. Suffice it to say that coarctation is an important cause of hypertension which, if not corrected, leads to death in 60 percent of patients before the age of forty years. With surgical treatment, complete remission of the hypertension occurs in 95 percent of patients. In our study of 1,070 hypertensive patients two adults and one teen-ager had coarctation of the thoracic aorta.

RENOVASCULAR HYPERTENSION

Renovascular hypertension may be defined as diastolic hypertension secondary to an occlusive lesion of a main renal artery or segmental renal artery which is sufficiently

Fig. 23-4. Aortogram showing left renal artery stenosis due to atherosclerosis involving orifice and proximal third of the renal artery. Poststenotic dilatation is common with such lesions.

severe to activate the renal pressor mechanism. Interest in renovascular hypertension was initiated by Goldblatt and colleagues in the early 1930s, when they produced persistent hypertension in dogs by constriction of the renal arteries. Thereafter Page, Helmer, and Braun Menendez, with their colleagues, independently described the renin-angiotensin system. For the next two decades attention was focused on the kidney in the etiology of hypertension, although renal artery stenosis was considered to be a relatively uncommon cause of hypertension. Adequate and safe methods of studying renal function and vascular anatomy were not available. Nephrectomy was frequently performed for hypertension with an associated small kidney seen on excretory urography, but remission of the hypertension was observed infrequently. In 1956 Homer Smith reviewed a series of 575 hypertensive patients treated by nephrectomy in which it was observed that only 26 percent were normotensive after 1 year. Smith concluded that nephrectomy should be done only for strict urologic indications and not with any hope of relieving hypertension. At that time vascular surgery was developing rapidly, and new and improved techniques of aortography were being introduced and used with increasing frequency. Renal artery stenosis was seen frequently, and usually in patients with hypertension. The demonstrations by De-Camp and Birchall, Morris et al., DeBakey et al., Dustan et al., and others that normal blood pressure could be restored in many hypertensive patients with obstructive disease of the renal artery by surgical relief of the stenotic lesion initiated the present interest in renovascular hypertension. Refinements in excretory urography and renal arteriography and the development of split renal function studies, isotope renography, better methods of renin-angiotensin assay, and improved surgical techniques followed. All these advances contributed materially to a better understanding of renovascular hypertension and to a better selection of those hypertensive patients who would benefit from surgical treatment.

PATHOLOGY. Arteriosclerosis has been the underlying cause in 60 to 70 percent of the proved cases of renovascular hypertension reported to date. The atherosclerotic lesions usually occur in older patients and more frequently in the male. There is usually an atheromatous plaque situated in the orifice or proximal third of the renal artery (Fig. 23-4). However, the presence of an arteriosclerotic plaque in a renal artery does not necessarily indicate a causal relationship to associated hypertension. Autopsy and arteriographic studies by Eyler et al., Holley et al., and Foster et al. show that over 50 percent of patients after fifty years of age have some degree of arteriosclerotic renal artery stenosis whether they are hypertensive or normotensive. Associated arteriosclerotic disease of other vascular systems is commonly encountered. Bilateral renal artery lesions are present in roughly one-third of patients with renovascular hypertension due to arteriosclerosis (Fig. 23-5). Complete occlusion of a renal artery, with filling of the distal segment of the artery via collaterals, is not uncommon in patients over fifty-five years of age (Fig. 23-6).

Fibromuscular hyperplasia or dysplasia of the renal

artery has been the underlying cause in 20 to 25 percent of the reported cases of renovascular hypertension. Significant series of cases have been reported by Wylie et al., by Hunt et al., by Ernst et al., and by Fry et al. It has usually been observed in young patients, especially women in the twenty-five to forty-five age range. The lesion is characterized by a thickening of the media with a myxomatous-appearing fibrous tissue, which separates and distorts the muscle fibers, and by degenerative and disruptive changes in elastic tissue and smooth muscle. These changes result in lesions of the arterial wall which have been termed *microaneurysms*. Dissecting aneurysms and hematomas have also been observed. The striking feature of fibromuscular hyperplasia is the corrugation of the internal surface of the renal artery caused by alternating zones of hyperplasia and disruption of the media and elastic tissue in the wall of the artery. This corrugation gives the "string of beads" effect seen on renal arteriography (Figs. 23-7 and 23-8).

Earlier it was thought the lesions were unilateral in the majority of cases. However, it has now become apparent that the vast majority are bilateral lesions. The reason for this turnabout is found in the improvements in renal arteriography during the past few years. Selective oblique arteriograms in several projections are demonstrating lesions which previously were undetected. This holds true for both atherosclerotic and fibrodysplastic lesions but most commonly for the latter. Hunt et al. believe that virtually 100 percent of the fibromuscular lesions are bilateral, and our recent experience tends to support this concept. An aortogram in the anteroposterior projection will not suffice to demonstrate many renal artery lesions. The reason for this is shown schematically in Fig. 23-9. The origin of the renal artery may be masked by the aorta in such a projection, and the distal renal artery courses in almost an antero-

Fig. 23-5. Aortogram showing bilateral renal artery stenosis due to atherosclerosis. About one-third of patients with renovascular hypertension due to atherosclerosis have bilateral lesions.

posterior direction. The lesion is usually located in the middle and distal thirds of the artery, frequently extending into the segmental branches. With multiple renal arteries to one kidney, more than one of the arteries may show fibromuscular hyperplasia. On serial arteriograms over a period of several years, the lesions have been seen to become progressively more severe in some patients.

A variant of fibromuscular hyperplasia called *subadventitial fibroplasia* by McCormack et al. consists of a dense collar of collagen located in the periphery of the media, which is often thinned and disorganized by the fibrous tissue (Fig. 23-10). These lesions also have been most commonly found in females in the twenty-to-forty age

Fig. 23-6. *A.* Aortogram showing complete atherosclerotic occlusion of the left renal artery in a fifty-three-year-old man. Arrow indicates proximal portion of left renal artery which is still patent. *B.* Later film in aortographic series showing filling of the distal portion of the left renal artery via collaterals. Arrow indicates patent distal left renal artery. Lesion is amenable to correction by either bypass grafting or thromboendarterectomy with a patch graft.

Fig. 23-7. Aortogram showing fibromuscular hyperplasia of the right renal artery with typical "string of beads" effect. Lesions often extend out to or even involve branch arteries. Selective left renal arteriography in this patient showed some lesions which had not been demonstrated by the aortogram.

range. A third variant is the occlusive lesion caused by an intimal fibrous proliferation producing either a discrete short area of stenosis or a long tubular stenosis; this has been called *single mural hyperplasia* (Fig. 23-11). It has been most commonly encountered in the very young patient, less than twenty years of age and as young as four months. Children with unilateral stenosis have been observed by Foster et al. to develop contralateral stenosis in subsequent years.

Harrison and McCormack, and Sheps et al. (1972), have devised a classification of the various fibromuscular lesions which allows recognition on radiograph and has some prognostic implications. These writers feel they can recognize whether the lesion will progress in severity.

The pathogenesis of the fibromuscular dysplasia group of lesions is not known. The lesion does occasionally occur in other arterial systems. Whether it is congenital or acquired is uncertain, and there may be more than one underlying cause. Suggested etiologic factors have been summarized by Hunt et al.; they include congenital anomaly, intrinsic defects in the elastic tissue, Erdheims' medial necrosis, healed arteritis, and abnormal stretching of arteries, especially in pregnancy.

Less common lesions causing renovascular hypertension are renal artery aneurysm, dissecting aneurysm of the renal artery, embolism with segmental infarction, primary thrombosis, and compression of the artery by a fibrous or muscular band (right crus of diaphragm) or a mass. In the author's experience, segmental infarction, presumably due either to an embolus or a segmental artery thrombosis, has been the third most common cause of proved renovascular hypertension.

PATHOPHYSIOLOGY. Reduction or dampening of the arterial pulse pressure in the renal artery beyond the obstruction is thought to be the stimulus which initiates the renal pressor mechanism. The manner in which this is brought about is not entirely understood. Both Crocker et al. and Tobian have shown that patients with renovascular hypertension frequently have hyperplasia and increased cellularity of the juxtaglomerular apparatus (JGA). The JGA surrounds the afferent arteriole of the cortical nephron and is thought to be the source of renin production. These observations have led to the hypothesis that the JGA contains a volume- or pressure-sensing mechanism which responds to reduced pulse pressure by liberating renin. Renin, a proteolytic enzyme, acts on the substrate angiotensinogen, a globulin produced by the liver and found in the α 2-globulin fraction of plasma, to produce a decapeptide which is designated *angiotensin I*. A plasmolytic converting enzyme splits off the last two amino acids from the apparently inert angiotensin I to produce an octapeptide called *angiotensin II*, which is the active pressor agent. Angiotensin II is an extremely powerful vasoconstrictive substance. On a weight basis, it is approximately ten times as potent a pressor agent as norepinephrine. The biologic properties of angiotensin II have been studied extensively, and it appears well established as the active vasoconstrictive factor in renovascular hypertension. Angiotensin II has other effects which are important in producing hyper-

Fig. 23-8. Resected right kidney with renal artery opened longitudinally to show fibrous septa forming corrugated internal surface.

tension. It potentiates the circulatory responses to norepinephrine, and it also stimulates secretion of aldosterone by the adrenal cortex. This latter effect may result in potassium depletion, sodium and water retention, and all the other features of aldosteronism in patients with renovascular hypertension. Recent studies by Louis and his associates have cast some doubt about the role the renin-angiotension system plays in the etiology of experimental renovascular hypertension.

CLINICAL MANIFESTATIONS. The incidence of renovascular hypertension in patients with diastolic hypertension is not known. In a study searching for patients with renovascular hypertension at Vanderbilt University Hospital during the years 1963 to 1972, the incidence was 16 percent. However, this cannot be considered a study of diastolic hypertension in unselected subjects, because of the bias introduced by the physician's referral of a patient to the study. At present it is estimated that 5 percent of patients with diastolic hypertension have renovascular hypertension.

There are no unique features in history, physical examination, or routine laboratory determinations which will differentiate renovascular hypertension from essential hypertension, although a number have been suggested. Most of the classic concepts about essential hypertension are based on patients in whom other causes of hypertension were not excluded. Table 23-4 shows a comparison of the clinical findings in a group of 57 patients with proved renovascular hypertension and a group of 260 patients with essential hypertension. These data still pertain to our larger experience with 1,070 hypertensive patients. Every one of these patients had a complete evaluation, including rapid-

Fig. 23-9. Diagram showing the course of the renal arteries. Lesions in the renal arteries may be masked in the anteroposterior projection. Oblique selective arteriograms are required to demonstrate these lesions.

sequence excretory urography, isotope renography, and renal arteriography. If a renal artery stenosis was found, split renal function study was performed, and in the later period of the study renal vein renin was assayed. The diagnosis of renovascular hypertension was based strictly on a favorable response to surgical treatment, the most critical of diagnostic criteria. In those cases designated as essential hypertension, all tests were normal. Patients with hypertension due to adrenal causes or renal parenchymal disease were eliminated. The reason for the disparate figures under the various clinical observations is that for some patients the pertinent information was not known.

Classic teaching has been that a family history of hypertension suggests essential hypertension, but renovascular hypertension was just as frequently associated with this

Fig. 23-10. A. Selective right renal arteriogram of patient with subadventitial fibroplasia; lesion is more disorganized and does not have the regularity of the "strings of beads" effect seen in Fig. 23-7. B. Photomicrograph of renal artery with subadventitial fibroplasia. In the upper and lower corners at the right the dense collar of collagen is seen in the peripheral media. Disorganization of the media and intima is also seen.

Fig. 23-11. *A.* Aortogram showing single mural hyperplasia of the right renal artery, in an eighteen-year-old girl. *B.* Photograph of the stenosis seen at operation. The vena cava has been retracted to the patient's right to expose the renal artery and the area of stenosis.

observation. A history of recent acceleration of hypertension, recent onset of hypertension, and flank pain or trauma in the hypertensive patient was equally frequent in the two groups. The mean duration of hypertension was but slightly longer in the patient with essential hypertension. Only the finding of an upper abdominal bruit on physical examination provided any differentiation between the two groups, since it was four times more frequent in the renovascular hypertension group. The eye ground changes on fundoscopic examination provided information as to the severity of the hypertension but not as to the origin.

It is commonly stated that hypertension in the young patient is more likely to have a renovascular cause. Figure 23-12 compares patients with renovascular hypertension and those with essential hypertension by decade of life. Again patients with renal parenchymal disease were eliminated, and the diagnoses of essential hypertension and renovascular hypertension were on the same basis as for Table 23-4. The highest incidence of renovascular hypertension was in the first decade of life, the next highest incidence was in the sixty- to sixty-nine-year age group, and surprisingly few instances were found in patients ten to nineteen years of age. It can only be concluded that renovascular hypertension occurs at all ages. Certainly the very young patient with severe hypertension is a

Table 23-4. CLINICAL FINDINGS IN RENOVASCULAR HYPERTENSION AND ESSENTIAL HYPERTENSION
(Vanderbilt University Hospital, 1963–1966)

	Renovascular hypertension		Essential hypertension	
	Number	*Percent*	*Number*	*Percent*
Family history of hypertension	26/51	51	130/245	53
Recent acceleration of hypertension.	7/48	15	31/225	14
Recent onset of hypertension (6 months). . . .	10/50	20	40/230	17
Hypertension associated with history of flank pain, hematuria, or renal trauma . . .	4/57	7	18/260	7
Upper abdominal bruit	22/57	40	24/260	9
Duration of hypertension, years:				
Range	0–23		0–28	
Mean	5.4		6.2	

prime suspect, but so is the older hypertensive patient.

LABORATORY FINDINGS. Routine laboratory determinations provide little help in the detection of renovascular hypertension. Only an occasional patient will have secondary aldosteronism with hypokalemic alkalosis. Tarazi et al. have noted an increased incidence of elevated hematocrit level in patients with hypertension secondary to renal artery stenosis, but this was found in only a small percentage (less than 20 percent) of the patients. The urinalysis, phenolsulfonphthalein excretion, and hemogram or serum electrolyte determinations provide few clues as to the cause of the hypertension. Azotemia occurs with equal frequency in renovascular and essential hypertension. The changes of left ventricular hypertrophy found on the chest x-ray or electrocardiogram are helpful in gauging the severity of the hypertension but not in determining the underlying cause.

SELECTION OF PATIENTS FOR INTENSIVE DIAGNOSTIC STUDY. As the foregoing discussion of the clinical characteristics of renovascular hypertension indicates and as will be seen in the discussion of some of the special screening tests, there is no simple way to predict which patient will be found to have renovascular hypertension. This has led to the author's principle that *any patient with significant diastolic hypertension in whom surgical correction would be recommended if a significant lesion were found should have intensive diagnostic study.* This approach eliminates the mildly hypertensive patient and the patient who is an unacceptable operative risk.

SPECIAL DIAGNOSTIC STUDIES. Rapid-Sequence Excretory Urography. This is a simple variation of the standard intravenous pyelogram described by Maxwell et al. The patient, having been dehydrated, receives a rapid intravenous injection of contrast medium, and roentgenograms are made at 1, 2, 3, 4, 5, 10, 15, and 30 minutes. Contrast medium should appear in the calyceal system of the normal kidney on the 2-minute film. Findings suggestive of renovascular hypertension include (1) unilateral delay in appearance of contrast medium, strongly suggesting renal artery stenosis (Fig. 23-13); (2) decrease in renal length greater than 1.5 cm as compared with the contralateral kidney (Fig. 23-14); (3) unilateral decreased concentration or density of the medium on the early films; (4) ureteral notching due to collateral arterial supply; and (5) unilateral hyperconcentration of the medium on the late films (Fig. 23-15), which is explained by the fact that the kidney with a significant renal artery stenosis displays increased tubular resorption of water and sodium, while the contrast medium is a fixed solute and is not resorbed, thus appearing in hyperconcentration on the late films. (This effect may be accentuated by hydrating the patient or even giving an intravenous infusion of a saline solution of urea, so-called "washout" intravenous pyelography.) This phenomenon is the basis of the split renal function tests described below. A further finding on the urogram, defects in the renal silhouette, may indicate segmental infarction (Fig. 23-16).

The urogram also provides important information re-

Fig. 23-12. Incidence of renovascular hypertension and essential hypertension in 317 hypertensive patients.

garding renal parenchymal disease, e.g., pyelonephritis and hydronephrosis. However, in the recent analysis by Foster et al. of 122 patients with proved renovascular hypertension, the urogram was judged to be normal in 31 percent of the patients. If, as some have advocated, the urogram had been used to determine whether to proceed with further studies (i.e., arteriography), we would have missed almost one-third of the patients with renovascular hypertension. The fact that one-half the false-negative results occurred in patients with bilateral lesions is of interest but does not alter the fact that they would have been missed. A urogram that is abnormal preoperatively but normal postoperatively is very reassuring. On many occasions we have seen a kidney increase in length by 1.5 to 2.0 cm

Fig. 23-13. Two-minute film from a rapid-sequence excretory urogram. Contrast medium is present in the calyceal system on the right; none is seen on the left. This is strongly suggestive of a left renal artery stenosis.

Fig. 23-14. Nephrographic phase of aortogram showing difference in renal size which suggests renal artery stenosis.

Fig. 23-16. Nephrographic phase of an aortogram showing defect in midportion of the right kidney. This was detected on the excretory urogram. Aortogram shows branch artery to midportion of right kidney completely occluded. Heminephrectomy resulted in remission of hypertension.

by the seventh day following successful operative treatment.

Isotope Renography. The ^{131}I orthoiodohippurate renogram has been widely used in screening hypertensive patients for renovascular hypertension. Tracer doses of the

Fig. 23-15. Late film in excretory urogram showing hyperconcentration of contrast medium in the right renal pelvis, a sign indicative of right renal artery stenosis.

15 MIN.

isotope are injected intravenously, and external scintillation counters, placed posteriorly over each kidney, simultaneously record timed uptake and excretion curves. Features characteristic of renal artery stenosis are reduced total height of curve, delayed time to maximal height, and delayed excretion. These abnormalities reflect the degree of reduced renal tubular function and the reduced volume of urine excreted by the ischemic kidney. The test is not specific and must be interpreted with the aid of the excretory urogram. Obstructive uropathy simulates renal ischemia. Pyelonephritis and other parenchymal renal diseases are also responsible for false-positive interpretations in perhaps 20 percent of patients with renovascular hypertension. As with excretory urography, the renogram compares one kidney with the other; hence bilateral renal artery stenosis may not be detected. We have not found the renogram to be particularly helpful in the diagnosis of renovascular hypertension. A triple isotope renogram study is currently being evaluated in the study of patients with hypertension.

Renal Arteriography. If one accepts stenosis of a main or segmental renal artery as part of the definition of renovascular hypertension, renal arteriography becomes the best screening test for renovascular hypertension. Hesitancy to apply arteriography in all patients with diastolic hypertension is related to the fact that the procedure involves a small but definite risk, is expensive, and ordinarily requires that the patient be hospitalized.

A number of methods of obtaining contrast angiographic demonstration of the renal arteries are available. The most widely accepted method is the percutaneous retrograde catheter technique via a femoral artery. Under fluoroscopic control the catheter tip is located in the aorta at the level of the L_1–L_2 interspace; a pressure injector is used to inject the contrast medium, and a rapid film changer is used to obtain serial films. The films will show the aorta, the main renal arteries, the segmental branch arteries, and the entire kidney in the nephrographic phase.

In recent years oblique aortograms and selective renal arteriography, with the catheter tip placed in the renal artery, have been used to obtain additional information. With a catheter selectively placed in a renal artery one

Fig. 23-17. *A.* Left selective renal arteriogram in straight antero-posterior projection; renal artery stenosis is not seen. *B.* Repeat arteriogram with same patient in oblique position shows severe stenosis of distal left renal artery and distal renal artery segment suitable for implantation of an aorticorenal bypass graft utilizing a segment of saphenous vein.

can rotate the patient in various oblique views to demonstrate a severe stenosis which may have appeared to be of questionable significance on straight posteroanterior projection (Fig 23-17). Similarly, in some patients with extensive fibromuscular hyperplasia which on the aortic-injection arteriogram did not appear amenable to surgical correction, a selective arteriogram may show a distal seg-

ment of the renal artery suitable for placement of a bypass graft (Fig. 23-18). Figure 23-9 shows why oblique arteriograms are required in these patients.

In patients with severe arteriosclerotic occlusive disease of the aortoiliac-femoral system it may not be possible or advisable to insert the catheter via a femoral artery. In this situation translumbar aortography or a catheter inserted via an axillary artery may be used to demonstrate the renal arteries.

In the Vanderbilt University Hospital study of 1,070 consecutive hypertensive patients, 1,423 renal arteriograms have been made in the course of initial and follow-up studies. There have been 10 serious complications (0.7 percent): three massive hematomas, one false aneurysm of the femoral artery, thrombosis of the femoral artery in six patients, and one death following aortic surgery for postaortogram thrombosis of the aorta in a patient with severe atherosclerotic occlusive disease.

Fig. 23-18. *A.* Aortogram showing fibromuscular hyperplasia which appears to extend into branch arteries and precludes satisfactory corrective surgery. *B.* Oblique left renal arteriogram in same patient showing distal segment suitable for implantation of a bypass graft (see Fig. 23-23).

Fig. 23-19. Aortogram showing stenosis of proximal right renal artery due to extrinsic compression of the artery. At operation the right crus of the diaphragm was found to be compressing the artery in this forty-two-year-old man.

Arteriosclerosis is the most common cause of renal artery stenosis, and the lesions are bilateral in about one-third of the cases (Fig. 23-4 and 23-5). The process usually involves the origin and the proximal third of the renal artery; poststenotic dilatation is common with severe lesions. Complete occlusion is not uncommon in patients over fifty years of age; in this circumstance the distal renal artery is usually seen to opacify on the later films via collateral arterial supply (Fig. 23-6).

Fibromuscular hyperplasia is the second most commonly encountered stenosis of the renal artery. The lesion usually involves the middle and distal thirds of the renal artery, and frequently the segmental branch arteries are involved. In women in the twenty-five to forty-five age range the lesion is that of multiple mural hyperplasia with the "string of beads" appearance (Fig. 23-7). In patients under twenty years of age and in the male in general a single mural hyperplasia (intimal hyperplasia) is more common (Fig. 23-11).

Less common lesions causing renal artery occlusion are aneurysm, embolism or thrombosis, and compression by a fibrous or muscular band or mass (Fig. 23-19).

Figure 23-20 shows the frequency of arteriographic demonstration of a renal artery stenosis in 317 hypertensive patients. Stenosis in patients under thirty years of age was almost exclusively due to fibromuscular dysplasia; arteriosclerosis was the predominant lesion in patients over fifty years of age. Between ages thirty and fifty the incidence of arteriosclerosis and fibromuscular dyplasia was about equal. Table 23-5 shows the arteriographic findings in the larger series of 1,070 patients.

A renal artery stenosis found on arteriogram in hypertensive patients does not establish a causal relationship. Two-thirds of patients over sixty years of age had a stenosis, but Fig. 23-12 shows that only half the stenoses were of proved functional significance. At present there are three ways of determining whether a stenosis is functionally significant: renal biopsy and histologic study of the juxtaglomerular apparatus, reninangiotensin assay, and split renal function study. The first (JGA study) is not very practical, and accumulated experience to date is quite limited. From our experience, if either of the latter two studies are positive, a good blood pressure response following operative treatment can be expected in 90 percent of the patients.

Split Renal Function Studies. In normal persons and persons with essential hypertension the two kidneys seldom vary significantly in their handling of water, sodium, or solutes. In renal artery stenosis a functionally ischemic kidney resorbs sodium and water excessively, while fixed solutes appear in the urine in increased concentration. These characteristics of the ischemic kidney led to the development of a number of tests to determine when a given stenosis is functionally significant. All the tests involve catheterizing the ureters, collecting urine specimens for successive controlled periods of time, and analyzing the urine specimens.

The Howard test was the first such test described. A reduction in urine volume of 50 percent and a reduction in urine sodium concentration of at least 15 percent or an increase of urinary creatinine concentration of at least 15 percent from the involved kidney have functional significance. The Rappaport test is based on sodium/creatinine ratios from each kidney. A tubular rejection fraction ration (TRFR) is obtained by multiplying the sodium/creatinine ratio on the left by that on the right. A ratio of less than 0.6 indicates significant left renal artery stenosis, and a ratio of more than 1.6 implicates the right renal artery. When the values are between 0.6 and 1.6, the test is negative. The Birchall test employs an infusion of hypertonic saline solution (0.25 Gm sodium chloride/100 ml/kg body weight in 45 minutes). Sodium/creatinine urinary concentration ratios from the two kidneys are compared. The larger sodium/creatinine ratio is divided by the smaller one; if the resultant value is 2 or more,

Fig. 23-20. Incidence of renal artery stenosis, demonstrated by arteriography, in 317 hypertensive patients.

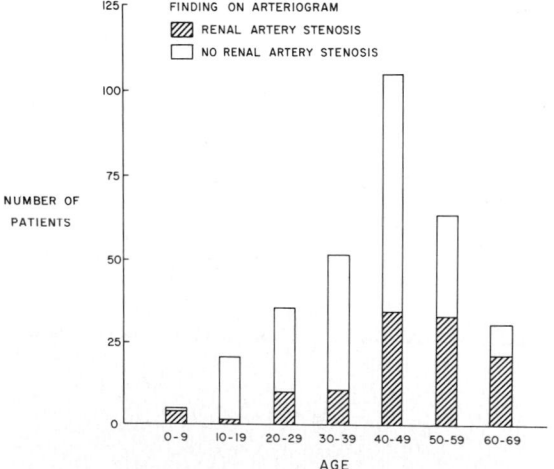

INCIDENCE OF ANGIOGRAPHIC RENAL ARTERY STENOSIS BY DECADE OF LIFE

Table 23-5. RESULTS OF EVALUATION OF 1,070 HYPERTENSIVE PATIENTS

	Renal arteriogram	Renovascular hypertension*
Normal	610 (57%)	—
Renal artery stenosis due to:		
Atherosclerosis	297 ⎫ (43%)	114 ⎫
Fibromuscular dysplasia . .	152 ⎬	51 ⎬ 39% ⎱ 16%
Miscellaneous	11 ⎭	11 ⎭

*Positive functional tests—split renal function studies or renal venous renin assays.

the test is positive. The smaller ratio indicates the involved kidney. The Stamey test involves osmotic diuresis by means of an intravenous infusion of urea. Para-aminohippurate (PAH), a fixed solute excreted by the kidney but not resorbed by the tubules, is added to the infusion. Functionally significant renal artery stenosis is suggested when the involved kidney shows a 66 percent smaller urine volume and a 100 percent greater PAH concentration than the uninvolved kidney. In the Stamey test one also determines the effective renal plasma flow (ERPF) in each kidney. This is valuable in assessing the function of the contralateral or normal kidney; severely impaired plasma flow usually indicates intrarenal small vessel disease. Table 23-6 shows the results of split renal function studies in patients with functionally significant right renal artery stenosis.

In bilateral renal artery stenosis, the split function studies are frequently difficult to interpret; however, in most cases of bilateral stenosis there is a marked discrepancy in the severity of stenosis on the two sides, and the split function studies demonstrate this functional difference.

The author's experience is limited to the use of the Howard and Stamey tests. The original criteria for the interpretation of these tests were based on a very small number of patients. In the beginning we adhered rigidly to those criteria in selecting patients for operative treatment. However, since 1966 liberalized criteria for a positive test have been used. A recent retrospective study of 41 patients who are unequivocally cured following unilateral

renal arterial surgery revealed that the following criteria seem to suffice for a positive test: (1) consistently lateralizing discrepancies in the triplicate samples; (2) Howard test—25 percent reduction in urine volume and 15 percent increase in creatinine from the involved kidney as compared with the contralateral kidney; and (3) Stamey test—25 percent increase in PAH concentration and 25 percent reduction in urine volume in the affected kidney.

Disadvantages of split renal function studies include patient discomfort and occasional complications secondary to the study, e.g., urinary tract infection, ureteral colic, and, rarely, transient ureteral obstruction secondary to edema. A more frequent problem is technical failure to obtain a satisfactory study in about 10 percent of the patients. This occurs most frequently in the male over fifty years of age with prostatic enlargement which interferes with ureteral catheterization.

Renal Venous Renin Assay. If the renin-angiotensin pressor system is the mechanism through which renal artery stenosis causes renovascular hypertension, assay of these substances should afford an accurate way of detecting the disorder. Reports by Fitz, by McPhaul et al., and by Michelakis et al. support this concept. Renin assays, using a radioimmunoassay technique, are now widely available and have proved to be extremely accurate in demonstrating renovascular hypertension. Peripheral venous renin assays are important in detecting primary aldosteronism or other conditions in which renin secretion is severely depressed. However, for the diagnosis of renovascular hypertension, comparative assays of the renin activity in the individual renal veins are usually required. In our initial report, Michelakis et al. stated that the criterion for a positive study was a 1.5 renin ratio when comparing the involved and uninvolved kidneys, and we have continued to use this criterion. Ernst and his associates have indicated that a 1.4 ratio is sufficient, and under certain circumstances (e.g., extensive collateralization) even a smaller ratio is significant.

Disadvantages of the renal vein renin assay are few. Thrombophlebitis subsequent to femoral vein catheterization is occasionally encountered. Catheterization of the renal veins under fluoroscopic control is simple and almost always feasible.

Table 23-6. RESULTS OF SPLIT RENAL FUNCTION STUDIES IN PATIENTS WITH RIGHT RENAL ARTERY STENOSIS

	Right kidney			Left kidney			Serum		
	Patient 1	Patient 2	Patient 3	Patient 1	Patient 2	Patient 3	Patient 1	Patient 2	Patient 3
Volume, ml/min	1.6	1.5	2.4	15.2	18.0	23.2			
Na, mEq/L	35.0	43.0	54.0	70.0	93.0	103.0	140.0		
Creatinine, mg/100 ml .	19.0	18.0	16.0	5.0	3.5	3.5	0.67	0.67	0.67
Creatinine clearance, ml/min	55.0	49.0	70.0	138.0	115.0	148.0			
PAH mg/100 ml	264.0	240.0	216.0	60.0	52.0	48.0	1.84	1.76	1.76
PAH cleared, mg/min . .	4.224	3.600	5.184	9.120	9.360	11.136			
ERPF, ml/min	281	250.0	360.0	605.0	649.0	772.0			
Osmolality, mOsm/kg . .	488	522	532	275	292	309	290	292	299

Relative Value of Split Renal Function Studies and Renal Venous Renin Assays in Renovascular Hypertension. Now that renin assays are fairly widely available, many physicians are using this test alone to determine when a renal artery stenosis is causing hypertension. As mentioned earlier, in our experience when either or both of the tests are positive, a good blood pressure response will follow operative treatment in 90 percent of the cases. We have persisted in using both tests whenever feasible and recommend operative treatment when either is positive. Retrospective analysis of patients who are unequivocally cured following operative treatment of unilateral lesions reveals that about 10 percent had negative or normal split function studies and the same number had negative or normal renin assays. In each of these patients the other test had been positive. There are a number of variables which influence the results of both tests, and these variables are often difficult to control. We think the two tests complement each other and, in addition, the renal function studies provide valuable information regarding the status of the contralateral, or uninvolved, kidney.

Preoperative Renal Biopsy. Vertes et al. have advocated percutaneous biopsy of the kidney in the assessment of patients with renovascular hypertension. They have correctly noted that there are degrees of intrarenal arterial and arteriolar nephrosis which *may* preclude a beneficial result following corrective surgery. The problem has been to determine when such changes exist. Schacht et al., Baker et al., and Strickler have reported patients with renovascular hypertension and a renal biopsy interpreted as moderate or severe who have been cured or unequivocally improved by corrective surgery. In the future a well-controlled retrospective study of a large group of patients with renovascular hypertension may validate the recommendation of Vertes et al. However, it must also be pointed out that the etiology of hypertension does not follow an "all-or-none" law. Patients with severe renovascular hypertension due to an ischemic kidney may also have an element of hypertension as the result of arteriolar nephrosclerosis. Correction of the renovascular lesion will often change such a patient from the category of malignant hypertension to a mild hypertensive categorized as improved in the results of treatment. This has been observed repeatedly in older patients with complete occlusion of a renal artery.

TREATMENT. Selection of Patients for Surgical Treatment. Patients who have significant diastolic hypertension secondary to a functionally significant rental artery stenosis, as demonstrated by split renal function study or renal vein renin assay, and who present a reasonable surgical risk should have corrective surgical treatment. The consideration of surgical risk is relative. A patient with severe or malignant renovascular hypertension, even though cardiac or central nervous system complications may have already occurred, should have corrective surgical treatment if at all possible because of the extremely poor prognosis if the hypertension is not brought under control. Stamey and others have stated that unless the contralateral, uninvolved kidney has a renal plasma flow of 200 ml/minute or more, as determined by split function study, the patient will not benefit from corrective surgery. As with Vertes' opinion regarding nephrosclerosis, future analysis of differential renal function studies in a large number of patients may provide accurate prognostic information of this sort. The author and others have seen patients with unilateral renovascular hypertension and contralateral renal plasma flow of less than 200 ml/minute who have been benefited by corrective surgery.

Preoperative Preparation. If at all possible the patient should be off antihypertensive medication for 10 days or 2 weeks before operation. These agents alter the vasomotor system so that when a general anesthetic is administered, profound vasomotor collapse may occur. Reserpine and other *Rauwolfia* drugs are notorious for this effect: it takes 10 to 14 days for patients on reserpine or guanethidine to become free of their effects. However, there are patients in whom the hypertension is so severe that antihypertensive medication must be continued up to and even during the surgical procedure. This has been demonstrated particularly in young children with malignant hypertension secondary to renal artery stenosis. In such instances control of the blood pressure with alpha-methyldopa, a relatively short-acting agent which does not deplete the nerve endings of norepinephrine stores, has been well tolerated, and vasomotor instability has not been a problem. In general, if the anesthetist knows that the patient has been receiving drugs, anesthesia can be administered safely.

Renal artery reconstruction or nephrectomy should not be undertaken after split renal function study or renal arteriography until it has been determined that these procedures have not caused any degree of renal injury. This is rarely a problem after arteriography, but after split renal function study some degree of ureteral edema is not infrequent. If one adds the trauma of a period of renal artery occlusion or removal of functioning kidney tissue, a disastrous result may ensue. Therefore a 2- or 3-day period should elapse between split renal function study and the surgical procedure, during which the patient's urine output and BUN levels should be monitored. If there is evidence of renal or ureteral injury, the operative procedure should be postponed until the patient has fully recovered.

A blood volume deficit of 500 to 1,740 ml is encountered in 31 percent of patients with renovascular hypertension. Preoperatively the blood volume should be determined, and appropriate correction of plasma or red blood cell deficits should be made to avoid postoperative hypotension and attendant thrombotic complications. In the occasional patient with secondary aldosteronism, metabolic aberrations must be corrected preoperatively.

Operative Treatment. In the selection of an operative procedure for renovascular hypertension, preservation of renal tissue is a prime consideration. Nephrectomy should be done only as a last resort. Patients with both fibromuscular and atherosclerotic lesions frequently have progression of insignificant lesions or develop new lesions in the contralateral renal artery. The younger the patient, the more important this consideration becomes. At present about the only indication for nephrectomy is a destroyed, virtually nonfunctioning kidney.

Adequate exposure for reconstruction of the renal arteries can be obtained through either a long midline incision from the pubic symphysis to the xiphoid or a supraumbilical transverse incision extending from flank to flank. When a coexisting lesion of the abdominal aorta, an aneurysm, or occlusive disease requires attention, the midline incision provides better exposure for dealing with the iliac arteries. Previously we performed bilateral renal biopsy and measurement of pressure gradients across the stenosis in every case. The value of these observations was quite limited, and now these determinations rarely are made. Any value judgment of bilateral renal biopsies must await the report of the pathologists of The Cooperative Study of Renal Arterial Hypertension. They are analyzing biopsy material from several hundred cases. As regards pressure gradients, as Thomas et al. have pointed out, if there is one present, it means the stenosis is significant, but the absence of a gradient is difficult to interpret.

To expose the left renal artery, the entire small bowel is retracted to the right, and the posterior peritoneum overlying the aorta is incised. With appropriate dissection of the surrounding retroperitonal fatty areolar tissue, the left renal vein crossing the aorta is displaced superiorly and the left renal artery exposed. To expose the right renal artery, the inferior vena cava is mobilized and retracted to the right to expose the origin and first portion of the artery. One or more pairs of lumbar veins may be divided in this dissection. To approach the distal right renal artery, the hepatic flexure of the colon and the second portion of the duodenum are mobilized and retracted to the left, and the dissection is carried down to expose the distal right renal vein and artery. This approach is now used in most cases of right renal artery stenosis. It provides the best exposure for an anastomosis between the graft and the renal artery.

The most applicable and most commonly used operative procedure is either a thromboendarterectomy, with or without a patch graft, or some form of bypass graft from the aorta to the renal artery distal to the stenosis (Fig. 23-21). Other operative procedures include splenorenal anastomosis, implantation of the renal artery into the side of the aorta; resection of the lesion with end-to-end anastomosis of the renal artery; and interposition of a graft into the renal artery (Fig. 23-22).

When thromboendarterectomy is performed, the remaining renal artery is usually an extremely delicate and thin-walled structure. A patch graft of autogenous vein or Dacron is often required to avoid narrowing of the renal artery lumen by the suture line. Sometimes a thromboendarterectomy can be performed transaortically after the aorta has been occluded above the renal artery, thus avoiding direct handling and suturing of the renal artery. Transaortic endarterectomy in patients with orificial atherosclerotic lesions has been strongly advocated by Wylie and Starney and their associates.

From a practical point of view, the bypass procedure is the most widely applicable. In dealing with a small renal artery, as in most cases of fibromuscular hyperplasia, a segment of saphenous vein or autologous hypogastric artery lends itself well to a precise, delicate anastomosis with the renal artery (Fig. 23-23). If the distal renal artery is

Fig. 23-21. The most commonly employed methods of correcting a renal artery stenosis. Saphenous vein or a Dacron prosthesis may be used for a bypass or patch graft.

large, as is often the case in arteriosclerotic lesions with poststenotic dilatation, a Dacron prosthesis works quite well (Fig. 23-24).

Prior to application of occluding vascular clamps the patient is given 50 mg of heparin intravenously. A mannitol solution is infused intravenously to stimulate osmotic diuresis prior to and during periods of renal artery occlusion. The graft is first anastamosed end to side to the renal artery. This is the more difficult anastomosis and is easier if done first. Occluding vascular clamps are then removed from the renal artery, and a small bulldog clamp is placed across the graft at the anastomotic site. The aortic anastomosis is then done. A recent improvement in technique has been the use of a monofilament polypropylene suture material (Prolene). Previously we had used a braided polyester suture and routinely encountered brisk bleeding from the suture lines requiring administration of 2 or more units of blood and reversal of the heparin with protamine. Since 1971 we have used the polypropylene suture; we have noted minimal anastomotic bleeding, blood transfu-

Fig. 23-22. Various operative procedures available to correct a renal artery stenosis.

Fig. 23-23. Aortogram showing left aorticorenal bypass graft 1 year after implantation (same patient as Fig. 23-18). The graft is a segment of saphenous vein.

sion rarely has been necessary, and we have not had to give protamine. A review of 38 comparable procedures showed over twice as much blood replacement was required with the braided suture. Examination of the braided suture under the microscope reveals that it is quite porous and has an irregular serrated surface when compared with smooth monofilament material. When the braided suture is pulled through an artery or vein, a sawing effect results which enlarges the hole created by the needle. We believe this is the cause of the greater suture line's bleeding with the braided suture. At any rate the polypropylene suture creates a watertight suture line. It has virtually no drag as it is pulled through the vessel wall. One must take care to avoid a purse-string effect with this suture. For this

Fig. 23-24. Aortogram showing bilateral aorticorenal bypass grafts of crimped Dacron. This aortogram was obtained 4 years after the operation (preoperative aortogram is shown in Fig. 23-5).

reason the suture line is interrupted in four places, and the arteriotomy is held open widely with traction sutures during the anastomosis.

In constructing an aorticorenal bypass great care must be taken in orienting the course of the graft so as to avoid kinking or twisting. Wylie et al. and Fry and his associates prefer an end-to-end anastomosis between the renal artery and the graft. This technique avoids angulation at the renal artery anastomosis which sometimes causes kinking. If a kink is encountered, the anastomosis must be redone. The best course for the graft from the renal artery to the aorta varies from patient to patient. On the left side the graft usually seems to course better behind the left renal vein. On the right side a retrocaval course usually works best.

If the aortic bifurcation has been resected, because of occlusive disease or aneurysm, and there is a coexisting significant renal artery stenosis, a side-arm bypass graft can be attached in the aortic prosthesis before the graft is interposed between the aorta and iliac arteries and subsequently anastomosed to the renal artery.

Renal transplantation experience has shown that if the vasculature of the donor kidney is washed out and the kidney cooled, tubular necrosis and renal dysfunction are minimized. This technique is now being employed in renal artery reconstructions. When the renal artery is opened, a cannula is inserted and the kidney perfused with 500 ml of a saline solution which has been cooled to 1 to 2°C. The perfusate is collected from the renal vein to prevent its entrance into the systemic circulation. Thereafter the arterial reconstruction is done. This technique produces a core kidney temperature of 16°C. The results with this technique are only preliminary, but they appear to show better tubular function in the early postoperative period, and no complications have attended the procedure. Prior to adoption of this technique, the triple isotope renogram done on the first postoperative day would show normal renal artery blood flow but poor tubular function. With this technique, tubular function appears to be normal or near normal on the first postoperative day. Again, these are preliminary results.

Another perplexing problem has been the patient with renovascular hypertension secondary to stenoses and/or aneurysm in the distal renal artery with extension into the branch renal arteries, usually fibromuscular lesions. A distal renal arterial segment suitable for conventional bypass is not present. In the past for many such patients nephrectomy was performed. However, the propensity for the development of bilateral severe lesions in these patients has dampened any enthusiasm for nephrectomy. In patients with stenoses involving the segmental branch arteries, Fry and his associates adopted a technique of using olive-tipped dilators to dilate these lesions and have presented interesting follow-up arteriographic data supporting the merits of the procedure.

Renal transplantation experience has led to an alternative technique that appears to be applicable in these patients: ex vivo reconstruction of the renal artery. Ota et al., Lim et al., and Belzer as well as others have reported use of this technique. The exact details of the operative procedure have varied from group to group, and the technique is still in the developmental stage. We have employed the procedure in five renal arterial reconstructions, anatomically successful in each instance. The renal artery and vein are divided close to the aorta and vena cava. The kidney is then rotated out on the abdominal wall onto a small operating platform. The ureter has been mobilized to allow this maneuver but has not been divided. The renal vasculature is flushed with 500 ml of a cold (1 to 2°C) saline solution. The artery is then attached to the Belzer apparatus and perfused with an acellular, oxygenated solution. Gravity is used to return the venous effluent to the Belzer pump. Using magnification and 7-0 arterial sutures, the multiple segmental renal artery lesions are repaired. In the case of terminal renal artery aneurysm the branch arteries are implanted into a saphenous vein graft. The artery or vein graft is then implanted into the common iliac artery and the renal vein into the distal vena cava. Ureteral collaterals, in cases of severe stenosis, can lead to significant renal blood flow which appears in the venous effluent. This can be avoided by application of atraumatic Potts ties to the ureteral artery. It is too early to judge this technique, but it appears to be an exciting development in renal artery surgery.

The problem of what to do in case of a severe functionally significant stenosis in one renal artery and a moderate nonsignificant stenosis in the other has not yet been answered objectively. In the opinion of some, performing a bypass on the side with the moderate stenosis adds little time or risk to the operative procedure, may be beneficial in avoiding future problems, and will improve renal blood flow. The evidence supporting this concept at the present time is tenuous.

Postoperative Care. Following renal artery reconstruction the patient is maintained on nasogastric suction and intravenous fluids for 3 to 5 days. Central venous pressure is monitored in the early postoperative period in older patients and in any patient with an impaired myocardial reserve. Most patients have some degree of diuresis following successful repair. In an occasional patient the diuresis may be massive, and severe electrolyte aberrations may ensue if the losses are not replaced. Urine output is monitored hourly via an indwelling catheter, and daily urinary output of sodium, potassium, and chlorides is determined, as are the serum levels of these electrolytes. Significant losses are replaced quantitatively. The patient is weighed daily to gauge fluid balance and to avoid overloading. It is difficult to overemphasize the importance of this simple observation. These patients often have an impaired myocardial reserve, and a fluid overload can result in congestive heart failure, pulmonary edema, and accelerated hypertension.

The blood volume should be determined early in the postoperative period, and the hematocrit should be monitored for several days. Postoperative hypotension and oliguria are usually related to an inadequate blood volume, due either to failure to expand a contracted blood volume preoperatively or to failure to replace operative blood losses.

Severe hypertension in the postoperative period is not an uncommon problem. There are a number of underlying causes: *Hypothermia* with peripheral vasoconstriction is managed by warming the patient and administering Thorazine. *Fluid overload* with increased central venous pressure and weight gain is managed with fluid restriction and judicious diuretic therapy. Finally, a number of patients will have *severe blood pressure elevations* that cannot be explained and must be treated with antihypertensive drugs; alpha-methyldopa is administered intravenously (500 mg every 4 to 6 hours) for several days. If hypertension becomes more severe than it was preoperatively, thrombosis of the reconstruction is to be strongly suspected. An excretory urogram or renogram is helpful in determining whether the kidney is functioning properly; if it is not, renal arteriography should be performed. Thrombosis of a renal artery reconstruction can result in malignant hypertension in a matter of a few days, as reported by Miller and Foster. Revision of the reconstruction or nephrectomy is usually required.

Some degree of transient azotemia is usually observed in patients who have undergone bilateral renal artery operations and in many patients who have had unilateral operation. This is probably due to renal tubular damage secondary to intraoperative renal artery occlusion which has been previously noted, and we are now reluctant to do bilateral simultaneous renal artery reconstructions. The degree of renal injury is usually minor, and with adequate hydration the BUN usually returns to normal by the time the patient is ready for discharge, ordinarily the eighth to tenth postoperative day. Renal failure secondary to tubular necrosis occasionally occurs after surgical treatment of renovascular hypertension. Other postoperative complications that have been recorded are those which might be expected in any seriously ill patient with hypertensive cardiovascular disease: myocardial infarction, congestive heart failure, cerebrovascular accident. Avoidance of hypotension or severe hypertension is the only means of preventing these complications.

RESULTS OF SURGICAL TREATMENT. The bulk of experience with operative treatment of renovascular hypertension has accumulated in the last decade. It is not surprising that there has been considerable variation in classifying the response to surgical treatment. Definition of the term "cure" presents the least problem: adults with documented diastolic hypertension who 3 or more months after surgical treatment have a diastolic blood pressure of less than 90 mm Hg are considered to be cured. It is more difficult to define a cure in children, especially children less than ten years of age.

The blood pressure response in the first 7 to 14 days after operative treatment is not a reliable index to the true response. The combination of the operation and strict bed rest may result in normal blood pressure levels which return to hypertensive levels when the patient resumes normal activity. On the other hand, some patients may remain hypertensive in the early postoperative period and become normotensive several weeks or months later. The greatest problem in defining response to treatment is in patients who are improved by operation but who continue to have a diastolic blood pressure above 90 mm Hg. These patients are largely the elderly, with atherosclerosis, who

Table 23-7. RESULTS OF OPERATIVE TREATMENT
OF RENOVASCULAR HYPERTENSION

Report	Period	Year of report	No. of patients	Cure, percent	Cure and improved, percent	Operative mortality, percent
Michigan	60–61	1962	43	40	82	4.0
Cleveland Clinic	57–61	1963	76	62	78	10.0
UCLA	59–64	1964	67	37	82	4.0
Baylor	56–64	1966	432	41	81	7.0
Vanderbilt	62–65	1966	35	46	77	6.0
Mayo Clinic*	58–65	1967	100	55	84	0.0
UCSF	52–66	1967	122	37	65	8.0
Virginia	61–67	1968	53	28	75	3.6
Columbia	64–69	1970	40	53	76	2.5
Mayo Clinic†	64–70	1970	46	46	66	6.0
Cooperative Study . . .	61–69	In press	502	47	61	6.8
Vanderbilt‡	62–72	1973	122	70	90	5.4
UCSF§	52–62	1969	41	22	56	15.0
UCSF§	63–68	1969	42	26	74	2.4
Michigan*	61–70	1972	66	62	94	0.0

   *None of these patients had simultaneous treatment of extrarenal atherosclerotic vascular lesions.
   †All patients had aortic occlusive disease or aneurysm in addition to renal artery stenosis and operative treatment of both.
   ‡All patients had positive split renal function studies and/or renal venous renin assays.
   §Atherosclerotic lesions only.

in addition to a renovascular cause for their hypertension have an underlying essential hypertension or arteriolar nephrosclerosis. "Improvement" has generally been defined as a persistent (i.e., at least 3 months) 20 mm Hg reduction in diastolic pressure. In the future, more rigid criteria for defining improvement should be forthcoming from such groups as The Cooperative Study of Renal Arterial Hypertension, which involves 13 institutions under U.S. Public Health Service sponsorship. The number of patients classified as failures or unimproved after surgical treatment will obviously be influenced by definition of the "improved" category; however, overt failures are quite obvious.

The time lapse between a successful operation for renovascular hypertension and a salutary blood pressure response has been variable. In most patients (perhaps 75 percent) the blood pressure recorded 1 month after operation accurately reflects the ultimate result; but some patients have required 3 months or more to become normotensive. The reasons for this are poorly understood.

Table 23-7 presents a composite view of the response to operative treatment of renovascular hypertension in a number of centers. Methods of selection of patients for operative treatment were varied, as were the criteria used to classify the operative result. The two reports with a 0 percent operative mortality omitted patients with simultaneous treatment of extrarenal atherosclerotic vascular lesions. A similar adjustment of our 1972 series would decrease the number of patients to 106 and the operative mortality to less than 3 percent. The Vanderbilt University Hospital series shows that more than 90 percent of the patients have a good result following operative treatment if the preoperative functional studies were positive. Figure

23-25 shows our yearly incidence of renal artery operations for renovascular hypertension since 1962.

Interest in renovascular hypertension varies widely from one center to another in the United States. In a few institutions the condition is being recognized frequently; however, in most centers it is identified only occasionally or is virtually unknown. There are several reasons for this difference: (1) A prime reason is that in the late 1950s and early 1960s many patients with hypertension and an associated renal artery stenosis had operative treatment but were not benefited. They did not have functional evidence of renovascular hypertension. This experience dampened or extinguished interest in renovascular hypertension. (2) There is widespread belief that renovascular hypertension is a rare condition. Our experience indicates that about 5 percent of patients with diastolic hypertension have renovascular hypertension. By conservative estimate there are at least 30 million patients with hypertension in the United States, or 1.5 million patients with renovascular hypertension. The condition can hardly be considered rare. (3) A multidisciplinary team approach to the study of the patient with hypertension is necessary if patients with renovascular hypertension are to be recognized. The internist is the key physician; if the experience of the 1950s and early 1960s has left him with little interest in renovascular hypertension (Item 1, above) or if he believes renovascular hypertension is rare (Item 2), he will probably treat his hypertensive patients with drugs and not try to find an underlying cause for the high blood pressure. Our group had a slow start, but the medical community has gradually adopted the philosphy of complete study of the patient with hypertension. While we have detailed data on 1,070 hypertensive patients, it is probable that an equal number of hypertensive patients have been evaluated according to the same protocol in our community. This explains the high frequency (16 percent) of renovascular hypertension in the 1,070 patients—many of the patients have been referred after a positive pyelogram or arteriogram.

In the past 15 years there have been tremendous advances in the drug therapy of hypertension. Freis and his associates have presented convincing evidence of the efficacy of antihypertensive drug treatment of hypertension and prevention of the complications attending hypertension. However, drug therapy has many untoward side effects. Most notable is postural hypotension. In many hypertensive patients effective control of the blood pressure is limited to the time spent in the upright position; hypertension during the hours spent in the supine position must be accepted. Control of the supine blood pressure may result in intolerable hypotension in the upright position.

Shapiro and his associates and others have stated that patients with renovascular hypertension who are over fifty years of age should not have operative treatment. From their experience it was felt that the risk is too great and the chance of a good result is too small. They advised drug therapy in this age group. Fifty-two of our patients were over fifty years of age, and 80 percent of them were either cured or improved following operative treatment. The operative mortality (10 percent) was higher in these older patients, but this was primarily because of patients who had simultaneous operative treatment of extrarenal vascular lesions such as an aortic aneurysm or occlusive disease.

A comparative study of drug treatment and operative treatment of renovascular hypertension has not yet been reported. Our group is presently doing such a prospective randomized study, but it is too early to report any results.

Figure 23-25 shows the number of patients a year since 1960 who have had renal artery operations. An analysis of the results of surgical treatment related to the type of renal artery lesion shows that patients with fibromuscular hyperplasia are cured more often (73 percent) than patients with an arteriosclerotic plaque (53 percent), although the improved group of patients contains a higher percentage of patients with arteriosclerosis. If the results of treatment are related to the type of surgical procedure, renal artery reconstruction has resulted in cure in 76 percent, while cure has been effected in 52 percent of nephrectomized patients. However, the nephrectomy series contains a larger proportion of the improved patients.

The severity of arteriolar nephrosclerosis, as determined by study of bilateral renal biopsies, has not correlated well with the response to operative treatment. There is a higher incidence of severe arteriolar nephrosclerosis in the unimproved group and of benign arteriolar nephrosclerosis in the cured group, but there are numbers of patients with severe changes who have been cured and of unimproved patients with benign changes.

Renovascular hypertension due to unilateral stenosis can so severely damage the contralateral kidney that it becomes the more powerful renin-secreting kidney. In this

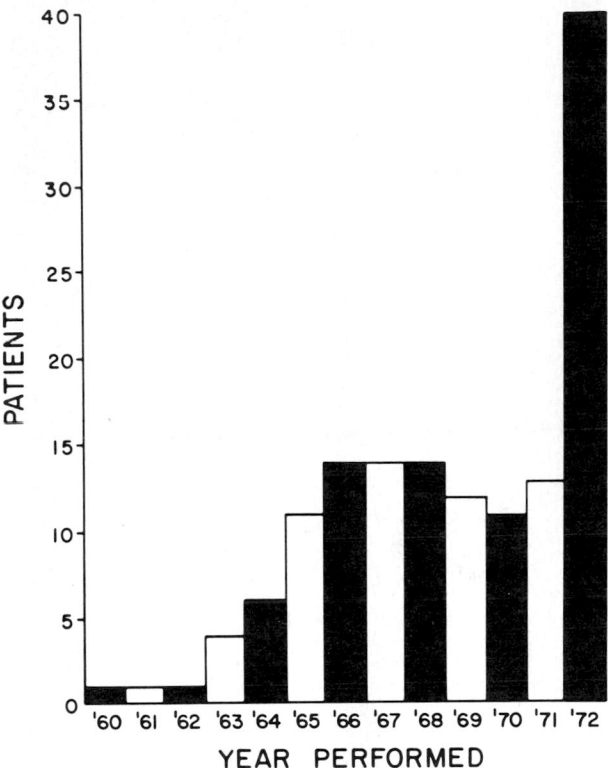

Fig. 23-25. Number of patients undergoing operative treatment for renovascular hypertension each year since 1960 at Vanderbilt University Hospital.

condition, the kidney with the renal artery stenosis is protected from the ravages of severe hypertension. Floyer demonstrated this experimentally in the 1950s, and there have been occasional reports providing human confirmation since that time (Thal et al., Marable et al., Morris et al., and others). We have encountered this situation in two patients, one of whom was reported by McAllister et al. Relief of the hypertension requires unilateral arterial reconstruction and contralateral removal of the kidney which has been destroyed by the hypertension (Fig. 23-26). An interesting observation has emerged from the treatment of these patients and of patients with a solitary kidney with renal artery stenosis—their blood pressure returns to normal immediately following successful operative treatment. This is in contradistinction to many patients with renovascular hypertension due to unilateral stenosis in whom it may require days, weeks, or even months before the blood pressure becomes normal. In these patients, as Alpert et al. have shown, it seems likely that the contralateral kidney has been damaged by hypertension. The ultimate result then depends on whether the damage is reversible; if reversible, considerable time may be required.

The reported incidence of thrombosis or stenosis of a renal artery reconstruction has ranged from 15 to 35 percent. In our experience and in that of Ernst et al. and Fry

Fig. 23-26. *A.* Dacron graft bypass to right renal artery. *B.* Photomicrograph showing destroyed left kidney which was removed. Arteriolar changes including fibrinoid necrosis are apparent.

et al., thrombosis usually occurs in the first few postoperative days and is due to technical errors in performing the reconstruction. With experience and improved operative technique it has been possible to reduce the frequency of this complication to less than 5 percent. Immediate postrepair arteriograms and flowmeter studies should help reduce this problem further.

Serious postoperative complications have occurred frequently in these patients. Many have compromised cardiac function, and congestive failure and pulmonary edema are common problems unless fluid balance is carefully managed. Table 23-8 lists the complications in 122 patients.

There have been few reported follow-up arteriographic

Table 23-8. POSTOPERATIVE COMPLICATIONS
OF OPERATIVE TREATMENT OF
RENOVASCULAR HYPERTENSION

Complication	*No. of Patients*
Congestive heart failure	4
Acute tubular necrosis	4
Intestinal obstruction	2
Aortic suture line disruption	1
Basilar artery thrombosis	1
Hemolytic crisis	1
Bracheal plexus stretch injury	1
Renal arteriovenous fistula	1
Abdominal angina	1

data on aorticorenal bypass. Exceptions are the reports of Kaufman et al. and of Ernst et al. Ernst and Fry and their associates have shown that the saphenous vein, used to construct an aorticorenal bypass, almost routinely undergoes uniform dilatation, sometimes progressing to aneurysmal proportions. We have noted these same changes, and vein graft aneurysm has occurred in 2 of 68 patients 4 to 6 years following implantation (Fig. 23-27). Arteriographic follow-up studies of aorticorenal bypass utilizing hypogastric artery are needed.

UNILATERAL RENAL PARENCHYMAL DISEASE

There is an ill-defined group of patients with hypertension who have a small atrophic kidney on one side, a normal or hypertrophic contralateral kidney, and no evidence of main or segmental renal artery stenosis on arteriography. The underlying etiologic factors have usually been unilateral pyelonephritis, congenital hypoplasia, radiation fibrosis, or posttraumatic fibrosis. The problem has been to determine when an atrophic kidney is responsible for the hypertension. For 20 years after Goldblatt's original studies, nephrectomy was frequently performed on the basis of hypertension and an associated small kidney. Although these patients were operated on because it was thought they might have a "Goldblatt kidney," remission in the hypertension was observed infrequently. Smith's review in 1956 of 575 patients indicated that only 26 percent were benefited.

A recent 5-year experience with hypertensive patients, involving careful study in search of an underlying cause, indicates that perhaps 5 percent have a small kidney on one side and no evidence of main or segmental renal artery stenosis on arteriography. The involved kidney may be anywhere from 3 to 7 cm shorter than its mate, and the renal cortex of the involved kidney is proportionately thinned. The uninvolved kidney may be normal in length or hypertrophic (less than 13.5 to 14 cm long). Renal artery stenosis can cause these same changes in kidney length. However, in unilateral parenchymal disease the main renal artery and its segmental branches are uniformly small throughout, without evidence of stenosis or occlusion. In unilateral pyelonephritis, calyceal clubbing is usually seen on the pyelogram. There are often areas in the parenchyma which suggest focal atrophy, and there is distortion of the small intrarenal arterial branches. In so-called "congenital hypoplasia" all the structures are small and may be diminutive but have no distortion or other abnormality.

Recent reports by McDonald, by Hickler, et al., and by Crocker et al. indicate that nephrectomy in patients with unilateral renal parenchymal disease has been accompanied by cure or improvement of their hypertension only if there was evidence of an ischemic pattern on split renal function study. The author's experience indicates that an increase in the renal vein renin from the involved side is equally valid. In the case of a totally nonfunctioning kidney, renal vein renin assays may be the only means of

Fig. 23-27. Arteriograms showing a saphenous vein aorticorenal artery bypass 1, 3, and 5 years after implantation. Aneurysmal dilatation is apparent at 5 years.

determining functional significance as regards the hypertension. Hypertension due to unilateral renal parenchymal disease is of unknown pathogenesis but is generally considered to result from activation of the renal pressor mechanism by intrarenal small artery disease.

SURGICAL TREATMENT OF ESSENTIAL HYPERTENSION

During the era 1940 through 1959, before effective antihypertensive drug therapy was available, thoracolumbar sympathectomy or splanchnicectomy was used frequently in the treatment of patients with severe diastolic hypertension. During the latter part of this period, bilateral total or subtotal adrenalectomy alone or in conjunction with thoracolumbar sympathectomy was advocated for control of severe hypertension. The effectiveness of these forms of treatment depends on interrupting the increased peripheral resistance so commonly present in most forms of diastolic hypertension. Beneficial and at times long-lasting results were obtained with these forms of treatment, as documented in reports by Grimson, Smithwick, Zintel, and Jeffers et al. During the following decade these forms of surgical treatment were largely abandoned, being replaced by the use of the potent antihypertensive drugs currently available.

Recently, baropacing of the carotid sinus nerve as a means of decreasing peripheral resistance and thereby lowering the blood pressure has been the subject of experimental and clinical studies reported by Schwartz and Griffith and by Bilgutay and Lillehei. The carotid sinus nerve, a branch of the glossopharyngeal nerve, is the afferent nerve of the carotid baroreceptor reflex and transmits to the medullary vasomotor centers action potentials which originate in the carotid sinus. Under normal conditions, an increase in the intraluminal pressure of the carotid baroreceptor reflexly lowers blood pressure, induces bradycardia, decreases cardiac output, and diminishes venous return. When pressure is lowered in the baroreceptor, the reverse occurs. Chronic neurogenic vasoconstriction is thought to occur when the baroreceptor mechanism loses its efficiency or is "reset" at elevated blood pressure levels. This resetting has been attributed to the development of refractoriness or elevation of the thresholds of the baroreceptors in chronic hypertensive states. McCubbin et al. hypothesized that either the vasomotor centers are altered by hypertension and unable to appreciate afferent stimuli from the baroreceptor organs or there is an adaptation within the baroreceptor, so that an insufficient number of impulses results from the hypertension stimulus. Using electroneurography, they demonstrated that the baroreceptors continued to function in hypertension but that the threshold stimulus required to trigger the receptor was significantly raised. These observations led to Warner's use of electrical stimulation of the carotid sinus nerve to lower systemic blood pressure in the dog. Subsequently, Griffith and Schwartz reported reversal of renal hypertension in dogs by electrical stimulation of the carotid sinus nerve, an observation confirmed by Bilgutay and Lillehei. Chronic electrical stimulation of the carotid sinus nerve as a method of treating hypertension has been applied clinically. The stimulator, or baropacer, was implanted in the neck and connected to the carotid sinus nerve; unilateral stimulation was initially employed, and more recently bilateral stimulation has been used. Schwartz and Griffith have reported encouraging results with treatment of 11 hypertensive patients, and Bilgutay and Lillehei have had favorable experiences with 2 patients.

At present, stimulation of the carotid sinus nerve in the treatment of hypertension must be considered an experimental approach. Two major unresolved questions are whether chronic stimulation will result in fibrosis and destruction of the nerve and whether the baroreceptor system will eventually reset itself so that hypertension will recur. Experience with baropacing continues to accumulate slowly. In addition to controlling hypertension, it has been reported to be useful in management of angina pectoris and paroxysmal supraventricular tachycardia. Recent reports have been summarized by Brest. More study of this method of treatment is needed. It may eventually prove to be a valuable addition to the treatment of hypertension.

Bilateral nephrectomy and renal transplantation for patients with severe essential hypertension and end-stage renal disease are discussed in Chap. 10.

References

Pheochromocytoma

Scott, H. W., Jr., Riddell, D. H., and Brockman, S. K.: Surgical Management of Pheochromocytoma, *Surg Gynecol Obstet,* **120:**707, 1965.
Van Way, C. W., III, Michelakis, A. M., Alper, B. J., Hutcheson, J. K., Rhamy, R. K., and Scott, H. W., Jr.: Renal Vein Renin Studies in a Patient with Renal Hilar Pheochromocytoma and Renal Artery Stenosis, *Ann Surg,* **172:**212, 1970.

Primary Aldosteronism

Conn, J. W.: Primary Aldosteronism: A New Clinical Syndrome, *J Lab Clin Med,* **45:**3, 1955.
———, Cohen, E. L., and Rovner, D. R.: Suppression of Plasma Renin Activity in Primary Aldosteronism, *JAMA,* **190:**125, 1964.
———, ———, ———, and Nesbit, R. M.: Special Communication: Normokalemic Primary Aldosteronism, *JAMA,* **193:**100, 1965.
———, Knoph, R. F., and Nesbit, R. M.: Primary Aldosteronism: Present Evaluation of Its Clinical Characteristics and the Results of Surgery, in E. E. Baulieu and P. Robel, *"Aldosterone,"* Blackwell Scientific Publications, Ltd., Oxford, 1964.
Egdahl, R. H., Kahn, P. C., and Melby, J. C.: Unilateral Adrenalectomy for Aldosteronomas Localized Preoperatively by Differential Adrenal Vein Catheterization, *Surgery,* **64:**117, 1968.
Fishman, L. M., Kuchel, O., Liddle, G. W., Michelakis, A. M., Gordon, R. D., and Chick, W. T.: Incidence of Primary Aldosteronism in Uncomplicated "Essential" Hypertension, *JAMA,* **205:**497, 1968.
Grim, C. E., McBryde, A. C., Glenn, J. F., and Gunnels, J. C., Jr.: Childhood Primary Aldosteronism with Bilateral Adrenocortical Hyperplasia: Plasma Renin Activity As an Aid to Diagnosis, *Pediatrics,* **71:**377, 1967.
Melby, J. C., Spark, R. F., Dale, S. L., Egdahl, R. H., and Kahn, P. C.: Diagnosis and Localization of Aldosterone-Producing Adenomas by Adrenal-Vein Catheterization, *N Engl J Med,* **277:**1050, 1967.
Silen, W., Biglieri, E. G., Slaton, P., and Galante, M.: Management of Primary Aldosteronism, *Ann Surg,* **164:**600, 1966.

Cushing's Syndrome

Cushing, H.: The Basophil Adenomas of the Pituitary Gland and Their Clinical Manifestations, *Bull Johns Hopkins Hosp,* **50:**137, 1932.
Hayes, M.: Operative Treatment of Adrenal Cortical Hyperfunctionary Disease, *Ann Surg,* **154:**33, 1961.
Liddle, G. W.: Tests of Pituitary-Adrenal Suppressibility in the Diagnosis of Cushing's Syndrome, *J Clin Endocrinol Metab,* **20:**1939, 1960.
———: "Cushing's Syndrome: The Adrenal Cortex," Little, Brown and Company, Boston, 1967.

Orth, D. N., and Liddle, G. W.: Results of Treatment in 108 Patients with Cushing's Syndrome, *N Engl J Med,* **285:**243, 1971.
Scott, H. W., Jr.: "Tumors of the Endocrine Glands: Tumors of the Adrenal Cortex and Cushing's Syndrome," Seventh National Cancer Conference Proceedings, p. 513, 1973.

Coarctation of the Aorta

Beattie, E. J., Jr., Cooke, F. N., Paul, J. S., and Orbison, J. A.: Coarctation of Aorta at Level of Diaphragm Treated Successfully with Preserved Human Blood Vessel Graft, *J Thorac Surg,* **21:**506, 1951.
Bjork, V. O., and Intonti, F.: Coarctation of Abdominal Aorta with Right Renal Artery Stenosis, *Ann Surg,* **160:**54, 1964.
Crafoord, C., and Nylin, G.: Congenital Coarctation of the Aorta and Its Surgical Treatment, *J Thorac Cardiovasc Surg,* **14:**347, 1945.
Glenn, F., Keefer, E. B. C., Speer, D. S., and Dotter, C. T.: Coarctation of the Lower Thoracic and Abdominal Aorta Immediately Proximal to the Celiac Axis, *Surg Gynec Obstet,* **94:**561, 1952.
Gross, R. E., and Hufnagel, C. A.: Coarctation of the Aorta: Experimental Studies Regarding Its Surgical Correction, *N Engl J Med,* **233:**287, 1945.
Morris, G. C., Jr., DeBakey, M. E., Cooley, D. A., and Crawford, E. S.: Subisthmic Aortic Stenosis and Occlusive Disease, *Arch Surg,* **80:**87, 1960.
Robicsek, F., Sanger, P. W., and Daugherty, H. K.: Coarctation of the Abdominal Aorta Diagnosed by Aortography: Report of Three Cases, *Ann Surg,* **162:**227, 1965.

Renovascular Hypertension

Belzer, F. O., Salvatierra, O., Palubinskas, A., and Stoney, R. J.: Ex Vivo Renal Artery Reconstruction, *Ann Surg,* **182:**456, 1975.
Dean, R. H., and Foster, J. H.: Criteria for the Diagnosis of Renovascular Hypertension, *Surgery,* **74:**926, 1973.
DeBakey, M. E., Morris, G. C., Jr., Morgen, R. O., Crawford, E. S., and Cooley, D. A.: Lesions of the Renal Artery: Surgical Technic and Results, *Am J Surg,* **107:**84, 1964.
DeCamp, P. T., and Birchall, R.: Recognition and Treatment of Renal Artery Stenosis Associated with Hypertension, *Surgery,* **43:**134, 1958.
Dustan, H. P., Page, I. H., and Poutasse, E. F.: Renal Hypertension, *N Engl J Med,* **261:**647, 1959.
———, ———, ———, and Wilson, L.: An Evaluation of Treatment of Hypertension Associated with Occlusive Renal Arterial Disease, *Circulation,* **27:**1018, 1963.
Ernst, C. B., Bookstein, J. J., Montie, J., Baumgartel, E., Hoobler, S. W., and Fry, W. J.: Renal Vein Renin Ratios and Collateral Vessels in Renovascular Hypertension, *Arch Surg,* **104:**496, 1972.
———, Marshall, F. F., Stanley, J. C., and Fry, W. J.: Autogenous Saphenous Vein for Aortorenal Bypass: A Ten Year Experience, *Arch Surg,* **105:**855, 1972.
Foster, J. H.: Surgically Correctible Hypertension, in S. Schwartz (ed.), "Principles of Surgery," 2d ed., p. 939, McGraw Hill Book Company, 1974.
———, Dean, R. H., Pinkerton, J. A., and Rhamy, R. K.: Ten

Years Experience with the Surgical Management of Renovascular Hypertension, *Ann Surg,* 1973.

———, Klatte, E. C., and Burko, H. C.: Arteriographic Pitfalls in the Diagnosis of Renovascular Hypertension, *Arch Surg,* **99:**792, 1969.

———, Oates, J. A., Rhamy, R. K., Klatte, E. C., Burko, H. C., and Michelakis, A. M.: Hypertension and Fibromuscular Dysplasia of the Renal Arteries, *Surgery,* **65:**157, 1969.

———, ———, ———, Pettinger, W. A., Burko, H. C., Younger, R. K., and Scott, H. W., Jr.: Detection and Treatment of Patients with Renovascular Hypertension, *Surgery,* **60:**240, 1966.

———, Pettinger, W. A., Oates, J. A., Rhamy, R. K., Klatte, E. C., Burko, H. C., Bolasny, B. L., Gordon, R., Puyau, F. A., and Younger, R. K.: Malignant Hypertension Secondary to Renal Artery Stenosis in Children, *Ann Surg,* **164:**700, 1966.

———, Rhamy, R. K., Oates, J. A., Klatte, E. C., Burko, H. C., and Michelakis, A. M.: Renovascular Hypertension Secondary to Atherosclerosis, *Am J Med,* **46:**741, 1969.

Fry, W. J., Brink, B. E., and Thompson, N. W.: New Techniques in the Treatment of Extensive Fibromuscular Disease Involving the Renal Arteries, *Surgery,* **68:**959, 1970.

———, Ernst, C. B., Stanley, J. C., and Brink, B.: Renovascular Hypertension in the Pediatric Patient, *Arch Surg,* **107:**692, 1973.

Goldblatt, H., Lynch, J., Hanzal, R. F., and Summerville, W. W.: Studies on Experimental Hypertension, *J Exp Med,* **59:**347, 1934.

Holley, K. W., Hunt, J. C., Brown, A. L., Kincaid, O. W., and Sheps, S. G.: Renal Artery Stenosis: A Clinical-Pathologic Study in Normotensive and Hypertensive Patients, *Am J Med,* **37:**14, 1964.

Howard, J. E., and Connor, T. B.: Use of Differential Renal Function Studies in the Diagnosis of Renovascular Hypertension, *Am J Surg,* **107:**58, 1964.

Hunt, J. C., Harrison, E. G., Jr., Kincaid, O. W., Bernatz, P. E., and Davis, G. D.: Idiopathic Fibrous and Fibromuscular Stenoses of the Renal Arteries Associated with Hypertension, *Proc Staff Meetings Mayo Clin,* **37:**181, 1962.

Leadbetter, W. F., and Burkland, C. E.: Hypertension in Unilateral Renal Disease, *J Urol,* **39:**611, 1938.

Michelakis, A. M., Foster, J. H., Liddle, G. W., Rhamy, R. K., and Kuchel, O.: Measurement of Renin in Both Renal Veins and Its Use in Diagnosis of Renovascular Hypertension, *Arch Intern Med,* **120:**444, 1967.

Morris, G. C., Jr., DeBakey, M. E., Crawford, E. S., Cooley, D. A., and Zanger, L. C. C.: Late Results of Surgical Treatment for Renovascular Hypertension, *Surg Gynecol Obstet,* **122:**1255, 1966.

Ota, K., Mori, S., Awane, Y., and Ueno, A.: Ex Situ Repair of Renal Artery for Renovascular Hypertension, *Arch Surg,* **94:**370, 1967.

Page, I. H., and Corcoran, A. C.: Hypertension: Review of Humoral Pathogenesis and Clinical Treatment, *Adv Intern Med,* **1.**103, 1942.

Shapiro, A. P., Perez-Stable, E., Scheib, E. T., Bron, K., Montsou, S. E., Bert, G., and Misage, J. R.: Renal Artery Stenosis and Hypertension. Observations on the Current Status of Therapy from a Study of 115 Patients, *Am J Med,* **47:**175, 1969.

Sheps, S. G., Hunt, J. C., and Bernatz, P. E.: Diagnosis of Hypertension Associated with Renal Artery Disease, *Manit Med Rev,* **45:**558, 1965.

Stamey, T. A.: Renovascular Hypertension—1965, *Am J Med,* **38:**829, 1965.

———, Nudelmon, I. J., Good, P. H., Schwentker, F. N., and Hendricks, F.: Functional Characteristics of Renovascular Hypertension, *Medicine (Baltimore),* **40:**347, 1961.

Stanley, J. C., Ernst, C. B., and Fry, W. J.: Fate of 100 Aortorenal Vein Grafts: Characteristics of Late Graft Expansion, Aneurysmic Dilatation and Stenosis, *Surgery,* **74:**931, 1973.

Vaughan, E. D., Jr., Buhler, F. R., Laragh, J. H., Sealey, J. E., Baer, L., and Bard, R. H.: Renovascular Hypertension: Renin Measurements to Indicate Hypersecretion and Contralateral Suppression, Estimate Renal Plasma Flow and Score for Surgical Curability, *Am J Med,* **55:**402, 1973.

Vertes, V., Grauel, J. A., and Stoney, R. J.: Autogenous Tissue Revascularization Technics in Surgery for Renovascular Hypertension, *Ann Surg,* **170:**416, 1969.

Vermeulen, F., Stas, F., Delegher, C., Buyssens, N., et al.: Surgical Correction of Renovascular Hypertension in Children, *J Cardiovasc Surg (Torino),* **16:**21, 1975.

Wylie, E. J., Perloff, D., and Stoney, R. J.: Autogenous Tissue Revascularization Techniques in Surgery for Renovascular Hypertension, *Ann Surg,* **170:**416, 1969.

———, Perloff, D., and Wellington, J. S.: Fibromuscular Hyperplasia of the Renal Arteries, *Ann Surg,* **156:**592, 1962.

Unilateral Renal Parenchymal Disease

McDonald, D. F.: Renal Hypertension without Main Arterial Stenosis: Function Tests Predict Cure., *JAMA,* **203:**130, 1968.

Vaughan, E. D., Jr., Buhler, F. R., Laragh, J. H., Sealey, J. E., Gavras, H., and Baer, L.: Hypertension and Unilateral Parenchymal Renal Disease: Evidence for Abnormal Vasoconstriction-Volume Interaction, *JAMA,* **223:**1177, 1975.

Essential Hypertension

Bilgutay, A. M., and Lillehei, C. W.: Treatment of Hypertension with an Implantable Electronic Device, *JAMA,* **191:**649, 1965.

Brest, A. N.: Carotid Sinus Nerve Stimulation, *Am J Cardiol,* **26:**328, 1970.

Gordon, T., and Devine, B.: "Hypertension and Hypertensive Heart Disease in Adults, United States—1960–62: Vital and Health Statistics Data from the National Health Survey," U.S. Department of Health, Education, and Welfare, National Center for Health Statistics ser. 11, no. 13.

Griffith, L. S. C., and Schwartz, S. I.: Reversal of Renal Hypertension by Electrical Stimulation of the Carotid Sinus Nerve, *Surgery,* **56:**232, 1964.

Grimson, K. S.: Total Thoracic and Partial to Total Lumbar Sympathectomy and Celiac Ganglionectomy in the Treatment of Hypertension, *Ann Surg,* **114:**753, 1941.

Jeffers, W. A., Sellers, A. M., Wolferth, C. C., Ross, A. M., and Blakemore, W. S.: Results of Sympathectomy and Adrenalectomy, *Am J Surg,* **107:**211, 1964.

McCubbin, J. W., Green, J. H., and Page, I. H.: Baroreceptor Function in Chronic Renal Hypertension, *Circ Res,* **4:**205, 1956.

Schwartz, S. I., and Griffith, L. S. C.: "Reduction of Hypertension by Electrical Stimulation of the Carotid Sinus Nerve, Baroreceptors and Hypertension," Pergamon Press, New York, 1967.

———, ———, Neistadt, A., and Hagfors, N.: Chronic Carotid Sinus Nerve Stimulation in the Treatment of Essential Hypertension, *Am J Surg,* **114:**5, 1967.

Smithwick, R. H.: Practical Treatment for Hypertension, Splanch-nicectomy, Adrenalectomy, and Nephrectomy, *Postgrad Med,* **34:**32, 1963.

Warner, H. R.: The Frequency-dependent Nature of Blood Pressure Regulation by the Carotid Sinus Studied with an Electric Analog, *Circ Res,* **6:**35, 1958.

Zintel, H. A.: Adrenalectomy versus Sympathectomy: Results of Surgery, in J. H. Moyer (ed.), "Hypertension," p. 695, W. B. Saunders Company, Philadelphia, 1959.

Chapter 24

Manifestations of Gastrointestinal Disease

by **Seymour I. Schwartz** and **Edward H. Storer**

Symptoms represent subjective manifestations of disturbance in function and are not specific for a disease but rather for a pathophysiologic state. In the gastrointestinal tract, the following changes in physiologic function may be implicated: altered secretion, altered motility, inadequate digestion, inadequate absorption, obstruction. The resultant symptoms of gastrointestinal disease include abdominal pain, dysphagia, anorexia, nausea and vomiting, bloating or distension, constipation, and diarrhea.

Signs of gastrointestinal disease are objective demonstrations of a pathologic process. These include tenderness, abdominal wall rigidity, palpable masses, altered bowel sounds, evidence of gastrointestinal bleeding, poor nutrition, jaundice, and stigmata of hepatic dysfunction.

PAIN

Pain (from the Latin *poena*, penalty, punishment, torment) is the predominant sensory experience by which man judges the existence of disease within himself. Like all subjective experiences, pain cannot be satisfactorily defined but is known to us by experience and described by illustration.

Most diseases of the abdominal viscera are associated with pain at some time during their course. Indeed, the correct diagnosis of acute abdominal disorders (the "acute abdomen") usually amounts to the correct identification of the cause of the abdominal pain.

There have been two opposing theories of the nature of pain. Proponents of the *intensity theory* held that pain is the consequence of excessive stimulation of any nerve endings, be they touch, temperature, sight, smell, or taste. Sensations of every order which in moderate degree are rather pleasant become unpleasant when their intensity grows too strong. In this intensity scheme, any nervous pathways are considered potential pain pathways and conduct the impulse patterns that are associated with the perceptions of pain. Integration at the thalamocortical level provides the possibility for impulses received from the same peripheral apparatus to be perceived as pain.

Although there is not yet unequivocal proof that each peripheral nerve fiber is devoted to but one type of sensory modality—pain, touch, cold, or warmth—most physiologists now subscribe to the *specificity theory*, which holds that pain is a separate sensory modality with its own specific neural apparatus. In 1965 Melzak and Wall proposed the *gate-control theory*. They indicated that the specificity theory was strongly supported but disagreed with the proposal that sensation is achieved by a fixed direct-line communication from skin to brain. Their contribution was the suggestion that the amount and quality of perceived pain are determined by many physiological and psychological variables. Modulation of nociceptive impulses occurs at the dorsal horn and at various levels of the ascending afferent systems. Appropriate stimuli initiate impulses in skin, muscle, or viscera. These sensory impulses are transmitted to the posterior horn of the spinal cord in the primary sensory neuron which has its cell body in the dorsal root ganglion. The secondary sensory neuron in the posterior horn transmits the impulses in the contralateral spinothalamic tract to the posterolateral nucleus of the thalamus. The tertiary sensory neuron transmits the impulses from the thalamus to the postcentral gyrus of the cerebral cortex (Fig. 24-1).

Three kinds of pain are recognized and designated: superficial, or cutaneous pain; deep pain from muscles, tendons, joints, and fascia; and visceral pain. The first two may be combined as somatic pain. Knowledge of visceral pain has lagged, in part because of the difficulty of the laboratory investigation of pain, but also because of some early theories which, by the strength of tradition and prestige, delayed progress.

PAIN PATHWAYS. Until well into the twentieth century,

Fig. 24-1. Schematic representation of pathways involved in abdominal pain.

the viscera were thought to be completely insensitive. The first important observer of visceral sensation was William Harvey in the seventeenth century. When the young son of Count Montgomery sustained a chest wound which on healing left the heart exposed, Harvey observed that touching the heart caused not the slightest sensation. After the discovery of local anesthesia, Lennander found that human abdominal viscera are insensitive to cutting, crushing, and even burning. He categorically stated in 1901 that the viscera are wholly insensitive and that only traction or irritation of the parietal peritoneum could cause abdominal pain. The record was set straight in 1911 by Hurst, who demonstrated that distension of any hollow viscus is painful. Ryle amplified this by emphasizing that contraction of smooth muscle of hollow viscera is an adequate physiologic stimulus.

The current and preferable terminology uses the term *visceral afferents* to denote all afferent fibers from the viscera including those which give rise to visceral reflexes as well as those which subserve pain. The terms *autonomic, sympathetic,* and *parasympathetic* are reserved for the visceral *efferent* fibers.

Pain impulses from the abdominal cavity reach the central nervous system by three routes: from the viscera via visceral afferents that travel with (1) the sympathetic and (2) the parasympathetic nerves, and from the parietal peritoneum, body wall, diaphragm, and root of mesenteries via somatic afferents that travel in (3) the segmental spinal nerves or phrenic nerves. Primary sensory neurons for pain, both visceral and somatic, are mostly small (1 to 2 μ), unmyelinated fibers but with some small (3 to 4 μ), myelinated fibers (Gasser classes C and A delta, or groups IV and III in Lloyd's terminology).

The route of a typical afferent from an abdominal viscus is as follows: the axons of nerve endings in the wall of the viscus follow the artery to the aorta and then through the collateral sympathetic ganglion without synapsing. They then enter the splanchnic nerve, traverse the paravertebral sympathetic ganglion, again without synapsing, and join the spinal nerve via the white ramus communicans. The cell body of this primary visceral afferent neuron is located in the spinal ganglion from which central processes are sent to the dorsal horn of the spinal cord via the dorsal root.

The central processes of the primary sensory neuron synapse with at least three distinct spinal tracts: (1) secondary pain neurons whose axons ascend for two or three segments and then cross in the anterior commissure to the anterolateral spinothalamic tract, (2) secondary sensory neurons whose processes ascend the posterior columns, and (3) many small neurons in the substantia gelatinosa which contribute to the tract of Lissauer. As the secondary sensory neurons ascend, collaterals are given off to the reticular substance forming the core of the brainstem, and to the hypothalamus. The role of these extraspinothalamic pathways is uncertain—they may be alternative pain pathways, may inhibit central pain responses, or may be involved in the affective aspects of pain. Sensory tracts synapse in the thalamus with tertiary neurons that project to the cortex. The cortical areas involved with pain are not completely known. Stimulation of various areas of the postcentral gyrus in conscious man produces contralateral paresthesias of small areas of the body, but even total hemispherectomy does not consistently abolish pain, though localization is defective. The functions of the thalamus in man, in contrast to animals, are largely expressed through the cortex. But one function that may have been retained in the evolutionary process is the expression of the affective aspects of sensation. Affectivity— pleasantness and unpleasantness—is considered a primitive function which has remained at the thalamic level despite development of the cerebral cortex.

Though the thalamus and frontal cortex are the principal areas of the brain involved with pain, they cannot be considered as *the* brain centers, since the hypothalamus, the limbic system, the brainstem reticular formation, and the parietal cortex are also involved in pain perception.

Abdominal Pain

Three distinct types of pain are involved in the general symptom complex of abdominal pain: visceral pain, (deep) somatic pain, and referred pain.

VISCERAL PAIN. True visceral pain, or splanchnic pain, arises in abdominal organs invested with visceral peritoneum via impulses conducted to the spinal cord over visceral afferent nerve fibers. As noted above, the viscera are normally insensitive to stimuli that produce pain when applied to the skin. But there is no reason for the viscera to react to these stimuli to which they are not normally exposed, and thus sensitivity has not evolved. Adequate stimuli for visceral pain are those arising from their own environment—pathologic conditions of the viscera. Stimuli that produce pain include increased tension in the wall of hollow viscera from either distension or spastic contraction, stretching of the capsules of solid viscera, ischemia, and certain chemicals. The threshold for pain is lowered by inflammation and by ischemia, so that normal muscular contractions that would ordinarily not be felt may produce pain.

The role of chemical substances in visceral pain is not clear at this time. Experimentally, pain can be produced by the intraarterial injection of acid, alkaline, or hypertonic solutions: lactate, potassium ions, or bradykinin. Potassium which is released from cells by injury or ischemia has long been known as a pain-producing agent, and it has been suggested that the release of intracellular potassium ions may be the actual physiologic stimulus for pain. Lim would classify some pain receptors as chemoceptors and attributes the pain of ischemia to increasing concentrations of hydrogen ions and the pain of inflammation to the accrual of algesic bradykinin peptides.

Visceral pain tends to be rather diffuse and poorly localized, has a high threshold, and exhibits an exceedingly slow rate of adaptation. The high threshold and poor localization are probably in part attributable to the relatively sparse distribution of sensory endings in the viscera. The pain is felt by the patient to be "deep" in those cutaneous areas or zones which correspond roughly to the segmental distribution of somatic sensory fibers which take origin from the same segments of the cord as the visceral afferent fibers from the viscus in question.

With severe visceral or deep somatic pain, concomitant responses, presumably due to autonomic reflexes, may be prominent. These include sweating; nausea, sometimes with vomiting; tachycardia or bradycardia; fall in blood pressure; cutaneous hyperalgesia, hyperesthesia, or tenderness; and involuntary spastic contractions of abdominal wall musculature. The muscular rigidity accompanying severe pain is most marked when the body wall is involved by the pain-inciting lesion, e.g., the boardlike rigidity associated with perforated peptic ulcer. The distribution is regional rather than segmental and thus involves sustained reflexes in several segmental nerves. Maintained muscular rigidity may of itself become painful, so that on occasion the deep muscular tenderness outlasts and outweighs the original visceral pain.

SOMATIC PAIN. Pain arising in the abdominal wall, particularly the parietal peritoneum, root of the mesenteries, and respiratory diaphragm, is mediated by somatic afferents in segmental spinal nerves. Pain from parietal structures is for the most part sharper and brighter than visceral pain; it is well localized close to the site of stimulation; and when the source is on one side of the midline, the pain is also lateralized. Acute appendicitis is a common visceral disease that well illustrates typical visceral and somatic abdominal pain. The visceral pain of early appendicitis is perceived diffusely and dully in the periumbilical and lower epigastric regions, and there is little or no rigidity of the abdominal musculature. Later, when parietal peritoneum becomes involved in the inflammatory process, the somatic component of pain is more severe and sharply localized in the right lower quadrant. There is also

cutaneous hyperesthesia, tenderness, and muscular rigidity in the right lower quadrant.

REFERRED PAIN. Visceral disease may give rise to pain localized to more superficial areas of the body, often at a considerable distance from the diseased viscus. The reference is usually dermatomic, but on occasion pain may be referred to the scar of a previous surgical operation, trauma, or localized pathologic process. This is called *habit reference* and implies that pain perception is influenced by the individual's prior pain experience.

There are two major hypotheses of the dermatomic reference of visceral pain: *convergence-facilitation* and *convergence-projection*. MacKenzie believed that visceral afferents have no direct connection to the spinothalamic tracts but can only set up an irritable focus in the spinal segment at which they enter the cord. According to his hypothesis, afferent impulses from surface areas which are arriving in insufficient numbers to be felt as pain by themselves are facilitated by the visceral impulses with the production of cutaneous pain and hyperalgesia. There is little evidence to support this hypothesis of referred pain; in general, neurophysiologists have found that one afferent volley tends to block another. As a matter of fact, in the gate-control hypothesis of Melzack and Wall, input of impulses into the substantia gelatinosa from surface afferents, along with corticospinal impulses, serves to inhibit the transmission of pain, not to facilitate it.

More consonant with current evidence is the convergence-projection hypothesis. Since the pain fibers in the posterior roots greatly outnumber the fibers in the spinothalamic tracts, several pain fibers must converge on one tract fiber. This same convergence may occur at thalmaic or cortical levels as well. When afferents from the skin and viscera converge on the same neuron at some point in the pain pathway, the resulting impulses, on projection to the brain, are interpreted as coming from the skin, an interpretation learned from previous experiences in which the same tract fiber was stimulated by cutaneous afferents.

INTRACTABLE PAIN

Fortunately, most abdominal pain is caused by pathologic processes that are amenable to medical or surgical treatment. The control of pain associated with diseases that cannot be satisfactorily treated is one of the most challenging and often frustrating problems the clinician has to face. Examples are unresectable carcinoma of the pancreas and chronic pancreatitis.

Opiate analgesics if given in sufficient dosage can usually control abdominal pain, but at the risk of addiction and negating the patient's ability to function as an effective person. This is probably the best therapy, however, for a patient with incurable disease and a life expectancy of a few weeks or months. It should not be used in patients with severe pain from nonmalignant causes with an unpredictable life expectancy.

Neurosurgical intervention on the pain pathways, though disappointing at times, is the treatment of choice for intractable pain in properly selected patients. Narcotic addiction prior to surgery usually compromises the result, as an addicted patient continues to be addicted even though his pain is relieved by the procedure.

Splanchnicectomy and celiac ganglionectomy can effectively control abdominal pain if somatically innervated structures are not involved in the pain-producing process. When both visceral and somatic pain fibers are involved, posterior rhizotomy or tract interruption is indicated. The spinothalamic tracts are usually interrupted, either by surgical incision or injection of sclerosing chemicals, in the spinal cord a few segments above the segments where the noxious impulses are entering. The interruption has also been done at medullary or mesencephalic levels. After anterolateral chordotomy, pain and temperature sensation are lost, while proprioception and touch are virtually unimpaired. Paresthesias often replace pain in the anesthetic areas, and in a significant number of patients, after about 1 year, the paresthesias become disagreeable and painful. For this reason, root or tract interruption is most useful in patients with intractable pain and a life expectancy of a year or so.

For patients with pain arising from areas too great to be controlled by peripheral interventions, prefrontal lobotomy may be considered. Such lesions do not abolish pain but diminish the reaction to pain. The price paid for such relief, however, includes inability to experience pleasure, as well; i.e., there is a flattening of all affect and the development of a more or less apathetic state.

It is obvious from the above that there is a need for a means to relieve intractable pain which would be nonaddicting, would not affect the patient's personality or mind, and would not destroy normal neural tissue. Recent developments in clinical research offer some hope. Shealy et al. have devised and successfully tested a dorsal column stimulator which is now commercially available. In theory, impulses arising from electrostimulation of descending dorsal column fibers are used to inhibit, in accordance with the gate-control theory, prolonged small-fiber afterdischarge which is uniquely related to pain. Electrodes are implanted four to eight segments above the pain input. The external transmitter is controlled by the patient. There is a buzzing or tingling sensation below the site of the stimulator, but pain is usually controlled without significant alteration of normal sensory function. Transcutaneous electrical stimulation has been used effectively to control postoperative pain. Whether this technique can be extended over prolonged periods remains to be evaluated.

ETIOLOGY. Abdominal pain may be caused by a great variety of gastrointestinal and intraperitoneal diseases, and, because of overlapping nerve distribution, the pain may be secondary to extraperitoneal disorders. Pain of intraabdominal origin (Table 24-1) may emanate from the peritoneum, hollow intestinal viscera, solid viscera, mesentery, or pelvic organs, and may be caused by inflammation, mechanical processes such as obstruction or acute distension, and vascular disturbances.

The extraperitoneal causes of abdominal pain are outlined in Table 24-2. Most of the intrathoracic diseases which cause abdominal pain are confused with upper abdominal disorders, since their segmental distribution is similar. The intraspinal diseases have pain patterns which

Table 24-1. GASTROINTESTINAL AND INTRAPERITONEAL CAUSES OF ABDOMINAL PAIN

I. Inflammation
  A. Peritoneum
    1. Chemical and nonbacterial peritonitis—perforated peptic ulcer, gallbladder, ruptured ovarian cyst, mittelschmerz
    2. Bacterial peritonitis
      a. Primary peritonitis—pneumococcal, streptococcal, tuberculous
      b. Perforated hollow viscus—stomach, intestine, biliary tract
  B. Hollow intestinal organs
    1. Appendicitis
    2. Cholecystitis
    3. Peptic ulceration
    4. Gastroenteritis
    5. Regional enteritis
    6. Meckel's diverticulitis
    7. Colitis—ulcerative, bacterial, amebic
    8. Diverticulitis
  C. Solid viscera
    1. Pancreatitis
    2. Hepatitis
    3. Hepatic abscess
    4. Splenic abscess
  D. Mesentery
    1. Lymphadenitis
  E. Pelvic organs
    1. Pelvic inflammatory disease
    2. Tuboovarian abscess
    3. Endometritis
II. Mechanical (obstruction, acute distension)
  A. Hollow intestinal organs
    1. Intestinal obstruction—adhesions, hernia, tumor, volvulus, intussusception
    2. Biliary obstruction—calculi, tumor, choledochal cyst, hematobilia
  B. Solid viscera
    1. Acute splenomegaly
    2. Acute hepatomegaly—cardiac failure, Budd-Chiari syndrome
  C. Mesentery
    1. Omental torsion
  D. Pelvic organs
    1. Ovarian cyst
    2. Torsion or degeneration of fibroid
    3. Ectopic pregnancy
III. Vascular
  A. Intraperitoneal bleeding
    1. Ruptured liver
    2. Ruptured spleen
    3. Ruptured mesentery
    4. Ruptured ectopic pregnancy
    5. Ruptured aortic, splenic, or hepatic aneurysm
  B. Ischemia
    1. Mesenteric thrombosis
    2. Hepatic infarction—toxemia, purpura
    3. Splenic infarction
    4. Omental ischemia
IV. Miscellaneous
  A. Endometriosis

are similar to the referred pain from abdominal pathologic conditions, but they are usually not accompanied by tenderness or muscular rigidity. Inflammation of peripheral nerves, as in the case of herpes zoster, may be accompanied

Table 24-2. EXTRAPERITONEAL CAUSES
OF ABDOMINAL PAIN

Cardiopulmonary
  Pneumonia
  Empyema
  Myocardial ischemia
  Active rheumatic heart
    disease
Blood
  Leukemia
  Sickle cell crisis
Neurogenic
  Spinal cord tumors
  Osteomyelitis of spine
  Tabes dorsalis
  Herpes zoster
  Abdominal epilepsy
Genitourinary
  Nephritis
  Pyelitis
  Perinephric abscesses
  Ureteral obstruction (calculi,
    tumors)
  Prostatitis
  Seminal vesiculitis
  Epidydimitis

Vascular
  Dissection, rupture, or ex-
    pansion of aortic aneurysm
  Periarteritis
Metabolic
  Uremia
  Diabetic acidosis
  Porphyria
  Addisonian crisis
Toxins
  Bacterial (tetanus)
  Insect bites
  Venoms
  Drugs
  Lead poisoning
Abdominal wall
  Intramuscular hematoma
Psychogenic

by tenderness and pain before the lesion becomes apparent. The pain usually has a distribution similar to myocardial infarction of biliary tract disease.

CLINICAL EVALUATION. Since pain is the subjective reaction to a stimulus which initiates transmission along nerve pathways to cortical centers, the patient's response is dependent upon both physical and psychologic factors. Physical requirements for response to pain include the patient's consciousness to permit perception, and integrity of the entire avenue along which impulses are transmitted to the brain. With repeated stimulation, the cortical threshold becomes lowered, and resistance is reduced along nerve pathways, which results in hypersensitivity and "facilitated pain." Hyperthyroidism, hyperadrenalism, and the menopausal syndrome are all associated with increased response to pain, while hypothyroidism is usually accompanied by an increased pain threshold. Sensitivity alters with age, increasing from infancy to adult life and then gradually diminishing in the elderly patient. The asthenic habitus is generally characterized by increased sensitivity, and the Anglo-Saxon and Nordic types are generally less sensitive and responsive to pain than Latins and Jews.

The physical responses to painful stimuli are also variable. While superficial pain is frequently associated with diffuse sympathetic nervous system stimulation and outpouring of epinephrine as part of a defense reaction, severe deep pain is more often accompanied by bradycardia, hypotension, nausea and vomiting, sweating, and, at times, syncope. Continued pain may cause a decrease in renal blood flow, renal clearance, and oliguria. Cardiac arrythmias may also occur, and, in the extreme case, neurogenic shock may result.

History. In eliciting a description of pain, the character, severity, location, timing, and factors which either augment or reduce the pain should all be defined. Certain pathologic states are associated with characteristic pain patterns.

Colic—biliary, ureteral, or intestinal—is intermittent, frequently occurring in waves, and is described as cramping, or the patient may use the very term "colicky." Pain of a penetrating ulcer is "burning," while pain accompanying expansion of an abdominal aneurysm is "boring and pounding." Tabes is manifested by "stabbing" pain, and the pain accompanying pleuritis or perforation of a viscus has also been described as "knifelike."

The severity of the pain is an expression of the intensity of stimuli plus the patient's physical and emotional response. Colicky pain related to acute distension of the biliary tract, intestine, or ureters and pain of neurologic origin such as herpes and tabes all have an extremely high intensity. Pain evoked by inflammatory stimuli is less marked. In patients with peritonitis, the degree of pain and muscular rigidity generally parallel each other. Severe pain may be manifested by physical responses, to which previous reference has been made.

In general, abdominal pains which persist for 6 hours are caused by conditions of surgical significance. However, it is rare for any pain to be absolutely constant. The pain resulting from distension of hollow viscera is generally intermittent, while the pain of peritonitis is most frequently continuous. Pain which awakens the patient from sleep is usually characteristic of organic disease. Ulcer pain frequently occurs at night or prior to a meal, whereas gallbladder pain may be stimulated by eating. Peptic ulcer pain also has a seasonal variation, occurring more frequently in the spring and fall. In addition to the effect of digestion of food on the pain, the effects of position, motion, and respiration have diagnostic importance.

The location of pain should include a description of original situation, any shifting, and radiation. The initial location may better define the visceral involvement, since once peritonitis occurs, pain becomes diffuse. Because of variation in location of the organs and the pathologic processes plus the vagueness of visceral pain, it is difficult to totally exclude diseases on the basic of location, but certain relationships generally pertain (Fig. 24-2). Visceral intestinal pain is usually experienced in the midportion of the abdomen. Duodenal pain is felt in the epigastrium, while the pain of the remainder of the small intestine is characteristically referred to the region of the umbilicus. Pain originating in the large bowel is less well localized and frequently experienced in the hypogastrium. Sigmoid dilatation may result in suprapublic or presacral pain.

The patient's age represents a factor which focuses attention on certain processes. Acute colicky pain in a child under two is suggestive of intussusception, whereas peptic ulcer is extremely uncommon in the young age group. Appendicitis is most frequently a disease of the young adolescent, cholecystitis is more commonly seen in the middle-age group, while diverticulitis rarely occurs before the age of thirty-five.

Vomiting is indicative of severe irritation of the peritoneum, stretching of the mesentery, obstruction, or absorbed toxins. The exact timing of vomiting in relation to the onset of pain is pertinent. Pain almost always precedes vomiting by several hours in patients with appendicitis. Vomiting may also occur early in relation to the onset of

PERITONITIS
PANCREATITIS
LEUKEMIA
SICKLE CELL CRISIS
EARLY APPENDICITIS
MESENTERIC ADENITIS
MESENTERIC THROMBOSIS
GASTROENTERITIS
ANEURYSM
COLITIS
INTESTINAL OBSTRUCTION
METABOLIC, TOXIC, AND
    BACTERIAL CAUSES

A

DIFFUSE PAIN

GALL BLADDER AND BILIARY TRACT
HEPATITIS
HEPATIC ABSCESS
HEPATOMEGALY DUE TO
    CONGESTIVE FAILURE
PEPTIC ULCER
PANCREATITIS
RETROCECAL APPENDICITIS
RENAL PAIN
HERPES ZOSTER
MYOCARDIAL ISCHEMIA
PERICARDITIS
PNEUMONIA
EMPYEMA

B

RIGHT UPPER QUADRANT PAIN

APPENDICITIS
INTESTINAL OBSTRUCTION
REGIONAL ENTERITIS
DIVERTICULITIS
CHOLECYSTITIS
PERFORATED ULCER
LEAKING ANEURYSM
ABDOMINAL WALL HEMATOMA
ECTOPIC PREGNANCY
OVARIAN CYST OR TORSION
SALPINGITIS
MITTELSCHMERZ
ENDOMETRIOSIS
URETERAL CALCULI
RENAL PAIN
SEMINAL VESICULITIS
PSOAS ABSCESS

C

RIGHT LOWER QUADRANT PAIN

DIVERTICULITIS
INTESTINAL OBSTRUCTION
APPENDICITIS
LEAKING ANEURYSM
ABDOMINAL WALL HEMATOMA
ECTOPIC PREGNANCY
MITTELSCHMERZ
OVARIAN CYST OR TORSION
SALPINGITIS
ENDOMETRIOSIS
URETERAL CALCULI
RENAL PAIN
SEMINAL VESICULITIS
PSOAS ABSCESS

D

LEFT LOWER QUADRANT PAIN

Fig. 24-2. Characteristic location of abdominal pain associated with various diseases.

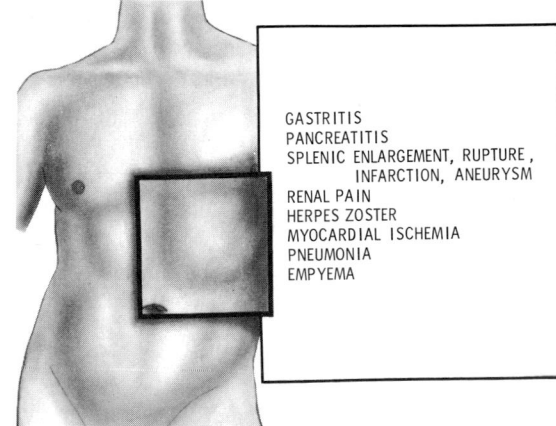

GASTRITIS
PANCREATITIS
SPLENIC ENLARGEMENT, RUPTURE,
    INFARCTION, ANEURYSM
RENAL PAIN
HERPES ZOSTER
MYOCARDIAL ISCHEMIA
PNEUMONIA
EMPYEMA

E   LEFT UPPER QUADRANT PAIN

pany biliary obstruction or diseases with pyloric obstruction.

An evaluation of bowel habits is particularly pertinent in patients with colon obstruction, and a menstrual history is imperative in women with lower abdominal or pelvic pain. Past history should be complete and include pertinent medical illnesses, previous surgical treatment, trauma, and drugs.

Physical Examination. Pain itself evokes physical changes which may be manifested on examination. Hyperalgesia may occur at the site of the original stimulus or in the area of referred pain. Muscle contraction may be a consequence of deep pain, or the muscle spasm itself may be responsible for pain. The autonomic responses to pain include pallor, sweating, nausea, vomiting, bradycardia, hypotension, and syncope. Regard for the patient's general appearance includes his attitude in bed, tissue turgor, respiratory rate, and temperature. Restricted motion in bed suggests peritonitis, whereas writhing is more frequently an accompaniment of biliary or ureteral colic.

The abdomen should be examined in a routine manner

pain in patients with peritonitis and biliary or ureteral colic. With intestinal obstruction, the interval between the onset of pain and vomiting provides some indication of the level of obstruction. Frequent vomiting is indicative of intestinal obstruction, while a clear emesis may accomwith inspection, auscultation, percussion, and palpation performed sequentially. On inspection, restricted motion of the abdominal wall during respiration suggests diffuse peritonitis. Maintenance of the hip in a position of flexion is suggestive of a psoas abscess, appendicitis, or a pelvic abscess. Auscultation for bowel sounds may reveal the borborygmi associated with mechanical intestinal obstruction, while an absence of bowel sounds is suggestive of diffuse peritonitis. Percussion is performed for the detection of free peritoneal fluid, distension, and the absence of liver dullness associated with a perforated viscus. Palpation should always begin away from the area of pain and include all possible sites for hernia. Superficial palpation may demonstrate hyperesthesia to pinprick or pinching in a segmental area of referred pain. Deep palpation may detect a mass. Muscle rigidity is a relative term, and its evaluation is dependent on the patient's cooperation. Pelvic and rectal examination are integral procedures for the evaluation of the acute surgical abdomen, as is a thorough examination of the chest for cardiac and pulmonary disease.

Laboratory Procedures. The hemogram with specific interest in the white blood cell count to define the presence of an inflammatory process and a hematocrit reading to determine if there is hemoconcentration or anemia should be routine. Urinalysis is directed toward evaluating diabetes, porphyria, the presence of infection, or red cells associated with calculi. An elevated serum amylase level is most frequently associated with acute pancreatitis but does occur with a variety of other intraabdominal processes including perforated viscera, cholecystitis, choledocholithiasis, and intraabdominal bleeding. A sickle cell preparation may be called for in Negroes. Emergency roentgenographic studies include supine films and upright or lateral decubitus films to determine the presence of air within the intestinal lumen or free within the peritoneal cavity. A chest x-ray is particularly applicable in patients over forty with upper abdominal pain, as is an electrocardiogram to rule out mycrocardial ischemia, which may mimic cholecystitis. The determination of the presence of free blood or significant amounts of peritoneal fluid may be accomplished by paracentesis with microscopic examination of the specimen or, in the case of lower abdominal or pelvic pain, culdocentesis and culdoscopy. It is to be emphasized that laparotomy may consitute an important tool in the diagnosis of acute abdominal pain.

DYSPHAGIA

Dysphagia refers to a difficulty in swallowing and is related to either a functional alteration in the mechanism of deglutition or physical encroachment upon the lumen of the esophagus. The term *odynophagia* is used when swallowing is painful

ACT OF SWALLOWING. This is classically divided into three stages. In the first stage the bolus of food or liquid is voluntarily moved into the pharynx by contraction of the mylohyoid muscle. In the second stage, the material is transported through the pharynx by waves of contractions which are involuntary, or reflex. This reflex is initiated by a stimulus from the base of the tongue, soft palate, uvula, and posterior pharyngeal wall and travels up the glossopharyngeal nerve, the second division of the trigeminal nerve, and the superior laryngeal nerve. The impulses terminate in the medulla and initiate a series of efferent stimuli which coordinate contraction of the pharyngeal constrictors. Elevation of the soft palate closes off the nasopharynx, and contraction of the suprahyoid muscles elevates the larynx and brings it forward, thus closing the entrance into the larynx and trachea. Respiration is inhibited, and the respiratory tract is completely sealed off by approximation of the vocal cords and posterior displacement of the epiglottis. The terminal phase of the second stage is relaxation of the cricopharyngeus muscles, which permits the bolus to enter the upper esophagus.

The third stage of deglutition transports the bolus through the esophagus into the stomach. Waves of positive pressure sweep down the body of the esophagus in an orderly fashion, and the wave of pressure may reach an intensity of 50 to 100 cm of water. This wave is effected by a reflex arc, the afferent impulses of which are carried through the glossopharyngeal nerve and the efferent impulses transported by the vagi. Auerbach's plexuses within the wall of the esophagus are also involved. When distension by a solid bolus of food occurs, secondary peristaltic contractions result in that segment. Nonperistaltic tertiary esophageal contractions are seen in the lower esophagus of normal people after the age of forty. They are important considerations in the differential diagnosis of esophageal varices.

Transport of the bolus through the esophagus is dependent upon the pressure gradient produced by the primary peristaltic contraction plus, in the case of liquids, the effect of gravity. The final phase of deglutition is the propulsion of the bolus from the esophagus into the stomach. This is dependent upon relaxation of the inferior esophageal sphincter, which reacts reflexly and autonomously in response to pressure or peristalsis in the lower esophagus.

ETIOLOGY. Dysphagia may be due to oropharyngeal or esophageal causes. The former includes disorders of the mouth, upper respiratory tract, and pharynx. Any painful lesion of the mouth or tongue including pharyngitis, retropharyngeal abscess, or oral carcinoma may be implicated. Acute thyroiditis is usually accompanied by pharyngeal dysphagia. Neuromuscular disturbances which may affect deglutition include poliomyelitis, syringomyelia, glossopharyngeal neuritis, and myasthenia. Alteration of the muscle itself, as is seen in amyloidosis and scleroderma, also results in dysphagia, which may be either oropharyngeal or esophageal in location.

Esophageal dysphagia is related to a great variety of causes, which are listed in Table 24-3. The level at which the patient localizes a sticking sensation usually corresponds well to the level of the responsible lesion. Dysphagia may be caused by disturbance in esophageal motility with either hypomotility or hypermotility implicated (see Chap. 25). The passage of fluid through the esophagus

Table 24-3. CAUSES OF ESOPHAGEAL DYSPHAGIA

Cause	Predominant sex	Age incidence		Salient historical and related characteristics
		10–45	*45 and over*	
Carcinoma	Male	Rare	Common	Duration of symptoms less than 2 years; painful swallowing occurs early, dysphagia later.
Peptic esophagitis	Male	Common	Common	Heartburn for years, often preceding dysphagia; odynophagia later.
Achalasia	Male-female	Common	Common	Liquids, especially cold, cause dysphagia early; regurgitation easy; odynophagia mild and late.
Contractile ring	Male	Rare	Common	Brief, intermittent attacks of dysphagia with no interval symptoms.
Diffuse spasm	Male	Rare	Rare	Affects elderly persons; multiple ringlike contractions along esophageal tube.
Zenker's diverticulum	Male	Rare	Rare	Sticking feeling in neck, gurgling on swallowing; occasional regurgitation of decayed food.
Scleroderma	Female	Common	Rare	Skin changes; Raynaud's phenomenon.
Paraesophageal hiatal hernia . . .	Female	Rare	Rare	Attacks of substernal pressure, pain, dysphagia, and belching during meals.
Extrinsic masses		Common	Rare	Symptoms of primary disorder.

SOURCE: After Ingelfinger, *Med Sci,* Apr. 10, 1960, pp. 451–470.

may also be impaired by encroachment upon the lumen. In the proximal esophagus, Zenker's pharyngoesophageal diverticulum, obstructing bands, and hypertrophic spurs of the anterior cervical vertebrae may be implicated. Dysphagia in the region of the cervical esophagus may also be due to esophageal carcinoma, cervical lymphadenopathy, stenosis secondary to ingestion of a caustic substance, or pressure from an enlarged thyroid. In the middle third of the esophagus carcinoma, stenosis, esophagitis, and traction diverticulum all may be causes. In addition, a wide variety of mediastinal inflammatory malignant lesions may encroach upon the lumen. Vascular lesions such as enlargement of the left atrium, aneurysm in the arch of the aorta, and anomalous right subclavian artery are rare causes of dysphagia in this region. In the lower third of the esophagus, primary carcinoma and carcinoma of the stomach with craniad extension represent common causes, particularly in the older age group. Other lower esophageal causes of dysphagia include reflux esophagitis, achalasia, contractile rings, and epiphrenic diverticula.

Dysphagia is a relatively common manifestation of emotional diseases. Inability to swallow accompanies anxiety states, conversion hysteria, and anorexia nervosa.

CLINICAL EVALUATION. History should include a precise description of the symptom with particular reference to the duration, location, and timing in relation to ingestion of food. True dysphagia occurs within 15 minutes of swallowing. The patient can usually pinpoint the site of obstruction. The determination of the amount of weight loss and the presence of associated vomiting are important. Physical examination is directed toward the detection of cervical nodes suggesting mediastinal or esophageal lesions, enlargement of the esophagus, and stigmata of scleroderma. Barium study of the esophagus is frequently diagnostic, and the use of cineroentgenography and/or

manometric motility studies are particularly applicable in determining disorders of motility. In the case of intrinsic esophageal lesions, the ultimate diagnostic study is esophagoscopy with biopsy.

ANOREXIA

Anorexia is the absence of the desire to eat and can be related to a variety of organic and psychologic disturbances. Since appetite is essentially a central phenomenon, anorexia is dependent upon central effects producing a loss of appetite. Animal experiments have demonstrated a feeding center in the lateral hypothalmus and a satiety center in the medial hypothalmus. In most instances, gastric hypofunction, with mucosal pallor and decrease in gastric motility and secretion, has been associated with anorexia, but the stomach itself plays a minor role. Anorexia may also occur when both the secretory and motor activity of the stomach and gastrointestinal tract are increased. Visceral stimuli are generally carried to the midbrain via the vagus, pelvic, and sympathetic nerves, but combined sympathetic and parasympathetic denervation may not alter appetite or preclude the possibility of anorexia. The absence of precise pathophysiologic explanation and the protean disorders associated with the symptom of anorexia make it of little diagnostic significance. Among the organic diseases associated with anorexia are inflammatory processes within the intestinal tract; carcinoma of the stomach, pancreas, and liver; hepatitis and alcoholism; advanced renal disease with uremia; congestive heart failure; and certain endocrine disorders such as panhypopituitarism, adrenal cortical insufficiency, and hyperparathyroidism. Many, if not most, drugs can cause anorexia; there is no medication which consistently increases appetite.

NAUSEA AND VOMITING

Nausea and vomiting may occur separately but are closely allied. Nausea usually refers to the feeling of an imminent desire to vomit. Vomiting may be defined as the forceful expulsion of gastrointestinal contents through the mouth. In most instances, nausea precedes vomiting.

In spite of the frequency and great clinical importance of vomiting, the nervous mechanism of the act and the physical and chemical stimuli are not well understood. Most physiologists have agreed to the existence of a vomiting center and to its location in the reticular core of the medulla oblongata. There are actually two medullary centers concerned with emesis: (1) a sensory "chemoreceptive trigger zone" and (2) an integrated center which is concerned directly with the production of vomiting. The former is implicated in the drug-induced emesis and also in the vomiting associated with uremia, infections, and radiation sickness.

Afferent pathways to the vomiting center emanate from almost all sites in the body. Impulses from the gastrointestinal system pass through the emetic center by way of afferent fibers in both the vagal and sympathetic nerves. Although neither vagotomy nor sympathectomy alone abolishes the vomiting of peritonitis, the vagus is considered the more important afferent pathway from this stimulus. The vomiting induced by intestinal distension is dependent upon afferent impulses transmitted in the sympathetic nerves as evidenced by the fact that denervation of the mesenteric pedicle prevents vomiting associated with distension of that segment. Distension of the gallbladder and extrahepatic biliary tract also causes vomiting which may be obviated by a combination of vagotomy and splanchnicectomy. Pyloric pouch distension vomiting is abolished by vagotomy alone. However, it is known that vomiting may be a consequence of surgical vagotomy and that the higher the vagotomy, the more frequent the incidence of vomiting. In this circumstance, the vomiting is related to esophageal stasis with regurgitation of esophageal content into the pharynx and subsequent pharyngeal irritation.

The act of vomiting is primarily a motor function involving the respiratory and somatic muscular systems in addition to the gastrointestinal tract. Vomiting occurs in the normal fashion following total denervation of the intestine. The efferent neuropathways involve the phrenic nerves to the diaphragm, spinal nerves to the abdominal and intestinal muscles, and efferent visceral fibers along the vagus and sympathetic nerves to the intestine and muscles of the pharynx and larynx. The act of vomiting depends upon the coordinated closure of the glottis, contraction and fixation of the diaphragm in the inspiratory position, closure of the pylorus, and relaxation of the rest of the stomach including the cardia. Relaxation of the upper half of the stomach and the esophageal cardia is followed by peristaltic contractions passing from the midstomach to the incisura angularis. Contraction at the incisura persists and prevents the contents of the stomach from passing into the gastric antrum. This is followed by forceful contraction of the abdominal, diaphragmatic, and intercostal muscles, which transmit a pressure to the stomach and cause regurgitation. Reverse peristalsis in the stomach plays no major role in the mechanism of vomiting. Reverse peristalsis of the small intestine frequently occurs and results in the passage of intestinal contents into the stomach and the presence of bile in the vomitus after repeated retching. However, this type of intestinal activity has been shown to occur normally in the duodenum and does not contribute to the act of vomiting. Vomiting is frequently associated with autonomic activity including pallor, sweating, increased salivation, and cardiovascular changes including irregularity, ectopic beats, heart block, and, rarely, arrest.

All organic diseases of the alimentary tract and its appendages as well as diseases of almost every organ of the body have been associated with vomiting. Derangements of the autonomic nervous system, psychogenic disturbances, and the ingestion of noxious materials may also cause vomiting. A broad spectrum of drugs are considered as emetic agents. These include morphine, cardiac glycosides, quinine and quinidine, veratrine alkaloids, pilocarpine, Pituitrin, Pitocin, acetylcholine, ergot alkalis, atropine, tartar emetic, ipecac, zinc sulfate, and bacterial endotoxins. With each of these causes of vomiting any combination of three major factors may be involved: impulses arising from the gastrointestinal tract, central or cerebral impulses, and chemical materials transported in the blood.

The vomiting associated with shock and severe pain may be related to a reduced blood supply in the cerebral medullary centers or vasoconstriction in the splanchnic areas. Reduction of oxygen supply to the vomiting center has been implicated in the vomiting associated with anemia, vascular occlusion, and increased intracranial pressure. Migraine may also induce vomiting by an effective increase in intracranial pressure with interference of blood supply to the cerebromedullary center. Emetic drugs act in one of two ways, either directly on the cerebrum, hypothalamus, or brainstem or by their irritative effect on the gastric and intestinal mucosa. These two factors may also be involved in vomiting induced by spoiled or contaminated food and the vomiting following the ingestion of alcohol. The vomiting associated with diabetic acidosis, uremia, and Addisonian crisis has been related to changes in electrolytes and, more specifically, acidosis and hyperkalemia affecting the emesis center. An augmented irritability of the emesis center is postulated as playing a significant role in the vomiting of thyrotoxicosis.

The gastrointestinal pathophysiologic processes which lead to vomiting are many and varied. Obstruction to passage of food at any level will eventually be accompanied by vomiting. The higher the obstruction, the more rapid the onset of vomiting. The rapidity is also related to the acuteness of onset, since a gradual obstruction is attended by compensation with stretching of muscle fibers and hypertrophy. Inflammatory diseases and malignant tumors of the stomach are frequent causes of vomiting and are usually preceded by anorexia and nausea. In the child under three months of age, vomiting of clear, non-bile-stained materials is highly suggestive of hypertrophic pyloric stenosis. Acute inflammatory diseases of the intestine and pelvic organs are associated with nausea and vomiting through visceral reflexes; the more common disorders include appendictis, cholecystitis, hepatitis, pancreatitis, and salpingitis.

The pattern of vomiting is of clinical significance. Vomiting without antecedent nausea suggests a central nervous system lesion with increased intracranial pressure, such as hemorrhage or brain tumor. In these cases vomiting is usually sudden in onset and often projectile. Projectile vomiting is also characteristic of hypertrophic pyloric stenosis. Emesis which follows and relieves epigastric pain is usually associated with intragastric lesions or pyloric spasm. Vomiting which immediately follows eating is noted with toxic causes, such as uremia and hyperemesis gravidarum, gastritis, high intestinal obstruction, and gastric neoplasms. Vomiting of large amounts of digested food at 12- to 48-hour intervals is suggestive of chronic pyloric obstruction. Vomiting of feculent material is associated with gastrocolic fistula. Continued retching and vomiting, especially in alcoholics, may lacerate the gastroesophageal mucosa and result in the Mallory-Weiss syndrome with severe bleeding and, at times, exsanguination. An extension of this process is the spontaneous rupture of the esophagus which occurs more frequently in vomiting by the patient with a full stomach.

CONSEQUENCES OF VOMITING. Depending upon the intensity and duration, vomiting may produce hypovolemia, hypokalemia, alteration in the acid-base balance, and the consequences of starvation. Vomitus, without admixture of ingested food, is isoosmotic with the extracellular fluid. However, the electrolyte composition is extremely variable and dependent upon the extent of hydrogen ion excretion.

When hydrogen ion is excreted into the gastric juice, there is a shift of bicarbonate ion into the plasma, and, to maintain electric neutrality of the blood, chloride is excreted into the gastric juice. Concentration of bicarbonate in the plasma is augmented by the loss of chloride and excessive sodium in the vomitus. In general, an inverse relation exists between the concentration of hydrogen ion and sodium ion in the vomitus. Even in the achlorhydric state, when vomiting results in a depletion of sodium chloride and potassium chloride, chloride is excreted in excess of the physiologic proportions of that existent in plasma, i.e., 145 mEq of sodium and 100 mEq of chloride. As the plasma bicarbonate rises, the body compensates by increasing renal excretion of bicarbonate and reducing the rate and depth of respiration to decrease the respiratory loss of $HHCO_3$ to maintain the acid/base ratio. These compensatory features may maintain the normal blood pH, while the urine is alkaline because of excretion of bicarbonate. Determination of plasma electrolytes is only partly informative, since it is dependent upon the relative loss of electrolytes and water and also upon the solutions ingested.

With continued vomiting, the plasma and extracellular potassium concentration becomes reduced as a result of the increased quantities of potassium excreted in the urine in exchange for sodium, which in turn is related to the lack of availability of hydrogen ions depleted by loss in the vomitus. Adrenal cortical stimulation intensifies the potassium loss and potentiates the absorption of bicarbonate by the renal tubular cell. The extracellular and subsequently intracellular potassium concentrations become reduced, sodium cations shift into the cell, and, in order to conserve sodium, an acid urine is formed in the face of generalized alkalosis. This intensifies the alkalosis and sets up a vicious cycle which includes shift of more potassium out of the cell in exchange for sodium.

The fluid loss results in reduction in the circulating blood volume, and in time the consequences of starvation such as cellular breakdown of protein and increased renal load of nitrogenous waste products cause a rise in the BUN (blood urea nitrogen) level. Fat stores are utilized. Ketone bodies are formed, and since they require sodium for excretion, this further depletes the body stores of sodium.

Therapy should be instituted early, correcting relatively minor defects, since advanced deficiencies are critical and difficult to reverse. Drugs used to treat vomiting include anticholinergics, antihistamines, phenothiazine derivatives, and orthopramides.

CONSTIPATION AND DIARRHEA

Alteration in bowel habits may be related to the type of food ingested, psychologic disorders, or lesions in the gastrointestinal tract.

INTESTINAL TRANSIT. The rate of gastric emptying varies with the amount and quality of food and the emotional state of the individual. Generally, the healthy stomach is emptied within 3 to 4 hours, and passage through the duodenum and jejunum is rapid. Digested food usually begins to traverse the ileocolic sphincter in 2 to 3 hours and completes its passage into the cecum in 9 hours. Some delay occurs almost constantly in the distal ileum, where "segmentation" of a radiopaque bolus can be noted. The contents of the small intestine travel at an average rate of 1 in./minute, or 22 ft in 4 hours.

The chyme which enters the cecum is semiliquid in consistency. Most of the absorption of water which occurs in the large intestine takes place in the cecum and ascending colon. The intensity and frequency of muscular contractions increase from the duodenum to the rectum. Mass peristalsis carries the bolus from the hepatic flexure onward. These waves occur at varying times but are known to be frequent after meals, the so-called "gastrocolic reflex." Although some food products are evacuated within 24 hours of ingestion, the major portion requires several days for disposition.

Normally, the fecal bolus does not pass beyond the sigmoid into the rectum until defecation is about to occur. The passage into the rectum is brought about by powerful peristaltic waves with concomitant relaxation of the smooth musculature at the rectosigmoid junction. Distension of the rectum initiates afferent nervous impulses conducted via hypogastric and pelvic nerves to the sacral cord, whence efferent impulses are discharged. The process of defecation may be entirely involuntary but is usually assisted by voluntary contractions of the muscles of the abdomen and diaphragm and voluntary relaxation of the external anal sphincter. The intraluminal pressure is increased, forcing the stool through the relaxed internal sphincter and the voluntarily relaxed external sphincter. The entire colon, distal to the splenic flexure, is usually emptied at one time.

Four types of wave action have been noted in the colon: Type 1 waves are small and of short duration, lasting 5 seconds, and are not propulsive in character. These are not observed roentgenographically and are only noted in a pressure-measuring system. Type 2 waves are characterized by an increase in pressure, and the duration varies between 12 and 120 seconds. They constitute the principal activity in the descending and pelvic segments of the colon. They may or may not be propulsive. Type 3 waves are of low intensity, affecting 10 cm of water pressure and last 1 to 4 minutes. They may play a role in absorption by increasing the luminal pressure. Type 4 waves are strong, propulsive contractions with pressures up to 100 cm of water and effect a mass movement of the fecal bolus. They are commonly noted in patients with ulcerative colitis.

Although intestinal motility continues after transection of the nerves, under normal conditions the vagi, splanchnics, and pelvic nerves do play a significant role. Parasympathetic efferent supply to the small intestine and proximal colon courses over the vagi, while the remainder of the colon innervation is carried over the lower sacral segment via the pelvic nerves. Splanchnic nerves supply sympathetic innervation. The intrinsic myenteric reflexes are the prime movers, but motility is augmented by parasympathetic stimulation, while sympathetic stimulation results in inhibition of tone. Sympathetic stimulation explains the reflex ileus which is known to accompany retroperitoneal trauma or dissection.

The external anal sphincter, a voluntary muscle, receives nerve fibers from the gray matter of the conus terminalis, where the reflex is located. Transection of the cord in this region does not affect reflex contraction. However, if the lower segment of the cord is destroyed, the external sphincter becomes relaxed and no longer contracts. If the afferent nerves are destroyed, the fecal bolus may accumulate without sensation. It has been suggested that the medullary center may be implicated in the act of defecation, since a central nervous system influence is capable of causing either diarrhea or constipation.

In addition to neurogenic factors, chemicals also influence defecation. Acetylcoholine-like drugs increase the tone and activity of the intestine. Pilocarpine causes smooth muscle contraction, while neostigmine and Mecholyl inhibit the destruction of cholinesterase and produce intestinal activity. Serotonin also alters intestinal motility with resultant increased activity. Guanethidine causes increased motility by its inhibitory effect on the sympathetic nerves, and reserpine acts by its effect on serotonin release. Vasopressin is strongly motor to the entire intestine. Potassium is implicated in intestinal motility, since the function of the muscle cell is dependent upon

its potassium level. Drugs may also delay the passage of intestinal contents. Morphine and codeine decrease the propulsive motility by resulting in a marked increase in tone. Atropine decreases motility by paralyzing the parasympathetic nerve endings.

Constipation

Constipation may be defined as an abnormal retention of fecal matter or undue delay in discharge when compared with the patient's usual bowel habits. However, the term is used in a variety of ways. It may refer to the fact that the stool occurs with relative infrequency, that the stool is insufficient in quantity, or that it is abnormally hard and dry.

ETIOLOGY. Constipation may be due to psychologic factors, dietary constituents, laxatives and drugs, neurogenic causes, decreased skeletal muscular power, and mechanical factors which are either intrinsic or extrinsic to the gastrointestinal tract.

Psychogenic constipation may be related to improper training, and the symptom frequently dates from early childhood. The end result may be a functional megacolon, which is considered to be more common than Hirschsprung's disease. *Dietary factors* include a lack of bulky foods and the use of laxatives which lead to overstimulation of the bowel with eventual fatigue. Drugs with constipating effects have already been referred to in the section on Intestinal Transit.

Decreased muscular power in the skeletal muscles of the diaphragm, abdominal wall, and pelvic floor may all cause constipation. Weakness of the diaphragm may be associated with a variety of chronic pulmonary diseases, while weakness of the abdominal wall may occur in pregnancy, in the presence of large, rapidly expanding intraabdominal masses, and in patients with marked ascites. Weakness of the pelvic floor is usually a consequence of pregnancy. The role of *atony of the intestinal muscle* is difficult to evaluate and may be of minimal importance. Hypokalemia results in ileus based on this cause. Collagen and endocrine disorders are thought to be associated with intestinal atony. *Neurogenic causes* include tabes dorsalis, multiple sclerosis, spinal cord tumors, and trauma. These lesions may result in deficient reflex activity or may directly destroy or depress the autonomic innervation of the intestine. In Hirschsprung's disease the neurologic deficit in the myenteric and submucosal plexuses interrupts the peristaltic action to that segment. *Factors which are intrinsic to the gastrointestinal tract* and contribute to the symptom of constipation include tumors, fecal impactions, intussusception, and volvulus. The mechanical factor is also implicated at the anal sphincter, when spasm and the voluntary avoidance of defecation because of pain occur in patients with hemorrhoids, fissures, or proctitis. *Extrinsic causes* consist of large intraabdominal masses such as ovarian cysts, fibroids, pregnancy, and obstructing adhesions.

ASSOCIATED SYMPTOMS AND EFFECTS. Obstipation, which is defined as the absence of passage of both flatus and feces, is suggestive of mechanical obstruction. Reflex symptoms accompanying constipation include back and hip pain, headache, and, occasionally, tachycardia. So-called "intestinal toxemia" in patients with chronic constipation remains unproved but probably occurs. Fecal accumulations within the rectum may reach large size and contribute to the formation of anal lesions such as hemorrhoids, fissures, and ulcers. Constipation also has a significant role in the development of colonic diverticula and sigmoid volvulus.

CLINICAL EVALUATION. The history should include complete elaboration of bowel habits and also the patient's dietary intake. Direct questioning concerning the color, consistency, and caliber of the stool, the presence of melena or unaltered blood, mucus, or undigested fats or foods, and the occurrence of tenesmus is indicated. Although abdominal examination may reveal a mass, the rectal is usually the most rewarding aspect of the physical examination. Proctosigmoidoscopy may define the presence of inflammation, tumors, or the melanosis coli of patients who take laxatives chronically. Roentgenographic examination with a barium enema is indicated in all patients with prolonged constipation.

Diarrhea

Diarrhea refers to an excessively rapid evacuation of excessively fluid stool. It may be acute, in which instance it is usually related to dietary, toxic, or infectious causes. When diarrhea is chronic or recurrent, it is more likely a manifestation of gastrointestinal disease.

ETIOLOGY. Even when discussion is limited to chronic diarrhea, classification is at best imperfect.

Functional enterocolonic disease represents the most common cause of chronic diarrhea, which is a relatively frequent manifestaton of emotional disorder. The mechanism has not been defined, and the spectrum of emotions which are associated with diarrhea is great. Emotional problems are major factors in the development of mucous colitis and may play a contributory role in ulcerative colitis.

Organic colonic disease is a frequent cause of diarrhea. Included in this group is ulcerative colitis and granulomatous colitis, diverticulitis, obstructive lesions such as malignancy or fecal impaction, and polyposis. Rarer causes are lymphogranuloma venereum, endometriosis of the colon, and colitis secondary to ingestion of toxic drugs such as the heavy metals. Orally ingested arsenic, mercury, and alcohol in high concentration induce hyperemia and edema of both the small intestine and colon. Villous adenoma is frequently associated with diarrhea because of the large quantity of fluid and mucus excreted by the tumor itself. Diarrhea, paradoxically, may be the presenting manifestation in patients with obstruction, particularly fecal impaction.

Small intestinal causes of diarrhea include regional ileitis, tuberculous enteritis, and a great variety of diseases associated with a defect in absorption. The absorption defect may be primary in such syndromes as sprue or may be secondary to intestinal tumors such as carcinoid, intestinal lipodystrophy, or the Zollinger-Ellison syndrome. Reduction of absorption may also be due to mechanical causes such as extensive enterectomy, fistulas, or entero-colostomy bypassing a significant proportion of the bowel. Malabsorption and diarrhea are also a consequence of the blind loop syndrome.

Gastric factors have been implicated as causes of diarrhea. Diarrhea may be an accompaniment of either hypo-chlorhydria, such as is seen in achylia gastrica or with gastric neoplasms, and also with the hyperchlorhydria of patients with the Zollinger-Ellison syndrome. Diarrhea is often a major symptom following surgical treatment for peptic ulceration. It is one of the manifestations of the dumping syndrome following gastrectomy, the afferent loop syndrome, gastrojejunal colic fistula, or the inadvertent performance of a gastroileostomy rather than a gastrojejunostomy. Diarrhea is also seen following vagotomy and drainage procedures because of changes in the innervation of the small intestine.

Disorders of the *solid viscera of the gastrointestinal system,* particularly the pancreas and hepatobiliary organs, are also causes of diarrhea. A deficiency of pancreatic juice, such as occurs with chronic pancreatitis and obstructive malignancy, is associated with diarrhea. As has already been mentioned, diarrhea is one of the major manifestations of the non-insulin-secreting islet cell tumor of Zollinger-Ellison. Diarrhea may be a symptom of obstruction of the extrahepatic biliary tract but is more frequently noted with extrahepatic biliary fistulas. It is a major manifestation of the syndrome of watery diarrhea, hypokalemia, and achlorhydria ascribed to secretion of vasoactive intestinal peptide.

Enteric infections and parasitic infestations are characteristically manifested by diarrhea. Included in this group are infections with the viruses, *Salmonella* and *Shigella* and some coliform organisms, and the ominous staphylococcal enterocolitis. The last occurs after antibiotics have eliminated the usual intestinal flora. Amebiasis and leishmaniasis are commonly accompanied by diarrhea, as are the infestations with helminths such as *Ascaris,* liver flukes, schistosomes, and *Trichinella.*

Metabolic disorders may also cause diarrhea. Thyrotoxicosis, with its excitation of the nervous system, results in a marked autonomic hyperactivity and is frequently associated with diarrhea. Parathyroid deficiency with its accompanying hypocalcemia increases neuromuscular excitability and results in a hyperirritable bowel. Medullary carcinoma of the thyroid is frequently associated with diarrhea related to increased secretion of calcitonin. Hypermotility is also noted in uremia. The pathophysiology explaining the diarrhea which is associated with diabetes has not been defined. In these patients, diarrhea has a tendency to occur at night, and antibiotic therapy has induced remission. Patients with Addisonian crisis may also have diarrhea.

A variety of *central nervous system stimulations* result in increased peristaltic contractions in both the small intestine and colon. Diarrhea is seen in patients with tabes dorsalis and intracranial space-occupying lesions and tumors.

Drugs act in different ways to produce diarrhea. Most cathartics result in loose stools because of their muscosal irritating effect or by a hygroscopic effect. Certain drugs administered parenterally cause intestinal hypermotility by their action on the autonomic nervous system. Acetylcholine, neostigmine, and Urecholine are all intestinal stimulants. Intravenously administered serotonin stimulates intestinal peristalsis, and its precursor, 5-hydroxytryptophan, is thought to be the etiologic factor in the diarrhea associated with the carcinoid syndrome.

CONSEQUENCES OF DIARRHEA. The consequences are dependent upon the intensity and duration of the symptom. Severe or prolonged diarrhea may result in dehydration, electrolyte loss, and acidosis. The fecal sodium and chloride concentrations are usually lower than the plasma levels, whereas the potassium and bicarbonate levels are higher. The villous adenoma excretes a fluid which is particularly high in potassium with concentrations many times that of plasma.

Acidosis may result because of a high bicarbonate content in the stool or may be related to the production of acid due to starvation or to the dehydration compromising renal function. Dehydration and acidosis accelerate the body depletion of potassium by a shift of the cation out of the cell in exchange for sodium and hydrogen ions. These factors coupled with the large amount of potassium lost in the stool because of excretion into the intestine in exchange for sodium absorption from the lower small intestine and colon may result in significant hypokalemia.

Plasma or electrolyte determinations do not represent a guide to the severity of volume loss, since this reflection is dependent upon the relative tonicity of the stool with respect to extracellular fluid and the amount of fluid lost. In the absence of associated bleeding, the hematocrit is the better index of the severity of dehydration.

CLINICAL EVALUATION. History. Direct questioning should elicit the duration of diarrhea, the time of day during which diarrhea occurs, the patient's description of the stool, the presence of accompanying pain or urge to defecate, and the presence of other manifestations of gastrointestinal disease such as anorexia, nausea, and vomiting. A family or community history of similar episodes suggests an infectious basis. Diarrhea which alternates with constipation occurs with colon lesions such as carcinoma, diverticulitis, partial intestinal obstruction, and chronic constipation treated with laxatives. Recurrent episodes of diarrhea are characteristic of ulcerative colitis, psychogenic causes, and amebic colitis. Ulcerative colitis may be associated with red stools, while the patient may recognize infestation by the presence of the offending organism in the stool. Large, pale, bulky stools suggest pancreatic deficiency. Large amounts of mucus in the stool are seen in patients with mucous colitis, ulcerative colitis, carcinoma of the colon, and villous adenoma.

Pain is a frequent factor with ulcerative colitis and diverticulitis, and may be present when diarrhea is due to carcinoma. Tenesmus commonly accompanies ulcerative colitis and carcinoma of the rectum and lymphogranuloma venereum. Anorexia, nausea, and/or vomiting are more characteristic symptoms of intestinal malignancy, ulcerative colitis, and severe bacillary or amebic dysentery.

Physical Examination. *Fever* may be present with a variety of inflammatory processes and occurs more rarely as an accompaniment of neoplastic disease with the exception of lymphoma. Arthritis is particularly common in ulcerative colitis, regional enteritis, and lipodystrophy. This also applies to other hypersensitivity reactions such as iritis and erythema nodosum. A palpable *abdominal mass* should be sought. In the left lower quadrant, this may suggest sigmoid carcinoma or diverticulitis with inflammatory obstruction. Granulomas of regional enteritis, amebic infection, and tuberculosis may all cause palpable masses. *Tenderness* suggests regional enteritis, diverticulitis, or intraabdominal inflammatory processes. *Digital examination* of the rectum may define the presence of lymphogranuloma venereum, carcinoma, granulomas, ulcerative colitis, diffuse polyposis, or a fecal impaction. *Proctosigmoidoscopy* should represent an integral part of the examination of the patient with diarrhea. A friable rectal mucosa may suggest ulcerative colitis or amebiasis. The overwhelming majority of patients with ulcerative colitis have lesions which may be visualized by this technique. Malignant lesions, polyps, and villous adenomas can usually be defined by proctosigmoidoscopy.

Stool. The stool should be evaluated for consistency and the presence of mucus and occult and unaltered blood. Fatty stools suggest pancreatic insufficiency or malabsorption. Carcinoma and diverticulitis may be associated with bloody stools. Microscopic examination for ova and parasites is particularly pertinent to the diagnosis of infestations.

Radiological Studies. Abdominal films may demonstrate intestinal obstruction, a mass, or calculi associated with chronic pancreatitis. Barium enema is an essential part of the examination and is frequently diagnostic for ulcerative colitis, tumors, and diverticulitis. Regurgitation at the terminal ileum may define the presence of regional enteritis or tuberculous enteritis. In rare instances, regurgitation of barium into the jejunum or stomach will demonstrate a fistula. The upper gastrointestinal series is also of importance, particularly in determining the presence of gastrocolic fistula, blind loop syndrome, and iatrogenic gastroileostomy. The barium meal may be utilized as a method of determining intestinal transit time in patients with massive resection. Primary malabsorption syndromes may be associated with a small bowel pattern which is quite characteristic. Pancreatography may be indicated.

Laparotomy. In some cases, laparotomy should be considered a diagnostic procedure. Small bowel biopsy is indicated in the differential diagnosis of malabsorption syndrome, regional enteritis, Whipple's disease, lymphomas, and small intestinal tumors.

INTESTINAL OBSTRUCTION

Intestinal obstruction exists when there is interference with the normal aboral progression of intestinal contents. The term *mechanical intestinal obstruction* is used if an actual physical barrier blocks the intestinal lumen. The term *ileus*, though properly a synonym for intestinal obstruction from whatever cause, by common usage now connotes failure of downward progress of bowel contents because of disordered propulsive motility of the bowel.

Gastric outlet obstruction is discussed in Chap. 26, esophageal obstruction in Chap. 25, and mesenteric vascular obstruction in Chap. 35. Discussion of specific entities causing intestinal obstruction in infancy and childhood will be found in Chap. 39.

ETIOLOGY. The causes of mechanical obstruction may be classified according to the manner in which the obstruction is produced: (1) by obturation of the lumen as in gallstone ileus, (2) by encroachment on the lumen by intrinsic disease of the bowel wall as in regional enteritis or carcinoma, or (3) by lesions extrinsic to bowel such as an adhesive band (Table 24-4).

Classification of intestinal obstruction on clinical and pathologic grounds is also necessary. In *simple mechanical obstruction* the lumen is obstructed, but the blood supply

Table 24-4. MECHANISMS OF INTESTINAL OBSTRUCTIONS

Mechanical obstruction of the lumen
  Obturation of the lumen
    Meconium
    Intussusception
    Gallstones
    Impactions—fecal, barium, bezoar, worms
  Lesions of bowel
    Congenital
      Atresia and stenosis
      Imperforate anus
      Duplications
      Meckel's diverticulum
    Traumatic
    Inflammatory
      Regional enteritis
      Diverticulitis
      Chronic ulcerative colitis
    Neoplastic
    Miscellaneous
      K^+-induced stricture
      Radiation stricture
      Endometriosis
  Lesions extrinsic to bowel
    Adhesive band constriction, or angulation by adhesion
    Hernia and wound dehiscence
    Extrinsic masses
      Annular pancreas
      Anomalous vessels
      Abscesses and hematomas
      Neoplasms
  Volvulus
Inadequate propulsive motility
  Neuromuscular defects
    Megacolon
    Paralytic ileus
      Abdominal causes
        Intestinal distension
        Peritonitis
        Retroperitoneal lesions
      Systemic causes
        Electrolyte imbalance
        Toxemias
    Spastic ileus
  Vascular occlusion
    Arterial
    Venous

is intact. If mesenteric vessels are occluded, then *strangulation obstruction* exists. *Closed-loop obstruction* results when both limbs of the loop are obstructed so that neither aboral progression nor regurgitation is possible. Obstruction is further delineated by classification as partial or complete, acute or chronic, high or low, small intestinal or colonic.

INCIDENCE. Because accurate vital statistics are still not universally available in the United States, the overall incidence of intestinal obstruction and the mortality therefrom can be only roughly estimated. Probably about 20 percent of surgical admissions for acute abdominal conditions are for intestinal obstruction.

Adhesive bands are now the most frequent cause of obstruction for all age groups combined. Strangulated groin hernia, formerly the most common cause, is now in second place, with neoplasm of the bowel in third place. In some recently reported series, neoplasm has taken over second place, with hernia now in third. These three etiologic agents account for more than 80 percent of all intestinal obstruction.

The order of frequency differs for different age groups. Hernia is by far the most common cause of obstruction in childhood. Colorectal carcinoma and diverticulitis coli are prominent etiologic agents in the older age group, and these lesions are becoming more prominent in the overall picture as more of the population is living into the geriatric age where these lesions prevail.

The mortality rate from intestinal obstruction was over 50 percent in the United States in the early part of this century. There has been a gradual reduction, the sharpest fall occurring in the decade after World War II. The mortality rate is now under 10 percent. The factors principally responsible for the reduction are (1) recognition of the role of fluid and electrolyte therapy, (2) gastrointestinal decompression by intubation, and (3) antibiotics. Probably equally responsible is the definitive marked rise in surgical standards that occurred in the United States after World War II.

Though the mortality rate is now but one-fifth of the rate in the early twentieth century, it is still distressingly and needlessly high. This death rate could be appreciably lowered if patients with hernias were urged to have their hernias repaired, since herniorrhaphy can now be done with only about a 0.1 to 0.2 percent mortality even in the presence of other chronic systemic disease. A further lowering of the death rate could be attained if a larger percentage of patients could be operated upon before simple mechanical obstruction has progressed to strangulation obstruction with its greatly increased morbidity and mortality.

PATHOPHYSIOLOGY. Though simple mechanical obstruction, strangulation obstruction, and ileus have much in common, there are important differences in pathophysiology and management. Also, colon obstruction differs in some aspects from small bowel obstruction.

Simple Mechanical Obstruction of the Small Intestine. The principal physiologic derangements of the mechanically obstructed intestine with intact blood supply are accumulation of fluid and gas above the point of obstruction and altered bowel motility, which lead also to systemic derangements. These will be considered separately, although such a division is somewhat artificial.

Fluid and Electrolyte Losses. Death from intestinal obstruction was for many years attributed to "toxins" that were absorbed from the intestine. In 1912 Hartwell and Hoguet were able to prolong the life of dogs with high intestinal obstruction by the daily parenteral administration of physiologic saline solution. Gamble later demonstrated that the "toxic" factor in simple mechanical obstruction was actually the loss of fluid and electrolytes from the body by vomiting and by sequestering in the obstructed bowel.

Accumulation of large quantities of fluid and gas within the lumen of the bowel above an obstruction is striking and progressive. Some have felt that the fluid is principally digestive secretions and that obstruction causes hypersecretion of digestive juices. Others have felt that the principal defect is not hypersecretion of digestive juices but rather the inability of the obstructed bowel to absorb water and electrolytes at the normal rate.

Availability of isotopes since about 1940 to measure movements of water and electrolytes in both directions across the intestinal mucosa has greatly simplified these measurements and has produced much quantitative data. It is now clear that the absorption of ingested fluid and of upper gastrointestinal digestive secretions are but a part of a much larger exchange of fluid between the body and the lumen of the gastrointestinal tract. For example, if a fasting adult ingests 1,000 ml of water, about 50 percent is absorbed in 30 minutes. When barium sulfate is mixed with the water, it can be seen fluoroscopically to be distributed throughout the small intestine within 2 or 3 minutes. If D_2O—heavy water—is placed in the intestine, 50 percent of the D_2O reaches the blood within 3 minutes. Thus during absorption there must be a flux of water from blood to intestinal lumen only slightly slower than the flux from the lumen into the blood. The above example suggests that in 30 minutes about 5,000 ml goes from blood to lumen while 5,500 ml is going from lumen to blood, giving a net absorption of 500 ml.

The movement of a substance across the intestinal mucosa (sorption) is equal to the difference between the unidirectional flux from intestinal lumen to blood (insorption) and the opposite flux from blood to lumen (exsorption).

Accumulation of fluid within the bowel—a negative net flux—will result if the flux from lumen to blood (insorption) is decreased or if the flux from blood to lumen (exsorption) is increased. Currently available evidence from animal experiments is conflicting on which mechanism is responsible for the accumulation of fluid within the lumen in intestinal obstruction—increased secretion or decreased absorption.

Shields studied the movement of water, sodium, and potassium across the ileal mucosa of dogs in which obstruction had been produced by transecting the distal ileum and closing both ends. He found that within 12 hours the ileum above the obstruction ceased to absorb (net) and began to secrete water at a steadily increasing rate. This resulted initially from a decrease in the flux from lumen to blood. The flux from blood to lumen continued at a normal rate initially, but after 48 hours the rate of entry

of water increased rapidly and significantly. The findings for sodium and potassium were parallel. At sacrifice, the obstructed bowel was heavier and shorter than the unobstructed bowel, and histologically the veins in the bowel wall were greatly congested and engorged. The part of the intestine distal to the obstruction did not react in the same way as the part of the intestine above. Although the volume of water absorbed by this segment was reduced to one-third of its original rate after 60 hours of obstruction, at no time did exsorption exceed insorption. And at sacrifice there was no edema or congestion of the bowel wall.

Davenport has reported similar studies in which the fluxes across the mucosa of an obstructed ileal segment were measured by placing a radioactive sodium chloride solution in the lumen. Normal fluxes were found in the direction of blood to lumen, but fluxes from lumen to blood were depressed or abolished. As a result, water, sodium, and chloride (and presumably other ions) moved into the obstructed intestinal segment but not out of it, distending it with fluid having approximately the electrolyte composition of plasma.

Further studies are obviously needed to clarify the pathophysiologic mechanism by which the obstructed bowel becomes progressively distended with fluid.

The bowel immediately above the obstruction is the most affected initially. It becomes distended with fluids and electrolytes, and circulation is impaired. With increasing intraluminal pressure the fluid is dispersed orad until it reaches bowel that is still capable of absorbing. When obstruction has been present for a long time, the proximal portions of the intestine also lose their ability to handle fluid and electrolytes, and the entire bowel proximal to the obstruction becomes distended.

A second route of fluid and electrolyte loss is into the wall of the involved bowel, accounting for the boggy edematous appearance of the bowel often seen at operation. Some of this fluid exudes from the serosal surface of the bowel, resulting in free peritoneal fluid. The extent of fluid and electrolyte loss into the bowel wall and peritoneal cavity depends on the extent of bowel involved in venous congestion and edema, and the length of time before the obstruction is relieved.

The most obvious route of fluid and electrolyte loss is by vomiting—or gastrointestinal tube after treatment is initiated. The aggregate of these losses (1) into the bowel lumen, (2) into the edematous bowel wall, (3) as free peritoneal fluid, plus (4) by vomiting or nasogastric suction rapidly depletes the extracellular fluid space, leading progressively to hemoconcentration, hypovolemia, renal insufficiency, shock, and death unless treatment is prompt and resolute. The blood chemistry values to be expected in intestinal obstruction will be found below under Clinical Manifestations.

Intestinal Gas. Much of the distension of the bowel above a mechanical obstruction can be accounted for by the fluid sequestered within the lumen. Intestinal gas is also responsible for distension.

The approximate composition of small intestine gas (Table 24-5) shows that the basic composition is that of air to which small amounts of gases not found in the atmosphere have been added.

Table 24-5. INTESTINAL GAS

Percent

Nitrogen	70
Oxygen	12
Carbon dioxide	8
Hydrogen sulfide	5
Ammonia and amines.	4
Hydrogen	1

Gases are absorbed from the intestine at rates that are directly related to the partial pressure of the particular gas in the intestine, in the plasma, and in the air breathed. Thus with nitrogen there is little diffusion, since the partial pressures of the gas are virtually the same in intestine, plasma, and air. On the other hand carbon dioxide diffuses very rapidly, because the partial pressure of carbon dioxide is high in the intestine, intermediate in plasma, and very low in air. For this reason, though carbon dioxide is produced in large amounts in the intestine, it contributes little to gaseous distension because of its rapid diffusibility.

Maddock et al. studied the accumulation of intestinal gas by serial roentgenography in patients who had been prepared for pyelography. He found that by continuous gastric suction, considerable volumes of air were aspirated from the stomach, and when it was kept empty, no increase in intestinal gas occurred. Patients without gastric suction rapidly accumulated gas on the serial x-rays. Nervous patients undergoing pyelography had three times as much air aspirated from their stomachs as calm patients. It is probable that air swallowing is increased in patients with the abdominal discomfort of intestinal obstruction.

Wangensteen produced simple mechanical obstruction of the lower ileum in dogs and found that an average of 328 ml of gas accumulated. Closed-loop obstructions, precluding swallowed air, contained but 12 ml of gas. To elucidate further the role of swallowed air, the cervical esophagus was divided, the proximal end brought to the skin, the distal end closed, and the ileum then divided. Parenteral fluids and electrolytes were given. The average survival was 35 days, and the amount of gas and fluid found in the intestine at autopsy was not great. The control animals—with obstruction but without esophageal transection—lived about 5 days.

On the basis of these and other studies, it is now felt that intestinal gases are principally derived from swallowed air.

Bowel Motility. With obstruction of the lumen, peristalsis becomes violent in an "attempt" to overcome the obstruction. After a short time, continuous peristalsis above the obstruction gives way to regularly recurring bursts of peristaltic activity interspersed with quiescent periods. The duration of the quiescent period is related to the level of the obstruction in the gastrointestinal tract—it is 3 to 5 minutes with high obstruction, 10 to 15 minutes with lower ileal obstruction. These muscular contractions may be of sufficient violence to traumatize the bowel and contribute to the swelling and edema of the bowel wall. As bowel above the obstruction distends, bowel below the obstruction becomes progressively more quiet. This results from an inhibitory reflex initiated by distension of the bowel above.

Strangulated Obstruction. Occlusion of the blood supply to a segment of bowel in addition to obstruction of the lumen is usually referred to as strangulated obstruction. Interference with the mesenteric blood supply is the most serious complication of intestinal obstruction. This frequently occurs secondary to adhesive band obstruction, hernia, and volvulus.

The accumulation of fluid and gas in obstructed loops and the altered motility seen in simple mechanical obstruction are rapidly overshadowed by the consequences of blockage of venous outflow from the strangulated segment—extravasation of bloody fluid into the bowel and bowel wall.

In addition to the loss of blood and plasma-like fluid, the gangrenous bowel leaks toxic materials (not to be confused with the pre-Gamble "toxins") into the peritoneal cavity. These have been variously identified as exotoxins or endotoxins, or toxic hemin breakdown products.

The pathophysiology of the strangulated loop was pointed out in a series of papers by Murphy, Brooks, et al. in the early part of this century. They showed (1) that the contents of an obstructed bowel are toxic; (2) that bacteria are necessary for the production of this toxin; (3) that neither living tissue nor mucous membrane, nor any of the secretions of the mucous membrane, are necessary for the formation of the toxin; (4) that the toxin does not pass through normal mucosa; (5) that absorption of the toxin is more important than its production, as the toxin is physiologically lost if it exists within a loop and is never absorbed; (6) that circulatory damage aids absorptions; and (7) that symptoms may be correlated with the toxin formed in the obstructed intestine.

Recent work by Barnett et al. has reemphasized the role of bacteria. A standard method of producing strangulation obstruction uniformly killed dogs in 24 to 36 hours. Peritoneal fluid from dogs succumbing to obstruction was lethal when injected intravenously into normal animals. If the strangulated segment was enclosed in a plastic bag so that the exuding fluid was kept separate from the abdominal cavity, survival was extended far past the usual lethal period. Furthermore, if the plastic bag with the accumulated fluid and the strangulated segment of intestine was removed, the dogs survived indefinitely. But if the bag was allowed to spill its contents into the peritoneal cavity, the animals died within 8 to 12 hours. The toxicity could be largely counteracted by instilling antibiotics into the obstructed loop of intestine or the plastic bag. Passage through a Seitz filter also removed the toxicity, indicating that bacteria played a major role in these experiments.

Cohn and Atik were able to lower the mortality rate in dogs with a closed loop of ileum from a control level of 91 to 13 percent by instilling antibiotics into the loop, again pointing to the importance of bacteria in strangulation obstruction.

Closed-Loop Obstruction. When both afferent and efferent limbs of a loop of bowel are obstructed, closed-loop intestinal obstruction exists. This is a clinically dangerous form of obstruction because of the propensity for rapid progression to strangulation of the blood supply before the usual manifestations of intestinal obstruction become obvious. Interference with blood supply may occur either from the same mechanism that produced obstruction of the intestine—twist of the bowel on the mesentery, extrinsic band—or from distension of the obstructed loop. The secretory pressure in the closed loop quite rapidly reaches a level sufficient to interfere with venous return from the loop. Widespread distension of the intestine usually does not occur, and so neither does abdominal distension.

Colon Obstruction. The effects on the patient with colon obstruction are usually less dramatic than the effects of small bowel obstruction. First, colon obstruction, with the exception of volvulus, usually does not strangulate. Second, because the colon is principally a storage organ with relatively minor absorptive and secretory functions, fluid and electrolyte sequestration progresses more slowly. Systemic derangements therefrom are of less magnitude and urgency than in small bowel obstruction.

Progressive distension is the most dangerous aspect of nonstrangulated colon obstruction. If the ileocecal valve is incompetent, then partial decompression of the obstructed colon may occur by reflux into the ileum. But if the ileocecal valve is competent, then the colon becomes essentially a closed loop—closed below by the obstructing lesion and above by the competent valve. If the obstruction is not relieved, distension progressing to rupture of the colon threatens. The cecum is the usual site of rupture, because it is the segment of the colon with the largest diameter. According to the law of Laplace, the pressure required to stretch the walls of a hollow viscus decreases in inverse proportion to the radius of curvature. Applying this law to the colon, given an equal pressure throughout the colon, we find that the greatest distension will occur in the portion of the colon with the largest radius (Fig. 24-3).

CLINICAL MANIFESTATIONS. The initial symptoms of simple mechanical intestinal obstruction are abdominal pain, vomiting, and failure to pass gas or feces by rectum. Abdominal distension is a later symptom.

As the bowel obstructs, severe *cramping pain* is felt synchronously with hyperperistalsis. Initially, the waves of cramps are unremitting, but after a short time attacks of pain alternate with quiescent periods during which the patient may feel quite well. The pain is diffuse, poorly localized, and is felt across the upper abdomen in high obstruction, at the level of the umbilicus in low ileal obstruction, in the lower abdomen in colon obstruction, and in the perineum as well as the abdomen in rectosigmoid obstruction. The period between attacks of pain is short with high intestinal obstruction (4 or 5 minutes) and is longer the lower the obstruction (15 to 20 minutes). When obstruction is not relieved, the characteristic colicky pain may cease (as distension becomes extreme) and be replaced by a steady generalized abdominal discomfort. There is no real pain in adynamic ileus, just a steady generalized abdominal discomfort similar to that seen in neglected simple mechanical obstruction. Steady severe

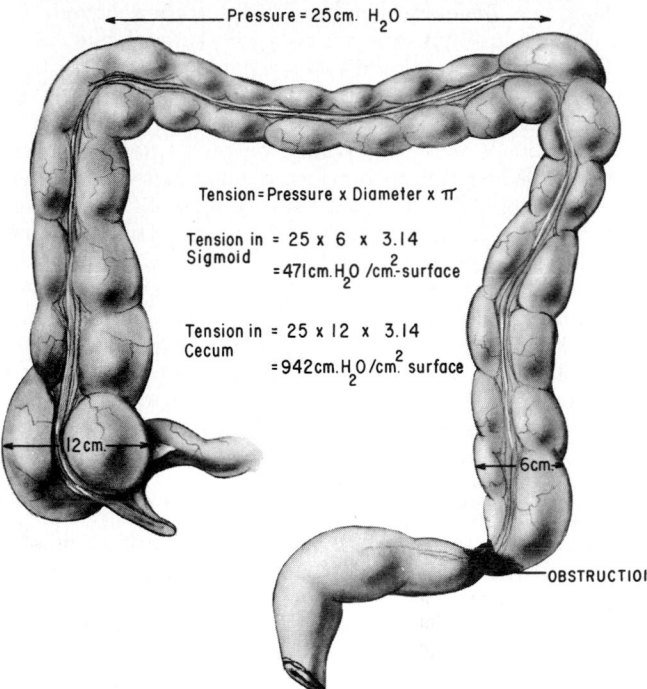

Fig. 24-3. Physics of cecal rupture in colon obstruction.

pain with no quiescent periods is usually indicative of strangulation.

Vomiting, like pain, usually occurs almost immediately after obstruction of the bowel. This early vomiting is "reflex" vomiting and is followed by a variable quiescent period before vomiting resumes. The quiet interval is short in high obstruction but may even be a day or two with low small bowel obstruction. The vomitus frequently becomes thick, dark, and malodorous (i.e., feculent) from stagnation and bacterial action but is not actually regurgitated feces. With high obstruction, vomiting is more frequent and copious and may effectively decompress the obstructed bowel. With low small bowel obstruction, vomiting is less frequent and less productive; little decompression of bowel occurs, because of the excessive length of bowel that the regurgitated material must traverse and because segmentation of the boggy loops prevents regurgitation. Reflex vomiting is unusual in colon obstruction. Thus, vomiting does not occur in most cases until retrograde distension involves the small bowel. When the ileocecal valve is competent, small bowel distension and vomiting may not occur in colonic obstruction.

Failure to pass gas or feces through the rectum is a valuable diagnostic symptom. Gas and feces distal to the obstruction may pass through the rectum after obstruction occurs, however, particularly if the obstruction is high in the jejunum. Cramping pain followed shortly by explosive diarrhea often indicates partial intestinal obstruction.

Abdominal distension is the result of fairly long-standing obstruction. There may be no generalized distension with high small bowel obstruction.

Physical examination of a patient with simple mechanical obstruction within the first 24 hours may yield surprisingly few abnormal findings except during periods of colicky pain. Vital signs are essentially normal, and dehydration and distension are not yet marked. Strangulation obstruction is likely if the patient appears seriously ill during this early period. *Palpation* during colic usually demonstrates muscle guarding; between attacks of pain only slight tenderness remains. A mass or localized area of tenderness usually indicates strangulation. *Auscultation* is of great value: in simple mechanical obstruction the abdomen is quiet except during attacks of colic, at which time the sounds become loud, high-pitched, and metallic and occur in bursts or rushes; in paralytic ileus an occasional isolated bowel sound is heard; gangrenous bowel produces complete silence. By the second or third day of obstruction serious illness is obvious. Dehydration and distension are marked, and vital signs are increasingly abnormal, though frank shock does not occur until very late in simple obstruction.

Laboratory Findings. The loss of large amounts of essentially isotonic extracellular fluid into the intestine is principally responsible for the laboratory findings in simple mechanical obstruction. The body responds to this sudden volume decrease by antidiuresis and renal sodium retention. In the early phases, in which the effects are predominantly those of extracellular fluid loss, the hematocrit rises roughly in proportion to the fluid loss. There is little change in the concentration of sodium, potassium, and chloride in the plasma. Acid-base changes, as manifested by the pH and carbon dioxide, are slight. The markedly reduced urine flow is reflected in a somewhat elevated BUN level. The dehydration and antidiuresis is often so marked that patients may not be able to produce a urine specimen until after intravenous fluid therapy has been started. Urinary specific gravity of 1.025 to 1.030 is the rule; mild proteinuria or acetonuria may also be present.

In the untreated patient, sodium-free water, derived from catabolism of cells and oxidation of fat, tends to restore the acute loss of extracellular fluid volume but at the expense of plasma osmolality. Thus, there is a gradual reduction of the plasma sodium and chloride concentration. Urine volume gradually increases, though not to normal, with excretion of potassium, including the potassium freed by cellular catabolism. The previously noted progressive increase in the hematocrit is halted or actually reversed by the ingress of endogenous water. Acid-base effects are determined by the nature of the fluid lost. Metabolic acidosis due to the combined effects of dehydration, starvation, ketosis, and loss of alkaline secretions is most common. Metabolic alkalosis is infrequent and is principally due to loss of highly acid gastric juice. With great distension of the abdomen, the diaphragm may be sufficiently elevated to embarrass respiration, resulting in carbon dioxide retention and respiratory acidosis.

The white blood cell count is useful in differentiating between different types of obstruction. In general, simple mechanical obstruction calls forth only modest numbers of leukocytes—white blood cell counts often to 15,000 with some shift to the left. White blood cell counts of 15,000 to 25,000/mm^3 and marked polymorphonuclear predominance with many immature forms strongly suggest that the

obstruction is strangulated. Very high white cell counts, such as 40,000 to 60,000/mm^3, suggest primary mesenteric vascular occlusion.

Serum amylase level elevations may occur in intestinal obstruction and compromise the differential diagnostic value of the test. Amylase gains entry to the blood by regurgitation from the pancreas because of back pressure in the duodenum, or by peritoneal absorption after leakage from dying bowel.

Radiologic Findings. When properly done, this is the most important diagnostic procedure. The films must be of good technical quality—not the type that are made in the emergency room by a substitute technician with a portable x-ray machine.

X-rays should be made as early in the hospitalization as the patient's condition permits—usually within the first hour. Plain films of the abdomen (without contrast medium) in the supine and upright positions, and posteroanterior and lateral views of the chest are obtained. If the patient is too weak to remain in the sitting position for the 15 minutes that is necessary to demonstrate air under the diaphragm (best seen on the posteroanterior chest film), then a left lateral decubitus film may be substituted.

The diagnostic features that enable one to distinguish in the majority of cases between simple mechanical obstruction, strangulation obstruction, and paralytic ileus are summarized in Table 24-6. Representative films of the three types of obstruction are shown in Fig. 24-4.

Gas-fluid levels are among the important criteria in the x-ray diagnosis of intestinal obstruction. Gas is normally visible in the colon and stomach on plain films of the abdomen in normal adults. Small bowel gas may be visible in infants and occasionally in apparently normal adults. The transit time of swallowed air is normally so rapid that there is an insufficient amount in any one place to show on the x-ray. But if the normal aboral progression of intestinal content is interfered with, then gas collects along with retained fluid and produces gas-fluid levels which are best seen on the upright film of the abdomen. Though gas-fluid levels are highly suggestive of intestinal obstruction (including ileus), they may be seen in other conditions such as extreme aerophagia, gastroenteritis, severe constipation, and sprue.

Additional radiographic studies are sometimes indicated. These are barium enema, intravenous urography, and occasionally administration of contrast medium by mouth or nasogastric tube.

Barium enema is indicated when the clinical picture and plain films suggest colon obstruction, to give information on the type and location of the obstruction. Barium enema is often helpful also when the distribution of gas is not clear on the plain films. Barium enema may be used therapeutically for attempted reduction of nonstrangulated intussusception in children.

The dangers of barium enema in obstruction are the possibility of perforating an inflammatory lesion such as diverticulitis or appendicitis and, secondly, changing a partial colon obstruction to a complete one by forcing barium up past a partially obstructing lesion to form an obstructing concretion of inspissated barium.

Table 24-6. RADIOLOGIC SIGNS IN INTESTINAL OBSTRUCTION

Sign	*Simple mechanical obstruction* (see Fig. 24-4A)	*Strangulation obstruction* (see Fig. 24-4B)	*Adynamic ileus* (see Fig. 24-4C)
Gas in intestine	Large bow-shaped loops in ladder pattern	Little distension, often only single loop	Copious gas diffusely through intestine
Gas in colon	Less than nomal	Less than normal	Increased, scattered through colon
Fluid levels in intestine	Definite	If present, small and localized	Often very large throughout
Tumor.	None	Rounded, smooth, C-shaped margin	None
Peritoneal exudate	None	Present; general haziness may obscure	Present with peritonitis; otherwise absent
Diaphragm	Somewhat elevated; free motion	Diminished motion	Elevated; diminished motion

SOURCE: Adapted from C. E. Welch and J. Frimann-Dahl (see References at end of chapter).

Intravenous urography may be indicated to look for ureteral calculi, which often produce marked paralytic ileus.

The principal indication for administration of contrast medium above an obstruction is to differentiate postoperative ileus from mechanical obstruction. The actual point of obstruction rarely can be demonstrated because of dilution of the contrast medium, but if some medium is seen to go through the gastrointestinal tract, the diagnosis of ileus is strengthened. Some surgeons are loath to give barium above an obstruction and prefer to use a liquid medium such as Hypaque. There is, however, little evidence that small amounts of barium are harmful in small bowel obstruction.

MANAGEMENT. The principles of treatment are fluid and electrolyte therapy, decompression of the bowel, and timed surgical intervention.

Essentially all patients with mechanical intestinal ob-

struction except in the immediate postoperative period should be operated upon. The decision to be made is *when* to operate—selection of the optimal time for the individual patient.

Patients with simple mechanical obstruction who can be operated upon within the first 24 hours of the disease do not need extensive preoperative preparation, because water and salt depletion and distension are usually not serious at this stage. After the history and physical examination have established the presumptive diagnosis, laboratory studies should be done, intravenous repletion initiated, decompression started with a nasogastric sump tube in the stomach, and abdominal and chest x-ray films taken on the way to the operating room. This whole process should take less than 2 hours. The mortality rate is less than 1 percent for patients with simple mechanical obstruction who are operated upon within the first 24 hours.

If the obstruction has been present for more than 24 hours when the patient is first seen, depletion and distension may be so severe that if strangulation or closed-loop obstruction seems unlikely, the patient's best interests are served by a period of preparation before the obstruction

Fig. 24-4. Plain films of the abdomen in intestinal obstruction. *A.* Simple mechanical obstruction of the small intestine. *B.* Closed-loop obstruction with strangulation. *C.* Postoperative adynamic ileus.

A   B   C

is surgically relieved. In general, the longer the obstruction has existed, the longer it will take to get the patient ready for surgical treatment. Patients with moderate derangements, particularly hypokalemia, usually require 6 to 12 hours; in those with severe problems, 24 to 36 hours may be necessary, mainly because of the hazard of giving intravenous potassium ion faster than it can equilibrate.

With the possible exception of patients with early simple mechanical obstruction, all patients with intestinal obstruction should have a plastic venous catheter threaded into the superior vena cava for frequent measurements of the central venous pressure, as well as for rapid administration of fluid, and an indwelling catheter inserted into the bladder for accurate continual measurement of the urinary output.

The initial hematocrit reading may be used to estimate the extent of extracellular fluid loss, and thus the volume necessary for restoration of this static debt. For example, if the hematocrit has risen to 55 percent, this indicates a loss of approximately 40 percent of the plasma and extracellular fluid volume. In a 70-kg man, this would amount to about 1,100 ml of plasma and 4,000 ml of electrolyte solutions.

Colloid replacement may be either as plasma per se or as human serum albumin, using 1 unit of 12.5 Gm for each 300 ml of plasma required. If acid gastric juice loss is prominent, then normal saline solution is used; otherwise lactated Ringer's solution and 5% dextrose in water in about equal proportions are preferred to replace the lost fluid and to cover maintenance fluid needs. Potassium chloride also will be necessary but should not be given until a good urinary output is established. Antibiotics should also be given in generous dosage and may be added to the intravenous fluids. The choice of antibiotics is a matter of individual preference: the authors currently use a tetracycline and ampicillin.

The rate of fluid administration is best controlled by monitoring the central venous pressure (CVP). Fluids may be given rapidly as long as the CVP remains below 10 to 12 cm of water. The end point of volume replacement is indicated by a sudden rise in the CVP. Other guides are return of skin turgor and the hourly rate of urine production.

The goal in terms of electrolyte concentration and acid-base balance is restoration of these to, or close to, the normal range by the time the volume deficit has been repaired. This is usually possible in patients with reasonably normal renal and pulmonary functions.

When the possibility of strangulation exists, preoperative treatment to fluid-electrolyte normality is not possible or advisable. This is an emergency situation requiring vigorous preparation with blood, plasma, fluids and electrolytes, massive antibiotics, nasogastric suction, and an operation at the earliest possible moment to remove the cause of the strangulation and/or nonviable bowel. Despite application of these principles, the mortality rate in strangulated obstruction is still about 25 percent.

Intubation. Tubes for gastrointestinal aspiration, available in bewildering variety, are basically of but two types: "short" tubes for gastric aspiration and "long" tubes for aspiration of the small intestine. The Levin tube, for nasogastric intubation, is preferred by many surgeons for preoperative gastrointestinal decompression in patients with obstruction. Complete decompression of the gastrointestinal tract is not accomplished, since only the intestinal gas and fluid from the upper intestine that regurgitates into the stomach is removed. The stomach is completely emptied, however, which prevents any possible aspiration during anesthesia, and progression of intestinal distension is halted, since all swallowed air is removed. Nasogastric tubes with a double lumen, one for aspiration plus a small second channel to allow ingress of air into the stomach—the "sump" tube, perform much more efficiently than the old single-lumen tubes.

Long intestinal tubes, of which the Miller-Abbott tubes is the prototype, have a lumen for aspiration plus a mercury-containing balloon or small bag at or near the distal end. When inflated in the intestine, the balloon is carried distad by peristalsis. The purpose of the mercury is to aid in getting the tube through the pylorus. After the tube is passed into the stomach, the patient lies on his right side with feet slightly elevated, so that gravity will help pull the tip of the tube through the pylorus.

In the past, intestinal intubation was advocated for the definitive treatment of simple mechanical intestinal obstruction, and a few surgeons still cling to the belief that a trial of suction therapy is warranted. There is now good evidence that the use of suction as definitive therapy (except as noted below) should be condemned—temporizing may lead to death from strangulation obstruction. For example, Becker analyzed 412 cases of acute intestinal obstruction due to old adhesions and showed that the usual criteria, presence or absence of fever, tachycardia, leukocytosis, a palpable mass, and peritoneal irritation, did not suffice to differentiate simple obstruction from strangulation obstruction. The overall mortality rate in the series was 11.8 percent; in the 52 cases in which tube decompression was abused, the mortality rate was 38.4 percent. Another reason for not using intubation as definitive therapy is an early recurrence rate of over 30 percent. The principal indications now for primary intubation therapy are obstruction in the immediate postoperative period, partial small bowel obstruction, or obstruction due to inflammation which is expected to subside under conservative therapy.

Some surgeons prefer to use a long intestinal tube for preoperative gastrointestinal decompression in patients with obstruction, feeling that decompression of the intestine per se is sufficiently important to warrant the extra time and trouble necessary to pass an intestinal tube as compared to the Levin nasogastric tube. Emptying of the stomach is inadequate with the long tube, however, and a second short tube is required for this purpose.

Operation. Proper timing of the operation for intestinal obstruction is essential. There are four types of obstruction in which the operation should be done as an emergency as soon as possible after admission: strangulation, closed-loop obstruction, colon obstruction, and early simple mechanical obstruction.

The principal hazard to life in strangulation is septic

shock from transperitoneal absorption of toxins spilled from dying bowel. In closed-loop obstruction, which cannot be decompressed by intubation, the hazard is that the loop will strangulate, and it must be treated with the same urgency as strangulation.

In colon obstruction, which also cannot be decompressed by tube, a competent ileocecal valve preventing regurgitation into the ileum converts the colon into a closed loop. Since fluid and electrolyte abnormalities progress slowly in colon obstruction, a brief period of hydration while laboratory studies are being done is all that is necessary before operation. And, as noted above, when patients with simple mechanical obstruction get to the surgeon early in the course of their disease, immediate surgical procedures may be carried out with essentially no mortality. Thus only in *late* simple mechanical obstruction of the small intestine does extensive preparation for operation take priority over immediate operation.

Anesthesia. General anesthesia is safest for the patient and the method of choice from the point of view of both surgeon and anesthesiologist. Endotracheal intubation, at times performed intially under local anesthesia, is particularly indicated to prevent aspiration of regurgitated gastric content. The surgeon should not be tempted to use local anesthesia for abdominal exploration on the assumption that local anesthesia is easier on the poor-risk patient than general anesthesia—it is not! Local anesthesia should be used only when the surgeon knows the cause of the obstruction and plans a limited procedure only, such as cecostomy.

Surgical Procedures. Surgical procedures for the relief of intestinal obstruction may be divided into five categories:

1. Procedures not requiring opening of bowel—lysis of adhesions, manipulation-reduction of intussusception, reduction of incarcerated hernia
2. Enterotomy for removal of obturation obstruction—gallstone, bezoars
3. Resection of the obstructing lesion or strangulated bowel with primary anastomosis
4. Short-circuiting anastomosis around an obstruction
5. Formation of a cutaneous stoma proximal to the obstruction—cecostomy, transverse colostomy (Figs. 24-5 and 24-6).

On opening the peritoneum, the presence or absence of free peritoneal fluid should be noted, as well as the appearance of the fluid. Bloody fluid denotes strangulation, whereas clear straw-colored fluid is found with simple obstruction. The point of obstruction is usually best found by starting in the right lower quadrant. If the cecum is grossly distended, the obstruction is in the colon. If collapsed small bowel is found, then this is followed back to the point of obstruction, thus avoiding evisceration of the proximal distended loops.

The surgeon is sometimes faced with the difficult decision of whether to resect or to replace in the abdomen a loop of intestine of questionable viability. Before release the strangulated loop has a dull purple-red appearance and is devoid of motion. After release there is a dramatic color change to bright red in the obviously viable loop as well as a return of peristalsis. Conversely, in obviously dead

bowel there is no color change and no motion after release of the strangulating obstruction. The loop that only partially pinks up and has little or no motion is the problem. It is usually best to wrap the questionable segment in moist laparotomy pads and leave it completely undisturbed for 10 minutes by the clock. If the circulation is obviously better at the end of this time, the loop is replaced in the abdomen. If the viability of the segment is still in doubt, resection should be done. But if a very long segment of bowel is involved, requiring a very extensive resection, then an attempt should be made to restore flow in the larger vessels supplying the segment. Even if this is unsuccessful, one should probably accept the risk of replacing nonviable bowel rather than make an intestinal cripple. The patient is observed very closely; if evidence of progressive toxicity develops, reoperation and resection are done. In any event, reexploration and reevaluation of the status of the bowel about 24 hours later may be advisable.

Decompression of grossly distended intestine during the operative procedure is sometimes necessary, particularly in late simple mechanical obstruction. Operative decompression is still a contentious point. There is no doubt that the operation is facilitated: the site of obstruction is more easily found, the uncontrolled eventration of distended loops through the incision is avoided, the bowel can be returned to the peritoneal cavity without the kinks that may cause segmentation and postoperative obstruction, and closure of the incision is possible without a struggle. Relief of distension also improves the blood supply to the intestine, and peristalsis returns sooner. It is also probable that removal of toxic bowel content is worthwhile. Whereas the normal mucosa is impermeable to these toxins, permeability is affected by impairment of the blood supply, and absorption may occur in compromised bowel.

Operative aspiration can be done in a variety of ways. Multiple needle aspirations are ineffective and definitely increase the morbidity, e.g., a wound infection rate of 20 percent versus a rate of 4 percent in a comparable group of patients without needle aspiration. Decompression with an ordinary suction tip through multiple enterotomies, though effective, is similarly attended by an increased infection rate, plus the risk of small bowel fistula. An effective, safe method of decompression is by passage of a tube from above downward, so that the entire gastrointestinal tract proximal to the obstruction is decompressed. A firm tube with generous lumen (Baker tube) is introduced through a proximal jejunostomy. The tube is advanced by manipulation through the intact bowel until the entire length of involved bowel down to the obstructed segment is pleated on the long tube. The tube is secured in that position for postoperative decompression.

Postoperative Care. The principles of postoperative care are the same as for the preoperative preparation of the patient with obstruction—fluids and electrolytes, antibiotics, and gastrointestinal decompression.

Fluid and electrolyte management is more difficult in the postoperative intestinal obstruction patient than in the usual postoperative abdominal surgical patient because of the large third space of sequestered, isotonic fluid. There is continued loss in the immediate postoperative period

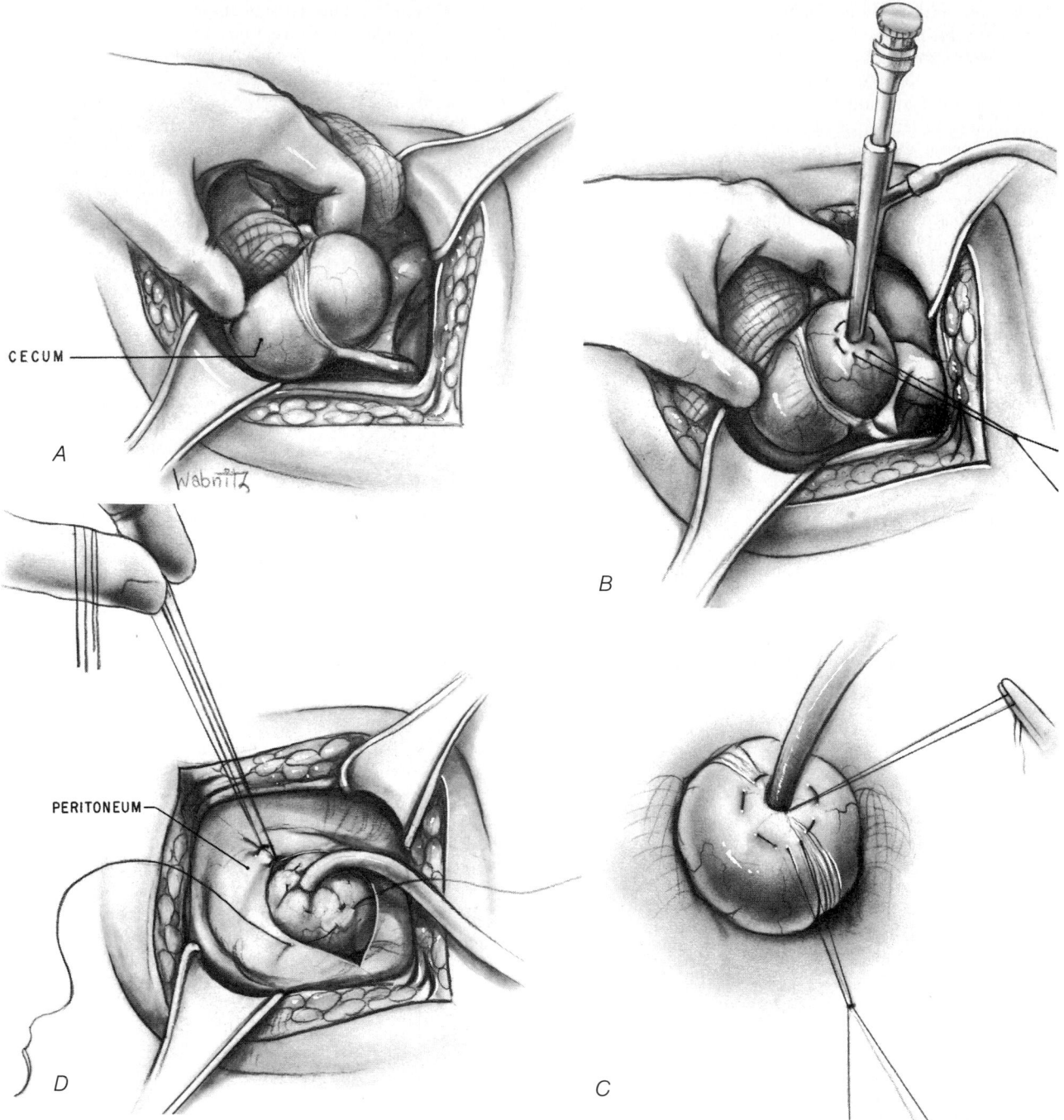

CECUM

A

Wabnitz

B

PERITONEUM

D

C

Fig. 24-5. Tube cecostomy. *A.* A McBurney incision is made in the right lower quadrant, the lateral peritoneal attachment of the cecum is divided, and the cecum is delivered into the wound, using a dry sponge. *B.* The distended cecum is held by the assistant, using gauze sponges, while the surgeon decompresses the cecum with a large trocar connected to suction. If distension is not great, this step may be omitted. *C.* A large rubber tube is then placed in the cecum by enlarging the opening made by the trocar, and the tube is secured in place with two concentric purse-string sutures. *D.* The peritoneum is sutured circumferentially to the cecum. Fascia is approximated; skin and subcutaneous tissues are packed open. The tube is connected to straight drainage.

into the sequestered fluid space. This loss slows in rate, however, and is reversed in direction after a variable period, usually about the third postoperative day. This large autoinfusion, as fluid is picked up by the vascular compartment from the sequestered fluid, must be allowed for in planning the daily ration of intravenous fluid therapy, lest the patient be watered into congestive failure.

Serum sodium and potassium levels must be watched very closely and kept in the normal range. A deficit of

Fig. 24-6. Transverse loop colostomy. *A.* A short transverse incision is made about midway between costal margin and umbilicus. Choice of right or left depends on the type of definitive surgical treatment planned for the future. *B.* After freeing the omentum, an opening is made in an avascular area of the transverse mesocolon close to the bowel. *The middle colic artery must be avoided. C.* A glass rod is inserted through the mesentery and secured in place by rubber tubing. The incision is closed in layers about the colon loop. No sutures are placed in the colon. *D.* If colon distension is extreme, trocar decompression may be done immediately after closing the incision. Otherwise the colostomy is opened with cautery about 24 to 36 hours after operation. *E.* Double-barrel colostomy may be performed initially using deMartel's clamps. A small catheter can be inserted into the proximal limb to achieve immediate decompression.

either or both of these ions is associated with prolonged paralysis of the gastrointestinal tract.

Decompression of the gastrointestinal tract is also harder to handle than in the usual postoperative patient, because restoration of normal propulsive intestinal motility is usually significantly delayed after release of intestinal obstruc-

tion. Whereas bowel function usually resumes on about the third day after abdominal operation, after intestinal obstruction it is often 5 or 6 days before gastrointestinal decompression can be discontinued. After 2 or 3 days of suction drainage it is often advisable to discontinue the suction and vent the intestinal tube to straight drainage only, to minimize fluid and electrolyte losses.

Ileus

Ileus may be divided into three groups: *adynamic, or inhibition, ileus,* in which there is diminished or absent motility because of inhibition of the neuromuscular apparatus; *spastic ileus,* in which the bowel musculature remains tightly contracted without coordinated propulsive motility; and the *ileus of vascular occlusion,* in which the bowel wall is incapable of coordinated motility, because it is dying from ischemia.

Spastic ileus, an uncommon form caused by uncoordinated hyperactivity of the intestine, is seen in heavy-metal poisoning, in prophyria, and sometimes in uremia. Therapy of the intestinal manifestations is usually not indicated—therapy should be aimed at the underlying disorder.

Adynamic ileus of some degree is extremely common, since it occurs after every abdominal operation. The rate of recovery of motor function is different in different segments of the gastrointestinal tract: small bowel motility returns within 24 hours and gastric motility within 48 hours, but colonic inertia persists for 3 to 5 days. Oral intake usually can be resumed on the third or fourth postoperative day. Only when postoperative ileus persists does it become a clinical problem. Common causes of serious degrees of inhibition ileus are many and varied and include intraperitoneal inflammation such as acute appendicitis or acute pancreatitis; retroperitoneal pathologic conditions such as ureteral colic, retroperitoneal hematoma, or fracture of the spine; thoracic lesions such as basal pneumonia or fractured ribs; and systemic causes such as severe toxemia, hyponatremia, or hypokalemia.

Overactivity of the sympathetic system appears to be the common denominator in inhibition ileus associated with many of the lesions listed above; alterations in the composition of the internal environment also playing an important role.

The mechanism by which sympathetic activity brings about inhibition of intestinal motility was studied extensively by Kock, using anesthetized cats. He concluded that centrally induced inhibition of motility is virtually exclusively dependent on the hormonal component of the sympathoadrenal system. Landman and Longmire studied the hormonal influences of peritonitis on paralytic ileus in conscious dogs. Jejunal loops were studied, then subjected to extrinsic denervation by division of the neurovascular pedicle. They found that induction of chemical peritonitis produced atony of the loop with or without innervation and so concluded that inhibition of motility in the denervated loop must be explained on the basis of a blood-borne substance.

CLINICAL MANIFESTATIONS. The primary disease causing the ileus may predominate in the clinical picture, or conversely, in some cases, abdominal findings may so predominate that the primary process is overlooked. In postoperative ileus, the division between physiologic ileus and the undue abnormal prolongation of bowel hypofunction is blurred. Instead of the patient's passing flatus and becoming hungry on about the third day, as expected following abdominal operation, he is noted to be distended and disinterested in food and his surroundings. Examination confirms that there is generalized abdominal distension with tympany and scattered, occasional bowel sounds.

Assistance from the laboratory is needed mainly in evaluating some of the causes of ileus such as acute anemia, sepsis, hyponatremia, hypokalemia, and hypoosmolarity.

As outlined above (Table 24-6 and Fig. 24-4), x-ray can often help in the differential diagnosis between postoperative adynamic ileus and postoperative mechanical obstruction. If the plain films are inconclusive, contrast medium is given by mouth or through a gastrointestinal tube. In inhibition ileus, some medium should reach the cecum in about 4 hours, whereas a stationary column of medium for 3 or 4 hours indicates complete obstruction of the small intestine.

Adynamic ileus characteristically involves both the small and large bowel to a greater or lesser degree. Occasionally, there is marked distension confined largely to the colon without evidence of mechanical obstruction of the bowel itself or interference with its blood supply—pseudoobstruction of the colon or Ogilvie's syndrome. Barium enema is indicated to rule out organic obstruction. Cecal perforation may occur even though mechanical intestinal obstruction is absent.

TREATMENT. The treatment of ileus is essentially the treatment of the primary lesion. Postoperative ileus is caused in the vast majority of patients either by focal inflammation—leaking anastomosis, abscess following contamination—or by gross fluid-electrolyte derangements. When these problems are promptly eradicated, the ileus will take care of itself.

Treatment of the distension is best done by passage of a long tube. Unfortunately it is much more difficult to pass than in mechanical ileus because of the difference in motility of the intestine. If the long tube will not pass the pylorus, then gastric suction should be used and will prevent further distension.

The availability of newer pharmacologic agents that affect gastrointestinal motility has led to renewed interest in this method of treating ileus. In the past, nonoperative techniques were either ineffective or dangerous. Gastrointestinal pacing by means of an electrode in the tip of the nasogastric tube through which physiologic electric currents are delivered appears to be of little value. Similarly, injections of d-pantothenyl alcohol (a component of coenzyme A which is necessary for the production of acetylcholine) have been shown to be ineffective in postoperative ileus.

Vasopressin which causes contraction of smooth muscle, and parasympathomimetic drugs such as neostigmine or Urecholine will often increase intestinal motility but are not safe to use, because perforation of the bowel can result if there is mechanical obstruction. Catchpole and others have shown that if the sympathetics are blocked pharmacologically, then small (and presumably safe) doses of parasympathomimetic drugs will produce effective propulsive gastrointestinal motility.

Rarely, paralytic ileus does not respond to conservative measures—the obstruction does not relent, and operation must be considered. In most such cases, mechanical obstruction will be found. If no mechanical factors are found, a long tube should be manipulated by the surgeon well down into the small bowel. If the ileocecal valve is competent and marked colon distension is present, then cecostomy should be added. The ileus will be made worse by the operation but can now be managed with adequate decompression.

GASTROINTESTINAL BLEEDING: HEMATEMESIS, MELENA, AND RECTAL BLEEDING

Bleeding may be a manifestation of a variety of diseases along the entire length of the gastrointestinal tract from the oropharynx to the anus. Bleeding represents the initial symptom of gastrointestinal disease in more than one-third of these patients, and in 70 percent there is no history of a previous bleeding episode.

DEFINITIONS. *Hematemesis* refers to the vomiting of blood which is either fresh and unaltered or digested by gastric secretion. It is a manifestation of a bleeding site located between the oropharynx and the ligament of Treitz and may be accompanied by simultaneous melena. The character of the specimen depends on the site of bleeding, the rate of hemorrhage, and the rate of gastric emptying. The presence of blood clots reflects massive bleeding, while a coffee-ground vomitus usually indicates a slower rate with retention in the stomach and alteration to form acid hematin.

Melena is usually defined as the passage of a black, tarry stool. Only 50 ml of blood is necessary to produce this sign and, following the cessation of a bleeding of 1,000 ml, the finding may persist for as long as 5 days. A guaiac-positive stool, indicative of occult blood, may persist for 3 weeks following hematemesis or melena. In general, blood from the distal colon is red and not thoroughly mixed with the stool, whereas blood from the upper gastrointestinal tract produces a tarry stool. However, massive bleeding from the upper gastrointestinal tract may be associated with red or currant jelly clots if the bleeding is rapid and the gastrointestinal motility is increased. Red or black stools may also result from the ingestion of food dye substances and iron. The tarry color, which accompanies upper gastrointestinal bleeding, is attributable to the production of acid hematin by action of gastric acid on the hemoglobin or the production of sulfide from heme by the action of hydrogen sulfide on the iron in the heme molecule. Melena without hematemesis generally indicates a lesion distal to the pylorus but has been associated with bleeding varices and gastritis.

CONSEQUENCES OF GASTROINTESTINAL BLEEDING. Hypotension and shock are dependent upon the rate of the bleeding and the patient's response to the blood loss. It is difficult to estimate the amount of blood loss in either the vomitus or stool, because both specimens contain a mixture of multiple components. The hematocrit and hemoglobin levels are unreliable until equilibration occurs, i.e., 6 to 48 hours subsequent to the bleeding, and estimations of blood volume have also proved unreliable, since the error associated with the technique is great and the range of normals for a given physical state is wide. Shortly after bleeding has begun, a vasovagal reaction is associated with bradycardia, whereas with the progression of time the heart rate increases and the cardiac output decreases. The clinical picture of shock may reflect a coronary occlusion or myocardial ischemia precipitated by hemorrhage rather than the consequences of massive blood loss per se. An-

other consequence of hypotension is reduced renal blood flow resulting in either oliguria or anuria.

Azotemia, which is characteristically associated with bleeding esophagogastric varices, also occurs in patients with other types of massive hemorrhage. Blood urea nitrogen levels of 30 mg/100 ml or more occur in two-thirds of patients with bleeding varices, and an elevation of 50 mg/100 ml or more occurs in one-fifth of the cases. Following cessation of the bleeding, normal levels are usually achieved within 3 days. Azotemia usually does not occur with hemorrhage originating in the colon, and since it is dependent upon bacterial action, normal levels may be associated with upper gastrointestinal tract bleeding in patients on antibiotics which sterilize the intestinal flora. The level to which the BUN rises parallels the extent of gastrointestinal bleeding, but it may be potentiated by shock, impairment of renal function, and increased catabolism. In the presence of blood in the intestinal tract renal function can be evaluated by clearance studies.

Upper Gastrointestinal Tract Bleeding

ETIOLOGY. Although a great variety of lesions above the ligament of Treitz have been implicated in the cause of upper gastrointestinal tract hemorrhage, in the vast majority it is due to peptic ulceration, acute mucosal lesions—gastritis and erosions, esophagogastric varices, diaphragmatic hernia, or gastric neoplasms (Table 24-7).

Peptic ulceration represents the most common cause and accounts for one-half to two-thirds of the cases. Hemorrhage from duodenal ulcer occurs four times more frequently than that from gastric ulcer, but since this represents the relative incidence of the two lesions, the two types have an equal tendency to bleed. Massive bleeding occurs in 10 to 15 percent of ulcer patients with hemorrhage and is the first symptom in 16 percent of the patients who bleed. The bleeding is generally caused by the inflammatory process eroding into the regional artery. In the case of duodenal ulcers, the gastroduodenal artery is involved, while the left and right gastric arteries and their branches are most frequently involved with gastric ulcers. Most bleeding ulcers are chronic lesions, and the adjacent arteries suffer from local inflammatory changes. Since hemostasis is dependent on the retraction of the walls of the vessel, persistent bleeding is more likely to occur with chronic lesions and in older patients with atherosclerotic vessels.

Peptic ulceration of the stomal mucosa at the site of a gastroenterostomy is to be considered in any patient who has had previous gastric surgical treatment. It is a more frequent occurrence when less than two-thirds of the stomach has been removed and an accompanying vagotomy has not been performed, especially if there is retained antrum.

The next most common cause of gross upper gastrointestinal tract hemorrhage after peptic ulcer is a diverse group of lesions that can best be collectively termed *acute mucosal lesions* until they are clearly delineated and separated into entities. The reported incidence (Table 24-7)

Table 24-7. ETIOLOGY OF UPPER GASTROINTESTINAL TRACT BLEEDING IN 10,554 CASES

Author	Year	Number of cases	Peptic ulcer percent	Acute mucosal lesions, percent	Esophageal varices, percent	Diaphragmatic hernia, percent	Gastric cancer, percent	Other, percent	Undetermined percent
Jones	1956	1,910	57	29	3	2	2	3	5
Ferguson	1962	1,124	62	4	7	1	4	1	20
Hirschowitz. . .	1963	216	58	22	1	1	1	5	12
Dorsey	1965	405	68	2	2	3	. . .	5	20
Katz	1970	800	24	33	17	. . .	. . .	10	16
Palmer	1970	1,400	45	12	19	8	. . .	11	7
Schiff	1970	640	53	1	13	2	2	8	21
Halmagyi	1970	199	65	1	7	6	1	15	5
Preston	1970	535	50	2	30	. . .	. . .	7	17
Schiller	1970	2,149	45	3	2	. . .	2	22	26
Foster	1971	296	67	13	9	. . .	3	4	4
Crook	1972	880	50	19	11	3	2	5	4
Average . . .	. . .	. . .	50	13	9	2	2	8	16

ranges from 1 to 33 percent. The true incidence will not be known until endoscopy is universally applied early in the course of upper gastrointestinal tract hemorrhage. Pathologically, these lesions are sometimes single but more often multiple, or the mucosa may be diffusely involved in hemorrhagic necrosis. The process usually does not extend through the muscularis mucosae, and therefore the lesions are technically *erosions,* not true ulcers. In contradistinction to chronic benign ulcers, which are characteristically located in the antrum or on the lesser curvature, the acute erosive lesions are found in the body and fundus of the stomach, sparing the antrum, and on the greater curvature as often as on the lesser.

"Stress ulceration" is a much abused term which if used at all should be confined to the acute gastroduodenal lesions that occur secondary to shock and sepsis following operation, trauma, or burns. McClelland et al. have shown in patients with trauma and hemorrhagic shock that gastric secretion is not increased but that splanchnic blood flow is significantly decreased. They conclude that "ischemic damage to the superficial gastric mucosa may induce stress ulceration." Sepsis also plays a prominent role. Altemeier et al. documented upper gastrointestinal tract bleeding in approximately one-third of surgical patients with septicemia and also implicated the coagulation abnormalities that attend sepsis. Nance et al. found that in germ-free rats subjected to restraint stress there is a marked reduction in the incidence and severity of gastric ulceration as compared to conventional animals and concluded that bacterial factors play a significant role in the pathogenesis of stress ulcers.

Probably closely related to stress erosions is the acute ulceration or erosion of the stomach and duodenum which occurs in burn patients. Such lesions are usually referred to as Curling's ulcers, after the man who described them in 1842. Curling's ulcers occur in about 12 percent of patients hospitalized for burns. The incidence increases with burn size—up to a 40 percent incidence in burns of 70 percent or more of the body surface. Sepsis is an additive stress. In two-thirds of patients with Curling's ulcer the presenting clinical sign is bleeding, and in 45 percent such bleeding is massive. Though there are many similarities between stress erosions and Curling's ulcers, their distribution is somewhat different: stress erosions are usually multiple and usually in the stomach; Curling's ulcers are about evenly divided between single and multiple, and between stomach and duodenum.

Another eponymic ulcer that is probably closely related to stress erosions is the *Cushing ulcer.* In 1932, Harvey Cushing described a variety of esophagogastroduodenal lesions in nine patients following craniotomy. Since then the belief has persisted that dysfunction in specific areas of the brain leads to gastrointestinal ulceration. In many of these patients, the etiologic factors are probably the same as for patients after any major operation, but there is some evidence that significant gastric hypersecretion may occur after certain intracranial operations or trauma.

Adrenal corticosteroids, given in large doses for prolonged periods, frequently lead to gastroduodenal erosions or ulcers, or to activation of preexisting quiescent peptic ulcers. Patients receiving steroids for rheumatoid arthritis or lupus erythematosus are more prone to this complication than patients with asthma or inflammatory bowel disease. Despite the fact that steroids do not increase the gastric acid output, antacid therapy is often efficacious. The distribution of "steroid ulcers" is much the same as that of postoperative "stress ulcers."

Aspirin and alcohol are the major offenders of a large group of ingested agents that may produce erosive, hemorrhagic gastritis and duodenitis. The incidence with which this lesion is diagnosed is directly related to the degree to which early endoscopic examination is employed. Alcohol is a known gastric secretagogue, but aspirin and similar agents are not; the latter presumably act by increasing back-diffusion of HCl through the gastric mucosa. The hemorrhage is generally mild to moderate but is sometimes massive. Since the gastric mucosa normally renews itself every 48 to 72 hours, the process is self-limited if symptoms can be controlled until mucosal regeneration occurs. Emergency operation for exsanguinating hemorrhage is sometimes necessary.

Esophagogastric varices constitute the most common cause of bleeding in patients with cirrhosis or extrahepatic obstruction of the portal vein. These account for approximately 10 percent of all cases of upper gastrointestinal tract bleeding, but the incidence varies widely, being significantly higher in the hospitals with a large indigent population. Bleeding varices constitute 95 percent of the cases of massive hematemesis in the child, and they are usually associated with extrahepatic obstruction of the portal vein. In cirrhotic patients, varices are the cause of bleeding in 53 percent of the cases, while gastritis is implicated in 22 percent and duodenal and gastric ulcers in 20 percent. Correlation of the lesions and severity of bleeding reveals that in the majority of cases (70 percent) patients with bleeding from varices have severe hemorrhage while 84 percent of patients with bleeding from gastritis demonstrate mild to moderate blood loss. The precipitation of the bleeding episode has been ascribed to two major factors: increased pressure within the varix and ulceration secondary to esophagitis. Although esophagogastric varices are almost always associated with portal hypertension, the diagnosis has been established in occasional patients with normal portal pressures. The veins responsible for the bleeding are usually opened laterally by transmural erosion, and any hemostasis which occurs is dependent upon occlusion of the opening by a thrombus. The bleeding is nearly always associated with hematemesis and is generally very profuse.

Hiatal hernia frequently may be associated with occult bleeding but is usually not a cause of gross upper gastrointestinal tract hemorrhage, accounting for approximately 2 percent of the cases. The bleeding in the sliding hernia is related to reflux peptic esophagitis. Bleeding is more commonly seen with paraesophageal hernias and is thought to be caused by the retention of acid contents within the incarcerated gastric pouch or congestion of the vascular supply of the herniated portion of the stomach.

A variety of miscellaneous lesions account for up to 8 percent of occasional upper gastrointestinal tract bleeding, while in 16 percent the diagnosis is never determined. Neoplasms are uncommonly implicated, and there is evidence that the incidence of carcinoma of the stomach is decreasing in the United States. Bleeding associated with gastric carcinoma is caused by erosion of the tumor into underlying vessels. It is usually mild to moderate, but if a large vessel is involved, massive bleeding can occur. Massive hemorrhage may be the initial symptom in a patient with gastric carcinoma. Other tumors occur less frequently. Leiomyoma and leiomyosarcoma of the stomach or esophagus may be manifested by profuse bleeding, usually in men in the third decade of life. Leukemia with intestinal infiltrates may cause significant gastrointestinal bleeding. Also, polyps, either single, familial, or associated with the Peutz-Jeghers syndrome are included as neoplastic lesions with a bleeding potential.

Vascular lesions, including angiomas, hereditary hemorrhagic telangiectasia (Rendu-Osler-Weber), and vasculitis,

have all been reported as etiologic factors in upper gastrointestinal tract bleeding. Spontaneous rupture of aortic, hepatic arterial, and splenic arterial aneurysms may produce alarming bleeding. Characteristically, aortic aneurysm is manifested by moderate bleeding which stops for a variable period of time only to recur as massive bleeding.

Inflammation of the mucosa with erosion of small or large vessels may accompany prolapsing gastric mucosa and duodenal diverticula. Prolapsing gastric mucosa, which is usually not considered a common source of bleeding, may be accompanied by moderate blood loss. Similarly, although duodenal diverticula are generally considered to be asymptomatic, massive hemorrhage has accompanied ulceration of this lesion. Hepatic trauma with development of a central or subcapsular hematoma which discharges into the biliary tree is responsible for the development of the syndrome known as hematobilia, which may represent a cause of moderate or massive bleeding. Hematobilia may also occur with cholecystitis, cholelithiasis, and passage of stones. The interval between trauma and the bleeding manifestation is variable. Another traumatic cause of upper gastrointestinal tract bleeding is the Mallory-Weiss syndrome, which consists of linear tears of the esophagogastric junction induced by severe vomiting, usually in alcoholic patients.

DIAGNOSIS. History and Physical Examination. The patient's own account of the amount of bleeding is frequently misleading. Vomiting of large amounts of blood is more suggestive of bleeding ulcer or esophagogastric varices. A history of active ulcer symptoms preceding the hemorrhage with cessation of the pain at the onset of bleeding suggests that the bleeding is originating from the peptic ulcer. However, 20 percent of patients with bleeding have no previous history of ulcer. Although there is an increased incidence of the ulcer diathesis in cirrhotic patients, esophagogastric varices represent the most common cause of bleeding in these patients and account for over 50 percent of the bleeding episodes. Violent retching and vomiting in alcoholics or pregnant women is characteristic of a Mallory-Weiss syndrome. The history should include questions directed toward the recent ingestion of drugs implicated as causes of gastrointestinal bleeding, particularly salicylates, Butazolidin, alcohol, anticoagulants, and steroids. A history regarding the bleeding tendency during childhood, in early adulthood, and in other members of the family focuses on the possibility of hematologic disorders. Previous gastric surgical treatment such as gastroenterostomy or partial gastrectomy directs one's thinking toward the possibility of a marginal ulcer. Heartburn, epigastric substernal pain accentuated by the recumbent position and the ingestion of large meals, suggests the presence of a hiatal hernia. A recent history of upper abdominal or chest trauma is most compatible with a diagnosis of hematobilia, particularly when the bleeding is accompanied by jaundice and intermittent colicky pain.

Examination of the patient with upper gastrointestinal tract bleeding is directed at determining stigmata of the various diseases considered in the etiology. The skin and mucous membranes should be examined for ictcrus, spider angiomas, liver palms, and decreased hair over the extremity, all suggestive of hepatic disease. The mucous membrane should be investigated for melanin spots of the Peutz-Jeghers syndrome. Hereditary telangiectasia lesions are most common on the lips, tongue, and ears. Lymphadenopathy, particularly in the left supraclavicular region, may suggest a malignant intraabdominal process. Abdominal palpation more commonly reveals tenderness when the bleeding is related to ulcer or gastritis, whereas a palpable liver, particularly when accompanied by splenomegaly and abdominal veins which fill in a centrifugal pattern from the umbilicus, is more indicative of bleeding varices. Examination should always include aspiration via nasogastric tube in order to determine presence of blood at this level and the extent of bleeding at the time of examination.

Special Diagnostic Procedures. The extent of anemia may be assessed by the hematocrit level. It should be appreciated that, with acute blood loss, the initial level may be normal, since the hematocrit reduction does not occur for 4 to 6 hours, during which time equilibration occurs. Repeat hematocrit readings taken at 4- to 6-hour intervals are more meaningful. Leukocytosis, with levels of 25,000, may accompany acute hemorrhage, but more marked increases are suggestive of leukemia. Both the neutrophils and platelets may be reduced in the case of hypersplenism secondary to primary hepatic disease, suggesting bleeding from esophagogastric varices.

Clinical chemistries are directed toward evaluating the extent of bleeding and, particularly, determining the presence of hepatocellular dysfunction. None of the tests define the site of bleeding. A rise in the BUN level parallels the extent of hemorrhage and is related to the absorption of blood products from the gastrointestinal tract, possible associated reduction in renal flow secondary to shock or dehydration, and, at times, the presence of preexisting renal disease. In the presence of marked hepatic dysfunction, the BUN level may not be elevated, since the liver is unable to synthesize urea. In this circumstance, the blood ammonia level is frequently elevated with bleeding varices, since it is related to the extent of portal collateralization and reduced hepatic function. The validity of this test, however, is not uniform. Normal values are present in patients with variceal bleeding. When this test is combined with the BSP (Bromsulphalein test), no diagnostic significance can be attributed if either level is elevated and the other normal. However, when both the blood ammonia and BSP retention levels are elevated, this represents strong evidence of cirrhosis. The BSP retention is particularly applicable to the diagnosis of cirrhosis in patients with massive hemorrhage. Abnormal BSP retention may be related either to liver disease or to shock from hemorrhage regardless of the site. In contrast, a normal value in association with massive bleeding suggests that the liver is not responsible.

Determination of the blood clotting factors is of great importance, particularly in patients bleeding from stress ulceration. Reduced platelet adhesiveness, thrombocytopenia, prolonged prothrombin time, and other clotting defects are common in such patients. The bleeding often stops, obviating emergency operation, following the administration of fresh platelet infusions, vitamin K, and fresh frozen plasma.

Rarely, bleeding is so rapid that immediate operation without preoperative diagnostic procedures is necessary to save life. More commonly, transfusions can easily allow time for diagnosis and preparation; further, many patients stop bleeding soon after admission. As the above tests are being done, the patient should be rapidly transfused to circulatory normality, with vital signs, central venous pressure, and urinary output as guides. The stomach should be completely evacuated using iced Ringer's lavage through a nasogastric tube; an Ewald tube may be advisable initially if many large clots are present.

Endoscopy is the first special diagnostic procedure to be considered; it is virtually mandatory if the bleeding is thought to be from esophagogastric varices or from an acute mucosal lesion. Esophagoscopy defines the bleeding point in the case of varices, since liver function tests, manometry, barium x-ray, and isotopic studies merely indicate the presence of portal hypertension or varices but do not determine if these lesions are actually bleeding. The reported esophagscopic accident rate is 0.25 percent, and an experienced endoscopist is required. A 33 percent disagreement rate between two experienced endoscopists evaluating a given group of patients is reported. This is related to the difficulty in differentiating varices and mucosal folds. Gastroduodenoscopy with fiberoptic instruments is particularly valuable in revealing acute gastritis, erosions, and small superficial ulcers that are not demonstrable on upper gastrointestinal tract x-ray.

Radiologic Studies. Selective arteriography of the celiac and superior mesenteric arteries and their branches is a relatively safe and accurate method of identifying active bleeding points in the upper gastrointestinal tract (Fig. 24-7). A skillful experienced radiologist using highly specialized, sophisticated equipment is essential to obtain reliable information. Angiography is usually done after endoscopy if that procedure has not identified the bleeding point. In any event, it must come before the upper gastrointestinal barium x-rays, which will obscure the field. Although bleeding at the rate of 1 to 2 ml/minute can be detected experimentally, bleeding must be at the rate of 3 to 5 ml/minute for accurate clinical angiographic diagnosis. The diagnostic accuracy of angiography in visualizing actively bleeding arterial lesions is about 90 percent; the accuracy in variceal bleeding, using the venous phase of the angiogram, is only about 20 percent.

In addition to diagnosis, selective arterial catheterization can be used for therapy of gastrointestinal bleeding. After the bleeding point is identified, a small therapeutic catheter is guided into the artery supplying the bleeding area, and vasoconstrictive agents, usually vasopressin at the rate of 0.1 to 0.2 units/minute, are infused. In the case of variceal bleeding, the main superior mesentric artery is infused in order to reduce splanchnic blood flow and thus decrease portal vein flow and pressure. In many patients (depending on the nature of the lesion), the bleeding is arrested; in some, bleeding is only partially controlled, and an operation is necessary but can be done under more orderly circumstances. In about 20 percent, vasopressin infusion does not control bleeding. Regional vasoconstrictive therapy should be used only in patients in whom the potential benefit justifies the very considerable risk; Conn et al. have reported a 35 percent complication rate. Also, several comparative studies of systemic intravenous vasopressin versus regional arterial vasopressin have not shown any advantage for the more difficult and dangerous arterial route.

An upper gastrointestinal tract series, the cornerstone of morphologic radiographic diagnosis, should be done next, if endoscopy and arteriography have not revealed the bleeding site. As with endoscopy, the stomach should be evacuated of clots prior to the examination.

In the case of bleeding ulcer, delaying for several days after hemorrhage has ceased does not increase the accuracy of diagnosis. The question of safety in the patient with bleeding has been raised, since the routine gastrointestinal series involves compression which may be attended by increasing hemorrhage. The Hampton technique for demonstration of bleeding ulcers obviates the use of palpation or compression and is attended by a diagnostic accuracy of 86 percent for demonstration of ulcers. The diagnostic accuracy in the case of bleeding varices is approximately 50 percent. Both the Valsalva and Müller maneuvers may occasionally show varices when other methods fail. Roentgenograms have proved of little value in the diagnosis of gastritis with a yield of approximately 25 percent.

Percutaneous splenoportography affords a high yield for the diagnosis of esophageal varices but is rarely performed on an emergency basis. Before carrying out this procedure, a platelet count greater than 50,000 and a prothrombin time greater than 35 percent should be demonstrated.

Splenic pulp manometry has been applied as an emergency test in the differential diagnosis of upper gastrointestinal tract bleeding. A 90 percent accuracy has been reported, but there is a zone of splenic pulp pressures which cannot differentiate variceal bleeding from other causes. In addition, isotopic and splenoportographic studies have demonstrated patients in whom portal hypertension is unaccompanied by the development of a collateral circulation. Finally, the admittedly rare situation of bleeding esophageal varices associated with normal portal pressure would not be diagnosed by this technique.

Balloon tamponade has been used as a diagnostic-therapeutic measure. However, varices are controlled even temporarily in only 65 to 75 percent of patients, and a peptic ulcer may coincidentally stop bleeding after a gastric balloon is inflated.

In some instances, an operation is performed on a patient with massive upper gastrointestinal tract bleeding in whom a diagnosis has not been established preoperatively. Laparotomy is to be considered as an important diagnostic tool. Once the peritoneal cavity has been opened, inspection of the liver may reveal cirrhosis, and distension of the omental vessels may suggest portal hypertension. In most cases, however, a determination of the source of bleeding requires a long gastrotomy which permits visualization of the gastric mucosa and the proximal portions of the duodenum. An attempt should be made to identify duodenal ulcer or a gastric lesion, and if these are not

Fig. 24-7. Selective angiography in upper gastrointestinal bleeding. Dye injection into the common hepatic artery has outlined a bleeding duodenal ulcer (arrow). Later films showed a persistent puddling of contrast medium in the duodenum after all intravascular contrast had disappeared.

apparent, traction on the lower end of the nasogastric tube which is brought out through the gastrotomy will often expose the cardiac end of the stomach and distal esophagus to inspection. Intraoperative esophagogastroscopy by the usual route also may be helpful. Occasionally, in the absence of a preopoerative diagnosis, no site of bleeding will be found at operation. In this situation, some surgeons do a vagotomy and drainage procedure; others simply close and hope that if bleeding recurs, the diagnosis can be made at that time and specific therapy instituted. The "blind" gastric resection which was formerly done in this situation has fallen into disfavor.

Lower Gastrointestinal Tract Bleeding

Bleeding distal to the ligament of Treitz is manifested by the passage of tarry stools or unaltered blood (hemochezia) and is characteristically unaccompanied by hematemesis. It is usually moderate or mild but may be massive.

ETIOLOGY. A great variety of lesions extending from the ligament of Treitz to the anus may be implicated as causes of lower gastrointestinal tract bleeding.

Jejunal and Ileal Bleeding. Meckel's diverticulitis, intussusception, and regional enteritis represent the most common causes. Meckel's diverticulitis with associated bleeding occurs most frequently in children, and the bleeding episode is related to gastric mucosa within the diverticulum stimulating ulceration of the adjacent ileum. Ileocecal intussusception is also a lesion of childhood, occurring most commonly before the age of two and attended by a characteristic currant jelly stool. The cause of this mechanical process in childhood is usually undetermined, while ileocecal intussusception in the adult is usually secondary to an intestinal polyp or tumor. Regional enteritis is accompanied by severe melena in approximately 5 percent of the cases, while some rectal bleeding is a common symptom in about 20 percent of the patients with this disease. Although tumors of the small intestine are rare, approximately half are accompanied by bleeding. The neoplasms include leiomyomas, polyps, either single or multiple (familial polyposis), and the polyps of the Peutz-Jegher syndrome. Carcinomas, sarcomas, and leukemias have all been reported to be associated with bleeding, whereas bleeding is an uncommon manifestation of a carcinoid tumor. Hemangiomas, hereditary telangiectasis, microaneurysms of blood vessels within the wall of the intestine, mesenteric thrombosis, drug reactions, and blood dyscrasias all represent rare causes of small intestinal bleeding.

Colonic Bleeding. The common causes include carcinoma, diverticula, colitis, and polyps (Table 24-8). Although carcinoma represents the most common cause of rectal bleeding, the bleeding associated with this lesion is rarely massive. Carcinoma of the right colon, particularly of the cecum, is usually accompanied by melena which may be so subtle that it is not considered until anemia has become established. Diverticulosis presents the most common cause of *massive* rectal bleeding. This is related to erosion of vessels within the neck of the diverticulum. In contrast, the bleeding which accompanies diverticulitis is mild to moderate and is caused by a superficial erosion of smaller vessels on the surface of the mucosa. Although the bleeding which accompanies ulcerative colitis is usually mild to moderate, massive hemorrhage may occur. Polyps

which may be single or multiple and may be located in any segment of the colon represent a relatively frequent source of rectal bleeding. Rarer causes include cecal ulceration, sarcomas, lymphomas, leukemia, hematologic disorders, and impairment of the vascular supply due to mesenteric thrombosis or ischemic colitis, or secondary to aortic resection with interruption of a functionally important inferior mesenteric artery.

Prior to angiography, bleeding lesions of the right colon were thought to be rare, but in the past decade many reports have emphasized that the right colon is a common site of bleeding. Diverticula were thought to be the responsible lesion. Boley and associates have shown that vascular ectasias are probably responsible for much of the right colon bleeding; they suggest that ectasias may be the commonest cause of major lower intestinal bleeding in the elderly. They present evidence that these vascular ectasias: (1) are degenerative lesions of aging and are not congenital or neoplastic; (2) occur in patients over 60 years of age; (3) are not associated with angiomatous lesions of the skin or other viscera; (4) occur in the cecum and proximal ascending colon; (5) are small, usually less than 5 mm in diameter; (6) can be diagnosed only by angiography; and (7) usually cannot be identified by the surgeon at operation or by the pathologist using standard techniques—injecting-clearing techniques must be used.

Rectal and Anal Bleeding. This is usually manifested by unaltered blood on the surface of the stool. The causes include hemorrhoids, and fissures, and proctitis. It is to be emphasized that the presence of hemorrhoids in a patient with rectal bleeding should not preclude investigation of other possible sources, particularly carcinoma.

DIAGNOSIS. A precise description of the bleeding episode and the nature of the stool is indicated. The question of familial polyposis and drug ingestion should be investigated. Physical examination includes a search for skin and mucosal lesions of the hemorrhagic telangiectasis (Rendu-Osler-Weber syndrome) or the Peutz-Jegher syndrome. Abdominal palpation may reveal a mass, tumor, or intussusception, the last frequently accompanied by absence of bowel in the right lower quadrant. Rectal ex-

Table 24-8. INCIDENCE OF RECTAL BLEEDING (1955–1960)

Characteristic lesion	All rectal bleeding, no. of cases	Moderate rectal bleeding, no. of cases	Severe rectal bleeding, no. of cases
Cancer, left colon	75	73	2
Diverticulosis.	62	45	17
Ulcerative colitis	39	39	
Polyps	25	23	2
Diverticulitis	16	16	
Cancer, right colon	14	13	1
Miscellaneous	14 (1 each)	12 (1 each)	2 (1 each)
Total	245	221	24

SOURCE: From R. J. Noer et al., Rectal Hemorrhage: Moderate and Severe, *Ann Surg,* 155:794, 1962, and from the Louisville General Hospital and Louisville Veterans Administration Hospital.

amination may be diagnostic for tumor, polyps, or anal lesions. Proctosigmoidoscopy should be done early in the hospital course.

Selective angiography is by far the most accurate method of diagnosis provided there is active bleeding at the rate of at least 2 or 3 ml/minute at the time of the examination. The small intestine and right half of the colon are examined by catheterization of branches of the superior mesenteric artery (Fig. 24-5). Examination of the left colon is sometimes more difficult, since the inferior mesenteric artery may be more difficult to catheterize. As with upper gastrointestinal tract bleeding, regional infusion of vasoconstrictive agents via a catheter in the artery supplying the bleeding site is often an effective method of controlling bleeding.

Barium contrast studies, if needed, should follow angiography so that the contrast material does not obscure the angiographer's field. Barium enema studies, including air contrast, represent a reliable, accurate method of diagnosing colon lesions but yield no information as to whether or not the lesions visualized are responsible for the bleeding. Gastrointestinal series with small bowel followthrough is less productive in the case of lesions of the small intestine. Every effort should be made to demonstrate the bleeding site prior to operation, since diagnosis at the operating table is often not possible.

JAUNDICE

The term *jaundice* is derived from the French word meaning "yellow" and refers to the presence of an excess of bile pigments in the tissues and the serum. It is the presenting sign of a number of hepatic and nonhepatic diseases. The differential diagnosis and management are dependent upon an appreciation of the normal and abnormal variants of bile pigment metabolism. A flow sheet analysis of hyperbilirubinemia is presented in Table 24-9.

NORMAL BILE PIGMENT METABOLISM. The bile pigment bilirubin (Fig. 24-8) is a tetrapyrrole which is formed to the greatest extent from hemoglobin and, to a lesser extent, from myoglobin breakdown and hepatic synthesis itself. When the red blood cell is destroyed by the reticuloendothelial system, either at the end of its natural life span or prematurely, the iron and globin are removed, and the heme ring is opened and transformed into biliverdin, which is green. The latter is reduced to become bilirubin, which is yellow (Fig. 24-9). The bilirubin combines with albumin to form a relatively stable protein-pigment complex and is transported as such to the hepatic parenchymal cell. This complex, which is referred to as *indirect-reacting* bilirubin, since it gives the van den Bergh diazo reaction only after treatment with alcohol and other substances which split the protein bond, is poorly soluble in water and is not excreted in the urine.

In the hepatic parenchymal cell the albumin is removed, and the bilirubin is conjugated with glucuronic acid to form a diglucuronide, which is water-soluble and is excreted into the bile canaliculi. This substance gives an

Fig. 24-8. Normal bile pigment metabolism.

Fig. 24-9. Conversion of heme to bilirubin.

Table 24-9. ANALYSIS OF A CASE OF HYPERBILIRUBINEMIA

Fractionate serum bilirubin and measure urine bilirubin and urobilinogen to determine whether:

I. Unconjugated hyperbilirubinemia

Determine mechanism on basis of age, clinical features, and laboratory findings:

A. Production of bilirubin beyond excretory capacity. Evidence of:
  1. Hemolysis
     a. Extracorpuscular
        (1) Immune body reactions
            (a) Transfusion reactions
            (b) Erythroblastosis
        (2) Infections and chemicals
        (3) Physical agents
        (4) Secondary hemolysis in pregnancy
     b. Intracorpuscular
        (1) Congenital hemolytic jaundice
        (2) Sickle cell anemia
        (3) Mediterranean anemia
  2. No hemolysis
     a. Pulmonary infarction
     b. Transfusion of aged red blood cells
     c. Hematomas
     d. "Shunt" hyperbilirubinemia

B. Deficient hepatic uptake of bilirubin:
  1. ? Gilbert's disease (normal biopsy, low-grade hyperbilirubinemia)
  2. ? Acquired liver disease

C. Deficient conjugation of bilirubin:
  1. Physiologic jaundice of newborn
  2. Crigler-Najjar syndrome (transferase deficiency)
     a. Inadequate bilirubin glucuronide synthesis
  3. Inhibition of glucuronyl transferase
     a. Large doses of vitamin K analogs in premature infants
     b. Increased level of pregnanediol
     c. Breast milk containing pregnane-3-(a), 20-(β)-diol
     d. Novobiocin
  4. Competitive inhibition
     a. Drugs detoxified as glucuronides

II. Conjugated hyperbilirubinemia
Determine mechanism on basis of age, clinical features, and laboratory findings:

A. Defect in bilirubin excretion
Confirm with serum alkaline phosphatase (elevated), cephalin flocculation (normal). In absence of rapid subsidence, exploratory surgery is desirable to differentiate:

1. Extrahepatic biliary obstruction
Identify by radiologic means and/or direct inspection during surgical intervention.
 a. Calculus
 b. Stricture
 c. Neoplasm

2. Intrahepatic biliary obstruction
Confirm absence of extrahepatic biliary obstruction with operative or T-tube cholangiography. Identify localization of lesion by surgical biopsy.
 a. Lesion of bile canaliculi
  (1) Drugs
  (2) Viruses
 b. Lesion of bile ductules
  (1) Drugs
  (2) Viruses
 c. Lesion of bile ducts
  (1) Drugs
  (2) Viruses

B. Deficient liver cell secretion of bilirubin
May need to differentiate from excretory defect by surgical exploration, cholangiography, or biopsy:

1. Persistence of excretory defect in immature liver after development of adequate glucuronide-synthesizing capacity
2. Dubin-Johnson syndrome (biopsy showing characteristic pigment)
3. Rotor syndrome (absence of characteristic pigment)

III. Combined unconjugated and conjugated hyperbilirubinemia
Determine mechanism on basis of clinical features and laboratory findings:

A. Familial defect or immature liver reflected in partial deficiency of glucuronide formation or excretion

B. Acquired liver cell damage
Confirm with liver function tests and determine primary abnormality:
1. Deficient hepatic uptake of bilirubin
2. Deficient conjugation of bilirubin
3. Deficient secretion or excretion of conjugated bilirubin

C. Hemolysis with secondary liver damage
Demonstrate presence of hemolysis:
1. Hepatic damage secondary to shock
2. Hepatic damage secondary to hemolysis

D. Biliary obstruction with secondary liver damage:
1. Bile stasis with secondary injury
2. Ascending cholangitis

SOURCE: Leevy, C. M.: "Evaluation of Liver Function in Clinical Practice," The Lilly Research Laboratories, Indianapolis, Ind., 1965, by permission.

immediate diazo reaction, is therefore termed *direct-reacting,* and is readily passed into the urine. Normally there is less than 1.2 mg of indirect-reacting serum bilirubin and less than 0.3 mg of direct-reacting serum bilirubin per 100 ml of serum.

The conjugated bilirubin, which is excreted via the bile into the intestine, is acted upon by bacteria and undergoes a series of reductive reactions leading to the formation of two groups of compounds, the colorless urobilinogens and the colored urobilin (Fig. 24-10). The normal daily fecal excretion ranges between 40 and 300 mg with an average of 100 to 200 mg. In children values are lower, and in newborn infants, because of the absence of bacterial flora, urobilinogen may be absent. A reduction in enteric bacteria is also responsible for the reduced pigment excretion that accompanies the use of intestinal antibiotics. Some of the urobilinogen is resorbed by way of the portal venous system and returns to the liver, where it is either removed or, to a small extent, excreted in the urine.

ABNORMAL BILE PIGMENT METABOLISM. No classification of jaundice is totally satisfactory. The classification most widely used distinguishes between hemolytic, obstructive, and hepatocellular jaundice. However, it is more reasonable to categorize (1) those disease states in which the bile flow is unimpeded and (2) those types which are associated with an impairment of bile flow (Fig. 24-11).

Normal Bile Excretion. The overproduction of bile pigment from excessive hemolysis creates a situation in which the normal liver is confronted with more pigment than it is able to remove. This occurs in the physiologic jaundice of infancy and all patholigic hemolytic states. However, the reserve capacity of the liver is great, and even when the bilirubin production is increased six times, there is only a 2- to 3-mg rise in the serum bilirubin level per 100 ml. In this situation, the increase in serum bilirubin is in the unconjugated indirect-reacting pigment. No bilirubin appears in the urine, but there is an increase in the fecal and urinary urobilinogen. An excess of bilirubin production also occurs in *shunt hyperbilirubinemia,* in which indirect-reacting bilirubin accumulates in the absence of any reduction in red cell life span.

Constitutional defects of liver function may also cause hyperbilirubinemia without impairment of bile flow. In Gilbert's disease, there is a defect in the bilirubin transport into the liver cell, while in the Crigler-Najjar syndrome the defect is an inability of the liver to conjugate the

bilirubin with glucuronic acid. In these states, the elevation of bile pigment is in the indirect-reacting fraction. All other hepatic function tests are normal, and no histologic abnormalities are noted. With all the above-mentioned diseases, the bilirubin pigment is attached to the albumin and cannot be excreted by the kidney, thus prompting the term *acholuric jaundice.*

Impaired Bile Excretion. All other lesions are associated with an accumulation of conjugated bilirubin in the blood and impaired excretion. The bilirubin pigment, which is water-soluble, is readily excreted into the urine, which becomes brown. Both the fecal urobilinogen and the urinary urobilinogen are decreased or absent, depending upon the degree of obstruction. Obstructive jaundice may be intrahepatic or extrahepatic.

Intrahepatic Obstructive Jaundice. In the Dubin-Johnson syndrome, which is associated with the appearance of iron-free pigment in the hepatic cells and normal liver function, the hepatic excretion of the conjugated bilirubin is impaired. Intrahepatic cholestasis has also been related to a variety of drugs and hepatocellular diseases. Methyltestosterone and norethandrolone damage the microvilli of the bile canaliculi and may cause jaundice. The phenothiazine drugs, such as chlorpromazine, may evoke a hypersensitivity reaction in a small percentage of patients and result in cholangiolitic hepatitis and intrahepatic cholestasis. A lesion along the excretory path within the liver is believed to cause the obstructive jaundice associated with primary biliary cirrhosis.

The jaundice from hepatocellular degeneration, such as occurs in hepatitis and cirrhosis, is associated with morphologic changes in the parenchymal cells and abnormal liver function tests. With these diseases, a Kupffer cell liver block has been proposed to result in regurgitation of bilirubin from the bile canaliculi into the tissue spaces. This defect, coupled with the reduction in the ability of the liver cell to convert the bilirubin protein to the bilirubin glucuronide, causes a rise in both bilirubin and its conjugates. In contrast to the pure obstructive jaundice, urinary urobilinogen may be increased, since the parenchyma is no longer capable of clearing the serum urobilinogen entering from the intestinal tract. However, the excretion of bile may be so suppressed that virtually no bilirubin reaches the intestine; under these conditions the stools are clay-colored, and the production and resorption of the bilirubin from the intestine is diminished, in which case the urine urobilinogen falls to a low level. In rare instances of intrahepatic bile duct atresia absolute obstruction of the bile conduits within the liver results in jaundice.

Extrahepatic Cholestasis. This is caused by an anatomic obstacle to the flow of bile from the liver to the intestine. The obstacle may be situated anywhere from the junction of the right and left hepatic ducts to the termination of the common bile duct in the duodenum. Atresia, stricture, gallstones, tumors of the bile duct and pancreas, choledochal cysts, and parasites have all been implicated. Obstruction of the extrahepatic ducts results in an increase in the serum bilirubin, particularly the direct-reacting type, the appearance of bile in the urine, and the passage of clay-colored stools. When the total bilirubin level is above

Fig. 24-10. Conversion of bilirubin to urobilin.

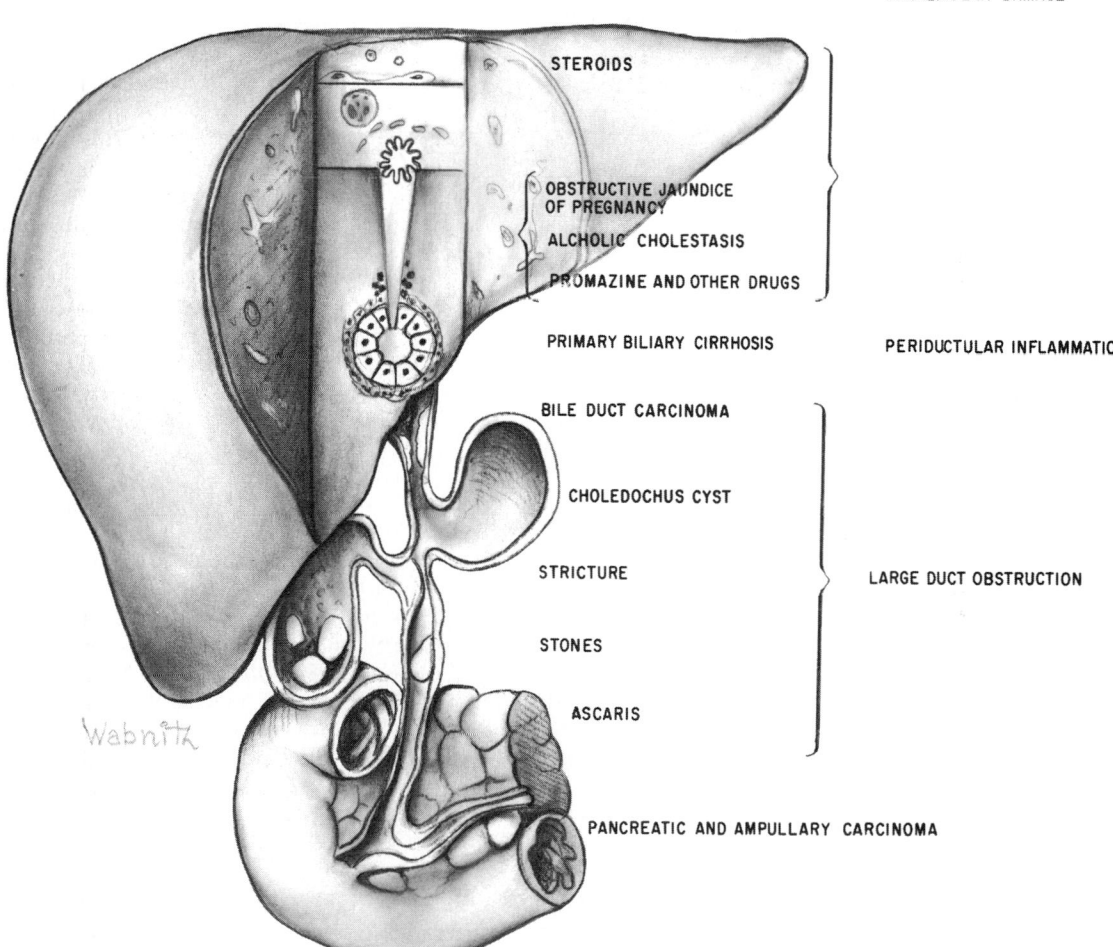

CAUSE OF JAUNDICE

HEMOLYSIS

SHUNT
        HYPERBILIRUBINEMIA
GILBERT

NEONATE, CRIGLER - NAJJAR

DUBIN-JOHNSON
HYPERBILIRUBINEMIA

POSTULATED DEFECT

EXCESS BILIRUBIN PRODUCTION

BILIRUBIN TRANSPORT

BILIRUBIN CONJUGATION

CONJUGATION TRANSPORT

CANALICULAR DAMAGE

STEROIDS

OBSTRUCTIVE JAUNDICE
OF PREGNANCY

ALCHOLIC CHOLESTASIS

PROMAZINE AND OTHER DRUGS

PRIMARY BILIARY CIRRHOSIS

PERIDUCTULAR INFLAMMATION

BILE DUCT CARCINOMA

CHOLEDOCHUS CYST

STRICTURE

STONES

ASCARIS

LARGE DUCT OBSTRUCTION

Wabnitz

PANCREATIC AND AMPULLARY CARCINOMA

Fig. 24-11. Abnormal bile pigment metabolism.

3 mg/100 ml, the increases in both the direct- and indirect-reacting fractions parallel one another. With complete and persistent obstruction, the serum bilirubin may plateau, while the fecal and urinary urobilinogen becomes zero. If the obstruction is fluctuating, the levels of these three determinations will change.

EVALUATION AND MANAGEMENT OF THE PATIENT WITH JAUNDICE. For a discussion of neonatal jaundice and biliary atresia see Chap. 31.

Jaundice is apparent when the serum bilirubin level

exceeds 2 mg/100 ml. Tissues rich in elastic fibers have a particular affinity for bilirubin, thus accounting for the earlier appearance and greater intensity in the sclerae and in the skin of the face and upper trunk. Jaundice is not a mere reflection of yellow light through the skin from underlying interstitial fluid but rather a deposition in the tissue fibers and cells. Tissues stain more readily with direct bilirubin than with the indirect-reacting fraction. There is a failure to stain in areas of marked edema and vitilligo.

The diagnosis of jaundice attempts to define the precise cause and also is directed toward the division into surgically correctable lesions, on one hand, and other types in which surgical intervention is not indicated.

Fig. 24-12. Postcholecystectomy jaundice in a sixty-four-year-old man with recurrent attacks of pancreatitis. Intravenous cholangiogram revealed a dilated common bile duct but no calculus. Note the demonstration by endoscopic retrograde choledochopancreatography of a normal pancreatic duct and dilated common bile duct with a large calculus at its lower end. (*By permission of Surgery, Gynecology & Obstetrics, 138:565, 1974.*)

History. Jaundice secondary to obstruction of the extrahepatic ducts usually starts insidiously and becomes progressively more pronounced. Gastrointestinal disturbances are uncommon, with the exception of those related to biliary calculi. Although, classically, carcinoma of the head of the pancreas is painless, some 20 to 30 percent of these patients do complain of deep epigastric distress or backache. Extrahepatic obstruction associated with ascending cholangitis is accompanied by spiking fevers and abdominal pain. A history of pruritus preceding the onset of jaundice occurs frequently with both extrahepatic biliary obstruction and intrahepatic obstruction secondary to primary cholangiolitis or primary biliary cirrhosis. A detailed family history and history of drug ingestion are imperative before subjecting a patient to surgical treatment, since both constitutional deficiencies and drug-induced jaundice result in a defect in excretion of bile. Loss of appetite, fever, and change of smoking habits are particularly suggestive of hepatitis, and history should be taken of possible contact with persons with known cases and of injections in the previous 6 months. Inquiry into chronic alcohol ingestion is important to rule out jaundice associated with cirrhosis.

Physical Examination. Physical examination also contributes to the diagnosis. Inspection of the skin may reveal a rash, typical of drug reactions, spider angiomas of cirrhosis, or excoriations suggestive of pruritus. Anemia and splenomegaly may be present with hemolytic jaundice. Hepatomegaly and hepatic tenderness are predominant findings with viral hepatitis. A palpable gallbladder in a patient with extrahepatic obstruction occurs more frequently when the obstruction is related to malignancy and less commonly when obstruction is due to biliary calculi. This axiom, known as Courvoisier's law, however, is not universal. Careful search for extrahepatic neoplasm should be made, and the stigmata of portal hypertension including prominent abdominal wall veins and ascites should be investigated.

Laboratory Studies. Hemolytic jaundice is accompanied by anemia and an increased reticulocyte count. Smears for sickle cells, spherocytes, and target cells should be made. The white blood cell count is usually not elevated in viral hepatitis, while it is frequently markedly increased with extrahepatic obstruction and accompanying ascending cholangitis. Stools should be studied for pigment and the presence or absence of guaiac, indicative of bleeding. With carcinoma of the pancreas, approximately one-third of the patients have guaiac-positive stools; this occurs more frequently in patients with obstructive jaundice secondary to carcinoma of the ampulla of Vater.

The so-called "liver function tests" are directed toward assessing the degree of functional impairment of the liver and differentiating between "medical" and "surgical" jaundice. The extreme functional reserve of the liver occasionally produces normal results in the face of significant lesions, and none of the tests provides a pathologic diagnosis. Recently, significant advances in the detection of hepatitis virus have been reported.

Icterus index is a colorimetric evaluation of the serum compared with a chemical standard. It is approximately ten times the value of the serum bilirubin, and jaundice becomes clinically apparent at a level of 16 units. The major application of this procedure is as a rapid screening test to determine whether a more precise measurement of the serum bilirubin is indicated. Serum bilirubin is normally present in concentrations up to 1.5 mg/100 ml and, as previously mentioned, appears both in water-insoluble unconjugated form, which gives the indirect van den Bergh reaction, and the water-soluble conjugated form, which reacts directly. Up to 1.2 mg/100 ml of unconjugated bilirubin is present in the normal serum. Increases in this fraction accompany hemolytic processes such as physiologic jaundice of the newborn, erythroblastosis, and hereditary and acquired hemolytic crises. This fraction is also elevated in the Crigler-Najjar syndrome and in Gilbert's disease. In patients with jaundice secondary to obstruction of the flow of bile or hepatocellular degeneration, the determination of the direct fraction is a more sensitive index of impairment than the total serum bilirubin.

Normally no bilirubin is present in the urine, and bilirubinuria does not accompany hemolytic jaundice or jaundice related to deficiency in the glucuronal transferase system, since the unconjugated fraction, which is increased in these situations, cannot be excreted by the kidney. An elevation in the direct-reacting bilirubin level is associated with bilirubinuria. The production of foam by shaking the urine suggests this elevation. Increased direct-reacting serum bilirubin may not appear in the urine of patients with severe renal failure.

Fecal urobilinogen and to a lesser extent urinary urobilinogen increase with hemolytic jaundice. With obstructive jaundice, the fecal urobilinogen approaches zero, and the urinary urobilinogen follows suit. With hepatocellular jaundice, a mild to moderate decrease in fecal urobilinogen may be associated with an increase in urinary urobilinogen because of a spillover of pigment absorbed from the intestine. A fluctuating fecal or urinary urobilinogen level is suggestive of intermittent hepatic obstruction, most commonly choledocholithiasis.

Enzyme studies are also applicable to the differential diagnosis of jaundice. A markedly elevated serum alkaline phosphatase level is usually associated with obstructive jaundice of either extrahepatic or intrahepatic origin. Elevations in SGOT and SGPT are indicative of hepatocellular disease.

Other laboratory findings, such as a reduction in serum albumin and a reduction in the esterified fraction of the cholesterol, and abnormal turbidity studies are altered with hepatocellular disease. Removal of foreign dye from the liver, either rose bengal or BSP, is dependent upon hepatic blood flow, hepatocellular function, and biliary excretion. The response of prothrombin time to injection of parenteral vitamin K is helpful in establishing a differential diagnosis between hepatocellular and obstructive jaundice. An increase in the prothrombin time within 48 hours of parenteral administration suggests the diagnosis of obstructive jaundice, while a lack of response is more compatible with hepatocellular disease.

Other Diagnostic Procedures. Radiological Studies. An x-ray of the abdomen is indicated, since 20 percent of gallstones are radiopaque (see Chap. 31). Oral cholecystography is rarely effective if the serum bilirubin level is above 1.8 mg/100 ml, while intravenous studies are unrewarding if the serum bilirubin level exceeds 3.5 mg/100 ml.

Recent advances which have contributed significantly in the differential diagnosis of jaundice include endoscopic retrograde cholangiopancreatography (ERCP), percutaneous transhepatic cholangiography (PTC) with the skinny Chiba needle, ultrasonography, and computed tomography (CT) scanning. In experienced hands 90 to 95 percent success rates for ERCP (Fig. 24-12) definition of the extrahepatic biliary system have been reported, but in most institutions the yield is less than 65 percent. Cholangitis and pancreatitis are uncommon complications. The technique is uniquely suited to the evaluation of sclerosing cholangitis. In a randomized trial comparing PTC with ERCP for bile duct visualization in deeply jaundiced patients, PTC (see Fig. 31-21) was demonstrated to be the procedure of choice when cholestasis had a surgical cause. PTC was successful in 95 percent of cases with extrahepatic cholestasis and in 25 percent of patients with intrahepatic cholestasis, while ERCP was successful in 62 percent of patients with extrahepatic and 76 percent with intrahepatic cholestasis. In the patient with extrahepatic obstructive jaundice, provision for early operation should be made if bile peritonitis, an uncommon complication, occurs. ERCP is preferred when coagulation defects preclude PTC.

Compound B scanning provides echographic patterns in patients who are deeply jaundiced and whose ducts cannot be visualized with contrast media. Dilated ducts, calculi, and tumors can be defined by serial laminographic scans. (Equipment capable of defining gray scale has increased the sensitivity of this technique.) CT employing the body scanner also will demonstrate dilatation of intrahepatic and/or extrahepatic portions of the biliary tract (Fig. 24-13).

Fig. 24-13. CT scan in a jaundiced woman, showing dilated intrahepatic bile ducts as linear and circular branching structures with an attenuation value approximating water radiating from the porta hepatis. Scans at lower levels showed an enlarged pancreatic head, which proved at operation to contain carcinoma. (*By permission of Radiology, 124:123, 1977.*)

Liver Biopsy. Percutaneous needle biopsy of the liver may, on one hand, prevent procrastination of surgical intervention and progressive parenchymal damage in patients with extrahepatic biliary obstruction; on the other hand, it may preclude laparotomy in patients with severe hepatocellular disease. Patients should be screened for deficiency in the clotting mechanism, and the risk is small. Characteristic lesions of viral hepatitis, cholangiolitic hepatitis, and bile laking suggestive of extrahepatic biliary obstruction can be defined by this technique.

Laparotomy. This is considered an important tool in the diagnostic armamentarium. Laparotomy for obstructive jaundice is never urgent unless there is an acute suppurative cholangitis. Surgical intervention is indicated when other diagnostic procedures have raised a suspicion of extrahepatic obstruction and when the danger of operating on a patient with possible hepatocellular jaundice is considered minimal.

References

Pain

Cope, Z.: "The Early Diagnosis of Acute Abdomen," 14th ed., Oxford University Press, London, 1972.

Lewis, T.: "Pain," The Macmillan Company, New York, 1942.

Lim, R. K. S.: Pain, *Annu Rev Physiol,* **32:**269, 1970.

Long, D. M.: Electrical Stimulation for the Control of Pain, *Arch Surg,* **112:**884, 1977.

Melzack, R., and Wall, P. D.: Pain Mechanisms: A New Theory, *Science,* **150:**971, 1965.

Nathan, P. W.: Pain, *Br Med Bull,* **33:**149, 1977.

Pflug, A. E., and Bonica, J. J.: Physiopathology and Control of Postoperative Pain, *Arch Surg,* **112:**773, 1977.

Ruch, T. C.: Pathophysiology of Pain, in T. C. Ruch and H. D. Patton (eds.), "Physiology and Biophysics," 19th ed., W. B. Saunders Company, Philadelphia, 1965.

Ryle, J. A.: "The Natural History of Disease," 2d ed., Oxford University Press, London, 1948.

Shealy, C. N., Mortimer, J. T., and Hagford, N. R.: Dorsal Column Electroanalgesia, *J Neurosurg,* **32:**560, 1970.

Sweet, W. H.: Pain, in H. W. Magoun (ed.), "Handbook of Physiology" sec. 1, vol. I, "Neurophysiology," American Physiological Society, Washington, 1959.

White, J. C., Smithwick, R. H., and Simeone, F. A.: "The Autonomic Nervous System: Anatomy, Physiology, Surgical Application," 3d ed., The Macmillan Company, New York, 1952.

—— and Sweet, W. H.: "Pain and the Neurosurgeon: A Forty-Year Experience," Charles C Thomas, Publisher, Springfield, Ill., 1969.

Wolff, H., and Wolf, S.: "Pain," 2d ed., Charles C Thomas, Publisher, Springfield, Ill., 1958.

Dysphagia

Davenport, H. W.: "Physiology of the Digestive Tract," 3d ed., Year Book Medical Publishers, Inc., Chicago, 1971.

Glass, G. B. J.: "Introduction to Gastrointestinal Physiology," Prentice-Hall, Inc., Englewood Cliffs, N.J., 1968.

Goyal, R. K., Bauer, J. L., and Spiro, H. M.: The Nature and Location of Lower Esophageal Ring, *N Engl J Med,* **284:**1175, 1971.

Hightower, N. C.: The Physiology of Symptoms: I. Swallowing and Esophageal Motility, *Am J Dig Dis,* **3:**562, 1958.

Ingelfinger, F. J.: Swallowing Disorders in Clinical Practice, *Med Sci,* Apr. 10, 1960, p. 451.

Spiro, H. M.: "Clinical Gastroenterology," The Macmillan Company, New York, 1970.

Anorexia, Nausea, and Vomiting

Borison, H. L., and Wang, S. C.: Physiology and Pharmacology of Vomiting, *Pharmacol Rev,* **5:**193, 1953.

Code, C. F., (sec. ed.): Control of Food and Water Intake, in W. Heidel (ed.), "Handbook of Physiology," sec. 6, vol. I, American Physiological Society, Washington, 1967.

Davenport, H. W.: "Physiology of the Digestive Tract," 3d ed., The Year Book Medical Publishers, Inc., Chicago, 1971.

Drucker, W. R., and Wright, H. K.: Physiology and Pathophysiology of Gastrointestinal Fluids, *Curr Probl Surg,* May, 1964.

Gregory, R. A.: Changes in Intestinal Tone and Motility Associated with Nausea and Vomiting, *J Physiol (Lond),* **105:**58, 1946.

——:The Nervous Pathways of Intestinal Reflexes Associated with Nausea and Vomiting, *J Physiol (Lond),* **106:**95, 1957.

Hawkins, C.: Anorexia and Loss of Weight, *Br Med J,* **2:**1373, 1976.

McGuigan, J. E.: Anorexia, Nausea and Vomiting, in C. M. MacBryde and R. S. Blacklow (eds.), "Signs and Symptoms," 5th ed., J. B. Lippincott Company, Philadelphia, 1970.

Constipation and Diarrhea

Chaudhary, N. A., and Truelove, S. C.: Colonic Motility: A Critical Review of Methods and Results, *Am J Med,* **31:**86, 1961.

Davenport, H. W.: "Physiology of the Digestive Tract," 3d ed., The Year Book Medical Publishers, Inc., Chicago, 1971.

Hurst, A. F.: "Constipation and Allied Intestinal Disorders," 2d ed., Oxford University Press, London, 1921.

Low-Beer, T. S., and Read, A. E.: Diarrhoea: Mechanisms and Treatment, *Gut,* **12:**1021, 1971.

Mellinkoff, S. M. (ed.): "The Differential Diagnosis of Diarrhea," McGraw-Hill Book Company, New York, 1964.

Morrison, A. B., Rawson, A. J., and Fitts, W. T., Jr.: The Syndrome of Refractory Watery Diarrhea and Hypokalemia in Patients with a Noninsulin-secreting Islet Cell Tumor, *Am J Med,* **32:**119, 1962.

Phillips, S. F.: Diarrhea, *Postgrad Med,* **57**(1):65, 1975.

Rabinowitz, R., Farber, M., and Friedman, I. S.: A Depletion Syndrome in Villous Adenoma of the Rectum, *Arch Intern Med,* **109:**265, 1962.

Intestinal Obstruction

Adams, J. T.: Adynamic Ileus of the Colon; an Indication for Cecostomy, *Arch Surg,* **109:**503, 1974.

Baker, J. W., and Ritter, K. J.: Complete Surgical Decompression for Late Obstruction of the Small Intestine, with Reference to a Method, *Ann Surg,* **157:**759, 1963.

Barnett, W. O., Oliver, R. I., and Elliott, R. L.: Elimination of the Lethal Properties of Gangrenous Bowel Segments, *Ann Surg,* **167:**912, 1968.

——, Petro, A. B., and Williamson, J. W.: A Current Appraisal of Problems with Gangrenous Bowel, *Ann Surg,* **183:**653, 1976.

Becker, W. F.: Acute Adhesive Ileus: A Study of 412 Cases with Particular Reference to the Abuse of Tube Decompression in Treatment, *Surg Gynecol Obstet,* **95:**472, 1952.

Berk, J. E., (ed.): "Gastrointestinal Gas," *Ann NY Acad Sci,* **150:**1, 1968.

Billig, D. M., and Jordan, P. H., Jr.: Hemodynamic Abnormalities Secondary to Extracellular Fluid Depletion in Intestinal Obstruction, *Surg Gynecol Obstet,* **128:**1274, 1969.

Boley, S. J., Agrawal, G. P., Warren, A. R., Veith, F. J., Levowitz, B. S., Treiber, W., Dougherty, J., Schwartz, S. S., and Gliedman, M. L.: Pathophysiologic Effects of Bowel Distention on Intestinal Blood Flow, *Am J Surg,* **117:**228, 1969.

Bussemaker, J. B., and Lindeman, J.: Comparison of Methods to Determine Viability of Small Intestine, *Ann Surg,* **176:**97, 1972.

Carmichael, M. J., Weisbrodt, N. W., and Copeland, E. M.: Effect of Abdominal Surgery on Intestinal Myoelectric Activity in the Dog, *Am J Surg,* **133:**34, 1977.

Catchpole, B. N.: Ileus: Use of Sympathetic Blocking Agents in Its Treatment, *Surgery,* **66:**811, 1969.

Clark, D. D., and Hubay, C. A.: Tube Cecostomy: An Evaluation of 161 Cases, *Ann Surg,* **175:**55, 1972.

Cohn, I., Jr., and Atik, M.: Strangulation Obstruction: Closed Loop Studies, *Ann Surg,* **153:**94, 1961.

Davenport, H. W.: "Physiology of the Digestive Tract," 4th ed., The Year Book Medical Publishers, Inc., Chicago, 1977.

Day, E. A., and Marks, C.: Gallstone Ileus, *Am J Surg,* **129:**552, 1975.

Dennis, C.: The Gastrointestinal Sump Tube, *Surgery,* **66:**309, 1969.

Drucker, W. R., and Wright, H. K.: Physiology and Pathophysiology of Gastrointestinal Fluids, *Curr Probl Surg,* May, 1964.

Ellis, H.: Collective Review: The Cause and Prevention of Postoperative Intraperitoneal Adhesions, *Surg Gynecol Obstet,* **133:**497, 1971.

Frimann-Dahl, J.: "Roentgen Examinations in Acute Abdominal Diseases," 3d ed., Charles C Thomas, Publisher, Springfield, Ill., 1974.

Gammill, S. L., and Nice, C. M., Jr.: Air Fluid Levels: Their Occurrence in Normal Patients and Their Role in the Analysis of Ileus, *Surgery,* **71:**771, 1972.

Heimbach, D. M., and Crout, J. R.: Treatment of Paralytic Ileus with Adrenergic Neuronal Blocking Agents, *Surgery,* **69:**582, 1971.

Hubbard, T. B., Jr., Khan, M. Z., Carag, V. R., Albites, V. E., and Hricko, G. M.: The Pathology of Peritoneal Repair: Its Relation to the Formation of Adhesions, *Ann Surg,* **165:**908, 1967.

Kock, N. G.: An Experimental Analysis of Mechanisms Engaged in Reflex Inhibition of Intestinal Motility, *Acta Physiol Scand,* vol. 47 (*Suppl 164*), 1959.

Landman, M. D., and Longmire, W. P., Jr.: Neural and Hormonal Influences of Peritonitis on Paralytic Ileus, *Am Surg,* **33:**756, 1967.

Larsen, E., and Pories, W. J.: Frequency of Wound Complications after Surgery for Small Bowel Obstruction, *Am J Surg,* **122:**384, 1971.

Levitt, M. D., and Bond, J. H., Jr.: Volume, Composition, and Source of Intestinal Gas, *Gastroent,* **59:**921, 1970.

Maddock, W. G., Bell, J. L., and Tremaine, M. J.: Gastrointestinal Gas: Observations on Belching during Anesthesia, Operations and Pyelography; and Rapid Passage of Gas, *Ann Surg,* **130:**512, 1949.

Miller, R. E., and Brahme, F.: Large Amounts of Orally Administered Barium for Obstruction of the Small Intestine, *Surg Gynecol Obstet,* **129:**1185, 1969.

Nachlas, M. M., Younis, M. T., Roda, C. P., and Wityk, J. J.: Gastrointestinal Motility Studies as a Guide to Postoperative Management, *Ann Surg,* **175:**510, 1972.

Nadrowski, L. F.: Pathophysiology and Current Treatment of Intestinal Obstruction, *Rev Surg,* **31:**381, 1974.

Norton, L., Young, D., and Scribner, R.: Management of Pseudo-obstruction of the Colon, *Surg Gynecol Obstet,* **138:**595, 1974.

Öhman, U.: Studies on Small Intestinal Obstruction, I–VI, *Acta Chir Scand,* **141:**413, 417, 536, 545, 763, 771, 1975.

Playforth, R. H., Holloway, J. B., and Griffen, W. O., Jr.: Mechanical Small Bowel Obstruction: A Plea for Earlier Surgical Intervention, *Ann Surg,* **171:**783, 1970.

Price, J. E., Michel, S. L., and Morgenstern, L.: Fruit Pit Obstruction, *Arch Surg,* **111:**773, 1976.

Raf, L.: Causes of Small Intestinal Obstruction, *Acta Chir Scand.,* **135:**67, 1969.

Saegesser, F., and Sandblom, P.: Ischemic Lesions of the Distended Colon: A Complication of Obstructive Colorectal Cancer, *Am J Surg,* **129:**309, 1975.

Schuffler, M. D., Rohrmann, C. A., Jr., and Templeton, F. E.: The Radiologic Manifestations of Idiopathic Intestinal Obstruction, *Am J Roentgenol,* **127:**729, 1976.

Shields, R.: The Absorption and Secretion of Fluid and Electrolytes by the Obstructed Bowel, *Br J Surg,* **52:**774, 1965.

Shin, C-S., Nimmannit, S., Hoff, A., and Enquist, I. F.: Body Fluid Compartments in Patients with Nonstrangulating Obstruction of the Small Intestine, *Surg Gynecol Obstet,* **132:**980, 1971.

Smith, J., Kelly, K. A., and Weinshilboum, R. M.: Pathophysiology of Postoperative Ileus, *Arch Surg,* **112:**203, 1977.

Sufian, S., and Matsumoto, T.: Intestinal Obstruction, *Am J Surg,* **130:**9, 1975.

Sullivan, M. A., Snape, W. J., Jr., Matarazzo, S. A., Petrokubi, R. J., Jeffries, G., and Cohen, S.: Gastrointestinal Myoelectrical Activity in Idiopathic Intestinal Pseudo-obstruction, *N Engl J Med,* **297:**233, 1977.

Sung, D. T. W., and Williams, L. F., Jr.: Intestinal Secretion after Intravenous Fluid Infusion in Small Bowel Obstruction, *Am J Surg,* **121:**91, 1971.

Sykes, P. A., Boulter, K. H., and Schofield, P. F.: The Microflora of the Obstructed Bowel, *Br J Surg,* **63:**721, 1976.

Tibblin, S.: Diagnosis of Intestinal Obstruction with Special Regard to Plain Roentgen Examination of the Abdomen, *Acta Chir Scand,* **135:**249, 1969.

Tinker, M. A., Teicher, I., and Burdman, D.: Cellulose Granulomas and Their Relationship to Intestinal Obstruction, *Am J Surg,* **133:**134, 1977.

Trippestad, A., and Midtvedt, T.: The Role of Hemoglobin for the Lethal Effect of Intestinal Strangulation Fluid, *J Surg Res,* **10:**465, 1970.

Wangensteen, O. H.: "Intestinal Obstruction," 3d ed., Charles C Thomas, Publisher, Springfield, Ill., 1955.

————: Historical Aspects of the Management of Acute Intestinal Obstruction, *Surgery,* **65:**363, 1969.

Weilbaecher, D., Bolin, J. A., Hearn, D., and Ogden, W., II.: Intussusception in Adults, *Am J Surg,* **121:**531, 1971.

Welch, C. E.: "Intestinal Obstruction," The Year Book Medical Publishers, Inc., Chicago, 1958.

Welch, J. P., and Donaldson, G. A.: Management of Severe Obstruction of the Large Bowel Due to Malignant Disease, *Am J Surg,* **127:**492, 1974.

Wojtalik, R. S., Lindenauer, S. M., and Kahn, S. S.: Perforation of the Colon Associated with Adynamic Ileus, *Am J Surg,* **125:**601, 1973.

Wright, H. K., O'Brien, J. J., and Tilson, M. D.: Water Absorption in Experimental Closed Segment Obstruction of the Ileum in Man, *Am J Surg,* **121:**96, 1971.

Yale, C. E.: Ischemic Intestinal Strangulation in Germ-free Rats, *Arch Surg,* **99:**397, 1969.

Gastrointestinal Bleeding

Altemeier, W. A., Fullen, W. D., and McDonough, J. J.: Sepsis and Gastrointestinal Bleeding, *Ann Surg,* **175:**759, 1972.

Athanasoulis, C. A., Baum, S., Rosch, J., Waltman, A. C., Ring, E. J., Smith, J. C., Jr., Sugarbaker, E., and Wood, W.: Mesenteric Arterial Infusions of Vasopressin for Hemorrhage from Colonic Diverticulosis, *Am J Surg,* **129:**212, 1975.

————, ————, Waltman, A. C., Ring, E. J., Imbembo, A., and Vander Salm, T. J.: Control of Acute Gastric Mucosal Hemorrhage: Intra-arterial Infusion of Posterior Pituitary Extract, *N Engl J Med,* **290:**597, 1974.

Bauer, J. J., Kreel, I., and Kark, A. E.: The Use of the Sengstaken Blakemore Tube for Immediate Control of Bleeding Esophageal Varices, *Ann Surg,* **179:**273, 1974.

Behringer, G. E., and Albright, N. L.: Diverticular Disease of the Colon: A Frequent Cause of Massive Rectal Bleeding, *Am J Surg,* **125:**419, 1973.

Boley, S. J., Sammartano, R., Adams, A., DiBiase, A., Kleinhaus, S., and Sprayregen, S.: On the Nature and Etiology of Vascular Ectasias of the Colon: Degenerative Lesions of Aging, *Gastroenterology,* **72:**650, 1977.

Conn, H. O., Ramsby, G. R., Storer, E. H., Mutshnick, M., Joshi, P. H., Phillips, M. M., Cohen, G. A., Fields, G. N., and Petroski, D.: Intraarterial Vasopressin in the Treatment of Upper Gastrointestinal Hemorrhage: A Prospective, Controlled Clinical Trial, *Gastroenterology,* **68:**211, 1975.

Crook, J. N., Gray, L. W., Jr., Nance, F. C., and Cohn, I., Jr.: Upper Gastrointestinal Bleeding, *Ann Surg,* **175:**771, 1972.

Drapanas, T., Woolverton, W. C., Reeder, J. W., Reed, R. L., and Weichert, R. F.: Experiences with Surgical Management of Acute Gastric Mucosal Hemorrhage: A Unified Concept in the Pathophysiology, *Ann Surg,* **173:**628, 1971.

Dronfield, M. W., McIllmurray, M. B., Ferguson, R., Atkinson, M., and Langman, M. J. S.: A Prospective, Randomized Study of Endoscopy and Radiology in Acute Upper-Gastrointestinal-Bleeding, *Lancet,* **1:**1168, 1977.

Eastwood, G. L.: Does Early Endoscopy Benefit the Patient with Active Upper Gastrointestinal Bleeding? *Gastroenterology,* **72:**737, 1977.

Fischer, R. P., Jelense, S., and Fulton, R. L.: The Maintenance of Gastric Mucosal Barrier during the Early Erosive Gastritis Component of Stress Ulceration, *Surgery,* **80:**40, 1976.

Foster, J. H.: Immediate Results of Emergency Operation for Massive Upper Gastrointestinal Hemorrhage, *Am J Surg,* **122:**387, 1971.

Grace, D. M., Pitt, D. F., and Gold, R. E.: Vascular Embolization and Occlusion by Angiographic Techniques as an Aid or Alternative to Operation, *Surg Gynecol Obstet,* **143:**469, 1976.

Halmagyi, A. F.: A Critical Review of 425 Patients with Gastrointestinal Hemorrhage, *Surg Gynecol Obstet,* **130:**419, 1970.

Hamlyn, A. N., Lunzer, M. R., Morris, J. S., Puritz, H., and Dick, R.: Portal Hypertension with Varices in Unusual Sites, *Lancet,* **2:**1531, 1974.

Harvey, R. F., and Langman, M. J. S.: Late Results of Medical and Surgical Treatment for Bleeding Duodenal Ulcer, *Q J Med,* **39:**539, 1970.

Johnson, W. C., Widrich, W. C., Ansell, J. E., Robbins, A. H., and Nabseth, D. C.: Control of Bleeding Varices by Vasopressin: A Prospective Randomized Study, *Ann Surg,* **186:**369, 1977.

Katon, R. M.: Experimental Control of Gastrointestinal Hemorrhage via the Endoscope: A New Era Dawns, *Gastroenterology,* **70:**272, 1976.

Knauer, C. M.: Mallory-Weiss Syndrome, *Gastroenterology,* **71:**5, 1976.

Langman, M. J. S.: Epidemiological Evidence for the Association of Aspirin and Acute Gastrointestinal Bleeding, *Gut,* **11:**627, 1970.

Le Gall, J. R., Mignon, F. C., Rapin, M., Redjemi, M., Harari, A., Bader, J. P., and Soussy, C. J.: Acute Gastroduodenal Lesions Related to Severe Sepsis, *Surg Gynecol Obstet,* **142:**377, 1976.

McClelland, R. N., Shires, G. T., and Prager, M.: Gastric Secretory and Splanchnic Blood Flow Studies in Man after Severe Trauma and Hemorrhagic Shock, *Am J Surg,* **121:**134, 1971.

Malt, R. A.: Control of Massive Upper Gastrointestinal Hemorrhage, *N Engl J Med,* **286:**1043, 1972.

Matsumoto, T., ed.: "Current Management of Acute Gastrointestinal Hemorrhage," Charles C Thomas, Publisher, Springfield, Ill., 1977.

Menguy, R., and Masters, Y. F.: Gastric Mucosal Energy Metabolism and "Stress Ulceration," *Ann Surg,* **180:**538, 1974.

Meyers, M. A., Alonso, D. R., Gray, G. F., and Baer, J. W.: Pathogenesis of Bleeding Colonic Diverticulosis, *Gastroenterology,* **71:**577, 1976.

Miller, R. D., Robbins, T. O., Tong, M. J., and Barton, S. L.: Coagulation Defects Associated with Massive Blood Transfusions, *Ann Surg,* **174:**794, 1971.

Milliser, R. V., Greenberg, S. R., and Neiman, B. H.: Exsanguinating Stercoral Ulceration, *Am J Dig Dis,* **15:**485, 1970.

Moody, F. G.: Rectal Bleeding, *N Engl J Med,* **290:**839, 1974

Moss, G.: Cause of Azotemia after Gastrointestinal Hemorrhage: Examining an Old Wives' Tale, *Am J Surg,* **130:**269, 1975.

Nance, F. C., Kaufman, H. J., and Batson, R. C.: The Role of the Microbial Flora in Acute Gastric Stress Ulceration, *Surgery,* **72:**68, 1972.

Netterville, R. E., Hardy, J. D., and Martin, R. S.: Small Bowel Hemorrhage, *Ann Surg,* **167:**949, 1968.

Northfield, T. C., and Smith, T.: Physiologic Significance of Central Venous Pressure in Patients with Hemorrhage, *Surg Gynecol Obstet,* **135:**267, 1972.

Novis, B. H., Duys, P., Barbecat, G. O., Clain, J., Bank, S., and Terblanche, T.: Fibreoptic Endoscopy and the Use of the Sengstaken Tube in Acute Gastrointestinal Hemorrhage in Patients with Portal Hypertension and Varices, *Gut,* **17:**258, 1976.

Nusbaum, M., and Conn, H. O.: Arterial Vasopressin Infusions: Science or Seance?, *Gastroenterology,* **69:**263, 1975.

Parsa, F., Gordon, H. E., and Wilson, S. E.: Bleeding Diverticulosis of the Colon, *Dis Colon Rectum,* **18:**37, 1975.

Pitcher, J. L.: Safety and Effectiveness of the Modified Sengstaken-Blakemore Tube: A Prospective Study, *Gastroenterology,* **61:**291, 1971.

Pruitt, B. A., Foley, F. D., and Moncrief, J. A.: Curling's Ulcer: A Clinical-Pathological Study of 323 Cases, *Ann Surg,* **172:**523, 1970.

Ritchie, W. P., Jr.: Bile Acids, the "Barrier," and Reflux-Related Clinical Disorders of the Gastric Mucosa, *Surgery,* **82:**192, 1977.

Safaie-Shirazi, S., Foster, L. D., and Hardy, B. M.: The Effect of Metiamide, an H_2-Receptor Antagonist, in the Prevention of Experimental Stress Ulcers, *Gastroenterology,* **71:**421, 1976.

Schiff, L.: Hematemesis and Melena, in C. M. MacBryde, (ed.), "Signs and Symptoms," 5th ed., J. B. Lippincott Company, Philadelphia, 1970.

Schiller, K. F. R., Truelove, S. C., and Williams, D. G.: Haematemesis and Melaena, with Special Reference to Factors Influencing the Outcome, *Br Med J,* **2:**7, 1970.

Silen, W.: New Concepts of the Gastric Mucosal Barrier, *Am J Surg,* **133:**8, 1977.

Simonian, S. J., and Curtis, L. E.: Treatment of Hemorrhagic Gastritis by Antacid, *Ann Surg,* **184:**429, 1976.

Sutherland, D., Frech, R. S., Weil, R., Najarian, J. S., and Simmons, R. L.: The Bleeding Cecal Ulcer: Pathogenesis, Angiographic Diagnosis, and Nonoperative Control, *Surgery,* **71:**290, 1972.

Wagner, M., Kiselow, M. C., Keats, W. L., and Jan, M. L.: Varices of the Colon, *Arch Surg,* **100:**718, 1970.

Wilson, W. S., Gadacz, T., Olcott, C., III, and Blaisdell, F. W.: Superficial Gastric Erosions: Response to Surgical Treatment, *Am J Surg,* **126:**133, 1973.

Villar, H. V., Fender, H. R., Watson, L. C., and Thompson, J. C.: Emergency Diagnosis of Upper Gastrointestinal Bleeding by Fiberoptic Endoscopy, *Ann Surg,* **185:**367, 1977.

Yajko, R. D., Norton, L. W., and Eiseman, B.: Current Management of Upper Gastrointestinal Bleeding, *Ann Surg,* **181:**474, 1975.

Jaundice

Blumgart, L. H., Salmon, P. R., and Cotton, P. B.: Endoscopy and Retrograde Choledochopancreatography in Diagnosis of Patient with Jaundice, *Surg Gynecol Obstet,* **138:**565, 1974.

Elias, E., Hamlyn, A. N., Jain, S., Long, R. G., Summerfield, J. A., Dick, R., and Sherlock, S.: A Randomized Trial of Percutaneous Transhepatic Cholangiography with the Chiba Needle versus Endoscopic Retrograde Cholangiography for Bile Duct Visualization in Jaundice, *Gastroenterology,* **71:**439, 1976.

Freimanis, A. T.: Intraabdominal Fluid Collections, in S. Gottlieb and M. Viamonte, Jr. (eds.), "Diagnostic Ultrasound," Chicago, Ill. The American College of Radiology, Committee on New Technology, 1976.

Leevy, C. M.: "Evaluation of Liver Function in Clinical Practice," The Lilly Research Laboratories, Indianapolis, Ind., 1965.

Levitt, R. G., Sagel, S. S., Stanley, R. J., and Jost, R. G.: Accuracy of Computed Tomography of the Liver and Biliary Tract, *Radiology,* **124:**123, 1977.

Popper, H., and Schaffner, F.: "Liver: Structure and Function," McGraw-Hill Book Company, New York, 1957.

Schwartz, S. I.: "Surgical Diseases of the Liver," McGraw-Hill Book Company, New York, 1964.

Thompson, R. P. H.: Recent Advances in Jaundice: Physiology, *Br Med J,* **1:**223, 1970.

Williams, R.: Recent Advances in Jaundice: Medical Aspects of Investigation and Treatment, *Br Med J,* **1:**225, 1970.

Chapter 25

Esophagus and Diaphragmatic Hernias

by W. Spencer Payne and F. Henry Ellis, Jr.

Anatomy

Physiology

Esophageal Motility Disturbances

Hypomotility
    Achalasia
    Hypotensive Lower Esophageal Sphincter
Hypermotility

Diverticula

Pharyngoesophageal Diverticulum
Epiphrenic Diverticulum
Parabronchial or Midesophageal Diverticulum

Esophageal Hiatal Hernia

Sliding Hernia
Paraesophageal Hernia

Complications of Gastroesophageal Reflux

Esophagitis
Short Esophagus
Lower Esophagus Lined by Columnar Epithelium (Barrett
    Esophagus)

Corrosive Esophagitis

Esophageal Perforation

Malignant Tumors

Benign Cysts and Tumors

Miscellaneous Esophageal Lesions

Plummer-Vinson (Paterson-Kelly) Syndrome
Lower Esophageal Ring
Mallory-Weiss Syndrome
Scleroderma and Related Diseases
Neuromuscular Disturbances
Acquired Fistulas

Other Diaphragmatic Hernias and Conditions

Posterolateral (Foramen of Bochdalek) Hernias
Foramen of Morgagni Hernias
Eventration of the Diaphragm
Rupture of the Diaphragm

Surgery of the esophagus is primarily a development of the twentieth century, and its major advances have paralleled those of thoracic surgery. Operations on the esophagus were carried out in earlier years, but they were concerned mainly with removal of foreign bodies or with local excision of malignant lesions or diverticula of the cervical esophagus. Transabdominal procedures for the relief of esophageal achalasia were done in the early 1900s, as were staged reconstructive operations for corrosive stricture and malignant lesions; but only later, after the development of techniques permitting intrathoracic operations, was the thoracic portion of this organ approached with confidence. The first successful one-stage transpleural esophagogastrectomy for carcinoma was performed in 1933 by Ohsawa. Marshall was the first to perform this operation successfully in the United States, in 1937. Thereafter, advances in all aspects of thoracic surgery came rapidly, and as a result the esophagus became accessible to the surgeon's knife. The reductions in surgical morbidity and mortality at first were not matched, however, by similar advances in the understanding of the function of the esophagus. Largely as a result of studies of esophageal motility carried out by Ingelfinger and by Code and Schlegel, the surgical approach to esophageal lesions now rests on sounder physiologic grounds.

ANATOMY

The esophagus is a long muscular tube extending downward from the pharynx at the C_6 level and terminating in a region commonly referred to as the "cardia," whose definition is highly variable (Fig. 25-1). In its course between these two points, it occupies in the neck a midline position immediately behind the trachea. In the thorax it inclines posteriorly behind the great vessels, curving slightly to the left to pass behind the left main bronchus, whence it inclines slightly to the right as it continues in the posterior mediastinum. It again deviates to the left behind the pericardial sac, where it runs anterior to the thoracic aorta, crossing it to the left of the midline. It reaches the abdomen through the esophageal hiatus, a noose of diaphragmatic muscle composed chiefly of the right crus of the diaphragm. An esophageal segment of variable length usually occupies an intraabdominal location before joining the stomach at the point referred to as the "cardia." In general, this term applies to a vague region including the lower esophagus, the esophagogastric junction, and the upper portion of the stomach. Identification of the esophagogastric junction by reference to the

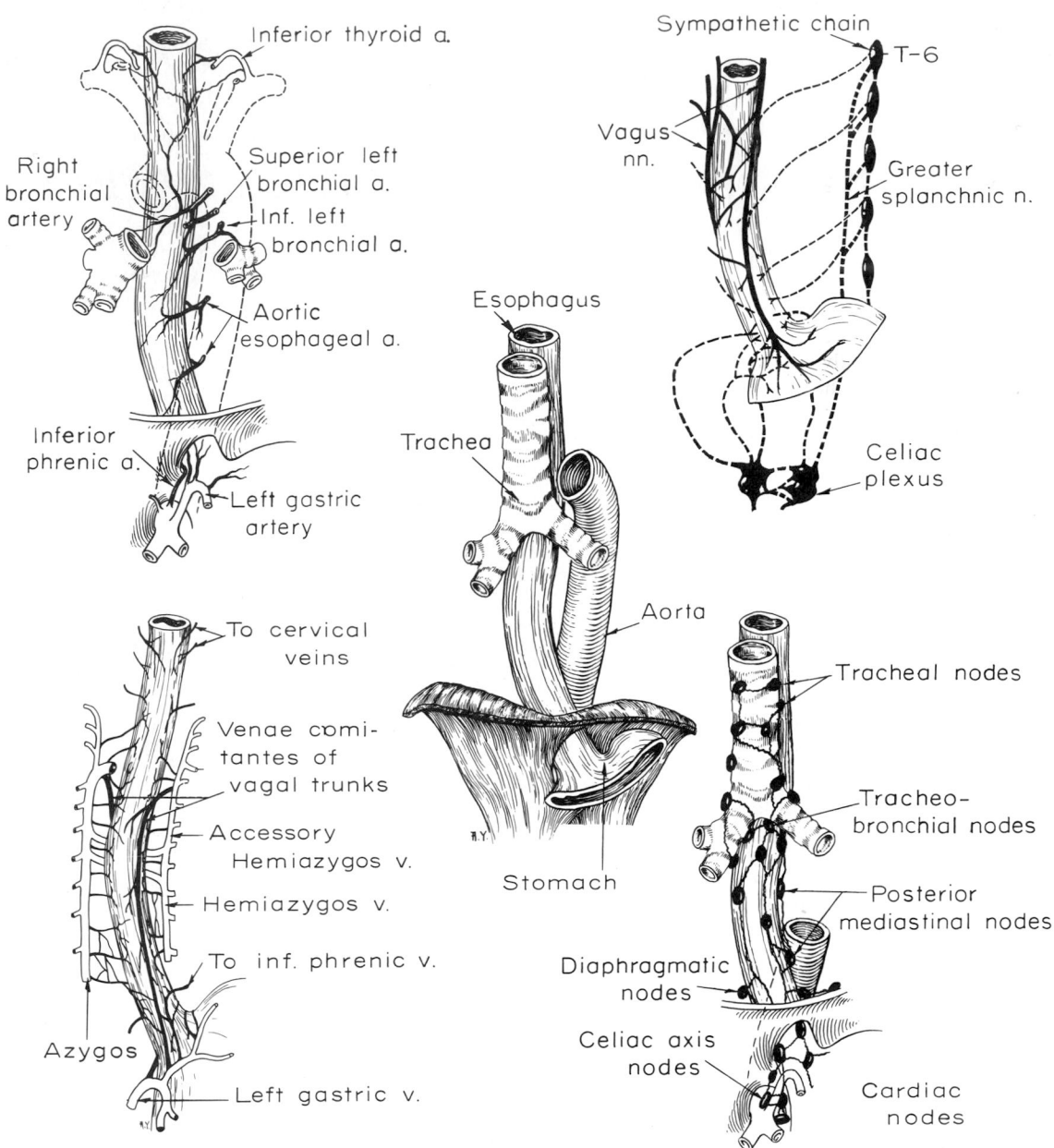

Fig. 25-1. Anatomy of the human esophagus. Upper Left: Arterial supply. Lower left: Venous drainage. Upper right: Innervation. Lower right: Lymphatic system. [*From F. H. Ellis, Jr., The Esophagus, in L. Davis (ed.), "Christopher's Textbook of Surgery," 8th ed., W. B. Saunders Company, Philadelphia, 1964, pp. 591–620.*]

mucosal lining is also difficult. From a practical standpoint, the junction can best be described as that point where the esophageal tube meets the gastric pouch.

There are important supporting structures in the region of the diaphragm and the esophagogastric junction. The anatomy of the diaphragmatic crura varies (Fig. 25-2). The muscle fibers which form the crura arise from the lateral aspects of the second, third, and fourth lumbar vertebrae and pass superiorly and anteriorly past the aorta to form the margins of the esophageal hiatus, inserting into the central tendon of the diaphragm. Many variations may be seen. In the most common, the right crus contributes all the fibers which form the esophageal hiatus and is reinforced by muscle from the left side (Fig. 25-2*A*). The

second most common type is quite similar, but a slip of muscle from the left crus passes behind the esophagus to form part of the right margin of the hiatus (Fig. 25-2*B*). These two variations account for four-fifths of the known variations. The phrenoesophageal membrane or ligament, another important anatomic structure, was described by Laimer in 1883. Composed of mature collagenous fibers, this structure is a continuation of the transversalis fascia of the abdominal parietes and inserts onto the circumference of the lower thoracic esophagus 2 to 3 cm above the true esophagogastric junction. A contribution to this structure is provided by fascia arising from the upper surface of the diaphragm. Further support is provided by the pleura above and the peritoneal reflection below. The fibers themselves fan out and insert into the lower esophagus over a relatively wide zone (Fig. 25-3A).

The blood supply of the esophagus is provided in its cervical portion by the inferior thyroid arteries and in its thoracic portion by the aorta itself and by esophageal branches of the bronchial arteries. Supplemental vessels come from arteries on the abdominal side of the diaphragm as well as branches from intercostal arteries. The venous drainage is more complex. Subepithelial and subvenous channels course longitudinally to empty above into the hypopharyngeal and below into the gastric veins. These channels also penetrate the esophageal muscle, from which they receive branches, and leave the esophagus to form a periesophageal plexus, the longest trunks of which accompany the vagus nerves. Drainage from the cervical portion of the esophagus empties ultimately into the inferior thyroid and vertebral veins, that from the thoracic portion into the azygos and hemiazygos veins, and that from the abdominal portion into the left gastric vein.

The lymphatic vessels run longitudinally in the wall of the esophagus before penetrating the muscle layers to reach regional lymph nodes. Thus malignant lesions of the middle or upper esophagus may metastasize first to the cervical nodes and lesions of the lower esophagus to gastric and celiac nodes. On leaving the esophagus, however, the lymphatic channels go to the nearest group of nodes, which within the thorax are usually identified by their location as tracheal, tracheobronchial, posterior mediastinal, or diaphragmatic nodes.

The esophagus receives both vagal and sympathetic nerves, its upper portion being supplied by the recurrent nerves and branches from the ninth and tenth cranial nerves and the cranial root of the eleventh and by sympathetic nerves. The vagal trunks send branches to the remaining voluntary muscles, and the parasympathetic preganglionic fibers to the smooth muscles. The vagus nerves lie on either side of the esophagus through most of its course, forming a plexus about it. At the hiatus, however, two major trunks emerge, the left one coming to lie anteriorly and the right one posteriorly. The vagal plexuses are joined by mediastinal branches of the thoracic sympathetic chain of the splanchnic nerves. The lower end of the esophagus and the esophagogastric junction zone also receive sympathetic branches from the periarterial plexus along the left gastric and left inferior phrenic arteries.

The esophageal wall is composed of an inner circular layer of muscle and an outer longitudinal layer without a surrounding serosal covering. Striated muscle fibers make a considerable contribution to the outer longitudinal coat in the upper portion of the esophagus, whereas smooth muscle predominates in the lower portion of the esophagus. Measurements of the thickness of the muscle layers of the distal esophageal wall reveal no consistent increase in the segment that corresponds to the physiologic gastro-

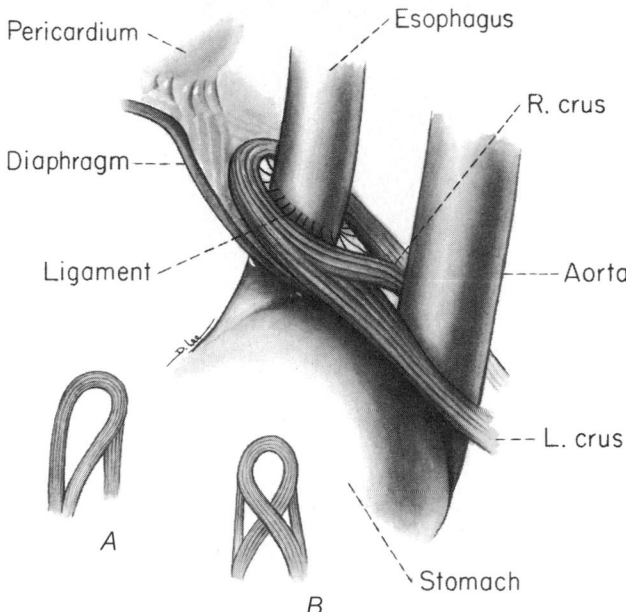

Fig. 25-2. The crura of the diaphragm. *A.* Most common anatomic variation. *B.* Next most common variation.

esophageal sphincter, but an area of thickened muscle known as the gastric sling fibers of Willis can be demonstrated partially encircling the proximal part of the stomach at the esophagogastric junction area (Fig. 25-3B).

There is a prominent submucosa containing mucous

Fig. 25-3. Gross anatomy of region of esophagogastric junction area. *A.* Details of origin and insertion of phrenoesophageal membrane or ligament. *B.* Cross section of distal esophagus and proximal stomach. *C.* Oblique gastric sling fibers.

Fig. 25-4. Microscopic anatomy of esophagogastric junction area. Left: Photomicrograph. (Hematoxylin and eosin; ×1.) Right: Schematic representation, showing origin and insertion of phrenoesophageal ligament, diaphragm, and mucosal lining.

glands, blood vessels, Meissner's plexus of nerves, and a rich network of lymphatic vessels. The mucosal lining is characteristically made up of squamous epithelium, although ectopic islands of gastric mucosa have been identified, particularly in the proximal portions of the esophagus. The distal 1 or 2 cm of the esophageal lumen is lined by columnar epithelium, the columnar-squamous junction lying not at the true esophagogastric junction but within the lower esophagus (Figs. 25-3 and 25-4).

PHYSIOLOGY

The esophagus provides a channel by which ingested material is conveyed from the pharynx to the stomach. At

Fig. 25-5. Balloon-covered differential transformer and open-tipped tubes (arrows) used in measurement of esophageal and sphincteric pressures. (From C. F. Code, M. L. Kelley, Jr., J. F. Schlegel, and A. M. Olsen, Detection of Hiatal Hernia during Esophageal Motility Tests, Gastroenterology, 43:521–531, 1962.)

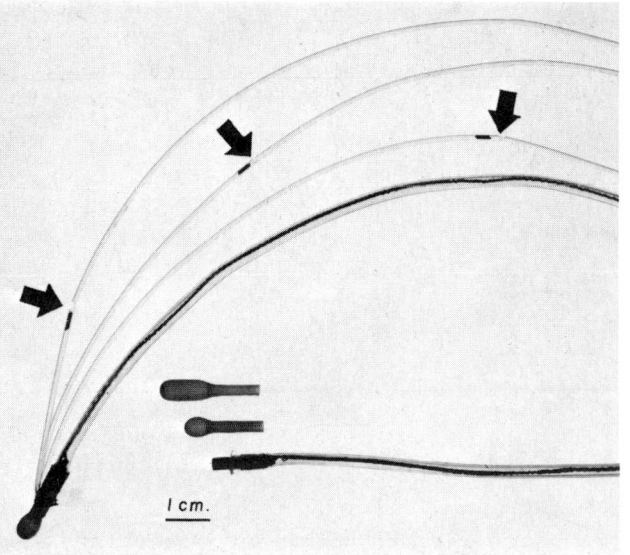

either end of the tube are regulatory mechanisms which assist in this function. Current knowledge of the physiology of the esophagus has been gained by the use of special recording techniques to detect and record intraesophageal pressures. In routine tests, three or four pressure-detecting units (fine water-filled polyethylene tubes attached to strain-gauge manometers) are positioned at various points in the esophagus. Some prefer to use a balloon-covered transducer in addition to tubes with lateral openings at 5-cm intervals (Fig. 25-5). The infusion of saline solution at a constant rate through the open-tipped tubes may provide more accurate pressure recordings. Measurements are made when the esophagus is at rest and after swallowing, the resting pressures being measured while the units are being withdrawn in stepwise fashion from the stomach into the esophagus prior to the recording of deglutition pressures.

At the upper end of the esophagus there is a zone, about 3 cm long, of increased pressure which relaxes promptly with swallowing and contracts thereafter as a wave of high pressure passes through it (Fig. 25-6). Contractions of this sphincter are in peristaltic sequence with those of the pharynx above and the esophagus below, and the primary peristaltic wave of the esophagus is thus initiated. The sphincter relaxes to allow the wave to pass and then closes more tightly. This wave of positive pressure sweeps in an orderly peristaltic fashion down the body of the esophagus, reaching an intensity of 50 to 100 cm H_2O and being somewhat more forceful in the lower esophagus. The resting pressures in the body of the esophagus are normally less than atmospheric pressure, reflecting negative intrathoracic pressure. There is also a zone of increased pressure at the lower end of the esophagus, somewhat longer than that at the upper end (3 to 5 cm long), which can be detected by withdrawing the recording units from the stomach into the esophagus (Fig. 25-7). It is located in the region of the hiatus; in response to a swallowing effort, relaxation of this zone of increased pressure can be identified, along with the immediately following sphincteric contraction in sequence with the peristaltic wave from the esophagus above (Fig. 25-8). This zone is the inferior sphincter of the esophagus.

The details of esophageal innervation remain to be clarified, but esophageal peristalsis seems to be under vagal control, because division of these nerves produces low simultaneous pressures in the body of the esophagus after deglutition. The inferior esophageal sphincter, however, continues to relax with swallowing even after complete denervation, suggesting a certain degree of autonomy.

In spite of the clear demonstration of a physiologic sphincter at the lower end of the esophagus, there remains considerable controversy concerning the exact mechanism by which gastroesophageal reflux is prevented under normal circumstances. Factors that have been suggested as important include the diaphragm, a valve flap mechanism, the gastric sling fibers and the oblique angle of entry, and the mucosal rosette. There is substantial evidence to suggest that the first three are not involved in gastroesophageal competence and that the musculature of the intrinsic sphincter, in combination with prominent folds of epithelial gastric lining at the cardia, comprise the main antireflux mechanisms.

Recent studies by Goyal indicate that the lower esophageal sphincter (LES) is controlled by neural, hormonal, myogenic, and mechanical influences.

In the past some observers believed that the basal sphincter pressure was maintained by continuous vagal tone and that sphincter relaxation was a result of a decrease of tonic vagal activity. However, it is now held that both relaxation and contraction of the LES are due to the vagal transmission of active inhibitory or excitatory impulses but that neither acts as the major determinant of basal LES pressure. The role of sympathetic innervation on the LES is less well understood. Stimulation of alpha-adrenergic receptors causes the LES to contract, and that of beta-adrenergic receptors causes it to relax. It is further hypothesized that sympathetic nerves act to modulate vagal activity on the LES. The fact that complete pharmacologic denervation of the LES does not influence basal sphincter pressure suggests that basal sphincter pressure is not due to tonic autonomic neural activity but that it may be due to tonic myogenic activity of the LES muscle itself.

Fig. 25-6. Response of pharynx and pharyngoesophageal sphincter to swallowing and to peristalsis and sphincteric relaxation. (*From C. F. Code and J. F. Schlegel, The Physiologic Basis of Some Motor Disorders of the Oesophagus, in A. N. Smith, "Surgical Physiology of Gastrointestinal Tract," Royal College of Surgeons, Edinburgh, 1963, pp. 1–19.*)

Many hormones have been known to modify basal pressure of the LES. It has been held that circulating gastrin is the major determinant of basal LES pressure and that this effect is modulated by interaction of secretin. However, recent studies do not support these views and suggest that the changes previously observed were obtainable only in response to unphysiologically high levels of these hormones. Other hormones such as prostaglandins, histamine, and serotonin produce less clear or variable effects on LES pressure, depending on experimental conditions.

Thus, at this time it appears that the basal LES pressure is due to background basal tone provided by intrinsic myogenic activity of the sphincter muscle itself and that this tone is modulated by a variety of excitatory and inhibitory neurohormonal influences. The sphincter relaxation is chiefly due to neural activity mediated by inhibitory vagal and extravagal pathways.

Loss of the LES basal tone can occur as a consequence of pregnancy (because of elevated levels of progesterone and estrogens), excessive ingestion of alcohol, smoking, and use of drugs that especially inhibit the LES (atropine, nitrites, beta-adrenergic agents, etc.). The LES basal tone can be enhanced by neutralization of gastric acid and by the administration of drugs such as bethanecol or metoclopramide.

Fig. 25-7. Pressure profiles of normal lower esophageal sphincter, detected by withdrawal of open-tipped tube and small balloon. (*From F. H. Ellis, Jr., The Esophagus, in L. Davis, "Christopher's Textbook of Surgery," 8th ed., W. B. Saunders Company, Philadelphia, 1964, pp. 591–620.*)

Fig. 25-8. Deglutitive response of inferior esophageal sphincter in healthy subject. Note that relaxation precedes arrival of peristaltic wave in the sphincter. (*From F. H. Ellis, Jr., and W. S. Payne, Motility Disturbances of the Esophagus and Its Inferior Sphincter: Recent Surgical Advances, Adv Surg, 1:179–246, 1965. Copyright 1965 by Year Book Medical Publishers Inc. Used by permission.*)

When the LES is challenged by an increase in intragastric pressure, its resting tone increases. This response is due to a vagus-mediated neural reflex that can be blocked by atropine or vagotomy, as shown by Cohen and Lipshutz. The ability to increase the LES pressure so that it is greater than the rise in intragastric pressure is one of the essential features of the competent LES.

ESOPHAGEAL MOTILITY DISTURBANCES

The development of techniques for physiologic evaluation of esophageal function has permitted the classification of esophageal motility disorders in two main categories: those characterized by hypomotility of the esophagus, such as esophageal achalasia, and those characterized by hyper-

motility, such as diffuse spasm of the esophagus with or without hypertensive gastroesophageal sphincter. Although the causes of these conditions remain in doubt, their clinical and physiologic manifestations are now well known, so surgical treatment can be undertaken on sound grounds in properly selected patients.

Hypomotility

ACHALASIA

Achalasia of the esophagus, or cardiospasm, as it is more commonly but inaccurately known, has been recognized by the medical profession for almost 300 years. As early as 1674, Thomas Willis in his *Pharmaceutice Rationalis* described the symptoms of this condition and advised forceful dilation as treatment. It is a disease characterized by a disturbance of esophageal motility, in which there is absence of peristalsis in the body of the esophagus and failure of the inferior esophageal sphincter to relax in response to swallowing.

The causes of the disease are unknown, although a variety have been suggested, including inherent weakness of the esophagus, spasm of the esophagus, mechanical factors such as external compression or trauma, and congenital factors. Most students of the subject now agree that the disease has a neurogenic basis, and pathologic evidence in support of this theory is provided by demonstration of degeneration or absence of the ganglion cells of Auerbach's plexus in the esophagus of many patients with the disease, a finding first reported by Rake in 1926. Subsequent studies have shown that the changes occur throughout the thoracic esophagus, particularly in the body of the organ, but one-third of the patients are unaffected.

The reason for these nerve cell changes remains obscure; infections due to bacteria or viruses, infestations by para-

Fig. 25-9. Esophageal roentgenograms of achalasia of the esophagus. Left: Mild. Center: Moderate. Right: Severe. (*From A. M. Olsen, S. W. Harrington, H. J. Moersch, and H. A. Andersen, The Treatment of Cardiospasm: Analysis of a Twelve-Year Experience, J Thorac Surg, 22:164–187, 1951.*)

sites, and vitamin deficiencies have all been incriminated. That the primary site of the disorder may be in the extra-esophageal nerve supply—either the vagus nerve itself or its central nuclei—has been suggested by pathologic studies of biopsy and autopsy material and by experiments involving the selective destruction of the motor nuclei of the vagus nerve in the medulla of the cat and the dog.

CLINICAL MANIFESTATIONS. Whatever the cause of the disease, its clinical manifestations are now well recognized. It occurs with equal frequency in men and in women, and although it may occur at any age, it is more frequently seen in persons between the ages of thirty and fifty years. The earliest and most constant symptom is obstruction to swallowing, which at first may be intermittent. However, as the condition progresses, difficulty is experienced with all efforts to swallow. As a rule, the patient experiences more difficulty with cold than with warm foods, and solids may at first seem to pass more easily than liquids. Pain is rare and is more likely to occur in the early stages of the disease than later; it becomes less noticeable as the esophagus dilates. Regurgitation of ingested food and liquids is a common symptom and may occur particularly at night when the patient is recumbent, leading to aspiration and the development of pulmonary complications. Carcinoma of the esophagus occurs approximately seven times as often in patients with esophageal achalasia as in the general population.

Roentgenographic studies are helpful in the diagnosis of the disease, because even in the early stages evidence of obstruction at the cardia and slight dilatation of the esophagus may be noted. As the disease progresses, the classic roentgenographic signs develop (Fig. 25-9), the esophagus becoming dilated and its lower portion projecting beaklike into the distal narrowed segment with very little, if any, barium present in the stomach. In some cases, the esophagus may reach huge proportions, so that it may be seen on the ordinary thoracic roentgenogram. Differentiation between early stages of esophageal achalasia and benign stricture or carcinoma of the cardia may be difficult, and esophagoscopy may be required for diagnosis.

PHYSIOLOGIC STUDIES. Confirmation of the clinical diagnosis can be provided by studies of esophageal motility. Such studies demonstrate that the pressure in the body of the esophagus is higher than normal, often being equal to atmospheric pressure, presumably because of esophageal dilatation with retention of food and fluid. In response to a swallowing effort, feeble, simultaneous, repetitive contractions occur throughout the esophagus, but there is no coordinated peristaltic wave (Fig. 25-10). Although relaxation of the upper esophageal sphincter occurs normally, in the majority of cases the lower sphincter fails to relax after swallowing, but the resting pressures within it are usually within normal limits. However, Cohen and Lipshutz carried out manometric studies using perfused polyvinyl catheters and suggested that the lower esophageal sphincter pressure at rest is increased in patients with achalasia to approximately twice that seen in normal subjects. Furthermore, when the sphincter does relax during swallowing, the relaxation is incomplete, and pressures remain higher than gastric pressures. Occasionally contrac-

Fig. 25-10. Response to deglutition in achalasia of the esophagus. Feeble simultaneous contractions in response to swallowing occur in the body of the esophagus, with failure of sphincteric relaxation. (*From F. H. Ellis, Jr., and W. S. Payne, Motility Disturbances of the Esophagus and Its Inferior Sphincter: Recent Surgical Advances, Adv Surg, 1:179–246, 1965. Copyright 1965 by Year Book Medical Publishers, Inc. Used by permission.*)

tions of the esophagus and the sphincter may be vigorous, and the term "vigorous achalasia" has been applied to this condition.

TREATMENT. Current knowledge does not permit restoration of the disordered esophageal motility to normal. Effective therapy, therefore, can be directed only to relief of the distal esophageal obstruction. Because diet and drugs are ineffective, this must be accomplished either by forceful dilation of the distal esophagus or by surgical means.

Mechanical, pneumatic, and hydrostatic dilators have been used with success. At the Mayo Clinic, hydrostatic dilation (Fig. 25-11) has been used extensively in the past and has been found to be a useful technique. Sanderson and associates reported good to excellent results in 65 percent of patients observed for an average of $9\frac{1}{2}$ years (Table 25-1). The method is not without risk—an esophageal perforation occurred in about 2 percent of cases.

Limitations of medical therapy, including the use of forceful dilation, have led to surgical efforts to relieve the symptoms of patients with esophageal achalasia. These techniques have included excisional or bypassing procedures and denervation procedures. The latter were ineffective, and the uniform development of severe esophagitis after any procedure which destroys or bypasses the inferior esophageal sphincter has rightly led to their abandonment.

Current surgical therapy stems historically from the double cardiomyotomy first proposed by Heller in 1913. It has been modified by a number of surgeons in subsequent years. The simplest and most effective modification involves an incision through the muscle layers of the distal esophagus, through a thoracic approach. The mucosa is exposed to free completely the narrowed distal esophageal segment of its circular musculature, but the incision is

Figure. 25-11. Method of performing hydrostatic dilation. *A.* Passage of #41 F olive-tipped bougie into stomach; *B.* Passage of #50 to 60 F sound guided by flexible wire spiral; *C.* Passage of hydrostatic dilator into esophagogastric junction; *D.* Distension of dilator. (*From A. M. Olsen, S. W. Harrington, H. J. Moersch, and H. A. Andersen, The Treatment of Cardiospasm: Analysis of a Twelve-Year Experience, J Thorac Surg, 22:164–187, 1951.*)

extended onto the stomach only far enough to ensure completeness of this portion of the procedure (Fig. 25-12). Damage to the vagus nerves and the supporting structures about the hiatus is avoided. An operation carried out in the manner described should relieve the distal esophageal obstruction in almost every patient and should rarely lead to esophageal reflux. The addition of such ancillary procedures as gastric drainage operations and vagotomy should not be necessary. Ellis and Olsen reported that 94 percent of 268 patients treated in this fashion were benefited by the operation, and approximately 83 percent had excellent or good results (Table 25-1). More recent reviews of other series confirm our favorable experience with surgical treatment of achalasia.

Because of the superior results obtainable by a properly performed esophagomyotomy, surgery is replacing all other forms of treatment for achalasia. Forceful dilation should be used only for selected patients whose general condition precludes major surgery or for patients who decline to undergo operation. Thus, myotomy should now be offered to all but extremely high-risk patients.

The late results of a properly performed esophagomyotomy are so satisfactory that it is neither advisable nor necessary to consider the performance of ancillary esophageal procedures in all patients at the time of myotomy.

Indeed, Peyton et al. have reported that the performance of an antireflux procedure at operation on all achalasia patients in the absence of a preexistent sliding esophageal hiatal hernia constitutes an overreaction to the 3 percent incidence of incompetence after myotomy alone. Further, the failure rate of antireflux procedures exceeds the failure rate which they are designed to prevent. Fewer than 6 percent of patients have poor results requiring reoperation for any cause. Indeed, the majority of patients requiring reoperation for achalasia require treatment for persistent obstruction at the distal esophagus due to achalasia, not for stricture or esophagitis. In the majority of these patients the previous myotomy is found to have healed and the patients respond rather well to performance of a properly designed procedure with attention to the details outlined.

HYPOTENSIVE LOWER ESOPHAGEAL SPHINCTER

A unified concept of the etiology of gastroesophageal incompetence gained credibility with the objective manometric studies of Cohen and Harris. These investigators were able to differentiate clearly among patients with and without hiatal hernia those with symptoms of reflux and those without, on the basis of level of lower esophageal sphincter pressure. Subsequently, Olsen, Schlegel, and Payne described a group of patients without demonstrable anatomic esophageal hiatal hernia in whom symptomatic reflux was occurring. They were able to differentiate these

Table 25-1. COMPARISON OF TWO METHODS USED IN TREATING ACHALASIA AT THE MAYO CLINIC, 1949 THROUGH 1967

	Hydrostatic dilation (*1950 through 1967*)	*Esophagomyotomy* (*1949 through 1966*)
Number of patients	408*	268
Ages, yr	1–85	4–80 (46.5 mean)
Operative mortality, %	0.5†	0.3 (1 of 300)
Follow-up:		
Percent	77	96
Number	313‡	256
Range, yr	1–18	1–17.5
Average, yr	9.5	5.5
Result:		
Excellent, %, (no.)	28 (88) ⎤ 65	47 (120) ⎤ 83
Good, %, (no.)	37 (115) ⎦ 81 improved	36 (91) ⎦ 94 improved
Fair, %, (no.)	16 (50)	11 (29)
Poor, %, (no.)	19 (58)	6 (16)
Complications:		
Percent	4.6	3.3
Number	19§	11 (11 of 300)¶

*Eighty-two percent (334 patients) dilated once; 16 percent (66 patients) dilated twice; 2 percent (8 patients) dilated three or more times.

†Two patients died from unrelated illness 5 days and 2 weeks, respectively, after dilation.

‡Fifty patients (12 percent) whose initial treatment was dilation subsequently underwent esophagomyotomy because of persistent or recurrent major symptoms.

§Ten patients (2.4 percent) required operation for rupture of distal esophagus; all recovered.

¶Mainly infections; all recovered.

SOURCE: W. S. Payne and F. E. Donoghue, Surgical Treatment of Achalasia, *Mod Treat,* 7:1229–1240, 1970. By permission of Harper & Row, Publishers, Incorporated, New York.

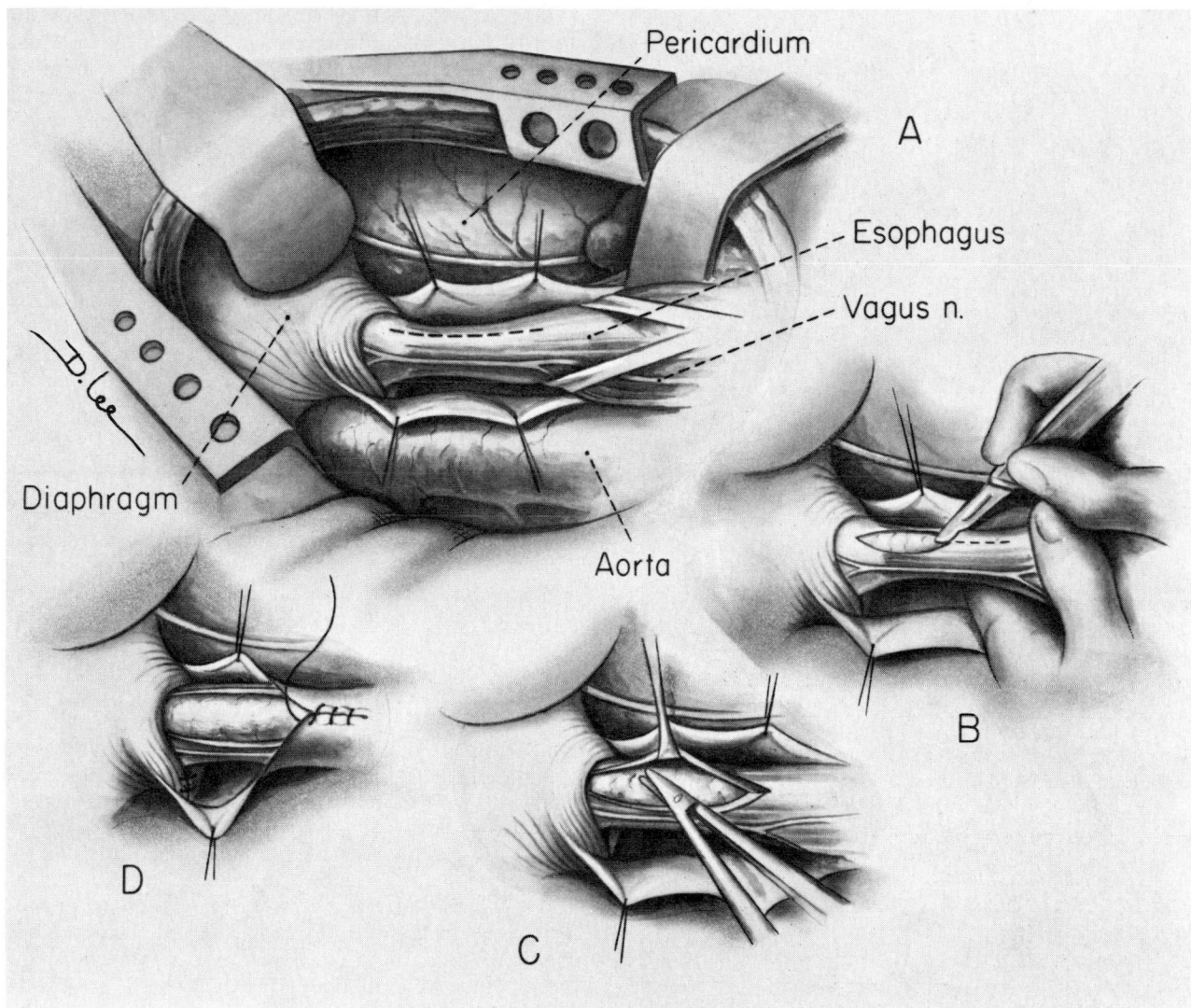

Fig. 25-12. Technique of modified Heller esophagomyotomy for achalasia of the esophagus. *A.* Transthoracic exposure of distal esophagus for esophagomyotomy. The esophagus has been mobilized and elevated from its bed by a Penrose drain. The intended incision is indicated by the dashed line. *B.* Beginning the incision. *C.* Dissection of mucosa from muscularis. *D.* Restoration of esophagogastric junction to intraabdominal position with suture narrowing of esophageal hiatus if necessary. (*From F. H. Ellis, Jr., J. C. Kiser, J. F. Schlegel, R. J. Earlam, J. L. McVey, and A. M. Olsen, Esophagomyotomy for Esophageal Achalasia: Experimental, Clinical, and Manometric Aspects, Ann Surg, 166:640–655, 1967.*)

patients from normal controls on the basis of the level of lower esophageal sphincter pressure. Thus, the concept of a hypotensive lower esophageal sphincter as an isolated clinical entity without hiatal hernia assumed respectability. Such studies have served to emphasize that the restoration of competence is dependent on restoration of sphincter pressure, not on correction of anatomic deformity—a concept that forms the basis of the modern treatment of reflux esophagitis and its complications. As enlightening as this

concept may be, the cause of sphincter failure remains obscure. The treatment of hypotensive lower esophageal sphincter with or without hiatal hernia is discussed further on in detail in the section Complications of Gastroesophageal Reflux.

Though the cause of hypotensive lower esophageal sphincter is unknown in most patients with or without hiatal hernia, it is widely appreciated that certain diseases, such as scleroderma, or certain operations which destroy or bypass the lower esophageal sphincter cause reflux esophagitis and its complications.

Among the postsurgical states that may interfere with the tone and responsiveness of the lower esophageal sphincter are truncal vagotomy, esophagogastrectomy with esophagogastrostomy, and esophagogastric myotomy. Esophagomyotomy may weaken the sphincter but not diminish it, while esophagogastric myotomy usually totally destroys sphincter tone. Other, largely obsolete procedures that destroy sphincter function include Wendel cardioplasty

Fig. 25-13. Esophageal roentgenograms of two patients with hypermotility disturbances. Above: Diffuse spasm of esophagus with epiphrenic diverticulum and small hiatal hernia. Below: Hypertensive gastroesophageal sphincter with small hiatal hernia. (*From F. H. Ellis, Jr., and W. S. Payne, Motility Disturbances of the Esophagus and Its Inferior Sphincter: Recent Surgical Advances, Adv Surg, 1:179–246, 1965. Copyright 1965 by Year Book Medical Publishers, Inc. Used by permission.*)

and the Heyrovsky and Gröndahl procedures. Total gastrectomy is usually associated with loss of competence of the lower esophageal sphincter, and special reconstruction of esophagointestinal continuity is required to prevent alkaline biliary reflux. In our experience, reconstruction with a long-limb Roux en Y provides reliable control of this problem. In other situations, though prevention is to be stressed, treatment is usually feasible through performance of one of the antireflux operations.

DIAGNOSTIC STUDIES. Though reflux symptoms are usually clear-cut, further objectivity is achievable through clinical diagnostic testing. Pope has emphasized the value of certain specific objective histologic changes seen in epithelial biopsies in patients with reflux. Such findings are of special diagnostic value in the evaluation of patients with reflux symptoms in whom macroscopic esophagitis is endoscopically absent. Esophageal manometric studies not only define sphincter tone but also identify associated motility disturbances that may require additional management. Introduced by Lind and associates, the abdominal compression test is important in identifying an incompetent sphincter. The procedure consists of raising intragastric pressure by exerting pressure on the abdomen and observing its effect on both the sphincter pressure and the intraluminal esophageal pressure above the sphincter. The normal response is a 1:1 or greater rise of sphincteric pressure in comparison to gastric pressure with no transmission of pressure to the esophagus above the sphincter. In patients with incompetence, there is little or no rise in sphincter pressure with free transmission of intragastric pressure into the esophagus—the so-called common cavity effect. As noted previously, this response is eliminated by vagotomy and use of atropine.

Although many have used radiography, acid perfusion and acid clearing tests, and measurements of pH levels on withdrawal of an electrode from the stomach to the esophagus, it is generally agreed that a far more sensitive test of gastroesophageal reflux is the pH reflux test in which a pH electrode is placed 5 cm above the esophagogastric junction and 0.1 N hydrochloric acid is injected intragastrically. A positive response, indicating free reflux, is a quick drop in pH as recorded on the intraesophageal pH meter. Whereas none of these tests is entirely diagnostic, when taken together they are extremely useful; they provide objective evidence of the existence of reflux. Undoubtedly, they will be used more extensively in the future, not only in the preoperative evaluation of patients with a hypotensive inferior esophageal sphincter but also in the postoperative evaluation of the effectiveness of medical or surgical treatment or both.

Hypermotility

The causes of hypermotility disorders are also unknown, although they too may be related to abnormalities affecting the vagus supply to the organ. Diffuse spasm of the esophagus and hypertensive gastroesophageal sphincter are the conditions under discussion, and there is little evidence that they may be precursors of esophageal achalasia.

CLINICAL MANIFESTATIONS. Differentiation of these conditions from esophageal achalasia can usually be made on clinical grounds. Pain and dysphagia are the predominant symptoms, pain being more pronounced and dysphagia occurring intermittently or not at all. The pain may manifest itself only as a sensation of discomfort under the lower half of the sternum, or it may be severe and colicky, with extension through to the back or into the neck, shoulders, or arms, mimicking cardiac pain. It may be provoked by eating, or it may come on spontaneously, even awakening the patient at night. Patients so afflicted tend to be high-strung and nervous, and the diagnosis of psychoneurosis may be entertained. The symptoms are intermittent and are more likely to be troublesome than incapacitating; even during an attack, the patient seldom appears to be seriously ill.

Abnormalities of the esophageal roentgenogram occur in fewer than half the cases. When present, however, they may be quite striking, ranging from simple narrowing to segmental spasm and finally to extreme changes, including pseudodiverticulosis (Fig. 25-13). A small diaphragmatic hernia is frequently present, and an epiphrenic diverticulum commonly exists. A localized area of obstruction may be detectable in patients with hypertensive gastroesophageal sphincter.

PHYSIOLOGIC STUDIES. Because esophageal roentgenograms may appear normal in patients with these disorders, the diagnosis usually rests on the results of esophageal motility studies. In patients with diffuse spasm, there is a specific abnormal pattern of the deglutitive pressures. A primary peristaltic wave can be recognized over the upper half or two-thirds of the esophagus, but in the lower half or third it is replaced by simultaneous, repetitive, and occasionally prolonged increases in pressure (Fig. 25-14). Evidence of hiatal herniation is common. In most patients, however, there is no evidence of abnormality of the two sphincters unless there is a hypertensive gastroesophageal sphincter, in which case resting pressures in that region are excessive and relaxation may be poor.

TREATMENT. The use of an extended esophagomyotomy for the treatment of patients with "diffuse nodular myomatosis of the esophagus" was suggested in 1950 by Lortat-Jacob. Although physiologic studies were not made in his patients, many probably had forms of esophageal hypermotility disturbances. A similar approach was initiated independently at the Mayo Clinic in 1956 in order to control the severe symptoms of hypermotility disturbance of the esophagus in carefully selected patients.

In many respects, the technique of the operation resembles that used for achalasia of the esophagus. However, the proximal limit of the esophageal muscular incision varies, depending on the preoperative estimate of the extent of the disease as defined by esophageal motility studies. It may occasionally extend as high as the aortic arch (Fig. 25-15). Surgical repair of an associated diaphragmatic hernia is essential. Henderson and associates have stressed the need for an antireflux procedure at operation on all patients with diffuse spasm and extension of the myotomy from the stomach to 10 cm above the aortic end. Flye and Sealy have reported similar good results with long esophagomyotomy, reserving antireflux operations for patients with manifest hernia or incompetence. This treatment is less effective than it is for achalasia; only 78 percent of the patients so treated are benefited. Patients should therefore be selected carefully for this operation, the ideal candidate being an emotionally stable person with serious disability from the disease but without evidence of associated gastrointestinal problems. There should be demonstrable evidence of the severity of the disease in the form of a markedly abnormal esophageal motility pattern, ideally

Fig. 25-14. Motility in esophagus and sphincter of patient with diffuse spasm. Note giant repetitive contractions. The sphincter relaxes normally. Peristalsis, although usually absent, is present in this case. (*From F. H. Ellis, Jr., C. F. Code, and A. M. Olsen, Long Esophagomyotomy for Diffuse Spasm of the Esophagus and Hypertensive Gastroesophageal Sphincter, Surgery, 48:155–169, 1960.*)

associated with roentgenographic evidence of esophageal spasm.

DIVERTICULA

Diverticula of the esophagus are among the more common lesions that cause esophageal dysfunction. They may have serious consequences if neglected, but current techniques of management offer a particularly rewarding opportunity for effective surgical treatment.

Typical diverticula of the esophagus are thought to be acquired lesions which result either from the protrusion of mucosa through a defect in the esophageal musculature (pulsion diverticula) or from the traction effect of adjacent inflamed parabronchial lymph nodes (traction diverticula). Such acquired lesions should be clearly differentiated from the rare congenital diverticulum of the esophagus and the occasional duplication, enterogenous cyst, or neoplasm which may have a fistulous communication with the esophageal lumen.

Pharyngoesophageal Diverticulum

The most common diverticulum of the esophagus arises at the pharyngoesophageal junction. Typically, it is located posteriorly in the midline, protruding between the oblique fibers of the inferior pharyngeal constrictor and the transverse fibers of the cricopharyngeus. Although first described in 1769 by the English surgeon Ludlow, Zenker's name has become intimately associated with the condition as the result of his studies on 27 collected cases in 1874.

INCIDENCE, PATHOPHYSIOLOGY, AND ANATOMY. Pharyngoesophageal diverticulum is definitely an acquired abnormality, since it is rarely encountered in patients less

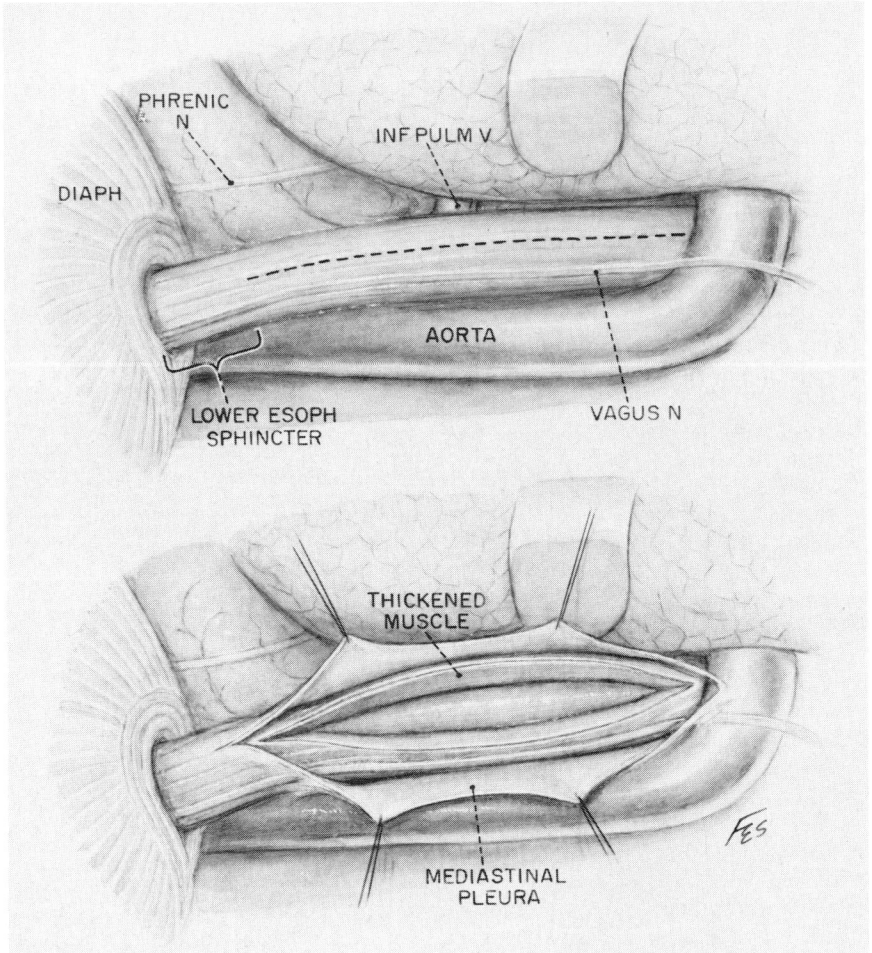

Fig. 25-15. Technique of long esophagomyotomy for diffuse spasm of esophagus. Note that incision extends to the aortic arch and spares the lower esophageal sphincter.

than thirty years old and usually occurs in those more than fifty. Esophageal motility studies have demonstrated premature contraction of the cricopharyngeus muscle in patients with pharyngoesophageal diverticulum. This occurs with sufficient frequency during swallowing that the partial obstructive effects of cricopharyngeal incoordination are implicated in the development of these diverticula. Because of the recurrent pressures involved and the effect of gravity and peristalsis, a globular dependent sac filled with ingested material gradually develops, insinuating itself posteriorly between the esophagus and the cervical vertebrae. In more advanced stages it may descend into the mediastinum.

Since the mouth of the diverticulum is located above the superior esophageal sphincter, there is no barrier to prevent spontaneous pharyngeal reflux and aspiration. Particularly in the sleeping or obtunded patient, this may result in recurrent episodes of airway contamination and aspiration pneumonitis.

CLINICAL MANIFESTATIONS. A sensation of high cervical obstruction to swallowing is the most common symptom. Such patients complain of a noisy, gurgling sound in their throats with drinking and the regurgitation of portions of recent meals into the mouth. Characteristically,

this food is undigested but may have an offensive odor due to decomposition. Frequently such regurgitation is associated with paroxysms of coughing, which may occur either immediately after meals or on reclining and may even awaken the patient from sleep.

The patient with a neglected pharyngoesophageal diverticulum may find eating to be a slow and laborious process, with dysphagia and interruptions by episodes of regurgitation and cough. In the extreme case, fatigue, malnutrition, hoarseness, and suppurative lung disease may further complicate the clinical course. Occasionally, patients with pharyngoesophageal diverticula are unaware of the abnormality until they experience some complication from it.

The diagnosis may be strongly suspected from the patient's history, but it can be firmly established only by roentgenographic examination of the esophagus with contrast medium (Fig. 25-16). Esophagoscopy usually is not necessary.

TREATMENT. In general, any diverticulum arising in the pharyngoesophageal region and producing symptoms warrants treatment. In a given patient, the minimal risks of intervention must be weighed against the severity of symptoms and the risk of present or potential complications arising from the diverticulum.

Currently, most patients with a pharyngoesophageal diverticulum seek medical assistance before severe complications have developed, and little or no preoperative preparation is required. Nonetheless, some effort should be made to ensure that the diverticulum is emptied of all secretions, food, and barium before anesthesia is induced.

If the patient is poorly nourished or dehydrated, appropriate measures should be employed to correct these abnormalities. In such patients it is often possible to give temporary preoperative palliation for dysphagia by performing esophageal dilation.

When aspiration pneumonitis or lung abscess has complicated a diverticulum, attempts should be made to resolve this before proceeding with operation. Occasionally, however, it is necessary to correct the esophageal problem before the pulmonary process will improve.

Although a wide variety of ingenious surgical procedures have been devised and many continue to be used in the treatment of this condition, one-stage diverticulectomy is the method most generally used at the present time. Cricopharyngeal myotomy also is an effective method of treatment. In our experience, dependable results with myotomy are confined to the smaller diverticula, which are less amenable to surgical excision. Therefore, we prefer diverticulectomy for the larger diverticula and myotomy for the smaller diverticula.

Technique of One-Stage Pharyngoesophageal Diverticulectomy. Either regional cervical block or general anesthesia can be used satisfactorily. Local anesthesia has also been particularly effective in elderly, debilitated patients who have complicating cardiovascular or respiratory disease. Because most diverticula tend to extend more to the left in the neck, in 80 percent of Mayo Clinic patients exploration has been from that side. Both the horizontal and the oblique lower cervical incision have been used (Fig. 25-17A). After the incision has been deepened, exposure of the retropharyngeal space and the diverticulum is obtained by retracting the sternocleidomastoid muscle and the carotid sheath and its contents laterally and the thyroid gland and larynx mediad (Fig. 25-17B). The apex of the diverticulum is grasped with an Allis forceps and elevated into the wound. The diverticulum must be thoroughly dissected, so that the neck of the mucosal sac and the surrounding ring of the muscular defect are clearly defined. A curved clamp is placed accurately across the neck of the mucosal sac at right angles to the long axis of the esophagus (Fig. 25-17B). The mucosal diverticular sac is amputated proximal to the clamp and flush with the neck of the sac. Amputation of the sac and suture closure of the esophagus are best accomplished in steps, by placing interrupted fine silk sutures in the mucosa as it is incised (Fig. 25-17B). When the diverticulum is completely excised and the mucosal cut edge is closed, the muscular and fascial layers of the hypopharynx are closed over the repair in a transverse direction (Fig. 25-17C). A small Penrose rubber drain is placed near the site of repair in the pre-

Fig. 25-16. Roentgenogram of the esophagus demonstrating a pharyngoesophageal diverticulum. Note that main lumen is angulated and compressed by this moderate-sized diverticulum. (*From W. S. Payne, and O. T. Clagett, Pharyngeal and Esophageal Diverticula, Curr Probl Surg, April 1965, pp. 1–31. Copyright 1965 by Year Book Medical Publishers, Inc. Used by permission.*)

vertebral space and brought to the outside through the lower end of the incision prior to closure (Fig. 25-17D).

Results of One-Stage Diverticulectomy. During the 28-year period ending December 31, 1971, 828 consecutive patients with pulsion diverticula of the hypopharynx were operated on at the Mayo Clinic by a one-stage procedure. In Clagett and Payne's 1960 review of 478 consecutive one-stage operations performed during the first 14 years of this experience, the surgical mortality was 0.8 percent. Esophagocutaneous fistulas developed postoperatively in 4 of the 478 patients. All fistulas closed spontaneously in 1 to 3 months. There were no instances of serious mediastinal infection. Unilateral paralysis of the vocal cords was noted postoperatively in 11 patients; in only 3 was this paralysis permanent. Symptoms or roentgenologic evidence of recurrence of the diverticulum developed in 6 of 250 patients restudied. All other patients were asymptomatic. In a recent 5- to 14-year follow-up of 164 patients, Welsh and Payne found that 93 percent had good or excel-

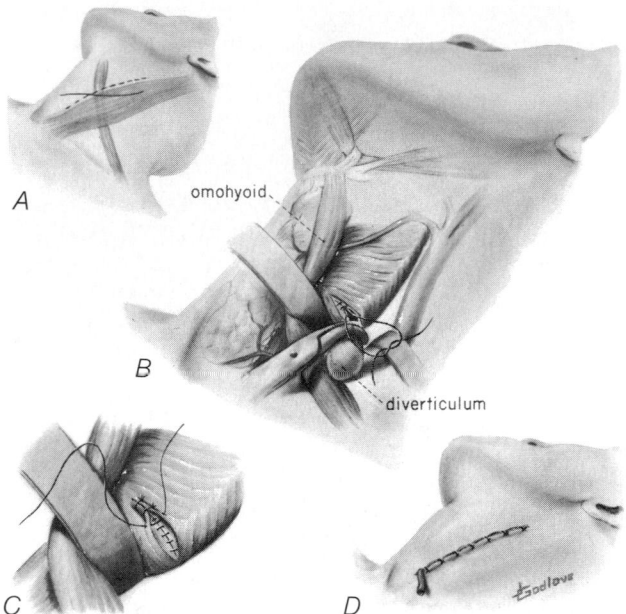

Fig. 25-17. Technique of one-stage pharyngoesophageal diverticulectomy. *A.* Surgical incisions employed when neck is explored from left. Note location of both oblique and horizontal incisions and their relationship to sternocleidomastoid and omohyoid muscles. *B.* Exposure obtained during removal of diverticulum. Note relationship of omohyoid to origin of diverticulum. Curved clamp has been placed across neck of sac, and sac has been amputated and esophageal mucosa closed in steps, with use of "cut-and-sew" technique. *C.* Layer closure of esophagus is completed with approximation of musculofascial tissues. *D.* Single soft-rubber drain is brought from prevertebral space and region of repair to outside through lower end of incision. Platysma and skin are closed in layers. (*From W. S. Payne, and O. T. Clagett, Pharyngeal and Esophageal Diverticula, Curr Probl Surg, April 1965, pp. 1–31. Copyright 1965 by Year Book Medical Publishers, Inc. Used by permission.*)

lent symptomatic results. The late recurrence rate was 3 percent.

Other Techniques. The two-stage diverticulectomy advocated by Lahey and Warren in 1954 is infrequently indicated today except in the late management of a neglected perforated diverticulum. In this procedure the sac is first freed and brought out through the wound. Two weeks later, after the fascial planes have sealed, the sac is removed much as in the one-stage procedure.

Extramucosal cricopharyngeal myotomy is a relatively new procedure in the management of pharyngoesophageal diverticulum. Cross and associates have suggested the use of such a myotomy as an adjunct to one-stage diverticulectomy to prevent recurrence. Belsey uses esophagomyotomy with diverticulopexy. Sutherland has reported the use of cricopharyngeal myotomy as the sole means of treating pharyngoesophageal diverticulum. The technique is certainly an effective means of dealing with smaller diverticula, not only because it reduces the tone of the partially obstructing sphincter, but also because it eliminates the distal support of the diverticular neck and obliterates the

septating spur. Dohlman and Mattsson have accomplished this same reentry effect by an endoscopic diathermic division of the spur formed by the diverticular esophageal wall. The total number of patients treated by cricopharyngeal myotomy, either alone or in conjunction with other techniques, has not been sufficient to permit valid statistical comparisons with diverticulectomy. Nonetheless, myotomy alone appears to be a satisfactory technique for the smaller diverticula. Whether its use in conjunction with diverticulectomy can effect further improvement remains unanswered.

Technique of Cricopharyngeal Myotomy. Surgical exposure is accomplished as described for diverticulectomy (Fig. 25-18).

After the diverticulum is freed to its neck, the transverse fibers of the cricopharyngeal muscle bordering the inferior margin of the neck of the diverticulum are easily identified and incised vertically. The incision is carried down to mucosa and is extended caudad onto the esophagus, the length of the incision averaging about 3 cm. After the myotomy, the esophageal and cricopharyngeal muscles are dissected for half the circumference of the mucosal tube to allow the mucosa to protrude freely through the incision. The cervical wound is then closed, with or without drainage.

Epiphrenic Diverticulum

Probably no other benign condition affecting the esophagus has been so poorly understood for so long as the epiphrenic diverticulum. Unfortunately, lack of basic knowledge concerning pathogenesis has all too often been equated with poor surgical results. Current surgical management permits a safe and often rational approach for most patients with this condition.

INCIDENCE, PATHOPHYSIOLOGY, AND ANATOMY. This diverticulum usually occurs among older persons. As its name implies, the epiphrenic diverticulum usually occurs in the lower thoracic esophagus—typically within 10 cm of the cardia—but may occur at higher levels in the thoracic esophagus. The pathologic anatomy is almost identical with that of pulsion diverticula in the pharyngoesophageal region in that the diverticulum is essentially a herniated sac of mucosa and submucosa protruding through the usual supporting sheath of esophageal musculature. The sac is covered by thin bands of attenuated muscle, which are often not discernible except on microscopic study.

The association of epiphrenic diverticula with motility disturbances and esophageal hiatal hernia was first appreciated by Vinson in 1934. Others since have noted the incidence of associated abnormal esophageal and diaphragmatic conditions to be as high as 75 percent. These and other data suggest that the majority of pulsion diverticula of the lower esophagus develop as the result of abnormal intraesophageal pressures. Allen and Clagett, in a review of 160 patients with epiphrenic diverticulum, found diffuse spasm of the esophagus in 39, esophageal achalasia in 16, esophageal hiatal hernia in 55, and esophagitis and a

Fig. 25-18. Technique of cricopharyngeal myotomy. *A.* Site of skin incision. *B.* Exposure of diverticulum. Dashed line indicates proposed myotomy site. *C.* Completed operation. (*From F. H. Ellis, Jr., J. F. Schlegel, V. P. Lynch, and W. S. Payne, Cricopharyngeal Myotomy for Pharyngoesophageal Diverticulum, Ann Surg, 170:340–349, 1969.*)

variety of other associated conditions in 18. Only 66 of the 160 patients had no apparent abnormality associated with the epiphrenic diverticulum.

CLINICAL MANIFESTATIONS. Because of the high incidence of abnormal conditions of the esophagus associated with epiphrenic diverticula, it is difficult to be certain which, if any, of a given patient's symptoms are due to the diverticulum. Certainly, as with pharyngoesophageal diverticula, dysphagia and regurgitation are the most frequent complaints, but many patients have no symptoms referable to the esophagus. Habein and associates, in a study of 149 nonsurgical cases, estimated that only 15 to 20 percent of pulsion diverticula in this region produce definite symptoms. As with other diverticula, the regurgitated food is undigested and is recognizable as retention

from a recent meal. The relatively low incidence of tracheobronchial aspiration and suppurative pneumonitis is understandable in view of the distance and the sphincteric and peristaltic barriers between the diverticulum and the pharynx.

The symptoms of epiphrenic diverticulum are less definite than those of pharyngoesophageal diverticulum and may be only suggestive of the diagnosis. Roentgenographic examination of the esophagus with contrast medium is the best means of determining the presence and location of a pulsion diverticulum and the associated conditions (Fig. 25-13, top). Esophagoscopy is not required to establish a diagnosis but should be performed to seek out and define associated esophageal disease. Studies of esophageal motility are essential in current surgical management of epiphrenic diverticulum.

TREATMENT. The management of most epiphrenic diverticula is largely symptomatic. The presence of a defect causing few or no symptoms does not warrant surgical intervention if more serious associated conditions can be excluded. Generally, operation is indicated only when symptoms are progressive and severe or when associated conditions require it.

Surgical Treatment. The chief preoperative consideration

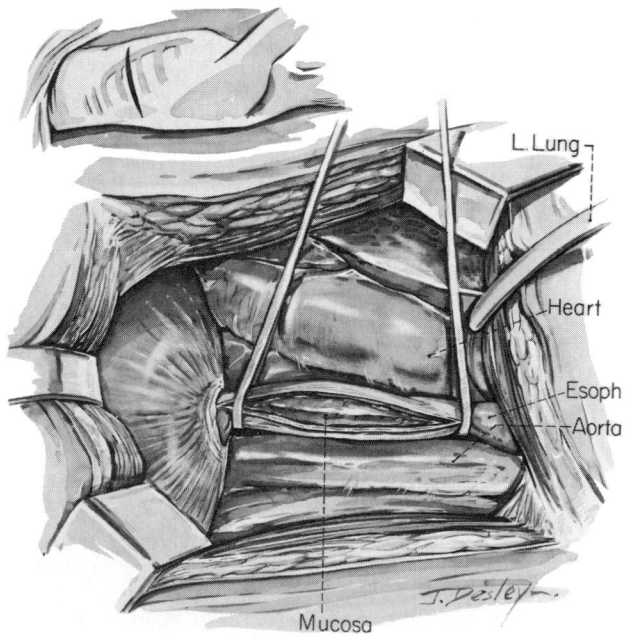

in the treatment of epiphrenic diverticulum is the prevention of aspiration during the induction of anesthesia. In addition to emptying the diverticulum, some consideration should be given to esophageal retention secondary to associated conditions. Occasionally, it is necessary to consider endoscopic evacuation. Often, preoperative esophageal bougienage will effect satisfactory emptying of the esophagus and diverticulum.

Left thoracotomy (Fig. 25-19) should be used almost routinely in the surgical treatment of epiphrenic diverticulum, since this incision provides the necessary exposure for excision of the diverticulum and, more important, is usually required to correct frequently associated esophageal and diaphragmatic conditions. Furthermore, the results of diverticulectomy are more satisfactory if a long, extramucosal esophagomyotomy is routinely performed in all such diverticulectomies along with correction of any other associated defects of the esophagus and diaphragm.

Results of Surgical Treatment. The significance of the present concept of the surgical treatment of pulsion diverticula of the lower esophageal region is clearly apparent on review of the Mayo Clinic experience from 1944 through 1963. Early in this experience, esophagomyotomy was not performed concomitantly with diverticulectomy and correction of associated diaphragmatic hernia. Of 29 patients so treated, 7 had significant postoperative complications (there were 4 recurrent epiphrenic diverticula in this group). Later, esophagomyotomy was performed routinely with diverticulectomy. Of the 11 patients so treated, only 1 had a postoperative complication and none died.

Parabronchial or Midesophageal Diverticulum

Granulomatous infections of mediastinal lymph nodes may cause traction diverticula. Although they occur typically in relation to subcarinal and parabronchial lymph nodes in the middle third of the esophagus, they can occur at any level. Generally these minute triangular esophageal deformities are of little or no clinical significance except as indications of a previous, often healed infection; they produce no esophageal symptoms and require no treat-

Fig. 25-19. Above: Surgical treatment of pulsion diverticulum of lower esophagus. Inset shows placement of left posterolateral thoracotomy incision. *A.* Exposure of diverticulum of esophagus obtained when chest is entered through bed of left eighth rib; note that tapes have been passed around esophagus and esophagus has been rotated to bring diverticulum into view. *B.* Removal of diverticulum and closure of mucosa; note that mucosal sutures are tied with knots within esophageal lumen. *C.* Closure of esophageal musculature over mucosal suture line. Below: Complete long esophagomyotomy, which should be performed concomitantly with diverticulectomy and through the same posterolateral thoracotomy incision. Site of diverticular excision has been rotated back to right and is not visible. A long myotomy incision, extending from cardia to aortic arch, is apparent, with underlying mucosa bulging through incision. If a diaphragmatic hernia is present, it too should be repaired through same incision. (*From W. S. Payne, and O. T. Clagett, Pharyngeal and Esophageal Diverticula, Curr Probl Surg, April 1965, pp. 1–31. Copyright 1965 by Year Book Medical Publishers, Inc. Used by permission.*)

ment. When symptoms are present, they are usually caused by some other, unrelated process.

In the presence of symptoms, the usual studies should be carried out to determine the cause and rule out more serious disease. These include roentgenographic examination, endoscopy, and occasionally motility studies. When active infection is suspected, appropriate skin tests and microbiologic studies are indicated.

Interest in traction diverticula is thus focused chiefly on differentiating them from more serious conditions. Such a diverticulum may, however, be the site of serious, although rare, complications. These include obstruction to swallowing, esophagitis, hemorrhage, perforation with empyema, pericarditis, and tracheobronchial-esophageal fistula. Usually the symptomatic traction diverticulum can be managed by simple excision. Fistulas between the esophagus and lower respiratory tract respond to excision and closure of the communication and interposition of normal tissues to prevent recurrence. Perforation with empyema or pericarditis often requires specific antibiotic

treatment as well as surgical drainage and temporary defunctionalization of the esophagus.

ESOPHAGEAL HIATAL HERNIA

Esophageal hiatal hernias are not only the most common hernias of the diaphragm but also are among the more common abnormalities affecting the upper gastrointestinal tract.

There are basically two main types of esophageal hiatal hernias: the sliding hernia and the paraesophageal hernia. A third type, the short esophagus hiatal hernia, is a complication of gastroesophageal reflux usually associated with a sliding hernia and will be discussed subsequently (Fig. 25-20).

Sliding Hernia

The most common is the sliding hernia, in which there is displacement of the esophagogastric junction and portions of the proximal part of the stomach through the esophageal hiatus into the posterior mediastinum. Although such herniations are known to move in and out of the thorax with changes in intrathoracic and intraabdominal pres-

Fig. 25-20. Two chief varieties of esophageal hiatal hernia. *Left:* Sliding esophageal hiatal hernia. *Right:* Paraesophageal hiatal hernia. (*From J. E. Mobley and N. A. Christensen, Esophageal Hiatal Hernia: Prevalence, Diagnosis and Treatment in an American City of 30,000, Gastroenterology, 30:1, 1956. By permission of Williams & Wilkins Company.*)

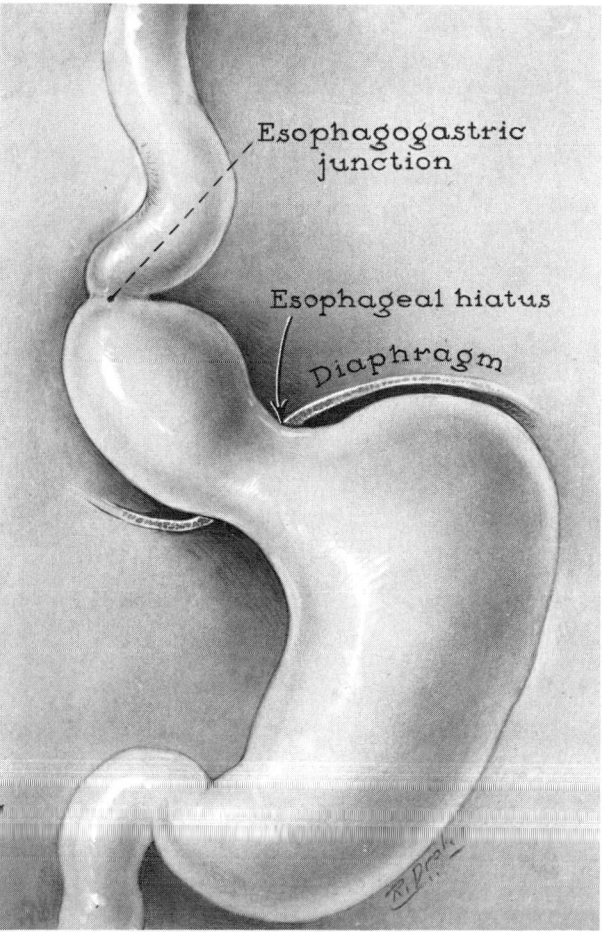

sures, the term *sliding* is applied not because of this behavior but because the hernia has a partial peritoneal sac, the stomach forming the other wall of the hernial sac. In the paraesophageal hiatal hernia, a portion or all of the stomach is displaced into the thorax through the esophageal hiatus alongside the esophagus. The esophagogastric junction is in its normal position while the fundus and successively greater portions of the remainder of the stomach ascend into the thorax.

Gastroesophageal reflux may or may not occur in patients with a sliding esophageal hiatal hernia. In view of the prevalence of the condition (5 per 1,000 population in one series), only a minority ever have significant symptoms of reflux. The presence or absence of reflux in hiatal hernia is directly related to the level of pressure at the inferior sphincter. In fact, Cohen and Harris have suggested that the abnormal anatomy is less important than the abnormal physiology consequent to a hypotensive inferior esophageal sphincter. Reflux is accentuated by certain postural or physiologic changes that are associated with increased intraabdominal or intragastric pressure: stooping, lifting, overeating, or straining.

Fig. 25-21. Belsey Mark IV transthoracic repair of sliding esophageal hiatal hernia. Exposure is gained through a left thoracotomy incision. After complete mobilization of the cardia, the lower 4 cm of esophagus is cleared of connective tissue. *A.* Mattress sutures are placed between gastric fundus and muscular layers of esophagus 1 to 2 cm above and below the esophagogastric junction. *B.* After these mattress sutures are tied, a second row of mattress sutures is placed to imbricate additional fundus onto the lower esophagus. Note that these sutures pass through the hiatus and out through the tendinous portion of the diaphragm. Before these sutures are tied, crural sutures are placed to narrow the esophageal hiatus. *C.* Completed repair after reduction of hernia and tying of sutures to maintain reconstruction. Previously placed crural sutures have been tied behind the esophagus to narrow the hiatus (not shown).

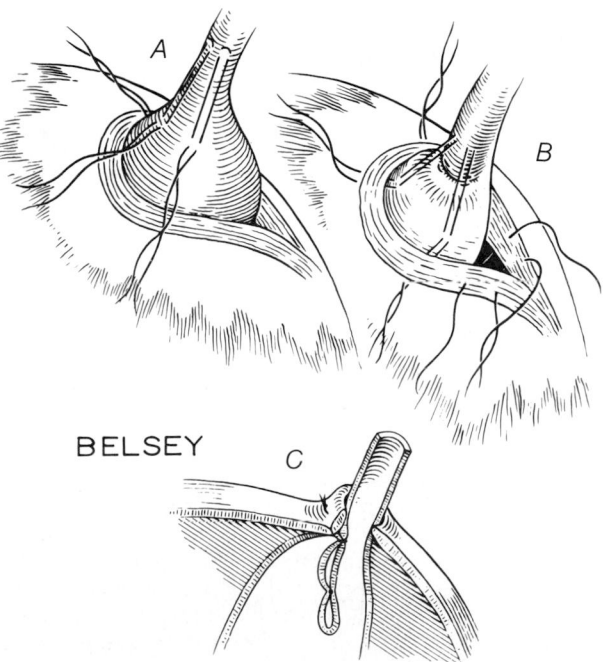

BELSEY

Gastroesophageal reflux in itself would not be deleterious if it were not for the presence of acidic gastric fluid, which in man is secreted continuously. The esophagus appears to be particularly susceptible to the corrosive effects of acidic secretions, as well as to the more alkaline biliary, pancreatic, and intestinal secretions. Fortunately, patients with sliding esophageal hiatal hernias rarely exhibit gastric hypersecretion.

CLINICAL MANIFESTATIONS. Symptoms and complications of gastroesophageal reflux are the major consequences of sliding esophageal hiatal hernia. The majority of these hernias, however, are asymptomatic.

The symptoms of uncomplicated gastroesophageal incompetence are heartburn and regurgitation. The retrosternal or epigastric burning distress is noted particularly after meals; typically, it is accentuated when the patient lies down, stoops, or strains. It is characteristically relieved by sitting and standing or by ingestion of water or antacids. Regurgitation of secretions into the mouth occurs with postural changes and is often described as a hot, bitter, or sour liquid coming into the throat or mouth. Food is regurgitated infrequently, but when it is, it is recent and partially digested and is mixed with gastrointestinal secretions. Dysphagia may occur even in the absence of demonstrable complications such as esophagitis, stricture, or spasm. Other symptoms may be present and may be difficult to differentiate from those due to associated conditions such as coronary artery disease, cholelithiasis, colonic diverticulosis, and duodenal ulcer.

The diagnosis of sliding esophageal hiatal hernia, with or without symptoms, depends almost entirely on demonstrating by roentgenographic examination the protrusion of gastric mucosa through the esophageal hiatus. Although a variety of diagnostic maneuvers have been suggested to aid the roentgenologist, in some patients a sliding hernia, with or without gastroesophageal reflux, may not be apparent unless specifically sought.

Esophagoscopy is indicated in symptomatic patients, particularly those considered for surgical treatment, both to assess esophageal complications and to exclude other, more serious disease. Occasionally studies of esophageal motility are advisable to assist in the diagnosis of sliding hernia, or pH studies may be required for objective evaluation of reflux.

TREATMENT. The treatment of sliding esophageal hiatal hernia with no complications is largely symptomatic. When symptoms are absent or only mild and transient, no therapy is indicated, since the condition is rarely progressive. In other cases the treatment is designed to eliminate gastroesophageal reflux and to minimize its deleterious effects. Such measures as weight reduction, ulcer diet, administration of antacids, elimination of constricting garments, avoidance of stooping, lifting, or straining, and elevation of the head of the bed for sleeping are instituted with these goals in mind. If these medical measures are unavailing or if there are complications, surgical measures may be required for relief of symptoms.

Surgical Treatment. The primary goal of the surgical treatment of sliding esophageal hernia is restoration of gastroesophageal competence. Because restoration of normal anatomy has been found to be an inadequate operation for restoration of normal pressures to the hypotensive sphincter, "antireflux" operations have been devised to accomplish this end more effectively. The operations associated with the names Belsey, Nissen, and Hill are typical of these procedures. All are variations of a basic "wrap-around" procedure, and their success in preventing reflux makes it unnecessary to perform concomitant vagotomy and pyloroplasty unless there is an active duodenal ulcer. The routine use of these additional procedures is discouraged because of their disagreeable side effects.

Belsey's operation (Fig. 25-21) is a transthoracic procedure that creates a segment of intraabdominal esophagus held in place by a buttress of plicated stomach which surrounds approximately 280° of the distal esophagus. Long-term results indicate that the procedure is successful in relieving symptoms in 85 percent of patients and that the recurrence rate varies between 10 and 15 percent, depending on the length of follow-up.

Nissen's fundoplication can be performed either transabdominally or transthoracically (Fig. 25-22). This operation, which totally surrounds the distal esophagus with the adjacent gastric fundus, also produces good clinical results and a low recurrence rate. A worldwide survey of the results of the Nissen operation indicated an overall success rate of 96 percent, failures being usually the result of either recurrent hernia or postoperative reflux. Some dissatisfaction with this procedure has been expressed by Woodward and associates, who found an unacceptably high rate of dysphagia and the so-called gas-bloat syndrome, complications that should be minimal or absent if the procedure is performed in the presence of an indwelling nasogastric tube of ample caliber to prevent excessive narrowing of the distal esophagus. Long-term follow-up, furthermore, showed a regression in the severity of these symptoms when they did occur.

Hill's operation (Fig. 25-23) is basically a posterior gastropexy performed transabdominally, but incorporating plicating sutures to narrow the esophagogastric junction. He reported the cases of 149 patients treated by this technique in an 8-year period, with no deaths and no anatomic recurrences during the follow-up period; 97 percent of the patients were improved.

In addition to these gratifying clinical and roentgenologic results, physiologic studies of postoperative sphincteric function are encouraging. Not only is the amplitude of the lower esophageal sphincteric pressure more than doubled, but also the high-pressure zone is lengthened and the normal neural and hormonal response at the sphincter is restored. Now both experimental and clinical evidence suggest that the 360° wrap afforded by the Nissen fundoplication is the most effective of the three antireflux procedures in restoring lower esophageal sphincter pressure and preventing reflux.

Paraesophageal Hernia

A paraesophageal hiatal hernia is a rare life-threatening entity. Unlike the symptoms of a sliding hernia, which are primarily the result of deranged physiology, the symptoms

Fig. 25-22. Technique of transabdominal Nissen fundoplication. Above: Abdominal exposure and mobilization of the distal esophagus and upper stomach in preparation for carrying out a fundoplication. *A.* Mobilized fundus is displaced behind the esophagus by the surgeon's right hand. *B.* Placement of sutures so as to encircle the distal esophagus with a generous portion of fundus. Note indwelling #40 F gastric tube. *C.* Completed procedure. (*From F. H. Ellis, Jr., Gastroesophageal Reflux: Indications for Fundoplication, Surg Clin North Am, 51:575–588, 1971.*)

of a paraesophageal hernia result from anatomic defect. Although it may occur in combination with sliding esophageal hernia, in its pure form it is not associated with gastroesophageal reflux. The major complications of paraesophageal hiatal hernia are obstruction and hemorrhage. With these hernias there may be hemorrhage from erosions of the mucosa of the herniated part of the stomach. When a large portion of the stomach or all of it is displaced into the thorax, obstruction, symptoms may occur on the basis of angulation and compression. Occasionally other viscera, including spleen, colon, and small bowel, may be involved as well as the stomach. Incarceration, hemorrhage, volvulus, and strangulation are major complications of massive

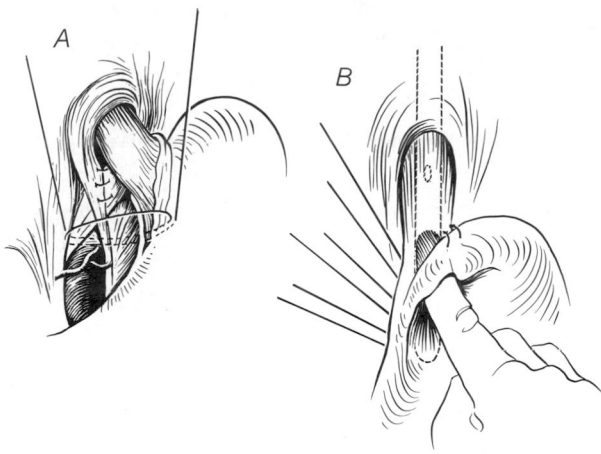

Fig. 25-23. Hill's transabdominal repair of sliding esophageal hiatal hernia. *A.* Reduced esophagogastric junction with crural sutures narrowing the hiatus in place behind esophagus. A single suture is shown incorporating gastrohepatic omentum along lesser curvature of stomach and preaortic fascia. Care is taken in placing sutures to avoid injury to adjacent vagal nerve trunks. Two or three additional sutures are similarly placed on lesser curvature, anchoring stomach posteriorly (posterior gastropexy). *B.* When these sutures are tied, gastric sling fibers should be sufficiently shortened to permit distal phalanx of index finger to invaginate snugly into terminal esophageal lumen alongside Levin tube. Angle of His is further accentuated by placement of sutures between gastric fundus and terminal esophagus. [*From W. S. Payne, and F. H. Ellis, Jr., Diaphragmatic Hernia, in F. H. Ellis, Jr., (ed.), "Lewis-Walters' Practice of Surgery," vol. 5, "Thoracic Surgery," Harper & Row, Publishers, Inc., New York, 1971, chap. 15, pp. 1–59.*]

paraesophageal hernias. Because of the high incidence of serious complications associated with paraesophageal hernia, surgical repair is generally indicated even in the absence of symptoms or complications. The method of repair differs from that described for sliding esophageal hernia. Since the lower esophageal sphincter functions normally, the esophagogastric junctional area is not disturbed. Rather, the herniated fundus is reduced through an abdominal incision, the hernial sac is excised, and the widened hiatus is narrowed by sutures placed in the limbs of the crus anterior to the esophagus as in the technique described by Hill and Tobias (Fig. 25-24). The results of repair of paraesophageal hernias are almost always satisfactory.

COMPLICATIONS OF GASTROESOPHAGEAL REFLUX

Esophagitis

Esophagitis represents a manifestation of the unusual sensitivity of the esophageal mucosa to a variety of agents, particularly strong acids and alkalies, which may be endogenous or exogenous. The most common cause of esophagitis is reflux of acidic gastric juice into the esophagus, a condition resulting from hypotension of the lower

esophageal sphincter (see above). Mucosal inflammation and ulceration occur, and if tissue destruction is severe, a stricture may form during the healing phase. Pathologic study of involved tissues has stressed the superficial nature of the inflammation in most cases, the muscularis propria rarely being involved. Localized marginal esophageal ulceration is common in the presence of a hiatal hernia, whereas extended areas of linear esophagitis are more common in patients with a history of vomiting or duodenal ulcer or both, in surgical patients, and in patients requiring a nasogastric tube.

CLINICAL MANIFESTATIONS. Dysphagia, odynophagia, regurgitation, substernal or epigastric pain, and heartburn are the common symptoms of esophagitis. Dysphagia is more prominent in the later stages of the disease when fibrosis and stricture have occurred. Occasionally, hematemesis or melena may be prominent, although massive gastrointestinal bleeding is rare. Roentgenography is of little value in diagnosing esophagitis but is helpful in excluding a malignant lesion. Since some patients with symptoms of heartburn and regurgitation have normal esophageal mucosa while others have severe esophagitis and even early stricture formation in the absence of typical symptoms, esophagoscopy is required in order to establish a definitive diagnosis.

TREATMENT. Treatment of reflux esophagitis is designed to eliminate gastroesophageal reflux or to minimize its

Fig. 25-24. Technique of surgical repair of paraesophageal hiatal hernia. *A.* Left lobe of liver mobilized and hernia exposed. *B.* Stomach reduced and apex of widened hiatus pulled anteriorly. Sac has been excised. *C.* Hiatus closed anterior to normally placed esophagus with interrupted sutures in crura. [*From F. H. Ellis, Jr., Paraesophageal Hiatus Hernia, in L. M. Nyhus (ed.), "Hernia," 2d ed., J. B. Lippincott Company, Philadelphia, 1977.*]

deleterious effects. In the absence of significant complications, a trial of medical treatment is often justified. Weight reduction, ulcer diet, use of antacids, elimination of constricting garments, and elevation of the head of the bed for sleeping all help to minimize reflux and to neutralize gastric acids. If medical measures fail or if there are complications, surgical measures may be required for relief of symptoms. The various operations that will prevent reflux and allow healing of esophagitis have been described previously.

Short Esophagus

If reflux esophagitis is not promptly and effectively managed in its early stages, complications such as fibrosis and scarring with esophageal shortening and, ultimately, stricture may develop.

Congenital shortening of the esophagus rarely if ever occurs, almost all examples of a shortened esophagus being the result of long-standing untreated gastroesophageal reflux, usually in the presence of a sliding esophageal hiatal hernia. Almost always the fibrosis leading to esophageal shortening also results in an esophageal stricture, usually localized to the esophagogastric junction (Fig. 25-25). Medical therapy, unfortunately, is usually ineffective at this stage of the disease, although it should be tried initially. Bougienage sometimes is successful in dilating the stricture and providing an adequate esophageal lumen. If, as often happens, medical treatment is unsuccessful, surgical treatment must be considered, but a complex procedure is frequently required, simple reduction of the hernia alone rarely being successful if there is prominent shortening of the esophagus.

A variety of ingenious operative procedures has been suggested over the years for the management of this severe complication of gastroesophageal reflux, yet agreement is lacking among surgeons as to the best. Though commonly undertaken in the recent past, resection of the stricture is now rarely used. Rather, an esophageal lengthening procedure, the Collis gastroplasty, coupled with an antireflux operation such as the Belsey (Fig. 25-26) or Nissen fundoplication, is preferred. Intraoperative and postoperative dilation of the stricture is performed as indicated until healing occurs. With acid reflux prevented, healing occurs within an adequate time in most cases. In those rare cases in which the stricture is too firm to permit dilation, one of the three procedures illustrated in Fig. 25-27 may be selected.

Lower Esophagus Lined by Columnar Epithelium (Barrett Esophagus)

In 1950, Barrett described a condition in which the lower end of the esophagus is lined by a continuous sheet of gastric epithelium; he postulated that this was of congenital origin. The designation *lower esophagus lined by columnar epithelium* was adopted after Allison and Johnstone demonstrated that the epithelial lining was similar to the columnar epithelium present at the junctional zone and did

Fig. 25-25. Short-esophagus hiatal hernia with stricture. Above: Esophageal roentgenogram. Below: Resected specimen showing ulceration and stricture.

not contain acid-producing cells. It is now generally agreed that the lesion is acquired rather than congenital in origin, the mucosal changes representing, in patients with esophageal hiatal hernia, a mucosal adaptation to the injurious effects of acidic gastric juice by which the squamous epithelium lining the distal portion of the esophagus is destroyed and replaced with columnar epithelium. It is as yet uncertain whether these epithelial changes are the result of metaplasia or of cephalad growth of functional epithelium from the distal esophagus. This abnormal esophageal lin-

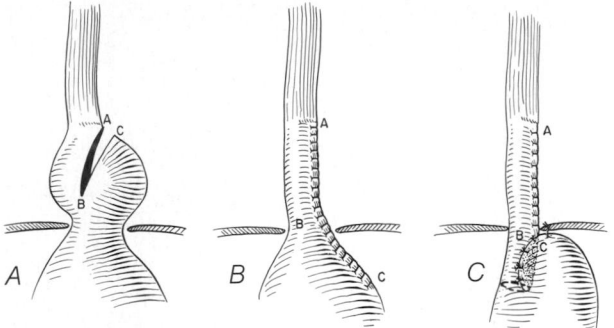

Fig. 25-26. Collis gastroplasty with Belsey hiatal hernia repair for irreversible short esophagus as suggested by Pearson et al. Procedure is effected through a left thoracotomy. *A*. After appropriate mobilization of esophagus and stomach, an incision (A, B, c) in herniated proximal stomach is made parallel with lesser curvature. *B*. Closure of the incision (A, B, C). *C*. Sufficient esophageal length and fundus are acquired to perform a Belsey Mark IV hiatal hernia repair (A, B, C). (*From W. S. Payne and A. M. Olsen, "The Esophagus," Lea & Febiger, Philadelphia. In press.*)

ing may extend to the level of the aortic arch, and ulcer formation may occasionally be demonstrated therein (Barrett's ulcer). A stricture at the columnar-squamous junction is common (Fig. 25-28). The risk of a carcinoma's developing in this abnormal epithelium is high, so that even after treatment the condition of such patients should be closely and carefully followed.

Controversy regarding the nature of this defect is not without therapeutic implications, because if it is an acquired condition secondary to a hiatal hernia, surgical reduction of the hernia should prevent reflux and relieve the symptoms without necessitating removal of the abnormal distal esophagus or of the stricture, which can be successfully dilated once reflux has been eliminated.

CORROSIVE ESOPHAGITIS

The ingestion of strong acid or alkali causes a severe inflammatory reaction of the affected mucosa, known as *corrosive esophagitis*. Lye, a strong cleaning agent containing sodium hydroxide and sodium carbonate, is most commonly responsible for such injuries, although a variety of other fluids, including mineral acids, strong bases, phenol, and organic solvents, can produce similar changes. The nature and concentration of the agent ingested determine the degree and extent of the injury, which may involve limited areas of the esophagus, the entire esophagus, or even the stomach.

PATHOLOGY. The pathologic changes after ingestion of lye have been shown experimentally to consist of edema and congestion of the submucosal layer associated with inflammation and thrombosis of its vessels. Sloughing of the superficial layers occurs, with varying degrees of necrosis of the muscularis, followed by fibrosis and delayed reepithelization. In severe cases the entire mucous membrane of the upper portion of the alimentary tract may slough, with subsequent development of an esophageal stricture.

CLINICAL MANIFESTATIONS. During the acute phase of the reaction, burns of the lips, tongue, mouth, and pharynx are apparent. Pain in the involved region is a common symptom, and there may be associated vomiting. Painful dysphagia is prominent during the acute phase, which lasts from several days to several weeks. As the chronic phase develops, dysphagia may become the predominant symptom as a stricture forms.

Fig. 25-27. Operative procedures for management of short-esophagus diaphragmatic hernia with stricture. Left: Esophagogastrectomy with Roux-en-Y esophagojejunostomy. Center: Esophagogastrectomy with colon interposition and pyloroplasty. Right: Gastric tube of Gavriliu.

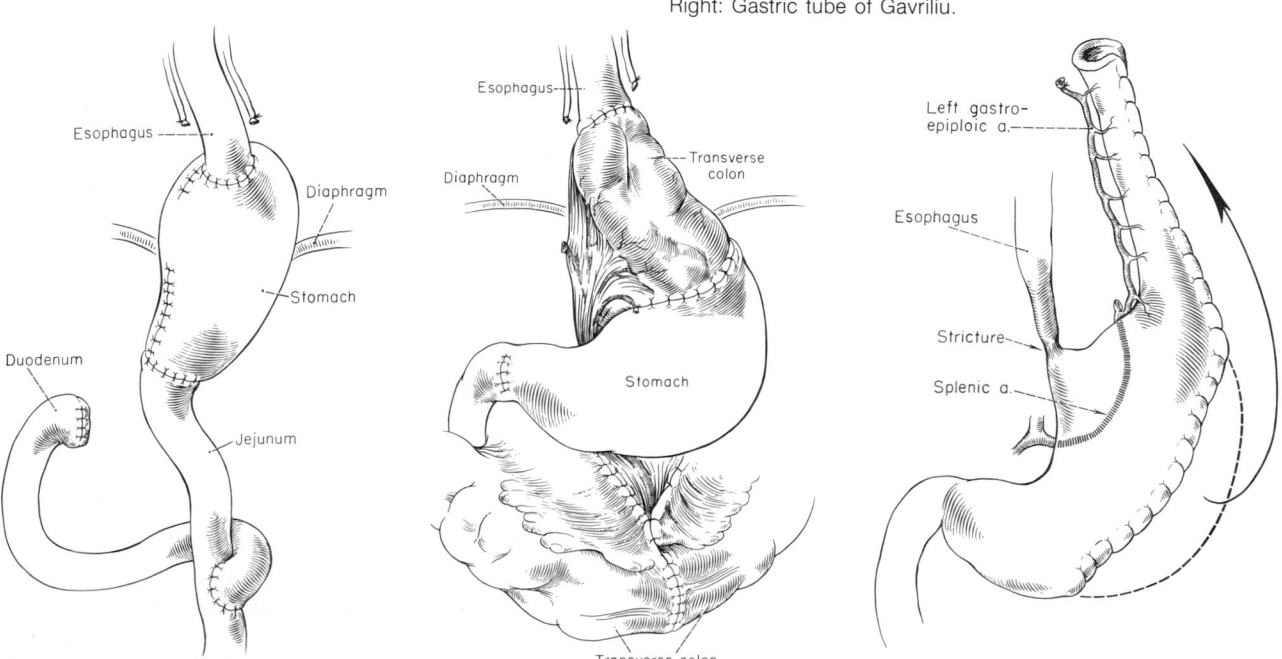

TREATMENT. During the initial period of the injury, appropriate neutralizing agents (such as dilute acidic or alkaline solutions) should be administered to minimize the local effect of the ingested material. Antibiotics are administered to counteract bacterial invasion, and administration of cortisone during the acute phase of the burn has been advocated in order to reduce the incidence and severity of the subsequent stricture formation. Early esophagoscopy is important to determine the extent of the injury and should be repeated every 10 days to 2 weeks to allow proper planning and evaluation of treatment. This can be done safely over a previously swallowed thread, which should be kept in place until the need for dilation has been determined.

Stricture formation is rare if prompt treatment as outlined is initiated. However, should esophagoscopy reveal evidence of stricture formation, dilation of the strictured zone by bougienage over the swallowed thread may be begun within a few weeks of the accident. In some patients, repeated dilation at intervals may be required for prolonged periods, sometimes a year or more. When patients are seen in the chronic phase of the disease and a string has not been ingested previously, it may be necessary to perform gastrostomy for feeding purposes and also for retrograde dilation of the esophageal stricture.

In a small percentage of cases it may become apparent that repeated dilation cannot maintain a satisfactory esophageal lumen. In such cases extensive reconstructive operative procedures are required to establish a satisfactory, functioning esophageal substitute. Many procedures have been devised, including use of skin-lined tubes and segments of intestine or stomach, as reported by Yudin; the Russian surgeons have had extensive experience with these. Total bypass of the strictured esophagus by a segment of right or left colon interposed substernally between the pharynx and stomach is currently preferred. For lesser degrees of stricture, the site of the disease may be approached transthoracically and either resected or bypassed with a segment of jejunum or colon.

ESOPHAGEAL PERFORATION

Irrespective of cause, esophageal perforation or rupture may initiate a virulent periesophageal infection. Prompt recognition and proper treatment may avert death or obviate a prolonged and difficult convalescence. In spite of all efforts, esophageal perforation continues to be associated with high mortality and morbidity.

INCIDENCE. Most esophageal perforations today occur after some form of esophageal instrumentation. The number of such perforations appears to have increased over the past 30 years as a result of the greater use of esophagoscopy, gastroscopy, esophageal dilation, tamponade, and even simple esophageal intubation for diagnosis or treatment.

Of equal interest are those less frequently encountered instances of noninstrumental perforation, which occur as the result of accidental ingestion of foreign bodies or as a consequence of the strain of emesis with or without

Fig. 25-28. Roentgenogram of esophagus in a patient with Barrett esophagus. Note presence of small diaphragmatic hernia (sliding type) and midesophageal stricture. The tubular structure between stricture and hernia is columnar epithelium-lined esophagus with typical esophageal motility. (*From J. N. Burgess, W. S. Payne, H. A. Andersen, L. H. Weiland, and H. C. Carlson, Barrett Esophagus: The Columnar-Epithelial-Lined Lower Esophagus, Mayo Clin Proc, 46:728–734, 1971.*)

predisposing esophageal disease. A variety of other conditions also have been implicated in the noninstrumental perforation of the esophagus, including "stress" associated with neurologic disease or following operations or burns remote from the esophagus. Infrequently, the esophagus may be perforated as the result of either penetrating or nonpenetrating external trauma.

ETIOLOGY. The wall of the esophagus can be breached in a number of ways by either an instrument or a foreign body: (1) simple penetration of the entire wall of the esophagus, (2) simple splitting or rupture of the esophagus by strain exceeding its circumferential tensile strength, (3) breaking down of the wall of the esophagus by a localized inflammatory process resulting from impacted bones, (4) perforation through pressure necrosis.

Instrumental and foreign body perforations can occur at any level of the esophagus; however, the sites of normal narrowing are the ones most frequently involved. The narrowest of these is the esophageal introitus and, indeed, accounts for the high incidence of perforations seen in this region. The impingement of the rigid scope on the bodies of hyperextended cervical vertebrae may result in a crushing effect on the mucosa, particularly in the presence of hypertrophic bony spurs.

The second most common site for instrumental and foreign body perforations has been the lower esophagus immediately above the point where the esophagus narrows to pass through the diaphragmatic hiatus. The incidence of perforation at this level is further contributed to by the increased occurrence of disease and the frequent need for endoscopic manipulations in this region. Perforations of the middle third and abdominal part of the esophagus occur infrequently.

The mechanism of postemetic perforation of the lower esophagus has evoked considerable interest. Mackler has shown that the inflation of fresh human cadaver esophagus resulted in simple splitting when the pressure exceeded its circumferential tensile strength. In 95 percent of the 65 specimens studied, such tears occurred in the distal portion of esophagus. Duval, as cited by Kinsella and coworkers,

Fig. 25-29. Lateral roentgenogram of cervical part of spinal column 2 hours after instrumental perforation of the cervical part of the esophagus. Note anterior displacement of trachea by an anterior bulging of the retrovisceral space, emphysema in tissue planes, and hypertrophic bony spurs on lower cervical vertebrae. (*From F. H. Ellis, Jr., and W. S. Payne, Complications of Esophageal and Diaphragmatic Surgery, in C. P. Artz, and J. D. Hardy, "Complications in Surgery and Their Management," 2d ed., W. B. Saunders Company, Philadelphia, 1967.*)

demonstrated that the rapidity of the increase in pressure rather than the amount of pressure per se may be a critical factor in such injuries. The fact that most postemetic perforations occur in adults rather than in children may be explainable by the higher incidence of predisposing factors in adults and especially by the fact that the strength of the esophagus is thirteen times greater in infants (less than one year old) and four times greater in children (less than twelve years old) than it is in adults.

PATHOPHYSIOLOGY. The consequences of esophageal perforation are due to contamination of periesophageal spaces with corrosive digestive fluids, food, and bacteria, which leads to a diffuse cellulitis with localized or extensive suppuration.

Anatomic considerations are important, both in the evolution of signs and symptoms and in treatment. The majority of cervical esophageal perforations are posterior and result in suppuration first in the retrovesical space and then extending along fascial planes into the mediastinum.

Perforations of the anterior wall of the cervical esophagus and those involving the lateral pharyngeal spaces and pyriform fossae enter the pretracheal space. The pretracheal space communicates with the mediastinum via the fascial attachment to the pericardium. The manifestations of perforation depend on the relation of the esophagus to the contiguous spaces. The upper two-thirds of the thoracic esophagus is in close proximity to the right pleural cavity. In its lower third, the esophagus lies adjacent to the left pleural space. In rare cases, the intraabdominal or subphrenic esophagus may be perforated, leading to peritonitis and intraabdominal abscess.

Although the perforation need not be extensive or impressive to produce marked local or systemic reaction, the consequent sequestration of body fluids in the adjacent spaces may add hypovolemia to bacteremic shock. In addition, the accumulation of fluid and leakage of free air from the perforated hollow viscus may significantly interfere with normal cardiorespiratory dynamics.

CLINICAL MANIFESTATIONS. The diagnosis of esophageal perforation depends on an awareness of the circumstances in which it may occur, the patient's symptoms, the presence of physical signs, and the demonstration of the perforation and its secondary manifestations by roentgenography.

Although the symptoms of perforation depend to a large degree on its site and the extent of inflammatory reaction, pain, fever, and dysphagia are the most frequent early complaints. Dyspnea is usually related to pleural space involvement, with or without pneumothorax. Cervical tenderness is an early and constant feature of cervical esophageal perforation. Cervical crepitation may be minimal but is an almost constant finding.

The physical findings with thoracic esophageal perforation are usually limited to the thorax; cervical crepitation may be a feature, but there is usually no cervical tenderness. Auscultation over the heart may elicit signs of mediastinal emphysema (Hamman's sign). Cardiorespiratory embarrassment with shock and cyanosis is more commonly seen early with thoracic and subphrenic esophageal perforations but may not be apparent until a late stage.

Roentgenographic studies are of great assistance in diagnosis. Anterior, posterior, and lateral views of the cervical part of the spinal column often demonstrate pathognomonic signs of cervical perforation (Fig. 25-29). Anterior displacement of the trachea, widening of the retrovisceral space, air in tissue spaces, and occasionally widening of the superior mediastinum are seen. Widening of the superior mediastinum is a common sign in perforation of the cervical or upper thoracic part of the esophagus. Mediastinal emphysema and pleural effusion with or without pneumothorax may be present with thoracic or subphrenic esophageal injuries. Studies with opaque medium are occasionally indicated to localize the site or sites of perforation and to detect associated abnormalities (Fig. 25-30). The medium should be nonirritating and, preferably, absorbable. Endoscopic procedures are rarely indicated in the diagnosis of esophageal perforations except when a foreign body is present.

TREATMENT. While there is wide agreement that most perforations of the esophagus are best treated by immediate surgical exploration, repair if necessary, and drainage, this is neither universally accepted nor always feasible. Parenteral antibiotic therapy plus parenteral fluid and electrolyte correction and support are appropriate measures for all patients with esophageal injury.

Simple surgical exploration and drainage of the retrovisceral space or, on rare occasions, of the pretracheal space is the treatment of choice for cervical esophageal perforations (Fig. 25-31). Suppuration extending as low as the fourth vertebra can be evacuated effectively by this route. The usually encountered early perforation may be small, and the inflammatory reaction may be slight; however, major lacerations occasionally are present and require suture closure, with drainage of considerable retrovisceral and mediastinal collections.

Instrumental and noninstrumental perforations of the thoracic and subphrenic parts of the esophagus are often large and require surgical exploration, repair, and drainage. The upper two-thirds of the esophagus is best approached transpleurally through a right midthoracotomy and the lower third through a lower left thoracotomy. The rare subphrenic lacerations are best explored transabdominally. Gastric decompression, either by nasogastric tube or, rarely, by gastrostomy, is indicated. On occasion, resection of the perforated region and associated esophageal lesion is required.

Late localized cervical and mediastinal abscesses are uncommon complications after adequate early surgical treatment of perforations. When present, they can be drained either by cervical mediastinotomy (Fig. 25-31) or,

Fig. 25-30. Extravasation of ingested contrast medium into neck and superior mediastinum, pathognomonic of cervical esophageal perforation. Note failure of distal part of esophagus to fill. (*From F. H. Ellis, Jr., and W. S. Payne, Complications of Esophageal and Diaphragmatic Surgery, in C. P. Artz, and J. D. Hardy, "Complications in Surgery and Their Management," 2d ed., W. B. Saunders Company, Philadelphia, 1967.*)

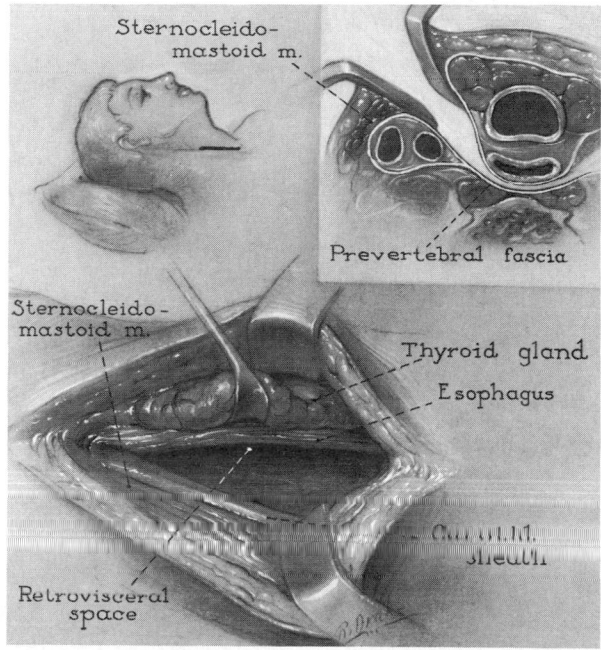

Fig. 25-31. Technique of cervical mediastinotomy. Upper left: Placement of skin incision in lower part of neck. Upper right: Incision is carried deep and mediad, with retraction of sternomastoid muscle and carotid artery laterally and trachea and thyroid mediad. Below: Note accessibility of pretracheal space. Collections as low as fourth thoracic vertebra are adequately drained through such an incision. (*From W. D. Seybold, M. A. Johnson, III, and W. V. Leary, Perforation of the Esophagus. An Analysis of 50 Cases and an Account of Experimental Studies, Surg Clin North Am, August, 1950, pp. 1155–1183.*)

Fig. 25-32. Posteroinferior mediastinotomy. This may be required for extrapleural drainage of a mediastinal abscess. (*From W. D. Seybold, M. A. Johnson, III, and W. V. Leary, Perforation of the Esophagus: An Analysis of 50 Cases and an Account of Experimental Studies, Surg Clin North Am, August, 1950, pp. 1155–1183.*)

if in the lower mediastinum, by posteroinferior mediastinotomy (Fig, 25-32). As a rule, the late development of empyema can be prevented by early and adequate closed intercostal-tube drainage of the pleural space. When empyema occurs, it usually responds to appropriate open or closed drainage; if it does not, thoracotomy may be required for pulmonary decortication.

Esophagopleural or esophagopleural-cutaneous fistulas may occur as a complication of any esophageal perforation. If the esophagus is not obstructed distad and good drainage is provided, such fistulas invariably close with time, provided that no local infection, foreign body invasion, malignant change, or epithelization of the tract is involved. When there is an esophageal fistula, it is best to seek out and treat any factors which may contribute to chronicity. Generally, it is wise to carry out repeated esophageal dilation over a previously swallowed thread during the healing stage of such chronic fistulas, even if no obstruction is demonstrated. With healing, cicatricial narrowing may occur after any perforation.

Tuttle and Barrett stressed the nutritional aspects in cases of esophageal fistula and noted the difficulties attending long-term intravenous maintenance of patients after esophageal perforation. They stressed not only the desirability but also the feasibility of resuming early oral feeding, even in the presence of a fistula. In a series of late perforations treated by them, the excellent survival rate was attributed to a policy of early intensive effort to confine draining mediastinal abscesses and esophageal fistulas to a small, localized, basal empyema pocket. With this accomplished, a full diet was given by mouth. If the fistula is not too large, most of the food passes to nourish the patient, and adequate drainage provides egress for the remainder.

RESULTS. The results of the surgical treatment of esophageal perforation depend not only on the cause, site, and severity of the reaction but also, to a large extent, on the lapse of time between perforation and treatment and on the type of treatment.

The results of treatment of cervical esophageal perforations, regardless of cause, have been excellent with early cervical exploration and drainage. Even with major injuries with marked contamination and delayed treatment, the results of surgical management have been satisfactory. Although the incidence of complications, secondary procedures, prolonged hospitalization, and late sequelae has been greater in this latter group, the mortality has been negligible.

The results of treatment for perforations involving the thoracic and subphrenic esophagus have been less satisfactory. Delay in diagnosis and treatment beyond 18 hours appears to be a major factor contributing to morbidity and mortality. Recent reports of series of thoracic esophageal perforations mention mortalities in excess of 60 percent with the usual surgical methods in late perforation and between 10 and 30 percent with early treatment.

Not all surgeons agree with the operative management outlined. There are instances of cervical and of thoracic esophageal perforation (usually instrumental) in which it may be possible to use successfully a nonoperative management (parenteral fluids and antibiotics and intercostal tube drainage), because of a late and benign course, or the patient may refuse treatment by other means. Neuhof and Jemerin reported in 1943 that surgical drainage alone resulted in 60 percent survival, whereas conservative nonsurgical management resulted in 16 percent survival. A decade later, Seybold and coworkers and Weisel and Raine reported greatly reduced mortality with early suture closure and drainage of esophageal perforation.

The high mortality associated with late diagnosis and treatment of intrathoracic esophageal perforations has led to the development of a variety of alternative methods of management (Fig. 25-33) which are applicable under a variety of circumstances.

In addition to the multiple procedures illustrated (Fig. 25-33), there is a number of effective technical variants. Thus, in lieu of the gastric patch technique shown, diaphragmatic (Rao et al.), pericardial (Millard), intercostal (Dooling and Zick), and parietal pleural (Grillo and Wilkins) pedicles have been used with success to buttress or augment surgical repair of esophageal perforation. Variations on the esophageal exclusion described by Johnson et al. include the partial exclusion and diversion techniques

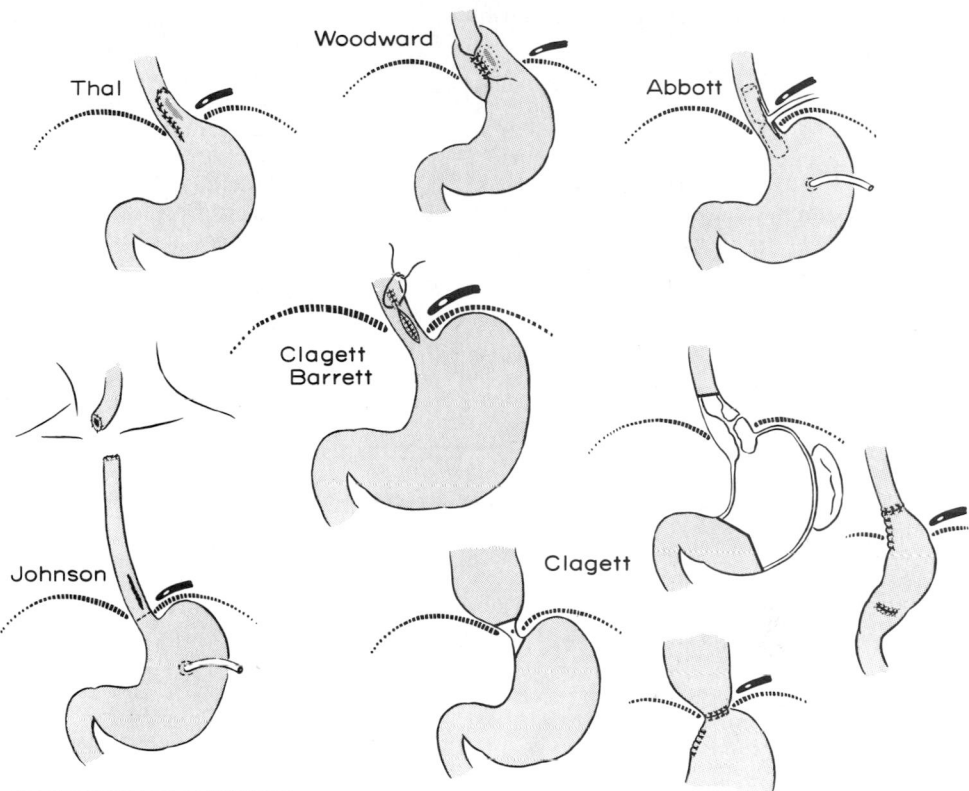

Fig. 25-33. Methods of managing distal esophageal perforations. *Clagett-Barrett:* In absence of delay or severe inflammation, it is usually possible to carry out a primary transthoracic layer closure of a distal esophageal tear with appropriate gastric and pleural space drainage. *Clagett:* In presence of associated cancer or other obstructive esophageal disease, some type of appropriate resection of lesions with esophagogastrostomy may be indicated, as shown by this procedure. *Thal:* Use of gastric fundus as patch for esophageal perforations. *Woodward:* Fundus completely wrapped around esophagus after insertion of fundal patch. *Johnson:* Complete defunctionalization of esophagus for late perforations by creation of proximal cervical esophagostomy, with closure of esophagus above and below. Colon interposition is employed after recovery to reestablish esophagogastric continuity. *Abbott:* Insertion of a Silastic T tube through an esophageal perforation with tube leading from esophagus to outside. With appropriate tube drainage of pleural space, T tube is removed after a few weeks, and resultant fistula closes spontaneously. Gastric decompression is an essential feature in all these repairs, and tube gastrostomy often is preferred. The proper placement of a double-lumen gastrostomy tube with one limb advanced through the pylorus to the jejunum while the other remains in the stomach may permit simultaneous tube feeding and gastric decompression during healing. (*From W. S. Payne and R. H. Larson, Acute Mediastinitis, Surg Clin North Am, 49:999–1009, 1969.*)

reported by Urschel et al. and by Menguy. It is, of course, impossible to prescribe a technique applicable to all thoracic esophageal perforations or even those of a given variety. It is essential however, to have a clear and concise understanding of the clinical problems and the rational application of multiple available techniques in planning the care of individual patients.

MALIGNANT TUMORS

Both benign and malignant tumors occur in the esophagus, but the vast majority are carcinomas which arise from the epithelial lining of the esophagus and cardia. While these are not the most commonly encountered visceral cancers, they are certainly among the most discouraging from the standpoint of control.

INCIDENCE AND ETIOLOGY. Carcinoma of the esophagus is predominantly a disease of males (male-to-female ratio, 3:1) between the ages of fifty and seventy years. The incidence varies widely throughout the world, being notably high in China, Japan, Scotland, Russia, and the Scandinavian countries. In South Africa incidence is high especially among the native Bantu. Although the basic cause of the disease is unknown, dietary and alcoholic habits, as well as tobacco use, have been implicated. A particularly high incidence has been reported in patients with achalasia and corrosive esophagitis. Joske and Benedict noted an unusually high incidence of cancer of the cervical esophagus in patients with Plummer-Vinson (Paterson-Kelly) syndrome. Other conditions associated with a high incidence of esophageal carcinoma include lye burns, diverticula of the esophagus, the columnar epithelial-lined lower esophagus of Barrett, and the syndrome known as tylosis palmaris et plantaris.

PATHOLOGY. Although almost all malignant tumors arising in the body of the esophagus are squamous cell carcinomas, most of those involving the esophagogastric

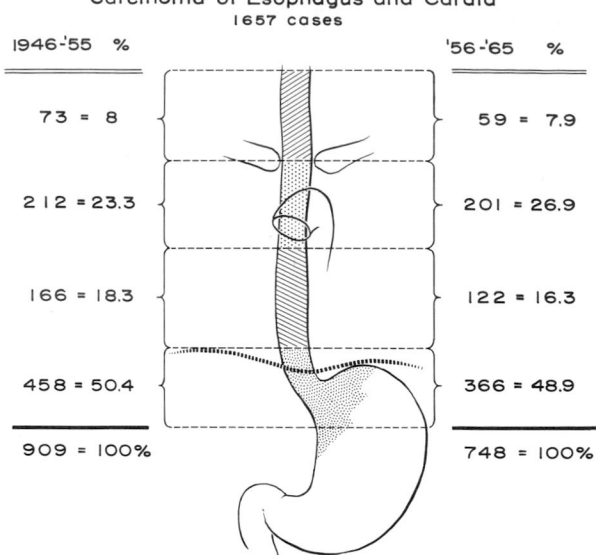

Carcinoma of Esophagus and Cardia
1657 cases

1946-'55	%		'56-'65	%
73 = 8			59 = 7.9	
212 = 23.3			201 = 26.9	
166 = 18.3			122 = 16.3	
458 = 50.4			366 = 48.9	
909 = 100%			748 = 100%	

Fig. 25-34. Distribution of 1,657 patients with carcinoma of the esophagus and cardia according to anatomic location. (*From G. H. Gunnlaugsson, A. R. Wychulis, C. Roland, and F. H. Ellis, Jr., Analysis of the Records of 1,657 Patients with Analysis of Carcinoma of the Esophagus and Cardia of the Stomach, Surg Gynecol Obstet, 130:997–1005, 1970. By permission of Surgery, Gynecology & Obstetrics.*)

junction are adenocarcinomas of gastric origin. Figure 25-34 shows the anatomic locations of 1,657 malignant lesions of the esophagus and cardia encountered at the Mayo Clinic from January 1946 through December 1965. It should be noted that almost as many tumors affected the cardia as affected the entire cervical and thoracic segments of the esophagus combined.

The remainder of the malignant tumors of the esophagus are rare sarcomas, mostly leiomyosarcomas. These are predominantly extramucosal, but in contrast to the benign leiomyomas, they tend to ulcerate and calcify. Carcinosarcoma is another uncommon malignant lesion of the esophagus; it is of interest because it appears to be associated with a better prognosis than other malignant neoplasms. Although melanoblasts have never been demonstrated in the human esophagus, there have been reports of primary malignant melanomas of the esophagus.

Some carcinomas develop as bulky, fungating, obstructive growths and others as superficially ulcerated, surface-spreading tumors producing little obstruction. These tumors spread via lymphatic vessels, by direct extension from the esophagus, and by vascular invasion. Tumors of the cervical esophagus disseminate through the lymphatic vessels to cervical nodes, particularly the anterior jugular and supraclavicular nodes. Those arising in the thoracic esophagus spread early to local mediastinal (peritracheal and esophageal) glands as well as supraclavicular and, occasionally, subdiaphragmatic nodes. Those occurring at the cardia may involve local mediastinal as well as subdiaphragmatic nodes. Metastasis through the bloodstream may produce liver, lung, or bone implants. Raven reported

that no lymph node metastases were present in 42 percent of cases in which autopsy was performed, but many of these cases showed extensive local infiltration of vital structures or distant spread which would have precluded complete removal.

CLINICAL MANIFESTATIONS. The earliest and almost constant feature of carcinoma of the esophagus is progressive dysphagia. Initially, it is noted with ingestion of solid foods, but ultimately, the swallowing of even liquids and saliva becomes difficult. Weight loss and weakness are the inevitable consequences of inanition. Aspiration pneumonitis is not infrequent as obstructive symptoms progress. The diagnosis of carcinoma of the esophagus can be made with a high degree of accuracy by the usual roentgenographic examination of the esophagus. This usually demonstrates an irregular, ragged mucosal pattern with annular luminal narrowing. Unlike the more chronic benign obstructive lesions, carcinoma usually is not associated with marked proximal dilatation of the esophagus.

Esophagoscopy should be performed in all patients suspected of having esophageal cancer, irrespective of the interpretation of the roentgenogram, both to establish a tissue diagnosis and to determine accurately the upper limit of the lesion. In lesions involving the upper esophagus, it is usually desirable to perform bronchoscopy to detect malignant involvement of the adjacent tracheobronchial tree. Cytologic study of smears made from suggestive lesions is a valuable diagnostic adjunct. Occasionally, study of esophageal motility may suggest malignant involvement, but this technique is of greater assistance in defining one of the more common motility disturbances as a cause for dysphagia. Occasionally surgical exploration is required to establish the presence or absence of malignant growth when results of diagnostic studies are not definitive.

A report from the Honan Province of China indicates that the application of special screening techniques to a high-risk population permits detection of carcinoma of the esophagus before symptoms develop and at a stage when nearly all cases are resectable, with more than a 70 percent chance of 5-year survival.

TREATMENT. There are only two methods of treatment which offer benefit to patients with carcinoma of the esophagus: surgical resection and irradiation. Neither of these methods is new; hence it is not surprising that there has been no recent notable improvement in survival statistics among patients with this condition.

Squamous cell carcinoma of the esophagus is a radiosensitive and theoretically radiocurable tumor. Unfortunately, although the primary lesion can be controlled, failures result from the presence of tumor outside the irradiated field, and few permanent cures are obtainable. Surgical resection, too, suffers from being a local form of therapy with a high incidence of failure from distant recurrences. Surgical ablation is more effective than radiotherapy in dealing with adenocarcinomas that occur around the distal esophagus and cardia. It is apparent that some form of systemic therapy is desperately needed to deal more effectively with the problem of esophageal malignancy. Combining surgical treatment and radiotherapy has been suggested as a possible means of improving the results of treatment. The main rationale for the use of radiotherapy before operation in a combined program is the local control of microscopic disease, particularly at the margins of the primary tumor and involved nodes. The suggestion also has been made that preoperative radiotherapy might convert a locally unresectable lesion to a resectable one. Unfortunately, existing data comparing different treatment modalities in esophageal carcinoma are far from conclusive. Many studies have been reported, but all of them compare different types of patients or different periods of time. None has been prospective or randomized to eliminate the effects of selection of patients. Thus Pearson's results with radiotherapy alone are far superior to any others yet reported with this method. Yet his report represents selected cases, since about half the patients who entered the study were unable to complete the planned treatment and were excluded from the final results. Furthermore, little emphasis has been placed on the complications of excessive radiotherapy, which, as shown in the series of some investigators, include radiation pneumonitis, myocardial injury, spinal cord injury, tracheoesophageal fistula, hemorrhage, and postradiation strictures.

Palliation in terms of relief of dysphagia is the goal of therapy for most patients; for the few with well-localized lesions there is the possibility of cure. Surgical resection is more effective than radiotherapy in relieving dysphagia (95 percent versus 20 percent) and in increasing mean survival time after treatment (11 months with surgery versus 5 months with radiotherapy).

Proponents of combined therapy cite the improved results in a recent decade compared to that of a previous era when combination therapy was not employed. Interpretation is rendered even more confusing by the fact that in at least one reported series only 25 percent of patients completed the combined protocol.

In a recent decade at the Mayo Clinic, 5-year survival with surgery alone improved 100 percent over that of an earlier period of similar duration simply as the result of increasing operability, higher resectability rates, and lowered hospital mortality.

It is our conclusion that cure is not generally obtainable for the majority of patients with cancer of the esophagus and cardia by currently available means, but that resection provides the most expedient and effective means of restoring function while retaining the possibility of cure. Radiotherapy should be reserved for lesions of the cervical portion of the esophagus that would require laryngectomy for removal. But here, too, the exact site and extent of invasion of the adjacent larynx, trachea, or hypopharynx may dictate palliation by combined or exclusively surgical means. Close collaboration between radiotherapist and esophageal and laryngeal surgeons is desirable. Certain lesions of the thoracic part of the esophagus that appear nonresectable may become resectable with radiotherapy.

In the interest of time, specifically the duration of the patient's disability, staged operations and time-consuming treatments should be minimized or avoided. Selection factors will continue to be used to define those patients who will derive the greatest benefit-to-risk ratio from treatment.

Indications and Preparation for Surgical Treatment. In general, the selection of patients for operation for carcinoma of the esophagus entails careful clinical evaluation to exclude those whose tumor has extended beyond the scope of total surgical excision. Patients with obvious distant metastasis or those showing obvious involvement of vital structures, such as heart, liver, trachea, or aorta, are not generally considered suitable candidates. Survival after incomplete excision under such circumstances usually is not long enough to justify the risk, discomfort, and expense of resective procedures, and other forms of palliation should be considered.

Because of the difficulty in accurately assessing the possibility of total excision of esophageal lesions prior to operation, alternative palliative procedures are not infrequently carried out after the extent of the lesion has been more accurately defined at the time of surgical exploration.

Before undergoing operation for the control of esophageal malignant growths, patients must be in satisfactory condition to tolerate the proposed procedure. Prolonged preoperative preparation usually is not justified, but efforts should be made to restore blood volume, fluid, and electrolyte balance. Swallowing may be temporarily improved by dilation over a thread as a guide. Oral alimentation is doubtless superior to intravenous, but preoperative feeding by gastrostomy or jejunostomy is rarely if ever indicated. It is reasonable to employ parenteral hyperalimentation in the severely nutritionally depleted patient before operation and to continue such nutritional support in the postoperative period until full oral intake is well established. However, operation should not be delayed in some vain hope of restoring body weight in a short time by this or any other means. At best it is aimed at minimizing further negative nitrogen balance in the early postoperative period. Associated pulmonary problems are frequent, particularly emphysema and bronchitis. Occasionally patients with obstructive carcinoma of the esophagus experience aspiration and subsequent suppurative pneumonitis, which should be resolved before definitive surgery.

Technique. The surgical procedure used in the treatment of carcinoma of the esophagus varies with the anatomic location of the tumor.

For carcinomas arising at or near the esophagogastric junction, esophagogastrectomy is usually used. At the Mayo Clinic, a technique similar to that described by Kirklin and Clagett is commonly used. The exposure obtained through a left thoracoabdominal incision (Fig. 25-35) usually permits wide resection of the distal esophagus and proximal part of the stomach, along with spleen, omentum, and regional nodes. When local extension demands it, portions of the pancreas, diaphragm, transverse mesocolon, and colon can be included in the en bloc resection. The point of gastric transection is selected to permit removal of most of the acid producing portion of the stomach. In creating a tubular gastric remnant or antrum for anastomosis to the esophagus, most of the lesser curvature, along with its lymph node–bearing tissue, is

Fig. 25-35. Esophagogastrectomy for lesions of distal esophagus and esophagogastric junction. *A.* Incision. *B.* Shading indicates tissue to be resected. *C.* Completed operation. Note gastric drainage procedure. *(From F. H. Ellis, Jr., Surgical Aspects of Malignant Lesions of the Esophagogastric Junction, in W. H. ReMine, J. T. Priestley, and J. Berkson, "Cancer of the Stomach," W. B. Saunders Company, Philadelphia, 1964, pp. 127–140.)*

excised. Esophagogastrectomy, as described, results in bilateral vagotomy. Gastric retention due to postvagotomy pylorospasm and gastric hypomotility may be minimized by pyloromyotomy or pyloroplasty. The avoidance of gastric retention is particularly desirable in patients in whom

Fig. 25-36. Esophagogastrectomy for lesions of lower and middle thirds of thoracic esophagus. *A.* Incision. Either thoracoabdominal incision or separate thoracic and abdominal incisions may be used. *B.* Shading indicates portion of esophagus to be resected. *C.* Completed operation with high intrathoracic anastomosis. Note gastric drainage procedure. *(From F. H. Ellis, Jr., Treatment of Carcinoma of the Esophagus and Cardia, Proc Staff Meetings Mayo Clin, 35:653–663, 1960.)*

the gastroesophageal sphincter mechanism is resected, because esophageal reflux occurs readily with its destruction. Bombeck and associates have suggested retention of sufficient stomach so that an end-to-side anastomosis between the esophagus and stomach can be effected and a valve-competent plication of stomach about the anastomosis can be developed. Some cardial cancers are found to involve the proximal portion of the stomach extensively, and these are best managed by total gastrectomy. Esophagointestinal continuity under these circumstances must be aimed at preventing reflux of erosive biliary and pancreatic secretions into the esophagus. Payne has found that a long-limb Roux en Y provides the best means of reconstruction to prevent this complication after total gastrectomy.

Although the majority of lesions in the lower half of the esophagus can be managed through a left thoracoabdominal incision, a right thoracotomy is preferred for excision of those lesions arising in the thoracic esophagus at sites above the cardia.

Reconstruction of esophagogastric continuity after resection for thoracic esophageal cancer again depends on the anatomic site of the lesion. For those resections involving the esophagus above the cardia but below the level of the azygos vein, the stomach may be brought into the thorax for anastomosis high in the thorax (Fig. 25-36). For resections for tumors at or above the level of the azygos vein, the colon may be interposed (Figs. 25-37 and 25-38). As with other procedures involving vagal resection, pyloromyotomy or pyloroplasty is a desirable adjunctive procedure.

Colon interposition can be accomplished with either the right or left half of the colon prepared on a pedicle of middle colic vessels. Since there appears to be no disadvantage to using an antiperistaltic segment of large bowel, the left colon is preferred because the length, lumen, and blood supply are more adequate and dependable. Belsey described the use of an isoperistaltic segment of left colon with an inferior mesenteric vascular pedicle.

The use of interposed colon has the advantage of a proximal cervical anastomosis, which, if anastomotic leakage should occur, is less dangerous. Such interposed large bowel may be passed from the abdomen to the neck, either subcutaneously through a presternal tunnel or retrosternally. Occasionally, the interposed colon can be placed in the posterior mediastinal bed of the resected esophagus. In recent years the stomach has gained increasing favor over the colon as the organ to be used to replace resected esophagus or to bypass an unresectable thoracic lesion. Griffen and associates favor a substernal reversed gastric tube of the Gavriliu type. Ong, Akiyama, Le Quesne, and their associates as well as others have favored bringing the gastric fundus to the neck for anastomosis either to the cervical esophagus or, after laryngectomy, to the pharynx. Sufficient length is available to bring the stomach either through the posterior mediastinal esophageal bed or substernally. Advantage over the colon is obvious since only one anastomosis is required.

Alternatives to the use of either colon or stomach after laryngopharyngocervical esophagectomy are locally developed pedicle skin grafts used to restore continuity between the pharynx and the thoracic esophagus. Wooky devised a unilateral, cervically based pedicle graft to create a skin-lined tube to bridge this defect. In more recent years, the medially based deltopectoral skin flap devised by Bakamjian has proved simpler and more reliable (Fig. 25-39).

Results. The results of surgical treatment of carcinoma of the esophagus depend largely on the anatomic site, extent, and type of the tumor. It is apparent from a 1970 review of patients treated at the Mayo Clinic (Table 25-2) that there was a significant increase in resection rates during the period when surgical techniques were being developed and standardized. The 3- and 5-year survival rates after resections for carcinoma at various sites in the esophagus and cardia during that period are shown in Table 25-3. The influence of cell type and of the lymph node metastasis on 5-year survival is clearly apparent on review of follow-up data on patients treated for cancer of the cardia (Table 25-4).

The reader is referred to the earlier section on treatment for a discussion of the results of other methods of definitive treatment.

Palliation. All too often, patients with cancer of the esophagus present with lesions which are not amenable to curative excision. Although malnutrition is related to inanition, patients with cancer of the esophagus cannot be made to live longer by establishing a means of feeding them. Furthermore, it appears that the greatest problem associated with high-grade obstructions of the esophagus is not inanition per se but the inability to cope with the normal salivary secretions, which tend to accumulate in the mouth and to be aspirated if the patient attempts to swallow them. Accordingly, gastrostomy or jejunostomy for feeding are rarely used in the management of these patients. Instead, methods which permit swallowing are preferred. Irradiation or simple bougienage or both may alleviate the esophageal obstruction temporarily in cases of frankly inoperable cancer. For patients found at opera-

Fig. 25-37. Esophagectomy with interposition of right colon. Procedure may be carried out in one or two stages. *A.* Incision. *B.* Shading indicates portion to be resected. *C.* Mobilization of right colon. *D.* Completed operation. (*From F. H. Ellis, Jr., Treatment of Carcinoma of the Esophagus and Cardia, Proc Staff Meetings Mayo Clin, 35:653–663, 1960.*)

Fig. 25-38. Esophagectomy with interposition of left colon. *A.* Incision. *B.* Shading indicates portion of esophagus to be resected. *C.* Mobilized portion of colon. *D.* Completed operation.

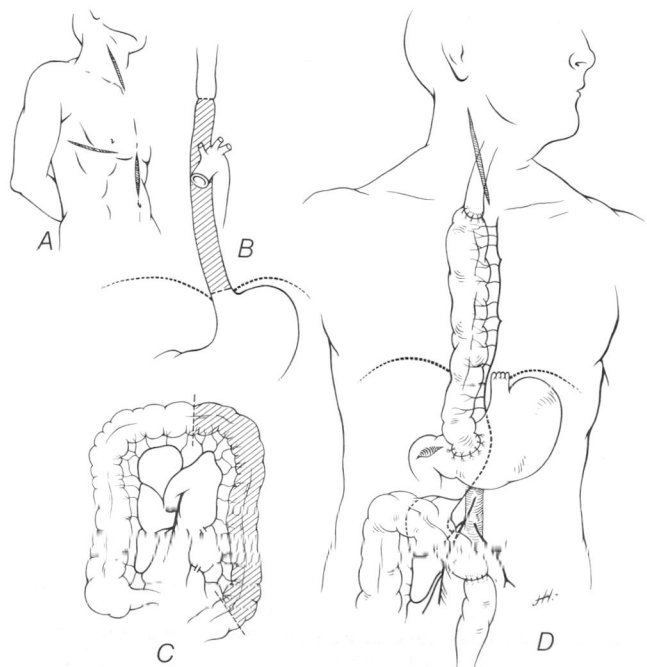

Table 25-2. OPERABILITY AND RESECTABILITY IN 1,657 PATIENTS WITH CARCINOMA OF ESOPHAGUS AND CARDIA

	Patients			
	1946–1955		*1956–1965*	
Operation	*No.*	*Percent*	*No.*	*Percent*
Resection	245	27	334	45
Exploration	169	19	165	22
None	495	54	249	33
Total	909	100	748	100
Hospital mortality after resection	39	16	39	12

SOURCE: Modified from G. H. Gunnlaugsson, A. R. Wychulis, C. Roland, and F. H. Ellis, Jr., Analysis of the Records of 1,657 Patients with Analysis of Carcinoma of the Esophagus and Cardia of the Stomach, *Surg Gynecol Obstet,* **130:**997–1005, 1970. By permission.

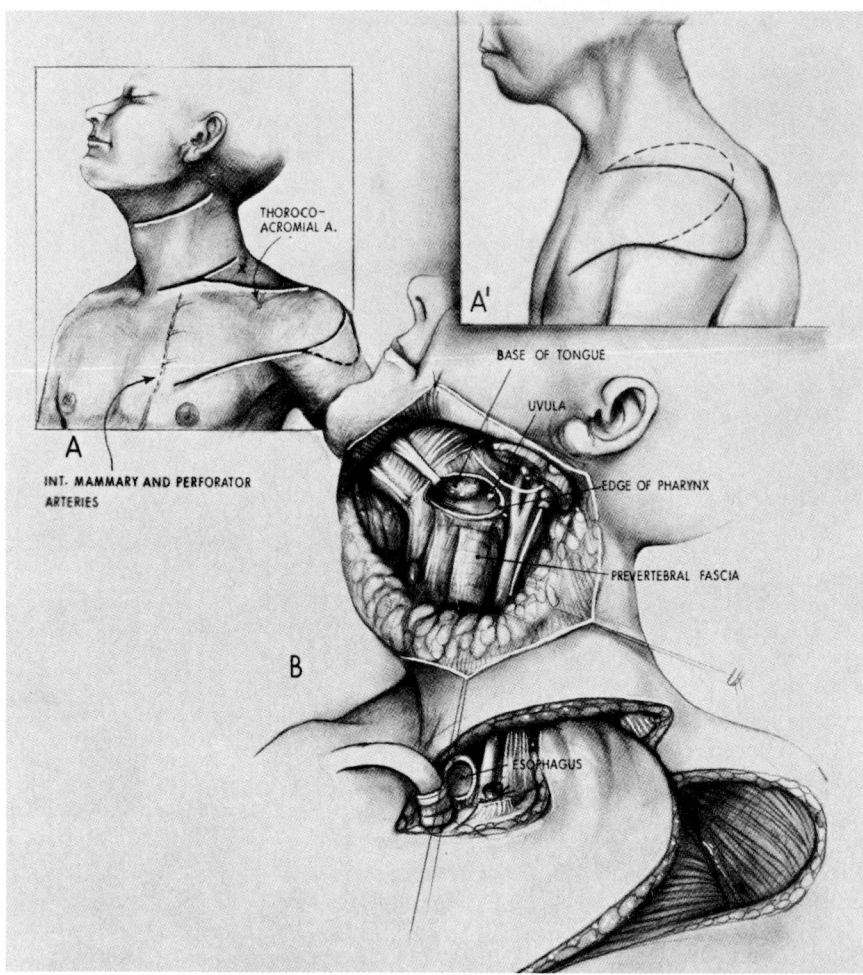

THOROCO-
ACROMIAL A.

A'

BASE OF TONGUE

UVULA

EDGE OF PHARYNX

PREVERTEBRAL FASCIA

A

INT. MAMMARY AND PERFORATOR
ARTERIES

B

ESOPHAGUS

Fig. 25-39. Bakamjian reconstruction of the pharynx and cervical esophagus after laryngectomy and radical neck dissection for pharyngoesophageal malignancy. A medially based deltopectoral skin flap is elevated, rotated, and folded into a tubular conduit between pharynx and esophagus, to which it is anastomosed. At a subsequent stage (not shown) the base of the pedicle is divided and the cervical fistula is closed. (*From J. M. Loré, Jr., "An Atlas of Head and Neck Surgery," vol 1, 2d ed., W. B. Saunders Company, Philadelphia, 1973.*)

tion to have nonexcisable lesions, a plastic tube may be inserted as a palliative measure. Satisfactory palliation occurs in the majority of patients in whom the Celestin tube is employed. Palliative intubation is particularly applicable in patients with obstructive lesions of the lower esophagus. The decision to bypass or exclude a nonresectable thoracic esophageal neoplasm must be decided on an individual basis. Certainly, the experience of Skinner and DeMeester with the Japanese extracorporeal esophagogastric tube suggests that esophageal exclusion can be made more tolerable without resorting to extensive surgical reconstruction. The suggestion of Orringer and Sloan and of Griffen and associates to employ stomach to restore swallowing in all patients with esophageal malignancy, though appealing, has not been widely applied.

BENIGN CYSTS AND TUMORS

Benign cysts and tumors of the esophagus are uncommon but are of clinical concern, not only because they must be differentiated from more serious conditions but also because on occasion they can produce significant clinical symptoms and even threaten life. More than half of

the 246 benign esophageal tumors and cysts seen at the Mayo Clinic before 1973 were surgically or endoscopically removed; the rest were encountered at autopsy (Table 25-5).

Leiomyomas are the most common benign tumors. Those less than 5 cm in diameter are rarely symptomatic. Most leiomyomas occur in the lower half of the esophagus, and the majority of these are extramucosal and can be treated by simple enucleation. Roentgenographic examination often suggests the diagnosis (Fig. 25-40). Those encountered in the region of the esophagogastric junction tend to be large, obstructive lesions and usually require esophagogastrectomy for successful removal.

Cysts are the second most common benign lesions of the esophagus. Most can be removed successfully by enucleation. Complete reduplication is extremely rare.

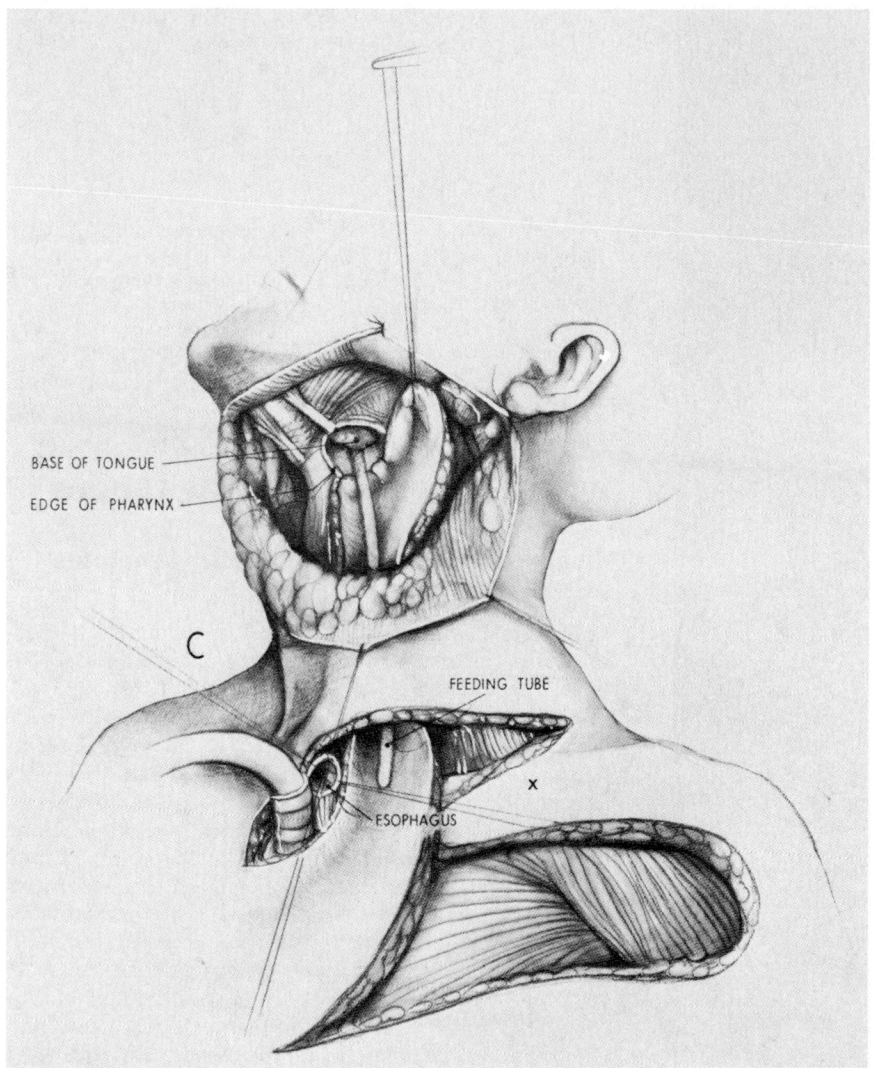

BASE OF TONGUE

EDGE OF PHARYNX

C

FEEDING TUBE

x

ESOPHAGUS

Fig. 25-39. Continued.

Table 25-3. SURVIVAL RATES FOR 3-YEAR AND 5-YEAR PERIODS
AFTER RESECTION FOR CARCINOMA OF THE ESOPHAGUS
AND CARDIA, MAYO CLINIC, 1946–1965

	3-year follow-up				5-year follow-up			
	Patients		Survival		Patients		Survival	
Site of resection	Total	Traced	No.	%	Total	Traced	No.	%
Esophagus:								
Cervical	17	17	3	18	13	15	1	7
Upper thoracic	103	94	17	18	86	82	7	9
Lower thoracic	92	90	30	33	82	79	21	27
Cardia.	367	358	76	21	322	315	40	13
Total	579	559	126	23	505	491	70	14

Fig. 25-40. Roentgenogram of esophagus, demonstrating presence of extramucosal filling defect which proved to be a leiomyoma that could be treated by simple enucleation.

A variety of polypoid intraesophageal tumors have been described, including mucosal polyps, chondromas, lipomas, fibrolipomas, and myxofibromas. The smaller lesions can be managed by endoscopic snare; others require esophagotomy for removal.

Table 25-4. 5-YEAR SURVIVAL RATES AFTER RESECTION FOR LESIONS INVOLVING THE ESOPHAGOGASTRIC JUNCTION, MAYO CLINIC, 1946–1963

Pathologic finding	No. of patients	Survival for 5 years or more after hospital dismissal*	
		No.	Percent
Squamous cell epithelium .	24	8	33.3
Negative lymph nodes . .	11	6	54.5
Positive lymph nodes . .	13	2	15.4
Adenocarcinoma.	238	31	13.0
Negative lymph nodes . .	67	18	26.9
Positive lymph nodes . .	171	13	7.6

*Based on traced patients; hospital deaths excluded in calculation of survival rates.
SOURCE: Data compiled from G. H. Gunnlaugsson, A. R. Wychulis, C. Roland, and F. H. Ellis, Jr., Analysis of the Records of 1,657 Patients with Analysis of Carcinoma of the Esophagus and Cardia of the Stomach, *Surg Gynecol Obstet*, **130**:997–1005, 1970.

Table 25-5. 246 BENIGN TUMORS AND CYSTS OF THE ESOPHAGUS SEEN AT THE MAYO CLINIC BEFORE 1973

Type	Total	Type	Total
Leiomyoma	145	Myxofibroma . . .	2
Cyst	55	Fibrolipoma . . .	2
Polyp	12	Neurofibroma . .	2
Papilloma	5	Fibroma	1
Lipoma	5	Lymphangioma .	1
Hemangioma	4	Mucocele	1
Adenoma	3	Duplication	1
Granular cell myoblastoma . .	3	Chondroma	1
Indeterminate	3		

MISCELLANEOUS ESOPHAGEAL LESIONS

Plummer-Vinson (Paterson-Kelly) Syndrome

In 1919, Paterson and Kelly independently described a clinical state with which the names of Plummer and Vinson later became associated in the United States. The typical patient is a middle-aged, edentulous woman with atrophic oral mucosa, spoon-shaped fingers with brittle nails, and a long-standing history of anemia and dysphagia. Because of the common finding of iron-deficiency anemia, the term *sideropenic dysphagia* has been used by some to describe the condition, which is more common in the Scandinavian countries than in the United States. The dysphagia is explained by the endoscopic and roentgenographic demonstration of a fibrous web partially obstructing the esophageal lumen in an eccentric fashion a few millimeters below the cricopharyngeus muscle. A dietary deficiency has been established as the cause, and the condition responds well to iron therapy and forceful dilation of the stricture. In approximately 10 percent of affected persons, a malignant lesion of the oral cavity, hypopharynx, or esophagus develops. The syndrome covers a broad spectrum of clinical entities, and not all patients exhibit hypochromic anemia, nor do they necessarily show evidence of malnutrition. Conversely, not all patients with the other clinical features of the Plummer-Vinson syndrome are found to have esophageal webs. Furthermore, some upper esophageal webs in younger patients who lack the clinical stigmata of the classic syndrome may have a congenital basis.

Lower Esophageal Ring

A ringlike constriction of the lower esophagus has been demonstrated roentgenographically by Schatzki and Gary in patients with hiatal hernia. The majority of patients in whom this abnormality is demonstrated are asymptomatic. However, some complain of dysphagia, and the symptom is directly related to the degree of narrowing produced by the ring. There is controversy as to the exact location of the narrowing, but most investigators believe it to be at the squamocolumnar mucosal junction. This abnormal roentgenographic finding has been related to the presence of a hypertonic inferior esophageal sphincter, an esophageal stricture, or the accordionlike or shortening effect on the esophagus of intrathoracic displacement of the esophagogastric junction in hiatal hernia. That it is truly an organic lesion is now generally accepted, although the cause remains obscure. Incision, resection, or partial excision of the ring should be done at the time of repair of the hiatal hernia in those patients with significant dysphagia not improved by dilation. The pathologic specimens from such procedures show little more than submucosal fibrosis.

Mallory-Weiss Syndrome

In 1929, Mallory and Weiss reported 15 cases of gastrointestinal bleeding after repeated emesis. Linear tears in the mucosa of the esophagogastric junction were demonstrated at postmortem examination in some of these patients. In subsequent years the condition has been noted more commonly and should be considered in the differential diagnosis of patients with unexplained hematemesis. The mechanism of the development of the lacerations is similar to that involved in the development of spontaneous rupture of the esophagus—namely, an explosive vomiting effort against a closed cardia or esophagus. A history of prolonged retching or vomiting, often but not always associated with alcoholism, is characteristic. Early diagnosis can be facilitated by roentgenographic studies to exclude the possibility of other lesions and by endoscopy to identify the site of bleeding. Bleeding may cease with conservative management, but surgical exploration may be required if it persists. The upper end of the stomach should be exposed through a long gastrotomy, and after manual evacuation of clots and the insertion of proper retractors for exposure, the lacerated areas should be repaired with sutures. Prompt arrest of bleeding can be expected with this technique.

Scleroderma and Related Diseases

Sometimes systemic diseases involve the esophagus, and scleroderma is probably the most common disease which gives rise to significant abnormalities of this organ. This disease affects the connective tissues of the body; when the esophagus becomes involved, the characteristic changes are fragmentation and homogenization of the submucosal connective tissue elements. The muscular layers usually are not involved. Motor failure of the esophagus is the characteristic finding on esophageal motility studies, and these findings may often precede the development of significant symptoms. When symptoms develop, dysphagia, regurgitation, and heartburn are common, and because the disease affects the inferior esophageal sphincter, gastroesophageal reflux with esophagitis may occur. At this stage of the disease, an antireflux operation such as the Nissen fundoplication may prove beneficial. As the disease process progresses, fibrosis and shortening of the esophagus ensue, with the development of a hiatal hernia. In advanced cases a stricture may be encountered, requiring forceful dilation for the relief of symptoms. The usual medical measures

to minimize the deleterious effects of gastroesophageal reflux should always be instituted. Resection of the strictured region may occasionally be required when dilation fails to relieve persistent dysphagia.

Dysphagia may occur in most of the so-called collagen diseases, but it is encountered most frequently in dermatomyositis, an incidence of 60 percent being reported by Donoghue and associates. A generalized muscular defect may be demonstrated by esophageal motility studies in patients with this disease. Weakness of the pharyngeal muscles predominates, but the abnormalities in the body of the esophagus resemble those seen in scleroderma. Usually, however, the integrity of the inferior sphincter is maintained. Remission of the disease may occur after administration of corticosteroids.

Neuromuscular Disturbances

Swallowing dysfunction is common in patients with neuromuscular disorders, and the details of these abnormalities can be demonstrated by esophageal motility studies. The most striking abnormalities can be seen in patients with disorders that are primarily myotonic in origin, such as myasthenia gravis and myotonia dystrophica. Rarely do esophageal motility studies give normal results in such patients. In myasthenia gravis, the amplitudes of the peristaltic waves are decreased, and they disappear in the lower esophagus during repetitive swallowing. Motor failure of the esophagus also occurs in myotonia dystrophica, a condition in which both smooth and striated muscles are affected.

A variety of nonspecific abnormalities may be seen in patients with central and peripheral neurologic disorders, usually involving changes in peristalsis. There may be an increase in the number of simultaneous waves, or esophageal spasm may be demonstrated. Some of these changes are seen even in patients with hemiplegia or Parkinson's disease. In amyotrophic lateral sclerosis, the most common finding is the occurrence of feeble peristaltic contractions in place of the vigorous contractions seen normally. Sometimes the contractions are simultaneous and may be repetitive; sphincteric changes are relatively less common. In multiple sclerosis, a variety of abnormalities may be noted, including poor relaxation of the pharyngoesophageal or gastroesophageal sphincter, simultaneous deglutition waves, incoordination of swallowing complexes, and diffuse spasm of the esophagus. Cricopharyngeal dysfunction has been implicated in the genesis of certain cervical dysphagia syndromes seen in a variety of neurologic conditions, especially bulbar poliomyelitis and amyotrophic lateral sclerosis, or after radical oral laryngeal surgery. The exact mechanism of dysphagia awaits clarification, but cricopharyngeal myotomy provides relief in properly selected patients. A similar problem has been described by Henderson and associates in patients with peripheral unilateral recurrent laryngeal nerve paralysis and in patients with gastroesophageal reflux. In classic idiopathic globus sensation, long thought to be a subjective emotional problem, there is demonstrable hypertonicity of the upper esophageal sphincter. The physiologic studies of Winans are particularly pertinent in interpreting reported observations in pharyngoesophageal function.

Acquired Fistulas

Occasionally, a fistulous communication requiring treatment may develop between the esophagus and the lower part of the respiratory tract. Other potential sites of fistulous communication include the aorta, the vena cava, and the heart. The commonest cause of acquired fistula is malignancy and usually represents a preterminal event in the course of incurable carcinoma of the esophagus, the lungs, or the neck structures.

Typically, a fistula between the esophagus and the tracheobronchial tree produces cough on eating or drinking, although it may present more subtly, with pulmonary symptoms alone. The basic principles of surgical treatment include division of the fistulous tract and suture closure of the defect in the esophagus and respiratory tree, with the interposition of viable tissue to prevent recurrence. Additionally, distal esophageal obstruction should be corrected.

The management of congenital tracheoesophageal fistula with and without atresia is discussed in the chapter dealing with pediatric surgery.

OTHER DIAPHRAGMATIC HERNIAS AND CONDITIONS

Although esophageal hiatal hernias are the most common type of diaphragmatic defect, a variety of other congenital and acquired defects and abnormalities may affect this structure and may cause considerable disability or even death unless promptly recognized and appropriately managed.

Posterolateral (Foramen of Bochdalek) Hernias

Congenital hernias through the posterolateral aspect of the diaphragm (pleuroperitoneal canal, or foramen of Bochdalek) are the most common diaphragmatic hernias in infants. This hernia often presents as an acute respiratory emergency at or shortly after birth, depending on the amount of herniated abdominal viscera present in the thorax. Rarely, such defects remain undetected until later childhood.

PATHOLOGY. The normal diaphragm results from the fusion of several anlagen, which completes the separation of the thoracic and abdominal cavities. Essentially, this type of hernia is thought to develop as the result of a failure, on either side, of complete fusion of the pleuroperitoneal folds during the first trimester of gestation. Normally the posterior portion of this embryonic membrane is the last to close; it is known as the *pleuroperitoneal canal,* or *foramen of Bochdalek.*

Initially the pleuroperitoneal folds consist of membranous pleura and peritoneum, between which later grow muscle fibers derived from cervical myotomes. Thus it may

be postulated that a foramen of Bochdalek hernia may or may not have a hernial sac, depending on whether the failure of fusion occurs during the late or the initial stage of development. Usually, however, the defect results in a primary failure of the membranous anlage, which results in a muscular defect without a sac. The fact that the left diaphragmatic anlage evolves more slowly than the right might account for the higher incidence of left-sided hernias.

The consequences of such a hernia depend on the mass of abdominal viscera that herniates into the thorax. Although severe respiratory insufficiency may be apparent at birth, an infant may appear to be normal initially and may not have symptoms until the ingestion of air and food causes distension of the herniated hollow viscera. Labored respiration with associated negative intrathoracic pressures may further increase the mass of herniated abdominal organs in the chest.

Usually, prolonged residence of abdominal viscera in the thorax during embryonic development results in severe hypoplasia of the lung on the affected side. Furthermore, the displacement of abdominal viscera into the thorax may result in an abdominal cavity that is too small to accommodate these normal structures. Finally, not uncommon concomitant abnormalities of gastrointestinal rotation and attachment, which may be associated with peritoneal bands, may affect intestinal patency or predispose to a volvulus.

CLINICAL MANIFESTATIONS. Usually, an infant with foramen of Bochdalek hernia presents in a state of acute respiratory emergency, with cyanosis and greatly increased respiratory rate and effort. The affected hemithorax is usually dull on percussion, and there is evidence of shift of mediastinal structures to the opposite side. The diagnosis is almost always apparent on standard roentgenograms of the thorax, which often clearly demonstrate gas-filled intestines. In rare cases, it is difficult to differentiate this process from various inflammatory conditions of the lung, enterogenous cysts, duplications, pneumothorax, lobar emphysema, or other anomalies. Under such circumstances, it is desirable to have the infant ingest an appropriate nonirritating contrast medium.

TREATMENT. Because of the severe, life-threatening respiratory distress associated with this condition, immediate surgical repair is indicated on an emergency basis. The passage of a small catheter into the stomach for decompression may provide temporary improvement and, more important, may prevent progressive distension. Accidental contamination of the respiratory tract may be minimized by keeping the infant in an upright position. A high-oxygen atmosphere may decrease respiratory distress and cyanosis.

Usually, not enough time has elapsed since birth for development of significant fluid and electrolyte problems, and little preoperative preparation is required except to provide an adequate intravenous route for administration of fluids. Peroral tracheal intubation for assisted ventilation may be necessary in severely ill infants.

Technique. Generally, the abdominal route is preferred

in the management of this type of hernia. It provides easy access to the defect, and viscera are more easily reduced and do not interfere with repair when reduced. Furthermore, this route provides easy access for the assessment of associated gastrointestinal anomalies and satisfies the frequent need for the creation of a ventral hernia (to accommodate the reduced viscera) and for gastrostomy. The reduction of the hernial contents from the thorax is often facilitated by the insertion of a catheter or finger through the diaphragmatic defect from below to allow air to enter the thorax as the viscera are removed.

Although commonly of relatively large size, the defect usually can be closed primarily with interrupted nonabsorbable sutures. Occasionally such defects are so large that complete closure by direct suture is difficult or impossible. Under such circumstances it may be necessary to use a patch of plastic material to fill the defect. Rosenkrantz and Cotton have suggested obliterating large diaphragmatic defects by using a flap of innervated muscle, fascia, and peritoneum from the anterior abdominal wall.

A hernial sac should be carefully sought for and removed if present. Repair of the diaphragmatic defect without excision of the sac may result in the formation of an expanding cystic structure that may be as life-threatening as an unrepaired hernia. If such a cyst should develop, simple aspiration will prevent respiratory embarrassment until excision can be accomplished.

It is often tempting to try forceful reexpansion of the hypoplastic lung on the affected side. Such efforts are not only fruitless but may cause irreparable damage and intractable postoperative pulmonary edema. After the abdominal contents are reduced, it seems preferable to adjust intrapleural pressures on the affected side as the defect is closed. This naturally results in a pneumothorax, which will be resorbed as the hypoplastic lung matures and expands during the ensuing days or even months. Fluids may accumulate in the pleural space and may require aspiration.

The occurrence of severe respiratory distress or recurrence of the hernia in the postoperative period can be minimized by appropriate gastrointestinal decompression, usually by tube gastrostomy. Often it is difficult to replace gas-distended intestines in the abdomen, particularly in infants in whom marked distension of the intestine has been allowed to develop. Under such circumstances, attempts at evacuating the intestinal contents may not be adequate, and it may be necessary to create a ventral hernia to provide space for the viscera and to minimize both tension on the repair and dyspnea. When such a hernia is created, one of the difficult postoperative decisions may be the timing of its repair.

Results. In spite of all efforts, severe respiratory and metabolic acidosis may occur in the postoperative period, requiring assisted ventilation and administration of sodium bicarbonate. In any event, postoperative management should include a moist atmosphere high in oxygen, frequent turning of the patient, and aspiration of secretions. Feeding is started when intestinal activity returns. In infants, although recurrences are rare, mortality has ranged

from 12 to 30 percent. However, Cerilli has noted that when the diagnosis was made at the age of two to thirty days, the mortality rate was about one-third that in the immediate neonatal period.

Foramen of Morgagni Hernias

This type of hernia has been called *anterior diaphragmatic, parasternal,* or *retrosternal* hernia but is best known by the eponym *foramen of Morgagni hernia.* The exact cause is unknown. Although generally thought to be due to a congenital defect in the fusion of sternal and costal elements of the diaphragmatic anlage, it is an uncommon hernia in infants and children; the majority of defects are detected in adults.

CLINICAL MANIFESTATIONS. When these hernias occur in infants and children, the manifestations are cardiorespiratory distress and the usual findings associated with foramen of Bochdalek hernia, but the vast majority of Morgagni hernias are detected incidentally as asymptomatic anterior cardiophrenic masses on routine roentgenographic examination of the thorax of adults. Approximately 20 percent of patients have symptoms referable to the hernia; these are predominantly vague, nonspecific gastrointestinal complaints. Almost all these hernias have a hernial sac. Although most contain herniated omentum or colon, portions of liver, small bowel, and stomach have been encountered.

The diagnosis is often obvious on standard roentgenograms of the thorax: gas and fluid are seen in the herniated large bowel. On lateral or stereoscopic views of the thorax, the anterior cardiophrenic location is apparent. In some patients, examination of the colon and, less frequently, of the upper gastrointestinal tract with appropriate contrast medium will establish the nature of such a defect.

TREATMENT. When a definitive clinical diagnosis can be established, it is usually desirable, even in the absence of severe symptoms, to advise repair as an elective prophylactic procedure unless other conditions preclude operation. Under usual circumstances, the simplest and most direct approach is through an upper transabdominal incision (Fig. 25-41). This permits easy access to either a right- or left-sided hernia or to bilateral hernias. Viscera are easily reduced by traction from below. The peritoneal sac is easily excised and the defect readily closed by this route.

When a definitive preoperative diagnosis cannot be established and more serious disease cannot be excluded, the transthoracic approach is indicated. This approach is more difficult technically but affords a better opportunity to deal with other unsuspected pulmonary, diaphragmatic, or paramediastinal conditions that may occur in this region.

Eventration of the Diaphragm

Unilateral elevation of the diaphragm may be a congenital or an acquired abnormality and may be seen in patients of any age. It may occur as the result of anomalous development of the diaphragm or its innervation or as a

Fig. 25-41. Bilateral foramen of Morgagni hernia as seen at operation from abdominal approach. (*From T. P. Comer, and O. T. Clagett, Surgical Treatment of Hernia of the Foramen of Morgagni, J Thor Surg, 52:461, 1966.*)

result of injury, at birth or later, to the phrenic nerve and diaphragm. This process may affect a portion or all of the hemidiaphragm on one side. It may be impossible to differentiate certain elevations of the diaphragm from congenital hernias, particularly from foramen of Bochdalek hernias. Irrespective of cause, which usually cannot

Fig. 25-42. Diaphragmatic eventration and operative procedures available for its correction. (*From F. H. Ellis, Jr., Eventration: Unilateral Elevation of the Diaphragm, in L. M. Nyhus and H. N. Harkins, "Hernia," J. B. Lippincott Company, Philadelphia, 1964, pp. 554–565.*)

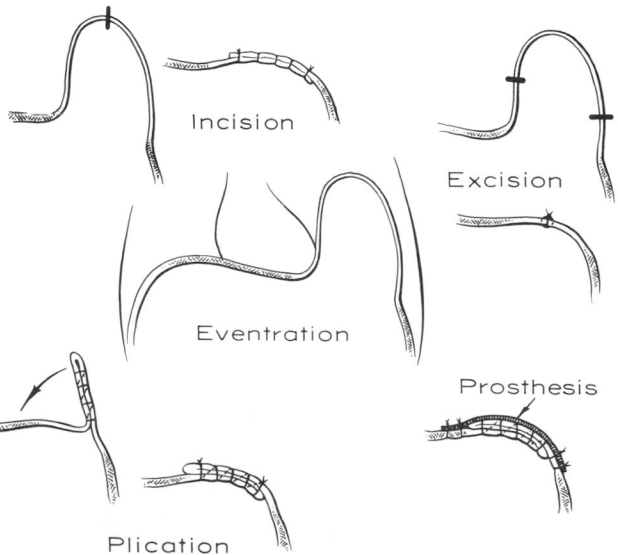

be established with certainty, such abnormalities of the diaphragm are of significance only when they are associated with symptoms or when they cannot be differentiated from more serious conditions.

CLINICAL MANIFESTATIONS. Eventration of the diaphragm causes symptoms as the result of interference with pulmonary ventilation. Typically, symptoms are encountered in infants and in old persons. When seen in the newborn, the symptoms and problems are identical to those of the massive congenital diaphragmatic hernias already described. In the fifth and sixth decades of life, when decreased cardiopulmonary reserve develops in combination with intraabdominal pressure secondary to obesity, digestive and respiratory symptoms related to this abnormality may appear for the first time.

TREATMENT. Prompt emergency treatment is indicated in the newborn infant who is dyspneic and cyanotic. Usually the transabdominal approach is preferred, for the reasons indicated for the repair of foramen of Morgagni hernias. Operation consists of imbrication of the eventrated leaf.

In patients of any age, and particularly in those in whom surgical treatment is contraindicated, if symptoms are not life-threatening, symptomatic palliation is indicated. These measures include restriction of activities, weight reduction, and avoidance of abdominal distension, lifting, or straining.

In older children and adults in whom symptoms are disabling, surgical treatment to restore the diaphragm to its normal position should be considered. Such procedures help to stabilize the mediastinum and permit more normal pulmonary ventilation. The procedure most commonly used is diaphragmatic plication (Fig. 25-42). In adults, the thoracic approach gives better exposure and greater ease of repair than the abdominal approach. When viscera are adherent to the undersurface of the diaphragm, a thoracoabdominal incision may be advantageous.

Rupture of the Diaphragm

Loss of anatomic continuity of the diaphragm may occur under a variety of circumstances and may permit the passage of abdominal contents into the pleural space.

The majority of such ruptures of the diaphragm occur as the result of severe blunt external trauma. Occasionally, some inflammatory process, such as a subphrenic abscess or empyema, will produce a diaphragmatic defect. Penetrating injuries, such as gunshot or stab wounds, are relatively infrequent causes of rupture of the diaphragm. Dehiscence of surgical incisions in the diaphragm may also result in hernia.

CLINICAL MANIFESTATIONS. Irrespective of cause, the majority of ruptures of the diaphragm are on the left, and the symptoms are almost invariably related to the type and amount of herniated abdominal viscera present in the thorax. Clinical manifestations vary from no symptoms to life-endangering problems immediately after injury. Late complications include gastrointestinal hemorrhage and obstructions. With massive herniation, rapidly progressive cardiorespiratory distress poses a life-threatening problem.

Extraneous shadows above the diaphragm, such as a gas-filled or homogeneous area, along with a shift of the mediastinum, are extremely suggestive of a ruptured diaphragm. Occasionally, roentgenographic examination of the gastrointestinal tract is required to establish a diagnosis. With massive herniation of the stomach into the thorax, the passage of a nasogastric tube both confirms the diagnosis and prevents progressive distension.

TREATMENT. Acutely traumatic diaphragmatic hernia is best managed via a transabdominal incision, since associated abdominal visceral injury is common and is best managed via abdominal exposure. Furthermore, acute herniation of abdominal viscera is not associated with adhesions to intrathoracic structures, and reduction is readily effected from below. Late operations are often difficult because of the presence of adhesions, and a transthoracic exploration provides the best exposure for their lysis in preparation for reduction and repair of the hernia. In either early or late intervention, primary suture repair of the diaphragmatic defect is usually possible, but on rare occasions adjacent tissue or even prosthetic material may be required for diaphragmatic closure.

References

General

Code, C. F., Creamer, B., Schlegel, J. F., Olsen, A. M., Donoghue, F. E., and Andersen, H. A.: "An Atlas of Esophageal Motility in Health and Disease," Charles C Thomas, Publisher, Springfield, Ill., 1958.

——— and Schlegel, J. F.: Motor Action of the Esophagus and Its Sphincters, in W. Heidel (ed.), "Handbook of Physiology," sec. 6: "Alimentary Canal," vol. 4, p. 1821, American Physiological Society, Washington, 1968.

Earlam, R.: "Clinical Tests of Oesophageal Function," Grune & Stratton, Inc., New York, 1975.

Ellis, F. H., Jr., and Olsen, A. M.: Achalasia of the Esophagus, *Major Probl Clin Surg,* **9:**1, 1969.

Henderson, R. D.: "Motor Disorders of the Esophagus," Williams & Wilkins Company, Baltimore, 1976.

Ingelfinger, F. J.: Esophageal Motility, *Physiol Rev,* **38:**533, 1958.

Marshall, S. F.: Carcinoma of the Esophagus: Successful Resection of Lower End of Esophagus with Reestablishment of Esophageal Gastric Continuity, *Surg Clin North Am,* **18:**643, 1938.

Ohsawa, T.: Surgery of the Oesophagus, *Arch Jap Chir,* **10:**605, 1933.

Payne, W. S., and Olsen, A. M.: "The Esophagus," Lea & Febiger, Philadelphia, 1974.

Postlethwait, R. W., and Sealy, W. C.: "Surgery of the Esophagus," Charles C Thomas, Publisher, Springfield, Ill., 1961.

Siewert, R., Blum, A. L., and Waldeck, F.: "Funktionsstörungen der Speiseröhre," Springer-Verlag KG, Berlin, 1976.

Skinner, D. B., Belsey, R. H. R., Hendrix, T. R., and Zuidema, G. D.: "Gastroesophageal Reflux and Hiatal Hernia," Little, Brown & Company, Boston, 1972.

Smith, R. A., and Smith, R. E.: "Surgery of the Oesophagus," Butterworth & Co. (Publishers) Ltd., London, 1972.

Vantrappen, G., and Hellemans, J.: "Diseases of the Esophagus," Springer-Verlag New York, Inc., New York, 1974.

Von Hacker, V., and Lotheissen, G.: "Chirurgie der Speiseröhre," vol. 34, Ferdinand Enke, Stuttgart, 1926.

Zaino, C., Jacobson, H. G., Lepow, H., and Ozturk, C. H.: "The Pharyngoesophageal Sphincter," Charles C Thomas, Publisher, Springfield, Ill., 1970.

Anatomy

Butler, H.: The Veins of the Oesophagus, *Thorax,* **6:**276, 1951.

Carey, J. M., and Hollinshead, W. H.: An Anatomic Study of the Esophageal Hiatus, *Surg Gynecol Obstet,* **100:**196, 1955.

Daniels, B. T.: The Phrenoesophageal Membrane, *Am J Surg,* **110:**814, 1965.

Hayward, J.: Phreno-oesophageal Ligament in Hiatal Hernia Repair, *Thorax,* **16:**41, 1961.

Higgs, B., Shorter, R. G., and Ellis, F. H., Jr.: A Study of the Anatomy of the Human Esophagus with Special Reference to the Gastroesophageal Sphincter, *J Surg Res,* **5:**503, 1965.

Laimer, E.: Beitrag zur Anatomie des Oesophagus, *Med Jahrb Wien,* 1883, p. 333.

Listerud, M. B., and Harkins, H. N.: Variations in the Muscular Anatomy of the Esophageal Hiatus: Based on Dissections of Two Hundred and Four Fresh Cadavers, *West J Surg,* **67:**110, 1959.

Swigart, L. L., Siekert, R. G., Hambley, W. C., and Anson, B. J.: The Esophageal Arteries: An Anatomic Study of 150 Specimens, *Surg Gynecol Obstet,* **90:**234, 1950.

Physiology

Botha, G. S. M.: Mucosal Folds at Cardia as a Component of the Gastro-oesophageal Closing Mechanism, *Br J Surg,* **45:**569, 1958.

Braasch, J. W., and Ellis, F. H., Jr.: The Gastroesophageal Sphincter Mechanism: An Experimental Study, *Surgery,* **39:**901, 1956.

Carveth, S. W., Schlegel, J. F., Code, C. F., and Ellis, F. H., Jr.: Esophageal Motility after Vagotomy, Phrenicotomy, Myotomy, and Myomectomy in Dogs, *Surg Gynecol Obstet,* **114:**31, 1962.

Castell, D. O., and Harris, L. D.: Hormonal Control of Gastroesophageal-Sphincter Strength, *N Engl J Med,* **282:**886, 1970.

———, and Levine, S. M.: Lower Esophageal Sphincter Response to Gastric Alkalinization: A New Mechanism for Treatment of Heartburn with Antacids, *Ann Intern Med,* **74:**223, 1971.

Code, C. F., Creamer, B., Schlegel, J. F., Olsen, A. M., Donoghue, F. E., and Andersen, H. A.: "An Atlas of Esophageal Motility in Health and Disease," Charles C Thomas, Publisher, Springfield, Ill., 1958.

———, and Schlegel, J. F.: The Physiologic Basis of Some Motor Disorders of the Oesophagus, in A. N. Smith, "Surgical Physiology of Gastrointestinal Tract," Royal College of Surgeons, Edinburgh, Scotland, 1963.

Cohen, S., and Lipshutz, W.: Anticholinergic Therapy: A Triple Threat to Lower Esophageal Sphincter Competence (Abstract), *Ann Intern Med,* **72:**792, 1970.

———, and ———: Hormonal Regulation of Human Lower Esophageal Sphincter Competence: Interaction of Gastrin and Secretin, *J Clin Invest,* **50:**449, 1971.

Dennish, G. W., and Castell, D. O.: Inhibitory Effect of Smoking on the Lower Esophageal Sphincter, *N Engl J Med,* **284:**1136, 1971.

Dillard, D. H., and Anderson, H. N.: A New Concept of the Mechanism of Sphincteric Failure in Sliding Esophageal Hiatal Hernia, *Surg Gynecol Obstet,* **122:**1030, 1966.

Goyal, R. K.: The Lower Esophageal Sphincter, *Viewpoints Dig Dis,* **8:**1, 1976.

Greenwood, R. K., Schlegel, J. F., Helm, W. J., and Code, C. F.: Pressure and Potential Difference Characteristics of Surgically Created Canine Hiatal Hernia, *Gastroenterology,* **48:**602, 1965.

Gryboski, J. D., Thayer, W. R., Jr., and Spiro, H. M.: Esophageal Motility in Infants and Children, *Pediatrics,* **31:**382, 1963.

Ingelfinger, F. I.: Esophageal Motility, *Physiol Rev,* **38:**533, 1958.

Lind, J. F., Crispin, J. S., and McIvor, D. K.: The Effect of Atropine on the Gastroesophageal Sphincter, *Can J Physiol Pharmacol,* **46:**233, 1968.

Mann, C. V., Ellis, F., H., Jr., Schlegel, J. F., and Code, C. F.: Abdominal Displacement of the Canine Gastroesophageal Sphincter, *Surg Gynecol Obstet,* **118:**1009, 1964.

———, Schlegel, J. F., Ellis, F. H., Jr., and Code, C. F.: Studies of the Isolated Gastroesophageal Sphincter, *Surg Forum,* **13:**248, 1962.

Meiss, J. H., Grindlay, J. H., and Ellis, F. H., Jr.: The Gastroesophageal Sphincter Mechanism: II. Further Experimental Studies in the Dog, *J Thorac Cardiovasc Surg,* **36:**156, 1958.

Vandertoll, D. J., Ellis, F. H., Jr., Schlegel, J. F., and Code, C. F.: An Experimental Study of the Role of Gastric and Esophageal Muscle in Gastroesophageal Competence, *Surg Gynecol Obstet,* **122:**579, 1966.

Esophageal Motility Disturbances

Barker, J. R., and Franklin, R. H.: Heller's Operation for Achalasia of the Cardia: A Study of the Early and Late Results, *Br J Surg,* **58:**466, 1971.

Benz, L. J., Hootkin, L. A., Margulies, S., Donner, M. W., Cauthorne, R. T., and Hendrix, T. R.: A Comparison of Clinical Measurements of Gastroesophageal Reflux, *Gastroenterology,* **62:**1, 1972.

Bombeck, C. T., Helfrich, G. B., and Nyhus, L. M.: Planning Surgery for Reflux Esophagitis and Hiatus Hernia, *Surg Clin North Am,* **50:**29, 1970.

Butin, J. W., Olsen, A. M., Moersch, H. J., and Code, C. F.: A Study of Esophageal Pressures in Normal Persons and Patients with Cardiospasm, *Gastroenterology,* **23:**278, 1953.

Butterfield, D. G., Struthers, J. E., Jr., and Showalter, J. P.: A Test of Gastroesophageal Sphincter Competence: The Common Cavity Test, *Am J Dig Dis,* **17:**415, 1972.

Cassella, R. R., Brown, A. L., Jr., Sayre, G. P., and Ellis, F. H., Jr.: Achalasia of the Esophagus: Pathologic and Etiologic Considerations, *Ann Surg,* **160:**474, 1964.

———, Ellis, F. H., Jr., and Brown, A. L., Jr.: Diffuse Spasm of the Lower Part of the Esophagus: Fine Structure of Esophageal Smooth Muscle and Nerve, *JAMA,* **191:**379, 1965.

Code, C. F., Schlegel, J. F., Kelley, M. L., Jr., Olsen, A. M., and Ellis, F. H., Jr.: Hypertensive Gastroesophageal Sphincter, *Proc Staff Meet Mayo Clin,* **35:**391, 1960.

Cohen, S., and Lipshutz, W.: Lower Esophageal Sphincter Dysfunction in Achalasia, *Gastroenterology,* **61:**814, 1971.

Creamer, B., Donoghue, F. E., and Code, C. F.: Pattern of Esophageal Motility in Diffuse Spasm, *Gastroenterology,* **34:**787, 1958.

Earlam, R. J., Ellis, F. H., Jr., and Nobrega, F. T.: Achalasia of the Esophagus in a Small Urban Community, *Mayo Clin Proc,* **44:**478, 1969.

Effler, D. B., Loop, F. D., Groves, L. K., and Favaloro, R. G.: Primary Surgical Treatment of Esophageal Achalasia, *Surg Gynecol Obstet,* **132:**1057, 1971.

Ellis, F. G.: The Natural History of Achalasia of the Cardia, *Proc R Soc Med,* **53:**663, 1960.

Ellis, F. H., Jr., Code, C. F., and Olsen, A. M.: Long Esophagomyotomy for Diffuse Spasm of the Esophagus and Hypertensive Gastroesophageal Sphincter, *Surgery,* **48:**155, 1960.

———, and Gibb, S. P.: Reoperation after Esophagomyotomy for Achalasia of the Esophagus, *Am J Surg,* **129:**407, 1975.

———, and Olsen, A. M.: Achalasia of the Esophagus, *Major Probl Clin Surg,* **9:**1, 1969.

———, and Payne, W. S.: Motility Disturbances of the Esophagus and Its Inferior Sphincter: Recent Surgical Advances, *Adv Surg,* **1:**179, 1965.

Ferguson, T. B., Woodbury, J. D., Roper, C. L., and Burford, T. H.: Giant Muscular Hypertrophy of the Esophagus, *Ann Thorac Surg,* **8:**209, 1969.

Flye, M. W., and Sealy, W. C.: Diffuse Spasm of the Esophagus, *Ann Thorac Surg,* **19:**677, 1975.

Grimes, O. F., Stephens, H. B., and Margulis, A. R.: Achalasia of the Esophagus, *Am J Surg,* **120:**198, 1970.

Heller, E.: Extramuköse Cardioplastik beim chronischen Cardiospasmus mit Dilatation des Oesophagus, *Mitt Grengeb Med Chir,* **27:**141, 1913.

———, ———, Schlegel, J. F., and Code, C. F.: Surgical Treatment of Esophageal Hypermotility Disturbances, *JAMA,* **188:**862, 1964.

Helsingen, N., Jr.: Oesophagitis following Total Gastrectomy: A Follow-up Study on 9 Patients 5 Years or More after Operation, *Acta Chir Scand,* **118:**190, 1960.

Henderson, R. D., Ho, C. S., and Davidson, J. W.: Primary Disordered Motor Activity of the Esophagus (Diffuse Spasm): Diagnosis and Treatment, *Ann Thorac Surg,* **18:**327, 1974.

———, and Rodney, K.: Tone of the Gastroesophageal Junction: Its Response to Abdominal Compression and to Swallowing, *Can J Surg,* **14:**328, 1971.

Hiebert, C. A.: Primary Incompetence of the Gastric Cardia, *Am J Surg,* **119:**365, 1970.

Higgs, B., Kerr, F. W. L., and Ellis, F. H., Jr.: The Experimental Production of Esophageal Achalasia by Electrolytic Lesions in the Medulla, *J Thorac Cardiovasc Surg,* **50:**613, 1965.

Ismail-Beigi, F., Horton, P. F., and Pope, C. E., II: Histological Consequences of Gastroesophageal Reflux in Man, *Gastroenterology,* **58:**163, 1970.

Jahadi, M. R., and Chandler, J. P.: Detecting Gastroesophageal Reflux by pH Recording and Acid Reflux Test, *Am Surg,* **38:**281, 1972.

Koberle, F.: Megaesophagus, *Gastroenterology,* **34:**460, 1958.

Lind, J. F., Cotton, D. J., Blanchard, R., Crispin, J. S., and Dimopolos, G. E.: Effect of Thoracic Displacement and Vagotomy on the Canine Gastroesophageal Junctional Zone, *Gastroenterology,* **56:**1078, 1969.

———, Warrian, W. G., and Wankling, W. J.: Responses of the Gastroesophageal Junctional Zone to Increases in Abdominal Pressure, *Can J Surg,* **9:**32, 1966.

Lipshutz, W. H., Gaskins, R. D., Lukash, W. M., and Sode, J.:

Pathogenesis of Lower-Esophageal–Sphincter Incompetence, *N Engl J Med,* **289:**182, 1973.

Lortat-Jacob, J.-L.: La Myomatose nodulaire diffuse de l'oesophage, *Acquis Med Recent,* 1950, p. 108.

Maillet, P., Micol, P., Parsal, J. P., Viard, H., and Favre, J.-P.: Les Résultats du traitement chirurgical du méga-oesophage (72 observations), *Ann Chir,* **27:**579, 1973.

Olsen, A. M., and Creamer, B.: Studies of Oesophageal Motility, with Special Reference to the Differential Diagnosis of Diffuse Spasm and Achalasia (Cardiospasm), *Thorax,* **12:**279, 1957.

————, Schlegel, J. F., and Payne, W. S.: The Hypotensive Gastroesophageal Sphincter, *Mayo Clin Proc,* **48:**165, 1973.

Patrick, D. L., Payne, W. S., Olsen, A. M., and Ellis, F. H., Jr.: Reoperation for Achalasia of the Esophagus, *Arch Surg,* **103:**122, 1971.

Peyton, M. D., Greenfield, L. J., and Elkins, R. C.: Combined Myotomy and Hiatal Herniorrhaphy: A New Approach to Achalasia, *Am J Surg,* **128:**786, 1974.

Pope, C. E., II: Pathophysiology and Diagnosis of Reflux Esophagitis, *Gastroenterology,* **70:**445, 1976.

Rapant, V., and Králik, J.: Die Problematik der Therapie der Achalasie der Speiseröhre, *Bruns Beitr Klin Chir,* **218:**12, 1970.

Sanderson, D. R., Ellis, F. H., Jr., Schlegel, J. F., Code, C. F., and Olsen, A. M.: "Syndrome of Vigorous Achalasia: Clinical and Physiologic Considerations," paper presented at meeting of American College of Chest Physicians, Chicago, June 23–27, 1966.

————, ————, and Olsen, A. M.: Achalasia of the Esophagus: Results of Therapy by Dilation, 1950–1967, *Chest,* **58:**116, 1970.

Skinner, D. B., and Booth, D. J.: Assessment of Distal Esophageal Function in Patients with Hiatal Hernia and/or Gastroesophageal Reflux, *Ann Surg,* **172:**627, 1970.

Windsor, C. W. O.: Gastro-oesophageal Reflux after Partial Gastrectomy, *Br Med J,* **2:**1233, 1964.

Diverticula

Allen, T. H., and Clagett, O. T.: Changing Concepts in the Surgical Treatment of Pulsion Diverticula of the Lower Esophagus, *J Thoracic Cardiovasc Surg,* **50:**455, 1965.

Belsey, R.: Functional Diseases of the Esophagus, *J Thorac Cardiovasc Surg,* **52:**164, 1966.

Clagett, O. T., and Payne, W. S.: Surgical Treatment of Pulsion Diverticula of the Hypopharynx: One-Stage Resection in 478 Cases, *Dis Chest,* **37:**257, 1960.

Cross, F. S., Johnson, G. F., and Gerein, A. N.: Esophageal Diverticula: Associated Neuromuscular Changes in the Esophagus, *Arch Surg,* **83:**525, 1961.

Dohlman, G., and Mattsson, O.: The Endoscopic Operation for Hypopharyngeal Diverticula: A Roentgencinematographic Study, *Arch Otolaryngol,* **71:**744, 1960.

Ellis, F. H., Jr., Schlegel, J. G., Lynch, V. P., and Payne, W. S.: Cricopharyngeal Myotomy for Pharyngoesophageal Diverticulum, *Ann Surg,* **170:**340, 1969.

Goodman, H. I., and Parnes, I. H.: Epiphrenic Diverticula of the Esophagus, *J Thorac Cardiovasc Surg,* **23:**145, 1952.

Habein, H. C., Jr., Kirklin, J. W., Clagett, O. T., and Moersch, H. J.: Surgical Treatment of Lower Esophageal Pulsion Diverticula, *Arch Surg,* **72:**1018, 1956.

————, Moersch, H. J., and Kirklin, J. W.: Diverticula of the

Lower Part of the Esophagus: A Clinical Study of 149 Nonsurgical Cases, *Arch Intern Med,* **97:**768, 1956.

Lahey, F. H., and Warren, K. W.: Esophageal Diverticula, *Surg Gynecol Obstet,* **98:**1, 1954.

Negus, V. E.: Pharyngeal Diverticula: Observations on Their Evolution and Treatment, *Br J Surg,* **38:**129, 1950.

Putney, F. J., and Clerf, L. H.: Epiphrenic Esophageal Diverticulum, *Ann Otol Rhinol Laryngol,* **62:**803, 1953.

Sutherland, H. D.: Cricopharyngeal Achalasia, *J Thorac Cardiovasc Surg,* **43:**114, 1962.

Vinson, P. P.: Diverticula of the Thoracic Portion of the Esophagus: Report of 42 Cases, *Arch Otolaryngol,* **19:**508, 1934.

Welsh, G. F., and Payne, W. S.: The Present Status of One-Stage Pharyngoesophageal Diverticulectomy, *Surg Clin North Am,* **53:**953, 1973.

Wychulis, A. R., Ellis, F. H., Jr., and Andersen, H. A.: Acquired Nonmalignant Esophagotracheobronchial Fistula: Report of 36 Cases, *JAMA,* **196:**117, 1966.

Esophageal Hiatal Hernia

Allison, P. R.: Reflux Esophagitis, Sliding Hiatal Hernia, and the Anatomy of Repair, *Surg Gynecol Obstet,* **92:**419, 1951.

Battle, W. S., Nyhus, L. M., and Bombeck, C. T.: Nissen Fundoplication and Esophagitis Secondary to Gastroesophageal Reflux, *Arch Surg,* **106:**588, 1973.

Behar, J., Sheahan, D. G., Biancani, P., Spiro, H. M., and Storer, E. H.: Medical and Surgical Management of Reflux Esophagitis: A 38-Month Report on a Prospective Clinical Trial, *N Engl J Med,* **293:**263, 1975.

Belsey, R.: Reconstruction of the Esophagus with Left Colon, *J Thorac Cardiovasc Surg,* **49:**33, 1965.

Bosher, L. H., Jr., Fishman, L., Webb, W. R., and Old, L., Jr.: Strangulated Diaphragmatic Hernia with Gangrene and Perforation of the Stomach, *Dis Chest,* **37:**504, 1960.

Bushkin, F. L., Neustein, C. L., Parker, T. H., and Woodward, E. R.: Nissen Fundoplication for Reflux Peptic Esophagitis, *Ann Surg,* **185:**672, 1977.

Cohen, S., and Harris, L. D.: Does Hiatus Hernia Affect Competence of the Gastroesophageal Sphincter? *N Engl J Med,* **284:**1053, 1971.

Collis, J. L.: An Appraisal of the Methods of Treating Hiatus Hernia and Its Complications, *Ann R Coll Surg Engl,* **46:**338, 1970.

Csendes, A., and Larrain, A.: Effect of Posterior Gastropexy on Gastroesophageal Sphincter Pressure and Symptomatic Reflux in Patients with Hiatal Hernia, *Gastroenterology,* **63:**19, 1972.

Culver, G. J., Pirson, H. S., and Bean, B. C.: Mechanism of Obstruction in Para-esophageal Diaphragmatic Hernias, *JAMA,* **181:**933, 1962.

DeMeester, T. R., Johnson, L. F., and Kent, A. H.: Evaluation of Current Operations for the Prevention of Gastroesophageal Reflux, *Ann Surg,* **180:**511, 1974.

DiMarino, A. J., Rosato, E., Rosato, E., and Cohen, S.: Improvement in Lower Esophageal Sphincter Pressure following Surgery for Complicated Gastroesophageal Reflux, *Ann Surg,* **181:**239, 1975.

Ellis, F. H., Jr., El-Kurd, M. F. A., and Gibb, S. P.: The Effect of Fundoplication on the Lower Esophageal Sphincter, *Surg Gynecol Obstet,* **143:**1, 1976.

Harrington, S. W.: Esophageal Hiatal Diaphragmatic Hernia, *Surg Gynecol Obstet,* **100:**277, 1955.

Hill, L. D.: An Effective Operation for Hiatal Hernia: An Eight Year Appraisal, *Ann Surg,* **166:**681, 1967.

————: Incarcerated Paraesophageal Hernia: A Surgical Emergency, *Am J Surg,* **126:**286, 1973.

————, and Tobias, J. A.: Paraesophageal Hernia, *Arch Surg,* **96:**735, 1968.

Leonardi, H. K., Lee, M. E., El-Kurd, M. F. A., and Ellis, F. H., Jr.: An Experimental Study of the Effectiveness of Various Anti-reflux Operations, *Ann Thorac Surg.* (In press.)

Lipshutz, W. H., Eckert, R. J., Gaskins, R. D., Blanton, D. E., and Lukash, W. M.: Normal Lower-Esophageal-Sphincter Function after Surgical Treatment of Gastroesophageal Reflux, *N Engl J Med,* **291:**1107, 1974.

Mobley, J. E., and Christensen, N. A.: Esophageal Hiatal Hernia: Prevalence, Diagnosis and Treatment in an American City of 30,000, *Gastroenterology,* **30:**1, 1956.

Nissen, R.: Eine einfache Operation zur Beeinflussung der Refluxoesophagitis, *Schweiz Med Wochenschr,* **86:**590, 1956.

Orringer, M. B., Skinner, D. B., and Belsey, R. H. R.: Long-Term Results of the Mark IV Operation for Hiatal Hernia and Analyses of Recurrences and Their Treatment, *J Thorac Cardiovasc Surg,* **63:**25, 1972.

Polk, H. C., Jr.: Fundoplication for Reflux Esophagitis: Misadventures with the Operation of Choice, *Ann Surg,* **183:**645, 1976.

————, and Zeppa, R.: Hiatal Hernia and Esophagitis: A Survey of Indications for Operation and Technic and Results of Fundoplication, *Ann Surg,* **173:**775, 1971.

Pridie, R. B.: Incidence and Coincidence of Hiatus Hernia, *Gut,* **7:**188, 1966.

Rex, J. C., Andersen, H. A., Bartholomew, L. G., and Cain, J. C.: Esophageal Hiatal Hernia: A Ten Year Study of Medically Treated Cases, *JAMA,* **178:**271, 1961.

Woodward, E. R., Thomas, H. F., and McAlhany, J. C.: Comparison of Crural Repair and Nissen Fundoplication in the Treatment of Esophageal Hiatus Hernia with Peptic Esophagitis, *Ann Surg,* **173:**782, 1971.

Complications of Gastroesophageal Reflux

Allison, P. R., and Johnstone, A. S.: The Oesophagus Lined with Gastric Mucous Membrane, *Thorax,* **8:**87, 1953.

Barrett, N. R.: Chronic Peptic Ulcer of the Oesophagus and "Oesophagitis," *Br J Surg,* **38:**175, 1950.

Behar, J., Biancani, P., and Sheahan, D. G.: Evaluation of Esophageal Tests in the Diagnosis of Reflux Esophagitis, *Gastroenterology,* **71:**9, 1976.

Benedict, E. B.: Esophageal Stenosis Caused by Peptic Esophagitis or Ulceration, *Surg Gynecol Obstet,* **122:**613, 1966.

Borrie, J., and Goldwater, L.: Columnar Cell-Lined Esophagus: Assessment of Etiology and Treatment; a 22 Year Experience, *J Thorac Cardiovasc Surg,* **71:**825, 1976.

Bremner, C. G., Lynch, V. P., and Ellis, F. H., Jr.: Barrett's Esophagus: Congenital or Acquired? An Experimental Study of Esophageal Mucosal Regeneration in the Dog, *Surgery,* **68:**209, 1970.

Bugden, W. F., and Delmonico, J. E., Jr.: Lower Esophageal Web, *J Thorac Cardiovasc Surg,* **31:**1, 1956.

Burgess, J. N., Payne, W. S., Andersen, H. A., Weiland, L. H., and Carlson, H. C.: Barrett Esophagus: The Columnar-Epithelial-Lined Lower Esophagus, *Mayo Clin Proc,* **46:**728, 1971.

Collis, J. L.: Gastroplasty, *Thorax,* **16:**197, 1961.

Gavriliu, D.: État actuel du procédé de reconstruction de l'oesophage par tube gastrique (138 malades opérés), *Ann Chir,* **19:**219, 1965.

Hawe, A., Payne, W. S., Weiland, L. H., and Fontana, R. S.: Adenocarcinoma in the Columnar Epithelial Lined Lower (Barrett) Oesophagus, *Thorax,* **28:**511, 1973.

Hill, L. D., Gelfand, M., and Bauermeister, D.: Simplified Management of Reflux Esophagitis with Stricture, *Ann Surg,* **172:**638, 1970.

Moersch, R. N., Ellis, F. H., Jr., and McDonald, J. R.: Pathologic Changes Occurring in Severe Reflux Esophagitis, *Surg Gynecol Obstet,* **108:**476, 1959.

Olsen, A. M., and Harrington, S. W.: Esophageal Hiatal Hernias of the Short Esophagus Type: Etiologic and Therapeutic Considerations, *J Thorac Cardiovasc Surg,* **17:**189, 1948.

Orringer, M. B., and Sloan, H.: Complications and Failings of the Combined Collis-Belsey Operation, *J Thorac Cardiovasc Surg.* (In press.)

Payne, W. S., Andersen, H. A., and Ellis, F. H., Jr.: Reappraisal of Esophagogastrectomy and Antral Excision in the Treatment of Short Esophagus, *Surgery,* **55:**344, 1964.

Pearson, F. G., and Henderson, R. D.: Long-Term Follow-up of Peptic Strictures Managed by Dilatation, Modified Collis Gastroplasty, and Belsey Hiatus Hernia Repair, *Surgery,* **80:**396, 1976.

————, Langer, B., and Henderson, R. D.: Gastroplasty and Belsey Hiatus Hernia Repair: An Operation for the Management of Peptic Stricture with Acquired Short Esophagus, *J Thorac Cardiovasc Surg,* **61:**50, 1971.

Radigan, L. R., Glover, J. L., Shipley, F. E., and Shoemaker, R. E.: Barrett Esophagus, *Arch Surg,* **112:**486, 1977.

Corrosive Esophagitis

Campbell, G. S., Burnett, H. F., Ransom, J. M., and Williams, G. D.: Treatment of Corrosive Burns of the Esophagus, *Arch Surg,* **112:**495, 1977.

Floberg, L. E., and Koch, H.: Effect of Cortisone on Scarification in Corrosive Lesions of Esophagus, *Acta Otolaryngol [Suppl.] (Stockh.),* **109:**33, 1953.

Ogura, J. H., Roper, C. L., and Burford, T. H.: Complete Functional Restitution of the Food Passages in Extensive Stenosing Caustic Burns, *J Thorac Cardiovasc Surg,* **42:**340, 1961.

Viscomi, G. J., Beekhuis, G. J., and Whitten, C. F.: An Evaluation of Early Esophagoscopy and Corticosteroid Therapy in the Management of Corrosive Injury of the Esophagus, *J Pediatr,* **59:**356, 1961.

Yudin, S. S.: The Surgical Construction of 80 Cases of Artificial Esophagus, *Surg Gynecol Obstet,* **78:**561, 1944.

Esophageal Perforation

Abbott, O. A., Mansour, K. A., Logan, W. D., Jr., Hatches, C. R., Jr., and Symbas, P. N.: Atraumatic So-called "Spontaneous" Rupture of the Esophagus: A Review of 47 Personal Cases with Comments on a New Method of Surgical Therapy, *J Thorac Cardiovasc Surg,* **59:**67, 1970.

Barrett, N. R.: Report of a Case of Spontaneous Perforation of the Oesophagus Successfully Treated by Operation, *Br J Surg,* **35:**216, 1947.

Dooling, J. A., and Zick, H. R.: Closure of an Esophagopleural Fistula Using Onlay Intercostal Pedicle Graft, *Ann Thorac Surg,* **3:**553, 1967.

Grillo, H. C., and Wilkins, E. W., Jr.: Esophageal Repair following Late Diagnosis of Intrathoracic Perforation, *Ann Thorac Surg,* **20:**387, 1975.

Johnson, J., Schwegman, C. W., and Kirby, C. K.: Esophageal Exclusion for Persistent Fistula following Spontaneous Rupture of the Esophagus, *J Thorac Cardiovasc Surg,* **32:**827, 1956.

Kinsella, T. J., Morse, R. W., and Hertzog, A. J.: Spontaneous Rupture of Esophagus, *J Thorac Cardiovasc Surg,* **17:**613, 1948.

McBurney, R. P., Kirklin, J. W., Hood, R. T., Jr., and Andersen, H. A.: One-Stage Esophagogastrectomy for Perforated Carcinoma in the Presence of Mediastinitis, *Proc Staff Meet Mayo Clin,* **28:**281, 1953.

Mackler, S. A.: Spontaneous Rupture of the Esophagus: An Experimental and Clinical Study, *Surg Gynecol Obstet,* **95:**345, 1952.

Mengoli, L. R., and Klassen, K. P.: Conservative Management of Esophageal Perforation, *Arch Surg,* **91:**238, 1965.

Menguy, R.: Near-Total Esophageal Exclusion by Cervical Esophagostomy and Tube Gastrostomy in the Management of Massive Esophageal Perforation: Report of a Case, *Ann Surg,* **173:**613, 1971.

Millard, A. H.: "Spontaneous" Perforation of the Oesophagus Treated by Utilization of a Pericardial Flap, *Br J Surg,* **58:**70, 1971.

Neuhof, H., and Jemerin, E. E.: "Acute Infections of the Mediastinum," The Williams & Wilkins Company, Baltimore, 1943.

Payne, W. S., and Larson, R. H.: Acute Mediastinitis, *Surg Clin North Am,* **49:**999, 1969.

Rao, K. V. S., Mir, M., and Cogbill, C. L.: Management of Perforations of the Thoracic Esophagus: A New Technic Utilizing a Pedicle Flap of Diaphragm, *Am J Surg,* **127:**609, 1974.

Seybold, W. D., Johnson, M. A., III, and Leary, W. V.: Perforation of the Esophagus: An Analysis of 50 Cases and an Account of Experimental Studies, *Surg Clin North Am,* **30:**1155, 1950.

Strauch, G. O., and Lynch, R. E.: Subphrenic Extrathoracic Rupture of the Esophagus: First Reported Case, *Ann Surg,* **161:**213, 1965.

Takaro, T., Walkup, H. E., and Okano, T.: Esophagopleural Fistula as a Complication of Thoracic Surgery, *J Thorac Cardiovasc Surg,* **40:**179, 1960.

Thal, A. P.: A Unified Approach to Surgical Problems of the Esophagogastric Junction, *Ann Surg,* **168:**542, 1968.

Tuttle, W. M., and Barrett, R. J.: Late Esophageal Perforations, *Arch Surg,* **86:**695, 1963.

Urschel, H. C., Razzuk, M. A., Wood, R. E., Galbraith, N. F., and Paulson, D. L.: An Improved Surgical Technique for the Complicated Hiatal Hernia with Gastroesophageal Reflux, *Ann Thorac Surg,* **16:**443, 1973.

Weisel, W., and Raine, F.: Surgical Treatment of Traumatic Esophageal Perforation, *Surg Gynecol Obstet,* **94:**337, 1952.

Worman, L. W., Hurley, J. D., Pemberton, A. H., and Narodick,
B. G.: Rupture of the Esophagus from External Blunt Trauma, *Arch Surg,* **85:**333, 1962.

Wychulis, A. R., Fontana, R. S., and Payne, W. S.: Instrumental Perforations of the Esophagus, *Dis Chest,* **55:**184, 1969.

——, ——, and ——: Noninstrumental Perforations of the Esophagus, *Dis Chest,* **55:**190, 1969.

Malignant Tumors

Akakura, I., Nakamura, Y., Kakegawa, T., Nakayama, R., Watanabe, H., and Kakegawa, T.: Surgery of Carcinoma of the Esophagus with Preoperative Radiation, *Chest,* **57:**47, 1970.

Akiyama, H., and Hiyama, M.: A Simple Esophageal Bypass Operation by the High Gastric Division, *Surgery,* **75:**674, 1974.

——, ——, and Miyazono, H.: Total Esophageal Reconstruction after Extraction of the Esophagus, *Ann Surg,* **182:**547, 1975.

——, Sato, Y., and Takahashi, F.: Immediate Pharyngogastrostomy following Total Esophagectomy by Blunt Dissection, *Jap J Surg,* **1:**225, 1971.

Andersen, H. A., McDonald, J. R., and Olsen, A. M.: Cytologic Diagnosis of Carcinoma of the Esophagus and Cardia of the Stomach, *Proc Staff Meet Mayo Clin,* **24:**245, 1949.

Bakamjian, V. Y.: Total Reconstruction of Pharynx with Medially Based Deltopectoral Skin Flap, *NY State J Med,* **68:**2771, 1968.

Bombeck, C. T., Coelho, R. G. P., and Nyhus, L. M.: Prevention of Gastroesophageal Reflux after Resection of the Lower Esophagus, *Surg Gynecol Obstet,* **130:**1035, 1970.

Clifton, E. E., Goodner, J. T., and Bronstein, E.: Preoperative Irradiation for Cancer of the Esophagus, *Cancer,* **13:**37, 1960.

Collis, J. L.: Surgical Treatment of Carcinoma of the Oesophagus and Cardia, *Br J Surg,* **58:**801, 1971.

Department of Surgery, Cancer Institute, Chinese Academy of Medical Sciences: Surgical Treatment of Carcinoma of Esophagus and Gastric Cardia: An Analysis of 1,432 Cases, *Chin Med J [Engl] n.s.,* **1:**60, 1975.

Dickson, R. J.: Radiation Therapy in Carcinoma of the Esophagus: A Review, *Am J Med Sci,* **241:**662, 1961.

Duvoisin, G. E., Ellis, F. H., Jr., and Payne, W. S.: The Value of Palliative Prostheses in Malignant Lesions of the Esophagus, *Surg Clin North Am,* **47:**827, 1967.

Ellis, F. H., Jr., and Salzman, F. A.: Carcinoma of the Esophagus: Surgery versus Radiotherapy, *Postgrad Med,* **61:**167, 1977.

Farrell, K. H., Devine, K. D., Harrison, E. G., Jr., and Olsen, A. M.: Granular Cell Myoblastoma of the Esophagus: Incidence and Surgical Treatment, *Ann Otol Rhinol Laryngol,* **82:**784, 1973.

Garfinkle, J. M., and Cahan, W. G.: Primary Melanocarcinoma of the Esophagus, *Cancer,* **5:**921, 1952.

Gavriliu, D.: Aspects of Esophageal Surgery, *Curr Probl Surg,* **12:**36, 1975.

Griffen, W. O., Jr., Daugherty, M. E., McGee, E. M., and Utley, J. R.: Unified Approach to Carcinoma of the Esophagus, *Ann Surg,* **183:**511, 1976.

Gunnlaugsson, G. H., Wychulis, A. R., Roland, C., and Ellis, F. H., Jr.: Analysis of the Records of 1,657 Patients with Analysis of Carcinoma of the Esophagus and Cardia of the Stomach, *Surg Gynecol Obstet,* **130:**997, 1970.

Hawe, A., Payne, W. S., Weiland, L. H., and Fontana, R. S.: Adenocarcinoma in the Columnar Epithelial Lined Lower (Barrett) Oesophagus, *Thorax,* **28:**511, 1973.

Hughes, R. O., and Price, J.: Tylosis and Oesophageal Carcinoma (Letter to the Editor), *Br Med J,* **3:**111, 1971.

Inberg, M. V., Scheinin, T. M., Voutilainen, A., Havia, T., and Nikkanen, T. A. V.: Management of Oesophageal Carcinoma: A Report of 267 Cases, *Scand J Thorac Cardiovasc Surg,* **8:**220, 1974.

Joske, R. A., and Benedict, E. B.: The Role of Benign Esophageal Obstruction in the Development of Carcinoma of the Esophagus, *Gastroenterology,* **36:**749, 1959.

Kirklin, J. W., and Clagett, O. T.: Some Technical Aspects of Esophagogastrectomy for Carcinoma of the Lower Part of the Esophagus and Cardiac End of the Stomach, *Surg Clin North Am,* **31:**959, 1951.

Kiviranta, U. K.: Corrosion Carcinoma of the Esophagus: 381 Cases of Corrosion and Nine Cases of Corrosion Carcinoma, *Acta Otolaryngol (Stockh),* **42:**89, 1952.

Le Quesne, L. P., and Ranger, D.: Pharyngolaryngectomy, with Immediate Pharyngogastric Anastomosis, *Br J Surg,* **53:**105, 1966.

Leverment, J. N., and Milne, D. M.: Oesophagogastrectomy in the Treatment of Malignancy of the Thoracic Oesophagus and Cardia, *Br J Surg,* **61:**683, 1974.

Lewis, I.: The Surgical Treatment of Carcinoma of the Oesophagus: With Special Reference to a New Operation for Growths of the Middle Third, *Br J Surg,* **34:**18, 1946.

McKeown, K. C.: Trends in Oesophageal Resection for Carcinoma: With Special Reference to Total Oesophagectomy, *Ann R Coll Surg Engl,* **51:**213, 1972.

Manning, P. C., Jr., Beahrs, O. H., and Devine, K. D.: Pharyngoesophagoplasty: Interposition of Right Colon; Surgical Treatment of Six Cases of Cancer of the Hypopharynx and Upper Part of the Esophagus, *Arch Surg,* **88:**939, 1964.

Marks, R. D., Jr., Scruggs, H. J., and Wallace, K. M.: Preoperative Radiation Therapy for Carcinoma of the Esophagus, *Cancer,* **38:**84, 1976.

Nakayama, K.: Preoperative Irradiation in the Treatment of Patients with Carcinoma of the Oesophagus and of Some Other Sites, *Clin Radiol,* **15:**232, 1964.

Ong, G. B.: Resection and Reconstruction of the Oesophagus in Oesophageal Cancer, *J Jap Assoc Thorac Surg,* **22:**769, 1974.

Orringer, M. B., and Sloan, H.: Substernal Gastric Bypass of the Excluded Thoracic Esophagus for Palliation of Esophageal Carcinoma, *J Thorac Cardiovasc Surg,* **70:**836, 1975.

Parker, E. F., and Gregorie, H. B.: Carcinoma of the Esophagus: Long-Term Results, *JAMA,* **235:**1018, 1976.

———, ———, Arrants, J. E., and Ravenel, J. M.: Carcinoma of the Esophagus, *Ann Surg,* **171:**746, 1970.

Payne, W. S.: Esophageal Reflux Ulceration: Causes and Surgical Management, *Surg Clin North Am,* **51:**935, 1971.

———, and Bernatz, P. E.: One-Stage Resection and Reconstruction for Carcinoma of the Esophagogastric Junction, in R. L. Varco and J. P. Delaney, "Controversy in Surgery," W. B. Saunders Company, Philadelphia, 1976.

Pearson, J. G.: The Value of Radiotherapy in the Management of Esophageal Cancer, *Am J Roentgenol,* **105:**500, 1969.

People's Republic of China: Surgical Treatment of Cancer of the Esophagus in the County and Commune Hospitals in the Rural Regions (Abstract), *Bull Soc Int Chir,* **34:**281, 1975.

Raven, R. W.: Carcinoma of the Oesophagus: A Clinicopathological Study, *Br J Surg,* **36:**70, 1948.

Skinner, D. B., and DeMeester, T. R.: Permanent Extracorporeal Esophagogastric Tube for Esophageal Replacement, *Ann Thorac Surg,* **22:**107, 1976.

Talbert, J. L., and Cantrell, J. R.: Clinical and Pathologic Characteristics of Carcinosarcoma of the Esophagus, *J Thorac Cardiovasc Surg,* **45:**1, 1963.

Wilson, S. E., Plested, W. G., and Carey, J. S.: Esophagogastrectomy versus Radiation Therapy for Midesophageal Carcinoma, *Ann Thorac Surg,* **10:**195, 1970.

Wooky, H.: Cited by V. Y. Bakamjian, Total Reconstruction of Pharynx with Medially Based Deltopectoral Skin Flap, *NY State J Med,* **68:**2771, 1968.

Wychulis, A. R., Gunnlaugsson, G. H., and Clagett, O. T.: Carcinoma Occurring in Pharyngoesophageal Diverticulum: Report of Three Cases, *Surgery,* **66:**979, 1969.

———, Woolam, G. L., Andersen, H. A., and Ellis, F. H., Jr.: Achalasia and Carcinoma of the Esophagus, *JAMA,* **215:**1638, 1971.

Wynder, E. L., and Bross, I. J.: A Study of Etiological Factors in Cancer of the Esophagus, *Cancer,* **14:**389, 1961.

———, Hultberg, S., Jacobsson, F., and Bross, I. J.: Environmental Factors in Cancer of the Upper Alimentary Tract: A Swedish Study with Special Reference to Plummer-Vinson (Paterson-Kelly) Syndrome, *Cancer,* **10:**470, 1957.

———, and Mabuchi, K.: Etiological and Environmental Factors, *JAMA,* **226:**1546, 1973.

Benign Cysts and Tumors

Johnston, J. B., Clagett, O. T., and McDonald, J. R.: Smooth-Muscle Tumours of the Oesophagus, *Thorax,* **8:**251, 1953.

Moersch, H. J., and Harrington, S. W.: Benign Tumor of the Esophagus, *Ann Otol Rhinol Laryngol,* **53:**800, 1944.

Schmidt, H. W., Clagett, O. T., and Harrison, E. G., Jr.: Benign Tumors and Cysts of the Esophagus, *J Thorac Cardiovasc Surg,* **41:**717, 1961.

Miscellaneous Esophageal Lesions

Adler, R. H.: Congenital Esophageal Webs, *J Thorac Cardiovasc Surg,* **45:**175, 1963.

Creamer, B., Andersen, H. A., and Code, C. F.: Esophageal Motility in Patients with Scleroderma and Related Diseases, *Gastroenterologia,* **86:**763, 1956.

Daly, D. C., Code, C. F., and Andersen, H. A.: Disturbances of Swallowing and Esophageal Motility in Patients with Multiple Sclerosis, *Neurology* (Minneap.), **12:**250, 1962.

Donoghue, F. E., Winkelmann, R. K., and Moersch, H. J.: Esophageal Defects in Dermatomyositis, *Ann Otol Rhinol Laryngol,* **69:**1139, 1960.

Ellis, F. H., Jr.: Upper Esophageal Sphincter in Health and Disease, *Surg Clin North Am,* **51:**553, 1971.

Fisher, R. A., Ellison, G. W., Thayer, W. R., Spiro, H. M., and Glaser, G. H.: Esophageal Motility in Neuromuscular Disorders, *Ann Intern Med,* **63:**229, 1965.

Henderson, R. D., and Pearson, F. G.: Surgical Management of Esophageal Scleroderma, *J Thorac Cardiovasc Surg,* **66:**686, 1973.

————, Boszko, A., and vanNostrand, A. W. P.: Pharyngoesophageal Dysphagia and Recurrent Laryngeal Nerve Palsy, *J Thorac Cardiovasc Surg,* **68:**507, 1974.

————, Woolf, C., and Marryatt, G.: Pharyngoesophageal Dysphagia and Gastroesophageal Reflux, *Laryngoscope,* **86:**1531, 1976.

Kelley, M. L., Jr.: Dysphagia and Motor Failure of the Esophagus in Myotonia Dystrophica, *Neurology* (*Minneap*), **14:**955, 1964.

Kelly, A. B.: Spasm at the Entrance of the Oesophagus, *J Laryngol Otol,* **34:**285, 1919.

Lam, C. R., Taber, R. E., and Arciniegas, E.: The Nature and Surgical Treatment of Lower Esophageal Ring (Schatzki's Ring), *J Thorac Cardiovasc Surg,* **63:**34, 1972.

Mallory, G. K., and Weiss, S.: Hemorrhages from Lacerations of the Cardiac Orifice of the Stomach Due to Vomiting, *Am J Med Sci,* **178:**506, 1929.

Orringer, M. B., Dabich, L., Zarafonetis, C. J. D., and Sloan, H.: Gastroesophageal Reflux in Esophageal Scleroderma: Diagnosis and Implications, *Ann Thorac Surg,* **22:**120, 1976.

Palmer, E. D.: Disorders of the Cricopharyngeus Muscle: A Review, *Gastroenterology,* **71:**510, 1976.

Paterson, D. R.: A Clinical Type of Dysphagia, *J Laryngol Otol,* **34:**289, 1919.

Payne, W. S., and Olsen, A. M.: "The Esophagus," Lea & Febiger, Philadelphia. (In press.)

Schatzki, R., and Gary, J. E.: Dysphagia Due to a Diaphragm-like Localized Narrowing in the Lower Esophagus ("Lower Esophageal Ring"), *Am J Roentgenol,* **70:**911, 1953.

Smith, A. W. M., Mulder, D. W., and Code, C. F.: Esophageal Motility in Amyotrophic Lateral Sclerosis, *Proc Staff Meet Mayo Clin,* **32:**438, 1957.

Stiennon, O. A.: The Anatomic Basis for the Lower Esophageal Contraction Ring: Plication Theory and Its Applications, *Am J Roentgenol,* **90:**811, 1963.

Treacy, W. L., Baggenstoss, A. H., Slocumb, C. H., and Code, C. F.: Scleroderma of the Esophagus: A Correlation of Histologic and Physiologic Findings, *Ann Intern Med,* **59:**351, 1963.

Watson, W. C., and Sullivan, S. N.: Hypertonicity of the Cricopharyngeal Sphincter: A Cause of Globus Sensation, *Lancet,* **2:**1417, 1974.

Wesselhoeft, C. W., Jr., and Keshishian, J. M.: Acquired Nonmalignant Esophagotracheal and Esophagobronchial Fistulas, *Ann Thorac Surg,* **6:**187, 1968.

Wilkins, E. W., Jr., and Bartlett, M. K.: Surgical Treatment of the Lower Esophageal Ring, *N Engl J Med,* **268:**461, 1963.

Winans, C. S.: The Pharyngoesophageal Closure Mechanism: A Manometric Study, *Gastroenterology,* **63:**768, 1972.

Wychulis, A. R., Ellis, F. H., Jr., and Andersen, H. A.: Acquired Nonmalignant Esophagotracheobronchial Fistula: Report of 36 Cases, *JAMA,* **196:**117, 1966.

Other Diaphragmatic Hernias and Conditions

Beck, W. C., and Motsay, D. S.: Eventration of Diaphragm, *Arch Surg,* **65:**557, 1952.

Bernatz, P. E., Burnside, A. F., Jr., and Clagett, O. T.: Problem of the Ruptured Diaphragm, *JAMA,* **168:**877, 1958.

Butsch, W. L., and Leahy, L. J.: A Technique for the Surgical Treatment of Congenital Eventration of the Diaphragm in Infancy: Report of a Case, *J Thorac Cardiovasc Surg,* **20:**968, 1950.

Cerilli, G. J.: Foramen of Bochdalek Hernia: A Review of the Experience at Children's Hospital of Denver, Colorado, *Ann Surg,* **159:**385, 1964.

Chin, E. F., and Duchesne, E. R.: The Parasternal Defect, *Thorax,* **10:**214, 1955.

Comer, T. P., and Clagett, O. T.: Surgical Treatment of Hernia of the Foramen of Morgagni, *J Thorac Cardiovasc Surg,* **52:**461, 1966.

Effler, D. B.: Allison's Repair of Hiatal Hernia: Late Complication of Diaphragmatic Counterincision and Technique to Avoid It, *J Thorac Cardiovasc Surg,* **49:**669, 1965.

Gross, R. E.: "The Surgery of Infancy and Childhood: Its Principles and Techniques," W. B. Saunders Company, Philadelphia, 1953.

Kenigsberg, K., and Gwinn, J. L.: The Retained Sac in Repair of Posterolateral Diaphragmatic Hernia in the Newborn, *Surgery,* **57:**894, 1965.

Kiesewetter, W. B., Gutierrez, I. Z., and Sieber, W. K.: Diaphragmatic Hernia in Infants under One Year of Age, *Arch Surg,* **83:**561, 1961.

Nylander, P. E. A., and Elfving, G.: Partial Eventration of Diaphragm, *Ann Chir Gynaecol Fenn,* **40:**1, 1951.

Rosenkrantz, J. G., and Cotton, E. K.: Replacement of Left Hemidiaphragm by a Pedicled Abdominal Muscular Flap, *J Thorac Cardiovasc Surg,* **48:**912, 1964.

Snyder, W. H., Jr., and Greaney, E. M., Jr.: Congenital Diaphragmatic Hernia: 77 Consecutive Cases, *Surgery,* **57:**576, 1965.

Stomach

by **René B. Menguy**

ANATOMY

The J-shaped organ lies between the esophagus and the duodenum, separated from the former by a multicomponent sphincter mechanism and from the latter by the anatomically well-defined pyloric sphincter. The stomach is described as having two borders, or curvatures, known as the lesser and greater curvatures, and two surfaces, anterior and posterior. The two curvatures of the stomach are important surgically, because of their relation to the major vascular and lymphatic arcades of the stomach. The arterial arcade along the lesser curvature is supplied by the left gastric artery, which originates from the celiac axis and divides into the left gastric artery proper, or descending branch, and the ascending esophageal branch, which supplies the cardiac portion of the stomach and the lower esophagus. The left gastric artery connects with the right gastric artery, a branch of the hepatic artery. Along the greater curvature of the stomach lies a vascular arcade formed by the right gastroepiploic artery, a branch of the gastroduodenal artery, sending gastric branches, each of which divides into anterior and posterior rami. At about the midportion of the greater curvature of the stomach, the right gastroepiploic artery connects with the left gastroepiploic artery, which rises from the splenic artery and reaches the greater curvature in the gastrosplenic ligament. The point at which the gastric branches of this vascular arcade change direction corresponds to the midportion of

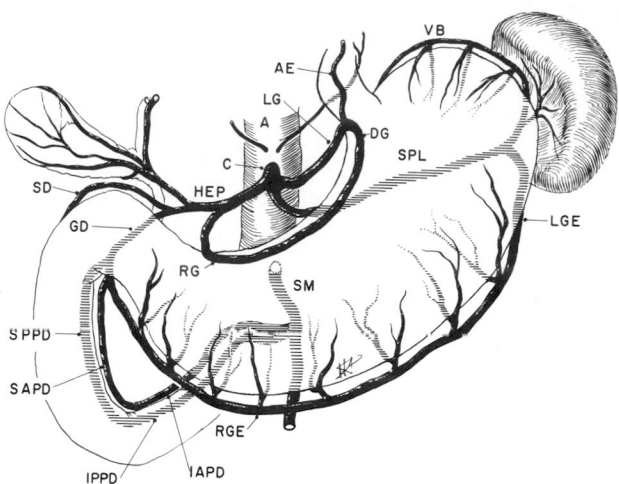

Fig. 26-1. Blood supply of the stomach. C, Celiac artery; LG, left gastric artery; AE, ascending esophageal artery; DG, descending gastric artery; RG, right gastric artery; GD, gastroduodenal artery; RGE, right gastroepiploic artery; LGE, left gastroepiploic artery; SPL, splenic artery; VB, vasa brevia.

the greater curvature. The left gastroepiploic also sends gastric branches to the greater curvature. The arterial arcade along the proximal segment of the greater curvature of the stomach is supplied by vasa brevia, which arise either from the splenic trunk or from the left gastroepiploic artery (Fig. 26-1).

Branches from these two arcades ramify through the entire submucosa, forming a plexus from which branches supply the mucosal membrane of the entire stomach, except for the lesser curvature; this receives its arterial supply directly from branches of the right and left gastric arteries. This anatomic arrangement of the arterial supply to the lesser curvature has been interpreted as rendering the lesser curvature more liable to ischemia. The veins and the lymphatics are distributed along the arterial arcades.

Knowledge of the autonomic nervous supply to the stomach by the vagus nerves is particularly important today because interruption of the parasympathetic supply to the stomach has become an essential part of the surgical treatment of duodenal ulcer. Distribution of vagus nerves

Fig. 26-2. Parasympathetic innervation of the stomach.

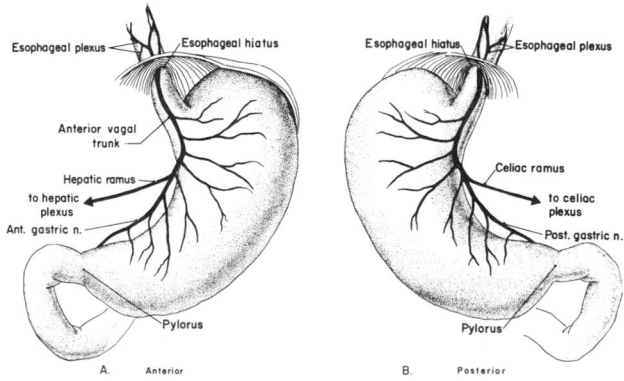

to the stomach is illustrated in Fig. 26-2. The preganglionic fibers in these nerves terminate by synapsing with ganglion cells of Auerbach's plexus located between the longitudinal and circular muscle layers of the stomach. Postganglionic fibers are distributed from these ganglion cells to the submucous (Meissner) network of nerve fibers. These postganglionic fibers are cholinergic. Postganglionic sympathetic fibers from the celiac plexus reach the stomach along the main gastric arteries.

GASTRIC FUNCTION

Three times a day the stomach discharges into the duodenum 500 to 1,000 ml of gastric chyme, a mixture of gastric juice and food subjected to gastric digestion. Actually, the digestive role of the stomach is rather unimportant. When food is chewed carefully, carbohydrates exposed to the action of salivary amylase are hydrolyzed as long as the gastric pH remains elevated, but as gastric pH falls, amylase becomes inactive. The contribution of the stomach to the digestion of dietary protein is minimal; only 10 to 15 percent is reduced to peptones. Although gastric pepsin is a powerful proteolytic enzyme, it can only initiate protein hydrolysis. It also disperses intracellular contents by digesting cell walls. However, denaturation of protein by gastric acid facilitates the action of other proteolytic enzymes of pancreatic and intestinal origin. The contribution of the stomach to lipolysis is negligible. In summary, the stomach decreases the particulate size of foodstuffs, denatures alimentary protein by acidification, and brings ingested materials to levels of temperature and osmolarity which will be tolerated by the mucosa of the proximal small bowel.

Motor Function

The musculature of the stomach differs from that of the remainder of the digestive tract by having three layers instead of two. An outer layer of longitudinal fibers continuous with the longitudinal coat of the esophagus is thickest along the two curvatures. The circular layer is continuous with the circular coat of the esophagus and is thickest over the prepyloric antrum. A deep layer of oblique fibers originates from the left side of the cardia and fans out toward the greater curvature. An important feature of the muscular coat of the stomach is its greater thickness in the prepyloric antrum.

The volume of the stomach fluctuates tremendously. When empty, its volume is 50 ml or less. As food enters its lumen the stomach wall relaxes and allows its volume to increase without a change in intragastric pressure until volumes of greater than 1,500 ml are reached. This ability of the stomach to accommodate a large increase in intraluminal volume without stretching of its walls is known as *receptive relaxation*. At rest, the stomach undergoes transient phases of nonpropulsive motor activity lasting for 5 to 10 minutes, separated by periods of 15 to 20 minutes of quiescence. When food enters the stomach, motor activity gradually increases. The characteristic manifestation of gastric motor activity is a peristaltic wave which originates near the cardia and travels toward the pylorus. At the beginning of a meal these waves are shallow and die out as they reach the antrum. Later, the waves become deeper and sweep over the antrum and pylorus.

The gastric peristaltic wave depends in part upon a reflex arc with afferent signals arising from sensory receptors in the stomach that are stimulated by gastric distension. Ascending fibers of this arc are carried in the vagus nerves, which also carry its efferent branches. During the height of digestion, peristaltic waves occurring at a rhythmic rate of approximately four per minute mix the gastric contents and force chyme into the antrum where gastric digestion occurs. Periodically, a portion of gastric chyme coming from the fundus of the stomach is propelled through the entire length of the antrum, where the greater thickness of the gastric wall increases the propulsive strength of the peristaltic wave. This portion of the stomach has the function of a pump. At rest, the pyloric muscle is relaxed, allowing its borders to be in apposition. Moreover, the absence of a pressure gradient between the stomach and the duodenum prevents the stomach from emptying its contents. As the antral peristaltic wave approaches the pylorus, its strength, as well as its speed, increases so that the antrum contracts almost as a unit; at the same time the pylorus relaxes because of the relaxation that precedes the peristaltic wave. In addition, the gastric peristaltic wave produces a positive pressure gradient from the stomach to the antrum which drives a small fraction of gastric chyme (2 to 6 ml) into the duodenum. At the end of the cycle the peristaltic wave traverses the pylorus, which contracts, and gastric emptying ends for that cycle. The fraction of gastric chyme evacuated into the duodenum is propelled distally by duodenal contractions and is prevented by the closure of the pylorus from refluxing into the stomach.

The entry of gastric chyme into the duodenum initiates "feedback" regulatory mechanisms which alter the rate of gastric emptying. Excessive variations of temperature, of tonicity, or a pH below 3.5 all reduce gastric motility and the rate of gastric emptying. These inhibitory influences are mediated by hormonal substances released from the mucosa of the proximal small intestine under the influence of one of the conditions listed above. These hormones are known as *enterogastrones*. Secretin may be involved in the inhibition of gastric motility occurring when the duodenal pH falls below 3.5 since secretin release from the duodenum is brought about, *inter alia,* by duodenal acidification and since secretin is known to inhibit gastric motility in addition to inhibiting gastrin-stimulated gastric acid secretion. A particularly strong inhibition of gastric motility takes place when the gastric chyme reaching the proximal small intestine has a high fat content. The hormonal substance for the mediation of this gastric inhibition by fat—the first enteric hormone to be called enterogastrone— unlike secretin and cholecystokinin, has not yet been defined as a distinct chemical entity.

Secretory Function

HISTOLOGY. The gastric mucosa is divided into three parts: the *cardiac gland area* forms a 1- to 3-cm-wide strip beginning at the esophagogastric junction; the *fundus or parietal cell area,* primarily responsible for secretion of acid and pepsin, occupies the proximal three-fourths of the gastric mucosa; the *antrum or pyloric gland area* occupies the distal one-fourth of the stomach. The mucosal surface consists of a columnar epithelium. Over the fundus the mucosa is thrown into numerous "rugal" folds which increase its secretory surface. The antral mucosa is almost completely flat. Microscopic examination of the mucosal surface reveals multiple pits or *foveolae* into which open three or four gastric glands. The types of cells lining the gland vary according to the region of the stomach. In the fundus the mucosal surface and the foveolae are lined by *surface mucous cells* containing numerous granules of mucin. At the junction of the body of the gland with the gastric pit, *mucous neck cells* also containing mucin granules are found. The function of these cells will be discussed below. In the upper portion of the gland the predominant cell type is the *parietal cell,* a large pyramidal-shaped cell with the base on the basement membrane of the gland with a centrally placed nucleus and a finely granular, eosinophilic cytoplasm. These cells have the function of producing HCl and, in humans, intrinsic factor. In the

Fig. 26-3. Schematic illustration of a gastric gland. (*From S. Ito et al., J Cell Biol, 16:541, 1963.*)

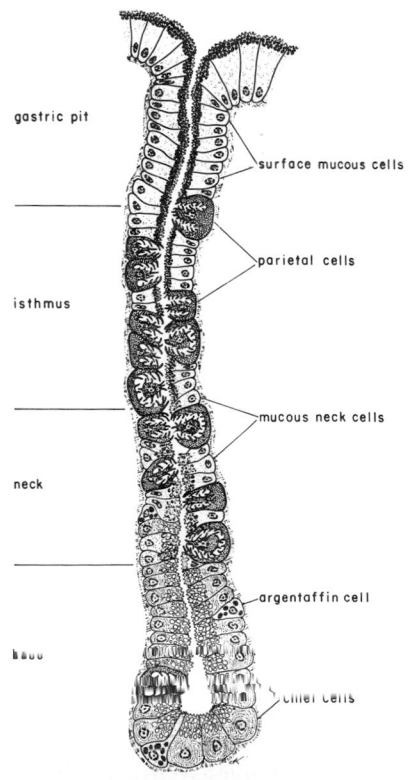

GASTRIC GLAND

deeper portion of the fundic glands the predominant cell type is the *chief cell,* a cuboidal-shaped cell with a basally situated nucleus and a basophilic cytoplasm which is responsible for the elaboration of *pepsinogen.* In addition, true argentaffin and argyrophilic cells, whose functions are not known, are found (Fig. 26-3). The *cardiac glands* are characterized by a shallow foveola and a short length. They are lined mainly by mucous cells. The *pyloric mucosa* is covered by surface mucous cells similar to those lining the remainder of the stomach. The glandular foveolae are deeper than in the fundus and the deeper portions of the glands are coiled. The cells lining the glands are similar to the mucous neck cells in the fundus. The major secretory product of these glands is mucus. Unidentified cells in the pyloric mucosa are responsible for the elaboration of the hormone *gastrin.*

In between the glands and foveolae lies the *lamina propria,* a loose aggregation of connective tissue, lymphocytes, plasma cells, and mast cells containing serotonin and histamine. The mucosa is separated from the submucosa by a thin layer of smooth muscle, the *muscularis mucosae.*

Renewal of the Surface Epithelium. The surface mucous cells lining the lumen undergo continuous renewal due to mitotic activity confined to mucous neck cells situated in the isthmus of the glands. The daughter cells migrate up the walls of the foveolae, reach the surface, and are eventually exfoliated into the lumen. The whole cycle covers approximately 36 hours in the rat, the animal in which this phenomenon, crucial to the health of the mucosa, has been most extensively studied. Although the neck mucous cells differentiate primarily into surface mucous cells, they appear also to contribute to a much slower renewal of chief and parietal cells.

The histology of the superficial duodenal mucosa resembles that of the remainder of the small intestine. The characteristic feature of the mammalian duodenum is the presence in the proximal duodenum of *glands of Brunner.* Situated in the submucosa they empty into the crypts of Lieberkühn via small secretory ducts. Their viscous, mucoid alkaline secretion probably contributes to the protection of the duodenal mucosa against the corrosive action of gastric juice.

METHODS OF STUDYING GASTRIC SECRETION. To study glandular function one must be able to collect the secretory product. For experimental purposes the collection of gastric juice uncontaminated by saliva and food is possible with the gastric pouch preparations devised by Heidenhain and Pavlov, illustrated in Fig. 26-4. A vagally denervated pouch is used to study humoral influences on gastric secretion, since the only systemic connections of the pouch are via its blood supply. A vagally innervated pouch serves to study neural influences on gastric secretion.

Human gastric secretion both in health and disease is measured by placing under radioscopic control the aspirating tip of a tube in the most dependent portion of the stomach. Gastric secretions are withdrawn, preferably by manual suction, for a determined period of time and under various conditions. It is important that the subject be instructed to spit his saliva continuously during the collection.

Fig. 26-4. Schematic illustration of (*A*) vagally denervated (Heidenhain) and (*B*) vagally innervated (Pavlov) gastric pouches. [*Reproduced from Ballinger (ed.), "Research Methods in Surgery," Little, Brown and Company, Boston, 1964.*]

COMPOSITION OF GASTRIC JUICE. Gastric secretion is not the simple hydrochloric acid solution often depicted in advertisements for antacids. The components for gastric juice can be divided into two parts: organic and inorganic.

Organic Constituents of Gastric Juice. *Mucus.* Gastric mucus, secreted predominantly by the prepyloric glands but also by the surface epithelial cells lining the stomach, is a heterogeneous mixture of several molecular species. Although their molecular structures are not known, several are glycoproteins of very high molecular weight. These mucoid secretions have characteristic properties of adhesiveness, cohesiveness, and high viscosity, allowing them to form a thin layer adherent to the mucosa. It has been postulated that this layer of mucus limits the access of gastric juice to the underlying epithelium. A corollary of this view is that a deficiency in the quantity of mucus or its quality could lead to peptic ulceration. In addition to these physicochemical properties, the glycoproteins comprising the major portion of gastric mucus are resistant to enzymatic proteolysis, a quality imparted to the molecule of glycoprotein by its carbohydrate prosthetic groups.

Pepsinogen. The important proteolytic enzyme, pepsin, is secreted by the chief cells of the fundus of the stomach in the form of an inactive precursor called *pepsinogen*. The latter is formed by the coupling of the active molecule of pepsin with a peptide called the *pepsin inhibitor.* Below a pH of 5, disassociation of the pepsin inhibitor liberates active pepsin. The activity of pepsin is greatest when the pH of the medium is 2. Above pH levels of 5 peptic activity gradually decreases. Recent studies have shown that human gastric juice contains several types of pepsin with different optimal pH levels.

Pepsinogen is also found in blood and urine. Uropepsinogen undoubtedly comes from the stomach, since it disappears from the urine after a total gastrectomy. Unfortunately, uropepsinogen levels cannot be utilized to measure gastric secretory activity because of a poor correlation between the two.

Intrinsic Factor. Intrinsic factor (IF), discovered by Castle, appears to be a mucoprotein which binds with vitamin B_{12}. The IF-vitamin B_{12} complex renders vitamin B_{12} unavailable to intestinal microorganisms. Dissociation of this complex occurs in the ileum, where vitamin B_{12} is absorbed. The fate of intrinsic factor is unknown. Malabsorption of vitamin B_{12} occurs in patients with pernicious anemia whose stomachs do not elaborate IF, and after total gastrectomy. Vitamin B_{12} deficiency appears only after 3 to 7 years following a total gastrectomy, since the daily needs of vitamin B_{12} are 1 to 2 μg and the normal liver stores approximately 2 mg.

Blood Group Substances. In about 75 percent of the population the stomach secretes into gastric juice the major blood group antigens A, B, and H(O) as well as minor blood group antigens such as the Lewis substances (Le^a and Le^b). Individuals who have the Le^{a+} substance on their red blood cells (about 25 percent of the population are Le^{a+}) in addition to their major blood group antigen do not secrete their major blood group antigens into their gastric juice or saliva, but secrete similar amounts of Lewis^a antigen. For unknown reasons, these individuals, called "nonsecretors," are more liable to duodenal ulceration than "secretors." These blood group antigens found in gastric juice, saliva, and other body fluids are *water-soluble* glycoproteins containing galactose, L-fucose, galactosamine, glucosamine, N-acetylneuraminic acid. The corresponding antigens extractable from red blood cell membranes are alcohol-soluble lipoglycoproteins.

Nonorganic Constituents of Gastric Juice. HCl, secreted by the parietal cells, is the important and characteristic nonorganic constituent of gastric juice. 0.167 N HCl from the parietal cells is admixed with varying amounts of secretions from the other gastric mucosal cells, so that aspirated gastric juice contains Na$^+$ and K$^+$, and HCO$_3$, in addition to HCl. Although the levels of the ions are constantly changing, the average concentrations are Na,

65 mEq; K, 13 mEq; Cl, 100 mEq; and H, 90 mEq. The molar concentration of Cl exceeds that of H$^+$, because a small amount of "neutral" Cl is secreted as KCl and NaCl. There is a reciprocal relationship between ions, so that as H$^+$ increases, Na$^+$ and K$^+$ decrease. A fundamental consideration in the study of gastric secretory function is the quantification of the concentration of HCl in gastric juice.

Measurement of Gastric Acidity. Juice is collected by one of the methods described above for fixed periods, usually 15 minutes. The H$^+$ concentration of each sample is estimated by pH measure and by titration to an end point of 7. Results are expressed as mEq HCl/15 minutes [volume of 15-minute sample (liters) $\times$ HCl concentration (mEq/L)].

Mechanism of HCl Secretion. The essential aspects of gastric juice secretion are well established. The parietal cells elaborate hydrogen ion, chloride, water, and intrinsic factor. The chief cells secrete pepsinogen, and chloride may come from other cells as well as from the parietal cells. The principal anion in gastric juice is chloride, and during slow rates of acid secretion, the other cation is sodium. The maximal concentration of acid in the gastric juice is between 140 and 160 mEq/L which represents a concentration gradient over two million times greater than that in the blood bathing the gastric cells. The important questions with respect to the mechanism of HCl secretion are the following: How does the parietal cell establish this concentration gradient? How does the stomach alter it? How does the stomach maintain it?

The actual secretion of hydrogen ion into the canaliculi of the parietal cells against an enormous concentration gradient is dependent upon a "pump" mechanism utilizing energy derived from high-energy substrates. During the secretion it is possible that sodium ion in the glandular tubule is exchanged for hydrogen ion.

It is almost certain that the secretion from a parietal cell always has a "maximal," constant acidity of about 160 to 170 mEq/L. Variations in the concentration of acid in the gastric juice appear due in part to dilution of the parietal cell secretion by alkaline secretions from the other cells. The more important regulatory mechanism may be the variable rate at which hydrogen ion diffuses back from lumen to mucosa. At low rates of acid secretion this back diffusion would be great and would be offset by an enhanced movement of sodium ion from plasma to lumen. The reverse would occur during high rates of secretion.

To explain how the stomach can maintain such an enormous concentration gradient of hydrogen ion between the lumen and the plasma, one must introduce the concept of a gastric mucosal *barrier.*

Gastric Mucosal Barrier. Hydrogen ion in gastric juice is separated from the interior of mucosal cells at two sites, the canaliculi of the parietal cells and the luminal border of the cells lining the glands and the mucosal surface. The two sites form a barrier which gives the stomach its unique property of "holding" a high concentration of HCl in its lumen. To this barrier one must attach a feature of *variable permeability.*

Studies conducted mainly in experimental animals have shown that natural (i.e., normal) differences in mucosal permeability occur from one animal to another and may account in part for individual variations in gastric acidity under standard conditions of gastric stimulation. Intraindividual variations of mucosal permeability to hydrogen ion *under physiologic conditions* remain to be studied. However, the classical studies of Davenport have shown that in contrast to the small permeability of the *normal* gastric mucosa to hydrogen ion, injury of the mucosa with agents such as eugenol, acetic acid, or aspirin in HCl increases its permeability to hydrogen ion enormously. Such an abnormally permeable mucosa can no longer generate or maintain a high concentration of hydrogen ion. It is reasonable to postulate that the stomach's capacity to retain digestive juices within its lumen and away from the mucosal tissues depends upon the integrity of this barrier. In all likelihood this relative impermeability to hydrogen ion results not from a static "barrier" (impervious membrane) but from an ATP(adenosine triphosphate)-dependent, energy-consuming process.

REGULATION OF GASTRIC SECRETION. Stimulation of Gastric Secretion. The mechanisms responsible for a secretory response to a meal have been divided into three phases: the cephalic, gastric, and intestinal phases of gastric secretion. For reasons that will be discussed below, a classification of the stimulatory mechanisms into two phases, vagal-antral and intestinal, is more in agreement with modern physiologic data.

Vagal-Antral Phase. The sight, thought, smell, and taste of food coinciding with the beginning of a meal provoke a strong secretory response. These stimuli are mediated to the stomach by the vagus nerves. This neural influence on gastric secretion is exerted via two mechanisms: a direct stimulating effect on the parietal cells, and an indirect stimulating influence on the parietal cells mediated by the vagally induced release of the hormone *gastrin* by the antrum. Vagal stimulation of gastric secretion can be induced by the administration of insulin (0.2 µg/Kg body weight). The resulting hypoglycemia stimulates vagal centers with a resulting increase in vagal tone. Characteristically, gastric juice secreted in response to vagal stimulation has a high concentration of pepsin.

When the bolus of food enters the stomach, distension of the antrum further enhances the elaboration of the stimulatory hormone *gastrin,* the release of which has already been initiated by vagal stimulation of the antrum.

Gastrin. Although the concept of a humoral phase of gastric secretion originated in 1906 with the work of Edkins, only recently has the concept been fully accepted; that occurred only after Gregory succeeded in extracting pure gastrin from the antral mucosa of man and animals, determined its structure, and synthesized it. Gastrin, the most potent known stimulant of gastric acid secretion, is a heptadecapeptide amide. The principal action of gastrin is a strong stimulation of the secretion of water, electrolytes, and intrinsic factor by the stomach; the secretion of pepsin is stimulated only weakly. Gastrin also stimulates water and electrolyte secretion of the liver, pancreas, and Brunner's glands. It inhibits absorption of water and electrolytes by ileal mucosa. It increases the tone of the lower esopha-

geal sphincter, reduces the tone of the sphincter of Oddi, and increases the motility of the stomach, intestine, and gallbladder. Gastrin also has a potent *trophic* action on the gastric mucosa. These physiologic properties are carried by the C-terminal tetrapeptide amide portion of the molecule (tryp-met-asp-phe-NH$_2$). It is interesting that *cholecystokinin,* a hormone released by the small intestine, has the identical amino acid sequence at its C-terminus. Although these two hormones act on the same targets, the intrinsic activities by which they act on a given site differ. Gastrin is a far more potent stimulus to gastric acid secretion than cholecystokinin. The latter stimulates acid secretion weakly and actually inhibits gastrin-stimulated acid secretion (competitive inhibition). On the other hand, cholecystokinin is a far more potent stimulant of gall bladder motility than gastrin. The structures of gastrins from various mammalian species (man, dog, sheep, hog, cat) are virtually identical. In all species gastrin occurs in two forms: gastrin I, in which a tyrosine residue is nonsulfated, and gastrin II, in which the tyrosine is sulfated. Both forms have the same potency on acid secretion. The gastrin produced by pancreatic islet-cell tumors (Zollinger-Ellison syndrome) and that produced by the human antrum are identical. Both occur as a mixture of gastrins I and II. In the blood gastrin circulates in the form of a larger molecule ("big gastrin") than the 17 amino acid residue polypeptide extractable from the antrum.

Although gastrin is formed in small amounts in the gastric fundus and the proximal small intestine, the principal site of gastrin formation is in the antral mucosa in as-yet-undetermined cells. The release of gastrin into the circulation by the antral mucosa occurs in response to vagal stimulation, to distension of the antrum and to the presence in its lumen of specific secretagogues such as peptone solutions. These factors potentiate each other so that a vagally denervated antrum releases less gastrin in response to a given degree of distension than when its vagal innervation was intact. These stimuli of gastrin release are strengthened when the antral contents are alkaline and are suppressed when the pH in the antrum falls below 2.0.

The release of gastrin from the antral mucosa is blocked by *secretin* and enhanced by *calcium.* In addition, secretin inhibits the action of gastrin on the parietal cell.

In addition to a synergism between vagal innervation of the antrum and gastrin release during mechanical or chemical stimulation of the antrum, gastrin and vagal stimuli act synergistically on the parietal cell. Denervated parietal cells respond less to exogenous gastrin. Therefore, separation of a cephalic, or neural, phase from a gastric, or humoral, phase of gastric secretion is no longer justified.

Synthetic derivatives of gastrin like the pentapeptide (*N-t*-butyloxycarbonyl-B ala-tryp-met-asp-phe-NH$_2$) "pentagastrin" have a potent stimulating effect on gastric secretion and have proved very useful in the experimental and clinical study of gastric acid secretion.

Intestinal Phase. Gastric secretory activity reaches a peak with each meal and then wanes. However, secretion never stops. The stimuli influencing the stomach between meals belong to the intestinal phase of gastric secretion. In an animal with a denervated total gastric pouch and an esophagoduodenal anastomosis, a weak secretory response lasting for 5 or 6 hours occurs several hours after a meal. The stimuli responsible for this phase of gastric secretion are not known. Possibly certain by-products of digestion of dietary substances, such as histamine, formed by the bacterial decarboxylation of histidine, may be involved. An active gastric secretory response follows the direct introduction of peptones or histamine into the small intestine.

Inhibition of Gastric Secretion. Several factors intervene at the end of gastric digestion to inhibit gastric secretory activity. It is convenient to classify these in the same categories considered for the stimulatory factors.

Vagal-Antral Phase. An important mechanism for the decrease in gastric secretion 2 to 3 hours after a meal relates to the decrease in vagal activity. This is an example of inhibition due to removal of a stimulus. The importance of this vagal cutoff can be demonstrated in the experimental animal with a vagally innervated gastric pouch and an esophageal fistula. Sham feeding causes prolonged gastric secretion due to continuous vagal stimulation of the pouch.

Antral distension, an important stimulus to gastrin release from the antrum, subsides with gastric emptying. Moreover, it has been shown that the low pH in the antrum at the end of gastric digestion interrupts gastrin release. This phenomenon of "acid inhibition" is activated when antral contents reach a pH level of 2. In addition, it has been postulated that the acidified antrum releases an inhibitory hormone. However, the existence of this inhibitory chalone remains unproved.

Intestinal Phase. The entry of acid gastric chyme into the duodenum lowers duodenal pH and triggers an important inhibitory mechanism. This phenomenon of duodenal acid inhibition was first demonstrated by Sokolov. Many investigators have confirmed the fact that acidification of the duodenum inhibits both gastric secretion and motility via neural and humoral pathways. Because the hormone secretin inhibits gastrin-stimulated gastric secretion in addition to stimulating pancreatic secretion, it is possible that this hormone, which is released by the acidified duodenum, may mediate duodenal acid inhibition of gastric secretion. In addition to duodenal acid inhibition, the presence of fat in the proximal small intestine decreases gastric secretion and motility. It has been postulated that the mucosa of the duodenum, when in contact with fat, releases a gastric inhibitory chalone known as "enterogastrone."

In addition, extreme variations in tonicity or temperature of chyme entering the duodenum also have a mild inhibitory influence on gastric function.

The cyclic waxing and waning of gastric secretory activity corresponding with meals is due to the smooth interplay of these stimulatory and inhibitory factors. Under certain conditions these physiologic mechanisms become deranged, and altered states of gastric function characteristic of disease occur.

PEPTIC ULCER DISEASE

A peptic ulcer is a mucosal defect located in an area adjacent to or in acid-secreting epithelium. Accordingly, it can be found in the lower esophagus, the body of the stomach, the duodenum, in the jejunum marginal to a surgically constructed gastrojejunostomy and in the ileum at the outlet of a Meckel's diverticulum containing aberrant gastric mucosa. By definition an *ulcer* penetrates beyond the muscularis mucosae whereas an *erosion* is superficial to this layer. Traditionally all "ulcerating" lesions in the gastroduodenal area have been called "peptic ulcers." Recent knowledge has enabled the separation of these lesions into several distinct entities.

1. Duodenal ulcer diathesis
   a. Duodenal ulcer
   b. Ulcer immediately proximal to the pylorus or in the pyloric canal
   c. Combined gastric and duodenal ulcer
2. Gastric ulcer
3. Acute gastric mucosal lesions (erosive gastritis)

At the turn of the century, peptic ulceration became an increasingly important cause of morbidity. Data from the National Center for Health Statistics indicated that the annual prevalence rate for peptic ulcer was 19 per 1,000 adults per year in 1965. This figure was 30 percent greater than the rate for 1959. The total deaths attributed to peptic ulcer were estimated to be 12,500 in 1965.

The incidence of gastroduodenal ulceration and the ratio of duodenal (DU) to gastric ulceration (GU) have changed considerably since the last century when "peptic" ulcers were usually gastric, duodenal ulceration being rarely mentioned by pathologists of the nineteenth century. Acute gastric ulceration in young women was a common clinical problem. At the turn of the century a commonly quoted DU:GU ratio was 1:20. Since then and until the mid-1960s, the incidence of duodenal ulceration has increased, and this, coupled with a decrease in the prevalence of gastric ulceration, has resulted in the generally accepted DU:GU ratio of 10:1. Since the mid-1960s the incidence of duodenal ulceration has, for unknown reasons, decreased by almost 40 percent. This evolution of peptic ulcer disease has not been uniform throughout the world. Certain areas such as Japan and parts of South America remain afflicted with a high incidence of gastric ulceration. Another interesting aspect of the evolution of peptic ulcer disease is the change brought about by violent social upheavals such as the two world wars, during which the incidence of gastric ulceration among the civilian European population on both sides of the conflict increased sharply.

DUODENAL ULCER DIATHESIS

The duodenal ulcer diathesis is characterized by the presence of a chronic ulcer in the duodenal mucosa usually in the base of the bulb on its anterior or posterior wall. Other locations are the superior or the inferior recess of the bulb, the postbulbar mucosa, or rarely, the second portion of the duodenum. As mentioned above, ulcerations located in the pyloric canal or immediately proximal to it belong to the duodenal ulcer diathesis, as do jejunal ulcers appearing at the margin of a gastrojejunostomy after a partial gastrectomy for duodenal ulcer.

Pathogenesis

The best explanation for this condition is that the ulceration results from a relative or absolute excess of acid-peptic gastric secretions. Several arguments support this view.

The average patient with duodenal ulcer has higher rates of gastric acid secretion than an ulcer-free subject of the same age and sex in the general population (Table 26-1).

Conditions producing extremely high rates of gastric acid secretion are associated with a very high incidence of duodenal ulceration.

Continuous stimulation of gastric acid secretion in dogs produces duodenal ulceration.

Constant infusion of acid gastric juice into the duodenum of experimental animals produces duodenal ulceration.

The production of a relative hyperacidity in the gastric outlet zone of dogs by diversion of the alkaline pancreatic secretion to another segment of the gut (Mann-Williamson preparation, Figs. 26-5 and 26-6) results in lesions similar to human duodenal ulcers.

The temporary reduction of gastric acidity by buffers alleviates the symptoms of duodenal ulceration, and healing of the ulcer follows permanent reduction of acidity by surgical means. However, some aspects of the relationship between acid output and duodenal ulceration remain unclear, suggesting

Table 26-1. BASAL AND HISTALOG-STIMULATED GASTRIC SECRETION IN NORMAL SUBJECTS AND IN PATIENTS WITH PEPTIC ULCER OR WITH GASTRIC CANCER

Condition	Basal acid output, mEq/hr	Histalog,* mEq/1 hr post-Histalog
Normal:		
Male	2.44 ± 2.85	11.64 ± 7.62
Female	1.33 ± 2.00	7.53 ± 5.20
Duodenal ulcer:		
Male	5.29 ± 4.63	19.91 ± 9.70
Female	2.87 ± 3.14	13.42 ± 6.87
Gastric ulcer:		
Male	1.45 ± 1.99	9.68 ± 6.97
Female	1.00 ± 1.49	7.95 ± 5.96
Gastric cancer:		
Male	0.45 ± 1.23	3.25 ± 4.79
Female	0.16 ± 0.47	1.46 ± 2.50

*Histalog given in a dose of 0.5 mg/kg of body weight.
SOURCE: Data from Grossman et al., *Gastroenterology,* **45:**14, 1963.

that some factor other than acid-peptic activity may intervene. Although *average* gastric output is higher in patients with duodenal ulcer than in ulcer-free subjects, the values overlap greatly; many patients with an ulcer have normal acid outputs. Even

Fig. 26-5. The similarity between the marginal ulceration that used to occur after a Roux en Y bypass of the duodenum and the ulcer occurring in animals after total diversion of duodenal secretions to the ileum. Both lesions result from hyperacidity of the gastric outlet zone.

GASTRO-JEJUNOSTOMY "EN Y"   MANN-WILLIAMSON PREPARATION

The basic mechanism of the two lesions, one clinical and one experimental, is diversion of alkaline duodenal secretions from the gastric outlet zone.

Fig. 26-6. Example of a Mann-Williamson ulcer from Mann's first experiment. (*Courtesy of Dr. Jesse Bollman.*)

more surprising is the absence of duodenal ulceration in some patients with gastric-producing pancreatic islet-cell tumors and enormously elevated levels of acid output.

Unless a serious complication supervenes, most duodenal ulcers heal spontaneously. *Healing is not accompanied by a decrease in gastric acid output.*

ROLE OF PEPSIN. The relation between duodenal ulceration and gastric acidity has evolved because acid output is easily quantified, whereas pepsin output can only be estimated as *peptic activity* in gastric juice. Its role is important since the tissue destruction characteristic of ulcerogenesis requires peptic activity. Yet pepsin cannot be considered separately, any more than can acid be. Human pepsins have acid pH optima. The longer the gastric outlet zone's pH remains within the range where pepsin is active (as when excessive acid output overwhelms the buffering capacity of duodenal secretions), the longer will the duodenal mucosa remain exposed to the proteolytic action of pepsin. Thus gastric acid and pepsins operate in concert, not only in the degradation of dietary protein but also in the mucosal destruction characteristic of ulcerogenesis. As a general rule, the gastric output of peptic activity parallels that of acid.

Because of the importance of the acid-peptic factor many studies of the etiology of duodenal ulceration have been directed at the mechanism of the acid hypersecretion so often present. Several possibilities have been explored.

MECHANISM OF GASTRIC HYPERACIDITY. Excessive Neural Stimulation of Gastric Secretion. It has been suggested that increased vagal impulses of subconscious origin may cause hypersecretion accompanying duodenal ulcer. This theory is based on the well-known fact that vagotomy, when complete, abolishes gastric hypersecretion. This observation, although correct, does not prove the theory, since another influence of the vagus nerves on gastric secretion, in addition to direct and indirect stimulation, is to render the parietal cell more reactive. Therefore, one would expect vagotomy to decrease HCl production regardless of the nature of the abnormal stimulus initially responsible for the hypersecretion.

Excessive Hormonal Stimulation of Gastric Secretion. The recent availability of serum gastrin assay based on radioimmunoassay with antibodies to synthetic human gastrin I has made it possible to estimate serum gastrin levels under various conditions in normal subjects and in patients with duodenal ulceration. McGuigan has found that fasting serum gastrin levels are not higher in patients with duodenal ulceration than in ulcer-free control subjects. However recent studies suggest that serum gastrin levels may reach higher levels than those in normal subjects in response to vagal stimulation. At present the role of gastrin output in the etiology of the common variety of duodenal ulcer (as distinguished from the Zollinger-Ellison syndrome) remains unclear.

Impairment of Physiologic Mechanism Responsible for Gastric Inhibition. This theory has received the least experimental support. Patients with duodenal ulcer appear to have a normal drop in gastric secretion upon acidification of the antrum or the duodenum. However, gastric emptying is more rapid in patients with a duodenal ulcer than in ulcer-free subjects. This, coupled with an augmented acid output, should have an adverse effect on the duodenal mucosa.

Excessive Capacity to Produce Acid. This hypothesis is an attractive one. It has been shown that stomachs of patients with duodenal ulcer contain more parietal cells than those of normal individuals. This in turn causes the greater maximal histamine response often found in patients with duodenal ulcer. Furthermore, the predominance of duodenal ulcer in males may be explained by the fact that, generally men have more parietal cells than women. It would be attractive to view the greater parietal cell mass in patients with duodenal ulcer as a genetically inherited trait, in turn responsible for hypersecretion and duodenal ulcer production. However, it could also represent the result of work hyperplasia in response to an unknown stimulus. The latter explanation appears more valid at present, since recent animal studies have shown that parietal cell hyperplasia accompanies constant gastric stimulation produced by chronic administration of histamine or following construction of an Eck fistula.

Genetic Aspects of Duodenal Ulceration. An excess of peptic ulcer disease exists among siblings of patients with this condition. Moreover, such studies have shown that this predisposition is type-specific; an excess of duodenal ulcer exists among the relatives of patients with a duodenal ulcer and the same is true for gastric ulcer among the relatives of patients with this lesion. In addition, it has been proven by several workers that subjects with blood group O are more prevalent among patients with a duodenal ulcer than in the control population. This relationship is particularly strong for duodenal ulceration complicated by bleeding. Another factor to consider is an individual's "secretor status." Approximately 75 percent of our population secrete into saliva, gastric juice, and urine, water-soluble blood group antigens immunologically identical to the blood group antigens on their red blood cells. They are "secretors." The remainder are all Le^{a+} and irrespective of their major blood group antigen, they secrete into these body fluids the Lewis antigen. These subjects are "nonsecretors," a state determined by the Le^{a+} phenotype. Nonsecretors are more liable to duodenal ulceration than secretors. It is interesting that the greater risk associated with the nonsecretor status and the risk associated with blood group

O are additive, so that an individual with type O blood who is also a nonsecretor of H(O) antigen in gastric and salivary secretions is almost three times more liable to duodenal ulceration than someone who is A or B and Le^{a-}. There is no explanation for this well-documented phenomenon.

ASSOCIATION OF PEPTIC ULCER WITH OTHER CLINICAL ENTITIES. Extragastric factors appear to influence the stomach in a way not always related to gastric secretion. The greater frequency of duodenal ulcer in association with certain disease entities suggests such relationships.

Pulmonary Disease. Carefully controlled clinical and autopsy studies have shown that in patients with pulmonary emphysema, peptic ulcer is at least three times more common than in the general population. Conversely, emphysema occurs three to four times more often in patients with peptic ulcer than would be expected from the normal incidence of emphysema in the general population. In all the clinical studies of this problem, duodenal ulcer was five times more common than gastric ulcer. The mechanism by which chronic lung disease predisposes to peptic ulceration is not known.

Liver Disease. A relationship between the liver and the stomach was suspected when it was noted that gastric hyperacidity occurred following the construction of an Eck fistula (end-to-side portacaval shunt) in dogs. However, *clinical* data have failed to show a pattern of hyperacidity in patients with Laennec's cirrhosis. In cirrhotics without coexisting duodenal ulcer, gastric hyposecretion and frequent anacidity in response to histamine prevail. In cirrhotics with duodenal ulcer, gastric acidity is higher than in those without an ulcer, but lower than in healthy individuals and much lower than the acidity usually accompanying duodenal ulcer. Gastric acidity is higher in cirrhotics with a portacaval shunt. Moreover, reports of an increased incidence of "peptic ulceration" in patients with cirrhosis have been misleading by their failure to define which type of ulceration is involved. More recent data indicate that cirrhotics are particularly liable to acute erosive gastritis and acute/or chronic gastric ulceration. Duodenal ulceration with its attendant hyperacidity is not appreciably more common in cirrhotics than in the general population.

Exocrine Pancreatic Disease. The evidence for a relationship between the exocrine pancreas and the stomach is based upon the frequency of peptic ulcer, particularly duodenal ulcer, in patients with chronic pancreatitis. Because the earliest manifestation of chronic pancreatitis is a decrease in the concentration of bicarbonate in pancreatic juice, ulceration could be due to a decreased buffering capacity of duodenal secretions. In addition, it has been theorized that patients with chronic pancreatitis may have increased gastric HCl production. This view is founded upon experimental observations of gastric hyperacidity in dogs after ligation of the pancreatic ducts, an experimental situation which simulates human chronic pancreatitis. However, one cannot extrapolate these data to the explanation of the human disease. Patients with chronic pancreatitis do not secrete more acid than healthy subjects.

ENDOCRINE DISORDERS. Zollinger-Ellison Syndrome. In 1955 Zollinger and Ellison described the syndrome now bearing their names. The important aspects of this syndrome are a markedly elevated rate of gastric acid secretion, a very severe duodenal ulcer diathesis, and a non-beta islet-cell tumor of the pancreas. Over half of the tumors are malignant. In 20 percent of cases there is diffuse microadenomatosis of the pancreas, a feature of this condition which prohibits the therapeutic use of tumor excision or partial pancreatectomy. In some instances the islet-cell tumor is found in an extrapancreatic location such as the wall of the first portion of the duodenum. Some cases of this syndrome result from a diffuse hyperplasia of the islets of Langerhans. In some instances the elevated serum gastrin levels may be caused by a hyperplasia of the antral gastrin-producing cells (G cells). It has been definitely proven that the hyperacidity and the ulcer diathesis are due to the release of gastrin by the tumor. Radioimmunoassay with antibodies to synthetic human gastrin I have shown large amounts of gastrin in tumor tissue and the blood of patients with this syndrome. In normal subjects serum gastrin concentrations are usually lower than 200 pg/ml whereas levels higher than 600 pg/ml are found in patients with this syndrome. Strangely, some patients with this syndrome do not develop an ulcer despite enormously elevated rates of acid secretion and instead present with diarrhea, malabsorption, and weight loss. In 20 percent of cases there are other endocrine tumors, often of the parathyroid glands (MEA I).

The ulcer disease associated with this syndrome has characteristic features listed below. It is important that the physician treating a patient with a duodenal ulcer disease recognize these features so that specific diagnostic procedures may be initiated. Although the proportion of duodenal ulcer patients with a Zollinger-Ellison syndrome is well below 1 percent, the consequences of improper treatment are so devastating that early, accurate diagnosis is essential.

1. Although most ulcers associated with this syndrome are in the usual location for duodenal ulcer disease, some may appear in a postbulbar location or even in the jejunum and may be associated with jagged and irregular mucosal folds (Fig. 26-7).
2. The basal acid output is very high, over 20 mEq/hour, and the ratio of the basal acid output to the maximal acid output (obtained with stimulation by Histalog) is usually greater than 60 percent.
3. This syndrome should be suspected when ulcer rapidly and severely recurs after adequate surgical treatment.
4. Severe diarrhea associated with hyperkalemia.
5. Duodenal ulcer in a patient with a functioning endocrine tumor such as a parathyroid adenoma.

The diagnosis may then be confirmed by one or more of the following tests:

Radioimmunoassay of serum gastrin levels. In normal subjects and in patients with the common form of duodenal ulcer, the fasting serum gastrin concentration does not exceed 200 pg/ml. The Zollinger-Ellison syndrome is associated with levels ranging from 200 to 300,000 pg/ml. Although comparable or even higher levels are found in patients with atrophic gastritis, the crucial point is that in this condition the high gastrin levels are associated with a very low gastric acid output: the high gastrin levels result from a lack of inhibition of gastrin release by HCl.

Secretin infusion test. During an intravenous infusion of secretin, both serum gastrin and gastric acid output of normal subjects and of patients with the common form of duodenal ulcer *diminish;* in patients with a Zollinger-Ellison syndrome they *increase* (Fig. 26-8).

Provocative calcium infusion test. In patients with the Zollinger-Ellison syndrome, an intravenous infusion of calcium (5 mg/hour) causes an excessive rise in serum gastrin levels (>500 pg/ml), as well as a greater rise in acid output than in normal subjects or patients with ordinary duodenal ulceration.

Arteriography. Selective celiac and superior mesenteric arteriography are capable of demonstrating a pancreatic lesion in a high percentage of cases of Zollinger-Ellison syndrome caused by a tumor.

Parathyroid Glands. Several clinical studies have demonstrated a slightly higher incidence of duodenal ulcer in patients with primary hyperparathyroidism. It is likely that some of these patients have gastrin-producing pancreatic tumor and Zollinger-Ellison syndrome; in these patients serum gastrin levels are increased by calcium infusions after removal of the parathyroid adenoma. In normal subjects gastric acid secretion is increased by intravenous calcium infusion and, conversely, hypocalcemia is accompanied by a reduction in gastric secretion. These relationships between serum calcium levels and gastric secretion may explain the occasional appearance of a duodenal ulcer in a patient with hypercalcemic hyperparathyroidism and no gastrin-producing pancreatic tumor.

Clinical Manifestations

An active duodenal ulcer reveals its presence by a symptom complex often described as "ulcer pain." The pain of duodenal ulcer is vague and often located in the mid-epigastrium to the right of the midline. The following characteristics should be determined in the evaluation of ulcer distress: the site of the pain, its quality, its radiation, the time of onset in relation to meals, aggravation of pain, relief of pain, and finally the chronology of painful attacks.

The quality of the pain is often the most difficult characteristic to elicit. Classically, it is described as a burning pain. In reality this is rarely accurate. Often, patients complain of a sensation of "pressure," of a "cramp," or of

Fig. 26-7. Zollinger-Ellison syndrome. Note large duodenal ulcer crater (1) and irregular appearance of the mucosa of the second portion of the duodenum (2).

"discomfort." Occasionally, a patient describes the sensation of being "hungry." When investigating complaints suggestive of duodenal ulcer, one should open the questioning by asking the patient whether or not discomfort rather than actual pain is experienced. The distinction may seem overly subtle, but to many patients pain is something akin to a toothache. Moreover, the distinction has physiologic relevance, since the painful impulses in visceral disease are carried by the autonomic nervous system and

Fig. 26-8. Strongly positive secretin infusion test in a patient with a presumptive diagnosis of Zollinger-Ellison syndrome based upon a high BAO/MAO. Diagnosis was confirmed surgically.

cause different subjective sensations from those mediated by the somatic nervous system.

The epigastric discomfort of duodenal ulcer radiates in a beltlike fashion across the upper abdomen. When the ulcer penetrates posteriorly into the pancreas, the pain radiates to the back at T8 to T10. Occasionally, posterior radiation of pain becomes the dominant symptom, and the author has encountered several patients with duodenal ulcer who were being mistakenly treated for a chronic backache.

Because the epigastric discomfort of active duodenal ulcer is aggravated by fasting, these patients often realize that they must eat frequently. Occasionally, rapid ingestion of excessively cold or excessively warm fluids may aggravate these symptoms. Aspirin is avoided by many patients with duodenal ulcer because of severe symptomatic exacerbation.

Ingestion of anything that dilutes or buffers gastric acid relieves the ulcer pain. Plain water, which dilutes gastric secretions, affords immediate, although very temporary, relief. Milk or antacids which have a buffering capacity give prompt and longer relief.

The symptoms of duodenal ulcer usually occur when the stomach is empty: late in the morning, in midafternoon, and during the middle of the night. This rhythmicity may be lacking in children. A useful symptom in distinguishing a peptic ulcer from psychosomatic gastrointestinal distress is a history of the patient's being awakened by discomfort. This rarely occurs in the absence of organic disease. Night pain reflects the high nocturnal secretion of HCl unbuffered by food.

An important trait of duodenal ulcer is its tendency to chronicity and periodicity. Symptomatic attacks lasting for several weeks are interspersed with months of complete or near-complete absence of symptoms. The relationship of these symptoms to climatic and seasonal variations is well known. In temperate zones, exacerbations and complications occur during fall and spring. This is not true in other parts of the world. This seasonal influence may be related to an increase in volume and acidity of gastric secretion occurring in animals and in man during the autumn and spring. It has also been noticed that exacerbations of the ulcer process are often associated with traumatic emotional experiences. During World War II, admissions for perforated duodenal ulcer in Great Britain increased sharply during heavy air raids.

Diagnosis

RADIOLOGY. Radiologic examination of the duodenum is the most important diagnostic tool available to the clinician. The radiologist looks for two important abnormalities: a crater and duodenal deformity (Figs. 26-9 and 26-10). A crater appears as a barium-filled defect in the duodenal bulb or more frequently as a persistent fleck of barium. The evolutionary pattern of duodenal ulcer is a succession of episodes of ulceration followed by healing; this is what eventually deforms the bulb. At the level of the ulcer a stricture forms, above which the bulb dilates into two or three irregular outpouchings called pseudodiverticula. In addition, the fibrotic and rigid duodenum fails to fill with barium when pressure is applied to the abdomen. Normally, pressure distends the bulb, because the pyloric sphincter prevents regurgitation of barium into the stomach. A deformed duodenal bulb in a patient with a history suggestive of duodenal ulcer is a reliable radiologic sign and is more often present than a crater.

ENDOSCOPY. With the refinement of fiberoptic instrumentation, this procedure has become a valuable adjunct to radiology. One can evaluate the condition of the esophageal mucosa for the presence of esophagitis, often associated with duodenal ulceration. Superficial gastric lesions such as erosions and antral gastritis may be demonstrated. Duodenal ulcers too shallow to be demonstrated radiologically may be detected, as well as the chronic inflammation of the duodenal mucosa—duodenitis—often found instead of a crater in patients with symptomatic gastric hyperacidity.

GASTRIC ANALYSIS. The value of gastric analysis is often questioned because at least half of the patients with a duodenal ulcer have normal rates of gastric secretion. However, a gastric analysis in patients with a peptic ulcer (including duodenal ulcer and gastric ulcer) may furnish the following information:

Recognition of patients with a duodenal ulcer diathesis due to a functioning endocrine tumor in the pancreas (Zollinger-Ellison syndrome).

Evaluation of the severity of the duodenal ulcer process. Obviously, patients with marked hyperacidity (without pyloric obstruction) have a more severe duodenal ulcer process with a greater expectancy of recurrence after therapy.

Evaluation of the results of therapy. It is useful to compare gastric analysis after surgical treatment for peptic ulcer or after treatment by anticholinergic drugs with control values. Gastric analysis is indispensable for the evaluation of the results of vagotomy.

Differentiation between benign and malignant ulcerations. When an ulcerating gastric lesion is accompanied by high rates of gastric secretion, the lesion may be considered and treated as belonging to a duodenal ulcer diathesis, whether or not a frank duodenal ulcer coexists. This is often true when a gastric ulcer is prepyloric or when a duodenal ulcer has caused pyloric stenosis with gastric stasis and subsequent gastric ulceration. It is very unusual to find gastric adenocarcinoma accompanied by frank hyperacidity.

Augmented Histamine Test. Gastric juice is aspirated in the morning after an overnight fast until the stomach is completely empty. During the test the subject is instructed to spit out his saliva. After removal of residual juice in the stomach, basal secretion is collected for 1 hour. At the end of an hour, Histalog (betazole, 3-β-aminoethylpyrazole dihydrochloride) is injected subcutaneously in a dose of 1.5 mg/kg of body weight. Gastric juice is collected in 15-minute periods for 2 hours after the injection.

Pentagastrin Stimulation Test. Pentagastrin is a synthetic polypeptide containing the five active terminal amino acids of gastrin. An injection of 6 mg/kg of pentagastrin produces a maximal acid output similar to that induced by histamine phosphate or Histalog without side effects. Since it is a more physiologic gastric stimulant, it will probably be used extensively in the future.

Hollander Insulin Test. The Hollander insulin test remains the most reliable method of determining the completeness of vagotomy. The test is based upon the fact that insulin-induced hypoglycemia stimulates gastric secretion only if there are intact vagal pathways to the stomach. The usual indication for the test is an investigation of the reasons for a recurrent ulcer in a patient previously treated by a vagotomy and drainage procedure. The test must be performed in the fasting patient. The stomach is intubated and after its contents have been evacuated, four 15-minute samples of basal secretion are collected. Following this the patient receives 20 units of regular insulin intravenously, and venous blood samples are taken for estimation of blood sugar at the time of the insulin injection and again 30 and 45 minutes later. For 2 hours after the insulin injection, 15-minute aspirates of gastric juice are collected and their volume, pH, and acid concentration are measured. A positive response is indicated by an increase in acid concentration greater than 20 mEq/L over the fasting concentration during the 2 hours following the injection of insulin, provided that the blood sugar falls to at least 35 mg/100 ml. When basal secretions are anacid, an increase in acid concentration greater than 10 mEq/L is considered to represent a positive response.

Management

The treatment of this condition has three aspects: long-term, or supportive, management; the management of an acute exacerbation; and the management of complications.

LONG-TERM MANAGEMENT

Therapy is aimed at decreasing gastric secretion and minimizing its effects on the duodenal mucosa. Many myths are attached to the dietary management of duodenal ulcer. Of these, that of a bland diet is particularly naive. With the exception of alcohol, foods ordinarily consumed by man do not irritate the gastroduodenal mucosa. It is the acid-peptic action of gastric juice that causes the tissue destruction characteristic of a duodenal ulcer. Food buffers gastric juice by accepting hydrogen ion; also, it binds the pepsin in gastric juice to the peptide bonds mobilized by digestion of protein and thus minimizes the ulcerogenic action of gastric juice. Therefore, the important aspect of the dietary management of duodenal ulcer is not what one eats but how one eats. A patient with a duodenal ulcer soon learns that discomfort accompanies an empty stomach. The reason for this must be explained to the patient when he is advised to follow a schedule of frequent feedings: breakfast, snack at midmorning, light lunch, snack at midafternoon, dinner, light snack before retiring. Skim milk rather than cream or half-and-half is taken between meals. Although alcohol in moderation may have beneficial sedative effects, its heavy consumption is harmful, and it should be completely avoided during acute exacerbations. Excessive consumption of fat, which retards gastric emptying and may thus increase gastric acidity by enhancement of the antral phase of gastric secretion, is harmful. Coffee and tea, because of their important secretagogue effects, should be left out.

Fig. 26-9. Small ulcer crater (arrow) in the duodenal bulb with minimal deformity of the bulb.

Anticholinergic agents may contribute to the long-term management of duodenal ulcer by decreasing the number of recurrences. Their beneficial effects are, at best, questionable, and because they reduce the tone of the lower esophageal sphincter, they should *never* be used in patients who have associated reflux esophagitis.

Although antacids are often used for the long-term management of duodenal ulcer, they have little value except during exacerbations of the process. The buffering capacity of nonabsorbable antacids is smaller than is usually realized, principally because they are emptied from the stomach rapidly. Absorbable antacids, which are more

Fig. 26-10. Characteristic radiologic findings in duodenal ulcer. Scarring of the bulb resulting in obliteration of the inferior recess of the bulb (1), large crater (2), and narrowing of the lumen at the level of the crater (3).

efficient buffers of HCl, may be hazardous when used for longer than a few weeks.

Conventional antihistaminic agents do not inhibit gastric acid secretion. It has been suggested that the action of histamine on secretion is mediated by H_2 receptors structurally different from the H_1 receptors which mediate those histamine effects blocked by conventional antihistaminics. *Metiamide,* a compound which inhibits effects mediated by H_2 but not by H_1 receptors, has been produced by side-chain modifications of histamine. In man, Metiamide inhibits gastric secretory responses to histamine, pentagastrin, insulin, and food. It has been used successfully abroad in the treatment of duodenal ulceration but has since been withdrawn because of its depressing action on the bone marrow. An analog of Metiamide, *Cimetidine,* has identical antisecretory properties but, at least so far, appears free of significant side effects. It has been used with success in Great Britain in the treatment of duodenal ulcer.

It is important that a patient with a duodenal ulcer lead a stereotyped existence, in addition to following the dietary schedule outlined above. Departures from the daily routine of life, whether they be physical or emotional, often precipitate symptomatic relapses. Patients should be warned against excessive smoking, and of course aspirin or aspirin-containing compounds are contraindicated.

MANAGEMENT OF AN ACUTE EXACERBATION

For a mild, symptomatic relapse, a simple intensification of the treatment often suffices. However, a severe relapse requires admission to the hospital for more intensive treatment, which includes (1) complete bed rest, (2) nasogastric suction, (3) antacid therapy, (4) anticholinergics, and (5) sedation.

A remarkable feature of duodenal ulcer is the rapidity with which intractable pain disappears when a patient is hospitalized and isolated from his usual environment. Keeping gastric juices away from the ulcer for 24 to 48 hours by constant suction accelerates healing of an intractable ulcer. After 24 to 48 hours of suction, a gastroduodenal series is obtained to rule out pyloric obstruction. If the stomach empties normally, the patient is given 150 ml of skim milk every 2 hours and 4 Gm of calcium carbonate every alternate 2 hours. The latter is a good buffer of HCl and is safe as long as the patient is free of renal disease and a high urinary output is maintained. Rising serum calcium and BUN (blood urea nitrogen) levels, accompanied by a falling urinary output, require immediate cessation of this antacid therapy and a change to a nonabsorbable antacid. This regimen should be continued for 72 hours or until complete disappearance of epigastric discomfort. It is important to awaken the patient at 3- to 4-hour intervals during the night for administration of milk and antacids. After 3 to 4 days the patient gradually returns to a soft diet with six small and equal feedings.

Anticholinergics are given up to tolerance as indicated by dryness of the mouth. Sedation is obtained with small doses of phenobarbital, which is a very helpful adjunct to the treatment.

At discharge, the patient is instructed to set his alarm for the middle of the night and take some milk and antacid

at this time. A month after the onset of the acute exacerbation, the therapeutic regimen can gradually be readjusted to that followed for the long-term management.

INDICATIONS FOR SURGERY

The usual indications for recommending an operation to patients with a duodenal ulcer are intractability, a complication such as uncontrollable bleeding or late-occurring obstruction, and perforation. As a general rule, approximately 20 percent of patients with a duodenal ulcer ultimately require an operation.

INTRACTABILITY. By contrast with massive bleeding, severe pyloric obstruction, and duodenal perforation, which represent incontrovertible indications for surgery, intractability is less readily defined and a less compelling guideline for the clinician. It may be defined as a situation where medical management cannot control the symptoms of the disease. Naturally, the interpretation of intractability as an indication for surgery depends not only on the physician's judgment and the patient's willingness to accept the disability of a chronic disease, but also on the individual patient's circumstances. If the exigencies of an adequate therapeutic regimen—a regular pattern of living and eating, the constant use of antacids, anticholinergic and sedative drugs—are not compatible with the patient's occupation, family status, or finances, surgery might be imposed sooner than the severity of the duodenal ulcer diathesis might otherwise indicate. It is important that the clinician be satisfied that all reasonable avenues of medical management have been properly followed before proceeding with surgery based on the indication of intractability. It is every surgeon's experience that the patients who spontaneously request an operation after an exhaustive trial of medical management, ultimately have the best symptomatic results from surgery.

BLEEDING. Hemorrhage from a duodenal ulcer is responsible for approximately 20 percent of all cases of upper gastrointestinal bleeding. There are two aspects to the management of this complication. First in importance is resuscitation with all the measures used in the treatment of blood loss. In addition the stomach must be decompressed by a large-bore gastric tube such as an Ewald tube and lavaged thoroughly with cold isotonic saline solution to evacuate blood and clots.

After hypovolemic shock, if present, has been controlled, the clinician can proceed with the diagnostic aspect of the management. Patients with bleeding duodenal ulcer often have a previous history of similar episodes. A history of duodenal ulcer distress with its characteristic rhythmicity and periodicity is usually present. Emergency fiberoptic gastroscopy is an important diagnostic maneuver as it helps to exclude bleeding from esophageal or gastric varices in patients with cirrhosis and bleeding from a gastric ulcer or gastric erosions. When a duodenal ulcer is the source of bleeding, the operator may actually see the bleeding lesions, or more often, see blood refluxing into the stomach through the pylorus.

Bleeding from peptic ulcer is often treated by a milk drip. This is superfluous and possibly harmful. The blood already in the stomach is a better buffer than milk. Moreover, distension of the stomach interferes with spontaneous hemostasis which results from contraction of the gastric wall. Usually bleeding subsides with medical measures, and the patient may return to a rigid ulcer regimen for several weeks. Beyond that, the long-term management varies. In a young patient with a short ulcer history, long-term medical management should be continued. However, when the bleeding has been preceded by a long history of ulcer disease or by previous bleeding episodes, an ulcer operation should be considered.

When the ulcer is bleeding actively, the clinician's major concern is to recognize early enough the failure of conservative therapy and recommend an operation. The criterion of massive bleeding is a good guide to follow in determining which cases are surgical. Gastrointestinal bleeding is "massive" when 30 percent of the patient's blood volume must be replaced during 12 hours to maintain stable vital signs. In practice this represents 1,500 to 2,000 ml of blood for an adult of average size. The surgical approach to bleeding peptic ulcer will be described below.

PYLORIC OBSTRUCTION. The management of pyloric obstruction by a chronic duodenal ulcer depends upon the length of the ulcer history. Pyloric obstruction preceded by a short history of peptic ulcer disease usually signifies that the obstruction is due to duodenitis and antral gastritis impairing the propulsive motility of the antrum and active relaxation of the pyloric sphincter. This process is reversible, and normal gastric emptying returns as the inflammatory reaction around the ulcer subsides. Treatment consists of the following:

Nasogastric Suction and Interdiction of Oral Intake. It is important to forbid drinking, which patients often think is permissible because of the relief after gastric decompression.

Fluid and Electrolyte Replacement. Pyloric obstruction often stimulates gastric secretion. Enough fluid and electrolytes may be lost by vomiting to cause *hypochloremic* and *hypokalemic alkalosis.* This metabolic abnormality results from the combined losses of hydrogen, chloride, and potassium ions in gastric juice. The resulting potassium depletion may, in addition, alter renal function so that tubular reabsorption of bicarbonate is increased, thus leading to the characteristic finding of an aciduria associated with the alkalosis. There may also be impairment of the sodium-cation exchange mechanism.

Anticholinergic agents should not be given to patients with pyloric obstruction since they may aggravate the gastric stasis by decreasing gastric motility. When fluoroscopic examination with small amounts of barium shows return of gastric emptying, the patient should resume the rigid ulcer program used for the management of an acute exacerbation. The long-term medical management should be continued. Often after such an episode many years elapse without further symptoms of ulcer.

Pyloric obstruction occurring after a long history of duodenal ulcer distress almost always results from severe cicatricial duodenal deformity, and little can be expected from further conservative management. It is advisable to operate after fluid and electrolyte replacement. Clinging stubbornly to nasogastric suction and fluid and electrolyte

Fig. 26-11. Perforated duodenal ulcer. Note inflammatory exudate around the perforation.

replacement for several weeks in the futile hope of overcoming a cicatricial pyloric stenosis only renders the ultimate and necessary surgical management more difficult. Details of the surgical approach to this problem will be discussed below.

PERFORATION. Free perforation into the peritoneal cavity is the most dramatic and potentially the most lethal complication of duodenal ulcer (Fig. 26-11). Its major symptom is sudden, generalized epigastric pain. The patient can often give the hour and the minute of onset. It is the perforated duodenal ulcer that usually causes the rigid, "boardlike," scaphoid abdomen described as the classic physical finding in acute peritonitis. The large amounts of air in the peritoneal cavity are revealed clinically by an absence of the normal liver dullness. These findings and a history of peptic ulcer disease suffice to make a diagnosis which can be confirmed by a chest x-ray (in preference to an upright view of the abdomen) showing air under one or both sides of the diagram (Fig. 26-12). Occasionally, a perforation is the first manifestation of peptic ulcer disease. The actual perforation is sometimes accompanied by bleeding which, if appreciable, may overshadow the more lethal event. Of crucial importance is the existence of hypovolemic shock. Although the blood pressure may initially be normal, peripheral vasoconstriction, an accelerated pulse, and a decreased urinary output are usually present. The parietal and serosal peritoneum exposed to gastric acid contents undergo a chemical "burn," and changes similar to those of thermal burns occur, i.e., a decrease of plasma volume, a rise in hematocrit and all the systemic abnormalities characteristic of hypovolemic shock.

The only safe way to treat a perforated duodenal ulcer is by surgical intervention. From time to time it is argued that a patient may be too ill to tolerate an operation. Patients are rarely too ill to tolerate surgical treatment. In this instance the intolerable insult is not the surgical treatment

Fig. 26-12. Perforated duodenal ulcer. Note the presence of air under both sides of the diaphragm on this chest film.

but the continued soiling of the peritoneal cavity. Rarely are patients so ill that they fail to improve with preoperative treatment of the hypovolemic shock. These measures are (1) restoration of blood volume by administration of colloid, (2) parenteral fluid and electrolyte therapy, (3) nasogastric suction, and (4) administration of antibiotics.

After these corrective measures the ulcer is sutured or, in selected cases, definitive surgical treatment of the duodenal ulcer diathesis may be carried out. The details of the procedure will be described below.

From time to time, nonoperative treatment of perforated ulcer has been advocated. This consists of nasogastric suction and administration of blood, fluid, and antibiotics. The rationale of this method rests upon the demonstrated ability of perforations to become sealed spontaneously. Unfortunately, this event is unpredictable. If spontaneous closure of small acute ulcers does happen, a chronic indurated ulcer lacks the same potential. Today the risk of a laparotomy is so low that it is safer to operate; operation for a perforated duodenal ulcer is indeed the conservative approach.

The patient's future after closure of a perforated duodenal ulcer depends in part upon the length of the ulcer history prior to the perforation. In young patients with a short ulcer history the perforation is often the first and last manifestation of ulcer disease. However, when a long ulcer history precedes the perforation, over half of the patients continue to suffer. Some patients have another perforation; the author has seen several patients who had three perforations over a period of several years. Recurrent duodenal ulcer distress after simple closure of a perforation is an indication for operation.

Elective Surgical Treatment of Duodenal Ulceration

HISTORICAL EVOLUTION

Operations on the stomach were first developed for gastric cancer during the latter part of the nineteenth century. *Posterior gastroenterostomy* was devised to overcome gastric outlet obstruction by gastric cancer. The applicability of this operation to the treatment of duodenal ulcer and its complications was then recognized. Since it was known that duodenal ulcer was due in part to the corrosive action of gastric juice on the duodenal mucosa, gastroenterostomy, which diverts secretions from the ulcer bed, appealed to physiology-minded surgeons. Its simplicity, at a time when the mortality and morbidity of intraabdominal operations was high, was also in its favor. This appeal was so great that gastroenterostomy was abandoned in this country only recently and after recognition of postoperative stomal ulceration. This complication was first reported in 1899. By 1930 it was obvious that stomal ulceration complicated 30 percent of posterior gastroenterostomies. As early as 1910, Austrian and German surgeons recognized this and adopted *partial gastrectomy* for duodenal ulcer. Except for a few isolated clinics, it was not until the late 1930s and early 1940s that gastroenterostomy was abandoned in favor of subtotal gastric resection in this country.

The rationale of partial gastrectomy was reduction of gastric acidity by removal of the parietal cell mass. Against this background were many controversial issues on details of technique, such as whether or not resection should encompass the ulcer or whether the reconstruction should be in the form of a gastroduodenostomy or gastrojejunostomy, and in the latter case whether the anastomosis should be antecolic or retrocolic. During the late 1930s, 1940s, and early 1950s, the trend moved toward more radical operations. However, it became evident that although 80 percent gastrectomy effectively cured duodenal ulcer, its sequelae were too frequent and too serious to be discounted. This prompted a search for operations equally effective and less costly in morbidity and mortality. In 1943 the rediscovery of the principle of vagus nerve section by Lester Dragstedt and his associates at the University of Chicago inaugurated a new era in the surgical treatment of ulcer disease. At first the principle of *vagotomy,* as applied by Dragstedt to the treatment of duodenal ulcer, sometimes failed, because the severe gastric stasis due to loss of the coordinated motor function of the pyloric muscle and the antrum produced intolerable side effects; recurrent ulcers, particularly gastric, were common. Addition of a gastric drainage procedure, namely, posterior gastroenterostomy designed to prevent gastric stasis, created an effective operation for duodenal ulcer. Subsequently the principle of vagotomy coupled with a gastric drainage operation—posterior gastroenterostomy, pyloroplasty, or antrectomy—became solidly established. Because of the possibility that some of the undesirable side effects of vagotomy, such as diarrhea, may be due to vagal denervation of the midgut, modifications of vagotomy designed to preserve all but the vagal supply to the stomach and known as *selective vagotomy* have been introduced during the past decade. Although selective vagotomy, which preserves the hepatic and celiac branches, appears to reduce the incidence of diarrhea, it still requires a drainage procedure and thus exposes the patient to the possibility of a postoperative *dumping syndrome*. In 1970, the concept of vagal denervation of the parietal cell area—*highly selective vagotomy, proximal gastric vagotomy*—without a drainage procedure was first tested clinically in Denmark and Great Britain. The early results appear encouraging.

In the ensuing paragraphs some of the advantages and disadvantages of these procedures will be discussed.

GASTROENTEROSTOMY

This operation should never be performed alone for the treatment of duodenal ulcer. Although a gastroenterostomy allows gastric juice to bypass the duodenal lesion, it also allows alkaline pancreatic and biliary secretions to flow into the antrum. Enhancement of antral gastrin mechanism by alkalinization of the antrum was the reason for this operation's frequent failure to cure the duodenal ulcer diathesis. In a dog prepared with a Heidenhain pouch, secretion from the pouch increases appreciably after a gastroenterostomy.

SUBTOTAL GASTRIC RESECTION

This procedure consists of removal of at least the distal 75 percent of the stomach (Fig. 26-13). Alimentary continuity is reestablished by anastomosing the entire section of the gastric pouch (Pólya) or a portion of its section after closure of the lesser curvature (Hofmeister) to the jejunum. The anastomosis may be antecolic or retrocolic. Anastomosis of the gastric remnant to the jejunum by any one of these methods is known as a "Billroth II operation." When the anastomosis joins the gastric remnant to the duodenal stump, the operation is termed "Billroth I." The latter procedure is best applied to the treatment of gastric ulcer and should not be used to treat duodenal ulceration unless supplemented by a vagotomy. The rationale of partial gastrectomy rests upon the assumption that removal of a large portion of the parietal cell mass diminishes gastric secretion. However, the anatomy of the gastric mucosal membrane is such that a 75 to 80 percent gastric resection removes the antrum and only a portion of the parietal cell mass. Moreover, the remaining parietal cells retain their vagal innervation and their responsiveness to other stimuli and therefore a secretory potential capable of causing recurrent ulcers. Recurrent ulceration after a partial gastrectomy for duodenal ulcer appears on the jejunal side of the gastrojejunostomy and is known as a "stomal," or "marginal," ulcer. When a partial gastrectomy alone has been done, the possible causes for the recurrence are (1) inadequate gastric resection; (2) excessively long afferent loop; (3) existence of a remnant of antrum left behind intentionally or inadvertently, resulting in excessive gastric

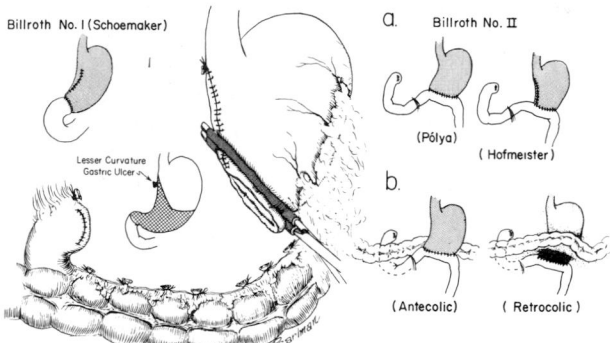

Fig. 26-13. Partial gastrectomy for benign disease. The larger sketch shows the Hofmeister closure of the lesser curvature. This is particularly applicable to the management of high-lying lesser curvature gastric ulcers. Gastrointestinal continuity is reestablished either by a gastroduodenostomy (Billroth I) technique, particularly applicable to gastric ulcer, or by a gastrojejunostomy (Billroth II). The latter may be performed with the full section of the gastric pouch (Pólya) or after resection and closure of the lesser curvature (Hofmeister). The anastomosis may be placed in front of or behind the transverse colon.

stimulation by gastrin released from the antrum bathed by alkaline juices; or (4) presence of a pancreatic islet-cell adenoma of the Zollinger-Ellison variety.

The recurrence rate is particularly high when patients are followed for more than 10 years after the operation. Gastric resection has other drawbacks. Primary is the mortality rate of gastric resection, which ranges from 1.0 percent to as high as 4 or 5 percent. The mortality rate is primarily related to circumferential dissection of the chronically inflamed duodenum, since half of the early postoperative deaths come from nonhealing of the duodenal stump with the formation of a duodenal fistula, with or without generalized peritonitis, or localized subphrenic and subhepatic abscesses.

Without question, a very radical subtotal gastric resection cures the ulcer diathesis. The reductio ad absurdum is the assurance of a zero incidence of recurrent ulcer after a total gastrectomy. However, time has shown that even after lesser resections of the stomach a host of undesirable sequelae related to loss of the reservoir function of the stomach and to impaired digestion and absorption follow in the wake of gastrectomy.

COMPLICATIONS OF PARTIAL GASTRECTOMY. Dumping Syndrome. The salient manifestation of the loss of the reservoir function of the stomach is known as the "dumping syndrome." The latter consists of some of or all the following postcibal symptoms: weakness, sweating, pallor, nausea and/or vomiting, epigastric discomfort, borborygmi, palpitations, dizziness, and diarrhea. These symptoms appear within 10 minutes after a meal and subside after 40 to 60 minutes. They may be accompanied by the following objective findings: tachycardia, tachypnea, elevation in blood pressure, increased small intestinal intraluminal pressure and motility, electrocardiogram changes in the T wave and the S-T segment, decreased plasma volume, decreased plasma potassium and phosphate, increased urinary excretion of uric acid, hyperglycemia, decreased cardiac output, increased digital blood flow, increased renal blood flow, and abnormal intestinal electrical activity. The syndrome is due in part to distension of the jejunum by an outpouring of extracellular fluid into the bowel lumen, which in turn results from the premature entry into the proximal small bowel of hypertonic chyme. Other manifestations, such as apprehension, sweating, and vascular instability, are due to autonomic or adrenomedullary corrective mechanisms. Some patients experience symptoms of hypoglycemia 60 to 90 minutes after a meal, particularly if it is high in carbohydrate content. The exact incidence of the dumping syndrome after gastric resection is unknown. It should be emphasized that some of or all these manifestations follow the administration of a hypertonic meal in virtually every individual who has had a gastric resection. However, only 5 to 10 percent of patients suffer from clinically significant dumping after a gastrectomy. In only 1 or 2 percent of the patients are the symptoms incapacitating. Often dumping is potentiated by the patient's emotional makeup.

Bilious Vomiting. Postoperative bilious vomiting may result from a chronic afferent loop syndrome or from alkaline reflux gastritis.

Chronic afferent loop syndrome is due to a partial obstruction of the afferent loop at, or close to, the stoma. Patients experience dull epigastric discomfort after meals. The distress is completely relieved by the vomiting of large amounts of bilious material which does not contain recently ingested food.

Alkaline reflux gastritis is a postgastrectomy condition due to reflux of bile into the stomach. This causes a chronic gastritis ("peristomal gastritis") which, in turn, leads to *constant* epigastric distress and frequent nausea and vomiting; the vomitus often contains food, since the gastritis impairs gastric emptying. The diagnosis is made by gastroscopy, which shows a fiery red, friable mucosa with superficial erosions. The changes are predominantly in the vicinity of the stoma.

Steatorrhea. Steatorrhea, defined as a fecal excretion greater than 7 percent of ingested fat, occurs more often after a Billroth II type of gastrectomy. The gastrojejunostomy allows gastric chyme to bypass the duodenum and escape the digestive action of pancreatic enzymes and the emulsifying action of bile salts. Undigested food stimulates intestinal motility and is propelled distad before pancreatic secretion and gallbladder emptying can occur. In other words, gastric emptying and pancreatobiliary digestion of dietary fat are out of phase. Steatorrhea occurs in approximately 50 percent of all patients who have had a gastric resection, is rare after gastrojejunostomy or vagotomy alone, but is almost the rule after total gastrectomy. Still another factor in steatorrhea after partial gastrectomy is the so-called "blind loop" syndrome. There may be sufficient stasis in the proximal loop of duodenum to cause bacterial proliferation. Bacterial enzymes are capable of deconjugating bile salts. In turn deconjugated bile salts are irritating to the intestinal mucosa and appear to be responsible for diarrhea. Moreover the altered bile salts are less able to contribute to the formation of lipid micelles essential for normal fat digestion and absorption and thus con-

tribute to the development of steatorrhea. The latter may be corrected by the administration of a broad-spectrum antibiotic.

Anemia. Chronic iron deficiency anemia is another facet of the postgastrectomy state. It occurs in at least 50 percent of patients who have had a partial gastrectomy. Although patients can absorb iron normally after gastrectomy, they cannot increase iron absorption in the face of increased iron losses. About 30 percent of patients have impaired absorption of vitamin B_{12} after a partial gastrectomy, and in about 6 percent megaloblastic anemia develops. The malabsorption usually comes from deficient secretion of intrinsic factor due to loss of gastric tissue and atrophy of the gastric remnant.

Calcium Deficiency. Deficient calcium absorption is another consequence of subtotal gastric resection. Balance studies have shown that as many as 30 percent of patients have an abnormal calcium metabolism 7 to 16 years after gastric resection. In some patients the defect in calcium absorption may lead to osteomalacia.

Small Bowel Obstruction. Small bowel obstruction is an occasional late complication of partial gastrectomy, particularly of the Billroth II variety. A loop of small bowel may herniate through the operative defect in the transverse mesocolon when it has been improperly closed, or a volvulus may form around the gastrojejunostomy.

Gastrocolic Fistula. The stomal ulcer that used to occur so often after gastroenterostomy (done alone without vagotomy) is a particularly virulent type of ulcer diathesis with a great propensity for perforation either into the peritoneal cavity or into the transverse colon, causing a gastrojejunocolic fistula responsible for severe diarrhea, emaciation, and anemia. In the absence of such specific aggravating circumstances as a Zollinger-Ellison syndrome, this particular complication rarely occurs after a gastrojejunostomy constructed in conjunction with an adequate partial gastrectomy. It is not the short-circuiting of gastric contents into the colon that causes the diarrhea, as one would expect, but rather the reflux of feces into the small bowel. The resulting increase in the bacterial population of the proximal gastrointestinal tract probably causes the diarrhea and malabsorption. The latter can be corrected rapidly by a proximal colostomy, which may be necessary to restore proper nutrition before undertaking definitive treatment of the gastrocolic fistula. A gastrocolic fistula is demonstrated much more readily by a barium enema than by an upper gastrointestinal series.

VAGOTOMY

The rationale of vagotomy has been described above. This operation interrupts vagal impulses to the parietal cell gland area and to the antrum. By inhibiting antral motility and rhythmic relaxation of the pyloric sphincter mechanism, it also causes gastric stasis. Many of the patients who had this operation in the 1940s were severely incapacitated by gastric distension, foul eructations, and gastric ulceration. For these reasons vagotomy alone was not a satisfactory operation. By adding an operation which relieves the gastric stasis, all its advantages are conserved without its disadvantages. At present, three types of gastric drainage operations are currently performed: pyloroplasty, gastroenterostomy, and antrectomy, followed by a Billroth I or II type of reconstruction.

The operation of vagotomy and pyloroplasty interrupts neural stimuli to the parietal cells and decreases the responsiveness of the parietal cells to other stimuli. In addition, the antrum is denervated and gastric emptying is enhanced, so that endogenous release of gastrin is depressed. All these factors lower gastric HCl production. Pyloroplasty which defunctionalizes the pyloric sphincter mechanism and corrects a duodenal stricture can be performed according to the Heineke-Mikulicz, Finney, or Jaboulay techniques (Fig. 26-14). Of these three techniques, the first, in the author's opinion, is the least desirable, since it is more prone to stenosis and dysfunction and is awkward to construct in the face of severe duodenal fibrosis (Fig. 26-15 and Fig. 26-16).

Gastroenterostomy has been proposed by some as the best method of decompressing the stomach in conjunction with a vagotomy. In the author's opinion, gastroenterostomy is less desirable than pyloroplasty, because the normal continuity of the gastroduodenal tract is not respected. The goal of surgery should be restoration, not alteration, of normal physiology. A gastrojejunostomy bypasses the important digestive and absorptive functions of the duodenum. Moreover, this type of anastomosis is subject to mechanical complications leading to gastric outlet obstruction and afferent loop stasis.

Others consider antrectomy the best method of decompressing the stomach with vagotomy, since it removes the source of gastrin. It should be pointed out that if the antrum is preserved, as is the case with a pyloroplasty and vagotomy, it is denervated, and gastrin release is diminished (but not as much as after antrectomy). Therefore, the argument supporting antrectomy is not entirely valid. However, it is true that the lowest rates of recurrence after surgery for duodenal ulcer (1 to 2 percent) have been provided by vagotomy and antrectomy. The "best" recurrence rates observed after vagotomy and simple drainage—pyloroplasty or gastrojejunostomy—have been around 5 percent. However, patients who have had a vagotomy and antrectomy are liable to postgastrectomy symptoms—dumping, etc.—in addition to *postvagotomy episodic diarrhea.*

The operative risk of vagotomy with pyloroplasty or gastroenterostomy is small; in the author's experience the mortality rate is less than 0.5 percent. Many patients experience diarrhea, which usually improves after a few weeks or months but in a few patients (1 to 2%) may persist and may be disabling. The mechanism of the diarrhea is unknown. It is distinguished from the diarrhea associated with the dumping syndrome by its tendency to occur episodically and without relation to meals. In addition it has been suggested that truncal vagotomy predisposes to gallstone formation. This belief is based on the observation that progressive enlargement of the gallbladder is a consequence of complete severance of the vagus nerves and on the impression of some authors that the incidence of cholelithiasis is greater among previously vagotomized pa-

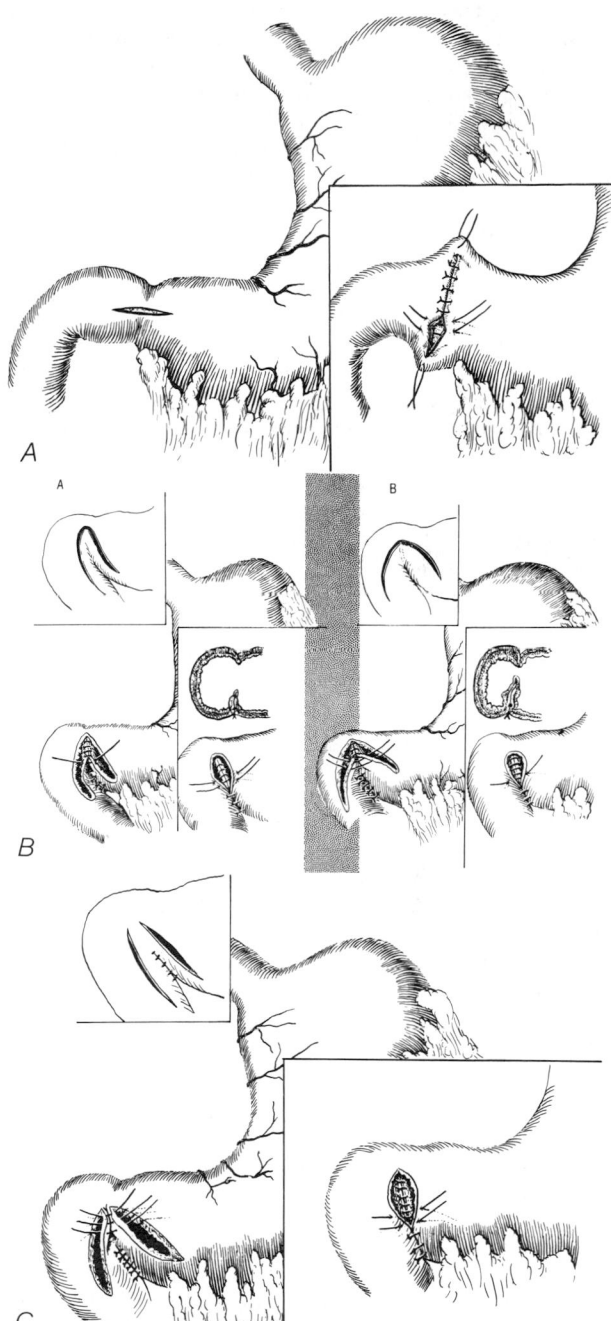

Fig. 26-14. *A.* Heinecke-Mikulicz pyloroplasty: vertical incision 3 cm in length centered on the pyloric ring and closed transversely with one layer of interrupted seromuscular sutures. *B.* Finney pyloroplasty. Insert B demonstrates the correct technique; note the wider septum turned. This leads to malfunction of the pyloroplasty. *C.* Jaboulay pyloroplasty. In reality this is a side-to-side gastroduodenostomy and is an excellent method of drainage when the duodenum is severely scarred.

tients than in the general population. Although the former appears valid, it is also true that in man contraction of the gallbladder is primarily hormone-dependent and that after a vagotomy the gallbladder contracts normally in response

Fig. 26-15. Severe gastric stasis after a vagotomy and a Heineke-Mikulicz pyloroplasty. Note that the stenosis from the patient's duodenal ulcer disease remains *distal* to the pyloroplasty (arrows).

to a test meal. Impressions of an abnormal incidence of cholelithiasis after vagotomy remain unconfirmed. Nevertheless, attempts to prevent postvagotomy diarrhea and biliary dysfunction have led to the introduction of selective vagotomy designed to preserve the celiac branches of the posterior vagus and the hepatic branches of the anterior trunk. Since a selective vagotomy results in complete vagal denervation of the stomach, the procedure requires a supplemental drainage procedure, i.e., pyloroplasty, gastrojejunostomy, or antrectomy with Billroth I or Billroth II reconstruction. Although there appear to be fewer instances of postvagotomy diarrhea after this operation than after truncal vagotomy, the incidence of other sequelae such as dumping and alkaline gastritis is not lessened. The rationale of *highly selective vagotomy* is to interrupt vagal pathways to the fundus and corpus while preserving vagal branches (anterior and posterior nerves of Latarjet) going to the antrum. The vagally innervated antrum maintains a normal pumping function, and, as amply demonstrated by clinical experience, a *drainage procedure is not necessary.* This eliminates the risk of any sequelae associated with a drainage procedure, as well as technical problems related

to invasion of the gastrointestinal lumen: leaking suture line, intraabdominal abscess, and wound infection (Fig. 26-17).

APPLICATION TO DUODENAL ULCERATION. Today fewer and fewer surgeons continue to treat duodenal ulceration with a two-thirds partial gastrectomy. The operations most commonly applied to the treatment of this condition are vagotomy—truncal or selective—*and drainage*—antrectomy, gastroenterostomy, or pyloroplasty. It is a surprising fact that whenever the worth of these various procedures has been subjected to rigorous clinical experimentation, no *significant* differences in results have been found among them. However, some generalizations regarding these procedures can be made. In general the operative mortality is higher for procedures involving resection of the stomach (distal partial gastrectomy or vagotomy and antrectomy) than for vagotomy and simple drainage. Weight loss or inability to maintain a preoperative weight, steatorrhea, and symptoms of "dumping" occur more often after partial gastrectomy and vagotomy with antrectomy than after vagotomy and simple drainage. However, recurrence is least common after vagotomy and antrectomy (approximately 2 percent) and greatest (approximately 7 percent) after vagotomy and simple drainage. The recurrence rate after two-thirds partial gastrectomy lies between these two extremes.

Some argue that the lower mortality of a vagotomy and simple drainage makes the slightly greater recurrence rate acceptable. Others believe that this benefit may be canceled by the mortality and morbidity of additional surgery for recurrent ulceration. Rather than adopting a rigid attitude, an experienced surgeon will select the operation best suited to an individual patient. He may perform a vagotomy and antrectomy in a good-risk patient with a severe ulcer diathesis and reserve vagotomy and simple drainage for cases where the risk of a resection is enhanced by very severe duodenal inflammation or advanced age and associated diseases. At the time of writing, highly selective vagotomy remains under clinical trial. Although the initial results have been almost uniformly good, it is still too early to compare recurrence rates with those of the other established procedures.

Surgical Treatment of Complications of Duodenal Ulceration

BLEEDING

The general management of a patient bleeding from a peptic ulcer has been discussed previously. Details of the surgical management follow.

The failure of medical measures to control the bleeding is the indication of laparotomy. The criterion usually followed is that of massive bleeding, i.e., bleeding which requires replacement of 30 percent of the patient's blood volume over a period of 12 hours to maintain stable vital signs. At the time of laparotomy the duodenum is inspected carefully for signs of scarring and inflammation. If none is found, the stomach is carefully palpated after opening the gastrocolic ligament. If the duodenum is scarred or the serosa of the anterior duodenal wall is stippled and edematous, a vertical incision extending 1 to $\frac{1}{2}$ cm on either side of the pylorus is made. A duodenal ulcer, if present, is usually located in the first portion of the duodenum. An arterial "spurter" may be seen in the base of the ulcer which should be carefully oversewn with two mattress sutures of 2-0 chromic catgut placed on either side of the arterial defect. If possible, one should try to undermine the mucosa so that it can be closed over the ulcer by one or two sutures after suture ligature of the bleeding artery. When suturing a very large ulcer, the author usually places a piece of muscle from the rectus into the base of the ulcer and holds it in place with a mattress suture. The vertical incision over the pylorus is incorporated into a Finney pyloroplasty, and a vagotomy is performed. Whether or not an ulcer is found in the duodenum, a vertical gastrotomy is then made in the midportion of the stomach. One should search for a bleeding gastric ulcer, even though a duodenal ulcer has been found, because of the frequent association of gastric and duodenal ulcer. Frequently hemorrhage from an ulcer ceases with the induction of anesthesia, and the finding of an active crater in the duodenum is not sufficient assurance that it was the source of bleeding. After the gastrotomy incision has been made, retractors are placed in the lumen of the stomach, and the entire mucosal surface is carefully examined. It is often necessary to irrigate the gastric lumen thoroughly to evacuate blood and clots. Some bleeding ulcers are small and easily hidden by a mucosal fold. If the fundic mucosa is not exposed, the greater curvature is mobilized so that by pushing on the anterior or posterior surface of the stomach the fundic mucosa may be turned inside out into the gastrotomy incision. A bleeding gastric ulcer should be oversewn carefully, after a four-quadrant biopsy of the lesion.

The superiority of the concept of vagotomy and simple drainage over partial gastrectomy has been most obvious when applied to the surgical treatment of massively bleeding duodenal ulcer. Under these conditions the operative mortality of gastrectomy approached 20 percent. The current experience is that massively bleeding duodenal ulcer can be managed by vagotomy and pyloroplasty with suture ligation of the ulcer, with a mortality rate close to that expected for elective surgery.

PYLORIC OBSTRUCTION

The proper timing of surgical treatment in the management of pyloric obstruction due to a duodenal ulcer has been discussed above. The obstruction is usually due to a duodenal ulcer, although a gastric ulcer in the pyloric canal ("channel ulcer") or a prepyloric ulcer can cause enough fibrosis of the antrum to obstruct the gastric outlet. The operation should relieve the obstruction and control the duodenal ulcer diathesis, goals which can be achieved by a vagotomy and pyloroplasty. Often the deformity of the duodenum is so severe that a Heineke-Mikulicz pyloroplasty is technically not feasible. Under these conditions, it is usually possible to construct a Finney or a Jaboulay type of pyloroplasty without difficulty. Faced with a severely deformed duodenum, some surgeons prefer a gas-

Fig. 26-16. Note by comparison with Fig. 26-15 the excellent gastric drainage obtained with a Jaboulay pyloroplasty. Arrows indicate the margins of the pyloroplasty.

trojejunostomy to a pyloroplasty. Occasionally a patient has such a severe distension of the stomach that the tone of the muscularis of the stomach has been lost. In these patients, the delay in gastric emptying often accompanying vagotomy may be more severe. When such far-advanced gastric distension is encountered, a subtotal gastric resection may be preferable to a vagotomy and drainage procedure.

Fig. 26-17. Diagram of the three types of vagotomy.

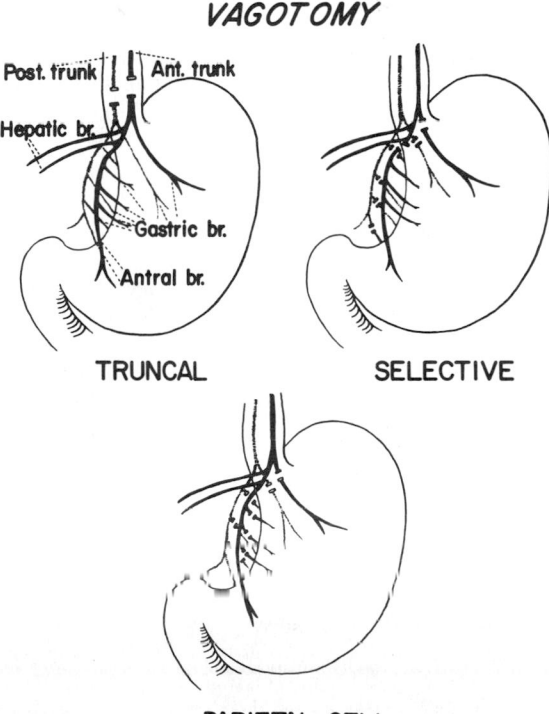

VAGOTOMY

TRUNCAL   SELECTIVE

PARIETAL CELL

PERFORATION

The goal of surgical treatment is to prevent further contamination of the peritoneal cavity. The exploration should be carried out through a short incision either in the upper midline or in the right upper quadrant. Over 75 percent of the perforations occur in the anterior wall of the first portion of the duodenum. Varying amounts of food debris and inflammatory exudate occupy the peritoneal cavity. The perforation should be closed with one or two mattress sutures of 2-0 silk, the ends of which are tied over a fold of omentum to reinforce the closure. After the perforation has been closed, the peritoneal cavity should be cleansed of debris and inflammatory exudate by repeated irrigation of the peritoneal cavity, of the subhepatic and suprahepatic spaces, of the paracolic gutters, and of the pelvic cavity with several gallons of normal saline solution. One can thus prevent localized intraperitoneal abscesses, formerly a frequent complication of perforated duodenal ulcer.

A controversial point is the one of definitive treatment of the duodenal ulcer diathesis at the time of exploration for perforation. This matter should be left to the judgment of the individual surgeon. However, a third of the patients remain symptom-free after the perforation has been closed; for them definitive treatment would not be justified. Experience has shown that the patients whose ulcer symptoms recur after closure of a perforation have long antecedent histories of ulcer. Therefore, in selected patients, i.e., those with long histories of ulcer distress in whom exploration is carried out a short time after the perforation, a vagotomy and pyloroplasty can be done safely. The pyloroplasty incision is carried through the perforation with excision of its margins.

MARGINAL ULCER

A marginal ulcer after partial gastrectomy is notoriously refractory to medical management and usually requires additional surgical procedures. Unless clinical evidence for a Zollinger-Ellison syndrome is present, a vagotomy, transabdominal or transthoracic, is the preferred treatment (Fig. 26-18). When a marginal ulcer occurs in a patient who has had a vagotomy and drainage operation (gastroenterostomy with or without antrectomy), one should first of all determine the completeness of the vagotomy by a Hollander test. Recurrence due to incomplete vagotomy is managed by re-vagotomy and antrectomy. Recurrence despite a complete vagotomy usually results from gastric stasis due to malfunction of the stoma and requires another abdominal exploration, at which time the findings dictate the choice of procedure, i.e., closure of gastrojejunostomy and construction of a pyloroplasty, antrectomy, etc. The possibility of endocrine adenomatosis, however, should always be considered when the clinician is confronted by recurrent ulcer disease. Should the proper diagnostic tests for a Zollinger-Ellison syndrome, including radioimmunoassay of serum gastrin, indicate that a recurrent ulcer is associated with a gastrin-producing pancreatic islet-cell tumor, the only course of management should be complete removal of the target organ: a total gastrectomy. It is futile to attempt to treat what is usually a fulminating ulcer diathesis by lesser resections since even minuscule gastric remnants may under these conditions secrete huge amounts of acid. Equally futile are attempts to reduce serum gastrin levels by searching for and removing these islet-cell tumors, because they are so often multiple and microscopic and/or malignant and have already metastasized. It is particularly important to remove the entire stomach when faced with a Zollinger-Ellison syndrome due to metastatic islet-cell tumor, because it has been shown that these tumors grow very slowly and may actually regress after the stomach has been removed. It is the fulminating ulcer diathesis, not the tumor, which is the lethal factor.

SURGICAL TREATMENT OF SEQUELAE OF ULCER SURGERY

Usually the undesirable side effects of ulcer operations become less noticeable as time goes by. But in a small percentage of patients (<5 percent), crippling symptoms persist. Fortunately, these are often amenable to surgical

Fig. 26-18. *A.* Large marginal ulcer crater 4 years after partial gastrectomy for duodenal ulcer (1). *B.* Seven days posttransthoracic vagotomy; the stoma (2) is now free of ulceration.

correction. The problems encountered most often are *alkaline reflux gastritis, dumping syndrome,* and *episodic* (postvagotomy) *diarrhea.*

Alkaline reflux gastritis is usually associated with a prior gastrectomy and gastrojejunostomy with or without vagotomy. It is corrected by converting the gastrojejunostomy to a Roux en Y arrangement, which effectively diverts bile-containing duodenal juices from the gastric pouch. If not already done, *vagi must be divided.*

A dumping syndrome which does not respond to conservative measures such as a dry, high-protein, low-carbohydrate diet and which persists for more than 2 years after the initial surgery, may be appreciably improved by interposing a *reversed loop* of jejunum, 6 to 8 cm in length, between the gastric pouch and the duodenum. The symptoms of episodic diarrhea may be corrected in a similar fashion by reversing a short (4 to 6 cm) segment of intestine at a point about 100 cm distal to the gastric outlet.

GASTRIC ULCERATIONS

Chronic Gastric Ulcer

Although the term gastric encompasses the antral, fundic, and cardiac segments of the stomach, it has been shown that most chronic gastric ulcers appear in antral mucosa.

DIFFERENCES BETWEEN DUODENAL AND GASTRIC ULCERATION

As will be pointed out below, some ulcers located in the *stomach* actually behave like *duodenal* ulcers. However, some important features separate duodenal ulceration from high-lying gastric ulcers.

SEX. Although both types of ulcer are more prevalent among men, the ratio of men to women is only 2:1 for gastric ulcer as compared with a ratio of 6 or 7:1 for duodenal ulcer. During the decade 1950–1960 the mortality rate for gastric ulcer among women increased by 26 percent and among men decreased by 20 percent.

AGE. By contrast with duodenal ulcer, a disease of middle-aged men (thirty-five to forty-five), the incidence of gastric ulcer increases steadily with age.

FAMILIAL FACTOR. There is an excess of peptic ulcer among the siblings of patients with peptic ulcer disease. Moreover, such studies have shown that the predisposition to an ulcer is type-specific. An excess of gastric ulcer exists among the relatives of patients with gastric ulcer and the same is true for duodenal ulcer among the relatives of patients with this lesion. In addition, there exists among patients with duodenal ulcer a preponderance of blood group O whereas high-lying gastric ulcers tend to be associated with blood group A.

EPIDEMIOLOGY. In most countries, including the United States, duodenal ulcer prevails over gastric ulcer by a ratio of 6:1 or 7:1. However, in some countries such as Japan, where gastric ulceration causes 90 percent of all peptic ulcer deaths, the reverse is true.

ENVIRONMENT. Duodenal ulcer tends to occur more often in individuals working under conditions of tension in positions of responsibility: skilled workers, foremen, executives, etc. Gastric ulcer, on the other hand, occurs more often in unskilled workers and is two to five times more prevalent in the poorer social classes than in the upper social strata.

GASTRIC SECRETORY ACTIVITY. Patients with a duodenal ulcer have higher average rates of gastric secretion than ulcer-free individuals. On the other hand, patients with gastric ulcer have normal or slightly lower than normal levels of HCl secretion (with exceptions to be discussed below).

RESPONSE TO TREATMENT. Duodenal ulcers usually respond well to medical management, whereas gastric ulcers require an operation more often. However, the recurrence rate after operations for duodenal ulcer is higher than is the case for gastric ulcer.

No longer is it believed that gastric ulcers can become malignant. Benign gastric ulcers remain benign and gastric cancers start de novo.

ETIOLOGY OF CHRONIC GASTRIC ULCERATION

The pathophysiology of chronic gastric ulcer is more complex than that of duodenal ulceration. In recent years several etiological factors have been studied.

CHRONIC GASTRITIS AND REDUCED MUCOSAL RESISTANCE. The presence of atrophic gastritis in the stomachs of patients with gastric ulcer, a phenomenon exhaustively studied by DuPlessis, is an important clue to the cause of chronic gastric ulcer. DuPlessis found atrophic gastritis in 61 of 75 stomachs with a gastric ulcer. The ulcer always appeared in chronically inflamed and atrophic mucosa and gastric ulcers located in the body of the stomach were always associated with gastritis extending into the fundus. It has been proposed that the chronic gastritis which appears to favor the formation of a gastric ulcer is due to the chronic reflux of bile into the stomach. Reflux of bile into the stomach can be demonstrated more often in patients with a chronic gastric ulcer than in patients with duodenal disease. Experimental preparations designed to allow bile to bathe the gastric mucosa continuously result in the development of a chronic gastritis which is strikingly similar to the human disease. The gastric mucosa near the stoma of a gastrojejunostomy always shows changes of chronic gastritis. These observations suggest that the reflux of bile-containing duodenal secretions into the stomach over a long time causes chronic gastritis which in turn lessens the resistance of the gastric mucosa to ulceration. Since chronic gastritis is associated with an atrophy of the acid-secreting apparatus, these changes also explain the reduced output of HCl associated with many (but not all) gastric ulcers.

DRUG-INDUCED CHRONIC GASTRIC ULCERATION. In about 20 percent of patients with gastric ulcer, chronic gastritis is absent and the etiological mechanism described in the previous paragraph is not applicable. Of the other possible etiological factors, drug-induced chronic gastric ulceration has received the most interest in recent years. This interest began when it was noticed that the incidence of chronic gastric ulcer in young women in New South Wales (Australia) began to increase in 1943. In subsequent studies a significant association was found between *gastric ulcers in women* and the chronic use of aspirin-containing preparations. No such association was found for duodenal ulcer in either sex or for gastric ulcer in men. Although aspirin, because of its universal use, is the most important of the "ulcerogenic drugs," this phenomenon was first noticed after the introduction of the adrenocorticosteroids. It is now a generally accepted fact that the therapeutic use of steroids particularly for rheumatoid arthritis may be complicated by the development of a chronic *gastric* ulceration. Phenylbutazone and Indomethacin are also occasionally responsible for causing a gastric ulcer. All the drugs—aspirin, steroids, Phenylbutazone, Indomethacin—known to be capable of producing an ulcer have similar antirheumatic, anti-inflammatory properties. The exact mechanisms by which these drugs cause gastric ulceration is not known. However, studies from the author's laboratory have shown that all of these drugs reduce substantially the ability of the gastric mucosa to secrete mucus, which may favor ulcer formation since the layer of mucus covering the gastric epithelium is believed to play a role in mucosal defense mechanisms against ulceration (Fig. 26-19).

HEREDITARY FACTORS. As previously mentioned there is an inherited predisposition to one type or the other of peptic ulceration. This phenomenon has received considerable support with respect to duodenal ulceration from the well-documented association between blood group O and duodenal ulceration. Unfortunately, a relationship between blood group phenotypes and *gastric* ulceration remained buried by the anatomical classification of peptic ulcers into duodenal and gastric. When Johnson separated gastric ulcers into three categories (lesions in the corpus

of the stomach without abnormalities of the duodenum, pylorus, or prepyloric region; gastric ulcers associated with an active duodenal ulcer or with a scarred duodenum; and gastric ulcers situated close to the pylorus), he found a significant excess of blood group A among the patients in the first category. Patients in the other two categories showed the strong association with blood group O characteristic of duodenal ulceration. Although these observations do not provide an explanation for the greater susceptibility to gastric ulceration associated with blood group A (any more than we understand the reason for the association between blood group O and duodenal ulceration) they at least have formed the basis for a more rational classification of gastric ulceration to be discussed below.

GASTRIC ACIDITY. As in the case of duodenal ulceration (DU), a *chronic* gastric ulcer (GU) does not occur in the absence of gastric secretion of HCl and pepsin. However, whereas duodenal ulceration is associated, on the average, with excessive gastric acidity, patients with gastric ulcer (anatomic classification) secrete, on the average, normal amounts of acid (Table 26-1). Nevertheless, a frequently cited theory of gastric ulceration attributes the process to gastric hyperacidity due to gastric stasis. This view is based on the frequency with which a gastric ulcer is associated with an active duodenal ulcer or a scarred duodenum. The incidence of combined GU-DU is approximately 25 percent of all chronic gastric ulcers. Because the duodenal ulcer usually precedes the appearance of the gastric lesion, it has been assumed that the gastric stasis produced by the duodenal ulcer increases antral release of gastrin, and the resulting hyperacidity would lead to the formation of the gastric ulcer.

Actually, much of the confusion surrounding the possible role of an augmented acid-peptic factor in the etiology of chronic gastric ulceration is cleared when one departs from a purely anatomic definition of a gastric ulcer. On the basis of physiologic data one may separate chronic ulcers located in the stomach into two categories. On the one hand, there are lesions located near the pylorus or in the pyloric canal or associated with an active duodenal ulcer. When these lesions are analyzed separately, one finds that they are associated with blood group O and *with rates of gastric secretion greater than those of normal subjects and close to the range commonly found in patients with a duodenal ulcer.* On the other hand, lesions located in the body of the stomach, in addition to being associated with blood group A, as previously mentioned, are characterized by a *reduced* gastric output of acid.

The following classification of chronic gastric ulcer summarizes the foregoing discussion of the etiological aspects of this lesion.

Fig. 26-19. Bars represent volume (in milliliters) of gastric antral mucus secreted during a daily 3-hour collection period. Note the decrease in the rate of secretion under the influence of cortisone. (*Reproduced from Menguy and Masters, Surgery, 54:19, 1963.*)

EFFECT OF CORTISONE ON SECRETION OF MUCUS BY GASTRIC ANTRUM

Type	Location	Etiological Relationship
I	High-lying, lesser curvature	Chronic gastritis, blood group A
II	Prepyloric or associated with a duodenal ulcer or scarred duodenum	Hyperacidity
III	Random, may be on greater curvature	Drug-induced: aspirin, steroids, Indomethacin, Phenylbutazone

CLINICAL MANIFESTATIONS

Symptomatic differences between gastric and duodenal ulcer are subtle. As with duodenal ulcer the distress of a gastric lesion occurs when the stomach is empty and is relieved by food and antacids. The astute physician may recognize some differences. The pain is often to the left of the midline. The patient with a gastric ulcer may experience discomfort ("burning," "pressure," "gas") immediately after drinking hot or cold liquids, alcohol or highly spiced foods, raw fruits, and vegetables. Sometimes, and this is characteristic of penetrating gastric ulcers, food does not relieve the distress (as it does with duodenal ulcer), but, on the contrary aggravates it. Sometimes, a gastric ulcer may remain asymptomatic until its presence is manifested by a serious complication such as bleeding or perforation.

The greater seriousness of gastric ulceration by comparison with duodenal ulceration is emphasized by the fact that gastric ulceration, although less common than the duodenal disease, is responsible for at least one-half of all ulcer deaths. Perhaps because patients with a gastric ulcer are older, the consequences of such ulcer-related complications as hemorrhage and perforation are compounded by associated age-related conditions. Moreover, even when the age factor is discounted, the mortality rate of perforated gastric ulcer is greater than that of perforated duodenal ulcer. The gravity of perforated gastric ulcer may result from a higher incidence of intraperitoneal septic complications caused by the heavy bacterial growth to be expected in the hypochlorhydric stomachs of patients with a gastric ulcer.

Another feature of chronic gastric ulceration is the tendency for it to recur after healing. One may expect that in at least 50 percent of cases the lesion will recur during the two years following initial healing of the lesion. This recurrence rate seems to be particularly high for gastric ulcers associated with a duodenal ulcer.

DIAGNOSIS

The roentgenographic demonstration of an ulcerating lesion in the stomach is the most important step in the diagnosis. Once the presence of an ulcerating lesion has been recognized, its benign or malignant nature must be established. It is vital that all of the information that roentgenography, gastroscopy, and cytology can provide be applied to this end.

ROENTGENOGRAPHY. Roentgenographic demonstration of a gastric ulceration is the first and most important step in the diagnosis. After its discovery, the benign or malignant nature of the ulceration must be determined. This diagnosis is based upon certain characteristic roentgenographic features.

The projection of the base of the ulcer with respect to the gastric wall is important. When the base lies in or outside the gastric contour, the ulcer is probably benign. If the base lies inside the gastric contour, and particularly if it is located in a space-occupying gastric mass, it is probably malignant. Rigidity of the gastric wall in the vicinity of the ulceration indicates malignancy. An ulcer

Fig. 26-20. Large benign gastric ulcer crater. Note that gastric mucosal folds radiate toward the ulcer.

with a regular round or oval shape has greater chance of being benign, whereas irregular or asymmetric craters are often malignant. When the mucosal folds in the vicinity of the ulcer radiate toward the ulcer, the latter is probably benign (Fig. 26-20). A gastric ulcer accompanied by a duodenal ulcer or a deformity of the duodenal bulb is probably benign. The size of the ulceration is of diagnostic importance only if it is small. A diameter of less than 1 cm probably indicates a benign lesion.

Without question, the most valuable roentgenologic feature is the relation of the ulceration to the contour of the gastric wall. As can be seen in Fig. 26-21, a benign gastric ulcer crater extends beyond the contour of the wall. The margin surrounding the ulcer is smooth and slightly rolled. The healing ulcer fills with granulation tissue and assumes a pyramidal shape as it gradually becomes smaller and

Fig. 26-21. Benign gastric ulcer. Sequential films at 2-week intervals on the same patient. A. The base of the ulcer extends beyond the contour of the gastric wall. Some edema surrounds the ulcer. B. Good healing of the crater is evidenced by the pyramidal shape it has assumed. Note mucosal folds radiating toward the crater. C. Complete healing with scarring and stellar configuration of mucosal folds.

closes. By contrast, Fig. 26-22 illustrates a malignant ulcer which has the appearance of a broad plateau projecting into the lumen of the stomach. Mucosal folds do not reach the mass because of infiltration of the mucosa around the ulcer by carcinomatous tissue. Digestion of the tumor mass by acid-peptic juice results in the formation of a crater in its center.

The accuracy with which a gastric carcinoma may be recognized varies with its location. The diagnosis of fundic

Fig. 26-22. Malignant gastric ulceration. Sequential films in a patient who refused surgical intervention. *A.* and *B.* The ulcer does not extend beyond the contour of the stomach but is contained in a broad plateau projecting into the lumen. Inexorable progression of the lesion is obvious.

lesions is unreliable because of the difficulty in filling this portion of the stomach with barium. Recognition of lesions in the antrum is more accurate. In general, the accuracy of radiologic interpretation approximates 90 percent.

GASTROSCOPY. Direct visualization of a gastric lesion is a very useful adjunct to the differential diagnosis, particularly since the introduction of the fiberoptic instrumentation which has made the procedure a simple and safe one. The endoscopic diagnosis of an ulcerating lesion is based on the gross features of the lesion: a smooth, regular, round punched-out lesion with a clean white base and radiating folds is likely to be benign, whereas an irregular lesion with a dirty-looking base and heaped-up edges is more likely to be malignant. The value of gastroscopy has been enhanced by the capability, provided by the newer instrumentation, of brushing cytology and biopsy under direct vision. Because of the small amount of material sampled, the latter techniques are associated with false negative results even in the hands of experienced operators.

Fig. 26-23. Single malignant cell demonstrated upon cytologic study of gastric aspirate from a patient with a small malignant ulceration.

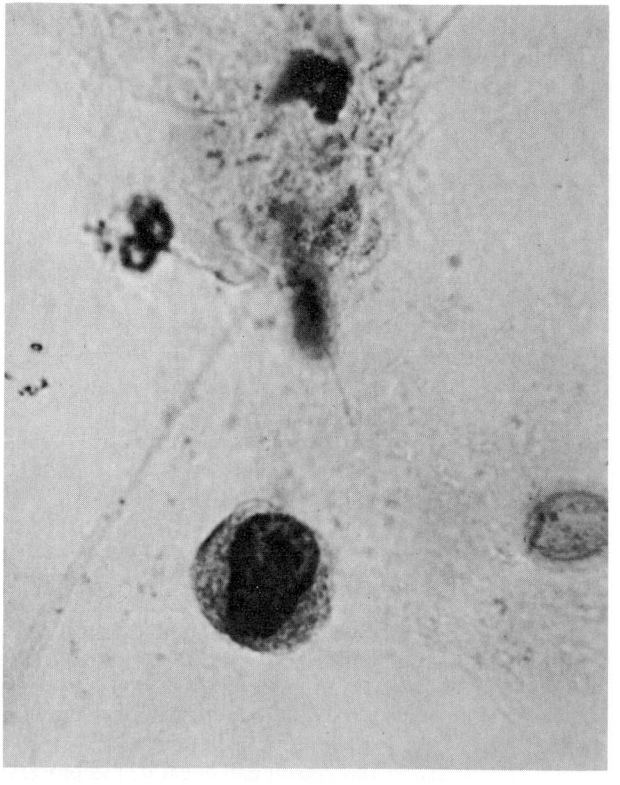

EXFOLIATIVE CYTOLOGY. The value of cytology in separating benign from malignant gastric ulcerations has been proved only in centers where the procedure has been applied as a research arm of medicine or pathology. The morphologic features of malignant exfoliated cells (Fig. 26-23) include increased nuclear-cytoplasmic ratio, hyperchromasia, irregular clumping of chromatin, increased number and size of nucleoli, and "signet ring" appearance of cells. It must be stressed that the value of the procedure depends upon the experience of the cytologist. A negative cytological study cannot stand alone and can serve only to reinforce an impression of benignancy provided by other methods. A positive result must of course be accepted as a formal indication of malignancy even though false-positive results do occur.

GASTRIC ANALYSIS. Approximately one-half of patients

with a gastric carcinoma are achlorhydric; i.e., the pH of gastric juice remains above 3.5 even during stimulation with secretagogues. However, because the presence of even high concentrations of HCl in gastric juice does not exclude the possibility of a malignant gastric ulcer, gastric analysis has only limited value in the differential diagnosis of gastric ulcerations.

ACCURACY OF DIFFERENTIAL DIAGNOSIS. It is often claimed that the combined use of roentgenography, gastroscopy, biopsy (endoscopic), and cytology provide the clinician with almost 100 percent accuracy in differentiating benign from malignant gastric ulcerations. It should be pointed out that because of the recent decrease in the incidence of gastric cancer only about 8 percent of ulcerating lesions in the stomach are malignant. In other words, if one were to approach all gastric ulcerations as being benign one would be "correct" in at least 90 percent of instances. In the author's opinion the "almost 100 percent accuracy" is due to the smaller number of cancers, some of which are all too obvious. It is with the small number of potentially curable gastric cancers associated with many of the features of a benign ulcer that the diagnostic tools described above may be severely taxed.

In clinical practice one often relies upon the test of healing to make this crucial diagnosis (Fig. 26-21). The test is based on the generally valid assumption that malignant ulcerations rarely show sustained healing. But, in fact, they can heal sufficiently to satisfy radiological criteria of healing. In a recent study of 638 patients with a gastric ulceration, 25 proved to have a cancer. In 4 of the 25 patients with gastric cancer, the initially detected ulceration had appeared benign radiologically and subsequently healed with medical treatment. The correct diagnosis was made only 9 to 19 months later.

MEDICAL TREATMENT OF CHRONIC GASTRIC ULCERATION

If all of the diagnostic procedures described above indicate that the lesion is benign, medical treatment based on the following measures is instituted.

ABSTINENCE FROM SMOKING. This—and bed rest—is the only measure which has been shown to accelerate healing.

ABSOLUTE BED REST. This is an important feature of the treatment and, at least initially, should be in-hospital, the best environment for the intense diagnostic and therapeutic program required for this potentially serious disease.

ANTACID THERAPY. Although gastric acidity is usually lower in patients with a gastric ulcer, it remains true that a peptic ulcer does not occur in the absence of HCl. If the already low levels of gastric acid accompanying gastric ulcer can be lowered even more, the ulcer often heals rapidly. As mentioned previously, effective antacid therapy is provided by absorbable antacids such as calcium carbonate in doses of 4 Gm every 2 hours (after excluding organic renal disease).

DIET. A multiple-feeding program keeps gastric juice buffered by food. There may be merit in avoiding foods with roughage such as raw fruit and vegetables.

AVOIDANCE OF GASTRIC STASIS. Anticholinergics are contraindicated because of their inhibitory action on gastric motility.

NEW MEASURES. Carbenoxolone sodium, a compound synthesized from an essential ingredient of licorice, has recently been found to accelerate the rate of healing of gastric ulcers in ambulatory patients. It has been postulated that this occurs via an enhanced secretion of gastric mucus. The main side effect of carbenoxolone is an aldosterone-like activity which may precipitate congestive heart failure in elderly patients.

INDICATIONS FOR SURGERY

If one excludes from this discussion obviously malignant lesions for which the decision to operate should not be in question, this decision is based upon the behavior of the lesion and its potential for complications, recurrence, or prolonged morbidity. The following features of gastric ulceration should suggest the advisability of an operation.

Gastric ulcers associated with a duodenal ulcer are more liable to recur after healing and deserve an early operation.

Pyloric canal "channel" ulcers are often severely symptomatic and respond poorly to medical treatment.

When there is evidence of deep penetration, the risk of a serious complication such as perforation or hemorrhage is higher and warrants early consideration of surgery.

Very large or so-called "giant" gastric ulcers should be treated surgically. In addition to the hazard of complications, the healing of these lesions often causes sufficient scarring to impair gastric emptying.

Ulcers failing to undergo a 50 percent reduction in size over a 3-week period of medical treatment are best treated surgically.

The recurrence of a gastric ulcer should, in the absence of a contraindication, be considered as an indication for surgery.

And above all, should there be *the slightest doubt* about the benignancy of the lesion, surgical intervention should be advised without undue delay.

Acute Gastric Mucosal Lesions

An *erosion* is a mucosal defect that does not penetrate deeper than the muscularis mucosae. A lesion extending beyond this layer is an *ulcer*. A condition characterized by profuse bleeding from multiple gastric *erosions* was described for the first time in 1898 by Dieulafoy who used the term of "exulceratio simplex" to describe it. Since then such terms as "acute erosive gastritis," "acute hemorrhagic gastritis," "Cushing's ulcer," "Curling's ulcer," and "stress ulcer" have been employed. Because the cause of these acute, superficial mucosal lesions remains poorly defined it seems preferable to refer to them as "acute gastric mucosal (AGM) lesions" which cause "acute gastric mucosal bleeding."

The true incidence of this condition was not appreciated until recently when the introduction of fiberoptic endoscopic instrumentation made it practically feasible to examine the gastric mucosa in most cases of upper gastrointestinal bleeding. As long as emergency radiological examination of the stomach was the mainstay of the workup of the "upper gastrointestinal bleeder," the importance of AGM lesions was not appreciated because erosions, when present, would result in a negative radiological study. The latter would often be interpreted as "bleeding probably due to peptic ulcer." It is now apparent that gastric erosions are responsible for at least 20 percent of all cases of upper gastrointestinal bleeding.

PATHOLOGIC ANATOMY

The main gross feature is the presence of mucosal erosions, usually multiple, ranging in size from barely visible petechiae, to round lesions about 1 cm in diameter (Fig. 26-24). In addition one may find acute penetrating ulcers often with an irregular "geographic" contour particularly when the condition complicates a stressful situation (see below). The lesions may involve any segment of the stomach and particularly after a "stress" may be found in the duodenum. The mucosal erosion is the main microscopic feature of this condition. It is preceded by the development of focal mucosal hemorrhagic and coagulative necrosis. As the foci of necrotic mucosa slough, erosions based on the muscularis mucosae are left. These erosions rapidly heal without scarring. Elsewhere, one finds mucosal and submucosal edema and hemorrhage. Antecedent chronic, atrophic gastritis may be present in some patients, particularly in those where AGM bleeding is not precipitated by one of the usual "causes" of this condition (see below).

ETIOLOGY

The appearance of acute gastric erosions is often preceded by one of the following situations:

Stress: trauma; burns; surgical operations. The complication of any one of these situations by *sepsis* is particularly conducive to the development of AGM lesions.

Alcohol.

Drugs: aspirin, steroids, Indomethacin, Phenylbutazone.

No apparent cause. Patients in whom AGM lesions do not appear to have been precipitated by one of the "causes" listed above often have an underlying chronic, atrophic gastritis which seems to predispose the gastric mucosa to this acute condition.

Although it is not known why stress or drugs should cause mucosal erosions, the following etiological mechanisms have been investigated.

GASTRIC HYPERSECRETION. Because of the role played by an excessive gastric output of acid in some types of ulceration, a similar relationship has been investigated for AGM lesions, but with scant success. Although gastric hyperacidity has been found in patients having undergone neurosurgical operations, operations particularly susceptible to this complication, a consistent pattern of hyperacidity has never been found in burned patients, who are most prone to AGM lesions. Moreover viable microorganisms have been found on the gastric mucosa of burned patients. This finding is not consistent with gastric acidity. Whenever this factor has been studied it has been found that stressful situations suppress rather than stimulate gastric acid secretion. Drug-induced AGM lesions are probably not acid related since these drugs have no important action on gastric secretion, except for the steroids which, when given over many days, increase acid secretion slightly. The development of AGM lesions in patients with atrophic gastritis and pernicious anemia suggests that mucosal erosions may appear in the absence of measurable amounts of gastric acid.

ABNORMAL GASTRIC MUCOSAL BARRIER. Normally the permeability of the gastric mucosal membrane to hydrogen ion is limited. This relative impermeability is responsible for the extremely high gradient in HCl concentration between the lumen of the stomach and the extracellular fluid compartment. Recent studies suggest that experimental conditions simulating those commonly associated with the clinical development of AGM lesions, such as hemorrhagic shock, increase the permeability of the gastric mucosa to hydrogen ion. It has been suggested that hypochlorhydria often found in critically ill patients may be due to this

Fig. 26-24. Gross appearance of gastric mucosal erosions. In this instance, the lesions were caused by aspirin.

Fig. 26-25. Endoscopic appearance of erosive gastritis.

loss of hydrogen ion by back diffusion rather than from an absolute reduction in gastric acid secretion. With respect to the mechanism of drug-induced erosive gastritis, Davenport found that after canine stomachs had been exposed to aspirin, mucosal damage with fluid and ionic diffusion into the lumen occurred. He postulated that the increased permeability of the mucosa to hydrogen ion leads to gross mucosal injury and bleeding. Other factors which may play a role in the development of mucosal erosions under the influence of stress and "ulcerogenic drugs" are related to the mucous layer lining the mucosa and the rate at which the mucosa is capable of renewing itself. Studies from the author's laboratory have shown that steroids reduce the rate of gastric mucous secretion as well as the rate of epithelial cell turnover in the canine stomach, changes which should affect adversely the ability of the mucosal membrane to maintain its integrity.

CLINICAL MANIFESTATIONS

It may be redundant to point out that the salient clinical feature of AGM lesions or "hemorrhagic gastritis" is bleeding. Some aspects of the bleeding merit discussion. The hemorrhage may be occult and discovered only at autopsy. Signs of hemorrhagic shock may be misinterpreted in a patient already burdened with several potentially lethal problems. One must be alert to this possibility in all severely stressed patients (particularly when sepsis enters the picture). The interval between the stressful incident (trauma, operation) and the appearance of bleeding seems to be approximately 6 days. When AGM lesions complicate a severe illness or multiple injuries, the patient's primary problems may completely overshadow the bleeding. There may be, particularly in burned patients, penetrating acute ulcers. A free perforation may be masked by the symptoms of the primary problems and by the bleeding.

DIAGNOSIS OF AGM LESIONS

The most important diagnostic step is early endoscopy (Fig. 26-25). It is important to realize that the shallow erosions which characterize this condition cannot be demonstrated by conventional barium meal roentgenographic studies; these can only serve to interfere with subsequent endoscopy. Moreover, endoscopy must be performed early, while the hemorrhage is active. If the examination is delayed, these lesions, which heal rapidly, may be completely missed. Selective arteriography is gaining favor as a diagnostic method for this condition. However, it provides less specific information on the source of bleeding, is more hazardous, and, in patients with severely diseased arteries, may be impossible to perform.

MEDICAL TREATMENT OF AGM LESIONS

As with any condition associated with blood loss, adequate replenishment of the blood volume is very critical. It is even more critical in stress-related AGM lesions because hypovolemia and inadequate tissue perfusion pose another burden on a patient already seriously ill. The replacement, although aggressive, must be accurate with due allowance for the patient's cardiac reserve, which in the cirumstances often surrounding AGM lesions may be marginal.

Gastric cooling, which may prevent further mucosal injury by reducing gastric secretion and peptic activity, appears to have some merit in this condition although it has only questionable value in arresting bleeding from gastric or duodenal ulcers. The best way to cool the stomach is to lavage it extensively with iced saline solution via an Ewald tube, a method which also allows one to empty the stomach of blood and thus facilitate endoscopy.

Recently some success in arresting hemorrhage from AGM lesions has been reported with selective catheterization of the celiac axis and infusion of Pitressin or epinephrine into the vascular bed of the stomach.

Surgical Treatment of Chronic Gastric Ulceration

The elective surgical management of a chronic gastric ulcer depends upon the type of gastric ulceration.

If the ulcer belongs to the type and category of high-lying gastric ulcerations associated with chronic gastritis and gastric acid hyposecretion (approximately 75 percent of chronic gastric ulcerations), the best method of treatment is a partial gastrectomy. It is especially important to carry the resection high on the lesser curvature of the stomach to remove all of the antral mucosa. The absence of duodenal scarring not only eliminates the technical problems associated with this operation when it is done for duodenal ulceration, but also allows one to reestablish gastrointestinal continuity by a Billroth I gastroduodenostomy. The limited extent of the resection and the gastroduodenal anastomosis reduce the incidence of the various symptoms associated with the postgastrectomy state. Experience accumulated over the past two decades indicates that the operative mortality of elective gastrectomy for chronic gastric ulceration is 1 percent or lower. The long-term results with respect to ulcer recurrence are excellent and it has been customary to compare the good results after gastrectomy for gastric ulcer with the accepted recurrence rate of about 5 percent after the same but more extensive operation for duodenal ulcer. Recurrence rates ranging from 0 to 1 percent are representative of the results that one has learned to expect after partial gastrectomy for chronic gastric ulcer.

When dealing with a Type II lesion characterized by associated duodenal ulceration or a scarred duodenal bulb and/or by an abnormally high rate of gastric acid secretion or by the location of the lesion in the pyloric canal or immediately proximal to it, the goal of therapy should be reduction of acid secretory activity rather than excision of all of the antral mucosa. Vagotomy and a drainage procedure such as a pyloroplasty, or a distal antrectomy are the procedures of choice. Naturally, a careful four-quadrant biopsy of the lesion should be carried out whenever the ulcer is to be left in situ. It should be mentioned at this juncture that during the early and mid-1960s there was a wave of interest in the application of vagotomy and pyloroplasty (with a four-quadrant biopsy of the ulcer) to *all* cases of gastric ulceration. The results published to date suggest that the recurrence rate is prohibitively high. However, as mentioned above, this approach has a sound rationale when reserved for those gastric ulcers which belong to the duodenal ulcer diathesis.

Chronic gastric ulcers associated with ulcerogenic drugs are often quite large when detected, are liable to severe complications, do not always respond promptly to removal of the responsible agent and in the author's experience are best treated by a partial gastrectomy.

Surgical Treatment of Acute Gastric Mucosal Lesions

As previously indicated, bleeding from multiple, superficial gastric erosions is one of the most common causes of upper gastrointestinal bleeding. Fortunately the hemorrhage ceases spontaneously in the majority of cases. But when surgery becomes necessary, the choice of an appropriate operation may be difficult. For many years the operation most commonly performed for this condition was a partial gastrectomy. An all-too-common sequela was persistent bleeding due to overlooked erosions or new lesions in the remaining gastric mucosa. Because of this problem, Sullivan and Waddel advocated vagotomy and pyloroplasty along with multiple-suture-ligatures of the bleeding lesions through a wide gastrotomy. This approach, initially satisfactory in their hands, has been used widely but with mixed results. As reported by various authors, the rate of rebleeding cases after this operation ranges from 15 to 100 percent. All too often patients with this condition are so desperately ill because of the condition which may have precipitated the erosive gastritis that they cannot tolerate the continued bleeding, much less the reoperation to control it. For this reason the author has suggested that when erosive gastritis requires an operation, it should be tailored to the individual patient. When the patient is desperately ill, usually because of the condition responsible for the erosive gastritis (severe burns, multiple injuries, sepsis), the operation performed should be one which precludes further bleeding, i.e. a near-total gastrectomy. But if the patient's condition is good enough to allow him to tolerate rebleeding (and, possible reoperation) after a more conservative procedure, a vagotomy and hemigastrectomy or vagotomy and pyloroplasty with suture-ligation of all visible bleeding points through a large gastrotomy should be carried out.

It is important to stress that fatalities from this condition often result from the primary precipitating illness and its complications, of which erosive gastritis and massive bleeding may be one of several. The least the surgeon can do is to ensure that bleeding isn't the last straw.

MISCELLANEOUS SURGICAL DISEASES

Acute Gastric Dilatation

This condition may occur after operations on the stomach or the upper abdomen and after certain types of trauma, particularly of the chest. It is especially common in women and children and is more likely to occur in patients who are partially conscious and receiving oxygen through a nasal catheter or artificial respiration without a properly cuffed tracheostomy tube. A particularly lethal combination is the administration of oxygen via a nasal catheter in a patient with an indwelling nasogastric tube. There are occurrences on record (and probably many more not on record) in which the oxygen line was inadvertently connected to the gastric tube, resulting in severe distension and bursting of the stomach. The error is obviously so easy to commit by nonprofessional personnel that one should never give oxygen therapy via a nasal catheter to a patient with a Levin tube in the stomach.

The usual mechanism of acute gastric dilatation is a vicious cycle of gastric distension compounded by the patient's efforts at belching, which result only in swallowing more air, which increases the distension, and so on. As the stomach becomes distended, interstitial fluid seeps into its lumen; in addition, gastric secretion is stimulated by the distension. In this manner, several liters (up to 4 or 5) may accumulate in the stomach. Distension of this degree can lead to death by dehydration and fall in plasma volume, and by interference with cardiac and pulmonary function from compression of the diaphragm. In any patient with the conditions described above, the onset of hiccuping, regurgitation of small amounts of fluid, a rise in pulse rate, and tympany over the epigastrium should lead to the recognition of acute gastric dilatation and indicate the need for immediate insertion of a nasogastric tube. Acute gastric dilatation can be rapidly fatal if not corrected. Death often results from acute pulmonary edema caused by sudden aspiration of gastric contents into the tracheobronchial tree.

Mallory-Weiss Syndrome

The pathologic basis of this syndrome is the development of longitudinal mucosal tears along the gastroesophageal junction. By definition, the tears involve only the mucosa and submucosa. They lie in the region of the cardia. Profuse gastric hemorrhage is the salient clinical manifestation. Most cases of this syndrome have been associated with acute alcoholic debauches, and it has been surmised that the lacerations result from violent retching motions forcing gastric contents against a contracted cardia. The laceration may involve the full thickness of the cardia with or without extension into the esophagus. Spontaneous rupture of the gastroesophageal junction (Boerhave's syndrome) is almost invariably fatal if not recognized and treated promptly. The perforation may cause signs of peritonitis when located below the phrenoesophageal ligament; when involving the esophagus above the latter structure, signs of mediastinitis with severe retrosternal pain, high fever, crunching precordial sounds, and a *characteristic air fluid level in the posterior mediastinum* may occur. Occasionally both the mediastinum and the peritoneal cavity may be involved.

Prolapse of Gastric Mucosa

The major clinical manifestations are delayed gastric emptying and episodes of vomiting, accompanied by epigastric fullness. Roentgenographic studies may show the prolapse of antral folds into the duodenum (Fig. 26-26). It should be pointed out that such a prolapse may be found in otherwise asymptomatic patients. Therefore, one should rule out very carefully the existence of other diseases before attempting specific treatment of a mucosal prolapse. This treatment consists of antrectomy and reconstruction of gastroduodenal continuity by a Billroth I anastomosis.

Fig. 26-26. Prolapse of gastric mucosa into the duodenum. Patient also has a small prepyloric gastric ulcer on the lesser curvature.

Gastritis

ATROPHIC GASTRITIS

The diagnosis of atrophic gastritis is usually a clinical one and is based upon demonstrated hypochlorhydria or achlorhydria. At gastroscopy one may see a thinning of the gastric mucosal membrane, through which vessels are visible, and flattening of the rugal folds. A decrease in number of the gastric glands with a chronic inflammatory reaction in the mucosa and intestinalization of the gastric mucosal membrane constitute the histologic picture. In some patients with this condition, circulating antibodies to parietal cells have been demonstrated. Malabsorption of vitamin B_{12} may or may not be present.

CORROSIVE GASTRITIS

Although the ingestion of caustic agents usually causes more damage to the esophagus than to the stomach, occasionally enough material may reach the stomach to cause acute gastritis. In extreme cases of this condition, the injury may involve the full thickness of the gastric wall with resulting perforation. Total gastrectomy becomes necessary as a lifesaving measure. In less severe instances of corrosive gastritis, the caustic material pooling in the more dependent portion of the stomach results in scarring and pyloric obstruction, requiring a gastrojejunostomy to relieve the obstructive process (Fig. 26-27).

EOSINOPHILIC GASTRITIS

This rare condition is characterized by a chronic inflammatory infiltrate in the wall of the stomach and sometimes of the proximal small bowel. The infiltrate is of the granulomatous variety, and eosinophilia may be present. Occasionally the chronic inflammation may cause sufficient scarring and thickening of the gastric wall to mimic the

Fig. 26-27. *A.* Corrosive gastritis due to ingestion of concentrated HCl. Healing with severe cicatricial contraction of the antrum. *B.* Obstruction relieved by a gastrojejunostomy.

gross appearance of a gastric carcinoma, particularly of the linitis plastica variety. Gastric ulceration may occur.

HYPERTROPHIC GASTRITIS

This condition was first described by Ménétrier (polyadénomes en nappe). The clinical significance of giant hypertrophic gastritis is poorly understood. It is often a roentgenographic finding of enlarged rugal folds requiring a diagnosis between hypertrophic gastritis and a gastric lymphoma. This diffuse enlargement of the rugal folds is often found in association with polyendocrine adenomatosis in the Zollinger-Ellison syndrome. Under these conditions, the enlarged rugal folds represent a hyperplasia of the gastric mucosal membrane. Hypertrophic gastritis is often associated with an increased permeability of the gastric mucosal barrier to serum proteins and loss of albumin into the lumen.

Gastric Volvulus

The symptomatic triad of gastric volvulus consists of the following: (1) severe nausea with a paradoxical inability to vomit, (2) localized epigastric pain, and (3) impossibility

of introducing a stomach tube. These lesions are idiopathic or secondary to such conditions as eventration of the diaphragm and paraesophageal hiatal hernia. Incarceration of the displaced stomach in a paraesophageal hernia sac may cause occult bleeding and anemia or massive bleeding. The treatment requires surgical reduction of the volvulus.

Foreign Bodies

Clinicians are frequently confronted with a patient, often a child, who has inadvertently or intentionally swallowed a foreign body. One should adopt an attitude of watchful expectation unless the object has sharp projections which could injure the mucosal membrane or is obviously too large to pass the pylorus. In patients with a duodenal ulcer, small gastric foreign bodies which might otherwise enter the duodenum are often retained in the stomach and may precipitate pyloric obstruction. When it becomes obvious that the foreign body is not passing through the pylorus or is causing symptoms, it should be removed surgically. Before opening the abdomen, it is worthwhile to pass a flexible gastroscope into the stomach under general anesthesia and attempt removal with the biopsy attachment.

BEZOARS

Bezoars are concretions formed by the swallowing of material retained in the stomach. They may be:

1. Trichobezoars (balls formed from hair eaten by children, usually girls)
2. Phytobezoars (balls formed from vegetable fibers, such as those of persimmons)

Symptomatic bezoars require surgical removal only when they cannot be broken down by the intragastric administration of a preparation of *cellulose.* Because of the reduced gastric acidity and motility produced by a vagotomy for duodenal ulcer, patients who have had this operation seem more prone to developing phytobezoars. They must be cautioned against eating large amounts of highly fibrous fresh fruits.

GASTRIC CANCER

INCIDENCE. For unknown reasons the incidence of gastric cancer has been falling during recent decades. In the United States the age-adjusted mortality rate from gastric cancer fell from 29 per 100,000 in 1930 to 20 per 100,000 in 1945, to 13 per 100,000 in 1955 and to 7 per 100,000 in 1966. During the same time, deaths from all cancers increased from 197,042 in 1948 to 245,070 in 1956. The same phenomenon has been observed in the Netherlands, Norway, and Great Britain. By contrast, gastric cancer has become more prevalent in Japan, Chile, Iceland, Finland, and the Scandinavian countries. In Japan, gastric cancer constitutes slightly more than one-half of all cases of cancer. It is interesting to note that as the decrease in gastric cancer was taking place in the United States, the incidence of colonic cancer increased, so that today the colon is the most common location of cancers of the gut.

ETIOLOGY. The cause of gastric cancer remains unknown. Nevertheless it is associated with several factors which may eventually provide a clue to its etiology.

Environmental Factors. In the United States, as well as in several other countries, the frequency of gastric cancer increases with the distance from the equator. It has already been pointed out that the incidence of gastric cancer is considerably higher in Japan than it is in the United States. However, it is appreciably lower in Japanese immigrants to the United States. The incidence of gastric cancer in Japanese born in the United States is no greater than in Caucasian Americans.

Elsewhere, the incidence of gastric cancer has been found to be higher in the city than in the surrounding rural areas. Moreover, in urban areas, gastric cancer was more prevalent among laborers than among artisans and white collar workers.

Diet. Although a possible correlation between diet and gastric cancer has been studied extensively, consumption of cabbage is the only dietary factor correlating with gastric cancer in the United States. Countries with a high incidence of gastric cancer also have a high consumption of fish. Whether it is the fish itself or whether it is the cooking in superheated oils and fats or smoking that is responsible remains to be proved. Others have incriminated the salty and spicy foods so characteristic of the Japanese diet.

Heredity. The risk of developing a gastric cancer is greater than expected among the male and female relatives of patients with gastric cancer.

The interaction between gastric cancers and ABO blood groups may be a related phenomenon. Many controlled studies have shown an excess of blood group A and a deficiency of blood group O in comparison with control patients from the same population. These studies indicate that blood group A increases the risk of gastric cancer by about 20 percent, a proportional increase which remains the same regardless of the local overall incidence of gastric cancer. There does not appear to be a correlation between ABO blood groups and the site of origin of the tumor in the stomach.

Sex. As with other tumors of the gut, gastric cancer is more prevalent among men than among women. This male predominance appears greater during the fifth, sixth, and seventh decades of life and greater for tumors originating in the fundus than for tumors growing in the antrum.

Atrophic Gastritis and Achlorhydria. Several prospective studies have shown that individuals with atrophic gastritis when followed over many years eventually proved to have an incidence of gastric cancer of about 10 percent. This is in comparison with similar prospective studies of subjects with a normal gastric mucosa in whom no gastric cancers developed during the same period. Studies such as these have shown conclusively that gastritis with intestinal metaplasia found in the mucosa around a carcinoma or in areas remote from the tumor represents a premalignant state rather than a secondary reaction induced by the

cancer. The atrophic gastritis accompanying gastric cancer may be of the diffuse, "autoimmune" type associated with pernicious anemia or of the multifocal "simple" variety. Recent studies suggest that the latter is numerically a more important precursor of gastric cancer than the former.

It is well known that achlorhydria exists in approximately one-half of patients with gastric cancer. The atrophic gastritis which almost invariably accompanies a gastric cancer is sufficient to account for this phenomenon.

Relationship between Gastric Ulcer and Gastric Cancer. In the past, one of the most controversial questions concerning gastric carcinoma was its relationship to benign gastric ulcer. For many years it was believed that benign ulcers often underwent malignant degeneration. This view has been discredited; it is now generally agreed that an ulcer either is malignant from the beginning or remains benign. The respective locations of benign gastric ulcers and gastric cancers argue against a common etiology. The majority of benign gastric ulcers occur on the lesser curvature. By contrast, 40 to 71 percent of cancers appear in the antrum. Occasionally, a pathologist discovers neoplastic cells in the margin of what appears to be a benign gastric ulcer. This may result from necrosis of carcinoma or may represent coincidental development of carcinoma in the vicinity of a benign gastric ulcer. At present, the important question raised by the finding of a gastric ulceration is not whether it may become malignant but whether it is, in fact, benign or malignant.

CLINICAL MANIFESTATIONS. The clinical manifestations of gastric carcinoma are so vague and misleading that a tumor may develop and become inoperable while a patient is being followed carefully. The most frequent symptom is weight loss. Lesions in the prepyloric antrum interfere with gastric emptying and cause gastric stasis and vomiting. The vomitus often has a characteristic coffee-ground appearance due to slow bleeding from the tumor. Anorexia, particularly pronounced for meat, postprandial fullness, and indigestion occur in one-fourth of the cases. As an early symptom pain is unreliable but is often present in far-advanced cases and under these conditions represents extragastric invasion by the tumor. The chronic slow bleeding from a fungating tumor often causes an iron deficiency anemia accompanied by weakness, dizziness, and dyspnea upon exertion. Occasionally, the first manifestation of a gastric carcinoma is an acute peritonitis due to a perforation of the malignant ulceration. A mass is present in one-third of the cases and, although an ominous sign, does not always signify inoperability. As a general rule, it can be said that when many of or all these symptoms are present, the chances for operative cure are minimal. Experience indicates that survival after curative operation is longer when the tumor has been asymptomatic.

LABORATORY AND DIAGNOSTIC STUDIES. Discussed previously under the heading Roentgenography in the section on Gastric Ulceration.

PATHOLOGY. Gross Appearance. According to their gross appearance, gastric carcinomas may be classified as follows.

Polypoid or Fungating. The lesion forms a bulky mass

protruding into the gastric lumen. This type is more often located in the cardia or the fundus. Most of these tumors have the histologic appearance of well-differentiated adenocarcinoma.

Ulcerative. Most of these malignant ulcerations are located on the lesser curvature or in the prepyloric antrum, and about half are moderately well-differentiated adenocarcinomas. This is the variety that may be confused clinically with a benign gastric ulcer.

Infiltrating. This type infiltrates the gastric wall diffusely and forms sessile intraluminal masses. The histologic appearance is more often that of a poorly differentiated adenocarcinoma. Linitis plastica, or "leather bottle stomach" (Fig. 26-28), is simply a variant of infiltrating gastric carcinoma. The lesion is characterized by a profound desmoplasia with sections of the gastric wall appearing thickened by a grayish white infiltrate. Histologic sections contain large amounts of fibrous tissue with rare signet ring cells often in "single file." Gland formation is sparse. The infiltrating *"diffuse"* form of gastric adenocarcinoma carries the worst prognosis.

Histology. The histologic classification of gastric carcinoma is based upon the degree of cellular anaplasia. This classification has some prognostic value. For instance, the

Fig. 26-28. Radiologic appearance of a stomach diffusely infiltrated with adenocarcinoma of the linitis plastica variety. This is the typical "leather-bottle stomach."

5-year survival after curative operation for low-grade carcinoma without nodes is approximately 50 percent. The 5-year survival rate for highly undifferentiated carcinomas is much lower.

One of the characteristics of gastric carcinoma is a tendency to intramural extension via lymphatic channels. In tumors involving the gastric antrum, submucosal invasion of the duodenum along subserosal lymphatics occurs in 43 percent of the cases. In tumors of the fundus and cardia, spread into the esophagus along submucosal lymphatics is frequent. Therefore, the lines of surgical transection should be placed well beyond the palpable margins of the tumor, since the distance involved by the intramural spread ranges from 3 to 6 cm. It seems to be greater for the esophagus than for the duodenum.

Lymphatic Spread. Invasion of the regional lymphatics in carcinoma of the stomach is often extensive and is present in 50 to 70 percent of the cases in which curative operation is attempted. If one includes cases in which surgical treatment is carried out for palliation, the incidence of lymph node metastasis is as high as 75 percent. Metastases to regional lymphatics from an adenocarcinoma of the stomach characteristically involve four zones of spread, listed below.

Infiltrating adenocarcinoma spreads to these regional lymph nodes more often than the polypoid variety. Recent studies have shown that the zone 2 groups of lymph nodes are involved in 30 percent of the cases of carcinoma involving the distal portion of the stomach. This finding has prompted some workers to include the spleen in the en bloc resection of the stomach and zones of lymphatic spread.

Zone 1 consists of nodes and lymphatic vessels located in the gastrocolic ligament around the right gastroepiploic vessels. Drainage to this group of lymph nodes comes from the pyloric portion of the greater curvature. Lymph flow from this area goes to the pylorus and then to the celiac and aortic nodes.

Zone 2 consists of nodes and lymphatic vessels situated in the gastrocolic and gastrosplenic ligaments around the left gastroepiploic vessels. This group of lymph nodes drains the cardia and fundus of the stomach. From here, lymph reaches the splenic vessels along the upper border of the pancreas and then the preaortic lymph nodes.

Zone 3 is situated around the left gastric artery along the proximal two-thirds of the stomach and drains the proximal portion of the lesser curvature of the stomach. From here, lymph reaches nodes around the celiac axis. Lymph from the nodes located around the cardia may drain into periesophageal nodes.

Zone 4 drains the pylorus and distal portion of the lesser curvature. Lymph from these nodes, situated above the pylorus and first portion of the duodenum, drains into hepatic nodes located around the hepatic artery, and from there to celiac and preaortic nodes.

Extramural Spread. Gastric adenocarcinoma also spreads by direct invasion of surrounding structures. Those most frequently involved are the liver, the pancreas, and the transverse colon. In addition, after the serosa of the stomach has been invaded, cells become seeded directly into the peritoneal cavity and form widespread serosal tumor implants. Implants occur with characteristic frequency in the rectovesical or rectouterine cul de sac (Blumer's shelf) and in the ovary (Krukenberg's tumor).

Staging of Gastric Cancer. The accurate staging of each gastric tumor is essential for prognosis in a given case and for the meaningful evaluation of various therapeutic modalities. A widely adapted staging scheme is the one recently proposed by the American Joint Committee for Cancer Staging and End Results Reporting. This staging system, known as the TNM system, is based upon the degree of penetration of the primary tumor into the wall of the stomach, upon spread to regional lymph nodes, and upon the presence or absence of metastatic tumor in distant organs. The size of the primary lesion, its location in the stomach, and its degree of histologic differentiation all have no weight in this staging scheme and in the ultimate prognosis of an individual lesion.

Three components comprise this TNM system:

1. The status of the primary tumor, designated by the letter "T," expressed by the degree of penetration of the tumor through the gastric wall.
   T1. Tumor confined to the mucosa.
   T2. Tumor involving all layers of the gastric wall including the serosa but not extending through the serosa.
   T3. Tumor extends through the serosa with or without invasion of adjacent structures.
   T4. Diffuse infiltration of all layers of the gastric wall. The lesion has no demonstrable boundaries (linitis plastica).
   TX. Degree of involvement of gastric wall not determined.
2. The status of the regional lymph nodes, designated by the letter N.
   N0. Lymph nodes free of tumor.
   N1. Metastatic deposits in the perigastric lymph nodes adjacent to the primary tumor.
   N2. Metastatic deposits in the perigastric lymph nodes remote from the tumor or on both gastric curvatures.
   NX. Presence or absence of lymph node metastases not determined.
3. The status of distant organs and tissues with respect to metastatic spread, designated by the letter M.
   M0. No distant metastasis.
   M1. Distant metastasis demonstrated clinically, radiologically, or surgically in remote tissues or organs and including nodes beyond the regional lymph nodes but excluding direct invasion by the primary tumor.

On the basis of the preceding classification of the extent of the disease in a given case the following scheme of staging is being widely adopted.

Stage I
   A. Tumor confined to the mucosa without tumor deposits in the regional lymph nodes or remote tissues. (T1, N0, M0.)
   B. Tumor extending to but not through the serosa without tumor deposits in the regional lymph nodes or remote tissues. (T2, N0, M0.)
   C. Tumor extending through the serosa with or without invasion of adjacent structures and without tumor deposits in the regional lymph nodes or remote tissues. (T3, N0, M0.)

Stage II
   Diffuse involvement of the gastric wall (linitis plastica) without node involvement or distant metastasis. (T4, N0, M0.)

Or, any degree of involvement of the gastric wall with tumor deposits in the regional lymph nodes but without distant metastasis. (T1, N1, M0; T2, N1, M0; T3, N1, M0; T4, N1, M0.)

Stage III
   Any degree of involvement of the gastric wall accompanied by metastatic deposits in perigastric lymph nodes remote from the tumor or on both gastric curvatures but without metastasis in remote tissues or organs. (T1, N2, M0; T2, N2, M0; T3, N2, M0; T4, N2, M0.)

Stage IV
   Any gastric carcinoma with distant metastasis regardless of the status of the primary tumor or the perigastric lymph nodes.

TREATMENT. At present the only way of curing carcinoma of the stomach is to remove the involved stomach before the advent of metastases or invasion extending beyond the confines of the stomach and the adjacent channels of lymphatic spread. The history of surgical operation for gastric cancer goes back to 1881, when the first successful partial gastrectomy was performed by Billroth. Schlatter, in 1897, performed the first total gastrectomy for gastric cancer. With perfection of surgical techniques and of preoperative and postoperative care, surgical operations for gastric carcinoma became more and more extensive. In the 1940s routine total gastrectomy for gastric carcinoma was employed in several clinics as the method of choice. Because of lymphatic spread to lymph nodes along the superior border of the pancreas and along the celiac axis, several writers have described inclusion of the body and tail of the pancreas, the spleen, the hepatic artery up to the junction of the gastroduodenal artery, the gastrocolic ligament, and the omentum in the block of tissue resected with the stomach. The mortality rate of such extensive procedures has been as high as 50 percent. However, technical improvements have reduced the mortality of extensive operations to below 10 percent. But time has shown that the 5-year survival rate after surgical treatment has not been appreciably increased by extending the scope of the operation. As a result, there has been a return to less extensive procedures, and the approach followed by many surgeons at present is as follows.

For carcinomas involving the distal portion of the stomach, which represents the majority of gastric carcinomas, the operation performed is a radical distal subtotal gastric resection, removing approximately 80 percent of the stomach. The operation is extended distally to include the first portion of the duodenum, so that lymph nodes and lymphatic channels in the pyloric region may be removed. Because of the frequent involvement of nodes in the gastrosplenic ligament, the spleen and the greater omentum are included in the bloc of resected tissue. The left gastric artery is divided at its origin, and the entire gastrohepatic omentum is removed in continuity with the specimen. Gastrointestinal continuity is reestablished by anastomosing the remaining gastric pouch either to the first portion of the duodenum as a Billroth I type of anastomosis or to the jejunum as a Billroth II procedure, which may be antecolic or retrocolic. A total gastrectomy including the omentum, the spleen, the first portion of the duodenum, and possibly the celiac artery if surrounded by involved nodes is reserved for more extensive tumors, particularly of the fundus. *Adjunctive* chemotherapy, preferably with several drugs, should be started as soon as possible after the patient's recovery from surgery. At present, this represents the only hope of improving the survival rate.

It is important that the operating surgeon thoroughly explore the abdomen before attempting to remove the gastric tumor. Hepatic metastases, ascitic fluid in the peritoneal cavity, visible serosal implants, implants in the rectouterine or rectovesical pouch preclude curative surgical operation. To attempt heroic resective surgical treatment under these conditions is simply a refusal to acknowledge that the tumor has extended beyond the limits where resection can be carried out with a reasonable expectation of a cure. Because of the frequency with which one of the reasons mentioned above renders a gastric carcinoma inoperable, palliation is a frequent consideration. The main indications for palliative surgery are pyloric obstruction, bleeding, or impending perforation.

Under these conditions a limited gastric resection, when technically feasible, appears to provide more satisfactory results than a bypass procedure such as a gastroenterostomy. From time to time one may have to consider palliative procedures for problems created by a recurrence following a previous curative resection. A particularly distressing problem is the severe dysphagia caused by massive local recurrence around an esophagojejunostomy after a previous total gastrectomy. This situation cannot be controlled by a feeding jejunostomy since one of the symptoms is the inability to swallow salivary secretions with consequent aspiration pneumonitis. We have achieved worthwhile palliation under these circumstances by bypassing the obstruction with a long jejunal loop brought up through the left leaf of the diaphragm and anastomosed to the esophagus above and to an unobstructed loop of small bowel below.

PROGNOSIS. Data indicating a slight improvement in the results of surgical treatment of gastric cancer are summarized in Fig. 26-29. It is quite obvious that although the results, expressed as 5-year survival rates of operated patients, may appear encouraging on the surface, they are in actuality quite dismal when one considers the 5-year survival rate of all patients with gastric cancer, which remains around 15 percent. This, of course, is due to the fact that only half of the patients with gastric cancer are operable with the goal of cure. The most significant factor in determining the prognosis of a patient with gastric carcinoma operated on for cure is the presence or absence of lymph node metastases. Only 7 percent of patients with metastases to regional lymph nodes survive for more than 5 years after the operation. By contrast, 35 percent of the patients can be expected to survive after gastrectomy if the regional nodes are uninvolved. More recent figures suggest that the 5-year survival rate in the absence of lymph node involvement in some hands may be as high as 45 percent.

Fig. 26-29. Ultimate survival rates for all patients with diagnosed gastric carcinoma. Note that from about 1910 to 1965 the greatest improvements have been in the rates of operability and resectability. (*Reproduced from W. H. ReMine, J. T. Priestley, and J. Berkson, "Cancer of the Stomach," W. B. Saunders Company, Philadelphia, 1964.*)

MISCELLANEOUS TUMORS

Malignant Tumors

LEIOMYOSARCOMA

These lesions comprise approximately 1 percent of all gastric malignant tumors. They usually form bulky intraluminal tumors, although they may infiltrate the gastric wall widely or grow extraluminally. A characteristic of intraluminal leiomyosarcomas is necrosis of the core of the tumor with formation of a huge ulceration within the tumor mass. The prognosis for 5-year survival following gastric resection is good (67 percent).

LYMPHOMA

Gastric lymphomas represent approximately 2 percent of gastric malignant tumors. Radiologically, they often present as ill-defined gastric masses, frequently with diffuse thickening of the rugal folds. The treatment of gastric lymphoma consists of a radical subtotal resection followed by postoperative radiation. The 5-year survival rate following this form of therapy is approximately 40 percent.

Benign Tumors

Polypoid adenomas or polyps of the stomach represent the most frequent benign gastric tumors. They are often single but may be multiple, and have demonstrated a propensity for malignant degeneration. There is an increased incidence of carcinoma with polyps above 3 cm. Treatment consists of resection of the polyp with a rim of normal mucosa around it. A partial gastrectomy should be performed for diffuse gastric polyposis. If the latter involves the entire stomach, a total gastrectomy should be considered, because of the malignant potential of these lesions. However, before resecting the stomach, it should be definitely ascertained that one is dealing with gastric polyps and not a giant hypertrophic gastritis. In the latter condition, the giant rugal folds often simulate polyps. Other common benign tumors of the stomach are, in order of decreasing frequency, aberrant pancreatic tumors, leiomyomas, neurogenic tumors, fibromas, and lipomas. The majority of these tumors are asymptomatic and usually are discovered incidentally during an upper gastrointestinal tract series.

References

Anatomy

Bentley, F. H., and Barlow, T. E.: Stomach: Vascular Supply in Relation to Gastric Ulcer, *Surg Prog, 1952,* Butterworth & Co., London, 1953.

Gastric Function

Anderson, S., and Olbe, L.: Gastric Acid Secretory Responses to Gastrin and Histamine in Dogs before and after Vagal Denervation of the Gastric Pouch, *Acta Physiol Scand,* **60:**51, 1964.

Brackney, E. L., Thal, A. P., and Wangensteen, O. H.: Role of duodenum in the control of gastric secretion, *Proc Soc Exp Biol Med,* **88:**302, 1955.

Brunschwig, A., Rasmussen, R. A., Camp, E. J., and Moe, R.: Gastric Secretory Depressant in Gastric Juice, *Surgery,* **12:** 887, 1942.

Card, W. I., and Marks, I. N.: The Relationship between the Acid Output of the Stomach following "Maximal" Histamine Stimulation and the Parietal Cell Mass, *Clin Sci,* **19:**147, 1960.

Code, C. F., and Watkinson, G.: Importance of Vagal Innervation in the Regulatory Effect of Acid in the Duodenum on Gastric Secretion of Acid, *J Physiol* (*Lond*), **130:**233, 1955.

Davenport, H. W., Warner, H. A., Code, C. F.: Functional Significance of Gastric Mucosal Barrier to Sodium, *Gastroenterology,* **47:**142, 1964.

Davenport, H. W.: Destruction of the Gastric Mucosal Barrier by Detergents and Urea, *Gastroenterology,* **54:**175, 1968.

Edkins, J. S.: The Chemical Mechanism of Gastric Secretion, *J Physiol* (*Lond*), **34:**133, 1906.

Gibson, R., Hirschowitz, B. I., and Hutchison, G.: Actions of Metiamide, an H_2-Histamine Receptor Antagonist on Gastric H^+ and Pepsin Secretion in Dogs, *Gastroenterology,* **67:**93, 1974.

Gregory, R. A.: The Effect of Portal Venous Occlusion on Gastric Secretion, *J Physiol* (*Lond*), **131:**100, 1957.

——— and Tracy, H. J.: The Constitution and Properties of Two Gastrins Extracted from Hog Antral Mucosa. I. The Isolation of Two Gastrins from Hog Antral Mucosa. II. The Properties of Two Gastrins Isolated from Hog Antral Mucosa. W. H.

Taylor: A Note on the Nature of the Gastrin-like Stimulant Present in Zollinger-Ellison Tumors, *Gut,* **5:**103, 1964.

Isenberg, J. I.: Gastric Secretory Testing, in M. H. Sleisenger and J. S. Fordtran (eds.), "Gastrointestinal Disease," pp. 536–554, W. B. Saunders Company, Philadelphia, 1973.

Lebedinskaja, S. I.: Über die Magensekretion bei Eckschen Fistelhunden, *Z Gesamte Exp Med,* **88:**264, 1933.

Max, M., and Menguy, R.: Influence of Adrenocorticotropin, Cortisone, Aspirin and Phenylbutazone on the Rate of Exfoliation and the Rate of Renewal of Gastric Mucosal Cells, *Gastroenterology,* **58:**329, 1970.

McGuigan, J. E.: Immunochemical Studies With Synthetic Human Gastrin, *Gastroenterology,* **54:**1005, 1968.

McGuigan, J. E., and Trudeau, W. L.: Serum Gastrin Concentrations in Pernicious Anemia, *N Engl J Med,* **282:**358, 1970.

McGuigan, J. E., and Trudeau, W. L.: Studies With Antibodies to Gastrin: Radioimmunoassay in Human Serum and Physiological Studies, *Gastroenterology,* **58:**139, 1970.

Menguy, R.: Studies on the Role of the Pancreatic and Biliary Secretion in the Mechanism of Gastric Inhibition by Fat, *Surgery,* **48:**195, 1960.

———: Effect of Biliary Diversion from the Small Intestine on Gastric Secretory Activity in Dogs, *Gastroenterology,* **41:**568, 1961.

———: Pathogenesis of Mann-Williamson Ulcer. III. Effect of Excluding Pancreatic or Biliary Secretions from the Intestine on Gastric Secretion and Liver Function, *Surgery,* **54:**495, 1963.

——— and Masters, Y. F.: Effect of Cortisone on Mucoprotein Secretion by Gastric Antrum of Dogs: Pathogenesis of Steroid Ulcer, *Surgery,* **54:**19, 1963.

Nyhus, L. M., Chapman, N. D., DeVito, R. V., and Harkins, H. N.: The Control of Gastrin Release: An Experimental Study Illustrating a New Concept, *Gastroenterology,* **39:**582, 1960.

Passaro, E. P., and Grossman, M. I.: Effect of Vagal Innervation on Acid and Pepsin Response to Histamine and Gastrin, *Am J Physiol,* **206:**1068, 1964.

Porter, R. W., Brady, J. V., Conrad, M. A., Mason, J. W., Galambos, R., and Rioch, D. M.: Some Experimental Observations on Gastrointestinal Lesions in Behaviorally Conditioned Monkeys, *Psychosom Med,* **20:**379, 1958.

Shay, H.: Stress and Gastric Secretion, *Gastroenterology,* **26:**316, 1954.

Silen, W., Hein, M. F., and Harper, H. A.: The Influence of the Liver upon Canine Gastric Secretion, *Surgery,* **54:**29, 1963.

———, Skillman, J. J., Hein, M., and Harper, H. A.: The Effect of Biliary Obstruction upon Canine Gastric Secretory Activity, *J Surg Res,* **2:**197, 1962.

Sircus, W.: The Intestinal Phase of Gastric Secretion, *Q J Exp Physiol,* **38:**91, 1953.

Skillman, J. J., Silen, W., Harper, H. A., Neely, J. C., and Simmons, F. I.: Effect of Hepatocellular Injury on Gastric Secretion in Dogs, *Surg Forum,* **12:**276, 1961.

Solntseff, A. F.: Analysis of the Secretory Work of the Stomach in the Dog, thesis, St. Petersburg, 1904.

Stavney, L. S., Kato, T., Savage, L. E., Harkins, H. N., and Nyhus, L. M.: Parietal Cell Reactivity, *Surg Gynecol Obstet,* **118:**1269, 1964.

Trudeau, W. L., McGuigan, J. E.: Relations between Serum

Gastrin Levels and Rates of Gastric Hydrochloric Acid Secretion, *N Engl J Med,* **284:**408, 1971.

Uvnas, B.: The Part Played by the Pyloric Region in the Cephalic Phase of Gastric Secretion, *Acta Physiol Scand,* **4**(Suppl. 13):1942.

Villarreal, R., Ganong, W. F., and Gray, S. J.: Effect of Adrenocorticotrophic Hormone upon the Gastric Secretion of Hydrochloric Acid, Pepsin and Electrolytes in the Dog, *Am J Physiol,* **183:**485, 1955.

Walsh, J. H., and Grossman, M. I.: Gastrin, *N Engl J Med,* **292:**1324, 1975.

Wolf, S., and Wolff, H. G.: "Human Gastric Function," Oxford University Press, London, 1943.

Woodward, E. R., Lyon, E. J., Landor, J., and Dragstedt, L. R.: The Physiology of the Gastric Antrum: Experimental Studies on Isolated Antral Pouches in Dogs, *Gastroenterology,* **27:**766, 1954.

———, Robertson, C., Fried, W., and Schapiro, H.: Further Studies on the Isolated Gastric Antrum, *Gastroenterology,* **32:**868, 1957.

Peptic Ulcer Disease

Brooks, J. R., and Eraklis, A. J.: Factors Affecting the Mortality from Peptic Ulcer, *N Engl J Med,* **271:**803, 1964.

Clarke, J. S., Costarella, R., and Ward, S.: Gastric Secretion in the Fasting State and after Antral Stimulation in Patients with Cirrhosis and Portacaval Shunts, *Surg Forum,* **9:**417, 1958.

———, McKissock, P. K., and Cruze, K.: Studies on the Site of Origin of the Agent Causing Hypersecretion in Dogs with Portacaval Shunt, *Surgery,* **46:**48, 1959.

———, Ozeran, R. S., Hart, J. C., Cruze, K., and Crevling, V.: Peptic Ulcer following Portacaval Shunt, *Ann Surg,* **148:**551, 1958.

Doll, R., and Buch, J.: Hereditary Factors in Peptic Ulcer, *Ann Eugenics,* **15:**135, 1950.

———, Swynnerton, B. F., and Newell, A. C.: Observations on Blood Group Distribution in Peptic Ulcer and Gastric Cancer, *Gut,* **1:**31, 1960.

Dragstedt, L. R.: The Etiology of Gastric and Duodenal Ulcers, *Postgrad Med,* **15:**99, 1954.

DuPlessis, D. J.: Some Aspects of the Pathogenesis and Surgical Management of Peptic Ulcers, *S Afr Med J,* **34:**101, 1960.

Flint, F. J., and Warrack, A. J.: Acute Peptic Ulceration in Emphysema, *Lancet,* **2:**178, 1958.

Grossman, M. I., Kirsner, J. B., and Gillespie, I. E.: Basal and Histalog-stimulated Gastric Secretion in Control Subjects and in Patients with Peptic Ulcer or Gastric Cancer, *Gastroenterology,* **45:**14, 1963.

Kammerer, W. H., Freiberger, R. H., and Rivelis, A. L.: Peptic Ulcer in Rheumatoid Patients on Corticosteroid Therapy: Clinical Experimental and Radiologic Study, *Arthritis Rheum,* **1:**122, 1958.

Katz, D., Douvres, P., Weisberg, H., McKinnon, W., Glass, G. B. Jerzy: Early Diagnosis of Upper Gastrointestinal Hemorrhage, *JAMA,* **188:**405, 1964.

Kern, F., Jr., Clark, G. M., and Lukens, J. G.: Peptic Ulceration Occurring during Therapy for Rheumatoid Arthritis, *Gastroenterology,* **33:**25, 1957.

Lambling, A., Gosset, J., Bertrand, I., and Viau, P.: Le genie

evolutif de la maladie ulcereuse avant et pendant la guerre, *Paris Med,* **36:**146, 1946.

Meltzer, L. E., Bockman, A. A., Kanenson, W., and Cohen, A.: Incidence of Peptic Ulcer among Patients on Long term Prednisone Therapy, *Gastroenterology,* **35:**351, 1958.

Menguy, R., and Masters, Y. F.: Effects of Aspirin on Gastric Mucous Secretion, *Surg Gynecol Obstet.,* **120:**92, 1965.

Muir, A., and Cossar, I. A.: Aspirin and Ulcer, *Br Med J,* **2:**7, 1955.

Ostrow, J. D., Timmerman, R. J., and Gray, S. J.: Gastric Secretion in Human Hepatic Cirrhosis, *Gastroenterology,* **38:**303, 1960.

Palmer, E. D.: Cyclic Dynamism in Ulcer Disease, *Surg Gynec Obstet,* **130:**709, 1970.

Spicer, C. C., Stewart, D. N., and Winser, D. M. deR.: Perforated Peptic Ulcer during the Period of Heavy Air Raids, *Lancet,* **1:**14, 1944.

Stolzer, B. L., Barr, J. H., Jr., Eisenbeis, C. H., Jr., Wechsler, R. C. and Margolis, H. M.: Prednisone and Prednisolone Therapy in Rheumatoid Arthritis: Clinical Evaluation with Emphasis on Gastrointestinal Manifestations in 156 Patients Observed for Periods of 4 to 14 months, *JAMA,* **165:**13, 1957.

Trudeau, W. L., and McGuigan, J. E.: Serum Gastrin Levels in Patients with Peptic Ulcer Disease, *Gastroenterology,* **59:**6, 1970.

Welsh, J. D., and Wolf, S.: Geographical and Environmental Aspect of Peptic Ulcer, *Am J Med,* **29:**754, 1960.

Winkelman, E. I., and Summerskill, W. H. G.: Gastric secretion in Relation to Gastrointestinal Bleeding from Salicylate Compounds, *Gastroenterology,* **40:**56, 1961.

Zasly, L., Baum, G. L., and Rumball, J. M.: A Study of Gastric Secretions in Chronic Obstructive Pulmonary Emphysema, *Dis Chest,* **38:**69, 1960.

Zollinger, R. M., Elliott, D. W., Endahl, G. L., Grant, G. N., Goswitz, J. T., and Taft, D. A.: Origin of the Ulcerogenic Hormone in Endocrine Induced Ulcer, *Ann Surg,* **156:**570, 1962.

——— and ———: Primary Peptic Ulcerations of the Jejunum Associated with Islet-cell Tumors of the Pancreas, *Ann Surg,* **142:**709, 1955.

Duodenal Ulcer Diathesis

Amdrup, B. M., and Griffith, C. A.: Selective Vagotomy of the Parietal Cell Mass. I. With preservation of the innervated antrum and pylorus, *Ann Surg,* **170:**207, 1969.

Bruce, J., Card, W. I., Marks, I. N., and Sircus, W.: The Rationale of Selective Surgery in the Treatment of Duodenal Ulcer, *J R Coll Surg Edinb,* **4:**85, 1959.

Burns, G. P., Cheng, F. C. Y., Cox, A. G., Payne, R. A., Spencer, J., and Welbourn, R. B.: Significance of Early and Late Positive Responses to Insulin Hypoglycaemia in Patients with Intact Vagi, *Gut,* **10:**820, 1969.

Cushing, H.: Peptic Ulcers and the Interbrain, *Surg Gynecol Obstet,* **55:**1, 1932.

Davies, R. E., and Longmuir, N. M.: Production of Ulcers in Isolated Frog Gastric Mucosa, *Biochem J,* **42:**621, 1948.

Desbaillets, L., and Menguy, R.: Influence of Corticotrophic Hormone on the Secretion of Gastric Mucus, *Surg Forum,* **17:**291, 1966.

Donegan, W. L., and Spiro, H. M.: Parathyroids and Gastric Secretion, *Gastroenterology*, **38**:750, 1960.

Dragstedt, L. R.: Pathogenesis of Gastroduodenal Ulcer, *Arch Surg*, **44**:438, 1942.

Dragstedt, L. R.: Vagotomy for Gastroduodenal Ulcer, *Ann Surg*, **122**:973, 1945.

——— and Owens, F. M., Jr.: Supradiaphragmatic Section of Vagus Nerves in Treatment of Duodenal Ulcer, *Proc Soc Exp Biol Med*, **53**:152, 1943.

———: The Role of the Nervous System in the Pathogenesis of Duodenal Ulcer, *Surgery*, **34**:902, 1953.

Elliott, D. W., Taft, D. A., Passaro, E., and Zollinger, R. M.: Pancreatic Influences on Gastric Secretion, *Surgery*, **50**:126, 1961.

Ellison, E. H., and Wilson, S. D.: Zollinger-Ellison Syndrome: Re-appraisal and Evaluation of 206 Registered Cases, *Ann Surg*, **160**:512, 1964.

Elman, R., and Hartmann, A. F.: Spontaneous Peptic Ulcers of Duodenum after Continued Loss of Total Pancreatic Juice, *Arch Surg*, **23**:1030, 1931.

Emas, S., and Grossman, M. I.: Effect of Truncal Vagotomy on Acid and Pepsin Responses to Histamine and Gastrin in Dogs, *Am J Physiol*, **212**:1007, 1967.

Evans, D. A. P.: The Fucose and Agglutinogen Contents of Saliva in Subjects with Duodenal Ulcers, *J Lab Clin Med*, **55**:386, 1960.

Evans, R., Zajtchuk, R., and Menguy, R.: Role of Vagotomy and Gastric Drainage in the Surgical Treatment of Duodenal Ulcer: Results of a 10-year Experience at the University of Chicago Hospitals, *Surg Clin North Am*, **47**:141, 1967.

Farris, J. M., and Smith, G. K.: Vagotomy and Pyloroplasty for Bleeding Duodenal Ulcer, *Am J Surg*, **105**:388, 1963.

Fox, P. S., Hofmann, J. W., DeCosse, J. J., and Wilson, S. D.: The Influence of Total Gastrectomy on Survival in Malignant Zollinger-Ellison Tumors, *Ann Surg*, **180**:558, 1974.

Garrido-Klinge, G., and Pena, L.: Gastroduodenal ulcer in High Altitudes (Peruvian Andes), *Gastroenterology*, **37**:390, 1959.

Gillespie, G., Gillespie, I. E., and Kay, A. W.: An Analysis of the Insulin Test after Vagotomy Using Single and Multiple Criteria, *Gut*, **9**:470, 1968.

Goligher, J. C., Pulvertaft, C. N., deDombal, F. T., Clark, C. G., Conyers, J. T., Duthie, H. L., Feather, D. B., Latchmore, A. J. C., Matheson, T. S., Shoesmith, J. H., Smiddy, F. G., and Willson-Pepper, J.: Clinical Comparison of Vagotomy and Pyloroplasty with Other Forms of Elective Surgery for Duodenal Ulcer, *Br Med J*, **2**:787, 1968.

Gregory, R. A., Tracy, H. J., French, J. M., and Sircus, W.: Extraction of a Gastrin-like Substance from a Pancreatic Tumor in a Case of Zollinger-Ellison Syndrome, *Lancet*, **1**:1045, 1960.

Grossman, M. I., Matsumoto, K. K., and Lichter, R. J.: Fecal Blood Loss Produced by Oral and Intravenous Administration of Various Salicylates, *Gastroenterology*, **40**:383, 1961.

Herrington, J. L., Sawyers, J. L., and Scott, H. W., Jr.: A Twenty-five Year Experience with Vagotomy-Antrectomy, *Arch Surg*, **106**:469, 1973.

Hollander, F.: Laboratory Procedures in the Study of Vagotomy, *Gastroenterology*, **11**:419, 1948.

Holle, F., and Andersson, S. (eds.): "Vagotomy: Latest Advances

with Special Reference to Gastric and Duodenal Ulcer Disease," Springer-Verlag, New York, 1974.

Johnston, D., and Wilkinson, A. R.: Highly Selective Vagotomy without a Drainage Procedure in the Treatment of Duodenal Ulcer, *Br J Surg*, **57**:289, 1970.

Kramer, P., and Markarian, B.: Gastric Acid Secretion in Chronic Obstructive Pulmonary Emphysema, *Gastroenterology*, **38**:295, 1960.

McGuigan, J. E., and Trudeau, W. L.: Serum Gastrin Levels Before and After Vagotomy and Pyloroplasty or Vagotomy and Antrectomy, *N Engl J Med*, **286**:184, 1972.

Myhill, J., and Piper, D. W.: Antacid Therapy of Peptic Ulcer, *Gut*, **5**:581, 1964.

Oberhelman, H. A., Jr., Nelson, T. S., Johnson, A. N., Jr., and Dragstedt, L. R., II: Ulcerogenic Tumors of the Duodenum, *Ann Surg*, **153**:214, 1961.

Ostrow, J. D., Blanshard, G., and Gray, S. J.: Peptic Ulcer in Primary Hyperparathyroidism, *Am J Med*, **29**:769, 1960.

Rogers, H. M., Keating, F. R., Morlock, C. G., and Braker, N. W.: Primary Hypertrophy and Hyperplasia of the Parathyroid Glands Associated with Duodenal Ulcer, *Arch Intern Med*, **79**:307, 1947.

Roth, J. L. A.: Clinical Evaluation of the Caffeine Gastric Analysis in Duodenal Ulcer Patients, *Gastroenterology*, **19**:199, 1951.

Sawyers, H. L., and Scott, H. W., Jr.: Selective Gastric Vagotomy with Antrectomy or Pyloroplasty, *Ann Surg*, **174**:541, 1971.

Schlaeger, R., LeMay, M., and Wermer, P.: Upper Gastrointestinal Tract Alterations in Adenomatosis of the Endocrine Glands, *Radiology*, **75**:517, 1960.

Spencer, J. A., Morlock, C. G., and Sayre, G. P.: Lesions in the Upper Portion of the G. I. Tract Associated with Intracranial Neoplasms, *Gastroenterology*, **37**:20, 1959.

Tompkins, R. K., Kraft, A. R., Zimmerman, E., Lichtenstein, J. E., and Zollinger, R. M.: Clinical and Biochemical Evidence of Increased Gallstone Formation after Complete Vagotomy, *Surgery*, **71**:196, 1972.

Weinberg, J. A.: Treatment of the Massively Bleeding Duodenal Ulcer by Ligation, Pyloroplasty and Vagotomy, *Am J Surg*, **102**:158, 1961.

Wormsley, K. G., and Grossman, M. I.: Maximal Histalog Test in Control Subjects and Patients with Peptic Ulcer, *Gut*, **6**:427, 1950.

Gastric Ulcerations

Billington, B. P.: Observations from New South Wales on the Changing Incidence of Gastric Ulcer in Australia, *Gut*, **6**:121, 1965.

Black, R. B., Roberts, G., and Rhodes, J.: The Effect of Healing on Bile Reflux in Gastric Ulcer, *Gut*, **12**:552, 1971.

Burge, H.: The Etiology of Lesser-Curve Gastric Ulceration. Its Treatment by Vagotomy and Pyloroplasty, *De Med Tuenda*, **1**:16, 1964.

Chapman, B. L., and Duggan, J. M.: Aspirin and Uncomplicated Peptic Ulcer, *Gut*, **10**:443, 1969.

Davenport, H. W.: Is the Apparent Hyposecretion of Acid by Patients with Gastric Ulcer a Consequence of a Broken Barrier to Diffusion of Hydrogen Ions into the Gastric Mucosa? *Gut*, **6**:513, 1965.

Dragstedt, L. R., Oberhelman, H. A., Jr., Evans, S. O., and Rigler,

S. P.: Antrum Hyperfunction and Gastric Ulcer, *Ann Surg,* **140:**396, 1954.

Duggan, J. M., and Chapman, B. L.: The Incidence of Aspirin Ingestion in Patients with Peptic Ulcer, *Med J Aust,* **7:**797, 1970.

DuPlessis, D. J.: Pathogenesis of Gastric Ulceration, *Lancet,* **1:**974, 1965.

Farris, J. M., and Smith, G. K.: Some Other Operations for Gastric Ulcer, *Surg Clin North Am,* **46:**329, 1966.

Farris, J. M., and Smith, G. K.: Treatment of Gastric Ulcer (in situ) by Vagotomy and Pyloroplasty. A Clinical Study, *Ann Surg,* **158:**461, 1963.

Flint, F. J., and Grech, P.: Pyloric Regurgitation and Gastric Ulcer, *Gut,* **11:**735, 1970.

Gear, M. W. L., Truelove, S. C., and Whitehead, R.: Gastric Ulcer and Gastritis, *Gut,* **12:**639, 1971.

Harvey, H. D.: Twenty-five Years Experience with Elective Gastric Resection for Gastric Ulcer, *Surg Gynecol Obstet,* **113:**191, 1961.

Henley, W. H., and Bowers, R. F.: Observations of Surgical Therapy for Gastric Ulcer, *Arch Surg,* **90:**205, 1965.

Johnson, H. D.: Gastric Ulcer: Classification Blood Group Characteristics, Secretion Patterns and Pathogenesis, *Ann Surg,* **162:**996, 1965.

Kraft, R. O., Myers, J., Overton, S., and Fry, W. J.: Vagotomy and the Gastric Ulcer, *Am J Surg,* **121:**122, 1971.

Lampert, E. G., Waugh, J. M., and Dockerty, M. D.: The Incidence of Malignancy in Gastric Ulcers Believed Preoperatively to Be Benign, *Surg Gynecol Obstet,* **91:**673, 1950.

Larson, N. E., Cain, J. C., and Bartholomew, L. G.: Prognosis of the Medically Treated Small Gastric Ulcer. I. Comparison of Follow Data in Two Series, *N Engl J Med,* **264:**119, 1961.

Lawson, H. H.: Gastritis and Gastric Ulceration, *Br J Surg,* **53:**493, 1966.

Lawson, H. H.: Effect of Duodenal Contents on the Gastric Mucosa Under Experimental Conditions, *Lancet,* **1:**469, 1964.

Levrat, M., Pasquier, J., Martin, F., and Truchot, R.: Les ulceres medicamentaux de la grande courbure, *Arch Mal App Dig Nut,* **54:**305, 1965.

Mauer, E. F.: Toxic Effects of Phenylbutazone (Butazolidin); Review of Literature and Report of Twenty-third Death Following Its Use, *N Engl J Med,* **253:**404, 1955.

Menguy, R., and Max, M.: Influence of Bile on the Canine Gastric-Antral Mucosa, *Am J Surg,* **119:**177, 1970.

Ruding, R.: Gastric Ulcer and Antral Border, *Surgery,* **61:**495, 1967.

Stemmer, E. A., Zahn, R. L., Hom, L. W., and Connolly, J. E.: Vagotomy and Drainage Procedures for Gastric Ulcer, *Arch Surg,* **96:**586, 1968.

Veterans Administration Cooperative Study on Gastric Ulcer, *Gastroenterology,* **61:**567, 1971.

Wanka, J., Jones, L. I., Wood, P. H. N. and Dixon, St. J.: Indomethacin in Rheumatic Diseases: A Controlled Clinical Trial, *Ann Rheum Dis,* **23:**218, 1964.

Weisberg, H., and Glass, G. B.: Coexisting Gastric and Duodenal Ulcers; A Review, *Am J Dig Dis,* **8:**992, 1963.

Woodward, E. R., Eisenberg, M. M., and Dragstedt, L. R.: Recurrence of Gastric Ulcer After Pyloroplasty, *Am J Surg,* **113:**5, 1967.

Zahn, H. L., Stemmer, E. A., Hom, L. W., and Connolly, J. E.: Delayed Recurrence of Gastric Ulcer Following Vagotomy and Drainage Procedures, *Am Surg,* **34:**757, 1968.

Acute Gastric Mucosal Lesions

Bryant, L. R., and Griffen, W. O.: Vagotomy and Pyloroplasty: An Inadequate Operation for Stress Ulcers, *Arch Surg,* **93:**16, 1966.

Davenport, H. W.: Damage to the Gastric Mucosa: Effects of Salicylates and Stimulation, *Gastroenterology,* **49:**189, 1965.

Davenport, H. W.: Gastric Mucosal Injury by Fatty and Acetylsalicylic Acids, *Gastroenterology,* **46:**245, 1964.

Dieulafoy, G.: Exulteratio Simplex: L'Intervention Chirurgicale dans les Hematemèses Foudroyantes Consécutives, *Bull Acad Med,* **39:**49, 1898.

Ferguson, H. L., and Clarke, J. S.: Treatment of Hemorrhage from Erosive Gastritis by Vagotomy and Pyloroplasty, *Am J Surg,* **112:**739, 1966.

Fletcher, D. G., and Harkins, H. N.: Acute Peptic Ulcer as a Complication of Major Surgery, Stress or Trauma, *Surgery,* **36:**212, 1954.

Flowers, R. S., Kyle, K., and Hoerr, S. O.: Postoperative Hemorrhage from Stress Ulceration of the Stomach and Duodenum, *Am J Surg,* **119:**632, 1970.

Gilchrist, R. K., and Chun, N.: Severe Hemorrhage in Presumed Peptic Ulcer: Surgical Treatment in the Absence of Demonstrable Lesion, *Arch Surg,* **69:**366, 1954.

Goodman, A. A., and Frey, C. F.: Massive Upper Gastrointestinal Hemorrhage Following Surgical Operations, *Ann Surg,* **167:**180, 1968.

Harjola, P. A., and Sivula, A.: Gastric Ulcerations Following Experimentally Induced Hypoxia and Hemorrhagic Shock, *Ann Surg,* **163:**21, 1966.

Kirtley, J. A., Scott, H. W., Sawyers, J. L., Graves, H. A., and Lawler, M. R.: The Surgical Management of Stress Ulcers, *Ann Surg,* **169:**801, 1969.

Langman, M. J. S., Hansky, J. H., Drury, R. A. B., and Avery Jones, F.: The Gastric Mucosa in Radiologically Negative Acute Gastrointestinal Bleeding, *Gut,* **5:**550, 1964.

Law, E. J., Day, S. B., and MacMillan, B. G.: Autopsy Findings in the Upper Gastro-Intestinal Tract of 81 Burn Patients, *Arch Surg,* **102:**412, 1971.

Lucas, C. E., Sugawa, C., Riddle, J., Rector, F., Rosenberg, B., and Walt, A. J.: Natural History and Surgical Dilemma of "Stress" Gastric Bleeding, *Arch Surg,* **102:**266, 1971.

Menguy, R., Desbaillets, L., and Masters, Y. F.: Mechanism of Stress Ulcer: Influence of Hypovolemic Shock on Energy Metabolism in the Gastric Mucosa, *Gastroenterology,* **66:**46, 1974.

Menguy, R., Gadacz, T., and Zajtchuk, R.: The Surgical Management of Acute Gastric Mucosal Bleeding, *Arch Surg,* **99:**198, 1969.

Nusbaum, M., Baum, S., and Kuroda, K.: Selective Intra-arterial Infusion of Vasoactive Agents in the Control of Gastrointestinal Bleeding, *Arch Surg,* **97:**1005, 1968.

O'Neill, J. A., Pruitt, B. A., and Moncrief, J. A.: Surgical Treatment of Curling's Ulcer, *Surg Gynecol Obstet,* **126:**40, 1968.

Palmer, E. D.: Hemorrhage from Erosive Gastritis and its Surgical Implications, *Gastroenterology,* **36:**856, 1959.

Skillman, J. J., Bushnell, L. S., Goldman, H., and Silen, W.: Respiratory Failure, Hypotension, Sepsis and Jaundice: A Clinical Syndrome Associated with Lethal Hemorrhage from Acute Stress Ulceration of the Stomach, *Am J Surg,* **117:**523, 1969.

Skillman, J. J., and Silen, W.: Acute Gastroduodenal "Stress" Ulceration: Barrier Disruption of Varied Pathogenesis, *Gastroenterology,* **59:**478, 1970.

Sullivan, R. C., and Waddell, W. R.: Accumulated Experience with Vagotomy and Pyloroplasty for Surgical Control of Hemorrhagic Gastritis, *Am J Surg,* **116:**745, 1968.

Winawer, S. J., Bejar, J., and Zamcheck, N.: Recurrent Massive Hemorrhage in Patients with Achlorhydria and Atrophic Gastritis, *Arch Intern Med,* **120:**327, 1967.

Miscellaneous Surgical Diseases

Booher, R. J., and Grant, R. N.: Eosinophilic Granuloma of the Stomach and Small Intestine, *Surgery,* **30:**388, 1951.

Bruno, M. S., Grier, W. R. N., and Ober, W. B.: Spontaneous Laceration and Rupture of Esophagus and Stomach: Mallory-Weiss Syndrome, Boerhaave Syndrome, and Their Variants, *Arch Intern Med,* **112:**574, 1963.

DeBakey, M., and Ochsner, A.: Bezoars and Concretions, *Surgery,* **4:**934, 1938; **5:**132, 1939.

Dobbins, W. O.: Mallory-Weiss Syndrome: A Commonly Overlooked Cause of Upper Gastrointestinal Bleeding: Report of Three Cases and Review of the Literature, *Gastroenterology,* **44:**689, 1963.

Feldman, M., Morrison, S., and Myers, P.: The Clinical Evaluation of Prolapse of the Gastric Mucosa into the Duodenum, *Gastroenterology,* **22:**80, 1952.

Fieber, S. S.: Hypertrophic Gastritis: Report of 2 Cases and Analysis of 50 Pathologically Verified Cases from the Literature, *Gastroenterology,* **28:**39, 1955.

Mallory, G. K., and Weiss, S.: Hemorrhages from Lacerations of the Cardiac Orifice of the Stomach Due to Vomiting, *Am J Med Sci,* **178:**506, 1929.

Gastric Cancer

Ackerman, N. B.: An Evaluation of Gastric Cytology: Results of a Nationwide Survey, *J Chronic Dis,* **20:**621, 1967.

Aird, I., Bentall, H. H., and Fraser-Roberts, J. A.: A Relationship between Cancer of the Stomach and the ABO Blood Groups, *Br Med J,* **1:**799, 1953.

Berkson, J., Walters, W., Gray, H. K., and Priestley, J. T.: Mortality and Survival in Cancer of the Stomach: A Statistical Summary of the Experience of the Mayo Clinic, *Proc Staff Meetings Mayo Clin,* **27:**137, 1952.

Blendis, L. M., Beilby, J. O. W., Wilson, J. P., Coles, M. J., and Hadley, G. D.: Carcinoma of the Stomach: Evaluation of Individual and Combined Diagnostic Accuracy of Radiology, Cytology and Gastrophotography, *Br Med J,* **1:**656, 1967.

Brown, P. M., Cain, J. C., and Dockerty, M. B.: Clinically "Benign" Gastric Ulcerations Found to Be Malignant at Operation, *Surg Gynecol Obstet,* **112:**82, 1961.

Eisenberg, H., and Shambaugh, E.: Cancer of the Gastrointestinal Tract: Trends in Incidence and Mortality Rates. In: "Proceedings of the Sixth National Cancer Conference," p. 417, J. B. Lippincott Company, Philadelphia, 1968.

Gilbertsen, V. A.: Results of Treatment of Stomach Cancer. An Appraisal of Efforts for More Extensive Surgery and a Report of 1,983 Cases, *Cancer,* **23:**1305, 1969.

Huppler, E. G., Priestley, J. T., Morlock, C. G., and Gage, R. P.: Diagnosis and Results of Treatment in Gastric Polyps, *Surg, Gynecol Obstet,* **110:**390, 1960.

Kennedy, B. J.: TNM Classification for Stomach Cancer, *Cancer,* **26:**971, 1960.

Scott, H. W., Jr., and Longmire, W. P., Jr.: Total Gastrectomy. Report of Sixty-three Cases, *Surgery,* **26:**488, 1949.

"Staging System for Carcinoma of the Stomach, 1971," American Joint Committee for Cancer Staging and End Results Reporting, Chicago, 1971.

Stout, A. P.: Tumors of the Stomach, in "Atlas of Tumor Pathology," sec. VI, fascicle 21, Armed Forces Institute of Pathology, Washington, 1953.

Strode, J. E.: Malignant Lesions of the Stomach in Hawaii: Experiences with 350 Patients, *Surgery,* **49:**573, 1961.

Walker, I. R., Strickland, R. G., Ungar, B., and MacKay, I. R.: Simple Atrophic Gastritis and Gastric Carcinoma, *Gut,* **12:**906, 1971.

Welch, C. E., and Wilkins, E. W., Jr.: Carcinoma of the Stomach, *Ann Surg,* **148:**666, 1958.

Zinninger, M. M.: Extension of Gastric Cancer in the Intramural Lymphatics and its Relation to Gastrectomy, *Am Surg,* **20:**920, 1954.

Chapter 27

Small Intestine

by Edward H. Storer

Inflammatory Diseases

Regional Enteritis
Tuberculous Enteritis
Typhoid Enteritis

Neoplasms

Benign Neoplasms
    Peutz-Jeghers Syndrome
Malignant Neoplasms
    Carcinoids

Diverticular Disease

Meckel's Diverticulum
Duodenal Diverticula
Jejunal and Ileal Diverticula

Miscellaneous Problems

Ulcer of the Small Intestine
Ingested Foreign Bodies
Fistula
Pneumatosis Cystoides Intestinalis
Blind Loop Syndrome
Short Bowel Syndrome
Intestinal Bypass
    Morbid Obesity
    Hyperlipidemia

The length of the human small intestine at autopsy, after separation from its mesentery, is 6 to 8 m. In life, however, the intestine is about 3 m long because of a constant base-line state of muscular contraction. Estimates of the absorbing surface vary from 2.2 m² to larger than a tennis court depending on whether the microvilli are included in the estimate. Despite this impressive length and surface area, the small intestine is much less susceptible to primary disease than the stomach or colon—except for its first 3 cm, the duodenal bulb. Disease is as frequent in the first 3 cm as in all of the remaining 300 cm combined.

The small intestine has been relatively inaccessible for nonoperative diagnostic procedures compared to stomach or colon. Recent additions to the diagnostic armamentarium are proving to be of value in selected types of small bowel disease. Mucosal biopsies obtained with the peroral biopsy capsule are often diagnostic in diffuse mucosal diseases. Selective mesenteric angiography is often helpful in cases of discrete lesions that have vascular abnormalities such as neoplasms, vascular malformations, or actively bleeding lesions. Fiberoptic endoscopy of the duodenum and proximal jejunum is now a feasible clinical procedure.

Some diseases affecting the small intestine are discussed in other chapters: intestinal obstruction, Chap. 24; mesenteric vascular disease, Chap. 35; diseases of the intestine in infancy and childhood, Chap. 39; the intestine in trauma, Chap. 6; duodenal and gastrojejunal peptic ulcer, Chap. 26; and carcinoma of the second part of the duodenum, Chap. 32.

INFLAMMATORY DISEASES

Regional Enteritis

This is a chronic, sclerosing granulomatous disease of the gastrointestinal tract of unknown cause. Soon after Crohn's separation, in 1932, of what he initially called "terminal ileitis" from other chronic granulomas of the intestine, it was recognized that the disease, though most common in the terminal ileum, may affect any segment of the small or large bowel, so the term "regional enteritis" is now used in the United States. The eponym "Crohn's disease" is commonly employed elsewhere.

INCIDENCE. Though regional enteritis is the most common surgical disease of the small intestine, it is quite uncommon compared to other gastrointestinal diseases such as peptic ulcer or actue appendicitis. The range of incidence in the United States and Europe was estimated in 1972 to be two to four new cases per year per 100,000 population. Crohn's disease has its highest incidence in the United States, followed by the United Kingdom and Scandinavia. It is infrequent in Central Europe and only occasionally seen in Africa, Asia, and South America. The incidence is about three times higher in Jews than in non-Jews, appreciably higher in whites than in nonwhites, and slightly higher in males. The disease is seen in all age groups but is most frequent in young adults; the average age at onset of symptoms is twenty-seven years.

PATHOLOGY, PATHOGENESIS, AND ETIOLOGY. The usual sequence in discussion of a disease entity is etiology, pathogenesis, pathology. This sequence is here reversed in order to relate pathologic findings, which are well known, to hypotheses concerning pathogenetic and etiologic factors, which are not known.

Intestinal segments involved in chronic regional enteritis present a very characteristic appearance at operation. Diseased segments are beefy, dull purple-red, thickened to two or three times normal diameter, and covered with strands and patches of thick gray-white exudate. Mesenteric fat tends to grow over the serosa so that it nearly encompasses the bowel in areas of maximal involvement. The thickened bowel wall is very firm, rubbery, and virtually incompressible. Involved segments are often adherent to adjacent loops or other viscera, or several loops may be matted together into a bulky conglomerate mass. Internal fistulas are frequently present in such adherent areas. The mesentery of the segment is characteristically greatly thickened, dull, and rubbery, and contains lymph node masses up to 3 or 4 cm in size. The uninvolved proximal bowel is often dilated because of the considerable degree of obstruction present in the diseased segment.

Three striking abnormalities are seen in areas of maximal involvement on opening a resected specimen: tremendous thickening of the bowel wall, the submucosa showing the greatest increase in breadth; marked narrowing of the lumen; and varying degrees of mucosal nodularity, ulceration, and destruction.

Diseased tissues are less strikingly abnormal in the acute phase of regional enteritis. Early changes are principally marked hyperemia, dullness and fine granularity of the serosal surface, edema and soft thickening of the bowel wall, and edema of the corresponding mesentery. Moderately enlarged soft mesenteric lymph nodes are frequently but not invariably present.

The relationship of "acute regional enteritis" to the classical chronic form is unclear. Acute enteritis is usually discovered at laparotomy for suspected appendicitis. Only a minority of these patients progress to chronic regional enteritis; in the majority the process subsides without medical or surgical therapy. Some acute regional enteritides may be attributable to specific agents such as enteroviruses or Yersinia species, and perhaps also to allergic phenomena.

Regional enteritis may involve any segment of the gastrointestinal tract from esophagus to rectum. Isolated involvement of esophagus, stomach, or duodenum are rare, however. Granulomatous disease limited to the colon occurs fairly frequently and is discussed in Chap. 28. There are three principal patterns of involvement of the small intestine that occur in about 95 percent of all patients with this disease. The most frequent site of involvement is the terminal ileum, and in nearly one-half this is the only segment involved. In the classic terminal ileitis pattern there is an abrupt demarcation at the ileocecal valve with minimal or no cecal abnormality. Maximal disease of bowel and mesentery extends proximally for 15 to 25 cm, beyond which the degree of involvement diminishes fairly rapidly to dilated but otherwise normal proximal small bowel and accompanying mesentery. In about one-third of patients both small and large bowel are involved. The disease is often continuous, since terminal ileum is the most frequently involved segment of small bowel, and cecum and right colon the most frequent site of colonic involvement. This is not invariable, however, and areas of disease may be separated by segments of essentially normal bowel—"skip areas." The third pattern, jejunoileitis, extensively involves the distal one-half of the jejunum and proximal one-half of ileum. Infrequently, multiple diseased segments of varying lengths involve the entire length of small bowel.

Microscopic features of regional enteritis are somewhat variable, but histologic features occur with sufficient consistency to create a pattern that, while not specific, is characteristic of the disease. Some understanding of pathogenesis may be gained by observing the progression of changes from early to late phases of regional enteritis.

The most striking finding in the early phase is a marked edema of the entire bowel wall, but especially the submucosa. The edema is accompanied by lymphangiectasis and hyperemia. Mucosa is essentially normal except for an increase in the proportion of goblet cells. A fibrinopurulent exudate is invariably present on the serosal surface. Granulomas are not found in the early phase.

In the intermediate phase, though edema and lymphangiectasis persist, thickening of the bowel wall is more attributable to fibrosis of submucosa and subserosa. Small focal ulcers that rarely penetrate the muscularis mucosa are numerous, and the lamina propria is infiltrated with lymphocytes, plasma cells, and variable numbers of eosinophils. In the submucosa, the extensive fibrosis is fine and fibrillar in character and is accompanied by diffuse infiltration of mononuclear cells and prominent hypertrophy and hyperplasia of lymphoid follicles. The muscularis propria also demonstrates hypertrophy, fibrosis, and cellular infiltrate but to a lesser degree than the submucosa. Granulomas may be present, particularly in the submucosa, subserosa, or regional lymph nodes. They resemble the epithelioid giant cell granulomas of tuberculosis but do not caseate and do not contain tubercle bacilli, and thus are often called "sarcoidlike granulomas."

Coarse dense fibrosis of submucosa and subserosa characterizes the late phase. The degree of fibrosis is disproportionate and suggests that it is not a simple process of repair and replacement of damaged tissue but rather an altered tissue reactivity that is peculiar to the disease process. The mucosa is denuded over wide areas. Where mucosal islands are present, villi are blunted or absent and glands atrophied, producing a picture resembling colonic mucosa. Small mucous glands deep in the mucosa resemble the glands of the pyloric region and are termed "aberrant pyloric glands," or "Brunner's gland metaplasia." Deep ulcers are often present, surrounded by focal areas of suppuration. Progression through the entire bowel wall may occur, producing a fistulous tract. Sarcoidlike granulomas are frequently but by no means invariably present.

The marked lymphangiectasia which is invariably present in regional enteritis has led to speculation that progressive obstructive lymphangitis is the principal primary pathogenetic mechanism, all other changes being secondary. Some have suggested that primary mesenteric adenitis initiates the process. Experimentally, lymphatic obstruction with lymphedema, chronic inflammatory changes, and fibrosis of the submucosa has been produced by feeding finely divided silicates to laboratory animals. Ulcerogranulomatous lesions similar to regional enteritis are not produced, however, nor is foreign material in significant amounts detectable in the diseased tissues of regional enteritis.

Until 1932, regional enteritis was probably most frequently misdiagnosed as hyperplastic tuberculosis. As noted above, the granulomas in regional enteritis do not caseate, and tubercle bacilli cannot be isolated. Antituberculosis chemotherapy has no beneficial effect in patients with regional enteritis.

Similarities between sarcoidosis and Crohn's disease suggest an etiologic relationship. Histologically, both diseases often have noncaseating epithelioid cell granulomas with Langhans' giant cells, both may respond to corticosteroid therapy, and both are associated with some depression of cell-mediated immune reactions. But sarcoid is thought to be a systemic disease with involvement of many sites, principally lungs, lymph nodes, skin, liver, and spleen, whereas, the granulomas of regional enteritis are found only in the gastrointestinal tract, mesenteric nodes, and occasionally the liver. The Kveim test, which is positive in about 80 percent of patients with active sarcoidosis, is nearly always negative in Crohn's disease. (In the early 1970s, there were several reports of positive Kveim tests in about 50 percent of patients with Crohn's disease. These were apparently false positives attributable to defective batches of Kveim antigen.)

Crohn, in his original paper, proposed that terminal ileitis may have a specific infectious causative agent, but despite countless investigations, no infectious agent has yet fulfilled Koch's postulates. Interest was rekindled in 1970 by Mitchell and Rees, who reported sarcoidlike granulomas in the footpads of mice which had been injected months earlier with homogenates of intestine and mesenteric lymph nodes from a patient with Crohn's disease. Some investigators have been unable to repeat this work, but others have confirmed and extended the observations. Granulomas have been induced in rabbit intestine by intraileal injection of tissue from a patient with Crohn's disease. These lesions can be serially passed by intravenous, footpad, or intraileal injection in both mice and rabbits. Tissues from patients without inflammatory bowel disease do not produce granulomas. The pathogenicity of Crohn's tissues is maintained after 220 nm filtration and freezing at $-70°C$, but is removed by autoclaving. This suggests a virus as the transmissible agent but does not rule out L-forms or mycoplasmas. Two groups have subsequently cultured viruses from intestinal tissues of patients with a variety of chronic gastrointestinal disorders including Crohn's disease. It is not clear at this point, however, what role, if any, these viruses play in Crohn's disease. They may be innocent passenger viruses in a diseased bowel.

The possibility that immune mechanisms play a role in the initiation and/or perpetuation of inflammatory bowel disease is also receiving considerable attention. Shorter has proposed that these diseases are the result of a local hypersensitivity reaction. Initial sensitization of the gut-associated lymphoid tissues is thought to occur in the neonatal period when the mucosal barrier is incomplete, permitting penetration of enterobacteria and macromolecules. Reexposure to bacteria and intestinal antigens may occur in later life if the normal mucosal integrity is damaged by gastroenteritis, bacillary dysentery, amebic colitis, ischemic episodes, or even metabolic alterations induced by psychologic stress. This reexposure then causes the local primary cellular, immune-mediated hypersensitivity reaction resulting in inflammatory bowel disease.

Whether or not immune phenomena are involved in the intestinal disease per se, it is entirely possible that some of the extraintestinal manifestations, such as erythema nodosum and peripheral arthritis, are mediated by circulating antigen-antibody complexes originating in the diseased bowel. The systemic manifestations usually improve following resection of the diseased bowel.

From 10 to 15 percent of patients with inflammatory bowel disease have a relative with the disease, which suggests genetic transmission. It now seems clear that these are not classic genetically transmitted disorders but may represent the combined interaction of several genes, the multifactorial type of inheritance, interacting with environmental influences in susceptible individuals.

Many clinicians feel that emotional stress is important in the initiation and perpetuation of inflammatory bowel disease—that these are psychosomatic phenomena. There is no convincing scientific evidence to date to support this. But evaluation of psychological influences is difficult when the patient already has the somatic disease when first seen. Cause and effect are difficult to identify at this point.

Crohn's statement that "the actual etiology is completely unknown" is still essentially true.

CLINICAL MANIFESTATIONS. The symptom pattern depends largely upon the anatomic site of involvement, extent of disease process, and presence or absence of complications. Onset is varied. Some patients present with only a febrile illness without localizing symptoms or signs. Careful questioning will usually elicit a history of abdominal discomfort that increases after eating, mild anorexia, and loose stools.

In about 10 percent of patients, more frequently in the young, the onset is acute and mimics acute appendicitis. There is midabdominal or right lower quadrant pain and tenderness, low-grade fever, leukocytosis, often nausea and vomiting, occasionally diarrhea. The correct diagnosis in acute regional enteritis is usually made only at operation.

In the majority of patients the onset is insidious, the course protracted and slowly progressive. Symptomatic periods are interspersed with symptom-free periods, but the symptomatic periods gradually become more frequent, more severe, and longer-lasting. Pain or discomfort is the most frequent and occasionally the only symptom. It is usually of an intermittent peristaltic type and early in the course is precipitated by dietary indiscretion. This cramping may gradually take on the characteristics of frank partial obstruction with distension and visible bowel loops. A second type of pain is a constant aching or soreness and usually implies advanced disease. Tenderness and a palpable mass nearly always accompany this type of pain.

Diarrhea is the next most frequent symptom and is

present, at least intermittently, in about 85 percent of patients. The frequency of stools is not great compared to ulcerative colitis, numbering two to five daily, and, unlike ulcerative colitis, the stools rarely contain mucus, pus, or blood.

Fever is present in about one-third of these patients; moderate weight loss, loss of strength, and easy fatigability, in over one-half. Frank nutritional disorders and steatorrhea are uncommon prior to surgical treatment. Extraintestinal manifestations, although quite rare, comprise a lengthy list: ankylosing spondylitis, migratory polyarthritis, erythema nodosum, pyoderma gangrenosum, pericholangitis, hepatic fatty infiltration, portal fibrosis, cholelithiasis, uveitis, periureteric fibrosis producing hydronephrosis, pancreatic fibrosis, and secondary amyloidosis.

Presenting symptoms in some patients may be those of a complication of regional enteritis: intestinal obstruction, confined perforation with abscess or internal fistula, free perforation with peritonitis, perianal abscesses or fistulas, or hemorrhage. About 40 cases of adenocarcinoma of the small bowel associated with regional enteritis have been reported. Though the number is small, it is probably significant because carcinoma of the ileum is a rare disease. Immunosuppression from chronic corticosteroid administration may play a role. The prognosis is poor: the 5-year survival rate is less than 10 percent, compared to about 21 percent for carcinoma of the ileum not associated with regional enteritis.

Complete obstruction is uncommon in contrast to partial obstruction. Emergency operation for obstruction per se

Fig. 27-1. Small bowel barium meal radiograph of a patient with regional enterocolitis. Arrows point to a string sign in the terminal ileum.

is usually not necessary, since most patients respond rather quickly to nonoperative measures. Elective operative treatment for the high-grade partial obstruction is usually indicated, however, as soon as the patient can be prepared.

Perforation as the result of an ulcer burrowing through the entire thickness of the bowel wall occurs in 15 to 20 percent of patients. Rarely, the perforation is into the free peritoneal cavity; confined perforation is the rule, resulting in abscesses or internal fistulas. Fistulization may be into another loop of intestine, small or large, urinary bladder, or vagina. Enterocutaneous fistulas do not occur in patients not operated upon but are common after operation. Perianal or perirectal abscesses and fistulas are also a common manifestation of regional enteritis with a reported frequency varying from 14 to 50 percent. The pathogenesis of this complication is not understood, since the abscesses or fistulas usually do not communicate with the diseased small bowel.

Frank hemorrhage producing hematochezia or melena is a rare complication of regional enteritis in contrast to ulcerative colitis. Occult bleeding sufficient to produce anemia is common, however.

ROENTGENOGRAPHIC FINDINGS. Barium enema with ileocecal reflux usually suffices to demonstrate involvement of the terminal ileum. Small bowel barium meal study should also be done to identify other possible sites of small bowel involvement.

With severe disease, the wall is thickened and rigid and encroaches on the lumen so that only a thin trickle of barium is seen, producing the string sign of Kantor (Fig. 27-1). Thickening of the wall and mesentery increases the space between the hoselike loops. In areas of lesser involvement, the mucosal pattern is grossly distorted with thick, irregular folds. Fistulas may be seen but are often obscured by overlapping loops.

TREATMENT. There is no curative therapy, either medical or surgical, for regional enteritis. Despite the fact that medical therapy is symptomatic and empiric, this form of therapy is indicated until a serious complication supervenes, because the recurrence rate after operation is so high. Medical therapy is directed at relieving abdominal pain, treating infection, controlling diarrhea, and correcting deficiencies in hemoglobin, protein, electrolytes, and vitamins.

Systemic antibiotics are often of value in the management of suppurative complications but have little or no effect on the primary disease process and should not be given for prolonged periods. Nonabsorbable antibiotics, particularly salicylazosulfapyridine, do sometimes exert a beneficial effect on the symptoms and should be tried. Results of treatment with corticotropin or corticosteroids have been disappointing. There is no clear evidence that they have exerted any favorable influence in mitigating the complications of stenosis, perforation, and fistula formation, and may increase the postoperative morbidity in patients who subsequently must have surgical therapy. Nevertheless some patients do appear to be benefited, so that a course of steroid therapy is probably worthwhile. Improvement of mood and appetite, more than antiinflammatory effect, are the principal benefits.

Despite the paucity of evidence implicating immune mechanisms in regional enteritis, immunosuppressive therapy is currently very popular. Azathiaprine, the antimetabolite used by most, has not caused serious toxicity when used in modest doses. Amelioration of the disease may be attributable to the anti-inflammatory effects of azathiaprine and not to immunosuppression. Hepatotoxicity, bone marrow depression, masking of infectious complications, and in the long run, increased oncogenesis are hazards. The usefulness of immunosuppressive therapy is still uncertain. Controlled studies have not provided clear-cut evidence to support its effectiveness, though some patients improve dramatically. It may be that there is a small subset of Crohn's patients, not yet identified, in whom immunosuppression will be the preferred mode of therapy.

A major advance in the nonoperative therapy of inflammatory bowel disease has been the elemental diet and total parenteral nutrition. The elemental diet provides a high-caloric, high-nitrogen, fat-free, zero-residue substrate which is absorbed in the upper part of the small bowel. This can be given to nearly all patients with Crohn's disease, even during acute exacerbations. Parenteral hyperalimentation, since it is not as safe as the oral elemental diet, should be reserved for patients with active upper intestinal disease or small bowel fistulas. Operation can often be avoided by the use of this nutrition therapy. It is also useful for getting patients in optimal shape for operation.

Failure of medical therapy results from progression of the disease process at the established existing sites of disease. Longitudinal extension along the bowel rarely occurs prior to surgical intervention.

Surgical Therapy. Indications. In general, failure of medical therapy to ameliorate the disease and prevent complications is the indication for operative intervention. Surgical treatment is used to correct complications that are themselves producing serious symptoms. The majority of patients with chronic regional enteritis will eventually require operation at least once in the course of their disease. Specific indications, in descending order of frequency, are obstruction; persistent, symptomatic abdominal mass or abscess; fistula, internal and/or external; perirectal fistulas that do not respond to local therapy; and intractability, or continued downhill course despite medical therapy. Uncommon indications are free perforation, hemorrhage, growth retardation in children, and blind loop syndrome. Contraindications for surgical therapy include acute regional enteritis, mucosal or superficial enteritis, and extensive jejunoileitis with involvement of all or a large part of the small bowel.

Procedure. Three surgical approaches are available: simple bypass of the diseased segment, bypass with exclusion, and resection of the diseased segment with primary anastomosis (Fig. 27-2). The choice of procedure depends on the findings at operation and the preference of the surgeon.

Simple bypass is rarely used now for a single short segment of disease because fecal diversion is incomplete, but it is the procedure of choice in extensive disease with several stenotic segments requiring surgical relief. Bypass in the form of a gastrojejunostomy instead of resection is also preferred for obstructive gastroduodenal Crohn's disease.

Bypass with exclusion was popular for a time, because it could be done with a lower mortality-morbidity rate than resection but with about the same recurrence rate as resection. It was also hoped that diversion of the fecal stream would permit healing in the excluded bowel, and that restoration of normal continuity might then be feasible. This has proved to be a forlorn hope most of the time. Disease in the excluded bowel does usually become quiescent but only rarely does the excluded segment "heal" sufficiently to permit restoration of continuity. On the contrary, active disease sometimes continues, with persistence of fistulas, bleeding, and symptoms and signs of continuing inflammation. Bypass with exclusion is now used in elderly, poor-risk patients; in patients who have had several prior resections and can ill afford to lose any more bowel; and in patients in whom resection would necessitate entering an abscess or endangering normal structures. It must be kept in mind that the proximal end of the bypassed segment can be brought out onto the abdominal wall as a mucous fistula, permitting introduction of topical therapy directly to the diseased area. If new, effective topical agents become available, bypass with exclusion will need to be resurrected.

The procedure now preferred by most surgeons is conservative resection of the grossly diseased intestine along with its mesentery. Current evidence indicates that results are not improved by increasing the margins of normal tissue proximal and distal to the diseased intestine. Thus the proximal margin should be through soft, pliable bowel—dilatation does not necessarily indicate disease—and microscopic control of margins with frozen sections is not helpful and is often confusing. The distal line of resection (with disease in the terminal ileum) should be in the ascending colon although the standard right colectomy is technically easier. Nor should any attempt be made to remove all enlarged mesenteric lymph nodes, since this does not change the rate of recurrence and may endanger the blood supply of otherwise normal intestine.

There has been considerable controversy in the past whether to do an appendectomy when enteritis is encountered at laparotomy done for suspected appendicitis because of the very appreciable incidence of postoperative enterocutaneous fistula through the incision. It now seems clear that appendectomy should be done except when the cecum at the base of the appendix is involved in the inflammation. Up to 90 percent of patients with acute regional enteritis do not progress to the chronic form, and it has been shown that postoperative fistulas, when they do occur, usually arise in the diseased ileum and not in the appendiceal stump,

Results. The operative mortality rate is now about 4 percent in most series and is about the same for all three procedures. The morbidity is appreciable and is higher in patients who have been on large doses of steroids for prolonged periods at the time of operation. Principal complications are enterocutaneous fistula, intraperitoneal or wound sepsis, and prolonged postoperative ileus.

The recurrence rate is from 35 to 50 percent overall. It is lower in elderly patients and higher in the young. Recurrences may be more frequent and occur sooner after each successive operation for regional enteritis. These postoperative recurrences characteristically develop in the neoterminal ileum and end abruptly at the colon. The fact that about one-half of surgically treated patients will at some time have a symptomatic or radiographic recurrence of disease does not negate the great benefit to be derived from properly timed surgical therapy. One-half do not have recurrence—they are completely rehabilitated. Many of the patients with recurrence have substituted a disabling life-threatening complication for a relatively mild recurrence that is managed very well by proper medical therapy.

Regional enteritis is not a particularly fatal disease ini-

Fig. 27-2. Operations for regional enteritis. *A.* Simple side-to-side ileocolostomy bypass. *B.* Bypass with exclusion. The ileum is divided proximal to any evidence of disease; the distal end is closed or brought out as a mucous fistula; the proximal end is anastomosed end-to-side into the colon. *C* through *G.* Resection with primary anastomosis. *C.* Extent of bowel and mesentery to be resected. *D.* Insert: Methods of increasing the diameter of end of ileum to be anastomosed. The clamp may be placed obliquely or an incision made on the antimesenteric border. *E.* Placing the posterior outer suture line. The discrepancy in diameter of the bowel ends is eliminated by placing the two end sutures first, then progressively bisecting intervening spaces with successive sutures. *F.* Placing the anterior inner suture line—an infolding, hemostatic running stitch. *G.* The anastomosis completed with interrupted sutures in the outer anterior row. The cut edges of mesenteries of ileum and colon are approximated.

tially or at any one time, but becomes progressively more dangerous as the years go by. In general the death rate of persons with this disease is about twice that for the normal population.

Tuberculous Enteritis

Tuberculosis of the gastrointestinal tract occurs in two forms. Primary infection is usually due to the bovine strain of *Mycobacterium tuberculosis* and results from ingesting infected milk. This is now rare in the United States but is still common in undeveloped countries. Secondary infection, due to the human strain, results from the swallowing of bacilli by patients with active pulmonary tuberculosis. Chemotherapy has markedly decreased the incidence of secondary tuberculous enteritis, so that it now occurs in only about 1 percent of patients with pulmonary tuberculosis.

The ileocecal region is the site of involvement in about 85 percent of patients with tuberculous enteritis, presumably because of the abundance of lymphoid tissue in this area.

Primary tuberculous enteritis often produces minimal symptoms unless dissemination to other organs occurs. Occasionally a hypertrophic reaction produces contracture and stenosis of the lumen of distal ileum, cecum, and ascending colon. Such involvement may produce symptoms, signs, and radiographic findings that are indistinguishable from those of carcinoma of the colon, and surgical exploration with biopsy may be advisable. If the diagnosis is suspected preoperatively, chemotherapy, consisting of isoniazid, 100 mg three times a day, and para-aminosalicylic acid (PAS), 3 Gm three times a day, should be administered for about 2 weeks. Streptomycin, 0.5 Gm, twice daily, is started the day before operation. If tuberculosis is found at operation, all drugs are continued—streptomycin for 1 to 2 weeks, isoniazid and PAS at the same dose for 1 year after the patient has become asymptomatic. Surgical therapy of hypertrophic tuberculous enteritis is usually inadvisable unless high-grade stenosis dictates immediate relief. Right colectomy is applicable if the involved segment is short and clearly defined, otherwise ileocolic bypass is the safer procedure.

Symptoms of the more common ulcerative form of tuberculous enteritis secondary to pulmonary disease are also variable, and the diagnosis may be made only by routine radiographic intestinal examination of patients with pulmonary tuberculosis. When present, symptoms consist of alternating constipation and diarrhea associated with crampy lower abdominal pain. In severe cases, diarrhea is persistent, and anemia and inanition are progressive. The diagnosis can usually be made by barium enema examination. Early in the disease, irritability of the terminal ileum and cecum causes rapid emptying of barium from the affected segment. Later, intestinal contours become spiculated as folds stiffen and thicken. Ulceration may be visible, followed by fibrosis, narrowing, and shortening of the area. Clinical confirmation of a presumptive diagnosis may be obtained by a prompt response to antituberculous chemotherapy. Surgical therapy is contraindicated except for the rare complications of perforation, obstruction, or hemorrhage. Chemotherapy which is prescribed for the pulmonary disease usually brings about healing of the intestinal lesions.

Typhoid Enteritis

This is an acute, systemic infection of several weeks' duration, caused by *Salmonella typhosa* and manifested by fever, headache, prostration, cough, maculopapular rash, abdominal pain, and leukopenia. There is hyperplasia and ulceration of Peyer's patches of the intestine, mesenteric lymphadenopathy, splenomegaly, and parenchymatous changes in the liver. Confirmation of diagnosis is obtained by culturing *S. typhosa* from blood or feces or by finding a high titer of agglutinins against the O and H antigens.

Typhoid fever is still a major disease in areas of the world that have not yet attained high public health standards, but the incidence has progressively declined in the United States since 1900. The death rate, which was formerly about 10 percent, is now about 2 percent, in large part because of the specific antimicrobial chloramphenicol, which was introduced in 1948.

Chloramphenicol is given orally in doses of 50 mg/kg of body weight per day in four divided doses until the temperature is normal, then reduced to 30 mg/kg/day for a total of 2 weeks. Ampicillin is also effective and should be given intravenously or intramuscularly in doses of 1 Gm every 6 hours for 2 weeks. Severely toxic patients who do not respond well within 1 week should also receive prednisone in doses of 15 mg four times a day the first day, 10 mg four times a day the second, and 5 mg four times a day the third day. When given with appropriate antibiotic therapy, prednisone does not increase the risk of complications.

Gross hemorrhage occurs in 10 to 20 percent of hospitalized patients, even while they are on adequate therapy. Transfusion therapy is indicated and usually suffices. Every effort should be made to avoid operation, since the bleeding is often from multiple ulcers and the bowel is exceedingly friable. Rarely, laparotomy must be done for uncontrollable, life-threatening hemorrhage.

Perforation, through ulcerated Peyer's patches, is usually in the terminal ileum, and occurs in about 2 percent of cases. Operative treatment is indicated unless the patient is moribund, since localization or walling-off of the perforation is uncommon. Simple closure of the perforation, along with appropriate toilette of the peritoneal cavity, usually suffices. With multiple perforations, which occur in about one-fourth of patients, resection with primary anastomosis is preferred. The mortality rate of those with free perforation is about 10 percent.

NEOPLASMS

Neoplasms of the small bowel are uncommon. Despite the much greater length and surface area of the small bowel, colonic neoplasms occur forty times as frequently.

Though the numbers are small, the variety is great, since virtually all the cells that histologically make up the small bowel give rise to benign and malignant neoplasms. Benign and malignant lesions are reported to occur with about equal frequency in clinical series, while benign lesions are more frequent in autopsy series. Two interesting clinical syndromes are associated with small bowel neoplasms: the Peutz-Jeghers syndrome and the malignant carcinoid syndrome.

Benign Neoplasms

Histologic types of small bowel benign tumors and their relative incidence are shown in Table 27-1. This information should be considered only as a rough approximation, since it is a compilation from many reports, some clinical, some necropsy, utilizing varied terminology. For example, adenomas are the most frequent tumor in one review but are not even mentioned in another review because of subclassification.

About 15 percent of benign tumors are found in the duodenum; about 25 percent in the jejunum, principally in the upper one-third; and about 60 percent in the ileum, principally the lower one-third. All ages are affected with the peak incidence, in clinical cases, in the fourth decade.

CLINICAL MANIFESTATIONS. An appreciable number of small bowel benign tumors apparently cause no serious symptoms during life and are incidental findings at autopsy. The diagnosis is delayed or missed in many clinical cases because symptoms may be absent or vague and nonspecific until significant complications have developed; physical examination rarely provides any clue unless intestinal obstruction is present; and roentgenographic small bowel studies and selective angiography, the only specific diagnostic aids, may fail to demonstrate an existing tumor even though it is suspected clinically. In only about one-half of small bowel tumors found at operation has the correct diagnosis been made preoperatively.

The two most common clinical manifestations of small bowel tumors are bleeding and obstruction. Rarely, perfo-

Table 27-1. TYPES AND RELATIVE FREQUENCY OF SMALL BOWEL BENIGN NEOPLASMS

Neoplasms	Percent
Leiomyomas	17
Lipomas	16
Adenomas	14
Polyps	14
Polyposis, Peutz-Jeghers	3
Hemangiomas	10
Fibromas	10
Neurogenic tumors	5
Fibromyomas	5
Myxomas	2
Lymphangiomas	2
Fibroadenomas	1
Others	1

ration of the bowel wall occurs, resulting in abscess or internal fistula formation, peritonitis, or pneumatosis cystoides intestinalis. Bleeding occurs in about one-third of patients but is rarely gross hemorrhage. More commonly bleeding is occult and intermittent, producing guaiac-positive stools and iron-deficiency anemia. Leiomyomas and hemangiomas are the lesions that most often cause bleeding. The differential diagnosis of small bowel bleeding should include hereditary hemorrhagic telangiectasia, or Osler-Rendu-Weber syndrome. This is transmitted as a simple dominant trait and is manifested by multiple telangiectases of bowel, skin, and mucous membranes.

Intestinal obstruction may be produced either by encroachment on the lumen by the tumor, in which case obstruction is usually chronic and partial, or by intussusception, with the tumor acting as the intussusceptum. Intussusception in adults differs from that seen in children. An organic cause is demonstrable in about 80 percent of adults; benign neoplasm is the organic cause in nearly one-half. Adults often have "chronic" intussusception with recurrent bouts that resolve by spontaneous reduction.

ROENTGENOGRAPHIC FINDINGS. Small bowel barium meal studies are indicated when clinical findings suggest small bowel neoplasms. Accuracy of diagnosis varies from 50 to 90 percent depending on the nature of the lesion and on the diligence with which the examination is done. Oral barium should not be given to patients with findings of complete or high-grade partial obstruction.

TREATMENT. Surgical removal of benign tumors is nearly always indicated because of the risk of complications if untreated and because the diagnosis of benignity can be made with certainty only by microscopic examination of the resected tumor. Segmental resection with primary anastomosis is usually necessary except in very small lesions. The entire bowel should be searched for other lesions, since they are often multiple.

PEUTZ-JEGHERS SYNDROME

This is an uncommon familial disease manifested by intestinal polyposis and melanin spots of the oral mucosa, lips, palms of the hands, and soles of the feet. Over 300 cases have been reported since Peutz first described the syndrome in 1921 and Jeghers et al. rediscovered it in 1949. Inheritance is as a simple mendelian dominant. Both males and females carry the factor, and there is a high degree of penetrance. A single pleiotropic gene is responsible for both the polyps and melanin spots. Pigmentation without polyposis and polyposis without pigmentation have been reported.

Jejunum and ileum are the most frequently involved portion of the gastrointestinal tract, polyposis being found in essentially all cases reported. Colon and rectum are also involved in about one-third, stomach in about one-fourth. The polyps were initially thought to be adenomas but are now thought by most to be hamartomas and thus without malignant potential (Fig. 27-3). There are several single-case reports of malignant tumors of the gastrointestinal tract in patients with the Peutz-Jeghers syndrome. In a few of these patients, the malignant process appeared to be related to Peutz-Jeghers polyps. It is not yet clear whether this represents coincidence or a malignant potential in the syndrome.

Recurrent colicky abdominal pain caused by transient intussusception is the most frequent symptom. Abdominal pain with a palpable mass is present in about one-third of patients. Hemorrhage occurs less frequently.

Surgical therapy is required for obstruction or bleeding, but the procedure should be limited to relieving the complication only, i.e., polypectomy or minimal resection. The wide distribution and large number of polyps usually preclude removal of all polyps, lest the patient be left a cripple from the short bowel syndrome.

Malignant Neoplasms

Malignant tumor of the small bowel is relatively infrequent, comprising about 2 percent of gastrointestinal malignant neoplasms. Adenocarcinoma is the most frequent, followed by carcinoid, lymphoma, and sarcoma, principally leiomyosarcoma. Adenocarcinoma occurs with about equal frequency in duodenum, jejunum, and ileum; the others occur predominantly in the ileum.

CLINICAL MANIFESTATIONS. Clinical manifestations fall roughly into three groups: diarrhea with large amounts of mucus, and tenesmus; obstruction with nausea, vomiting, and cramping abdominal pain; and chronic blood loss with anemia, weakness, guaiac-positive stools, and occasionally melena or hematochezia. As with benign neoplasms, symptoms of malignant neoplasms are often present for many months before the diagnosis is made, emphasizing the insidious nature of small bowel lesions.

TREATMENT. The therapy of choice is wide resection including regional lymph nodes. This requires pancreatoduodenectomy in duodenal lesions. If spread of disease precludes curative resection, short-circuiting procedures usually offer worthwhile palliation. The overall resectability rate of small bowel malignant neoplasms is about 40 percent. The 5-year survival of all diagnosed cases is about 20 percent in adenocarcinoma, 35 percent in lymphoma, and 40 percent in leiomyosarcoma. Carcinoids are discussed below. Postoperative irradiation is indicated in the lymphomas but is of no value in the other lesions. Similarly chemotherapy has little to offer except in the lymphomas.

Two variant lymphomas of the small intestine are of special interest. After many years of malabsorption due to celiac sprue, a small percentage of patients develop lymphoma. The cell type is most frequently histiocytic lymphoma (formerly called reticulum cell sarcoma), followed by Hodgkin's sarcoma and mixed-cell lymphoma. The second variant, so-called Mediterranean-type lymphoma, was first found in non-European Jews and Arabs in the Middle Eastern countries; hence the name. Patients with this lymphoma have monoclonal alpha heavy chains of immunoglobulin in the serum and urine, and a high percentage also have a heavy plasma-cell infiltration of the intestinal mucosa and lymph nodes away from the areas of lymphoma. The prognosis in both the celiac-associated and Mediterranean lymphomas is much worse than in the conventional small intestine lymphoma.

Fig. 27-3. Low-power photomicrograph of a Peutz-Jeghers jejunal polyp. Instead of one predominant cell as seen in most intestinal polyps, these contain all cells of normal intestinal mucosa interspersed within bands of smooth muscle—a hamartoma.

CARCINOIDS

Carcinoids are of particular interest because of their great variability in malignant potential and because of an unusual clinical syndrome associated with them.

The first histologic description of these tumors was published in 1808. Ninety-nine years later the term "carcinoid" was applied to emphasize biologic benignity (erroneously) despite morphologic resemblance to carcinoma. Their true potential for biologic malignancy was first recognized in 1911 but has only recently been generally accepted. Masson identified the cell of origin of carcinoids as the Kultschitzky cell because of a similar affinity of cytoplasmic granules for silver and named these lesions "argentaffin tumors." Masson also suggested that argentaffin tumors are endocrine in nature. Between 1953 and 1954, three groups independently described the malignant carcinoid syndrome, and shortly thereafter the biochemical abnormalities responsible for the syndrome were elucidated.

Carcinoid tumors can occur anywhere in the gastrointestinal tract that Kultschitzky cells occur—from gastric cardia to anus. The appendix is most frequently involved (46 percent), followed by ileum (28 percent) and rectum (17 percent). Other locations are shown in Table 27-2. Outside the gastrointestinal tract, carcinoid tumor is found in the bronchus and has been reported in ovarian and sacrococcygeal teratoma.

The malignant potential and the ability to metastasize appear to be related to the site of origin and size of the primary. Only about 3 percent of appendiceal carcinoids metastasize, but about 35 percent of ileal carcinoids do (Table 27-2). Seventy-five percent of gastrointestinal carcinoids are less than 1 cm in diameter, and only 2 percent of this group have metastasized. About 20 percent of the primary tumors are 1 to 2 cm in diameter, and about half of this group have metastasized. Only about 5 percent are over 2 cm in diameter; 80 to 90 percent of these have metastasized. No primary carcinoid of the gastrointestinal tract exceeding 3 cm in diameter has been reported. Carcinoids of the small bowel are multiple in 30 percent of cases, rarely so in the appendix. This tendency to multicentricity exceeds that of any other malignant neoplasm of the gastrointestinal tract. Another unusual and, to date, unexplained feature of carcinoids of the bowel is the frequent coexistence of a second primary malignant neoplasm of a different histologic type. A second primary neoplasm was found in 29 percent of patients in one large series.

Carcinoids present grossly as slightly elevated, smooth, rounded yellow-gray or tan nodules. They are apt to be overlooked by radiologist and surgeon unless carefully searched for because of their small size and submucosal location. The mucosa over carcinoids is usually intact but may ulcerate. Narrowing of the lumen is produced, not by the bulk of the tumor per se, but by a fibrous reaction around the tumor. Also, metastasis to mesentery usually results in kinking and fixation of the bowel both by an extensive desmoplastic reaction and by very large secondary tumor masses—in contrast to the characteristically small primary.

Symptomatology is similar to that seen in other small bowel tumors as outlined above unless the malignant carcinoid syndrome is present. The radiographic picture may resemble regional enteritis if infiltration of the bowel wall and mesentery has caused narrowing and fixation of a loop. Small, noninfiltrating carcinoids are difficult to detect.

TREATMENT. The magnitude of the indicated surgical resection of small bowel carcinoids is determined by the presence or absence of metastases and the size of the primary tumor. If the primary is less than 1 cm in diameter and no extension or metastasis is demonstrable, local excision is adequate therapy. A standard cancer operation is indicated for lesions of less than 1 cm with demonstrable spread of disease, for multiple primaries, and for all primary lesions of the intestine that exceed 1 cm in diameter. Since most of the tumors are in the distal ileum, adequate resection of node-bearing tissue usually requires right colectomy with the accompanying mesentery in addition to distal ileum. Even with widespread metastatic disease that precludes resection for cure, removal of all resectable tumor tissue is usually indicated, since very significant palliation often results. Bypass procedures are used in poor-risk patients with disseminated disease. Streptozotocin and 5-fluorouracil, singly or in combination, are sometimes helpful.

The overall 5-year survival rate following resection of malignant carcinoids of the small bowel is about 50 percent. If a "curative resection" is done, about 70 percent live 5 years. Even with palliative therapy, about 25 percent live 5 years. One patient is reported who lived in comfort for 14 years with known unresectable tumor in mesenteric and aortic nodes, only to die of unrelated disease.

Malignant Carcinoid Syndrome

This syndrome comprises a group of striking and debilitating symptoms, involving six different organ systems, that can be divided into episodic and permanent manifestations (Fig. 27-4). Episodic manifestations include cutaneous flushing, hyperperistalsis and diarrhea, asthma, and hemodynamic alterations that may result in vasomotor collapse. Permanent manifestations are facial hyperemia, peripheral edema, cutaneous lesions of pellagra, and valvular heart disease. The syndrome was initially thought to be due to excessive amounts of circulating serotonin that was being produced by functioning carcinoid tumors. Some recent observations indicate, however, that this simple hypothesis is inadequate and the biochemical aspects of the malignant carcinoid syndrome are much more complex than first thought.

Serotonin, one of the biologically active peptides, was first isolated in 1948, the formula of 5-hydroxytryptamine was applied in 1949, and it was synthesized in 1951. Serotonin secretion by Kulschitzky cells was demonstrated in 1952, and in 1953 serotonin was extracted from a carcinoid tumor found at autopsy. Shortly thereafter, the clinical

Table 27-2. DISTRIBUTION OF GASTROINTESTINAL CARCINOIDS: INCIDENCE OF METASTASES AND OF CARCINOID SYNDROME

Site	Cases	Average % metastasis	Cases of carcinoid syndrome
Esophagus	1	. . .	0
Stomach	93	23	8
Duodenum	135	20	4
Jejunoileum	1,032	34	91
Meckel's diverticulum	42	19	3
Appendix	1,686	2	6
Colon	91	60	5
Rectum	592	18	1
Ovary	34	6	17
Biliary tract	10	30	0
Pancreas	2	. . .	1
	3,718		136

SOURCE: From Wilson, Cheek, Sherman, and Storer, 1970.

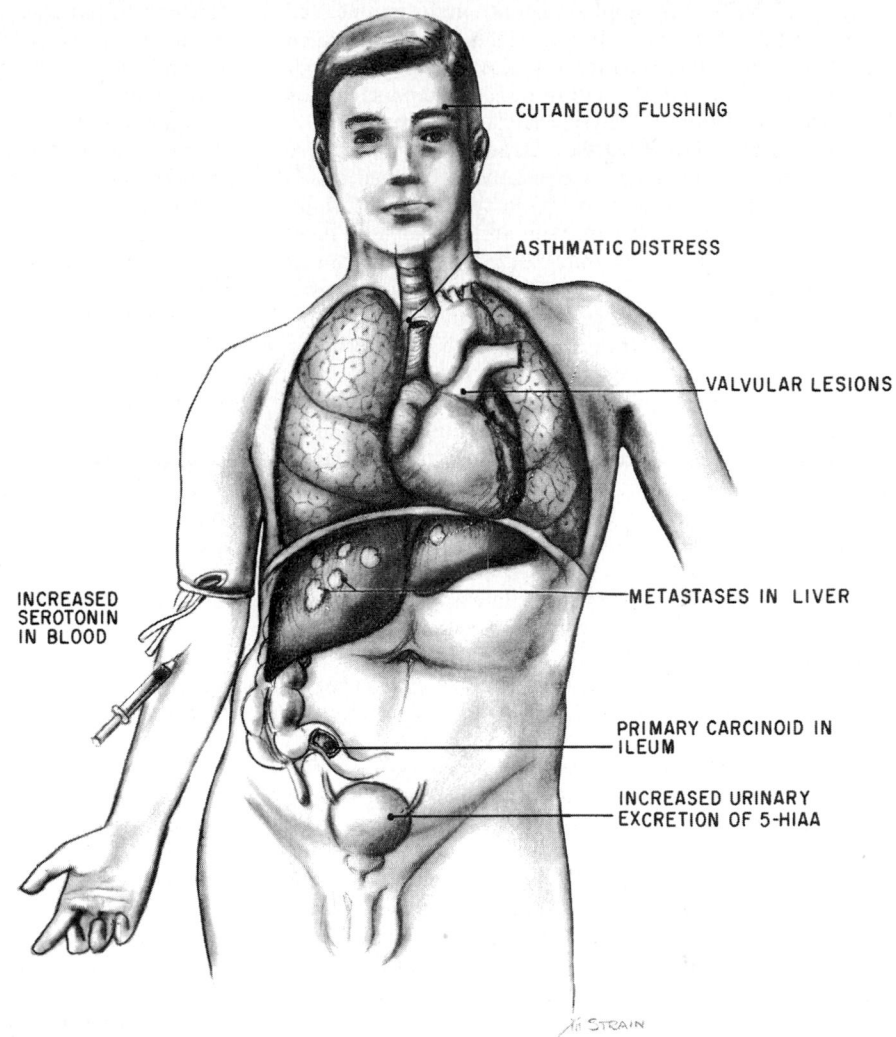

CUTANEOUS FLUSHING

ASTHMATIC DISTRESS

VALVULAR LESIONS

METASTASES IN LIVER

PRIMARY CARCINOID IN ILEUM

INCREASED URINARY EXCRETION OF 5-HIAA

INCREASED SEROTONIN IN BLOOD

STRAIN

Fig. 27-4. Clinical manifestations of malignant carcinoid syndrome.

syndrome of functioning malignant carcinoids was described and overproduction of serotonin implicated in the pathogenesis of the syndrome.

Serotonin is derived in the body from the essential amino acid tryptophan:

Tryptophan

Hydroxylase

5-Hydroxytryptophan

Decarboxylase

5-Hydroxytryptamine
(Serotonin)

Monoamine oxydase
Aldehyde dehydrogenase

5-Hydroxyindole acetic acid
(5-HIAA)

Normally only about 1 percent of dietary tryptophan is metabolized in this manner. Functioning carcinoid tumors may divert as much as 60 percent into the serotonin pathway, leaving less tryptophan available for the formation of other substances such as niacin and body protein, which, along with diarrhea and decreased food intake, contribute to development of pellagra and protein deficiency.

Serotonin is broken down in the liver to 5-HIAA, which is excreted in the urine. This is the basis of a test for the presence of functioning carcinoid tumors: 5-HIAA excretion in normal persons is 2 to 10 mg/day. With functioning tumors the excretion is greatly increased, being 50 to 600 mg/day.

5-HIAA is biologically inactive. Thus carcinoids drained by the portal vein may elaborate tremendous amounts of serotonin without producing the malignant carcinoid syndrome. Release of serotonin into the systemic circulation occurs most frequently with carcinoid metastases in the liver, occasionally with metastases in other sites drained by systemic veins, or from primary carcinoids outside the portal area, such as ovary or bronchus.

Functioning carcinoids may produce, in addition to

serotonin, 5-hydroxytryptophan, kallikrein, histamine, and ACTH. Also, a functioning tumor of the duodenum which morphologically and functionally has features of both foregut carcinoids and islet-cell tumors of the pancreas has been implicated in the Zollinger-Ellison syndrome.

CLINICAL MANIFESTATIONS. Cutaneous phenomena are the most characteristic and frequently recognized manifestations of the malignant carcinoid syndrome. Flushing is the most common early symptom and is present in most but not all patients. It is characteristically episodic and of short duration initially. During the flush, the face, neck, arms, and upper trunk are involved by a dusky red hyperemia, often with a cyanotic hue. This may be accompanied by pruritus, sweating, edema of face and hands, paresthesias, tachycardia, and occasionally vasomotor collapse. Vascular collapse and death occurring during induction of anesthesia have been reported. The flushing episodes usually occur spontaneously but may be precipitated by emotional stress, ingestion of food or alcohol, or defecation. As the syndrome progresses, permanent reddening of the skin occurs and telangiectases appear on the cheeks, nose, and forehead. A permanent cyanotic hue is often seen even in patients without valvular heart disease and with normal arterial oxygen saturation.

Diarrhea is a significant complaint in over 80 percent of patients with the carcinoid syndrome. This is characteristically sudden in onset, watery, not bloody, and more frequent in the morning. Audible borborygmus and cramping abdominal pain frequently accompany the stools. Abdominal symptoms may or may not be related to episodes of flushing. Malabsorption is occasionally seen with severe, long-continued diarrhea.

Peripheral edema is present in about 70 percent of patients and may occur in the absence of valvular heart disease or hypoaluminemia. Periodic increases in venous pressure during flushing and the antidiuretic effect of serotonin may play a role.

Asthmatic attacks, usually concurrent with flushing attacks, have been reported in about 25 percent of patients with the syndrome. Severe bronchoconstriction has occurred during anesthetic induction.

Cardiac involvement is a late development in the syndrome and occurs in about one-half of cases. This peculiar form of valvular disease affects primarily the tricuspid and pulmonic valves; mitral and aortic valve lesions also occur but much less frequently. The valve cusps are progressively thickened, shortened, and narrowed, producing stenosis of the pulmonic valve and usually both stenosis and insufficiency of the tricuspid valve.

The role of serotonin as the sole mediator of all of the varied manifestations has been placed in doubt by some recent observations. Some patients with the carcinoid syndrome have normal levels of 5-HIAA in the urine. Conversely, some patients with grossly elevated levels of serotonin in peripheral blood do not exhibit any of the manifestations of the syndrome. Further, intravenous infusion of pure serotonin does not elicit all the manifestations of the clinical syndrome. Considerable work has been done on the pathogenesis of cutaneous flushing. The levels of circulating serotonin do not correlate with episodes of flushing in patients with the syndrome, and only atypical flushing is produced by infused serotonin. Typical attacks of flushing can usually be induced by intravenous administration of small doses of epinephrine. There is evidence that the flush is not caused by a local response to epinephrine but is mediated through the release of other substances, probably bradykinin. Typical flushing in carcinoid syndrome patients can also be produced by giving synthetic bradykinin. Kallikrein, an enzyme that catalyzes the formation of kinin peptides, as well as kininogen and histamine, has been found in carcinoid tumors. It would appear that carcinoid tumors have multiple endocrine capacities and that several biologically active peptides and amines may be involved. This could account for the variability of clinical syndromes encountered as well as for the discrepancies in the serotonin hypothesis.

DIAGNOSTIC FINDINGS. The syndrome is easily recognized when fully manifest, but a single symptom or sign may be the only clinical evidence of a functioning carcinoid. Knobby hepatomegaly is often present, since the syndrome is nearly always produced by massive liver metastases. Radioisotope scan is useful to document the presence of space-occupying lesions in the liver. Needle biopsy of one of the palpable nodules frequently establishes a histologic diagnosis. Flush induction by intravenous epinephrine is a useful bedside test. The initial dose is 1 μg, with subsequent doses of 2 μg, 5 μg, and 10 μg if necessary. Appearance of a flush, usually associated with hypotension and tachycardia, between 45 and 90 seconds after injection is considered positive. A negative result consists of no reaction or transient facial blanching or transient hypertension.

A 4-hour intravenous infusion of calcium also has been used successfully to provoke attacks in patients suspected of having the carcinoid syndrome.

The most practical laboratory test is the quantitative determination of urinary 5-HIAA. Patients with the syndrome excrete more than 40 mg/day compared to a normal excretion of less than 10 mg/day. A negative test makes the diagnosis of functioning carcinoid unlikely, but there are occasional patients who excrete increased amounts of serotonin instead of 5-HIAA. The qualitative test for urinary 5-HIAA is of some value as a screening procedure, but false positives and false negatives can occur after the ingestion of certain drugs.

TREATMENT. Surgical removal of all neoplastic tissue is rarely possible, except for solitary bronchial or ovarian carcinoids or fortuitously located liver metastases. Exploration is indicated, however, in essentially all patients with malignant carcinoid syndrome. Removal of as much tumor, primary and metastatic, as possible should be attempted even though the line of resection crosses gross tumor. Very remarkable amelioration of symptoms for prolonged periods is the rule rather than the exception when subtotal resection of tumor can be done. Ligation of the hepatic artery in an attempt to deprive the metastases of blood supply has also been reported to be effective.

Drug therapy is of some value for controlling symptoms. The antiserotonin agents methysergide, cyprohepadine, and p-chlorophenylalanine have proved to be helpful in controlling the bowel symptoms, but not flushing, in some patients. Methyldopa is occasionally effective. Empirically, opiates can usually control the diarrhea. Flushing attacks sometimes are ameliorated by the phenothiazines or by α-adrenergic blocking agents such as phentolamine or phenoxybenzamine. Rather marked decreases in carcinoid syndrome symptomatology have been obtained occasionally with corticosteroid therapy. Cancer chemotherapy with the combination of 5-fluorouracil and streptozotocin has yielded some palliation of the syndrome in a small group of patients. Since streptozotocin has little hematologic toxicity, it can be combined with 5-FU at essentially full doses of each agent. Such treatment should be initiated cautiously lest tumor necrosis produce a fatal carcinoid crisis.

DIVERTICULAR DISEASE

Meckel's Diverticulum

The most frequently encountered diverticulum of the small intestine is named for Johann Meckel, who described this structure in 1809. The embryology of Meckel's diverticulum and related anomalies, and diseases of these structures occurring in infancy and childhood, are discussed in Chap. 39.

Meckel's diverticulum is found on the antimesenteric border of the ileum about 2 ft, rarely more than 3 ft, from the ileocecal valve. A persistent band or sinus may connect with the umbilicus. Many of these diverticula are incidental findings at laparotomy or necropsy. Clinically important manifestations are found primarily in childhood, over 60 percent occurring before age ten.

The most common complication of Meckel's diverticulum in the adult, in contrast to the child, is intestinal obstruction. This may result from volvulus or kinking around a band running from the tip of the diverticulum to umbilicus, abdominal wall, or mesentery; or it may be caused by intussusception with the diverticulum as the intussusceptum.

Bleeding is also a common manifestation. This is due to peptic ulceration produced by secretion of acid-pepsin by ectopic gastric mucosa in the diverticulum. Melena is usual, but frank hemorrhage with passage of dark red clots also occurs. Preoperative diagnosis is sometimes possible utilizing abdominal scanning following the administration of radiotechnicium which has an affinity for gastric parietal cells.

Meckel's diverticulitis, clinically indistinguishable from appendicitis, is the third complication in the adult. The incidence of perforation and peritonitis is about 50 percent.

Meckel's diverticulum as a primary lesion should be considered in patients who present with mechanical obstruction of the ileum, with low small bowel hemorrhage, or with signs of inflammation or peritonitis in the midabdomen or lower abdomen. Treatment is prompt surgical intervention with removal of the offending diverticulum by diverticulectomy or resection of the segment of ileum bearing the diverticulum.

Soltero and Bill have challenged the time-honored dictum that incidentally encountered Meckel's diverticula should be removed prophylactically. They estimate that only about 4 percent of diverticula ever become diseased and that thus the morbidity of incidental removal outweighs the potential disease prophylaxis.

Duodenal Diverticula

This is an uncommon lesion, seen in about 1 percent of patients studied by upper gastrointestinal roentgenography. These diverticula, composed only of mucosa and submucosa, are usually single and project mediad from the concavity of duodenum in the region of the head of the pancreas. Nonspecific epigastric symptoms are present in about 10 percent of patients; bleeding and perforation occasionally occur. The morbidity and mortality of these complications is high because of difficulty in diagnosis leading to delay in treatment.

The clinical manifestations of perforated duodenal diverticula are those of other acute gastrointestinal diseases so that the diagnosis is usually made at laparotomy. The inflammatory mass may obstruct the common bile duct and/or the major pancreatic duct producing jaundice and/or pancreatitis. Enteroliths are sometimes found and may be the proximal cause of the inflammation. The perforation is usually walled-off in the retroperitoneal space producing an abscess or phlegmon. Drainage of the collection and gastrojejunostomy is the procedure of choice. Decompression of biliary and pancreatic ducts also may be necessary.

In patients with bleeding or with symptomatic but uncomplicated diverticula, diverticulectomy is indicated. This can usually be done by rolling the duodenum and pancreas forward by the Kocher maneuver. Excision is performed in such a manner as to leave a transverse opening, which is closed with interrupted inverting nonabsorbable sutures. Diverticula imbedded in the pancreas are more safely approached through an anterior duodenotomy. The sac is invaginated and amputated, and the defect closed from within the lumen. Removal of asymptomatic or incidentally encountered diverticula is not advisable.

Jejunal and Ileal Diverticula

Diverticula of the small intestine are distinctly uncommon lesions, being seen in from 0.1 to 0.5 percent of small bowel barium studies. Most are found in the jejunum and are usually multiple. Like duodenal diverticula, these are composed only of mucosa and submucosa. They lie on the mesenteric border, often projecting between the leaves of the mesentery.

Symptoms of partial upper small bowel obstruction may be produced by pressure from a distended or inflamed diverticulum or by adhesions from the diverticulum to surrounding viscera. Acute diverticulitis and hemorrhage from ulceration in a diverticulum have been reported.

Since diverticula are usually limited to the upper small bowel, resection of the segment is usually advisable for obstruction or hemorrhage. Drainage and bypass may be done for diverticulitis with perforation if primary resection appears hazardous. Blind-loop symptoms can usually be controlled with broad-spectrum antibiotics. Asymptomatic diverticula require no treatment.

MISCELLANEOUS PROBLEMS

Ulcer of the Small Intestine

Ulcer of the small intestine of unknown cause has been the subject of sporadic reports since it was first described by Baillie in 1795. A total of 76 cases were reported in the American and European literature between 1936 and 1955. Perforation was the most frequent complication; stenosis occurred in 32 percent.

In 1964, two reports suggested a possible relationship between the administration of thiazide diuretics in combination with enteric-coated potassium chloride and the development of small intestinal ulceration and stenosis. Accordingly a survey of 440 hospitals was made and data obtained on 484 patients with ulcers of the small intestine. Fifty-seven percent of the patients had received diuretics or potassium chloride. The typical ulcerations were reproduced in dogs and monkeys by oral administration of enteric-coated potassium chloride, but not by thiazides. Accordingly, enteric-coated potassium preparations were withdrawn from the United States drug market. A new, slow-release wax matrix formulation of potassium chloride has greatly decreased but has not eliminated gastrointestinal ulceration.

Potassium chloride ulcers are strikingly uniform. There is a circumferential, sharply limited mucosal ulceration overlying a zone of cicatricial narrowing. The width of the ulcerated zone averages 1 cm. Potassium chloride locally in concentrations exceeding 10 percent causes, sequentially, venous spasm and stasis, submucosal edema, segmental hemorrhagic infarction, ulceration, and stenosis.

Symptoms produced by potassium chloride ulcers are most frequently due to stenosis and consist of postprandial cramping abdominal pain, nausea, vomiting, and intermittent fullness. Hemorrhage and perforation are occasionally seen.

Once symptomatic, these lesions nearly always require surgical therapy. Resection of the involved segment with primary anastomosis is the procedure of choice.

Ingested Foreign Bodies

A wide variety of objects, potentially capable of penetrating the wall of the alimentary tract, are swallowed, usually accidentally but sometimes intentionally by the mentally deranged. These include glass and metal fragments, pins, needles, cocktail toothpicks, fish bones, coins, whistles, toys, and broken razor blades.

Treatment is expectant, since the vast majority pass without difficulty. If the object is radiopaque, progress can be followed by serial plain films. Catharsis is contraindicated.

Sharp, pointed objects such as sewing needles, may penetrate the bowel wall. If abdominal pain, tenderness, fever, and/or leukocytosis occur, immediate surgical removal of the offending object is indicated. Abscess or granuloma formation are the usual outcome without surgical therapy.

Fistula

Enterocutaneous fistulas of the mesenteric small intestine are nearly always secondary to operation—less than 2 percent of fistulas result from bowel disease or trauma per se. In some patients there are contributing factors, such as: preoperative radiotherapy, intestinal obstruction, inflammatory bowel disease, mesenteric vascular disease, and intraabdominal sepsis. But in the majority surgical misadventures are the primary cause. These include anastomotic leak, inadvertent injury of bowel or blood supply at operation, laceration of bowel by wire mesh or retention sutures, and retained sponges.

Diagnosis of small bowel fistula is usually not difficult. When the damaged area of the small bowel breaks down and discharges its contents, dissemination may occur widely in the peritoneal cavity producing the picture of generalized peritonitis. More commonly, however, the process is more or less walled-off to the immediate area of the leak, with formation of an abscess. This in turn presents at the operative incision, so that when a few skin sutures are removed to ascertain why the incision is becoming red and tender, contents of the abscess are discharged and the fistula established. Initially the discharge may be purulent or bloody, but this is followed in a day or two by drainage of obvious small bowel contents. If the diagnosis is in doubt, confirmation can be obtained by oral administration of a nonabsorbable marker such as charcoal or Congo red.

Small bowel fistulas are classified according to their location and daily volume flow, since these factors dictate treatment, as well as morbidity and mortality rates. In general, the higher the fistula in the intestine, the more serious the problem. Proximal fistulas have a greater fluid and electrolyte loss, the drainage has a greater digestive capacity, and an important segment is not available for food absorption. It is important therefore, as soon as the patient's condition is stabilized, to identify the site of the fistula, and secondly, to ascertain if there is distal obstruction, since fistulas will not close in the presence of distal obstruction. Upper gastrointestinal series with small bowel follow-through and barium enema studies usually yield this information. Fistulograms may also be helpful not only to delineate the fistula but also to determine the extent of the associated abscess cavity.

Initial priorities in management are concerned with fluid and electrolyte replacement, control of the fistula, and control of sepsis. Fluid losses in high fistulas, particularly if the patient is still febrile and has a persistent ileus with attendant high nasogastric suction losses, may require heroic volumes of replacement fluids. A central venous catheter with around-the-clock therapy is usually in order.

Fistula care consists of cleaning up any residual sepsis, protecting the skin, and measuring the output. Early on, a soft rubber sump works well but should be abandoned as soon as possible in favor of a cement-on collection device lest the bowel opening be kept open by the tube. Occasionally a circular-frame bed can be used allowing gravity drainage when the patient is prone. The skin surrounding the fistula must be protected from excoriation by the digestive enzymes particularly in high jejunal fistulas. This is usually best accomplished by the frequent application of karaya powder. Aluminum paste or zinc oxide are also useful. Control of sepsis requires administration of appropriate antibiotics plus establishment of free drainage of the process at the site of the fistula. Some patients may have additional pockets of suppuration apart from the fistula site. The peritoneum often can handle these, but surgical drainage may also be necessary.

Nutrition rapidly becomes a major consideration in patients with small bowel fistulas. Fortunately two recent developments now allow effective therapy: intravenous hyperalimentation, and elemental oral diets. The oral route is to be preferred whenever possible because of the hazard of prolonged intravenous therapy in the presence of sepsis and antibiotics. If the fistula is in the ileum or lower jejunum, oral elemental diets work well even though the fistula output may be increased. With proximal jejunal fistulas, feeding can often be carried out via a tube which has been threaded past the fistula.

With proper supportive care, and in the absence of distal obstruction, up to 40 percent of small bowel fistulas can be expected to close spontaneously. But if the fistula is not closing satisfactorily in 2 or 3 weeks, then operative intervention likely will be necessary and should not be delayed. Hopefully, by this time the patient's condition is stable; sepsis is under control and he is in anabolic phase as the result of vigorous nutritional therapy.

The preferred procedure is resection of the portion of bowel containing the fistula(s) with primary anastomosis. Distal obstruction, if present, must also be corrected at the same time. Simple closure of the fistulous openings is almost invariably unsuccessful and should not be attempted, but closure may be successful if a loop of uninvolved jejunum is used as a serosal patch to buttress the repair. If resection or serosal patch technique is not possible or is felt to be unduly hazardous, then a staged procedure should be elected. The fistula is not disturbed; afferent and efferent loops are found and divided, and an anastomosis made between proximal and distal ends, thus completely excluding the fistula (Fig. 27-5). The bowel ends on the fistulous segment are oversewn, or brought to the skin as mucous fistulas. The diseased segment is left in place to be removed at a later, safer time. Bypass with proximal exclusion only (Fig. 27-5) is inferior to complete bypass but may be indicated in very poor-risk patients or where the distal bowel cannot be mobilized. Simple side-to-side bypass without exclusion is without merit.

The overall mortality rate in enterocutaneous fistulas of the small bowel is still more than 20 percent. It is higher in jejunal fistulas and significantly lower in ileal fistulas.

Pneumatosis Cystoides Intestinalis

This is an uncommon condition manifested by multiple gas-filled cysts of the gastrointestinal tract. The cysts are either submucosal or subserosal and vary in size from microscopic to several centimeters in diameter. The jejunum is most frequently involved, followed by the ileocecal region and colon. Gas cysts are associated with other lesions of the gastrointestinal tract in about 85 percent of cases. Pneumatosis not associated with other lesions (15 percent) is called "primary."

Grossly the cysts resemble cystic lymphangiomas or hydatid cysts. On section, the involved portion has a honeycomb appearance. The cysts are thin-walled and break easily. Spontaneous rupture gives rise to pneumoperitoneum.

Symptoms are nonspecific and in "secondary" pneumatosis may be those of the associated disease. In primary pneumatosis, symptoms, when present, resemble those of irritable bowel syndrome. Diagnosis is usually made radiographically (Fig. 27-6). No treatment is necessary unless one of the very rare complications supervenes, such as rectal bleeding, cyst-induced volvulus, or tension pneumoperitoneum. Prognosis in most patients is that of the underlying disease. The cysts may disappear spontaneously or may persist for prolonged periods without serious symptoms.

Blind Loop Syndrome

This is a rare clinical syndrome manifested by diarrhea, steatorrhea, anemia, weight loss, abdominal pain, multiple vitamin deficiencies, and neurologic disorders. The underlying cause is not a blind loop per se but stagnation of small intestinal contents by stricture, stenosis, fistulas, blind pouch formation, or diverticula. The bacterial flora are altered in the stagnant area, both in number and in kind. The bacteria successfully compete for vitamin B_{12}, producing a systemic deficiency of B_{12} and megaloblastic anemia. Steatorrhea also occurs; bacteria in the stagnant area deconjugate bile salts, causing disruption of micellar solubilization of fats. There may also be absorptive defects of other macro- and micronutrients. The mechanism of these defects is not clear at this time.

The syndrome can be confirmed by a series of laboratory investigations. First, a Schilling test (cobalt 60—labeled B_{12} absorption) is performed; this should reveal a pernicious anemia type of urinary excretion of vitamin B_{12} (0 to 6 percent, compared with the normal of 7 to 25 percent). The test is then repeated with the addition of intrinsic factor. In true pernicious anemia the excretion should rise to normal; in the blind loop syndrome, the addition of intrinsic factor will not increase the excretion of B_{12}. Next, the patient is given a course of tetracycline for 3 to 5 days, and the Schilling test is repeated. With blind loop syndrome, absorption of cobalt 60—labeled B_{12}—returns to normal; this does not occur in the macrocytic anemia due to steatorrhea. Whereas patients with the blind loop syndrome respond to tetracyclines and parenteral B_{12} therapy,

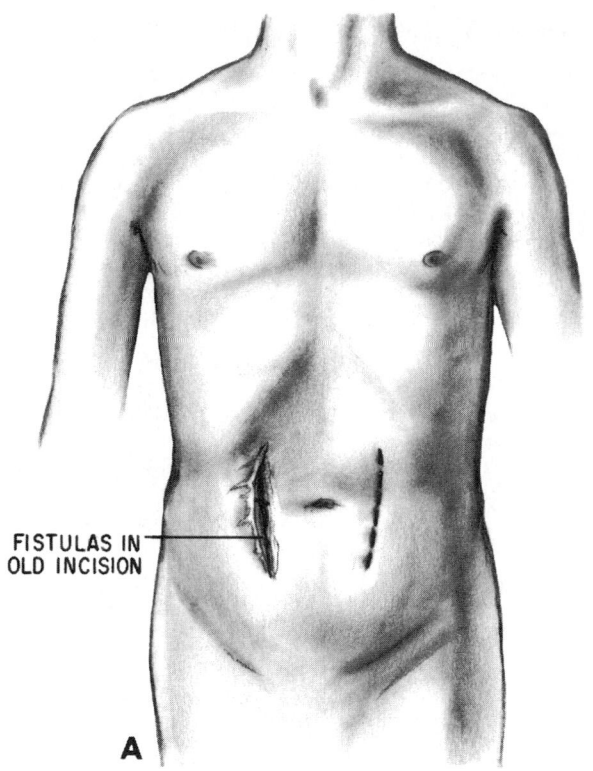

FISTULAS IN OLD INCISION

A

B

surgical correction of the condition producing stagnation and blind loop syndrome effects a permanent cure and therefore is indicated.

Short Bowel Syndrome

Emergency massive resection of small bowel must sometimes be done when extensive frank gangrene precludes revascularization. Mesenteric occlusion, midgut volvulus, and traumatic disruption of the superior mesenteric vessels are the most frequent causes. Short bowel syndrome may also be the end result in patients with severe recurrent regional enteritis in whom several bowel resections have been done.

No nutritional deficits are produced by resection of the entire jejunum. Loss of the entire ileum is compatible with essentially normal nutrition, though B_{12} replacement will always be necessary since the sole site of absorption is the lower ileum and adaptation does not occur. Though there is considerable individual variation, in general, resection of up to 70 percent can be tolerated if the terminal ileum and ileocecal valve can be preserved. If these are resected, nutrition can be severely impaired by a 50 to 60 percent small bowel resection. A few patients with resections of 95 to 100 percent of the small bowel have survived. Until recently it was possible for such patients to live only in the hospital. It is now possible, by use of the Scribner technique of parenteral nutrition with an implanted right atrial catheter, for selected anenteric patients to live outside the hospital.

PATHOGENESIS. Absorption defects in short bowel syn-

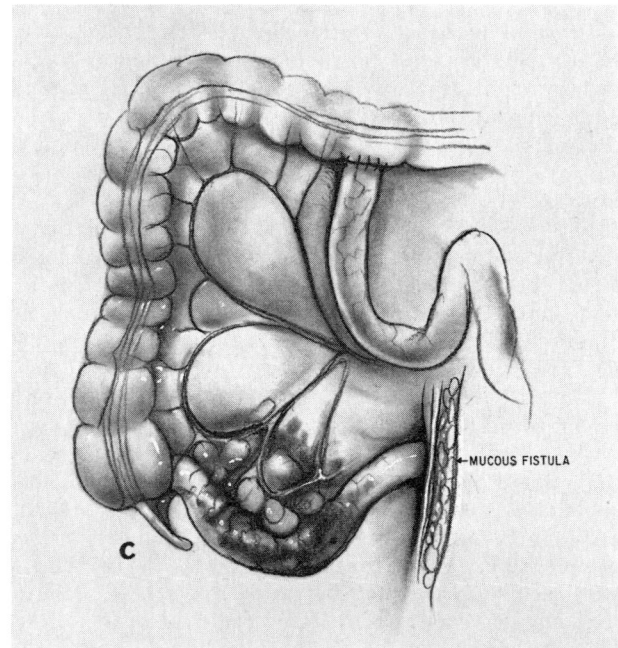

MUCOUS FISTULA

C

Fig. 27-5. Exclusion of a fistula. *A.* Placement of incision in uninvolved area of abdomen. *B.* Complete exclusion. Intestinal loops leading to and from the fistulous areas are divided and anastomosed end-to-end. The ends of the fistulous loop are oversewn or brought out as mucous fistulas. *C.* Exclusion with bypass. The intestine is divided above the fistula, and continuity is restored by anastomosis of proximal bowel to normal bowel distal to the fistula. Both procedures avoid dissection in inflamed tissue. A second operation to excise the diseased loop is necessary.

drome may be divided into three categories: vitamin B_{12}, fat, and water and electrolytes.

Fat presents the absorbing mechanism with its greatest problem, since it, of the three major nutrients, is least efficiently absorbed. Fat can be absorbed, however, by both jejunum and ileum. Three reasons for fat malabsorption have been elucidated recently. Gastric hypersecretion of hydrochloric acid is produced by massive intestinal resection. A low pH in the bowel interferes with digestion and shortens the transit time, thus shortening digestion-absorption time. A second factor is interruption of the normal enterohepatic circulation of bile salts. Absorption of bile salts occurs in the ileum. If the ileum is missing or diseased, bile salts are lost instead of recirculating, producing a relative bile-salt deficiency and a defect in the intraluminal phase of fat absorption. The third factor is a corollary of the second. Soaps and fatty acids formed during fat digestion, if not absorbed, are very irritative to the colonic mucosa, further increasing diarrhea and steatorrhea. Castor oil and soapsuds enemas are effective by virtue of this same chemical mechanism.

Fluid and electrolyte depletion are a function of short transit time and watery diarrhea. These are all rapidly absorbed in all segments of the small intestine.

TREATMENT. The key to treatment of the short bowel syndrome is control of diarrhea and steatorrhea. This requires patient trial and error, since what works in one may be of no value in another.

Pullan has divided the course of patients after partial

Table 27-3. SUMMARY OF TREATMENT OF THE SHORT GUT SYNDROME

Stage	Signs	Treatment
First Stage	Diarrhea exceeds 7–8 bowel movements per day or more than 2½ liters per day	(a) Only intravenous fluids (b) Control diarrhea (c) Maintain fluid and electrolyte balance
Second Stage	Diarrhea less than 2 liters per day	(a) Continue intravenous fluids to give calories (b) Start hypotonic oral fluids to maintain fluid and electrolyte volume, consider space diets, add carbohydrates and proteins, medium chain triglycerides
Third Stage	Stabilization of diarrhea on fat-free diet	(a) Add fat (b) Adjust weight to gut length (c) Consider adjunctive surgical procedures to control gastric hypersecretion and motility

SOURCE: From H. K. Wright and M. D. Tilson: The Short Gut Syndrome; Pathophysiology and Treatment, *Curr Probl Surg*, June, 1971. Copyright © 1971 by Year Book Medical Publishers. Used by permission.

Fig. 27-6. Barium enema radiograph of an infant with pneumatosis cystoides coli. Arrows point to several submucosal gas cysts.

enterectomy into three stages. Wright and Tilson use these clinical stages as a basis for treatment (Table 27-3).

Drugs to slow intestinal motility, such as Lomotil or codeine, are usually helpful. Oral calcium carbonate decreases diarrhea by neutralizing hydrochloric acid and free fatty acids. Dietary fat is restricted to 30 to 50 Gm daily to minimize steatorrhea. Medium chain triglycerides, which are water-soluble and thus absorbed into the portal vein instead of lacteals, are worthwhile in some patients but poorly tolerated by others. Similarly, oral bile salts to increase fat absorption help some patients but increase diarrhea by their cathartic effect in others. Cholestyramine, an agent that sequesters bile acids, is often useful in patients with resections of less than 100 cm, but is of no value in patients with greater resections. Electrolyte losses, particularly calcium and potassium, must be closely watched and replaced parenterally as needed.

A number of surgical procedures have been tried in an attempt to ameliorate the short bowel syndrome. This includes reversal of a segment of intestine, recirculating loops, artificial sphincters, and vagotomy-pyloroplasty. The usefulness, if any, of the procedures is certainly unclear at this time. It is certain, however, that no accessory procedures should be done at the time of the initial surgery, but should only be considered 6 to 12 months after resection in patients who cannot maintain weight within 30 percent of normal without intravenous supplementation. Vagotomy-pyloroplasty may be required in a few patients for demonstrated gastric hypersecretion that is producing severe steatorrhea out of proportion to the length of bowel resection because of acid inhibition of lipase activity.

The hope of the future is probably allotransplantation of a segment of intestine. The procedure is technically feasible as shown by the studies of Ruiz et al. (in association with Lillehei). Four human allotransplants have been unsuccessful with no patient surviving a month. The major unsolved problem at present is control of the immunologic response. When the entire small bowel is allotransplanted in dogs, the grafted intestine remains viable, but the host is killed by a massive graft-versus-host reaction, presumably because of the massive amount of lymphoid tissue in the intestine. The group of Holmes et al. (in association with Fortner) has suggested that intestinal segments 4 to 5 feet in length should provide adequate function and that rejection may be easier to control.

Fig. 27-7. Bypass operations. *A.* Payne-DeWind operation. The proximal 35 cm of jejunum is anastomosed end-to-side to the ileum 10 cm above the ileocecal valve. *B.* Scott operation. The proximal 30 cm of jejunum is anastomosed end-to-end to the distal 15 cm of ileum. The proximal end of the divided ileum is anastomosed to the transverse colon. *C.* Mason operation. The distal 90 percent of the stomach is surgically excluded; the proximal pouch is anastomosed by a narrow stoma to the jejunum. *D.* Buchwald-Varco operation. The distal one-third of the small intestine is excluded; the proximal intestine is anastomosed end-to-side to the ascending colon.

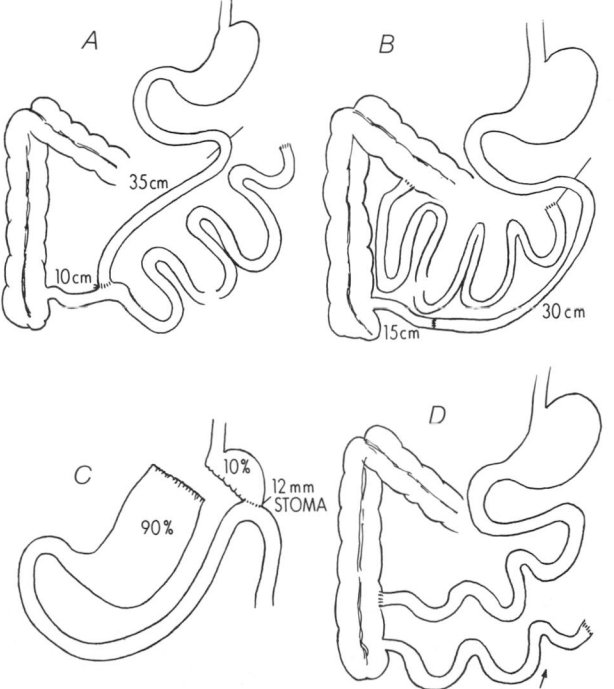

Intestinal Bypass

MORBID OBESITY

A surgically created short-gut malabsorption syndrome has become a rather widely used method of treating massive exogenous obesity that has proved refractory to all other efforts at control. The original operation, anastomosis of the proximal jejunum to the transverse colon, had to be abandoned because of an unacceptable rate of complications. The two most popular operations currently are diagramed in Fig. 27-7*A* and *B.* An alternate method of surgical therapy of obesity is the gastric exclusion operation (Fig. 27-7*C*). This operation limits food intake by reducing the reservoir capacity of the stomach to 10 percent of normal.

Before operative management of obesity is considered, a fully informed patient and his internist must agree that operation is now the logical next step in the management of the patient's problem—that all else has been tried and has failed. In addition to massive obesity per se, other indications for weight-reduction surgery are Pickwickian syndrome, adult-onset diabetes, and essential hypertension. The best results have been in patients between the ages of eighteen and thirty years. Jejunoileal bypass should not be done in growing patients since intellectual, skeletal, and reproductive growth may be adversely affected.

Satisfactory weight loss without serious complications is attained in about 80 percent of patients, with the most overweight patients losing the most weight. Weight loss goes on for 12 to 18 months; the weight then usually plateaus at a level still considerably above the ideal but well below the preoperative weight. Adaptation of the gut, as described above under Short Bowel Syndrome, is the principal reason for the plateau.

The operative mortality rate of jejunoileostomy is 2 to 5 percent. The morbidity, as always in operations on very obese patients, is appreciable and includes atelectasis, pneumonia, wound infection and dehiscence, and thromboembolism. These must be weighed, however, against the risks of untreated massive obesity.

The late mortality rate has been about 10 percent, one-half the deaths being from liver failure. Late complications are many and formidable; they include hepatic steatosis, cirrhosis, and failure; hyperoxaluria and calcium oxalate urinary tract calculi; hyperbilirubinemia and gallstones; electrolyte imbalances including hypocalcemia, hypomagnesemia, and hypokalemia; avitaminoses; psychologic problems and emotional upsets; loss of hair; polyarthropathy; pancreatitis; blind loop syndrome; pneumatosis cystoides intestinalis; colonic pseudoobstruction; intussusception of bypassed jejunum; and bypass enteritis.

Hepatic failure has been the most serious of the late complications of jejunoileal bypass for obesity. Essentially all massively obese patients have slight to moderate hepatic steatosis prior to operation—the steatosis of hyperphagia. The amount of fat in the liver usually increases postoperatively, particularly in those patients who are losing weight rapidly, then decreases as the patient's weight plateaus. Frank cirrhosis has developed in a few patients. The majority of investigators feel that this post-bypass hepatic dysfunction is a form of kwashiorkor, i.e., protein malnutrition in the presence of adequate or high carbohydrate intake. There is also some evidence from the laboratory that overgrowth of bacteria, particularly bacteroides, in the excluded intestine contributes to the hepatic dysfunction. As noted above, the hepatic dysfunction spontaneously ameliorates as the patient's weight stabilizes in most cases, but in a small percentage of patients (the exact number not yet known) a severe liver failure syndrome intervenes which is fatal if not promptly diagnosed and vigorously treated. It is particularly dangerous because the ordinary liver function tests do not herald the incipient crisis. The diagnosis, at present, is made on clinical grounds. The failure is manifested by marked anorexia, nausea, vomiting, and crampy abdominal pain. Fluid retention is manifested by weight gain, peripheral edema, and ascites. The most striking laboratory findings are profound hypoalbuminemia and hypokalemia. Liver function tests, including conjugated bilirubin, become markedly abnormal. The immediate treatment is massive infusions of albumin and potassium plus parenteral alimentation with amino acid solutions containing little or no carbohydrate. Reversal of the shunt after the patient's condition is stabilized is usually advisable unless the hepatic dysfunction can be managed with amino acid supplements.

Most of the weight lost by these morbidly obese persons after a shunt represents lost fat and water. Whether or not significant lean body mass is also lost is not yet settled. Most investigators who have done body composition studies have found that lean body mass is also lost, but some others have found that such loss is insignificant. The reasons for the differences are not apparent at this time. If it is confirmed that lean tissue is lost, then the validity of the procedure will be in question.

In some 10 or 15 percent of patients in whom jejunoileal bypass has been performed it becomes necessary to revise or to reverse the shunt. The principal indications have been hepatic failure, unmanageable electrolyte and metabolic imbalances, persistent uncontrollable diarrhea or associated severe anorectal problems, excessive or excessively rapid weight loss, and inadequate weight loss. It is imperative that the patient be carefully prepared for the reversal operation by vigorous appropriate parenteral therapy. Several weeks in the hospital may be required to attain the optimum state for reoperation.

Griffen and associates have conducted a prospective comparison of gastric and jejunoileal bypass for morbid obesity. In patients examined one year after operation, they found that the jejunoileal bypass resulted in a somewhat greater weight loss—average of 69 kg versus 51 kg, the risk of immediate operative complications was equal, but the gastric bypass led to fewer late complications, less need for rehospitalization, less medication requirement, and no increase in liver disease. If these results hold up with time and are confirmed by others, then gastric bypass should be the preferred operation for treatment of morbid obesity.

HYPERLIPIDEMIA

Surgical bypass of a portion of the small intestine is also a useful method of treating hypercholesterolemia and hypertriglyceridemia. The operation (Fig. 27-7D), designed by Buchwald and Varco, short-circuits the distal 200 cm or one-third the small intestine length, whichever is greater. This operation, though associated with diarrhea at times, does not cause significant weight loss and is not associated with the undesirable side effects of the jejunoileal bypass.

This procedure lowers serum cholesterol level by two mechanisms: by interfering with the absorption of cholesterol by short-circuiting the usual site of absorption, and secondly, by increasing cholesterol and bile acid excretion, which accelerates cholesterol turnover.

Clinical metabolic studies have demonstrated a 60 percent decrease in cholesterol absorption, a 40 percent reduction in serum cholesterol, and more than a 50 percent reduction in plasma triglycerides. About 70 percent of patients with angina have had improvement or total remission of symptoms after this operation. Thus partial ileal bypass appears to be an effective method of lipid reduction. It is obligatory in its actions, safe, and associated with minimal side effects.

References

General

Broido, P. W., Gorbach, S. L., and Nyhus, L. M.: Microflora of the Gastrointestinal Tract and the Surgical Malabsorption Syndromes, *Surg Gynecol Obstet*, **135**:449, 1972.

Christensen, J.: The Controls of Gastrointestinal Movements: Some Old and New Views, *New Engl J Med*, **285**:85, 1971.

Colcock, B. P., and Braasch, J. W.: Surgery of the Small Intestine in the Adult, in "Major Problems in Clinical Surgery," vol. VII, W. B. Saunders Company, Philadelphia, 1968.

Creamer, B. (ed.): "The Small Intestine," Year Book Medical Publishers, Inc., Chicago, 1974.

Gangl, A., and Ockner, R. K.: Intestinal Metabolism of Lipids and Lipoproteins, *Gastroenterology*, **68**:167, 1975.

Grand, R. J., Watkins, J. B., and Torti, F. M.: Development of the Human Gastrointestinal Tract, *Gastroenterology*, **70**:790, 1976.

Kagnoff, M. F.: Induction and Paralysis: A Conceptual Framework from Which to Examine the Intestinal Immune System, *Gastroenterology*, **66**:1240, 1974.

Mallory, A., Kern, F., Jr., Smith, J., and Savage, D.: Patterns of Bile Acids and Microflora in the Human Small Intestine, *Gastroenterology*, **64**:26, 1973.

Pearse, A. G. E., Polak, J. M., and Bloom, S. R.: The Newer Gut Hormones. Cellular Sources, Physiology, Pathology, and Clinical Aspects, *Gastroenterology*, **72**:746, 1977.

Scott, B. B., and Losowsky, M. S.: Peroral Small-Intestine Biopsy: Experience with the Hydraulic Multiple Biopsy Instrument in Routine Clinical Practice, *Gut*, **17**:740, 1976.

Trier, J. S.: Diagnostic Value of Peroral Biopsy of the Proximal Small Intestine, *N Engl J Med*, **285**:1470, 1971.

Inflammatory Diseases

Beeken, W. L., Mitchell, D. N., and Cave, D. R.: Evidence for a Transmissible Agent in Crohn's Disease, in "Clinics in Gastroenterology," vol. 5, p. 289, W. B. Saunders Company, Philadelphia, 1976.

Block, G. E., Enker, W. E., and Kirsner, J. B.: Significance and Treatment of Occult Obstructive Uropathy Complicating Crohn's Disease, *Ann Surg,* **178:**322, 1973.

————, Moossa, A. R., and Simonowitz, D.: The Operative Treatment of Crohn's Disease in Childhood, *Surg Gynecol Obstet,* **144:**713, 1977.

Cave, D. R., Mitchell, D. N., and Brooke, B. N.: Experimental Animal Studies of the Etiology and Pathogenesis of Crohn's Disease, *Gastroenterology,* **69:**618, 1975.

Crohn, B. B., Ginzburg, L., and Oppenheimer, G. D.: Regional Ileitis: Pathological and Clinical Entity, *JAMA,* **99:**1323, 1932.

Das, P., and Shukla, H. S.: Clinical Diagnosis of Abdominal Tuberculosis, *Br J Surg,* **63:**941, 1976.

DeDombal, F. T., Burton, I. L., Clamp, S. E., and Goligher, J. C.: Short-term Course and Prognosis of Crohn's Disease, *Gut,* **15:**435, 1974.

Dunne, W. T., Cooke, W. T., and Allan, R. N.: Enzymatic and Morphometric Evidence for Crohn's Disease as a Diffuse Lesion of the Gastrointestinal Tract, *Gut,* **18:**290, 1977.

Eade, M. N., Cooke, W. T., and Williams, J. A.: Clinical and Hematologic Features of Crohn's Disease, *Surg Gynecol Obstet,* **134:**643, 1972.

Farmer, R. G., Hawk, W. A., and Turnbull, R. B., Jr.: Indications for Surgery in Crohn's Disease: Analysis of 500 Cases, *Gastroenterology,* **71:**245, 1976.

Freeman, J. B., Egan, M. C., and Millis, B. J.: The Elemental Diet, *Surg Gynecol Obstet,* **142:**925, 1976.

Gitnick, G. L., Arthur, M. H., and Shibata, I.: Cultivation of Viral Agents from Crohn's Disease: A New Sensitive System, *Lancet,* **2:**215, 1976.

Glass, R. E., and Baker, W. N. W.: Role of the Granuloma in Recurrent Crohn's Disease, *Gut,* **17:**75, 1976.

Glotzer, D. J., and Silen, W.: Surgical Management of Regional Enteritis, *Gastroenterology,* **61:**751, 1971.

Gump, F. E., Sakellariadis, P., Wolff, M., and Broell, J. R.: Clinical-Pathological Investigation of Regional Enteritis as a Guide to Prognosis, *Ann Surg,* **176:**233, 1972.

Kewenter, J., Hulten, L., and Kock, N. G.: The Relationship and Epidemiology of Acute Terminal Ileitis and Crohn's Disease, *Gut,* **15:**801, 1974.

Kim, J.-P., Oh, S.-K., and Jarrett, F.: Management of Ileal Perforation due to Typhoid Fever, *Ann Surg,* **181:**88, 1975.

Kirsner, J. B.: Genetic Aspects of Inflammatory Bowel Disease, in "Clinics in Gastroenterology," vol. 2, p. 557, W. B. Saunders Company, Philadelphia, 1973.

Klein, M., Binder, H. J., Mitchell, M., Aaronson, R., and Spiro, H.: Treatment of Crohn's Disease with Azathioprine: A Controlled Evaluation, *Gastroenterology,* **66:**916, 1974.

MacPherson, B. R., Albertini, R. J., and Beeken, W. L.: Immunological Studies in Patients with Crohn's Disease, *Gut,* **17:**100, 1976.

Marshak, R. H., and Lindner, A. E.: Roentgen Features in Crohn's Disease, in "Clinics in Gastroenterology," vol. 1, p. 411, W. B. Saunders Company, Philadelphia, 1972.

Menguy, R.: Surgical Management of Free Perforation of the Small Intestine Complicating Regional Enteritis, *Ann Surg,* **175:**178, 1972.

Mitchell, D. N., and Rees, R. J. W.: Agent Transmissible from Crohn's Disease Tissue, *Lancet,* **2:**168, 1970.

Morson, B. C.: Pathology of Crohn's Disease, in "Clinics in Gastroenterology," vol. 1, p. 265, W. B. Saunders Company, Philadelphia, 1972.

Mottet, N. K.: Histopathologic Spectrum of Regional Enteritis and Ulcerative Colitis, in "Major Problems in Pathology," vol. II, W. B. Saunders Company, Philadelphia, 1971.

Nesbit, R. R., Jr., Elbadawi, N. A., Morton, J. H., and Cooper, R. A., Jr.: Carcinoma of the Small Bowel, a Complication of Regional Enteritis, *Cancer,* **37:**2948, 1976.

Nugent, F. W., Richmond, M., and Park, S. K.: Crohn's Disease of the Duodenum, *Gut,* **18:**115, 1977.

Reilly, J., Ryan, J. A., Strole, W., and Fischer, J. E.: Hyperalimentation in Inflammatory Bowel Disease, *Am J Surg,* **131:**192, 1976.

Rocchio, M. A., MoCha, C.-J., Haas, K. F., and Randall, H. T.: Use of Chemically Defined Diets in the Management of Patients with Acute Inflammatory Bowel Disease, *Am J Surg,* **127:**469, 1974.

Sachar, D. B., Taub, R. N., and Janowitz, H. D.: A Transmissible Agent in Crohn's Disease? New Pursuit of an Old Concept, *N Engl J Med,* **293:**354, 1975.

Senewiratne, B., and Senewiratne, K.: Reassessment of the Widal Test in the Diagnosis of Typhoid, *Gastroenterology,* **73:**233, 1977.

Shorter, R. G., Huizenga, K. A., and Spencer, R. J.: A Working Hypothesis for the Etiology and Pathogenesis of Non-specific Inflammatory Bowel Disease, *Am J Dig Dis,* **17:**1024, 1972.

Simonowitz, D., Block, G. E., Riddell, R. H., Kraft, S. C., and Kirsner, J. B.: The Production of an Unusual Tissue Reaction in Rabbit Bowel Injected with Crohn's Disease Homogenates, *Surgery,* **82:**211, 1977.

Smith, L. H., and Hofmann, A. F.: Acquired Hyperoxaluria, Urolithiasis, and Intestinal Disease: A New Digestive Disorder? *Gastroenterology,* **66:**1257, 1974.

Steinberg, D. M., Cooke, W. T., and Williams, J. A.: Abscess and Fistulae in Crohn's Disease, *Gut,* **14:**865, 1973.

Tandon, H. D., and Prakash, A.: Pathology of Intestinal Tuberculosis and Its Distinction from Crohn's Disease, *Gut,* **13:**260, 1972.

Thayer, W. R., Jr.: Are the Inflammatory Bowel Diseases Immune Complex Diseases? *Gastroenterology,* **70:**136, 1976.

Truelove, S. C., and Penn, A. S.: Course and Prognosis of Crohn's Disease, *Gut,* **17:**192, 1976.

Vantrappen, G., Ponette, E., Geboes, K., and Bertrand, P.: Yersinia Enteritis and Enterocolitis: Gastroenterological Aspects, *Gastroenterology,* **72:**220, 1977.

Walker, W. A., and Isselbacher, K. J.: Uptake and Transport of Macromolecules by the Intestine, Possible Role in Clinical Disorders, *Gastroenterology,* **67:**531, 1974.

Weakley, F. L., and Turnbull, F. L.: Recognition of Regional Ileitis in the Operating Room, *Dis Colon Rectum,* **14:**17, 1971.

Whorwell, P. J., and Wright, R.: Immunological Aspects of Inflammatory Bowel Disease, in "Clinics in Gastroenterology," vol. 5, p. 303, W. B. Saunders Company, Philadelphia, 1976.

Neoplasms

Barry, R. E., and Read, A. E.: Coeliac Disease and Malignancy, *Q J Med,* **42:**665, 1973.

Brown, N. K., and Smith, M. P.: Neoplastic Diathesis of Patients with Carcinoid, *Cancer,* **32:**216, 1973.

Bussey, H. J. R.: Gastrointestinal Polyposis, *Gut,* **11:**970, 1970.

Calman, K. C.: Why Are Small Bowel Tumours Rare? An Experimental Model, *Gut,* **15:**552, 1974.

Davis, Z., Moertel, C. G., and McIlrath, D. C.: The Malignant Carcinoid Syndrome, *Surg Gynecol Obstet,* **137:**637, 1973.

Fu, Y.-S., and Perzin, K. H.: Lymphosarcoma of the Small Intestine, *Cancer,* **29:**645, 1972.

Gardner, B., Dollinger, M., Silen, W., Back, N., and O'Reilly, S.: Studies of the Carcinoid Syndrome: Its Relationship to Serotonin, Bradykinin, and Histamine, *Surgery,* **61:**846, 1967.

Jeghers, H., McKusick, V. A., and Katz, K. H.: Generalized Intestinal Polyposis and Melanin Spots on the Oral Mucosa, Lips and Digits, *N Engl J Med,* **241:**993, 1949.

Kaplan, E. L., Jaffe, B. M., and Peskin, G. W.: A New Provocative Test for the Diagnosis of the Carcinoid Syndrome, *Am J Surg,* **123:**173, 1972.

Lewin, K. J., Kahn, L. B., and Novis, B. H.: Primary Intestinal Lymphoma of "Western" and "Mediterranean" Type, Alpha Chain Disease and Massive Plasma Cell Infiltration, *Cancer,* **38:**2511, 1976.

McDermott, W. V., and Hensle, T. W.: Metastatic Carcinoid to the Liver Treated by Hepatic Dearterialization, *Ann Surg,* **180:**305, 1974.

McKittrick, J. E., Lewis, W. M., Doane, W. A., and Gerwig, W. H.: The Peutz-Jeghers Syndrome, *Arch Surg,* **103:**57, 1971.

Masson, P.: Carcinoids (Argentaffin-Cell Tumors) and Nerve Hyperplasia of Appendicular Mucosa, *Am J Pathol,* **4:**181, 1928.

Moertel, C. G.: Clinical Management of Advanced Gastrointestinal Cancer, *Cancer,* **36:**675, 1975.

Postlethwait, R. W.: Gastrointestinal Carcinoid Tumors: A Review, *Postgrad Med,* **40:**445, 1966.

Ranchod, M., and Kempson, R. L.: Smooth Muscle Tumors of the Gastrointestinal Tract and Retroperitoneum, *Cancer,* **39:**257, 1977.

Reid, J. D.: Intestinal Carcinoma in the Peutz-Jeghers Syndrome, *JAMA,* **229:**833, 1974.

Sheahan, D. G., Martin, F., Baginsky, S., Mallory, G. K., and Zamcheck, N.: Multiple Lymphomatous Polyposis of the Gastrointestinal Tract, *Cancer,* **28:**408, 1971.

Teitelbaum, S. L.: The Carcinoid. A Collective Review, *Am J Surg,* **123:**564, 1972.

Wilson, H., Cheek, R. C., Sherman, R. T., and Storer, E. H.: Carcinoid Tumors, in "Current Problems in Surgery," The Year Book Medical Publishers, Inc., Chicago, 1970.

Wilson, J. M., Melvin, D. B., Gray, G. F., and Thorbjarnarson, B.: Primary Malignancies of the Small Bowel: A Report of 96 Cases and Review of the Literature, *Ann Surg,* **180:**175, 1974.

———, ———, ———, and ———: Benign Small Bowel Tumor, *Ann Surg,* **181:**247, 1975.

Diverticular Disease

Altemeier, W. A., Bryant, L. R., and Walsh, J. H.: The Surgical Significance of Jejunal Diverticulosis, *Arch Surg,* **86:**732, 1963.

Economides, N. G., McBurney, R. P., and Hamilton, F. H., III: Intraluminal Duodenal Diverticulum in the Adult, *Ann Surg,* **185:**147, 1977.

Herrington, J. L., Jr.: Spontaneous Asymptomatic Pneumoperitoneum: A Complication of Jejunal Diverticulosis, *Am J Surg,* **113:**567, 1967.

Kellum, J. M., Boucher, J. K., and Ballinger, W. F.: Serosal Patch Repair for Benign Duodenocolic Fistula Secondary to Duodenal Diverticulum, *Am J Surg,* **131:**607, 1976.

Kilpatrick, Z. M., and Aseron, C. A.: Radioisotope Detection of Meckel's Diverticulum Causing Acute Rectal Hemorrhage, *N Engl J Med,* **287:**653, 1972.

Localio, S. A., and Stahl, W. M.: Diverticular Disease of the Alimentary Tract. II. The Esophagus, Stomach, Duodenum and Small Intestine, in "Current Problems in Surgery," The Year Book Medical Publishers, Inc., Chicago, 1968.

Roses, D. F., Gouge, T. H., Scher, K. S., and Ranson, J. H. C.: Perforated Diverticula of the Jejunum and Ileum, *Am J Surg,* **132:**649, 1976.

Soltero, M. J., and Bill, A. H.: The Natural History of Meckel's Diverticulum and Its Relation to Incidental Removal, *Am J Surg,* **132:**168, 1976.

Ulcer of the Small Intestine

Guest, J. L.: Nonspecific Ulceration of the Intestine: Collective Review, *Surg Gynecol Obstet,* **117:**409, 1963.

McMahon, F. G., and Akdamar, K.: Gastric Ulceration after "Slow-K," *N Engl J Med,* **295:**733, 1976.

Foreign Bodies

Maleki, M., and Evans, W. E.: Foreign-body Perforation of the Intestinal Tract, *Arch Surg,* **101:**475, 1970.

Fistula

Aguirre, A., Fischer, J. E., and Welch, C. E.: The Role of Surgery and Hyperalimentation in Therapy of Gastrointestinal-Cutaneous Fistulae, *Ann Surg,* **180:**393, 1974.

Gross, E., and Irving, M.: Protection of the Skin around Intestinal Fistula, *Br J Surg,* **64:**258, 1977.

Hill, G. L., Mair, W. S. J., Edwards, J. P., Morgan, D. B., and Goligher, J. C.: Effect of a Chemically Defined Liquid Diet on Composition and Volume of Ileal Fistula Drainage, *Gastroenterology,* **68:**676, 1975.

Jones, S. A., and Steedman, R. A.: Management of Chronic Infected Intestinal Perforations by the Serosal Patch Technic, *Am J Surg,* **117:**731, 1969.

MacFadyen, B. V., Jr., Dudrick, S. J., and Ruberg, R. L.: Management of Gastrointestinal Fistulas with Parenteral Hyperalimentation, *Surgery,* **74:**100, 1973.

MacFarlane, M., and Frawley, J. E.: A Technique for Drainage of Enterocutaneous Fistulas, *Surg Gynecol Obstet,* **141:**263, 1975.

Roback, S. A., and Nicoloff, D. M.: High Output Enterocutaneous Fistulas of the Small Bowel, *Am J Surg,* **123:**317, 1972.

Sheldon, G. F., Gardiner, B. N., Way, L. W., and Dunphy, J. E.: Management of Gastrointestinal Fistulas, *Surg Gynecol Obstet,* **133:**385, 1971.

Pneumatosis Cystoides Intestinalis

Feinberg, S. B., Schwartz, M. Z., Clifford, S., Buchwald, H., and Varco, R. L.: Significance of Pneumatosis Cystoides Intestinalis after Jejunoileal Bypass, *Am J Surg,* **133:**149, 1977.

Reyna, R., Soper, R. T., and Condon, R. E.: Pneumatosis Intestinalis, *Am J Surg,* **125:**667, 1973.

Blind Loop Syndrome

Aabakke, J., and Schjonsby, H.: Value of Urinary Simple Phenol and Indican Determinations in the Diagnosis of the Stagnant Loop Syndrome, *Scand J Gastroentol,* **11**:409, 1976.

Ellis, H., and Smith, A. D. M.: The Blind-loop Syndrome, in "Monographs in the Surgical Sciences," The Williams & Wilkins Company, Baltimore, 1967.

Fromm, D.: Ileal Resection, or Disease, and the Blind Loop Syndrome: Current Concepts of Pathophysiology, *Surgery,* **73**:639, 1973.

Short Bowel Syndrome

Binder, H. J.: Fecal Fatty Acids—Mediators of Diarrhea? *Gastroenterology,* **65**:847, 1973.

Dowling, R. H.: Intestinal Adaptation, *N Engl J Med,* **288**:520, 1973.

Hofmann, A. F.: Bile Acid Malabsorption Caused by Ileal Resection, *Arch Intern Med,* **130**:597, 1972.

Mackby, M. J.: The Short Bowel Revisited, *Surgery,* **79**:1, 1976.

Riella, M. C., and Scribner, B. A.: Five Years' Experience with a Right Atrial Catheter for Prolonged Parenteral Nutrition at Home, *Surg Gynecol Obstet,* **143**:205, 1976.

Weser, E.: The Management of Patients after Small Bowel Resection, *Gastroenterology,* **71**:146, 1976.

Winchester, D. P., and Dorsey, J. M.: Intestinal Segments and Pouches in Gastrointestinal Surgery, *Surg Gynecol Obstet,* **132**:131, 1971.

Wright, H. K., and Tilson, M. D.: The Short Gut Syndrome. Pathophysiology and Treatment, in "Current Problems in Surgery," The Year Book Medical Publishers, Inc., Chicago, 1971.

Intestinal Bypass

Brown, R. G., O'Leary, J. P., and Woodward, E. R.: Hepatic Effects of Jejunoileal Bypass for Morbid Obesity, *Am J Surg,* **127**:53, 1974.

Buchwald, H., Moore, R. B., and Varco, R. L.: Ten Years Clinical Experience with Partial Ileal Bypass in Management of the Hyperlipidemias, *Ann Surg,* **180**:384, 1974.

Cegielski, M. M., Organ, C. H., Jr., and Saporta, J. A.: Revision of Intestinal Bypass Procedures, *Surg Gynecol Obstet,* **142**:829, 1976.

DeWind, L. T., and Payne, J. H.: Intestinal Bypass Surgery for Morbid Obesity, *JAMA,* **236**:2298, 1976.

Dudrick, S. J., Daly, J. M., Castro, G., and Akhtar, M.: Gastrointestinal Adaptation following Small Bowel Bypass for Obesity, *Ann Surg,* **185**:642, 1977.

Griffen, W. O., Jr., Young, V. L., and Stevenson, C. C.: A Prospective Comparison of Gastric and Jejuno-ileal Bypass for Morbid Obesity, *Ann Surg,* **186**:500, 1977.

Holmes, J. T., Yeh, S. D. J., Winawer, S. J., Kawano, N., and Fortner, J. G.: Absorption Studies in Canine Jejunal Allografts, *Ann Surg,* **174**:101, 1971.

Mason, E. E., Printen, K. J., Hartford, C. E., and Boyd, W. C.: Optimizing Results of Gastric Bypass, *Ann Surg,* **182**:405, 1975.

Malt, R. A., and Guggenheim, F. G.: Surgery for Obesity, *N Engl J Med,* **295**:43, 1976.

Moxley, R. T., III, Pozefsky, T., and Lockwood, D. H.: Protein Nutrition and Liver Disease after Jejunoileal Bypass for Morbid Obesity, *N Engl J Med,* **290**:921, 1974.

Ruiz, J. O., Uchida, H., Schultz, L. S., and Lillehei, R. C.: Problems in Absorption and Immunosuppression after Entire Intestinal Allotransplantation, *Am J Surg,* **123**:297, 1972.

Scott, H. W., Jr.: Metabolic Surgery for Hyperlipidemia and Atherosclerosis, *Am J Surg,* **123**:3, 1972.

———, Dean, R., Shull, H. J., Abram, H. S., Webb, W., Younger, R. K., and Brill, A. B.: New Considerations in Use of Jejunoileal Bypass in Patients with Morbid Obesity, *Ann Surg,* **177**:723, 1973.

Spanier, A. H., Kurta, R. S., Shibata, H. R., MacLean, L. D., and Shizgal, H. M.: Alterations in Body Composition following Intestinal Bypass for Morbid Obesity, *Surgery,* **80**:171, 1976.

Toledo-Pereyra, L. H., Simmons, R. L., and Najarian, J. S.: Prolonged Survival of Canine Orthotopic Small Intestinal Allografts Preserved for 24 Hours by Hypothermic Bloodless Perfusion, *Surgery,* **75**:368, 1974.

Chapter 28

Colon, Rectum, and Anus

by **Edward H. Storer, Stanley M. Goldberg, and Santhat Nivatvongs**

The principal functions of the colon are water absorption and storage of feces. The cecum receives about 500 ml of chyme from the ileum daily. This is dehydrated in the right half of the colon to about 150 ml—the daily volume of feces. Thus only about 5 percent of water absorption in the intestinal tract occurs in the colon. The left colon functions principally as a storage organ. Voluntary control of defecation is regulated by rectum and anus. Their principal function in our society is to allow defecation only at socially convenient times. The colon, rectum, and anus therefore play a relatively unimportant role in the bodily economy; completely normal biologic existence is possible following total proctocolectomy. They are indispensable, however, for a comfortable life in society without the constant risk of embarrassment.

Though the colon, rectum, and anus are relatively unimportant biologically, they are one of the most important organ systems clinically because of the high incidence and variety of diseases associated with these organs. About 10 million persons now living in the United States have diverticulosis coli; about 20 million harbor *Endamoeba histolytica* in their colons. Primary chronic ulcerative colitis is fortunately uncommon, for it is one of the most miserable chronic diseases known to mankind. A diagnosis of carcinoma of the colon or rectum was made for the first time in 101,000 Americans in 1977. This is the most common internal cancer in the United States and causes 51,300 deaths annually—about 13 percent of all cancer deaths. Some 11 million Americans have colonic polyps, which are thought to be premalignant lesions. The number of persons with hemorrhoids and anorectal fissures and fistulas cannot even be estimated—there are countless millions.

INFLAMMATORY DISEASES

Ulcerative Colitis

Idiopathic nonspecific ulcerative colitis is an uncommon inflammatory disease involving primarily mucosa and submucosa of the colon. Both acute and chronic forms are seen. Though colitis (segmental colitis, right-sided colitis, Crohn's disease of the colon) was recognized as an entity distinct from ulcerative colitis in 1932, the distinction has gradually gained acceptance only since about 1959. Thus reports prior to 1959 are of limited value. Strenuous efforts were aimed for a time at clear separation of the two forms of idiopathic colitis, but there is now a growing tendency to emphasize their similarities and to refer to them together as "inflammatory bowel disease."

INCIDENCE. Most information on incidence and prevalence of ulcerative colitis has been derived from hospital admission records. This data may be misleading, because patients with chronic ulcerative colitis tend to gravitate to large teaching centers and because the composition of the population from which the patients were drawn is not known. Ulcerative colitis has been studied recently in four populations of known composition in Baltimore, Maryland, in Rochester, Minnesota, in Oxford, England, and in Norway. The average annual incidence rate (the number of patients affected by the disease for the first time in a given year divided by the number of people at risk in that year) for idiopathic ulcerative colitis in white adults was 4.6 per 100,000 in Baltimore, 3.4 in Rochester, 6.5 in Oxford, and 2.1 in Norway.

The incidence of ulcerative colitis in Jews is about three times the rate in non-Jews; females are affected more than males by a ratio of about 5:4. Blacks probably have a significantly lower incidence than whites, but valid large-scale studies are not available. The disease affects all age groups, with the highest incidence in the third and fourth decades. In the United States, ulcerative colitis is seen more frequently in the North and East—more frequently than can be accounted for by differences in Jewish and black populations.

The familial incidence of ulcerative colitis is higher than would be expected from chance alone, but the rate is not striking and may be due to environmental factors, not heredity. In a study of 2,000 patients with ulcerative colitis, 26 had positive family histories; in another study of 1,084 patients, 66 reported colitis in other family members.

ETIOLOGY. Ulcerative colitis is still idiopathic despite many years of study and voluminous publications by persons of diverse interests and backgrounds. Clinical investigation is difficult, because the course of the disease is unpredictable and characterized by spontaneous and unexplained remissions.

Laboratory investigation of ulcerative colitis is handicapped because there is still no disease of other animals,

either spontaneous or experimentally induced, that closely resembles the human disease. A form of colitis occurs infrequently in boxer dogs that has some of the characteristics of ulcerative colitis but also some of the characteristics of Crohn's colitis and of Whipple's disease. The cause of canine colitis is unknown, and the condition cannot be induced at will. Ulcerative colitis-like lesions of the cecum and colon have been induced in small laboratory animals by the feeding of carrageenan, a hydrocolloid extracted from seaweed, and by the feeding of two pepsin inhibitors, sodium lignosulfonate and sulfated amylopectin. This is a convenient laboratory model but unfortunately appears to have little or no relationship to the human disease. Carrageenan is widely used as a food additive and as a medicine; the pepsin inhibitors are commercially available for the treatment of peptic ulcer.

The similarity of the clinical picture in idiopathic ulcerative colitis to that of the specific dysenteries has led to attempts to implicate specific microorganisms. There are a few documented cases of chronic ulcerative colitis following proved *Shigella* or amebic dysentery, but such cases are the exception and not the rule. Specific therapy directed against *Shigella* or *E. histolytica* rarely exerts any beneficial effect on the course of the ulcerative colitis. Furthermore, the incidence of ulcerative colitis is low where these specific dysentery infections are endemic. Other organisms that have been proposed as specific etiologic agents include an enteric diplostreptococcus and *Bacterium necrophorum*. New evidence for a transmissible infectious factor has been presented by Cave and associates, who injected filtered homogenates of ulcerative colitis tissues into rabbits and produced histologic changes in the rabbit colon that resemble those in the human disease. These data suggest a virus but do not rule out L forms or mycoplasmas.

The generally favorable influence of adrenal corticosteroids on the course of chronic ulcerative colitis has led to a revival of the thesis that allergy or hypersensitivity plays a role in the genesis of the disease. Occasional patients have a remarkable remission of symptoms following omission of milk and milk products from their diets. Antibodies to cow's milk proteins can be demonstrated in some patients with ulcerative colitis, and it has been suggested that this may be attributable to early weaning with ingestion of cow's milk formula before fourteen days of age. This exposes the infant to foreign proteins at a time of immunologic tolerance and permissive absorption of whole proteins. But circulating antibodies to cow's milk protein can be found in control patients with the same frequency as in patients with ulcerative colitis. Furthermore, circulating antibodies to milk proteins are not correlated with the presence or absence of clinical intolerance to milk. The occasional intolerance to milk may be related to a secondary deficiency in intestinal lactase rather than to a specific allergy.

Shorter and associates have proposed that the inflammatory bowel diseases are produced by local hypersensitivity reactions. Initial sensitization of the gut-associated lymphoid tissues is thought to occur in the neonatal period before the mucosal barrier is complete, permitting penetration of enterobacteria and macromolecules. Reexposure to bacteria and intestinal antigens may occur in later life if the mucosal integrity is damaged by infection, ischemia, or even metabolic alterations induced by emotional stress. Antigen reexposure then causes the local primary cellular immune-mediated hypersensitivity reaction, with the production of inflammatory bowel disease.

Hemorrhagic colitis somewhat resembling the human disease has been produced in several different laboratory animals by the administration of anticolonic antisera. These experimental immune lesions of the colon do not completely reproduce human ulcerative colitis, and their occurrence does not necessarily imply any connection with the natural genesis of human ulcerative colitis. They demonstrate only that the colon can generate autoimmune reactions. Immunosuppressive drugs, particularly azathioprine, might be expected to exert a beneficial effect if ulcerative colitis is truly an autoimmune disease. The results to date are inconclusive: some but not all patients are improved, and the benefit is slower and less marked than with corticosteroids.

Studies indicate that sensitized lymphocytes play an important role in autoimmunity in ulcerative colitis and suggest that a more fruitful approach would be via the cellular factors of hypersensitivity rather than circulating antibodies. It has been clearly demonstrated that circulating lymphocytes, but not sera, from patients with ulcerative colitis are cytotoxic for human fetal or adult colon epithelial cells. Lymphocytes from normal controls are not cytotoxic.

Mast cells, in the connective tissue of the colon, have been shown to contain histamine, serotonin, heparin, chymase, tryptase, and other biologically active substances. Sommers has proposed that mucosal hyperemia and persistent edema in ulcerative colitis are attributable to local excesses of histamine released by an increased colonic population of mast cells and that release of stored serotonin by mast cells is an exacerbating factor. This hypothesis has not yet received experimental confirmation; indeed one study reported normal levels of histamine in the blood, urine, and colonic mucosa of patients with ulcerative colitis.

The left colon has been shown in the laboratory to respond to parasympathomimetic drugs, to serotonin, and to emotional tension by sustained high-tension contractions that shorten and narrow the organ. Extravasation of blood is the first change one might expect in a mucosa rendered turgid because of impedance of venous outflow by sustained muscle contraction.

Numerous attempts to implicate mental disorders in the etiology of ulcerative colitis have produced no convincing evidence. Patients with psychoses or depressive reactions are not prone to develop ulcerative colitis, nor has functional bowel distress been observed to lead to ulcerative colitis. Whereas it is certainly true that ulcerative colitis patients manifest abnormalities of the psyche, such abnormalities may well be the effect, not the cause, of the disease—a somatopsychic rather than a psychosomatic disorder. Esler and Goulston have assessed the levels of

anxiety and neuroticism in patients with ulcerative colitis and in general medical patients; there was no significant difference in these dimensions of personality. Mendeloff and associates compared life stresses in patients with ulcerative colitis and control subjects drawn from the same population group. They concluded that "this and other studies fail to support the thesis that ulcerative colitis is a paradigm of psychosomatic illness."

Despite these observations, many clinicians still have the impression that emotional stress, particularly if the patient's reaction is one of hopelessness and helplessness, often seems to trigger exacerbations of chronic ulcerative colitis, and in a small but definite percentage emotional stress appears to precipitate the disease. Conversely, emotional stress, hopelessness, and helplessness are virtually ubiquitous in our society, and yet ulcerative colitis remains an uncommon disease.

The search for a single cause of ulcerative colitis may be unrealistic. The colon can respond to injury (in the broad sense) in a limited number of ways. Several etiologic factors may have in common the initial injury to colonic mucosa in biologically predisposed individuals. Perpetuation of the process could well be due to a different mechanism(s).

PATHOLOGY. The rectum is the most frequently involved portion of the bowel in idiopathic ulcerative colitis. It is the earliest site of involvement in patients in whom the disease spreads proximally and in some is the only site of involvement. In more than half, the entire colon is diseased. With less than total involvement, disease is always in continuity—there are no skip areas, in contrast to Crohn's colitis—and the lesion is usually in the left colon, rarely the right colon alone. The terminal ileum is involved for a short distance in continuity with cecal involvement in up to 10 percent—so-called "backwash ileitis." Involvement is segmental in more than 50 percent in Crohn's colitis and affects the proximal colon more frequently than the distal. A comparison of the two forms of colitis will be found in Table 28-1.

Grossly, the serosal surface is probably essentially normal early in the disease, since ulcerative colitis initially involves the mucosa and submucosa. In advanced cases, as seen at operation or at necropsy, the bowel is greatly shortened, the sigmoid redundancy is lost, and the right and left colon segments occupy a more medial position than normal. The mesentery is contracted, edematous, and somewhat thickened, but this is much less marked than with Crohn's colitis, and large lymph node masses are conspicuously absent in ulcerative colitis. The serosal surface of the bowel is dull and grayish but with little or no exudate unless perforation has occurred. The wall is moderately thickened and firm. Contained perforations on the mesenteric margin are frequent, with abscess formation. Abscesses are also frequently encountered at the sites of stricture formation. Fistulas, except perianal, are rare in ulcerative colitis compared to Crohn's colitis. With fulminating acute colitis, the entire bowel wall is hemorrhagic and very friable, with numerous areas of necrosis.

The mucosal surface in advanced chronic ulcerative

Table 28-1. DIFFERENTIATION OF ULCERATIVE COLITIS FROM CROHN'S
DISEASE OF THE COLON

Features	Ulcerative colitis	Crohn's disease
Pathology	Essentially mucosal	Transmural
Rectal involvement and distribution of the disease	Rectal involvement almost invariable (95%); spread is in continuity to the rest of the colon	Rectum frequently (50%) spared; distribution often segmental
Cobblestoning of mucosa	Unusual	Common
Extensive small bowel involvement	Never	May occur
Anorectal complications (e.g., perineal fistulas, rectovaginal fistulas, anal fissures)	Uncommon	Common
Abdominal wall or interfistulas	Never	Frequent
Granulomatous foci	Absent	Present in two-thirds
Lymph nodes	Reactive hyperplasia	Often granulomatous foci
Ulceration	Diffuse distribution	Longitudinal or serpiginous ulcers with normal mucosa in between
Benign colonic or rectal strictures	Rare (about 10%)	Common
Bleeding	Very common	Less common
Inflammatory abdominal mass	Never	Sometimes
Sigmoidoscopy	Diffuse involvement	Submucosal edema with heaping up of the mucosa to give a cobblestone appearance; discrete ulcerations with normal intervening mucosa

SOURCE: L. Wise, G. Efron, D. G. Glotzer, and R. B. Turnbull, Jr.: Symposium: Ulcerative Colitis and Crohn's Disease, *Contemp Surg*, **2**:95, 1973.

colitis is even more strikingly abnormal than the serosa. Bloody pus covers the ragged, moth-eaten-appearing surface. Irregular, shallow, linear, often anastomosing ulcers interspersed with islands of swollen mucosa—"pseudo polyps"—account for the characteristic appearance.

Biopsies of the rectal mucosa afford the opportunity to observe the disease histologically in all stages. The earliest lesion develops in the bases of the crypts of Lieberkühn, where neutrophils can be seen passing between the lining cells to accumulate inside the crypt lumen or lamina propria. The accumulation of neutrophils, plus eosinophils, red blood cells, and serum, forms the microscopic "crypt abscess" which is a characteristic feature of the disease. These may rupture through the mucosal surface, forming a microulcer, or into the submucosa. Whereas crypt abscesses may be seen in other inflammatory diseases of the bowel, they are always present in ulcerative colitis and in much greater numbers. With progression, numerous crypts are involved, and large areas of their walls break down, liberating exudate into the submucosa and producing widespread ulceration. As the disease becomes chronic, lymphocytes, plasma cells, and macrophages infiltrate the mucosa and submucosa. Eosinophils and increased numbers of mast cells also may be present. In advanced cases, all layers of the bowel wall are involved in acute and chronic inflammation and in fibrosis. The mucosa is absent over wide areas and replaced by granulation tissue. Pseudopolyps between the denuded areas consist of inflamed edematous mucosa or vegetative proliferations of granulation tissue.

CLINICAL MANIFESTATIONS. Idiopathic ulcerative colitis may be divided into three forms according to the clinical course: acute, fulminant; chronic, continuous; and chronic-relapsing-remitting.

The disease has an abrupt onset in about one-third of patients but fortunately runs a fulminant course in less than 10 percent. Rarely fulminant colitis is superimposed as an exacerbation upon the chronic form. Unrelenting diarrhea, preceded by severe lower abdominal cramps, continues day and night. Incontinence is frequent; tenesmus and urgency are marked. Stools are small in amount but may number 30 to 40 per day and consist of bloody mucus, pus, and watery fecal material. Systemic toxicity is striking, with fever spiking to 39 or 40°C. The malignant diarrhea rapidly produces extreme dehydration, hypokalemia, anemia, hypoproteinemia, and marked weight loss with gaunt facies and sunken eyeballs. Heroic nonoperative therapy brings the process under control in some patients, but many require urgent operative therapy because of failure to respond or for a complication—hemorrhage, colonic perforation, or toxic megacolon. The mortality rate in fulminant colitis is still about 20 percent.

The relapsing-remitting form is much more common and is seen in over two-thirds of all patients with chronic ulcerative colitis. The course is variable and characterized by almost unpredictable exacerbations and remissions. Recurrences are often associated with emotional stress, physical fatigue, respiratory infections and other acute illnesses, dietary indiscretions, use of antibiotics and cathartics, and, in women, menses and pregnancy. Bloody diarrhea is the predominant symptom. The onset is acute in some, but more commonly the diarrhea has gradually become worse for a considerable period, recurring periodically, with essentially normal bowel habits during remissions. Lower abdominal cramping is nearly always present in the earlier phases, but when the bowel becomes scarred, thickened, and shortened, cramping is less marked. Cramping is followed shortly by urgency and tenesmus, and the painful passage of a small watery stool consisting of an admixture of stool, mucus, blood, and pus. In later stages, cramping may not be present to warn of impending defecation, which then occurs unexpectedly, accounting for some of the anxiety and insecurity that colitis patients often exhibit. Anorexia is marked during relapses. This, combined with the considerable continuing caloric loss by diarrhea, causes rapid and appreciable weight loss and malnutrition.

COMPLICATIONS. Complications of chronic ulcerative colitis are numerous and varied, and are frequently of sufficient gravity of themselves to require definitive surgical therapy of the primary colonic disease. Systemic complications include electrolyte deficiencies, microcytic anemia, hypoproteinemia, avitaminoses, amyloidosis, osteoporosis, amenorrhea, retarded sexual development, and retarded growth. Serious complications in other organs or systems include arthritis, ankylosing spondylitis, and sacroileitis; conjunctivitis, iritis, and episcleritis; gallstones, fatty liver, hepatitis, pericholangitis, cirrhosis, and carcinoma of the bile ducts; erythema nodosum, pyoderma gangrenosum, aphthous stomatitis, and clubbing of the fingers; pyelonephritis and urolithiasis; interstitial pancreatitis; peripheral neuropathy and vascular thromboses. Colonic complications include gross hemorrhage; stricture formation with partial obstruction; perforation, either free, producing peritonitis, or confined, with abscess or fistula formation; perianal and perirectal abscesses and fistulas; malabsorption; carcinoma of the colon; and toxic megacolon.

Toxic Megacolon. Toxic megacolon is a dreaded complication of ulcerative colitis that fortunately occurs in only 2 to 5 percent of patients with the disease. It is a manifestation of fulminant colitis and usually occurs with the initial acute episode, less frequently during a relapse of the remitting type, rarely in the chronic, continuous form of ulcerative colitis.

The cause of toxic dilatation is not known. The loss of tone, contractility, and propulsive motility have been attributed by some to necrotizing inflammation of the smooth muscle of the bowel and by others to damage of the myenteric plexus. Barium enema during a period of severe diarrhea is almost surely a precipitating factor. Other factors that may play a role include hypokalemia, hypomagnesemia, hypoproteinemia, opiates, and anticholinergics. Corticosteroids apparently do not play an etiologic role but may mask symptoms, particularly those of perforation of the megacolon.

The diagnosis should be immediately suspected in any patient with active colitis who has a sharp decrease in the number of daily stools without a corresponding amelioration in general status. Bloody rectal discharges may continue but with little gas or feces. The patient is obviously severely toxic, febrile, apathetic, and obtunded. Abdominal distension is progressive, and bowel sounds are hypoactive or absent. Plain abdominal roentgenograms show marked gaseous distension, particularly of the transverse colon.

Since toxic megacolon is a reversible process, a trial of intensive nonoperative therapy is indicated, with the patient watched very closely for actual or impending perforation. Therapy consists of intestinal decompression, antibiotics, correction of electrolyte deficits, discontinuance of opiates and anticholinergics, blood and albumin transfusions, and intravenous alimentation. If the patient has been receiving steroids, these are continued; if not, it is not clear whether initiation of steroid therapy is helpful or harmful.

Efficacy of therapy is measured by frequent plain films of the abdomen to evaluate the diameter of the dilated colon and watch for free air or intraabdominal collections, resumption of bowel function, fever, leukocytosis, and frequent physical examination of the abdomen. If the patient improves or at least the rapid downhill course is arrested, then medical therapy is continued. Operative intervention is indicated for perforation, deterioration in clinical status, or failure to improve after several days of intensive therapy. Most surgeons have preferred total or subtotal colectomy and ileostomy. The mortality rate has been at least 20 percent and much higher in some series, but recent studies indicate that much lower mortality rates are attainable if the patients are operated upon early in the course before colonic perforation and progressive metabolic deterioration have occurred. Turnbull and associates prefer the operation of ileostomy-colostomy, particularly if sealed-off perforations are suspected at laparotomy. They have reported a series of 42 patients so treated with only one death. If the patient with toxic megacolon has been treated medically or by Turnbull's procedure, definitive total colectomy–permanent ileostomy should be carried out electively as soon as the patient's condition warrants.

Carcinoma of the Colon. Carcinoma of the colon is a late complication of chronic ulcerative colitis, particularly of the smoldering, chronic, continuous form of the disease. Reported frequency of cancer in ulcerative colitis ranges from 0.7 to 17 percent but is usually about 3 percent. The most reliable current estimate would indicate that cancer in patients with chronic ulcerative colitis is about ten times as common as in the general population.

Factors affecting the frequency of cancer in colitis include extent of colonic involvement, duration of disease, and age at onset. In patients with total colitis cancer develops much more frequently than in those with left-sided colitis or ulcerative proctitis. Duration of the disease is also important, since most studies indicate that the risk of cancer is very low in the first 10 years of colitis but then rises to a risk of about 4 percent per year. Age at onset of colitis is the third factor; the incidence of cancer in colitis beginning before the age of twenty-five years is twice as great as in those with symptoms beginning after age twenty-five. The average age at the time of diagnosis of cancer in patients with ulcerative colitis is about thirty-seven years; in patients with idiopathic colon cancer, sixty-five years.

Carcinomas arising in ulcerative colitis are distributed more evenly throughout the colon as compared with the usual high incidence in the sigmoid and rectum. The growths are often multiple and commonly flat and infiltrating, and there is a high incidence of poorly differentiated and mucus-secreting types. These carry a poor prognosis. Neoplasia occurs in abnormal regenerated mucosa—the malignant potential of pseudopolyps is universally regarded as almost nil.

The most frequent symptoms of neoplasm simulate those of an exacerbation of ulcerative colitis—diarrhea, abdominal pain, rectal bleeding, and weight loss. Symptoms different from colitis—abdominal pain unrelated to defecation, and constipation—are unfortunately usually associated with far advanced cancer.

The prognosis for cancer arising in ulcerative colitis is much worse than for idiopathic colon cancer, probably because of the more frequent occurrence of more malignant histologic varieties and because of difficulty in diagnosis. The overall 5-year survival in idiopathic cancer is about 40 percent; for colitic cancer, it is less than 20 percent.

Diagnosis continues to be difficult and uncertain before the carcinoma is quite extensive. Morson proposed that certain premalignant histologic changes in rectal biopsies herald the development of carcinoma elsewhere in the ulcerative colitis colon—but this has not yet proved to be reliable. Nor is the carcinoembryonic antigen test reliable; the test is sometimes positive in patients with ulcerative colitis alone without carcinoma and sometimes negative in patients with early carcinomas. Fibercolonoscopy is emerging as an accurate diagnostic modality and will probably become the preferred method. Visual identification of carcinoma in a universally diseased mucosa is difficult, but most lesions can be detected by biopsy permitting histologic verification. Barium enema roentgenography is still the standard diagnostic tool but is considerably less accurate in diagnosing carcinoma in the presence of ulcerative colitis than in the otherwise normal colon.

The specter of carcinoma must influence the management of patients with chronic ulcerative colitis of many years' duration. The diagnosis of cancer in the ulcerative colitis colon is difficult, and the required studies are not without hazard. At present, any patient who has had active universal colitis for 10 years should be strongly urged to have a total colectomy–permanent ileostomy.

DIAGNOSIS. The diagnosis of nonspecific ulcerative co-

litis is one of exclusion of the specific causes of diarrhea and ulcerative colitis. Diseases to be evaluated by appropriate bacteriologic, serologic, chemical, radiologic, and sigmoidoscopic techniques include amebiasis, bacillary dysentery, intestinal tuberculosis, diverticulitis, lymphogranuloma venereum, carcinoma coli, malignant carcinoid syndrome, celiac disease, nontropical sprue, malabsorption syndrome, and ischemic colitis.

Sigmoidoscopy and colonoscopy, including biopsy, are the most reliable procedures for establishing the diagnosis of nonspecific ulcerative colitis. The endoscopic appearance of the rectal mucosa, while characteristic, is not pathognomonic for nonspecific ulcerative colitis. For this reason, bacteriologic and histologic examination of biopsy material is essential. Hyperemia, edema, and small, scattered, pinpoint ulcerations are seen in the early stages. The mucosa is friable and bleeds easily when touched. Later, the pinpoint ulcerations enlarge and coalesce to form larger ulcers which are usually covered with bloody pus. After several exacerbations and healing, the mucosa develops a finely granular appearance. Healing is also evidenced by submucosal scarring with small, irregular pearly plaques visible through the mucosa. With advanced disease, gross areas of ulceration are surrounded by irregular pseudopolypoid islands of abnormal mucosa. Additional findings include stricture formation, carcinoma, perianal abscesses and fistulas, and stenosis and fissures, and thrombosed hemorrhoids.

Barium enema is also helpful but should be given with caution, if at all, during acute exacerbations of the disease. Extensive preparation is unnecessary; a single low-pressure saline enema usually suffices; oral laxatives should not be given. Early in the disease, barium enema examination may be within normal limits, or irritability may be noted. With established disease there is some loss of haustration; fine ulcerations and alterations of the reticular mucosal pattern are seen on the postevacuation films. When the ulcers become larger and more numerous, the colon appears characteristically stippled and serrated. With moderately advanced disease, pseudopolyposis shows as multiple lucencies in the barium column—the "cobblestone" picture. In far advanced disease the lumen is narrowed, the bowel is rigid and shortened, haustra are absent, and the mucosal pattern is completely disorganized—the hose-like colon (Fig. 28-1).

TREATMENT. The primary treatment of nonspecific ulcerative colitis is medical. Since the specific cause of the disease is not known, there is no specific treatment. The components of therapy are antidiarrheal agents, antimicrobials, corticosteroids, diet, vitamin and mineral supplements, and general support.

Antidiarrheal agents are of some value in most patients but should be used with caution, since they may be implicated in the genesis of toxic megacolon. Most frequently used are diphenoxylate hydrochloride with atropine (Lomotil), codeine, paregoric, and calcium carbonate powders. Kaolin and pectin are of little value.

Salicylazosulfapyridine (Azulfidine), an oral nonabsorbable sulfonamide, is the antimicrobial of choice and should be tried in all patients on nonoperative therapy. It is not clear whether the benefit is derived from the antimicrobial action of the sulfa portion or the anti-inflammatory action of the salicylic acid component. Antibiotics are of no value in uncomplicated ulcerative colitis and should be used only for purulent complications such as abscesses or impending perforation.

Corticosteroid therapy of ulcerative colitis is controversial. There is no doubt that many patients are significantly benefited. This has been shown by serial rectal biopsies to be truly organic and not merely due to the sense of well-being, increased appetite, and reduction of fever which occur as a by-product of steroid therapy. On the other hand, some patients are not helped; morbidity is significantly higher in patients who subsequently require operative therapy; symptoms of perforation and peritonitis may be masked; and Cushing's syndrome is produced by prolonged therapy. In seriously ill patients, steroid therapy should be initiated with intravenous ACTH, 40 I.U. every 12 hours, or continuous intravenous prednisolone, 100 mg/day. If remission is achieved, oral prednisolone can be used after a few days. If there is no significant improvement in 7 to 10 days, colectomy must be seriously considered, since it is unlikely that nonoperative therapy will be successful.

Maintenance steroid therapy is with oral prednisone, starting at 60 mg daily in divided doses and tapering as rapidly as possible to 15 mg or less. The principal role of maintenance therapy is the control of symptoms; maintenance steroids do not abort exacerbations. Therefore every effort should be made to wean the patient completely. If a daily maintenance level of more than 15 mg prednisone is required to control symptoms for any length of time, then operative therapy should be advised. Retention enemas containing water-soluble corticosteroids are often beneficial in patients with disease limited to the rectum or left colon.

Rigid dietary restrictions have not been shown to be worthwhile. Every effort should be made to offer these patients a balanced diet of foods that appeal to them—served expeditiously and not allowed to stand on a cart until both hot foods and cold foods have reached room temperature. A milk-free diet should be tried, to observe possible benefit.

Vitamins A, C, and D and calcium are usually necessary. With very active disease and inadequate alimentation parenteral B complex should be given daily. Supplemental iron is given for iron-deficiency anemia. Potassium supplements are used during steroid therapy.

Supportive therapy consists of physical and emotional rest. Formal psychiatric therapy is rarely indicated and is sometimes harmful. The indicated psychotherapy should be given by a trusted sympathetic physician with a sincere interest in all the patient's problems.

Immunosuppressive therapy, based on the hypothesis that ulcerative colitis is an autoimmune disease, has had very limited success. Further trials, under rigidly controlled conditions, are indicated, but immunosuppressive therapy certainly cannot be recommended for general use at this time. These drugs may interfere with normal immunologic homeostasis, enhance oncogenic viruses, and repress im-

Fig. 28-1. Barium radiograph of chronic idiopathic ulcerative colitis. Note shortening of colon, absence of haustrations, destruction of mucosal pattern. Ileum is not affected.

munologic mechanisms for the surveillance and rejection of malignant cells. Thus there may be an added neoplastic risk in patients with ulcerative colitis who are already more vulnerable to colonic carcinoma.

Operative Therapy. Seventy-five to eighty percent of patients with idiopathic ulcerative colitis are more or less satisfactorily managed medically. Surgical therapy cures the disease, but because proper surgical therapy necessitates a permanent ileostomy, physicians and patients are understandably reluctant to agree to definitive surgical therapy until absolutely necessary.

Indications for emergency surgical intervention include uncontrollable hemorrhage, complete intestinal obstruction, free perforation with peritonitis, and toxic megacolon. Elective indications include partial intestinal obstruction; confined perforation with abscess formation; failure of medical management to control the disease; carcinoma; developmental retardation, either somatic or sexual; and serious systemic or distant complications that do not respond to nonoperative measures. An indication for prophylactic operation is long-continued colitis, which carries a high risk of colonic cancer.

Preparation for operation, as time permits, is intensive and consists of blood and albumin transfusions to restore blood volume, hematocrit, and plasma proteins to normality; correction of electrolyte abnormalities; correction of avitaminoses; and preoperative broad-spectrum antibiotics. If the patient has received corticosteroids within the past year, a slow intravenous drip of 100 mg of hydrocortisone is given the night before operation and a similar infusion started in the morning prior to, and continued through, the operation. Steroids are gradually tapered off over several days postoperatively. An important part of preoperative preparation is a frank discussion with the patient and his family as to exactly what the procedure entails.

The definitive procedure of choice is total proctocolectomy and ileostomy. This is preferably done in one stage, though some surgeons prefer a subtotal colectomy at the first stage with removal of the rectal stump at a later date. Permanent urinary dysfunction and impotence are uncommon after proctectomy for ulcerative colitis, as compared to abdominoperineal resection for rectal cancer, because the dissection is kept close to the rectal wall.

Ileostomy was formerly made by simply exteriorizing the terminal several centimeters of the divided ileum. This was often followed by a stormy several months of ileostomy dysfunction while the ileostomy "matured." It is now known that the problems with the old form of ileostomy were caused by a local peritonitis on the short segment of exteriorized ileostomy. This trouble can be avoided by fashioning an immediately "matured" ileostomy. The mucosa of the exteriorized segment is turned back over the remainder, either with or without excision of a distal ring of the seromuscular layers, and sutured circumferentially to the skin (Fig. 28-2). The ileum should be brought out through a separate elliptical incision, not the operative

Fig. 28-2. Creation and maturation of ileostomy. *A.* Excision of distal ring of seromuscular layers. (1) Seromuscular layer dissected off distal ileum. (2) Remaining muscularis and mucosa turned back. (3) Sutures placed between mucosa and skin. *B.* Maturation without excision of seromuscular layers. (1) Inner layers everted. (2) Mucosa sutured directly to skin.

incision, so placed that the 10-cm disc of the ileostomy appliance will not encroach on the umbilicus or anterior superior iliac spine. The individually fitted ileostomy bag should be applied early in the postoperative period to avoid digestion and excoriation of the skin.

Kock has devised a "continent" ileostomy which, when successful, permits the patient to dispense with external appliances. An internal reservoir to hold 100 ml or more is made from a doubled loop of ileum just proximal to the cutaneous ileostomy. The ileostomy is made continent by intussuscepting a 5-cm segment of the distal limb back into the pouch. The internal pouch is emptied two or three times a day with a catheter and is continent not only of liquid but of gas as well. Revision procedures are necessary in about one-third of cases, but the procedure ultimately functions satisfactorily in about 80 percent of patients. Causes of failure are recurrence of inflammatory bowel disease, ileal stomatitis, and incontinence of the stoma.

Subtotal colectomy with ileoproctostomy has been championed by Aylett, but most surgeons are less enthusiastic about it. The procedure may be tried in patients who have refused operation because of the ileostomy if the rectal segment is not severely diseased or strictured, the sphincter function is not deficient, and there is no perianal infection. One-half to two-thirds of patients have acceptable results; the remainder have to be converted to total colectomy-ileostomy because of continuing severe ulcerative proctitis or because of cancer in the rectal stump.

The mortality rate for emergency operations for ulcerative colitis, including the fulminant type, is 15 to 20 percent; for elective operations, 3 to 5 percent. Morbidity is appreciable and is significantly higher in steroid-treated patients. Complications include severe wound infection, intraabdominal abscess, septicemia, wound dehiscence, retraction of mucous fistulas, severe electrolyte imbalance, hemorrhage, and postoperative psychosis.

The long-term outlook for patients with ulcerative colitis treated by proctocolectomy-ileostomy is quite favorable. Some 10 to 15 percent of these patients will require revision of their ileostomy, usually within the first year, and most of them have to watch their diets to avoid diarrhea of the ileostomy. But over the long term, fully 95 percent are in excellent or good health.

Crohn's Colitis

The disease that Crohn described in 1932 as "terminal ileitis" may also involve the colon either alone or in association with small bowel disease. Terminology has been confused, but there are now hopeful signs that consensus is close. Terms which have been used include granulomatous colitis, segmental colitis, Crohn's disease of the colon, regional colitis, cicatrizing colitis, regional enteritis of the colon, right-sided regional colitis, regional migratory ulcerative colitis, and transmural colitis. The preferred terminology for disease limited to the colon is Crohn's colitis; for disease of both small and large bowel, Crohn's enterocolitis.

INCIDENCE. Available information suggests that perhaps one-third of cases of primary ulcerative disease of the colon are Crohn's colitis; the remainder are idiopathic ulcerative colitis except for a small percentage that cannot be clearly classified. A recent report of colitis patients who had been operated upon revealed that 58 percent had Crohn's colitis and 32 percent, idiopathic ulcerative colitis; 10 percent could not be classified. This probably means that a larger percentage of patients with Crohn's colitis require surgical therapy and does not reflect the true incidence of the disease.

Most of the discussion of the etiology and pathogenesis of regional enteritis in Chap. 27 is applicable to Crohn's colitis and will not be repeated.

PATHOLOGY. The distribution of the disease is somewhat different in the two forms of primary ulcerative colitis. Total involvement of the colon is seen in both but is more frequent with idiopathic ulcerative colitis. With partial involvement, Crohn's colitis more often involves the right colon, while idiopathic ulcerative colitis generally affects the left colon and rectum. Rectal involvement is found in about 95 percent of patients with ulcerative colitis and in about 50 percent with Crohn's colitis. Ulcerative colitis involves the colon in continuity, whereas skip areas are common in Crohn's disease. The small bowel is involved, often extensively, in about one-half of patients with Crohn's colitis, i.e., enterocolitis, whereas "backwash ileitis" occurs in perhaps 10 percent of patients with idiopathic ulcerative colitis (Table 28-1).

The gross appearance of the colon is usually pathognomonic of Crohn's disease. The serosal surface is dull, thickened, hyperemic and granular, and fat partially envelops the bowel wall. Tiny, gray-white nodules may be visible in the subserosa. Shortening of the colon is minimal. The wall is thickened and rubbery hard—the fibrotic thickening of the wall producing stenosis of the lumen. The appearance of the mucosal surface of the opened specimen is also pathognomonic. In some areas, the mucosa, which appears knobby and swollen from lymphedema, remains intact. In other areas there are deep, serpiginous or undermined longitudinal furrow ulcerations with a characteristic shape—the "bear-claw" ulcer. Microscopically the two distinguishing features of Crohn's colitis are transmural inflammation and fibrous thickening of the bowel wall. This is due initially to submucous edema but later to extensive fibrosis. The inflammatory exudate consists of lymphocytes, often with prominent follicle formation; plasma cells; and sarcoidlike granulomas. Fully formed granulomas consist of collections of epithelioid cells, multinucleated giant cells predominantly of the Langhans type, but without any caseation. These granulomas are an important diagnostic feature when present but are not found in 20 to 25 percent of cases that otherwise fit the classification of Crohn's colitis.

CLINICAL MANIFESTATIONS. Symptomatically, the two types of colitis are similar—patients present with chronic diarrhea associated with abdominal cramps, fever, and weight loss. Grossly bloody stools which are the hallmark of idiopathic ulcerative colitis, however, are rarely seen in Crohn's colitis. The correct diagnosis may also be suspected at sigmoidoscopy—if the mucosa is essentially normal or just edematous but without bleeding, then the

presumptive diagnosis of Crohn's colitis is made, since this tends to spare the rectum.

The relative incidence of some complications also is quite different. Fistulas between the diseased colon and other segments of bowel, bladder, vagina, and skin as well as perianal fistulas are common in Crohn's colitis—more than 40 percent have perianal fistulas versus less than 10 percent in mucosal colitis. Fistulization except in the perianal area is rare in chronic ulcerative colitis. Carcinomas and toxic megacolon are seen much more often in ulcerative colitis. Gross hemorrhage is rarely a problem in Crohn's colitis, in contrast to ulcerative colitis.

The radiographic features usually serve to distinguish the two forms of ulcerative colitis (Figs. 28-1 and 28-3). In Crohn's colitis, shortening is not conspicuous, and there is often segmental involvement with intervening normal segments. Haustration is only partially obliterated; the wall is rigid and the lumen is stenotic. Fistulas are common. Intramural fissures or tracts appear as tiny radiating spikes extending from the lumen. The normal mucosal pattern is lost, replaced in some areas by gross ulcerations but in others by a coarse cobblestoning that can usually be distinguished from the irregular pseudopolyposis of ulcerative colitis.

Fig. 28-3. Barium radiograph of Crohn's enterocolitis with involvement of terminal ileum, cecum, ascending and transverse colon; left colon is normal. Colon is a little shortened, and haustra are present but abnormal. Mucosal pattern is altered but not destroyed.

TREATMENT. Nonoperative therapy of Crohn's colitis is essentially the same as for idiopathic ulcerative colitis. The therapy, particularly corticosteroids, seems to be less effective in controlling Crohn's colitis or enterocolitis, with the result that a higher proportion require operative therapy. Azathioprine is also being tried for Crohn's colitis. Its use in this disease is certainly more justified than in ulcerative colitis. A curative operation is not available as it is in ulcerative colitis, and there is much less hazard of carcinoma. The principal use of azathioprine in Crohn's disease may well be in the postoperative patient to prevent recurrences.

In contrast to ulcerative colitis where ileostomy–total colectomy is clearly the procedure of choice, there is little unanimity of opinion as to the proper role of the various procedures that are available for the surgical therapy of the various problems encountered in Crohn's colitis.

Emergency operation is necessary much less frequently in Crohn's colitis than in ulcerative colitis; massive hemorrhage is rare, and toxic megacolon and free perforation are distinctly uncommon. The indications for elective operative therapy are also somewhat different for colonic disease than for Crohn's disease of the small intestine. Obstruction, abdominal abscess, or fistula formation are uncommon indications. The indication for most patients is chronic disabling symptoms that cannot be controlled by conservative means. Symptoms include chronic blood loss, hypoalbuminemia, chronic cramping abdominal pain and diarrhea, weight loss, and general ill health. Uncontrollable perianal disease is also a frequent indication.

With total involvement of the colon including the rectum most surgeons do a total proctocolectomy and permanent ileostomy. Reported recurrence rates vary from 3 to more than 50 percent. The reason for this wide variation is not apparent. The recurrence is nearly always just proximal to the stoma, and many but not all patients will require resection of the juxtastomal ileum and a new ileostomy. Oberhelman and Kohatsu, and others, have proposed the use of a diverting ileostomy without resection. The terminal ileum is transected and both ends brought out, the proximal as a functioning ileostomy and the distal as a defunctionalized mucous fistula. In many patients so treated the colonic disease becomes quiescent. A few patients have had intestinal continuity restored at a later time without exacerbation of the colonic disease; others have had flare-ups after restoration and have then required colectomy. Diverting ileostomy is also a useful first-stage procedure in patients whose conditions are so precarious as to preclude one-stage total colectomy. When general health has improved after diversion, colectomy can be done electively under more favorable circumstances.

When the colon is extensively diseased but without rectal involvement, total proctocolectomy and ileostomy are still preferred by most, but some would do total abdominal colectomy and leave the rectum. Ileoproctostomy can be done primarily or an ileostomy with oversewing the rectal stump, with expectation of restoring continuity at a later time. The recurrence rate after ileoproctostomy for Crohn's disease is about 50 percent.

Segmental colonic involvement would appear to invite segmental resection with primary anastomosis. Unfortunately, the extent of disease found at operation is often greater than appeared on barium enema. If disease is limited to the right colon, or right colon and terminal ileum, primary resection and ileo-transverse colostomy are preferred. If disease involves the left colon, proctocolectomy with ileostomy is advisable, since the results of left hemicolectomy have been poor.

The long-term outlook after definitive surgery in Crohn's colitis is less favorable than in ulcerative colitis. Recurrence of disease is a continuing problem and requires further surgery in about one-third of patients. Despite this, about 70 percent are sufficiently rehabilitated so that their health can be classified as excellent or good.

Ischemic Colitis

Although infarcts of the colon have been described from time to time, usually as single-case reports, only in the past decade has ischemic colitis emerged as a clearly defined clinicopathologic entity. Ischemic colitis is not primarily an inflammatory disease but is included in this section because of its importance in the differential diagnosis of inflammatory bowel disease as well as diverticular disease.

Ischemic colitis presents as three quite different clinical syndromes depending upon (1) the extent of the vascular occlusion, (2) the duration of the occlusion, (3) the efficiency of the collateral circulation, and (4) the extent of secondary bacterial invasion. With transitory impairment of arterial supply which is soon compensated by collateral flow there is a partial mucosal slough that is healed by mucosal regeneration within 2 or 3 days—reversible or *transient ischemic colitis* (Table 28-2). Gross impairment of arterial supply results in hemorrhagic infarction of the mucosa, which ulcerates, allowing invasion of bowel bacteria. Healing is by fibrosis, which often produces stenosis —*stricturing ischemic colitis*. With complete loss of arterial flow, there is full-thickness infarction, gangrene, and, if untreated, perforation with peritonitis and death—*gangrenous ischemic colitis*.

Early reports stressed that the splenic flexure is the most vulnerable segment, presumably because this is the area at the periphery of both superior and inferior mesenteric artery supply and because in this area the marginal artery of Drummond is at its greatest distance from the bowel wall. It is now clear, however, that ischemic colitis can affect any segment from the cecum to the rectosigmoid. Major vascular occlusion does not correlate with ischemic colitis; many patients, particularly those with abdominal aneurysms, have occlusion of the inferior mesenteric artery without bowel symptoms. Conversely, some patients with frank ischemic colitis have demonstrably patent major mesenteric arteries. Experimentally, ligation of the inferior mesenteric artery in the dog has no deleterious effect on the colon; it is only when the small vessels between the mesenteric arcade and the bowel are ligated that colonic ischemia is produced.

Most patients with ischemic colitis are in the older age group; it is rarely seen under age forty-five. The majority also have associated medical problems such as cardio-

Table 28-2. ISCHEMIC COLON DISEASE

	Form 1	Form 2	Form 3
Synonyms.........	Nonspecific colitis; ulcerative colitis of aged; reversible ischemia of colon	Ischemic stricture	Colonic infarction; necrotizing colitis; gangrene of colon; irreversible ischemia
Symptoms	Cramping abdominal pain; bloody diarrhea	Cramping abdominal pain; abdominal distension; decreased bowel movements	Diffuse abdominal pain; obtundation; bloody diarrhea
Signs	Localized tenderness; hyperactive intestinal sounds; mild pyrexia; leukocytosis	Abdominal distension, hyperactive intestinal sounds; normal temperature; normal white blood count	Diffuse direct and rebound tenderness; rigid abdomen; hypoactive or absent intestinal sounds; abdominal distension; pyrexia, leukocytosis, taciycardia, hypotension
Barium enema	Mucosal irregularity; thumbprinting; local narrowing	Stricture; intestinal obstruction	Mucosal irregularity; dilatation of colon; thickening of intestinal wall; perforation
Treatment.........	Medical	Resection of involved intestine	Correction of predisposing factors; immediate operation
Results	Resolution	Correction of symptoms	High mortality rate due to associated diseases or complications of colonic gangrene

SOURCE: From O'Connell, Kadell, and Tompkins, 1976.

vascular disease, rheumatoid arthritis, or diabetes. The onset of ischemic colitis is characteristically acute with mild to moderate generalized or lower abdominal cramping pain followed by passage of blood per rectum. Vomiting is uncommon. Further symptoms depend on which of the three types of ischemic colitis is developing. With the gangrenous type, the abdominal pain becomes more severe until it is constant. Systemic symptoms of an abdominal catastrophe ensue. On physical examination, abdominal tenderness is usually generalized but is often most marked over the ischemic segment. Voluntary guarding and involuntary spasm are present but are not marked. Bowel sounds, which are hyperactive early, gradually cease. Later, with progression of infarction to gangrene, necrosis, and perforation, the findings are those of spreading bacterial peritonitis and septic shock. Diagnosis can usually be made from the clinical picture alone. Sigmoidoscopy reveals only a normal distal segment with blood coming from above unless the rectosigmoid is the segment involved, in which case a blue-black, sloughing mucosa oozing blood is seen.

Barium enema is contraindicated in gangrenous colitis, and arteriography is unnecessary and delays proper treatment. Plain abdominal roentgenograms are often confirmatory and reveal adynamic ileus with the gaseous distension stopping at the involved segment. Occasionally small bubbles of gas may be detected in the wall of the infarcted bowel. Treatment is emergency operation as soon as the patient's condition is stabilized by vigorous preparatory therapy. Under favorable circumstances, the involved segment is resected and primary anastomosis performed.

More frequently, however, this disease in this age group dictates exteriorization of the involved segment.

With impairment but not complete loss of blood supply, the patient's symptoms do not progress, but neither do they disappear promptly. Mild to moderate abdominal pain continues, as does rectal bleeding, which, however, is usually not massive. There may also be symptoms and signs of partial intestinal obstruction. Barium enema radiography is diagnostic. Marginal "thumbprinting," or "pseudotumors," due to submucosal hemorrhage and pericolic fat inflammation is seen. Spasm and ulceration also may be present. Conservative therapy is indicated at this point since the process may be self-limited and reversible. Anticoagulants should not be used. After several days the barium enema findings revert toward normality, but repeat barium enema in a few weeks often reveals stricture formation at the ischemic site. The strictured colon should be electively resected with primary anastomosis.

In the transient or reversible form of ischemic colitis, symptoms are mild and last only 2 to 4 days. Barium enema, if done promptly, usually reveals thumbprinting or superficial ulceration but promptly reverts to normal. Follow-up barium enema is also within normal limits. No specific therapy is necessary.

Radiation Enterocolitis

That roentgen rays have deleterious effects on the intestine has been known since 1897, 2 years after their discovery, when Walsh described a self-limited instance of diarrhea and cramps which was resolved by placing a metal shield between the observer and the source of radiation. Radiation enterocolitis has become a major problem in recent years because of the higher radiation doses employed in the therapy of uterine, bladder, and prostatic malignancies and, perhaps, because the newer external radiation sources deliver large visceral doses with little or no skin reaction to alert the therapist.

The incidence of radiation injury to the bowel is very roughly dose-dependent. At tissue doses below 4,000 rads, significant bowel injury is quite uncommon. With 5,000 rads, essentially all patients will have some demonstrable damage; in 5 to 10 percent the damage will be significant and ongoing. Other factors that increase the likelihood of problems include asthenia, advanced age, hypertension, arteriosclerotic vascular disease, diabetes, and previous abdominal surgery with resulting adhesions that fix the bowel.

The rapidly proliferating intestinal epithelium is most sensitive to ionizing radiation and shows changes early in the course. There are mucosal hyperemia and edema, an extensive inflammatory cell infiltrate, and crypt abscesses. With higher doses there are areas of ulceration because of failure of epithelial regeneration. After cessation of therapy, reepithelization is the rule but with a thin mucosa with shortened villi. Of more serious import is the long-term effect of radiation on blood vessels. Beginning several weeks after radiation exposure and continuing for years is a progressive vasculitis, affecting principally the small arterioles in the submucosa with marked thickening of the vessel wall and leading to luminal occlusion and thrombosis. Large foam cells seen beneath the intima are said to be pathognomonic of radiation vasculitis. The progressive ischemia is accompanied by progressive thickening and fibrosis, principally of the submucosa. As ischemia progresses, ulceration supervenes. This in turn leads to abscess and fistula formation, also on an ischemic basis.

At least 75 percent of patients undergoing radiotherapy with exposure of the gastrointestinal tract will have nausea and vomiting, and often diarrhea with cramping. With high doses of radiation there may also be rectal bleeding and tenesmus. Most patients can be managed symptomatically, but in some the reaction is so severe that the therapy has to be stopped for a time or prolonged. These acute symptoms subside fairly promptly after completion of therapy.

Late symptoms of radiation damage to the intestines appear from several months to many years after exposure. The clinical presentation is determined by the segment of bowel involved as well as by the type of lesion: atrophic mucosa, ulcer, stricture, abscess, fistula, or perforation. The rectum is by far the most common site of involvement because of its proximity to the cervix and its fixed position. Rectal ulcers are most commonly seen on the anterior wall at 4 to 6 cm above the dentate line and cause the passage of bloody mucus and tenesmus. Symptomatic rectal strictures are usually found at the 8- to 12-cm level and produce the picture of partial colonic obstruction. A particularly distressing complication is a postradiation fistula from rectum into bladder or vagina producing feculent vaginal dis-

charge or pneumaturia. With small intestine involvement, symptoms of malabsorption may be prominent. Extensive fibrosis also produces the bacterial stasis syndrome and intestinal obstruction.

Diagnosis may be difficult because of the difficulty in distinguishing between radiation changes and recurrent tumor. Barium contrast radiographic studies usually demonstrate rather characteristic changes, but these are not specific. Similarly, angiography also usually demonstrates changes that are characteristic of, but not specific for, radiation damage. Endoscopy with biopsy yields a specific diagnosis in some cases but not in all. If a positive histologic diagnosis is not possible prior to treatment, the patient should be given the benefit of the doubt and not denied maximal therapy because his lesion may be recurrent cancer.

Management of radiation injuries is difficult and often unsatisfactory. Conservative measures should be used as long as they are effective. Ischemic fibrotic tissues make for poor wound healing, anastomotic disruption, infection, and occult perforation. Morgenstern and associates have well summarized several caveats for the surgeon: (1) Avoid entry into the abdomen for radiation injury unless absolutely forced to operate. (2) Avoid extensive resections and multiple anastomoses. Short isolated segments are best resected, but long segments are most safely treated by side-to-side bypass. (3) Avoid extensive adhesiolysis. Lysis of adhesions in damaged intestine produces minute openings into the intestine which lead to postoperative perforation or fistulas. (4) Use frozen-section control of the intestinal ends to be anastomosed to rule out unsuspected radiation changes. (5) Protect anastomoses. Colon anastomoses should be protected with a proximal colostomy; small bowel anastomoses, with a long tube.

The outlook in radiation enterocolitis is grim. Many patients are spared this travail because they die of their primary diseases before radiation damage supervenes. But many more will die as a result of the treatment that cured their cancer. DeCosse and associates followed 94 patients with radiation enterocolitis. Of these, 27 were living, 28 died from cancer, 13 died from other causes, and 22 died from complications of radiation enterocolitis.

Pseudomembranous Enterocolitis

Shortly after the introduction of antibiotics, there were several reports of a presumably new syndrome that had occurred postoperatively in patients receiving antibiotics. These patients developed severe diarrhea, abdominal pain and distension, circulatory collapse, and death. Necropsy revealed severe enteritis with extensive pseudomembrane formation under which pure cultures of *Staphylococcus aureus* could usually be isolated. It was reasoned that the antibiotics had altered the normal flora of the bowel and allowed overgrowth of resistant pathogenic staphylococci. Doubt was soon cast on this hypothesis by finding that the syndrome had first been reported in 1893, noting that the syndrome sometimes occurred in patients who had not been operated upon and had not received antibiotics, finding patients with the syndrome whose stool culture did not grow staphylococci. Mucosal ischemia, rather than bacterial overgrowth, is currently the prime suspect in this condition.

PATHOLOGY. The intestine in pseudomembranous enterocolitis grossly resembles that found in uremia, bacillary dysentery, or heavy-metal poisoning. The entire gastrointestinal tract may be involved, or changes may be limited to one or more segments. In man the ileum is the most commonly affected part, followed by small and large bowel together, and by colon alone. The edematous bowel is usually distended with fluid and may contain as much as 5,000 ml. Serosa is hyperemic and edematous but otherwise not remarkable. The open bowel presents a shaggy yellow-green pseudomembrane, loosely adherent to the mucosa, and arranged in large patches or diffusely covering entire segments. The pseudomembrane consists of a fibrin mesh and mucus, containing inflammatory cells, and cellular debris of desquamated mucosal cells, leukocytes, erythrocytes, and bacteria. A severe inflammatory process affects principally mucosa and submucosa, occasionally extending into the muscularis. The inflammatory infiltrate consists chiefly of polymorphonuclear leukocytes, lymphocytes, and plasma cells. Necrosis of superficial mucosal cells is prominent. With deeper necrosis, mucosal ulcerations and fragmentation of villi are produced. Full-thickness necrosis with perforation of the bowel does not occur in pseudomembranous enterocolitis.

CLINICAL MANIFESTATIONS. Initial symptoms of pseudomembranous enterocolitis usually develop between the third and seventh postoperative days, and so may be masked by the general postoperative state. First noted are lethargy, weakness, and abdominal pain out of proportion to that usually due to the operative procedure. If diarrhea occurs, the diagnosis becomes obvious, but diarrhea is by no means a constant accompaniment of the enteritis. A valuable physical sign is abdominal distension despite audible peristalsis. The typical diarrheal stool is green and resembles rice water. The liquid stool contains suspended fragments, occasionally large sheets of pseudomembrane. If the disease pursues a severe course, then weakness, nausea, and mild abdominal distension are soon followed by vomiting, marked distension, copious diarrhea, tachycardia, fever to 40 or 41°C, disorientation, shock, and oliguria. The volume of stool passed in 24 hours may amount to 10,000 ml. Shock dominates the terminal phase, and death occurs in circulatory collapse. Less severe forms of the disease occur, but the incidence is not known, since the disease may not be recognized and mild forms may not be included in published reports. The incidence of circulatory collapse is low in the less severe forms.

TREATMENT. To be successful, therapy must be immediate and aggressive. The extensive water, electrolyte, and plasma deficits must be replaced rapidly, guided by monitoring vital signs and control venous pressure. All antibiotics that the patient has been receiving are immediately discontinued. Antibiotics specific for resistant staphylococci should be administered intravenously in large doses. Glucocorticosteroids in pharmacologic doses are given as in septic shock (Chap. 4).

The outcome is usually apparent within 24 or, at most,

48 hours. If the patient is going to respond to treatment, the response is rapid; if not, the continuing downhill course is also rapid.

CLINDAMYCIN-ASSOCIATED COLITIS

A condition related to but probably distinct from pseudo-membranous enterocolitis should be called *antibiotic-associated enterocolitis,* since it has been reported with aureomycin and other tetracyclines, streptomycin, chloramphenicol, ampicillin, and cephazolin as well as lincomycin and clindamycin. The reported incidence has been highest with the latter two agents; hence the name *clindamycin-associated colitis,* which is now in common usage.

In its mildest form, occurring in up to 20 percent of patients receiving lincomycin or clindamycin, there is bloodless, watery diarrhea without fever or leukocytosis. Proctoscopy reveals only some edema, hyperemia, and slight friability, but no ulceration or plaques. Bacteriological studies do not reveal single species overgrowth; the flora is qualitatively normal, though there is some quantitative reduction in anaerobes. The diarrhea subsides within a few days after administration of the antibiotic has been stopped, and only symptomatic treatment is indicated. The antibiotic need not be stopped if it is essential to the patient's care, but the patient's condition should be monitored by frequent proctoscopy to determine if progression to a more severe form of colitis is occurring which would require that the antibiotic be stopped.

In the severe forms, occurring in up to 10 percent of patients receiving lincomycin or clindamycin, there are severe diarrhea, abdominal cramping, high fever, and leukocytosis. Two different pictures are found on examination. In the more common one, proctoscopy reveals an erythematous friable mucosa studded with white-yellow plaques. The plaques when confluent form a pseudomembrane. Biopsy shows acute inflammation and microscopic ulceration covered by a layer of fibrin and mucus containing leukocytes and necrotic cells. Both in its symptoms and in the proctoscopic and barium enema radiographic findings, the less common form closely mimics an acute attack of idiopathic ulcerative colitis. In some patients the plain x-ray alone is adequate for diagnosis (Fig. 28-4). Bacteriologic studies of the colonic microflora in these severe forms have shown a striking decrease, both quantitatively and qualitatively, in the number of anaerobes present. The process is usually reversible, but recovery may be prolonged. The offending antibiotic must be stopped immediately and vigorous supportive therapy given. The role of corticosteroids is unclear; many feel they are beneficial but this is not based on solid evidence. A few patients have not responded to therapy: several have succumbed, and several more have required total colectomy-ileostomy.

Amebiasis

Amebiasis is an infection produced by the protozoan *E. histolytica,* involving the colon primarily and other organs secondarily, especially the liver. The infestation is an asymptomatic carrier state in most individuals with the incidence of carrier state ranging from about 10 percent

Fig. 28-4. Plain x-ray of the abdomen in a patient with fatal clindamycin colitis. Arrows point to "thumbprinting." Submucosal edema causes mucosal projections into the gas-filled lumen.

in the United States and Europe to over 60 percent in some undeveloped countries and some mental institutions.

ACUTE AMEBIC DYSENTERY

Acute amebic dysentery is unusual and is seen principally with massive contamination of the water supply. Onset is abrupt, with high fever, abdominal cramps, and profuse bloody diarrhea with tenesmus. Extensive ulceration of the rectum is usually seen at proctoscopy. Numerous trophozoites, containing ingested erythrocytes, can usually be found in warm saline preparations of fresh stool, exudate, or scrapings from the ulcers. Serological tests for *E. histolytica* antibodies should be used if the diagnosis is uncertain. It is imperative that amebic colitis be distinguished from idiopathic ulcerative colitis or Crohn's colitis, which it may closely resemble; because of systemic dissemination of the amebas, the usual corticosteroid therapy of these diseases can be lethal to the patient with amebic colitis. Administration of metronidazole, 750 mg three times daily for 10 days, is the preferred treatment. If the patient is unable to take oral medication, the conventional emetine-tetracycline-diiodohydroxyquin followed by chloroquin should be used.

Perforation of the colon is rare and is difficult to diagnose unless free intraperitoneal air is demonstrated, because acute amebic colitis is associated with diffuse abdominal tenderness often so severe that peritonitis is suspected. Exteriorization of the perforated segment is the preferred operation. Resection with primary anastomosis is dangerous because of the friability of the bowel.

CHRONIC AMEBIC DYSENTERY

Chronic amebic dysentery is the common form. Onset is gradual. There is usually intermittent diarrhea with two to four foul-smelling stools daily often containing blood and mucus, vague abdominal cramps, weight loss, and low-grade fever. Symptomatic periods may alternate with asymptomatic periods lasting for many weeks or months. Positive diagnosis may be difficult, since cysts or trophozoites are not always demonstrable in patients strongly suspected of having chronic amebiasis. The diagnostic yield is increased by looking for the organisms in rectal biopsies. Sigmoidoscopy is within normal limits in about 30 percent of cases, but organisms may be found in grossly normal mucosa. *E. histolytica* antibodies are detectable in the serum in over 90 percent of patients with active amebiasis. Asymptomatic or mild infestations should be treated with diiodohydroxyquin, 650 mg three times daily for 21 days. More severe infections are best treated by metronidazole followed by diiodohydroxyquin. Relapse is common; therefore monthly examination of stools should be carried out for at least a year, with retreatment as necessary.

Amebic abscess of the liver is the most common serious complication of amebic colitis. Hepatic abscesses may rupture into the pleura, pericardium, or peritoneum (see Chap. 30).

An uncommon complication of chronic amebic colitis of interest to surgeons is the ameboma, a mass of granulation tissue in the colon. Partial obstruction may be produced, and a tender, sausage-shaped mass is often palpable. Granulomas are most frequent in the cecum, where radiologic demonstration of ragged encroachment upon the lumen may lead to an erroneous diagnosis of carcinoma, tuberculosis, or actinomycosis. It is important therefore to search for amebas in the stools or rectal mucosa of patients with this finding. Surgical intervention in untreated ameboma can lead to peritonitis or to pericecal abscess and fecal fistula.

Actinomycosis

Actinomycosis is an uncommon suppurative infection produced by the anaerobic fungus *Actinomyces israelii*, a normal resident of the mouth. Clinical disease is characterized by chronic inflammatory induration and sinus formation. The cervicofacial area is the most frequently involved site, followed by thoracic and abdominal involvement.

The cecal area is most frequently the site of abdominal actinomycosis. An indurated, tumorlike pericecal mass sometimes develops. If the condition is untreated, abscesses develop and burst, forming indolent sinuses. More typically the history begins with an attack of acute appendicitis with perforation. After appendectomy, a persistent draining sinus forms, or, less commonly, an indurated mass forms under the incision which then results in a persistent sinus after surgical drainage.

The diagnosis of actinomycosis is made by demonstration of sulfur granules or the ray fungus in the purulent sinus discharge.

Treatment consists of surgical drainage and antibiotics. Both penicillin and tetracyclines are effective.

DIVERTICULAR DISEASE

Two types of diverticula of the colon are recognized: One is very common, an acquired disease which consists of multiple false diverticula principally in the left colon —*diverticulosis*. The other is very uncommon, is probably a congenital disease, and consists of a single true diverticulum of the cecum or ascending colon.

Diverticulosis Coli

INCIDENCE. The incidence of diverticulosis of the colon on barium enema examination or at necropsy is about 5 percent. Thus, about 11 million persons in the United States have the disease. Diverticulosis is rarely seen in persons under age thirty-five. The incidence rises with age, so at age fifty about 15 percent are affected; at sixty-five, about 35 percent; and at eighty-five, about 65 percent.

ETIOLOGY AND PATHOGENESIS. The sigmoid is the sole site of diverticula in about 50 percent of patients with diverticulosis; sigmoid and descending colon are the sites in 80 percent; sigmoid plus other colonic sites, in 95 percent. The cecum is involved in 2 percent; ascending colon and rectum, 4 percent each; and transverse colon, 10 percent.

Diverticula of the colon are herniations of mucosa and submucosa through the circular muscular layer and so are classified as false diverticula, since they lack a muscular coat. Diverticula characteristically break through the circular muscle on either side of the colon between the mesenteric and the respective antimesenteric taeniae. Radiographs of injected normal colon segments demonstrate a large circumferential vessel coursing around the bowel outside the muscular coat on each side with branches penetrating the muscularis on the mesenteric side of each antimesenteric taenia. This penetrating vessel is thought to create the *locus minoris resistentiae* through which mucosal herniation can occur. Injection studies of colon segments bearing diverticula also demonstrate that the penetrating vessel is in close relation to the neck of the diverticulum where it breaks through the circular muscle. The proximity of this vessel presumably accounts for the propensity of diverticula to bleed.

The mechanism(s) furnishing the pulsion force to herniate the mucosa through the weak spot in the circular muscle that has not been clearly delineated. Contributing factors are thought to be chronic constipation, tissue degeneration associated with age and obesity, and an inherited predisposition. Hypertrophy of the bowel musculature is often demonstrable in diverticular disease but has been considered to be secondary to fully developed diver-

ticulitis. Morson has found hypertrophy of the sigmoid musculature in some specimens with only microscopic intrusions of mucosa—a prediverticular state—and suggests that the muscular abnormality is primary. Some investigators have confirmed this finding, but others have not. Painter et al. studied the colons of patients by means of simultaneous cineradiography and intraluminal pressure recordings. Contraction rings form in the sigmoid colon. These close the lumen, creating a series of "bladders" each of which has its outflow obstructed at each end. With contraction of the colonic muscle forming the wall of the segments, intraluminal pressures up to at least 90 mm Hg are generated. Contraction of these closed segments creates a pulsion force that was observed to distend existing diverticula. The investigators conclude that this mechanism may well be responsible for the initial mucosal herniation. Similar motility and pressure abnormalities have been demonstrated in the irritable colon syndrome, which is thought by some to predispose to diverticular disease.

Diet appears to play a prominent role in the causation of diverticulosis, since it is almost entirely a disease of industrial societies. Diverticulosis is rare in Asia and Africa but is relatively frequent among United States residents of African origin. Diverticulosis coli has been produced in the rat and rabbit by feeding a low-residue diet, a diet similar to that of industrial societies. Only four mammals have teniae coli—horse, guinea pig, rabbit, and man; three of these are herbivores. Was the human colon designed for a bulky herbivorous diet?

Diverticulosis per se does not cause symptoms. The majority of persons with this condition never have trouble enough to require medical attention. Only 1 in 70 will require hospital treatment, and only 1 in 200 will require operation for a symptomatic complication. Complications of diverticulosis are bleeding, and inflammation, i.e., diverticulitis.

BLEEDING IN DIVERTICULAR DISEASE

The reported incidence of bleeding in diverticular disease varies from 3 to 48.5 percent. This large variation is attributable to the following: (1) some writers have reported the incidence of bleeding in patients hospitalized for diverticular disease, whereas others have reported the incidence in all patients, clinic and hospital, in whom the diagnosis has been made; (2) some have included all bleeding, overt and occult, whereas others have reported only gross bleeding; and (3) until recently, many writers refused to believe that diverticulosis without frank diverticulitis could bleed. It is now recognized that gross rectal hemorrhage is caused more frequently by diverticulosis than by diverticulitis, that bleeding from diverticulosis is massive in about one fourth of the patients, and that diverticulosis is responsible for about two-thirds of all cases of massive lower gastrointestinal bleeding. Colorectal carcinoma is the most frequent cause of rectal bleeding, but the bleeding is nearly always mild to moderate in degree, rarely severe and exsanguinating (see also Chap. 24).

DIAGNOSIS. Bleeding due to diverticular disease of the colon is characteristically sudden, unexpected, and often profuse from the onset, and occurs more frequently in older individuals and in those with arteriosclerotic and/or hypertensive cardiovascular disease. Bleeding is often the only symptom of diverticulosis. Many patients with massive rectal bleeding will have had a previous episode suggesting diverticulitis but usually do not have frank symptoms of inflammation at the time of the hemorrhage.

Some patients bleed so massively that immediate operation must be done to prevent death from exsanguination. Most, however, will respond, at least temporarily, to vigorous transfusion therapy. Every effort should be made, after the patient is clinically stable, to ascertain the nature of the bleeding lesion and its location. The known presence of diverticula does not guarantee that they are the source of the bleeding. The diagnostic steps to be taken are discussed in Chap. 24 under Lower Gastrointestinal Tract Bleeding. The use of selective angiography in recent years for detection of the bleeding point has demonstrated, unexpectedly, that although most diverticula are in the left colon, most major diverticular bleeding is from diverticula in the right colon. The use of aortography to demonstrate the bleeding point is illustrated in Fig. 28-5.

TREATMENT. The majority of patients with lower gastrointestinal hemorrhage will stop bleeding spontaneously with adequate transfusions and supportive therapy. Selective infusion of vasoconstrictive substances such as vasopressin into the visceral artery supplying the bleeding site, after identification by selective angiography, has been shown by several groups to be a quite effective and safe nonoperative method of controlling diverticular bleeding. In some patients the bleeding is controlled and does not recur; in others bleeding is only temporarily slowed or stopped but time is gained for a more orderly approach to the operative procedure. In a few, the selective infusion is completely ineffective and immediate operation is necessary. Adams has reported the use of the barium enema as therapy for massive diverticular bleeding; 47 of 49 bleeding episodes were arrested, possibly due to tamponade of the bleeding point by barium. If bleeding continues, after correction of hypovolemia, at a rate of more than 500 ml/8 hours or if massive hemorrhage recurs during the hospital course, then immediate operative therapy is indicated. Opinion is divided on whether a single massive hemorrhage in a patient who is found on work-up to have nothing but diverticulosis is sufficient reason for elective colon resection. Nearly all agree, however, that a second massive hemorrhage in such a patient is an indication for surgical intervention.

In elective operations for bleeding, the entire gastrointestinal tract should be minutely examined for lesions that might have been missed in the diagnostic work-up. If no other lesions are found, then all colon bearing diverticula is resected with primary anastomosis. This usually requires sigmoid or sigmoid and descending colon resection but may require removal of the entire colon down to the rectum. The mortality rate for elective resections is less than 5 percent.

Emergency surgical treatment for massive bleeding when the presumptive source of bleeding has not been identified preoperatively is often a frustrating, difficult

Fig. 28-5. Aortogram in bleeding diverticulosis. Arrow on left side of illustration points to the bleeding diverticulum in the right colon.

problem. The entire colon is usually grossly distended with blood, even though the bleeding point is in the sigmoid. Segmental colotomies with operative endoscopy is rarely rewarding. Isolation of segments with clamps is sometimes helpful. The colon is emptied of blood by "milking" it downward through a rectal tube; then several noncrushing clamps are applied to isolate the different colon segments. If active bleeding is present, the involved segment or segments will be seen to fill with blood, and the appropriate resection can then be done. For patients in whom the bleeding point cannot be located with assurance, total abdominal colectomy with ileoproctostomy is gaining favor as the procedure of choice. There is currently an unresolved difference of opinion between angiographers and surgeons as to the preferred operation when a bleeding diverticulum has been identified angiographically. Many surgeons feel that all diverticula-bearing colon should be resected. Angiographers, however, feel that this is unnecessarily radical. In their opinion a segmental resection of the bleeding area is sufficient, since they believe that the chance of bleeding from remaining diverticula is slight. The mortality rate of emergency surgical measures for massive rectal bleeding is over 20 percent.

DIVERTICULITIS

Inflammation is the most frequent complication of diverticulosis coli. Diverticulitis is more frequent in patients with widespread diverticulosis, and the frequency increases with age. The inflammation may remain localized as a simple diverticulitis or extend to produce secondary complications such as intestinal obstruction, confined perforation with abscess or fistula formation, free perforation with spreading peritonitis, and hemorrhage. These grave complications supervene in about 15 percent of patients with diverticulitis and usually require operative therapy.

PATHOGENESIS. Diverticula readily fill with colonic contents, as can be seen at barium enema examination, but emptying is often slow because of the narrow neck and the lack of musculature of the diverticulum. If an inspissated fecal plug obstructs the neck of the diverticulum, continued mucus secretion and proliferation of everpresent bacteria distend the flask-shaped diverticulum and produce inflammation at the apex. This focal diverticulitis often resolves by discharge of the contents into the colonic lumen, but if the obstructing plug remains in place, inflammation spreads to peridiverticular tissues. Initial spread is to the pericolic fat between the muscularis propria and serosa. Extension is usually longitudinal in this plane, giving rise to intramural fistulas, which are one of the diagnostic signs of diverticulitis on barium enema (Fig. 28-6). Diverticulitis is thought to start as inflammation of a single diverticulum; other diverticula may become secondarily involved as edema from the initial diverticulitis narrows their necks, preventing emptying and thus initiating another inflammatory focus. Berman and associates have presented evidence that actual perforation of a single diverticulum is the initiating event, followed by an inflammatory focus in the pericolic fat.

CLINICAL MANIFESTATIONS. The diagnosis of acute diverticulitis is aided by a history of previous demonstration of diverticulosis with barium enema radiography. The clinical picture of sigmoid diverticulitis so resembles appendicitis that it is often called "left-sided appendicitis." Pain is nearly always the most prominent symptom. It is mild to moderate and felt deep in the left lower quadrant or suprapubic area. The pain is usually dull, aching, and constant; less frequently, it is intermittent and crampy. Anorexia and mild nausea are common, but vomiting is uncommon. An associated change in bowel habits frequently is noted, i.e., diarrhea, constipation, or irregularity. Urinary symptoms are sometimes present as a result of inflammation close to bladder or ureter. On examination, low-grade fever and mild leukocytosis are usually found. Tenderness and some rigidity in the left lower quadrant and/or suprapubic area are the rule. A tender mass representing the inflamed, feces-filled colon may be palpable. Mild distension is common, but bowel sounds are usually within normal limits in uncomplicated diverticulitis. Sigmoidoscopy should be done if only to rule out other causes for the symptoms. Mucosal edema and erythema may be seen, but the most characteristic finding in acute diverticulitis is inability to introduce the scope beyond about 15 cm because of immobility of the bowel and fixed angulation at that point. It is advisable to defer the barium enema until the process has cooled off somewhat with conservative therapy. Barium enema then should be done, with caution, to attempt to differentiate diverticulitis from carcinoma of the colon, which can cause the same clinical picture. Differential diagnostic criteria are as follows: (1) Diverticulitis usually involves a long segment, carcinoma a much shorter one. (2) Normal bowel contour above and below diverticulitis tapers smoothly and gradually into the involved area to form a funnel-shaped transition; in carcinoma the transition is abrupt. (3) The bowel is spastic in diverticulitis. (4) The mucosa is intact, although it may show a picket-fence contour in diverticulitis, but it is destroyed in carcinoma. (5) Finally, diverticula in other areas of the bowel favor but do not prove diverticulitis, since carcinoma and diverticulosis may coexist. A typical radiograph of sigmoid diverticulitis is shown in Fig. 28-6 and of sigmoid carcinoma in Fig. 28-7.

TREATMENT. Nonoperative therapy should be tried for first attacks of acute uncomplicated diverticulitis. Operative therapy is indicated, if the patient does not respond promptly, for recurrent acute diverticulitis, for diverticulitis with complications, and if carcinoma cannot be ruled out. Initial nonoperative treatment consists of parenteral fluids, broad-spectrum antibiotics, and nasogastric suction. Pain is controlled with pentazocine or meperidine, but not morphine, to avoid increasing intracolonic pressure. Significant amelioration of all symptoms and signs should occur within 48 hours. If not, or if symptoms progress, operation should be considered. After subsidence of acute symptoms, treatment is aimed principally at avoiding constipation. Bulk-forming hemicellulose laxatives are taken as needed to keep the stool soft and bulky. In the past, low-residue diets have been prescribed. It is now recognized that bulky high-residue diets should be advised since low-residue diets have been implicated in the etiology of diverticulosis coli.

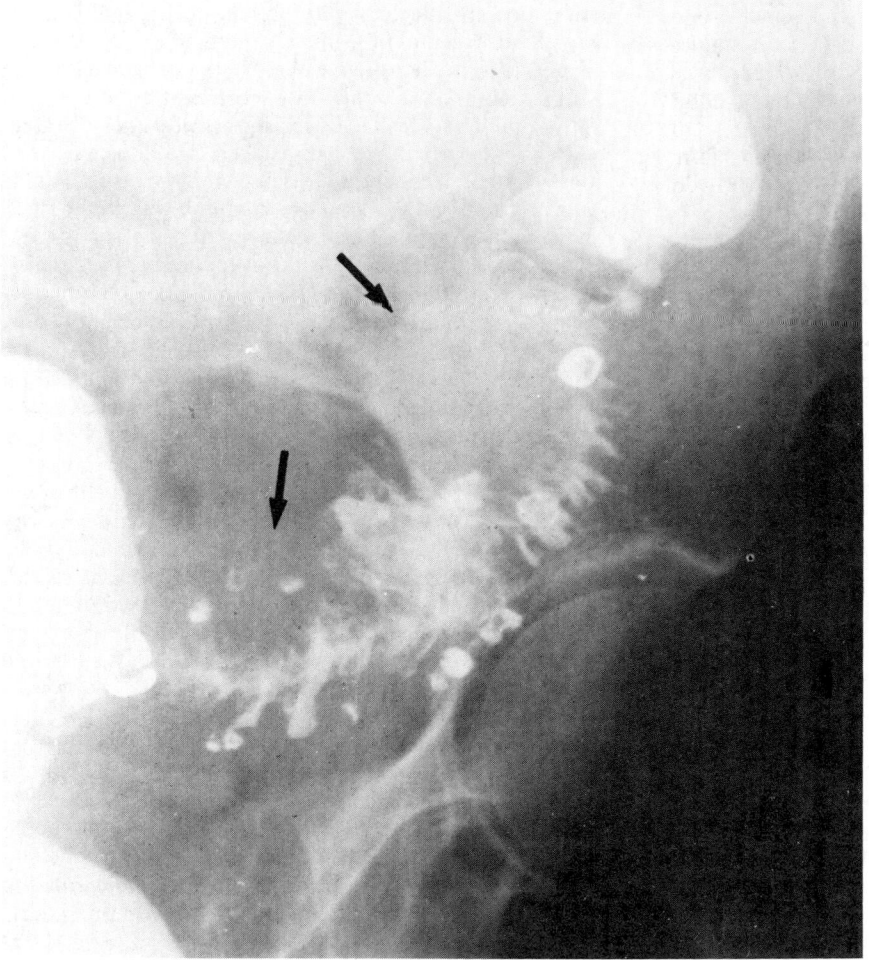

Fig. 28-6. Barium radiograph of diverticulitis of sigmoid colon. Note long length of involvement. Arrows point to intramural abscesses.

Fig. 28-7. Oblique view, barium radiograph of annular carcinoma of sigmoid colon. Note sharp transition from normal to abnormal area, short length of involvement.

Colomyotomy has been advocated for the treatment of chronic persistent diverticular disease that is a nuisance to the patient but has not yet progressed to a complication that would require resective therapy. The operation interrupts the muscle coats of the colon by a longitudinal incision between the two antimesenteric teniae. It is designed to lower intraluminal pressure and thus diminish the threat of complications. Results to date are equivocal.

If attacks of diverticulitis recur despite medical therapy, elective resection is indicated. With proper preparation, single-stage resection of all diverticulum-bearing colon with primary anastomosis is usually possible.

Complications of Diverticulitis

Obstruction. Some degree of colonic obstruction occurs in about two-thirds of patients with acute diverticulitis. This is usually partial obstruction due to inflammation with spasm and edema, plus an element of adynamic ileus. Complete obstruction occurs in about 10 percent and is the second most frequent cause of acute colonic obstruction. Complete obstruction usually implies abscess formation with encroachment on the lumen or repeated episodes of diverticulitis with fibrosis and stenosis. Small bowel obstruction also occurs secondarily to involvement in an inflammatory mass or to adhesions. Clinical manifestations of intestinal obstruction are discussed in Chap. 24. Obstructive symptoms in diverticulitis usually respond fairly promptly to nonoperative therapy. Plain films of the abdomen are valuable to differentiate small and large bowel obstruction by delineation of the gas pattern. If there is doubt about the locus of the obstruction, barium enema, though somewhat hazardous in acute diverticulitis, should be done. Adynamic ileus secondary to free perforation and peritonitis must be kept in mind. If complete colon obstruction does not open up within a few hours, operative therapy is indicated lest cecal rupture occur.

Most surgeons still feel that the combination of acute inflammation and obstructed unprepared bowel interdict primary resection and consider diverting transverse colostomy to be the procedure of choice. A few advocate primary resection, feeling that the morbidity and mortality, though appreciable, is less than the combined morbidity and mortality of the two- or three-stage procedures. After colostomy, an interval of about 3 months is allowed for inflammation to subside before resection is done. If there is a question about the presence of carcinoma, however, the second-stage operation is done in 2 or 3 weeks. The colostomy may be closed at the time of the resection or may be left to decompress the colon anastomosis and closed later as a third-stage procedure.

Perforation. The inflammatory process of uncomplicated diverticulitis is confined to the colonic wall by the serosa; a breach in the integrity of this layer constitutes perforation. The inflammation is ordinarily localized to the area adjacent to the perforation by the body's walling-off mechanism, thus forming a pericolic abscess. The abscess may in turn burrow into one of the viscera contributing to the walling-off process with formation of an internal fistula. Less frequently, the pericolic abscess bursts into the free peritoneal cavity producing purulent peritonitis. Also infrequently, the initial perforation is not walled off, so that free communication is established between the colonic lumen and the peritoneal cavity with gross fecal spillage and generalized fecal peritonitis. About 10 percent of patients with diverticulitis requiring operative therapy have spreading peritonitis either from free perforation or from secondary rupture of an abscess. The clinical manifestations and the principles of management of peritonitis are discussed in Chap. 34. With small free perforations that appear to be walling off quickly, thus localizing the peritonitis, nonoperative therapy with very close observation is justified. Resectional therapy can then be done electively after subsidence of the acute inflammation. With spreading peritonitis or if a previously stabilized and subsiding abdomen shows evidence of enlargement with increasing peritoneal signs, urgent operative therapy is mandatory.

There continues to be a difference of opinion as to which surgical procedure should be used. There is agreement that drainage alone, closure of perforation and drainage, or colostomy alone are inadequate. The procedure still preferred by many consists of closure of the perforation to

prevent further peritoneal soiling, drainage, and proximal diverting colostomy. Three stages are required to complete the treatment—resection at the second stage and colostomy closure as the third stage. A more radical and direct approach consists of resection of diseased bowel and primary anastomosis, usually with a proximal decompressing colostomy. Primary resection has the advantage of being a two-stage procedure or even a single stage if colostomy has not been necessary at the time of resection. Enthusiasm for this approach seems to be waning as more surgeons realize that primary anastomosis in the presence of peritonitis is foolhardy.

A third approach (preferred by the authors) has the advantage of completing therapy in two stages but without the hazard of performing a colonic anastomosis in the presence of pus and feces. All diseased colon is mobilized and resected. The proximal bowel is brought out as an end colostomy. The distal bowel is brought out as a mucous fistula if this is possible, but if the distal segment is short, the end is closed and left in place (Hartmann procedure). The peritoneal cavity is copiously irrigated, the last wash containing cephalothin or kanamycin. Drains are placed in the pelvis and gutter. At a second stage, in 2 or 3 months, continuity is reestablished by end-to-end anastomosis.

Fistulas. In about 5 percent of patients with complicated diverticulitis fistulas develop between the involved segment of colon and adjacent organs, i.e., bladder, uterus, vagina, ileum, and ureter. Colocutaneous fistulas rarely occur spontaneously but are a common postoperative complication, discharging through the incision or drain site. Fistulas develop when adjacent organs wall off acute diverticulitis, with subsequent burrowing of the disease process into the lumen of the adjacent viscus. Urinary urgency and frequency, and dysuria occur with inflammation of the bladder or ureter before fistulization has occurred. After the process has broken through to form a fistula, pneumaturia and fecaluria are diagnostic. Chills and fever are also frequent. Sigmoidoscopy is of no value in demonstrating fistulas. Barium enema often, but not always, demonstrates the tract. Cystoscopy and cystography are also useful. If the actual opening is not demonstrated, its location can be suspected by finding localized edema, ulceration, and granulations. Fistulas into the uterus or vagina offer little difficulty—passage of flatus and feces per vaginam establishes the diagnosis; speculum examination, the location. Coloenteric fistulas may cause no symptoms in addition to those of the primary disease, or there may be fecal urgency and frequency.

The choice of operative procedure for diverticulitis complicated by fistula depends on the extent of the inflammatory process and whether the correct diagnosis has been made preoperatively. With proper preoperative preparation, a one-stage procedure is often feasible. Fistulas into the bladder are dissected out, the bladder wall closed, diseased colon resected with primary anastomosis, and suprapubic drainage instituted. Hysterectomy en bloc with involved colon is done for colouterine fistulas. Similarly, the involved ileal loop is resected en bloc with colon for coloenteric fistulas. If the inflammatory process is extensive or if the bowel has not been prepared, staged procedures are indicated. If possible, diseased tissue is resected, the proximal colon is brought out as an end colostomy, and the distal end is brought out as a mucous fistula or is dropped back as a Hartmann pouch. The anastomosis is done as a second stage. If inflammation is so extensive as to preclude resection, a diverting proximal colostomy only is done as the initial stage, with completion in one or two more stages.

Diverticulum of the Right Colon

The cecum and ascending colon infrequently are involved in diverticulosis coli. Even more uncommon is a solitary true diverticulum, usually called *cecal diverticulitis,* that is found only in the cecum and ascending colon. In contrast to the false diverticula of diverticulosis coli, solitary cecal diverticula contain all layers of the bowel wall and are, therefore, true diverticula. Because of this and because these lesions are found in younger individuals, they are considered to be congenital in origin.

Symptoms are produced in the same manner as in diverticulitis coli or acute appendicitis. The ostium of the diverticulum becomes obstructed by a plug of feces or fecalith, creating a miniature closed loop. Inflammation ensues from continued secretion within the diverticulum and infection by resident bacteria.

CLINICAL MANIFESTATIONS. Clinical manifestations of acute cecal diverticulitis are essentially identical to those of acute appendicitis. The true nature of the lesion may be suspected if there is a history of numerous frequent episodes of similar attacks. The correct diagnosis is made preoperatively in only about 5 percent of patients, nearly always by barium enema demonstration of the diverticulum. The preoperative diagnosis is acute appendicitis in about 80 percent, tumor in about 5 percent.

TREATMENT. The operative procedure is determined by the findings. If inflammation is limited to the diverticulum, then simple diverticulectomy with inversion of the stump is done as for appendicitis. Ruptured diverticulum with abscess is treated by drainage and removal of the diverticulum if it can easily be done; otherwise only drainage is performed, and interval diverticulectomy is carried out later. When inflammation involves the cecum also, resection of diverticulum and adjacent cecum is indicated if the cecal closure is through healthy tissue, and the ileocecal valve is not encroached upon. When the cecum is extensively involved, terminal ileum and cecum are resected with ileo-ascending colon anastomosis. If frank peritonitis is present, ileo-ascending colectomy, cutaneous ileostomy, and creation of a transverse colon mucous fistula should be done because of the risk of primary anastomosis in this situation. Chronic diverticular disease with extensive productive inflammation and fibrosis may be indistinguishable from neoplasm at the operating table. Right colectomy with ileo-transverse colostomy as for cancer is indicated.

No treatment is indicated for asymptomatic cecal diverticula that are an incidental finding on barium enema. Diverticula found incidentally at operation should be re-moved if their removal does not add significantly to the risk of the primary procedure.

NEOPLASMS OF THE COLON AND RECTUM

Although a broad spectrum of neoplasms occurs in the colon and rectum, there are essentially only two important types of tumors: polyps, which may cause symptoms in themselves but more importantly may develop into, or be associated with, adenocarcinoma, and adenocarcinoma itself. Thus emphasis will be placed on these two lesions and their discussion followed by a brief discussion of some of the less common tumors. Neoplasms of the anus are quite different from those of colon and rectum and will be considered separately.

Polyps

The term *polyp* refers to any circumscribed mass of tissue that arises from mucosa and protrudes into the lumen of the gastrointestinal tract. It is a clinical term and should imply no histopathologic significance. After removal and histologic diagnosis, polyps are classified as: inflammatory—benign lymphoid polyps and pseudopolyps (ulcerative colitis); hamartomas—juvenile and Peutz-Jeghers polyps (Chap. 27); neoplastic—adenomatous (tubular) polyps, villous adenomas (papillomas); or unclassified—the hyperplastic (metaplastic) polyp.

JUVENILE POLYPS

This lesion, also called *mucous polyp* or *retention polyp,* technically should not be included under "neoplasms," since it is probably a hamartoma or possibly an inflammatory, polypoid, retention cyst.

INCIDENCE. As the name implies, juvenile polyps occur principally in children, but they also are found in young adults. They have not been reported in infants under age one. The peak incidence is about age five; they are uncommon after about age sixteen and very rare after age thirty-five. The incidence in children is probably about 1 percent. The polyps are single in 70 percent of patients. When multiple, there are usually only three or four polyps, but in rare instances the polyps may be so numerous that familial polyposis is simulated. This is now thought to represent an inherited polyposis syndrome. Inheritance is autosomal dominant with complete penetrance. Polyps are usually in the colon and rectum but may involve the small intestine and stomach. Some investigators consider these as variations of one syndrome, others divide them into juvenile polyposis coli and juvenile gastrointestinal polyposis.

PATHOLOGY. Grossly, juvenile polyps are nearly always pedunculated, rarely sessile, from 3 to 10 mm in diameter, smooth, spherical, reddish brown, and often covered with mucus. Histologically, the slender stalk is covered with essentially normal colonic mucosa that is continuous with adjacent mucosa. The bulbous portion is covered by a single layer of goblet cells, frequently with ulceration and chronic inflammation. In the tissue are numerous cystic spaces lined by mature, columnar, mucus-secreting cells, a heavy infiltration of leukocytes and plasma cells, and abundant granulation tissue. Strands of fibrous tissue from the stalk fan out into the bulbous portion.

CLINICAL MANIFESTATIONS. The usual symptom of colorectal polyps is blood streaking of the stool, less frequently rectal bleeding. Anemia is the presenting symptom in some patients. Rectal polyps may protrude through the rectum and be described as a small cherry by the parent. Rarely, a colonic polyp initiates intussusception. Diagnosis is by sigmoidoscopy, by air-contrast barium enema, or by colonoscopy for polyps beyond the reach of the sigmoidoscope.

TREATMENT. Treatment should take into account the fact that juvenile polyps have no malignant potential. All polyps within reach of the sigmoidoscope should be removed by excision biopsy, since this is so easily done. Polyps in the colon that would require laparatomy and colotomy for removal may be observed safely unless they are causing serious symptoms or unless they are so numerous that the possibility of familial polyposis exists. Autoamputation is common. New polyps, not recurrences, appear in about 10 percent after polypectomy.

HYPERPLASTIC POLYPS

These tiny mucosal excrescences—usually from 1 to 3 mm in diameter, very rarely over 5 mm, and never over 10 mm—can be found in 50 percent of adult colons if searched for diligently enough. Since they arise as the result of localized minor imbalances between cell division and desquamation (see Malignant Potential of Polyps, page 1214), the terms *hyperplastic* and *metaplastic* are appropriate. Hyperplastic polyps cause no symptoms and of themselves are of no consequence; they are important only because they arise in the same locations in the colorectum and in the same age groups as do neoplastic polyps. Removal is indicated only for histologic diagnosis. Distinction between adenomatous and hyperplastic polyps is usually easy. Differential features are summarized in Table 28-3.

ADENOMATOUS POLYPS

INCIDENCE. This is by far the most common neoplasm of the colon and rectum. Adenomatous polyps, except with familial polyposis, are rare under age twenty-one, and then the incidence gradually increases with age throughout life, perhaps indicating that the lesions do not spontaneously regress. The incidence in adults is variously reported as from 1 to 50 percent. There are several possible explanations for this great variation. Some writers include any and all lesions that are elevated above the surrounding mucosa, so that hyperplastic polyps and lymphoid polyps are counted. Others have reported only lesions found at sigmoidoscopy or on barium enema. The best available estimate is that about 5 percent of adults harbor at least one adenomatous polyp in the colon or rectum. There is also considerable variation in reports on the distribution of polyps within the different segments of the colon and rectum. In clinical studies, based on sigmoidoscopy and

Table 28-3. DIFFERENTIAL FEATURES OF ADENOMATOUS AND HYPERPLASTIC POLYPS

	Adenomatous polyp	Hyperplastic polyp
A. Tinctorial quality	Basophilic	Acidophilic
B. Glands per unit area	Greater than normal	Similar to normal
C. Cell number	Marked increase	Moderate increase
D. Papillary infolding of epithelium	Usually absent; gland lumen has smooth tubular profile	Present; lumen appears sawtooth, corkscrew, stellate
E. Cell crowding	Marked; narrowed, pencil-shaped cells	Minimal
F. Nuclei	Crowded, elongated, hyperchromatic	Inconspicuous, vesicular, basal
G. Cell types	Often only one type at any random level of adenomatous tubule	Usually two types: near-surface, absorptive cells adjacent to mature or distended goblet cells
H. Secretion	Unpredictable; may be absent; may be abundant, even in depth of tubule	Uniformly present in all tubules; generally most marked in upper one-half of gland
I. Over-all mitotic activity	Usually increased	Usually increased
J. Mitotic activity in:		
Surface	May be present	Absent
Neck and mouth of crypt	May be maximal	Absent
Midportion of crypt	Present	May be present
Depth of crypt	Present	Present
K. Thickness of basement membrane (collagen and mucopolysaccharide)		
Surface	Less than normal	Greater than normal
Depth of crypt	Minimal	Minimal

SOURCE: From Lane, Kaplan, and Pascal, 1971.

barium enema, about 73 percent are in the rectum, rectosigmoid, and lower sigmoid within reach of the sigmoidoscope; 20 percent in the middle and upper sigmoid; 3 percent in the descending colon; 2 percent each in transverse and ascending colon. In autopsy studies, only 27 percent are found in the rectum and sigmoid, 11 percent in descending colon, 25 percent in transverse colon, and 37 percent in cecum and ascending colon.

PATHOLOGY. Adenomatous polyps are usually pedunculated firm tumors varying from 1 mm to several centimeters in diameter. Two-thirds are less than 1 cm. The bulbous head is irregularly lobulated. Microscopically, the vascular connective tissue stalk is covered by mucosa that appears to be an extension of the normal adjacent mucosa, suggesting that the stalk is not part of the neoplasia but rather a pedicle pulled out by traction exerted on the polyp by peristalsis. The microscopic characteristics are summarized in Table 28-3. About 15 percent of polyps demonstrate villous elements as well as the adenomatous or tubular architecture. The frequency of the villous admixture increases with the size of the polyp. Not infrequently, circumscribed areas of adenomatous polyps demonstrate the cytologic criteria of malignancy, i.e., marked pleomorphism and atypia of glands and cells, hyperchromatism, and frequent mitoses. This is carcinoma in situ. Truly invasive cancer can be diagnosed only if definite invasion beneath the muscularis mucosae is demonstrated. True invasion of the stalk or base by malignant glands is extremely rare; apparent invasion of the stalk may be seen when oblique sectioning of a polyp appears to project glands into the submucosa while actually they lie above the muscularis mucosae. Serial sectioning is necessary to clarify this pseudoinvasion.

CLINICAL MANIFESTATIONS. Adenomatous polyps may produce symptoms such as hematochezia, bleeding per rectum, anemia, prolapse of polyp through the anus, and, rarely, intussusception. Much more commonly they are asymptomatic and are an incidental finding by sigmoidoscopy, colonoscopy, or barium enema. Treatment is discussed below under Malignant Potential of Colorectal Polyps.

VILLOUS ADENOMA

These polypoid lesions, also called *papillary adenomas,* are so named because of their characteristic frondlike projections. The separation of villous adenomas from adenomatous polyps was first made in 1948 because of the marked difference in malignant propensity of the two lesions. It is now thought by many that they represent different points on the spectrum of abnormal cell division in the colonic mucosa.

INCIDENCE. Villous adenomas are found with about one-eighth the frequency of adenomatous polyps and represent from 1 to 3 percent of surgically removed neoplasms of the colon. One institution, however, reported that 10.3 percent of intestinal carcinomas in their material arose in villous tumors. About 60 percent of villous adenomas arise in the rectum, 20 percent in the rectosigmoid, 10 percent in the sigmoid, and 10 percent in all other segments of the colon. The average age of the patients is sixty-three;

for adenomatous polyp, fifty-four. Villous adenoma is rarely seen in patients under age forty-five.

PATHOLOGY. Grossly, villous tumors are poorly demarcated, bulky, broad-based lesions. They are smooth, soft, and velvety, and therefore are difficult to detect by palpation. Areas of firmness usually represent malignancy. On inspection, these polyps may be pale or may be similar in color to adjacent normal mucosa but can be detected because of the numerous characteristic frondlike projections. Microscopically, there are numerous long villous projections with narrow stroma covered by a single layer of cylindrical epithelial cells. The cells are elongated, with nuclei compressed and usually in a basal position, and contain less mucus than normal mucosal cells. The histologic abnormalities that characterize malignancy are often found. If subjacent tissues are included in the section and show invasion, the diagnosis of invasive villous adenocarcinoma is established. Invasive malignancy is present at the time of first treatment in about one-third of patients; cytologic evidence of malignancy but without frank invasion, in another one-third.

CLINICAL MANIFESTATIONS. Presenting symptoms are usually discharge of blood and mucus from the rectum and a feeling of incomplete evacuation. About one-half the patients have some obstruction with constipation and lower abdominal colic. A minority present with an interesting syndrome consisting of passage of numerous watery mucoid stools, severe muscle weakness, and weight loss. This is attributable to the secretion of very large quantities, i.e., up to 3 liters/day, of electrolyte-rich mucus by the tumor. Serum electrolyte determinations reveal a severe hypokalemia and hypochloremia, and often hyponatremia and uremia. Heroic therapy of this severe desalting water loss is necessary to prepare for operation. One writer has given as much as 1,000 mEq of potassium chloride daily, orally and parenterally, in order to restore normal values.

Diagnosis can be made in over 80 percent by sigmoidoscopy because of the usual fortuitous location of villous tumors. Several biopsies should be taken from several areas of the tumor including the base at the junction with "normal" colon in an attempt to establish histologically whether invasive cancer is present. Lesions above the sigmoidoscope can usually be seen on barium enema. They produce an irregular filling defect with wrinkled margins due to penetration of barium between the villous projections. Some alteration in shape is noted during compression or on the postevacuation film. Colonoscopic diagnosis has the advantage that the lesion can be biopsied.

TREATMENT. The operative procedure is determined by the location and size of the tumor and whether invasive malignancy is present. Colonoscopic removal is indicated for small tumors without invasive malignancy above the peritoneal reflection. Anterior resection is indicated for large tumors and for tumors of any size with demonstrated invasive malignancy located more than 7 cm above the dentate line. With lesions in the rectum proper, i.e., less than 7 cm above the dentate line, a combined abdominoperineal resection is done for those lesions with invasive cancer proved by biopsy. When invasive cancer is not demonstrable on biopsy, the lesion is locally completely excised after wide dilatation or division of the anal sphincter. The entire specimen is examined histologically. If invasive malignancy is not found, nothing further is done, but with demonstrable *invasive* malignancy, immediate abdominoperineal resection should be done. Frequent follow-up proctoscopy is mandatory after local excision; recurrence is common even though the lesion is histologically benign.

FAMILIAL POLYPOSIS

INCIDENCE AND PATHOGENESIS. This is a rare hereditary disease characterized by the appearance, early in life, of large numbers of adenomatous polyps in the colon and rectum. If untreated, it is almost invariably fatal because of carcinoma of colon or rectum. Estimates of the incidence vary from 1 in 8,300 live births to 1 in 29,000.

The mode of inheritance is not clear, though much of the evidence suggests a single dominant pleiotropic gene with variable penetrance. Males and females are equally affected, and either may transmit the disease. Marriage between a heterozygote (affected) and a homozygote (unaffected) results in one-half the children being affected, and only those who have inherited polyposis can transmit it to the next generation. Solitary, nonfamilial cases are probably a manifestation of gene mutation; these individuals can transmit the disease. The severity of the polyposis coli and the liability to carcinoma vary considerably in different families.

Colonic polyps are probably not present at birth but usually start appearing at about age thirteen, then appear with increasing frequency, until by about age twenty-one the entire colon and rectum are carpeted by hundreds—even thousands—of polyps ranging in size from 1 mm to several centimeters. The small bowel is not involved. The distal segments of the colon and the rectum are involved initially, and the polyps are mostly sessile in younger patients with a shift to pedunculated forms later. Though the above is the usual pattern, typical familial polyposis has been reported in 75 patients under age fourteen with the youngest a thirteen-month-old infant. The incidence of carcinoma in this group was 6.6 percent. Carcinoma of the colorectum will develop in essentially 100 percent of patients with familial polyposis unless treated or unless death from another cause supervenes. If untreated, most die of carcinoma before age fifty. The average age of death from cancer of the large bowel is 41.5 years, compared with 68 years of age for death from cancer of the large bowel in the general population. Cancer associated with familial polyposis is often multiple and presumably of multicentric origin.

Microscopically the polyps are adenomatous polyps that appear in no way different from the common adult-type single adenomatous polyp. Villous elements mixed with adenomatous glands—"intermediate" or "mixed" polyps—are seen, but true villous tumors are very rare.

It is logical to assume that carcinoma in familial polyposis arises in one of the myriad of adenomatous polyps; though the malignant potential of each individual polyp is very small, one chance in a thousand, if there are more than a thousand polyps in the colon, cancer is inevitable.

The association of polyps and cancer does not necessarily indicate a polyp-cancer sequence but may represent varying degrees of genetically dominated large bowel proneness both to cancer and to adenoma, so that an increased propensity to one may be reflected by an increased proclivity for the other.

CLINICAL MANIFESTATIONS. Symptoms may be absent or consist only of vague intermittent abdominal discomfort. In some, the first symptoms may be those of colorectal carcinoma. More commonly, however, rather marked symptoms develop consisting of frequent bouts of abdominal pain, passage of loose, blood-stained stools and much mucus, weight loss, anemia, and general debility. Occasionally, large polyps may prolapse through the anus, causing symptoms of intestinal obstruction, partial or complete, or initiate intussusception. Diagnosis is apparent on sigmoidoscopy and barium enema. Biopsy of one of the polyps, with histologic examination, should be done to be sure one is not dealing with multiple juvenile polyps. Any lesion in the rectum suspected of being malignant is also biopsied.

TREATMENT. If carcinoma is found in the rectum and is determined to be operable, total abdominal colectomy, abdominoperineal resection of rectum and anus, and terminal cutaneous ileostomy are done. Otherwise total abdominal colectomy with ileoproctostomy is usually done. After recovery from the operation, all polyps in the rectum are removed through the proctoscope, and the base is fulgurated. Proctoscopy at frequent intervals with removal of any polyps nearly always adequately controls the rectal polyposis. There are several reports of spontaneous regression of rectal polyps following subtotal colectomy. Some surgeons advise total coloproctectomy and cutaneous ileostomy for all patients with familial polyposis because of the possibility of cancer developing in the rectal stump.

The prognosis for patients with familial polyposis in whom invasive carcinoma of the colorectum develops is not good: the 5-year survival is probably about 20 percent compared to 40 percent for idiopathic colorectal carcinoma.

GARDNER'S SYNDROME

This inheritable disease, even more rare than familial polyposis, is characterized by polyposis coli, plus any combination of osteomas or exostoses, principally of the mandible, skull, and sinuses; multiple epidermoid or sebaceous cysts; desmoid tumors, principally in abdominal incisions; and postoperative mesenteric fibromatosis. The associated manifestations may appear before polyposis is present.

The intestinal polyposis pattern is somewhat different in Gardner's syndrome and familial polyposis. The colon polyps are more scattered in Gardner's syndrome, and polyps may occur also in the small bowel. Polyps may not develop in Gardner's syndrome until after age thirty or even forty years. The age of onset of colorectal cancer is also later in life. Possibly because of this, cancer has been found in only 36 percent of reported cases.

Gardner's syndrome is rather definitely thought to be determined by a single pleiotropic gene, transmitted as an autosomal dominant. This gene is thought to be distinct from that determining familial polyposis, but it is possible that it is all one syndrome with variable expressivity, and that patients with familial polyposis simply do not have the extracolonic abnormalities expressed. The Turcot syn-

Fig. 28-8. *A.* The normal colonic mucosa has a simple structure. There are no villi—only simple test tube glands (crypts of Lieberkühn). They contain fully differentiated goblet and absorptive cells. Cell division (shown in heavy shading) is restricted to the deepest third of the gland. *Mm,* muscularis mucosa; *Sm,* submucosa. *B.* In the hyperplastic polyp, excess cell production leads to crowding of cells, with resultant papillary infoldings of the epithelium. Full differentiation to goblet and absorptive cells also occurs. This combination of features imparts a distinctive and readily recognizable microscopic pattern. A key point indicating that this is a hyperplastic rather than a neoplastic process is that cell division remains restricted to the lower portion of the crypt (shaded area). *C.* In the adenomas, cell division is unrestricted, so that mitotic activity is observed at all levels of the adenomatous tissue (shaded area). This uncontrolled cell production elongates the crypts and, with further proliferation, leads ultimately to adenomas of all sizes and shapes. The unrestricted replication plus failure of orderly differentiation into mature goblet and absorptive cells indicate the neoplastic nature of this process. The resulting characteristic microscopic appearance of an adenoma is readily distinguishable from that of a hyperplastic polyp.

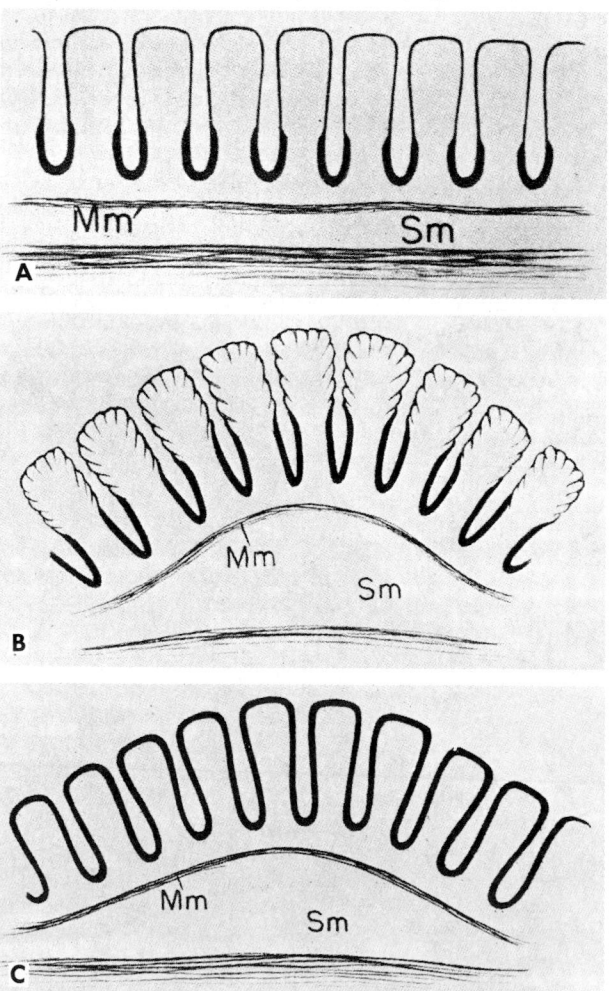

drome—central nervous system tumors and polyposis coli—may also be a variation of Gardner's syndrome.

The extraintestinal abnormalities of Gardner's syndrome are managed as they would be if they were idiopathic lesions. The treatment of the intestinal polyposis is essentially the same as outlined for familial polyposis.

MALIGNANT POTENTIAL OF COLORECTAL POLYPS

The hazard of malignancy in villous adenomas, familial polyposis, and Gardner's syndrome is clearly established, as described above, and generally accepted. Until 1958, it was nearly unanimously agreed that adenomatous polyps were also premalignant lesions. In 1958, Spratt and associates evaluated the evidence and concluded that "the theory of the origin of adenocarcinomas of the colon within adenomatous polyps has little to support it." Since then there has been a continuing vigorous controversy concerning the role of adenomatous polyps. Published conclusions have ranged from "Probably no benign process exists in which a greater incidence of malignant change occurs than that seen in colonic polyps. Eventually, 100 percent of these lesions become malignant" to "The adenomatous polyp is a lesion of negligible malignant potential."

Part of the difficulty is inherent in the available methods of study. It is impossible to examine a given tissue by present techniques without destroying its viability. A tissue that is excised, fixed, stained, and sectioned does not live out its natural course and disclose its destiny. Histologic examination of a polyp reveals only the situation obtaining at a given point in its development and maturation. Therefore what might have happened if the polyp had been left in place can only be surmised.

Studies of normal and abnormal cell division in the colonic mucosa have explained to the satisfaction of many investigators the natural history of neoplastic polyps. In the normal mucosa, cell division is restricted to the deepest one-third of the crypts of Lieberkühn (Fig. 28-8*A*). As the cells migrate up the crypt toward the surface, they differentiate into mature goblet and absorptive cells and after a life-span of 3 or 4 days are exfoliated from the free mucosal surface. Normally exfoliation just balances cell division. If exfoliation is slowed or cell division increased, cells will accumulate locally and form a protrusion. Both mechanisms are involved in the formation of a hyperplastic polyp.

In hyperplastic polyps there is a minor imbalance in the cycle of cell renewal. Cell division in the crypts is slightly expanded, but complete differentiation into goblet and absorptive cells occurs as the cells migrate to the surface (Fig. 28-8*B*). Migration of the cells is slower than normal, and desquamation from the surface is also delayed, leading some to call these polyps *hypermaturation* or *senescent* polyps. It is clear that these are not neoplastic lesions—cell division occurs only in its normal location, and there is complete cellular differentiation.

In neoplastic polyps, cell division is no longer restricted to its normal locus in the depths but is found at all levels in the crypts and on the mucosal surface as well (Fig. 28-8*C*). Cell differentiation into mature goblet and absorptive cells is incomplete. These are two of the hallmarks of neoplasia:

unrestricted cell division and incomplete cell differentiation.

The above-described mechanisms have been well worked out for adenomatous polyps. It is probable that villous adenomas arise in the same way, though there is much less evidence for this at present. Possible growth patterns are diagramed in Fig. 28-9.

There is still no agreement on the potential of adenomatous polyps to become carcinomatous. Morson says it is 5 percent; Grinnell and Lane, 2.9 percent; and Ackerman, from 0.2 to 0.8 percent. There is general agreement on the factors that correlate with incidence of malignancy in neoplastic polyps, however. These are size, histologic type, and epithelial atypia. Only 1 percent of adenomatous polyps under 1 cm are malignant; this rises to 10 percent for 1- to 2-cm polyps. Three histologic types are recognized: adenomatous polyp or tubular adenoma, villous adenoma, and an intermediate type which has an admixture of both. The malignancy rate for adenomatous polyps (all sizes) is about 5 percent; for villous adenomas, about 35 percent; and for the intermediate type, about 20 percent. Epithelial atypia is graded into mild, moderate, and severe. As might be expected, mild atypia is common in small adenomatous polyps and severe atypia in large villous adenomas.

Two clinical studies have shed some light on the polyp-cancer problem. Knoernschild followed the course of 213 patients with asymptomatic benign polyps by serial proctosigmoidoscopy for 3 to 5 years. A cytologic smear from the surface of the lesion was taken each time and the site of the lesion identified by a permanent tattoo mark. He showed that 18 percent of the lesions completely disappeared, 8 percent decreased in size, 70 percent showed no change, and 4 percent increased in size. Two polyps developed into histologically proved invasive carcinoma.

Gilbertsen has evaluated the role of proctosigmoidoscopy and polypectomy in reducing the incidence of lower bowel cancer. Over 18,000 patients participated in this 25-year study. During the years of the study, statistically 75 to 80 cancers could have been expected; only 11 were found.

It seems obvious that neoplastic polyps do become cancerous and so should be removed if this can be done safely. Colonoscopy has revolutionized the management of colonic polyps. In times past all polyps within reach of the sigmoidoscope were removed. Those above the reach of the scope were watched if they were less than 1.2 cm in diameter, since the risk of the operation was greater than the risk of cancer. Colonoscopic polypectomy can be done with a mortality of about 0.1 percent, a colonic perforation rate of 1 to 2 percent, and a serious hemorrhage rate of 2 to 4 percent. The most experienced colonoscopists report mortality-morbidity figures well below these levels. Large lesions and invasive carcinoma, whatever the size, should be removed at laparotomy after diagnosis is established by colonoscopic biopsy.

Carcinoma of the Colon and Rectum

INCIDENCE. Cancer of the colon and rectum is now the most common visceral cancer in the United States, exceeded in frequency only by skin cancer. In 1977, in about 101,000 Americans a diagnosis of colonic or rectal cancer was made for the first time, as mentioned earlier, and 51,300 died of the disease—13.3 percent of all cancer deaths. Lung cancer, with 98,000 cases in 1977, is the leading cause of cancer deaths in the United States, with 89,000 deaths in 1977, because the results of treatment of lung cancer are even poorer than the results for colorectal cancer. Cancer of the stomach, formerly the most common internal cancer and the leading cause of cancer deaths, has shown a steady significant unexplained decrease in incidence in both sexes since the early 1930s. Carcinoma of the lung has shown a steady increase in incidence in both sexes probably due to cigarette smoking. Colorectal carcinoma has shown a slight decrease in frequency in both sexes.

Females are affected by colonic cancer more than males in a ratio of 1.2:1; the sex ratio is reversed for rectal cancer with males predominating 1.1:1. Colorectal carcinoma is usually a disease of older persons with the peak incidence in the seventh decade. About 8 percent of colorectal cancers are diagnosed before age forty, however, and the disease is seen before age twenty, particularly in association with familial polyposis.

Fig. 28-9. Mechanism of carcinogenesis appears to involve induction of cell division in cells of the surface epithelium. Proliferating cells are seen on the periphery rather than in the depths of the crypts, indicating a centrifugal growth pattern. Increasing numbers of cells accumulate on the advancing edge of the tumor, but since not all are dividing at the same rate, lobulations may form and the same carcinogenic agent may produce different gross tumor forms, depending on the number of cells affected. A few cells protruding into the lumen could become pedunculated, but if a broad area is affected, a villous papilloma may develop.

ETIOLOGY. Colorectal carcinoma develops in patients affected by familial polyposis, Gardner's syndrome, villous tumors, and chronic ulcerative colitis. The extent of the contribution of adenomatous polyps is still speculative. Genetic factors have been suggested because of a very high incidence of colorectal cancer in some families, but no convincing evidence for the hereditary transmission of the disease can be found in the vast majority. There are striking variations in the incidence of colorectal cancer in different parts of the world; the rate is very low in sub-Saharan Africa, low in Japan, and very high in the United States. Studies of migrant populations indict environmental factors, since colon cancer mortality in migrants shifts from the rate characteristic of the country of origin and tends to rise to the rate characteristic of their adopted country. Some epidemiologic data suggest a correlation between a high intake of fats and cancer of the colon. Metabolic products of bile acids or cholesterol are known to be carcinogenic in animals and are known to be degraded in the colon by certain bacteria, particularly a group of *Clostridia* and bacteroides. Populations with a high fat intake have a colonic bacterial flora of the type that metabolizes bile acids, and an increased fecal excretion of bile acid metabolites.

Burkitt has also implicated diet in the etiology of several colonic diseases. He has pointed out that rural blacks in Africa eat a diet of raw fruits and vegetables and unrefined grains, and produce large bulky stools with a rapid transit time. They have a very low incidence of polyps, cancer, and diverticulosis. Whites living in England consume a diet consisting largely of processed and refined foods and have much smaller stools and slower transit time. The English have a high incidence of polyps, cancer, and diverticulosis.

Recent animal studies tend to support the idea that ingestion of carcinogenic substances may be responsible for induction of colorectal cancer. Adenomatous polyps and adenocarcinoma of the colon can regularly be produced in laboratory animals by the administration of 4-aminobiphenyl derivatives or 1,2-dimethylhydrazine derivatives including the plant product cycasin.

PATHOLOGY. Carcinomas of the colon and rectum occur with different frequencies in the various segments of the colon. The relative segmental distribution is cecum, 11 percent; ascending colon, 9 percent; transverse colon, 12 percent; descending colon, 6 percent; sigmoid, 26 percent; rectosigmoid, 11 percent; and rectum, 25 percent. Thus 62 percent of colorectal cancer is found in the distal colon and rectum, with 25 percent of all cancers within reach of the examining finger and 50 percent within reach of the sigmoidoscope. A second or even a third primary colon carcinoma, either synchronously or metachronously, occurs in about 4 percent of patients with colorectal carcinoma. The incidence is higher in familial polyposis coli. Extracolonic malignant tumors also occur with increased frequency in patients with colorectal cancer.

Grossly, colorectal carcinomas are described as polypoid, nodular, ulcerating, scirrhous, or colloid. More than one descriptive term is often necessary, such as ulcerated, nodular carcinoma. Bulky exophytic tumors occur principally in the cecum. Colloid, or mucinous, carcinoma, which has a soft gelatinous consistency, occurs in the cecum, ascending colon, and rectum. Nodular and scirrhous tumors may be found anywhere in the colon but are more frequent in the left half. Scirrhous tumors are often associated with an exuberant desmoplastic reaction, as is seen in the napkin-ring lesion; they usually occur in the left colon and often produce obstruction. Gross characteristics do not correlate well with prognosis except for polypoid carcinomas on a stalk, which have a very good prognosis, and the rare linitis plastica type of infiltrating carcinoma, which carries a very poor prognosis.

Microscopically, colon carcinomas resemble the parent tissue in varying degrees, according to the degree of differentiation of the neoplastic cells. In well-differentiated tumors the cells are grouped in acinar clusters simulating normal glands. In poorly differentiated or anaplastic tumors, cells with little or no resemblance to colonic mucosa cells are dispersed in irregular sheets or cords with no suggestion of gland formation. Malignant cells are characterized by pleomorphism; hyperchromatism; large vesicular nuclei of various sizes, shapes, and position in the cytoplasm; and frequent mitoses, often with bizarre configurations. The Broders grading system classifies tumors numerically, based on increasing degrees of cytologic departure of individual cells from the glandular elements from which they derived. This system is of some value in predicting biologic behavior but does not correlate as well with prognosis as the Dukes system (see below).

Carcinoma spreads by direct extension, by lymphatic or bloodstream dissemination, by gravitational seeding, and by implantation at operation.

The significant extension by continuity is by penetration of the bowel wall. Some intramural extension, principally in the submucosa, may occur but is nearly always limited to less than 4 cm of grossly normal bowel distal to the tumor and 7 cm proximally.

Regional lymph node involvement is the most common form of metastasis in colorectal carcinoma. When carcinoma has extended through the bowel wall, lymph node involvement exceeds 90 percent; with lesions still confined to the bowel wall, the incidence of positive nodes is about 45 percent. Positive nodes are frequently found some distance from the primary site with normal nodes intervening. It is for this reason, rather than possible intramural extension, that long segments of colon are removed with accompanying blood and lymphatic channels in order to offer the best chance of eradicating the disease. The finding of retrograde nodal metastases due to lymphatic block in the normal drainage area is a grave prognostic sign; the 5-year survival rate is essentially zero.

Hematogenous metastases occur when tumor cells invade venous channels. The usual route is via the portal system to the liver. Lung and bone are next most frequently involved by metastasis, with cells reaching them either by passage through the liver into the inferior vena cava or by extension of tumor into tissues drained by systemic veins. Circulating tumor cells may be detected in the blood of some cancer patients, but the technique has not proved to be of significant value clinically either to diagnose malignancy or predict prognosis. The technique is hampered by the great difficulty in distinguishing between tumor cells and benign nucleated cells that are found normally in the bloodstream.

Gravitational metastases occur when the carcinoma has penetrated the bowel to involve the serosal surface; cells may become detached and seeded to distant points in the peritoneal cavity. Eventually peritoneal carcinomatosis results. Early sites of involvement by seeding are omentum and the rectovesical or rectouterine pouches with production of Blumer's shelf. Another frequent site is the ovary, occasionally resulting in large bilateral Krukenberg tumors. Bilateral oophorectomy should be a part of operations for colorectal cancer unless definitely contraindicated.

Recurrence after operations for carcinoma of the colorectum is frequently at or near the anastomosis even though the operation was considered to be curative and the cut ends of the resected specimen were histologically free of tumor. Recurrence is attributed to implantation of malignant cells spilled at operation. Newer operative techniques attempt to minimize this unfortunate complication.

The Dukes classification of colorectal cancer as modified by Astler and Coller is based on the extent of the malignant process and predicts prognosis reasonably well. It is particularly valuable to the surgeon, since he can perform the appropriate operation for the individual on the basis of findings at the operating table, which is not possible with grading systems based on gross configuration or degree of cellular dedifferentiation of the cancer. Dukes typing at the operating table is an approximation; final classification is done on the permanent histologic sections: Dukes type A, lesion confined to mucosa; type B-1, lesions extending into, but not through, muscularis propria, negative lymph nodes; type B-2, lesions penetrating the muscularis propria, negative nodes; type C-1, lesions limited to the wall, positive nodes; type C-2, lesions through all layers, positive nodes. There should also be added a type D, lesions with distant, unresectable metastases (liver, lung, spine).

Size of primary tumor does not correlate well with either incidence of metastasis or survival. Grinnell found a 23 percent incidence of metastasis from cancers 1.5 to 2.9 cm in diameter. The incidence rose to a peak of 53 percent in the 5 to 6.9-cm range and then decreased somewhat in larger tumors. Spratt and Ackerman found that single cancers of the colon are associated with the same frequency of metastasis to regional nodes whether they measure 2 to 3 cm in diameter or 7 to 12 cm in diameter. They also found that survival is independent of size with cancers larger than 1.5 cm in diameter. They made two significant observations: (1) even the very large colonic cancers are curable with a frequency comparable to that of small tumors provided that a circumscribing resection including contiguously involved organs together with the perirectal and mesocolic lymph nodes can be performed, and (2) the limited resection of a small invasive cancer is unwarranted, because 30 percent of the cancers of 3.12 cm diameter or smaller had lymph nodal metastases.

Despite advances in methods of diagnosis and techniques of treatment, the mortality rate in colorectal cancers has declined only very modestly over the past three decades. The chief cause of failure to achieve cure is presumed to be the occurrence of distant metastases beyond the area accessible to resection before the time of diagnosis and treatment. It is usually stated that the answer to the problem is earlier diagnosis—detection of malignant tumors prior to symptoms or signs which herald their presence. How much earlier would be early enough? When do distant metastases occur? How long are colon cancers present before they can be detected? Welin and associates determined the doubling time of colon tumors by serial barium enema radiography and found doubling times of colon cancer to range from 139 to 1,155 days. This probably gives a false impression, however, of the growth rate throughout the life of the tumor. The growth of microscopic tumors is thought to proceed exponentially until the tumor size approaches the limitations of nutrition, at which time apparent deceleration of net growth occurs. The doubling time of pulmonary metastases from colonic cancer may more closely reflect the true growth rate, since tumor necrosis is much less in the metastases than is often found in the primary growths. When the series of Welin et al. and of Collins were combined, the doubling time ranged from 34 days to infinity with a mean doubling time of 109 days. A minimum of 30 doublings is required for a single $10\text{-}\mu$ malignant colonic mucosa cell to become a tumor 1 cm in diameter—the minimum size that can be detected clinically. Assuming a doubling time of 109 days, a 1-cm tumor would have been growing for over 9 years before detection as a small "early" cancer. Even the fastest growing tumor with a doubling time of 34 days would have been present for $2\frac{1}{2}$ years. The 1-cm nodule is small but not early. Tumors with long doubling times permit uncured patients to live clinically free of evidence of the disease and to contribute to "survival" figures.

CLINICAL MANIFESTATIONS. Symptoms of colorectal carcinoma depend on several factors including the anatomic location of the lesion, its size and extent, and the presence of complications such as obstruction, hemorrhage, or perforation. Some carcinomas are detected while patients are asymptomatic as part of a routine sigmoidoscopic and barium enema examination. Carcinomas arising in the right colon, left colon, and rectum produce characteristic, somewhat different symptom complexes.

The caliber of the cecum and ascending colon is about $2\frac{1}{2}$ times that of the left colon, and the fecal content is fluid. Thus obstructive symptoms are unusual despite the bulky polypoid lesions that are the most common type of tumor in this site. Dull, nagging, persistent right lower quadrant pain is frequent, as are symptoms of anemia. These include pallor, easy fatiguability, weakness, dizziness, dyspnea on exertion, and cardiac palpitation. Anorexia, indigestion, and weight loss are often presenting complaints. A mass in the right side of the abdomen is the first sign of disease in about 10 percent of patients with right colonic cancer. Obstructive symptoms are uncommon but do occur, particularly with hepatic flexure lesions. Severe symptoms such as excessive weight loss, cachexia, jaundice, and hepatomegaly usually imply far advanced cancer.

For purposes of grouping the symptom complexes of colorectal cancer, the left colon is considered to extend from the hepatic flexure to the rectosigmoid. The caliber of the lumen is smaller and the fecal content more solid in the left colon than the right. Cancers in the left colon are usually of the scirrhous or annular type, so that obstructive symptoms predominate. A change in bowel habits may be the first symptom noted with a progressive decrease in the caliber of the stools. Blood and mucus are seen in or on the stool. Severe anemia is uncommon but if present portends a poor prognosis. Tumors of the transverse colon and splenic flexure tend to invade adjacent structures. With gastric involvement, gastrocolic fistula may result. Complete intestinal obstruction may be the presenting picture in some patients.

Passage of bright red blood, often with mucus, is the most common symptom of rectal cancer. Since it frequently is the only symptom, the bleeding is often incorrectly attributed to hemorrhoids. With low rectal lesions there is often tenesmus and a feeling of incomplete evacuation. Obstructive symptoms are uncommon because of the large caliber of the rectal ampulla. Mild abdominal cramping may occur, but severe rectal pain usually means extensive local disease.

Examination of the abdomen of patients with colorectal cancer may disclose a palpable mass, extension to or involvement of the abdominal wall, umbilical metastasis, hepatomegaly, ascites, and a caput medusae. The general physical examination should include a thorough search for distant metastasis. If questionably involved nodes are found, they should be excised for histologic examination.

Digital examination of the rectum and sigmoidoscopy are done sequentially. If a rectal lesion is suspected, no preparation is indicated; for higher lesions, the colon is prepared as described later in this chapter. Carcinoma is usually easily diagnosed on digital examination because of the characteristic hard, rough, irregular surface. If no lesion is felt, the patient is asked to strain to bring higher lesions against the examining fingertip. Proctosigmoidoscopy is then done to the full length of the scope if possible. An adequate biopsy should be obtained from all suspicious lesions seen. Colitis cystica profunda may be confused with invasive carcinoma of the rectum, since mucus-filled glandular structures are seen microscopically in and below the muscularis. This rather rare entity, thought to be inflammatory but in any event not carcinomatous, occurs in a generalized form throughout the colon and in a localized form in the rectum.

DIAGNOSTIC STUDIES. Barium enema radiographic examination or colonoscopy is done next even though a lesion has been found on sigmoidoscopy, inasmuch as other lesions such as multiple polyps or a second primary tumor may be present at a higher level. Repeated examinations using air-contrast studies and oblique projections may be necessary. The "difficult" areas are the cecum, redundant sigmoid loop, and splenic flexure. A radiograph of a typical sigmoid carcinoma is shown in Fig. 28-7. The criteria for distinguishing carcinoma from diverticulitis are presented on page 1207. Colonoscopy has the advantage that a histologic diagnosis can be made by either biopsy or exfoliative cytology.

Patients with a histologic or clinical diagnosis of colo-

rectal cancer who are not categorically inoperable because of far advanced disseminated metastatic disease require further procedures to attempt to demonstrate any metastatic spread; to evaluate cardiac, pulmonary, and renal status; and to prepare the patient physically and mentally for operative therapy. The work-up should include determinations of serum electrolytes, plasma proteins and A/G ratio, blood urea nitrogen, 2-hour postprandial blood sugar, serum bilirubin, alkaline phosphatase, lactic dehydrogenase, and prothrombin time; radioisotope liver scan; electrocardiogram and radiography of the chest. Intravenous pyelography is done in patients with sigmoid colon lesions or any lesion elsewhere that is suspected of involving the urinary tract. Pulmonary function studies are done if indicated by clinical findings. Hemoglobin and plasma protein deficits are corrected by appropriate transfusion therapy.

TREATMENT. It is imperative that the surgeon have a frank discussion with the patient prior to operation, particularly if a colostomy will have to be done. A former patient who is well rehabilitated after cancer operation with colostomy can be very helpful.

Preoperative Preparation. There is unanimous agreement that preoperative mechanical cleansing of the gastrointestinal tract is important and desirable, and there is beginning to be some consensus on the role of preoperative intestinal antisepsis. Prospective, randomized, double-blind studies by Clarke, Condon, and associates, and by Washington and associates have clearly demonstrated that a preoperative oral antibiotic preparation significantly reduces the risk of septic complications after elective colorectal operations. Pseudomembranous enterocolitis from overgrowth of resistant species was not a problem. Many different antibiotic regimens are in use. One of the most popular consists of neomycin sulfate, 1 Gm, and erythromycin base, 1 Gm, at 1 P.M., 2 P.M., and 11 P.M. the day before operation.

Mechanical cleansing may be accomplished in 2 days unless significant obstruction exists. The patient is placed on a liquid or elemental diet, given a strong oral cathartic on each of two mornings before the operation, and given a saline enema the night before the operation. Nasogastric suction is usually not necessary.

Foley catheter drainage is instituted just prior to operation in all patients with lesions of the sigmoid or rectum. If ureteral involvement is suspected, then ureteral catheters may be inserted prior to operation, though this can be done during the procedure if it becomes necessary. The presence of the catheters facilitates identification of the ureters and thus avoidance of injury to them.

Operative Treatment. The abdomen is first thoroughly explored to determine the extent of intraabdominal spread if any. On the basis of these findings the decision is made as to whether a curative operation should be attempted.

After operability is determined, all lesions of the peritoneal colon are resected by the no-touch isolation technique with primary anastomosis (Fig. 28-10). This technique is designed to minimize hematogenous dissemination of cancers by the trauma of surgical removal. Turnbull and associates have reported a 5-year survival of 61 percent of patients resected for cure by this technique

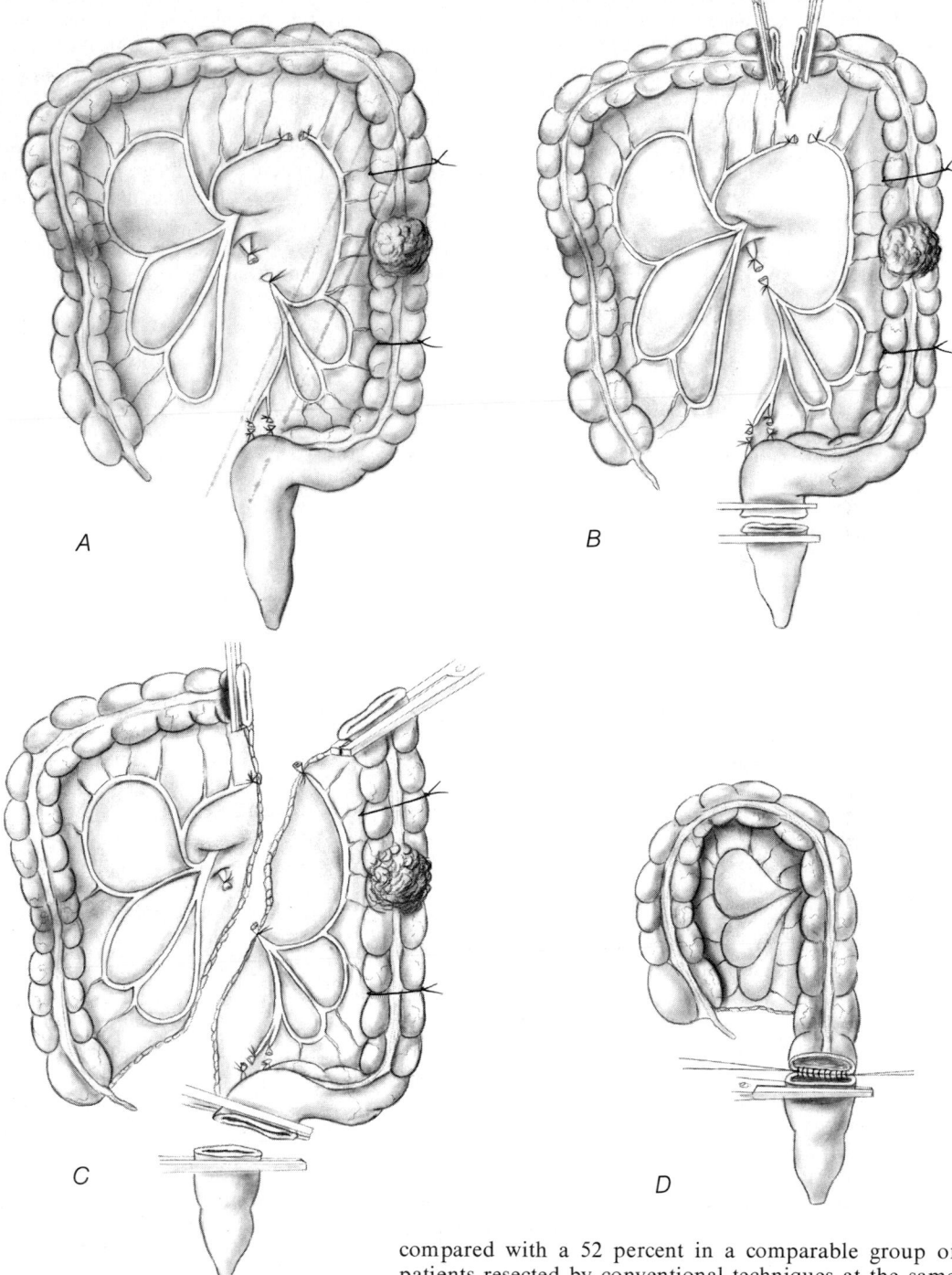

Fig. 28-10. No-touch isolation technique of anterior resection. *A.* Major vascular pedicles are isolated and divided and tapes tied tightly around colon and bowel lumen. *B.* Colon is divided at elected sites of resection. *C.* Cancer-bearing segment is removed last. *D.* End to end anastomosis is made. Posterior row is shown. (*After R. B. Turnbull, R. Kyle, F. H. Watson, and J. Spratt, Ann Surg, 166:420, 1967.*)

compared with a 52 percent in a comparable group of patients resected by conventional techniques at the same clinic. When corrected for age, the 5-year survival rate of the patients of Turnbull and associates is 78 percent.

Recurrences due to implantation may be minimized by the use of closed anastomosis, iodized suture, and copious irrigation of the operative field with saline solution.

Extent of Resection. In an attempt to improve the results of surgical therapy of colonic cancer, there was considerable enthusiasm in the late 1940s and early 1950s for more radical operations. For example, radical left hemicolectomy instead of segmental resection was advised for left colon lesions. In this operation, the inferior mesenteric artery is divided at the aorta, thus achieving a wider resection of the lymph drainage area. The anticipated improvement was not forthcoming. Apparently, when metastases to lymph nodes near the origin of the inferior mesenteric artery has occurred, cancer cells have already spread beyond the reach of surgical procedures. Most surgeons then reverted to the former practice of segmental resection. There is now some renewed interest in wider resections, even subtotal colectomy, prompted by different considerations. First, a significant number of patients will have disease—second primaries, polyps, or diverticula—in segments other than that bearing the primary lesion. Second, Wright and associates found suture line recurrences in only 0.7 percent of patients with ileocolic anastomosis versus a 12 percent rate in patients with colocolic anastomosis. The mechanism is not known but may be related to the disappearance of rectal polyps after ileoproctostomy in patients with familial polyposis.

Now, more than ever, the well-worn cliché that the operation should be appropriate to the individual situation is applicable. The following list of resections applies to the majority of patients; greater or lesser procedures may be indicated in some patients. For cancers arising in the cecum, ascending colon, or hepatic flexure, the resection includes a short segment of terminal ileum, cecum, ascending colon, right half of the transverse colon, and ileocolic, right colic, and right branch of middle colic vessels with accompanying mesentery and greater omentum en bloc. Ileo-transverse colostomy restores gastrointestinal continuity.

Lesions in the mid-transverse colon are segmentally removed with the middle colic vessels. Both flexures must be mobilized to allow anastomosis. For cancers of the distal transverse colon or splenic flexure, the resection includes the transverse and descending colons along with middle colic and left colic vessels. The distal ascending colon is anastomosed to the proximal sigmoid colon. A more conservative resection would leave the right branch of the middle colic artery and join proximal transverse colon to distal descending colon.

For cancers of the descending colon, the segment supplied by the left colic vessels is removed, from distal transverse colon to proximal sigmoid colon.

For cancers of the sigmoid and most proximal rectosigmoid the resection includes distal descending colon, sigmoid and proximal rectosigmoid, with sigmoidal and superior hemorrhoidal vessels. The left colic vessels remain; the inferior mesenteric vessels are skeletonized to remove as much lymphatic tissue as possible. Distal descending colon is anastomosed to rectosigmoid. Mobilization of the splenic flexure may be necessary to be able to bring the ends together without tension. A temporary proximal colostomy or cecostomy is advisable when there is any question about a low anastomosis.

Emergency Operations. When surgical treatment must be carried out on unprepared bowel because of obstruction, perforation, or hemorrhage or when a colorectal cancer is encountered unexpectedly, most surgeons prefer to pro-

ceed with the definitive resection if the lesion is in the right half of the colon. Some surgeons are also doing emergency primary resections of left colon lesions. With lesions of the left half of the colon, most surgeons prefer to resect the lesion and bring both cut ends of the colon out—the proximal as an end colostomy, the distal as a mucous fistula. If the distal end is too short to exteriorize, the Hartmann procedure is used. Proximal diverting colostomy alone is the procedure of choice for obstruction in poor-risk patients. The 5-year survival rate is low in patients with perforating cancers in all segments and in those with obstructing cancers of the right colon.

Palliative Operations. If unresectable metastases preclude curative resection, a palliative resection should be done if the lesion is locally resectable. This does not lengthen survival but greatly improves the quality of survival. If the primary lesion is locally unresectable, a short-circuiting anastomosis around the lesion offers worthwhile palliation. Even a colostomy is usually preferable to death from intestinal obstruction.

Operations for Rectal Carcinoma. There is general agreement that lesions above the posterior peritoneal reflection, which is about 15 cm above the dentate line, can and should be treated by anterior resection with primary anastomosis (Fig. 28-10). There is also general agreement that lesions at or below 5.5 cm in women and 7 cm in men should be treated by the Miles procedure, combined abdominoperineal resection (Fig. 28-11). This is because it

Fig. 28-11. Abdominoperineal resection. *A.* Peritoneal cavity is entered through a paramedian or oblique incision. *B.* Lateral attachment of sigmoid colon is incised, taking care to avoid the ureter. *C.* Medial reflection of transverse mesocolon is incised. Inferior mesenteric artery and vein are transected. *D.* Peritoneal reflection between bladder and rectum is transected, and an anterior plane between these two organs is established. *E.* Posterior dissection is carried out in midline digitally. The finger establishes a plane just anterior to the anterior surface of the sacrum and continues the dissection as far caudad as possible. *F.* The lateral attachment of the rectum, including the middle hemorrhoidal vessels, is transected. These vessels are, at times, of sufficient size to require individual ligatures. G_1. Pelvic floor is reperitonealized. The distal colon and rectum are now caudad to the peritoneal floor. The proximal colon is mobilized so that a colostomy may be established without undue tension. G_2. Sagittal section demonstrating that distal colon resides below reperitonealized pelvic floor. *H.* With the patient in lithotomy position or on his side, the anal orifice is closed with a purse-string suture and a circumferential elliptical incision made in the perianal region. I_1. Dissection carried down to coccyx and the posterior dissection is continued until it communicates with the space anterior to the sacrum which has been established previously transabdominally. The levator muscles are then transected on each side. I_2. Distal colon is brought down into the anal wound and dissection carried between it and the prostate or bladder. *J.* Specimen resected and drain inserted into depth of wound. Multiple Penrose drains may be used, or a Foley catheter may be inserted and the deep tissues closed around it. K_1. Abdominal incision is closed and colostomy brought out through separate stab wounds. K_2. Perineal incision closed with Foley catheter brought out through depth of wound.

The abdominal and perineal portions of this operation may be carried out simultaneously with two teams. The patient is initially positioned on his back with the legs out in stirrups. This approach has resulted in a reduction in operating time and blood loss.

B

AFTER A. FEINBERG

C

A

D

E

is not possible to resect with the promontory 1 cm distal margin of normal tissue, perform an anastomosis, and have rectal continence postoperatively. Though abdominoperineal resection was first done by Czerny in 1883, it was Miles who perfected and popularized the procedure. It is the standard by which all other procedures for rectal cancer must be measured. The principal drawback is of course,

the permanent colostomy. It is also attended by a significant morbidity (see below). A simultaneous abdominal and perineal approach utilizing two surgical teams is widely used in England and is gaining favor in the United States, because it shortens operative time and also decreases blood loss. Abdominoperineal resection in the female should probably include in-continuity resection of the posterior

F

G₁

G₂

H

wall of the vagina, broad ligaments, cul-de-sac, uterus, tubes, ovaries, and cardinal ligaments, because of the abundant lymphatic connections from the rectum to the female genitalia.

Carcinoma of the rectum involving the lower urinary tract should be treated in good-risk patients by complete pelvic exenteration. The preferred procedure is left-sided colostomy and urinary diversion to an ileal segment draining through the right side of the abdomen. The mortality rate is under 20 percent; the 5-year survival rate is 30 percent in those surviving the procedure. Electrocoagulation has been advocated as an alternative to abdomino-perineal resection for low-lying rectal cancer. Madden and Kandalaft have treated 77 patients by this method. The number followed for 5 years is too small to be significant, but earlier results at least equal and may surpass those of resection. Crile and Turnbull have carried on the electrocoagulation studies of Jones. Their 5-year survival rate is 68 percent in 62 patients, compared to 46 percent in a roughly comparable group treated by resection. Mucosal

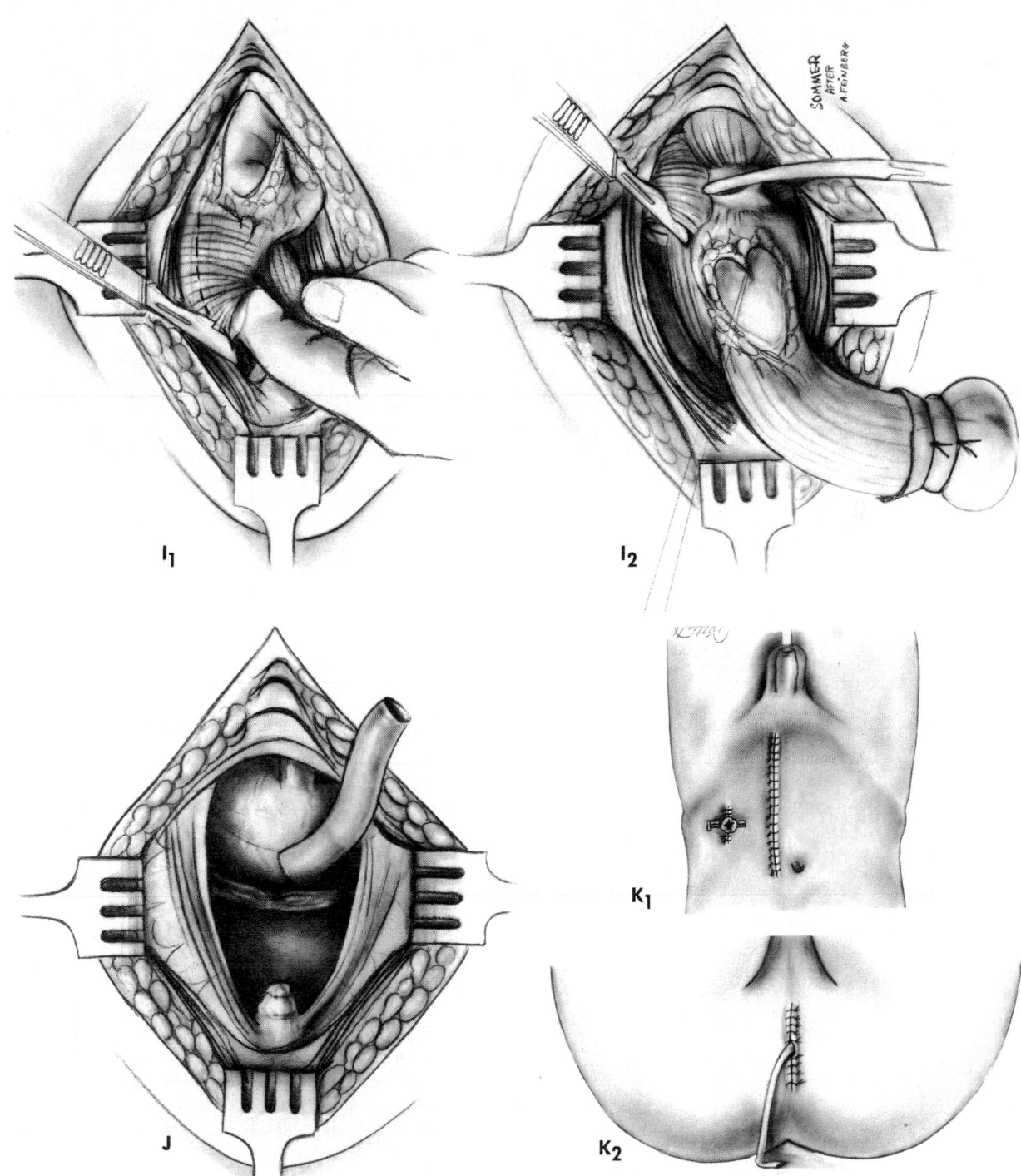

I₁

I₂

J

K₁

K₂

and polypoid lesions are most amenable to electrocoagulation. Annular wall lesions in women should be resected because of the threat of rectovaginal fistula. Similarly, annular lesions are rarely controlled by local treatment, and stricture may result. If repeated electrocoagulation does not control the lesion within 6 months, abdominoperineal resection can still be done with as good prospects of cure as if it had been resected initially.

Radiotherapy administered directly to the lesion through a sigmoidoscope-like device has been used by Papillon. This technique is applicable as definitive therapy in small superficial lesions or as preoperative therapy in more invasive lesions.

The proximal rectum and the rectosigmoid lesions—from about 6 to 15 cm—constitute a gray zone where there is no unanimity of opinion as to the best operative procedure. Many surgeons still prefer abdominoperineal resection, feeling that the alternative procedures do not offer the patient an adequate "cancer operation." Statistical results do not confirm this; in general, the 5-year survival is about the same for low anterior resection and pull-through as for the Miles procedure.

Low anterior resection below the peritoneal reflection is technically difficult, particularly in the narrow male pelvis. The side-to-end technique described by Baker is often technically easier than end-to-end anastomosis. Aside from the technical aspects the principal drawback of low anterior resection is an incidence of anastomotic leak of about 25 percent; thus a proximal decompressing temporary colostomy is often advisable.

The pull-through operation has never attained popularity even though results equal the Miles procedure and permanent colostomy is avoided. A principal drawback is the fact that some patients do not regain fecal continence, and a perineal colostomy is much worse than an abdominal colostomy. Also, a surgeon who does not do a large volume of rectal surgery probably cannot attain the technical proficiency required to perform this procedure with consistent success. The modified Soave and Boley pull-through operation described by Gardner and associates may well prove to be the preferred pull-through technique.

Localio has described a combined approach to midrectal cancer. The abdominal dissection is done as in the Miles procedure. The rectum is then approached through a posterior transacral route. After resection of the lesion, the proximal colon is anastomosed primarily to the distal rectal stump. He has reported on 50 patients, with one operative death, seven anastomotic leaks, and fecal continence in all.

Several randomized, controlled prospective studies are now being conducted to evaluate the usefulness of preoperative radiation therapy in the treatment of carcinoma of the rectum. These studies were stimulated, in large part, by the report of a retrospective analysis of 971 patients who underwent resection for carcinoma of the rectum, one-half of whom had received from 1,200 to 2,000 rads, tissue dose of x-radiation, preoperatively. Patients with Dukes A and B lesions were not benefited; irradiated patients with Dukes C lesions had a 37 percent 5-year survival rate as compared to 23 percent for Dukes C controls. The same authors could not confirm this in a later randomized study.

A cooperative, prospective study by Higgins and collaborators randomized 700 patients with carcinoma of the rectum or rectosigmoid to be given either radiotherapy prior to operation (2,000 to 2,500 rads in 2 weeks) or the operation alone. Five-year survival was 48.5 percent in the radiated group, compared to 38.8 percent in controls. With low-lying lesions requiring abdominoperineal resection, survival was 46.9 in the treated group versus 34.3 percent in the controls. Although suggestive of a treatment benefit, neither finding is statistically significant.

There have been several trials of adjuvant chemotherapy with operation utilizing triethylenethiophosphoramide, 5-fluorouracil, or 5-fluorodeoxyuridine. No significant benefit was shown in any of the trials. Current trials of adjuvant therapy are evaluating combination drug therapy or combined postoperative radiotherapy-chemotherapy.

Mortality and Morbidity. The operative mortality of abdominoperineal resection varies in large reported series from 4 to 20 percent, with a mean of about 8 percent. The mortality of anterior resection is somewhat less, ranging from 2.4 to 20 percent, with a mean of about 5 percent. The morbidity of both procedures is formidable: from 25 to 68 percent for the Miles procedure, and from 15 to 56 percent for anterior resection. Morbidity in anterior resection is inversely proportional to the level at which it is done: the lower the resection, the higher the morbidity. It also correlates with whether or not proximal colostomy is done. Significant urinary tract obstruction or infection occurs in about 35 percent of patients after the Miles procedure, in about 15 percent after anterior resection. Aside from the cardiovascular and pulmonary complications that attend major surgery in this age group, septic complications loom large. The perineal wound is the principal site in the combined procedure, followed by the abdominal incision. Inadvertent perforation during the pelvic dissection contributes to the septic problems. Breakdown of the anastomosis is the principal source of sepsis after anterior resection. The incidence is higher than generally realized. Goligher and associates studied 73 patients in the early postoperative period by digital examination, sigmoidoscopy, and barium enema. Anastomotic dehiscence was detected in 40 percent after high anterior resection and in 69 percent after low anterior resection! Many of these were not serious, but Slanetz and associates had 35 symptomatic leaks in 247 patients after anterior resection—a rate of 17 percent. The use of drains near the anastomosis increases the incidence of dehiscence. Goldstein and Duff found an incidence of 23.1 percent in patients in whom the anastomosis was drained, but only 7.8 percent if no drain was used. Intestinal anastomoses must fulfill three criteria: no tension on the suture line, adequate blood supply, and minimal encroachment on the lumen. Whenever anastomosis is performed under less than ideal conditions, such as in the presence of infection or significant contamination, or low in the pelvis, a proximal decompressing colostomy or cecostomy should be done even though this means that another procedure may be necessary for closure. If anastomotic leak occurs or is strongly suspected, immediate reoperation is often indicated, though minor leaks may close with nonoperative therapy.

Pseudomembranous enterocolitis is an infrequent, serious complication. Preoperative bowel sterilization and systemic broad-spectrum antibiotics increase the hazard of this postoperative complication developing.

Wound complications, i.e., hemorrhage or hematoma, infection, and dehiscence, are fairly frequent. These may be minimized by meticulous hemostasis; changing gowns, gloves, drapes, and instruments before closing the incision; irrigating the wound, layer by layer, with a dilute antibiotic solution; and the use of retention sutures.

Urinary complications occur in at least 35 percent of patients after abdominoperineal resection. Nearly all have difficulty in voiding in the immediate postoperative period. After removal of the retention catheter, residual urine volume after voiding should be determined to make certain the bladder is emptying adequately. Transurethral resection is sometimes required if inadequate voiding persists. Most men are impotent after abdominoperineal resection for carcinoma secondary to injury of the autonomic nerve supply to the genital organs.

PROGNOSIS. The 5-year survival rates following curative resection are essentially the same for all segments of the colon. Rectal cancer has a somewhat lower overall survival rate because of a lower resectable-for-cure rate.

The 5-year survival rate in patients with carcinomas limited to the bowel wall and with no demonstrated metastases is 80 percent. The rate with disease extending through the bowel wall but with no evidence of metastasis is 71 percent. With disease in the bowel wall and lymph node metastases, the rate drops to 32 percent. With disseminated disease, only 1.2 percent live 5 years. Considering all stages of disease together, the absolute 5-year survival rate is 34 percent, and the determinate 5-year survival rate is 40 percent.

The above prognosis figures are from a compilation of published reports. They may be somewhat optimistic because of the human tendency to publish more favorable results.

Recurrent Disease. Since only 30 to 40 percent of patients with colorectal cancer are relieved of the disease by surgical therapy, it follows that 60 to 70 percent have recurrent disease. This is a very trying problem for patient and physician because of the often painful, debilitating, demoralizing symptoms produced by recurrent disease, and the lack of any really effective palliative therapy.

Wangensteen et al. and Griffen and associates have attempted to improve the outlook in colorectal cancer with lymph node metastases by routine abdominal exploration in asymptomatic patients at 6-month intervals. Seven percent of the patients found to have cancer at second-look operations were freed of the disease. However, the operative mortality (by patient) was also 7 percent, and there was often difficulty in detecting residual cancer.

Local recurrence in the bowel, usually at or near the anastomosis, can occasionally be resected with reanastomosis. Unresectable disease should be bypassed if possible; with distal lesions that preclude anastomosis below the lesion, proximal colostomy usually gives worthwhile symptomatic palliation.

The efficacy of the chemotherapeutic agents 5FU, 5FUDR, and methotrexate in the palliation of disseminated colorectal carcinoma has been evaluated by a cooperative group study. The results give small comfort. Requirements for admission to the study were stringent in order to obtain valid results, thus often excluding patients who most needed help. Overall response rate was about 15 percent with some very gratifying remissions. But drug toxicity was a major problem and was seen in 93 percent of the 134 patients with seven fatalities. Furthermore, harm (in addition to fatality) may have been done to some of the 85 percent of the nonresponders. The response rates are just about as good and the toxicity much less on an ambulatory treatment schedule of one dose weekly. Current trials involve multiple drug therapy or combined chemotherapy-radiotherapy.

Metastases from colorectal carcinoma to the liver, too extensive to be resected, have been treated with modest success by chronic infusion of 5FU into the hepatic artery.

Radiation therapy is usually not helpful in treating recurrences, because colorectal carcinomas are only moderately radiosensitive tumors whereas the liver and normal gastrointestinal mucosa do not tolerate radiation very well; anorexia, severe nausea, and diarrhea often result. Radiotherapy, however, sometimes gives good symptomatic relief in localized painful perineal recurrences after abdominoperineal resection and very often relieves pain in solitary skeletal metastases.

EARLY DETECTION. Sixty to seventy percent of persons who develop carcinoma of the colon or rectum will die of the disease. Most investigators agree that it is unlikely that changes in operative technique, chemotherapy, or radiotherapy will lead to a dramatic improvement in prognosis. But there is also agreement that improvement could be attained if presently available treatment modalities could be applied to localized disease, if the diagnosis could be made before clinical symptoms are obvious and the disease far advanced. Routine sigmoidoscopy of asymptomatic patients has been advocated; recent reports, however, are disenchanting. In seven published series, sigmoidoscopic examination of 50,727 asymptomatic patients detected invasive carcinoma in 0.11 percent. The incidence of polyps was 5 to 7 percent. If one holds that polyps have a negligible malignant potential, then it would appear that a yield of 1 cancer per 900 sigmoidoscopies would hardly justify the time, expense, and patient discomfort. If, however, one feels that all polyps will eventually undergo malignant change, then a 5 to 7 percent yield would certainly make the procedure worthwhile. On the basis of currently available evidence the authors feel that the use of sigmoidoscopy as a screening method is unrealistic. It should, however, continue to be done as an essential part of a complete physical examination for all patients over age forty.

Gold and Freedman in 1965 described an antigen present in the serum of patients with colorectal cancer, in extracts of the carcinomas and in fetal colonic mucosa, but absent from extracts of normal colonic mucosa. This carcinoembryonic antigen (CEA) can be detected in serum in the millimicrogram (nanogram) range by radioimmune assay. It was hoped that at last a blood test for colorectal cancer would be available. Gold and Freedman's findings have been confirmed by several groups, but the findings are not specific for colorectal cancer and not invariably positive in all patients with colorectal cancer. The results vary from about 20 percent positive with localized colorectal cancer to 100 percent with advanced metastatic cancer. Cancers of the pancreas, lung, breast, and other areas sometimes give positive results, certain nonneoplastic diseases such as uremia or cirrhosis also give some positive results, and, most significant, there have been some false positives in persons with no detectable disease. Thus the CEA cannot be used as a screening test because of the considerable number of false positives. Its principal use now is to monitor patients who have had a curative resection. Reversion to normal after operation is a hopeful sign that all tumor was removed. A rising CEA titer usually means recurrent disease. Serial determinations are of value in monitoring the efficacy of palliative therapy.

Chemical determination of occult blood in the stool is a simple, inexpensive screening method for lesions involving the gastrointestinal mucosa. If three consecutive stools are negative for occult blood in patients on meat-free, high-residue diets, nothing further need be done. All patients with positive reactions should undergo complete gastrointestinal work-up. Greegor, in a recent study, did stool studies for 900 patients, 5 percent of whom had positive stools. One percent of the entire group had an asymptomatic colon cancer, 2 percent had diverticulosis, and 1 percent had nonmalignant polyps. Greegor feels that every adult should have this screening test annually. The aesthetic problem of having patients bring stool specimens to the office is solved by the use of commercially available test slides that the patients can prepare at home and mail to the office. If properly done, stool examination is a much more realistic screening procedure for gastrointestinal carcinoma than is sigmoidoscopy.

Uncommon Neoplasms of the Colon and Rectum

CARCINOID

These interesting tumors are rare in the colon and uncommon in the rectum, about 2 percent of all gastrointestinal carcinoids occurring in the colon and 17 percent in the rectum. This probably does not represent true frequency, because small asymptomatic lesions are easily found in the rectum by sigmoidoscopy. Carcinoids of the colon and rectum very rarely cause the malignant carcinoid syndrome, which is usually associated with carcinoids of the ileum (Chap. 27).

Carcinoids smaller than 1 cm in diameter in the colon rarely cause symptoms, are very rarely malignant, and, because they are submucosal, rarely can be seen on barium enema. If found incidentally, they may safely be removed by wedge excision. The incidence of invasive malignancy in carcinoids, unlike adenocarcinoma of the colon, correlates well with size. Most carcinoids larger than 1 cm that produce symptoms are malignant, and more than half have nodal metastases at the time of diagnosis. Clinical and radiographic manifestations of symptomatic carcinoids are essentially the same as in adenocarcinoma of the colon. A definitive cancer resection is done if liver metastases are not demonstrable. Worthwhile palliation is often attained in patients with unresectable disease by resection of the primary. Some have lived in relative comfort for many years with residual disease.

Most rectal carcinoids are small, asymptomatic, yellow-gray nodules found incidentally at sigmoidoscopy. Larger lesions may bleed and cause rectal pain. Rectal lesions, unless frankly malignant clinically, should be completely excised transanally with the deep margin extending into the muscularis propria. The diagnosis of malignancy is based on invasion; cytologic criteria are unreliable. If invasive malignancy is found, abdominoperineal resection is indicated.

LYMPHOMA AND LYMPHOSARCOMA

Benign lymphoma occurs in the rectum and rectosigmoid as a polypoid circumscribed proliferation of the lymphoid tissue of the mucosa. These polyps, often mistaken grossly for adenomatous polyps, are generally single, but about 15 percent of patients have two or more. These lesions have no known malignant potential. Simple excision is adequate therapy.

Lymphosarcoma may involve the colon and rectum as part of generalized disease or as the dominant organ in "localized" disease. Reticulum cell and giant follicular lymphosarcoma predominate, though all cell types are seen. Longitudinal extent of involvement varies from a localized tumor to diffuse disease of the entire large bowel. Symptoms are abdominal pain, marked weight loss, and change in bowel habits. An abdominal mass is usually palpable. The radiologic diagnosis is frequently carcinoma unless involvement is extensive. If colonic involvement is part of widespread disease, no surgical therapy is indicated. The colonic lesions respond to irradiation and/or chemotherapy. Disease grossly limited to the bowel should be widely resected along with as much node-bearing mesentery as possible, since nodal involvement is common. The optimal timing for postoperative irradiation is not clear. Some feel that it should be given routinely in the immediate postoperative period; others prefer to wait. If and when the disease recurs, then irradiation therapy is given. The disease is unresectable for cure in the majority of patients, but when it is localized, the 5-year survival rate is about 50 percent.

LEIOMYOMA, LEIOMYOSARCOMA, AND OTHER TUMORS

Leiomyomas and leiomyosarcomas are very rare tumors of the colon and rectum, occurring much less frequently than in the stomach or small intestine. Leiomyomas are more frequent in reported series than their malignant counterpart by a 2:1 ratio. When symptomatic, they cause obstruction and bleeding. Deep ulceration with massive hemorrhage, such as occurs with lesions in the stomach or small intestine, has not been reported in lesions of colon or rectum. So few of these tumors are seen that rules of treatment are not yet formulated. Local excision of leiomyomas and small low-grade leiomyosarcomas is probably sufficient. Frank leiomyosarcomas are usually treated by the same procedures as carcinomas of the same area. The 5-year survival in lesions resected for cure is 30 to 40 percent.

Other rare sarcomas of the colon include rhabdomyosarcoma, fibrosarcoma, and hemangiopericytoma. Rare benign tumors include neurofibroma, eosinophilic granuloma, granular cell myoblastoma, lymphangioma, hemangioma, and lipoma. Their principal importance is that they may be mistaken for malignant lesions and are widely resected needlessly.

ENDOMETRIOSIS

Though not a neoplasm, endometriosis is included in this section because it may simulate cancer of the distal colon. The term *endometriosis* implies the occurrence of endometrial tissue at sites other than the lining of the corpus uteri. Ectopic endometrial tissue is found at the time of pelvic operation in 8 to 20 percent of women between the age of twenty and the menopause. The earliest reported case was in a sixteen-year-old; the oldest was seventy-eight years old. About 25 percent of patients with endometriosis have colonic involvement.

Endometrial ectopia is thought by most to result from influx of endometrial tissue through the fallopian tubes during menstruation. This hypothesis has been questioned, because menstrual endometrium may not be viable tissue—it has not been successfully transplanted. The hypothesis of lymphatic dissemination of endometrial emboli has some adherents. Others believe that serosal cells of the peritoneum, derived from the same embryonic tissue as the endometrium, undergo metaplasia and produce tissue identical with endometrium.

PATHOLOGY. The lesions of endometriosis, grossly and microscopically, essentially are identical to the normal uterine lining. These lesions also menstruate with the uterus, but since there is no cervix to drain off the effluvium, glands and cysts filled with menstrual blood are formed. Rupture of the cysts, with spillage of its irritating contents, produces dense reactive fibrosis. Spillage of viable cells produces new implants and spread of the fibroplastic process.

The frequency of endometrial implants varies with distance from the uterus. Most frequently and most heavily involved are external surface of the uterus, broad ligaments, ovaries, cul-de-sac, rectosigmoid, rectovaginal septum, rectum, and sigmoid colon. Colonic lesions may be a single discrete implant (endometrioma) in or on the wall of the bowel, or involvement may be diffuse and extensive, and completely surround the bowel.

CLINICAL MANIFESTATIONS. Symptoms may be present only at the time of menstruation or, if present throughout the cycle, are exacerbated at or just before the period. More common symptoms include gradually increasing dysmenorrhea, menstrual irregularities, rectal discomfort or pain on defecation, rectal tenesmus, lower abdominal cramps, constipation or diarrhea, abdominal distension, nausea, and dysuria. Less common are rectal bleeding and symptoms of intestinal obstruction, usually partial but occasionally complete. There is increased incidence of infertility in these patients.

Vaginal examination often reveals a general matting and nodular thickening of the pelvic organs. Speculum examination frequently discloses purplish submucosal nodules of varying size, which should be biopsied. Rectovaginal examination often demonstrates the same somewhat tender nodular thickening of the septum. On digital rectal examination, tenderness may be felt anteriorly at the fingertip, representing cul-de-sac lesions. Pelvic and rectal examinations should be repeated at different phases of the menstrual cycle, since cyclic changes in the findings help confirm the diagnosis.

Sigmoidoscopy is usually unrewarding except to note that the procedure causes more discomfort than usual and that intrinsic lesions are absent. It is usually impossible to introduce the sigmoidoscope beyond about 15 cm; some narrowing of the lumen may be seen.

The roentgenographic manifestations of endometriosis of the colorectum are not pathognomonic. Any lesion, benign or malignant, which seeds the pelvic peritoneum can mimic endometriosis. Changes in the rectosigmoid and sigmoid are those of extrinsic pressure with the picture of invasion of the outer layers without mucosal distortion or infiltration. A solitary endometrioma may be indistinguishable from neoplasm, particularly if located in a part of the bowel that is difficult to visualize adequately.

TREATMENT. If symptoms are mild, no treatment is necessary. With more severe symptoms, suppression of menstruation with gradually increasing doses of a combination birth-control pill, given continuously without cycling, for 6 to 9 months usually causes regression of the lesions and relief of symptoms. Exploratory laparotomy is indicated if the clinical evaluation does not exclude the possibility of neoplasm. Bowel resection is very rarely indicated. Solitary endometriomas that encroach on the lumen can be removed by anterior resection. If the disease is so severe and extensive that bowel function is compromised, a temporary colostomy is done and the patient placed on hormonal therapy as outlined above. After regression of lesions, the colostomy is closed. If lesions do not regress satisfactorily, however, then hysterectomy and bilateral salpingo-oophorectomy should be done. Abdominoperineal resection and permanent colostomy are not justified.

VOLVULUS

Volvulus of the colon results from rotation of a segment of bowel about its mesenteric axis sufficient to produce partial or complete obstruction of the lumen. Varying degrees of circulatory impairment of the twisted segment are produced by the twisting of the root of the mesentery and secondarily by progressive distension of the involved loop. Volvulus can occur only in a freely movable segment of bowel with its points of fixation in close approximation and thus is seen principally (90 percent) in the sigmoid colon, less frequently (10 percent) in the cecum. Volvulus of the transverse colon is very rare and usually a complication of megacolon. In the United States, volvulus is the third most common cause of colonic obstruction, is the leading cause of strangulated obstruction of the colon, and accounts for about 4 percent of all colonic obstructions.

Sigmoid Volvulus

A redundant sigmoid loop attached by a narrow mesenteric root is the *sine qua non* of sigmoid volvulus. In Eastern Europe, where volvulus is common, barium studies have shown that the sigmoid redundancy is present at an early age and so is presumed to be a congenital rather than an acquired condition. Congenital megacolon (Hirschsprung's disease), which is due to congenital absence of ganglion cells in the rectosigmoid, may be present in subclinical form throughout life. This probably accounts

Fig. 28-12. Plain film of sigmoid volvulus, showing the greatly distended, horseshoe-shaped sigmoid loop (*right*) and distended cecum and ascending colon (*left*).

for only a small percentage of cases of sigmoid volvulus, however. In some parts of the world, acquired megacolon is a complication of Chagas' disease.

A history of severe chronic constipation can be elicited in nearly all patients with sigmoid volvulus in the United States. Dilatation and lengthening of the chronically distended colon occurs. This is most marked in the sigmoid colon. Chronic constipation of this magnitude and sigmoid volvulus are seen principally in two groups: The first includes patients of any age with severe psychiatric or neurologic diseases, such as parkinsonism; in some series, over one-half of the patients with sigmoid volvulus were inmates of mental institutions. The second group consists of the elderly, more often men than women, many with serious cardiovascular and pulmonary disease attendant upon their advanced age, who are now leading lives of inactivity. It is distinctly uncommon for sigmoid volvulus to occur in a person who leads an active life and who has no serious mental or physical illness.

CLINICAL MANIFESTATIONS. Symptoms of acute sigmoid volvulus are intermittent, cramping lower abdominal pain, progressive marked abdominal distension, complete obstipation, and absence of flatus. Nausea, vomiting, and dehydration occur after several hours. The majority of patients have had similar episodes in the past that spontaneously terminated by passage of large amounts of flatus and stool with relief of pain and distension. Marked abdominal distension and tympany are the most striking

physical findings. Respiratory embarrassment may be present because of extreme distension and elevation of the diaphram. Severe, constant abdominal pain and a shock syndrome usually mean strangulated obstruction.

DIAGNOSTIC FINDINGS. Plain film of the abdomen nearly always shows a spectacularly distended single loop occupying the left half of the abdomen with both ends in the pelvis and the bow at or near the diaphragm (Fig. 28-12.) This was called "bent inner-tube sign" before the advent of tubeless tires. The right half of the abdomen shows variable distension of the colon proximal to the obstruction and of small bowel, depending on the duration of the obstruction. Barium enema radiography is usually not necessary, unless the findings on plain films are atypical. The barium column ends at the level of the distal sigmoid torsion in a pathognomic twisted bird's beak or ace-of-spades deformity.

TREATMENT. General principles of management are discussed in Chap. 24. There are two specific problems in sigmoid volvulus: management of the acute episode and definitive management of the megasigmoid. Until about 1950, preferred management of nonstrangulated volvulus was operative detorsion of the sigmoid loop followed as soon as possible by elective sigmoid resection, because when only detorsion was performed, the volvulus recurred in up to 90 percent of patients. The combined mortality of the two-stage detorsion-resection management was 20 to 30 percent. Primary resection of sigmoid volvulus was tried by some but was attended by a mortality rate of at least 50 percent. Gradually, nonoperative detorsion followed by elective resection has emerged as the preferred management for nonstrangulated sigmoid volvulus. Sigmoidoscopy is done to visualize the site of distal sigmoid obstruction; only rarely is this beyond the reach of the 25-cm scope. If frank mucosal ulceration, or slough, or dark blood are seen, strangulation obstruction is probable, and emergency operative intervention is indicated. But if no signs of strangulation are seen, a well-lubricated long rectal tube is gently advanced via the sigmoidoscope through the obstructing twist into the distended sigmoid loop. Dramatic deflation usually results. (The sigmoidoscopist must be alert, or the result will be dramatic for him too!) The tube is secured in place in the loop by taping to the buttocks and left in place for 2 or 3 days, until bowel function resumes. Patients must be closely watched for signs of gangrenous bowel, which occasionally is present but unrecognized at the time of tube deflation. There is a small but definite risk of perforating the weakened sigmoid wall with the tube. Attempted tube deflation is successful in 80 to 90 percent of patients; the mortality rate is about 2 percent. Elective resection with primary anastomosis should be done as soon as the patient can be properly prepared, preferably within a week or so, because the risk of recurrent volvulus is so great. Not infrequently, the volvulus recurs while the patient is being prepared for elective resection. The mortality rate of elective resection is 8 to 10 percent. This higher rate for elective resection of volvulus than for other colonic problems is chiefly attributable to the age, debility, and concomitant disease that so many of these patients have.

When strangulation of the twisted loop exists or is suspected, emergency operation is required. If strangulation is not found, simple operative detorsion is done, but if strangulation is found, the nonviable bowel must be resected, and the proximal end brought out as a colostomy. When the distal limb is too short to allow exteriorization, a Hartmann procedure is preferred: normal bowel below the nonviable loop is divided, the distal end is oversewn and dropped back. The mortality rate for emergency resection of strangulated sigmoid volvulus is about 50 percent.

Cecal Volvulus

Volvulus of the sigmoid and of the cecum have in common only the pathogenetic mechanism of twisting of a mobile segment of bowel. Their etiology, clinical manifestations, and treatment are quite different.

Hypofixation of the cecum, terminal ileum, and proximal ascending colon is the prerequisite for cecal volvulus. Normally, the attachments to the posterior abdominal wall preclude volvulus. Rotation of the hypermobile cecum, usually 360° or up to 720° around the mesenteric pedicle of the ileocolic artery, produces a closed-loop obstruction. Circulatory impairment of the loop is frequent and occurs early in the course. A second mechanism has been suggested and may play a role in patients with partial intermittent cecal obstruction. This is a simple folding instead of twisting, with the mobile cecum pointing toward the left upper quadrant, producing partial obstruction of terminal ileum proximally and ascending colon distad.

Volvulus of the cecum is seen at all ages but is most frequent in the twenty-five to thirty-five age group.

CLINICAL MANIFESTATIONS. The clinical manifestations are essentially those of acute small bowel obstruction. Onset is rapid and characterized by severe midabdominal colicky pain, nausea, and vomiting, followed by moderate abdominal distension. The pain, intermittent and cramping early, may become a constant, severe burning pain within a few hours. Some gas and feces may be passed after onset of pain as the existing contents of the colon are eliminated, but complete obstipation and absence of flatus ensue. Physical findings may be only those of acute small bowel obstruction (Chap. 24), or there may be, in addition, hyperresonance of percussion in the right lower quadrant. Severe peritoneal signs indicate that strangulation is present.

DIAGNOSTIC FINDINGS. An abdominal plain film is often pathognomic but may be confusing unless one remembers that lack of lateral fixation allows the mobile cecum to be seen anywhere in the abdomen. Characteristically a large midabdominal ovoid dilated segment is seen, with distended small bowel loops and a relatively empty large bowel. Barium enema is usually not necessary and is not diagnostic, although it does indicate where the obstruction is located.

TREATMENT. Operation is indicated as soon as the patient can be prepared. Conservative measures cannot untwist the loop, and the hazard of strangulation in the closed-loop obstruction is great. Detorsion of the segment and suture fixation of the mobile cecum to the lateral gutter suffices if the cecum is viable. Right colectomy with ileo-

transverse colostomy is done for strangulation obstruction and for recurrent volvulus. Exteriorization obstructive resection is justified in moribund patients with gangrenous bowel.

The mortality rate for cecal volvulus is still about 10 percent, principally because of delay in diagnosis and treatment until strangulation obstruction with gangrenous bowel has supervened.

MEGACOLON

The term *megacolon,* meaning large colon, should also imply chronic dilation, elongation, and hypertrophy of the colon. Megacolon may be congenital or acquired. Acquired megacolon may be due to organic causes or may be idiopathic. The common denominator in megacolon is chronic partial colon obstruction with associated chronic constipation. In general the degree of megacolon is proportional to the duration of the partial obstruction. Megacolon is of interest to surgeons not only because many patients require surgical correction but also because of the propensity for volvulus in patients with megacolon.

Congenital Megacolon (Hirschsprung's Disease)

This disease is due to congenital absence of ganglion cells in the myenteric plexus of the bowel. The rectosigmoid is frequently involved, but the aganglionosis is sometimes more extensive, even involving the entire colon. The functional defect is the inability of the aganglionic segment to relax to allow a peristaltic wave to pass, thus producing a functional partial obstruction with proximal retention of feces, which in turn causes megacolon above the aganglionic segment. This is primarily a disease of infants and children (Chap. 39) but occasionally may not become manifest until later in life. It is therefore advisable, whenever performing operations for megacolon or volvulus, to have a frozen section of colon examined for ganglion cells.

A different form of megacolon that may be congenital has been reported to occur in certain areas of the world such as Eastern Europe and Okinawa where the vegetable diets are high in roughage and residue. It is not clear whether the unusually large, long colon is acquired by the individual as an adaptation of the high-residue diet or whether this is a hereditary characteristic that was selected in the evolutionary process because of its adaptive significance. It would be interesting to determine if children of immigrants to the United States from Eastern Europe have large colons when raised on the relatively low-residue diets of the United States.

Acquired Megacolon

Chagas' disease is caused by infection with a protozoan, *Trypanosoma cruzi,* and is endemic in South and Central America. Megacolon, one of the complications of the chronic form of the disease, is attributable to widespread destruction of the intramural nervous system. Surgical therapy is sometimes necessary for severe constipation, recurring fecal impaction, or volvulus. Subtotal colectomy with ileoproctostomy is probably the procedure of choice, though some surgeons prefer abdominoendoanal recto-sigmoidectomy.

Acquired organic megacolon results also from partial mechanical obstruction of the lower colon, rectum, or anus. More common causes are postoperative anorectal stricture; lymphogranuloma venereum (lymphopathia venereum); endometriosis; radiation proctitis; and anorectal injury, either accidental or from sexual perversion. Treatment is aimed at the offending stricture; the secondary megacolon regresses toward, but not to, normal when the primary cause is removed.

Megacolon is also seen in association with neurologic disorders such as paraplegia or poliomyelitis. Constipation is a problem, because the contribution of the voluntary muscles to the defecatory act is lost. If constipation is avoided by the use of enemas and stool softeners, mega-colon is avoided.

Acute dilatation of the colon, as seen in fulminating colitis, septic shock, prolonged adynamic ileus, or diabetes, has no relationship to chronic megacolon.

Megacolon is frequent in institutionalized psychotic patients. No organic cause has been found, so it is referred to as psychogenic or idiopathic megacolon. Severe constipation, because of extreme inactivity and perhaps voluntary inhibition of defecation, is presumed to be the principal cause. Better nursing care would avoid the problem if only it were possible to provide this. Psychogenic megacolon has also been seen in young children, presumably as an extension of problems with bowel training. Colectomy for megacolon is occasionally justified in these patients. If sigmoid volvulus occurs in patients with mega-colon, subtotal colectomy to "straighten out" the colon is preferable to sigmoid segmental colectomy.

Fecal Impaction

Impaction is the arrest and accumulation of feces in the rectum or colon. Feces are progressively dehydrated by the colonic mucosa the longer they remain in the colon. When normal progression of feces does not occur, the hard dry fecal mass is increased in size as more feces are pushed downward from above. Retained barium after radiographic studies and calcium carbonate used as ulcer therapy frequently contribute to fecal impactions. With dehydration these substances attain a consistency resembling concrete.

Many of the patients with chronic constipation discussed above under Acquired Megacolon frequently have impactions. A frequent cause in otherwise healthy persons is an acute painful lesion of the anus—fissures, fistulas, thrombosed external hemorrhoid, or recent anorectal surgical therapy.

CLINICAL MANIFESTATIONS. The most common symptoms of a rectal impaction is the passage of frequent loose stools but without relief of the sense of rectal urgency and fullness. This is "overflow" evacuation around a partial obstruction. Marked rectal urgency but inability to defe-

cate is also common. In patients who have lost rectal sensation, as occurs in paraplegia or spina bifida, or in psychotics, there may be no symptoms of fecal impactions until a complication supervenes.

Infrequently, full-blown mechanical obstruction of the colon is the presenting picture. A fortunately rare but serious complication may occur when the fecal impaction does not obstruct completely and allows overflow evacuation to occur. The unmoving hard mass eventually erodes the mucosa with production of a stercoraceous ulcer. If the ulcer is in the rectum, serious bleeding may ensue; if in the abdominal colon, perforation with spreading fecal peritonitis. Management of this complication is the same as for perforated diverticulitis.

Diagnosis is usually easily made by digital rectal examination. If the impaction is higher, large, hard fecal masses can be palpated in the colon. These masses can also be seen on plain radiographs of the abdomen.

TREATMENT. Unless a complication is present, fecal impaction is treated by instillation of 5 ml of a 1% solution of dioctyl sodium sulfosuccinate in 60 ml of mineral oil into the rectum and left overnight. This will usually soften the stool sufficiently that it can be passed. If not, a saline enema may be given. If defecation still does not occur, then the impaction must be broken up and delivered digitally. It is helpful in female patients to exert gentle digital pressure on the rectal mass through the rectovaginal septum with two fingers in the vagina while the mass is delivered through the anus with the other hand. If a painful anal condition is present, hot sitz baths and an anesthetic ointment often relieve the spasm and permit defecation.

RECTUM AND ANUS

Anatomy

The rectum, measuring 12 to 15 cm, is the distal portion of the large intestine (Fig. 28-13), beginning at the level of the third sacral vertebra and ending at the anal canal. The rectum differs from the sigmoid colon in that it lacks haustra, teniae coli, and appendices epiploicae. The rectal valves of Houston represent folds of mucosa, submucosa, and circular musculature but contain no elements of longitudinal muscle. The upper one-third of the rectum is covered by peritoneum anteriorly and laterally; the middle one-third is covered anteriorly only; the lower one-third is devoid of peritoneum. On the average the anterior peritoneal reflection in the male is 7.5 to 8.5 cm from the anal verge, while in females it is 5.0 to 7.5 cm. The posterior peritoneal reflection is usually 12 to 15 cm from the anal verge.

The anal canal is the terminal portion of the large intestine. The "surgical anal canal" begins at the anorectal ring, terminates at the anal verge, and is about 4 cm long. The circular muscle of the large intestine continues downward and thickens to form the *internal sphincter.* The *external sphincter,* which is striated muscle, loops around the entire length of the anal canal. It has three components: the *subcutaneous, superficial,* and *deep portions.* Recently, it

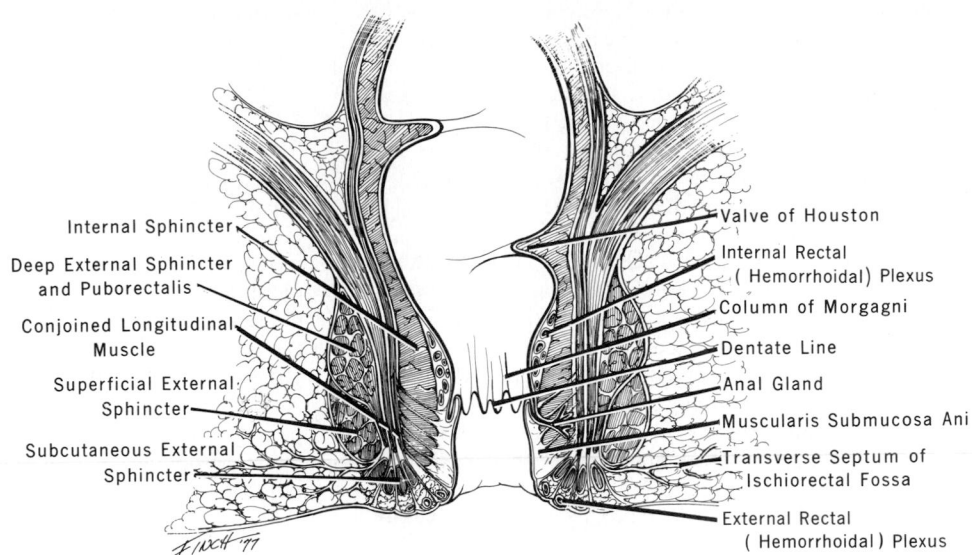

Fig. 28-13. Coronal section of the rectum and anal canal, showing sphincter muscles and the lining of anal canal.

was determined that the puborectalis is fused with the deep portion of the external sphincter and is not part of the levator ani muscles. Between the internal and external sphincter is the longitudinal smooth muscle. This muscle continues from the rectum to where it receives fibers from the levator ani and puborectalis muscles to form the *conjoined longitudinal muscle.* These muscle fibers pass down and break up into a series of septums and ultimately attach to the anal and perianal skin. Some of the longitudinal muscle fibers traverse the internal sphincter into the submucosa and are called *muscularis submucosa ani;* some fibers traverse the external sphincter to form the *transverse septum of the ischiorectal fossa.* The role of the longitudinal muscle is to affix the anal canal and to evert the anus during defecation.

The puborectalis, the deep part of the external sphincter, the longitudinal muscle layer, and the upper part of the internal sphincter form a palpable "anorectal ring."

ANAL SPHINCTER MECHANISM. The recent concept by Shafik of the anal sphincter as three distinct U-shaped loops simplifies the understanding of its mechanism (Fig. 28-14).

In the *top loop* the deep portion of the external sphincter and the puborectalis are fused into one muscle. This attaches to the lower part of the symphysis pubis and loops around the upper part of the anal canal with a downward inclination.

The *intermediate loop* is the superficial external sphincter which arises from the tip of the coccyx as a tendon and gives rise to strong muscle bundles passing forward to encircle the anal canal below the top loop.

The *base loop* is the subcutaneous external sphincter. It attaches anteriorly to the perianal skin in the midline and passes backward with an upward inclination to loop around the lower part of the anal canal.

During voluntary anal contraction the three loops contract in the direction of their origin. The top and the base

loops, innervated by the inferior hemorrhoidal branch of the pudendal nerve, will bring the posterior anal wall anteriorly, whereas the intermediate loop, supplied by the fourth sacral nerve, will pull the anal canal posteriorly. Thus, each loop is a separate sphincter and complements the other loops to maintain complete continence.

SURGICAL ANAL CANAL LINING (Fig. 28-13). The surgical anal canal is lined above by mucosa and below by anoderm, which is modified skin. The anal crypts are in the upper part of the anoderm. A line at the level of the crypts is the pectinate, or dentate, line. Above this line are a number of vertical mucosal folds, the columns of Mor-

Fig. 28-14. U-shaped anal sphincters.

gagni, which overlie the internal hemorrhoidal plexus. Immediately above the dentate line is a zone of transitional epithelium, measuring 0.5 to 1.0 cm.

The pectinate, or dentate, line is an important landmark for surgeons. The epithelium above this line is supplied by sensory fibers from the autonomic nervous system and therefore is insensitive to painful stimuli such as cutting or cauterizing. The epithelium below this line is innervated by spinal nerves and has somatic sensation.

Anal glands are vestigial structures lined by stratified, mucus-secreting columnar epithelium and squamous epithelium. Normally there are 6 to 10 glands in the circumference of the anus. Each gland has a duct and discharges into an anal crypt at the dentate line. Some of the glands penetrate the internal sphincter, extending into the conjoined longitudinal muscle fibers, but not beyond them. Infection originating in these glands is the primary cause of perianal abscess and fistula-in-ano.

ARTERIAL SUPPLY OF THE RECTUM AND ANAL CANAL (Fig. 28-15)

1. The superior rectal (hemorrhoidal) artery is the continuation of the inferior mesenteric artery and descends posteriorly to the rectum, where it bifurcates to supply the rectum and upper portion of the anal canal.
2. The middle rectal (hemorrhoidal) arteries arise from the internal iliac artery on each side and enter the lower portion of the rectum anterolaterally at the level of the levator ani muscle; they do not enter the lateral stalks, as previously believed. These arteries anastomose with the branches of the superior rectal artery.
3. The inferior rectal arteries arise on each side from the internal pudendal artery, a branch of the internal iliac artery, and traverse the ischiorectal fossa on each side to supply the anal sphincter muscles. There is no evidence of anastomosis between the superior and inferior rectal arteries.

4. The middle sacral artery provides an insignificant amount of blood supply to the rectum. It arises posteriorly, just above the bifurcation of the aorta, descends over the lumbar vertebrae, sacrum, and coccyx, and gives only small branches to the posterior wall of the lower portion of the rectum.

VENOUS DRAINAGE OF THE RECTUM AND ANAL CANAL
(Fig. 28-16). Return of blood from the rectum and the anal canal is via two systems: portal and systemic. The superior rectal (hemorrhoidal) vein drains the rectum and upper part of the anal canal into the portal system via the inferior mesenteric vein. Primarily, the middle rectal veins drain the lower part of the rectum and the upper part of the anal canal. They accompany the middle rectal arteries and terminate in the internal iliac veins. The inferior rectal veins, following the corresponding arteries, drain the lower part of the anal canal via the internal pudendal veins, which empty into the internal iliac veins. Dilatation of the inferior rectal veins leads to external hemorrhoids.

The superior, middle, and inferior rectal veins converge to form the internal rectal (hemorrhoidal) plexus in the submucosa of the columns of Morgagni. Dilatation of this plexus gives rise to internal hemorrhoids.

LYMPHATIC DRAINAGE OF THE RECTUM AND ANAL CANAL.
The lymph from the upper and middle parts of the rectum ascends along the superior rectal lymphatics and subsequently to the inferior mesenteric nodes. The lower part of the rectum and the upper part of the surgical anal canal drain cephalad via the superior rectal lymphatics and laterally via the middle rectal lymph vessels. The lymph from the anal canal, below the dentate line, can drain to the superior rectal lymph nodes, to the nodes on the lateral wall of the pelvis, or to the inguinal nodes.

Fig. 28-15. Arterial supply of the rectum and anal canal.

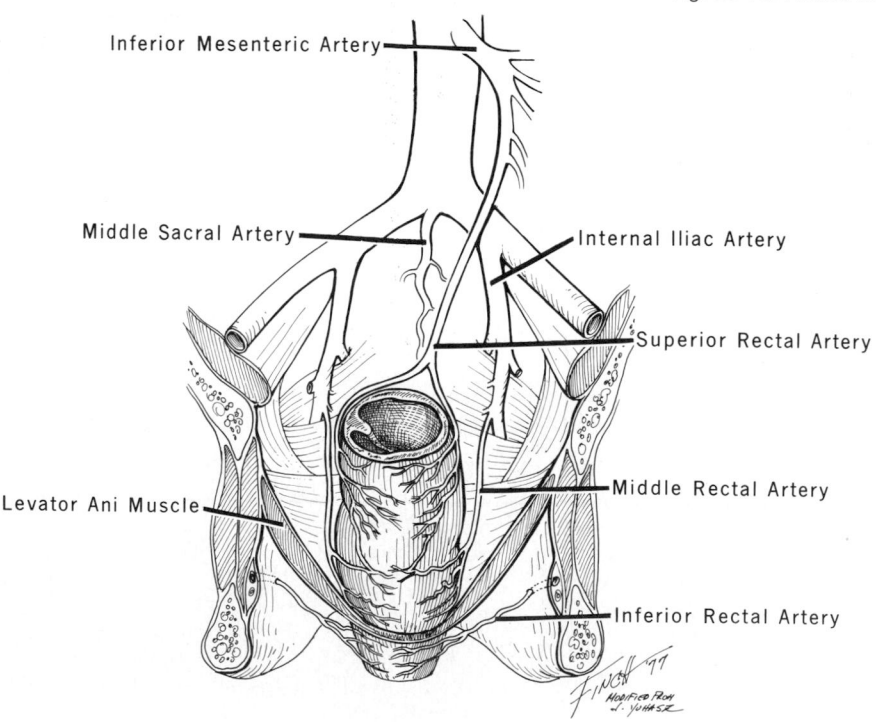

Inferior Mesenteric Artery

Middle Sacral Artery

Internal Iliac Artery

Superior Rectal Artery

Middle Rectal Artery

Levator Ani Muscle

Inferior Rectal Artery

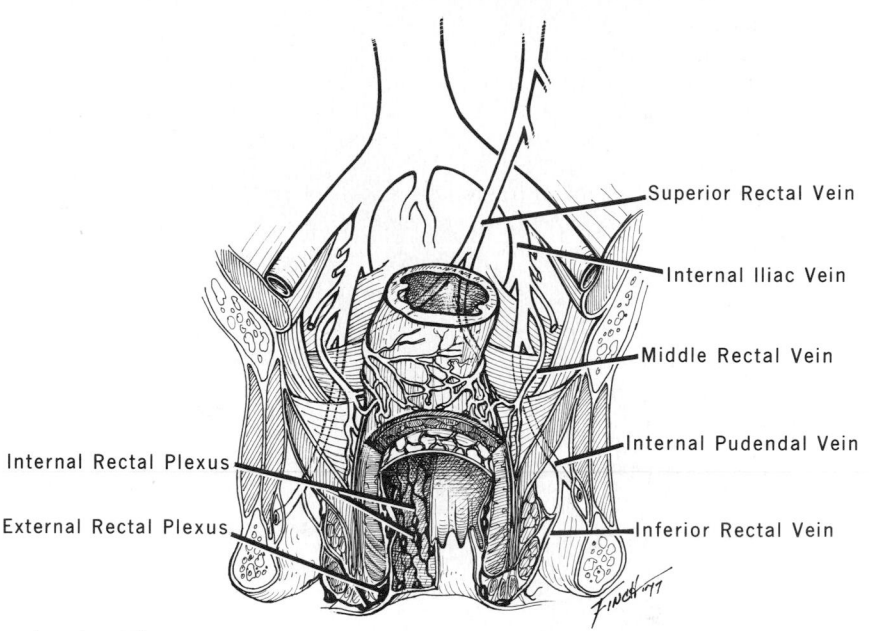

Fig. 28-16. Venous drainage of the rectum and anal canal.

PERIANAL AND PERIRECTAL SPACES (Figs. 28-17 and 28-18). Around the rectum and anal canal are several spaces filled with connective tissue or fat, which may become sites of abscesses. The *supralevator (pelvirectal) space* is situated on each side of the rectum above the levator ani. It is bound superiorly by the pelvic peritoneum, laterally by the pelvic wall, and medially by the rectum. The space is filled with fibroareolar tissue. The *retrorectal space* lies between the rectum and sacrum, above the levator ani muscles. It communicates with the supralevator space on each side. The *ischiorectal space* lies inferiorly to the levator ani muscle and is bound superiorly by the pelvic diaphragm (levator ani muscle), medially by the external sphincters, laterally by the pelvic wall, and inferiorly by the transverse septum of the ischiorectal fossa. It is filled com-

pletely with fat and contains the inferior rectal vessels and lymphatics. The space on each side communicates through the posterior space between the levator ani and tendinous portion of the superficial external sphincter (*deep postanal space*). With this communication, infection on either side of the ischiorectal space can lead to a horseshoe abscess or fistula. The *perianal space,* containing fat, inferior rectal vessels, and lymphatics, is located between the perianal skin and the transverse septum of the ischiorectal fossa. Posteriorly, this space lies inferiorly to the superficial external sphincter muscle and is called the *superficial postanal space.* The perianal space is the most common site of abscess in this region. The *intersphincteric space* lies within the conjoined longitudinal muscle between the internal and external anal sphincters. This space surrounds the anal canal.

Fig. 28-17. Coronal section of the perianal and perirectal spaces.

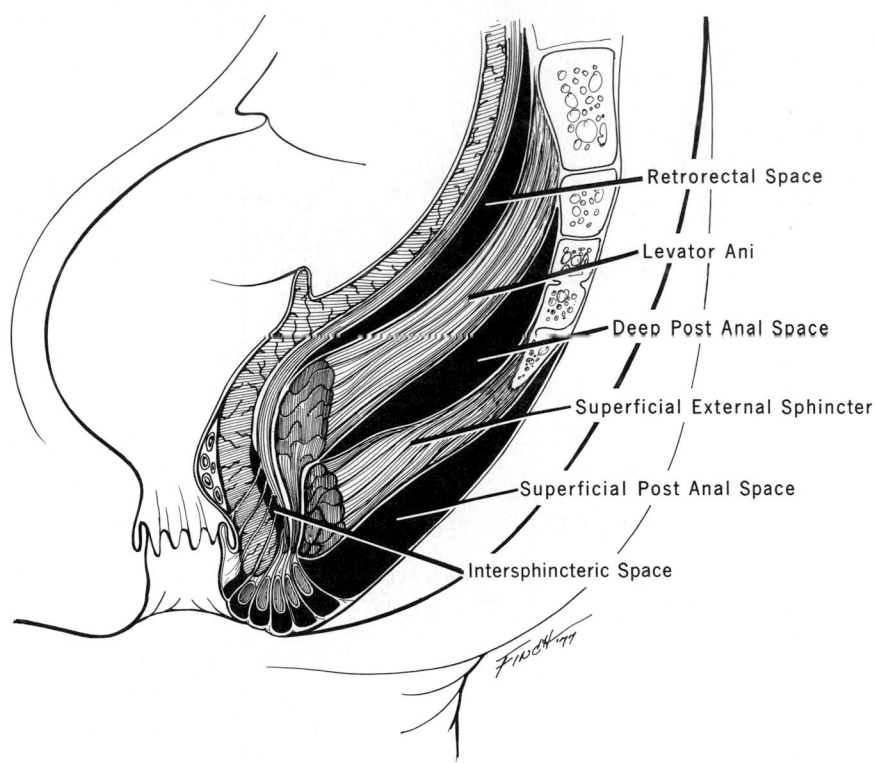

Fig. 28-18. Sagittal section of the perianal and perirectal spaces.

Labels on figure:
- Retrorectal Space
- Levator Ani
- Deep Post Anal Space
- Superficial External Sphincter
- Superficial Post Anal Space
- Intersphincteric Space

Examination

Patients with painful anal lesions are apprehensive about any examination; thus it is important they be approached gently and be informed of every step of the procedure. This "vocal anesthesia" should be applied to both digital and sigmoidoscopic examinations.

PREPARATION. Opinions vary with respect to the need for special preparation of the rectum prior to routine sigmoidoscopic examination. The most common preparation is one 4-oz packaged phosphate enema given 20 minutes prior to the examination. However, the majority of ambulatory patients can be examined adequately without prior enemas. This is particularly pertinent for the patient with a history suggestive of inflammatory bowel disease. In this circumstance, adding an irritating preparatory enema can often mask the salient early findings. Conversely, patients have been diagnosed as having inflammatory bowel disease when, actually, the mucous membrane appeared inflamed from the irritating enema. Evaluation of the patient with rectal bleeding should always be made without a preparatory enema in order to eliminate the possibility of washing away important clues such as bloody mucus streaked on the bowel wall, an indication of a lesion higher in the intestine. Proctosigmoidoscopic examination should not be carried out just prior to a barium enema unless there is an emergency, since the insufflation of air at the time of sigmoidoscopy can create artifacts simulating polyps or other filling defects on the barium enema examination.

SIGMOIDOSCOPIC EXAMINATION. This procedure can be performed on a proctosigmoidoscopic table which places the patient in an inverted position, allowing the viscera to slide cephalad and create a negative pressure, thus minimizing the need for insufflation to distend the bowel. Examination also may be carried out with the patient on a flat table in the prone or knee-chest position. In the latter position, the knees should be 6 to 8 in. apart to relax the gluteal musculature. For the elderly or seriously ill patient who cannot tolerate the knee-chest or prone positions, the lateral, or Sims' position may be used. After turning the patient on the side, the lower leg is extended while the upper leg is flexed at the knee and hip in order to spread the buttocks and lend some stability to the position. By positioning the buttocks 10 to 12 cm over the edge of the bed, a complete rotation of the sigmoidoscope is facilitated.

A variety of sigmoidoscopes is available. There are proximally lighted scopes, distally lighted scopes, and fiberoptic scopes. Advocates of the proximally lighted sigmoidoscopes claim that the distally lighted scopes become coated with bowel contents or blood, obscuring visibility. By contrast, advocates of the distally lighted scopes claim that better illumination is possible with this instrument. A recent advance in fiberoptics has led to the development of a flexible colonoscope which can be advanced throughout the entire colon in 70 to 90 percent of patients (Fig. 28-19). This instrument may be used diagnostically and therapeutically, since lesions throughout the colon may be biopsied and pedunculated polyps may be removed.

Fig. 28-19. Fiberoptic colonoscope introduced to the cecum.

Principles of Anorectal Surgery

PREPARATION. In preparing a patient for an anorectal operation, a general evaluation is mandatory. Procto-sigmoidoscopy should be carried out preoperatively and is deferred only if the patient has an extremely painful condition, in which cases it is carried out under anesthesia. Contrast roentgenographic examinations of the large and small intestine are indicated when neoplastic lesions and/or inflammatory bowel diseases are suspected. Any patient presenting with a history of bleeding requires a complete roentgenographic assessment of the lower intestinal tract. If the patient gives a history of diarrhea or other symptoms suggestive of inflammatory bowel disease, both the small and large intestine should be studied roentgeno-graphically prior to the performance of any anorectal operation. If a rectal lesion suggests the possibility of systemic diseases, such as leukemia, syphilis or Crohn's disease, these should be evaluated completely prior to surgery.

The preoperative preparation of the patient should take into consideration specific anxieties related to rectal surgery; these include fear of pain, incontinence, recurrence, and malignancy. Preparation of the bowel for most ano-rectal operations requires only a packaged phosphate enema the evening before and the morning of surgery. No specific antibiotic is given except when perforation of the bowel is a significant possibility, e.g., when sessile adenomas are excised from high in the rectum or a polyp in the sigmoid colon is snared with electrocautery. Laxatives or stool softeners are not administered routinely, although they are not contraindicated. No special diets are instituted preoperatively, since a bowel movement on the second or third postoperative day is desirable. Shaving the perianal skin, which has been a long-standing tradition, is totally unnecessary. Regrowth of hair adds to the postoperative pruritus and irritation, and the presence of hair does not complicate the healing process.

Most of the common rectal operations can be carried out under local anesthesia with regional field block, epidural anesthesia, spinal anesthesia or general anesthesia with or without endotracheal intubation, depending on the position of the patient. Many surgeons prefer to use supplemental local anesthesia combined with epinephrine solution to aid hemostasis and facilitate identification of the anatomy. Long-acting oil-soluble anesthetics have been used to assist in controlling postoperative pain, but these have been associated with a high incidence of postoperative suppuration.

TECHNIQUE. The three commonly used positions for anorectal operations are prone-jackknife, dorsal lithotomy, and Sims' position. The techniques should all be characterized by minimal handling of the tissue, sharp dissection, primary closure of wounds when possible, and the use of fine absorbable sutures *without tension* on the suture lines. In all circumstances, normal skin should be conserved, and injury to the sphincteric mechanism should be avoided.

POSTOPERATIVE CARE. Packing of the anorectum is rarely necessary to effect hemostasis, but some surgeons use a small amount of oxidized cellulose. Bulky, painful pressure dressings should be avoided so that spontaneous voiding can occur, and the need for catheterization is minimized. A bulk-producing compound and a lubricant are administered orally, starting on the day of operation. If the patient has not had a spontaneous bowel movement by the third postoperative day, a tap water enema is administered through a soft rubber catheter. Dilatation and irrigations of the anal canal are not used postoperatively. The patient is placed on a regular diet early in the postoperative course, usually on the first hospital day. Hospital dismissal is indicated following the first spontaneous bowel movement and when intramuscular injections of analgesics are no longer required. A psyllium seed bulk producer is prescribed, and the patient is instructed to keep a cotton dressing in the anal area to collect discharge and drainage. Sitz baths are encouraged as often as necessary for cleanliness and comfort. The patient is seen postoperatively approximately 10 days following hospital discharge and at regular intervals until complete healing has occurred.

COMPLICATIONS. Bleeding is one of the most common complications following anorectal surgery. This complication can be reduced by the use of electrocautery or suture ligature techniqe at the time of operation. In most instances, postoperative bleeding is related to either ineffective hemostasis at the time of operation or to heavy packing of the anal canal. The latter is unnecessary and should be discouraged, since it only adds to the patient's discomfort.

Direct suture of the bleeder is the treatment of choice to control postoperative hemorrhage during the first 24 hours. Thus, any patient who begins to bleed postoperatively and does not respond to light packing should be taken to the operating room, where, under the proper anesthetic, the site of bleeding can be demonstrated and sutured.

Secondary hemorrhage, or late bleeding, occurs in 1.0 to 1.5 percent of anorectal procedures. The most common time for this complication is the seventh or tenth postoperative day when the catgut suture is dissolved almost completely. The management is similar as for an acute bleeder, viz., examination under anesthesia, evacuation of clots, and suture of the bleeding point.

Abnormal pain accompanies a variety of complications related to rectal surgery. Pressure-like pain associated with fecal impaction must be differentiated from the usual postoperative pain related to the surgical procedure itself. This distressing complication can be avoided by or treated with simple tap water enemas administered through a soft rubber catheter. The pain associated with perianal suppuration, such as intersphincteric abscess, is usually described as a "toothache" type of pain and characteristically appears on the fourth or fifth postoperative day. The sharp, searing pain of an anal fissure, which persists long into the healing phase following rectal surgery, heralds the complication of anal stenosis. This usually occurs in the midline posteriorly or in one of the posterolateral quadrants and rarely responds to conservative management; a second operation is generally indicated. Similar pain may represent the first symptom of undiagnosed Crohn's disease. Approximately 20 percent of patients with Crohn's disease have, as their initial symptom, a fissure or suppurative process in the anorectum or a slowly healing anorectal wound.

Anal stricture is a dreaded complication of anorectal surgery. It is an infrequent complication of closed hemorrhoidectomy since this technique precludes the excessive removal of anoderm. Since treatment is difficult, efforts are best directed at prevention. Dilatation has been used for many years, but this is painful and often unsuccessful. The use of a bulk producer, such as psyllium seed compound, following rectal surgery is a simple and physiologic method for dilating the anal canal. It is far superior to forceful, painful dilatation with a finger or anal dilator. If stricture persists and is painful, anoplasty is indicated.

In certain anorectal operations, where the mucous membrane is advanced to form a new dentate line, an *ectropion* may result. This condition, in which the mucous membrane has been advanced beyond the anal verge, results in a "wet anus," and has been referred to as a *Whitehead deformity*. Ectropion is best treated by excision of the offending mucous membrane and application of a sliding skin graft.

Incontinence following anorectal procedures can arise from several causes. The most common cause, fecal impaction, allows liquid stool to bypass the impaction while the pressure of the impaction holds the sphincteric mechanism open. This may be corrected with tap water enemas. During the first few weeks following an anorectal operation, there may be some fecal staining, and the patient may report loss of ability to distinguish between flatus and feces. This is usually a temporary, self-limited situation due to the disruption of proprioceptive nerve endings in the anoderm. The use of large amounts of mineral oil compound to lubricate the stool following surgery results in a "leakage" of mineral oil which is often interpreted as incontinence. Severe forms of incontinence generally are related to division of the sphincteric muscles.

In operative procedures for anal fissures when a concomitant superficial partial sphincterotomy is carried out, a slight degree of fecal staining may result, but this is rarely permanent. In extensive fistula surgery, where a great deal of the sphincteric mechanism is transected, incontinence may persist; sphincteroplasty may be indicated if improvement is not effected with sphincteric exercises. Preservation of the sphincteric mechanism is a most important consideration in the treatment of deep or high fistulas and when fistulas involve the anterior sphincter mechanism, especially in females.

Anal pruritus is not a true complication of rectal surgery. Most patients notice a degree of anal pruritus during the healing phases, similar to that noted in the healing of any cutaneous wound. If anal pruritus persists, it may be a sign of an anal fissure or may be due to a particular sensitivity to one of the anesthetic ointments used following rectal surgery.

Urinary tract symptoms, particularly retention and infection, were frequent complications following anorectal operations in the past. The incidence of urinary retention recently has been reduced to 5 percent by decreasing fluid administration during operation and postoperatively, resorting to catheterization only when the patient is distended. When catheterization is to be repeated, the catheter should be left in place for several days.

Hemorrhoids

In the human being, the upper anal canal is lined by separate, bulky cushions of specialized submucosal vascular tissue, likened to erectile tissue, composed of a stroma of elastic connective tissue containing smooth muscle fibers derived from the outer longitudinal muscle coat of the colon. This supports the normally large and dilated veins of the internal hemorrhoidal venous plexus, which also have demonstrable arteriovenous shunts. Such cushions are discrete and separated so that the anal canal lumen is seen to form a triradiate slit. The stem of the "Y," so formed, invariably approaches the midline posteriorly, so that its arms separate three cushions lying in constant sites—left lateral, right anterior, right posterior. Secondary folds are present in each of these large cushions. This anatomical arrangement is remarkably constant; however, it bears no relationship, as previously thought, to the terminal branching of the superior rectal vessels, which is quite inconstant. That this arrangement of anal cushions is the normal state is borne out by its presence in children; it can also be demonstrated in the fetus and even in the embryo. The function of these cushions is speculative; however, many reasonable theories have been advanced. By their bulk, they must aid in anal continence, and, during the act of defecation when they become engorged with blood, they cushion the anal canal and support the lining. Being separate structures, rather than a continuous ring of vascular tissue, allows the anal canal to dilate during defecation.

ETIOLOGY. Hemorrhoidal disease exists only when this situation becomes exaggerated and the patient develops symptoms. Many factors have been implicated in the causation of hemorrhoids, including the erect position of the human being, the absence of venous valves, obstruction of venous return, and hereditary weakness of the vessels. Since these factors are all present in the normal physiologic status of the vascular arrangement of the anal canal, they

bear no direct relationship to the disease state. Straining during defecation and the passage of hard, small-volume stools, however, results in tense engorgement of the anal cushions. This may cause injury to the mucous membrane, resulting in bright red bleeding from the capillaries of the lamina propria. With repeated straining, the anal cushions are damaged so that the normal supports are stretched and the tendency to prolapse outside the anal canal develops. Early in the evolution of the disease, the cushions reduce spontaneously; however, with repeated episodes, the situation becomes irreversible, so that manual replacement is necessary. In the prolonged state of the disease, the normally lax rectal mucosa above the anal cushions eventually is dragged with the prolapsing anal cushion so that it adds to the bulk of what now could be described as a classical hemorrhoid. The prolapsed hemorrhoids lying outside the normally contracted anal sphincter ring may become strangulated, with resulting thrombosis of the venous plexus. This, in turn, may result in gangrene and sloughing.

Recent epidemiologic studies have implicated the low-roughage "Western" diet as the cause of many diseases, including hemorrhoids. Adding bulk, in the form of cereal fiber or bulk-forming compounds, can prevent hemorrhoidal disease and, in many cases, reverse the early stages.

For clarity of surgical description, the various states of hemorrhoidal disease should be defined. *Internal hemorrhoids* are exaggerated vascular cushions, normally located above the dentate line, and are covered by the mucous membrane of the anal canal. *External hemorrhoids* are mainly the dilated venules of the inferior hemorrhoidal plexus, which are located below the dentate line and are covered by squamous epithelium. A *mixed hemorrhoid* is a combination of an external and internal hemorrhoid. *Prolapsing hemorrhoids* are internal hemorrhoids which protrude beyond the dentate line and lie outside the anal canal. They are always associated with redundant rectal mucosa. A *thrombosed hemorrhoid* is one in which the blood has clotted, both intravascularly and, to some degree, extravascularly. An *external skin tag* is an area of fibrous connective tissue, covered by skin, which is usually the result of a previously thrombosed hemorrhoid or anal surgery.

CLINICAL MANIFESTATIONS. External hemorrhoids are usually asymptomatic. Perianal irritation and pruritus rarely result from external hemorrhoids. The patient's first awareness of an external hemorrhoid may be the pain which accompanies thrombosis. Thrombosis may recur in the same or in a different hemorrhoidal complex. Internal hemorrhoids most commonly are manifested by painless, bright-red rectal bleeding associated with defecation. The patient commonly describes the bleeding episode by stating, "The blood drips into the toilet bowl." Prolapse of an internal hemorrhoid may be accompanied by a feeling of moisture in the anal region. Early in its course, the prolapse reduces spontaneously; but as the condition becomes chronic, the internal hemorrhoids prolapse permanently, a situation frequently accompanied by inflammation and thrombosis. Other sequelae of internal hemorrhoids are anemia, edema, suppuration, ulceration, fibrosis, strangulation, and, rarely, pylephlebitis with gangrene. Pain is not

Fig. 28-20. Excision of thrombosed external hemorrhoid demonstrating elliptical skin incision.

a symptom of hemorrhoids, unless associated with thrombosis or infection, but indicates other anal disease which may accompany hemorrhoids; viz., anal fissure, proctalgia fugax, proctitis, or, occasionally, anal cancer. Likewise, discharge, with or without pruritus, is not a symptom of hemorrhoids unless chronic prolapse is present, but is indicative of other diseases, such as fistula, proctitis, procidentia, and neoplasm.

Uncomplicated internal hemorrhoids usually are not palpable, but having the patient strain at the completion of the digital examination will reveal prolapse of an internal hemorrhoid and the rectal mucosa. The anoscope is particularly suitable for viewing internal hemorrhoids, but proctosigmoidoscopy must be performed to rule out neoplastic or inflammatory disease, which may present with similar

Fig. 28-21. Ligation technique for internal hemorrhoids.

Elastic Bands

symptoms. In patients with an atypical history or in the older age group, a barium enema is mandatory to exclude colonic disease.

TREATMENT. Usually, the treatment of a painful thrombosed hemorrhoid is an outpatient procedure. Anesthesia is achieved by a subcutaneous injection of 3.5 ml of 1% procaine or lidocaine solution containing 1:200,000 epinephrine. Incision alone frequently does not suffice. It is preferable to excise the entire thrombosed hemorrhoid and electrocoagulate the bleeding points (Fig. 28-20). Adequate treatment by total excision of a single thrombosed external hemorrhoid prevents further thrombosis in that area and usually obviates the need for subsequent hemorrhoidectomy. If the thrombosed hemorrhoid is unassociated with pain, nonoperative therapy will suffice. Pain associated with thrombosis lasts only 2 to 3 days; resolution usually requires 10 to 14 days.

Initial treatment for bleeding internal hemorrhoids should be nonoperative, with emphatic dietary education of the patient to correct any underlying bowel disturbance attributed to constipating food, especially dairy products, inadequate hydration, and lack of high-fiber food, such as bran. The use of hydrophilic bulk stool–forming additives may be contemplated. Injection therapy of 5% phenol in vegetable oil or quinine urea hydrochloride to sclerose the submucosal tissue above the hemorrhoid may afford temporary, symptomatic relief but should be used only for uncomplicated bleeding internal hemorrhoids.

Another nonoperative technique is rubber band ligation of uncomplicated bleeding internal hemorrhoids. This is an effective, simple procedure and has gained in popularity, now superseding injection. In this outpatient procedure, a constricting rubber band is placed high in the anal canal on the most redundant portion of the rectal mucosa immediately above the internal hemorrhoid (Fig. 28-21). Incorporated tissue sloughs in approximately 7 days, leaving an area of inflammation which results in fibrosis and fixation. This technique does not require anesthesia. Any excessive discomfort indicates that the band has been placed too low and should be removed immediately. The technique provides a more permanent result than injection therapy, since there is precisely controlled loss of redundant mucosa. Repeated applications may be carried out at 6- to 8-week intervals until the patient's symptoms are improved. Occasionally, two to three areas can be banded per visit. The procedure has been performed without incident on patients receiving anticoagulant therapy. The contraindications are the same as for surgical hemorrhoidectomy, viz., inflammatory bowel disease, leukemia, and portal hypertension.

Hemorrhoidal tissue can be frozen with a specialized probe, activated by carbon dioxide, nitrous oxide, or, preferably, liquid nitrogen. With care, the final results of cryosurgery are anatomically satisfactory, and the procedure may be accomplished without anesthesia and with minimal discomfort to the patient. The aftertreatment period is characterized by profuse anal discharge and delayed wound healing, taking as long as 6 to 8 weeks for complete resolution. Moreover, a relatively high incidence of secondary hemorrhage is being reported. Because of these disadvantages and since the results of such treatment do not equal those of formal surgical hemorrhoidectomy, this technique has failed to gain widespread acceptance and use.

Hemorrhoidectomy. Principal indications for hemorrhoidectomy are prolapse, pain, bleeding, and large hemorrhoids associated with other anorectal pathologic conditions requiring operative management. In general, hemorrhoidectomy is reserved for patients having severe symptoms related to multiple thrombosed hemorrhoids or marked redundant protrusion which cannot be handled by the ligature technique. Hemorrhoidectomy may be indicated in the immediate postpartum period in women who have had difficulties prior to pregnancy and in whom prolapse of thrombosed hemorrhoids occurred at the time of delivery. In most instances, hemorrhoids which appear to intensify during delivery resolve, but there is a small group of women in whom the problem is of such magnitude as to indicate operation.

The principles for all operative procedures include removing diseased tissues (i.e., internal-external hemorrhoids and redundant rectal mucosa), leaving minimal scarring of the anal canal, avoiding interference with the sphincteric mechanism, and leaving an anal orifice ample for a normal bowel movement without discomfort. Although there are many variations, all hemorrhoid operations basically employ the ligature and excision technique; the method of handling the perianal skin differentiates various techniques. In some techniques, the mucous membrane is closed up to the dentate line, and the external wounds are left open. Other techniques employ primary closure of the hemorrhoidectomy wound.

The technique of *closed hemorrhoidectomy* offers (1) effective removal of hemorrhoidal tissue, (2) prompt healing of wounds, (3) elimination of mucous drainage by lining the anal canal with stratified squamous epithelium, (4) minimal inpatient and virtually no outpatient care, (5) less postoperative discomfort, (6) no loss of continence, and (7) no need for anal dilatation. An adequate dissection-type closed hemorrhoidectomy may be carried out on the acute, prolapsed, thrombosed, edematous hemorrhoid without fear of anal stenosis or stricture if meticulous dissection and preservation of anoderm are accomplished. This technique may be combined with other operative procedures, such as fissurectomy, internal sphincterotomy, fistulotomy, or excision of hypertrophied anal papillae.

Operative Technique (Fig. 28-22). The hemorrhoidal tissue and the extent of the redundant mucosa are demonstrated by grasping the redundant mucosa with tissue forceps. Although every case does not conform to the classic three-quadrant distribution, the most frequently involved quadrants are left lateral, right posterior, and right anterior. Removal of every hemorrhoidal plexus is unnecessary, since the symptoms usually are related to the prolapsing hemorrhoids.

After exposure is accomplished with an operating anoscope, dissection is started on the perianal skin, and the hemorrhoidal mass is dissected carefully off the sphincteric mechanism without injury to the internal sphincter. The redundant rectal mucosa is excised well above the internal hemorrhoid, to correct the redundancy. The mucous mem-

Fig. 28-22. Operative technique for a closed hemorrhoidectomy (see text for description).

brane and anoderm are elevated, and the hemorrhoidal tissue is dissected from beneath the flaps to remove the secondary hemorrhoidal complexes adequately. Anoderm is preserved, bleeding points are electrocoagulated or ligated with catgut sutures, and the mucous membrane is approximated and sutured to the underlying sphincteric mechanism with running fine chromic catgut suture. Edges of the perianal skin are trimmed, and the wound is closed *without tension*. This procedure is repeated in as many areas as necessary. At the completion of the operation it is imperative that the anal canal admit two fingers readily. An intraanal dressing is seldom used.

PROGNOSIS. Symptoms rarely reappear following adequate hemorrhoidectomy. Reappearance of bleeding and prolapse following a hemorrhoidectomy is related to inadequate removal of redundant rectal mucosa or hemorrhoidal tissue. The opponents of primary closure technique express concern for the possible complications of infection and abscess formation, with consequent pain and stenosis. The postoperative infection rate for closed hemorrhoidectomy, as reported by Ferguson et al., was 0.2 percent, and postoperative bleeding occurred in 1.3 percent of patients.

Anal Fissure

Anal fissure is a tear of the skin-lined part of the anal canal. Distribution is equal between males and females. In 80 to 90 percent of the females and over 90 percent of the males, fissures occur in the posterior midline, and the remainder are in the anterior midline. The relatively im-

COMMON LOCATIONS OF CHRONIC ANAL FISSURE AND OTHER ANORECTAL CONDITIONS

Posterior Anus

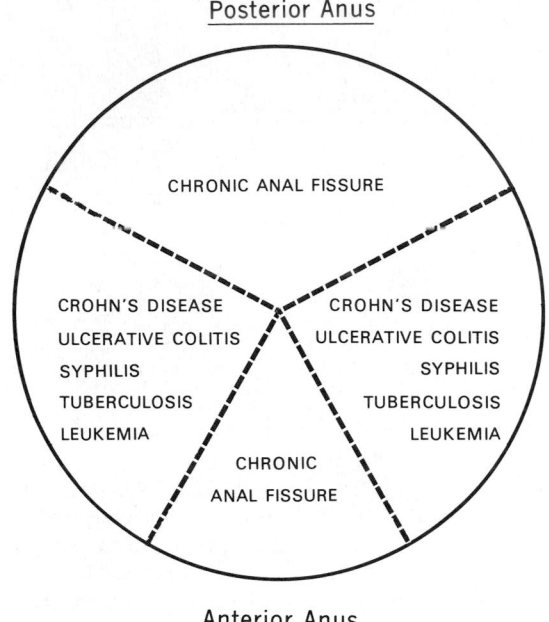

Anterior Anus

Fig. 28-23. Common locations of chronic anal fissure and other anorectal conditions.

mobile skin overlying the posterior area and the angulation of the anal canal cause the stool to traumatize the fissure-bearing area.

Acute fissure is invariably superficial and is extremely painful, especially during and after a bowel movement. Edematous skin edges and induration are absent. With proper conservative management, consisting of use of stool softeners and lubricants, most of these fissures will heal.

Chronic fissure is the result of repeated trauma to the fissure-bearing area. It is deep, with exposure of the underlying circular fibers of the internal sphincter muscle. The chronicity of anal fissure may be due to an abnormality of the internal sphincter. Anal pressure studies have provided conflicting findings. A tight anal sphincter observed in these patients makes it logical to assume that defecation stimulates the sensitive fissure and causes severe reflex spasm. This would draw the anal canal cephalad during anal contraction, and the stool traumatizes the fissure repeatedly.

Diagnosis of anal fissure presents no problem. The history of pain during and after defecation, bright spotted blood on the cleansing tissue after bowel movement, and the location of the fissure in the posterior or anterior midline are suggestive of the diagnosis. Indolent-looking fissures, or fissures located off the midline area, suggest possible inflammatory bowel disease. Anal fissure may represent the initial manifestation of Crohn's disease (Fig. 28-23).

Care should be taken to make the examination as painless as possible. It is advisable to apply a topical anesthetic to the fissure before examining the patient. Gentle spreading of the buttocks usually is all that is necessary to reveal the fissure. In some chronic cases, the triad consists of anal fissure, sentinel pile, or edematous skin tag, and hypertrophied anal papillae may be present.

Digital anoscopic proctosigmoidoscopic examination should be performed if this can be carried out without causing too much discomfort, mainly to exclude other lesions of the anal canal and rectum. In certain patients, excessive pain necessitates delayed examination, and an occasional patient may require examination under anesthesia.

The differential diagnosis for anal fissures includes:

1. Abrasion of the anal canal by trauma. This invariably heals with conservative management.

Table 28-4. ALTERNATIVE PROCEDURES FOR CHRONIC ANAL FISSURE

Type of procedure	Approximate days in hospital	Advantage	Disadvantage
Lateral sphincterotomy	1	Minimal operation	Skin tag remains, if present
Sliding V-flap	2–3	Eliminate skin tag Early primary healing	More extensive operation Possible slough of flap
Fissurectomy and sphincterotomy	3–5	None	"Key-hole" deformity Prolonged wound healing
Anal-sphincter stretching	1	No incision required	Uncontrolled tearing of sphincters Hematoma

2. Anal fissures secondary to ulcerative colitis and, more commonly, Crohn's disease. These are usually situated off the midline, frequently are multiple, and are more edematous or indolent in appearance. They should be treated conservatively. Definitive operation for these fissures should be deferred until the underlying condition has been quiescent for a long time.

3. Epidermoid carcinoma of the anal canal.

4. Tuberculous ulcer is a rare lesion. It is always associated with pulmonary tuberculosis.

5. Syphilitic fissure is usually a "mirror image" lesion which can be established by dark-field examination; serologic studies are necessary to confirm the diagnosis.

6. Leukemic infiltration of the perianal area is extremely painful. Treatment is drainage of the associated abscess.

7. Perianal fissuring, commonly associated with anal pruritus, responds to simple measures of anal hygiene.

TREATMENT. The objectives of treatment are to reduce pain and associated sphincter spasm. When this is accomplished, a superficial fissure will heal readily. Conservative treatment includes stool lubricants, preferably simple cocoa butter suppositories, bulk stool softeners, such as psyllium seed, and warm baths for comfort. To date, unequivocal studies establishing the advantage of steroid suppositories for this condition have not been conducted.

Anal fissures in children are generally superficial and rarely require an operation. Increased fluid intake and decreased consumption of dairy products are directed toward correcting the constipation problem. If these methods do not suffice, stool softeners and a sphincter stretch, without anesthesia, may be done.

Operative treatment of anal fissure is indicated if conservative measures fail (see Table 28-4). The concept of treatment is to enlarge the skin-lined portion of the anal canal and to relieve spasm during and after defecation. The classical fissurectomy and sphincterotomy at the posterior midline area should be avoided, since healing is delayed. Posterior sphincterotomy is associated with a high

Fig. 28-24. Lateral partial internal sphincterotomy.

incidence of soiling from the "key-hole" deformity. Anal-sphincter stretching has been practiced since the nineteenth century and has become popular in the United Kingdom. The disadvantage of stretching is the uncontrolled amount of sphincter muscle torn. Additionally, it requires an anesthetic, during which a better-controlled internal sphincterotomy could be performed. Our treatment of choice is the lateral partial internal sphincterotomy (Fig. 28-24). If there is a redundant external skin tag, a partial internal sphincterotomy at the fissure site with a V-shaped sliding skin flap is used (Fig. 28-25). The procedure can be done under local, regional, or general anesthesia.

Perirectal Suppuration

Abscess formation in the tissues of the anal canal, rectum, and perirectal area is common. Most often no pre-existing lesion can be found. The pathophysiology likely relates to abscess formation in the anal glands lying between the internal sphincter and the longitudinal inter-

Fig. 28-25. V-shaped sliding skin flap for anal fissure. 1 and 2. The 90° V-shaped flap with the apex at the fissure. 3. Full-thickness flap has been mobilized, the edges of the wound undermined, and the internal sphincterotomy made over the fissure. 4. The flap advanced to cover the entire wound.

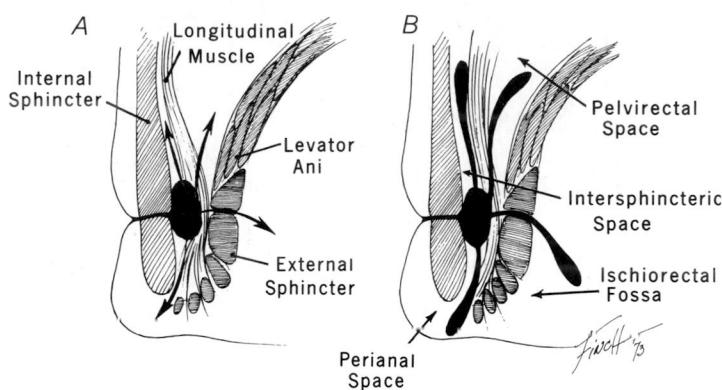

Fig. 28-26. Pathways of infection in perirectal spaces.

sphincteric muscle fibers. From this origin, the infection may spread downward, upward, circumferentially, or laterally to involve the various perianal and perirectal spaces (Fig. 28-26). At times, the cause of the infectious process is identifiable. These conditions include pilonidal abscess, hidradenitis suppurativa, infected sebaceous cyst, folliculitis, periprostatic abscess, Bartholin gland abscess, intraabdominal inflammatory disease with extraabdominal perforation, and, rarely, actinomycosis or tuberculosis.

Perirectal suppuration characteristically presents with pain, often with a palpable inflammatory process, and commonly with a high fever. The diagnosis of the more common perianal and ischiorectal abscesses is apparent. The throbbing pain in the perianal region is acute and aggravated by sitting, coughing, sneezing, and straining. Swelling, induration, and tenderness define the area of involvement. The horseshoe abscess, which begins in an infected, posterior midline anal gland and spreads to both ischiorectal spaces, presents with bilateral perineal findings. The infrequent intersphincteric abscess causes a dull, aching pain in the rectum rather than in the perianal region. There is no swelling or induration of the perianal skin, but excessive tenderness frequently precludes adequate examination without anesthesia. Rectal examination may reveal a soft, tender mass, and in the patient with a ruptured abscess, there may be passage of purulent material per rectum.

The rare supralevator abscess is difficult to diagnose. The patient may present with fever of unknown origin and no

history of anal or rectal pain. Rectal or vaginal examination may reveal tenderness in the pelvis, and signs of peritonitis may be present, suggesting an intraabdominal process. In addition to extension of infralevator inflammatory processes, supralevator abscesses can result from a perforated intraabdominal viscus which has extended downward. Also, injudicious probing of a simple fistula-in-ano, creating a false infected passage in the previously uninfected supralevator space, accounts for some of these abscesses (Fig. 28-27).

TREATMENT. Standard treatment of perianal and perirectal suppuration is incision and drainage, even in the absence of evident fluctuation. Antibiotics should never represent principal therapy but may be used adjunctively. Drainage of most perianal abscesses using local anesthesia can be an outpatient procedure (Fig. 28-28). Many of these abscesses, properly drained, will heal primarily without subsequent formation of fistula-in-ano. Ischiorectal and horseshoe abscesses should be drained in the operating room under general or regional block anesthesia. Since a

Fig. 28-27. Iatrogenic tract created by injudicious probing of a fistula-in-ano.

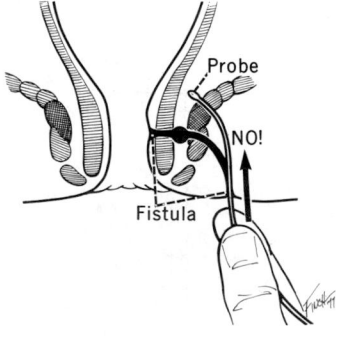

Fig. 28-28. Drainage of perirectal abscess with cruciate incision.

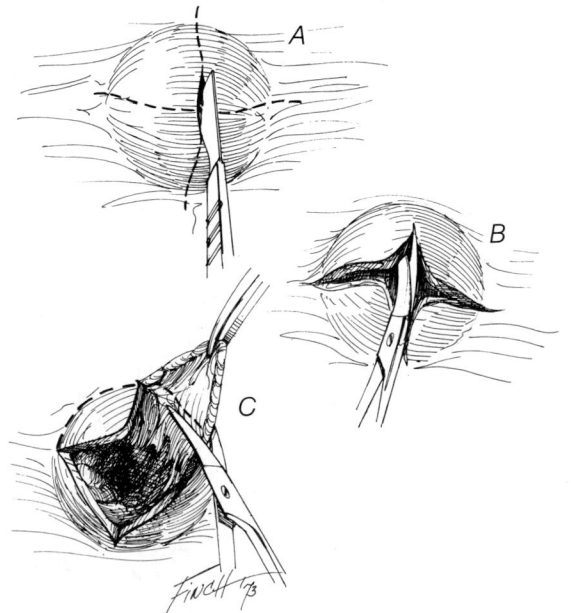

primary opening rarely can be defined, the initial approach should be limited to drainage. The presence of an acute process obviates definitive fistula operation (fistulectomy), since normal sphincter muscle may be sacrificed unnecessarily. A recent study by Scoma, Salvati, and Rubin documented primary healing in over one-third of 232 patients who had incision and drainage alone as their initial therapy for perianal suppuration.

The intersphincteric abscess is best treated in the operating room under general or regional anesthesia. The bulging area is visualized using an operating anoscope, and an internal sphincterotomy is performed directly over the abscess. Subsequent to incision, the abscess should be palpated digitally to establish complete drainage and to break up any loculations. Likewise, the supralevator or pelvirectal abscess should be treated in the operating room under anesthesia. The abscess may be drained through the appropriate ischiorectal space or through the rectum (Fig. 28-29). It is important that the aperture be enlarged to admit two fingers and to ensure continued drainage. A recent controlled study by Leaper et al. demonstrated excellent results in the treatment of idiopathic anorectal abscess by incision, curettage, and primary suture under systemic antibiotic cover. In selected patients, this technique offers shortened hospitalization and decreased morbidity.

Fistula-in-ano

Fistula-in-ano is an inflammatory tract with a *secondary* opening (external opening) in the perianal skin and a *primary* opening (internal opening) in the anal canal at the dentate line. The fistula originates in an abscess in the intersphincteric space of the anal canal. Goodsall's rule relates the location of the internal opening to the external opening (Fig. 28-30). If the external opening is anterior to an imaginary line drawn across the midpoint of the anus, the fistula usually runs directly into the anal canal. If the external opening is posterior to that line, the tract usually will curve to the posterior midline of the anal canal. An exception to this rule is an external opening anterior to this imaginary line and greater than 3 cm from the anus, in

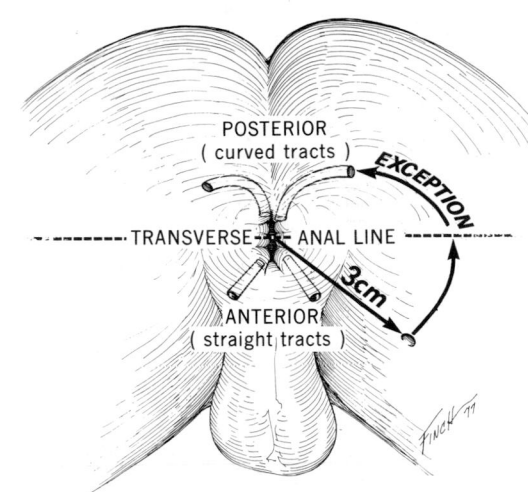

Fig. 28-30. Goodsall's rule.

which case the tract may curve posteriorly and end in the posterior midline.

A more precise classification of fistula-in-ano has been offered recently by Parks, Gordon, and Hardcastle. It consists of four categories: intersphincteric, transsphincteric, suprasphincteric, and extrasphincteric (Fig. 28-31).

Most patients present with previous history of anorectal abscess associated with intermittent drainage. Recurrence of a perianal abscess suggests the presence of a fistula-in-ano. The external opening is usually visible as a red elevation of granulation tissue with purulent or serosanguineous drainage on compression. In the simple or superficial fistula, the tract can be palpated as an indurated cord (Fig. 28-32). Deep, high, or horseshoe fistulas usually are not palpable.

Several disorders must be considered in the differential diagnosis of a fistula-in-ano. It is important to rule out fistulas associated with ulcerative colitis and Crohn's disease, in which case one would refrain from extensive operative procedures for fistula-in-ano because of poor secondary healing. This differential can be established by proctosigmoidoscopy, upper gastrointestinal examination with small bowel follow-through, and barium enema. Di-

Fig. 28-29. Proper route of drainage in supralevator abscess.

Fig. 28-31. The four main anatomical types of fistula: (1) intersphincteric, (2) transsphincteric, (3) suprasphincteric, and (4) extrasphincteric.

Fig. 28-32. Bidigital palpation for locating the indurated fistulous tract.

Fig. 28-33. Fistulotomy. 1. The probe is in the fistulous tract. 2 and 3. Unroofing of the fistulous tract over the probe. 4. Redundant skin is excised. 5. The wound is marsupialized.

verticulitis of the sigmoid colon, with perforation and fistulization to the perineum, occurs rarely. Hidradenitis suppurativa is differentiated by the presence of multiple perianal skin openings. A pilonidal sinus with perianal extension and infected perianal sebaceous cysts must be considered. Rarely, carcinomas, mostly low-grade, may develop in long-standing fistulas. Low rectal and anal canal carcinomas rarely present as a fistula in the perineum.

TREATMENT. The first step in the management is the identification of the opening of the primary fistulous tract. About 50 percent of patients do not have clinically detectable openings. Positive identification is best accomplished in the operating room under anesthesia. Bidigital palpation, using the index finger and the thumb, delineates the indurated tract to the primary opening (Fig. 28-32). Probing the tract from the external opening is successful in 50 percent of cases, but care must be taken to avoid creating an artificial opening and seeding infected material into clean tissue, thus risking iatrogenic extensions above or beyond the original fistula (Fig. 28-27). The injection of methylene blue and/or other chemicals into the secondary opening is unsatisfactory and unnecessary. However, fistulography, utilizing water-soluble contrast solutions, is a valuable method to identify and to manage high, complicated fistulas. If definition of the primary opening is impossible at operation, the crypt-bearing area suspected of harboring the infected duct and gland must be excised.

The principles of fistulotomy include unroofing all fistulas, eliminating the primary opening (infective source), and establishing adequate drainage. The tracts are unroofed from the primary source at the dentate line through the secondary opening or openings by excising all overlying tissue, including sphincter (Fig. 28-33). Failure to unroof the entire tract and divide the necessary amount of sphincter may lead to recurrence. The wound is allowed to heal by secondary intention. Fistulectomy is the excision of the entire fistulous tract and is rarely necessary.

Occasionally, a patient may present with an acute perianal abscess associated with an obvious fistula-in-ano. Incision and drainage of the abscess and primary fistulotomy are indicated. If the fistula is high in relation to the anorectal ring, a two-stage procedure may be indicated. In the first stage, a seton of heavy black silk or a rubber band is placed loosely around the sphincter muscle as a marker (Fig. 28-34). This stimulates fibrosis adjacent to the sphincter muscle so that when the second stage, which involves laying open the intersphincteric portion of the fistulous tract, is completed, the sphincter will not gape. Incontinence is the most serious complication of operations for fistula. Concern that the patient may become incontinent postoperatively is the criterion for seton insertion.

Horseshoe fistula, an uncommon form of fistula-in-ano, is a direct extension of an intersphincteric abscess, and usually starts in the posterior midline. Radical unroofing procedures are seldom necessary. A posterior midline internal sphincterotomy combined with lateral tract curetting and drainage, as recommended by Hanley and Parks, has proved effective (Fig. 28-35).

Fig. 28-34. Use of seton in high fistula. 1. The probe is in the fistulous tract. 2 and 3. A seton or suture is inserted into the fistulous tract and tied loosely over the sphincter to create fibrosis. The fistulous tract will be laid open in the second stage 6 to 8 weeks later.

Anal Incontinence

Anal incontinence results when there is loss of control of the anal sphincter. The term actually covers a broad spectrum of anal function impairment, ranging from simple involuntary passage of flatus to complete loss of sphincter tone with involuntary passage of formed stool.

The external sphincter and puborectalis muscles are primarily responsible for voluntary control. The internal sphincter muscle maintains continence at rest.

Total anal incontinence, with complete loss of sphincter muscle control, is due to physical loss of muscle mass, sensory innervation damage, or central nervous system disease.

Partial anal incontinence is intermittent soiling or passage of flatus involuntarily. This occurs if either the internal sphincter or the external sphincter muscle is defective. Trauma, obstetrical procedures, and anorectal surgery are the three main identifiable causes of partial incontinence. Other causes are inflammatory bowel disease, rectal carcinoma, or rectal prolapse.

Overflow anal incontinence is found in patients with fecal impaction or chronic constipation with prolonged laxative abuse. These patients are either the elderly (bedridden or chronically debilitated) or young children with acquired constipation and/or megacolon. The sphincter muscle mechanism is intact, but the large bolus of feces distends the rectal ampulla, causing relaxation of the internal sphincter, and is responsible for loss of the defecation reflex.

Correction consists of evacuation of the impaction with enemas and, occasionally, manually. Prevention is dietary alteration, the use of bulk-forming stool softeners, in-

Fig. 28-35. Internal sphincterotomy at the site of the intrasphincteric abscess and drainage of the limbs of a horseshoe abscess.

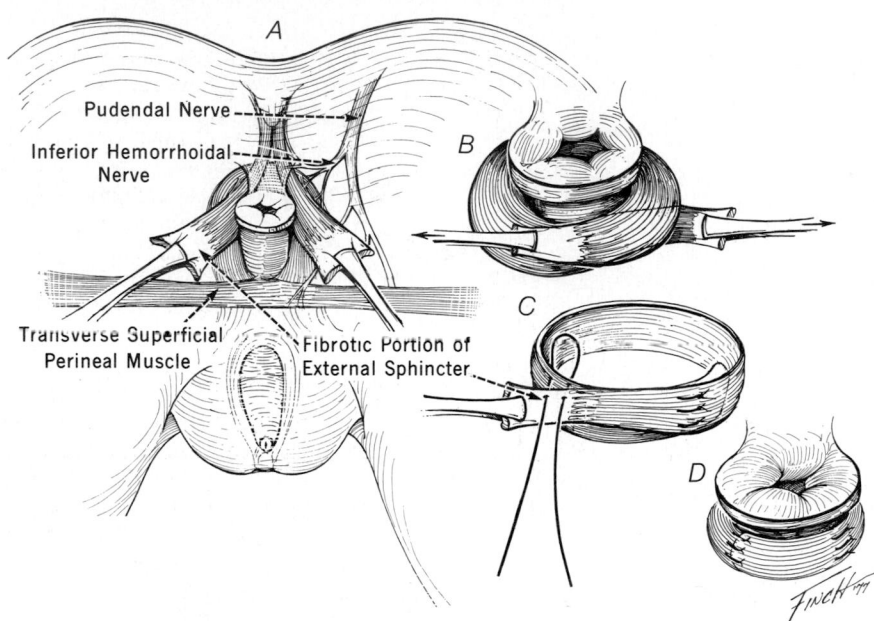

Fig. 28-36. Sphincteroplasty: *A.* The external sphincter muscle is mobilized along with the fibrotic ends. Care should be taken not to injure the inferior hemorrhoidal nerve. *B.* The well-mobilized external sphincter muscle is wrapped around the anal canal. *C.* Mattress sutures of 2-0 polyglycol inserted into the fibrotic ends. *D.* At completion, the anal canal should admit only an index finger.

creased fluid intake, and reestablishment of regular bowel habits. This may require the frequent use of enemas over a long period of time.

TREATMENT. Therapy must be based on consideration of the etiologic factors and judicious selection of patients for operative correction. Only patients with incontinence where there is a muscle defect secondary to trauma, obstetrical tears, or operative procedures should be treated operatively. There are varying types of sphincter repair, and the cause and extent of sphincter loss determine the procedure of choice.

Sphincteroplasty involves mobilization of the divided sphincteric muscle and reapproximation *without tension* (Fig. 28-36). This procedure has become the preferred treatment, because restoration of sphincter continence is achieved. In perineorrhaphy, the puborectalis sling is tightened by a row of sutures anterior or posterior to the rectum. Sphincter-reefing operations are designed to take a tuck in the sphincter to reduce patulousness. Fascial grafts

have been inserted as a sling around the anus to achieve some constriction. Also, the gracilis muscle has been transferred to encircle the anus in an attempt to substitute a segment of innervated muscle, which may be trained as a sphincter. The levator ani muscle group also has been substituted for the puborectalis sling in an attempt to gain voluntary control. Recently, electrical implants have been tried experimentally to provide exogenous electrical stimulation to atonic sphincter muscles. The results are not encouraging to date. Finally, if local operation is futile, a colostomy may be advisable, since an abdominal colostomy is more easily cared for than a "perineal colostomy."

Rectal Prolapse

Prolapse of the rectum is a rare condition in which some or all of the layers of the rectum extrude through the anus. There are two classes of prolapse: true procidentia and rectal mucosal prolapse (false procidentia). The true procidentia extrudes through the anus and is seen as concentric circular rings of mucosa (Fig. 28-37). Rectal mucosal prolapse is seen extruding through the anus in radial folds. True rectal prolapse can occur at any age; however, it seems to be prevalent in institutionalized patients with irregular bowel habits.

There are two predominant theories of the etiology of prolapse: sliding hernia and intussusception. Moschcowitz in 1912 put forth the theory that it is a sliding hernia of the peritoneum of the cul-de-sac of Douglas. The hernia slides through a defect in the pelvic diaphragm, invaginates the anterior wall of the rectum, and intussuscepts the rectum

Fig. 28-37. True rectal procidentia with concentric circular rings of mucosa.

and the rectosigmoid, which protrudes through the anal sphincter. More recently, others have shown the prolapse is not a hernia but an intussusception of the rectosigmoid. It has been shown that the intussusception begins at the rectosigmoid junction. The intussusception pulls the rectosigmoid from its attachments, and, with repeated straining, the rectum pulls away distally. As the intussusception proceeds downward, it reaches the area of the lateral neurovascular stalks, where there are stronger fascial attachments, and hesitates for variable time periods. Eventually, repeated pressure from above, by straining, weakens this barrier and the bowel further descends and protrudes from the anus. In advanced cases, loss of sphincter tone may be due to a neuromuscular deficit. The anatomic defects associated with procidentia of the rectum are a diastasis of the levator ani muscles, weakened endopelvic fascia, loss of the normal horizontal position of the rectum, abnormally deep cul-de-sac, and a weak anal sphincter.

In all these theories, the common characteristic is marked redundancy of the rectosigmoid and loss of the normal angle the rectum makes with the puborectalis sling. Correction entails reestablishment of the proper angle, whether by closing the pelvic floor defect or securing the rectum to the hollow of the sacrum posteriorly.

TREATMENT. Irrespective of one's view of etiologic factors, the operative approach is to correct anatomic defects. Various technical aspects utilized in the repair are correction of the pelvic wall defect by endopelvic fascia repair, approximation of the levator ani muscles and the perineal body in the female, establishment of a normal angle between the rectum and anal canal by securing the rectum in the sacral hollow, obliteration of the cul-de-sac, and removal of the redundant sigmoid colon. The operative approach may be abdominal, abdominoperineal, perineal, or posterior to the rectum through the bed of the coccyx. Each and every procedure has advantages and disadvantages, and none is suitable for all patients.

Altemeier and associates employ resection via a perineal approach, thus avoiding an abdominal operation. This is surprisingly well tolerated in the elderly. It involves excising the protruding bowel, closing the pouch of Douglas as high as possible, and approximating the levator ani muscles anteriorly.

Thomas advocates another approach in which the deep cul-de-sac of Douglas is obliterated, the rectum is affixed to the sacral periosteum, and the mobile redundant sigmoid colon is resected through a sacral approach. This is a satisfactory procedure, but the morbidity and mortality are much higher than with Altemeier's technique.

Those who feel that prolapse is due to intussusception favor a technique by which the rectum is secured to the sacrum, thus restoring the normal horizontal position. Ripstein simply is a sling of synthetic mesh to hold the rectum firmly in the sacral concavity and thus prevent prolapse. Beahrs feels that an anterior resection, removing the redundant sigmoid and rectosigmoid colon, produces the best results. He fully mobilizes the rectum to take advantage of the postoperative scarring that normally takes place, thereby securing the rectum to the sacrum and avoiding the use of a foreign material.

Goldberg and associates use an intraabdominal repair, fully mobilizing the rectum posteriorly but leaving the lateral stalks intact. The lateral stalks are sutured posteriorly to the sacral periosteum. A convenient sigmoid resection with primary anastomosis is performed to eliminate any redundant colon (Fig. 28-38).

In the elderly, if conditions preclude definitive repair, the Thiersch wire procedure may be used, i.e., the anus is encircled with wire or other suture material. The procedure is well tolerated, but success rate is poor, with a high incidence of fecal impaction and suture breakage.

Generally, an intraabdominal repair of anatomic defects is indicated whenever the patient can tolerate the procedure. Reported recurrence rates following the various operative procedures vary from 4 to 35 percent. The principal postoperative problem is anal incontinence. When compared with the perineal approach, the intraabdominal procedure to remove the redundant colon, combined with fixation of the colon to the sacrum, gives a better result, with a lower recurrence rate.

Pruritus Ani

Pruritus ani is a common problem, but a difficult one to solve. The perianal area is sensitive, and any condition causing soiling or moisture to the area can produce itching. The surgically correctable conditions contributing to this condition are prolapsing hemorrhoids, ectropion, anal fissure, fistula-in-ano, condylomata acuminata, and neoplasm of the anal canal and perineum. Other conditions include diabetes mellitus, dermatitis, jaundice, diarrhea, and leukorrhea. Fungous infections, most commonly due to *Monilia* and *Epidermophyton* organisms, are mainly secondary invaders. In children, *Enterobius vermicularis* (pinworm) is a common cause. When no specific causes are found, the pruritus is called "idiopathic" and can be very difficult to treat.

At the present time, there is no specific treatment for idiopathic pruritus ani. Anal hygiene, consisting of gentle cleansing of the anal canal with moist tissue or water, is the cornerstone of successful control. All other possible causes (e.g., sensitivity to toilet paper, various dyes in underclothing, allergy to soap, cream, and ointment) should be excluded. Hydrocortisone, 0.5% preparation, applied locally, gives temporary symptomatic relief. Topical fungicides have also been used successfully for symptomatic control of pruritus ani.

The undercutting operation described for idiopathic pruritus ani is to be condemned, since it provides only temporary relief. Similarly, the subcutaneous injection of alcohol, tattooing with mercury sulfate, and topical irradiation have been abandoned, since they are ineffective or hazardous and give temporary relief.

Condylomata Acuminata

Anal condylomata acuminata, or warts, are caused by a papilloma virus. Condylomata occur in the perianal area or the squamous epithelium of the anal canal. Occasionally, the mucosa of the upper part of the anal canal or the lower

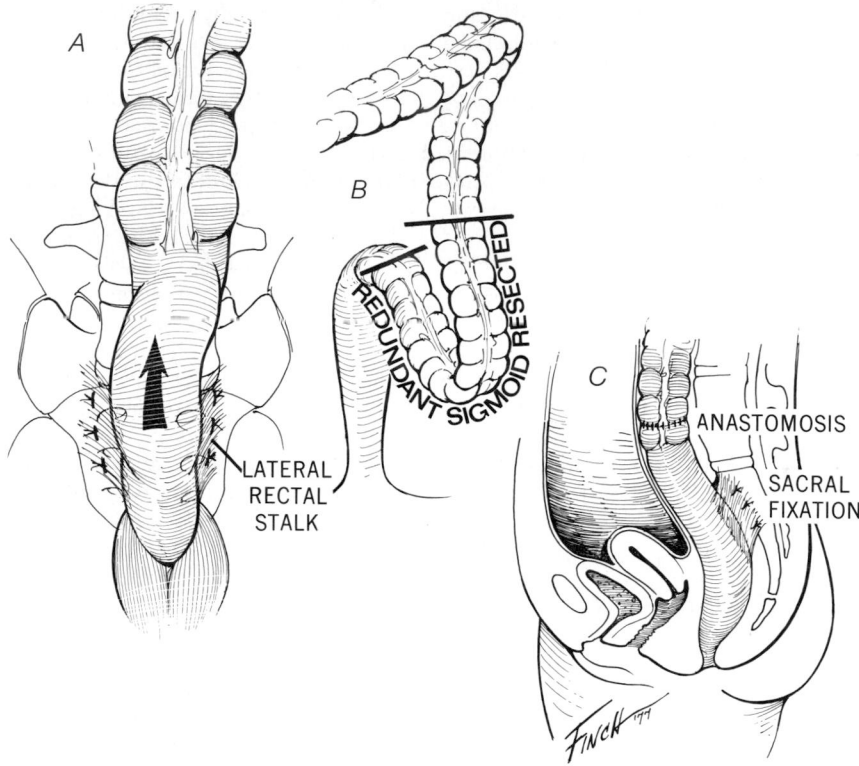

Fig. 28-38. Transabdominal repair of rectal prolapse. 1. Lateral stalks fixed to periosteum of sacrum with 2-0 silk, after rectum has been fully mobilized. 2. Resection of the redundant sigmoid colon. 3. Lateral view after completion.

part of the rectum is involved. The extent of the disease varies from a few small warts to an extensive mass, occluding the anal canal. Bleeding, itching, and irritation are common symptoms. The diagnosis is based on the characteristically soft, papillary appearance. Since most cases are transmitted by sexual contact, other coexisting venereal diseases, especially syphilis and gonorrhea, should be excluded. Multiple biopsies and histologic examination should be done in the extensive warts, since a few cases of squamous cell carcinoma arising from the condylomata acuminata have been reported.

TREATMENT. Small perianal warts can be destroyed by applying 25% podophyllin solution. Extensive warts in the perianal area or in the anal canal require fulguration and excision under anesthesia. Frequent postoperative follow-up is necessary, since recurrence is common. Recently, Abcarian reported encouraging results with immunotherapy, using autogenous wart tissue vaccine. This approach should be used with caution, since vaccines containing oncogenic viruses are potentially dangerous.

Gonococcal Proctitis

Gonococcal proctitis is found most commonly among homosexuals. In the female, the rectum may be infected by the spread of discharge from the gonococcal cervicitis or urethritis. Patients are generally asymptomatic but may have mild anal burning, pain, or discharge in the acute phase. Proctoscopic examination reveals hyperemic and edematous rectal mucosa with purulent discharge in the anal crypt. In the chronic phase, examination of the anal canal and rectum may show them to be normal. Diagnosis

is confirmed by gram smears of the discharge and culture in the appropriate media, Thayer-Martin or Stuart.

Penicillin remains the antibiotic of choice. Kanamycin is used if patients are sensitive to penicillin. Whether the cure is complete is determined by smears and cultures taken at regular intervals after treatment.

Lymphogranuloma Venereum

Lymphogranuloma venereum (lymphogranuloma inguinale) is either an acute or a chronic venereal disease caused by a minute chlamydial bacterium. Transmission of the disease is by intercourse or contact with contaminated exudate from active lesions. In the male, the most common sites are the coronal sulcus, prepuce, glans penis, and urethra. In the female, the primary lesion may appear on any part of the external genitalia, but the most common site is the posterior vaginal wall. The lesion usually is single, consisting of a small erosion, blister, or ulcer, without induration or infiltration. The primary focus is painless and so transient that few patients with lymphogranuloma venereum are aware of it. Adenitis develops in the lymphatic drainage area soon after the primary lesion disappears, although, at times, several months elapse.

Rectal stricture is the sequela to perirectal lymphatic involvement or direct anorectal mucosal infection. The stricture usually is several centimeters above the anal orifice and is 4 to 10 cm in length. Involvement of the perirectal tissues causes perirectal abscess or chronic anal fistulas. Diagnosis is confirmed by the Frei intradermal test and the lymphogranuloma venereum complement fixation test. A cross-reaction with organisms of psittacosis and other chlamydiae may take place. Once positive, the test remains positive for life, and a persistent negative result in the presence of the disease is rare.

Tetracycline or chloramphenicol is the drug of choice. In early stricture, dilatation by finger or dilator is recommended. Colostomy is indicated for complete obstruction. Biopsy for possible malignancy is mandatory.

Proctalgia Fugax

Proctalgia fugax is a severe, spasmodic rectal pain lasting a few minutes or longer. The exact cause is unknown, but the condition may be due to levator ani muscle spasm. The symptom generally occurs in patients who are anxious and overworked. The characteristic history is that of severe pain awakening the patient. The pain usually is located in the midrectum and disappears spontaneously without residual symptoms. Complete proctosigmoidoscopic examination should be performed to rule out anorectal disease.

Treatment to relieve the spasm during an acute attack consists of warm baths or a heating pad applied to the perineum. Since many of these patients are anxious and have cancer phobia, reassurance is an important aspect of therapy.

Neoplasms of the Anus

EPIDERMOID CARCINOMA

Epidermoid carcinoma of the anal canal is uncommon, representing 1 to 2 percent of rectal and colonic carcinomas. The two common varieties are squamous cell carcinoma and transitional cell carcinoma (cloacogenic, basosquamous or basaloid). Squamous cell carcinoma occurs both above and below the dentate line of the anal canal. Transitional cell carcinoma originates from the transitional zone above the dentate line. Since the clinical behavior and prognosis are similar to those of squamous cell carcinoma, transitional cell carcinoma is considered a variant of epidermoid carcinoma.

Early carcinoma of the anal canal presents as an indurated or ulcerated nodule. Rectal pain and bleeding are the most common symptoms. Many cases are misdiagnosed as benign anorectal problems, such as hemorrhoids and anal ulcers, and, consequently, treatment is delayed. Early diagnosis is made by careful examination of the anal canal and confirmed by biopsy.

TREATMENT. Carcinoma of the anal canal spreads to the superior rectal nodes, pelvic nodes, and inguinal nodes. Abdominoperineal resection, with wide evulsion of the perineal tissues, is the treatment of choice. In selected small tumors distal to the dentate line, local excisions have been adequate, provided the sphincter muscles are not involved. The 5-year survival of the operatively treated patients is 55 to 60 percent.

Recently, Papillon used radium implantation to treat epidermoid carcinoma of the anal canal. The 5-year survival, with no evidence of disease, was 68 percent. He selected patients who had no palpable nodes in the rectal wall. Those with clinically palpable nodes should have abdominoperineal resection. Modern techniques of supervoltage irradiation also offer good results. Williams treated 32 patients who were not suitable for surgery. The 5-year survival was 37.5 percent, and there was no irradiation necrosis. Prophylactic inguinal node dissection is not advisable. However, prompt radical groin dissection should be carried out when clinical metastases have developed. Frequent and careful follow-up examinations are essential, since the incidence of inguinal node involvement is 35 to 40 percent. Inguinal node metastases occur synchronously in 15 percent of patients and subsequently develop in 20 to 25 percent.

Generally, prognosis is poor in patients with anal epidermoid carcinoma with simultaneous groin metastases. Those with subsequent groin metastases have a much better prognosis. Stearns and Quan reported that 15 of 20 patients survived 5 years after groin dissection for subsequent metastases.

MALIGNANT MELANOMA

Melanoma, a rare malignant tumor of the anal canal, accounts for 0.5 to 1.0 percent of anal canal malignant tumors. The anal canal, however, represents the third most common site for melanomas, preceded only by the skin and eyes. Almost all the tumors arise from the epidermoid lining of the anal canal. Most melanomas occur adjacent to the dentate line, although there are a few reports of these tumors arising in the rectum.

Rectal bleeding is the most common symptom. Melanoma is suspected when a deeply pigmented lesion is noted, but this can be confused with thrombosed hemorrhoids. The majority of tumors, however, are pigmented lightly or nonpigmented, and they often are misdiagnosed as polyps or epidermoid carcinoma. In the amelanotic malignant melanoma, tissue biopsy can be misdiagnosed as an undifferentiated epidermoid carcinoma.

Anal canal melanomas have a marked tendency to spread submucosally into the rectum, but they rarely invade adjacent organs. Lymphatic spread to the mesenteric nodes occurs in about one-third of the patients; spread to the inguinal nodes is less common. Hematogenous spread to the liver and lung is early and rapid, accounting for most of the deaths.

Melanomas are radioresistant and do not respond well to chemotherapy. The only chance for cure, therefore, is early diagnosis followed by radical operation. Abdominoperineal resection represents the approach of choice, but the prognosis remains extremely poor.

References

Inflammatory Bowel Disease

Barker, W. F., Benfield, J. R., deKernion, J. B., Fonkalsrud, E. W., and Fowler, E.: "The Creation and Care of Enterocutaneous Stomas," *Curr Probl Surg,* Year Book Medical Publishers, Inc., Chicago, 1975.

Beahrs, O. H.: Creating an Ileal Reservoir with a Continent Ileostomy, *Contemp Surg,* **8:**43, 1976.

Binder, S. C., Patterson, J. F., and Glotzer, D. J.: Toxic Megacolon in Ulcerative Colitis, *Gastroenterology,* **66:**909, 1974.

Brooke, B. N. (ed.): Crohn's Disease, in "Clinics in Gastroenterology," vol 1, part 2, W. B. Saunders Company, Ltd., London, 1972.

Burch, P. R. J., DeDombal, F. T., and Watkinson, G.: Aetiology of Ulcerative Colitis: A New Hypothesis, *Gut,* **10:**277, 1969.

Buzzard, A. J., Baker, W. N. W., Needham, P. R. G., and Warren, R. E.: Acute Toxic Dilatation of the Colon in Crohn's Colitis, *Gut,* **15:**416, 1974.

Cave, D. R., Mitchell, D. N., and Brooke, B. N.: Evidence of an Agent Transmissible from Ulcerative Colitis Tissue, *Lancet,* **1:**1311, 1976.

Devroede, G., and Taylor, W. F.: On Calculating Cancer Risk and Survival of Ulcerative Colitis Patients with the Life Table Method, *Gastroenterology,* **71:**505, 1976.

Dissanayake, A. S., and Truelove, S. C.: A Controlled Therapeutic Trial of Long-Term Maintenance Treatment of Ulcerative Colitis with Sulphasalazine (Salazopyrin), *Gut,* **14:**923, 1973.

Eade, M. N., Cooke, W. T., and Brooke, B. N.: Liver Disease in Ulcerative Colitis: II. The Long-Term Effect of Colectomy, *Ann Intern Med,* **72:**489, 1970.

Esler, M. D., and Goulston, K. J.: Levels of Anxiety in Colonic Disorders, *N Engl J Med,* **288:**16, 1973.

Farmer, R. G., Hawk, W. A., and Turnbull, R. B., Jr.: Clinical Patterns in Crohn's Disease: A Statistical Study of 615 Cases, *Gastroenterology,* **68:**627, 1975.

Fawaz, K. A., Glotzer, D. J., Goldman, H., Dickerson, G. R., Gross, W., and Patterson, J. F.: Ulcerative Colitis and Crohn's Disease of the Colon—A Comparison of the Long Term Postoperative Courses, *Gastroenterology,* **71:**372, 1976.

Foglia, R., Ament, M. E., Fleisher, D., and Fonkalsrud, E. W.: Surgical Management of Ulcerative Colitis in Childhood, *Am J Surg,* **134:**58, 1977.

Gadacz, T. R., Kelly, K. A., and Phillips, S. F.: The Continent Ileal Pouch: Absorptive and Motor Features, *Gastroenterology,* **72:**1287, 1977.

Goodman, M. J., Kirsner, J. B., and Riddell, R. H.: Usefulness of Rectal Biopsy in Inflammatory Bowel Disease, *Gastroenterology,* **72:**952, 1977.

Greenstein, A. J., Sachar, D. B., and Kark, A. E.: Stricture of the Anorectum in Crohn's Disease Involving the Rectum, *Ann Surg,* **181:**207, 1975.

———, Sachar, D. B., Pasternack, B. S., and Janowitz, H. D.: Reoperation and Recurrence in Crohn's Colitis and Ileocolitis, *N Engl J Med,* **293:**685, 1975.

Keighley, M. R. B., Thompson, H., and Alexander-Williams, J.: Multifocal Colonic Carcinoma and Crohn's Disease, *Surgery,* **78:**534, 1975.

Kirsner, J. B.: Toxic Megacolon Complicating Ulcerative Colitis: Current Therapeutic Perspectives, *Gastroenterology,* **66:**1088, 1974.

———: Problems in the Differentiation of Ulcerative Colitis and Crohn's Disease of the Colon: The Need for Repeated Diagnostic Evaluation, *Gastroenterology,* **68:**187, 1975.

———, and Shorter, R. G.: "Inflammatory Bowel Disease," Lea & Febiger, Philadelphia, 1975.

Kock, N. G.: Present Status of the Continent Ileostomy: Surgical Revision of the Malfunctioning Ileostomy, *Dis Colon Rectum,* **19:**200, 1976.

Lefton, H. B., Farmer, R. G., and Fazio, V.: Ileorectal Anastomosis for Crohn's Disease of the Colon, *Gastroenterology,* **69:**612, 1975.

Margulis, A. R., Goldberg, H. I., Lawson, T. L., Montgomery, C. K., Rambo, O. N., Noonan, C. D., and Amberg, J. R.: The Overlapping Spectrum of Ulcerative and Granulomatous Colitis, *Am J Roentgenol Radium Ther Nucl Med,* **113:**325, 1971.

Mendeloff, A. I., Monk, M., Siegel, C. I., and Lilienfeld, A.: Illness Experience and Life Stresses in Patients with Irritable Colon and with Ulcerative Colitis, *N Engl J Med,* **282:**14, 1970.

Morson, B. C.: Rectal Biopsy in Inflammatory Bowel Disease, *N Engl J Med,* **287:**1337, 1972.

Mottet, N. K.: "Major Problems in Pathology," vol. II, "Histopathologic Spectrum of Regional Enteritis and Ulcerative Colitis," W. B. Saunders Company, Philadelphia, 1971.

Nugent, F. W., Veidenheimer, M. C., Meissner, W. A., and Haggitt, R. C.: Prognosis after Colonic Resection for Crohn's Disease of the Colon, *Gastroenterology,* **65:**398, 1973.

Rosenberg, J. L., Wall, A. J., Levin, B., Binder, H. J., and Kirsner, J. B.: A Controlled Trial of Azathioprine in the Management of Chronic Ulcerative Colitis, *Gastroenterology,* **69:**96, 1975.

Schachter, H., and Kirsner, J. B.: Definitions of Inflammatory Bowel Disease of Unknown Etiology, *Gastroenterology,* **68:**591, 1975.

Shorter, R. G., Huizenga, K. A., and Spencer, R. J.: A Working Hypothesis for the Etiology and Pathogenesis of Non-specific Inflammatory Bowel Disease, *Am J Dig Dis,* **17:**1024, 1972.

Sommers, S. C.: Mast Cells and Paneth Cells in Ulcerative Colitis, *Gastroenterology,* **51:**841, 1966.

Steinberg, D. M., Allan, R. N., Brooke, B. N., Cooke, W. T., and Alexander-Williams, J.: Sequelae of Colectomy and Ileostomy: Comparison between Crohn's Colitis and Ulcerative Colitis, *Gastroenterology,* **68:**33, 1975.

Teague, R. H., and Read, A. E.: Polyposis in Ulcerative Colitis, *Gut,* **16:**792, 1975.

Thayer, W. R., Jr.: Are the Inflammatory Bowel Diseases Immune Complex Diseases? *Gastroenterology,* **70:**136, 1976.

Tompkins, R. K., Weinstein, M. H., Foroozan, P., Marx, F. W., and Barker, W. F.: Reappraisal of Rectum-retaining Operations for Ulcerative and Granulomatous Colitis, *Am J Surg,* **125:**159, 1973.

Turnbull, R. B., Jr., Hawk, W. A., and Weakley, F. L.: Surgical Treatment of Toxic Megacolon, *Am J Surg,* **122:**325, 1971.

Veidenheimer, M. C., Nugent, F. W., and Haggitt, R. C.: Ulcerative Colitis of Crohn's Colitis: Is Differentiation Necessary? *Surg Clin North Am,* **56:**721, 1976.

Warshaw, A. L., Welch, J. P., and Ottinger, L. W.: Acute Perforation of the Colon Associated with Chronic Corticosteroid Therapy, *Am J Surg,* **131:**442, 1976.

Watt, J., and Marcus, R.: Progress Report. Experimental Ulcerative Disease of the Colon in Animals, *Gut,* **14:**506, 1973.

Watts, J. McK., and Hughes, E. S. R.: Ulcerative Colitis and Crohn's Disease: Results after Colectomy and Ileorectal Anastomosis, *Br J Surg,* **64:**77, 1977.

Wright, H. K.: The Functional Consequences of Colectomy, *Am J Surg,* **130:**532, 1975.

———, and Tilson, M. D.: A Method for Testing the Functional Significance of Tight Ileostomy Stomas, *Am J Surg,* **123:**417, 1972.

Yudin, I. Y., Sergevnin, V. V., Krasmova, A. I., and Ginsburg, S. A.: The Feasibility of Ileorectal Anastomosis for Nonspecific Ulcerative Colitis, *Contemp Surg,* **6:**73, 1975.

Ischemic Colitis

Marston, A. (ed.): Vascular Diseases of the Alimentary Tract, in "Clinics in Gastroenterology," vol 1, part 3, W. B. Saunders Company, Ltd., London, 1972.

O'Connell, T. X., Kadell, B., and Tompkins, R. K.: Ischemia of the Colon, *Surg Gynecol Obstet,* **142:**337, 1976.

Williams, L. F., Jr., and Wittenberg, J.: Ischemic Colitis: An Useful Clinical Diagnosis, but Is It Ischemic? *Ann Surg,* **182:**439, 1975.

Radiation Enterocolitis

Cram, A. E., Pearlman, N. W., and Jochimsen, P. R.: Surgical Management of Complications of Radiation-Injured Gut, *Am J Surg,* **133:**551, 1977.

DeCosse, J. J., Rhodes, R. S., Wentz, W. B., Reagan, J. W., Dworken, H. J., and Holden, W. D.: The Natural History and Management of Radiation Induced Injury of the Gastrointestinal Tract, *Ann Surg,* **170:**369, 1969.

Green, N., Iba, G., and Smith, W. R.: Measures to Minimize Small Intestine Injury in the Irradiated Pelvis, *Cancer,* **35:**1633, 1975.

Morgenstern, L., Thompson, R., and Friedman, N. B.: The Modern Enigma of Radiation Enteropathy: Sequelae and Solutions, *Am J Surg,* **134:**166, 1977.

Palmer, J. A., and Bush, R. S.: Radiation Injuries to the Bowel Associated with the Treatment of Carcinoma of the Cervix, *Surgery,* **80:**458, 1976.

Swan, R. W., Fowler, W. C., Jr., and Boronow, R. C.: Surgical Management of Radiation Injury to the Small Intestine, *Surg Gynecol Obstet,* **142:**325, 1976.

Pseudobranous Enterocolitis

Birnbaum, D., Laufer, A., and Freund, M.: Pseudomembranous Enterocolitis, *Gastroenterology,* **41:**345, 1961.

Gorbach, S. L., and Bartlett, J. G. (eds.): The Role of Clindamycin in Anaerobic Bacterial Infections. A Symposium, *J Infect Dis,* **135** (suppl), 1977.

Tedesco, F. J., Barton, R. W., and Alpers, D. H.: Clindamycin-associated Colitis, a Prospective Study, *Ann Intern Med,* **81:**429, 1974.

Amebiasis

Grigsby, W. P.: Collective Review: Surgical Treatment of Amebiasis, *Surg Gynecol Obstet,* **128:**609, 1969.

Mahmoud, A. A. F., and Warren, K. S.: Algorithms in the Diagnosis and Management of Exotic Diseases: XVII. Amebiasis, *J Infect Dis,* **134:**639, 1976.

Pittman, F. E., El-Hashimi, W. K., and Pittman, J. C.: Studies of Human Amebiasis, *Gastroenterology,* **65:**581 1973

Actinomycosis

Davies, M., and Keddie, N. C.: Abdominal Actinomycosis, *Br J Surg,* **60:**18, 1973.

Diverticular Disease

Adams, J. T.: The Barium Enema as Treatment for Massive Diverticular Bleeding, *Dis Colon Rectum,* **17:**439, 1974.

Athanasoulis, C. A., Baum, S., Rosch, J., Waltman, A. C., Ring, E. J., Smith, J. C., Jr., Sugarbaker, E., and Wood, W.: Mesenteric Arterial Infusions of Vasopressin for Hemorrhage from Colonic Diverticulosis, *Am J Surg,* **129:**212, 1975.

Behringer, G. E., and Albright, N. L.: Diverticular Disease of the Colon: A Frequent Cause of Massive Rectal Bleeding, *Am J Surg,* **125:**419, 1973.

Berman, L. G., Burdick, D., Heitzman, E. R., and Prior, J. T.: A Critical Reappraisal of Sigmoid Peridiverticulitis, *Surg Gynecol Obstet,* **127:**481, 1968.

Botsford, T. W., Zollinger, R. M., Jr., and Hicks, R.: Mortality of the Surgical Treatment of Diverticulitis, *Am J Surg,* **121:**702, 1971.

Canter, J. W., and Shorb, P. E., Jr.: Acute Perforation of Colonic Diverticula Associated with Prolonged Adrenocorticosteroid Therapy, *Am J Surg,* **121:**46, 1971.

Casarella, W. J., Kanter, I. E., and Seaman, W. B.: Right-sided Colonic Diverticula as a Cause of Acute Rectal Hemorrhage, *N Engl J Med,* **286:**450, 1972.

Classen, J. N., Bonardi, R., O'Mara, C. S., Finney, D. C. W., and Sterioff, S.: Surgical Treatment of Acute Diverticulitis by Staged Procedures, *Ann Surg,* **184:**582, 1976.

Colcock, B. P.: Diverticular Disease of the Colon, in "Major Problems in Clinical Surgery," W. B. Saunders Company, Philadelphia, 1971.

———, and Stahmann, F. D.: Fistulas Complicating Diverticular Disease of the Sigmoid Colon, *Ann Surg,* **175:**838, 1972.

Drapanas, T., Pennington, D. G., Kappelman, M., and Lindsey, E. S.: Emergency Subtotal Colectomy: Preferred Approach to Management of Massively Bleeding Diverticular Disease, *Ann Surg,* **177:**519, 1973.

Eng, K., Ranson, J. H. C., and Localio, S. A.: Resection of the Perforated Segment: A Significant Advance in Treatment of Diverticulitis with Free Perforation or Abscess, *Am J Surg,* **133:**67, 1977.

Fleischner, F. G.: Diverticular Disease of the Colon: New Observations and Revised Concepts, *Gastroenterology,* **60:**316, 1971.

Havia, T.: Diverticulosis of the Colon: A Clinical and Histological Study, *Acta Chir Scand [Suppl],* 415, 1971.

Magness, L. J., Sanfelippo, P. M., van Heerden, J. A., and Judd, E. S.: Diverticular Disease of the Right Colon, *Surg Gynecol Obstet,* **140:**30, 1975.

Meyers, M. A., Alonso, D. R., Gray, G. F., and Baer, J. W.: Pathogenesis of Bleeding Colonic Diverticulosis, *Gastroenterology,* **71:**577, 1976.

Miller, D. W., Jr., and Wichern, W. A., Jr.: Perforated Sigmoid Diverticulitis: Appraisal of Primary versus Delayed Resection, *Am J Surg,* **121:**536, 1971.

Morson, B. C.: Pathology of Diverticular Disease of the Colon, in A. N. Smith (ed.), "Clinics in Gastroenterology," vol 4, part 1, W. B. Saunders Company, Ltd., London, 1975.

Nahrwold, D. L., and Demuth, W. E.: Diverticulitis with Perforation into the Peritoneal Cavity, *Ann Surg,* **185:**80, 1977.

Nicholas, G. G., Miller, W. T., Fitts, W. T., and Tondreau, R. L.: Diagnosis of Diverticulitis of the Colon: Role of the Barium

Enema in Defining Pericolic Inflammation, *Ann Surg,* **176:**205, 1972.

Painter, N. S., Truelove, S. C., Ardran, G. M., and Tuckey, M.: Segmentation and the Localization of Intraluminal Pressures in the Human Colon, with Special Reference to the Pathogenesis of Colonic Diverticula, *Gastroenterology,* **49:**169, 1965.

Parks, T. G., and Connell, A. M.: The Outcome in 455 Patients Admitted for Treatment of Diverticular Disease of the Colon, *Br J Surg,* **57:**775, 1970.

Parsa, F., Gordon, H. E., and Wilson, S. E.: Bleeding Diverticulosis of the Colon, *Dis Colon Rectum,* **18:**37, 1975.

Ranson, J. H. C., Lawrence, L. R., and Localio, S. A.: Colomyotomy: A New Approach to Surgery for Colonic Diverticular Disease, *Am J Surg,* **123:**185, 1972.

Reilly, M.: Sigmoid Myotomy, in A. N. Smith (ed.), "Clinics in Gastroenterology," vol 4, part 1, W. B. Saunders Company, Ltd., London, 1975.

Rugtiv, G. M.: Diverticulitis: Selective Surgical Management, *Am J Surg,* **130:**219, 1975.

Walker, J. D., Gray, L. A., Sr., and Polk, H. C., Jr.: Diverticulitis in Women: An Unappreciated Clinical Presentation, *Ann Surg,* **185:**402, 1977.

Polyps and Polyposis

Alm, T.: Surgical Treatment of Hereditary Adenomatosis of the Colon and Rectum in Sweden during the Last 20 Years: II. Patients with Prophylactic Operations, Primary and Late Results, *Acta Chir Scand,* **141:**228, 1975.

Bussey, H. J. R.: "Familial Polyposis Coli," The Johns Hopkins University Press, Baltimore, 1975.

Cole, J. W.: Carcinogens and Carcinogenesis in the Colon, *Hosp Pract,* **8:**123, 1973.

———, and Holden, W. D.: Postcolectomy Regression of Adenomatous Polyps of the Rectum, *Arch Surg,* **79:**385, 1959.

———, and McKalen, A.: Studies on the Morphogenesis of Adenomatous Polyps in the Human Colon, *Cancer,* **16:**998, 1963.

DeCosse, J. J., Adams, M. B., and Condon, R. E.: Familial Polyposis, *Cancer,* **39:**267, 1977.

Erbe, R. W.: Current Concepts in Genetics. Inherited Gastrointestinal-Polyposis Syndromes, *N Engl J Med,* **294:**1101, 1976.

Fenoglio, C. M., and Lane, N.: The Anatomical Precursor of Colorectal Carcinoma, *Cancer,* **34** [suppl], 819, 1974.

Gilbertsen, V. A.: Proctosigmoidoscopy and Polypectomy in Reducing the Incidence of Rectal Cancer, *Cancer,* **34** [suppl], 936, 1974.

Knoernschild, H. E.: Growth Rate and Malignant Potential of Colonic Polyps: Early Results, *Surg Forum,* **14:**137, 1963.

Lane, N., Kaplan, H., and Pascal, R. R.: Minute Adenomatous and Hyperplastic Polyps of the Colon: Divergent Patterns of Epithelial Growth with Specific Associated Mesenchymal Changes. Contrasting Roles in the Pathogenesis of Carcinoma, *Gastroenterology,* **60:**537, 1971.

Lipkin, M.: Phase 1 and Phase 2 Proliferative Lesions of Colonic Epithelial Cells in Diseases Leading to Colonic Cancer, *Cancer,* **34** [suppl], 878, 1974.

Lynch, H. T., Harris, R. E., Organ, C. H., Jr., Guirgis, H. A., Lynch, P. M., Lynch, J. F., and Nelson, E. J.: The Surgeon, Genetics, and Cancer Control: The Cancer Family Syndrome, *Ann Surg,* **185:**435, 1977.

Moertel, C. G., Hill, J. R., and Adson, M. A.: Surgical Management of Multiple Polyposis: The Problem of Cancer in the Retained Bowel Segment, *Arch Surg,* **100:**521, 1970.

Morson, B. C., and Bussey, H. J. S.: Predisposing Causes of Intestinal Cancers, *Curr Probl Surg,* February, 1970.

Muto, T., Bussey, H. J. R., and Morson, B. C.: The Evolution of Cancer of the Colon and Rectum, *Cancer,* **36:**2251, 1975.

Nivatvongs, S., and Goldberg, S. M.: Results of 100 Consecutive Polypectomies with the Fiberoptic Colonoscope, *Am J Surg,* **128:**347, 1974.

Shinya, H., and Wolff, W.: Flexible Colonoscopy, *Cancer,* **37** [suppl], 462, 1976.

Spratt, J. S., Ackerman, L. V., and Moyer, C. A.: Relationship of Polyps of the Colon to Colonic Cancer, *Ann Surg,* **148:**682, 1958.

Watne, W. L., Lai, H.-Y., Carrier, J., and Coppula, W.: The Diagnosis and Surgical Treatment of Patients with Gardner's Syndrome, *Surgery,* **82:**327, 1977.

Welch, C. E., and Hedberg, S. E.: "Polypoid Lesions of the Gastrointestinal Tract," 2d ed., W. B. Saunders Company, Philadelphia, 1975.

Welch, J. P., and Welch, C. E.: Villous Adenomas of the Colorectum, *Am J Surg,* **131:**185, 1976.

Carcinoma

Bengmark, S., and Hafström, L.: The Natural History of Primary and Secondary Malignant Tumors of the Liver: I. The Prognosis for Patients with Hepatic Metastases from Colonic and Rectal Carcinoma by Laparotomy, *Cancer,* **23:**198, 1969.

Berge, T., Ekelund, G., Mellner, C., Pihl, B., and Wenckert, A.: Carcinoma of the Colon and Rectum in a Defined Population, *Acta Chir Scand* [suppl], 438, 1973.

Burkitt, D. P.: Large-Bowel Cancer: An Epidemiologic Jigsaw Puzzle, *J Natl Cancer Inst,* **54:**3, 1975.

Cass, A. W., Million, R. R., and Pfaff, W. W.: Patterns of Recurrence following Surgery Alone for Adenocarcinoma of the Colon and Rectum, *Cancer,* **37:**2861, 1976.

Clark, J., Hall, W. W., and Moossa, A. R.: Treatment of Obstructing Cancer of the Colon and Rectum, *Surg Gynecol Obstet,* **141:**541, 1975.

Clarke, J. S., Condon, R. E., Bartlett, J. G., Gorbach, S. L., Nichols, R. L., and Ochi, S.: Preoperative Oral Antibiotics Reduce Septic Complications of Colon Operations: Results of Prospective, Randomized, Double-blind Clinical Study, *Ann Surg,* **186:**251, 1977.

Cole, W. H.: Collective Review: The Mechanisms of Spread of Cancer, *Surg Gynecol Obstet,* **137:**853, 1973.

Collins, V. P.: Time of Occurrence of Pulmonary Metastases from Carcinoma of Colon and Rectum, *Cancer,* **15:**387, 1962.

Crapp, A. R., and Cuthbertson, A. M.: William Waldeyer and the Rectosacral Fascia, *Surg Gynecol Obstet,* **138:**252, 1974.

Crile, G., Jr., and Turnbull, R. B., Jr.: The Role of Electrocoagulation in the Treatment of Carcinoma of the Rectum, *Surg Gynecol Obstet,* **135:**391, 1972.

Ekelund, G. R., and Pihl, B.: Multiple Carcinomas of the Colon and Rectum, *Cancer,* **33:**1630, 1974.

Gardner, B., Kottmeier, P., and Harshaw, D.: The Surgeon at Work: A Modified One Stage Pull Through Operation for Carcinoma or Prolapse of the Rectum, *Surg Gynecol Obstet,* **136:**95, 1973.

Goldsmith, H. S.: Protection of Low Rectal Anastomosis with Intact Omentum, *Surg Gynecol Obstet,* **144:**585, 1977.

Goldstein, M., and Duff, J. H.: Reconsideration of Colostomy in Elective Left Colon Resection, *Surg Gynecol Obstet,* **134:**593, 1972.

Goligher, J. C., Graham, N. G., and DeDombal, F. T.: Anastomotic Dehiscence after Anterior Resection of Rectum and Sigmoid, *Br J Surg,* **57:**109, 1970.

Greegor, D. H.: Occult Blood Testing for Detection of Asymptomatic Colon Cancer, *Cancer,* **28:**131, 1971.

Griffen, W. O., Jr., Humphrey, L. J., and Sosin, H.: The Prognosis and Management of Recurrent Abdominal Malignancies, *Curr Probl Surg,* April, 1969.

Grinnell, R. S.: The Chance of Cancer and Lymphatic Metastasis in Small Colon Tumors Discovered on X-ray Examination, *Ann Surg,* **159:**132, 1964.

Herrera, M. A., Chu, T. M., Holyoke, E. D., and Mittelman, A.: CEA Monitoring of Palliative Treatment of Colorectal Carcinoma, *Ann Surg,* **185:**23, 1977.

Higgins, G. A., Jr., Conn, J. H., Jordan, P. H., Jr., Humphrey, E. W., Roswit, B., and Keehn, R. J.: Preoperative Radiotherapy for Colorectal Cancer, *Ann Surg,* **181:**624, 1975.

———, Humphrey, E., Juler, G. L., LeVeen, H. H., McCaughan, J., and Keehn, R. J.: Adjuvant Chemotherapy in the Surgical Treatment of Large Bowel Cancer, *Cancer,* **38:**1461, 1976.

Irvin, T. T., and Goligher, J. C.: A Controlled Clinical Trial of Three Different Methods of Perineal Wound Management following Excision of the Rectum, *Br J Surg,* **62:**287, 1975.

Johnson, R. J. R.: The Role of Radiation Therapy in the Management of Rectosigmoid Cancer, *Cancer,* **40:**595, 1977.

Keighley, M. R. B.: Prevention of Wound Sepsis in Gastro-intestinal Surgery, *Br J Surg,* **64:**315, 1977.

Lawrence, W., Jr., Terz, J. J., Horsley, S., III, Donaldson, M., Lovett, W. L., Brown, P. W., Ruffner, B. W., and Regelson, W.: Chemotherapy as an Adjuvant to Surgery for Colorectal Cancer, *Ann Surg,* **181:**616, 1975.

Localio, S. A., and Eng, K.: Malignant Tumors of the Rectum, *Curr Probl Surg,* September, 1975.

Lockhart-Mummery, H. E., Ritchie, J. K., and Hawley, P. R.: The Results of Surgical Treatment for Carcinoma of the Rectum at St. Mark's Hospital from 1948 to 1972, *Br J Surg,* **63:**673, 1976.

Madden, J. L., and Kandalaft, S.: Electrocoagulation in the Treatment of Cancer of the Rectum: A Continuing Study, *Ann Surg,* **174:**530, 1971.

Nadler, S. H., and Phelan, J. T.: The Surgeon at Work: Abdominoperineal Resection, *Surg Gynecol Obstet,* **128:**119, 1969.

Oh, C., and Kark, A. E.: The Transsphincteric Approach to Mid and Low Rectal Villous Adenoma: Anatomic Basis of Surgical Treatment, *Ann Surg,* **176:**605, 1972.

Papillon, J.: Intracavitary Irradiation of Early Rectal Cancer for Cure, *Cancer,* **36:**696, 1975.

Polk, H. C., Jr., Ahmad, W., and Knutson, C. O.: Carcinoma of the Colon and Rectum, *Curr Probl Surg,* January, 1973.

Reddy, B. S., Mastromarino, A., and Wynder, E.: Diet and Metabolism: Large-Bowel Cancer, *Cancer,* **39:**1815, 1977.

Schrock, T. R., Deveney, C. W., and Dunphy, J. E.: Factors Contributing to Leakage of Colonic Anastomoses, *Ann Surg,* **177:**513, 1973.

Silverman, D. T., Murray, J. L., Smart, C. R., Brown, C. C., and

Myers, M. H.: Estimated Median Survival Times of Patients with Colorectal Cancer Based on Experience with 9,745 Patients, *Am J Surg,* **133:**289, 1977.

Slanetz, C. A., Herter, F. P., and Grinnell, R. S.: Anterior Resection versus Abdominoperineal Resection for Cancer of the Rectum and Rectosigmoid, *Am J Surg,* **123:**110, 1972.

Spjut, H. J., and Noall, M. W.: Experimental Induction of Tumors of the Large Bowel of Rats, *Cancer,* **28:**29, 1971.

Tank, E. S., Ernst, C. B., Woolson, S. T., and Lapides, J.: Urinary Tract Complications of Anorectal Surgery, *Am J Surg,* **123:**118, 1972.

Turnbull, R. B., Jr.: The No-Touch Isolation Technique of Resection, *JAMA,* **231:**1181, 1975.

Wallack, M. K., Brown, A. S., Rosato, E. F., and Rosato, F. E.: Collective Reviews: The Treatment of Cancer of the Large Intestine, *Surg Gynecol Obstet,* **142:**97, 1976.

Washington, J. A., II, Dearing, W. H., Judd, E. S., and Elveback, L. R.: Effect of Preoperative Antibiotic Regimen on Development of Infection after Intestinal Surgery: Prospective, Randomized, Double-Blind Study, *Ann Surg,* **180:**567, 1974.

Weinstein, M., and Roberts, M.: Sexual Potency following Surgery for Rectal Carcinoma, *Ann Surg,* **185:**295, 1977.

Welch, J. P., and Donaldson, G. A.: Perforative Carcinoma of Colon and Rectum, *Ann Surg,* **180:**734, 1974.

Welin, S., Youker, J., and Spratt, J. S., Jr.: The Rates and Patterns of Growth of 375 Tumors of the Large Intestine and Rectum Observed Serially by Double Contrast Enema Study (Malmo Technique), *Am J Roentgenol Radium Ther Nucl Med,* **90:**673, 1963.

Whittaker, M., and Goligher, J. C.: The Prognosis after Surgical Treatment for Carcinoma of the Rectum, *Br J Surg,* **63:**384, 1976.

Winawer, S. J., Sherlock, P., Schottenfeld, D., and Miller, D. G.: Screening for Colon Cancer, *Gastroenterology,* **70:**783, 1976.

Wright, H. K., Thomas, W. H., and Cleveland, J. C.: The Low Recurrence Rate of Colonic Carcinoma in Ileocolic Anastomosis, *Surg Gynecol Obstet,* **129:**960, 1969.

Other Tumors

Freni, S. C., and Keeman, J. N.: Leiomyomatosis of the Colon, *Cancer,* **39:**263, 1977.

Gray, L. A.: Endometriosis of the Bowel: Role of Bowel Resection, Superficial Excision and Oophorectomy in Treatment, *Ann Surg,* **177:**580, 1973.

Orloff, M. J.: Carcinoid Tumors of the Rectum, *Cancer,* **28:**175, 1971.

Scott, J. E.: Carcinoid Tumours of the Colon, *Br J Surg,* **60:**684, 1973.

Wychulis, A. R., Beahrs, O. H., and Woolner, L. B.: Malignant Lymphoma of the Colon: A Study of 69 Cases, *Arch Surg,* **93:**215, 1966.

Volvulus and Related Problems

Andersson, Å., Bergdahl, L., and Van der Linden, W.: Volvulus of the Cecum, *Ann Surg,* **181:**876, 1975.

Arnold, G. J., and Nance, F. C.: Volvulus of the Sigmoid Colon, *Ann Surg,* **177:**527, 1973.

Caplan, L. H., Jacobson, H. G., Rubenstein, B. M., and Rotman, M. Z.: Megacolon and Volvulus in Parkinson's Disease, *Radiology,* **85:**73, 1965.

Childress, M. H., and Martel, W.: Fecaloma Simulating Colonic Neoplasm, *Surg Gynecol Obstet,* **142:**664, 1976.

da Silveira, G. M.: Chagas' Disease of the Colon, *Br J Surg,* **63:**831, 1976.

Fairgrieve, J.: Hirschsprung's Disease in the Adult, *Br J Surg,* **50:**506, 1963.

Flanigan, R. C., and Barry, F.: Dual Cecostomy as an Approach to Volvulus of the Cecum, *Surg Gynecol Obstet,* **141:**775, 1975.

Hines, J. R., Guerkink, R. E., and Bass, R. T.: Recurrence and Mortality Rates in Sigmoid Volvulus, *Surg Gynecol Obstet,* **124:**567, 1967.

Huttunen, R., Heikkınen, E., and Larmi, T. K. I.: Stercoraceous and Idiopathic Perforations of the Colon, *Surg Gynecol Obstet,* **140:**756, 1975.

Maglietta, E. D.: Congenital Aganglionic Megacolon in Adults, *Arch Surg,* **18:**598, 1960.

Peterson, H.: Volvulus of the Cecum, *Ann Surg,* **166:**296, 1967.

String, S. T., and DeCosse, J. J.: Sigmoid Volvulus: An Examination of the Mortality, *Am J Surg,* **121:**293, 1971.

Watkins, G. L., and Oliver, G. A.: Giant Megacolon in the Insane: Further Observation on Patients Treated by Subtotal Colectomy, *Gastroenterology,* **48:**718, 1965.

Rectum and Anus

Abcarian, H.: Lateral Internal Sphincterotomy—a New Technique for Treatment of Chronic Fissure-in-ano, *Surg Clin North Am,* **55:**143, 1975.

————: Acute Suppuration of the Anorectum, *Surg Annu,* **8:**305, 1976.

————, Smith, D., and Sharon, N.: The Immunotherapy of Anal Condyloma Acuminata, *Dis Colon Rectum,* **19:**237, 1976.

Abrams, A. J.: Lymphogranuloma Venereum, *JAMA,* **205:**199, 1968.

Alexander, R. M., and Cone, L. A.: Malignant Melanoma of the Rectal Ampulla: Report of a Case and Review of the Literature, *Dis Colon Rectum,* **20:**53, 1977.

Alexander, S.: Dermatological Aspects of Anorectal Disease, *Clin Gastroenterol,* **4:**651, 1975.

Alexander-Williams, J.: Fistula-in-ano: Management of Crohn's Fistula, *Dis Colon Rectum,* **19:**518, 1976.

————, and Crapp, A. R.: Conservative Management of Haemorrhoids. Part I: Injection, Freezing and Ligation, *Clin Gastroenterol,* **4:**595, 1975.

Altemeier, W. A., Culbertson, W. R., Schowengerdt, C., and Hunt, J.: Nineteen Years' Experience with the One-stage Perineal Repair of Rectal Prolapse, *Ann Surg,* **173:**993, 1971.

Ani, A. N., and Solanke, T. F.: Anal Fistula: A Review of 82 Cases, *Dis Colon Rectum,* **19:**51, 1976.

Barron, J.: Office Ligation Treatment of Hemorrhoids, *Dis Colon Rectum,* **6:**109, 1963.

Beahrs, O. H., and Wilson, S. M.: Carcinoma of the Anus, *Ann Surg,* **184:**422, 1976.

Bennett, R. C., and Goligher, J. C.: Results of Internal Sphincterotomy for Anal Fissure, *Br Med J,* **2:**1500, 1963.

Bevans, D. W., Jr.: Perirectal Abscess: A Potentially Fatal Illness, *Am J Surg,* **126:**765, 1973.

Block, I. R., and Enquist, I. F.: Lymphatic Studies Pertaining to Local Spread of Carcinoma of the Rectum in Female, *Surg Gynecol Obstet,* **112:**41, 1961.

————, Rodriquez M. S., and Calva P. C.: Levator Ani as Substi-

tute Puborectalis Sling in Treatment of Anal Incontinence, *Surg Gynecol Obstet,* **141:**611, 1975.

Boxall, T. A., Smart, P. J. G., and Griffiths, J. D.: The Blood Supply of the Distal Segment of the Rectum in Anterior Resection, *Br J Surg,* **50:**399, 1962.

Brocklehurst, J. C.: Management of Anal Incontinence, *Clin Gastroenterol,* **4:**479, 1975.

Burkitt, D. P.: Hemorrhoids, Varicose Veins and Deep Vein Thrombosis: Epidermologic Features and Suggested Causation Factors, *Can J Surg,* **18:**483, 1975.

Catterall, R. D.: Sexually Transmitted Diseases of the Anus and Rectum, *Clin Gastroenterol,* **4:**659, 1975.

Cram, A. E., Pearlman, N. W., and Jochimsen, P. R.: Surgical Management and Complications of Radiation Injured Gut, *Arch Surg,* **133:**551, 1977.

Crapp, A. R., and Alexander-Williams J.: Fissure-in-ano and Anal Stenosis, *Clin Gastroenterol,* **4:**619, 1975.

DeCosse, J. J., Rhodes, R. S., Wentz, W. B., Reagan, J. W., Dworken, H. J., and Holden, W. E.: The Natural History and Management of Radiation Induced Injury of the Gastrointestinal Tract, *Ann Surg,* **170:**369, 1969.

Deveney, C. W., Lewis, F. R., and Schrock, T. R.: Surgical Management of Radiation Injury of the Small and Large Intestine, *Dis Colon Rectum,* **19:**25, 1976.

Douthwaite, A. H.: Proctalgia Fugax, *Br Med J,* **2:**164, 1962.

Duthie, J. L., and Bennett, R. C.: Anal Sphincteric Pressure in Fissure-in-ano, *Surg Gynecol Obstet,* **119:**19, 1964.

Editorial: To Tie; to Stab; to Stretch; Perchance to Freeze, *Lancet,* **2:**645, 1975.

Eisenhammer, S.: The Surgical Correction of Chronic Anal (Sphincteric) Contracture, *S Afr Med J,* **25:**486, 1951.

Ferguson, J. A., Mazier, W. P., Ganchrow, M. I., and Friend, W. G.: The Closed Technique of Hemorrhoidectomy, *Surgery,* **70:**480, 1971.

Fitzgerald, D. M., and Hamit, H. F.: The Variable Significance of Condylomata Acuminata, *Am J Surg,* **179:**328, 1974.

Frykman, H. M., and Goldberg, S. M.: The Surgical Treatment of Rectal Procidentia, *Surgery,* **129:**1225, 1969.

Gabriel, W. B.: Theirsch's Operation for Anal Incontinence, *Proc R Soc Med,* **41:**467, 1948.

Ganchrow, M. I., Bowman, E., and Clark, J. F.: Thrombosed Hemorrhoids: A Clinico-pathologic Study, *Dis Colon Rectum,* **14:**331, 1971.

————, Mazier, W. P., Friend, W. G., and Ferguson, J. A.: Hemorrhoidectomy Revisited: A Computer Analysis of 2038 Cases, *Dis Colon Rectum,* **14:**128, 1971.

Goldberg, S. M., and Gordon, P. H.: Treatment of Rectal Prolapse, *Clin Gastroenterol,* **4:**489, 1975.

Golden, G. T., and Horsley, J. S., III: Surgical Management of Epidermoid Carcinoma of the Anus, *Am J Surg,* **131:**275, 1976.

Goligher, J. C.: Cryosurgery for Hemorrhoids, *Dis Colon Rectum,* **19:**213, 1976.

————, Leacock, A. G., and Brossy, J. J.: The Surgical Anatomy of the Anal Canal, *Br J Surg,* **43:**51, 1955.

Gordon, P. H., and Hoexter, B.: Complications of Ripstein Procedure, Presented at 76th Annual Meeting, ASC&RS, Orlando, Fl, May 1977. To be published in *Dis Colon Rectum.*

Graham-Stewart, C. W.: The Etiology and Treatment of Fissure-in-ano, *Int Abstr Surg,* **115:**511, 1962.

Hagihara, P. F., and Griffen, W. O.: Delayed Correction of Ano-rectal Incontinence Due to Anal Sphincteral Injury, *Arch Surg,* **111:**63, 1976.

Hancock, B. D.: The Internal Sphincter and Anal Fissure, *Br J Surg,* **64:**92, 1977.

Hanley, P. H., Ray, J. E., Pennington, E. E., and Grablowsky, O. M.: Fistula-in-ano: A Ten Year Follow-up Study of Horseshoe Abscess Fistula-in-ano, *Dis Colon Rectum,* **19:**507, 1976.

Hawley, P. R.: Anorectal Fistula, *Clin Gastroenterol,* **4:**635, 1975.

Homan, W. P., Tang, C., and Thorbjarnarson, B.: Anal Lesions Complicating Crohn's Disease, *Arch Surg,* **111:**1333, 1976.

Jones, C. B., and Schofield, P. F.: Comparative Study of Methods of Treatment for Haemorrhoids, *Proc R Soc Med,* **67:**51, 1974.

Kheir, S., Kichey, R. C., Martin, R. G., MacKay, B., and Galla-gher, H. S.: Cloacogenic Carcinoma of the Anal Canal, *Arch Surg,* **104:**407, 1972.

Klein, E. J., Fisher, L. S., Chow, A. W., and Guze, L. B.: Ano-rectal Gonococcal Infection, *Ann Int Med,* **86:**340, 1977.

Klotz, R. G., Pamukcoglu, T., and Souilliard, D. H.: Transitional Cloacogenic Carcinoma of the Anal Canal, *Cancer,* **20:**1727, 1967.

Leaper, D. J., Page, R. E., Rosenberg, I. L., Wilson, D. N., and Goligher, J. C.: A Controlled Study Comparing the Conven-tional Treatment of Idiopathic Anorectal Abscess with That of Incision, Curettage and Primary Suture under Systemic Anti-biotic Cover, *Dis Colon Rectum,* **19:**46, 1976.

Lockhart-Mummery, H. E.: Anal Canal Perineal Ulceration in Crohn's Disease, *Proc R Soc Med,* **57:**897, 1964.

McColl, I.: The Comparative Anatomy and Pathology of Anal Glands, *Ann R Coll Surg,* **40:**36, 1967.

Mason, J. K., and Helwig, E. B.: Anorectal Melanoma, *Cancer,* **19:**39, 1966.

Morson, B. C.: The Pathology and Results of Treatment of Squa-mous Cell Carcinoma of the Anal Canal and Anal Margin, *Proc R Soc Med,* **53:**416, 1960.

———, and Volkstadt, H.: Malignant Melanoma of the Anal Canal, *J Clin Pathol,* **16:**126, 1963.

Moschcowitz, A. V.: The Pathogenesis, Anatomy, and Cure of Prolapse of the Rectum, *Surg Gynecol Obstet,* **15:**7, 1912.

Northman, B. J., and Schuster, M. M.: Internal Anal Sphincter Derangement with Anal Fissures, *Gastroenterology,* **67:**216, 1974.

Notaras, M. J.: The Treatment of Anal Fissure by Lateral Subcu-taneous Internal Sphincterotomy—a Technic and Results, *Br J Surg,* **58:**96, 1971.

O'Connor, J. J.: The Role of Cryosurgery in Management of Anorectal Disease: A Study of Cryosurgical Techniques, *Dis Colon Rectum,* **18:**298, 1975.

Oh, C., and Kark, A. E.: Anatomy of the External Anal Sphincter, *Br J Surg,* **59:**717, 1972.

Pack, G. T., and Oropeza, R.: A Comparative Study of Melanoma and Epidermoid Carcinoma of the Anal Canal: A Review of 20 Melanomas and 29 Epidermoid Carcinomas, *Dis Colon Rectum,* **10:**161, 1967.

Palmer, J. A., and Bush, R. S.: Radiation Injuries to the Bowel Associated with the Treatment of Carcinoma of the Cervix, *Surgery,* **80:**458, 1976.

Papillon, J.: Radiation Therapy in the Management of Epidermoid Carcinoma of the Anal Region, *Dis Colon Rectum,* **17:**181, 1974.

Paradis, P., Douglass, H. O., Jr., and Holyoke, E. D.: The Clinical Implications of a Staging System for Carcinoma of the Anus, *Surg Gynecol Obstet,* **141:**411, 1975.

Parks, A. G.: Anatomical Causes of Rectal Prolapse, *Proc R Soc Med,* **66:**26, 1975.

———: Fistula-in-ano: Perineal Fistula of Intra-abdominal or Intrapelvic Origin Simulating Fistula-in-ano—Report of 7 Cases, *Dis Colon Rectum,* **19:**500, 1976.

———, Goligher, J. C., Alexander-Williams, J., and Hanley, P. H.: Symposium (Moderator: S. M. Goldberg): Treatment of High Fistula-in-ano, *Dis Colon Rectum,* **19:**487, 1976.

———, Gordon, P. H., and Hardcastle, J. D.: A Classification of Fistula-in-ano, *Br J Surg,* **63:**1, 1976.

———, Porter, N. H., and Melyath J.: Experimental Study of the Reflex Mechanism Controlling the Muscles of the Pelvic Floor, *Dis Colon Rectum,* **5:**407, 1962.

Pilling, L. F., Swenson, W. M., and Hill, J. R.: The Psychologic Aspects of Proctalgia Fugax, *Dis Colon Rectum,* **8:**372, 1965.

Ripstein, C. B., and Lanter, B.: Etiology and Surgical Therapy of Massive Prolapse of the Rectum, *Ann Surg,* **157:**259, 1963.

Ross, S. T., and Bernstein, W. C.: The Role of Cryosurgery in Management of Anorectal Disease: The Loyal Opposition, *Dis Colon Rectum,* **18:**301, 1975.

Samson, R. B., and Stewart, W. R. C.: Sliding Skin Grafts in the Treatment of Anal Fissures, *Dis Colon Rectum,* **13:**372, 1970.

Schottler, J. L., Balcos, E. G., and Goldberg, S. M.: Postpartum Hemorrhoidectomy, *Dis Colon Rectum,* **16:**395, 1973.

Scoma, J. A., Salvati, E. P., and Rubin, R. J.: Incidence of Fistulas Subsequent to Anal Abscesses, *Dis Colon Rectum,* **17:**357, 1974.

Shafik, A.: A New Concept of the Anatomy of the Anal Sphincter Mechanism and the Physiology of Defecation:—The External Anal Sphincter: A Triple-loop System, *Invest Urol,* **12:**412, 1975.

———: A New Concept of the Anatomy of the Anal Sphincter Mechanism and the Physiology of Defecation: II. Anatomy of the Levator Ani Muscle with Special Reference to Puborec-talis, *Invest Urol,* **13:**175, 1975.

———: A New Concept of the Anatomy of the Anal Sphincter Mechanism and the Physiology of Defecation: III. The Lon-gitudinal Anal Muscle: Anatomy and Role in Anal Sphincter Mechanism, *Invest Urol,* **13:**271, 1976.

Sinclair, D. M., Hannah, G., McLaughlin, I. S., Patrick, R. S., and Slavin, G.: Malignant Melanoma of the Anal Canal, *Br J Surg,* **57:**808, 1970.

Slade, M. S., Goldberg, S. M., Schottler, J. L., Balcos, E. G., and Christenson, C. E.: Sphincteroplasty for Acquired Anal In-continence, *Dis Colon Rectum,* **20:**33, 1977.

Stearns, M. N., Jr., and Quan, S. H. Q.: Epidermoid Carcinoma of the Anorectum, *Surg Gynecol Obstet,* **131:**953, 1970.

Theuerkauf, F. J., Beahrs, O. H., and Hill, J. R.: Rectal Prolapse: Causation and Surgical Treatment, *Ann Surg,* **171:**819, 1970.

Thomson, W. H. F.: The Nature of Haemorrhoids, *Br J Surg,* **62:**542, 1975.

Wolfe, H. R. I., and Bussey, H. J. R.: Squamous Cell Carcinoma of the Anus, *Br J Surg,* **55:**295, 1968.

Chapter 29

Appendix

by **Edward H. Storer**

FUNCTION AND DEVELOPMENT

The human vermiform appendix is usually referred to as "a vestigial organ with no known function." This implies a more fully developed organ in an earlier stage of the individual or in earlier stages in the evolution of the species. There is little evidence that this is the case. On the contrary, currently available evidence suggests that the appendix is a highly specialized part of the alimentary tract. As the evolutionary scale is ascended, the lymphoid tissue of the large intestine becomes concentrated in the cecum, later in the apex of the cecum, and finally, in the higher anthropoids and man, as a vermiform appendix.

Lymphoid tissue first appears in the human appendix about 2 weeks after birth. The number of lymph follicles gradually increases to a peak of about 200 between the ages of twelve and twenty. After thirty there is an abrupt reduction to less than half and then to a trace or total absence of lymphoid tissue after sixty. Concurrent with lymphoid atrophy is fibrosis, which partially or totally obliterates the lumen in many older persons.

The role of the lymphoid aggregates in the appendix of higher mammals is still incompletely defined. Tonsils, Peyer's patches, and vermiform appendix together may well be the immunologic analog of the avian bursa of Fabricius and thus play an important role in immunoglobulin production.

A possible role for the appendix in human disease was suggested by McVay in 1964. In a retrospective study of autopsy data he found that the incidence of previous appendectomy in patients dying of carcinoma of the colon was significantly higher than in a comparable control group. He hypothesized that the appendix may act as a protective device against enteric viruses that may initiate malignant change in the colon and possibly at other sites.

He urged further studies since if his findings be confirmed, then incidental appendectomy in the course of another operation should not be proscribed. Several subsequent studies have been about evenly divided in supporting or denying an appendectomy-cancer relationship. All the above studies were designed to answer the question: "How many patients with cancer have had a previous appendectomy?" Moertel and associates designed a prospective study to answer the question: "In how many patients who have undergone appendectomy will cancer develop?" They studied 1,779 residents of Rochester, Minnesota, who had undergone appendectomy at the Mayo Clinic from 1925 through 1944, and a comparable control group. They found no evidence of a predisposition to cancer overall or to any specific cancer in patients who had undergone previous appendectomy, regardless of the age at which appendectomy was performed. Thus on the basis of currently available evidence, the practice of incidental appendectomy seems advisable since acute appendicitis and its complications continue to be significant sources of morbidity and mortality which removal of the appendix effectively prevents.

At birth the cecum and appendix have the so-called infantile contour—the appendix arising from the inferior tip of the cecum, which is shaped like an inverted pyramid. The cecum becomes bilaterally sacculated in early childhood but with the appendix still at the inferior tip. Further growth of the cecum is unequal, rapid growth of the right side and anterior aspects rotating the appendix to its adult position on the posteromedial aspect, below the ileocecal valve. The relation of the base of the appendix to the cecum is essentially constant, whereas the free end is found in a variety of locations—pelvic, retrocecal, retroileal, left lower quadrant, as well as right lower quadrant. The three taeniae coli meet at the junction of cecum with appendix and form the outer longitudinal muscle layer of the appendix. Thus the taeniae, particularly the anterior taenia, may be used as a landmark to identify an elusive appendix.

INFLAMMATION OF THE APPENDIX

Congenital defects of the appendix such as diverticula, duplication, or congenital absence are rare and of little clinical importance. The appendix occasionally gives rise to tumors, such as carcinoid or adenocarcinoma, and may be involved in inflammatory diseases of the cecum and ileum, such as tuberculosis, typhoid fever, or regional enteritis. However, by far the most important disease of the appendix is acute inflammation.

Acute Appendicitis

HISTORICAL BACKGROUND. There are isolated reports of appendectomy from 1736 on, when Amyand successfully removed from a hernial sac an appendix that had been perforated by a pin. There are also many reports, from 1581 on, of fatal suppurative disease of the cecal region, usually referred to, however, as "perityphlitis." The recognition of appendicitis as a clinical and pathologic entity for which surgical therapy is essential dates from 1886 when Reginald Fitz, Professor of Pathologic Anatomy at Harvard, gave a paper at the first meeting of the Association of American Physicians entitled "Perforating Inflammation of the Vermiform Appendix: with Special Reference to Its Early Diagnosis and Treatment." Soon thereafter McBurney described the clinical manifestations of early acute appendicitis prior to rupture, including the point of maximal abdominal tenderness, and an incision "made in the abdominal wall in cases of appendicitis."

INCIDENCE. Acute appendicitis is the most common acute surgical condition of the abdomen. The disease occurs at all ages but is most frequent in the second and third decades of life. It is quite rare in the very young, probably because the configuration of the appendix at this age makes obstruction of the lumen unlikely. There is a rough parallel between the amount of lymphoid tissue in the appendix and the incidence of acute appendicitis, the peak for both occurring in the middle teens.

The sex ratio in acute appendicitis is about 1:1 prior to puberty. At puberty the frequency in males increases, so that the male-to-female ratio is about 2:1 between the ages of fifteen and twenty-five, after which the male incidence gradually declines until the sex-related incidences are again equal.

The incidence of acute appendicitis requiring appendectomy has significantly decreased over the past 3 or 4 decades, and the trend appears to be continuing. The decline has been noted in many countries, particularly United States, Great Britain, and Scandinavia. Some of the decrease in the number of primary appendectomies is attributable to better diagnosis (and perhaps the advent of tissue committees): acute appendicitis is being reported in 75 to 80 percent of primary appendectomies in the 1970s, as opposed to 50 to 60 percent in the 1940s. But the declining incidence is much greater than can be accounted for by better diagnosis alone. No reason for the declining incidence of appendicitis has been established. Speculation has included changing dietary habits, changing intestinal flora, better nutrition, higher vitamin intake, antibiotics, and many other reasons.

ETIOLOGY AND PATHOGENESIS. Obstruction of the lumen is the dominant factor in the production of acute appendicitis. Fecaliths are the usual cause of appendiceal obstruction. Less common are hypertrophy of lymphoid tissue; inspissated barium from previous x-ray studies; vegetable and fruit seeds; and intestinal worms, particularly ascarids.

The frequency with which appendiceal obstruction is found is proportional to the diligence with which it is looked for. Only the more obvious obstructions are noted on "routine" surgical pathology reports. The frequency of obstruction also rises with the severity of the inflammatory process. Fecaliths are found in about 40 percent in simple acute appendicitis, in about 65 percent in gangrenous appendicitis without rupture, and in about 90 percent in gangrenous appendicitis with rupture.

The sequence of events following occlusion of the lumen is probably as follows: A closed-loop obstruction (Chap. 24) is produced by the proximal block, and continuing normal secretion of the appendiceal mucosa very rapidly produces distension. The luminal capacity of the normal appendix is only about 0.1 ml—there is no real lumen. Secretion of as little as 0.5 ml distal to a block raises the intraluminal pressure to about 60 cm H_2O. The human being is one of the few animals with an appendix capable of secreting at pressures high enough to lead to gangrene and perforation. Distension stimulates nerve endings of visceral afferent pain fibers, producing vague, dull, diffuse pain in the midabdomen or lower epigastrium. Peristalsis is also stimulated by the rather sudden distension, so that some cramping may be superimposed on the visceral pain early in the course of appendicitis.

Distension continues, not only from continued mucosal secretion, but also from rapid multiplication of the resident bacteria of the appendix. As pressure in the organ increases, venous pressure is exceeded. Capillaries and venules are occluded, but arteriolar inflow continues, resulting in engorgement and vascular congestion. Distension of this magnitude usually causes reflex nausea and vomiting, and the diffuse visceral pain becomes more severe. The inflammatory process soon involves the serosa of the appendix and in turn parietal peritoneum in the region, producing the characteristic shift in pain to the right lower quadrant.

The mucosa of the gastrointestinal tract, including the appendix, is very susceptible to impairment of blood supply. Thus its integrity is compromised early in the process, allowing bacterial invasion of the deeper coats. Fever, tachycardia, and leukocytosis develop as a consequence of absorption of dead tissue products and bacterial toxins. As progressive distension encroaches on the arteriolar pressure, the area with the poorest blood supply suffers most—ellipsoidal infarcts develop in the antimesenteric border. As distension, bacterial invasion, compromise of vascular supply, and infarction progress, perforation occurs, usually through one of the infarcted areas on the antimesenteric border.

This sequence is not inevitable—some episodes of acute appendicitis apparently subside spontaneously. Many patients who are found at operation to have acute appendicitis give a history of previous similar but less severe attacks of right lower quadrant pain. Pathologic examination of the appendices removed from these patients often reveals thickening and scarring, suggesting old healed acute inflammation. Presumable obstruction of the lumen when due to lymphoid hypertrophy or soft fecalith can be spontaneously relieved, allowing subsidence of appendiceal inflammation and attendant symptoms.

CLINICAL MANIFESTATIONS. Symptoms. Abdominal pain is the prime symptom of acute appendicitis. Classically the pain initially is diffusely centered in the lower epigastrium or umbilical area, is moderately severe, and is steady—sometimes with intermittent cramping superimposed. After a period varying from 1 to 12 hours, but usually within 4 to 6 hours, the pain localizes in the right lower quadrant. This classic pain sequence, though usual, is not invariable. In some patients the pain of appendicitis begins in the right lower quadrant and remains there. Variations in the anatomic location of the appendix account for many of the variations in the principal locus of the somatic phase of the pain. For example, a long appendix with the inflamed tip in the left lower quadrant causes pain in that area; a retrocecal appendix may cause principally flank or back pain; a pelvic appendix, principally suprapubic pain; and a retroileal appendix may cause testicular pain, presumably from irritation of the spermatic artery and ureter. Malrotation is also responsible for puzzling pain patterns. The visceral component is in the normal location, but the somatic component is felt in that part of the abdomen where the cecum has been arrested in rotation.

Anorexia nearly always accompanies appendicitis. It is so constant that the diagnosis should be questioned if the patient is not anorectic. Vomiting occurs in about 75 percent of patients but is not prominent or prolonged, most patients vomiting only once or twice.

Most patients give a history of obstipation from before the onset of abdominal pain, and many feel that defecation would relieve their abdominal pain. Diarrhea occurs in some patients, however, particularly children, so that the pattern of bowel function is of little differential diagnostic value.

The sequence of symptom appearance has great differential diagnostic significance. In over 95 percent of patients with acute appendicitis, anorexia is the first symptom, followed by abdominal pain, which is followed in turn by vomiting (if vomiting occurs). If vomiting precedes the onset of pain, the diagnosis should be questioned.

Signs. Physical findings are determined principally by the anatomic position of the inflamed appendix as well as by whether the organ has already ruptured when the patient is first examined.

Vital signs are not changed very much by uncomplicated appendicitis. Temperature elevation is rarely more than 1°C; the pulse rate is normal or slightly higher. Changes of greater magnitude usually mean that a complication has occurred or that another diagnosis should be considered.

Patients with appendicitis usually prefer to lie supine with the thighs, particularly the right, drawn up, because any motion increases pain. If asked to move, they do so slowly and gingerly.

The classic right lower quadrant physical signs are present when the inflamed appendix lies in the anterior position. Tenderness is often maximal at or near the point described by McBurney as being "located exactly between an inch and a half and two inches from the anterior spinous process of the ileum on a straight line drawn from that process to the umbilicus." Direct rebound tenderness usually, and referred or indirect rebound tenderness frequently, are present and are also felt maximally in the right lower quadrant, indicating peritoneal irritation. Rovsing's sign—pain in the right lower quadrant when palpatory pressure is exerted in the left lower quadrant—also indicates the site of peritoneal irritation. Cutaneous hyperesthesia in the area supplied by the spinal nerves on the right at T_{10}, T_{11}, and T_{12} is a frequent but not a constant accompaniment of acute appendicitis. In patients with obvious appendicitis, this sign is superfluous, but in some early cases it may be the first positive sign. It is elicited either by needle prick or, better, by gently picking up the skin between forefinger and thumb. This ordinarily is not unpleasant but is painful in areas of cutaneous hyperesthesia.

Muscular resistance to palpation of the abdominal wall roughly parallels the severity of the inflammatory process. Early in the disease, resistance, if present, consists mainly of voluntary guarding. As peritoneal irritation progresses, muscle spasm increases and becomes largely involuntary—true reflex rigidity as opposed to voluntary guarding.

Variations in the position of the inflamed appendix produce variations from the usual in physical findings. With a retrocecal appendix, the anterior abdominal findings are less striking, and tenderness may be most marked in the flank. When the inflamed appendix hangs into the pelvis, abdominal findings may be entirely absent, and the diagnosis may be missed unless the rectum is examined. As the examining finger exerts pressure on the peritoneum of the cul-de-sac of Douglas, pain is felt in the suprapubic area as well as locally. Signs of localized muscle irritation may also be present. The *psoas* sign indicates an irritative focus in proximity to that muscle. The test is performed by having the patient lie on his left side; the examiner then slowly extends the right thigh, thus stretching the iliopsoas muscle. The test is positive if extension produces pain. Similarly, a positive *obturator* sign of hypogastric pain on stretching the obturator internus indicates irritation at that locus. The test is performed by passive internal rotation of the flexed right thigh with the patient supine.

LABORATORY FINDINGS. Moderate leukocytosis, ranging from about 10,000 to 18,000 per cubic millimeter and accompanied by a moderate polymorphonuclear predominance, is the rule in acute uncomplicated appendicitis. With normal total and differential white blood cell counts, the diagnosis of appendicitis is in question though not ruled out. If the white cell count is greater than about 18,000 per cubic millimeter or if the shift to the left is extreme, perforated appendicitis or an acute inflammatory disease of greater magnitude than appendicitis is probable.

Urinalysis, except for the high specific gravity of dehydration, is normal unless the inflamed appendix lies near the ureter or bladder, in which case white cells and occasionally even red cells may be seen. Bacilluria in a fresh catheterized urine is not seen in appendicitis, however, allowing differentiation from urinary tract infection.

Roentgenography. The diagnosis of acute appendicitis is usually based on history and clinical findings. X-rays are used, therefore, only in differential diagnosis and to demonstrate complications of appendicitis.

Plain films of the abdomen in acute appendicitis often reveal a distended loop or two of small bowel in the right lower quadrant, less often a distended cecum. Visualization of a gas-filled appendix usually, but not invariably, indicates acute appendicitis with proximal appendiceal obstruction. A radiopaque fecalith when present in the right lower quadrant is nearly always associated with gangrenous appendicitis. Barium enema examination may be helpful in selected patients, particularly children, in whom the diagnosis remains unclear and operation is thought to be hazardous. It is done cautiously and gently, without prior preparation of the colon and without external manipulation or pressure. Complete filling of the appendix and absence of mucosal changes in both the appendix and ileocecal region rule out acute appendicitis. Pathognomonic findings of acute appendicitis on barium enema consist of nonfilling of the appendix, mass effect on the medial and inferior borders of the cecum, and mass effect or mucosal irregularities of the terminal ileum.

Chest films are sometimes necessary to rule out disease in the right lower lung field, since lesions that irritate nerves at T_{10}, T_{11}, and T_{12} may simulate appendicitis.

COMPLICATIONS—APPENDICEAL RUPTURE. Though some patients with acute appendicitis have spontaneous subsidence of the acute process, there is no way of predicting in which patients this will occur. The only safe course of action in uncomplicated acute appendicitis is immediate appendectomy. Ideally, every patient would have the offending organ removed before complications, particularly rupture, supervene. Some progress has been made, but too many patients still are seen first only after rupture has occurred, and some physicians still are needlessly indecisive. The use of antibiotic therapy in an attempt to avoid or postpone operative therapy ignores the obstructive etiology of acute appendicitis, is dangerous, and is ill-advised.

Pathogenesis. Unrelenting obstruction of the appendiceal lumen leads inexorably to gangrene and rupture of the pus-filled organ. Among the sequelae are appendiceal phlegmon, abscesses, spreading peritonitis, suppurative pylephlebitis, and intestinal obstruction.

Rupture of the appendix nearly always is distal to an occluding fecalith. The contents of the distended distal appendix spill through the necrotic rent, but this is rarely more than a few milliliters because of the small capacity of the appendix. Retrograde spill of cecal contents is ordinarily prevented by the occluding fecalith, unless the fecalith becomes dislodged through the rupture site or the necrotic area involves the base of the appendix and contiguous cecum.

During the several hours elapsing between onset of acute appendicitis and rupture, nature's walling-off process is able to quarantine the inflammation in about 95 percent of patients and confine the spill to the periappendiceal area.

A phlegmon is produced consisting of a mass of inflamed, matted intestines and omentum but with little or no discrete collection of pus. This process may slowly resolve spontaneously or may be hastened in resolution by timely surgical intervention. In some patients, however, a progressive suppurative process produces an expanding collection of pus contained by the walling-off process—a periappendiceal abscess.

If the walling-off process has not been completed by the time appendiceal rupture occurs, contamination spreads beyond the right lower quadrant. The two sites of predilection are the pelvic cul-de-sac via gravity drainage, and the right subhepatic space, which is reached via the right gutter (see also Chap. 34). With indiscriminate centrifugal contamination, virulent bacteria thus seeded initiate spreading diffuse peritonitis. An even more lethal form of peritonitis is produced by secondary rupture of intraabdominal abscesses that were produced by ruptured appendicitis. Ascending septic thrombophlebitis of the portal venous system—pylethrombophlebitis—is a very grave but fortunately rare complication of gangrenous appendicitis. It is heralded by chills and spiking fever, followed by right upper quadrant pain and jaundice. Septic clots from the involved mesenteric radicles embolize the liver, producing multiple pyogenic abscesses (Chap. 30).

Incidence. The proportion of patients with acute appendicitis who already have ruptured appendicitis when they are first seen varies with the age of the patients and with the type of hospital reporting. Twenty-five to thirty percent of charity hospital patients have ruptured appendicitis on admission versus about 15 percent in private hospitals. The rupture incidence is also significantly higher in the pediatric and geriatric age groups.

Diagnosis. Diagnosis usually is not difficult after rupture has occurred. The patient is obviously quite ill, prostrated, toxic, dehydrated, and distended. Right lower quadrant pain increases in severity and spreads over a somewhat larger area. Abdominal pain has been said to lessen dramatically at the moment of perforation and to be diminished for a few hours thereafter. This was attributed to sudden relief of the pain-producing distension of the obstructed appendix. Temporary relief of pain is rarely seen, however, occurring in only 4 percent in one series. In the vast majority, pain continues unabated—apparently local peritonitis is as effective in producing pain as distension of the appendix.

Physical findings are also more definite after rupture. With periappendiceal phlegmon or abscess, a tender, boggy mass with ill-defined margins usually can be felt. Tenderness, which is fingerpoint with simple acute appendicitis, now encompasses the whole right lower quadrant. Rebound tenderness and muscular rigidity are usually marked and correspond in extent to the extent of the local peritonitis. As in simple acute peritonitis, however, physical findings depend on the position of the appendix. For example, the only physical finding with a pelvic abscess secondary to a ruptured pelvic appendix may be a boggy tender mass on rectal examination. With spreading peritonitis, the physical signs advance with the spread of the inflammation (see also Chap. 34). Abdominal distension and paralytic ileus roughly parallel the severity and duration of the inflammatory process.

Fever and pulse also parallel the severity of the process. The temperature, which is rarely over 38°C in simple acute appendicitis, rises to about 39°C with localized peritonitis and often spikes over 40°C with diffuse peritonitis. Leuko-cytosis increases to 20,000 to 30,000 per cubic millimeter with extreme polymorphonuclear predominance and marked shift to immature forms. Hemoconcentration and desalting are variable and reflect the amount of fluid sequestered in the inflamed area as well as loss of oral intake.

DIFFERENTIAL DIAGNOSIS. The differential diagnosis of acute appendicitis is essentially the diagnosis of the "acute abdomen" (see Chap. 24). This is because clinical manifestations are not specific for a given disease but are specific for disturbance of a physiologic function or functions. Thus an essentially identical clinical picture can result from a wide variety of acute processes within or near the peritoneal cavity that produce the same alterations of function as acute appendicitis.

Accuracy of preoperative diagnosis should be about 80 to 85 percent. If it is consistently less than 75 percent, some unnecessary operations are probably being done, and a more rigorous preoperative differential diagnosis is in order. On the other hand, an accuracy consistently greater than 90 percent should also cause concern, since this usually means that some patients with atypical but bona fide acute appendicitis are being "observed" when they should have prompt surgical intervention. There are a few conditions in which operation is contraindicated, but in general the disease processes that are confused with appendicitis are also surgical problems or, if not, are not made worse by operation. The more frequent error is to make a preoperative diagnosis of acute appendicitis only to find some other condition (or nothing) at operation; much less frequently, acute appendicitis is found after a preoperative diagnosis of another condition. Most common erroneous preoperative diagnoses—accounting for more than 75 percent—in descending order of frequency are acute mesenteric lymphadenitis, no organic pathologic condition, acute pelvic inflammatory disease, twisted ovarian cyst or ruptured graafian follicle, and acute gastroenteritis.

Differential diagnosis of appendicitis depends upon three major factors: the anatomic location of the inflamed appendix, the stage of the process—whether simple or ruptured, and the age and sex of the patient.

Diseases to be considered in the differential diagnosis of appendicitis in children include primary acute mesenteric lymphadenitis; acute gastroenteritis, usually "green-apple colic" or "viral" gastroenteritis but occasionally paratyphoid or typhoid infections; acute pyelonephritis; Meckel's diverticulitis; intussusception; regional enteritis; primary peritonitis; and Henoch-Schönlein purpura.

Acute Mesenteric Adenitis (Chap. 35). This is the disease most often confused with acute appendicitis in children. Almost invariably an upper respiratory infection is present or has recently subsided. The pain is usually less or more diffuse, and tenderness is not as sharply localized as in appendicitis. Voluntary guarding is sometimes present, but true rigidity is rare. Generalized lymphadenopathy may be noted. Laboratory procedures are of little help in differentiating, though a relative lymphocytosis, when present, suggests mesenteric adenitis. Observation for several hours to allow the clinical picture to clarify is in order if the diagnosis of mesenteric adenitis seems likely, since this is

a self-limited disease, but if the differentiation is in doubt, then immediate operation is the only safe course.

Acute Gastroenteritis. This is very common in childhood but usually can easily be differentiated from appendicitis. Viral gastroenteritis, an acute self-limited infection of diverse causes, is characterized by profuse watery diarrhea, nausea, and vomiting. Hyperperistaltic abdominal cramps precede the watery stools. The abdomen is relaxed between cramps, and there are no localizing signs. Laboratory values are normal.

Salmonella gastroenteritis results from ingestion of contaminated food. Abdominal findings are usually similar to those in viral gastroenteritis, but in some the abdominal pain is intense, localized, and associated with rebound tenderness. Chills and fever are common. Leukocyte count is usually normal. The causative organisms can be isolated from essentially 100 percent of patients, but this may take too long to help the clinician in differential diagnosis of abdominal pain. Similar attacks in other persons eating the same food as the patient greatly strengthen the presumptive diagnosis of salmonella gastroenteritis.

Typhoid fever is now a rare disease. This probably accounts for the frequency of missed diagnosis—it is rarely seen and rarely thought of. The onset is less acute than appendicitis, with a prodrome of several days. Differentiation is usually possible because of the prostration, maculopapular rash, inappropriate bradycardia, and leukopenia. Diagnosis is confirmed by culture of *Salmonella typhosa* from stool or blood. Intestinal perforation, usually in the lower ileum, develops in about 1 percent of cases and requires immediate surgical therapy.

Yersiniosis. Human infection with *Yersinia enterocolitica* or *Y. pseudotuberculosis,* though reported frequently in Europe, has only recently become generally recognized in the United States. It is probable that the recent increase in the incidence of *Yersinia* infections is attributable to increased awareness and laboratory skill, not to actual spread of the disease in human beings and animals. These zoonotic organisms are not members of the indigenous biota of man and are probably transmitted through food contaminated by feces or urine.

Yersinia infections cause a variety of clinical syndromes, including mesenteric adenitis, ileitis, colitis, and acute appendicitis. Many of the infections are mild and self-limited, but some lead to a systemic septic course with a high fatality rate if untreated. The organisms are usually sensitive to tetracyclines, streptomycin, ampicillin, and kanamycin. A preoperative suspicion of the diagnosis should not delay operative intervention, since appendicitis caused by *Yersinia* cannot be clinically distinguished from appendicitis of other causation.

Recent studies in Europe indicate that about 5 percent of cases of mesenteric adenitis and 5 percent of cases of acute appendicitis are caused by *Yersinia* infection.

Urinary Tract Infection (Chap. 40). Acute pyelonephritis on the right side particularly may mimic a retroileal acute appendicitis. Chills, right costovertebral angle tenderness, pus cells, and particularly bacteria in the urine usually suffice to differentiate the two.

Meckel's Diverticulitis (Chap. 39). This causes a clinical picture very similar to acute appendicitis. Preoperative differentiation is academic and unnecessary, since Meckel's diverticulitis is attended by the same complications as appendicitis and requires the same treatment—prompt surgical intervention. Diverticulectomy can nearly always be done through a McBurney incision, extended if necessary. If the base of the diverticulum is broad, so that removal would compromise the lumen of the ileum, then resection of the segment of ileum bearing the diverticulum with end-to-end anastomosis is done.

Intussusception (Chap 39). In contrast to Meckel's diverticulitis, it is extremely important to differentiate intussusception from acute appendicitis, because the treatment may be quite different. The age of the patients is important: appendicitis is very uncommon under age two, whereas nearly all idiopathic intussusceptions occur under age two. Intussusception occurs typically in a well-nourished infant who is suddenly doubled up by apparent colicky pain. Between attacks of pain the infant appears quite well. After several hours, the patient usually passes a bloody mucoid stool. A sausage-shaped mass may be palpable in the right lower quadrant. Later, as the intussusception progresses distad, the right lower quadrant feels abnormally empty. The preferred treatment of intussusception, if seen before signs of peritonitis supervene, is reduction by barium enema. Treatment of acute appendicitis by barium enema might well be catastrophic.

Regional Enteritis (Chap. 27). The manifestations of acute regional enteritis—fever, right lower quadrant pain and tenderness, and leukocytosis—often simulate acute appendicitis. Diarrhea and the infrequency of anorexia, nausea, and vomiting favor a diagnosis of enteritis but are not sufficient to exclude acute appendicitis without celiotomy. In an appreciable percentage of patients with chronic regional enteritis, the diagnosis has been first made at the time of operation for presumed acute appendicitis.

Primary Peritonitis (Chap. 34). This situation rarely mimics simple acute appendicitis but presents a picture very similar to diffuse peritonitis secondary to a ruptured appendix. The diagnosis is made by peritoneal aspiration. If nothing but cocci are seen on the Gram-stained smear, peritonitis is primary and treated medically; if the flora are mixed, secondary peritonitis is indicated.

Henoch-Schönlein Purpura. This syndrome usually occurs 2 to 3 weeks after a streptococcal infection. Abdominal pain may be prominent, but joint pains, purpura, and nephritis are nearly always present also.

Gynecologic Disorders. Diseases of the female internal generative organs (Chap. 41) that may be erroneously diagnosed as appendicitis are, in approximate descending order of frequency, pelvic inflammatory disease, ruptured graafian follicle, twisted ovarian cyst or tumor, endometriosis, and ruptured ectopic pregnancy.

Pelvic Inflammatory Disease ("Pus Tubes"). The infection is usually bilateral but if confined to the right tube may mimic acute appendicitis. Pain and tenderness are usually lower, and motion of the cervix is exquisitely painful. Intracellular diplococci may be demonstrable on smear of the purulent vaginal discharge.

Ruptured Graafian Follicle. Not uncommonly ovulation results in spill of sufficient blood and follicular fluid to produce brief, mild lower abdominal pain. If the fluid is unusually copious and from the right ovary, appendicitis may be simulated. Pain and tenderness are rather diffuse. Leukocytosis and fever are minimal or absent. Since this occurs at the midpoint of the menstrual cycle, it is often called *mittelschmerz.*

Ruptured Ectopic Pregnancy. This is manifested by lower abdominal pain and symptoms of hypovolemia. A tubo-ovarian mass is usually palpable on pelvic examination. Culdocentesis yields nonclotting blood.

Diseases of the Male. Two diseases of males (Chap. 40) must be considered in differential diagnosis of appendicitis, torsion of the testis and acute epididymitis, since epigastric pain may overshadow local symptoms early in these diseases. The correct diagnosis is easily made if one remembers to include the genitalia in the physical examination.

Other Diseases. Diseases occurring in patients of all ages and both sexes, not mentioned above, that must be considered in differential diagnosis are perforated peptic ulcer (Chap. 26); diverticulitis coli, particularly cecal (Chap. 28); perforating carcinoma of the colon, particularly cecal (Chap. 28); foreign body perforations of the bowel; closed-loop intestinal obstruction (Chap. 24); mesenteric vascular occlusion (Chap. 35); pleuritis of the right lower chest (Chap. 24); acute cholecystitis (Chap. 31); acute pancreatitis (Chap. 32); right ureteral calculus (Chap. 40); infarcted epiploic appendage (Chap. 35); hematoma of abdominal wall (Chap. 35); and many others too numerous and too rare to mention.

Perforated Peptic Ulcer. This closely simulates appendicitis if the spilled gastroduodenal contents gravitate down the right gutter to the cecal area and if the perforation spontaneously seals fairly soon, thus minimizing upper abdominal findings.

Diverticulitis or Perforating Carcinoma of the Cecum or of That Portion of the Sigmoid That Lies on the Right Side. These lesions may be impossible to distinguish from appendicitis. Extensive diagnostic studies in an attempt to make a preoperative differentiation are not warranted.

Ureteral Stone. If the calculus is lodged near the appendix, it may simulate a retrocecal appendicitis. Pain referred to the labia, scrotum, or penis, hematuria, or absence of fever or leukocytosis suggests stone. Pyelography usually confirms the diagnosis.

Epiploic Appendicitis. Epiploic appendicitis probably results from infarction of the appendage(s) secondary to torsion. Symptoms may be minimal, or there may be continuous abdominal pain in an area corresponding to the contour of the colon, lasting several days. Pain shift is unusual, and there is no diagnostic sequence of symptoms. The patient does not look ill, nausea and vomiting are unusual, and unlike in appendicitis appetite is commonly unaffected. Localized tenderness over the site is usual and is often marked on rebound but without rigidity. In 25 percent of reported cases pain has persisted or recurred until the infarcted epiploic appendages were removed.

TREATMENT. There is but one treatment for acute appendicitis and its complications. Thus the only question to be resolved is when—the timing of surgical intervention.

Immediate appendectomy is indicated in acute appendicitis without rupture just as soon as the minimal work-up compatible with good medical practice is completed. Ruptured appendicitis with local peritonitis or phlegmon formation also should be operated upon early in the hospital course. A brief period of preparation is advisable during which nasogastric suction is instituted and sufficient intravenous fluids, usually Ringer's lactate solution and 5% dextrose in water, are given to correct systemic fluid and electrolyte deficits. Systemic antibiotics in large doses are administered: since bacteroides organisms play such a major role in appendiceal infections, clindamycin should be one of the antibiotics used pending culture-sensitivity data. (See also Chap. 5.)

Patients with ruptured appendicitis producing spreading peritonitis should similarly be prepared with "all deliberate haste" for early surgical intervention. Preparation (Chap. 34) may take somewhat longer than with localized peritonitis because of the greater magnitude of the physiologic derangements caused by the more extensive process but rarely requires more than 3 or 4 hours. It is essential to remove the necrotic appendix to prevent continued contamination of the peritoneum.

There is general agreement on the timing of the operation for the three categories of appendicitis mentioned above—acute appendicitis without rupture, ruptured appendix with local peritonitis or phlegmon formation, and ruptured appendix with spreading peritonitis. There is still a difference of opinion, however, concerning the optimal timing of the operation for ruptured appendicitis with frank periappendiceal abscess formation. "Expectant treatment" was advocated by A. J. Ochsner in 1901. As now practiced this consists of intravenous fluids, nasogastric suction, and large doses of antibiotics. Vital signs, leukocytosis, and size of the mass are followed closely. If progression occurs, the abscess is drained. If the patient improves, conservative treatment is continued. With these measures the majority of appendiceal abscesses resolve satisfactorily, although many days of hospital treatment are required. An elective appendectomy 6 weeks to 3 months later is strongly advised, since the recurrence rate is very high. Proponents of conservative treatment feel that operation in the acute phase of the abscess is dangerous, because the protective walling-off barrier may be broken down by the procedure.

Advocates of prompt operation for ruptured appendicitis with abscess as soon as the patient can be prepared feel that, with the supportive measures now available, drainage of the abscess and removal of the appendix, if possible, can be done with a lower mortality and morbidity than with expectant treatment. They point out that the mortality rate following secondary rupture of a periappendiceal abscess is about 90 percent. Expectant treatment also necessitates two hospitalizations, the first often prolonged.

Nearly all surgeons favor prompt operation for all categories of acute appendicitis in children, since expectant treatment of ruptured appendicitis has been less successful than in adults.

Conduct of the Operation (Fig. 29-1). Many surgeons (including the author) prefer a McBurney incision in all patients with suspected appendicitis, while others use a McBurney incision in clear-cut appendicitis but use a right paramedian incision if the diagnosis is in doubt, particularly in females. The principal argument against the McBurney incision is that a second incision may be necessary if a procedure other than appendectomy has to be done. The principal argument against the paramedian incision is that if the patient does indeed have appendicitis, the diseased organ can be removed only by traversing the previously unsoiled peritoneal cavity.

When a periappendiceal abscess is suspected, paramedian incision is contraindicated. The abscess is approached from a laterally placed McBurney incision without entering the free peritoneal cavity. The abscess is evacuated, with care to avoid breaking down any of the walling-off process. Most surgeons attempt to remove the appendix in this situation. If the appendix is in the surgical field, it should be removed, but if extensive dissection is necessary to expose the organ, appendectomy is hazardous. Interval appendectomy should be done some weeks later.

There are several methods of managing the appendiceal stump. The traditional method of ligation-inversion has the advantage that peritonealization and hemostasis are secured, but the disadvantage of inverting an infected stump into a closed cavity is the risk of an intramural abscess of the cecum. However, if the ligation is done with fine plain catgut this risk is minimal. Inversion without ligation obviates the risk of abscess, but hemostasis of the intramural branch of the appendiceal artery may not be secure. Ligation without inversion avoids burying the stump and secures hemostasis but is unsurgical because there remains free in the peritoneal cavity a contaminated raw surface. Contamination of the peritoneal cavity may result from the ligated stump either from bacteria on the stump or from the slipping of the ligature or necrosis of the stump as a result of the ligation. Total inversion of the normal appendix after division of the mesoappendix has been revived recently as an alternative to stump closure at the time of incidental appendectomy. It is technically more difficult but has the advantage that the gastrointestinal tract is not opened. Intussusception of the cecum has not been a significant problem.

If appendicitis is not found, an orderly investigation for the cause of the symptoms must be done. This should include gross examination and immediate Gram stain of any peritoneal fluid or exudate. With the assistant elevating the anterior abdominal wall by retraction, the pelvic organs are examined. Next the gallbladder and gastroduodenal areas are visualized. The mesentery is examined for nodes. The small intestine is then "run" in a retrograde manner, starting at the cecum, looking particularly for regional enteritis and Meckel's diverticulum. Finally, palpation of the colon and kidneys is done as well as is possible through a McBurney incision. It is axiomatic that if the cause of the acute abdomen is found, exploration

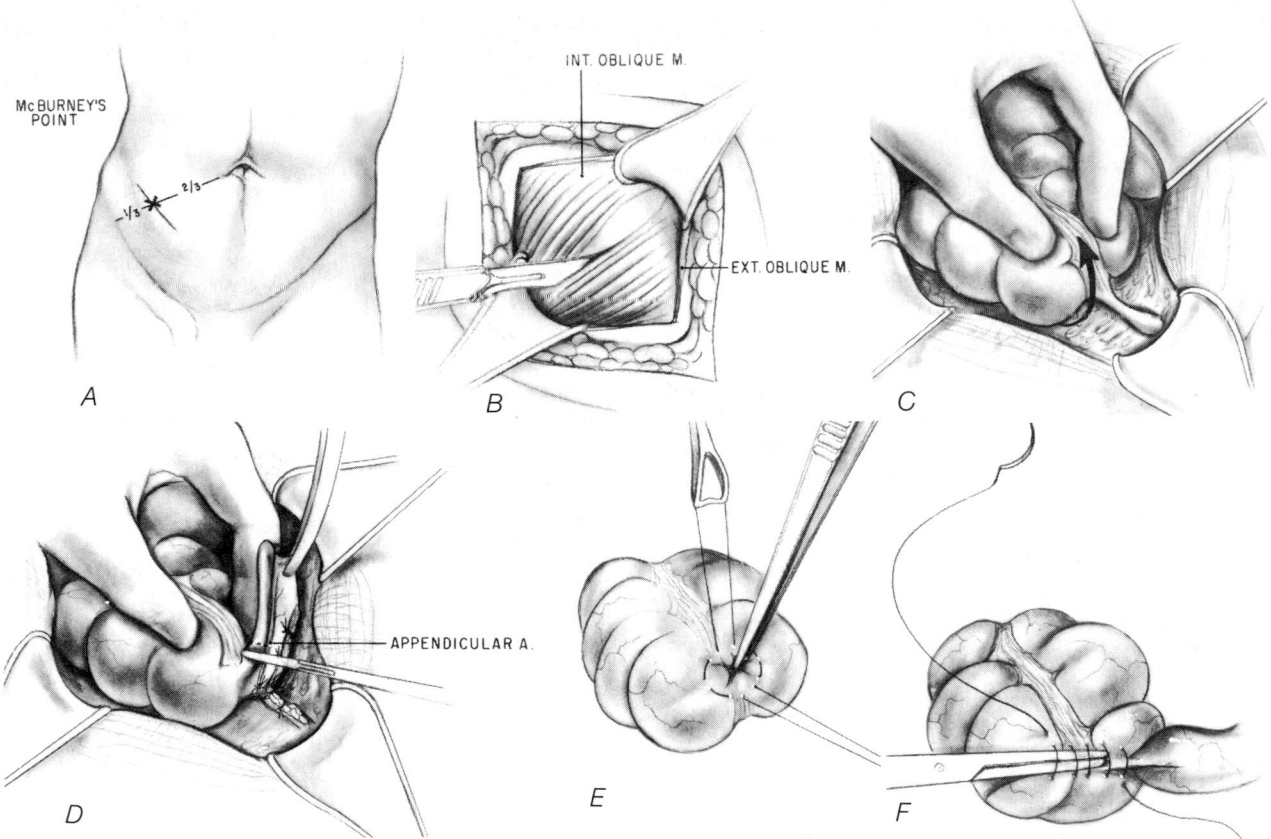

Fig. 29-1. Appendectomy. *A.* McBurney incision passing through McBurney's point, which is located one-third of the distance from the anterior superior iliac spine to the umbilicus. *B.* The incision has been carried through skin and subcutaneous tissue, and has divided the aponeurosis of the external oblique muscle in the course of its fibers. The internal oblique muscle is being separated in the direction of its fibers. *C.* The peritoneum has been incised and the peritoneal cavity entered. The appendix is delivered into the wound by rotation of the cecum up and out. *D.* The vessels within the mesoappendix have been doubly ligated and transected with particular attention directed toward the appendicular artery. A crushing clamp is applied to the base of the appendix and then moved distad (to dotted line), so that a ligature may be placed in the resulting groove. *E.* The stump of the appendix may or may not be tied with a ligature. It is customary to invert the stump and place a purse-string suture through the seromuscular layers of the cecum. *F.* An alternate method of inverting the appendiceal stump is demonstrated with a continuous seromuscular suture. A Z suture can also be used to achieve this end.

is terminated and appropriate therapy for the offending process undertaken.

The question of when to drain has been contentious for many years. Some have followed the dictum "When in doubt, drain." Others, with equal vehemence have said, "When in doubt, don't drain." The following is based on collected currently available evidence:

Drainage of localized collections of pus is indicated and should be done with one or more soft rubber drains to each collection, brought out through the McBurney incision. If a paramedian incision has been used, then a separate stab wound is preferred to avoid incisional hernia. A sump drain is more effective in large collections. Drainage of diffuse peritonitis is unwarranted, because it is physically impossible and physiologically undesirable. If an intact though inflamed appendix has been removed, all layers of the incision should be closed without drainage. However, if a ruptured appendix has been removed, then each anatomic layer is washed with a dilute antibiotic solution such as kanamycin or neomycin as it is closed. A small drain is placed in the subcutaneous tissues and the skin loosely approximated or left open for secondary closure in 4 or 5 days.

Appendicitis in the Young

Acute appendicitis is a more serious disease in infants and children than in adults, because the rupture rate is higher, which in turn produces higher morbidity and mortality rates.

Diagnostic accuracy for acute appendicitis is considerably lower than in adults. Contributing to this are a clinical picture that is less "typical"—a fever which is often higher and more vomiting; the unavoidable fact that infants cannot give a history of present illness; and the failure of physicians to consider appendicitis because of its relative infrequency in the very young.

The disease progresses more rapidly than in adults—

gangrene and rupture occur earlier in the course of acute appendicitis in children. The rupture rate varies from 15 to 50 percent in reported series. In preschool children it is even higher, ranging from 50 to 85 percent. Because of the frequency of "bellyaches" in children, parents may think that an attack of appendicitis is just another "belly-ache" and not seek medical advice until after rupture has occurred and the child is obviously very ill. Too many parents still administer harsh cathartics to children with abdominal discomfort and/or constipation. The resulting increase in bowel motility hastens perforation.

Rupture of gangrenous appendicitis is more frequently followed by diffuse peritonitis and distant intraabdominal abscesses than in adults. The walling-off process is less efficient because of the small, incompletely developed greater omentum and because, as noted above, the interval between onset and rupture may be short. Cathartics are also implicated: the induced writhing of the bowel not only hastens rupture but after rupture smears contamination widely about the peritoneal cavity.

Appendicitis in the Elderly

Acute appendicitis in the older age group, as in the very young, is a much more serious disease. The mortality rate is many times that for younger adults. This is attributable to delay of definitive treatment, greater frequency of progressive uncontrolled infection, and a high incidence of concomitant disease.

Appendicitis is often very deceptive in the aged, because the clinical manifestations are much milder than might be expected from the gravity of the disease process. The usual symptoms are present but subtle and difficult to elicit; abdominal pain is often mild and causes little concern. Similarly, physical findings, with the exception of tenderness, may be minimal or absent. The fever and leukocyte response, which as a rule are very helpful in diagnosis, are less than expected and in some elderly patients are within normal limits. Because of the deceptively mild clinical course of the disease, from 67 to 90 percent of elderly patients are found to have a ruptured appendix at the time of operation.

Concomitant diseases, which dangerously lower physiologic reserve in this group, are present in significant degree in from one-half to two-thirds of the patients. These are principally cardiac disease, pulmonary insufficiency, pneumonia, and diabetes.

PROGNOSIS. Mortality. The mortality from appendicitis in the United States has steadily decreased from a rate of 9.9 per 100,000 in 1939 to 0.4 per 100,000 in 1975. Among the factors responsible are the significantly decreasing incidence of appendicitis; better diagnosis and treatment, attributable to the now available antibiotics, intravenous fluids, blood, and plasma, but particularly to the greatly improved training of most surgeons; and a higher percentage of patients receiving definitive treatment before rupture (though the rate of improvement is discouragingly slow).

Principal factors in mortality are whether or not rupture occurs prior to surgical treatment, and the age of the patient. The overall mortality rate in unruptured acute appendicitis is little higher than the rate for a general anesthetic (0.06 percent) and is now about 0.1 percent. The overall mortality rate in ruptured acute appendicitis is about 3 percent—a thirtyfold increase. The mortality rate of ruptured appendicitis in the elderly is about 15 percent—a fivefold increase from the overall rate.

Death is usually attributable to uncontrolled sepsis—peritonitis, intraabdominal abscesses, or gram-negative septicemia. Sepsis may impose metabolic demands of such magnitude on the cardiovascular or respiratory systems that they cannot be met, in which case cardiac or respiratory insufficiency is the direct cause of death. Pulmonary embolism continues to account for some deaths. Aspiration producing drowning in the patient's vomitus is a prominent mode of death in the older age group.

Morbidity. Morbidity rates parallel mortality rates, being precipitously increased by rupture of the appendix and to a lesser extent by old age. Most of the serious early complications are septic and include abscess (Chap. 34) and wound infection. Wound infection is common but is nearly always confined to the subcutaneous tissues and promptly responds to wound drainage, which is accomplished by reopening the skin incision. Wound infection predisposes to wound dehiscence also. The type of incision is relevant, since complete dehiscence rarely occurs in a McBurney incision.

Fecal fistula is an annoying but not particularly dangerous complication of appendectomy. This may be produced by sloughing of that portion of the cecum inside a constricting purse-string suture, by the ligature's slipping off a tied but not inverted appendiceal stump, by necrosis from an abscess encroaching on the cecum, or by a cecotomy produced by removing a cigarette drain that is adherent to the cecum—a cogent reason for removing the wick from the rubber drain before insertion.

Intestinal obstruction, initially paralytic but sometimes progressing to mechanical, may occur with slowly resolving peritonitis with loculated abscesses and exuberant adhesion formation.

Late complications are quite uncommon. Adhesive band intestinal obstruction after appendectomy does occur but much less frequently than after pelvic surgical therapy. Incisional hernia is analogous to wound dehiscence—infection predisposes to it, and it rarely occurs in a McBurney incision but is not uncommon in a lower right paramedian incision.

TUMORS

Neoplasms of the appendix are very uncommon and are usually diagnosed at operation or autopsy. Three histologic types of malignant tumors occur: carcinoid, adenocarcinoma, and malignant mucocele. Various benign tumors also occur but are of no clinical significance except as a very rare etiologic agent in the production of acute appendicitis from appendiceal obstruction. In a study of 50,000 appendices the incidence of carcinoid was 0.5 percent, primary adenocarcinoma 0.08 percent, and mucocele

0.2 percent. Carcinoid tumors of the gastrointestinal tract and the malignant carcinoid syndrome are discussed in Chap. 27.

Carcinoid

Forty-five percent of all reported carcinoid tumors of the gastrointestinal tract have been found in the appendix. The true incidence probably exceeds 75 percent, since carcinoids of the appendix are not sufficiently unusual to elicit the urge to publish while carcinoids elsewhere more often are. Although cytologic criteria of malignancy are not uncommonly present, biologic malignancy evidenced by mestastasis has been demonstrated in only 2.9 percent of appendiceal carcinoids. There are but six reported cases of malignant carcinoid of the appendix producing the malignant carcinoid syndrome.

Carcinoids of the appendix are typically small, firm, circumscribed, yellow-brown tumors. About three-fourths occur in the distal third of the appendix; less than 10 percent occur at the base. They are nearly always an incidental finding at the time of appendectomy (or autopsy), though rarely they may initiate acute appendicitis. Simple appendectomy with wide excision of the mesoappendix is adequate treatment unless invasion beyond the line of resection and/or nodal metastasis is demonstrated, in which case right colectomy with excision of the node-bearing mesentery is indicated.

Adenocarcinoma

This is often referred to as "colonic" type of carcinoma of the appendix because of the resemblance in behavior and in gross and microscopic appearance to colonic cancer. It also serves to distinguish it from the mucocele. Preoperative diagnosis may be based on the visualization of an extracecal mass on barium enema, but usually the appendiceal tumor is not suspected prior to operation, which is usually an appendectomy. In a few instances the lesion is unrecognized at appendectomy and is detected on pathologic examination of the specimen. Treatment is right colectomy including mesentery. The prognosis is probably about the same as for carcinoma of the cecum.

Mucocele

This is a cystic dilatation of the appendix containing mucoid material. Histologically, mucoceles are divided into a benign type, which results from noninflammatory occlusion of the proximal lumen of the appendix and thus is not a neoplasm, and a malignant type, which is a grade 1 mucous papillary adenocarcinoma. Appendectomy is adequate treatment, but care should be taken to avoid rupture, since pseudomyxoma peritonei has been reported to occur following rupture and peritoneal dissemination of the appendiceal contents.

References

Function and Development

Berry, R. J. A.: The True Caecal Apex, or the Vermiform Appendix: Its Minute and Comparative Anatomy, *J Anat Physiol,* **35:**83, 1900.

Buschard, K., and Kjaeldgaard, A.: Investigation and Analysis of the Position, Fixation, Length and Embryology of the Vermiform Appendix, *Acta Chir Scand,* **139:**293, 1973.

Mavligit, G. M., Jubert, A., Gutterman, J. U., Reed, R. C., and Hersh, E. M.: Subpopulations of Thymus Dependent and Thymus Independent Lymphocytes in Human Gut Associated Lymphoid Tissues, *Surg Gynecol Obstet,* **140:**397, 1975.

McVay, J. R. Jr.: The Appendix in Relation to Neoplastic Disease, *Cancer,* **17:**929, 1964.

Moertel, C. G., Nobrega, F. T., Elveback, L. R., and Wentz, J. R.: A Prospective Study of Appendectomy and Predisposition to Cancer, *Surg Gynecol Obstet,* **138:**549, 1974.

Perey, D. Y., Cooper, M. D., and Good, R. A.: The Mammalian Homologue of the Avian Bursa of Fabricius, *Surgery,* **64:**614, 1968.

Inflammation of the Appendix

Amyand, C.: Of an Inguinal Rupture with a Pin in the Appendix Caeci Encrusted with Stone: Some Observations on Wounds in the Guts, *Philosoph Trans,* **39:**329, 1736.

Bowers, W. F.: Appendicitis: With Special Reference to Its Pathogenesis, Bacteriology, and Healing, *Arch Surg,* **39:**362, 1939.

Burkitt, D. P.: The Aetiology of Appendicitis, *Br J Surg,* **58:**695, 1971.

Castleman, K. B., Puestow, C. B., and Sauer, D.: Is Appendicitis Decreasing in Frequency? *Arch Surg,* **78:**794, 1959.

Deschenes, L., Couture, J., and Garneau, R.: Diverticulitis of the Appendix, *Am J Surg,* **121:**706, 1971.

Fernel, J.: Universa Medicina, BK 6, 1554, in R. H. Major, "Classic Descriptions of Disease," Charles C Thomas, Publisher, Springfield, Ill, 1932.

Fitz, R. H.: Perforating Inflammation of the Vermiform Appendix: With Special Reference to Its Early Diagnosis and Treatment, *Trans Assoc Am Physicians,* **1:**107, 1886.

Gierup, J., and Karpe, B.: Aspects on Appendiceal Abscess in Children with Special Reference to Delayed Appendectomy, *Acta Chir Scand,* **141:**801, 1975.

Gilmore, O. J. A., Brodribb, A. J. M., Browett, J. P., Cooke, T. J. C., Griffin, P. H., Higgs, M. J., Ross, I. K., and Williamson, R. C. N.: Appendicitis and Mimicking Conditions. A Prospective Study, *Lancet,* **2:**421, 1975.

Grosfeld, J. L., and Solit, R. W.: Prevention of Wound Infection in Perforated Appendicitis: Experience with Delayed Primary Wound Closure, *Ann Surg,* **168:**891, 1968.

Haller, J. A., Jr., Shaker, I. J., Donahoo, J. S., Schnaufer, L., and White, J. J.: Peritoneal Drainage versus Non-drainage for Generalized Peritonitis from Ruptured Appendicitis in Children, *Ann Surg,* **177:**595, 1973.

Hobson, T., and Rosenmann, L. D.: Acute Appendicitis: When Is It Right to Be Wrong? *Am J Surg,* **108:**306, 1964.

Howie, J. G. R.: Death from Appendicitis and Appendectomy. An Epidemiological Survey, *Lancet,* **2:**1334, 1966.

Jepsen, O. B., Korner, B., Lauritsen, K. B., Hancke, A.-B., Andersen, L., Henrichsen, S., Brenøe, E., Christiansen, P. M., and Johansen, A.: *Yersinia enterocolitica* Infection in Patients with Acute Surgical Abdominal Disease, *Scand J Infect Dis,* **8:**189, 1976.

Jona, J. Z., Belin, R. P., and Selke, A. C.: Barium Enema as a Diagnostic Aid in Children with Abdominal Pain, *Surg Gynecol Obstet,* **144:**351, 1977.

Law, D., Law, R., and Eiseman, B.: The Continuing Challenge of Acute and Perforated Appendicitis, *Am J Surg,* **131:**533, 1976.

Leigh, D. A., Simmons, K., and Norman, E.: Bacterial Flora of the Appendix Fossa in Appendicitis and Post-operative Wound Infection, *J Clin Pathol,* **27:**997, 1974.

————, Pease, R., Henderson, H., Simmons, K., and Russ, R.: Prophylactic Lincomysin in the Prevention of Wound Infection following Appendicectomy: A double-blind study, *Br J Surg,* **63:**973, 1976.

Lewis, F. R., Holcroft, J. W., Boey, J., and Dunphy, J. E.: Appendicitis. A Critical Review of Diagnosis and Treatment in 1,000 Cases, *Arch Surg,* **110:**677, 1975.

Longland, C. J., Gray, J. G., Lees, W., and Garrett, J. A. M.: The Prevention of Infection in Appendicectomy Wounds, *Br J Surg,* **58:**117, 1971.

McBurney, C.: Experience with Early Operative Interference in Cases of Diseases of the Vermiform Appendix, *NY State Med J,* **50:**676, 1889.

————: The Incision Made in the Abdominal Wall in Cases of Appendicitis, *Ann Surg,* **20:**38, 1894.

McDonald, J. C.: Nonspecific Mesenteric Lymphadenitis: Collective Review, *Surg Gynecol Obstet,* **116:**409, 1963.

Magarey, C. J., Chant, A. D. B., Rickford, C. R. K., and Magarey, J. R.: Peritoneal Drainage and Systemic Antibiotics after Appendicectomy, *Lancet,* **2:**179, 1971.

Marchildon, M. B., and Dudgeon, D. L.: Perforated Appendicitis: Current Experience in a Children's Hospital, *Ann Surg,* **185:**84, 1977.

Mason, L. B., and Deyden, W. R.: Primary Appendectomy, *Am Surg,* **42:**239, 1976.

Meade, R. H.: The Evolution of Surgery for Appendicitis, *Surgery,* **55:**741, 1964.

Noer, T.: Decreasing Incidence of Acute Appendicitis, *Acta Chir Scand,* **141:**431, 1975.

Raftery, A. T.: The Value of the Leukocyte Count in the Diagnosis of Acute Appendicitis, *Br J Surg,* **63:**143, 1976.

Sherman, J. O., Luck, S. R., and Borger, J. A.: Irrigation of the Peritoneal Cavity for Appendicitis in Children: A Double-blind Study, *J Pediatr Surg,* **11:**371, 1976.

Thomas, D. R.: Conservative Management of the Appendix Mass, *Surgery,* **73:**677, 1973.

Thomas, E. J., and Mueller, C. B.: Appendectomy: Diagnostic Criteria and Hospital Performance, *Hosp Pract,* **4:**72, 1969.

Thorbjarnarson, B.: Acute Appendicitis in Patients over the Age of Sixty, *Surg Gynecol Obstet,* **125:**1277, 1967.

Wangensteen, O. H., and Dennis, C.: Experimental Proof of the Obstructive Origin of Appendicitis in Man, *Ann Surg,* **110:**629, 1939.

Weber, J., Finlayson, N. B., and Mark, J. B. D.: Mesenteric Lymphadenitis and Terminal Ileitis due to *Yersinia pseudotuberculosis,* *N Engl J Med,* **283:**172, 1970.

White, J. J., Santillana, M., and Haller, J. A., Jr.: Intensive In-hospital Observation: A Safe Way to Decrease Unnecessary Appendectomy, *Am Surg,* **41:**793, 1975.

Willis, A. T., Ferguson, I. R., Jones, P. H., Phillips, K. D., Tearle, P. V., Berry, R. B., Fiddian, R. V., Graham, D. F., Harland, D. H. C., Innes, D. B., Mee, W. M., Rothwell-Jackson, R. L., Sutch, I., Kilbey, C., and Edwards, D.: Metronidazole in Prevention and Treatment of Bacteroides Infections after Appendectomy, *Br Med J,* **1**(6005):318, 1976.

Tumors

Aho, A. J., Heinonen, R., and Laurén, P.: Benign and Malignant Mucocele of the Appendix. Histological Types and Prognosis, *Acta Chir Scand,* **139:**392, 1973.

Godwin, J. D., II: Carcinoid Tumors. An Analysis of 2837 Cases, *Cancer,* **36:**560, 1975.

Higa, E., Rosai, J., Pizzimbono, C. A., and Wise, L.: Mucosal Hyperplasia, Mucinous Cystadenoma, and Mucinous Cystadenocarcinoma of the Appendix: A Re-evaluation of Appendiceal "Mucocele," *Cancer,* **32:**1525, 1973.

Steinberg, M., and Cohn, I., Jr.: Primary Adenocarcinoma of the Appendix, *Surgery,* **61:**644, 1967.

Wilson, H., Cheek, R. C., Sherman, R. T., and Storer, E. H.: Carcinoid Tumors, in "Current Problems in Surgery," Year Book Medical Publishers, Inc., Chicago, 1970.

Wolff, M., and Ahmed, N.: Epithelial Neoplasms of the Vermiform Appendix (Exclusive of Carcinoid): I. Adenocarcinoma of the Appendix, *Cancer,* **37:**2493, 1976.

Wolff, M., and Ahmed, N.: Epithelial Neoplasms of the Vermiform Appendix (Exclusive of Carcinoid): II. Cystadenomas, Papillary Adenomas, and Adenomatous Polyps of the Appendix, *Cancer,* **37:**2511, 1976.

Liver

by Seymour I. Schwartz

ANATOMY

The liver constitutes approximately one-fiftieth of the total body weight. Its size reflects the complexity of its functions. The anatomic division with respect to biliary drainage and vascular supply differs from the classic description in which the organ was divided into right and left lobes by the falciform ligament. True division is to the right of the falciform ligament, in line with the fossa for the inferior vena cava above and the gallbladder fossa below (Fig. 30-1). A right segmental fissure divides the right lobe into anterior and posterior segments, while the falciform ligament divides the left lobe into medial and lateral segments. The left lateral segment corresponds to the left lobe in the classic description. This segmental division can be observed only in cast specimens in which the Glissonian structures, i.e., hepatic artery, portal vein, and bile ducts, have been injected.

BILIARY DRAINAGE. Each segment is drained by a major segmental duct formed by the confluence of subsegmental draining structures. The anterior and posterior segmental ducts in the right lobe join to form the right hepatic duct, while the medial and lateral segmental ducts in the left lobe terminate in the left hepatic duct, which joins the right duct to form a common hepatic duct in the porta hepatis. This lies anteriorly in relation to other structures in the area. The common hepatic duct descends for a variable distance in the hepatoduodenal ligament and is joined by the cystic duct which enters from the right at an angle. These two structures and the liver form the cystohepatic triangle of Calot, which is extremely important surgically, since it frequently contains the cystic and right hepatic arteries as well as aberrant segmental hepatic arteries and ducts.

BLOOD SUPPLY. The afferent blood supply to the liver arises from two sources: (1) the hepatic artery, which carries oxygenated blood and accounts for approximately 25 percent of hepatic blood flow and (2) the portal vein, which accounts for approximately 75 percent of hepatic blood flow and drains the splanchnic circulation. The common hepatic artery originates from the celiac axis and, after contributing the right gastric artery, ascends in the hepatoduodenal ligament to the left of the common bile duct and anterior to the portal vein. It bifurcates into a right and left branch to the left of the main lobar fissure. The major right hepatic artery originates from the superior mesenteric artery in 17 percent of people. Intrahepatic anastomoses between the right and left hepatic arteries do not occur. The cystic artery is usually an extrahepatic branch of the right hepatic artery.

The portal venous system contains no valves (Fig. 30-2). It returns to the liver the blood that the celiac, superior mesenteric, and inferior mesenteric arteries supply to the gastrointestinal tract, pancreas, and spleen. The vessel is formed behind the pancreas, at the level of L_1 to L_2, by the confluence of the superior mesenteric and splenic veins and, at times, the inferior mesenteric vein. The portal vein resides posteriorly in relation to the hepatic artery and bile duct in the hepatoduodenal ligament but, in rare instances,

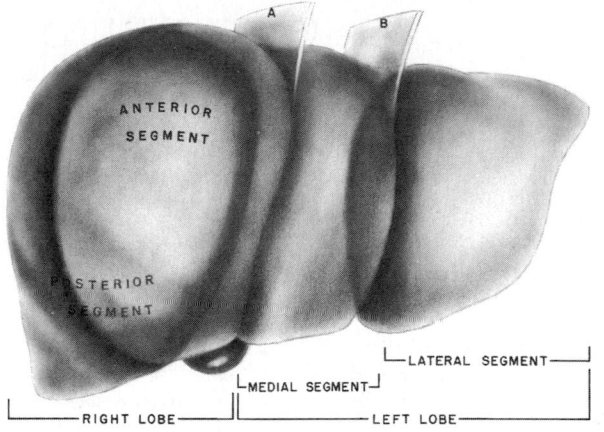

Fig. 30-1. Lobar and segmental divisions of the liver. *A.* Lobar fissure. *B.* Left segmental fissure. A right segmental fissure divides the right lobe into its anterior and posterior segments. (*From Seymour I. Schwartz, "Surgical Diseases of the Liver," McGraw-Hill Book Company, 1964.*)

is located anterior to the pancreas and first portion of the duodenum, in which circumstance it is frequently associated with a partial or complete situs inversus and is subject to injury during cholecystectomy or gastrectomy. In the porta hepatis the vein divides into two branches, which

Fig. 30-2. Anatomy of the extrahepatic portal venous system, anterior aspect. The termination of each vein is shown as it was encountered most frequently in 92 dissections. The pancreas is represented by the shaded area. *A.P.,* accessory pancreatic vein; *C.,* coronary vein; *Cystic,* cystic vein; *I.,* intestinal veins; *I.C.,* ileocolic vein; *I.M.,* inferior mesenteric vein; *I.P.D.,* inferior pancreaticoduodenal vein; *L.,* liver; *L.B.P.,* left branch of portal vein; *L.C.,* left colic vein; *L.G.E.,* left gastroepiploic vein; *M.C.,* middle colic vein; *O.,* omental vein; *P.,* pancreatic veins; *Pyloric,* pyloric vein; *R.C.,* right colic vein; *R.G.E.,* right gastroepiploic vein; *R.B.P.,* right branch of portal vein; *S.,* splenic vein; *S.G.,* short gastric veins; *S.H.,* superior hemorrhoidal vein; *S.M.,* superior mesenteric vein; *S.P.D.,* superior pancreaticoduodenal vein; *S.T.,* splenic trunks. (*From Douglass et al., Surg Gynecol Obstet, 91:562, 1950.*)

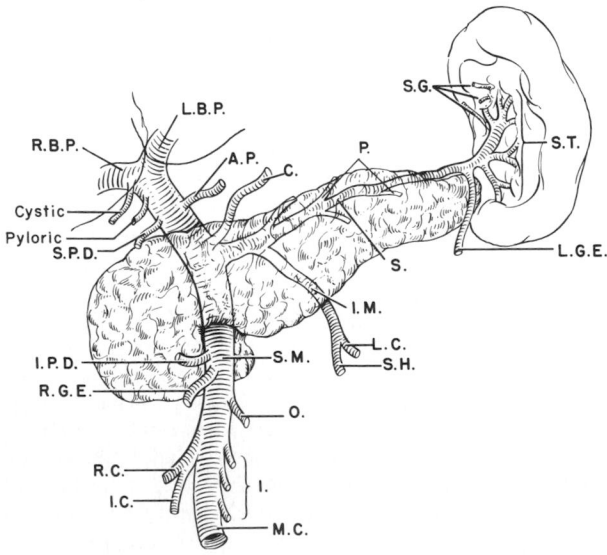

course to each lobe. The average length of the main portal vein is 6.5 cm, and the average diameter is 0.8 cm. Much has been written concerning the streaming phenomenon within the portal vein accounting for preferential metastases to the right and left lobe depending on the venous drainage of the primary site. Recent experimental and clinical findings have refuted this concept.

The hepatic venous system (Fig. 30-3) begins as a central vein of the liver lobule and represents the only vessel in man into which the sinusoids empty. The central veins unite to form sublobular veins, which in turn fuse to form collecting veins. The collecting veins gradually increase in size by joining other large intrahepatic collecting channels, which coalesce to form the three major hepatic veins. The hepatic venous tributaries occupy the fissures and are intersegmental in position. The major hepatic veins are classified as right, left, and middle. The right hepatic vein drains the entire posterior segment as well as the superior area of the anterior segment of the right lobe. The left hepatic vein drains the entire lateral segment and the superior area of the medial segment of the left lobe. The inferior areas of the medial and anterior segments of the two lobes are drained by the middle vein. In man there are no valves in the hepatic venous system, whereas the dog has a sphincteric action in the hepatic veins which constitutes an important difference experimentally. Total hepatic blood flow can be measured by means of hepatic vein catheterization and the use of the Fick principle. The average value is 1,500 ml/minute/1.73 m^2 of body surface.

LIVER FUNCTION

The liver consists of four physiologic-anatomic units which are interrelated:

1. The circulatory system. A dual blood supply nourishes the liver and acts as a vehicle for material absorbed from the intestinal tract to be utilized in the metabolic pool. Blood vessels are accompanied by lymphatics and nerve fibers which contribute to the regulation of blood flow and intrasinusoidal pressure.
2. Biliary passages. These serve as channels of exit for materials secreted by the liver cells, including bilirubin, cholesterol, and detoxified drugs. This system originates with the Golgi apparatus adjacent to the microvilli of the bile canaliculi and eventually terminates in the common bile duct.
3. The reticuloendothelial system. This system has 60 percent of its cellular elements in the liver and includes the phagocytic Kupffer cells and endothelial cells.
4. The functioning liver cells, which are capable of a wide variation of activity. The metabolic pool in the liver serves the needs of the entire body. The cell performs both anabolic and catabolic activities, secretes, excretes, and stores. The large amount of energies required for these transformations result from the conversion of adenosine triphosphate (ATP) to adenosine diphosphate (ADP). A second source is the aerobic oxygenation in the metabolic pool via the tricarboxylic acid cycle of Krebs.

Function Tests (Table 30-1)

The so-called liver "function" tests evaluate liver activity by assessing the degree of functional impairment. They do not provide a pathologic diagnosis, and the extreme functional reserve of the organ occasionally produces normal results in the face of significant lesions. Many of these tests do not measure a specific function of the liver, and other organ systems may be implicated. False positives for each of the tests are found in about 2.5 percent of normal controls and in about 10 percent of hospital controls. False-negative tests also occur in about 10 percent of most tests.

PROTEINS. Hepatic cells are responsible for the synthesis of albumin, fibrinogen, prothrombin, and other factors involved in blood clotting. A reduction of serum albumin is one of the most accurate reflections of the extent of liver disease and the effects of medical therapy. Because the half-life of albumin is slightly more than 10 days, impairment of hepatic synthesis must be present for over 2 weeks before abnormalities are noted. The correlation between total protein and disease of the liver is not as close as that between the serum albumin level and liver disease, since albumin is produced only by hepatic cells and a reduction is frequently compensated for by an increase in the level of globulin.

CARBOHYDRATES AND LIPIDS. Glycogenesis, glycogen storage, glycogenolysis, and the conversion of galactose into glucose all represent hepatic functions. Hypoglycemia is a rare accompaniment of extensive hepatic disease, but the amelioration of diabetes in patients with hemochromatosis is considered an indication of neoplastic change. The more common effect of hepatic disease is a deficiency of glycogenesis with resultant hyperglycemia. A hepatic enzyme system is responsible for the conversion of galactose into glucose, and abnormal galactose tolerance tests are seen in hepatitis and active cirrhosis. In rare instances, a familial deficiency in this enzyme system accounts for spontaneous galactosemia accompanied by an obstructive type of jaundice which appears after the first week of life and subsides when lactose is removed from the diet.

Synthesis of both phospholipid and cholesterol takes place in the liver, and the latter serves as a standard for the determination of lipid metabolism. The liver is the major organ involved in the synthesis, esterification, and excretion of cholesterol. In the presence of parenchymal damage, both the total cholesterol and percentage of esterified fraction decrease. Biliary obstruction results in a rise in cholesterol, and the most pronounced elevations are noted with primary biliary cirrhosis and the cholangiolitis accompanying toxic reactions to phenothiazine derivatives.

ENZYMES. The three enzymes which achieve abnormal serum levels in hepatic disease that have been widely studied are alkaline phosphatase, serum glutamic oxylactic transaminase (SGOT), and serum glutamic pyruvic transaminase (SGPT). The SGOT is present in the liver, myocardium, skeletal muscles, kidney, and pancreas. Cellular damage in any of the above-mentioned tissues results in elevation of the serum level. In reference to the liver, the most marked increases accompany acute cellular damage regardless of cause and extremely high levels are noted in patients with hepatitis. The SGOT is only moderately increased in cirrhosis and biliary obstruction. The SGPT is more particularly applicable to the evaluation of liver disease, since the hepatic content greatly exceeds myocar-

Fig. 30-3. Prevailing pattern of drainage of hepatic veins in the human liver. (*From Seymour I. Schwartz, "Surgical Diseases of the Liver," McGraw-Hill Book Company, 1964.*)

dial concentration. Elevations accompany acute hepatocellular damage. Lactic acid dehydrogenase (LDH) levels also may be elevated.

A variety of methods of assaying the serum alkaline phosphatase are currently in use, and in all notations of results normal values should be parenthetically indicated. Serum alkaline phosphatase provides an evaluation of the patency of the bile channels at all levels, intrahepatic and extrahepatic. Elevation is demonstrated in 94 percent of

Table 30-1. NORMAL VALUES FOR HEPATIC "FUNCTION" TESTS

Test	*Normal value*
Serum albumin	4.6–6.7 Gm/100 ml
Total protein	6.0–8.0 Gm/100 ml
Albumin/globulin	1.5–3.6
Cholesterol	135–325 mg/100 ml
Esters	65% of total
Alkaline phosphatase:	
Bodansky	1.5–4.0 units
King-Armstrong	3–13 units
Shinowara-Jones-Reinhart	2.8–8.6 units
Bessey-Lowry-Brock	1.8 × Bodansky units
Serum glutamic oxalacetic transaminase	40 units
Serum glutamic pyruvic transaminase	45 units
Lactic acid dehydrogenase	90–200 units
Bromsulphalein retention	0–6% at 45 minutes
Prothrombin time	90–100%
Fibrinogen	200–400 mg/100 ml
Blood "ammonia"	40–60 μg/100 ml
Icterus index	3–8 units
Serum bilirubin:	
Total	Less than 1.5 mg/100 ml
Direct	Less than 0.3 mg/100 ml
Indirect	Less than 1.2 mg/100 ml
Urinary bilirubin	0
Urobilinogen:	
Urinary	0.2–3.0 mg/day
Fecal	40–300 mg/day

patients with obstruction of the extrahepatic biliary tract due to neoplasm and 76 percent of those in whom the obstruction is caused by calculi. Intrahepatic biliary obstruction and cholestasis also cause a rise in the enzyme level. In the presence of space-occupying lesions such as metastases, primary hepatic carcinoma, and abscesses, the alkaline phosphatase is also increased. The overall correlation between metastatic carcinoma of the liver and an elevated enzyme level is as high as 92 percent. Sixty percent of patients with primary hepatic carcinoma also demonstrate a significant increase. Granulomatous and infiltrative lesions such as sarcoidosis, tuberculosis, and lymphoma are irregularly associated with mild to moderate increases in the alkaline phosphatase. Elevation of the serum level of this enzyme is also associated with diseases that have as a common denominator increased osteoblastic activity.

DYE EXCRETION. The hepatic removal of dyes from the circulation is dependent upon hepatic blood flow, hepatocellular function, and biliary excretion. Sulfobromophthalein (Bromsulphalein, or BSP) provides an assessment of hepatic function, although 20 percent is removed by an extrahepatic means. The presence of jaundice produces a disproportionate BSP retention, and fever, shock, hemorrhage, and recent surgical treatment may all result in increased levels. An increased retention is associated with acute cellular damage and is also noted in patients with cirrhosis, carcinoma, and chronic passive congestion. Since the rate of disappearance from the blood is constant, hepatic blood flow can be determined by injecting the dye at a rate which will maintain a constant blood level and applying Fick's principle to the blood removed from a catheterized hepatic vein.

Indocyanine green now is used more frequently to determine hepatic blood flow. More recently an intestinal xenon technique has been shown to provide an accurate method of measuring portal vein and total hepatic blood flow.

Rose bengal is another phthalein dye which, when labeled with radioactive iodine, has been useful in the evaluation of liver disease. Since all of this material is removed by the hepatic parenchymal cell, it provides a more accurate estimate of hepatic blood flow. Determination of the fecal excretion of the radioactive material has been applied to the differential diagnosis of obstructive jaundice, particularly in the establishment of the diagnosis of congenital atresia of the bile ducts.

COAGULATION FACTORS. In liver disease, multiple coagulation defects may occur. Two mechanisms contribute to the deficiency of coagulation factors: (1) in obstructive jaundice, the bile source required for the absorption of the fat-soluble vitamin K results in a decreased synthesis of prothrombin, and (2) hepatocellular dysfunction is accompanied by an inability of the liver to synthesize the prothrombin. Abnormal values for prothrombin time have been noted in a variety of hepatic diseases with parenchymal damage, and determination is particularly applicable in the evaluation of patients undergoing liver biopsy or surgical procedures. Values above 40 percent are generally not associated with excessive bleeding. An increase in

prothrombin time subsequent to the injection of parenteral vitamin K is used as an indication of hepatic function and suggests obstructive jaundice. Decreases in factor V (proaccelerin), Christmas factor, factor VII (proconvertin), and fibrinogen have also been noted in hepatic disease.

BILE PIGMENT METABOLISM. See the section on Jaundice in Chap. 24.

SPECIAL STUDIES

NEEDLE BIOPSY OF THE LIVER. This is the one study which provides a pathologic diagnosis. It is dependent on an area of tissue measuring 1 to 4 cm in length and containing approximately 5 to 20 lobules representing a general anatomic change. Close to 100 percent accuracy has been demonstrated for both posthepatitic and postnecrotic cirrhosis. Intrahepatic cholestasis, hepatitis, and cellular degeneration resulting from toxicity are all diffuse lesions and readily diagnosed. Focal lesions, such as neoplasm, granulomas, and abscess may be missed, but the correlation between needle biopsy and operative and autopsy findings is high. A mortality rate of 0.08 percent has been determined, and pain, pneumothorax, hemorrhage, and bile peritonitis are the complications to be considered.

SCINTILLATION SCANNING. This technique has been used as a method of evaluating liver size, shape, and position, and also to determine the presence and location of intrahepatic neoplasms or focal lesions. Either ^{131}I-tagged rose bengal, which is absorbed and excreted by the parenchymal cells of the liver, or ^{198}Au or preferably technetium-sulfur colloid (^{99m}Tc), which is deposited in the reticuloendothelial system, may be utilized. The scan is limited in detection to small lesions. For lesions over 1.5 cm, the correlation with autopsy and operative findings is excellent and is over 83 percent for metastatic lesions.

ANGIOGRAPHY. Since hepatic tumors, both primary and metastatic, are dependent on an arterial circulation, unusual vascular patterns are also detected by injection of the hepatic artery with the radiopaque material. Unusual arrangements of the arteries and "tumor staining," analogous to that found in cerebral and osseous neoplasms, may be noted.

MEASUREMENTS OF PORTAL PRESSURE, SPLENOPORTOGRAPHY, ISOTOPIC EVALUATION OF PORTAL CIRCULATION. See Portal Hypertension, later in this chapter.

TRAUMA

INCIDENCE. The liver ranks high on the list of intra-abdominal organs involved by injury (Table 30-2). The rapid increase in motor traffic has resulted in an increasing incidence and in a change of pattern from one with a predominance of penetrating wounds to the present higher incidence of blunt traumatic injuries. The frequency of traumatic rupture of the liver was 1 in 1,300 accident admissions to a general hospital. Seventy-four percent had additional abdominal organs involved, and 45 percent also had thoracic injuries.

Table 30-2. RELATIVE FREQUENCY OF
VISCERAL INJURY FROM BLUNT TRAUMA

Viscera involved	Series I	Series II	Series III	Series IV	Series V	Series VI
Spleen........	56	20	53	37	20	38
Intestine......	14	3	27	13	4	19
Liver	6	9	45	5	14	19
Kidneys......	8	25	Not incl.	26	27	91
Bladder	11	9	Not incl.	4		8
Others, including pancreas, the diaphragm, and mesentery ...	46	8	8	39	7	25
Total	141	74	183	124	72	200

SOURCE: From McCort, *Radiology,* **78:**49, 1962.

Rupture of the liver also occurs spontaneously in pathologic organs. It occurs in approximately 8 percent of patients with primary carcinoma and has been reported with increasing frequency for benign hepatic adenoma and in association with toxemia of pregnancy. Rupture of the liver in the newborn infant is related to the trauma of birth and is more common in infants who are larger than average and classified as "postmature."

PATHOLOGY. Liver injuries are classified as transcapsular, subcapsular, or central (Fig. 30-4). When rupture of the liver extends through Glisson's capsule, extravasated blood and bile are found in the peritoneal cavity. If the capsule remains intact, the collection of blood between the capsule and parenchyma is usually found on the superior surface of the organ. Central rupture consists of interruption of the parenchyma of the liver. Blunt trauma may be associated with hepatic parenchymal emboli to the right heart and lungs, causing death.

Persons with injury about the hilus rarely survive long enough for surgical exploration. Nonpenetrating injuries result in a tear in the anteroposterior portion. The dome of the liver is frequently involved, particularly in older patients. With penetrating lesions of the lower thorax, the dome is also most frequently involved, and the ratio of right lobe to left lobe involvement is 7:1.

CLINICAL MANIFESTATIONS. These are determined by the pathologic types. With rupture of Glisson's capsule, signs and symptoms are related to shock and peritoneal irritation. Shock is present in over three-quarters of the cases, and abdominal pain, spasm, and rigidity are usual accompaniments.

DIAGNOSTIC STUDIES. Shortly after trauma, an increased leukocyte count is more consistent than a reduced hemoglobin. Hematuria is frequently coexistent. The SGOT and SGPT levels are elevated, but this usually occurs several hours subsequent to trauma. Infrequently mild elevation of the serum bilirubin level occurs on the third or fourth day. X-ray may reveal evidence of fluid in the peritoneum and pelvis or a wide right flank stripe indicating blood accumulated between the ascending colon and the peritoneal line. Paracentesis is useful in verifying the presence of hemoperitoneum, but a negative tap does not exclude the diagnosis. Celiac angiography may precisely define hepatic rupture and will distinguish between hepatic splenic rupture in a patient with a positive tap (Fig. 30-5).

TREATMENT. Shock is corrected and associated thoracic lesions are treated first. Surgical procedures are directed at the control of bleeding, the removal of necrotic devitalized tissue, and the establishment of external drainage. These should be initiated early, because time has proved to be a definite factor in morbidity and mortality statistics. With penetrating wounds of the liver, particularly knife wounds, the bleeding has usually stopped at the time of exploration and simple drainage is all that is required. Such is usually not the case with blunt trauma and shotgun wounds. Hemorrhages are controlled preferably by exposing individual bleeders within the parenchyma of the liver and ligating these vessels. The technique of placing a row of interlocking through-and-through mattress sutures parallel to the surfaces of the laceration should be avoided, since this adds to the amount of tissue necrosis. In general, hepatic resection is not carried out along precise anatomic lines

Fig. 30-4. Diagram of three types of liver rupture. *A.* Transcapsular. *B.* Subcapsular. *C.* Central. (*From Seymour I. Schwartz, "Surgical Diseases of the Liver," McGraw-Hill Book Company, 1964.*)

Fig. 30-5. Celiac angiogram demonstrating normal spleen and hepatic rupture.

Hematobilia

The pathologic *sine qua non* for this condition is free communication between a blood vessel and the biliary tree. It is a consequence of central or subcapsular hematomas and also capsular wounds which have been primarily closed or packed. The triad of abdominal injury, subsequent gastrointestinal hemorrhage, and colicky pain should raise a high index of suspicion. This may occur within few days after injury or, more characteristically, after a period of weeks. Multiple episodes of bleeding with some suggestion of periodicity occur. Melena is more frequent than hematemesis, and jaundice of mild to severe proportion is present in some cases. Diagnosis is established and the lesion located by angiographic techniques. Operations have been varied and have included resection of the lesion, which is preferable, debridement and unroofing, or ligation of the contributing hepatic artery.

Hepatorenal Syndrome

The term *hepatorenal syndrome* was introduced to describe the fatal combination of renal and hepatic dysfunction occurring in patients after biliary tract surgery. Shortly thereafter, the association of this syndrome with traumatic necrosis of the liver was proposed. It was theorized that the damaged liver cells released into the circulation a toxin capable of destroying kidney cells. There is no question that renal failure often is associated with massive hepatic injury, but the so-called "hepatic nephrotoxin" has not been identified. In this regard, recent animal experiments have demonstrated abnormal renal function and increased exchangeable sodium in animals subjected to hepatic damage.

PROGNOSIS. The improvement in mortality statistics accompanying hepatic injuries is evident from war experience. During World War II with the institution of routine drainage and the elimination of gauze packs the mortality rate dropped from 30 to 17 percent. During the Korean war, penetrating injuries were associated with a mortality rate of 14 percent, whereas in the Vietnam war a mortality rate of 4.2 percent has been reported for United States military personnel. The mortality rate associated with blunt trauma is consistently higher than that accompanying penetrating injuries. In a large series, extending from 1963 to 1971, the overall mortality was 13 percent. Blunt trauma and shotgun wounds had a significantly higher mortality rate than penetrating wounds. In patients requiring a sublobar resection the mortality rate was 47 percent; associated damage to the hepatic veins or inferior vena cava raised the rate to 85 percent.

MAJOR VASCULAR INJURIES. The effects of ligation of the major vessels are diagrammed in Fig. 30-6. When the common or proper hepatic artery is ligated, collateral supply is apparent roentgenographically within 4 hours and it is unusual for major dysfunction caused by hepatic ischemia to occur. However, primary repair of a surgically traumatized artery and restoration of flow are indicated.

Hepatic vein injuries represent a significant factor in the high mortality accompanying blunt liver trauma. Fifteen

unless the injury demands it. Most resections are best regarded as sublobar debridements, with as much tissue preserved as possible. All the devitalized tissue and markedly traumatized tissue is removed to avoid subsequent autolysis, abscess formation, and secondary hemorrhage.

Packing with gauze is contraindicated, since it is attended by a high incidence of secondary hemorrhage and infection. Recently, there has been enthusiasm for hepatic artery ligation to control bleeding. This is appropriate when it can be demonstrated that bleeding is reduced by temporarily cross-clamping the hepatic artery. In most circumstances of extensive bleeding, it is venous in character and requires a direct approach. The most vigorous bleeding associated with hepatic trauma is usually caused by deep lacerations of the posterior portions of the right lobe with involvement of the hepatic veins. The use of an internal stent passed either from the atrium down to the infrahepatic vena cava or from the infrahepatic vena cava up to the suprahepatic vena cava may facilitate control of the bleeding while maintaining caval flow.

External drainage should be carried out in almost all cases and is directed at the prevention of abscess and bile peritonitis. The drains are brought out from the subphrenic and subhepatic spaces, depending upon the lesion. There is controversy regarding the appropriateness of routinely draining the common bile duct. An increased complication rate has been reported for T-tube drainage in patients with hepatic trauma. This includes infections and an increased incidence of upper gastrointestinal bleeding. Although common duct drainage does not prevent the development of a hematobilia, it does permit postoperative cholangiography, which may aid in the diagnosis of this complication and which also can be used to determine the status of hepatic regeneration.

COMPLICATIONS. The incidence of complications is well over 50 percent and is related to the extent of injury to other organs. Hemorrhage is the most important cause of death, and recurrent bleeding may occur secondarily to necrosis and sequestration of infected tissue.

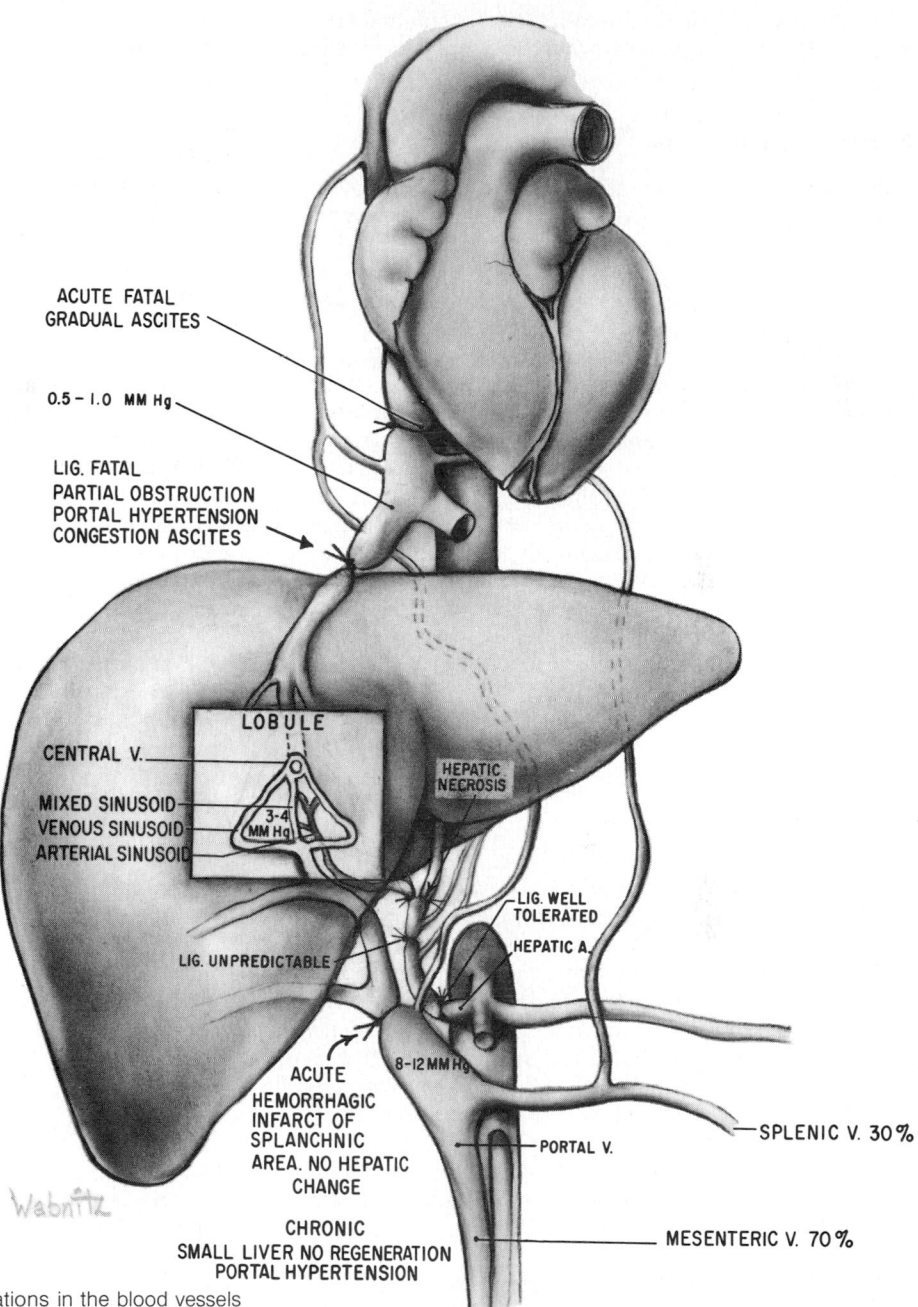

ACUTE FATAL
GRADUAL ASCITES

0.5 - 1.0 MM Hg

LIG. FATAL
PARTIAL OBSTRUCTION
PORTAL HYPERTENSION
CONGESTION ASCITES

LOBULE

CENTRAL V.

MIXED SINUSOID
VENOUS SINUSOID
ARTERIAL SINUSOID

3-4
MM Hg

HEPATIC
NECROSIS

LIG. WELL
TOLERATED

HEPATIC A.

LIG. UNPREDICTABLE

8-12 MM Hg

ACUTE
HEMORRHAGIC
INFARCT OF
SPLANCHNIC
AREA. NO HEPATIC
CHANGE

PORTAL V.

SPLENIC V. 30%

CHRONIC
SMALL LIVER NO REGENERATION
PORTAL HYPERTENSION

MESENTERIC V. 70%

Wabnitz

Fig. 30-6. Pressures and effects of ligations in the blood vessels of the liver. (*From H. Popper and F. Schaffner, "Liver: Structure and Function," McGraw-Hill Book Company, 1957.*)

percent of patients with blunt hepatic trauma have sustained injury to the hepatic veins, and most of these patients die from uncontrollable hemorrhage either in the operating room or prior to operation. Because the hepatic veins are multiple, often forming connecting channels, the safe approach is to expose all the veins and the entire retrohepatic inferior vena cava. Control of the bleeding vein or veins is best accomplished by occluding the porta hepatis and inserting a catheter via either the inferior vena cava or the right atrium in such a fashion that umbilical

tapes may be placed above and below the area of the hepatic veins. A review of portal vein injury reported that 16 of 17 patients survived ligation but that reconstruction should be attempted.

HEPATIC ABSCESSES

Hepatic abscesses are related to two distinct groups of pathogens, pyogenic bacteria and *Entamoeba histolytica*.

Distinctive features in the clinical manifestations and therapy of these two variations necessitate separate consideration.

Pyogenic Abscesses

INCIDENCE. The lesion is present in 0.36 percent of autopsies. Prior to the widespread use of antibiotic therapy, this incidence was 0.44 percent as contrasted with 0.28 percent in autopsies since 1945. The highest percentage of cases occur in the sixth, seventh, and eighth decade, and there is no predilection for either sex.

ETIOLOGY. Pyogenic abscesses of the liver result from (1) ascending biliary infection, (2) hematogenous spread via the portal venous system, (3) generalized septicemia with involvement of the liver by way of the hepatic arterial circulation, (4) direct extension from intraperitoneal infection, and (5) other causes, including hepatic trauma. Recently, the most frequent antecedent cause has been cholangitis secondary to calculi or carcinoma in the extrahepatic biliary duct system. The second most common cause is related to generalized septicemia, while the portal venous route of infection has decreased in importance. Pylephlebitis occurs in 0.05 percent of cases of acute appendicitis and 3 percent of patients with perforated appendicitis. No segment of the intestine drained by the portal venous system can be excluded as a possible cause, and the incidence associated with acute diverticulitis is as high as that of appendicitis. There has been an increase in the percentage in which no cause is apparent. In one series these accounted for over half the cases.

Positive cultures are obtained from pyogenic abscesses in only 50 percent of cases. *Escherichia coli* has been the only microorganism demonstrated in abscesses secondary to biliary tract infection and infection along the portal venous route. By contrast, the cocci, particularly *Staphylococcus aureus* and hemolytic streptococcus, are usually isolated from abscesses related to systemic infection. *Bacteroides* and other anaerobes have become increasingly prevalent as a cause, thus emphasizing the need to culture anaerobically at the time of drainage.

Pyogenic abscesses may be solitary, multiple, and multilocular. The greatest proportion are multiple small abscesses. When a single abscess is present, it is usually located in the right lobe.

CLINICAL MANIFESTATIONS. Since most pyogenic hepatic abscesses are secondary to other significant infections, it is difficult to delineate a pathognomonic symptom. Fever is the most common symptom, and a "picket fence" configuration of the temperature chart generally has been noted. Fever is frequently accompanied by chills, profuse sweating, nausea, vomiting, and anorexia. Pain is a late symptom and is more common with large solitary abscesses. Enlargement of the liver and tenderness have been considered almost constant findings. However, in more recent series liver enlargement was noted in 30 to 60 percent of cases. Hepatic tenderness was absent in one-third of the patients. Jaundice is a relatively uncommon finding.

DIAGNOSTIC STUDIES. Leukocytosis with white blood cell counts ranging between 18,000 and 20,000 is usual.

Most patients are anemic. Positive blood cultures are demonstrated in approximately 30 percent of patients, the most significant yields accompanying abscesses secondary to systemic septicemia. Liver function tests are not diagnostic, but elevation of the alkaline phosphatase level is the most frequent abnormality. Hypoalbuminemia is common. Characteristically, x-rays reveal an elevation and immobility or restriction of motion of the right leaf of the diaphragm. There is also obliteration of the right cardiophrenic angle on the posteroanterior chest film and the anterior costophrenic angle on the lateral film. Abscesses produced by gas-forming microorganisms are associated with air-fluid levels in the liver. Cholangiography is of little value. The lesions generally can be defined by hepatic arteriography or ^{99m}Tc-sulfur colloid scan.

TREATMENT. This is based on appropriate antibiotic therapy combined with surgical drainage in selected cases. Either chloramphenicol or gentamycin should be given until cultures and sensitivities are reported. Drainage is particularly indicated for solitary abscesses or for large multiple abscesses. The route of access depends on the position of the abscess and may be transthoracic or transabdominal (Figs. 30-7 and 30-8). Because of the availability of antibacterial agents, transperitoneal drainage is no longer associated with prohibitive morbidity or mortality.

PROGNOSIS AND COMPLICATIONS. The prognosis is significantly better in patients with single or multilocular abscesses than in those with multiple abscesses. Similarly, there is a much higher mortality rate associated with patients in whom complications including subphrenic abscess, empyema, or pyopericardium have developed. The mortality rate approaches 100 percent in undrained patients; 66 percent of the drained patients survive, and over 90 percent of patients with a solitary abscess which is drained survive. Subphrenic abscess occurs in approximately 5 percent of cases, and rupture of the hepatic abscess into the free peritoneal cavity may cause a diffuse peritonitis.

Amebic Abscesses

INCIDENCE. *Entamoeba histolytica* has been found wherever surveys have been made on the human population from Northern Canada to the Straits of Magellan. It has been estimated that at least 10 percent of the population of this country is infected with the parasite. The incidence of amebic involvement of the liver is more difficult to assess. An average involvement of 3.6 percent of autopsy cases and 1 to 25 percent of clinical cases have been reported. Much of this disparity is related to the lack of clinical recognition. Amebic abscess of the liver is a

Fig. 30-7. Extraserous transthoracic drainage. *A.* Incision is made posteriorly over right twelfth rib. *B.* Latissimus dorsi muscle exposed. *C.* Periosteum of twelfth rib incised. *D.* Twelfth rib removed subperiosteally and bed incised. *E.* Diaphragm is detached and peritoneum is reflected from the inferior surface of diaphragm. *F.* Schematic drawing of position of drain. (*From Seymour I. Schwartz, "Surgical Diseases of the Liver," McGraw-Hill Book Company, 1964.*)

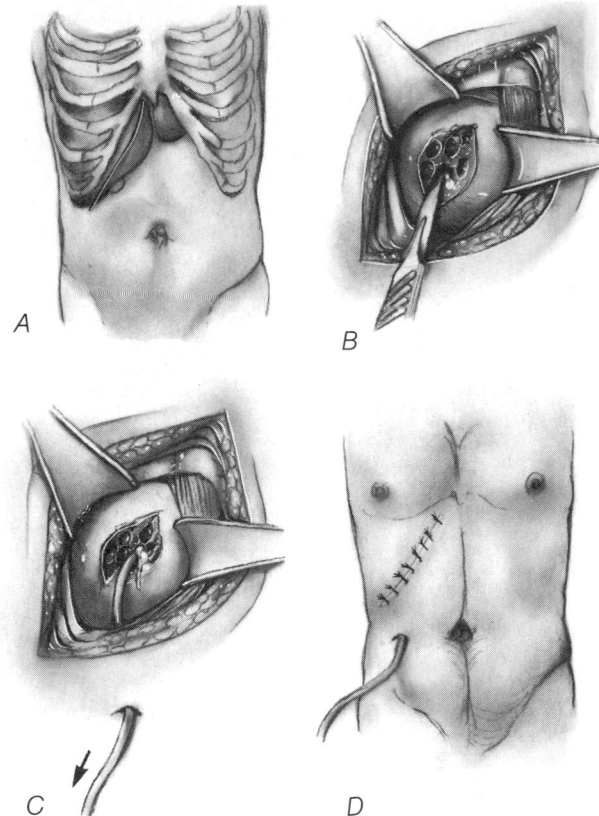

Fig. 30-8. Transabdominal drainage. *A.* Subcostal incision. *B.* Peritoneum has been entered and abscess incised. *C.* Drain is positioned in abscess and brought out through the stab wound. *D.* Closure of wound and position of stab wound. (*From Seymour I. Schwartz, "Surgical Diseases of the Liver," McGraw-Hill Book Company, 1964.*)

disease of the middle-aged adult and predominates in the male with a 9:1 ratio. The concept of racial immunity is no longer considered valid.

PATHOLOGY. Amebas reach the liver by way of the portal venous system from a focus of ulceration in the bowel wall. Hepatic involvement is usually a large single abscess containing liquefied material with a characteristic reddish brown "anchovy paste" fluid. The lesions are usually single and occur in the right lobe of the liver either near the dome or on the inferior surface in juxtaposition to the hepatic flexure. The wall is only a few millimeters thick and consists of granulation tissue with little or no fibrosis. Microscopically, three zones are recognized: a necrotic center, a middle zone with destruction of parenchymal cells, and an outer zone of relatively normal hepatic tissue in which amebas may be demonstrated. The concept of amebic hepatitis or presuppurative hepatitis has been challenged, since it is not certain that biliary abscesses or even larger central hepatic abscesses do not exist.

CLINICAL MANIFESTATIONS. Abscesses become evident when they cause generalized systemic disturbances coupled with symptoms and signs of hepatic involvement. The chief complaints are fever and liver pain. Pain is present in 88 percent of patients, and the pattern is related to the lo-

cation of the hepatic abscess. With pain and tenderness over the right lower intercostal spaces, there may be associated bulging and pitting edema of the subcutaneous tissue. Superior surface abscesses result in pain referred to the right shoulder, while abscesses in the bare area, which have no contact with the serosal surface, are latent as far as pain is concerned. Left lobe abscesses present as a painful epigastric swelling.

Fever accompanied by chills and sweating is present in over three-quarters of the patients, but the temperature does not reach the levels resulting from pyogenic abscesses unless there is secondary infection. One-third to one-half of the adults offer a history of antecedent diarrhea, while in children grossly bloody mucous stool occurs more frequently. Tender hepatomegaly is an almost constant feature. Clinical jaundice is relatively rare, and abnormal pulmonary findings are present in about one-quarter of the patients.

DIAGNOSTIC STUDIES. Patients with acute disease show no anemia but an appreciable degree of leukocytosis, whereas those with prolonged illness have anemia with less marked leukocytosis. Examination of the stool does not provide a high diagnostic yield. Although DeBakey and Ochsner demonstrated amebas in the stools of 47 percent of their own patients, these were found in only 15.4 percent of cases collected from the literature. Liver function tests are not helpful in establishing the diagnosis, although the BSP retention may be increased and the alkaline phosphatase level may be elevated. A specific complement-fixation test has been more reliable than a history of diarrhea, stool examination, and proctoscopy. However, a negative test does not exclude the diagnosis. Roentgenographic findings are similar to those described for pyogenic abscesses. Scintillography and angiography have also helped to localize the lesion.

Diagnosis is frequently established by aspiration of the abscess cavity, a relatively innocuous procedure. Although the "anchovy paste" aspirate is considered pathognomonic, the abscess content may be creamy white even though there is no secondary bacterial infection. Amebic trophozoites are demonstrated in the aspirate of fewer than one-third of the patients.

COMPLICATIONS. The most common complication is secondary infection, which occurs in approximately 22 percent of patients. Rupture of the amebic abscess accounts for the next most common group of complications. The direction of rupture is reproduced in Fig. 30-9. Pleuropulmonary complications occur in 20 percent of patients. This is usually the result of direct extension of the hepatic process. The most serious route of rupture is into the pericardial cavity, and this is usually secondary to extension of an abscess in the left lobe. Rupture into the peritoneal cavity or into an intraabdominal viscus occurs in 6 to 9 percent of the patients.

TREATMENT. This consists of administration of amebicidal drugs combined with aspiration or surgical drainage when indicated. The initial approach is usually conservative and directed toward eradicating the parasite from the intestinal tract, liver, and abscess itself. In general, the patient is not considered for surgical treatment until the intestinal phase is controlled. Metronidazole, which acts in both the hepatic and intestinal sites, has replaced emetine and chloroquine. Both the hepatic and intestinal infections have generally been cured by 400 mg three times a day for 4 days combined with closed aspiration. A single dose of 2.5 Gm combined with aspiration also has had dramatic results. Since both emetine, which may be cardiotoxic, and chloroquine act mainly on the hepatic phase, following completion of therapy with these drugs, intestinal amebicidals such as Diodoquin, chiniofon, and tetracycline must be administered to control the intestinal phase.

Surgical Procedures. The indications for aspiration are (1) the persistence of clinical manifestations following a course of amebicidal drugs, (2) clinical or roentgenographic evidence of a hepatic abscess, and (3) absence of findings which would suggest secondary infection of a liver abscess. Drug therapy should be instituted several days prior to aspiration. There is no indication for injection of any drug directly into the abscess cavity. In the absence of localizing signs, the preferred route is through the ninth or tenth interspace between the anterior and posterior axillary line. More recently, there has been renewed enthusiasm for frequent open drainage of amebic abscesses of the liver. Once an abscess has been demonstrated to be secondarily infected, open drainage is the treatment of choice. Although there is an obvious advantage to the extraserous approach, antibiotics have obviated the prohibitive mortality or morbidity associated with transserous drainage (Figs. 30-7 and 30-8).

PROGNOSIS. This is dependent upon the relative virulence of the organism and the resistance of the host, the stage of infection, the multiplicity of abscesses, and the presence of complications. In uncomplicated cases, the mortality rate is only 7 percent, whereas with complications a 43 percent mortality has been reported.

CYSTS AND BENIGN TUMORS

Nonparasitic Cysts

These lesions may be single, multiple, diffuse, localized, unilocular, or multilocular. They include (1) blood and degenerative cysts, (2) dermoid cysts, (3) lymphatic cysts, (4) endothelial cysts, (5) retention cysts, consisting of (*a*) solitary retention cysts and (*b*) multiple retention cysts (polycystic disease), and (6) proliferative cysts (cystadenomas). Autopsy incidences of approximately 0.15 percent have been reported. The clinically apparent cystic disease and nonparasitic solitary cysts occur more frequently in the fourth, fifth, and sixth decades, at an average age of fifty-three. Solitary cysts occur more commonly in females (4:1). Traumatic cysts are more common in children whereas cystadenomas occur at an average age of fifty two years. Polycystic hepatic disease also occurs much more frequently in the female.

PATHOLOGY. Solitary nonparasitic cysts are usually located on the anteroinferior surface of the right lobe of the liver. The cyst content is a clear, watery, yellowish brown material, and characteristically the cysts have a low inter-

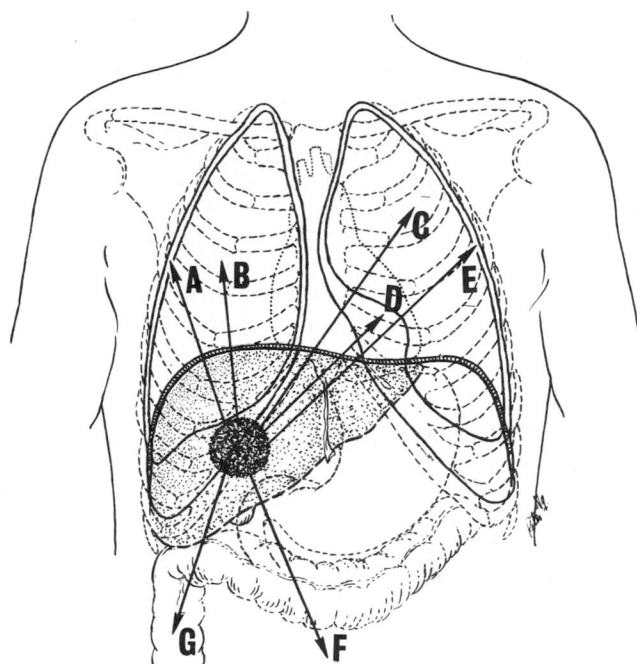

Fig. 30-9. Directions of rupture in 44 cases of amebic liver abscess: A. 8 cases, right pleural cavity. B. 13 cases, right lung. C. 4 cases, left lung. D. 7 cases, pericardium. E. 1 case, left pleural cavity. F. 10 cases, peritoneal cavity. G. 1 case, colon. (*After Lamont, Q J Med, 27:389, 1958.*)

nal pressure in contrast to the high tension in parasitic cysts. Polycystic disease of the liver has a honeycomb appearance with multiple cavities, and the lesions are commonly distributed throughout the entire liver, but at times one lobe, more frequently the right, is preferentially involved. Unlike the solitary nonparasitic cyst, polycystic disease of the liver is frequently associated with cystic involvement of other organs; 51.6 percent of polycystic livers are associated with polycystic kidneys. Conversely, the incidence of hepatic cysts in patients with known polycystic renal disease varies between 19 and 34 percent. Polycystic livers have been implicated as a rare cause of portal hypertension and also have been associated with atresia of the bile ducts, cholangitis, and hemangiomas.

Traumatic cysts are usually single, are filled with bile, and contain no epithelial lining. Cystadenomas are grossly smooth, encapsulated, and lobular, and contain a mucoid material. They are lined by a proliferative columnar epithelium.

CLINICAL MANIFESTATIONS. Both solitary and polycystic lesions grow slowly and are relatively asymptomatic. A painless right upper quadrant mass is the most frequent complaint, and when symptoms occur they are usually related to pressure on adjacent viscera. Acute abdominal pain may accompany the complications of torsion, intracystic hemorrhage, or intraperitoneal rupture. Physical examination may reveal the mass, and the kidneys may be palpable. Jaundice is rare. Liver function tests are of little diagnostic aid. Scintillography and arteriography have been used to define the intrahepatic position of the mass, and peritoneoscopy may be diagnostic.

TREATMENT. With the exceptions of rupture, torsion, and intracystic hemorrhage, the treatment is elective. Ideally, complete extirpation is the treatment of choice, but few cysts are resectable. Solitary cysts which are superficial should be resected, but resection of a large cyst extending deep into the parenchyma may be hazardous. When the cyst contents are sterile and contain no bile, unroofing the cyst and establishing a free connection with the peritoneal cavity is satisfactory. When bile is present, internal drainage into a Roux en Y jejunal limb is preferable, while the presence of purulent contents indicates external drainage or marsupialization. With polycystic disease of the liver and serious renal involvement, excisional therapy for the hepatic cyst is contraindicated. Also, if the patient has been asymptomatic and excision is deemed to be technically difficult, resection should not be carried out. However, if the patient is in good health and there is a possibility of complete surgical extirpation, wide excision is justifiable.

PROGNOSIS. The prognosis of polycystic disease is essentially that of the accompanying renal disease. Hepatic failure, jaundice, and the manifestations of portal hypertension are rare. The mortality rate for surgically treated nonparasitic cysts of the liver is approximately 5 percent. The morbidity is usually related to the development of a persistent sinus.

Hydatid Cysts

Hydatid disease (echinococcosis) is characterized by worldwide distribution and frequent hepatic involvement. The incidence among human beings is dependent on the incidence in intermediate hosts including sheep, pigs, and cattle. The southern half of South America, Iceland, Australia, New Zealand, and southern parts of Africa are regarded as intensive endemic areas. Fewer than 1,000 cases have been reported in the United States, most of these occurring in immigrants.

PATHOLOGY. The most common unilocular hydatid cyst is caused by *Echinococcus granulosis,* while the alveolar type is caused by *Echinococcus multilocularis.* Approximately 70 percent of hydatid cysts are located in the liver, and in one-quarter to one-third of these cases there are multiple cysts. The right lobe is affected in 85 percent of patients. Cysts are usually superficial and are composed of a two-layer laminated wall, an inner germinative membrane, and an outer adventitia. The two membranes are in close contact with each other but are not linked. The fluid in the hydatid cyst has a high pressure of approximately 300 ml of water and is colorless, opalescent, and slightly alkaline. Inside the main hydatid vesicle daughter cysts are usually found. Extension is commonly into the peritoneal cavity, but progressive intrahepatic expansion may result in the replacement of liver parenchyma.

In contrast to the unilocular hydatid cysts, the alveolar hydatid is a growth without a capsule and with a tendency toward multiple metastases. As growth progresses, the center becomes necrotic, and the peripheral portion invades the blood vessels and lymph channels. The causative agent of this lesion is found more frequently in the colder regions of Alaska, Russia, and the Alps.

COMPLICATIONS. Intrabiliary rupture represents the most common complication and occurs in 5 to 10 percent of cases. Suppuration, the second most common complication, is caused by bacteria from the biliary tract. The formation of the purulent material results in the death of the parasite and conversion into a pyogenic abscess. Intraperitoneal rupture results in the showering of hydatid fluid, brood capsules, and scolices into the peritoneum, leading to transient peritoneal irritation of varying intensity. Usually, the reproductive elements survive and initiate the formation of new cysts, "secondary echinococcosis of the peritoneum." Cysts located in the superior portion of the liver tend to grow craniad into the pleural cavity and become intrathoracic. These can be differentiated from primary pulmonary cysts by the presence of daughter cysts and bile pigments. Empyema and bronchopleural fistula may result.

CLINICAL MANIFESTATIONS. Patients with simple or uncomplicated multivesicular cysts are usually asymptomatic. When symptoms occur, they are caused by pressure on adjacent organs. A tumor, which is palpable in 70 percent of the patients, or diffuse hepatic enlargement in a patient who has lived in an endemic region is cause for suspicion. The so-called "hydatid thrill" and "fremitus" are quite rare. Jaundice and ascites are uncommon. With secondary infection, tender hepatomegaly, chills, and spiking temperatures occur. Urticaria and erythema offer evidence of a generalized anaphylactic reaction. With biliary rupture, the classic triad of biliary colic, jaundice, and urticaria may be noted. Vomiting with passage of hydatid membranes in the emesis (hydatidemesia) and passage of membranes in the stool (hydatidenteria) may also occur. The complication of intraperitoneal rupture is heralded by abdominal pain and signs of anaphylactic shock. Intrathoracic rupture is associated with shoulder pain and cough initially productive of a frothy blood-stained fluid that subsequently becomes bile-stained. Membranes are intermittently expectorated in 80 percent of the cases.

DIAGNOSTIC STUDIES. Roentgenographically, an unruptured cyst presents as a round, reticulated calcified shadow in the liver (Fig. 30-10). Secondary infection with gas-producing organisms may demonstrate as daughter cysts. With intrabiliary rupture, gas is noted in the remaining cyst cavity. Liver scans furnish useful information and correlate well with operative findings. Eosinophilia is the least reliable of immunologic responses, being present in only 25 percent of all patients. Complement-fixation tests have been positive in up to 93 percent of patients with living cysts. This reaction becomes negative 2 to 6 months after removal of the cyst. Casoni's skin test is positive in approximately 90 percent of patients, and the reaction may be obtained years after surgical removal of the cyst or after the parasite has died. Diagnosis may also be made by demonstrating the elements of the hydatid cyst in the excreta or during biopsy.

TREATMENT. Small calcified cysts in patients with negative serologic test results need no treatment. Treatment is surgical, since there is no response to drug administration or radiation therapy. Therapy consists of removal of the cyst without contaminating the patient, followed by appropriate management of any remaining cavity. Since the hydatid fluid is under high tension, evacuation and sterilization are carried out initially using hydrogen peroxide or hypertonic saline solution. The classic approach using Formalin has fallen into disrepute. Removal of the parasite is accomplished by excision of the hydatid vesicle using the natural cleavage plane which exists between the germinative layer and adventitia. Total removal of the cysts, including the adventitial layer, may also be performed. Partial hepatectomy with controlled hepatic resection has been advised for larger and multiple cysts. When a hepatic cavity remains, this may be treated by (1) suture without drainage, (2) marsupialization and drainage, and (3) omentoplasty (Fig. 30-11). Omentoplasty is the treatment of choice in these cases since the incidence of biliary leakage is reduced. Marsupialization or partial hepatectomy are the alternatives for large or infected cysts. In uncomplicated cases, the results of surgical treatment are excellent, and the postoperative mortality is less than 5 percent. With intrabiliary rupture, marsupialization should be accompanied by drainage of the bile duct if there is associated obstruction. Rupture into the peritoneal cavity is treated by laparotomy and thorough cleansing, although it is frequently impossible to prevent secondary contamination. Intrathoracic, rupture generally can be controlled by evacuating and draining the hepatic cysts. Alveolar disease of the liver was inevitably fatal, but, more recently, satisfactory results have been obtained with extensive hepatic resection.

Benign Tumors

HAMARTOMA. Hamartomas are composed of tissues normally present in the organ but arranged in a disorderly fashion. The lesions vary from minute nodules to large tumors and are rarely of clinical significance. Grossly, the tumors are firm, nodular, and located immediately beneath the surface of the liver, and may be solitary or multiple. On cut section, they are grayish brown and frequently contain a central element of connective tissue arranged in a stellate fashion. With lesions of clinical significance, surgical excision is generally indicated. However, deeply located lesions should be left alone after histologic diagnosis has been established, since they do not grow rapidly and do not undergo malignant transformation.

ADENOMA AND FOCAL NODULAR HYPERPLASIA. In the past hepatic adenomas were extremely rare. In a 47-year-period only four cases were seen at the Mayo Clinic. In 1973 Baum and associates brought attention to a possible relationship between oral contraceptives and these tumors. Many subsequent reports have appeared, and an association with focal nodular hyperplasia also has been noted. Many of the reported patients with liver cell adenoma presented with massive intraperitoneal hemorrhage as an

Fig. 30-10. Hydatid cyst of liver, demonstrating calcification. (*From Seymour I. Schwartz, "Surgical Diseases of the Liver,"* McGraw-Hill Book Company, 1964.)

initial manifestation. This has not occurred in patients with focal nodular hyperplasia. A liver scan and arteriogram aid in diagnosis. Resection of the lesion and discontinuance of contraceptives are generally indicated. Recently regression of the lesions following cessation of contraceptives has been documented, and an operation may be avoided in a patient with a lesion which has not ruptured.

HEMANGIOMA. Hemangioma is the most common nodule in the liver, and the liver is the internal organ most frequently affected with this lesion. Of 126 benign tumors treated at Memorial Sloan-Kettering Cancer Center, 106 were hemangiomas. The tumor occurs five times more frequently in the female than in the male, and this has been related to the hormonal influence. There are two types, capillary and cavernous. Almost all liver lesions are cavernous. These are frequently associated with cysts of the liver and pancreas. Malignant degeneration does not occur, but the hemangioma must be distinguished from a hemangioendothelioma or diffuse hemangiomatosis. The latter consists of widespread multicentric lesions accompanied by vascular involvement of the skin and occurs in children with clinical manifestations in the first week of life.

When a mass is apparent, it is most commonly felt in the epigastrium or left upper quadrant, since the majority of lesions arise in the left lobe. A bruit is heard only rarely. Hepatic arteriography is frequently diagnostic. The major complication is rupture with intraperitoneal hemorrhage, which occurs more commonly in children. In this circumstance, the mortality rate has been over 80 percent. Large tumors in infants may be associated with high-output cardiac failure.

The management in infants is determined by the cardiac output. With high output and congestive failure, supportive therapy including steroids is effective and the lesions generally regress. In rare cases hepatic artery ligation may

Fig. 30-11. Methods of handling residual hepatic cavity. *A.* Suture without drainage (capsulorraphy). Cavity is filled with sterile saline solution, and adventitia is closed without drainage. *B.* Same as *A* but peripheral peritoneum of anterior abdominal wall is sutured to periphery of capsule to facilitate extraperitoneal drainage of secondary infection, if one arises. *C.* Marsupialization. Edges of cavity are sutured to abdominal wall, and several drains are inserted in depths of wound. *D.* Variant of marsupialization. Catheter is inserted into cavity, and closed drainage is used. *E.* Omentoplasty. Omentum is used to fill remaining cavity and is sutured to periphery of fibrous capsule. Vascular omental pedicle absorbs effusion. (*From Seymour I. Schwartz, "Surgical Diseases of the Liver," McGraw-Hill Book Company, 1964.*)

be required to reverse the cardiac failure. Large lesions in any age group may necessitate resection, which is also indicated for a hemangioma with free intraperitoneal rupture. Radiation therapy using up to 2,000 rads in 15 days in adults and 600 rads in children may significantly reduce the size of the tumor.

MALIGNANT TUMORS

Primary Carcinoma

INCIDENCE. Although the disease is rare in people of Western Europe and North America, it is remarkably common among the aboriginal inhabitants of Africa and certain parts of Asia. Postmortem rates in the United States average 0.27 percent, whereas in Africa the postmortem rate is 1.1 percent, hepatic carcinomas representing 17 to 53 percent of all cancers.

Primary carcinoma of the liver occurs with greater frequency in the male sex. In the Caucasian it is rare before the age of forty, while in the African and Indonesian the affection is primarily one of youth, usually occurring before the age of forty. Although it has been suggested that the American Negro still exhibits a distinct predisposition toward the disease, recent statistics do not substantiate this. In contrast, a higher incidence is present in Chinese subjects even after they have changed their habitation. In children, the first appearance of the neoplasm is usually before the age of two, and primary carcinoma of the liver represents the most common carcinoma in the first few years of life.

ETIOLOGY. A variety of etiologic factors have been implicated. Aflatoxins of the mold *Aspergillus flavus* contaminate the diet in African and Asian communities with high incidences of hepatocellular carcinoma. Low protein intake and consequent kwashiorkor also may be factors. Just as almost every type of experimentally induced cirrhosis may be followed by carcinoma of the liver, so a definite association between cirrhosis and primary carcinoma has been noted in the human being. Postnecrotic cirrhosis is the type most commonly preceding hepatocellular carcinoma; cirrhosis is present in 60 percent of cases. Hepatic malignant tumors occur in 4.5 percent of cirrhotic patients, and the incidence is increased in patients with hemochromatosis. Parasitic infestation with the liver fluke *Clonorchis sinensis* has been considered a factor in the development of cholangiocarcinoma, but this is open to question. There is no increased risk for hepatic carcinoma following infectious hepatitis. In the pediatric age group cirrhosis is noted only rarely.

PATHOLOGY. Three types based on the prevalent cell have been defined: (1) liver cell carcinoma (hepatocellular), resembling the parenchymal cell and occurring most frequently, (2) bile duct carcinoma (cholangiocarcinoma), in which the cell is apparently derived from bile duct epithelium, and (3) a mixture of these two types. The term embryoma or hepatoblastoma has been used to represent an immature variant of the hepatic cell carcinoma.

Grossly, each of these types may present as a single large nodule, as extensive nodularity, or as a diffuse permeation throughout the organ. The hepatocellular carcinomas have a trabecular structure, and vascularity is a prominent feature. These lesions frequently invade branches of the portal vein and occasionally the hepatic veins. The formation of giant cells is a feature of hepatocellular carcinoma and aids in distinguishing this lesion from the secondary carcinoma of the liver. The cell type of the bile duct carcinoma is columnar, and its microscopic appearance may be impossible to distinguish from that of carcinoma of the gallbladder or extrahepatic biliary duct system. Bile is never seen in the acini or the cells, whereas mucus formation is common.

Hepatic tumors extend by four methods:

1. Centrifugal growth, which indicates nodular expansion leading to compression of the surrounding hepatic tissue.
2. Parasinusoidal extension, which refers to tumor invasion into the surrounding parenchyma, either through the parasinusoidal spaces or through the sinusoids themselves.
3. Venous spread, which is the extension of tumor from small branches of the portal system in a retrograde fashion into larger branches and eventually into the main portal vein. Invasion of hepatic vein tributaries is less common but may extend up to the inferior vena cava or right atrium.
4. Distant metastases, which are the result of invasion of lymph channels and vascular systems. The most frequently involved locations are regional lymph nodes and the lungs.

Metastases occur in 48 to 73 percent of cases.

CLINICAL MANIFESTATIONS. A correct antemortem diagnosis at one time was extremely rare, but recent figures represent significant improvement. Weight loss and weakness occur in 80 percent of cases, while abdominal pain is present in half. The pain is usually dull and persistent, but dramatic sudden onset may occur in patients with intraperitoneal hemorrhage secondary to rupture of a necrotic nodule or erosion of a blood vessel. This was the initial manifestation in 14 percent of one series. Bleeding varices are infrequent, but foreboding symptoms and delirium have almost always represented a terminal event (Table 30-3).

The liver is almost always enlarged but not tender. Splenic enlargement is present in one-third of the cases,

as are other signs of portal hypertension. The incidence of jaundice varies from 20 to 58 percent. Ascites develops in one-half to three-quarters of patients. A rapid increase in the symptoms and signs associated with cirrhosis or hemachromatosis is highly suggestive of superimposed hepatic carcinoma. In these cases, the amelioration of diabetes and occasional hypoglycemic intervals also indicate neoplastic change.

DIAGNOSTIC STUDIES. Erythrocytosis has been associated with hepatomas. The most consistently altered liver function tests are the BSP and alkaline phosphatase. An increase in alkaline phosphatase, in the absence of bone disease and significant hepatic dysfunction, is considered presumptive evidence of a liver tumor. The serum bilirubin level is usually normal, as are other liver function tests.

The demonstration of α-fetoprotein (AFP) in the serum by immunodiffusion, immunoelectrophoresis, and immunoassay techniques is useful in differential diagnosis and epidemiologic studies. This protein is normally present in the fetus but disappears a few weeks after birth. Positive AFP tests are noted in about 75 percent of Africans but in only 30 percent of patients in the United States and Europe. False-positive results occur with embryonic tumors of the ovary and testis. Resection of the tumor converts the test to "negative"; recurrence may be detected by the reappearance of AFP in the serum.

Selective hepatic arteriography has been utilized to demonstrate an arterial pattern within the tumor, characterized by pooling and increased vascularity (Fig. 30-12).

Fig. 30-12. Hepatic arteriogram demonstrating vascularity of hepatocellular carcinoma.

Table 30-3. PRIMARY EPITHELIAL CANCER IN ADULTS: 1974 LIVER TUMOR SURVEY— SYMPTOMS AND SIGNS ON HOSPITAL ADMISSION

Mass	60
Pain	51
Weight loss	29
Epigastric distress	16
Intraperitoneal hemorrhage	15
Hepatomegaly	14
Fever	9
Incidental at laparotomy for other disease	7
Diarrhea	6
Anorexia	6
Nausea and vomiting	6
Weakness, malaise	5
Misdiagnosis—cholecystitis	5
Endocrine symptoms	3
Pruritus	3
Jaundice	2
Calcification on x-ray	1
Needle biopsy for benign disease	1
Abnormal liver function tests	1
Abnormal scan	1

SOURCE: James Foster and Martin Berman, "Solid Liver Tumors," vol XXII, W. B. Saunders Company, Philadelphia, 1977.

Scintillation scanning may also identify the space-occupying lesion within the liver. A recent review has shown that even when angiography and scans are combined there are significant incidences of false positives and negatives. Percutaneous needle biopsy can provide a definitive diagnosis. Most investigators have been unable to find any evidence to support the view that the presence of hepatic tumor enhances the hazard of liver biopsy.

TREATMENT. The only definitive treatment is surgical excision. The criteria which should be met before resection include:

1. The carcinoma must be solitary or localized.
2. There must be no evident lymph node, blood vessel, or bile duct involvement.
3. There should be no distant metastases.

The recent appreciation of segmental anatomy of the liver coupled with improvements in surgical technique, anesthesia, and blood replacement have placed hepatic resection on an acceptable level. The overall operative mortality in a 1974 Liver Tumor Survey was 21 percent, with 12 percent in noncirrhotic patients.

Total hepatectomy with orthotopic liver transplantation has been performed in more than 48 patients. The results to date have not been encouraging, since only three patients survived longer than 1 year. Starzl's four patients with hepatoma who lived long enough to permit observation of the course of malignant disease all demonstrated diffuse metastases in addition to involvement of the homograft.

Radiation therapy is considered of little value, and extensive radiation damage to the liver, including suppurative cholangitis and abscesses, has been described. Systemic chemotherapy generally has not prolonged survival. However, one patient with disseminated hepatoma survived 10 years with continued 5-fluorouracil systemic therapy, and no tumor was noted at autopsy. Direct arterial infusion is reported to have obtained response in 25 percent of cases, but the response has been temporary. Hepatic artery ligation or more complete dearterialization has been applied, with minimal temporary success. Distal intraarterial infusion coupled with hepatic artery ligation has achieved similar results.

PROGNOSIS. The outlook for primary carcinoma of the liver is extremely poor, and the duration of the disease is rarely longer than 4 months from the time of onset of symptoms. Death is the result of cachexia, hepatic failure, sequelae of portal vein thrombosis, intraperitoneal hemorrhage, and metastases. In the 1974 Liver Tumor Survey 20 of 59 patients with epithelial liver carcinomas who survived the operative procedure lived 5 years or more. In children under age two years with hepatoblastoma, 21 of 27 who survived operation were alive and well with no evidence of disease for a mean of 53 months. In children over age two with the same lesion, 4 in 10 were alive without evidence of disease for a mean of 81 months. Five-year survival following dearterialization or chemotherapeutic regimens is extremely rare and difficult to evaluate, since spontaneous regression has been recorded.

Other Primary Neoplasms

A review in 1947 collected fewer than 100 cases of sarcoma of the liver. Twenty-five percent of these were combined with cirrhosis. The three major lesions are sarcoma, mesenchymoma, and infantile hemangioendothelioma. All hepatic mesenchymal lesions are considered malignant. Angiosarcoma is the most common primary sarcoma of the liver. Recently exposure to vinyl chloride has been implicated as an etiologic factor.

Angiosarcoma is characterized by short illness, jaundice, and coma progressing rapidly to death. Thorotrast also has been implicated as an etiologic factor. Infantile hemangioendotheliomas occur in children under the age of five and are associated with skin lesions and cardiac failure secondary to arteriovenous shunts within the tumor. Although most of these pediatric lesions are fatal, spontaneous regression has been recorded, as has success with partial hepatectomy.

Metastatic Neoplasms

These represent the most common malignant tumor of the liver. The liver is second only to regional lymph nodes as a site of metastases for tumors, and 25 to 50 percent of all patients dying of cancer have been found to have hepatic metastases. Fifty percent of patients with gastrointestinal tumors have hepatic metastases when autopsied. The relative proportion of primary to secondary neoplasms is estimated to be 1:20, and there is no statistical difference between those with and those without cirrhosis.

Metastatic neoplasms reach the liver by four routes: (1) portal venous circulation, (2) lymphatic spread, (3) hepatic arterial system, and (4) direct extension.

Metastases appear in the liver at varying times in relation to primary lesions: (1) Precocious metastasis is evident when the primary lesion is not suspected (carcinoid of the ileum). (2) Synchronous metastases occur when the hepatic neoplasm is detected at the same time as the primary lesion. (3) Metachronous metastasis is one in which appearance is delayed following the successful removal of a primary tumor (ocular melanoma). The growth pattern of the metastatic tumor is frequently more rapid than the original lesion, and the mitotic count of the metastatic hepatic neoplasms has been shown to be five times greater than that of the extrahepatic primary lesion.

CLINICAL MANIFESTATIONS. Symptoms referable to the liver are present in 67 percent of patients with proved metastases. These include hepatic pain, ascites, jaundice, anorexia, and weight loss. On examination, hepatic nodularity is apparent in half the cases, and a friction rub is audible in 10 percent. Jaundice, ascites, and the signs of portal hypertension are present in approximately one-quarter to one-third of the patients. With carcinoid tumors, hepatic metastases are of major importance in the pathogenesis of the flushing syndrome.

DIAGNOSTIC STUDIES. The BSP retention test and alkaline phosphatase level are the most sensitive indices of hepatic involvement. The former is increased in almost 100 percent of the patients, while the serum alkaline phospha-

Table 30-4. RESECTION OF METASTATIC CANCER—1974 LTS:
PRIMARY COLON AND RECTUM: OPERATION VERSUS SURVIVAL

Operation	Patients	Operative deaths	Survival*	
			Mean, mo	5-yr
Extended right lobectomy	4	1	70	1/2
Right lobectomy	25	4	29	2/16
Left lobectomy	10	0	9	0/8
Left lateral segmentectomy	20	0	24	3/12
Wedge	67	3	31	10/50

*Excludes operative deaths.
SOURCE: From James Foster and Martin Berman, "Solid Liver Tumors," vol XXII, W. B. Saunders Company, Philadelphia, 1977.

tase is increased in over 80 percent of patients. The SGOT level is elevated in approximately two-thirds of the patients, but the serum α-fetoprotein determination is negative. Hepatic arteriography, biphasic splenoportography, and scintillation scanning may prove diagnostic. All are associated with significant incidences of false positives and negatives.

TREATMENT. This may be directed toward palliation or cure. Only surgical treatment has the possibility of curing. Encouraging results have been noted with involvement of the liver by direct extension from carcinoma of the stomach, colon, or gallbladder. Right hepatic lobectomy at the time of cholecystectomy has been advised for treatment of carcinoma of the gallbladder, but the data argue against a major hepatic resection, since cures are extremely rare. Surgical treatment of hepatic metastases should be considered only if (1) control of the primary tumor is accomplished or anticipated, (2) there are no systemic or intraabdominal metastases, (3) the patient's condition will tolerate the major operative procedure, and (4) the extent of hepatic involvement is such that resection and total extirpa-

tion of the metastasis is feasible. In a collective review, 21 percent of patients who survived curative resection of metastatic liver tumors lived 5 years. The results of resection of metastatic tumors in the liver are shown in Tables 30-4 and 30-5. Palliative surgical measures are indicated for marked pain associated with hepatic neoplasm and for the excision of metastases in patients with the flushing syndrome or carcinoid tumor.

Most tumors are not responsive to irradiation. The one exception is the neuroblastoma. Hepatic arterial infusion of chemotherapeutic agents, with or without dearterialization, has been applied to therapy of metastatic tumors. Although the response has been better than that noted for primary tumors of the liver (see above), improvement has been brief.

HEPATIC RESECTION

The present indications for hepatic resection include (1) trauma with resultant necrosis of hepatic tissue, (2) cysts,

Table 30-5. LIVER RESECTION FOR METASTATIC CANCER FROM PRIMARY TUMORS OTHER THAN COLON AND RECTUM—1974 LTS: OPERATION VERSUS SURVIVAL

	Patients	Operative deaths	Survival*		
			Mean, mo	Median, mo	5-yr
Extended right lobectomy	2	0	21	—	0/1
Right lobectomy . .	11	2	19	9	1/9
Left lobectomy . . .	2	0	6	—	0/2
Left lateral segmentectomy	9	3	13	8	0/4
Wedge	18	1	17	10	1/16
	50	6	17	9	2/32†

*Excludes operative deaths.
†Both 5-year survivors dead with disease at 105 months after liver resection.
SOURCE: From James Foster and Martin Berman, "Solid Liver Tumors," vol XXII, W. B. Saunders Company, 1977.

(3) granulomas, (4) primary neoplasms of the liver, and (5) secondary malignant tumors which involve the liver either by direct extension or as metastatic lesions.

Up to 80 percent of the liver can be removed with little or no alteration in hepatic function. There is experimental evidence for hepatotropic substances in portal venous blood. Insulin may represent the major anabolic factor and may be counterbalanced by glucagon. Following excision of this amount, patients maintain normal blood ammonia levels and normal prothrombin times. Fibrinogen production is usually unimpaired, and clinical jaundice is a transient phenomenon. Immediately postoperatively, there may be an increase in alkaline phosphatase, transaminase, and BSP retention. However, by the fifth postoperative day, 95 percent of patients show clinical improvement in function, with the bilirubin and alkaline phosphatase returning to normal by the end of the third week. The most profound changes are noted in serum proteins, particularly the albumin fraction, which by the third week is usually restored to normal levels. Regeneration results from marked hypertrophy of the remaining lobe. The remaining portion of the liver responds as rapidly and completely after second and third partial hepatectomies as after an initial insult. It is now felt that portal venous blood flow is an important contributory factor in liver regeneration. Very little restoration occurs after partial hepatectomy of the cirrhotic liver.

MANAGEMENT OF THE PATIENT. Approximately 25 percent demonstrate significant dysfunction related to underlying cirrhosis or a critically positioned tumor. Preoperative therapy is directed at maintaining optimal liver function and correcting any defects which may be present.

Fig. 30-13. Nomenclature for hepatic resection.

SUBSEGMENTAL RESECTION

LEFT LATERAL SEGMENTECTOMY

LEFT MEDIAL SEGMENTECTOMY

TOTAL LEFT HEPATIC LOBECTOMY

RIGHT LOBECTOMY

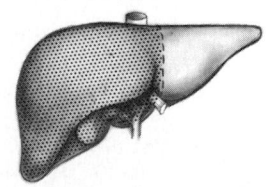

EXTENDED RIGHT LOBECTOMY

A diet high in calories, proteins, and carbohydrates is utilized, and the administration of serum albumin may be required to achieve normal levels. Vitamin K is given routinely until a normal prothrombin time results. In the presence of jaundice, other fat-soluble vitamins are added. Since many patients have a reduced hematocrit, transfusion with fresh whole blood rich in platelets and coagulation factors is indicated. Major hepatic resection is attended by a prohibitive mortality rate in the patient with BSP retention greater than 35 percent, a serum albumin level lower than 2.5 Gm, and an increased prothrombin time which does not respond to parenteral vitamin K.

Postoperatively, infusion of 10% glucose or fructose is continued until the patient maintains an adequate oral intake to obviate severe hypoglycemia, which has been reported. Daily administration of 25 to 50 Gm of albumin is usually required for 7 to 10 days to maintain the serum level above 3 Gm. Vitamin K and antibiotics which achieve a high biliary concentration are indicated. Analgesics and hypnotics which are detoxified by the liver are used only sparingly.

OPERATIVE PROCEDURES. Control of Bleeding. This may be accomplished by (1) compression of blood vessels within the substance of the remaining liver segment, (2) efforts directed at the raw surface, and (3) control of the main blood vessels entering the porta hepatis. Omental grafts, split-thickness grafts, peritoneal grafts, Gelfoam, micronized collagen, and rapidly polymerizing adhesives have been applied to the raw surface as local hemostatic agents. However, their effects are temporary, and generally are associated with high incidences of secondary hemorrhage and infection. Compression of the main vessels entering the liver facilitates the demonstration of bleeding sites along the raw surface. The hepatic artery and portal vein may be compressed for 15 minutes without affecting hepatic structure and function. Moderate hypothermia has extended the time safety factor.

Technique of Resection. On the basis of new concepts of segmental anatomy, the following classification of hepatic resection is applicable (Fig. 30-13): (1) Subsegmental or wedge resection is the removal of an area of the liver that is less than a segment and without an anatomic dissection plane. (2) Left lateral segmentectomy ("left lobotomy" in old nomenclature) is the excision of the liver mass to the left of the left segmental fissure along an anatomic plane. (3) Left medial segmentectomy is resection between the main interlobar fissure and the left segmental fissure. (4) Left lobectomy is the excision of all hepatic tissue to the left of the main lobar fissure. (5) Right lobectomy is the removal of the liver to the right of the main lobar fissure. (6) The extended right lobectomy is the excision of the entire right lobe plus the medial segment of the left lobe (trisegmentectomy), i.e., excision of all tissue to the right of the umbilical fossa, fossa for the ligamentum venosum, and the ligamentum teres.

Segmental resection is applicable for biopsy of the liver and for the removal of small localized benign tumors. Left lateral segmentectomy is performed for extensive trauma to that segment and for tumors or cysts confined to that portion of the liver. Left medial segmentectomy may be performed for benign tumors, particularly hemangiomas localized to this segment, and also as an en bloc dissection for direct extension of carcinoma of the gallbladder. Total left hepatic lobectomy is indicated for tumors of the left medial or lateral segments encroaching upon the lateral segmental plane and thus precluding a segmentectomy. Total excision of the right lobe of the liver is considered for massive injuries, large primary tumors residing in that lobe, metastatic tumors involving only the right lobe, and en bloc dissection of tumors extending from the gallbladder, colon, or stomach.

The liver is initially mobilized by dividing the appropriate ligamentous attachments, i.e., ligamentum teres and triangular ligament (Fig. 30-14A). It is then possible to rotate the liver to the side to expose its inferior surface at the porta hepatis. Dissection of the porta hepatis identifies the branches of the hepatic artery, portal vein, and biliary duct system supplying the segment or lobe to be removed (Fig. 30-14B). These are individually doubly ligated and transected. Glisson's capsule is then incised along the surgical plane (Fig. 30-14C), and the cleavage plane of the hepatic parenchyma itself is best established by means of a scalpel handle or finger to permit exposure of the larger ducts and vessels, which may be individually clamped and ligated as they are encountered. This incision is continued posteriorly until the major hepatic vein or veins are identified, doubly ligated, and transected. By rotating the liver, the hepatic veins may be isolated at their junctions with the inferior vena cava and ligated (Fig. 30-14D and E). The specimen is removed, and the duodenum area is covered with a flap of peritoneum provided by the transected ligament (Fig. 30-14F). The blood flow to and from the remaining segments of the liver must be carefully preserved.

The majority of lobar resections, even right lobe resections, can be carried out transabdominally, and it is not necessary to proceed along the outlined sequence of events for surgical excision. Finger fracture is employed for trauma but is also applied in many instances for tumor. One can reduce the blood flow into the liver by temporarily cross clamping the hepatoduodenal ligament; this procedure can be carried out for 20 minutes using a bulldog clamp intermittently. Glisson's capsule is then incised anteroinferiorly, and the incision is carried down to the region of the porta hepatis. The vessels in the porta hepatis are then picked up in the parenchyma as they enter the liver. The parenchymal dissection is continued along anatomic planes, picking up vessels and ducts as they traverse the liver, until the hepatic venous structures are also picked up in the hepatic parenchyma. The operative time is significantly reduced by this technique, and the blood loss is only moderately increased. Trisegmentectomy necessitates anatomic dissection in order to avoid interrupting veins from the remaining segment.

TRANSPLANTATION

Since the first orthotopic liver transplant was performed, approximately 13 years ago, about 275 patients have un-

dergone the procedure. Of these transplants, 40 percent were carried out by Starzl and his associates. His last report indicates an overall 1-year survival of 29 percent, and half of all the 1-year survivors are still alive. There are four 5-year survivors.

Favorable indications for liver transplantation include biliary atresia, chronic aggressive hepatitis, inborn errors of metabolism, and certain other benign hepatic diseases. Alcoholic cirrhosis is regarded as a less favorable indication, and primary hepatic malignancy is now considered a relative contraindication. It is interesting that the immunologic criteria for donor recipients are less rigid than those for renal transplant. Biliary reconstruction at present is the principal technical problem encountered with orthotopic transplantation.

Another approach to the problem is the use of heterotopic (auxillary) liver transplantation. Fortner et al. have recently reported on six heterotopic liver transplants—three in patients with congenital biliary atresia, one with idiopathic cholestasis syndrome, and two with postnecrotic liver cirrhosis. One patient is alive and well 4 years after transplantation.

PORTAL HYPERTENSION

Hypertension within the portal vein and its tributaries may accompany hepatic disease or disturbance in the anatomy of the extrahepatic vascular system. As a consequence of this elevated pressure or in association with it, congestion of collateral pathways is established and may be manifested by esophagogastric varices, ascites, hypersplenism, or encephalopathy.

ETIOLOGY. The etiologic factors implicated in portal hypertension are listed in Table 30-6. Increased hepatope-

Table 30-6. ETIOLOGY OF PORTAL HYPERTENSION

A. Increased hepatopetal flow without obstruction
  1. Hepatic arterial–portal venous fistula
  2. Splenic arteriovenous fistula
  3. Intrasplenic origin
B. Extrahepatic outflow obstruction
  1. Budd-Chiari syndrome
  2. Failure of right side of heart
C. Obstruction of extrahepatic portal venous system
  1. Congenital obstruction
  2. Cavernomatous transformation of portal vein
  3. Infection
  4. Trauma
  5. Extrinsic compression
D. Intrahepatic obstruction
  1. Nutritional cirrhosis
  2. Postnecrotic cirrhosis
  3. Biliary cirrhosis
  4. Other diseases with hepatic fibrosis
     a. Hemochromatosis
     b. Wilson's disease
     c. Congenital hepatic fibrosis
  5. Infiltrative lesions
  6. Venoocclusive diseases
     a. *Senecio* poisoning
     b. Schistosomiasis

tal flow is an infrequent cause of portal hypertension. Hepatic arterial–portal venous fistula has been reported 10 times and the diagnosis established by aortography. Successful treatment has been effected by ligation of the hepatic artery or aneurysmorraphy. Splenic arteriovenous fistula is also a relatively uncommon lesion. This has a predilection for females between the ages of twenty and fifty and may become symptomatic during pregnancy. Calcification in the left upper quadrant is suggestive, and aortography may be diagnostic. Resection of the fistula is therapeutic. An increase in forward blood flow in the portal venous system has also been proposed as the cause of portal hypertension in patients with Boeck's sarcoid, Gaucher's disease, and myeloid metaplasia. The pathophysiology is related to an intrasplenic arteriovenous fistula. A small group of well-documented cases of bleeding esophageal varices with portal hypertension in the absence of demonstrable intrahepatic or extrahepatic obstruction may be related to a similar intrasplenic pathology. These include tropical splenomegaly and represent the rare circumstances in which splenectomy alone may be therapeutic.

Since the hepatic veins constitute the sole efferent vascular drainage of the liver, obstruction or increased pressure within these vessels or their radicles results in an increased sinusoidal and portal pressure. This outflow obstruction (Budd-Chiari) syndrome is most frequently associated with an endophlebitis of the hepatic veins, which may be isolated or part of a generalized thrombophlebitic process. A web in the suprahepatic vena cava has been reported to cause the syndrome in Japanese people. The clinical picture depends on the rapidity and degree of venous

obstruction. With sudden and complete obstruction, the presentation is that of an abdominal catastrophe with severe abdominal pain, nausea, vomiting, and rapid enlargement of the abdomen by ascites. This rarely occurs. More commonly, obstruction to the hepatic venous tract appears to be gradual and is associated with mild to moderate abdominal discomfort and ascites. The therapy is a side-to-side portal systemic anastomosis, since the portal vein must act as an efferent hepatic conduit.

Portal hypertension secondary to impaired flow in the extrahepatic portal venous system is unique in that the hypertension usually is not complicated by hepatocellular dysfunction. Congenital atresia or hypoplasia, as an extension of the obliterative process of the umbilical vein and ductus venosus, is rare. More commonly, there is a cavernomatous transformation of the portal vein which probably represents organization and recanalization of thrombi within the vessel. The most common etiologic factor in the development of extrahepatic portal venous obstruction

Fig. 30-14. *A.* Right thoracoabdominal incision with division of right leaf of diaphragm is used. Ligamentum teres is transected and used for traction. *B.* After ligamentous attachments have been divided, dissection of hepatoduodenal ligament and porta hepatis is carried out. Cystic artery is traced to its origin from right hepatic artery, which is then doubly ligated and transected, and finally portal vein is treated in similar fashion. *C.* Glisson's capsule is incised and the hepatic parenchyma divided, ligating individual vessels and ducts. *D.* Right lobe is rotated clockwise, and inferior vena cava and right hepatic vein are demonstrated. *E.* Exposure of inferior vena cava with ligation of right hepatic vein and middle hepatic vein. *F.* Denuded surface of liver is covered by flap of falciform ligament. (*From Seymour I. Schwartz, "Surgical Diseases of the Liver," McGraw-Hill Book Company, 1964.*)

DIAPHRAGM

LIG. TERES

OVERSEWN RT. PORTAL V.

CYSTIC A.

RT. HEPATIC A.

RT. HEPATIC DUCT

A   *B*

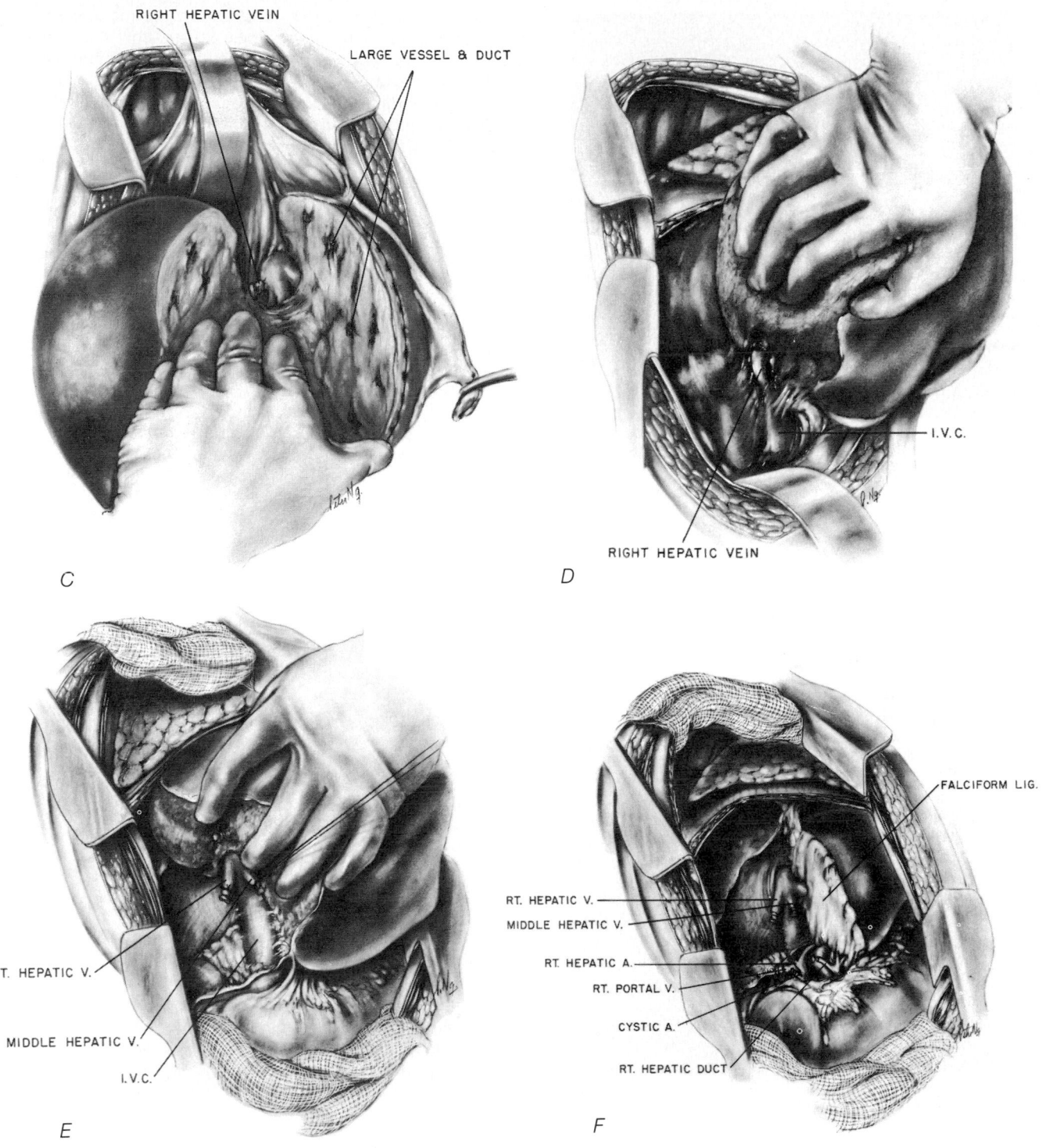

RIGHT HEPATIC VEIN   LARGE VESSEL & DUCT

C

D   I.V.C.

                                      RIGHT HEPATIC VEIN

RT. HEPATIC V.   FALCIFORM LIG.

MIDDLE HEPATIC V.   RT. HEPATIC V.

I.V.C.   MIDDLE HEPATIC V.

                                      RT. HEPATIC A.

                                      RT. PORTAL V.

                                      CYSTIC A.

                                      RT. HEPATIC DUCT

E   *F*

Fig. 30-14 C–F. (See legend on facing page.)

in childhood may be some form of infection. Bacteria may be transmitted via a patent umbilical vein, but a history of neonatal omphalitis is rarely obtainable. Extrahepatic obstruction also may be secondary to trauma and extrinsic compression caused by adhesions, inflammatory processes, and tumors. Isolated splenic vein thrombosis, usually a consequence of alcoholic pancreatitis, may cause esophagogastric varices. In this case splenectomy cures the portal hypertension.

The overwhelming majority of cases of portal hypertension are related to an intrahepatic obstruction. This accounts for 90 percent of patients with portal hyper-

Fig. 30-15. Normal splenoportogram. Note site of injection in spleen and diffusion of radiopaque material through organ. Main splenic vein and two hilar veins are visualized. Portal vein, major branches, and intrahepatic arborization can be seen. No collateral veins are present. Note radiolucency at junction of splenic and superior mesenteric veins. (*From Seymour I. Schwartz, "Surgical Diseases of the Liver," McGraw-Hill Book Company, 1964.*)

Fig. 30-16. Splenoportogram: portal hypertension secondary to intrahepatic obstruction. Note large tortuous coronary vein and inferior mesenteric vein. Intrahepatic arborization is minimal. (From Seymour I. Schwartz, "*Surgical Diseases of the Liver,*" *McGraw-Hill Book Company, 1964.*)

tension in most large series. A variety of hepatic diseases have been implicated, but no single explanation of pathogenesis has proved totally satisfactory. The implicated pathogenic factors include (1) hepatic fibrosis with compression of portal venules, (2) compression by regenerative nodules, (3) increased arterial blood flow, (4) fatty infiltration and acute inflammation, and (5) intrahepatic vascular obstruction. The hepatic diseases associated with portal hypertension include nutritional cirrhosis, postnecrotic cirrhosis, biliary cirrhosis, hemochromatosis, Wilson's disease, congenital hepatic fibrosis, and infiltrative lesions.

Nutritional cirrhosis is the most common and has a worldwide distribution. In the Western countries, it is frequently associated with chronic alcoholism. As is true with all intrahepatic lesions, with the exception of congenital hepatic fibrosis and schistosomiasis, the major resistance to the flow of portal blood is located on the hepatic venous side of the sinusoid (postsinusoidal). Postnecrotic cirrhosis accounts for 5 to 12 percent of the cases and represents progression of an acute viral hepatitis or toxic hepatic injury. Frequently a history of viral infection is not obtainable. Biliary cirrhosis may be due to extrahepatic obstruction and secondary cirrhosis or to a primary hepatic lesion. Advanced portal cirrhosis is an almost invariable feature of hemachromatosis. Wilson's disease (hepatolenticular degeneration) is characterized by alteration of hepatic function and structure and by mental deterioration. Congenital hepatic fibrosis is related to cystic disease of the liver. Clinical features include gross enlargement and firm consistency of the liver, accompanied by manifestations of portal hypertension. Hepatic function is not disturbed. As hepatic infestation with *Schistosoma mansoni* results in presinusoidal obstruction, there is no consequent impairment of hepatic function until late in the course of the disease.

PATHOPHYSIOLOGY. Portal hypertension refers to an elevated pressure within the portal venous system. This pressure reflects a dynamic, constantly fluctuating force. In addition to diurnal fluctuations, the pressure varies with changes of position, phases of respiration, and intraabdominal pressure. The normal portal pressure is less than 250 mm of water with a mean value of 215 mm of water. Portal pressure can be assessed by a variety of techniques. During an operative procedure, cannulation of an omental vein or the portal vein itself provides a direct recording. The pressure can also be determined by occlusive catheterization of a hepatic venule (OHVP). This procedure is analogous to determination of pulmonary capillary pressure, in that it is based on the assumption that the occluding catheter creates a static column of blood extending from the hepatic vein to the junction of the hepatic arterial and portal venous streams as they converge in the sinusoidal bed. The procedure is carried out by cardiac catheterization technique and is particularly valuable in the diagnosis of extrahepatic portal obstruction. In this situation, the presinusoidal obstruction is associated with a normal OHVP and an elevated splenic pulp pressure.

In all instances of portal hypertension, splenic pulp pressure is elevated. Intrasplenic pressure is essentially uniform throughout the pulp and is unrelated to the size of the organ. The pressure is usually 2 to 6 mm Hg higher than the pressure within the portal vein per se, a function of the direction of venous flow. Splenic pulp manometry is carried out under local anesthesia but is contraindicated in patients with a bleeding tendency or severe jaundice.

Splenoportography or the venous phase of celiac and superior mesenteric angiography defines the pathologic features of the portal circulation. The studies provide a demonstration of collateral veins, particularly esophagogastric varices. They also provide graphic demonstration of the site of obstruction, i.e., intrahepatic or extrahepatic. Under normal circumstances no collaterals are visualized and a good arborization is noted in the liver (Fig. 30-15). Whenever collaterals are apparent, the diagnosis of portal hypertension is suggested. Usually one can define the coronary vein contributing to esophageal varices by this technique (Fig. 30-16).

The umbilical vein also has been used to outline the portal system. In 80 percent of these cases the obliterated vein can be isolated and dilated to permit passage of a catheter and injection of radiopaque material into the left portal vein.

The injection of radioactive isotopes into the spleen with simultaneous external monitoring of the areas over the liver, right side of the heart, and esophagus have been used to define the dynamics of the portal circulation. The system employs the same equipment as that used for radioactive renography. Distinctive patterns for normal circulation, esophageal varices, portal vein thrombosis, and both natural and surgically created portal systemic shunts have been defined.

PATHOLOGIC ANATOMY. The collateral vessels (Fig. 30-17) which become functional in cases of portal hypertension are classified in two groups:

1. Hepatopetal circulation occurs only when the intrahepatic vasculature is normal and obstruction is limited to the portal vein. In this situation, the accessory veins of Sappey, the deep cystic veins, the epiploic veins, the hepatocolic and hepatorenal veins, the diaphragmatic veins, and the veins of the suspensory ligaments carry a limited amount of portal venous blood to the liver.
2. Hepatofugal flow is the type most commonly provided by the collateral circulation.

The vessels of the hepatofugal circulation include:

1. The coronary vein, which courses to the esophageal veins and thence to the azygos and hemiazygos veins with eventual termination in the superior vena cava.
2. The superior hemorrhoidal veins, which communicate by way of the hemorrhoidal plexus with hemorrhoidal branches of the middle and inferior hemorrhoidal veins and ultimately drain into the inferior vena cava.
3. The umbilical and paraumbilical veins, which communicate with superficial veins of the abdominal wall and anastomose freely with the superior and inferior epigastric veins. Dilatation occurs in 22 percent of patients with portal cirrhosis, and the advanced stage is known as the *caput Medusae.* The cephalad portion of the obliterated umbilical vein may remain patent in adult life or become recanalized, contributing to the Cruveilhier-Baumgarten syndrome.
4. Retroperitoneally, the veins of Retzius, which from an anastomo-

Fig. 30-17. Collateral circulation. 1, Coronary vein; 2, superior hemorrhoidal veins; 3, paraumbilical veins; 4, veins of Retzius; 5, veins of Sappey; A, portal vein; B, splenic vein; C, superior mesenteric vein; D, inferior mesenteric vein; E, inferior vena cava; F, superior vena cava; G, hepatic veins; a, esophageal veins; a¹, azygos system; b, vasa brevia; c, middle and inferior hemorrhoidal veins; d, intestinal; e, epigastric veins. (*From Seymour I. Schwartz, "Surgical Diseases of the Liver," McGraw-Hill Book Company, 1964.*)

sis between the mesenteric and peritoneal veins and empty directly into the inferior vena cava.

In general, the collateral circulation does not effectively decompress the portal system, and the amount of blood shunted is relatively insignificant. Assuming the cross-sectional diameter of the normal portal vein to be 2 cm, then, according to Poiseuille's law, over 4,000 collateral veins ½ cm in diameter will be needed to provide equivalent flow. Collateral circulation in the veins of the portal system occurs in 97 percent of patients with elevated pressure, but this diversion does not produce any demonstrable alleviation of portal hypertension. On the contrary, the highest values of portal pressure are recorded in the group in which collateralization is more marked. In rare instances, spontaneous portal systemic shunts have effectively decompressed the portal system.

Esophagogastric Varices

As the veins become engorged, vessels in the submucosal plexus of the esophagus increase in size and become dilated. In the later stages, the overlying submucosa may disappear and the walls of the vein actually form a lining of the esophagus. The submucosal veins in the fundus and subfundal regions of the stomach also become varicose. Gastric varices occur predominantly in the cardiac end of the stomach but have also been found along the lesser curvature. Varices also have been demonstrated in the duodenum and ileum.

Although the presence of esophagogastric varices is, in itself, of minor consequence, rupture and bleeding from these vessels constitute the most alarming and serious complication of portal hypertension. The varices are almost always associated with portal hypertension but infrequently have occurred in patients with normal pressure. Ninety percent of adult patients demonstrate intrahepatic disease, whereas in childhood the varices are usually related to extrahepatic portal obstruction. Precipitation of the bleeding episode has been ascribed to two factors, increased pressure within the varix and ulceration secondary to esophagitis. Regurgitation of gastric juice into the esophagus has been implicated, and ulcers of the esophagus have been demonstrated in 25 percent of nonintubated and 50 percent of intubated patients. The frequency and severity of bleeding also is related to the degree of hepatic damage and ingestion of salicylates.

NATURAL COURSE. Bleeding is to be anticipated in approximately 30 percent of cirrhotic patients with demonstrable varices. The elapsed time from the diagnosis of varices to the first hemorrhage varies between 1 and 187 weeks. Almost all hemorrhages occur within 2 years of the initial observation. Survival of patients who have not bled at the time of discovery of varices is identical to the survival of the overall group of patients whose varices are discovered before death. Etiology is a prime consideration. Varices secondary to extrahepatic portal obstruction must be considered separately, since it is rare for these patients to die of hemorrhage. By contrast, the mortality risk of repeated hemorrhage in patients with esophageal varies secondary to cirrhosis is extremely high. Approximately 70 percent of these patients die within 1 year of the first hemorrhage. Sixty percent of cirrhotic patients who have hemorrhaged once rebleed massively within 1 year.

A prophylactic shunt is not advised for a patient with varices which have not bled, since one cannot predict which patients will bleed; the survival is not improved and encephalopathy may be induced.

ACUTE BLEEDING. In children, massive hematemesis almost always emanates from bleeding varices. Acute hemorrhage is usually the first manifestation of portal hypertension in children. Seventy percent of patients experience their first bleeding episode before the age of seven, and almost 90 percent hemorrhage before the age of ten.

In the adult, bleeding varices comprise one-quarter to one-third of the cases of massive upper gastrointestinal tract bleeding. In cirrhotic patients, varices are the source of bleeding in approximately 50 percent, whereas gastritis is implicated in 30 percent and duodenal ulcers in 9 percent. It is now felt that peptic ulcer does not occur more frequently in cirrhotic patients. Correlation of the lesion with the severity of bleeding reveals that in the majority of cases bleeding from varices is severe hemorrhage whereas bleeding from gastritis involves only mild to moderate blood loss.

Since the management of bleeding varices differs significantly from that of bleeding due to other causes, it is important to establish a diagnosis on an emergency basis. Physical examination may reveal the stigmata of cirrhosis. Splenomegaly is particularly suggestive of portal hypertension. Tests of hepatic function have been used but do not have uniform reliability. Abnormal BSP retention may be related to underlying liver disease or to shock from hemorrhage. A normal BSP value is more significant and in association with massive bleeding suggests that the liver is not responsible. The qualitative test for hyperammonemia is rarely performed, and pretreatment with antibiotics, glutamic acid, and arginine will negate the value of this test. The presence of any large portal-systemic collateral vessel will result in a positive test. Barium-swallow has a significantly high percentage of false-negative results. In a series of patients with proved varices, roentgenographic demonstration was present in only half. Selective angiography is replacing upper gastrointestinal series as a primary diagnostic procedure. Celiac angiography will rule out an arterial bleeding site, and the venous phase of the superior mesenteric arteriogram will demonstrate collateral venous circulation. Bleeding from a varix is not visualized. A 90 percent correlation has been reported for splenic pulp manometry, but there is a zone of splenic pulp pressures which may be characteristic of patients bleeding from varices or from other causes. The isotopic evaluation of the portal circulation has been applied with success to the differential diagnosis of acutely bleeding varices. Esophageal balloon tamponade has also been used as a diagnostic measure. However, varices are controlled in only two-thirds of the patients, and, moreover, peptic ulcer may stop bleeding after the gastric balloon is inflated. Esophagoscopy represents the single most reliable technique, since it alone defines the bleeding point. On the other hand, esophagoscopy may fail to reveal varices because of variations in transvariceal blood flow. In addition, there is a significant observer variation in the endoscopic evaluation of varices.

TREATMENT. The therapeutic regimen is directed at promptly controlling bleeding without further disturbing an already impaired hepatic function. Rapid control is critical in order to avoid the injurious effects of shock on hepatic function and also the toxic effects of absorption of blood from the gastrointestinal tract. The therapeutic approaches may be divided into methods which directly approach the bleeding site and techniques which act indirectly by decreasing portal pressure (Table 30-7).

Table 30-7. CONTROL OF ACUTE BLEEDING

A. Nonoperative
　1. Direct: control of bleeding site
　　a. Tamponade
　　b. Local hypothermia
　　c. Esophagoscopic injection of sclerosing solution
　　d. Transhepatic sclerosis of coronary vein
　2. Indirect: reduction of portal pressure
　　a. Vasopressin
　　b. Arfonad
　　c. Paracentesis
B. Operative
　1. Direct: control of bleeding site
　　a. Transesophageal ligation
　　b. Esophageal transection
　　c. Gastroesophageal resection: colon or jejunum interposition
　2. Indirect: reduction of portal pressure
　　a. Portal-systemic shunt
　　b. Drainage of thoracic duct ⎫
　　c. Hepatic artery ligation　　⎬ No longer advised
　　d. Splenectomy　　　　　　　 ⎭

Balloon tamponade has been the most popular nonoperative method, and the Sengstaken-Blakemore tube has been used most frequently. This technique has reduced the mortality and morbidity from bleeding varices in good-risk patients, particularly those in whom the varices were secondary to extrahepatic portal hypertension or compensated cirrhosis. Little change has been noted in the mortality rate for poor-risk patients, and reports have indicated failure to control hemorrhage in 25 to 55 percent of cases. Increasing awareness of the complications associated with this technique, including aspiration, asphyxiation, and ulceration at the site of the tamponade, has reduced its use.

Hypothermia has been used, either in combination with tamponade or alone, to produce local vasoconstriction and thus control bleeding. Both general hypothermia and local gastric hypothermia have been employed. A special balloon with a long esophageal neck, which permits cooling of the distal half of the esophagus and the upper gastric fundus, has been devised for more effective application. Generalized hypothermia is ineffective, since it does not reduce hepatic flow until the core temperature drops below 35°C. Endoscopic injection of a sclerosing solution into varices has also successfully controlled bleeding. In a large series, bleeding was controlled in 93 percent of patients. Recently, transhepatic catheterization and obliteration of the coronary vein using thrombin, sclerosing solution, or microspheres have been applied to the control of bleeding.

Drug therapy to reduce portal hypertension has employed surgical vasopressin, which acts by constricting the splanchnic arterial circulation and consequently reducing portal pressure and flow by approximately 40 percent. The drug is contraindicated in patients with angina, since generalized vasoconstriction results. Effective control has as compared direct infusion of vasopressin, 0.2 unit/ml/minute, into the superior mesenteric artery. Equal efficacy has been achieved with the same dosage administered into a peripheral vein. Isoproterenol may be given to reduce the hemodynamic hazards of vasopressin related to its potential effect on the cardiac output. Arfonad also has been used to induce a predictable decrease in portal hypertension by establishing a generalized arterial hypotension. Paracentesis in a patient with bleeding varices and tense ascites will immediately and significantly reduce portal pressure.

Surgical therapy includes transesophageal ligation, gastric resection, cannulation of the thoracic duct, and emergency portacaval shunt. The results of transesophageal ligation have not been uniformly encouraging, and in cirrhotic patients the procedure has been accompanied by a high incidence of recurrent bleeding. Other methods directed at the site of bleeding have been concerned with interrupting the blood supply of the esophagus by extensive gastroesophageal resection. Cannulation with drainage of the thoracic duct has also been applied as a method of reducing portal hypertension and controlling bleeding from the varices, but these effects have been inconsistent. Reduction of portal pressure by transumbilical decompression using an extracorporeal shunt has been applied with rare instances of success.

A more liberal use of emergency portacaval shunts to stop bleeding has been advised for the cirrhotic patients whose bleeding cannot be controlled by tamponade or vasopressin. The base figure which serves as a frame of reference for comparison is the mortality for patients with bleeding varices not subjected to emergency portacaval shunts, and this ranges between 66 and 73 percent. There is little question that an effective portal-systemic decompressive procedure almost always stops bleeding. A review of reported experiences indicates that so-called emergency shunts are associated with survival for immediate hospitalization in 50 to 71 percent of cases, despite a more liberal attitude toward acceptability of patients in reference to their liver profile. Orloff and his associates have reported an operative survival of 48 percent and an actuarial 7-year survival of 42 percent in consecutive, unselected patients with alcoholic cirrhosis and bleeding varices operated on within 8 hours of admission to hospital. In regard to selection of patients, reported results could not be correlated with the patient's liver function profile in some series. No significance could be attributed to the presence or absence of jaundice, but ascites, when present, was associated with a marked reduction of survival rate.

It is the author's personal opinion that in the absence of controlled and randomized trials an emergency portacaval shunt should be performed in selected patients, since it offers greater survival than a more conservative form of therapy. There has been a gradual liberalization of criteria for selection of patients, and there is an obvious advantage in the logistics of managing patients in reference to depletion of blood banks.

In the pediatric age group, despite the fact that the bleeding is often alarming, spontaneous cessation almost always occurs, and esophageal tamponade or vasopressin is rarely necessary. Hospitalization, bed rest, blood replacement, and sedation almost always suffice for patients with bleeding secondary to extrahepatic portal obstruction.

The majority of patients with acute bleeding varices are not in shock at the time of admission to the hospital, although the hematocrit is often reduced and blood replacement may be necessary. Fresh blood should be employed for transfusing cirrhotic patients. This provides the clotting factors which are frequently diminished in the presence of hepatic disease and avoids the increased ammonia content and diminished platelet and prothrombin supply characteristic of old bank blood. There is a linearly progressive daily increment of 35 μg/100 ml of ammonia nitrogen in banked blood, which can be responsible for exogenous hepatic coma. Therapy directed at preventing hyperammonemia and hepatic coma consists primarily of removing blood from the gastrointestinal tract. Catharsis, gastric lavage, and enemas are employed. If vasopressin has been administered, it will induce intestinal motility and effect a catharsis. A reduction in intestinal bacterial flora also contributes to the prevention of coma, and nonabsorbable antibiotic therapy is used to accomplish this.

Protocol for Acute Bleeding Episodes. *Treatment of Shock.* Intravenous administration of 10% dextrose in water and fresh blood are begun immediately.

Nursing Care. Special nursing care is advisable, particularly if balloon tamponade is employed. Repeated endotracheal suction is indicated, and tracheostomy may be necessary.

Control of Hemorrhage. A soft nasogastric tube is inserted into the stomach, or if the patient is in incipient or established coma or uncooperative, a gastrostomy tube is inserted under local anesthesia. Suction is established to monitor the extent of bleeding while the stomach is lavaged with iced saline solution. Vasopressin is administered via either the superior mesenteric artery or a peripheral vein. If bleeding is not controlled by these measures, balloon tamponade is applied. A conservative, nonsurgical regimen is relied upon to control bleeding in patients with a serum bilirubin level above 3 mg/100 ml, a serum albumin level below 2.5 Gm/100 ml, and a prothrombin time reduced to less than 30 percent of normal. Patients with minimally impaired liver function or portal hypertension secondary to extrahepatic obstruction who continue to bleed should be prepared for surgical intervention, and a portacaval shunt is performed as an emergency procedure.

Control of Hepatic Coma. Intestinal catharsis is accomplished by vasopressin or 15 ml of magnesium sulfate instilled via the nasogastric tube. Tap-water enemas are administered twice daily. Neomycin sulfate, 1 Gm every hour for 4 hours followed by 1 Gm every 4 hours, is administered via the nasogastric tube. Analgesics and hypnotics, which are detoxified by the liver, are avoided.

Diet. A diet high in carbohydrates and low in fat and protein with vitamin supplements, including vitamin K, is used. Atropine and antacids are administered to reduce gastric acidity.

Elective Surgical Treatment for Prevention of Recurrent Hemorrhage. The case for surgical intervention is based on the precept that a patient who has bled from esophageal varices is likely to rebleed and that subsequent bleeding episodes are associated with a higher mortality than an elective operative procedure. It is important to define the role of surgical procedure in relation to the factors implicated in the cause of portal hypertension.

A difference of opinion exists regarding the role of decompressive procedures in children with portal hypertension due to extrahepatic portal venous thrombosis. Some children can be treated satisfactorily and safely without operation despite repeated episodes of variceal bleeding. The results of operation in terms of survival are significantly more encouraging in this population than in adults. Therefore, most series have suggested an aggressive approach in children with recurrent bleeding episodes. The central splenorenal shunt or an anastomosis between the inferior vena cava and superior mesenteric vein is applicable to this group of patients. The incidence of postoperative encephalopathy has been negligible.

Presinusoidal obstruction (hepatic fibrosis, extrahepatic portal venous thrombosis, schistosomiasis) is characterized by portal hypertension and may be associated with normal hepatic function. In patients with hepatic fibrosis and extrahepatic portal venous obstruction the results are gratifying; the surgical procedure will generally prevent subsequent bleeding and provide the patient with an essentially normal life expectancy. The patients with schistosomiasis are a unique group in that they are extremely liable to postshunt encephalopathy.

Postsinusoidal portal hypertension is invariably complicated by impaired hepatic function. The role of decompressive procedures is least well defined for this group of cirrhotic patients. Elective procedure should be considered when the presence of an active intrahepatic process such as hyaline necrosis or acute fatty infiltration has been ruled out. Ascites which fails to respond to medical therapy, a prothrombin time which remains prolonged following parenteral administration of vitamin K, a serum bilirubin above 3 mg/100 ml, a BSP retention greater than 20 percent, and a serum albumin level less than 2.5 Gm/100 ml are all associated with a poor postoperative prognosis. In these patients there is immediate deterioration following portacaval shunting, but this is actually no greater than after other operations of comparable severity. Child's criteria and other assessments of hepatic function are not completely predictive.

Two randomized series have been reported. The Cooperative Study of the Veterans Administration randomized cirrhotic patients who had at least one major gastrointestinal hemorrhage and were considered suitable for an operative procedure. Increased survival rate was noted in the group of patients who were operated upon. By contrast, the Boston Interhospital Liver Group's study of patients on whom a therapeutic portacaval shunt had been performed showed that recurrent variceal bleeding could be prevented but that greater longevity could not be expected for these patients. Increased survival following shunting procedures in patients with a single major variceal hemorrhage remained a statistical possibility. Recently it has been shown that better results are to be anticipated in patients with biliary cirrhosis than in those with nutritional, alcoholic, or cryptogenic cirrhosis.

Ascites

ETIOLOGY. The mechanisms contributing to the formation of ascites are complex and incompletely understood.

Portal hypertension is regarded as a contributory but minor factor, since there is no correlation between the degree of portal hypertension and the extent of ascites. Ascites is not a usual accompaniment of extrahepatic portal venous obstruction but has been noted occasionally. Impairment of hepatic venous outflow with subsequent congestion of the liver is the experimental method most consistently used to produce ascites. This lesion is accompanied by an increase in the size of lymphatic vessels and increased production of hepatic lymph which extravasates through the capsule of the liver into the peritoneal cavity. In clinical cirrhosis, there is an increase in the size of hepatic channels and an augmented flow of thoracic duct lymph. Two distinct patterns of intrahepatic vasculature have been correlated with the presence or absence of ascites. With irreversible ascites, there is an absolute decrease in the hepatic venous bed and a concomitant increase in both the portal venous and hepatic arterial beds. By contrast, when cirrhosis is unaccompanied by ascites, there is a deficit in all vascular systems. Obstruction of the hepatic venous outflow fails to explain the development of ascites in patients with portal vein obstruction and also the relief of ascites following end-to-side portacaval shunt.

Reduced serum osmotic pressure related to hypoalbuminemia does exert some influence. However, the response of patients to albumin infusion is variable, and the reduced osmotic pressure may represent the result rather than the cause of fluid accumulation. The most profound biochemical change which accompanies the formation of ascites is the retention of sodium and water. There is evidence that the adrenal cortical hormone is a factor in the renal retention of sodium, and higher concentrations of antidiuretic substances have been noted in the urine of patients with cirrhosis and ascites.

TREATMENT. Bed rest is prescribed, since it reduces the functional demand on the liver. A diet high in calories with an excess of carbohydrates and proteins, supplemented by vitamins, is directed toward improving hepatic function, while low sodium (10 to 20 mEq daily) intake is essential. Fluid is usually not restricted, and potassium supplements are routinely provided to treat the potassium depletion which accompanies the formation of ascites. A negative sodium balance may be achieved by the use of ion-exchange resins. The administration of salt-poor albumin is directed at raising colloidal pressure. This may be provided by an intravenous infusion of antogenous ascitic fluid.

Chlorothiazide is usually used to initiate diuretic therapy, and approximately two-thirds of patients will respond to this medication. Potassium supplements are required, because the diuresis is accompanied by depletion. For patients refractory to chlorothiazide the aldosterone antagonists are employed, while for those patients with incipient or frank hepatic coma mercury diuretics are considered safer. Abdominal paracentesis as an initial procedure has diagnostic value, but repeated procedures are contraindicated, since they deplete the body of protein and contribute to the development of systemic hyponatremia. Furosemide (Lasix) and ethacrynic acid are recently introduced powerful diuretics.

Emphasis on the importance of obstruction of hepatic venous outflow led to the proposal of side-to-side portacaval shunts as a method of therapy. These procedures were based on the hypothesis of providing a second outflow tract with the portal vein acting as a hepatofugal conduit. At present, the operation is limited to those patients who cannot be managed on a strict low-sodium diet and diuretic therapy, an unusual circumstance. A variety of procedures has been proposed to augment internal drainage of the ascitic fluid. These include omentopexy, drainage into the subcutaneous tissue, drainage directly into the venous system, and ileoentectropy. None has been effective. Drainage of the lymph from the cannulated cervical thoracic duct also reduces the ascites, which reappears as soon as the drainage ceases. Bilateral adrenalectomy combined with sodium restriction has enjoyed some success. Recently Leveen and associates have reported success with a peritoneal-venous shunt which employs a one-way valve.

Umbilical herniorraphy in a cirrhotic patient with marked ascites presents a significant risk, with hazards of leakage of ascitic fluid, infection, necrosis of the abdominal wall, and variceal bleeding due to interruption of collateral veins.

Hypersplenism

Splenomegaly, with engorgement of the vascular spaces, frequently accompanies portal hypertension. There is little correlation between the size of the spleen and the degree of hypertension. When hematologic abnormalities occur, they have been related to sequestration and destruction of the circulating cells by immune mechanisms mediated by the enlarged spleen or secretion by the hyperactive spleen of a substance which inhibits bone marrow activity. The patient may demonstrate reduction of any or all of the cellular elements of blood. The usual criteria are a white blood cell count below 4,000 and a platelet count below 100,000/mm³. Schistosomal fibrosis frequently induces hypersplenism, which is best determined by the size of the spleen. No correlation exists between the degree of anemia or leukopenia and the 5-year survival rate in patients. Decompression of the portal venous system is rarely indicated for treatment of hypersplenism alone. Significant hypersplenism in a patient undergoing elective surgical treatment for bleeding varices favors a splenorenal anastomosis, but portacaval anastomosis has been accompanied by reduction of the spleen and correction of the hypersplenism in about two-thirds of the cases.

Hepatic Coma

The development of neuropsychiatric symptoms and signs is related to natural and surgically created portal-systemic shunts and is identified by the term *portal-systemic encephalopathy.* This rarely occurs in patients with obstruction of the extrahepatic portal venous system. The neuropsychiatric syndrome usually is associated with cirrhosis and occurs in patients with marked hepatic dysfunction. Hepatic coma or precoma is a clinical manifesta-

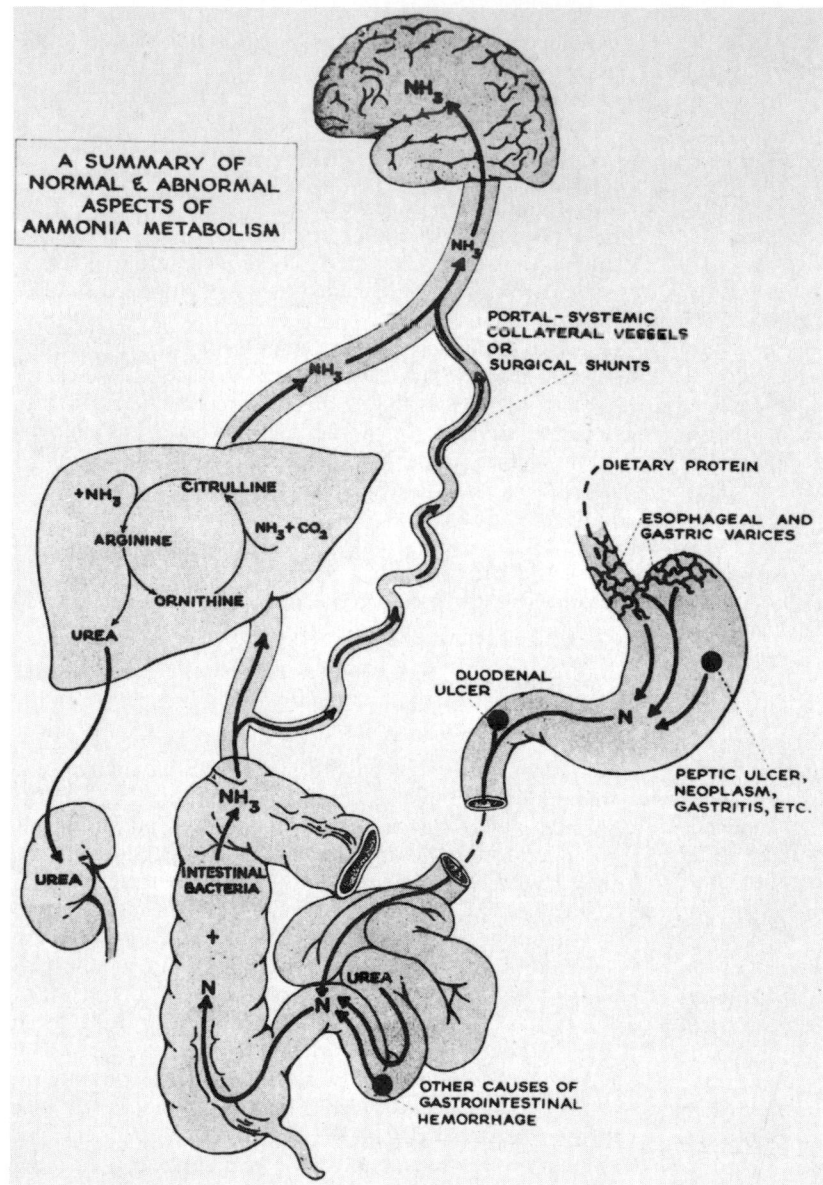

A SUMMARY OF
NORMAL & ABNORMAL
ASPECTS OF
AMMONIA METABOLISM

Fig. 30-18. A summary of normal and abnormal aspects of ammonia metabolism. Dietary protein is the normal primary source of intestinal nitrogen. However, when gastrointestinal bleeding occurs, the blood that accumulates within the intestine may become an important source of intestinal nitrogen. Urea, which is excreted in part into the gastrointestinal tract, also adds to the intestinal nitrogen pool. All these nitrogen-containing compounds are converted into ammonia by the numerous bacteria within the colon. This ammonia is absorbed into the portal circulation and, under normal conditions, is rapidly removed in the liver by the formation of urea, which is excreted by the kidneys. This mechanism of detoxification of ammonia is so efficient that little or no ammonia can be found in the peripheral blood. Because of the important role of the liver in the detoxification of ammonia, (1) a decrease in hepatic function or (2) a bypass of the liver associated with (a) the development of portal systemic collaterals or (b) surgical shunting procedures will result in an increase in concentrations of ammonia in the peripheral blood, which will exert its toxic effects on the central nervous system. (*From Najarian et al., Am J Surg, 96:172, 1958.*)

tion in approximately two-thirds of patients with varices and is most prominent in cirrhotic patients who bleed. Coma and exsanguination are responsible for an almost equal percentage of deaths in cirrhotic patients with gastrointestinal varices. Operative procedures which decompress the portal system have also been associated with varying incidences of encephalopathy. With splenorenal anastomoses, the syndrome is demonstrated in 5 to 19 percent, while it has been reported in 11 to 38 percent following a portacaval anastomosis. The Warren distal splenorenal shunt has been associated with a negligible incidence of postoperative coma.

Hepatic coma has been related to hyperammonemia and ammonia intoxication (Fig. 30-18). Both exogenous and endogenous sources contribute to the blood ammonia level. Dietary protein is the usual source of intestinal am-

monia. In patients who bleed, blood within the intestinal tract is also converted into ammonia by bacteria. In the patient with hepatic disease, the ammonia formed within the intestine is carried to the liver but because of hepatic dysfunction cannot enter the Krebs-Henseleit (ornithine-citrulline-arginine) cycle. Endogenous urea produced within the gastrointestinal tract also represents an important source of ammonia, and gastric ammonia production from urea is a significant factor in patients with azotemia and cirrhosis. Galambos and associates have reported a randomized trial in which there was less deterioration of maximum urea synthesis following a selective splenorenal shunt than after total shunts.

In the cirrhotic patient with portal hypertension, the two factors implicated in the disturbed ammonia metabolism are impairment of hepatocellular function and portal-systemic collateralization. The blood ammonia level is raised by (1) ingested protein, (2) gastrointestinal bleeding, (3) increased ammonia production by the kidneys, and (4) increased ammonia production by muscles which are actively contracting during delirium tremens. The problem of an increased load is compounded by deficiencies in the removal mechanism caused by portal-systemic shunts which bypass the liver and hepatocellular disease which interferes with the functional activity of the liver. The neuropsychiatric manifestations involve the state of consciousness, motor activity, and deep tendon reflexes. These have been divided into three stages, delirium, stupor, and coma. In the early stages there is mental confusion and exaggerated reflexes. The characteristic "liver flap" may be elicited. In the second stage, there is an accentuation of muscular hypertonicity, to the extent of rigidity, and in the final stage there is complete flaccidity. The electroencephalogram is a sensitive indicator of portal-systemic encephalopathy, and the changes antedate clinical manifestations. Blood ammonia level does not define precisely the nature of material measured by standard tests. In patients with hepatic coma, the concentration of ammonia in the blood has correlated well with the clinical progress in over 90 percent of the cases. An elevated level, over 125 μg/100 ml, is usually associated with the clinical features of hepatic coma. Treatment with antibiotics negate the value of the test.

TREATMENT. Treatment is directed at (1) reducing nitrogenous material within the intestinal tract, (2) reducing the production of ammonia from this nitrogenous material, and (3) increasing ammonia metabolism. Since ammonia is an end product of protein metabolism, dietary protein must be drastically reduced to 50 Gm daily or less. Glucose is included in the diet, since it inhibits ammonia production by bacteria. Gastrointestinal hemorrhage frequently precipitates portal-systemic encephalopathy with blood acting as a source of ammonia. Therefore, a major factor in the prophylaxis of hepatic coma is prompt control of active bleeding. Potassium supplements are administered, particularly in patients who are receiving thiazide diuretics, since the rise in blood ammonia which accompanies diuresis has been related to hypokalemia.

The protein substrate on which bacteria can act may be initially reduced by using cathartics and enemas to purge the gastrointestinal tract. If active bleeding has occurred, infused vasopressin plays a dual role in temporarily stopping the bleeding as well as stimulating motility and evacuation of the intestine. Bacteria within the bowel are reduced by administering nonabsorbable antibiotics such as neomycin or kanamycin. In the presence of renal disease, kanamycin is preferred since there is less associated renal toxicity. For patients with severe renal impairment, chlortetracycline is more appropriate since it is not excreted primarily by the kidneys. Lactulose acts as a mild cathartic, and the products of its oxidation by bacteria include lactic and acetic acids, which lower the colonic pH and interfere with ammonia transfer across colonic mucosa. This drug has produced encouraging results in the treatment of hepatic encephalopathy.

Since the colon is the site of most ammonia absorption

into the portal circulation, partial colectomy has been suggested as treatment of intractable encephalopathy. Resnick and associates studied a matched group of patients, randomly selecting half the group for colon bypass. The longevity figures for the two groups were identical, and the dietary protein tolerance and encephalopathy control only slightly favored the bypass group.

The possibility of stimulating the liver's intrinsic mechanism for detoxifying ammonia has fostered the use of glutamic acid and arginine. Although success has been reported, most studies have not been impressive. Recently, the pathophysiology of hepatic failure has been related to the accumulation of false neurochemical transmitters in the presynaptic storage sites of the peripheral and central adrenergic nervous system. L-Dopa, which represents normal precursor material in the central nervous system, is administered to permit restoration of central nervous system stores of norepinephrine and dopamine. An awakening effect of L-Dopa has been reported by Parkes and associates and by Fischer and James, but recent series have not been encouraging.

Attempts to dilute or remove toxic substances from the bloodstream will be discussed in the section on acute fulminant hepatic failure.

Surgery of Portal Hypertension

The surgical therapy of portal hypertension may be divided into two major categories: (1) procedures which directly attack a manifestation of portal hypertension, such as bleeding varices or ascites, and (2) procedures aimed at decreasing the portal hypertension and/or portal venous flow (Table 30-8).

TRANSESOPHAGEAL LIGATION OF VARICES. Using either a transthoracic or transabdominal approach, transesophageal ligation of varices and esophageal transection have been directed at controlling bleeding varices. The procedures do provide temporary control, particularly in children with extrahepatic portal block who are too small to be considered for splenorenal anastomosis. However, control is not prolonged. In patients without cirrhosis, recurrent bleeding has been reported in 28 percent, while among the cirrhotic group approximately 50 percent of survivors have recurrent bleeding. The operative mortality rate associated with this procedure is 43 percent, but it must be appreciated that the technique generally is applied to the poorest-risk patients.

Technique. Transthoracic ligation (Fig. 30-19) is performed through the eighth left intercostal space. The lower esophagus is freed, but the esophageal hiatus of the diaphragm is not disturbed. An umbilical tape is tightened around the esophagus just above the hiatus in order to minimize bleeding. A 7-cm longitudinal incision is made through all layers and three tortuous columns of veins, coursing longitudinally and communicating with one another, are obliterated with continuous locking sutures of 3-0 chromic catgut. The esophagotomy is closed in two layers with interrupted silk sutures and the edges of the defect in the mediastinal pleura are reapproximated. Direct ligation of varices can be performed transabdominally.

Table 30-8. OPERATIVE PROCEDURES

I. Control of manifestation
    A. Bleeding varices
        1. Ligation of varices
            a. Transthoracic
            b. Transabdominal
        2. Transection procedures
            a. Gastric
            b. Esophageal
        3. Resection of varix-bearing area–esophagogastrectomy
            a. Roux en Y
            b. Jejunal interposition
            c. Colonic interposition
            d. Reversed gastric tube
    B. Ascites
        1. Crosby-Cooney button: subcutaneous drainage
        2. Ileoentectropy
        3. Peritoneal cavity–venous shunt
        4. Drainage of thoracic duct
        5. Adrenalectomy
II. Reduction of portal pressure and flow
    1. Splenectomy
    2. Hepatic and splenic arterial ligation
    3. Omentopexy
    4. Mediastinal packing
    5. Supradiaphragmatic transposition of spleen
    6. Portacaval shunt
        a. End-to-side
            (1) End-to-side shunt with arterialization of the portal
                vein stump
        b. Side-to-side
        c. Double end-to-side
    7. Splenorenal shunt
        a. End-to-end
        b. End-to-side
        c. Distal (selective)
    8. Superior mesenteric–inferior vena cava shunt

TOTAL OR NEAR-TOTAL GASTRECTOMY. This has been proposed in order to interrupt communication between the portal and esophageal veins and to remove the acid-peptic factor implicated in the initiation of bleeding from varices. To reduce the incidence of postoperative esophagitis, a variety of interposition procedures have been employed (Fig. 30-20). In the pediatric age group, esophagogastrectomy with colon interposition has successfully prevented recurrence of bleeding.

PROCEDURES FOR REDUCTION OF PORTAL PRESSURE. The operations directed at portal hypertension are based on the consideration that any reduction in portal pressure should decrease the potential for bleeding from varices. Splenectomy and hepatic arterial ligation have been offered as methods of reducing portal venous flow, but such an effect has not been documented. Splenectomy alone, unaccompanied by a concomitant splenorenal anastomosis, is now disapproved. Similarly, hepatic and splenic arterial ligation no longer enjoys a popularity. Reduction of portal pressure by diffuse shunts between a high-pressure portal venous system and low-pressure systemic circulation has also been attempted. These procedures include omentopexy, posterior mediastinal packing, and transposition of the spleen into the thoracic cavity. Encouraging results have been reported for the last procedure, but application of Poiseuille's law would suggest that

any diffuse shunting would be less effective than a major portal systemic shunt.

Functionally, portal-systemic shunts have been categorized as either totally or partially diverting portal venous flow away from the liver and also as decompressing or failing to decompress intrahepatic venous hypertension (Fig. 30-21). The end-to-side portacaval shunt prevents blood from reaching the liver by providing complete drainage of the splanchnic venous circulation to the vena cava. Controversy exists over whether this shunt deprives the liver of an important source of blood, and the associated alteration of hepatic blood flow is extremely variable, ranging from an increase of 34 percent to a decrease of 53 percent. This shunt also prevents the portal vein from serving as an efferent conduit from the liver. However, it has been shown that following the end-to-side shunt, the wedged hepatic vein pressure declined in all of a small series of patients. Proponents of the end-to-side shunt have indicated this as the best method of preventing recurrent bleeding from varices, since it most completely decompresses the portal venous system's splanchnic circulation. In refutation, it has been shown that end-to-side and side-to-side portacaval shunts demonstrate equal portal flow increases and equivalent reductions of portal pressure.

The concept that the side-to-side portacaval shunt provides the liver with portal venous flow is erroneous in most circumstances. Injection of radioisotope into the distal portal vein results in minimal recovery in the portal vein cephalad to a side-to-side anastomosis. Accumulated evidence indicates that the side-to-side portacaval shunt converts the cephalad portion of the portal vein to an outflow tract from the liver. Whether decompression of sinusoidal hypertension is greater with the side-to-side shunt than with the end-to-side shunt has not been defined. There is also concern whether the portal vein is beneficial or harmful as an efferent conduit, because of a possible siphon effect which may reduce the blood available to the hepatic cell.

The classic end-to-side splenorenal shunt using the central end of the splenic vein also prevents the flow of portal venous blood to the liver if it adequately performs its prescribed function of decompressing esophagogastric varices. In addition, the splenorenal shunt less completely decompresses portal venous hypertension. The other functional side-to-side shunts, including the end-to-side inferior vena cava–superior mesenteric shunt and the interposition of an H graft between these vessels, do not permit significant portal venous flow to enter the liver. This would be expected hemodynamically, since the flow within the cephalad portion of the portal vein should be away from high-pressure hepatic venous sinusoids into the low-pressure inferior vena cava if the functioning shunt is adequately decompressing esophagogastric varices.

The distal splenorenal shunt proposed by Warren and associates is the one procedure which can be classified as truly selective, because it decompresses esophagogastric varices while maintaining portal hypertension within the portal veins and hepatic sinusoids. Portal perfusion has been demonstrated in over 90 percent of patients with selective distal splenorenal shunts; the total hepatic blood

Fig. 30-19. Transthoracic transesophageal ligation. *A.* Left eighth intercostal space incision. Patient in right lateral decubitus position. *B.* Pulmonary ligament has been divided to permit retraction of lung, and line of incision in mediastinal pleura is outlined. *C.* Mediastinal pleura is incised, esophagus is mobilized, and line of incision in esophagus is outlined. *D.* Umbilical tape is tightened around esophagus just above hiatus to minimize bleeding, and edges of esophageal incision are retracted by stay sutures. *E.* The tortuous columns of esophageal veins are obliterated with continuous locked suture of 3-0 chromic catgut swaged on an atraumatic needle. (*From Seymour I. Schwartz, "Surgical Diseases of the Liver," McGraw-Hill Book Company, 1964.*)

flow has been shown to be unchanged, while the splenic venous circulation and esophagogastric veins have been reasonably decompressed.

Selection of Procedure. To date, selection of a surgical decompressive procedure has not been based on statistically valid data. Before performing a major shunt, the presence of portal hypertension should be defined manometrically, and a splenoportogram or a selective superior mesenteric arteriogram with a venous phase should be obtained to determine the status of the major veins. Portal vein thrombosis occurs as a complication in approximately 2 percent of the patients with portal cirrhosis. But lack of visualization of the portal vein in and of itself does not establish this diagnosis, and collateral veins of Sappey must be visualized. In order to obviate increasing hepatic dysfunction and portal-systemic encephalopathy, comparison with preoperative estimations of hepatic blood flow has been implied. But these estimations are fraught with errors in interpretation, particularly in cirrhotic patients. In reference to the role of blood flow and pressure determinations as factors in selection of the type of shunt, data can be offered to substantiate almost any argument. Large series have shown that pressure determinations and differentials within the portal venous system, measurements of the

estimated hepatic blood flow, and splenoportographic findings did not approximate true flow and these findings could not be related to the subsequent development of postshunt encephalopathy. Concerning the expressed advantage of side-to-side shunts for a cirrhotic patient in whom there is spontaneous reversal of flow in the portal vein, actual measurement in 273 cirrhotics showed no instance of spontaneous reversal. Recently, one factor, the increase in hepatic arterial flow subsequent to the creation of a portacaval shunt, has offered a hemodynamic correlate with the patient's prognosis.

The end-to-side portacaval shunt is the procedure most commonly performed, since it is technically easiest and has been associated with the lowest incidence of thrombosis. The presence of a large caudate lobe is less compromising to this procedure than to a side-to-side shunt. Rarely a large caudate lobe encroaches upon the inferior vena cava and causes caval hypertension, which precludes any portal-systemic decompressive procedure. Therefore, the workup of the cirrhotic patient should include determination of infrahepatic caval pressure. For some patients with extensive adhesions from previous operative procedures in the right upper quadrant, the splenorenal and mesocaval shunts are preferred. Thrombosis with or without recanali-

Fig. 30-20. Resection of varix-bearing area with or without interposition. *A.* and *B.* Total or near-total gastrectomy with excision of distal third of esophagus. *C.* Roux en Y isoperistaltic esophagojejunostomy. *D.* Interposition of isoperistaltic isolated segment of jejunum. *E.* Interposition of segment of colon. *F.* Reversed gastric tube. (*From Seymour I. Schwartz, "Surgical Diseases of the Liver," McGraw-Hill Book Company, 1964.*)

zation of the portal vein (cavernomatous transformation) generally precludes a portacaval anastomosis. The Budd-Chiari syndrome, whether related to a web in the inferior vena cava or to endophlebitis of the hepatic veins, dictates a side-to-side shunt to decompress the liver.

To define whether the portal vein has been acting as a significant hepatic outflow, one can determine the portal pressure, apply a vascular clamp, and then remeasure the pressure on the cephalad limb. In the event that the portal vein is serving as a natural decompressive channel for the liver, the portal pressure in the cephalad limb would be significantly increased, but this is extremely rare.

In reference to the factor of ascites as a determinant of the decompressive procedure, Voorhees and associates indicated that 39 percent of patients with end-to-side

shunts who had preoperative ascites experienced postoperative relief; in 12 percent, ascites appeared after the shunt, while all patients with side-to-side shunts and ascites had permanent relief. Interestingly, the splenorenal shunt, which is a functional side-to-side shunt, failed to relieve ascites in 12 percent of the cases, and ascites appeared after the shunt in 16 percent. It is therefore felt that ascites per se cannot be considered a significant factor in determining the shunt to be performed. Similarly, whether previous encephalopathy or the presence of asterixis are important determinants of the type of shunt has not been resolved. The only procedures which specifically attack the problem of encephalopathy are the selective splenorenal shunt or the portacaval shunt with arterialization of the distal portal vein. In the case of the selective splenorenal shunt, coupled with ligation of the coronary vein, right gastroepiploic vein, and inferior mesenteric vein, randomized series have

Fig. 30-21. Diagrammatic representation of major portal-systemic shunts. (*From Seymour I. Schwartz, "Surgical Diseases of the Liver," McGraw-Hill Book Company, 1964.*)

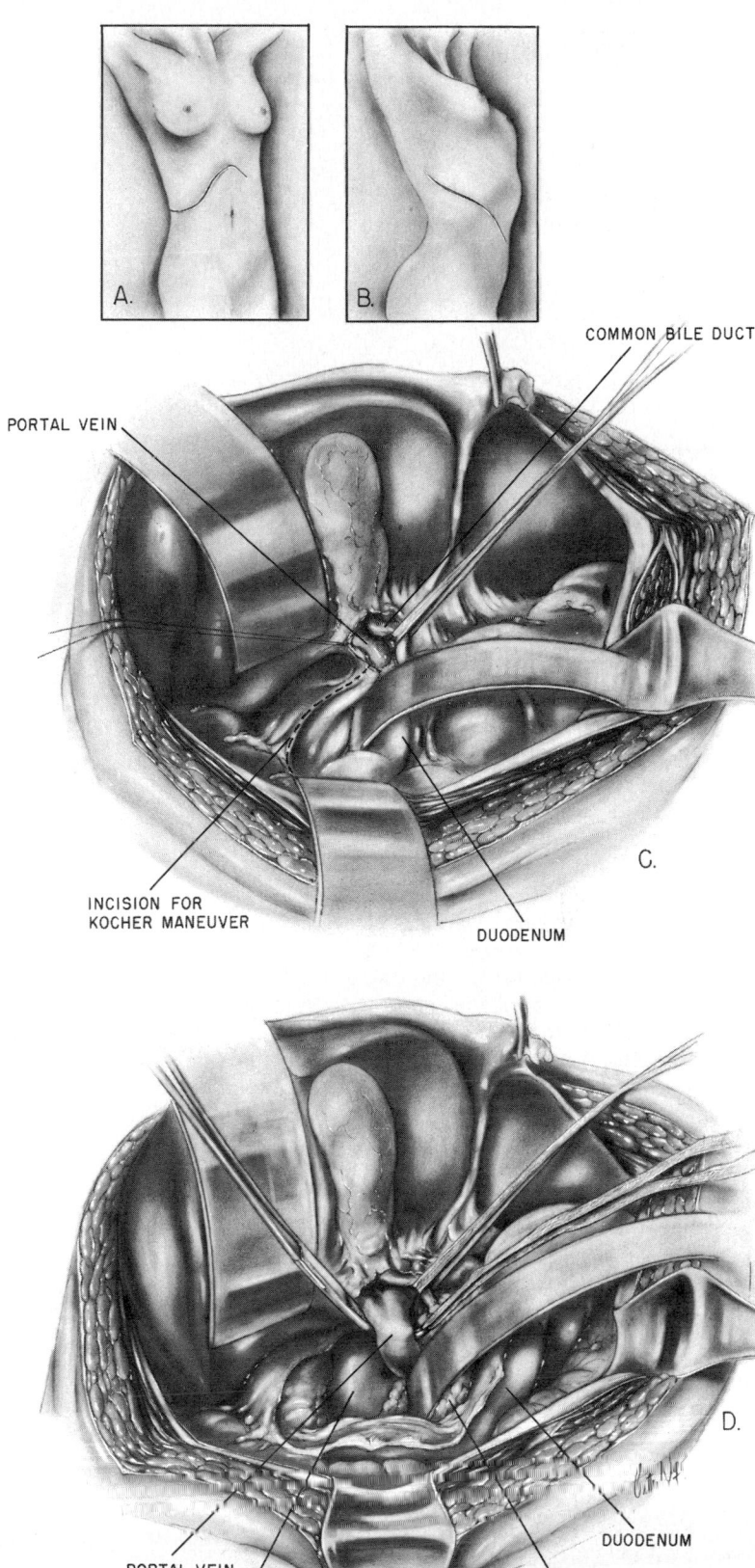

Fig. 30-22. Three kinds of portacaval shunt. (1) End-to-side portacaval shunt: *A.* Subcostal transabdominal incision. *B.* Thoracoabdominal incision over ninth intercostal space. *C.* Line of incision for Kocher maneuver. Initial dissection of hepatoduodenal ligament, with isolation and retraction of common bile duct and exposure of portal vein. *D.* Completion of dissection of portal vein, with demonstration of bifurcation in porta hepatis. Dissection of retroperitoneum to clear inferior vena cava. *E.* Technique for end-to-side anastomosis. Note partially occluding clamp on anteromedial aspect of inferior vena cava. Atraumatic clamps are applied to proximal and distal portions of portal vein. *F.* An ellipse has been removed from inferior vena cava. This should measure 1½ times diameter of portal vein. Portal vein has been transected. *G.* Distal end of portal vein has been oversewn with continuous silk sutures. (This may be handled by ligature and transfixion ligature.) Portal vein has been approximated to stoma of inferior vena cava. Two stay sutures are initially tied, and posterior layer is in place. *H.* Placement of posterior layer of sutures is facilitated by passing cranial suture into lumen of portal vein and continuing this suture to caudal limb of portal vein, where it is then passed to outside and tied. *I.* Closure of anterior row is accomplished with interrupted horizontal mattress sutures. (A continuous suture may also be employed.) *J.* Completed anastomosis. (2) Side-to-side portacaval shunt: *K.* Beginning of side-to-side anastomosis. Use of rubber-shod bulldog clamps is preferable. An ellipse has been removed from both anteromedial aspect of inferior vena cava and anterolateral aspect of portal vein. Posterior row of sutures is shown in place. This is accomplished in a manner similar to that described for end-to-side anastomosis. *L.* Completed side-to-side anastomosis. Anterior row of sutures is placed in horizontal mattress fashion. (0) Double end-to-side shunt: *M.* Upper shunt is placed on anterior aspect of inferior vena cava; lower shunt is positioned on anteromedial aspect. Pancreas is split to facilitate lower shunt. (*From Seymour I. Schwartz, "Surgical Diseases of the Liver," McGraw-Hill Book Company, 1964.*)

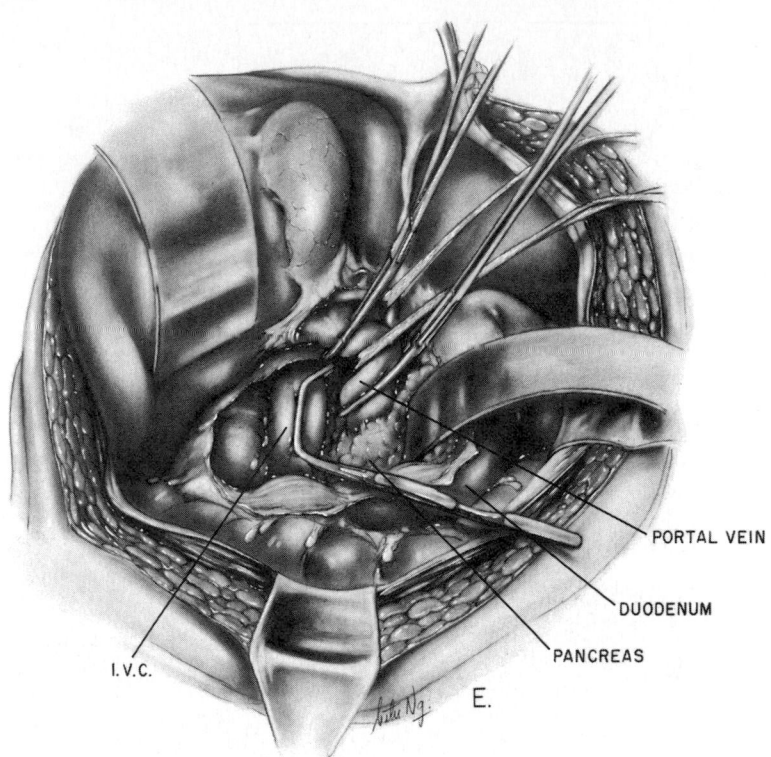

PORTAL VEIN

DUODENUM

PANCREAS

I.V.C.

E.

Fig. 30-22. Continued.

shown reduction in size of varices. The incidence of encephalopathy was less than that following total shunts. There are few long-term data for the arterialization procedure, and there is concern regarding the deleterious effects related to increased pressure.

Selection of Patients. Linton was one of the first to emphasize the importance of the status of liver function on the patient's ability to tolerate portal-systemic decompressive procedures. Ascites which failed to respond to medical therapy, a prothrombin time which remained prolonged after parenteral administration of vitamin K, serum albumin less than 3, serum bilirubin greater than 1, and BSP retention greater than 10 percent were all associated with poor postoperative prognosis. Child divided patients into three groups including those with good hepatic function (A), those with moderate hepatic function (B), and those with advanced disease and poor reserve (C). In group A are patients with a serum bilirubin below 2, albumin above 3.5, no ascites, no neurologic disorders, and excellent nutrition. Patients in the B group have bilirubin between 2 and 3, albumin between 3 and 3.5, easily controlled ascites, minimum neurologic disorder, and good nutrition. In the C group, bilirubin is above 3, the albumin is below 3, and the ascites is poorly controlled with advanced coma and wasting. Operative mortality following portacaval shunts in the A group was zero, in the B group was 9 percent, and in the C group was 53 percent. There is general agreement that hepatic function is more important than the type of shunt in determining prognosis.

Portacaval Shunt Technique. This shunt (Fig. 30-22) generally is performed through a subcostal incision, but in the presence of extreme hepatomegaly or obesity a thoracoabdominal approach may be used. The liver is retracted craniad and a Kocher maneuver performed to permit mobilization of the duodenum. Dissection is begun in the hepatoduodenal ligament, and the portal vein, which resides posteriorly in relation to the common bile duct, is dissected free along the entire course. Small tributaries of the main portal vein may be encountered, and they are doubly ligated and transected. Attention is then directed to the dissection of the inferior vena cava. The incision in the retroperitoneum is extended, and the anterior and lateral aspects of the inferior vena cava are exposed from the renal veins inferiorly to the point where the vessel passes retrohepatically. Atraumatic clamps are applied to the portal vein just above its origin and just below its bifurcation, after which the vein is transected as far craniad as possible. The hepatic end is either ligated or oversewn. A sidearm, nonocclusive clamp is positioned along the anterior aspect of the inferior vena cava and an incision is made in the inferior vena cava wall. This should be approximately $1\frac{1}{2}$ times as long as the diameter of the portal vein. Employing vascular suture techniques, an anastomosis is made between the portal vein and the side of the inferior vena cava, utilizing a continuous suture which is interrupted at the two ends. After completing the anastomosis, the clamp is removed from the inferior vena cava, and then the clamp occluding the portal vein is

Fig. 30-22. Continued.

removed. Pressure should be recorded directly from the portal vein in order to define the efficacy of the shunt.

Splenorenal Shunt. In the cirrhotic patient with post-sinusoidal obstruction, the splenorenal anastomosis is not as hemodynamically efficient as the portocaval shunt and is associated with a higher incidence of recurrent bleeding. However, proponents of this procedure indicate that in their experience the prevention of recurrent bleeding is similar to that resulting from a portacaval shunt, and the incidence of portal-systemic encephalopathy and persistent hypersplenism is reduced. The operation is generally employed in patients with obstruction of the extrahepatic portal venous system in which the portal vein is not available for shunting. In the pediatric age group, it is preferable to postpone this procedure until the child is ten years old and the splenic vein is large enough to maintain its patency.

Technique (Fig. 30-23). An oblique subcostal incision or thoracoabdominal approach may be used. The transverse colon and splenic flexure are mobilized and retracted caudad, and the short gastric vessels are doubly ligated and transected. The splenophrenic and splenorenal ligaments are then transected and dissection continued in the hilus until an ultimate pedicle of splenic artery and vein remains. The splenic vein is freed as it courses along the pancreas. The posterior peritoneum is incised just medial to the hilus of the kidney and the left renal artery and vein dissected free. Tapes are passed around the main renal vein and the major branches in the hilus of the kidney. Traction on these tapes establishes control of bleeding and minimizes the number of clamps interfering with the anastomosis. The splenic artery is doubly ligated and transected, and an atraumatic clamp is applied to the central end of the splenic vein. The splenic vein is then transected as close to the hilus of the spleen as possible and brought down to an appropriate site on the anterosuperior aspect of the renal vein. The renal artery is occluded temporarily with a bulldog clamp, and an incision made in the renal vein.

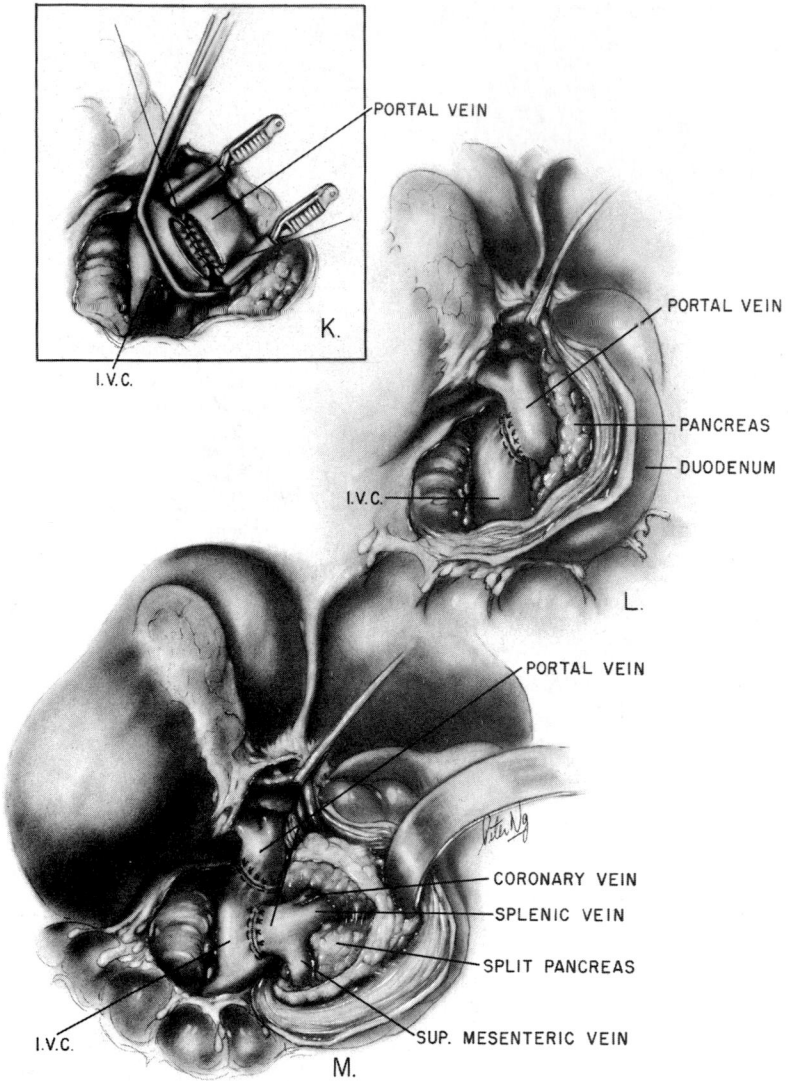

PORTAL VEIN

I.V.C.

K.

PORTAL VEIN

PANCREAS

DUODENUM

I.V.C.

L.

PORTAL VEIN

CORONARY VEIN

SPLENIC VEIN

SPLIT PANCREAS

SUP. MESENTERIC VEIN

I.V.C.

M.

Fig. 30-22. Continued.

An end-to-side anastomosis is performed by initially securing two stay sutures and completing the posterior layer as a continuous suture. Anastomosis of the anterior layer is accomplished with either horizontal mattress sutures or a continuous suture.

Superior Mesenteric–Inferior Vena Cava Shunt. This operation is generally employed for patients with extrahepatic vein obstruction and is particularly applicable to the patient in whom a previous splenorenal shunt failed or to a small child in whom a splenorenal anastomosis is doomed to failure because of the size of the splenic vein. The operation is also advised for patients with cirrhosis if there is associated thrombosis of the portal vein or extensive scarring in the right upper quadrant which precludes safe dissection of the portal vein or marked enlargement of the caudate lobe of the liver. Interruption of the inferior vena cava results in venous stasis in the lower extremity, and in the immediate postoperative pe-

riod the foot of the bed must be elevated to reduce potential edema. The procedure is well tolerated by young patients in whom postoperative chronic dependent edema of the legs is uncommon. In older patients, any edema may be readily controlled with elastic stockings. The report of prevention of recurrent bleeding in all 31 survivors of a large series has been encouraging.

Technique (Fig. 30-24). The peritoneal cavity is entered through a midline or right paramedian incision extending from the xiphoid process to well below the umbilicus. A branch of the superior mesenteric vein is cannulated and portal pressure determined manometrically. An operative phlebogram is then performed to define the patency of the superior mesenteric vein. Upward traction on the transverse colon exposes the superior mesenteric vessels. The peritoneum is incised in the region of the superior mesenteric arterial pulse, and the superior mesenteric vein is identified and dissected free. The lateral reflection of

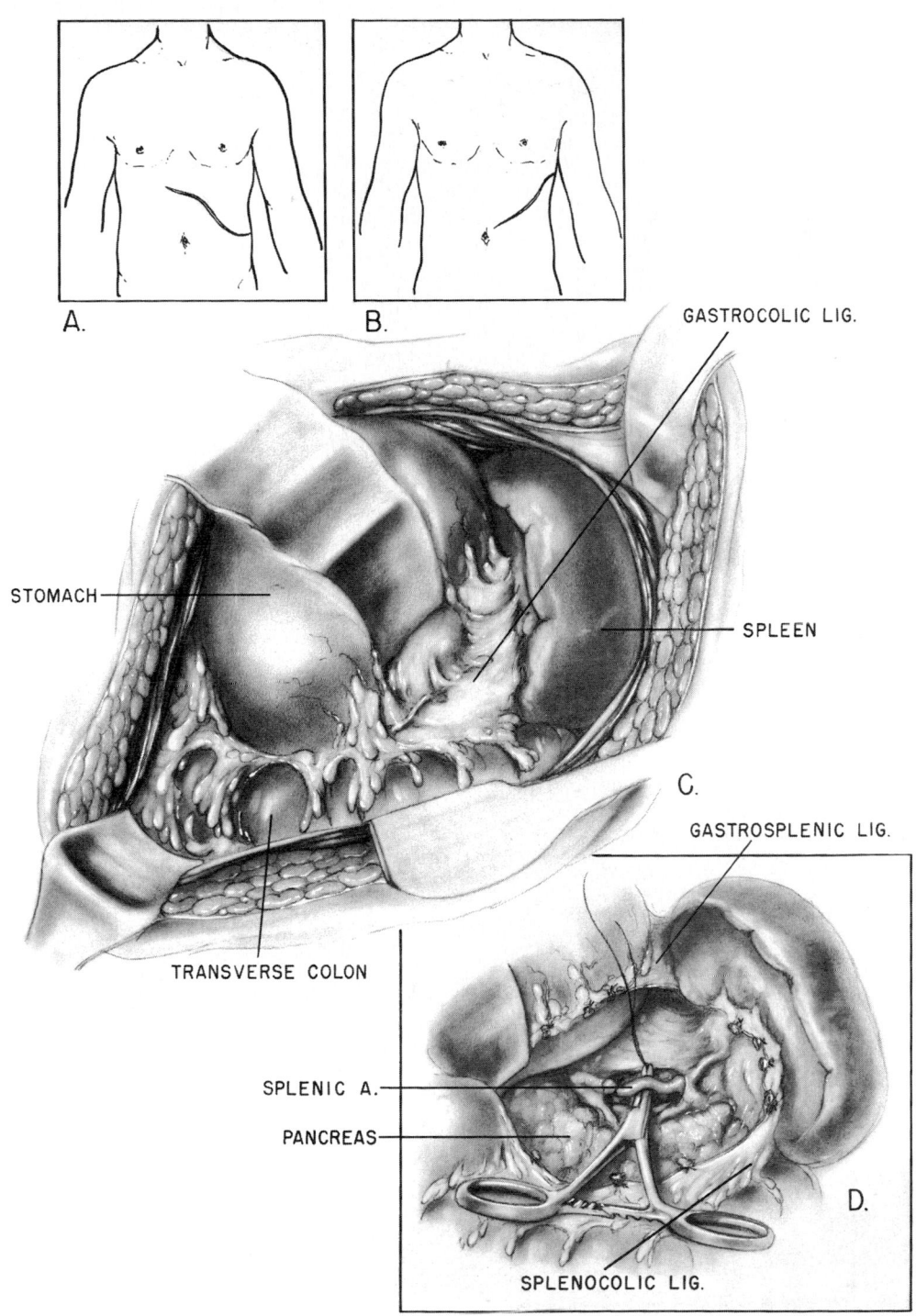

Fig. 30-23. Splenorenal anastomosis. *A.* Subcostal transabdominal incision. *B.* Thoracoabdominal incision overlying ninth intercostal space. *C.* Retraction of stomach medially. *D.* Vasa brevia have been transected. Splenic artery is ligated. Gastrosplenic and splenocolic ligament are to be transected. *E.* Colon is mobilized so that an ultimate pedicle of splenic vein remains. *F.* Retroperitoneum has been incised, and tapes are placed around renal artery and renal vein. *G.* Tapes are placed around major tributaries of renal vein within hilus of kidney and around main renal vein. Renal artery is occluded with bulldog clamp, and traction is applied to tapes around renal vein to secure control. An ellipse is then removed from anterosuperior aspect of renal vein. This should be 1½ times diameter of splenic vein. Vascular clamp has been applied to splenic vein, and spleen is removed, as long a segment of splenic vein as possible is retained. *H.* Splenic vein is brought down and anastomosed to stoma which has been created in main renal vein. Occlusive tapes have been removed from splenic vein and renal artery. (*From Seymour I. Schwartz, "Surgical Diseases of the Liver," McGraw-Hill Book Company, 1964.*)

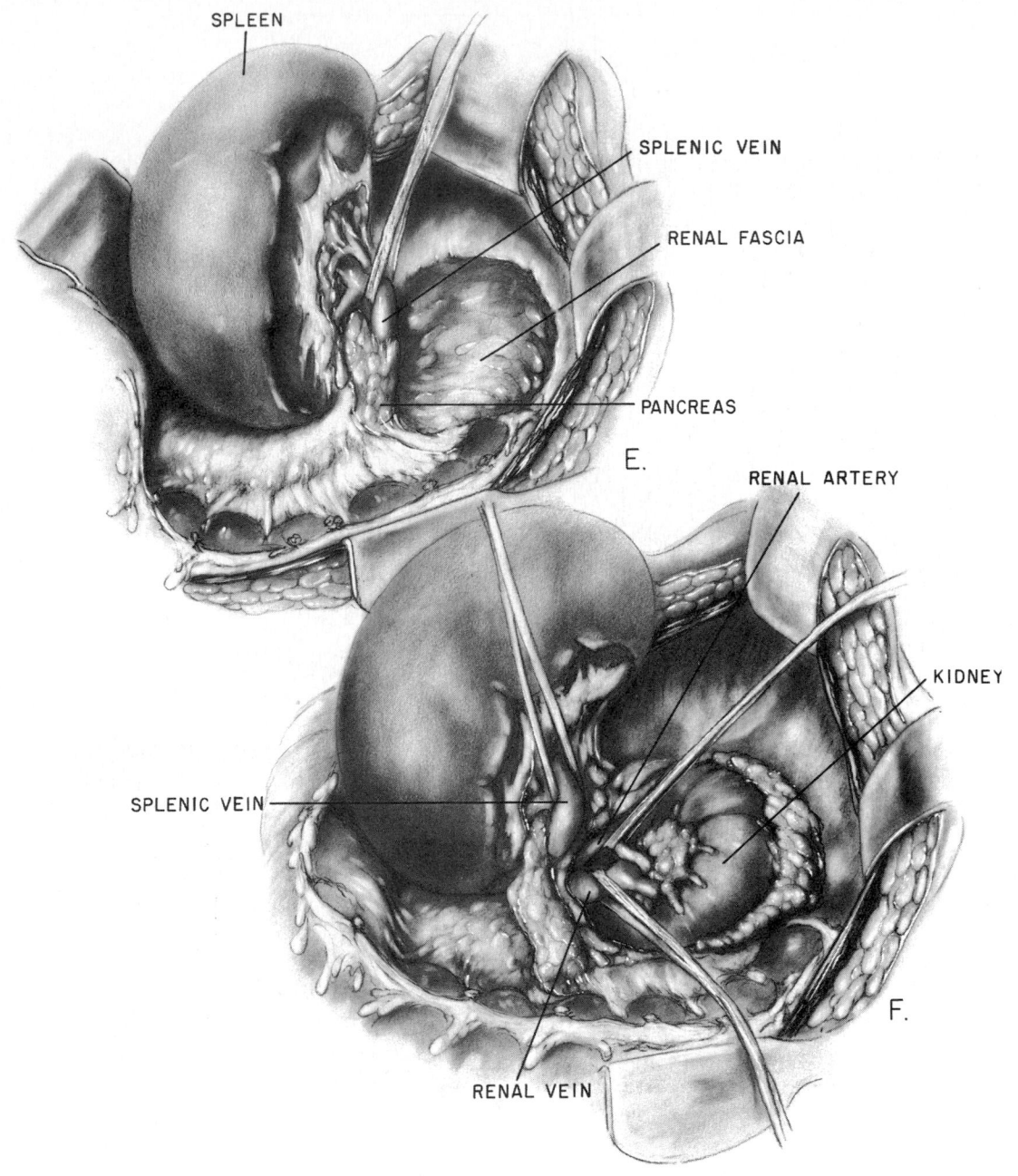

SPLEEN

SPLENIC VEIN

RENAL FASCIA

PANCREAS

E.

RENAL ARTERY

KIDNEY

SPLENIC VEIN

F.

RENAL VEIN

Fig. 30-23. Continued.

the ascending colon is then incised along its entire length
to permit medial displacement of the transverse and ascending colons and the medial reflection of the ascending
mesocolon. This exposes the inferior vena cava and the
third portion of the duodenum. The inferior vena cava is
mobilized from its origin up to the entrance of the right
renal vein. The paired lumbar veins are ligated and transected. After the entire inferior vena cava has been freed,
vascular clamps are applied immediately below the renal
veins and at the junction of the iliac veins. The inferior
vena cava is transected as far distad as possible and the

caudal stump ligated. The right iliac vein may be left
attached to the vena cava to achieve greater length. A
window is created in the mesentery of the small intestine
between the ileocolic vessels and the origin of the main
ileal trunk to permit approximation of the end of the
inferior vena cava to the right posterolateral aspect of the
superior mesenteric vein. The anastomosis between the
inferior vena cava and the superior mesenteric vein is
usually performed proximal to the right colic vein, utilizing
a continuous arterial suture interrupted at both ends.
Decompression also can be accomplished by the con-

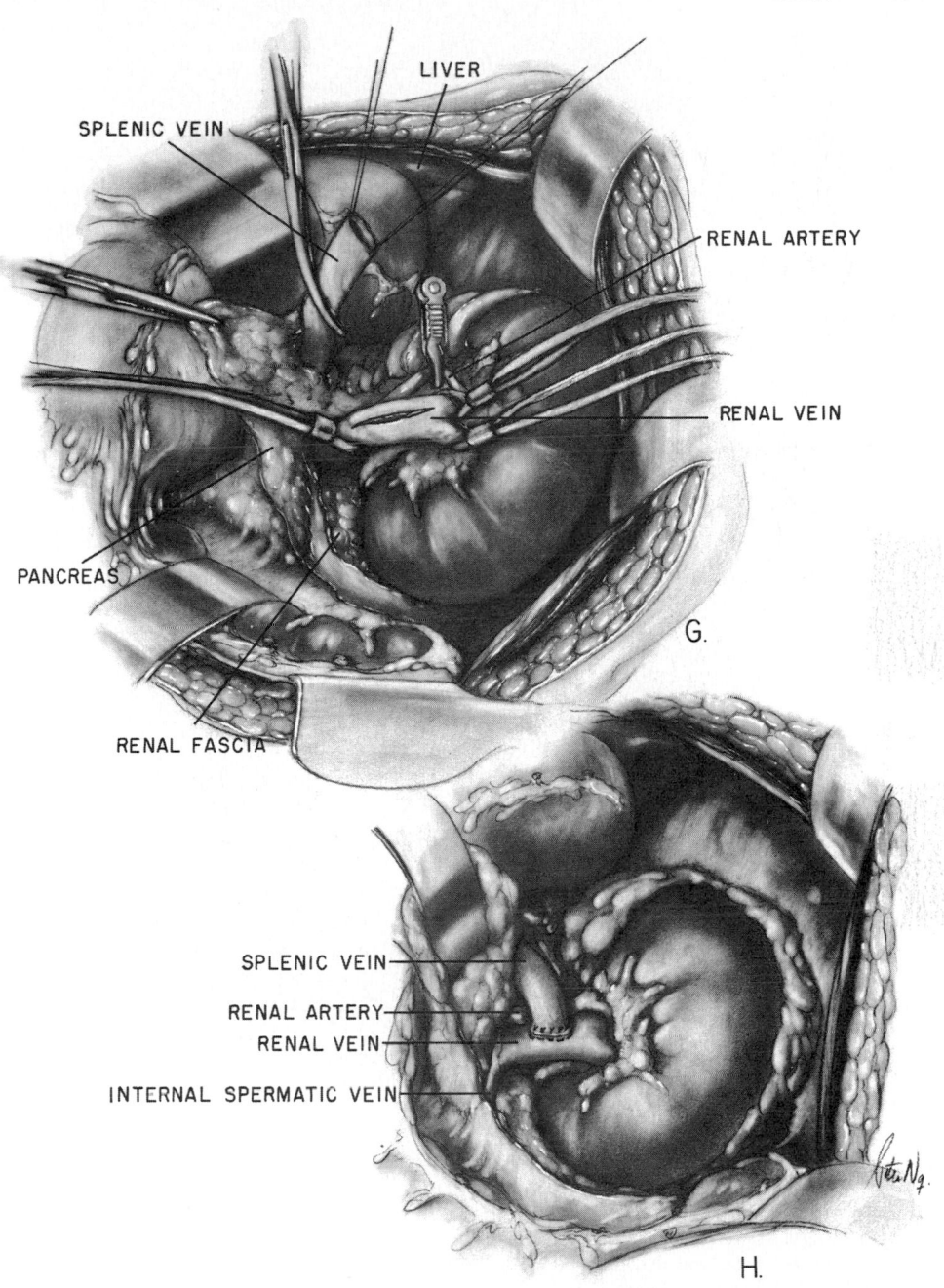

SPLENIC VEIN

LIVER

RENAL ARTERY

RENAL VEIN

PANCREAS

RENAL FASCIA

G.

SPLENIC VEIN

RENAL ARTERY

RENAL VEIN

INTERNAL SPERMATIC VEIN

H.

Fig. 30-23. Continued.

struction of an H-graft using a 19 to 22 mm prosthesis interposed between the superior mesenteric vein and the inferior vena cava (see Fig. 30-25).

Selective Splenorenal Shunt. The indications for the selective distal splenorenal shunt include a substantial portal venous flow to the liver, favorable anatomic features related to the site and patency of the splenic vein and the site and size of the left renal vein, and satisfactory liver function in the absence of ascites.

Technique. The operative procedure is shown in schematic fashion in Fig. 30-26. Decompression is effected through the short gastric vessels in the spleen. The spleen is not removed, and the distal or splenic side of the splenic vein is used for an anastomosis to the left renal vein. This technique can be modified by transecting the left renal vein close to the hilus of the kidney, turning and anastomosing the caval side of the renal vein to the side of the splenic vein, and ligating the splenic vein close to the confluence with the superior mesenteric vein. Included in the procedure is ligation of the coronary vein and devascularization of the stomach by ligating of all vessels with the exception of the right gastric artery and the short gastric veins.

SUP. MESENTERIC VEIN

SUP. MESENTERIC ARTERY

A.

Complications of Portal-Systemic Shunts. The complications uniquely associated with portal-systemic shunting procedures occur intraoperatively or during the postoperative period. The intraoperative complications include bleeding and a nonshuntable situation, while the postoperative complications include rebleeding, hepatic failure, changes in cardiorespiratory dynamics, the hepatorenal syndrome, plus delayed complications of hemosiderosis, peptic ulcer, and portal-systemic encephalopathy.

The complication of intraoperative bleeding can be reduced by correction of coagulation defects and by continuing the infusion of vasopressin during the operative procedure. A nonshuntable situation may be related to extension of cavernomatous transformation of the portal vein to involve the superior mesenteric vein and the splenic vein. In these patients, the so-called makeshift shunt, using large collaterals, is generally doomed to failure. The circum-

Fig. 30-24. Superior mesenteric-inferior vena cava shunt, right route. *A.* Insert: right paramedian incision. Traction applied to transverse colon exposes superior mesenteric artery and vein. Peritoneum over vessels has been incised. Right side of superior mesenteric vein is dissected carefully to preserve colic branches. *B.* Lateral reflection of ascending colon has been incised, and colon is reflected medially. This has exposed inferior vena cava and third portion of duodenum. Inferior vena cava is mobilized from convergence of two common iliac veins up to entrance of right renal vein. In course of this dissection, paired lumbar veins are ligated in continuity and transected. *C.* Inferior vena cava has been transected. Stay sutures are inserted into adventitia of proximal vena cava, to be used for traction and orientation. Window has been created in small intestinal mesentery between ileocolic vessels and origin of main ileal trunk. *D.* Distal end of inferior vena cava has been oversewn. Proximal inferior vena cava is passed anterior to third portion of duodenum and through window in mesentery. Anastomosis is made between end of inferior vena cava and right posterolateral aspect of superior mesenteric vein. (*From Seymour I. Schwartz, "Surgical Diseases of the Liver," McGraw-Hill Book Company, 1964.*)

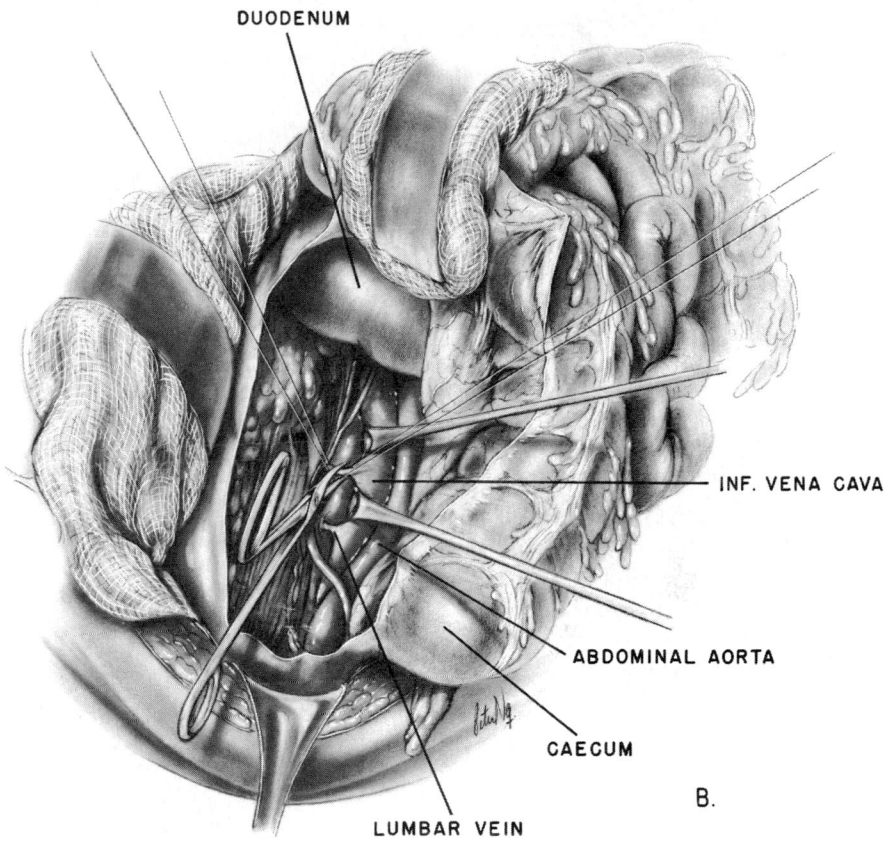

DUODENUM

INF. VENA CAVA

ABDOMINAL AORTA

CAECUM

B.

LUMBAR VEIN

Fig. 30-24. Continued.

stance of caval hypertension caused by hypertrophy and nodularity of the caudate lobe encroaching on the infrahepatic vena cava has been referred to previously. Attempts have been made to shunt between the portal system and the pulmonary artery, but they have not provided long-term decompression.

Early postoperative bleeding is usually related to thrombosis of a reconstructed shunt. This can be defined by splenoportography in the case of a portacaval shunt. The rapid onset of ascites during the early postoperative period may be managed by restriction of sodium intake and the administration of diuretic agents. In this circumstance the early institution of a peritoneal-venous shunt has provided dramatic relief. Renal failure following a portal-systemic shunt is not predictable, and treatment consists of supportive measures. Recently the use of essential amino acids and hypertonic glucose hyperalimentation has added another factor in management. The early postoperative development of hepatic coma is an ominous sign, and the various treatments for fulminant hepatic failure are not applicable in these patients.

Portacaval Shunt for Glycogen Storage Disease and Hypercholesterolemia

In 1963, Starzl and associates performed a portacaval transposition on an eight-year-old child with type III gly-

cogen storage disease, which resulted in resumption of weight gain and growth rate. Since then, several investigators have reported clinical improvement following an end-to-side portacaval shunt in children with type I glycogen storage disease in which the enzyme glucose 6-phosphatase is deficient or absent. This represents the most severe and most common form of inherited disorders of glycogen metabolism. Intravenous hyperalimentation for 2 to 3 weeks prior to surgery is advised to reduce the liver size, restore the bleeding time to normal, correct acidosis and hypoglycemia, and promote a favorable outcome of the shunting procedure. Children who have undergone diversion of portal flow have shown no evidence of encephalopathy so far. Recently, portacaval shunts have been applied to a few patients with homozygous hypercholesterolemia.

FULMINANT HEPATIC FAILURE

This refers to the clinical syndrome characterized by sudden, severe impairment of hepatic function generally as a consequence of massive necrosis of liver cells. In most instances, the cause is acute hepatitis of viral origin. Massive necrosis and dysfunction have been reported with Reye's syndrome, as a rarity in pregnancy, and following exposure to drugs such as carbon tetrachloride and di-

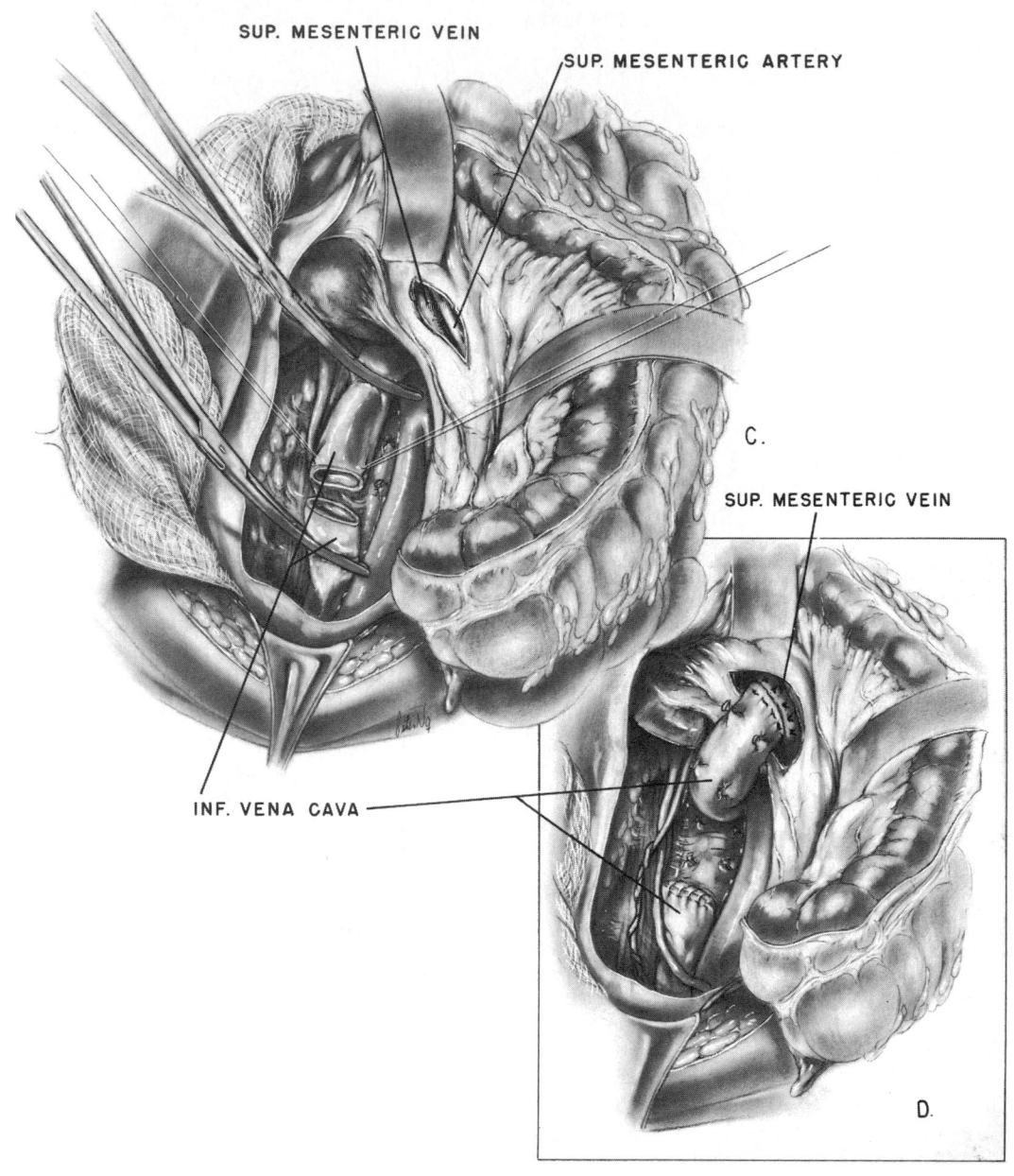

SUP. MESENTERIC VEIN

SUP. MESENTERIC ARTERY

C.

SUP. MESENTERIC VEIN

INF. VENA CAVA

D.

Fig. 30-24. Continued.

methyl nitrosamine. Circulatory necrosis of hepatic cells has been reported following vasopressor therapy and following the inadvertent intraarterial infusion of vasopressin into the hepatic artery. Halothane, particularly in cases of multiple exposures, has been indicted, but evaluation of its role awaits more statistically significant data.

The manifestations are essentially those described for hepatic encephalopathy, frequently accompanied by renal failure. The treatment can be considered in two major categories: The first is related to general supportive therapy plus regimens directed at reducing hyperammonemia which have been described in the section on encephalopathy, under Hepatic Coma, earlier in this chapter. The

second category consists of a series of intercessions, all aimed at removing so-called noxious elements from the affected patient and preserving life long enough for the liver to regenerate sufficiently. Included in this category are hemodialysis and peritoneal dialysis, exchange transfusion, plasmapheresis, asanguinous hypothermic total body perfusion, ex vivo perfusion of a liver of the same or different species, and cross circulation with a human being or a subhuman primate.

Patients in fulminant hepatic failure who are categorized at the comatose level with spasticity have a mortality of between 85 and 90 percent; this approaches 100 percent when the flaccidity stage is reached. The effect of any form

Fig. 30-25. H-graft (interposition mesocaval shunt). The transverse colon is elevated, and the superior mesenteric vein is dissected free at the route of the small bowel mesentery. A partially occlusive clamp is applied to the infrarenal vena cava, and an anastomosis is made between the vena cava and a 19- to 22-mm Dacron prosthesis. Occlusive clamps are then placed on the superior mesenteric vein, and the graft is anastomosed in an end-to-side fashion to the superior mesenteric vein. Heparinization is unnecessary.

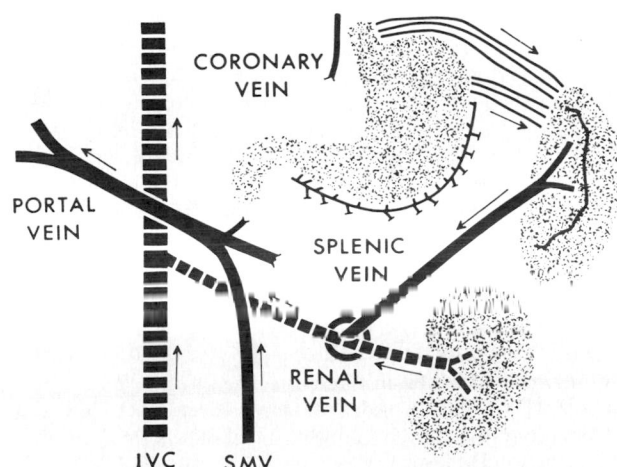

Fig. 30-26. Diagrammatic illustration of the selective distal splenorenal shunt. Note coronary vein ligation and gastric devascularization which protects the vasa brevia and other collateral vessels from esophagus and diaphragm. (*From A. A. Salam et al., Ann Surg, 173:827, 1971.*)

of therapy is difficult to evaluate since spontaneous recovery occurs in 10 to 20 percent of the cases. The difficulty in managing these patients is that recovery depends on hepatocyte regeneration, which usually takes several days, while the treatment only lasts for hours or fractions of days. To date, the results generally have been unsatisfactory.

References

General

Foster, J. H., and Berman, M. M.: "Solid Liver Tumors," W. B. Saunders Company, Philadelphia, 1977.

Popper, H., and Schaffner, F.: "Liver: Structure and Function," McGraw-Hill Book Company, New York, 1957.

Schwartz, S. I.: "Surgical Diseases of the Liver," McGraw-Hill Book Company, New York, 1964.

Sherlock, S.: "Diseases of the Liver and Biliary System," 5th ed., Blackwell Scientific Publications, Ltd., Oxford, 1977.

Anatomy

Douglass, B. E., Baggenstoss, A. H., and Hollinshead, W. H.: The Anatomy of the Portal Vein and Its Tributaries, *Surg Gynecol Obstet*, **91**:562, 1950.

Dreyer, B.: Streamlining in the Portal Vein, *Q J Exp Physiol*, **39**:305, 1954.

Healey, J. E., Jr., and Schroy, P. C.: Anatomy of the Biliary Ducts within the Human Liver: Analysis of the Prevailing Pattern of Branching and the Major Variations of the Biliary Ducts, *Arch Surg*, **66**:599, 1953.

Michels, N.: The Hepatic, Cystic and Retroduodenal Arteries and Their Relations to the Biliary Ducts, *Ann Surg*, **133**:503, 1951.

Liver Function

Faloon, W. W., Eckhardt, R. D., Murphy, T. L., Cooper, A. M., and Davidson, C. S.: An Evaluation of Human Serum Albumin in the Treatment of Cirrhosis of the Liver, *J Clin Invest*, **28**:583, 1949.

Gutman, A. B.: Serum Alkaline Phosphatase Activity in Diseases of the Skeletal and Hepatobiliary Systems: A Consideration of Current Status, *Am J Med*, **27**:875, 1959.

Leevy, C. M.: "Evaluation of Liver Function in Clinical Practice," The Lilly Research Laboratories, Indianapolis, Ind., 1965.

West, M., and Zimmerman, H. J.: Serum Enzymes in Disease. I. Lactic-Dehydrogenase and Glutamic Oxaloacetic Transaminase in Carcinoma, *Arch Intern Med*, **102**:103, 1958.

Special Studies

Braunstein, H.: Needle Biopsy of the Liver in Cirrhosis: Diagnostic Efficiency as Determined by Postmortem Sampling, *Arch Pathol*, **62**:87, 1956.

Greenway, C. V., and Stark, R. D.: Hepatic Vascular Bed, *Physiol Rev*, **51**:23, 1971.

Nagler, W., Bender, M. A., and Blau, M.: Radioisotope Photoscanning of the Liver, *Gastroenterology*, **44**:36, 1963.

Shizgal, H. M., and Goldstein, M. S.: Measurement of Portal and Total Hepatic Blood Flow by the Intestinal Xenon Technique, *Surgery*, **72**:83, 1972.

Zamcheck, N., and Klausenstock, O.: Liver Biopsy (Concluded). II. The Risk of Needle Biopsy, *N Engl J Med*, **249**:1062, 1953.

Trauma

Amerson, J. R., and Stone, H. H.: Experiences in the Management of Hepatic Trauma, *Arch Surg*, **100**:150, 1970.

Brittain, R. S., Marchioro, T. L., Hermann, G., Waddell, W. R., and Starzl, T. E.: Accidental Hepatic Artery Ligation in Humans, *Am J Surg*, **107**:822, 1964.

Carroll, C. P., Cass, K. A., and Whelan, T. J.: Wounds of the Liver in Vietnam: Critical Analysis of 254 Cases, *Ann Surg*, **177**:385, 1973.

Crosthwait, R. W., Allen, J. E., Murga, F., Beall, A. C., Jr., and DeBakey, M. E.: The Surgical Management of 640 Consecutive Liver Injuries in Civilian Practice, *Surg Gynecol Obstet*, **114**:650, 1962.

Fish, J. C.: Reconstruction of the Portal Vein. Case Reports and Literature Review, *Am Surg*, **32**:472, 1966.

Koehler, R. E., Korobkin, M., and Lewis, F.: Arteriographic Demonstration of Collateral Arterial Supply to Liver after Hepatic Artery Ligation, *Radiology*, **117**:49, 1975.

Lewis, F. R., Lim, R. C., Jr., and Blaisdell, F. W.: Hepatic Artery Ligation: Adjunct in Management of Massive Hemorrhage from the Liver, *J Trauma*, **14**:743, 1974.

Lim, R. C., Jr., Knudson, J., and Steele, M.: Liver Trauma, Current Method of Management, *Arch Surg*, **104**:544, 1972.

Lucas, C. E., and Ledgerwood, A. M.: Controlled Biliary Drainage for Large Injuries of the Liver, *Surg Gynecol Obstet*, **137**:585, 1973.

——— and Walt, A. J.: Critical Decisions in Liver Trauma: Experience Based on 604 Cases, *Arch Surg*, **101**:277, 1970.

McGhee, R. N., Townsend, C. M., Jr., Thompson, J. C., and Fish, J. C.: Traumatic Hemobilia, *Ann Surg*, **179**:311, 1974.

Madding, G. F.: Injuries of the Liver, *Arch Surg*, **70**:748, 1955.

Monafo, W. W., Ternberg, J. L., and Kempson, R.: Accidental Ligation of the Hepatic Artery, *Arch Surg*, **92**:643, 1966.

Moss, L. K., and Hudgens, J. C., Jr.: Spontaneous Rupture of the Liver Associated with Pregnancy: Case Report and Review of the Literature, *Am Surgeon*, **26**:763, 1960.

Trunkey, D. D., Shires, G. T., and McClelland, R.: Management of Liver Trauma in 811 Consecutive Patients, *Ann Surg*, **179**:722, 1974.

Hepatic Abscesses

Altemeier, W. A., Schowengerdt, C. G., and Whiteley, D. H.: Abcesses of the Liver: Surgical Considerations, *Arch Surg*, **101**:258, 1970.

Brodine, W. N., and Schwartz, S. I.: Pyogenic Hepatic Abscesses: Review of Representative Literature and Presentation of Ten Cases, *NY State J Med*, **73**:1657, 1973.

Crane, P. S., Lee, Y. T., and Seel, D. J.: Experience in Treatment of 200 Patients with Amebic Abscess of the Liver in Korea, *Am J Surg*, **123**:332, 1972.

DeBakey, M. E., and Ochsner, A.: Hepatic Amebiasis: A Twenty Year Experience and Analysis of 263 Cases, *Surg Gynecol Obstet*, **92**:209, 1951.

Lee, J. F., and Block, G. E.: The Changing Clinical Pattern of Hepatic Abscesses, *Arch Surg*, **104**:465, 1972.

Pitt, H. A., and Zuidema, G. D.: Factors Influencing Mortality in

Treatment of Pyogenic Hepatic Abscess, *Surg Gynecol Obstet,* **140:**228, 1975.

Powell, S. J., Wilmot, A. J., and Elsdon-Dew, R.: Further Trials of Metronidazole in Amoebic Dysentery and Amoebic Liver Abscess, *Ann Trop Med Parasitol,* **61:**511, 1967.

Rubin, R. H., Swartz, M. N., and Malt, R.: Hepatic Abscess: Change in Clinical, Bacteriologic and Therapeutic Aspects, *Am J Med,* **57:**601, 1974.

Cysts and Benign Tumors

Arce, J.: Hydatid Disease (Hydatidosis): Pathology and Treatment, *Arch Surg,* **42:**1, 1941.

Baum, J. K., Brockstein, J. J., Holtz, F., et. al: Possible Association between Benign Hepatomas and Oral Contraceptives, *Lancet,* **2:**926, 1973.

Christopherson, W. M., Mays, E. T., and Barrows, G. H.: Liver Tumors in Women on Oral Contraceptive Steroids, *Obstet Gynecol,* **46**(2):221, 1975.

Feldman, M.: Polycystic Disease of the Liver, *Am J Gastroenterol,* **29:**83, 1958.

Geist, D. C.: Solitary Nonparasitic Cyst of the Liver, *Arch Surg,* **71:**867, 1955.

Katz, A. M., and Pan, C.-T.: Echinococcus Disease in the United States, *Am J Med,* **25:**759, 1958.

Lewis, J. W., Koss, N., and Kerstein, M. D.: A Review of Echinococcal Disease, *Ann Surg,* **181:**390, 1975.

Longmire, W. P., Jr., Mandiola, S. A., and Earl, G. H.: Congenital Cystic Disease of the Liver and Biliary System, *Ann Surg,* **174:**711, 1971.

Magath, T. B.: The Antigen of Echinococcus, *Am J Clin Pathol,* **31:**1, 1959.

Melnick, P. J.: Polycystic Liver: Analysis of Seventy Cases, *Arch Pathol,* **59:**162, 1955.

Papadimitriou, J., and Mandrekas, A.: The Surgical Treatment of Hydatid Disease of the Liver, *Br J Surg,* **57:**431, 1970.

Park, W. C., and Phillips, R.: The Role of Radiation Therapy in the Management of Hemangiomas of the Liver, *JAMA,* **212:**1496, 1970.

Rake, M. O., Liberman, M. M., Dawson, J. L., Evans, R., Raftery, E. B., Laws, J., and Williams, R.: Ligation of the Hepatic Artery in the Treatment of Heart Failure Due to Hepatic Haemangiomatosis, *Gut,* **11:**512, 1970.

Sewell, J. H., and Weiss, K.: Spontaneous Rupture of Hemangioma of the Liver: A Review of the Literature and Presentation of Illustrative Case, *Arch Surg,* **83:**105, 1961.

Malignant Tumors

Adam, Y. G., Huvos, A. G., and Hajdu, S. I.: Malignant Vascular Tumors of Liver. *Ann Surg,* **175:**375, 1972.

Almersjö, O., Bengmark, S., Hafström, Lo., and Rosengren, K.: Accuracy of Diagnostic Tools in Malignant Hepatic Lesions: Comparative Study Using Serum Tests, Angiography, Scintiscanning and Laparotomy *Am J Surg* 127:666, 1974.

Alrenga, D. P.: Primary Angiosarcoma of the Liver: Review Article, *Int Surg,* 60:190, 1975.

Curutchet, H. P., Terz, J. J., Kay, S., and Lawrence, W., Jr.: Primary Liver Cancer, *Surgery,* **70:**467, 1971.

Edmondson, H. W., and Steiner, P. E.: Primary Carcinoma of the Liver: A Study of 100 Cases among 48,900 Necropsies, *Cancer,* **7:**462, 1954.

Fenster, L. F., and Klatskin, G.: Manifestation of Metastatic Tumors of the Liver: A Study of 81 Patients Subjected to Needle Biopsy, *Am J Med,* **31:**238, 1961.

Fortner, J. G., Mulcare, R. J., Solis, A., Watson, R. C., and Golby, R. B.: Treatment of Primary and Secondary Liver Cancer by Hepatic Artery Ligation and Infusion Chemotherapy, *Ann Surg,* **178:**162, 1973.

Foster, J. H.: Survival after Liver Resection for Cancer, *Cancer,* **26:**493, 1970.

Gulesserian, H. P., Lawton, R. L., and Condon, R. W.: Hepatic Artery Ligation and Cytotoxic Infusion in Treatment of Liver Metastases, *Arch Surg,* **105:**280, 1972.

Kew, M. C., Dos Santos, H. A., and Sherlock, S.: Diagnosis of Primary Cancer of the Liver, *Br Med J,* **4:**408, 1971.

Lin, T.-Y., Chu, S.-H., Chen, M.-F., and Chen, C.-H.: Serum Alpha-Fetoglobulin and Primary Cancer of the Liver in Taiwan, *Cancer,* **30:**435, 1972.

Purves, L. R., Bersohn, I., and Geddes, E. W.: Serum Alpha-Feto-Protein and Primary Cancer of the Liver in Man, *Cancer,* **25:**1261, 1970.

Ramirez, G., Ansfield, F. J., and Curreri, A. R.: Hepatoma: Long-Term Survival with Disseminated Tumor Treated with 5-Fluorouracil, *Am J Surg,* **120:**400, 1970.

Rosenthal, S., and Kaufman, S.: Liver Scan in Metastatic Disease, *Arch Surg,* **106:**656, 1973.

Shallow, T. A., and Wagner, F. B.: Primary Fibrosarcoma of the Liver, *Ann Surg,* **125:**439, 1947.

Starzl, T. E.: "Experience in Hepatic Transplantation," W. B. Saunders Company, Philadelphia, 1969.

Warvi, W. N.: Primary Neoplasms of the Liver, *Arch Pathol,* **37:**367, 1944.

Hepatic Resection

Lin, T.-Y., and Chen, C.-C.: Metabolic Function and Regeneration of Cirrhotic and Non-cirrhotic Livers after Hepatic Lobectomy in Man, *Ann Surg,* **162:**959, 1965.

Starzl, T. E., Bell, R. H., Beart, R. W., and Putnam, C. W.: Hepatic Trisegmentectomy and Other Liver Resections, *Surg Gynecol Obstet,* **141:**429, 1975.

Transplantation

Fortner, J. G., Kinne, D. W., Shiu, M. H., Howland, W. S., Kim, D. K., Castro, E. B., Yeh, S. D. J., Benua, R. S., and Krimins, S.: Clinical Liver Heterotopic (Auxiliary) Transplantation, *Surgery,* **74:**739, 1973.

Putnam, C. W., Halgrimson, C. G., Koep, L., and Starzl, T. E.: Progress in Liver Transplantation, *World J Surg,* **1:**165, 1977.

Starzl, T. E.: "Experience in Hepatic Transplantation," W. B. Saunders Company, Philadelphia, 1969.

Portal Hypertension

Appel, G. H., and Wollaeger, E. E.: Portal Hypertension Due to Chronic Occlusion of the Extrahepatic Portion of the Portal Vein: Its Relation to Ascites, *Am J Med,* 21:16, 1956.

Baker, L., Smith, C., and Lieberman, G.: The Natural History of Esophageal Varices, *Am J Med,* **26:**228, 1959.

Bauer, J. J., Gelernt, I. M., and Kreel, I.: Portosystemic Shunting in Patients with Primary Biliary Cirrhosis: A Good Risk Disease, *Ann Surg,* **183:**324, 1976.

Bismuth, H., and Franco, D.: Portal Diversion for Portal Hypertension in Early Childhood, *Ann Surg,* **183**:439, 1976.

Brown, H., Trey, C., and McDermott, W. V., Jr.: Lactulose Treatment of Hepatic Encephalopathy in Outpatients, *Arch Surg,* **102**:25, 1971.

Burchell, A. R., Moreno, A. H., Panke, W. F., and Nealon, T. F., Jr.: Hemodynamic Variables and Prognosis following Portacaval Shunts, *Surg Gynecol Obstet,* **138**:359, 1974.

Child, C. G. III: "Hepatic Circulation and Portal Hypertension," W. B. Saunders Company, Philadelphia, 1954.

Conn, H. O., Smith, H. W., and Brodoff, M.: Observer Variation in the Endoscopic Diagnosis of Esophageal Varices, *N Engl J Med,* **272**:830, 1965.

Eisenmenger, W. J., Blondheim, S., Bongiovanni, A. M., and Kunkel, H. G.: Electrolyte Studies on Patients with Cirrhosis of the Liver, *J Clin Invest,* **29**:1491, 1950.

Fischer, J. E., and James, H. J.: Treatment of Hepatic Coma and Hepatorenal Syndrome: Mechanism of Action of L-dopa and Aramine, *Am J Surg,* **123**:222, 1972.

Galambos, J. T., Warren, W. D., Rudman, D., Smith, R. B., III, and Salam, A. A.: Selective and Total Shunts in the Treatment of Bleeding Varices: A Randomized Controlled Trial, *N Engl J Med,* **295**:1089, 1976.

Garrett, J. C., Voorhees, A. B., Jr., and Sommers, S. C.: Renal Failure following Portasystemic Shunt in Patients with Cirrhosis of the Liver, *Ann Surg,* **172**:218, 1970.

Jackson, F. C., Perrin, E. B., Felix, W. R., and Smith, A. G.: A Clinical Investigation of the Portacaval Shunt: V. Survival Analysis of the Therapeutic Operation, *Ann Surg,* **174**:672, 1971.

Johnston, G. W., and Rodgers, H. W.: Review of 15 Years' Experience in Use of Sclerotherapy in Control of Acute Hemorrhage from Esophageal Varices, *Br J Surg,* **60**:797, 1973.

Langer, B., Stone, R. M., Colapinto, R. F., Meindok, H., Phillips, M. J., and Fisher, M. M.: Clinical Spectrum of the Budd-Chiari Syndrome and Its Clinical Management, *Am J Surg,* **129**:137, 1975.

Leveen, H. H., Christoudias, G., Ip, M., Luft, R., Falk, G., and Grosberg, S.: Peritoneo-Venous Shunting for Ascites, *Ann Surg,* **180**:580, 1974.

Linton, R. R.: The Selection of Patients for Portacaval Shunts, *Ann Surg,* **134**:433, 1951.

Lunderquist, A., and Vang, J.: Transhepatic Catheterization and Obliteration of the Coronary Vein in Patients with Portal Hypertension and Esophageal Varices, *N Engl J Med,* **291**:646, 1974.

Madden, J. L., Lore, J. M., Jr., Gerold, F. P., and Ravid, J. M.: The Pathogenesis of Ascites and a Consideration of Its Treatment, *Surg Gynecol Obstet,* **99**:385, 1954.

Maillard, J.-N., Rueff, B., Prandi, D., and Sicot, C.: Hepatic Arterialization and Portacaval Shunt in Hepatic Cirrhosis: Assessment, *Arch Surg,* **108**:315, 1974.

Malt, R. A.: Portasystemic Venous Shunts (First of Two Parts), *N Engl J Med,* **295**:24, 1976.

———: Portasystemic Venous Shunts (Second of Two Parts), *N Engl J Med,* **295**:80, 1976.

Merigan, T. C., Jr., Hollister, R. M., Gryska, P. F., Starkey, G. W. B., and Davidson, C. S.: Gastrointestinal Bleeding with Cirrhosis: A Study of 172 Episodes in 158 Patients, *N Engl J Med,* **263**:579, 1960.

Moreno, A. H., Burchell, A. R., Reddy, R. V., Steen, J. A., Panke, W. F., and Nealon, T. F., Jr.: Spontaneous Reversal of Portal Blood Flow: Case for and against Its Occurrence in Patients with Cirrhosis of the Liver, *Ann Surg,* **181**:346, 1975.

Nusbaum, M. S., Baum, S., Kuroda, K., and Blakemore, W. S.: Control of Portal Hypertension by Selective Mesenteric Arterial Drug Infusion, *Arch Surg,* **97**:1005, 1968.

Orloff, M. J., Charters, A. C., III, Chandler, J. G., Gordon, J. K., Grambort, D. E., Modafferi, T. R., Levin, S. E., Brown, N. B., Sviokla, S. C., and Knox, D. G.: Portacaval Shunt as Emergency Procedure in Unselected Patients with Alcoholic Cirrhosis, *Surg Gynecol Obstet,* **141**:59, 1975.

Owens, J. C., and Coffey, R. J.: Aneurysm of Splenic Artery including a Report of Six Additional Cases, *Surg Gynecol Obstet,* **97**:313, 1953.

Parkes, J. D., Sharpstone, P., and Williams, R.: Levodopa in Hepatic Coma, *Lancet,* **2**:1341, 1970.

Resnick, R. H., Chambers, T. C., Ishibara, A. M., Garceau, A. J., Callow, A. D., Schimmel, E. M., and O'Hara, E. T.: A Controlled Study of the Prophylactic Portacaval Shunt: A Final Report, *Ann Intern Med,* **70**:675, 1969.

———, Iber, F. L., Ishihara, A. M., Chalmers, T. C., Zimmerman, H., and the Boston Inter-Hospital Liver Group: Controlled Study of Therapeutic Portacaval Shunt, *Gastroenterology,* **67**:843, 1974.

Reynolds, T. B., Freedman, T., and Winsor, W.: Results of the Treatment of Bleeding Esophageal Varices with Balloon Tamponage, *Am J Med Sci,* **224**:500, 1952.

———, Redeker, A. G., and Davis, P.: Controlled Study of Effects of L-A ginine on Hepatic Encephalopathy, *Am J Med,* **25**:359, 1958.

Salam, A. A., Warren, W. D., and Tyras, D. H.: Splenic Vein Thrombosis: Diagnosable and Curable Form of Portal Hypertension, *Surgery,* **74**:961, 1973.

Schwartz, S. I.: Complications of Portal-Systemic Shunting Procedures, in H. Beebe (ed.), "Complications of Vascular Disease," J. B. Lippincott Company, Philadelphia, 1973.

———, Bales, H. W., Emerson, G. L., and Mahoney, E. B.: The Use of Intravenous Pituitrin in Treatment of Bleeding Esophageal Varices, *Surgery,* **45**:72, 1959.

——— and Greenlaw, R. H.: Evaluation of Portal Circulation by Percutaneous Splenic Isotope Injection, *Surgery,* **50**:833, 1961.

Sokhi, G. S., Morrice, J. J., McGee, J. O'D., and Blumgart, L. H.: Congenital Hepatic Fibrosis: Aspects of Diagnosis and Surgical Management, *Br J Surg,* **62**:621, 1975.

Starzl, T. E., Putnam, C. W., Porter, K. A., Halgrimson, C. G., Corman, J., Brown, B. L., Gotlin, R. W., Rodgerson, D. O., and Greene, H. L.: Portal Diversion for Treatment of Glycogen Storage Disease in Humans, *Ann Surg,* **178**:525, 1973.

Thompson, J. C.: Alterations in Gastric Secretion after Portacaval Shunting, *Am J Surg,* **117**:854, 1969.

Tisdale, W. A., Klatskin, G., and Glenn, W. W.: Portal Hypertension and Bleeding Esophageal Varices: Their Occurrence in the Absence of Both Intrahepatic and Extrahepatic Obstruction of the Portal Vein, *N Engl J Med,* **261**:209, 1959.

Turcotte, J. G., and Lambert, M. J., II: Variceal Hemmorhage, Hepatic Cirrhosis and Portacaval Shunts, *Am J Surg,* **126**:748, 1973.

Voorhees, A. B., Jr., Price, J. B., Jr., and Britton, R. C.: Portasystemic Shunting Procedures for Portal Hypertension: 26-

Year Experience in Adults with Cirrhosis of the Liver, *Am J Surg,* **119:**501, 1970.

Warren, W. D., Salam, A. A., Hutson, D., and Zeppa, R.: Selective Distal Splenorenal Shunt: Technic and Results of Operation, *Arch Surg,* **108:**306, 1974.

Glycogen Storage Disease and Hypercholesterolemia

Folkman, J., Philippart, A., Tze, W.-J., and Crigler, J., Jr.: Portacaval Shunt for Glycogen Storage Disease: Value of Prolonged Intravenous Hyperalimentation before Surgery, *Surgery,* **72:**306, 1972.

Starzl T. E., Brown, B. I., Blanchard, H., and Brettschneider, L.: Portal Diversion in Glycogen Storage Disease, *Surgery,* **65:**504, 1969.

Stein, E. A., Peltifor, J., Mieny, C., et al.: Portacaval Shunt, in Four Patients with Homozygous Hypercholesterolaemia, *Lancet,* **1:**832, 1975.

Fulminant Hepatic Failure

Abouna, G. M., Cook, J. S., Fisher, L. McA., Still, W. J., Costa, G., and Hume, D. M.: Treatment of Acute Hepatic Coma by Ex Vivo Baboon and Human Liver Perfusions, *Surgery,* **71:**537, 1972.

Klebanoff, G., Hollander, D., Cosimi, A. B., Stanford, W., and Kemmerer, W. T.: Asanguineous Hypothermic Total Body Perfusion (TBW) in the Treatment of Stage IV Hepatic Coma, *J Surg Res,* **12:**1, 1972.

Trey, C., and Davidson, C. S.: The Management of Fulminant Hepatic Failure, *Prog Liver Dis,* **3:**282, 1970.

Chapter 31

Gallbladder and Extrahepatic Biliary System

by **Seymour I. Schwartz**

ANATOMY

DUCT SYSTEM. The extrahepatic biliary system begins with the hepatic ducts and ends at the stoma of the common bile duct in the duodenum. The right hepatic duct is approximately 1 cm in length, while the left duct is somewhat larger. Both are approximately 3 mm in diameter. The two ducts join to form a common hepatic duct which resides in the porta hepatis and is 3 to 4 cm in length. It, in turn, is joined at an acute angle by the cystic duct from the gallbladder to form the common bile duct.

The common bile duct is approximately 8 cm in length and 6 mm in diameter. The upper portion is situated in the free edge of the lesser omentum, to the right of the hepatic artery, and anterior to the portal vein. The middle third of the common duct curves to the right behind the first portion of the duodenum, where it diverges from the portal vein and hepatic arteries. The lower third of the common bile duct curves more to the right behind the head of the pancreas, which it grooves, and enters the duodenum at the ampulla of Vater, where it is frequently joined by the pancreatic duct. The portions of the duct have also been named according to their relationships to intestinal viscera: the terms *suprapancreatic, intrapancreatic,* and *intraduodenal* have been applied.

The union of the bile duct and the main pancreatic duct follows one of three patterns. The structures may (1) unite outside the duodenum and traverse the duodenal wall and papilla as a single duct, (2) join within the duodenal wall and have a short, common, terminal portion, or (3) exit independently into the duodenum. The common channel has been considered important in permitting reflux from the pancreas into the biliary tract and the reverse. Separate orifices have been demonstrated in 29 percent of autopsied specimens, while injection into cadavers reveals reflux from the common bile duct into the pancreatic duct in 54 percent. Radiographically, reflux from the common bile duct into the pancreatic duct is present in about 16 percent of the cases. The sphincter of Oddi surrounds the common bile duct and pancreatic ducts at the papilla of Vater, and although some fibers are derived from the duodenal muscle, there are additional, intrinsic muscles of the duct in the ampulla. These provide a control of the flow of bile and pancreatic juice. An ampullary sphincter which is present in one-third of adults may produce a common channel effect.

GALLBLADDER. The gallbladder is located in the bed of the liver in line with the anatomic division of that organ into right and left lobes. It represents an outpouching of the extrahepatic biliary duct system and has an average capacity of 50 ml. It is a pear-shaped organ which is divided into four anatomic portions: fundus; corpus, or body; infundibulum; and neck. The fundus represents the rounded, blind end which normally extends beyond the liver margin behind the tip of the right costal cartilage. It may be unusually kinked and present the appearance of a "phrygian cap." It contains most of the smooth muscle of the organ, in contrast to the corpus, or body, which is the major storage area and contains most of the elastic tissue. The body tapers into a neck, which is funnel-shaped and connects with the cystic duct. The neck usually follows a gentle curve, the convexity of which may be distended into a dilatation known as the *infundibulum,* or *Hartmann's pouch.*

The wall of the gallbladder is made up of smooth muscle and fibrous tissue, and the lumen is lined with a high columnar epithelium which contains cholesterol and fat globules. The mucus secreted into the gallbladder originates in the tubular alveolar glands in the globular cells of the mucosa lining the infundibulum and neck.

The gallbladder is supplied by the cystic artery, which normally branches from the right hepatic artery behind the cystic duct. It is approximately 2 mm in diameter and courses above the cystic duct for a variable distance, until it passes down the peritoneal surface of the gallbladder and branches. Venous return is carried through small veins, which enter directly into the liver from the gallbladder, and a large cystic vein, which carries blood back to the right portal vein. Lymph flows directly from the gallbladder to the liver and drains into several nodes along the surface of the portal vein. The nerves of the gallbladder arise from the celiac plexus and lie along the hepatic artery. Motor nerves are made up of vagus fibers mixed with postganglionic fibers from the celiac ganglion. The preganglionic sympathetic level is at T_8 and T_9. Sensory supplies are provided by fibers in the sympathetic nerves coursing to the celiac plexus through the posterior root ganglion at T_8 and T_9 on the right side.

The gallbladder enters the common duct system by means of the cystic duct, which has a variable length, averaging 4 cm. It joins the common hepatic duct at an

Fig. 31-1. Variations of the cystic duct. *A.* Low junction between cystic duct and common hepatic duct. *B.* Cystic duct adherent to common hepatic duct. *C.* High junction between cystic and common hepatic duct. *D.* Cystic duct drains into right hepatic duct. *E.* Long cystic duct which joins common hepatic duct behind duodenum. *F.* Absence of cystic duct. *G.* Cystic duct crosses anterior to common hepatic duct and joins it posteriorly. *H.* Cystic duct courses posteriorly to common hepatic duct and joins it anteriorly. (*After W. H. Hollinshead, "Anatomy for Surgeons," vol. II, Hoeber Medical Division, Harper & Row, Publishers, Inc., New York, 1956.*)

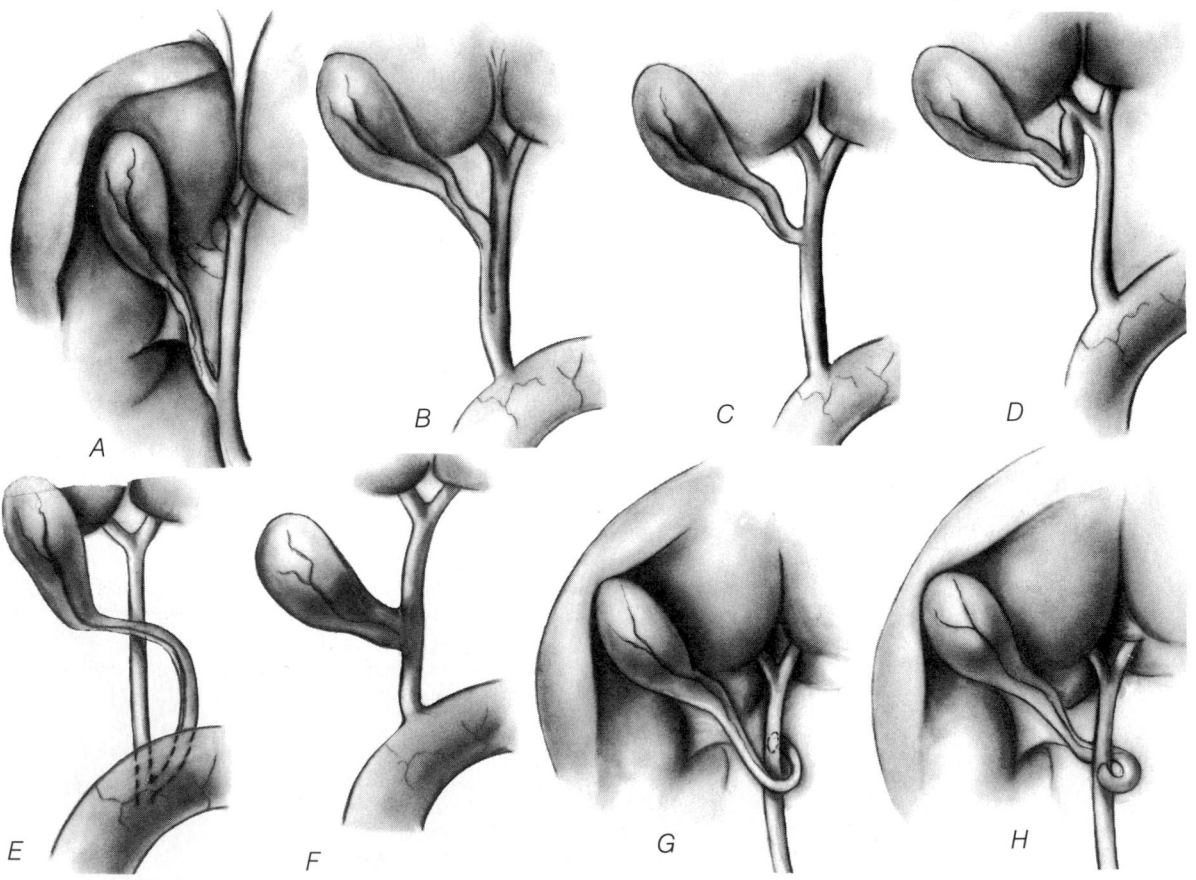

acute angle, and the right branch of the hepatic artery resides immediately behind it. Variations of the cystic duct are surgically important, relating to the point of union with the common hepatic duct (Fig. 31-1). The cystic duct may run parallel to the common hepatic duct and actually be adherent to it, or it may be extremely long and unite with the hepatic duct in the duodenum. On the other hand, the cystic duct may be absent or very short, and there may be an extremely high union with the hepatic duct. In some instances, the cystic duct may spiral either anteriorly or posteriorly in relation to the hepatic duct and join the common hepatic duct on the left side. The segment of the cystic duct adjacent to the gallbladder bears a variable number of mucosal folds which have been referred to as the "valves of Heister" but do not have valvular function.

Anomalies

The classic description of the extrahepatic biliary passages and their arteries applies in only about one-third of the patients. An appreciation of the great frequency of anomalies is critical to avoid errors in surgical technique. Important anomalies of the gallbladder relate to number, position, and form (Fig. 31-2). Isolated congenital absence of the gallbladder is extremely rare; autopsy incidences of 0.03 percent have been computed. Before the diagnosis is made, the presence of an intrahepatic vesicle or a left-sided organ must be ruled out. Duplication of the gallbladder with two separate cavities and two separate cystic ducts has an incidence of approximately 1 in 4,000. The accessory gallbladder may be situated on the left side, and its cystic duct may empty into the left hepatic duct rather than the common duct. Pathologic processes such as cholelithiasis and cholecystitis may involve one organ while the other is spared.

The gallbladder may be found in a variety of abnormal positions. The so-called "floating gallbladder" occurs when there is an increase in the peritoneal investment. The organ may be completely invested by peritoneum with no mesentery, in which case only the cystic duct and artery connect it to the liver. In other instances, the gallbladder may be suspended from the liver by a complete mesentery, or

the neck may have a mesentery in which the cystic artery lies, while the fundus and body are free. This condition is relatively common, occurring in about 5 percent of the cases. This anomaly predisposes to torsion and resulting gangrene or perforation of the viscus. Left-sided gallbladder with the cystic duct entering directly into the left hepatic duct or common duct is extremely rare, as is the situation known as *retrodisplacement,* in which the fundus extends backward in the free margin of the gastrohepatic omentum. The gallbladder may also be totally intrahepatic, a situation occurring in many animals. In man, the partial or completely intrahepatic gallbladder is associated with an increased incidence of cholelithiasis.

The anomalies in the cystic duct have been referred to (Fig. 31-1). Accessory hepatic ducts are present in approximately 15 percent of cases. Large ducts are usually single and drain a portion of the right lobe of the liver joining the right hepatic duct, common hepatic duct, or infundibulum of the gallbladder. Small ducts (Luschka) may drain directly from the liver into the body of the gallbladder. It is the frequent incidence of the accessory hepatic ducts and the fact that they are overlooked during cholecystectomy that impel many surgeons to drain the hepatorenal pouch routinely following this operation.

Anomalies of the hepatic artery and cystic artery are very common (Fig. 31-3). The large accessory left hepatic artery, originating from the left gastric artery, occurs in about 5 percent of cases. In about 20 percent of cases, the right hepatic artery originates from the superior mesenteric artery, and in about 5 percent of cases there are two hepatic arteries—one originating from the common hepatic and the other from the superior mesenteric artery. The right hepatic artery is vulnerable during surgical procedures, particularly when it parallels the cystic duct and is adherent to it or when it resides in the mesentery of the gallbladder. In 10 percent of cases, the cystic artery originates from the left hepatic artery or from the junction of the left or right hepatic arteries with the common hepatic artery. In about 15 percent of cases, the cystic artery passes in front of the common hepatic duct, rather than to the right of or posterior to this duct. Double cystic arteries occur in about 25 percent of cases, and they may both arise from the right hepatic artery, or one may have an abnormal origin.

Fig. 31-2. Anomalies of the gallbladder. *A.* Double gallbladder with single cystic duct. *B.* Bilobed gallbladder. *C.* Intrahepatic gallbladder. *D.* Left-sided gallbladder.

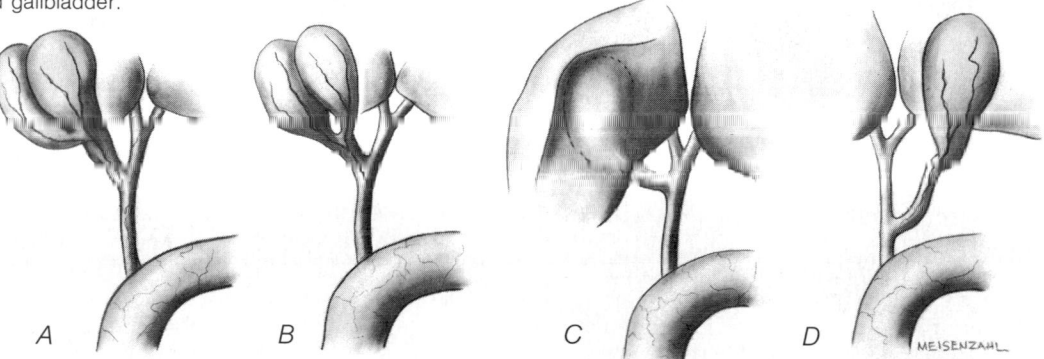

A   B   C   D   MEISENZAHL

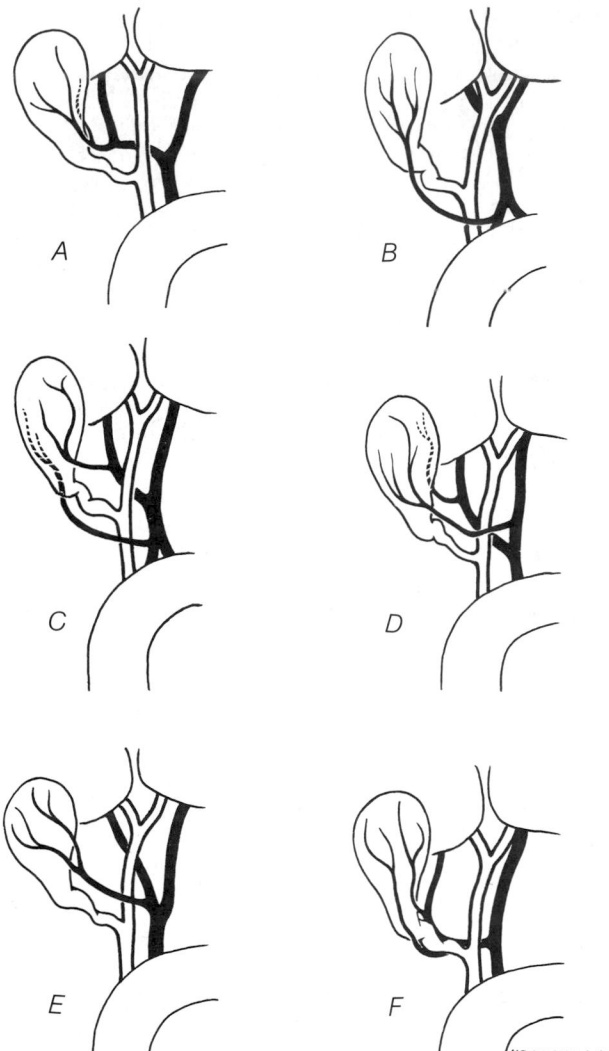

Fig 31-3. Anomalies of the arteries to the gallbladder. *A*. Cystic artery arises from right hepatic artery in 95 percent of cases. *B*. Cystic artery arises from gastroduodenal artery. *C*. Two cystic arteries, one arising from right hepatic artery and the other from common hepatic artery. *D*. Two cystic arteries. Abnormal one arises from left hepatic artery and crosses common hepatic duct anteriorly. *E*. Cystic artery arises from right hepatic artery but courses anterior to common hepatic duct. *F*. Two cystic arteries arising from right hepatic artery. Right hepatic artery is adherent to cystic duct and neck of gallbladder. Posterior cystic artery is very short (a common finding).

CYSTIC DISEASE OF THE EXTRAHEPATIC BILIARY TRACT (CHOLEDOCHAL CYST)

Congenital cystic abnormalities may occur throughout the entire biliary system, i.e., from intrahepatic biliary radicals to the terminal common duct. Intrahepatic cystic dilatation is discussed in Chap. 30, Liver. The present discussion is limited to extrahepatic cystic disease according to the original classification of Alonso-Lej et al. and the more recent classic review of Longmire et al.

Choledochal cyst (Alonso-Lej type A), the most common congenital cyst of the extrahepatic biliary tract, occurs four times more frequently in females. There are three major varieties: cystic dilatation involving the entire common bile duct and common hepatic duct with the cystic duct entering the choledochal cyst; a small cyst usually localized to the distal common bile duct; and diffuse fusiform dilatation of the common bile duct. Over 30 percent of cases are diagnosed within the first decade of life. The clinical manifestations include pain, jaundice, and a palpable epigastric mass. The pain and jaundice are frequently intermittent and are generally progressive in severity. Diagnosis is occasionally established by cholangiography. But the highest diagnostic yield is associated with ^{131}I rose Bengal and other isotopic scans. Untreated cases may progress to complete biliary obstruction, cholangitis, secondary biliary cirrhosis, or spontaneous rupture, which occurs frequently during pregnancy. Early operation is therefore indicated.

A variety of operative procedures have been prescribed, but the preferable approach is cystojejunostomy, employing either a long antecolic limb with enteroenterostomy or the Roux en Y procedure (Fig. 31-4). Decompression may also be effected by a cystoduodenostomy (Fig. 31-5). Longmire et al. have advised cholecystectomy at the time of cyst drainage to obviate postoperative cholecystitis. Although a higher mortality rate is associated with the operation, some have advised excision of the cyst followed by hepatodochojejunostomy.

Congenital diverticulum (Alonso-Lej type B) is a rare disorder in which the cyst is connected by a stalk to the common duct, a hepatic duct, or the gallbladder and can be totally excised. The choledochocele (Alonso-Lej type C) is the least common cystic dilatation and involves only the intraduodenal portion of the common bile duct. Other cystic anomalies include multiple cystic dilatations of the common and hepatic ducts and unexplained diffuse ductal dilatations, usually manifested by repeated bouts of jaundice and cholangitis, pigment stones, and sludged bile. Choledochoduodenostomy has not been uniformly satisfactory, and at times hepaticojejunostomy may be required.

CONGENITAL BILIARY ATRESIA

Congenital atresia of the extrahepatic bile ducts is the most common cause of prolonged obstructive jaundice in the neonatal period. Although the entity was first described by Aristotle, it was not until 1916 that an operative approach was suggested.

INCIDENCE. It is estimated that biliary atresia may be expected to occur once in every 20,000 to 30,000 births. There are an equal number of males and females, and all races are represented in numbers proportional to their frequency in the population. A familial occurrence has been reported. Of 156 cases of prolonged obstructive jaundice seen at the Children's Medical Center in Boston from 1940 to 1951, 61 percent were due to biliary atresia.

PATHOLOGY. Coexistence of atresia of the extrahepatic and intrahepatic ducts supports the belief that a developmental anomaly is the basic defect. The developing bile ducts pass through a solid stage analogous to that of the intestine, becoming obliterated by epithelial concrescence or proliferation. In the course of normal development, this solid core becomes vacuolated, and the vacuoles coalesce to reestablish the lumen. The order of succession and appearance of the lumen is common bile duct, hepatic duct, cystic duct, and gallbladder. An arrest in this solid stage affords the best explanation for the malformation, and innumerable anomalies are possible (Fig. 31-6).

Stowens reported that 10 percent of the cases had complete absence of all extrahepatic ducts, 64 percent had partial absence, 11 percent had total atresia of the hepatic bile ducts associated with normal common ducts, 7 percent had atresia of the visible larger intrahepatic ducts, 5 percent had atresia of the intrahepatic bile canaliculi, and 3 percent demonstrated only stenosis. The atretic segment may not be identifiable or may appear as a thin, fibrous cord.

The obliterative process may involve the common duct, cystic duct, one or both hepatic ducts, and the gallbladder in a variety of combinations. With atresia of the distal portion of the common duct system, dilatation of the proximal portion and the gallbladder may be noted. The liver is usually enlarged, dark green, and in the late stages of disease diffusely nodular. Histologically, there is an increased amount of fibrous tissue in the periportal areas and proliferation of the bile duct with intraductal stasis. The signs of biliary cirrhosis may be apparent. Coexisting intrahepatic atresia is present in 3 to 5 percent of the cases. Approximately one-quarter of the patients have coincidental malformations including congenital heart disease, imperforate anus, duodenal atresia, mongolism, and, most commonly, urinary tract involvement.

CLINICAL MANIFESTATIONS. Jaundice, a constant finding, is usually present at birth or shortly thereafter but does not become marked until the child is two to three weeks old, after which it becomes progressively more intense. Initially, the growth and weight gains of the children are within normal limits, but in later stages of disease malnutrition and retarded growth may be apparent. Abdominal enlargement is frequent and may be related to hepatomegaly or, rarely, accumulation of ascites. In extended cases, the spleen may also be enlarged, and the anteroabdominal wall veins may be apparent, reflecting portal hypertension. Later in the course of the disease, the effects of limited absorption of fat-soluble vitamins may become apparent with bone changes and other signs of deficiency. Petechiae and subcutaneous hemorrhages are uncommon but suggest a reduction in prothrombin time secondary to vitamin K deficiency.

LABORATORY STUDIES. A mild anemia may be noted in the later course of the disease. The urine is dark and positive for bile, and contains no urobilinogen. The stools are acholic with pasty consistency. The initial stool may have a normal green color, since it is formed at the fourth month of fetal development and the obstruction of the biliary tract may occur after that time. Later, the occasional appearance of a yellow color in the stool and a positive test for bile may be explained by the excretion of small amounts of pigment by the glands of the intestinal tract. The serum bilirubin progressively increases with ultimate establishment of extremely high levels. Weekly determi-

Fig. 31-4. Decompression of choledochal cyst by Roux en Y procedure.

nations for a period of 1 month is considered to be the single most valuable laboratory aid. High levels of alkaline phosphatase are common. Elevations in the serum transaminase levels with serum glutamic oxaloacetic transaminase (SGOT) between 400 and 500 have been reported.

DIFFERENTIAL DIAGNOSIS. Neonatal jaundice may also be due to (1) physiologic changes, (2) constitutional deficiency, (3) hemolytic disease, (4) sepsis, (5) neonatal hepatitis, or (6) the inspissated bile syndrome. Physiologic jaundice occurs in approximately two-thirds of full-term

Fig. 31-5. Decompression of choledochal cyst by cystoduodenostomy.

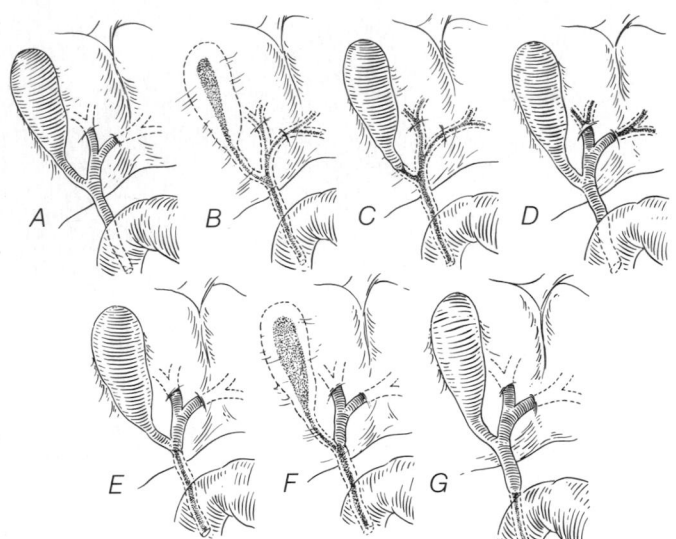

Fig. 31-6. Variations of extrahepatic bile duct atresia. *A.* Normal. *B.* Total atresia of all ducts. *C.* Atresia of all ducts with exception of gallbladder. *D.* Intrahepatic ductal atresia. *E.* Atresia of common bile duct. *F.* Atresia of common bile duct and gallbladder. *G.* Segmental atresia of distal common bile duct. (*From Seymour I. Schwartz, "Surgical Diseases of the Liver," McGraw-Hill Book Company, New York, 1964.*)

infants and more frequently in premature infants. It is due to the destruction of fetal red cells which are no longer required after birth and the normal functional immaturity of the liver at birth, which is unable to excrete the excessive load of pigment presented to it. The jaundice reaches its peak within 2 to 5 days after delivery and then gradually disappears. The serum bilirubin levels rarely exceed 10 mg/100 ml.

Of the constitutional deficiencies causing hyperbilirubinemia, only the rare Crigler-Najjar syndrome manifests itself early. The total serum bilirubin is usually over 10 mg/100 ml, and the greater proportion is unconjugated. There is always an associated hepatomegaly, and kernicterus is a common complication. The patients usually die early, although some may survive without neurologic deficit. Another hepatic disturbance with familial tendency is related to the ingestion of lactose in infants with galactosemia. An obstructive type of jaundice appears after the first week of life and subsides immediately when lactose is removed from the diet. If the lactose is not withheld, the jaundice spontaneously subsides over a period of several weeks. Examination of the urine for reducing substances provides the diagnosis.

Hemolysis due to blood grouping incompatibility between fetus and mother may result in neonatal jaundice. Jaundice may intensify until death ensues or until a gradual recovery takes place in several weeks. The increase in the bilirubin is in the unconjugated portion, the urine contains bilirubin and urobilinogen, and a positive Coombs test confirms the diagnosis for Rh incompatibility but may be negative with ABO incompatibility. Overwhelming sepsis can cause damage to the liver and jaundice. Recent interest has been directed toward cytomegalic inclusion disease with jaundice occurring in the first week or later and accompanied by hepatomegaly and splenomegaly, microcephaly and mental retardation, motor disability, and petechiae.

Twenty-five percent of cases of prolonged obstructive jaundice in infancy have been ascribed to neonatal hepa-

titis. The usual clinical picture is that of a fluctuating jaundice which appears during the early weeks of life. Liver function tests contribute little to the differential diagnosis, but liver biopsy may be diagnostic by demonstrating the microscopic picture of local necrosis and large multinucleated liver cells. Neonatal jaundice may also be caused by the "inspissated bile syndrome," which accounted for 15 percent of the cases in one large series. The term is applied to patients with normal biliary tracts who have had persistent signs of obstructive jaundice. Increased viscosity of bile and obstruction of the canaliculi are implicated as causes. Most cases are related to hemolytic disease, but in some instances no etiologic factor can be defined. It is now felt that many of the cases which were classified as the "inspissated bile syndrome" were, in fact, instances of prolonged hemolytic disease, hepatitis, cirrhosis, or cholangitis.

The clinical approach to persistent obstructive jaundice in infancy is directed at defining the cause and, more particularly, determining whether operative intervention is indicated and, if so, optimal timing. Several criteria are used to establish the diagnosis of biliary atresia. The conventional liver function tests are of little value, since they are normal in patients with either biliary atresia or "inspissated bile syndrome" and also frequently normal in patients with neonatal hepatitis. The alkaline phosphatase level is of little value, since it is elevated in all types of obstructive jaundice. Examination of the serum bilirubin level is helpful in that a slowly rising serum bilirubin level is to be expected with biliary atresia. Needle biopsy may be indicated to establish the diagnosis of neonatal hepatitis. The radioactive rose bengal test measuring the excretion of radioactivity in the stool has made it possible to differentiate between severe biliary obstruction of hepatitis and complete obstruction associated with biliary atresia. The maximal radioactivity consistent with the diagnosis of biliary atresia is between 2 and 4 percent. Higher levels may be reached with hepatitis. Determination of indocyanine green also has been used. Lipoprotein X is

present in the serum of patients with cholestasis. An increase after administration of cholestyramine is evidence
that an operation should be performed; a decrease suggests
nonoperative management of the jaundice.

TREATMENT. Timing of the surgical operation is critical.
This should be deferred if there is any evidence of bile in
the duodenal fluid or stool or if the bilirubin has shown a
tendency to decrease. However, surgical intervention is
indicated if there is a consistent absence of bile in the stool,
a continued rise in the serum bilirubin level, and no urobilinogen in the urine. Most investigators have advised early
operative intervention, since biliary atresia may give rise to
irreparable damage to the liver within 2½ months. Well-
established cirrhosis has been noted at six weeks, and
almost all successfully treated patients have been operated
on under the age of two months.

After the peritoneal cavity has been entered, liver biopsy
should be performed, and a frozen section may be examined in order to rule out the possibility of intrahepatic bile
duct atresia or neonatal hepatitis. Dissection is initiated
in the region of the gastrohepatic ligament in an attempt
to define the common hepatic ducts and/or atresic segments. If a proximal filled bile duct is not encountered,
attention is directed toward the gallbladder. If the gallbladder contains a lumen, the fundus is opened to determine the characteristics of the fluid within (white bile
indicates obstruction of the cystic duct; normal-appearing
bile in the gallbladder implies that both the hepatic and
cystic ducts are patent). The free flow of saline solution
injected into the gallbladder suggests that the cystic and
common duct are patent. An operative cholangiogram is
useful in defining the pathologic anatomy in this situation.
If no gallbladder is found, exploration is continued in the
region of the porta hepatis with efforts directed at delineating the hepatic duct stump. During dissection possible
residual or rudimentary structures which appear as tiny
cords without lumens should be handled with great care

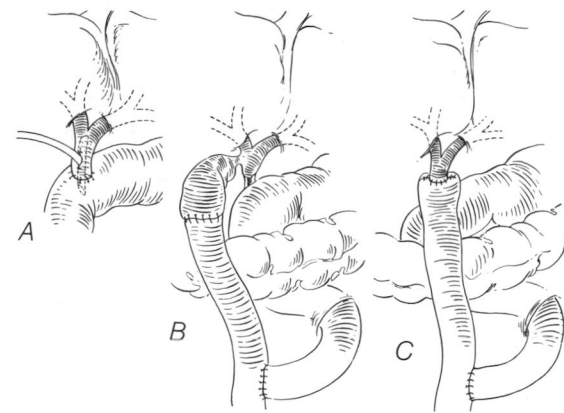

Fig. 31-7. Decompression of biliary tract. *A.* Choledochoduodenostomy. *B.* Cholecystojejunostomy (Roux en Y); *C.* Hepaticodochojejunostomy (Roux en Y). (*From Seymour I. Schwartz,
"Surgical Diseases of the Liver," McGraw-Hill Book Company,
New York, 1964.*)

and preserved, since there is evidence that bile ducts continue to grow after birth.

If a proximal segment of the extrahepatic bile duct
system is patent, this can be decompressed by choledochoduodenostomy, cholecystojejunostomy, or hepaticodocho-
duodenostomy, depending on the circumstance (Fig. 31-7).
In those cases without an identifiable extrahepatic biliary
system, in which liver biopsy demonstrates the presence
of intrahepatic ducts, transhepatic drainage should be attempted. Ksai has popularized the hepatic portoenterostomy with a double Roux en Y anastomosis, including an
external vent to prevent ascending cholangitis. A single
Roux en Y portoenterostomy is also used (Fig. 31-8).

A few patients who had been considered noncorrectible
have been salvaged at a "second look" operation, since
there is some evidence that the development of bile ducts
is merely retarded and growth continues after birth, providing a situation which becomes correctible. Orthotopic
total liver transplantation has been applied in patients with
biliary atresia involving the intrahepatic duct, with result-

Fig. 31-8. Transhepatic drainage. *A.* Cholangiojejunostomy with
partial left hepatic lobectomy. *B.* Cholangiojejunostomy through
main interlobar plane. (*From Seymour I. Schwartz, "Surgical
Diseases of the Liver," McGraw-Hill Book Company, New York,
1964.*)

ant reduction in bilirubin levels and normal liver function extending for several years.

In general, the operative results have been poor. Even when good bile drainage has been established, cholangitis, cirrhosis, and portal hypertension eventually develop.

PHYSIOLOGY

BILE SECRETION. The normal adult with an intact hepatic circulation and consuming an average diet secretes from the hepatic cells 250 to 1,100 ml bile per day. This is an active process which is dependent upon hepatic blood flow and an oxygen supply available to the hepatic cell. The secretion of bile is responsive to neurogenic, humoral, and chemical control. Vagal stimulation increases secretion, whereas stimulation of the splanchnic nerves results in vasoconstriction and decreased bile flow. The release of secretin from the duodenum following the stimulus of hydrochloric acid, breakdown products of protein, and fatty acids results in an increased bile flow. Bile salts are very effective choleretics, acting directly on the liver to augment secretion.

COMPOSITION OF BILE. The main constituents of bile include electrolytes, bile salts, proteins, cholesterol, fats, and bile pigments. Sodium, potassium, calcium, and chloride have approximately the same concentration in bile as in plasma. There is a direct relation between the volume rate of secretion and the electrolyte concentration. As the former increases, there is an increase in bicarbonate and pH and a slight increase in chloride. The pH of liver bile, which usually ranges between 5.7 and 8.6, tending to the alkaline side, varies with the diet, an increase in protein ingestion shifting the pH to the acid side.

Bile salts act as anions which are balanced by sodium. The major salts, cholic, deoxycholic, and chenodeoxycholic acids, conjugate with taurine or glycine and are present in the bile in concentrations of 10 to 20 mEq/L. The bile salt anion has extremly weak osmotic activity because of its tendency to form large molecular aggregates. Proteins are present in lesser concentrations than in plasma, with the exception of mucoproteins and lipoproteins, which contribute to the composition of bile but are not present in plasma. Liver bile contains 0.6 to 1.7 Gm/L unesterified cholesterol, 1 to 5 Gm/L lecithin, and 3 Gm/L neutrofat, which in turn consists of palmitic, oleic, and linoleic acids. The concentrations of both cholesterol and phospholipids are lower in liver bile than in plasma.

The color of the bile secreted by the liver is related to the presence of the pigment bilirubin diglucuronide, which is the metabolic product of hemoglobin and is secreted into the bile in concentrations 100 times greater than that present in the plasma. After this pigment has been acted upon by the bacteria in the intestine and converted into urobilinogen, a small fraction of the urobilinogen is absorbed and also secreted into the bile. A variety of dyes foreign to the body, such as sulfobromophthalein (BSP), rose bengal, and indocyanine green, are removed from the blood by the liver, concentrated, and secreted into the bile.

GALLBLADDER FUNCTION. The gallbladder provides storage and concentration of bile, using the mechanisms of absorption, secretion, and motor activity. Sodium, chloride, and water are selectively absorbed, while the absorption of potassium and calcium is less complete and the concentration of bicarbonate in the gallbladder bile is twice that in plasma. This absorption of water and electrolytes results in a tenfold concentration of bile salts, bile pigments, and cholesterol in relation to levels present in liver bile. The gallbladder mucosa has the greatest absorptive power per unit area of any structure in the body, and this rapid absorption prevents a rise in pressure within the biliary system under normal circumstances.

Secretion of mucus in amounts approximating 20 ml/24 hr, protects the mucosa from the lytic action of bile and facilitates the passage of bile through the cystic duct. This mucus makes up the colorless "white bile" present in hydrops of the gallbladder resulting from obstruction of the cystic duct. The gallbladder also secretes calcium in the presence of inflammation or obstruction of the cystic duct.

Motor activity is a critical function, since the passage of bile into the duodenum requires the coordinated contraction of the gallbladder and relaxation of the sphincter of Oddi. In addition to rhythmic contractions occurring two to six times per minute and mediating of pressure less than 30 mm water, tonic contractions lasting 5 to 30 minutes increase the pressure within the gallbladder up to 300 mm water. Since the hepatic secretory pressure is 375 mm water and is greater than the maximal pressure mediated within the gallbladder, the passage of bile is dependent upon the relaxation of the sphincter of Oddi. The gallbladder empties following humoral or nervous stimulation. The main stimulus in man is cholecystokinin, which is released from the intestinal mucosa in response to food, particularly fat entering the duodenum. Following the intravenous injection of cholecystokinin, the gallbladder begins to contract in 1 to 2 minutes and is two-thirds evacuated within 30 minutes. Evacuation of the gallbladder occurs a half hour after a fatty meal. Cholecystokinin also relaxes the terminal bile duct, the sphincter of Oddi, and the duodenal musculature. Splanchnic sympathetic stimulation is inhibitory to the motor activity of the gallbladder, while the vagus stimulates contraction. Although vagotomy for duodenal ulcer will increase the size and volume of the gallbladder, the rate of emptying is unchanged. A gallbladder which contains calculi should be removed concomitantly with vagotomy in view of a significant incidence of early postoperative cholecystitis in this circumstance reported by Schein. Parasympathomimetic drugs such as pilocarpine and neostigmine contract the gallbladder, whereas atropine tends to relax the organ. Magnesium sulfate acts as a potent evacuator of the gallbladder. Hydrochloric acid and bile salts have little direct effect on motor activity.

The common bile duct was generally regarded as an inert tube until recent cineradiographic studies demonstrated waves of peristalsis. The sphincter of Oddi is a major factor in the evacuation of bile. During starvation, the sphincter maintains an intraductal pressure approximating the maximal expulsive power of the gallbladder, i.e., 300 mm water, and thus prevents evacuation. Following the ingestion of food, this is reduced to 100 mm water. When pressures within the biliary system are greater than 360 mm water, there is suppression of bile secretion. Following obstruction or occlusion of the common bile duct, the time required to reach this pressure level and to result in jaundice is dependent upon the presence and function of the gallbladder. When the gallbladder is absent, the bilirubin levels are raised within 6 hours of total occlusion, while with a functioning gallbladder jaundice may not occur for 46 to 48 hours.

Motor Dysfunction. Biliary dyskinesia, a term introduced by Westphal in 1923, lacks objective findings. It was originally used to describe functional disturbances of biliary tract motility which occurred in the absence of anatomic changes and were related to alterations in autonomic reflex activity. Subsequently, the term has been applied to both this primary condition and situations secondary to other biliary tract diseases, such as cholecystitis and cholelithiasis, and following biliary tract surgical treatment. However, the origin of biliary tract pain itself has not been precisely defined. Experiments inducing gallbladder contraction by fatty foods and cholecystokinin in the presence of a closed sphincter of Oddi have demonstrated that pain can result from motor incoordination. The factor of distension remains suspect, but this is difficult to implicate, since above pressures of 300 to 360 mm water bile secretion ceases. Acute distension of the common bile duct produced by inflation of a balloon-tipped catheter results in colicky pain. When identical pressures are used but dilatation is increased gradually, distress rather than colic results. Biliary tract pain has also been related to spasm of the sphincter of Oddi per se. Recently, Jutras has introduced the concept of hyperplastic cholecystoses, characterized by a functional abnormality manifested by hyperconcentrating and excessive emptying of the gallbladder on cholecystogram. Cholecystectomy is reported to be curative in symptomatic patients, but results are difficult to evaluate.

DIAGNOSIS OF BILIARY TRACT DISEASE

(See also Jaundice, in Chap. 24.)

Radiologic Studies

ROUTINE ABDOMINAL X-RAYS (Fig. 31-9). Plain films of the abdomen prior to the administration of any radiopaque material are indicated, since biliary calculi have been demonstrated in up to 15 percent of cases, and faintly calcified stones may be rendered invisible when contrast materials surround them. Demonstration of calculi on plain films is dependent upon the presence of calcium. Bile pigment calculi, which are characteristically associated with hemolytic disorders, are nonradiopaque, but in 10 percent of the cases they contain sufficient amounts of calcium to be noted on routine x-ray. Similarly, the pure cholesterol calculus is nonradiopaque, whereas calcium carbonate calculi are all visible. Gallstones formed in association with infection or inflammation are generally

Fig. 31-9. Routine abdominal x-ray demonstrating radiopaque biliary calculi in gallbladder.

mixed and contain two or all elements. Their visibility is dependent upon the amount of calcium present.

CHOLECYSTOGRAPHY. In 1924, Graham and Cole introduced the use of contrast media for visualizing the gallbladder. There has been a gradual improvement in the radiopacity and toxicity of the contrast media, and the radiologic examination which was limited to the gallbladder has been extended to visualization of the bile ducts. In the 1950s, biligrafin and cholegrafin were administered intravenously to provide for rapid visualization of the biliary tract independent of the gallbladder's ability to concentrate. These drugs outline the major intrahepatic and extrahepatic ducts, and occasionally the gallbladder will visualize with cholegrafin after failure to do so with an orally administered agent such as Telepaque.

Successful visualization of the gallbladder by a radiopaque iodine-containing compound is dependent upon blood flow to the liver, functional ability of the liver cell to excrete the dye into the bile, patency of the hepatic and cystic duct system, and water absorption by the gallbladder to concentrate the excreted dye. Most diseases of the gallbladder reduce the absorptive capacity in the mucosa; an exception is cholesterosis, in which the dye may concentrate beyond normal. The primary examination of the gallbladder should be performed with an oral medium, while intravenous examination is used to define the common duct and extrahepatic bile duct, particularly in the absence of the gallbladder.

Oral Cholecystography. This procedure (Fig. 31-10) provides visualization of the normal gallbladder. Subsequent to the ingestion of a fatty meal, contraction begins promptly, and within 40 minutes the gallbladder should be reduced to at least one-third or one-fourth of its normal size. The abnormal cholecystogram may demonstrate poor visualization or nonvisualization of the gallbladder or may indicate the presence of filling defects such as calculi or

Fig. 31-10. Oral cholecystogram. *A.* Normal filled gallbladder. *B.* Normal emptying subsequent to fatty meal. This film also shows cystic duct and common bile duct and entrance of dye into duodenum. *C.* Calculi present in gallbladder as evidenced by radiolucent areas.

tumors. Reliability of the Telepaque examination has been reported as 98 percent accurate when compared with surgical findings. Nonvisualization with the use of the dye may be caused by failure to retain the oral medication, faulty absorption such as with pyloric obstruction, hepatic dysfunction, hepatic or cystic duct obstruction, loss of concentrating ability of the gallbladder mucosa, or faulty x-ray technique. Oral cholecystography is seldom effective if the serum bilirubin is over 1.8 mg/100 ml. Approximately 2 percent of nonopacifying gallbladders have been found to be normal at operation with no obvious reason for failure to concentrate the oral dye. Oral cholecystography is the best method of demonstrating calculi, either by direct visualization of filling defects or by demonstration of a nonopacifying gallbladder, which is associated with a 90 percent incidence of calculi. This technique has also been applied to the differential diagnosis of acute cholecystitis. If the gallbladder fills, the lesion can be excluded, but failure to fill is of little significance, since it may be related to vomiting and the patient's inability to retain or absorb contrast medium. Examination of the extrahepatic bile ducts by oral cholecystography can be accomplished in approximately 80 percent of patients whose gallbladders are visualized. Recently cholecystoki-

nin (CCK) cholangiography has been used to define gallbladder disease in patients with suggestive pain and a normal cholecystogram. 75 Ivy units of CCK are instilled intraduodenally or intravenously. The normal gallbladder will demonstrate a volume reduction greater than 50 percent in 20 minutes.

Intravenous Cholecystography. This technique (Fig. 31-11) is applied when there is failure of the gallbladder to visualize after oral cholecystography or there is inability of the patient to retain or absorb the orally administered medication. The technique is particularly applicable to the visualization of bile ducts in cholecystectomized patients, since oral administration of Telepaque results in demonstration of the ducts in only about 40 percent of the cases. The test is preferable to oral cholecystography to evaluate the status of the gallbladder in a patient with an acute condition in the abdomen. Intravenous cholecystography is of little value if the serum bilirubin is greater than 3.5 mg/100 ml, with the exception of the situation of hemolytic jaundice, in which case there is no impairment of gallbladder visualization. The standard dose of 20 ml of 52 percent Cholagrafin is associated with fewer adverse reactions than the infusion technique. The SGOT is elevated in 9 percent of patients receiving the single dose and in 18 percent of those receiving a double dose.

PERCUTANEOUS TRANSHEPATIC CHOLANGIOGRAPHY. See also Jaundice, in Chap. 24.

Fig. 31-11. Intravenous cholangiogram showing normal common duct and arborization of ducts in the liver. There is no evidence of ductal obstruction or choledocholithiasis.

Operative Cholangiography (T-tube Cholangiography). This procedure (Fig. 31-12) is frequently performed in the operating room at the time of exploration of the biliary tract, with injection of radiopaque material either into the cystic duct or into the T tube placed in the common duct. The main application of cystic duct cholangiography is to avoid common bile duct exploration. It is also used to identify calculi which have escaped palpation in order to avoid a subsequent common duct exploration. The technique may contribute to confusion because of failure of the opaque medium to enter the duodenum despite the fact that there is no abnormality present in the sphincter of Oddi and no obstruction within the common duct. Postoperative cholangiography is usually performed in the x-ray suite prior to removal of a T tube to demonstrate the patency of the common duct, the absence of retained stones, and free passage of bile into the duodenum. The most rewarding technique employs 10 to 15 ml 50 percent Hypaque diluted to 30 ml with saline solution and administered slowly.

Isotopic Scans (Fig. 31-13)

A variety of isotopes which are secreted in the bile have been used to define gallbladder function and pathology. [131]I rose Bengal, ^{99m}Tc-dihydrothiotic acid, and ^{99m}Tc-pyridoxylideneglutamate are among the preparations employed. Accumulation of activity in the gallbladder has been recorded by a gamma camera. The isotopic technique has also been combined with computer axial tomography. The advantage of the technique is that the isotopes are administered intravenously and are not associated with the adverse reactions which occasionally accompany intravenous cholecystography. The absence of visualization of the gallbladder is highly suggestive of cholecystitis.

Cholangiomanometry

This procedure, which frequently combines determination of bile duct pressure (normal is 12 ± 3 cm) and flow of an infused solution (normal is 23.0 ± 7 ml/min), is widely used by the European surgeon but rarely used in North America. Proponents of the method suggest that the additional 5 minutes of operative time increases the yield for diagnoses of abnormalities in the common duct, stones in the distal end of the duct, and most particularly organic changes in the sphincter which cause functional changes.

TRAUMA

Penetrating and Nonpenetrating Injuries of the Gallbladder

Injuries of the gallbladder are uncommon, as evidenced by Penn's collective review of 5,670 abdominal injuries in which there was an incidence of 1.9 percent. However, in one series, an incidence of 8.6 percent was recorded for involvement of the gallbladder in war injuries of the abdo-

Fig. 31-12. T-tube cholangiogram demonstrating normal caliber of duct with absence of choledocholithiasis. Liver arborization is normal. Tapering at terminal portion of common bile duct is normal, and radiopaque material is noted in duodenum.

men. Penetrating injuries are usually due to gunshot wounds or stab wounds and occur rarely during attempted needle biopsy of the liver, particularly in patients with obstructive jaundice. Nonpenetrating injuries are most frequently caused by automobile accidents, kicks, blows, and falls. They are extremely rare; only about 50 cases have been reported. The associated visceral damage with both penetrating and nonpenetrating gallbladder injuries includes involvement of the liver in 72 percent, small bowel in 36 percent, colon in 32 percent, and in only 20 percent of the cases the gallbladder alone. Although it is very uncommon for the gallbladder to be the only organ involved with nonpenetrating injuries to the abdomen, isolated involvement of the gallbladder due to penetrating injuries is relatively frequent.

The types of injuries include (1) contusions, (2) avulsion, (3) rupture, and (4) traumatic cholecystitis. Contusion is difficult to verify but may be associated with vague or temporary symptoms which require no specific therapy. The contused area may undergo necrosis and perforate. Avulsion of the gallbladder from its liver bed occurs as a result of nonpenetrating injury. When the gallbladder's attachments are torn, the organ usually hangs by its neck but may be attached only by the cystic duct and artery. Volvulus of the gallbladder may result. Traumatic cholecystectomy, in which the cystic duct, cystic artery, and gallbladder attachments are transected, has been reported. An acutely inflamed gallbladder may be avulsed from the liver as a result of minor trauma. Laceration is the most common type of injury following penetrating wounds but also may result from blunt trauma. Cases of delayed rupture of the gallbladder occur days to weeks following injury. Traumatic cholecystitis is an unusual condition which occurs as a result of blunt trauma. Bleeding into

Fig. 31-13. Normal study in patient with pancreatitis. Thirty minutes before study, patient received 75 units of cholecystokinin. Then 150 uCi ^{131}I-rose Bengal was injected; sequential gamma camera images show accumulation, then slow decline of radioactivity in liver. Gallbladder is discernible by 60 minutes, providing evidence that cystic duct is patent. Some bowel activity is apparent by 60 minutes. At 90 minutes additional injection of cholecystokinin is associated with decrease in gallbladder activity and increase in bowel activity on images. Time-activity curves of liver and gallbladder are graphed below images. Characteristics of these curves varied from patient to patient but were unnecessary for diagnosis in this series. (*After Edward A. Eikman, Ann Int Med, 82:308, 1975.*)

the gallbladder, due to injury either of the gallbladder or of the liver, precipitates cholecystitis and, at times, gangrene of the gallbladder. The retained blood may clot and block the cystic duct, and the patient presents with the manifestations of hematobilia, including intermittent jaundice, colicky pain, hematemesis, and melena.

EFFECTS OF INTRAPERITONEAL BILE. Effects of extravasation of bile into the peritoneal cavity depend upon whether or not the bile is infected. When infected bile escapes into the peritoneal cavity, a fulminating and frequently fatal peritonitis results. On the other hand, when bile is sterile, it is well tolerated and results in a chemical peritonitis which may be relatively mild. In the majority of gallbladder injuries, the organ is normal and the bile is sterile. The fact that sterile bile is relatively innocuous is borne out by the very low mortality rate associated with nonpenetrating wounds of the gallbladder. Penetrating wounds are potentially more serious because of the danger of secondary infection. Continuous leakage of noninfected bile, however, is not innocuous. The extravasated bile may produce ascites or become encysted, and extensive chemical peritonitis causes an outpouring of fluid into the peritoneal cavity from the general circulation which may result in shock. There is also some evidence to indicate that absorption of large amounts of bile salts may be toxic.

CLINICAL MANIFESTATIONS. The diagnosis of involvement of the gallbladder or extrahepatic biliary tract is frequently entertained preoperatively in patients with penetrating injuries, in contrast to a low incidence of diagnosis associated with blunt trauma. Bile leakage through the penetrating wound suggests the possibility of damage to the biliary system, but duodenal laceration may have a similar manifestation. With blunt trauma, manifestations may be delayed for 36 hours or more. This has been related to the fact that there are other serious injuries which mask injury of the biliary tract and that the sterile bile causes only minimal symptoms. The presence of severe shock and pain in the right upper quadrant or lower part of the right side of the chest should make one suspicious. The manifestations of bacterial peritonitis may ensue, or if the bile leakage is minimal, the patient may recover only to subsequently develop ascites or an intraperitoneal cyst. The finding of bile-stained fluid during diagnostic paracentesis is suggestive, but a negative tap does not exclude gallbladder injury. In most instances, the diagnosis is made at laparotomy, emphasizing the necessity for careful examination of the biliary system following abdominal trauma.

TREATMENT. The injured gallbladder has been success-

fully treated by simple suture of the laceration, cholecystostomy, and cholecystectomy. In general, it is preferable
to remove the traumatized gallbladder. Cholecystectomy
is usually quite easy to perform, since the gallbladder is
rarely diseased, and must be performed if the gallbladder
has been avulsed or the cystic artery torn. In the severely
ill patient, cholecystostomy may be used for treatment of
the extensive laceration or traumatic cholecystitis in order
to reduce the time of operative procedure and avoid injury
to the common duct. Although suture of the clean laceration has been successfully used, this should be applied only
infrequently. Prognosis is directly related to the incidence
of associated injuries. In the Korean conflict of the 1950s
there was no mortality in 33 cases of gallbladder injury.

Injury of the Extrahepatic Bile Ducts

Rare cases of solitary penetrating wounds involving the
bile duct have been reported, but there is usually associated trauma to other viscera. Approximately 100 cases of
traumatic rupture of the extrahepatic bile duct have been
reported, and in 15 cases complete transection occurred.
The clinical manifestations are similar to those described
for gallbladder injury, and diagnosis is extremely difficult.

Treatment consists initially of meticulous exploration,
particularly if injury to the gallbladder has been excluded
and bile has been demonstrated retroperitoneally or within
the peritoneal cavity. A Kocher maneuver should be performed to rule out perforation of the common duct behind
the duodenum. The presence of hematoma in this region
should make one suspicious. Complete transection by a
knife of either the common hepatic duct or common bile
duct is best treated by debridement and an end-to-end
anastomosis over a T tube, which should be left in place
for several weeks. If the lower end of the common bile duct
is severely traumatized, and in most cases of blunt trauma,
the proximal end of the duct should be anastomosed to a
Roux en Y of jejunum. The patient should be placed on
antibiotics, such as ampicillin or tetracycline, which
achieve high levels in the bile.

Operative Injury of the Bile Ducts

The great majority of injuries of the extrahepatic biliary
duct system are iatrogenic, occurring in the course of gallbladder surgical procedures. In a 15-year period, the Lahey
Clinic managed 501 patients with stricture of the bile ducts
subsequent to surgical treatment. In over 70 percent of the
cases, the cholecystectomy had apparently been carried out
without incident. In the remaining 20 percent, a variety
of factors were implicated. These included cholecystectomy for contracted gallbladder, intimate association between the ampulla of the gallbladder and the common
hepatic duct, massive hemorrhage at the time of operation
with attempted "blind control," during which the duct was
occluded and traumatized, and excessive tension when
ligating a cystic duct. Lack of appreciation of anatomy and
possible anomalies in the region increase the incidence
of surgical trauma of the common duct.

DIAGNOSIS. In approximately 15 percent of the cases,
ductal injuries are recognized and treated at the time of
operation. The remaining 85 percent become manifest by
either increasing obstructive jaundice or profuse and persistent drainage of bile through a fistula. Jaundice usually
becomes manifest in 2 to 3 days but, in some instances,
does not develop for weeks. It may be continuous or intermittent; if intermittent, it is frequently accompanied by
attacks of chills and fever suggesting ascending cholangitis.
Hepatomegaly almost always accompanies jaundice if it
has been persistent for a period of time, and splenomegaly
may also occur if secondary biliary cirrhosis has evolved.
Some patients do not display the signs or symptoms of
partial or complete blockage until months or years after
surgical treatment. This is related to increasing fibrosis and
narrowing of the channel and repeated episodes of cholangitis, which, in turn, leads to fibrosis. The intravenous
cholangiogram usually fails to demonstrate the stricture.
Percutaneous transhepatic cholangiography may clearly
define the site of obstruction and is a helpful procedure.
When this is performed on patients with prolonged extrahepatic obstructive jaundice, the bile should be removed
before the radiopaque material is injected, and operation
should be carried out shortly after the procedure to prevent
the consequences of extravasated blood and bile.

TREATMENT. Patients with jaundice or persistent fistula
require a vigorous preoperative regimen including a high-
protein, low-fat diet and intravenous administration of
fat-soluble vitamins, particularly vitamin K. If there is
concomitant portal hypertension with bleeding varices, this
preempts repair of the common duct, and the portal hypertension is usually best treated by a splenorenal shunt
because of extensive scarring of the right upper quadrant.
Sedgwick and associates have described 12 such patients,
5 of whom were salvaged.

Operative Approach. Injury of the bile duct recognized
during surgical operation should be corrected with an immediate reconstructive procedure. Restoration of the continuity of the duct with an end-to-end anastomosis over a
T tube may be feasible. Chronic strictures are also preferably treated by axial anastomosis to preserve sphincteric
mechanism, employing a choledocho-choledochostomy or
a hepaticocholedochostomy as indicated. However, direct
anastomosis is usually impractical, in which case the proximal end of the duct should be anastomosed to a Roux en Y
of jejunum. In most instances, the anastomosis is performed over a T or U tube which may be brought out
through either the common duct or the intestine. The
Longmire operation, with transection of the left lobe of the
liver and anastomosis of the jejunum to a large intrahepatic bile duct, has been associated with discouraging
results.

In general, the prognosis is good if the initial repair is
carried out at the time of injury. The operative mortality
of patients with chronic stricture is reported to be 8 percent, and approximately 10 percent of patients die of liver
failure or its attendant complications after leaving the
hospital. A satisfactory result is obtained in about 70 percent of patients after one or more operative procedures.
If the patients are symptom-free 4 years after reconstruction, the cure is almost always permanent.

Fig. 31-14. Three major components of bile (bile salts, lecithin, and cholesterol) plotted on triangular coordinates. Point *P* represents bile consisting of 80 mol percent bile salt, 5 percent cholesterol, and 15 percent lecithin. Line *ABC* represents the maximal solubility of cholesterol in varying mixtures of bile salt and lecithin. Because point *P* falls below line *ABC* and within the zone of a single phase of micellar liquid, this bile is less than saturated with cholesterol. Bile with a composition that would place it above line *ABC* would contain excess cholesterol in supersaturated or precipitated form. (After D. M. Small, Gallstones, N Engl J Med, 279:588, 1968.)

GALLSTONES

COMPOSITION. The major elements involved in the formation of gallstones are cholesterol, bile pigment, and calcium. Other constituents include iron, phosphorus, carbonates, proteins, carbohydrates, mucus, and cellular debris. In Europe and the United States, most stones are made up of the three major elements and have a particularly high content of cholesterol, averaging 71 percent. These stones have a characteristic central nucleus which was initially thought to consist of epithelial desquamation from the inflamed gallbladder wall, but recently it has been shown that the constituents of the nucleus cannot be distinguished from the rest of the stone. Womack has demonstrated that a prosthesis of mucus is essential, and he suggests that crystal growth in gel may be critical. Surrounding the nucleus are layers of cholesterol and pigment. Most mixed stones are not radiopaque, and radiopacity is dependent upon the amount of calcium.

Pure cholesterol stones are uncommon, usually large with smooth surfaces, and solitary. Bilirubin pigment stones are also uncommon, with a characteristic smooth, glistening green or black surface. The pigment stones may be "pure" or consist of calcium bilirubinate. The "pure" pigment stones are usually associated with hemolytic jaundice or situations in which the bile is abnormally concentrated. Increased red blood cell destruction following cardiac valve replacement has resulted in production of

gallstones. Calcium bilirubinate stones are prevalent in Asia, where they constitute 30 to 40 percent of all gallstones. The bilirubinate content of these stones varies between 40 and 50 percent in contrast to the 0.2 to 5 percent bilirubin present in mixed stones. Cholesterol is also present in the calcium bilirubin stone in concentrations of 3 to 26 percent.

FORMATION. Gallstones form as a result of solids settling out of solution. The recent contribution of Small and his associates provides a working model of this process. The solubility of cholesterol (the predominant crystal in westernized countries) depends on the concentrations of conjugated bile salts, phospholipids, and cholesterol in bile. Lecithin is the predominant phospholipid in bile and, although insoluble in aqueous solutions, is dissolved by bile salts in micelles. Cholesterol is also insoluble in aqueous solution but becomes soluble when incorporated into the lecithin–bile salt micelle. By plotting the percentages of cholesterol, lecithin, and bile salts on triangular coordinates (Fig. 31-14), the limits of micellar liquid in which bile is less than saturated with cholesterol may be defined. Above these limits, the bile is either a supersaturated liquid or a two-phase system of liquid bile and solid crystalline cholesterol. When crystals achieve macroscopic size during a period of entrapment in the gallbladder, gallstones form.

Factors which have been implicated in the formation and precipitation of cholesterol include constitutional elements, bacteria, fungi, reflux of intestinal and pancreatic fluid, hormones, and bile stasis. Constitutional elements are best exemplified in the Pima Indians, of whom 70 percent of females by age 30 and 70 percent of males by age 60 have gallstones. The Masai of Africa, on the other hand, do not have gallstones. Evidence in favor of infection as a cause includes the isolation of such organisms as *Escherichia coli, Bacterium typhosum,* and *Streptococcus* from gallbladder walls and centers of stones in a high percentage of cases and the demonstration of slow-growing actinomyces recovered from over half the stones examined in one series. However, the development of gallstones in the absence of infection or inflammation argues against infection as a universal factor. In Oriental people, concretions are known to form about liver flukes and other parasites within the bile ducts.

The reflux factor receives support from the findings of Chaimoff and Dintsman, who demonstrated pancreatic enzymes in the gallbladders of patients with cholelithiasis. Trypsin disturbs colloidal balance, and pancreatic phospholipase A can convert lecithin into toxic lysolecithin. Hormones have been implicated in an unproved correlation between calculi and parity, diabetes, hyperthyroidism, and the predominance in females. It is known that prolonged administration of progesterone and estradiol to rabbits results in the formation of stones, and that symptoms frequently develop in patients during pregnancy.

Stasis, which includes temporary cessation of bile flow into the intestine and stagnation in the gallbladder, has also been assigned a major role. Temporary bile stasis may be due to functional disorders or to a mechanical blockage in the region of the choledochoduodenal junction or gallbladder. The interruption of bile flow to the intestine is associated with an interruption in enterohepatic circulation, which, in turn, is accompanied by a decrease in the output of bile salts and phospholipids, reducing the solubility of cholesterol. When over 20 percent of bile is diverted, the bile salt pool cannot be maintained. Bile salt secretion is also diminished by reduction of the distal third of the intestine, explaining the development of stones in patients with ileal resection or disease.

Solubility has been investigated as a possible regimen to prevent the development of stones in patients at risk and also to dissolve stones already formed. Chenodeoxycholic acid, which replenishes the bile acid pool and reduces cholesterol synthesis and secretion, administered to potential stone formers may return supersaturated bile to its normal composition, preventing stone formation. Oral administration of bile salts can be predicted to dissolve 15 small stones with a cumulative weight of 1 mg in 1 year and one large stone of similar weight in 3 years, according to Small. A question has been raised concerning hepatotoxicity, and the argument is advanced that even if stones disappear, a diseased gallbladder remains.

Asymptomatic Gallstones

Asymptomatic cholelithiasis is rare. Of 3,012 patients with cholecystitis and cholelithiasis, only 134 had no symptoms attributable to gallbladder disease. The liberal use of cholecystography has resulted in the diagnosis of calculi in patients without symptoms referable to the biliary tract. The question has been raised as to whether surgical intervention is indicated in this situation. In several large series of asymptomatic patients with gallstones who were followed without surgical treatment, symptoms developed in 50 percent, and serious complications occurred in 20 percent. An operative mortality of 0.7 percent has been reported for asymptomatic patients, in contrast with 5 percent in cases of acute cholecystitis. The relationship of cholelithiasis and carcinoma of the gallbladder is also of some significance. A review of several series showed that the incidence of calculi in cancer of the gallbladder varied between 65 and 100 percent with a mean of 90 percent. Conversely, the incidence of cancer of the gallbladder in patients with symptomatic gallstones ranged between 1 and 15 percent with a mean of 4.5 percent. However, Comfort et al. reported no carcinoma among 112 patients with asymptomatic cholelithiasis. Based on the high incidence of ultimate development of symptoms or complications and the small risk of carcinoma, it is generally felt that unless there is strong contraindication, the presence of cholelithiasis with or without symptoms is indication for cholecystectomy.

Cystic Duct Obstruction

Calculi, usually of the cholesterol type, may become impacted in the cystic duct or neck of the gallbladder, resulting in a hydrops. The bile is absorbed, and the gallbladder becomes filled and distended with mucinous material. The gallbladder is generally palpable and tender, and the impacted stone with the resulting edema may encroach upon the common duct and cause mild jaundice. Although hydrops may persist with few consequences, early cholecystectomy is generally indicated to avoid the complications of biliary tract infection or perforation of the gallbladder. In questionable cases, isotopic scanning of the gallbladder, following intravenous CCK (cholecystokinin) can define cystic obstruction or patency.

Choledocholithiasis

Common duct stones may be single or multiple and are found in approximately 12 percent of cases subjected to cholecystectomy. Most common duct calculi are formed within the gallbladder and migrate down the cystic duct into the common bile duct. Madden et al. have described stones which are thought to form within the ducts. In patients infected with tropical parasites such as *Clonorchis sinensis* and in other rare instances, stones may form within the hepatic ducts or the common bile duct itself. Although small stones may pass via the common duct into the duodenum, the distal duct with its narrow lumen (2 to 3 mm) and thick wall frequently obstructs their passage. Edema, spasm, or fibrosis of the distal duct secondary to irritation by the calculi contribute to biliary obstruction. The extrahepatic bile ducts become dilated, and there is evidence of laking in the biliary radicals of the liver. There is also thickening of the duct walls and inflammatory cell infiltration. Chronic biliary obstruction may cause secondary biliary cirrhosis with bile thrombi, bile duct proliferation, and fibrosis of the portal tracts. Also associated with chronic obstruction is the development of infection within the bile duct giving rise to ascending cholangitis and occasionally extending up to the liver, resulting in hepatic abscesses. The offending organism is almost always *E. coli*.

CLINICAL MANIFESTATIONS. The manifestations of calculi within the common duct are variable. Stones may be present within the extrahepatic duct system for many years without causing symptoms. Characteristically, the symptom complex consists of colicky pain in the right upper quadrant radiating to the right shoulder with intermittent jaundice accompanied by pale stools and dark urine. Biliary obstruction is usually chronic and incomplete but may be acute or complete. If obstruction is complete, jaundice progresses but is rarely intense. In contrast to patients with neoplastic obstruction of the common bile duct or ampulla of Vater, the gallbladder is usually not distended because of associated inflammation (Courvoisier's law). Liver function tests demonstrate the pattern of obstructive jaundice, and the alkaline phosphatase level usually becomes elevated earlier and remains abnormal for longer periods of time than the icterus index. The prothrombin time is frequently prolonged because the absorption of vitamin K is dependent upon bile entering the intestine, but a normal level can usually be achieved with parenteral vitamin K. Tests of hepatocellular function are generally normal. In patients with ascending cholangitis, Charcot's intermittent fever accompanied by intermittent abdominal pain and jaundice is characteristic.

TREATMENT. The question of stones within the common bile duct is usually resolved surgically. When surgical operation is performed to establish the cause of obstructive jaundice, there is little question whether the duct should be explored, since there is dilatation and thickening of the duct and stones are usually palpable. Criteria for exploration of the common bile duct during cholecystectomy for cholelithiasis have been proposed. The three obvious indications are (1) palpable stones within the common bile duct, (2) dilated common bile duct, and (3) significant jaundice or a definite history of jaundice. Other indications are recurrent chills and fever suggestive of cholangitis, pancreatitis, multiple small stones within the gallbladder, and inflamed gallbladder which is empty of stones in a patient with biliary tract symptoms.

The optimal time for exploration of the common bile duct is during the initial procedure of cholecystectomy, provided acute inflammation does not obscure the anatomy. Recently one large prospective series showed that exploration of the common bile duct in the presence of acute cholecystitis carried no greater risk than during elective cholecystectomy. The higher the incidence of duct exploration at the time of cholecystectomy, the lower the incidence of residual stones but the higher the incidence of negative exploration. Considering all patients, including those with jaundice, the performance of a concomitant choledochostomy at the time of cholecystectomy increases the operative mortality by 0.2 to 1.2 percent. If one excludes the jaundiced patients, there is little difference in operative mortality between cholecystectomy alone and cholecystectomy plus concomitant choledochostomy. But there is a significant increase in postoperative morbidity and hospital stay. In order to avoid the negative duct explorations, an operative cholangiogram via a catheter inserted into the cystic duct has been used. This study will demonstrate the caliber of the duct, and a duct greater than 12 mm in diameter should be considered pathologic. The technique will also indicate the presence or absence of filling defects, in which case air bubbles within the ductal system must be differentiated before applying a diagnosis of choledocholithiasis. With this technique, the incidence of concomitant exploration of the common bile duct has been reduced from 65 to 29 percent, while the incidence of positive exploration has been increased from 23 to 66 percent in one large series. The treatment for stones within the common bile duct or hepatic ducts is surgical removal. Preoperatively, patients with common duct stones should be prepared with fat-soluble vitamins, particularly vitamin K, and if there is evidence of ascending cholangitis, a broad spectrum of antibiotics which achieve high levels in the bile should be administered. At the time of exploration, all stones and sludge should be removed, and free passage into the duodenum should be demonstrated. Removal of stones from the common and hepatic ducts may be facilitated by the use of balloon-tipped catheters. As instrumentation was refined, choledochoscopic techniques have been more widely applied. After exploring the common duct, a T tube is inserted prior to closure and drainage maintained for approximately 1 week, at which time a T tube cholangiogram is performed in order to demonstrate patency of the duct and absence of retained stones. If these criteria are met, the T tube then can be removed. If there is obstruction of the distal duct, transduodenal sphincteroplasty and

removal of the stone may be performed, or choledochoduodenostomy may be carried out. Choledochoduodenostomy has become increasingly popular for patients, particularly the elderly, with enlarged ducts and multiple retained stones. A wide sphincteroplasty is preferred by others.

RETAINED COMMON DUCT STONES. If stones are noted to be present when a T-tube cholangiogram is performed postoperatively, there are four general approaches which can be entertained. Small stones, particularly those located in the branches of the hepatic duct, may be disregarded since the majority will remain asymptomatic and if symptoms ensue, operative extraction is not associated with significantly increased morbidity. A second approach employs either flushing or chemical dissolution. Sodium cholate, 100 mmol in saline solution buffered to a pH of 7.5, is continuously infused into the T tube over a 14-day period at a rate of 30 ml/hour. Way and Dunphy have reported success in about two-thirds of the cases, but others have had less satisfying experiences. This approach is associated with diarrhea, which can be controlled by administering cholestyramine; there is also some suggestion of damage to the duct wall. Another approach of dissolution employs heparin, which acts by altering the zeta potential of particles. Heparin, 25,000 units in 250 ml saline solution, is infused every 8 hours as a continuous drip into the T tube. Complete dissolution of stones has been observed in a few cases within five days.

The most encouraging approach employs mechanical extraction of the retained stone under radiographic control. Mazzariello achieved success in 92.7 percent of 220 cases, while Burhenne and associates, reporting on 612 patients managed at 38 hospitals, reported no deaths and no significant complications, coupled with a 91 percent success rate. The T tube is generally left in place for at least 4 weeks after the operation; it is then extracted and a polyethylene catheter is used to instill radiopaque material into the common duct. A Dormia basket is then advanced through the catheter to entrap the stone (Fig. 31-15).

If the T tube had been removed and a common duct stone demonstrated cholangiographically, transduodenal papillotomy with extraction of the stone under endoscopic visualization has been reported. Operative intervention is indicated in some cases if there is evidence of obstruction and/or cholangitis, or if nonoperative methods fail.

Gallstone Ileus

Mechanical obstruction of the gastrointestinal tract caused by gallstones is a relatively infrequent occurrence. Gallstone ileus causes 1 to 2 percent of mechanical small intestinal obstructions and has been associated with high mortality rates. Recently, mortality rates of less than 10 percent have been reported.

Since cholelithiasis occurs three to six times more commonly in the female than in the male, the higher incidence of gallstone ileus in the female is to be anticipated. Preponderance in the female is actually higher than one would expect, and in several series all patients were female. It is characteristically a disease of the aged, with an average

Fig. 31-15. Technical steps for retained common duct stone extraction. 1. Repeat T-tube cholangiogram is obtained on the day of stone extraction 4 to 5 weeks after choledochotomy. 2. After the location of the retained stone has been ascertained, the T tube is withdrawn. 3. Using the sinus tract of the T tube, the steerable catheter is guided into the bile duct, and its movable tip is advanced beyond the retained stone. 4. The basket is inserted through the steerable catheter, the catheter is withdrawn, and the basket is opened. 5. The open basket is withdrawn in order to engage the stone. The basket is only retracted, never advanced, outside the enclosure of the steerable catheter. 6. The stone is extracted through the drain tract. (*After H. J. Burhenne, Radium Therapy and Nuclear Medicine, Amer J Roentgenol, 117:388, 1973.*)

age of sixty-four, and is unusual under the age of fifty. Associated diseases are common, diabetes occurring in 50 percent and major cardiovascular disorders in 58 percent.

The process usually begins with formation of the stone within the gallbladder, but cases have been reported in which the gallbladder was not present, having been removed several years prior to the intestinal obstruction. After the gallstone has left the gallbladder, it may obstruct the alimentary tract in one of two ways: rarely, it enters the peritoneal cavity, causing kinking or inflammation and extrinsic obstruction of the intestine; more commonly, the blockage is caused by the entrance of the stone into the gastrointestinal tract, producing an intraluminal type of obstruction. The stone may enter the duodenum via the common duct, but this is unusual, and almost always the offending calculus enters through a cholecystoenteric fistula. The fistulous tract may connect the gallbladder with the stomach, duodenum, jejunum, ileum, or colon. In addition, internal biliary fistulas may communicate with the pleural or pericardial cavities, tracheobronchial tree, pregnant uterus, ovarian cyst, renal pelvis, and urinary bladder. In a series of 176 fistulas caused by gallstones, the duodenum was involved in 101, the colon in 33, the stomach in 7, and multiple sites in 11.

The fistula probably originates with a stone obstructing the cystic duct, acute cholecystitis, empyema, and the formation of adhesions between the gallbladder and adjacent viscera. Perforation then occurs between the intimately adherent organs, and the stone traverses the fistula. The cholecystoenteric fistula then frequently closes, and only a fibrous remnant remains. Having entered the alimentary tract, the gallstone, which is usually single, may be vomited or passed spontaneously per rectum. The size of the stone is important, since stones smaller than 2 to 3 cm usually pass. When obstruction occurs, the site is usually at the terminal ileum, which is the narrowest portion of the small intestine. Of 154 collective cases, the duodenum was obstructed in 6, the jejunum in 14, the proximal ileum in 6, the middle ileum in 31, the terminal ileum in 88, the colon in 3, and the rectum in 2. When a gallstone blocks the small intestine, the morbid anatomic and physiologic effects of a mechanical obstruction pertain. There are extremely large losses of fluid into the intestine. Edema, ulceration, or necrosis of the bowel may occur, and perforation may result.

CLINICAL MANIFESTATIONS. A past history suggestive of cholelithiasis is present in 50 to 75 percent of patients. Symptoms of acute cholecystitis immediately preceding the onset of gallstone ileus are extremely uncommon, occurring in one-quarter to one-third of the cases. A history of jaundice is present in about 10 percent of the cases. Occasionally, there may be an initial episode of pain suggestive of biliary colic, but major pain is usually not experienced until the intestinal colic results. There is associated cramping, nausea, and vomiting which may be intermittent. When complete small intestinal obstruction occurs, the vomiting increases and the patient becomes obstipated. Analysis of the incidence of varying symptoms indicates that vomiting is present in almost 100 percent, cramps in 90 percent, distension in 90 percent, obstipation in 78 percent, and feculent vomiting in 67 percent. Serum electrolytes reveal the pattern of lower intestinal obstruction with marked hypochloremia, hyponatremia, hypokalemia, and an elevated carbonate level.

The correct preoperative diagnosis is infrequently made, ranging between 13 to 30 percent in several series. The usual diagnosis is that of intestinal obstruction of unknown cause. Radiologic examination may be diagnostic if air is demonstrated within the biliary tract (Fig. 31-16). Flat, upright, and lateral films plus spot films over the liver are indicated if the diagnosis is considered. The plain x-ray reveals the pattern of small intestinal obstruction, and in less than 20 percent of the cases a stone is visualized. The diagnosis has also been based on the migration of a previously observed radiopaque gallstone.

TREATMENT. The patient often requires vigorous fluid and electrolyte replacement in order to correct deficiency, and a nasogastric tube is used to decompress the stomach. Definitive therapy consists of locating the stone or stones, enterotomy proximal to the stone, and removing the offending calculi with closure of the intestine. The recurrence rate of gallstone ileus is 5 to 9 percent, and it is important

Fig. 31-16. Gallstone ileus. *A.* Radiopaque calculus present in right lower quadrant; suggestion of air in biliary tract within liver. *B.* Demonstration of air in intrahepatic biliary system.

to palpate the intestine, gallbladder, and common duct for retained stones, particularly if the obstructing stone is faceted. Either concomitant or planned interval cholecystectomy and closure of the fistula, if patent, is indicated, since recurrent symptoms or complications develop in one-third of the patients and in eight cases carcinoma of the gallbladder was either present or developed 5 to 16 years after removal of the obstructing gallstone. Performance of concomitant cholecystectomy is determined by the patient's general condition, and since many of these patients are extremely ill and depleted, prolongation of the operative procedure is contraindicated.

INFLAMMATORY AND OTHER BENIGN LESIONS

Cholecystitis

In 85 to 95 percent of the cases, inflammation of the gallbladder is associated with calculi. Whether the stones represent cause or effect has not been defined, but they are generally implicated as a cause of the acute inflammatory process. Stasis of the gallbladder with consequent maintenance of contact between stagnant bile and the gallbladder wall is also considered a cause of cholecystitis. A bacterial cause of cholecystitis has been proposed, and positive bile cultures have been noted in 60 percent of patients with acute cholecystitis. A variety of organisms have been cultured both in acute and chronically inflamed gallbladders. *E. coli,* streptococci, *Aerobacter aerogenes, Salmonella,* and clostridia have all been implicated, but in many cases of both acute and chronic cholecystitis cultures of the bile are negative. In addition to bile, which in its concentrated or desiccated form is known to cause acute cholecystitis, pancreatic juice with its enzymatic properties is also considered a chemical irritant. Since pressures developed in the pancreatic duct are generally greater than those in the biliary tract, the presence of a common channel permits entrance of pancreatic juice into the gallbladder; the frequent finding of amylase in the bile supports this assumption.

ACUTE CHOLECYSTITIS

In the overwhelming majority of cases, acute cholecystitis is associated with an obstruction of the neck of the gallbladder or cystic duct due to stones impacted in Hartmann's pouch. Direct pressure of the calculus on the mucosa results in ischemia, necrosis, and ulceration with swelling, edema, and impairment of venous return. These processes, in turn, increase and extend the intensity of the inflammation. The ulceration may be so extensive that the mucosa is frequently hard to define on microscopic examination and there are segmented leukocytes infiltrating all layers. The results of necrosis are perforation with pericholecystic abscess formation, fistulization, or bile peritonitis. In the past, acute cholecystitis secondary to systemic infection occurred most commonly with typhoid fever, but this is now rare. Acute cholecystitis, due either to generalized sepsis or to stasis and/or impaction of a calculus, may occur while the patient is recovering from trauma or an operation. Among other causes of acute cholecystitis are the vascular effects of collagen disease, terminal states of hypertensive vascular disease, and thrombosis of the main cystic artery. Less than 1 percent of acutely inflamed gallbladders contain a malignant tumor which may play a role in causing obstruction. The incidence of common duct calculi is similar in acute and chronic cholecystitis, averaging 7 to 15 percent.

CLINICAL MANIFESTATIONS. Most attacks of acute cholecystitis occur in patients who give a past history compatible with chronic cholecystitis and cholelithiasis. Acute cholecystitis can occur at any age, but the greatest incidence is between the fourth and eighth decades, and patients over sixty comprise between one-quarter and one-third of the group. Caucasians are afflicted much more frequently than blacks.

The onset of acute symptoms is frequently related to a vigorous attempt of the gallbladder to empty its contents, usually after a heavy, fatty, or fried meal. Moderate to severe pain is experienced in the right upper quadrant or epigastrium and may radiate to the back in the region of the angle of the scapula or in the interscapular area. The patient is often febrile, and vomiting may be severe. Tenderness, usually along the right costal margin, often associated with rebound tenderness and spasm, is characteristic. The gallbladder is palpable in about one-third to three-quarters of the cases. Mild icterus may be present and can be related to calculi within the ampulla and edema encroaching upon the common duct. Moderate to marked icterus suggests the presence of associated choledocholithiasis but can occur with isolated cholecystitis.

The differential diagnosis includes perforation or penetration of peptic ulcer, appendicitis, hepatitis, myocardial ischemia or infarction, pneumonia, pleurisy, and herpes zoster involving an intercostal nerve.

The hemogram usually demonstrates leukocytosis with a shift to the left. Roentgenograms of the chest and abdomen are indicated to rule out thoracic processes. A radiopaque calculus is noted in less than 20 percent of the cases. The icterus index or serum bilirubin levels may determine the presence of common duct obstruction. Although the elevated amylase level is generally regarded as evidence of acute pancreatitis, levels as high as 1,000 Somogyi units have been associated with acute cholecystitis uncomplicated by pancreatitis. To rule out myocardial ischemia, an electrocardiogram should be made on any patient over the age of forty-five being considered for surgical treatment. However, acute cholecystitis may be responsible for some changes. Intravenous cholecystography and isotopic scans have been used diagnostically in patients presenting with acute abdominal pain. If the cholecystogram is normal, it is highly unlikely that cholecystitis is present. An abnormal oral cholecystogram is not necessarily diagnostic of biliary tract disease, since the oral Telepaque may not be absorbed in a patient with acute abdominal pain.

TREATMENT. Conflicting opinions concerning the management of acute cholecystitis, with particular reference to the optimal time for surgical intervention, persist. For the purpose of discussion, early operation is defined as one performed within 72 hours after the onset of the acute process; intermediate operation is one carried out between 72 hours and the cessation of clinical manifestations; delayed operative management permits the acute inflammatory process to subside; and scheduled elective surgery is performed at an interval of 6 weeks to 3 months.

The proponents of the conservative treatment, i.e., delayed operative management, base their thesis on the following premises: (1) Most cases of acute cholecystitis subside on conservative management without significant complications. (2) Surgery performed in the presence of inflammation with vascular congestion may be injurious as a result of spreading infection. (3) The acute inflammatory changes obscure the anatomy and lead to technical errors. In the presence of intense inflammatory process, exploration of the common duct for stones is compromised. (4) Many of the patients with acute cholecystitis have associated diseases and do not represent optimal risk for surgical intervention.

Nonoperative management is directed at creating a situation of functional rest for the gallbladder and upper gastrointestinal tract and relaxing spasm of the sphincter of Oddi. The regimen includes restriction of fluid and food intake and continuous nasogastric suction. Anticholinergic drugs are administered in an effort to decrease spasm of the sphincter. Pain is treated with small amounts of Demerol, while morphine is withheld, because it causes sphincteric spasm. Antibiotics which achieve high levels in bile are advised by many physicians.

The proponents of nonoperative management of acute cholecystitis argue against the importance of perforation and bile peritonitis. In one series of 679 patients subjected to laparotomy, although perforation was noted in 9 percent of the patients, only 3 percent demonstrated free perforation into the peritoneal cavity. In another series of 441 patients treated surgically, there were only 2 instances of free perforation, while 11 patients had pericholecystic abscesses. In several series, there was no serious morbidity associated with perforation.

The arguments for early or intermediate cholecystectomy point out that about 5 percent of patients fail to respond to medical management and more than half of the patients who respond initially experience an exacerbation. Unless there is a medical contraindication, eventual surgical intervention is indicated for almost all patients with cholecystitis and cholelithiasis. Low mortality rates have been reported for early cholecystectomy, and these rates are quite comparable with those reported for the elective procedure. The risk of operating in an area of inflammation, in the early stages of acute cholecystitis, is refuted. In the first 2 to 3 days after the onset of symptoms, although edema may be significant, there is usually little difficulty in displaying the duct system. If the structures can be safely defined, exploration of the common duct for stones can be carried out without increased risk. If early operation is performed and the inflammatory process has progressed to obscure the structures, cholecystostomy, which can be carried out with a low mortality rate, speeds the patient's recovery. Acute cholecystitis in the diabetic is associated with higher incidences of complications and

Fig. 31-17. Emphysematous cholecystitis. Gallbladder is shown as gas-filled organ.

mortality than in the nondiabetic. Schein reports significant improvement in these statistics with early cholecystectomy.

In the United States the majority of surgeons favor early operation, whereas in Great Britain it is more customary to treat the condition conservatively, unless there is specific indication for surgical intervention.

The mortality rate for emergency cholecystectomy ranges from near zero to 5 percent and, in several series, is comparable to the mortality rate for elective cholecystectomy. In one series, the mortality rate for cholecystectomy was 3.9 percent, while the nonoperative patients had a mortality of 5.5 percent. In the first truly randomized series, van der Linden and Sunzel showed that early cholecystectomy was as safe as the nonoperative approach and that the period of morbidity and disability was shortened. Cholecystostomy for extremely ill patients was accompanied by a mortality rate of 15 percent in one series, in contrast to the 1.5 percent mortality rate reported by Dunphy and Ross.

Author's Approach. If the diagnosis of acute cholecystitis is relatively unequivocal and the patient presents within 3 days of the onset of symptoms, early operation is performed. Immediate *emergency* cholecystectomy is rarely indicated, and the patient should be thoroughly investigated and prepared prior to operation. If the patient is extremely ill with a palpable gallbladder, surgical treatment is usually carried out within 24 hours of admission.

If possible, cholecystectomy is performed. However, if the patient will not tolerate this procedure because of extreme toxicity or otherwise complicating medical illness, a cholecystostomy, under local anesthesia, is carried out. If a cholecystectomy has been planned but the inflammatory process is so marked that it compromises the dissection, cholecystostomy terminates the procedure. Patients whose symptoms continue to progress under medical management are operated upon. With associated cholangitis, a course of antibiotics is initiated, and early operation is performed for relief of obstruction. If the patient presents 72 hours after the onset of symptoms and shows signs of improvement during the early periods of hospitalization, surgical intervention is deferred, and an elective operation is planned in approximately 6 weeks in most instances, but there is no hesitation in operating after the "golden" 72 hours.

At the time of surgical treatment for acute cholecystitis, the indications for common bile duct exploration are the same as those which pertain during elective cholecystectomy. Patients with obstructive jaundice due to stones or ascending cholangitis require early surgical relief of obstruction and drainage of the common bile duct. Palpable stones and ductal dilatation demonstrated at operation constitute indications for common duct exploration. Pancreatitis is not, in itself, an indication in the presence of acute cholecystitis, since the yield is small, and it is best to leave a catheter in the cystic duct for future study. If indications for exploration of the common duct are present but the inflammatory process compromises dissection, cholecystostomy is performed and the stones are removed from the gallbladder. An attempt may be made to pass a catheter via the cystic duct into the common bile duct.

Emphysematous Cholecystitis. This is a rare form of acute, usually gangrenous, cholecystitis, caused by gas-forming organisms and characterized radiologically by the presence of gas in the gallbladder (Fig. 31-17). Approximately 100 cases have been reviewed in this century. Unlike ordinary acute cholecystitis, which is more prevalent among women, emphysematous cholecystitis is more often found in men, with a sex incidence of 75 percent for males and 25 percent for females. Pathogenesis is related to acute inflammation of the gallbladder, which often begins aseptically, complicated by a secondary infection with gas-forming bacilli. These may reach the gallbladder by bile ducts, bloodstream, or lymphatic channels and grow in an anaerobic environment. The clinical manifestations are similar to those present in acute cholecystitis. In approximately half the patients, a history of previous gallbladder attacks can be elicited. Cholelithiasis is also present in half the patients, who are frequently diabetic. The diagnosis is usually made on the basis of roentgenographic findings which show a globular shadow, distended with gas, in the region of the gallbladder. Later, intramural or submucosal gas may appear, and gas may also appear in the pericholecystic area denoting extension of the pathologic process outside the confines of the gallbladder. The treatment of choice is early operation, since the incidence of free perforation is reported to be 40 to 60 percent. Cholecystectomy is indicated, but if this is not feasible, cholecystostomy should be performed. In 9 percent of cases, choledocholithiasis is present, and exploration of the common duct may be required. Although positive bile cultures are found in only half the cases, antibiotics directed toward the clostridial and coliform organisms are indicated. The mortality rate is significantly greater than that for nonemphysematous cholecystitis.

CHRONIC CHOLECYSTITIS

Chronic inflammation of the gallbladder is generally associated with cholelithiasis and consists of round cell infiltration and fibrosis of the wall. Buried crypts of mucosa (Rokitansky-Aschoff sinuses) may be seen dipping into the mucosa (Fig. 31-18). Obstruction by gallstones of the neck of the cystic duct may produce a mucocele of the gallbladder (hydrops). The bile is initially sterile but may be secondarily infected with coliform bacilli, streptococci, and occasionally clostridia or *Salmonella* (typhoid). Secondary effects of cholecystitis include obstruction of the common duct, cholangitis, perforation of the gallbladder with formation of a pericholecystic abscess or a cholecystoenteric fistula, bile peritonitis, pancreatitis, and carcinoma of the gallbladder.

CLINICAL MANIFESTATIONS. The patients generally present with moderate intermittent abdominal pain in the right upper quadrant and epigastrium, occasionally radiating to the scapula and interscapular region. There is usually a history of intolerance of fatty and/or fried foods, and the patient may have noted intermittent nausea and anorexia. If the patient is not experiencing acute pain, there may be no diagnostic findings on physical examination. Occasionally tenderness is elicited over the gallbladder. This is usually maximal during inspiration. The diagnosis is usually established by an oral cholecystogram, which demonstrates either the absence of filling of the gallbladder or the presence of stones.

TREATMENT. The treatment of chronic cholecystitis and cholelithiasis is cholecystectomy, and the results are usually excellent. Early cholecystectomy is particularly important for the diabetic patient. Operative mortality of less than 1 percent has been reported for large series. Seventy-five percent of patients undergoing cholecystectomy for cholelithiasis are completely relieved of all preoperative symptoms, and the remaining 25 percent have only mild symptoms which are apparently unrelated to the biliary system.

POSTCHOLECYSTECTOMY SYNDROME. This ill-defined syndrome refers to symptoms which either develop subsequent to or continue in spite of cholecystectomy. In patients with abdominal symptoms subsequent to cholecystectomy for chronic cholecystitis and cholelithiasis, these symptoms are usually related to an extrabiliary cause such as hiatal hernia, peptic ulceration, or pancreatitis. However, symptoms may also be due to a residual stone in the common bile duct, residual cystic duct stones, or spasm of the sphincter of Oddi.

The *cystic duct stump* is rarely responsible for clinical manifestations similar to those of cholecystitis. It has been thought that the residual stump becomes a diseased gallbladder undergoing changes of inflammation and capable of forming calculi which may pass into the common duct.

However, cholangiographic studies have recently demonstrated that abnormalities in the insertion of the cystic duct are quite common, and it is probable that, in many instances, a significant length of cystic duct remains after cholecystectomy. Since many of the patients with the "cystic duct syndrome" have demonstrated calculi in the extrahepatic biliary system, it is difficult to determine which factor is responsible for postcholecystectomy symptoms.

ACALCULOUS CHOLECYSTITIS

Acute and chronic inflammatory disease of the gallbladder can occur without stones. Mackey reported recurrent symptoms after cholecystectomy in 36 percent of 264 cases in which stones were not present, while Glenn and Mannix reported poor results in 24 percent of patients from whom an acalculous gallbladder was removed. CCK-cholecystography has been helpful in determining which patients will benefit from cholecystectomy.

The incidence of acalculous cholecystitis is difficult to establish. It is present in over 50 percent of children and 35 percent of Nigerians with gallbladder disease, and the accepted incidence for adults in the United States is between 5 and 10 percent. Postoperative acute cholecystitis is frequently acalculous. Possible causes include (1) anatomic conditions such as kinking, fibrosis, and obstruction of the cystic duct due to tumor or anomalous vessels; (2) throm-

Fig. 31-18. Rokitansky-Aschoff sinuses presenting as a halo effect, a finding present in chronic cholecystitis.

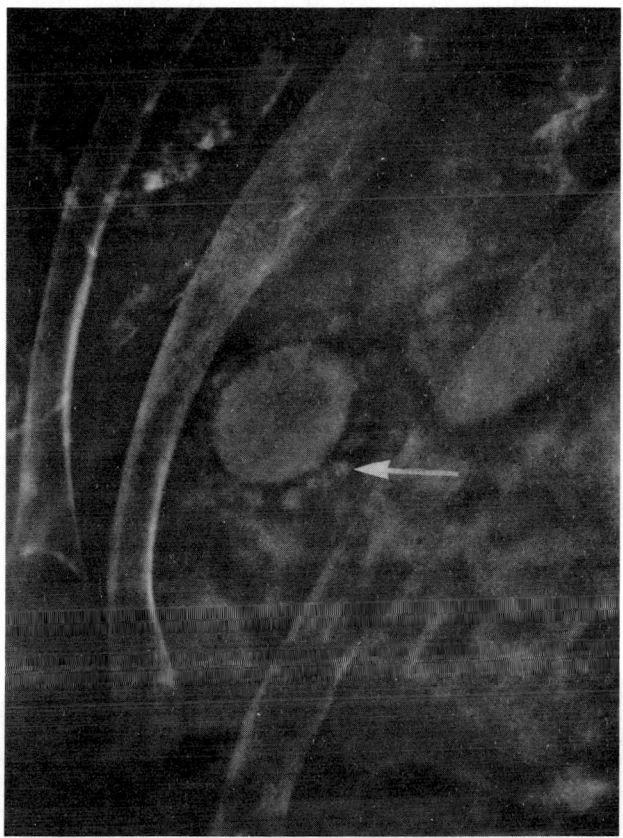

bosis of major blood vessels producing ischemia and gangrene; (3) spasm or fibrosis of the sphincter of Oddi in patients with a "common channel" with or without associated pancreatitis; (4) systemic diseases such as diabetes mellitus and collagen diseases; (5) specific infections such as typhoid fever, actinomycoses, and parasitic infestation; and (6) scarlet fever and a wide variety of febrile illnesses in young children.

TREATMENT. Cholecystectomy is generally carried out because of classic symptoms attributed to the gallbladder. An effort should be made to determine the presence of etiologic or associated conditions, and these should be corrected. The liver should be biopsied in any patient with a history of jaundice, and bacteriologic culture of the gallbladder wall should be carried out. Spasm or obstruction of the sphincter of Oddi due to papillitis or fibrosis should be ruled out. Postoperatively, the stool should be cultured for *Salmonella,* and serial estimations of the serum amylase level and a lupus erythematosus (LE) test are indicated.

Cholangitis

Infection within the biliary duct system is most frequently associated with choledocholithiasis but has also accompanied choledochal cysts and carcinoma of the bile duct, and has followed sphincteroplasty. Infection and inflammatory changes may extend up the duct system into the liver and give rise to multiple hepatic abscesses. Clinically, the condition is characterized by intermittent fever, upper abdominal pain, exacerbation of jaundice, pruritus, and at times rigor.

In patients with common duct stones in whom there is ascending cholangitis, a broad-spectrum antibiotic directed particularly at *E. coli,* which is the most common offending organism, should be given for several days prior to surgical treatment. Antibiotics usually control the infection, but if the temperature does not fall, surgical intervention should

not be delayed. Occasionally, the patient may be so ill as to allow only insertion of a T tube into the common duct, and when cholangitis has subsided, a second operation can be performed to remove the stone.

ACUTE SUPPURATIVE CHOLANGITIS. Suppurative cholangitis, in which there is gross pus within the biliary tract, merits special consideration, since it constitutes one of the most urgent causes for laparotomy in patients with obstructive jaundice. The entity was first described in 1877 by Charcot, who suggested a diagnostic triad of jaundice, chills and fever, and pain in the right upper quadrant. To these, Reynolds and Dargan added shock and central nervous system depression as specific identifying features of the condition.

The disease occurs almost exclusively in patients over seventy years. All patients are febrile, and a majority are jaundiced. Hypotension, confusion, or lethargy occur in about 20 percent of cases. A white blood cell count of less than 12,000 has been reported in over half the patients, probably related to the age and lack of response. Bilirubin, SGOT, and alkaline phosphatase levels are characteristically elevated, but the serum amylase is usually normal. The correct diagnosis has been made in less than a third of the patients.

At operation, all patients demonstrate gross distension of the common bile duct, with frank pus, frequently under considerable pressure, and choledocholithiasis. If the gallbladder is present, it is invariably distended and inflamed. Spontaneous perforation of the bile ducts has been reported. Surgical treatment is directed at rapid decompression of the duct system and is combined with large doses of antibiotics, particularly those which achieve high levels in the bile. In a review of the literature, it was reported that all patients who were not operated upon died while mortality following surgical procedures ranged between zero and 88 percent, averaging 33 percent.

Cholangiohepatitis

Cholangiohepatitis, which is also known as "recurrent pyogenic cholangitis," is found almost exclusively among the Chinese, with the largest number of cases seen among Cantonese living in the Pearl River delta in China. In Hong Kong it is the most commonly encountered disease of the biliary passages and is the third most common abdominal emergency after appendicitis and perforated ulcer. It has also been encountered in Great Britain, in Australia, and in the Chinese population in the United States. Cholangiohepatitis occurs most frequently in the third and fourth decades but has been reported at all ages and has an equal sex frequency.

The etiology is summarized in Fig. 31-19. The pyogenic element probably originates from the bowel and is caused by *E. coli* or *Streptococcus fecalis.* In most instances, positive cultures are obtainable from the bile and portal venous blood. The Chinese liver fluke, *C. sinensis,* is thought to be an important contributing factor. Ova have been found in the feces or bile of 91 percent of cases, but in some instances there has been no evidence of infestation. It has been postulated that in the presence of the pyogenic infec-

Fig. 31-19. Schema of etiologic factors implicated in cholangiohepatitis. (*After F. E. Stock and J. H. Y. Fung, Oriental Cholangiohepatitis, in R. Smith and S. Sherlock, "Surgery of the Gall Bladder and Bile Ducts," Butterworth & Co. [Publishers] Ltd., London, 1964.*)

tion the fluke may die. *C. sinensis* has been shown to cause severe irritation of the bile passages and has been implicated as a cause of bile duct tumors. Other factors which have been implicated as contributing causes for cholangiohepatitis include ascariasis and hemolysis associated with malaria.

PATHOLOGY. The gallbladder is usually distended with viscous, dark bile. The wall is thickened but not grossly inflamed. The common bile duct is also usually grossly distended and contains large stones. The stones are produced by precipitation of bile pigments, desquamation of epithelium, and products of inflammation, and, not infrequently, the nucleus of the stone may contain an adult *Clonorchis* worm, an ovum, or an ascarid. Acute or hemorrhagic pancreatitis occurs in less than 1 percent of the cases. The most marked changes occur in the liver, where the intrahepatic bile ducts are both dilated and constricted. Inflammatory changes are present in the periductal tissue and may progress to frank abscess formation. With time, additional liver tissue is destroyed as abscesses are formed.

CLINICAL MANIFESTATIONS. In highly endemic areas, cholangiohepatitis is the first consideration in patients with jaundice, pain, and pyrexia. In almost all cases, pain is present at some stage and is frequently severe. It is usually located in the right upper quadrant and epigastrium and may be colicky or constant. As is typical with biliary tract disease, it radiates frequently to the back or shoulder tip. In most acute attacks, there is fever accompanied by chills and rigors, and 50 percent of the patients are jaundiced, while the remainder have an elevation of the serum bilirubin level. Recurrence of symptoms is one of the most characteristic features of the disease.

Most patients appear toxic, with temperatures up to 40°C. There is tenderness and guarding in the right upper quadrant. The white blood cell count is usually in about 15,000, and the serum bilirubin level is generally above 2 mg/100 ml with accompanying bilirubinuria. The alkaline phosphatase is increased, and there may be evidence of impairment of hepatocellular function. In the majority of cases calculi are not demonstrable on routine x-rays. An occasional finding of significance is the presence of air in the biliary tree, which may be due to a secondary gas-forming organism or a fistula between the duct and duodenum. Cholecystography and intravenous cholangiography rarely produce diagnostic findings. Endoscopic retrograde cholangiopancreatography (ERCP) may establish the diagnosis. Operative cholangiography also is helpful in revealing intrahepatic stones, constrictions of intrahepatic ducts, and small filling defects due to the liver fluke. Manifestations of portal hypertension may be present.

TREATMENT. Patients are generally prepared with antibiotics. Vitamin K should be administered, and anemia, if present, should be corrected. Surgical therapy, however, should not be delayed for the patient who is jaundiced and has pain and pyrexia.

Treatment is directed at providing an adequate permanent drainage of the biliary tree. Cholecystostomy is reserved for the seriously ill patient showing signs of rupture of the gallbladder. The definitive operative procedure, however, consists of removal of stones and debris from the extrahepatic bile ducts and providing an improved communication between the duct system and the intestine. Transduodenal sphincteroplasty has been performed in cases where the common duct was not grossly dilated, but wide choledochoduodenostomy is the treatment of choice. T-tube drainage represents a temporizing procedure, since obstruction frequently recurs after the tube has been removed. The gallbladder is usually removed, although it is rarely acutely inflamed and never represents the primary site of disease.

If large hepatic abscesses are noted, drainage should be performed. Left hepatic lobectomy has been carried out on occasion, when there has been gross dilatation of the ducts and abscess formation in the left lobe while the right was apparently normal.

The prognosis is generally guarded, since recurrence is not uncommon. In advanced cases, particularly with multiple abscesses, the prognosis is poor, and the patient eventually succumbs to liver failure, septicemia, or cholangiocarcinoma.

Sclerosing Cholangitis

Sclerosing cholangitis is an uncommon disease which involves either all or part of the extrahepatic biliary duct system and, occasionally, affects the intrahepatic biliary radicles. The disease has also been called *obliterative cholangitis* and *stenosing cholangitis,* in reference to a progressive thickening of the bile duct walls encroaching upon the lumen. It may be associated with gallstones, but several series have been presented in which there were no stones in either the gallbladder or the common duct. A significant number of cases have been associated with ulcerative colitis, Riedel's struma, retroperitoneal fibrosis, and porphyria cutanea tarda.

Schwartz and Dale reviewed the literature prior to 1958, and only 13 cases satisfied their criteria of generalized extrahepatic bile duct stenosis in the absence of previous biliary surgical treatment and gallstones. Manesis and Sullivan reviewed the literature for a 40-year period from 1924 to 1964 and found only 24 cases which they considered acceptable. By contrast, Warren et al. have been less restrictive in the diagnosis and reported a group of 42 cases seen at the Lahey Clinic including 15 with a history of gallstones or previous surgical treatment. A follow-up period long enough to exclude sclerosing carcinoma of the biliary tree is essential to the diagnosis.

Most patients present with symptoms during the fourth, fifth, and sixth decades of life, and the disease appears to occur more often in males, in contrast to acute cholecystitis.

The cause of sclerosing cholangitis is unknown. Histologic sections in several cases failed to reveal any granulomatous lesion, metaplasia, or neoplasia. In several series, none of the patients had had previous surgical treatment, and therefore trauma was excluded as an etiologic agent; irritation of the common duct by passage of calculi is refuted by the fact that there are usually no stones present either in the common duct or gallbladder. It has been suggested that the disease may be caused by local response to viral infection, since a relative lymphocytosis with atypical lymphocytes has been noted. Allergic reaction and collagen disease have also been considered as possible etiologic factors.

PATHOLOGY. Grossly there is diffuse thickening of the wall of the extrahepatic biliary tract with a concomitant encroachment upon the lumen, resulting in marked luminal narrowing. The duct system may be completely involved, or the hepatic ducts may be spared and the disease restricted to the entire length of the common duct. The gallbladder is usually not involved, but the lymph nodes in the region of the common duct and foramen of Winslow are usually markedly enlarged and succulent. Microscopic analyses of the affected duct show that the walls are as much as eight times thicker than normal. The areas of inflammation and fibrosis are in the submucosal and subserosal portions with an edematous field between them. The mucosa is intact throughout. Biopsy of the liver may reveal bile stasis or, in long-standing cases, biliary cirrhosis. The histologic evaluation is critical, since it is difficult to differentiate this disease from sclerosing carcinoma of bile ducts.

CLINICAL MANIFESTATIONS. The diagnosis is to be considered in patients, particularly those in middle age, with a clinical and laboratory picture of extrahepatic jaundice. Jaundice is usually associated with intermittent pain in the right upper quadrant, nausea, vomiting, and occasionally chills and fevers. In long-standing cases with biliary cirrhosis, the manifestations of portal hypertension, such as bleeding varices and ascites, may be apparent. The diagnosis has been established by ERCP. At operation a dense inflammatory reaction in the region of the gallbladder and gastrohepatic ligament is noted. Palpation of the duct reveals a cordlike structure which may feel like a thrombosed blood vessel, but the wall of the common duct is obviously thickened and cuts with difficulty. The edges of the incision characteristically pout out. Usually, only a fine

probe or small Bâkes dilator can be inserted into the lumen. Operative cholangiography may vividly demonstrate the extensive narrowing of the lumen (Fig. 31-20).

TREATMENT. Treatment has varied and is dictated by the extent of involvement of the extrahepatic biliary duct system. It is usually preferable to drain the common duct by means of a T tube. If the gallbladder is normal, it should not be removed, because it may be required subsequently to shunt bile from the biliary tract to the intestine. Postoperatively, the patient is treated with bile salts, such as dehydrocholic acid, to increase the fluidity of bile; a broad-spectrum antibiotic, which achieves a high level in bile; and corticoids. Prednisone (40 to 50 mg daily) is preferred for long-term use, since its anti-inflammatory effect is four to five times as great as that of cortisone with less salt-retaining potential. Recurrence of symptoms or icterus is indication for reinstitution of steroid therapy.

A T-tube drainage is maintained until a satisfactory lumen is demonstrated throughout the duct system by cholangiogram and it is apparent that the bile flows readily into the duodenum. The combination of surgical decompression of the biliary tract and administration of corticoids, bile salts, and antibiotics has reduced the overall mortality, but the prognosis is guarded because of the difficulty in differentiating primary sclerosing cholangitis from sclerosing carcinoma of bile ducts.

Fibrosis or Stenosis of the Sphincter of Oddi

In 1884, Langenbuch, only 2 years after reporting the first successful removal of a gallbladder, suggested trans-

Fig. 31-20. *A.* Operative cholangiogram of patient with sclerosing cholangitis showing markedly narrow common cystic and hepatic ducts. *B.* Cholangiogram on twenty-fourth postoperative day showing increased diameter of lumen of common, cystic and hepatic ducts in same patient. Patient had received cortisone from first postoperative day.

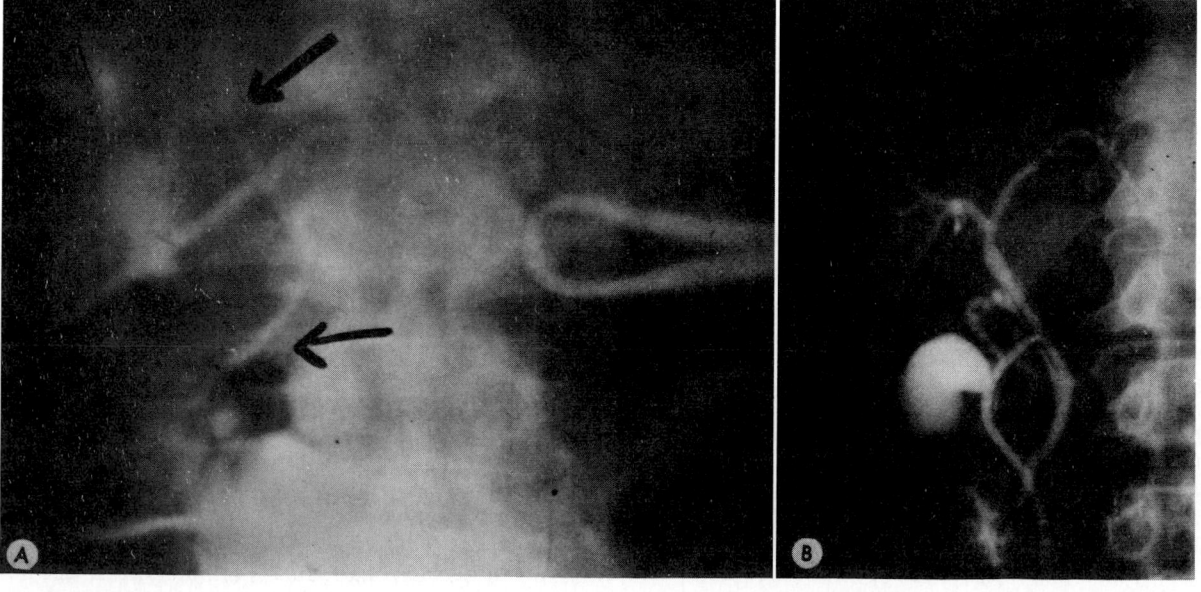

duodenal division of the "diverticulum" of Vater in cases of cicatricial stenosis for chronic inflammation. In 1901, Opie called attention to the "common channel" theory as the cause of pancreatitis, and in 1913 Archibald suggested sphincteroplasty as the treatment for pancreatitis.

The pathogenesis of fibrosis or stenosis of the sphincter of Oddi and the papilla of Vater is not fully understood. Long-standing spasm may play an important role, and infection of the biliary tract or pancreas have also been implicated. Irritation from stones within the common duct may also lead to fibrosis. In a series of 50 patients in whom sphincteroplasty was performed because of inability to pass a small Bâkes dilator, biopsies revealed no abnormalities in 18, while 18 showed inflammatory infiltration, 17 had minimal fibrosis, and 2 had diffuse fibrosis. Glandular dilatation was seen in seven cases, and squamous metaplasia and pyogenic granuloma were each seen in one case. No definite correlation could be found between the various manifestations of biliary tract disease and the histologic changes.

CLINICAL MANIFESTATIONS. The main symptom is abdominal pain, which is usually colicky and frequently associated with nausea and vomiting. The pain begins in the right upper quadrant and radiates to the shoulder, and it may be intermittent in nature. Over half the patients give a history of intermittent jaundice, and many indicate that they have had previous cholecystectomy without relief of symptoms.

TREATMENT. The diagnosis is generally made at operation when there is difficulty in passing a 3-mm Bâkes dilator through the ampulla of Vater into the duodenum. Operative cholangiography and pressure studies on the common bile duct have theoretical application but are generally not used. If a 3-mm dilator cannot be easily passed through the ampulla, a transduodenal exploration should be carried out. Thomas et al. compared the results of transduodenal sphincteroplasty and choledochoduodenostomy in 30 patients with stenosis or stricture of the sphincter. The procedures were equally and highly effective, and neither was associated with a significant incidence of subsequent cholangitis. Sphincteroplasty is preferable if the common duct is small, and a transduodenal approach is indicated if an ampullary tumor is suspected. Choledochoduodenostomy appears preferable if the stenosis is long, if it is difficult to identify the sphincter, or if exposure is difficult.

PAPILLITIS

In 1926, DelValle first described a benign inflammatory and fibrous process of the ampulla of Vater and indicated that it was a factor in producing stenosis. It was postulated that acute and subacute inflammatory changes occur and that stenosis is the final and irreversible result of these changes. Acosta and Nardi have presented 61 cases of papillitis, 21 of which were chronic ulcerative papillitis, 20 chronic sclerosing papillitis, 15 chronic granulomatous papillitis, and 5 chronic adenomatous papillitis. The acute stage, which is characterized by edema, papillary dilatation, hemorrhage, and infiltration, may be reversible, while sclerosing papillitis and chronic granulomatous papillitis

are considered irreversible in view of their inevitable evolution into scar tissue.

The clinical and pathologic features associated with papillitis include the postcholecystectomy syndrome in 30 percent, dilatation of the common duct in 50 percent, biliary disease without stones in 25 percent, obstructive jaundice in 60 percent, pancreatitis in 70 percent, and liver damage in 25 percent. There has been no correlation between the specific clinical syndromes and the pathologic changes. A pancreatic evocative test, utilizing morphine-prostigmine or secretin-CCK, has been used. Elevation of at least one serum pancreatic enzyme by a factor of 4 over the normal, coupled with reproduction of the patient's pain, is considered a positive test result. Since the majority of patients with papillitis have irreversible lesions, sphincteroplasty is generally employed.

TUMORS

Carcinoma of the Gallbladder

Carcinoma of the gallbladder represents the fifth most common type of carcinoma involving the gastrointestinal tract and accounts for 4 percent of all carcinomas. Its occurrence in random autopsy series averages approximately 0.4 percent, while approximately 1 percent of patients undergoing biliary tract operations are noted to have carcinoma. Approximately 80 percent of patients in most series are female. The lesion usually presents after the age of sixty.

PATHOLOGY. The relationship between gallstones and carcinoma has been emphasized for many years. Approximately 90 percent of patients with carcinoma have associated cholelithiasis. Five to ten percent of patients over the age of sixty-five with symptomatic gallstones have carcinoma of the gallbladder. However, it has been stressed that in patients with asymptomatic cholelithiasis the frequency of occurrence is extremely low.

Approximately 80 percent of the tumors are adenocarcinomas, while the remainder are either undifferentiated or squamous cell carcinomas. Of the adenocarcinomas, 70 percent are scirrhous, 20 percent are papillary, and 10 percent are mucoid. The routes of metastases include spread along the lymphatics to the choledochal and pancreatic or duodenal nodes, localized involvement of the venules and veins of the gallbladder, and invasion of the liver. In approximately one-third of the cases the disease spreads directly to the liver, an important consideration as far as therapy is concerned. In patients with metastases, the liver is involved in two-thirds of the cases, the regional lymph nodes in about one-half, and the omentum, duodenum, colon, or porta hepatis in about one-fourth. Pulmonary metastases are relatively uncommon.

CLINICAL MANIFESTATIONS. Signs and symptoms of carcinoma of the gallbladder are generally indistinguishable from those associated with cholecystitis and cholelithiasis. Most patients present with abdominal distress, epigastric and right upper quadrant pain, nausea, and vomiting. About half the patients are jaundiced, and in two-thirds there is a palpable right upper quadrant mass. Less than 10 percent present with normal findings on abdominal examination.

Laboratory findings are of little assistance. The liver function tests are diagnostic of obstructive jaundice, and the gallbladder is usually not visualized by cholecystography. A correct preoperative diagnosis has been made in less than 20 percent of patients, and in many patients the gallbladder carcinoma is found incidentally during routine cholecystectomy.

TREATMENT. Surgical treatment offers the only, albeit small, hope for cure. Most of the reported long-term survivors are patients who underwent surgical treatment for acute and chronic cholecystitis and in whom an incidental localized microscopic focus of neoplasia was detected in the specimen. The best results in patients with grossly visible carcinoma have been achieved with cholecystectomy and regional lymphadenectomy. When the lymph nodes are removed, the portal vein, hepatic artery, hepatic duct, and common bile duct should be skeletonized from the pylorus to the porta hepatis. The minimal liver resection which should be performed consists of removal of the wedge of hepatic tissue comprising the gallbladder bed. A formal right hepatic lobectomy has been suggested, but the 5-year survival rate has not been improved by this approach.

The prognosis for 5-year survival is extremely poor, however, approximating 2 percent. Ninety percent of patients die before the end of 1 year and 50 percent within 3 months.

Fig. 31-21. Transhepatic cholangiogram demonstrating a tumor of the common bile duct.

Carcinoma of the Extrahepatic Bile Ducts Exclusive of the Periampullary Region

This lesion has an average autopsy incidence of approximately 0.3 percent. The ratio of incidence of carcinoma of the extrahepatic bile duct exclusive of the periampullary region to that of carcinoma of the gallbladder ranges from 1:2 to 1:5 in various series, while the ratio of this lesion to carcinoma of the ampulla is 3:2. The tumor occurs more frequently in males and has the highest incidence in the sixth and seventh decades.

PATHOLOGY. The primary lesion is often small but so located as to cause symptoms early. Approximately one-third of the cases occur in the common bile duct, one-fifth are at the junction of the cystic and common hepatic ducts, and one-fourth are higher in the common hepatic duct. Ten percent occur in either the right or left hepatic duct, and about 13 percent are located in the cystic duct. The tumor usually involves the whole thickness of the duct, resulting in complete anatomic obstruction in about one-third of the cases. Grossly, the tumor presents as a firm, circumscribed, grayish tan mass which causes a "napkin ring" obstruction. In rare instances, the growth projects into the lumen of the duct in the form of a polypoid mass. Histologically, all lesions are adenocarcinomas. Metastatic spread has been reported in about three-fourths of autopsy cases, liver and regional lymph nodes being most frequently involved. Spread to adjacent structures accounts for 20 percent of metastases. Recently a series employing operative choledochoscopy has demonstrated that multicentric lesions in the duct are common. The extent of liver involvement is variable. In some instances there is severe bile stasis, while in others there are suppurative cholangitis and hepatic abscesses. The incidence of metastases at operation was reported to be approximately 50 percent.

Cholelithiasis has been implicated as a contributing factor just as in carcinoma of the gallbladder. However, the incidence of stones is not as high, ranging from 20 to 57 percent in several series. The incidence of calculi within the bile ducts themselves is extremely low.

CLINICAL MANIFESTATIONS. The symptoms are variable, and the correct preoperative diagnosis is seldom made. Characteristically, there is a rapid onset of jaundice, which is present in almost all patients. This is frequently preceded by pruritus. Nearly always there is weight loss, and abdominal pain occurs in over half the patients. The liver is palpable in about 80 percent of the cases and is usually nontender and rarely nodular. The gallbladder is palpable in about one-third of the patients who have not undergone previous cholecystectomy. The serum bilirubin is usually elevated, often to an extremely high level, and fluctuation of the bilirubin level has been recorded in about 60 percent of the cases. Intravenous cholangiography rarely visualizes the ducts because of the high degree of obstructive jaundice, but transhepatic cholangiography may provide a diagnosis (Fig. 31-21). At the time of surgical treatment, an operative cholangiogram is very helpful in establishing the diagnosis and choledochoscopy should be performed to assess multicentricity.

TREATMENT. The surgical procedure may be either a

potentially curative one or palliative and is dependent upon the location of the tumor. Tumors located within the common bile duct or common hepatic duct may be resected or bypassed by anastomosing the dilated proximal duct system to a segment of intestine, preferably by a Roux en Y procedure. Tumors occurring high in the hepatic duct system can rarely be removed, and palliative procedures are also difficult. The jejunum may be anastomosed to a dilated duct in the hilus or on the inferior surface of the left lobe of the liver. Recently Terblanche et al. have achieved prolonged palliation by decompressing the distended intrahepatic duct with a tube passed through the obstruction via the common duct and out the surface of the liver as a U tube (Fig. 31-22). The results either with or without surgical treatment are discouraging, and the patients survive an average of 4 months after operation or 6 months after the onset of their symptoms. Radical dissection has rarely proved curative and has been associated with a high operative mortality.

SCLEROSING CARCINOMA OF THE HILAR DUCTS

This lesion usually arises from the major hepatic ducts near the hilus of the liver and extends into the intrahepatic ducts, developing slowly and often mimicking a chronic inflammatory process. As the tumor obstructs the bile ducts, progressive jaundice, cholestasis, suppurative cholangitis, and hepatic abscess may result. The average age at diagnosis is about sixty-five, and the ratio of male to female has been reported at 8:1.

The signs and symptoms are variable. There is characteristically insidious and progressive jaundice, and there is usually associated marked weight loss. Fever is noted in over half the patients. The syndrome may progress to hepatic coma, renal failure, or septicemia. Laboratory and preoperative roentgenographic findings are inconclusive, but operative cholangiography has been helpful in establishing the diagnosis.

Surgical treatment is directed at establishing biliary drainage and has been accomplished by a T tube passed as a stent through the tumor, hepaticodochojejunostomy, and the Longmire procedure. If transhepatic cholangiography demonstrates high obstruction and no accessible segment for reanastomosis, percutaneous transhepatic catheter drainage can relieve the jaundice at least temporarily and at times for prolonged periods. In spite of the fact that metastases are frequently present in the regional lymph nodes, liver, and omentum, in several instances there has been a surprisingly long survival: the difficulty in establishing a diagnosis of sclerosing cholangitis is thus emphasized.

OPERATIONS ON THE BILIARY TRACT

ANTIBIOTIC THERAPY. The infectious complications after biliary surgery are more frequent in patients with infected bile than in those with sterile bile. It has been shown that patients over the age of seventy who have acute cholecystitis, common bile duct stones, jaundice, or diabetes have a significantly higher incidence of positive bile cultures and therefore are at risk for postoperative infec-

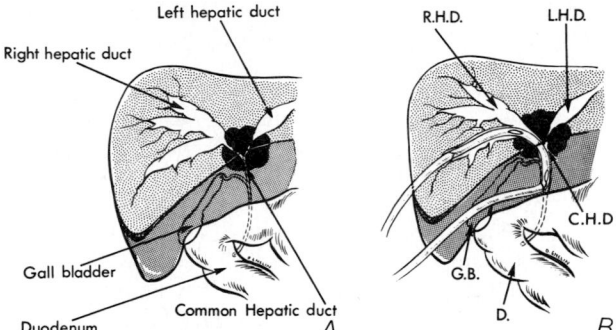

Fig. 31-22. The U-tube procedure. *A.* The carcinoma situated at the main hepatic duct junction. *B.* The U tube in situ after dilatation. (*From J. Terblanche et al., Surgery, 71:720, 1972.*)

tion. This group of patients should receive antibiotics preoperatively. In all cases, the gallbladder bile should be cultured at the time of the operative procedure. The selection of antibiotics should be based on appreciation of the fact that most organisms are *E. coli* or *Klebsiella*. One study has shown that half the bacteria cultured from the bile was resistant to ampicillin.

CHOLECYSTOSTOMY. The procedure accomplishes decompression and drainage of the distended, hydroptic, or empyematous gallbladder. It is particularly applicable if the patient's general condition is such that it precludes prolonged anesthesia, since the operation may be performed under local anesthesia. It is also performed for the situation in which marked inflammatory reaction obscures the anatomic relation of critical structures. Cholecystostomy may be a definitive procedure, particularly if a postoperative tube cholangiogram is normal.

Technique (Fig. 31-23). A circumferential purse-string suture is placed in the fundus of the gallbladder, and a small incision is made through the serosa within the suture. A trochar is inserted into the lumen of the gallbladder, which is then decompressed. After the gallbladder has been emptied, a stone forceps may be introduced to the junction of the ampulla and cystic duct, and obstructing calculi may be removed. A mushroom or Foley catheter is inserted into the lumen of the gallbladder, and a second purse-string suture is placed concentrically in relation to the first one. The sutures are tied, inverting the serosa. Unless a small, oblique incision was employed initially, the drainage tube should be brought out through a stab wound.

If the fundus of the gallbladder is necrotic, the gangrenous portion should be excised and the remainder of the gallbladder closed around the catheter, using purse-string sutures as previously described.

CHOLECYSTECTOMY. A principal aim of the technique is to avoid injury to the common duct while transecting the cystic duct close to its junction with the common bile duct to obviate a long cystic duct remnant.

Technique (Fig. 31-24). The gallbladder may be approached through an oblique right upper quadrant incision (Kocher or Courvoisier), through a vertical right paramedian incision, or through the upper midline. There are frequently adhesions between the gallbladder, particularly

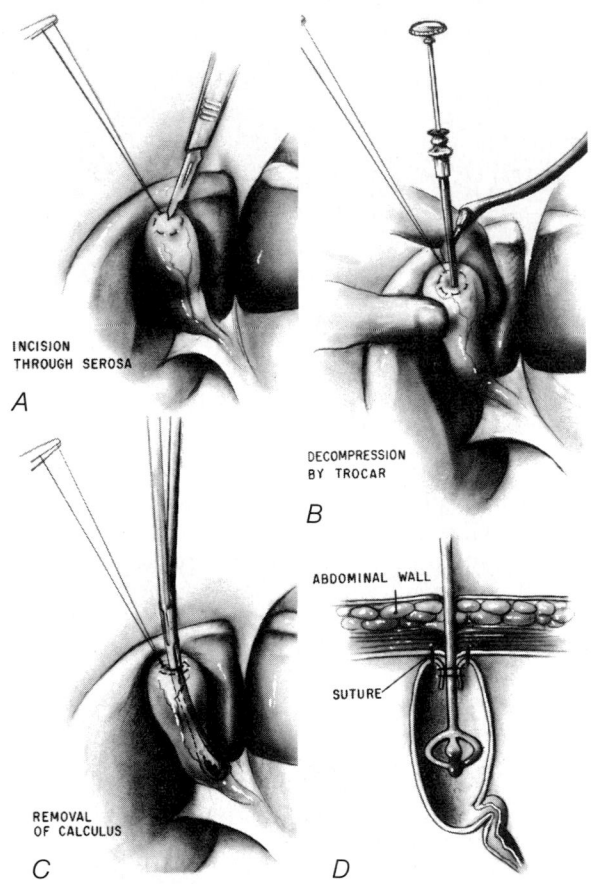

INCISION
THROUGH SEROSA

A

DECOMPRESSION
BY TROCAR

B

ABDOMINAL WALL

SUTURE

REMOVAL
OF CALCULUS

C   *D*

Fig. 31-23. Cholecystostomy. *A.* Placement of purse-string suture in fundus of gallbladder, and incision through serosa. *B.* Trochar decompression. *C.* Removal of calculus from ampulla. *D.* Sagittal section demonstrating two concentric purse-string sutures, intraluminal catheter, and suturing of serosa of gallbladder to peritoneum.

the ampulla, and the duodenum and colon. These should be lysed by sharp dissection. By applying traction laterally to the ampulla and retracting the duodenum medially, the veil of peritoneum running from ampulla to hepatoduodenal ligament may be accentuated and incised. The cystic duct is identified and a silk ligature passed around it. Traction is applied to the ligature to prevent passage of a stone down the cystic duct during dissection of the gallbladder. Dissection is then continued craniad in this peritoneal fold, and the cystic artery is identified. The course of this artery to the gallbladder should be demonstrated to avoid ligating the right hepatic artery. The cystic artery should be doubly ligated and transected. If bleeding occurs from the cystic artery, it is best controlled by applying pressure on the hepatic artery within the hepatoduodenal ligament. The artery is compressed between the index finger, which is inserted into the foramen of Winslow posteriorly, and the thumb anteriorly. The peritoneum overlying the gallbladder is then incised close to the liver, and dissection is begun from the fundus of the gallbladder down to an ultimate pedicle of cystic duct. During this dissection, blood vessels coursing from the liver may require ligation, and the gallbladder bed should be inspected

for large draining ducts, which should also be ligated. Attention is then directed toward visualization of the junction of the cystic duct with the common duct. The cystic duct is transected and ligated 3 mm from the common bile duct. It is not necessary to close the bed of the gallbladder, but a drain should be brought out from the hepatorenal pouch, which is the most dependent portion of the upper abdomen with the patient in the supine position, via a separate stab wound. Several series have shown that in the absence of specific indications, drainage is not required.

The above-described method is directed at facilitating demonstration of the junction between the cystic duct and common bile duct. The gallbladder may also be removed in a so-called "retrograde" fashion, in which the cystic duct is ligated close to the junction with the common duct as the initial part of the procedure. Then, after the cystic duct and artery have been transected, dissection is begun from the cystic duct and continued outward toward the fundus (Fig. 31-25).

OPERATIONS ON THE COMMON BILE DUCT. The situations necessitating operative procedure on the common bile duct include exploration for calculi, repair of a surgically interrupted or injured common duct, stenosis of the sphincter of Oddi, and bypass procedures for obstructive jaundice secondary to trauma, tumors, and atresia. The indications for concomitant exploration of the common bile duct during cholecystectomy have been enumerated in the section of choledocholithiasis.

Initial Exploration for Choledocholithiasis. When the procedure (Fig. 31-26) is being performed at the time of cholecystectomy, the cystic duct should be identified initially. Traction is applied to a ligature passed around this duct to avoid passage of stones from the gallbladder into the common duct. The gallbladder is generally removed after the common duct has been thoroughly explored and distal patency demonstrated. After the common duct has been visualized, aspiration with a fine needle provides confirmation. Two fixation sutures are placed distal to the junction of the cystic and common bile duct, and a vertical incision is made between these through the anterior wall. Calculi are removed by a combination of stone forceps, scoops, balloon-tipped catheters, and irrigation. These procedures should first be applied to the common bile duct toward the ampulla of Vater and subsequently to each of the main hepatic ducts. After the stones have been removed, a #6 Bâkes dilator should pass readily into the duodenum, and the tip of the dilator should be visualized through the wall of the intestine. After free passage of the dilator has been demonstrated, a T tube, with the ellipse removed from the junction of the horizontal and vertical limbs of the T to facilitate removal of the tube postoperatively, is inserted into the common duct. The limbs of the T should be short, so that the distal limb does not pass through the ampulla of Vater and the proximal limb does not obstruct either of the hepatic ducts. The common duct is then closed with interrupted sutures, and saline solution is injected into the T tube to demonstrate absence of leaks. At this stage an operative cholangiogram may be performed to rule out retained stones and demonstrate free passage of the radiopaque medium into the duodenum.

A *B* *C* Wabnitz

D *E* *F* Wabnitz

Fig. 31-24. Cholecystectomy (preferred approach.) *A.* Veil of peritoneum coursing from ampulla to hepatoduodenal ligament is transected, and cystic duct is identified. *B.* Ligature is passed around cystic duct and traction applied to prevent passage of calculi from gallbladder into common duct during the course of subsequent dissection. Dissection is continued along same fold of peritoneum, and cystic artery is doubly ligated and transected. Incision is made in peritoneum overlying gallbladder. *C.* Gall-bladder is removed from its bed, and if large vessels or bile ducts are encountered, they are ligated. Dissection continues from fundus toward junction between cystic duct and common bile duct. *D.* Ultimate pedicle of cystic duct is established, and junction between cystic duct and common bile duct is defined. *E.* Cystic duct is ligated and transfixed and then transected approximately 3mm from its junction with the common bile duct. *F.* Drain is brought out via stab wound from the hepatorenal (Morison's) pouch

The T tube should be brought out through a stab wound to prevent dislodgment when the major incision is dressed. If there is no evidence of choledocholithiasis or obstruction at the ampulla of Vater, some surgeons advise primary closure of the choledochotomy without T-tube drainage. Postoperative cholangiogram is performed on the seventh

to eighth day, and if absence of stones plus clear passage of radiopaque into the duodenum is demonstrated, the tube can be removed.

Transduodenal Choledochotomy: Sphincteroplasty (Fig. 31-27). In the event that a stone is impacted at the ampulla of Vater or that a Bâkes dilator cannot be passed into the duodenum thus suggesting fibrosis of the sphincter of Oddi, a duodenotomy is performed. The lateral peritoneal reflection of the second portion of the duodenum is incised (Kocher maneuver) to facilitate exposure. A longitudinal duodenotomy is performed on the anterior aspect of the duodenum and, with the Bâkes dilator in place in the common duct to facilitate demonstration of the sphincter, the sphincter is incised, and the impacted calculus is removed. If there is evidence of fibrosis of the sphincter, a V segment should be removed. Free passage of a #6 Bâkes dilator into the duodenum from the common bile duct should then be demonstrated and a T tube inserted into the common duct. The duodenotomy is preferably closed in two layers. The longitudinal incision may be converted into a transverse closure to prevent stenosis. The

RETROGRADE DISSECTION OF GALLBLADDER FROM ITS CAPSULE

Fig. 31-25. Retrograde dissection of gallbladder. After cystic duct has been identified, its junction with common bile duct is defined, and cystic duct is transected. Cystic artery is also doubly ligated and transected, and gallbladder is removed from its bed with dissection progressing from the cystic duct and ampulla outward toward fundus.

procedure is also applicable to the problem of multiple or recurrent stones.

Operative Procedures for Recurrent Choledocholithiasis: Choledochoduodenostomy (Fig. 31-28). Common duct exploration is carried out as described above. If the surgeon is concerned about the possibility of subsequent reexplorations, either because of the patient's age or the fact that the surgeon is not totally satisfied that all stones have been removed, a choledochoduodenostomy may be performed.

The incision in the common duct should be enlarged, and after all apparent stones have been removed, a Kocher maneuver is performed on the duodenum, and a side-to-side anastomosis between the common duct and the duodenum is carried out. One or two layers may be used for this anastomosis, but it is imperative that the stoma be large enough so that subsequent scarring does not result in spontaneous closure.

Repair of Injured or Strictured Common Duct (Fig. 31-29). If transection of the common bile duct is noted at operation, an end-to-end anastomosis over a T tube stent is indicated. A single layer of sutures is sufficient, and the results are usually excellent.

If the stricture has developed subsequent to injury of the common duct, the preferable method of treatment is direct repair of the common bile duct over a T tube. The strictured area may be excised and the common duct mobilized so that an end-to-end anastomosis is possible. If the area of stricture is extensive and if the distal common bile duct cannot be identified, a proximal decompressive procedure is indicated.

Decompressive Procedures. A great variety of procedures are applicable, and the selection is primarily dependent upon the availability of the gallbladder or proximal ducts.

Fig. 31-26. Exploration of the common bile duct. *A.* Ligature has been placed around cystic duct to prevent passage of stones from gallbladder into common duct. After common bile duct has been identified by dissection and aspiration, two stay sutures are placed on either side. A longitudinal incision is made in the common duct. *B.* Duct is explored with stone forceps and scoops, and irrigated in both directions, i.e., toward liver and toward ampulla of Vater. Prior to insertion of a T tube, a #6 Bâkes dilator should pass readily into duodenum. *C.* An ellipse is removed from junction of horizontal and vertical limbs of the T tube, and a T tube is inserted into common duct via choledochotomy. Distal limb of T tube should be short and should not pass through ampulla of Vater. Proximal limb should also be short and positioned so that it does not obstruct either of hepatic ducts. *D.* Choledochostomy is closed tightly around T tube, which is irrigated to demonstrate absence of leakage.

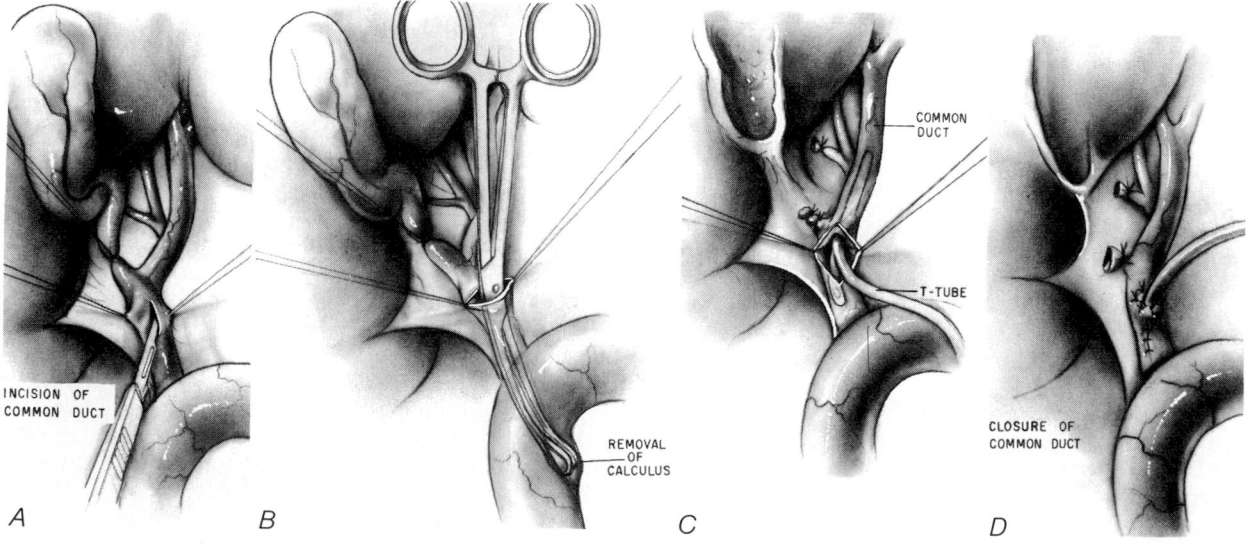

INCISION OF COMMON DUCT

REMOVAL OF CALCULUS

COMMON DUCT

T-TUBE

CLOSURE OF COMMON DUCT

A   *B*   *C*   *D*

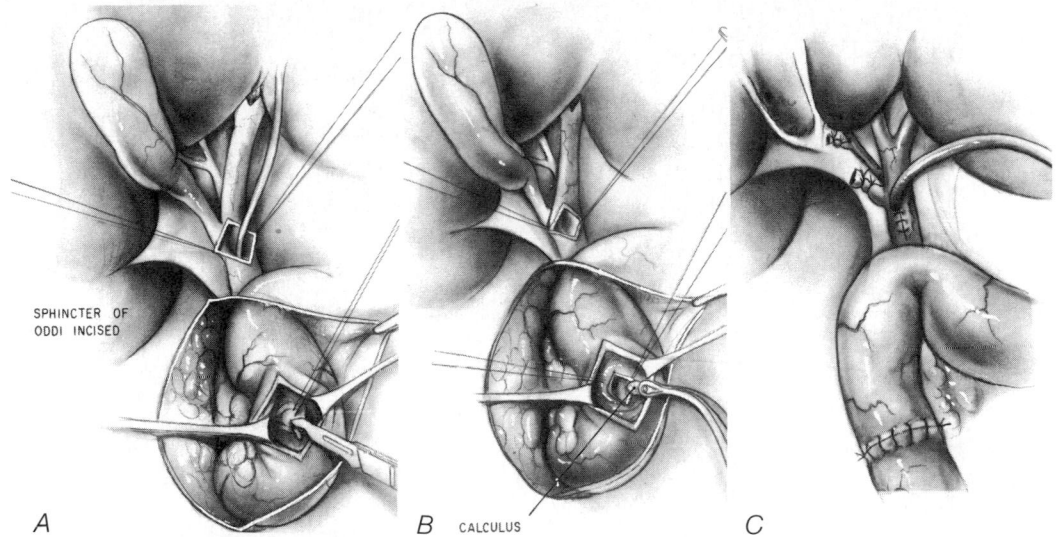

A　　　*B* CALCULUS　　　*C*

Fig. 31-27. Transduodenal choledochotomy: sphincterotomy. *A.* Kocher maneuver is performed on second portion of duodenum, and longitudinal duodenotomy is carried out. With Bâkes dilator inserted in common duct in order to define ampulla of Vater, stay suture is placed in ampulla, which is incised. *B.* Wedge of tissue should be removed from sphincter, and calculus impacted in this region can readily be excised. *C.* T tube is inserted into the common bile duct, and duodenotomy is closed transversely.

If obstruction is at the level of the distal common duct, an anastomosis between proximal common duct and intestine is indicated. The common duct may be anastomosed to the side of the jejunum or preferably to a Roux en Y jejunal segment 30 cm in length. The latter has the theoretic advantage of decreasing the incidence of ascend-

ing cholangitis. With obstruction of the proximal common bile duct, the gallbladder, if present, can be anastomosed to the jejunum (Fig. 31-7*B*), or the common hepatic duct may be anastomosed as a Roux en Y (Fig. 31-7*A*). If obstruction is at the confluence of the hepatic ducts, in the porta hepatis, decompression is more difficult, but a single hepatic duct may be anastomosed to the Roux en Y of the jejunum, or the liver may be split along its anatomic plane (Fig. 31-8*B*) and the confluence anastomosed to the intestine. With high ductal obstruction, the Longmire procedure, i.e., transection of the left lateral segment of the liver and identification of a duct with an anastomosis of the duct-bearing area of the liver to the side of the jejunum, has been applied (Fig. 31-8*A*). The results of this procedure have not been generally encouraging. The jejunal mucosal graft, as introduced by Smith (Fig. 31-30), and the U tube popularized by Terblance and associates (Fig. 31-22), have been applied with increasing frequency.

Fig. 31-28. Choledochoduodenostomy. *A.* Kocher maneuver is performed on second portion of duodenum, and common bile duct has been isolated. *B.* Seromuscular suture approximates duodenum to common bile duct. Longitudinal incision is made in distal common bile duct and in duodenum. *C.* Anterior row of anastomosis is completed, and wide stoma between duodenum and common bile duct is created.

A　　　*B*　　　*C*

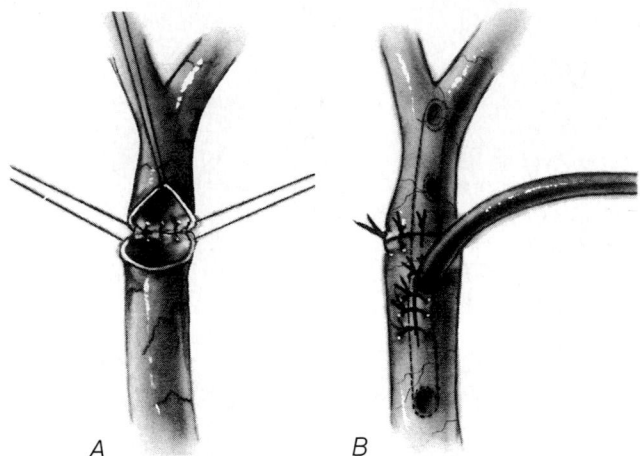

A   B

Fig. 31-29. Immediate repair of injured common duct. *A.* End-to-end anastomosis using interrupted suture is effected after cut ends of duct have been debrided. This procedure can also be carried out if there is stricture of common duct and both proximal and distal segments are identifiable. *B.* Anastomosis is complete, and T tube has been inserted as a stent via separate choledochostomy.

Fig. 31-30. Decompression of intrahepatic ducts by jejunal mucosal graft (Smith). *A.* Jejunal Roux en Y established and elipse of serosa removed. *B.* Catheter passed through liver parenchyma and into jejunal limb, where it is secured with catgut sutures. *C.* Jejunal limb pulled up so that mucosal patch abuts stoma of hepatic duct.

References

General

Glenn, F.: "Atlas of Biliary Tract Surgery," The Macmillan Company, New York, 1963.

Smith, R., and Sherlock, S.: "Surgery of the Gall Bladder and Bile Ducts," Butterworth & Co. (Publishers) Ltd., London, 1964. ●

Anatomy

Ahrens, E. H., Jr., Haris, R. C., and MacMahon, H. E.: Atresia of the Intrahepatic Bile Ducts, *Pediatrics,* **8:**628, 1951.

Alonso-Lej, F., Rever, W. B., and Pessagno, D. J.: Congenital Choledochal Cyst, with a Report of 2, and an Analysis of 94 Cases, *Surg Gynecol Obstet,* **108:**1, 1958.

Barlow, B., Tabor, Ed, Blanc, W. A., Santullo, T. V. and Harris, R. C.: Choledochal Cyst: A Review of 19 Cases, *J Pediatr,* **89:**934, 1976.

Benson, E. A., and Page, R. E.: A Practical Reappraisal of the Anatomy of the Extrahepatic Bile Ducts and Arteries, *Br J Surg,* **63:**853, 1976.

Bill, A. H., Brennom, W. S., and Huseby, T. L.: Biliary Atresia: New Concepts of Pathology, Diagnosis and Management, *Arch Surg,* **109:**367, 1974.

Boyden, E. A.: The Anatomy of the Choledochoduodenal Junction in Man, *Surg Gynecol Obstet,* **104:**641, 1957.

Campbell, D. P., and Williams, G. R.: Identification of the Jaundiced Infant Who Is Likely to Recover without Surgical Intervention, *Ann Surg,* **184:**89, 1976.

Gellis, S. S., and Hsia, D. Y.-Y.: Jaundice in Infancy, *Pediatr Clin North Am,* May, 1955, p. 446.

Hsia, D. Y.-Y., Patterson, P., Allen, F. H., Jr., Diamond, L. K., and Gellis, S. S.: Prolonged Obstructive Jaundice in Infancy: I. General Survey of 156 Cases, *Pediatrics,* **10:**243, 1952.

Ladd, W. E.: Congenital Atresia and Stenosis of the Bile Ducts, *JAMA,* **91:**1082, 1928.

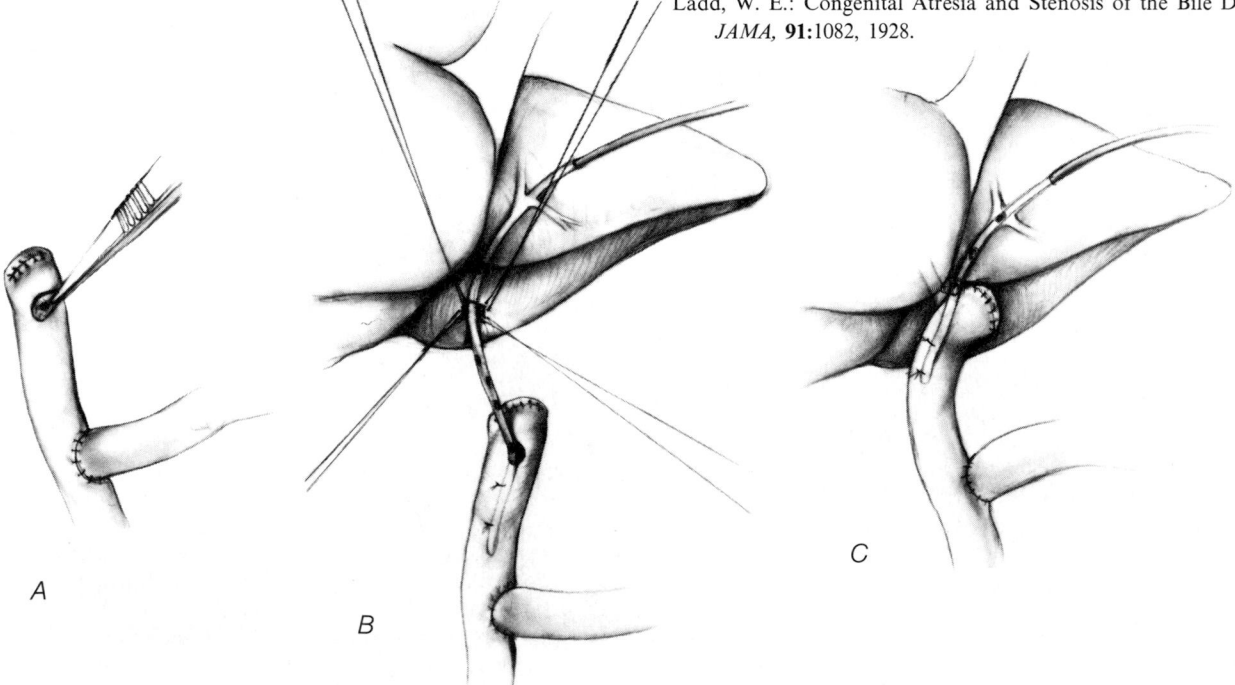

A   B   C

Leevy, C. M., Bender, J., Silverberg, M., and Naylor, J.: Physiology of Dye Extraction by the Liver: Comparative Studies of Sulfobromophthalein and Indocyanine Green, *Ann NY Acad Sci,* **111:**161, 1963.

Lilly, J. R., and Altman, R. P.: Hepatic Portoenterostomy (Kasai Operation) for Biliary Atresia, *Surgery,* **78:**76, 1975.

Longmire, W. P., Jr., Mandiola, S. A., and Gordon, H. E.: Congenital Cystic Disease of the Liver and Biliary System, *Ann Surg,* **174:**711, 1971.

Michels, N. A.: "Blood Supply and Anatomy of the Upper Abdominal Organs," J. B. Lippincott Company, Philadelphia, 1955.

Miyata, M., Satani, M., Ueda, T., and Okamoto, E.: Long-Term Results of Hepatic Portoenterostomy for Biliary Atresia: Special Reference to Postoperative Portal Hypertension, *Surgery,* **76:**234, 1974.

Odievre, M., Valayer, J., Razemon-Pinta, M., Habib, E.-C., and Alagille, D.: Hepatic Porto-cntcrostomy or Cholecystostomy in the Treatment of Extrahepatic Biliary Atresia. A Study of 49 Cases, *J Pediatr,* **88:**774, 1976.

Physiology

Davenport, H. W.: "Physiology of the Digestive Tract: An Introductory Text," The Year Book Medical Publishers, Inc., Chicago, 1961.

Ivy, A. C., and Goldman, L.: Physiology of Biliary Tract, *JAMA,* **113:**2413, 1939.

Jacobs, L. A., DeMeester, T. R., Eggleston, J. C., Margulies, S. I., and Zuidema, G. D.: Hyperplastic Cholecystoses, *Arch Surg,* **104:**193, 1972.

Johnson, F. E., and Boyden, E. A.: Effect of Double Vagotomy on Motor Activity of Human Gall Bladder, *Surgery,* **32:**591, 1952.

Jutras, J. A.: Hyperplastic Cholecystoses, *Am J Roentgenol Radium Ther Nucl Med,* **83:**795, 1960.

Kjellgren, K.: Persistence of Symptoms following Biliary Surgery, *Ann Surg,* **152:**1026, 1960.

Tanturi, C. A., and Ivy, A. C.: Study of Effect of Vascular Changes in Liver and Excitation of Its Nerve Supply on Formation of Bile, *Am J Physiol,* **121:**61, 1938.

Diagnosis of Biliary Tract Disease

Baker, H. L., Jr., and Hodgson, J. R.: Further Studies on the Accuracy of Oral Cholecystography, *Radiology,* **74:**239, 1960.

Eikman, E. A., Cameron, J. L., Colman, M., Natarajan, T. K., Dugal, P., and Wagner, H. N., Jr.: Test for Patency of Cystic Duct in Acute Cholecystitis, *Ann Intern Med,* **82:**318, 1975.

Freeman, J. B., Cohen, W. N., and Den Besten, L.: Cholecystokinin Cholangiography and Analysis of Duodenal Bile in Investigation of Pain in Right Upper Quadrant of the Abdomen without Gallstones, *Surg Gynecol Obstet,* **140:**371, 1975.

Graham, E. A., and Cole, W. H.: Roentgenologic Examination of Gallbladder: New Method Utilizing Intravenous Injection of Tetrabromphenolphthalein, *JAMA,* **82:**613, 1924.

Nora, P. F., Berci, G., Dorazio, R. A., Kirshenbaum, G., Shore, G. M., Tompkins, R. K., and Wilson, S. D.: Operative Choledochoscopy, *Am J Surg,* **133:**105, 1977.

Schein, C. J., and Beneventano, T. C.: Biliary Manometry: Its Role in Clinical Surgery, *Surgery,* **67:**255, 1970.

———, Stern, W. Z., and Jacobson, H. G.: The Common Bile Duct: Operative Cholangiography, Biliary Endoscopy and Choledocholithotomy," Charles C Thomas, Publisher, Springfield, 1966.

Scholz, F. J., Johnston, D. O., and Wise, R. E.: Intravenous Cholangiography: Optimum Dosage and Methodology. *Radiology,* **114:**513, 1975.

Shehadi, W. H.: "Clinical Radiology of the Biliary Tract," McGraw-Hill Book Company, New York, 1963.

White, T. T., Waisman, H., Hopton, D., and Kavlie, H.: Radiomanometry, Flow Rates, and Cholangiography in the Evaluation of Common Bile Duct Disease, *Am J Surg,* **123:**73, 1972.

Williams, J. A. R., Baker, R. J., Walsh, J. F., and Marion, M. A.: The Role of Biliary Scanning in the Investigation of the Surgically Jaundiced Patient, *Surg Gynecol Obstet,* **144:**525, 1977.

Trauma

Cattell, R. B., and Braasch, J. W.: General Considerations in the Management of Benign Strictures of the Bile Duct, *N Engl J Med,* **261:**929, 1959.

Cole, W. H., Ireneus, C., and Reynolds, J. T.: Strictures of the Common Duct, *Ann Surg,* **133:**684, 1951.

Diethrich, E. B., Beall, A. C., Jr., Jordan, G. L., Jr., and DeBakey, M. E.: Traumatic Injuries to the Extrahepatic Biliary Tract, *Am J Surg,* **112:**756, 1966.

Ellis, H., and Cronin, K.: Bile Peritonitis, *Br J Surg,* **48:**166, 1960.

Glenn, F.: Postoperative Strictures of the Extrahepatic Bile Ducts, *Surg Gynecol Obstet,* **120:**560, 1965.

Longmire, W. P., Jr.: Early Management of Injury to the Extrahepatic Biliary Tract, *JAMA,* **195:**623, 1966.

Manlove, C. H., Quattlebaum, F. W., and Ambrus, L.: Nonpenetrating Trauma to the Biliary Tract, *Am J Surg,* **97:**113, 1959.

Penn, I.: Injuries of the Gall-Bladder, *Br J Surg,* **49:**636, 1961–1962.

Rubenstone, A. I., Mintz, S. S., and Meranze, D. R.: Case of Fatal Bile Peritonitis following Liver Needle Biopsy, *Ann Intern Med,* **36:**166, 1952.

Schwartz, S. I., Adams, J. T., Cockett, A. T. K., and Morton, J. H.: Blunt Trauma to the Upper Abdomen, *Surg Annu,* **3:**273, 1971.

Sedgwick, C., Poulantas, J., and Kune, G.: Management of Portal Hypertension Secondary to Bile Duct Strictures: Review of 18 Cases with Splenorenal Shunt, *Ann Surg,* **163:**949, 1966.

Smith, S. W., and Hastings, T. N.: Traumatic Rupture of Gallbladder, *Ann Surg,* **139:**517, 1954.

Turney, W. H., Lee, J. P., and Raju, S.: Complete Transection of Common Bile Duct Due to Blunt Trauma, *Ann Surg,* **179:**440, 1974.

Gallstones

Adams, R., and Stranahan, A.: Cholecystitis and Cholelithiasis: Analytical Report of 1,104 Operative Cases, *Surg Gynecol Obstet,* **85:**776, 1947.

Bartlett, M. K., and Waddell, W. R.: Indications for Common-duct Exploration: Evaluation in 1,000 Cases, *N Engl J Med,* **258:**164, 1958.

Berliner, S. D., and Burson, L. C.: One-Stage Repair for Cholecyst-Duodenal Fistula and Gallstone Ileus, *Arch Surg,* **90:**313, 1965.

Bogren, H.: The Composition and Structure of Human Gallstones, *Acta Radiol Suppl,* 226, 1964.

Burhenne, H. J.: Complications of Nonoperative Extraction of Retained Common Duct Stones, *Am J Surg,* **131:**260, 1976.

Chaimoff, C., and Dintsman, M.: Presence of Pancreatic Juice in the Gallbladder of Patients with Cholelithiasis, *Isr J Med Sci,* **6:**313, 1970.

Colcock, B. P.: Stenosis of the Sphincter of Oddi, *Surg Clin North Am,* **38:**663, 1958.

———, Killen, R. B., and Leach, N. G.: The Asymptomatic Patient with Gallstones, *Am J Surg,* **113:**44, 1967.

Comfort, M. W., Gray, H. K., and Wilson, J. M.: Silent Gallstone: 10 to 20 Year Follow-up Study of 112 Cases, *Ann Surg,* **128:**931, 1948.

Cotton, P. B., Chapman, M., Whiteside, C. G., and LeQuesne, L. P.: Duodenoscopic Papillotomy and Gallstone Removal, *Br J Surg,* **63:**709, 1976.

Coyne, M. J., Bonorris, G. C., Chung, A., Goldstein, L. I., Lahana, D., and Schoenfield, L. J.: Treatment of Gallstones with Chenodeoxycholic Acid and Phenobarbital, *N Engl J Med,* **292:**604, 1975.

Day, E. A., and Marks, C.: Gallstone Ileus: Review of Literature and Presentation of 34 New Cases, *Am J Surg,* **129:**552, 1975.

Deckoff, S. L.: Gallstone Ileus, *Ann Surg,* **142:**52, 1955.

Degenshein, G. A.: Choledochoduodenostomy: An 18-Year Study of 175 Consecutive Cases, *Surgery,* **76:**319, 1974.

Fung, J.: Liver Fluke Infestation and Cholangio-Hepatitis, *Br J Surg,* **48:**404, 1961.

Henzel, J. H., and DeWeese, M. S.: Common Duct Exploration with and without Balloon-Tipped Biliary Catheters, *Arch Surg,* **103:**199, 1971.

Kleeberg, J.: Experimental Studies on the Colloid Chemical Mechanism of Gallstone Formation, *Gastroenterologia,* **80:** 313, 1953.

Large, A. M.: On the Formation of Gallstones, *Surgery,* **54:**928, 1963.

Madden, J. L., Chun, J. Y., Kandalaft, S., and Parekh, M.: Choledochoduodenostomy: An Unjustly Maligned Surgical Procedure?, *Am J Surg,* **119:**45, 1970.

Maki, T.: Pathogenesis of Calcium Bilirubinate Gallstone: Role of *E. coli,* β-Glucuronidase and Coagulation by Inorganic Ions, Polyelectrolytes and Agitation, *Ann Surg,* **164:**90, 1966.

Merendino, K. A., and Manhas, D. R.: Man-Made Gallstones: New Entity following Cardiac Valve Replacement, *Ann Surg,* **177:**694, 1973.

Method, H. L., Mehn, W. H., and Frable, W. J.: "Silent" Gallstones, *Arch Surg,* **85:**338, 1962.

Räf, L., and Spangen, L.: Gallstone Ileus, *Acta Chir Scand,* **137:** 665, 1971.

Rains, A. J. H.: Researches concerning the Formation of Gallstones, *Br Med J,* **2:**685, 1962.

Small, D. M.: Gallstones: Diagnosis and Treatment, *Postgrad Med,* **51:**187, 1972.

Thistle, J. L., and Schoenfield, L. J.: Lithogenic Bile among Young Indian Women: Lithogenic Potential Disease with Chenodeoxycholic Acid, *N Engl J Med,* **284:**177, 1971.

Thureborn, E.: Formation of Gallstone in Man, *Arch Surg,* **91:**952, 1965.

Van Der Linden, W.: Some Biological Traits in Female Gallstone-disease Patients, *Acta Chir Scand [Suppl],* vol. **269,** 1961.

Warshaw, A. L., and Bartlett, M. K.: Choice of Operation for Gallstone Intestinal Obstruction, *Ann Surg,* **164:**1051, 1966.

Way, L. W., Admirand, W., and Dunphy, J. E.: The Management of Choledocholithiasis, *Ann Surg.,* **176:**347, 1972.

Womack, N. A.: The Development of Gallstones, *Surg Gynecol Obstet,* **133:**937, 1971.

Zollinger, R. M., Boles, E. T., and Crawford, G. B.: The Diagnosis and Management of Biliary-Tract Disease, *N Engl J Med,* **252:**203, 1955.

Inflammatory and Other Benign Lesions

Acosta, J., and Nardi, G. L.: Papillitis of the Ampulla of Vater, *Arch Surg,* **92:**354, 1966.

Adams, J. T., Libertino, J. A., and Schwartz, S. I.: Significance of an Elevated Serum Amylase, *Surgery,* **63:**877, 1968.

Bartlett, M. K., and Dreyfuss, J. R.: Residual Common Duct Stones, *Surgery,* **47:**202, 1960.

Becker, W. F., Powell, J. I., and Turner, R. J.: A Clinical Study of 1,060 Patients with Acute Cholecystitis, *Surg Gynecol Obstet,* **104:**491, 1957.

Bisgard, J. D., and Baker, C. P.: Studies Relating to the Pathogenesis of Cholecystitis, Cholelithiasis, and Acute Pancreatitis, *Ann Surg,* **112:**1006, 1940.

Burnett, W.: The Management of Acute Cholecystitis, *Aust New Zeal J Surg,* **41:**25, 1971.

———, and Shields, R.: Symptoms after Cholecystectomy, *Lancet,* **1:**923, 1958.

Cattell, R. B., and Colcock, B. P.: Fibrosis of the Sphincter of Oddi, *Ann Surg,* **137:**797, 1953.

Charcot, J. M.: "Leçons sur les maladies du foie des voies filiares et des reins," Faculté de Médecine de Paris, 1877.

Chetlin, S. H., and Elliott, D. W.: Biliary Bacteremia, *Arch Surg,* **102:**303, 1971.

Colcock, B. P., and Perey, B.: Exploration of the Common Bile Duct, *Surg Gynecol Obstet,* **118:**20, 1964.

Danzi, J. T., Makipour, H., and Farmer, R. G.: Primary Sclerosing Cholangitis: A Report of Nine Cases and Clinical Review, *Am J Gastroenterol,* **65:**109, 1976.

DeCamp, P. T., Ochsner, A., Baffes, T. G., Bancroft, H., and Bendel, W.: Timing in the Surgical Treatment of Acute Colecystitis, *Ann Surg,* **135:**734, 1952.

Dunphy, J. E., and Ross, F. P.: Studies in Acute Cholecystitis, *Surgery,* **26:**539, 1949.

Ellison, E. H.: Early Operation for Acute Cholecystitis, in J. H. Mulholland, E. H. Ellison, and S. R. Friesen (eds.), "Current Surgical Management," W. B. Saunders Company, Philadelphia, 1957.

Friesen, S. R.: Management of Acute Cholecystitis by Selection of Patients for Early or Delayed Operation, in J. H. Mulholland, E. H. Ellison, and S. R. Friesen (eds.), "Current Surgical Management," W. B. Saunders Company, Philadelphia, 1957.

Garlock, J. H., and Hurwitt, E. S.: The Cystic Duct Stump Syndrome, *Surgery,* **29:**833, 1951.

Glenn, F.: Common Duct Exploration for Stones, *Surg Gynecol Obstet,* **95:**431, 1952.

——— and Moody, F. C.: Acute Obstructive Suppurative Cholangitis, *Surg Gynecol Obstet,* **113:**265, 1961.

——— and Whitsell, J. C., II: The Surgical Treatment of Cystic Duct Remnants, *Surg Gynecol Obstet,* **113:**711, 1961.

Goldstein, F., Grunt, R., and Margulies, M.: Cholecystokinin Cholecystography in Differential Diagnosis of Acalculous Gallbladder Disease, *Am J Dig Dis,* **19**:835, 1974.

Grage, T. B., Lober, P. H., Imamogly, K., and Wangensteen, O. H.: Stenosis of the Sphincter of Oddi, *Surgery,* **48**:304, 1960.

Haupert, A. P., Carey, L. C., Evans, W. E., and Ellison, E. H.: Acute Suppurative Cholangitis: Experience with 15 Consecutive Cases, *Arch Surg,* **94**:460, 1967.

Havard, C.: Non-malignant Bile Duct Obstruction, *Ann R Coll Surg Engl,* **26**:88, 1960.

Hinchey, E. J., Elias, G. L., and Hampson, L. G.: Acute Cholecystitis, *Surg Gynecol Obstet,* **120**:475, 1966.

Hoerr, S. O., and Hazard, J. B.: Acute Cholecystitis without Gallbladder Stones, *Am J Surg,* **111**:47, 1966.

Keighley, M. R. B., Lister, C. M., Jacobs, S. I., and Giles, G. R.: Hazards of Surgical Treatment Due to Microorganisms in Bile, *Surgery,* **75**:578, 1974.

Lindenauer, S. M.: Surgical Treatment of Bile Duct Strictures, *Surgery,* **73**:875, 1973.

McCubbrey, D., and Thieme, E. T.: Perforation of the Gallbladder, *Arch Surg,* **80**:204, 1960.

Mackey, W. A.: Cholecystitis without Stone, *Br J Surg,* **22**:274, 1934.

Mage, S., and Morel, S.: Surgical Experience with Cholangio-hepatitis (Hong Kong Disease), *Ann Surg,* **162**:187, 1965.

Manesis, J. G., and Sullivan, J. F.: Primary Sclerosing Cholangitis, *Arch Intern Med,* **115**:137, 1956.

Massie, J. R., Coxc, J. W., III, Parker, C., and Dietrick, R.: Gallbladder Perforations in Acute Cholecystitis, *Ann Surg,* **145**:825, 1957.

Mentzer, R. M., Jr., Golden, G. T., Chandler, J. G., and Horsley, J. S., III: Comparative Appraisal of Emphysematous Cholecystitis, *Am J Surg,* **129**:10, 1975.

Mulholland, J. H.: "Delayed Operative Management of Acute Cholecystitis," in J. H. Mulholland, E. H. Ellison, and S. R. Friesen (eds.), "Current Surgical Management," W. B. Saunders Company, Philadelphia, 1957.

Munster, A. M., and Brown, J. R.: Acalculous Cholecystitis, *Am J Surg,* **113**:730, 1967.

Ong, G. B.: A Study of Recurrent Pyogenic Cholangitis, *Arch Surg,* **84**:199, 1962.

Ostermiller, W., Thompson, R., Carter, R., and Hinshaw, D.: Acute Obstructive Cholangitis, *Arch Surg,* **90**:392, 1965.

Ottinger, L. W.: Acute Cholecystitis as a Postoperative Complication, *Ann Surg,* **184**:162, 1976.

Pheils, M. T., and Duraiappah, B.: Exploration of Common Bile Duct in Presence of Acute Cholecystitis, *Aust NZ J Surg,* **43**:136, 1973.

Reynolds, B. M., and Dargan, E. L.: Acute Obstructive Cholangitis, *Ann Surg,* **150**:299, 1959.

Rosoff, L., and Meyers, H.: Acute Emphysematous Cholecystitis: An Analysis of Ten Cases, *Am J Surg,* **111**:410, 1966.

Ruskin, R. B., Katon, R. M., Bilbao, M. K., and Smith, R.: Evaluation of Sclerosing Cholangitis by Endoscopic Retrograde Cholangiopancreatography, *Arch Intern Med,* **136**:232, 1976.

Schein, C. J.: "Acute Cholecystitis," Harper & Row, Publishers, Incorporated, New York, 1972.

Schwartz, S. I., and Dale, W. A.: Primary Sclerosing Cholangitis: Review and Report of Six Cases, *Arch Surg,* **77**:439, 1958.

Stefanini, P., Carboni, M., Patrassi, N., Basoli, A., Bernardinis, G. de, and Negro, P.: Roux en Y Hepaticojejunostomy: Reappraisal of Its Indications and Results, *Ann Surg,* **181**:213, 1975.

Stock, F. E., and Fung, J. H. Y.: Oriental Cholangiohepatitis, *Arch Surg,* **84**:409, 1962.

——— and Tinckler, L.: Choledochoduodenostomy in Treatment of Cholangiohepatitis, *Surg Gynecol Obstet,* **101**:599, 1955.

Ternberg, J. L., and Keating, J. P.: Acute Acalculous Cholecystitis: Complication of Other Illnesses in Childhood, *Arch Surg,* **110**:543, 1975.

Tinckler, L.: Primary Sclerosing Cholangitis, *Postgrad Med,* **47**:666, 1971.

Van der Linden, W., and Sunzel, H.: Early Versus Delayed Operation for Acute Cholecystitis: Controlled Clinical Trial, *Am J Surg,* **120**:7, 1970.

Warren, K., Athanassiades, S., and Monge, J.: Primary Sclerosing Cholangitis: A Study of 42 Cases, *Am J Surg,* **111**:23, 1966.

Watkins, D. F. L., and Thomas, G. G.: Jaundice in Acute Cholecystitis, *Br J Surg,* **58**:570, 1971.

Welch, J. P., and Donaldson, G. A.: The Urgency of Diagnosis and Surgical Treatment of Acute Suppurative Cholangitis, *Am J Surg,* **131**:527, 1976.

——— and Malt, R. A.: Outcome of Cholecystostomy, *Surg Gynecol Obstet,* **135**:717, 1972.

Womack, N. A., and Crider, R. L.: Persistence of Symptoms following Cholecystectomy, *Ann Surg,* **126**:31, 1947.

Tumors

Altemeier, W. A., Gall, E. A., Culbertson, W. R., and Inge, W. W.: Sclerosing Carcinoma of the Intrahepatic (Hilar) Bile Ducts, *Surgery,* **60**:191, 1966.

Beltz, W. R., and Condon, R. E.: Primary Carcinoma of the Gallbladder, *Ann Surg,* **180**:180, 1974.

Brasfield, R. D.: Right Hepatic Lobectomy for Carcinoma of the Gallbladder: A Five-Year Cure, *Ann Surg,* **153**:563, 1961.

Comfort, M. W., Gray, H. K., and Wilson, J. M.: Silent Gallstone: A 10 to 25 Year Follow-up Study of 112 Cases, *Ann Surg,* **128**:931, 1948.

Donaldson, L. A., and Busuttil, A.: Clinicopathologic Review of 68 Carcinomas of the Gallbladder, *Br J Surg,* **62**:26, 1975.

Fahim, R. B., McDonald, J. R., Richards, J. C., and Ferris, D. O.: Carcinoma of the Gallbladder: A Study of Its Modes of Spread, *Ann Surg,* **156**:114, 1962.

Kirshbaum, J. D., and Kozoll, D. D.: Carcinoma of the Gallbladder and Extrahepatic Bile Ducts: A Clinical and Pathological Study of 117 Cases in 13,330 Necopsies, *Surg Gynecol Obstet,* **73**:740, 1941.

Kuwayti, K., Baggenstoss, A. H., Stauffer, M. H., and Priestley, J. T.: Carcinoma of the Intrahepatic and Extrahepatic Bile Ducts Exclusive of the Papilla of Vater, *Surg Gynecol Obstet,* **104**:357, 1957.

Litwin, M. S.: Primary Carcinoma of the Gallbladder, *Arch Surg,* **95**:236, 1967.

Molnar, W., and Stockum, A. E.: Relief from Obstructive Jaundice through Percutaneous Transhepatic Catheter: New Therapeutic Method, *Am J Roentgenol Radium Ther Nucl Med,* **122**:356, 1974.

Mori, K., Misumi, A., Sugiyama, M., Okabe, M., Matsuoka, T.,

Ishii, J., and Akagi, M.: Percutaneous Transhepatic Bile Damage, *Ann Surg,* **185:**111, 1977.

Neibling, H. H., Dockerty, M. B., and Waugh, J. M.: Carcinoma of the Extrahepatic Bile Ducts, *Surg Gynecol Obstet,* **89:**429, 1949.

Pemberton, L. B., Diffenbaugh, W. F., and Strohl, E. L.: The Surgical Significance of Carcinoma of the Gallbladder, *Am J Surg,* **122:**381, 1971.

Quattlebaum, J. K., and Quattlebaum, J. K., Jr.: Malignant Obstruction of the Major Hepatic Ducts, *Ann Surg,* **161:**876, 1965.

Robertson, W. A., and Carlisle, B. B.: Primary Carcinoma of the Gallbladder: Review of Fifty-two cases, *Am J Surg,* **113:**738, 1967.

Sheinfeld, W.: Cholecystectomy and Partial Hepatectomy for Carcinoma of the Gallbladder with Local Liver Extension, *Surgery,* **22:**48, 1947.

Terblanche, J., Saunders, S. J., and Louw, J. H.: Prolonged Palliation in Carcinoma of the Main Hepatic Duct Junction, *Surgery,* **71:**728, 1972.

Thomas, C. G., Jr., Nicholson, C. P., and Owen, J.: Effectiveness of Choledochoduodenostomy and Transduodenal Sphincter-otomy in the Treatment of Benign Obstruction of the Common Duct, *Ann Surg,* **173:**845, 1971.

Thorbjarnarson, B.: Carcinoma of the Bile Ducts, *Cancer,* **12:**708, 1959.

Tompkins, R. K., Johnson, J., Storm, F. K., and Longmire, W. P., Jr.: Operative Endoscopy in the Management of Biliary Tract Neoplasms, *Am J Surg,* **132:**174, 1976.

Vaittinen, E.: Carcinoma of the Gallbladder: Study of 390 Cases Diagnosed in Finland, 1953–67, *Ann Chir Gynaecol Fenn,* Vol. 59, suppl, 168, 1970.

Whelton, M. J., Petrelli, M., George, P., Young, W. B., and Sherlock, S.: Carcinoma at Junction of Main Hepatic Ducts, *Q J Med,* **38:**211, 1969.

Operations on the Biliary Tract

Kambouris, A., Carpenter, W. S., and Allaben, R. D.: Cholecystectomy without Drainage, *Surg Gynecol Obstet,* **137:**613, 1973.

Wexler, M. J., and Smith, R.: Jejunal Mucosal Graft: Sutureless Technic for Repair of High Bile Duct Strictures, *Am J Surg,* **129:**204, 1975.

Pancreas

by **William Silen**

ANATOMY

The pancreas extends transversely across the upper abdomen behind the stomach. The junction of the upper left portion of the head of the pancreas with the body is called the "neck," or "waist," a constricted and narrowed area rarely more than 3 to 4 cm wide. The superior mesenteric vein and artery lie just behind the neck and are enclosed behind by a posterior extension of the lower left portion of the head (uncinate process).

DUCTAL SYSTEM. The main pancreatic duct (duct of Wirsung) begins at the tail of the pancreas and extends to the right at, or slightly superior to, a point halfway between the superior and inferior borders of the pancreas. It lies somewhat closer to the posterior than to the anterior surface of the organ, and its tributaries enter almost at right angles along its entire course. In the head of the pancreas the major duct turns inferiorly and joins the common bile duct at the papilla of Vater. The minor duct, or duct of Santorini, lies in the head of the pancreas in a much more ventral plane and therefore in a surgically more vulnerable plane than the duct of Wirsung. This duct begins at its junction with the main duct in the neck of the pancreas and terminates in the minor papilla, located about 2 cm proximal to the major papilla and 7 cm distal to the pylorus. Tiny accessory ducts emptying directly from the pancreas into the intrapancreatic portion of the common bile duct have been described.

Many variations in the normal anatomy of the ductal system have been described (Fig. 32-1). Configuration of the ducts is "normal" in only 60 to 70 percent of the population. In about 30 percent of cases, although a duct of Santorini exists, it does not communicate with the duodenum. Reich has recently found that this anatomic arrangement is more frequent in patients with duodenal ulcer, and he has suggested that the lack of alkaline pancreatic juice in this region may make the duodenum more susceptible to peptic ulceration. In 5 to 10 percent of human beings, the duct of Santorini is the sole duct draining the pancreas into the duodenum. In such cases injury to the duct of Santorini, especially during gastrectomy, may cause severe hemorrhagic or recurrent pancreatitis. Since the gastroduodenal artery always passes behind the duodenum proximal to the minor papilla, this vascular landmark may be useful as an indication that further distal dissection of the duodenum may be extremely hazardous.

In the second decade of life the major pancreatic duct is 3 to 4 mm in diameter. As aging progresses, the ducts become larger, and in persons over the age of seventy, ducts 5 to 6 mm in diameter are commonly encountered in the normal pancreas.

BLOOD SUPPLY. The arterial supply to the pancreas is remarkably constant (Fig. 32-2). Anterior and posterior arcades supply the head of the pancreas; each arcade derives a superior component from the gastroduodenal artery and an inferior component from the superior mesenteric artery. The anterosuperior pancreaticoduodenal and anteroinferior pancreaticoduodenal arteries join to form the anterior arcade; the posterosuperior pancreaticoduodenal and posteroinferior pancreaticoduodenal arteries form the posterior arcade. This arrangement occurs in almost 100 percent of cases. The anterior arcade constitutes virtually the only major group of blood vessels on the anterior surface of the pancreas, an important surgical consideration.

The inferior pancreatic artery, which is nearly always constant, runs along the posteroinferior surface of the pancreas in intimate contact with the organ. Its origin is variable; it may start from the superior mesenteric artery, anterosuperior or anteroinferior pancreaticoduodenal artery, or superior pancreatic artery.

The superior pancreatic artery is present in from 50 to 90 percent of patients and arises from the splenic, hepatic, superior mesenteric, or celiac arteries. It lies along the posterosuperior portion of the neck and body of the pan-

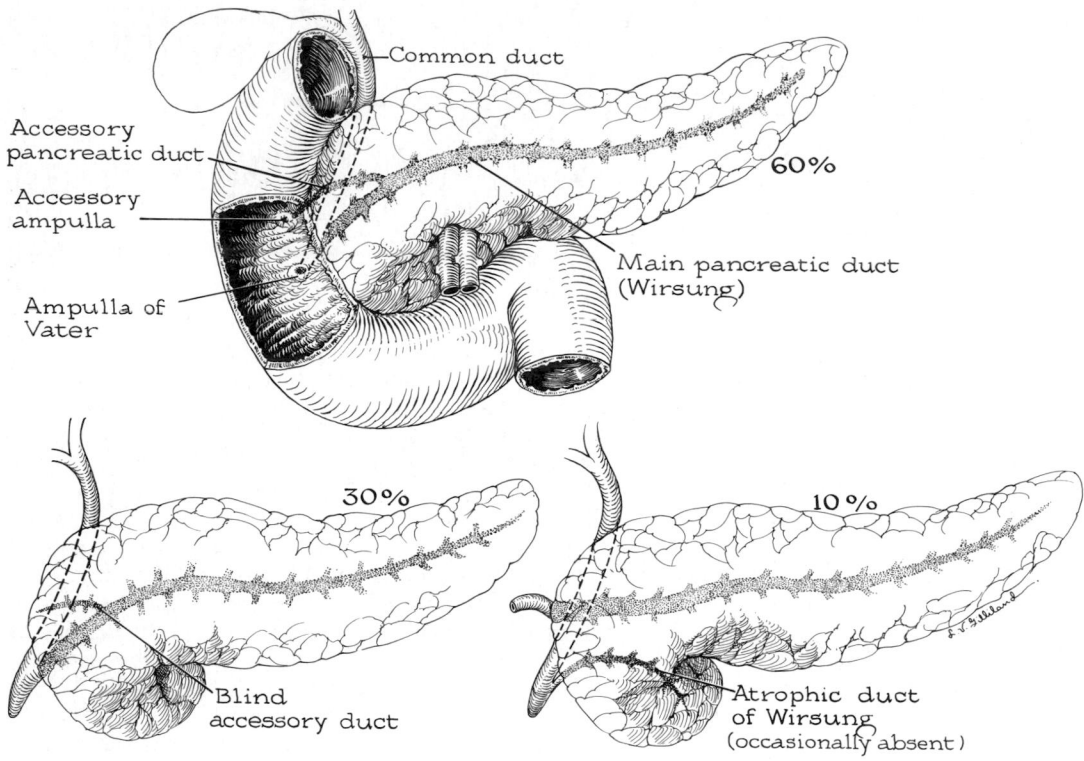

Common duct

Accessory
pancreatic duct

Accessory
ampulla

Ampulla of
Vater

60%

Main pancreatic duct
(Wirsung)

30%

10%

Blind
accessory duct

Atrophic duct
of Wirsung
(occasionally absent)

creas. The body and tail of the pancreas are also supplied
by branches from the splenic and left gastroepiploic arteries.

The venous drainage of the pancreas follows the course
of the arteries quite closely, but the veins lie superficial
to their arterial counterparts. Anterior and posterior venous arcades are always present around the head of the
pancreas. The confluence of the right gastroepiploic vein,
anterosuperior pancreaticoduodenal vein, and middle colic
vein forms the gastrocolic trunk, which empties directly
into the superior mesenteric vein at the inferior border of

Fig. 32-1. Anatomic configuration of the intrapancreatic ductal
system. Note the lack of communication between the two ducts in
10 percent of cases. (*From W. Silen, Surg Clin North Am,
44:1253, 1964.*)

the neck of the pancreas. This provides an important landmark for location of the superior mesenteric vein when
the pancreas is mobilized to determine operability of pancreatic tumors.

From the surgical standpoint it is important to remem-

Fig. 32-2. Arterial supply and venous drainage of the pancreas.
Note particularly the anatomic importance of the gastrocolic
venous trunk in defining the inferior portion of the neck. (*From
W. Silen, Surg Clin North Am, 44:1253, 1964.*)

Portal vein

Post. superior
pancreatico-duodenal
a. & v.

Right gastro-
epiploic a. & v.

Subpyloric
vein

Gastro-
colic
trunk

Ant. superior
pancreatico-
duodenal a. & v.

Splenic a. & v.

Inf. pancreatic vein

Sup. mesenteric a. & v.

Inferior pancreatico-
duodenal communis artery

Common stem of anterior
& posterior inf. pancreaticoduodenal veins

ber that occasionally the hepatic artery may arise from the superior mesenteric artery and pass behind the pancreas and common bile duct. An unusually long and tortuous hepatic artery may lie close to the superior border of the head of the pancreas, or in some cases it may be within the pancreas itself. Under these circumstances, the hepatic artery may be injured during resection of the body and tail of the pancreas and may require ligation. Pierson has pointed out that the distal duodenum and proximal jejunum receive their arterial supply from one of the inferior pancreaticoduodenal arteries, so that interruption of these vessels probably will necessitate resection of the proximal 3 to 5 cm of jejunum.

Anatomy textbooks usually state that the anterior surface of the superior mesenteric and portal veins is free of tributaries in the region of the pancreas. However, the superior pancreaticoduodenal vein often joins the portal vein at the anterior surface of the pancreas, and the gastrocolic vein almost always joins the anterior surface of the superior mesenteric vein inferior to the neck. Other small venous tributaries from the pancreas to the portal and superior mesenteric veins are often present, although hidden from view. The posterosuperior pancreaticoduodenal vein may be the source of severe hemorrhage during mobilization of the portal vein for portacaval shunt.

LYMPHATIC DRAINAGE AND NERVE SUPPLY. The lymphatic capillaries from the tail drain into the nodes at the hilus of the spleen. From the right side of the pancreas the lymphatics drain into the pancreaticoduodenal lymph nodes lying in the groove between the duodenum and pancreas and into the subpyloric nodes. Anteriorly the drainage is to the superior pancreatic, superior gastric, and hepatic nodes along the hepatic artery. Posteriorly the lymphatics pass to the inferior pancreatic, mesocolic, mesenteric, and aortic nodes.

The sympathetic nerve supply to the pancreas is derived from the greater, lesser, and lowest splanchnic nerves via the celiac ganglia and plexus. These fibers conduct the afferent pain fibers from the pancreas. The sympathetic nerves intermingle with branches of the right vagus nerve to form the splenic plexus from which most of the nerve supply to the pancreas emanates. The celiac branch of the right, or posterior, vagus nerve provides parasympathetic supply to the pancreas. This branch can be spared during selective gastric vagotomy for duodenal ulcer.

Annular Pancreas

Annular pancreas is a rare anatomic abnormality which results when two limbs of pancreatic tissue encircle the second portion of the duodenum because of incomplete migration of the ventral anlage of the gland. A variable degree of duodenal obstruction occurs, and associated anomalies, particularly complete atresia of the duodenum, are common. Histologically, the lesion presents as normal pancreatic tissue.

Frequently there are no symptoms, and the finding is incidental. When symptoms occur, they are related to acute and recurrent duodenal obstruction and include abdominal pain, nausea, and vomiting. The onset of symptoms ap-

Fig. 32-3. Roentgenogram demonstrating annular pancreas.

pears at all ages, but one-third present under the age of one. The diagnosis is suggested by the roentgenographic finding of partial or complete duodenal obstruction with notching of the right lateral duodenal wall (Fig. 32-3). A variety of surgical procedures have been proposed, including partial resection of the annular portion of the gland or bypassing the area of obstruction. The former is frequently followed by pancreatic fistula, and it is the consensus that duodenojejunostomy is the least hazardous and most effective way of relieving the obstruction.

PHYSIOLOGY

Exocrine Pancreas

PANCREATIC JUICE. The human pancreas daily produces from 1,500 to 2,500 ml of a colorless, odorless fluid which has a pH of 8.0 to 8.3. Pancreatic juice is isosmotic with the plasma, and its osmolality is independent of the rate of flow, both in health and disease. The bicarbonate of pancreatic juice is secreted by an active transport mechanism, and as the solution moves down the collecting system, exchange with chloride ion takes place. The sum of the concentrations of bicarbonate and chloride is constant under all conditions of secretion, although bicarbonate concentration rises with increasing rates of secretion. The secretion of bicarbonate is under the catalytic influence of carbonic anhydrase. The isosmotic reabsorption of water and electrolytes from the ductal lumen may be governed by antidiuretic hormone. The concentration of sodium and potassium is similar to that in plasma, which indicates that these ions are moved passively rather than actively.

Pancreatic juice contains between 1 and 3 percent protein, 90 percent of which is enzymatic. Since the metabolic turnover of protein in the acinar cells of the pancreas is the highest of any cells in the body, the pancreas is dependent upon a constant supply of amino acids. It is not surprising, therefore, that protein deficiency may be associated with severe defects in exocrine pancreatic function, as in kwashiorkor. Proteolytic, lipolytic, and amylolytic enzymes are present in the pancreatic juice; the optimal pH for activity of all three enzyme systems is greater than 7. These enzymes are formed within the mitochondrial apparatus of the secreting cells, at the site of the attached ribosomes of the endoplasmic reticulum. Pancreatic trypsinogen and chymotrypsinogen are activated to trypsin and chymotrypsin by the intestinal enzyme enterokinase, as well as by trypsin itself. These enzymes hydrolyze proteins to peptones and peptides.

Recently, other proteolytic enzymes such as procarboxypeptidases, carboxypeptidase, ribonuclease, and deoxyribonuclease have been discovered in porcine and bovine pancreatic juice, and it is probable that at least some are present in human pancreatic juice. The fat-splitting enzymes of the pancreas are lipase, which splits fat into glycerol and fatty acids in the presence of bile salts; phospholipases A and B; and cholesterol esterase. Pancreatic amylase splits starch to dextrins and disaccharides, principally maltose.

CONTROL OF PANCREATIC SECRETION (Fig. 32-4). The vagus nerve is the secretory nerve to the pancreas and plays a role in the "cephalic phase" of pancreatic secretion somewhat analogous to its relationship to the cephalic phase of gastric secretion. Sham feeding of an unanesthetized dog causes a scant flow of juice rich in enzymes, beginning 1 to 2 minutes after feeding and lasting for 30 minutes, provided that gastric juice is prevented from entering the duodenum. This response is abolished by atropine or by vagotomy. Although the splanchnic nerves may contain secretory fibers to the pancreas, the importance of these fibers is probably minimal.

White et al. have presented evidence for the existence of a gastropancreatic reflex by demonstrating that distension of the fundus of the stomach increases the volume and enzyme output of pancreatic juice, but this reflex can be temporarily abolished by vagotomy. Further evidence is required before the existence of such a reflex is definitely

Fig. 32-4. Schema of neurohumoral influences on external pancreatic secretion.

BLOCKS OR DECREASES ACTION OF 2 HORMONES

ATROPINE

REGULATION OF EXTERNAL PANCREATIC SECRETION

BLOOD STREAM

VAGUS NERVE POTENTIATES ACTION OF 2 HORMONES

VAGUS NERVE STIMULATES ENZYME OUTPUT

VAGUS NERVE POTENTIATES ANTRAL GASTRIN

VAGUS NERVE TO DUODENUM POTENTIATES RELEASE OF 2 HORMONES

PANCREOZYMIN

SECRETIN

ANTRAL GASTRIN

PANCREOZYMIN
STIMULATES ENZYME OUTPUT

STIMULATES VOLUME & ENZYME OUTPUT

SECRETIN
STIMULATES SECRETION OF H₂O & ELECTROLYTES

ACID PROTEIN FAT SOAP

INTRINSIC AUTONOMIC REFLEXES MAY POTENTIATE RELEASE OF 2 HORMONES confirmed. Even though gastrin is capable of stimulating volume and enzyme output in the pancreatic juice of cats and dogs, it remains moot as to whether physiological amounts of gastrin can produce a humoral gastric phase of pancreatic secretion.

Quantitatively, the intestinal phase of pancreatic secretion is probably the most important. When gastric contents enter the duodenum, the volume and enzyme outputs of the pancreas greatly increase. This response is mediated by the release of secretin and cholecystokinin (pancreozymin) from the duodenal mucosa. These hormones may be produced in response to the introduction of a number of substances into the duodenum, including hydrochloric acid, acid peptone, sodium oleate, and a solution of amino acids. The release of secretin by intraduodenal acid has recently been shown to be directly related to the quantity of acid entering the duodenum per unit time. Small but significant amounts of secretin can be released even between pH 3.5 and 4.5 when the quantity of acid exposed to the duodenal mucosa per unit time is high.

Cholecystokinin potentiates pancreatic volume and bicarbonate output stimulated by small amounts of endogenous or exogenous secretin. The release of both secretin and cholecystokinin from the duodenal mucosa is now known to be substantially diminished by total abdominal vagotomy, although the response of the vagotomized pancreas to exogenous secretin is not altered.

The most important physiologic effect of secretin is stimulation of flow of water and electrolytes from the pancreas. There is a short latent period (about 20 seconds) between the injection of secretin or the instillation of acid into the duodenum and the onset of the secretory response. Cholecystokinin profoundly stimulates the output of enzymes; that is, its effects are similar to those of vagal stimulation. The response of the pancreas to both the intraduodenal instillation of hydrochloric acid and to secretin is considerably decreased by administration of anticholinergic drugs.

Pituitary and adrenal hormones affect pancreatic secretion, but their exact influence on the physiologic regulation of such secretion is not known. Serotonin seems to decrease food-stimulated pancreatic secretion and possibly that stimulated by secretin. Glucagon diminishes volume and bicarbonate output.

EFFECTS OF LOSS OF PANCREATIC JUICE. The functional consequences of loss of pancreatic juice may be considerable. Exclusion of pancreatic juice from the gastrointestinal tract by pancreatectomy, by ligation of the pancreatic ducts, or by total external pancreatic fistula results in severe impairment of the digestion and absorption of various foodstuffs, particularly fat. Excessive losses of fat in the stool occur in patients in whom pancreatic juice is completely excluded from the intestine. Fat digestion is probably only slightly impaired if but a fraction of normal pancreatic juice enters the duodenum.

Profound gastric hypersecretion always occurs experimentally whenever pancreatic secretions are diverted from the intestine. It is likely that the absence of pancreatic juice from the intestine prevents normal fat inhibition by enterogastrone and that the nutritional consequences of in-

adequate digestion cause hepatic damage, which may also enhance gastric hypersecretion. Two conclusions of surgical importance can be reached: (1) if the head of the pancreas is resected, digestion is better, and the chances of marginal ulceration are less if the remaining pancreatic remnant is anastomosed to the gastrointestinal tract rather than being ligated; and (2) pancreatic extracts should be used freely whenever postoperative deficiency of external pancreatic secretion exists.

Impaired absorption of vitamin B_{12}, seemingly associated with a low duodenal pH, has been observed in patients with pancreatic insufficiency. Improved absorption of vitamin B_{12} occurred after administration of sodium bicarbonate, pancreatic extract, or both. Apparently, normal secretion of pancreatic juice is essential for unimpaired absorption of vitamin B_{12}. Conversely, pancreatic extracts may depress the abnormally high absorption of iron in hemochromatosis or pancreatitis. These findings provide further strong reasons for administering pancreatic extract to patients with pancreatic insufficiency.

PANCREATICOBILIARY PRESSURE RELATIONSHIPS. Studies of intrabiliary pressure in patients in whom T tubes have been placed in the common duct after cholecystectomy indicate that responses are similar to those observed in dogs. Menguy et al. have shown in dogs that resting pancreatic pressures consistently exceed those in the biliary tree, although the pressure in the bile duct rises after cholecystectomy. The pressure in both ductal systems rises after a meal. When the rate of flow of pancreatic juice is increased by injecting secretin, the pressure in the pancreatic ducts does not rise, although intravenous administration of sodium dehydrocholate definitely increases biliary pressure. Acid instilled into the duodenum causes little change in pancreatic intraductal pressure, in contrast to alcohol, which uniformly increases both pancreatic and biliary pressure. Morphine, codeine, and meperidine hydrochloride increase intrapancreatic pressure but raise biliary pressure only in the absence of the gall bladder. Atropine consistently lowers pancreatic intraductal pressure, and pilocarpine increases pressure. Infected bile, probably as a result of bacterial deconjugation of bile salts, causes a marked rise in resistance of the sphincter of Oddi.

Endocrine Pancreas

The internal secretions of the pancreas are formed by the islets of Langerhans, which approximate 1 million in number yet represent only about 1.5 percent of the normal pancreas by weight. The individual islets are 75 to 150 μ in diameter. The alpha cells are probably the source of glucagon. The beta cells manufacture, store, and secrete insulin, and comprise 60 to 80 percent of the cells of each islet. The function of C cells and delta cells is unknown, although gastrin-producing ulcerogenic tumors of the pancreas may arise from them. Delta cells may give rise to islet tumors which release VIP (vasoactive intestinal peptide).

Glucagon is composed of 20 amino acids arranged in a straight chain and has a molecular weight of 3,485. It causes glycogenolysis in the liver and release of glucose into the bloodstream. A decreased response to glucagon occurs in diseases of the liver. Purified glucagon, 1 mg given intravenously, will usually raise the blood sugar by 50 to 80 mg/100 ml, a gradual return to normal following in about 90 minutes. Glucagon is also secreted by the intestinal mucosa.

Insulin has a molecular weight of about 6,000 and consists of two polypeptide chains. The prime function of insulin is to promote the transfer of glucose and other sugars across certain cell membranes. The transfer of sugars into muscle cells, fibroblasts, and adipose tissue requires insulin, but neurons, erythrocytes, hepatic cells, and intestinal cells can accomplish this process without it. In the absence of glucose, fat is utilized, and ketosis and acidosis occur. Amino acids may be oxidized to provide energy and may cause a negative nitrogen balance when glucose is not being used properly. Insulin may also play a part in the conversion of glucose to glycogen in the liver.

Regulation of insulin secretion does not seem to depend upon trophic support, since neither vagotomy nor ablation of the anterior pituitary gland has an effect upon insulin secretion. The primary stimulus to the secretion of insulin is the blood sugar itself; an increase in blood sugar causes degranulation of the beta cells. Various hormones which increase the blood sugar, such as growth hormone, glucocorticoids, thyroid hormone, and epinephrine, may secondarily increase the secretion of insulin.

It has recently been demonstrated that all three of the major nutrient substrates, namely, glucose, amino acids, and fatty acids, stimulate varying degrees of insulin secretion. Gastrin, secretin, and cholecystokinin all produce a rise in insulin after injection, but the response to gastrin is quantitatively trivial while that to secretin is modest. Cholecystokinin elicits substantial release of both insulin and glucagon and augments the release of these two hormones by amino acids. Leucine and the sulfonureas used in the treatment of diabetes are known to produce their effects by releasing insulin from the beta cell granules.

It is possible that other humoral agents are produced by the islets of the normal pancreas. Certain islet-cell tumors produce gastrin, and others may secrete glucagon. Whether small amounts of gastrin are secreted by the normal pancreas remains conjectural, although gastrin-producing cells have now been identified in the normal pancreas by immunofluorescent techniques.

PANCREATITIS

Acute Pancreatitis

ETIOLOGY. There are two main types of pancreatitis, acute and chronic. Reference is frequently made in the literature to a form of "chronic relapsing pancreatitis" which is discussed as a third form of the disease. Most of these cases are actually recurrent attacks of acute pancreatitis or are simply acute exacerbations in the course of chronic pancreatitis.

Pancreatitis Associated with Gallstones. Approximately two-thirds of patients with pancreatitis in private hospitals have gallstones, but in charity hospitals only one-third or less prove to have gallstone pancreatitis. For many years, a common channel between the common bile duct and the duct of Wirsung was thought to be of great importance in the pathogenesis, not only of gallstone pancreatitis, but also of pancreatitis due to many other causes. It is true that, on occasion, a calculus impacted at the ampulla of Vater may produce pancreatitis. Yet this is a rare occurrence. Only about 18 percent of patients with gallstone pancreatitis have choledocholithiasis, and in only a small number of these is there impaction of a stone at the ampulla. Although a clear association exists between gallstones and acute pancreatitis and treatment of the biliary tract disease almost always cures the pancreatitis, the mechanism by which the pancreatitis is produced remains an enigma. Recent studies show that a high proportion of patients with gallstone pancreatitis have recoverable biliary calculi in the stools.

The classic experimental method for production of pancreatitis is injection of bile into the ductal system, but many facts militate against this mechanism in human gallstone pancreatitis. Continuous perfusion of the unobstructed pancreatic ductal system with bile in dogs and goats has not led to acute pancreatitis. In experimental biliary pancreatitis the bile is usually injected with sufficient pressure to rupture the pancreatic acini. The normal secretory pressure relationships argue against reflux, since pancreatic secretory pressure is generally higher than that of the liver. Radiocinemonometric studies have shown that contraction of the sphincter of Oddi often occludes both the biliary and the pancreatic ducts and isolates them from each other rather than producing an open common channel. Furthermore, reflux into the pancreatic duct occurs quite often during operative or T-tube cholangiography without apparent ill effects. Nevertheless, the bile factor cannot be discarded completely. Elliott et al. have shown that resistance to the flow of bile into the pancreatic duct greatly decreases after incubation of bile with pancreatic juice. Two components of bile, deconjugated bile salts and lysolecithins, have recently been found to be extremely toxic to the pancreas during experimental reflux. Deconjugated bile salts may be formed by bacterial action on conjugated bile salts, and lysolecithin results from the conversion of biliary lecithin by phospholipase A of pancreatic juice. It has been demonstrated that bile in the pancreas may cause vascular injury, stasis, and spasm, which may initiate pancreatitis.

Alcoholic Pancreatitis. About two-thirds of patients with pancreatitis in charity hospitals, but only one-third of such patients in private hospitals, have alcoholic pancreatitis. Alcohol is now known to cause an increase in protein concentration in pancreatic juice, precipitation of which may form a nidus upon which subsequent calcification occurs, and intraduodenal instillation of alcohol also causes a profound and sustained rise in pancreatic ductal pressure in dogs.

Duodenal inflammation may produce some degree of ductal obstruction in a gland actively secreting in response to the acid-secretin mechanism. Experimental ductal obstruction alone does not cause pancreatitis, but if hypersecretion induced by food, secretin, or vascular injury is also present, severe pancreatitis ensues. Persistent vomiting may cause regurgitation of duodenal contents into the pancreatic ducts. Dietary-induced hypertriglyceridemia has now been shown to produce a clinical syndrome of acute pancreatitis in about half of alcoholic patients who previously exhibited alcoholic pancreatitis. Pancreatic calculi and multiple stenoses within the ductal system late in the course of chronic pancreatitis are probably the sequelae of pancreatitis rather than the cause. As important as the mechanical factors may be, nutritional factors may ultimately prove to be more crucial. Since the turnover of protein by the pancreas is the greatest of any organ, it is not surprising that protein deficiency states have been associated with degeneration, atrophy, and fibrosis of the pancreas.

Postoperative Pancreatitis. Pancreatitis occasionally occurs after intraabdominal operations, especially those on the biliary tract and stomach. Rarely, it may develop after operations remote from the pancreas. It is clear that the pancreatitis which follows biliary operations occurs only when the common bile duct has been explored, especially if a long-armed T tube has been placed through the sphincter of Oddi. Pancreatitis is also likely to follow a gastrectomy in which the region of the head of the pancreas has been dissected. Direct ligation or laceration of the duct of Santorini may provide the insult that triggers the pancreatitis. Vascular injury, together with the damage to the duct, may set the stage for this serious disease. The interaction of obstruction and vascular factors is demonstrated by the development of experimental pancreatitis when the second part of the duodenum is converted into a closed loop. The clinical counterpart of this experiment is the occurrence of pancreatitis in a patient with afferent loop obstruction after a Billroth II gastrectomy. The mortality of postoperative pancreatitis is approximately 50 percent. After splenectomy, postoperative pancreatitis is usually the direct result of operative injury to the tail of the pancreas.

Metabolic Factors. An association exists between hyperparathyroidism and pancreatitis. Not only may repeated attacks of acute pancreatitis be one of the first signs of hyperparathyroidism, but occasionally a severe episode may follow removal of a parathyroid adenoma. Calcium markedly enhances the conversion of trypsinogen to trypsin, and its presence in high ionic concentration may produce a mass action effect that precipitates calcium phosphate in the ducts. Parathyroid function should always be investigated in any patient with pancreatitis of obscure cause.

A small group of patients with a hereditary type of pancreatitis have been described in whom aminoaciduria is a fairly consistent finding. Lysinuria and cystinuria are frequently observed, but the metabolic defect that produces the pancreatitis is not known. The disease usually begins in childhood, and inheritance follows the pattern of an autosomal gene. Some of these patients have calcification of the pancreas. The prognosis is generally good.

It has been known for many years that *transient* hyperlipemia may occur during the course of clinical and experimental acute pancreatitis. Release of an inhibitor of the

"clearing factor," lipoprotein lipase, by the diseased pancreas is the most likely cause of the hyperlipemia. This secondary type of hyperlipemia is to be distinguished from an idiopathic form in which the pancreatitis is probably caused by the hyperlipemia. In the idiopathic form, the neutral fats usually increase immediately before the onset of abdominal symptoms and return to normal when the attack is over. Klatskin and Gordon have suggested that the pancreatitis may be caused by fat emboli. The differentiation between the primary and secondary types of hyperlipemia is extremely important, because the attacks of pancreatitis may be prevented by a low-fat diet in the primary group. Dietary-induced hypertriglyceridemia can also cause attacks of acute pancreatitis in alcoholic patients.

Hemochromatosis has been thought to produce pancreatic fibrosis and atrophy because of the irritating properties of the deposited iron. However, iron absorption often increases after pancreatic damage caused by several diseases, and siderosis may in fact be secondary to the pancreatic disease.

Vascular, Toxic, Allergic, and Other Factors. Vascular stasis is an important factor in experimental pancreatitis. The process may be diffuse, probably at the arteriolar level, since ligation of major vessels to the pancreas alone causes only small infarcts. Occasionally, older patients who have widespread vascular obstruction are seen with severe hemorrhagic pancreatitis. The role of vascular spasm and obstruction in other forms of pancreatitis is not clear.

Various toxins, such as methyl alcohol, zinc oxide, cobaltous chloride, and chlorothiazide, have been known to produce pancreatic injury. Although Thal and others have implicated autoimmune mechanisms in the pathogenesis of pancreatitis, there is little evidence to suggest that these are of any particular importance in human pancreatitis.

Despite frequent reports of pancreatitis during mumps, no fatalities or complications have been recorded. The serum amylase may increase in patients with mumps, but whether this results from the parotitis or pancreatitis is unknown.

CLINICAL MANIFESTATIONS. Acute pancreatitis is sometimes divided into the acute edematous type and a hemorrhagic or necrotic form. This is a purely arbitrary distinction by the clinician which can be made only at operation or autopsy.

Attacks of acute pancreatitis often occur after a heavy meal or an episode of acute alcoholism. The pain usually begins suddenly but may start gradually. The pain is frequently located in the midepigastrium and often radiates to the back. The patient's discomfort is in many instances improved by sitting and aggravated by lying. The character of the pain is extremely variable, ranging from steady, knifelike distress to an agonizing intermittent cramping pain. Pain in the left or right upper quadrants is not uncommon and is caused by particularly severe involvement of the tail or the head of the gland.

Persistent and repeated vomiting without nausea but often to the point of extreme retching is common. The character of the vomitus is unremarkable, and the vomiting occurs with an empty stomach. Physical examination usually shows upper abdominal tenderness and guarding, sometimes far greater than what might be expected for the amount of pain the patient seems to have. About 90 percent of patients with proved pancreatitis have fever, tachycardia, and leukocytosis. Shock may be present, depending upon the amount of fluid and blood lost in the retroperitoneal area and peritoneal cavity, as well as the volume deficit incurred by persistent vomiting. Dissection of irritating exudate from the pancreas into the lower quadrants of the abdomen or even into the chest may produce signs and symptoms in these areas, as well as even greater volume deficits because of the local outpouring of fluid in response to the exudate. Adynamic ileus with intraluminal sequestration of fluid also contributes to extracellular fluid deficit. Lefer, with Wangensteen and others, has recently demonstrated a myocardial depressant factor (MDF) released from the pancreas during pancreatitis which may also contribute to the shock. Acute renal insufficiency often occurs in these patients. Mild jaundice occurs in 20 to 30 percent of the patients. This is partly due to swelling of the head of the pancreas and perhaps also to hemolysis of red blood cells, which become more fragile in acute pancreatitis. Carpopedal spasm may occur if enough fat necrosis is present in the abdomen and retroperitoneal area to remove large amounts of calcium from the blood to form calcium soaps. Recent studies indicate that an increased release of glucagon occurs in pancreatitis, which in turn stimulates the release of thyrocalcitonin, a factor which may also contribute to the development of hypocalcemia. It has been proposed recently that a substantial degree of hypocalcemia may be caused by the hypoalbuminemia found in patients with acute pancreatitis.

LABORATORY STUDIES. Acute pancreatitis is largely diagnosed by clinical history and findings rather than by laboratory studies. Disastrous outcomes have occurred when elevated serum amylase values have led the physician or surgeon immediately to eliminate from consideration any diagnosis but acute pancreatitis. Not only is simple elevation of the serum amylase level an inadequate diagnostic test of acute pancreatitis, but also there is ample evidence that serum amylase values of over 1,000 units are frequently caused by conditions other than acute pancreatitis. Blood drawn during the course of proved pancreatitis, when the amylase might be expected to be elevated, has indicated that approximately one-third of the patients had values of less than 200 Somogyi units, one-third had levels between 200 and 500 units, and one-third had more than 500 units.

Apart from acute pancreatitis, the most frequent causes of marked elevations of the serum amylase level are acute cholecystitis, common duct stone with or without cholangitis, perforated peptic ulcer, and strangulating obstruction of the small intestine. Other conditions in which the serum amylase level is elevated include acute alcoholism without pancreatitis, afferent loop obstruction after gastrectomy, ectopic pregnancy, perforated duodenal diverticulum, renal failure, carcinoma of the pancreas, and mumps. Although frequently claimed to have more diagnostic value than the serum amylase test, serum lipase not only

is a difficult determination to perform but also has proved to be disappointingly inaccurate.

Estimation of the total amount of amylase in a 2-hour urine sample is far more accurate than the concentration of the enzyme in the urine, blood, or the serum lipase. The number of positive diagnoses of pancreatitis is doubled when the amylase output in the urine exceeds 300 units in 1 hour. Recent studies show that the renal clearance of amylase in acute pancreatitis is much greater, relative to the creatinine clearance, than in any other condition. A ratio of amylase/creatinine clearance of >5 has recently been shown to be of greater diagnostic accuracy than either the serum or urinary amylase. Exceptions to this have been found in burned patients and in diabetic ketoacidosis. Elevated amylase values in pleural fluid are diagnostic of pancreatitis. Abdominal paracentesis may provide useful information, but increased amylase in abdominal fluid has been reported in other conditions as well. Estimations of trypsin levels in the blood and the separation of various organ-specific isoenzymes of the blood, especially those of amylase, seem to be encouraging but are not as yet sufficiently well evaluated to warrant widespread use.

Serum calcium values of less than 7.5 mg/100 ml generally indicate a poor prognosis and reflect the extensiveness of the disease process. Transient hyperglycemia and glycosuria have formerly been attributed to inadequate production of insulin by the injured pancreas, but recent work has shown that injection of amylase into the bloodstream converts glycogen to glucose in the liver, and that glucagon is released during the course of pancreatitis.

Radiologic examinations have only occasional value. The so-called "sentinel loop" of distended jejunum in the left upper quadrant is extremely nonspecific. Oral cholecystography during, or immediately following, an episode of acute pancreatitis frequently fails to produce visualization of the biliary tree, even when it is completely normal. Nonvisualization may persist for as long as 6 weeks after an attack. In contradistinction, intravenous cholangiography is often of great value in differentiating acute pancreatitis from acute cholecystitis, since the gallbladder can usually be visualized in most cases of acute pancreatitis.

The diagnosis of acute pancreatitis is usually made from clinical findings, although intelligent use of serum and urinary amylase tests and intravenous cholangiography may provide useful if not clearly diagnostic information. Frequent clinical reassessment of the patient is of the utmost importance. On occasion, laparotomy may be necessary in a carefully prepared patient as a purely diagnostic maneuver in order to avoid missing a strangulating obstruction of the small intestine or another potentially lethal but curable condition.

TREATMENT. Meticulous replacement of losses of colloid, fluid, and electrolytes, and adequate maintenance therapy are of the utmost importance. Constant attention to the urinary output, alterations in the hematocrit, blood volume, and central venous pressure, and estimation of the occult losses into the peritoneum and retroperitoneal area are mandatory. Blood transfusion may be required in hemorrhagic pancreatitis. Small doses of insulin may be necessary if hyperglycemia is marked and diabetic acidosis is imminent. Calcium gluconate should be given intravenously if the serum calcium level is depressed. Steroids should probably not be used, since they have been known to cause pancreatitis.

In addition to proper metabolic management, continuous aspiration of the stomach and withholding ingestion of food or fluids often relieves discomfort immediately. Parasympatholytic drugs may be used in moderate dosage. These maneuvers are designed to put the pancreas to rest by diminishing the acid-secretin mechanism of pancreatic stimulation, by eliminating gastric distension, which in turn invokes the gastropancreatic reflex and the production of antral gastrin, and by preventing the flow of pancreatic juice stimulated by foodstuffs in the duodenum. Adynamic ileus is also favorably affected by intubation. Such therapy is continued until the patient no longer has pain and tenderness. Suppression of pancreatic secretion by Diamox, propylthiouracil, or hypothermia has not been evaluated sufficiently in human pancreatitis to assess its true value. Trasylol, a trypsin inhibitor which also inhibits kallikrein, has received attention, but controlled clinical studies have not convincingly demonstrated the efficacy of this drug. Glucagon has recently been advocated in the treatment of acute pancreatitis, but no solid evidence to support its use has been forthcoming.

Although many authorities advocate the routine administration of antibiotics to patients with acute pancreatitis, we use these agents only in the occasional severe fulminating case, since these patients are the ones in whom secondary abscesses are most likely to develop. There is no evidence to support the belief that infection is an important contributing factor in the development of pancreatitis or that antibiotics can actually prevent the development of an abscess.

Meperidine is usually used to relieve pain, because it has less effect on the sphincter of Oddi than morphine and other opiates, although it does not relax this muscle, as was formerly believed. It is unnecessary to use paravertebral sympathetic blockade, since intubation usually provides marked relief of pain.

The patient with persistent or lingering acute pancreatitis secondary to acute or chronic biliary tract disease may require operation on the biliary tree with the expectation that the pancreatitis will subside. Recently Salzman and Bartlett have advocated transduodenal pancreatic duct exploration in certain patients with acute pancreatitis who did not respond to vigorous supportive measures. In fulminant hemorrhagic pancreatitis Watts and Smith have carried out total pancreatectomy with gratifying results, but the place of radical resection in the treatment of severe, acute pancreatitis is not yet clear. In some patients who fail to respond to all conservative means, it is probably more prudent to institute peritoneal lavage, which may produce profound improvement in selected instances.

COMPLICATIONS, MORBIDITY, AND MORTALITY. Pseudocyst is the most common complication of acute pancreatitis. Abscesses are rare but mortality is high, approaching 100 percent if clostridial organisms are the cause of the infection. Pseudocysts rarely appear before the second week of the disease and abscesses not usually before the third week. Obstruction of the common bile duct and duodenum is not common in the acute cases. The remaining complications of acute pancreatitis may be grouped together, since they are caused by the necrotizing effects of the process itself. These include rupture or thrombosis of the splenic, mesenteric, or portal vessels, necrosis and perforation of the common bile duct or colon, and perforation of the stomach and duodenum.

Just as important as the early complications of acute pancreatitis and perhaps even more so is the insidious development of sequelae of repeated attacks. Pancreatic calcification, secondary diabetes, and steatorrhea are far more common in alcoholic pancreatitis than in gallstone pancreatitis, in which these phenomena are almost nonexistent. Pseudocysts too are rarely encountered in the course of gallstone pancreatitis.

The overall mortality rate from acute pancreatitis in the past 10 years has been 10 to 15 percent. Twenty years ago most patients died during the first week of the disease, but now the vast majority do not succumb for several weeks after the onset, probably because of better early metabolic management. The mortality rate of alcoholic pancreatitis is approximately three times that of gallstone pancreatitis in most series, but reverse incidences have been recorded in a few reports. It is virtually impossible to determine the true mortality rate of hemorrhagic pancreatitis, since a clinical diagnosis may be impossible without operative or postmortem observation. Operation is generally regarded as detrimental to the outcome of the disease unless specific indications, as outlined above, are present. Paradoxically, operation has not increased the mortality rates in most reports. Secondary hemorrhage from major vessels, fulminating uncontrollable shock without hemorrhage, and infection are the most common causes of death.

Chronic Pancreatitis

This diagnosis usually refers to a clinical entity rather than a specific pathologic process. This is especially true during its early stages, when repeated attacks of acute pancreatitis of varying severity are likely to occur, whether alcoholism or biliary tract disease is the precipitating factor. As the disease progresses, however, the edges of the pancreas become rounded, and the organ becomes smaller, indurated, and nodular. Histologically, lobules of functional acinar and islet tissue are surrounded by thick bands of fibrous tissue. Alternating areas of stricture and dilatation of the main ductal system occur late in the disease. In the very last stages calcification occurs. It is almost always intraductal and rarely interstitial (Figs. 32-5 and 32-6). These severe changes are confined largely to patients with alcoholic pancreatitis and are extremely rare in gallstone pancreatitis. Calcification and ductal distortion have also been seen in familial or hereditary pancreatitis. Occasionally in chronic alcoholic pancreatitis, progressive fibrosis of the gland without ductal dilatation or calcification seems to be the primary pathologic process.

CLINICAL MANIFESTATIONS. The typical patient with

Fig. 32-5. Calcifications presenting within the duct of the opened pancreas. The guide probe is advanced into the head of the gland. Note alternate stenoses and dilatations of the main duct and the calcifications which occlude the ductal tributaries. (*From W. Silen, J. Baldwin, and L. Goldman, Am J Surg, 106:243, 1963.*)

chronic pancreatitis is in his late thirties or early forties and has a long history of alcoholism and repeated attacks of acute pancreatitis, often with delirium tremens. After approximately 10 years, the pain changes from intermittent to persistent and continuous. It is located in the epigastrium but radiates to the back and is often partially relieved if the patient sits in a hunched position. Anorexia and weight loss are common, and nausea and vomiting

Fig. 32-6. Example of amount of calcification removed from the ductal system of a patient with chronic pancreatitis.

occur if an exacerbation has been precipitated by an acute bout of alcoholism. Diabetes and steatorrhea with foul, bulky, greasy stools are common. At this stage, addiction to narcotics as well as alcohol is extremely common. Strangely, cirrhosis of the liver and its stigmata are not often present. Pseudocysts are frequently found in these patients.

This picture is in sharp contrast to the patient who has recurrent pancreatitis in association with biliary tract disease. Such persons generally have episodic bouts of acute pancreatitis, sometimes in association with attacks of acute cholecystitis or cholangitis caused by common duct calculi. Severe pancreatic fibrosis and insufficiency almost never occur in association solely with biliary tract disease. Hyperparathyroidism is often associated with recurrent attacks of acute pancreatitis, as in patients who have severe ductal stenosis resulting from major trauma to the pancreas. Occasionally the picture of familial pancreatitis may be similar to that seen in alcoholic chronic pancreatitis, but these cases are rare, and at times severe damage to the pancreas and calcification may be present without any symptoms at all and in the absence of a known cause.

LABORATORY STUDIES. Many psychoneurotic patients with abdominal pains are labeled as having chronic pancreatitis without adequate substantiation for such a serious diagnosis. Documentation is difficult, but in these instances thorough roentgenologic examinations of the biliary tree and upper gastrointestinal tract are mandatory. The recent advent of endoscopic retrograde cannulation of the pancreatic duct has proved of great value in these cases, since abnormalities of the ductal system are readily detected. Determination of serum or urinary amylase or serum lipase may not be fruitful, especially if the pancreas has been seriously damaged. The presence of calcification in the pancreas virtually establishes the diagnosis.

TREATMENT. The wide variety of operative procedures devised for chronic pancreatitis are a reflection of the generally unsatisfactory results of treatment. However, some confusion has been created by our own inability, or refusal, to differentiate clearly among the various types of chronic pancreatitis.

It is evident that definitive and corrective biliary tract operations are almost always curative in gallstone pancreatitis. Whether this implies simple cholecystectomy or common duct exploration, with or without sphincteroplasty, is dictated by the local and cholangiographic findings at operation. Sporadic initial success with biliary operations led to their widespread, indiscriminate use without due regard for the precipitating cause of the pancreatitis. Large numbers of patients with alcoholic pancreatitis were subjected to cholecystectomy and a variety of other biliary tract procedures, only to find that relief was not obtained. Even when biliary calculi are present in the alcoholic patient, correction of the biliary tract disease will not alter the course of the pancreatic disease, especially if the ingestion of alcohol is continued.

In the case of chronic alcoholic pancreatitis, the only logical and effective therapy is complete abstinence from alcohol before the stage of fibrosis, calcification, steatorrhea, and diabetes is reached, but rarely can this be achieved. Once the severe complications of chronic pancreatitis has developed, consideration should be given to pancreaticojejunostomy, originally advocated by Puestow and Gillesby. This procedure is based on the fact that multiple areas of stricture within the pancreatic ductal system often occur in patients with severe chronic pancreatitis, so that simple retrograde drainage of the pancreas via its tail, as originally proposed by DuVal, does not adequately decompress the pancreatic ducts. The limb of jejunum may be anastomosed, side to side, to the pancreas after wide incision of almost the entire pancreatic duct but without removal of the spleen or mobilization of the pancreas (Fig. 32-7). This procedure can be carried out rather simply, with an extremely low mortality and little morbidity. The relief of pain is dramatic, particularly if the duct is dilated at operation. The most accurate preoperative indication of a dilated duct is the presence of calcification.

Lateral pancreaticojejunostomy also provides for the return of pancreatic juice to the intestine, offers the potential for pancreatic regeneration if it is to occur, and preserves pancreatic tissue. In addition, the adequacy of ductal exploration, removal of calculi, and drainage is far greater than that which can be accomplished through a transduodenal sphincterotomy, advocated by some. If the pancreatic duct is small, without evidence of stricture, yet severe chronic pancreatitis is present, the best procedure is that of 95 percent distal pancreatectomy, proposed by Fry and Child. This is associated with a high incidence of diabetes and exocrine pancreatic insufficiency, both of which may be excessively morbid in the nonresponsible alcoholic patient. Relief of pain occurs in the majority of patients.

Sphincterotomy, ligation of the pancreatic ducts, and lumbodorsal sympathectomy and splanchnicectomy have all failed to provide lasting relief in patients with chronic pancreatitis. On occasion, the Whipple pancreaticoduodenal resection may be indicated if stricture of the common bile duct or stenosis of the duodenum is the result of chronic pancreatitis localized to the head of the pancreas.

TRAUMA

MECHANISMS OF INJURY. Penetrating trauma, caused by gunshot or stab wounds, is more common than blunt injury to the pancreas and constitutes from 70 to 80 percent of pancreatic injuries, even in civilian practice. Penetrating injuries, especially knife wounds, usually cause less destruction and disruption of the organ than does blunt

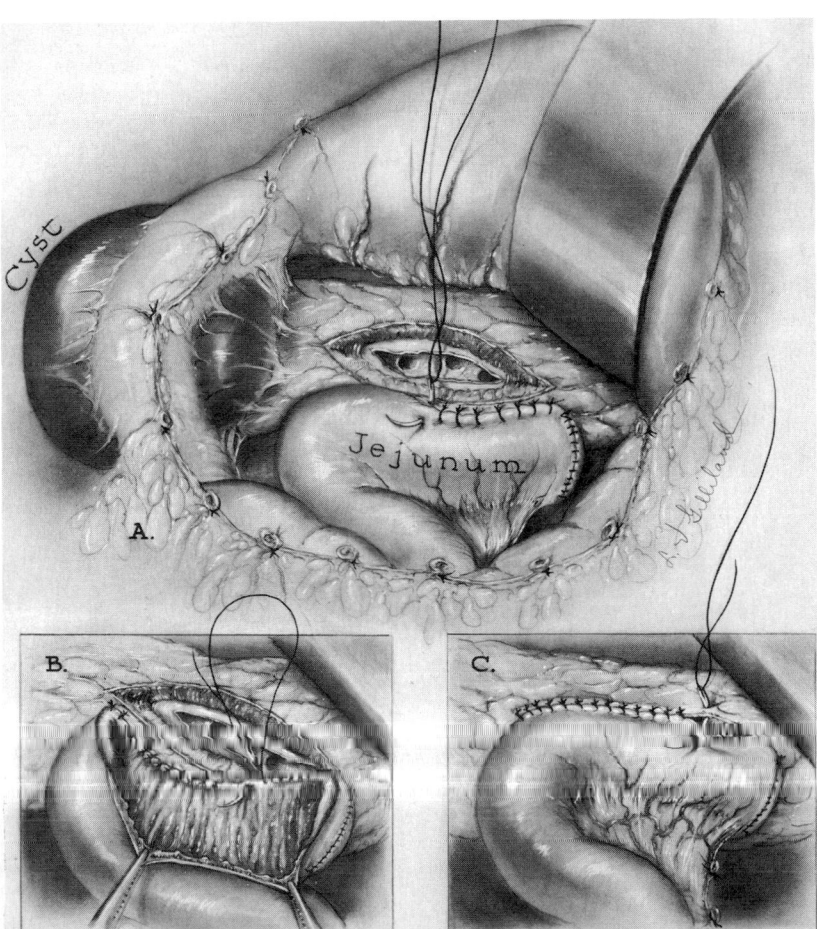

Fig. 32-7. Side-to-side pancreaticojejunostomy with preservation of the tail of the pancreas and spleen. An exploring needle is used to locate the dilated pancreatic duct, which is then incised. The end of the defunctionalized jejunum is closed and brought up for anastomosis with the opened pancreas in side-to-side fashion. The posterior row of sutures is placed first (A). The jejunum is then opened, and an inner layer of continuous sutures is placed, uniting jejunal mucosa and pancreatic duct (B). An anterior row of interrupted sutures completes the anastomosis (C). A Roux en Y is then constructed to complete intestinal continuity. (From W. Silen, J. Baldwin, and L. Goldman, Am J Surg, 106: 243, 1963.)

trauma. In gunshot wounds an area of contusion usually surrounds the track of the missile. Injury to adjacent structures is exceedingly common (70 to 96 percent). The stomach, liver, small intestine, spleen, colon, kidney, and duodenum are the most frequently wounded. These organs are usually the source of the most significant hemorrhage.

The immobility of the pancreas accounts for its vulnerability to blunt trauma, which may fracture it posteriorly across the rigid vertebral column. Usually the disruption occurs at the neck of the pancreas overlying the mesenteric vessels, although occasionally the gland may become completely separated from the duodenum. Associated injury to other organs is not as frequent as in penetrating trauma.

Although frequently referred to as "traumatic pancreatitis," the consequences of these injuries, such as fistula, pseudocyst, or death, are usually the result of disruption of the organ itself or its ductal system rather than pancreatitis per se. Crushing injury to the pancreas in itself does not seem to produce extensive inflammation in the remainder of the gland.

CLINICAL MANIFESTATIONS. It is significant that the interval between injury and surgical exploration is considerably longer after blunt trauma to the pancreas, often being many days. Adequate awareness of the possibility of this type of injury may shorten delay and reduce morbidity and mortality. Abdominal pain and findings on examination may be surprisingly minimal, which partly explains the frequent procrastination in undertaking laparotomy. Clinical and laboratory evidence of continuing hemorrhage makes the decision for operation an easy one. Continued abdominal pain, tenderness, fever, and ileus should immediately arouse suspicion of pancreatic injury.

Roentgenologic examinations, with or without contrast media, are rarely helpful. Paracentesis may provide a clear-cut indication for operation if the fluid is positive for blood or is rich in amylase, but a negative result should not deter the surgeon from exploration. Although frequently forgotten in cases of blunt trauma, serum amylase determination and amylase/creatinine clearance ratio may be of great help. These are elevated in over 80 percent of the patients with pancreatic injuries in whom they are measured. Possibly of greater surgical importance is the fact that persistent elevations of the serum amylase usually mean inadequate drainage of the injured pancreas.

TREATMENT. The high incidence of complications and the excessive mortality suggest that the treatment leaves much to be desired.

It is generally agreed that early operation is necessary in both penetrating wounds and in blunt injury.

Proper evaluation of the extent of the pancreatic injury is the key to adequate surgical therapy. It is impossible to explore the pancreas without widely exposing it by division of the gastrocolic omentum, as far as is necessary to provide adequate assessment of the major portion of the gland (Fig. 32-8). Care must be taken to protect the middle colic vessels during the procedure. If the injury is in the region of the head of the pancreas, the duodenum must be mobilized by the method of Kocher (Fig. 32-9) so that the full extent of the damage can be ascertained and the duodenum, common bile duct, and adjacent structures can be examined. If a hematoma is found over the pancreas, it should not be treated by drainage alone, but must be examined carefully, since it may hide major vascular or ductal injury. Vascular instruments should always

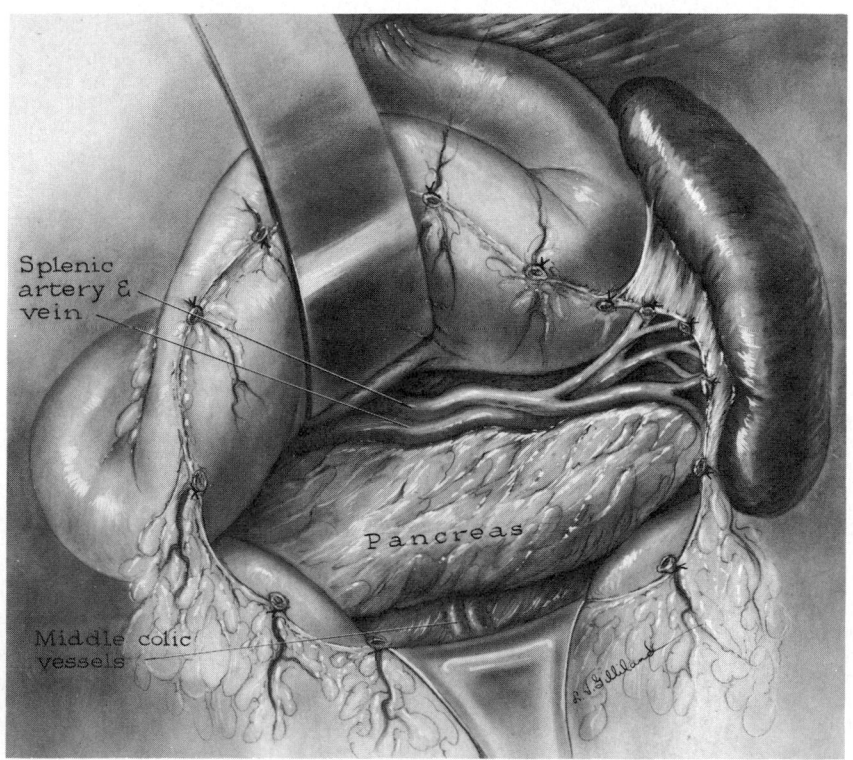

Fig. 32-8. Wide exposure of the pancreas obtained by the gastrocolic omental route. The middle colic vessels must be located and preserved. (*From W. Silen, Surg Clin North Am, 44:1253, 1964.*)

Fig. 32-9. Operative exposure of the head of the pancreas after the Kocher maneuver. Note that portal or superior mesenteric veins are covered posteriorly by the uncinate process, preventing direct vision of these structures inferiorly. (*From W. Silen, Surg Clin North Am, 44:1253, 1964.*)

Gastroduodenal a.
Portal vein
Common bile duct
Inferior vena cava
Pancreas
Duodenum

be readily available in the operating room when operations of this type are being performed.

During exploration of the hematoma, attention should be first directed toward hemostasis. Blind clamping in the depths of the pancreas or deep, carelessly placed sutures may injure the pancreatic ductal system, leading to pancreatitis or fistula. Damaged tissue should be thoroughly debrided; carefully placed nonabsorbable suture ligatures permit adequate hemostasis. If the ductal system is uninjured, these procedures, together with sump suction drainage, may be sufficient to treat small penetrating injuries. Complications with simple drainage or no drainage at all are considerably greater than when the more adequate sump drainage is used.

A much more aggressive approach is probably necessary when the pancreas is badly lacerated. Should the severely injured area involve only the tail or distal body of the pancreas, the simplest procedure is resection. Mobilization of the spleen and distal pancreas is easily carried out (Fig. 32-10). Since the gastrocolic omentum has already been opened, only a few vasa brevia remain to be ligated and divided; the distal pancreas and spleen can easily be delivered into the wound after division of the lienorenal and splenocolic ligaments and the thin posterosuperior and posteroinferior peritoneal attachments of the pancreas. After the splenic artery and vein are ligated and divided, the injured pancreas may be removed. The distal end of the pancreas remaining in situ should be carefully inspected for adequate hemostasis. If possible, the duct of Wirsung should be ligated with nonabsorbable sutures, and the area is then drained.

If the pancreas is transected near its neck or even farther to the right, preservation of pancreatic tissue may be important. The lacerated proximal segment is managed as

outlined above. The distal transected portion of the organ can be anastomosed end to end with a Roux en Y limb of jejunum. Generally, the limb of jejunum is placed in a retrocolic position. The transected proximal pancreas can also be implanted into the same limb of jejunum used for the distal end, but this is unduly complicated and probably is not necessary.

Although these procedures might appear too involved to be used in seriously injured patients, less adequate therapy results in a high incidence of severe complications and death. Furthermore, ductal obstruction and the late development of chronic pancreatitis in inadequately recognized and treated injuries support an aggressive approach to such lesions. Thal and Wilson have recently proposed that pancreaticoduodenal resection be carried out for severe lesions of the head of the pancreas. Berne advocates distal Billroth II gastrectomy with careful local repair of the badly injured duodenum and pancreas, coupled with adequate drainage, for injuries of this area. The choice between this procedure and the Whipple operation is determined by the extent of the injury. Should the pancreas be sheared away from the duodenum, disrupting pancreatic and biliary ductal continuity, careful reanastomosis to the duodenum may be carried out if the blood supply to the pancreas and duodenum has not been disrupted. The importance of recognizing major ductal injury in any case of pancreatic injury cannot be overemphasized. Cannulation of the pancreatic duct can sometimes be facilitated by intubation through a transduodenal sphincterotomy, as suggested by Doubilet and Mulholland. Although drainage of the ductal system can undoubtedly be achieved in this manner, definitive therapy by splinting of the duct alone by this method will not prevent subsequent ductal stricture and pancreatitis.

Fig. 32-10. Mobilization of tail and body of pancreas with spleen. (*From W. Silen, Surg Clin North Am, 44:1253, 1964.*)

MORBIDITY AND MORTALITY. The most serious complications of pancreatic injury are fistulization, pseudocyst formation, infection, and delayed hemorrhage. Fistula and pseudocyst are the result of disruption of a duct of significant size. Doubilet and Mulholland have suggested that the resistance to the flow of pancreatic juice into the duodenum by the duodenal musculature and sphincter of Oddi is sufficiently great so that in cases of injury the juice will preferentially flow into the retroperitoneal area. The incidence of complications in most series averages 30 percent. Pancreatic complications seem to occur much more frequently after blunt trauma than in penetrating injuries.

The overall mortality rate in recent years, like the complication rate, has averaged 20 percent. Usually the death rate after penetrating injuries is higher than that after blunt trauma, probably because adjacent organs are often injured. The most frequent causes of death are shock, renal failure, and sepsis.

CYSTS AND PSEUDOCYSTS

True cysts of the pancreas are filled with fluid and have an epithelial lining. These cysts are to be distinguished from the much more common pseudocysts, which have fibrous lining rather than epithelium.

True Cysts

A simple classification of true cysts of the pancreas is presented in Table 32-1.

Congenital cysts of the pancreas are extremely rare, and parasitic cysts of the pancreas have not been reported in the United States. Retention cysts are cystic dilatations of the pancreatic ducts and are almost always caused by pancreatitis. Although not as rare as the congenital cysts, neoplastic cysts of the pancreas are relatively uncommon. Cystadenoma and cystadenocarcinoma are important, since they may be confused with the much more common pseudocyst. The benign lesion (cystadenoma) is somewhat more common than its malignant counterpart.

CLINICAL MANIFESTATIONS. The benign tumors are very slow-growing, and even cystadenocarcinomas do not grow very rapidly. These tumors occur far more frequently in women than in men (9:1) and are most common in the sixth and seventh decades of life. They may be present for many years without causing symptoms. An abdominal mass is usually the only symptom. Minor discomfort,

Table 32-1. CLASSIFICATION OF TRUE CYSTS OF THE PANCREAS

A. Congenital
  1. Single cyst
  2. Multiple (polycystic disease)
  3. Dermoid cyst
  4. Fibrocystic disease
B. Acquired
  1. Retention cysts
  2. Parasitic cysts
  3. Neoplastic cysts
    a. Benign cystadenoma
    b. Cystadenocarcinoma

vague dyspepsia, and jaundice may be present. The diagnosis may be suggested if radiologic examination shows a mass in the region of the pancreas. Because of the profuse vascularity of these tumors, a loud bruit is occasionally heard over the lesion, and an arteriogram may visualize the profuse vascularity of the mass.

TREATMENT. Marsupialization or internal drainage are to be condemned. The tumor invariably recurs and presents far greater difficulties at a second operation. The importance of distinguishing between these lesions and pseudocysts becomes obvious. Whether the lesion is benign or malignant, complete excision is the preferred method. This is a simple matter when the lesion is located in the tail or body, since distal pancreatectomy, usually with splenectomy, is readily accomplished. If the lesion is in the head of the pancreas, simple resection of the lesion alone can be done if it has a small pedicle. However, pancreaticoduodenal resection may be necessary if the common bile duct is involved. Recurrences should not be anticipated if the entire lesion is removed.

Pseudocysts

More than three-quarters of all cystic lesions of the pancreas are pseudocysts. The fibrous wall of a pseudocyst surrounds a collection of pancreatic juice (with or without blood clot) and necrotic or suppurative pancreatic tissue. Most pseudocysts are unilocular and are located in the lesser sac. However, they occasionally occur within the pancreas (retention cysts), transverse mesocolon, or omentum and even more rarely may be found behind the pancreas or within the mediastinum. Since a pseudocyst usually results from disruption of the ductal system of the pancreas, the ultimate form and location of the lesion are dependent upon the position and the extent of pancreatic injury and the secretory pressure of the pancreas distal to the point of ductal damage. The fluid within a pseudocyst varies from clear and colorless to a brown or green murky material, depending upon the amount of blood or necrotic pancreas present.

Pancreatitis and trauma are the most important causes of pseudocysts, accounting for about 75 percent and 25 percent of cases, respectively. Neoplasm and parasites are extremely rare causes, and occasionally pseudocysts develop without any demonstrable cause whatever. In patients with pseudocysts caused by pancreatitis, alcoholism is more common than cholelithiasis. For this reason, pseudocysts appear most frequently in the fourth and fifth decades of life and are more common in men.

CLINICAL MANIFESTATIONS. The usual clinical findings in patients with pseudocysts are persistent pain, fever, and ileus, appearing 2 to 3 weeks after an attack of pancreatitis or trauma to the pancreas. Although a pseudocyst may develop after one attack of pancreatitis, the patient usually has had several previous attacks. Pain, in the epigastrium or the left upper quadrant with occasional radiation to the back, is the most common symptom. A mass, nausea, vomiting, and anorexia occur in approximately 20 percent of the patients. Rarely, gastrointestinal hemorrhage from gastroesophageal varices occurs from compression of the

portal venous system by the pseudocyst. Narrowing of the common bile duct may cause jaundice.

A mass is found on physical examination in about 75 percent of patients and is usually nontender or only slightly tender. The amount of movement of the mass is variable, depending upon the degree of surrounding inflammatory reaction and fixation to adjacent structures. The mass often changes in size, probably because of partial drainage into the ductal system of the pancreas. The complete and prolonged disappearance of the mass in some patients may be explained by the fact that these masses develop after attacks of acute pancreatitis and may represent small fluid collections, matted omentum, and enlarged pancreas, all of which resolve after the acute attack has subsided. Occasionally the mass may be confused with an aortic aneurysm because of the pulsations transmitted by the aorta immediately posterior to the pancreas. Patients may present with pleural effusion as the sole finding, undoubtedly caused by transdiaphragmatic drainage of pancreatic lymph. Pleural or pulmonary manifestations are common.

The diagnosis of pseudocyst is not particularly difficult. In addition to persistent pain, fever, and ileus during or after an attack of pancreatitis, continued elevation of the serum amylase level should suggest the development of a pseudocyst. The most helpful radiologic examination is the upper gastrointestinal tract barium study, which usually shows an extrinsic mass displacing the stomach anteriorly and superiorly. Occasionally the lesser curvature of the stomach may be flattened by a high-lying pseudocyst (Figs. 32-11 and 32-12). If located in the head of the pancreas, the duodenal loop may be widened. Barium enema may show inferior displacement of the colon. Ultrasonography has recently been shown to be of value in detecting a pseudocyst, and endoscopic retrograde cannulation of the pancreatic duct may show either obstruction of the duct of Wirsung or extravasation of dye into the pseudocyst.

The development of a pancreatitic abscess is detected by accentuation of fever and toxicity, usually at least 3 weeks after the onset of an attack of acute pancreatitis. The presence of gas bubbles on a plain film of the abdomen and bacterial growth in the bloodstream may help establish the diagnosis. The clinician should also be alert to the syndrome of pancreatic ascites, which is caused by leakage of pancreatic juice from a pseudocyst or actual pancreatic ductal disruption. The demonstration of high amylase content of ascitic fluid which also has the characteristics of an exudate serves to differentiate this condition from ascites of hepatic origin.

TREATMENT. Surgical treatment is recommended for pseudocyst of the pancreas, for two reasons: first, complications such as secondary infection, severe hemorrhage, or rupture into an adjacent viscus or into the free peritoneal cavity may occur if a pseudocyst remains untreated; second, these lesions rarely resolve once a thick fibrous wall has developed. If a patient develops a mass during an attack of acute pancreatitis and his condition remains satisfactory, he should be observed for several weeks. Should the mass enlarge or the patient become more ill during this period, immediate operation is indicated. If

Fig. 32-11. Flattening of the upper portion of the lesser curvature of the stomach by a pseudocyst of the tail of the pancreas.

Fig. 32-12. Roentgenogram taken after injection of contrast material into the dilated and tortuous pancreatic duct. Note the large pseudocyst of the tail of the pancreas in communication with the ductal system which produced the compression of the lesser curvature seen in Fig. 32-11. There is a smaller pseudocyst in the head of the pancreas.

physical and radiologic examination show complete disappearance of the mass, operation may be postponed indefinitely. True intrapancreatic pseudocysts often vary greatly in size and frequently disappear completely only to reappear at a later date.

No single operative procedure is appropriate for every pseudocyst of the pancreas. Simple external drainage or marsupialization should be used in extremely ill patients requiring urgent drainage in whom more extensive procedures might endanger life. If the pseudocyst has a thin flimsy wall, external drainage may be the only means of treatment. The mortality rate of this procedure is low (about 4.5 percent), but the morbidity (prolonged drainage, loss of electrolytes, and a relatively high rate of recurrence) is about 17 percent. Extensive and early drainage is mandatory for pancreatic abscess. In these instances, the lesser sac should be opened widely and all necrotic areas should be debrided and widely drained. Repeated operations may be necessary to accomplish complete cure.

Extirpation theoretically is an ideal method of therapy. Yet only the rare, very small pseudocyst located in the distal pancreas and unattached to vital structures lends itself to excision. Extirpation is not recommended except in these special circumstances, since the mortality is high.

Internal drainage of some type is the best treatment for most pseudocysts. Transgastric cystogastrostomy when the lesion is adherent to the stomach or transduodenal cystoduodenostomy if the cyst is located in the head of the pancreas have produced mortality rates of 2.5 to 5 percent with approximately the same low rate of recurrence. They are almost as easily accomplished as external drainage is. Suturing of the edges of the stomach and cyst or excision of a large ellipse of tissue may predispose to regurgitation. Pancreatic abscesses and gastric ulcer have also been sequelae of cystogastrostomy, and therefore cystojejunostomy to a Roux en Y of jejunum is preferred. A small piece of the wall of the cyst should always be excised and submitted for microscopic examination to exclude the possibility of a neoplastic cyst. Anastomosis of a Roux en Y jejunum to the wall of the pseudocyst requires a thick fibrous wall and results in the same mortality and recurrence rates as cystogastrostomy or cystoduodenostomy.

Drainage through the duct of Wirsung after transduodenal sphincterotomy has been advocated by Doubilet and Mulholland, based on the principle that pseudocysts have major ductal communications. There is little question that drainage of the ductal system will accomplish decompression of most pseudocysts, but the procedures mentioned above would seem to be simpler and more direct in most cases. The primary indication for transphincteric drainage is in patients with gallstone pancreatitis who are undergoing corrective biliary tract operation. In these cases, common duct exploration is frequently performed, making transphincteric drainage a rather simple matter, and recurrence of the pancreatitis is unlikely.

For cases of pancreatic ascites, internal drainage of the offending pseudocyst or resection of the pancreas distal to a ductal disruption is curative.

TUMORS

Carcinoma of the Pancreas and Periampullary Area

The manifestations of carcinoma of the pancreas and other malignant tumors of the periampullary areas (see Chap. 31 for carcinoma of the bile ducts) are so frequently indistinguishable that it seems reasonable to consider these neoplasms as a group. The relative frequency of these lesions in a series of 159 patients is shown in Table 32-2.

The average age of patients with carcinoma of the pancreas, duodenum, and common bile duct is sixty years, but in carcinoma of the ampulla the average age is about five years less. Males are more frequently affected by all these lesions, but there is no special racial predilection. The cause is unknown. Biliary lithiasis has been suspected as a cause of carcinoma of the common bile duct, but not all such patients have cholelithiasis.

PATHOLOGY. Carcinoma of the pancreas arises from the ductal system in 90 percent of the cases and from the acini in the remainder. Adenocarcinoma is the predominant lesion, often accompanied by extreme fibrous connective tissue stromal proliferation. The lesion itself is frequently small, in many instances one-third to one-half of the bulk of the gross lesion, the remainder consisting of a zone of pancreatitis. These tumors are most frequently found within the head of the pancreas and compress the pancreatic and common bile ducts. The pancreatic duct may become extremely dilated and tortuous and is often easily palpable at operation, especially if the surrounding pancreas is somewhat atrophic and firmer than usual. Other adjacent structures, such as the portal vein, stomach, duodenum, and vena cava, may be invaded by tumor. Regional lymph node metastasis is present in 90 percent of patients, and perineural invasion is extremely common. About 80 percent of the patients have liver metastases.

Carcinomas of the ampulla of Vater and the duodenum are frequently impossible to differentiate. Grossly and microscopically, they are columnar cell adenocarcinomas. Frequently, a large area of pancreatitis in the head of the pancreas will not only obscure the small primary lesion but may also be erroneously interpreted as the primary neoplasm itself. Some tumors of the ampulla are so small that they are not readily detected at operation, since biliary obstruction may have occurred very early. In both these neoplasms, intermittent jaundice is caused by recurrent sloughing of the central portion of the tumor. The pattern of metastatic spread is similar to that of carcinoma of the pancreas. Carcinomas of the common bile duct occasionally are fleshy fungating growths but more frequently form a hard mass which may be mistaken for a stone or stricture. In the absence of previous operation, a stricture should be considered to be carcinoma even though biopsies may not initially confirm this. Metastases generally follow the same route as other tumors in this region.

CLINICAL MANIFESTATIONS. Weight loss is the single most common symptom in carcinoma of the pancreas, no matter where the lesion is located. Pain is extremely frequent (70 to 80 percent), although it is rarely of the dramatic type caused by biliary colic resulting from a stone in the common bile duct. The pain is usually dull and aching and is most often confined to the midepigastrium. Radiation to the back is frequent, although the pain may extend to both lower quadrants. A helpful diagnostic feature of the pain is that it is relieved by sitting in a hunched position and accentuated by lying supine. Eating may aggravate the pain, which often antedates jaundice by many weeks or months, depending upon the proximity of the primary lesion to the common bile duct. Distension of the common bile duct, and especially of the pancreatic duct, and perineural invasion by tumor, are usually responsible for pain in carcinoma of the pancreas.

Progressive jaundice occurs in about 75 percent of patients with carcinoma of the head of the pancreas; the incidence of jaundice decreases as the location of the lesion progresses to the left. Occasionally a tumor may deform the second part of the duodenum without obstructing the common bile duct. Anorexia and weakness are common (about 50 percent of cases). Diarrhea, constipation, nausea, and vomiting are inconstant symptoms. Chills and fever are rare. Pruritus is frequent and may be an extremely trying symptom for the patient. The liver is palpable in 50 to 70 percent of patients with carcinoma of the head of the pancreas, but the gallbladder can be palpated in only one-third to one-fourth of the cases. These findings are obviously much less frequent in lesions of the body and tail of the pancreas. An enlarged palpable gallbladder in a jaundiced patient without chills or fever is most certainly a reliable diagnostic criterion for malignant choledochal obstruction, but no diagnostic inference is justified if the gallbladder cannot be palpated. Tenderness, ascites, the presence of an abdominal mass, a rectal shelf, or Virchow's nodes are all less frequent findings.

Pancreatic malignant tumors occur at least twice as frequently in diabetic as in nondiabetic patients, but diabetes is rarely the first sign of pancreatic cancer. Approximately 10 percent of patients with carcinoma of the pancreas are overtly diabetic, and 20 percent have asymptomatic glycosuria or hyperglycemia. It has often been stated that because of the high incidence of thrombosis in carcinoma of the pancreas, it must be seriously

Table 32-2. RELATIVE FREQUENCY OF PERIAMPULLARY NEOPLASMS

	Percent
Pancreas	83
Ampulla of Vater	10
Duodenum	4
Common bile duct	3

SOURCE: Taken with permission from G. L. Jordan, Jr., Benign and Malignant Tumors of the Pancreas and the Periampullary Region, in J. M. Howard and G. L. Jordan, Jr. (eds.), "Surgical Diseases of the Pancreas," J. B. Lippincott Company, Philadelphia, 1960.

considered in all patients who have a spontaneous onset of venous or arterial thrombosis. In fact, clinically detectable thromboses are quite rare in patients with carcinoma of the pancreas.

The clinical signs of carcinoma of the ampulla of Vater, common bile duct, and duodenum are similar to those of carcinoma of the head of the pancreas. Yet, a few distinguishing features may allow differentiation of these lesions from carcinoma of the pancreas. Pain is somewhat less frequent; when present it is apt to be more colicky in nature than the pain of pancreatic cancer. The jaundice is usually less intense when the patient is admitted to the hospital and is more likely to be intermittent (25 percent). Chills and fever are also somewhat more common. In carcinoma of the duodenum, duodenal obstruction and gastrointestinal hemorrhage are more common than in carcinoma of the pancreas.

LABORATORY AND DIAGNOSTIC STUDIES. The most important laboratory studies in periampullary and pancreatic carcinoma are tests for obstructive jaundice. No great significance can be attached to the relationship between the direct and indirect fractions of bilirubin, since they are nearly equal even in only moderately advanced obstructive jaundice. The serum bilirubin almost never rises above 30 to 35 mg/100 ml in pancreatic cancer, whereas acute hepatic necrosis may be associated with much higher levels. The alkaline phosphatase is almost always increased, occasionally even before the onset of jaundice. Quantitative tests of fecal urobilinogen over a 72-hour period are valuable in demonstrating complete or almost complete biliary obstruction if less than 5 mg of urobilinogen is excreted per 24 hours. Impaired bilirubin excretion to this degree is almost never seen in intrahepatic jaundice. Serum transaminase is of value in ruling out hepatitis, since in this disease the serum transaminase often rises to more than 1,000 units. In mechanical biliary obstruction, values below 500 are the rule. Exfoliative cytology and the response of the pancreas to secretin and pancreozymin are time-consuming and rarely of real diagnostic help.

Fifty to sixty percent of patients with pancreaticoduodenal cancer will have some radiologic abnormality, such as distortion and flattening of the gastric antrum or second and third parts of the duodenum, anterior displacement of the stomach, gross distortion of the duodenum and "reverse 3" sign, or widening of the duodenal loop. Yet, the normal variation is so great and these findings are so nonspecific that a definitive radiologic diagnosis is usually impossible. Hypotonic duodenography may provide a more accurate assessment of the duodenal loop in some instances. Positive radiologic findings in a patient whose history and physical examination are compatible with a diagnosis of carcinoma should be considered as strong confirmatory evidence. The biliary ducts cannot be visualized on oral or intravenous cholangiography when the bilirubin exceeds 4 mg/100 ml, especially if it is rising, and these tests are of little value.

Transhepatic cholangiography using a fine needle has been proposed as a means of differentiating between carcinoma and calculus. Carcinoma produces a smooth, tapering, complete obstruction, but calculi cause a typical convex deformity. This technique may be extremely helpful, especially in poor-risk patients, when preoperative assessment might permit a more rapid and less manipulative procedure. However, since hemorrhage and bile peritonitis may occur, it should only be done when the patient is thoroughly prepared for operation. Retrograde cannulation of the common bile duct and pancreatic duct by means of an endoscopic approach has recently received a great deal of well-deserved acclaim and has entered into competition with transhepatic cholangiography.

Splenoportography, retroperitoneal gas insufflation, and celiac angiography do not provide sufficient information to warrant the added risk and discomfort to the patient except in very special circumstances.

DIAGNOSIS. In patients without jaundice, diagnosis of carcinoma of the pancreas may be virtually impossible, despite all possible radiologic and laboratory studies. Many of these patients are thought to be psychoneurotic and are sent from one physician to another, often ending up in the care of a psychiatrist. It is for these cases that angiography and retrograde cannulation may be of special value. The diagnosis of carcinoma of the head of the pancreas and other periampullary lesions, on the other hand, is far easier. Differentiation between the various types of pancreaticoduodenal carcinoma is an interesting intellectual exercise and is to be encouraged, but definitive diagnosis from clinical and laboratory examination may be impossible. Hepatitis can usually be excluded by its tendency to affect younger persons; the 1- to 2-week prodromal period of malaise, anorexia, and fever which precedes the onset of jaundice; the presence of diffuse hepatic tenderness; and a marked increase in serum transaminase. Profound weight loss in a jaundiced patient almost always means carcinoma. Cholestatic jaundice due to viral hepatitis or drugs may be difficult to differentiate from obstruction caused by tumors, because the hepatic function tests show similar abnormalities. In these instances, needle biopsy of the liver should be done and may be invaluable.

TREATMENT AND PROGNOSIS. Once the diagnosis of obstructive jaundice has been established, early operation is advised. Procrastination can only lead to further deterioration of hepatic function and increased operative risk as the patient continues to lose weight. Adequate nutrition and correction of anemia should be accomplished as rapidly as possible. Preoperative evaluation of renal function is essential, since postoperative renal failure is common in severely jaundiced patients. Adequate hydration immediately prior to operation is mandatory for the same reason.

The only definitive and potentially curative therapy for pancreaticoduodenal carcinoma is adequate surgical resection. This implies pancreaticoduodenal resection of the type first successfully performed by Whipple in 1935. During the early years after this formidable operation was first introduced, mortality and morbidity were extremely high, often 40 to 50 percent. Because of these dismal statistics, many surgeons developed a fatalistic attitude toward the therapy of pancreaticoduodenal carcinoma, regarding surgical treatment as merely palliative. Recent improvements in preoperative and postoperative care as well as meticulous attention to technical details have markedly reduced mortality rates, in one instance to 0 percent in forty-one consecutive cases, making this operation a feasible therapeutic technique.

Most surgeons agree that pancreaticoduodenectomy should be performed for localized carcinoma of the ampulla of Vater, duodenum, or common bile duct in good-risk patients who have not been jaundiced for prolonged periods. Although many surgeons do not advocate excision of primary carcinoma of the pancreas, if the lesion is relatively confined and there is no evidence of spread to the liver, resection should be carried out. Additional reasons for resection in those cases which are locally removable include the surgeon's inability to differentiate between a primary lesion of the head of the pancreas and a tumor of the ampulla or the lower end of the common bile duct and also a longer, more comfortable survival after resection even for those who ultimately succumb to their disease.

A 5-year survival rate as high as 18.2 percent has recently been reported after resection for carcinoma of the head of the pancreas, and the 5-year survival rate for carcinoma of the ampulla of Vater and the duodenum may be twice as high. Twenty-five percent of patients who survived resection for cancer of the head of the pancreas have lived for 5 years or more.

The major problem confronting the surgeon at operation is accurate diagnosis, especially before he embarks upon a procedure as large as pancreaticoduodenectomy. Carcinoma of the ampulla of Vater and duodenum can usually be diagnosed rather easily by biopsy of the lesion through a duodenotomy. Establishing the existence of carcinoma of the head of the pancreas or lower end of the common bile duct is often impossible; repeated biopsies not only may be hazardous but are usually unrewarding because of the inflammation surrounding the primary lesion. The decision for resection must be made on the basis of the clinical and operative findings of a mass in the region of the head of the pancreas in a patient in the sixth or seventh decade of life, very frequently with dilatation of the duct of Wirsung. If a calculus can be ruled out by exploration of the common bile duct and cholangiography, the surgeon can take solace in the fact that he will rarely be wrong in the diagnosis of malignancy. Furthermore, if pancreatitis has progressed to the point of obstructing the common bile duct and if the resection can be performed with a reasonably low mortality rate, then successful resection for this benign lesion cannot be too strongly criticized.

Although the resectability rate of carcinoma of the ampulla and duodenum is between 65 and 75 percent, only 10 to 15 percent of patients with carcinoma of the pancreas have resectable lesions. The surgeon's role in palliation is, therefore, an important one though the average survival after diagnosis in patients with unresectable neoplastic obstructions of the biliary tract is approximately 6 months. Rarely do these patients live longer than 1 year. However, the relief of the jaundice, with its attendant pruritus, and possibly alleviation of obstruction, will often provide significant palliation for these unfortunate patients. A simple cholecystojejunostomy to a loop of jeju-

num without enteroenterostomy is easily performed and is rarely followed by cholangitis. Choledochojejunostomy may be necessary when the gallbladder is absent or the cystic duct is obstructed by tumor. Anastomosis of the biliary tree to the duodenum has been done successfully but is unwise if duodenal obstruction is likely. Invasion of the duodenum and stomach produces gastrointestinal obstruction in 20 percent of patients with carcinoma of the pancreas, and for this reason gastroenterostomy may be advisable.

Cattell and Warren advocate anastomosis of the dilated duct of Wirsung to the jejunum to improve digestion and possibly relieve the pain of ductal distension, but this adds to the extent of operation in an often already debilitated patient and may increase mortality and morbidity. Recently, Merendino has shown that vagotomy relieves the pain of pancreatic cancer. Combined radiation therapy and 5-fluorouracil have recently been shown to significantly prolong comfortable survival of patients with carcinoma of the head of the pancreas.

Pancreaticoduodenal Resection (Fig. 32-13). Pancreaticoduodenectomy is almost always performed in one stage. The two-stage procedure decreases the operative risk in only a small number of deeply jaundiced patients with prolonged obstruction and consequent hepatic injury.

A vertical or a transverse abdominal incision may be used, depending upon the habitus of the patient. The duodenum should have been thoroughly mobilized by the maneuver of Kocher, not only in its second part, but also in the third portion to the superior mesenteric vessels. This usually requires prior mobilization of the hepatic flexure. Gentle dissection between the vessels and the neck of the pancreas with a blunt-nosed clamp is performed once the gastrocolic trunk and pancreatic tributaries have been divided and the posterosuperior pancreaticoduodenal vein has been located. At this point, the surgeon may still turn back, before he has performed an irrevocable maneuver, but excellent assessment of the entire area is still available to him.

The gastrocolic omentum may also be divided at this point to allow better evaluation or so that resection can be continued. The right gastric, gastroduodenal, and descending branch of the left gastric arteries are divided and ligated. The stomach is transected between Payr clamps, leaving the entire antrum with the specimen. The pancreas is transected, usually at its neck. Large vessels are transfixed with fine nonabsorbable sutures. The uncinate process is mobilized by dividing numerous vessels to it between ligatures. Varying amounts of pancreas, or even the entire organ, may be removed with this procedure, at the discretion of the surgeon. The jejunal mesentery and jejunum are divided to allow removal of a few inches of jejunum distal to the ligament of Treitz; the jejunum is withdrawn from beneath the mesenteric vessels. The entire specimen may now be removed by division of the common bile duct. A concomitant cholecystectomy is not always necessary but is usually performed.

Many methods of reconstruction are available. The end of the jejunum is brought into the upper abdomen in a retrocolic position but anterior to the mesenteric vessels.

Fig. 32-13. A. Pancreaticoduodenectomy. Extent of resection. B. Anastomosis of pancreatic duct. C. Retrocolic method of reconstitution. D. Antecolic method of reconstitution.

Of prime importance is the anastomosis of the biliary and pancreatic ducts above, or proximal to, the gastrojejunal anastomosis, to prevent marginal ulceration. Vagotomy is not generally performed, although it has been recommended by some. If the common duct and jejunum are of equal size, they are joined end to end. When the jejunum is larger than the common bile duct, the end of the jejunum is closed, and end-to-side anastomosis is carried out. The pancreaticojejunostomy is performed between the end of the pancreas and the side of the jejunum several inches distal to the choledochojejunostomy, suturing the duct of Wirsung to jejunal mucosa, as suggested by Cattell and Warren. A gastrojejunostomy completes the operative procedure. A single soft Penrose drain is left in place close to, but not in apposition with, the pancreaticojejunal anastomosis.

Hemorrhage and renal failure are the most common complications in the early postoperative period. Meticulous hemostasis during operation and the administration of vitamin K will generally prevent hemorrhage and later renal failure. The importance of adequate replacement of blood, fluids, and electrolytes cannot be overemphasized. Pancreatic fistula is the third most common complication and is particularly apt to occur if the stump of the pancreas is closed. Careful pancreaticojejunostomy with anastomosis of the duct of Wirsung to the mucosa of the jejunum over a fine tube has largely obviated this complication. Should a pancreatic fistula occur, sump drainage should be instituted. The fistula will close in 2 to 3 weeks if adequate nutrition and electrolyte balance are maintained.

Metabolic Consequences of Pancreaticoduodenectomy. Most patients tolerate pancreaticoduodenectomy relatively well. Although some patients gain weight and thrive, the majority tend to lose some weight and may have varying degrees of malabsorption. The management of these problems is not unlike that in the postgastrectomy patient, but exocrine pancreatic substitution therapy is often necessary. Viokase in divided doses, up to 20 Gm daily, is preferred. Whether resection of the head, uncinate process, and neck of the pancreas or closure of the pancreaticojejunostomy causes the pancreatic insufficiency often seen after pancreaticoduodenectomy is unknown.

The nutritional and metabolic picture is quite different in the case of total pancreatectomy. The postoperative diabetes, even though mild and rarely requiring more than 30 units of insulin daily, is exceedingly difficult to manage because of the patient's extreme sensitivity to insulin. Diabetic retinopathy and glomerulosclerosis have been reported but are rare. Loss of nitrogen in the stool increases, and fat absorption is severely impaired. Iron absorption is very poor, and negative calcium and phosphorus balance is common. Theoretically, total pancreatectomy should improve the results of surgical therapy for carcinoma of the pancreas, since the tumor may spread via the pancreatic duct; the lesion is often multifocal; and the gross extent of the tumor may be difficult to ascertain at operation. However, the extreme metabolic derangements produced by total pancreatectomy and the absence of data to indicate that this operation increases survival in cancer of the pancreas make its use debatable at the present time.

Islet-Cell Tumors and Hyperinsulinism

Roscoe Graham achieved the first recorded cure of organic hyperinsulinism by removing an islet-cell adenoma. In a review of the literature published between 1929 and 1958, Moss and Rhoads found 766 cases, of which only 93 were malignant.

PATHOPHYSIOLOGY. The beta cells of the pancreatic islets secrete insulin, and tumors that cause hyperinsulinism arise from these cells. Bioassays of these tumors have usually shown large quantities of insulin, and recent studies of plasma insulin in patients harboring beta cell tumors have indicated markedly elevated levels after islet-cell stimulation by a variety of means.

The excessive circulating insulin causes profound hypoglycemia. Since the brain depends primarily on glucose for its metabolism and cannot store either glucose or glycogen in significant amounts, the hypoglycemia may cause convulsions, severe cerebral depression, and coma, which if allowed to persist for a prolonged period will be followed by death within 3 to 20 days. Mental deterioration, ataxia, hemiparesis, and a wide variety of neurologic sequelae may result from repeated minor hypoglycemic episodes. Early diagnosis and prompt treatment are of importance in the prevention of these irreversible changes.

Administration of glucose promptly reverses the hypoglycemia and relieves the symptoms. The spontaneous recovery which is so frequent in patients with organic hyperinsulinism has not been adequately explained. However, it has been suggested that hypoglycemia stimulates the release of epinephrine and glucagon, which in turn mobilize sufficient glycogen to elevate the blood sugar.

PATHOLOGY. Approximately 75 percent of patients with pancreatic organic hyperinsulinism have benign adenomas; 12.9 percent have suspiciously malignant lesions, and in 12.1 percent the lesions are clearly malignant. About 15 percent of the patients have multiple adenomas, but only a few cases of diffuse adenomatosis involving the entire pancreas have been described. Most of the adenomas measure between 1 and 3 cm, but the size of the tumor seems to have little relationship to the severity of the clinical symptoms. Metastases from malignant beta cell tumors may be functional or nonfunctional.

CLINICAL MANIFESTATIONS. Most of the patients with this syndrome are in the fourth to seventh decades of life. The sex incidence is approximately equal. Functioning islet-cell tumors are rare in childhood, but spontaneous hypoglycemia occasionally occurs without tumor. This type of hypoglycemia usually subsides spontaneously as the child grows older; its cause is unknown.

The symptoms may take one of two general forms, but between the two extremes many combinations of clinical signs may occur. The absolute level of blood sugar often bears little relationship to the severity or character of the symptoms, even in the same patient on different days. If the blood sugar falls rapidly, the primary symptoms may be referable to the release of epinephrine caused by the hypoglycemia. Sweating, hunger, weakness, tachycardia, and "inward trembling" result from this mechanism. A slower decrease in blood sugar produces "cerebral" symptoms, such as headache, mental confusion, visual disturbances, convulsions, and coma. Symptoms may last for a few weeks or as long as 20 years. Signs and symptoms of progressive muscular atrophy have been reported in these cases. The widest possible variety of bizarre neurologic or psychiatric disorders may be mimicked by organic hyperinsulinism. Fear of attacks leads many patients to consume large quantities of food, especially carbohydrates, and they often become extremely obese.

LABORATORY AND DIAGNOSTIC STUDIES. Whipple's triad consists of (1) attacks precipitated by fasting or exertion, (2) fasting blood sugar concentrations below 50 mg/100 ml, and (3) symptoms relieved by oral or intravenous administration of glucose. These criteria should always be met before considering operation. Three types of spontaneous hypoglycemia account for about 80 percent of all such cases: (1) functional hyperinsulinism, (2) organic hyperinsulinism due to pancreatic islet-cell tumor, and (3) hepatogenic hypoglycemia. Functional and alimentary hypoglycemia are usually easily ruled out, because they never occur in the fasting state and invariably occur 2 to 4 hours after eating. Hepatogenic hypoglycemia may be almost impossible to differentiate from insulinoma. Abnormal hepatic function and a high-plateau type of glucose tolerance curve which does not respond to a high-carbohydrate diet are the keystones to diagnosis of hepatogenic hypoglycemia. Abnormalities of the pituitary, adrenal, and central nervous system may also cause organic hypoglycemia but can usually be ruled out.

Apart from satisfying the conditions of Whipple's triad, prolonged fasting with or without exercise is the single most valuable test in the diagnosis of insulinoma. The blood sugar will invariably decrease to below 50 mg/100 ml under these circumstances, and fasting for longer than 30 hours is almost never necessary. Simultaneous measurement of serum insulin and blood sugar levels with the finding of an insulin level inappropriately high for the level of the blood sugar is diagnostic of insulinoma. Other aids to diagnosis are the response of the blood sugar to tolbutamide (oral or intravenous) and leucine. These drugs stimulate the release of insulin by the tumor; patients with insulinoma have a much greater and more prolonged depression in the blood sugar level than normal and for that reason these tests may be dangerous. The glucose tolerance test has been unduly deprecated because of the wide variation in the responses. However, if care is taken to restore the sensitivity of the islets in the nontumorous portion of the pancreas by feeding carbohydrates for a few days, the typical flat low curve will almost always be seen. Once the diagnosis has been established by biochemical means, pancreatic angiography may be extremely helpful in localizing the lesion for the surgeon, especially in patients who have undergone unsuccessful exploration before.

TREATMENT. Although dietary therapy has been attempted, the only permanent cure of organic pancreatic hyperinsulinism is by removal of the offending lesion. Streptozotocin, a potent antibiotic which destroys islets, is useful in treating patients with far-advanced metastatic islet-cell carcinoma but should be reserved for these patients because of the antibiotic's toxic side effects. The preoperative management is concerned mainly with the provision of adequate quantities of glucose, usually in the form of 10 percent dextrose solutions. ACTH and cortisone have been recommended, presumably to prevent hyperthermia during, or immediately after, operation. However, it is not necessary to use these drugs, and there is no sound physiologic reason for them.

Surgically, every portion of the pancreas must be carefully examined. The entire anterior aspect of the body, tail, and a portion of the head of the pancreas should be exposed. Then the entire body and tail of the pancreas with the spleen must be mobilized into the wound by division of the splenocolic and lienorenal ligaments and incision of the parietal peritoneum along the inferior and superior aspects of the pancreas. The entire posterior surface of the organ as far right as the superior mesenteric vessels may then be palpated and visualized. The head of the pancreas must be completely mobilized by the Kocher maneuver. Particular attention should be paid to exposure of the neck of the pancreas by division and ligation of the gastrocolic venous trunk and to the uncinate process. The latter is best seen after meticulous clearing of the superior mesenteric vessels. Adenomas in the stomach, duodenum, jejunum, ileum, mesentery, and omentum are aberrant locations in 1 to 2 percent of cases, and these areas should be carefully searched.

Simple excision of the adenoma is sufficient in most cases, since the majority are benign. If malignancy is suspected, a pancreatic resection should be done. Complete exploration should be performed even if a single tumor is found, since about 14 percent are multiple.

The greatest current controversy concerns proper procedure when the tumor cannot be found after thorough examination. Classically, a distal subtotal pancreatectomy to the left of the mesenteric vessels has been advocated under these circumstances, with the hope that a small adenoma might be present in this tissue (21 percent chance) or that hyperplasia of the islets might be ameliorated. It is doubtful whether there are any authenticated cases of hyperplasia of the islets in adults. Yet Moss and Rhoads have found that 42.6 percent of 129 patients were cured and 10.9 percent were improved after "blind" distal pancreatectomy when no tumor was found. The original diagnosis in those who were improved is questionable. Fonkalsrud et al. have suggested that pancreaticoduodenal resection with preservation of the tail of the pancreas should be done when the pancreatic tumor cannot be found after thorough exploration. These investigators feel that a small tumor is much more easily overlooked in the head and uncinate process than in the tail or body. They believe that distal pancreatectomy would be far easier technically after "blind" pancreaticoduodenectomy when no tumor has been found than the reverse sequence of operations. We are reluctant to advocate "blind" pancreaticoduodenectomy because of the higher morbidity and mortality and would still choose distal resection. The distal pancreatectomy can be extended to a 90 percent resection or more if necessary, more easily and with less morbidity than pancreaticoduodenectomy. However, it cannot be stressed strongly enough that all of the pancreas, and especially the head and uncinate process, must be seen and felt. A marked increase in blood glucose within 30 minutes of removal of tissue suspected of being responsible for the hyperinsulinism is confirmatory evidence that the disease has been eradicated. Subsequent determination of serum insulin levels on the same blood taken at operation will provide postoperative substantiation of cure.

The child with organic hypoglycemia can usually be managed with diet and ACTH or cortisone. If a response is not evident and if the patient seems to be deteriorating, operation is indicated, even though tumors are exceedingly rare in children. If no tumor is found, distal subtotal pancreatectomy in a child is much more logical procedure than in adults, since hyperplasia of the islets does occur and is responsive to partial resection.

The overall operative mortality for removal of a localized islet-cell tumor is 8.2 percent, and for partial resection (distal) of the pancreas it is 9.6 percent.

Ulcerogenic and Nonulcerogenic Tumors of the Islets

In 1955, Zollinger and Ellison reported two patients with coincidental fulminant peptic ulceration and non-beta cell tumors of the pancreas. Since then, many cases of ulcerogenic tumors of the pancreas have been described.

CLINICAL MANIFESTATIONS. The triad described originally by Zollinger and Ellison remains extremely useful today: (1) fulminant and often complicated peptic ulceration, frequently found in atypical locations, (2) extreme gastric hypersecretion, and (3) non-beta cell tumor of the pancreatic islets. The symptoms are similar to those caused by ordinary peptic ulceration. Some patients with this syndrome have had explosive and unrelenting ulceration from onset; others have had symptoms for several years which suddenly become fulminant. Perforation, hemorrhage, obstruction, internal fistulization, and intractability may occur. The ulceration, although often present in the first portion of the duodenum, occasionally is found in unusual locations, such as the third and fourth parts of the duodenum or the jejunum. Perforation or any other complication of jejunal ulceration should always make one suspect the presence of an ulcerogenic pancreatic tumor, since peptic ulceration of the jejunum rarely occurs when no tumor is present.

Fulminant ulceration often recurs within weeks after ordinarily effective surgical therapy. Subtotal gastrectomy with or without vagotomy, vagotomy with a drainage procedure, radiation therapy, and prodigious doses of alkalinizing and anticholinergic agents have generally been ineffective in controlling the ulcer diathesis. H_2 receptor antagonists have recently proved to be effective in selected patients who may have inoperable situations. Many patients have undergone several of these procedures before the true nature of the process was discovered.

The syndrome is slightly more common in males, the ratio being approximately 6:4. Most of the patients are in the third to fourth decade of life, although a few cases have occurred in the first decade and a rare case in the ninth. Two to three liters of fluid in a 12-hour nocturnal secretion is common even in the absence of pyloric obstruction. The overnight resting secretion often contains 200 to 300 mEq of free acid, although some patients have less than 100 mEq of free hydrochloric acid. Even the smallest remnants of gastric mucosa can cause extreme hypersecretion and recurrent ulceration in these patients. Since the secretory rates are already close to their maximum, further stimulation with histamine generally produces very little response. Marks et al. have suggested that a ratio of basal acid output to histamine-stimulated output of greater than 60 percent is virtually diagnostic of the Zollinger-Ellison syndrome, but exceptions are more common than generally recognized.

The extreme gastric hypersecretion is associated with distressing watery diarrhea in about a third of the reported cases. Some patients have excreted between 2 and 8 liters of liquid stool daily, and in many cases profound diarrhea has preceded the onset of peptic ulceration. In some cases in which diarrhea is the sole symptom, the patient has had gastric hypersecretion without peptic ulceration. Steatorrhea may also occur and probably is caused by three mechanisms: (1) inactivation of pancreatic and intestinal lipase by the abnormally acid environment of the upper small intestine, (2) precipitation of bile salts, and (3) irritative and inflammatory action of the acid environment upon the mucosa of the small bowel. Aspiration of the gastric secretion often temporarily relieves the diarrhea.

A sharp distinction should be made between the diarrhea of the Zollinger-Ellison syndrome and another syndrome of watery diarrhea and non-beta cell tumors of the pancreas which is much less common than the former, only about fifty cases having been reported. This latter group of patients is usually free from ulcers; gastric secretion is normal or low; the hypokalemia and alkalosis are almost always present. Hyperglycemia is common, and alternating hypercalcemia and normocalcemia are frequently encountered in the same patient. Total removal of the tumor results in cure of the disabling watery diarrhea, although steroid therapy may be temporarily beneficial for those with malignant tumors where all tumor could not be extirpated and the metastatic malignancy is functional. Although Kraft, Tompkins, and Zollinger originally proposed that secretin produced by the tumor was responsible for the observed effects, more recent studies indicate that the responsible agent is vasoactive intestinal peptide (VIP).

In addition to the usual radiologic findings of peptic ulceration, duodenal ileus with enlargement of rugal folds, hypertrophy of the gastric mucosa, and an abnormal feathery pattern of the small bowel are frequently found in patients with the Zollinger-Ellison syndrome.

PATHOLOGY AND PATHOPHYSIOLOGY. The origin of these tumors is as yet unknown, although histologic studies indicate that they do not arise from the alpha or beta cells of the islets. The typical tumor is composed of rather uniform cuboidal cells arranged mainly in strands and ribbons or occasionally in sheets and clumps. The nucleus is oval and has one or more round nucleoli. The cytoplasm usually contains fine stippling and irregular vacuoles, but no secretory granules have been identified. These tumors often bear a striking resemblance to argentaffin tumors (carcinoids) but do not react to silver stains. The growth pattern of these two tumors is remarkably similar in that both tend to grow slowly, metastasize late, and exhibit little correlation between the microscopic appearance and growth propensities. The patient with an islet-cell tumor often dies from the unremitting peptic ulceration rather than from metastasis, although recent long-term follow-up indicates an increasing and unexpected incidence of death from metastatic disease. Grossly, the tumors are slate gray to red-brown and vary from 2 mm to 10 cm. Most are solid, although a few cystic tumors have been reported.

In 249 collected cases, 61 percent of the patients had malignant tumors, and 44 percent of these had metastases, usually to the regional lymph nodes. The tumors are located with equal frequency in the head and tail of the pancreas. Diffuse microadenomatosis has been observed in 19 percent of the cases. A significant number of patients have had lesions in the duodenal wall. This is of particular interest because removal of the tumor alone in these cases has frequently sufficed to eradicate the disease, in contradistinction to the radical treatment by total gastrectomy usually advocated in this syndrome.

Associated endocrine disease has been found in 21 percent of the patients with the Zollinger-Ellison syndrome. This usually consists of adenomas of other endocrine glands, such as the pituitary, parathyroid, pancreatic islets (beta cells), and adrenal cortex, in that order of frequency. These patients usually do not have family histories of similar disturbances; therefore most of these cases can be distinguished from the group described by Wermer in 1954. He pointed out that some patients with polyendocrine adenomas and peptic ulceration often have giant gastric rugae (Ménétrier's disease) and that an abnormal gene may be responsible. Ellison and Wilson have found that only 3 percent of the patients with the Zollinger-Ellison syndrome fall into this classification. Gastrin is secreted by these tumors, and that extracted from tumors has physiologic effects identical to those of synthesized pure gastrin. Thus, the diagnosis can be substantiated by the detection of extremely high levels of gastrin in the serum. Sometimes the levels of serum gastrin are borderline elevated in patients with gastrinoma, especially if prior vagotomy without resection has been carried out. An exaggerated response of the serum gastrin to the intravenous infusion of calcium and a paradoxical rise of the serum gastrin level after intravenous infusion of secretin serve to elucidate the diagnosis in doubtful cases. These findings, together with the absence of a rise in serum gastrin level after a meal, are helpful in differentiating patients with gastrinoma from those who have the recently described antral G cell hyperplasia.

TREATMENT AND PROGNOSIS. It is attractive to hypothesize that removal of the pancreatic islet-cell tumor alone should suffice to alleviate the potent ulcerogenic stimulus in patients with this disease. Although a few patients with fulminant peptic ulceration have responded to removal of the pancreatic tumor alone or to excision of the tumor with concomitant subtotal gastrectomy, these procedures are usually destined for failure. The high incidence of malignancy with functioning metastases as well as the possibility of multiple pancreatic tumors or islet hyperplasia are responsible for these failures. Even the smallest amount of gastric mucosa is capable of secreting huge quantities of highly acid gastric juice in the presence of the ulcerogenic tumor. Thus, the safest and most conservative treatment of these patients is total gastrectomy, usually with Roux en Y jejunal reconstruction, and removal of the pancreatic tumor if possible.

Experience has repeatedly indicated that lesser operations or radiation therapy usually invite disaster in the form of recurrent ulceration, internal fistulization, hemorrhage, perforation, and death. The relatively protracted course of the tumor, even when it has metastasized, justifies the more radical procedure. Repeated determinations of serum gastrin levels may be of some prognostic value following total gastrectomy since disappearance of metastases and return of serum gastrin to normal have been reported in some cases. Persistently high levels of serum gastrin probably indicate lack of primary or metastatic tumor regression, whereas elevation of a posttherapeutic low level of serum gastrin suggests the development of metastatic disease. Oberhelman et al. have had good results from removal of the tumor alone without total gastrectomy when the tumor has been located in the wall of the duodenum. We have had similar results, but only in these cases would we consider procedures of less than total

gastrectomy. Whether these duodenal tumors differ materially from those in the pancreas is not known, although the microscopic appearance is similar.

References

Anatomy

Kleitsch, W. P.: Anatomy of the Pancreas: A Study with Special Reference to the Duct System, *Arch Surg*, **71:**795, 1955.

Payne, R. L., Jr.: Annular Pancreas, *Ann Surg*, **133:**754, 1951.

Pierson, J. M.: The Arterial Blood Supply of the Pancreas, *Surg Gynecol Obstet*, **77:**426, 1943.

Reemtsma, K.: Embryology and Congenital Anomalies of the Pancreas, in J. M. Howard and G. L. Jordan (eds.), "Surgical Diseases of the Pancreas," J. B. Lippincott Company, Philadelphia, 1960.

Reich, H.: Relation of the Duct of Santorini to the Pathogenesis of Duodenal Ulcer, *N Engl J Med*, **269:**1119, 1963.

Physiology

Albo, R., Silen, W., Hein, M. F., and Harper, H. A.: Relationship of the Acinar Portion of the Pancreas to Gastric Secretion, *Surg Forum*, **14:**316, 1963.

Christodoulopoulos, J. B., Jacobs, W. H., and Klotz, A. P.: Pharmacologic Inhibition of Humoral-stimulated Pancreatic Secretion, *Gastroenterology*, **40:**671, 1961.

Drapanas, T., Pollack, E. L., and Shim, W. K.: The Regulation of Pancreatic Secretion by Serotonin, *Arch Surg*, **83:**462, 1961.

Gregory, R. A.: "Secretory Mechanisms of the Gastro-intestinal Tract," The Williams & Wilkins Company, Baltimore, 1962.

—— and Tracy, H. J.: The Constitution and Properties of Two Gastrins Extracted from Hog Antral Mucosa, *Gut*, **5:**103, 1964.

—— and ——: A Note on the Nature of the Gastrin-like Stimulant Present in Zollinger-Ellison Tumors, *Gut*, **5:**115, 1964.

Janowitz, H. D., and Dreiling, D. A.: The Pancreatic Secretion of Fluid and Electrolytes, in *Ciba Found Symp Exocrine Pancreas Normal Abnormal Functions*, 1962.

Konturek, S. J., Radecki, T., Biernat, J., and Thor, P.: Effect of Vagotomy on Pancreatic Secretion Evoked by Endogenous and Exogenous Cholecystokinin and Caerulein, *Gastroenterology*, **63:**273, 1972.

McIlrath, D. C., Kennedy, J. A., and Hallenbeck, G. A.: Relationship between Atrophy of the Pancreas and Gastric Secretion: An Experimental Study, *Am J Digest Diseases*, **8:**623, 1963.

Menguy, R. B., Hallenbeck, G. A., Bollman, J. L., and Grindlay, J. H.: Intraductal Pressures and Sphincteric Resistance in Canine Pancreatic and Biliary Ducts after Various Stimuli, *Surg Gynecol Obstet*, **106:**306, 1958.

Meyer, J. H., Spingola, L. J., and Grossman, M. I.: Endogenous Cholecystokinin Potentiates Exogenous Secretin on Pancreas of Dog, *Am J Physiol*, **221:**742, 1971.

Meyer, J. H., Way, L. W., and Grossman, M. I.: Pancreatic Response to Acidification of Varying Lengths of Proximal Intestine in Dog, *Am J Physiol*, **219:**971, 1970.

Moreland, H. J., and Johnson, L. R.: Effect of Vagotomy of

Pancreatic Secretion Stimulated by Endogenous and Exogenous Secretin, *Gastroenterology,* **60:**425, 1971.

Perks, A. M., Schapiro, H., and Woodward, E. R.: The Influence of Antidiuretic Hormone on Pancreatic Exocrine Secretion, *Acta Endocrinol,* **45:**340, 1964.

Poncelot, P. R., and Thompson, A. G.: Role of Infected Bile in Spasm of Sphincter of Oddi, *Am J Surg,* **126:**387, 1973.

Routley, E. F., Mann, F. C., Bollman, J. L., and Grindlay, J. H.: Effects of Vagotomy on Pancreatic Secretion in Dogs with Chronic Pancreatic Fistula, *Surg Gynecol Obstet,* **95:**529, 1952.

Thomas, J. E.: Mechanism of Action of Pancreatic Stimuli Studied by Means of Atropine-like Drugs, *Am J Physiol,* **206:**124, 1964.

Unger, R. H., and Eisentraut, A. M.: Enteroinsular Axis, *Arch Intern Med,* **123:**261, 1969.

Unger, R. H., Ketterer, H., Dupre, J., and Eisentraut, A. M.: The Effects of Secretin, Pancreozymin, and Gastrin on Insulin and Glucagon Secretion in Anesthetized Dogs, *J Clin Invest,* **46:** 630, 1967.

Veeger, W., Abels, J., Hellemans, N., and Nieweg, H. O.: Effect of Sodium Bicarbonate and Pancreatin on the Absorption of Vitamin B_{12} and Fat in Pancreatic Insufficiency, *N Engl J Med,* **267:**1341, 1962.

Wang, C. C., and Grossman, M. I.: Physiological Determination of Release of Secretin and Pancreozymin from Intestine of Dogs with Transplanted Pancreas, *Am J Physiol,* **164:**527, 1951.

Warshaw, A. L., and Lesser, P. B.: Amylase Clearance in Differentiating Acute Pancreatitis from Peptic Ulcer with Hyperamylasemia, *Ann Surg,* **181:**314, 1975.

White, T. T., Hayama, T., and Magee, D. F.: Alternate Nervous Pathways for the Gastropancreatic Reflex, *Gastroenterology,* **39:**615, 1960.

——, Lundh, G., and Magee, D. F.: Evidence for the Existence of a Gastropancreatic Reflex, *Am J Physiol,* **198:**725, 1960.

Acute Pancreatitis

Adams, J. T., Libertino, J. A., and Schwartz, S. I.: Significance of an Elevated Serum Amylase, *Surgery,* **63:**877, 1968.

Albo, R. J., Silen, W., and Goldman, L.: A Critical Clinical Analysis of Acute Pancreatitis, *Arch Surg,* **86:**1032, 1963.

Avioli, L. V., Birge, S. J., Scott, S., and Shieber, W.: Role of the Thyroid Gland During Glucagon-induced Hypocalcemia in the Dog, *Am J Physiol,* **216:**939, 1969.

Bernard, H. R., Criscione, J. R., and Moyer, C. A.: The Pathologic Significance of the Serum Amylase Concentration: An Evaluation with Special Reference to Pancreatitis and Biliary Lithiasis, *Arch Surg,* **79:**311, 1959.

Bradley, E. L., III, and Clements, L. J.: Spontaneous Resolution of Pancreatic Pseudocysts: Implications for Timing of Operative Intervention, *Am J Surg,* **129:**23, 1975.

Cameron, J. L., Zuidema, G. D., and Margolis, S.: A Pathogenesis for Alcoholic Pancreatitis, *Surgery,* **77:**754, 1975.

Elliot, D. W., Williams, R. D., and Zollinger, R. M.: Alterations in the Pancreatic Resistance to Bile in the Pathogenesis of Acute Pancreatitis, *Ann Surg,* **146:**669, 1957.

Gambill, E. E., and Mason, H. L.: One-hour Value for Urinary Amylase in 96 Patients with Pancreatitis: Comparative Diagnostic Value of Tests of Urinary and Serum Amylase and Serum Lipase, *JAMA,* **186:**24, 1963.

Gross, J. B., and Comfort, M. W.: Hereditary Pancreatitis, *Proc Staff Meetings Mayo Clinic,* **32:**354, 1957.

Haverback, B. J., Dyce, B., Bundy, H., and Edmondson, H. A.: Trypsin, Trypsinogen, and Trypsin Inhibitor in Human Pancreatic Juice: Mechanism for Pancreatitis Associated with Hyperparathyroidism, *Am J Med,* **29:**424, 1960.

Howard, J. M.: The Causes of Death from Pancreatitis, in J. M. Howard and G. L. Jordan, Jr., "Surgical Diseases of the Pancreas," J. B. Lippincott Company, Philadelphia, 1960.

—— and Ehrlich, E. W.: The Etiology of Pancreatitis: A Review of Clinical Experience, *Ann Surg,* **152:**135, 1960.

Howes, R., Zuidema, G. D., and Cameron, J. L.: Evaluation of Prophylactic Antibiotics in Acute Pancreatitis, *J Surg Res,* **18:**197, 1975.

Kessler, J. I., Kniffen, J. C., and Janowitz, H. D.: Lipoprotein Lipase Inhibition in the Hyperlipemia of Acute Alcoholic Pancreatitis, *N Engl J Med,* **269:**943, 1963.

Klatskin, G., and Gordon, M.: Relationship between Relapsing Pancreatitis and Essential Hyperlipemia, *Am J Med,* **12:**3, 1952.

Lefer, A. M., Glenn, T. M., O'Neill, T. J., Lovett, W. L., Geissinger, W. T., and Wangensteen, S. L.: Inotropic Influence of Endogenous Peptides in Experimental Hemorrhagic Pancreatitis, *Surgery,* **69:**220, 1971.

Levitt, M. D., Rapoport, M., and Cooperbrand, S. R.: The Renal Clearance of Amylase in Renal Insufficiency, Acute Pancreatitis, and Macroamylasemia, *Ann Intern Med,* **71:**919, 1969.

Ranson, J. H. C., Rivkind, K. M., Roses, D. F., Fink, S. D., Eng, K., and Spencer, F. C.: Prognostic Signs and Role of Operative Management in Acute Pancreatitis, *Surg Gynecol Obstet,* **139:**69, 1974.

Robinson, T. M., and Dunphy, J. E.: Continuous Perfusion of Bile and Protease Activators through the Pancreas, *JAMA,* **183:**530, 1963.

Salzman, E. W., and Bartlett, M. K.: Pancreatic Duct Exploration in Selected Cases of Acute Pancreatitis, *Ann Surg,* **158:**859, 1963.

Schmidt, H., and Creutzfeld, W.: The Possible Role of Phospholipase A in the Pathogenesis of Acute Pancreatitis, *Scand J Gastroenterol,* **4:**39, 1969.

Smith, R. B., III, Warren, W. D., Rivard, A. A., Jr., and Amerson, J. R.: Pancreatic Ascites: Diagnosis and Management with Particular Reference to Surgical Technics, *Ann Surg,* **177:**689, 1973.

Watts, G. T.: Total Pancreatectomy for Fulminant Pancreatitis, *Lancet,* **2:**384, 1963.

Chronic Pancreatitis

Child, C. G., III, Frey, C. F., and Fry, W. J.: A Reappraisal of Removal of 95% of the Distal Portion of the Pancreas, *Surg Gynecol Obstet,* **129:**49, 1969.

Dreiling, D. A., and Janowitz, H. D.: Measurement of Pancreatic Secretory Function, in *Ciba Found Symp Exocrine Pancreas Normal Abnormal Functions,* 1962.

DuVal, M. K., Jr.: Caudal Pancreatico-jejunostomy for Chronic Relapsing Pancreatitis, *Ann Surg,* **140:**775, 1954.

Howard, J. M.: The Etiology of Acute Pancreatitis: Facts and Fancies, in J. M. Howard and G. L. Jordan, Jr. (eds.), "Surgical Diseases of the Pancreas," J. B. Lippincott Company, Philadelphia, 1960.

Joffe, B. I., Bank, S., Jackson, W. P. V., and Keller, P.: Insulin Reserve in Patients with Chronic Pancreatitis, *Lancet,* **2:**890, 1968.

Kalser, M. H., Leite, C. A., and Warren, W. D.: Fat Assimilation After Massive Distal Pancreatectomy, *N Engl J Med,* **279:**570, 1968.

Owens, J. L., and Howard, J. M.: Pancreatic Calcification: A Late Sequel in the Natural History of Chronic Alcoholism and Alcoholic Pancreatitis, *Ann Surg,* **147:**326, 1958.

Puestow, C. B., and Gillesby, W. J.: Retrograde Surgical Drainage of Pancreas for Chronic Relapsing Pancreatitis, *Arch Surg,* **76:**898, 1958.

Silen, W., Baldwin, J., and Goldman, L.: Treatment of Chronic Pancreatitis by Longitudinal Pancreaticojejunostomy, *Am J Surg,* **106:**243, 1963.

White, T. F., and Keith, R. G.: Long-term Follow-up Study of 50 Patients with Pancreaticojejunostomy, *Surg Gynecol Obstet,* **136:**353, 1973.

Trauma

Anderson, M. C., and Bergan, J. J.: An Experimental Study of Pancreatic Trauma and Its Relationship to Pancreatic Inflammation, *Arch Surg,* **86:**1044, 1963.

Baker, R. J., Dippel, W. F., Freeark, R. J., and Strohl, E. L.: The Surgical Significance of Trauma to the Pancreas, *Arch Surg,* **86:**1038, 1963.

Berne, C. J., Donovan, A. J., White, E. J., and Yellin, A. E.: Duodenal "Diverticulization" for Duodenal and Pancreatic Injury, *Am J Surg,* **127:**503, 1974.

Cleveland, H. C., Reinschmidt, J. S., and Waddell, W. R.: Traumatic Pancreatitis: An Increasing Problem, *Surg Clin North Am,* **43:**401, 1963.

Doubilet, H., and Mulholland, J. H.: Some Observations on the Treatment of Trauma to the Pancreas, *Am J Surg,* **105:**741, 1963.

Freeark, R. J., Kane, J. M., Folk, F. A., and Baker, R. J.: Traumatic Disruption of the Head of the Pancreas, *Arch Surg,* **91:**5, 1965.

Howard, J. M.: Pancreatic Trauma, in J. M. Howard and G. L. Jordan, Jr. (eds.), "Surgical Diseases of the Pancreas," J. B. Lippincott Company, Philadelphia, 1960.

Howell, J. F., Burrus, G. R., and Jordan, G. L., Jr.: Surgical Management of Pancreatic Injuries, *J Trauma,* **1:**32, 1961.

Stone, H. H., Stowers, K. B., and Shippey, S. H.: Injuries to the Pancreas, *Arch Surg,* **85:**525, 1962.

Thal, A. P., and Wilson, R. F.: A Pattern of Severe Blunt Trauma to the Region of the Pancreas, *Surg Gynecol Obstet,* **119:**773, 1964.

Cysts and Pseudocysts

Balfour, J. F.: Pancreatic Pseudocysts: Complications and Their Relation to the Timing of Treatment, *Surg Clin North Am,* **50:**395, 1970.

Cullen, P. K., Jr., ReMine, W. H., and Dahlin, D. C.: A Clinicopathological Study of Cystadenocarcinoma of the Pancreas, *Surg Gynecol Obstet,* **117:**189, 1963.

Doubilet, H., and Mulholland, H. J.: Pancreatic Cysts, *Surg Gynecol Obstet,* **96:**683, 1953.

Evans, F. C.: Pancreatic Abscess, *Am J Surg,* **117:**537, 1969.

Finley, J. W.: Respiratory Complications of Acute Pancreatitis, *Ann Surg,* **169:**420, 1969.

Jordan, G. L., Jr.: Pancreatic Cysts, in J. M. Howard and G. L. Jordan, Jr. (eds.), "Surgical Diseases of the Pancreas," J. B. Lippincott Company, Philadelphia, 1960.

Kaiser, G. C., King, R. D., Kilman, J. W., Lempke, R. E., and Shumacker, H. B.: Pancreatic Pseudocysts: An Evaluation of Surgical Management, *Arch Surg,* **89:**275, 1964.

Murphy, R. F., and Hinkamp, J. F.: Pancreatic Pseudocysts: Report of Thirty-five Cases, *Arch Surg,* **81:**564, 1960.

Piper, C. E., ReMine, W. H., and Priestley, J. T.: Pancreatic Cystadenomata: Report of 20 Cases, *JAMA,* **180:**648, 1962.

Polk, H. C., Zeppa, R., and Warren, W. D.: Surgical Significance of Differentiation Between Acute and Chronic Pancreatic Collections, *Ann Surg,* **169:**444, 1969.

Schindler, S. C., Schaefer, J. W., Hull, D., and Griffen, W. O., Jr.: Chronic Pancreatic Ascites, *Gastroenterology,* **59:**453, 1970.

Varriale, P., Bonanno, C. A., and Grace, W. J.: Portal Hypertension Secondary to Pancreatic Pseudocysts, *Arch Intern Med,* **112:**191, 1963.

Carcinoma of the Pancreas and Periampullary Area

Buckwalter, J. A., Lawton, R. L., and Tidrick, R. T.: Bypass Operations for Neoplastic Biliary Obstruction, *Am J Surg,* **109:**100, 1965.

Cattell, R. B., and Warren, K. W.: "Surgery of the Pancreas," W. B. Saunders Company, Philadelphia, 1954.

Eaton, S. B., Fleischli, D. J., Pollard, J. J., Nebesar, R. A., and Potsaid, M. S.: Comparison of Current Radiologic Approaches to the Diagnosis of Pancreatic Disease, *New Engl J Med,* **279:**389, 1968.

Guynn, V. L., Overstreet, R. J., and Reynolds, J. T.: Reduction of Mortality and Morbidity in Pancreatoduodenectomy, *Arch Surg,* **85:**260, 1962.

Howard, J. M.: Pancreatico-duodenectomy. Forty-one Consecutive Whipple Resections Without an Operative Mortality, *Ann Surg,* **168:**629, 1968.

Jordan, G. L., Jr.: Benign and Malignant Tumors of the Pancreas and Periampullary Region, in J. M. Howard and G. L. Jordan, Jr. (eds.), "Surgical Diseases of the Pancreas," J. B. Lippincott Company, Philadelphia, 1960.

———— and Grossman, M. I.: Pancreaticoduodenectomy for Chronic Relapsing Pancreatitis, *Arch Surg,* **74:**871, 1957.

Madden, J. L.: Technique for Pancreaticoduodenectomy, *Surg Gynecol Obstet,* **118:**247, 1964.

Merendino, K. A.: Vagotomy for the Relief of Pain Secondary to Pancreatic Carcinoma, *Am J Surg,* **108:**1, 1964.

Moertel, C. G., Reitemeier, R. J., Childs, D. S., Colby, M. Y., and Hallbrook, M. A.: Combined 5-fluorouracil and Supervoltage Radiation Therapy of Locally Unresectable Gastrointestinal Cancer, *Lancet,* **2:**865, 1969.

Monge, J. J., Dockerty, M. B., Wollaeger, E. E., Waugh, J. M., and Priestley, J. T.: Clinicopathologic Observations on Radical Pancreatoduodenal Resection for Peripapillary Carcinoma, *Surg Gynecol Obstet,* **118:**275, 1964.

ReMine, W. H., Priestley, J. T., Judd, E. S., and King, J. N.: Total Pancreatectomy, *Ann Surg,* **172:**595, 1970.

Silen, W.: Surgical Anatomy of the Pancreas, *Surg Clin North Am,* **44:**1253, 1964.

Warren, K. W.: The Surgical Exposure in the Differential Diagnosis of Pancreatic Disorders at Operation, *Surg Clin North Am,* **38:**799, 1958.

Islet Cell Tumors and Hyperinsulinism

Conn, J. W., and Seltzer, H. S.: Spontaneous Hypoglycemia, *Am J Med,* **19:**460, 1955.

Fajans, S. S., and Conn, J. W.: An Intravenous Tolbutamide Test as an Adjunct in the Diagnosis of Functioning Pancreatic Islet Cell Adenomas, *J Lab Clin Med,* **54:**811, 1959.

Flanagan, G. C., Schwartz, T. B., and Ryan, W. G.: Studies on Patients with Islet-cell Tumor, Including the Phenomenon of Leucine-induced Accentuation of Hypoglycemia, *J Clin Endocrinol Metab,* **21:**401, 1961.

Floyd, J. C., Fajans, S. S., Knopf, R. F., and Conn, J. W.: Plasma Insulin in Organic Hyperinsulinism: Comparative Effects of Tolbutamide, Leucine and Glucose, *J Clin Endocrinol,* **24:**747, 1964.

Fonkalsrud, E. W., Dilley, R. B., and Longmire, W. P., Jr.: Insulin Secreting Tumors of the Pancreas, *Ann Surg,* **159:**730, 1964.

Graham, R. R.: Quoted in G. Howland, W. R. Campbell, E. J. Maltby, and W. L. Robinson: Dysinsulinism: Convulsions and Coma Due to Islet-cell Tumor of the Pancreas, with Operation and Cure, *JAMA,* **93:**674, 1929.

Harrison, T. S., Child, G. C., III, Fry, W. J., Floyd, J. C., Jr., and Fajans, S. S.: Current Surgical Management of Functioning Islet Cell Tumors of the Pancreas, *Ann Surg,* **178:**485, 1973.

Moss, N. H., and Rhoads, J. E.: Hyperinsulinism and Islet-cell Tumors of the Pancreas, in J. M. Howard and G. L. Jordan (eds.), "Surgical Diseases of the Pancreas," J. B. Lippincott Company, Philadelphia, 1960.

Porter, M. R., and Frantz, V. K.: Tumors Associated with Hypoglycemia: Pancreatic and Extrapancreatic, *Am J Med,* **21:**944, 1956.

ReMine, W. H., Scholz, D. A., and Priestley, J. T.: Hyperinsulinism: Clinical and Surgical Aspects, *Am J Surg,* **99:**413, 1960.

Schnelle, N., Molnar, G. D., Ferris, D. O., Rosevear, J. W., and Moffitt, E. A.: Circulating Glucose and Insulin in Surgery for Insulinomas, *JAMA,* **217:**1072, 1971.

Whipple, A. O., and Frantz, V. K.: Adenoma of Islet Cells with Hyperinsulinism: A Review, *Ann Surg,* **101:**1299, 1935.

Ulcerogenic and Nonulcerogenic Tumors of the Islets

Ellison, E. H., and Wilson, S. D.: The Zollinger-Ellison Syndrome: Re-appraisal and Evaluation of 260 Registered Cases, *Ann Surg,* **160:**513, 1964.

Espiner, E. A., and Beaven, D. W.: Non-specific Islet-cell Tumor of the Pancreas with Diarrhea, *Q J Med,* **31:**447, 1962.

Friesen, S. R., Bolinger, R. E., Pearse, A. G. E., and McGuigan, J. E.: Serum Gastrin Levels in Malignant Zollinger-Ellison Syndrome After Total Gastrectomy and Hypophysectomy, *Ann Surg,* **172:**504, 1970.

Gjone, E., Fretheim, B., Nordoy, A., Jacobsen, C. D., and Elgjo, K.: Intractable Watery Diarrhoea, Hypokalaemia, and Achlorhydria Associated with Pancreatic Tumor Containing Gastric Secretory Inhibitor, *Scand J Gastroenterol,* **5:**401, 1970.

Hofmann, J. W., Fox, P. S., and Wilson, S. D.: Duodenal Wall Tumors and Zollinger-Ellison Syndrome: Surgical Management, *Arch Surg,* **107:**334, 1973.

Kraft, A. R., Tompkins, R. K., and Zollinger, R. M.: Recognition and Management of the Diarrheal Syndrome Caused by Nonbeta Islet Cell Tumors of the Pancreas, *Am J Surg,* **119:** 163, 1970.

Oberhelman, H. A., Jr., Nelsen, T. S., Johnson, A. N., Jr., and Dragstedt, L. R., II: Ulcerogenic Tumors of the Duodenum, *Ann Surg,* **153:**214, 1961.

Silen, W.: Personal observations.

Singleton, J. W., Kern, F., Jr., Waddell, W. R.: Diarrhea and Pancreatic Islet-cell Tumor: Report of a Case with Severe Jejunal Mucosal Lesion, *Gastroenterology,* **49:**197, 1965.

Summerskill, W. H. J.: Malabsorption and Jejunal Ulceration Due to Gastric Hypersecretion with Pancreatic Islet-cell Hyperplasia, *Lancet,* **1:**120, 1959.

Wermer, P.: Genetic Aspects of Adenomatosis of Endocrine Glands, *Am J Med,* **16:**363, 1954.

Zollinger, R. M., and Ellison, E. H.: Primary Peptic Ulcerations of the Jejunum Associated with Islet-cell Tumors of the Pancreas, *Ann Surg,* **142:**709, 1955.

Chapter 33

Spleen

by **Seymour I. Schwartz**

ANATOMY

The spleen arises by mesenchymal differentiation along the left side of the dorsal mesogastrium in the 8-mm embryo. The weight of the spleen in the healthy adult ranges between 75 and 100 Gm, decreasing somewhat with age. The organ is located in the left upper quadrant, having a superior relationship to the under surface of the left leaf of the diaphragm and protected anteriorly, laterally, and posteriorly by the lower portion of the rib cage. Its position is maintained by several suspensory ligaments, the major ones being the splenophrenic, splenorenal, splenocolic, and gastrosplenic ligaments (Fig. 33-1). The gastrosplenic ligament normally contains the short gastric vessels, while the remaining ligaments are generally avascular, except in patients with portal hypertension and myeloproliferative disorders. Arterial blood enters the spleen via the splenic artery, a branch of the celiac artery. The major venous drainage courses through the splenic vein, which joins the superior mesenteric vein to form the portal vein.

Accessory spleens have been reported in 14 to 30 percent of patients, with a higher incidence occurring in patients operated on for hematologic disorders. These accessory organs, which receive their vascular supply from the sple-

nic artery, are present, in decreasing order of frequency, in the hilus of the spleen, the gastrosplenic and splenocolic ligaments, the gastrocolic ligament, the splenorenal ligament, and the greater omentum (Fig. 33-2). They also may occur in the pelvis of the female, and functioning splenic tissue has been removed from the scrotum in juxtaposition to the left testicle.

The spleen consists of a capsule which is normally 1 to 2 mm thick and trabeculae which enclose the pulp. The pulp, itself, has conventionally been divided into three zones: white, marginal, and red. The white pulp consists of lymphocytes, plasma cells, and macrophages and is analogous to the lymph node, even to the extent that the follicles contain germinal centers. The marginal zone contains elements of blood plasma and also sequestered foreign material. The red pulp is made up of splenic cords and sinuses which interrelate to form a vascular space.

The spleen is the most vascularized organ in the body, and the splenic circulation has been the subject of disagreement for almost 300 years. Three major concepts of splenic circulation have been proposed. The "closed circulation" theory holds that the blood in the spleen follows endo-

Fig. 33-1. Ligaments of the spleen. (*From A. J. Erslev and W. F. Ballinger, II, Splenectomy, Curr Probl Surg, 1965. Copyright 1965, Year Book Medical Publishers, Inc., Chicago. Used by permission.*)

Fig. 33-2. Location of accessory spleens. *A.* Splenic hilus. *B.* Along splenic vessels; tail of pancreas. *C.* Splenocolic ligament. *D.* Greater omentum; perirenal regions. *E.* Mesentery. *F.* Presacral region. *G.* Adnexal region. *H.* Peritesticular region. (*From S. I. Schwartz, J. T. Adams, and A. W. Bauman, Splenectomy for Hematologic Disorders, Curr Probl Surg, May, 1971. Copyright 1971, Year Book Medical Publishers, Inc., Chicago. Used by permission.*)

thelialized pathways throughout. This theory generally has been abandoned because of the proven nature of the sinus walls, which as early as 1686 were shown by Malpighi to contain perforations in the finest ramifications of the intrasplenic veins. The "open circulation" theory, which can be credited to Billroth in 1860, suggests that the arteries empty into tissue spaces or that sheathed capillaries pour their blood directly into pulp cords from which the blood can then pass through sinus wall stomata and enter the veins. The theory of "divided circulation," as proposed by

Knisely, suggests that whole blood enters the sinuses from the afferent capillaries and that deplasmatization occurs through the sinus walls.

Electron microscopic studies have resolved some of the controversy. It has been established that blood which is brought to the spleen via the splenic arteries courses through branches, the trabecular arteries, which leave the trabeculae and enter the white pulp as central arteries (Fig. 33-3). These central arteries give off at right angles many arterioles, some of which terminate in the white pulp. Other branches cross the white pulp and end in the marginal zone or in the red pulp, itself. The branch of the central artery which terminates in the red pulp, known as the "artery of the pulp," breaks up into many arterioles or branches. Within the red pulp, the blood is collected in venous sinuses known as the "splenic sinuses." These large, thin-walled vascular spaces drain into the pulp veins which, in turn, drain into the trabecular veins and then into the main splenic veins to enter the portal circulation. Thus splenic pulp pressure reflects pressure throughout the portal venous system. The tissue between the splenic sinuses is a reticular, connective tissue meshwork which appears as cords on histologic section, hence designated the "splenic cords." Whether the splenic circulation is truly open or closed may not be of great importance with respect to functional capability since, even if the blood flows in a closed system, the presence of many fenestrations in the basement membranes facilitates passage from cord to sinus. Although these fenestrations are of small diameter (0.5 to 5.0 μ), they are traversed by normal red cells, which easily adjust to these dimensions. Under normal conditions, red cells pass from terminal arterioles directly into splenic sinuses (physiologic shunt) as well as from terminal arterioles into pulp cords and into splenic sinuses after traversing the cordal–sinus wall apertures.

PHYSIOLOGY AND PATHOPHYSIOLOGY

Galen is credited with the phrase "The spleen is an organ full of mystery"; to date this mystery has been only minimally unraveled. During the fifth to eighth month of fetal life, the spleen contributes actively to the production of both red cells and white cells which enter the circulation. This function does not continue in the normal adult, and both the qualitative and quantitative effects of splenic extramedullary hematopoeisis seen in myeloproliferative disorders have not been consistent. The role of the spleen in the immunologic processes of the body is discussed in Chap. 10, Transplantation. The splenic function, which is the focus of surgical attention, is determined by the organ's organization as a large mass of reticuloendothelial tissue which contributes to the removal of cellular elements from the circulating blood. Approximately 350 liters of blood pass through the spleen daily, and a variety of transsplenic circulation times have been demonstrated. Normally, cells pass through the spleen rapidly, but in the presence of splenomegaly and other disease states, the flow patterns become circuitous, contain more obstacles, and result in pooling of cells within the cords. Motulsky and associates, using ^{51}Cr studies, have demonstrated that the slow-circulating component may have a half-life of 30 minutes.

Abnormal and aged erythrocytes, abnormal granulocytes, normal and abnormal platelets, and cellular debris may be cleared by the spleen, which apparently is capable of discriminating between these and normal cellular components. In the normal adult, the spleen is the most important site of selective erythrocyte sequestration and, during its 120-day life cycle, the red cell spends an estimated minimum of 2 days within the spleen. The action of the spleen which results in the pathological reduction of circulating cellular elements of blood has been attributed to three possible mechanisms: (1) excessive splenic destruction of cellular elements, (2) splenic production of an antibody which results in the destruction of cells within the circulating blood, and (3) splenic inhibition of the bone marrow causing failure of maturation and cell release. The last proposal is not important in most circumstances. The production of antibodies may be important in certain circumstances, but, as this is not an exclusive function of splenic immunocytes, antibody production would continue in the absence of the spleen. Overactivity of splenic function leading to accelerated removal of any or all of the circulating cellular elements of the blood has been referred to as *hypersplenism*. This condition accounts for most of the splenic removal of apparently normal cells and may result in anemia, leukopenia, or thrombocytopenia, alone or in combination.

The normal adult spleen contains about 25 ml of red blood cells, but relatively few of these are removed during one passage through the organ. The spleen is capable of removing nuclear remnants from circulating erythrocytes (Howell-Jolly bodies) leaving the intact parent erythrocyte and cytoplasmic siderotic granules. The postsplenectomy blood smear may show the presence of circulating erythrocytes with Howell-Jolly bodies and Pappenheimer bodies (siderotic granules which stain with Wright's stain) as a result of the loss of the pitting function of the spleen. In addition, during the course of a day, approximately 20 ml of aged red blood cells are removed.

The alterations in the red cell which makes it sensitive to splenic destruction after 105 to 120 days in circulation have not been established with certainty. It appears that aging changes the biophysical properties of the red cell, making splenic entrapment more likely. In parallel, the enzyme activity and, therefore, the metabolic capacity of the red cell wanes with cell aging. Delay in splenic transit of aged or abnormal cells can lead to further cell injury because of the relatively hypoxic, acidic, and substrate (glucose)-deprived environment which is present in non gested splenic red pulp cords. These environmental conditions lead to further physical and chemical deterioration of the erythrocyte, making it more susceptible to phagocytosis by splenic macrophages and reticuloendothelial cells or to intrasinusoidal disintegration. The central event in cytolysis may be the fall in cellular adenosine triphosphate (ATP) to very low levels and the loss of vital cellular functions dependent on ATP, such as sodium and calcium

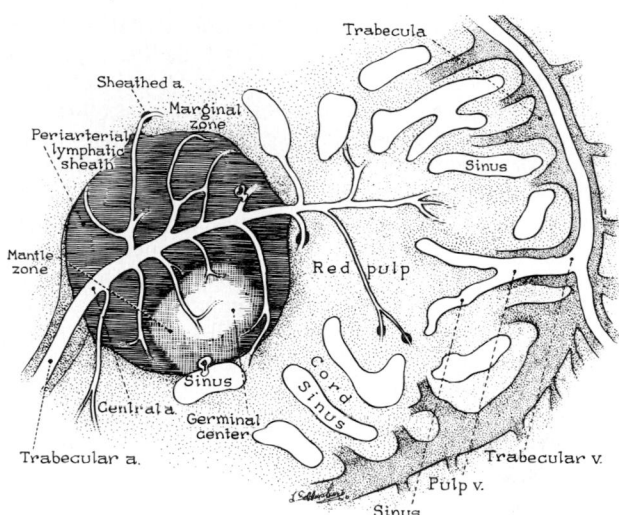

Fig. 33-3. Microcirculation of the spleen. (*From L. Weiss, The Spleen, in R. O. Greep (ed.), "Histology," McGraw-Hill Book Company, New York, 1966.*)

efflux, priming of glycolysis, and maintenance of membrane integrity. To what extent repeated passages through the spleen contribute to normal red cell aging is not certain, but evidence that the red cell loses surface area with aging, combined with the ability of the spleen to remove bits of red cell with surgical precision, raises this possibility. On the other hand, the presence of a normal red cell life span in splenectomized subjects suggests that red cell aging occurs independently of splenic presence and at approximately the normal rate. A variety of erythrocytes altered by intrinsic factors (membrane, hemoglobin, or enzymic abnormalities) or extrinsic factors (antibody and nonantibody injury) may be prematurely removed by the spleen. Severely damaged cells may be removed by the reticuloendothelial system at a variety of sites. Minimally altered erythrocytes may require the specific rigors of the splenic circulation for premature destruction and, therefore, may have normal or near-normal survival after splenic removal. In the dog and cat, unlike man, the spleen may contract significantly in response to hypovolemia or catecholamines, resulting in an autotransfusion; this is an important consideration in studies of experimental shock.

The neutrophil is removed from the circulation with a half-life of about 6.0 hours, hence 85 percent of neutrophils either emigrate at random into tissues or are destroyed within 24 hours. Although the role of the spleen in the destruction of neutrophils under normal conditions is not well quantified, in some hypersplenic states the spleen's role is augmented, with resulting neutropenia. This augmented removal can occur because of splenic enlargement and accelerated sequestration of granulocytes or because of enhanced splenic removal of altered granulocytes, as seen in immune neutropenias.

The platelet (thrombocyte), under normal circumstances, has a finite survival of about 10 days in the circulation. One-third of the total platelet pool is normally sequestered in the spleen, but the role of the spleen in the final removal of normal platelets has not been precisely defined. With splenomegaly, a larger proportion of platelets is sequestered in the spleen (up to 80 percent), and this and accelerated platelet destruction in the spleen account for thrombocytopenia. Splenectomy results in an increase in platelets, which at times reach levels greater than 1 million cells per cubic millimeter. Postsplenectomy thrombocytosis is often transient but may persist. This is particularly notable in congenital hemolytic states which do not respond well to splenectomy. In these circumstances, continued hemolysis in the absence of the splenic removal mechanism can lead to persistent, extreme thrombocytosis and intravenous thrombosis.

DIAGNOSTIC CONSIDERATIONS

EVALUATION OF SIZE. Normally the spleen is not palpable on abdominal examination, but the organ may be felt in about 2 percent of healthy adults. In healthy subjects, no significant dullness is elicited by percussion over the spleen either anteriorly or laterally. As the organ enlarges, dullness may be detected at the level of the ninth intercostal space in the left anterior axillary line especially on expiration. Thereafter, it becomes first percussible and then palpable below the left costal margin. With increasing splenomegaly, notching may be palpable on the anteromedial surface, distinguishing the spleen from other abdominal masses.

Routine radiologic examination of the abdomen usually provides an accurate estimate of the size of the spleen. Although splenomegaly may be suggested by medial or caudad displacement of the stomach bubble, frequently accompanied by caudad displacement of air in the splenic flexure, the organ's outline can often be clearly demarcated in the left upper quadrant, corroborating enlargement. Radioisotopic scanning of the spleen has provided a more precise method of outlining the organ and differentiating it from other masses in the left upper quadrant. The technetium (^{99m}Tc-sulfur colloid) scan (Fig. 33-4) is dependent upon the ability of the spleen to retain the radiocolloid; thus, "functional asplenia," in which vascular shunts allow blood to bypass splenic phagocytes, complicates radioisotopic estimate of splenic size.

EVALUATION OF FUNCTION. The functional abnormality of hypersplenism may be manifested by a reduction in the number of red cells, neutrophils, or platelets in the peripheral blood. An increase in the rate of red cell destruction will always result in a compensatory rise in the rate of production unless disease of the marrow coexists. The hallmark of increased red cell turnover (hemolysis) is reticulocytosis in the absence of blood loss. Other tests such as the plasma bilirubin, haptoglobin, and hemoglobin are less sensitive, dependent on the rate of hemolysis, the sites of hemolysis, and liver function, and are therefore only of adjunctive value.

Reduced red blood cell survival in patients with hemo-

Fig. 33-4. Scan of normal adult human spleen. (*Courtesy of Henry N. Wagner, Jr., M. D.*)

Fig. 33-5. ^{51}Cr-labeled red cell determination of hemolytic anemia and splenic sequestration. Top, disappearance of ^{51}Cr-labeled normal autogenous red cells from the bloodstream and accumulation by the tissues in normal subjects and in patients with hemolytic anemia. Bottom, accumulation of radioactivity in liver and spleen of normal subjects and patients with hemolytic anemia and splenic sequestration. (*After J. Jandl et al., J Clin Invest, 35:842, 1956.*)

lytic anemia may be more precisely demonstrated by measuring the disappearance of blood radioactivity after the patient's erythrocytes are labeled with $Na_2^{51}CrO_4$ (Fig. 33-5). With this technique, the normal half-life of the red cells is about 30 days, i.e., 50 percent of the cells remain in the circulation at that time. A half-life of 15 days or less indicates significantly increased hemolysis. The spleen's role in a hemolytic anemia may be assessed by determining the relative uptakes of ^{51}Cr-tagged erythrocytes by the spleen and the liver. A spleen/liver ratio greater than 2:1 indicates significant preferential splenic sequestration and anticipates a beneficial effect of splenectomy. Radioisotopic labeling also has been used to evaluate the survival of neutrophils and platelets. Presently there is no entirely practical method of assessing the decreased longevity of neutrophils or of measuring the role of the spleen in the destruction of these cells. The role of the spleen as a major offending organ has been precisely defined in patients with hypersplenism or immune thrombocytopenia. Platelet destruction in the spleen is such a common mechanism in thrombocytopenia that radioisotopic studies are not often done if the bone marrow aspirate indicates an abundance of megakaryocytes, suggesting adequate platelet production.

RUPTURE OF THE SPLEEN

The term "rupture" has been applied to splenic injuries in which there is disruption of the organ's parenchyma, capsule, or blood supply.

ETIOLOGY. The causes of splenic rupture include either transabdominal or transthoracic penetrating trauma, nonpenetrating trauma, operative trauma, and spontaneous rupture.

Penetrating Trauma. Rupture of the spleen may occur as a consequence of large gunshot wounds or small puncture lacerations due to stabbing or missiles traveling at high speeds. The trajectory of the penetrating wound may pass through the anterior abdominal wall, through the flank, or transthoracically, piercing the pleural space, the lung, and the diaphragm. Isolated splenic injury may be present. With penetrating trauma, the associated organs most frequently injured include the stomach, the left kidney, the pancreas, and vascular structures at the root of the mesentery. Percutaneous splenic puncture to perform splenic pulp manometry and splenoportography may be associated with persistent bleeding, but this is uncommon in patients whose platelet counts are above 100,000 and prothrombin times are greater than 35 percent.

Nonpenetrating Trauma. The spleen, alone or in combination with other viscera, is the most frequently injured organ following blunt trauma to the abdomen or the lower thoracic cage. Automobile accidents provide the predominating cause, while falls, sledding and bicycle injuries, and blows incurred during contact sports are frequently implicated in children. Splenic rupture which follows blunt trauma is an isolated event in only 30 percent of patients. The other organs which may be injured, in decreasing order of incidence, include (1) chest (rib fracture), (2) kidney, (3) spinal cord (fracture), (4) liver, (5) lung, (6) craniocerebral structures, (7) small intestine, (8) large intestine, (9) pancreas, and (10) stomach.

Operative Trauma. Operative trauma to the spleen most commonly occurs during operations on adjacent viscera. The spleen has been injured in about 2 percent of patients whose operations involved viscera of the left upper quadrant. Injury usually results from retractors placed against the organ in order to obtain exposure. This injury may permit repair or require splenectomy.

Spontaneous Rupture. Although spontaneous rupture of the normal spleen has been reported, it is a much more common event when the spleen is involved with a hematologic disorder. It is likely that the majority of patients classified as experiencing spontaneous rupture had trauma which was not appreciated. Spontaneous rupture or rupture associated with minor trauma is the most common cause of death for patients with infectious mononucleosis, which is second only to malaria as a cause of spontaneous splenic rupture. In patients with infectious mononucleosis, this complication occurs most frequently in the second to fourth weeks of the disease. Splenic rupture has also been reported in patients with sarcoidosis, acute and chronic leukemia, hemolytic anemia, congestive splenomegaly, and polycythemia vera.

Pathology. The spectrum of lesions associated with trauma to the spleen include linear and stellate lacerations, capsular tears secondary to traction from adhesions or suspensory ligaments, puncture wounds caused by penetrating objects or fractured ribs, subcapsular intrasplenic hematomas, avulsion of the organ from its vascular pedicle, and laceration of the short gastric vessels within the gastrosplenic omentum. In view of the extreme friability and vascularity of the organ, even minor trauma may result in significant bleeding, particularly if the spleen is enlarged or diseased.

Splenic rupture may be acute, delayed, or occult. *Acute rupture* which is attended by immediate intraperitoneal bleeding occurs in about 90 percent of the cases of blunt trauma to the spleen. *Delayed rupture,* with an interval of days or weeks between the injury and intraperitoneal bleeding, is reported in 10 to 15 percent of the cases of blunt trauma. The quiescent period, referred to as the "latent period of Baudet," persists for less than 7 days in half of these patients and less than 2 weeks in three-quarters of them. This is probably related to a temporary tamponade of a minor laceration or the presence of a slowly enlarging subcapsular hematoma which eventually ruptures. *Occult splenic rupture* is the term applied to traumatic pseudocysts of the spleen when injury to the organ previously has not been diagnosed. These appear in less than 1 percent of patients sustaining trauma and are generally caused by organization of an intrasplenic or parasplenic hematoma. Another pathologic lesion related to splenic trauma is *splenosis,* which is the result of autotransplantation of fragments of the traumatized spleen onto the peritoneal surfaces. Patients with splenosis are generally asymptomatic, but the lesions may stimulate adhesions which, in turn, lead to intestinal obstruction.

CLINICAL MANIFESTATIONS. The signs and symptoms produced by trauma to the spleen vary according to the severity and rapidity of intraabdominal hemorrhage, the presence of other organ injuries, and the interval between the injury and examination. The majority of patients present with some degree of hypovolemia, and tachycardia is almost always present. The latter is particularly evident when the pulse is recorded with the head of the patient elevated. A slight reduction of the blood pressure is characteristic. The patient usually complains of generalized upper abdominal pain, which in one-third of the cases is localized in the left upper quadrant. Pain at the tip of the shoulder (Kehr's sign) is evidence of diaphragmatic irritation but occurs in less than half the patients. If the patient is placed in the Trendelenburg position, left shoulder pain may be produced to accentuate it. Tenderness of the left upper quadrant or left flank is a frequent physical sign. A mass or a percussible area of fixed dullness in this region (Ballance's sign), secondary to subcapsular hematoma or omentum surrounding an extracapsular hemotoma, is rarely detected.

DIAGNOSTIC STUDIES. The hematocrit may be reduced if there is major bleeding, but the initial determination may be normal, emphasizing the fact that serial hematocrits are more meaningful. Increases of the white blood cell count to levels frequently greater than 15,000 per cubic milliliter are to be anticipated. Routine abdominal roentgenograms may demonstrate fractured ribs which should arouse suspicion of injury to the spleen. More specific findings which may be noted on abdominal films include: (1) elevated immobile left diaphragm, (2) an enlarged splenic shadow, (3) medial displacement of the gastric shadow with serration of the greater curvature due to dissection of blood into the gastrosplenic omentum, and (4) widening of the space between the splenic flexure and the properitoneal fat pad. Abdominal paracentesis yields a positive tap, i.e., return of blood which does not clot, in about 50 percent of the cases. A scan or celiac angiogram may define the lesion. The diagnosis may be established angiographically by visualization of (1) the disruption, (2) radiopacity in the peritoneal cavity, or (3) early filling of the splenic vein.

TREATMENT. Once the diagnosis of splenic rupture has been made, operation should not be delayed. Splenectomy is generally the recommended treatment, but efforts at preserving the spleen in children have become popular. An upper midline incision is generally preferred since this may be performed rapidly and can be extended to manage other intraabdominal injuries. The posterior approach to the splenic pedicle, emphasized by Dunphy, offers the most rapid means of controlling hemorrhage. Manual compression of the pedicle usually controls the bleeding and permits transection of the splenic ligaments and mobilization of the spleen forward and medially. Under adequate exposure lacerations may be sutured over omentum, oxidized cellulose, or micronized collagen. A damaged pole or segment may be excised and the raw edges compressed using sutures tied over the same hemostatic materials. The operative mortality for isolated penetrating injuries of the spleen is less than 1 percent. Operative mortality for blunt trauma to the spleen alone ranges between 5 and 15 percent, while the rates are between 15 and 40 percent when other serious concomitant injuries occur.

HEMATOLOGIC DISORDERS FOR WHICH SPLENECTOMY IS POTENTIALLY THERAPEUTIC

In 1887, Spencer-Wells performed a therapeutic splenectomy in a patient with what subsequently proved to be hereditary spherocytosis. Since then, as a consequence of appreciation of the physiology and pathophysiology of the spleen, the application of splenectomy for hematologic disorders has been extended.

Hemolytic Anemias

This category includes a broad spectrum of disorders in which there is accelerated destruction of mature red blood cells. Hemolytic anemias are generally classified as congenital or acquired. The congenital anemias are due to an intrinsic abnormality of the erythrocytes, and the acquired anemias are related to an extracorpuscular factor acting on an intrinsically normal cell. In both types of disorder, the reduced red blood cell survival may be demonstrated by measuring the disappearance of the patient's radioactive erythrocytes (labeled with ^{51}Cr), and the spleen's role may be evaluated by determining the relative uptakes of this radioactivity by the spleen and liver (Fig. 33-5).

HEREDITARY SPHEROCYTOSIS. Hereditary spherocytosis is transmitted as an autosomal dominant trait and is the most common of the symptomatic familial hemolytic anemias. The fundamental abnormality stems from a defective erythrocyte membrane which causes the cell to be smaller than normal, unusually thick, and almost spherical in shape. These cells also demonstrate increased osmotic fragility, i.e., lysis occurs at a higher concentration of sodium chloride than normal. The role of the spleen in this disorder is related to the inability of the spherocytic cells to pass through the splenic pulp. The cells that escape from the spleen are more susceptible to trapping and disintegration during each successive passage, until cell loss ensues. The precise pathogenesis of the cell injury may relate to a decreased availability of red cell ATP in the environment of the spleen, combined with a cell membrane which has been shown in in vitro studies to be more susceptible to reduction in ATP levels.

The salient clinical features of the disease are anemia, reticulocytosis, jaundice, and splenomegaly. It is unusual for the anemia to be extremely severe, and the jaundice usually parallels the severity of the anemia. Periodic and sudden increases in the intensity of the anemia and jaundice may occur, and rare, fatal crises have been reported. Cholelithiasis with gallstones of the pigmented variety has been reported in 30 to 60 percent of the patients but is rare in children under the age of ten. Leg ulcers, although emphasized in texts, are extraordinarily uncommon.

Diagnosis is generally established by the peripheral blood smear, which demonstrates the spherocytic-shaped erythrocyte with a mean diameter less than normal and a thickness greater than normal. The degree of spherocytosis varies from case to case, but usually more than 60 percent of the red cells demonstrate this characteristic. Increased osmotic fragility of the red blood cells provides diagnostic confirmation, but this test rarely is performed.

Splenectomy is the sole therapy for hereditary spherocytosis. It is generally recommended that the operation be delayed until the fourth year of life. Intractable leg ulcers indicate early splenectomy, as they heal only after the spleen is removed. The results of splenectomy have been uniformly good. Although an inherent membrane abnormality persists and the spherocytosis and increased osmotic fragility of the cells are not altered, in vivo hemolysis virtually ceases and, following removal of the spleen, the erythrocytes achieve a normal life span and the jaundice, if present, disappears. It is appropriate to perform an oral cholecystogram prior to splenectomy, and the gallbladder should always be examined at the time of operation. If gallstones are present, the gallbladder should be removed during the operation.

HEREDITARY ELLIPTOCYTOSIS. This usually exists as a harmless trait, but occasionally, when oval and rod-shaped forms constitute 50 to 90 percent of the red cell population, clinical manifestations indistinguishable from those noted with hereditary spherocytosis may occur. Splenectomy is indicated for all symptomatic patients since removal of the organ often is followed by decreased hemolysis and corrected anemia, although the morphologic abnormality of the red blood cell remains unchanged. Associated cholelithiasis should be managed as in hereditary spherocytosis.

HEREDITARY NONSPHEROCYTIC HEMOLYTIC ANEMIA. Included in this category are: (1) enzyme deficiencies in anaerobic glycolytic pathways, the prototype of which is the pyruvate-kinase deficiency (PK), and (2) enzyme deficiencies in the hexose monophosphate shunt, the prototype of which is the glucose-6-phosphate deficiency (G-6-PD). These deficiencies render the cells susceptible to increased hemolysis. Splenic enlargement occurs more frequently with PK deficiency, and the spleen is rarely enlarged in patients with G-6-PD deficiency. Specific enzyme assays are employed to define the deficiency.

The majority of patients maintain hemoglobins greater than 8 Gm/100 ml, are asymptomatic, and do not require therapy. With significant anemia, blood transfusions are indicated, and the transfused cells survive normally. ^{51}Cr-tagged red cell studies have demonstrated that the spleen serves as a major site for hemolysis in some patients with PK deficiency, and recent reports have suggested limited improvement following removal of the spleen from these patients. Splenectomy is not indicated for patients with G-6-PD deficiency.

THALASSEMIA. Thalassemia (Mediterranean anemia) is transmitted as a dominant trait and primarily derives from a defect in hemoglobin synthesis. The disease is classified as alpha, beta, and gamma types, determined by the specific defect in synthesis rate of the peptide chain. In the United States, most patients are of Southern European origin and suffer from beta thalassemia, i.e., a quantitative reduction in the rate of beta chain synthesis, resulting in a decrease in hemoglobin A (Hb-A). Thalassemia occurs in two major degrees of severity; homozygous thalassemia (thalassemia major), a severe disorder in which the affected child receives a gene for thalassemia from each parent, and heterozygous thalassemia (thalassemia minor), a mild disorder in which the affected child receives a gene from only one parent. Gradations of thalassemia range from heterozygous thalassemia (minor), often not detected until examination of the blood for an unrelated problem, to homozygous thalassemia, a severe, chronic anemia, with icterus, splenomegaly, and death early in life. In thalassemia minor, Hb-A_2 is always increased, and slight increases in Hb-F occur in 50 percent of patients. In both types of thalassemia, the hemoglobin-deficient cells are small, thin, and misshapen. These cells appear washed out and have a characteristic resistance to osmotic lysis.

The clinical manifestations of thalassemia major usually occur in the first year of life and consist of pallor, retarded body growth, and enlargement of the head. Intractable leg ulcers may be noted, intercurrent infections are common, and gallstones are reported in about 24 percent of patients. The manifestations of thalassemia minor may vary. Most patients with thalassemia minor lead normal lives, but some patients have a more severe expression of their disease (referred to as thalassemia intermedia) and generally present with signs and symptoms attributable to mild anemia, chronic mild jaundice, and moderate splenomegaly.

The diagnosis of thalassemia major is established by the smear revealing the hypochromic, microcytic anemia with markedly distorted red cells of various sizes and shapes. Nucleated red cells invariably are present, and the reticulocyte count is elevated, as is the white blood count. The characteristic feature of the disease is the persistence of Hb-F and a reduction in Hb-A, demonstrated by the alkali denaturation study. Importantly, both parents should have evidence of thalassemia minor.

Treatment is directed only at symptomatic patients. Transfusions are usually required at regular intervals, but as most patients accommodate to low hemoglobin levels, the transfusions should be directed at maintaining the hemoglobin level at 10 Gm/100ml. Although splenectomy does not influence the basic hematologic disorder, it may reduce both the hemolytic process and the transfusion requirements.

SICKLE CELL DISEASE. Sickle cell anemia is a hereditary hemolytic anemia seen predominantly in Negroes and characterized by the presence of sickle- and crescent-shaped erythrocytes. In this hereditary hemoglobinopathy, the normal Hb-A is replaced by the abnormal form of hemoglobin, sickle hemoglobin (Hb-S). Hb-F is also usually mildly increased. Combinations of Hb-S with other hemoglobin variants also occur as a result of an abnormal trait inherited from each parent, e.g., Hb-S/Hb-C or Hb-S/thalassemia.

Under conditions of reduced oxygen tension, Hb-S molecules undergo crystallization within the red cell, which elongates and distorts the cell. The sickling phenomenon occurs more readily with higher percentages of Hb-S, with a reduced pH, and under conditions of circulatory stasis which tend to exaggerate hemoglobin deoxygenation. The sickle cells, themselves, contribute to increased blood viscosity and circulatory stasis, thus establishing a vicious cycle. The primary consequence of this stagnation is thrombosis, which leads to ischemia, necrosis, and organ fibrosis.

The role of the spleen in this disorder is not clear. Early in the course of the disease, splenomegaly occurs, but following varying intervals in most patients, the spleen undergoes infarction and marked contraction with eventual autosplenectomy.

Although the sickle cell trait occurs in approximately 9 percent of the Negro population, the majority of patients are asymptomatic. However, sickle cell anemia has been observed in 0.3 to 1.3 percent of Negroes, who often show remarkable adaptation to the state of chronic anemia and jaundice. This adaptive state may be interrupted at intervals by acute symptoms or crises which are related to vascular occlusion. Depending on the vessels involved, the patient may have bone or joint pain, hematuria, priapism, neurologic manifestations, or ulcers over the malleoli. Abdominal pain and cramps due to visceral stasis are frequent, simulating an acute surgical abdomen. Thrombosis of the splenic vessels may result in an unusual complication of splenic abscess, manifested by splenomegaly, splenic pain, and fever. Most patients with sickle cell anemia die in the first decade of life, but a few survive to the fifth decade. Death may be the result of intercurrent infections or cardiac or renal failure.

The diagnosis is established by the presence of anemia, characteristic sickle cells on smear, hemoglobin electrophoresis showing 80 percent or more Hb-S, and the presence of the trait in both parents. Leukocytosis is often noted, and the platelets are frequently increased in number. There may be modest elevation of the serum bilirubin, and cholelithiasis is a frequent accompaniment.

For most patients only palliative treatment is possible. Recently, studies have shown that sodium cyanate will prevent sickling of Hb-S. Transfusions may be required to maintain adequate hemoglobin levels. Adequate hydration and partial exchange transfusion may help during a crisis. In the circumstance of splenic abscess, incision and drainage of the abscess cavity within the parenchyma of the spleen may be necessitated, since removal of the organ is hindered by marked inflammatory and adhesive processes. Splenectomy may be of benefit in a very few patients in whom excessive splenic sequestration of red cells can be demonstrated, although the operation does not affect sickling process. In general, splenectomy is most effective in children with large spleens but is not indicated for the trait.

IDIOPATHIC AUTOIMMUNE HEMOLYTIC ANEMIA. This is a disorder in which the life span of a presumably normal erythrocyte is shortened when exposed to an endogenous hemolytic mechanism. The etiology has not been defined, but an autoimmune process appears to be fundamental. In such patients, antibodies reacting with the patient's normal red cells have been defined, and there is evidence that the spleen may serve as a source of antibody. Both "warm" and "cold" antibodies have been described. Some "warm" antibodies have Rh specificity. Since most of these antibodies are hemagglutinins rather than hemolysins, the means by which hemolysis is initiated in vivo is not clear, but it is believed that the reticuloendothelial system traps and destroys the immunologically altered cells. Sequestration studies have demonstrated that this process sometimes occurs primarily in the spleen.

Although autoimmune hemolytic anemia may be encountered at any age, it occurs more frequently after the age of fifty and twice as often in females. Mild jaundice is often present. The spleen is palpably enlarged in half the cases, and gallstones have been demonstrated in a quarter of the cases. The extent of anemia varies, and hemoglobinuria and tubular necrosis have been reported in severe cases. In this circumstance, the prognosis is serious, as the mortality rate is 40 to 50 percent.

The diagnosis of hemolysis is made by demonstrating anemia and reticulocytosis accompanied by the products of red cell destruction in the blood, urine, and stool. The bone marrow is hypercellular with a predominance of erythroid precursors. A distinguishing feature of the disease is the demonstration by direct Coombs' test of an autoantibody on the patient's red cells.

In some patients, the disorder tends to run an acute, self-limiting course, and no treatment is necessary. If the anemia becomes severe, corticosteroids or blood transfusions may be required. Splenectomy should be considered in the following circumstances: (1) if steroids have been ineffective, (2) if excessive doses of steroids are required to maintain remission, (3) if toxic manifestations of steroids become apparent, and (4) if steroids are contraindicated for other reasons. Excessive splenic sequestration of ^{51}Cr-tagged red cells offers a guide for the selection of patients who may respond to splenectomy. A favorable response is to be anticipated in about 80 percent of selected splenectomized patients, with either complete hematologic remission or a significant decrease in the rate of hemolysis and alleviation of anemia.

Idiopathic Thrombocytopenic Purpura

Idiopathic thrombocytopenic purpura (immune thrombocytopenic purpura) (ITP) has no established etiology. Many cases are felt to represent the results of autoimmunity. The term ITP should be reserved for a hemorrhagic disorder characterized by a subnormal platelet count in the presence of bone marrow containing normal or increased megakaryocytes and in the absence of any systemic disease or history of ingestion of drugs capable of inducing thrombocytopenia. The spleen may be implicated either as a source of antibody production or as the major sequestering site for sensitized platelets.

Female patients outnumber males at a ratio of 3:1. The most common presenting signs are petechiae and/or ecchymoses. In the majority of patients, these signs are accompanied by one or several other symptoms which in order of frequency are: bleeding gums, vaginal bleeding, gastrointestinal bleeding, and hematuria. In some patients,

the clinical manifestations take an almost cyclic course with exacerbations occurring at the time of menses. The incidence of central nervous system bleeding ranges between 2 and 4 percent and usually occurs early in the course of the disease. The spleen is palpable in approximately 2 percent of cases, and its enlargement should evoke suspicion of the presence of another disease causing thrombocytopenia.

The characteristic laboratory findings include a platelet count generally reduced to 50,000 or less and at times approaching zero. Associated with reduced platelet count, the bleeding time may be prolonged, but the clotting time remains normal. There is usually no significant anemia or leukopenia. Platelet survival following the transfusion of ^{51}Cr-labeled normal platelets is short, but this test is not necessary for establishing the diagnosis of ITP. Bone marrow examination reveals megakaryocytes either normal or increased in number, with or without a relative increase in small forms. Qualitative changes in the megakaryocytes are characterized by degranulation of the cytoplasm, rounding of cytoplasmic edges, the disappearance of the usual pseudopodia containing granular-free platelets, and a varying degree of vacuolization of the cytoplasm.

Acute ITP has an excellent prognosis in children under the age of 16; approximately 80 percent of these patients will make a complete and permanent recovery without specific therapy. Much of the discussion regarding therapy for ITP centers around the relative values and disadvantages of steroid therapy and splenectomy. In 1916, Kaznelson, then a fourth-year medical student in Prague, suggested that splenectomy could induce an increase in circulating platelets and reported good results following splenectomy performed by Schloffer. The advent of steroid therapy provided the impetus for reevaluating the efficacy of splenectomy. In most series, the results achieved by splenectomy are significantly more impressive than are the responses to steroids (Fig. 33-6). Between 75 and 85 per-

Fig. 33-6. Idiopathic thrombocytopenic purpura. Comparative responses to steroids and splenectomy. (*From S. I. Schwartz, J. T. Adams, and A. W. Bauman, Splenectomy for Hematologic Disorders, Curr Probl Surg, May, 1971. Copyright 1971, Year Book Medical Publishers, Inc., Chicago. Used by permission.*)

cent of the total number of patients subjected to splenectomy respond permanently and require no further steroid therapy. A long-term follow-up of splenectomized patients does not support the contention that disseminated lupus erythematosus develops after this procedure. Reported series disagree regarding a correlation between response to steroids and splenectomy.

At present, the generally accepted protocol for managing patients with diagnosed ITP includes an initial 6-week to 2-month period of steroid therapy. If the patient does not respond with elevation of the platelet count, splenectomy is performed. If the patient does respond, the steroid therapy is tapered off, and, if thrombocytopenia recurs, splenectomy is carried out. Any manifestation suggestive of intracranial bleeding demands emergency splenectomy.

The majority of patients are seen by the surgeon after they have been taking steroids for weeks or months. Consequently, these patients require a booster dose of cortisone acetate during the evening prior to the splenectomy and intravenous cortisone during the surgical procedure. For patients with platelet counts approaching zero, platelet packs should be available for the operative procedure but should not be administered preoperatively. Platelet transfusion is reserved for patients who continue bleeding following removal of the spleen. Occasional patients in whom signs of the disease recurred months or years following splenectomy achieved permanent cure following removal of an accessory spleen, the presence of which may be defined by technetium scan.

Thrombotic Thrombocytopenic Purpura

Although thrombotic thrombocytopenic purpura (TTP) is a disease of arterioles or capillaries, there are significant accompanying hematologic changes for which the response to splenectomy may be striking. The etiology has not been precisely defined, but immune mechanisms have been suggested. Approximately 5 percent of reported cases occurred during pregnancy. TTP in pregnancy must be distinguished from an idiopathic thrombocytopenia which may develop in the third trimester and is reversed by termination of the pregnancy. Histologically, there is widespread occlusion of multiple arterioles and capillaries by hyaline membranes, with minimal inflammatory change and limited infarction.

The pentad of clinical features of virtually all cases consists of fever, purpura, hemolytic anemia, neurologic manifestations, and signs of renal disease. The pertinent laboratory findings include anemia with reticulocytosis, thrombocytopenia, and leukocytosis, at times accompanied by elevated serum bilirubin, proteinuria, hematuria, casts, or azotemia. The peripheral blood smear reveals pleomorphic, normochromic red cells that are fragmented and distorted. The degree of thrombocytopenia varies during the course of the illness, but a profound decrease often develops within hours of onset. The bone marrow usually reveals erythroid and myeloid hyperplasia with a normal or increased number of megakaryocytes.

In the majority of cases, the disease has a rapid onset, fulminating course, and fatal outcome usually due to intracerebral hemorrhage or renal failure. Recovery has been reported for patients treated with heparin, exchange transfusion of fresh blood, dextran, antimetabolites, and massive doses of steroids. However, the combination of steroid therapy and splenectomy has achieved the highest degree of success. Of approximately 350 cases reported, 44 patients were alive at the time of reporting, and 65 percent of the survivals had been treated with steroid therapy and splenectomy.

Primary Hypersplenism

In 1939, Doan and Wiseman described a disease consisting primarily of splenomegaly and neutropenia for which splenectomy is curative. A few years later, the concept of splenic neutropenia was enlarged to include some patients with anemia, thrombocytopenia, or pancytopenia. The etiology has not been determined, but ^{51}Cr-tagged red cell sequestration studies indicate that the spleen is a major site of phagocytosis. In some patients, lymphoproliferation of the spleen is so marked as to suggest the development of premalignant lymphoma. The spleen is almost always enlarged and the histologic features vary.

The overwhelming majority of patients are female, and the clinical manifestations are related to the depressed cell type. Fever, frequent and recurring infections, and oral ulcerations may be noted with neutropenia. Petechiae and ecchymoses predominate with thrombocytopenia, and pallor may indicate depression of the red cells. The peripheral blood smear is devoid of any of the diagnostic features of leukemia or myeloproliferative disorders. The bone marrow reveals a pancellular hyperplasia. The diagnosis is essentially one of exclusion, confirmed by clinical response to splenectomy.

Corticosteroids rarely affect the disease process, but splenectomy facilitates hematologic improvement in almost all patients. Disturbingly, occasional patients followed for long periods of time have subsequently developed reticulum cell sarcoma or histiocytic lymphoma.

Secondary Hypersplenism

Pancytopenia, thrombocytopenia, and leukopenia or anemia may stem from portal hypertension due either to hepatic disease or extrahepatic portal vein obstruction. Splenomegaly with engorgement of the vascular spaces accompanies portal hypertension, and accelerated destruction of the circulating cells within the spleen results. The clinical manifestations of thrombocytopenia, i.e., petechiae and spontaneous bleeding, are extremely uncommon in patients with portal hypertension. As no correlation exists between the degree of anemia, leukopenia, or thrombocytopenia and the long-term survival of patients with cirrhosis, hypersplenism per se rarely indicates operative intervention in a patient with portal hypertension. Percutaneous transfemoral arterial embolization has been performed in some of these patients. Although splenic hyperfunction was controlled, the development of painful infarction of the spleen and septic splenitis suggests that such an approach has limited value. The more common surgical situation relates to the patient with bleeding esophagogastric varices accompanied by significant secondary thrombocytopenia. In the experience of Child and Turcotte with more than 300 shunts, it was necessary to perform only one splenectomy for persistent, clinically significant hypersplenism. Thrombocytopenia is generally improved by a portacaval shunt, and, in the few instances in which the platelet count does not return to normal, complications are rarely attributable to thrombocytopenia. Splenectomy alone should not be performed in a patient with portal hypertension and secondary hypersplenism as there is no long-term effect on the elevated portal pressure. In the rare circumstance that splenectomy is required for a severe degree of hypersplenism in such a patient, it should be combined with a splenorenal shunt to decompress the portal circulation.

Myeloid Metaplasia

Myeloid metaplasia is a panproliferative process manifested by increased connective tissue proliferation of the bone marrow, liver, spleen, and lymph nodes and simultaneous proliferation of hemopoietic elements in the liver, spleen, and long bones. The disease is closely related to polycythemia vera, myelogenous leukemia, and idiopathic thrombocytosis. The etiology remains unclear. The spleen may be markedly enlarged, and portal hypertension has been described in some patients, due either to hepatic fibrosis of sufficient degree to be obstructive to the portal circulation or to increased forward blood flow through the splenoportal system in the absence of hepatic involvement.

Clinical manifestations generally become apparent in middle-aged and older adults. The presenting symptoms usually are related to anemia and increasing splenomegaly. Symptoms related to the spleen include the intermittent pain of splenic infarction, generalized abdominal discomfort, and a feeling of fullness after meals. Other symptoms include spontaneous bleeding, secondary infection, bone pain, pruritus, hypermetabolism, and complications associated with hyperuricemia. The most common physical findings are pallor and splenomegaly. Hepatomegaly is present in about three-quarters of the patients.

The laboratory hallmark of myeloid metaplasia is the peripheral blood smear. The red cells are characterized by fragmentation and immature forms and poikilocytosis with numerous teardrop and elongated shapes. Characteristically, the patients have anemia of the normochromic type. The white blood count is under 50,000 in the majority of the cases but may reach extremely high levels. Immature myeloid cells are found in the peripheral smear. The platelet counts are normal in about a quarter of the patients; thrombocytopenia is present in about one-third, and marked thrombocytopenia is present in 5 percent. Thrombocytosis over 1 million per cubic millimeter is observed in one-quarter of the patients. The platelets frequently are enlarged and bizarre in appearance. The leukocyte alkaline phosphatase usually is high, and hyperuricemia frequently is present. Roentgenograms of the bone demonstrate increased density in approximately 50 percent of the patients, particularly in the pelvic region. Marrow biopsy sections show varying degrees of bone marrow replacement by fibrous tissue interposed with small foci of megakaryocytes, erythropoiesis, and myeloid cells. ^{51}Cr-tagged red cell scan may be used to indicate the degree of splenic sequestration and to evaluate the applicability of splenectomy.

Treatment is generally directed at the anemia and splenomegaly. It usually consists of transfusions, hormones, chemotherapy, and radiotherapy. Male hormone preparations may be of value in patients with anemia due to marrow failure. Alkalating agents may be effective in reducing splenic size and transfusion requirements as well as for patients whose predominant clinical problem is hypermetabolism. Busulfan is the most commonly used alkalating agent, but cyclophosphamide may also be used in thrombocytopenic subjects since it is less likely to suppress platelet production. Since patients with myelofibrosis are very sensitive to chemotherapy, such agents must be used very cautiously.

Although splenectomy does not alter the general course of the disorder, the procedure is indicated for control of anemia, thrombocytopenia, and for symptoms attributable to splenomegaly. Thrombocytopenia associated with sufficiently reduced megakaryocytes to contraindicate chemotherapy is also a frequent indication for splenectomy, as is the large spleen which causes digestive difficulties or is symptomatic because of multiple infarctions despite chemotherapy and/or local irradiation. In patients with esophagogastric varices portal pressures should be determined before and after splenectomy. In most instances splenectomy alone will effect significant reduction in pressure and obviate the need for a concomitant splenorenal or portacaval shunt.

Splenectomy rarely has a deleterious effect on the hematologic status of the patient, and the old concept that splenectomy resulted in the removal of a significant hemopoietic element does not pertain. The incidence of the mortality and morbidity rates for patients with myeloid metaplasia undergoing splenectomy are higher than those reported for other hematologic disorders. Postoperative thrombocytosis and/or thrombosis of the splenic vein extending into the portal and mesenteric vein occur more commonly in these patients. The incidence of this complication can be reduced by correction of the thrombotic state preoperatively using alkylating agents and the use of drugs to prevent platelet aggregation during the perioperative period.

Hodgkin's Disease, Lymphoma, Reticulum Cell Sarcoma, and Chronic Leukemia

Splenectomy for patients with these disorders has been recently brought into focus for two reasons: first, the need for a more aggressive therapeutic approach in patients with advanced disease and hypersplenism, and, second, the introduction of laparotomy, including splenectomy, as a method of staging Hodgkin's disease in order to determine appropriate therapy.

PALLIATIVE SPLENECTOMY. Chemotherapy and/or radiation therapy are the major approaches to the treatment of these disorders. Splenectomy may be considered for patients with symptomatic splenomegaly and/or hypersplenism. Many of the older series report extremely high mortality rates, but review of these cases indicates that the patients were in a terminal phase. Recent series have reported more favorable results, with improvement in hematologic pattern although the eventual outcome of the primary disease was in no way altered. Crosby and associates suggested that splenectomy should be performed at the first sign of hypersplenism with Hodgkin's disease, before the patient becomes a hematologic cripple.

The results associated with palliative splenectomy for patients with lymphoma and chronic lymphatic leukemia who have symptomatic hypersplenism and/or splenomegaly uniformly are more encouraging. The hematologic responses are favorable in the majority of patients, and many have long periods of survival.

A favorable hematologic response has been reported for about half the patients with chronic myelogenous leukemia, while the results for patients with reticulum cell sarcoma generally are poor.

SPLENECTOMY IN THE STAGING OF HODGKIN'S DISEASE AND NON-HODGKIN'S LYMPHOMA. The diagnosis of Hodgkin's disease is generally established by histologic evaluation of a clinically suspect area of lymphadenopathy or splenomegaly. Demonstration of the typical, large, multinuclear cell, the Sternberg-Reed cell, is regarded as essential for the diagnosis. However, these cells do not form the bulk of the tumor. Four major histologic types have been defined: lymphocyte predominance, nodular sclerosis, mixed cellularity, and lymphocyte depletion. Survival with Hodgkin's disease is related in part to the histologic type and also to the distribution of disease and the presence or absence of specific symptoms. Stage I disease is defined as limited to one anatomic region; Stage II disease is limited to two or more contiguous or noncontiguous regions on the same side of the diaphragm; Stage III disease refers to disease on both sides of the diaphragm with involvement limited to lymph nodes, spleen, and Waldeyer's ring; and Stage IV refers to involvement of the bone marrow, lung, liver, skin, gastrointestinal tract, and any organ or tissue other than the lymph nodes or Waldeyer's ring.

The application of laparotomy, splenectomy, liver biopsy, and retroperitoneal node biopsy as diagnostic tools is based on the following considerations: (1) the lesion generally begins as a single focus and spreads in a predictable manner along adjacent lymph channels, (2) prognosis is related to clinical stage, (3) therapy may be dictated by clinical stage, and (4) previous methods of evaluating the clinical stage, including the physical examination, laboratory studies, and roentgenographic studies have significant degrees of inaccuracy. The procedure begins with a wedge biopsy of the liver performed before retractors are applied to avoid confusion of white cell migration. Splenectomy is then performed, the entire periaortic chain of lymph nodes is examined, and representative nodes are removed. The sites of lymph node removal are chosen according to preoperative lymphangiogram and surgical evaluation. Examination of the upper aortic chain, facilitated by transecting the ligament of Treitz, has proved most rewarding in regard to positive lymph node findings. Representative mesenteric and hepatoduodenal nodes should also be biopsied. A liberal iliac crest marrow biopsy is generally included.

The concept of surgical staging as a routine procedure for untreated patients with Hodgkin's disease was initiated at Stanford University Medical Center in July of 1968. A collation of reported series is presented in Fig. 33-7. The error for patients with preoperative diagnoses of splenic involvement based on palpability, roentgenographic, and/or scintillation scan studies which suggested enlargement was 38 percent, while the error for patients with preoperative diagnoses of normal spleens was 36 percent. The liver is suspected of being infiltrated by Hodgkin's disease if there is evidence of hepatomegaly, if liver function tests demonstrate abnormalities, or if liver scans define a space-occupying lesion. Preoperative suspicion of Hodgkin's disease of the liver was incorrect in 45 percent of the cases, whereas clinical judgment that the liver was not involved was incorrect in only 4 percent. Abdominal lymphangiography has been shown to be superior to both inferior vena cavography and intravenous pyelography for defining retroperitoneal node involvement. Thirty percent of positive lymphangiograms were not confirmed by laparotomy, while 15 percent of patients whose lymphangiograms were considered normal were shown to have Hodgkin's involvement of the retroperitoneal nodes. Summary of the reported cases indicates that surgical staging upgraded the clinical stage in about 27 percent of cases and decreased it in 15 percent, for a total alteration of 42 percent.

The applicability of surgical staging in patients with Hodgkin's disease has not been resolved. It is generally agreed that the procedure is indicated for a patient with Hodgkin's disease who presents evidence or suggestion of disease in the upper part of the abdomen, providing that the patient is not jaundiced and does not have other evidence of significant hepatic dysfunction. Other generally accepted indications include the presence of systemic symptoms in clinical Stage I and II patients, and a mixed cellularity or lymphocyte depletion type of histology. By

Fig. 33-7. Correlation between operative staging and clinical assessment. (*From S. I. Schwartz and R. A. Cooper, Jr., Surgery in the Diagnosis and Treatment of Hodgkin's Disease, Adv Surg, vol 6. Copyright 1972, Year Book Medical Publishers, Inc., Chicago. Used by permission.*)

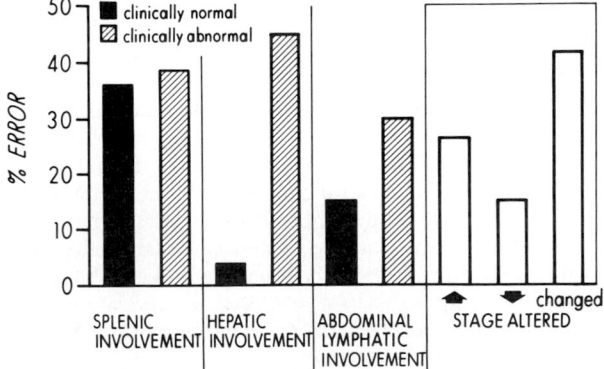

contrast, in patients with high cervical, lymphocyte-predominant lesions and no evidence of mediastinal involvement, staging is not indicated, since these lesions rarely involve the subdiaphragmatic nodes.

The argument regarding the role of staging centers around patients with clinical Stage I-A or II-A (asymptomatic). Those in favor base their opinion on negligible mortality and morbidity rates coupled with the additional "bonus" that splenectomy has facilitated radiation therapy and reduced the potential radiation pneumonitis and/or nephritis as well as leukopenia and thrombocytopenia which may complicate either radiotherapy or chemotherapy. The objections to routine staging in these patients relate to the facts that (1) some series do include perioperative deaths, and (2) the problem of susceptibility to infection subsequent to splenectomy has not been resolved. It has also been pointed out that ablation of the spleen can be accomplished by radiation therapy; many therapists advocate prophylactically treating all infradiaphragmatic areas in patients with Stage I and II Hodgkin's disease.

In reference to the routine staging for non-Hodgkin's lymphoma, a difference of opinion also pertains. Veronesi and associates conclude that diagnostic laparotomy and staging should be carried out in centers in which the information can be translated into aggressive treatment, but feel that it should not have the wide adoption which Hodgkin's staging has had. Chabner et al. reported that percutaneous and peritoneoscopically directed biopsies were reasonable alternatives to staging for non-Hodgkin's lymphoma and that the presence or absence of subdiaphragmatic disease could be established in over 80 percent of the patients by nonsurgical procedures, including lymphangiography, marrow biopsy, and percutaneous liver biopsy. The yield of staging procedures was highest in patients with nodular lymphomas and lowest in patients with histiocytic lymphomas.

Miscellaneous Diseases

FELTY'S SYNDROME. The triad of rheumatoid arthritis, splenomegaly, and neutropenia is referred to as Felty's syndrome. Mild anemia and/or thrombocytopenia have been noted in some cases, and gastric achlorhydria is common. An antibody specifically directed against neutrophil nuclei is nearly always demonstrable by fluorescent stains. Corticosteroids and splenectomy have been used to reverse the neutropenia in order to reduce susceptibility to infection. The response to steroids is usually not long-lasting, but the hematologic effects of splenectomy generally are excellent. There is a sharp rise in the total number of leukocytes in the first 24 hours, reaching a peak at about the third postoperative day. Although relative neutropenia may persist, the neutrophilic response to infection in the postsplenectomy state becomes normal. However, the clinical course of the arthritis is rarely altered.

SARCOIDOSIS. This disease affects young adults. There are few constitutional symptoms, and fever is unusual, although night sweats have been noted. Cough and shortness of breath may attend mediastinal or pulmonary involvement. Skin lesions appear in about 50 percent of

patients, and generalized lymphadenopathy is frequent. Involvement of the liver and spleen may produce hepatomegaly and splenomegaly in about 25 percent of the cases. About 20 percent of the patients with splenomegaly develop manifestations of hypersplenism, particularly thrombocytopenic purpura. Hemolytic anemia, neutropenia, pancytopenia, and spontaneous splenic rupture have all been observed.

There is no specific treatment, and spontaneous recovery can be anticipated in the majority of cases. Splenectomy should be considered for patients with splenomegaly when there are complications of hypersplenism, since the operation has been almost uniformly followed by correction of the hematologic abnormality.

GAUCHER'S DISEASE. This is a familial disorder characterized by abnormal storage or retention of glycolipid cerebrosides in reticuloendothelial cells. Proliferation and enlargement of these cells produces enlargement of the spleen, liver, and lymph nodes. The disease is generally discovered in childhood, but may become evident either early in infancy or late in adult life.

The sole clinical manifestation may be awareness of a progressively enlarging abdominal mass, primarily due to splenomegaly and, to a lesser extent, to hepatomegaly. The yellowish-brown pigmentation of the head and extremities occurs in about 45 to 75 percent of cases. Bone pain and pathologic fracture may develop in long-standing cases. Many patients develop the hematologic manifestations of hypersplenism as a result of excessive sequestration of formed blood elements. Moderate to severe thrombocytopenia and normocytic anemia are almost always present, and often there is mild leukopenia. In the patients with hypersplenism, splenectomy almost uniformly has been beneficial in correcting the hematologic disorder, but there is no evidence that the operation influences the course of the basic disease.

FANCONI SYNDROME (ANEMIA). This rare, hereditary condition is characterized by pancytopenia, bone marrow hypoplasia, and a variety of developmental abnormalities and is somewhat more common in males than in females. Anemia, often severe, is the most prominent of the hematologic abnormalities. Mild or moderate leukopenia and thrombocytopenia occur. The bone marrow is usually hypocellular and fatty but occasionally may be normal and even hypercellular.

Most patients die early in life. Splenectomy has been performed in a few patients with severe anemia and increasing transfusion requirements, but the results have been inconsistent.

PORPHYRIA ERYTHROPOIETICA. This is a congenital disorder of erythrocyte pyrrole metabolism which is transmitted as a recessive trait and characterized by the excessive deposition of porphyrins in the tissues. In the skin this results in pronounced photosensitization and severe bullous dermatitis. Premature red cell destruction within the spleen contributes to severe anemia. When the disease is complicated by hemolysis or splenomegaly, splenectomy is followed by marked improvement in the anemia and decreased concentrations of porphyrins in the red cells, bone marrow, and urine.

MISCELLANEOUS LESIONS

ECTOPIC SPLEEN. This unusual condition is ascribed to lengthening of the splenic ligaments which results in extreme mobility of the organ so that the spleen of normal size may be palpable in the lower abdomen or in the pelvis. In some cases, acute torsion of the pedicle occurs, necessitating surgical intervention.

SPLENIC ARTERY ANEURYSM. The splenic artery is the most common site of intraabdominal aneurysm other than the aorta. The incidence of splenic artery aneurysm ranges between 0.02 and 0.16 percent in autopsy series. The lesions occur more frequently in females, and the most common predisposing factor is atherosclerosis. Splenic artery aneurysms are usually discovered as incidental findings on an abdominal x-ray, and a bruit is rarely heard in the left upper quadrant. The frequency of rupture ranges between less than 10 percent to 46 percent, with about 20 percent of ruptures having occurred during pregnancy. Excision of the aneurysm, with or without splenectomy, is recommended for enlarging or symptomatic aneurysms, and in women in the child-bearing age. In many asymptomatic patients close observation is justified.

CYSTS AND TUMORS. Cysts of the spleen are unusual. Parasitic cysts are usually due to echinococcal involvement, while the nonparasitic cysts may be categorized as dermoid, epidermoid, epithelial, and pseudocysts. Pseudocysts occur after occult rupture of the spleen.

Primary and malignant tumors of the spleen are sarcomatous. Recent autopsy series have refuted the concept that metastases to the spleen are rare. However, laparotomy for undiagnosed splenomegaly which reveals unsuspected metastatic deposit in the absence of known generalized metastases is extremely uncommon.

ABSCESSES. Splenic abscess is an uncommon cause of abdominal sepsis. Primary splenic abscesses occur much more often in the Tropics, where they are frequently related to thrombosis of the splenic vessels with infarction in patients with sickle cell anemia. Clinical manifestations include fever, chills, splenomegaly, and left upper quadrant tenderness. Diagnosis may be established by scan or angiography. Removal of the spleen is the operation of choice, but some cases have been treated with splenotomy and drainage when there were gross adhesions or the condition of the patient did not permit splenectomy.

SPLENECTOMY

The operation for splenic rupture frequently requires the administration of whole blood. When elective splenectomy is performed for hematologic disorders, other specific considerations arise. Patients with malignant lymphoma and leukemia may develop cryoglobulinemia and, therefore, the blood should be administered at room temperature. For patients with thalassemia and, more particularly, acquired hemolytic anemia, typing and cross matching may be difficult, and sufficient time should be allotted during the preoperative period to accumulate the blood that may be required during the operation. For patients

with marked immune thrombocytopenia (ITP), platelet packs are not usually administered preoperatively since the platelets are rapidly destroyed by the spleen and, therefore, not very effective.

TECHNIQUE. Although the midline incision is generally employed for a ruptured spleen, the left subcostal incision is preferred for elective resection. The spleen is mobilized initially by dividing the ligamentous attachments, which are usually avascular but may contain large vessels in patients with secondary hypersplenism and myeloid metaplasia. The short gastric vessels then are doubly ligated and transected, taking care not to traumatize the stomach itself. If compromise of blood supply to the fundic portion of the greater curvature of the stomach is a concern, enfolding of this area should be performed to prevent the development of a gastric fistula. This permits ultimate dissection of the splenic hilus with individual ligation and division of the splenic artery and vein. During the course of hilar dissection, care should be taken to avoid injury to the tail of the pancreas in order to obviate pseudocyst formation. The technique of initial ligation of the splenic artery by exposure through the gastrosplenic omentum is applicable to the small spleen but not appropriate when there is marked splenomegaly or when large lymphomatous lymph nodes encircle the splenic vessels. Whenever splenectomy is performed for hematologic disorder, a careful search should be made for accessory spleens. The splenic bed is not drained routinely, but drains are used in patients with myeloid metaplasia.

POSTOPERATIVE COURSE AND COMPLICATIONS. Following splenectomy, characteristic changes in blood composition occur. Howell-Jolly bodies are present in almost all patients, and siderocytes are common. Generally, leukocytosis and increased platelet counts are observed. In patients with marked thrombocytopenia, the platelet count often returns to normal within two days, but peak levels may not be reached for two weeks. The white blood cell count usually is elevated the first day and may remain persistently elevated for several months. The most frequent complication is that of left lower lobe atelectasis. Other complications include subphrenic hematoma and abscess, injury to the pancreas causing fistula, or pancreatitis. Excessively elevated platelet counts, particularly in patients with myeloid metaplasia, and increased platelet adhesiveness have been reported. Although these factors have been implicated in the greater incidence of thrombophlebitis following splenectomy, many series can show no good correlation between these complications and the platelet counts.

There has been increasing concern regarding infection and sepsis in splenectomized patients. In a large review Singer reported that deaths from sepsis in splenectomized patients were 200 times as prevalent as in the population at large. Eraklis and Filler felt that overwhelming infection in splenectomized patients was mainly related to the primary disease and that the higher risk of sepsis occurred in patients with thalassemia, malignancies, and aplastic anemia. When the risk of infection in childhood Hodgkin's disease was assessed in 181 consecutive, previously untreated patients, the episode did not correlate with splenectomy alone, but appeared to be related more to the treatment with chemotherapy and radiotherapy.

It has been shown that splenectomy results in a variety of immunologic defects, including a poor response to intravenous immunization with particulate antigens, a deficiency in phagocytosis-promoting peptide, decreased serum Igm, and decreased properdin. The organisms most frequently isolated from septic splenectomized children are those of diplococcus pneumonia and H-influenza. It is therefore reasonable to delay splenectomy for hematologic disorders in very young children, especially those under the age of two years, to attempt to preserve the traumatized spleen in the pediatric patient and to maintain patients with "at-risk" diseases on long-term oral antibiotic therapy.

References

General

Schwartz, S. I., Adams, J. T., and Bauman, A. W.: Splenectomy for Hematologic Disorders, *Curr Probl Surg,* May, 1971.

Anatomy

Burke, J. A., and Simon, G. T.: Electron Microscopy of the Spleen. I. Anatomy and Microcirculation. II. Phagocytosis of Colloidal Carbon, *Am J Pathol,* **58:**127, 1970.

Knisely, M. H.: Spleen Studies: I. Microscopic Observations of the Circulatory System of Living Unstimulated Mammalian Spleens, *Anat Rec,* **65:**23, 1936.

Weiss, L.: The Structure of Intermediate Vascular Pathways in the Spleen of Rabbits, *Am J Anat,* **113:**51, 1963.

Wennberg, E., and Weiss, L.: The Structure of the Spleen and Hemolysis, *Ann Rev Med,* **20:**29, 1969.

Physiology and Pathophysiology

Doan, C. A.: The Spleen: Its Structure and Functions, *Postgrad Med,* **43:**126, 1968.

Harris, J. W.: "The Red Cell: Production, Metabolism, Destruction, Normal and Abnormal," Harvard University Press, Cambridge, Mass., 1963. (Published for the Commonwealth Fund.)

Motulsky, A. G., Casserd, F., Giblett, E. R., Broun, G. O., and Finch, C. A.: Anemia and the Spleen, *N Engl J Med,* **259:**1164 and 1215, 1958.

Diagnostic Considerations

Jandl, J. H., Greenberg, M. S., Yonemoto, R. H., and Castle, W. B.: Clinical Determination of the Sites of Red Cell Sequestration in Hemolytic Anemias, *J Clin Invest,* **41:**1628, 1962.

Samuels, L. D., and Stewart, C.: Estimation of Spleen Size in Sickle Cell Anemia, *J Nucl Med,* **11:**12, 1970.

Wagner, H. N., Jr., McAfee, J. G., and Winkelman, J. W.: Splenic Disease Diagnosis by Radioisotope Scanning, *Arch Intern Med,* **109:**673, 1962.

Rupture of the Spleen

Ayala, L. A., Williams, L. F., Widrich, W. C.: Occult Rupture of Spleen: Chronic Form of Splenic Rupture, *Ann Surg,* **179:**472, 1974.

Burrington, J. D.: Surgical Repair of a Ruptured Spleen in Children, *Arch Surg,* **112:**417, 1977.

Cioffino, W., Schein, C. J., and Gliedman, M. L.: Splenic Injury during Abdominal Surgery, *Arch Surg,* **111:**167, 1976.

Dunphy, J. E.: Splenectomy for Trauma, *Am J Surg,* **71:**450, 1946.

Lieberman, R. C., and Welch, C. S.: A Study of 248 Instances of Traumatic Rupture of the Spleen, *Surg Gynecol Obstet,* **127:**961, 1968.

Orloff, M. J., and Peskin, G. W.: Collective Review. Spontaneous Ruptures of the Normal Spleen: A Surgical Enigma, *Intern Abstr Surg,* **106:**1, 1958.

Schwartz, S. I., Adams, J. T., Cockett, A. T. K., and Morton, J. H.: Blunt Trauma to the Upper Abdomen, *Surg Ann,* **3:**273, 1971.

Widman, W. D., and Laubscher, F. A.: Splenosis: Disease or Beneficial Condition? *Arch Surg,* **102:**152, 1971.

Hematologic Disorders

Adler, A., Stutzman, L., Sokal, J. F., and Mittelman, A.: Splenectomy for Hematologic Depression in Lymphocytic Lymphoma and Leukemia, *Cancer,* **35:**521, 1975.

Bernard, R. P., Bauman, A. W., and Schwartz, S. I.: Splenectomy for Thrombotic Thrombocytopenic Purpura, *Ann Surg,* **169:**616, 1969.

Bertino, J., and Myerson, R. M.: The Role of Splenectomy in Sarcoidosis, *Arch Intern Med,* **106:**213, 1960.

Cannon, W. B., and Nelson, T. S.: Staging of Hodgkin's Disease: A Surgical Perspective, *Am J Surg,* **132:**224, 1976.

Chabner, B. A., Johnson, R. E., Young, R. C., Canellos, G. P., Hubbard, S. P., Johnson, S. K., and DeVita, V. T., Jr.: Sequential Nonsurgical and Surgical Staging of Non-Hodgkin's Lymphoma, *Ann Intern Med,* **85:**149, 1976.

Cooper, I. A., Ironside, P. N. J., Madigan, J. P., Morris, P. J., and Ewing, M. R.: Role of Splenectomy in Management of Advanced Hodgkin's Disease, *Cancer,* **34:**408, 1974.

Dacie, J. V.: "The Haemolytic Anaemias, Congenital and Acquired," vol. 2, pt. 1, Grune & Stratton, Inc., New York, 1960.

DeWeese, M. S., and Coller, F. A.: Splenectomy for Hematologic Disorders, *West J Surg,* **67:**129, 1959.

Doan, C. A.: Hypersplenism, *Bull NY Acad Med,* **25:**625, 1949.

——, Bruce, M. D. and Wiseman, B. K.: Hypersplenic Cytopenic Syndromes: A 25 Year Experience with Special Reference to Splenectomy, in "Proceedings of the Sixth International Congress of the International Society of Hematology," Grune & Stratton, Inc. New York, 1958.

——, Bouroncle, B. A., and Wiseman, B. K.: Idiopathic and Secondary Thrombocytopenic Purpura: Clinical Study and Evaluation of 381 Cases over a Period of 28 Years, *Ann Intern Med,* **53:**861, 1960.

Fahri, P. J., Metz, E. N., Nick, W. V., and Zollinger, R. M.: A Quarter Century with Splenectomy: Changing Concepts, *Arch Surg,* **100:**301, 1970.

Gendel, B. R.: Chronic Leg Ulcers in Diseases of the Blood, *Blood,* **3:**1283, 1948.

Glatstein, E., Guernsey, J. M., Rosenberg, S. A., and Kaplan, H. S.: The Value of Laparotomy and Splenectomy in the Staging of Hodgkin's Disease, *Cancer,* **24:**709, 1969.

Gruenberg, H., and Penner, J. A.: Gaucher's Disease: Observations on Its Clinical Course, *Mich Med,* **74:**323, 1975.

Liebowitz, H. R.: Splenomegaly and Hypersplenism Pre- and Post-portacaval Shunt, *NY J Med,* **63:**2631, 1963.

Lipton, E. I.: Elliptocytosis with Hemolytic Anemia: The Effects of Splenectomy, *Pediatrics,* **15:**67, 1955.

Meilleur, P. A., and Myers, M. C.: Thrombocytosis: A Postsplenectomy Complication in Agnogenic Myeloid Metaplasia, *Am J Med Sci,* **241:**68, 1961.

Mitchell, R. I., and Peters, M. V.: Lymph Node Biopsy during Laparotomy for Staging of Hodgkin's Disease, *Ann Surg,* **178:**698, 1973.

Necheles, T. F., Allen, D. M., and Gerald, P. S.: The Many Forms of Thalassemia: Definition and Classification of the Thalassemia Syndromes, *Ann NY Acad Sci,* **165**(Art. 1):5, 1969.

O'Brien, P. H., Hartz, W. H., Derlacki, D., and Graulich, K.: Splenectomy for Hypersplenism in Malignant Lymphoma, *Arch Surg,* **101:**348, 1970.

O'Neill, J. A., Jr., Scott, H. W., Jr., Billings, F. T., and Foster, J. H.: The Role of Splenectomy in Felty's Syndrome, *Ann Surg,* **167:**81, 1968.

Reynolds, P. M., Jackson, J. M., Brine, M. A. S., and Vivian, A. B.: Thrombotic Thrombocytopenic Purpura—Remission Following Splenectomy, *Am J Med,* **61:**439, 1976.

Schwartz, S. I.: Myeloproliferative Disorders, *Ann Surg,* **182:**464, 1975.

———, Adams, J. T., and Bauman, A. W.: Splenectomy for Hematologic Disorders, *Curr Probl Surg,* May, 1971.

———, Adesola, A. O., Elebute, E. A., and Rob, C. B.: "Tropical Surgery," McGraw-Hill Book Company, Inc., New York, 1971.

——— and Cooper, R. A., Jr.: Surgery in the Diagnosis and Treatment of Hodgkin's Disease, in "Advances in Surgery," vol. 6, Yearbook Medical Publishers, Inc., Chicago, 1972.

Veronesi, U., Musumeci, R., Pizzetti, F., Gennari, L., and Bonadonna, G.: Value of Staging Laparotomy in Non-Hodgkin's Lymphomas (with Emphasis on the Histiocytic Type), *Cancer,* **33:**446, 1974.

Wintrobe, M. M.: "Clinical Hematology," 6th ed., Lea & Febiger, Philadelphia, 1967.

Yam, L. T., and Crosby, W. H.: Early Splenectomy in Lymphoproliferative Disorders, *Arch Intern Med,* **133:**270, 1974.

Miscellaneous Lesions

Chulay, J. D., and Lankerani, M. R.: Splenic Abscess, *Am J Med,* **61:**513, 1976.

Gadacz, T., Way, L. W., and Dunphy, J. E.: Changing Clinical Spectrum of Splenic Abscess, *Am J Surg,* **128:**182, 1974.

Saw, E. C., Arbegast, N., Schmalhorst, W. R., and Comer, T. P.: Splenic Artery Aneurysms, *Arch Surg,* **106:**660, 1973.

Splenectomy

Ein, S. H., Shandling, B., Simpson, J. S., Stephens, C. A., Bandi, S. K., Biggar, W. D., and Freedman, M. H.: The Morbidity and Mortality of Splenectomy in Childhood, *Ann Surg,* **185:**307, 1977.

Eraklis, A. J., and Filler, R. M.: Splenectomy in Childhood: A Review of 1413 Cases, *J Pediatr Surg,* **7:**382, 1972.

Glatstein, E., Vosti, K. L., Donaldson, S. S., et al.: Serious Bacterial Infections in Pediatric Hodgkin's Disease: Relative Risks of Radiotherapy, Chemotherapy and Splenectomy, *Proc Am Soc Clin Oncol,* **17:**252, 1976.

Haller, J. A., Jr., and Jones, E. L.: Effect of Splenectomy on Immunity and Resistance to Major Infections in Early Childhood: Clinical and Experimental Study, *Ann Surg,* **163:**902, 1966.

Olsen, W. R., and Beaudoin, D. E.: Increased Incidence of Accessory Spleens in Hematologic Disease, *Arch Surg,* **98:**762, 1969.

Singer, D. B.: Postsplenectomy Sepsis, in Perspectives in Pediatric Pathology. Chicago, Year Book Medical Publishers Inc., 1973, vol. 1, pp. 285–311.

CHAPTER 34

Peritonitis and Intraabdominal Abscesses

by **Robert E. Condon**

PERITONEUM

STRUCTURE. The peritoneum is a single layer of flat mesothelial cells resting on a bed of looser connective tissue containing fat cells, macrophages, and some collagen and elastic fibers. The parietal peritoneum lines all of the abdominal cavity, covering the abdominal wall, diaphragm, and pelvis. Parietal peritoneum everywhere is reinforced by the endoabdominal (transversalis) fascia, which lies external to it. The visceral peritoneum covers all the intraabdominal viscera and mesenteries, and is identical with the serosa or capsule of the several intraabdominal organs. Excepting the ends of the fallopian tubes, the peritoneum is a completely closed sac.

The abdominal cavity is divided into the general peritoneal cavity, or greater sac, and the lesser sac. The lesser sac arises in the upper half of the abdomen during fetal development because of persistence of the embryologic ventral mesentery and rotation of the upper abdominal viscera. As a consequence, the embryologic right upper peritoneal cavity becomes isolated from the remainder of the peritoneal cavity, remaining in communication only at the foramen of Winslow.

INNERVATION. The parietal peritoneum is innervated by both somatic and visceral afferent nerves and is quite sensitive, responding to various stimuli somewhat as the skin does. As is true of the skin, there are regional differences in ability of the peritoneum to localize pain. The anterior parietal peritoneum is the most sensitive, and the pelvic peritoneum is relatively the least sensitive. The ability to localize a noxious stimulus affecting the parietal peritoneum, particularly that of the anterior abdominal wall, underlies much of our ability to diagnose acute intraabdominal illness.

In addition to perception of pain as localized tenderness and rebound tenderness, local injury or inflammation of the parietal peritoneum leads to protective voluntary muscular guarding and then to reflex muscular spasm, signs which are very useful in determining the presence and state of progression of intraabdominal disorders.

In contrast to the parietal peritoneum, the visceral peritoneum receives afferent innervation only from the autonomic nervous system and is relatively insensitive. Stimuli are perceived as poorly localized pain, often with the character of a toothache or of colic. Visceral afferent nerves respond primarily to traction or distension, less well to pressure, and apparently have no receptors capable of mediating pain and temperature sensation.

The root of the small-bowel mesentery and the biliary tree are relatively better innervated, accounting for more intense and more localized responses to stimulation of these areas. The small bowel, itself, is not well innervated, so that stimulation of its visceral afferents produces only a vague, dull ache in the midabdomen. Somatic reflex responses to visceral peritoneal stimulation are uncommon, but with maximal stimulation may result in bradycardia or hypotension. By contrast, visceral reflex responses serve to produce ileus early after the onset of peritoneal irritation or inflammation.

MEMBRANE FUNCTION. The surface area of the peritoneum is nearly 2 m², approximately identical to the area of the skin, and is appreciably larger than the filtering surface area of the renal glomeruli. Unlike the skin, the peritoneum acts as a semipermeable membrane and permits bidirectional transport of water, electrolytes, peptides, and similar small molecules.

The peritoneal cavity normally contains only about 100 ml of fluid to serve as lubrication between the abdominal viscera and the parietes. Since the peritoneum permits bidirectional fluid movement, the peritoneal cavity functions as a part, albeit a small one, of the total body extracellular fluid compartment. Hydraulic and osmotic concentration forces control the movement and the direction of transport across the peritoneum. In addition to these passive processes, there is evidence that active absorption also occurs, both intercellularly and transcellularly across the peritoneum.

Fluid tagged with heavy water or another marker and placed in the peritoneal cavity rapidly equilibrates with the interstitial fluid and the plasma. Albumin, electrolytes, and urea are freely transported bidirectionally across the peritoneum. Antibiotics also are easily absorbed. Endogenous and exogenous toxic substances, including bacterial toxins, are freely absorbed as well, and may produce systemic effects. Because of the tremendous surface available, the bidirectional transfer of substances across the peritoneal membrane is rapid and potentially large in volume. The membrane transfer properties of the peritoneum are used to advantage in peritoneal dialysis for acute renal insufficiency, but also may be a fatal disadvantage if spill of toxic bowel content occurs, as in strangulation obstruction.

In addition to fluid exchange across the peritoneal membrane, transdiaphragmatic lymphatic channels also play a role in fluid transport from the peritoneal cavity. These lymphatic channels probably are responsible for the appearance of so-called sympathetic pleural effusions whenever an intraabdominal inflammatory process involves the undersurface of the diaphragm. These lymphatic channels also provide a route by which amylase-rich abdominal fluid is transported into the pleural space, particularly on the left side, in patients suffering from pancreatitis.

RESPONSE TO INJURY. The peritoneum heals very rapidly following injury. Even large defects can be restored in a matter of hours. Unlike the skin, which heals only by regeneration of epithelial cells from the margins of a defect, a peritoneal defect is restored everywhere simultaneously, usually without adhesion formation. The majority of cells involved in healing of a peritoneal wound are derived by differentiation of stem cells present within the subperitoneal tissues. Transperitoneal migration of mesothelial cells shed by intact peritoneum to implant in the area of injury, and ingrowth of mesothelial cells from the margins of a defect, are additional mechanisms which play a minor role in peritoneal healing.

If normal peritoneal healing is delayed or incomplete, adhesions form. The adhesions may be transient in nature, eventually resolving as delayed healing becomes complete, or they may be more permanent in nature. Fibrin elaborated from the inflamed peritoneal mesothelium is the scaffold upon which adhesions are built. Agglutination of fibrin strands during the course of acute peritonitis leads to the formation of soft, fibrinous adhesions. In most instances, deposited fibrin is absorbed if functioning and intact mesothelium is present in the immediately adjacent area. If the fibrinous adhesions are not absorbed for any reason, they are invaded by fibroblasts between 5 and 10 days after the initial insult. Fibroblast invasion is followed by ingrowth of capillaries and further organization into true fibrous tissue.

The factors which favor development of fibrous adhesions following peritonitis include continuing action of an intraperitoneal irritant, necrosis extending through the mesothelium to involve the subperitoneal tissues, and a predisposition in certain persons that is not well understood. Fortunately, even fibrous adhesions become attenuated and may disappear with time.

Formation of adhesions is both a protective response, helping to localize a peritoneal insult, and an adaptive healing response which helps to bring additional blood supply to ischemic injured areas of perineum. These beneficial effects of adhesions are sometimes overlooked by surgeons.

PERITONITIS: GENERAL CONSIDERATIONS

Peritonitis is inflammation of a portion or all of the parietal and visceral surfaces of the abdominal cavity. The classical division of peritonitis into primary and secondary forms has little clinical utility. When a surgeon refers to "peritonitis" without qualification, the clinical situation is acute suppurative bacterial peritonitis. Other forms of peritonitis are less common, although nonetheless important.

Every case of peritonitis, of whatever cause, initiates a sequence of responses involving the peritoneal membrane, the bowel, and the body fluid compartments, which then produce secondary endocrine, cardiac, respiratory, renal, and metabolic responses (Fig. 34-1). In certain forms of peritonitis, most notably acute suppurative peritonitis, additional responses due to the presence of infection also occur. The general responses, found to some degree whenever peritonitis occurs, are described here; additional reactions specific to the various forms of peritonitis are described later.

Primary Responses in Peritonitis

MEMBRANE INFLAMMATION. The peritoneum responds to insult with hyperemia followed by transudation. Edema and vascular congestion occur in the subperitoneal tissues immediately external to the peritoneal membrane. Absorption across inflamed peritoneum is somewhat impaired while at the same time the peritoneal membrane permits passage of larger molecules than when in its normal state. Transudation of fluid with a low protein content from the extracellular interstitial compartment into the abdominal cavity is accompanied by diapedesis of large numbers of polymorphonuclear leukocytes. During the early vascular and transudative phase of engorgement, the peritoneum acts as a "two-way street," so that toxins and other materials which may be present in peritoneal fluid are readily absorbed, enter the lymphatics and bloodstream, and may lead to systemic symptoms.

Transudation of interstitial fluid into the peritoneal cavity across the inflamed peritoneum is followed shortly by

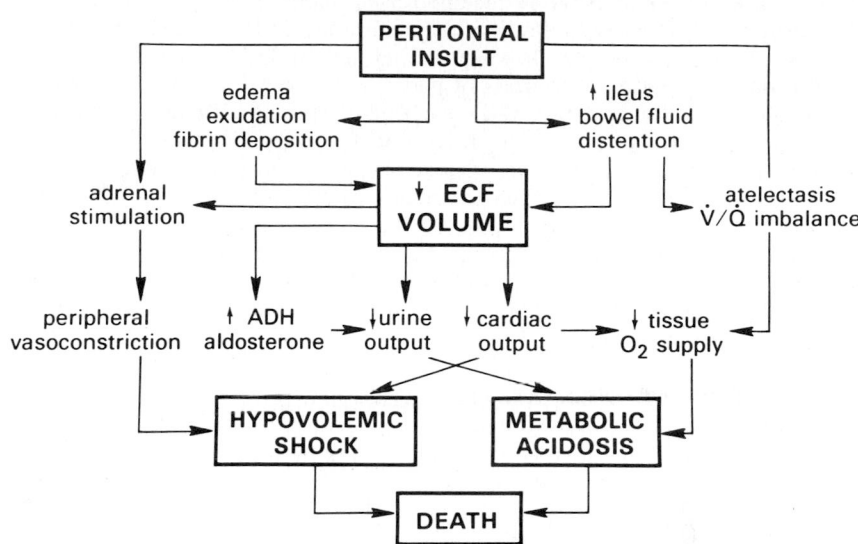

GENERAL RESPONSES TO PERITONITIS

Fig. 34-1. The major general responses to peritonitis are mediated by a decreased extracellular fluid volume, which, if not corrected, leads to metabolic acidosis, hypovolemic shock, and death.

exudation of protein-rich fluid. The fluid exudate in the peritoneal cavity contains large amounts of fibrin and other plasma proteins in concentrations sufficient to bring about clotting, which, in turn, results in agglutination of loops of bowel, other viscera, and the parietes in the area of peritoneal inflammation. This response helps to confine the source of peritoneal contamination.

Dermal inflammation causes a rapid local decrease in the concentration of collagen and a marked increase in the concentration of hexosamine and noncollagenous nitrogen in the skin. The inflamed human peritoneum behaves in a similar manner. Within the peritoneal membrane, the concentration of uronic acids and noncollagenous nitrogen increases markedly in peritonitis, while the concentration of hydroxyprolene and the hydroxyprolene-nitrogen ratio decreases. The content of uronic acid in the peritoneum is proportional to the extent and severity of the peritonitis.

The RNA/DNA ratio, which is an index of the protein synthetic capability of tissue, is decreased in peritonitis, and the defect progresses if peritonitis persists for longer than 24 hours. These changes have not been fully elucidated but could be due to tissue hypoxia inhibiting the synthesis of collagen, the action of bacterial collagenase, or the release of proteolytic lysozymal enzymes. The increase in uronic acid concentration probably reflects increased formation of glycosaminoglycans because of activation of fibroblasts and mesothelial cells.

BOWEL RESPONSE. The initial response of the bowel to peritoneal irritation is transient hypermotility. After a short interval, motility becomes depressed and nearly complete adynamic ileus soon follows. The bowel distends, and both air and fluid accumulate in the lumen. The source of the accumulating gas is largely swallowed air. Fluid secretion (exsorption) into the bowel lumen is enhanced in ileus, while resorption (insorption) is relatively impaired, pro-

moting sequestration of fluid in the bowel lumen. If the patient continues to ingest food or fluid, vomiting eventually occurs.

HYPOVOLEMIA. As noted above, the peritoneum reacts to irritation by vascular dilation and an outpouring of plasmalike fluid from the extracellular vascular and interstitial compartments into the peritoneal space as an exudate. The loose connective tissue beneath the mesothelium of the viscera, the mesenteries, and the parietes traps extracellular fluid as edema. The atonic, dilated gastrointestinal tract also accumulates fluid in the bowel lumen which is derived from the extracellular fluid volume. This translocation of water, electrolytes, and protein into a sequestered "third space" functionally removes this volume temporarily from the body economy. The rate of functional extracellular fluid loss is proportional to the surface area of peritoneum involved in the inflammatory process. With extensive peritonitis, fluid translocation of 4 to 6 liters, or more, in 24 hours is not uncommon.

Secondary Responses to Peritonitis

ENDOCRINE RESPONSE. Peritonitis acts as a stimulus to many endocrine organs. There is an almost immediate adrenal medullary response, with an outpouring of epinephrine and norepinephrine, producing vasoconstriction, tachycardia, and sweating. The adrenal cortex is stimulated to increased secretion of cortical hormones during the first 2 to 3 days following peritoneal injury. Originally thought to be the cause of increased nitrogen excretion in peritonitis, it has now been shown that the increase in adrenocortical hormones persists only for about 72 hours. Circulating concentrations of these hormones have returned to normal long before nitrogen losses cease to occur.

Secretion of both aldosterone and antidiuretic hormone also is increased as a response to the hypovolemia of peritonitis, resulting in enhanced renal conservation of sodium and water. In fact, water retention may be greater than sodium retention, so that there is dilution of plasma sodium (hyponatremia). Thyroid metabolism probably is unaltered despite increased rates of energy utilization and increased heat production by the body during peritonitis.

CARDIAC RESPONSE. The effects of peritonitis on cardiac function are a reflection both of the decrease in extracellular fluid volume and of progressing acidosis. The volume deficit results in decreased venous return and diminished cardiac output. The heart rate increases in an attempt to maintain cardiac output, but compensation usually is incomplete. Progressing acidosis brings about secondary dysfunction in cardiac contractility and a further decrease in cardiac output that compounds the problem of maintaining adequate tissue perfusion and aerobic metabolism.

RESPIRATORY RESPONSE. Abdominal distension, primarily due to adynamic ileus, coupled with restriction of both diaphragmatic and intercostal respiratory movements, results in a decrease in ventilatory volume and the early appearance of basilar atelectasis. Early in the course of peritonitis, an increase in respiratory rate may be noted, stimulated both by the hypoxia of diminished ventilation and by beginning accumulation of acidic end products of anaerobic tissue metabolism. Ventilation-perfusion imbalances result from continued pulmonary perfusion of underventilated or nonventilated alveoli and produce functional intrapulmonary shunting of blood and peripheral hypoxemia.

RENAL RESPONSE. Hypovolemia, reduced cardiac output, and increased secretion of antidiuretic hormone and of aldosterone in peritonitis all act synergistically on the kidney. Renal blood flow is diminished, resulting in a decrease in the volume of glomerular filtrate and in tubular urine flow. Reabsorption of both sodium and water is increased, often in imbalance; potassium is wasted. Urine volume output is diminished, and renal capacity to handle excess solutes is impaired. A tendency to development of metabolic acidosis is enhanced.

METABOLIC RESPONSE. The metabolic rate generally is increased, with a corresponding increase in peripheral oxygen demand. Simultaneously, the capacity of the lungs and the heart to deliver oxygen is diminished. Poor circulation leads to a shift from aerobic to anaerobic metabolism in muscle and other peripheral tissues. As a result, anaerobic end products of carbohydrate metabolism accumulate and lactic acidosis begins to develop.

Under normal circumstances, local tissue perfusion is controlled by regional metabolic requirements. If anaerobic metabolic end products begin to accumulate, local arteriolar dilation occurs. Cardiac output, in the absence of hypovolemia, increases to maintain circulatory homeostasis. Perfusion in the periphery improves, the acidic metabolic end products are cleared, and the tissues return to aerobic metabolism. This fine balance is upset by circulatory insufficiency due to the hypovolemia which accompanies peritonitis. Cardiac output may be inadequate to maintain normal arterial blood pressure and to supply required perfusion of all body tissues.

Compensatory vasoconstriction results in increased total peripheral resistance, which, in turn, maintains essential perfusion to the heart and brain. The skin, muscles, the splanchnic bed, and, to some degree, the kidneys are denied a portion of their normal circulatory volume. As a result of decreased tissue perfusion and oxygenation, anaerobic glycolysis persists and leads to a progressive increase in lactic acid and other acidic metabolic end products. Decreased renal clearance of these acidic solutes, secondary to reduced renal perfusion, contributes to the metabolic acidosis. The body attempts to compensate with increased respiratory effort to excrete carbon dioxide, but the increased respiratory effort, in turn, places an additional demand on the already inadequate circulation to perfuse the muscles of respiration.

The appearance, in some cases of peritonitis, of lactic acidosis before systemic hypotension or hypoxemia suggests the existence of a primary cellular insult which makes cells unable to use available oxygen and substrate. This hypothesis was investigated in isolated hepatic mitochondria harvested following induction of peritonitis by cecal ligation. In these experiments, hepatic cellular hypoxia followed the development of peritonitis even while systemic oxygenation was adequate and hypotension had not yet developed. Mitochondrial respiration, however, was unaltered in these experiments, suggesting that primary cellular injury does not occur in peritonitis but that alterations in oxygen delivery are responsible for reduced oxygen consumption and lactic acidosis.

Hepatic glycogen stores are utilized promptly in peritonitis. Insulin secretion by islet cells increases, promoting mobilization of fat as an energy source. Nonetheless, relative insulin resistance to muscle utilization of glucose uptake is unchanged, and an energy deficit persists.

Protein catabolism begins early in peritonitis and becomes progressively more severe. However, some data indicate that the rate of synthesis of plasma proteins is increased in terms of concentration and turnover. Plasma proteins preferentially are synthesized while muscle proteins preferentially are catabolized. Weight loss of 25 to 30 percent of lean body mass can occur if peritonitis persists. Albumin synthesis also is apparently increased during peritonitis, as judged by increased uptake of radioactive label, but the increased synthesis occurs in the face of a decreasing concentration of circulating albumin. The reason for this disparity is that a considerable amount of albumin accumulates in the peritoneal cavity and thus is lost to the general circulation.

Clinical Manifestations

The appearance of a patient with advanced peritonitis was described by Hippocrates: ". . . hollow eyes, collapsed temples; the ears cold, contracted and their lobes turned out; the skin about the forehead being rough, distended, and parched; the color of the whole face being brown, black, livid, or lead-colored." Patients with peritonitis which is so advanced as to present this classic Hippocratic facies are usually in a preterminal state. But even much earlier in the clinical course of peritonitis, patients quite obviously are gravely ill. Characteristically, they lie quietly in bed, supine, with knees flexed and with frequent limited intercostal respirations since any other motion intensifies the abdominal pain.

Abdominal pain almost always is the predominant symptom, unless its perception is masked by the administration of anodynes or the presence of a fresh surgical wound. The pain may have been sudden in onset, associated with rupture of a viscus, or more insidious. When fully developed, pain is steady, unrelenting, burning, and aggravated by any motion. Pain usually is most intense in the area of most advanced peritoneal inflammation. Decreasing intensity and extent of pain with time suggest localization of the inflammatory process, while increasing intensity and extent imply the presence of a spreading peritonitis.

Anorexia almost always is present. Nausea is frequent and may be accompanied by vomiting. The patient usually complains of thirst and of feeling feverish, often with intermittent chills. Body temperature elevation in peritonitis usually is in the range of 38 to 40°C. Fever is usually higher and more spiking in character in younger and healthier patients, while older and debilitated patients may exhibit only a modest febrile response.

Tachycardia and a diminished palpable peripheral pulse volume are early signs of hypovolemia. The blood pressure is maintained in the early stages of peritonitis, but, as hypovolemia progresses, compensatory vasoconstrictive responses may be overcome, with the rapid appearance of hypovolemic shock. Respirations typically are rapid and shallow; rapid because of progressively greater tissue demands for oxygen and a need to correct developing acidosis, and shallow because deep respirations intensify the perception of abdominal pain.

The abdomen is distended, quiet to auscultation, and tender to palpation. Tenderness is present over the entire extent of the peritoneum involved in the inflammatory process. Maximal tenderness usually is noted in the region of the organ in which the process originated, but in some cases, maximal tenderness is found over the advancing edge of the peritoneal inflammation. Direct, percussive, and referred rebound tenderness confirms the presence of peritoneal irritation. Percussion tenderness sometimes is more accurate than direct palpation in locating the point of maximal tenderness as well as in delineating the extent of peritoneal irritation.

Rigidity of the abdominal muscles is produced initially by voluntary guarding and, following involvement of the parietal peritoneum by inflammation, also by reflex muscular spasm. As peritonitis advances, reflex spasm may become so severe that boardlike abdominal rigidity is produced. Hyperresonance due to accumulating gas in the paralyzed, distended intestines usually can be demonstrated easily by percussion. If a pneumoperitoneum has resulted from rupture of a hollow viscus, gas accumulating under the right side of the diaphragm may produce a decrease in the vertical extent of liver dullness to percussion.

Some bowel sounds may be audible on auscultation early in peritonitis, but as inflammation spreads, the nearly silent abdomen of adynamic ileus supervenes. Rectal examination and vaginal examination of female patients are essential steps in establishing the diagnosis. The location and extent of tenderness, and the possible presence of a pelvic mass, permit assessment of the degree of involvement of pelvic peritoneum. Vaginal examination of the cervix may provide clues to the origin of an inflammatory process within the female generative organs.

Leukocytosis is usual in acute peritonitis, but the total white cell count, taken alone without a differential count, can be very misleading. Massive peritoneal inflammation may mobilize sufficient numbers of leukocytes into the diseased area so that only 3,000 to 4,000 white cells per cubic millimeter remain behind in the circulating blood. The differential count shows a moderate to a marked left shift in peritonitis, and the predominance of polymorphonucleocytes in the differential provides evidence of the presence of inflammation even when the total leukocyte count is not markedly elevated. Blood chemistry determinations are quite variable but usually will reflect hemoconcentration due to dehydration (increased hematocrit) as well as metabolic acidosis.

The radiologic picture of generalized peritonitis is that of paralytic ileus with distension of both small intestine and colon. Inflammatory exudate and edema of the intestinal wall may produce widening of the spaces between adjacent bowel loops noted on a flat film of the abdomen. Peritoneal fat lines and the psoas shadows may be obliterated. Free air may be visible on an upright abdominal or lateral decubitus film if a ruptured viscus is the cause of peritonitis. Air beneath the diaphragm also may be noted on x-rays of the chest.

In general, the importance of laboratory work in the diagnosis of peritonitis has been overemphasized, a statement which also holds true for almost every other acute intraabdominal disease. Though laboratory determinations undoubtedly are of occasional help, the major emphasis in both the diagnosis and management of peritonitis should be on clinical examination of the patient. Amelioration of symptoms and restoration of the patient's physical state toward normal are the best indicators that treatment is effective. Laboratory and radiologic examinations should be employed only to help rule out other causes of abdominal pain such as pneumonia. In an occasional obscure case, confirmation of the presence of peritonitis may require such diagnostic measures as a peritoneal tap or lavage.

ACUTE SUPPURATIVE PERITONITIS

Any breach in the integrity of a hollow abdominal viscus or of the abdominal parietes which permits peritoneal contamination is a potential catastrophe. Loss of integrity may be due to direct contamination from a traumatic abdominal wound, to perforation of an inflamed or traumatized hollow abdominal viscus, to functional loss of bowel integrity secondary to ischemia; may occur retrogradely via the fallopian tubes in pelvic infections; or may be iatrogenic, such as an improperly executed bowel anastomosis.

While no longer the overwhelming clinical problem it once was, suppurative peritonitis still is the most common cause of death following an abdominal operation. The mortality risk of septic peritonitis ranges from 24 percent in acute perforated diverticulitis to 90 percent with acute perforated ischemic colitis, particularly if treatment is delayed. About half of all cases of septic shock which terminate fatally are secondary to peritonitis. In 5 to 7 percent of autopsies, peritonitis is the primary or a contributory cause of death.

Although there is some degree of peritoneal inflammation (from mechanical and desiccation injury of exposed peritoneum as well as intraoperative bacterial contamination from room air or spillage during manipulation of viscera and minor breaks in aseptic technique) every time the peritoneal cavity is entered surgically, such contamination usually is not so great that clinically significant peritonitis ensues. Peritonitis following an operation is due most commonly to bile leakage, less commonly to breakdown of an anastomotic suture line; on occasion it follows ill-advised attempts at peritoneal drainage. The integrity of an anastomosis is endangered by tension on the suture line, ischemia, hemorrhage, mucosal eversion, infection, or the presence of a drain in apposition to the suture line, as well as all the systemic factors which interfere with wound healing (see Chap. 8).

Perforated peptic ulcer is the most common cause of peritonitis due to visceral rupture. Appendicitis, formerly the most common cause, is now less frequent because of a recent overall decline in the incidence of appendicitis. Pancreatitis is a frequent cause of peritonitis in certain hospitals. Gangrene of the bowel from strangulation obstruction, acute mesenteric vascular occlusion, or nonocclusive, low-perfusion states involving the bowel also is an important cause of peritonitis. Other common visceral diseases that may lead to peritonitis due to rupture of an inflamed organ are acute gangrenous cholecystitis and colonic diverticulitis. Gonorrheal salpingitis is a common cause of pelvic peritonitis, although this disease does not often progress to a generalized peritonitis.

Trauma to the abdomen may produce peritonitis by contamination of the abdominal cavity with foreign material, such as shotgun wadding or clothing, or disruption of a hollow abdominal viscus as the result of severe blunt, nonpenetrating trauma or the penetrating trauma of a stab or gunshot wound. Blunt abdominal trauma also may disrupt the vascular supply to abdominal viscera, leading to gangrene or rupture of the involved organ.

Interactions of Bacteria and the Peritoneum

The presence of bacteria within the peritoneal cavity by no means invariably results in spreading diffuse peritonitis. On the contrary, peritoneal defense mechanisms contain the insult in most instances; invading microorganisms are destroyed, and the peritoneum is restored to a relatively normal state.

If peritoneal defenses are successful in localizing the infectious process but the interaction between invading microorganisms and body defense mechanisms does not result in early elimination of the bacteria, confined suppuration and abscess formation ensues (see further on). On occasion, however, initial defense reactions are insufficient

and a more diffuse peritonitis ensues. The general responses to peritonitis then follow. They are mediated largely by translocation of extracellular fluid into the peritoneal cavity, with both the local and systemic consequences enumerated above.

In suppurative peritonitis, in addition, a group of specific responses due to the presence of overwhelming numbers of bacteria is superimposed on the general responses to peritonitis (Fig. 34-2). The magnitude of the specific responses to generalized spreading peritonitis is, in part, determined by (1) the virulence of the contaminating bacteria, (2) the extent and duration of contamination, (3) the presence or absence of an adjuvant, and (4) the appropriateness of initial therapy. If treatment fails to bring about prompt control of peritoneal infection, endotoxemia and septic shock may ensue.

VIRULENCE OF CONTAMINATING BACTERIA. A mixed, or polymicrobial, bacterial flora usually is present in patients suffering acute suppurative peritonitis secondary to contamination of the abdominal cavity from the gastrointestinal tract. The most common offending organisms include aerobic coliform bacilli, anaerobic *Bacteroides* species, anaerobic and aerobic streptococci, enterococci, and *Clostridia* (Table 34-1). These bacteria are significant pathogens for human beings.

Experiments of Nichols and colleagues in which the entire range of peritonitis, from overwhelming sepsis to resolution with an abscess, was produced, indicate that mortality risk is a dose-related phenomenon and correlates directly with the total number of pathogenic bacteria present in the peritoneal cavity. Experimental evidence also indicates that the mixed fecal flora usually found in peritonitis acts synergistically, so that total virulence is greater than the sum of its parts. Experimentally, injection of massive numbers of single species of fecal pathogens may

Table 34-1. BACTERIA IN PERITONITIS

	Percent of recovery of organisms	
	Bartlett, 1977*	Lorber, 1975*
No. of patients studied . .	21	76
Aerobes		
Escherichia coli	100	57
Proteus	24	11
Klebsiella	24	8
Pseudomonas	24	3
Other bacilli	33	6
Streptococci	33	47
Staphylococci	0	0
Anaerobes		
Bacteroides fragilis	90	93
Other *Bacteroides*	24	59
Peptostreptococci	38	29
Peptococci	19	28
Fusobacteria	24	20
Clostridia	52	9
Other anaerobes	. . .	23

*First author; full citations will be found in the references at the end of the chapter.

not produce a fatality, whereas mixtures of organisms, in the same total numbers, particularly combinations of aerobes and anaerobes, result in overwhelming peritonitis and death. Further, there is evidence to indicate that apparently nonpathogenic microorganisms may increase the virulence of pathogenic bacteria with which they are associated.

Although the frequency with which anaerobic bacteria are present in peritoneal infections probably has not changed over the years, modern methods have greatly improved the rate at which these organisms are recovered. Thus, the importance of anaerobic bacteria in peritonitis recently has become more widely recognized. Years ago, Meleney and Altemeier emphasized the frequency of recovery of anaerobic organisms in peritonitis. Experimental evidence indicates not only that the presence of anaerobic microorganisms enhances the virulence of aerobic pathogens, but that it is the presence of anaerobes or their degradation products which is responsible for the resolution of acute peritonitis by formation of an abscess rather than by complete healing.

Stone and colleagues recently demonstrated in patients undergoing operation that the recoverability of anaerobic organisms from a soiled peritoneal cavity showed a progressive decline with the passage of time. If the abdomen was open for 3 hours or longer, anaerobes could no longer be recovered. Although Stone suggested that in some cases, exposure to room air might be sufficient to manage the anaerobic component of peritoneal sepsis, specific antibiotic therapy obviously is more certain therapy.

EXTENT AND DURATION OF CONTAMINATION. Massive sudden contamination, as from a burst carcinoma of the cecum, often disseminates bacteria rapidly throughout the peritoneal cavity. Dissemination occurs widely before localization mechanisms have time to be effective. Experimentally, bacteria or liquid radiopaque media injected intraperitoneally at one locus can be demonstrated to spread throughout the entire peritoneum within 3 to 6 hours. Spread is produced by normal intestinal and abdominal movements, by movement of the diaphragm during respiration (which establishes a cyclic negative pressure differential between the subphrenic space and the rest of the peritoneal cavity, promoting upward flow of fluid and particulate matter), and by the effect of gravity related to body position, which tends to promote flow into the pelvic cavity. Even though infection spreads diffusely throughout the peritoneal cavity, if the source is controlled by early surgical intervention, peritonitis usually responds to vigorous antibiotic and supportive therapy. On the other hand, if the source of contamination persists, death nearly always results because of continuing peritoneal soiling.

The severity and extent of peritonitis secondary to spontaneous or traumatic perforation of the gastrointestinal tract vary not only with the size of the perforation but also with its location. Spillage of distal ileal or cecal content is associated with greater morbidity than a perforation proximally or distally in the gastrointestinal tract. Proximally there are few bacteria; distally the fecal content is more solid and tends to be more easily localized. But ileal and cecal content is fluid and contains high concentrations of

Fig. 34-2. The specific responses to suppurative peritonitis begin with septicemia, which initiates tachypnea, respiratory alkalosis, anxiety, and moderate hypotension in most cases. Continuing responses depend on the status of total body fluid volume. In most cases of peritonitis, patients are hypovolemic and a hypodynamic response pattern is seen. Successful early fluid resuscitation may convert the hypodynamic response to a hyperdynamic one. If sepsis continues uncontrolled, major functional deficits appear in the vital organ systems which are essential to survival, and death ensues.

bacteria as well as residual active enzymes which increase the severity of peritonitis and prevent effective local sequestration.

INFLUENCE OF ADJUVANTS. The virulence of peritonitis not only is determined by the nature of the contaminating mixture of bacteria and the duration of peritoneal soiling, but is importantly influenced by the presence of adjuvant substances such as mucus and hemoglobin. Trauma or any foreign body will retard the clearance of bacteria from the peritoneal cavity and can act as an adjuvant. Foreign substances which are proteinaceous in nature seem to be particularly associated with enhanced virulence.

Experimentally, the presence of an adjuvant nearly always is necessary to produce lethal peritonitis. Intraperitoneal injections of bacteria can be made lethal by the addition of such foreign substances as bile salts, talc, gum tragacanth, gastric mucin, or blood. The enhancement of virulence is attributed to the adverse effect of these adjuvant substances on defense mechanisms, particularly phagocytosis. The body apparently does not differentiate between contaminating bacteria and the contaminating adjuvant, attacking both with vigor. The presence of the adjuvant dilutes the net effectiveness of phagocytosis, since a proportion of leukocytes is diverted to phagocytosis of the adjuvant, retarding clearance of bacteria from the peritoneal cavity.

Hemoglobin seems to be a particularly noxious adjuvant in both experimental and clinical peritonitis. Hemoglobin, certainly as is true of any adjuvant, retards clearance of bacteria from the peritoneal cavity. However, there also is evidence that hemoglobin exerts an additional toxic effect, possibly because of the action of pigments or of ferrous iron liberated when hemoglobin is degraded.

Experimentally, if a pure suspension of *Escherichia coli* containing 10^9 organisms per milliliter is injected intraperitoneally into experimental animals in a dose of 5 ml/kg, all animals survive. But if 3 to 4 mg/100 ml of hemoglobin is combined with the same dose of *E. coli* organisms, lethal peritonitis is produced in 90 percent of animals. These observations are pertinent to the problem of peritonitis in human beings, since hemoglobin frequently is present in peritoneal fluid in clinical peritonitis.

Recently, Hau and coworkers have shown that hemoglobin inhibits the normal chemotactic responses of polymorphonuclear neutrophils and, therefore, might inhibit either migration of polymorphs into the peritoneal cavity or their subsequent attachment to and lysis of bacteria.

INAPPROPRIATE THERAPY. Peritonitis may be spread by errors of omission as well as by errors of commission. A frequently fatal error of omission is failure to diagnose the presence of a ruptured viscus and to undertake surgical control of the source of contamination of the peritoneum in timely fashion. Another error of omission occurs in efforts to control a persisting or expanding intraabdominal infection by administration of antibiotics without adequate surgical debridement or drainage. Subsequent rupture of an undrained abscess will broadcast highly virulent contents throughout the abdomen, often with fatal consequences. Conversely, an error of commission may occur if laxatives or enemas are administered to patients suffering abdominal pain. This practice seems to be on the wane, although occasional cases of injudicious catharsis are still seen. The bowel, stimulated to motility when otherwise it would be becoming quiescent, interferes with the walling-off process of localization which body defense mechanisms otherwise would dictate.

Pathophysiology of Sepsis

The presence of bacteria in suppurative peritonitis leads to a number of both local and systemic responses which are related directly to the effects of the microorganisms or their products. These responses are in addition to and superimposed on the general pathophysiologic responses which occur in all cases of peritonitis.

TOXIC ABSORPTION. The inflamed peritoneum acts as a bidirectionally permeable membrane, not only secreting fluid into the peritoneal cavity in the presence of peritonitis but also permitting ready absorption of both bacteria and bacterial toxins from peritoneal fluid. Endotoxins derived from the cell wall of aerobic gram-negative bacilli, such as *Escherichia coli,* are most frequently involved and are the most important in these systemic responses, although absorption of preformed exotoxins, elaborated by gram-positive organisms such as *Clostridia,* are the dominant influence in occasional cases.

Endotoxin is a lipopolysaccharide. It acts primarily on blood vessels, producing arteriolar and venular dilation and loss of endothelial integrity. Capillary leakage, accumulation of fluid in tissues, and intraorgan shunting are some of the consequences of endotoxin action which lead to the clinical features of septic shock. Exotoxins, in contrast, are proteins. They cause hemolysis of red cells or destruction of other body cells, or interfere with metabolic or other cellular processes. Exotoxins also cause peripheral arteriolar dilation, but the effects of exotoxins tend to be more cellularly specific and less totally pervasive compared with endotoxins.

Gram-negative sepsis of major proportions often begins with chills, rapid elevation of the temperature above 38.5°C, and moderate hypotension. Because of predominant peripheral vasodilation, the clinical picture often is characterized as "warm" shock unless the effects of hypovolemia predominate, in which case the clinical picture is of more typical "cold" shock.

The severity of septic shock varies depending on the amount and duration of exposure of body tissues to circulating gram-negative organisms and their endotoxins. Transient, self-limited bacteremia may produce minimal adverse systemic effects, whereas persisting or repetitive episodes of septicemia overwhelm the vital cardiorespiratory and renal support systems and, obviously, result in a much poorer prognosis. The presence of underlying disease of the cardiac, pulmonary, hepatic, or renal systems renders the patient more susceptible to development of septicemia and also impairs responses to the endotoxemic insult.

There are considerable species differences in the response to endotoxemia. Though the use of experimental animal models has contributed a great deal to our understanding of this entity, direct extrapolation of findings in animals to human septic shock cannot be made. For example, injection of lipopolysaccharide endotoxin in a dog causes splanchnic pooling as a consequence of hepatic venous constriction. Decreased venous return, reduction in cardiac output, and an abrupt fall in blood pressure follow immediately after injection of endotoxin. This pattern is very different from that seen in subhuman primates and in human beings, in whom injection of endotoxin produces chills, fever, transient vasoconstriction, then peripheral vasodilation; cardiac output initially rises and then declines.

There also are differences in response to experimental injection of preformed endotoxin as compared with septicemia produced by injection of live bacteria. Hypoglycemia and hypoinsulinemia are regularly observed after live E. coli–induced shock; hyperglycemia is a consistent hallmark in endotoxin-infused models. Renal fibrin thrombi (DIC) are present after live E. coli administration, while tubular necrosis is found following both organism and endotoxin infusions. Liver dysfunction is indicated by elevation of blood levels of hepatic enzymes and morphologic alterations in both models. The condition of the live E. coli–injected baboon appears to bear a closer similarity to the clinical entity of septic shock than does the endotoxin-treated animal.

Renal morphologic changes induced during experimental septic shock can be prevented by administration of heparin, although in all other respects, heparin-treated animals are identical to unheparinized animals in their reactions to injection of live organisms or endotoxin and suffer the same mortality risk. In particular, abnormal renal function, as reflected in rising BUN, creatinine, and uric acid levels, is not modified by administration of heparin.

INFLUENCE OF HYPOVOLEMIA IN SEPSIS. Septic shock in normovolemic patients begins with a hyperdynamic response associated with increased cardiac output, normal or high central venous pressure, low peripheral resistance, warm extremities despite a low blood pressure, hyperventilation, and respiratory alkalosis.

When sepsis is superimposed on hypovolemia, the typical situation in peritonitis, an initial hypodynamic pattern usually is present characterized by low cardiac output, low central venous pressure, vasoconstriction with high peripheral resistance, cold extremities, and low blood pressure. Expansion of venous capacitance vessels, together with the accumulation of fluid in the tissues as a result of capillary leakage (both effects of endotoxin), creates an additional functional "third-space" loss of fluid.

Hypovolemic septicemia is an unstable situation, since the peripheral vasoconstriction which is maintaining circulation to the heart and brain may, at any time, yield to the vasodilating effect of endotoxin, resulting in sudden loss of peripheral resistance and deep shock out of proportion to the degree of measurable hypovolemia. This form of combined shock does not respond completely to replenishment of fluid volume, but in the absence of overt cardiac failure, conversion to a hyperdynamic state despite continuing hypotension may be seen and is associated with a more favorable prognosis. If treatment is delayed or unsuccessful, circulatory failure, a low, fixed cardiac output, resistant metabolic acidosis, and death ensue.

RESPIRATORY RESPONSES IN SEPSIS. Compromise of vascular endothelial integrity in the lung as a consequence of the actions of endotoxin results in leakage of fluid from pulmonary arterioles and capillaries into the interstitial pulmonary space. The accumulating fluid makes the lungs stiffer (loss of compliance) and also results in pulmonary vascular hypertension. Interstitial edema also acts, in effect, as a barrier between pulmonary capillaries and adjacent alveoli, retarding uptake of oxygen and producing mild hypoxemia. Compensatory hyperventilation and respiratory alkalosis result. At this stage, there is little clinical or x-ray evidence of pulmonary compromise. It is worth emphasizing that the development of mild hyperventilation, respiratory alkalosis, and an altered sensorium may be the earliest signs of gram-negative sepsis; this triad may precede more obvious signs of sepsis or shock by many hours.

As pulmonary edema progresses, protein-rich fluid accumulates in alveoli. Directly or indirectly, endotoxemia also leads to a loss of pulmonary surfactant, promoting alveolar collapse and progressive pulmonary consolidation. The chest x-ray now shows patchy infiltrates diffusely in the lungs. Maintenance of circulation to areas of the lung which have lost effective capacity for oxygen uptake produces a ventilation-perfusion inequality. In addition, excessive beta-adrenergic stimulation is common in sepsis and causes opening of splanchnic and pulmonary arteriovenous shunts.

The effect of both functional and actual intrapulmonary shunting is entry of poorly oxygenated pulmonary blood into the general arterial circulation. This leads to tissue hypoxia, further compensatory hyperventilation, and respiratory alkalosis. "Respiratory distress syndrome," "septic lung," "shock lung," and "white lung" are some of the terms which have been used to describe the clinical and radiologic effects of this process. Subsequently, the picture frequently is one of rapid deterioration of pulmonary function, confluence of patchy infiltrates, and severe hypoxemia.

RENAL RESPONSE. The decrease in glomerular perfusion and filtration brought about by hypovolemia in peritonitis is reinforced by the endotoxin-induced opening of intrarenal shunts at the corticomedullary level. The blood circulating to the kidneys now preferentially perfuses more central renal tissues, while the cortex receives little blood flow at all. This phenomenon of "corticomedullary disconnection" produces a profound decrease in glomerular perfusion and results, when fully elaborated, in formation of little glomerular filtrate. As a consequence, urine flow is greatly diminished; this is recognized clinically by failure of urine output accompanied by progressive accumulation of unexcreted acidic end products of metabolism and metabolic acidosis. Recent evidence also indicates that prolonged sepsis in some cases may be accompanied by development of proliferative glomerulonephritis leading not only to acute renal failure but also to chronic renal insufficiency in survivors.

LEUKOCYTE FUNCTION. Both neutrophil and lymphocyte function are abnormal in patients suffering severe sepsis. Skin test anergy in septic patients is associated both with defects in cellular function and with the presence in serum of inhibitors of white cell function. These effects are reflected in abnormal neutrophil chemotactic responses and in decreased ability of lymphocytes to form rosettes. Severe infections also are associated with consumption of large amounts of antibody, decreases in concentration of complement in serum, and consumption of opsonic proteins which further hampers neutrophil responses to invading bacteria.

END-ORGAN FAILURE. The interaction of hypovolemia and endotoxemia in suppurative peritonitis is particularly vicious. Unless prompt and effective therapy is instituted, the multiple deleterious organ effects reinforce one another in a progressively worsening cycle of events. The elevated metabolic rate and great caloric expenditure, as well as local circulatory effects of extensive inflammation in peritonitis, contribute to a need for a greatly increased cardiac output. Increased respiratory efforts to correct acidosis are incapacitated by the inability of the already inadequate circulation to provide additional perfusion and oxygenation required by the muscles of respiration. Administration of fluid and electrolytes, respiratory support, reduction of body temperature, and maintenance of nutrition all may contribute to survival, but if these measures are not successful, pulmonary failure is followed rapidly by cardiorenal failure and death.

Clinical Manifestations

The patient with suppurative peritonitis presents all the features which characterize peritonitis in general: a distended, tender, painful abdomen; rapid, shallow respiration; fever; and tachycardia. The acute symptoms are of short duration and rapid progression, although occasional patients report symptoms suggesting past subacute or chronic disease.

The history and location of pain in the abdomen may provide clues to the possible organ source of peritonitis. Pain may increase or decrease at the time of viscus rupture. Thereafter, the story is one of progressively worse pain, initially diffuse but tending to localize if peritoneal defense mechanisms can contain the spillage. Tenderness increases, percussion tenderness appears or worsens, bowel sounds diminish and disappear, muscular rigidity replaces guarding, distension worsens. Leukocytosis with a left shift is usual but may not be marked in elderly or debilitated patients, or in patients with advanced peritonitis in whom trapping of neutrophils in the peritoneal cavity has occurred. Abdominal x-ray films may show paralytic ileus, free air, or atelectatic changes in the lung bases.

In some cases of septic peritonitis, fever may be misleading. Subnormal temperatures may occur, particularly later in the course of sepsis, because body compensatory mechanisms are unable to prevent hypothermia consequent upon peripheral vasodilation. Shock, due to accumulation of fluid in peripheral tissues as well as failure of compensatory vasoconstrictive mechanisms, is out of proportion to the degree of measurable hypovolemia.

In patients with generalized peritonitis, serum bilirubin and alkaline phosphatase levels demonstrate an irregular relationship. Sepsis is known to be associated with jaundice; it has been shown that some endotoxins inhibit mitochondrial respiration in human liver preparations. Among 44 fatal cases of peritonitis, 31 patients had an elevated bilirubin and 34 an elevated alkaline phosphatase level. When jaundice appeared after the ninth postoperative day or bilirubin exceeded 15.5 mg%, the outcome invariably was fatal. In 13 out of 14 patients, the reason for late onset of jaundice was traced to unsuspected peritoneal soiling from a leaking anastomosis. The presence of persisting or recurring hyperbilirubinemia is a warning sign of an intraabdominal abscess or leaking anastomosis.

Management

Initially, both therapeutic and diagnostic efforts are conducted simultaneously. Therapeutic efforts are directed to restoration of an effective total body fluid volume. Diagnosis is directed to the cause of the peritoneal sepsis. The objective is to determine the need for and the timing of operation.

Nonsurgical conditions simulating peritonitis should be considered and excluded. Pneumonia, particularly in the aged, often is accompanied by abdominal distension and ileus simulating a slowly progressive peritonitis. Diaphragmatic pleurisy may be associated with abdominal pain suggestive of acute cholecystitis or a perforated ulcer. Uremia commonly is associated with abdominal distension and ileus. A variety of other conditions, including acute gastroenteritis, ureteral calculi, and various female pelvic disorders such as twisted ovarian cyst, ectopic pregnancy, and ruptured ovarian follicle, may produce abdominal pain simulating early acute peritonitis.

PREOPERATIVE PREPARATION. The essential features of preoperative treatment of suppurative peritonitis involve (1) fluid resuscitation, (2) antibiotics, (3) oxygen and, if needed, ventilator support, and (4) nasogastric intubation, urinary catheterization, and monitoring of vital signs and biochemical and hemodynamic data. Additional measures which may need to be considered in an individual case are requirements for steroids, digitalis, and vasopressor drugs.

Patients are better served if major metabolic derangements and fluid deficits are corrected prior to operation, although inordinantly long periods of time cannot be taken in this exercise. Certain causes of peritonitis require more urgent intervention than others. For example, intestinal infarction demands nearly immediate intervention, whereas inflammatory perforation of the sigmoid colon with a developing fecal peritonitis will permit 1 or 2 hours of resuscitative effort prior to laparotomy.

Fluid Resuscitation. Large volumes of fluids may need to be administered very rapidly until blood volume and urine output are restored. In patients whose central venous pressure is less than 10 cm of water, fluid volume administration may go forward at as rapid a rate as can be achieved;

when the central venous pressure rises to 10 cm, the infusion rate can be slowed.

The most frequent mistake made in resuscitation of patients with advanced peritonitis and a major circulating blood volume deficit is that the rate of initial fluid administration is too slow. The slow rate is undertaken for fear of precipitating congestive heart failure. If the central venous pressure is monitored and the rate of infusion adjusted appropriately, congestive heart failure will not occur simply because initial fluid resuscitation is undertaken at rapid rates of administration. Fluids administered must include crystalloids for replacement of water and electrolytes functionally lost into "third-space" collections in the peritoneal cavity and bowel lumen. Whole blood or packed red blood cells are administered, if needed, to correct anemia and to maintain an adequate red cell mass (hematocrit, 30 to 35). The administration of colloid (albumin or plasma) is more controversial.

Crystalloid or Colloid. There is agreement that deficits in the interstitial fluid volume in patients with peritonitis should be replaced with a crystalloid solution, preferably Ringer's lactate. But controversy exists about replacement of the deficient plasma volume. Some authorities advocate administration of more crystalloid, others argue for administration of colloid.

The controversy over the relative merits of colloid versus large volumes of crystalloid solution as a replacement for plasma volume has raged for years. Proponents of each type of solution can cite evidence to support their view. The argument turns on the applicability of Starling's law to the pulmonary circulation, the liability to develop pulmonary edema, and the comparative efficiency of the two forms of therapy.

Though it is clear that albumin will restore an effective volume efficiently in terms of the total volume administered, the same end can be achieved if one gives three to four times as much crystalloid solution. The theoretical advantages of administering albumin in resuscitation of patients suffering peritonitis are that salt overload, peripheral edema, and weight gain are less likely. Administering balanced salt solutions in excess might result in interstitial fluid accumulation in the lung because of a reduction in the colloid osmotic pressure–pulmonary capillary wedge pressure gradient. This hypothesis is based on Starling's law of fluid movement across a semipermeable membrane, which, in essence, indicates that net movement of fluid is governed by the algebraic sum of the hydrostatic and colloid osmotic pressures on the two sides of the membrane.

However, it appears from experimental evidence that the oncotic pressure gradient as it relates to the alveolar-capillary membrane is not an important factor in the development of pulmonary edema. In studies in which pulmonary capillary wedge pressure has been measured, no relationship between colloid osmotic pressure or intrapulmonary pressure gradients and the development of pulmonary edema has been identified. Liability to development of pulmonary interstitial edema is related primarily to the degree of endothelial leakiness resulting from the actions of endotoxin, rather than being related to the type of resuscitation fluid. Colloid solutions are theoretically more efficient but also are more expensive and less readily available. Crystalloid solutions are readily available and more economical but require administration of a large volume excess which must later be excreted by the kidneys. Both types of solution are equally liable to be associated with pulmonary edema due to leakage from endotoxin-injured pulmonary capillaries; exclusive crystalloid resuscitation is more likely to be associated with pulmonary edema due to volume overload. We usually rely mainly on crystalloid solutions for resuscitation of most patients with septic peritonitis, but do employ partial colloid resuscitation in patients known to have preexisting cardiopulmonary disease.

Antibiotic Therapy. Although the actual organisms may not be known, intraabdominal infection should be presumed in every case of suspected septic peritonitis. Antibiotics which are effective against the full spectrum of aerobic and anaerobic gastrointestinal bacteria should be started as soon as feasible, either as a direct intravenous injection or rapidly instilled intravenously in a small volume of fluid from a subsidiary reservoir. Therapeutic levels of antibiotics should be present in the tissues at the time of operation. We currently administer gentamicin and clindamycin in full dosage to all patients suspected of having suppurative peritonitis.

Experimental evidence indicates that antibiotics which are effective against *Escherichia coli* are most important in reducing the mortality risk of experimental fecal septicemia. Drugs effective against *E. coli* include the cephalosporins, aminoglycosides, and chloramphenicol; tetracyclines and ampicillin also are active against many coliforms. Control of later liability to abscess formation, on the other hand, requires the additional administration of an antibiotic effective against anaerobic *Bacteroides fragilis*. Drugs effective against *B. fragilis* include clindamycin, chloramphenicol, metronidazole, and erythromycin; tetracycline and carbenicillin also may be active against this bacterium.

Oxygen and Ventilator Support. Oxygen is administered to help the response to the increased metabolic demands of peritonitis which are so often associated with impairment of pulmonary ventilatory function that mild hypoxia is common. A nasal catheter supplying oxygen at about 5 liters/minute usually is sufficient prior to induction of anesthesia. Assessment of respiratory function should be made clinically, noting apparent tidal volume and work of breathing. If impairment is suspected, measurement of ventilatory volume and arterial blood gases is indicated.

Ventilatory support, with an inspired gas concentration of 40 percent oxygen, should be initiated in patients whose arterial oxygen pressure falls below 70 mmHg. Addition of positive end-expiratory pressure (PEEP) to ventilator support is indicated in patients whose F_{O_2} is below 60 mmHg or who develop other evidence of more severe respiratory embarrassment. Efforts to maintain a normal or even rightward-positioned oxygen-hemoglobin dissociation curve are worthwhile, since red blood cell organic phosphates are reduced in sepsis.

Intubation, Catheterization, and Monitoring. Nasogastric intubation is performed to evacuate the stomach, prevent further vomiting, and, most importantly, reduce accumulation of additional air in the paralyzed bowel. Urinary catheterization is utilized to record initial volume and to monitor subsequent urinary output.

A central venous catheter should be placed to assess current hydration and intravenous replacement. Percutaneous subclavian vein catheterization is preferred except in infants, where it is easier and safer to place an internal jugular catheter. A chest roentgenogram after subclavian or jugular catheter placement is imperative to assure correct placement of the catheter tip and the absence of a pneumothorax or other complication. If pulmonary insufficiency or cardiac failure exists, placement of a Swan-Ganz catheter for direct measurement of pulmonary artery and wedge pressures is very helpful in precise fluid administration and avoidance of pulmonary edema.

Vital signs such as temperature, blood pressure, pulse and respiration rates are recorded every 4 hours, and more often if need be. Preoperative biochemical evaluation should include measurement of serum electrolytes, creatinine, glucose, bilirubin, and alkaline phosphatase, and a urinalysis.

Steroids. Administration of pharmacologic doses of steroids to septic patients has been advocated on the basis of experimental work in dogs but its advisability in the treatment of patients remains controversial. Recent clinical studies support the idea that large doses of potent steroids reduce the mortality risk in sepsis, particularly if given before or early after the onset of shock.

Steroids are not needed preoperatively in most cases of suppurative peritonitis. But if the patient's condition seems unstable or the symptomatic history is relatively long, consideration should be given to steroid administration. An initial intravenous dose of 30 mg methylprednisolone, or 5 mg dexamethasone, is given over 5 to 10 minutes, and may be repeated in 2 to 3 hours. If a beneficial response is obtained, additional injections usually are not needed. If no response is seen after two doses, continued administration of steroids is unlikely to have any effect.

Vasoactive Drugs. Experimentally, the effects of intraperitoneal injection of *E. coli* are not altered by the administration of alpha or beta blockers, phentolamine, propranolol, reserpine, or serotonin. By contrast, when *Staphylococcus aureus,* an exotoxin-producing organism, is used for challenge, administration of reserpine, serotonin, or the combination of phentolamine and propranolol significantly prolongs life.

Drugs with predominant alpha-adrenergic effects are of limited value in the treatment of sepsis secondary to peritonitis, since artificial attempts to maintain blood pressure by inducing vasoconstriction without thought to its consequences on tissue blood flow are potentially harmful. When volume replacement and other measures have failed to restore an adequate circulation, administration of isoproterenol may be helpful. Isoproterenol has potent inotropic and chronotropic effects on the heart. One or two milligrams of isoproterenol diluted in 500 ml of 5% dextrose in water may be administered by intravenous drip at a rate of 1 to 2 μg/minute, depending on the response. The infusion should be slowed or stopped completely if significant tachycardia (above 140 beats per minute) or cardiac arrhythmias occur. A fall in blood pressure in the absence of cardiac arrhythmia resulting from administration of isoproterenol indicates a need for additional volume replacement to maintain cardiac filling. The combination of isoproterenol stimulation of the heart together with effective volume resuscitation may restore tissue blood flow even though the blood pressure remains low.

Digitalis. Cardiac status should be assessed preoperatively in middle-aged or older patients by interpretation of a current electrocardiogram. Digitalis is not administered routinely. But gram-negative sepsis and shock frequently are superimposed on congestive failure in older patients or may precipitate early congestive failure in patients with limited cardiac reserve. In these instances, digitalis should be administered cautiously, with attention to its potential for toxicity if the patient is hypokalemic or also receiving isoproterenol.

Fever. A temperature above 38.5°C may be associated with difficulties in administration of anesthesia. Patients with such hyperthermia, and also those with hypothermia, should have their temperature corrected toward normal prior to operation. Administration of salicylates often will be effective in reducing fever. If not, or if the patient is hypothermic, a cooling-warming mattress should be employed.

Narcotics. Analgesic drugs should not be administered to patients with suspected peritonitis until a diagnosis has been made or, at least, a decision to operate has been made. The reason is that analgesia may obscure abdominal findings and hamper establishment of a diagnosis of peritonitis. Equally, once a decision to operate has been made, pain should be relieved with potent narcotics. Morphine is preferred to other drugs and should be given in small intravenous doses of 1 to 3 mg, frequently repeated, to maintain the patient's comfort. Small intravenous doses are safer than the traditional larger intramuscular doses, particularly in patients whose condition is unstable.

OPERATIVE MANAGEMENT. The incision of choice in adults is vertically in the midline. This incision can be extended from xiphoid to pubis, provides ready access to all quadrants of the abdomen, and is the quickest to open and to close. Transverse incisions are safer in patients under two years of age because of a propensity for postoperative dehiscence in infants. Another exception to the general recommendation for use of a vertical midline incision occurs in the presence of localized peritonitis, in which the objective is to open directly over the inflammatory process, avoiding contamination of other quadrants of the abdomen.

Objectives. The fundamental objective of the operation is to control the source of peritoneal contamination. The general principles of operative management include closure of perforations of the stomach and small bowel but exteriorization with fecal diversion of colonic perforations. As an example, management of acute perforated diverticulitis with generalized peritonitis by resection of the involved segment of sigmoid colon, temporary end colostomy, and peritoneal toilet is associated with survival of 9 of 10 patients. Alternative forms of management of this disorder, particularly attempts at a colonic anastomosis in the presence of peritonitis, are associated with a higher mortality risk.

Odor and Staining of Peritoneal Pus. Immediately on opening the abdomen, any odor should be noted and a representative sample of peritoneal pus sent for Gram stain and culture. An immediate report of the results of the Gram stain should be requested.

The odor of peritonitis pus is of diagnostic importance in relation to the bacteriology of suppurative peritonitis. Altemeier studied the ability of *E. coli* to produce a putrid odor when grown on sterile human pus and found that no odor resulted, although good growth of bacteria was obtained. On the other hand, when similar sterile pus was inoculated with anaerobic streptococci and *Bacteroides meleninogenicus,* a marked, penetrating foul odor was produced after 3 days of incubation under anaerobic conditions. In addition to these two organisms, other anaerobic bacteria, particularly members of the *Clostridium* group, recovered from pus of peritonitis are capable of producing strong odors.

The general rule is that aerobic infections do not produce a marked odor, whereas infections containing anerobes do. Combining information provided by the odor of the pus in peritonitis with the structure of bacteria noted on a Gram stain of the same material will permit a presumptive diagnosis of the infecting organisms.

Debridement of Exudate. All peritoneal pus, pseudomembranes, fibrin, and other exudates, as well as the content of any localized collections or abscesses, should be completely excised once the source of the peritonitis has been controlled. Gentle dissection of all adhesions and plications of bowel and mesentery should be done together with excision of pus and exudate from the subhepatic, subdiaphragmatic, and pelvic cavities. Although debridement has been a controversial issue, it is now clear that it has a salutary effect on mortality risk in peritonitis. For example, debridement was associated with no mortality in a group of 92 patients with peritonitis reported by Hudspeth.

Lavage. Debridement is followed by irrigation with saline solution of all parts of the peritoneal cavity until the effluent is clear. Washing the contaminated peritoneal cavity with large volumes of irrigant was first advocated by Price in 1905. The next year, Torek reported that the large-volume irrigation technique reduced mortality in general peritonitis following appendicitis to 14 percent, an extremely good experience at the time of this report. The procedure later fell into disrepute because of the fear, still widely held but never clinically proved, that lavage disseminates peritoneal contamination.

Burnett reintroduced peritoneal lavage in the management of suppurative peritonitis, and reported a two-thirds reduction in mortality. The modern concept of peritoneal lavage views the contaminated peritoneum in the same way as a contaminated dermal wound: copious irrigation is

a major component of therapy and involves the use of large volumes, up to 10 liters, of saline solution and occasionally more, with the objective of diluting and removing all the contaminated peritoneal content.

Antibiotic Lavage. The addition of antibiotics to peritoneal lavage solutions is associated with decreased mortality and a lower incidence of infected wounds in cases of purulent peritonitis. Under usual circumstances, antibiotics are used only in the final "rinse" of the peritoneum, plain normal saline solution or Ringer's lactate being used for lavage to clear most of the peritoneal exudate. A variety of antibiotic solutions has been demonstrated to be effective. We prefer the kanamycin-bacitracin solution recommended by Noon and associates.

Reports concerning the effectiveness of noxytiolin or povidone-iodine solutions for peritoneal lavage have been mixed. The most recent controlled clinical studies indicate that neither agent is as effective as solutions containing antibiotics.

Patients with severe peritonitis who fail to improve despite correction of the source of infection and appropriate therapy with fluids and systemic antibiotics may benefit from postoperative peritoneal lavage with an antibiotic solution. Experience with multiple instillations of intraperitoneal kanamycin or cephalosporins in patients who had perforated appendicitis or generalized peritonitis confirms that this is a rational form of treatment.

Antibiotic lavage can be conducted using a single catheter for infusion and subsequent drainage, or an infusion catheter can be used simultaneously with another catheter or other drains to provide egress of lavage solution. Irrigation catheters should be placed during laparotomy if the need for postoperative antibiotic lavage can be anticipated. Lavage will result in absorption of some variable fraction of the antibiotic employed; this effect needs to be taken into account in managing overall antibiotic administration.

Closure. If a midline wound has been used, the fascia may be closed as a single layer with running monofilament suture (Prolene, nylon, or wire), taking generous bites of tissue on either side. Some surgeons recommend use of interrupted fascial suture technique and also favor placement of additional retention sutures; the reason advanced for recommending these more tedious suture techniques is a supposed reduction in the incidence of wound dehiscence. However, the occurrence of dehiscence in suppurative peritonitis is primarily due to infection in the wound; septic wounds are likely to fail to heal whatever suture technique is used for closure; interrupted or retention sutures will not prevent subsequent dehiscence.

The skin and subcutaneous portions of the wound usually should be left open. A few layers of fine gauze soaked in antibiotic irrigating solution are used to cover the subcutaneous tissues, but the wound should not be tightly packed. Dry gauze dressings then lightly cover the wound. All dressings, including those within the wound, are removed in about 48 hours and replaced with a simple covering bandage. Secondary closure with adhesive strips can be done 4 or 5 days later if the wound remains healthy.

POSTOPERATIVE MANAGEMENT. The general principles

of postoperative care include continued administration of intravenous fluids and antibiotics. Complications of sepsis —particularly respiratory failure, renal failure, and disseminated intravascular coagulation—should be expected and searched for continuously by monitoring ventilatory volumes, urine output, blood gases, serum creatinine, and coagulation factors. A rise in bilirubin level may indicate the presence of a persistent or recurrent intraabdominal abscess which requires prompt reoperation and drainage.

When the results of antibiotic sensitivity studies done on the operative specimen of peritoneal pus are available, consideration should be given to changing antibiotic therapy to the most specific and least toxic of the drugs which appear to be effective (see Chap. 5). Antibiotic treatment should not be stopped until the patient is clinically well enough to be consuming a regular diet, or other clinical evidence indicates that residual infection is unlikely.

ASEPTIC (CHEMICAL) PERITONITIS

This form of peritonitis develops whenever irritant materials gain entry into the peritoneal cavity, usually because of rupture of a solid or upper abdominal viscus. The soilage initially is sterile or nearly so, a feature by which chemical peritonitis differs from suppurative peritonitis. The aseptic inflammatory reaction gives rise to the general clinical symptoms and physiologic sequellae of peritonitis. Translocation of plasma volume into the peritoneal cavity with the secondary systemic responses to hypovolemia, discussed above under general responses to peritonitis, is the major initial reaction.

Secondary bacterial invasion commonly occurs, sometimes as early as 12 hours after the initial peritoneal insult, even when no bacteria enter the peritoneal cavity via a perforated viscus or from the environment through a traumatic wound. In fact, presumably because episodes of transient bacteremia are relatively common though ordinarily innocuous, an initially aseptic peritonitis cannot be expected to remain sterile. Most of the substances which cause aseptic peritonitis are capable of acting as adjuvants whenever secondary bacterial contamination occurs, promoting proliferation of microorganisms and, later, the onset of the systemic effects of suppurative peritonitis.

Symptoms typically are sudden, severe pain, and tenderness and rigidity of the abdominal muscles. Backache occurs if the retroperitoneal area is involved. During the next few hours, peritoneal fluid dilution and neutralization of the irritant may produce a deceptive sense of improvement. Leukocytosis is present. Plain abdominal and chest films are useful in showing specific injuries after trauma, bowel distension, and intraabdominal fluid accumulation. The most helpful diagnostic test in some situations, apart from exploratory laparotomy itself, is a peritoneal tap.

The principles of surgical management in cases of aseptic peritonitis include preoperative resuscitation with fluids and similar measures; control of the source of contamination during laparotomy by suture closure or excision, as appropriate; debridement of foreign substances; copious lavage; and administration of antibiotics to combat the risks of existing infection.

GASTRIC CONTENTS. Gastric juice is highly irritating to the perineum, not only because of its hydrochloric acid content but also because of the presence of mucin and digestive enzymes. If gastric juice gains access to the peritoneal cavity through a perforated duodenal ulcer, spilled material initially is sterile in the majority of cases because the normal "acid barrier" of the stomach effectively kills swallowed microorganisms. It must be remembered, however, that in cases of perforated gastric ulcer, in which a high proportion of patients have a defective gastric acid barrier to bacteria, the spilled gastric juice regularly is contaminated with swallowed aerobic and anaerobic organisms chiefly originating in the oral (mouth) flora.

In gastroduodenal perforation, the interval between the occurrence of the perforation and its closure is viewed by many surgeons as the primary determinant of postoperative morbidity and mortality. But Hamilton and Harbrecht, in a review of patients with perforated ulcer, found the degree of peritoneal contamination and the incidence of contaminating virulent pathogens greater when operation was performed 6 hours or less after perforation than in operations done after 24 hours. The incidence of negative cultures in this study (about 50 percent) was the same whether spillage was light or marked. Postoperative complications (64 percent of which were septic) were related only to the presence of marked spillage. This apparent paradox must be due partially to peritoneal fluid dilution which occurs during the initial inflammatory response to the peritoneal insult. Unfortunately, the use and duration of antibiotic therapy in these patients was not recorded.

The findings in this study are in contrast to the usually accepted surgical wisdom which indicates that the incidence of peritoneal contamination by virulent pathogens is less when operation is performed within 6 hours of perforation compared with later operative times. The important point illustrated by this study is that taking sufficient time preoperatively to complete fluid resuscitation and otherwise prepare the patient for operation is rewarded by a reduction in mortality risk.

PANCREATIC JUICE. Pancreatic secretions enter the peritoneal cavity during episodes of acute pancreatitis or following pancreatic trauma. If the mode of entry is due to rupture of a pancreatic duct or pseudocyst, with release of relatively large volumes of activated pancreatic juice, pancreatic ascites ensues. Because the pancreatic juice is diluted in the ascites, the overall peritoneal reaction varies considerably, from mild to relatively severe inflammation. Alternatively, pancreatic juice may transude through the retroperitoneum in acute pancreatitis. In these cases, typically, the volume of accumulating intraperitoneal fluid is less. If the pancreatic exudate is combined with blood and breakdown products of pancreatic necrosis, as is true in cases of hemorrhagic pancreatitis, secondary infection occurs in a higher proportion of instances.

BILE. Most commonly bile enters the peritoneal cavity as a result of leakage following exploration of the common bile duct or other operation on the biliary system. Rupture of the gallbladder during acute cholecystitis, perforation of a gallbladder carcinoma, or, infrequently, rupture of the common duct due to necrosis from a common duct stone also may lead to spill of bile into the peritoneal cavity. Although bile peritonitis follows rupture of an inflamed gallbladder, biliary peritonitis can occur without detectable gallbladder perforation. In such cases, presumably, the mechanism for leakage of bile involves transudation through an ischemic portion of the acutely inflamed gallbladder wall.

Sterile bile is a chemical irritant in its own right. Frequently, bacterial contamination, either associated with the rupture itself or having been acquired secondarily, leads to a particularly virulent form of septic biliary peritonitis. Experimental studies of bile peritonitis have shown that both inflammation and lethality in animals are reduced if therapeutic serum levels of antibiotics have been achieved at the time of biliary leakage.

URINE. Intraperitoneal rupture of the bladder usually is a sequella of severe trauma. Sterile urine is an extremely irritating substance, and the chemical insult frequently is followed by secondary infection. Spontaneous intraperitoneal perforation of the urinary bladder also occurs in neurologically handicapped patients. Necrosis of the bladder wall in these patients, secondary to chronic intramural infection, results in spill of infected urine into the peritoneal cavity.

ACUTE HEMOPERITONEUM (ABDOMINAL APOPLEXY). Intraperitoneal blood is not irritating at all. If red cells lyse, the released cell contents act as a mild hyperosmolar irritant. Blood can be transfused intraperitoneally; the rate at which red cells subsequently enter the general circulation is slow, but the fraction of a transfused unit of blood detectable in the circulating blood volume 48 to 96 hours after intraperitoneal injection is the same as after an intravenous transfusion. It is not blood, per se, which is of concern in relation to peritonitis, but the fact that blood or, more particularly, hemoglobin and ferrous iron act as adjuvants of a particularly noxious sort should subsequent bacterial infection of the peritoneal cavity occur.

Spontaneous rupture of a visceral artery, most frequently the splenic and less commonly a gastroepiploic artery, or rupture of the spleen, liver, or a hepatic tumor, may produce a massive acute hemoperitoneum. The clinical symptoms are of abdominal pain accompanied by tenderness, absent bowel sounds, and other clinical signs suggestive of peritonitis. The leukocyte count may be elevated. Treatment consists of early laparotomy and control of the bleeding source.

MECONIUM. Intrauterine perforation of the bowel with leakage of sterile meconium produces a marked sterile peritonitis, resulting in matted adhesive obliteration of the abdominal cavity. If the bowel perforation remains uncontrolled after birth of the infant, secondary bacterial infection is the rule, the outlook in such cases is grim (see Chap. 39).

CHYLE. Chronic chylous effusions either into the peritoneal cavity as chylous ascites or into the chest as chylothorax are not rare; acute symptoms are unusual. Acute chylous peritonitis, on the other hand, which results from a sudden outpouring of chylous fluid into the free peritoneal cavity may produce signs and symptoms suggestive of an acute abdominal catastrophe but is a distinctly rare clinical syndrome.

MUCUS AND SIMILAR SUBSTANCES. Mucus from intestinal secretions released in small-bowel rupture or the contents from a ruptured ovarian cyst induce a sterile inflammatory reaction of the peritoneum. Rupture of a dermoid cyst of the ovary can produce a severe peritonitis, presumably because of the cyst content of cholesterol, hair, and other irritant materials.

ENDOTOXIC PERITONITIS. Under certain circumstances, constriction or occlusion of intestinal vessels produces sufficient ischemia that there is increased permeability of the bowel wall, permitting transudation of preformed endotoxin generated by the intestinal flora within the bowel lumen into the peritoneal cavity. Transperitoneal absorption of endotoxin then produces systemic symptoms of gram-negative sepsis. The degree of peritoneal inflammation, per se, in such instances ordinarily is not great unless bowel wall necrosis or perforation ensues. The vascular obstruction leading to this syndrome can involve either large or small bowel and may be segmental or extensive. A history of symptoms or episodes suggestive of arrhythmia or heart failure should be sought.

Generalized crampy abdominal pain, tenderness, low-grade fever, mental apathy or agitation, abdominal distension, and bowel hypomotility may be accompanied by vomiting, anorexia, and mucoid or bloody diarrhea. Leukocytosis with a left shift is consistently present. The serum amylase level is elevated, since amylase also escapes from the bowel into the peritoneal cavity and is absorbed. Plain films of the abdomen show only ileus. When mesenteric occlusion is suspected, arteriography may establish the diagnosis and also permits intraarterial vasodilator perfusion before and during laparotomy.

Episodes of aseptic endotoxic peritonitis also have been reported among patients undergoing chronic peritoneal dialysis. These cases are due to contamination of dialysis fluid by preformed coliform endotoxin. Onset of symptoms occurs on the average 7 hours after initiation of dialysis with the contaminated fluids. Diffuse abdominal pain and rebound tenderness are the predominant findings; fever is present in only about half the patients. Discontinuation of dialysis usually relieves the pain promptly, and the symptoms rapidly clear.

FOREIGN BODIES. A foreign body may be deposited in the peritoneal cavity during an operative procedure (sponge or instrument inadvertently left behind) or may result from penetrating injuries, with the penetrating missile itself or material carried with it (clothing, earth) acting as a foreign body. Foreign bodies such as fish bones, wood splinters, needles, pins, and glass may perforate the gastrointestinal or genitourinary tracts to enter the peritoneal cavity.

The relative amounts of acute exudation and later fibrosis vary greatly depending on the nature of the foreign body and the degree of bacterial contamination which occurs in conjunction with it. A foreign body may lead to formation of an abscess with an interval course of fever, chills, and toxicity, and the eventual appearance of an intraabdominal mass. On the other hand, small foreign bodies, such as shrapnel, simply may be walled off by fibrous tissue and give rise to few if any significant clinical manifestations.

BARIUM. Barium may be spilled into the peritoneal cavity during radiologic investigation of perforated bowel disease. The barium is extremely irritating and sets up a granulomatous peritoneal reaction similar to that of talc (see below). Simultaneous bacterial contamination occurs in every case if the perforation is in the colon, and in many cases if the perforation is in the stomach or duodenum. The association of barium and bacteria is more deleterious than either alone. Viable bacteria tend to be caught up in the granulomatous peritoneal reaction to barium, resulting in persisting foci of sepsis. The presence of these microabscesses increases the density and number of adhesions. In addition, any one may act as a nidus for development of a larger abscess.

Some years ago, by means of a mail survey of approximately 100 teaching institutions, Zheutlin and colleagues collected 53 cases of peritoneal contamination by barium following rupture of the colon. They found a relatively high percentage of perforation in barium enema examinations performed via a colostomy, with use of an inflatable rectal balloon, or immediately after proctoscopic examination.

Because the barium crystals used for radiologic investigation are so fine, it is practically impossible to remove all spilled barium from the peritoneal cavity. The best therapy, as in other situations, is prevention. If a perforation is suspected and radiologic investigation is essential, the initial study should be made with soluble contrast media. If the soluble contrast examination shows no evidence of perforation, careful barium contrast examination may be undertaken. The examination should be terminated at the first sign of perforation and the residual barium within the gastrointestinal lumen aspirated to reduce further spill. The patient should undergo an urgent laparotomy to control the site of perforation by exteriorization or suture closure.

Nonoperative management of barium peritonitis recently has been suggested; it relies on administration of broad-spectrum antibiotics and vigorous fluid therapy. The rationale in recommending nonoperative management of barium peritonitis is that it is impossible to remove all the barium. However, the degree of peritonitis is related only in part to the barium present in the peritoneal cavity; the perforation through which the barium leaked also needs to be controlled. Therefore, laparotomy seems the more reasonable management for most patients suffering intraperitoneal rupture of the bowel and barium spill.

GRANULOMATOUS PERITONITIS

This group of diseases is characterized by a peritoneal reaction which includes formation of granulomas and is associated with a markedly increased incidence of adhesion formation compared with other forms of peritonitis.

TUBERCULOUS PERITONITIS. Formerly quite common, the incidence of tuberculous peritonitis has declined, as has the incidence of all forms of human tuberculosis over the past several decades. This now is a rare disease; it usually occurs in patients who are malnourished or who have cirrhosis. The primary focus from which secondary involvement of the peritoneal cavity occurs in tuberculous peritonitis may not be clinically apparent. Although nearly all patients dying with tuberculous peritonitis have a primary focus identified at autopsy, in only about a third of cases currently being seen clinically is the primary focus readily diagnosed. In cases in which the primary focus remains obscure, almost always it is later demonstrated to be in the lung. Most cases are due to reactivation of latent peritoneal tuberculosis which had been established by hematogenous spread from a pulmonary focus during an earlier episode of acute disease. In the past, the disease has been classified into wet and dry phases. The "wet" phase refers to the early, subacute, ascitic stage of the disease, while the "dry" phase refers to later resolution, during which dense adhesions are formed.

Clinically, tuberculous peritonitis is insidious, presenting with fever, anorexia, weakness, and weight loss. Ascites almost always is present, and more than half of affected patients have dull, diffuse abdominal pain. On examination, the abdomen is modestly tender, but the classically described "doughy abdomen" is rarely found today. Clinical manifestations of generalized tuberculous infection are seen in about one-third of patients, and include anorexia, weight loss, and night sweats.

Tuberculous organisms can be retrieved 80 percent of the time from ascitic fluid if more than 1 liter of fluid is cultured. The ascitic fluid has an increased protein concentration, lymphocytic pleocytosis, and a glucose concentration below 30 mg/dl. Blind peritoneal biopsy is positive in about 60 percent of cases. If these measures do not establish the diagnosis, peritoneoscopy and guided direct biopsy of the peritoneum are recommended. The peritoneoscopic appearance of tuberculous peritonitis is quite characteristic. Typical stalactite-like fibrinous masses hang from the parietal peritoneum in the lower part of the abdomen. A directed, percutaneous needle biopsy of a granulomatous lesion, as well as samples of peritoneal fluid for direct smear examination and injection into a guinea pig, is obtained. As a last resort, exploratory laparotomy may be undertaken to establish the diagnosis. If laparotomy is carried out, a peritoneal biopsy should be obtained; the placement of drains or the exteriorization of bowel should be avoided.

Tuberculous peritonitis, formerly frequently fatal as a manifestation of uncontrolled generalized tuberculosis, now is arrested in nearly all patients. Triple antituberculous drug therapy, instituted early in the course of the disease, is associated with a good prognosis. Chemotherapy should continue for at least 2 years after the patient becomes asymptomatic. Since tuberculous peritonitis may heal with formation of dense fibrous adhesions, patients suffering this disease always are liable to the future development of an intestinal obstruction. Treatment with prednisone during the initial few months of antituberculous drug therapy reduces the incidence of adhesion formation and the subsequent development of obstruction.

OTHER GRANULOMATOUS PERITONEAL INFECTIONS. These are excessively rare diseases and occur under special circumstances. The organisms involved may be *Candida* or *Histoplasma* (fungi), or amebas or *Strongyloides* (parasites). *Candida* peritonitis seems to be associated with prolonged administration of broad-spectrum antibiotics to extremely debilitated patients who also are receiving parenteral alimentation or who have a prosthetic cardiac valve. Amebic peritonitis usually follows rupture of a hepatic amebic abscess, but a few cases have been due to perforation of amebic colitis. The prognosis is grave, but operative debridement results in a better outcome than nonoperative management.

IATROGENIC GRANULOMATOUS PERITONITIS. Peritoneal inflammation, exudation, formation of granulomas, and healing by formation of dense adhesions all may follow contamination of the peritoneal cavity by glove lubricants (talc, lycopodium, mineral oil, cornstarch, rice starch), or cellulose fibers from disposable gauze pads, drapes, and gowns. The reaction, particularly that to rice starch, is largely a hypersensitivity response.

The clinical features include migratory abdominal pain, fever, physical signs of peritonitis and, often, the presence of an abdominal mass, all developing within 3 weeks after an otherwise uncomplicated abdominal operation. The surgical wound may appear normal or may be moderately indurated. Plain abdominal films are nonspecific. The total white blood cell count is normal; eosinophilia of 4 to 9 percent sometimes is identified.

Laparoscopy may be helpful in establishing the diagnosis. If recognized with assurance, reoperation should be avoided and corticosteroids administered. Eventually, the acute peritonitis resolves. If laparotomy is undertaken because the diagnosis is obscure, a thickened peritoneum studded by white nodules is found. Histologically, the nodules, which contain starch granules, are doubly refractile under polarized light and are surrounded by granulomatous foreign body inflammation.

The cornerstone of management of this problem is prevention. Current techniques of wiping and washing gloves do not remove all the starch from their surface. Nonetheless, gloves should be washed or wiped off before hands are put into the peritoneal cavity and care should be taken to avoid spillage of glove contents should a glove be torn during an operation. The search for an acceptable and risk-free glove lubricant continues. Sodium bicarbonate has been used successfully as a gloving agent, but requires special sterilization measures; silicones also have been suggested.

SPONTANEOUS (PRIMARY) PERITONITIS

Spontaneous, or primary, peritonitis is a diffuse bacterial peritonitis without any apparent intraabdominal source of infection. Although still uncommon, the incidence of spontaneous peritonitis seems to be increasing. The currently reported prevalence is 3 percent in hospitalized cirrhotics and 8 percent in ascitic cirrhotics in pre-coma or coma.

The spectrum of bacteria causing this syndrome and the population primarily affected have changed during the last decade or so. Formerly, this disease occurred primarily in children; today, adults more often are affected. Formerly, females developed spontaneous peritonitis four times as frequently as males; today, there is no differential sex incidence. Formerly, gram-positive organisms caused most of these infections; today, gram-negative bacteria predominate.

Children with nephrosis and adults with cirrhosis or systemic lupus are the populations primarily affected. It appears that impairment of body immunological defense mechanisms is related to development of spontaneous peritonitis. The mortality risk is of the order of 20 to 40 percent in cirrhotic adults but lower in children. The relevance of preexisting ascites is not clear; ascites certainly provides an ideal culture medium. Any abnormal fluid collection appears to be at risk to develop infection in patients who are constitutionally predisposed; both spontaneous empyema and pericarditis have been reported in association with spontaneous peritonitis. On the other hand, adult patients have been described who had no preceding ascites, and the great majority of patients who develop spontaneous peritonitis in childhood do not have ascites.

This form of peritonitis is a monomicrobial infection; i.e., there is only a single species of bacteria present, in contrast to the polymicrobial infection of typical suppurative peritonitis. Though pneumococci formerly were the most frequent infecting organisms, coliform organisms now are the chief pathogens, accounting for over half of cases. Streptococcal infections still occur but are uncommon. In an increasing number of current cases, no bacteria are recovered but high viral titers are found in the serum. The bacterial spectrum also is broadening, recent single cases due to *Hemophilus*, *Clostridia*, *Pasteurella*, and *Bacteroides* species having been recorded.

The route by which organisms are transmitted to the peritoneal cavity is not known. Evidence favoring transmural migration of bacteria from the intestine is derived from the fact that systemic endotoxemia and the presence of endotoxin in ascitic fluid can be demonstrated by limulus assay in many decompensated cirrhotics, even though no bacteria are present in the ascites and the patients do not have clinical evidence of peritonitis. Evidence favoring the hematogenous route stems from the frequent clinical association of spontaneous peritonitis with urinary tract infections harboring the same organism and from cases of simultaneous spontaneous empyema and pericarditis.

Clinical symptoms usually are of short duration in children; the onset of symptoms is more insidious in ascitic adults. Most patients complain of some abdominal pain and distension; vomiting, lethargy, and fever are more prominant in children. Diarrhea is usual in neonates but seldom seen in adults. Bowel sounds are variable. A brisk leukocytosis usually is present. No free air is seen on abdominal x-rays. All in all, the clinical picture may be quite desultory and never appears to be as severe as in suppurative peritonitis.

A peritoneal tap is the most useful diagnostic test. The ascitic fluid has the character of an "infected transudate," i.e., the protein content is not abnormally high, but the fluid does contain leukocytes. If more than 300 polymorphonuclear cells per cubic millimeter are seen, peritonitis of some variety is sure to be present. If the Gram stain shows gram-negative bacteria, the presence of a surgically correctable intraabdominal lesion cannot be excluded. If a Gram stain shows only gram-positive cocci, the presence of spontaneous peritonitis is possible; however, the fallacy of assuming that an apparent monomicrobial gram-positive infection always is spontaneous peritonitis is illustrated by a case reported by Dimond and Proctor in which pneumococcal peritonitis was secondary to rupture of an acute pneumococcal appendix.

Differentiation of truly spontaneous peritonitis, in which early operative intervention is unnecessary, from suppurative peritonitis, in which an early operation may be essential to a successful outcome, is the essential diagnostic exercise. Exploratory laparotomy should be undertaken, because, as a practical matter, in most cases the possibility of an intraabdominal lesion requiring surgical correction is sufficiently great and the relative risk of operation is sufficiently small. Little harm is done by a negative exploration in the presence of spontaneous peritonitis, and, in particular, the prognosis is not worsened. Only in a nephrotic child or a cirrhotic adult in advanced hepatic decompensation, in whom all diagnostic criteria for the presence of spontaneous peritonitis are present, should operation be withheld and antibiotic therapy alone undertaken.

Once the abdomen has been opened and the diagnosis of spontaneous peritonitis confirmed, a specimen of peritoneal exudate is obtained for Gram stain, culture, and sensitivity studies. Appendectomy, even in the presence of spontaneous peritonitis, does not increase morbidity or mortality risk and should be performed. Accomplishment of appendectomy will eliminate one source of diagnostic confusion, should recurrent episodes occur. Drains should not be placed because their presence retards resolution of the peritonitis.

OTHER FORMS OF PERITONITIS

SCLEROSING PERITONITIS (PRACTOLOL). During the past 4 years, a number of cases have been reported of patients who developed striking thickening of the visceral peritoneum weeks to months after treatment with the beta-blocking drug, practolol. The most frequent clinical presentation is with a typical small-bowel obstruction, often insidious in onset, associated with profound weight loss and with a prominent abdominal mass on physical examination. At laparotomy, the visceral peritoneum is greatly thickened and encases the small bowel, usually from the duodenojejunal flexure to the ileocecal valve. The operative findings are striking: the whole of the small bowel usually is caught up in a thick sac, which sometimes

can be lifted as a single mass from the peritoneal cavity. This agglomeration of small intestine produces the mass that is palpable preoperatively. Psoriasis-like skin lesions and conjunctivitis also have been reported to occur in association with administration of practolol.

OTHER DRUG-RELATED PERITONITIS. The sudden occurrence of severe acute abdominal symptoms as a manifestation of drug sensitivity is distinctly unusual. Isoniazid has been reported to cause such an acute syndrome, and erythromycin estolate has been reported on occasion to produce abdominal distress.

PERIODIC PERITONITIS. Recurrent episodes of abdominal pain, fever, and leukocytosis occur in certain population groups in and around the Mediterranean Basin, notably Armenians, Jews, and Arabs. The disease appears to be familial. The major point for the surgeon is that the episodes do not require laparotomy, so the diagnosis should be kept in mind if dealing with patients from the Levant. Laparotomy often is performed for the first episode, since an acute intraabdominal process requiring surgical cure cannot be ruled out. At operation, the peritoneal surfaces may be inflamed and there is free fluid, but smears and cultures reveal no bacteria. Even though it is normal, the appendix should be removed to eliminate the possibility of acute appendicitis in the differential diagnosis of future episodes. Colchicine is highly effective in preventing recurrent attacks, and, in fact, a favorable response to chronic administration of colchicine is a definitive diagnostic test.

INTRAABDOMINAL ABSCESSES

Intraabdominal abscesses are localized collections of pus walled off from the rest of the peritoneal cavity by inflammatory adhesions between the parietes, loops of bowel, other intraabdominal viscera, the mesenteries, or omentum. An abscess may be solitary or multiple and may be located within the peritoneal cavity proper, within a viscus, or in the adjacent retroperitoneum. Abscesses arise during resolution and healing of more generalized peritonitis, or during situations in which a perforation of the gastrointestinal or biliary tracts occurs which is successfully walled off in the acute state by peritoneal defense mechanisms. Abscesses within solid viscera usually arise following hematogenous or lymphatic dissemination of infection to these organs from a septic focus elsewhere in the body. Retroperitoneal abscesses typically arise as a consequence of primary infection or of inflammation of one of the retroperitoneal viscera followed by secondary bacterial contamination.

Resolution of peritonitis with formation of a pelvic or subphrenic abscess is a reflection of the anatomy of the peritoneal cavity (Fig. 34-3). The upper part of the abdomen is divided nearly in half by the vertebral column. Both the pelvis and the subphrenic spaces on either side form deep and dependent cavities into which infected material is directed by gravity. In addition, the suction effect of respiration tends to draw infected peritoneal fluid up under the diaphragm. In a clinical investigation conducted in patients

Fig. 34-3. The posterior attachments of the upper abdominal viscera subdivide the major right and left subphrenic spaces into a series of smaller spaces, as indicated by the labels.

undergoing cholecystectomy or appendectomy, Autio found that x-ray contrast media injected at the operative site became widely disseminated within a few hours after operation. Whether the contrast material originally had been placed in the upper or the lower part of the abdomen seemed to make little difference in its liability to spread; material was noted to move initially along the pericolic gutters in both directions and to collect primarily in the pelvis and in the subphrenic spaces.

Intraabdominal abscesses generally are polymicrobic (Table 34-2). Anaerobic organisms usually are the predominant flora, with bacteroides species and anaerobic streptococci being found most commonly. In part, the predominance of anaerobes in intraabdominal abscesses is

Table 34-2. BACTERIOLOGY OF SUBPHRENIC ABSCESS

	Percent recovery of organisms	
	1950–1970 (60 patients)	1970–1975 (24 patients)
Aerobes		
E. coli	60	96
Streptococci	49	67
Staphylococci	31	8
Klebsiella	17	21
Proteus	11	38
Pseudomonas	8	8
Anaerobes		
Bacteroides spp.	11	83
Anaerobic cocci	0	50
Clostridia	6	50
Fusobacteria	0	38
Eubacteria	0	8

SOURCE: From Wang and Wilson, 1977.

related to the metabolic conditions existing within an abscess cavity, but also may be a reflection of the fact that aerobic organisms previously present in a more generalized peritoneal infection have been reduced in numbers or eradicated as a result of interactions of antibiotics and host defense mechanisms.

Symptoms of an intraabdominal abscess often are desultory, particularly early in the clinical course or with deep-seated infections. Recurring or persisting fever is seen in nearly all patients. Fever typically is intermittent or spiking in character at first, then becomes progressively more persistent as the abscess matures. The fever spikes, which often are accompanied by chills and tachycardia, are the result of transient episodes of bloodstream invasion from the abscess. On occasion, septicemia may be sufficiently persistent that septic shock ensues. Paralytic ileus, abdominal distension, and anorexia are frequent symptoms, and sometimes there is vomiting.

The intensity of symptoms may be modified by administration of antibiotics which tend to suppress the infection, although antibiotic therapy rarely cures an abscess once a phlegmonous infection has proceeded to the formation of fluid pus. Continued administration of antibiotics may only lead to a process which smolders for many weeks. Because continued administration of antibiotics may hamper diagnosis of an abscess, it often is preferable to discontinue antibiotic therapy when the presence of an intraabdominal abscess is suspected, and direct efforts toward establishing a precise diagnosis of the location of the abscess.

Abdominal tenderness and pain may be present with a visceral or midabdominal abscess, but are less commonly seen with subphrenic or retroperitoneal abscesses. Pain involving the anterior abdominal wall usually is absent with a pelvic abscess. When present, signs of pain and tenderness tend to be geographically related to the location of the abscess. Recurring or worsening jaundice also is an important clinical hallmark of the presence of an intraabdominal abscess.

Patients harboring an abscess invariably have leukocytosis accompanied by a left shift in the differential white cell count. The sedimentation rate is elevated, reflecting the presence of inflammation. Blood cultures will document septicemia and may identify one or several of the organisms involved in the abscess. Plain abdominal films may show localized gas bubbles or an air fluid level in the abscess. Barium contrast studies of the gastrointestinal tract may show organ displacement because of the abscess itself and, on occasion, may demonstrate a sinus tract or other extravasation which indicates the cause of the abscess. An intravenous pyelogram may indicate malfunction or displacement of genitourinary structures when the abscess is located in the retroperitoneum. Abdominal ultrasound scans are useful, particularly in thin patients, in localizing an abscess located in the upper part of the abdomen or retroperitoneum. Computer-assisted tomographic studies are most useful in patients who are moderately obese, since the presence of fat within the abdomen aids this examination in delineating the location of both normal and abnormal structures.

Diagnostic scans using gallium (^{67}Ga) also have been reported by some authors to be helpful in localizing an intraabdominal abscess. Radio-gallium collects and persists in areas of inflammation; in the presence of an intraabdominal abscess, the radioisotope tends to collect in the inflammatory membrane surrounding the abscess cavity. However, gallium scans are limited by the fact that the radioisotope also is excreted in the colon and the colon content must be evacuated before residual collections in the abdomen can be accurately localized. Because ileus so often accompanies an intraabdominal abscess, colonic emptying sometimes is incomplete or delayed, limiting the usefulness of this diagnostic test. Gallium scans, as is generally true of diagnostic scans directed at acute intraabdominal problems, have an indifferent record as regards accuracy, being subject to both false-positive and false-negative results in a significant proportion of cases.

The essential feature of surgical management of an intraabdominal abscess is to establish adequate drainage. Since many patients suffering an intraabdominal abscess are nutritionally depleted and septic, judicious, though urgent, preparation with attention to fluid resuscitation, parenteral nutrition, administration of antibiotics, and ap-

propriate monitoring measures should be instituted preoperatively. If the abscess is in contact with the abdominal parietes or the diaphragm, a direct and, insofar as possible, extraperitoneal approach is preferred. When the abscess is suspected clinically but cannot be accurately localized preoperatively, general abdominal exploration is needed. Abscesses in the lesser sac and in the midabdomen are best handled through transabdominal approaches. Abscesses in the pelvis, on the other hand, often can be drained through the rectum or vagina, obviating the need for an abdominal operation.

As the pyogenic membrane is encountered during exploration, confirmation of the presence of pus is obtained by needle aspiration. It is essential to obtain specimens of the abscess contents for Gram stain, culture, and sensitivity studies. All of the abscess contents should be evacuated by suction. The cavity should be thoroughly explored and all loculations within it broken down to create a single residual space. The cavity is irrigated and debrided of nonviable tissue. Multiple soft (Penrose) drains then should be brought from the abscess cavity to the exterior as directly and dependently as possible. If the abscess cavity is particularly large, or if thorough dependent drainage cannot be established, sump suction drains should be employed in addition to soft drains. Drains are left in place until external drainage stops or is clear; the drainage tract should then be irrigated, and a sinogram obtained to document collapse of the cavity before the drains are moved. It may take several weeks for a large cavity to become small enough to permit drains to be slowly advanced, allowing the drainage tract to seal as they are withdrawn.

Antibiotic therapy should be continued postoperatively, guided by the sensitivity studies obtained from the intraoperative specimen. Antibiotic administration should continue until all systemic signs of sepsis have been resolved and the patient's appetite and sense of well-being have returned. It is not, however, necessary to continue antibiotic therapy simply because drains remain in place.

Fig. 34-4. A combined liver-lung scan. Anterior view (*left*) suggests a defect laterally between the right lung and the liver. Lateral view (*right*) shows a posteriorly loculated abscess (arrow) with indentation of the liver and an increase in space between the liver and the lung. (*From White, Hayes, and Benfield, 1972.*)

Recently there has been some recurrent enthusiasm for the management of suspected intraabdominal abscesses by antibiotic therapy without drainage. This form of therapy will be successful in a proportion of cases if instituted at the time when there is localized phlegmonous inflammation but before the appearance of fluid pus. But once a localized collection of pus is formed, it must be drained. If not, the risk of complications related to delayed rupture of the abscess cavity increases markedly. Such secondary abscess rupture may result in recurrent generalized peritonitis, dissection through the diaphragm with production of an empyema or bronchopleural fistula, rupture into an adjacent hollow or solid viscus with marked worsening of the clinical state of the patient, and, on occasion, necrosis of a major blood vessel with consequent rupture and exsanguination. Once an abscess forms, failure to drain only produces a prolonged course of illness that nearly always culminates in death of the patient.

Right Subphrenic Abscess

The right subphrenic space is only a potential space between the liver and the diaphragm, lying above the attachments of the coronary and triangular ligaments to the posterior parietes and extending anteriorly to the costal margin. Abscesses within this space are most frequently secondary to rupture of a hepatic abscess or to operations on the stomach or duodenum; less frequently, they are due to contamination of the subphrenic space during the course of a generalized peritonitis, and, least frequently, right subphrenic abscesses are related to operations on the appendix or biliary system. Because the potential space is so limited in vertical dimension, right subphrenic abscesses tend to be localized to only a portion of the total potential space, loculating either anteriorly or posteriorly.

Clinical signs and symptoms may be quite minimal. Pain is occasionally reported in the upper part of the abdomen or lower part of the chest, sometimes referred to the back or to the right shoulder. Chest x-rays show a pleural effusion or platelike atelectasis in the right lower lung in 9 out of 10 patients, and the diaphragm is elevated and shows reduced motion on sniffing in two out of three patients. An air fluid level can be demonstrated in about 25 percent of patients, and establishes the diagnosis. A combined liver and lung isotopic scan is an important diagnostic study with a high accuracy rate; it demonstrates an increase in space, which is occupied by the abscess, between the perfused lung, above, and the perfused liver, below (Fig. 34-4).

The surgical management of right subphrenic abscesses was confused for years by a misunderstanding of the relevant anatomy. Barnard (1907) had described the triangular and coronary ligaments of the liver as arising from the dome of the diaphragm. This error, perpetuated by surgical authors for the next half century, resulted in the recommendation that abscesses loculated in the posterior part of the right subphrenic space should be drained posteriorly through the bed of the twelfth rib. This anatomic error was corrected by Boyd, who pointed out that the coronary and triangular ligaments attach posteriorly rather than superi-

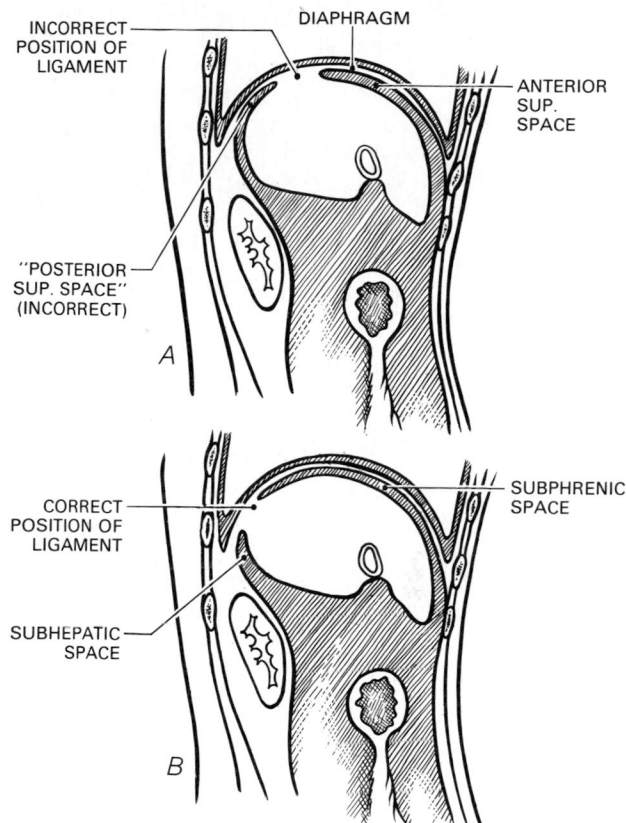

Fig. 34-5. *A.* The anatomic error that "created" a nonexistent postero superior subphrenic space was related to incorrect superior placement of the attachments of the liver (coronary and triangular ligaments) to the diaphragm. *B.* The correct anatomic relationships: the liver attaches posteriorly, separating the subphrenic from the subhepatic space.

orly (Fig. 34-5). It should be emphasized that abscesses in the right subphrenic space cannot be drained through a posterior approach unless the route of drainage transgresses the pleural space, a step which obviously is not desirable.

Right subphrenic abscesses preferably are drained using a lateral subcostal approach (Fig. 34-6). The incision is made beginning at the tip of the eleventh rib and carried obliquely anteriorly, paralleling the costal margin. The dissection is largely extraperitoneal until the abscess cavity, either anteriorly or posteriorly located, is approached. The advantage of the lateral approach is that it is possible to drain all the subphrenic and subhepatic spaces while avoiding contamination of the remainder of the peritoneal cavity.

Right Subhepatic Abscess

The right subhepatic space lies under the liver, is bounded inferiorly by the hepatic flexure and the transverse mesocolon, medially by the duodenum and hepatoduodenal ligament, and laterally by the body wall. The most posterior (deepest) part of this space is called *Morison's pouch.*

Fig. 34-6. Drainage of all subphrenic and subhepatic abscesses on the right side is done most easily through a lateral subcostal approach (DeCosse). *A.* The incision follows the costal margin anteriorly from the tip of the eleventh rib. *B.* The abscess is approached by blunt extraperitoneal dissection; the figure illustrates drainage of a high anterior subphrenic abscess; the arrows indicate the routes of approach to a posteriorly loculated subphrenic and to a subhepatic abscess. The principle of this approach also applies to drainage of a subphrenic abscess on the left side.

Gastric surgery, especially emergency operations for complications of ulcer disease, is the most common antecedent event. Biliary tract procedures are second in frequency. Appendicitis has now declined in importance and accounts for only 8 percent of cases of right subhepatic abscess. Complications of colonic surgery are increasing in importance. A right subhepatic abscess usually produces some tenderness in the right upper quadrant, and the patient may complain of pain, particularly exacerbated by coughing or similar activities which produce visceral motion in the region.

Halasz emphasized the serious problem of failure to recognize synchronous or multiple abscesses and recommended transperitoneal exploration for subphrenic abscess as preferable to more limited exploration. In his series of 43 patients, one-fourth had synchronous abscesses elsewhere in the abdomen. Failure to find and drain the concomitant abscess resulted in therapeutic failure. Our indications for use of a transabdominal exploration in the management of intraabdominal abscesses are limited to those situations in which the presence of an abscess in the midabdomen or in the lesser sac is suspected, and those situations in which the geographic location of the abscess is obscure. Whenever a well-localized pelvic, subphrenic, or subhepatic abscess is diagnosed, a direct approach for drainage should be made. The expectation is that the patient will promptly improve; should this not occur, consideration then should be given to transabdominal exploration to find and drain additional abscesses. Such a program will keep the risks of contamination of the general peritoneal cavity as a consequence of abscess drainage at a minimum, and yet should not result in excess mortality due to lingering, undrained, unrecognized abscesses.

Left Subphrenic Abscess

Formerly uncommon, these are now the commonest variety of upper abdominal abscess residual after peritonitis or leakage from a viscus. Left subphrenic abscesses follow splenectomy, particularly when the splenic fossa is drained; they also are a consequence of pancreatitis. The

physical signs are costal tenderness on the left, sometimes pain in the shoulder (Kehr's sign), the presence of a left pleural effusion, and limitation of diaphragmatic motion noted by x-ray. Unlike the subdiaphragmatic space on the right, which is divided by the liver into a suprahepatic (or subdiaphragmatic) space and a subhepatic space, on the left side all these areas are contiguous.

A left subhepatic abscess is best drained through a lateral extraserous approach, using fundamentally the same technique as recommended on the right side (Fig. 34-6). Alternatively, abscesses in the left subphrenic space may be drained posteriorly through the bed of the twelfth rib (Fig. 34-7). Via either route, the point at which the abscess is encountered during dissection is usually much deeper than might be expected. It is important in approaching a left subphrenic abscess to avoid injury to the spleen, should it still be present, and to ensure that the entire space has been explored by palpating the aorta, the esophagus and the region of the esophageal hiatus, the caudate lobe of the liver, and the anterior margin of the left lobe of the liver during exploration; such anatomic identification by palpation of the structures at the borders of the left subphrenic space will assure that no loculation of pus goes undrained to form a residual or recurrent abscess.

Lesser Sac Abscess

Technically, this is a variety of left subhepatic-subphrenic abscess, since the lesser peritoneal sac anatomically is a portion of the left subhepatic space. However, the anatomic features of this form of abscess, and the surgical maneuvers required for drainage, are distinctly different; hence its consideration as a separate entity. Lesser sac abscesses are unusual complications of diseases of the stomach, duodenum, or pancreas. The most common cause is a pancreatic abscess or a secondarily contaminated pancreatic pseudocyst which involves the lesser sac by direct extension. Perforation of a gastric ulcer or, less commonly, of a duodenal ulcer also may result in formation of a lesser sac abscess. Occasionally, rupture of an ulcerating malignant gastric tumor produces an abscess in the lesser sac.

Clinical diagnosis of a lesser-sac abscess can be extremely difficult, since much of this space is overlapped anteriorly by the liver. Tenderness to palpation in the midepigastrium usually is present but is such a nonspecific sign that it is not diagnostically very helpful. Ultrasonography is a most useful diagnostic test. Radiographic studies may show displacement of the stomach, but often appear quite normal; very occasionally, plain roentgenograms show fine gas bubbles within the lesser sac, indicative of the presence of purulent material.

Because of its anatomic location, extraperitoneal drainage of this variety of abscess is impossible. Lesser-sac abscesses should be approached through an upper abdominal incision, either vertical or transverse. If a transverse incision is chosen, it should be confined within the rectus sheath; rectus muscle should not be transected, only retracted. Drainage should be accomplished as dependently as possible. Theoretically, this would involve placement of drains inferior to the stomach, above the transverse mesocolon. However, it is usual for the lower portion of the lesser sac to be obliterated in cases of lesser-sac abscess, with the stomach densely adherent both to the transverse mesocolon and to the pancreas; attempts at dissection are

fraught with considerable difficulty. The commonly utilized route of drainage is along the superior border of the antrum, the drains being exteriorized through the operative wound.

Interloop (Midabdominal) Abscess

These abscesses arise as loculations between loops of bowel, mesentery, the abdominal wall, and omentum. The right and left gutters also are common sites. The transverse mesocolon acts as a barrier to superior extension so that, as a group, interloop abscesses do not involve the upper part of the abdomen. Quite commonly, they may be associated with a simultaneous abscess in the pelvis.

Diagnosis of a midabdominal abscess is one of the most difficult exercises in abdominal surgery. There are no reliable symptoms or signs. Huge abscesses containing more than a liter of pus may occur without any significant physical findings. The surgeon must suspect the possible presence of an interloop abscess whenever the clinical context is appropriate, i.e., a preceding episode of peritonitis with incomplete clinical resolution and recurring signs of sepsis. Occasionally, abdominal films may show either edema in the wall of loops of bowel involved in the loculation, or separation or fixation of involved structures. Very occasionally an interloop abscess may produce a palpable, enlarging abdominal mass.

Midabdominal interloop abscesses are multiple more often than not. Because of the need for general exploration, and because extraserous drainage cannot be arranged in any case, transabdominal exploration is utilized. All abscesses should be opened, aspirated, and debrided. Unless the abscess cavity is in contact with the abdominal wall, insertion of drains is not indicated. Rather, reliance is placed on thorough debridement and irrigation of the peritoneal cavity with copious amounts of saline solution followed by antibiotic irrigation, as outlined above in the

Fig. 34-7. Drainage of a left subphrenic abscess through the bed of the twelfth rib. Resecting the rib greatly improves exposure but is not essential; if the twelfth rib is not excised, the incision is carried deeply along its inferior margin. The pararenal space is entered and the dissection continued bluntly upward and medially on the undersurface of the diaphragm to locate and enter the abscess cavity.

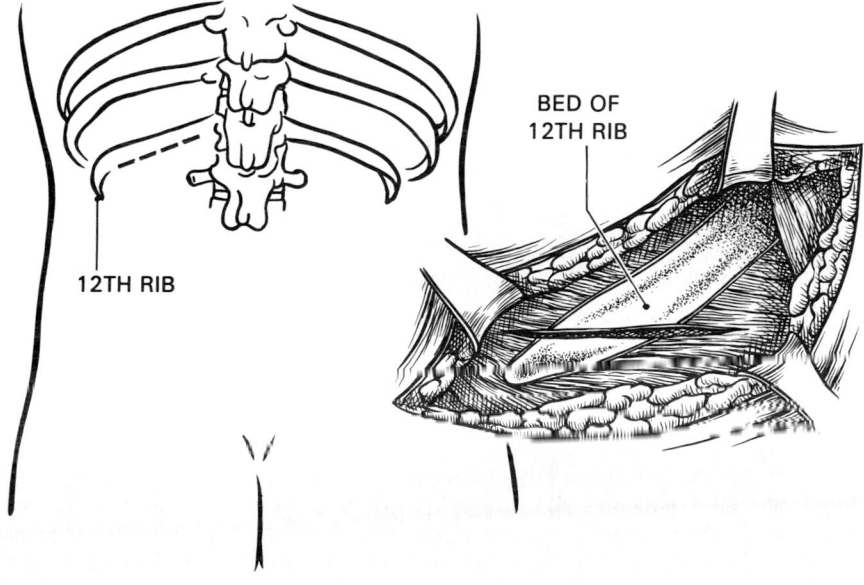

12TH RIB

BED OF 12TH RIB

management of suppurative peritonitis. Recurrence is common, and clinical evidence of such an event should be sought and treated vigorously.

Pelvic Abscess

These abscesses most often follow ruptured colonic diverticulum, pelvic inflammatory disease, ruptured appendix, or drainage into the pelvis during resolution of generalized peritonitis. Unless the abscess involves the anterior abdominal wall, few symptoms or physical signs are present on examination of the abdomen. The patient may complain of poorly localized, dull, lower abdominal pain. Irritation of the urinary system and the rectum produces symptoms of urgency and frequency or diarrhea and tenesmus.

Fortunately, localized purulent collections in the pelvis are the easiest of intraabdominal abscesses to diagnose. The abscess usually can be palpated directly by rectal or vaginal examination. The typical pelvic abscess bulges as a tender mass into the anterior rectal wall. It is important to distinguish between an inflammatory mass involving the pelvic organs and a true pelvic abscess. In general, pelvic inflammatory masses involving the fallopian tubes do not bulge into the rectum, and tend to become less tender and to resolve on serial examination, whereas a true pelvic abscess tends to enlarge and finally to rupture.

Drainage should be accomplished through either the rectum or the vagina. Incision for drainage should be delayed until formation of the pyogenic membrane has effectively excluded all of the small bowel and other intraabdominal viscera. If serial examinations have been done, readiness for drainage is apparent when the most prominent aspect of the abscess presenting vaginally or rectally begins to soften. Using a speculum or anoscope, the abscess should be exposed and the presence of pus confirmed by needle aspiration. The needle is left in place as a guide; sharp incision with a knife is made into the abscess cavity. The abscess cavity should be explored digitally, loculations broken down, and the cavity thoroughly irrigated. Drains are difficult to retain in a pelvic abscess cavity. To ensure continued drainage and obliteration of the cavity, daily dilations of the tract digitally or with an instrument should be done until the cavity becomes obliterated over the following few days.

Pancreatic Abscess

Acute pancreatitis is the antecedent cause of pancreatic abscess in the majority of cases. Secondary infection of a pancreatic pseudocyst is the only other important cause. Abdominal pain, nausea, vomiting, and swinging fever usually are present. Anterior abdominal tenderness may be present, although pain in the back is more common.

Pancreatic abscesses are polymicrobial in nature, the common organisms being aerobic representatives of the fecal flora, predominantly *E. coli* and aerobic hemolytic streptococci. Staphylococci usually are not involved in primary pancreatic abscesses but are frequently recovered

in those abscesses which follow inadvertent early abdominal exploration in the presence of pancreatitis.

Surgical drainage of a pancreatic abscess using largebore sump suction and soft drains is the essential feature of therapy. This treatment should be supported by administration of appropriate antibiotics, fluids, and similar measures. The mortality is 26 percent with sump drainage; all alternative forms of treatment carry a higher mortality risk.

REFERENCES

Peritoneum

Allen, L., and Vogt, E.: Mechanism of Lymphatic Absorption from Serous Cavities, *Am J Physiol,* **119:**776, 1937.

Cascarano, J., Rubin, A. D., Chick, W. L., and Zweifach, B. W.: Metabolically Induced Permeability Changes across Mesothelium, *Am J Physiol,* **206:**373, 1964.

Courtice, F. C., and Simmonds, W. J.: Physiological Significance of Lymph Drainage of the Serous Cavities and Lung, *Physiol Rev,* **34:**419, 1954.

Raftery, A. T.: Regeneration of Parietal and Visceral Peritoneum. A Light Microscopical Study, *Br J Surg,* **60:**293, 1973.

———: Regeneration of Parietal and Visceral Peritoneum: An Electron Microscopical Study, *J Anat,* **115:**375, 1973.

General Responses in Peritonitis

Davis, J. H.: Current Concepts of Peritonitis, *Am Surg,* **33:**673, 1967.

Duff, J. H., Groves, A. C., McLean, A. P. H., LaPointe, E. R., and MacLean, L. D.: Defective Oxygen Consumption in Septic Shock, *Surg Gynecol Obstet,* **128:**1051, 1969.

Fry, D. E., Silver, B. B., Rink, R. D., and Flint, L. M.: Hepatic Mitochondrial Function in Intraperitoneal Sepsis, *Rev Surg,* **34:**214, 1977.

Kukral, J. C., Riveron, E., Tiffany, J. C., Vaitys, S., and Barrett, B.: Plasma Protein Metabolism in Patients with Acute Surgical Peritonitis, *Am J Surg,* **113:**173, 1967.

Renvall, S.: Peritoneal Reaction in Acute Appendicitis. A Biochemical Study, *Acta Chir Scand,* **142:**407, 1976.

Interactions of Bacteria and the Peritoneum

Altemeier, W. A.: The Pathogenicity of the Bacteria of Appendicitis Peritonitis, *Ann Surg,* **114:**158, 1941.

Bartlett, J. G., Miao, P. V. W., and Gorbach, S. L.: Empiric Treatment with Clindamycin and Gentamicin of Suspected Sepsis due to Anaerobic and Aerobic Bacteria, *J Infect Dis,* **135**(Suppl), 80, 1977.

Davis, J. H., and Yull, A. B.: Possible Toxic Factor in Abdominal Injury, *J Trauma,* **2:**291, 1962.

——— and ———: A Toxic Factor in Abdominal Injury, II. The Role of the Red Cell Component, *J Trauma,* **4:**84, 1964.

Filler, R. M., and Sleeman, H. K.: Pathogenesis of Peritonitis. I. The Effect of *Escherichia coli* and Hemoglobin on Peritoneal Absorption, *Surgery,* **61:**385, 1967.

Hau, T., Nelson, R. D., Fiegel, V. D., Levenson, R., and Simmons, R. L.: Mechanisms of the Adjuvant Action of Hemoglobin in Experimental Peritonitis. 2. Influence of Hemoglobin on

Human Leukocyte Chemotaxis in Vitro, *J Surg Res,* **22:**174, 1977.

Holland, J. W., Hill, E. O., and Altemeier, W. A.: Numbers and Types of Anaerobic Bacteria Isolated from Clinical Specimens since 1960, *J Clin Microbiol,* **5:**20, 1977.

Lorber, B., and Swenson, R. M.: The Bacteriology of Intra-abdominal Infections, *Surg Clin North Am,* **55:**1349, 1975.

Meleney, F. L.: Bacterial Synergism in Disease Processes, *Ann Surg,* **94:**961, 1931.

Nichols, R. L., Condon, R. E., Bentley, D. W., and Gorbach, S. L.: Ileal Microflora in Surgical Patients, *J Urol,* **105:**351, 1971.

————, Smith, J. W., and Balthazar, E. R.: Peritonitis and Intra-abdominal Abscess: An Experimental Model for the Evaluation of Human Disease, *J Surg Res,* accepted for publication, 1977.

Simmons, R. L., Diggs, J. W., and Sleeman, H. K.: Pathogenesis of Peritonitis. III. Local Adjuvant Action of Hemoglobin in Experimental *E. coli* Peritonitis, *Surgery,* **63:**810, 1968.

Sleeman, H. K., Diggs, J. W., Hendry, W. S., and Filler, R. M.: Pathogenesis of Peritonitis. II. The Effect of *Escherichia coli* and Adjuvant Substances on Peritoneal Absorption, *Surgery,* **61:**393, 1967.

Stone, H. H., Kolb, L. D., and Geheber, C. E.: Incidence and Significance of Intraperitoneal Anaerobic Bacteria, *Ann Surg,* **181:**705, 1975.

Weinstein, W. M., Onderdonk, A. B., Bartlett, J. G., and Gorbach, S. L.: Experimental Intra-abdominal Abscesses in Rats: Development of an Experimental Model, *Infect Immunol,* **10:**1250, 1974.

Pathophysiology of Sepsis

Alexander, J. W., McClellan, M. A., Ogle, C. K., and Ogle, J. D.: Consumptive Opsoninopathy: Possible Pathogenesis in Lethal and Opportunistic Infections, *Ann Surg,* **184:**672, 1976.

Beaufils, M., Morel-Maroger, L., Sraer, J.-D., Kanfer, A., Kourilsky, O., and Richet, G.: Acute Renal Failure of Glomerular Origin during Visceral Abscesses, *N Engl J Med,* **295:**185, 1976.

Berk, J. L., Hagen, J. F., and Dunn, J. M.: The Role of Beta-adrenergic Blockade in the Treatment of Septic Shock, *Surg Gynecol Obstet,* **130:**1025, 1970.

Clowes, G. H. A., Jr., Hirsch, E., Williams, L., Kwasnik, E., O'Donnell, T. F., Cuevas, P., Saini, V. K., Moradi, I., Farizan, M., Saravis, C., Stone, M., and Kuffler, J.: Septic Lung and Shock Lung in Man, *Ann Surg,* **181:**681, 1975.

————, Vucinic, M., and Weidner, M. G.: Circulatory and Metabolic Alterations Associated with Survival or Death in Peritonitis: Clinical Analysis of 25 Cases, *Ann Surg,* **163:**866, 1966.

Hill, H. R., Gerrard, J. M., Hogan, N. A., and Quie, P. G.: Hyperactivity of Neutrophil Leukotactic Responses during Active Bacterial Infection, *J Clin Invest,* **53:**996, 1974.

Hinshaw, L. B., Benjamin, B., Holmes, D. D., Beller, B., Archer, L. T., Coalson, J. J., and Whitsett, T.: Responses of the Baboon to Live *Escherichia coli* organisms and Endotoxin, *Surg Gynecol Obstet,* **145:**1, 1977.

Holcroft, J. W., Blaisdell, F. W., Trunkey, D. D., and Lim, R. C.: Intravascular Coagulation and Pulmonary Edema in the Septic Baboon, *J Surg Res,* **22:**209, 1977.

MacLean, L. D., Mulligan, W. G., McLean, A. P. H., and Duff,

J. H.: Patterns of Septic Shock in Man—a Detailed Study of 56 Patients, *Ann Surg,* **166:**543, 1967.

Meakins, J. L., Pietsch, J. B., Bubenrek, O., Kelly, R., Rode, H., Gordon, J., and MacLean, L. D.: Delayed Hypersensitivity: Indicator of Acquired Failure of Host Defenses in Sepsis and Trauma, *Ann Surg,* **186:**241, 1977.

Ollodat, R. M., Hawthorne, I., and Altar, S.: Studies in Experimental Endotoxemia in Man, *Am J Surg,* **113:**599, 1967.

Postel, J., and Schloerb, P.: Metabolic Effects of Experimental Bacteremia, *Ann Surg,* **185:**475, 1977.

Schumer, W., Das Gupta, T. K., Moss, G. S., and Nyhus, L. M.: Effect of Endotoxemia on Liver Cell Mitochondria in Man, *Ann Surg,* **171:**875, 1970.

Skillman, J. J., Bushnell, L. S., and Hedley-Whyte, J.: Peritonitis and Respiratory Failure after Abdominal Operations, *Ann Surg,* **170:**122, 1969.

Management of Suppurative Peritonitis

Altemeier, W. A.: The Cause of the Odor of Peritonitis Pus, *Ann Surg,* **107:**634, 1938.

Aune, S., and Notman, N. E.: Diffuse Peritonitis Treated with Continuous Peritoneal Lavage, *Acta Chir Scand,* **136:**401, 1970.

Burnett, W. E., Brown, G. R., Jr., Rosemond, G. P., Caswell, H. T., Buchor, R. B., and Tyson, R. R.: The Treatment of Peritonitis Using Peritoneal Lavage, *Ann Surg,* **145:**675, 1957.

Condon, R. E.: Rational Use of Prophylactic Antibiotics in Gastrointestinal Surgery, *Surg Clin North Am,* **55:**1309, 1975.

————: Management of the Acute Complications of Diverticular Disease: Peritonitis and Septicemia, *Dis Colon Rectum,* **19:**296, 1976.

Fowler, R.: A Controlled Trial of Intraperitoneal Cephaloridine Administration in Peritonitis, *J Pediatr Surg,* **10:**43, 1975.

Ger, R., Salazar, C., and Stratford, F.: Prognostic Factors in Generalized Peritonitis, *J R Coll Surg (Edinb),* **21:**173, 1976.

Halasz, N. A.: Wound Infection and Topical Antibiotics: The Surgeon's Dilemma, *Arch Surg,* **112:**1240, 1977.

Holcroft, J. W., Trunkey, D. D., and Carpenter, M. A.: Sepsis in the Baboon: Factors Affecting Resuscitation and Pulmonary Edema in Animals Resuscitated with Ringer's Lactate versus Plasmanate, *J Trauma,* **17:**600, 1977.

Hudspeth, A. S.: Radical Surgical Debridement in the Treatment of Advanced Generalized Bacterial Peritonitis, *Arch Surg,* **110:**1233, 1975.

Hunt, J. A.: An Assessment of Antibiotic Peritoneal Lavage in the Treatment of Severe Bacterial Peritonitis, *S Afr J Surg,* **14:**31, 1976.

Moss, G. S., Das Gupta, T. K., Newson, B., and Nyhus, L. M.: The Effect of Saline Solution Resuscitation on Pulmonary Sodium and Water Distribution, *Surg Gynecol Obstet,* **136:**934, 1973.

Nahrwold, D. L., and Demuth, W. E.: Diverticulitis with Perforation into the Peritoneal Cavity, *Ann Surg,* **185:**80, 1977.

Nelson, J. L., Kuzman, J. H., and Cohn, I., Jr.: Intraperitoneal Lavage and Kanamycin in the Contaminated Abdomen, *Surg Clin North Am,* **55:**1391, 1975.

Noon, G. P., Beall, A. C., Jr., Jordan, G. L., Jr., Riggs, S., and DeBakey, M. E.: Clinical Evaluation of Peritoneal Irrigation with Antibiotic Solution, *Surgery,* **62:**73, 1967.

Peloso, O. A., Floyd, V. T., and Wilkinson, L. H.: Treatment of

Peritonitis with Continuous Postoperative Peritoneal Lavage Using Cephalothin, *Am J Surg,* **126:**742, 1973.

Price, J.: Surgical Intervention in Cases of General Peritonitis from Typhoid Fever and Acute Gonococcus Infection, *Am Med,* **9:**769, 1905.

Robin, E. D., Cross, C. E., and Zelis, R.: Pulmonary Edema, *N Engl J Med,* **288:**239, 1973.

Schumer, W.: Steroids in the Treatment of Clinical Septic Shock, *Ann Surg,* **184:**333, 1976.

Smith, I. M., Kennedy, L. R., Regne-Karlsson, M. H., Johnson, V. L., and Burmeister, I. F.: Adrenergic Mechanisms in Infection. III. α and β-Receptor Blocking Agents in Treatment, *Am J Clin Nutr,* **30:**1285, 1977.

Torek, F.: The Treatment of Diffuse Suppurative Peritonitis following Appendicitis, *Med Rec,* **70:**849, 1906.

Tullis, J. L.: Albumin 1. Background and Use, *JAMA,* **237:**355, 1977.

Virgilio, R. W., Smith, D. E., Rice, C. L., Hobelmann, C. L., Zarins, C. K., James, D. R., and Peters, R. M.: Effect of Colloid Osmotic Pressure and Capillary Wedge Pressure on Intrapulmonary Shunt, *Surg Forum,* **27:**168, 1976.

Aseptic (Chemical) Peritonitis

Carter, R., and Gosney, W. G.: Abdominal Apoplexy: Report of 6 Cases and Review of the Literature, *Am J Surg,* **111:**388, 1966.

Cochran, D. Q., Almond, C. H., and Shucart, W. A.: An Experimental Study of the Effects of Barium and Intestinal Contents on the Peritoneal Cavity, *Am J Roentgenol,* **89:**883, 1963.

Dale, G., and Solheim, K.: Bile Peritonitis in Acute Cholecystitis, *Acta Chir Scand,* **141:**746, 1975.

Dinner, M.: Biliary Peritonitis due to Idiopathic Perforation of the Common Bile Duct, *S Afr J Surg,* **13:**207, 1975.

Gardiner, H., and Miller, R. E.: Barium Peritonitis, *Am J Surg,* **125:**350, 1973.

Garfinkle, S. E., Chiu, G. W., Cohen, S. E., and Wolfman, E. F., Jr.: Spontaneous Perforation of the Neurogenic Urinary Bladder, *West J Med,* **124:**64, 1976.

Hamilton, J. E., and Harbrecht, P. J.: Growing Indications for Vagotomy in Perforated Peptic Ulcer, *Surg Gynecol Obstet,* **124:**61, 1967.

Kent, S. J., and Menzies-Gow, N.: Biliary Peritonitis without Perforation of the Gallbladder in Acute Cholecystitis, *Br J Surg,* **61:**960, 1974.

Krizek, T. J., and Davis, J. H.. Acute Chylous Peritonitis, *Arch Surg,* **91:**253, 1965.

Michas, C. A., Pollack, E. W., and Wolfman, E. A., Jr.: Hemoperitoneum due to Spontaneous Gastroepiploic Artery Rupture, *JAMA,* **237:**2526, 1977.

Moore, T. C.: Massive Bile Peritonitis in Infancy due to Spontaneous Bile Duct Perforation with Portal Vein Occlusion, *J Pediatr Surg,* **10:**537, 1975.

Nahrwold, D. L., Isch, J. H., Benner, E. A., and Miller, R. E.: Effect of Fluid Administration and Operations on Mortality Rate in Barium Peritonitis, *Surgery,* **70:**778, 1971.

Westfall, R. H., Nelson, R. H., and Musselman, M. M.: Barium Peritonitis, *Am J Surg,* **112:**760 1966.

Zheutlin, N., Lasser, E. C., and Rigler, L. G.: Clinical Studies on Effect of Barium in the Peritoneal Cavity following Rupture of the Colon, *Surgery,* **32:**967, 1952.

Granulomatous Peritonitis

Bayer, A. S., Blumenkrantz, M. J., Montgomerie, J. Z., Galpin, J. E., Coburn, J. W., and Guze, L. B.: Candida Peritonitis. Report of 22 Cases and Review of the English Literature, *Am J Med,* **61:**832, 1976.

Cromartie, R. S., III: Tuberculous Peritonitis, *Surg Gynecol Obstet,* **144:**876, 1977.

Dimmick, J. E., Bove, K. E., McAdams, A. T., and Benzing, G., III,: Fiber Embolization—A Hazard of Cardiac Surgery and Catheterization, *N Engl J Med,* **292:**685, 1975.

French, M. L. V., Ritter, M. A., Eitzen, H. E., and Hart, J. B.: Microbial Evaluation of Reusable and Disposable Laparotomy Sponges, *Surg Gynecol Obstet,* **137:**465, 1973.

Lintermans, J. P.: Fatal Peritonitis, an Unusual Complication of *Strongyloides stercoralis* Infestation, *Clin Pediatr (Phila),* **14:**947, 1975.

Monga, N. K., Sood, S., Kaushik, S. P., Sachdeva, H. S., Sood, K. C., and Datta, D. V.: Amebic Peritonitis, *Am J Gastroenterol,* **66:**366, 1976.

Singh, M. M., Bhargava, A. N., and Jain, K. P.: Tuberculous Peritonitis: An Evaluation of Pathogenic Mechanisms, Diagnostic Procedures and Therapeutic Measure, *N Engl J Med,* **281:**1091, 1969.

Sturdy, J. H., Baird, R. M., and Gerein, A. N.: Surgical Sponges: A Cause of Granuloma and Adhesion Formation, *Ann Surg,* **165:**128, 1967.

Tinker, M. A., Burdman, D., Deysine, M., Teicher, I., Platt, N., and Aufses, A. H., Jr.: Granulomatous Peritonitis due to Cellulose Fibers from Disposable Surgical Fabrics: Laboratory Investigation and Clinical Implications, *Ann Surg,* **180:**831, 1974.

Warshaw, A. L.: Management of Starch Peritonitis without the Unnecessary Second Operation, *Surgery,* **73:**681, 1973.

Spontaneous (Primary) Peritonitis

Brown, R. L., and Peter, G.: Clostridial Spontaneous Peritonitis, *JAMA,* **236:**2095, 1976.

Conn, H. O., and Fessel, J. M.: Spontaneous Bacterial Peritonitis in Cirrhosis, *Medicine,* **50:**161, 1971.

Correia, J. P., and Conn, H. O.: Spontaneous Bacterial Peritonitis in Cirrhosis: Endemic or Epidemic?, *Med Clin North Am,* **59:**963, 1975.

Curry, N., McCallum, R. W., and Guth, P. H.: Spontaneous Peritonitis in Cirrhosis Ascites: A Decade of Experience, *Am J Dig Dis,* **19:**685, 1974.

Dimond, M., and Proctor, H. J.: Spontaneous Pneumococcal Appendicitis, Peritonitis, and Meningitis, *Arch Surg,* **111:**888, 1976.

Flaum, M. A.: Spontaneous Bacterial Empyema in Cirrhosis, *Gastroenterology,* **70:**416, 1976.

Fowler, R.: Primary Peritonitis: Changing Aspects, 1956–1970, *Aust Paediatr J,* **7:**73, 1971.

Gerding, D. N., Khan, M. Y., Ewing, J. W., and Hall, W. H.: *Pasteurella multocida* Peritonitis in Hepatic Cirrhosis with Ascites, *Gastroenterology,* **70:**413, 1976.

McDougal, W. S., Izant, R. J., Jr., and Zollinger, R. M., Jr.: Primary Peritonitis in Infancy and Childhood, *Ann Surg,* **181:**310, 1975.

Murray, H. W., and Marks, S. J.: Spontaneous Bacterial Empyema, Pericarditis, and Peritonitis in Cirrhosis, *Gastroenterology,* **72:**772, 1977.

Rubin, H. M., Balu, E. B., and Michaels, R. H.: *Hemophilus* and Pneumococcal Peritonitis in Children with the Nephrotic Syndrome, *Pediatrics,* **56:**598, 1975.

Taraok, S. O. K., Moroi, T., Ikeuchi, T., Suyama, T., Endo, O., and Fukushima, K.: Detection of Endotoxin in Plasma and Ascitic Fluid of Patients with Cirrhosis: Its Clinical Significance, *Gastroenterology,* **73:**539, 1977.

Targan, S. R., Chow, A. W., and Guze, L. B.: Spontaneous Peritonitis of Cirrhosis due to *Campylobacter fetus, Gastroenterology,* **71:**311, 1976.

———, ———, and ———: Role of Anaerobic Bacteria in Spontaneous Peritonitis of Cirrhosis: Report of Two Cases and Review of the Literature, *Am J Med,* **62:**397, 1977.

Other Forms of Peritonitis

Brown, P., Baddeley, H., Read, A. E., Davies, J. D., and McGarry, J.: Sclerosing Peritonitis, an Unusual Reaction to a Beta-Adrengeric-Blocking Drug (Practolol), *Lancet,* **2:**1477, 1974.

Eltringham, W. K., Espiner, H. J., Windsor, C. W., Griffiths, D. A., Davies, J. D., Baddeley, H., Read, A. E., and Blunt, R. J.: Sclerosing Peritonitis due to Practolol: A Report on 9 Cases and Their Surgical Management, *Br J Surg,* **64:**229, 1977.

Kvale, P. A., and Parks, R. D.: Acute Abdomen. An Unusual Reaction to Isoniazid, *Chest,* **68:**271, 1975.

Reimann, H. A.: Periodic Peritonitis—Heredity and Pathology. Report of Seventy-two Cases, *JAMA,* **154:**1254, 1954.

———: Colchicine for Periodic Peritonitis, *JAMA,* **231:**64, 1975.

Robinson, M. M.: Antibiotics Increase Incidence of Hepatitis, *JAMA,* **178:**188, 1961.

Intraabdominal Abscesses

Autio, V.: The Spread of Intraperitoneal Infection: Studies with Roentgen Contrast Medium, *Acta Chir Scand* **321**[Suppl]:5, 1964.

Barnard, H. L.: Address on Surgical Aspects of Subphrenic Abscess, *Br Med J,* **1:**371 and 429, 1908.

Boyd, D. P.: The Subphrenic Spaces and the Emperor's New Robes, *N Engl J Med,* **275:**911, 1966.

DeCosse, J. J., Poulin, T. L., Fox, P. S., and Condon, R. E.: Subphrenic Abscess, *Surg Gynecol Obstet,* **138:**841, 1974.

Halasz, N. A.: Subphrenic Abscesses: Myths and Facts, *JAMA,* **214:**724, 1970.

Laing, F. C., and Jacobs, R. P.: Value of Ultrasonography in the Detection of Retroperitoneal Inflammatory Masses, *Radiology,* **123:**169, 1977.

Monk, R. S., and Wilson, S. D.: The Abdominal Cavity: An Observation, *Am J Surg,* **111:**854, 1966.

Owens, B. J., III, and Hamit, H. F.: Pancreatic Abscess and Pseudocyst, *Arch Surg,* **112:**42, 1977.

Perez, J., Rivera, J. V., and Bermudez, R. H.: Peritoneal Localization of Gallium-67, *Radiology,* **123:**695, 1977.

Ransom, J. H. C., and Spencer, F. C.: Prevention, Diagnosis and Treatment of Pancreatic Abscess, *Surgery,* **82:**99, 1977.

Wang, S. M. S., and Wilson, S. D.: Subphrenic Abscess: The New Epidemiology, *Arch Surg,* **112:**934, 1977.

White, P. H., Hayes, M. H., and Benfield, J. R.: Combined Liver-Lung Scanning in the Management of Subdiaphragmatic Abscess, *Am J Surg,* **124:**143, 1972.

Chapter 35

Abdominal Wall, Omentum, Mesentery, and Retroperitoneum

by **James T. Adams**

ANTERIOR ABDOMINAL WALL

General Considerations

The abdominal parietes contain and protect the abdominal viscera. Topographically, the anterior abdominal wall is bounded by the flare of the costal margins and the xiphoid process of the sternum above and by the iliac crests, inguinal ligaments, and pubis below. The principal structures that comprise the anterior abdominal wall are the rectus, external and internal oblique, and transversus abdominis and lower intercostal muscles together with their enveloping fascial sheaths and aponeuroses. The linea alba, a tendinous raphe formed by a blending of the aponeuroses of the oblique and transversus muscles in the midline, divides the anterior abdominal wall into two parts and thus restricts the medial extension of pathologic processes that may arise within it. Deep to the muscles is the continuous transversalis fascia, considered to be the strongest layer of the abdominal wall, and peritoneum.

The blood supply is furnished by the superior and inferior epigastric, lower intercostal, lumbar, and iliac circumflex arteries. The venous drainage corresponds to the arteries. Lymphatics in the upper half of the abdominal wall drain to the axillary nodes and those in the lower abdomen to the inguinal and thence to the iliac nodes. Lymph flow around the umbilicus may also ascend around the ligamentum teres (obliterated umbilical vein) to reach the porta hepatis. The nerve supply is via the intercostal and upper lumbar nerves.

In addition to protecting the abdominal viscera, the muscles function as an accessory respiratory apparatus and also aid in defecation by increasing intraabdominal muscle pressure with contraction.

Surgical diseases of the anterior abdominal wall include (1) hernia, (2) infection, (3) primary and metastatic tumors of soft tissue and muscle, (4) rectus sheath hematoma, and (5) desmoid tumor. With the exception of rectus sheath hematoma and desmoid tumor, these conditions are covered in other chapters of this textbook.

Rectus Sheath Hematoma

Bleeding into the rectus sheath produces a clinical picture which may simulate the acute surgical abdomen. The bleeding is usually the result of rupture of the epigastric artery or veins rather than a primary tear of the rectus muscle fibers. In a review of the entity by Jones and Merendino in 1962, reports were found on only 250 patients. The condition is probably more common than this, however, since minor degrees of bleeding can occur without causing significant symptoms.

ANATOMY (Fig. 35-1). The rectus abdominis muscle is crossed by three transverse tendinous intersections on its anterior aspect, so that its contractile force is divided into

Fig. 35-1. Rectus abdominis muscle and rectus sheath. From the rib margin to a point midway between the umbilicus and the pubis (linea semicircularis of Douglas), the posterior sheath is made up of the posterior leaf of the internal oblique aponeurosis, the aponeurosis of the transversus abdominis muscle, and the transversalis fascia. Below this level, the posterior wall is formed by transversalis fascia alone. The deep epigastric arteries and veins course along the posterior surface of the rectus muscle so that below the linea semicircularis they are separated from the peritoneum by only transversalis fascia.

three parts. The lowermost part is the longest, and hence its shortening with contraction is the greatest. There may be a difference of as much as 18 cm in length between extreme contraction and relaxation.

A strong fascial sheath, made up of the aponeuroses of the oblique and transversus abdominis muscles and transversalis fascia, contains the muscle. Anteriorly, the sheath is complete throughout; however, midway between the umbilicus and the pubis, the posterior sheath ends, forming an arched border, the linea semicircularis (of Douglas). Cephalad to this level, the internal oblique aponeurosis splits into two leaves, one passing on either side of the rectus, while below it no such division takes place, and, together with the aponeurosis of the transversus abdominis, it passes anteriorly. This leaves the rectus muscle below the linea semicircularis separated from the abdominal viscera only by transversalis fascia and peritoneum. The anterior leaf of the sheath is adherent to the transverse tendons and also to the lateral and medial margins of the muscle, while posteriorly the muscle is free. As a consequence of this anatomic arrangement, when there is bleeding within the rectus sheath below the umbilicus, the free blood may lie against the peritoneum, producing irritation and pain suggesting an acute intraabdominal disease.

The blood supply to the rectus muscle is from the superior and inferior epigastric arteries. The superior epigastric enters the rectus sheath from above as a terminal branch

of the internal mammary artery and passes caudad behind the muscle to anastomose with the larger inferior epigastric artery coming from below. The inferior epigastric artery, a branch of the external iliac artery, enters the rectus sheath just above the inguinal canal and courses upward along the posterior surface of the rectus muscle. Both arteries give off numerous muscular branches. Two veins accompany each artery. As the rectus muscle contracts, the epigastric vessels must glide beneath it to avoid injury.

ETIOLOGY. Rectus sheath hematoma may follow direct trauma to the epigastric blood vessels or occur spontaneously in association with several diseases. It has also been noted following a convulsive seizure. Spontaneous bleeding from the smaller muscular arteries has been reported in (1) infectious diseases, notably typhoid fever, (2) debilitating diseases, (3) collagen diseases, (4) blood dyscrasias such as hemophilia and leukemia, and (5) patients on anticoagulation therapy.

Frequently, however, bleeding occurs without obvious trauma or disease. In these patients the hematoma usually follows minor straining as in coughing or sneezing. Presumably the underlying factor is an inelasticity of the artery or vein which prevents the vessel from accommodating itself to the sudden marked variation in length which the rectus muscle undergoes during contraction and relaxation. Spontaneous rectus hematoma has also been described in pregnancy and in the puerperium. It is not known whether the hematoma is due to venous or arterial bleeding. However, stretching of the epigastric vessels by a distended abdomen during pregnancy or sudden relaxation after delivery are probably factors causing vessel injury. In the elderly, atheroma of an epigastric artery may predispose the vessel to rupture following minor exertion.

CLINICAL MANIFESTATIONS. Rectus sheath hematoma is three times more frequent in women than in men. The condition is rare in children and has a peak age incidence in the fifth decade. A prior history of trauma, sudden muscular exertion, generalized vascular disease, or anticoagulation suggests the diagnosis. Hematomas related to anticoagulation therapy usually become apparent 4 to 14 days after treatment is instituted. The first symptom is pain. This is sudden in onset, sharp, and progressively severe. The pain is felt in the side of the abdomen where the bleeding occurs and remains localized, since the hematoma in the rectus muscle is limited by the confines of its sheath. Usually this is the lower abdomen and more often on the right side. Anorexia, nausea but rarely vomiting, tachycardia, low-grade fever, and a moderate leukocytosis are frequent findings. With severe bleeding, signs of peripheral vascular collapse may develop. This is more apt to occur with bleeding below the linea semicircularis, where the peritoneum is only loosely adherent to the rectus muscle and thus cannot tampon the ruptured epigastric vessel. Tenderness and spasm are frequently present over the site of the hemorrhage. The bowel sounds are usually not altered. There may or may not be a palpable mass, depending on the extent of the bleeding. If present, the mass is tender, does not cross the midline, and remains palpable when the patient tenses the rectus muscle (Fothergill's sign). A bluish discoloration of the overlying skin is virtually diagnostic; however, this finding does not usually occur until 3 or 4 days after the patient is first seen.

The differential diagnosis may include almost every acute disease of the abdomen or pelvis. Notably, it has been mistaken for incarcerated interstitial hernia, acute appendicitis, acute cholecystitis, twisted ovarian cyst, diverticulitis, and ruptured aortic aneurysm. Teske, in a review of 100 cases, found that in only 17 percent was the correct diagnosis made preoperatively.

TREATMENT. If the correct diagnosis can be made and the rectus hematoma is small and not causing severe symptoms, the condition may be managed nonoperatively with bed rest and analgesics. Anticoagulants should be discontinued. It is rarely necessary to reverse a coagulation deficit when operation is not undertaken. Surgical intervention is necessary to rule out other, more serious diseases or to relieve symptoms of the hematoma. With a parame-

dian incision, the situation will become obvious as soon as the rectus sheath is opened and free blood is found. The hematoma may be diffuse throughout the rectus muscle or may be a localized clot. Bleeding arteries may or may not be present. Ideally, the hematoma is evacuated without entering the peritoneal cavity. Bleeding points are then ligated and the wound closed with or without drainage. The prognosis is dependent upon the underlying or concurrent disease but is generally good, and a full recovery can be anticipated. A poorer prognosis has been reported in pregnant patients in whom there is also a high fetal mortality.

Desmoid Tumor

Desmoid tumors are essentially benign, hard fibromas. It is probable, however, that they are not true neoplasms but an aggressive variant within a group of conditions referred to as "fibromatoses." The tumor is of aponeurotic origin and usually is found within or deep to the flat muscles of the anterior abdominal wall. Extraabdominal desmoid tumors involving skeletal muscles of the extremities, chest, and buttocks have also been reported but occur less frequently.

Desmoid tumors account for 3 to 4 percent of all tumefactions (7 percent of benign tumors) of the anterior abdominal wall. They usually occur in women in the child-bearing age group, often after a recent gestation. Occasionally they are seen in children.

ETIOLOGY. The cause of the tumor is unknown. It has been thought to be the result of hemorrhage following muscular injury from external trauma or sustained during pregnancy or parturition. Desmoids have also been reported arising in laparotomy scars. However, microscopic evidence of previous trauma, such as hemosiderin pigmentation, is usually absent. The finding of a high assay of gonadotropic substance in the tumor has prompted a sex-linked concept in explaining its cause.

PATHOLOGY. Desmoids are benign tumors that have the malignant property of local invasiveness. They grow slowly but progressively and can reach huge proportions. Rarely, they may penetrate the abdominal cavity or retroperitoneum and may even invade the periosteum of the pelvic bones. With such aggressive growth, they may not be totally resectable. Occasionally the tumor undergoes malignant transformation to a low-grade fibrosarcoma, but metastases from desmoids have never been reported. A striking feature of the tumor is its tendency to recur following local excision. The incidence of local recurrence is particularly high after excision of extraabdominal desmoids.

Grossly, the tumor is circumscribed or diffusely infiltrating yet characteristically unencapsulated and it invades as well as compresses muscle. It has a hard rubbery consistency which cuts with a creaking sensation and has a glistening whitish pink color. The microscopic appearance varies from an acellular fibroma to that of a cellular, low-grade fibrosarcoma. Masses of fibrous tissue can be seen that infiltrate, compress, and often destroy muscle bundles. In this respect, the tumor differs from the more commonly occurring benign fibroma of soft tissue. The absence of mitotic figures and the well-differentiated fibrous tissue are features which differentiate it from the malignant fibrosarcoma.

CLINICAL MANIFESTATIONS. There are no special clinical features characteristic of desmoid tumors. They usually present as a painless, deeply situated mass that is solitary and may be fixed. Its deep location allows it to assume a large size before it is recognized. Usually the tumor is located in the lower abdomen and rarely crosses the midline. It must be differentiated from other tumors of soft tissue and muscle, particularly sarcomas.

TREATMENT. The ideal treatment of desmoid tumors is wide surgical excision. This often necessitates resection of a large portion of the abdominal wall including skin, muscle, and peritoneum. The resulting defect may require fascia, skin, or a sliding muscle graft for closure. The excision, however, should not sacrifice major blood vessels, nerves, or an extremity. Even though recurrences are frequent, they can still be successfully treated by reexcision. In spite of its tendency to recur, the tumor is rarely fatal. Drugs that affect the metabolism of cyclic 3',5'-adenosine monophosphate, such as theophylline and chlorothiazide, have recently been shown to promote tumor shrinkage and may be worthy of use as an adjunct to surgery.

DISEASES OF THE OMENTUM

General Considerations

The greater omentum consists of a double sheet of flattened endothelium; between the folds the epiploic vessels, lymphatics, and nerves pass in areolar tissue enmeshed with a variable amount of fat. The structure hangs in a double fold, or sling, between the greater curvature of the stomach and the transverse colon. At birth, an agglutination of the two layers occurs, creating an apron-like shield overlying the intestinal coils. The right border attaches to the pylorus or first portion of the duodenum, while the left border forms the gastrosplenic ligament. The right side is usually longer and heavier and may possess tonguelike processes extending into the pelvis. Occasionally, accessory omenta exist attached to the main portion. The size of the greater omentum is related to the amount of fat which it contains, so that often it is huge in obese individuals and very thin and small in emaciated persons. The omentum in infants is usually underdeveloped and may be almost nonexistent. With growth of the individual, there is elongation and thickening of the organ due to the deposition of fat within its layers.

As a peritoneal fold, the omentum assumes the mechanical function of a mesentery, that is, the fixation of viscera and the transmission of a vascular supply. It is otherwise not a vital organ. Furthermore, it can be removed without appreciable disturbance to the individual.

It has long been held that the omentum possesses an inherent motility which allows it to seek out and arrest

trouble that may arise within the peritoneal cavity. In this regard, it has been referred to as the "policeman of the abdomen." While it is true that the omentum is often found at the site of an intraabdominal pathologic condition, yet objective evidence, summarized by Rubin, shows that it has no spontaneous or ameboid activity and that displacement occurs as a result of intestinal peristalsis, diaphragmatic excursions, and postural changes of the individual. The areolar tissue is rich in macrophages which have been shown to rapidly remove injected bacteria or foreign particles. Draper and Johnston concluded that the usefulness of the omentum in inflammatory processes is related to its bactericidal and absorptive properties and also its ability to form adhesions.

Surgical diseases of the omentum include torsion, infarction, cysts, and solid tumors.

Torsion of the Omentum

Torsion of the omentum is a condition in which the organ twists on its long axis to an extent causing vascular compromise. This may vary from mild vascular constriction producing edema to complete strangulation leading to infarction and frank gangrene. For torsion to occur, two situations must exist: first, a redundant and mobile segment and, secondly, a fixed point around which the segment may twist.

ETIOLOGY. Omental torsion has been classified as primary or secondary. Primary, or idiopathic, omental torsion is relatively rare. It was first described by Eitel in 1899, and since then less than 200 cases have been reported in the literature. The cause is obscure. Leitner et al. group the causes of primary torsion into predisposing factors and precipitating factors. Among the suggested predisposing factors are a variety of anatomic variations including tonguelike projections from the free edge of the omentum, bifid omentum, accessory omentum, a large and bulky omentum with a narrow pedicle, and obesity associated with irregular distribution of fat within the organ. Venous redundancy relative to the omental arterial blood supply has also been cited as a predisposing factor. The omental veins are larger and more tortuous than the arteries, allowing venous kinking and thus offering a point of fixation around which twisting may occur. The higher incidence of right-sided omental torsion is related to the greater size and mobility of the right omentum.

Precipitating factors are those which cause displacement of the omentum. These include heavy exertion, sudden change in body position, coughing, straining, and hyperperistalsis with overeating. Primary omental torsion is always unipolar in that there is only one locus of fixation.

Secondary omental torsion is that which is associated with adhesions of the free end of the omentum to cysts, tumors, foci of intraabdominal inflammation, postsurgical wounds, or scarring, or to internal or external hernias. It is more common than the primary type and is usually bipolar; that is, torsion of the central portion occurs between two fixed points. About two-thirds of these cases are found in patients with hernias, usually of the inguinal variety. The precipitating factors which incite secondary torsion are the same as those for primary torsion.

PATHOLOGY. The omentum in both the primary and secondary varieties twists a variable number of turns around a pivotal point, usually in a clockwise direction (Fig. 35-2). Either the whole omentum or more often a small portion may undergo torsion. The right side is involved more frequently. Venous return is restricted, and the distal omentum becomes congested and edematous. Hemorrhagic extravasation results in a characteristic serosanguineous effusion into the peritoneal cavity. If the process is of sufficient duration, acute hemorrhagic infarction and eventual necrosis of the segment occur. If not excised, the mass becomes atrophied and fibrotic, and on rare occasions is autoamputated.

CLINICAL MANIFESTATIONS. The clinical features of primary and secondary omental torsion are similar. The condition usually occurs in the fourth or fifth decades of life. Males are affected twice as frequently as females. Pain is the initial and predominant symptom. The onset of pain is usually sudden, and it is constant with a gradual increase in severity. Occasionally the pain is first experienced in the periumbilical region or is generalized. However, invariably it becomes localized to the right side of the abdomen, usually the right lower quadrant. This is in keeping with the more frequent involvement of the right side of the omentum. Movement intensifies the pain. Nausea and vomiting occur in less than half the patients. There is a moderate leukocytosis and a fever which rarely exceeds a rise of 1°C. Tenderness is invariably present, and rebound tenderness and voluntary spasm are also frequent findings. A mass may be palpable if the involved omentum is sufficiently large.

The symptoms and signs are not usually sufficient to allow an accurate preoperative diagnosis. Secondary torsion of the hernial type, however, can be suspected if a tender mass is palpable in the groin. The clinical impressions, in order of frequency, are acute appendicitis, acute cholecystitis, and twisted ovarian cyst. Actually, a preoperative diagnosis is of academic interest only, since the clinical manifestations warrant exploration. The finding of free serosanguineous fluid at the time of laparotomy in the absence of a pathologic condition in the appendix, gallbladder, or pelvic organs should alert the surgeon to the possibility of omental torsion.

TREATMENT. Treatment consists of resection of the involved omentum. In patients with secondary torsion, the underlying etiologic condition, that is, hernia, cysts, adhesions, etc., should also be corrected. The operative mortality and morbidity are virtually nil.

Idiopathic Segmental Infarction of Omentum

Idiopathic segmental omental infarction is an acute vascular disturbance of the omentum of unknown cause. The criteria for diagnosis of this condition are that it not be accompanied by omental torsion, that there be no associated cardiovascular disease or local intraabdominal patho-

Fig. 35-2. Surgical specimen of primary torsion of the omentum. A small segment of normal-appearing omentum can be seen above the pivotal point (arrow), where it has twisted several times. The omentum below this is congested and hemorrhagic.

logic condition, and that there be no history of external abdominal trauma, situations which produce secondary omental infarction. The condition is rare, less than 70 cases having been reported.

ETIOLOGY AND PATHOLOGY. The condition is precipitated by thrombosis of omental veins secondary to endothelial injury. Halligan and Rabiah summarized the several proposed causes of endothelial damage and thrombosis. These include (1) stretching or primary rupture of the omental veins by a sudden increase in intraabdominal pressure as with coughing, sneezing, or lifting, especially after the ingestion of a heavy meal; (2) gravitational pull of an extremely fatty omentum on the omental veins, causing their rupture; and (3) an anatomic peculiarity of the venous drainage of the omentum which predisposes to thrombosis.

The right lower segment of the omentum, which is the most mobile and richest in fat, is the portion usually involved. The area of infarction may vary from 2 to 20 cm in its greatest diameter. Grossly, the involved segment is well demarcated, edematous, and hemorrhagic or gangrenous. It is usually closely adherent to the parietal peritoneum or adjacent abdominal viscera. A variable amount of serosanguineous fluid in the free peritoneal cavity is a constant finding. Microscopically, the picture is that of a hemorrhagic infarction with thrombosis of the omental veins and infiltration of the omentum with inflammatory cells.

CLINICAL MANIFESTATIONS. The majority of patients are young or middle-aged adults, and there is a 3:1 predilection for males. The clinical features are nonspecific. Most patients present with a gradual onset of abdominal pain which is steady and virtually always on the right side of the abdomen. Anorexia and nausea are frequent, but vomiting is rare. Diarrhea or constipation is unusual. There is always tenderness and often rebound tenderness over the region of infarction. Voluntary guarding and occasionally spasm are also common. The infarcted segment, if large enough, may be palpable. A slight fever (rarely over 38.5°C) and a moderate leukocytosis are usual.

TREATMENT. Treatment of this condition is resection of the infarcted area to prevent the possible complications of gangrene and adhesions. A correct preoperative diagnosis is unusual, and most patients are explored for acute appendicitis or acute cholecystitis. The finding of serosanguineous fluid in the abdomen and a normal appendix or gallbladder should make the surgeon suspect disease in the omentum. The operative mortality is nil.

Cysts of the Omentum

PATHOLOGY. Cysts of the omentum are rare. The pathogenesis of these lesions is unclear, but presumably most true cysts are caused by obstruction of lymphatic channels or by growth of congenitally misplaced lymphatic tissue that does not communicate with the vascular system. They contain serous fluid and may be unilocular or multilocular. The cysts have an endothelial lining similar to cystic lymphangiomas found elsewhere. Their size may vary from a few centimeters to over 30 cm in diameter. Dermoid cysts, which are very rare, are lined with squamous epithelium and may contain hair, teeth, and sebaceous material.

Pseudocysts of the omentum result from fat necrosis, trauma with hematoma, or foreign body reaction. These have a fibrous and inflammatory lining and usually contain cloudy or blood-tinged fluid.

CLINICAL MANIFESTATIONS. True omental cysts are discovered most frequently in children or young adults but have been reported in the aged. Small cysts are generally asymptomatic and discovered incidentally at laparotomy or at autopsy. Large cysts present as a palpable abdominal mass or produce diffuse abdominal swelling. These may cause symptoms of heaviness or pain or manifestations of possible complications of omental cysts such as torsion, infection, rupture, or intestinal obstruction. Complications are more frequent in children and often produce a clinical picture of an acute surgical condition of the abdomen. The uncomplicated omental cyst usually lies in the lower midabdomen and is freely movable, smooth, and nontender.

Plain roentgenograms sometimes show a circumscribed soft tissue haziness in the abdomen, or, following a barium meal, there may be displacement of intestinal loops with pressure on adjacent bowel. The presence of bone or teeth is diagnostic of dermoid cyst.

Differential diagnosis includes cysts and solid tumors of the mesentery, peritoneum, and retroperitoneal region. An absolute diagnosis can be made only at the time of exploratory surgical procedures. Treatment consists of local excision.

Solid Tumors of the Omentum

The most common solid tumor of the omentum is metastatic carcinoma, which generally involves the omentum by tumor implant. The primary source is usually the colon, stomach, pancreas, or ovaries. Frequently there is associated ascites, presumably from "weeping" of serous or blood-tinged fluid from the metastatic implants.

Primary solid tumors of the omentum are exceedingly rare. They may be benign or malignant. Stout et al. recorded only 24 seen over a 55-year period at a major tumor institution. Most are tumors of smooth muscle, and about one-third are malignant. Benign tumors consist of lipomas, leiomyomas, fibromas, and neurofibromas. The malignant tumors are leiomyosarcoma, fibrosarcoma, liposarcoma, and hemangiopericystomas. The malignant tumors spread by direct extension or tumor implants and kill by involvement of vital abdominal organs.

The only treatment is surgical excision. Primary malignant tumors are highly invasive and often require resection of adjacent organs as well as total omentectomy. The prognosis for these is very poor. Resection of benign tumors is curative, and recurrences have not been reported. Palliative omentectomy for metastatic tumor implants in the omentum has been suggested to control any associated ascites.

MESENTERY AND MESENTERIC CIRCULATION

Anatomy

The mesentery is essentially a reflection of the posterior parietal peritoneum onto the surface of the intestine, where it becomes visceral peritoneum. It connects the intestine to the posterior abdominal wall and carries blood vessels and nerves.

The mesentery proper serves primarily as a suspensory ligament of the jejunum and ileum. It is fan-shaped, its root extending downward and obliquely from the ligament of Treitz (duodenojejunal flexure) at the level of L_2 to the right sacroiliac articulation (ileocecal junction) (Fig. 35-3). The entire root is only about 6 in. long and allows free motion of the small intestine in any direction, limited only by the length of the mesentery. Within its two fused layers of peritoneum run the intestinal branches of the superior mesenteric artery and accompanying vein. It also contains lymph vessels, mesenteric lymph nodes, visceral nerve fibers, and a variable amount of adipose tissue.

Following the embryonic formation of a distinct intestinal loop, torsion of the loop takes place about the superior mesenteric artery. At about the third or fourth fetal month, posterior peritoneal fixation of the colon takes place. The leaves of the mesentery to the ascending colon fuse with

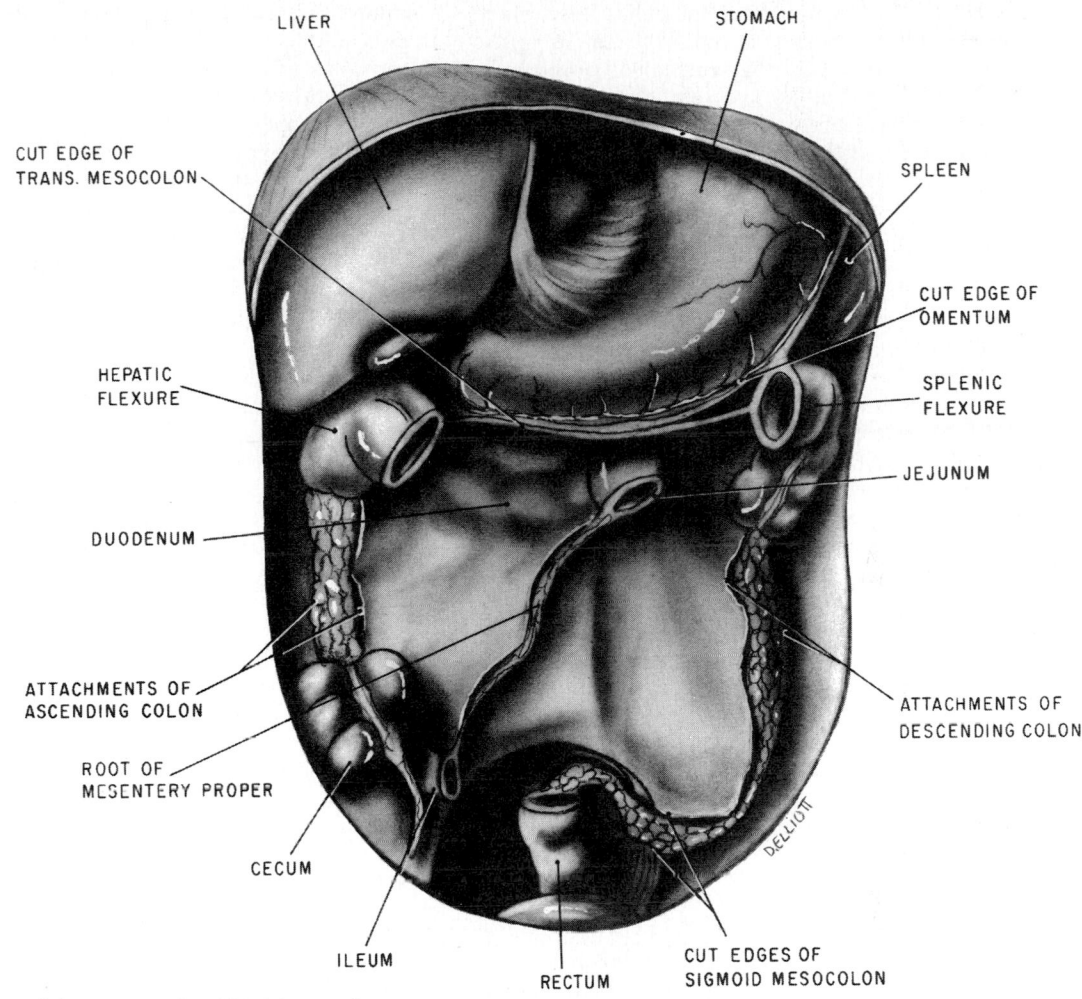

LIVER

STOMACH

CUT EDGE OF
TRANS. MESOCOLON

SPLEEN

CUT EDGE OF
OMENTUM

HEPATIC
FLEXURE

SPLENIC
FLEXURE

DUODENUM

JEJUNUM

ATTACHMENTS OF
ASCENDING COLON

ATTACHMENTS OF
DESCENDING COLON

ROOT OF
MESENTERY PROPER

CECUM

ILEUM

RECTUM

CUT EDGES OF
SIGMOID MESOCOLON

Fig. 35-3. Attachments of the mesenteries. The jejunum, ileum, and ascending, transverse, and descending colons have been removed.

the right parietal peritoneum, and those to the descending colon fuse with the left parietal peritoneum. The lateral posterior parietal peritoneum then passes directly from the abdominal wall over the ascending and descending colon respectively toward the midline and the root of the mesentery proper. For this reason, the mesentery to these portions of the large intestine is usually short or nonexistent. These fusions, however, form surgical cleavage plains allowing bloodless mobilization of the colon with its vascular supply. Within the embryonic mesentery to the ascending colon are the colonic arteries and veins from the superior mesenteric vessels, while those to the descending colon are derived from the inferior mesenteric vessels. On occasion, posterior fusion of the ascending or descending colon is incomplete or does not occur, leaving a well-developed mesentery and allowing free mobility of the bowel segment. This anomaly is more frequent with the right colon, thus predisposing to torsion with resulting intestinal obstruction.

The mesenteries of the transverse colon and sigmoid colon, in contrast to those of the ascending and descending colon, do not fuse with the posterior parietal peritoneum. These remain well developed and are referred to as the "transverse mesocolon" and "sigmoid mesocolon," respectively. The segment to the transverse colon extends obliquely across the posterior abdominal wall just below the pancreas, remaining fixed at the hepatic and splenic flexures of the bowel (Fig. 35-3). The fixation of the splenic flexure is higher than that of the hepatic flexure because of the presence of the liver on the right side. The mesocolon allows the transverse colon to hang over the small intestine. This sagging may be so marked that the transverse colon occasionally reaches the symphysis pubis. Within the transverse mesocolon run branches of the middle colic artery and accompanying vein. Fusion between the mesocolon and the undersurface of the greater omentum from the stomach offers stability which prevents the transverse colon from undergoing torsion.

The sigmoid mesocolon originates at the end of the descending colon in the left iliac fossa and has an inverted V-shape course (Fig. 35-3). It runs diagonally upward along the left iliac artery toward the aortic bifurcation and then bends directly downward into the pelvic fossa, where it is reflected off the rectum. It contains sigmoid vessels and branches of the superior hemorrhoidal vessels from the inferior mesenteric artery and vein. The length of the sigmoid mesocolon determines the location and mobility of the pelvic colon. If the sigmoid mesocolon is long, the bowel may cross the midline. Such a mobile pelvic colon may twist upon itself. The sigmoid colon is the most frequent site of torsion producing volvulus of the intestinal tract.

The lateral fixations of the ascending and descending colon and the superior origin of the transverse mesocolon serve to confine the small intestine within the midabdomen. The transverse mesocolon and greater omentum also restrict the small bowel from entering the upper abdomen to become adherent to inflammatory lesions of the stomach, duodenum, gallbladder, or liver.

Defects in the mesenteries are potential sites for internal hernia. Most defects are created inadvertently by the surgeon during the course of intraabdominal operations. On rare occasions congenital defects occur in areas of the mesentery that are thin and avascular. These are usually found in the mesenteries of the lower ileum, the sigmoid mesocolon, and the transverse mesocolon, the last through a wide avascular space just to the left of the middle colic artery (space of Riolan, Fig. 35-6).

The mesenteries share with the omenta bactericidal and absorptive properties as well as the ability to form adhesions. In this regard, they function to localize and combat intraperitoneal infection and to seal off intestinal perforations.

MESENTERIC CIRCULATION

In addition to serving as a system for the transport of nutriments, the mesenteric vascular bed is of major importance in the maintaining of bodily homeostasis. Under resting conditions, the splanchnic (visceral) vascular bed receives 25 to 30 percent of cardiac output and contains as much as one-third of total blood volume. It has been suggested that this reservoir of blood produces a mechanism for "autotransfusion" during periods of hypovolemia, when a relatively large volume of blood can be rapidly released into the circulation by active constriction of the splanchnic vessels. Control of the mesenteric vascular bed is primarily neural via sympathetic autonomic elements carried by the splanchnic nerves. These nerves accompany the celiac, superior mesenteric, and inferior mesenteric arteries which contain both alpha- and beta-adrenergic receptors. Stimulation of the splanchnic nerves produces vasoconstriction, with an increase in regional resistance. The mesenteric vasculature is also responsive to a number of pharmacological agents. Norepinephrine, an alpha-adrenergic stimulator, produces vasoconstriction, and epinephrine elicits a classic dose-dependent beta- or alpha-adrenergic response, low concentrations producing vasodilatation and higher concentrations producing vasoconstriction. Isoproterenol, a beta-adrenergic stimulator, effects a dilator response which can be blocked by propranolol. Tolazoline hydrochloride and papaverine hydro-

chloride elicit a direct vasodilatory effect, and the digitalis glycosides have been shown to produce mesenteric vasoconstriction, also presumably by a direct action on the mesenteric vasculature.

Knowledge of the anatomy of the mesenteric circulation is important in the performance of safe and adequate operations on the intestine and in the management of patients with occlusive mesenteric vascular disease and portal hypertension. In resections for malignant lesions, it is necessary to excise a wide segment of adjacent mesentery in order that real or potential sites of tumor spread to the mesenteric lymphatics and lymph nodes are removed.

ARTERIES. With the exception of the stomach and duodenum and the distal rectum, the arterial supply to the entire intestinal tract is derived from the superior and inferior mesenteric arteries.

The superior mesenteric artery arises from the aorta just below the celiac artery opposite the level of L_2. It passes behind the neck of the pancreas but in front of the uncinate process and crosses in front of the third portion of the duodenum to enter the root of the mesentery proper. The acute angle which the superior mesenteric artery makes at its origin from the aorta may compress the transverse portion of the duodenum between it and the aorta, causing partial intestinal obstruction, a condition referred to as the "superior mesenteric artery compression syndrome."

As the superior mesenteric artery continues downward between the two leaves of the mesentery, it gives off 12 or more major branches from its left side which supply the jejunum and ileum (Fig. 35-4). These jejunal and ileal arteries divide and then reunite within the mesentery to form groups, or arcades. Two to five such anastomotic arches are formed and allow collateral pathways for blood to reach the intestinal wall should occlusion of short arterial segments occur. The arcades become more numerous as the terminal ileum is reached. From the terminal arcades, straight branches (vasa recta) alternately pass to opposite sides of the jejunum and ileum. Within the intestinal wall, the vessels run parallel to the circular muscle coat and perpendicular to the direction of the lumen traversing successively the serous, muscular, and submucosal layers. Each of these terminal arteries supplies only 1 or 2 cm of bowel length. For this reason, they must be preserved as close to the cut margins of the intestine as is technically possible when performing a bowel resection to avoid necrosis and breakdown of the subsequent anastomosis. The terminal straight arteries do not anastomose until reaching the submucous plexuses, where their ramifications anastomose freely. This situation predisposes to serious compromise of the blood supply to the antimesenteric border of the intestine following segmental small bowel resection. Therefore, to ensure adequate circulation to the antimesenteric portion, it is customary to transect the small intestine obliquely rather than at a right angle (Fig. 35-5).

Arising from the right side of the superior mesenteric artery is the inferior pancreaticoduodenal artery and then successively, the middle colic, the right colic, and the ileo-

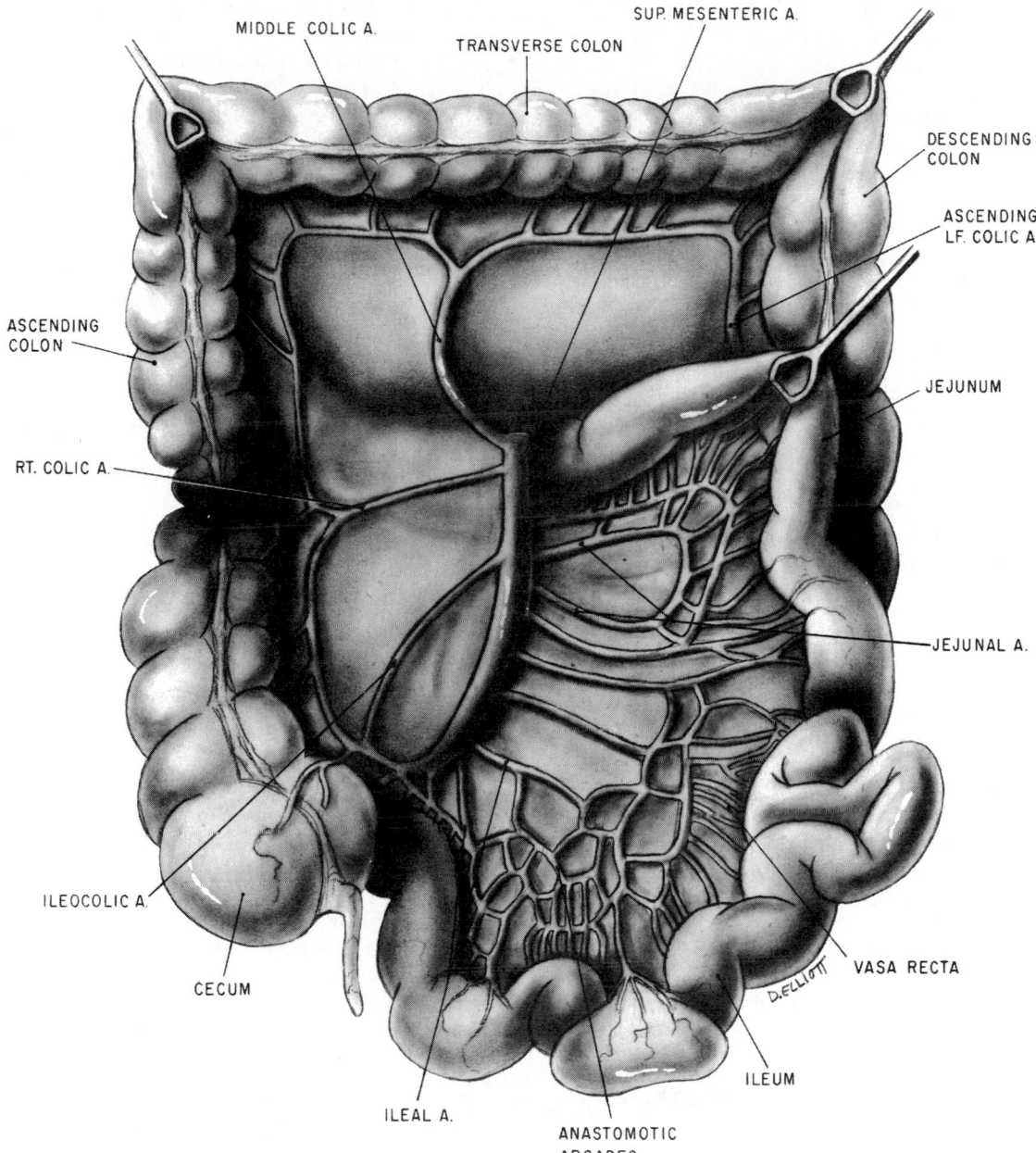

Fig. 35-4. Superior mesenteric artery and its branches. The artery supplies the distal duodenum, jejunum, ileum, ascending colon, and proximal two-thirds of the transverse colon.

colic arteries (Fig. 35-4). Except for the ileocolic artery, these vessels do not form anastomotic arcades until nearly reaching the bowel wall.

The middle colic artery arises below the pancreas, enters the transverse mesocolon, and passing to the right divides into a right and left branch. The right branch connects with the superior branch of the right colic artery and the left branch with the ascending branch of the left colic artery from the inferior mesenteric. It supplies the transverse colon. The location of the main arterial trunk to the

right of the midline allows the left side of the transverse mesocolon to be opened through a relatively avascular area (space of Riolan) when performing a retrocolic gastrojejunal anastomosis.

The right colic artery arises just below the middle colic and passes to the right just behind the peritoneum. On reaching the mid-ascending colon, it divides into superior and inferior branches, which anastomose close to the bowel wall, with branches from the middle colic and ileocolic arteries, respectively. The right colic artery supplies the ascending colon.

The ileocolic artery is the terminal branch of the superior mesenteric artery. It supplies the distal few inches of

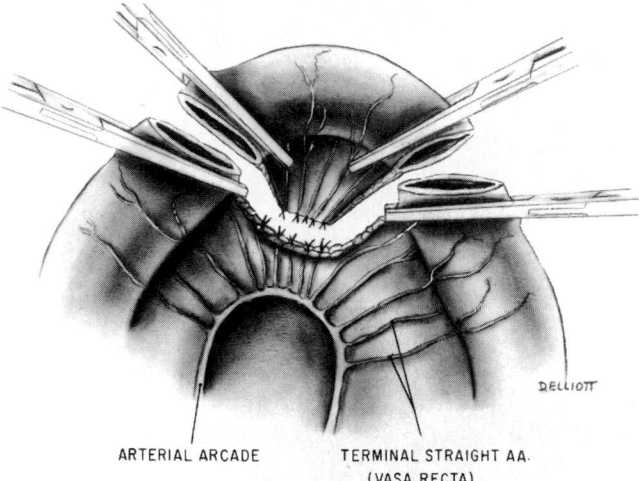

ARTERIAL ARCADE   TERMINAL STRAIGHT AA.
                              (VASA RECTA)

Fig. 35-5. Straight arteries (vasa recta) entering the wall of the small intestine perpendicular to the direction of its lumen. The arteries alternately pass to either side of the intestinal wall. In performing a segmental resection of the small intestine, transecting the bowel obliquely, as indicated, ensures an adequate blood supply to the antimesenteric border.

the ileum, the cecum, the appendix, and the lower portion of the ascending colon. It terminates by dividing into ascending and descending branches. The ascending branch anastomoses with the inferior branch of the right colic artery, while the descending branch forms secondary and tertiary arcades by anastomosing with terminal branches of the superior mesenteric artery within the mesentery proper. From these arcades arise the appendicular artery to the appendix, and cecal and ileal branches.

The superior mesenteric artery supplies the intestinal tract from the third portion of the duodenum to the midtransverse colon. Collaterals between the inferior pancreaticoduodenal artery and the superior pancreaticoduodenal artery from the gastroduodenal, a secondary branch of the celiac artery, enable the third part of the duodenum and proximal 4 or 5 in. of jejunum to survive when the superior mesenteric artery is occluded.

The inferior mesenteric artery supplies the left transverse colon, descending colon, sigmoid colon, and proximal part of the rectum. It arises from the anterior aorta opposite the body of the third lumbar vertebra and passes downward and to the left, entering the pelvis as the superior hemorrhoidal artery (Fig. 35-6). As it descends, it gives off the left colic and sigmoidal arteries. The left colic artery is the principal branch. It divides into ascending and descending limbs which anastomose with branches from the middle colic and sigmoid arteries, respectively. The sigmoid artery passes into the sigmoid mesocolon and divides into branches which anastomose with one another, forming several arcades. The lowest sigmoid arcade joins with arcades from the superior hemorrhoidal artery. The superior hemorrhoidal artery continues downward behind the rectum, where it communicates with branches from the middle and inferior hemorrhoidal arteries from the inter-

nal iliac artery, giving the rectum a dual source of arterial supply.

The anastomoses between primary branches of the superior and inferior mesenteric arteries form an arcade which passes along the margin of the colon and is referred to as the "marginal artery of Drummond" (Fig. 35-6). It is situated about $\frac{1}{2}$ in. from the margin of the bowel and extends from the end of the ileum to the end of the sigmoid colon. Through its anastomoses, it is capable of supplying the bowel even though one of the major arteries is ligated.

VEINS. The venous drainage of the small intestine and colon is through tributaries of the inferior and superior mesenteric veins, which in turn ultimately terminate in the portal vein (Fig. 35-7). The portal circulation begins within the mucosa of the intestine. Small venules coalesce, and the confluent veins pass through the wall of the intestine, emerging alternately in a similar manner to that of the straight arteries entering the bowel wall. These then converge to form a system of venous arcades within the mesentery from which blood enters the main tributaries to the superior and inferior mesenteric veins.

The inferior mesenteric vein is a continuation of the superior hemorrhoidal vein. It passes upward to the left side of the inferior mesenteric artery, receiving tributaries which correspond in name and location to the branches of the artery. However, the main trunk of the vein does not accompany the artery but rather courses over the duodenojejunal flexure just lateral to the ligament of Treitz and, passing over the body of the pancreas, joins with the splenic vein (Figs. 35-6, 35-7). It drains the left side of the large intestine from the upper rectum to the left midtransverse colon. A plexus of anastomoses around the midrectum between the superior hemorrhoidal vein and the middle and inferior hemorrhoidal veins to the internal iliac veins form a collateral pathway between the portal and systemic circulation.

The superior mesenteric vein runs within the mesentery proper lateral to the superior mesenteric artery. It receives tributaries which accompany corresponding branches of the superior mesenteric artery and which drain the entire small intestine and right half of the colon. As it passes over the third portion of the duodenum and behind the neck of the pancreas, it receives the confluence of the inferior mesenteric and splenic veins to become the portal vein (see Chap. 30).

The venous drainage from the entire gastrointestinal tract passes through the liver via the portal circulation before returning to the heart. Together with the mesenteric lymphatics, it represents the sole means by which ingested food products find their way into the circulation. The normal portal venous pressure is between 12 and 15 cm of water; that within the inferior vena cava (systemic pressure) varies between a positive pressure of about 3 cm during the expiratory phase of respiration to a negative pressure of 1 to 3 cm during inspiration. Like the vena cava, the portal system does not contain valves, and therefore the blood can flow in the direction of reduced venous pressure.

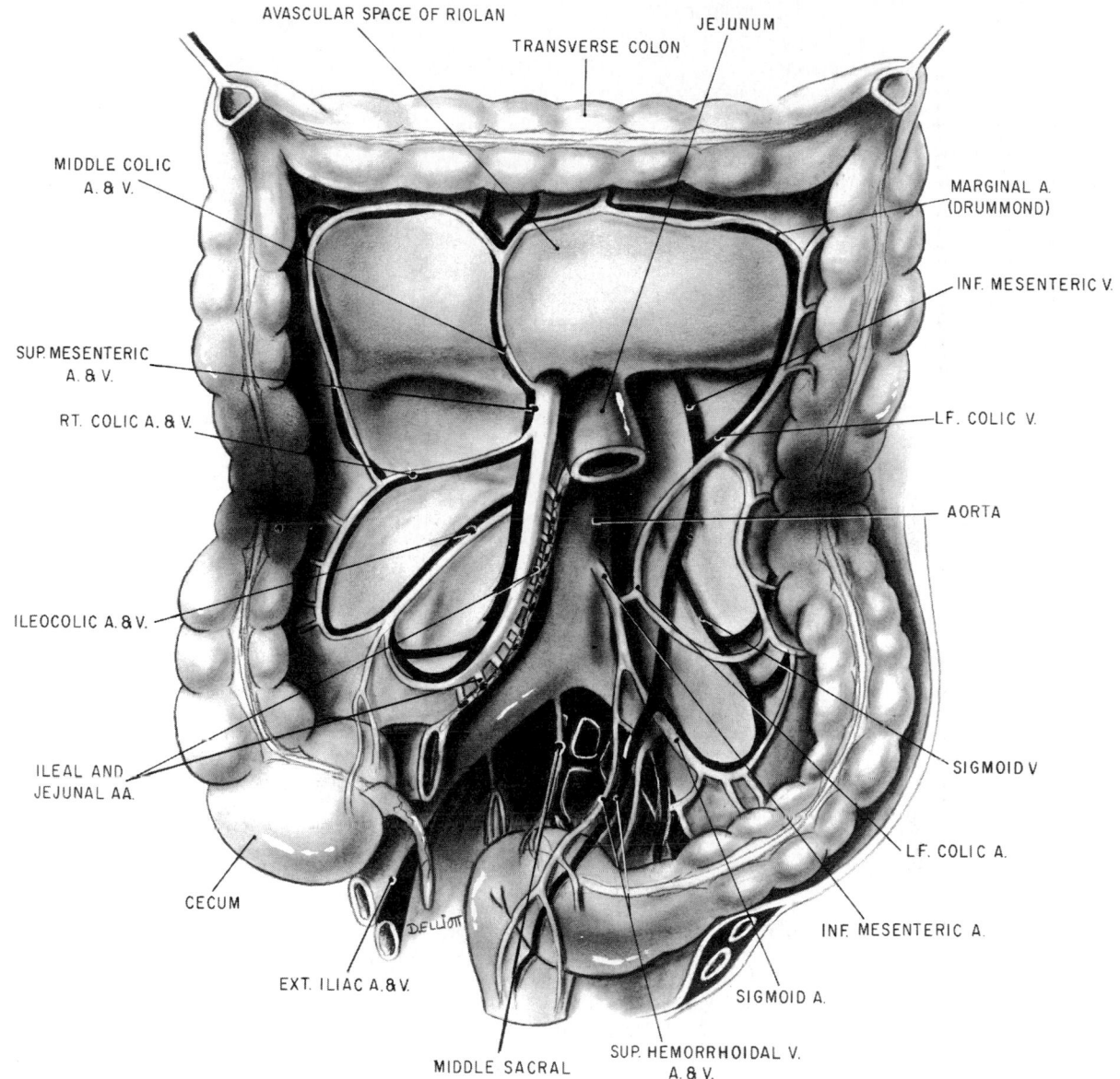

Fig. 35-6. Blood supply to the large bowel. An arterial arcade, formed by anastomoses between branches of the colic arteries, runs along the margin of the large intestine and is referred to as the *marginal artery of Drummond*. This vessel is the major collateral supplying blood to the colon when a main stem mesenteric or colic artery is occluded.

MESENTERIC LYMPHATICS AND LYMPH NODES. The lymph drainage of the small intestine and colon follow the course of the main blood vessels. Those accompanying the inferior mesenteric artery drain to perinortic nodes and thence to the superior mesenteric nodes before entering the cisterna chyli of the thoracic duct. Those accompanying branches of the superior mesenteric artery drain into the mesenteric glands within the mesentery proper, where they are closely related to the vascular arcades. The mesenteric nodes are distributed in three locations: (1) juxtaintestinal,

at the last anastomotic branch of the mesenteric arteries before they enter the intestines; (2) intermediate, in the region of the larger anastomosing branches; and (3) central, at the root of the mesentery near the origin of the main mesenteric artery. The nodes are more numerous in the right half of the mesentery, and they increase in size and number as they approach its root. These nodes are the usual site for mesenteric adenitis, tuberculosis, and other inflammatory as well as neoplastic conditions. From the mesenteric nodes, lymph drains into the superior mesenteric and celiac nodes and then to the thoracic duct.

Mesenteric Vascular Disease

Mesenteric vascular disease is not a single entity but rather a syndrome that includes (1) complete occlusion or

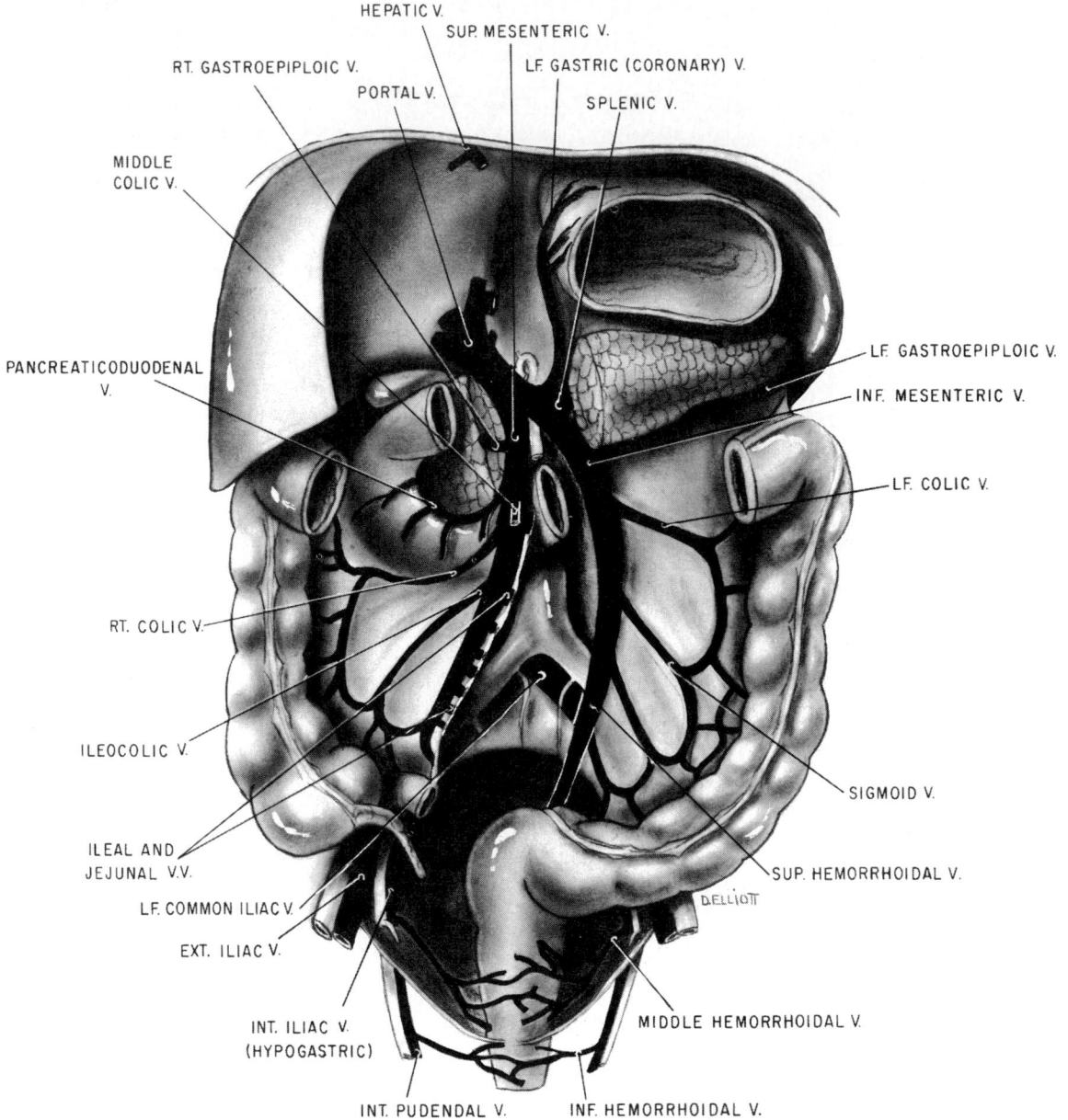

Fig 35-7. Mesenteric (portal) venous circulation, showing the communication with the systemic circulation through the middle and inferior hemorrhoidal veins. A similar communication (not shown) exists between the left gastric vein and the azygos system of veins.

stenosis of mesenteric arteries by embolism, thrombosis, or obliterative disease; (2) thrombosis of mesenteric (portal) veins; (3) extraluminal obstruction of mesenteric arteries by aortic aneurysm, dissecting aneurysm, fibrous and ligamentous bands, or tumors; (4) spontaneous rupture of visceral blood vessels (abdominal apoplexy); and (5) traumatic injury to visceral vessels. These conditions produce vascular insufficiency or infarction of the affected intestine. Intestinal disease due to impaired circulation is relatively uncommon when compared to the more frequently occurring mechanical obstructions of the mesenteric vessels by adhesive bands, strangulated hernia, or intestinal volvulus.

Occlusions of the mesenteric arteries may be acute and complete (those due to emboli or thrombosis), gradual and partial (those due to obliterative arterial disease), or acute and complete superimposed upon a previously narrowed

or stenotic vessel. The superior mesenteric artery at its origin or close to the takeoff of its middle colic branch is the usual site of both acute and chronic mesenteric arterial occlusions. Complete occlusion of the inferior mesenteric artery usually produces symptoms only if there is compromise of collateral blood flow from the superior mesenteric or internal iliac (hypogastric) arteries. Clinically apparent venous occlusions are sudden and complete and invariably due to thrombosis. Partial mesenteric venous occlusion is usually due to external compression and is asymptomatic.

The relative incidence of mesenteric arterial as opposed to venous occlusions is not known. When intestinal infarction occurs, it is not unusual to find thrombosis of both sides of the splanchnic circulation at laparotomy or autopsy, since initial occlusion of one eventuates in clot formation in the other. Moreover, the clinical distinction between the two is often difficult. It has been variously estimated that 15 to 20 percent of all clinically significant mesenteric vascular accidents are due to primary venous thrombosis and approximately 50 percent to primary arterial occlusion. In the remaining cases, intestinal infarction occurs in the absence of major arterial or venous occlusion.

ACUTE OCCLUSION OF SUPERIOR MESENTERIC ARTERY

ETIOLOGY. Embolism. Sudden, complete occlusion of the superior mesenteric artery is due more often to an embolus than to thrombosis. The anatomic characteristics of this artery make it more susceptible than the inferior mesenteric artery to symptomatic embolic occlusion. Its main stem leaves the aorta at an acute angle which runs parallel to the aorta, thus maintaining a straight-line connection with the heart. Moreover, the smaller orifice of the inferior mesenteric artery allows only small emboli to enter it, and when this occurs, lodgment is more likely at a site beyond the division of the artery into its major branches.

Most emboli come from the heart, either from a mural thrombus in a patient with early postcoronary heart disease or from an auricular thrombus in a patient with atrial fibrillation. Less frequently, vegetative endocarditis, thrombi at the site of atheromatous plaques within the aorta, or dislodgment of atheromatous plaques during translumbar or retrograde femoral arteriography are the sources of the emboli. The embolus may occlude the main orifice of the artery, particularly if it has been previously narrowed by an atheromatous plaque. More often, however, it lodges near a major branch where the artery narrows, usually at the egress of the middle colic artery. It may then remain at its initial location or fragment and be carried more distad. The initial effect of the embolus on the artery is to cause spasm of its distal branches. This and the rapid closure of the main trunk do not usually allow time for the development of a collateral circulation. Secondary thrombosis of the distal artery then occurs, probably within a few hours. Frequently the artery proximal to the embolus dilates. Sudden occlusion of the main stem superior mesenteric artery produces ischemia of the entire small intestine distal to the ligament of Treitz and also ischemia of the proximal half of the colon. Only rarely, when there are exceptional collateral channels through the celiac axis and inferior mesenteric artery, does the bowel survive. Acute occlusion of short arterial segments or of smaller branches may or may not eventuate in infarction, depending on the status of the collateral circulation.

Thrombosis. Acute, complete thrombosis of the superior mesenteric artery nearly always occurs in an artery partially occluded by atherosclerosis. Less frequently, it is superimposed on a vessel narrowed by aortic aneurysm or involved by thromboangitis obliterans or periarteritis nodosa. A sudden decrease in cardiac output, as occurs in acute congestive failure or myocardial infarction, often precedes the final thrombotic episode. The extent of intestinal ischemia or infarction is dependent on the site of thrombosis and the status of collateral channels. Sudden thrombosis of the main stem artery, as in embolic occlusion, usually results in infarction of the entire small intestine and right colon. However, slowly developing stenosis may allow time for the development of adequate collaterals so that bowel viability is preserved when acute occlusion supervenes. In inflammatory vascular diseases, the smaller visceral branches are usually affected, and intestinal infarction occurs in shorter segments.

PATHOLOGY. Sudden, complete arterial occlusion first causes an ischemic infarct in which the bowel is pale. This is the result of intense vasospasm of the intramural vessels, and it produces mucosal ulceration. At this stage, the bowel becomes hypertonic and contracted. Within 1 to 2 hours, the initial vessel spasm subsides, and the capillaries in the anoxic bowel wall become engorged with blood. As subsequent thrombosis of the artery beyond the site of occlusion occurs, the intestinal musculature becomes fatigued, and contractility is lost. Thrombosis of the visceral veins follows, and the bowel wall becomes inert, boggy, and cyanotic as a result of regurgitant flow from the veins or seepage of blood into the mural tissues of the ischemic intestine. As the infarction progresses to full-thickness necrosis of the intestine, the bowel wall becomes blood-soaked and cyanotic, and "weeps" serosanguineous fluid into the peritoneal cavity. The appearance is that of hemorrhagic infarction and is the end result of either primary arterial or venous occlusion.

CLINICAL MANIFESTATIONS. Sudden, complete occlusion of the superior mesenteric artery presents as a surgical emergency with all the manifestations of paralysis of the peristaltic mechanism as well as loss of viability of the affected intestine. The result is a form of strangulated intestinal obstruction and includes all the hazards associated with this condition (see Chap. 24).

The clinical features are usually the same whether occlusion is the result of embolism or thrombosis. Males are affected more often than females. The peak age incidence is in the fifth and sixth decades. Frequently the patient has coronary artery disease, with or without atrial fibrillation, and other manifestations of generalized atherosclerosis. A prior history of repeated episodes of cramping abdominal pain following the ingestion of food (intestinal angina) may be elicited from as many as one-third of these patients.

The most striking and constant complaint is extreme abdominal pain, often unresponsive to narcotics and initially out of proportion to the physical findings. The pain comes on suddenly and is first colicky but soon becomes steady and continuous. The early localization of the pain is to the segment of bowel involved. With acute main stem artery occlusion, the pain is first experienced in the mid-abdomen or epigastrium but later becomes generalized. Vomiting follows, is protracted, and may contain blood. Diarrhea and later constipation occur, and often the stool contains occult or gross blood. A peculiar, mottled cyanosis of the abdomen and flanks has been observed in about one-fifth of patients, a manifestation of low cardiac output accompanying extensive bowel infarction. The abdomen does not usually become distended until late. Voluntary and involuntary muscle spasm will be present, but the rigidity is almost never boardlike. Tenderness and rebound tenderness become severe as intestinal infarction occurs and are most marked over the ischemic segment of bowel. The presence of a mass is more usual with infarction of short intestinal segments. Bowel sounds are at first hyperactive, but within a short time the abdomen becomes silent. At the onset, temperature, pulse, and blood pressure may not be significantly altered. However, as infarction of the intestine progresses, the patient becomes febrile, the pulse rate increases, and the patient becomes hypotensive. Not infrequently, main stem artery occlusion initially produces acute circulatory collapse which is readily reversible but then recurs as gangrene of the bowel with peritonitis supervenes. Once bowel necrosis and perforation occur, the findings are those of generalized peritonitis and sepsis.

A correct diagnosis is sometimes difficult to make, especially with occlusions of short arterial segments. The most important early diagnostic feature is the severity of the abdominal pain relative to the physical findings and its unresponsiveness to narcotics. This finding in a patient with a recent myocardial infarction or atrial fibrillation or in one who has previously suffered emboli to extremity arteries should make the physician highly suspicious of an acute mesenteric vascular accident.

DIAGNOSTIC STUDIES. The leukocyte count may be normal early in the course of the disease but is increased to over 20,000 as hemorrhagic infarction occurs. Most patients have normal or high hematocrit levels. Often the serum amylase level is elevated. This has been related to seepage of the enzyme through the ischemic bowel wall. Roentgenograms of the abdomen are not often of significant diagnostic value. Frequently they show moderate to slight distension of both small and large intestine. The presence of gas in the right half of the colon which stops abruptly in the midtransverse colon has been considered a valuable finding; however, this is infrequent and occurs late. An abdominal paracentesis may be helpful in making the diagnosis, anticipating the recovery of serosanguineous fluid in which staining does not reveal bacteria.

TREATMENT. The treatment of acute mesenteric vascular occlusion is emergency surgical intervention, preferably before necrosis and perforation of the bowel have occurred. Until recently, the only surgical procedure considered was resection of the involved intestine. This operation was first successfully performed by Elliot in 1895. It was not until over 50 years later, in 1957, that Shaw and Rutledge reported the first successful superior mesenteric artery embolectomy not requiring associated bowel resection. Yet, the number of patients who present with a situation amenable to arterial reconstruction is small. This is because embolectomy (or emergency thrombectomy) must be performed within a few hours after the acute occlusion, before irreversible bowel changes have occurred.

At laparotomy, the ischemic intestine will be pale and thin (anemic infarction) or more often in the stage of hemorrhagic infarction. In either case, the mesentery will be pulseless. If short segments are affected, they are best handled by resection with primary end-to-end anastomosis. From previous experience, it has been learned that as much as 70 percent of the small intestine can be removed without creating serious digestive disturbances. Such extensive resections are tolerated better by adults than children.

In the situation where the main stem superior mesenteric artery is occluded, the decision to reestablish arterial flow is based on whether the process in the ischemic intestine is reversible. Although outwardly appearing nonviable, the deeply cyanotic and dull surface of the intestinal wall is at times deceiving. An attempt should be made to stimulate peristalsis, since its presence is indicative of viable and potentially salvageable bowel. In the absence of peristalsis, the only surgical procedure which can be considered is removal of all infarcted intestine. This will usually require resection of the entire small intestine distal to the ligament of Treitz and resection of the right half of the colon. Although this extensive resection is associated with a high operative mortality and late morbidity, it is worthy of consideration in an otherwise hopeless situation.

If the ischemia of all or part of the intestine is felt to be reversible, an attempt at arterial reconstruction is indicated. The superior mesenteric artery is traced proximally, and the location of the embolus or thrombus determined by finding a bounding pulse proximal to the occlusion with no pulsations distad. The artery is isolated between clamps and the occluding lesion removed through a longitudinal arteriotomy incision. An embolus is usually easily extracted, while a thrombus in a sclerotic vessel will require thromboendarterectomy. Proximal "milking" of the distal vessels may be necessary if fresh thrombus is present. The incision in the artery is then closed, preferably using a patch graft of synthetic material or autogenous vein. With resumption of arterial flow, pulsations will be felt in the mesenteric vessels, and color will return to the bowel within a few minutes provided the ischemia is reversible. The intestine should be visualized for 10 to 15 minutes and all obviously nonvascularized segments resected. If there is any question about the viability of the intestine, it is best to leave it and then reexamine it at a second operation 24 to 36 hours later. The advantage of this two-stage procedure is that it conserves intestine by confining resection to those segments which are necrotic.

The preoperative preparation and postoperative care of patients with acute mesenteric infarction is particularly important. Most of these patients will have a depleted circulating blood volume resulting from loss of plasma and whole blood into the bowel lumen, bowel wall, and peritoneal cavity. This loss can be considerable, and rapid replacement should be started while readying the patient for operation. Added intravenous fluids are necessary postoperatively to combat the reactive hyperemia that occurs after revascularization of the intestine. Since the ischemic bowel wall allows passage of bacteria into the peritoneal cavity even before frank necrosis has occurred, broad spectrum antibiotics should be administered in large doses beginning preoperatively and continuing throughout the postoperative period. Anticoagulation, preferably with heparin, has been recommended for patients following arterial reconstructive procedures. Nasogastric decompression of the stomach and intestine are necessary until bowel function returns.

The overall mortality rate following sudden superior mesenteric artery occlusion varies between 65 and 85 percent. The cause of death is usually peritonitis with septicemia. Frequent atherosclerotic involvement of the heart, kidneys, and other organs contributes to the high mortality rates.

NONOCCLUSIVE MESENTERIC INFARCTION

ETIOLOGY. In about 20 percent of patients with mesenteric infarction, careful examination will reveal no gross arterial or venous occlusion. Ottinger and Austen found this situation to be the most frequent cause of intestinal gangrene on a circulatory basis. It produces diffuse intestinal necrosis and is invariably fatal. It has been related to a sustained decrease in cardiac output such as in prolonged circulatory collapse and hypoxic states that may accompany septicemia, congestive heart failure, cardiac arrhythmia, acute myocardial infarction, and profound hypovolemia. The common denominator appears to be a low cardiac output state. Very frequently it is a terminal event in these illnesses. Its occurrence has been explained on the basis of persistent compensatory splanchnic vasoconstriction which becomes intractable. Sludging of blood due to erythrocytic agglutination follows as blood flow through the small arterioles slows down, and ultimately intestinal anoxia and infarction occur. Vasopressor therapy for shock may prolong the vasoconstriction and hasten the onset of gangrene. Additionally, the majority of patients presenting with nonocclusive mesenteric infarction have received digitalis, an agent which has been shown to induce mesenteric vasoconstriction. The genesis of acute nonocclusive mesenteric infarction has been explained by applying the law of Laplace. According to this law, the tension in the wall of the vessel must be less than the hydrostatic pressure exerted by the column of blood, or the vessel will collapse. It has been shown in dogs that when the blood pressure in the vasa recta drops below 15 mm of mercury with a blood flow below 10 ml/100 Gm of intestinal tissue for 8 consecutive hours, irreversible intestinal ischemia develops.

PATHOLOGY. The gross pathologic picture seen in patients with nonocclusive mesenteric infarction is essentially that of hemorrhagic necrosis. The mucosa is ulcerated and edematous, and the submucosal vessels are grossly dilated and packed with erythrocytes. The outer surface of the bowel is initially mottled with segmental areas of cyanosis distributed throughout the length of the intestine. In the late stages of the disease, gangrenous changes become advanced and lead to perforation.

CLINICAL MANIFESTATIONS. The clinical picture may be identical to that of patients with acute arterial or venous mesenteric occlusions. The patients, however, are usually older, and the infarction develops slowly over a period of several days, during which time there may be prodromal symptoms of malaise and vague abdominal discomfort.

Associated congestive heart failure, with or without arrythmia, is frequent. An unusually large number of patients have been found to be overdigitalized. Infarction of the intestine is heralded by the sudden onset of severe abdominal pain and vomiting. The patient usually becomes acutely hypotensive and develops a rapid pulse. Watery diarrhea is frequent, and the stools may be grossly bloody. The abdomen becomes diffusely tender and rigid. Bowel sounds are diminished and later absent. Fever and leukocytosis are usual, and frequently there is a thrombocytopenia related to intravascular thrombosis. A characteristic early laboratory finding is a markedly elevated hematocrit, which is apparently due to "trapping" of serum in the bowel wall and seepage into the peritoneal cavity.

In disorders in which the sphanchnic circulation is thought to be diminished, unexplained abdominal signs and symptoms should be viewed with the possibility of mesenteric vascular insufficiency and intestinal necrosis in mind. The single most important aid in establishing the diagnosis is abdominal angiography. A diagnostic selective superior mesenteric arteriogram will demonstrate patent major vessels with multiple segmental areas of narrowing of both small and medium-sized branches and diminution or absence of a mural intestinal circulation.

TREATMENT. The initial approach to the treatment of this condition is to correct the underlying disorder producing the low flow state. At the same time, it has been suggested that an attempt be made to improve mesenteric artery flow. This can be accomplished by direct infusion of vasodilating drugs such as isoproterenol, tolazoline hydrochloride, or papaverine hydrochloride into a catheter positioned in the superior mesenteric artery, or by a continuous epidural block. The response can be assessed by obtaining sequential mesenteric angiograms. Antibiotics have been shown to delay or diminish loss of intestinal viability and should be administered early and in large doses.

If, despite mesenteric vasodilatation, the abdominal signs and symptoms persist or reappear, operation is mandatory. With intractable hypotension and congestive failure, the gangrenous changes in the bowel wall are usually segmental; areas of anemic infarction are found interspersed with those of hemorrhagic infarction. Pulses can be felt in the superior and inferior mesenteric arteries and their major branches extending almost to the bowel wall. Serosanguineous fluid is a constant finding in the peritoneal cavity. The process usually extends throughout the entire large and small intestine and may also involve the stomach. For this reason, resection is not usually feasible. With involvement of lesser portions of the intestine, primary resection with end-to-end anastomosis should be attempted, although too often the remaining intestine will subsequently become infarcted in the immediate postoperative period. Massive fluid replacement and support of cardiac function combined with interruption of splanchnic vasoconstriction by continuous epidural block have been recommended postoperatively to help prevent progression following intestinal resection. The reported mortality rates approach 100 percent, a reflection primarily of the frequent occurrence of this type of mesenteric infarction in terminal illnesses.

Fig. 35-8. Lateral view of a retrograde visceral arteriogram showing a normal celiac axis and superior mesenteric artery.

CHRONIC OCCLUSION OF VISCERAL ARTERIES (INTESTINAL ANGINA)

Three possible sequelae may follow gradual occlusion of the main stem visceral arteries: (1) establishment of an adequate collateral circulation; (2) intestinal infarction; and (3) intestinal ischemia without infarction, due to collateral blood supply sufficient for life but not for function of the affected bowel. The last of these three sequelae produces a now well-recognized syndrome termed "intestinal angina." This entity is analogous to angina pectoris and intermittent claudication due to, respectively, arterial insufficiency to the heart and to the extremities.

ETIOLOGY. Collateral anastomoses among the three main gastrointestinal arteries from the aorta (celiac axis, superior mesenteric, and inferior mesenteric) provide for maintenance of intestinal viability and function when one of these branches is gradually occluded (Fig. 35-6). For this reason, most patients with isolated chronic occlusion of the superior mesenteric artery are completely asymptomatic. However, when blood flow through one of the surviving vessels then becomes (or has been) compromised, the now relatively ischemic intestine is unable to respond to the demands of digestion for an increased blood supply. This explains the "food-pain" sequence that characterizes intestinal angina.

As a major visceral artery becomes critically narrowed, the others dilate in order to carry more blood. This finding is of practical significance when the inferior mesenteric artery must be sacrificed in patients undergoing surgical treatment for aortic aneurysm or colon resection for carcinoma. In these circumstances, patency of the superior mesenteric artery should be ascertained before an unusually large inferior mesenteric is sacrificed. Otherwise, infarction of the intestine may be precipitated when the latter vessel is ligated. This complication can be prevented either by reimplanting the inferior mesenteric artery into the aortic graft or by restoring blood flow through the superior mesenteric artery.

PATHOLOGY. Chronic occlusion of the visceral arteries is most often due to atherosclerosis. The atheromatous plaques are invariably located at or near the origin of these large vessels, thus in a segment which anatomically is suitable for arterial reconstruction. Most of these patients also have evidence of generalized arteriosclerosis. Less frequently, the stenosis is due to compression of the celiac axis by a celiac ganglion or arcuate ligament of the diaphragm, by involvement of the arteries in an expanding aortic aneurysm or dissecting aneurysm, or by thromboangiitis obliterans or periarteritis nodosa.

CLINICAL MANIFESTATIONS. The dominant clinical feature of intestinal angina is generalized cramping abdominal pain which comes on soon after eating and lasts as long as 3 hours. The severity and duration of the distress depends on the amount of food ingested. Occasionally it is merely a sense of distension, or bloating, with a constant abdominal ache. If the pain is severe, nausea and vomiting often occur. Initially the patient will complain of constipation and later of diarrhea. There is usually a steady progression in the frequency and duration of symptoms. The food-pain relationship soon leads to a reluctance on the part of the patient to eat. The subsequent rapid and severe weight loss characterizes the syndrome. As the intestinal ischemia progresses, a form of malabsorption syndrome occurs which contributes to the weight loss, and is manifest by bulky, foamy stools high in fat and protein content. Symptoms of intestinal angina may exist for months or years before the visceral circulation becomes critically curtailed. Morris et al. estimate that histories of prodromal symptoms of intestinal angina may be obtained from as many as one-third of patients with mesenteric infarction.

On physical examination, weight loss will be obvious. Usually there are varying degrees of disability associated with generalized arteriosclerosis. A bruit is often heard over the epigastrium, although this may be transmitted from the aorta or sites other than the stenotic visceral artery. Laboratory studies and routine roentgenographic studies are not often contributory except to rule out other abdominal conditions. The differential diagnosis includes peptic ulcer disease, cholecystitis, abdominal neoplasm, and pancreatitis.

An awareness of the syndrome is perhaps the most important factor in making the diagnosis, which is then best confirmed by a selective visceral angiogram using a Seldinger catheter (Fig. 35-8). Lateral views are essential, because the standard anteroposterior view does not show the origin of the celiac or mesenteric arteries. The catheter is passed via a left brachial or femoral artery puncture to a level just above the origin of the celiac axis. After a small test dose has established the proper position of the catheter, 30 to 40 ml of 50% Hypaque is injected rapidly while taking multiple films using a rapid cassette changer. This outlines both the celiac axis and superior mesenteric arteries. Diagnostic arteriograms will show stenosis or complete occlusion of one or both these vessels, usually within 1 cm of the aortic orifice (Fig. 35-9). The catheter is then repositioned just above the origin of the inferior mesenteric artery and the arteriogram repeated. The demonstration of a markedly dilated and elongated inferior mesenteric artery which fills the superior mesenteric through collaterals is indicative of a superior mesenteric artery occlusion (Fig. 35-10).

TREATMENT. Once stenosis of the celiac and mesenteric arteries has been demonstrated in a symptomatic patient, surgical correction is advised if the patient will tolerate the procedure. Arterial reconstruction not only corrects the symptoms of intestinal angina but also prevents the eventual progression to intestinal infarction. At laparotomy, critical stenosis of the involved arteries is obvious, because there will be no palpable pulsations distal to the stenosis. Surgical treatment may be one of three types: (1) thromboendarterectomy; (2) synthetic or autogenous vein bypass graft circumventing the stenotic segment; or (3) excision of the stenotic segment and reimplantation of the superior mesenteric artery into the aorta. Since exposure of the origins of the superior mesenteric and celiac arteries is difficult, Morris et al., Rob, and others prefer improving the circulation with a bypass graft. For a lesion in the celiac artery, the graft is inserted between a major branch of the celiac artery, usually the splenic, and the aorta. Occasionally, the splenic artery itself may be mobilized and anastomosed to the side of the aorta. Bypass of a

Fig. 35-9. Lateral view of retrograde visceral arteriogram showing a high-grade stenosis (arrow) of the superior mesenteric artery close to its origin from the aorta. (Compare with Fig. 35-8.)

Fig. 35-10. Left: Retrograde inferior mesenteric arteriogram showing a prominent marginal artery of Drummond filling from a dilated and tortuous inferior mesenteric artery. Right: Later film showing filling of the superior mesenteric artery (arrow) through collaterals. The patient had complete occlusion of the celiac axis and superior mesenteric artery at their origins from the aorta.

superior mesenteric artery stenosis is best handled by inserting a graft to the side of the artery just beyond the egress of the middle colic artery and to the aorta below the origin of the renal arteries. When endarterectomy is performed, care should be taken to tack the distal intima to the artery wall in order to prevent dissection.

OCCLUSION OF INFERIOR MESENTERIC ARTERY

ETIOLOGY. Sudden occlusion of the inferior mesenteric artery is usually due to thrombosis superimposed on an atheromatous plaque and less often to embolism or a dissecting aneurysm. External compression by an expanding aortic aneurysm or involvement by atherosclerosis produces gradual occlusion. On occasion, obliterative arteritis, as associated with thromboangiitis obliterans and periarteritis nodosa, will involve the main artery or its branches.

Normally, the inferior mesenteric artery can be ligated at any point without interfering with bowel function or producing symptoms. This is because the extensive collateral circulation through anastomoses with branches of the middle colic artery (superior mesenteric) and lower hemorrhoidal arteries (internal iliac) are able to sustain the left colon (Fig. 35-6). When infarction of the descending colon follows thrombosis or ligation of the inferior mesenteric artery, there is almost always impairment of this collateral network. Usually this is due to advanced atheromatous narrowing or thrombosis of the superior mesenteric and internal iliac arteries. Such an event occasionally occurs when the inferior mesenteric artery is sacrificed during operations on the aorta for occlusive disease or aneurysm. Previous left colectomy with interruption of the marginal artery also predisposes to colon ischemia following occlusion of the inferior mesenteric artery.

CLINICAL MANIFESTATIONS. Circulatory infarction of the descending colon usually has a more insidious onset than infarction of other portions of the intestine. Since the inferior mesenteric supplies a shorter segment of bowel, occlusion produces less extensive disruption of circulating blood volume and fluid balance than when the superior mesenteric artery is occluded. Steady, slowly progressive lower abdominal pain is usually followed by loose, bloody stools and then constipation. The abdomen becomes distended and tender over the course of the descending colon. Occasionally a tubular mass may be felt in the left side of the abdomen. Some degree of circulatory collapse occurs. This is initially mild but becomes profound as the bowel becomes necrotic. The temperature and white blood cell count are only moderately elevated unless perforation has occurred. Roentgenograms of the abdomen may show an absence of gas in the descending colon, suggesting a mechanical obstruction of the transverse colon. Edema, cyanosis, and ulceration of the mucosal membrane of the sigmoid colon can often be detected by sigmoidoscopy. Unexplained diarrhea, with or without rectal bleeding, which comes on after operations on the abdominal aorta, suggests vascular impairment of the left colon and prompts immediate sigmoidoscopic evaluation.

TREATMENT. Early recognition of the intestinal ischemia and prompt surgical intervention is important for survival. Treatment consists of resection of the infarcted colonic segment. A temporary proximal end colostomy is safer than a primary anastomosis. The preexisting generalized arteriosclerotic disease afflicting most of these patients renders them poor operative risks. The overall mortality rate is about 70 percent.

MESENTERIC VENOUS OCCLUSION

ETIOLOGY. When occlusion of a visceral vein produces symptoms, they are almost always due to acute thrombosis. Mesenteric venous thrombosis may be idiopathic or evolve secondarily as a complication of several clinical disorders. The predisposing factors in secondary mesenteric venous thrombosis are (1) infection, usually intraabdominal suppuration such as appendicitis, diverticulitis, or pelvic abscess; (2) hypercoagulable states such as polycythemia vera and carcinomatosis; (3) local venous congestion and stasis, as with hepatic cirrhosis with portal hypertension or extrinsic obstruction of portal venous radicles by tumor masses; and (4) accidental or operative trauma to the mesenteric veins, particularly during or following a portacaval surgical procedure. In approximately 25 percent, no associated factor may be implicated; these cases are classified as primary, or idiopathic. A significant number of patients in this last group will give a past history of peripheral thrombophlebitis, suggesting a common cause.

PATHOLOGY. Sudden occlusion of the main stem superior mesenteric vein in the dog leads to rapid sequestration of splanchnic venous circulation, stagnation shock, and hemorrhagic infarction of the bowel progressing to necrosis and gangrene. However, in man, ligation of the portal vein or superior mesenteric vein does not produce infarction unless secondary thrombosis extends to the bowel wall and involves the venous arcades and vasa recta. Primary thrombotic occlusion of the visceral veins usually begins in the smaller tributaries. Depending on the extent and location of the propagating clot, the bowel lesion may be represented by small localized areas or extensive segments of infarction. With extensive venous occlusion, thrombosis of the arterial side of the splanchnic circulation often follows, so that it becomes impossible to determine accurately whether the occlusion was initially arterial or venous.

Phlebitis secondary to inflammatory diseases of the bowel may extend to involve the entire portal system (pyelophlebitis) or give rise to septic emboli that lodge within the liver, causing intrahepatic abscess. This complication of mesenteric venous thrombosis has become less frequent with the advent of antibiotics, and the bowel symptoms are usually overshadowed by those due to the infection.

Acute thrombosis of mesenteric veins is followed promptly by hyperemia, edema, and subserosal hemorrhages in the affected segment of intestine. The bowel wall becomes markedly thickened and cyanotic, and the lumen fills with dark bloody fluid. Serosanguineous fluid seeps from the surface of the congested mesentery and also from the intestinal loop. The picture is that of hemorrhagic infarction.

CLINICAL MANIFESTATIONS. The clinical manifestations are similar to those following acute visceral artery occlusion. Not infrequently, the patient complains of vague abdominal discomfort, anorexia, and change in bowel habits a few days or even weeks prior to the onset of severe symptoms. This prodromal period is more evident when the venous thrombosis is idiopathic. The early symptoms are then followed by sudden severe abdominal pain, vomiting, and circulatory collapse. Narcotics usually do not relieve the pain. Bloody diarrhea is more frequent than with arterial occlusions. The bowel sounds will be hypoactive or absent. Generalized abdominal tenderness, guarding, and distension are usual; however, true rigidity is not present unless gangrene and perforation of the bowel have occurred. A marked leukocytosis and elevated hematocrit are characteristic findings in venous thrombosis. The latter reflects the trapping of plasma in the occluded bowel segment as arterial blood continues to flow into a splanchnic bed without adequate venous drainage. Plain roentgenograms of the abdomen usually show dilated loops of small bowel with air fluid levels which, however, are not specific. Abdominal paracentesis invariably yields serosanguineous fluid, which, if foul-smelling, makes immediate laparotomy mandatory.

TREATMENT. The definitive treatment of mesenteric venous infarction is surgical. Without operation the mortality approaches 100 percent. Preparation of the patient for operation includes correcting the usually severe circulating volume deficit with blood and a balanced salt solution and decompression of the stomach via a nasogastric tube. Broad-spectrum antibiotics and penicillin in large doses should be started and should be continued in the postoperative period.

As soon as possible and when his condition permits, the patient is taken to the operating room. In contrast to acute mesenteric arterial occlusion, venous thrombosis tends to occur more frequently in peripheral tributaries than in the main stem vessel. For this reason, shorter segments of intestine are usually involved than if occlusion is primarily arterial. All devitalized intestine is resected and a primary end-to-end anastomosis performed. Frequently the thrombosis extends beyond the limits of gross infarction. Therefore, resection should include adjacent normal bowel and mesentery until all grossly thrombosed veins are encompassed. Otherwise, extension of residual clot postoperatively will lead to subsequent infarction. Intestinal infarction associated with acute thrombosis of the portal vein is usually not amenable to resection because of the wide extent of involved intestine.

Anticoagulation should be started 12 to 24 hours postoperatively. Naitove and Weismann reported no deaths in their cases of idiopathic mesenteric venous thrombosis in which anticoagulants were administered, in contrast to a 50 percent mortality in the group in which the drugs were not used. A second-look operation 24 to 36 hours later should be performed in this form of mesenteric infarction because of the frequent recurrence of thrombosis or extension of residual clots. In general, the prognosis is somewhat better than in mesenteric infarction due to arterial occlusion. This is probably a reflection of the shorter bowel segments usually involved, which make it more amenable to surgical treatment. The most important factor in prognosis is early operative intervention before extensive thrombosis has occurred throughout the splanchnic venous circulation.

MEDIAN ARCUATE LIGAMENT SYNDROME

In 1965, Dunbar and his associates reported 15 patients with abdominal complaints who were found to have partial occlusion of the celiac artery by fibers of the median arcuate ligament, since referred to as the median arcuate ligament syndrome. All of their patients had relief of symptoms following division of the diaphragmatic fibers which were compressing the artery. The basis of the constriction appears to be either a high origin of the celiac artery, with resultant compression as it passes through the aortic hiatus beneath the median arcuate ligament, or an abnormally low crossing of the ligament causing compression of a normally located artery. However, there are some who doubt whether the syndrome is a true clinical entity, because the arterial narrowing which is presumed to cause the syndrome is often encountered in patients without symptoms.

CLINICAL MANIFESTATIONS. The condition is most likely to occur in the fourth and fifth decades of life, with a three-to-one predominance of females. The principal and usually only symptom is abdominal pain which may vary from a vague periumbilical or epigastric aching discomfort to a severe postprandial pain. It has been inferred that the pain is related to intestinal ischemia, but true, chronic ischemia of the gastrointestinal tract generally requires interference with the blood flow in at least two of the three major visceral arteries. Irritation of visceral autonomic nerve fibers by the constricting fibers of the diaphragm has also been considered as the basis of the pain, but perivascular sympathectomy or ganglionectomy is not consistently palliative. Diarrhea and nausea with occasional vomiting also may occur, and weight loss because of voluntary avoidance of food is characteristic of patients with postprandial pain. A significant physical finding is a bruit invariably present in the upper midabdomen.

The diagnosis is made by arteriography demonstrating the entrapment of the celiac artery by the diaphragmatic fibers. The lateral film is the most reliable and, characteristically, will show eccentric compression of the celiac artery along its superior border with caudal displacement of the artery so that it lies adjacent to the superior mesenteric artery (Fig. 35-11). A presumptive diagnosis may be entertained if the selective superior mesenteric arteriogram demonstrates collateral filling of the celiac system. (In the true syndrome, both the superior mesenteric and inferior mesenteric arteries are of normal caliber radiographically.) Stanley and Frey believe that the demonstration of impaired absorption of xylose is useful in diagnosis as well as in selecting patients for surgery.

TREATMENT. Normal blood flow in the celiac artery can usually be restored by transecting the constricting median arcuate ligament. The results have generally been excellent: Marable et al. reported complete relief or marked improvement of symptoms in 24 of 30 patients following this operation. Direct arterial reconstruction may be necessary if the stenosis persists and the patient remains symptomatic after division of the ligament.

SPONTANEOUS RUPTURE OF VISCERAL BLOOD VESSELS (ABDOMINAL APOPLEXY)

The term "abdominal apoplexy" has been applied to the situation of massive abdominal hemorrhage from spontaneous rupture of visceral blood vessels. It is an unusual

Fig. 35-11. Lateral abdominal aortography showing compression of the superior border of the celiac artery (arrow) by the median arcuate ligament.

and very rare form of mesenteric vascular disease that is the abdominal counterpart of cerebral hemorrhage. In a recent review of the literature, Kleinsasser noted only 83 patients whose diagnoses could be substantiated.

ETIOLOGY. The occurrence of abdominal apoplexy in older patients has been related to localized arteriosclerotic disease causing weakness or aneurysmal formation of mesenteric vessels which later spontaneously rupture. In younger patients, congenital defects in the medial coat of the visceral arteries and veins have been incriminated. Necrotizing arteritis associated with certain autoimmune diseases may on rare occasion be the etiologic factor. Most of the patients have hypertension, which is believed to be of etiologic significance.

PATHOLOGY. The bleeding comes from an arterial source far more frequently than from a venous one. Multiple sites of rupture have been reported. Although it does not fulfill the exact criteria for abdominal apoplexy, rupture of a splenic artery aneurysm is perhaps the best-known source. This usually occurs during pregnancy or the puerperium. Of the intestinal vessels, rupture occurs most often in the superior mesenteric artery or its major colic branches. Not infrequently, no site of bleeding can be found at laparotomy or autopsy despite the loss of several liters of blood.

Bleeding may initially be intraperitoneal or, by extending between the leaves of the mesentery, retroperitoneal. The latter situation often secondarily produces a tear in the peritoneum, thus giving the picture of both retroperitoneal and intraperitoneal bleeding. The severity of hemorrhage will depend on the size of the ruptured vessel.

CLINICAL MANIFESTATIONS. With confined retroperitoneal bleeding, the clinical features will include steady back or testicular pain, pallor, tachycardia, and occasional vomiting. When bleeding is into the peritoneal cavity, there is sudden, severe abdominal pain rapidly followed by circulatory collapse. The pain is generalized and often referred to the left shoulder. Abdominal distension, spasm, and generalized tenderness are present. Bowel activity will be depressed or absent. The temperature is usually normal, but generally the white blood cell count will be increased. The hematocrit may or may not be low, depending on whether hemodilution has taken place. The vital signs following the initial bleeding may improve for a period of several hours and then be followed by a second, usually massive episode of bleeding which is fatal without prompt surgical intervention.

The above clinical findings in an older patient with hypertension and generalized arteriosclerosis or in a pregnant patient should lead one to suspect abdominal apoplexy. It must be differentiated from such abdominal catastrophes as perforated peptic ulcer, hemorrhagic pancreatitis, strangulated intestinal obstruction, ruptured abdominal aneurysm, and mesenteric vascular occlusion. An abdominal paracentesis with the recovery of nonclotting blood is diagnostic of intraabdominal bleeding from any source. Selective mesenteric arteriography may help to localize the bleeding site, but usually surgery cannot be delayed.

TREATMENT. Treatment of abdominal apoplexy is immediate blood replacement and surgical intervention as soon as the patient's condition permits. At times the bleeding may be so brisk that it will be necessary to take the patient to the operating room while still in shock. However, the chances of finding an open vessel are better if the blood pressure can be elevated. Bleeding from the smaller visceral arteries and most venous bleeding are the best treated by ligation. Splenectomy will facilitate exposure for ligation of a ruptured splenic artery aneurysm. A ruptured hepatic artery or main stem superior mesenteric artery should be reconstructed, if possible. This will usually require excision of the segment and replacement with a graft, preferably of autogenous vein. Following ligation of visceral arteries or reconstruction of the superior mesenteric artery, adequate circulation to the bowel must be assured and all obviously ischemic intestine resected. If there is a question of viability of a long segment, a second-look operation in 24 to 36 hours may avoid an extensive resection. When it is necessary to ligate the hepatic artery, protection should be afforded the liver with large doses of broad-spectrum antibiotics postoperatively.

The outlook for recovery is good, even with massive bleeding, if the patient is operated upon early and a definite bleeding point located. The overall mortality rate in a collected review by Carter and Gosney was 47 percent. However, of those coming to the operating room, the rate fell to 15 percent when the ruptured vessel could be identified.

TRAUMA TO VISCERAL BLOOD VESSELS

ETIOLOGY. Mesenteric arteries and veins may be injured by either penetrating or nonpenetrating abdominal trauma or accidentally during abdominal operations. In most cases, the vessels are lacerated. Less frequently, contusion of an artery by blunt trauma eventuates in thrombosis or later aneurysmal formation with rupture.

Most penetrating injuries of the mesenteric vessels are due to stabbings or gunshot wounds. In these circumstances, associated injury to other organs is frequent. Isolated injury to mesenteric vessels following blunt abdominal trauma is rare and usually involves vessels in the mesentery proper or porta hepatis.

CLINICAL MANIFESTATIONS. Depending on the size of the vessel lacerated, the rapidity of the bleeding, and associated organ injury, the patient will present with varying degrees of shock, abdominal pain, tenderness, distension, and spasm. Pain referred to the left shoulder is a particularly valuable diagnostic symptom. X-rays of the abdomen are not helpful unless associated visceral rupture has occurred, in which case free air may be seen.

TREATMENT. It is generally held that all gunshot wounds of the abdomen and most stab wounds should be explored early regardless of the physical findings. In nonpenetrating injury, a paracentesis yielding nonclotting blood prompts early surgical intervention. Basically, treatment consists of controlling the bleeding vessel. Lacerations of the inferior mesenteric artery or smaller mesenteric arteries and most mesenteric veins can usually be successfully treated by ligation. In the past, few patients with injury to the main trunk of the superior mesenteric artery survived. Most died from infarction of the intestine or because of complications arising from associated organ injury. Today, if the patient can be resuscitated and reaches the operating room, then arterial repair may be possible. This can be accomplished by either primary suture or interposition of a vascular graft between the severed ends of the vessel. Every attempt should also be made to repair lacerations of the hepatic artery or portal vein. Whether treatment is by ligation or reconstruction, it is important that adequate circulation to the intestine be established and any obviously ischemic bowel resected before closing the abdomen. Long segments of small intestine that are of questionable viability are best left in place and reexamined at a second operation 24 hours later.

Nonspecific Mesenteric Lymphadenitis

Nonspecific mesenteric lymphadenitis is one of the common causes of acute abdominal pain in children. Its existence as a distinct clinicopathologic entity is now well accepted, although the condition received little attention in early medical texts following its initial description by Wilensky and Hahn in 1926. An extensive review of the disease has been reported by McDonald.

Since the condition is invariably self-limiting and can be accurately diagnosed only at laparotomy, its true incidence is unknown. Yet, it is probably the most common cause of inflammatory enlargement of abdominal lymph glands, far surpassing that due to tuberculosis, with which it has been confused in the past. Consideration of the disease is important because of its clinical similarity to several abdominal conditions requiring surgical intervention, notably acute appendicitis.

PATHOLOGY AND PATHOGENESIS. The lymph nodes primarily involved in nonspecific mesenteric lymphadenitis are those that drain the ileocecal region. Undoubtedly this is due to the concentration of mesenteric nodes in this area and because the most abundant lymphatic drainage in the intestinal tract is in the lower ileum. Moreover, stasis of intestinal contents in the terminal ileum favors absorption of toxic or bacterial products from the bowel lumen, agents which may have a bearing on the pathogenesis of the disease.

In the early stages, the juxtaintestinal glands are predominantly affected. Later, there is involvement of the intermediate and terminal or central glands at the root of the mesentery. The nodes are enlarged, discrete, and soft and pink at first; later they may become firm and white. It is uncertain whether calcification ever occurs in nontuberculous adenitis, and suppuration is rare unless specific bacterial infection is present. The gross appearance of the intestine and appendix is normal, although often there is slight vascular congestion of the mesentery. A small amount of clear serous fluid is frequently present within the peritoneal cavity. Histologically, the involved nodes present a pattern of reactive hyperplasia similar to that found in inflammatory and allergic affections of lymph nodes in other parts of the body. The nodes and free peritoneal fluid, with rare exception, prove to be sterile on culture or on animal inoculation.

Although the appearance of the glands grossly and histologically suggests a response to infection, experimental and clinical studies have failed to support a specific bacterial or viral agent as the causal factor. Occasionally, specific mesenteric adenitis due to beta hemolytic streptococcal infection occurs. In these instances, there is an acute febrile illness with signs of peritoneal involvement, and the organism can be cultured from the glands. Only rarely have coliform organisms been isolated. Parasitic mesenteric adenitis secondary to ascariasis occurs in endemic areas; however, the lymph nodes contain numerous eosinophils, and worms are present within the intestine. The disease is distinct from the mesenteric node enlargements which accompany bowel diseases in which there are associated changes in the intestine.

It seems likely that nonspecific mesenteric adenitis represents a reaction to some type of material absorbed from the small intestine. The stimulating substance could reach the nodes via either lymph channels or the bloodstream, although the usual absence of generalized lymphadenopathy would make the latter route unlikely. The possibility that the disease represents a hypersensitive reaction to a foreign protein has also been suggested.

CLINICAL MANIFESTATIONS. The disease most commonly occurs in patients under eighteen years of age. There is no sex predilection. The clinical signs and symptoms are not particularly characteristic. Very often there has been a recent sore throat or upper respiratory tract infection. Pain is usually the first symptom. It varies in intensity from an ache to a severe colic. The mechanism responsible for producing pain is not completely understood. Lymph nodes have not been shown to have sensory innervation, and therefore enlargement of the node by itself should not produce pain. It is probable that the pain is referred from the mesentery, which has an abundance of sensory end organs that are stimulated when the mesentery is stretched during peristalsis. The initial pain is usually in the upper abdomen, but it may also begin in the lower right quadrant or be generalized. Eventually the pain localizes to the right side; however, an important point in differentiating the disease from acute appendicitis is that the patient is unable to indicate the exact site of the most intense pain. Between spasms of colic, the patient feels well and moves about without difficulty. Nausea and vomiting occur in about one-third of patients, while malaise and anorexia are inconstant symptoms. A previous history of one or more similar attacks is frequently obtained from the patient or the parents.

The patient often appears flushed, and an associated rhinorrhea or acute pharyngitis is not unusual. Approximately 20 percent of patients will have lymphadenopathy elsewhere, most often in the cervical region. The usual finding on examination of the abdomen is tenderness in the lower aspect of the right side, which is somewhat higher and more medial and considerably less severe than in acute appendicitis. The point of maximal tenderness often varies from one examination to the next. An appreciable number of patients will have diffuse or periumbilical tenderness as well. Rebound tenderness may or may not be demonstrated. Voluntary guarding is sometimes present; however, true muscular rigidity is rare. The enlarged abdominal lymph glands are seldom palpable. On rectal examination, there may be tenderness on the right side of the pelvis. Early in the attack, the temperature is moderately elevated, to 38 or 38.5°C, and at least half of the patients will have leukocyte counts over 10,000 per cubic millimeter.

DIFFERENTIAL DIAGNOSIS. The disease is most often confused with acute appendicitis but must also be differentiated from regional enteritis, intussusception, specific bacterial and granulomatous adenitis, and other forms of mesenteric glandular enlargement such as with infectious mononucleosis or lymphoma. The clinical similarity to acute appendicitis is such that, in several large series, as many as 20 percent of patients coming to the operating room for appendectomy were found to have nonspecific mesenteric adenitis and a normal appendix. Important differentiating factors are the more localized and constant location of the pain and tenderness, the presence of muscle rigidity, and the frequent occurrence of nausea and vomiting in children with appendicitis.

Tuberculous mesenteric adenitis has been rare since the almost universal use of pasteurized milk and the advent of antituberculous chemotherapeutic drugs. It is most often due to ingestion of milk containing bovine tubercle bacilli, which gain entry to the lymph nodes by way of a Peyer patch, or lymph follicle, in the terminal ileum. The patient usually complains of a less constant aching pain; abdominal tenderness is slight; and enlarged, matted glands are usually palpable in the root of the mesentery. At operation, the diagnosis can be suspected if there are surface tubercles on the nodes which may be caseous. Biopsy of the node

and acid-fast stain or guinea pig inoculation will be diagnostic.

Differentiation from *acute regional ileitis* is at times difficult. Mesenteric adenitis is an almost constant feature of regional ileitis, and indeed the adenitis is often nonspecific in this disease. Inflammatory edema or induration of the serous coat of the ileum with thickening and induration of the mesentery are characteristic of regional enteritis.

The low incidence of lymphadenopathy in other parts of the body and the brief course of nonspecific mesenteric adenitis are factors in excluding lymphomas and infectious mononucleosis. A peripheral blood smear and a Paul-Bunnell test for sheep red cell agglutinins are also helpful.

TREATMENT. The prognosis of nonspecific mesenteric adenitis is excellent, and complete recovery from an individual attack can be expected without specific treatment. Death from the disease is extremely rare and occurs only when secondary specific bacterial infection, usually caused by hemolytic streptococci, causes suppuration of the nodes with rupture leading to abscess or peritonitis.

If the condition is mistaken for acute appendicitis, as it frequently is, laparotomy should be undertaken. In such an instance, it is far safer to find a normal appendix than to run the risk of allowing acute appendicitis to go on to rupture. The diagnosis is readily established at the time of operation with the finding of enlarged mesenteric nodes in the absence of disease in the appendix or elsewhere in the intestinal tract or abdomen. In view of the tendency for recurrence and the difficulty of differentiating it from appendicitis, appendectomy should be performed. Approximately 25 percent of patients will have further bouts of abdominal pain during the childhood years. Apparently, generalized involution of lymphoid tissue with maturity leads to atrophy of many of the nodes, accounting, perhaps, for the rarity of the disease in adult life.

Mesenteric Panniculitis

"Mesenteric panniculitis" is a term applied by Ogden et al. in 1960 to describe a process of extensive thickening of the mesentery by a nonspecific inflammatory process. It has also been variously designated "retractile mesenteritis," "mesenteric lipodystrophy," "lipogranuloma of the mesentery," and "mesenteric manifestations of Weber-Christian disease." Many consider it a variant of retroperitoneal fibrosis.

ETIOLOGY AND PATHOLOGY. The cause of the condition is unknown; however, the process apparently results from an insult to the fatty tissue of the mesentery. Trauma, allergy, and subacute infection have all been implicated. The process usually involves the mesenteric root of the small bowel. Grossly, the normal fat lobulations of the markedly thickened and firm mesentery are lost. Scattered throughout are irregular areas of discoloration, which vary from reddish brown plaques to pale yellow foci resembling fat necrosis. The superior mesenteric vessels, though surrounded by the tumorlike mass of tissue, pass through it unaltered. Histologic sections show inflammatory involvement of the fibroadipose tissue with round cells, foam cells, and giant cells and various degrees of necrosis, fibrosis, and calcification.

CLINICAL MANIFESTATIONS. Men are affected more often than women. It is rarely described in children, in whom mesenteric fat is usually scant. The clinical features are nonspecific. Recurrent episodes of moderate to severe abdominal pain, nausea, vomiting, malaise, and low-grade fever are the usual complaints. In over 60 percent of patients, there is a palpable tender mass, usually in the right side of the abdomen. Roentgenograms are helpful only if the mass displaces or compresses viscera.

TREATMENT. Laparotomy is necessary to establish the diagnosis and to rule out other tumefactions of the abdomen. The widespread involvement of the mesentery precludes doing more than obtaining a biopsy. Since neoplasms of the mesenteric lymph nodes may present a similar gross appearance, several biopsies from different sites should be obtained. Rarely, colostomy or bypass will be necessary to relieve symptoms of obstruction. Treatment of the disease with steroids and irradiation has been suggested. However, the benefits from these are difficult to evaluate, because the inflammatory process is self-limiting and seldom causes any serious complications.

Tumors of the Mesentery

Tumors originating between the leaves of the mesentery are quite rare. In contrast, malignant implants from intraabdominal or pelvic tumors or metastases to mesenteric lymph nodes are relatively common. Tumors arising from mesenteric lymph nodes occur; however, these are not generally included in a discussion of primary mesenteric tumors.

Historically, primary mesenteric tumors were recognized as early as 1507, when Benivieni, a Florentine anatomist, described at autopsy a cyst originating in the small bowel mesentery. The first successful removal of a mesenteric tumor is credited to Tillaux in 1880. Isolated reports and a few large series have appeared in the literature subsequently. More recently, Rankin and Major, Hart, Fowler, and Yannopoulos and Stout have reviewed these tumors. Excepting tumors arising in lymph nodes, no more than 500 cases of primary mesenteric tumors have been described to date.

PATHOLOGY. Primary tumors of the mesentery may be cystic or solid. Of these, cystic growths occur more frequently than solid ones in a ratio of 2:1. A variety of tissues, including lymphatic, vascular, nervous, and connective tissue, are the source of these tumors. In addition, cystic tumors may arise from embryonic rests (enteroceles or dermoids), from developmental defects (chylous or serous retention cysts), or following trauma (hemorrhagic cysts). A classification of these tumors is shown in Table 35-1.

The majority of cystic mesenteric tumors are benign. Rare exceptions are lymphangiosarcomas, which are true neoplasms arising from lymph channels, and malignant teratomas arising from multipotential embryonic rests.

Table 35-1. CLASSIFICATION OF PRIMARY MESENTERIC TUMORS

Origin	*Benign*	*Malignant*
Cystic tumors:		
Developmental defects	Chylous cyst	
	Serous cyst	
Lymphatic tissue . . .	Lymphangioma	Lymphangiosarcoma
Trauma	Traumatic cyst	
Embryonic rests	Enteric cyst	
	Dermoid	Malignant teratoma
Solid tumors:		
Adipose tissue	Lipoma	Liposarcoma
Fibrous tissue	Fibroma	Fibrosarcoma
Nerve elements	Neurilemoma	Malignant schwannoma
	Neurofibroma	
Smooth muscle	Leiomyoma	Leiomyosarcoma
	Fibromyoma	Fibromyosarcoma
Vascular tissue	Hemangioma	Hemangiopericytoma

Rankin and Major contend that chylous or lymphatic cysts are the most frequently encountered benign mesenteric masses. These are thought to arise from developmental defects in mesenteric lymphatics creating closed spaces within which fluid accumulates. They may be unilocular or multilocular, have an endothelial lining, contain a grossly cloudy fluid resembling chyle, and often grow to extremely large size. A similar cause has been ascribed to serous cysts, which are differentiated from chylous cysts in that they contain clear fluid, are invariably unilocular, and may or may not have an endothelial lining. Lymphangioma of the mesentery is apparently a true neoplasm of lymphatics similar to those found in other parts of the body (cystic hygroma). Grossly and histologically, it is often difficult to differentiate this tumor from a chylous cyst, and in many series the two are grouped in a single category. Traumatic cysts follow external or surgical injury to the mesentery. They are lined with fibrous tissue and usually contain bloody fluid. It is probable that many serous retention cysts are in reality traumatic cysts which have evolved from disruption of mesenteric lymph channels. Enteric cysts are lined with intestinal mucosa and represent duplications of the intestinal tract that do not communicate with the bowel lumen. These and dermoid cysts of the mesentery are exceedingly rare.

Benign solid tumors of the mesentery are more common than malignant ones, and of these, lipomas and fibromas predominate. However, recurrence after incomplete excision of histologically benign mesenteric tumors has been reported and malignant degeneration also suggested. Moreover, histologically benign tumors can kill by local invasion with mechanical compression of adjacent viscera. The benign tumors of nerve elements and smooth muscles are uncommon. Vascular tumors of the mesentery are very rare, and of these, hemangiopericytomas dominate the picture. Ackerman states that liposarcoma is the most frequently encountered malignant tumor of this area,

Fig. 35-12. Small intestinal series showing displacement of bowel loops by a mass lesion in the lower right side of the abdomen. The patient proved to have a large benign fibroma in the mesentery of the terminal ileum. (*J. Adams and F. Kutner, Am J Surg, 111:735, 1966.*)

whereas Yannopoulos and Stout report leiomyosarcoma to be the most frequent. Few malignant mesenteric tumors have embolic metastases until very late. They spread by local extension or by peritoneal implants, which occurs most often with leiomyosarcomas. As a rule, the malignant solid tumors arise near the root of the mesentery, whereas solid benign tumors have a greater tendency to develop peripherally near the intestine.

Approximately two-thirds of mesenteric tumors, either cystic or solid, are located in the mesentery of the small intestine, usually that of the ileum. Less frequently, they arise in the transverse or sigmoid mesocolon or in the gastrohepatic ligament. In the greater number of cases, the tumor is located peripherally in the mesentery, where it is often adherent to the adjacent intestine. The mobility of the mesentery permits both benign and malignant tumors to grow to very large sizes before causing symptoms.

CLINICAL MANIFESTATIONS. The early clinical features do not usually differentiate benign tumors from malignant ones. There is an equal sex incidence, although benign cystic tumors are somewhat more common in women and malignant tumors occur more frequently in men. These tumors have been described in children and also the very aged; however, the average age of patients with benign tumors is forty-five years, while those with malignant tumors average fifty-five years old.

The manifestations of mesenteric tumors are dependent upon the size, location, and mobility of the growth. In the vast majority of patients, symptoms are few or nonexistent, and the tumor is detected during a routine examination. Symptoms appear sooner when the tumor is situated in the periphery of the mesentery near the intestine than when located at its root. The patient may merely experience a sensation of fullness or pressure in the abdomen, particularly after eating. Less frequently, there are frank abdominal complaints. About one-half of patients with malignant tumors complain of abdominal pain, weakness, and weight loss, and one-third have diarrhea, cramps, anorexia, and nausea. Only rarely will the patient present with symptoms of complete intestinal obstruction or symptoms resulting from complications of the tumor per se such as torsion, hemorrhage, or infarction of the tumor mass. In the absence of intestinal obstruction or these complications, the sole clinical finding will be the presence of a nontender, intraabdominal mass, usually in the lower right part of the abdomen. The mass varies in size from a few inches in diameter to one which may literally fill the entire abdomen. The extremely large masses are usually cystic, in which case they are tense and fluctuant. Both cystic and solid tumors of the mesentery are mobile; they can be easily moved from side to side but only slightly in an upward and downward direction.

The differential diagnosis takes into consideration all tumefactions of the abdominal cavity and retroperitoneum. Roentgenograms are helpful only when the mesenteric mass is sufficiently large to cause compression and displacement of the bowel or ureters (Fig. 35-12). They do not differentiate a benign tumor from a malignant one, and in most instances the x-ray studies are not helpful. Calcification in the mass is suggestive of a dermoid or teratoma. Routine laboratory studies are usually uninformative.

Since there are no pathognomonic symptoms or signs, a high index of suspicion is necessary for the diagnosis to be made preoperatively. A mesenteric tumor may be suggested by a movable abdominal mass extrinsic to the gastrointestinal and urinary systems; however, final diagnostic confirmation can be made only during laparotomy.

TREATMENT. Surgical excision is the only treatment for both benign or malignant lesions. All mesenteric cysts of a size sufficient to be palpated should be removed if at all possible, since even benign lesions eventually cause pain and compression of neighboring structures. Benign cystic tumors can be removed by enucleation or local excision, although resection in continuity with the adjacent intestine is often necessary because of possible compromise to the vascularity of the bowel or difficulty in separating the tumor from the intestine. Wide excision together with resection of adjacent intestine are recommended for benign solid tumors, since these have a tendency toward local recurrence and malignant degeneration. Prognosis after adequate excision of both cystic and solid benign tumors of the mesentery is excellent.

The outlook for malignant mesenteric tumors is dependent upon whether complete removal is possible and is generally poor. Since malignant growths tend to occur in the root of the mesentery and often involve the great vessels and vasculature to most of the small intestine and colon, curative resection is usually prohibitive. Resectable lesions invariably will require removal of a portion of bowel; however, fewer than one-third of the malignant tumors are totally resectable. Nevertheless, since these growths may enlarge slowly and embolic metastases occur late, it is worthwhile to partially remove them to relieve obstructions, and prolonged survival has been recorded in a few instances. Irradiation therapy offers little if any benefit, since the tumors are invariably radioresistant. Few patients with malignant primary mesenteric tumors are alive after 5 years. Death results from invasion with obstruction of the gastrointestinal tract leading to perforation and hemorrhage or from metastases to liver and lung.

RETROPERITONEUM

General Considerations

The retroperitoneum consists of that portion of the body which is bounded anteriorly by the peritoneum, posteriorly by the spine and psoas and quadratus lumborum muscles, superiorly by the twelfth ribs and attachments of the diaphragm, and inferiorly by the brim of the pelvis. The lateral margins of the space correspond to the lateral borders of the quadratus lumborum muscles. These limits define both an actual and a potential space, the actual space containing solid organs and major blood vessels while the potential space includes soft tissues, nerve elements, and small blood vessels. Since there are no anatomic barriers in this area, pathologic processes may extend easily throughout it and therefore are often bilateral.

Contained within the retroperitoneum are the kidneys, ureters, adrenal glands, portions of the autonomic and peripheral nervous systems, pancreas, abdominal aorta, inferior vena cava, spermatic or ovarian vessels, lymphatics and lymph nodes, and certain portions of the intestinal tract, notably the duodenum. The space also contains fatty and areolar tissue and fibrous connective tissue.

The diagnosis of diseases involving the retroperitoneum has been enhanced by the application of such radiocontrast roentgenographic studies as pyelography, venography, arteriography, lymphangiography, and presacral air insufflation. Nevertheless, it remains an obscure area of the body, enabling pathologic processes to become advanced before producing symptoms.

The multiplicity of structures within the retroperitoneum gives rise to a variety of pathologic conditions. This chapter will deal with the relatively uncommon entities of (1) idiopathic retroperitoneal fibrosis and (2) primary tumors of the retroperitoneal space.

Idiopathic Retroperitoneal Fibrosis

Idiopathic retroperitoneal fibrosis is a nonspecific, nonsuppurative inflammation of fibroadipose tissue of unknown cause which produces symptoms by the gradual compression of the tubular structures in the retroperitoneal space. It is currently believed that the disease represents one of the manifestations of a widespread entity termed "systemic idiopathic fibrosis." Idiopathic mediastinal fibrosis, Riedel's struma, sclerosing cholangitis, mesenteric panniculitis, Peyronie's disease, pseudotumor of the orbit, and perhaps desmoid tumor are other fibromatoses which are considered to be localized forms of systemic idiopathic fibrosis. A factor common to all these diseases is an inflammatory fibrotic process involving areolar and adipose tissue.

Retroperitoneal fibrosis was first described in 1905 by Albarran, a French urologist, who performed ureterolysis for ureteral compression produced by the disease. The first report in English is credited to Ormond in 1948. It has since been referred to as Ormond's syndrome but has also been labeled "idiopathic fibrous retroperitonitis," "periureteritis plastica," and "sclerosing retroperitonitis." Retroperitoneal lipogranulomatosis (xanthogranulomatosis), which can produce a similar clinical picture, may be a granulomatous, prefibrotic stage of retroperitoneal fibrosis.

ETIOLOGY. Attesting to the obscure etiology of retroperitoneal fibrosis are the many theories which have been advanced to explain its origin. Hackett, in finding hemosiderin deposits in biopsy specimens, felt that the cause might be previous trauma that produced a retroperitoneal hematoma which subsequently underwent organization. The possibility that extravasated urine might cause a fibrotic reaction in the retroperitoneum was mentioned by Ormond, and both he and Hackett also suggested that an abortive infection elsewhere, only partially treated with antibiotics, might later start an inflammatory reaction in the lymphatic and perivascular tissues of the retroperitoneum. Others have speculated that the disease may be an autoimmune reaction to interstitial protein. Hache et al. proposed the concept that the fibrosis was the end result of an ascending lymphangitis, adenitis, or periadenitis in the retroperitoneum with the infection arising from chronic or recurrent genitourinary infections or inflammatory diseases of the gastrointestinal tract or pelvic organs. Reports of retroperitoneal fibrosis occurring in patients taking the antiserotonin drug methysergide for headache prompted the theory that the disease may be due to a hypersensitivity reaction to the drug. Suby reported a reversal of the fibrotic process after discontinuing the medication and speculated that other drugs may be similarly at fault.

It is probable that no single factor is responsible for causing the disease in all cases and that perhaps multiple factors may be implicated in any one case.

PATHOLOGY. The gross appearance of retroperitoneal fibrosis is usually that of a plaque of woody, white fibrous tissue which is distributed along the course of the periaortic lymphatics. In about one-third of the cases, it is bilateral. The diseased tissue, which may be 2 to 12 cm thick, extends from the sacral promontory to the renal pedicles and laterally to cover the iliopsoas muscles. It is sharply demarcated but not encapsulated. The mass surrounds and constricts but does not invade the regional structures in the retroperitoneum, primarily the blood vessels, nerves, and ureters to which it becomes adherent.

A localized form has been observed as a circumscribed fibrous reaction surrounding only the ureters, and exten-

Fig. 35-13. Retrograde pyelogram in a patient with retroperitoneal fibrosis showing bilateral hydronephrosis without organic obstruction of the ureters. The medial displacement of the ureters is a characteristic roentgenographic finding which differentiates this disease from retroperitoneal tumefactions.

sive involvement of the entire retroperitoneum with compression of the duodenum, common bile duct, and pancreas has also been seen. A similar fibrotic process has been described penetrating the diaphragm along the great vessels into the mediastinum causing superior vena cava obstruction and also extending into the root of the mesentery, causing intestinal obstruction.

Microscopically, the pattern varies from a subacute cellular process with polymorphonuclear cells, lymphocytes, fibroblasts, and fat cells to a completely hyalinized, relatively acellular sclerosis. Eosinophils, foreign body giant cells, and small areas of calcification may also be present. Suppuration with abscess formation does not occur. The amount of fat and cellular infiltration and the degree of fibrosis vary between patients and in different biopsy specimens from the same patient. The more cellular picture is usually seen in the early stages of the disease, when there may be systemic signs of inflammation, whereas the dense fibrotic process is found late.

CLINICAL MANIFESTATIONS. Retroperitoneal fibrosis is two to three times more common among men than among women. It may occur in children and also the aged; however, about two-thirds of the patients are between forty and sixty years old.

The protean manifestations of the disease are related to the phase and extent of the process and the structures secondarily involved. Ormond divided the natural history of the disease into three periods: (1) the period of incidence and development; (2) the period of activity, that is, spread of the cellular and fibrotic process to envelopment of the retroperitoneal structures; and (3) the period of contraction of the fibrotic mass with compression of the involved structures. The disease is apparently self-limiting once the fibrotic stage is reached, a factor of major importance in considering types of therapy.

Early symptoms are vague and nonspecific, but the first complaint is invariably pain. This is dull, noncolicky, and insidious in onset. It usually originates in the flank or low back and often radiates to the lower abdomen, groin, genitalia, or anteromedial aspect of the thigh. The pain is unilateral at first but may become bilateral later, as the fibrotic process spreads. Anorexia, nausea, diarrhea, generalized malaise, and weight loss variably occur in the early and late phases of the disease. Features of a subacute inflammation such as lower abdominal or costovertebral tenderness, moderate fever, leukocytosis, and an elevated sedimentation rate are often present early. A transabdominal or pelvic mass is palpable in about one-third of the patients during some phase of the disease.

Symptoms due to compression of the tubular retroperitoneal structures may follow the initial complaints by 1 month to 2 years and reflect the late fibrotic phase of the disease with sclerotic contraction. The major structures involved are the ureters, aorta, and inferior vena cava. These all lie within the same fascial compartment. However, the aorta is resistant to compression, and the inferior vena cava has abundant collaterals, so that the symptoms are generally related to ureteral involvement. Partial or complete ureteral obstruction occurs in 75 to 85 percent of patients. The usual site of obstruction is in the lower third of the ureter. Excretory urograms will show a hydroureter and hydronephrosis on one or both sides with medial deviation of the ureter in contrast to lateral displacement that is characteristically associated with retroperitoneal tumors. Retrograde studies may be required if there is complete ureteral obstruction with nonfilling of the kidney (Fig. 35-13). The ureteral obstruction is usually functional, rather than organic, as a consequence of cessation of peristalsis in the incarcerated ureteral segment. In the majority of cases, a ureteral catheter can still be passed in a retrograde manner.

Dysuria, frequency of urination, and chills and fever occur with secondary infection of a hydronephrotic kidney. These symptoms may be intermittent for years, or a single attack may culminate in sudden anuria from bilateral obstruction. As many as 40 percent of patients will have oliguria or anuria with laboratory evidence of azotemia. Clinically, the enlarged kidneys may be palpable, and the urine, if infected, will contain white blood cells and bacteria. Hematuria, in the absence of infection, is rare.

Lower extremity edema, presumably from lymphatic as well as venous obstruction, occasionally occurs and may be unilateral. The level of obstruction in most cases will correspond to that of the ureteral obstruction and can be demonstrated on phlebograms.

Arterial insufficiency due to fibrous constriction of the aorta or iliac arteries is uncommon but can occur and may constitute the major problem. The intermittent claudication, rest pain, and limb ischemia are indistinguishable clinically and radiographically from those of atherosclerotic occlusion.

Rarely, the fibrotic process will involve the retroperitoneal duodenum and common bile ducts, causing duodenal and biliary obstruction. Mechanical or functional intestinal obstruction due to extension into the root of the mesentery or sigmoid mesocolon is also a rare manifestation.

The diagnosis of retroperitoneal fibrosis may be suspected from the clinical features and the contrast roentgenograms of the urinary and vascular systems. Intravenous pyelography is the most definitive noninvasive diagnostic test. The triad that is highly suggestive of retroperitoneal fibrosis is (1) hydronephrosis with a dilated, tortuous upper ureter; (2) medial deviation of the ureter; and (3) extrinsic ureteral compression. However, a variety of conditions can produce a similar picture, and final confirmation can be made only following exploratory surgical procedures and biopsy of the fibrotic mass. The differential diagnosis includes the primary retroperitoneal tumors,· notably Hodgkin's disease, and metastatic tumor from the kidneys, pancreas, or pelvic organs. Inflammatory conditions to be excluded include tuberculosis, pancreatitis and intraabdominal inflammation of the intestine tract.

TREATMENT. Once the diagnosis is established, the patient should be carefully followed and surgical intervention timed properly. Improvement may be anticipated in some patients with supportive measures alone. However, with the onset of urinary infection or depression of renal function, surgical intervention becomes necessary.

The discontinuance of methysergide is sometimes followed by a reversal of the fibrotic process with an improvement in symptoms. Steroids, antibiotics, and x-ray therapy have been used with inconsistent results. The self-limiting nature of the disease and the reports of spontaneous resolution in untreated patients make it difficult to evaluate the results of any of these therapeutic modalities. Steroids are of theoretical use in the early inflammatory stages to diminish the generation of fibrosis or control a hyperimmune reaction if one exists. For patients in the prefibrotic stage of the disease with renal insufficiency and prominent constitutional symptoms, steroid-induced regression of the inflammatory edema may reestablish urinary patency and thus facilitate elective, rather than emergency, surgery. However, usually an advanced stage of fibrosis has been reached before the diagnosis is made.

Surgical treatment is directed toward relief of the tubular obstructions, which are usually urinary, less often vascular, and rarely intestinal. Since the disease is fundamentally a midline process which is often bilateral, a midtransabdominal approach offers the best exposure. Several deep biopsies of the mass should be obtained to rule out the possibility of an underlying neoplasm, since these may produce a similar picture, particularly tumors of lymphatic origin. The aorta, inferior vena cava, small bowel mesentery, and sigmoid mesocolon as well as the ureters should be adequately examined for possible involvement.

Ureterolysis with intraperitoneal transplantation is currently the most effective means of relieving obstruction of the involved ureter. This consists of freeing the ureter from the enveloping mass of fibrous tissue and transferring it into the peritoneal cavity, closing the posterior peritoneum behind it. Lateral reposition of the ureter within the retroperitoneal space has been reported to yield equally good results. A preliminary nephrostomy may be indicated if bilateral ureteral obstruction has resulted in severe renal impairment with uremia. On rare occasion, it will be necessary to reimplant the mobilized ureter into the bladder or to replace it with a vascularized segment of small intestine.

Aortic or iliac artery obstruction can be treated by arteriolysis or bypass with a synthetic vascular graft.

Symptoms due to venous obstruction are best treated with elevation and elastic support to the lower limbs until a sufficient collateral venous system develops. The extent of any permanent venous insufficiency will depend upon the availability of collateral pathways and the competency of deep vein valves. Release of the obstructed vein from its fibrous encasement may be difficult and hazardous, and bypass procedures for obstruction of the inferior vena cava have been uniformly unsuccessful.

The prognosis of the disease is generally good, provided that appropriate treatment has been instituted prior to the development of irreversible renal damage. Ormond, in 1960, reviewed 64 cases and reported 10 deaths, most from renal failure secondary to unrecognized obstructive uropathy which presumably could have been corrected with earlier diagnosis. In 1977 a combined series of 481 cases reported by Koep and Zuidema showed the cumulative mortality to be 9 percent.

Retroperitoneal Tumors

Primary tumors of the retroperitoneum include those neoplasms arising from tissues which occupy the potential retroperitoneal space. These tumors develop independently and have no apparent connection with any organs or major vessels except by areolar tissue. Tumors of the retroperitoneal solid organs, such as the pancreas, adrenal, or kidney, and tumefactions of the great blood vessels, therefore, are not included in this category.

The first description of retroperitoneal tumors is credited to Morgagni in 1761. Several large series have been reported by Ackerman, Braasch, Donnelly, Melicow, and Pack and Tabah. Although they are uncommon, nonetheless, they are not rare and must always be considered in the differential diagnosis of an unexplained abdominal mass. The majority occur in the fifth or sixth decades with a peak incidence at about sixty years, although approximately 15 percent are found in children under ten years of age.

PATHOLOGY. The several theories relating to the histogenesis of these tumors have been summarized by Donnelly and by Pack and Tabah. Tumors in this locale may arise from fat, areolar connective tissue, fascia, muscle, vascular tissue, somatic and sympathetic nervous tissue, and lymph vessels and lymph nodes. Less frequent neoplasms are smooth muscle tumors, complex teratomas, embryonal carcinomas, and certain bizarre cysts of unknown origin. These rarer tumors are believed to arise from remnants of the embryonal urogenital apparatus, which includes tissue of both epithelial and mesothelial origin. A classification of the benign and malignant tumors according to tissue type is given in Table 35-2. Malignant tumors outnumber those which are benign in a ratio of 4:1.

The tumors may be solid, cystic, or a combination of both. Their color varies from white (fibroma), yellow (lipoma), or pinkish to red (sarcoma), depending on the predominant tissue. They may be single or multiple and vary in size from small outgrowths to tumors weighing as much as 40 lb. As a rule, the predominantly cystic tumors are benign, whereas the solid tumors are usually malignant.

CLINICAL MANIFESTATIONS. Early symptoms of retroperitoneal tumors are characteristically vague or lacking. The loose retroperitoneal areolar tissue allows the tumor to grow unrestricted in all directions except posteriorly. For this reason, it may attain an extremely large size before producing symptoms. As the tumor grows, it compresses, obstructs, or invades adjacent organs or structures, so that the presenting symptoms are often referable to these organs.

The initial manifestations include an enlarging abdomen, backache, a sense of fullness or heaviness, and vague indefinite pain which later may become severe and radicular. Nausea, vomiting, change in bowel habits, and other symptoms suggestive of bowel obstruction result from compression of portions of the gastrointestinal tract. Later,

the malignant tumors cause anorexia, weight loss, weakness, fever, and, less frequently, hematemesis. Genitourinary complaints include hematuria, dysuria, and urgency and frequency of urination. Rarely, there is oliguria or anuria. Pain radiating into one or both thighs is usually late and due to involvement of lumbar and sacral nerve routes; it invariably denotes a malignant tumor. Swelling and varicosities of the lower extremities are usually due to obstruction of lymphatics and venous return. Hormonally active tumors of extraadrenal chromaffin tissue (pheochromocytoma) produce symptoms referable to hypertension. Rarely, hypoglycemia and its associated symptoms may be seen with retroperitoneal sarcomas.

The predominant physical finding is the presence of an abdominal mass. This is usually nontender and may fill the entire abdomen. A fixed, hard mass suggests malignancy, whereas a soft or tense and ballottable one may be a benign neoplasm or cyst. The mass usually occupies the midline and extends into one or both flanks or may be deep-seated in the pelvis, where it can be felt through the rectum. Ascites due to compression of the portal or hepatic veins, edema of the lower extremities, scrotal varicosities, and dilated superficial abdominal veins are infrequently present. Enlarged hemorrhoids or rectal tenesmus are symptoms in patients with presacral neoplasms.

The diagnosis of primary retroperitoneal tumors is mainly one of exclusion of other abdominal tumefactions. Differential diagnosis includes lesions of the kidney, such as hydronephrosis, polycystic disease, or hypernephroma; pancreatic cysts and tumors; splenomegaly; neoplasms of the liver; tumors of the gastrointestinal tract; ovarian tumors; abdominal aortic aneurysms; and cysts of the omentum and mesentery. To aid in this differentiation,

Table 35-2. CLASSIFICATION OF RETROPERITONEAL TUMORS

Tissue type	Benign tumors	Malignant tumors
Lymphatic tissue	Lymphangioma	Lymphangiosarcoma
Lymph nodes	. . . .	Lymphosarcoma
		Hodgkin's disease
		Reticulum cell sarcoma
Adipose tissue	Lipoma	Liposarcoma
Fibrous tissue	Fibroma	Fibrosarcoma
Smooth muscle	Lieomyoma	Lieomyosarcoma
Nerve elements	Neurilemoma	Malignant schwannoma
	Neurofibroma	
	Ganglioneuroma	Sympathicoblastoma (neuroblastoma)
		Chordoma
Striated muscle	Rhabdomyoma	Rhabdomyosarcoma
Mucoid tissue	Myxoma	Myxosarcoma
Vascular tissue	Hemangioma	Malignant hemangiopericytoma
Mesothelial tissue	. . . .	Mesothelioma
Mesenchyme		Mesenchymoma
Extraadrenal chromaffin tissue	Benign pheochromocytoma	Malignant pheochromocytoma
Gland tissue	Adenoma	Carcinoma
Embryonic remnants	Nephrogenic cysts	Urogenital ridge tumor
Cell rests	Dermoid	Teratoma
Miscellaneous	Xanthogranuloma	Synovioma
		Dysgerminoma
		Undifferentiated malignant tumor

Fig. 35-14. Right retrograde pyelogram (anteroposterior film) showing displacement of the right kidney into the left side of the abdomen with distortion of the renal pelvis. At laparotomy, the patient was found to have a very large liposarcoma completely filling the right retroperitoneal space.

roentgenographic studies of the genitourinary and gastrointestinal tracts are particularly useful in addition to an ordinary flat plate of the abdomen, abdominal aortography, inferior vena cava phlebography, and special scanning techniques. The intravenous and retrograde pyelogram is the most valuable of these studies. Typically with malignant tumors, anteroposterior films will show distortion and displacement of the ureters laterally, partial or complete obstruction of the ureter, or distortion of the kidney pelvis (Fig. 35-14). Lateral films may demonstrate anterior ureteral displacement. Displacement of the ureter without distortion is seen with benign neoplasms (Fig. 35-15).

The main value of a gastrointestinal series and barium enema is the exclusion of gastrointestinal tumors. However, if the tumor is of sufficient size, it will show displacement or distortion of the stomach or intestines (Fig. 35-16). Calcification is not unusual in certain retroperitoneal tumors, while the finding of teeth or other recognizable bony structures is diagnostic of teratoma.

Lowman and associates reported in detail the diagnostic use of retroperitoneal angiography. The lumbar arteries supply a large segment of the retroperitoneal space, and stretching or displacement of these vessels or displacement of the aorta by the tumor mass can give precise localization of the tumor and exclude primary visceral tumors (Fig. 35-17). Neovascularity often indicates malignant disease, but most retroperitoneal tumors lack this feature.

Beta-scan ultrasonography is a safe, noninvasive technique which will differentiate solid tumors from cysts. Recently, computerized axial tomography has also been used for diagnosing retroperitoneal tumors. Retroperitoneal pneumography, although widely discussed in the literature, is now rarely used, having been replaced by safer diagnostic techniques.

Positive histologic diagnosis can be made only with biopsy of the tumor at the time of laparotomy. At least 75 percent of the malignant tumors are sarcomas. In order of frequency, these are malignant lymphomas, liposarcomas, leiomyosarcomas, rhabdomyosarcomas, and fibrosarcomas. Sympathicoblastomas or neuroblastomas also comprise a large group of the malignant tumors. The most frequent benign tumors are cystic and include lymphatic or chylous cysts, cysts of urogenital origin, dermoids, and enterogenous cysts. Other relatively common benign tumors are xanthogranulomas, lipomas, and benign pheochromocytomas.

TREATMENT. Some retroperitoneal tumors are benign and can be cured by simple excisions; some are histologi-

Fig. 35-15. Right retrograde pyelogram in a patient with a benign retroperitoneal neurofibroma causing partial obstruction of the kidney. The right ureter is displaced laterally, which is the usual finding with retroperitoneal tumors.

Fig. 35-16. Barium enema in the patient depicted in Fig. 35-14 showing marked displacement of the ascending colon to the left by the retroperitoneal tumor.

cally benign but clinically malignant; others grow slowly but tend to recur and invade locally; and still others are rapidly malignant from the start.

Treatment of these growths consists of surgical or irradiation therapy, or a combination of the two. With the exception of lymphomas, chemotherapy has only limited therapeutic application. Surgical treatment is the most effective and offers the greatest prospect for cure. In some cases, it is imperative because of intestinal or urinary obstructions or because of hemorrhage.

As many as one-third of patients with malignant tumors may be inoperable because of multiple peritoneal tumor implants or distant metastases to liver, lung, and bone, in order of frequency.

In operable patients, initial biopsy of the tumor with frozen section will usually determine its malignant or benign nature. A cure may be anticipated following complete resection of benign tumors. On occasion, however, a tumor previously considered benign will recur, and this is especially true of retroperitoneal lipomas, which may undergo sarcomatous change.

For a malignant tumor, the initial operation offers the best chance for cure. These tumors are quite invasive and

often become adherent to vital organs or structures. Adequate exposure is extremely important to enable safe dissection of the tumor and avoid injury to major blood vessels. For this reason, a generous transperitoneal abdominal incision is preferred over an extraperitoneal flank approach. It is estimated that fewer than 25 percent of malignant tumors can be completely resected with anticipation of cure. Fixation of the tumor to the parietes does not contraindicate an attempt at resection, since partial excision can often give satisfactory palliation. At times, nephrectomy or partial intestinal resection may be required. Operative mortality is high, with reports varying between 10 and 25 percent.

Malignant retroperitoneal tumors have a high recurrence rate, from 30 to 50 percent in most large series. The tumors become more malignant with each recurrence, and reoperation becomes more hazardous. Nevertheless, long-term survival has been reported after multiple resections.

Radiotherapy, although rarely curative, may relieve pain, and obstruction and prolong life. As many as 75 percent of patients will benefit from irradiation therapy even though most retroperitoneal tumors are not radiocurative. Indications for irradiation include (1) inoperable tumors; (2) tumor recurrence following previous resection; (3) residual tumor following partial surgical resection; (4) certain radiosensitive tumors, particularly the malignant lymphomas; and (5) as an adjunct to surgery for some malignant tumors such as neuroblastomas, liposarcomas, rhabdomyosarcomas, and undifferentiated anaplastic sarcomas. Radiotherapy is the treatment of choice for malignant lymphomas, since the multicentric origin of these tumors makes surgical extirpation difficult.

The overall prognosis for malignant retroperitoneal tumors is poor. Five-year survival free of tumor is less than 10 percent and can be anticipated only in those patients in whom complete surgical removal is possible. Rare cures following irradiation therapy of neuroblastoma or lymphosarcoma have also been reported. However, since many of the tumors are slow-growing or responsive to irradiation, long-term survival with existing tumor is possible in as many as 15 percent of patients. Neuroblastoma and liposarcoma offer the best prognosis with average survivals of 4 and 5 years, respectively. Most patients with other malignant retroperitoneal tumors are dead in 2 years, death resulting from widespread metastases, intestinal or urinary obstruction, or hemorrhage from invasion of major blood vessels.

References

Abdominal Wall

Ackerman, L. V.: "Surgical Pathology," p. 964, The C. V. Mosby Company, St. Louis, 1964.

Brasfield, R. D., and Das Gupta, T. K.: Desmoid Tumors of the Anterior Abdominal Wall, *Surgery,* **65**:241, 1969.

Cullen, T. S., and Brodel, M.: Lesions of the Rectus Abdominus Muscle Simulating an Acute Intra-abdominal Condition, *Bull Johns Hopkins Hosp,* **61**:295, 1937.

Das Gupta, T. K., Brasfield, R. D., and O'Hara J.: Extra-

Fig. 35-17. Abdominal aortogram showing lateral displacement of the aorta and lumbar arteries by a large right retroperitoneal tumor.

abdominal Desmoids: A Clinicopathological Study, *Ann Surg,* **170:**109, 1969.

Geschickter, C. F., and Lewis, D.: Tumors of Connective Tissue, *Am J Cancer,* **25:**630, 1935.

Hildreth, D.: Anticoagulant Therapy and Rectus Sheath Hematoma, *Am J Surg,* **124:**80, 1972.

Jones, T. W., and Merendino, K. A.: The Deep Epigastric Artery: Rectus Muscle Syndrome, *Am J Surg,* **103:**159, 1962.

Pack, G. T., and Ehrlich, H. E.: Neoplasms of the Anterior Abdominal Wall with Special Consideration of Desmoid Tumors, *Surg Gynecol Obstet,* **79:**177, 1944.

Sheehan, V.: Spontaneous Hematoma of the Rectus Abdominis Muscle in Pregnancy, *Br Med J,* **2:**1131, 1951.

Stiles, Q. R., Raskowski, H. J., and Henry, W.: Rectus Sheath Hematoma, *Surg Gynecol Obstet,* **12:**331, 1965.

Stout, A. P.: Fibrosarcoma: The Malignant Tumor of Fibroblasts, *Cancer,* **1:**30, 1948.

Teske, J. M.: Hematoma of the Rectus Abdominis Muscle: Report of a Case and Analysis of 100 Cases from the Literature, *Am J Surg,* **71:**689, 1946.

Waddell, W. R.: Treatment of Intra-abdominal and Abdominal Wall Desmoid Tumors with Drugs that Affect the Metabolism of Cyclic 3',5'-Adenosine Monophosphate, *Ann Surg,* **181:**299, 1975.

Omentum

Anton, J. E., Jennings, J. E., and Spiegel, M. B.: Primary Omental Torsion, *Am J Surg,* **68:**303, 1945.

Beahrs, O. H., Judd, E. J., Jr., and Dockerty, M. B.: Chylous Cysts of the Abdomen, *Surg Clin North Am,* **30:**1081, 1950.

Brown, H. J., and Noone, R. B.: Primary Omental Torsion, *J Okla State Med Assoc,* **64:**177, 1971.

Draper, J. W., and Johnston, R. K.: The Pathologic Omentum, *JAMA,* **88:**376, 1927.

Eitel, G. G.: A Rare Omental Tumor, *Med Rec,* **55:**715, 1899.

Halligan, E. J., and Rabiah, F. A.: Primary Idiopathic Segmental Infarction of the Greater Omentum, *Arch Surg,* **79:**738, 1959.

Leitner, M. J., Jordan, C. G., Spinner, M. H., and Reese, E. C.: Torsion, Infarction and Hemorrhage of the Omentum as a Cause of Acute Abdominal Distress, *Ann Surg,* **135:**103, 1952.

Mainzer, R. A., and Simoes, A.: Primary Idiopathic Torsion of the Omentum, *Arch Surg,* **88:**974, 1964.

Rubin, I. C.: The Functions of the Great Omentum, *Surg Gynecol Obstet,* **12:**117, 1911.

Stout, A. P., Hendry, J., and Purdie, F. J.: Solid Tumors of the Great Omentum, *Cancer,* **16:**231, 1963.

Walker, A. R., and Putnam, T. C.: Omental, Mesenteric and Retroperitoneal Cysts, *Surgery,* **178:**13, 1973.

Wrzesinski, J., and Firestone, S.: Primary Idiopathic Segmental Infarction of the Omentum, *Surgery,* **39:**663, 1965.

Mesentery

Ackerman, L. V.: "Surgical Pathology," The C. V. Mosby Company, St. Louis, 1964.

Adams, J. T., and Kutner, F. R.: Pure Fibroma of the Mesentery, *Am J Surg,* **111:**734, 1966.

Aird, I.: Acute Non-specific Mesenteric Lymphadenitis, *Br Med J,* **2:**680, 1945.

Anane-Safah, J. C., Blair, E., and Reckler, S.: Primary Mesenteric Venous Occlusive Disease, *Surg Gynecol Obstet,* **141:**740, 1975.

Beahrs, O. H., Judd, E. S., Jr., and Dockerty, M. B.: Chylous Cysts of the Abdomen, *Surg Clin North Am,* **30:**1081, 1950.

Bergan, J. J., Dean, R. H., Conn, J., Jr., and Yao, J. S. T.: Revascularization in Treatment of Mesenteric Infarction, *Ann Surg,* **182:**430, 1975.

Bernatz, P. E.: Necrosis of Colon following Resection for Abdominal Aortic Aneurysm, *Arch Surg,* **81:**373, 1960.

Berry, F. B., and Bougas, J. A.: Agnogenic Venous Mesenteric Thrombosis, *Ann Surg,* **132:**450, 1950.

Britt, L. C., and Cheek, R. C.: Nonocclusive Mesenteric Vascular Disease: Clinical and Experimental Observations, *Ann Surg,* **169:**704, 1969.

Carey, J. P., Stemmer, E. A., and Connolly, J. E.: Median Arcuate Ligament Syndrome, *Arch Surg,* **99:**441, 1969.

Caropreso, P. R.: Mesenteric Cysts, A Review, *Arch Surg,* **108:**242, 1974.

Carter, R., and Gosney, W. G.: Abdominal Apoplexy: Report of Six Cases and Review of the Literature, *Am J Surg,* **111:**388, 1966.

Connolly, J. E., Abrams, H. L., and Kieraldo, J. H.: Observations on the Diagnosis and Treatment of Obliterative Disease of the Visceral Branches of the Abdominal Aorta, *Arch Surg,* **90:**596, 1965.

Crile, G., Jr., and Newell, E. T., Jr.: Abdominal Apoplexy: Spontaneous Rupture of Visceral Vessel, *JAMA,* **114:**1155, 1940.

Donhauser, J. L.: Primary Acute Mesenteric Lymphadenitis, *Arch Surg,* **74:**528, 1957.

Dunbar, J. D., Molnar, W., Beman, F. F., and Marable, S. A.: Compression of the Celiac Trunk and Abdominal Angina: Preliminary Report of 15 Cases, *Am J Roentgenol Radium Ther Nucl Med,* **95:**731, 1965.

Dunphy, J. E.: Abdominal Pain of Vascular Origin, *Am J Med Sci,* **192:**109, 1936.

Durst, A. L., Freund, H., Rosenmann, E., and Birnbaum, D.: Mesenteric Panniculitis: Review of the Literature and Presentation of Cases, *Surgery,* **81:**203, 1977.

Fogerty, T. J., and Fletcher, W. S.: Genesis of Nonocclusive Mesenteric Ischemia, *Am J Surg,* **111:**130, 1966.

Fowler, E. F.: Primary Cysts and Tumors of the Small Bowel Mesentery, *Am Surg,* **27:**653, 1961.

Fry, W. J., and Kraft, R. O.: Visceral Angina, *Surg Gynecol Obstet,* **117:**417, 1963.

Grossman, L. A., Kaplan, H. J., Preuss, H. J., and Herrington, J. L., Jr.: Mesenteric Panniculitis, *JAMA,* **183:**318, 1963.

Habbooshe, F., Wallace, H. W., Nusbaum, M., Baum, S., Dratch, P., and Blakemore, W. S.: Nonocclusive Mesenteric Vascular Insufficiency, *Ann Surg,* **180:**819, 1974.

Handelsman, J. C., and Shelly, W. M.: Mesenteric Panniculitis, *Arch Surg,* **91:**842, 1965.

Hart, J. T.: Solid Tumors of the Mesentery, *Ann Surg,* **104:**184, 1936.

Jackson, B. B.: "Occlusion of the Superior Mesenteric Artery," Charles C Thomas, Publisher, Springfield, Ill., 1963.

Kleinsasser, L. J.: Abdominal Apoplexy: Report of Two Cases and Review of the Literature, *Am J Surg,* **120:**623, 1970.

Laufman, H., Nora, P. F., and Mittelpunkt, A. I.: Mesenteric Blood Vessels: Advances in Surgery and Physiology, *Arch Surg,* **88:**1021, 1964.

Levinsky, R. A., Lewis, R. M., Bynum, T. E., and Hanley, H. G.: Digoxin Induced Intestinal Vasoconstriction: The Effects of Proximal Arterial Stenosis and Glucagon Administration, *Circulation,* **52:**130, 1975.

Loeb, M. J.: Mesenteric Cysts, *NY State J Med,* **41:**1564, 1941.

McCort, J. J.: Infarction of the Descending Colon Due to Vascular Occlusion, *N Engl J Med,* **262:**168, 1960.

McDonald, J. C.: Nonspecific Mesenteric Lymphadenitis, *Surg Gynecol Obstet,* **116:**409, 1963.

Madore, P., Kahn, D. S., Webster, D. R., and Skoryna, S.: Nonspecific Mesenteric Lymphadenitis, *Can J Surg,* **5:**59, 1962.

Marable, S. A., Kaplan, M. F., Beman, F. M., and Molnar, W.: Celiac Compression Syndrome, *Am J Surg,* **115:**97, 1968.

Morris, G. C., Crawford, E. S., Cooley, D. A., and DeBakey, M. E.: Revascularization of the Celiac and Superior Mesenteric Arteries, *Arch Surg,* **84:**95, 1962.

——— and DeBakey, M. E.: Abdominal Angina: Diagnosis and Treatment, *JAMA,* **176:**91, 1961.

Naitove, A., and Weismann, R. E.: Primary Mesenteric Venous Thrombosis, *Ann Surg,* **161:**516, 1965.

Ogden, W. W., Bradburn, D. M., and Rives, J. D.: Mesenteric Panniculitis, *Ann Surg,* **161:**864, 1965.

Ottinger, L. W., and Austen, W. G.: A Study of 136 Patients with Mesenteric Infarction, *Surg Gynecol Obstet,* **124:**251, 1967.

Pierce, G. E., and Brockenbrough, E. C.: The Spectrum of Mesenteric Infarction, *Am J Surg,* **119:**233, 1970.

Rankin, F. W., and Major, S. G.: Tumors of the Mesentery, *Surg Gynecol Obstet,* **54:**809, 1932.

Reul, G. J., Jr., Wukasch, D. C., Sandiford, F. M., Chiarillo, L., Hallman, G. L., and Cooley, D. A.: Surgical Treatment of Abdominal Angina: Review of 25 Patients, *Surgery,* **75:**682, 1974.

Rob, C. G.: The Indications for Operation in Occlusive Disease of the Visceral Arteries, *J Thorac Cardiovasc Surg,* **3:**223, 1962.

———: Surgical Diseases of the Celiac and Mesenteric Arteries, *Arch Surg,* **93:**21, 1966.

Seldinger, S. I.: Catheter Replacement of Needle in Percutaneous Arteriography: New Technique, *Acta Radiol (Stockholm),* **39:**368, 1953.

Shaw, R. S., and Maynard, E. P., III: Acute and Chronic Thrombosis of Superior Mesenteric Arteries Associated with Malabsorption: Report of Two Cases Successfully Treated by Thromboendarterectomy, *N Engl J Med,* **258:**874, 1958.

——— and Rutledge, R. H.: Superior Mesenteric Artery Embolectomy in the Treatment of Massive Mesenteric Infarction, *N Engl J Med,* **257:**595, 1957.

Smith, R. F., Szilagyi, D. E., and Pfeifer, J. R.: Arterial Trauma, *Arch Surg,* **86:**825, 1963.

Stanley, J. C., Thompson, N. W., and Fry, W. J.: Splanchnic Artery Aneurysms, *Arch Surg,* **101:**689, 1970.

—— and Fry, W. J.: Median Arcuate Ligament Syndrome, *Arch Surg,* **103:**252, 1971.

Thorek, P.: "Anatomy in Surgery," 2d ed., J. B. Lippincott Company, Philadelphia, 1963.

Van Way, C. W., Brockman, S. K., and Rosenfeld, L.: Spontaneous Thrombosis of the Mesenteric Veins, *Ann Surg,* **173:**561, 1971.

Watson, W. O., and Sadikali, F.: Celiac Axis Compression: Experience with 20 Patients and a Critical Appraisal of the Syndrome, *Ann Intern Med,* **86:**278, 1977.

Wilensky, A. O., and Hahn, L. J.: Mesenteric Lymphadenitis, *Ann Surg,* **83:**812, 1926.

Yannopoulos, K., and Stout, A. P.: Primary Solid Tumors of the Mesentery, *Cancer,* **16:**914, 1963.

Retroperitoneum

Ackerman, L. V.: Tumors of the Retroperitoneum, Mesentery and Peritoneum, in "Atlas of Tumor and Pathology," Armed Forces Institute of Pathology, sec. VI, Washington, 1954.

—— and delRegato, J. A.: "Cancer: Diagnosis, Treatment and Prognosis," The C. V. Mosby Company, St. Louis, 1962.

Albarran, J.: Rétention rénale par périuretèrite libération externe de l'uretère, *Assoc Franc Urol,* **9:**511, 1905.

Armstrong, J. R., and Cohn, I.: Primary Malignant Retroperitoneal Tumors, *Am J Surg,* **110:**937, 1965.

Braasch, J. W.: Primary Retroperitoneal Tumors, *Surg Clin North Am,* **47:**663, 1967.

Donnelly, B. A.: Primary Retroperitoneal Tumors, *Surg Gynecol Obstet,* **83:**705, 1946.

Duncan, R. E., and Evans, A. T.: Diagnosis of Primary Retroperitoneal Tumors, *Urology,* **117:**19, 1977.

Gow, J. G.: An Appraisal of Inflammatory Strictures of the Ureter, *Ann R Coll Surg Engl,* **51:**177, 1972.

Hache, L., Utz, D. C., and Woolner, L. B.: Idiopathic Fibrosing Retroperitonitis, *Surg Gynecol Obstet,* **115:**737, 1962.

Hackett, E.: Idiopathic Retroperitoneal Fibrosis: A Condition involving the Ureters, the Aorta, and the Inferior Vena Cava, *Br J Surg,* **46:**3, 1948.

Harbrecht, P. J.: Variants of Retroperitoneal Fibrosis, *Ann Surg,* **165:**388, 1967.

Hewitt, C. B., Nitz, G. L., Kiser, W. S., Straffon R. A., and Stewart, B. H.: Surgical Treatment of Retroperitoneal Fibrosis, *Ann Surg,* **169:**611, 1969.

Hoffman, W. W., and Trippel, O. H.: Retroperitoneal Fibrosis: Etiologic Considerations, *J Urol,* **86:**222, 1961.

Koep, Lawrence, and Zuidema, G. D.: The Clinical Significance of Retroperitoneal Fibrosis, *Surgery,* **81:**250, 1977.

Longmire, W. P., Jr., Goodwirs, W. E., and Buckberg, G. D.: Management of Sclerosing Fibrosis of the Mediastinal and Retroperitoneal Areas, *Ann Surg,* **165:**1013, 1967.

Lowman, R. M., Peck, D. R., Love, L., and Dubash, D.: Lumbar Angiography in the Diagnosis of Primary Retroperitoneal Tumors, *Surg Gynecol Obstet,* **132:**597, 1971.

Melicow, M. M.: Primary Tumors of the Retroperitoneum, *J Intern Coll Surg,* **19:**401, 1953.

Mitchell, R. J.: Alimentary Complications of Non-malignant Retroperitoneal Fibrosis, *Br J Surg,* **58:**254, 1971.

Neistadt, A., Jones, T., and Rob, C.: Vascular System Involvement by Idiopathic Retroperitoneal Fibrosis, *Surgery,* **59:**950, 1966.

Ormond, J. K.: Bilateral Ureteral Obstruction Due to Envelopment and Compression by Inflammatory Retroperitoneal Process, *J Urol,* **59:**1072, 1948.

——: Idiopathic Retroperitoneal Fibrosis, *JAMA,* **174:**1561, 1960.

——: Idiopathic Retroperitoneal Fibrosis: Ormond's Syndrome, *Henry Ford Hosp Med Bull,* **10:**13, 1962.

Pack, G. T., and Tabah, E. J.: Primary Retroperitoneal Tumors, *Surg Gynecol Obstet,* **99:**209, 1954.

Ross, J. C., and Goldsmith, H. J.: The Combined Surgical and Medical Treatment of Retroperitoneal Fibrosis, *Br J Surg,* **58:**411, 1971.

Schneider, C. F.: Idiopathic Retroperitoneal Fibrosis Producing Vena Caval, Biliary Ureteral and Duodenal Obstructions, *Ann Surg,* **94:**316, 1964.

Suby, H. I., Kerr, W. S., Graham, J. R., and Fraley, E.: Retroperitoneal Fibrosis: A Missing Link in the Chain, *J Urol,* **93:**144, 1965.

Wagenknecht, L. V., and Auvert, J.: Symptoms and Diagnosis of Retroperitoneal Fibrosis, *Urol Int,* **26:**185, 1971.

Chapter 36

Abdominal Wall Hernias

by John H. Morton

DEFINITION

Although hernia is one of the most common ailments with which mankind is afflicted, there continues to be debate among physicians about many points ranging from etiology to proper management. Even the definition of a hernia remains a matter of discussion. Some writers define a hernia in terms of a weakness or abnormal opening in an enclosing layer. Others emphasize a protrusion through the opening rather than the opening itself. Still others stress a combination of both. Clearly, for herniation to occur there must be a defect in supporting structures through which a contained organ or tissue *may* protrude—but the organ need not be present within the weakness for a hernia to exist. The contents of many hernias will reduce readily when the patient is recumbent, but the basic anatomic defect persists. However, it is important to stress that a peritoneal diverticulum, such as a patent processus vaginalis, does not per se constitute a hernia. There must, in addition, be an associated weakness large enough to permit passage of a viscus into the sac before a hernia is truly present.

By far the larger number of hernias occur in the inguinal or femoral region, and these are usually classified together under the term *groin hernia.* If a contained viscus can be returned from the hernia to its normal domain, the hernia is *reducible.* A hernia from which a contained organ cannot be reduced is said to be *incarcerated;* this may be either an acute, painful condition or a long-standing, asymptomatic one. If, in addition to incarceration, there is a compromise of the blood supply of the contained organ, this is called a *strangulated hernia.* The term is a poor one since the contents of the hernia, not the sac itself, are strangulated. When a portion of the wall of the hernia sac is composed of an organ such as the cecum or the sigmoid colon, a *sliding hernia* is present. Rarely, the sac in a groin hernia spreads out between the layers of the abdominal wall instead of following the course of the inguinal canal. Under these circumstances the hernia is known as an *interparietal hernia.* These hernias may be preperitoneal, when the sac lies between peritoneum and transversalis fascia; interstitial, when it extends between the various muscle layers; or superficial, when it is found between external oblique aponeurosis and skin.

A *ventral hernia* occurs in the abdominal wall at some site other than the groin. The umbilical hernia and the incisional hernia, which develops in a previous laparotomy incision, are the most common ventral hernias. The epigastric hernia, another frequent ventral hernia, presents through a defect in the linea alba above the umbilicus. The linea semicircularis below the umbilicus marks the level below which the rectus abdominis muscle lies behind the aponeurosis of the oblique and transversus abdominis muscles rather than within the layers of the internal oblique aponeurosis. The point where the vertical linea semilunaris along the lateral border of the rectus muscle joins the linea semicircularis is a potential weak area. The rare hernia which protrudes at this site is known as a *Spigelian hernia.*

Hernias from the abdominal cavity may also develop through the lateral abdominal wall, the so-called lumbar hernias. The most common of these relatively unusual hernias is the postoperative hernia developing in an incision made to expose the kidney. The most frequent naturally occurring hernia in this area is the Petit's triangle hernia. Petit's triangle is bounded by the external oblique anteriorly, the iliac crest inferiorly, and the latissimus dorsi posteriorly. The internal oblique forms the floor of the triangle, and it must be weakened or absent for herniation to develop. Cystoceles, urethroceles, and rectoceles are common hernias in women, but perineal hernias through the levator ani area and sciatic hernias through either the greater or the lesser sciatic foramen are exceedingly rare. The obturator hernia is another rare defect, with herniation of a peritoneal sac into the medial thigh through the obturator foramen.

In addition to these abdominal wall hernias and to diaphragmatic hernias a number of internal hernias—all of them rare—may occur. In these instances a loop of intestine enters an opening, either congenital or acquired, and becomes obstructed. This may occur through the foramen of Winslow, at the junction of duodenum and jejunum, around the cecum or sigmoid colon in association with malrotation, through a defect in the mesentery following bowel resection, or between the urinary bladder and the anterior abdominal wall. These conditions are usually discovered during an exploration for intestinal obstruction. They are not true hernias in the sense of this discussion, and they will not be considered further here.

INCIDENCE

For several reasons the prevalence of abdominal hernias is difficult to estimate. If a hernia is small, it may not be readily detected on any one examination. If findings from anatomic dissections are used, the incidence will be higher than if figures are drawn from routine physical examinations. In certain borderline lesions, not all physicians will agree as to whether or not a hernia is present. For instance, some pediatric surgeons equate a patent processus vaginalis with an indirect inguinal hernia, but most surgeons and anatomists do not accept this proposition without qualification. However, it is generally agreed that the most common hernia in either sex is the indirect inguinal variety, that direct hernias are very unusual in females, that femoral hernias as a class are more common in females than in males, and that hernias in general are over five times more common in males. Summarizing available evidence, Zimmerman and Anson in their excellent monograph on hernias conclude that the frequency of hernia can be placed at 5 percent of the total male adult population. Regardless of the exact figure, the magnitude of the problem is readily appreciated.

ANATOMY

All hernias of the abdominal wall involve the same tissue layers. Under the skin lies the subcutaneous fat. In the inguinal area particularly, this fat includes a well-defined condensation of connective tissue, identified as *Scarpa's fascia*. Although this layer is not true fascia, the term is undoubtedly too ingrained in the literature to be altered. The external oblique, internal oblique, and transversus abdominis are encountered in order, either as muscle fibers laterally or as layers of aponeurosis medially. The longitudinal rectus abdominis muscle lies within layers of the aponeurosis down to the semilunar line and is placed entirely behind them in the lower abdomen. The important inner investing layer of the transversus abdominis, the

transversalis fascia, and parietal peritoneum complete the abdominal wall. With an abdominal hernia at any level, the parietal peritoneal sac either passes through a defect in some of the layers of the abdominal wall or is covered with attenuated remnants of these layers.

Inguinal Region

In the descent of the testicle from its original retroperitoneal site into the scrotum, it passes through the abdominal wall in the inguinal region. A diverticulum of parietal peritoneum, the processus vaginalis, accompanies the testicle, although normally this connection with the peritoneum is obliterated before birth or in early infancy. The spermatic cord contains layers representative of each abdominal wall layer as follows:

Abdominal wall layer	*Spermatic cord layer*
Parietal peritoneum	Obliterated processus vaginalis
Transversalis fascia ⎱ . . . . . Transversus abdominis ⎰	Internal spermatic fascia
Internal oblique	Cremaster muscle
External oblique	External spermatic fascia
Subcutaneous tissue	Dartos muscle (in scrotum)
Skin	Skin

The spermatic cord passes obliquely downward through the inguinal canal from the internal inguinal ring, an opening in the transversalis fascia and transversus abdominis aponeurosis where they extend onto the spermatic cord as internal spermatic fascia. The medial margin of the internal ring is defined by the inferior epigastric artery, coursing from the external iliac artery medially and superiorly into the rectus sheath. The cord lies superior to the inguinal ligament and anterior to the inguinal canal floor. After running obliquely downward, it emerges through the external inguinal ring, an opening in the external oblique aponeurosis just above the pubic spine, to pass into the scrotum. The tubular external spermatic fascia joins the cord at the external inguinal ring, the cremaster fibers having enveloped the cord along the course of the inguinal canal.

An indirect inguinal hernia (Fig. 36-1) leaves the abdominal cavity at the internal ring and passes with the structures of the spermatic cord either a variable distance down the inguinal canal or all the way into the scrotum. Thus the indirect hernia must lie within the fibers of the cremaster muscle. Except in infants an indirect hernia is associated with an enlargement of the internal ring. The opening in the transversus abdominis aponeurosis medial to the spermatic cord is dilated and the peritoneal sac enters the spermatic cord at this point. The edge of the sac is recognized as a readily defined grayish white membrane found inside these fibers, anteromedial to the vas deferens and the other structures of the cord. Should the hernia be of the sliding variety (Fig. 36-2), the intestinal component makes up a part or all of the posterior wall of the sac. A sliding hernia in the right groin may incorporate the cecum in this fashion. On the left, the lateral leaf of the meso-

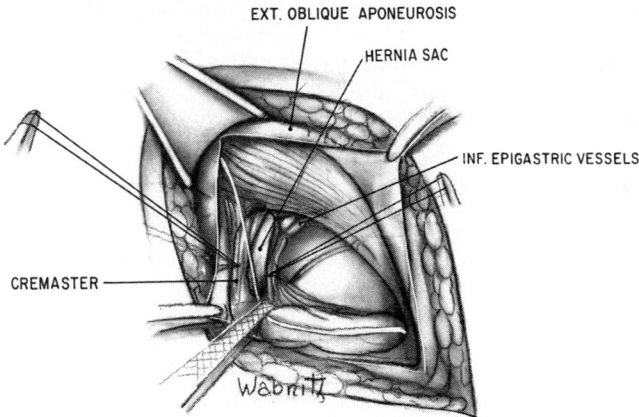

Fig. 36-1. Indirect inguinal hernia. Sac projects through internal inguinal ring anteromedial to vas deferens and inside cremaster fibers.

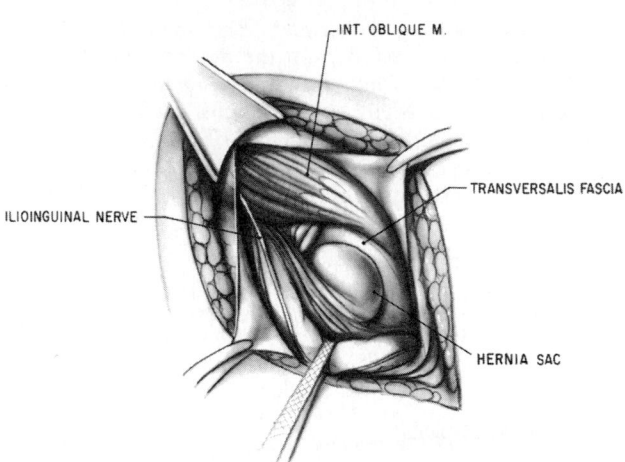

Fig. 36-3. Direct inguinal hernia. Weakness involves medial inguinal canal floor and lies behind structures of spermatic cord.

sigmoid and occasionally the sigmoid itself may be involved.

A direct hernia (Fig. 36-3) protrudes through the floor of the inguinal canal in Hesselbach's triangle, an area bounded laterally by the inferior epigastric artery, inferiorly by the inguinal ligament, and medially by the lateral margin of the rectus sheath. In Hesselbach's triangle the inguinal canal floor is formed by transversalis fascia reinforced by aponeurotic fibers from the transversus abdominis. In Hesselbach's triangle the aponeurotic reinforcement is discontinuous. Hence, the area is a potential site of weakness. When a direct hernia develops, either the entire canal floor in Hesselbach's triangle becomes attenuated and stretched out over the peritoneum, or, less commonly, a rent develops through the canal floor. Since the direct hernia projects through the medial canal floor, it cannot lie within the cremaster muscle fibers; rather, it is behind the cremaster and the rest of the spermatic cord. Thus this type of hernia is not guided through the external inguinal ring and is unlikely to reach the scrotum. On the rare occasion when a direct hernia does enter the scrotum, it must pass through the external ring separate from and behind the spermatic cord. In contrast to the other groin hernias, in which a diverticulum of peritoneum with a relatively narrow neck is present, the direct hernia usually presents as a diffuse weakness and general bulging in Hesselbach's triangle. The absence of this narrow neck makes incarceration unusual in direct inguinal hernia. When incarceration does occur, it is usually at the level of the external inguinal ring in those rare situations where a direct sac passes through this area. With a large direct hernia it is not unusual for a portion of the wall of the urinary bladder to be incorporated in a sliding fashion in the medial portion of the sac.

The third groin hernia, the femoral type (Fig. 36-4), also depends for its development upon a defect in the transversalis fascia in Hesselbach's triangle. In this type of hernia, however, there is a peritoneal sac which passes under the inguinal ligament into the femoral triangle rather than following the course of the direct hernia ante-

Fig. 36-4. Femoral hernia. Although sac projects beneath inguinal ligament into femoral triangle, basic defect making hernia possible is weakness in attachment of transversalis fascia and transversus abdominis aponeurosis to Cooper's ligament.

Fig. 36-2. Evolution of sliding hernia. A. Leading peritoneal sac "pulls" mobile cecum or sigmoid. B. Sliding hernia is established with colon or cecum as part of wall of sac.

riorly into the inguinal canal. The inguinal ligament stretches as a tight band from the anterior superior iliac spine to the spine of the pubis, and beneath it the femoral vessels enter the thigh. Medial to the femoral vein is a small empty space through which a femoral hernia may project. The resulting sac will have, perforce, a very narrow neck. Once the sac enters the thigh, however, it may assume quite large proportions in the loose connective tissue. It may even double back on top of the external oblique aponeurosis, coming to lie over the groin, where it can be mistaken for an inguinal hernia. Because of the narrow neck in this type of hernia, incarceration with strangulation of the contents of the hernia is a strong possibility.

Umbilical Region

During the embryonic period before completion of intestinal rotation there is a herniation of abdominal contents through the umbilicus into the extraembryonic coelomic cavity. At about the tenth week of fetal life the viscera normally return to the abdominal cavity, the intestine completing its rotation in the process. The defect in the abdominal wall closes slowly during subsequent fetal development, until at birth only the space occupied by the umbilical cord remains patent. Following ligation of the cord, the umbilical stump heals by granulation and organization, with epithelialization from the margins of the defect. Abdominal wall closure at this level thus consists of the fusion of skin, a single fascial layer, and peritoneum.

At birth many infants will show a small umbilical hernia (Fig. 36-5) because this process has not been carried through to completion. In most of these children spontaneous closure of the fascial defect occurs within the first four years of life in a fashion identical with that described above. An umbilical hernia which is still present in a four-year-old will usually persist, but bowel strangulation in these congenital umbilical defects is unusual.

Occasionally, however, the process of abdominal wall closure is much less complete at birth, and several interesting congenital anomalies may be encountered. An omphalocele is present when at birth there is a defect at the umbilicus covered only by a peritoneal sac. Within such a sac virtually any abdominal organ may be encountered, but small bowel, colon, and liver are the most common viscera present.

If the embryologic duct from small bowel to yolk sac remains attached to the umbilical cord at birth, it is likely to be included in the tie placed by the obstetrician. This duct, although extremely narrow, amounting to no more than a cord, may be lined with bowel epithelium. When the umbilical remnant sloughs later under these circumstances, a fistula into the small gut is created. This anomaly is known as a patent omphalomesenteric or viteline duct. On occasion the fibrous cord is not lined with epithelium, and the umbilicus then heals normally after ligation, usually without an umbilical hernia. The cord, however, may persist, connecting the umbilicus to the small gut, and it may be encountered in later life as one of the congenital bands leading to volvulus and intestinal obstruction. One patient in the author's experience was found to have a thin band of this type at abdominal exploration during adult life. The patient had never experienced drainage from the umbilicus, but the band was excised. A fecal fistula promptly developed. On further investigation it was evident that this band contained an epithelial lining at its intestinal end, although it had not extended far enough toward the umbilicus to create problems when cord ligature was performed following birth.

A sinus tract from the bladder, the urachus, enters the umbilical area from below, between the umbilical arteries, during fetal life. This tract, the remnant of the cephalic portion of the embryonic urinary bladder, is usually obliterated before birth, but should it remain patent, it may become incorporated in the umbilical cord ligature. Thus a later draining umbilical sinus may represent a patent urachus as well as a patent omphalomesenteric duct.

Umbilical hernias may also develop during adult life. This occurs more commonly in women, usually after childbirth. The hernia may become a large one, and strangulation of intestine or omentum within the defect is not uncommon.

ETIOLOGY

Hernias may result from congenital anomalies or may develop secondarily during later life. Although congenital

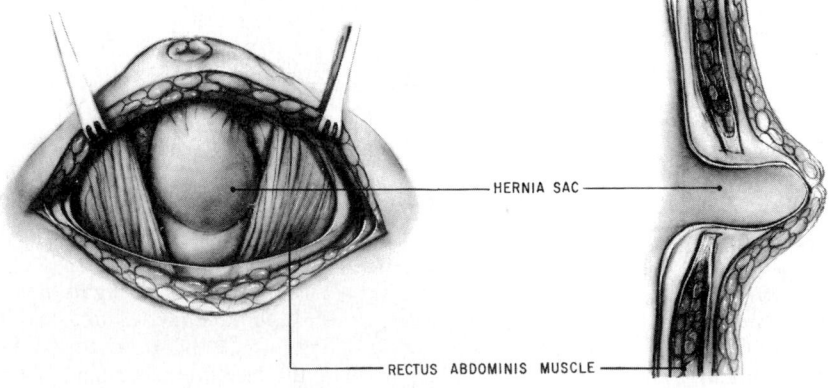

HERNIA SAC

RECTUS ABDOMINIS MUSCLE

Fig. 36-5. Umbilical hernia. Peritoneal sac is attached directly to underside of umbilical skin, with only thin attenuated fascia covering sac.

umbilical hernias are more common in black infants, other congenital hernias occur with equal frequency in blacks and whites. Inguinal hernias are more common in males, and femoral hernias occur primarily in females. When a hernia develops secondarily in later life, it is frequently the result of trauma. Hence it is compensable if the injury occurs when the patient is at work. It should be pointed out, however, that the traumatic explanation for these hernias is not entirely satisfying. In many instances, for example, the patient is not aware of any specific event which precipitated the hernia. Rather, a bulge develops gradually after years of hard work. In other circumstances, a similar hernia may develop in a sedentary individual who has not changed his habits before herniation occurred. In any case, many men never develop a hernia despite a lifetime of vigorous physical activity. In evaluating the direct hernia of later life, Zimmerman and Anson concluded that this lesion also results from a congenital anatomic defect—the absence of adequate muscular support for the lower portion of the inguinal canal. They find the lowermost fibers of the internal oblique lacking, so that a larger triangle without muscular reinforcement is present in the individual who is prone to hernia formation. As a result of his dissections Condon concluded that a direct hernia resulted from the lack of adequate reinforcement of transversalis fascia in Hesselbach's triangle.

In considering the development of a hernia in the groin during middle life, it is wise to remember that increased intraabdominal pressure is at least as important a predisposing factor as external trauma. Chronic cough or symptoms of genitourinary tract or gastrointestinal tract obstruction may precede herniation. Benign prostatic hypertrophy and carcinoma of the left colon are two important entities which should be considered in an adult seeking medical attention because of a hernia. Cirrhosis of the liver with ascites, massive splenomegaly, and uterine enlargement during pregnancy are other possible etiologic factors of this type.

Recently, several investigators have suggested that a connective tissue abnormality may be involved in adult-onset hernias. Abnormalities in the ultrastructure and the physicochemical properties of collagen in patients with direct hernias suggest that the hernia is one manifestation of a generalized abnormality in collagen metabolism.

From the legal point of view a hernia is an important condition about which a physician must frequently testify, and the wording or interpretation of a workmen's compensation law can be important. Many young adult males first discover a hernia after some vigorous physical labor; this type of hernia is usually indirect. The physician is aware that such a defect is almost always congenital, and it would be difficult to testify that the traumatic incident produced the hernia. On the other hand, it is hard to convince a young man that the hernia has been present all his life and that he was unaware of it because no intraabdominal organ had previously entered the sac. This uncomfortable situation is satisfactorily avoided in jurisdictions where exacerbation of preexisting disease is sufficient evidence of a compensable injury. In these circum-stances the surgeon can bear witness that a hernia is present and that its appearance may be related to the injury in question.

SYMPTOMS AND SIGNS

A hernia may be an asymptomatic defect, discovered incidentally during a routine physical examination. The individual may or may not have been aware of its presence. The usual reducible hernia produces no symptoms of importance other than pain. The type and degree of pain vary considerably from one individual to another. If the hernia is first recognized after an acute traumatic episode, local pain of a muscular type may be quite severe for several days. This pain occurs when, in the presence of a preexisting patent processus vaginalis, sudden enlargement of the internal inguinal ring permits development of a true hernia.

In a few days the discomfort subsides without specific treatment. In a long-standing hernia occasional twinges of local discomfort may be present, usually in association with straining or with the temporary entry of an intraperitoneal organ into the sac. Another type of discomfort may occur when a loop of small intestine enters the hernia. Epigastric or paraumbilical pain may then develop, representing visceral pain in the superior mesenteric distribution as a result of mesenteric stretching.

The physical signs of an uncomplicated hernia vary with the contents of the sac. When there are no peritoneal contents present, the sac is collapsed and its presence is difficult to identify. It is said that the opposing peritoneal surfaces may be rubbed one over the other to detect a sensation of gliding, but this is an unreliable sign. When an organ occupies the sac, the findings vary with the organ involved. If bowel is present, crepitation will be noted on palpation because of the presence of gas and fluid within the lumen. If a solid organ such as an ovary is present, a movable firm regular mass will be felt. When omentum is within the sac, an ill-defined irregular rubbery mass will be palpable. When an organ enters an inguinal hernia sac, reduction may be attempted by gentle pressure with a finger through the invaginated scrotal skin. This should be done with the patient supine and relaxed. If the organ is not readily reduced, a sliding hernia should be suspected, especially if the bulge is a large one.

A hernia may be particularly difficult to identify in an infant, who cannot cooperate during examination. If the mother gives a suggestive history and no hernia can be found, she should be instructed to bring the infant back when a bulge is obvious or to return later with the youngster for a second examination under any circumstance. If a hydrocele of the cord is present in an infant, an indirect hernia is almost invariably present as well, and it should be repaired at the time of hydrocelectomy.

If no hernia is obvious when examination is begun, one may become apparent if the patient is requested to strain. A sustained contraction of the muscles of the abdominal wall is more effective than the traditional cough as a method of raising intraabdominal pressure, thus demonstrating the hernia. Position during the examination is important. When a ventral hernia is suspected, the supine patient should be asked to raise head and shoulders from the bed. When a male is being examined for a groin hernia, he should be standing in a relaxed position, and the physician should invaginate the scrotum with the examining finger. The finger should be introduced through the external ring into the inguinal canal while the patient strains. It is harder to examine a female for a groin hernia. She should be standing and the labia majora examined while she strains. A definite bulge and mass should be palpated before the diagnosis of a hernia can be considered secure. The presence of a dilated external inguinal ring is of no significance per se as regards the presence of a hernia and does not predispose to the later development of a hernia. With groin hernias the location of the mass should be helpful in distinguishing the femoral hernia. However, an obese individual may be unaware of a mass in the groin, and the groin should be carefully palpated for evidence of an incarcerated hernia when a patient presents with intestinal obstruction.

The clinical distinction between direct and indirect hernia by physical examination is academic, since the operative approach for repair is the same for both. This is fortunate since accurate distinction is often difficult to make. When the examining finger has been advanced well into the inguinal canal, the indirect hernia should strike the fingertip and the direct hernia the ball of the finger— but this difference is frequently hard to appreciate. A thumb placed over the internal inguinal ring should keep an indirect hernia reduced when the patient strains while permitting a direct hernia to appear; again, it is not always possible to locate the internal ring accurately enough to make this technique foolproof.

The predominant finding with an incarcerated or strangulated hernia is a tender mass at one of the hernial sites.

Fig. 36-6. Richter's hernia. Strangulation of antimesenteric portion of the bowel may lead to abscess without intestinal obstruction.

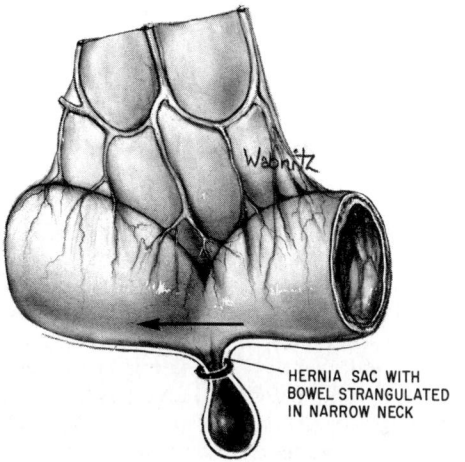

HERNIA SAC WITH
BOWEL STRANGULATED
IN NARROW NECK

A testicular torsion may be mistaken for an incarcerated inguinal hernia and an acute femoral lymphadenitis for an incarcerated femoral hernia.

COMPLICATIONS

The risk is that an intraperitoneal organ may become incarcerated or strangulated within the hernia sac. The small intestine is the organ most frequently affected, and acute incarceration or strangulation within a hernia sac remains one of the two most frequent causes for small bowel obstruction. This complication changes a simple situation into one which may prove fatal. A mass incarcerated in the inguinal hernia of a female infant is commonly an ovary, although incarceration of the appendix has been reported.

Occasionally only a portion of the antimesenteric wall of the intestine becomes strangulated within a hernia sac, producing a so-called Richter's hernia (Fig. 36-6). In this special situation there is not complete bowel obstruction, but the entrapped portion of bowel wall may become gangrenous. An abscess results if the strangulation is not recognized and treated early. An abscess of the medial thigh in an elderly female which, on incision and drainage, releases pus with a feculent odor suggests the presence of an obturator hernia with a partially strangulated bowel.

The development of complications in a hernia is not predictable. When complications do occur, an elective situation becomes an emergency, and a simple problem becomes more difficult. The rationale for elective herniorrhaphy is to prevent this situation.

TREATMENT

General

A hernia may be approached in three ways: expectantly, nonoperatively, or by surgical repair. Expectant treatment is based on the hope of spontaneous cure; in most situations this is not realistic. However, with the congenital umbilical hernia spontaneous cure does occur in most children before the age of four. This is a natural process which is not enhanced by the use of adhesive strapping. The physician should not advise operation until the patient reaches age four unless the hernia has incarcerated—a most unusual event in a hernia of this type—or unless it is a very large defect of the proboscis type. Expectant management of uncomplicated groin hernias is also reasonable in patients severely ill from some other cause. In most other circumstances an expectant attitude is not warranted.

The nonoperative treatment of a hernia involves the use of some external device or truss to maintain hernial reduction. These devices are a nuisance to the patient, and they are expensive to construct and to fit. In the groin they are almost universally unsuccessful in maintaining satisfactory reduction. A properly fitting corset may be an excellent remedy, however, for a ventral hernia, particularly when a large defect develops in an abdominal wound which became infected following initial laparotomy. Surgical repair of these defects is difficult, and a trial with external support is certainly justified before operation is recommended. With this exception external support has little to recommend it. The injection of sclerosing solutions into the tissues around a hernia, at one time a popular method of therapy, is mentioned only to be condemned.

Once the decision is made to perform an elective herniorrhaphy, it is a general rule that the operation should not be delayed. However, the presence of some other illness, such as an infection of the upper respiratory tract or a recent myocardial infarction, warrants delay. With premature infants it is wise to wait until the child is making satisfactory progress nutritionally so that the risk of anesthesia is decreased. With other infants many surgeons would prefer not to operate before the infant is ten weeks of age, since by this time the hemoglobin level is returning from its postnatal dip. Whenever operation is delayed for any reason, however, it should be realized that there is always the possibility of strangulation, which changes an elective situation into an emergency. Elderly patients with hernias are just as prone to strangulation as younger, more vigorous individuals, and old age per se should not be considered a contraindication to an elective herniorrhaphy.

When the patient has no systemic signs such as fever or leukocytosis, one preoperative effort to reduce an acutely incarcerated hernia is permissible. An ice bag should be applied to the local area and an appropriate dose of morphine given parenterally. With a groin hernia the patient should be placed in the Trendelenburg position as well. After 30 to 40 minutes, gentle sustained pressure over the mass may effect reduction without undue difficulty. The sensation that some gas has moved within the intestine frequently presages successful reduction. No more than one such effort should be attempted prior to emergency surgery—and the presence of systemic symptoms and signs contraindicates even this effort. Because of the small area below the inguinal ligament and medial to the femoral vein, reduction of an incarcerated femoral hernia is virtually impossible and should not be attempted. If these rules are followed, the reduction of a hernia en masse—that is, with the contained organ still strangulated—should not occur. The advantage of reducing an incarcerated hernia is that a repair 2 or 3 days later can be done at a time when edema has been reduced, thus permitting a better herniorrhaphy. Also, if other medical problems are present, the patient's general condition may be improved preoperatively, thus permitting a safer operative and postoperative course.

Operative Repair

PRINCIPLES. In any herniorrhaphy there are two essential steps to consider: (1) the management of the peritoneal sac and its contents, and (2) the repair of the fascial defect. If the sac is a narrow-necked diverticulum, it is usually excised and the neck closed. If it is a broadbased bulge, the peritoneum is usually not opened; rather, it is reduced intact beneath the fascia and held there by the fascial repair. Management of the sac is complicated when a sliding hernia is present or when intraperitoneal organs are fixed within the sac by adhesions. If the latter situation is suspected, it is vital to make certain that the situation is not in reality a sliding hernia. Once the surgeon is convinced that adhesions are holding an organ *within* the peritoneal sac, these adhesions must be carefully divided to effect reduction of the incarcerated contents. The sac itself is then managed in the usual fashion. The presence of a sliding hernia requires that the organ forming part of the wall of the sac be returned to the abdomen before the sac is excised. If this condition is anticipated and recognized, direct reduction of the sliding organ from the groin through the fascial defect is usually possible. The peritoneal sac is then excised without injury to the bowel or its blood supply. Rarely, an adjacent separate incision into the peritoneal cavity may be required to reduce the viscus from above, but the need for this has been overemphasized in the literature (Fig. 36-7).

Once the peritoneal sac has been satisfactorily managed, attention is turned to the associated fascial defect. When the patient is a youngster with a congenital indirect inguinal hernia, the opening in the transversalis fascia around the internal inguinal ring may not be dilated, and repair may not be required. In almost all other circumstances, however, closing or decreasing the size of this defect is vital. In certain circumstances the fascial margins of the defect can be approximated satisfactorily after adequate mobilization; this technique is applicable to most umbilical hernias, congenital or acquired, which require repair. In other instances an adjacent fascial relaxing incision makes possible a primary closure which would not otherwise be feasible. In some circumstances, especially when a large defect is present, repair will require the use of some substance introduced from elsewhere. An autogenous fascial graft, usually from the fascia lata, or an inert foreign body may be used for this purpose. A solid sheet of foreign material cannot be effectively organized by the body. Rather, it tends to become incorporated in a loose pocket or rejected altogether. Consequently, if an inert foreign material is selected, it should be in the form of a mesh which can be invaded and incorporated by the host's fibroblasts during the organization phase of wound healing. Screens of this type have been constructed of a metal such as tantalum or synthetic substances such as polypropylene (Marlex) or Dacron (Mersilene).

Following satisfactory repair of any hernia, it is traditional for the surgeon to advise against heavy lifting and other vigorous effort for 4 to 8 weeks. The rationale for this advice is to permit proper healing of the repaired tissue. Dunphy's studies indicate that collagen maturation and gain in tensile strength of the wound continue over many months, and this process is not complete within 4 weeks even under ideal circumstances. Studies by Lichtenstein and colleagues suggest that for at least the first 2 months strength of a repaired wound depends primarily

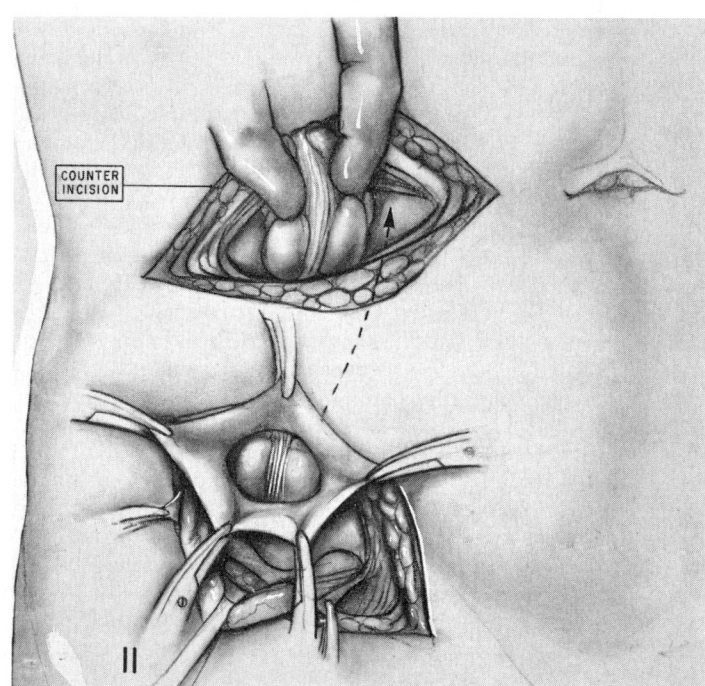

Fig. 36-7. Repair of sliding hernias. I. In simplest method, intestine, forming part of posterior wall of hernia sac, is directly reduced into abdomen, permitting closure of peritoneum and reconstruction of internal ring below it. II. Rarely, counterincision entering peritoneum above sac is needed to permit reduction of intestine by traction. III. *A,B,C.* Some surgeons free the sliding organ from the peritoneal sac (*A*). The posterior surface of the organ is then peritonealized (*B*), and the peritoneum is then closed at the internal ring (*C*). This procedure seems time-consuming and unnecessary.

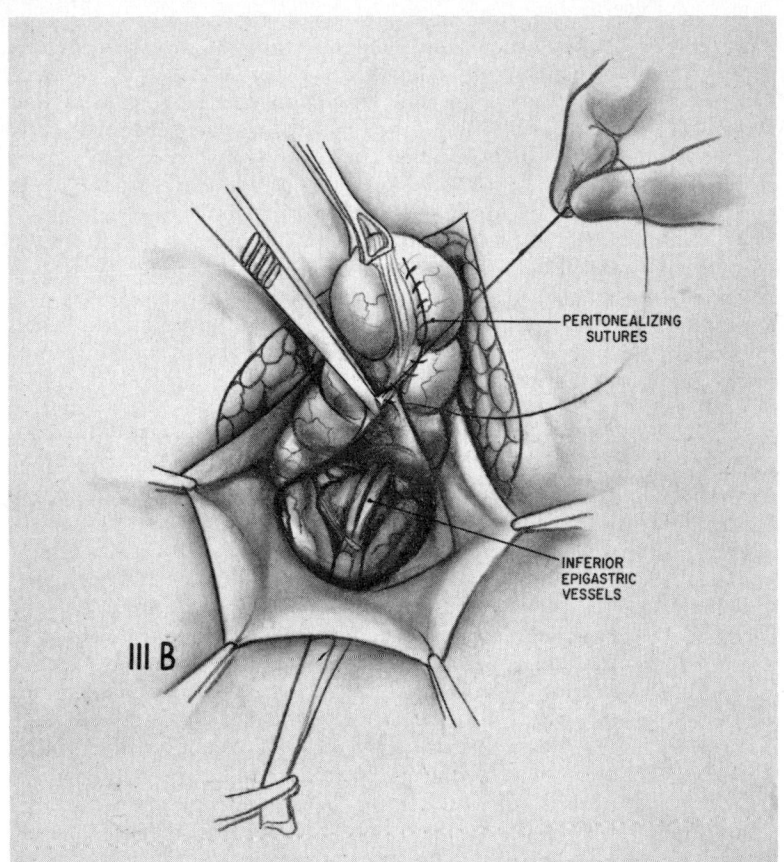

PERITONEALIZING
SUTURES

INFERIOR
EPIGASTRIC
VESSELS

III B

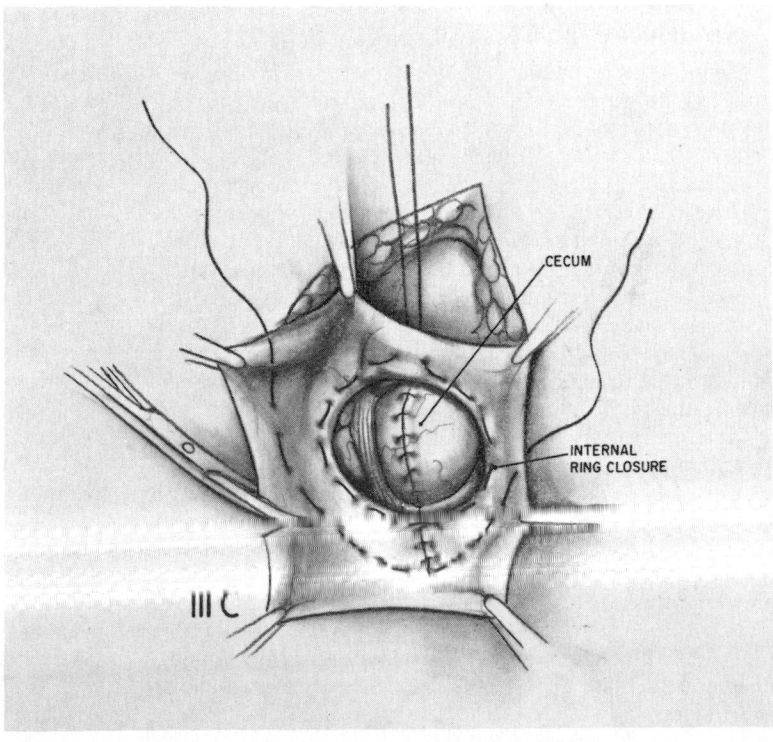

CECUM

INTERNAL
RING CLOSURE

III C

upon an intact suture line. In their experiments, the sutured wound showed 70 percent of intact tissue strength immediately, and there was no appreciable gain in strength during the next 8 weeks. The 4-week period of inactivity is perhaps a satisfactory compromise, postponing vigorous effort until some degree of healing has occurred, but it should be recognized that the basis for the recommendation is empiric rather than scientific.

STRANGULATED HERNIAS

When emergency operation is undertaken for a hernia with strangulated contents, it is vital that the operation be performed so that the contents of the sac can be inspected before reduction. To achieve this, it is necessary to open the sac early in the dissection and gain control of the structures within it. If operation has been done early enough, the prompt return of circulation to strangulated tissue indicates viability. Reduction is then effected and routine repair carried out. When gangrene has already developed, all gangrenous tissue must be resected. When strangulated intestine is present, this entails the construction of an anastomosis between normal bowel sections proximal and distal to the necrotic area. In some circumstances tissue viability is not so easily defined. Bowel of doubtful viability should be covered with a warm moist towel and reinspected after 5 minutes. Improved color of the bowel wall, passage of a peristaltic wave through the strangulated segment, or pulsation in the arcuate arteries usually indicate that the intestine will survive if returned to the peritoneal cavity. Intestine of questionable viability should be resected, since reduction of bowel which is not viable may lead either to early perforation with peritonitis or to late stricture. However, unnecessary intestinal resection increases morbidity and mortality.

GROIN HERNIAS

Many surgeons make the mistake of performing the same operation for all hernias in the groin. A proper evaluation of the anatomy in the area would make it evident that indirect, direct, and femoral hernias are different anatomic problems requiring different repairs.

Groin hernias can be successfully repaired with general, spinal, or local anesthesia. When local anesthesia is employed, the ilioinguinal and iliohypogastric nerves should be blocked just above and medial to the anterior superior iliac spine. The nerves lie deep to the external oblique aponeurosis at this level. In addition, subcutaneous infiltration of the incision site and deeper injection of the area around the pubic spine are required.

Certain authors suggest that the femoral hernia be repaired through a vertical incision over the femoral triangle. However, it is generally agreed that a better anatomic repair can be achieved through the groin. All groin hernias therefore should be approached through an incision above the inguinal ligament. Most frequently the incision is made above and parallel to the medial portion of the inguinal ligament; some surgeons extend this incision laterally almost to the iliac spine, but the lateral portion of the wound does not facilitate exposure and should be omitted. The subcutaneous tissue is incised and the external oblique

aponeurosis exposed. The external oblique is then opened through the external inguinal ring, the ilioinguinal nerve being carefully identified and preserved. The nerve is most frequently adherent at the external ring; hence the aponeurosis should be opened from above downward to prevent nerve injury. The nerve is readily identified as a grayish white structure with a small red blood vessel on its surface, running roughly parallel to the external oblique fibers. Moosman and Oelrich have found that the nerve lies inside the cremaster fibers in direct contact with spermatic cord structures in 35 percent of patients. By dividing those cremaster fibers which join the spermatic cord from the inguinal ligament, the cord is freed from the inguinal canal floor and a tape passed around it at the level of the pubic spine. This step facilitates lifting the cord away from Hesselbach's triangle. The major portion of the cremaster muscle is then divided all the way around the cord at the internal inguinal ring, and it becomes possible to identify the type of hernia and isolate the structures required for fascial repair.

INDIRECT HERNIA. When an indirect hernia is present, the sac will be visible as a translucent white structure lying inside the cremaster fibers and anteromedial to the cord structures at the level of the internal inguinal ring. The sac may be obscured by a lobulated mass of fatty tissue, often incorrectly referred to as a "lipoma of the cord." In reality it represents a projection of fat from the retroperitoneal area. Typically the fat extends through the dilated internal inguinal ring lateral and inferior to the cord structures. Rarely, this retroperitoneal fat may be present without an associated peritoneal sac. In either instance it should be removed as part of the indirect hernia repair. Once the sac is identified, it is separated from the spermatic cord by sharp or blunt dissection back to the internal ring. The vas deferens, which is usually adherent to the sac at the level of the internal ring, is the only cord structure which does not separate easily once the proper plane for dissection is entered. When the sac is adequately freed, it can be opened and any intraperitoneal contents reduced, with lysis of adhesions as necessary. If the hernia has a sliding component, it will form part or all of the posterior wall of the sac. This component should be manually replaced into the abdominal cavity before the hernia sac is excised.

A palpating finger can then be introduced into the peritoneal cavity through the open sac. The finger is brought up beneath the inguinal canal floor in Hesselbach's triangle to test the possibility of an associated direct hernia. Palpation beneath the inguinal ligament medial to the femoral vessels will disclose a femoral hernia if one is present. Directly behind this area the obturator membrane can be felt and an obturator hernia sought where the obturator artery and vein leave the true pelvis.

The sac can then be transected at the level of the internal inguinal ring. In doing this it is well to remember that the parietal peritoneum is quite elastic and that by traction a good deal of peritoneum from the abdominal wall can be pulled through the ring. Depending upon the size of the peritoneal defect, it is closed with either a purse-string suture or a series of interrupted sutures of some nonabsorbable suture material.

Except in infants, in whom this step may be omitted because the internal ring is not dilated, the transversus abdominis aponeurosis below the spermatic cord should be reapproximated with a series of interrupted sutures (Fig. 36-8). This repair should be continued until it is barely possible to insert a small clamp through the internal ring alongside the cord. The external oblique muscle, subcutaneous tissue, and skin are then united over the cord, which occupies its usual location, passing obliquely through the inguinal canal. It is unnecessary to transplant the neck of the hernial sac up beneath the abdominal muscles and unwise to move the cord into a subcutaneous location by closing the external oblique aponeurosis underneath it. If the medial inguinal canal floor is strong, this area should not be repaired. Indeed, Glassow suggests that in women direct recurrences may result from unnecessary dissection in Hesselbach's triangle during the initial operation. In closing the external oblique aponeurosis it is important to avoid passing a suture around the ilioinguinal nerve. Incorporating the nerve in a suture may lead to the development of a troublesome, painful neuroma.

When an indirect hernia has been neglected for a prolonged period, it may become very large, and the inferior epigastric vessels may be displaced medially all the way to the pubic spine. In effect such a hernia is direct as well as indirect, and the area in Hesselbach's triangle should be managed in the manner adopted for a direct hernia. For large or recurrent indirect hernias it may be possible to achieve a more secure repair by dividing the cord at the internal ring and closing the defect completely at that level. Orchiectomy is usually performed along with cord transection. However, if the scrotum is not disturbed during operation and is handled gently after surgery, the testicle may be left in place with little likelihood that gangrene will occur.

SLIDING HERNIA. The most important step in operative management of a sliding hernia is recognition of the situation. On the right side the cecum and on the left the sigmoid colon may make up part of the posterior wall of an indirect sac, and failure to recognize this may lead to fecal contamination or to injury to colonic blood supply. The urinary bladder may be similarly involved in a direct sac, but since this type of sac is reduced unopened, the presence of bladder does not create a technical problem. Because a sliding component is present in only about 3 percent of groin hernias, the surgeon tends to forget the possibility. However, certain circumstances increase the likelihood of a sliding component, and the surgeon should be wary when dealing with any large indirect hernia, especially one of long standing in an elderly male.

Most sliding hernias can be managed without undue difficulty. The peritoneal sac is identified and opened anteriorly away from the bowel which makes up its posterior wall. The entire anterior portion of the sac is removed. Posteriorly as much sac as possible is removed without injuring the sliding bowel or its mesentery. The bowel is then reduced manually into its original retroperitoneal position and the defect in peritoneum closed. The defect in the transversalis fascia at the internal inguinal ring is then closed in the same manner used for any indirect

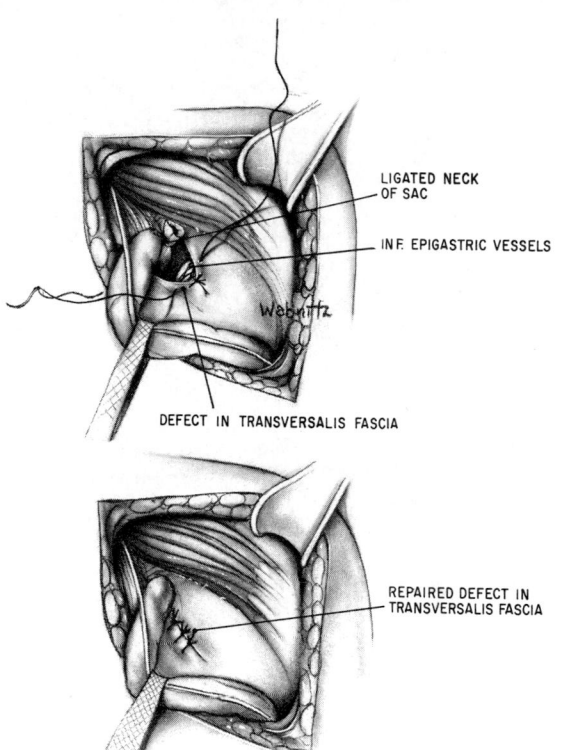

LIGATED NECK OF SAC

INF. EPIGASTRIC VESSELS

DEFECT IN TRANSVERSALIS FASCIA

REPAIRED DEFECT IN TRANSVERSALIS FASCIA

Fig. 36-8. Indirect inguinal hernia repair. High ligation of sac is followed by closure of defect in transversus abdominis aponeurosis at internal inguinal ring.

hernia, producing a snug internal ring. The herniorrhaphy is completed in whatever fashion is most appropriate to the remaining anatomic defect (Fig. 36-7I).

Rarely, when a large amount of colon is involved in the wall of the hernia, it may prove difficult to reduce the colon into its retroperitoneal position by manipulation from below. In these circumstances it is appropriate to enter the abdomen through a higher transverse incision so that the colon can be moved superiorly by traction from above, a procedure described by LaRoque. The abdomen may be entered through a fresh skin incision or by an extension of the groin incision, retracting the external oblique aponeurosis superiorly to facilitate the counterincision through the internal oblique, transversus abdominis, and peritoneum. In either event the colon is displaced from the internal ring by gentle traction and repair effected by excising the residual sac and carefully closing the internal ring (Fig. 36-7II).

Some surgeons consider it important to enter the abdomen in all cases and to dissect the herniated colon away from the peritoneal sac (Fig. 36-7IIIA). When the cecum is involved, these surgeons form a posterior peritoneal investment for this portion of the bowel by closing the margins of the peritoneal sac behind the cecum. In effect, this procedure makes an intraperitoneal organ out of one which previously lay retroperitoneally (Fig. 36-7IIIB). When the sliding hernia is on the left side involving the sigmoid, this procedure leaves a raw surface on the lateral aspect of the sigmoid mesocolon, and, again, closure of this

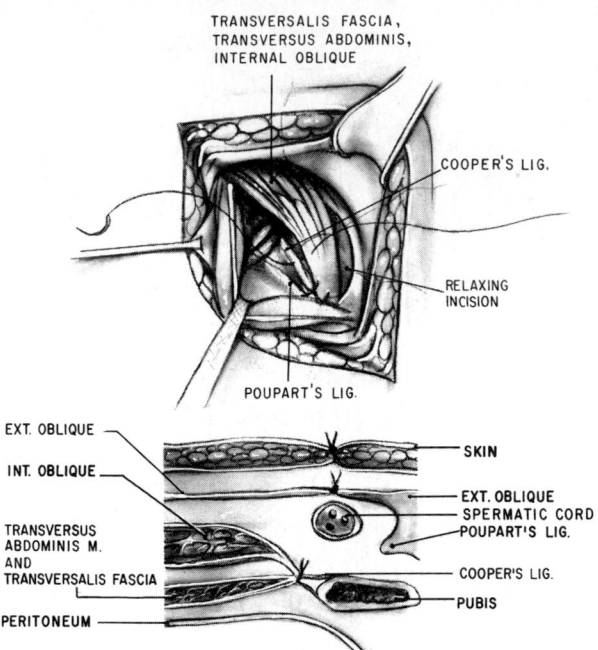

Fig. 36-9. Cooper's ligament repair. Cross section demonstrates level of repair; operative drawing shows placement of sutures in Cooper's ligament.

Fig. 36-10. Repair at level of inguinal ligament. Bassini operation remains standard against which other herniorrhaphies for direct inguinal hernia are judged; transversus abdominis aponeurosis as well as transversalis fascia should be incorporated in repair layer.

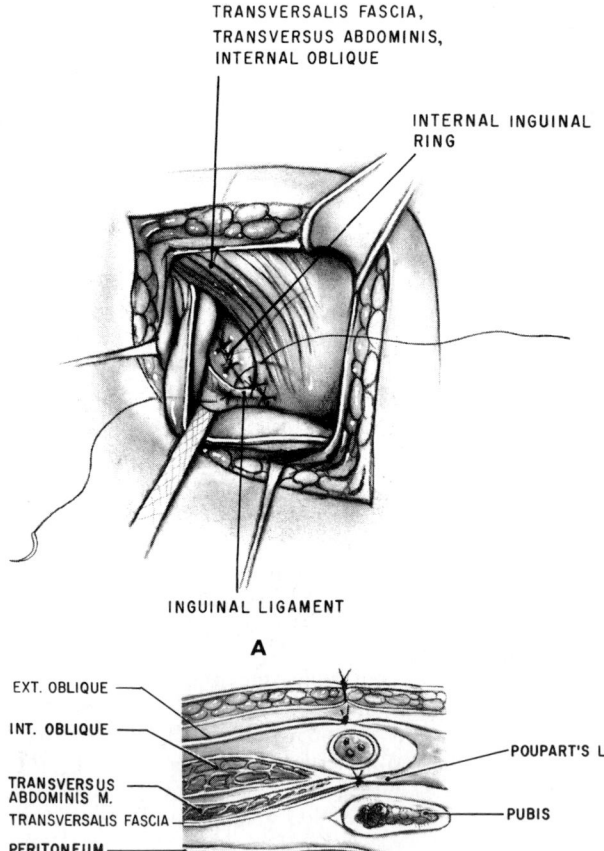

area is advised. In addition, surgeons who advocate an abdominal approach to sliding hernias sometimes fix this freed colon higher in the abdomen by some kind of colopexy. Both these procedures are designed to decrease the incidence of recurrence when this type of hernia is repaired. However, both procedures are cumbersome, the peritonealization of the posterior surface of the cecum is unsound anatomically, and the hernia should not recur in any case if the internal ring is properly closed (Fig. 36-7IIIC).

DIRECT HERNIA. When a direct hernia is present instead of or in addition to an indirect hernia, a different type of repair is required. Here the weakness lies in the inguinal canal floor medial to the inferior epigastric artery. In most instances there is a general ballooning out in the area, and the peritoneum should be reduced beneath the reconstituted inguinal canal floor without being opened. In the unusual instances where a narrow-necked diverticulum of peritoneum is present, it should be managed in the same way as an indirect sac.

To restore the inguinal canal floor requires removal of attenuated fascia and reconstruction with a new and stronger layer. In most instances this layer can be developed from the strong aponeurotic portion of the transversus abdominis muscle which is found just superior to the weakness in the inguinal canal floor. If a curved relaxing incision is made in the inner layer of the rectus sheath where the internal oblique and transversus abdominis form a fused aponeurosis, it is not difficult to bring the transversus abdominis aponeurosis down across Hesselbach's triangle. This layer can then be approximated to Cooper's ligament (Fig. 36-9), to the iliopubic tract, an aponeurotic band superficial to Cooper's ligament, or to the shelving edge of Poupart's ligament (Fig. 36-10), depending upon the preference of the surgeon. If Poupart's ligament is used for the repair, there are several levels at which the spermatic cord may be placed. The cord lies beneath the repaired inguinal canal floor as far as the external inguinal ring in the Ferguson repair (Fig. 36-11) and in the later technique described by Halsted. In the Bassini herniorrhaphy (Fig. 36-10B) the cord lies on top of the repaired canal floor. In the Andrews operation (Fig. 36-12) the superior leaf of the incised external oblique aponeurosis is sutured to Poupart's ligament beneath the cord to reinforce the repair of the inguinal canal floor, and the inferior leaf of the external oblique is then sutured up over the cord. In the original Halsted operation (Fig. 36-13) the external oblique aponeurosis is closed underneath the cord as far laterally as the internal ring, thus transplanting the cord into the subcutaneous tissue. Halsted himself later abandoned his technique, and most surgeons today employ some form of the Bassini operation. A properly done Bassini repair involves bringing transversus abdominis aponeurosis rather than muscle fibers from transversus abdominis and internal oblique down to Poupart's ligament. Bassini emphasized this point, although it has often been unwisely ignored by surgeons doing this type of repair. Bassini's technique—the first modern herniorrhaphy, originally described in 1887—has stood the test of time and remains today the standard against which the repair of direct inguinal hernias is judged.

McVay demonstrated that transversalis fascia normally attaches to Cooper's ligament, and theoretically transversalis fascia should be reapproximated to this ligament in direct hernia repairs. The procedure was first described by Lotheissen in 1898, and it is used in modified form by many surgeons today. However, this operation is technically more difficult than a repair to Poupart's ligament, and an adequate reconstruction based on Poupart's ligament will prevent recurrence of a direct hernia. Anatomically it is possible for a femoral hernia to develop below a Poupart's ligament repair, but if this actually occurs, it must be most unusual. If a Cooper's ligament repair is done, the surgeon is faced with a problem when he reaches the femoral vein, which passes in front of the ligament. From this point laterally the repair must be done at the more superficial Poupart's ligament level. Where the repair moves from Cooper's ligament to Poupart's ligament, there is a potential weakness, and recurrent herniation at this point is a distinct possibility. To prevent this weakness, McVay recommends suturing transversalis fascia to the medial side of the femoral sheath with one or two stitches as an intermediate step between the two levels of repair. The management of this area, and the greater danger of injury to the femoral vein with a Cooper's ligament repair, continue to be problems in the opinion of many surgeons. Hence the majority of surgeons continue to prefer repair at the level of the inguinal ligament, and many good results have been reported with this technique. Other surgeons feel that a Cooper's ligament repair for direct hernias is to be preferred whenever possible. A careful repair using strong tissue to cover the inguinal canal floor is probably more important than the level of the suture line. Glassow emphasized excision of all weak tissue from the inguinal canal floor and the construction of a multilayered, overlapping floor repair using continuous sutures of an inert material. He believed that recurrent hernias could develop between stitches if interrupted sutures were used for the herniorrhaphy.

Whichever level is selected for repair, it must be remembered that the hernia developed through a weakened transversalis fascia initially. Therefore, although McVay does nothing further to the canal floor, most surgeons agree that the newly constituted transversalis fascia repair should be reinforced in some manner. The technique suggested by Zimmerman and Anson, employing the inferior portion of the incised external oblique aponeurosis as a pedicle flap brought underneath the cord and sutured to transversalis fascia superior to the free edge of the internal oblique muscle, is probably the best anatomically. Another technique involves turning down a flap from the inner layer of the rectus sheath beneath the cord and uniting it to Poupart's ligament, thus reversing the procedure advocated by Zimmerman (Fig. 36-14). Still other surgeons prefer to place a free graft of autogenous fascia lata over the transversalis fascia repair. The graft is applied either as a single fascial sheet or as a mesh woven from fascial strips. In place of fascia lata, reinforcement can be done with a sheet of tantalum gauze or with a synthetic mesh sutured over the repaired Hesselbach's triangle beneath the cord. Because tantalum may break, leaving sharp metallic

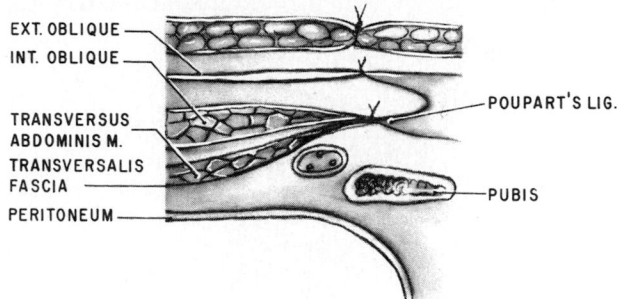

Fig. 36-11. Ferguson operation. Spermatic cord is placed deep to reconstructed inguinal canal floor.

ends to traumatize neighboring structures, a synthetic material is preferred. Once the inguinal canal floor is adequately repaired, the cord is replaced in the canal. External oblique aponeurosis, subcutaneous tissue, and skin are closed over it exactly as in the repair for indirect hernia.

FEMORAL HERNIA. The femoral hernia protrudes from the groin underneath the inguinal ligament between the

Fig. 36-12. Andrews operation. This involves suturing superior leaf of external oblique aponeurosis to shelving edge of Poupart's ligament beneath spermatic cord, with inferior leaf of external oblique sutured up over it.

lacunar ligament medially and the femoral vein laterally. If transversalis fascia is strongly attached to Cooper's ligament, as is normally the case, this creates a curtain which effectively prevents the peritoneum or any intraperitoneal structure from reaching the femoral ring. Thus the femoral hernia is a groin hernia and should be treated as such, with an incision above the inguinal ligament. When the inguinal

Fig. 36-13. Halsted's original repair. Spermatic cord is transplanted subcutaneously and inguinal canal closed beneath it. Halsted later abandoned this operation, and it is little used today.

EXT. OBLIQUE APONEUROSIS

INCISION INTO INNER LAYER OF RECTUS SHEATH

RECTUS ABDOMINIS M.

FLAP OF RECTUS SHEATH SUTURED TO INGUINAL LIG.

Fig. 36-14. Reinforcement of canal floor repair using flap of rectus sheath. Some technique for reinforcement of Hesselbach's triangle should be part of any repair done for direct hernia.

canal is opened and the spermatic cord or the round ligament retracted, a bulge will be evident beneath the transversalis fascia near the pubic spine. When the transversalis fascia is incised, the peritoneal neck of the hernia sac will be visible, and the surgeon thus has control of the sac and its contents. This is important especially when there may be strangulation of bowel in the sac, for the hernia should not be permitted to reduce before the viability of its contents has been ascertained. Attention may then be turned safely to the femoral triangle, where the peritoneal sac is dissected free from the subcutaneous tissues. Once the sac is freed, it is frequently possible to reduce it beneath the inguinal ligament by traction from above. Since the neck of the sac is quite narrow, however, this reduction may not be possible without dividing the inguinal ligament transversely at the level of the hernia, thus releasing the sac. The continuity of the inguinal ligament is of little consequence, and it need not be restored.

After inspecting the contents of the sac and returning them to the peritoneal cavity, the sac itself is removed and its neck closed with a nonabsorbable purse-string suture. Anatomically, the best method of preventing recurrent herniation is to bring transversalis fascia down to Cooper's ligament exactly as described for the direct hernia. With the femoral hernia, repair must be at the level of Cooper's ligament rather than of the inguinal ligament, since herniation into the femoral triangle may recur beneath an inguinal ligament repair. Further reinforcement of the inguinal canal floor is then carried out, using the same approach described for the direct hernia.

Two other general methods for preventing recurrence

of a femoral hernia have been advocated. In the first of these, the Moschcowitz technique, the femoral ring is obliterated by suturing Poupart's ligament to Cooper's ligament. In the second a pedicle of aponeurosis from the inferior margin of the external oblique incision is sutured down to Cooper's ligament. Both these methods effectively obliterate the femoral ring, but they do not strengthen the inguinal canal floor, so that development of a direct hernia through the weakened floor remains possible. Strengthening the inguinal canal floor through a femoral triangle incision is difficult or impossible; hence the incision above the inguinal ligament is preferred.

BILATERAL HERNIAS. It is possible to operate on bilateral groin hernias through two separate groin incisions as described above. Most surgeons feel that in adults it is better to stage these operations, rather than doing both simultaneously. The recurrence rate when bilateral repairs are done simultaneously in adults seems unacceptably high. If both groins are to be repaired at one time, it is more expeditious to use a Cheatle-Henry incision. In this approach a vertical lower-midline incision is made and carried down to the peritoneum, which is then reflected away from the lower abdominal wall. By traction upward on the abdominal wall it is possible to dissect down to the inguinal triangle easily, and good exposure of Cooper's ligament is readily obtained. Transversalis fascia from the inner surface of the transversus abdominis can then be sutured down to Cooper's ligament under excellent direct vision to provide a satisfactory repair for either a direct or a femoral hernia. Reinforcement of the inguinal canal floor repair is not readily possible through this approach, and this represents a distinct disadvantage to its routine use. It is also somewhat more inconvenient, although not impossible, to deal with an indirect hernia. The major advantage of this approach is that bilateral hernias can be repaired much more rapidly. With a patient who is a poor anesthetic risk the resultant saving of time may be an important factor.

When an infant presents with a unilateral indirect inguinal hernia, there is perhaps 1 chance in 5 that a second undetected hernia is present on the opposite side. In the view of certain surgeons, this is sufficient reason for exploring the opposite side in all infants. Since right-sided hernias are somewhat more common than those on the left, this argument is advanced most strongly when a left-sided hernia is detected preoperatively. Since exploring the second side is a simple undertaking once the patient is under anesthesia, the argument seems superficially attractive. However, to carry out four negative explorations in the hope of finding one undetected hernia seems on reflection an unjustified meddling with normal tissues. Rather, a careful examination of both groins should precede any elective herniorrhaphy, and the second side should be explored only if there is reasonable suspicion of a defect on physical examination. It has been suggested recently that infant groin hernias may be identified preoperatively by injection of a radiopaque dye into the abdominal cavity followed by the exposure of an upright abdominal roentgenogram. If this technique proves safe and reliable, it will offer a reasonable solution to this debate.

UMBILICAL HERNIAS

When it has been decided that an umbilical hernia warrants surgical repair, a curved incision is made below the umbilicus and carried through subcutaneous fat to expose the anterior rectus sheath (Fig. 36-15). By dissecting toward the inferior margin of the defect, the surgeon delineates the peritoneal sac projecting through the fascial opening. Continued dissection at this level around the umbilicus defines the fascial defect and isolates the sac. The sac is then freed from the undersurface of the umbilical skin, and excess peritoneum is removed. Following closure of the peritoneum, the fascia above and below the defect is united by a series of nonabsorbable sutures. This repair is traditionally done by bringing the fascia above the defect down over the fascia from below to effect a two-layer closure—the so-called "vest over pants" type of repair (Fig. 36-16). These two fascial layers fuse, but there is no convincing proof that the resulting repair is any stronger than that produced by a careful approximation of fascial margins without undue tension. The umbilicus is then tacked down to the fascial repair and the skin incision closed. When a large hernia has been repaired in an obese adult, it is desirable to drain the resulting dead space to prevent formation of a seroma in the incision; otherwise drainage is not employed. Formerly it was customary to excise the umbilicus during umbilical herniorrhaphy. This is unnecessary except when a proboscis-type defect is present, and the loss of the umbilicus is psychologically disturbing to many children and even to some adults. When, for technical reasons, removal of the umbilicus is desirable, the patient should be clearly informed of this preoperatively.

VENTRAL HERNIAS

The hernia which develops in an old operative incision may present a vexing problem in repair; many hernias of this type can be successfully managed by a good external support. When operative repair is undertaken, the defect should be closed with local tissue if possible. The old operative scar can be excised or a fresh incision made perpendicular to it (Fig. 36-17A). In either event the first aim of the surgeon should be to dissect down to normal fascia all around the herniation. Dissection is then continued to separate the peritoneal sac from the margins of the fascial defect (Fig. 36-17B). The peritoneum is opened, the contents of the sac are appropriately managed, and excess peritoneum is removed. After closure of the incision into the peritoneum, the fascia is approximated to obliterate the hernia. If the initial defect was a small one, it may be possible to close it without undue tension by the use of interrupted sutures of some nonabsorbable material. With a larger defect, two relaxing incisions, one to either side of the original hernia, may make closure practical. This technique is particularly useful in the situation where the incisional hernia developed in a vertical midline or paramedian incision. The relaxing incisions are then made in the anterior rectus sheath, and midline approximation does not result in herniation laterally where the relaxing incisions were done (Fig. 36-17C). There is usually weak

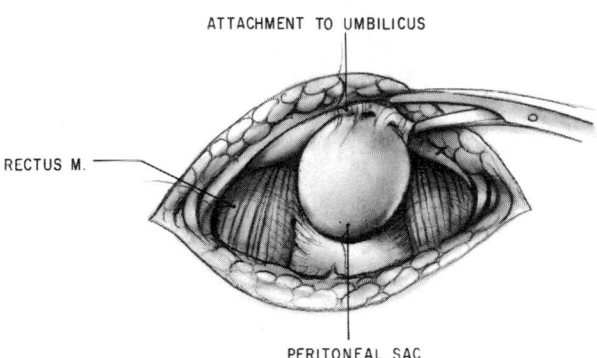

Fig. 36-15. Umbilical hernia repair. Curvilinear incision below the umbilicus gives excellent exposure. Sac must be freed by sharp dissection from undersurface of umbilicus.

attenuated fascia surrounding the actual defect, and failure to extend the repair through this area is one of the common technical errors which frequently results in recurrence. When no local tissue can be found for this type of repair, an artificial substitute of metallic or synthetic mesh may be employed. Although Koontz has reported very good results

Fig. 36-16. Umbilical hernia repair. "Vest over pants" type of imbrication is traditionally used, but single layer, well opposed without imbrication, is equally effective.

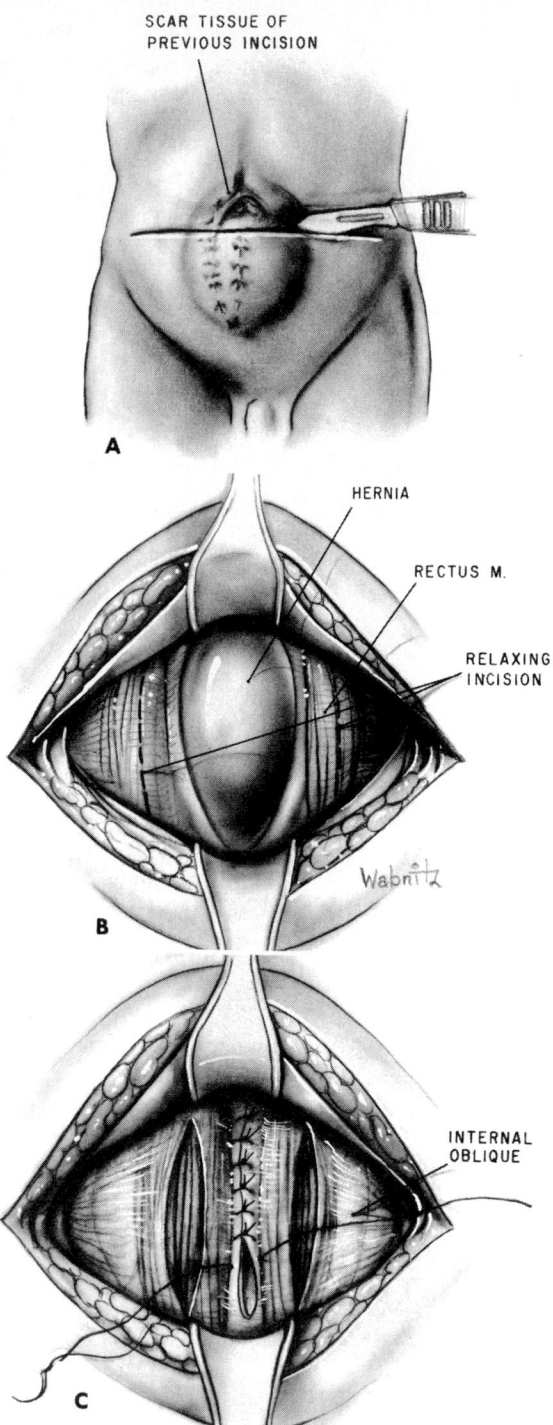

SCAR TISSUE OF
PREVIOUS INCISION

A

HERNIA

RECTUS M.

RELAXING
INCISION

Wabnitz

B

INTERNAL
OBLIQUE

C

Fig. 36-17. Ventral hernia repair. *A.* It is frequently desirable to make fresh incision perpendicular to old hernia scar. *B.* Closure of fascial defect may be facilitated by making relaxing incision in rectus sheath to either side of hernia sac. *C.* Relaxing incisions permit good fascial approximation over defect without producing significant weakness in areas of relaxation.

from the use of tantalum for this purpose, most surgeons have not been happy with the use of any foreign material for these repairs.

RESULTS

Uncomplicated herniorrhaphies have a negligible operative mortality, and results must be evaluated in terms of recurrence rate. Acutely incarcerated or strangulated hernias remain even today significant causes for morbidity and mortality.

The literature gives no basis for dogmatic statements about the results of herniorrhaphy. Most hernias can be satisfactorily treated, but a small number of recurrences can be expected. If patients undergoing herniorrhaphy are followed carefully for a long enough period of time, the number of known recurrences will, of course, increase.

As a general rule, hernias treated early yield better results, and recurrence following repair of an indirect inguinal hernia in an infant is quite unusual. Indirect hernias at any age have a lower recurrence rate than direct or femoral hernias. A rather high recurrence rate is to be anticipated following repair of postoperative ventral hernias, because they usually develop following some wound complication such as infection or dehiscence, with consequent weakness of the tissues available for repair.

It is axiomatic that the first repair has the greatest chance of success and that recurrence is frequent following any secondary repair of a recurrent hernia. Glassow, reporting extensive experience at Shouldice Hospital in Toronto, indicates that the recurrence rate for primary inguinal or femoral hernias in women should be less than 1 percent. On the other hand, their rate for recurrent femoral hernias after secondary surgery in women was 6.5 percent. Since the most frequent cause for recurrence would appear to be improper technique during the original operation, the importance of a proper initial approach is obvious. All too frequently a hernia is treated by a junior member of the staff without adequate supervision. No surgeon should undertake herniorrhaphy until he is thoroughly conversant with the anatomy of the area and the theory behind the technique of repair.

Although McVay has reported recurrence rates as low as 0.6 percent for groin hernias, nationwide results do not approximate this degree of success. Zimmerman and Anson report from the literature recurrence rates varying between 2 and 30 percent for indirect hernias and between 4 and 33 percent for direct hernias. The recurrence rate for femoral hernias is harder to evaluate, but it probably approximates that for direct hernias. Certainly these results permit no ground for complacency. They emphasize the need for continued careful technique, with attention to detail and a proper evaluation of the type of repair appropriate for the hernia in question.

SUMMARY

Hernias are among the most common afflictions of mankind. Although the operative results are not perfect, repair of an uncomplicated hernia prevents the possibility of intestinal obstruction or gangrene secondary to hernial incarceration. Both these complications remain potentially lethal and entail a prolonged convalescence at best. Therefore it is a general rule that—save for the congenital umbilical hernias, which are likely to close spontaneously, and certain postoperative incisional hernias—all hernias of the abdominal wall should be subjected to prompt surgical correction. When it is elected for medical reasons not to repair other abdominal hernias, it must be remembered that, with a poor-risk patient, the danger of emergency surgery for strangulation is greatly increased. If good results are to be anticipated from operation, the surgeon must have a thorough knowledge of the involved anatomy and a respect for tissues. A repair which is appropriate to the type of defect present must be selected, and the patients must be followed carefully so that the surgeon can profit from his or her mistakes.

References

Carlson, R. I.: The Historical Development of the Surgical Treatment of Inguinal Hernia, *Surgery,* **39:**1031, 1956.

Condon, R. E.: Surgical Anatomy of the Transversus Abdominis and Transversalis Fascia, *Ann Surg,* **173:**1, 1971.

———— and Nyhus, L. M.: Complications of Groin Hernia and of Hernial Repair, *Surg Clin North Am,* **51:**1325, 1971.

Dunphy, J. E.: Wound Healing, in C. Rob and R. Smith (eds.), "Clinical Surgery," vol. 1, pp. 219–232, Butterworth & Co. (Publishers), Ltd., London, 1964.

Glassow, R.: The Surgical Repair of Inguinal and Femoral Hernias, *Can Med Assoc J,* **108:**308, 1973.

Halverson, K., and McVay, C. B.: Inguinal and Femoral Hernioplasty: 22-Year Study of Authors' Methods, *Arch Surg,* **101:**127, 1970.

Heifetz, C. J.: Age and the Testis after Resection of the Spermatic Cord in the Repair of Inguinal Hernia, *Am J Surg,* **121:**634, 1971.

Koontz, A. R.: "Hernia," Appleton-Century-Crofts, Inc., New York, 1963.

Lichtenstein, I. L., Herzikoff, S., Shore, J. M., Jiron, M. W., Stuart, S., and Mizuno, L.: The Dynamics of Wound Healing, *Surg Gynecol Obstet,* **130:**685, 1970.

Margoles, J. S., and Braun, R. A.: Properitoneal versus Classical Hernioplasty, *Am J Surg,* **121:**641, 1971.

Mizrachy, B., and Kark, A. E.: The Anatomy and Repair of the Posterior Inguinal Wall, *Surg Gynecol Obstet,* **137:**253, 1973.

Moosman, D. A., and Oelrich, T. M.: Prevention of Accidental Trauma to the Ilioinguinal Nerve during Inguinal Herniorrhaphy, *Am J Surg,* **133:**146, 1977.

Ravitch, M. M., and Hitzrot, J. M., II: The Operations for Inguinal Hernia, *Surgery,* **48:**439, 1960.

Rowe, M. I., and Clatworthy, H. W., Jr.: The Other Side of the Pediatric Inguinal Hernia, *Surg Clin North Am,* **51:**1371, 1971.

Shackelford, G. D., and McAlister, W. H.: Inguinal Herniography, *Am J Roentgenol Radium Ther Nucl Med,* **115:**399, 1972.

Thompson, W., Longerbeam, J. K., and Reeves, C.: Herniograms, an Aid to the Diagnosis and Treatment of Groin Hernias in Infants and Children, *Arch Surg,* **105:**71, 1972.

Wagh, P. V., Leverich, A. P., Sun, C. N., White, H. J., and Read, R. C.: Direct Inguinal Herniation in Men: A Disease of Collagen, *J Surg Res,* **17:**425, 1974.

Zimmerman, I. M., and Anson, B. J.: "The Anatomy and Surgery of Hernia," The Williams & Wilkins Company, Baltimore, 1953.

Chapter 37

Pituitary and Adrenal

by **Richard M. Bergland and Timothy S. Harrison**

PITUITARY

(by Richard M. Bergland)

Historical Background

Harvey Cushing, near the end of his career, wrote:

I was once told by Professor Kocher, who I suppose had his experiences with the thyroid in mind, that no satisfactions in medicine were so great as those which came from concentration upon and the mastery of a small subject, and that this necessitated an approach from all aspects; diagnostic, experimental, pathological, and therapeutic, not the least important part of which at one time or another in the history of the subject was likely to be surgical.

Cushing must have heeded Kocher's advice and could surely have been satisfied with his lifelong productive involvement with the pituitary gland. He was the first to describe the syndrome of chiasmal compression, the first to demonstrate the usefulness of radiographs in the diagnosis of pituitary tumors, the first to emphasize that the pituitary holds the dominant position in the endocrine orchestra, the first to describe the hyposecretion associated with chromophobe tumors and the hypersecretion of both eosinophilic and basophilic tumors, and the first surgeon to operate successfully on a large series of patients with pituitary problems.

Remarkably, Harvey Cushing proposed in 1910 that pituitary secretions were released into the ventricle. This proposal has not been generally accepted, but Cushing maintained this belief throughout his career and in 1930 studied the physiological effects of pituitrin injected into the ventricles of humans. The discovery of the tanycyte ependyma, coupled to the reassessment of the vascular anatomy of the pituitary, lends credibility to Cushing's hypothesis. If pituitary secretions are indeed secreted directly to the brain, most of what we now know about the pituitary, and about the brain, will require rethinking.

Cushing's contributions to the understanding of the pituitary are of eternal significance; no other surgeon has made such a profound and lasting impact on any other organ system. The biography of this remarkable man should be read by every student of surgery; predictably some students reading this chapter will enter surgical research and carry on the rewarding tradition passed from Kocher to Cushing.

Gross Anatomy

The pituitary and its parts are schematically illustrated in Fig. 37-1. Unfortunately, pituitary nomenclature is not well standardized, but that of Wislocki is recommended. In his terminology, the *neurohypophysis* is composed of three parts: the infundibulum (which is often termed the median eminence), the infundibular stem (which is often termed the pituitary stalk), and the infundibular process (which is variably designated posterior lobe, posterior pituitary, or pars nervosa).

Wislocki separated the *adenohypophysis* into the pars distalis (often called the anterior lobe or anterior pituitary), the pars intermedia, and the pars tuberalis.

In clinical medicine the terms "median eminence," "pituitary stalk," "anterior pituitary," and "posterior pituitary" have gained general acceptance. But in basic research in other species, Wislocki's terminology is employed more often; an understanding of terms is essential if one is to apply laboratory observations to the understanding of clinical problems.

Fig. 37-1. A schematic illustration of the parts of the human pituitary, as well as the projection of parvicellular and magnocellular neurons into the neurohypophysis.

Fig. 37-2. A midline sagittal section of the human pituitary in situ within the sella. The height of the pituitary does not match the depth of the sella.

HUMAN ANATOMICAL VARIATIONS. The adult human pituitary does not have a distinct pars intermedia (Fig. 37-2); the basophils that invade the human posterior pituitary might be considered the functional counterpart of the pars intermedia found in other species.

The pars tuberalis varies in human beings; sometimes the entire pituitary stalk is surrounded by secreting adenohypophyseal cells, but in other instances, the surface of the stalk is totally devoid of adenohypophyseal cells.

In 50 percent of human beings, the sella turcica is covered by the dura of the diaphragma sella, and the intrasellar space is thus separated from the intracranial space. In 40 percent of human beings the opening in the diaphragma that surrounds the pituitary stalk is greater than 5 mm (Fig. 37-3), and in 10 percent of human beings the diaphragma is extremely thin. Without the sturdy barrier of the diaphragma sella, a pituitary tumor may preferentially extend into the suprasellar region; with a sturdy, complete diaphragma, a growing tumor will preferentially enlarge and balloon the sella.

The height of the human pituitary does not match the depth of the sella (Fig. 37-2), and the width of the pituitary does not match the width of the sellar floor (Fig. 37-4); thus plain x-rays permit assessment of the length of the pituitary but not of its height or its width.

Not infrequently the lateral margins of the pituitary are indented by the carotid arteries, and during stereotaxic pituitary procedures the carotids may be damaged. For this reason, some surgeons advocate carotid angiography before any stereotaxic procedure.

VASCULAR ANATOMY. The neurohypophysis is one of the five areas of brain that does not have a blood brain barrier. Its capillaries have a fenestrated endothelium (brain capillaries have no fenestrations) and are surrounded by a double basement membrane (brain capillaries have a single basement membrane). A distinct plane can be drawn between the neurohypophysis and the hypothalamus by the characteristics of the capillaries of each. No neuronal cell bodies are found within the neurohypophysis; all the axons projecting to the neurohypophysis are derived from hypothalamic neurons.

All the elements of the neurohypophysis (the median eminence, stalk, and posterior pituitary) are joined by a common capillary bed, and the direction of blood flow within that capillary bed is variable. The adenohypophysis does not receive a direct arterial supply; all blood reaching it must pass first through the capillary bed of the neurohypophysis.

Adenohypophyseal capillaries resemble those of the neurohypophysis. No nerves terminate within the adenohypophysis, but neurosecretory material is conveyed by pituitary portal vessels from the neurohypophysis to the adenohypophysis. Recently it has been established that some portal vessels carry adenohypophyseal secretions back to the neurohypophysis (Figs. 37-5 and 37-6).

Fig. 37-3. The chiasm has been removed to expose the diaphragma sella. The opening in the diaphragm is about 7 mm in diameter (black arrow), much greater than the penetrating pituitary stalk (white arrow). In 40 percent of human beings, this opening is greater than 5 mm.

Fig. 37-4. A dissection of the human pituitary resting in situ on the floor of the sella. The width of the pituitary is greater than the width of the sella.

In other species the secreting cells within the pars inter-media have a limited capillary bed but are well innervated; in the human being those basophils that invade the posterior pituitary are also directly innervated.

The distortion of the normal vascular relationships of the pituitary by tumor growth may play an important role in the endocrine disturbances that develop with pituitary tumors, but the current techniques of angiography do not allow the visualization of pituitary vascular anatomy.

Cellular Physiology

THE NEUROHYPOPHYSIS

Hypothalamic neurons with large cell bodies (the *magnocellular neurons* of the supraoptic and paraventricular nuclei) project to the neurohypophysis, and most of them terminate near capillaries within the posterior pituitary (Fig. 37-1). The dense-core neurosecretory granules in these neurons measure about 2,000 Å in diameter and are

Fig. 37-5. A vascular cast of the monkey pituitary. Very few connections are found between the capillary bed of the adeno-hypophysis (*A*) and the cavernous sinus (*CS*). This suggests that some blood must exit from the adenohypophysis via other routes.

Fig. 37-6. The vascular relationships of the primate pituitary; arrows indicate the potential directions of blood flow. (1) In some portal vessels, flow may be *into* or *out of* the adenohypophysis. (2) Flow reversal may occur within the neurohypophysis. (3) Flow may occur from the posterior pituitary directly to the cavernous sinus. (4) Recent evidence suggests that flow reversal may occur in certain hypophyseal arteries. (5) Tanycytes may carry pituitary secretions into the ventricle. (6) Capillaries may carry hypophyseal blood directly to the hypothalamus. (7) Fenestrations within endothelial cells of the pituitary portal vessels may allow hormones access to the subarachnoid cerebrospinal fluid.

composed of octapeptides coupled to the carrier protein neurophysin. At the nerve terminals the octapeptides are uncoupled from neurophysin and released into the capillary bed of the neurohypophysis. Two kinds of octapeptides are present: vasopressin and oxytocin. Vasopressin has many systemic actions, but most interest has focused on its antidiuretic effect. Oxytocin has few established physiological effects in the human male, but a profound effect on the pregnant uterus. Like the octapeptides, the carrier protein neurophysin is released into the neurohypophyseal capillary bed, but its physiological role is uncertain.

Hypothalamic neurons with small cell bodies (the *parvicellular neurons* of the arcuate and other hypothalamic nuclei) project to the neurohypophysis, and most of them terminate near capillaries within the median eminence (Fig. 37-1). The dense-core neurosecretory granules in these neurons are smaller (about 800 to 1,000 Å in diameter) and are composed of releasing and inhibiting factors that are destined for the adenohypophysis. No carrier protein similar to neurophysin has been found for the releasing and inhibiting hormones. Many pituitary releasing and inhibiting substances have been isolated from hypothalamic extracts, and their chemical structure has been determined; three have been synthesized (TRH, somatostatin, and GNRH). By tradition, hypothalamic releasing and inhibiting substances have been called "factors" (such as prolactin-inhibiting factor, or PIF) until their chemical structure is identified; then they are termed "hormones" (such as thyrotropin-releasing hormone, or TRH).

Many other substances are found in the neurohypophysis. These include epinephrine, norepinephrine, dopamine, histamine, angiotensin, neurotensin, and substance P. Why these substances are released and/or stored in the neurohypophysis is uncertain; of the group, only dopamine has an established role in adenohypophyseal function.

THE ADENOHYPOPHYSIS

It is appropriate to recall that the chromophobe/eosinophil/basophil cellular classification was introduced in 1892, preceding the birth of endocrinology. There was no need at that time to link the histological appearance of pituitary cells to their secretory function, but as the several secretory functions of the adenohypophysis were established, an effort was made to link cell structure to cell function. For many decades, both histochemistry and electron microscopy were employed in an effort to determine which cells secreted which hormones. These techniques were not very successful and produced a nomenclature of such complexity that clinicians had little choice but to employ the chromophobe/basophil/eosinophil system of classification.

The development of immunohistochemistry brought order to the study of pituitary histology, and for the first time, pituitary cells could be described according to their secretory function (Fig. 37-7). Remarkably, this technique has established that some pituitary cells secrete more than one hormone. The use of the functional classification of pituitary cell types allows the simultaneous consideration of the biochemistry and physiology of each different trophic hormone.

GROWTH HORMONE CELLS (SOMATOTROPES). Growth hormone–secreting cells are found in the lateral aspect of the adenohypophysis; these cells appear eosinophilic with traditional stains. Growth hormone (GH) is a large peptide (190 amino acids) that effects the growth of bone, muscle, and visceral organs; it also elevates blood glucose level. GH is species-specific; human GH has not been synthesized and currently can be obtained only by extraction from human pituitaries recovered at autopsy.

Between 5 and 10 percent of the weight of the adenohypophysis is accounted for by GH; the pituitary glands of children and adults have a similar GH content. The resting level of serum GH is 1 to 5 ng/ml, but secretory surges occur six to eight times daily; the largest surge occurs during sleep in the early morning hours. During adolescence the total amount of GH secreted per 24 hours increases, largely because the secretory surges occur more frequently.

Secretions from the parvicellular hypothalamic neurons influence GH secretion; growth hormone–releasing factor (GRF) stimulates secretion, and growth hormone–inhibiting factor (somatostatin) limits secretion. GRF has been isolated from hypothalamic extracts, but its chemical structure has not been determined. Somatostatin, found during the search for GRF, has been isolated, chemically identified as a tetradecapeptide, and synthesized. Somatostatin has other biological effects, including the inhibition of glucagon release from the pancreatic islet cells and the inhibition of gastrin secretion from the stomach; somatostatin is produced in the pancreas and the intestine as well as within the hypothalamus.

Fig. 37-7. A schematic illustration of the Nakane horseradish peroxidase immunohistochemical staining technique. Antibodies to specific trophic hormones are produced in vivo, harvested, and conjugated with horseradish peroxidase. Serial sections of the pituitary are obtained, washed with the various antibody-horseradish peroxidase conjugates, and reacted with lead. The lead precipitate (brownish-black) is visible over the cell containing the appropriate antigen. The technique allows a functional designation of pituitary cells, i.e., somatotrophic cell, thyrotrophic cell, etc. Note that follicle-stimulating hormone (FSH) and luteinizing hormone (LH) are formed in a common "gonadotroph." This technique may be employed with the light microscope or the electron microscope. *GH,* growth hormone; *TSH,* thyroid-stimulating hormone; *ACTH,* adrenocorticotrophic hormone.

Exercise, stress, or hypoglycemia physiologically stimulate GH secretion. Insulin, arginine, epinephrine, L-dopa, and apomorphine can be infused pharmacologically to effect GH release.

PROLACTIN CELLS (MAMMOTROPES). Prolactin-secreting cells also are found in the lateral aspect of the adenohypophysis and also are eosinophils by traditional histochemical staining. Prolactin is a large peptide structurally similar in many ways to GH. In humans, prolactin promotes lactation, but in lower species the hormone has many different and profound effects on behavior. Synthetic prolactin is not available for therapeutic use.

The normal daytime levels of prolactin are 15 to 25 ng/ml; during sleep, prolactin levels increase two- or threefold by episodic surges of secretion. Men have circulating levels that equal those of nonpregnant women.

Hypothalamic control of prolactin secretion is achieved by the transport of prolactin-inhibiting factor (PIF) and prolactin-releasing factor (PRF) to the adenohypophysis. The net effect of the hypothalamic influence on prolactin secretion is inhibition. The chemical nature of PIF is not firmly established; some evidence suggests that dopamine may be PIF: for instance, L-dopa, the precursor of dopamine, limits prolactin secretion. No distinct prolactin-releasing factor (PRF) has been found, yet both TRH and somatostatin (along with their other established functions) increase prolactin levels, and either or both of them may serve as PRF.

Pregnancy, lactation, stress, and exercise are associated with high levels of prolactin; stimulation of the breast in both males and females activates reflex secretion of prolactin. Reserpine, synthetic TRH, and oral contraceptives all increase prolactin levels.

Prolactin levels are diminished by water loading and by the administration of L-dopa, apomorphine, and bromergocryptine.

THYROID-STIMULATING HORMONE CELL (THYROTROPE). The cells which make thyroid-stimulating hormone (TSH) are located in the central portion of the adenohypophysis and would be termed *basophils* by an older classification. TSH is a glycoprotein that increases thyroid growth and the synthesis of thyroid hormones.

Episodic secretory surges maintain a normal serum daytime level of TSH between 1 and 10 ng/ml; during the late stages of sleep (between 4 A.M. and 8 A.M.), a larger surge of secretion occurs which lasts 2 to 3 hours.

Hypothalamic control of TSH secretion is achieved in part by the delivery of thyrotropin-releasing hormone (TRH) to the adenohypophysis; TRH is a tripeptide (perhaps the smallest peptide) which effects TSH release. Thyroid hormones also inhibit TSH release by a direct effect on thyrotropes.

Cold, stress, and electrical stimulation of the hypothalamus cause TSH release; TRH administration has become a convenient pharmacological way to increase TSH levels and to test TSH secretory reserve.

Age, hyperthyroidism, L-dopa, adrenal steroids, somatostatin, and bromergocryptine all result in diminished TSH levels.

ADRENOCORTICOTROPIC HORMONE CELL (CORTICO-TROPE). Adrenocorticotropic hormone (ACTH) is formed by cells within the adenohypophysis as well as by those basophils which have invaded the neurohypophysis. ACTH is a peptide (39 amino acids) which promotes growth of the adrenal cortex and the synthesis of the adrenal steroid hormones.

The biological half-life of ACTH is about 10 minutes; throughout the day, from six to ten secretory surges occur, but circulating levels are highest during sleep. The nocturnal rise of ACTH is not the consequence of sleep and occurs in a circadian rhythm even in sleep-deprived subjects.

Hypothalamic stimulation, stress, fear, trauma, hemorrhage, and extreme cold cause ACTH release. The search for a hypothalamic corticotropin-releasing hormone (CRH) has to date been unsuccessful, but it is well established that the hypothalamus plays an important stimulatory role in ACTH release. Some investigators have postulated that vasopressin may function as CRH, since high levels of vasopressin cause ACTH release.

The feedback relationships between ACTH and the adrenal are discussed later in this chapter.

THE GONADOTROPES. Cells which produce follicle-stimulating hormone (FSH) and luteinizing hormone (LH) collectively have been termed *gonadotropes*. These cells would have been termed *basophils* by an earlier histological classification. Both FSH and LH are glycoproteins, and a single cell secretes both hormones. FSH promotes spermatogenesis in males and promotes the maturation of ovarian follicles and the production of ovarian steroids in females. LH stimulates the male's testes to produce testosterone and promotes the development of the corpus luteum in the female.

The basal levels of FSH and LH are maintained by small secretory surges that occur at hourly intervals. In the mid-cycle of menstruating women, a larger ovulatory surge of both hormones (the surge of LH is greater) occurs, which results in ovulation. During puberty, LH levels rise dramatically during sleep and are associated with REM (rapid eye movement) sleep.

The hypothalamus influences both FSH and LH secretion via a single releasing hormone which has been termed *gonadotropin-releasing hormone* (GNRH), a decapeptide which has been synthesized. Some have termed this substance *luteinizing hormone–releasing hormone* (LHRH), since its action is more pronounced on LH secretion than on FSH secretion.

The cyclical release of FSH and LH in females results from complex ovarian events, and although the hypothalamus controls gonadotropin release, the rhythm of the cycle is derived from cyclical changes in ovarian function.

Gonadotropin secretion is increased by electrical stimulation of the hypothalamus, stress, certain visual or olfactory stimuli, and castration; in lower forms, dopamine causes FSH and LH release, but this has not been demonstrated in human beings. Synthetic GNRH can be employed to stimulate gonadotropin release and to test gonadotropin reserve.

BETA-LIPOTROPIN CELLS. The pituitary produces beta-lipotropin (LPH), a peptide containing 91 amino acids. In other species this substance is found in both the pars intermedia and the pars distalis. The structural peptide sequence of LPH contains amino acid groups which are identical to ACTH, beta MSH, endorphine, and enkephalin; thus LPH may serve as a mother molecule which can be cleaved in various places to produce smaller peptides.

Melanocyte-stimulating hormone (MSH), one of the constitutents of LPH, is produced in the pars intermedia in other species and promotes melanin production by the melanophores in the skin; some evidence suggests that MSH functions as a neurotransmitter which enhances memory.

The endorphines (alpha and beta) are moderately large peptides which also are part of the LPH molecule; both have been found in brain and spinal cord. Endorphines are bound by the same opiate receptors that bind morphine, and their physiological effects are blocked by naloxone. There is increasing physiological evidence that these substances are involved in the modulation of pain perception.

Enkephalin is a pentapeptide that has part of the molecular sequence of LPH and some of the physiological properties of the endorphines; it too has been found in brain. The intraventricular injection of enkephalin into rats results in a catatonic stupor.

FOLLICULAR CELLS. The pituitary gland in many species, including the human, contains stellate-shaped cells which form PAS-positive follicles within the adenohypophysis. These cells are difficult to visualize with light microscopy, since their thin processes are below the level of optical resolution, but they are readily seen with the electron microscope.

To date, no function has been linked to follicular cells; they are the only cells within the pituitary that still must be designated by their structure rather than their function. Unfortunately, *follicular cells* (an anatomic designation) are often confused with *follicular-stimulating hormone cells* (a functional designation).

CELL RESTS. Frequently, large PAS-positive follicles or cysts are found in the cleft between the pars distalis and pars nervosa of the human pituitary; these cysts do not resemble the pars intermedia in lower species, and their function is unclear.

In the vicinity of the pars tubralis, squamous cell rests are frequently found in the human being. These cells resemble those contained in a craniopharyngioma and may be the embryological remnant of Rathke's pouch.

Pituitary Disorders

TRAUMA

The pituitary stalk traverses the subdural space and may be partially or even totally disrupted during the deacceleration of head trauma. As many as 10 percent of patients with fatal head trauma have a divided pituitary stalk. Since the adenohypophysis derives all of its blood supply from the pituitary portal vessels and has no independent arterial supply, pituitary necrosis and panhypopituitarism result.

POSTPARTUM PITUITARY ISCHEMIA

During pregnancy the weight of the pituitary increases by as much as 50 percent, and should postpartum hemorrhage result in shock, the pituitary becomes necrotic. This syndrome, variously described as Sheehan's syndrome or Simmonds' disease, generally results in panhypopituitarism. Treatment must focus on prevention, but once present, the condition can be treated with endocrine substitution therapy.

CHROMOPHOBE ADENOMAS

Nonsecreting pituitary tumors, first described by Cushing, are the most common kind of pituitary tumor; these tumor cells have very few cytoplasmic granules and are commonly classified by the old nomenclature as *chromophobe adenomas*.

As chromophobe tumors enlarge, the adjoining secreting cells within the sella turcica are compressed, and diminished secretion results; most often growth hormone secretion is affected first, gonadotropic secretion next, thyrotropic secretion third, and ACTH secretion last. These functions are often lost in sequence, and patients who have lost adrenal function usually have had an earlier loss of thyroid and gonadal function. Despite the distortion of the

Fig. 37-8. *Left,* the normal arterial supply to the human optic chiasm. While the lateral portions of the chiasm receive a superior *and* an inferior arterial supply, the central portion of the chiasm receives only an inferior supply. *Right,* distortion of the inferior vascular supply by a pituitary tumor causes ischemia of the central portion of the chiasm, which results in a bitemporal hemianopsia.

neurohypophysis that is caused by chromophobe adenomas, diabetes insipidus seldom occurs.

The visual system may be distorted by larger chromophobe adenomas, and typically a bitemporal hemianopsia develops. Although large tumors may compress the inferior aspect of the optic nerves, optic chiasm, and optic tract, a horizontal altitudinal defect rarely ensues; the peculiarities of the vasculature of the chiasm (Fig. 37-8) make the central portion of the chiasm (containing the crossing fibers from the mesial retina) more vulnerable.

Rarely, chromophobe adenomas may enlarge laterally to compress those cranial nerves within the cavernous sinus (the oculomotor, the trochlear, the first division of the trigeminal, and the abducent); this is more commonly noted when the tumors outgrow their vascular supply and "pituitary apoplexy" results. This sudden hemorrhage within the tumor occurs in 5 percent of chromophobe adenomas, usually in large tumors, and is associated with sudden visual loss, severe headache, hyposecretion of trophic hormones, and subarachnoid hemorrhage.

The largest of the suprasellar chromophobe adenomas will extend into the third ventricle to cause hydrocephalus and/or hypothalamic dysfunction.

Although radiotherapy is effective in treating chromophobe adenomas, surgical procedures (either via a transfrontal or transsphenoidal route) are generally indicated, both to decrease the bulk of the tumor and to verify the histopathology. Surgery can be accomplished with a mortality rate of 1 percent.

ACROMEGALY

The hypersecretion of growth hormone results in gigantism in adolescents (before the epiphyses have closed) and acromegaly in adults (after the epiphyses have closed). Growth hormone causes excessive bone growth, excessive muscle growth (with weight gain), diabetes (with elevation of blood sugar level), and organomegaly. Enlargement of the face, hands, and feet often permits a bedside diagnosis (Fig. 37-9). The enlargement of the heart may result in valvular dysfunction and cardiomyopathy; patients with acromegaly commonly die of cardiac complications.

Some hypersecreting growth hormone tumors are large and cause hypofunction of other secreting cells, visual symptoms, and hydrocephalus. Although the first tumors associated with acromegaly were small eosinophilic microadenomas, the majority of acromegalic pituitary tumors removed at surgery are chromophobe tumors, not eosinophilic tumors. Even so, immunohistochemical analysis of the chromophobe tumors found in acromegaly will demonstrate GH within the cytoplasm of the tumor cells (Fig. 37-10).

The goal of therapy in acromegaly or gigantism is a reduced level of GH. In smaller, well-circumscribed tumors, the so-called microadenomas (Fig. 37-11), this can be accomplished by tumor removal alone, but in larger tumors a radical hypophysectomy is necessary, with postoperative endocrine replacement therapy.

The development of the proton beam, which has added a new dimension to the therapy of acromegaly, may supplant invasive surgical approaches.

Fig. 37-9. Patient with acromegaly. Note the large broad hands, stubby thumbs, thick lips, and prominent jaw. The classic full-blown features of acromegaly are seldom seen at present, since treatment is instituted at a much earlier stage than formerly.

Fig. 37-10. Acidic-basic stains may show the tumor from an acromegalic patient to be chromophobic. The horseradish peroxidase immunohistochemical techniques can be used on serial sections of tumor tissue to reveal the presence of growth hormone within the cells. This allows a functional designation of the tumor, i.e., somatotrophic.

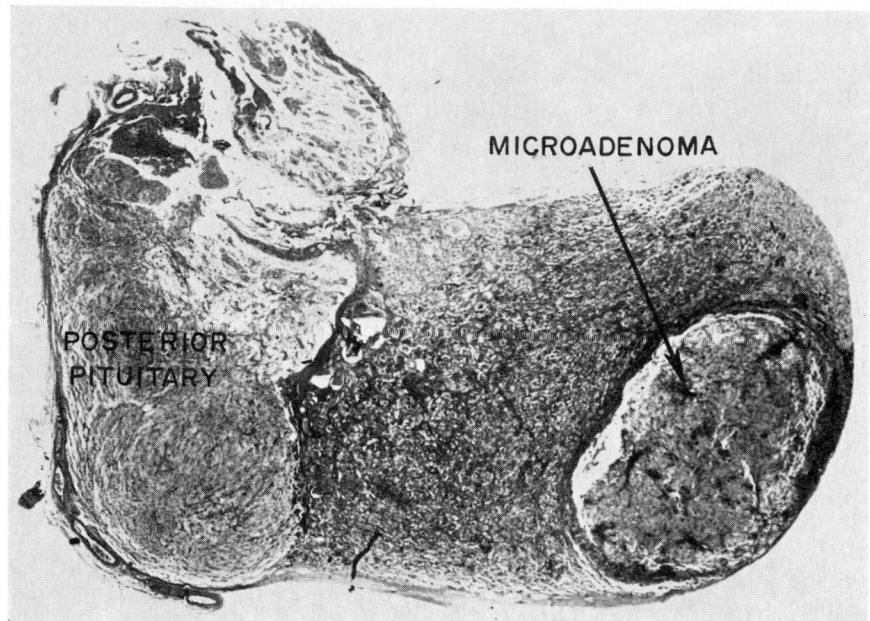

MICROADENOMA

POSTERIOR PITUITARY

Fig. 37-11. A microadenoma of the pituitary. (*Courtesy of Dr. J. Hardy.*) These tumors may secrete large amounts of hormones, yet not enlarge the sella. Their presence may be determined by radioimmune assay; they are perhaps best removed by the trans-sphenoidal approach.

CUSHING'S DISEASE

Hypersecretion of ACTH by the pituitary results in hypersecretion of steroid hormones from the adrenal cortex. Not all patients with excessive levels of adrenal steroid hormones have ACTH-producing tumors; the cause of the steroid excess can be determined only by the measurement of pituitary and adrenal secretions and by manipulating the pituitary/adrenal axis with dexamethasone and/or metapyrone.

Many of the ACTH-producing tumors are small, and a normal-sized sella turcica does not exclude the presence of a pituitary tumor; patients with the signs and symptoms of Cushing's disease must have a variety of hormone determinations before a pituitary tumor is excluded. Many small ACTH-producing tumors have been removed from normal-sized sella turcicas.

If excessive secretion of ACTH from a pituitary tumor is the cause of Cushing's disease, most investigators would agree that the pituitary tumor should be treated, rather than the adrenal hyperplasia.

The diagnosis and therapy of Cushing's disease is discussed more fully later in this chapter.

PROLACTIN-SECRETING TUMORS

Since a suitable assay for prolactin has been developed, it has been ascertained that 30 percent of all pituitary tumors originate in prolactin-secreting cells. Many of these grow to a large size and were previously termed *chromophobe adenomas,* but immunohistochemical analysis may demonstrate prolactin within the cytoplasm of the pale chromophobe cells.

In females, tumors which produce excessive prolactin cause amenorrhea as well as galactorrhea. The amenorrhea/galactorrhea syndrome (the "A/G syndrome") often results from microadenomas which do not enlarge the sella. With increasing frequency, surgeons are exploring the sella turcica to discover and remove small tumors that could not be visualized by radiography.

In males, excessive levels of prolactin may result in impotence; the removal of the offending prolactin-secreting tumor may return sexual function to normal.

Most patients with prolactin-secreting adenomas come to operation, and the surgical removal of a prolactin-secreting microadenoma can improve female fertility and give afflicted males a return of sexual vigor. Yet the systemic disturbances of prolactin excess are not known to be life threatening (in contrast to GH excess or ACTH excess), and a more conservative course often is indicated.

OTHER HYPERSECRETING TUMORS

Hypersecreting tumors of the gonadotropic cells or the thyrotropic cells are rare but have been reported.

CRANIOPHARYNGIOMAS

In both children and adults, remnants of Rathke's pouch may produce a squamous cell tumor of the pituitary, which has been termed a *craniopharyngioma.* Those tumors that develop within the sella turcica result only in hypofunction of the adenohypophysis, but the majority of craniopharyngiomas develop above the diaphragma sella and affect the neurohypophysis, the hypothalamus, the visual system, and the ventricular system. This tumor is a common cause of dwarfism. Many of these tumors are cystic, and many are calcified; not all these tumors are well encapsulated.

Once diagnosed, craniopharyngiomas may be totally

excised (if they are well encapsulated), but often cyst drainage with partial resection is preferable. Some degree of palliation may be achieved by radiotherapy.

OTHER TUMORS

Meningiomas of the tuberculum sella, ependymomas, gliomas, and pinealomas may distort the hypothalamus and/or pituitary and cause signs and symptoms not easily distinguished from those produced by primary pituitary tumors.

Metastases to the pituitary are not infrequent. Since all blood reaching the pituitary initially passes through the neurohypophysis, most metastases occur in the neurohypophysis, not the adenohypophysis.

Diagnostic Studies

RADIOLOGICAL PITUITARY STUDIES

Skull films should be obtained in patients whose signs and symptoms lead to the suspicion of a pituitary disorder. Lateral films will demonstrate the sagittal profile of the sella turcica, and anteroposterior films, properly taken, will demonstrate the floor of the sella. But only the posterior, anterior, and inferior aspects of the pituitary can be evaluated by these films. Tomograms provide a more certain assessment of the sella turcica and are especially helpful for the study of small microadenomas. The lateral aspect of the pituitary can be assessed only by angiography, and the superior aspect can be visualized only by pneumoencephalography. Since patients will often develop some degree of malaise following pneumoencephalography, angiograms usually are performed first. These radiological studies may be stressful, and patients with a disordered pituitary-adrenal axis should be protected with supplementary adrenal steroids during their radiographic studies.

Not all patients with enlargement of the sella turcica have pituitary tumors; fully 10 percent of this group have the empty sella syndrome, in which pneumoencephalography results in filling of the sella with air. The etiology of this syndrome is unclear. Should endocrine studies point to a hypersecreting tumor, the sella nonetheless should be explored as a moderate number of microadenomas have been removed from so-called empty sellas.

FUNCTIONAL PITUITARY STUDIES

Increasingly, endocrine studies of pituitary function are replacing anatomical studies in the diagnosis of hypersecreting tumors. Since patients with pituitary disorders may have hyperfunction of some cell populations and hypofunction of other cell populations, a full battery of assays is usually essential to understand the functional derangements caused by the tumor.

Therapeutic Modalities

TRANSCRANIAL SURGERY

Before the era of antibiotics, surgeons were reluctant to open the frontal sinus to reach the pituitary; the intracra-nial route was via a lateral subfrontal or temporal approach. Antibiotics made it possible for surgeons to remove the frontal bone and, if needed, to open the frontal sinus without fear of meningitis. Working through the frontal sinus (Fig. 37-12) permits less retraction of the frontal lobe and better exposure of the pituitary and chiasm; the unilateral anosmia that results is seldom noticed by patients.

Experienced surgeons can perform transfrontal pituitary surgery for hypophysectomy and for tumors with little morbidity or mortality. This approach allows the surgeon to visualize the anatomical variations that frequently surround the pituitary and to assay the distortions of the surrounding neural and vascular structures that result from tumor growth.

TRANSSPHENOIDAL APPROACHES

Early in the history of pituitary surgery, the advantages of the transsphenoidal approach to the pituitary were recognized; yet the high incidence of infection in the pre-antibiotic era worked against this approach. After opening the frontal sinus during pituitary surgery was proved safe, the transnasal approach through the sphenoid sinus was again employed (Fig. 37-13).

Although this approach does not allow the surgeon to visualize intracranial anatomical variations or the variable distortions that occur with large tumors, it is cosmetically superior, since the incision is hidden in the gingival mucosa of the upper lip. Experience has verified that this approach to the pituitary is safe, and in recent years it has supplanted the transfrontal intracranial approach in most clinics. This procedure demands an operative microscope and intraoperative fluoroscopy.

By this approach the normal sella turcica can be opened and microadenomas which were not visible by x-ray but whose presence was ascertained by functional endocrine assays can be removed. The sella turcica can be explored, much as the abdomen or chest is explored in troublesome diagnostic cases.

STEREOTAXIC TECHNIQUES

Because the sella turcica is such a convenient radiographic target, the pituitary has been treated by a variety of stereotaxic techniques. Many of these techniques were developed for the purpose of hypophysectomy in the treatment of metastatic cancer, but in selected cases, the same techniques have been employed in the treatment of pituitary tumors.

In most instances, the cannula employed in stereotaxic pituitary surgery is introduced by the transsphenoidal or transethmoidal route. Radiographic control is essential, but these procedures can be performed under local anesthesia.

Radioactive gold, radioactive yttrium, cryosurgery, and radiofrequency generators have been employed with good success to destroy the normal pituitary and to treat certain pituitary tumors. A major problem with stereotaxic procedures has been the high incidence of cerebrospinal fluid rhinorrhea.

PROTON BEAM

The development of the linear accelerator led to efforts to treat certain pituitary diseases by the proton beam (only two clinics in this country have this capability). As in the stereotaxic procedures, the radiographic shadow of the sella turcica allows the surgeon to aim the proton beam at the pituitary and to destroy the normal pituitary or certain pituitary tumors. This procedure is performed without an incision and may be the first of many surgical procedures that will be done by noninvasive techniques.

Fig. 37-12. An illustration from Cushing of the transcranial approach to the pituitary. Note the unopened frontal sinus; Cushing's efforts preceded the development of antibiotics, and meningitis often ensued if the frontal sinus was opened. Modern surgeons often open the frontal sinus, since the lower exposure provides better visualization of the pituitary.

Fig. 37-13. Another illustration from Cushing of the transsphenoidal approach to the pituitary. Because of the high incidence of infection, Cushing gave up this approach. Since the advent of antibiotics, it has gained favor.

HYPOPHYSECTOMY

The beneficial effect of oophorectomy for patients with metastatic breast cancer was known before the discovery of the endocrine system. The discovery that ovarian function was largely controlled by the pituitary, coupled to the realization that some estrogen was formed by the adrenals, suggested that hypophysectomy might be a more effective method for treating patients with far-advanced breast cancer. Since hypophysectomy also causes hypoadrenalism, it could not be employed until 1952, when adrenal replacement therapy became available.

There is little doubt that hypophysectomy is effective in the palliation of metastatic breast cancer (and prostatic cancer), but not all patients achieve a beneficial response and none is cured. Perhaps 40 percent of patients with metastatic breast cancer are benefited; their objective remission is usually measured in months, not years.

The demonstration of estrogen receptor sites in the pathological evaluation of the cancerous breast tissue has aided in predicting which patients will benefit from hypophysectomy, but proper selection of patients is still critical in the recommendation of hypophysectomy for breast cancer.

Hypophysectomy has also been employed in the therapy of diabetic retinopathy; the serendipitous observation that retinopathy improved following postpartum necrosis of the pituitary led to this form of treatment. It has not been established which hormone is involved in the response, and selection of patients remains a problem; generally patients with hemorrhagic complications respond better than those with proliferative disease. It has been verified that the benefits of the procedure are enduring.

ADRENAL

(*by Timothy S. Harrison*)

Historical Background

ADRENAL CORTEX

Early confusion surrounding adrenal cortical hyperfunction has been largely resolved as the individual adrenal cortical hormones and their specific effects have been recognized. In this brief account early reports will be separated into the hormonal syndrome categories which they seem now in retrospect to have represented.

ADRENOGENITAL AND VIRILIZING. DeCrecchio in 1865 first reported congenital adrenal hyperplasia in a female pseudohermaphrodite. Phillips in 1887 reported four cases of female pseudohermaphroditism in one family, with adrenal hypertrophy and death, apparently from salt wasting. Marchand in 1891 suggested that the adrenal hyperplasia was the cause of pseudohermaphroditism, and Butler et al. in 1939 related the salt wasting to adrenal insufficiency. Fibiger in 1905 reported four siblings with the adrenogenital syndrome, including the first male, who apparently died of salt wasting. The first postnatal adrenogenital syndrome was reported by Cooke in 1811—in a four-year-old girl with marked virilization and some ele-

ments of Cushing's syndrome associated with an adrenal tumor. Linser in 1903 reported the first male, a five-year-old boy, with pseudoprecocious puberty and an adrenal tumor. Gallais in 1912 separated adrenal hyperplasia from virilizing tumors and tumors producing obesity and diabetes (Cushing's syndrome). Wilkins et al. in 1950 first demonstrated the therapeutic use of cortisone in congenital adrenal hyperplasia.

ESTROGEN-SECRETING TUMORS. Tilesius in 1803 described a four-year-old girl with pseudoprecocious puberty, breast development, hirsutism, and obesity with an adrenal carcinoma and metastases. This was probably an estrogen-secreting tumor with some cortisol secretion as well. Birtorf in 1919 reported the first case in an adult male, the most common circumstance with this tumor.

CUSHING'S SYNDROME. Guthrie and Emery in 1907 reported a boy of four with the clinical features of Cushing's syndrome and a large adrenal tumor, and a girl of three with an identical clinical picture and no endocrine abnormalities noted at autopsy. Apert in 1910 collected 31 cases from the literature with obesity, amenorrhea and hirsutism, often associated with adrenal cortical tumors, and Achard and Thiers in 1921 described a woman with Cushing's syndrome and adrenal hyperplasia.

Parkes-Weber in 1926 reported a case with the clinical findings of Cushing's syndrome and a basophil adenoma of the pituitary. Cushing gathered 12 cases from the literature with clinical features of the syndrome subsequently named after him. Eight of these cases had autopsies, but only two had basophil adenomas. Two others had chromophobe adenomas, but one of these had an adrenal adenoma as well. Moehlig and Bates in 1933 suggested that the pituitary changes were secondary. Oppenheimer et al. in 1935 and 1937 demonstrated that basophilic adenomas of the pituitary were associated with Cushing's syndrome only when adrenal hyperplasia was also present, and they felt that the adrenal changes were primary. Albright in 1942 suggested that Cushing's syndrome was due to an overproduction of "S hormone" while adrenal virilism was due to an overproduction of "N hormone." Crooke in 1935 thought that the hyaline changes of the basophils, present in all patients with Cushing's syndrome, were the cause of the syndrome, but Laqueur in 1950 showed that these changes were secondary to overproduction of corticosteroid.

Christy, Bornstein et al., Holub and Katz, and Meador et al. in 1961 first reported cases of Cushing's syndrome secondary to ectopic ACTH production by a nonadrenal carcinoma, and Marks et al. 1963 demonstrated the presence of corticotropic activity in the tumor and its absence in the pituitary.

ALDOSTERONISM. Greep and Deane in 1949 showed that hypophysectomy caused atrophy of the zona fasciculata and zona reticularis but not the zona glomerulosa (see under Anatomy, below) and postulated that the mineralocorticoids were made in the zona glomerulosa. Tait and Simpson identified aldosterone in 1952. The clinical syndrome of primary aldosteronism was first described in 1955 by Conn and by Foye and Feichtmeier and others.

ADRENAL MEDULLA

PHEOCHROMOCYTOMA. The first case of pheochromocytoma associated with hypertension was reported by Frankel in 1886. Manasse was the first, in 1896, to demonstrate the chromaffin reaction of the cells comprising the tumor. Kohn, in 1902, described the sites at which chromaffin tissue could be found in the body. Labbé, Tinel, and Doumer, in 1922, first described the typical paroxysmal attacks of hypertension and vasomotor phenomena in a twenty-eight-year-old woman found to have a pheochromocytoma at autopsy. The first pheochromocytoma to be removed at operation was in the case of Masson and Martin in 1923, but the patient died. The first clinical diagnosis was made in 1926 by Vaquez and Donzelot. The first successful removals of pheochromocytomas were by Roux in Lausanne in February, 1926, and by Charles Mayo in the United States in October of the same year, but in neither of these cases was a preoperative diagnosis made. Pincoffs, in 1929, made the first correct preoperative diagnosis of pheochromocytoma in a patient whose tumor

Fig. 37-14. Location of ectopic adrenal tissue. The location of ectopic adrenal medullary tissue is shown in black, while the cortical tissue is shown in the shaded areas. The incidence of extraadrenal medullary tissue is very high compared with the incidence of extraadrenal cortical tissue, and while functioning extraadrenal medullary tissue occurs in about 1 out of every 8 cases of medullary hyperfunction, it occurs in less than 1 out of 1,000 cases of adrenocortical hyperfunction.

was successfully removed by Shipley on a second exploration.

The first patients in whom a pheochromocytoma was noted to be associated with sustained, as contrasted to paroxysmal, hypertension were those described by Binger and Craig and by Palmer and Castleman in 1938. Rabin, in 1929, demonstrated that a pheochromocytoma contained epinephrine in amounts greater than that seen in the normal adrenal medulla and suggested that this was the cause of the hypertension. Beer, King, and Prinzmetal, in 1937, first demonstrated a pressor agent, assumed to be epinephrine, in the blood of a patient with a pheochromocytoma during a hypertensive crisis. Holton, in 1949, reported the occurrence of norepinephrine in pheochromocytomas, and Engel and Von Euler, in 1950, demonstrated that large amounts of norepinephrine were secreted in the urine of two patients proved to have pheochromocytomas, in one of whom there was also an increased output of epinephrine.

Embryology

The adrenal cortex and medulla have separate embryologic origins. The medullary portion is derived from the chromaffin ectodermal cells of the neural crest. These cells are split off very early from the sympathetic ganglion cells, and migrate further ventrally, so as to lie ventrolateral to the aorta, where they form the paraganglia. Several such nodules near the cranial end of the gonads combine into a larger mass of cells lying between the dorsal aorta and the dorsomedial border of the mesinephros. Here they come into approximation with a group of mesodermal cells destined to become the adrenal cortex. These latter cells derive principally from a narrow strip of coelomic mesothelium lying between the dorsal mesentery and the genital ridge. These cells, arising in numerous places in the suprarenal ridge, lose their connection with the mesothelium and form a complete layer of mesoderm around the ectodermal cells derived from the sympathetic ganglia. The chromaffin cells thus become enclosed within the cortex to form the medulla.

In lower forms of vertebrates the adrenal cortex and medulla may remain completely separate. During the course of development medullary or cortical tissue may be left behind in various locations to form accessory collections of cells. The most common locations for this accessory tissue are shown in Fig. 37-14. Pheochromocytomas frequently develop in these accessory sites, particularly in the paraganglia around the aorta at the level of the kidney, anterior to the inferior aorta at the level of the organs of Zuckerkandl, in the mediastinum, in the bladder, and occasionally even in the neck or the sacrococcygeal, anal, or vaginal areas.

Adrenocortical rests are most commonly found close to the adrenal, within the kidney, in the ovarian pedicle, in the ovary itself, in the broad ligament, and in the testis. In the adrenogenital syndrome in the male there is often a well-developed adrenocortical rest in the testis that is sometimes mistaken for a normal-sized testis. Actually the

C7

ADRENAL MEDULLARY TISSUE
ADRENAL CORTICAL TISSUE

testis is atrophic, and the adrenal cortical tissue is hyperplastic. Cushing's syndrome has resulted from the hyperplasia of an intrarenal rest and persisted after bilateral adrenalectomy. Adrenocortical rests are said to occur in 50 percent of newborn infants and to atrophy and disappear in a few weeks. Their persistence in the adrenogenital syndrome is due to continued ACTH stimulation.

It has been pointed out by Schechter that the anomalous locations of the adrenal cortex are clinically important for the following reasons: hyperplasia in the accessory adrenal tissue may produce continued adrenal activity after adrenalectomy for Cushing's syndrome or for metastatic cancer; adrenal insufficiency occasionally develops when misplaced normal adrenal glands are inadvertently ablated during nephrectomy; and neoplastic transformation of heterotopic or accessory adrenal tissue may take place.

Anatomy

The adrenal glands lie along the anteromedial border of the superior pole of the kidney reaching caudad at times almost as far as the renal vessels at the hilus of the kidney. The base of the gland is thicker and broader, while the apex of the gland is thin and narrow and along the diaphragm. The general anatomy of the gland is shown in Fig. 37-15.

The arterial blood supply of the glands is variable, although generally it comes from the three sources, the phrenic artery superiorly, the aorta medially, and the renal artery inferiorly. The extreme variability of the arterial supply of the glands has been recognized in recent years, since arteriography of the glands has been performed so frequently. Variation from the classic blood supply is said to be the rule rather than the exception. Some arteriograms of the blood supply of adrenal tumors are shown in Figs. 37-48 and 37-49.

The venous supply is more constant, there usually being one large vein on the left which drains into the left renal vein and a single vein on the right which drains into the inferior vena cava. There may occasionally be small accessory veins which drain into the inferior vena cava on the left and the renal vein on the right, but these are responsible for little of the circulation of the gland unless they increase in size and number, as with the development of an adrenal tumor. Coupland has emphasized the importance of the adrenal portal venous system. This delivers blood high in glucocorticoid content to the adrenal medulla, creating conditions favorable for the induction of the enzyme phenylethanolamine-*N*-methyl transferase (PNMT). PNMT is responsible for the methylation of norepinephrine to form epinephrine. This is why over 95 percent of epinephrine originates from the adrenal medulla.

Despite the vascularity of the adrenal the blood flow of the normal adrenal in man is only about 10 ml/minute. With large adrenal tumors, however, this blood flow is magnified many times. It has been assumed by some writers that constriction of the adrenal medullary blood supply takes place in trauma to provide a better blood

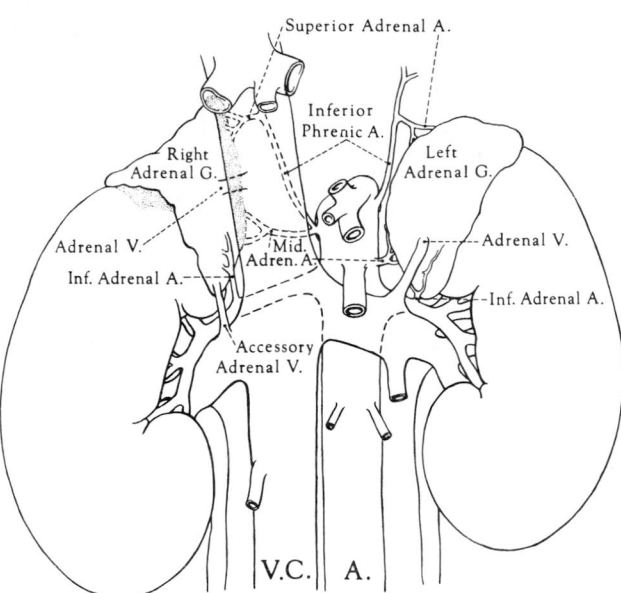

Fig. 37-15. Location and blood supply of the adrenal glands. There is great variation in the arterial blood supply of the glands, but this generally comes from three sources: a branch from the renal artery, a branch from the aorta, and a branch from the inferior phrenic artery. There is usually only one main vein on each side, the left adrenal vein opening into the left renal vein while the one on the right opens into the inferior vena cava. On occasion there may be very small accessory adrenal veins such as that illustrated for the right adrenal.

supply to the cortex. It was found by Kramer and Sapirstein in rats, however that the blood supply to both medulla and cortex increased under stress. ACTH produces an immediate marked increase in blood flow to the adrenal in dogs and man.

Microscopically the adrenal cortex is divided into three zones: the zona glomerulosa, or outer zone, the zona fasciculata—a wide intermediate zone—and the zona reticularis, a narrow inner zone closely applied to the medulla. The zona glomerulosa is responsible for the production of aldosterone, while the zona fasciculata and zona reticularis manufacture cortisol and other glucocorticoids. There is still some debate as to whether the androgens and estrogens are manufactured by cells distributed throughout the zona fasciculata and zona reticularis or whether their manufacture is primarily related to cells concentrated in or near the reticularis.

Adrenal Cortex

PHYSIOLOGY

The general structure of the steroids secreted by the adrenal cortex is shown in Fig. 37-16. The corticosteroids, or corticoids, include both the glucocorticoids and mineralocorticoids and are C-21 compounds, the androgens are C-19 steroids, and the estrogens are C-18 steroids.

The entire adrenal cortex normally contains 11- and 21-hydroxylating enzymes for the production of cortisol

STERANE

CORTICOID
NUCLEUS
(C-21 Steroids)

ANDROGEN
NUCLEUS
(C-19 Steroids)

ESTROGEN
NUCLEUS
(C-18 Steroids)

and similar glucocorticoids, while only the zona glomeru-losa contains 18-oxidase, an enzyme capable of oxidating the 18 carbon atom to produce aldosterone, the principal mineralocorticoid, as shown in Fig. 37-17. The principal active compounds of each class secreted by the adrenal are shown in Fig. 37-18. The relative secretion rates of the adrenal compounds are shown in Table 37-1. The two most important adrenal corticosteroids by far are cortisol, the major glucocorticoid, and aldosterone, the major miner-alocorticoid.

Fig. 37-16. Basic adrenal steroid structure. The numbering system for the carbon atoms in the steroid nucleus is shown at the top. The basic steroid nucleus (Sterane) is modified to form the C-21, C-19, and C-18 steroids, as shown in the lower line.

CORTISOL. Secretion. Normally the hypothalamus se-cretes CRF, which promotes the release of ACTH from the anterior pituitary. ACTH in turn stimulates the adrenal cortex to produce and release cortisol. Rising blood levels of cortisol then serve to inhibit the further release of CRF from the hypothalamus and thus effect a feedback regula-tory mechanism (Fig. 37-19). After trauma this feedback

Fig. 37-17. Enzymes of the adrenal cortex. The entire adrenal cortex contains 11- and 21-hydroxylating enzymes, while the zona fasciculata and zona reticularis contain 17-hydroxylating enzymes in addition. The zona glomerulosa lacks 17-hydroxylat-ing but contains 18-oxidase, which is necessary for the formation of aldosterone. The androgens are also formed in the zona fas-ciculata and zona reticularis, particularly in the latter.

Fig. 37-18. Principal active compounds of the adrenal cortex. The structural formulas are shown for the principal glucocorticoids, mineralocorticoid, androgens, and estrogen.

Table 37-1. SECRETION RATES OF ADRENAL
STEROIDS IN MAN

Compound	24-hour secretion
Cortisol	30 mg
Corticosterone	5 mg
Aldosterone	150 mg
Androstenedione	5 mg
11-β-Hydroxyandrostenedione	5 mg
Estradiol	Trace

SOURCE: From Forsham and Melmon, 1968.

mechanism is overcome by other central nervous system mechanisms, when CRF and ACTH are secreted in spite of rising levels of cortisol to bring about an acute increase in the blood level of cortisol. Normally there is a diurnal variation in the release of CRF, ACTH, and therefore cortisol. This diurnal variation, or circadian rhythm, is shown in Fig. 37-20. It occurs even in blind people or people who work at night and is independent of sleep. It shifts with changes in latitude but is not changed by travel from north to south. An important feature of Cushing's syndrome seems to be a failure of this diurnal variation, so that ACTH is secreted constantly around the clock, presumably in response to a continued CRF stimulus.

The normal feedback mechanism can be disturbed by metyrapone (Metopirone). This compound interferes with 11-β-hydroxylation in the adrenal cortex. The synthesis of cortisol therefore ceases, and there is thus no opposition to continued pituitary secretion of ACTH, as shown in Fig. 37-21. This is used as a test of pituitary activity, to determine whether the pituitary is capable of secreting increased amounts of ACTH. The 11-desoxycortisol which is produced instead of cortisol under these circumstances is incapable of inhibiting the release of CRF and ACTH. Since there is an oversecretion of ACTH, other adrenal substances such as the androgens are also produced in large quantities, since they are incapable of inhibiting the release of ACTH. This produces a situation similar to that seen in the adrenogenital syndrome.

Binding and Transport. Once secreted, the cortisol exists in three states in the blood—free, bound, and conjugated. In the free state cortisol is a metabolically active compound available to the tissues. For transport and protection from degradation it is bound to a substance known as corticosteroid-binding globulin (CBG), or transcortin, which is an α-globulin. This makes it somewhat more soluble and protects it from conjugation. When large amounts of cortisol are secreted, the binding sites become saturated, and the levels of free cortisol rise in the plasma. Under these circumstances some free cortisol will be excreted in the urine, although ordinarily only very tiny amounts of unconjugated cortisol appear in the urine.

Metabolism. Cortisol is metabolized in the liver by conversion to tetrahydrocortisol and conjugation with glucuronide and sulfate. Once the cortisol is conjugated, it becomes water-soluble and is easily excreted in the urine (Fig. 37-22A and B).

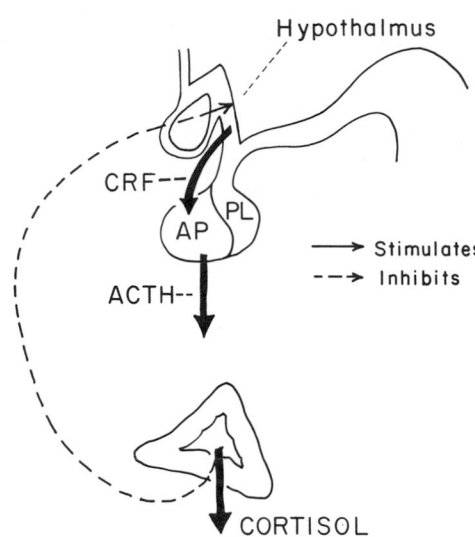

Fig. 37-19. Feedback regulation of cortisol secretion. CRF manufactured in the hypothalamus stimulates the anterior pituitary to release ACTH. ACTH stimulates the adrenal cortex to release cortisol and androgens. Cortisol, but not the androgens, act on the hypothalamus to inhibit release of CRF and thus of ACTH. In trauma the feedback mechanism is temporarily overcome as the hypothalamic centers secrete an increased amount of CRF leading to pituitary-adrenal stimulation and increased blood levels of cortisol.

Fig. 37-20. Diurnal variation in cortisol plasma levels in response to a circadian hypothalamic rhythm. There is a daily variation in CRF and ACTH secretion which is reflected in the plasma cortisol levels. Thus blood cortisol (or ACTH) has its lowest rate of secretion around midnight with its highest secretion coming around 6 A.M. In Cushing's syndrome this rhythm is lost, and while the plasma cortisol level may not be greatly elevated beyond that seen in the normal patient in the early morning, it continues at the same level throughout the day and fails to show the decline in plasma cortisol levels seen normally during the late afternoon and evening. A good way to diagnose Cushing's disease is to compare the 12 midnight and 8 A.M. plasma cortisol levels. In Cushing's disease these are very nearly the same, while in normal patients the 8 A.M. level is two or three times as high as the midnight level.

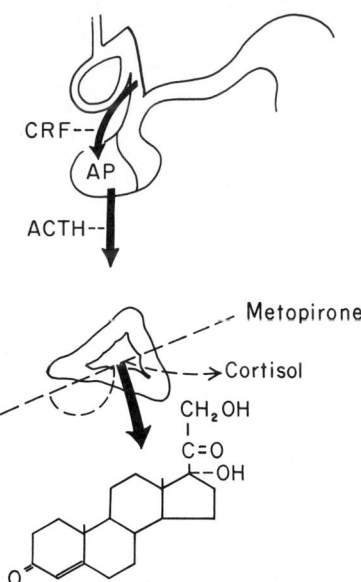

Fig. 37-21. Effect of metyrapone (Metopirone, SU-4885) on ACTH secretion. Metyrapone interferes with 11-hydroxylation in the adrenal cortex, and 11-desoxycortisol is formed instead of cortisol. Since cortisol is not present in the plasma to inhibit the release of CRF from the hypothalamus, there is a markedly increased CRF and ACTH secretion which stimulates the adrenal cortex to secrete more and more 11-desoxycortisol. This substance is measured in the urine by methods designed to measure 17-hydroxycorticosteroids. An increase in these substances following the administration of metyrapone indicates a function of both the anterior pituitary and adrenal cortex. If there is a response to ACTH but not to metyrapone, this indicates a decreased pituitary reserve.

Fig. 37-22. Metabolism and excretion of cortisol. *A*. The degradation of cortisol takes place in the liver. In the first step dihydrocortisol is formed by a saturation of the double bond between carbons 4 and 5, adding a hydrogen to each of these carbon atoms. Further reduction takes place to the tetrahydrocortisol configuration by the substitution of a hydroxyl group for the ketone group on the 3 carbon atom. The tetrahydrocortisol is then conjugated with glucuronide through the hydroxyl group on the 3 carbon atom. Some conjugation with sulfates also takes place. The conjugated tetrahydrocortisol is then excreted in the urine. *B*. The free cortisol secreted by the adrenal cortex becomes largely bound to transcortin, an α-globulin manufactured in the liver. This carrier protein prevents the rapid breakdown of cortisol but makes it available to the tissues as needed. As the cortisol passes through the liver, it becomes reduced and conjugated and thus inactivated. The conjugated corticosteroids are water-soluble and are excreted in the urine. A small amount of free cortisol is also excreted in the urine. At any given time the peripheral blood contains free, bound, and conjugated cortisol. If there is a marked increase in cortisol secretion, the transcortin-binding sites become saturated, and the amount of free cortisol increases greatly. In renal failure the conjugated corticosteroids are not excreted normally, and they pile up in the bloodstream. In hepatic failure there is very little conjugation of the corticosteroids, and a proportionately greater amount of free cortisol is present in the plasma.

METABOLISM OF CORTISOL

CORTISOL

DIHYDROCORTISOL

TETRAHYDROCORTISOL

TETRAHYDROCORTISOL
3α GLUCURONIDE

A

EXAMPLES

	PLASMA µg %		URINE mgm/D	
	Free + Bound	Conj.	Free + Bound	Conj.
Normal	22	22	10	0.1
Liver Disease	22	2	3	0.1
Kidney Disease	22	900	2	0
Cushing's Disease	34	45	20	0.3

NORMAL

PLASMA
50% Conjugated (22 µg%)
40% Bound (20 µg%)
10% Free   (2 µg%)

URINE
99% Conjugated CS (10 mg/D)
1% Free CS (<100 µg/D)

B

ANDROGENS. The androgens are conjugated and excreted in the same fashion as cortisol. While the androgens, like cortisol, are dependent upon ACTH secretion for their release, they are not capable of inhibiting ACTH secretion in a feedback fashion.

ALDOSTERONE. Secretion. Roughly 30 percent of aldosterone secretion is influenced by ACTH. The remainder depends primarily on the secretion of renin and angiotensin II for regulation. In response to a fall in blood volume there is a fall in pressure in the afferent renal arteriole. This produces a release of renin by the juxtaglomerular cells. The renin combines with angiotensinogen manufactured in the liver to form angiotensin I, which is converted by a converting enzyme in the pulmonary circulation into angiotensin II. Angiotensin II stimulates the zona glomerulosa of the adrenal cortex to release aldosterone. The feedback mechanism for the regulation of aldosterone production under normal circumstances depends upon the aldosterone-induced renal retention of sodium, which raises the blood volume and turns off the production of renin. This regulatory mechanism can be overcome by any situation in the kidney, e.g., renal artery stenosis, which produces a permanent fall in afferent arteriolar pressure. This gives rise to hypertrophy of the juxtaglomerular cells and a markedly increased secretion of renin, thus producing the increased aldosterone secretion which is seen in secondary aldosteronism. The normal mechanism for the regulation of aldosterone secretion is shown in Fig. 37-23.

The mechanism for aldosterone release is probably more complicated than this, but it seems certain that in man it proceeds without the stimulus of ACTH. Some experimental animals seem to require a pituitary factor other than ACTH for aldosterone release to be normally responsive to a fall in the plasma sodium level. In the rat this may be GH, whereas in the dog it may be some other, unnamed substance. Other workers have found that GH does not restore the response of aldosterone to hyponatremia in hypophysectomized rats and postulate an unnamed hormone in this species as well.

Because a low sodium intake stimulates an increased aldosterone production in the normal individual, it is essential that aldosterone excretion measurements to determine whether or not primary aldosteronism is present be made while the patients are on diets which are normal in sodium. Low-sodium diets appear to produce renal vascular constriction even when significant changes in serum levels are not seen, and this is postulated as one of the mechanisms whereby a low-sodium diet brings about renin release.

It is established that the sympathetic nervous system plays a role in aldosterone secretion. Plasma renin activity and aldosterone secretion in normal patients have been shown to increase in response to an infusion of catecholamines or electrical stimulation of the sympathetic nervous system. The stimulation of upright posture and of sodium depletion, which normally results in an increase of renin and aldosterone secretion, fails to do so when autonomic insufficiency is present. In such patients the injection of catecholamines produces an increase in the secretion of

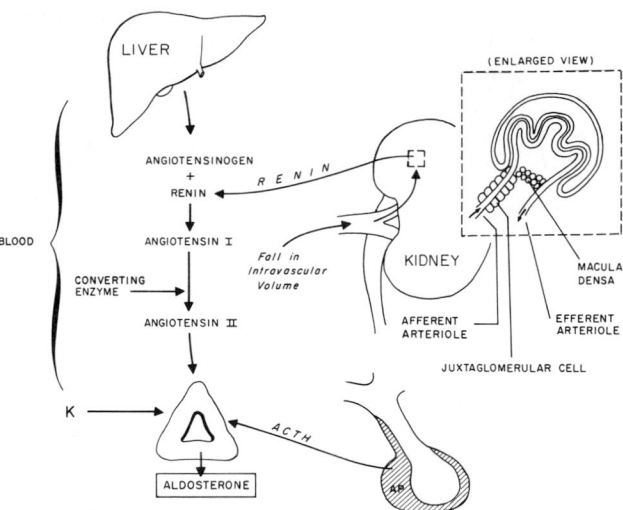

Fig. 37-23. Regulation of aldosterone secretion. A fall in blood volume, a fall in blood pressure, or vasoconstriction of the renal arteries due to norepinephrine produces a decrease in pressure in the afferent arteriole leading to a release of renin from the juxtaglomerular cells. The renin converts angiotensinogen manufactured in the liver to angiotensin I. This substance is further converted in the bloodstream by an enzyme in angiotensin II which stimulates the zona glomerulosa of the adrenal cortex to release aldosterone. Aldosterone, in turn, leads to sodium retention and a rise in blood pressure, which acts as a feedback mechanism to shut off the further release of renin. Secondary aldosteronism results when there is an obligatory secretion of renin as with an anatomic stricture of the renal arteries.

these two substances, presumably by producing renal afferent arteriolar constriction, thus leading to an increase in renin output. Renal transplantation with complete denervation of the kidney does not prevent the response to sodium depletion or the upright position, so that circulating, rather than locally formed, catecholamines may be responsible for this change. A review of this subject has been published by Gross. Marusic and Mulrow have studied isolated mitochondria from rat adrenal glands and have found that the mitochondria from rats on a low-sodium diet have a greater capacity for converting corticosterone to aldosterone than do mitochondria from rats fed a normal diet.

Metabolism. Aldosterone is metabolized in the same fashion as cortisol. Since it is such an active compound, it is excreted in the urine in minute quantities, and its chemical determination was, therefore, difficult until a radioimmunoassay for aldosterone became available.

SYNTHETIC ADRENOCORTICAL COMPOUNDS. Synthetic adrenocortical compounds are commonly used in clinical practice. Some common ones are shown in Fig. 37-24. Their relative potencies with respect to cortisol and aldosterone are shown in Table 37-2.

CUSHING'S SYNDROME

Cushing's syndrome refers to the changes seen with excess cortisol secretion. It may be produced as a consequence of excessive ACTH production either by the normal pituitary, presumably in response to a hypothalamic

Prednisone
(Δ₁ Cortisone)

Prednisolone
(Δ₁ Cortisol)

Dexamethasone
(9 – α Fluoro 16–α
Methylprednisolone)

9– α Fluorohydrocortisone
(9 – α   Fluorocortisol; 9α FF)

Desoxycorticosterone

Fig. 37-24. Synthetic compounds. Structural formulas are shown for the synthetic glucocorticoids prednisone, prednisolone, and dexamethasone, and the mineralocorticoids, 9-α-fluorocortisol and deoxycorticosterone acetate (DCA).

stimulus, by a pituitary tumor, or by an ectopic ACTH-producing malignant tumor. Cushing's syndrome may result from increased cortisol production from an adrenal cortical carcinoma, an adrenal adenoma, or nodular hyperplasia of the adrenal cortex. Adrenal hyperplasia is the most common, followed by adrenal adenoma, adrenal carcinoma, an ectopic ACTH source, pituitary tumors secreting ACTH, and nodular dysplasia, in that order.

PATHOLOGY. The pathologic features of Cushing's syndrome vary, depending upon the cause, as shown in Fig. 37-25.

Hyperplasia, Adenoma, Carcinoma, Pituitary Tumor. Cushing in 1932 ascribed the syndrome to a basophilic adenoma

of the anterior pituitary. This is actually a very rare cause of this disease. Adrenal cortical hyperplasia, shown in Fig. 37-26 is the most common cause of Cushing's syndrome, and it is customary to refer to patients with adrenocortical hyperplasia as having Cushing's disease. Cushing's disease is due to increased production of ACTH, usually associated with loss of the normal diurnal variation of ACTH release.

Fig. 37-25. Causes of Cushing's syndrome. Hyperplasia of the adrenal cortex is brought about by an increased secretion of ACTH which may result either from a continual stimulation of the pituitary by CRF (1), an ACTH-secreting tumor of the anterior pituitary (2), or an ectopic malignant tumor secreting ACTH (3). The increased cortisol production can also come about as a consequence of an adrenal carcinoma (4), an adrenal adenoma (5), or nodular dysplasia (6).

Table 37-2. RELATIVE ANTI-INFLAMMATORY POTENCIES OF SOME THERAPEUTIC CORTICOIDS

Compound	Relative potency compared to cortisol	Relative sodium-retaining activity
Cortisol	1	+ +
Cortisone acetate	0.8	+ +
Prednisolone (1-2-dehydrocortisol) . .	4	+
Prednisone (1-2-dehydrocortisone) . .	3.5	+
Triamcinolone (9-α-fluoro-16-α-hydroxyprednisolone).	5	0
6-Methylprednisolone (9-α-fluoro-6-α-methylprednisolone)	5	0
Haldranolone (6-α-fluoro-16-α-methylprednisolone)	10	0
Betamethasone (9-α-fluoro-16-β-methylprednisolone)	25	0
Dexamethasone (9-α-fluoro-16-α-methylprednisolone)	30	0
9-α-Fluorohydrocortisone*	15	+ + + + +

*Used chiefly topically or as a sodium retainer.
SOURCE: From Forsham and Melmon, 1968.

(1)   (2)   (3)

CRF--

ACTH--   ACTH --   ACTH--   ectopic tumor

CORTISOL   CORTISOL   CORTISOL

(4)   (5)   (6)   ACTH

adrenal Ca.   adrenal adenoma   nodular dysplasia

CORTISOL   CORTISOL   CORTISOL

This in turn is presumed to be brought about by an increased hypothalamic stimulation of the pituitary. Cortical pathways subserving a wide variety of emotional and psychic stimuli can then influence the hypothalamic regulation of CRF and of pituitary ACTH release. Hyperplasia can also be caused by any excessive ACTH secretion either from a tumor of the pituitary or an ectopic tumor. Under any of these circumstances both adrenal glands are hyperplastic, and the usual sharp edge of the gland is rounded by the thickened cortices. Microscopically the widening of the cortex occurs primarily in the zona fasciculata. It may sometimes be difficult to distinguish hyperplasia, either grossly or microscopically, from the normal gland, but it is always easy to distinguish hyperplasia from an atrophic gland.

An adrenal adenoma causing Cushing's syndrome is shown in Fig. 37-27 and an iodocholesterol scan is presented in Fig. 37-28. The cortex of the remainder of the adrenal is extremely thin and atrophic, as was the cortex on the opposite side. This atrophy is due to inhibition of ACTH secretion by the large amounts of cortisol secreted by the autonomous tumor.

Adrenocortical carcinomas occur in about 10 percent of patients with Cushing's syndrome. They usually give rise to florid signs of the disease and sometimes occur in young children. Widespread metastases may occur, and the metastases are frequently hyperfunctioning.

It is sometimes difficult to make the diagnosis of malignancy in an adrenal cortical tumor, because the presence of bizarre cells and blood vessel invasion are not necessarily indicators of true malignancy. However, the histologic criteria which tend to suggest malignancy include pleomorphism, giant and bizarre nuclei, frequent and sometimes atypical mitoses, hemorrhage, necrosis, and calcification. The absolute criteria of malignancy are said by Heinbecker et al. to be invasion of veins, invasion into and through the capsule, and distant metastases.

Nodular Dysplasia. The syndrome of nodular dysplasia of the adrenal has been reported in recent years by Kirschner et al. and Meador et al., who named it. This strange type of hyperplasia, of which fewer than 10 cases

Fig. 37-27. Adrenocortical adenoma causing Cushing's disease. The oval-shaped adenoma can be easily seen beneath the retractor. Note the extreme thinning of the rest of the adrenal cortex. This severe adrenocortical atrophy is due to inhibition of ACTH release by the cortisol manufactured by the adenoma.

have been reported, behaves like an autonomous adenoma rather than hyperplasia, since the secretion is not suppressible with large doses of dexamethasone and does not respond to ACTH. Endogenous ACTH secretion is suppressed. The characteristic appearance on cut section is of numerous nodules 2 mm or less in diameter. Microscopically the nodules contain large oval or polyhedral

Fig. 37-28. An adrenal photoscan from a patient with Cushing's syndrome due to a hyperfunctioning adenoma of the right adrenal cortex. Viewed from the posterior aspect, the uptake seen is in a solitary lesion of the right adrenal gland. The remainder of the right adrenal and the entire left adrenal are suppressed by the exaggerated release of glucocorticoids and therefore do not take up the iodocholesterol.

Fig. 37-26. Adrenal cortical hyperplasia causing Cushing's disease. The cut section of the gland shows marked thickening of adrenal cortex.

Fig. 37-29. Cushing's disease caused by nodular dysplasia: gross appearance of the gland.

cells with small, dark, round nuclei and slightly granular, heavily eosinophilic cytoplasm. In the case of Meador et al. the cells contained pigment and appeared black to the naked eye. The adrenal cortical cells adjacent to the nodules appear normal, not atrophic.

A gland involved in nodular hyperplasia is shown in Fig. 37-29. This case was complicated by the fact that bilateral adrenal hemorrhages developed following adrenal venograms. The patient made an uneventful recovery from surgical treatment.

Ectopic-ACTH Syndrome. It occasionally may be difficult

Fig. 37-30. Cushing's disease. *A.* Note the round face and the increase in preauricular fat pads. Despite the marked obesity and protuberance of the abdomen the extremities are disproportionately thin. There are a few striae over the lower abdomen. *B.* A side view of the same patient, again showing the marked protuberance of the abdomen and central fat, with thin extremities.

to make a definitive diagnosis of an ectopic ACTH-secreting tumor preoperatively. Clinically such patients often have chemically severe Cushing's syndrome without the typical distribution of fat, or even with weight loss. Chemically the diagnosis rests upon the demonstration of increased cortisol excretion, which is not suppressible with dexamethasone, coupled with elevated levels of ACTH in the plasma. Patients with the pituitary type of adrenal hyperplasia have ACTH in the plasma but generally show suppression of cortisol production with large doses of dexamethasone, while those patients with adrenocortical adenoma or carcinoma fail to show suppression of cortisol production by dexamethasone but have no measurable ACTH in the plasma. Since MSH is usually secreted in conjunction with ACTH, patients with ectopic ACTH syndrome may show hyperpigmentation, but this is usually not prominent until after adrenalectomy.

The primary source of these carcinomas is usually an oat cell carcinoma of the lung, but the syndrome has also been seen with tumors of the parotid, liver, pancreas, thymus, thyroid, esophagus, and the adrenal medulla.

General Considerations. Systemically, patients with Cushing's disease show marked muscle wasting and severe osteoporosis. There is disappearance of elastic fibers in the skin leading to thinning and fragility of the skin and production of striae. Marked atherosclerosis of the vessels occurs, and there may be nephrosclerosis of the kidneys and sometimes nephrocalcinosis. The ovaries and testes may show some atrophy, and the pancreas may show fatty necrosis and islet cell hyperplasia.

In the untreated case the cause of death is usually related to the sequelae of hypertension, but another common cause of death is infection, frequently with fungal organisms.

CLINICAL MANIFESTATIONS. Incidence. The peak incidence of Cushing's disease is found in the third and fourth decades. The syndrome has been known to occur in children less than a year of age and also to have its onset in patients as old as seventy. Some observers have been impressed that an experience with great emotional impact often precedes by several weeks the onset of Cushing's disease. Cushing's syndrome is considerably more common in women than in men, in a ratio of 4:1. Adenomas are also far more common in women than men, occurring particularly following pregnancy. Cushing's disease is a relatively rare condition, occurring in fewer than 1 of 1,000 autopsies.

Signs and Symptoms. The signs and symptoms of Cushing's syndrome are listed in Table 37-3. Most of these are due to an excess secretion of cortisol, and almost all of them, including hirsutism, hypokalemia, hypertension, and the typical moon face appearance, can be produced in normal patients by the exogenous administration of cortisol. At times, however, a tumor of the adrenal cortex may produce an increased secretion both of cortisol and of androgen, thus giving a mixed picture of Cushing's disease and the adrenogenital syndrome. This is discussed later on. The moon face, acne, hirsutism, striae, buffalo hump, ecchymoses, truncal obesity, and thin extremities are illustrated in Fig. 37-30*A* and *B*.

Table 37-3. SYMPTOMS AND SIGNS OF
CUSHING'S SYNDROME

Moon facies	Acne
Truncal obesity	Fungal infections
Hypertension	Back pain
Plethora	Headache
Amenorrhea or impotence	Emotional lability
Weakness and fatigue	Pathologic fractures
Hirsutism	Polyuria
Striae	Renal calculi
Easy bruising and ecchymoses	Hypokalemic alkalosis
Osteoporosis	Atherosclerosis
Edema	Possibly tumor shown on IVP
Diabetes, latent or overt	With malignant tumors, pos-
Supraclavicular fat pads	sibly metastases detected by
Buffalo hump	x-ray
Muscle wasting	

As the disease progresses, the patients undergo marked muscle wasting and osteoporosis, with collapse of vertebrae, backache, buffalo hump, easy fatigability, and weakness. Spontaneous rib fractures may also occur. Arteriosclerosis develops, and the patients have a diabetic glucose tolerance curve, or occasionally frank diabetes. There is marked emotional lability or even frank psychosis.

Cushing's disease is potentially fatal, death usually occurring within 5 years of the first evidences of the disease.

DIAGNOSTIC FINDINGS. The diagnostic tests for Cushing's syndrome which have proved to be of most value are listed in Table 37-4.

Diurnal Variation of Blood Cortisol Levels. There is normally a diurnal variation in the blood ACTH and cortisol level, such that the cortisol level is at its highest around 6 A.M. and then gradually falls off during the day, hitting its lowest point around midnight (see Fig. 37-20). In some cases of Cushing's syndrome the blood cortisol level may not be elevated above normal, but the diurnal variation is gone, and the secretion of cortisol and ACTH remain constant throughout the day. Absence of the diurnal variation can easily be detected by taking blood samples for cortisol at midnight and at 8 A.M. The one taken at 8 A.M. should be two to three times as high as the one obtained at midnight. If they are the same, this is strong evidence for Cushing's syndrome. The normal values are listed in Table 37-5.

Diurnal Variation of Urinary Corticosteroid Levels. Vagnucci et al., Martin and Hamman, and Jefferies et al. have demonstrated a circadian cycle and characteristic patterns of urinary cortisol excretion which are helpful in

Table 37-4. TESTS FOR CUSHING'S SYNDROME

Diurnal variation of blood cortisol
Diurnal variation of urine cortisol
Blood cortisol response to ACTH with conjugates
Dexamethasone suppression
Rapid dexamethasone suppression
Metyrapone (Metopirone)
Blood ACTH measurement
Urinary, free cortisol, cortisol secretory tests, etc.
X-ray of sella turcica
Adrenal angiography
Iodocholesterol scan of the adrenal

Table 37-5. NORMAL STEROID VALUES

Steroid	Values
Plasma	
Cortisol:	
8 A.M.	6–28 µg/100 ml
Midnight	2–12 µg/100 ml
Urinary estrogens	
Ages 0–10 years	0–1 µg/day
Premenopausal females . . .	5–20 µg/day
Men	0.1–2 µg/day
Urinary pregnanetriol	
Ages 0–6 years	0.02–0.2 mg/day
Ages 7–15 years	0.6–1.2 mg/day
Over 16 years	0.5–2.5 mg/day

Urine	Male	Female
Urinary 17-OH corticoids. . . .	4–11 mg/day	3–11 mg/day
Urinary 17-ketosteroids	10–20 mg/day	5–15 mg/day

SOURCE: Modified from Forsham and Melmon, 1968.

the diagnosis of Cushing's disease. This is said to be useful in differentiating between hyperplasia, tumor, and normal adrenal cortical function.

Blood Cortisol Response to ACTH. Patients with adrenocortical hyperplasia have a greater responsiveness to ACTH than do normal patients. Thus the administration of ACTH intravenously over a 4- to 6-hour period produces a greater rise in plasma cortisol levels than one would expect in the normal patient. We have found it useful to measure the conjugated corticosteroids as well as the free, since the differential between adrenal cortical hyperplasia and the normal is even greater when the conjugated corticosteroids are measured. Patients with functioning adrenocortical adenomas as the cause of the Cushing's syndrome fail to show a rise in cortisol with ACTH administration, because the secretion is autonomous and not dependent upon ACTH production. This test is not always capable of differentiating between hyperplasia and tumor, since the adrenals of some patients with tumors will respond to ACTH stimulation, but it is usually possible to differentiate between the normal patient and one with Cushing's syndrome.

Dexamethasone Suppression Test. Dexamethasone is a synthetic corticosteroid of great potency. Small quantities of this drug are capable of blocking ACTH release in the normal patient, as demonstrated by a fall in urinary cortisol excretion (Fig. 37-31). The test, which was originally devised by Liddle et al., is usually done as follows: The patient is put on continuous 24-hour urinary collections for corticosteroids during the 6 days of the test. The first 2 days are control periods, the second two days the patient received 0.5 mg of dexamethasone by mouth every 6 hours for a total of 2 mg/day, and on the final 2 days the patient receives 2 mg of dexamethasone by mouth every 6 hours for a total of 8 mg/day. The normal patient will show a suppression of 17-hydroxycorticosteroid excretion of 50 percent or more on the 2 mg/day dose of dexamethasone. Patients with Cushing's syndrome do not. Patients with

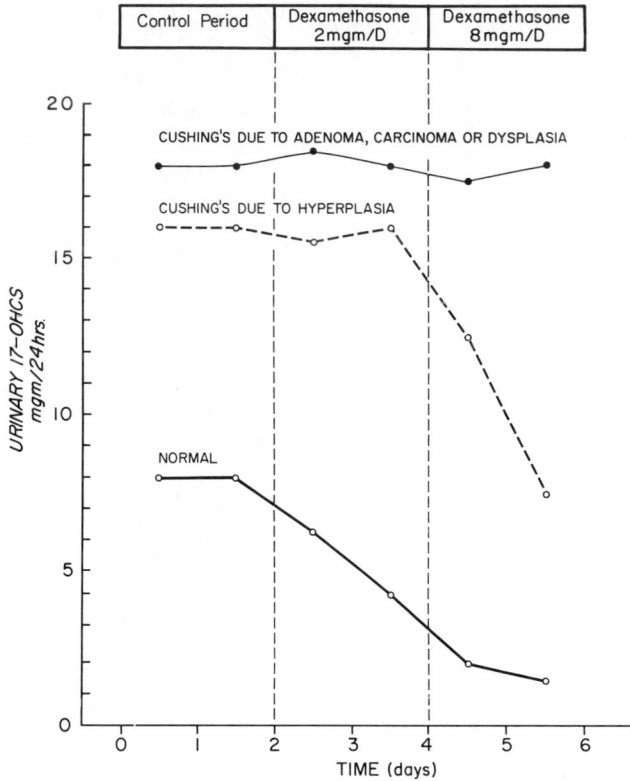

Fig. 37-31. Dexamethasone suppression test: the effect of a low and high dose of dexamethasone on urinary 17-hydroxycorticosteroid excretion. The normal patient shows suppression on both the low and the high dose, whereas in Cushing's disease due to hyperplasia there is no suppression with the low dose but there is suppression with the high dose. In Cushing's disease due to adenoma, cancer, or dysplasia, there is no suppression with either the low or the high dose.

Fig. 37-32. Metyrapone test. With adrenal cortical hyperplasia there is an increased urinary 17-hydroxycorticosteroid excretion in response to metyrapone, while there characteristically is no such response with adrenal cortical adenoma, dysplasia, or carcinoma.

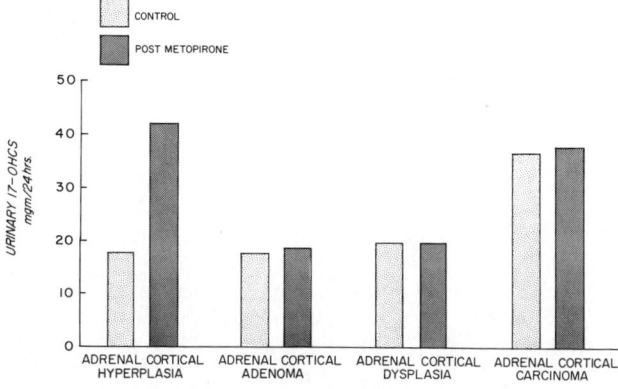

Cushing's disease due to bilateral adrenal hyperplasia show a suppression on 8 mg/day of dexamethasone, whereas those with an adrenal cortical adenoma or carcinoma do not. Unfortunately this test is not completely reliable, since it fails to show suppression in some cases of hyperplasia and does show suppression in some cases of cortical adenoma. It also fails to show suppression in patients with nodular adrenal dysplasia.

Rapid Dexamethasone Suppression Test. This test is better than the regular dexamethasone suppression test mentioned above and, along with the test for diurnal variation, is probably the best overall test for adrenocortical function. The test can be carried out either with plasma cortisol measurements or with urine corticosteroid and creatinine measurements. In the simplest form of the test the patient received 1 mg of dexamethasone by mouth at 11 P.M., and after adequate sedation with barbiturate a plasma cortisol sample is drawn the next morning at 8 o'clock. If the level of 17-hydroxycorticosteroids in the plasma is above $10 \mu g/100$ ml, this suggests nonsuppressibility of ACTH secretion and is diagnostic of Cushing's syndrome. In the normal patient the level falls nearly to zero. In order to perform the test, the patient must not be taking birth control pills containing estrogen, since this raises the transcortin level and produces high levels of plasma hydroxycorticosteroids. It would be satisfactory to take two morning samples, one the day before and one the day after dexamethasone administration, since the normal patient even on birth control pills would be expected to show a very marked suppression of the cortisol level on the second day. The ratio of urinary corticosteroid to creatinine can be used in lieu of a plasma cortisol level to indicate suppression by dexamethasone.

Tucci et al. have extended the rapid dexamethasone suppression test by obtaining not only a plasma value the morning after the dexamethasone administration but also a 5-hour urinary collection from 7 A.M. until noon. Both 17-hydroxycortisteroids and creatinine are calculated. A steroid/creatinine ratio of less than 4 makes the diagnosis of Cushing's syndrome highly likely, whereas a ratio greater than 4 suggests either that the patient is normal or that further studies will have to be carried out to establish the diagnosis of Cushing's disease. Although the test is highly reliable, both false negatives and false positives have occasionally been found.

Metyrapone (Metopirone) Test. This test was devised by Liddle to test pituitary as well as adrenal function (Fig. 37-32). As noted previously, metyrapone blocks $11-\beta$-hydroxylation in the adrenal cortex, resulting in a fall in cortisol production and therefore a release of ACTH inhibition. This leads to an increased output of ACTH in normal individuals, with an increased output of non-11-β-hydroxylated corticosteroids from the adrenal. Since these hormones are 17-hydroxycorticosteroids, they can be measured in the urine by the usual test. In patients with Cushing's disease due to adrenal hyperplasia there is a markedly increased output of corticosteroids in the urine, greater than that seen in the normal person. Patients with Cushing's syndrome due to autonomously functioning adrenal cortical adenomas do not show an increase. This test probably has no real advantage over ACTH stimulation in the detection of Cushing's disease, but it is very helpful in detecting inadequate pituitary reserve. Insulin and vasopressin can also be used to test pituitary adrenal cortical reactivity but are not of any value in diagnosing Cushing's disease.

Blood ACTH Measurements. The measurement of blood ACTH levels may be helpful in the diagnosis of Cushing's disease. The ACTH level is elevated in adrenal hyperplasia, and the characteristic diurnal variation of ACTH is absent. ACTH is absent in patients with adrenal adenomas, carcinomas, or nodular dysplasia. Thus the immunoassay of ACTH can be a helpful tool for the definitive diagnosis of Cushing's disease.

Other Tests. Various other tests may be useful in the diagnosis of Cushing's disease. Among these is the measurement of free cortisol. Although most of the urinary cortisol is conjugated, there is normally a very small amount of the free compound in the urine. The values in Cushing's disease increase from the normal level of 30 to 60 μg to levels of 200 or more per 24 hours. An increased cortisol secretion is diagnostic of Cushing's syndrome.

Some patients with a mixed syndrome will have a normal output of 17-hydroxycorticosteroids but an increased output of 17-ketogenic steroids. The measurement of 17-hydroxysteroids by the Porter-Silber method measures the usual conjugates of cortisol, but in some cases cortisol metabolism is greatly altered so that compounds are secreted that are not usually measured by the Porter-Silber method, largely cortolone. Cortolone and some of the other end products of corticosteroid metabolism are measured by the 17-ketogenic technique.

X-ray of the Sella Turcica and Angiography of the Adrenal. X-ray of the sella turcica should be made in all patients with Cushing's syndrome, particularly those with pigmentation, since a pituitary tumor is more likely under these circumstances. X-ray of the bones will frequently demonstrate pathologic fractures and osteoporosis.

Arteriograms or venograms of the adrenal are often used to localize adrenal tumors or to demonstrate hyperplasia of the adrenal in Cushing's syndrome. More recently [131]iodocholesterol emission photoscanning has been highly effective in demonstrating the adrenal lesion in Cushing's syndrome (Fig. 37-28). Occasionally an adrenal tumor can be seen on the intravenous pyelogram.

DIFFERENTIAL DIAGNOSIS. Obesity. Simple obesity can usually be differentiated from Cushing's disease because of the differences in the distribution of the fat, as shown in Fig. 37-30. Furthermore patients with Cushing's disease are seldom extremely obese; they rarely exceed 200 lb. Although obese people may have a slightly increased cortisol secretion, they show the normal diurnal variation, and their cortisol secretion is easily suppressed with dexamethasone.

Diabetes Mellitus and Hypertension. Patients with diabetes mellitus and hypertension may superficially resemble Cushing's syndrome but are easily differentiated by the various tests described above.

TREATMENT. Medical Treatment. The primary application of medical treatment in Cushing's syndrome is to inoperable carcinoma of the adrenal cortex with metastases. There may be an occasional patient, however, who is so sick that he would be an extremely poor surgical risk without a period of medical preparation.

At the present time there are four drugs which have received clinical trial. These are metyrapone, SU-9055, aminoglutethimide, and o,p'-DDD. The action of these drugs has been summarized by Lipsett.

When given by mouth in doses of 2 to 6 Gm/day in divided doses metyrapone is capable of lowering the plasma cortisol level considerably. This has been shown both for adrenocortical hyperplasia and for adrenocortical carcinoma. In metastatic adrenal cancer the response even to 6 Gm/day usually has not been good. There is relatively little toxicity. When present, the symptoms of toxicity have consisted of anorexia, nausea, and skin rash.

SU-9055 is a 17-hydroxylase and 18-hydroxylase inhibitor. It produces inhibition of aldosterone but has not been used clinically to inhibit cortisol production.

Aminoglutethimide is an anticonvulsant with the trade name of Elipten. It was withdrawn from the market because it tended to produce hirsutism and goiter. In patients with Cushing's syndrome doses of 1 to 2 Gm/day have caused significant decreases in cortisol secretion. The drug acts by blocking steroid synthesis at some point between cholesterol and pregnenolone. Benefit has also been observed in patients with Cushing's syndrome due both to adrenocortical carcinoma and to adenoma. It was not effective, however, in a case of Cushing's syndrome due to an ACTH-producing oat cell carcinoma. Fever, skin rashes, and somnolence may be permanent side effects.

The drug o,p'-DDD is unlike any of the previously mentioned drugs, since it is not an enzyme blocker and does not interfere with steroid synthesis but instead produces direct cellular damage to adrenocortical cells. There is marked species variation in the effectiveness of the drug, so that although it causes adrenocortical necrosis in the dog, it is inactive in the mouse, rat, monkey, and other animals. Some cytolytic changes have been observed in man. It has been used primarily to treat metastatic adrenocortical carcinoma. There has been some evidence of regression in 25 percent of the patients with steroid-producing carcinoma, and rarely in patients with nonfunctioning adrenocortical carcinomas.

O,p'-DDD is given in doses of 10 to 20 Gm/day for prolonged periods of time and has not produced a cure in any patient, although regressions of 3 to 5 years have been seen. The side effects of the drug are quite severe, including intolerable nausea, skin rashes, pigmentation, somnolence, nystagmus, blurring of vision, and slurring of speech. If the drug is effective in attacking the tumor, it may be necessary to give glucocorticoids to prevent adrenal insufficiency from developing. The drug has been used in doses of 2 to 5 Gm/day to treat Cushing's syndrome due to hyperplasia or adenoma.

Recently Krieger et al. have shown remission of Cushing's disease after treatment with the antiserotonin agent cyproheptadine. Effective in about 30 percent of the patients in whom it has been tried, cyproheptadine acts by inhibiting hypothalamic serotoninergic mechanisms which usually promote ACTH release.

Pituitary Irradiation. While the treatment of Cushing's disease due to adrenocortical adenoma or carcinoma is immediate surgical intervention, patients with adrenocortical hyperplasia and Cushing's syndrome may first be treated by pituitary irradiation. It is our feeling that unless the patient has a rapidly progressing Cushing's syndrome or is quite ill with hypotension (in which case immediate surgical treatment should be carried out), pituitary irradiation should be tried first. Pituitary irradiation takes at least 6 months to produce an effect, so the patient must be well enough to tolerate a 6- to 12-month wait, during or after which he may receive no benefit.

Since Cushing's syndrome due to adrenal hyperplasia is secondary to overproduction of ACTH, the objective of pituitary irradiation is to reduce ACTH secretion and perhaps prevent the development of pituitary tumors which sometimes follow bilateral adrenalectomy for Cushing's disease. The usual radiation dose is 4,000 to 5,000 r to the pituitary fossa using a ^{60}cobalt or other high-energy source. The remission rate with this technique has been variously stated to be from 10 to 60 percent but is probably somewhere in the neighborhood of 25 percent in most clinics. Proton beam irradiation has also been tried and may offer some advantages.

Fraser and Wright have recently summarized their experience with ^{90}yttrium implantation in the pituitary for Cushing's disease. Using doses up to 50,000 rads, they treated 18 patients, with death of 1 patient, satisfactory remission in 9, and partial remission in 8. Four of the eighteen patients needed a second implant. Long-term follow-up of these patients has not yet been achieved, however, and the likelihood that marked depression of other pituitary function will ensue lessens the appeal of this technique.

Since it seems probable that the increased ACTH secretion in this type of Cushing's disease comes about as a consequence of increased hypothalamic stimulus to the anterior pituitary, it is possible that in the future the disease will be treated by making discrete hypothalamic lesions in the CRF area or by increasing sophistication in the use of cyproheptadine.

At the present time it seems wise to use temporary medical management for those patients too sick to tolerate operation at once, to employ immediate surgical intervention for those patients with adenoma or nonmetastatic adrenal carcinoma, to administer ^{60}cobalt irradiation to the pituitary for those patients with adrenocortical hyperplasia in whom the disease is mild enough to tolerate a 6- to 12-month waiting period, to operate immediately on those patients with adrenocortical hyperplasia who are too sick to wait 6 months but not too sick to survive surgical treatment, and to operate on those patients who have been given a trial of x-ray therapy to the pituitary and have failed to respond. Many feel it is advisable to irradiate the pituitary following surgical treatment in all patients undergoing total bilateral adrenalectomy for Cushing's syndrome, without waiting for the possible development of a pituitary tumor. Those patients with metastatic adrenocortical carcinoma producing Cushing's disease should receive combined medical management, and those patients with ectopic tumors producing ACTH should have the tumor excised if possible. If this is not possible, adrenalectomy should be done. Patients with a pituitary tumor producing ACTH should have ^{90}yttrium or cold probe destruction of the tumor, or surgical excision of the pituitary.

Molinatti et al. have treated 24 patients with Cushing's syndrome by intrasellar implantation of ^{90}yttrium. He noted rhinorrhea in seven and fatal meningitis in two. Optic nerve injury, cerebral necrosis, and fibrosarcoma have also been noted following pituitary radiotherapy.

Preoperative Preparation. Preoperative preparation for Cushing's disease is unnecessary, as the patient already has an excess of cortisol. If the patient has received treatment with cortisol inhibitors prior to surgical treatment, it may be necessary to begin treatment with corticosteroids the night before the operation. Under ordinary circumstances, however, no particular preparation is necessary, except to correct hypokalemia if it exists. If bilateral adrenalectomy is carried out, intravenous cortisol administration is begun after removing the second adrenal, and postoperative therapy is given according to the schedule in Table 37-6.

Operative Technique. Although the transabdominal, back, and flank approaches have all been used to perform adrenalectomy for Cushing's syndrome, we prefer the posterior approach. It is our practice to take out the twelfth rib on the left and the eleventh rib on the right; this gives excellent exposure.

In most instances the presence of a tumor has been established preoperatively and has been localized by ap-

Table 37-6. SCHEDULE FOR INTRAOPERATIVE AND POSTOPERATIVE CORTICOSTEROID ADMINISTRATION AFTER ADRENALECTOMY

Day	Intravenous cortisol,* mg	Intramuscular cortisone,† mg	Oral cortisone,‡ mg
Day of operation	300	100	
First day	200	100	
Second day	100	100	
Third day	...	100	50
Fourth day	...	50	50
Fifth day	...	50	50
Sixth day	...	...	75
Thereafter	...	...	50–37.5

*Intravenous cortisol given by continuous infusion through plastic cannula. On the operative day, 100 mg is given in the first 4 hours, 100 in the next 8 hours, and 100 in the next 12 hours.

†Intramuscular cortisone acetate given in two divided doses every 12 hours.

‡Oral cortisone given in divided doses every 12 hours. Reduction from 50 to 37.5 mg should be done slowly and cautiously. Some patients have to be maintained on 50 or even 75 mg/day.

propriate angiographic studies or by the radiocholesterol scan. The side where the tumor is located is operated upon, and the entire gland containing the tumor is excised. If the patient is thought to have bilateral adrenal hyperplasia, the left side is operated upon first, because exposure here is somewhat easier and faster. If the gland appears normal or enlarged, it is removed. If the gland appears atrophic, it is biopsied but is otherwise left undisturbed, and the wound is closed. This means that the diagnosis was incorrect and that the patient has adrenocortical adenoma or carcinoma on the opposite side. In either event a similar procedure is carried out on the second side. This is easy to do and has not led to any problems. When the second side is then exposed, if bilateral adrenal hyperplasia is present, the second adrenal is also totally removed. If an adrenocortical adenoma is present, the adrenal and the adenoma on that side are totally removed.

A great deal of controversy has evolved in the past about whether a subtotal adrenalectomy or total adrenalectomy should be done, but most people now feel that a total adrenalectomy is preferable in every case. The reasons for this are that with subtotal adrenalectomy there is a high recurrence rate, difficulty in adjusting the dose of steroid replacement therapy, a high incidence of failure to cure, uncertain function of the remnant, and a likelihood of development of adrenal insufficiency. In the Mayo Clinic series there was a recurrence rate of 30 percent after subtotal adrenalectomy, and in the Massachusetts General Hospital series of 30 patients having adrenal surgical treatment other than total adrenalectomy for adrenocortical hyperplasia 10 had no relief, and of the 20 who were relieved, 9 needed further surgical treatment for recurrence. Furthermore, adrenal insufficiency has developed in patients having subtotal adrenalectomy months or years after surgical treatment despite the presence of seemingly normal adrenal function early after surgical treatment.

As one might expect, the abnormal pituitary-adrenal relationship which gave rise to the adrenal hyperplasia in the first place still persists, and Drucker et al. have noted no ACTH response and no diurnal variation in plasma cortisol levels after subtotal adrenalectomy, the stage thus being set either for recurrent Cushing's disease or adrenal insufficiency during stress. Similar findings have been reported by Egdahl and Melby. Their patients were treated either by removal of the adrenal remnant or pituitary irradiation, which greatly facilitated the maintenance of the patients with exogenous steroid therapy.

Some surgeons have advised doing a subtotal adrenalectomy and making an adrenal autotransplant of the remaining fragment in some convenient location, such as the groin, so that the fragment can easily be removed if the disease recurs. Unfortunately the fragment usually fails to function, and this procedure, while ingenious, probably is not helpful in the treatment of Cushing's disease.

When the patient has a large adrenocortical carcinoma, it may be wise to use an abdominal approach to search for metastases and, if none is found, to extend the incision into a thorocoabdominal approach to achieve a wide margin around the tumor.

Operation for Ectopic-ACTH Syndrome. If the ACTH-producing tumor is resectable, this is the procedure of choice. If not, appropriate antitumor therapy should be carried out.

Postoperative Complications. Following bilateral total adrenalectomy for Cushing's syndrome due to adrenal hyperplasia, in about 10 to 15 percent of the patients an ACTH-secreting chromophobe adenoma of the pituitary develops. This is accompanied by marked hyperpigmentation and, if the adenoma becomes large, visual symptoms. The development of these tumors is usually seen about 3 years after surgical treatment. In order to attempt to avoid this difficulty some centers give 4,000 r of irradiation of the pituitary of all patients undergoing bilateral adrenalectomy for Cushing's syndrome, unless they have had irradiation prior to the operation. Once a tumor has developed, it may be treated by irradiation, cold probe hypophysectomy, ^{90}yttrium implantation, or surgical hypophysectomy.

Although it would appear that such tumors have arisen postoperatively *in response to* the bilateral adrenalectomy, they have occasionally been detected before the operation or after partial adrenalectomy. These tumors are accompanied by very high levels of blood ACTH, as shown in Fig. 37-33*A* and *B*, and the levels are usually not easily suppressible by the administration of large amounts of corticosteroids.

Patients with Cushing's disease are more prone to infection than the average patient, and wound infections must be guarded against. The patients are also particularly prone to fungus infection. Because of the involvement of the cardiovascular system and kidney from long-standing hypertension, failure of these systems may occur in the postoperative period.

As the corticosteroid replacement dose is gradually tapered, severe corticosteroid withdrawal symptoms will sometimes develop—including fever, depression, psychosis, and sometimes even suicidal attempts. These symptoms usually disappear after the patient becomes adjusted to the lower dosage level.

Patients having bilateral adrenalectomy for Cushing's disease usually require a higher maintenance level of corticosteroids than patients having adrenalectomy for carcinoma of the breast or for other conditions in which pre-existing hyperfunction was not present.

Despite these potential complications the operative mortality in Cushing's syndrome is low, and unless metastatic neoplasm is present most patients do very well.

ADRENOGENITAL SYNDROME

The adrenogenital syndrome may appear at three different times in life—at birth, in childhood, or in adult life. The congenital adrenogenital syndrome showing symptoms at birth is by far the most common variety. Congenital adrenal hyperplasia in the female produces a pseudohermaphrodite, while in the male it produces macrogenitosomia praecox. The treatment is not operative, except for the occasional ultimate need to carry out plastic procedures on the genitalia of female pseudohermaphrodites.

The postnatal adrenogenital syndrome is usually the

result of an adenoma or carcinoma of the adrenal cortex. In the female it produces masculinization and in the male sexual precocity.

The adrenogenital syndrome appearing in adult life is usually due to a tumor and is much more common in

Fig. 37-33. Plasma ACTH levels in patients undergoing adrenalectomy. The technique used was a rather insensitive one, which is not usually capable of detecting levels in the unstressed normal individual or the patient with Cushing's disease prior to operation. *A.* There were uniformly low levels in the normal patient, in the patient undergoing adrenalectomy for carcinoma of the breast, and in Cushing's disease prior to operation. Following total adrenalectomy there was a marked increase in plasma ACTH levels, and this was particularly marked in those patients developing pigmentation postoperatively presumably on the basis of the development of the pituitary adenoma. The plasma ACTH levels in two patients having subtotal adrenalectomy for Cushing's disease was somewhat lower than those seen after total adrenalectomy, particularly for the patient who was pregnant. Pregnancy produces increased levels of corticosteroids, presumably because of the increased production of transcortin, which is produced in pregnancy, thus elevating the levels of bound cortisol. *B.* The plasma ACTH levels on a patient at various stages after total adrenalectomy. By 2 years postoperatively the patient had begun to develop pigmentation, presumably due to the formation of an ACTH-secreting chromophobe adenoma of the pituitary. This was accompanied by marked increases in the plasma ACTH level. These levels could be inhibited by the administration of intravenous cortisol but could not be inhibited by increasing the maintenance dose of cortisone from 37.5 to 50 mg/day.

women than in men. In women it produces virilism with male habitus, with or without signs of Cushing's syndrome. In the male it produces feminization or Cushing's syndrome without virilism. Mixed patterns are very common in both sexes.

In broad terms the adrenogenital syndrome refers to any situation in which there is an overproduction of androgens resulting in virilization. For this reason the symptoms of the syndrome are much more marked and distressing in the female than in the male, with the solitary exception of the salt-losing form of the syndrome, which is often overlooked in males because of the apparent lack of physical stigmata of the syndrome.

CONGENITAL ADRENAL HYPERPLASIA. Congenital adrenal hyperplasia is thought to be familial, the inheritance being by an autosomal recessive gene. The incidence has been variously estimated at from $1:5,000$ to $1:67,000$.

Classification. There are six variants of congenital adrenal hyperplasia, although by far the most common type is that seen in patients with a block of C-21 hydroxylation. The defects present in the different types are shown in Fig. 37-34.

C-21 Hydroxylation Block. This is by far the most common type of congenital adrenal hyperplasia. It results in virilization due to androstenedione secreted by the adrenal cortex and converted into testosterone. In the incomplete syndrome female infants with C-21 hydroxylation defect are pseudohermaphrodites, while the males have macrogenitosomia praecox. In about a third of the cases the defect is more complete, and subnormal amounts of aldosterone are formed, leading to a salt-losing syndrome with vascular collapse and death unless treatment with mineralocorticoids is promptly stated.

C-11 Hydroxylation Block. This produces virilization with hypertension because of the production of 11-desoxycorticosterone and 11-desoxycortisol, in addition to adrenal androgens.

3-β-Hydroxysteroid Dehydrogenase Deficiency. This produces a male or female pseudohermaphrodite with adrenal insufficiency. Since both the adrenal and the gonads require 3-β-hydroxysteroid dehydrogenase for the synthesis of their active hormones, there is a defective production of androgen by the fetal interstitial cells. Females show less masculinization than with the preceding types of adrenal hyperplasia, but males exhibit varying degrees of male pseudohermaphroditism because of the lack of androgen. These patients frequently have severe salt losing, and most of them die in early life.

C-20 Block. This block prevents the production of any active steroids, and there have been no survivors. Males exhibit pseudohermaphroditism. The patients die from adrenal insufficiency, although it is possible that with the early institution of therapy survival might be achieved. The pseudohermaphroditism of the male is caused by the failure to produce any differentiation of the female external genitalia as a consequence of the lack of androgens. The adrenals characteristically show lipoid hyperplasia.

C-18 Hydroxylation Block. This produces severe salt losing because of the absence of aldosterone and is generally fatal.

C-17 Hydroxylation Block. This produces sexual infantilism, hypertension, and hypokalemic alkalosis. The patients are unable to make androgens, estrogens, or cortisol. The hypertension and hypokalemic alkalosis result from the secretion of large quantities of corticosterone and 11-desoxycorticosterone.

Clinical Manifestations. The first two types of congenital adrenal hyperplasia produce virilism, while the rest are usually fatal and do not produce virilism. In the male the virilism produces enlargement of the penis, usually with testicular atrophy and inhibition of spermatogenesis. Short stature due to closure of the epiphyses will occur unless treatment is instituted early. Adrenal rests are often present in the testes and are sometimes mistaken for Leydig cell adenomas. If early treatment with corticosteroids is instituted, normal sexual development will usually follow.

The female with a C-21 or C-11 defect is a pseudohermaphrodite. If the diagnosis is not made at birth, it can be made later on by the early appearance of pubic hair, clitoral hypertrophy, occasional presence of pigmentation due to the high ACTH levels, and an increase in 17-ketosteroids and pregnanetriol in the urine. Premature closure of the epiphyses will lead to dwarfism unless early treatment is instituted.

The cause of the virilism is the failure of the adrenal to produce cortisol, so that ACTH secretion is unopposed, thus causing adrenal hyperplasia and the production of large quantities of androgens.

The females have masculinization varying from simple enlargement of the clitoris to complete labioscrotal fusion with a normal appearing penis. However, the uterus, tubes, and ovaries are always normal. The problem is that the severely masculinized females are often mistaken for boys at birth and raised in this sex until the mistake is discovered. Before the advent of corticosteroids this was preferable, because the virilism persisted throughout adult life. It is impossible, of course, for the patient to function sexually as a male. With adequate substitution therapy the child can grow up as a perfectly adequate female capable of full sexual activity and procreation. It is thus mandatory that affected females be reared as girls. Female pseudohermaphrodites are much more apt to be tomboys than normal female infants and also tend to have higher intelligence than average. If corrective surgical treatment for clitoral hypertrophy is not undertaken at a very early age, the question in the child's mind as to whether she is a girl or a boy may be very difficult to resolve at a later date, and some of these children—though genetically and sexually female—may elect to remain males.

Differential Diagnosis. Female pseudohermaphroditism must be differentiated from true hermaphroditism where both ovary and testes are present. Determination of chromosomal sexing (Barr bodies) with a buccal smear will confirm the female genotype in female pseudohermaphroditism. A male pseudohermaphrodite with testes and female external genitalia may resemble this syndrome but can be differentiated by genotyping. An estrogen-secreting tumor of the adrenal occasionally will produce female genitalia in a male infant.

In the male, macrogenitosomia praecox must be differ-

CORTISOL

Fig. 37-34. Alterations in the cortisol molecule seen in the adrenogenital syndrome. (1) C-21 hydroxylation block. A partial block produces simple virilization (female pseudohermaphrodite); a complete block produces virilization plus salt losing. (2) C-11 hydroxylation block. This produces virilization plus hypertension. (3) 3-β-hydroxysteroid dehydrogenase deficiency. This produces a male or female pseudohermaphrodite with adrenal insufficiency. (4) C-20 block. This produces a male pseudohermaphrodite with lipoid hyperplasia of the adrenal cortex, and no survivals. (5) C-18 hydroxylation block. This produces profound salt losing. (6) C-17 hydroxylation block. This produces sexual infantilism, hypertension, and hypokalemic alkalosis.

entiated from precocious puberty that is either idiopathic or secondary to a tumor around the third ventricle. Testicular biopsy will easily provide the differential, since in the child with precocious puberty the testicular tissue demonstrates early maturity whereas in macrogenitosomia praecox there is testicular atrophy or replacement of much of the testicular tissue with masses of adrenocortical cells.

Treatment. It is generally agreed that the child with female pseudohermaphroditism should be operated upon before she is four years of age and usually sometime after the first year. If the clitoris has not diminished significantly in size on medical management, the operation should be undertaken. It is preferable not to amputate the clitoris, although this has been advocated by some. A better procedure is to relocate it by removing the skin of the phallus, creating a tunnel leading to a buttonhole, severing the suspensory ligaments, pulling the phallus through the buttonhole, and suturing the skin around it to the edges of the hole. The skin defect at the base of the phallus is then closed over. Labioscrotal fusion is also corrected when present. The urogenital sinus is opened in the midline, the vaginal mucosa is freed on the rectal side, and the externalization of the vaginal orifice is completed by suturing the mucosa to the skin.

Even with early diagnosis by sex chromatin studies and immediate treatment with cortisone the clitoris still almost always requires plastic surgical procedures. The operation of recession and relocation of the enlarged clitoris was originally described by Lattimer and has been well illustrated by Seymour and Kinch.

POSTNATAL AND PREPUBERTAL ADRENOGENITAL SYNDROME. The postnatal and prepubertal adrenogenital syndrome is usually caused by an adenoma or carcinoma of the adrenal cortex. In the female masculinization occurs without change in the genitalia except for enlargement of the clitoris. Hirsutism, amenorrhea, short stature, and advanced bone age are characteristic. In the male pseudo-precocious puberty is seen. Signs include pubic hair, phallic enlargement, short stature, advanced bone age, and normal-sized testes, in contradistinction to congenital hyperplasia of the adrenal.

If the adrenogenital syndrome is produced by a tumor of the adrenal cortex instead of hyperplasia, there is a much-increased urinary 17-ketosteroid excretion, and this usually fails to be suppressed with corticoid administration. There is an excess production of urinary dehydroepiandrosterone rather than α-pregnanetriol, which is typical of congenital adrenal hyperplasia. No further increase in 17-ketosteroid excretion is usually seen with ACTH administration, since the tumor is already autonomous and functioning maximally.

ADULT ADRENOGENITAL SYNDROME. The adult form of the adrenogenital syndrome is usually produced by a tumor, although on occasion it may result from acquired hyperplasia. When a tumor is present, there is a large increase in the urinary excretion of 17-ketosteroids which is not suppressed with cortisol. The tumors can usually be distinguished from hyperplasia by the failure to respond to ACTH, the failure of 17-ketosteroid excretions to be suppressed by dexamethasone, and the preponderance of dehydroepiandrosterone rather than pregnanetriol in the urine. A single case has been reported in which an adult woman with a virilizing syndrome due to an adrenocortical tumor showed good suppression of 17-ketosteroid excretion by dexamethasone. The tumor was therefore dependent upon ACTH, unlike other reported cases.

In hyperplasia, ACTH produces a marked increase in 17-ketosteroid excretion in contrast to the findings when an adenoma or carcinoma is present.

The adult adrenogenital syndrome is much more common in women than in men. It produces virilism in the female, with or without some of the changes of Cushing's syndrome. Hirsutism, scanty or absent menses, decreased libido, atrophy of the breasts, male habitus, and hypertrophy of the clitoris are characteristic.

In the male the syndrome is very rare. It has been discovered only by chance and has been confirmed by the presence of an excess of androgen excretion, sometimes accompanied by testicular atrophy.

When the diagnosis of virilism due to an adrenocortical tumor is made, the tumor should be localized by arteriography, venography, and iodocholesterol scanning, and the adrenal on that side should be removed.

EXCESSES IN ANDROGEN PRODUCTION

There are a variety of situations in young women, including the Stein-Leventhal syndrome, in which there is a mild overproduction of androgens, leading to hirsutism, acne, and occasionally amenorrhea. There may be a slight increase in 17-ketosteroid excretion. Treatment is by the administration of corticosteroids or of estrogens.

ESTROGEN-SECRETING TUMORS

Feminizing adrenocortical tumors are rare. In the male the presenting sign is usually gynecomastia, occasionally with lactation. The prevalence of the various signs and symptoms are shown in Table 37-7.

The tumors are usually large and can be palpated in at least 50 percent of the cases. In the 52 cases of Gabrilove et al. there were 41 with carcinoma, 7 adenomas, and 4 of questionable nature.

The peak incidence for feminizing tumors is between ages of twenty-five and forty-five, and they occur only rarely in young boys. When the tumor occurs in young girls, it results in striking premature female sexual development. The signs of Cushing's syndrome are frequently present as well.

There is a marked increase in urinary estrogens, and often in 17-hydroxycorticosteroids and 17-ketosteroids as well. The steroids cannot be suppressed by dexamethasone or stimulated by ACTH in most cases.

In the adult male the testes show marked atrophy, and the diagnosis is based on gynecomastia and diminished libido, while in women the diagnosis is usually not apparent unless the patient has a mixed secretion and presents as a case of Cushing's syndrome.

The patient is treated by surgical excision as soon as the diagnosis is made, and this is followed by radiotherapy if the tumor is malignant. In most instances, in men, metastases are present by the time the patient is first seen, and the patient usually dies within a matter of 2 or 3 years. Metastases occur in the liver, lungs, bones, brain, and local lymph nodes and are usually hyperfunctioning. For a time after the operation libido and spermatogenesis return toward normal. Because estrogen-secreting tumors of the

Table 37-7. INCIDENCE OF SIGNS AND SYMPTOMS OF FEMINIZING TUMORS IN THE MALE (52 PATIENTS)

Sign or symptom	Percent
Gynecomastia	98
Palpable tumor	58
Atrophy of testis	52
Diminished libido and/or potency	48
Pain at site of tumor	44
Tenderness of breast	42
Pigmentation of areolae	27
Obesity	27
Feminizing hair change	23
Atrophy of the penis	20
Elevation of the blood pressure	16
Increasing skin pigmentation	12
Varicocele	11
Acne	8

SOURCE: From J. L. Gabrilove, D. C. Sharma, H. H. Wotiz, and R. I. Dorfman, *Medicine,* **44**:37, 1965.

adrenal cortex in men are so malignant and relatively insensitive to irradiation and chemotherapy, radical thoracoabdominal resection and lymphadenectomy have been advocated. Half the patients with this tumor are dead within 18 months, and the 3-year survival rate is only 20 percent. Stewart et al. pointed out that almost all the feminizing adrenal neoplasms in adult men have been malignant, whereas all those in children have been benign. However, malignant tumors occasionally have been reported in children. This is in sharp contrast to the general picture of adrenal tumors causing Cushing's syndrome, which are usually benign in adults and often malignant in children.

ADRENOCORTICAL CARCINOMAS AND TUMORS WITH MIXED SECRETIONS

MacFarlane has reported on 55 patients with adrenocortical carcinoma, and Lipsett et al. have reported on 38 such patients. In this latter series the patient's ages varied between twelve months and sixty-two years. Twenty-three of the thirty-eight patients were females, which is similar to the increased incidence of Cushing's syndrome in women. Of those adrenocortical carcinomas producing Cushing's syndrome in the adult 87 percent were in women. In the non-hormone-secreting tumors the incidence was higher in men (60 percent). Adrenocortical carcinoma occurs more often on the left side than on the right. The tumor is highly malignant, 50 percent of the patients dying within 2 years of the onset of symptoms.

The presenting complaints in most instances are those associated with virilization, Cushing's syndrome, or precocious puberty. Women usually complain of hirsutism, acne, virilism, truncal obesity, and menstrual irregularity. In patients without endocrine symptoms abdominal discomfort, pain, distension, and the presence of a mass lead to the diagnosis. Mixed pictures are common, particularly those of Cushing's syndrome and virilization. Only one woman had Cushing's syndrome alone. In addition to producing Cushing's syndrome and feminizing and virilizing syndromes adrenocortical carcinomas can produce hypokalemic alkalosis and hypoglycemia. Villee et al. reported a case of virilizing adrenocortical carcinoma in a sixteen-year-old girl which eventually produced overt Cushing's syndrome.

Adrenal cortical cancer is almost always accompanied by large amounts of 17-ketosteroids in the urine. This appears to be true whether the tumor causes Cushing's syndrome, virilization, or even feminization. It is often true even if the tumor does not have any obvious endocrine manifestations. Since excessive virilization is difficult to pick up in men, the tumor usually appears nonfunctioning in the adult male.

After surgical excision of the tumor it is important to follow the urinary excretion of steroids at frequent intervals, so that the metastases can be detected early and treatment instituted. Adrenocortical carcinomas have been treated with o,p'-DDD. Hutter and Kayhoe reported the results of the treatment of 138 patients with adrenocortical carcinoma with o,p'-DDD. A marked reduction in urinary hormone excretion occurred in 69 percent of the patients and was often associated with a reduction in endocrine symptoms. The mean duration of response was 4.8 months. Thirty-four percent of the patients had objective tumor regression, with a mean duration of about 7 months. It was felt that this type of chemotherapy should be instituted for both functioning and nonfunctioning adrenal carcinoma.

DISORDERS OF SEXUAL DEVELOPMENT

Feminizing and virilizing tumors of adrenal origin can sometimes produce changes which can be confused with disorders of sexual development. It is therefore wise to have some idea about the diagnosis of these disorders (see Chap. 41). A summary presented by Federman is reproduced in Table 37-8. Sexual development can be divided into three phases:

1. Intrauterine genital differentiation, in which an inducer of testicular origin causes the otherwise female genitalia to differentiate into the male form. In the absence of this inducer at the proper time embryologically, regardless of the genetic sex, the duct system will differentiate along female lines. Androgen, in the absence of the inducer, does not suppress the development of female structures and has an incomplete effect on male development.

Table 37-8. SUMMARY OF THE DISORDERS OF SEXUAL DEVELOPMENT

Disorders of gonadogenesis	Klinefelter's syndrome Turner's syndrome	Infertility without ambiguity
	True hermaphroditism Mixed gonadal dysgenesis Male pseudohermaphroditism (dysgenetic)	Infertility with ambiguity
Disorders of endocrinology: Androgen deficiency in the male	Male pseudohermaphroditism (familial)	
Androgen excess in the female	Female pseudohermaphroditism Congenital adrenal hyperplasia Others	Ambiguity with infertility

SOURCE: From D. D. Federman, Disorders of Sexual Development, *N Engl J Med*, **277**:353, 1967.

2. The gradual development of the secondary sex characteristics in the male brought about by androgens.
3. Fertility, which occurs at puberty.

The disorders of sexual development can be divided into three types: infertility without ambiguity in genital development, infertility with ambiguity in genital development, and ambiguity without fertility.

The patients with *Klinefelter's syndrome* are phenotypic males, with no obvious abnormality before puberty. At the time of puberty pubic hair and some body hair develops, but the beards are sparser than normal, and the patients usually have gynecomastia. The body build ranges from rather feminine to eunuchoid to normal male. A key to the diagnosis is that despite development of the pubic hair and penis, the testes are extremely small, 1.5 cm or less in longest diameter. The urinary 17-ketosteroids are normal, while the gonadotropins are increased. Plasma testosterone levels are lower than in normal males but higher than in females. The patients are almost always genotypic females with chromatin-positive nuclei. The patients with chromatin-positive Klinefelter's syndrome have at least two X chromosomes and a Y chromosome in at least some of their cells.

In *Turner's syndrome* the patients are phenotypic females with short stature, amenorrhea, lack of estrogen effect, congenital anomalies consisting of low-set ears and hairline, coarctation of the aorta, congenital lymphedema, and other changes. The patients have female external and internal genitalia, but the gonad is an undifferentiated "streak" without true germinal secretory elements. After puberty the urinary gonadotropins are increased. About 60 percent of the patients with Turner's syndrome are chromatin-negative like the normal male, but unlike Klinefelter's syndrome, where there are more chromosomes than normal, in Turner's syndrome there are fewer, usually only a single X without a Y and no second X. The remainder of the patients are chromatin-positive, but in many of these there are fewer of the female markers than one sees in the normal woman.

The *true hermaphrodites* have both ovarian and testicular tissue. They may have a testes on one side and an ovary on the other or an ova-testis on one or the other side, or combinations of these two. Both gonads are usually intra-abdominal, but the testes occasionally descend toward a scrotal position. The true hermaphodite almost invariably has a uterus and at least one tube on the ovarian side, while the other side may have some male structures. Most of these patients have been raised as males, but external virilization is seldom complete, and hypospadias and cryptorchidism are clues to the diagnosis. Gynecomastia usually develops at puberty, and about two-thirds of the patients menstruate, and half of them ovulate. The ovarian function is more nearly normal than the testicular, and an occasional true hermaphrodite may be potentially fertile. Eighty percent of hermaphrodites are chromatin-positive, or genetic females. Some of them may have mixtures of normal male and female cells, and they apparently develop from a double fertilization of the ovum, wherein the patient represents a fused fraternal twin.

Those patients with *mixed gonadal dysgenesis* have a "streak" gonad on one side similar to that of the Turner's syndrome and a testis on the other side. Other patients have a testis or a "streak" on one side and a gonadal tumor on the other. All these patients have a uterus and at least one tube but may have some male structures as well. There is an extreme variation in external appearance. A few have been normal females, others have been females with enlargement of the clitoris, while still others have graded off into male appearances with hypospadias and cryptorchidism. A very few have had the male phenotype and are normal except for unilateral cryptorchidism. At puberty the patients undergo virilism, and breast development occurs only in those who have a gonadal tumor.

These patients are always chromatin-negative, or males, which makes it easy to differentiate them at an early stage from female pseudohermaphrodites secondary to the adrenogenital syndrome. The dysgenetic male pseudohermaphrodite has two testes but incomplete virilization. Since the testes are abnormal, they fail to suppress female development, and the result is a female, or inadequate male, phenotype.

The *familial male pseudohermaphrodites* are genetic and gonadal males, with a defect in genital virilization, so that the testes secrete estrogens. They are chromatin-negative male genotypes with normal-appearing female external genitalia and breast development. At puberty they get normal breast development but no menstrual period. The vagina ends blindly, and there is no uterus. If the testes are removed before puberty, normal female breast development does not occur, and urinary estrogen levels fall immediately after orchiectomy. A patient has been reported in whom the urinary estrogen output remained normal after orchiectomy, which was considered as evidence for adrenal origin of the estrogens. The testes probably should not be removed.

ADRENALECTOMY FOR METASTATIC CANCER OF THE BREAST OR PROSTATE AND FOR HYPERTENSION

Adrenalectomy for Metastatic Breast or Prostatic Cancer

Cancer of the breast is sometimes responsive to estrogenic stimulation, and when this is the case, oophorectomy may provide a prolonged remission. Although the ovaries are the principal source of estrogen, the adrenal cortex also manufactures estrogenic substances. For this reason Dao and Huggins proposed and carried out adrenalectomy for metastatic carcinoma of the breast and, because the adrenals also manufacture androgens, for metastatic carcinoma of the prostate in patients who had previously had an orchiectomy. Dao and Huggins in 1953 reported 100 cases of patients with metastatic breast cancer who had undergone bilateral adrenalectomy. Adrenalectomy has been reported to ameliorate symptoms from metastatic carcinoma of the male breast as well.

Symptomatic improvement in metastatic carcinoma of the breast following either adrenalectomy or hypophysectomy is about 30 percent. Patients with bony or skin metastases do the best, those with lung metastases do not fare quite so well, and those with liver metastases seem to do most poorly. Block et al. in 1959 suggested that patients with cancer of the breast be selected for bilateral adrenalectomy only if they did not have liver metastases, had had a previous response to oophorectomy, had a high estrogen secretion, and had a relatively prolonged duration of the primary disease, i.e., over 3 years. Several workers have since emphasized that better results are obtained with adrenalectomy if the patient has had a positive response to oophorectomy.

In recent years it has been helpful to measure estrogen binding in tumor cells of the breast carcinoma. Only those patients demonstrating binding of estrogen to receptors on the tumor cell should receive hormonal therapy. In those patients without estrogen receptor activity the results of hormonal manipulation have been poor.

Dao and Nemoto have advocated the use of adrenalectomy as the primary therapy in patients with disseminated metastases and have claimed that involvement of over 30 percent of the liver is necessary before bilateral adrenalectomy is contraindicated.

Fracchia et al. in a report of 500 consecutive cases of adrenalectomy for metastatic cancer of the breast achieved an objective remission of 35.6 percent of the cases for 6 months or longer. Again, those patients did better the longer the interval between mastectomy and recurrence, if they were premenopausal and had shown a previous response to oophorectomy or if they were postmenopausal and vaginal smears showed a high level of estrogenic activity.

Fig. 37-35. Comparison of primary and secondary aldosteronism. In primary aldosteronism there is an obligatory secretion of aldosterone, which produces sodium retention, increased plasma volume, increased renal artery pressure, and inhibition of renin secretion. In secondary aldosteronism there is a primary decrease in renal artery pressure which stimulates the juxtaglomerular cells to secrete an increased amount of renin, thus leading to the production of angiotensin and stimulation of the adrenal cortex to produce increased amounts of aldosterone.

Bilateral Adrenalectomy for Essential Hypertension

Bilateral adrenalectomy either alone or combined with splanchnicectomy or thoracoabdominal sympathectomy used to be advocated for the treatment of hypertension. This is seldom practiced any longer.

PRIMARY ALDOSTERONISM

Primary hyperaldosteronism is characterized by hypertension, ADH-resistant polyuria, and muscle weakness due to hypokalemic alkalosis. Secondary aldosteronism has some of the same features and must be differentiated from the primary disease. There is little doubt that ACTH plays a minor but interesting role in aldosterone secretion. The chief stimulus to aldosterone production is angiotensin II.

The hormone secretion patterns in primary versus secondary aldosteronism are shown in Fig. 37-35. In the typical cases the principal endocrinologic difference is an increased renin and angiotensin secretion in secondary aldosteronism and inhibition of renin and angiotensin secretion in primary aldosteronism.

PATHOLOGY. At least 90 percent of patients with primary aldosteronism have a benign solitary adrenocortical adenoma, more commonly on the left than on the right side. These adenomas are sometimes so small that they cannot be seen or felt until the gland is sectioned. Unlike hyperparathyroidism, where the size of the tumor is roughly proportional to the degree of hypersecretion, the size of the tumor in aldosteronism has very little relation to the degree of hypersecretion. Very small tumors sometimes produce a profound hypokalemia and hypersecretion of aldosterone. The adenomas are bilateral in 5 percent of the cases or less. Bilateral adrenal glomerulosa cell hyperplasia can cause primary aldosteronism, and in these patients with hyperplasia plasma renin activity tends to be normal, rather than suppressed as it is with aldosterone-secreting adenomas. Nodular hyperplasia has also been said to cause primary aldosteronism occasionally. Rarely, primary aldosteronism is produced by an adrenocortical carcinoma.

SECONDARY ALDOSTERONISM | PRIMARY ALDOSTERONISM

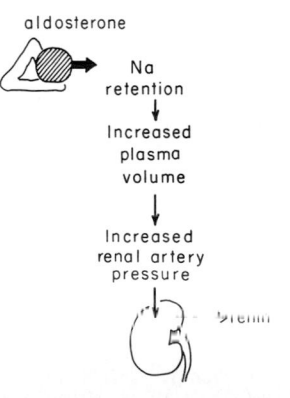

1. High aldosterone output
2. High renin output

1. High aldosterone output
2. Low renin output

A heterotopic adrenocortical adenoma has been reported to cause primary aldosteronism in one case. In a few cases mixed patterns of excessive aldosterone and excessive glucocorticoid or androgenic secretion have been observed. In some cases the excessive secretion of aldosterone can be inhibited by 2 mg/day of dexamethasone, suggesting that the stimulus to excess aldosterone secretion must have been ACTH in those patients.

Grossly the tumors are discrete, circumscribed, and sharply demarcated from the normal cortex. On cut section they are characteristically bright canary yellow. The normal cortex is not atrophic (Fig. 37-36). The microscopic pathologic features of primary aldosteronism have been summarized by Neville and Symington, who observed that the cells often do not look like the zona glomerulosa while at other times they are composed largely of zona glomerulosa–type cells. They are said to be composed of "hybrid" cells with the biochemical features of both the zona glomerulosa and the zona fasciculata. The normal zona glomerulosa is hyperplastic.

CLINICAL MANIFESTATIONS. The most common incidence is between the ages of thirty and fifty, but the disease has been seen in children as young as three and adults as old as seventy-five. It is twice as common in women. Conn originally thought that the incidence of the disease might be as high as 20 percent of patients with essential hypertension, but it is now clear that only about 1 to 2 percent of the hypertensive population have primary aldosteronism.

Kaplan studied 75 patients with thiazide-induced hypokalemia and hypertension and found that none of them had primary aldosteronism. Furthermore the content of aldosterone in small adenomas seen in some patients with essential hypertension is similar to that seen in normal adrenal tissue and much less than the amounts present in adenomas of patients with primary aldosteronism. It seems likely, therefore, that many of the incidental adrenal tumors which were found in patients with hypertension and which Conn speculated were the cause of the hypertension did not actually function. This contention is further borne out by an autopsy study of Kokko et al. indicating that the incidence of hypertension was the same in patients who had adrenal adenomas, adrenal hyperplasia, or no adrenal disease. Fishman et al. found that subnormal plasma renin was characteristic of certain patients with essential hypertension and that primary aldosteronism rarely occurred in hypertensive patients with normal serum potassium levels.

Fig. 37-36. Section cut through an aldosterone-producing tumor and a portion of the normal cortex. The tumor was a rather large one which was well circumscribed. The cut surface was bright yellow, and there was no atrophy of the normal adrenal cortex.

Table 37-9. SIGNS AND SYMPTOMS OF PRIMARY ALDOSTERONISM

Causes	Signs and symptoms
Hypertension and Na retention ..	Hypertension
	Headache
	Cardiac enlargement
Hypokalemia and K deficit	Muscle weakness and paralysis
	Tetany
	Paresthesias and muscle cramps
	Diabetic glucose tolerance curve
	Hypokalemic renal damage
Hypokalemic renal damage	Polyuria
	Polydipsia
	Nocturia
	Proteinuria
Hypernatremia	Increased blood volume (edema rare)

The symptoms and signs of primary aldosteronism are shown in Table 37-9, and the incidence of the major symptoms in Table 37-10. The most common symptoms and signs of primary aldosteronism are hypertension, muscle weakness, polydipsia, headache, nocturnal polyuria, and hypokalemic alkalosis.

Hypertension is frequently mild, and the retinal and renal changes of malignant hypertension are almost never seen. In contrast to pheochromocytoma, where there may be a contracted blood volume and severe, often episodic hypertension, in primary aldosteronism there is expanded blood volume and relatively mild sustained hypertension.

The disease is thus characterized by hypertension without grade IV retinopathy, hypokalemic alkalosis, overwhelming of the kidney's ability to conserve sodium, an increased aldosterone excretion, increased plasma aldosterone, decreased or undetectable levels of plasma renin, normal corticosteroid secretion, the absence of hyponatremia, and a normal renal arteriogram.

It is usually not difficult to differentiate secondary from

Table 37-10. FREQUENCY OF SYMPTOMS AND SIGNS IN CLASSIC PRIMARY ALDOSTERONISM

Symptoms and signs	Percent
Hypertension	100
Hypokalemia	100
High aldosterone	95
Polyuria	92
Polydipsia	84
Alkalosis	76
Albuminuria	68
Paresthesias	58
Periodic paralysis	38
Edema	Less than 10

SOURCE: After Conn.

primary aldosteronism, even though both may be accompanied by hypertension, increased aldosterone secretion, hypokalemia, and alkalosis. The plasma sodium level is usually lower in secondary hyperaldosteronism, the plasma renin levels are elevated rather than low, and a cause for the secondary aldosteronism—usually renal artery stenosis or malignant hypertension—can be demonstrated by the proper tests, including renal arteriograms.

A variant of classic primary aldosteronism has been described by Conn et al. under the title of "normokalemic primary aldosteronism." In these patients there is hypertension with increased aldosterone secretion and low plasma renin levels with normal serum potassium and cure of the hypertension by removal of an adrenal cortical tumor. This can be viewed as an early or prehypokalemic phase of the disease.

Proteinuria may be present as a consequence of the renal damage brought about by hypokalemia, and this is also the cause of the nocturnal polyuria.

There are some other rather rare variants of aldosteronism, including normotension with primary hyperaldosteronism in the early stages, and primary aldosteronism in patients who have become so potassium-depleted that they are secreting normal amounts of aldosterone. After restoration of normal potassium stores a very high level of aldosterone secretion can be demonstrated.

DIAGNOSTIC TESTS. The tests for primary aldosteronism may be divided into two categories, the first designed to establish the presence of hyperaldosteronism and the second to distinguish between primary and secondary hyperaldosteronism (Table 37-11).

Diagnostic Tests to Establish the Presence of Hypersecretion of Aldosterone. *Plasma Potassium and Sodium.* In primary aldosteronism there is typically a low potassium level and a high normal or elevated plasma sodium level, although normokalemic primary aldosteronism has been reported by Conn et al. The plasma potassium level is also low in secondary aldosteronism, but the sodium concentration is normal or low. Brown et al. found a good inverse correlation between plasma sodium and renin levels. Thus the greater the degree of secondary aldosteronism and renin secretion, the lower the sodium. Schacht and Frame have advocated the use of chlorothiazide to intensify the hypokalemia as a diagnostic aid. Chlorothiazide does produce more profound depression of the plasma potassium level in patients with primary aldosteronism than it does in other patients, and indeed in one of our patients it brought on paralysis, but Kaplan has shown that in many patients with essential hypertension hypokalemia develops on thiazide medication, and therefore it is probably not a discriminating test.

ECG. Severe hypokalemia produces *ECG* changes that may be helpful in establishing the diagnosis. The *ECG* changes in a patient with primary aldosteronism before and after operative removal are shown in Fig. 37-37. The changes characteristic of hypokalemia were present preoperatively and reverted to normal after removal of an aldosterone-secreting tumor.

Urinary Potassium (K) and Sodium (Na) Measurements. The patients suspected of having primary aldosteronism should be placed on normal sodium intake and taken off diuretics before coming into the hospital, since a low so-

Table 37-11. DIAGNOSTIC TESTS FOR ALDOSTERONISM

Test	Primary aldosteronism	Secondary (renal) aldosteronism	Normal or essential hypertension
To detect hyperaldosteronism:			
Serum K	3 mEq/100 ml or less	3 mEq/100 ml or less	Over 3 mEq/100 ml
Serum Na	High normal or high	Normal or low	Normal
Urine K on high-Na diet	Often exceeds intake <20 mEq/day rules out >30 mEq/day likely >50 mEq/day diagnostic	20–40 mEq/day	Less than intake, usually <20 mEq/day
Urine K on low-Na diet	Falls	Falls	Increases
Aldosterone excretion in urine	>10 μg/day, often 15–50 μg/day	>10 μg/day, often 25–100 μg/day	10 μg/day or less
Aldosterone secretion rate	>170 μg/day	>170 μg/day	60–170 μg/day
Spironolactone test	Rise in serum K 1 mEq/L or more	Rise in serum K 1 mEq/L or more	Low K does not rise
To differentiate primary from secondary hyperaldosteronism:			
Plasma renin on high-Na diet	Low or absent	High	Normal
Plasma renin on low-Na diet	Low or absent	Very high	High
Aldosterone response to DCA administration	No change	Falls	Falls
Renal vein renin	Low	High	Normal
Adrenal vein aldosterone	High on side with tumor	High both sides	Normal
Renal arteriography	Normal	Arterial lesion	Normal
Adrenal angiography	Tumor present	No tumor	No tumor
Angiotensin infusion	Blood pressure rises	No blood pressure change	Blood pressure rises

Na 143
K 1.2

Na 147
K 2.2

Na 143
K 3.6

Na 139
K 4.3

Fig. 37-37. ECG of a patient with primary aldosteronism. All the tracings are from lead V$_2$. The top strip was taken just after stopping the chlorothiazide diuretic which the patient had been receiving for some time. There are marked signs of hypokalemia including ST depression, inversion of the T wave, a prolonged ST interval, and U waves. The second strip was taken a week after cessation of the diuretic therapy and, despite some improvement in the plasma potassium level, still shows a markedly prolonged ST interval and well-developed U waves. The third strip shows tracing taken in the early postoperative period. There is marked improvement in the tracing with upright T waves, a shortening of the ST interval, and the absence of U waves. The last tracing was taken 10 days after the operation and is essentially a normal tracing.

dium intake will produce increased aldosterone secretion even in normal people. The patient with hyperaldosteronism and normal or elevated sodium intake loses excessive amounts of potassium in the urine, while salt restriction produces an immediate fall in urinary potassium excretion (Fig. 37-38). Postoperatively a high salt intake no longer produces excessive potassium loss. The patient should be on a constant potassium intake throughout the 6 days of the test, with 3 days of increased salt intake and 3 days of low salt intake.

Urinary Specific Gravity with Pitressin. Patients with hyperaldosteronism characteristically have large volumes of urine with a low specific gravity. This is resistant to ADH, so that the failure to increase the urinary concentration with the administration of Pitressin can be used as a further diagnostic test.

Aldosterone Excretion in the Urine. If a patient has been on chlorothiazide diuretics or a low-sodium diet, these should be stopped for at least a month before measuring the urinary aldosterone excretion. Under circumstances of normal salt intake the normal patient will excrete less than 10 μg/day in the urine, while the patient with primary aldosteronism will excrete greater amounts, often between 15 and 50 μg/day. The patient with secondary aldosteronism will also excrete increased amounts of aldosterone, and often even greater amounts than are commonly seen in primary aldosteronism.

Espiner et al. have proposed the measurement of urinary aldosterone produced in response to an infusion of saline solution as a diagnostic test for aldosteronism. Patients are placed on a diet of 10 mEq of sodium and 60 mEq of potassium daily. After 5 days of this diet the patients are given 2,000 ml of physiologic saline solution over a 4-hour period on 2 consecutive days. Normal persons show a profound fall of aldosterone excretion, while patients with primary aldosteronism show only very small changes.

Induction of Hypokalemia by Oral Sodium Loading. It is helpful to give oral sodium chloride, 8 Gm/day for 4 days, to low-normokalemic patients suspected of having primary aldosteronism. At the end of this period the serum potassium may be distinctly low in the patients with hyperaldosteronism.

Aldosterone Secretion Rate. Although this test is still not available for general use, the rate of aldosterone secretion can be computed by giving the patient a small amount of radioactive aldosterone and measuring the amount of radioactivity and aldosterone excreted in the urine. The normal patient secretes between 60 and 170 μg/day, while patients with aldosteronism secrete greater amounts.

Spironolactone Test. The spironolactone test developed by Biglieri et al. consists of giving 100 Gm of Aldactone four times a day for 3 days while the patient is on normal sodium intake. The serum potassium level should rise by at least 1 mEq/L if aldosterone excess is present. Patients with hypokalemia from other causes will not show an increase. We have not found this to be a particularly useful test.

Tests to Differentiate Primary from Secondary Aldosteronism. Differentiation between primary and secondary aldosteronism is usually not difficult, since advanced renal disease is easy to detect and is usually accompanied by severe eye ground changes which are almost never seen in primary aldosteronism.

Plasma Renin Activity. Plasma renin levels are measured in the supine patient who is on a normal sodium intake. If primary aldosteronism is present, the values will be normal, low, or not measurable, while in secondary aldosteronism they will be high.

Aldosterone Excretion Response to DCA Administration. Biglieri et al. have developed a test in which the patient is given deoxycorticosterone acetate (DCA), 5 mg twice daily, for 3 consecutive days. If primary aldosteronism is

Fig. 37-38. The urinary and plasma sodium and potassium findings in primary aldosteronism. *A.* On a regular diet with an adequate intake of salt and potassium there is marked urinary potassium wasting, with daily urinary potassium excretions exceeding 50 mEq/L. When a low-sodium diet is instituted, there is an immediate sharp decline in urinary potassium excretion. On resumption of a normal sodium intake there is an immediate increase in urinary potassium excretion to levels which equal or exceed the intake. The plasma potassium level shows a fall during high-salt-intake periods and a rise during low-salt-intake periods. *B.* Same patient as in *A.* There is a striking urinary potassium wasting on a regular diet with a sudden and striking decrease on a low-salt diet. During the first period there is an increase in the plasma potassium level despite the high salt intake in response to stopping the diuretic. *C.* Same patient as in *A* and *B.* The patient was prepared for operation with a low-salt diet and adequate amounts of potassium. This produced a fall in the plasma sodium level and a rise in the plasma potassium level. Following excision of the adenoma there is a steady increase in the plasma potassium level.

present, the urinary aldosterone excretion will be unchanged, while if the patient has secondary aldosteronism, there will be a marked fall in the urinary aldosterone output.

Arterial and Venous Catheter Studies. Catheters may be inserted into the renal veins or into either adrenal vein. An elevated renin level in the renal venous blood establishes the diagnosis of secondary aldosteronism, and if the level is elevated on only one side, this pinpoints the site of the pathologic change. Catheterization of the adrenal vein reveals an elevated aldosterone level in primary aldosteronism. This is elevated only on the side of the tumor. In secondary aldosteronism levels may be elevated on both sides. In the instances of primary aldosteronism due to bilateral adrenal hyperplasia, elevated aldosterone levels will be found on both sides.

Angiography of the adrenal gland, both venous and arterial, can be used to demonstrate the location of the tumor. Venous angiography is not without hazard in hyperaldosteronism because the adrenal veins are notoriously fragile in this condition and adrenal hemorrhage may occur even with gentle retrograde injection of the contrast medium. Renal arteriography demonstrates the site of the

lesion in renal artery stenosis and may demonstrate disease of the intrarenal vessels in malignant hypertension due to intrinsic renal disease.

[131]*Iodocholesterol Adrenal Scan.* Beierwaltes and his coworkers have recently developed a photoscan of the adrenals. This technique images tissue in which iodinated cholesterol is concentrated. The adrenal cortex is such a tissue. Conn et al. have applied this technique, with good success, to the study of patients with primary hyperaldosteronism. Hyperfunctioning aldosteronomas appear as "hot spots" which are not suppressed with dexamethasone; in patients in whom adrenocortical hyperplasia causes the hyperaldosteronism, iodocholesterol uptake will be suppressed with administration of dexamethasone (Fig. 37-39). Conn has recently shown clear separation of these two groups using this technique. As we shall see later, it is an important distinction to make.

Angiotensin Infusion. An indirect measurement of renin-angiotensin activity in plasma using an intravenous infusion of angiotensin has been developed. In patients with secondary aldosteronism and increased levels of renin and angiotensin in the plasma there will be no blood pressure response to the infusion of angiotensin, while in

Fig. 37-39. A radio-cholesterol scan from a patient with primary hyperaldosteronism. In the right adrenal, imaged on the right side of the print-out, is an obvious area of focal increased uptake. The scan in the right half of the photograph was exposed after dexamethasone suppression. Normal adrenal tissue has been suppressed, but the increased uptake of the aldosterone-secreting tumor of the right adrenal persists.

patients with primary aldosteronism the infusion will produce a rise in blood pressure, as it will in the normal person.

SPECIAL CONSIDERATIONS. Normokalemic Primary Aldosteronism. This can be diagnosed with the routine tests used for any patient with primary aldosteronism, except that it is more difficult to recognize initially, and the urinary potassium studies are less apt to be diagnostic unless careful balance studies are done. These normokalemic patients characteristically have hypertension, increased aldosterone excretion, and suppressed plasma renin levels. Oral sodium loading, mentioned previously, may uncover their hypokalemia.

Bilateral Adrenal Hyperplasia. In a few cases typical primary aldosteronism is produced by bilateral adrenal hyperplasia. Adrenalectomy has not produced good resolution of the hypertension in the hyperplasia patients. For this reason many patients with hyperplasia are being treated medically with spironolactone, an aldosterone antagonist. In two cases of hyperplasia reported in a father and son, the entire clinical syndrome was relieved by the administration of 2 mg dexamethasone a day.

Normotensive Primary Aldosteronism. In the early phases of primary aldosteronism patients will sometimes be found who are hypokalemic and have all the other features of aldosteronism without hypertension. A high-sodium diet will sometimes reveal the hypokalemia.

Primary Aldosteronism with Normal Aldosterone Output. If the patient has undergone profound potassium depletion over a long period of time, aldosterone secretion may be diminished to normal levels. The diagnosis can be made by replenishing the potassium stores, after which markedly elevated levels of aldosterone can be detected.

Congenital Aldosteronism. There have been some patients described by Conn as having congenital aldosteronism who probably have malignant hypertension and secondary hyperaldosteronism. Some of these patients, however, may have bilateral adrenal hyperplasia.

DIFFERENTIAL DIAGNOSIS (Table 37-12). **Secondary Aldosteronism.** The differential diagnosis of secondary aldosteronism has been defined above. The differential can usually be established by plasma renin measurements.

Juxtaglomerular Cell Hyperplasia. Bartter et al. described the syndrome of juxtaglomerular hyperplasia with hyperaldosteronism and hypokalemia. At least 20 such patients have been detected. The cause of the syndrome is apparently impairment of the vascular response to angiotensin. The decrease in pulse pressure acts as a constant stimulus to the release of renin from the juxtaglomerular apparatus and leads to hypertrophy of these cells. Secondary aldosteronism develops as a consequence of the effects of angiotensin on the adrenal. Aldosterone levels are increased, the plasma renin level is markedly elevated, and the blood pressure is normal.

Cushing's Syndrome. Cushing's syndrome may be associated with hypertension and marked hypokalemia but can easily be differentiated by its physical features and the high levels of cortisol.

Potassium-wasting Renal Disease. Although many patients originally thought to have potassium-losing nephritis

Table 37-12. DIFFERENTIAL DIAGNOSIS OF ALDOSTERONISM

Clinical state	Aldosterone production	Plasma renin	Hypertension	Hypokalemia	Special features
Primary aldosteronism	High	Low	Yes—benign	Yes	
Normokalemic primary aldosteronism (Conn)	High	Low	Yes	No	High Na intake produces hypokalemia.
Normoaldosteronal primary aldosteronism (Biglieri)	Normal	Low	Yes	Severe	Aldosterone output increases with K replacement.
Normotensive primary aldosteronism	High	Low	No	Yes	
ACTH-dependent aldosteronism (Sutherland)	High	Low	Yes	Yes	Aldosterone output suppressed with dexamethazone.
Congenital aldosteronism (Conn)	High	....	Yes—usually malignant	Yes	Probably secondary to renal disease.
Secondary aldosteronism:					
Renal artery stenosis	High or normal	High	Yes—benign or malignant	Occasional	
Intrinsic renal ischemia	Usually high	High	Malignant	Frequent	
Juxtaglomerular hyperplasia (Bartter)	High	High	No	Yes	Impaired vascular response to angiotensin.
Secondary aldosteronism without renin (Laragh)	High	Low	Yes	Yes	Hypoplasia of juxtaglomerular cells. Nonrenin stimulus to aldosterone secretion.
Renal K wasting	Variable	....	No or benign	Yes	Acidosis, hyponatremia, hypovolemia.
With hypomagnesemia	Variable	High	No	Yes	Mg loss in urine.
With Na conservation	Low	Low	Yes	Yes	
Cushing's syndrome	Normal	Low or normal	Yes—benign	Occasional	Cortisol secretion increased.

have since been shown to have primary aldosteronism, there continue to be some patients who waste potassium because of a primary renal defect. The hypokalemia is associated with metabolic acidosis rather than alkalosis, hyponatremia rather than hypernatremia, and hypovolemia rather than hypervolemia. The production of aldosterone may be increased because of the impairment of the resorption of sodium. The plasma renin activity may be high.

Familial Disorders Mimicking Aldosteronism. Two familial disorders have recently been reported which could be confused with primary aldosteronism. In the first of these there is hypomagnesemia resulting from impaired conservation of magnesium by the kidney. These patients secondarily developed hypokalemia but are normotensive. The second disorder consists of a renal tubular defect characterized by increased reabsorption of sodium and thus excessive loss of potassium leading to hypokalemia. There is low renin activity in the plasma but decreased, rather than increased, production of aldosterone. These patients are hypertensive.

Other Causes of Hypokalemia. There are many other causes of hypokalemia including diarrhea, hypoparathyroidism, licorice addiction (the glycyrrhizic acid acts like aldosterone), small bowel fistula, chronic thiazide diuretic therapy, cirrhosis, and amyloidosis. The differentiation of primary aldosteronism from these causes is usually fairly easy.

TREATMENT. Medical Management. Spironolactone is an antagonist of aldosterone at the level of the kidney tubule but does not alter the production of aldosterone by the adrenal. The use of this substance to treat patients with primary aldosteronism has been summarized by Melby. As the spironolactone reduces serum sodium and elevates serum potassium levels, the hypertension is reduced. This substance does not have a similar effect in patients with secondary aldosteronism. The headaches and nocturnal polyuria vanish.

There are other drugs which act as antagonists to aldosterone, including progesterone and its derivatives. Recently a new heparinlike compound, heparinoid RO1-8307, has been utilized. This compound depresses aldosterone secretion rather than inhibiting its action on the kidney. Since surgical treatment in primary aldosteronism is primarily to correct the hypokalemia and thus prevent continuing damage to the kidney and other organs, these substances may find a place in the permanent treatment of this disease. At present it seems that their chief usefulness might be in patients with primary aldosteronism and mild hypertension who are found to have adrenal hyperplasia rather than a tumor. At the moment, however, the ideal treatment for an adrenal cortical adenoma producing primary aldosteronism is surgical removal, since this is safe and curative, and does not require substitution therapy.

Surgical Therapy. Preoperatively the patient with hyperaldosteronism should be placed on low-sodium, high-potassium intake. The serum potassium level should be raised to 3 mEq/L or more prior to surgical treatment.

Some have advocated the use of spironolactone as pre-operative preparation to aid in raising the plasma potassium level, though we have usually not found this necessary.

Operative Technique. Many prefer a simultaneous bilateral posterior approach for primary aldosteronism. The patients are usually thin, and exposure of the glands is easy. The adenomas are usually relatively small, discrete, smooth, and rounded. The entire gland is removed. The adenomas are seldom bilateral, but the other adrenal should be explored, with care not to injure its blood supply. On rare occasions a heterotopic adrenocortical adenoma causing primary aldosteronism may occur. One such case, in which the adenoma was located in the kidney, has been reported by Flanagan et al.

If no adrenal tumor is palpable at surgery, the adrenal which yielded the higher aldosterone content in its venous blood should be removed. Microscopic adenomas have been found in meticulous serial sections of such glands, and in one of our patients hypertension has resolved. If the sections should ultimately show hyperplasia, spironolactone therapy can easily be instituted.

The importance of obtaining adrenal venous blood samples for the localization of aldosteronomas has been stressed by Melby et al. Egdahl, Kahn, and Melby, using this technique, have been able to localize the site of the tumor in eight consecutive patients prior to operation and in two instances to localize two adenomas which were less than 0.3 cm in diameter. These were not palpable at operation, and could not be identified with certainty until the gland was sectioned after its removal. The increased rate of aldosterone production by these tumors was indicated by incubation studies after removal, which showed that the tumor was producing much more aldosterone than the normal zona glomerulosa of the remainder of the gland. This would certainly seem to be an important adjuvant to the surgical treatment of aldosteronomas, particularly in patients in whom the disease has been discovered very early in its course.

Postoperative Complications. Some writers have described hypoadrenocorticism after removal of one adrenal and exploration of the other. However, this can be avoided at operation by careful handling of the gland.

The blood pressure usually returns to normal in a matter of weeks unless severe renal changes have been present. The serum sodium levels may be low for a time in the postoperative period, but this can be counteracted by giving the patient large amounts of sodium immediately postoperatively (see Fig. 37-38).

ADRENOCORTICAL INSUFFICIENCY (ADDISON'S DISEASE)

Adrenocortical insufficiency is a relatively rare occurrence in the surgical patient, but since failure to recognize it may lead to the death of the patient, it is extremely important that it be kept in mind and recognized early.

ETIOLOGY. Classic Addison's disease in the past has frequently been due to bilateral adrenal tuberculosis, but in recent years with a general decline in tuberculosis bilateral atrophy is a somewhat more common cause. The most frequent cause for the atrophy is apparently an autoimmune mechanism which brings about a self-destruction of the adrenal cortex. Autoantibodies against adrenal tissue can usually be identified in this disease, and other glands are sometimes simultaneously involved with a similar process. There are also other agents which can bring about adrenal destruction, including fungus infection, amyloidosis, vascular lesions, and adrenal hemorrhage. Classic Addison's disease develops slowly and is usually not recognized until it has reached the chronic state.

The combination of Addison's disease and hypothyroidism, presumably on an immunologic basis, has been called "Schmidt's syndrome," although it was described many years earlier. The rather frequent coexistence of Addison's disease and diabetes mellitus has been thought to be due to antibodies to both the corticosteroid-secreting cells of the adrenal and the insulin-secreting islet cells of the pancreas. The frequency of extraadrenal endocrine deficiencies in patients with Addison's disease has recently been studied and in 32 patients was found to be 41 percent. Nineteen percent had diabetes, and 23 percent had primary gonadal disease. While this association is present in idiopathic adrenal insufficiency, presumably due to autoantibodies, it is not present in Addison's disease due to tuberculosis. Hereditary Addison's disease is sometimes associated with hypoparathyroidism or diabetes.

Hereditary, familial, and congenital Addison's disease has been reported, as has congenital absence or marked hypoplasia of the pituitary gland with secondary atrophy of the adrenal. Familial Addison's disease is sometimes associated with spastic paraplegia with or without gliosis of the cerebral hemispheres and with hypoparathyroidism, diabetes, and moniliasis. Hereditary familial adrenal atrophy and fibrosis also occur as an isolated autosomal recessive genetic defect. The adrenogenital syndrome is another congenital defect which may be associated with adrenal insufficiency.

Patients have been reported who show none of the usual stigmata of Addison's disease and who have relatively normal urinary 17-hydroxycorticosteroid excretion but who nonetheless fail to respond normally to ACTH. A 1-hour response of plasma corticosteroids to 25 units of ACTH has recently been reported as a method to detect such patients. A taste test has also been advocated to detect adrenal insufficiency. This is based on the fact that patients with Addison's disease are hypersensitive to the taste of salt and can detect the difference between a 1 mM/L saline solution and distilled water, whereas none of the normal subjects could detect less than 6 mM/L. The patients with Addison's disease also have a hypersensitivity to galvanic current applied to the tongue.

Isolated hypoaldosteronism, a reflection of a renin deficiency syndrome, has been reported by Schambelan et al. In these patients other aspects of adrenal cortical function were normal.

Some toxic substances, such as o,p'-DDD, interfere with adrenal production of corticosteroids and may produce adrenocortical insufficiency. Infection can cause adrenal insufficiency by hemorrhage into the glands or by tubular degeneration of the adrenals. Bilateral adrenal hemorrhage as a consequence of infection, the so-called Waterhouse-Friderichsen syndrome, is usually produced by meningococcal septicemia, and is usually seen in children under the age of two, although it has been described in adults. There is some question whether the patients actually die of adrenal insufficiency or of the effects of the meningococcal septicemia, the adrenal hemorrhage simply being a terminal manifestation of the disease. It seems likely that the latter is more often the case, the adrenal hemorrhage and consequent insufficiency developing so close to the terminal phase as to have little effect on the course of the disease. In adults with severe infection degeneration of the adrenal cortex can occur even without hemorrhage. This again is most commonly seen with meningococcal infections, but it is also occasionally seen with pneumococcal, streptococcal, and diphtherial infections. Adrenal insufficiency is occasionally seen in the severely burned patient with invasive sepsis.

There are four circumstances in which the adrenal can be occasionally destroyed by hemorrhage in addition to sepsis. Bilateral adrenal hemorrhage has been seen in the newborn infant as a consequence of asphyxia, syphilis, or eclampsia of the mother. Hemorrhage and necrosis of the maternal adrenals will occasionally occur during pregnancy, the cause being unknown. Bilateral adrenal hemorrhage has occurred as a consequence of anticoagulant therapy and in some instances has led to the death of the patient from adrenal insufficiency. It has been seen with both Coumadin and heparin. Hemorrhage into an adrenal tumor will occasionally produce destruction of the remainder of the gland; this can produce adrenal insufficiency if the opposite adrenal has been removed or is involved in a similar destructive process. Bilateral adrenal hemorrhage and adrenal insufficiency sometimes occur spontaneously for no discernible reason in patients with chronic illness or with cancer.

The adrenal is not infrequently the site of metastases, particularly from carcinoma of the lung or breast, but it is very rare for these metastases to produce sufficient destruction to lead to adrenal insufficiency.

Surgical excision of the pituitary or adrenal may lead to adrenal insufficiency if the patient's maintenance dose of corticosteroids is too low, if the patient forgets to take his medication, or if the patient is subject to an intercurrent infection or trauma without an increase in the maintenance dose. Patients with Cushing's disease and bilateral total adrenalectomy require more corticosteroid maintenance than patients who have had adrenalectomy for cancer of the breast. The development of adrenal insufficiency in patients who have had subtotal adrenalectomy for Cushing's disease, with uncertain or variable function of the remaining fragment, is one of the reasons why this operation has been largely abandoned in favor of total adrenalectomy with total replacement.

In bilateral pheochromocytoma, a fragment of one or both adrenal cortices, if left behind, will usually maintain the patient. However, temporary Addison's disease may develop until this occurs, and the patient has to be closely watched.

Pituitary insufficiency leads to secondary adrenal insufficiency which is not as severe as that seen in classic Addison's disease. Since aldosterone secretion depends only partially on ACTH stimulation, urinary salt wasting is less likely to occur in patients with pituitary insufficiency than in those with primary adrenal disease. Nevertheless these patients are often hypoglycemic, and they withstand trauma poorly without adequate adrenocortical support therapy. By far the most common cause of adrenal insufficiency at the present time is that secondary to the administration of adrenal corticosteroids. This suppresses the secretion of ACTH and leads to atrophy of the adrenal. After discontinuance of the corticosteroid therapy it may take a long time for adrenal reactivity to return. The patient may therefore have relative adrenal insufficiency if he is operated upon without supportive therapy. If operation is contemplated and the facilities are available, it is wise to carry out an ACTH stimulation test with plasma corticosteroid levels to determine whether the adrenal is reactive or not. If such facilities are not available, it is wise to put the patient on corticosteroid therapy during the acute phase of the operation.

CLINICAL MANIFESTATIONS. Adrenal cortical insufficiency may become apparent in any of four clinical patterns, depending on the time of development. The first of these is adrenal insufficiency appearing shortly after birth as a consequence of the salt-wasting variant of the adrenogenital syndrome. The insufficiency, of the salt-losing type, is manifested by fever, weight loss, vomiting, hyponatremia, shock, and marked salt loss in the urine. Symptoms often appear within the first week after birth and sometimes may not become noticeable for 5 or 6 weeks.

Chronic adrenocortical insufficiency due to classic Addison's disease which has been present for many months or years before operation or trauma is usually recognizable by the characteristic pigmentation, weakness, weight loss, hypotension, easy fatigability, and sometimes nausea, vomiting, abdominal pain, hypoglycemia, hyponatremia, and hyperkalemia. An x-ray of the abdomen may show adrenal calcification if the disease is caused by tuberculosis but will not be suggestive if the disease is due to an autoimmune mechanism. A chest x-ray will usually show reduced heart size. The diagnosis is confirmed by demonstration of reduced urinary corticosteroid excretion and the failure of plasma corticosteroids to increase in response to an infusion of ACTH. If such a patient is operated upon without establishing the diagnosis, death will usually occur within a matter of 3 to 6 hours.

The third form of adrenal insufficiency is acute Addisonian crisis. This may occur in response to injury or operative trauma, or it may occur spontaneously and mimic some other type of acute illness. It is accompanied by fever, shock, lethargy, somnolence or coma, nausea, vomiting, and abdominal pain. If unrecognized and untreated, it may lead to death in a short time. The diagnosis is confirmed by low levels of blood corticosteroid. Hypoglycemia, hyponatremia, and hyperkalemia will usually be present. The electrolyte changes are more apt to occur in the chronic Addisonian patient, whereas if the patient has adrenal insufficiency as a consequence of steroid administration ending in the recent past, the electrolyte changes and shock may not manifest themselves until the preterminal or terminal period.

The fourth type of adrenal insufficiency which is seen surgically is that of semiacute adrenal insufficiency. This is not present prior to operation but develops during surgery or in the immediate postoperative period. It has been seen when anticoagulants are begun in the immediate postoperative period producing bilateral adrenal hemorrhage which destroys the adrenals. It is also occasionally seen in the severely burned patient in whom invasive infection leads to adrenal insufficiency. When the adrenal insufficiency begins with, or immediately after, the operative insult, the symptoms are much slower to develop than when the patient has had preexisting adrenal insufficiency and is then operated upon. Instead of the patient's dying in a matter of hours, the development of symptoms takes place in a matter of days. Insufficiency is usually manifested in convalescence by weakness, abdominal distension, decreased peristalsis, anorexia, nausea, and general lassitude out of proportion to that expected. These symptoms usually begin to appear on the third or fourth postoperative day and gradually become worse during the next 3 or 4 days. If the condition is unrecognized and untreated, death is apt to ensue in about 7 to 10 days. There is a progressive hypoglycemia and hyponatremia, and the hyponatremia continues in spite of the intravenous administration of large amounts of saline solution. It is accompanied by massive urinary sodium loss. The diagnosis is made by measuring the 24-hour urinary sodium to document the marked salt wasting. This can be immediately corrected by deoxycorticosterone, and the response to this drug is a diagnostic finding. The further demonstration that the patient is unresponsive to ACTH clinches the diagnosis. The adrenal insufficiency is usually permanent.

Adrenal hemorrhage and infarction are sometimes seen as a consequence of adrenal vein thrombosis after adrenal venograms. A review of bilateral adrenal hemorrhage has been published by Jagatic and Rubnitz. The hemorrhages have occurred in response to involution and destruction of the glands in newborn babies, capillary wall damage, accompanying toxemia, various hemorrhagic disorders, adrenal vein thrombosis, electric shock therapy, pregnancy and delivery, anticoagulant therapy, exogenous corticosteroid therapy, and aortic aneurysms with arterial and venous thromboses of the adrenal vessels. The suggestion also has been made that irritation of the hypothalamus due to intracranial surgical procedures might lead to adrenal hemorrhage.

SURGICAL COMPLICATIONS OF ADRENAL STEROID THERAPY

At the other extreme of the scale from Addison's disease are the problems that arise not from too little adrenal secretion but from the administration of excessive doses of adrenal steroids. The surgical complications of massive adrenal steroid therapy have been summarized by Glenn and Grafe. These writers reported 53 patients who required surgical treatment for a total of 109 complications. Rheumatoid arthritis, ulcerative colitis, and disseminated lupus erythematosus were the most common diseases under treatment. Ten percent of the total did not have valid indications for adrenal steroid therapy.

Ulcers of the stomach and duodenum were the lesions most frequently encountered, 41 of the 53 patients having developed this complication. The ulcers were gastric in 23, of which 12 were single and 11 multiple. All occurred in the antrum. Eighteen patients had duodenal ulcers all in the first portion of the duodenum except for one. Fourteen females and nine males had gastric ulcers, and twelve males and six females had duodenal ulcers. There were 11 perforations of gastroduodenal ulcers, 2 of esophageal ulcers, 5 of small bowel ulcers, and 3 of large bowel ulcers. Acute pancreatitis was seen in two patients activation of pulmonary tuberculosis in two, and empyema in one. There were seven small bowel ulcers and three large bowel ulcers.

Although it has been claimed that the incidence of peptic ulcer is no higher in patients being treated with steroids for rheumatoid arthritis than it is in the general population, others have found a considerably higher incidence. This experience certainly points up the necessity for the withholding of corticosteroid therapy unless there is a specific well-established reason for it. It is of particular note that none of the patients in this series had complications within the first week of corticosteroid therapy.

Adrenal Medulla

The adrenal medulla gives rise primarily to two types of tumors, the pheochromocytomas, which are well differentiated, are metabolically mature, and occur primarily in adults, and the neuroblastomas, which are immature, are metabolically primitive, are virtually always malignant, and occur primarily in early childhood.

PHYSIOLOGY

Three catecholamines are found in adrenergically innervated human tissues—epinephrine, norepinephrine, and dopamine. These compounds are found in chromaffin cells of the sympathetic nervous system, which includes the adrenal medulla, aberrant tissue along the sympathetic chain, and paraganglia. Norepinephrine and dopamine are found at the endings of the postganglionic fibers of the sympathetic system and in the central nervous system. Dopamine is found in several other locations, notably the kidney, liver, and lungs.

In the embryo the chromaffin cells are widely distributed in the adrenal medulla, the sympathetic ganglia, the paraganglia, which lie along the sympathetic chain, and the organs of Zuckerkandl, which are paraganglia lying along the abdominal aorta with particular concentration in the region of the inferior mesenteric artery. The organs of Zuckerkandl usually degenerate shortly after birth. The fetal adrenal and the organs of Zuckerkandl contain norepinephrine only, epinephrine appearing some time after birth. In the adult the great majority of chromaffin cells are concentrated in the adrenal medulla, although small collections may be found along the aorta, particularly in the remnants of the organs of Zuckerkandl, in the walls of blood vessels, and scattered through various organs—especially the heart, prostate, and ovary. Aberrant collections of chromaffin tissue may persist in the adult and may be the site for the development of a pheochromocytoma.

The principal pathway for the production of epinephrine from phenylalanine and tyrosine is shown in Fig. 37-40. Norepinephrine is the immediate precursor of epinephrine and thus has a dual role, as a hormone and neurotransmitter and as an intermediate in the production of epinephrine. The proximity of adrenal cortex and medulla is functionally important. The N-methylation of norepinephrine to form epinephrine is promoted by the enzyme phenylethanolamine-N-methyltransferase (PNMT). PNMT requires adrenal steroids for its physiologic function. In man and in some other species there is an adrenal portal venous drainage system. This delivers large quantities of cortical steroids to the adrenal medulla. Norepinephrine and dopamine are therefore the catecholamines principally found in extraadrenal locations. Thus while norepinephrine is present in normal or slightly increased amounts in the urine of patients who have undergone bilateral adrenalectomy, epinephrine is markedly reduced. The epinephrine still present is presumed to come from chromaffin cells located in various organs and, over a period of time, can begin to produce increasing amounts of epinephrine as well as norepinephrine. Therefore, whereas the urine of patients who have undergone bilateral adrenalectomy is virtually devoid of epinephrine in the early postoperative period, it may contain appreciable but subnormal amounts of epinephrine from 6 months to 3 years later.

All three catecholamines are found in the adrenal medulla (epinephrine and norepinephrine being present usually in amounts of 0.5 to 1 mg/Gm of tissue) and physiologically are released in response to a wide variety of sensitive reflex stimuli, including body tilting, blood volume contraction, psychic arousal, and consciousness.

It has been recognized that when epinephrine and norepinephrine are injected intravenously, only small amounts appear in the urine, most of the urinary excretion consisting of various metabolites—primarily metanephrine, normetanephrine, and VMA (vanilmandelic acid, or 4-hydroxy-3-methoxymandelic acid). A simplified scheme of epinephrine and norepinephrine metabolism together with the relative amounts of these substances usually found in the blood and urine is shown in Fig. 37-41. Most commonly urinary catecholamines are measured for the diagnosis of benign pheochromocytoma. Epinephrine, norepinephrine, and VMA formerly were used for this purpose. More recently determinations of metanephrine and normetanephrine have been the most useful diagnostic adjuncts. Recently rare cases of pheochromocytoma have been found in which no convincing elevation of urinary catecholamine and metanephrine levels have appeared. Repeated study on different days, measurement of plasma norepinephrine and epinephrine before and after glucagon stimulation, and rarely abdominal exploration are necessary to resolve the problem.

While the metabolism of dopamine regularly leads to

Fig. 37-40. Main pathway for the formation of epinephrine and norepinephrine. (*After Blaschko et al.*)

the production of norepinephrine, epinephrine, and their metabolites, an alternative route is available by means of which 3-methoxytyramine and homovanillic acid (HVA) are formed, as shown in Fig. 37-42. It was first suggested in 1956 that malignant pheochromocytomas may selectively secrete dopamine, though this was not confirmed by studies in 1961 of the primary growth of a malignant pheochromocytoma. Robinson et al. found large amounts of dopamine metabolites in the urine of a patient with a malignant pheochromocytoma. Increased secretion of dopamine metabolites was not found in patients with benign pheochromocytoma, and their presence was thought to be a valuable indication of malignancy. Subsequently many benign pheochromocytomas have been found to secrete dopamine and its metabolites.

Functionally active neuroblastomas secrete catecholamine metabolites which are very similar to those seen in the patient with the malignant pheochromocytoma, thus reflecting both their biochemical immaturity and their malignancy. These patients secrete large amounts of dopamine metabolites as well as norepinephrine metabolites. Neuroblastoma patients almost never form epinephrine in their tumors.

In addition to the well-known ability of epinephrine to promote glycogenolysis in muscle and liver it has a profound effect on lipid metabolism. Although the carbohydrate effects of catecholamines are limited primarily to epinephrine, both epinephrine and norepinephrine have the ability to release free fatty acids from adipose tissue by means of lipolysis, thus markedly increasing the blood level of nonesterified fatty acids. In patients with pheochromocytoma the blood levels of nonesterified fatty acids may be several hundred times normal, and serum cholesterol and phosphatide levels also may be high. The lipid mobilizing effects of epinephrine and norepinephrine are opposed by the prostaglandins.

The effects of epinephrine on blood pressure, uterine motility, heat production, and glucose metabolism are all increased by thyroid hormone. The α- and β-adrenergic

Fig. 37-41. Some of the principal metabolites of epinephrine and norepinephrine, with the urinary values for the commonly measured ones. MNO stands for monoamine oxidase, and CMT stands for catecholamine methyl transferase. (*After Kopin et al., Res Publ Assoc Res Nerv Ment Dis. 43:343, 1966.*)

effects of the catecholamines are outlined in Table 37-13. Some conditions characterized by altered sensitivities to catecholamines are shown in Table 37-14.

PHEOCHROMOCYTOMA

Pheochromocytomas are functionally active chromaffin tumors which may be located in the adrenal medulla or other sites where sympathetic ganglia or chromaffin tissue are known to exist. They are of particular interest because of their tendency to produce large amounts of catecholamines, primarily norepinephrine with or without epinephrine and, uncommonly, predominantly epinephrine.

CLINICAL PICTURE. Incidence. The incidence of pheochromocytoma in autopsy cases was reported by Minno et al. to be 15 out of 15,934, or 0.1 percent. In one study, eight unsuspected pheochromocytomas were found in the course of 1,700 splanchnicectomies performed for hypertension, an incidence of 0.7 percent. In three additional cases the diagnosis was made preoperatively. On the basis of this observation, Graham suggested that there should be about 600 to 800 new cases a year in the United States. Kvale et al. reported an incidence of 2 percent in 900 patients studied for hypertension and also reported the discovery of 51 patients with pheochromocytoma in 7,993 patients screened with pharmacologic tests and blood catecholamines for hypertension, an incidence of 0.64 percent. Hume found one pheochromocytoma in 317 hypertensive patients screened with urinary catecholamines, an incidence of 0.32 percent, and subsequent to this the incidence has been 0.4 percent, nine pheochromocytomas having been found in 2,386 patients screened for hypertension with urinary catecholamine determination (Table 37-15).

Folger et al. found 21 pheochromocytomas in 31,227 autopsies at the Johns Hopkins Hospital, an incidence of 0.07 percent. In Holland the autopsy incidence was found to be 0.02 percent, while the incidence in hypertensive patients was thought to be roughly 0.6 percent.

Pheochromocytomas have been reported in persons from five months to eighty-two years of age. The maximal incidence is between the ages of twenty and fifty. A pheochromocytoma should be suspected and searched for in hypertensive patients who show any of the findings listed in Table 37-16.

Location of Tumors. A predilection for the right adrenal

Table 37-13. CLASSIFICATION OF α- AND β-ADRENERGIC EFFECTS OF
CATECHOLAMINES

Effects	*Alpha** (*norepinephrine*)	*Beta†* (*isoproterenol*)	*Epinephrine*	*Dopamine*
Vasoconstriction	0	+	+	
Vasodilatation	0	+	−	+
Increase in systolic blood pressure . .	+	±	+	
Increase in diastolic blood pressure . .	+	0	0	
Vascular:				
Increase in hepatic and muscle blood flow.	0	+	+	
Cardiac:				
Increase in coronary flow	+	+	0	
Increase in heart rate	0	+	+	
Increase in atrial contracility and conduction rate	0	+	+	
Increase in conduction velocity of AV node.	0	+	+	
Increase in cardiac output	0	+	+	+
Pulmonary:				
Dilatation of bronchial musculature	0	+	+	
Metabolic:				
Increase in fasting blood glucose and free fatty acid levels	±	+	+	0
Increase in BMR	±	+	+	0

*α blockers: phenoxybenzamine (Dibenzyline), dibenamine, phentolamine (Regitine).

†β blockers: dichloroisoproterenol, pronethalol, and propranalol.

Fig 37-42. Some of the metabolites of dopamine. MAO stands for monoamine oxidase, and CMT stands for catecholamine methyl transferase.

Table 37-14. SOME CONDITIONS CHARACTERIZED
BY ALTERED SENSITIVITY TO
CATECHOLAMINES

Conditions associated with increased sensitivity:
  Cardiomegaly
    Congestive heart failure
    Hypertrophy—secondary to physical obstruction or increase
      in peripheral vascular resistance
    Myocardiopathy of various causes
  Thyrotoxicosis
  Sympathetic denervation
    Diabetes mellitus
    Surgical or anesthetic procedures
    Orthostatic hypotension
  Nutritional abnormalities
    Scurvy
  Unclassified diseases
    β-Adrenergic hyperresponders
    Familial dysautonomia
  Drugs
    Imipramine
    Some antiadrenergic drugs (e.g., guanethidine and reserpine)
Conditions associated with decreased sensitivity:
  Acidosis—metabolic or respiratory
  Myxedema
  Adrenal insufficiency
Conditions associated with paradoxical effects:
  Diseases
    Carcinoid syndrome
  Drug administration
    Phenothiazine and congeners

Table 37-15. MEAN FREE URINARY LEVELS IN NONPHEOCHROMOCYTOMA
HYPERTENSIVE PATIENTS AND IN PHEOCHROMOCYTOMA

	Normal (n = 100)	*Pheochromocytoma* (n = 63)
Norepinephrine	28.9* ± 29.0† (P < 0.001)	1250 ± 2456
Epinephrine	7.6 ± 7.4 (P < 0.001)	238 ± 408
	Normal (n = 37)	*Pheochromocytoma* (n = 29)
Normetanephrine	44.2 ± 38.9 (P < 0.001)	1127 ± 842
Metanephrine	32.9 ± 16.4 (P < 0.001)	1305 ± 1708

* All urinary values in micrograms per 24 hr.
† ± 1 Standard deviation.
SOURCE: From Freier and Harrison, *J Surg Res,* **14:**177, 1973.

is a constant finding. This predilection for the right side
is even more pronounced in children, in whom the right
adrenal is involved twice as often as the left.

Seven percent of tumors are bilateral in adults, while
twenty-four percent are bilateral in children (Table 37-17).
Nine percent of all tumors, in adults and children, are
bilateral. When the familial cases are excluded (one-half
are bilateral), only 5.3 percent are bilateral in adults.
Abdominal pheochromocytomas are commonly located in
the adrenal medulla, the extraadrenal paraganglia, the
organs of Zuckerkandl, and the bladder, in that order.
Extraabdominal tumors may be located in the thorax or
neck (Fig. 37-43). The tumors range in size from tiny
nodules up to 3,600 Gm. Some large tumors have relatively
little function.

Malignant Pheochromocytomas. The incidence of malignancy in pheochromocytoma is about 10 percent or less.
Many of these tumors appear malignant histologically,
even with venous invasion, without ever subsequently
demonstrating a true malignant potential. Some arise from
multicentric though benign origins. The only acceptable
criterion of malignancy, therefore, is definitive evidence of
metastases to sites not usual for chromaffin tissue. Using

Table 37-16. CONDITIONS WHICH SUGGEST
PHEOCHROMOCYTOMA IF PRESENT IN
THE HYPERTENSIVE PATIENT

1. Any sort of "attack," with or without precipitating stress
2. Diabetes or elevated fasting blood sugar level, especially between the ages of twenty and fifty
3. An elevated BMR (and normal RAI)
4. Childhood—in the absence of renal disease or coarctation
5. Postural hypotension, excessive sweating, an elevated temperature, frequent headaches, or vasomotor phenomena
6. Pregnancy with sweating, vomiting, and headaches or shock
   or hypertension during delivery
7. Neurofibromatosis
8. Familial history of pheochromocytoma
9. A previously removed pheochromocytoma
10. Weight loss or failure to gain weight if patient is already
    thin
11. Recent onset of hypertension with severe retinopathy

this criterion the incidence has varied from 2.8 to 14.5
percent.

The metastases are frequently functional, and the symptoms of pheochromocytomas recur as the lesions spread.
The metastases may be more primitive than the primary
tumor and produce metabolic products of dopamine in
addition to those of epinephrine and norepinephrine. The
presence, therefore, of large amounts of 3-methoxytyra-
mine and HVA in addition to VMA is highly suggestive
of the presence of metastases.

The incidence of malignancy in childhood is not low,
which is of interest in view of the almost complete restriction to childhood of neuroblastomas—a highly malignant
neural crest tumor closely related to pheochromocytoma
even in regard to the secretion of catecholamines or their
metabolic products. Malignant tumors can occur in pheochromocytomas of the organs of Zuckerkandl or bladder
as well as in those of adrenal origin and may be nonfunctioning. Malignant pheochromocytomas are relatively
radioresistant, and prognosis is generally poor.

Signs, Symptoms, and Pathophysiology. The hypertension
associated with pheochromocytomas may be paroxysmal,
sustained, or absent. In adult patients the hypertension is
sustained in about 65 percent, paroxysmal in about 30
percent, and absent in about 5 percent, whereas in children
about 92 percent show sustained hypertension and 8 percent paroxysmal.

Typical paroxysmal attacks usually consist of severe
headaches, palpitation, profuse sweating, nausea and vomiting, pallor, epigastric or substernal pain, dyspnea, vertigo,
apprehension or fear of impending death, and visual
difficulties, in that order. Sometimes only one or two of
these symptoms are present.

A list of the symptoms and signs is shown in Table 37-18.
The general symptom complexes with pheochromocytoma
are shown in Table 37-19. Nausea, weight loss, abdominal
pain, visual changes, and convulsions are more common
in children. Attacks may last from a few moments to many
hours, and they may occur several times a day or only
once every year or two. They are often precipitated by
emotional upsets, change in position, intercourse, physical

Table 37-17. LOCATION OF TUMORS

Location	Adult*		Child	
	No.	Percent	No.	Percent
Total cases	207		76	
Right adrenal	92	44.5	25	33
Left adrenal	70	33.8	11	14.5
Bilateral	18	8.7	15	19.7
Bilateral plus extraadrenal	...	....	3	4.0
Right side, extraadrenal . .	7	3.4	1	1.3
Left side, extraadrenal . . .	5	2.4	6	7.9
Adrenal and extraadrenal .	1	0.5	7	9.2
Multiple	3	1.5	4	5.3
Aorta (organs of Zuckerkandl)	8	3.8	3	3.8
Intrathoracic	2	0.9	1	1.3
Celiac ganglion	1	0.5		

	Adult, percent	Child† percent	Familial† percent
Bilateral	9 ⎫	24 ⎫	50
Multiple	1.5 ⎬ 10.5	15 ⎬ 39	9
Extraadrenal	11.5	15	14
Total percent	22	54	73

Bilateral, familial, neurofibromatosis† (1960)

	Adult		Child	
	No.	Percent	No.	Percent
Total cases	543		83	
Bilateral	38	7	18	24
Familial	14	2.6	8	10
Familial bilateral	9	1.7	2	2.4
Bilateral, not familial . . .	29	5.3	16	21
Neurofibromatosis	26	4.8	1	1.4

*From J. B. Graham, *Int Abstr Surg,* **92**:105, 1951.
†See D. M. Hume, *Am J Surg,* **99**:458, 1960.

thyroid crisis, toxemia, tumors of the brain, and diencephalic epilepsy. Recently monamine oxidase inhibitors have been shown occasionally to produce attacks simulating pheochromocytoma, including headaches, pallor, vomiting, and blood pressure elevation. These attacks are precipitated or exacerbated by cheese, which contains tyramine, a strong stimulant to catecholamine secretion, the effect of which is potentiated by monoamine oxidase inhibitors.

Most functioning pheochromocytomas secrete increased amounts of norepinephrine. About one-half of these secrete epinephrine as well. Uncommonly, most (80 percent) of the secreted catecholamine is epinephrine. These lesions are almost exclusively confined to the adrenal medulla.

Because epinephrine is a more metabolically active compound than norepinephrine, it has commonly been assumed that those patients with pheochromocytoma having marked metabolic manifestations and cardiac arrhythmias are epinephrine secretors. However, this assumption is incorrect. While the BMR is elevated in 50 percent of patients with pheochromocytoma, it is significant that Gifford et al. found it to be elevated nearly three times as

Fig. 37-43. Location of pheochromocytomas in ectopic sites. About 10 to 15 percent of pheochromocytomas are located in ectopic sites with principal concentration in the areas shown.

effort, trauma, sneezing, eating, urination, or anesthesia and operation. The attack often ends with profuse diaphoresis and a feeling of fatigue or even prostration. Attacks are usually accompanied by increases in blood sugar, body temperature, and blood and urinary catecholamines. The first sign may be sudden death, or the patient may have symptoms for as long as 32 years or more. Some patients with paroxysmal attacks early in their course may develop sustained hypertension later on or may continue to have only paroxysmal attacks for many years. If the hypertension is sustained, very advanced hypertensive retinopathy may develop.

There are other conditions which may produce paroxysms of hypertension not unlike those seen with pheochromocytoma. The most common among these include renovascular hypertension, angina pectoris, anxiety states, eclampsia, hysteria, migraine, neurosis, periarteritis nodosa,

Table 37-18. SYMPTOMS AND SIGNS
OF PHEOCHROMOCYTOMA

	Approximate percent	
	Adult	*Child*
Symptoms:		
Persistent hypertension	65	92
Paroxysmal hypertension	30	8
Headache	80	81
Sweating	70	68
Palpitation, nervousness	60	34
Pallor of face	40	27
Tremor	40	
Nausea	30	56
Weakness, fatigue	25	27
Weight loss	15	44
Abdominal or chest pain	15	35
Dyspnea	15	16
Visual changes	10	44
Constipation	5	8
Raynaud's phenomenon	5	
Convulsions	3	23
Polydipsia, polyuria	..	25
Puffy, red, cyanotic hands	..	11
Signs:		
BMR over +20 percent	50	83
Fasting blood sugar over 120 mg/100 ml	40	40
Glycosuria	10	3
Eye ground changes	30	70

SOURCE: From D. M. Hume, E. B. Astwood, and C. E. Cassidy,
Grune & Stratton, Inc., 1968.

Table 37-19. SYMPTOM COMPLEXES
OF PHEOCHROMOCYTOMA

1. Symptom-free patients, with pheochromocytoma an incidental or accidental finding
2. Symptom-free patients who die suddenly after minor trauma
3. Patients with typical attacks
4. Patients with sustained hypertension indistinguishable clinically from essential or renal vascular hypertension
5. "Diabetics," with or without hypertension
6. Patients with headaches (migraine or other), fever, and nausea, or the metabolic changes of pheochromocytoma, without either sustained or paroxysmal hypertension
7. Patients who present with "hyperthyroidism," especially if BMR does not fall with treatment, RAI and PBI are normal, and patient has hypertension
8. Patients with unexplained shock during anesthesia or minor trauma
9. Patients with cardiac irregularities, tachycardia, or arrest with induction of anesthesia or beginning of operation
10. Patients whose symptoms simulate an acute anxiety attack
11. Patients who have attacks when voiding—occasionally occurs with pheochromocytoma in bladder

SOURCE: From D. M. Hume, E. B. Astwood, and C. E. Cassidy,
Grune & Stratton, Inc., 1968.

often in patients with persistent hypertension as in those with paroxysmal hypertension. Furthermore, children with pheochromocytomas, who usually have sustained hypertension and in whom the tumors are primarily norepinephrine-secreting, have an elevated BMR in 83 percent of cases. The PBI and uptake of radioiodine (RAI) are usually normal, even when the BMR reaches extremely high levels, and this can be an important diagnostic sign. The fasting blood sugar is elevated in 41 percent of the patients, while during an attack it is elevated in 75 percent. About 10 percent of the patients have frank "diabetes." On rare occasions the metabolic changes of a pheochromocytoma can occur in the absence of hypertension.

It is of note that pheochromocytoma patients demonstrate an increased release of catecholamines in response to the reflex stimulus of the tilt test (Fig. 37-44). We believe this represents release from adrenergic stores that contain greater than normal quantities of catecholamines because of increased uptake from prolonged elevations in circulating catecholamine levels which are seen in pheochromocytoma patients. Hepatic catecholamine content was significantly increased in four of five pheochromocytoma patients in whom we measured it when compared to the hepatic content of catecholamines in patients undergoing uncomplicated cholecystectomy.

From these facts one can form a dynamic picture in pheochromocytoma in which catecholamines are synthesized and released into the circulation with no restraint from the tumor. They are then taken up and stored in greatly increased quantities in adrenergic storage pools, from which they can be released in response to reflex stimulation (Fig. 37-45). The mechanisms no doubt account, at least in part, for the day-to-day variation in catecholamine excretion that occurs in many pheochromocytoma patients.

Patients with pheochromocytoma are usually thin or give a history of having recently lost weight. An occasional obese patient is noted, but this is almost always when paroxysmal rather than sustained hypertension is present.

DIAGNOSTIC FINDINGS. Prior to the advent of techniques for measuring urinary catecholamines several drug tests were developed for the detection of pheochromocytoma. These were based upon a fall in blood pressure with adrenolytic drugs and a rise in blood pressure with drugs which stimulated catecholamine release. For the most part these have been discarded. The phentolamine (Regitine) tests can be used only in patients with sustained hypertension. A positive test consists of a 35/25 mm Hg fall of pressure within 3 to 10 minutes after the intravenous injection of 5 mg of Regitine. False-positive reactions are common, and false-negative reactions are also seen. Deaths have been recorded in pheochromocytoma patients overreacting to the Regitine test.

The histamine test as it was originally described probably no longer has a place. A modification of this test to include the measurement of blood catecholamines is helpful in the rare patient with paroxysmal hypertension who does not have elevated levels of urinary catecholamines. The test is performed between paroxysms, when the blood pressure is fairly normal. After the intravenous injection

INCREASE IN FREE NOREPINEPHRINE EXCRETION AFTER TILT

Fig. 37-44. Change in body posture with tilting is an easily repro-duced reflex stimulus for catecholamine release. As is apparent in this study, the response is greatly exaggerated in pheochromo-cytoma. We believe this reflects release of catecholamines from increased peripheral adrenergic stores, and have demonstrated significant increases in hepatic catecholamines in four of five liver biopsies from pheochromocytoma patients. Of added interest is the exaggerated release of α-methyl norepinephrine in a patient re-ceiving α-methyl-dopa treatment. (*By permission from the New England Journal of Medicine, 277:725, 1967.*)

mocytoma the catecholamines are rapidly metabolized, methods have been developed for the measurement of the metabolites of catecholamines in the urine. α-Methyldopa (Aldomet) is a specific interfering drug in catecholamine determination and must be stopped for at least 3 weeks before collecting urine for analysis. It can interfere with metanephrine and normetanephrine measurements.

Urinary epinephrine and norepinephrine excretion re-mains a reliable method for the detection of pheochro-mocytoma, but less so for neuroblastoma or the occasional tumor in which the catecholamines are largely methylated in the tumor or consist principally of dopamine metabo-lites. The separate detection of urinary epinephrine and norepinephrine is diagnostically helpful and not difficult. The measurement of conjugated epinephrine and norepi-nephrine extends the usefulness of this determination, since some patients with pheochromocytomas excrete mainly conjugated catecholamines. Urinary VMA is less sensitive, is nonspecific for epinephrine and norepine-phrine, requires strict dietary control to avoid interference,

Fig. 37-45. Findings from a pheochromocytoma patient with distinct elevations of urinary norepinephrine (NE) and epineph-rine (E) secretion. The caval catheterization values show the highest NE content, 4.9 μg/liter, in the sample representing the tumor, and the highest E content, 4.8 μg/liter, from the left (nor-mal) adrenal. The tumor itself contains only NE. After removal of the tumor, both NE and E excretion returned to normal, 17 and 7 μg/24 hours, respectively. The findings are compatible with release of NE from the tumor, uptake and methylation of NE to form E in the normal left adrenal gland, and subsequent release of increased quantities of E from the left adrenal gland into the circulation and ultimately into the urine. (*By permission from the Johns Hopkins Medical Journal, 139:137, 1976, The Johns Hop-kins University Press, Md.*)

CAVAL CATHETERIZATION

of 0.025 to 0.050 mg of histamine base, blood samples are taken 4 and 6 minutes later. No increase in blood catechol-amine levels occurs levels hypertensive patients, while a striking increase occurs in patients with pheochromocy-toma. A stimulating test using tyramine has been advo-cated, but its error rate is unacceptably high. Tyramine proved to have fewer side effects than histamine, but to have only a disappointing 50 percent positive result in patients with pheochromocytoma and paroxysmal hyper-tension. A glucagon-provocative test advocated by Law-rence produced positive responses in 3 pateints with pheo-chromocytoma and negative responses in 126 hypertensive patients, but Sheps and Maher found positive responses in only 6 of 11 patients with pheochromocytoma.

It is far better to make the diagnosis of pheochromocy-toma by measurement of urinary catecholamines or their metabolites. This was first demonstrated by von Euler, and since then a flood of articles has been published confirming his observations and developing scores of new ways to detect catecholamines in urine. The results of catechola-mine determinations in screening hypertensive patients are shown in Table 37-15.

Because the amount of epinephrine and norepinephrine in the urine represents only 4 percent of the secretion of these substances and because in some cases of pheochro-

and gives rise to more equivocal results. Tumors other than pheochromocytomas or neuroblastomas can sometimes secrete catecholamines, and increased secretion of these substances may be seen in the absence of tumors. Thus elevated urinary excretion of VMA has been seen in ganglioneuroma, ganglioneuroblastoma, retinoblastoma, carotid body tumor, malignant carcinoid chemodectoma (a glomic tissue tumor which is a "nonchromaffin" paraganglioma), and acrodynia.

HVA, the major end product of dopamine metabolism, is useful primarily in the detection of malignant or dopamine-secreting pheochromocytoma or neuroblastoma. It may also be increased in ganglioneuroma, melanoma, Parkinson's disease, and Wilson's disease. Normal values are frequently found in pheochromocytoma. Elevated levels of metanephrine (M) and/or normetanephrine (NM) are a highly reliable sign of pheochromocytoma, and the measurement of conjugated metanephrines further improves the value of the test.

Although epinephrine, norepinephrine, metanephrine, normetanephrine, and 3-methoxy-4-hydroxyphenylglycol have been detected in tissue from pheochromocytomas, VMA has not, and studies by Sunderman suggest that the liver is the major site for the production of this metabolite.

Patients with neuroblastomas may not have hypertension, despite the excretion of large amounts of catecholamine metabolites. Although an occasional patient with nonmalignant pheochromocytomas will excrete dopamine metabolites, this is unusual, whereas the patients with neuroblastoma characteristically do. Furthermore the patients with neuroblastoma demonstrate a great fluctuation in day-to-day excretion rates, which may be related to the poorer function of cytoplasmic granules than is the case with pheochromocytomas. Gjessing and Hjermann have described three secretion patterns: (1) epinephrine and norepinephrine metabolites in benign pheochromocytoma, (2) dopamine metabolites in ganglioneuroma, and (3) dopa, dopamine, and norepinephrine-epinephrine metabolites in neuroblastoma, with increasing dopa metabolites excretion with increasing malignancy.

As mentioned earlier, a few cases have been reported of pharmacologically active pheochromocytomas in which the urinary epinephrine and norepinephrine, metanephrines, or VMA were near the upper limit of normal. Fre-

quently this dilemma can be resolved by repeated study of resting urinary catecholamine and metanephrine excretion. Also, these patients usually exhibit paroxysmal hypertension and will nearly always show elevated catecholamine levels in plasma after histamine or glucagon stimulation. Forced ventilation will sometimes stimulate an increase in catecholamines, even under these circumstances.

In cases with minimally secreting tumors the excretion of free catecholamines may provide the greatest relative increase over normal values, while in patients in whom catecholamines are being methylated within the tumor metanephrines or VMA may show the greatest relative increase.

Localization. There are four circumstances in which localization of pheochromocytomas may be of importance: extraadrenal (or multiple) pheochromocytomas, which may be difficult to locate, tumors producing narrowing of the renal artery, extraabdominal pheochromocytomas, and functioning metastases.

Localization by retroperitoneal O_2 or CO_2 insufflation has been generally abandoned in the United States because of inconsistency of results, and the combination of this with aortography seems unnecessarily cumbersome. Retroperitoneal CO_2 insufflation with excretory nephrotomography is still used frequently in many European clinics. The intravenous pyelogram may occasionally show the tumor if it is in an adrenal location but is usually of no help in extraadrenal locations, unless the ureter is blocked by the tumor or stenosis of the renal artery results. Photoscanning with iodocholesterol has proved helpful in locating six adrenal pheochromocytomas recently under our care. The lack of uptake and dispersion of the adrenal cortical uptake on the involved side were clear (Fig. 37-46).

Fig. 37-46. *Left,* a typical retrograde venogram of an 11-year-old school boy with hypertension whose brother had multiple pheochromocytomas. This right adrenal tumor measured 5 cm in diameter. *Right,* a radio-iodocholesterol scan of the same patient. Because the image is made from a posterior orientation of the patient to the counter, the image of the right adrenal is that seen to the right of the photo. Dispersion of the adrenocortical tissue on the right indicates a mass in that adrenal which does not take up iodocholesterol. The image of the left adrenal gland is normal, indicating that physiological function of the left adrenal has been preserved.

Fig. 37-47. A 16-year-old school girl with episodic hypertension. *Left,* a subselective middle adrenal arteriogram showing a lesion of the inferior portion of the adrenal which displaces the normal gland superiorly. *Right,* a retrograde venogram at a slightly higher magnification showing a beautifully delicate outline of the right adrenal tumor's venous silhouette. The lesion measured 4 cm in diameter and was removed without difficulty. The patient's attacks have completely subsided. *(By permission from T. S. Harrison, D. S. Gann, A. J. Edis, and R. H. Egdahl, "Surgical Disorders of the Adrenal Gland," p. 102, Grune & Stratton, Inc., New York, N.Y., 1975.)*

A chest x-ray will virtually always show the tumor if it is intrathoracic. The peculiar symptomatology of hematuria and hypertensive attacks with micturition may suggest the location of bladder pheochromocytomas, or they may be detected by cystoscopy. Occasionally a plain abdominal x-ray will show calcification in the tumor, or a venacavagram will show infringement by a bulky mass. A palpable mass may be noted in a few abdominal pheochromocytomas and may simplify the location of tumors in the neck. The first pheochromocytoma to be successfully removed (by Roux in February, 1926) was a palpable right adrenal mass the size of "a croquet ball."

It was originally suggested by von Euler that pheochromocytomas secreting epinephrine most likely were located in the adrenal, while those secreting norepinephrine were extraadrenal. Von Euler and Strom reviewed 35 cases of pheochromocytoma and noted several exceptions to this themselves. Actually, if the tumor is producing epinephrine as well as norepinephrine, it often will be located in the adrenal, the only exceptions being a rare epinephrine-producing tumor of the organs of Zuckerkandl, in the mediastinum, or pulmonary metastases secreting epinephrine. If it produces only norepinephrine, a pheochromocytoma will be located in the adrenal in about two-thirds

of the cases and extraadrenal (including the organs of Zuckerkandl) in about one-third. In about 6 percent it will be extraabdominal.

Localization of the primary tumor, recurrences, or metastases can sometimes be achieved by passing a catheter up the inferior vena cava and obtaining blood samples at various levels for catecholamine determination. The highest concentration is seen in relation to the tumor. This is not true for plasma VMA measurements, where the highest concentration is seen in relation to the hepatic veins, presumably because a large fraction of oxidative deamination of the catecholamines occurs in the liver.

Retrograde adrenal venography can often be done in conjunction with inferior vena caval sampling. Blood samples are taken first, and then 3 or 4 ml contrast medium is gently injected retrograde in the adrenal vein. The venous silhouette of the tumor is often clear. Ordinarily there is only a mild pressure response to the injection (Fig. 37-47).

Aortography, often with subtraction techniques, provides another means of localizing pheochromocytomas and has the advantage that it is equally as good for extraadrenal as adrenal tumors (Figs. 37-48 and 37-49). Although deaths have been reported with aortography, the newer methods, which include retrograde aortic catheterization, selective arteriograms, initial injection of small amounts of contrast material, and the availability of drugs to control a hypertensive reaction, appear to be safe in experienced hands.

SPECIAL CONSIDERATIONS. Familial Relationships. Some pheochromocytomas are definitely familial, being inherited by simple mendelian dominance with varying but usually high penetrance. Familial cases differ from sporadic ones in the following ways: They are much more

A

B

Fig. 37-48. Aortography for localization of pheochromocytoma. *A.* Retrograde femoral arteriogram in a patient with a pheochromocytoma of the left adrenal. There is a network of blood vessels supplying the tumor of the left adrenal gland and filling the space just above the left kidney, an arteriogram of which is also shown. *B.* A later picture of the same patient showing contrast material in vessels of the tumor as indicated by the arrows. The blood supply from the aorta and that from the left renal artery can be clearly seen. *S,* splenic artery; *L.R.,* left renal artery; *H,* hepatic artery; *G.D.,* gastroduodenal artery. The patient had congenital absence of the right kidney.

apt to be bilateral and multiple and somewhat more apt to be extraadrenal or extraabdominal (see Table 37-17). They affect children more frequently, and the mean age for familial cases is 26 compared to 37.1 years for sporadic cases. There is a striking predilection for the organs of Zuckerkandl in familial cases, several examples having been reported. Familial adrenal pheochromocytomas are more apt to be on the left, whereas sporadic ones are more

apt to be on the right. Familial cases are associated more frequently with neurocutaneous syndromes, other neural tumors, medullary carcinoma of the thyroid (Sipple's syndrome), and other polyglandular syndromes.

Pheochromocytoma in Pregnancy. Pheochromocytomas become symptomatic during pregnancy, about 80 cases having been reported. The symptoms appear as (1) severe or fatal preeclampsia; (2) typical attacks of paroxysmal hypertension with headache, restlessness, apprehension, sweating, and tachycardia; (3) headaches without hypertension; (4) sudden shock and death in the antepartum period; (5) hyperpyrexia after delivery; or (6) shock after delivery with or without previous symptoms, either spontaneous or induced by anesthesia or delivery.

A patient reported by Pickles had symptoms during three pregnancies, each time, and died immediately after the third delivery. In the patient of Parbossingh and Tate symptoms developed in the last trimester of her sixth pregnancy at twenty-five years of age. She aborted an incarcerated fetus and died. A previous successful pregnancy, with or without symptoms, does not, therefore, preclude the presence of a pheochromocytoma during a subsequent pregnancy. Patients with toxemia, preeclampsia, headaches, or unexplained attacks should be screened for the presence of a pheochromocytoma. Pregnancy per se does not increase urinary catecholamine excretion.

The outcome of pheochromocytoma in pregnancies has been poor, a 48 percent overall mortality being recorded. Walker reported four cases, all with survival of the mother and two with survival of the fetus as well. In three cases of 28, 29, and 30 weeks the tumor was removed during the pregnancy, and two of the patients went on to deliver normal infants by the vaginal route. The fourth patient had a Cesarean section with removal of the tumor. Walker feels that the tumor should be removed as soon as the diagnosis is made, instead of waiting if the diagnosis is made during the last trimester. An alternative approach is the intelligent use of α- and β-adrenergic receptor blockade through delivery until elective postpartum pheochromocytoma excision is carried out.

Barzel et al. measured norepinephrine in maternal and cord blood and noted results which suggested a placental barrier, presumably enzymatic, to norepinephrine transfer. Five times more VMA and ten times less norepinephrine have been noted in cord blood than in maternal blood. This also suggests that the placental barrier is enzymatic in nature, and, indeed, monoamine oxidase has been demonstrated in the human placenta.

Malignant tumors may occur in pheochromocytomas during pregnancy, and the tumors may be familial or bilateral. Several of the cases have been located in the organs of Zuckerkandl.

Neurocutaneous Syndromes. Multiple neurofibromatosis (von Recklinghausen's disease) occurs in about 5 percent of patients with pheochromocytoma. Other neurocutaneous syndromes are related to the occurrence of pheochromocytoma, including café au lait spots, tuberous sclerosis (Bourneville's disease), meningofacial angiomatosis (Sturge-Weber disease). Other neural tumors such as ependymoma of the cord, meningioma of the foramen magnum, and schwannoma have also been reported in patients with pheochromocytoma.

Shocket and Teloh reported a patient in whom there was an association of pheochromocytomas with several neural abnormalities including aganglionic megacolon, megalo-ureter, and neurofibroma. Megacolon has been seen by others. Williams and Pollack reported two cases with multiple unusual neuromas, pheochromocytoma, and thyroid cancer.

Congenital Heart Disease. Folger et al. first reported the association of pheochromocytoma and congenital heart disease, although the association of other endocrine tumors with congenital heart disease had previously been noted. They rejected a congenital cause for the pheochromocytomas associated with congenital heart disease on the basis that clinical manifestations of the tumor did not appear until the ages of twelve to forty-one years. However, there would seem to be strong evidence for a familial (genetic) rather than chronic stimulatory cause for these cases. This has been detailed by Hume.

Pheochromocytoma and Medullary Carcinoma of the Thyroid. In 1961 Sipple first published an article drawing attention to the association of pheochromocytomas with thyroid carcinoma—a syndrome now associated with his name. Since then other features of the syndrome have become apparent: (1) the thyroid cancer is virtually always a medullary cancer of the type described by Hazard et al.; (2) the adrenal tumors are frequently bilateral (65 percent), as they are in familial cases; (3) there is a strong familial history of pheochromocytoma (35 percent) and of medullary carcinoma of the thyroid (35 percent); (4) there is sometimes an association with multiple neural tumors or parathyroid adenomas, suggesting a relation to the multiple endocrine adenoma syndrome, although Williams points out that "multiple adenomas," which is taken to mean the association of pituitary, pancreatic, parathyroid, and occasionally adrenal cortical adenomas, have never been associated either with medullary carcinoma of the thyroid or pheochromocytoma. The parathyroid adenomas associated with thyroid carcinoma and pheochromocytoma do not, therefore, constitute a part of the former syndrome, which seems to originate from a diffuse neoplasia of the involved glands, with adenoma formation. In general the hyperparathyroidism of Sipple's syndrome (MEA-II) is milder than that seen in MEA-I.

Nourok found bilateral pheochromocytomas and medullary cancer in both mother and daughter, and Huang and McLeish reported three members of the same family with pheochromocytomas (two of them bilateral) and medullary thyroid cancer. Sapira et al. points out that the thyroid and adrenal medulla appear at similar periods, embryologically, and that both require tyrosine as the precursor of their respective hormones. The above findings taken together strongly suggest a common familial cause for medullary cancer of the thyroid and the associated pheochromocytoma.

It is felt by Schimke and Hartmann that the association of thyroid cancer and pheochromocytomas may depend upon a single gene, and the occasional additional association of parathyroid adenoma may represent pleiotropism.

A

B

Fig. 37-49. Pheochromocytoma producing renal artery stenosis. *A.* Aortogram showing a marked constriction of the terminal portion of the right renal artery indicated between the two arrows. The patient had severe hypertension. *B.* Cut section of the kidney in pheochromocytoma showing the tumor closely applied to the terminal portion of the right renal artery.

These writers mention an unpublished case where bilateral pheochromocytoma, neurofibromatosis, and medullary cancer of the thyroid all coexisted, lending some credence to the genetic or embryologic theories.

Relation of Pheochromocytoma to Other Glands. Apart from the relation to thyroid cancer just discussed, pheochromocytomas may occasionally be associated with other endocrine abnormalities. Thus pheochromocytomas have been seen in association with acromegaly, adrenocortical hyperplasia, Cushing's disease and hyperaldosteronism, and parathyroid adenoma. Pheochromocytomas occasionally have been observed to produce cortisol, to inhibit insulin secretion, and to metabolize 17 β-estradiol.

Although the hypermetabolism seen in patients with pheochromocytoma is characteristically associated with an elevated BMR and normal RAI and PBI, a case has been reported in which the RAI was increased.

Pheochromocytoma, Cholelithiasis, and Increase in Free Fatty Acids. There have been a series of reports from the Mayo Clinic mentioning the high incidence (40 percent) of cholelithiasis in patients with pheochromocytoma. No explanation is offered, and this finding is not stressed by other writers. A possible explanation is that both epinephrine and norepinephrine stimulate the release of free fatty acids from adipose tissue, and elevated levels of free fatty acids are regularly seen in patients with pheochromocytoma. These elevations are directly correlated with the BMR.

Pheochromocytoma and Renovascular Hypertension. Extraadrenal pheochromocytomas, which constitute only 10 to 15 percent of the total group, are most commonly located in proximity to the kidneys, the organs of Zuckerkandl, the mediastinum, and the bladder, in that order. Those located on, or adjacent to, the renal artery may be associated with, or produce, renovascular hypertension. Harrison et al. reported a case in which renal hypertension persisted after excision of three pheochromocytomas, ultimately requiring a nephrectomy on that side for relief of hypertension. Rosenheim et al. reported two patients with unilateral renal ischemia due to compression of the renal artery by the pheochromocytoma. Both were treated by removal of the tumor and simultaneous nephrectomy. Hume had an identical case treated in the same manner (Fig. 37-49). Garret et al. reported a case treated by excision of the tumor and patch grafting of the renal artery stenosis, but there was no compression of the artery in his patient. It was postulated that the proximity of a norepinephrine-secreting tumor might have accounted for the changes in the arterial wall, though this seems somewhat unlikely, particularly in that case.

Straube and Hodges reported a case in which the tumor surrounded the renal artery. A portion of the artery was sacrificed and replaced by a Dacron graft. Kerzner et al. reported a patient treated by nephrectomy in an identical twin, the other twin being completely normal.

It is now established that plasma renin activity is raised in many pheochromocytoma patients who do not have renal artery lesions. This phenomenon is believed to be related to intense intrarenal vasoconstriction caused by high levels of circulating catecholamines. In one series renin elevation was most marked in patients with norepinephrine-secreting tumors and is decreased toward, but not all the way to, normal by α-adrenergic receptor blockade in pheochromocytoma patients. In a recent report from Germany, elevated plasma renin activity has been correlated with epinephrine-secreting lesions. In a case of malignant hypertension from pheochromocytoma we found the course of hypertension followed the plasma renin activity more closely than it did increased urinary norepinephrine excretion.

Hypotension, Shock, and Sudden Death. Some functional pheochromocytomas are characterized by lack of hypertension, hypotension, or shock and sudden death. These are usually epinephrine-secreting tumors.

In the case described by Parkinson the patient developed attacks of palpitations, headache, sweating, nausea, dyspnea, and abdominal pain on standing. Her initial blood pressure was 100/70, and this later declined to 70/50. She continued to be hypotensive with an occasional hypertensive episode, one of which was precipitated by metaraminol given to raise her blood pressure. At operation she was found to have a left adrenal pheochromocytoma containing large amounts of epinephrine and lesser amounts of norepinephrine.

In the case described by Richmond et al. the patient had recurrent attacks of *hypo*tension down to 70/0, associated with abdominal pain and vomiting. The attacks were preceded by aura of fear and apprehension, and accompanied by pallor and tachycardia, effects characteristic of epinephrine, rather than norepinephrine, excess. The patient had an epinephrine-secreting tumor of the right adrenal.

Abdominal pain and shock may occur as a consequence of sudden hemorrhage into a pheochromocytoma. Huston and Stewart reviewed the cases reported in the literature of four patients who died and one of their own who survived. There was no direct evidence of hyperfunction in this latter case, however, and the patient was obese, the tumor was located in the left paravertebral gutter, and the blood supply was thrombosed. There were no signs or symptoms to suggest functioning pheochromocytoma, except the degree of shock and the difficulty in maintaining blood pressure postoperatively. The other reported cases were all adrenal in origin. McAlister and Koehler reported a case of hemorrhage into a functioning right adrenal pheochromocytoma with shock, in a patient on anticoagulants. The patient was operated upon and survived.

In one group of hospitals two deaths have followed surgical treatment over a 10-year period (about 60,000 operations) in which the patients were found to have unsuspected pheochromocytomas, and these were the only two cases of pheochromocytoma found in those hospitals in that entire time. One patient was a forty-four-year-old thin woman with migraine (which might have been the clue) and a blood pressure of 120/80. She had a benign mass removed from her breast, using thiopentone and suxamethonium induction and nitrous oxide and halothane anesthesia. The pulse was 80, and the anesthesia and operation were uneventful. Fifteen minutes after the end of the operation she became restless and cyanotic, and marked tachycardia developed. Ten minutes later she was seen to be in collapse with pallor, sweating, dyspnea, dilated pupils, tachycardia, and pulmonary edema. Despite supportive measures she died 30 minutes later and was found to have a right adrenal pheochromocytoma at postmortem. An almost identical case has been reported in which the patient also had migraine, took ergotamine, had no hypertension, and died with dyspnea, tachycardia, pupillary dilatation, and peripheral vasoconstriction.

Two contrasting cases were reported by Crockett et al., in which marked hypertension and bradycardia developed upon induction, with subsequent tachycardia, shock, pulmonary edema, ventricular fibrillation, and death. Cyclopropane anesthesia was used for both cases. The pheochromocytoma was in the adrenal in each case.

Pheochromocytoma in Children. There have been about 140 cases of pheochromocytoma reported in children. Hypertension was sustained in 85 percent, the tumors were bilateral in 25 percent, and over 50 percent had bilateral, multiple, or extraadrenal tumors.

The high incidence of bilateral, multiple, and ectopic pheochromocytomas in children, the rapid and intense course often seen, and the preponderance of females (in adults the reverse is true), suggest a pathogenesis in childhood involving factors which are not operative in the adult. The most likely suspects are the advent of puberty and the influence of GH. The cases in females appear to be concentrated around the menarche, 62 percent occurring between the ages of eleven and fifteen, whereas in males the cases were more randomly distributed. Moon et al. injected GH into male rats over a 15-month period. They found that in 9 of 16 rats so injected pheochromocytomas developed, while this tumor was not seen in any of the controls. The tumor formation in the injected rats differed from the controls only with respect to the adrenal medulla. Of the nine pheochromocytomas, five were bilateral. Pheochromocytomas have been seen in association with acromegaly. Thus both the onset of puberty and the presence of GH may be factors leading to the appearance of pheochromocytoma in childhood. Ten percent of childhood cases are familial, while this is true for only 2.6 percent of adult cases (Table 37-17), so that a genetic cause is more commonly seen in the young.

Special Locations. There are four locations for pheochromocytoma about which specific references are often made: (1) bilateral, (2) intrathoracic, (3) the organs of Zuckerkandl, and (4) the bladder.

Bilateral Pheochromocytomas. Bilateral adrenal pheochromocytoma is an important entity because of its frequent occurrence in childhood (one-fourth of cases), its relatively high mortality, its familial relationship, and the surgical problems it poses, particularly the decision as to whether adrenal cortical substitution therapy is needed.

The hazards of bilateral pheochromocytoma are illustrated by two early papers reporting death from attempted aortography in one and death in a six-year-old boy from urethral dilation under anesthesia in the other. The operative mortality in bilateral pheochromocytomas in childhood was high, but this has been greatly improved with

preoperative adrenergic receptor blockade, better anesthesia, and better operative methods, especially the abandonment of the flank approach for an abdominal exploration. Through the abdominal approach the second tumor can be easily detected and removed.

Successive bilateral pheochromocytomas have been detected by aortography, but strict precautions should be taken if this technique is utilized.

The anesthetic precautions referred to later should be particularly adhered to in operations for bilateral tumors.

Although some patients have been subjected to total adrenalectomy for bilateral pheochromocytomas, thus requiring lifetime corticosteroid administration, this is seldom necessary. A portion of the adrenal on both sides almost always can be left. Recurrent pheochromocytoma, although not uncommon (about 10 percent in our series), has not occurred in or near the adrenocortical remnant.

Hume had a case in which a total right adrenalectomy was done for a pheochromocytoma on that side. Several years later a large tumor developed in the left adrenal. A fragment of normal adrenal was left behind at the time that the tumor was removed, and its blood supply from the phrenic artery was left intact. An ACTH test postoperatively showed an excellent blood 17-OH corticosteroid response, and no replacement therapy was necessary. It may be necessary to use intravenous administration of cortisol during the operation if the blood supply of the fragment is in doubt and until its function can be demonstrated.

The Organs of Zuckerkandl. These vestigial organs are paraganglia which lie on the aorta with greatest concentration in the region of the inferior mesenteric artery. Pheochromocytomas affecting these "organs" are found on the aorta from beneath the third portion of the duodenum to the bifurcation. They are important because they can be missed if the abdominal approach is not used. Tumors of the organs of Zuckerkandl tend to be familial and may on rare occasions produce epinephrine in addition to norepinephrine. On occasion the tumor will displace the duodenum and be visible by gastrointestinal series.

Pheochromocytoma of the Bladder. Pheochromocytomas of the bladder are often, though not always, characterized by hematuria, headache, and hypertensive attacks on micturition. Micturition may precipitate attacks, however, from pheochromocytomas not associated with the bladder. Bladder pheochromocytomas are usually benign but may be malignant and are apt to occur in childhood. They are sometimes seen on excretory urography and are usually confirmed by cystoscopy. They may block the ureteral orifice, producing a picture of hydronephrosis and nonfunction of the kidney. Partial cystectomy is the treatment of choice. One pheochromocytoma of the bladder produced some epinephrine as well as norepinephrine.

Intrathoracic and Mediastinal Pheochromocytoma. Intrathoracic pheochromocytomas are often not diagnosed prior to surgical intervention. Only 50 percent of these patients have elevated blood pressure, and some of these tumors are nonfunctioning. They generally occur in the sympathetic ganglia and may be malignant. They can always be found on chest x-ray, and when functioning the localization can be confirmed by vena cava catheter sampling for plasma catecholamines. Some intrathoracic and mediastinal pheochromocytomas have produced epinephrine.

TREATMENT. Medical Treatment. *α-Adrenergic Receptor Blockade.* Medical treatment of a patient with a pheochromocytoma is often employed in preparation for operation, for patients who have functioning metastases, or for patients who refuse surgical treatment.

The usefulness of the prolonged oral administration of phentolamine (Regitine) was first described by Iseri et al. It has been used for as long as eight years in one patient who refused surgical treatments. Despite control of symptoms on 25 mg every 3 hours this patient's blood pressure was not well controlled, and she had a marked hypertensive reaction to minor surgical treatment, followed by shock. The addition of reserpine was said to help control the hypertension, though other writers have failed to note an effect on blood pressure with this drug in patients with pheochromocytomas. Furthermore reserpine and guanethidine release peripheral stores of catecholamines and can precipitate hypertensive crises or arrhythmias.

More recently phenoxybenzamine (Dibenzyline), an α-adrenergic receptor blocking agent, has been used to achieve chronic blood pressure reduction in patients with pheochromocytomas, with excellent results. In one case of malignant pheochromocytoma α-methyldopa was tried without success.

β-Adrenergic Receptor Blockade. Recently the β-adrenergic receptor blocking agent propranolol has been used to prepare patients for surgical treatment or to treat malignant pheochromocytomas chronically. It provides control of the tachycardia and helps to prevent arrhythmias intraoperatively.

Propranolol can be a valuable asset but must be used carefully. We are aware of two preoperative deaths in pheochromocytoma patients in whom overdoses of propranolol were directly responsible for death. The dose necessary for effective preoperative β-adrenergic receptor blockade is generally around 60 mg/day by mouth in three or four divided doses. This is a smaller dose of propranolol than that used for indications other than pheochromocytoma. The end point of treatment is resolution of tachycardia to a pulse rate near 90 beats per minute.

Anesthesia and Surgical Therapy. Although pheochromocytomas have been successfully removed under adverse circumstances, there is sufficient operative risk, particularly in children with bilateral tumors, to justify attempts to provide an ideal anesthetic and operative environment. The intraoperative use of phentolamine, first described by Grimson et al., has markedly improved operative results.

Whether medical pretreatment is desirable is still being debated, the opponents pointing out that sometimes ineffective, detrimental, or even fatal results have followed the administration of phentolamine (Regitine). Furthermore, it is said that with pretreatment one cannot use the rise in blood pressure on palpation of a tumor to localize it. Actually this is seldom necessary and in fact can still be done whenever desired, even with pretreatment. It is further said that the pretreatment renders the patient un-

responsive to norepinephrine after the tumor is removed, although this is usually not true. This unresponsiveness can be overcome when present by using angiotensin II, a drug which is not affected by phentolamine. Furthermore, resistance to norepinephrine sometimes occurs even when phentolamine has not been used.

The advocates point out that the operative course is apt to be a great deal smoother with preoperative adrenergic receptor blockade. Epinephrine and norepinephrine reduce the blood volume by causing peripheral vasoconstriction, and plasma volume is decreased in many patients with pheochromocytoma. This is more apt to be true in some but not all patients with sustained hypertension. Therefore, preoperative vasodilatation with phenoxybenzamine will expand the blood volume and will help to correct the marked swings of blood pressure that characterize operation in the unprepared patient. The preparation of the patient may be further enhanced by the administration just prior to and during surgical treatment of β-receptor blockers, such as propranalol, to prevent or treat arrhythmias if such are present. Patients with very high plasma catecholamines or with very high basal metabolic rates are said to be the poorest anesthetic risks.

Premedication should consist of Demerol and a small dose of scopolamine, which is preferable to atropine because it produces less tachycardia. Furthermore atropine can produce arrhythmias and hypertension. Barbiturates are apt to cause arrhythmias in the presence of hypoxia.

The anesthetic agents to be avoided are cyclopropane, halothane, trichloroethylene, and chloroform. Halothane has been advocated as the anesthetic agent of choice by some because of its tendency to suppress circulating catecholamine levels. However, halothane may lead to arrhythmias in the presence of an excess of circulating catecholamine, and if used it should be in conjunction with a β-receptor blocker. We generally prefer not to use it. The safest anesthetic appears to be Pentothal-nitrous oxide-Demerol-muscle relaxant, preferably succinylcholine. The soda lime canister should be fresh and changed during the operation to provide for optimal absorption of carbon dioxide. Arterial and venous pressure monitors are helpful and an ECG monitor mandatory. Phentolamine or nitroprusside should be used to control hypertension, and blood and norepinephrine or angiotensin II to control hypotension after removal of the tumor. Postresection hypotension has been uncommon since the preoperative use of phenoxybenzamine has become widespread. Postexcision hypotension was apparently due to acute catecholamine withdrawal vasodilatation, chronically decreased blood volume, residual phentolamine effect, if this substance was used, and occasionally insensitivity to norepinephrine. Transfusion and vasoconstrictors are the treatment.

In addition to blocking the α receptors, inhibition of the β receptors during surgical treatment, as mentioned above, may be important to prevent cardiac arrhythmias—the usual cause of operative death. In patients whose increased catecholamine excretion is more than 80 percent epinephrine, we believe it is wise to use preoperative β-receptor blockade routinely. If a patient is receiving β-receptor blockade, it is wise to use α blockade as well, to diminish the vascular resistance against which the β-blocked heart is pumping.

Though the question of corticosteroid administration is often raised, the function of the adrenal cortex is usually normal, except in some cases of bilateral pheochromocytoma, where corticosteroids should be employed until the function of the adrenal fragment has been established.

It is generally accepted now that an abdominal approach with complete exploration is indicated in all cases (Fig. 37-50).

Despite the precision in diagnostic accuracy created by the advent of catecholamine measurements, cases are still occasionally missed for want of consideration of this diagnosis, and sudden death may eventuate. In recent years the operative mortality has been considerably reduced, but there remains the occasional case, especially in children, where survival may depend upon the employment of all possible adjuncts, particularly those designed to reduce the incidence of cardiac arrhythmias.

Recurrent Pheochromocytoma. Important but still underemphasized features of pheochromocytoma are the frequency and pathological diversity of recurrences after a seemingly successful primary operation.

In our total experience with 49 patients, 10 had recurrent disease. Six of those had been referred to us as having problems in recurrent pheochromocytoma, making the incidence of recurrence from our own primary operations approximately 10 percent. In three cases surgery could not be carried out. In the most extreme case under our care, 17 years elapsed before the recurrences became symptomatic.

They may be regional recurrences near the bed of the original tumor dissection, they may be diffusely occult occurrences in the lungs (as in two patients who died because we did not appreciate this), or the recurrences may be obviously malignant pheochromocytomas with metastases to bone, liver, and lung.

If the disease cannot be removed, effective palliation may be achieved with chronic α- and β-receptor blockade. Tyrosine hydroxylase inhibition, though theoretically appealing, has depended on agents such as α-methyl-paratyrosine which are too nephrotoxic to permit their extended use. Radiation therapy and chemotherapy have not been helpful to date.

NEUROBLASTOMA

Neuroblastomas are malignant tumors occurring primarily in children, usually under the age of five. They usually present with abdominal masses, often first noted by the mother or by the pediatrician on routine physical examination. The five recognized symptom complexes are shown in Table 37-20.

Neuroblastomas metastasize to bone (30 percent), regional lymph nodes (26 percent), liver (20 percent), skull or brain (11 percent), lungs (9 percent), or cervical lymph nodes (5 percent). They are more common on the left, as are adrenocortical carcinomas. While usually arising from the adrenal they can arise from the sympathetic chain or

Table 37-20. SYMPTOM COMPLEXES
OF NEUROBLASTOMA

Abdominal mass and liver enlargement are the most common symptoms, with or without pallor, weight loss, diffuse adenopathy, leukocytosis, vomiting, and abdominal pain.
Swelling of head, exophthalmos with ecchymosis of eyelids, blindness, increased intracranial pressure, and palpable abdominal tumor.
Extensive bony metastases, pallor, and severe anemia, without other findings.
Abdominal distension and diarrhea with or without mass.
Hypertension may be an additional finding with any of the above.

paraganglia. On rare occasions they have been found in the pelvis or neck.

Liver function tests are usually not of great value even with hepatic metastases, because of the general unreliability of the liver function tests in very young children. There is often a severe anemia. The urinary excretion of catecholamines or the metabolites of catecholamines may be elevated. Since neuroblastomas are more embryonic than the better-differentiated pheochromocytomas, they tend to secrete epinephrine precursor rather than epinephrine itself. They may secrete large amounts of dopamine, and as a consequence the most common urinary metabolite to be found in neuroblastomas is HVA. The urinary VMA level is quite frequently elevated, whereas the urinary catecholamines are only occasionally increased. Postoperative elevation in level of those catecholamines or metabolites elevated preoperatively is often the earliest and most sensitive indicator of recurrence. When the urinary catecholamines are increased, hypertension may be present.

The great problem in operating for neuroblastoma is hemorrhage. These are extremely vascular tumors and very difficult to remove completely. Fresh blood should be available to help counteract the bleeding. Radiation should be given postoperatively, and Cytoxan has been added for the treatment of metastases. New combined chemotherapy protocols are under investigation now and give promise of more effective chemotherapeutic control of this tumor.

Familial neuroblastoma has been reported by Chatten and Voorhess. In this study neuroblastomas were observed in three of four siblings. During one pregnancy the mother was noted to be excreting abnormal amounts of urinary catecholamines during her sixth month of pregnancy. The infant born of this pregnancy was followed and became the fourth affected sibling, when she was discovered to have a mediastinal neuroblastoma at five months of age. The inheritance is thought to be by autosomal dominance. Despite this, there have been three examples of discordant twin pairs in which only one member of the pair had the disease. It is probable, therefore, that many sporadic cases arise by mutation and represent lethal genes or that the dominant gene has variable penetrance or expression. Neuroblastoma in situ is found in 1 in 200 autopsies on infants, while the incidence in live-born children is 1 in 10,000. Therefore, many in situ lesions may have regressed. While other congenital anomalies do not usually accom-

Fig. 37-50. Transabdominal exposure for operations for pheochromocytoma. *A.* A bilateral subcostal incision is made. A variety of other abdominal incisions can be used to good advantage depending on the patient's age, size, and abdominal configuration. *B.* The left adrenal gland is exposed by dividing the gastrocolic ligament and lifting the stomach upward. An incision is made in the posterior peritoneum along the lower border of the pancreas. *C.* The pancreas is elevated, exposing the renal and adrenal veins, and the adrenal gland is easily identified. *D.* An alternative exposure to the left adrenal can be obtained by dividing the peritoneum lateral to the splenic flexure of the colon and mobilizing the colon mediad. An incision is then made through the perirenal fascia, and the adrenal is exposed. *E.* Exposure of the right adrenal gland is obtained by doing a Kocher maneuver with a short lateral extension in the peritoneal incision. The liver is elevated upward, and the adrenal is exposed. The lateral border of the vena cava is rolled mediad to facilitate exposure of the gland, which is partially tucked under the vena cava.

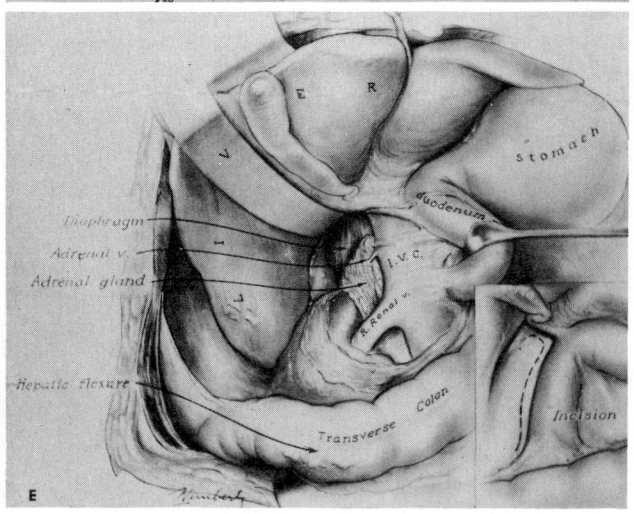

pany neuroblastoma, multiple developmental anomalies have been reported.

Although the mortality of neuroblastoma is high, there is a better prognosis if the diagnosis is made before the infant is one year of age, if the tumor is located in the mediastinum, if the tumor is more mature, and if metastases are not present at the time of treatment. Total removal followed by radiotherapy can be associated with an excellent prognosis.

The natural history of the disease and the results of treating 133 cases have been reported by Fortner et al. The degree of differentiation of the tumor is extremely important in the negative sense, in that without differentiation of the tumor beyond rosettes only one patient survived 5 years. Most of the patients in this series had advanced disease when first seen, only 4.5 percent of them having disease confined to the primary site. This has an extremely important prognostic implication, since in Gross' series 88 percent of patients whose tumors can be totally excised are cured while palliative excision resulted in a 64 percent cure rate and biopsy alone in 10 percent. In the patients of Fortner et al., many of whom had metastases when operated upon, there was a 36.3 percent 5-year survival rate in those with complete removal of the primary lesion and an 18.5 percent 5-year survival in those with partial removal. Because of the greatly improved prognosis with removal of the primary tumor, the writers advise reoperation after radiation therapy if the tumor is not removed when first explored. The exception to this is in those patients with a diffuse retroperitoneal spread of the malignancy over to the other side without massing of tumor at the primary site. This type is impossible to remove.

GANGLIONEUROMA

This is a rare tumor almost always occurring in the adult in contradistinction to neuroblastoma. It is benign and usually discovered as an asymptomatic incidental finding. There are no diagnostic laboratory findings.

References

PITUITARY

Historical Background

Bergland, R. M., Davis, S. L., and Page, R. B.: Pituitary Secretes to Brain, *Lancet*, **2:**276, 1977.

Cushing, H.: Basophil Adenomas of the Pituitary Body, *Bull Johns Hopkins Hosp*, **50:**137, 1932.

———: The Reaction of Posterior Pituitary Extract When Introduced into the Cerebral Ventricles, *Proc Natl Acad Sci*, **17:**163 and 239, 1931.

———: "Studies in Intracranial Physiology and Surgery," Oxford University Press, Fair Lawn, N.J., 1926.

———: The Functions of the Pituitary Body, *Am J Med Sci*, **139:**473, 1910.

———: "The Pituitary Body and Its Disorders," J. B. Lippincott Company, Philadelphia, 1912.

———: The Hypophysis Cerebri: Clinical Aspects of Hyperpituitarism and Hypopituitarism, *JAMA*, **53:**249, 1909.

——— and Davidoff, L.: The Pathological Findings in Acromegaly, Rockefeller Institute Monograph 22, pp. 1–131, 1927.

——— and Goetsch, E.: Concerning the Secretion of the Infundibular Lobe of the Pituitary Body and Its Presence in Cerebrospinal Fluid, *Am J Phys*, **27:**60, 1910.

Fulton, J.: "Harvey Cushing, A Biography," Charles C Thomas, Publisher, Springfield, Ill., 1946.

Henderson, W. R.: The Pituitary Adenomata, *Br J Surg*, **26:**809, 1939.

Page, R. B., Munger, B. L., and Bergland, R. M.: Scanning Microscopy of Pituitary Vascular Casts, *Am J Anat*, **146:**273, 1976.

Rodriguez, E. M.: Ependymal Specializations, *Z Zellforsch*, **102:**153, 1969.

Gross Anatomy

Bergland, R. M., Ray, B. S., and Torack, R. M.: Anatomical Variations in the Pituitary Gland, *J Neurosurg*, **28:**93, 1968.

Harris, G. W.: Neural Control of Pituitary Gland, *Physiol Rev*, **28:**139, 1948.

Lewis, D., and Lee, F. L.: On the Glandular Elements in the Posterior Lobe of the Human Hypophysis, *Bull Johns Hopkins Hosp*, **41:**240, 1927.

Oliver, C., Renon, S. M., and Parter, J. C.: Hypothalamic Pituitary Evidence Vasculature: Evidence for Retrograde Blood Flow in the Pituitary Stalk, *Endocrinol*, **101:**598, 1977.

Page, R. B., and Bergland, R. M.: The Neurohypophyseal Capillary Bed, *Am J Anat*, **148:**345, 1977.

Wislocki, G. B., and King, L. S.: The Permeability of the Hypophysis and Hypothalamus of Vital Dyes, *Am J Anat*, **58:**421, 1936.

Cellular Physiology

Bergland, R. M., and Torack, R. M.: An Electronmicroscopic Study of the Human Infundibulum, *Z Zellforsch*, **99:**1, 1969.

——— and ———: An Ultrastructural Study of Follicular Cells in the Anterior Pituitary, *Am J Pathol*, **57:**273, 1969.

Bloom, F., Segal, D., Ling, N., and Guillemin, R.: Endorphins: Profound Behavioral Effects in Rats Suggest New Etiological Factors in Mental Illness, *Science*, **194:**630, 1976.

deWied, D., and Bohus, B.: Retention of Continued Avoidance Response in Rats by Treatment with Pitressin or a-MSH, *Nature* (Lond.), **212:**1484, 1966.

Goldstein, A.: Endorphins in Pituitary and Brain, *Science*, **193:**1081, 1976.

Martin, J. B., Reichlin, S., and Brown, S.: "Clinical Neuroendocrinology," F. A. Davis Company, Philadelphia, 1977.

Nakane, P. K.: Classifications of Anterior Pituitary Cell Types with Immunoenzyme Histochemistry, *J Histochem Cytochem*, **18:**9, 1970.

Phifer, R. F., Midgley, A. R., and Spicer, S. S.: Histology of Human Hypophyseal Gonadotropin Secreting Cells, in "Gonadotropins," B. B. Saxena and C. G. Beling (eds.), John Wiley & Sons Inc., New York, 1972, pp. 9–24.

Rasmussen, A. T.: The Percentage of Different Cells in Male Adult Human Hypophysis, *Am J Pathol*, **5:**263, 1929.

Schonemann, A.: Hypophysis and Thyreoida, *Arch Pathol*, **129:**310, 1892.

Snyder, S.: Opiate Receptors in the Brain, *N Engl J Med*, **296:**266, 1977.

Pituitary Disorders

Bergland, R. M., and Ray, B. S.: The Arterial Supply of the Human Optic Chiasm, *J Neurosurg,* 31:327, 1966.

Ceballos, R.: Pituitary Changes in Head Trauma, *Alabama J Med Sci,* 3:185, 1966.

Hardy, J.: Transsphenoidal Microsurgical Removal of Pituitary Micro-adenoma, *Prog Neurosurg* (Karger), 6:200, 1975.

Hoff, J. T., and Patterson, R. H.: Craniopharyngiomas in Children and Adults, *J Neurosurg,* 36:299, 1972.

Kjellberg, R. N., and Kliman, B.: Bragg Peak Proton Treatment for Pituitary-Related Conditions, *Proc R Soc Med,* 67:32, 1974.

Malarkey, W. B., and Johnson, J. C.: Pituitary Tumors and Hyperprolactinia, *Arch Int Med,* 136:40, 1976.

Ray, B. S., and Horwith, M.: Surgical Treatment of Acromegaly, *Clin Neurosurg,* 10:31, 1964.

——— and Patterson, R. H.: Surgical Experience with Chromophobe Adenomas, *J Neurosurg,* 34:726, 1971.

Rovitt, R., and Fein, J. M.: Pituitary Apoplexy: A Review, *J Neurosurg,* 37:280, 1972.

Sheehan, H. L., and Whitehead, R.: The Neurohypophysis in Postpartum Hypopituitarism, *J Pathol Bacteriol,* 85:145, 1963.

Teears, R. J., and Silverman, E. M.: Review of 88 Cases of Carcinoma Metastatic to the Pituitary Gland, *Cancer,* 36:216, 1975.

Young, D. G., Bohn, R. C., and Randall, R. V.: Pituitary Tumors Associated with Acromegaly, *J Clin Endocrinol,* 25:249, 1965.

Diagnostic Studies

Lee, W. M., and Adams, J. E.: The Empty Sella Syndrome, *J Neurosurg,* 28:351, 1968.

Therapeutic Modalities

Beatson, G. T.: On the Treatment of Inoperable Cases of Carcinoma of the Mamma, *Lancet,* 2:104, 1896.

Fraser, T. R., and Joplin, G. F.: Subtotal or Total Pituitary Ablation by Implantation of Radioactive Rods, *Mod Treat,* 3:189, 1966.

Luft, R., and Oliverona, H.: Experiences with Hypophysectomy in Man, *J Neurosurg,* 10:301, 1953.

Maas, H., et al.: Estrogen Receptors in Human Breast Cancer Tissue, *Am J Obstet Gynecol,* 113:377, 1972.

Mundinger, F.: Interstitial Curie-Therapy in the Treatment of Pituitary Adenomas, *Prog Neurol Surg* (Karger), 6:326, 1975.

Poulsen, J. E.: Recovery from Retinopathy in a Case of Diabetes with Simmonds' Disease, *Diabetes,* 2:7, 1953.

Rand, R. W., Dashe, A. M., Paglia, D. E., et al: Stereotactic Cryohypophysectomy, *JAMA,* 189:255, 1964.

Ray, B. S.: Intracranial Hypophysectomy, *J Neurosurg,* 28:180, 1968.

——— et al.: Pituitary Ablation for Diabetic Retinopathy, *JAMA,* 203:79, 1968.

Zervas, N.: Stereotaxic Thermal Hypophysectomy, *Prog Neurol Surg* (Karger), 6:217, 1975.

Zimmerman, B. R., and Molnar, G. D.: Prolonged Followup in Diabetic Retinopathy, *Mayo Clin Proc,* 52:233, 1977.

ADRENAL

General

Bajusz, E. (ed.), "An Introduction to Clinical Neuro-endocrinology," The Williams & Wilkins Company, Baltimore, 1967.

Blizzard, R. M.: in L. Wilkins (ed.), "The Diagnosis and Treatment of Endocrine Disorders in Childhood and Adolescence," Charles C Thomas, Publisher, Springfield, Ill., 1965.

Cope, C. L.: "Adrenal Steroids and Disease," J. B. Lippincott Company, Philadelphia, 1964.

Dorfman, R. I., and Ungar, F.: Metabolism of Steroid Hormones, Academic Press, Inc., New York, 1965.

Forsham, P. H., and Melmon, K. L.: The Adrenals, in R. H. Williams (ed.), "Textbook of Endocrinology," 4th ed., p. 287, W. B. Saunders Company, Philadelphia, 1968.

Soffer, L. J., Dorfman, R. I., and Gabrilove, J. L.: "The Human Adrenal Gland," Lea & Febiger, Philadelphia, 1961.

Van Wyk, J. J., and Grumbach, M. M.: Disorders of Sex Differentiation, in R. H. Williams (ed.), "Textbook of Endocrinology," 5th ed., p. 423, W. B. Saunders Company, Philadelphia, 1976, 1,138 pages.

Embryology

Schechter, D. C.: Aberrant Adrenal Tissue, *Ann Surg,* 167:421, 1968.

Anatomy

Kramer, R. K., and Sapirstein, L. A.: Blood Flow to the Adrenal Cortex and Medulla, *Endocrinology,* 81:403, 1967.

ADRENAL CORTEX

Physiology

Fraser, T. R., and Wright, A. D.: Treatment of Acromegaly and Cushing's Disease by [90]Y Implant for Partial Ablation of the Pituitary, in E. B. Astwood and C. E. Cassidy (eds.), "Clinical Endocrinology II," Grune & Stratton, Inc., New York, 1968.

Gordon, R. D., Kuchel, O., Liddle, G. W., and Island, D. P.: Role of the Sympathetic Nervous System in Regulating Renin and Aldosterone Production in Man, *J Clin Invest,* 46:599, 1967.

Gross, F.: The Regulation of Aldosterone Secretion by the Renin-Angiotensin System under Various Conditions, *Acta Endocrinol [Suppl] (Kbh),* 124:41, 1968.

Luetscher, J. A., and Cheville, R. A.: Measurement of Secretion Rates of Adrenal Cortical Hormones, in E. B. Astwood and C. E. Cassidy (eds.), "Clinical Endocrinology II," p. 444, Grune & Stratton, Inc., New York, 1968.

Marusic, E. T., and Mulrow, P. J.: Stimulation of Aldosterone Biosynthesis in Adrenal Mitochondria by Sodium Depletion, *J Clin Invest,* 46:2101, 1967.

Palmore, W. P.: Control of Aldosterone Secretion by the Pituitary Gland, *Science,* 157:1482, 1967.

Cushing's Syndrome

Pathology

Hyperplasia, Adenoma, Carcinoma, Pituitary Tumor

Chaffee, W. R., Moses, A. M., Lloyd, C. W., and Rogers, L. S.: Cushing's Syndrome with Accessory Adrenocortical Tissue, *JAMA,* 186:799, 1963.

Heinbecker, P., O'Neal, L. W., and Ackerman, L. V.: Functioning and Nonfunctioning Adrenal Cortical Tumors, *Surg Gynecol Obstet,* **105:**21, 1957.

Hunder, G. G.: Pathogenesis of Cushing's Disease, *Proc Staff Meetings Mayo Clin,* **41:**29, 1966.

Neville, A. M., and Symington, T.: The Pathology of the Adrenal Gland in Cushing's Syndrome, *J Pathol Bacteriol,* **93:**19, 1967.

O'Neal, L. W.: Pathologic Anatomy in Cushing's Syndrome, *Ann Surg,* **160:**860, 1964.

Rovit, R. L., and Berry, R.: Cushing's Syndrome and the Hypophysis: A Re-evaluation of Pituitary Tumors and Hyperadrenalism, *J Neurosurg,* **23:**270, 1965.

Nodular Dysplasia

Cohen, R. B.: Observations on Cortical Nodules in Human Adrenal Glands: Their Relationship to Neoplasia, *Cancer,* **19:**552, 1966.

Kirschner, M. A., Powell, R. D., Jr., and Lipsett, M. B.: Cushing's Syndrome: Nodular Cortical Hyperplasia of Adrenal Glands with Clinical and Pathological Features Suggesting Adrenocortical Tumor, *J Clin Endocrinol Metab,* **24:**947, 1964.

Meador, C. K., Bowdoin, B., Owen, W. C., Jr., and Farmer, T. A., Jr.: Primary Adrenocortical Nodular Dysplasia: A Rare Cause of Cushing's Syndrome, *J Clin Endocrinol Metab,* **27:**1255, 1967.

Ectopic ACTH Syndrome

Feldman, F., Mitchell, W., and Soll, S.: Psychosis, Cushing's Syndrome and Hyperparathyroidism, *Can Med Assoc J,* **98:**508, 1968.

Gault, M. H., Bilefsky, R., Kinsella, T. D., and Aronoff, A.: Adrenocortical Hyperfunction Associated with Bronchogenic Carcinoma: Report of Five Cases, *Can Med Assoc J,* **93:**1243, 1965.

Goldberg, W. M., and McNeil, M. J.: Cushing's Syndrome Due to an ACTH-producing Carcinoma of the Thyroid, *Can Med Assoc J,* **96:**1577, 1967.

Harris, P. W. R., and El-Katib, M. B.: Cushing's Syndrome and Myelolipomatosis with Carcinoma of the Thymus, *Br J Surg,* **55:**472, 1968.

Hills, E. A.: Adrenocarcinoma of the Bronchus with Cushing's Syndrome, Carcinoid Syndrome, Neuromyopathy and Urticaria, *Br J Dis Chest,* **62:**88, 1968.

Liddle, G. W., Givens, J. R., Nicholson, W. E., and Island, D. P.: Ectopic ACTH Syndrome, *Proc Int Congr Endocrinol 2d London 1964,* International Congress ser., no. 83, 1965, pp. 1063–1067.

Marks, L. J., Russfield, A. B., and Rosenbaum, D. L.: Corticotropin-secreting Carcinoma, *JAMA,* **183:**115, 1963.

Sayle, B. A., Lang, P. A., Green, W. O., Jr., Bosworth, W. C., and Gregory, R.: Cushing's Syndrome Due to Islet Cell Carcinoma of the Pancreas: Report of Two Cases, One with Elevated 5-Hydroxyindole Acetic Acid and Complicated by Aspergillosis, *Ann Intern Med,* **63:**58, 1965.

Schteingart, E., Conn, J. W., Orth, D., Fox, J. E., Bookstein, J. J., and Harrison, T. S.: Secretion of ACTH and B/-MSH by an Adrenal Medullary Paraganglioma, *J Clin Endocrinol Metab,* **34:**676, April, 1972.

Strott, C. A., Nugent, C. A., and Tyler, F. H.: Cushing's Syndrome Caused by Bronchial Adenomas, *Am J Med,* **44:**97, 1968.

Biochemical or Physiological Diagnostic Tests

Baylink, D. J., and Hurxthal, L. M.: Assessment of Adrenocortical Function, *Postgrad Med,* **33:**20, 1963.

Cassidy, C. E., Rosenfeld, P. S., and Bokat, M. A.: Suppression of Activity of Adrenal Cortex by Dexamethasone in Cushing's Syndrome, *J Clin Endocrinol Metab,* **26:**1181, 1966.

Cope, C. L.: The Adrenal Cortex in Internal Medicine, pt. 1, *Br Med J,* **2:**847, 1966.

——— and Mattingly, D.: Some Recent Advances in Adrenal Diagnosis, *Postgrad Med J,* **44:**235, 1968.

Givens, J. R., Ney, R. L., Nicholson, W. E., Graber, A. L., and Liddle, G. W.: The Absence of a Normal Diurnal Variation of Plasma ACTH in Cushing's Disease, *Clin Res,* **12:**267, 1964.

James, V. H. T., Landon, J., and Wynn, V.: Oral and Intravenous Suppression Tests in Diagnosis of Cushing's Syndrome, *J Endocrinol,* **33:**515, 1965.

Jefferies, W. M., Michelakis, A. M., and Price, J. W.: Urinary Cortisol Metabolites in Adrenocortical Hyperfunction, *J Clin Endocrinol Metab,* **26:**219, 1966.

Liddle, G. W.: Tests of Pituitary-Adrenal Suppressibility in the Diagnosis of Cushing's Syndrome, *J Clin Endocrinol Metab,* **20:**1539, 1960.

———, Estep, H. L., Kendall, J. W., Jr., Williams, W. C., Jr., and Townes, A. W.: Clinical Application of a New Test of Pituitary Reserve, *J Clin Endocrinol Metab,* **19:**875, 1959.

Martin, M. M., and Hamman, B. L.: Patterns of Urinary Excretion of Steroids in Cushing's Syndrome, *J Clin Endocrinol Metab,* **26:**257, 1966.

Maynard, D. E., et al.: Rapid Test for Adrenocortical Insufficiency, *Ann Intern Med,* **64:**552, 1966.

Musa, B. U., and Dowling, J. R.: Rapid Intravenous Administration of Corticotropin as Test of Adrenocortical Insufficiency, *JAMA,* **201:**633, 1967.

Nelson, D. H., Sprunt, J. G., and Mims, R. B.: Plasma ACTH Determinations in 58 Patients before or after Adrenalectomy for Cushing's Syndrome, *J Clin Endocrinol,* **26:**722, 1966.

Paris, J.: On Diagnosis of Addison's Disease and Cushing's Syndrome by Laboratory Methods, *Proc Staff Meetings Mayo Clin,* **39:**26, 1964.

Tucci, J. R., Jagger, P. I., Lauler, D. P., and Thorn, G. W.: Rapid Dexamethasone Suppression Test for Cushing's Syndrome, *JAMA,* **199:**379, 1967.

Vagnucci, A. I., Hesser, M. E., Kozak, G. P., Pauk, G. L., Lauler, D. P., and Thorn, G. W.: Circadian Cycle of Urinary Cortisol in Healthy Subjects and Cushing's Syndrome, *J Clin Endocrinol Metab,* **25:**1331, 1965.

Angiographic or Vascular Catheter Studies

Kahn, P. C., and Nickrosz, L. V.: Selective Angiography of the Adrenal Glands, *Am J Roentgenol Radium Ther Nucl Med,* **101:**739, 1967.

Lagergren, C.: Angiographic Changes in the Adrenal Glands, *Am J Roentgenol Radium Ther Nucl Med,* **101:**132, 1967.

Starer, F.: Percutaneous Suprarenal Venography, *Br J Radiol,* **38:**675, 1965.

Selection of Treatment

Nelson, D. H.: Treatment of Cushing's Syndrome, *Mod Treat,* **3:**1421, 1966.

Soffer, L. J., Iannaccone, A., and Gabrilove, J. L.: Cushing's Syndrome: A Study of Fifty Patients, *Am J Med,* **30:**129, 1961.

Pituitary Irradiation

Levene, M. B.: Pituitary Radiotherapy, *Radiol Clin North Am,* **5:**333, 1967.

Molinnati, G. M., Massara, C. F., and Messina, M.: Implantation of the Sella Turcica with ^{90}Yttrium in the Treatment of Cushing's Syndrome of Pituitary Origin, *J Clin Endocrinol Metab,* **27:**861, 1967.

Medical Treatment

Coll, R., Horner, I., Kraiem, Z., and Gafni, J.: Successful Metyrapone Therapy of the Ectopic ACTH Syndrome, *Arch Intern Med,* **121:**549, 1968.

Hutter, A. M., and Kayhoe, D. E.: Adrenal Cortical Carcinoma: Results of Treatment with *o,p'*DDD in 138 Patients, *Am J Med,* **41:**581, 1966.

Krieger, D. T., Amorosa, L., and Linick, F.: Cyproheptadine-Induced Remission of Cushing's Disease, *N Engl J Med,* **293:**893, 1975.

Lipsett, M. B.: Rationale for Chemotherapy of Cushing's Syndrome, in E. B. Astwood and C. E. Cassidy (eds.), "Clinical Endocrinology II," p. 489, Grune & Stratton, Inc., New York, 1968.

Operative Approach and Results

Coone, H. W., and Humphreys, J. W., Jr.: Subtotal Adrenalectomy in Cushing's Syndrome, *Ann Intern Med,* **44:**188, 1956.

Drucker, W. D., Roginsky, M. S., and Christy, N. P.: Persistence of Abnormal Pituitary-Adrenal Relationship in Patients with Cushing's Disease Partially Corrected by Bilateral Subtotal Adrenalectomy, *Am J Med,* **38:**522, 1965.

Egdahl, R. H., and Melby, J. C.: Recurrent Cushing's Disease and Intermittent Functional Adrenal Cortical Insufficiency following Subtotal Adrenalectomy, *Ann Surg,* **166:**586, 1967.

Herrera, M. G., Cahill, C. F., Jr., and Thorn, G. W.: Cushing's Syndrome: Diagnosis and Treatment, *Am J Surg,* **107:**144, 1964.

Ledingham, J. G. G., Nabarro, J. D. N., and Le Quesne, L. P.: Adrenal Autografts in the Treatment of Cushing's Syndrome Caused by Adrenal Hyperplasia, *Br J Surg,* **53:**1057, 1966.

Raker, J. W., Cope, O., and Ackerman, I. P.: Surgical Experience with the Treatment of Hypertension of Cushing's Syndrome, *Am J Surg,* **107:**153, 1964.

Scott, H. W., Jr., Foster, J. H., Liddle, G., and Davidson, E. T.: Cushing's Syndrome Due to Adrenocortical Tumor: 11-Year Review of 15 Patients, *Ann Surg,* **162:**505, 1965.

————, Liddle, G. W., Harris, A. P., and Foster, J. H.: Diagnosis and Treatment of Cushing's Syndrome, *Ann Surg,* **155:**696, 1962.

Total Adrenalectomy for Treatment of Cushing's Syndrome, *JAMA,* **175:**130, 1961. (Editorial.)

Complications of Surgery

Montgomery, D. A. A., Welbourn, R. B., McCaughey, W. T. E., and Gleadhill, C. A.: Pituitary Tumors Manifested after Adrenalectomy for Cushing's Snydrome, *Lancet,* **2:**707, 1959.

Nelson, D. H., and Sprunt, J. G.: Pituitary Tumors Postadrenalectomy for Cushing's Syndrome, *Proc Int Congr Endocrinol 2d London 1964,* International Congress ser., no. 83, 1965, p. 1053.

Adrenogenital Syndrome, Feminizing Syndromes

Adrenocortical Carcinomas, and Inter-sex Problems

Adrenogenital

Congenital Adrenal Hyperplasia

Bongiovanni, A. M., and Root, A. W.: Adrenogenital Syndrome, *N Engl J Med,* **268:**1283, 1963.

Ehrhardt, A. A., Epstein, R., and Money, J.: Fetal Androgens and Female Gender Identity in the Early-treated Adrenogenital Syndrome, *Bull Johns Hopkins Hosp,* **122:**160, 1968.

Hamilton, W.: Surgical Procedures in Congenital Adrenal Hyperplasia, *Dev Med Child Neurol,* **10:**106, 1968.

Huffstadt, A. J. C.: Surgical Correction of Female Pseudohermaphroditism Due to Adrenal Hyperplasia, *Br J Plast Surg,* **20:**359, 1967.

Lattimer, J. K.: Relocation and Recession of the Enlarged Clitoris with Preservation of the Glans: An Alternative to Amputation, *J Urol,* **86:**113, 1961.

Seymour, R. J., and Kinch, R. A. H.: Recession and Relocation of the Enlarged Clitoris in Congenital Adrenogenital Syndrome, *Can J Surg,* **9:**365, 1966.

Postnatal

Cooper, J. D., Maldonado, L., and Earll, J. M.: Adrenocortical Carcinoma with Virilism in an Infant under 1 Year of Age, *Am J Dis Child,* **113:**730, 1967.

Adult

Brooks, R. V., Mattingly, D., Mills, I. H., and Prunty, F. T. G.: Postpubertal Adrenal Virilism with Biochemical Disturbance of the Congenital Type of Adrenal Hyperplasia, *Br Med J,* **1:**1294, 1960.

Gabrilove, J. L., Sharma, D. C., and Dorfman, R. I.: Adrenocortical 11β-Hydroxylase Deficiency and Virilism First Manifest in the Adult Woman, *N Engl J Med,* **272:**1189, 1965.

Hutter, A. M., Jr., and Kayhoe, D. E.: Adrenal Cortical Carcinoma: Clinical Features of 138 Patients, *Am J Med,* **41:**572, 1966.

——— and ———: Adrenal Cortical Carcinoma: Results of Treatment with *o,p'*DDD in 138 Patients, *Am J Med,* **41:**581, 1966.

Serge, E. J.: Androgens, Virilization and the Hirsute Female, Charles C Thomas, Publisher, Springfield, Ill., 1967.

Mild Excesses in Androgen Production

Jacobs, J. P.: Hirsutism and Benign Androgenic Hyperplasia of the Adrenals, *Am J Obstet Gynecol,* **101:**37, 1968.

Prunty, F. T. G.: Androgen Metabolism in Man: Some Current Concepts, *Br Med J,* **2:**605, 1966.

Estrogen-secreting Tumors

Gabrilove, J. L., Sharma, D. C., Woitz, H. H., and Dorfman, R. I.: Feminizing Adrenocortical Tumors in Male: Review of 52 Cases including Case Report, *Medicine,* **44:**37, 1965.

Stewart, W. K., Fleming, L. W., and Wotiz, H. H.: The Feminizing Syndrome in Male Subjects with Adrenocortical Neoplasms, *Am J Med,* **37:**455, 1964.

Adrenocortical Carcinomas and Tumors with Mixed Secretions

Lipsett, M. B., Hertz, R., and Ross, G. T.: Clinical and Pathophysiologic Aspects of Adrenocortical Carcinoma, *Am J Med,* **35:**374, 1963.

MacFarlane, D. A.: Cancer of the Adrenal Cortex, *Ann R Coll Surg Engl,* **23:**155, 1958.

Villee, D. B., Rotner, H., Kliman, B., Briefer, C., Jr., and Federman, D. D.: Androgen Synthesis in a Patient with Virilizing Adrenocortical Carcinoma, *J Clin Endocrinol Metab,* **27:**1112, 1967.

Disorders of Sexual Development

Federman, D. D.: Disorders of Sexual Development, *N Engl J Med,* **277:**351, 1967.

Adrenalectomy for Metastatic Cancer of the Breast or Prostate

Block, G. E., Jensen, E. V., and Polley, T. Z.: The Prediction of Hormonal Dependency of Mammary Cancer, *Ann Surg,* **182:**342, 1975.

———, Vial, A. B., McCarthy, J. D., Porter, C. W., and Coller, F. A.: Adrenalectomy in Advanced Mammary Cancer, *Surg Gynecol Obstet,* **108:**651, 1959.

Cade, S.: Adrenalectomy for Disseminated Breast Cancer, *Br Med J,* **2:**613, 1966.

Dao, T. L-Y., and Huggins, C.: Bilateral Adrenalectomy in the Treatment of Cancer of the Breast, *Arch Surg,* **71:**645, 1955.

——— and Nemoto, T.: An Evaluation of Adrenalectomy and Androgen in Disseminated Mammary Carcinoma, *Surg Gynecol Obstet,* **121:**1257, 1965.

Fairgrieve, J.: Selective Criteria for Surgical Removal of the Endocrine Glands in Advanced Breast Cancer, *Surg Gynecol Obstet,* **120:**371, 1965.

Fracchia, A. A., Randall, H. T., and Farrow, J. H.: The Results of Adrenalectomy in Advanced Breast Cancer in 500 Consecutive Patients, *Surg Gynecol Obstet,* **125:**747, 1967.

Huggins, C. B.: Adrenalectomy as Palliative Treatment, *JAMA,* **200:**973, 1967.

Nemoto, T., and Dao, T. L.: Significance of Liver Metastasis in Women with Disseminated Breast Cancer Undergoing Endocrine Ablative Surgery, *Cancer,* **19:**421, 1966.

Adrenalectomy for Hypertension

Sellers, A. M., Barrett, J. S., Wolferth, C. C., Sr., Lopez, R., Itskovitz, H. D., Blakemore, W. S., and Zintel, H. A.: Adrenalectomy and Sympathectomy for Hypertension, *Arch Surg,* **89:**880, 1964.

Smithwick, R. H.: Practical Treatment for Hypertension: Splanchnicectomy, Adrenalectomy and Nephrectomy, *Postgrad Med,* **34:**32, 1963.

Aldosteronism

Symptoms and Signs and Review

Conn, J. W.: Hypertension, the Potassium Ion and Impaired Carbohydrate Tolerance, *N Engl J Med,* **273:**1135, 1965.

———, Knopf, R. F., and Nesbit, R. M.: Clinical Characteristics of Primary Aldosteronism from an Analysis of 145 Cases, *Am J Surg,* **107:**159, 1964.

Kaplan, N. M.: Primary Aldosteronism, in E. B. Astwood and C. E. Cassidy (eds.), "Clinical Endocrinology II," p. 467, Grune & Stratton, Inc., New York, 1968.

Incidence

Conn, J. W., Rovner, D. R., Cohen, E. L., and Nesbit, R. M.: Normokalemic Primary Aldosteronism: Its Masquerade as "Essential" Hypertension, *JAMA,* **195:**21, 1966.

Fishman, L. M., Kuchel, Olo, Liddle, G. W., Michelakis, A. M., Gordon, R. D., and Chick, W. T.: Incidence of Primary Aldosteronism Uncomplicated "Essential" Hypertension, *JAMA,* **205:**497, 1968.

Kokko, J. P., Brown, T. C., and Berman, M. M.: Adrenal Adenoma and Hypertension, *Lancet,* **1:**468, 1967.

Pathology

Crane, M. G., Harris, J. J., and Herber, R.: Primary Aldosteronism Due to an Adrenal Carcinoma, *Ann Intern Med,* **63:**494, 1965.

Davis, W. W., Newsome, H. H., Wright, L. D., Hammond, W. G., Easton, J., and Bartter, F. C.: Bilateral Adrenal Hyperplasia as a Cause of Primary Aldosteronism with Hypertension, Hypokalemia and Suppressed Renin Activity, *Am J Med,* **42:**642, 1967.

Flanagan, M. J., and McDonald, J. H.: Heterotropic Adrenocorticol Adenoma Producing Primary Aldosteronism, *J Urol,* **98:**133, 1967.

Neville, A. M., and Symington, T.: Pathology of Primary Aldosteronism, *Cancer,* **19:**1854, 1966.

Biochemical or Physiologic Tests

Biglieri, E. G., Slaton, P. E., Jr., Kronfield, S. J., and Deck, J. B.: Primary Aldosteronism with Unusual Secretory Pattern, *J Clin Endocrinol Metab,* **27:**715, 1967.

———, ———, ———, and Schambelan, M.: Diagnosis of an Aldosterone-producing Adenoma in Primary Aldosteronism, *JAMA,* **201:**510, 1967.

Brown, J. J., Davies, D. L., Lever, A. F., and Robertson, J. I. S.: Plasma Renin Concentration in Human Hypertension: I. Relationship between Renin, Sodium, and Potassium, *Br Med J,* **2:**144, 1965.

Conn, J. W., and Cohen, E. L.: Primary Aldosteronism: Importance of the Level of Plasma Renin as an Adjunct in Diagnosis, in Bumpus, F. M., and Page, I. H., "Handbook of Experimental Pharmacology," Springer-Verlag, 1973.

Cope, C. L.: The Adrenal Cortex in Internal Medicine, pt. II, *Br Med J,* **2:**914, 1966.

Espiner, E. A., Tucci, J. R., Jagger, P. I., and Lauler, D. P.: Effect of Saline Infusions on Aldosterone Secretion and Electrolyte Excretion in Normal Subjects and Patients with Primary Aldosteronism, *N Engl J Med,* **277:**1, 1967.

Kaplan, N. M.: Hypokalemia in the Hypertensive Patient with Observations on the Incidence of Primary Aldosteronism, *Ann Intern Med,* **66:**1079, 1967.

Lauler, D. P.: Preoperative Diagnosis of Primary Aldosteronism, *Am J Med,* **41:**855, 1966.

Relman, A. S.: Diagnosis of Primary Aldosteronism, *Am J Surg,* **107:**173, 1964.

Salti, I. S., Stiefel, M., Ruse, J. L., and Laidlaw, J. C.: Non-tumorous "Primary" Aldosteronism: Type Relieved by Gluco-Corticoid, *Can Med Ass J,* **101:**1, 1969.

Schacht, R. A., and Frame, B.: Infusion of Chlorothiazide in a Patient with Primary Aldosteronism: Observations on Potassium Clearance, *JAMA,* **201:**323, 1967.

Localization Techniques

Conn, J. W., Beierwaltes, W. H., Liegerman, L. M., Ansari, A. N., Cohen, E. L., Bookstein, J. J., and Herwig, K. R.: Primary Aldosteronism: Preoperative Tumor Visualization by Scintillation Scanning, *J Clin Endocrinol Metab,* **33:**713, 1971.

Egdahl, R. H., Kahn, P., and Melby, J. C.: Unilateral Adrenalectomy for Aldosteronomas, Localized Preoperatively by Differential Adrenal Vein Catheterization, *Surgery,* **64:**117, 1968.

Melby, J. C., Spark, R. F., Dale, S. L., Egdahl, R. H., and Kahn, P. C.: Diagnosis and Localization of Aldosterone-producing Adenomas by Adrenal-Vein Catheterization, *N Engl J Med,* **277:**1050, 1967.

Sutton, D.: Diagnosis of Conn's and Other Adrenal Tumours by Left Adrenal Phlebography, *Lancet,* **1:**453, 1968.

Medical Treatment

Abbott, E. C., Gornall, A. G., Sutherland, D. J., Stiefel, M., and Laidlaw, J. C.: Influence of Heparin-like Compound on Hypertension, Electrolytes and Aldosterone in Man, *Can Med Assoc J,* **94:**1155, 1966.

Melby, J. C.: Aldosterone Inhibitors, in E. B. Astwood, and C. E. Cassidy (eds.), "Clinical Endocrinology II," p. 477, Grune & Stratton, Inc., New York, 1968.

Preoperative Treatment

Flanagan, M. J., Gantt, C. J., and McDonald, J. H.: Primary Aldosteronism, *J Urol,* **88:**111, 1962.

Mobley, J. E., Headstream, J. W., and Melby, J.: Primary Aldosteronism: Preoperative Preparation with Spironolactone, *JAMA,* **180:**1056, 1962.

Operative Technique and Results

Nesbit, R. M.: Primary Aldosteronism: Its Diagnosis and Surgical Management, *J Urol,* **97:**404, 1966.

Rhamy, R. K., McCoy, R. M., Scott, H. W., Fishman, L. M., Michelakis, A. M., and Liddle, G. W.: Primary Aldosteronism: Experience with Current Diagnostic Criteria and Surgical Treatment in Fourteen Patients, *Ann Surg,* **167:**718, 1968.

Silen, W., Biglieri, E. G., Slaton, P., and Galante, M.: Management of Primary Aldosteronism: Evaluation of Potassium and Sodium Balance, Technic of Adrenalectomy and Operative Results in 24 Cases, *Ann Surg,* **164:**600, 1966.

Smithwick, R. H., Harrison, J. H., Unger, L., and Whitelaw, G. P.: Surgical Treatment of Aldosteronism: Combined Experiences at the Massachusetts Memorial and the Peter Bent Brigham Hospitals, *Am J Surg,* **107:**178, 1964.

Complications and Postoperative Course

Bartter, F. C., Pronove, P., Gill, J. R., Jr., and MacCardle, R. C.: Hyperplasia of the Juxtaglomerular Complex with Hyper-aldosteronism and Hypokalemic Alkalosis: A new Syndrome, *Am J Med,* **33:**811, 1962.

Biglieri, E. G., Slaton, P. E., Jr., Silen, W. S., Galante, M., and Forsham, P. H.: Postoperative Studies of Adrenal Function in Primary Aldosteronism, *J Clin Endocrinol. Metab,* **26:**553, 1966.

Adrenocortical Insufficiency (Addison's Disease)

Autoimmunity in Idiopathic Addison's Disease, *Lancet,* **1:**1040, 1967.

Donnelly, W. J.: Unexplained Addison's Disease, *Postgrad Med,* **42:**339, 1967.

Jagatic, J., and Rubnitz, M. E.: Massive Bilateral Adrenal Bleeding: Five-Year Review of Cases, *Ill Med J.,* **132:**273, 1967.

Maynard, D. E., et al.: Rapid Test for Adrenocortical Insufficiency, *Ann Intern Med,* **64:**552, 1966.

Schambelan, M., Stockigt, J. R., and Biglieri, E. G.: Isolated Hypoaldosteronism in Adults, *N Engl J Med,* **287:**573, 1972.

Turkington, R. W., and Lebovitz, H. E.: Extra-adrenal Endocrine Deficiencies in Addison's Disease, *Am J Med,* **43:**499, 1967.

Surgical Complications of Adrenal Steroid Therapy

Glenn, F., and Grafe, W. R., Jr.: Surgical Complications of Adrenal Steroid Therapy, *Ann Surg,* **165:**1023, 1967.

ADRENAL MEDULLA

Pheochromocytoma

Glenn, F., and Mannix, H., Jr.: The Surgical Management of Chromaffin Tumors, *Ann Surg,* **167:**619, 1968.

Hume, D. M.: Pheochromocytoma in the Adult and in the Child, *Am J Surg,* **99:**458, 1960.

Scott, H. W., Riddell, D. H., and Brockman, S. K.: Surgical Management of Pheochromocytoma, *Surg Gynecol Obstet,* **120:**707, 1965.

Physiology and Pharmacology of Epinephrine and Norepinephrine

Axelrod, J.: Metabolism of Epinephrine and Other Sympathomimetic Amines, *Physiol Rev,* **39:**751, 1959.

——— and Weinshilboum, R.: Catecholamines, *N Engl J Med,* **287:**237, 1972.

Blaschko, H.: The Development of Current Concepts of Catecholamine Formation, *Pharmacol Rev,* **11:**307, 1959.

Von Euler, U. S. Noradrenaline: Chemistry, Physiology, Pharmacology and Clinical Aspects, Charles C Thomas, Publisher, Springfield, Ill., 1956.

Voorhess, M. L.: The Catecholamines in Tumor and Urine from Patients with Neuroblastoma, Ganglio-neuroblastoma and Pheochromocytoma, *J Pediat Surg,* **3:**147, 1968.

Wurtman, R. J., and Axelrod, J.: Control of Enzymatic Synthesis of Adrenaline in the Adrenal Medulla by Adrenal Cortical Steroids, *J Biol Chem,* **241:**2301, 1966.

Incidence

Graham, J. B.: Collective Review: Pheochromocytoma and Hypertension: An Analysis of 207 Cases, *Int Abstr Surg,* **92:**105, 1951.

Kvale, W. F., Roth, G. M., Manger, W. M., and Priestly, J. T.: Pheochromocytoma, *Circulation,* **14:**622, 1956.

Minno, A. M., Bennett, W. A., and Kvale, W. F.: Pheochromcytoma: Study of 15 Cases Diagnosed at Autopsy, *Proc Staff Meet Mayo Clin,* **30:**394, 1955.

Symptoms, Signs, and Pathophysiology

Harrison, T. S., Bartlett, J. D., Jr., and Seaton, J. F.: Exaggerated Urinary Norepinephrine Response to Tilt in Pheochromocytoma, *N Engl J Med,* **277:**725, 1967.

Vallance, W. B.: Sudden Death from an Asymptomatic Pheochromocytoma, *Br Med J,* **23:**686, 1957.

Simulation of Pheochromocytoma Attack

Plass, H. F.: Monoamine-Oxidase Inhibitor Reactions Simulating Pheochromocytoma Attacks, *Ann Intern Med,* **61:**924, 1964.

Location

Cahill, G. F.: Pheochromocytoma, *Bull NY Acad Med,* **29:**749, 1953.

Symington, T., and Goodall, A. L.: Studies in Pheochromocytoma: Pathological Aspects, *Glasgow Med J,* **34:**75, 1953.

Malignant Pheochromocytoma

Holsti, L. R.: Malignant Extra-adrenal Phaeochromocytoma, *Br J Radiol,* **37:**944, 1964.

Palmieri, G., Ikkos, D., and Luft, R.: Malignant Pheochromocytoma, *Acta Endocrinol, (Kbh),* **36:**549, 1961.

Diagnostic Tests

Bogaert, M. G., and Vermuelen, A.: Pheochromocytoma of the Urinary Bladder, with Inconclusive Chemical and Pharmacologic Tests, *Am J Med,* **53:**797, 1972.

Crout, J. R., Pisano, J. J., and Sjoerdsma, A.: Urinary Excretion of Catechol Amines and Their Metabolites in Pheochromocytoma, *Am Heart J,* **61:**375, 1961.

Engelman, K., Horwitz, D., Amerose, I. M., and Sjoerdsma, A.: Further Evaluation of the Tyramine Test for Pheochromocytoma, *N Engl J Med,* **278:**705, 1968.

Freier, D. T., and Harrison, T. S.: Rigorous Biochemical Criteria for the Diagnosis of Pheochromocytoma, *J Surg Res,* **14:**177, 1973.

Gifford, R. W., and Tweed, D. C.: Spurious Elevation of Urinary Catecholamines during Therapy with Alpha-Methyldopa, *JAMA,* **182:**493, 1962.

Gitlow, S., Mendlowitz, M., and Bertani, L. M.: The Biochemical Techniques for Detecting and Establishing the Presence of a Pheochromocytoma, *Am J Cardiol,* **26:**270, 1970.

Gjessing, L. R., and Hjermann, I.: Difficulties in Chemical Diagnosis in Phaeochromocytoma, *Lancet,* **2:**1014, 1964.

Lawrence, A. M.: Glucagon Provocative Test for Pheochromocytoma, *Ann Intern Med,* **66:**1091, 1967.

Robinson, R., Ratcliffe, J., and Smith, P.: A Screening Test for Pheochromocytoma, *J Clin Pathol,* **12:**541, 1959.

———, Smith, P., and Whittaker, S.: Secretion of Catecholamines in Malignant Phaeochromocytoma, *Br Med J,* **1:**1422, 1964.

Sheps, S. G., and Maher, F. T.: Histamine and Glucagon Tests in Diagnosis of Pheochromocytoma, *JAMA,* **205:**895, 1968.

Sunderman, G. W.: Measurements of Vanilmandelic Acid for the Diagnosis of Pheochromocytoma and Neuroblastoma, *J Clin Pathol,* **42:**481, 1964.

Wolf, R. L., Mendlowitz, M., Raboz, J., and Gitlow, S. E.: New Rapid Test for Pheochromocytoma, *JAMA,* **188:**859, 1964.

Localization

Epinephrine versus Norepinephrine

Von Euler, U. S.: Increased Urinary Excretion of Noradrenaline and Adrenaline in Cases of Pheochromocytoma, *Ann Surg,* **134:**929, 1951.

Inferior Vena Cava Sampling

Harrison, T. S., Seaton, J. F., Cerny, J. C., Bookstein, J. J., and Bartlett, J. D., Jr.: Localization of Pheochromocytoma by Caval Catheterization, *Arch Surg,* **95:**339, 1967.

Von Euler, U. S., and Strom, G.: Present Status of Diagnosis and Treatment of Pheochromocytoma, *Circulation,* **15:**5, 1957.

Arteriography and X-ray

Boijsen, E., Williams, C. M., and Judkins, M. P.: Angiography and Pheochromocytoma, *Am J Roentgenol Radium Ther Nucl Med,* **98:**225, 1966.

Kahn, P. C.: Radiologic Identification of Functioning Adrenal Tumors, *Radiol Clin North Am,* **5:**221, 1967.

Meaney, T. F., and Buonocore, E.: Selective Arteriography as a Localizing and Provocative Test in the Diagnosis of Pheochromocytoma, *Radiology,* **87:**309, 1966.

Meyers, M. A.: Characteristic Radiographic Shapes of Pheochromocytomas and Adrenocortical Adenomas, *Radiology,* **87:**889, 1966.

Rossi, Plinio, Young, I. S., and Panke, W. F.: Techniques, Usefulness and Hazards of Arteriography of Pheochromocytoma, *JAMA,* **205:**547, 1968.

Familial

Carman, C. T., and Brashear, R. E.: Pheochromocytomas as an Inherited Abnormality: Report of 10th Affected Kindred and Review of the Literature, *N Engl J Med,* **263:**419, 1960.

Tisherman, S. E., Gregg, F. J., and Danowski, T. S.: Familial Pheochromocytoma, *JAMA,* **182:**152, 1962.

Pregnancy

Barzel, U. S., Bar-Ilan, Z., and Rumney, G.: Pheochromocytoma and Pregnancy: Simultaneous Delivery by Caesarean Section and Resection of Tumor, *Am J Obstet Gynecol,* **89:**519, 1964.

Blair, R. G.: Phaeochromocytoma and Pregnancy: Report of a Case and Review of 51 Cases, *J Obstet Gynaecol Br Commonw,* **70:**110, 1963.

Parbossingh, I. S., and Tate, J.: Pheochromocytoma and Pregnancy: Case Report, *West Indian Med J,* **4:**265, 1955.

Pickles, B. G.: Phaeochromocytoma Complicating Pregnancy, *J Obstet Gynaecol Br Commonw,* **65:**1010, 1958.

Walker, R. M.: Phaeochromocytoma in Relation to Pregnancy, *Br J Surg,* **51:**590, 1964.

Neurocutaneous Syndromes

Shocket, E., and Teloh, H. A.: Aganglionic Megacolon, Pheochromocytoma, Megaloureter, and Neurofibroma: Co-occurrence of Several Neural Abnormalities, *Am J Dis Child,* **94:**185, 1957.

Williams, E. D., and Pollack, D. J.: Multiple Mucosal Neuromata with Endocrine Tumors: A Syndrom Allied to von Recklinghausen's Disease, *J Pathol Bacteriol,* **91:**71, 1966.

Congenital Heart

Folger, G. M., Jr., Roberts, W. C., Mehrizi, A., Shah, K. D., Glancy, D. L., Carpenter, C. C. J., and Esterley, J. R.: Cyanotic Malformations of the Heart with Pheochromocytoma, *Circulation,* **29:**750, 1964.

Lees, M. H.: Catecholamine Metabolic Excretion of Infants with Heart Failure, *J Pediat,* **69:**259, 1966.

Reisman, M., Goldenberg, E. D., and Gordon, J.: Congenital Heart Disease and Neuroblastoma, *Am J Dis Child,* **111:**308, 1966.

Pheochromocytoma and Thyroid Carcinoma

Hazard, J. B., Hawk, W. A., and Crile, G.: Medullary (Solid) Carcinoma of the Thyroid: A Clinicopathologic Entity, *J Clin Endocrinol Metab,* **19:**152, 1959.

Huang, S., and McLeish, W. A.: Familial Pheochromocytoma and Amyloid-producing Medullary Carcinoma of Thyroid, *Laval Med,* **39:**22, 1968.

Nourok, D. S.: Familial Pheochromocytoma and Thyroid Carcinoma, *Ann Intern Med,* **60:**1028, 1964.

Sapira, J. D., Althan, M., Vandyk, K., and Shapiro, A. P.: Bilateral Adrenal Pheochromocytoma and Medullary Thyroid Carcinoma, *N Engl J Med,* **273:**140, 1965.

Schimke, R. N., and Hartmann, W. H.: Familial Amyloid Producing Medullary Thyroid Carcinoma and Pheochromocytoma: Distinct Genetic Entity, *Ann Intern Med,* **63:**1027, 1965.

Sipple, J. H.: The Association of Pheochromocytoma with Carcinoma of the Thyroid Gland, *Am J Med,* **31:**163, 1961.

Williams, E. D.: A Review of 17 Cases of Carcinoma of the Thyroid and Phaeochromocytoma, *J Clin Pathol,* **18:**288, 1965.

Pheochromocytoma, Cholelithiasis, and Increase in Free Fatty Acids

Gifford, R. W., Jr., Kvale, W. F., and Maher, F. T.: Clinical Features, Diagnosis and Treatment of Pheochromocytoma: A Review of 76 Cases, *Proc Staff Meetings Mayo Clin,* **39:**281, 1964.

Pheochromocytoma and Renovascular Hypertension

Assaykeen, T. A., and Ganong, W. F.: The Sympathetic Nervous System and Renin Secretion, in W. F. Ganong and L. Martini (eds.), "Frontiers in Neuroendocrinology," Oxford University Press, New York, 1971.

Garrett, H. C., Scott, R., Jr., Howell, J. F., and DeBakey, M. E.: Pheochromocytoma and Renal Artery Stenosis: Surgical Treatment of Secondary Hypertension, Case Report, *Arch Surg,* **90:**97, 1965.

Harrison, J. H., Gardner, F. H., and Dammin, G. J.: Note on Pheochromocytoma and Renal Hypertension, *J Urol,* **79:**173, 1958.

Harrison, T. S., Birbari, A., and Seaton, J. F.: Malignant Hypertension in Pheochromocytoma: Correlation with Plasma Renin Activity, *Johns Hopkins Med J,* **130:**329, 1972.

Kerzner, M. S., Reeves, J. A., DeNyse, D., and Claunch, B. C.: Pheochromocytoma with Renal Artery Compression in an Identical Twin, *Arch Intern Med,* **121:**91, 1968.

Maebashi, M., Miura, Y., and Yoshinaga, K.: Plama Renin Activity in Pheochromocytoma, *Jap Circ J,* **32:**1427, 1968.

Rosenheim, M. L., Ross, E. J., Wong, O. M., Hudson, C. L., Davies, D. R., and Smith, J. F.: Unilateral Renal Ischaemia Due to Compression of Renal Artery by Phaeochromocytoma, *Am J Med,* **34:**735, 1963.

Straube, K. R., and Hodges, C. V.: Pheochromocytoma Causing Renal Hypertension, *Am J Roentgenol Radium Ther Nucl Med,* **98:**222, 1966.

Tanigawa, H., Allison, D. J., and Assaykeen, T. A.: A Comparison of the Effects of Various Catecholamines on Plasma Renin Activity Alone and in the Presence of Adrenergic Blocking Agents, in J. Genest and E. Koiw (eds.), "Hypertension—1972," Springer Verlag New York, Inc., New York, 1972.

Vetter, H., Vetter, W., Warnholz, C., Bayer, J.-M., Käser, H., Vielhaber, K., and Krück, F.: Renin and Aldosterone Secretion in Phenochromocytoma, *Am J Med,* **60:**866, 1976.

Hypotension, Shock, or Sudden Death

Hypotension or Shock

Huston, J. R., and Stewart, W. R.: Hemorrhagic Pheochromocytoma with Shock and Abdominal Pain, *Am J Med.,* **39:**502, 1965.

McAlister, W. H., and Koehler, P. R.: Hemorrhage into a Pheochromocytoma in a Patient on Anticoagulants, *J Can Assoc Radiol,* **18:**404, 1967.

Parkinson, T.: Phaeochromocytoma Presenting as Postural Hypotension, *Proc R Soc Med,* **57:**673, 1964.

Richmond, J., Frazer, S. C., and Miller, D. R.: Paroxysmal Hypotension Due to an Adrenalin-secreting Phaeochromocytoma, *Lancet,* **2:**904, 1961.

Sudden Death

Coates, P. A., and Rigal, W. M.: Post Anesthetic Death from Pheochromocytoma without Hypertension, *Lancet,* **1:**1374, 1961.

Crockett, K. A., Snow, E., and Rees, V. L.: Pheochromocytoma as Cause of Unexpected Operating Room Deaths, *Am Surg,* **27:**395, 1961.

Mitchell, L.: An Unusual Cause of Sudden Death, *Practitioner,* **193:**205, 1964.

Childhood

Insley, J., and Smallwood, W. C.: Pheochromocytoma in Children, *Arch Dis Child,* **37:**606, 1962.

Moon, H. D., Koneff, A. A., Li, C. H., and Simpson, M. E.: Pheochromocytomas of Adrenals in Male Rats Chronically Injected with Pituitary Growth Hormone, *Proc Soc Exp Biol Med,* **93:**74, 1956.

Stackpole, R. H., Melicow, M. M., and Uson, A. C.: Pheochromocytoma in Children: Report of 9 Cases and Review of the First 100 Published Cases with Followup Studies, *J Pediatr,* **63:**314, 1963.

Special Locations

Bilateral

Baker, N. H., Swindell, H. F., Rollins, L. T.: The Surgical Treatment of Bilateral Pheochromocytomas, *Ann Surg,* **159:**456, 1964.

Zuckerkandl

Van Zyl, J. J. W., van Zyl, F. D. dT, and Wicht, C. L.: Phaeochromocytoma of the Organ of Zuckerkandl, *Suid-Afrikaanse Tydskr Chir,* **4:**43, 1966.

Bladder

Besser, M. I. B., and Pfau, A.: Pheochromocytoma of the Urinary Bladder, *Br J Urol,* **40:**245, 1968.

Intrathoracic

Engelman, K., and Hammond, W. G.: Adrenaline Production by an Intrathoracic Phaeochromocytoma, *Lancet,* **1:**609, 1968.

Cervical

Fries, J. G., and Chamberlin, J. A.: Extra-adrenal Pheochromocytoma: Literature Review and Report of a Cervical Pheochromocytoma, *Surgery,* **63:**268, 1968.

Medical Treatment

Bellos, J.: Non Surgical Treatment of Pheochromocytoma, *JAMA,* **185:**601, 1963.

Crago, R. M., Eckholdt, J. W., and Wiswell, J. G.: Pheochromocytoma: Treatment with α- and β-Adrenergic Blocking Drugs, *JAMA,* **202:**870, 1967.

Egdahl, R. H., and Chobanian, A. V.: Acute Pheochromocytoma, *Surg Clin North Am,* **46:**645, 1966.

Harrison, T. S., Dagher, F. J., Beck, L., and Bartlett, J. D., Jr.: Rationale and Indications for Preoperative Adrenergic Receptor Blockade in Pheochromocytoma, *Med Clin North Am,* **53:**1349, 1969.

Iseri, L. T., Henderson, H. W., and Derr, J. W.: Use of Adrenolytic Drug, Regitine, in Pheochromocytoma, *Am Heart J,* **42:**129, 1951.

Surgical and Anesthetic Considerations

Buist, N. R. M., Mijer, F., and O'Brien, D.: Treatment of a Phaeochromocytoma with a β-Adrenergic Blocking Agent, *Arch Dis Child,* **41:**435, 1966.

Glenn, F., and Mannix, H. Jr.: The Surgical Management of Chromaffin Tumors, *Ann Surg,* **167:**619, 1968.

Grimson, K. S., Longino, F. H., Kernodle, C. E., and O'Near, H. B.: Treatment of a Patient with a Pheochromocytoma: Use of an Adrenolytic Drug before and during Operation, *JAMA,* **180:**1273, 1949.

Priestley, J. T., Kvale, W. F., and Gifford, R. W., Jr.: Pheochromocytoma: Clinical Aspects and Surgical Treatment, *Arch Surg,* **86:**778, 1963.

Schnelle, N., Carney, F. M., Didier, E. P., and Faulconer, A., Jr.: Anesthesia Surgical Treatment of Pheochromocytoma, *Surg Clin North Am,* **45:**991, 1965.

Recurrent Pheochromocytoma

Harrison, T. S., Freier, D. T., and Cohen, E. L.: Recurrent Pheochromocytoma, *Arch Surg,* **108:**450, 1974.

Neuroblastoma

Bohuon, C.: Catecholamine Metabolism in Neuroblastoma, *J Pediat Surg,* **3:**114, 1968.

Brown, W. G., Owens, J. B., Berson, A. W., and Henry, S. K.: Vanilmandelic Acid Screening Test for Pheochromocytoma and Neuroblastoma, *Am J Clin Pathol,* **46:**599, 1966.

Chatten, J., and Voorhess, M. L.: Familial Neuroblastoma, *N Engl J Med,* **277:**1230, 1967.

Fortner, J., Nicastri, A., and Murphy, M. L.: Neuroblastoma: Natural History and Results of Treating 133 Cases, *Ann Surg,* **167:**132, 1968.

James, D. H., Jr.: Proposed Classification of Neuroblastoma, *J Pediat,* **71:**764, 1967.

Keep, C. E.: The Role of Surgery in Resectable, and Metastatic Neuroblastoma, *JAMA,* **205:**57, 1968.

Rubin, P.: Urogenital Tract: Wilms' Tumor and Neuroblastoma, *JAMA,* **205:**153, 1968.

Chapter 38

Thyroid and Parathyroid

by **Seymour I. Schwartz and Edwin L. Kaplan**

THYROID

(by Seymour I. Schwartz)

Historical Background

The thyroid gland, previously referred to as the "laryngeal" gland, was so named by Wharton in 1646 because of either its own shieldlike (*thyreos,* shield) shape or the shape of the thyroid cartilage, with which it is closely associated. Classic descriptions of hyperthyroidism, or exophthalmic goiter, were presented by Parry (1825), Graves (1835), and von Basedow (1840), and hypothyroidism, or myxedema, was described by Curling (1850) and Gull (1875). Schiff, in the middle of the nineteenth century, conducted experiments demonstrating the importance of the thyroid. Excision in dogs resulted in fatality which could be prevented by a previous graft of the gland. In 1882, Reverdin produced experimental myxedema by total or partial thyroidectomy. In the 1890s, Murray and Howitz successfully treated myxedema with thyroid extract. Although Hedenus performed a total thyroidectomy for goiter in 1800, Theodor Kocher is regarded as the father of thyroid surgery. He was the first to successfully excise the thyroid for goiter (1878), and he performed this operation over 2,000 times with only a 4.5 percent mortality. He also described "cachexia strumipriva," i.e., myxedema, which he noted as a sequel in 30 of his first 100 thyroidectomies. For his pioneering efforts in the field of thyroid surgery, he received the Nobel prize in 1909. The first successful transplantation of thyroid was reported by Payr in 1906, who transplanted a portion of the gland from a woman into the spleen of a myxedematous daughter with "successful" results. Isolation of the hormone thyroxine (T4) was accomplished by Kendall in 1914.

Anatomy

The thyroid gland, which has an average weight of 20 Gm, is convex anteriorly and concave posteriorly as a result of its relation to the anterolateral portions of the trachea and larynx, around which it is wrapped and to which it is firmly fixed by fibrous tissue. The lateral lobes extend along the sides of the larynx, reaching the level of the middle of the thyroid cartilage. They reside in a bed between the trachea and larynx mediad and the two carotid sheaths and the sternocleidomastoid muscles laterally. The thyroid gland is enveloped by a thickened fibrous capsule which sends septa into the gland substance to produce an irregular and incomplete pseudolobulation. No true lobulation exists. The deep cervical fascia divides into an anterior and posterior sheath, creating a loosely applied false capsule for the thyroid. Anteriorly, the thyroids are in relation to the infrahyoid muscles. Situated on the posterior surface of the lateral lobes of the gland are the parathyroid glands, which reside within the surgical capsule, and the recurrent nerves, which lie in a cleft between the trachea and esophagus just medial to the lateral lobes. The lateral lobes are joined by the isthmus which crosses the trachea. The pyramidal lobe is a long, narrow projection of thyroid tissue extending upward from the isthmus lying on the surface of the thyroid cartilage usually to the left of the prominence of that structure. It represents a vestige of the embryonic thyroglossal duct and can be demonstrated in about 80 percent of patients at operation.

The thyroid has an abundant blood supply with a normal flow rate of about 5 ml/Gm/minute. The four major arteries are the paired superior thyroid arteries, which arise from the external carotid arteries and descend several centimeters in the neck to reach the upper poles of the thyroid glands, where they branch, and the paired inferior thyroid arteries, which arise from the thyrocervical trunks of the subclavian arteries and enter the lower poles from behind. A fifth artery, the thyroidea ima, arises from the arch of the aorta and enters the thyroid in the midline. A venous plexus forms under the capsule and contributes to confluences forming the superior thyroid vein at the upper pole and the middle thyroid vein at the lower pole, both of which enter the internal jugular vein. Also occasionally arising from the lower pole are the inferior thyroid veins, which drain directly into the innominate vein.

The gland receives its innervation from sympathetic and parasympathetic divisions of the autonomic nervous system. The sympathetic fibers arise from the cervical ganglion and enter with blood vessels, while the parasympathetic fibers are derived from the vagus and reach the gland via branches of the laryngeal nerves.

Microscopically, the thyroid is composed of follicles, or acini. The follicles are roughly spherical and have an average diameter of 30μ. They represent storage depots which receive and store the products of the lining epithelial cells. These are usually cuboidal. Under the influence of thyrotropin stimulation, the height of the cells increases, changing the shape to a columnar one, and the lumen decreases proportionally.

The thyroid gland's relation to the recurrent laryngeal and external laryngeal nerves is of major surgical significance. Riddell indicated that among cases in which surgeons "avoid" rather than expose the recurrent laryngeal nerve there is a 4 percent incidence of vocal cord damage. Hunt et al. reported the anatomy of the recurrent laryngeal nerves in 100 cases. The right recurrent laryngeal nerve resided in the tracheoesophageal groove in 64 percent of cases, whereas the left nerve was similarly located on the left side in 77 percent of cases. The nerve was lateral to the trachea in 33 percent of cases on the right side and 22 percent on the left side. In six cases on the right side and four on the left, the nerve was anterolateral to the trachea and in danger of division during subtotal lobectomy. On one occasion, a direct recurrent laryngeal nerve was given off in the neck without looping around the subclavian artery. The inferior thyroid artery is often used as a landmark for demonstration of the recurrent laryngeal nerve. The vessel was absent in five instances on the left and twice on the right in the above series. The recurrent laryngeal nerve passed anterior to the inferior thyroid artery in 37 percent of cases on the right side and 24

percent on the left. In 50 percent of cases, the nerve was embedded in the ligament of Berry, which is of importance because traction on the gland would put the nerve on stretch and make it subject to section. Damage to the recurrent laryngeal nerve results in paresis or paralysis of the intrinsic musculature of the larynx.

The superior laryngeal nerves innervate the cricothyroid muscle. There is dispute as to whether the innervation of the interarytenoid muscle is supplied by the superior or inferior laryngeal nerves. In 85 percent of cases, the superior laryngeal nerves lie immediately adjacent to the vascular pedicles of the superior poles of the thyroid glands, requiring that the vessels be ligated with care to avoid injury. In 18 percent of cases, the nerve is intimately related to the vessels lying parallel and just deep to them in the pretracheal fascia. In 7 percent, the nerve passes through the division of the superior thyroid vessels, coursing over the anterosuperior portion of the gland. In only 15 percent of cases does the superior laryngeal nerve enter the thyropharyngeal muscle before reaching the region of the superior pole of the thyroid gland, thus protecting it from manipulation by the surgeon.

ANOMALIES

The thyroid is embryologically an offshoot of the primitive alimentary tract, from which it later becomes separated. A median anlage arises from the pharyngeal floor in the region of the foramen cecum of the tongue. The main body of the thyroid descends into the neck from this origin and is supposedly joined by a pair of lateral components originating from the ultimobranchial bodies of the fourth and fifth branchial pouches. The contribution of these lateral components presently is considered to be small.

The median thyroid anlage may fail to develop, with the rare situation of athyreosis as a result, or it may differentiate in abnormal locations. The most common of these is the pyramidal lobe, which has been reported in as many as 80 percent of patients in whom the gland was surgically exposed. Other variations involving the median thyroid anlage represent an arrest in the usual descent of part or all of the thyroid-forming material to its normal location in front of the second to sixth tracheal rings. These include the development of a lingual thyroid, suprahyoid, infrahyoid, and prethyroid tissue, and persistence of the thyroglossal duct, which is the most common of the clinically important anomalies of thyroid development (see Chap. 39). Infrequently, the entire gland or parts of it descend more caudad, which results in thyroid tissue located in the superior mediastinum behind the sternum, adjacent to the aortic arch or between the aorta and pulmonary trunk, within the upper portion of the pericardium, and even in the interventricular septum of the heart. Most intrathoracic goiters, however, are not true anomalies but rather extensions of pathologic elements of a normally situated gland into the superior or posterior mediastinum.

LATERAL ABERRANT THYROID RESTS. True lateral aberrant thyroid tissue is rare, since the lateral anlagen are normally incorporated into the expanding lateral lobes of the median thyroid anlage. Lateral aberrant thyroid tissue has not been shown to function in man. It is now felt that the so-called "lateral aberrant thyroid" is a metastasis from the gland proper. Carcinoma, which has been noted so frequently in "lateral rests," actually represents metastatic disease within cervical lymph nodes from a primary site and does not arise independently.

LINGUAL THYROID. Lingual thyroid is relatively rare and estimated to occur in 1 in 3,000 cases of thyroid disease. It does, however, represent the most common form of functioning ectopic thyroid tissue which achieves clinical significance. Lingual thyroids are associated with cervical athyreosis in 70 percent of cases and occur much more commonly in females.

Clinical Manifestations. The diagnosis may be made by discovery of an incidental posterior lingual mass in an asymptomatic patient. The mass may enlarge and cause dysphagia, dysphonia, dyspnea, or sensation of choking. Lingual thyroid has been known to cause complications during induction of anesthesia. Hypothyroidism is frequently present, but hyperthyroidism, which is unusual, can occur. The incidence of malignancy is extremely low, occurring in 4 of 144 patients with symptomatic lingual thyroid. The diagnosis should be suspected when a mass is detected in the region of the foramen cecum of the tongue. The diagnosis is readily established by scanning with [131]I.

Treatment. Unless there is immediate surgical indication, treatment should be instituted with replacement thyroid hormone to suppress the lingual thyroid and reduce its size. Radioactive ^{131}I may also be used to reduce the size and is particularly appropriate if there is associated hyperthyroidism.

Indications for surgical intervention include difficulty in swallowing, speech, or breathing; hemorrhage; degeneration and necrosis; uncontrolled hyperthyroidism; and, occasionally, the suspicion of malignancy. A preliminary tracheostomy may be indicated with large or hemorrhagic lesions to obviate the consequences of postoperative tracheal edema. The lingual thyroid may be removed by an intraoral route, by drawing the tongue forward and incising directly over the growth, which is completely or partially removed. Lateral pharyngotomy, in some instances, may represent a preferential approach. Autotransplantation of the excised lingual thyroid has been recommended to avoid the development of hypothyroidism, and success has been reported by several writers.

Physiology

The function of the thyroid gland is to synthesize and secrete thyroid hormone, which is necessary for overall metabolism. This function is dependent upon an interplay between several processes, including (1) iodine metabolism, (2) the production, storage, and secretion of thyroid hormone by the thyroid gland, and (3) the effects of this hormone on various organ systems. The production of thyroid hormone is influenced by intricate regulatory mechanisms and responds to multiple and diverse physiologic, pathologic, and pharmacologic alterations.

IODINE METABOLISM. The formation of thyroid hormone depends upon the availability of exogenous iodine which is normally satisfied by dietary sources and is thus dependent upon the iodine content of water and soil. Ingested iodine is rapidly absorbed from the gastrointestinal tract, usually within 1 hour. It is then distributed through the extracellular space in the form of iodides and is progressively extracted from the plasma both by the thyroid and kidneys until essentially all the iodine is either bound in organic form within the thyroid or excreted as urinary iodides (Fig. 38-1). Ninety percent of the body iodine stores are present within the thyroid, predominantly in the organic form. Studies employing labeled iodine have demonstrated that approximately two-thirds of the administered dose ultimately appears in the urine, while the thyroid collects the remaining third. The partitioning of the ingested iodide between thyroid and kidney is complete within 48 hours, and the plasma and tissues are almost cleared of iodide. The subsequent appearance of labeled iodine within the circulation is the result of the secretion of thyroid hormone and is concomitant with a decrease in activity within the thyroid gland. A small fraction of the iodine which had been removed from the extracellular fluid by the thyroid gland is ultimately secreted back into the circulation as inorganic iodide. Renal disease such as nephrosis and marked proteinuria may be associated with a significant urinary loss of iodide affecting the body economy. Gastrointestinal malabsorption may be accompanied by significant augmentation of the usually small amounts of iodine lost in the stool.

SYNTHESIS AND SECRETION OF THYROID HORMONE. The steps in the synthesis of thyroid hormone are (1) the concentration of iodide within the gland, (2) the formation of precursor amino acids, 3-monoiodotyrosine (MIT) and 3-5-diiodotyrosine (DIT), (3) the coupling of these inactive iodotyrosines to form the hormonally active iodothyronines, triiodothyronine (T3) and thyroxine (T4).

The production of thyroid hormone begins with the active transport of iodine from the plasma into the thyroid cells. The iodine transfer mechanism is influenced by thyroid-stimulating hormone (TSH), which stimulates every step in thyroid hormone synthesis and secretion, and is also modified by an internal autoregulatory system so that its responsiveness to TSH stimulation varies inversely with the glandular content of organic iodine. When iodine transport is defective, because of either pharmacologic inhibitors or spontaneous disease, goiter and/or hypothyroidism results. However, this can be overcome by increasing the plasma iodine concentration and allowing quantities to enter the gland by diffusion.

The iodide which enters the thyroid remains in its free state only briefly before it is further metabolized. It is rapidly incorporated into thyroglobulin, and it has been shown that 24 hours after administration of labeled iodine, 99 percent is bound to protein. Tyrosine radicals of proto thyroglobulin molecules are iodinated to form MIT and DIT. Organic iodinations are conditioned to some extent by the stimulation of TSH and may be inhibited by a great number of pharmacologic agents, including the usual antithyroid drugs, or by defects in the organ-binding mechanism with resultant hypothyroidism and/or goiter. The

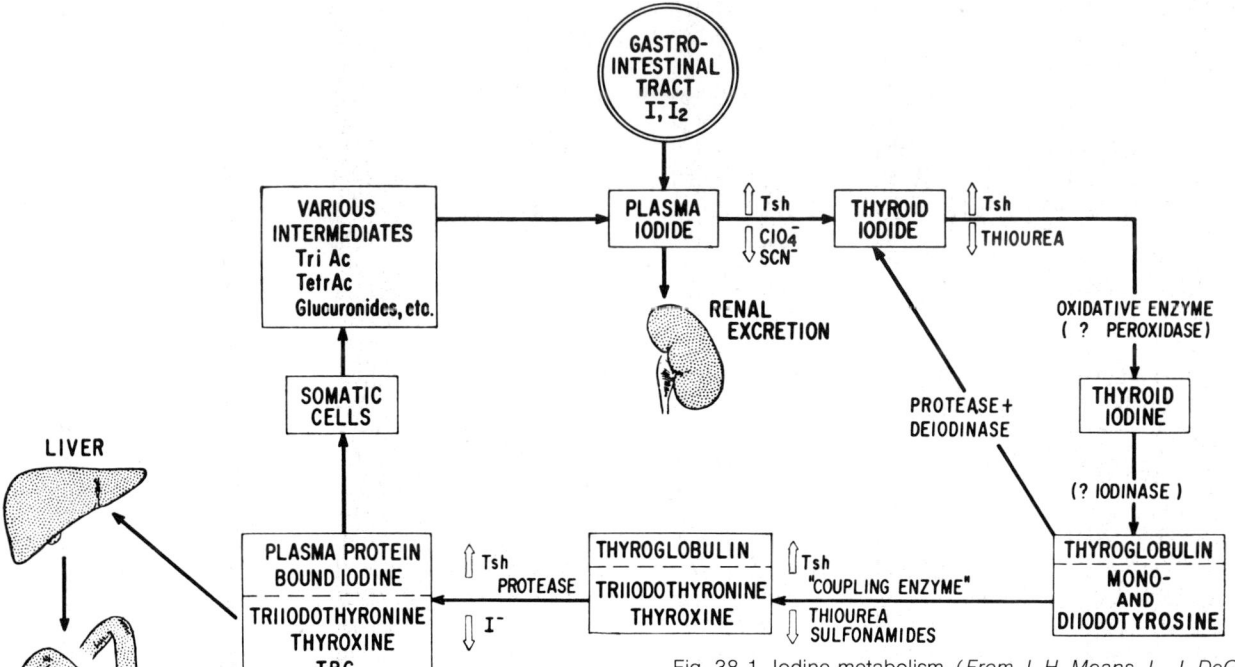

Fig. 38-1. Iodine metabolism. (*From J. H. Means, L. J. DeGroot, and J. B. Stanbury, "The Thyroid and Its Diseases," 3d ed., chap. 2, McGraw-Hill Book Company, New York, 1963.*)

coupling of two iodotyrosine molecules leads to the formation of iodothyronine, a process in which a variety of enzymatic systems have been implicated. T4 is formed by the coupling of two DIT radicals, while T3 is formed by the coupling of one MIT and one DIT radical. The proportion of T3 to T4 synthesized and secreted is dependent on the degree of iodination of intrafollicular thyroglobulin.

STORAGE, SECRETION, AND METABOLISM OF THYROID HORMONE. The hormonally active iodothyronines, T4 and T3, are held in peptide linkage with a specific thyroprotein, thyroglobulin, which forms the major component of intrafollicular colloid. The storage is of such magnitude that the administration of antithyroid blocking agents for as long as 2 weeks results in only minimal decrease of T4 and T3. The normal human thyroid gland contains enough preformed T4 to maintain the euthyroid state for 2 months without synthesis, thus forming an excellent buffer against the changes in dietary intake of iodine.

Release of the active hormones into the circulation involves hydrolysis of the thyroglobulin by proteases and peptidases, resulting in T4 and T3. The activity of these enzymes is enhanced by the administration of TSH. At the same time, some metabolically inert iodine amino acids enter the circulation and are deiodinized, and the iodine is reutilized in the metabolic cycle. The active thyroid hormones become attached to plasma protein, the best known of which is the thyroxine-binding globulin (TBG) and the more recently recognized thyroxine-binding prealbumin (TBPA).

Disorders related to the storage-and-release mechanism occur in subacute thyroiditis, in Hashimoto's disease, and

after surgical manipulation of the gland. Also, iodides and iodotyrosines may be found in the blood, associated with several types of nontoxic goiter and hyperplastic tissue.

In the plasma, the ratio of T4 to T3 is 10–20:1. T3 is bound less firmly to protein and thus enters the peripheral tissues more rapidly. It is three to four times more active than T4 per unit weight and accounts for approximately half the metabolic effect of the secreted hormone. The free hormone available to the tissue is responsible for its metabolic action. The half-life of T3 is 2 to 3 days, while the half-life of T4 is 6 to 11 days, and both hormones leave the blood in an exponential fashion. A significant amount of T4 is converted to T3, which may be the only active hormone intracellularly. As they lose iodine atoms, the iodine returns to the blood to reenter the metabolic pool. T3 and T4 are conjugated in the liver with glucuronic acid and excreted into the bile. In the intestine, these conjugates are disrupted, and a portion of the free hormones is reabsorbed. In man, less than 5 percent of the circulating T4 is involved in the enterohepatic circulation. In acute hepatitis, the functional hepatic turnover of T4 is retarded, while in chronic diarrhea and nephrosis there may be excessive loss. Large amounts of hormone and iodide may appear in the milk of lactating females.

The metabolic impact of thyroid hormone on peripheral tissue is widespread and accompanied by an increased oxygen consumption and calorigenesis. Thyroid hormone stimulates protein synthesis and affects all aspects of carbohydrate metabolism, regulating the magnitude of the glycogenolytic and hyperglycemic effects of epinephrine and potentiating the effects of insulin on glycogen synthesis and glucose utilization. Thyroid hormone also influences the processes of lipid metabolism, as evidenced by the fact that the serum cholesterol and phospholipid vary inversely with the state of thyroid function.

REGULATION OF THYROID ACTIVITY. The function of the thyroid gland is closely regulated by the central nervous system and by the level of circulating iodine. As a consequence of these regulatory mechanisms, thyroid activity responds to a variety of physiologic and pathologic changes as well as pharmacologic agents.

The suspicion that the central nervous system is involved in the stimulation and inhibition of thyroid hormone is an old one, but scientific support is relatively recent. The anterior pituitary basophil cells secrete TSH, which regulates thyroid function. Absence or reduction of TSH secretion is accompanied by decreased synthesis and secretion of thyroid hormone, flattening of the thyroid epithelium, and reduction in vascularity of the gland. Conversely, increased TSH secretion accelerates the production and release of thyroid hormone while anatomically increasing the cellularity and vascularity of the thyroid gland. TSH stimulates all processes leading to the synthesis and secretion of thyroid hormone. When the target gland is responsive, the basal metabolic rate (BMR) is increased within a few hours of TSH administration, and there is an associated increase in the T4 and T3.

It is now felt that the cerebral cortex acts on the hypothalamus, which secretes a thyrotropin-releasing hormone (TRH), which in turn acts on the pituitary and induces the release of TSH. The secretion of TSH is also controlled in a "feedback" manner by the level of thyroid hormone in the blood (Fig. 38-2). TSH secretion is inhibited by an excess of circulating thyroid hormone and augmented by thyroid hormone deprivation. When antithyroid substances of the thiourea type cause hypothyroidism, the pituitary responds by increasing TSH secretion with resultant hyperplasia and increased vascularity of the thyroid gland.

The concentration of intrathyroidal iodide inversely influences responsiveness to TSH, thus effecting an intrinsic regulatory system. When small doses of iodine are administered, there is an increase in thyroid hormone synthesis for a short time. With progressively larger doses, there is a biphasic response, at first increasing and then decreasing, due to a relative blockade in organic binding. With moderate or large doses administered repeatedly, the relative inhibition of organic binding eventually escapes, representing an adaptation phenomenon. Pharmacologic doses of iodide decrease the rate of release of glandular iodine and the formation of active hormone. Concentration of T4 in the serum is reduced, and thyrotoxicity in patients with diffuse toxic goiter is rapidly relieved. The vascularity and hyperplasia of the gland are reversed through the action of iodine on TSH, thus facilitating surgical excision.

In addition to these pharmacologic effects of iodine, the biosynthesis of thyroid hormone may be altered by agents known as *antithyroid drugs*. There are two major categories: The first, represented by perchlorate and thiocyanate, prevent the concentration of iodine by the thyroid. In the presence of high iodine intake, however, the blood iodine can rise to a level at which the concentrating mechanism

Fig. 38-2. Schema of the homeostatic regulation of thyroid function. Secretion of TSH is regulated by a negative feedback mechanism acting directly on the pituitary and is normally inversely related to the concentration of unbound hormone in the blood. Release of TSH is induced by TRH, secretion of which appears to set the level of the pituitary feedback mechanism. Factors regulating secretion of TRH are uncertain but may include the free hormone in the blood and stimuli from higher centers. Autoregulatory control of thyroid function is also shown. High concentrations of intrathyroidal iodide decrease the rate of release of thyroidal iodine. In addition, the magnitude of the organic iodine pool inversely influences the iodide transport mechanism and the response to TSH. [*From S. H. Ingbar and K. A. Woeber, The Thyroid Gland, in R. H. Williams (ed.), "Textbook of Endocrinology," 4th ed., W. B. Saunders Company, Philadelphia, 1968.*]

is not required and the drugs lose their effect. The second group of antithyroid drugs include organic substances which prevent the binding of iodine to tyrosine radicals. The best known of this group are the thiourea derivatives. The action of this group of drugs is characteristically independent of the level of blood iodide.

The regulatory mechanisms contribute to the alterations in thyroid function associated with physiologic and pathologic changes in the organism. From childhood through senescence, the T4 and T3 are essentially unchanged, while the thyroidal ^{131}I uptake, clearance, and turnover rate tend to decrease slightly with age. In pregnancy, the thyroid becomes enlarged, and there is evidence of increased vascularity. Thyroidal uptake is increased, and the T4 and T3 levels rise and remain elevated until after delivery. All changes in thyroid function which accompany normal pregnancy are exaggerated in molar pregnancy, which may be associated with excess "placental thyrotropin." Ectopic TSH activity also has been described with choriocarcinomas. However, in general, thyroid function in human beings appears to be independent of sex. In women thyroid disorders do occur more frequently during puberty, pregnancy, and the menopause. ACTH and cortisone reduce thyroidal iodine uptake and slightly decrease the T4 and T3, while epinephrine and norepinephrine increase the BMR in thyrotoxic patients unassociated with a measurable alteration in T4 and T3.

Since the hepatobiliary system is an important site for

degradation of thyroid hormone, liver disease may cause an alteration in protein-bound iodine (PBI). With infectious hepatitis and obstructive jaundice, there may be an associated increase in PBI due to regurgitation of iodine from the bile to the blood. With cirrhosis there is a decrease in PBI and an increase in the proportion of the free T4 and T3, and the ^{131}I uptake is often increased. With reduced glomerular filtration and cardiac disease, there is an elevation in the PBI level and a lowered rate of thyroidal clearance of ^{131}I. A nephrotic syndrome may be associated with the stigmata of hypothyroidism, while in cardiac failure the increased work in breathing results in an elevated basal metabolic rate. Several anesthetic agents, particularly ether, increase the circulating thyroid hormone, and surgical treatment may be associated with an increased concentration of free T4 in the plasma due to a decrease in the binding by protein.

Evaluation of Patients with Thyroid Disease

Interview of the patient is directed at determining whether there is evidence of hyperfunction or insufficient function of the thyroid gland. Symptoms in this regard include gross changes in appearance, skin texture, hair, temperature tolerance, and perspiration. Inquiry should also evaluate changes in mental activity, irritability, emotional lability, lethargy, muscular strength, and endurance. Other evidences of abnormal thyroid activity include change in sleep habits, weight, appetite, bowel habits, and muscular strength. The specific signs and symptoms of thyrotoxicosis and myxedema will be presented in subsequent sections of this chapter.

Symptoms related to pressure of the thyroid on neighboring structures in the neck include dysphagia, dysphonia, dyspnea, and a choking sensation. When a thyroid mass is apparent, the duration, rate of growth, and presence of accompanying pain should be determined. A history of exposure to ionizing radiation is pertinent. In the patient with a nontoxic goiter, diet, possible ingestion of goiterogenic drugs, and family history are all relevant.

Physical examination requires a precise evaluation of the thyroid gland and adjacent cervical structures. The neck should be inspected while it is slightly extended. In thin patients, a normal thyroid, particularly in the region of the isthmus, may be visible. If the thyroid is visible, it will rise with deglutition unless it is adherent to adjacent structures because of invasive malignant disease or thyroiditis. A goiter which fills the suprasternal notch may be seen to rise out of the chest with swallowing. Asymmetry and large masses within the gland may be apparent. Palpation should be performed from two vantage points, in front of and behind the seated patient, applying the tips of the fingers in a gentle fashion. In most thin people, it is possible to outline the gland, whereas the normal thyroid is not palpable in obese individuals and in those with short necks. Palpation of the cricoid cartilage serves to orient the examiner, since the superior border of the isthmus lies just below this level.

The normal gland has a rubbery consistency. The diffuse goiter and hyperplastic gland is softer. In Hashimoto's disease the gland is firmer, while with carcinoma or Riedel's struma the thyroid may be stony hard. Nodules may be identified, and transillumination should be used to distinguish between cystic and solid masses. The thyroid should be auscultated to identify bruits which are indicative of a hyperactive gland but must be differentiated from murmurs transmitted from the base of the heart and venous hums. The regional lymph nodes should be examined in the anterior triangles of the neck. A node, known as the Delphian node, may be palpable on the trachea just above the thyroid isthmus. This is frequently associated with malignant disease or thyroiditis. If there is suggestion of retrosternal goiter, the arms should be raised in an attempt to elicit respiratory distress.

Radiologic examination of the upper neck and mediastinum may demonstrate evidence of compression or displacement of the trachea. Miliary calcification may be noted in papillary carcinoma, while more extensive calcification is suggestive of nodular goiter. An electrocardiogram is indicated if there is suggestion of thyrotoxicosis. If carcinoma is considered, the vocal cords should be visualized for mobility.

THYROID FUNCTION TESTS

A variety of laboratory tests have been developed to assess thyroid function and thyroid lesions. Each test has specific indications, none is uniformly reliable, and all are subject to alteration by exogenous and endogenous factors.

RADIOACTIVE ISOTOPE STUDIES. These are widely employed to evaluate the state of thyroid function and hormonal synthesis. Several radioactive isotopes of iodine, ^{131}I, ^{132}I, and ^{125}I, are available. ^{131}I is the most widely used, but ^{132}I is particularly applicable when repeated doses are required, because it has a shorter half-life. By contrast, ^{125}I is recommended for localization of functioning thyroid tissues with scanning procedures. Recently ^{99m}Tc has been used for scanning, since a reduced radiation is used and a more rapid readout is possible.

Thyroidal Uptake and Urinary Excretion. When iodine isotopes are administered either orally or intravenously, they are cleared by the thyroid and kidney. Within 24 hours, the mean value in the plasma is extremely low, and it is essentially undetectable by 72 hours. Measurements of the percentage of thyroidal uptake of radioactive iodine are therefore generally made at 24 hours and are directed at establishing or excluding a diagnosis of hyperthyroidism or hypothyroidism. When doses of 2 to 50 μc are given orally, the normal mean 24-hour thyroidal uptake is 25 percent, with a range of 9 to 35 percent. Values lower than 8 percent indicate hypothyroidism, while values higher than the normal range indicate hyperfunction. In states of severe hyperfunction the thyroidal uptake peak may be reached within a few hours, and it may be appropriate to measure the uptake several hours after administration. The normal uptake at 3 hours rarely exceeds 25 percent.

The expansion of the body stores of iodine is probably the most common exogenous cause of lowering of thyroidal ^{131}I uptake. This is seen following the administration of organic iodinated dyes as used in radiologic studies such as pyelography and cholecystography. While the dyes employed in pyelography are usually cleared rapidly, those used for cholecystography may last for several months. The reduction in renal iodide clearance may be due to renal failure or cardiac failure. Decreased thyroidal iodine accumulation follows the administration of replacement doses of thyroid hormone which suppress the secretion of TSH and also occurs in patients with nephrosis and excessive hormonal loss in the urine.

Thyroid Scanning. Scintillation scanning localizes the site of radioiodine accumulation in the thyroid gland or in ectopic thyroid tissue. ^{131}I is the time-honored isotope which has been utilized, but more recently ^{125}I with a softer gamma energy appears to be superior in resolving small areas and in defining some "cold" nodules. ^{125}I is inferior to ^{131}I when part of the thyroid is retrosternal because of the significant absorption of the soft radiation by the overlying bone. The technique employs a mechanical device which moves a columnated detector back and forth and determines the location of activity (Fig. 38-3).

The indications for thyroid scanning can be divided into three general categories: (1) patients with solitary or multiple nodules in whom clinical findings are insufficient, (2) thyrotoxicotic patients, and (3) patients with suspected or proved cancer of the thyroid. Nodules of the thyroid may be classified as hyperfunctional, that is, with more radioactivity than the normal portion of the gland (Fig. 38-4); functional, that is, nodules which concentrate radioactivity equal to the remainder of the gland (Fig. 38-5); hypofunctional, or nodules which concentrate less activity than the remainder of the gland; and finally nonfunctional, or "cold" nodules, which concentrate no radioactivity (Fig. 38-6). Caution must be exercised in interpreting the scintillation scan of nodules less than 1.5 cm in diameter. In hyperthyroidism, the scintillation scan may be of value in determining the presence of abnormally positioned hyperfunctioning tissue, such as substernal thyroid (Fig. 38-7) or lingual thyroid. In patients with recurrent thyrotoxicosis following thyroidectomy, remnants which are not palpable may be visualized by the scan.

Many feel that a scintogram should be routine before an operation on the thyroid is performed because of suspicion of carcinoma. A preoperative scan is of value in differentiating functioning metastatic carcinoma (Fig. 38-8). However, in patients with metastatic disease from an unknown primary lesion, the results are rarely helpful, because metastases from thyroid glands fail to pick up ^{131}I when normal thyroid is present.

T4 AND T3 DETERMINATIONS. The old standard measurement of PBI and butanol-extractable iodine in patients receiving large amounts of iodine has been replaced by specific measurements of T4 and T3. The PBI has been compromised by the widespread use of estrogen-containing oral contraceptives, which increase binding power, and also by the contamination of our environment with iodine, as well as the liberal use of iodinated compounds for radiologic procedures.

Fig. 38-3. ^{131}I scintillation scan. Normal thyroid.

The competitive binding (Murphy-Pattee) method measures T4 specifically and is unaffected by iodine-containing substances. However, oral contraceptives increase TBG and, therefore, increase total serum T4, while testosterone and anticonvulsants decrease this level. An absolutely free T4 test is uninfluenced by binding proteins or iodine, but it is too complex and not widely available. T3 resin uptake is readily determined and has been combined with the PBI to result in normal values in euthyroid patients with abnormal levels of binding proteins. Also, the serum T4 determination has been combined with a resin uptake test using labeled T4 to define the absolute free T4 value. Kits are available for these studies. Methods for determining T3 are also available commercially.

Normal ranges for these determinations are:

Total T4—4 to 11µg/100 ml
Free T4—0.8 to 2.9 mg/100 ml
      T3—160 to 320 mg/100 ml

Fig. 38-4. ^{131}I scintillation scan. Hyperfunctional nodule, left lobe. (Palpable mass enclosed in circle.)

Fig. 38-5. ^{131}I scintillation scan. Functional nodule, left lobe. (Palpable mass enclosed in circle.)

Simplistically, the patient's T4/normal × patient's T3/normal = 1. For euthyroid state

$$>1.2 = \text{hyperthyroidism}$$
$$<0.8 = \text{hypothyroidism}$$

TESTS OF REGULATION. Autonomy of thyroid function may be demonstrated by lack of suppression when T3 is administered in amounts to meet peripheral requirements. One hundred micrograms of T3 are given for 5 days. Lack of suppression is manifested by no decrease of thyroid-labeled iodine uptake. An abnormal suppression test oc-

Fig. 38-6. ^{131}I scintillation scan. Nonfunctional (cold) nodule, right lobe.

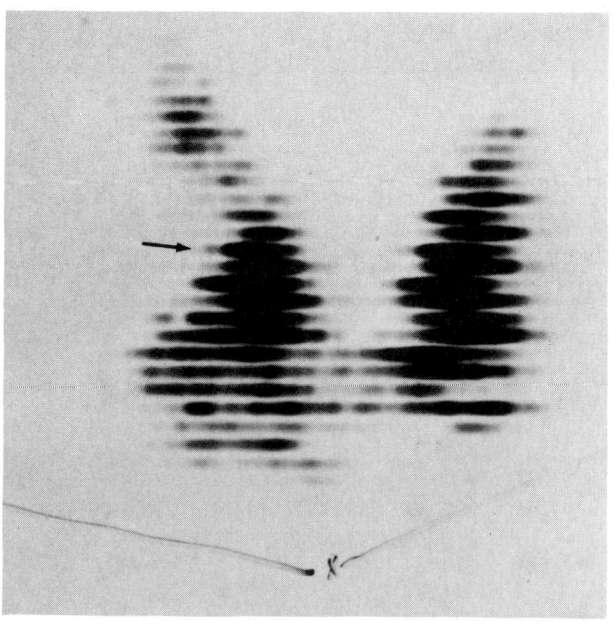

curs in thyrotoxicosis, since there is a disruption of the normal homeostatic mechanism. An abnormal suppression test in the absence of thyrotoxicosis is indicative of diffusely active goiter with opthalmopathy (Graves' disease). Recently, euthyroid patients with Graves' disease have shown a failure of serum TSH to increase in response to TRH. Tests of TSH stimulation have been supplanted by radioimmunoassay for TSH in serum.

BMR AND SERUM CHOLESTEROL. These determinations are directed at assessing the metabolic response to circulating thyroid hormone. They are particularly applicable when other indices are complicated by iodine injection and for patients on therapy.

The BMR is a measure of the calorogenic effect of thyroid hormone and the associated energy expenditure in heat production. The test specifically measures oxygen consumption, and standard values have been established for surface areas of normal patients of varying ages and sexes. The normal range of the BMR is −10 to +10 percent. The evaluation of the result is dependent upon the patient's being in a truly basal state, having fasted for at least 12 hours. The BMR is elevated with thyrotoxicosis and reduced during hypothyroidism. Extrathyroidal factors which increase the BMR include anxiety, food ingestion, smoking, perforated eardrums, and mechanical errors of testing such as leakage of oxygen. The BMR is also elevated in cardiovascular disease, leukemia, lymphoma, pheochromocytoma, adrenal hyperfunction, pregnancy, starvation, malnutrition, shock, skin diseases associated with increased heat loss, and fever.

The serum cholesterol is usually increased in primary myxedema, while the value is characteristically normal when hypothyroidism is due to pituitary failure. The concentration is influenced by age, sex, and dietary intake, but measurements are helpful in determining the response to therapy.

CIRCULATING ANTITHYROID ANTIBODIES. The work of Witebsky and associates has focused attention on the antigenic properties of thyroid protein and the importance of autoantibodies in the development of certain types of thyroid disease. Antibodies have been demonstrated in patients with Hashimoto's thyroiditis and spontaneous hypothyroidism. Circulating antithyroid antibodies are often found in high titers in patients with Graves' disease and in their relatives. Long-acting thyroid stimulator (LATS) is an immunoglobulin (IgG) with many qualities of an antibody.

THYROID BIOPSY. Biopsy of the thyroid is useful in establishing a diagnosis of thyroiditis and differentiating between nodular goiter and carcinoma. Histologic evidence of glandular hyperplasia can also result. Biopsy may be performed with a Vim-Silverman needle for diffuse disease, but if the diagnosis of malignancy is entertained, it is felt that excisional biopsy is preferable.

Thyrotoxicosis

Thyrotoxicosis refers to a spectrum of clinical manifestations which are related to primary excess secretion of active thyroid hormone or increased secretion of hormones

Fig. 38-7. ^{131}I scintillation scan. Substernal thyroid. *A.* Anteroposterior. *B.* Lateral.

which act on the thyroid to stimulate secretion. There are three types of pathologic processes associated with thyrotoxicosis: Graves' disease (toxic diffuse goiter), toxic multinodular goiter, and a single toxic adenoma. In rare instances, the pathologic process is located in ectopic thyroid tissue such as lingual thyroid or struma ovarii. Since the distinctions between these three pathologic processes are not absolute, thyrotoxicosis will be considered as an inclusive entity, and characteristic features of each of the three pathologic types will be presented.

ETIOLOGY AND PATHOLOGY. Graves' Disease. The cause of Graves' disease is unknown. In general, hyperthyroidism is currently regarded either as an autoimmune cell-mediated delayed hypersensitivity induced by thymic-dependent lymphocytes situated within the thyroid and acting directly on thyroid cells or as an intrinsic thyroid cellular disorder with secondary autoimmune phenomena as contributory factors. An LATS has been shown to be capable of inducing thyroid hyperplasia and increased

iodine accumulation independent of the pituitary gland. LATS is now thought to play an important role in the pathogenesis of Graves' disease, even though the titer in the serum does not correlate closely with the severity of thyrotoxicosis and LATS may be present when the thyrotoxicotic state has been relieved. Contributory factors include heredity, sex, and emotional disturbances. There is a tendency for Graves' disease to be present in several members of the same family, and the incidence of thyroid disorders other than Graves' disease, particularly Hashimoto's thyroiditis, is also increased in these families. Abnormalities of iodine metabolism have been demonstrated in euthyroid relatives of patients with Graves' disease. The proportion of nontasters of phenylthiourea is very low among patients with Graves' disease and families of these patients, which suggests an inherited predisposition. The incidence of females to males affected by Graves' disease is 6 : 1 to 7 : 1. The psychosomatic aspects have been stressed in many series, but although they modify the manifestations, their etiologic importance has not been defined.

Fig. 38-8. ^{131}I scintillation scan. Functional thyroid pulmonary metastases not demonstrated roentgenographically.

The term "Graves' disease" has been extended to include patients showing certain extrathyroid manifestations, even if goiter and/or hyperthyroidism are absent. In general, however, the thyroid of the patient with Graves' disease is enlarged and uniformly affected, and the surface is characteristically smooth but may be slightly nodular. Microscopically, the thyroid is hyperplastic, the epithelium is columnar, and only a minimal amount of colloid is evident in the gland. The nuclei may exhibit mitoses, and papillary projections of the hyperplastic epithelium are common. There may be aggregates of lymphoid tissue, and vascularity is markedly increased. These pathologic characteristics are associated with an overproduction of thyroid hormones, hypersecretion, an increased clearance of thyroidal iodine, an enhanced uptake of iodine, and an increased turnover of iodine. The thyroid hormone-protein interaction is also disturbed, and there is an increase in unbound circulating T4.

Toxic Multinodular Goiter. This is usually superimposed on a long-standing nontoxic multinodular goiter. The factors leading to alteration in function are unknown, but the hyperfunctioning cells are probably a somatic mutation resulting in units which function and grow unrelated to TSH. Genetic studies suggest a distinction between Graves' disease and toxic nodular goiter. Grossly, the gland contains multiple nodules, many of which contain aggregates of irregularly large cells and scant amount of colloid. These areas are capable of function independent of stimulation by TSH. The amount of overproduction of thyroid hormone is characteristically less than that associated with Graves' disease.

Toxic Adenoma. The solitary toxic adenoma is a follicular tumor of unknown cause. Like the multinodular toxic adenoma, it is capable of function independent of TSH and LATS, and the administration of exogenous thyroid fails to suppress the secretion of T3 and T4.

CLINICAL MANIFESTATIONS. The clinical manifestations of excessive secretion of thyroid hormone will be considered initially, since these pertain to Graves' disease, toxic multinodular goiter, and toxic adenoma, with minor individual variations. Subsequently, thyroidal and specific extrathyroidal manifestations of these three pathologic processes will be considered.

Hyperthyroidism. The onset of symptoms and signs related to an excess amount of circulating thyroid hormone differs for the three pathologic processes. Graves' disease most commonly becomes clinically apparent in patients in the third to fifth decade of life in the United States, but the age group with the highest prevalence in Great Britain is forty-five to sixty-five years. Although the disease can occur at all ages from infancy on, it is rare before the age of ten and in the elderly patient. The male/female ratio of 1 : 6 pertains in all geographic areas. The thyrotoxicosis of toxic multinodular goiter usually becomes manifest after the age of fifty and is more common in women than men. Toxic adenoma occurs in a younger age group, usually in the thirties to forties.

Many of the characteristic features of thyrotoxicosis in the adult are related to increased calorogenesis. The patient feels warmer than other people in the same environment and becomes intolerant of heat. There may be minimal to moderate temperature elevations, depending on the degree of thyrotoxicosis, and there is increased sweating and consequent thirst, due to the need of dissipating the excess heat. As a result of increased calorogenesis, weight loss associated with an increased appetite is generally noted. At times the intake of food may be sufficiently increased to prevent this loss. Increased appetite is more characteristic of younger patients, while anorexia is frequently noted in the elderly patients. These manifestations of increased calorogenesis are more marked in patients with Graves' disease than in those with toxic multinodular goiter or toxic adenoma.

By contrast, the cardiovascular manifestations of thyrotoxicosis are more prominent in patients with toxic adenomas. These include marked tachycardia, frequent atrial fibrillation, congestive heart failure, and poor response to digitalis. Hyperthyroidism increases the force and rate of the heartbeat, but this is probably related to the body's attempt to meet the general metabolic needs rather than a direct action. Sleeping pulse rate is characteristically over 80, and marked tachycardia may be apparent during the physical examination. Patients commonly experience palpitations. The marked cutaneous and peripheral vasodilatation results in an increased pulse pressure. Atrial fibrillation initially may be paroxysmal but eventually becomes continuous and is a common finding among older patients. In this group, it may be the only clinically detectable sign of hyperthyroidism. Congestive heart failure with ankle edema and dyspnea is seldom seen unless there is an underlying heart disease, which explains the increased incidence of these manifestations in patients with toxic nodular goiter who represent an older age group.

Patients with thyrotoxicosis frequently are extremely excitable, restless, hyperkinetic, and emotionally unstable, and complain of insomnia. Frank psychosis may develop, but this is not specific, and depression is as common as mania. The response of psychosis to therapy directed at relief of hyperthyroidism is unpredictable, and about half the cases return to normal. Muscle wasting, muscle weakness, and fatigue are common manifestations of thyrotoxicosis. There is usually no objective evidence of local disease of the muscle. Myopathy affects men more frequently, and the clinical picture may be confused by the fact that thyrotoxicosis occurs in 3 to 6 percent of patients with myasthenia gravis. The muscle weakness is most evident in the proximal limb muscles. Physical examination of patients with hyperthyroidism may demonstrate a tremor of the extended and abducted fingers and hyperactive Achilles tendon reflex. The emotional, neurogenic, and myopathic manifestations are more marked in patients with Graves' disease.

The changes of the skin and its appendages related to thyrotoxicosis include warm, moist skin, facial flushing, and perspiration. There also may be nail changes, which include softening, increased fragility, and separation of the distal margins from the nail bed. With advanced thyrotoxicosis and Graves' disease, clubbing of the fingers may become apparent. The hair is fine and readily falls out with combing. Pretibial myxedema occurs in 3 to 5 percent of patients with Graves' disease, is frequently present when the patient is euthyroid, and is almost always associated with eye signs. Gynecomastia occurs in 3 to 5 percent of males. Breast enlargement may be noted in females with diffuse toxic goiter. This has been related to hepatic dysfunction and incomplete metabolism of circulating estrogen. Menstrual periods are often scant or absent but return when thyroid function is controlled. Libido may be increased, but fertility is reduced, and the rate of miscarriages is reportedly high.

The effects on the gastrointestinal tract are variable. Diarrhea or increased frequency of defecation is the most characteristic symptom and may occur intermittently or chronically. Increased secretion of thyroid hormone results in increased excretion of calcium in both the feces and urine, with consequent diminution of the radiologic density of bones. There is no increased incidence of renal calculi. The relations between the thyroid gland and bone and mineral metabolism is complex. Although the thyroid gland secretes the hormone thyrocalcitonin, which is antagonistic to parathyroid hormone, alterations of thyrocalcitonin in thyrotoxicosis have not been established.

Graves' Disease. Clinically, Graves' disease is characterized by the classic triad of goiter, thyrotoxicosis, and exophthalmos. These features may occur singly or in any combination. The thyroid is nearly always diffusely enlarged and symmetric; the pyramidal lobe may be enlarged to the extent of becoming readily palpable. The gland is characteristically smooth but may be irregular. The extreme vascularity is evidenced by an audible bruit, best heard over the superior poles on either side. Obstructive symptoms, related to the size of the gland or encroachment on the trachea or esophagus, are rare. In about 3 percent of the patients with Graves' disease and thyrotoxicosis, the thyroid is normal in size. The eye signs vary from minimal to severe and, fortunately, are mild in most patients. Excess thyroxine per se will not produce exophthalmos. Severe thyrotoxicosis may be unaccompanied by exophthalmos, and, conversely, exophthalmos may be the only manifestation of Graves' disease. In about one-third of the cases, the ocular manifestations and the signs and symptoms of thyrotoxicosis begin coincidentally. Exophthalmos infrequently progresses after thyrotoxicosis has been relieved by surgical treatment or radioactive iodine.

The eye signs of Graves' disease include (1) spasm of the upper lid with lid retraction, (2) external ophthalmoplegia, (3) exophthalmos with proptosis, (4) supraorbital and infraorbital swelling, and (5) congestion and edema. Spasm of the upper lid may be manifested by lid lag and excessively apparent sclerae. Weakness of the extrinsic ocular muscles is present in about 40 percent of patients with Graves' disease. Upper rotation is the most common abnormality, while lateral rotation also occurs frequently. The extent of exophthalmos, or proptosis, can be measured with an exophthalmometer, which provides determination of the distance in a horizontal plane between the anterior convexity of the cornea and the bony margin of the orbit.

The appearance of venous congestion and edema is a sign of severity and has been described as "malignant exophthalmos." It occurs more commonly in the male and is associated with increased lacrimation and pain in the eye. In extreme cases, the eyesight may be lost.

Toxic Multinodular Goiter. The thyroid in these patients contains several palpable nodules, and in some instances the rings of the trachea may be felt because of the involution of the overlying glandular tissue. On palpation, the characteristics of the goiter cannot be distinguished from those of nontoxic multinodular goiter. Symptoms related to obstruction of the trachea and/or esophagus occur more commonly than with Graves' disease. Exophthalmos is rarely present.

Toxic Adenoma. There is frequently a history of a long-standing, slowly growing mass in the neck. Recent rapid growth may be associated with central necrosis and hemorrhage. Palpation reveals a solitary tumor within the thyroid. Thyrotoxicosis is uncommon unless the lesion is at least 3 cm in diameter. A toxic adenoma which undergoes hemorrhagic necrosis may be accompanied by spontaneous remission of the manifestations of thyrotoxicity. With larger lesions, cervical compression symptoms may be present. Exophthalmos is absent. As in the case of toxic multinodular goiter, no bruit is discernible.

DIAGNOSTIC FINDINGS. Thyrotoxicosis is characterized by an elevated T4 and/or T3 level (see the preceding section, Thyroid Function Tests).

Graves' Disease. The thyroidal ^{131}I uptake is characteristically markedly elevated with 45 to 90 percent of the administered dose localizing in the gland. If the thyroidal ^{131}I studies are equivocal, a 2-hour ^{132}I uptake with greater than 25 percent of the administered dose demonstrable in the gland confirms the diagnosis. The T3 suppression test is also applicable to the patient with an equivocal diagnosis. In normal patients the radioactive iodine uptake is decreased by 80 percent, and, for practical purposes, if the decrease is 50 percent or less, the diagnosis of hyperthyroidism can be made. The urinary excretion of nitrogen, phosphorus, calcium, and creatine is increased. The BMR is generally markedly elevated to levels of +35 to +70 percent. With severe thyrotoxicosis, hepatic dysfunction may be marked, in which case there will be associated hypoproteinemia, Bromsulphalein (BSP) retention, and increased serum alkaline phosphatase. About 1 percent of patients with Graves' disease have pernicious anemia, and 30 percent are reported to have circulating antibodies against gastric parietal cells. A high titer of thyroid autoantibodies is also found in about one-third of patients with Graves' disease.

Toxic Multinodular Goiter and Toxic Adenoma. In these patients, the thyroidal ^{131}I uptake is generally less than that in Graves' disease, 10 to 55 percent localizing in the functioning tissue. The BMR is elevated to +25 to +30 percent. The increase in urinary excretion of nitrogen, phosphorus, calcium, and creatine is less significant than that noted in patients with Graves' disease. In the case of a multinodular gland, ^{131}I thyroidal uptake and T4 and T3 determinations may be of little value unless they are distinctly elevated. The thyroid suppression test may provide the diagnosis but should not be performed in a patient with overt heart disease. In some instances, a therapeutic trial with an antithyroid agent constitutes the diagnostic test.

In the case of a toxic adenoma, much of the laboratory data also is determined by the extent of thyrotoxicosis. When thyrotoxicosis is clinically manifest, the thyroidal ^{131}I uptake and T4 and/or T3 are usually greatly increased. The scintillation scan is particularly critical, since it will indicate the functional status of the nodule (see Fig. 38-4).

TREATMENT. Definitive treatment may be effected with antithyroid drugs, radioactive iodine, or surgical excision of thyroid tissue. The approach to a given patient must be individualized and depends on the patient's age, general health, and the pathologic process involved.

Antithyroid Drugs. The majority of the presently employed antithyroid drugs interfere with the organic binding of thyroidal iodine and inhibit the coupling of iodotyrosines. They have no effect on the underlying cause of disease, and the thyroidal ^{131}I uptake remains elevated during treatment and when there is return to a euthyroid state. The drugs cross the placenta and inhibit fetal thyroid function and are also excreted in breast milk. Usually, some improvement in the degree of thyrotoxicosis is noted within the first 2 weeks of therapy, and a euthyroid thyroid state can be restored in 6 weeks. Treatment is generally regulated on a clinical basis, following the patient's weight and pulse. The size of the goiter and the eye changes should be recorded. The T4 and/or T3 levels and BMR may be helpful in assessing treatment, while radioiodine tests offer no guide.

The majority of patients are treated in the hope that a natural remission will occur within 1 to 2 years, at which time drug therapy can be stopped. A normal suppression test indicates that the disease is inactive. In Trotter's experience, one-third of the patients had remission lasting 10 years or more following a course of treatment with drugs of not more than 2 years' duration. The patients' response could not be identified prospectively. It has been reported that 54 percent of patients with diffuse or multinodular goiter had remissions lasting 10 to 20 years and no significant difference was noted in respect to the drugs which are commonly applied at the present time, i.e., propylthiouracil and methimazole (Tapazole).

Methimazole has a potency about 10 times that of propylthiouracil, and therefore one-tenth the dose is required: 100 to 300 mg of propylthiouracil every 6 to 8 hours or 10 to 40 mg of methimazole every 12 hours. The side effects of drug therapy include skin rash, fever, peripheral neuritis, and polyarteritis. Propylthiouracil has been associated with prothrombin deficiency responsive to vitamin K therapy. The serious complications of antithyroid drugs are agranulocytosis and aplastic anemia, which occur in less than 1 percent of the treated cases. Leukocyte counts are of little help, since agranulocytosis comes on so rapidly. When a significant reduction in the white blood cell count is noted, the drug should be stopped promptly, and the prognosis is good. Aplastic anemia is a much rarer complication, and the prognosis is poorer.

Antithyroid drugs are also employed in the preparation of thyrotoxicotic patients for surgical treatment. Propylthiouracil or methimazole is administered to establish a normal metabolic state. These drugs, however, increase the vascularity of the thyroid gland. Therefore, in order to facilitate surgical excision, iodine, in the form of Lugol's solution or potassium iodide, is added for a period of 10 days to 2 weeks immediately prior to the operation. Iodine inhibits hormonal release and results in a firmer and less vascular gland. Historically, iodine was used as a major chemotherapeutic agent, but since escape from its effects occurs in 2 to 3 weeks, long-term therapy is not advisable. In addition to the application of iodine in the preoperative preparation of the patient, the drug is used as treatment for impending or established thyroid storm.

Radioactive Iodine. This represents the treatment of choice in many large series. The average dose for diffuse toxic goiter was 7 to 9 mc of ^{131}I and for toxic nodular goiter 12 to 15 mc. This is intended to deliver approximately 8,500 rads to the thyroid. About 20 percent of patients treated with ^{131}I will require more than one dose. The advantages of radioactive therapy are the avoidance of a surgical procedure, with its attendant rare complications of recurrent nerve paralysis or hypoparathyroidism, and reduced cost. The major disadvantages of radioactive iodine treatment are the time required to gain control of the disease, the incidence of permanent myxedema, and the development of nodules. Remission rates ranging from 80 to 98 percent have been reported. Exacerbations are extremely uncommon. In most series, the results have been less satisfactory for hyperthyroidism associated with nodular toxic goiter than with diffuse toxic goiter. T4 and T3 determinations are less valuable in assessing thyroid functions after radioactive iodine therapy. Clinical criteria and BMR correlate better. Nofal et al. indicated a 70 percent incidence of hypothyroidism at the end of 10 years. The absence of a plateau in the slope of the curve suggests that hypothyroidism is a potentiality in almost 100 percent of the patients if they live long enough subsequent to therapy.

An objection to radioactive iodine therapy in the young patient is based on a subsequent development of carcinoma or leukemia. Many reports have indicated an increased incidence of benign and malignant tumors of the thyroid in patients subjected to irradiation of the thymic area or cervical lymphatics during infancy. Although there is a tendency for thyroid nodules to develop following radioactive iodine therapy, the incidence of thyroid carcinoma is not increased. Most centers have restricted the use of radioactive iodine to adults over the age of thirty-five and will not treat pregnant women or nursing mothers, since the isotope crosses the placenta and enters the milk. Review of the expected incidence of leukemia in the general population as compared to its occurrence in patients treated with radioactive iodine has led to the conclusion that the incidence of leukemia is little, if at all, increased by this therapeutic modality.

Subtotal Thyroidectomy. Prior to the advent of radioactive iodine, subtotal thyroidectomy was accepted as the treatment of choice for thyrotoxicosis. The operative procedure, which is generally planned to leave a remnant of 3 to 6 Gm, eliminates both the hyperthyroidism and the goiter. Patients with active hyperthyroidism require pre-operative preparation. Antithyroid drugs are used initially in order to establish a euthyroid state. Iodine is added to the regimen 10 days to 2 weeks prior to the operation, to decrease the vascularity of the gland.

The mortality rate associated with the procedure is extremely low. Gould et al. reported 1,000 thyroidectomies for all causes with no deaths, while Colcock and King reported 1,246 consecutive thyroidectomies with no mortality. In a collected review of major series, the mortality rate was less than 0.1 percent. Subtotal thyroidectomy provides rapid correction of the thyrotoxicotic state in about 95 percent of patients.

The incidence of complications varies with the series. Permanent recurrent laryngeal nerve paralysis has been reported in 0 to 3 percent of the cases. Damage to the parathyroid gland resulting in tetany has been reported in about 3 percent of patients subjected to thyroidectomy for thyrotoxicosis. In 4 to 9 percent of patients subjected to thyroidectomy for thyrotoxicosis permanent hypothyroidism developed, while in 2 to 12 percent hyperthyroidism recurred. Thus, the major advantages of surgical therapy are prompt control of disease and a lowered incidence of myxedema as compared with radioactive iodine therapy. Surgical thyroidectomy also makes possible the simultaneous removal of an incidental papillary carcinoma, which was noted in 2 percent of the cases in one series. The patients usually leave the hospital within 4 to 5 days and resume work within 6 weeks.

Selection of Therapy. In patients with Graves' disease (diffuse toxic goiter) either antithyroid drug therapy or radioactive iodine is used initially. Antithyroid drugs are used in the younger age group and in pregnant or lactating females. Radioactive iodine is employed in patients over the age of thirty-five. If prolonged drug therapy is required, i.e., for more than 2 years, or if recurrence of thyrotoxicosis follows the discontinuance of drugs, thyroidectomy or radioactive iodine is used. Subtotal thyroidectomy occasionally represents the treatment of choice in young adults with severe disease and large goiters or in patients in whom a rapid response is desirable. Radioactive iodine is the treatment of choice in most patients with toxic multinodular goiter, but in regions where goiter tends to be endemic, such as the Great Lakes, there is an increased resistance to radioactive iodine therapy. In these regions, subtotal thyroidectomy may represent the procedure of choice. The preferable treatment for hyperfunctioning adenoma is surgical excision.

Because of the questionable carcinogenic potential of radioactive iodine in childhood, the choice of treatment is between surgical excision and antithyroid therapy. However, there is usually a lower incidence of remission following antithyroid therapy in adults, and recurrences are frequent. If sustained remission does not follow a 2-year course of antithyroid therapy in a child, surgical intervention is indicated. Thyrotoxicosis in pregnancy is best treated with antithyroid drugs. Surgical therapy may be required, but it is best not to use iodine in preparation because of the likelihood of an induced goiter in the fetus.

Hyperfunctioning thyroid tissue in the ovary should be treated by oophorectomy. Hyperfunctioning tissue within aberrant thyroid tissue, such as a lingual thyroid, may be treated by radioactive iodine or surgical excision. The uncommon situation of metastatic tumor with hyperfunctioning tissue is best treated by radioactive iodine.

RESULTS. Antithyroid drugs effect a remission of 10 years or more in one-third to one-half of the patients with diffuse or multinodular goiter. Radioactive iodine effectively controls hyperthyroidism in about 90 percent of patients, although some require one or more subsequent doses. Failure to control the hyperthyroidism occurs more frequently with nodular toxic goiter as compared to diffuse toxic goiter. This modality of therapy is associated with a high incidence of myxedema, which is greater than 60 percent at 10 years and increases each year by an additional 2 to 3 percent. Subtotal thyroidectomy is also associated with 90 percent good results in respect to control of thyrotoxicosis. In 2 to 12 percent of the patients, goiter and/or hyperthyroidism recurs at some time following the operation. In this group of patients, radioactive iodine is indicated. Permanent hypothyroidism occurs in 4 to 18 percent of the patients following subtotal thyroidectomy. Unlike the situation with radioactive iodine therapy where there is a continuous increase with time in the percentage of hypothyroid patients, hypothyroidism following subtotal thyroidectomy occurs within 1 year.

The effects of treatment on the eye signs are variable. The stigmata of exophthalmos may gradually improve or may deteriorate as the thyrotoxicosis is controlled. In general, the changes in the eye signs are biphasic. During the acute phase lasting some months, the signs progress fairly rapidly. Following this, there is a chronic phase lasting years during which the lid retraction tends to disappear while the exophthalmos increases slightly. The treatment of hyperthyroidism affects this pattern. The lid retraction disappears in about two-thirds of the patients who become euthyroid, while the exophthalmos increases by an average of 1 mm, partly because of the gain in body fat, when hyperthyroidism is removed. In most instances, treating the thyrotoxicosis improves the eye signs. In those instances in which the treatment seems to precipitate rapid deterioration of the eyes, this may represent the acute phase or the development of exophthalmos and should not necessarily be attributed to the therapy.

TREATMENT OF EXOPHTHALMOS. The severe form of exophthalmos is fortunately rare. The control of thyrotoxicosis has no appreciable effect on the progression of eye signs. The earliest symptom of development of the so-called "malignant exophthalmos" is increased lacrimation. The earliest signs consist of venous congestion and chemosis. Treatment is essentially symptomatic, since no therapeutic measure has been demonstrated to have a decisive influence on the progression of the disorder. The eyes should be protected against the wind and sun. The patients should sleep in a sitting position to reduce venous congestion. If chemosis is severe, tarsorrhaphy to oppose the lids and prevent corneal ulceration may be indicated. If the intraorbital tension increases to the extent of threatening vision, a trial of massive doses of prednisone (120 to 140 mg daily) is indicated. Steroids have been particularly effective in managing pain, tearing, and irritation. Other methods of therapy include external irradiation to the orbit or the pituitary gland, implantation of ^{90}yttrium into the pituitary, stalk section, or cryosurgical treatment of the pituitary gland. In cases where the intraorbital pressure immediately threatens vision, lateral decompression was generally used in the past, but the results were disappointing in that only half the patients were improved. Transfrontal craniotomy and transantral decompression have provided good results.

Hypothyroidism

Hypothyroidism is the term applied to a failure of the thyroid gland to maintain an adequate plasma level of hormone. A brief discussion is included in this chapter for three reasons: (1) the treatment of hyperthyroidism by subtotal thyroidectomy and, more commonly, by radioactive iodine represents one of the causes of hypothyroidism, (2) some of the clinical manifestations of hypothyroidism mimic a variety of surgical diseases, and (3) a recognition of the hypothyroid state in the preoperative patient is important, since major surgical treatment in the hypothyroid patient is associated with an increased mortality. The reader is referred to the general texts listed in the references for a more complete consideration of hypothyroidism.

ETIOLOGY. Spontaneous hypothyroidism, or myxedema, may result from aplasia of the thyroid or replacement of the gland by nonfunctional goiter, adenoma, or thyroiditis. In the presence of functioning thyroid tissue, hypothyroidism may be secondary to hypopituitarism. This is termed *pituitary myxedema.* Hypothyroidism following subtotal thyroidectomy or radioactive iodine therapy for hyperthyroidism accounts for about one-fourth of cases. Kocher recognized the importance of this disorder and referred to it as "cachexia strumipriva." In 4 to 18 percent of patients subjected to thyroidectomy hypothyroidism develops. The occurrence is related to the histologic state, being more common in patients with Hashimoto's disease and lymphadenoid changes. However, as far as absolute figures are concerned, postoperative hypothyroidism most frequently follows subtotal resection of a diffuse goiter in a patient with Graves' disease. Autoantibodies against thyroid cytoplasm are frequently present in patients who become hypothyroid. The incidence varies inversely with the incidence of recurrent hyperthyroidism. In most of these patients, the hypothyroidism becomes manifest during the first year after the operation, usually within the first few months. Following ablation of diffuse toxic goiter using radioactive iodine, there is a progressive rising incidence of hypothyroidism.

CLINICAL MANIFESTATIONS. Functional failure of the thyroid in the newborn is termed *cretinism.* This is not seen at birth because of the transplacental passage of hormone and becomes manifest later in infancy. Mental retardation is marked and frequently irreversible. Children demonstrate a poor growth pattern, are difficult to nurse, and present with a typical appearance which must be distinguished from mongolism and dwarfism. The remaining manifestations are similar to those which will be described below for adult hypothyroidism but are more pronounced.

Thyroid failure during childhood or adolescence is known as *juvenile hypothyroidism,* and the extent and degree of symptoms and signs are intermediate between cretinism and adult hypothyroidism. The child appears younger than his chronologic age. Intellectual performance is poor, but severe mental deficiency is not present. In children, abdominal distension, umbilical hernia, and prolapse of the rectum are all common.

Spontaneous hypothyroidism in the adult is a rare disease. About one case of adult hypothyroidism is admitted for every eight cases of thyrotoxicosis. Eighty percent of adults with spontaneous hypothyroidism are female. Both spontaneous hypothyroidism and hypothyroidism which follows ablative procedures on the thyroid gland have an insidiously progressive course in the adult, with protean manifestations. There is increasing fatigue and apathy. Mental and physical processes are generally slowed. Intellectual function and speech may be impaired. Headaches occur frequently and dementia may develop. Weight gain is a characteristic feature. The skin becomes thickened and puffy; the nonpitting bogginess of the skin is most apparent around the eyes, hands, and feet. The secretion of sweat glands is reduced. The hair becomes dry and brittle, and tends to fall out. The tongue is enlarged and tends to fill the mouth, and the voice is hoarse. Muscle cramps are common and represent one of the early symptoms of hypothyroidism following ablative therapy. The cramps may be precipitated by slight motion, such as turning in bed or lifting of the arms, and may be accompanied by paresthesias.

The cardiovascular manifestations are related to a reduced cardiac output and hemodynamic alterations which resemble those of congestive heart failure. There is a narrowing in pulse pressure, a prolonged circulation time, and a decrease in cutaneous circulation resulting in coolness and pallor of the skin and intolerance to cold. There is widening of cardiac dullness due to dilatation of the heart or pericardial effusion, and the heart sounds are distant. The resting pulse is slow, and at times the blood pressure is elevated to hypertensive levels. As the disease progresses, shortness of breath and pulmonary effusions become more common.

Abdominal symptoms may represent the outstanding complaint. Most frequently, these consist of constipation and changes in bowel habits. Abdominal distension due to intraintestinal gases or ascites may be present. When pain is present, it is generally of a dull, nonperistaltic character and occasionally colicky. Achlorhydria occurs in about half the patients, and there is also an impairment of absorption of vitamin B$_{12}$. Pernicious anemia may be present in 12 percent of the cases.

In women, diminished libido, failure of ovulation, and menorrhagia may occur, and in men there may be decreased libido, impotence, and oligospermia.

DIAGNOSTIC FINDINGS. The hemogram may demonstrate anemia. The electrocardiogram is characterized by sinus bradycardia, diminished voltage, and inverted or flattened T waves; the electroencephalogram shows slow alpha activity and loss of amplitude. The tests of thyroidal function and the effects of thyroid hormone may be variable and contradictory. In general, the BMR and ^{131}I uptake are decreased in proportion to the extent of the disease. Early in the course of the disease, the BMR is only moderately lowered and with progression falls to about −35 to −45 percent. There is a decreased serum T4 and/or T3, and the serum cholesterol is frequently in excess of 300 mg/100 ml.

TREATMENT. Treatment of adult hypothyroidism is extremely effective and is directed at producing a normal metabolic state with the smallest possible dose of drugs. The choice of therapeutic agent is most frequently determined by the preference of the physician, and either synthetic hormones or thyroid extracts from animal glands may be employed. The approximate equivalence of biologic potency for the commonly used medications is 60 mg of thyroid extract = 100 μg of *l*-thyroxine = 25 μg of *l*-triiodothyronine.

The untreated patient with hypothyroidism is sensitive to small doses, and therefore caution is exercised in initiating replacement therapy. Treatment may be begun with 15 to 30 mg of thyroid extract daily, and the dose is increased by 15 to 30 mg at 2-week intervals until a satisfactory metabolic rate is obtained. The replacement therapy is augmented slowly to avoid cardiac problems related to an increased demand on the myocardium. Most patients perform well with a BMR of −20 to −10. The maintenance dose for thyroid extract is usually 60 to 120 mg. The maintenance dose for *l*-thyroxine is approximately 300 μg daily, and the maintenance dose for *l*-triiodothyronine is about 75 μg daily. In the infant or child, treatment may be begun with 25 μg of *l*-thyroxine (or its equivalent) and increased by 25 μg at weekly intervals, so that a daily dose of 100 μg is achieved in 3 to 4 weeks. Thereafter the dose is increased slowly in order to keep the total T4 at about 10 μg/100 ml.

Thyroiditis

Inflammatory processes of the thyroid may be acute or chronic. Acute thyroiditis is further subdivided into the suppurative and nonsuppurative varieties. Chronic thyroiditis includes Hashimoto's disease, granulomatous (giant cell) thyroiditis, and Riedel's thyroiditis.

ACUTE SUPPURATIVE THYROIDITIS

Acute suppurative thyroiditis is the most uncommon form of thyroiditis. Hendrick reviewed 1,309 consecutive operations on the thyroid of which 117 were on patients who had thyroiditis of various forms. Twenty-eight patients were classified as having acute thyroiditis, and of these only six had the suppurative form. Acute suppurative thyroiditis, with abscess formation, almost invariably follows an acute upper respiratory tract infection. The disease is characterized by the sudden onset of severe pain in the thyroid and anterior neck, accompanied by dysphagia, fever, and chills. The suppurative process usually remains unilateral, but there may be extension into the deep spaces of the neck with invasion of the trachea and/or esophagus, or tracking into the chest. Treatment consists of drainage of the abscess. There is no persistent effect on thyroid function.

HASHIMOTO'S DISEASE (LYMPHADENOID GOITER)

Hashimoto's disease is the most common form of chronic thyroiditis, and the incidence apparently has been increasing. The frequency with which this lesion is identified in specimens of removed thyroid glands varies with geographic location. In England, 1.5 percent of thyroidectomies demonstrate Hashimoto's disease. In the United States, in the Southern Gulf states 11 percent of glands contain the lesion, whereas in New England lymphadenoid goiter is present in only 0.3 percent of thyroidectomies. An increasing frequency which is greater in younger age groups recently has been reported in Minnesota. The disease occurs at least five to ten times more frequently than subacute thyroiditis.

ETIOLOGY. Hashimoto's disease is an autoimmune process in which the thyroid gland is sensitive to its own thyroglobulin. In 1957, Doniach and Roitt first discovered antithyroid antibodies in the serum of most patients with this disease. Four autoantigens have been detected: thyroglobulin, nonthyroglobulin colloid, thyroid cell microsomes, and nuclear component. Thyroglobulin antigen may be demonstrated by a precipitant test or agglutination of specifically treated red cells. Autoantibodies formed against nonthyroglobulin colloid may be demonstrated by the fluorescent technique of Coons and Kaplan. This technique can also be applied to the demonstration of antibody to thyroid intracellular microsomes and antinuclear antibody. The sera of patients with Hashimoto's disease also contain an abnormal iodinated protein distinct from thyroglobulin and apparently related to albumin. This is used as a diagnostic test. There is some evidence of genetic predisposition for Hashimoto's disease. Members of the family of patients with this disease have an increased incidence of Hashimoto's disease, goiter, spontaneous hypothyroidism, and thyrotoxicosis.

A statistically significant relationship has been demonstrated for the coexistence of papillary carcinoma of the thyroid and Hashimoto's disease. The data of Hirabayashi and Lindsay suggest that chronic thyroiditis occurs secondarily with papillary carcinoma and that there is a possibility that antigens from the neoplasm may be implicated in the formation of thyroiditis. In 92 percent of the specimens of papillary carcinoma which Hirabayashi and Lindsay studied, thyroiditis was found in the neoplasm, in the remaining thyroid parenchyma, or in both regions. The presence of thyroiditis was uncommon with other forms of thyroid carcinoma.

PATHOLOGY. In 80 percent of the cases, the thyroid is symmetrically enlarged, pale, and semifirm. In the remaining cases, the enlargement may be asymmetric, and the nodularity and firmness suggest colloid goiter and, at times, carcinoma. The disease is focal in the beginning but extends to involve one or both lobes and the isthmus. Lymphoid tissue predominates (Fig. 38-9). There is dis-

Fig. 38-9. Hashimoto's disease.

ruption of epithelial cells with degeneration and fragmentation of the follicular basement membrane. The remaining epithelial cells are larger and demonstrate oxyphilic changes (Askanazy cells). The lymphocytic infiltration may be focal or diffuse, and as the disease progresses, the thyroid tissue may degenerate or be replaced by fibrous tissue.

CLINICAL MANIFESTATIONS. The overwhelming majority of patients are women, and the disease occurs from age twenty to sixty-nine, with an average of fifty years. The most frequent complaints are enlargement of the neck with pain and tenderness in the region of the thyroid. There may be associated difficulty in breathing and swallowing caused by compression of the trachea and esophagus. Coughing is a common symptom. Shortness of breath, increasing fatigue, and increase in weight are related to a hypothyroid state when this is present. In the series reported by Linden and Clark, 22 percent presented with symptoms of hyperthyroidism, while 4 percent were myxedematous. Palpation generally reveals a diffusely enlarged gland, and enlargement of the pyramidal lobe is common. In about 20 percent of cases, the gland is nodular rather than diffusely enlarged.

Several investigators have indicated an increased incidence of autoimmune diseases such as rheumatic fever and rheumatoid arthritis, disseminated lupus, hemolytic anemia, purpura, myasthenia gravis, and pernicious anemia in these patients. On occasion Hashimoto's disease is part of a generalized endocrine organ failure syndrome which may include idiopathic Addison's disease, diabetes mellitus, and ovarian or testicular insufficiency. In contrast, Mulhern et al. could demonstrate no association between Hashimoto's disease and other autoimmune disorders, with the possible exception of rheumatoid arthritis and the presence of false-positive tests for syphilis.

DIAGNOSTIC FINDINGS. Early in the course of the disease, tests of thyroidal function occasionally indicated thyroidal hyperfunction without overproduction of metabolically active hormones. The thyroidal ^{131}I uptake may be increased. As the disease progresses, the thyroidal uptake and T4 reach subnormal levels, and the response to TSH reveals diminished thyroid reserve. In a majority of patients, however, tests of thyroidal function and clinical manifestations suggest a euthyroid state. Diagnosis is confirmed by demonstrating high titers of thyroid antibodies in the serum. Almost all patients with Hashimoto's disease have circulating antibody as determined by the tanned red cell agglutinin and complement-fixation tests. The various immunologic tests are not specific for Hashimoto's disease and occur in other disorders of the thyroid gland, such as spontaneous myxedema, hyperthyroidism, nontoxic goiter, and thyroid carcinoma.

Biopsy may be indicated in the case of asymmetric and nodular glands, to rule out the diagnosis of carcinoma. Crile and Hazard performed needle biopsy in 119 patients with Hashimoto's disease, and only one patient subsequently proved to have a malignant tumor, a reticulum cell sarcoma. Beahrs et al. also feel that needle biopsy of the thyroid has a role in the diagnosis and management of Hashimoto's disease. By contrast, others, for example Block et al., feel that whenever a nodule is suspicious, excisional biopsy is indicated.

TREATMENT. There is almost universal agreement that if the thyroid is symmetric and nonnodular and if there are no symptoms of compression, the patient should be managed with suppressive doses of thyroid hormone. Three hundred milligrams of thyroid extract may be required, and triiodothyronine in daily doses of 75 to 100 μg is also effective. Surgical intervention is indicated if there are marked pressure symptoms, such as difficulty in swallowing, for suspected malignant tumor, and for cosmetic reasons, in the case of an extremely enlarged gland. The surgical procedure usually performed consists of near-total thyroidectomy with clearing of the trachea. The treatment of a nodular form of Hashimoto's disease is controversial. Most writers prefer the use of suppressive hormone. Block et al. represent the other approach, which consists of surgical excision. They feel that if nodules are present in one lobe, lobectomy, isthmusectomy, and superficial contralateral lobectomy should be performed. Nodules within the isthmus should be treated by resection of the isthmus and the superficial portion of both adjacent lobes. Since most carcinomas associated with Hashimoto's disease are of the papillary type, concomitant radical neck dissection is not indicated. Suppressive therapy with thyroid hormones should be continued postoperatively.

SUBACUTE THYROIDITIS

In 1904 de Quervain described the pathology (Fig. 38-10) of subacute thyroiditis and reviewed the literature. Many synonyms, including granulomatous (giant cell), epidemic, and de Quervain's thyroiditis, have confused the diagnosis. In 1948, Crile clearly established subacute thyroiditis as an entity separate from Hashimoto's thyroiditis and Riedel's struma.

The disease occurs widely in over half of the United States but infrequently along the Eastern seaboard, in England, and in Japan. The age of onset ranges from three to seventy-six, with a mean in the forties. Females outnumber males in every series, the proportion varying between 60 and 100 percent.

Subacute thyroiditis is generally not felt to be of viral origin, but there is no definitive proof, and no epidemiologic pattern has been demonstrated. Recent studies have led to the conclusion that the disease is not autoimmune.

The gland is usually adherent to surrounding tissues but, unlike Riedel's struma, can be dissected free without difficulty. There is enlargement of the follicles with infiltration by large mononuclear cells, lymphocytes, and neutrophils. Giant cells of the epitheloid foreign body type containing many nuclei characterize the lesion.

Volpé et al. classified subacute thyroiditis into four stages:

Stage I—acute toxicity with a painful, swollen gland and thyrotoxic symptoms lasting 1 to 2 months.
Stage II—the transition or euthyroid stage with an enlarged, hard, nontender gland. The BMR is normal, but the sedimentation rate is still elevated.
Stage III—the compensation or hypothyroid phase, occurring 2 to 4 months after onset.
Stage IV—remission or recovery, which may occur in 1 to 6 months.

Almost all patients manifest thyroid swelling and pain which may radiate to parts of the head, neck, or anterior chest. The onset is usually sudden. About two-thirds of patients are febrile, and fatigue, weakness, malaise, menstrual irregularities, and weight loss are characteristic. White blood cell counts usually are normal, but the erythrocyte sedimentation rate (ESR) is almost always elevated during the first month. α_2- and γ-globulin levels are elevated. The latter is also elevated in Hashimoto's disease, but the colloidal gold reaction which is positive in Hashimoto's disease is negative in subacute thyroiditis. In the acute stage there is a characteristically low ^{131}I uptake. Needle biopsy may aid in establishing the diagnosis, as may cytodiagnosis by aspiration, but these techniques are not always reliable.

ACTH and corticosteroids effectively relieve the symptoms but do not alter the disease. Therapy should be initiated with 40 mg of prednisone daily, tapering the drug over 1 to 2 months. Radiation in doses of 200 to 400 rads has been used to treat thyroid pain, but steroids are generally more effective. Salicylates and desiccated thyroid (1 to 3 Gm daily) have provided successful therapy. Thyroidectomy is not applicable because of the high incidence of postoperative myxedema.

RIEDEL'S (STRUMA) THYROIDITIS

Riedel's thyroiditis is a rare chronic inflammatory process involving one or both lobes of the thyroid, frequently extending to the surrounding fascia, trachea, muscles, nerves, and blood vessels. It was formerly thought to be a terminal stage of Hashimoto's disease or granulomatous thyroiditis, but this thesis is no longer popular.

Microscopically, the follicles are small and few in number, and a dense fibrous tissue permeates the gland (Fig. 38-11). There is firm attachment to the trachea by scar tissue, resulting in constriction and narrowing of the tracheal lumen.

When involvement is unilateral, the disease is clinically indistinguishable from carcinoma. The disease occurs more

Fig. 38-10. Acute nonsuppurative thyroiditis. Note infiltration of inflammatory cells.

frequently in women but not to the same extent as Hashimoto's disease. The average age of patients is about fifty. Symptoms are generally due to compression of the trachea, esophagus, and recurrent laryngeal nerve. Consequently, there is difficulty in swallowing and hoarseness. Vocal cord paralysis may be demonstrable on indirect laryngoscopy. Thyroidal ^{131}I uptake may be normal or depressed, and in advanced disease tests of thyroidal function may indicate hypothyroidism. Some patients have circulating thyroid autoantibodies, but this occurs less frequently and in lower titers than in patients with Hashimoto's disease.

Treatment consists of thyroid hormones. Surgical intervention is justified to relieve symptoms of tracheal or esophageal constriction. The operation may be dangerous, resulting in damage to the trachea, carotid sheath, or recurrent laryngeal nerve. When only one lobe is involved, unilateral lobectomy and isthmusectomy are indicated. When there is bilateral involvement, the technique advocated by Lahey is applicable. This consists of removal of

Fig. 38-11. Riedel's thyroiditis.

the isthmus and as much of each lobe as possible. The prethyroid muscles are sutured to the lateral wall of the trachea to cover the severed ends of the lobe and prevent fibrous thyroid tissue from uniting. The medial borders of the "strap" muscles are then sutured together to prevent the trachea from becoming adherent to the skin.

Goiter

The term *goiter* is derived from the French word *goitre,* which in turn comes from the Latin *guttur,* meaning "throat." In general, the term is applied to benign enlargement of the thyroid gland, usually associated with a normal production of thyroid hormone.

ETIOLOGY. The development of a goiter may be related to a variety of factors, including inherited enzyme defects and extrinsic causes, or it may be idiopathic. Goiters associated with thyrotoxicosis, thyroiditis, and benign and malignant neoplasms are excluded from this discussion.

Familial Goiter. Goiters caused by inherited enzyme defects are usually associated with hypothyroidism, but many patients remain euthyroid. The inborn error in metabolism is generally inherited as an autosomal recessive trait, but inheritance as a dominant characteristic also has been reported. The metabolic defect may impair iodine accumulation organification, coupling of iodotyrosine into iodothyronine, or dehalogenation of iodotyrosine, or it may be related to a disorder affecting the serum iodoprotein.

Endemic Goiter. The distinction between endemic and "sporadic" goiter is statistical and arbitrary. Endemic goiter is defined as thyroid enlargement affecting a significant number of inhabitants of a particular locale. Most major countries have goiter belts. In the United States, the prevalent regions are in mountainous areas, the upper Northwest, and around the Great Lakes. The extrinsic factors implicated in the etiology include iodine deficiency and the ingestion of goitrogens. Genetic factors may play a contributory role. Iodine deficiency is particularly important, and in the endemic areas the iodine content of the drinking water is extremely low. Surveys of patients in endemic goiter regions have demonstrated an augmented average uptake of radioiodine. No clearly defined biochemical abnormalities have been detected in the thyroid glands of these patients. The administration of iodine as prophylaxis prevents endemic goiter, and the preferable method has been iodination of table salt. Excess iodide ingestion may lead to goiter with hypothyroidism. Some opponents of this measure have suggested that it has also led to a higher incidence of toxic goiter. In patients with endemic goiter who receive daily supplemental doses of iodine, the adjustment period is slow. It takes several weeks for the level of iodine balance to be achieved and the thyroidal avidity for radioiodine to return to normal. Experiments in animals have demonstrated a goitrogenic property of yellow turnips, cabbage, kale, and other vegetables. However, the final proof implicating the goitrogenic factors in the etiology of endemic goiter in human beings is still lacking on epidemiologic grounds. Certain proprietary medications such as Felsol and therapeutic drugs such as paraaminosalicylic acid are goitrogenic. Patients administered very large doses of iodide daily may develop goiter with thyrotoxicosis, known as "jodbasedow" disease.

Sporadic Goiter. This term is applied to an enlargement of the thyroid for which a definite cause cannot be established. The diagnosis is one of exclusion in which thyroiditis and tumor and the possibility of endemic goiter are ruled out. It is thought that the goiter represents a compensatory response to an impaired efficiency of the thyroid gland. Hypersecretion of TSH may lead to stimulation of glandular growth and morphologic changes.

PATHOLOGY. The thyroid gland may be diffusely enlarged and smooth, or it may be grossly nodular. In the early stages of development, the gland is hyperplastic. The hyperplastic state may be reversed by the ingestion of iodine. Subsequently, hyperinvolution occurs forming enlarged follicles filled with colloid. At this stage, the administration of iodine fails to have an effect, but thyroid or thyroxine in replacement doses may cause reduction in size of the gland.

The nontoxic nodular goiter is grossly a multinodular structure in which the nodules vary in number and size. There is also variation in the extent of encapsulation, from sharp to poorly defined margins, and in the histology, from nonfollicular areas to gelatinous colloid-rich nodules. Scattered between the nodules are areas of normal thyroid tissue and focal areas of lymphocytic infiltration. There may be gross or microscopic evidence of degeneration of the nodules with cyst formation, recent or old hemorrhage, or calcification.

CLINICAL MANIFESTATIONS. In totally goitrous endemic regions, there is no difference in incidence related to sex. However, as one proceeds to areas diminishing in intensity, the ratio of females to males increasingly rises until in mildly endemic areas the ratio is 8 : 1. The age incidence varies with the amount of iodine available in the diet. Goiter may be observed in 20 percent of children at age five to six in some regions, while in others almost 100 percent of children have thyroids two to three times normal size. In females, the size increases up to age seventeen or eighteen, and although some glands become smaller, few disappear. In males, the number of presenting goiters declines after the age of fourteen, and there is a higher incidence of significant decrease in size and disappearance. In women, an increase in size may be noted during pregnancy with reduction in size after delivery to the antepartum level.

Most patients with goiter are asymptomatic and do not consult a physician. Those patients who are referred to the hospital, therefore, represent a selected group. The manifestations of hospitalized patients are related to the physical effects of the goiter, associated symptoms, or psychologic effects.

The most common symptom related to the thyroid gland itself is an awareness of increasing size of the neck or the presence of a mass. Pressure effects may cause embarrassment of the respiration with tracheal compression or dysphagia due to pressure on the esophagus. The tracheal compression is frequently associated with a goiter extending into the thorax. Distension of the jugular veins in these cases, indicative of impedance of return of blood, may be noted by the patient. The patients may achieve relief by flexing the neck to relieve the pressure on the trachea. Paralysis of the recurrent laryngeal nerve rarely is due to stretching across the surface of an expanding goiter and is more frequently related to a malignant tumor. Similarly, pressure on the superior sympathetic ganglion may produce a Horner's syndrome, but this is more suggestive of involvement by a neoplastic lesion. The patients may experience sudden pain in the neck associated with a rapid increase in size. This is generally related to hemorrhage into part of the goiter, either a cyst or a degenerating lesion. These symptoms usually subside spontaneously, and the gland reverts to its previous size. In rare instances, with large hemorrhage, the resulting pressure may obstruct the airway and be life-threatening.

The characteristic physical finding associated with an enlarged thyroid is a palpable mass which moves on swallowing. If the thyroid fails to move on swallowing, this suggests either goiter with intrathoracic extension, carcinoma of the thyroid with invasion of surrounding tissues, or thyroiditis extending into adjacent structures. An enlarged thyroid in a patient who is euthyroid generally is softer than the gland in a patient with Graves' disease. Marked discrepancy in the size of the two lobes of the gland is presumptive evidence that the goiter is nodular. The distinct presence or absence of nodularity and whether there is a single nodule or multiple nodules is frequently difficult to determine. Tracheal compression is difficult to recognize clinically. It may be detected by listening to the patient as he breathes with the mouth open, or displacement of the trachea may be apparent on inspection or palpation.

The history of a goiter and hypothyroidism which is manifest at birth or in childhood is evidence that some kind of inherited defect is present. In these patients, a family history is important. If the patient has been deaf since birth and goitrous since infancy or middle childhood, the diagnosis of a genetic entity known as *Pendred's syndrome* can be made. In this group of patients, the audiogram reveals a characteristic loss of hearing for high tones in those who are not totally deaf, and the diagnosis is confirmed by showing that perchlorate will result in a discharge of the radioiodine accumulated within the thyroid during the first few hours after administration.

One-third of patients with endemic cretinism have appreciable enlargement of the thyroid gland. Some children are born with marked enlargement. Endemic cretins are usually not deaf-mute but are more likely to suffer from neurologic disorders causing spasticity.

Simple and nontoxic nodular goiters rarely progress to hypothyroidism. By contrast, thyrotoxicosis develops in a large percentage of patients with a long-standing history of goiter. In the series at the Mayo Clinic, 60 percent of patients with nodular goiter over the age of sixty were thyrotoxicotic. The average duration of goiter before the onset of thyrotoxicosis was seventeen years. As indicated

in the discussion of thyrotoxicosis, exophthalmos is a rare manifestation of toxic nodular goiter, whereas congestive heart failure and atrial fibrillation may dominate the picture.

DIAGNOSTIC FINDINGS. A radiogram of the chest and neck is important to visualize the trachea in order to establish its position and the diameter of the lumen. The study will also reveal whether the goiter has extended into the thorax. Barium swallowing is indicated only if the patient has dysphagia. In most patients with simple or endemic goiter, the thyroidal ^{131}I uptake, T4, and T3 are normal. The thyroidal iodine uptake may be increased if there is iodine deficiency. In patients with familial and drug-induced goiters, the 2-hour radioiodine uptake is in the hyperthyroid range, even though the patient is clinically euthyroid or hypothyroid. Since the iodine leaves the thyroid rapidly, the 24-hour uptake is lower than normal. When the goiter is caused by excess iodide or iodopyronine, the thyroidal 2-hour uptake of radioiodine is low. Return to normal can be effected by stopping the preparation and repeating the test in 1 week. At this stage, the thyroidal radioiodine uptake at 2 hours will be in the hyperthyroid range. A goiter retains its capacity to respond to TSH, indicating that the gland is not under maximal stimulation.

Differentiation from diffuse thyroiditis may be established by needle biopsy. The diagnostic findings in patients with goiters becoming hyperthyroid are discussed in the section on Thyrotoxicosis. Consideration of the differential diagnosis of the nodular thyroid is presented in the section on treatment that follows.

TREATMENT. The therapeutic approach to a patient with a goiter takes into account the etiology, symptoms, and the presence or absence of nodularity.

Diffuse (Nonnodular) Goiter. Goiters caused by inherited enzyme defects characteristically respond well to the administration of thyroxine. The drug eliminates hypothyroidism, if present, and diminishes the size of the gland by depressing TSH stimulation. The required dosage may be established by trial and error using ^{132}I thyroidal uptake as a method of control. The minimal dose needed to abolish ^{132}I uptake is employed, and treatment is continued indefinitely. Patients with Pendred's syndrome usually manufacture an adequate or nearly adequate amount of hormone. They have normal physical and mental development, but thyroid hormone should be administered to prevent growth of goiter.

Treatment of drug-induced goiter requires the discontinuance of the offending drug, if possible. If continued drug therapy, such as para-aminosalicylic acid for tuberculosis, is required, thyroxine should be administered. Occasionally goiters in newborn children can be attributed to drugs taken by the mother during pregnancy. The enlargement disappears spontaneously during the first months of life. Endemic goiter is prevented by the administration of iodine. Occasionally, when an endemic goiter is in a hyperplastic state, iodine therapy results in decrease in size. After hyperinvolution or colloid accumulation has occurred, the administration of iodine therapy fails to have an effect. Desiccated thyroid or thyroxine in replacement doses may result in a dramatic decrease in size. This is particularly true of the diffusely enlarged, nonnodular gland.

The possible coexistence of thyroid carcinoma is not a significant problem in the nonnodular goiter. The indications for operation are (1) signs and symptoms of pressure effects, (2) pain and rapid increase in size of the gland related to intraglandular bleeding, and (3) cosmetic needs. Low-lying goiters, intrathoracic goiters, and goiters which encircle the trachea are most likely to produce symptoms of respiratory obstruction. The rare circumstance of tracheal obstruction caused by congenital goiter in the newborn is best treated by resection of the thyroid isthmus rather than tracheostomy. Hemorrhage or rapid development of an intrathyroidal cyst may cause pain and an alarming mass. Crile has reported 50 patients treated with aspiration followed by administration of desiccated thyroid. There were only three failures. Others prefer surgical excision of the cyst and a rim of surrounding tissue. Surgical procedures for cosmesis must be individualized, but it is to be emphasized that partial thyroidectomy further restricts the ability of the gland to meet hormonal requirements. Therefore, whenever a significant segment of goiter is removed, supplemental hormone therapy is indicated.

Multinodular Goiter. The results achieved by suppressive therapy, 120 to 180 mg of thyroid extract or its equivalent daily, are variable. Astwood and associates noted reduction in size of multinodular goiters in over 50 percent of their cases, whereas most other investigators report favorable effects in less than one-quarter of the patients. In most instances, although there is a decrease in overall size, the nodularity remains unchanged. The indications for operation, which have been considered in the treatment of nonnodular goiter, pertain to the nodular gland. The major argument concerning the management of the nodular thyroid is related to the likelihood that carcinoma is present within the gland and the effects of excision on the course of the disease.

It is estimated that 4 percent of inhabitants of the United States have nodules which are clinically detectable, i.e., greater than 1 cm. In Boston, routine postmortem examinations demonstrated that 8 percent of the population had one or more nodules at least 1 cm in diameter, and in women over the age of fifty a 15 percent incidence was noted. Most series have demonstrated that benign nodular goiter occurs nine times more frequently in females than males and generally becomes manifest after the age of forty.

The incidence of malignant tumors within nodular goiters ranges between 4 and 17 percent. Cole et al., evaluating a large series of thyroidectomy specimens, noted that cancer was found in 24 percent of glands with solitary nodules as compared with 10 percent in those with multiple nodules. The distinction between uninodular and multinodular goiters is extremely difficult, and it has been shown in several series that at least 50 percent of cases diagnosed preoperatively as a single nodule proved to be multinodular at the time of surgical exploration. The incidence of carcinoma within nodular thyroids varies with criteria used by pathologists and the selection of patients. The incidence of malignant thyroid tumors is related to the incidence of goiter in that area. A particularly pertinent but unresolved question is: "What percentage of lesions which satisfy the criteria for malignancy are potentially lethal?"

The mortality for thyroid cancer in 1955 was five per million for men and eight per million for women. In England and Wales, carcinoma of the thyroid accounts for 0.2 and 0.5 percent of all cancer deaths in males and females respectively. These figures emphasize the discrepancy between the mortality from thyroid carcinoma and its reported incidence in surgical specimens of multinodular goiters. The discrepancy is in part related to the factor of selectivity of patients. Those patients with multinodular goiter subjected to surgical treatment represent a group in which clinically there is a greater likelihood of carcinoma. In the experience of Shimaoka et al., which is representative of other specialty clinics, the overall incidence of carcinoma in surgical specimens was approximately 7 percent. Fifteen percent of 235 patients were suspected of having a malignant lesion preoperatively, and 40 percent proved to have thyroid carcinoma. Only 2 percent of those classified as benign preoperatively proved to be malignant.

The possibility that a multinodular goiter contains carcinoma is difficult to exclude, but there are certain criteria which increase the diagnostic accuracy. The incidence of carcinoma within a multinodular gland is greater in patients less than forty years of age and in men. The increased incidence in truly solitary nodules has been referred to. Fixation of the gland, vocal cord paralysis, Horner syndrome, and involvement of the cervical nodes are suggestive of carcinoma. A history of recent rapid and painless growth also increases the index of suspicion. A roentgenogram of the neck may reveal localized deposits of calcium arranged in concentric layers (psammoma bodies). These are characteristics of papillary carcinoma. They also have been seen subsequent to hemorrhage in a benign lesion. Radioiodine scintillation scan of the thyroid gland may contribute to the diagnosis. Nodules in which the concentration of iodine is greater than, or equal to, the remainder of the gland are less likely to harbor malignant disease. "Cold" nodules with decreased concentration of iodine have a high incidence of malignancy. In operative cases, Robinson et al. reported an incidence of carcinoma for warm or hot nodules of 6.8 and 6.4 percent, respectively, while 31.5 percent of the cold nodules contained malignant tumor.

Therapeutic Approach. Operation is indicated if there is a high index of suspicion of carcinoma based on clinical findings or diagnostic studies. Solitary nodules in patients of either sex under the age of forty and particularly in children should be removed. Solitary nodules in men over forty should also be removed. In women over forty, if the nodule is functioning as evidenced by radioiodine scan, a trial of suppressive drug therapy may be undertaken. If this induces regression, drug therapy should be continued indefinitely. If the nodule fails to regress after several months or enlarges, surgical intervention is indicated. It is also indicated if there is evidence of thyrotoxicosis associated with the nodule.

The above-mentioned criteria pertain if two or three nodules are felt. If the gland obviously contains many nodules and the patient is asymptomatic, treatment with thyroid hormone in suppressive doses is indicated.

When an operation is performed for excision of nodular goiter and only one lobe is affected, a lobectomy and isthmusectomy is the procedure of choice. Frozen section should be performed to define any questionable lesion. The treatment of proved carcinoma is discussed later in this chapter. Following surgical treatment for nodular goiter, patients are placed on replacement doses of thyroid hormone to depress TSH production and prevent regeneration. The incidence of recurrence of benign nodules varies from 5 to 15 percent depending on the period of follow-up. Subtotal thyroidectomy for nodular goiter should not be regarded as prophylaxis against carcinoma of the thyroid, since abnormal tissue is left in the neck and has a tendency to grow.

Benign Tumors

Benign tumors of the thyroid are classified as embryonal, fetal, follicular, Hürthle cell, and papillary adenomas according to their predominant histologic pattern. Grossly, the lesions are enveloped by a discrete capsule surrounded by a thin zone of compressed thyroid tissue. Microscopically, the architecture is orderly, mitoses are rare, and there is no lymphatic or blood vessel invasion. In some series, papillary adenoma is considered as a low-grade carcinoma. Several series have indicated that 80 percent of surgical specimens which proved to contain a solitary nodule are benign tumors, while 20 percent are malignant growths.

CLINICAL MANIFESTATIONS. Patients usually present with a history of a slowly growing mass which must reach the size of 1 cm to be palpable. The lesions are rarely symptomatic. Bleeding into the mass is manifested by sudden onset of localized pain. There is no evidence of cervical node involvement. Radiogram of the neck may demonstrate encroachment on the trachea. Radioiodine may indicate concentration of iodine equal to, greater than, or less than normal thyroid tissue. The criteria of differential diagnosis from malignant lesion have been referred to under Multinodular Goiter.

TREATMENT. Although some writers report treatment of solitary nodules with thyroid hormone, the majority have had no success with this approach. Since malignancy cannot be ruled out, excisional biopsy is indicated. The lesion and a margin of normal tissue should be removed and a frozen section performed to establish the diagnosis. Excision is usually achieved by subtotal or total lobectomy and isthmusectomy. The postoperative mortality approaches zero; the hospitalization is 3 to 5 days, and the postoperative morbidity is extremely low.

Malignant Tumors

GENERAL CONSIDERATIONS

INCIDENCE. The number of new cases of thyroid cancer in the United States has been estimated as 25 per 1 million population. Annual mortality from thyroid cancer is five deaths per 1 million men and eight deaths per 1 million women. The incidence of malignant tumor within the thyroid observed at routine autopsy ranges between 0.08 and 0.11 percent. There is a disputed slight association of follicular carcinoma with endemic goiter, but this does not pertain for papillary carcinoma. Ionizing radiation in childhood, usually directed at the thymus or cervical lymph nodes, has been shown to be definitely carcinogenic for the human thyroid. There is no firm evidence of increased incidence of thyroid cancer in autoimmune thyroiditis.

Clinically significant thyroid carcinoma is two to four times more common in females than in males. This sex discrepancy is less marked than that noted for other thyroid diseases. The lesions can occur at any age. The mean age for men is fifty-three years and for women forty-eight years. There has been an increasing incidence in children related to ionizing radiation in childhood, as mentioned above.

PATHOLOGY. The American Thyroid Association has accepted the classification proposed by Hazard and Smith. The four major classes are (1) papillary adenocarcinoma, (2) follicular adenocarcinoma, (3) medullary adenocarcinoma or solid adenocarcinoma with amyloid stroma, and (4) anaplastic adenocarcinoma. In addition, the thyroid may be involved with lymphosarcoma and metastatic carcinoma.

CLINICAL MANIFESTATIONS. Patients generally present with enlargement or nodularity of the thyroid. Direct questioning should determine if there is a history of irradiation to the thymus or radiation therapy for cervical adenitis in infancy. Occasionally there is a history of recent rapid growth of the lesion. Hoarseness, dysphagia, and dyspnea are late symptoms. Physical examination in the case of an early lesion frequently reveals only a thyroid mass. This may be a diffusely enlarged firm gland, a discrete nodule, or an unusually hard and dominant nodule in a multinodular gland. Regional lymph nodes may be enlarged and firm, which is suggestive of metastatic involvement. Horner's syndrome may be present, and indirect laryngoscopy may reveal paralysis of the vocal cords in advanced cases. Limitation of movement of the thyroid on swallowing suggests fixation and extension of the tumor through the capsule. Most early lesions cannot be differentiated from nodular goiter.

In general, patients with thyroid carcinoma are euthyroid, and the indices of function are normal. However, an incidence of thyroid carcinoma in Graves' disease of 9 percent has been reported. The lesions may secrete an abnormal iodoprotein with the properties of serum albumin. A similar protein has been found in other types of thyroid disease, such as thyrotoxicosis and thyroiditis. Thyroid carcinomas, in general, lose their ability to accumulate iodide as evidenced by the scintiscan, which demonstrates a reduction or absence of radioiodine in the region of the lesion. Follicular carcinomas tend to retain the ability to accumulate iodide more completely than other tumors, and radioiodine scanning is therefore less diagnostic in these cases.

An association between thyroid carcinoma and other endocrine abnormalities has been noted. The medullary-type tumor of the thyroid may occur concomitantly with pheochromocytoma. Solid carcinomas with amyloid stroma also have been associated with Cushing's syndrome due to overproduction of ACTH and symptoms of the carcinoid syndrome. An increased incidence of thyroid cancer also has been reported in patients with hyperparathyroidism.

The differential diagnosis includes the thyroidites, benign adenomas, and nodular goiter. Although needle biopsy of the thyroid has been applied to establish the diagnosis, it is not generally recommended, since a negative biopsy may not be representative.

TREATMENT. Treatment generally consists of surgical excision of the lesion. There is a great difference of opinion concerning the extent of the procedure. This will be expanded in the discussion of the therapy of the various types of pathologic lesions. Radioiodine has been employed, but effectiveness is limited by the fact that almost all cancers of the thyroid have a relative to absolute lack of avidity for iodine. High-voltage and supervoltage local radiation therapy is used in some instances when the tumor is obviously not resectable.

PAPILLARY CARCINOMA

Papillary carcinoma is the most common of the malignant tumors of the thyroid. It accounts for approximately half the thyroid malignant tumors in adults and three-quarters of those in children. Over half the cases are clinically manifest before the age of forty, with a peak incidence in the third and fourth decades. The tumors occur three times more frequently in females than males. In some patients, radiation therapy which was administered during childhood for cervical lymphadenitis or thymic enlargement has been implicated. As papillary carcinoma grows slowly, follow-up periods of at least 10 years are required to assess mortality rates.

PATHOLOGY. Papillary carcinoma is composed of columnar thyroidal epithelium arranged in papillary projections with connective tissue and vascular stalks. Outside the papillae, there may be a homogeneous material resembling colloid. The tumor may contain localized deposits of calcium arranged in concentric layers (psammoma bodies). The papillary pattern may predominate in mixed lesions containing follicular elements, and, at times, Hürthle cells.

Papillary carcinoma is the most slowly growing of the malignant tumors of the thyroid and has a tendency to become more malignant with advancing age. It has been suggested that anaplastic carcinoma may develop from a preexisting low-grade papillary carcinoma. There is some evidence that the growth of papillary carcinoma is dependent on TSH stimulation. Spread of the lesion is usually intraglandular and via pericapsular regional lymph

nodes, where it may remain localized for a long period of time. This spread, overshadowing the primary lesion, may occur when a primary tumor is of microscopic size, a circumstance now felt to be responsible for the so-called "lateral aberrant thyroid rest." The acceptable terminology is now *occult papillary carcinoma,* referring to small papillary tumors with or without deposits in cervical lymph nodes. Within the thyroid gland itself, the tumor is multicentric in about 20 percent of the cases. Although the carcinoma may persist in the neck for decades without further spread, distant metastases may occur. These are potentially functional and may accumulate radioiodine, particularly if there is a follicular element.

CLINICAL MANIFESTATIONS. The lesion usually presents as an asymptomatic nodule within the thyroid gland or as enlargement of the regional lymph nodes. Fixation of the thyroid, manifestations of pressure on adjacent structures, and distant metastases all occur late. A radiogram of the neck may reveal calcium flecks suggesting psammoma bodies. Radioiodine scan of the palpable nodule frequently demonstrates a lack of iodine uptake.

TREATMENT. All agree that the treatment of choice for contained lesions is surgical excision, but debate centers around the extent of resection. Most feel that if the tumor is apparently contained within the thyroid and there are no obvious cervical lymph node metastases, the entire lobe containing the tumor and the isthmus should be removed. Others feel that more radical surgical treatment is indicated. The latter thesis is based on the fact that several investigators have demonstrated that as many as two-thirds of the patients without clinical evidence of metastatic adenopathy have histologically apparent lymph node involvement. In addition, the multicentric origin of some of the papillary carcinomas suggests that the thyroid resection should be more extensive. In rebuttal to these histologic findings, definite proof that radical neck dissection or extensive thyroidectomy increases survival is difficult to obtain. Medina and Elliott demonstrated that more radical procedures, including neck dissection, produced no greater survival than lobectomy with or without excision of the opposite lobe. On the other hand, the more extensive procedures were associated with a higher incidence of serious complications including hypoparathyroidism, recurrent nerve injury, and airway obstruction. Crile has emphasized the fact that thyroidectomy and radical neck dissection does not meet the criteria for en bloc continuity, since the thyroid lies in the visceral compartment of the neck. In appreciation of this fact, Crile and others advise excision of cervical nodes only when they are apparently involved. Marchetta and Sako advise a modified neck dissection which preserves the sternocleidomastoid muscle, spinal accessory nerve, and internal jugular vein.

Our approach to papillary carcinoma of the thyroid is determined by the extent of the lesion. If the diagnosis of papillary carcinoma is made on frozen section and there is no apparent extension to cervical lymph nodes, a total lobectomy of the involved lobe plus isthmusectomy with subtotal lobectomy on the opposite side is performed. The node-bearing tissue adjacent to the gland is removed, and enlarged lymph nodes are excised. If there is bilateral involvement but no apparent extension outside the gland, a total thyroidectomy is performed. Solitary cervical node metastases at a distance from the gland are removed individually. If multiple nodes are involved on one side, a modified neck dissection which preserves the sternocleidomastoid muscle, spinal accessory nerve, and internal jugular vein is performed.

The prognosis for advanced lesions is usually not improved by extensive surgical treatment. Because of the chronic course of many of these tumors, solitary distant metastases, particularly in the mediastinum, which can be removed surgically should be so treated. If multiple metastases occur, treatment with radioactive iodine may be employed, but the results are frequently disappointing. Response to radioiodine therapy is more favorable when the lesion consists of an orderly arrangement of cells in the direction of an acinar pattern. Accumulation of radioactive iodine by metastases can be enhanced by total thyroidectomy or by the administration of thyroid hormone coupled with large doses of TSH. The administration of mannitol to induce acute iodine depletion has also increased the radioactive iodine uptake of metastases. Since many of the follicular carcinomas are TSH-dependent, suppressive doses of thyroid hormone should be administered to all patients with metastatic disease or locally invasive involvement on a long-term basis.

PROGNOSIS. The prognosis for long-term survival of patients with papillary carcinoma is excellent. In Crile's experience of 307 patients followed for at least 5 years 16 patients died of cancer. The prognosis is definitely worse in patients older than forty years of age. In this series, total thyroidectomy was employed only in patients with gross involvement of both lobes, and no clinically apparent cancer developed in the remaining contralateral lobe. There were no prophylactic neck dissections in patients who did not have gross evidence of nodal involvement. Black et al. analyzed 418 cases of papillary carcinoma. The 10-year survival rates for occult and contained intrathyroidal lesions were 89.5 and 83.9 percent respectively. None of the patients with occult lesions had metastases to distant sites or died of thyroidal cancer. Of 270 patients with clinically apparent but contained intrathyroidal cancer 6 died. Some patients with papillary carcinoma will die of the disease. In these cases, the originally dominant papillary elements become less prominent, and the histologic appearance becomes more anaplastic. Hirabayashi and Lindsay reported that 11 percent of their patients died of disease and that 40 percent of the deaths resulted from uncontrollable disease within the neck. Since many of the patients with papillary carcinoma are young, the effects of pregnancy on the prognosis has been of some concern. Hill et al., analyzing 70 patients, could demonstrate no difference in the overall recurrence rate subsequent to pregnancy and concluded that pregnancy had no effect on the course of disease.

FOLLICULAR CARCINOMA

Follicular carcinoma is the predominant element of one-quarter of malignant tumors of the thyroid. The lesion tends to occur in older age groups, with a peak incidence in the fifth decade. It is three times more common in females than in males.

PATHOLOGY. Grossly, the tumor may appear encapsulated. Histologically, the lesion resembles the acinar structure of normal thyroid tissue and is recognizable as an adenocarcinoma. The lumen of the acini may be devoid of colloid. The lesions contain varying numbers of large eosinophilic cells arranged in columns, Hürthle cells. The malignant potential exceeds that of papillary carcinoma. Although there may be spread to regional lymph nodes, hematogenous spread to distant sites such as bone, lung, and liver predominates and often occurs early. Occasionally, a follicular tumor with an extremely benign histologic appearance is coupled with distant metastases resembling normal thyroid. The term *benign metastasizing goiter* has been applied to these lesions.

CLINICAL MANIFESTATIONS. In many patients there is a long history of goiter with recent change in the gland, such as diffuse enlargement or the development of a single firm nodule. Pain and invasion of adjacent structures are late manifestations. Regional lymph nodes are seldom enlarged, but distant metastases are frequent. In the Massachusetts General Hospital series, one-half of the patients had evidence of distant metastases at the time that the diagnosis was established. Pulmonary and bony lesions, which are usually osteolytic, represent the most frequent sites of metastases. The metastases may possess an ability to retain iodine but are rarely responsible for thyrotoxicosis.

TREATMENT AND PROGNOSIS. In the case of an apparently contained lesion, hemithyroidectomy and isthmusectomy are usually the procedures employed. If local metastases are apparent, dissection includes these nodes. Since lymph node metastases are less common than hematogenous spread, concomitant radical neck dissection is rarely indicated. Metastases sometimes regress under the influence of suppressive thyroid hormone. Radioiodine may accumulate within the metastases and have a therapeutic effect. Total thyroidectomy has been performed in order to increase the avidity of metastases for radioiodine. Isolated metastases may be removed surgically.

Follicular tumors have the biologic behavior of a low-grade malignant tumor. The histologically more benign lesions (benign metastasizing goiter) have a better prognosis. The prognosis of follicular tumors in which the Hürthle cell predominates is similar to other follicular tumors but has a stronger propensity for recurrence. Black et al. reported 10-year survival rate of 72 percent for follicular tumors. In those lesions without marked invasiveness, the 10-year survival rate was 86 percent, whereas when invasiveness was apparent, the 10-year survival rate was 44 percent.

MEDULLARY CARCINOMA

PATHOLOGY. These lesions comprise about 7 to 10 percent of the cases of thyroid carcinoma and usually occur after the age of fifty. The diagnosis is based on specific microscopic features. The cell type varies from small and round to large and ovoid or polyhedral. At times, spindle cells are palisaded and show pleomorphism. Mitotic figures are not conspicuous. The stroma contains greater or lesser amounts of amyloid which may dominate the picture. The tumor tends to spread via the bloodstream to distant sites, particularly lung, bone, and liver. In some instances, medullary thyroid carcinoma can simulate papillary carcinoma with predominant cervical node metastases. Sixty to seventy-five percent of cases have cervical node metastases, and in thirty-eight percent mediastinal nodes are involved.

CLINICAL MANIFESTATIONS. The lesions are slightly more common in women. The first manifestation may be a hard nodular mass in the thyroid, at times accompanied by enlargement of the lymph nodes. Occasionally, symptoms attributable to a distant metastasis constitute the chief complaint. Both lobes of the thyroid are usually involved. Pain and tenderness may be severe. Thyroidal radioiodine scan demonstrates that the lesions accumulate iodine poorly. Clinically apparent regional lymph node metastases are present in over half the patients.

The lesion has evoked a great deal of interest because of its association with other endocrine abnormalities and is part of the multiple endocrine neoplasia (MEN-II) syndrome. The most commonly associated lesion is pheochromocytoma. This is thought to have a genetic basis in view of its familial occurrence. Block et al. reported personal experience with 18 patients, 10 of whom were members of two families. Either lesion, i.e., the medullary carcinoma or the pheochromocytoma, may predominate. Nonfamilial coexistence of these lesions also occurs. The frequency of bilateral thyroidal lesions in patients with medullary carcinoma combined with pheochromocytoma is greater than in those patients without pheochromocytoma (80 versus 8 percent). Other abnormalities occurring in families exhibiting the medullary carcinoma–pheochromocytoma syndrome include hyperparathyroidism, Cushing's syndrome, diabetes mellitus, carcinoid syndrome with flushing, mucosal neuromas, and unexplained diarrhea. It is thought that the syndrome may represent a disturbance in amine metabolism, and elevated serotonin calcitonin, and prostaglandin levels have been demonstrated in these patients. The diagnosis can be made by demonstration of hypocalcemia and assay of calcitonin. Determination of peak thyrocalcitonin response to pentagastrin provides a method for diagnosing medullary carcinoma in asymptomatic family members who are related to a patient with the MEN-II syndrome. Pheochromocytoma diagnostic studies must be performed in all patients with suspected medullary carcinoma.

TREATMENT AND PROGNOSIS. Pheochromocytomas, if present, should be removed first. The frequent involvement of both lobes of the thyroid and cervical lymph nodes makes an extensive excision advisable. Total or near-total thyroidectomy and modified neck dissection on one or both sides are justified if metastases are suspected. In some cases, pain emanating from the thyroid gland is so severe as to warrant palliative resection.

During the thyroid operation the parathyroid glands should be explored. If there is hypocalcemia or normocalcemia, the parathyroids should be left intact. If there is hypercalcemia, a single large gland should be removed if the remaining three are normal. This is the most common circumstance when there is hyperparathyroidism. If more than one gland is enlarged, the three largest glands and part of the fourth should be removed. Subtotal parathyroidectomy should not be routine in these patients, since hyperparathyroidism does not always occur and when present is mild.

The tumor does not respond to treatment with radioactive iodine, external radiation, or thyroid hormone. The prognosis is poorer than that noted for papillary and follicular carcinoma. Black et al. reported a 61 percent 10-year survival rate in 49 patients who underwent resection. Thirteen of twenty-five patients without involvement of the lymph nodes died during the follow-up period. However, the ultimate outcome appeared to depend more on the extent of disease than on the surgical procedure. In the experience of Black et al., recurrences within unresected remnants of the thyroid were not found.

ANAPLASTIC CARCINOMA

Undifferentiated carcinomas make up about 10 percent of malignant tumors of the thyroid and usually occur after the age of fifty. In some instances, the lesion represents a transformation of a low-grade differentiated tumor. Frazell and Foote reviewed 393 papillary tumors and reported 6 in which such a transformation occurred. Wychulis et al. reported 16 patients with mixed anaplastic and papillary carcinoma. The ratio of men to women is 1.3 : 1, and 50 percent are in the seventh and eighth decades of life, with an average age of sixty-six years.

Grossly, the tumor is unencapsulated and may extend widely outside the confines of the gland, invading adjacent structures. Histologically, the cell structure is variable, ranging from spindle-shaped to multinucleated giant cells. There are numerous mitoses, and the appearance is similar to that of a lymphosarcoma. In some cases, areas of follicular or papillary carcinoma may be present.

Patients generally present with painful enlargement of the thyroid, which is often fixed and moves poorly on swallowing. Regional lymph nodes are frequently enlarged, and signs and symptoms of pressure effects are common. Metastases are usually located in the lungs rather than the bones. The disease is characterized by an extremely rapid progress. Total thyroidectomy and modified neck dissection is the treatment of choice, but in many patients the lesion is not resectable. In one series of 130 cases, resection was attempted in only 49, and only one patient was known to be alive at the time of the report. Seventy-five percent of the deaths occurred within 1 year. External radiation may afford palliation for pain. Radioactive iodine is ineffective, since the tumors do not concentrate the material.

LYMPHOMA AND SARCOMA

The thyroid is a rare site for primary lymphoma. Mikal, in a review of the literature, indicated that 165 cases had been reported, with tumors arising from reticular cells, lymphoblasts, and lymphocytes. Only 13 cases of Hodgkin's disease arising primarily in the thyroid have been documented. At times the lesions are difficult to differentiate from Hashimoto's disease.

Treatment is determined by the extent of disease. When the tumor is localized, a total or near-total thyroidectomy followed by deep x-ray therapy to the cervical nodes is indicated. If the disease has metastasized to cervical nodes or invaded the capsule, a total thyroidectomy and radical neck dissection should be performed and followed by radiation. Disseminated lymphoma may be treated by Cytoxan or chlorambucil, or prednisone may be used in patients who cannot tolerate chemotherapy because of bone marrow depression. The 5-year survival rate is approximately 50 percent.

METASTATIC CARCINOMA

Metastases are present in the thyroid in 2 to 4 percent of the patients dying of malignant disease. Bronchogenic carcinomas account for 20 percent of secondary thyroid metastases. Three percent of all bronchogenic carcinomas autopsied demonstrate metastases to the thyroid. Wychulis et al. reported that among more than 20,000 surgical specimens 10 represented metastatic involvement of the thyroid gland. The most common primary lesion in that series was hypernephroma, with the average age of the patient fifty-six years. Freund reported two 5-year survivals following thyroidectomy in which there were metastatic lesions from bronchogenic carcinoma and lipomyxosarcoma.

Surgery of the Thyroid

Surgical treatment of the thyroid is performed (1) to establish the diagnosis in a patient with diffuse enlargement of, or a mass within, the thyroid gland; (2) to remove benign and malignant tumors; (3) as therapy for thyrotoxicosis; and (4) to alleviate pressure symptoms attributable to the thyroid. Preoperative preparation of patients with thyrotoxicosis is important to obviate the complication of thyroid storm during the operation and in the immediate postoperative period. The patients should be made euthyroid by the administration of an antithyroid drug. Seven to ten days prior to the operative procedure, potassium iodide or Lugol's solution is administered to decrease the vascularity and cause involution of the gland. Propanalol provides an alternative method of preparation.

OPERATIVE TECHNIQUE. The procedure (Fig. 38-12) is almost always performed under endotracheal anesthesia, although there was a time when local anesthesia was popular in some clinics. The patient's neck is extended by inflating a pillow beneath the shoulders. An equilateral low collar incision is made in the line of a natural skin crease approximately 2 cm above the clavicle. The incision is carried through skin, subcutaneous tissue, and platysma down to the dense cervical fascia that overlies the pretracheal muscles and anterior jugular veins. The upper flap is raised to the level of the thyroid cartilage, with care to avoid cutting sensory nerves, in order to obviate unnecessary paresthesias during convalescence. The lower flap is elevated to the level of the manubrial notch. If dissection of the flap is performed in the plane between the platysmal

muscle and the fascia overlying the strap muscles, the bleeding is minimal. The cervical fascia is then incised vertically in the midline from the upper margin of the thyroid cartilage to the manubrium.

Exposure of the superior and lateral aspects of the thyroid gland generally is achieved by retracting the sternohyoid and sternothyroid muscles or by dividing these muscles. Division of these muscles is associated with little or no disability, but is not necessary unless the gland is markedly enlarged. High transection is preferable, since the ansa hypoglossi nerve innervates the muscles from below. This diminishes the amount of muscle paralyzed.

Digital dissection frees the thyroid from surrounding fascia. We then prefer to rotate one lobe medially in order to identify the middle thyroid veins, which vary in number. These are doubly ligated in continuity and transected. This maneuver facilitates exposure of the superior and inferior poles of the thyroid. The suspensory ligaments are transected craniad to the isthmus, and the cricothyroid space is opened in order to separate the superior pole from surrounding tissue. During dissection of the superior lobe care is taken to avoid injury to the superior laryngeal nerve. The internal branch of the nerve, which provides sensory fibers to the epiglottis and larynx, is rarely in the operative field. It is the external branch, which supplies motor innervation to the inferior pharyngeal constrictor and cricothyroid muscles, which must be protected. This is accomplished by dissecting the nerve away from the superior pole vessels, which are then clamped and ligated separately.

The lobe is then retracted mediad to permit identification of the inferior thyroid artery and the recurrent laryngeal nerve. The inferior thyroid artery is isolated to avoid trauma to the recurrent laryngeal nerve and doubly ligated in continuity as it passes beneath the common carotid artery. The recurrent laryngeal nerve is identified along its course. At the junction of the trachea and larynx, it is in its most anterior position and relatively fixed. At this point, the lobe may be totally mobilized, as is indicated for tumor and *recurrent* hyperthyroidism, or a remnant of approximately 1 to 2 Gm of posterior thyroid tissue may be left in those patients in whom the operation is being performed for primary hyperthyroidism.

During exposure of the posterior surface of the thyroid gland, the parathyroids should be identified and preserved along with their vascular pedicle. Using sharp dissection, the lobe is then dissected clear from the lateral aspect of the trachea, and dissection is continued in order to separate the isthmus from the anterior trachea. If a pyramidal lobe is present, it is removed at this time. It is important that the entire anterior trachea be cleared in order to avoid development of a mass due to hypertrophy of the thyroid in this region. When the operation is being performed for a unilateral lesion, it is terminated at this point by approximating the anterior and posterior aspects of the cut end of the medial portion of the remaining lobe. When subtotal or total thyroidectomy is performed, the remaining lobe is removed in the same manner.

The remnants of thyroid are folded in and sutured to the trachea to complete hemostasis. The entire wound is

SUP. THYROID
VESSELS

MID. THYROID V.

INF. THYROID A.

PARATHYROID
RECURRENT N.
INF. THYROID A.

Fig. 38-12. Thyroidectomy. *A.* Collar incision made. Subplatysmal flaps developed. *B.* High transection of strap muscles (optional). *C.* Middle thyroid vein divided. *D.* Superior and inferior pole vessels divided. *E.* Identification of recurrent laryngeal nerve and parathyroids. *F.* Remnants of thyroid sutured to trachea to effect hemostasis.

inspected, and it is mandatory that the operative field show no evidence of bleeding. Some surgeons prefer to drain the bed of the thyroid lobes, employing a small, soft rubber drain which is split at one end to achieve a "Y" effect with the drain brought out through the incision. Others feel that little is accomplished by this maneuver, since rapid bleeding leading to respiratory distress cannot be decompressed by the small drain. The midline fascial incision is closed, and if the sternothyroid and sternohyoid muscles have been transected, they are reapproximated. The platysma and superficial fascia are then sutured with fine silk, and skin closure may be accomplished with fine silk or clips.

A tracheostomy set is left at the patient's bedside for 24 hours, so that the wound can be opened rapidly if there is significant distension, or a tracheostomy can be performed if there is evidence of respiratory obstruction.

Intrathoracic Goiter. In about 1 percent of patients undergoing thyroidectomy part or all of the thyroid tissue is intrathoracic. Intrathoracic goiter usually represents the extension of cervical thyroid tissue into the chest rather than aberrant glandular tissue. Since the lesion usually

retains its connection to the cervical thyroid and receives its blood supply from the inferior thyroid artery, it generally can be removed through the conventional collar incision described above. In the case of a very large mass the semiliquid colloid and degenerated portions may be evacuated to permit delivery of the remainder of the tissue and the capsule in the neck. The indications for transsternal or transpleural thyroidectomy include (1) an inability to remove the tumor totally through a cervical approach, (2) large masses with extensive blood supply within the mediastinum, (3) evidence of superior vena cava obstruction, and (4) undiagnosed superior mediastinal lesions.

Transsternal thyroidectomy (Fig. 38-13) can be performed as an extension of a cervical exploration by "T-ing" the cervical incision over the sternum. The sternum is transected horizontally at the level of the third interspace and vertically from the suprasternal notch down to the level of the horizontal transection. This permits extrapleural resection of the gland and provides excellent visualization of the recurrent laryngeal nerves and the vascular supply.

A thoracic extension of a cervical goiter may also be removed through a combined cervical-anterior thoracic approach using two incisions, the standard cervical incision and an incision in the second interspace. In the case of an intrathoracic goiter in the posterior portion of the mediastinum, some have advised a posterolateral thoracotomy. The disadvantage of this approach is that the position of the recurrent laryngeal nerve is difficult to determine and the major blood supply from the inferior thyroid artery is harder to control.

COMPLICATIONS

The mortality rate accompanying thyroidectomy is very low. Gould et al. reviewed 1,000 patients, operated on consecutively by a large group of surgeons over a 5-year period, and reported no hospital deaths. The mortality rate reported by Colcock was 0.12 percent, with no deaths since 1954. The morbidity is about 13 percent when all complications, including those of the most minor types, are considered. Pulmonary problems and infections are relatively uncommon. Four major complications classically have been associated with thyroidectomy. These include (1) thyroid storm, which is related to the patient's thyrotoxicosis, (2) wound hemorrhage, (3) recurrent laryngeal nerve injury, and (4) hypoparathyroidism. The latter three are regarded as complications of technique.

THYROID STORM. Thyrotoxicotic storm occurs in patients with preexisting thyrotoxicosis who either have not been treated at all or have been treated incompletely. It usually occurs in patients with Graves' disease but may be related to toxic multinodular goiter. In the past, before adequate preparation with antithyroid drugs, surgical treatment was the most common precipitating factor. Presently thyrotoxicotic crisis is a rare complication of surgical treatment and is more frequently precipitated by trauma, infection, diabetic acidosis, or toxemia of pregnancy.

When thyroid storm is related to surgical treatment, the manifestation may develop during the operative procedure or in the recovery room. The patient becomes markedly hyperthermic with profuse sweating and tachycardia. Nausea, vomiting, and abdominal pain are common. Initial tremor and restlessness may progress to delirium with eventual coma.

Treatment is directed at inhibiting the production of thyroid hormone and antagonizing effects of the hormone. Large doses of sodium or potassium iodide, i.e., to 1 to 2.5 Gm, should be administered intravenously and supplemented with 100 mg of cortisol. Oxygen and large amounts of glucose should be administered intravenously as therapy for the hypermetabolic state. Fluid and electrolytes must be maintained in view of the losses. A hypothermia blanket may be applied to reduce the temperature. Propranolol has replaced guanethidine and reserpine to antagonize

A   *B*

Fig. 38-13. Transsternal thyroidectomy. *A.* Incision. *B.* Transection of sternum. "T-ing" incision into second interspace.

sympathetic effects, since it is not complicated by congestive heart failure. Exchange transfusion is a last, but perhaps effective, resort. The mortality rate for this complication is approximately 10 percent.

WOUND HEMORRHAGE. This is a problem of the early postoperative period, i.e., within the first few hours. It has been reported in 0.3 to 1 percent of consecutive thyroidectomies. Hemorrhage in the neck is a significant problem, since small amounts of blood may obstruct the airway and result in respiratory death. The complication is usually caused by bleeding from branches of the inferior thyroid or superior thyroid artery, and the rate of bleeding is such that the commonly employed drains do not afford protection. Holl-Allen has reported four cases of postthyroidectomy hemorrhage due to hypoprothrombinemia with deficiency of factors VII and X. The deficiency was ascribed to carbimazole therapy for thyrotoxicosis. These patients required reoperation despite routine drainage at the time of the initial procedure, and vitamin K_1 corrected the deficiency.

The patients are rarely in shock. The initial manifestation is swelling of the neck and bulging of the wound, which demands immediate attention. If untreated, respiratory obstruction due to compression eventually ensues. Treatment consists of opening the incision, evacuating the clot, and securing the bleeding vessel. This constitutes an emergency procedure and frequently should be performed at the patient's bedside. Tracheostomy is not required, and is in fact contraindicated, if the wound is decompressed early. Only if there is a question of severe and potentially prolonged tracheal compression should tracheostomy be performed. Hemostasis should be complete prior to the tracheostomy to obviate bleeding into the tracheostomy tube and encrustation.

RECURRENT LARYNGEAL INJURY. Damage to the recurrent laryngeal nerve may be unilateral or bilateral and temporary or permanent. Injury occurs more commonly when thyroidectomy is being performed for malignant disease. In a series of 1,011 thyroidectomies there were 28 examples of vocal cord paralysis, three of which proved to be permanent. The incidence of recurrent nerve injury in another series of 1,000 patients reported by Gould et al. was 0.2 percent. Colcock and King, evaluating 1,246 thyroid operations, noted one bilateral recurrent laryngeal nerve paralysis. Recently Thompson and Harness reported an incidence of 4.8 percent for accidental unilateral nerve injury in total thyroidectomy for carcinoma.

Loss of function of the recurrent laryngeal nerve may result from excessive trauma to the nerve during exposure, inclusion of the nerve in a ligature, or an inadvertent sectioning of the nerve. Recurrent laryngeal nerve injury produces an abductor laryngeal paralysis, and the vocal cord assumes a median or paramedian position, which is identifiable on postoperative laryngoscopy. The involved cord or cords are initially flaccid, but with the passage of time the flaccidity is replaced by spasticity. If the injury is related to dissection and the nerve is intact, function should return usually within 3 months and invariably within 9 months. In the immediate postoperative period, cord paralysis results in narrowing of the glottic aperture, but this is not sufficient to produce obstruction of the airway unless it is accompanied by glottic edema due to hematoma in the cervical space or trauma to the larynx, or related to the cuffed endotracheal tube. Because of the initial flaccidity, bilateral or cord paralysis may not be apparent for several hours. As the laryngeal muscles atrophy, the cords contract and the glottic aperture narrows, causing airway obstruction. Paralysis of one cord results in disturbance of the voice with varying degrees of hoarseness.

The incidence of this complication can be markedly reduced by identifying the nerve or nerves routinely during thyroidectomy. The recurrent laryngeal nerve is in greatest jeopardy at the level of the two upper tracheal rings, where the middle third of the thyroid lobe is in closest contact with it. The lobe is attached by a strong process of pretracheal fascia (the suspensory ligament of Berry) to the cricoid cartilage and trachea, which must be severed before it can be removed. Although the recurrent laryngeal nerve usually runs posteriorly to this adherent connective tissue zone, in 25 percent of patients it courses through the ligament of Berry. Asymptomatic paralysis does not require treatment. In some instances, reexploration of the wound is indicated, since removal of a ligature often reestablishes function. Once the diagnosis of bilateral cord paralysis, a rarity, is established, tracheostomy should be performed, since airway obstruction eventually occurs, frequently related to a respiratory tract infection. Subsequently the glottic aperture can be widened by arytenoidectomy or arytenoidopexy, which displaces the posterior portion of the vocal cord laterally. These procedures provide an adequate airway but cause further deterioration of the voice. Six to nine months should be allowed to pass between the time of thyroidectomy and these procedures in order to be certain that there is no returning function. Direct repair of the transected recurrent laryngeal nerve as late as 2 to 3 months postinjury has been successful in some cases. Splitting the vagus nerve and anastomosing it to the distal end of the recurrent laryngeal nerve or burying the nerve in the posterior cricoarytenoid muscle are being evaluated.

HYPOPARATHYROIDISM. Overt manifestations of hypoparathyroidism occur in 2 to 3 percent of patients following thyroidectomy. This is usually a temporary syndrome related to dissection in the region of the parathyroid glands. There is an increased incidence of temporary hypoparathyroidism following thyroidectomy for hyperthyroidism. It is necessary to leave only one gland in situ with an adequate blood supply to avoid the complication. Postoperative permanent hypoparathyroidism occurred in 0.6 percent of the 1,000 thyroidectomies reviewed by Gould et al. and in 2.8 percent of the total thyroidectomies in that series. Persik and Catz, in a review of 210 consecutive total thyroidectomies, noted that permanent hypoparathyroidism resulted in none of the patients with nonmalignant disease and in 9 percent of those with malignant disease. In the series of Thompson and Harness permanent hypoparathyroidism occurred in 5.4 percent of all patients undergoing total thyroidectomy for carcinoma, in 1.6 percent of those having primary procedures, and in 7.4 percent of those having secondary operations. An incidence of 8.2 percent was noted when there was an associated neck dissection.

Postthyroidectomy hypoparathyroidism may be due to the inadvertent removal of the parathyroid glands but more frequently is caused by damage to the blood supply. The parathyroid end arteries have to be damaged in order to infarct the gland. The anastomotic arterial network is so extensive that if proximal arteries are injured, there is sufficient collateralization. The clinical manifestations usually occur within the second 24 hours after operation and almost invariably within the first week. The initial symptoms are circumoral numbness, tingling, and intense anxiety. The Chvostek sign appears early, followed by Trousseau's sign and carpopedal spasm. As the disease progresses, muscle cramps and frank tetany develop. Prolonged hypoparathyroidism may cause cataracts, convulsive episodes, and psychoses. The diagnostic findings consist of reduced serum calcium, increased serum phosphorus, and decreased or absent calcium in the urine as evidenced by the Sulkowitch test.

Recently an occult type of hypoparathyroidism has been described. The symptoms are those of general ill health and mental depression. The serum calcium is within normal limits, but there is a lack of parathyroid reserve which can be demonstrated by the calcium deprivation test. When the serum calcium is depressed in the normal patient, the parathyroid glands are stimulated to increase secretion of parathyroid hormone in order to restore the calcium to normal levels. In patients with occult hypoparathyroidism this response is inadequate. EDTA (edetic acid) is infused for 2 hours, and the serum calcium level falls in both normal and abnormal cases. In normal patients a rise to 8.5 mg occurs within 24 hours, while the rise is markedly delayed in patients with occult hypoparathyroidism. Abnormal response to calcium load also has been observed in patients following a thyroid operation with extensive removal of tissue. This has been interpreted as evidence of calcitonin deficiency, but no clinical significance has been ascribed to this situation.

Postoperative hypoparathyroidism must be differentiated from tetany caused by alkalosis associated with anxiety and hyperventilation. This causes a reduction in ionized calcium, but the manifestations can be promptly reversed by inhalation of carbon dioxide or breathing through an increased dead space.

The treatment of hypoparathyroidism should be initiated promptly. When the diagnosis has been made, 10 ml of a 10 percent solution of calcium chloride or gluconate should be administered intravenously and usually results in immediate improvement of symptoms. Continued therapy includes 5 to 15 Gm of calcium lactate powder daily or calcium syrup, and 50,000 to 200,000 units of vitamin D_2 daily. The dosage of these drugs is regulated by following the patient's clinical course and serum calcium and phosphorus levels. The intake of certain meat, fish, and dairy products which are high in phosphorus should be limited, since it results in a depression of serum calcium levels. Parathyroid hormone (PTH) and dihydrotachysterol (AT 10) should be reserved for the exceptional case when usual measures fail. Watkins et al. have employed autotransplantation of parathyroid tissue at the time of operation with questionable evidence of take. Because of the factor of vascular deficiency these writers employed aortic vascular pedicle transplantation of neonatal parathyroid tissue in eight patients. Clinical improvement was noted despite histologic evidence of graft rejection. The efficacy of parathyroid transplantation in this situation remains to be proved.

PARATHYROID

(by Edwin L. Kaplan)

Historical Background

HYPERPARATHYROIDISM. Von Recklinghausen, in 1891, first described the fibrocystic disease of bone produced by hyperparathyroidism but did not recognize the association. In 1903 Askanazy suggested a relation between tumors of the parathyroid and the bone disease described by von Recklinghausen. Erdheim in 1907 correctly surmised that parathyroid enlargement in osteomalacia, rickets, and pregnancy was *secondary* to the bone changes, and from this observation the concept grew that parathyroid enlargement was secondary in other types of bone disease as well. Schlagenhaufer in 1915 suggested that the parathyroid enlargement might be the cause of the bone disease and recommended excision of the parathyroid tumor as the treatment. The first parathyroidectomy was carried out by Mandl in Vienna in 1925 in a patient with classic von Recklinghausen's disease of bone. The patient's calcium level fell abruptly, and the bone lesions improved.

In 1926 a case referred by Du Bois for study by Aub at the Massachusetts General Hospital was diagnosed as probable hyperparathyroidism, and the neck was explored on two occasions, but no parathyroid tumor was found. These workers were at this time unaware of Mandl's experience, which had not yet been published. A third unsuccessful operation was carried out in New York. The patient ultimately returned to Boston, where, in 1932 at his seventh

operation, the adenoma was found in the mediastinum. The patient died 6 weeks later in tetany after another operation for a renal stone producing anuria. The first successful operation in America was that reported by Barr and Bulger in 1930.

The bone tumors of hyperparathyroidism were emphasized by Hunter and Turnbull, who called them "osteoclastomas" and in 1931 reported a case of successful removal of a parathyroid adenoma.

Hall and Chaffin reported the first parathyroid carcinoma in 1934. Water-clear cell (*wasserhellen Zellen*) hyperplasia was first described by Albright et al. in 1934 and primary chief cell hyperplasia by Cope et al. in 1958. Secondary chief cell hyperplasia in renal disease had been described by Pappenheimer and Wilens in 1935.

Albright recognized the association between parathyroid adenomas and renal stones, and in August 1932 the first patient to undergo excision of a parathyroid adenoma for renal stones without bone disease was operated upon. Albright emphasized that hyperparathyroidism was much more common than previously supposed, and often associated with renal stones. The frequency of the disease was further underscored by Cope, who in 1942 published a series of 67 cases from the Massachusetts General Hospital.

The association of hyperparathyroidism with peptic ulcer was first described by Rogers et al. (1946–1947) and the association with pancreatitis by Cope et al. (1957).

HYPOPARATHYROIDISM. Sanström (1880) first described the parathyroid glands. Gley (1891) showed that tetany following thyroidectomy in the dog was due to parathyroid removal. Vassale and Generali (1900) removed the parathyroids in the dog and produced tetany. Loeb (1901) showed that the injection of agents which bound calcium produced tetany. MacCallum and Voegtlin (1908) recognized that the function of the parathyroids was to regulate calcium metabolism and were able to relieve the tetany which followed parathyroidectomy by the administration of calcium.

Hanson (1924) and Collip (1925) prepared the first stable crude parathyroid hormone extracts. Collip (1926) correctly observed that parathyroid hormone (PTH) acted directly on bone to increase resorption. This view was challenged by Albright and Ellsworth (1929), who thought the bone effect was secondary to the effect of PTH on renal phosphate excretion. It is now clear that PTH acts both on bone and kidney.

Embryology

The upper parathyroids arise embryologically from the fourth branchial pouch along with the anlage of the thyroid (Fig. 38-14). They descend only slightly during embryologic life along with the thyroid and continue to remain in close association with the upper portion of the lateral thyroid lobes. Because of their relatively circumscribed migration their position in adult life remains quite constant. When they become adenomatous, they enlarge and tend to be displaced downward somewhat, dragging their blood supply with them. They may on occasion descend as far down as the superior portion of the posterior mediastinum. When they do descend into the mediastinum, they tend to be more posterior than the lower parathyroids.

The lower parathyroids arise from the third branchial pouch along with the thymus and descend with the thymus (Fig. 38-15). Because they travel so far in embryologic life, they have a very wide range of distribution in the adult. They may be found all the way from just beneath the mandible to the pericardium. When the lower parathyroid does descend into the mediastinum, it is almost always anterior and usually supplied by the inferior thyroid artery, which is dragged behind it (Fig. 38-16). A mediastinal parathyroid gland can be found by tracing the branch of the inferior thyroid artery which supplies it even in its abnormal location.

Anatomy

Gilmour, in a study of 527 autopsies, found that roughly 80 percent had four glands, 6 percent had five, and 13 percent had three. Two glands or six glands were present very rarely. These data are shown in Table 38-1.

In 1938 Gilmour described the position of the glands in 787 autopsy cases. The locations with the relative percentages found are shown diagrammatically in Figs. 38-17 and 38-18. In nearly 75 percent of the cases the upper gland lay on the posterior portion of the middle third of the thyroid, usually toward the superior part of this area, either in a groove on the thyroid or on a projecting nodule. It usually lay above the inferior thyroid artery but occasionally behind it or between it and the thyroid gland.

The inferior parathyroid glands were of course more

Fig. 38-14. Embryology of the parathyroid glands. The upper parathyroid has its origin in the fourth branchial pouch and moves to a position in adult life adjacent to the middle third of the lateral thyroid lobe. It thus travels little from its site of embryologic origin. The lower parathyroid, by contrast, arises from the third branchial pouch and travels down past the upper parathyroid to come to rest opposite the lower pole of the thyroid. Because of this embryologic mobility the lower parathyroid is more likely to lie in some ectopic location, either left behind high up in the neck or moving far down past the upper parathyroid into the mediastinum along with the thymus.

I-4 CLEFTS

I-V ARCHES

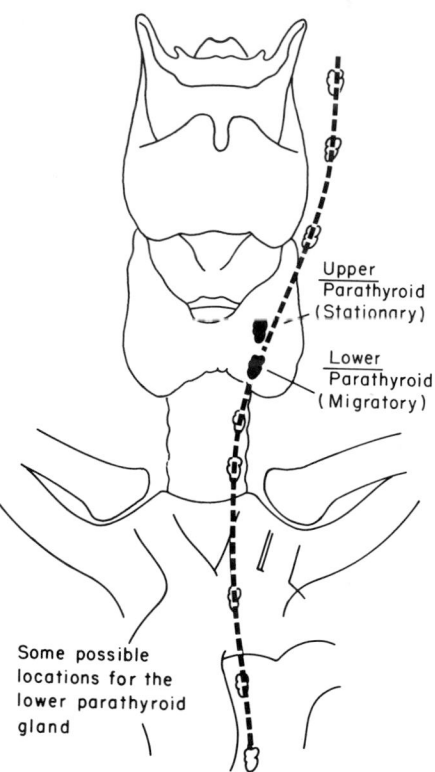

Fig. 38-15. Descent of the lower parathyroid. While the upper parathyroid occupies a relatively constant position in relation to the middle or upper third of the lateral thyroid lobe, the lower parathyroid normally migrates in embryonic life and may end up anywhere along the course of the dotted line. When this gland is in the chest, it is nearly always in the anterior mediastinum.

variable. In somewhat more than 50 percent of the cases the lower parathyroid was found on the lateral or posterior surface of the lower pole of the thyroid gland, or not more than 0.5 cm below the lower pole. The next most common location, in 12.8 percent, was 1 cm below the lower pole of the thyroid.

Gilmour, while examining 1,713 parathyroid glands in 428 patients, found that the parathyroids were occasionally included within the thyroid capsule or lay beneath it and

Table 38-1. NUMBER OF PARATHYROIDS IN 527 AUTOPSY CASES

Number of parathyroid glands	Number of patients	Percentage of patients with this number
6	2	0.4
5	31	5.9
4	419	79.5
3	69	13.1
2	6	1.1
Total.	527	100

SOURCE: Gilmour, 1937.

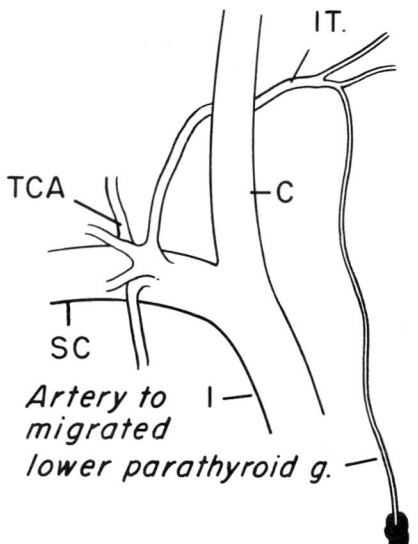

Fig. 38-16. Migration of the adenomatous parathyroid gland. If an adenoma develops in the parathyroid gland, the gland may gradually descend into the chest. Under these circumstances, it is always supplied with blood from the inferior thyroid artery. If the lower parathyroid has descended into the mediastinum during embryonic life, it may then receive its blood supply from the branches of the thymic arteries. *C,* carotid artery; *SC,* subclavian artery; *I,* innominate artery; *IT,* inferior thyroid artery.

that they were sometimes carried partially into the substance of the thyroid by the thyroid vessels but that they were never completely covered by thyroid tissue. In two other dissections, however, he did find a parathyroid completely covered by the thyroid, and in both instances these were the inferior parathyroid glands. Other writers have described normal parathyroids lying within the thyroid. Not only have we seen instances in which the normal gland has been entirely within the thyroid, but we have seen a parathyroid adenoma or a hyperplastic parathyroid gland which lay completely within the thyroid. This has been reported by others.

The upper parathyroids have been shown to be slightly larger than the lower in some studies. The average weight of a normal parathyroid gland is about 30 mg, but some authors think that normal glands may be heavier if they contain a great deal of fat. The total weight of four normal parathyroids is about 120 to 140 mg.

The usual positions for the superior and inferior thyroid arteries, the recurrent laryngeal nerve, and the parathyroids are shown in Figs. 38-51 and 38-52. The superior gland is usually supplied by the superior thyroid artery, while the inferior gland is almost always supplied by the inferior thyroid artery, though in rare instances it may be supplied by the superior thyroid artery. The inferior gland which descends into the mediastinum because of the development of an adenoma is always supplied by the inferior thyroid artery, while an adenoma which develops in a gland that has come to be located in the mediastinum embryologically may be supplied by branches from the internal mammary or thymic vessels, or rarely from the aorta.

Physiology

CALCIUM METABOLISM. The body contains somewhat over 1,000 Gm of calcium, of which 1 Gm is in the extracellular fluid, 4 Gm is exchangeable in bone, 1,000 Gm is stable in bone, and 11 Gm is in cells. The average daily dietary intake is 0.5 to 1 Gm. Urinary calcium excretion varies with the dietary calcium intake and may be as high as 300 to 400 mg/day on an unrestricted diet. Usually, however, it is about 100 to 200 mg/day. On a low-calcium diet containing 200 mg calcium, less than 175 mg calcium should be excreted in the urine. Small amounts of calcium, up to 100 mg/day, are also excreted in sweat; the remainder is excreted in the feces. About 600 mg of calcium is secreted into the intestines from various glands and most of it is resorbed. Calcium absorption takes place principally in the duodenum and upper jejunum. It is an active process involving vitamin D metabolites.

In plasma about 47 percent of the calcium is ionized, 47 percent is protein-bound, and the remainder is complexed to organic anions such as citrate and phosphates.

The ionized calcium is the important one physiologically. It is well known that calcium ion plays a critical role in determining the excitability of nerve function and in the contractility of skeletal and cardiac muscle. More

Fig. 38-17. Most frequent locations for the normal parathyroid (anterior view). The locations for the upper parathyroid are shown at the left and for the lower at the right. The relative frequency with which the glands are found in the various locations is indicated on the diagram. (*From J. R. Gilmour, J Pathol, 45:507, 1937.*)

Fig. 38-18. Most frequent locations for normal parathyroid glands (lateral view). (*From J. R. Gilmour, J Pathol, 45:507, 1937.*)

recently it has been demonstrated that calcium ion is important in the structure and function of cell membranes and organelles, and in numerous cellular metabolic events including hormone release. In fact, it is postulated by Rasmussen that there is a close relation between calcium ion and the actions of cyclic adenosine monophosphate (cAMP). Ideally we would like to measure the ionized calcium concentration in serum. Since this is difficult to determine, we utilize the total serum calcium concentration, instead. Total serum calcium concentrations correlate

Fig. 38-19. The relationship of total calcium, ionized calcium, and protein-bound calcium in the serum. *A.* Normal serum. *B* and *D*. An elevated total calcium, due to an increase of ionized calcium, as found in cases of primary hyperparathyroidism. *C.* An elevated total calcium concentration due to an increase of serum proteins and hence of protein-bound calcium. This may be incorrectly interpreted as compatible with primary hyperparathyroidism if serum proteins are not determined.

very well clinically as long as the serum protein concentrations are normal. However, in abnormal states, the total calcium must be considered in relation to plasma protein levels, especially albumin. Though there is not an invariable relationship between the amount of protein-bound calcium and total protein levels, in general for each gram of alteration of total protein above or below 6.5 Gm/100 ml there is an 0.8- to 1-mg/100 ml increase or decrease in protein-bound calcium and hence in total serum calcium as well (Fig. 38-19). Normal total serum calcium concentration ranges from 9 to 10.5 mg/100 ml in many laboratories, but this varies with the technique used.

The calcium in the extracellular pool exchanges forty to fifty times a day with that in the intracellular fluid, the glomerular filtrate, and the exchangeable bone (Fig. 38-20). The kidneys normally resorb 99 percent of the filtered calcium. Even with marked hypercalcemia the urinary calcium excretion rarely exceeds 500 mg/day. With rapid bone destruction from metastatic tumor or increased secretion of PTH the kidney is unable to excrete enough calcium to keep up with the rising serum levels, particularly if some renal damage is present, and a state of serious or fatal hypercalcemic crisis may ensue.

PHOSPHORUS METABOLISM. The body contains about 500 Gm of phosphate, the extracellular fluid 0.4 Gm, the bone 425 Gm, and the cells about 75 Gm. The diet contains about 1,000 mg/day.

In plasma about 15 percent is protein-bound, and a considerable amount exists as complexes with monovalent and divalent cations. In contrast to calcium, the serum phosphate value changes markedly with diet, age (it is higher in children), and hormone secretion (other than

Fig. 38-20. Calcium metabolism. The diet contains approximately 1,000 mg of calcium each day. The intestinal glands secrete approximately 600 mg into the intestine. Of this 1,600 mg, 800 is absorbed, and 800 is excreted in the feces. The extracellular fluid contains about 1,000 mg of calcium. This is constantly being exchanged with calcium in other pools. Each day 10,000 mg are filtered through the glomerulus, and 9,900 mg of this are resorbed. There is a slow exchange from stable bone and a rapid exchange from exchangeable bone. Calcium is constantly being resorbed and added to bone, and this activity is under hormonal control.

PTH). The serum value varies between 3 and 4.5 mg/100 ml in adults and between 5 and 6 mg/100 ml in children.

About 70 percent of the dietary phosphate is absorbed from the intestine, the absorption primarily taking place in the midintestine. Absorption is increased by PTH, growth hormone (GH), vitamin D, and a low-calcium diet. It is decreased by a high calcium intake, beryllium poisoning, aluminum hydroxide ingestion, and factors which diminish calcium absorption.

Almost all of the absorbed phosphate is excreted in the urine. With a 1,000-mg diet 700 mg will be absorbed and 670 mg excreted in the urine. Urinary excretion is increased in hyperparathyroidism, vitamin D excess, vitamin D deficiency with secondary hyperparathyroidism, osteoporosis, bone metastases, sarcoidosis, acidosis, and various renal tubular disorders. It is decreased by GH, hypoparathyroidism, Addison's disease, chronic renal failure, lacta-

tion, dietary phosphate deficiency, osteopetrosis, and osteoblastic tumors of bone.

MAGNESIUM METABOLISM. The body contains about 200 mEq of magnesium. Half of this is in the skeleton, and most of the rest is intracellular, only 1 percent being in the extracellular fluid. The normal serum magnesium level is 1.6 to 2.5 mg/100 ml in our laboratory.

The daily dietary intake is about 25 mEq. About 8 to 10 mEq is absorbed and excreted in the urine. Absorption is increased by vitamin D and decreased by calcium. The renal excretion of magnesium closely follows that of calcium, and PTH increases the resorption of both.

The various factors regulating magnesium metabolism are not well known, but PTH certainly plays a role. Hypomagnesemia occurs in hyperparathyroidism, alcoholism, malnutrition, and chronic intravenous hyperalimentation if magnesium is not added to the feeding regimen. A low plasma magnesium level stimulates the secretion of PTH and an elevated level inhibits it, as with calcium. Plasma magnesium is also decreased in hyperthyroidism and increased in hypothyroidism.

While hypomagnesemia is present in many patients with hyperparathyroidism, the plasma levels may be normal if the dietary intake is good and intestinal absorption is not

Fig. 38-21. Microradiograph of a cross section of a normal human cortical bone, showing regions of resorption, formation, and inactivity. (*Taken from J. Jowsey, Am J Med, 40:485, 1966.*)

thus serves as an index of the degree of bone resorption taking place. Hydroxyproline is not a perfect indicator of bone resorption, however, because not all collagen is in bone and various rate-limited factors affect hydroxyproline metabolism before it is excreted.

PTH increases degradation of collagen and increases urinary hydroxyproline excretion. Calcitonin decreases bone resorption in patients with Paget's disease of bone. A decrease in urinary hydroxyproline accompanies this response.

BONE. Bone is made up of a matrix (osteoid) which is nearly all collagen, and inorganic crystals of hydroxyapatite $[Ca_{10}(Po_4)_6(OH)_2]$. The matrix makes up 30 percent and the mineral 70 percent of the dry weight.

The metaphysis of the bone is the most active part metabolically and the first to respond to PTH excess.

The collagen matrix of the bone is covered by a layer of bone cells, some of which are engaged in osteoblastic activity, laying down new bone, and some in osteoclastic activity, resorbing bone. Osteocytes, which are located within the substance of compact cortical bone, have been demonstrated by Belanger also to be important in bone resorption. This process, called *osteocytic osteolysis*, may be the principal mechanism for rapid mobilization of calcium from bone particularly in response to the initial action of PTH. The osteoclast may be more important in bone remodeling and also in the chronic stimulation of bone resorption in hyperparathyroidism. Some measure of the metabolic activity of the bone has been gained by a study of the number and appearance of these cells. Recently, however, new techniques have permitted a quantitation of bone activity by a study of the bone tissue itself, in a calcified state, rather than of the cells which make or destroy it.

Microradiography has been used by Jowsey and others to avoid some of the difficulties inherent in other methods. This technique is used to study the distribution of minerals in bone. A section of bone is ground down, and an x-ray is made of the section with a low-energy beam and fine-grain film. The x-ray film (rather than the section) is then examined under the microscope, as shown in Figs. 38-21 and 38-33. Areas of active resorption and formation can be delineated and measured, to quantitate bone turnover. The percent of the total area of the section undergoing resorption and that undergoing bone formation are calculated.

Additional information concerning bone formation may be obtained by tetracycline labeling. When tetracycline is administered, it is incorporated in osteoid at the site of new mineral deposition. The tetracycline is located by its characteristic fluorescent emission. A rate of bone formation may be obtained by giving two doses of tetracycline at intervals of several weeks. Two discrete lines of deposition may be determined in subsequent biopsy specimens, and a measurement of the area between the lines gives a measure of growth rate.

The rates of bone formation and resorption are normally equal and low, and do not change significantly between the ages of twenty and forty. In young growing people the rates of formation and resorption are high, while in older people the rate of resorption increases, and the rate of

interfered with by anorexia or vomiting. After resection of the parathyroid adenoma temporary hypomagnesemia frequently occurs even when the plasma level has been normal preoperatively. The serum magnesium level rises to normal values in a few days because of the marked increase in tubular resorption of this ion after parathyroidectomy. The variation in the magnesium balance probably relates to (1) variations in dietary intake, to which magnesium levels are very sensitive, (2) the degree of bone disease present—significant bone disease increasing the likelihood that postoperative hypomagnesemia will occur, and (3) the marked increase in renal magnesium resorption which occurs after removal of the adenoma. Some cases of tetany are caused by hypomagnesemia and cannot be corrected until serum magnesium levels are returned to normal.

HYDROXYPROLINE. Bone matrix is made up largely of collagen, which is the only major source of hydroxyproline in the body. When collagen is destroyed, most of it is hydrolyzed to amino acids or further degraded and then reused. However, about 5 to 8 percent of it is only partially degraded to hydroxyproline-containing peptides which are excreted in the urine. The urinary hydroxyproline content formation remains the same as in the young adult, with a resultant net loss of bone.

Jowsey has compared bone taken in disease states to normal individuals of the same age and charted the results on the basis of the number of standard deviations from the normal for that age. In hyperparathyroidism (Fig. 38-22) the amount of resorption was increased to over 2 standard deviations above normal in all but one case—presumably because of the stimulation of the osteoclasts by PTH. This was true even when the bones appeared perfectly normal on standard skeletal x-rays. In three cases bone formation was also increased, which may account for the absence of gross bone changes. In hypoparathyroidism both formation and resorption are reduced.

In osteoporosis there is loss of bone mass. Osteoporosis may be primary (idiopathic) or secondary to hyperparathyroidism, hyperthyroidism, Cushing's syndrome, or many other causes. In primary osteoporosis there is an increase in bone resorption, while bone formation remains normal. In Cushing's syndrome there is a marked increase in bone resorption accompanied by a decrease in bone formation.

Bed rest reduces bone formation, while resorption is increased more in the osteoporotic patient than in the normal. In Paget's disease both resorption and formation are high, the first somewhat more than the second, while in hyperthyroidism there is also increased resorption and formation, but to a lesser degree. In osteomalacia and rickets little or no bone formation occurs.

PARATHYROID HORMONE, VITAMIN D, CALCITONIN. Parathyroid Hormone. In recent years, PTH has been purified from bovine and porcine parathyroid glands. The amino acid sequence of both molecules has been determined; the bovine molecule is shown diagrammatically in Fig. 38-23. Both molecules have a molecular weight of about 9,500 and contain 84 amino acid residues. Synthesis of a biologically active fragment of the bovine molecule containing the 1 to 34 residues from the amino terminal has now been achieved. Purification of human glandular PTH has been hampered by the relatively small amount of human parathyroid tissue available for study. Recently, Brewer et al. purified human PTH from parathyroid adenomas and have determined the sequence of the 34 amino acids at the amino terminal of the molecule; this fragment has been shown to be biologically active. A comparison of the structure of these human and animal N-terminal fragments of PTH is shown in Fig. 38-24.

Within the parathyroid glands, larger precursor molecules of parathyroid hormone have now been identified. These are called *pro PTH* and *pre-pro PTH* (Fig. 38-25). It seems unlikely, at this time, that these larger molecules circulate in peripheral blood.

Vitamin D. Largely due to the work of DeLuca and associates many significant advances in vitamin D metabolism recently have been made. The natural form of vitamin D is called vitamin D_3, or cholecalciferol (Fig. 38-26). It is produced by the irradiation of 7-dihydrocholesterol in the skin. To be metabolically active D_3 is first hydroxylated in the liver to 25-hydroxyvitamin D_3 (25-OH D_3). The 25-OH D_3 is further hydroxylated in the kidney to 1,25-dihydroxy-

Fig. 38-22. Bone turnover in hypoparathyroidism and hyperparathyroidism. Open circles indicate resorption; solid circles indicate formation. (*From J. Jowsey, Am J Med, 40:485, 1966.*)

vitamin D_3 [1,25-(OH)$_2$D$_3$]. This latter metabolite is believed to be the metabolically active form of vitamin D which carries out the well-known functions of this substance—namely, mobilizing calcium and phosphorus from bone and enhancing intestinal absorption of calcium and phosphorus. Nephrectomized animals and human beings, for example, are insensitive to administration of both vita-

Fig. 38-23. Amino acid sequence of bovine parathyroid hormone. (*From J. T. Potts, Jr., et al., Am J Med, 50:639, 1971.*)

HUMAN PARATHYROID HORMONE

BOVINE PARATHYROID HORMONE

PORCINE PARATHYROID HORMONE

Fig. 38-24. Comparison of the amino acid sequence of the amino terminal 34 residues of human, bovine, and porcine PTH. (*From H. B. Brewer, Jr., et al., Proc Natl Acad Sci USA, 69:3585, 1972.*)

min D_3 and 25-OH D_3, since they cannot convert this to the active 1,25-$(OH)_2D_3$ form.

It is now suggested that vitamin D acts as a physiologic hormone which has feedback control mechanisms in animals and human beings. In the presence of parathyroid hormone, when serum calcium or serum phosphorus levels are low, there is an increased synthesis of 1,25-$(OH)_2D_3$, which then makes calcium and phosphorus available from the bone and intestines. Thus the serum calcium concen-

tration returns toward normal. When the serum calcium concentrations are normal, less 1,25-$(OH)_2D_3$ and more 24,25-$(OH)_2D_3$ are produced. This latter metabolite is relatively inactive, and therefore less calcium and phosphorus are mobilized.

These findings not only are of interest physiologically but may be important clinically in the treatment of renal osteodystrophy and hypoparathyroidism. In both these conditions, microgram quantities of 1,25-$(OH)_2D_3$ or its analogue, 1 α-hydroxy vitamin D_3, have proved effective. When they become available, they may well be the treatment of choice for these and other conditions, such as malabsorption states.

Recently, methods for measurement of serum 25-OH D_3 and 1,25-$(OH)_2D_3$ in human beings have become available. These should lead to a better understanding of normal and abnormal states of vitamin D metabolism.

Calcitonin (Thyrocalcitonin). Calcitonin, a calcium-lowering polypeptide, was originally described by Copp (1962) and Hirsh and Munson (1963). It was originally shown to be present in the epifollicular or parafollicular cells of the mammalian thyroid gland. These cells are now commonly referred to as *C cells*. It has now been demonstrated that C cells come from the neural crest and are part of the APUD system of peptide- or amine-secreting cells described by Pearse. They migrate to the ultimobranchial bodies, glandular structures derived from the lowest branchial pouches embryologically. In man and other mammals these structures are vestigial; they fuse with and are incorporated into the lateral thyroid lobes during embryologic development. In lower animals C cells are found within the ultimobranchial bodies which remain as separate structures. Medullary carcinomas of the thyroid gland are C cell, calcitonin-producing tumors.

Calcitonin has been purified from the thyroid glands of pigs, sheep, and cows, from medullary carcinomas in man

Fig. 38-25. Partial amino acid sequence of bovine pre-proparathyroid hormone (Pre-proPTH). In the parathyroid glands, preproPTH, a molecule containing 115 amino acids, is converted to proPTH, a 90–amino acid molecule. Then six additional molecules are cleaved, leaving the 84 amino acids of PTH. PTH = amino acids 1 to 84. ProPTH = 6 amino acids added to the NH$_2$ terminus of PTH: −6 to 84. Pre-proPTH = 25 amino acids added to the NH$_2$ terminus of proPTH: −31 to 84. (*From B. Kemper et al., Biochemistry, 15:15, 1975.*)

Fig. 38-26. Summary of vitamin D metabolism. (*From H. F. DeLuca, Ann Intern Med, 85:367, 1976.*)

(called *calcitonin M*), and from salmon ultimobranchial glands. Each of these has a molecular weight of 3,500 and 32 amino acids, and they have the same molecular configuration. However, as shown in Fig. 38-27, wide variations of amino acid sequences occur within these molecules. Radioimmunoassay systems for measurement of the different calcitonins have added greatly to our knowledge of the physiology of calcitonin and are important in the diagnosis of occult medullary carcinoma of the thyroid in man.

Calcitonin lowers the serum calcium concentration by inhibiting bone resorption. In pharmacologic doses, salmon calcitonin has been successfully utilized in the treatment of Paget's disease of bone.

Serum Calcium Homeostasis

Serum calcium concentration in man has long been recognized to vary only minimally from day to day (Fig. 38-28). Its regulation is primarily by the parathyroid glands through a negative feedback system. A fall in serum calcium (or serum magnesium) concentration stimulates secretion of PTH which then acts peripherally to raise the serum calcium concentration to normal. Hypocalcemia also results in increased formation of $1,25\text{-}(OH)_2D_3$.

An elevation of the serum calcium level reduces both PTH secretion and also the formation of $1,25\text{-}(OH)_2D_3$. Both effects tend to lower serum calcium concentration. Calcitonin may also be important in the control of hypercalcemia, especially in animals. In mammals other than man in whom it can be measured, secretion of calcitonin is directly related to the serum calcium concentration. Hypercalcemia results in increased calcitonin release from the thyroid gland. Calcitonin lowers both the serum calcium and serum phosphorus concentrations primarily by an inhibition of bone resorption. Thus it seems to play an important protective role against hypercalcemia in these animals. Arnaud et al. hypothesize that in mammals calcitonin acts as a potent rapid-acting factor suppressing oscillations in the serum calcium *above* physiologic levels and that PTH acts as the major controlling factor of serum calcium *below* physiologic levels. In normal man, however, there is little or no evidence that calcitonin functions as a physiologic hormone responsible for regulation of serum calcium homeostasis.

The infusion of PTH into experimental animals or man results in hypercalcemia, hypophosphatemia, and phosphaturia. These effects are the result of three mechanisms:

1. Direct action on bone leading to increased bone resorption
2. Increased calcium absorption from the intestine
3. Decreased tubular resorption of phosphate (TRP) and increased tubular resorption of calcium by the kidney

In addition, PTH effects on the kidney lead to increased excretion of potassium, bicarbonate, amino acids, and, under some circumstances, sodium, while decreasing the excretion of magnesium, ammonia, and titratable acid. Vitamin D and its metabolites are not necessary for the renal tubular effects of PTH. However, vitamin D is necessary for the action of PTH on bone. Vitamin D also appears to have a direct action on bone resorption as well. Finally a major action of vitamin D is intestinal absorption of calcium. Recent studies suggest that $1,25\text{-}(OH)_2D_3$ plays

Fig. 38-27. Comparison of amino acid sequences of porcine, bovine, ovine, salmon, and human calcitonin. Solid bars indicate sequence positions homologous among all five molecules; cross-hatched bars indicate salmon and human calcitonin. [*From J. T. Potts, Jr., et al., in R. V. Talmage and P. L. Munson (eds.), "Calcium Parathyroid Hormone and the Calcitonins," Proceedings of Fourth Parathyroid Conference, Excerpta Medica, Amsterdam, 1972.*]

the most important direct role in intestinal absorption of calcium; PTH may act by regulating the formation of this metabolite.

The action of PTH on kidney and bone has been demonstrated to be mediated through the adenyl cyclase system. PTH stimulates adenyl cyclase activity and raises cyclic 3′,5′-AMP levels in bone and kidney. Urinary excretion of cyclic AMP is a potentially useful test of parathyroid function.

Primary Hyperparathyroidism

PATHOLOGY. Parathyroid. Primary hyperparathyroidism may be due to a parathyroid adenoma, hyperplasia of the parathyroid glands, carcinoma, or a nonparathyroid tumor which is producing a parathyroidlike substance. The symptoms are similar whatever the actual cause of the primary hyperparathyroidism. It is also possible for a patient with secondary hyperparathyroidism due to renal, bone, or metabolic disease to develop hypercalcemia without any therapy. This condition is referred to as *tertiary hyperparathyroidism.*

The relative frequency of entities producing primary hyperparathyroidism is shown in Table 38-2. Several points are important to note. Primary chief cell hyperplasia was described by Cope in 1958. Hence studies which include data prior to 1958 can be misleading. Cope, for example, who reviewed his data of 343 cases at the Massachusetts General Hospital in 1966, carefully pointed out that in his

last 100 cases 25 percent had hyperplasia. This apparent trend toward increased primary chief cell hyperplasia is thought by some to be due in part to the fact that primary hyperparathyroidism is diagnosed and operated upon at a much earlier stage today. Several other trends are also evident. Water-clear hyperplasia is rarely diagnosed any longer. Multiple adenomas are less frequently diagnosed at the present time. More often these are thought to be part of chief cell hyperplasia. Finally, the incidence of carcinoma of the parathyroid glands is misleading when one is looking only at the larger referral series. As described below, carcinoma of the parathyroid makes up 1 percent or less of all cases of primary hyperparathyroidism.

It is apparent that the frequency of adenoma versus hyperplasia varies greatly in these series. Goldman, for example, reported that single glands were diseased in 92 percent of his patients, while Paloyan and coworkers found that almost two-thirds of all patients had more than one gland involved.

These discrepancies undoubtedly are due to several factors—the operative approach, the pathologic interpretation of the glands, and the incidence of patients with familial hyperparathyroidism or multiple endocrine adenomatosis in each series.

Paloyan performs a subtotal parathyroidectomy so that each gland can be examined. Others remove only any enlarged gland which is encountered. When a single enlarged gland is sent to a pathologist it is most likely to be called an adenoma. However, there is no uniform agreement among pathologists at this time as to what constitutes an adenoma and what represents chief cell hyperplasia. The condition described by the classical definition of an adenoma—an enlarged gland with a rim of normal tissue—is found in cases of hyperplasia as well. Roth and other pathologists state that they can not tell the difference between hyperplasia and adenoma from looking at only one gland. The greatest differences of opinion relate to what constitutes *mild* hyperplasia. Some pathologists feel that normal-sized or mildly enlarged glands are hyperplastic if they do not contain enough fat. Others do not feel that these glands are abnormal. Knowledge of the normal development of parathyroid glands is imperative.

From birth through three months of age, mean weight of the four parathyroid glands is 5 to 9 mg. There is then an almost linear increase in mean total parathyroid gland weight until the third to fourth decades, when it levels off at a mean of 117.6 mg for males and 131.3 mg for females. These changes in weight are accompanied by changes in histology of the gland. In children the gland is composed of fairly uniform sheets and cords of chief cells. The stroma has little or no mature fat cells, and oxyphil cells are absent. At puberty some mature fat cells appear. These increase in number through the remainder of life, and in older persons they may occupy 60 to 70 percent of the gland volume. Obese individuals have larger numbers of fat cells than one would expect for their age. Oxyphil cells also appear at puberty and show an increase with age. Chief cells and water-clear cells are thought to actively secrete PTH. Oxyphil cells are thought of as inactive but have been shown to be rich in mitochondria.

Thus to evaluate whether or not a parathyroid gland is normal, one must evaluate its size and weight, the number of chief cells, and the amount of fat which it contains in relation to the age of the individual.

The major problem for both the surgeon and the pathologist is to differentiate an adenoma caused by chief cell hyperplasia or single gland disease from multiglandular disease of the parathyroids. Perhaps the ultimate proof that a lesion is an adenoma is the lack of recurrence of hyperparathyroidism after its removal.

Adenomas. The sine qua non for the diagnosis of a parathyroid adenoma has been the presence of an enlarged parathyroid gland with a rim or fragment of normal parathyroid which is being compressed by the adenoma. This is shown in Fig. 38-29. Another previously demanded criterion was the presence of a normal or atrophic parathyroid elsewhere. However, since we now know that parathyroid adenomas and hyperplasias can coexist and that hyperplasia occasionally appears to spare one gland, this criterion no longer seems to be absolute. Furthermore, as Black has shown, chief cell hyperplasia may give the appearance of compression of normal gland beneath the capsule. Thus an

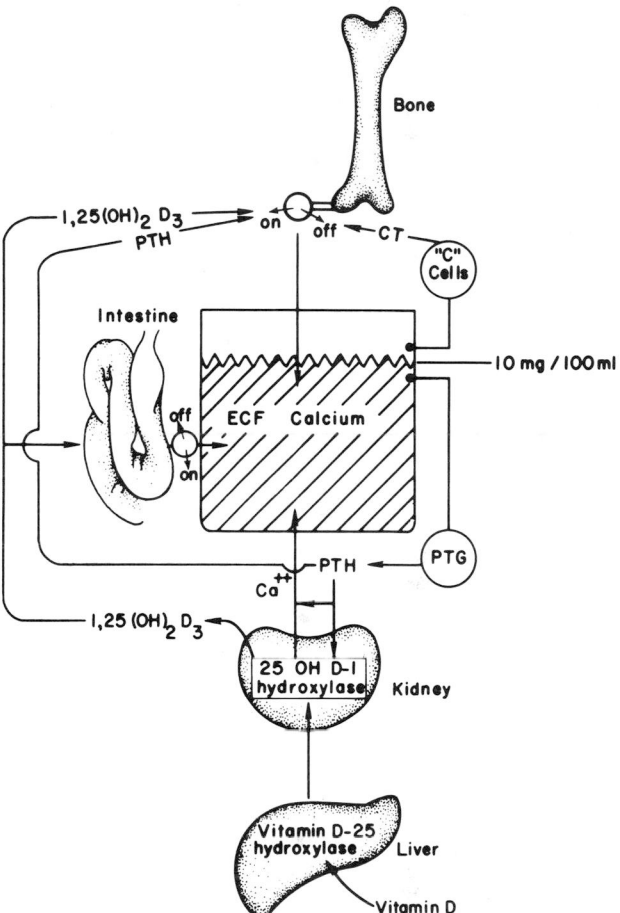

Fig. 38-28. Mechanism of calcium homeostasis. *Hypocalcemia* results in increased parathyroid hormone (PTH) secretion from the parathyroid glands (PTG). PTH acts directly on bone and on the kidney. PTH also results in an increase in the formation of 1,25-$(OH)_2D_3$ by the kidney, which acts on bone and promotes intestinal absorption of calcium as well. Each of these effects tends to raise the serum calcium concentration toward normal. *Hypercalcemia* results in a decrease in PTH secretion, a lesser production of 1,25-$(OH)_2D_3$, and an increase in calcitonin (CT) secretion. Calcitonin inhibits bone resorption and is important in animals other than human beings. These changes tend to decrease serum calcium levels to normal. (*From H. F. DeLuca, Ann Intern Med, 85:367, 1976.*)

adenoma should be diagnosed only when one or, rarely, two glands are enlarged, the others being normal in size and on histologic section. Any gland larger than 40 to 60 mg should be suspected of being abnormal.

Grossly adenomas are usually reddish brown, though they may be yellow-brown, particularly in older people. At times they may be very difficult to distinguish grossly from thyroid tissue, particularly when imbedded in the thyroid. They are usually soft and smooth, and the surface is very vascular, bleeding easily when rubbed. They are generally not adherent to the surrounding structures. On occasion they contain cysts, hemorrhage, or areas of calcification. Areas of necrosis are sometimes seen. The location of the tumors is given later under Operative Technique.

Table 38-2. RELATIVE FREQUENCY (PERCENT) OF ENTITIES PRODUCING HYPERPARATHYROIDISM

Author	Date	Institution	Adenomas		Hyperplasia		Carcinoma	Unknown	Total cases
			1 adenoma	2 or more adenomas	Chief cell*	Water-clear			
Norris	1947	Collected	94	6	...	...	...	...	322
Cope et al	1958	Massachusetts General Hosp.	76	5	4	7	4	4	206
Black, B. M.	1961	Mayo Clinic	92	2.5	...	5	0.5	...	385
Cope	1966	Massachusetts General Hosp.	77	4	11	4	4	...	343
Straus and Paloyan	1969	University of Chicago	46	7	10	9	4	...	58
Haff et al	1970	Washington Univ., St. Louis	41	Mixed adenoma and hyperplasia—24	49	...	...	11	47
Goldman et al	1971	Univ. of Calif., San Francisco	92	4	3	...	<1	...	300
Paloyan et al	1973	University of Chicago	33	Multiglandular disease—65‡			2	...	84
Wang et al	1975	Massachusetts General Hosp.	81	2	12	2	3	...	525

*Since chief cell hyperplasia was described by Cope in 1958, there are no reports of this entity before that date.
†Of his last 100 cases, 25% had chief cell hyperplasia.
‡More than one gland involved with disease.

Fig. 38-29. Normal parathyroid compared with a chief cell adenoma. *A.* Photomicrograph of a normal parathyroid, below, adjacent to the thyroid gland, shown above. Note the abundant fat present in the normal gland. (×75.) *B.* Photomicrograph of a chief cell adenoma compressing the normal parathyroid beneath the capsule. The adenoma is the large mass shown to the right. The open spaces are blood vessels. The normal gland is the small rounded object shown to the left. The open spaces are fat cells. (×35.) *C.* Photomicrograph of a parathyroid adenoma shown below with the capsule separating it from the rim of normal parathyroid shown above. Note the fat in the normal parathyroid and the absence of fat cells in the adenoma. (×150.)

Microscopically chief cell adenomas are composed of closely packed small cells which resemble the cells of the normal parathyroid except that they are more tightly packed and there is little or no fat seen. The chief cells are of two types: the light cells, which are rich in glycogen and are thought to be inactive, and the dark cells, which are poor in glycogen and rich in secretory granules with a prominent Golgi apparatus and endoplasmic reticulum. The dark cells are thought to be the main source of PTH. A glandular pattern is sometimes seen with small uniform acini whose lumina are empty or filled with acidophilic colloid. These adenomas sometimes resemble fetal adenomas of the thyroid gland.

The water-clear, or *wasserhellen,* adenomas have large vacuolated cells with clear cytoplasm arranged in a uniform pattern. In the rare oxyphil adenomas the cells have a pink cytoplasm. Undoubtedly oxyphil cells can also secrete PTH, since adenomas of oxyphil cells, while rare, can also cause hyperparathyroidism.

The chief importance for the histologic differentiation into adenoma or hyperplasia has to do with what operation is performed. If one adopts the policy of exploring all four parathyroids in each case, the microscopic differentiation between adenoma and hyperplasia in a single gland becomes far less important.

Carcinoma. Carcinoma of the parathyroid is rare. Many cases which have originally been thought to represent carcinoma have been discarded on review, since benign adenomas can sometimes have cells with bizarre nuclear

patterns. Black reviewed the literature to the end of 1953 and found only 20 cases which he thought were acceptable, using the diagnostic criteria of hyperfunction with local tissue invasion or metastases. Rapaport et al. in 1960 collected 8 more cases to make a total of 28 and found records of only 8 with visceral metastases. Holmes et al. found 46 cases of hyperfunctioning parathyroid cancer and 4 cases of apparent nonfunctioning cancer when they reviewed the literature in 1969. In these 50 patients, 85 percent presented with hypercalcemia. Bone disease was present in 73 percent, a palpable neck mass in 52 percent, and renal disease in 32 percent. Thus, hypercalcemia and a palpable neck mass should alert one to the possibility of parathyroid carcinoma. Cervical metastases were found in 32 percent and distant metastases (liver, lung, bone, pancreas, and adrenal) in 21 percent. Cervical recurrences following surgery occurred in 65 percent of patients. Typically hypercalcemia recurred several months after surgery in many instances and was the first sign of recurrent tumor.

It is apparent that a diagnosis of malignant disease cannot be made by the histologic features of the tumor, a situation which also obtains in pheochromocytoma. Very wild-looking tumors may pursue a completely benign course. The reverse is also true, as exemplified by a case reported by Rapaport et al. in which histology of the original tumor appeared to be that of an adenoma but in which the tumor recurred 22 months after operation, with pulmonary metastases confirmed at autopsy. Capsular infiltration is a particularly inadequate sign of malignancy, since this is often seen in benign adenomas and even the neoplastic cells can occur within blood vessels in benign tumors. The only completely acceptable criteria for malignancy are recurrence of the tumor following removal, distant metastases, or invasion of adjacent structures. Some carcinomas can be identified grossly because they are attached to adjacent tissues by a thick fibrous capsule which gives the gland a whitish hue. Fifty percent of reported cases were adherent to or invading into adjacent structures at the time of surgery.

Though some individuals die because of tumor growth and spread, more commonly morbidity and mortality are related to the complications related to the persistent and progressive hypercalcemia, which is very difficult to control chronically. Schantz and Castleman collected 70 cases of proved parathyroid carcinoma in their review in 1973.

Hyperplasia. Although it is stated in most older texts that the most common type of hyperplasia is the water-clear cell type, this no longer is true. Almost all incidences of hyperplasia in our experience have been of the chief cell type. Primary chief cell hyperplasia cannot be differentiated by light microscopy from the chief cell hyperplasia which is always present in secondary hyperparathyroidism, although there are ultrastructural differences. It seems likely that a number of instances previously thought to be multiple adenomas because of their predominant chief cell structure were in fact instances of chief cell hyperplasia.

Grossly the glands with *water-clear cell hyperplasia* show diffuse enlargement and are usually unequal in size. The color is a striking chocolate brown, and the parathyroids are often very large. They tend to be lobulated and irregular in shape, with pseudopods extending from the surface, in contrast to the generally smooth contour of adenomas or glands with chief cell hyperplasia.

Histologically they are composed of large clear cells arranged in a relatively uniform alveolar or acinary pattern.

The glands may be very large in water-clear hyperplasia, the total weight of all four glands ranging up to as much as 70 Gm. Their huge size plus the striking color and characteristic appearance makes them very easy to recognize.

Primary Chief Cell Hyperplasia. This condition was first described by Cope et al. in 1958. The incidence of this disease entity is becoming more common as it is being recognized that many cases thought to be multiple parathyroid adenomas are in reality chief cell hyperplasia. This disease entity is almost invariably encountered when surgical treatment of the parathyroid glands is carried out in patients with familial hyperparathyroidism and in patients with multiple endocrinopathies.

It may sometimes be extremely difficult to differentiate chief cell hyperplasia from the typical parathyroid adenoma if only one gland is examined (Fig. 38-30). Roth and other pathologists believe that grossly and histologically a single hyperplastic gland is *indistinguishable* from an adenomatous gland. Classically, one expects each of the glands to be enlarged; however, it is known that the size of glands may be very asymmetrical, and one or more glands may appear relatively normal. It is frequently stated in the literature that the presence of a single normal parathyroid is diagnostic of a parathyroid adenoma, since hyperplasia always involves all four glands. This is not true, however, because we and others have seen instances in which one gland was the site of a very clear-cut parathyroid adenoma, while two other glands showed hyperplasia and the fourth appeared normal. It is true, however, that the presence of a single normal parathyroid *usually* indicates that the enlarged gland represents an adenoma rather than hyperplasia.

Microscopically the cells appear identical to those of an adenoma (Fig. 38-31). There is a greater tendency, however, toward the appearance of many fibrous tissue septa, and the gland appears to have been composed of a number of nodules coalescing with each other. There are very few fatty cells, which are common in the normal gland. Although parathyroid adenomas are characterized by having a well-developed capsule and by the presence of an area where normal gland is compressed by the developing adenoma, a very similar appearance can be seen in chief cell hyperplasia. It is said that this develops when a hyperplastic area of the gland grows out into the surrounding fat and appears to be compressed normal gland or when one portion of the gland is simply separated from the rest of the gland by a well-developed septum in the course of development of nodular hyperplasia. It has been stressed

Fig. 38-30. Comparison of adenoma and hyperplasia. *A.* Detail of a chief cell adenoma adjacent to the capsule. Note the solid grouping of uniform chief cells, with absence of fat. (×200.) *B.* Chief cell hyperplasia. The cellular morphology is similar to that of the adenoma. Note the small focus of water-clear cells in the left central portion of the field. (×150.) *C.* Chief cell hyperplasia. Note the cords and small acinary groupings. (×200.)

Fig. 38-31. Comparison of water-clear and chief cell hyperplasia. *A.* Chief cell hyperplasia. The cells are small and uniform, with finely granular and transparent cytoplasm. (×400.) *B.* Water-clear cell hyperplasia. The tubules are well formed, and the cells are large and clear. (×200.) *C.* Water-clear cell hyperplasia: a higher magnification of *B.* (×400.) (*Photograph courtesy Saul Kay.*)

by Black and Utley that the final diagnosis of adenoma or chief cell hyperplasia can sometimes be made only several years after the original operation and will occasionally have to be based on the subsequent course of the patient rather than on any absolute histologic diagnostic criteria. They feel, however, that the presence of a single normal or atrophic parathyroid is diagnostic of an adenoma, but, as mentioned above, this is not necessarily so. Although the differential diagnosis between chief cell hyperplasia and parathyroid adenoma is an extremely interesting and somewhat important one, its importance is diminished by inspecting all four parathyroid glands at operation for hyperparathyroidism, which is our practice. The difficulty in distinguishing between the two does add considerable impetus to the adoption of this practice.

While the chief cell is the predominant cell type in chief cell adenomas and in chief cell hyperplasia, the other cell types are frequently represented. In chief cell adenomas a mixture of water-clear and oxyphil cells is frequently seen, while in chief cell hyperplasia the oxyphil cell is the second most frequent type of cell seen. Occasional water-clear cells may also be seen, however, and multinucleated giant cells are occasionally present.

Hypercalcemia Associated with Nonparathyroid Malignancies. It has long been known that on occasion neoplasms can produce a variety of polypeptide hormones identical or biologically similar to ACTH, melanocyte-stimulating hormone (MSH), follicle-stimulating hormone (FSH), antidiuretic hormone (ADH), insulin, and chorionic gonadotropin. It is now clear that some tumors also produce PTH-like circulating hormones or prostaglandin E_2, each of which may result in hypercalcemia.

The most common cause of hypercalcemia of malignant disease is osseous metastasis. Normal radiographs do not always exclude the presence of bone metastases. Bachman and Sproul in a series of autopsies found that only one-half of the cases with histologically documented skeletal metastases had radiographic findings indicative of metastatic cancer. One hopes that the use of bone scans will help to diagnose some of these occult metastases.

Recent studies have shown that one cause of hypercalcemia associated with malignant tumor without apparent skeletal metastases is the synthesis and secretion of a PTH-like substance by the malignant tumor. This clinical syndrome of a nonparathyroid tumor associated with hypercalcemia and hypophosphatemia has been referred to as *pseudohyperparathyroidism,* or *ectopic hyperparathyroidism.*

Goldberg et al. in 1964 found reports in the literature of 18 patients with hypercalcemia associated with neoplasm in the absence of bony metastases. They explored the neck of one patient with hypercalcemia and found only atrophic parathyroid glands. At autopsy this was confirmed, and the patient was found to have a hypernephroma. Bioassays of both the tumor and a pulmonary metastasis revealed a substance indistinguishable from PTH. The removal of tumors of this type has been associated many times with a prompt fall of serum calcium concentration to normal as demonstrated in the case of hypernephroma reported by Plimpton and Gelhorn. The reappearance of metastases may be associated with an elevation of the serum calcium level.

Although a number of tumors can produce ectopic hyperparathyroidism, the most common are squamous cell and small cell carcinomas of the lung, and hypernephromus. Other less common neoplasms include hepatoma and cancer of the ovary, stomach, pancreas, parotid gland, and colon.

The hypercalcemia of breast cancer has not been demonstrated to be due to ectopic hyperparathyroidism. It has been postulated, but never proved, that a *vitamin D–like sterol* is responsible for hypercalcemia in patients with this tumor in whom no bone metastases are found. Most cases of hypercalcemia of breast cancer do not have hypophosphatemia. When a low serum phosphorus level is present with hypercalcemia, one should consider the possibility of a coincident parathyroid adenoma. Samaan and coworkers recently reported that 35 percent of patients with different types of malignancy and hypercalcemia were subsequently proved to have *coexistent primary hyperparathyroidism.* Thus, this diagnostic possibility should not be excluded because the patient has a malignancy.

In addition to ectopic PTH secretion, several other humoral factors have been associated with the hypercalcemia of some malignancies. Tashjian has demonstrated that *prostaglandin E$_2$* infused into animals causes hypercalcemia. In a rat sarcoma system, he has demonstrated that metabolites of prostaglandin increased before hypercalcemia occurred, and thus appeared to be the cause of the increased serum calcium concentrations. Seyberth and associates demonstrated that patients with various malignant tumors and hypercalcemia had elevated concentrations of metabolites of prostaglandins. In several of their patients, treatment with aspirin or indomethacin (which decreases prostaglandin production) resulted in a lowering of the serum calcium levels to normal. Prostaglandin E$_2$ appears to result in hypercalcemia by stimulating bone resorption. These data suggest that prostaglandin E$_2$ may be an important causative agent for the hypercalcemia of malignancy in some patients.

Finally, Mundy and associates have described a factor which they call *osteoclast activating factor* (O.A.F.). This is produced by myeloma and other lymphoid cells and causes bone resorption. It may be the cause of hypercalcemia in some patients with hematologic diseases. A great deal of investigation is continuing in the area of hypercalcemia in neoplastic diseases.

The differentiation of ectopic hyperparathyroidism from primary hyperparathyroidism due to parathyroid gland disease is often difficult. Lafferty suggests that ectopic hyperparathyroidism is more likely when the serum calcium concentration exceeds 14 mg/100 ml, when serum alkaline phosphatase activity is increased, when osteitis fibrosa is absent, and when there is a significant degree of anemia. Conversely, primary hyperparathyroidism is more likely with a long-standing history of repeated renal lithiasis or with radiographic evidence of osteitis fibrosa.

Skeletal Changes. The full-blown skeletal changes of hyperparathyroidism are rarely seen today, since most patients are operated upon at an early stage before such changes have had a chance to develop. The principal skeletal pathologic changes consist of osteitis fibrosa cystica, cysts, giant cell tumors, and osteoporosis.

When the skeletal changes become sufficiently pronounced, they can be detected by conventional x-rays, although it seems likely from recent studies that the skeleton is always involved even when the x-rays reveal no detectable change. The skeletal changes can be most easily demonstrated in the long bones, spine, skull, pelvis, hands, clavicles, and jaw.

Osteitis fibrosa cystica is brought about by an overactivity of the osteoclasts which causes resorption of cortical and cancellous bone. The bone is replaced by vascularized cellular connective tissue in which there may be abortive bone formation. As the condition progresses, there is an increasing loss of mature bone with the development of multiple soft cystic areas. These changes are histologically entirely similar to those seen in fibrous dysplasia.

The bone cysts may be small or large, single or multiple; they may have a solitary cavity or be multilocular. They contain brownish fluid or mucoid material and are lined by connective tissue. The giant cell tumors, or brown tumors, are frequently partly cystic and are brown or reddish on section. Histologically they consist of numerous large osteoclasts in a cellular stroma. They are commonly found in the long bones and in the jaw, where they may constitute the presenting symptom. In the jaw the lesion consists of an area of bony destruction with an expansion of the cortical contour of the bone which may erupt beneath the gum and is often confused with an epulis. Hemorrhage into the area may occur, followed by the appearance of multinucleated giant cells and organization of the area with the formation of delicate trabeculae of osteoid tissue. The brown tumors therefore grossly and microscopically resemble the osteoclastomas which are not of parathyroid origin.

CLINICAL MANIFESTATIONS. Incidence. Hyperparathyroidism very rarely occurs under the age of puberty, although a very few instances of neonatal familial hyperparathyroidism have been reported. Of those cases which were not familial the youngest to have been diagnosed and operated upon was a boy aged three. The most common age is between thirty and sixty. Those having prominent skeletal lesions tend to develop the disease at an earlier age, usually between ten and thirty, while those with renal calculi alone are much more common in the thirty-to-sixty age group. Hyperparathyroidism in children and in neonates is discussed in later sections.

Hyperparathyroidism is more common in women than in men, in a ratio of 2:1.

The incidence of skeletal and renal changes in patients with hyperparathyroidism reported prior to 1965 is shown in Table 38-3. It is interesting to note that in the earlier series of Norris, in 1947, when all cases of hyperparathyroidism that had been reported to that date were collected, only 5 percent of the patients had renal changes without skeletal changes while 61 percent of the patients had skeletal changes only. In a more recent series of published cases up to 1965 it was found that 59 percent had renal changes only while 16 percent had skeletal changes only. Thus 78 percent of all cases had renal involvement, and 35 percent of all cases had skeletal involvement. Ninety-four percent had renal or skeletal involvement, while only six percent had neither renal nor skeletal involvement.

Since 1965 marked changes in our understanding of the incidence and symptomatology of primary hyperparathyroidism have occurred. These changes are due largely to the fact that primary hyperparathyroidism is being diagnosed in many relatively asymptomatic individuals who are found to have an elevated serum calcium level on routine multiphasic serum chemistry screening programs which are being carried out in most hospitals today. The efficacy and importance of this screening can be seen in the

Table 38-3. INCIDENCE OF RENAL AND OSSEOUS INVOLVEMENT
IN EARLIER COLLECTED SERIES

	Skeletal only	Skeletal plus renal	Renal only	No skeletal or renal	Total
Norris (1947)	191 (61%)	101 (32%)	17 (5%)	5 (2%)	314
1953–1965	83 (16%)	99 (19%)	308 (59%)	31 (6%)	521

	Percent
Renal only	59
Renal and osseous	19
Total renal involvement	78
Osseous only	16
Renal and osseous	19
Total osseous involvement	35
Renal *or* osseous involvement	94
Neither renal nor osseous involvement	6

following study conducted by a Mayo Clinic team. Automated screening of serum calcium resulted in the diagnosis of as many new cases of proved primary hyperparathyroidism in residents of the Rochester, Minnesota, area during a 1½-year period (1974–1975) as had occurred during the previous 9½ years. The minimum incidence of primary hyperparathyroidism in this geographical area now exceeds 0.1 percent of the population. In other series, an incidence of primary hyperparathyroidism as high as 0.5 percent of the general population has been noted. Many patients in this recent group have only mild symptoms.

The incidence of hyperparathyroidism in patients who have had urinary calcium stones is variously estimated to be between 2.5 and 15 percent. The mean figure is somewhere around 5 percent.

Symptoms. When the disease of hyperparathyroidism was first recognized, it was thought to be a skeletal disease, and it was not until 7 years after the first patient had been operated upon that it was recognized that the disease could occur only with renal manifestations. Now the disease is seldom seen with marked skeletal involvement, because it is usually recognized long before this occurs. Today the disease is sometimes diagnosed and treated in the absence of either skeletal or renal involvement. With the widespread application of multiphasic blood screening such as the SMA-12, more asymptomatic or mildly symptomatic (anxiety, depression, abdominal pain) patients are being discovered. In the Rochester, Minnesota, group, 49 percent had one or more of these serious complications possibly attributable to primary hyperparathyroidism: hypertension, 35 percent; renal stone disease, 25 percent; psychiatric symptoms, 21 percent; decreased renal function, 16 percent, and subperiosteal bone resorption, 5 percent.

Though some patients with only mild disease will be diagnosed as having primary hyperparathyroidism, it is important that the symptoms and signs of the classical clinical presentation of this disease be recognized.

The clues which first led to the diagnosis in 343 cases of the Massachusetts General Hospital series are shown in Table 38-4. As expected, renal stones head the list, with bone disease a distant second. Peptic ulcer and pancreatitis

form a small but important minority, while 20 of the patients complained only of fatigue, mental disturbance, or central nervous system signs. Familial cases are sometimes diagnosed after diagnosis of one member of the family and subsequent screening of the kindred, and some cases are discovered through routine laboratory tests. A careful study of patients who are recurrent renal stone formers will establish the diagnosis of hyperparathyroidism in 2.5 to 12.5 percent of the cases. The causes of the symptomatology of hyperparathyroidism are shown in Table 38-5.

Symptoms Related to Hypercalcemia. Since virtually all the patients with hyperparathyroidism demonstrate hypercalcemia, it is not surprising that many of the symptoms and signs relate directly to this alteration.

Renal Damage. The renal damage which occurs in this disease is a consequence both of the hypercalcemia and of the increased secretion of PTH. Hypersecretion of PTH results in increased excretion of phosphate and in relative urinary alkalosis, both of which may predispose to calcium precipitation. Renal damage can occur, however, as a consequence of hypercalcemia from any source. The length

Table 38-4. CLUES TO THE DIAGNOSIS OF HYPERPARATHYROIDISM IN THE FIRST 343 CASES AT THE MASSACHUSETTS GENERAL HOSPITAL

Clue	*Number of cases*
Renal stones	195
Bone disease	80
Peptic ulcer	27
Fatigue	10
Pancreatitis	9
Central nervous system signs	7
Hypertension	6
Mental disturbance	3
Multiple endocrine abnormalities	3
No symptoms (routine laboratory test)	2
Lump in neck	1

SOURCE: From Cope, 1966.

Table 38-5. CAUSES OF SYMPTOMS OF HYPERPARATHYROIDISM

Cause	*Symptoms and signs*
Hypercalcemia	Renal damage
	Mental: Depression, fatigue, delerium, coma
	Muscle: General muscle weakness, and hypotonia, walking with cane, hypoactive reflexes
	Gastrointestinal: Peptic ulcer, constipation, gastric disturbance, loss of appetite, pancreatitis (?)
	Eye changes: Band keratitis, calcium in palpebral fissure
	Ectopic calcification
	Hypercalcemic crisis: Profound muscle weakness, nausea and vomiting, lethargy and drowsiness, confusion, bone pain, abdominal pain, thirst, polyuria, constipation, coma, hypertension, fever, ECG changes, short Q-T interval and nearly absent ST segment, azotemia with increased PO_4, hypokalemia
Increased urinary calcium	Polyuria, polydipsia, and hypokalemia
Hypomagnesemia	Paresthesias, hyperreflexia
Direct action of PTH	Demineralization of the skeleton due to bone resorption: Bone pain, cysts, known tumors, fractures
	Renal damage
	Peptic ulcer (?)
	Pancreatitis (?)
Renal damage	Hypertension
	Renal stones, nephrocalcinosis

of time required for hypercalcemia to produce renal damage depends upon the degree of hypercalcemia. The renal damage is worse in those patients who have skeletal changes demonstrable by x-ray and in those patients with nephrocalcinosis than in those with renal calculi alone.

Mental Changes. Patients with hypercalcemia frequently complain of mental symptoms consisting of depression, fatigue, listlessness, and occasionally confusion. The patients may be irritable or regressive, subject to crying spells, or simply depressed. In some individuals with severe hypercalcemia, delirium and even coma may occur, while others tolerate the same increase in serum calcium with few symptoms. Correction of the hyperparathyroidism and hypercalcemia results in a reversion to a normal mental state in many but not all persons.

Muscle Weakness. Generalized muscle weakness is common in hypercalcemia and is associated with hypotonia and hyporeflexia. The joints are often extremely flexible, and the weakness may lead to difficulty in walking.

Gastrointestinal Symptoms. Some type of gastric disturbance, loss of appetite, nausea, vomiting, and/or constipation are common in hypercalcemia. There is a questionable increased incidence of peptic ulcer in patients with hyperparathyroidism, and this is probably related to the hypercalcemia, though direct action of PTH on the gastric mucosa may contribute as well. Duodenal ulcer is much more common than gastric ulcer. This entity will be discussed more fully below, under Peptic Ulcer. Pancreatitis may also be related to hypercalcemia, though direct action of PTH on the pancreatic cells may be more likely. Calcium salts are apt to be precipitated out in the pancreatic ducts in the presence of hypercalcemia, and this may contribute to pancreatitis. The increased calcium in the pancreatic juice which is present in hypercalcemia is said to accelerate the conversion of trypsinogen to trypsin, and the activated

enzyme may lead to pancreatitis. Pancreatitis has been noted only rarely in patients with hypercalcemia from causes other than hyperparathyroidism.

Eye Changes. Band keratitis and calcium in the palpebral fissure are seen in hypercalcemia of various causes.

Ectopic Calcification. Ectopic calcification occasionally occurs in primary hyperparathyroidism, almost always in association with gross pathologic changes in bone. It occurs in only a small percentage of patients and is not a particularly valuable sign of this disease.

Hypercalcemic Crisis. This is sometimes called "acute hyperparathyroidism," but since the signs and symptoms are common to those of hypercalcemia of any origin (for example, breast cancer), it seems best to refer to it as *acute hypercalcemic crisis.* In hyperparathyroidism this usually does not eventuate until the serum calcium level rises to 16 mg/100 ml or above. It is equally common in males and females, while hyperparathyroidism itself is twice as common in females as in males. It is much more apt to occur in the presence of severe renal damage, and at least 90 percent of the patients have some degree of renal failure. The patient has usually had a long-standing history of skeletal or renal involvement with more recent symptoms of loss of appetite and weight, nausea and vomiting, constipation, thirst and polyuria, and generalized muscular weakness. The relative frequency of the symptoms is shown in Table 38-6.

If the early symptoms of hypercalcemic crisis are ignored, they may progress to the more serious ones of lethargy and drowsiness, confusion, severe muscular weakness, prostration, and coma. The electrocardiographic changes of hypercalcemia do not usually make their appearance until the calcium levels are quite high, but they may be seen in hypercalcemic crisis and consist of a short Q-T interval and a nearly absent ST segment. Fever and tachycardia may be present. Occasionally there is an association of acute pancreatitis with hypercalcemic crisis. A rising blood urea nitrogen (BUN) level is common.

In hypercalcemic crisis due to hyperparathyroidism there is a very high incidence of renal failure, nearly 90 percent, and a much greater percentage of the patients have bone involvement, nephrocalcinosis, and peptic ulcer than is true for hyperparathyroidism in general.

Hypercalcemic crisis was reviewed by Lemann and Donatelli, who collected 42 cases in 1964. Some of their findings are reproduced in Table 38-6. Payne and Fitchett collected 70 cases in 1965 in a review of the literature, and 16 cases were added by MacCleod and Holloway in 1967, including one of their own. In these 86 cases the age range was from five to seventy-seven years with a median age of fifty-one. The greatest incidence occurred in the three decades between forty and sixty-nine. Forty percent of the patients survived, and sixty percent died. Of the 45 patients undergoing operation, 33 survived. All patients not operated upon died, except for one who was a five-year-old child in whom the crisis was precipitated by injections of PTH. The crisis abated when the PTH was stopped. Since 1967, the medical treatment of hypercalcemia has improved greatly. Now parathyroidectomy as initial treatment is rarely indicated, even when primary hyperparathyroidism is diagnosed as the probable cause of the hypercalcemic crisis. The drug regimens which are useful in treating acute hypercalcemia will be discussed later in this chapter.

Symptoms Related to Increased Urinary Calcium. The symptoms of hyperparathyroidism due to increased urinary calcium loss are those of polyuria and polydipsia. The hypokalemia which is sometimes seen in this disease, particularly in cases of hypercalcemic crisis, is apparently due to excessive potassium loss in the urine, which may be related to the increased urinary calcium loss. Hypomag-

nesemia is sometimes seen in hyperparathyroidism. This appears to be more common when the serum calcium level is very high or when the intake of magnesium has been poor because of gastrointestinal disturbances. When present this may give rise to paresthesias or hyperreflexia.

Symptoms Related to Direct Action of PTH. *Demineralization of the Skeleton.* As a consequence of the increased bone resorption brought about by PTH the skeleton becomes demineralized and bone cysts, brown tumors, and pathologic fractures eventuate. The recent microradiographic studies of Jowsey and others have suggested that some degree of pathologic change in bone is present in virtually every case of hyperparathyroidism. This is frequently not detectable by the usual clinical means, however, and in many instances the patients do not have symptoms relating to the bones. The presence of demonstrable bony changes relates more to the severity of the disease, the duration of the disease, and the size of the adenoma than to anything else.

Cysts and tumors of the jaw are sometimes the presenting complaint. This appears as a swelling of the gum very similar to that seen with epulis and usually brings the patient to the dentist. Vague pains in the back, hip, or shoulder, often thought by the patient to be arthritis, are sometimes present, while in other instances the pain may be quite marked and related to a particular bone which is tender on palpation. In the more long-standing cases the stature may decrease, and a bowing of the spine may be apparent to the patient and his relatives. Sometimes local swelling of the bone or deformity of the bone may be noted. A pathologic fracture may be the first bone symptom of which the patient complains.

Renal Damage. Some of the renal damage in hyperparathyroidism is due to a direct effect of the PTH on the proximal tubular cell and is not related specifically to hypercalcemia. The most common symptom of renal

Table 38-6. SYMPTOMS AND SIGNS IN 42 PATIENTS WITH HYPERCALCEMIC CRISIS DUE TO HYPERPARATHYROIDISM

Symptoms	Percent of cases	Signs	Percent of cases
Muscular weakness	80	Hypotonia	44
Nausea and vomiting	80	Neck mass	42
Weight loss	65	Hypertension	35
Fatigue	65	Dehydration	31
Lethargy and drowsiness	65	Tachycardia	26
Confusion	57	Fever	22
Bone pain	55	Abdominal tenderness and distension	15
Abdominal pain	48	Band keratopathy	9
Polyuria	40	Tracheal deviation	4
Constipation	37		
Coma	26		
Polydipsia	24		
Renal colic	22		
Neck swelling	9		
Dysphagia and neck pain	4		

SOURCE: From Lemann and Donatelli, 1964.

damage is the presence of renal calculi. Symptoms related to the renal calculi are by far the most common presenting complaint of patients with hyperparathyroidism.

Peptic Ulcer (Questionable). Though it was originally thought that patients with primary hyperparathyroidism have a greatly increased incidence of peptic ulcers, this view has been recently challenged. It is well known that patients with severe ulcer diatheses and hyperparathyroidism are often markedly improved by parathyroidectomy and the return of their serum calcium level to normal. In these patients after parathyroidectomy, the gastric acid secretion falls dramatically and the ulcer may even heal. However, many of these individuals later prove to have a Zollinger-Ellison syndrome (gastrinoma) and their hyperparathyroidism is part of the multiple endocrine neoplasia, type 1, syndrome. If this group of Zollinger-Ellison patients with hypercalcemia is eliminated from consideration, it is difficult to demonstrate a truly increased incidence of peptic ulcer disease in patients with primary hyperparathyroidism.

Recent studies have demonstrated that calcium infusion with production of hypercalcemia results in (1) a small rise of basal gastric acid secretion in about one-half of normal patients, (2) a mean rise in basal acid in duodenal ulcer patients to about 30 percent of maximal Histalog (betazole) stimulation, and (3) a rise of gastric acid output in Zollinger-Ellison patients equal to that produced by maximal stimulation by Histalog. These changes are accompanied by a statistically significant increase in circulating gastrin in duodenal ulcer patients and a marked increase of serum gastrin in most patients with Zollinger-Ellison syndrome. To date, in fact, calcium infusion with measurement of gastrin and gastric acid output is one of the most reliable provocative tests for Zollinger-Ellison tumors. Calcium ion appears to play a significant role in release of gastrin and other polypeptide hormones.

Patients with parathyroid disease and hypercalcemia without the Zollinger-Ellison syndrome have been demonstrated to have mildly elevated serum gastrin concentrations which return to normal after parathyroidectomy and restoration of normocalcemia. On the other hand, it has *not* been conclusively demonstrated that patients with primary hyperparathyroidism have statistically increased acid secretion as a group. We and others have noted basal achlorhydria, in fact, in some of these patients. Some patients with severe chronic renal disease and secondary hyperparathyroidism have been shown to have increased serum gastrin levels as well, which appears to be due to the fact that the kidneys play an essential role in the metabolism of gastrin.

The incidence of peptic ulcer and hyperparathyroidism is probably somewhere around 10 percent. Incidences as high as this have been reported in some groups of normal population, and doubt has been expressed as to whether there really is an association between peptic ulcer and hyperparathyroidism.

Our view is that it is uncertain that hyperparathyroidism directly causes duodenal ulcer disease. In individuals who have an ulcer diathesis, however, this may be worsened by the hypercalcemia of parathyroid disease. Because of the fact that 20 percent of patients with Zollinger-Ellison syndrome have associated parathyroid gland abnormalities, this islet cell tumor must be ruled out in any hypercalcemic individual with an ulcer by obtaining a serum gastrin determination and making other appropriate tests. In both routine duodenal ulcers and those associated with the Zollinger-Ellison syndrome parathyroidectomy may be of benefit if primary hyperparathyroidism is present.

Pancreatitis (Questionable). The relation between hyperparathyroidism and pancreatitis seems less secure. If the relationship does exist, it is probably due either to the effect of hypercalcemia or of PTH on the precipitation of calcium salts from the pancreatic juice. Although calcification of the pancreas occurs in some patients with hyperparathyroidism, it is frequently only an incidental finding. Pyrah et al. suggest that the cases in which pancreatitis and hyperparathyroidism are associated fall into six groups:

1. One or more attacks of acute pancreatitis following which the diagnosis of hyperparathyroidism is established. With removal of the parathyroid adenoma there are no further attacks of pancreatitis, and the serum amylase returns to normal.
2. Acute pancreatitis occurring as a complication of operation for the removal of a parathyroid adenoma.
3. Acute pancreatitis occurring as a complication of some unrelated operation in a patient with hyperparathyroidism, as, for example, the removal of a renal calculus.
4. Acute pancreatitis occurring as a complication of acute hypercalcemic crisis due to hyperparathyroidism.
5. Chronic pancreatitis manifested by recurring attacks of abdominal pain and associated with pancreatic calculi in patients with hyperparathyroidism.
6. Development of hypercalcemia (tertiary hyperparathyroidism) in a patient with known chronic pancreatitis, steatorrhea, and secondary hyperparathyroidism.

One might add to the list above hereditary pancreatitis associated with familial hyperparathyroidism.

Paloyan et al. have demonstrated an increase in circulating glucagon in acute pancreatitis and postulate that this may be the cause of the hypocalcemia which frequently accompanies this disease. Glucagon infusions result in hypocalcemia in experimental animals and increased serum PTH in man. Thus it is possible but not yet proved that secondary hyperparathyroidism may occur in patients with pancreatitis and that hypercalcemia in these individuals may represent a form of tertiary hyperparathyroidism.

The incidence of pancreatitis associated with hyperparathyroidism has not been definitely established, but in the series reported by Mixter et al. it was about 7 percent. In carcinoma of the parathyroid and familial hyperparathyroidism the incidence of pancreatitis is somewhat higher.

Symptoms Related to Renal Damage. *Hypertension.* Although the association of hypertension with hyperparathyroidism is well known, it is likely that in almost all instances this is due to the renal damage brought about by the disease and not to any direct effect of PTH itself. In the study by Hellstrom et al. of 95 cases of hyperparathyroidism submitted to parathyroidectomy and followed afterward, 44 patients had a normal blood pressure preoperatively, but in 15 of them hypertension developed postoperatively. Forty-seven patients had preoperative hypertension, and in seventeen of these the blood pressure returned to normal following parathyroidectomy, but it remained elevated in thirty. Furthermore, the patients in whom the blood pressure became normal after the operation with a single exception had had only moderate hypertension preoperatively. In many patients with only moderate hypertension preoperatively increasing hypertension had developed in the postoperative period. There was a lower incidence of hypertension in those patients with renal stones or nephrocalcinosis only than in those patients who had bone changes preoperatively. There was a good correlation, however, between the degree of hypertension and the degree of renal damage. Hypertension and cardiac failure are important causes of death in hyperparathyroidism.

A role of serum renin in the pathogenesis of the hypertension of primary hyperparathyroidism has also been postulated.

Renal Stones, Nephrocalcinosis. Renal colic, of course, is frequently seen in patients with hyperparathyroidism. Nephrocalcinosis does not usually produce any symptoms. Hellstrom and Ivemark showed that the incidence of renal damage was high in patients with gross skeletal changes and in patients with nephrocalcinosis but much less so in patients with renal calculi alone. In a high proportion of patients there is an inability to concentrate the urine normally which is probably due to a direct physiologic action of PTH rather than to anatomic calcification.

Nephrocalcinosis refers to diffuse calcification of the kidney as demonstrated roentgenographically. These collections of radiopaque material are usually in the renal pyramids and the medulla. There are many other conditions which can give rise to nephrocalcinosis besides hyperparathyroidism. If one examines all cases of nephrocalcinosis, only about 20 percent or less are due to hyperparathyroidism, the next most common causes being tubular acidosis, medullary sponge kidney, and idiopathic causes. The patient with nephrocalcinosis usually has renal stones as well, so that renal colic or hematuria is a frequent complaint. Lumbar pain or aching may also be present. The nephrocalcinosis does not improve after removal of the parathyroid adenoma.

Other Manifestations. In some patients hyperparathyroidism manifests itself primarily in terms of mental changes consisting of depression, irritability, forgetfulness, confusion, and vague complaints. The diagnosis under these circumstances may be very difficult to make unless one is thinking of it.

Patients with nonparathyroid PTH-secreting tumors may have any of the usual symptoms of hyperparathyroidism due to parathyroid disease. Since these tumors are frequently malignant, they may have symptoms relating to the local or distant spread of the disease. Because of the rather frequent, and sometimes fatal, elevation of serum calcium levels in patients with malignant tumors with or without bone metastases, it is extremely important to follow blood calcium and phosphorous levels in such patients.

Physical Findings. Some of the physical findings and signs were discussed in the preceding section on symptoms, and others will be mentioned under diagnostic tests.

Hypotonia of the muscles can be detected in many patients. This hypotonicity leads to flexibility of the limbs, which develops to a marked degree in some patients. A decreased excitability of the neuromuscular apparatus can be demonstrated by nerve stimulation. It takes about twice as much galvanic current to stimulate the nerve in hyperparathyroidism as in the normal state. There is a decrease in auditory sensitivity, and some patients are quite deaf. The eyes show calcium phosphate crystals in the palpebral fissure, and band keratitis can be demonstrated with a slit lamp. There is sometimes difficulty in focusing the eyes. Metastatic calcification is rare, in contrast to the situation seen in secondary hyperparathyroidism and vitamin D intoxication, where it is quite common.

It is seldom possible to palpate the parathyroid adenoma, except in patients with hypercalcemic crisis, where the adenoma is usually very large and can be felt in 40 percent of the cases. Apart from this circumstance, the adenoma can be felt in only about 5 percent of the cases or less. A large parathyroid malignant tumor may be palpable.

When bone disease is present, it may be possible to detect bending of the long bones, vertebral deformity, a decrease in stature, fractures of the bones, or the appearance of an epulislike growth in the lower gum.

DIAGNOSTIC FINDINGS. Calcium, Phosphate, Alkaline Phosphatase, and Chloride Measurements. The diagnosis of hyperparathyroidism in most cases rests upon biochemical determinations. The most important of these is the *serum calcium level.* The normal range varies in different laboratories depending on the techniques used. In our own the normal range is generally considered to be between 8.5 and 10.5 mg/100 ml. There are some cases of early hyperparathyroidism in which the calcium level may be very close to the normal range or may fluctuate from the normal levels to slightly elevated levels. Although some writers have stated that a single normal value, if obtained with proper techniques, makes a diagnosis of hyperparathyroidism unlikely, others, including McGeown and Morrison, have suggested that measurements should be repeated over a period of months or even years in borderline cases. Our own experience would fit with this latter concept. Hodgkinson and Edwards found that large fluctuations in serum calcium levels were not common but that variations of 1 to 2 mg/100 ml did occur occasionally over a period of weeks or months and that this could be misleading when the calcium level was only slightly elevated. They felt that such patients should be reexamined at intervals of several weeks until the diagnosis is firmly established (Fig. 38-32). Bartter and associates have popularized the concept of "normocalcemic hyperparathyroidism" in which renal stones occur in patients with borderline or totally normal serum calcium concentrations. Whether or not these patients have *primary* hyperparathyroidism has not yet been resolved.

An additional reason for following the blood calcium and phosphorous levels in patients who are suspected of having or who have once had the disease is shown in Fig. 38-54. This patient had three separate episodes of hypercalcemia and hypophosphatemia covering a 9-year period. The interim values were normal. While this was originally

A

B

Fig. 38-32. Serum calcium and phosphate values. *A.* Serum calcium and phosphate values before and after excision of a parathyroid adenoma. The serum calcium values were only minimally elevated. The tubular resorption of phosphate (TRP) was depressed preoperatively and rose following the operation. Postoperatively the serum calcium level fell to the point where the patient required a brief intravenous treatment with calcium. *B.* Urine calcium and phosphate values of the same patient. During 1952, the patient was on a low-calcium diet, and urinary calcium excretion was never very high. In April-May, 1958, the patient was on a 350-mg calcium diet for the first half of the period charted and a 137-mg calcium diet for the second half. Apart from two determinations in the early part of this period the calcium excretion was never strikingly increased. The calcium excretion did not change appreciably following excision of the parathyroid adenoma, while the phosphate excretion decreased strikingly.

thought to represent the formation and removal of three separate parathyroid adenomas, it is much more likely that this represents unrecognized parathyroid hyperplasia treated by removal of a single grossly enlarged gland on each occasion.

In order to interpret the calcium level adequately it is helpful to get a serum total protein determination and electrophoretic pattern. Since it is only the *ionized calcium* which is physiologically active, it has been suggested that measurements of the ionized calcium would be more valuable than measurements of the total calcium. Ionized calcium recently has become much easier to measure because of the new electrode systems which are available. Ionized calcium concentrations are occasionally elevated in primary hyperparathyroidism when total calcium is normal. It is of course essential to rule out other possible causes for the elevated serum calcium level before concluding that the patient has hyperparathyroidism.

The *serum phosphate level* is a somewhat less reliable guide to the diagnosis of hyperparathyroidism. A normal

value does not rule out primary hyperparathyroidism. Low values may occur in several other diseases, e.g., idiopathic hypercalcinuria and renal calculi. Furthermore, it may rise considerably in patients with hyperparathyroidism in whom significant renal damage has developed. Nonetheless it remains a valuable test and in light of our experience should be taken cognizance of when it consistently runs below 3 mg/100 ml, especially if occasional values are below 2.5 mg/100 ml.

The *serum alkaline phosphatase level* usually is elevated in hyperparathyroidism only when there is x-ray evidence of bone disease, and it is frequently elevated in other conditions. This has not proved to be a helpful diagnostic test in our experience.

Wills and McGowan have reported that the *plasma chloride level* is elevated in patients with primary hyperparathyroidism. It was found to be higher than 102 mEq/L in all except 1 of 33 patients with hyperparathyroidism, whereas it was less than 102 mEq/L in all 28 patients with hypercalcemia due to other causes. Pyrah et al. surveyed their cases and confirmed this finding. Rasmussen has also noted an elevated chloride level in hyperparathyroidism but finds that it may be elevated in vitamin D intoxication and osteomalacia as well, although not as consistently so. It is probably a valuable additional test to determine.

Determination of *arterial pH* also may be helpful diagnostically. Barzel has demonstrated that patients with primary hyperparathyroidism have a hyperchloremic metabolic acidosis while those with hypoparathyroidism are slightly alkalotic. Hypercalcemia of nonparathyroid hormone origin results in suppression of the parathyroid glands and a mildly alkaline arterial blood pH.

Urinary Hydroxyproline and Calcium Excretion. The *urinary hydroxyproline level* is a rough measurement of collagen breakdown, and since most collagen is contained in bone, it is to that extent a measure of bone destruction. It is elevated in hyperparathyroidism but also in many other conditions. In general urinary hydroxyproline determinations have not been of much value in establishing the diagnosis of hyperparathyroidism. An elevated *urinary calcium level* may suggest a diagnosis of hyperparathyroidism but is certainly not diagnostic of it. Furthermore hypercalcinuria is not a constant finding in this disease, as may be seen in Fig. 38-32.

Tubular Resorption of Phosphate (TRP) Tests. Since one of the actions of PTH is to decrease the tubular absorption of phosphate, the TRP would seem to be a valuable determination to help establish the diagnosis of hyperparathyroidism. However, the test has not proved to be as useful as it was hoped. The formula for computing the TRP is

$$1 - \frac{UP \times SC}{SP \times UC} \times 100 = TRP$$

where UP = urinary phosphorus
　　　 SC = serum creatinine
　　　 SP = serum phosphorus
　　　 UC = urinary creatinine

The normal value is somewhere between 85 and 95 percent, whereas with hyperparathyroidism it falls to 35 to 85 percent. Although the TRP test is certainly not without error, it provides additional information which may help to confirm the diagnosis. Following a successful parathyroidectomy and correction of the hyperparathyroid state, the urinary excretion of phosphate decreases markedly and the tubular resorption of phosphate rises to normal (Fig. 38-32).

Cortisone Administration (Dent Test). The oral administration of 150 mg of cortisone daily for 10 days was found to reduce the serum calcium to normal levels in patients with hypercalcemia due to vitamin D intoxication or sarcoidosis, whereas the hypercalcemia of hyperparathyroidism was often unaltered. Cortisone also usually reduces the hypercalcemia due to carcinomatosis, multiple myeloma, and the milk-alkali syndrome, but this is not always the case, and hypercalcemia has been reduced in several patients with hyperparathyroidism. Although the test has its limitations, it may be of some value in differentiating between the various causes of hypercalcemia.

Strott and Nugent have emphasized that none of these indirect measurements of PTH hypersecretion is diagnostic of hyperparathyroidism with an accuracy greater than 88 percent.

Bone Biopsy. Even when no gross bone changes are discernible on x-ray, changes in the bone in hyperparathyroidism can almost always be detected by microradiography. These changes have been discussed in an earlier section. A bone biopsy specimen can be taken out of the iliac crest under local anesthesia and subjected to microradiography (Fig. 38-33). The findings, while not completely diagnostic, may help to establish the diagnosis when added to all other evidence.

Bone Densitometry. Cameron and Sorenson recently introduced photon beam scanning of bone. This method appears to be very promising and is being tested in a number of centers. Changes in bone density as small as 5 to 10 percent may be measured by this means. In hyperparathyroidism there is frequently a loss of bone density which returns to normal after parathyroidectomy.

Plasma PTH Measurements. Measurement of PTH in serum by radioimmunoassay has been one of the most exciting recent developments. It has been shown to be the most important and valuable tool for the diagnosis of hyperparathyroidism, since it provides a direct measurement of the hormone whose hypersecretion causes the disease.

Measurement of PTH by immunoassay has proved to be more difficult than that of most other polypeptides. Very useful assays have been developed in the laboratories of Arnaud, Potts, Reiss, and others. However, some results appear to differ from one laboratory to another. The reasons for these difficulties are now beginning to emerge. Circulating PTH in hyperparathyroidism is heterogeneous. At least three distinct fragments of PTH ranging in molecular weight from 4,000 to 10,000 have been identified. The various antisera used in detecting PTH at this time have been produced by injection of bovine or porcine PTH into animals. Different antisera detect different parts of the PTH molecule and hence measure all or only some of these PTH fragments; hence the differences in results. The

Fig. 38-33. Microradiography of a bone biopsy specimen in a patient with hyperparathyroidism due to an adenoma. The area labeled *S* is a static bone surface, the one labeled *F* is a bone formation area, and those labeled *R* are bone resorption areas. There is markedly increased bone resorption. (*Courtesy R. W. Bright.*)

Fig. 38-34. Relationships between serum calcium and serum iPTH values in normal subjects (●) and patients with proved primary hyperparathyroidism (○) using GP IM (anti-C) and CH 14M (anti-N) antisera. (*From C. D. Arnaud et al., Am J Med, 56:785, 1974.*)

amino (NH$_2$) terminal end of the PTH molecule (Fig. 38-24) confers the biological effects of parathyroid hormone. Antisera directed against this part of the molecule measure physiological secretion rates. However, it has been clearly demonstrated that antisera directed against the carboxyl fragments (C-terminal) of PTH are much better for diagnosing clinical primary hyperparathyroidism. In Fig. 38-34 the same blood samples from normal and hyperparathyroid patients were examined; the anti-C assay discriminates very well between normal subjects and patients with hyperparathyroidism, while in the anti-N assay there is a considerable overlap between these groups. Thus, C-terminal assays for PTH are excellent and aid greatly in our ability to diagnose primary hyperparathyroidism.

Another example of the value of direct measurement of plasma PTH is demonstrated in Fig. 38-35. Reiss and Canterbury were able to differentiate normal patients from those with primary hyperparathyroidism and others with hypoparathyroidism. In secondary hyperparathyroidism the serum PTH level is also elevated. In chronic renal failure, for example, circulating PTH varies inversely with the creatinine clearance; as renal function deteriorates, the PTH level rises. Therefore, one must know the serum calcium and serum PTH concentrations and correlate these two parameters. Elevation of both the serum calcium and PTH levels is diagnostic of primary or tertiary hyperparathyroidism or less commonly of ectopic secretion of PTH from a tumor; all other causes of hypercalcemia are associated with low PTH concentrations.

Other tests utilizing the measurement of PTH may have diagnostic applicability in primary hyperparathyroidism.

Calcium, EDTA, and sodium bicarbonate infusions have been utilized to try to differentiate adenomas from hyperplasia preoperatively. An adenoma, it was thought, would be autonomous and not change its PTH secretion when the serum calcium was raised or lowered. Since hyperplasia is

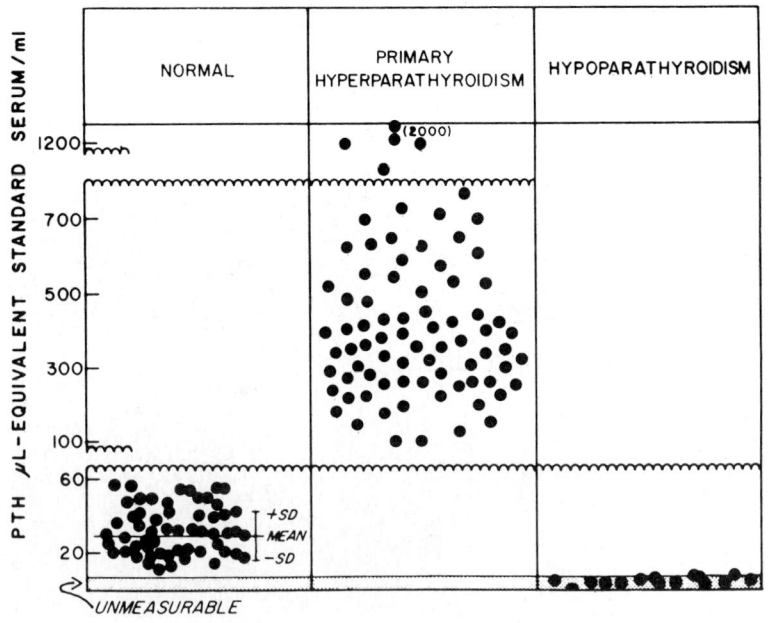

Fig. 38-35. Results of radioimmunoassy of PTH in normal subjects and patients with primary hyperparathyroidism and with hypoparathyroidism. The units of PTH in this figure relate the potency of test serums to that of an arbitrarily selected hyperparathyroid serum. In the hyperparathyroid group, the presence of disease was confirmed surgically in all instances. (*From E. Reiss and J. M. Canterbury, Am J Med, 50:679, 1971.*)

not a neoplasm, these parathyroid glands would be responsive to serum calcium changes, it was postulated. Unfortunately this differentiation has not proved to be as complete as originally thought. Many adenomas have been demonstrated to resemble hyperplasia in secreting more PTH when the calcium ion is lowered and in suppressing their secretion of PTH when serum calcium is elevated. Thus, it is difficult to differentiate adenomas from hyperplasia physiologically as well as histologically.

Roentgenography of Bones. The x-ray appearance of advanced hyperparathyroidism is characteristic. At times this will greatly aid in the diagnosis of primary hyperparathyroidism. X-rays of the skull may show the typical "moth-eaten" ground-glass skull of hyperparathyroidism, with either a thin or thick calvarium (Fig. 38-36). In osteogenesis imperfecta there is a thin, well-calcified skull, while in Paget's disease there is an overgrown fuzzy skull. In multiple myeloma there are many sharp, punched-out areas, and metastatic cancer, especially that from the breast, can give a similar appearance (Fig. 38-37). X-rays of the lamina dura are best taken on dental film. The lamina dura is frequently absent in patients with hyperparathyroidism, but it may also be absent in other conditions and present in hyperparathyroidism. Furthermore it is of no use in the edentulous patient. It is no longer regarded as a very valuable sign.

Chest x-rays may show multiple bony lesions (Fig. 38-38*A*). X-rays of the clavicle are sometimes helpful, since in hyperparathyroidism there is often a marked absorption of the distal third of the clavicle (Fig. 38-38*B*). The spine may show marked decalcification and wedging of the vertebrae (Fig. 38-39). The jaws are a favorite place for the development of bone tumors (Fig. 38-40*A*), and these may be seen in the metacarpals, metatarsals, and the ends of the long bones (Fig. 38-40*B*). On x-ray a bone tumor and a cyst look the same.

X-rays of the hands are particularly useful in diagnosis of hyperparathyroidism, since they may show the characteristic subperiosteal bone resorption in the middle and terminal phalanges of the fingers (Fig. 38-41). An x-ray of the pelvis may show the presence of metastatic malignancy, the decalcification of primary hyperparathyroidism, bone cysts in the femur, pathologic fractures, or other changes.

X-rays of the bones may show soft tissue calcification, which is much more common in secondary than in primary hyperparathyroidism and still more common in vitamin D intoxication (Fig. 38-42). It is uncommon in primary hyperparathyroidism.

In summary, in primary and secondary hyperparathyroidism bone changes may occur. Subperiosteal bone resorption of the middle and distal phalanges of the fingers and resorption of the distal end of the clavicle are the most common and useful diagnostic abnormalities noted. To be useful, hand films must be taken on high-grade industrial-type film. These abnormalities are pathognomonic of PTH excess.

Roentgenography of the Kidneys. A plain film of the kidneys will sometimes show renal calculi or nephrocalcinosis. Staghorn calculi may be present, as shown in Fig.

Fig. 38-36. Skull x-rays in patients with hyperparathyroidism. *A.* Lateral view of the skull in a child with secondary hyperparathyroidism due to renal failure. Note the punched-out lesions resembling multiple myeloma. *B.* Secondary hyperparathyroidism. Note the moth-eaten appearance of the skull *C.* Primary hyperparathyroidism. Note the similarity between this and the patients with secondary hyperparathyroidism.

Fig. 38-37. Skull x-rays in patients with hypercalcemia but without hyperparathyroidism. *A.* This patient was admitted in a semicomatose state with a serum calcium level of 21 mg/100 ml. The x-ray shows multiple small metastatic lesions. A bone biopsy showed metastatic squamous cell carcinoma. The metastases were ultimately demonstrated to have come from a squamous cell carcinoma of the esophagus. *B.* Skull metastases in carcinoma of the breast. *C.* Paget's disease. This disease is most often confused with hyperparathyroidism because of the bone changes. It can on occasion produce hypercalcemia.

38-39. An example of nephrocalcinosis is shown in Fig. 38-43. An intravenous pyelogram may confirm this diagnosis and may also give some idea as to the functional capacity of the kidney and the presence or absence of hydronephrosis. An intravenous pyelogram may also reveal the presence of a renal neoplasm producing the hypercalcemia, just as x-ray of the chest may reveal metastatic cancer or the presence of a mediastinal parathyroid adenoma.

Localization of Hyperfunctioning Parathyroid Glands. A parathyroid adenoma is rarely palpable preoperatively. In about 5 percent of patients the hyperfunctioning gland is found in the chest, not in the neck at all. Furthermore, occasionally an enlarged parathyroid gland is difficult even for the experienced neck surgeon to find. For these reasons many attempts have been made to localize the enlarged overactive parathyroid gland or glands before operation. Until recently, most attempts have met with little success.

A chest x-ray will occasionally be helpful by demonstrating a mass in the mediastinum. On very rare occasions a barium swallow may demonstrate an indentation due to an enlarged parathyroid gland. Thermography, ultrasonography, and computerized tomography have had only limited trials and limited success thus far. An isotope scan is an attractive idea; however, the use of ^{75}selenium methionine scanning, either preoperatively or at the operating table, has not proved to be of great value. We have recently visualized an oxyphil adenoma using a gallium scan. Further tests are necessary to determine if this technique has greater applicability; however, other procedures utilizing PTH secretion have been of considerable help in some instances. Reiss has described the *parathyroid squeeze test.* Massage of the side of the neck harboring the parathyroid adenoma results in a rise of the peripheral serum PTH level. Massage of normal glands results in no change in serum PTH. In the presence of hyperplastic glands, a rise in peripheral serum PTH follows the massage of both sides of the neck, since this disease is bilateral. Catheterization of the large veins of the neck and mediastinum (the jugulars, innominate, and superior vena cava) with sampling of blood for serum PTH from various sites has successfully localized the site of abnormal parathyroid glands in some patients (Fig. 38-44). The serum PTH level will be highest at the site of drainage from a hyperfunctioning gland or glands.

A recent modification of this technique is more efficacious. The small veins draining the thyroid gland, as well as the large veins of the neck and chest, are catheterized and sampled for serum PTH (Fig. 38-45). An elevation of serum PTH on one side of the neck signifies an adenoma, while a gradient of PTH on neck veins of both sides signifies the presence of bilateral hyperplasia. Often this examination has been performed with arteriography (Fig. 38-46). Arteriography by itself may be helpful in localizing an enlarged parathyroid gland, since in some cases a vascular tumor blush is seen, or one inferior thyroid artery may be deviated from its normal position or may be larger than the other. However, several cases of hemiplegia and quadriplegia have followed highly selective inferior thyroid artery arteriography, presumably because of spinal

Fig. 38-38. Typical lesions of hyperparathyroidism. *A.* Multiple lesions of bones demonstrated on chest x-ray. *B.* Resorption of the outer end of the clavicle in a patient with secondary hyperparathyroidism. Similar lesions are seen in the primary disease.

cord injury. Hence, this technique should be used with the utmost of caution and only after careful consideration of alternative approaches.

Most endocrinologists and surgeons agree that venous catheterization studies should *not* be done routinely on all patients before their initial parathyroid exploration. We reserve the use of this procedure for patients who have already had a negative neck exploration performed by a highly competent parathyroid surgeon. Its greatest potential usefulness is in the preoperative localization of a mediastinal parathyroid adenoma.

SPECIAL CONSIDERATIONS. Familial Hyperparathyroidism. The familial occurrence of hyperparathyroidism was first reported by Goldman and Smyth in 1936, who described a case in siblings. All told, at least 15 families have been reported in which more than one member has had hyperparathyroidism. A distinction is made between these families and those in whom tumors of multiple endocrine glands have been encountered. This latter group of familial endocrinopathy is discussed later. Although the mode of inheritance has not been completely worked out, it has been assumed to be one of autosomal dominance with incomplete penetrance.

In familial hyperparathyroidism there is a high incidence of involvement of the glands by chief cell hyperplasia, and recurrence of the disease after operation is quite common. In the four cases reported by Stevens et al., however, the parathyroid involvement was by solitary adenomas in each case.

Familial hyperparathyroidism has been reported in conjunction with pancreatitis and with peptic ulceration. In one of the most convincing instances of familial hyperparathyroidism Cutler et al. reported a kindred involving 11 patients with hyperparathyroidism in two families in which the mothers were sisters and the fathers were brothers. Hillman et al. reported neonatal familial hyperpara-

thyroidism in two siblings born to first-cousin parents. One child died and the second was successfully operated upon.

Several of the cases of familial hyperparathyroidism have been asymptomatic, having been discovered when the members of an affected family were screened for hyper-

Fig. 38-39. X-ray of the abdomen of a patient with primary hyperparathyroidism, showing bilateral staghorn calculi with severe osteoporosis, scoliosis, and splenic calcification. The patient's chemical studies are shown in Fig. 38-32. A parathyroid adenoma was removed, and this was followed by chemical and clinical improvement.

Fig. 38-40. Bone cysts and tumors in hyperparathyroidism. *A.* Bone cyst of the lower jaw. *B.* Cysts of long bones.

calcemia. In a recent study, in 11 percent of families, other members were proved to have primary hyperparathyroidism as well. Thus, a familial occurrence of primary hyperparathyroidism may be more common than previously considered.

Hyperparathyroidism in Children. Hyperparathyroidism is a rare occurrence before puberty. A few such cases have been reported, including the neonates mentioned above under Familial Hyperparathyroidism.

Fig. 38-41. X-rays of the fingers in primary and secondary hyperparathyroidism. *A.* Secondary hyperparathyroidism. Note the intense subperiosteal resorption of bone. This usually is most prominent on the radial side of the middle and distal phalanges of the index and middle fingers. *B.* Primary hyperparathyroidism. Many patients with primary hyperparathyroidism have normal hand films with conventional radiographic techniques. With *fine-detail* radiography, subtle cases of subperiosteal bone resorption can be recognized. Mild subperiosteal bone resorption (arrows) of middle phalanx in a patient with a parathyroid adenoma. (*From H. K. Genant et al., Radiology, 109:513, 1973.*)

A   *B*

Fig. 38-42. X-ray studies of a child with chronic renal failure and vitamin D intoxication. Note the severe ectopic calcification in the soft tissues. *A.* The olecranon bursa and subcutaneous tissues of the left arm. *B.* The subcutaneous tissues and muscle of the lower leg. *C.* The patellar bursa and the popliteal and tibial arteries.

Apart from the neonates, there have been over 35 cases of hyperparathyroidism in children reported in the literature. The ages have ranged from three to sixteen. Over 80 percent of them have been between the ages of ten and fourteen, the disease being very rare before the age of ten.

The symptoms are the same as those recorded in the adult, including those referable to severe bone involvement. Duodenal ulcer has been reported, and joint abnormalities have occurred in 17 percent of the patients. Blindness was recorded in one case.

Acute hypercalcemic crisis has been recorded in neonates and in older children, with serum calcium values of over 20 mg/100 ml. The serum calcium values in children have generally been somewhat higher than those seen in adults.

Pregnancy. Fertility does not seem to be greatly depressed in hyperparathyroidism, and labor and delivery are not influenced by it. The birth weight of infants born to mothers who are suffering from hyperparathyroidism is low, being less than 3,000 Gm in 50 percent of the cases. There is a high frequency of stillbirth, neonatal death, and neonatal tetany.

In 1962, Ludwig reviewed the literature and described the clinical course of 40 gestations of the 21 women who were recognized at that time as having primary hyperparathyroidism while they were pregnant. Serious fetal complications were noted in half these pregnancies. Stillbirths, spontaneous abortions, and neonatal deaths occurred in 31 percent and neonatal tetany in 19 percent of these instances. Delmonico and associates, analyzing the 15 pregnancies of 13 hyperparathyroid women reported since that time who were not operated upon, found that 80 percent of these gestations were complicated. Spontaneous abortions and neonatal deaths occurred in 27 percent; 55 percent of the newborns suffered significant hypocalcemia soon after birth.

It appears that the diagnosis of primary hyperparathyroidism associated with pregnancy is rarely made. It is not uncommon, in fact, for this disease to be recognized in the mother only retrospectively following the appearance of hypocalcemia in the newborn infant. A potential difficulty in diagnosis may be the fact that during the normal pregnancy a physiologic decrease of maternal serum calcium concentration occurs. Thus, even borderline high values of serum calcium obtained from the pregnant woman should be considered to be of utmost significance.

Perhaps of even greater importance is the apparent lack of awareness by many physicians that hyperparathyroidism can occur during pregnancy. Serial calcium concentrations should be performed as part of all routine prenatal care. The diagnosis of maternal primary hyperparathyroidism can be made with virtual certainty when an elevated serum

Fig. 38-43. X-ray of the abdomen showing nephrocalcinosis. While this change sometimes occurs in hyperparathyroidism, it is not diagnostic of this condition.

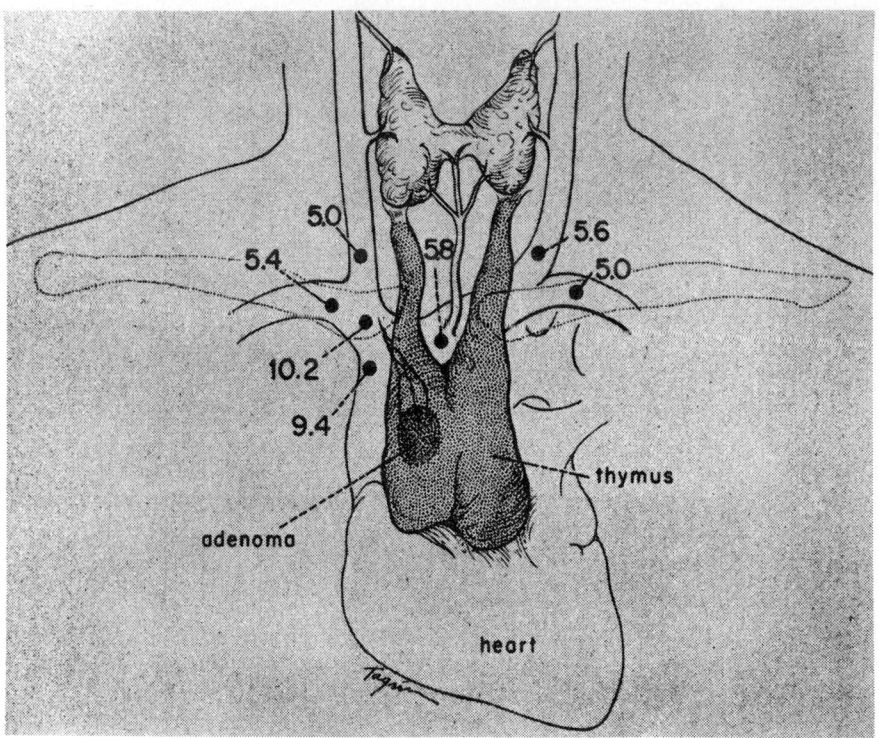

Fig. 38-45. Plasma PTH concentrations in samples obtained at different points in the circulation. Veins are jugular (*J*), innominate (*I*), superior vena cava (*SVC*), superior thyroid veins (*STV*), and inferior thyroid veins (*ITV*). Samples also were obtained from the medial and lateral branches of the right inferior thyroid vein (*ITV—M* and *ITV—L*). Sites of sampling are indicated by • ; adjacent numbers indicate PTH concentration in mµg/ml. These data indicate an adenoma of the right lower parathyroid gland. Elevated PTH concentrations in samples from both sides of the neck indicate parathyroid hyperplasia. (*From J. T. Potts, Jr., et al., Am J Med, 50:639, 1971.*)

Fig. 38-44. Radioimmunoassay of blood samples obtained during venous catheterization of a patient with primary hyperparathyroidism. Localized increases in PTH values are demonstrated in the right innominate vein and the superior vena cava (10.2 and 9.4 mµg/ml). At operation a parathyroid adenoma was found in the thymus gland. Its venous drainage was to the right innominate vein and corresponded to the area of elevated PTH levels. (*From R. E. Reitz et al., N Engl J Med, 281:349, 1969.*)

calcium concentration is accompanied at the same time by an elevated serum parathyroid hormone level, since ectopic hyperparathyroidism from occult malignancy is rare in these young women.

When maternal hyperparathyroidism is diagnosed during pregnancy, Kaplan feels that the proper therapy is parathyroidectomy. Optimally, the operation should be performed during the second trimester of pregnancy, since accidental abortion is lessened during this period. Furthermore, with correction of the hypercalcemic state at this early time, parathyroid development of the fetus can proceed normally.

The results in patients so managed are far better than those reported without operation. Only one instance of neonatal death and another of neonatal hypocalcemia occurred. Several recent studies clarify the pathophysiology of maternal hyperparathyroidism. It is known that both ionized and total calcium concentrations are somewhat higher in the fetal than in the maternal circulation. While calcium ion moves freely across the placenta, serum parathyroid hormone cannot cross from mother to fetus. In primary hyperparathyroidism the elevated serum calcium concentration of the mother results in an increased circulating serum calcium concentration in the fetus. Hypercalcemia, per se, may result in toxicity to the fetus. Also, it clearly causes suppression of fetal parathyroid function and possibly of parathyroid development. Following birth, hypocalcemia will occur in the newborn if its own parathyroid function is inadequate. Parathyroidectomy performed during early pregnancy permits restoration of the normal fetal calcium homeostasis and thus should eliminate this neonatal hypocalcemia.

Although there are other conditions which can cause neonatal tetany besides hyperparathyroidism in the mother, it is extremely important to obtain serum calcium and phosphorus values on mothers of children with neonatal tetany. This may be the best way that this cause for neonatal tetany can be definitely established, since the calcium level in neonates with tetany will be low whatever the cause of the tetany.

Multiple Endocrinopathies, Type 1 (M.E.A.-Type 1). The glands involved in the *endocrine polyglandular syndrome, Type 1,* are the parathyroid, the pancreatic islets, and the pituitary. The syndrome tends to fall into four main classifications: pancreatic beta cell tumor, hypercalcemia, Zollinger-Ellison syndrome, and acromegaly.

Pancreatic Beta Cell Tumor. In these patients the pancreatic beta cell tumor secretes insulin and produces symptoms of hypoglycemia. Rarely, there also may be parathyroid hyperfunction which gives rise to an elevated serum calcium level and renal stones in some patients. The pituitary tumors are usually asymptomatic. Peptic ulcers are sometimes present in these patients, but they are rarely intractable and usually respond to the resection of the parathyroid and pancreatic tumors. For those which do not respond, the usual ulcer treatment is effective. Total gastrectomy is not required.

Hypercalcemia. The second most frequent group is composed of patients in whom the pancreatic and pituitary tumors are nonfunctioning and who have symptoms of mild hyperparathyroidism. Peptic ulcers also occur in this group of patients and, again, respond readily to the usual therapy.

Zollinger-Ellison Syndrome. The third group of patients have pancreatic islet cell tumors of the non-beta cell type and are associated with severe enteritis or intractable ulceration. The parathyroid tumors are usually functionally hyperactive when present, and the patients may have hypercalcemia, whereas the pituitary tumors generally tend to be asymptomatic. Total gastrectomy is required for control of the severe ulcer diathesis.

Wilson (1973) has found that 27 percent of 677 patients with sufficient data for study in the Zollinger-Ellison Tumor Registry have one or more manifestations of multiple endocrine adenomatosis. Twenty percent have parathyroid disease documented either at neck operation or at autopsy. Our group has reported that some patients with the Zollinger-Ellison syndrome have elevated PTH levels despite normal or low serum calcium concentrations. We postulate that the parathyroid disease associated with Zollinger-Ellison syndrome may be due to secondary hyperparathyroidism (malabsorption) in some cases.

The pituitary tumors in the foregoing types of endocrine

Fig. 38-46. Arteriogram of the inferior thyroid arteries, both sides being visualized simultaneously. The vessels are in their normal position. The patient was found to have hyperparathyroidism due to chief cell hyperplasia. Neither artery is larger than the other, and no displacement seems to have occurred. The arteries are indicated by the arrows. In some cases arteriograms result in a "tumor blush" because of the vascularity of the enlarged parathyroid glands.

polyglandular syndrome are generally made up of more than one cell type or else are chromaphobe adenomas and usually are nonfunctioning. The parathyroid glands show a variety of pathologic features and are characterized by having multiple gland involvement. Most cases of MEA-1 are found to have chief cell hyperplasia of the parathyroids when all glands are examined. Despite the elevated serum calcium levels which frequently accompany this disease the patients rarely show skeletal involvement, and renal complications are uncommon.

Acromegaly. There is a fourth type of multiple adenomas which consists of a pituitary tumor producing acromegaly with parathyroid and pancreatic islet cell tumors. Patients with this syndrome have died with perforated peptic ulcers, and there have been cases of acromegaly in which there was clinical hyperparathyroidism with impaired renal function. The early cases are well summarized by Underdahl et al.

General Considerations. The first account of chronic polyglandular syndrome, type 1, was given by Erdheim in 1903 and consists of a rather sketchy mention of a patient with acromegaly, eosinophilic adenoma of the pituitary, and four enlarged parathyroids. The first report of pituitary, parathyroid, and pancreatic islet cell tumors in combination was by Cushing and Davidoff in 1927, whereas the first report of acromegaly and clinical hyperparathyroidism was in 1948. Involvement of pituitary, parathyroids, and islet cells occurs in 34 percent, pituitary and parathyroids in 25 percent, pituitary and islet cells in 19 percent, parathyroids and islet cells in 22 percent. Twenty-five percent of the patients have peptic ulcer.

The syndromes of polyglandular disease are almost always associated with chief cell hyperplasia of the parathyroids but at times may consist of almost every conceivable combination of adenomas and hyperplasia. A dominant inheritance pattern seems to be characteristic of both chief cell hyperplasia and polyendocrine disease. Familial hyperparathyroidism is not uncommonly a part of the endocrine polyglandular syndrome, as evidenced by a large number of cases collected by Jackson and Boonstra.

Multiple Endocrinopathies, Type 2. Medullary carcinoma of the thyroid may be associated with all or part of a syndrome called *multiple endocrine neoplasia,* type 2, *familial medullary carcinoma syndrome,* or sometimes *Sipple's syndrome.* In its entirety it consists of pheochromocytomas (often bilateral), typical mucosal neuromas, and parathyroid gland abnormalities. Occasional individuals also have a Marfanoid habitus, coarse features, and ganglioneuromatous changes of the plexuses of Meissner and Auerbach.

The serum calcium level is almost always normal in these individuals but occasionally may be high or low. The parathyroid glands in this familial form of medullary carcinoma almost always demonstrate chief cell hyperplasia if they are abnormal. While it is attractive to think of the parathyroid gland abnormalities as compensatory for the calcitonin secreted by the medullary cancers, recent evidence suggests that they may be genetic in origin. Serum PTH is often elevated in cases of familial medullary carcinomas, but it is normal in sporadic cases of this same tumor despite similar high circulating levels of calcitonin. Renal stones have been noted occasionally in both normocalcemic and hypercalcemic individuals with this syndrome.

Hyperparathyroidism, Gout, Pseudogout, and Arthralgia. Gout has been observed from time to time in association with hyperparathyroidism. In most of the patients there has been some renal damage which might have interfered with the excretion of uric acid and thus produced the hyperuricemia. Uric acid calculi have been seen in hyperparathyroidism.

Other types of joint disease also occur in association with hyperparathyroidism. Sharp and Kelly have reported an acute monoarticular arthralgia occurring after the surgical correction of hyperparathyroidism. In each of their two cases the right knee was involved, and the patient had a leukocytosis, joint infusion, and low-grade fever. Sharp and Kelly felt that they had ruled out rheumatoid and infectious arthritis. This kind of arthralgia seems to occur when the serum phosphorous is at its highest, and it is associated with hyperuricemia, presumably because the tubular mechanisms for the excretion of phosphorus and uric acid are similar. Hyperuricemia can thus occur both

in hyperparathyroidism and in hypoparathyroidism. The arthritis described here is a transient one and disappears in a few days. It seems clear that some cases of hyperuricemia and gout in hyperparathyroidism are coincidental or due to renal failure and not related directly to the hyperparathyroidism. Some patients with hyperparathyroidism have symptoms of gout without hyperuricemia.

It has recently been noted that *pseudogout*—the intraarticular deposition of calcium pyrophosphate crystals—is seen in association with hyperparathyroidism. In three of six patients with pseudogout and hyperparathyroidism, pseudogout was the initial clinical manifestation of the hyperparathyroidism. This suggests that all patients with pseudogout should be carefully screened for hyperparathyroidism.

DIFFERENTIAL DIAGNOSIS. Some of the features of the differential diagnosis of hypercalcemia are shown in Table 38-7.

Parathyroid Disease versus Extraparathyroid PTH-producing Tumor. It may be very difficult to make the differential diagnosis between a parathyroid adenoma and an extraparathyroid PTH-producing tumor, since the effects on the patient are identical. The known presence of tumors which are likely to produce this syndrome—bronchogenic or small cell carcinomas of the lung, hypernephromas, hepatomas, epidermoid cancer, bladder, ovary, uterus, vulva, pancreas, liver, and lymphatic malignant tumors—should suggest this possibility. The history, physical findings, and appropriate x-ray studies may establish the diagnosis. As discussed earlier, ectopic production of PTH-like fragments may be diagnosed by radioimmunoassay by certain antisera which react with these substances. The ultimate diagnosis may require neck exploration and the demonstration of normal or atrophic parathyroid glands. In cases in which the differential diagnosis cannot be made with certainty it may be better, at times, to explore the neck than to miss the diagnosis of primary parathyroid overactivity.

Secondary Hyperparathyroidism. What usually distinguishes secondary hyperparathyroidism from the primary disease is that the serum calcium level is not elevated and the patient demonstrates an underlying condition which has caused the hyperparathyroidism, frequently chronic renal failure. In secondary hyperparathyroidism, the serum calcium is usually low, in fact. If this parameter becomes elevated, this is referred to as tertiary hyperparathyroidism (see further on). It may be extremely difficult or impossible to distinguish primary hyperparathyroidism with advanced renal failure from tertiary hyperparathyroidism, in which the renal failure was primary and led to secondary hyperparathyroidism and later to hypercalcemia. In both instances either chief cell hyperplasia alone or an adenoma and chief cell hyperplasia may be present.

When a patient with secondary hyperparathyroidism is operated upon and the parathyroids are removed, they invariably show chief cell hyperplasia, often with nests of oxyphil cells interspersed throughout the gland.

Vitamin D Poisoning. Vitamin D intoxication can be suspected when this vitamin has been administered in excess. The patients tend to have an increased, rather than de-

Table 38-7. THE DIFFERENTIAL DIAGNOSIS OF SOME DISEASES PRODUCING HYPERCALCEMIA, HYPERCALCINURIA, OR BONE CHANGES

Disease	Serum			Urine		Special tests and criteria	Parathyroid hormone
	Calcium	Phosphate	Alkaline phosphatase	Calcium	Phosphate		
Primary hyperparathyroidism	Increased	Decreased*	Normal or increased	Increased	Increased	TRP measurements	Increased
Secondary hyperparathyroidism (renal failure)	Decreased	Increased	Normal or increased	Decreased	Decreased	Chronic renal failure present	Increased
Vitamin D intoxication	Increased	Increased	Decreased	Increased	Increased	Ectopic calcification present	Decreased
Metastatic carcinoma	Increased	Normal	Normal or increased	Increased	Normal	X-rays showing metastases	Decreased†
Multiple myeloma	Increased	Normal	Normal	Normal or increased	Normal or decreased	X-rays showing lesions Bence-Jones protein present Increased plasma globulin	Decreased
Sarcoidosis	Increased	Normal or decreased	Normal or increased	Increased	Increased	Increased plasma globulin Hepatomegaly—biopsy Splenomegaly Kveim test positive	Decreased
Idiopathic hypercalcemia of infancy	Increased	Increased	Normal	Increased	Decreased	Presence of mental retardation Increased blood cholesterol Hypersensitivity to vitamin D	Decreased
Milk-alkali syndrome	Increased	Normal*	Normal	Normal or decreased	Normal or decreased	History of milk and alkali intake Renal insufficiency often present	Decreased
Paget's disease	Normal or increased	Normal	Increased	Increased	Normal	Bone changes on x-ray Serum calcium reduced by mobilization	Normal or decreased
Idiopathic hypercalciuria	Normal	Decreased	Normal	Increased	Normal or increased	Renal calculi may be present	Normal

*Increased when renal failure supervenes.

†In ectopic hyperparathyroidism, PTH is also elevated.

creased, phosphate level in the serum. Metastatic calcification is much more common in vitamin D intoxication than in hyperparathyroidism (see Fig. 38-42). It is somewhat more apt to occur in the presence of renal failure. In vitamin D intoxication small yellowish deposits may be present underneath the fingernails, along the outer borders of the lips, in the skin, and in the corneal conjunctiva. Serum PTH level is low.

Metastatic Cancer. In metastatic cancer the phosphate level in the serum is usually not depressed. The cancer is usually of breast, kidney, lung, thyroid, or prostatic origin and may already have been established by previous procedures. Serum PTH is low unless the tumor secretes ectopic parathyroid hormone-like fragments. The bony involvement usually can be detected by x-ray. The plasma calcium level will usually fall in response to cortisone infusion. Sometimes the lesions in the bone may look quite similar to those seen with primary or secondary hyperparathyroidism as shown in Figs. 38-36 and 38-37.

Multiple Myeloma. This entity usually shows sharp, punched-out areas of destruction in the bone, generally well seen in the skull. At times rather similar lesions can be produced by hyperparathyroidism (see Fig. 38-36). The Bence-Jones protein is present in about 50 percent of the patients, and the plasma globulin level is high. Plasma cells are present in the bone marrow. The alkaline phosphatase level is usually not elevated. Serum PTH is low and the plasma calcium level is decreased with cortisol infusion.

Sarcoidosis. Hypercalcemia in sarcoidosis was first described by Harrell and Fisher. It occurs in about a third of the cases. Although bone destruction may be present in sarcoidosis, it is apparently not the basis for the hypercalcemia. There appears instead to be a hypersensitivity to vitamin D in some individuals with sarcoid, and exposure to sunlight or administration of vitamin D will produce hypercalcemia in the patients manifesting this phenomenon. Since band keratopathy of the eyes, bone cysts, renal calculi, nephrocalcinosis, and polyuria can occur, the incorrect diagnosis of hyperparathyroidism is sometimes made and neck exploration carried out.

The presence of an increased plasma globulin, hepatomegaly, and splenomegaly should suggest the correct diagnosis. In over 50 percent of the patients with sarcoidosis the Kveim reaction will be positive. This test consists of the intracutaneous injection of a heat-sterilized suspension of spleen or lymph node from patients with sarcoid. A positive test is indicated by the production of a papulonodular lesion with epithelioid tubercles demonstrated by biopsy 4 to 6 weeks after the initial injection. The administration of 150 mg of cortisone daily for 10 to 14 days reduces the serum calcium to normal (Dent test). A positive diagnosis may be established by biopsy of the liver, lymph nodes, or, when present, skin nodules. Serum PTH level is low.

Sarcoidosis and hyperparathyroidism may coexist in the same patient, the diagnosis being suspected when the serum calcium level fails to fall with cortisone administration.

Idiopathic Hypercalcemia of Infancy. This syndrome is believed to be due to a hypersensitivity to vitamin D, such as that seen in sarcoidosis. It occurs in infants who have mental retardation, an elevated serum cholesterol level, and hypercalcemia. The serum calcium level falls with the administration of cortisone.

The Milk-Alkali Syndrome. Burnett et al. described a syndrome in which hypercalcemia developed in patients ingesting large amounts of milk and absorbable alkali—such as sodium bicarbonate, usually for peptic ulcer. This is most apt to occur when there is some degree of renal insufficiency. The serum phosphate level is normal or elevated rather than low. Renal calculi and nephrocalcinosis may be present. Patients with primary hyperparathyroidism may develop renal failure, an elevated serum phosphate level, and peptic ulceration, at which point the picture may be difficult to distinguish from the milk-alkali syndrome. The history of ingestion of large amounts of milk and alkali, the improvement noted when these are stopped, and the absence of hypercalcinuria distinguish the latter condition. Serum PTH is low in this condition.

Paget's Disease (Osteitis Deformans). Paget's disease may occasionally be associated with an elevated serum calcium level. X-rays will show the characteristic lesion, usually in the pelvis, lower extremities, or skull. The blood calcium concentration may be normal, but hypercalcemia can develop, particularly if the patient is immobilized. Immobilization leads to disuse atrophy and osteoporosis with a diminished use of calcium for bone repair. Since the localized bone destruction which is the primary underlying feature of this disease continues, there is a net loss of calcium from the bone. The rate at which calcium enters the plasma may exceed the rate at which the kidney can excrete it, thus leading to hypercalcemia.

Paget's disease and primary hyperparathyroidism may coexist, making it difficult to establish the latter diagnosis. The measurement of PTH (not elevated in Paget's disease) and the failure of cortisone and mobilization to reduce the blood calcium should suggest the correct diagnosis.

Idiopathic Hypercalcinuria. This syndrome is characterized by hypercalcinuria, hypophosphatemia, and stone formation in the presence of a normal serum calcium value. It occurs almost exclusively in men. The bones are normal, and the alkaline phosphatase level is not elevated. The cause is unknown. However, hyperabsorption of calcium from the intestine may be responsible for some cases. If an elevated serum calcium level develops, studies for hyperparathyroidism should be carried out. This condition has been treated successfully by thiazide administration, which lowers the urinary calcium output.

Hyperthyroidism. Hypercalcemia occurs on rare occasions in association with hyperthyroidism. The serum calcium may return to normal when the hyperthyroidism is cured. Since hyperparathyroidism may coexist with hyperthyroidism, it is important to determine whether this may not be the cause of the hypercalcemia in any particular case.

Osteomalacia. In osteomalacia there is a failure to mineralize the skeletal matrix, leading to bone changes that might be confused with hyperparathyroidism. Since in osteomalacia the serum calcium level is not elevated and the urinary calcium and phosphate excretion is low rather than high, the conditions are fairly easily differentiated.

Thiazides. Hypercalcemia has been reported with increasing frequency in patients receiving benzothiadiazine diuretics. Hypercalcemia resulting solely from these diuretics is almost always mild. After cessation of the diuretic the serum calcium value usually returns to normal in less than 1 month. The thiazide diuretics can aggravate hypercalcemia in primary hyperparathyroidism. Thus when possible these diuretics should be stopped and the patient studied 1 to 2 months later. In patients with hypercalcemia greater than 12 mg/100 ml, this may not be practical, especially if the cause of the hypercalcemia is clear.

TREATMENT. Indications for Operation. Patients with primary hyperparathyroidism in whom the diagnosis has been established with relative certainty should definitely be subjected to parathyroid surgical treatment if they have either bony or renal manifestations of the disease, since these will almost inevitably become worse with time. The urgency is greater the higher the calcium level, the most impelling example being the patient with hypercalcemic crisis. Treatment is also indicated if peptic ulcer or pancreatitis is secondary to the hyperparathyroidism. Hypertension may or may not be benefited by parathyroidectomy, depending upon its relation to permanent renal damage which has been incurred by long-standing hypercalcemia.

As newer methods for establishing the diagnosis of hyperparathyroidism have developed, more and more cases are operated upon at an earlier stage. There is no question that it is advantageous to prevent the severe renal and bone changes which will eventuate if the patient is not operated upon. There may be an occasional case, however, in which the elevation of serum calcium level is so slight as to make a definitive diagnosis of the disease difficult. There is probably no harm in watching such cases for a few years until such time as the diagnosis can be established. The ability to measure PTH in the blood by immunoassay in an accurate and predictable fashion will facilitate early establishment of the diagnosis and will effect an improvement in the criteria for selection for operation. The mortality for this operation is so extremely low that unless the patient presents an unusually poor risk, operation should be undertaken when any of the indications listed above present themselves.

Some completely asymptomatic patients with minimal hypercalcemia (<11 mg/100 ml) are now being followed without surgery at the Mayo Clinic even though the diagnosis of primary hyperparathyroidism has been definitively made. At the end of a 5-year study period, 20 percent of these patients were operated upon because of complications attributable to the disease or a rise in serum calcium levels to above 11.0 mg/100 ml. Another 20 percent were dropped from the study because of lack of cooperation in the follow-up program. No criteria are evident that would permit identification of those patients who will ultimately require parathyroid operation. They have concluded that surgical treatment is correct in this asymptomatic group in most cases. We follow this same recommendation.

Treatment of Hypercalcemic Crisis. Hypercalcemia is a serious and potentially lethal complication of many diseases. The approach to therapy must be tempered by an appreciation of the underlying disease state and whether or not emergency reduction of serum calcium is required. Individual tolerance to hypercalcemia is variable and may reflect the rapidity with which the concentration of serum calcium rises. It is not uncommon, for example, to observe nearly asymptomatic patients with hyperparathyroidism with a serum calcium of 15 mg/100 ml yet virtually moribund patients with rapidly progressive cancer have a similar serum calcium. A very good review of this subject was written by Goldsmith.

General Support. Since patients with hypercalcemia often have had anorexia, nausea, and vomiting for some time prior to seeking medical assistance, severe dehydration and oliguria are common presenting features. Thus perhaps the most important treatment is restoration of the extracellular fluid volume with 0.9% sodium chloride. Hypokalemia is frequently present and may require replacement of large amounts of potassium for correction.

Calcium and digitalis are synergistic in effect on the myocardium and conducting system. Hence the fully digitalized patient may manifest digitalis toxicity if he becomes hypercalcemic. Thus it may be necessary to reduce or stop digitalis. Similarly, if digitalization is necessary in a hypercalcemic patient, a lower dose is generally required.

Treatment of the Underlying Disorder. An early assessment of the underlying disorder is essential so that specific therapy may be begun. Because of the increased hazard of general anesthesia in the ill, severely hypercalcemic patient it is unwise to rush into emergency surgery. Since specific medical therapy for hypercalcemia is generally adequate, it is no longer necessary to perform parathyroidectomy as an emergency procedure. Rather, dangerous levels of hypercalcemia should be controlled prior to surgery. Specific therapy after control of hypercalcemia would include surgical removal of neoplasms, radiation, cytotoxic drugs, corticosteroids, or withdrawal of milk and alkali, estrogens, thiazides, or vitamin D as appropriate.

Therapy of the Hypercalcemia Per Se (See Table 38-8). *Gastrointestinal Measures.* Attempts to lower intestinal absorption of calcium by use of a low-calcium diet are reasonably effective only for sarcoidosis or vitamin D intoxication. Cortisone appears to inhibit calcium absorption, which is related to vitamin D mechanisms.

Renal Excretion and Dialysis. In most instances, calcium excretion parallels sodium excretion. Hence mechanisms which increase sodium excretion are effective in lowering serum calcium levels. Isotonic saline solution is excellent in this regard but is limited by the cardiac and renal status of the patient. The use of furosemide or ethacrynic acid gives excellent results alone or with saline infusion. At present, furosemide with saline infusion is the treatment of choice for hypercalcemia. Fluid and electrolyte balance must be carefully monitored when these agents are used. Sodium sulfate does not seem to be better than sodium chloride and may be more dangerous. Therefore, it is rarely used.

EDTA chelates ionized calcium and also increases urinary excretion of calcium by forming soluble complexes. Its effects are difficult to monitor, and it produces pain at the site of infusion. It should be used only for emergency

Table 38-8. USUAL DOSES OF HYPOCALCEMIC AGENTS

Drug	Route	Dosage	Reported complications	Contraindications
Sodium chloride solution (isotonic)	Intravenous	1 liter every 3–4 hr	Pulmonary edema	Congestive heart failure, renal insufficiency, hypertension
Sodium sulfate solution (isotonic)	Intravenous	3 liters over 9 hr	Pulmonary edema, hypernatremia	Congestive heart failure, renal insufficiency, hypertension
Furosemide	Intravenous	100 mg/hr	Volume depletion, hypokalemia	Renal insufficiency
EDTA	Intravenous	50 mg/kg body weight over 4–6 hr	Renal failure, hypotension	Renal insufficiency
Cortisone	Oral or parenteral	150 mg/day	Hypercorticism	Emergency reduction of serum calcium required
Mithramycin	Intravenous	25 µg/kg body weight	Hemorrhage, thrombocytopenia, nausea, vomiting	Bleeding disorder, renal insufficiency, liver impairment
Phosphate	Intravenous	1 mM*/kg body weight over 6–8 hr	Extraskeletal calcification, hypocalcemia	Renal insufficiency, hyperphosphatemia
	Oral	1–2 mM*/kg body weight daily		
Calcitonin	Parenteral	1–5 MRC units/kg body weight/day	Nausea, vomiting	Thrombotic disorders

*1 mM of phosphate is equivalent to 31 mg of phosphorus.
SOURCE: Modified from W. N. Suki, J. J. Yium, M. Von Minden et al., Acute Treatment of Hypercalcemia with Furosemide, *N Engl J Med,* **283:**836–840, 1970.

reduction of life-threatening hypercalcemia, since doses in excess of 3 Gm have produced renal insufficiency.

If renal function is poor, temporary reduction of hypercalcemia may be obtained by peritoneal or hemodialysis.

Skeletal Factors—Reduction of Bone Resorption. Cortisone is especially useful in treatment of sarcoidosis, vitamin D intoxication, myeloma, and various leukemias or lymphomas. The effect is often slow; a lag period of 7 to 10 days is not exceptional. One of the major drawbacks to long-term therapy is the production of osteoporosis.

Phosphate given orally or intravenously has been demonstrated to be effective in lowering serum calcium levels. Intravenously administered phosphate may be risky;

when not used precisely as directed, death has resulted. Phosphate given orally is safe and efficacious but slower in effect. When given in excess, diarrhea will occur.

Calcitonin, by inhibiting bone resorption, should be the ideal emergency drug for treatment of hypercalcemia. Porcine calcitonin has proved far less effective than was predicted. Salmon calcitonin, which is available commercially, is more efficacious in human beings but has not been very useful in this regard.

Finally, mithramycin, a cytotoxic drug originally used

Fig. 38-47. Incision for parathyroidectomy. The dotted lines indicate the extension of the incision used for mediastinal exploration. The deep fascia is divided in the midline, and the strap muscles are divided.

Strap muscles divided midline

Sternomastoid m. being freed up

Line of skin incision

Fig. 38-48. Strap muscles are cut and retracted, and the gland is exposed. This may facilitate the exposure.

for therapy of testicular tumors, is very effective in reducing serum calcium concentrations but takes 12 to 24 hours to do so. Side effects are few when given as an infusion every 5 days at a dose of $25\mu g/kg$. In a recent study this schedule was shown to be effective in controlling the hypercalcemia of breast cancer. At present, we reserve this drug for cases of malignant tumor, although others have used it for benign disease.

Operative Technique. In general, parathyroid surgery requires an unrushed, meticulous dissection with a bloodless field. Intratracheal anesthesia with the neck somewhat hyperextended by means of a small pad between the shoulder blades is usually preferred for parathyroid exploration. The entire operating table may be tilted so that the head is somewhat elevated, thus diminishing bleeding.

The platysma muscle is elevated with the skin flap, and the superior flap is dissected to the hyoid superiorly and the upper border of the sternum inferiorly. The skin flaps may be held apart by a self-retaining retractor or by sutures, and the deep cervical fascia is divided longitudinally in the midline from the hyoid bone to the suprasternal notch. Others prefer to divide the sternohyoid and sternothyroid muscles routinely at the junction of the upper and middle third to facilitate exposure of the gland (Figs. 38-47 and 38-48); however, we usually do not find this necessary.

Locating the Parathyroid Glands. The thyroid gland is mobilized by dividing the middle thyroid veins and rolling the lobe of the thyroid anteriorly and mediad. The recurrent laryngeal nerve is then identified. The landmarks for this are the groove between the trachea and esophagus, and the inferior thyroid artery. The recurrent nerve may also be identified at the inferior cornu of the thyroid cartilage, as described by Wang. The areolar tissue is cleared from around the nerve, and the inferior thyroid artery is cleaned off and preserved at the same time. The best place to begin the search for a parathyroid adenoma is at the point where the recurrent laryngeal nerve crosses behind the inferior thyroid artery. The adenomas are very frequently tucked down under the lateral lobe of the thyroid in a little space alongside the esophagus lying just slightly posterior to the groove between the esophagus and the trachea or thyroid cartilage (Figs. 38-49 and 38-50). Tracing the branches of the inferior thyroid artery may sometimes be helpful in locating the hyperfunctioning parathyroid gland, since this vessel supplies the parathyroid adenoma with blood in

nearly 90 percent of the cases (Figs. 38-51 and 38-52). The adenoma can sometimes be located by tracing a branch of the inferior thyroid artery to its termination in the gland. After a preliminary search in this area the inferior parathyroid will usually be found just below the point at which the recurrent laryngeal nerve intersects the inferior thyroid artery. The superior parathyroid will often be found within 1 or 2 cm above this point, usually on a little prominence of the posterior surface of the thyroid.

An adenoma, particularly one of the lower gland, can be tucked well behind the thyroid or between the trachea and esophagus, so that it is not readily apparent until the thyroid has been rotated forward and the fatty tissue in this area has been gently teased away (Fig. 38-53). The adenoma is not usually bound down to the surrounding tissues, however, and usually can be popped out of its hiding place. It is generally red-brown, at times yellow-brown, smooth, and with a surface which is vascular and bleeds easily when rubbed or cut. On rare occasions, particularly when it lies beneath the capsule of the thyroid, it may look extremely similar to thyroid tissue itself.

Once the provisional location of the glands has been established, the procedure is repeated on the other side. We

Fig. 38-49. The middle thyroid veins are divided, and the lateral lobe of the thyroid is retracted anteriorly and mediad. The recurrent laryngeal nerve is exposed in the tracheoesophageal groove, and the inferior thyroid artery is dissected out and preserved. The inferior parathyroid is usually located just below the intersection of these two structures and is supplied by a branch of the inferior thyroid artery.

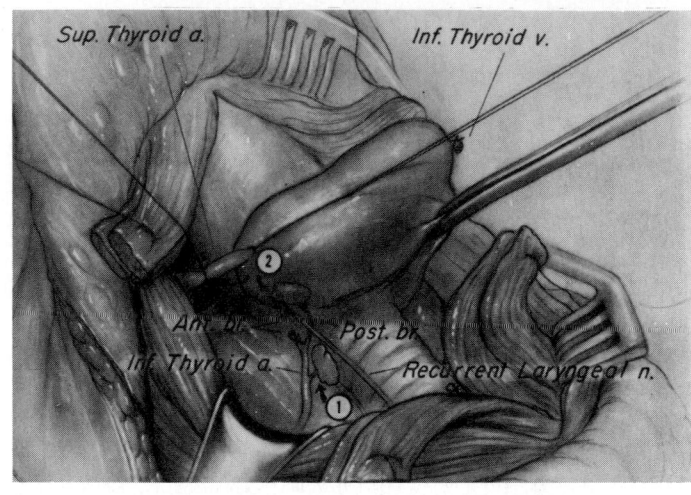

Fig. 38-50. It may be necessary to divide a branch of the inferior artery or to divide the superior thyroid artery to identify the upper parathyroid (2). The lower parathyroid gland (1) is not infrequently opposite the lower pole of the thyroid or below this and can sometimes be identified in the fatty tissue just behind the divided strap muscles.

make it a policy to identify by biopsy and frozen section all parathyroid glands which are questionable in appearance before removing any of them. This is to protect against circumstances which have been reported in which three enlarged parathyroid glands were resected as they were encountered, only to find that the patient had no fourth gland. When all the parathyroids cannot be found adjacent to the thyroid gland, further search is facilitated by dividing the superior pole vessels on the side on which the upper gland has not been identified and following the branch which joins the inferior artery to identify the blood supply of this gland. The lower parathyroid is not infrequently located below the lower pole of the thyroid, and it may be

found by pulling the divided sternothyroid muscle superiorly and laterally and looking in the areolar tissue along the posterior surface of the muscle. The entire space leading down to the superior mediastinum should be carefully searched in order to find a missing inferior gland. The upper part of the thymus should also be removed if possible, since the lower parathyroid may be embedded in this tissue.

The upper gland may sometimes be found in unusual positions as well. It may be several centimeters above the upper pole of the thyroid gland. Furthermore, the retro-

Fig. 38-51. A. Blood supply of the parathyroids. B. The relation of the inferior thyroid artery to the recurrent laryngeal nerve.

esophageal space of the lower neck and upper mediastinum should be explored, since adenomas of the superior parathyroid glands occasionally may be found in this location.

Most parathyroid glands can be found by utilizing a systematic, meticulous dissection. We have not found the injection of toluidine blue at operation to be helpful. This dye is said to selectively color the parathyroid glands blue or purple and thus to aid in their identification. Unfortunately, occasional cardiac arrhythmias and bone marrow depression have been reported. Furthermore, most experienced parathyroid surgeons have learned to recognize parathyroid glands, so that this technique does not add greatly to their efficiency.

Extent of Operation. Several different approaches regarding the extent of parathyroid resection for primary hyperparathyroidism have been proposed. Wang feels that a normal parathyroid gland in addition to an enlarged parathyroid gland is diagnostic of an adenoma and that the other side of the neck should not be explored. Paloyan, on the other hand, feels that the only way to prevent recurrent hyperparathyroidism is to perform a subtotal parathyroidectomy in each patient.

Our practice has been to take an intermediate approach—to try to identify all the parathyroid glands, to biopsy them at the time of operation, and then to decide which gland or glands should be removed. If only one gland is enlarged and the others are normal both in size and histologically on frozen section, only the enlarged gland is removed. If more than one gland is involved, a subtotal parathyroidectomy is performed, since we consider this to represent multiglandular disease. It is apparent that the surgeon must play a diagnostic as well as a therapeutic role at the time of exploration, regardless of which technique is chosen.

If hypoparathyroidism is to be prevented, a subtotal parathyroidectomy should be performed with the greatest of care. It is essential that the remnant of parathyroid tissue left behind have an intact blood supply. Generally, 40 to 60 mg of the smallest gland is left in place. It is first examined and seen to be viable before the other glands are removed. We mark it either with a metal clip or a suture to permit it to be found at a subsequent exploration, if necessary.

If three normal parathyroid glands have been found and the hyperfunctioning gland has not been identified, it is wise to resect the thyroid lobe on the side of the missing gland, since 3 percent of parathyroid adenomas have been reported by Goldman to be totally intrathyroidal.

If the possibility of *carcinoma of the parathyroid gland* is entertained at operation, the lesion should be completely removed with an adequate margin of surrounding tissue, including the thyroid lobe on that side. Great care should be exercised not to enter the lesion or to spill tumor cells, since recurrent disease in the neck is very common. With good surgical technique and an *en bloc* resection much of this local recurrence is avoidable.

Mediastinal Exploration. When a patient has been referred with an established diagnosis of hyperparathyroidism and neck exploration done elsewhere has failed to reveal a tumor, the neck operation should always be re-

Fig. 38-52. Lateral view with the thyroid retracted anteriorly and mediad to show the surgical landmarks for locating the parathyroids.

peated, since in nearly every instance the tumor will be discovered there, rather than in the mediastinum. Increased difficulty with second or third operations is an added incentive to perform a satisfactory procedure the first time.

Since at least 95 to 98 percent of the parathyroid adenomas can be reached from the neck, mediastinal exploration is seldom necessary. We do not recommend a mediastinal exploration at the time of initial neck exploration, even if three normal glands have been found and the thyroid lobe on the side of the missing gland has been demonstrated to contain no parathyroid tissue. Even when four normal glands are found in the neck we do not recommend immediate exploration of the mediastinum, despite our realization that a fifth gland may be the culprit. Rather, we explore the superior mediastinum as carefully as possible from the neck, explore all other areas again, and then close.

Prior to reexploration and possible mediastinal exploration we feel that it is appropriate to reconfirm the diagnosis of primary hyperparathyroidism and then, if possible, to perform selective venous catheterization with PTH measurement to try to further localize the gland. This has been helpful in several instances.

If mediastinal exploration is necessary, the mediastinotomy may be done by splitting the sternum in the midline down to the level of the third interspace and making a short cut out into this interspace on each side. It is often easier to divide the entire sternum in the midline. The sternum is then held apart with a retractor, and the mediastinum is explored. If one is searching for the superior gland on that side, it may be located in the posterior part of the mediastinum, while if one is looking for the inferior parathyroid, it is generally located in the anterior mediastinum. It may be embedded in the thymus itself, or it may lie against the pericardium. One case of an intrapericardial parathyroid gland has been reported. In most instances it is in the upper portion of the mediastinum. The mediastinal exploration is usually carried out for a tumor which has arisen from a mediastinal parathyroid, rather than a tumor which has arisen from a parathyroid in the neck and descended during growth into the mediastinum—since these

Fig. 38-53. Parathyroid exploration. *A.* The normal right lower parathyroid has been exposed and is identified by the end of the instrument. It is embedded in fat. It lies on top of the recurrent laryngeal nerve just below the inferior thyroid artery. An adenoma of the upper parathyroid gland is indicated by the arrow. *B.* Another adenoma is indicated by the arrow. The hemostat on the right side points to a normal-appearing parathyroid gland.

can usually be reached from the neck. The blood supply therefore will usually be from a mediastinal vessel (see Fig. 38-51).

In the Massachusetts General Hospital series only 19 of 400 parathyroid tumors (5 percent) required mediastinal exploration for removal. In the Mayo Clinic series, only 14 of 1,000 (1.4 percent) of patients with primary hyperparathyroidism were cured by a sternal splitting operation. Thus, a careful neck exploration is imperative at the initial operation.

Postoperative Complications. The postoperative complications consist of hypoparathyroidism, hemorrhage, recurrent laryngeal nerve damage, and persistent or recurrent disease.

Hypoparathyroidism can occur because of excision of all parathyroid tissue or because of permanent or temporary damage to the blood supply of the remaining parathyroid tissue. In thyroid and parathyroid operations, the inferior thyroid artery should *not* be ligated laterally, since this can devascularize the parathyroid glands. A temporary hypoparathyroidism often follows the excision of large parathyroid adenomas, and temporary calcium treatment may have to be instituted. This will usually correct itself in a week or two. The treatment of hypoparathyroidism is discussed in another section.

Hypocalcemia in the postoperative period is more apt to occur when a large adenoma has been removed, when there is impaired renal function, or when there is considerable bone disease. In the latter two cases the calcium level is depressed as a response to an elevated serum phosphorus level or by calcium deposition in calcium-starved bones. In this latter circumstance it may take many weeks for the calcium level to become normal. Examination of the serum phosphorus level is helpful postoperatively. If hypoparathyroidism is present, the phosphorus level is elevated; in "bone hunger" the phosphorus level may be low if renal function is not impaired.

It is our practice always to drain the wound after parathyroid exploration. The drain is brought out through one side of the incision and is usually removed in 24 hours. A loose dressing is applied so that if *hemorrhage* does occur, it will be less apt to compress the trachea and cause respiratory embarrassment. The wound is inspected frequently in the immediate postoperative period. A severe

hemorrhage will necessitate reopening the wound or re-exploration.

Damage to the recurrent nerve will rarely be a problem if the location of the nerve is determined as the first step in the surgical procedure as outlined above. Temporary malfunction of the nerve may occur if the nerve is stretched during the performance of the operation. The nerve will occasionally lie on top of the parathyroid adenoma. If the nerve is inadvertently divided, it should be resutured. Injury to the nerve is most apt to occur when there is a large adenoma located in the superior mediastinum pushing up into the neck, where it may displace the nerve anteriorly. If the recurrent laryngeal nerves are injured bilaterally, severe respiratory difficulty may occur, sometimes necessitating a tracheostomy.

Persistent disease means that hypercalcemia remains after operation. This occurs when the diagnosis of hyperparathyroidism is incorrect, or when the hyperfunctioning gland or glands have not been adequately removed. In the hands of experienced neck surgeons, this should occur only infrequently. *Recurrent disease* means that the calcium returns to normal postoperatively but that months to years later, hypercalcemia due to hyperparathyroidism returns. This condition is most commonly seen if primary chief cell hyperplasia is not recognized and one or two enlarged glands are removed because they are diagnosed as adenomas. When recurrent hyperparathyroidism does occur, the parathyroid disease should be treated as hyperplasia with subtotal parathyroidectomy. A lesser procedure, illustrated in Fig. 38-54, will be once more doomed to failure. Hyper-

Fig. 38-54. Recurrent hyperparathyroidism. In this patient, hypercalcemia and hypophosphatemia developed three separate times. On each occasion a single enlarged gland was removed. After removal of three glands, the patient has remained normocalcemic. While each of these glands was originally diagnosed as an adenoma, it is very likely that this process represents undiagnosed primary chief cell hyperplasia which was finally cured by the cumulative subtotal parathyroidectomy.

calcemia recurring several months after an apparently successful parathyroidectomy should alert the physician to the possibility of a parathyroid carcinoma, although inadequately treated hyperplasia is more likely. It is necessary to follow patients for many years following parathyroidectomy if the results of therapy are to be truly assessed.

Results of Therapy. In Table 38-9, the incidence of severe hypoparathyroidism and that of recurrent hyperparathyroidism are tabulated from some of the recent series of primary hyperparathyroidism. Note that although the recognition of multiglandular disease varied greatly from series to series, the incidence of recurrent hyperparathyroidism is low. Thus, when performed by an experienced surgeon, parathyroidectomy is generally successful. The series of Clark et al. points out clearly that those patients with multiple endocrine adenomatosis (MEA) or familial hyperparathyroidism (FHP) are most likely to get a recurrence. This may occasionally occur even following a subtotal parathyroidectomy. When these conditions were not present, recurrent disease occurred in only 0.4 percent of patients; when MEA or FHP was present, recurrent disease occurred in 33 percent of patients. Long-term follow-up studies are essential.

Severe hypoparathyroidism may occur more frequently following subtotal parathyroidectomy than after lesser operations if great care is not exercised in performing this operation. When done by experienced surgeons, however, the incidence of permanent hypoparathyroidism necessitating vitamin D therapy is quite low.

Secondary Hyperparathyroidism

In primary hyperparathyroidism there is an oversecretion of PTH which does not cease even in the presence of an elevated serum calcium level. In secondary hyperparathyroidism there is also an increased secretion of PTH but this is in response to a *lowered blood calcium* level which has been brought about by some factors, often renal disease or malabsorption syndromes. These diseases are associated with abnormalities in vitamin D metabolism [lack of production of $1,25\text{-}(OH)_2D_3$] and by poor calcium and vitamin D absorption from the intestines, respectively. The response of the parathyroids is thus a compensatory one, as the body attempts to raise the serum calcium level to the normal range. In secondary hyperparathyroidism there is a chief cell hyperplasia of the parathyroids, which is quite commonly accompanied by nests of oxyphil cells.

Other causes of secondary hyperparathyroidism include rickets and osteomalacia, where there is a deficient absorption of calcium from the intestine.

In secondary hyperparathyroidism the serum calcium level is usually low or low-normal. In rickets and osteomalacia the serum phosphate level is reduced, as it is in primary hyperparathyroidism, whereas in chronic renal failure it is usually elevated. The intestinal absorption of calcium is increased in primary hyperparathyroidism, and the fecal excretion is reduced, whereas the reverse is true in secondary hyperparathyroidism.

At times there may be some difficulty in differentiating between secondary and primary hyperparathyroidism be-

cause primary hyperparathyroidism can lead to renal failure through nephrocalcinosis and the effects of PTH and calcium on the kidney, thus producing an elevated serum phosphate level which may in turn lower the serum calcium level to some degree. The renal failure may lead to hyperplasia of the uninvolved parathyroid glands, thus leading to the coexistence of an adenoma and hyperplasia. This course of events is further discussed under Tertiary Hyperparathyroidism. The most significant differentiation between secondary (dependent) versus primary (autonomous) hyperparathyroidism depends upon the serum calcium level, which is seldom elevated in the former and almost always elevated in the latter. In parathyroid hypercalcemic crisis, in fact, there is usually a markedly elevated serum calcium level despite renal failure, azotemia, and an elevated serum phosphate level.

The skeletal changes of secondary hyperparathyroidism are identical to those of primary hyperparathyroidism except that ectopic calcification in the arteries, muscles, etc., is much more common in secondary hyperparathyroidism, especially if the patient has been given large doses of vitamin D (Fig. 38-42). Today severe bone disease associated with hyperparathyroidism is rare in primary hyperparathyroidism but is not infrequently seen in patients with chronic renal failure maintained on chronic hemodialysis.

The bone disease in chronic renal failure, commonly called *renal osteodystrophy,* is caused by at least several factors: Hyperphosphatemia results in a decreased serum calcium. Hypocalcemia results in secondary hyperparathyroidism. Impaired calcium absorption due to vitamin D insensitivity results in osteomalacia. Systemic acidosis may also contribute to bone resorption.

Recent advances in the treatment of renal osteodystrophy appear to be significant. By elevating the calcium in the dialysis bath, Arnaud and associates have demonstrated a decrease in serum PTH and a decreased incidence of bone disease in patients on chronic hemodialysis.

Patients with chronic renal failure may have an impaired ability to convert vitamin D_3 to its active metabolite $1,25\text{-}(OH)_2D_3$. This results in decreased calcium absorption from the intestine. In these patients, physiologic doses of vitamin D are usually ineffective, but improvement following administration of large pharmacologic doses of this vitamin may occur. The $1,25\text{-}(OH)_2D_3$ metabolite promises to be very effective. In a recent study it was given to uremic patients. Significant improvement in intestinal absorption of calcium and elevation of calcium concentrations were noted on a dose of only 100 units/day for 6 to 10 days. The same individuals were insensitive to 40,000 units of vitamin D_3. Thus administration of $1,25\text{-}(OH)_2D_3$ or other similar metabolites may be useful in the prevention and treatment of renal osteodystrophy. Medical therapy for the bone disease should be tried in all patients with secondary hyperparathyroidism before surgery is contemplated.

Stanbury et al. have advocated parathyroidectomy for patients in chronic renal failure with severe bone change who have developed intractable bone pain. The pain and severe itching, which is also sometimes present in patients on chronic dialysis, are often relieved in a dramatic fash-

Table 38-9. INCIDENCE OF RECURRENT HYPERPARATHYROIDISM AND SEVERE HYPOPARATHYROIDISM FOLLOWING OPERATION FOR PRIMARY HYPERPARATHYROIDISM

Author and year	Total no. of patients	Multiple gland involvement, %	Recurrent hyperparathyroidism, %	Severe hypoparathyroidism, %	Follow-up
Paloyan et al. (1969)	I 27	18	15	19	7 mo.-3 yr.
	II* 26	58	0	8	
Haff and Ballinger (1971)	I 38	50	3	5	18 mo. or longer
Bruining (1971)	I 267	45	0	1.2	3½ yr. (average)
	II* 11	...	0	27	
Clark and Taylor (1971)	99	15	1	2	
Johanssen et al. (1972)	203	18	0	3.8	
Paloyan et al. (1973)	98	65	1	2	
Romanus et al. (1973)	274	20	1	7	4 yr. average
Hines and Suker (1973)	51	10	0	...	To 15 yr.
Wang (1973)	256	...	0.8	...	10 mo.-15 yr.
Davies (1974)	350	10	3	5	mo.-38 yr.
Myers (1974)	82	13	1	...	1-6.5 yr.
Purnell et al. (1974)	475	13	0.6	0.2	4½ yr. (average)
Block et al. (1974)	121	20	1	4	
Muller et al. (1975)	352	50	1	...	
Palmer et al. (1975)	250	15	0.5	2	15 yr.
Farr (1976)	100	5	2	4	
Block (1976)	182	20	0	0	
Clark et al. (1976)	263	12	2.7	4	6 mo.-40 yr.
MEA or FHP‡	21	71	33	24†	
Without MEA or FHP	242	6	0.4	2.6	

*Subtotal parathyroidectomy.
†None permanent.
‡MEA, multiple endocrine adenomatosis; FHP, familial hyperparathyroidism.
SOURCE: Adapted from O. H. Clark, L. H. Wang, and T. K. Hunt, *Ann Surg,* **184:**391, 1976.

Fig. 38-55. Secondary hyperparathyroidism. Chief cell hyperplasia with four enlarged parathyroid glands was found in this patient with chronic renal failure and bone disease. Arrows point to two of the hyperplastic parathyroid glands. *T,* retracted thyroid lobe.

ion. Remineralization of the skeleton can be hastened by the administration of vitamin D postoperatively.

Patients with secondary hyperparathyroidism due to chronic renal failure are dialysed 1 day before surgery to reduce serum potassium. Before or during surgery washed frozen red cells may be administered. A subtotal parathy-

roidectomy is routinely performed leaving only 40 to 60 mg of vascularized parathyroid tissue behind (Fig. 38-55). Lesser operations may result in a reexacerbation of bone symptoms. Drains are always used. Postoperatively, the first dialysis is often accomplished with regional heparinization.

PARATHYROID TRANSPLANTATION. Following subtotal parathyroidectomy for secondary hyperparathyroidism, the remaining remnant of tissue is subjected to a continuing hypocalcemic stimulus. Thus, it is likely to hypertrophy and to cause symptoms again. To avoid reoperation in the neck, which is always more dangerous, Wells et al. have proposed that the parathyroid remnant be minced into small pieces and implanted into the muscles of the forearm. All other parathyroid tissues are removed. This technique has worked successfully in 29 patients with secondary hyperparathyroidism. Histologically viable parathyroid tissue has been biopsied in the arm, and the antecubital veins draining the grafted tissue have higher serum PTH

Fig. 38-56. The clinical course of a 19-year-old male who had undergone a total parathyroidectomy for severe bone pain in 1973 and then received a renal transplant 6 months later. Because of severe symptoms of hypocalcemia in the patient, two parathyroid glands were removed from his father (who had also contributed donor kidney) and implanted in the patient's forearm in November 1973. Thereafter serum calcium rose to normal values and calcium and vitamin D therapy was stopped. Serum PTH levels returned to normal and were higher in the antecubital veins on the side of the transplant. The patient remains on prednisone and cyclophosphamide (Cytoxan) therapy. (*From S. A. Wells, Jr., et al., Surgery, 78:34, 1975.*)

levels than do veins of the opposite, nongrafted arm. If hyperparathyroidism recurs, some of the tissue can be removed from the forearm using local anesthesia (a much safer procedure).

Parathyroid tissue which has been quick-frozen and stored at −196°C for as long as 9 months has been successfully reimplanted in the arm. This could lead some day to a "parathyroid bank," in which some tissue is saved from each patient who undergoes a parathyroidectomy. In the event of hypoparathyroidism, some of his own parathyroid could be reimplanted.

Wells has suggested that patients with *primary* chief cell hyperplasia be treated by total parathyroidectomy and transplantation of tissue to the arm as well. We have not done this routinely but have successfully used this technique in one patient who developed recurrent hyperparathyroidism 3 years after a subtotal parathyroidectomy done elsewhere for hyperplasia.

Finally, one immunosuppressed, aparathyroid patient received a parathyroid allograft from a parent who previously had been his renal transplant donor (Fig. 38-56). This technique has only limited application, however, since most patients do well with vitamin D therapy.

Tertiary Hyperparathyroidism

Tertiary hyperparathyroidism is the term which has been employed to describe the situation in which secondary hyperparathyroidism with chief cell hyperplasia appears to have become "autonomous." The diagnosis is made when an elevated serum calcium level develops in the patient with chronic renal failure and secondary hyperparathyroidism or in a patient with known intestinal malabsorption who previously had hypocalcemia. Tertiary hyperparathyroidism may be present even when the blood calcium level is not grossly elevated but is simply in the upper normal range when it should have been low.

When renal transplantation is carried out in a patient with renal failure and secondary hyperparathyroidism, three patterns are characteristically seen: In the first the calcium level rises and the phosphorous level falls for a period of a week or two, after which they both return to normal levels. This is illustrated in Fig. 38-57. In the second pattern the elevated calcium and lowered phosphorus levels may persist for several weeks before gradually returning to normal (Fig. 38-58A). In the third pattern, hypercalcemia with hypophosphatemia persists for long periods of time. In the patient illustrated in Fig. 38-58B a staghorn calculus developed in the transplanted kidney within 6 months. Parathyroidectomy was carried out at this point, and the function of the kidney has remained excellent up to the present time, 5 years after transplantation.

Recent studies suggest that true parathyroid autonomy rarely occurs in patients with so-called tertiary hyperparathyroidism. It has been demonstrated that the hyperplastic glands found in chronic renal failure do suppress their secretion but cannot completely shut off their secretion of PTH despite the presence of hypercalcemia. Furthermore, because of their bulky size it may take a long time for them to involute. Johnson et al. have demonstrated that,

REVERSAL OF SECONDARY HYPERPARATHYROIDISM FOLLOWING RENAL HOMOTRANSPLANTATION

Fig. 38-57. Serum calcium and phosphate values in a patient with secondary hyperparathyroidism who received a kidney transplant. Preoperatively the serum calcium level was low and the phosphate level high. After an initial rise in calcium level and fall in phosphate level to levels outside the normal range the values quickly returned to normal levels. No parathyroid exploration was carried out.

following renal transplantation, PTH concentrations in these patients slowly return toward normal within several months if renal function is good (see Fig. 38-59). Hypercalcemia posttransplantation may also be the result of increased end organ responsiveness, since abnormalities in vitamin D metabolism are corrected.

Some workers have a considerable fear that renal damage may occur very rapidly in the presence of hypercalcemia and advocate doing parathyroidectomy prior to renal transplantation in those patients suspected of having severe secondary or tertiary hyperparathyroidism. In view of the fact that in most of these cases normal serum calcium concentrations will return in a reasonable period after transplantation, it would seem a more appropriate policy to wait and watch the patient carefully posttransplantation for at least 6 months. Oral phosphate administration has been useful in restoring the elevated serum calcium level to normal if the serum phosphorus is low and should be tried. Only rarely will parathyroidectomy be necessary. Subtotal parathyroidectomy was only necessary in 3 of 111 patients following transplantation at the Mayo Clinic.

Hypoparathyroidism

ETIOLOGY. The most common cause of hypoparathyroidism is surgical removal of the parathyroids either during parathyroid surgical treatment or, more commonly, during operations on the thyroid. Postoperative tetany after thyroidectomy for goiter was first described by Reverdin and Kocher in 1882, although of course it was not recognized that this was due to parathyroid deficiency. Primary idiopathic hypoparathyroidism is extremely rare and is usually first noted in patients under the age of sixteen.

As mentioned earlier, transient hypoparathyroidism can

Fig. 38 58. Serum calcium and phosphate values in patients with secondary hyperparathyroidism who received kidney transplants. *A.* Patient with secondary hyperparathyroidism whose serum phosphate level took somewhat longer to return to normal after renal homotransplantation. The calcium level remained in the high normal range for many days. *B.* Another patient with renal failure and secondary hyperparathyroidism. In this patient the preoperative serum calcium level was nearly in the normal range, whereas the phosphorus level was markedly elevated. After transplantation the serum calcium value steadily rose, while the phosphate value declined to abnormally low levels. No spontaneous return toward normal occurred, and it was apparent that tertiary hyperparathyrodism had developed. A parathyroidectomy was carried out on the 275th day after transplantation, and the patient was found to have chief cell hyperplasia with very large glands. By this time calcium deposits had developed in the walls of the calcyceal system of the transplanted kidney. After parathyroidectomy the serum calcium and phosphate values returned to normal. (*From D. M. Hume et al., Ann Surg, 164:352, 1966.*)

be noted after removal of a parathyroid adenoma or a resection of most of the tissue in parathyroid hyperplasia. This is made worse when the patient has some degree of renal disease which tends to lower the calcium level by itself or when the patient has serious bone disease, when the calcium tends to be deposited in the bone, thus producing hypocalcemia. In some instances the transient hypocalcemia is due to trauma to the remaining glands or to interference with the blood supply.

Idiopathic hypoparathyroidism is an uncommon disease of unknown cause. Recent evidence would suggest that in some cases it is due to the presence of antibodies against parathyroid tissue. The patients may also have antibodies against adrenal, thyroid, and gastric parietal cells. One hypothesis is that the parathyroid disease is part of a generalized autoimmune disease. Other diseases sometimes associated with this include monilial infection, Hashimoto's thyroiditis, and steatorrhea.

CLINICAL MANIFESTATIONS. Symptoms. The symptoms of hypoparathyroidism are those of hypocalcemia and are related to the greatly increased neuromuscular excitability brought about by a decrease in the plasma ionized calcium. The most striking manifestation is tetany. This may consist of carpopedal spasm in which the fingers at the metacarpal phalangeal joint and the wrist are flexed and the elbow, legs, and feet are extended. Tonic and clonic convulsions and laryngeal stridor may be present and may even prove fatal. In the milder forms paresthesias, muscle cramps, numbness, dysphagia, and dysarthria may be present. There may be some degree of anxiety. In chronic hypoparathyroidism cataracts and mental changes may occur.

Physical Signs. Chvostek's sign consists of a contraction of the facial muscles in response to a tap over the facial nerve in front of the ear. Occluding the circulation at the arm by inflation of a blood pressure cuff above the level of systolic pressure induces carpopedal spasm within 3 minutes. This is Trousseau's sign, a less reliable sign than Chvostek's sign.

The electrocardiogram shows a prolongation of the Q-T interval. The plasma calcium level is low, and the phosphate is increased.

Differential Diagnosis. Tetany can be caused by factors other than hypoparathyroidism. Alkalosis can produce tetany even in the presence of a normal blood total calcium level by lowering the ionized calcium level. Rickets in the child, osteomalacia in the adult, steatorrhea, and renal insufficiency all produce hypocalcemia. In rickets, osteomalacia, and steatorrhea there is a low plasma calcium level with a normal or low plasma phosphate level. This differentiates it from hypoparathyroidism, where the plasma phosphate level is generally elevated. Chronic renal insufficiency is associated with hypocalcemia with a markedly elevated plasma phosphate level—higher than that usually seen in hypoparathyroidism. This can further be distinguished from hypoparathyroidism by the elevated BUN level.

A low plasma magnesium level can also produce tetany. In some cases of tetany, hypomagnesemia and hypocalcemia are both present. The tetany often cannot be corrected until the circulating magnesium level is brought to normal. Renal tubular acidosis (the Fanconi syndrome) can also produce tetany. In these circumstances there is a failure of resorption of certain amino acids.

TREATMENT. Postoperative Hypocalcemia. When mild, no treatment is needed, but careful, watchful waiting should be employed. Serum calcium levels should be determined every 12 hours for the first few days and then daily thereafter. If the patient becomes symptomatic, 1 Gm calcium gluconate can be given intravenously, and then 1 to 2 Gm/8 hours of this preparation may be dripped continuously in an intravenous bottle to alleviate all symptoms. Within several days all calcium therapy can usually be stopped.

For more persistent hypocalcemia, oral calcium is also begun in a dose of 1.5 to 2.0 Gm calcium ion per day. It is

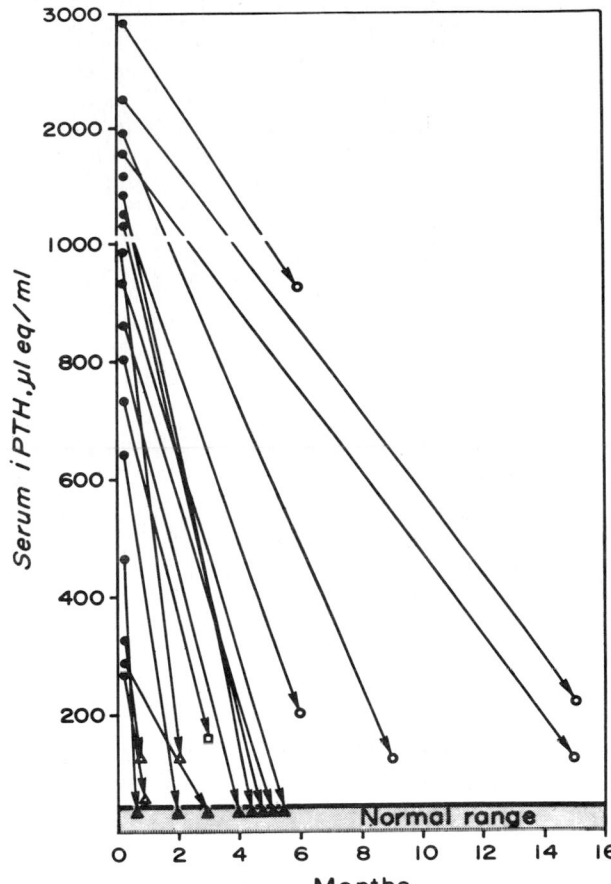

Fig. 38-59. Serum PTH concentrations before and after successful renal transplantation in patients with endogenous creatinine clearance of 60 ml/min/1.73 m² or greater. (*From W. J. Johnson et al., Med Clin North Am, 56:961, 1972.*)

important to note that to provide 1 Gm elemental calcium one must administer 5.5 Gm hydrated calcium chloride, 8 Gm calcium lactate, 11 Gm calcium gluconate, or 4 Gm calcium acetate. Calcium gluconate is palatable and therefore preferred. The patient may be sent home on oral calcium therapy when asymptomatic, and this can usually be discontinued after several weeks. It is preferable not to add vitamin D to this early regimen unless one strongly suspects that permanent hypoparathyroidism has occurred (or unless a parathyroid transplant has been performed).

If *permanent hypoparathyroidism* has occurred, in addition to the oral calcium therapy the patient is started on vitamin D_3, 50,000 to 100,000 units/day (1.25 to 2.5 mg/day). Others prefer to use dihydrotachysterol, 0.125 to 1.0 mg/day. In the future, metabolites of vitamin D_3 may prove more efficacious; however, they are not generally available at this time. The serum calcium concentration must be checked frequently, since some patients are insensitive to these preparations and need larger doses, whereas others develop vitamin D intoxication with severe hypercalcemia on relatively small dosages.

Serum PTH concentrations should be checked at intervals in patients being treated for permanent postoperative hypoparathyroidism. Several patients whom we have seen have been treated unnecessarily with vitamin D for many years because postoperative tetany had occurred. When serum PTH levels are detectable, vitamin D therapy should be slowly tapered and finally stopped if possible.

Other nonspecific factors may tend to influence the treatment of hypocalcemia. A diet high in phosphate or oxalate content should be avoided, since it may impair calcium absorption. Concomitant ingestion of anticonvulsants and tranquilizers may lower intestinal absorption of calcium both directly and by interfering with vitamin D metabolism. Estrogen and oral contraceptive therapy lower serum calcium level by suppressing bone resorption. Diuretics, such as furosemide, result in increased calcium excretion in the urine. Hypomagnesemia should be avoided since this leads to resistance to vitamin D therapy. Finally, the role of emotional stress in vitamin D resistance and hypocalcemia may be important.

Pseudohypoparathyroidism

Pseudohypoparathyroidism was first described by Albright et al. in 1942. This is a genetic disease in which the clinical and chemical features of hypoparathyroidism are present in association with the genetic stigmata of a round face, a short, thick body, and short, stubby fingers. There is a shortening of some of the metacarpal and metatarsal bones as a result of early epiphyseal closure, so that a dimple rather than a knuckle shows when the fist is clenched. Mental deficiency may be present, and there are sometimes areas of subcutaneous ossification. The manifestations are not due to lack of parathyroid secretion but to unresponsiveness of the end organ, the renal phosphaturic mechanism. The parathyroids are normal or hyperplastic, and serum PTH concentration is raised in these patients. There are hypocalcemia and hyperphosphatemia. Patients with this syndrome may show evidence of increased bone resorption and even osteitis fibrosa cystica, since PTH appears to act appropriately on bone but not on the kidney.

Pseudohypoparathyroidism can be distinguished from hypoparathyroidism not only by the characteristic physical picture of the patient but also because individuals with hypoparathyroidism respond to parathyroid extract while those with pseudohypoparathyroidism usually do not. The Ellsworth-Howard test has been designed to demonstrate this difference. The patient is slowly given 200 units of parathyroid extract intravenously, and the urinary phosphate excretion is determined for 3 hours before and 3 hours after the administration. The parathyroid extract produces a fivefold increase in urine phosphate excretion in normal persons, a tenfold increase in patients with hypoparathyroidism, and less than a twofold increase in patients with pseudohypoparathyroidism.

Recently it has been demonstrated that patients with pseudohypoparathyroidism have a deficient renal adenyl cyclase system. This offers a new diagnostic test for differentiating patients with idiopathic hypoparathyroidism from those with pseudohypoparathyroidism. In the former group, PTH administration results in increased urinary cyclic 3'5'-AMP, while in pseudohypoparathyroid patients PTH gives no change or only a slight increase in urinary cyclic AMP.

A high concentration of calcitonin has been found in the thyroid gland of some patients with this disease. This, however, appears to be the result of the hypocalcemia rather than its cause.

The treatment of pseudohypoparathyroidism is the same as that for hypoparathyroidism: low-phosphate diet, alumina gel, and vitamin D or its new metabolites.

Pseudopseudohypoparathyroidism

Pseudopseudohypoparathyroidism is also a genetic defect with the same physical features as pseudohypoparathyroidism. It differs from pseudohypoparathyroidism in that the plasma calcium and phosphate levels are normal and Chvostek's and Trousseau's signs are absent. The administration of PTH in one patient resulted in a normal rise in urinary cyclic AMP.

References

Thyroid: Anatomy

Durham, C. F., and Harrison, T. S.: The Surgical Anatomy of the Superior Laryngeal Nerve, *Surg Gynecol Obstet,* **118:**38, 1964.

Fish, J., and Moore, R. M.: Ectopic Thyroid Tissue and Ectopic Thyroid Carcinoma, *Ann Surg,* **157:**212, 1963.

Hung, W., Randolph, J. G., Sabatini, D., and Winship, T.: Lingual and Sublingual Thyroid Glands in Euthyroid Children, *Pediatrics,* **38:**647, 1966.

Hunt, P. S., Poole, M., and Reeve, T. S.: A Reappraisal of the Surgical Anatomy of the Thyroid and Parathyroid Glands, *Br J Surg,* **55:**63, 1968.

Riddell, V. H.: Injury to Recurrent Laryngeal Nerves during Thyroidectomy, *Lancet,* **2:**638, 1956.

Sloan, L. W.: Normal and Anomalous Development of the Thyroid, in S. C. Werner (ed.), "The Thyroid," chap. 19, Hoeber Medical Division, Harper & Row, Publishers, Incorporated, New York, 1955.

Ward, G. E., Cantrell, J. R., and Allan, W. B.: The Surgical Treatment of Lingual Thyroid, *Ann Surg,* **139:**536, 1954.

Thyroid: Physiology

Acland, J. D.: The Nature, Determination and Clinical Importance of Blood Iodine: A Review, *J Clin Pathol,* **2:**195, 1958.

Astwood, E. B., and Solomon, D. H.: Mechanisms of Action of Antithyroid Drugs, Iodides, and Other Thyroid Inhibitors, in S. C. Werner (ed.), "The Thyroid," chap. 6, Hoeber Medical Division, Harper & Row, Publishers, Incorporated, New York, 1955.

Burke, G.: Thyroid Stimulators and Thyroid Stimulation, *Acta Endocrinol (Kbh)* **66:**558, 1971.

DeGroot, L. J.: Current Views on the Formation of Thyroid Hormones, *N Engl J Med,* **272:**243, 1963.

———: Kinetic Analysis of Iodine Metabolism, *J Clin Endocrinol Metab,* **26:**149, 1966.

Greer, M. A.: Factors Regulating Triiodothyronine (T3) and Thyroxine (T4) in Blood, *Mayo Clin Proc,* **47:**944, 1972.

Hershman, J. M.: Hyperthyroidism Induced by Trophoblastic Thyrotropin, *Mayo Clin Proc,* **47:**913, 1972.

Hoch, F. L.: Biochemical Actions of Thyroid Hormones, *Physiol Rev,* **42:**605, 1962.

Ingbar, S. H.: Autoregulation of the Thyroid: Response to Iodide Excess and Depletion, *Mayo Clin Proc,* **47:**814, 1972.

――― and Woeber, K. A.: The Thyroid Gland, in R. H. Williams (ed.), "Textbook of Endocrinology," chap. 4, W. B. Saunders Company, Philadelphia, 1968.

Maloof, F., and Soodak, M.: Intermediary Metabolism of Thyroid Tissue and the Action of Drugs, *Physiol Rev,* **15:**43, 1963.

Means, J. H., DeGroot, L. J., and Stanbury, J. B.: "The Thyroid and Its Diseases," 3d ed., chaps. 2–4, McGraw-Hill Book Company, New York, 1963.

Reichlin, S.: Control of Thyrotropic Hormone Secretion, in L. Martini and W. F. Ganong (eds.), "Neuroendocrinology," Academic Press, Inc., New York, 1966.

Werner, S. C., and Ingbar, S. H.: "The Thyroid: A Fundamental and Clinical Text," 3d ed., Harper & Row, Publishers, Incorporated, New York, 1971.

Evaluation of Patients with Thyroid Disease

Alexander, W. D., Harden, R. McG., and Shimmins, J.: Thyroidal Suppression by Triiodothyronine as a Guide to Duration of Treatment of Thyrotoxicosis with Antithyroid Drugs, *Lancet,* **2:**1041, 1966.

Andrews, G. A., Sitterson, B. W., and Ross, D. A.: The Use of Scanning in Thyroid Cancer, in R. M. Kniseley, G. A. Andrews, and C. C. Harris (eds.), "Progress in Medical Radioisotope Scanning," chap. 15, Oak Ridge Institute of Nuclear Studies, Oak Ridge, Tenn., 1963.

Atkins, H. L., and Richards, P.: Assessment of Thyroid Function and Anatomy with Technetium-99m as Pertechnetate, *J Nucl Med,* **9:**7, 1968.

Becker, D. V., and Hurley, J. R.: The Impact of Technology on Clinical Practice in Graves' Disease, *Mayo Clin Proc,* **47:**835, 1972.

Boehme, E. J., Winship, T., Lindsay, S., and Kypridakis, G.: Evaluation of Needle Biopsy of Thyroid Gland, *Surg Gynecol Obstet,* **119:**831, 1964.

Gharib, H., Ryan, R. J., and Mayberry, W. E.: Triiodothyronine (T3) Radioimmunoassay: A Critical Evaluation, *Mayo Clin Proc,* **47:**934, 1972.

Mayberry, W. E., Gharib, H., Bilstad, J. M., and Sizemore, G. W.: Radioimmunoassay for Human Thyrotrophin: Clinical Value in Patients with Normal and Abnormal Thyroid Function, *Ann Intern Med,* **74:**471, 1971.

Meadows, P.: Thyroid Nodules, in R. M. Kniseley, G. A. Andrews, and C. C. Harris (eds.), "Progress in Medical Radioisotope Scanning," chap. 14, Oak Ridge Institute of Nuclear Studies, Oak Ridge, Tenn., 1963.

Means, J. H., DeGroot, L. J., and Stanbury, J. B.: "The Thyroid and Its Diseases," 3d ed., chap. 5, McGraw-Hill Book Company, New York, 1963.

Ormston, B. J., Garry, R., Cryer, R. J., Besser, G. M., and Hall, R.: Thyrotrophin-releasing Hormone as a Thyroid-Function Test, *Lancet,* **2:**10, 1971.

Riccabona, G.: "I^{125} in the Clinical Evaluation of Thyroid Disease," *N Engl J Med,* **273:**126, 1965.

Selenkow, H. A.: Tests for Circulating Thyroid Hormones, International Congress Series No. 227, Diagnosis and Treatment of Common Thyroid Diseases, in H. A. Selenkow and F. Hoffman (eds.), "Proceedings of a Symposium Held in San Francisco, California, U.S.A., March 6, 1970," Excerpta Medica Foundation, Amsterdam, 1971.

Solomon, D. H., Benotti, J., DeGroot, L. J., Greer, M. A., Pileggi, V. J., Pittman, J. A., Robbins, J., Selenkow, H. A., Sterling, K., and Volpe, R.: A Nomenclature for Tests of Thyroid Hormones in Serum: Report of a Committee of the American Thyroid Association, *J Clin Endocrinol Metab,* **34:**884, 1972.

Hyperthyroidism

Beahrs, O. H., Ryan, R. F., and White, R. A.: Complications of Thyroid Surgery, *J Clin Endocrinol Metab,* **16:**1456, 1956.

――― and Sakulsky, S. B.: Surgical Thyroidectomy in the Management of Exophthalmic Goiter, *Arch Surg,* **96:**512, 1968.

Bowers, R. F.: Hyperthyroidism: Comparative Results of Medical (I^{131}) and Surgical Therapy, *Ann Surg,* **162:**478, 1965.

Caswell, H. T., Robbins, R. R., and Rosemond, G. P.: Definitive Treatment of 536 Cases of Hyperthyroidism with I^{131} or Surgery, *Ann Surg,* **164:**593, 1966.

Goldsmith, R. E.: Radioisotope Therapy for Graves' Disease, *Mayo Clin Proc,* **47:**953, 1972.

Gould, E. A., Hirsch, E., and Brecher, I.: Complications Arising in the Course of Thyroidectomy, *Arch Surg,* **90:**81, 1965.

Green, M., and Wilson, G. M.: Thyrotoxicosis Treated by Surgery or Iodine 131 with Special Reference to Development of Hypothyroidism, *Br Med J,* **1:**1005, 1964.

Hales, I. B., and Rundle, F. F.: Ocular Changes in Graves' Disease: A Long-Term Follow-up Study, *Quart J Med,* **29:**113, 1960.

Hedley, A. J., Flemming, C. J., Chesters, M. I., Michie, W., and Crooks, J.: Surgical Treatment of Thyrotoxicosis, *Br Med J,* **1:**519, 1970.

Hollander, C. S., Nihei, N., Mitsuma, T., Scovill, C., and Gershengorn, M. C.: Elevated Serum Triiodothyronine in Association with Altered Available Iodide in Normal (NL) and Hyperthyroid Subjects, *Clin Res,* **19:**560, 1971.

Karlan, M. S., and Snyder, W. H.: Carcinoma of Thyroid following Treatment of Hyperthyroidism with I^{131}, *Calif Med,* **101:**196, 1964.

Michie, W., Pegg, C. A. S., and Bewsher, P. D.: Prediction of Hypothyroidism after Partial Thyroidectomy for Thyrotoxicosis, *Br Med J,* **1:**13, 1972.

Nofal, M. M., Beierwaltes, W. H., and Patno, M. E.: Treatment of Hyperthyroidism with Sodium Iodide I^{131}: A 16-year Experience, *JAMA,* **197:**695, 1966.

Ogura, J. H.: Transantral Orbital Decompression for Progressive Exophthalmos: A Follow-up of 54 Cases, *Med Clin North Am,* **52:**399, 1968.

Plested, W. G., III, and Pollock, W. F.: Radioactive Iodine, Antithyroid Drugs, and Surgery in Treatment of Hyperthyroidism, *Arch Surg,* **94:**517, 1967.

Riley, F. C.: Surgical Management of Ophthalmopathy in Graves' Disease: Transfrontal Orbital Decompression, *Mayo Clin Proc,* **47:**986, 1972.

Saenger, E. L., Thoma, G. E., and Tompkins, E. A.: Incidence of Leukemia following Treatment of Hyperthyroidism, *JAMA*, **205:**855, 1968.

Shapiro, S. J., Friedman, N. B., Perzik, S. L., and Catz, B.: Incidence of Thyroid Carcinoma in Graves' Disease, *Cancer*, **26:**1261, 1970.

Sheline, G. E., Lindsay, S., McCormack, K. R., and Galante, M.: Thyroid Nodules Occurring Late after Treatment of Thyrotoxicosis with Radioiodine, *J Clin Endocrinol Metab*, **22:**8, 1962.

Stanbury, J. B., and DeGroot, L. J.: Problems of Hypothyroidism after I^{131} Therapy of Hyperthyroidism, *N Engl J Med*, **271:**195, 1964.

Trotter, W. R.: "Diseases of the Thyroid," Blackwell Scientific Publications, Ltd., Oxford, 1962.

Volpé, R., Edmonds, M., Lamki, L., Clarke, P. V., and Row, V. V.: The Pathogenesis of Graves' Disease: A Disorder of Delayed Hypersensitivity? *Mayo Clin Proc*, **47:**824, 1972.

Wahner, H. W.: T3 Hyperthyroidism, *Mayo Clin Proc*, **47:**938, 1972.

Hypothyroidism

Ingbar, S. H., and Woeber, K. A.: The Thyroid Gland, in R. H. Williams (ed.), "Textbook of Endocrinology," 4th ed., chap. 4, W. B. Saunders Company, Philadelphia, 1968.

Means, J. H., DeGroot, L. J., and Stanbury, J. B.: "The Thyroid and Its Diseases," 3d ed., McGraw-Hill Book Company, New York, 1963.

Van Welsum, M., Feltkamp, T. E. W., DeVries, M. J., Doctor, R., Van Zijl, J., and Hennemann, G.: Hypoparathyroidism after Thyroidectomy for Graves' Disease: Search for an Explanation, *Br Med J*, **4:**755, 1974.

Thyroiditis

Altemeier, W. A.: Acute Pyogenic Thyroiditis, *Arch Surg*, **61:**76, 1950.

Beahrs, O. H., Woolner, L. B., Engel, S., and McConahey, W. M.: Needle Biopsy of the Thyroid Gland and Management of Lymphocytic Thyroiditis, *Surg Gynecol Obstet*, **114:**636, 1962.

Block, M. A., Horn, R. C., Jr., and Miller, J. M.: Unilateral Thyroid Nodules with Lymphocytic Thyroiditis, *Arch Surg*, **87:**118, 1963.

Coons, A. H., and Kaplan, M. H.: Localization of Antigen in Tissue Cells: Improvements in Method for Detection of Antigen by Means of Fluorescent Antibody, *J Exp Med*, **91:**1, 1950.

Crile, G., Jr., and Hazard, J. B.: Incidence of Cancer in Struma Lymphomatosa, *Surg Gynecol Obstet*, **115:**101, 1962.

Greene, J. N.: Subacute Thyroiditis, *Am J Med*, **51:**97, 1971.

Hagan, A. D., Goffinet, J., and Davis, J. W.: Acute Streptococcal Thyroiditis, *JAMA*, **202:**842, 1967.

Hashimoto, H.: Zur Kenntriss der lymphomatösen Veränderung der Schilddrüse (Struma lymphomatosa), *Langenbecks Arch Klin Chir*, **97:**219, 1912.

Heimann, P.: Treatment of Thyroiditis, *Acta Med Scand*, **187:**323, 1970.

Hendrick, J. W.: Diagnosis and Treatment of Thyroiditis, *Ann Surg*, **144:**176, 1956.

Hirabayashi, R. N., and Lindsay, S.: The Relation of Thyroid Carcinoma and Chronic Thyroiditis, *Surg Gynecol Obstet*, **121:**243, 1965.

Linden, M. C., Jr., and Clark, J. H.: Indications for Surgery in Thyroiditis, *Am J Surg*, **118:**829, 1969.

Mikal, S.: Hashimoto's Disease, *Surg Gynecol Obstet*, **121:**131, 1965.

Mulhern, L. M., Masi, A. T., and Shulman, L. E.: Hashimoto's Disease: A Search for Associated Disorders in 170 Clinically Detected Cases, *Lancet*, **2:**508, 1966.

Persson, P. S.: Cytodiagnosis of Thyroiditis: A Comparative Study of Cytological, Histological, Immunological, and Clinical Findings in Thyroiditis, Particularly in Diffuse Lymphoid Thyroiditis, *Acta Med Scand [Suppl]* 483, 1968.

Pollack, W. F., David, H., and Sprong, O. H., Jr.: The Rationale of Thyroidectomy for Hashimoto's Thyroiditis, *Western J Surg Obstet Gynecol*, **66:**17, 1958.

Quervain, F. de: Die akute, nicht eiterige Thyroiditis, *Mitt Grenzgeb Med Chir [Suppl]*, **2:**1, 1904.

Roitt, I. M., Doniach, D., Campbell, P. N., and Hudson, R. V.: Auto-antibodies in Hashimoto's Disease, *Lancet*, **2:**820, 1956.

Rudman, I., Novota, O. J., and Keener, R. L.: Complications of Hashimoto Thyroiditis Surgery, *Arch Surg*, **83:**822, 1961.

Swann, N. H.: Acute Thyroiditis: A Clinical Report of Twelve Cases within a Four-Month Period, *Ann Intern Med*, **56:**68, 1962.

Volpé, R., Johnston, M. W., and Huber, N.: Thyroid Function in Subacute Thyroiditis, *J Clin Endocrinal Metab*, **18:**65, 1958.

Witebsky, E., Rose, N. R., Terplan, K., Paine, J. R., and Egan, R. W.: Chronic Thyroiditis and Autoimmunization, *JAMA*, **165:**1439, 1957.

Goiter

Astwood, E. B., Cassidy, C. E., and Aurbach, G. D.: Treatment of Goiter and Thyroid Nodules with Thyroid, *JAMA*, **174:**459, 1960.

Cole, W. H., Majarakis, J. D., and Slaughter, D. P.: Incidence of Carcinoma of the Thyroid in Nodular Goiter, *J Clin Endocrinol Metab*, **9:**1007, 1949.

Crile, G., Jr.: Treatment of Thyroid Cysts by Aspiration, *Surgery*, **59:**210, 1966.

Dobyns, B. M.: Goiter, *Curr Probl Surg*, January 1969.

Glassford, G. H., Fowler, E. F., and Cole, W. H.: The Treatment of Nontoxic Nodular Goiter with Dessicated Thyroid: Results and Evaluation, *Surgery*, **58:**621, 1965.

Ingbar, S. H., and Woeber, K. A.: The Thyroid Gland, in R. H. Williams (ed.), "Textbook of Endocrinology," W. B. Saunders Company, Philadelphia, 1968.

Jenny, H., Block, M. A., Horn, R. C., and Miller, J. M.: Recurrence following Surgery for Benign Thyroid Nodules, *Arch Surg*, **92:**525, 1966.

Liechty, R. D., Graham, M., and Freemeyer, P.: Benign Solitary Thyroid Nodules, *Surg Gynecol Obstet*, **121:**571, 1965.

Robinson, E., Horn, Y., and Hochmann, A.: Incidence of Cancer in Thyroid Nodules, *Surg Gynecol Obstet*, **123:**1024, 1966.

Shimaoka, K., Badillo, J., Sokal, J. E., and Marchetta, F. C.: Clinical Differentiation between Thyroid Cancer and Benign Goiter, *JAMA*, **181:**179, 1962.

Sokal, J. E.: The Incidence of Thyroid Cancer and the Problem of Malignancy in Nodular Goiter, in E. B. Astwood (ed.),

"Clinical Endocrinology," vol. I, Grune & Stratton, Inc., New York, 1960.

Benign Tumors

Ackerman, L. V.: "Surgical Pathology," The C. V. Mosby Company, St. Louis, 1964.

Means, J. H., DeGroot, L. J., and Stanbury, J. B.: "The Thyroid and Its Diseases," 3d ed., McGraw-Hill Book Company, New York, 1963.

Malignant Tumors

Beahrs, O. H., and Pasternak, B. M.: Cancer of the Thyroid Gland, *Curr Probl Surg,* December 1969.

Black, B. M., YaDeau, R. E., and Woolner, L. B.: Surgical Treatment of Thyroidal Carcinomas, *Arch Surg,* **88:**610, 1964.

Block, M. A., Horn, R. C., Jr., Miller, J. M., Barrett, J. L., and Brush, B. E.: Familial Medullary Carcinoma of the Thyroid, *Ann Surg,* **166:**403, 1967.

———, and ———: Medullary Carcinoma of the Thyroid: Surgical Implications, *Arch Surg,* **96:**521, 1968.

———, and ———: Thyroid Carcinoma with Cervical Lymph Node Metastasis: Effectiveness of Total Thyroidectomy and Node Dissection, *Am J Surg,* **122:**458, 1971.

———, Jackson, C. E., and Tashjian, A. H., Jr.: Medullary Thyroid Carcinoma Detected by Serum Calcitonin Assay, *Arch Surg,* **104:**579, 1972.

Buckwalter, J. A., and Thomas, C. G., Jr.: Selection of Surgical Treatment for Well Differentiated Thyroid Carcinomas, *Ann Surg,* **176:**565, 1972.

Crile, G., Jr.: The Fallacy of the Conventional Radical Neck Dissection for Papillary Carcinoma of the Thyroid, *Ann Surg,* **145:**317, 1957.

———: Papillary Carcinoma of the Thyroid, in E. B. Astwood (ed.), "Clinical Endocrinology," vol. I, Grune & Stratton, Inc., New York, 1960.

———: Late Results of Treatment for Papillary Cancer of the Thyroid, *Ann Surg,* **160:**178, 1964.

———: Lymphosarcoma and Reticulum Cell Sarcoma of the Thyroid, *Surg Gynecol Obstet,* **116:**449, 1963.

———: Changing End Results in Patients with Papillary Carcinoma of the Thyroid, *Surg Gynecol Obstet,* **132:**460, 1971.

———, Suhrer, J. G., Jr., and Hazard, J. B.: Results of Conservative Operations for Malignant Tumors of the Thyroid, *J Clin Endocrinol Metab,* **15:**1422, 1955.

Doniach, I.: Aetiological Consideration of Thyroid Carcinoma, in D. Smithers (ed.), "Tumours of the Thyroid Gland," p. 55, E. & S. Livingstone, London, 1970.

Duffy, B. J.: Can Radiation Cause Thyroid Cancer? *J Clin Endocrinol Metab,* **17:**1383, 1957.

Frazell, E. L., and Duffy, B. J.: Invasive Papillary Cancer of the Thyroid, *J Clin Endocrinol Metab,* **14:**1362, 1954.

——— and Foote, F. W.: Papillary Cancer of the Thyroid: A Review of 25 Years of Experience, *Cancer,* **11:**895, 1958.

Freund, H. R.: Surgical Treatment of Metastases to the Thyroid Gland from Other Primary Malignancies, *Ann Surg,* **162:**285, 1965.

Glass, H. G., Waldron, G. W., Allen, H. C., Jr., and Brown,

W. G.: A Rational Approach to the Thyroid Malignancy Problem, *Am Surg,* **26:**81, 1960.

Gowing, N. F. C.: The Pathology and Natural History of Thyroid Tumours, in D. Smithers (ed.), "Tumours of the Thyroid Gland," p. 103, E. & S. Livingstone, London, 1970.

Harness, J. K., Thompson, N. W., Sisson, J. C., and Beierwaltes, W. H.: Differentiated Thyroid Carcinomas: Treatment of Distant Metastases, *Arch Surg,* **108:**410, 1974.

Hill, C. S., Clark, R. L., and Wolf, M.: The Effect of Subsequent Pregnancy on Patients with Thyroid Carcinoma, *Surg Gynecol Obstet,* **122:**1219, 1966.

Hirabayashi, R. N., and Lindsay, S.: Carcinoma of the Thyroid Gland: A Statistical Study of 390 Patients, *J Clin Endocrinol Metab,* **21:**1596, 1961.

Kaplan, E. L., and Peskin, G. W.: Physiologic Implications of Medullary Carcinoma of the Thyroid Gland, *Surg Clin North Am,* **51:**125, 1971.

Klopp, C. T., Rosvoll, R. V., and Winship, T.: Is Destructive Surgery Ever Necessary for Treatment of Thyroid Cancer in Children? *Ann Surg,* **165:**745, 1967.

McDermott, W. V., Jr., Morgan, W. S., Hamlin, E., Jr., and Cope, O.: Cancer of the Thyroid, *J Clin Endocrinol Metab,* **14:**1336, 1954.

Marchetta, F. C., and Sako, K.: Modified Neck Dissection for Carcinoma of the Thyroid Gland, *Surg Gynecol Obstet,* **119:**551, 1964.

Medina, R. G., and Elliott, D. W.: Thyroid Carcinoma: An Analysis of 130 Cases, *Arch Surg,* **97:**239, 1968.

Mikal, S.: Primary Lymphoma of the Thyroid Gland, *Surgery,* **55:**233, 1964.

Sedgwick, C. E., and Konvolinka, C. W.: Management of Carcinoma of the Thyroid, *Surg Clin North Am,* **47:**607, 1967.

Shapiro, S. J., Friedman, N. B., Perzik, S. L., and Catz, B.: Incidence of Thyroid Carcinoma in Graves' Disease, *Cancer,* **26:**1261, 1970.

Silverberg, S. G., and Vidone, R. A.: Carcinoma of the Thyroid in Surgical and Postmortem Material: Analysis of 300 Cases at Autopsy and Literature Review, *Ann Surg,* **164:**291, 1966.

Sipple, J. H.: The Association of Pheochromocytoma with Carcinoma of the Thyroid Gland, *Am J Med,* **31:**163, 1961.

Smithers, D. W.: Malignant Lymphomas of the Thyroid Gland, in D. Smithers (ed.), "Tumours of the Thyroid Gland," p. 141, E. & S. Livingstone, London, 1970.

Tollefsen, H. R., and DeCosse, J. J.: Papillary Carcinoma of the Thyroid: Recurrence in the Thyroid Gland after Initial Surgical Treatment, *Am J Surg,* **106:**728, 1963.

Wells, S. A., Jr., Ontjes, D. A., Cooper, C. W., Hennessy, J. F., Ellis, G. J., McPherson, H. T., and Sabiston, D. C., Jr.: Early Diagnosis of Medullary Carcinoma of the Thyroid Gland in Patients with Multiple Endocrine Neoplasia Type II, *Ann Surg,* **182:**362, 1975.

Williams, E. D.: The Origin and Associations of Medullary Carcinoma of the Thyroid, in D. Smithers (ed.), "Tumours of the Thyroid Gland," p. 130, E. & S. Livingstone, London, 1970.

Wychulis, A. R., Beahrs, O. H., and Woolner, L. B.: Metastasis of Carcinoma to the Thyroid Gland, *Ann Surg,* **160:**169, 1964.

———, ———, and ———: Papillary Carcinoma with Associated Anaplastic Carcinoma in the Thyroid Gland, *Surg Gynecol Obstet,* **120:**28, 1965.

Surgery of the Thyroid

Adams, H. D.: Transthoracic Thyroidectomy, *J Thorac Cardiov Surg,* **19:**741, 1950.

Block, M. A., Jackson, C. E., and Tashjian, A. H.: Management of Parathyroid Glands in Surgery for Medullary Thyroid Carcinoma, *Arch Surg,* **110:**617, 1975.

Buckwalter, J. A., Soper, R. T., Davies, J., and Mason, E. E.: Postoperative Hypoparathyroidism, *Surg Gynecol Obstet,* **101:**657, 1955.

Chamberlin, J. A., Fries, J. G., and Allen, H. C., Jr.: Thyroid Carcinoma and the Problem of Postoperative Tetany, *Surgery,* **55:**787, 1964.

Colcock, B. P.: Surgery of Primary Hyperthyroidism, *Surg Clin North Am,* **40:**595, 1960.

——— and King, M. L.: The Mortality and Morbidity of Thyroid Surgery, *Surg Gynecol Obstet,* **114:**131, 1962.

Cope, O.: Surgery of the Thyroid, in J. H. Means, L. J. DeGroot, and J. B. Stanbury, "The Thyroid and Its Diseases," 3d ed., McGraw-Hill Book Company, New York, 1963.

Doyle, P. J., Everts, E. C., and Brummett, R. E.: Treatment of Recurrent Laryngeal Nerve Injury, *Arch Surg,* **96:**517, 1968.

Gould, E. A., Hirsch, E., and Brecher, I.: Complications Arising in the Course of Thyroidectomy, *Arch Surg,* **90:**81, 1965.

Halsted, W. S., and Evans, H. M.: The Parathyroid Glandules: Their Blood Supply and Preservation in Operations upon the Thyroid Gland, *Ann Surg,* **46:**489, 1907.

Hawe, P., and Lothian, K. R.: Recurrent Laryngeal Nerve Injury during Thyroidectomy, *Surg Gynecol Obstet,* **110:**488, 1960.

Holl-Allen, R. T. J.: Haemorrhage following Thyroidectomy for Thyrotoxicosis, *Br J Surg,* **54:**703, 1967.

Johnston, J. H., and Twente, G. E.: Surgical Approach to Intrathoracic (Mediastinal) Goiter, *Ann Surg,* **143:**572, 1956.

Lahey, F. H.: Routine Dissection and Demonstration of Recurrent Laryngeal Nerve in Subtotal Thyroidectomy, *Surg Gynecol Obstet,* **66:**775, 1938.

———: Intrathoracic Goiters, *Surg Clin North Am,* **25:**609, 1945.

——— and Hoover, W. B.: Tracheotomy after Thyroidectomy, *Ann Surg,* **133:**65, 1951.

Lee, T. C., Coffey, R. J., Mackin, J., Cobb, M., Routon, J., and Canary, J. J.: Use of Propranolol in Surgical Treatment of Thyrotoxic Patients, *Ann Surg,* **177:**643, 1973.

Perzik, S. L.: "Surgery in Thyroid Disease," Stratton Intercontinental Medical Book Corporation, New York, 1976.

Pimstone, B., and Joffe, B.: Use and Abuse of β-Adrenergic Blockade in Surgery of Hyperthyroidism, *S Afr Med J,* **44:**1059, 1970.

Smith, R. N., and Laljee, H. C. K.: Thyrocalcitonin Deficiency after Treatment of Thyroid Disorders by Surgery or Radioiodine, *Br Med J,* **4:**589, 1967.

Thompson, N. W., and Harness, J. K.: Complications of Total Thyroidectomy for Carcinoma, *Surg Gynecol Obstet,* **131:**861, 1970.

———, Olsen, W. R., and Hoffman, G. L.: The Continuing Development of the Technique of Thyroidectomy, *Surgery,* **73:**913, 1973.

Wade, J. S. H.: Three Major Complications of Thyroidectomy, *Br J Surg,* **52:**727, 1965.

Watkins, E., Jr., Bell, G. O., Snow, J. C., and Adams, H. D.: Incidence and Current Management of Post-thyroidectomy Hypoparathyroidism: Histologic Evidence of Rejection of Neonatal Aortic Pedicle Parathyroid Gland Homotransplants, *JAMA,* **182:**138, 1962.

Parathyroid: Embryology and Anatomy

Block, M. A., Miller, M., and Horn, R. C.: Minimizing Hypoparathyroidism after Extended Thyroid Operations, *Surg Gynecol Obstet,* **123:**501, 1966.

Durham, C. T., and Harrison, T. S.: The Surgical Anatomy of the Superior Laryngeal Nerve, *Surg Gynecol Obstet,* **118:**38, 1964.

Gilmour, J. R.: The Embryology of the Parathyroid Glands, the Thymus and Certain Associated Rudiments, *J Pathol,* **45:**507, 1937.

———: The Weight of the Parathyroid Glands, *J Pathol Bacteriol,* **44:**431, 1937.

———: The Gross Anatomy of the Parathyroid Glands, *J Pathol Bacteriol,* **46:**133, 1938.

Hunt, P. S., Poole, M., and Reeve, T. S.: A Reappraisal of the Surgical Anatomy of the Thyroid and Parathyroid Glands, *Br J Surg,* **55:**63, 1968.

State, D.: The Enlarged Inferior Thyroid Artery: A Valuable Guide in Surgery of Parathyroid Adenomas, *Surgery,* **56:**461, 1964.

Parathyroid Hormone: Chemistry

Brewer, H. B., Fairwell, T., Ronan, R., Sizemore, G. W., and Arnaud, C. D.: Human Parathyroid Hormone: Amino-Acid Sequence of the Amino-Terminal Residues 1–34, *Proc Nat Acad Sci USA,* **69:**3585, 1972.

———, and Ronan, R.: The Amino Acid Sequence of Bovine Parathyroid Hormone, *Proc Nat Acad Sci USA,* **67:**1862, 1970.

Habener, J. F., Potts, J. T., Jr., and Rich, A.: Pre-Proparathyroid Hormone. Evidence for an Early Biosynthetic Precursor of Proparathyroid Hormone, *J Biol Chem,* **251:**3893, 1976.

Kemper, B., Habener, J. F., Ernst, M. D., Potts, J. T., Jr., and Rich, A.: Pre-proparathyroid Hormone Analysis of Radioactive Tryptic Peptides and Amino Acid Sequence, *Biochemistry,* **15:**15, 1976.

Keutmann, H. T., Aurbach, G. D., Dawson, B. F., Niall, H. D., Deftos, L. J., and Potts, J. T., Jr.: Isolation and Characterization of Bovine Parathyroid Isohormones, *Biochemistry,* **10:**2779, 1971.

Niall, H. D., Keutmann, H. T., Sauer, R., Hogan, M. L., Dawson, B. F., Aurbach, G. D., and Potts, J. T., Jr.: The Amino Acid Sequence of Bovine Parathyroid Hormone I, Hoppe-Seyler's Z, *Physiol Chem,* **351:**1586, 1970.

Potts, J. T., Jr., Murray, T. M., Peacock, M., et al.: Parathyroid Hormone: Sequence, Synthesis, Immunoassay Studies, *Am J Med,* **50:**639, 1971.

———, Tregear, G. W., Keutmann, H. T., Niall, H. D., Sauer, R., Deftos, L. J., Dawson, B. F., Hogan, M. L., and Aurbach, G. D.: Synthesis of a Biologically Active N-terminal Tetratriacontapeptide of Parathyroid Hormone, *Proc Nat Acad Sci USA,* **68:**63, 1971.

Parathyroid: Vitamin D

Brickman, A. S., Coburn, J. W., and Norman, A. W.: Action of 1,25-dihydroxycholecalciferol: A Potent, Kidney Produced

Metabolite of Vitamin D_3 in Uremic Man, *N Engl J Med,* **287**:891, 1972.

DeLuca, H. F.: Vitamin D: The Vitamin and the Hormone, *Fed Proc,* **33**:2211, 1974.

————: Vitamin D Endocrinology, *Ann Intern Med,* **85**:367, 1976.

Kodicek, E.: The Story of Vitamin D, from Vitamin to Hormone, *Lancet,* **1**:325, 1974.

Lawson, D. E. M., Fraser, D. M., Kodicek, E., et al.: Identification of 1,25-dihydroxycholecalciferol: A New Kidney Hormone Controlling Calcium Metabolism, *Nature (Lond),* **230**:228, 1971.

Teitelbaum, S. L., Bone, J. M., Stein, P. M., Gilden, J. J., Bates, M., Boisseau, V. C., and Avioli, L. V.: Calcifediol in Chronic Renal Insufficiency, *JAMA,* **235**:164, 1976.

Calcitonin and Medullary Carcinoma of the Thyroid

Aliapoulios, M. A., Goldhaber, P., and Munson, P. L.: Thyrocalcitonin Inhibition of Bone Resorption Induced by Parathyroid Hormone in Tissue Culture, *Science,* **151**:330, 1966.

Arnaud, C. D., Littledike, T., and Tsao, H. S.: Calcium Homeostasis and the Simultaneous Measurement of Calcitonin and Parathyroid Hormone in the Pig, in S. Taylor (ed.): "Calcitonin 1969: Proceedings of the Second International Symposium, London, 1970," pp. 95–101, William Heinemann Medical Books, Ltd., 1970.

————, ————, and Kaplan, E. L.: Radioimmunoassay for Calcitonin: A Preliminary Report, *Proc Staff Meetings Mayo Clin,* **43**:496, 1968.

Beahrs, O. H., and Pasternak, B. M.: Cancer of the Thyroid Gland, *Curr Probl Surg,* December 1969.

Copp, D. H., Cameron, E. C., Cheney, B. A., Davidson, A. G. F., and Henze, K. G.: Evidence for Calcitonin: A New Hormone from the Parathyroid That Lowers Blood Calcium, *Endocrinology,* **70**:638, 1962.

————, Cockcroft, D. W., and Kueh, Y.: Calcitonin from Ultimobranchial Glands of Dogfish and Chickens, *Science,* **158**:924, 1967.

Deftos, L. J., Bury, A. E., Habener, J. F., Singer, F. R., and Potts, J. T., Jr.: Immunoassay for Human Calcitonin: II. Clinical Studies, *Metabolism,* **20**:1129, 1971.

Gonzalez-Licea, A., Hartmann, W. H., and Yardley, J. H.: Medullary Carcinoma of the Thyroid: Ultrastructural Evidence of Its Origin from the Parafollicular Cell and Its Possible Relation to Carcinoid Tumors, *J Clin Pathol,* **49**:512, 1968.

Hazard, J. B., Hawk, W. A., and Crile, G., Jr.: Medullary (Solid) Carcinoma of the Thyroid: Clinicopathological Entity, *J Clin Endocrinol Metab,* **19**:152, 1959.

Hennessy, J. F., Wells, S. A., Jr., Ontjes, D. A., and Cooper, C. W.: A Comparison of Pentagastrin Injection and Calcium Infusion as Provocative Test for the Detection of Medullary Carcinoma of the Thyroid, *J Clin Endocrinol Metab,* **39**:487, 1974.

Hirsch, P. F., Gauthier, G. F., and Munson, P. L.: Thyroid Hypocalcemic Principle and Recurrent Laryngeal Nerve Injury as Factors Affecting the Response to Parathyroidectomy in Rats, *Endocrinology,* **73**:244, 1963.

Kaplan, E. L.: Recent Advances in Calcium Metabolism: Application to Medullary Carcinoma of Thyroid and Hyperparathyroidism, *Surg Annu,* 1973.

————, and Peskin, G. W.: Physiologic Implications of Medullary

Carcinoma of the Thyroid Gland, *Surg Clin North Am,* **51**:125, 1971.

Ljungberg, O.: On Medullary Carcinoma of the Thyroid, *Acta Patholog Microbiol Scand [A] Suppl* 231, 1972.

Melvin, K. E. W., Tashjian, A. H., Jr., and Miller, H. H.: Studies in Familial (Medullary) Thyroid Carcinoma, *Recent Prog Horm Res,* **28**:399, 1972.

Pearse, A. G. E., and Polak, J. M.: Cytochemical Evidence for the Neural Crest Origin of Mammalian Ultimobranchial C cells, *Histochemie,* **27**:96, 1971.

Potts, J. T., Jr., Niall, H. D. Keutmann, H. T., and Lequin, R. M.: Chemistry of the Calcitonins: Species Variation plus Structure-Activity Relations, and Pharmacologic Implications, in R. V. Talmage and P. L. Munson (eds.), "Calcium, Parathyroid Hormone and the Calcitonins," pp. 121–127. Excerpta Medica, Amsterdam, 1972.

Queener, S. F., and Bell, N. H.: Calcitonin: A General Survey, *Metabolism,* **24**:555, 1975.

Tashjian, A. H., Jr., Howland, B. G., Melvin, K. E. W., and Hill, C. S., Jr.: Immunoassay for Human Calcitonin: Clinical Measurement, Relation to Serum Calcium and Studies in Patients with Medullary Carcinoma, *N Engl J Med,* **283**:890, 1970.

Wells, S. A., Jr., Ontjes, D. A., Cooper, C. W., Hennessy, J. F., Ellis, G. J., McPherson, H. T., and Sabiston, D. C., Jr.: The Early Diagnosis of Medullary Carcinoma of the Thyroid Gland in Patients with Multiple Endocrine Neoplasia, Type II, *Ann Surg,* **182**:362, 1975.

Wolfe, H. J., Melvin, K. E. W., Cervi-Skinner, S. J., Al Saadi, A. A., Juliar, J. F., Jackson, C. E., and Tashjian, A. H., Jr.: C-Cell Hyperplasia Preceding Medullary Thyroid Carcinoma, *N Engl J Med,* **289**:437, 1973.

Parathyroid: Pathology

Black, W. C., III.: Correlative Light and Electron Microscopy in Primary Hyperparathyroidism, *Arch Pathol,* **88**:225, 1969.

———— and Haff, R. C.: The Surgical Pathology of Parathyroid Chief Cell Hyperplasia, *Am J Clin Pathol,* **53**:565, 1970.

Castleman, B.: Tumors of the Parathyroid Glands, in "Atlas of Tumor Pathology," Fascicle 15, p. 1, Armed Forces Institute of Pathology, Washington, 1952.

Cope, O., Keynes, W. M., Roth, S. I., and Castleman, B.: Primary Chief-Cell Hyperplasia of the Parathyroid Glands: A New Entity in the Surgery of Hyperparathyroidism, *Ann Surg,* **148**:375, 1958.

Hall, E. M., and Chaffin, L.: Final Report of a Case of Malignant Adenoma of the Parathyroid Glands, *Western J Surg,* **48**:685, 1940.

Hellstrom, J., and Ivemark, B. I.: Primary Hyperparathyroidism: Clinical and Structural Findings in 138 Cases, *Acta Chir Scand [Suppl],* **294**:1, 1962.

Holmes, E. C., Morton, D. L., and Ketcham, A. S.: Parathyroid Carcinoma: A Collective Review, *Ann Surg,* **169**:631, 1969.

Holzmann, K., and Lange, R.: Zur Zytologie der Glandula parathyroeidea des Menschen: Weitere Untersuchungen an Epithelkörperadenomen, *Z. Zellforsch* **58**:759, 1963.

Roth, S. I.: Pathology of the Parathyroids in Hyperparathyroidism: Discussion of Recent Advances in the Anatomy and Pathology of the Parathyroid Glands, *Arch Path (Chicago)* **73**:495, 1962.

———: The Ultrastructure of Primary Water-clear Cell Hyperplasia of the Parathyroid Glands, *Amer J Path,* **61**:233, 1970.

———: Recent Advances in Parathyroid Gland Pathology, *Amer J Med,* **50**:612, 1971.

——— and Marshall, R. B.: Pathology and Ultrastructure of the Human Parathyroid Glands in Chronic Renal Failure, *Arch Intern Med,* (*Chicago*) **124**:397, 1969.

Schantz, A., and Castleman, B.: Parathyroid Carcinoma: A Study of 70 Cases, *Cancer,* **31**:600, 1973.

Steiner, A. L., Goodman, A. D., and Powers, S. R.: Study of a Kindred with Pheochromocytoma, Medullary Thyroid Carcinoma, Hyperparathyroidism and Cushing's Disease: Multiple Endocrine Neoplasia, Type 2, *Medicine* (*Balt*) **47**:371, 1968.

Utley, J. R., and Black, W. C.: Hyperparathyroidism: A Clinicopathologic Evaluation, *Amer J Surg,* **114**:788, 1967.

Wermer, P.: Endocrine Adenomatosis and Peptic Ulcer in a Large Kindred: Inherited Multiple Tumors and Mosaic Pleiotropism in Man, *Amer J Med,* **35**:205, 1963.

Primary Hyperparathyroidism

Arnaud, C. D., Goldsmith, R., Bischoff, J., Sizemore, G., Oldham, S., and Larsen, J.: Antibody Specificity, Immunochemical Heterogeneity and the Interpretation of Measurements of Plasma Parathyroid Hormone by Radioimmunoassay, *J Clin Invest,* **51**:5a, 1972.

———, Sizemore, G. W., Oldham, S. B., Fischer, J. A., Tsao, H. S., and Littledike, E. T.: Human Parathyroid Hormone: Glandular and Secreted Molecular Species, *Am J Med,* **50**:630, 1971.

———, Tsao, H. S., and Littledike, T.: Radioimmunoassay of Human Parathyroid Hormone in Serum, *J Clin Invest,* **50**:21, 1971.

Aurbach, G. D., and Chase, L. R.: Cyclic 3′5′-Adenylic Acid in Bone and the Mechanism of Action of Parathyroid Hormone, *Fed Proc,* **29**:1179, 1970.

Ballard, H. S., Frame, B., and Hartsock, R. J.: Familial Multiple Endocrine Adenoma-Peptic Ulcer Complex, *Medicine* (*Baltimore*), **43**:481, 1964.

Barreras, R. F., and Donaldson, R. M., Jr.: Role of Calcium in Gastric Hypersecretion, Parathyroid Adenoma and Peptic Ulcer, *N Engl J Med,* **276**:1122, 1967.

Barzel, U. S.: Parathyroid Hormone and the Buffering Function of Bone, *Hosp Practice,* **6**:131, 1971.

Bélanger, L. F., Robichon, J., Migicovsky, B. B., et al.: Resorption without Osteoclasts (Osteolysis), in R. F. Sognnaes, (ed.), "Mechanisms of Hard Tissue Destruction," p. 531, American Association for the Advancement of Science, Washington, 1963.

Bernstein, D. S.: Hypercalcemia Associated with Sarcoidosis, Hypernephroma, and Parathyroid Adenoma, *J Clin Endocrinol Metab,* **25**:1436, 1965.

Black, B. K.: Carcinoma of the Parathyroid, *Ann Surg,* **139**:355, 1954.

Black, W. C., III, and Utley, J. R.: The Differential Diagnosis of Parathyroid Adenoma and Chief Cell Hyperplasia, *Am J Clin Pathol,* **49**:761, 1968.

Block, M. A., Frame, B., Jackson, C. E., et al.: The Extent of Operation for Primary Hyperparathyroidism, *Arch Surg,* **109**:798, 1974.

———, ———, ———, et al.: Primary Diffuse Microscopical Hyperplasia of the Parathyroid Glands, *Arch Surg,* **111**:348, 1976.

Bruining, H. A.: "Surgical Treatment of Hyperparathyroidism," Assen, The Netherlands, Charles C Thomas, Publisher, Springfield, Ill., 1971.

Buckle, R. M., Smith, F. G., and Alexander, D. P.: Assessment of Parathyroid Glandular Activity in the Foetus, in R. V. Talmadge and P. L. Munson (eds.), "Calcium, Parathyroid Hormone and the Calcitonins," p. 127, Excerpta Medica, Amsterdam, 1972.

Cameron, J. R., and Sorenson, J.: Measurement of Bone Mineral In Vivo: An Improved Method, *Science,* **142**:230, 1963.

Canterbury, J. M., and Reiss, E.: Fractionation of Circulating Parathyroid Hormone (PTH) in Man, *J Lab Clin Med,* **78**:814, 1971.

Chase, L. R., and Aurbach, G. D.: Renal Adenyl Cyclase: Anatomically Separate Sites for Parathyroid Hormone and Vasopressin, *Science,* **159**:545, 1968.

Chaves-Carballo, E., and Hayles, A. B.: Parathyroid Adenoma in Children, *Am J Dis Child,* **112**:553, 1966.

Clark, O. H., and Taylor, S.: Persistent and Recurrent Hyperparathyroidism, *Br J Surg,* **59**:555, 1972.

———, Way, L. W., and Hunt, T. K.: Recurrent Hyperparathyroidism, *Ann Surg,* **184**:391, 1976.

Clunie, G. J. A., Gunn, A., and Robson, J. S.: Hyperparathyroid Crisis, *Br J Surg,* **54**:538, 1967.

Condon, R. E., Granville, G. E., Jordon, P. H., and Helgason, A. H.: Hypercalcemic Crisis and Intractable Gastrointestinal Ulceration in a Patient with Endocrine Polyglandular Syndrome, *Ann Surg,* **167**:185, 1968.

Cope, O.: The Study of Hyperparathyroidism at the Massachusetts General Hospital, *N Engl J Med,* **274**:1174, 1966.

Cushing, H., and Davidoff, L. M.: "The Pathological Findings in Four Autopsied Cases of Acromegaly with a Discussion of Their Significance," Monograph 22, The Rockefeller Institute for Medical Research, New York, 1927.

Cutler, R. E., Reiss, E., and Ackerman, L. V.: Familial Hyperparathyroidism: A Kindred Involving Eleven Cases with a Discussion of Primary Chief-Cell Hyperplasia, *N Engl J Med,* **270**:859, 1964.

Davies, D. R.: The Surgery of Primary Hyperparathyroidism, *Clin Endocrinol Metab,* **3**:253, 1974.

Delmonico, F., Neer, R. M., Cosimi, A. B., Barnes, A. B., and Russell, P. S.: Hyperparathyroidism during Pregnancy, *Am J Surg,* **131**:328, 1976.

Dent, C. E.: Cortisone Test for Hyperparathyroidism, *Br Med J,* **1**:120, 1956.

DiGiulio, W., and Beierwaltes, W. H.: Parathyroid Scanning with Selenium 75 Labeled Methionine, *J Nucl Med,* **5**:417, 1964.

Egdahl, R. H., Canterbury, J. M., and Reiss, E.: Measurement of Circulating Parathyroid Hormone Concentration Before and After Parathyroid Surgery for Adenoma or Hyperplasia, *Ann Surg,* **168**:714, 1968.

Farr, H. W.: Hyperparathyroidism and Cancer, *Cancer,* **26**:66, 1976.

Friderichsen, C.: Tetany in a Suckling, *Lancet,* **1**:85, 1939.

Gaeke, R. F., Kaplan, E. L., Lindheimer, M. D., Coe, F., and Shen, K-I.: Successful Treatment of Maternal Primary

Hyperparathyroidism of Pregnancy by Parathyroidectomy, *JAMA,* **238**(6):508, 1977.

Goldberg, M. F., Tashjian, A. H., Jr., Order, S. E., and Dammin, G. J.: Renal Adenocarcinoma Containing a Parathyroid Hormone-like Substance and Associated with Marked Hypercalcemia, *Am J Med,* **36**:805, 1964.

Graber, A. L., and Jacobs, K.: Familial Hyperparathyroidism, *JAMA,* **240**:542, 1968.

Haff, R. C., and Ballinger, W. F.: Causes of Recurrent Hypercalcemia after Parathyroidectomy for Primary Hyperparathyroidism, *Ann Surg,* **173**:884, 1971.

———, Black, W. C., and Ballinger, W. F., II: Primary Hyperparathyroidism: Changing Clinical, Surgical and Pathologic Aspects, *Ann Surg,* **171**:85, 1970.

Hartenstein, H., and Gardner, L. I.: Tetany of the Newborn Associated with Maternal Parathyroid Adenoma, *N Engl J Med,* **274**:266, 1966.

Hellstrom, J.: Hyperparathyroidism and Gastroduodenal Ulcer, *Acta Chir Scand,* **116**:207, 1959.

———, Birke, G., and Edvall, C. A.: Hypertension in Hyperparathyroidism, *Br J Urol,* **30**:13, 1958.

——— and Ivemark, B. I.: Primary Hyperparathyroidism: Clinical and Structural Findings in 138 Cases, *Acta Chir Scand [Suppl],* **294**:1, 1962.

Hillman, D. A., Scriver, C. R., Pedris, S., and Shragovitch, I.: Neonatal Familial Primary Hyperparathyroidism, *N Engl J Med,* **270**:483, 1964.

Hines, J. R., and Suker, J. R.: Some Unusual Manifestations of Parathyroid Disease, *Surg Clin North Am,* **53**:221, 1973.

Jackson, C. E.: Hereditary Hyperparathyroidism Associated with Recurrent Pancreatitis, *Ann Intern Med,* **49**:829, 1958.

———: The Association of Peptic Ulcer with Hereditary Hyperparathyroidism, *Gastroenterology,* **37**:35, 1959.

——— and Boonstra, C. E.: The Relationship of Hereditary Hyperparathyroidism to Endocrine Adenomatosis, *Am J Med,* **43**:727, 1967.

Jackson, W. P.: Gout Hyperparathyroidism: Report of a Case with Examination of the Synovial Fluid, *Br Med J,* **2**:211, 1965.

Johansson, H., Thoren, L., and Werner, I.: Hyperparathyroidism, *Upsala J Med Sci,* **77**:41, 1972.

Jowsey, J.: Quantitative Microradiography, *Am J Med,* **40**:485, 1966.

Lafferty, F. W.: Pseudohyperparathyroidism, *Medicine,* **45**:247, 1966.

Low, J. C., Schaaf, M., Earll, J. M., Piechocki, J. T., and Li, T. K.: The Value of Serum Ionized Calcium in the Diagnosis of Normocalcemic and Hypercalcemic Primary Hyperparathyroidism, *Clin Res,* **19**:375, 1971.

Ludwig, G. D.: Hyperparathyroidism in Relation to Pregnancy, *N Engl J Med,* **267**:637, 1962.

MacLeod, W. A. J., and Holloway, C. K.: Hyperparathyroid Crisis: A Collective Review, *Ann Surg,* **166**:1012, 1967.

Maurer, W. J., Johnston, J. R., and Mendenhall, J. T.: Mediastinal Parathyroid Adenoma, *J Thorac Cardiovasc Surg,* **49**:637, 1965.

Mintz, D. H., Canary, J. J., Carreon, G., and Kyle, L. H.: Hyperuricemia in Hyperparathyroidism, *N Engl J Med,* **265**:112, 1961.

Mixter, C. G., Jr., Keynes, W. M., and Cope, O.: Further Experience with Pancreatitis as a Diagnostic Clue to Hyperparathyroidism, *N Engl J Med,* **266**:265, 1962.

Muller, H.: True Recurrence of Hyperparathyroidism: Proposed Criteria of Recurrence, *Br J Surg,* **62**:556, 1975.

Myers, R. T.: Followup Study of Surgically-Treated Primary Hyperparathyroidism, *Ann Surg,* **179**:729, 1974.

Nathaniels, E. K., Nathaniels, A. M., and Wang, C.-A.: Mediastinal Parathyroid Tumors: A Clinical and Pathological Study of 84 Cases, *Ann Surg,* **171**:165, 1970.

Nolan, R. B., Hayles, A. B., and Woolner, L. B.: Adenoma of the Parathyroid Gland in Children: Report of Case and Brief Review of the Literature, *Am J Dis Child,* **99**:622, 1960.

Norris, E. H.: Collective Review: Parathyroid Adenoma; Study of 322 Cases, *Int Abstr Surg,* **84**:1, 1947.

Palmer, J. A., Brown, W. A., Kerr, W. H., Rosen, I. B., and Watters, N. A.: The Surgical Aspects of Hyperparathyroidism, *Arch Surg,* **110**:1004, 1975.

Paloyan, E., Lawrence, A. M., Baker, W. H., and Straus, F. H.: Near-Total Parathyroidectomy, *Surg Clin North Am,* **49**(1):43, 1969.

———, ———, and Straus, F. H.: "Hyperparathyroidism," Grune & Stratton, New York and London, 1973.

———, ———, Straus, F. H., II, Paloyan, D., Harper, P. V., and Cummings, D.: Alpha Cell Hyperplasia in Calcific Pancreatitis Associated with Hyperparathyroidism, *JAMA,* **200**:757, 1967.

———, Paloyan, D., and Pickleman, J. R.: Hyperparathyroidism Today, *Surg Clin North Am,* **53**:211, 1973.

Plimpton, C. H., and Gelhorn, A.: Hypercalcemia in Malignant Disease without Evidence of Bone Destruction, *Am J Med,* **21**:750, 1956.

Purnell, D. C., Scholz, D. A., Smith, L. H., Sizemore, G. W., Black, B. M., Goldsmith, R. S., and Arnaud, C. D.: Treatment of Primary Hyperparathyroidism, *Am J Med,* **56**:800, 1974.

———, Smith, L. H., Scholz, D. A., Elveback, L. R., and Arnaud, C. D.: Primary Hyperparathyroidism: A Prospective Clinical Study, *Am J Med,* **50**:670, 1971.

Pyrah, L. N., Hodgkinson, A., and Anderson, C. K.: Primary Hyperparathyroidism, *Br J Surg,* **53**:245, 1966.

Rapaport, A., Serp, A. H., and Brown, W. A.: Carcinoma of the Parathyroid Gland with Pulmonary Metastases and Cardiac Death, *Am J Med,* **28**:443, 1960.

Rasmussen, H.: Ionic and Hormonal Control of Calcium Homeostasis, *Am J Med,* **50**:567, 1971.

Reiss, E., and Canterbury, J. M.: Application of Radioimmunoassay to Differentiation of Adenoma and Hyperplasia and to Preoperative Localization of Hyperfunctioning Parathyroid Glands, *N Engl J Med,* **280**:1381, 1969.

——— and ———: Genesis of Hyperparathyroidism, *Am J Med,* **50**:679, 1971.

Riggs, B. L., Kelly, D. J., Jowsey, J., and Keating, F. R., Jr.: Skeletal Alterations in Hyperparathyroidism: Determination of Bone Formation, Resorption and Morphologic Changes by Microradiography, *J Clin Endocrinol Metab,* **25**:777, 1965.

Romanus, R., Heimann, O., and Hansson, G.: Surgical Treatment of Hyperparathyroidism, *Prog Surg,* **12**:22, 1973.

Roof, B. S., Carpenter, B., Fink, D. J., and Gordan, G. S.: Some Thoughts on the Nature of Ectopic Parathyroid Hormones, *Am J Med,* **50**:686, 1971.

Scholz, D. A., Purnell, D. C., Goldsmith, R. S., Smith, L. H.,

Riggs, B. L., and Arnaud, C. D.: Diagnostic Considerations in Hypercalcemic Syndromes, *Med Clin North Am,* **56:**941, 1972.

————, Purnell, D. C., Woolner, L. B., and Clagett, O. T.: Mediastinal Hyperfunctioning Parathyroid Tumors: Review of 14 Cases, *Ann Surg,* **178:**173, 1973.

Seldinger, S. I.: Localization of Parathyroid Adenomata by Arteriography, *Acta Radiol (Stockh),* **42:**353, 1954.

Selzman, H. M., and Fechner, R. E.: Oxyphil Adenoma and Primary Hyperparathyroidism, *JAMA,* **199:**359, 1967.

Sharp, W. V., and Kelly, T. R.: Acute Arthritis: A Complication of Surgically Induced Hypoparathyroidism, *Am J Surg,* **113:**829, 1967.

Sherwood, L. M., Lundberg, W. B., Targovnik, J. H., Rodman, J. S., Seyfer, A.: Synthesis and Secretion of Parathyroid Hormone In Vitro, *Am J Med,* **50:**658, 1971.

Smallwood, R. A.: Effect of Intravenous Calcium Administration on Gastric Secretion of Acid and Pepsin in Man, *Gut,* **8:**592, 1967.

State, D.: The Enlarged Inferior Thyroid Artery: A Valuable Guide in Surgery of Parathyroid Adenomas, *Surgery,* **56:**461, 1964.

Steiner, R. E., Fraser, R., and Aird, I.: Operative Parathyroid Arteriography for Location of Parathyroid Tumor, *Br Med J,* **2:**400, 1956.

Stevens, A. C., and Jackson, C. E.: Localization of Parathyroid Adenomas by Esophageal Cineroentgenography, *Am J Roentgenol Radium Ther Nucl Med,* **99:**233, 1967.

Stevens, L. E., Bloomer, A., and Castleton, K. B.: Familial Hyperparathyroidism, *Arch Surg,* **94:**524, 1967.

Underdahl, L. O., Woolner, L. B., and Black, B. M.: Multiple Endocrine Adenomas: Report of Eight Cases in Which the Parathyroids, Pituitary and Pancreatic Islets Were Involved, *J Clin Endocrinol Metab,* **13:**20, 1953.

Wang, C. A., Potts, J. T., Jr., and Neer, R. M.: Controversy of Parathyroid Surgery in Calcium Regulating Hormones, in R. V. Talmage (ed.), Excerpta Medica, p. 82, Amsterdam, 1975.

Wells, H., and Lloyd, W.: Hypercalcemic and Hypophosphatemic Effects of Dibutyryl Cyclic AMP in Rats after Parathyroidectomy, *Endocrinology,* **84:**861, 1969.

Wermer, P.: Genetic Aspects of Adenomatosis of Endocrine Glands, *Am J Med,* **16:**363, 1954.

————: Endocrine Adenomatosis and Peptic Ulcer in a Large Kindred, *Am J Med,* **35:**205, 1963.

Wills, M. R., and McGowan, G. K.: Plasma-chloride Levels in Hyperparathyroidism and Other Hypercalcemic States, *Br Med J,* **1:**1153, 1964.

Wilson, R. E., Bernhard, W. F., Polet, H., and Moore, R. D.: Hyperparathyroidism: The Problem of Acute Parathyroid Intoxication, *Ann Surg,* **159:**70, 1964.

Wilson, S. D.: Zollinger-Ellison Tumor Registry, University of Wisconsin at Milwaukee. (Personal communication.)

Hypercalcemia: Differential Diagnosis

Albright, F.: Cited in Case Records of the Massachusetts General Hospital: Case 27461, *N Engl J Med,* **225:**789, 1941.

Bachman, A. L., and Sproul, E. E.: Correlation of Radiographic and Autopsy Findings in Suspected Metastases in the Spine, *Bull NY Acad Med,* **31:**146, 1955.

Bekerman, C., Schulak, J., Shen, K.-L., and Kaplan, E. L.: Locali-

zation of a Parathyroid Adenoma by Gallium Scan, *J Nucl Med,* 1977. In press.

Berson, S. A., and Yalow, R. S.: Parathyroid Hormone in Plasma in Adenomatous Hyperparathyroidism, Uremia, and Bronchogenic Carcinoma, *Science,* **154:**907, 1966.

Boonstra, C. E., and Jackson, C. E.: Serum Calcium Survey for Hyperparathyroidism: Results in 50,000 Clinic Patients, *Am J Clin Pathol,* **55:**523, 1971.

Duarte, C. G., Winnacker, J. L., Becker, K. L., et al.: Thiazide-induced Hypercalcemia, *N Engl J Med,* **284:**828, 1971.

Genant, H. K., Heck, L. L., Lanzl, L. H., Rossmann, K., Vander Horst, J., and Paloyan, E.: Primary Hyperparathyroidism, *Radiology,* **109:**513, 1974.

Goldsmith, R. S., and Forland, M.: Rapid Calcium Infusion Test for Hyperparathyroidism: Further Experiences, *Arch Intern Med,* **113:**550, 1964.

Knill-Jones, R. P., Buckle, R. M., Parsons, V., et al.: Hypercalcemia and Increased Parathyroid-Hormone Activity in a Primary Hepatoma: Studies Before and After Hepatic Transplantation, *N Engl J Med,* **282:**704, 1970.

Koppel, M. H., Massry, S. G., Shinaberger, J. H., et al.: Thiazide-induced Rise in Serum Calcium and Magnesium in Patients on Maintenance Hemodialysis, *Ann Intern Med,* **72:**895, 1970.

Lafferty, F. W.: Pseudohyperparathyroidism, *Medicine (Baltimore),* **45:**247, 1966.

Monchik, J. M., Doppman, J. L., Earll, J. M., and Aurbach, G. D.: Localization of Hyperfunctioning Parathyroid Tissue. Radioimmunoassay of Parathyroid Hormone on Samples from the Large Veins of the Neck and Thorax and Selectively Catheterized Thyroid Veins, *Am J Surg,* **129:**413, 1975.

Moore, E. W.: Ionized Calcium in Normal Serum, Ultrafiltrates, and Whole Blood Determined by Ion-Exchange Electrodes, *J Clin Invest,* **49:**318, 1970.

O'Riordan, J. L. H., Kendall, B. E., and Woodhead, J. S.: Preoperative Localisation of Parathyroid Tumours, *Lancet,* **2:**1172, 1971.

Parfitt, A. M.: Chlorothiazide-induced Hypercalcemia in Juvenile Osteoporosis and Hyperparathyroidism, *N Engl J Med,* **281:**55, 1969.

Purnell, D. C., Smith, L. H., Scholz, D. A., et al.: Primary Hyperparathyroidism: A Prospective Clinical Study, *Am J Med,* **50:**670, 1971.

Reece, R. L.: An Analysis of 4000 Chemistry Graphs: Comments on Disease Patterns, *Minn Med,* **51:**351, 1968.

Reitz, R. E., Pollard, J. J., Wang, C-A., et al.: Localization of Parathyroid Adenomas by Selective Venous Catheterization and Radioimmunoassay, *N Engl J Med,* **281:**348, 1969.

Riggs, B. L., Arnaud, C. D., Reynolds, J. C., et al.: Immunologic Differentiation of Primary Hyperparathyroidism from Hyperparathyroidism Due to Nonparathyroid Cancer, *J Clin Invest,* **50:**2079, 1971.

Roof, B. S., Carpenter, B., Fink, D. J., et al.: Some Thoughts on the Nature of Ectopic Parathyroid Hormones, *Am J Med,* **50:**686, 1971.

Samuels, B. I.: The Present Status of Parathyroid Thermography, *JAMA,* **223:**907, 1975.

Seitz, H., and Jaworski, Z. F.: Effect of Hydrochlorothiazide on Serum and Urinary Calcium and Urinary Citrate, *Can Med Assoc J,* **90:**414, 1964.

Sherwood, L. M., O'Riordan, J. L. H., Aurbach, G. D., et al.:

Production of Parathyroid Hormone by Nonparathyroid Tumors, *J Clin Endocrinol Metab*, **27**:140, 1967.

Strott, C. A., and Nugent, C. A.: Laboratory Tests in the Diagnosis of Hyperparathyroidism in Hypercalcemic Patients, *Ann Intern Med*, **68**:188, 1968.

Yendt, E. R., and Gagne, R. J. A.: Detection of Primary Hyperparathyroidism, with Special Reference to Its Occurrence in Hypercalciuric Females with "Normal" or Borderline Serum Calcium, *Can Med Assoc J*, **98**:331, 1968.

Ectopic Hyperparathyroidism

Benson, R. C., Jr., Riggs, B. L., Pickard, B. M., and Arnaud, C. D.: Immunoreactive Forms of Circulating Parathyroid Hormone in Primary and Ectopic Hyperparathyroidism, *J Clin Invest*, **54**:175, 1973.

Drezner, M. K., Neelon, F. A., Curtis, H. B., and Lebovitz, H. E.: Renal Cyclic Adenosine Monophosphate: An Accurate Index of Parathyroid Function, *Metabolism*, **25**:1103, 1976.

Levine, R. J., and Metz, S. A.: A Classification of Ectopic Hormone-Producing Tumors, *Ann NY Acad Sci*, **230**:533, 1974.

Mundy, G. R., Luben, R. A., Raisz, L. G., Oppenheim, J. J., and Buell, D. N.: Bone-resorbing Activity in Supernatant from Lymphoid Cell Lines, *N Engl J Med*, **290**:867, 1974.

Samaan, N. A., Hickey, R. C., Hill, C. S., Jr., and Medellin, H.: Parathyroid Tumors: Their Preoperative Localization and Association with Other Tumors, Atlanta Endocrine Society (Abstr) A-298, 1974.

Seyberth, H. W., Segre, G. V., Morgan, J. L., Sweetman, B. J., Potts, J. T., Jr., and Oates, J. A.: Prostaglandins as Mediators of Hypercalcemia Associated with Certain Types of Cancer, *N Engl J Med*, **293**:1278, 1975.

Shaw, J. W., Oldham, S. B., Rosoff, L., Bethune, J. E., and Fichman, M. P.: Urinary Cyclic AMP Analyzed as a Function of the Serum Calcium and Parathyroid Hormone in the Differential Diagnosis of Hypercalcemia, *J Clin Invest*, **59**:14, 1977.

Treatment of Hypercalcemia

Albright, F., Bauer, W., Claflin, D., et al.: Studies in Parathyroid Physiology: III. The Effect of Phosphate Ingestion in Clinical Hyperparathyroidism, *J Clin Invest*, **11**:411, 1932.

Brewer, R. I., and LeBauer, J.: Caution in the Use of Phosphates in the Treatment of Severe Hypercalcemia, *J Clin Endocrinol Metab*, **27**:695, 1967.

Chakmakjian, Z. H., and Bethune, J. E.: Sodium Sulfate Treatment of Hypercalcemia, *N Engl J Med*, **275**:862, 1966.

Goldsmith, R. S.: Treatment of Hypercalcemia, *Med Clin North Am*, **56**:951, 1972.

——— and Ingbar, S. H.: Inorganic Phosphate Treatment of Hypercalcemia of Diverse Etiologies, *N Engl J Med*, **274**:1, 1966.

Henneman, P. H., Dempsey, E. F., Carroll, E. L., et al.: The Cause of Hypercalcuria in Sarcoid and Its Treatment with Cortisone and Sodium Phytate, *J Clin Invest*, **35**:1229, 1956.

Kennedy, B. J.: Metabolic and Toxic Effects of Mithramycin during Tumor Therapy, *Am J Med*, **49**:494, 1970.

Lazor, M. Z., and Rosenberg, L. E.: Mechanism of Adrenal-Steroid Reversal of Hypercalcemia in Multiple Myeloma, *N Engl J Med*, **270**:749, 1964.

Nolph, K. D., and Stoltz, M. L.: Treatment of Hypercalcemia with Calcium Free Peritoneal Dialysis (CFPD), *Clin Res*, **19**:481, 1971. (Abstract.)

Pak, C. Y. C., Wortsman, J., Bennett, J. E., et al.: Control of Hypercalcemia with Cellulose Phosphate, *J Clin Endocrinol Metab*, **28**:1829, 1968. (Letter to the Editor.)

Strauch, B. S., and Ball, M. F.: Hemodialysis in the Treatment of Severe Hypercalcemia, *JAMA*, **235**:1347, 1976.

Suki, W. N., Yium, J. J., VonMinden, M., et al.: Acute Treatment of Hypercalcemia with Furosemide, *N Engl J Med*, **283**:836, 1970.

West, T. E. T., Joffe, M., Sinclair, L., et al.: Treatment of Hypercalcemia with Calcitonin, *Lancet*, **1**:675, 1971.

Secondary and Tertiary Hyperparathyroidism

Bricker, N. S., Slatopolsky, E., Reiss, E., et al.: Calcium, Phosphorus and Bone in Renal Disease and Transplantation, *Arch Intern Med*, **123**:543, 1969.

Curtis, J. R., DeWardener, H. E., Gower, P. E., et al.: The Use of Calcium Carbonate and Calcium Phosphate without Vitamin D in Management of Renal Osteodystrophy, *Proc Eur Dialysis Transplant Assoc*, **7**:141, 1970.

Davies, D. R., Dent, C. E., and Watson, L.: Tertiary Hyperparathyroidism, *Br Med J*, **3**:395, 1968.

Easson, L. H., Faulds, J. S., and Hartley, J. N.: Van Recklinghausen's Disease of Bone Associated with Idiopathic Steatorrhoea, *J R Coll Surg Edinb*, **3**:193, 1958.

Fournier, A. E., Johnson, W. J., Taves, D. R., et al.: Etiology of Hyperparathyroidism and Bone Disease during Chronic Hemodialysis: I. Association of Bone Disease with Potentially Etiologic Factors, *J Clin Invest*, **50**:592, 1971.

Gittes, R. F., and Radde, I. C.: Experimental Model for Hyperparathyroidism: Effect of Excessive Numbers of Transplanted Isologous Parathyroid Glands, *J Urol*, **95**:595, 1966.

Glanville, H. J., and Bloom, R.: Case of Renal Tubular Osteomalacia (Dent Type 2) with Later Development of Autonomous Parathyroid Tumours, *Br Med J*, **2**:26, 1965.

Goldsmith, R. S., Furszyfer, J, Johnson, W. J., et al: Control of Secondary Hyperparathyroidism during Long-Term Hemodialysis, *Am J Med*, **50**:692, 1971.

Johnson, W. J., Goldsmith, R. S., and Arnaud, C. D.: Prevention and Treatment of Progressive Secondary Hyperparathyroidism in Advanced Renal Failure, *Med Clin North Am*, **56**:961, 1972.

———, ———, Beabut, J. W., Jowsey, J., Kelly, P. J., and Arnaud, C. D.: Prevention and Reversal of Progressive Secondary Hyperparathyroidism in Patients Maintained on Hemodialysis, *Am J Med*, **56**:827, 1974.

Jowsey, J., Johnson, W. J., Taves, D. R., et al.: Effects of Dialysate Calcium and Fluoride on Bone Disease during Regular Hemodialysis, *J Lab Clin Med*, **79**:204, 1972.

———, Massry, S. G., Coburn, J. W., et al.: Microradiographic Studies of Bone in Renal Osteodystrophy, *Arch Intern Med*, **124**:539, 1969.

Katz, A. I., Hampers, C. L., and Merrill, J. P.: Secondary Hyperparathyroidism and Renal Osteodystrophy in Chronic Renal Failure: Analysis of 195 Patients, with Observations on the Effects of Chronic Dialysis, Kidney Transplantation and Subtotal Parathyroidectomy, *Medicine (Baltimore)*, **48**:333, 1969.

Kaye, M., Chatterjee, G., Cohen, G. F., et al.: Arrest of Hyperparathyroid Bone Disease with Dihydrotachysterol in Patients

Undergoing Chronic Hemodialysis, *Ann Intern Med,* **73:**225, 1970.

McPhaul, J. J., Jr., McIntosh, D. A., Hammond, W. S., and Park, O. K.: Autonomous Secondary (Renal) Parathyroid Hyperplasia, *N Engl J Med,* **271:**1342, 1964.

Mallick, N. P., and Berlyne, G. M.: Arterial Calcification after Vitamin-D Therapy in Hyperphosphatemic Renal Failure, *Lancet,* **2:**1316, 1968.

Messner, R. P., Smith, H. T., Shapiro, F. L., et al.: The Effect of Hemodialysis, Vitamin D, and Renal Homotransplantation on the Calcium Malabsorption of Chronic Renal Failure, *J Lab Clin Med,* **74:**472, 1969.

Ogg, C. S.: Total Parathyroidectomy in Treatment of Secondary (Renal) Hyperparathyroidism, *Br Med J,* **3:**31, 1967.

Oldham, S. B., Fischer, J. A., Capen, C. C., et al.: Dynamics of Parathyroid Hormone Secretion In Vitro, *Am J Med,* **50:**650, 1971.

Recker, R. R., and Saville, P.: Calcium Absorption in Renal Failure: Its Relationship to Blood Urea Nitrogen, Dietary Calcium Intake, Time on Dialysis, and Other Variables, *J Lab Clin Med,* **78:**380, 1971.

Reiss, E., and Canterbury, J. M.: Parathyroid Hormone in Renal Insufficiency, in Berglund, and B. Josephson (eds.), "Endocrinology: Metabolic Aspects (Proceedings of the Fourth International Congress of Nephrology, Stockholm, 1969)," vol. 2, pp. 164–174, S. Karger A. G., Basel, 1970.

Sherwood, L. M., Herrmann, I., and Bassett, C. A.: In Vitro Studies of Normal and Abnormal Parathyroid Tissue, *Arch Intern Med,* **124:**426, 1969.

Stanbury, S. W., Lumb, G. A., and Nicholson, W. F.: Elective Subtotal Parathyroidectomy for Renal Hyperparathyroidism, *Lancet,* **1:**793, 1960.

Hypoparathyroidism, Pseudohypoparathyroidism, and Parathyroid Transplants

Alvioli, L. V.: The Therapeutic Approach to Hypoparathyroidism, *Am J Med,* **57:**34, 1974.

Blizzard, R. M., Chee, D., and Davis, W.: The Incidence of Parathyroid and Other Antibodies in the Sera of Patients with Idiopathic Hypoparathyroidism, *Clin Exp Immunol,* **1:**119, 1966.

Chase, L. R., Nelson, G. L., and Aurbach, G. D.: Metabolic Abnormality in Pseudohypoparathyroidism: Defective Renal Excretion of Cyclic 3′5′-AMP in Response to Parathyroid Hormone, *J Clin Invest,* **47:**18a, 1968.

Costello, J. M., and Dent, C. E.: Hypohyperparathyroidism, *Arch Dis Child,* **38:**397, 1963.

Dimich, A., Bedrossian, P. B., and Wallach, S.: Hypoparathyroidism: Clinical Observations in 34 Patients, *Arch Intern Med,* **120:**449, 1967.

Fisher, B., Fisher, E., Feduska, N., and Sakai, A.: Thyroid and Parathyroid Implantation: An Experimental Reevaluation, *Surgery,* **62:**1025, 1967.

Franz, A. G., and Lee, J. B.: Pseudohypoparathyroidism: Assays of Parathyroid Hormone and Thyrocalcitonin, *Proc Natl Acad Sci USA,* **56:**1138, 1966.

Jordan, G. L., Jr., Erickson, E., Gordon, W. B., Jr., and Rose, R. G.: The Treatment of Hypoparathyroidism by Parathyroid Transplantation, *Surgery,* **52:**134, 1962.

Kenney, F. M., and Holliday, M. A.: Hypoparathyroidism, Moniliasis and Hashimoto's Disease, *N Engl J Med,* **271:**708, 1964.

Kolb, F. O., and Steinberg, H. L.: Pseudohypoparathyroidism and Secondary Hyperparathyroidism and Osteitis Fibrosa, *J Clin Endocrinol Metab,* **22:**59, 1962.

Tashjian, A. H., Frantz, A. G., and Lee, J. B.: Pseudohypoparathyroidism: Assays of Parathyroid Hormone and Thyrocalcitonin, *Pathology,* **56:**1138, 1966.

Wells, S. A., Jr., Ellis, G. J., Gunnells, J. C., et al.: Parathyroid Autotransplantation in Primary Parathyroid Hyperplasia, *N Engl J Med,* **295:**57, 1976.

———, Gunnells, J. C., Shelburne, J. D., et al.: Transplantation of the Parathyroid Glands in Man: Clinical Indications and Results, *Surgery,* **78:**34, 1975.

Williams, E., and Wood, A. O. C.: The Syndrome of Hypoparathyroidism and Steatorrhea, *Arch Dis Child,* **34:**302, 1959.

Chapter 39

Pediatric Surgery

by R. Peter Altman, Judson G. Randolph, and Kathryn D. Anderson

GENERAL CONSIDERATIONS

The normal adaptive demands upon infants and young children are enormous. Add to these the compensatory requirements imposed by illness and by operation, and the role of the children's surgeon is brought into perspective. As the size of the patient is scaled down, the period of time in which a state of well-being turns to a surgical catastrophe becomes shorter. Thus, patients on a children's surgical unit must be guarded unceasingly against subtle changes in clinical signs.

In addition to the technical performance of an operation, pediatric surgery encompasses all phases of care, including the diagnosis, preoperative preparation, postoperative management, and long-term rehabilitation of the child.

This requires an appreciation of the unique physiologic and emotional requirements of infants, children, and adolescents. Most of all, pediatric surgery demands that the surgeon care about children, about their fears, about their expectations for themselves, and about the impact of surgical illness on the child and the family.

FLUID AND ELECTROLYTE BALANCE. In an infant or child the margin between dehydration and fluid overload is small. The infant is born with a surplus of body water, but within a few days this is excreted. At birth and for the first 10 days of life, fluid requirements are between 65 and 150 ml/kg (750 to 1,000 ml/m^2). Thereafter the maintenance fluid requirement approaches 1,500 to 2,000 ml/m^2/day. For infants and children with normal renal function, fluid calculations based on a rough guideline of 75 ml/kg generally fall within the limits of safe replacement. For short-term intravenous therapy, sodium 5 mEq/kg/day and potassium 2 mEq/kg/day will satisfy the daily need. Fluid and electrolyte losses secondary to protracted vomiting or diarrhea are corrected by modifying this formula according to the measured losses. An additional parameter for assessment of hydration is measurement of the serum and urine osmolarities. The normal serum osmolarity lies between 280 and 290 mOsm/liter. Because of the inability of the immature kidney to concentrate, it is not always possible to utilize the urine osmolarity as a guideline for fluid replacement in neonates. Even in a dehydrated infant the urine osmolarity rarely exceeds 400 mOsm/liter. No matter what formula is used to calculate the fluid replacement, there is no substitute for recording and analyzing all fluid losses, including the insensible depletion, then replacing the depleted constituents precisely.

ACID-BASE EQUILIBRIUM. The serum pH and P_{CO_2} reflect the respiratory and metabolic status of the patient. Their measurement permits estimation of the base excess and recognition of derangement in metabolic or respiratory status. These data are essential during the resuscitation of critically ill patients and constitute an integral part of the intraoperative and postoperative monitoring. Metabolic acidosis is usually corrected by the administration of sodium bicarbonate. In a fragile infant the risks of excessive sodium administration, hyperosmolarity, and cardiovascular overload are appreciable. Thus, for infants requiring extensive metabolic manipulation (such as those with congenital diaphragmatic hernia), all intravenous sodium solution should be as Na HCO$_3$. This maximizes the amount of buffer provided while restricting Na administered.

Fluid and electrolyte losses from the upper gastrointestinal tract in infants are generally equivalent to 0.45 N saline solution. Adjustments for ileostomy or biliary losses are made when these are significant by analyzing the individual drainage.

BLOOD VOLUME AND BLOOD REPLACEMENT. Replacement of volume with whole blood, blood components, plasma, and plasma substitutes is an integral part of pediatric surgical therapy. Because of the risks of immunologic sensitization, transfusion reactions, or hepatitis, blood or its fractions are administered only when absolutely indicated. Volume expansion with 5% or 25% albumin solutions is often chosen over the administration of blood. For transfusion in infants and children, whole blood can be subdivided into smaller packets of 125 ml. A useful guideline for blood replacement in the infant is to consider 10 ml/kg roughly equivalent to a 500-ml unit in the 70-kg adult. Replacement with packed red blood cells is calculated at 5 ml/kg.

Platelet transfusions are indicated in special circumstances, such as thrombocytopenia secondary to hypersplenism. Clotting is restored to normal when the platelet count is raised to 50,000 per milliliter. This is accomplished by transfusion of multiple platelet packs prepared from whole blood. The biologic half-life of platelets is limited, and therefore transfusion of platelets must be carried out promptly after their preparation.

In the child, as in the adult, coagulation deficiencies assume clinical significance after extensive blood transfusion. It is advisable to alternate whole blood transfusion with administration of fresh frozen plasma in order to replace the labile clotting factors, especially V and VIII.

HYPERALIMENTATION AND NUTRITION. The techniques of total parenteral nutrition have now been refined and are especially beneficial to infants, translating formerly hopeless clinical problems into situations where there is a good chance for survival.

When the gastrointestinal tract is not usable, because of mechanical, ischemic, or inflammatory disorders, several options for nutritional support are available. The original technique makes use of an indwelling central venous catheter for delivery of the nutritional substrate. The fundamental principle involves the provision of a source of calories (hypertonic glucose) in combination with a source of nitrogen (protein hydrolysate or amino acid solution). Since energy requirements are satisfied, the exogenous nitrogen is converted into body protein and an anabolic state is achieved. Essential fatty acid supplements, minerals, and vitamins are provided in the infusate, and long-term growth can be sustained even in the rapidly developing infant.

The risks, however, are not trivial. The concentration of infusate approaches 25 percent and therefore requires that administration be carried out through a major channel with rapid flow. Most often the superior vena cava is utilized. Sepsis, caval thrombosis, pneumothorax, hydrothorax, and hypertonic crises are constant threats. For these reasons, alternative techniques to central venous hyperalimentation have been developed. Peripheral alimentation, utilizing less concentrated but greater volume of solutions, has been used successfully to achieve positive nitrogen balance. Lipid emulsions prepared from soy extract (Intralipid) have largely eliminated the need for central alimentation techniques. The caloric yield from fat solution (11 kcal/Gm) reduces reliance upon hypertonic glucose. Positive nitrogen balance can thus be accomplished by the administration of isotonic solutions, which are provided through a peripheral vein. Advances in the techniques of parenteral nutrition have had a greater impact on survival for pediatric surgical patients than any other surgical development in the past decade.

THERMOREGULATION. Infants or children compromised by illness are exceedingly thermolabile. Premature infants are particularly susceptible to changes in environmental temperature. Unable to shiver, and lacking stores of fat, their potential for thermogenesis is severely impaired. Since these patients lack adaptive mechanisms to cope with the environment, the environment must itself be carefully regulated. This is true before, during, and after surgery. During transfer of an infant, attention to heat conservation is essential. The simple expedient of wrapping the infant in aluminum foil during transportation will diminish radiant heat loss. In the operating room the ambient temperature should approach thermal neutrality *for the patient.* This is 73°F. Supplementary heat is provided by means of direct warming lights during positioning and intubation when much of the body surface is exposed. Warm solutions are utilized for "prepping" the operative field. Excess preparatory solutions must be avoided to minimize evaporation with concomitant body surface cooling. Irrigation solutions employed during surgery should also be warmed. Intraoperative temperature is monitored by placement of a thermister probe in the axilla or esophagus.

After operation, a heated isolette should be immediately available to receive the baby. It has been demonstrated that infants have a better survival rate when temperatures are maintained above 95°F than when temperatures are permitted to fall below this level. Complications of hypothermia include increased blood viscosity, cardiorespiratory depression, and metabolic acidosis. Most of the currently available isolettes are provided with thermoregulatory devices which respond to constant recordings of the infant's temperature.

INTRAOPERATIVE MONITORING. The same physiologic parameters are monitored during a major surgical procedure in an infant or child as for an adult patient. The basic minimum requirements for conducting a safe pediatric surgical procedure include a temperature thermister, Doppler flow sensor, ECG, and a stethoscope placed either on the chest or in the esophagus. When necessary, ready access is obtained for central venous pressure monitoring, even in the neonate, by means of a catheter placed in the superior vena cava through the jugular vein or subclavian vein. Arterial access is available through radial or temporal artery cut-down or by percutaneous technique. Scrupulous attention to these detailed preparations is essential if the infant is to be guided safely through major operative procedures.

LESIONS OF THE NECK

Cystic Hygroma

ETIOLOGY AND PATHOLOGY. Cystic hygroma occurs as a result of imperfect formation of the lymphatic channels. The majority occur in the neck, posterior to the sternocleidomastoid muscle (Fig. 39-1). Other sites are the mediastinum, axilla, and groin. The term *hygroma* implies

watery fluid contained within endothelial-lined spaces. The cyst may be unilocular, but more often there are multiple cysts which permeate the surrounding structures and distort the local anatomy. Supporting connective tissue shows extensive lymphocytic infiltration. Except in the case of single large cysts, no clear-cut cleavage plane is found between the hygroma and normal tissue. The lesion is usually apparent at birth. Occasionally, the mass occupies the entire submandibular region, distorting the subglottic tissues and compromising the airway. Local disfigurement may be severe. Not infrequently, an associated supraclavicular mass is seen which may become prominent with the Valsalva maneuver. This usually implies association with a mediastinal component.

CLINICAL MANIFESTATIONS. Symptoms are related to the location and size of the mass. Sudden enlargement of a hygroma generally indicates hemorrhage into a cyst. Infection in the mass may lead to dangerous regional cellulitis, but when the infection subsides, the resultant intracystic fibrosis and scar may significantly reduce the size of the mass.

TREATMENT. Surgical excision offers the best chance of cure. Total excision is often impractical because of the extent of the hygroma and its proximity to vital structures. Important nerves and vascular structures should not be sacrificed in an attempt to achieve total excision of this benign lesion; rather, repeated partial excisions of the residual hygroma are preferable. Some have favored repeated aspiration of the cysts with injections of sclerosing agents, but this approach has limited usefulness and is not recommended.

Thyroglossal Duct Remnants

PATHOLOGY AND CLINICAL MANIFESTATIONS. The thyroglossal duct originates as a diverticulum of the foregut, beginning at the base of the tongue in the foramen cecum and passing downward and forward through the hyoid bone to the normal anatomical position of the thyroid gland (Fig. 39-1). Persistence of a portion of the thyroglossal duct results in a midline cervical mass known as a *thyroglossal duct cyst.* These cysts can be troublesome because of repeated infection. The mass is usually discovered in the two- to four-year-old child when the baby fat subsides and irregularities in the neck are more readily apparent. The cyst is almost always found in the midline, but repeated infection and scarring may cause lateral displacement, which can lead to diagnostic confusion.

TREATMENT. Infected thyroglossal duct cysts should be treated with antibiotics; when an abscess is present, drainage is necessary. Removal of the cyst and thyroglossal duct tract, including the central portion of the hyoid bone, is carried out when infection subsides. The cyst occasionally presents in the mouth at the base of the tongue. A midline mass in the neck or at the base of the tongue which is thought to be a thyroglossal duct cyst may, in rare instances, be ectopic thyroid tissue. Therefore, if a normal thyroid cannot be palpated with certainty, a thyroid scan should be performed.

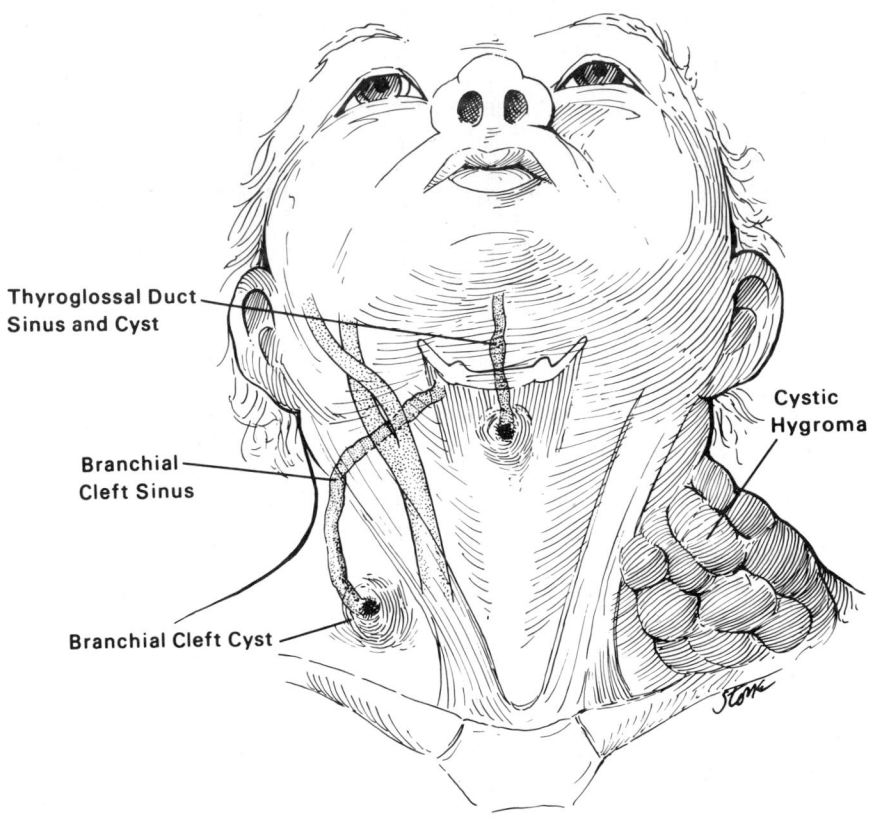

Fig. 39-1. Typical locations of lesions of the neck. Cystic hygroma—multilocular cysts in posterior triangle of neck. Thyroglossal duct cyst and sinus—usually a midline cyst with a sinus tract passing through the hyoid bone to the foramen cecum. Branchial cleft cyst and sinus. The sinus tract passes through the bifurcation of the carotid artery, ending in the pharynx.

Branchial Cleft Anomalies

Branchial clefts are those embryological grooves that ultimately evolve into the lower part of the face and neck. Persistence of various portions of the branchial apparatus leads to specific anomalies about the face and neck. A fistula or cyst orginating low in the anterior lateral region of the neck usually results from a malformation of the second branchial cleft. Typically the fistula extends from the skin of the lower part of the neck upward along the anterior border of the sternocleidomastoid muscle, then inward between the bifurcation of the carotid artery to enter the posterolateral pharynx just below the tonsillar fossa (Fig. 39-1). Cysts are typically found only in the lower end of the tract just above the clavicle. The presenting complaint is usually related to persistent or intermittent drainage onto the neck. Complete surgical extirpation is necessary for cure. Transverse "stair-step" incisions are preferred to a long incision encompassing the entire tract.

RESPIRATORY SYSTEM

Subglottic Stenosis

As more infants are being sustained with ventilatory support, acquired subglottic stenosis is assuming greater clinical importance (Fig. 39-2). Mild or moderate stenosis will usually respond to one or two tracheal dilatations. Severe tracheal stenosis may require tracheostomy, often

Fig. 39-2. Air tracheogram showing subglottic stenosis following protracted endotracheal intubation.

for a year or longer, with periodic dilatations. Tracheoplasty is reserved for the most severe stenoses, which do not respond to dilatation.

Subglottic Hemangioma

Hemangiomas in the subglottic area can compromise the airway and cause stridor. These tumors can often be demonstrated on a high-kilovolt neck film and confirmed by laryngoscopy and bronchoscopy. In some patients tracheostomy may be required, but the natural history of hemangioma is to increase in size during the first few months of life, after which there is a gradual involution and disappearance of the lesion. In critical circumstances involution of the hemangioma can be hastened by the systemic administration of steroids in combination with direct x-ray therapy (150 rads × three doses).

Diaphragmatic Hernia

PATHOLOGY. During formation of the diaphragm, the pleural and coelomic cavities remain in continuity via the pleuroperitoneal canal. Failure of this defect to close results in the congenital anomaly known as *Bochdalek hernia.* This anomaly has a predilection for the left side.

With incomplete closure of the posterior diaphragm, bowel fills the chest cavity during embryonic life. The abdominal cavity remains small and undeveloped. The presence of the intestinal loops in the chest interferes with the development of the lung, and prevents its expansion after birth. As the baby's bowel fills with air, further shift of the mediastinum occurs. Any newborn infant in respiratory distress who shows a scaphoid abdomen should be suspected of having a congenital diaphragmatic hernia (Fig. 39-3). Chest x-ray will confirm the diagnosis (Fig. 39-4).

TREATMENT. Diaphragmatic hernia is one of the most urgent surgical emergencies of the newborn infant. However, some severely compromised infants may benefit from a brief period of resuscitation with bicarbonate and 100 percent oxygen prior to surgical correction. Improved survival has been observed in infants in whom the pH can be partially corrected and the P_{CO_2} lowered toward normal.

Operative repair is best performed through a subcostal incision. There are advantages to the abdominal approach; withdrawing the bowel from the chest is technically simpler than pushing it from above, and a ventral hernia is usually necessary to accommodate the bowel which has lost its "right of domain" in the abdominal cavity. As a rule the anterior leaf of the diaphragm is well developed, since the defect is posterolateral. The posterior rim of the diaphragm is usually covered by a layer of peritoneum which is continuous with the parietal pleura. This must be incised and the diaphragm unrolled so that it can be sutured to the anterior diaphragmatic leaf. A single layer of nonabsorbable sutures is used to close the defect. A chest tube is positioned in the thoracic cavity and placed on gentle suction.

Fig. 39-3. Newborn with left congenital Bochdalek diaphragmatic hernia. Note scaphoid abdomen.

Fig. 39-4. X-ray showing left Bochdalek hernia. Intestine occupies the left side of the chest. Note the extreme mediastinal displacement.

A "prophylactic" chest tube is inserted on the opposite side, because pneumothorax, on the contralateral side, is a common life-threatening complication. Both chest tubes can be removed after the infant is weaned from the ventilator. The ventral hernia is repaired 10 days to 2 weeks after the abdominal cavity has expanded to accommodate the intestine. In spite of improvement in neonatal pulmonary support, diaphragmatic hernia is still associated with a 50 percent mortality. Perhaps technical developments in extracorporeal membrane oxygenation will be adapted to neonates and result in improved survival.

Congenital Lobar Emphysema

Hyperexpansion of a single lobe of the lung can produce a life-threatening respiratory crisis. Inspired air trapped in the affected lobe results in compression of the adjacent lung and displacement of the mediastinum. The right middle and left upper lobes are most frequently involved. In 10 percent of the cases the disease is bilateral. A chest x-ray which shows hyperaeration of the involved lobe and compression of adjacent lung parenchyma with mediastinal displacement to the contralateral side is diagnostic. In some patients, the lobar emphysema may pose a true surgical emergency and the affected lobe must be removed promptly. A bronchial abnormality is not usually identified in the resected specimen.

Pulmonary Sequestration

Accessory lung tissue may be present, either completely separate from adjacent lung parenchyma (extralobar sequestration) or invested within the visceral pleura of the adjoining normal lung tissue (intralobar sequestration). The former condition occurs most commonly in the left side of the chest, adjacent to the diaphragm. Typically there is no bronchial connection and the blood supply to the anomalous lobe emanates from the abdominal aorta. Symptoms are uncommon and this malformation is usually discovered on routine chest film. Arteriography is helpful in demonstrating the systemic arterial supply. Elective thoracotomy with excision is advisable.

Intralobar sequestration occurs in intimate association with normal lung parenchyma, usually in the lower lobes and more commonly in the left side of the chest. Unlike the asymptomatic extralobar sequestration, the intralobar sequestration may present with cough, hemoptysis, or pulmonary infection. The chest x-ray is usually diagnostic. There is no connection with the bronchus, but the sequestration may contain air which enters from adjacent alveoli. The sequestration may necessitate a lobectomy of the affected lobe, though segmental resection may be all that is required.

Bronchiectasis

Bronchiectasis is rare in children but can occur as a result of congenital cystic fibrosis. The condition also accompanies Kartagener's syndrome, with sinusitis drainage as the underlying cause. Bronchiectasis may result from infection secondary to a neglected bronchial foreign body.

Symptoms include chronic cough, which may be productive, and recurrent respiratory infection. Hemoptysis is not uncommon. The diagnosis is suggested on chest x-ray, and the saccular fusiform distortion of the peripheral bronchi can be confirmed by bronchography. Lobectomy or segmental resection is indicated if the disease is localized to a single lobe or portion of a lobe.

Foreign Bodies

Foreign objects aspirated into the larynx, trachea, and bronchi represent a major cause of respiratory difficulty in toddlers. Peanut aspiration is common, and severe lipid pneumonia secondary to the arachitic acid in the nut may result.

The history of choking while eating, often when the child is playing or laughing, should alert one to the possibility of foreign body aspiration. The coughing may then resolve and the only sign of the foreign body in the bronchus may be a unilateral wheeze. Fluoroscopy of the chest will often reveal air trapping and a swing of the mediastinum toward the side of the foreign body during expiration. Hyperaeration may involve a whole lung or be localized to a single lobe. In neglected cases where a foreign body is allowed to remain in the bronchus, atelectasis may ensue. Bronchiectasis is a late consequence of unrecognized bronchial foreign body.

A   B   C   D   E

Fig. 39-5. Five major varieties of esophageal atresia and tracheoesophageal fistula. *A.* Esophageal atresia without associated fistula. *B.* Esophageal atresia with tracheoesophageal fistula between proximal segment of esophagus and trachea. *C.* Esophageal atresia with tracheoesophageal fistula between distal esophagus and trachea. *D.* Esophageal atresia with fistula between both proximal and distal ends of esophagus and trachea. *E.* Tracheoesophageal fistula without esophageal atresia (H-type fistula).

Endoscopic removal of the foreign body under general anesthesia is recommended, although some foreign bodies are expelled by treatment with vigorous pulmonary physiotherapy.

Pneumothorax, Pneumomediastinum

The improved salvage of premature infants with respiratory distress syndrome has inevitably resulted in long-term maintenance on mechanic ventilation. Diminished compliance of lungs combined with positive-pressure ventilation has resulted in an increased incidence of pneumomediastinum and pneumothorax. The development of pulmonary interstitial emphysema (air surrounding the minor bronchi) precedes dissection of the air extrapleurally into the mediastinum or the pleural cavity. Pneumomediastinum is not usually clinically significant, but may contribute to respiratory distress and require needle aspiration. This can be safely accomplished by inserting a needle into the mediastinum beneath the xyphoid. Pneumothorax in neonates is almost always under tension and thus is life-threatening. Sudden deterioration of the infant's clinical status with a decrease in the arterial oxygen saturation and an increase in the P_{CO_2} may signal a pneumothorax. Chest x-rays are confirmatory, and the pneumothorax must be aspirated as an emergency. Even if immediate relief of the pneumothorax is obtained by needle aspiration, it is prudent to introduce a small chest tube for a few days. The tube is connected to suction of approximately 10 ml water since the infant is generally unable to generate the positive pressure necessary to evacuate the pneumothorax under unmodified water seal.

ESOPHAGUS

Tracheoesophageal Fistula and Esophageal Atresia

ESOPHAGEAL ATRESIA WITH LOWER-SEGMENT TRACHEOESOPHAGEAL FISTULA

PATHOLOGY. Esophageal atresia associated with distal tracheoesophageal fistulae (Vogt-Gross type C) (Fig. 39-5) accounts for 90 percent of the anomalies of the esophagus. The upper esophageal segment terminates as a blind pouch, and the proximal end of the lower segment of the esophagus joins the trachea, just above the carina. The fistula transmits inspired air to the stomach, and also allows acidic gastric secretions to reflux into the lungs. Associated anomalies are common. In nearly 20 percent of the infants born with esophageal atresia, some variant of congenital heart disease occurs; imperforate anus is found in about 12 percent.

CLINICAL MANIFESTATIONS. The earliest and most obvious clinical sign of esophageal atresia is regurgitation of saliva at the first offered feeding. The aspiration of feedings is soon followed by pneumonia. The pulmonary problem is magnified by refluxing gastric juice, and by the atelectasis which occurs consequent to aspiration secondary to gastric distension. When esophageal atresia is suspected, an attempt should be made to pass a catheter through the nose into the stomach (Fig. 39-6). Diagnosis of esophageal atresia is suggested if the catheter meets an obstruction and fails to advance. A lateral chest x-ray with 1 ml contrast media instilled in the upper pouch will outline the blind upper esophagus and confirm the diagnosis.

TREATMENT. Once the diagnosis of esophageal atresia with tracheoesophageal fistula has been established, one of the following is instituted: (1) infant warmer, in 30° head-up position; (2) sump catheter suction in the upper pouch (Repfogle tube); (3) parenteral antibiotics even if pneumonia is not clinically manifest. Gastrostomy is a useful, often vital, adjunct in the management of these infants and can be performed before operative repair of the esophagus,

Fig. 39-6. Type C esophageal atresia with tracheoesophageal fistula. Catheter is coiled in upper pouch. Gas below diaphragm confirms the presence of a tracheoesophageal fistula.

if necessary. The gastrostomy accomplishes gastric decompression, improves ventilatory mechanics, and minimizes reflux of gastric contents through the fistula into the tracheobronchial passages (Fig. 39-7).

If the infant is full-term and has no pneumonia or other major congenital anomaly, then primary esophageal repair can be safely undertaken (Fig. 39-8). The approach is made through a right thoracotomy in the retropleural plane. The lower segment of the esophagus is detached from the trachea, and the tracheal fistula is meticulously sutured closed. The blind upper pouch is mobilized, and its end opened; a union between the two esophageal segments is then carried out. The classic repair described by Haight in 1941 continues to be popular. However, when utilizing a retropleural approach, a single-layer anastomosis using nonabsorbable sutures has also been successful.

If the patient has pneumonia, cardiac disease, or other serious anomaly, these clinical circumstances take precedence, and surgical correction is deferred. In this group of patients a gastrostomy is performed, often under local anesthesia. Up to a week is then spent employing upper-pouch suction, head-up position, antibiotics, intravenous feeding, and gastrostomy drainage. Thoracotomy with repair is carried out after the infant's condition has been stabilized, the heart assessed, and appropriate treatment instituted. With this approach, high-risk infants become more satisfactory candidates for general anesthesia and definitive surgery.

For infants with overwhelming pneumonia, prematurity, or severe congenital heart disease, a staged approach may prove the wisest course. This involves temporary gastrostomy and fistula division, with complete repair of the esophagus weeks or months later.

The most frequent complication following surgical repair of esophageal atresia is stenosis at the site of the anastomosis. This may occur weeks after operation and is manifest by increasing difficulty in swallowing, followed by aspiration and pneumonia. Most patients with esophageal strictures can be managed by esophageal dilatation during the first year or two of life. In such instances, general anesthesia is preferred, and graduated tapered dilators can be guided down the esophagus with safety. When frequent repetitive dilations are needed, the gastrostomy should be maintained so that linked graduated rubber dilators (Tucker) can be pulled retrograde through the gastrostomy and up the esophagus to accomplish dilatation. In rare instances, when strictures are refractory to repeated dilatations, resection may be advisable.

Overall survival for babies with esophageal atresia and tracheoesophageal fistula is approximately 80 percent in most reported series.

Fig. 39-7. Supportive measures for an infant with esophageal atresia and tracheoesophageal fistula include use of sump catheter in upper pouch, intravenous fluids and antibiotics, and gastrostomy for gastric decompression. (From Randolph et al., J Thorac Cardiovasc Surg, 74:335, 1977, by permission.)

ISOLATED ESOPHAGEAL ATRESIA

Among those babies born with esophageal anomalies, 8 percent have isolated esophageal atresia. Characteristically, infants with isolated esophageal atresia present with a scaphoid abdomen, since the gastrointestinal tract is devoid of air. The x-ray finding of a blind upper pouch and the absence of air below the diaphragm is pathognomonic of isolated esophageal atresia without fistula.

Prompt esophagostomy with the upper esophageal pouch brought to the skin of the left side of the neck allows drainage of saliva and prevents aspiration. A gastrostomy is performed and serves for feeding in the early months of life. Esophageal replacement with colon or gastric tube is then recommended at a year of age. Some authors have shown that the esophageal ends can be dilated over a period of several months, allowing end-to-end union and avoiding esophageal replacement.

ISOLATED (H-TYPE) TRACHEOESOPHAGEAL FISTULA

In rare instances (3 percent), an isolated congenital fistula connecting the trachea to the esophagus may exist. In this anomaly both the trachea and the esophagus are otherwise normal, with no narrowing or obstruction. Infants with this condition seem to swallow normally. The clinical features are subtle; weeks or months may elapse before a correct diagnosis is made. The presence of an H-type tracheoesophageal fistula is suggested by the following triad of symptoms: (1) choking when feeding, (2) gaseous distension of the bowel, and (3) recurrent aspiration pneumonia. Diagnosis can usually be confirmed by cine contrast x-ray studies or by bronchoesophagoscopy using the recently available fiberoptic lens system. Definitive treatment consists of dividing the fistula. Surgical closure of the esophagus and trachea must be meticulous, and encroachment on the lumen of the trachea avoided. The fistula is usually accessible to surgical repair through an incision just above the clavicle.

Corrosive Injury of the Esophagus

Commercial cleaners stored in areas accessible to the toddler are commonly swallowed. These agents often contain a strong alkali which is hygroscopic and becomes firmly attached to the moist mucosal surface of the esophagus. The burn thus sustained coagulates protein and can involve the entire thickness of the esophagus. Children suspected of having swallowed corrosive materials should be admitted to the hospital and studied by esophagoscopy

Fig. 39-8. Primary repair of Type C tracheoesophageal fistula. *A.* Right thoracotomy incision. *B.* Azygos vein transected: proximal and distal esophagus demonstrated and fistula identified. *C.* Tracheoesophageal fistula transected and defect in trachea closed. *D.* End-to-end anastomosis between proximal and distal esophagus (posterior row). *E.* Anastomosis completed.

within 24 hours of injury. A burn will be seen as a whitish coagulum on the surface mucosa, surrounded by an area of hyperemia. If the esophageal injury is circumferential, it has been our practice to perform a gastrostomy for feeding, and to insert a string for subsequent dilatation.

Steroids seem to decrease the mucosal scarring and are therefore administered for 6 weeks. Antibiotics are used routinely for 3 weeks. After this interval, esophageal dilatation is begun. Dilatations are continued as often as twice weekly until either the stricture is resolved or it becomes apparent that esophageal substitution will be required. This latter decision is deferred for at least 6 to 12 months until healing is complete and the resulting esophageal injury can be fully assessed.

Esophageal Substitution

Esophageal substitution is required in children for two major conditions: severe esophageal strictures and isolated esophageal atresia. The colon has been the most widely used organ for esophageal substitution, reaching easily into the neck on the marginal artery of Drummond. It can be placed in a substernal tunnel or in the left side of the chest behind the lung root (Fig. 39-9). Since the colon acts as an aperistaltic conduit, antiperistaltic and isoperistaltic segments function equally well. An alternative method of esophageal substitution gaining popularity is the reversed gastric tube. This is fashioned from a flap cut from the greater curvature of the stomach, with a vascular pedicle based on the left gastroepiploic artery. The results of both

these methods of esophageal substitution are satisfactory. Children so treated are able to maintain normal growth and development, and the long-term complications are manageable.

Gastroesophageal Reflux

CLINICAL MANIFESTATIONS. Relentless vomiting in infants from pathologic gastroesophageal reflux is often caused by abnormal relaxation of the cardia ("chalasia"). Poor weight gain and recurrent aspiration pneumonia characterize the clinical course if esophageal reflux goes untreated.

Barium swallow is diagnostic for this condition. Recently, esophageal manometry has been adapted to young subjects. This has provided an important diagnostic adjunct in quantitating reflux. Esophagoscopy is helpful in those patients whose symptoms or x-ray studies suggest esophagitis.

TREATMENT. Upright propping of the infant in an infant seat and administration of small, frequent, thickened feedings constitute the conservative therapeutic approach. This is successful in relieving symptoms in the majority of patients. Many infants with gastroesophageal reflux recover function of the gastroesophageal junction spontaneously at about a year of age. Conservative measures fail in approximately 15 percent of infants and children, and

Fig. 39-9. Diagram showing coloesophagoplasty. Note that the colon can be placed in a substernal position or behind the root of the left lung. The vascular pedicle is supplied by the marginal artery of Drummond from the middle colic artery.

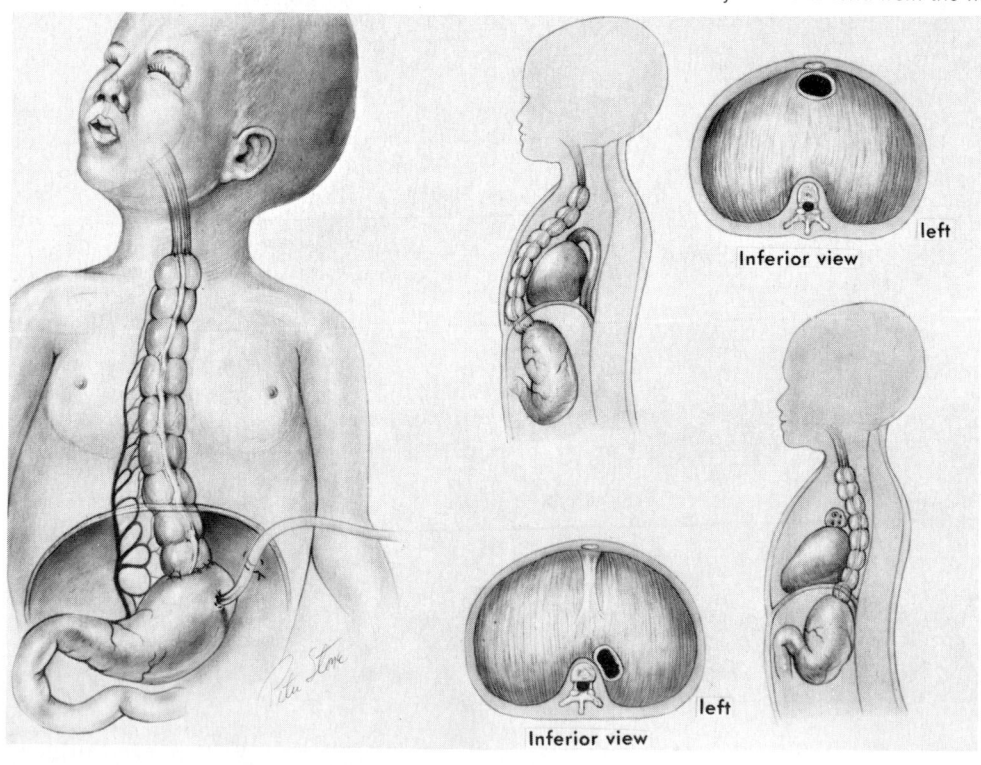

surgical correction is then necessary. The principal indications for surgery are (1) intractable vomiting despite conservative treatment, (2) failure to gain weight and grow normally, (3) recurrent aspiration pneumonia, (4) symptomatic esophagitis, (5) the formation of esophageal stricture. It is not necessary to demonstrate a hiatal hernia for the patient to be a candidate for surgical correction of esophageal reflux.

Both thoracic and abdominal approaches have been successful for surgical correction. Currently the most popular operation in infants and children is the Nissen fundoplication. Surgical correction is usually followed by gratifying clinical improvement and return toward normal growth and developmental parameters.

GASTROINTESTINAL TRACT

Pyloric Stenosis

CLINICAL MANIFESTATIONS. Hypertrophic pyloric stenosis affects male infants predominantly, often the firstborn. The typical history is one of projectile vomiting in an infant from three to ten weeks of age. The vomitus contains only ingested formula, never bile. The enlarged pyloric "olive" can usually be felt on abdominal examination but occasionally it may be necessary to confirm the diagnosis by upper gastrointestinal series. X-ray study shows a narrowed elongated pyloric channel with increased volume and peristaltic effort of the stomach.

TREATMENT. The extent of preoperative preparation depends upon the clinical status of the infant. If the diagnosis is recognized before electrolyte depletion has occurred, the infant may be operated on without elaborate preoperative preparation. Patients who have experienced days of vomiting, however, will show a metabolic alkalosis with a high serum pH and low chloride level. In this group of infants, there is a profound depletion of total body potassium. Correction is achieved by the administration of normal saline solution intravenously with added potassium, 2 to 4 mEq/kg, given over a 12- to 18-hour period. After resuscitation, surgical correction by the Fredet-Ramstedt pyloromyotomy is performed (Fig. 39-10). Postoperatively, cautious, small, frequent feedings are offered using dilute formula; feedings are gradually increased in strength and volume. In a few days a normal feeding schedule is resumed.

Pneumoperitoneum—Gastric Perforation

Pneumoperitoneum in the neonate usually constitutes a surgical emergency. Elevation of the diaphragm as a result of massive intraperitoneal accumulation of air can produce acute respiratory embarrassment. This air may be quickly and safely aspirated by abdominal-wall puncture, performed to the left or right of the midline. This simple maneuver can be lifesaving, as it improves respiratory dynamics until operative repair of the perforated viscus can be undertaken.

Fig. 39-10. Fredet-Ramstedt pyloromyotomy. *A.* Pylorus delivered into wound and seromuscular layer incised. *B.* Seromuscular layer separated down to submucosal base to permit herniation of mucosa through pyloric incision. *C.* Cross section demonstrating hypertrophied pylorus, depth of incision, and spreading of muscle to permit mucosa to herniate through incision.

Gastrostomy

A gastrostomy is a useful adjunctive procedure for neonates undergoing major abdominal surgery. It is preferred to an indwelling nasogastric tube, which has the potential for causing respiratory embarrassment and permitting gas-

Fig. 39-11. Air-contrast study of an infant with congenital duodenal obstruction. Note size of stomach and distended duodenum, forming the "double bubble."

troesophageal reflux and aspiration. The gastrostomy is also useful to gain access to the gastrointestinal tract in infants who are too weak to take adequate calories by mouth or in infants with complicated oropharyngeal anomalies whose swallowing is impaired.

A Stamm gastrostomy is preferred, employing a Malecot catheter brought out through a separate stab wound in the abdominal wall. It can be removed without difficulty when it is no longer required, and the abdominal defect will usually close spontaneously.

Intestinal Obstruction in the Newborn

The hallmark of intestinal obstruction in the newborn is bilious vomiting. A mechanical obstruction in the intestine must be presumed before assigning this event to other causes such as sepsis or renal disease. Abdominal distension may not be a prominent feature if the obstruction is in the duodenum or the proximal jejunum. Flat and upright abdominal films will frequently indicate the level of the obstruction. A contrast enema will yield information about

intestinal rotation and the caliber of the colon. Contrast material given by mouth is avoided if possible. The upper part of the gastrointestinal tract can be well visualized by instilling air into the stomach.

DUODENAL MALFORMATIONS

Duodenal obstruction may be complete, as in duodenal atresia, or partial, as seen with duodenal stenosis, duodenal web, annular pancreas, and malrotation of the colon. Anomalous entry of the common bile duct and pancreatic duct may be associated with duodenal anomalies; thus, caution must be exercised in the surgical approach to the duodenum.

Duodenal atresia is characterized on x-ray by a "double bubble" (Fig. 39-11). Incomplete obstruction may show this double bubble as well as small amounts of air distally in the gastrointestinal tract. The surgical treatment of congenital duodenal obstruction varies according to the cause. Duodenal atresia is bypassed by either a duodenoduodenostomy or a duodenojejunostomy. An intraluminal web may be excised completely. Obstruction caused by annular pancreas is best treated by a bypass anastomosis, with the pancreas itself left undisturbed. Gastric decompression is accomplished by the insertion of a gastrostomy which should complement any of these procedures.

JEJUNO-ILEAL ATRESIA

Intestinal atresia probably results from intrauterine interruption of the vascular supply to a portion of the bowel. The defect can be reproduced experimentally in the laboratory by ligating branches of the mesenteric artery in the developing fetus. Atresias of the small intestine may be single or multiple. When there has been extensive vascular deficiency there is complete discontinuity of the bowel and a large mesenteric defect. These infants may be subject to the short-gut syndrome after surgical reconstruction.

The clinical presentation of newborn infants with atresia of the jejunum or ileum is similar to that found in other types of intestinal obstruction. Bilious vomiting is an early sign. Abdominal distension is progressive as crying and air swallowing result in dilatation of the bowel proximal to the atretic segment. An abdominal upright film then shows the characteristic stepladder picture of air and fluid in the distended loops. The number of obstructed loops and distribution of air-fluid levels on the x-ray offer some indication of the level of obstruction in the small bowel (Fig. 39-12). It is helpful to obtain a barium enema to determine the size of the colon and to demonstrate whether or not normal bowel rotation has occurred. The finding of a "microcolon" is indicative of distal small-bowel obstruction. The association of abdominal distension, bilious vomiting, and radiographic evidence of obstruction demands urgent surgical intervention unless there is a strong deterrent, such as overwhelming sepsis, severe dehydration, or cardiac failure. In the latter circumstance a limited period of resuscitation is warranted.

The technical problem in the surgical correction of intestinal atresia results from the enormous disparity in lumen size between the proximal distended bowel and the unused distal limb (Fig. 39-13). Anastomosis may be accomplished by (1) end-to-back technique, (2) tapering the proximal dilated limb preparatory to end-to-end union, (3) Bishop-Koop end-to-side anastomosis, (4) Mikulicz exteriorization (Fig. 39-14), or (5) simple temporary ileostomy and delayed anastomosis.

MECONIUM ILEUS

The bowel obstruction in meconium ileus results from impaction of tenacious meconium in the distal ileum. It is always associated with cystic fibrosis of the pancreas (mucoviscidosis). The abdomen of an infant with meconium ileus becomes progressively more distended, although bile vomiting is a relatively late feature. The failure to pass meconium is also a characteristic. The contrast enema will show the tiny caliber of the unused colon (Fig. 39-15). On the plain abdominal film there are dilated small-bowel loops and a "ground-glass" appearance in the right lower quadrant, representing small bubbles of gas trapped in the meconium. The air fluid levels typical of most mechanical obstructions are not seen, a feature which distinguishes meconium ileus. Until Noblett's report all infants with this condition required emergency surgical intervention. It is now standard practice to attempt a Gastrografin enema under fluoroscopic control. In a high percentage of cases this hygroscopic agent permeates the sticky meconium so that it can be evacuated through the rectum, thereby obviating surgery. Because of its powerful osmotic effect, Gastrografin instillation must be done under controlled conditions with an intravenous infusion running.

MALROTATION AND MIDGUT VOLVULUS

PATHOLOGY. During early fetal development, the diminutive abdominal cavity cannot accommodate the rapidly elongating intestine. The midgut, supplied by the

Fig. 39-12. Newborn intestinal obstruction showing several loops of distended bowel with air-fluid levels characteristic of jejunal atresia.

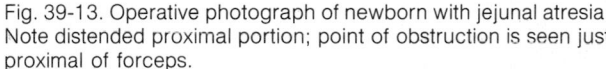

Fig. 39-13. Operative photograph of newborn with jejunal atresia. Note distended proximal portion; point of obstruction is seen just proximal of forceps.

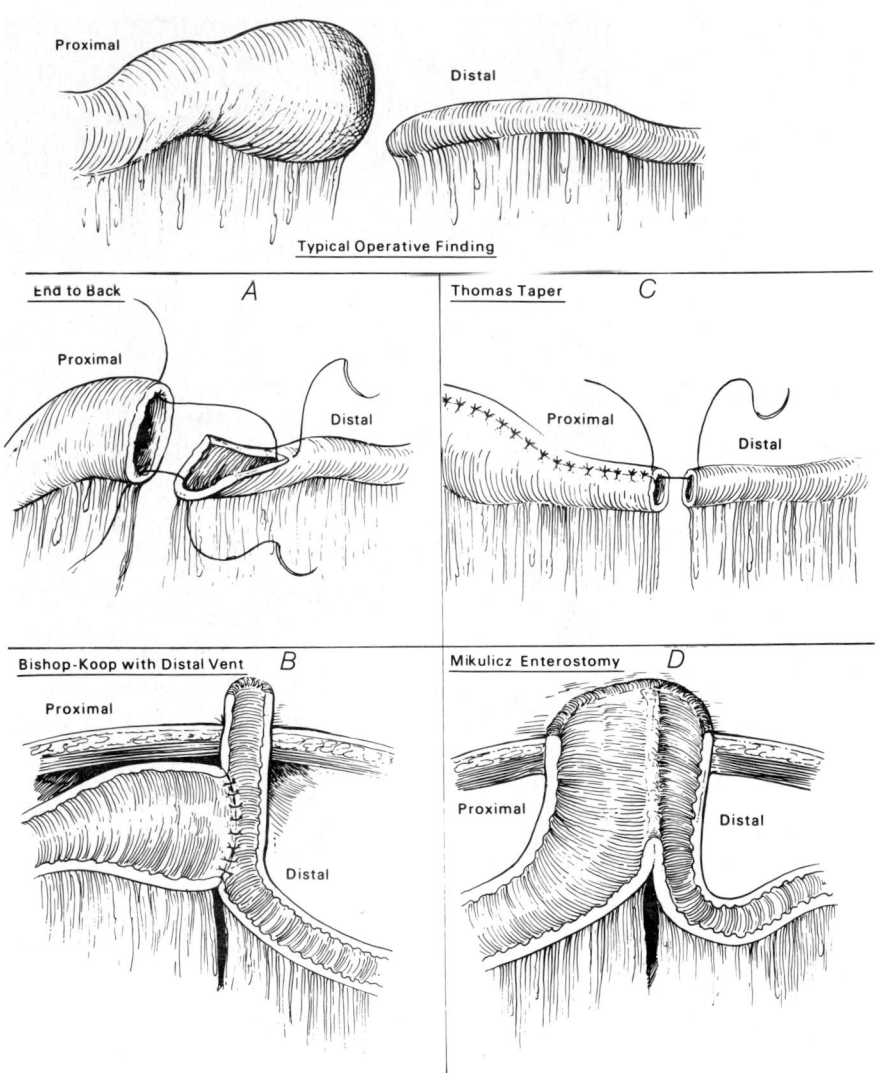

Fig. 39-14. Techniques of intestinal anastomosis for infants with small-bowel obstruction. (Typical operative findings: Proximal distension and discrepancy between ends of intestine to be anastomosed.) A. End to back distal limb has been Incised, creating "fishmouth" to enlarge lumen. B. Bishop-Koop: Proximal distended limb joined to side of small distal bowel, which is vented by "chimney" to the abdominal wall. C. Tapering: Portion of antimesenteric wall of proximal bowel excised, with longitudinal closure to minimize disparity in the limbs. D. Mikulicz double-barreled enterostomy is constructed by suturing the two limbs together, then exteriorizing the double stoma. The common wall can be crushed with a special clamp to create one large stoma. The stoma can be closed in an extraperitoneal manner.

superior mesenteric artery, therefore prolapses into the umbilical cord. As the intestinal loops return to the abdominal cavity during the tenth week of fetal life, final rotation and fixation occur. The duodenum rotates to form a C loop, terminating in the left upper quadrant, and the cecum assumes its final position in the right lower quadrant. When the usual rotation process does not occur, bands extending from the abnormally positioned cecum to the right lateral abdominal wall may cause extrinsic duodenal obstruction. If the cecum remains in the epigastrium, the mesentery is foreshortened and the entire midgut may undergo torsion around the superior mesenteric artery, thereby severely compromising circulation to the bowel.

CLINICAL MANIFESTATIONS. Midgut volvulus may occur at any time during life but is common in the first postnatal week. Characteristically the infant vomits bile and later may begin to pass bloody stools. An abdominal film will often show a paucity of gas in the small bowel. The abnormally placed cecum is demonstrated definitively by barium enema.

TREATMENT. Immediate surgical intervention is mandatory. The intestine must be untwisted to relieve vascular obstruction to the midgut. The bands between the cecum and abdominal wall (Ladd's bands) are then divided. At the completion of this procedure the duodenum is positioned vertically on the right side of the abdomen and the cecum is placed in the left lower quadrant (Fig. 39-16). The appendix is removed. When the viability of the midgut is in doubt, then the volvulus is reduced and all compromised intestine returned to the abdomen. Twenty-four to thirty-six hours later a "second look" is carried out, and only then is a decision made to resect that portion of the bowel judged irretrievably necrotic. This approach will result in maximum salvage of intestine and avoid an irretrievable short-bowel syndrome.

NECROTIZING ENTEROCOLITIS (NEC)

CLINICAL MANIFESTATIONS. Advances in management of high-risk premature infants have introduced a population of neonates at risk from an ischemic bowel disease of uncertain cause. Necrotizing enterocolitis most frequently affects a premature infant with a compromised status. Those with respiratory distress syndrome requiring mechanical ventilation are at greatest risk. It has been observed that symptoms do not develop until feedings are offered.

NEC begins as an ischemic insult to the mucosa of the small and large bowel with invasion of the intestinal wall by gas-producing bacteria. The radiologic finding of air in the wall of the intestine is typical (Fig. 39-17). The ischemic process may progress to involve all layers of the bowel wall, and perforation is common (Fig. 39-18). The afflicted infant shows signs of generalized sepsis and disseminated intravascular coagulation. The abdomen is distended, tense, shiny, erythematous, and tender. Air in the portal vein is a late sign and associated with a grim prognosis.

TREATMENT. The indications for surgery in NEC include physical signs of peritonitis or the x-ray finding of free intraabdominal air. Resection of frankly gangrenous areas of bowel should be carried out and the viable margin ends of the bowel exteriorized. A decompressing gastrostomy should also be carried out.

For at least 2 weeks after surgery, the infant is maintained on total parenteral nutrition, following which oral alimentation is cautiously reintroduced. Although adequate length of the intestine may be preserved, there may be prolonged intestinal malfunction, with malabsorption and diarrhea. Parenteral nutrition may therefore be required for a prolonged period of time.

The formation of strictures in areas of intestine compromised but not frankly gangrenous is not unusual. Therefore, before closing intestinal ostomies a complete evaluation of the gastrointestinal tract by contrast x-ray is mandatory.

Intussusception

Intussusception is an important cause of intestinal obstruction in pediatric patients. The highest incidence is observed in infants eight to twelve months of age. Intussusception occurs when one segment of the bowel (intussusceptum) invaginates into the lumen of the intestine distal to it (intussuscipiens). The most frequent type of intussusception occurs as prolapse of the distal ileum into the cecum, or the ileocolic type. Less commonly, ileoileal and colocolic intussusceptions occur. In these instances a polyp or Meckel's diverticulum may act as a leading point. In many cases of intussusception, no specific lead point is identified.

Fig. 39-15: Barium enema in an infant with meconium ileus. Microcolon is demonstrated. Colonic rotation is normal.

Frequently, intussusception is preceded by a viral syndrome characterized by abdominal pain, vomiting, and diarrhea. The symptoms merge into those of intussusception, thereby presenting a very difficult diagnostic dilemma for the physician. It was this association that led Zachary to the discovery that the adenovirus was frequently associated with intussusception. He reasoned that the intestinal inflammation caused enlargement of the ileal lymphoid tissue, or Peyer's patches, and that these tissues projected into the lumen of the ileum, forming the lead point of the intussusception.

Between paroxysms of intermittent crampy abdominal pain, the infant rests quietly, only to be awakened in 15 or 30 minutes with a recurrence of pain. Vomiting and the passage of bloody mucus per rectum (currant-jelly stool) are later signs. Unless the diagnosis is appreciated, and therapy instituted, serious vascular compromise of the bowel ensues, leading to infarction, peritonitis, and sepsis.

The pathognomonic physical finding in the infant with intussusception is an oblong mass in the right or midupper part of the abdomen and an absence of bowel in the right lower quadrant (Dance's sign). Bloody stool in the rectum is a late sign and indicates that venous compromise has already occurred.

The most important diagnostic procedure is the barium enema (Fig. 39-19). By this technique the intussusception is visualized as an obstructing filling defect preventing retrograde filling of the colon; typically, barium outlines the leading portion of the intussusceptum, giving an x-ray

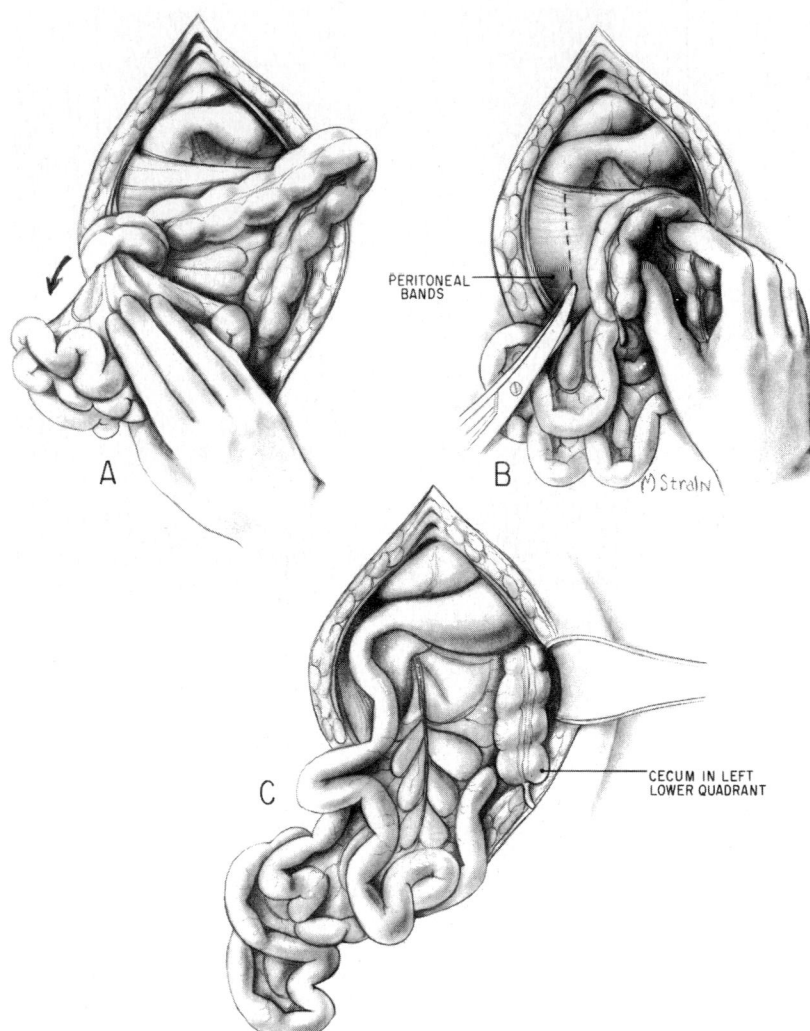

PERITONEAL
BANDS

CECUM IN LEFT
LOWER QUADRANT

Fig. 39-16. Operative procedure for incomplete rotation of cecum and midgut volvulus. *A.* Unwinding of intestine to correct volvulus. *B.* Transection of peritoneal bands extending from cecum in right upper quadrant. *C.* Cecum relocated in left lower quadrant.

appearance of a coiled spring. The barium enema is diagnostic only for ileocolic intussusception; the results will be completely normal if the intussusception is confined to the ileum.

In the majority of patients hydrostatic reduction by barium enema will succeed. Reduction of the intussusception by this modality is not attempted if there are signs of peritonitis or peripheral collapse. Barium is instilled into the rectum under fluoroscopic control (from a height no more than 3 ft 6 in. above the table). Gradually the intussusception is pushed retrograde until the intussusceptum is reduced completely and contrast medium refluxes freely into the terminal ileum. Unless reflux into the ileum is observed unequivocally, the intussusception is regarded as unreduced and immediate surgery is advised.

When hydrostatic reduction fails, or is only partially successful, or when signs of systemic toxicity preclude reduction by this method, surgical exploration is mandatory. The operation is performed through a right lower quadrant transverse incision, through which the involved mass representing the intussusception is delivered. The intussusceptum is reduced by distal compression, pushing

the ileum from within the lumen of the colon until the prolapse is completely reduced. Unless the cecal wall is compromised, the appendix can be removed after reduction. It has recently been shown that the intravenous administration of the biologically active peptide, glucagon, will enhance the chances for successful hydrostatic reduction by its action on the smooth muscle in the intestinal wall. The recurrence rate is low whether the intussusception is reduced by hydrostatic or surgical means, and when the bowel is viable, the prognosis is excellent.

When serious circulatory compromise results in intestinal infarction, the intussusception will not reduce and ileocolic resection is required. Primary reconstruction is carried out, and the infant is given intravenous fluids and antibiotics for 5 to 7 days postoperatively.

Duplications and Mesenteric Cysts

DUPLICATIONS

Duplications can occur at any level in the gastrointestinal tract. They are most common in the small bowel and

Fig. 39-17. X-ray study showing characteristic findings of necrotizing enterocolitis. There are distended, separated loops of bowel. Air is seen in the wall of the bowel (pneumotosis). The arrow depicts free air above the liver and below the diaphragm, signifying perforation.

affect primarily the ileum. These cystic masses are located on the mesenteric aspect of the intestine and lie within the leaves of the mesentery. They share a common wall with the contiguous small bowel. The duplications may be long and tubular, but more commonly are large, single cystic masses over which the normal intestinal tract is stretched. Duplications may cause obstruction by effacement of the adjacent small bowel; they may also undergo torsion, with gangrene and perforation. Bleeding into the lumen of the intestine occurs when ectopic gastric mucosa is present in the duplication. Although rare, these anomalies are troublesome and difficult to diagnose, since they are often mobile within the abdomen. Treatment consists of resection of the duplication and attached bowel. If extirpation is not possible, excision of a window from the septum between the cyst and intestine should be performed.

MESENTERIC CYSTS

Mesenteric cysts are similar to duplications in their location within the mesentery. However, they do not possess the muscular wall characteristic of duplications, and are not lined with mucosa. Chylous cyst is an unusual form of mesenteric cyst which develops secondary to congenital obstruction of the intestinal lymphatic drainage (Fig. 39-20). Mesenteric and chylous cysts can cause partial or complete intestinal obstruction, or may present as an abdominal mass. It is often necessary to resect a segment of involved intestine to circumscribe the mass surgically. Excision is curative, and there are no known malignant com-

ponents to these cysts. When these cystic structures involve a large portion of the intestinal mesentery they are best treated by partial surgical excision and marsupialization.

Hirschsprung's Disease

PATHOLOGY. The defect underlying this condition is congenital absence of ganglion cells in the rectum and rectosigmoid. Though the aganglionosis may involve the

Fig. 39-18. Operative photograph showing distended small bowel in an infant with necrotizing enterocolitis. Air is demonstrated beneath the serosa in the wall of the bowel.

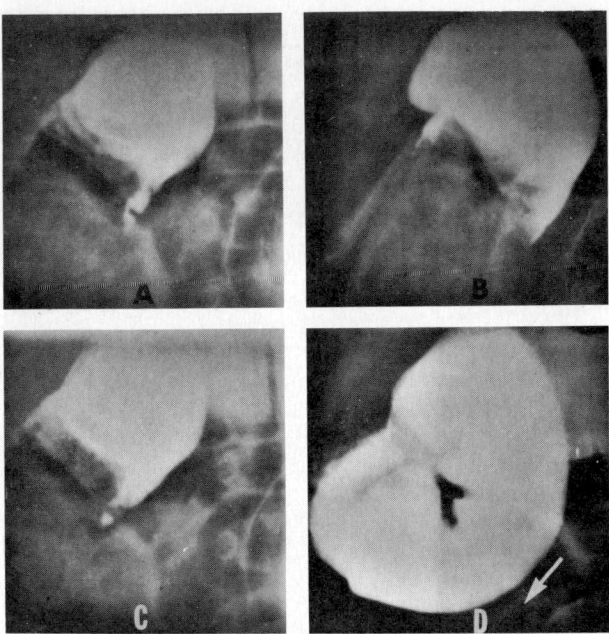

Fig. 39-19. Barium enema diagnosis and reduction of intussusception. *A* to *C*. Various stages of reduction. *D*. Reduction complete and radiopaque material noted in ileum.

entire colon, such extensive involvement is rare. Although this condition was originally described by Hirschsprung in 1888, appropriate surgical treatment was not devised until the classic work of Swenson in 1948. The absence of ganglion cells modifies the neuromuscular conduction. The area of aganglionosis in the bowel is inert and acts as an obstructing lesion. It is, however, the normally innervated proximal colon which dilates, distends, and undergoes muscular hypertrophy.

CLINICAL MANIFESTATIONS. The consequences of aganglionosis may be of such magnitude as to be life-threatening in the newborn period (Fig. 39-21). On the other hand the clinical presentation of Hirschsprung's disease may be subtle and in fact go unrecognized for months or years until the classic symptoms of constipation, abdominal distension, and secondary malnutrition become unmistakable. It is important to note, however, that the history of constipation almost always goes back to the early days of life in most patients with Hirschsprung's disease. Abdominal distension or debilitating enterocolitis brings the infant to the attention of the physician.

When an infant fails to pass meconium spontaneously in the first 24 hours of life, Hirschsprung's disease becomes a consideration. Though other forms of intestinal obstruction may be confused with Hirschsprung's disease, appropriate efforts will lead to a correct diagnosis.

In older children there are striking clinical findings. The abdomen is immense and out of proportion to the extremities, which are usually spindly. Children with long-standing megacolon are typically pale and cheerless. Growth and development are impeded. The major differential diagnosis in children with chronic constipation is Hirschsprung's disease or some form of habit constipation (psychogenic megacolon, chronic constipation, encopresis). The finding on physical examination of a dilated rectum, with stool well down against the anus, argues against the diagnosis of Hirschsprung's disease, since the aganglionic segment usually does not contain stool.

DIAGNOSTIC STUDIES. The barium enema in the newborn is not always a reliable study, since the characteristic disparity between the aganglionic distal segment and the

Fig. 39-20. Operative photograph depicting loops of ileum with a large chylous cyst in the mesentery. Note the relationship of the vascular supply to the bowel as it courses over the cyst. In most instances resection of the involved intestine is necessary.

Fig. 39-21. Abdominal distension in a four-month-old infant with Hirschsprung's disease. The faint outline of an enlarged colon can be seen in the upper abdomen. Immediate decompressing colostomy is advised in such circumstances.

distended ganglionic segment proximal to it may not be seen early in life. In older children the barium enema is diagnostic. Typically there is a distal narrow segment, aganglionic bowel, with greatly distended colon proximal to this.

Rectal biopsy affords the definitive diagnosis in Hirschsprung's disease. There are several techniques of biopsy. The purpose of biopsy is to obtain a specimen of the rectal wall in which the ganglion cells can be evaluated. Experienced pathologists can interpret the more superficial biopsies which include only the submucosal tissue. The advantage of a partial-thickness rather than a full-thickness biopsy is that intramural scarring is minimized—a factor which is important to the subsequent performance of corrective surgical procedures. A suction biopsy technique is available and has particular application for infants. This bedside procedure usually provides adequate submucosal tissue for interpretation by an experienced pediatric pathologist.

TREATMENT. Treatment is surgical in all cases. Colostomy is appropriate for almost all children with the diagnosis of Hirschsprung's disease. After a period of months with adequate diet, the distended bowel returns to normal caliber. A definitive operation designed to eliminate the aganglionic segment is then possible. There are now three generally applied operations, based on the principal developed by Swenson, which are used for the definitive treatment of Hirschsprung's disease. The first is the original Swenson pull-through procedure. In this operation the rectosigmoid is carefully dissected in the pelvis and the distal anorectal junction is joined to the colon by an anastomosis carried out through a perineal approach (Fig. 39-22B). Variations of Swenson's technique have been devised by Duhamel and Soave (Fig. 39-22). In the former

procedure the ganglionic bowel is brought into the retrorectal space and anastomosed just above the anus posteriorly, with preservation of the anterior aganglionic rectal wall. In Soave's operation, the dissection is completely intramural, with removal of the mucosa of the rectum and anastomosis within the seromuscular sleeve of aganglionic rectum (Fig. 39-23). Following any of these repairs the outlook for most patients is for normal or near-normal bowel function.

TOTAL COLONIC AGANGLIONOSIS

An infrequent variant, total colonic aganglionosis presents special problems in diagnosis and management. The barium enema does not show the typical transition area characteristic of low-segment Hirschsprung's disease. Diagnosis is based upon a series of biopsies taken at the time of laparotomy which prove the entire colon to be aganglionic, back to and sometimes including the ileum. Surgical therapy is predicated upon transposing normally innervated distal ileum to the anus by end-to-side suture technique, or by low anterior resection with ileorectal anastomosis. The latter converts the patient's condition to a short-segment Hirschsprung's disease, which, with the low ileal anastomosis, can be compensated.

Imperforate Anus

Imperforate anus affects males and females with equal frequency and occurs in approximately one of every 20 000 live births. The anomaly results from a failure of differentiation of the urogenital sinus and cloaca. Imperforate anus is classified as high or low, depending upon the level to which the rectal pouch has descended. High imperforate anus in either sex implies that the rectal pouch is at or above the levator musculature. Low imperforate anus implies that the rectum has descended through this muscle complex and resides in a normal anatomical relationship to the levator sling and the puborectalis muscle. In an infant

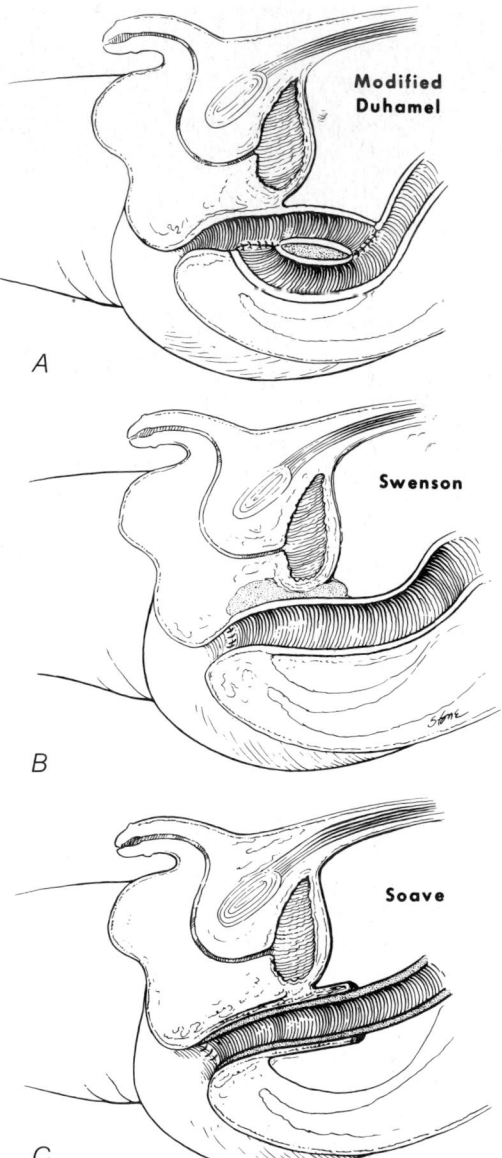

Fig. 39-22. The three basic operations for surgical correction of Hirschsprung's disease. *A.* The Duhamel procedure leaves the rectum in place and brings ganglionic bowel into the retrorectal space. The common wall, indicated by lines, is crushed to eliminate the septum. *B.* Classic Swenson operation (1948) is a resection with end-to-end anastomosis performed by exteriorizing bowel ends through the anus. *C.* The Soave operation is performed by endorectal dissection and removal of mucosa from the aganglionic distal segment and bringing the ganglionic bowel down to the anus within the seromuscular tunnel.

with low imperforate anus, the relationship of the rectum to the muscles of continence is normal, whereas patients with high imperforate anus will require a pull-through operation to establish the normal relationship between the levator muscles and the rectum.

Ninety percent of afflicted female infants will have imperforate anus of the low type. In these patients the rectum terminates by means of a fistula which presents anterior to

the normal location of the anus on the perineum, in the vaginal fourchette or low in the vagina. An emergency colostomy is not necessary in these infants, since satisfactory decompression can be accomplished through the fistula. Although it is technically feasible to perform an anoplasty in the newborn period, it is not necessary. In females with low imperforate anus and a vaginal fistula, dissection of the fistula and mobilization of the distal rectum from the vagina is optimally performed at three to six months of age. This dissection is performed entirely below the levator sling; thus continence should be assured. When the fistula is located high in the vagina, it is not accessible to dilation or surgical revision in the newborn period. For these infants, a colostomy is necessary. Definitive surgical therapy for high imperforate anus in the female is deferred until the baby weighs 15 to 20 lb.

In the male, the distribution of high and low imperforate anus is roughly equal. About half present with a fistula which opens on the perineum anterior to the normal location of the anus. In some the fistula terminates as far forward as the ventral surface of the penis. At birth, the opening of the fistula is not always apparent, and an interval of 12 to 24 hours may be required until meconium reaches the distal-most point in the gastrointestinal tract. For these infants, a perineal anoplasty supplemented by local dilatation will accomplish decompression of the bowel, and emergency colostomy is not needed.

When no fistula is visible on the perineum, the male infant must be presumed to have high imperforate anus with a fistulous connection to the posterior urethra. A colostomy is needed for decompression, and the definitive pull-through operation is generally deferred until the infant is about a year old. The colostomy should be placed high in the sigmoid colon. The definitive pull-through procedure can be performed through a sacroperineal or abdominosacroperineal approach, without taking down the colostomy. Urine refluxed through the urethral fistula is not exposed to excessive colonic surface and is not associated with reabsorption of urinary chloride and consequent acidosis. Even after the restoration of normal anatomic relationships the functional result may not be optimal. Analysis of long-term follow-up data has shown that in almost 50 percent of patients it is difficult to accomplish toilet training, and occasional soiling or minimal incontinence is not infrequent. In 50 percent continence is never achieved. Therefore, the families must be counseled truthfully, so that their expectations will be realistic.

JAUNDICE

General Considerations

PATHOLOGY. The primary surgical consideration in the evaluation of a jaundiced neonate is the differentiation between obstructive and nonobstructive causes. In addition to the physiologic jaundice of the newborn, other nonobstructive causes of hyperbilirubinemia include excessive red cell destruction from blood incompatibility, intrauterine infections such as toxoplasmosis, herpes, cytomegalic

Fig. 39-23. Operative photograph of Soave procedure for Hirschsprung's disease. The seromuscular tunnel has been developed, and the circular muscle of the rectum is clearly seen. The mucosa has been stripped away from this tunnel and can be seen below the normally innervated sigmoid colon. The mucosal sleeve will be pulled through the rectum and the normal sigmoid colon drawn into the seromuscular tunnel for anastomosis at the anus.

inclusion disease, and syphilis; and genetically determined metabolic disorders such as alpha$_1$ antitrypsin deficiency. Additionally, there is a heterogeneous group of conditions labeled "neonatal hepatitis" which result in severe intrahepatic cholestasis. In addition to these medical causes of jaundice in the neonate, there are anatomic derangements which result in obstructive forms of jaundice. The most common of these is biliary atresia.

DIAGNOSTIC STUDIES. In the laboratory evaluation of an infant with hyperbilirubinemia, no single test is diagnostic. Laboratory studies should include measurement of prothrombin time, PTT, alkaline phosphatase, transaminases, and serologic evaluation to rule out intrauterine infection. The most useful evaluations are the rose Bengal scan and percutaneous needle biopsy. Although the isotope scan will not discriminate between intrahepatic cholestasis and extrahepatic obstruction, the presence of isotope in the gastrointestinal tract confirms patency of the extrahepatic bile ducts. Severe intrahepatic cholestasis may result in complete retention of the isotope within the liver. The percutaneous needle biopsy is diagnostic in about 85 percent of the cases. When the laboratory information is overlapping or unclear, it may be necessary to undertake surgical exploration, with biopsy of the liver and operative cholangiogram. Today, surgical exploration of the jaundiced neonate can be carried out in such a way as not to prejudice adversely the recovery of those infants who will be diagnosed as having a neonatal cholestatic syndrome with normal extrahepatic biliary structures. However, delay in the diagnosis of an infant with biliary atresia may eliminate any chance for surgical correction by the portoenterostomy procedure. This operative approach, pioneered by Kasai, should be performed before the twelfth week of life, after which, the microscopic biliary ductules seem to lose their patency. At the time of surgical exploration and operative cholangiography, if no gallbladder is present, it is justifiable to enlarge the incision and carry out formal exploration of the porta hepatis.

Extrahepatic Biliary Atresia

TREATMENT. In the vast majority of infants with extrahepatic biliary atresia, the entire extrahepatic biliary tree is affected. About 5 to 10 percent of these patients will have a patent hepatic or common hepatic duct with distal atresia; this is the so-called favorable type, which lends itself to reestablishment of biliary continuity in the gastrointestinal tract by means of Roux-en-Y choledochojejunostomy or choledochoduodenostomy. The portoenterostomy procedure now offers a chance of surgical relief of jaundice in some of those infants for whom there was formerly no hope (Fig. 39-24). Biliary atresia does not imply an absence of the extrahepatic biliary system; rather these structures are present as fibrous cords. Kasai's work demonstrates that the cords at the porta hepatis contain microscopically patent ductules.

It is to these channels that the jejunal conduit is anastomosed. When the operation is carried out before the twelfth week of life, bile drainage can be accomplished in many infants. It has been shown, however, that bile drainage is not tantamount to cure, for cirrhosis may continue even when bile drainage is achieved. However, a significant salvage rate has been accomplished in this group of infants, who formerly died usually by the end of the first year of life.

Biliary Hypoplasia

At the time of surgical exploration and operative cholangiography, the extrahepatic bile ducts may appear anatomically normal in distribution but have only a minute

Fig. 39-24. Operative diagram of the Kasai portoenterostomy for biliary atresia. An isolated limb of jejunum has been brought to the porta hepatis and anastomosed to the transected ducts. The Roux-en-Y principle has been used to reconstitute intestinal continuity.

lumen. This has been termed *biliary hypoplasia* and is associated with a variety of hepatobiliary disorders resulting in intrahepatic cholestasis, including neonatal hepatitis and alpha₁ antitrypsin deficiency. Portoenterostomy is not applicable for this category of patients.

Choledochal Cyst

Extrahepatic biliary obstruction from choledochal cyst probably results from a localized obliterative process in the distal common duct. This disorder may be a more generalized alteration of the biliary drainage system, since many infants develop liver failure despite surgical relief of the obstructed bile flow. Diagnosis is often possible by palpation of the cyst. Barium studies of the upper gastrointestinal tract show displacement of the viscera by the cysts. Ultrasound echograms are also useful in defining cystic structures in the porta hepatis. The surgical options include drainage of the cyst to the duodenum or jejunum, or resection of the cyst with anastomosis of the bowel to the hepatic duct proximal to the origin of the choledochal cyst. The latter surgical approach is preferable, since malignant neoplasms may occur in the cyst wall and also the incidence of cholangitis is reduced.

ABNORMALITIES OF THE ABDOMINAL WALL

Umbilical Hernia

Most children with umbilical hernia heal spontaneously by about four years of age. Surgical repair is usually indicated if the hernia persists beyond this time. In younger patients, massive enlargement and distortion of the umbilicus dictate the need for earlier repair. Incarceration of umbilical hernia is extremely uncommon but has been seen in patients who have a small fascial defect associated with a large sac. A simple repair of the fascia is all that is required to correct this form of hernia. This can be done through a small curving infraumbilical incision which leaves an unobtrusive scar. Complicated fascial flap repairs are not necessary for children. The umbilicus is never excised.

Patent Urachus

During the development of the coelomic cavity, there is free communication between the urinary bladder and the abdominal wall through the urachus, which exits adjacent the omphalomesenteric duct. Persistence of this tract results in a communication between the bladder and the umbilicus (Fig. 39-25B). The first sign of a patent urachus is moisture or obvious urine emission from the umbilicus. Recurrent urinary tract infection may result. The urachus may be partly obliterated, with a remnant remaining beneath the umbilicus in the extraperitoneal position as an isolated cyst. Diagnosis of patent urachus is most reliably made by a cystogram in the lateral projection. Surgical correction is carried out via extraperitoneal exposure of the infraumbilical area. Identification and excision of the urachal tract with closure of the bladder is curative. Urachal cysts are also easily excised from this approach.

Patent Omphalomesenteric Duct

In fetal life, the omphalomesenteric duct is connected through the central wall of the coelomic cavity to the intestinal tract. Normally this duct involutes, but its persistence results in a tubular attachment between the ileum and the umbilicus (Fig. 39-25A). Liquid ileal content refluxes through the umbilical defect, soiling the abdominal wall. Diagnosis of a congenital fistula at the umbilicus is made by inspection, probing of the tract, and introduction of radiopaque material into the ostium. Proper surgical treatment consists of elective abdominal exploration with closure of the fistula on the antimesenteric border of the ileum and total excision of the fistulous tract, including its attachment to the undersurface of the umbilicus. Though not an emergency, this procedure should not be postponed, since there is a potential for intestinal volvulus to occur around this intraabdominal structure. Occasionally the peristaltic activity of the bowel will cause eversion of the intestine through this patent duct. The extruded intestine resembles a small ruptured omphalocele, and the lesion requires careful inspection at the neck of the defect to

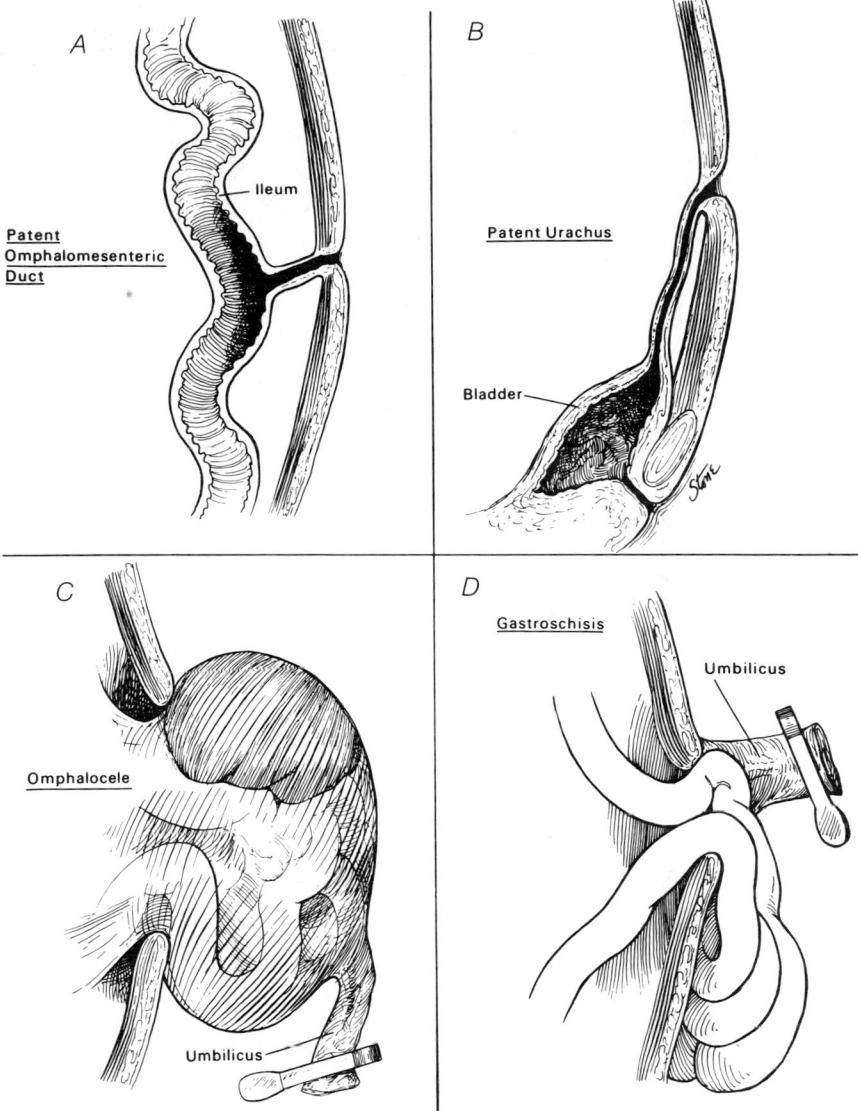

Fig. 39-25. Abnormalities at the umbilicus: *A.* Patent omphalo-mesenteric duct: persistent patent tract from ileum to abdominal wall, through which intestinal contents can be discharged or bowel can prolapse. *B.* Patent urachus: tract to umbilicus from bladder. Partial patency results in urachal cyst. *C.* Omphalocele: large abdominal wall defect with intestine and solid viscera within an intact sac. *D.* Gastroschisis: intestine prolapsing through small abdominal wall defect at the base of the umbilicus.

determine its true nature. In such cases the bowel has, in effect, turned inside out and prolapsed through the patent duct, forming an external intussusception. In this instance, immediate operation with reduction and correction is necessary.

Omphalocele

Interruption of normal formation of the abdominal wall can result in a central defect termed *omphalocele* (Fig 39-25C). In the newborn, the defect appears as a variable-sized mass of bowel and solid viscera in the center of the abdomen, covered by a translucent membrane. The size varies from 1 to 2 cm (Fig. 39-26) to a huge defect containing all the abdominal viscera. Usually the sac remains intact, but occasionally it is ruptured during delivery. The diagnosis of this anomaly is made by inspection, for it is readily apparent immediately after the birth. No pressure should be placed on the omphalocele sac in an effort to reduce it. This is not only hazardous to the integrity of the sac, but may interfere with abdominal venous return or impede the respiratory effort.

Small omphaloceles are usually amenable to complete one-stage reduction and anatomic surgical repair of the abdominal wall. For omphaloceles larger than 6 cm, a sheet of silastic with interwoven Marlex mesh is sewed around the edge of the defect to envelope the prolapsing viscera (Fig. 39-27). Continuous pressure on this prosthetic covering over a period of days brings about gradual reduc-

Fig. 39-26. Small omphalocele or hernia into the umbilical cord. Note that formation of the abdominal wall is nearly complete.

tion of the omphalocele, such that complete surgical closure of the abdominal wall can be accomplished as a staged procedure. The temporary use of a prosthetic covering allows gradual enlargement of the abdominal cavity, which then accommodates the extraneous viscera without compromising venous return or ventilatory dynamics. Intestinal atresia, congenital heart disease, and renal anomalies occur in approximately 30 percent of infants with omphalocele. The overall prognosis for these infants is affected by the existence and severity of associated anomalies.

Gastroschisis

Gastroschisis was originally thought to be a form of ruptured omphalocele, but now is recognized as a distinct embryologic phenomenon in which the abdominal wall has completed its development. There is no central defect, nor

Fig. 39-27. Close-up of silastic prosthesis for temporary covering of gastroschisis. The remnant of the umbilicus is seen in the center of the photograph. A gastrostomy tube is seen.

is there any significant separation of the rectus muscles. There is a small defect at the base of the umbilicus through which part or all of the intestine herniates (Fig. 39-25D). The escape of intestine into the amniotic fluid can occur at different times in fetal life. Thus the bowel of some infants born with gastroschisis is glistening and normal-appearing, suggesting a recent onset, just prior to birth, while others show edematous and matted intestinal loops which appear to have been exposed to the amniotic fluid for many weeks or months (Fig. 39-28).

Immediately upon recognition of gastroschisis, the prolapsed intestine should be wrapped with a dressing soaked in warm sterile saline solution and an outer dry layer. Prompt surgical repair should be undertaken. In about half the cases, the viscera can be returned to the abdomen and secure closure obtained. It is usually necessary to enlarge the defect in order to accomplish this. When the bowel is matted and edematous it may take many weeks before recovery of intestinal function. In such instances, support by total parenteral nutrition is lifesaving. If the abdominal wall cannot be closed without undue tension, then an extra abdominal prosthetic compartment is fashioned from silastic-covered Marlex (Fig. 39-27). Once the prosthesis is in place, the capacity of the prosthetic envelope is gradually reduced over 7 to 10 days until complete surgical closure is obtained.

Exstrophy of the Cloaca (Vesicointestinal Fissure)

Exstrophy of the cloaca represents one of the severest forms of embryologic derangement. In infants with cloacal exstrophy, the normal ventral closure of the pelvis and the wall is imperfect. Major components of the cloacal exstrophy are (1) omphalocele, (2) exstrophy of the bladder, (3) external intestinal fistula through the bladder (ompha-

Fig. 39-28. Newborn with gastroschisis. The intestine has escaped through a defect just to the right of the umbilicus. The intestine is edematous and matted, indicating that these loops have been floating freely in the amnion for some period of time.

lomesenteric duct), (4) epispadias in the males, (5) imperforate anus, and (6) foreshortened colon (Fig. 39-29). In addition there is often an associated orthopedic deformity of the distal leg and foot. The summation of these physical defects is such that many of the newborns are not hardy enough to survive.

Early surgical intervention in these patients becomes necessary when extensive intestinal prolapse through the fistula causes intestinal obstruction. In such circumstances

Fig. 39-29. Close-up of baby with exstrophy of the cloaca. Note large omphalocele with clamp on the umbilical cord. Two halves of the exstrophied bladder are readily seen, with a prolapsed intestinal defect in the center. The imperforate anus is also shown. Pubic bones are widely separated.

an ileostomy is required. The colon is temporarily exteriorized as a mucous fistula. The omphalocele is closed primarily or treated with a topical agent which promotes epithelialization. There is no urgency about repairing the exstrophied bladder, and reconstruction of the urinary system need not be completed until the patient is two or three years of age. While most patients suffer a number of physical limitations, many have the potential for functional rehabilitation, which justifies aggressive surgical efforts on their behalf.

Congenital Deficiency of the Abdominal Musculature (Eagle-Barrett Syndrome; Prune-Belly Syndrome)

Congenital deficiency of the abdominal musculature is a rare anomaly occurring in males. In severely affected in-

Fig. 39-30. Eagle-Barrett (prune-belly) syndrome. Baby with congenital absence of the abdominal musculature, showing lax, flaccid abdomen. This syndrome occurs in males and is associated with severe malformations of the urinary collecting system.

fants, there is marked wrinkling of the skin of the lower part of the abdomen and little or no muscular substance detectable beneath it (Fig. 39-30). In addition to the absent abdominal muscles, the bladder is large and the ureters are dilated and tortuous. The kidneys may be hypoplastic, but there is usually adequate renal parenchyma.

Advances in techniques of urinary reconstruction have improved the prognosis for this group. Temporary urinary diversion with subsequent stage reconstruction, by shortening, tapering, and reimplantation of the ureters, and reduction in the size of the bladder has been successful in rehabilitating the urinary tract. Various surgical procedures have been devised to tighten the lax abdominal musculature and reduce the redundancy of the abdominal wall, thereby providing adequate support. This approach has changed materially the dismal outlook that most of these children faced a decade age.

Inguinal Hernia

Inguinal hernia results from a failure of closure of the processus vaginalis, which is normally obliterated in males by two or three months of age. The processus is a fingerlike projection of the peritoneum which accompanies the testicle as it descends into the scrotum. Infants are at particular risk from incarceration of a hernia. The internal inguinal ring is narrow; therefore, intestine finding its way into the hernial sac in the inguinal canal can become trapped within the hernial sac. When there is diagnostic confusion between an incarcerated hernia and a hydrocele, a rectal examination with simultaneous abdominal palpation of the internal inguinal ring will delineate the structures passing through the internal ring into the inguinal canal. Using the vas deferens as a constant reference point, the presence of intestine adjacent to the vas between the examining fingers confirms the diagnosis of a hernia. Most often the hernia can be reduced. The infant is sedated, and moderate, bimanual pressure is applied by compressing the sac from below while a gentle counterforce downward is provided from the examiner's hand above the inguinal ring. Occasionally, these hernias will reduce spontaneously after sedation is given and the continuous struggling and crying are terminated. Surgery should be delayed 48 hours, until the local edema secondary to incarceration has resolved. If the hernia cannot be reduced, or, in cases of obvious intestinal obstruction, emergency operation, with reduction and repair, is necessary.

An inguinal hernia in the female usually is indicated by the appearance of a nontender groin mass. The mass represents an ovary herniated into the patent sac. Although the gonad can usually be reduced into the abdomen by gentle pressure, it often prolapses in and out until surgical repair is carried out. In some patients the ovary and fallopian tube constitute one wall of the hernial sac (sliding hernia), and in these cases the ovary can be effectively reduced only at the time of operation. Because of the frequency of bilaterality, contralateral exploration is recommended for all infants under one year of age except those in whom it is precluded by a coexisting medical condition or in whom the operation on the symptomatic side is unduly difficult.

Hydrocele is often associated with inguinal hernia. The hydrocele may communicate with the peritoneal cavity via the patent processus vaginalis and, therefore, wax and wane in size. Alternatively the hydrocele may be encysted and confined to the scrotum or to the inguinal canal. Usually a simple hydrocele does not require operation unless it is shown after 1 to 2 years of observation that it is not undergoing spontaneous regression.

GENITALIA

Undescended Testicle

One or both testicles may be absent from the scrotum of a newborn baby, or this finding may be noticed in the male child of any age. The empty scrotum can mean incomplete descent of the gonad or congenital absence. Confusion pervades the medical literature regarding the endocrinologic function and surgical treatment of the undescended testicle. The decision to operate is ideally made when the child is four to five years old. If the testicle can be drawn into the upper scrotum, then surgical therapy is delayed in favor of a period of observation, with the expectation that it will descend spontaneously. If the testicle cannot be brought into the scrotum by manual manipulation then it is unlikely that it will ever descend spontaneously. Operative repair cannot be delayed indefinitely, because spermatogenesis is reduced significantly when the testicle resides in the inguinal canal or within the abdomen where it is exposed to the normal body temperature. If the testicle cannot be palpated in the inguinal canal, it may occasionally be found in the perineum or medial thigh (ectopic testis). If an accompanying hernia is symptomatic, the surgical treatment of the undescended testicle and hernia should be performed as a combined procedure whenever the hernia manifests itself, even in infancy. Five specific reasons are generally advanced for operative replacement of an undescended testicle. These are (1) decreased or absent spermatogenesis; (2) embarrassment and concern to the boy with the empty scrotum, (3) increased incidence of malignancy, (4) increased incidence of torsion of the testicle, and (5) increased vulnerability to trauma (to the testicle which lies on the pubis).

Operative Technique. The operative approach to the undescended testicle is made through a groin incision exposing the retroperitoneum. The hernial sac is dissected from the cord and vascular pedicle. These structures are then freed of all connective tissue investments, which usually affords adequate length to allow the testicle to be placed in the scrotum. The testicle is brought through a new opening of the transversalis fascia immediately lateral to the pubic tubercle. In this way the internal ring is moved medially just behind the external ring. This shortens the distance that the cord and vessels must travel, thereby assuring adequate length. A scrotal pouch is dissected to accommodate the testicle outside the Dartos fascia. This maneuver ensures that the testicle remains in the scrotum without retraction into the inguinal canal.

In about 5 percent of patients an *abdominal testicle* will be found. In this group the artery and vein are short, precluding placement of the testicle in the scrotum even with a series of staged operations. In this circumstance it has been recommended that the artery and vein be divided and the testicle placed in the scrotum still attached to the vas deferens and its accompanying deferential artery. The deferential artery will supply enough blood to allow the testicle to remain viable. This approach is an attractive alternative to orchiectomy.

Intersexual Abnormalities (Ambiguous Genitalia; Hermaphrodite Syndromes)

The infant born with ambiguous external genitalia demands an urgent diagnostic workup (Fig. 39-31). Correct sex assignment must be made in the early days of life to avoid embarrassment and confusion on the part of the parents and the inevitable social stigma that results. Diagnostic procedures, including laparotomy when indicated, should be completed by the time the infant is a week old. However, hurried assignment of sex, without adequate understanding of the patient's anatomy, endocrine physiology, and chromosomes can lead to a mistaken diagnosis with tragic consequences.

Patients with ambiguous genitalia may be grouped into four categories:

1. True hermaphrodite (coexisting testicular and ovarian tissue)
2. Male pseudohermaphrodite (testicular gonads only) with hypospadias, one or both testes undescended, and persistent Müllerian duct remnants
3. Female pseudohermaphrodites (ovarian gonads only)
4. Absent or deficient gonads

Fig. 39-31. Ambiguous genitalia, manifest as enlarged clitoris and labioscrotal folds in a baby with the adrenogenital syndrome. This configuration can be confused with a normal penis and undescended testicles.

MOST COMMON SITES OF CANCER IN CHILDREN

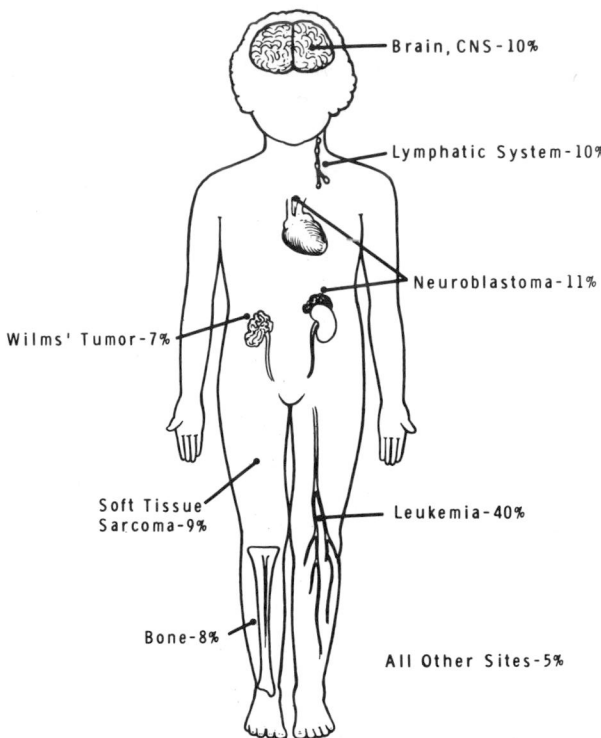

Brain, CNS - 10%

Lymphatic System - 10%

Neuroblastoma - 11%

Wilms' Tumor - 7%

Soft Tissue Sarcoma - 9%

Leukemia - 40%

Bone - 8%

All Other Sites - 5%

Fig. 39-32. Most common sites of cancer in children.

Securing a full family history, including details of the pregnancy with special attention to drug ingestion, is the first diagnostic step. Then the genitalia should be inspected and all orifices carefully defined. Rectal examination is helpful in detecting the uterus and cervix. Radiologic examination of the kidneys, urinary tract, and vagina discloses the presence and size of these structures. Chromosomal studies offer important information about genotypic sex, but this information alone should never constitute the basis for a final sex assignment without consideration of the anatomical and endocrine status of the patient. Elevated urinary excretion of pregnanetriol and 17 ketosteroids is diagnostic of congenital adrenal hyperplasia. When all other diagnostic maneuvers have been completed, a few patients will require laparotomy for identification of internal structures and biopsy of gonadal tissue. The laparotomy is for diagnosis only; excision of contradictory sexual structures is avoided at this stage until full disclosure of all the facts has been made before the family, and alternatives have been thoroughly discussed.

TREATMENT. Except for the diagnostic laparotomy, operative correction is usually begun at one or two years of age. Males require hypospadias repair and excision of remnants of the Müllerian ducts. In the case of true hermaphrodites, removal of the contradictory gonad is indicated. For many females, surgical revision of the enlarged clitoris may be necessary. A revision of the vaginal introitus may be needed in infancy to eliminate urinary

infection; a second surgical procedure may then be required in the premarital years. In some masculinized females, the distal vagina is congenitally absent and extensive reconstruction to unite the perineal skin and the proximal vagina is required.

Severe penile hypoplasia occurs in a small number of males. In these patients the testicles are histologically normal, albeit undescended; chromosome analysis reveals normal male genotype, but the phallus is a tiny clitoris-like structure. The phallus is inadequate for the male role, and there is presently no satisfactory medical or surgical treatment to alter the hypoplastic penis. Consequently, male patients in this small group are more successfully reared as females. The intersexual anomalies require effective teamwork between neonatologist, endocrinologist, geneticist, and surgeon to achieve the most satisfactory rehabilitation of these children.

MALIGNANT DISEASE

Approximately 12 percent of deaths in children is attributed to malignant disease. Of these, solid tumors account for 55 percent, while leukemia is responsible for death in the remaining children afflicted with cancer (Fig. 39-32).

Fig. 39-33. IVP from a patient with bilateral Wilms' tumor. Note bilateral distortion of calyceal systems.

Wilms' Tumor (Nephroblastoma)

Approximately 500 new cases of Wilms' tumor are recorded in the United States each year. The discovery of an asymptomatic mass in the abdomen is the usual presentation of this malignant tumor. The incidence is greatest in the first 2 years of life. Males and females are affected equally. Intravenous pyelography is diagnostic in most cases. The collecting system typically shows a marked distortion, with the calyces appearing to be pulled apart (Fig. 39-33). Unless the tumor has invaded the renal pelvis obstructing the ureter, drainage appears normal. Renal function is generally unimpaired. Prompt nephrectomy with ipsilateral lymph node dissection is the preferred treatment. Some centers advocate preoperative radiation and/or chemotherapy to shrink the tumor, thus making subsequent resection technically easier. This necessarily reduces the amount of radiation that can be delivered to the tumor bed postoperatively. Chemotherapy with actinomycin D and vincristine has changed the outlook remarkably for patients with residual or recurrent disease. Actinomycin D has a synergistic effect when coupled with radiation therapy. Results obtained in the National Wilms' Tumor Study show 95 percent cure rate when the tumor is confined to the kidney or regional nodes (Stage I, II). Even when the tumor has spread to distant sites, the combination of radiation chemotherapy and, when appropriate, repeated excisional therapy has resulted in a cure rate of 80 percent of all children with Wilms' tumor.

Neuroblastoma

Following leukemia and tumors of the central nervous system, neuroblastoma is the third most frequent tumor of childhood, accounting for approximately 11 percent of all malignant disease. Neuroblastomas arise from the sympathetic nervous system, the typical sites being the adrenal glands and the posterior mediastinum. Some 50 percent of neuroblastomas occur in patients under a year of age, and 85 percent occur by age three. The younger children have a better prognosis. Patients seen before the age of one year have an overall survival rate of approximately 75 percent. This favorable survival is realized even when the bone marrow, liver, or adjacent lymph nodes are involved. Evidence is accumulating that immune mechanisms conferred by the mother are responsible for the extraordinary spontaneous regression rate seen when neuroblastoma appears in the early months of life.

Abdominal neuroblastoma is characteristically an irregular and hard mass which often crosses the midline. An intravenous pyelogram will show lateral or inferior displacement of the kidney but almost never calyceal distortion (Fig. 39-34), an important differentiation from Wilms' tumor. Thoracic tumors of neural origin are located in the posterior mediastinum, a distinguishing feature which is readily determined on the lateral chest film. Surgical excision is the treatment for neuroblastoma, regardless of the site of origin. In the abdomen and retroperitoneum this may be impossible because the tumor often invades adjacent organs surrounding the celiac axis and mesenteric artery. If it is feasible, the bulk of the tumor should be surgically excised. X-ray therapy offers only temporary control of this tumor's growth. Chemotherapy in the form of cytoxian, vincristine, and Carboximide has prolonged life, but these agents have not altered survival to the extent accomplished with other childhood tumors.

Teratoma

Teratomas are comprised of tissue from all three embryonic germ layers, although one cell type may predominate. Dermoids arising exclusively from ectodermal precursors are usually benign. Though teratomas may arise in any part of the body, a predilection for certain sites is well recognized. Those tumors arising in the chest are usually found in the anterior mediastinum and are generally benign. Teratoma arising in the retroperitoneum may present as a mass in the abdomen or flank. Such tumors may mimic other abdominal tumors in clinical presentation. The goal of therapy is complete surgical removal. If contiguous spread has not occurred, the cure rate for retroperitoneal teratoma is high.

SACROCOCCYGEAL TERATOMA

Sacrococcygeal teratoma usually appears as a mass originating from the buttocks and projecting forward to distort

Fig. 39-34. IVP from a patient with retroperitoneal neuroblastoma. Note that both kidneys are pushed aside and rotated by adjacent mass.

Fig. 39-35. Newborn with huge sacrococcygeal teratoma.

the perineum. The mass may vary in size from a few centimeters to a grapefruit-sized tumor (Fig. 39-35). Myelomeningocele, lipoma, and neural tumors with intraspinal extension should be considered in the differential diagnosis. The potential for malignant degeneration is high in these tumors, but this rarely occurs if operation is carried out in the early days of life. Complete excision is essential and usually can be accomplished without damaging the rectum or genital structures. If the tumor is completely excised the cure rate is excellent.

A form of sacrococcygeal teratoma exists which is not evident externally but projects inward into the retrorectal

Fig. 39-36. Operative photographs of hepatoblastoma in the right lobe of the liver in an eight-month-old child. Extended right hepatic lobectomy was curative.

space and pelvis. Discovery of these tumors is often delayed until symptoms of rectal obstruction appear. The late discovery of this variant of sacrococcygeal teratoma allows malignant degeneration, and thus the cure rate is considerably decreased in this form.

Rhabdomyosarcoma

Once thought to originate only from striated muscle, rhabdomyosarcoma is now recognized as an embryonic tumor which can arise from a variety of mesenchymal tissues. The commonest sites of origin are the head and neck, the extremities, and the genitourinary system. This rapidly growing neoplasm invades surrounding structures. Metastases occur to regional nodes and the lungs. Wide local excision is now recognized as optimal surgical treatment for localized forms of rhabdomyosarcoma. Radical extirpation in the form of amputation does not improve survival. This latter change in concept has followed the extraordinary success of combined chemotherapy with actinomycin D, vincristine, and Adriamycin for this disease.

Hepatoma

Two main forms of liver disease occur in children, hepatoblastoma and hepatocellular carcinoma. Hepatoblastoma is slightly more frequent (Fig. 39-36), and its prognosis is considerably better than that of hepatic carcinoma. The child usually has an abdominal mass, often associated with anemia, low-grade fever, and anorexia. The patients are rarely jaundiced, and most tests of liver

Table 39-1. DEATHS IN CHILDREN AGED
1 TO 14 YEARS, UNITED STATES, 1974

Accidents	12,448
Cancer	2,961
Congenital anomalies	2,148
Pneumonia	1,277
Homicide	767
Heart disease	680
Cerebrovascular disease	375
Total all deaths	26,825

SOURCE: U. S. Bureau of Vital Statistics.

function are normal. Alpha fetoprotein, a protein usually not detectable in the serum after the first few weeks of life, is present in patients with hepatoblastoma and is a useful biologic marker. Prior to surgery complete radiologic evaluation, including selective hepatic angiography, is essential. Hepatic resection offers the only hope for cure, since no effective chemotherapy is known at present. The value of radiotherapy is limited, although some tumors have been reduced in size by x-ray therapy, making them surgically accessible. Extended radical hepatic surgery has increased the survival of children with primary liver tumors. For hepatoblastoma, approximately 60 percent of the children have a surgically accessible tumor, and of these patients, half are curable, for an overall survival of 30 percent. With respect to hepatocellular carcinoma, the outlook is much more dismal, with only 15 percent being cured by any surgical procedures.

TRAUMA

Accidents are the leading cause of death in children. Of the more than 26,000 deaths in 1974 in children from 1 to 14 years, almost one-half (12,448) were accidental (Table 39-1). Of the 12,448 deaths, 5,796 occurred as a direct result of motor vehicle accidents, 2,440 were drowning victims, and 1,218 children died of burns. Clearly the injured child needs immediate and expert management at the scene, prompt transport to a major pediatric trauma facility, and sophisticated surgical care in the hospital.

References

Fluid and Electrolyte Balance

Adamsons, K., Jr., and Towell, M. E.: Thermal Homeostatis in the Fetus and Newborn, *Anesthesiology,* **26:**531, 1965.

Altman, R. P., and Randolph, J. G.: The Applications and Hazards of Total Parenteral Nutrition in Infants, *Ann Surg,* **174:**85, 1971

Arch, M. J., Shu, J. M. Ph. D., and Trays, O. M.: Evaluation of Different Nitrogen Sources in High Calorie Parenteral Therapy, *J Pediatr Surg,* **7:**213, 1972.

Bill, A. H.: Immune Aspects of Neuroblastoma, *Am J Surg,* **122:**142, 1971.

Coran, A. G., and Nesbakken, R.: The Metabolism of Intravenously Administered Fat in Adult and Newborn Dogs, *Surgery,* **66:**922, 1969.

————: The Long-Term Total Intravenous Feedings of Infants Using Peripheral Vein, *J Pediatr Surg,* **8:**801, 1973.

Filler, F. M., Eraklis, A. J., Rubin, V. G., et al.: Long-Term Parenteral Nutrition in Infants, *N Engl J Med,* **281:**589, 1969.

Goudsouzian, N. G., Morris, R. H., and Ryan, J. F.: The Effect of a Warming Blanket on the Maintenance of Body Temperature in Anesthetized Infants and Children, *Anesthesiology,* **39:**351, 1973.

Groff, D. B.: Complications of Intravenous Hyperalimentation in Newborns and Infants, *J Pediatr Surg,* **4:**460, 1969.

Ikeda, K., and Suita, S.: Total Parenteral Nutrition Using Peripheral Veins in Surgical Neonates, *Arch Surg,* **112:**1045, 1977.

Knutrud, O.: The Water and Electrolyte Metabolism in the Newborn Child after Major Surgery, Norwegian Monographs on Medical Science, Olso, Scandinavian University Books, Universitets Forlaget, 1965.

Roe, C. F., Santulli, T. V., and Blair, C. S.: Heat Loss in Infants during General Anesthesia and Operations, *J Pediatr Surg,* **1:**266, 1966.

Rowe, M. I.: The Role of Serial Serum Osmolality Measurements in the Management of the Neonatal Surgical Patient, *Surg Gynecol Obstet,* **133:**93, 1971.

————, Lankau, C., and Newmark, S.: Evaluation of Methods to Clinically Monitor Colloid Oncotic Pressure in the Pediatric Surgical Patient, *Surg Gynecol Obstet,* **139:**889, 1974.

Wilmore, D. W., and Dudrick, S. J.: Growth and Development of an Infant Receiving All Nutrients Exclusively by Vein, *JAMA,* **203:**860, 1968.

Lesions of Neck

Bill, A. H., Jr., and Sumner D. S.: Unified Concept of Lymphangioma and Cystic Hygroma, *Surg. Gynecol Obstet.,* **120:**79, 1965.

———— and Vadheim, J. L.: Cysts, Sinuses, and Fistulas of the Neck Arising from the First and Second Branchial Clefts, *Ann Surg,* **142:**904, 1955.

Brown, P. M., and Judd, E. S.: Thyroglossal Cysts and Sinuses: Results of Radical (Sistrunk) Operation, *Am J Surg* **102:**494, 1961.

Gross, R. E., and Connerly, M. L.: Thyroglossal Cysts and Sinuses, *N Engl J Med,* **223:**616, 1940.

Randolph, J. G.: On the Treatment of Lymphangioma in Children, *Surgery,* **49:**289, 1961.

Sistrunk, W. E.: The Surgical Treatment of Cysts of Thyroglossal Tract, *Ann Surg,* **71:**121, 1920.

Respiratory System

Aberdeen, E.: Tracheostomy and Tracheostomy Care in Infants, *Proc R Soc Med,* **58:**900, 1965.

Adelman, S., and Benson, C. D.: Bochdalek Hernias in Infancy Factors Determining Mortality, *J Pediatr Surg,* **11:**560, 1976.

Anderson, K. D., and Chandra, R.: Pneumothorax as a Complication of Endotracheal Suction, *J Pediatr Surg,* **11:**687, 1976.

Boix-Ochoa, J., Peguero, G., Seijo, G., et al.: Acid-Base Balance and Blood Gases in Prognosis and Therapy of Congential Diaphragmatic Hernia, *J Pediatr Surg,* **9:**49, 1974.

Boles, E. T., Schiller, M. and Weinberger, M.: Improved Management of Neonates with Congenital Diaphragmatic Hernia, *Arch Surg,* **103:**344, 1971.

Gans, S. L., and Berci, G.: Advances in Endoscopy of Infants and Children, *J Pediatr Surg,* **6:**199, 1971.

Haller, J. A., Jr., and Talbert, J. L.: Clinical Evaluation of a New Silastic Tracheostomy Tube for Respiratory Support of Infants and Children, *Ann Surg,* **171:**915, 1970.

Hendren, W. H., and McKee, D. M.: Lobar Emphysema of Infancy, *J Pediatr Surg,* **1:**24, 1966.

Louhimo, I., Grahne, B., Pasila, M., et al.: Acquired Laryngotracheal Stenosis in Children, *J Pediatr Surg,* **6:**730, 1971.

McNamara, J. J., Eraklis, A. J., and Gross, R. E.: Congenital Posterolateral Diaphragmatic Hernia of the Newborn, *J Thorac Cardiovasc Surg,* **55:**55, 1968.

Mattila, M. A. K., Suutarinen, T., and Sulamaa, M.: Prolonged Endotracheal Intubation or Tracheostomy in Infants and Children, *J Pediatr Surg,* **4:**674, 1969.

Rowe, M. I., and Uribe, F.: Diaphragmatic Hernia in the Newborn Infant: Blood Gas and pH Considerations, *Surgery,* **70:**758, 1971.

Steele, R. W., Metz, J. R., Bass, J. W., et al.: Pneumothorax and Pneumomediastinum in the Newborn, *Radiology,* **98:**629, 1971.

White, J. J., Andrews, H. G., Risemberg, H., et al.: Prolonged Respiratory Support in Newborn Infants with a Membrane Oxygenator, *Surgery,* **70:**288, 1971.

Malformation of Esophagus

Anderson, K. D., and Randolph, J. G.: The Gastric Tube for Esophageal Replacement in Children, *J Thorac Cardiovasc Surg,* **66:**333, 1973.

Howard, R., and Myers, N. A.: Esophageal Atresia: A Technique for Elongating the Upper Pouch, *Surgery,* **58:**725, 1965.

Mahour, G. H., Woolley, M. M., and Gwinn, J. L.: Elongation of the Upper Pouch and Delayed Anatomic Reconstruction in Esophageal Atresia, *J Pediatr Surg,* **9:**373, 1974.

Mellins, R. B., and Blumenthal, S.: Cardiovascular Anomalies and Esophageal Atresia, *Am J Dis Child,* **107:**160, 1964.

Randolph, J. G., Lilly, J. R., and Tunell, W. P.: Gastric Division in the Critically Ill Infant with Esophageal Atresia and Tracheoesophageal Fistula, *Surgery,* **63:**496, 1968.

Waterston, D. J., Bonham, A., Carter, R. E., and Aberdeen, E.: Oesophageal Atresia: Tracheoesophageal Fistula. A Study of Survival in 218 Infants, *Lancet,* **1:**819, 1962.

Corrosive Injury of Esophagus

Anderson, K. D., and Randolph, J. G.: The Gastric Tube for Esophageal Replacement in Children, *J Thorac Cardiovasc Surg,* **66:**33, 1973.

Burrington, J. D., and Stephens, C. A.: Esophageal Replacement with a Gastric Tube in Infants and Children, *J Pediatr Surg,* **3:**246, 1968.

Ein, S. H., Shandling, B., Simpson M., et al.: A Further Look at the Gastric Tube as an Esophageal Replacement in Infants and Children, *J Pediatr Surg,* **6:**859, 1973.

German, J. C., and Waterston, D. J.: Colon Interposition for the Replacement of the Esophagus in Children, *J Pediatr Surg,* **11:**227, 1976.

Haller, J. A., Andrews, H. G., White, J. J., et al.: Pathophysiology and Management of Acute Corrosive Burns of the Esophagus:

Results of Treatment in 285 Children, *J Pediatr Surg,* **6:**578, 1971.

Sherman, C. D., Jr., and Waterston, D.: Oesophageal Reconstruction in Children Using Intrathoracic Colon, *Arch Dis Child,* **32:**11, 1957.

Webb, W. R., Koutras, P., Ecker, R. R., et al.: An Evaluation of Steroids and Antibiotics in Caustic Burns of the Esophagus, *Ann Thorac Surg,* **9:**95, 1970.

Weisskopf, A.: Effects of Cortisone on Experimental Lye Burn of the Esophagus, *Ann Otol Rhinol Laryngol,* **61:**681, 1952.

Gastroesophageal Reflux

Berenberg, W., and Neuhauser, E. B. D.: Cardioesophageal Relaxation (Chalasia) as a Cause of Vomiting in Infants, *Pediatrics,* **5:**414, 1950.

Cahill, J. L., Aberdeen, E., and Waterston, D. J.: Results of Surgical Treatment of Esophageal Hiatal Hernia in Infancy and Childhood, *Surgery,* **66:**597, 1969.

Carcassonne, M., Bansoussan, A., and Aubert, J.: The Management of Gastroesophageal Reflux in Infants, *J Pediatr Surg,* **8:**575, 1973.

Follette, D., Fonkalsrud, E. W., Euler, A., and Ament, M.: Gastroesophageal Fundoplication for Reflux in Infants and Children, *J Pediatr Surg,* **11:**757, 1976.

Johnson, D. G., Herbst, J. J., Oliveros, M. A., and Stewart, D. R.: Evaluation of Gastroesophageal Reflux Surgery in Children, *Pediatrics,* **59:**62, 1977.

Randolph, J. G., Lilly, J. R., and Anderson, K. D.: Surgical Treatment of Gastroesophageal Reflux in Infants, *J Thorac Cardiovasc Surg,* **55:**42, 1968.

Gastrointestinal Conditions

Bell, M. J., Kosloske, A. M., Martin, L. W., et al.: Neonatal Necrotizing Enterocolitis: Prevention of Perforation, *J Pediatr Surg,* **8:**601, 1973.

——, Ternberg, J. L., Askin, F. B., McAlister, W., and Shackelford, G.: Intestinal Stricture in Necrotizing Enterocolitis, *J Pediatr Surg,* **11:**319, 1976.

Clatworthy, H. W., Jr., Saleebe, R., and Lovingood, C.: Extensive Small Bowel Resection in Young Dogs: Its Effect on Growth and Development, *Surgery,* **32:**341, 1952.

deLorimier, A. A., Fonkalsrud, E. W., and Hayes, D. M.: Congenital Atresia of the Jejunum and Ileum in the Newborn, *Ann Surg,* **142:**478, 1955.

Ein, S.: Leading Points in Childhood Intussusception, *J Pediatr Surg,* **11:**209, 1976.

Gross, R. E., and Chisolm, T. C.: Annular Pancreas Producing Duodenal Obstruction, *Am Surg,* **119:**759, 1944.

Jackson, J. M.: Annular Pancreas and Duodenal Obstruction in the Neonate, a Review, *Arch Surg,* **87:**379, 1963.

Krasna, I. H., Becker, J. M., Schneider, K. M., et al.: Colonic Stenosis Following Necrotizing Enterocolitis of the Newborn, *J Pediatr Surg,* **5:**200, 1970.

Leonidas, J. C., Berdon, W. E., Baker, D. H., et al.: Meconium Ileus and Its Complications: A Reappraisal of Plain Film Roentgen Diagnostic Criteria, *Am J Roentgenol Radium Ther Nucl Med,* **108:**598, 1970.

Louw, J. H.: Jejunoileal Atresia and Stenosis, *J Pediatr Surg,* **1:**8, 1966.

Marks, R. M., Sieber, W. K., and Girdany, B. R.: Hydrostatic

Pressure in the Treatment of the Ileocolic Intussusception in Infants and Children, *J Pediatr Surg,* **1:**566, 1966.

Martin, L. W., and Zerella, J. T.: Jejunoilial Atresia: A Proposed Classification, *J Pediatr Surg,* **11:**399, 1976.

Nixon, H. H., and Tawes, R.: Etiology and Treatment of Small Intestinal Atresia: Analysis of a Series of 127 Jejunoileal Atresias and Comparison with 62 Duodenal Atresias, *Surgery,* **69:**41, 1971.

Noblett, H. R.: Treatment of Uncomplicated Meconium Ileus by Gastrografin Enema: A Preliminary Report, *J Pediatr Surg,* **4:**190, 1969.

Ravitch, M. M.: Intussusception, in W. T. Mustard, M. M. Ravitch, and W. H. Snyder, Jr., (eds.), "Pediatric Surgery," 2d ed., vol. 2, p. 914, Year Book Medical Publishers, Inc., Chicago, 1969.

Rowe, M. I., Furst, A. J., Altman, D. H., et al.: The Neonatal Response to Gastrografin Enema, *Pediatrics,* **48:**29, 1971.

Santulli, T. V., and Blanc, W. A.: Congenital Atresia of the Intestine: Pathogenesis and Treatment, *Ann Surg,* **154:**939, 1961.

Touloukian, R. J., Berdon, W. E., Amoury, R. A., et al.: Surgical Experience with Necrotizing Enterocolitis in the Infant, *J Pediatr Surg,* **2:**389, 1967.

——, Posch, J. N., and Spencer, R.: The Pathogenesis of Ischemic Gastroenterocolitis of the Neonate: Selective Gut Mucosal Ischemia in Asphyxiated Neonatal Piglets, *J Pediatr Surg,* **7:**194, 1972.

Intussusception

Hay, G. R., Boles, E. T., Jr., and Dunbar, D.: Use of Glucagon in the Diagnosis and Management of Ileocolic Intussusception, *J Pediatr Surg,* 1977. (In press.)

Ravitch, M. M., and McCune, R. M., Jr.: Reduction of Intussusception by Hydrostatic Pressure: An Experimental Study, *Bull Johns Hopkins Hosp,* **82:**550, 1948.

Zachary, R. B.: Acute Intussusception in Childhood, *Arch Dis Childhood,* **30:**32, 1955.

Hirschsprung's Disease

Asch, M. J., Weitzman, J. J., Hays, D. M., et al.: Total Colon Aganglionosis, *Arch Surg,* **105:**74, 1972.

Boley, S. J., Lafer, D. J., Kleinhaus, S., et al.: Endorectal Pull-Through Procedure for Hirschsprung's Disease with and without Primary Anastomosis, *J Pediatr Surg,* **3:**258, 1968.

Campbell, P. E., and Noblett, H. R.: Experience with Rectal Suction Biopsy in the Diagnosis of Hirschsprung's Disease, *J Pediatr Surg,* **4:**410, 1969.

Coran, A. G., Bjordal, R., Eek, S., et al.: The Surgical Management of Total Colonic and Partial Small Intestinal Aganglionosis, *J Pediatr Surg,* **4:**531, 1969.

Duhamel, B.: Retrorectal and Transanal Pull-Through Procedure for the Treatment of Hirschsprung's Disease, *Dis Colon Rectum,* **7:**455, 1964.

James, A. E., Jr., Greenfield, J. B., Pfister, R. C., et al.: The Roentgenologic Appearance of Postoperative Congenital Megacolon (Hirschsprung's Disease), *Am J Roentgenol Radium Ther Nucl Med,* **109:**351, 1970.

Martin, L. W.: Surgical Management of Hirschsprung's Disease Involving the Small Intestine, *Arch Surg,* **97:**183, 1968.

——: Surgical Management of Total Colonic Aganglionosis, *Ann Surg,* **176:**343, 1972.

Prevot, J., Bodart, N., Babut, J. M., et al.: Hirschsprung's Disease with Total Colonic Involvement: Therapeutic Problems, *Prog Pediatr Surg,* **4:**63, 1972.

Soave, F.: Hirschsprung's Disease: Technique and Results of Soave's Operation, *Br J Surg,* **53:**1023, 1966.

Soper, R. T., and Miller, F. E.: Modification of Duhamel Procedure: Elimination of Rectal Pouch and Colorectal Septum, *J Pediatr Surg,* **3:**376, 1968.

Swenson, O., and Bill, A. H., Jr.: Resection of Rectum and Rectosigmoid with Preservation of the Sphincter for Benign Spastic Lesions Producing Megacolon: An Experimental Study, *Surgery,* **24:**212, 1948.

——, Sherman, J. O., and Fisher, J. H.: Diagnosis of Congenital Megacolon: An Analysis of 501 Patients, *J Pediatr Surg,* **8:**587, 1973.

——, ——, ——, and Cohen, E.: Treatment and Postoperative Complications of Congenital Megacolon: A 25 Year Follow-up, *Ann Surg,* **182:**266, 1975.

Imperforate Anus

Kiesewetter, W. B.: Imperforate Anus. II. The Rationale and Technique of the Sacroabdominoperineal Operation, *J Pediatr Surg,* **2:**106, 1967.

Potts, W. J., Riker, W. L., and DeBoer, A.: Imperforate Anus with Recto-Vesical-Urethral-Vaginal and Perineal Fistula, *Ann Surg,* **140:**381, 1954.

Rehbein, F.: Imperforate Anus: Experiences with Abdomino-Perineal and Abdomino-Sacral-Perineal Pull-Through Procedures, *J Pediatr Surg,* **2:**99, 1967.

Santulli, T. V., Kiesewetter, W. B., and Bill, A. H., Jr.: Anorectal Anomalies: A Suggested International Classification, *J Pediatr Surg,* **5:**281, 1970.

Stephens, F. D.: "Congenital Malformations of the Rectum, Anus and Genitourinary Tract," E. and S. Livingstone, Edinburgh, 1963.

Wangersteen, D. H., and Rice, C. O.: Imperforate Anus: A Method of Determining the Surgical Approach, *Ann Surg,* **92:**77, 1930.

Jaundice

Adievre, M., Martin, J. P., Hadchouel, M., et al.: Alpha₁—Antitrypsin Deficiency and Liver Disease in Children: Phenotypes, Manifestations, and Prognosis, *Pediatrics,* **57:**226, 1976.

Altman, R. P., and Chandra, R.: Biliary Hypoplasia Consequent to Alpha₁ Antitrypsin Deficiency, *Surg Forum,* **37:**377, 1976.

—— and Lilly, J. R.: Technical Details or Surgical Correction of Extrahepatic Biliary Atresia, *Surg Gynecol Obstet,* **140:**952, 1975.

——, ——, and Chandra, R.: Ongoing Cirrhosis after Successful Porticoenterostomy in Infants with Biliary Atresia, *J Pediatr Surg,* **10:**685, 1975.

Clatworthy, H. W., Wall, T., and Watman, R. N.: A New Type of Porto to-Systemic Venous Shunt for Portal Hypertension, *Arch Surg* **71:**588, 1955.

Fonkalsrud, E. W.: Choledochal Cysts *Surg Clin North Am,* **53:**1275, 1973.

Kasai, M., Kimura, S., Asakura, Y., et al.: Surgical Treatment of Biliary Atresia, *J Pediatr Surg,* **3:**665, 1968.

Landing, B. H.: "Considerations of the Pathogenesis of Neonatal Hepatitis, Biliary Atresia, and Choledochal Cyst—the Concept of Infantile Obstructive Cholangiography," University Park Press, Baltimore, 1972.

Lilly, J. R.: The Surgery of Biliary Hypoplasia, *J Pediatr Surg,* **11:**815, 1976.

Suruga, K., Nagashima, K., Hirai, Y., et al.: A Clinical and Pathological Study of Congenital Biliary Atresia, *J Pediatr Surg,* **2:**558, 1967.

Portal Hypertension

Altman, R. P.: Portal Decompression by Interposition Mesocaval Shunt in Patients with Biliary Atresia, *J Pediatr Surg,* **11:**809, 1976.

Clatworthy, H. W., Jr., Wall, T., and Watman, R. M.: A New Type of Portal-to-Systemic Venous Shunt for Portal Hypertension, *Arch Surg,* **71:**588, 1955.

Drapanas, T.: Interposition Mesocaval Shunt for Treatment of Portal Hypertension, *Ann Surg,* **176:**435, 1972.

Marion, P.: Mesoenteric-Caval Anastomosis, *J Cardiovasc Surg,* **70**(Suppl):70, 1966.

Martin, L. W.: Changing Concepts of Management of Portal Hypertension in Children, *J Pediatr Surg,* **7:**559, 1972.

Tyson, K. R. T., Schuster, S. R., and Schwachman, H.: Portal Hypertension in Cystic Fibrosis, *J Pediatr Surg,* **3:**271, 1968.

Spleen

Eraklis, A. J., Kevy, S. V., Diamond, L. K., et al.: Hazard of Overwhelming Infection after Splenectomy in Childhood, *N Engl J Med,* **276:**1225, 1967.

Kiesewetter, W. B.: Pediatric Splenectomy: Indications, Technique, Complications and Mortality, *Surg Clin North Am,* **55:**449, 1975.

King, H., and Schumacker, H. B., Jr.: Splenic Studies: Susceptibility to Infection after Splenectomy Performed in Infancy, *Ann Surg,* **136:**239, 1952.

O'Mara, R. E., Hall, R. C., and Dombroski, D. L.: Scintiscanning in the Diagnosis of Rupture of the Spleen, *Surg Gynecol Obstet,* **131:**1077, 1970.

Pancreas

Cooney, D. R., and Grosfeld, J. L.: Operative Management of Pancreatic Pseudocysts in Infants and Children: A Review of 75 Cases, *Ann Surg,* **182:**590, 1975.

Filler, R. M., AvRuskin, T. W., Crigler, J. F., and Haryen, A. H.: The Role of "Total" Pancreatectomy in the Treatment of Unremitting Hypoglycemia of Infancy, *J Pediatr Surg,* **6:**284, 1971.

Hamilton, J. P., Baker, L., Kaye, R., and Koop, C. E.: Subtotal Pancreatectomy in the Management of Severe Idiopathic Hypoglycemia in Children, *Pediatrics,* **39:**49, 1967.

Miller, R. E.: Pancreatic Pseudocysts in Infants and Children, *Arch Surg,* **89:**517, 1964.

Otherson, H. B., Moore, F. T., and Boles, E. P.: Traumatic Pancreatitis and Pseudocyst in Children, *J Trauma,* **8:**535, 1968.

Abdominal Wall Abnormalities

Allen, R. G. and Wrenn, E. L., Jr.: Silon as a Sac in the Treatment of Omphalocele and Gastroschisis, *J Pediatr Surg,* **4:**3, 1969.

Gilbert, M. G., Mencia, L. F., Brown, W. T., et al.: Staged Surgical Repair of Large Omphaloceles and Gastroschisis, *J Pediatr Surg,* **3:**702, 1968.

Gross, R. E.: A New Method for Surgical Treatment of Large Omphaloceles, *Surgery,* **24:**277, 1948.

Mahour, G. H., Weitzman, J. J., and Rosencrantz, J. G.: Omphalocele and Gastroschisis, *Ann Surg,* **177:**478, 1973.

Raffensberger, J. G., and Jona, J. Z.: Gastroschisis, *Ann Surg,* **177:**478, 1973.

Schuster, S. R.: A New Method for the Staged Repair of Large Omphaloceles, *Surg Gynecol Obstet,* **125:**837, 1967.

Exstrophy

Marshall, V. F., and Muecke, E. C.: Variations in Exstrophy of the Bladder, *J Urol,* **88:**766, 1962.

Rosencrantz, J. G., Bailey, W. C., and Dumars, K. W., Jr.: Incomplete Exstrophy of the Cloaca, *J Urol,* **91:**549, 1964.

Williams, D. I., and Savage, J.: Reconstruction of the Exstrophied Bladder, *Br J Surg,* **53:**168, 1966.

Inguinal Hernia

Clatworthy, H. W., Jr., Gilbert, M., and Clement, A.: The Inguinal Hernia, Hydrocele and Undescended Testicle Problem in Infants and Children, *Postgrad Med,* **22:**122, 1957.

Gilbert, M., and Clatworthy, H. W., Jr.: Bilateral Operations for Inguinal Hernia and Hydrocele in Infancy and Childhood, *Am J Surg,* **97:**255, 1959.

Undescended Testicle

Gilbert, J. B., and Hamilton, J. B.: Studies in Malignant Testes Tumors: Incidence and Nature of Tumors in Ectopic Testes, *Surg Gynecol Obstet,* **71:**731, 1940.

Gross, R. E., and Jewett, T. C., Jr.: Surgical Experiences from 1,222 Operations for Undescended Testes, *JAMA,* **160:**634, 1956.

Koop, C. E.: Observations on Undescended Testes: I. Significance of Empty Scrotum, Indication for Orchiopexy, *Arch Surg,* **75:**801, 1957.

MacCollum, D. W.: Clinical Study of the Spermatogenesis of Undescended Testicles, *Arch Surg,* **31:**290, 1935.

Intersexual Abnormalities

Gross, R. E., Randolph, J. G., and Crigler, J. F.: Clitorectomy for Sexual Abnormalities: Indications and Techniques, *Surgery,* **54:**300, 1966.

Hendren, W. H., and Crawford, J. D.: Adrenogenital Syndrome: The Anatomy of the Anomaly and Its Repair: Some New Concepts, *J Pediatr Surg,* **4:**49, 1969.

Jones, H. W., Jr.: Clinical Significance of Anomalies of the Sex Chromosomes, *Am J Obstet Gynecol,* **93:**335, 1965.

Money, J., Hampson, J. G., and Hampson, J. L.: Hermaphroditism: Recommendations Concerning Assignment of Sex, Change of Sex and Psychologic Management, *Bull Johns Hopkins Hosp,* **97:**284, 1955.

Randolph, J. G., and Hung, W.: Reduction Clitoroplasty in Females with Hypertrophied Clitoris, *J Pediatr Surg,* **5:**224, 1970.

Rickman, P. P.: Vesico-intestinal Fissure, *Arch Dis Childhood,* **35:**97, 1960.

Wilkins, L.: The Diagnosis of Adrenogenital Syndrome and Its Treatment with Cortisone, *J Pediatr,* **41:**1952.

———: "The Diagnosis and Treatment of Endocrine Disorders in Childhood and Adolescence," 3d ed., Charles C Thomas, Publisher, Springfield, Ill., 1966.

Malignant Disease in Children

Altman, R. P., Randolph, J. G., and Lilly, J. R.: Surgical Treatment of Sacrococcygeal Teratoma, *J Pediatr Surg,* **9:**389, 1974.

Beckwith, J. B., and Martin, R. F.: Observations of the Histopathology of Neuroblastomas, *J Pediatr Surg,* **3:**106, 1968.

Bill, A. H., and Morgan, A.: Evidence for Immune Reactions to Neuroblastoma and Future Possibilities for Investigation, *J Pediatr Surg,* **5:**111, 1970.

Conference on the Biology of Neuroblastoma, *J Pediatr Surg,* **3:**101, 1968.

D'Angio, G. J.: Management of Children with Wilms's Tumor, *Cancer,* **30:**1528, 1972.

———, Evans, A. E., and Koop, C. E.: Special Pattern of Widespread Neuroblastoma with a Favorable Prognosis, *Lancet,* **1:**1046, 1971.

Evans, A. E.: Treatment of Neuroblastoma, *Cancer,* **30:**1595, 1972.

———, Heyn, R. M., Newton, W. A., et al.: Vincristine Sulfate and Cyclophosphamide for Children with Metastatic Neuroblastoma, *JAMA,* **207:**1325, 1969.

Farber, S.: Chemotherapy in the Treatment of Leukemia and Wilms's Tumor, *JAMA,* **198:**826, 1966.

Grosfeld, J. L., Smith, J. P., and Clatworthy, H. W., Jr.: Pelvic Rhabdomyosarcoma in Infants and Children, *J Urol,* **107:**673, 1972.

Hellstrom, I., Hellstrom, K. D., Bill, A. H., et al.: Studies on Cellular Immunity to Human Neuroblastoma Cell, *Int J Cancer,* **6:**172, 1970.

Holder, T. M., Stuber, J. L., and Templeton, A. W.: Sonography as a Diagnostic Aid in the Evaluation of Abdominal Masses in Infants and Children, *J Pediatr Surg,* **7:**532, 1972.

Koop, C. E.: Neuroblastoma: Two Year Survival and Treatment Correlations, *J Pediatr Surg,* **3:**178, 1968.

Towne, B. H., Mahour, G. A., Woolley, M. M., et al.: Ovarian Cyst and Tumors in Infancy and Childhood, *J Pediatr Surg,* **10:**311, 1975.

Trauma

Haller, A. J., Signer, R. D., Golladay, E. S., Shaker, I. J., and White, J. J.: Use of a Trauma Registry in the Management of Children with Life-Threatening Injuries, *J Pediatr Surg,* **11:**381, 1976.

Chapter 40

Urology

by **Irwin N. Frank and Donald F. McDonald**

ANATOMY

Knowledge of the anatomy of the genitourinary system and its anatomic relationships is a prerequisite to the accurate diagnosis and correct therapy of diseases involving these structures. Slight deviation of the axis of the kidney or the course of the ureter from normal may indicate a pathologic condition in adjacent organs. Disease within the genitourinary system may manifest itself in the form of gastrointestinal symptoms. Examples of this are the nausea and vomiting which so often occur with renal colic and ureteropelvic junction obstruction. Pathologic enlargement of structures situated in the pelvis commonly produces obstruction of the lower ureter and often leaves characteristic impressions on the bladder contour seen on a cystogram.

KIDNEY. The kidneys are paired retroperitoneal organs which weigh approximately 160 Gm each in the healthy adult. They are situated within the fascia of Gerota, and a variable amount of perinephric fat is present between the capsule of the kidney and this fascial envelope. Further protection of the kidneys is provided dorsally by their relationship to the lower ribs, the quadratus lumborum, and the psoas muscles. The ventral relationships of the kidney are illustrated in Fig. 40-1. They lie beneath the diaphragm, with the left kidney usually 1 to 2 cm. lower than the right kidney.

The renal arteries originate from the aorta at the upper level of the second lumbar vertebra, and the right artery is considerably longer than the left, since it crosses the midline behind the vena cava. About two-thirds of kidneys have a single renal artery, while multiple renal arteries are more prevalent in congenitally malformed or malpositioned kidneys. The main renal artery divides into five major branches, each of which represents an end artery. Partial occlusion of any branch produces ischemia, and complete occlusion produces infarction of the involved segment. However, the ureteral and capsular vessels can provide significant blood flow in the presence of marked renal artery occlusion. The renal veins are often multiple

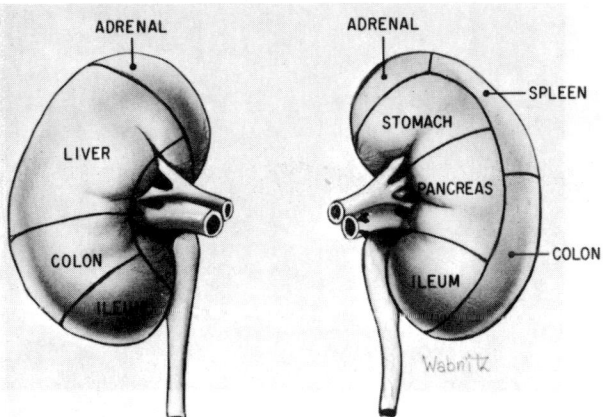

Fig. 40-1. Ventral relationships of the kidneys to adjacent organs.

and freely intercommunicate. The left renal vein crosses the midline ventral to the aorta after it has received blood from the left adrenal and gonadal veins. The renal lymphatics empty through a half-dozen hilar trunks in the region of the renal artery and vein. Capsular lymphatics travel through the perinephric fat to infradiaphragmatic periaortic nodes. The renal nerves, which receive contributions from T_4 to T_{12}, from the vagus nerve via the celiac axis, and from the splanchnics, contain vasomotor and pain fibers. Following total renal denervation, such as occurs with transplantation, no persistent abnormalities in renal function occur. The renal pelvis, which usually contains 5 ml of urine, lies dorsal to the renal vessels and has a transitional cell epithelium. The kidney's position with respect to the vertebral bodies and the axis of a line drawn through the upper and lower calyces offers a clue to focal diseases of the kidney and adjacent organs. The axis of the kidney often parallels that of the psoas muscle edge as noted on x-rays of the abdomen.

URETER. The ureters are muscular tubes which connect the renal pelvis to the bladder, traversing the retroperitoneal space in a linear course just lateral to the transverse processes of the lumbar vertebrae and crossing the common iliac arteries at their bifurcation. The lower ureter

Fig. 40-2. Posterior relationships of prostate, seminal vesicles, ureter, and bladder.

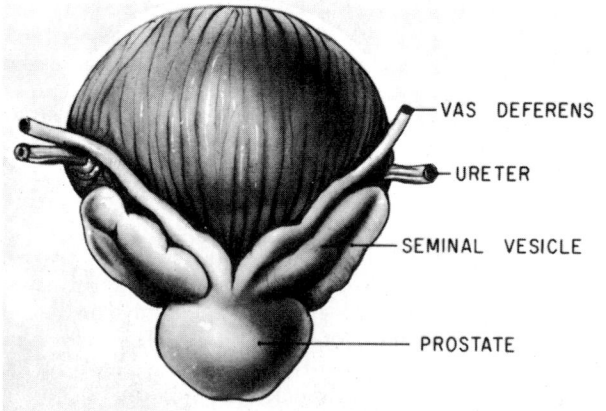

follows the contour of the pelvis and deviates laterally and then medially in a gentle curve to reach the trigone of the bladder above a line drawn between the spinous processes. The ureter is 28 to 30 cm long and about 5 mm in diameter. Its oblique course through the wall of the bladder measures 2 cm. The ureteral orifice is an oblique slit in the trigone. The function of the ureter is to transmit the urine from the renal pelvis to the bladder. Ordinarily urine is not modified in the ureter. However, during severe oliguria and dehydration the transitional epithelium acts as a semipermeable membrane which permits water and electrolyte changes in response to gradients. Normally, there are about four peristaltic waves per minute developing pressures of about 30 mm Hg. The ureteral blood supply originates from the renal, vesical, and lumbar arteries. Free intercommunication between these vessels permits extensive ureteral mobilization and transposition. Pain fibers refer stimuli to the T_{12} through L_2 segments, while the autonomic innervation is associated with intrinsic parasympathetic motor and sympathetic vasomotor ganglia. The lymphatic drainage is to segmental periaortic and caval nodes. The ureter may be drawn medially in retroperitoneal fibrosis and laterally as a result of enlargement of periaortic node involvement with tumor or an aortic aneurysm. It is essential to be aware of the course of the ureter during pelvic surgery and in difficult dissections of adjacent organs.

BLADDER. The urinary bladder is a muscular pelvic organ lined with transitional cell epithelium. It is related to the peritoneum superiorly, the sigmoid colon and rectum posteriorly in the male, and the uterus, cervix, and vagina in the female. In the male, the bladder is spherical, while in the female the uterus indents the dome. The smooth muscle (detrusor) is capable of stretching to a marked degree. The major blood supply originates from the superior, middle, and inferior branches of the hypogastric arteries. The lymphatics drain to the perivesical, hypogastric, and periaortic nodes. The autonomic nerve supply to the bladder is derived from the sacral cord and from the presacral and epigastric plexuses of nerves.

PROSTATE AND SEMINAL VESICLES. The chestnut-shaped prostate, which weighs approximately 25 Gm, surrounds the proximal male urethra. It is firmly attached to the bladder neck and symphysis pubis. Posteriorly, the fascia of Denonvilliers intervenes between the rectal ampulla and prostate (Fig. 40-2). Caudad, the prostate rests on the pelvic diaphragm, which contains the voluntary external sphincter. The blood supply derives from the inferior vesical and middle hemorrhoidal arteries, while the venous drainage communicates with an extensive pelvic plexus which empties into the hypogastric veins. This plexus also communicates with Batson's veins, thus explaining the common metastatic spread of prostatic carcinoma to the sacrum, ileum, and lumbar spine. The prostate receives secretory and motor (parasympathetic) innervation from S_3 and S_4 and vasomotor (sympathetic) fibers from the hypogastric plexus. The lymphatics drain into the external, internal, and common iliac nodes and then to the periaortic nodes. The seminal vesicles lie behind the bladder, lateral to the ampullae of the vasa deferentia. They are closely related to the ureters. Their secretions are rich in fructose, which may be of importance to survival of the spermatozoa.

PENIS AND URETHRA. The penis is composed of two lateral erectile bodies (corpora cavernosa) and a single ventral spongy erectile body (corpus spongiosum urethrae) through which the urethra passes. The latter terminates in the glans penis, which is also composed of erectile tissue. As the urethra emerges from the pelvic diaphragm, it enlarges to become the bulbous urethra which is invested by the bulbocavernosis muscle. The urethra continues as the pendulous urethra, which terminates in the fossa navicularis within the glans penis. The female urethra corresponds to the prostatic and membranous urethra in the male. It averages 4 cm in length and 32 mm in circumference. The principal blood supply to the penis and urethra originates from the internal pudendal arteries. Somatic sensory innervation of the penis is from S_3 and S_4 via the ilioinguinal and genitofemoral nerves. Sympathetic vasomotor innervation derives from the hypogastric plexus, while the parasympathetic innervation originates from S_2, S_3, and S_4 via the nervi erigentes. The lymphatic drainage is to the superficial and deep inguinal nodes and then to the external iliac and hypogastric nodes.

TESTIS AND EPIDIDYMIS. The testis is an ovoid firm scrotal organ which measures $4 \times 2.5 \times 2.5$ cm. The left testis commonly resides in the scrotum 2 to 4 cm lower than the right. The testis, which weighs approximately 20 Gm, is covered by a tough membrane, the tunica albuginea, except at its dorsal aspect where the epididymis and vascular pedicle are attached. The epididymis is a crescent-shaped body which curves around the dorsal portion of the testis. The vas deferens is a 4-mm thick-walled firm tubular structure which originates at the inferior pole of the epididymis and follows a cranial course with the spermatic vessels. The arterial blood supply to the testis and epididymis originates from the aorta just below the renal arteries. The left spermatic vein empties into the left renal vein, while the right spermatic vein empties directly into the inferior vena cava. The primary lymphatic drainage from the testis is to the periaortic nodes in the vicinity of the kidney. Crossover from these nodes to the opposite side is frequently observed.

DIAGNOSIS

SEQUENCE IN UROLOGIC DIAGNOSIS. Precision of diagnosis is a characteristic feature of the practice of urology. In order to maintain the achievable degree of accuracy, it is essential that a clinical problem be approached in a logical sequence. When so conducted, the diagnosis should be 95 percent accurate.

History

A variety of symptoms and signs are characteristic and often diagnostic of pathologic conditions involving the genitourinary system. The patient may spontaneously offer these clues, but in most instances it is necessary to ask them the proper questions to obtain this information. A brief discussion of some of the more significant signs and symptoms follows, and suggestions for evaluating them are discussed.

GROSS HEMATURIA. The presence of gross blood in the urine is a significant sign which is quite alarming to the patient and warrants further evaluation. Even small amounts of blood in the urine occurring on one occasion may be the only indication of a malignant process in the urinary tract. Intermittent bleeding is common, and large tumors may manifest themselves with only a small amount of bleeding while small tumors may produce considerable loss of blood. The bleeding originates from lesions which cause erosion or disruption of blood vessels or from inflammatory changes which in turn lead to erosions and diapedesis of red cells.

In a series of 1,000 cases in all age groups, almost three-quarters of the patients were over forty, and two-thirds were male (Fig. 40-3). Gross hematuria was the sole complaint in only 18.8 percent, while associated symptoms in order of frequency were those due to bladder infections, 37 percent; renal colic, 27.3 percent; obstructive symptoms, 15.6 percent; urethral discharge, 5 percent; and urethral pain, 3 percent. The origin of bleeding and etiologic factors in this series are also represented in Fig. 40-3. Other factors implicated to a lesser extent include congenital abnormalities, medical causes, and idiopathic hematuria. Hemophilia, thrombocytopenic purpura, uremia, and drug-induced hypothrombinemia represented rare causes.

Infections, predominantly acute cystitis and urethritis,

Fig. 40-3. Gross hematuria: sex incidence, site of origin, and etiology.

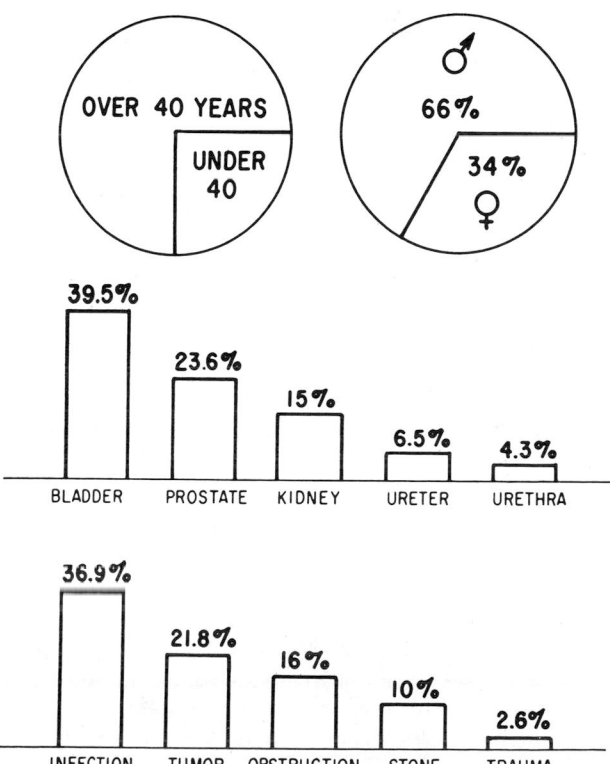

caused bleeding in 70 percent of male patients between the ages of eighteen and forty-one referred for a urologic consultation. Although 50 percent of the patients were referred with a diagnosis of glomerulonephritis none of them had it. Calculi were responsible for 4.9 percent; trauma, 6.1 percent; bladder tumors, 3.7 percent; medical, renal, and polycystic disease, 3 percent; and undiagnosed causes, 5.5 percent. In young individuals, gross hematuria is more likely to be the result of infection, while in older patients it is more likely to be related to tumors and prostatic disease. Three-quarters of patients with otherwise *asymptomatic* gross hematuria have bladder tumors.

It is important to determine whether hematuria appears at the beginning or end of voiding. Initial hematuria suggests lesions distal to the bladder neck, namely, the prostatic and membranous urethra. Predominantly terminal hematuria usually indicates involvement of the bladder neck and trigone. Uniform hematuria occurs with lesions of the ureter or kidney. The passage of blood clots suggests that the bleeding is quantitatively great, since urine inhibits coagulation of blood by the presence of citrate. Long, wormlike clots are apt to have been formed in the ureter. Reddish clots occur with recent bleeding, while brownish or grayish white clots indicate a time lapse between the bleeding episode and their passage.

ACUTE POSTRENAL RETENTION OF URINE. This term applies to an inability to empty a full bladder and is one of the most distressing symptoms. It should not be referred to as "anuria," since the latter indicates that urine is not being formed. The patient usually complains of lower abdominal distress, and the bladder is palpable as a tender suprapubic mass. A variety of afflictions may cause this condition.

Benign prostatic hypertrophy is the most common cause of acute retention in men. The vast majority have a long-standing history of increasing difficulty in voiding with gradually increasing nocturia. In contrast, *carcinoma of the prostate* is accompanied by a much shorter duration of symptoms. The history may be of months rather than years, and the urinary difficulties increase more rapidly. The patient with carcinoma of the prostate seldom presents with urinary retention when the lesion is early and amenable to surgical treatment. The presence of retention therefore suggests advanced disease, and symptoms of malignancy such as malaise, weight loss, anorexia, and sciatica are likely to be encountered. In young males, a *prostatic inflammation* is the most common cause of acute retention. This results from acute urethritis and prostatitis which have not been promptly or effectively treated. There is usually an antecedent history of frequent urination and dysuria progressing to acute retention. Fever, chills, and symptoms of systemic infection are common, and abscess formation occasionally occurs. Acute urinary retention may be the first manifestation of *urethral stricture* or may represent a recurrent problem related to the patient's unwillingness to undergo sufficiently frequent dilations. These patients usually give an antecedent history of gonorrhea, transurethral instrumentation, trauma, or radiation therapy. Many will have noted a gradual decrease in the force of the stream.

Neurogenic bladder dysfunction may lead to progressive increase in residual urine and eventual retention. This may be the first indication of spinal cord disease. In other patients, the retention may be preceded by difficulty in initiating voiding and overflow incontinence related to changes in abdominal pressure exerting force on a markedly distended bladder. Acute retention on a neurogenic basis may follow the administration of general anesthetics, spinal anesthesia, or the administration of certain drugs which influence the innervation of the bladder, bladder neck, proximal urethra, or external sphincter. Acute urinary retention in women is unusual and may be caused by neurogenic and psychogenic factors or urethral obstructions secondary to carcinoma, stricture, vaginal lesions, or cervical fibroids. A cystocele is seldom associated with acute retention.

INCONTINENCE. This is the situation in which a patient is unaware of the loss of urine until there is a sensation of wetness of the lower garments. The term is not a synonym for unintentional nocturnal bed wetting (enuresis) or urgency, where the patient knows he is going to wet himself but is unable to reach a suitable place to empty his bladder before the bladder empties itself. Patients with true incontinence have no residual urine. *True, or stress, incontinence* is the result of ineffective sphincter muscles which have been weakened by childbirth, stretched by an enlarged prostate, or traumatized by surgical procedures. A vesicovaginal or vesicoperineal fistula may also produce incontinence. Occasionally an ectopic ureter will open into the vagina, and this also will produce a constant leakage of urine. *Overflow, or paradoxical, incontinence* represents a second type, in which the bladder retains a large amount of residual urine. With each movement or breath the increased abdominal pressure causes overflow of a small amount of urine from a distended bladder. This condition may accompany neurogenic diseases of the spinal cord, or it may be the result of long-standing obstructive uropathy with detrusor decompensation. These patients may never really void, intermittently passing small quantities of urine without control. Incontinence of urine is a common manifestation of various neurologic diseases and spinal cord trauma.

URETERAL COLIC. This is related to a sudden increase in luminal pressure. Typically, there is sudden unilateral severe crescendo pain in the posterior subcostal region (lumbar triangle). The localization is frequently so precise that it can be defined by fingertip palpation. Obstruction at the ureteropelvic junction is associated with pain at the costovertebral angle, while obstruction lower in the ureter may have the added component of pain in the ipsilateral lower abdomen. With obstruction of the intramural ureter, pain, in addition to the above-mentioned sites, may be referred to the corresponding side of the scrotum or labia majora. Ureteral colic related to intramural obstruction is often associated with a sudden onset of urgency and frequency. Subsidence of these symptoms suggests that the stone has passed into the bladder and may be voided shortly. Narcotic addicts often simulate renal colic to procure drugs. Their deception may include fixing a radiopaque body to the skin in an appropriate area or placing blood from a finger prick in the urine sample.

FREQUENCY. This refers to the patient's voiding an excessive number of times. However, frequency of urination should not be confused with polyuria where the patient excretes large volumes of urine at more frequent intervals than normal. The correct term for frequency of urination with small volumes is pollakiuria. Most normal well-hydrated individuals void three to four times daily and do not arise from sleep to empty the bladder. Frequency may be related to reduction in bladder capacity associated with inflammation of the urinary passages or effective reduction in bladder capacity by increased residual urine, such as occurs with obstructive prostatic hypertrophy. Frequency is also a symptom of psychologic stress.

When patients complain of frequency, it is essential to question them carefully regarding fluid and caffeine intake. It is sometimes of value to have the patient record accurately the time and volume of the amounts of fluid ingested as well as the amount excreted in a 24-hour period. It is also essential to note the medications the patient is taking, since this may influence urinary frequency considerably. Further information regarding the relationship of urinary frequency to work, stress, weekend activity, and vacations is extremely helpful. Many patients have sought help from other physicians for this disturbing symptom, which may limit their activities because of the need to be close to a bathroom at all times. A careful history may lead to the information which will allow simple modification of habits, intake, and drug therapy to bring relief of this distressing and sometimes incapacitating problem.

NOCTURIA. Never normal, this condition may, however, be caused by consumption of an excessive amount of fluids prior to retiring, or it may be an expression of generalized restlessness. With cardiac decompensation, fluids which have accumulated in dependent portions of the body during the day are restored to the circulating blood when the patient maintains a horizontal position, thus causing nocturia. Patients with chronic renal disease who excrete large volumes because of an inability to concentrate the urine and patients on diuretics frequently experience nocturia. Prostatic hypertrophy and acute or chronic infection of the urinary tract cause nocturia by means of the same mechanisms described for frequency.

URGENCY. This is a symptom of vesical outlet inflammation and is most commonly due to prostatitis, urethritis, or cystitis. However, it may be a normal consequence of postponement of voiding for prolonged periods of time. The symptom may be so severe that the patient cannot restrain voiding.

DYSURIA. Difficult or painful urination is known as "dysuria." The sensation is commonly described as burning and may be referred to the glans penis or perineum. The symptom may be caused by urinary infection and the passage of clots, calculi, or crystals. However, it may also result from passage of highly concentrated urine. Pain at the termination of, or subsequent to, voiding is referred to as a "strangury" and may be associated with presence of a bladder calculus. Difficulty of urination is usually the result of an obstructive uropathy. "Hesitancy," indicating delayed voiding in response to mental command, is another symptom of chronic obstructive uropathy.

URINARY STREAM. The stream may lack force and have reduced projection in patients with obstructive uropathy. Stenosis of the meatus, which determines the caliber of the urinary stream, may be evidenced by a thin or duplicated stream.

IMPOTENCE AND EJACULATORY DYSFUNCTION. History taking in this area may prove to be quite difficult for the physician who has had little training in dealing with these problems. A careful history regarding medications is essential, since certain drugs will produce impotence and ejaculatory disturbances. However, in most situations, the underlying factor is situational or psychogenic, and this may become apparent during careful history taking. It is important to realize that in many instances patients wish to discuss their problems with a physician or have unsuccessfully attempted to do so before their present evaluation. In some instances, a physical or anatomic abnormality may be found to account for impotence.

Physical Examination

RENAL AREAS. The kidney regions may first be examined with the patient in the upright position. Observation may reveal obvious bulging or asymmetry of the costovertebral region. Scoliosis may be present from guarding in the presence of unilateral pain. Herpetic lesions occasionally may be encountered on the skin surface of this area and may be a clue to the etiology of pain in this area. Gentle palpation of the costovertebral angle areas may be followed by sharp percussion, disclosing an underlying obstructed or infected kidney. If the patient complains of pain in the flank region prior to examination, it is wise to start the evaluation on the contralateral side. Further examination of the kidney areas should be carried out with the patient supine, knees flexed, and arms at the side.

The examiner should stand on the side being examined. The posterior hand is placed parallel to the twelfth rib and below it. The anterior hand is placed 4 cm below the anterior rib cage and parallel to the posterior hand. Renal and retroperitoneal masses can be ballotted between the two hands. In slender individuals, the lower pole of the right kidney is often palpable. In others, the kidney may be palpable with deep inspiration. With unusually mobile kidneys (nephroptosis) the entire organ may be palpated. A solitary cyst may be distinguishable, while an irregular mass suggests a polycystic organ. Tenderness is usually related to obstruction or inflammation and is uncommon with uncomplicated tumors or cysts. The examiner again looks for evidence of asymmetry, rigidity of the costovertebral angle, tenderness, or bulging, which may suggest the presence of an underlying abscess, obstructed kidney, inflammation, or retroperitoneal extravasation of urine or blood.

URETERS. The deep retroperitoneal location of the ureters does not lend itself to palpation. It is unusual to be able to feel them when they are grossly dilated or to be able to localize a pathologic area within them.

BLADDER. The patient is examined in the supine position. The empty bladder is neither percussible nor palpable. In the markedly distended condition occurring with chronic obstruction, the bladder may be visible as a large abdominal mass rising out of the pelvis. However, under ordinary circumstances, the bladder is not percussible until it contains approximately 150 ml of urine. Persistence of a low abdominal mass following emptying of the bladder by catheterization documents the extravesical nature of the lesion.

PENIS. The penis may be examined with the patient in the upright position facing the examiner, who is sitting in a chair, or with the patient in a supine position on the examining table. If the patient is not circumcised, the foreskin should be retracted so that the underlying glans, urethral meatus, and inner aspect of the foreskin can be visualized. It is at this point in the examination that the patient may volunteer information regarding underlying fears, fantasies, or facts related to sexual dysfunction, erection, or impotence. If the patient does not do so, the examiner may utilize this opportunity to ask questions related to these topics. Further evaluation of the meatal caliber may be carried out with appropriate instrumentation, if indicated. A valid and recommended means of evaluating the presence of a meatal obstruction is observation of the patient voiding.

SCROTUM. Examination of the scrotum is carried out in conjunction with examination of the penis and with the patient in the positions noted above. Some patients are extremely sensitive to examination of this area, and the

Fig. 40-4. Differential diagnosis of scrotal lesions. *A.* Normal. *B.* Hydrocele. *C.* Spermatocele. *D.* Epididymitis. *E.* Tuberculous epididymitis and vasitis. *F.* Testis tumor. *G.* Hernia.

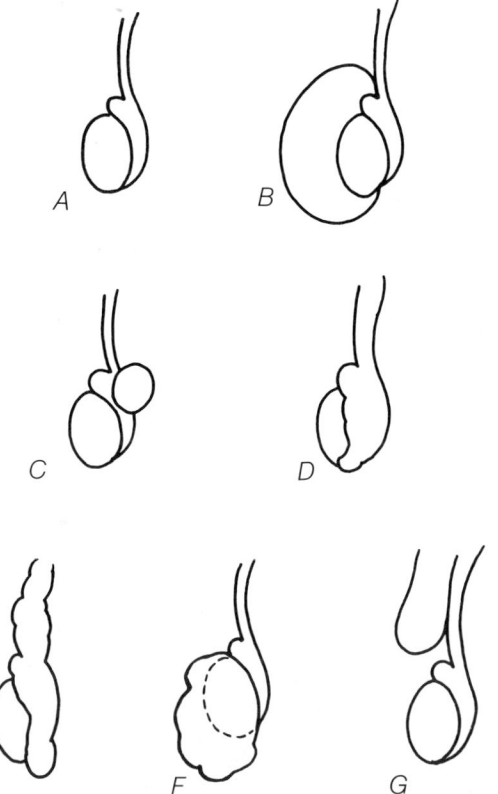

examiner may elicit a vasovagal response from the patient who is in the standing position. The examiner should be aware of this, since he may not appreciate that it is occurring while he is focusing his attention on the genital area. A knowledge of the normal scrotal contents and relationships is essential to the differential diagnosis of a variety of pathologic entities which occur in this area. Careful observation and palpation of this region and the use of a small flashlight to transilluminate lesions offer the only means of making an accurate diagnosis.

Scrotal Masses (Fig. 40-4)

As noted elsewhere in this text, an indirect *inguinal hernia* may present as a scrotal mass. The enlargement extends up into the inguinal region and may often be reduced with the patient in the supine position.

Epididymitis. Acute nonspecific pyogenic epididymitis is commonly a result of retrograde extension via the vas deferens from a focus of infection in the prostate or bladder. It may follow prostatic massage or instrumentation. The patient is frequently febrile and has a typical straddling gait to minimize contact with the inflamed scrotal contents. The scrotum is exquisitely tender and may contain a mass. The overlying skin is red and edematous. Nonspecific chronic epididymitis, which is a result of incompletely resolved acute epididymitis, presents with an indurated tender mass. Tuberculous epididymitis is characteristically nontender, stony hard, and may be associated with irregular indurated beadings of the vas deferens. It is the most common cause of scrotal fistulae. A sterile or chemical epididymitis may occur with the retrograde extravasation of fluid into the epididymis secondary to marked increase in intraabdominal pressure associated with heavy lifting while the bladder is distended. The urine is usually sterile in this situation, in contrast to the pyuria which is often present with epididymitis due to infection.

Varicocele. There is a predilection for the left side, because the left pampiniform plexus and spermatic vein drain into the left renal vein, which is usually 10 cm higher than the point at which the right spermatic vein enters the inferior vena cava. It is characteristically a lesion of puberty and becomes less obvious with age, usually disappearing after thirty-five. Acute onset of a left varicocele after the age of forty suggests left renal vein occlusion, commonly related to renal tumor. A varicocele on the right side may be secondary to vena caval obstruction or occlusion. This occasionally occurs with tumor thrombus from a hypernephroma invading and involving the lumen of the vena cava. The usual type of left varicocele is observed best with the patient in the standing position facing the examiner. The characteristic "bag of worms" appearance and feeling of the scrotum is noted. With the patient in the supine position, the varicocele collapses and usually cannot be palpated. Failure of drainage in the supine position is suggestive of left renal vein occlusion as noted above. The presence of a varicocele in a patient who is being examined for infertility may be a significant finding. This is especially true if the patient has a low sperm count with reduced motility of the sperm.

Hydrocele. Primary idiopathic hydrocele may be unilateral or bilateral and represents an increased collection of fluid between the tunica vaginalis and its contents. It is manifested as a large nontender mass which is translucent and obscures palpation of the testis and epididymis. It is ventral, superior, and inferior to the testis and frequently reaches the size of 25 cm in greatest dimension. Secondary hydroceles are the consequence of serous effusion in the vicinity of a disease process. Epididymitis, tuberculosis, trauma, and mumps are among the common causes. Twenty percent of acute hydroceles are secondary to testicular tumors. Aspiration of the hydrocele on the anterior ventral surface of the mass permits more precise palpation and differentiation from testicular tumors. A *communicating hydrocele* is a result of ascites in a patient with a patent processus vaginalis. In this situation, the scrotal mass fills and empties with varying positions.

Spermatocele. This is a cyst of an efferent ductule of the rete testis. It originates at the head of the epididymis and presents as a transilluminable cystic mass discrete from the testis. Spermatoceles are often bilateral and may be multiple. They are of no consequence except when they reach large proportions.

Testicular Tumor. A palpable nodule on or within the testis represents a potential malignant tumor until proved otherwise. The lesion is usually firm and nontender and is not transilluminable. It is often first noted by the patient or on a routine examination of this area. Prompt surgical exploration through an inguinal incision is indicated. One cannot stress enough the importance of being able to detect small lesions of the testis by careful palpation and the significance and urgency of proper management. The scrotal mass is usually hard, nontender, and irregular, and is not translucent. There is rarely associated pain, but the presentation of such a mass is regarded as surgical emergency requiring prompt inguinal exploration.

Mumps Orchitis. The lesion usually occurs in postpubertal males with acute parotitis. It commonly becomes apparent as the parotitis subsides, 7 to 10 days following the onset of the illness. Patients experience high fever, malaise, and marked testicular swelling which, unlike acute pyogenic epididymitis, is unaccompanied by scrotal edema.

Torsion of the Testis or Appendages. Torsion of the testis generally refers to torsion of the spermatic cord with a characteristic 540° rotation of the testis and an anterior presentation of the epididymis. The patient presents with sudden onset of pain accompanied by scrotal enlargement and edema. The testis, which appears to be elevated because the cord is shortened by twisting, is exquisitely tender. The differential diagnosis between acute epididymitis and torsion of the testis may be difficult. Since prompt treatment of the latter is important to save the testis from infarction, it may be necessary occasionally to explore patients with acute epididymitis to prevent loss of testis in patients with torsion. Four hours of torsion appears to be the limit after which the testis is irreversibly damaged. Because of the high incidence of bilateral anatomic predisposition to torsion, bilateral orchiopexy should be performed when surgical treatment for unilateral torsion is undertaken.

Torsion of the testis, per se, can occur only when there is a long mesorchium connecting it to the epididymis. In such a case, the testis, which is likened to a clapper in a bell, can twist inside the tunica vaginalis and undergo infarction. In this circumstance, the epididymis lies in its normal position, and the testis, which is enlarged, tender, and hard, is not drawn up high in the scrotum. A third condition of torsion involves the appendix testis. This normally present embryologic remnant lies at the upper pole of the testis. When it undergoes torsion, the patient presents with a painful lump on the surface of the testis. Transillumination before major swelling occurs may reveal a characteristic "black dot" sign, which is visualization of the infarcted appendage. Since testicular tumors are rarely tender, they are not likely to be confused with torsion of the appendix testis.

PROSTATE. The gland can best be evaluated after the patient has emptied his bladder, and it is preferable for the patient to be bending forward over the examining table or bed during the examination. If the patient is unable to stand, he should be examined while lying on his side with knees flexed and facing the standing examiner. If the examiner is right-handed, the patient should lie on his right side. Rectal examination should be carried out carefully, with very little pressure exerted while passing the finger through the anus and while the examining finger is on the prostate gland. It is seldom necessary to press hard on the prostate. Furthermore, exertion of pressure in this area may produce considerable discomfort and limit the examination. The normal prostate is two fingerbreadths wide with a 0.5 cm-deep sulcus between the two lobes. It is about 2.5 cm from apex to base. However, rectal examination is inadequate to define the precise size and must be combined with cystoscopy.

The consistency of both the normal prostate and the prostate with benign hypertrophy is similar to that of the thenar eminence. In contrast, carcinoma of the prostate feels stony hard, similar to the interphalangeal joint. Crepitations are related to multiple prostatic calculi. With benign hyperplasia, the gland can be delineated from surrounding tissues, and the contours are smooth. With carcinoma of the prostate, the surrounding tissues are frequently fixed to the gland, thus eliminating the usual discreteness of prostatic contour. Extension of the tumor may proceed into the seminal vesicle area superior and lateral to the prostate. Since 90 percent of carcinomas arise in the posterior portion of the gland, they are readily detectable on rectal examination as a single lump or a nodular mass. Acute suppuration of the prostate is accompanied by tenderness or fluctuation and dictates an atraumatic examination to avoid dissemination of the infection.

FEMALE URETHRA. Pelvic examination of the female patient in the lithotomy position is essential for evaluation of the lower urinary tract. Careful visualization and calibration of the urethral meatus can be carried out in this position. The presence of a cystocele or urethrocele can be determined with the patient bearing down. A urethral diverticulum may be detected by gentle pressure against the anterior vaginal wall, milking the urethra from the bladder to the meatus. Pressure in this region against the symphysis may result in release of purulent material or urine from a diverticulum of the urethra.

Urinalysis

A fresh two-glass specimen from the male or a catheterized specimen from the female provides optimal results. However, a carefully obtained, clean-voided midstream specimen from the female is useful. A midstream specimen from the circumcised male is usually satisfactory for culture and microscopic examination without any prior cleansing of the penis. The specimen should be examined while fresh, since refrigeration leads to sedimentation of phosphates and storage in a warm environment results in deterioration of formed elements and growth of bacteria.

A clear urine is usually normal. A cloudy urine may be normal if a few drops of dilute acetic acid render it clear, as in phosphaturia. The color may indicate disease, ingestion of certain foods, or administration of medications. Pyridium results in an orange-red color. Methylene blue incorporated in urinary medications leads to varying shades of green and blue. Pink urine may be due to food dyes or to medications like Serenium. Various degrees of bluish gray and brown may be associated with acute porphyria. The degree and timing of bleeding can often be best estimated by examination of the gross urine specimen.

The odor is often characteristic. A mousy odor which accompanies *Escherichia coli* infection is related to formation of ammonia. A pungent odor is characteristic of either necrotic bladder tumors or calculous pyonephrosis. Certain medications, such as ampicillin, have a characteristic and readily identifiable odor in the urine.

Chemical examination routinely includes tests for the presence of albumin, reducing sugars, acetone, and pH. Since there are no proteins in the secretions of the male

Fig. 40-5. Commonly used urologic instruments.

OLIVE TIPPED COUDÉ CATHETER

SELF RETAINING CATHETER

URETHRAL SOUND

FILIFORM

FILIFORM CATHETER FOLLOWER

PESSAR CATHETER

genital organs, albuminuria cannot be ascribed to them. The various paper-dip tests are usually quite reliable but do have some limitation in the detection of hematuria.

Casts, crystals, and clumps of epithelial cells are identified under low-power *microscopic examination,* while the nature of cells, crystals, and bacteria are determined under higher powers. When the urine sediment is heavy, both the centrifuged and uncentrifuged specimens should be examined. Staining with methylene blue facilitates the diagnosis of bacteriuria. Exfoliative cytologic examination of urine may be helpful, but there is often a greater yield from study of the wet preparation, which may demonstrate clusters of cells with nucleocytoplasmic disparity characteristic of malignancy. The identification of bacteria in an unspun urine specimen is strongly suggestive of the presence of a urinary tract infection rather than contamination.

Genital Secretions

URETHRAL DISCHARGE. Collection is accomplished on a glass slide before the patient urinates. A heat-fixed and Gram-stained specimen identifies responsible organisms. Gonococcal urethritis is diagnosed by the presence of gram-negative diplococci within epithelial cells and leukocytes. In mimae infection, the cocci are quite similar. They are frequently polychromatic and are predominantly extracellular. Examination of the wet specimen is helpful in identifying the presence of trichomonads. Confirmation of the presence of infection is established by adequate culture of the urethral discharge.

PROSTATIC SECRETION. The specimen is obtained by gentle massage of the gland. Examination of the normally opalescent fluid reveals three to five white cells per high-power field and tiny refractile cephalin bodies. Epithelial cells are present in small numbers. Seminal vesicle secretion presents as a gelatinous and fibrinous tree-shaped cast of the seminal vesicle containing strands and granules. In the presence of prostatic infection, the secretions become granular, and large clumps of white cells are readily seen. An increased amount of prostatic secretion with the presence of very few white blood cells is suggestive of prostatic congestion.

SEMEN ANALYSIS. For purposes of standardization, the specimen should be obtained by masturbation and collected in a dry container after 5 days of sexual abstinence. Examination, performed less than 1 hour after ejaculation, normally notes a volume of 3 to 5 ml with liquefaction complete within 1 hour. There should be over 20 million spermatozoa per milliliter with at least 60 percent demonstrating motility and 80 percent appearing morphologically normal.

Instrumentation

The insertion of any foreign body or instrument into the urethra carries a risk of trauma, introduction of infection, sepsis, and the possibility of exacerbation of preexisting inflammatory or obstructive conditions. Figure 40-5 illustrates commonly used urologic instruments. Instruments are designated by the French numbering system relating to the circumference of the instrument in millimeters, i.e., a #24 French sound is 24 mm in circumference.

CYSTOURETHROSCOPY. This investigative procedure should be performed in most cases of gross or microscopic hematuria and in selected cases of patients with symptoms of lower urinary tract obstruction or infection. It can often be performed as an office procedure. Instillation of a local anesthetic agent into the male urethra makes the procedure tolerable. The smallest caliber instrument that will provide adequate visualization of the bladder and urethra is used. No anesthetic is usually required for female cystourethroscopy. The presence of very small lesions of the bladder measuring 1 or 2 mm in diameter can readily be detected, as well as small calculi, the configuration and location of the ureteral orifices, prostatic size, urethral strictures or valves, and other pathologic conditions which may be present in the bladder or the urethra.

THERAPEUTIC INSTRUMENTATION. An indwelling catheter affords temporary relief of the obstruction. However, since maintenance for over 3 days is almost always attended by ascending infection, an external collecting device, such as a sheath, is more appropriate to improve nursing care of the incontinent patient who has no obstruction. Relative contraindications to instrumentation include acute cystitis, urethritis, prostatitis, pyelonephritis, and epididymitis. In these instances, it is best to pretreat the patient for the organism present. An exception to the rule is that if obstruction is the predisposing cause of infection, i.e., prostatic hypertrophy with retention and acute cystopyelitis, immediate instrumentation is necessary. Temporary drainage during the acute infection stage may be carried out by suprapubic tap and the insertion of a small polyethylene or plastic tube connected to constant drainage. Therapeutic instrumentation may be applied in the endoscopic removal of calculi or foreign bodies, biopsy or excision of tumors, cysts, or other obstructive lesions, drainage of prostatic abscesses, and transurethral removal of the prostatic obstruction. Institution of transurethral drainage may represent the most important therapeutic factor in obstructions secondary to prostatic hypertrophy or impacted ureteral calculus associated with cystopyelitis or pyelonephritis.

Catheterization should be performed with aseptic technique and minimal trauma. For routine stat catheterization, a #16 or #18 olive-tip coudé rubber catheter is the easiest to pass and the least traumatic. For indwelling drainage in the absence of gross bleeding or clots, a #18 Foley catheter is usually satisfactory. If one plans to allow the catheter to remain for several days, it should not be a tight fit which leads to ischemic changes of the urethra and subsequent stricture. Closed system drainage should be instituted; periodic instillation of an antibacterial irrigating solution left in contact with the bladder mucosa may help prevent infection during this period of constant drainage.

The operator should wear sterile gloves or use a sterile clamp, and the patient should be prepped with germicidal soap and draped. For dilatation or instrumentation of the male urethra, a topical anesthetic is instilled. After the catheter, which has been lubricated with a water-soluble lubricant, is inserted into the urethra, the latter is drawn upward to straighten the curves and folds. Resistance of the sphincter is best overcome by gentle pressure. In the case of acute retention, complete bladder decompression should be effected. However, with chronic and prolonged distension, rapid decompression of the bladder may lead to distressing vesical spasm and hemorrhage. Therefore, gradual decompression over a period of 72 hours is indicated.

Special Diagnostic Studies

EXCRETORY UROGRAPHY. Certain intravenously administered organic substances are filtered and excreted by the kidney. When rendered opaque by iodinization, they opacify the renal parenchyma and collecting system. Hypaque (sodium orthoiodohippurate) and Conray (meglumine iothalamate) are two examples. These agents are potent osmotic diuretics and may lead to dehydration, especially in children. Therefore it is important to compensate for this effect by encouraging copious fluid intake following examination. Occasionally the study is followed by anuria and renal failure in elderly, dehydrated, debilitated patients who have evidence of renal dysfunction. Satisfactory hydration of these patients is essential to decrease the risk of this occurring.

If time permits, a 3-day low-residue diet and oral laxatives should be administered to eliminate fecal and gas shadows. Also, the patient should be dehydrated for 12 hours prior to the examination to concentrate the opacified urine. However, dehydration should not be carried out in the uremic patient, and in this situation the quantity of opaque can be doubled or tripled to improve the quality of films. Patients with reduced renal function and BUN (blood urea nitrogen) in the neighborhood of 60 mg/100 ml can excrete a sufficient concentration of opaque to give clinically useful information. Pyelograms with inadequate preparation may give useful information in emergencies. They may be adequate to determine the presence of obstruction, extravasation, or nonfunction.

Renal Size, Location and Axis. The adult male kidney averages 13 by 6.2 cm on pyelography. The left kidney is usually several millimeters longer and broader. The kidneys of females are 5 mm smaller in both dimensions. The upper pole of the left kidney lies at mid T_{12}, while the right kidney is a half vertebral body lower. In the upright position, the kidney descends one vertebral body. If lines are drawn through the uppermost and lowermost calyces of the two kidneys, they should converge at T_9 (Fig. 40-6). Any deviation from this axis is considered abnormal. The calyces should be adequate in number and delicately cupped. The infundibulae are straight and fine. The pelvis points medially and describes a smooth curve without redundancy or tortuosity. There may be several areas of incomplete ureteral visualization due to peristalsis. The diameter of the ureter usually does not exceed 4 mm. Late upright films should demonstrate emptying of the collecting system and visualization of the urinary bladder. On supine films the contrast may pool in the fundus of the bladder and lead to the erroneous interpretation of an outlet filling defect. A postvoiding film is helpful in reveal-

ing the lower ureter and indicating the amount of residual urine.

NEPHROTOMOGRAPHY. More detailed and accurate visualization of the kidney and pelvocalyceal system is available by this technique. Several "slices" of the kidneys are obtained beginning posteriorly and advancing anteriorly. This eliminates the overlying gas and fecal material in the bowel. Lucent areas such as fat and cysts are more readily identifiable. The poorly prepared patient may be evaluated more satisfactorily.

RETROGRADE PYELOURETEROGRAPHY. This study is indicated to further evaluate lesions of the pelvocalyceal system and ureter. "Filling defects" of these structures may not be evaluated adequately by excretory urography. Urine may be collected from the pelves for cytologic study and also to determine differential renal function. Instillation of contrast medium provides a more detailed visualization of these structures and is best done under fluoroscopic control. Improved techniques of excretory urography and nephrotomography have significantly decreased the need for retrograde pyeloureterography.

CYSTOURETHROGRAPHY. The patient's bladder and urethra may be evaluated by antegrade or retrograde studies. Fluoroscopic examination of the patient voiding may reveal the dynamics of micturition and evidence of obstruction or reflux of urine. Voiding cystourethrography is a useful diagnostic tool in the evaluation of children with voiding problems or recurrent urinary tract infections. Isotopic cystograms may be employed for the evaluation of reflux in children and offer decreased radiation exposure.

ANTEGRADE PYELOGRAPHY. Percutaneous insertion of a small catheter into the pelvocalyceal system may be a valuable diagnostic and therapeutic tool. The procedure is performed with local anesthesia and with fluoroscopic control. Once the small tube is placed properly within the drainage structures of the kidney, adequate drainage of an obstructed, infected pyohydronephrosis may be instituted and adequate x-ray visualization of the upper urinary tract may be obtained. Occasionally a ureter cannot be catheterized from below and may have to be visualized by this technique. It is an extremely valuable technique to use in the seriously ill, toxic patient. Adequate drainage may convert the situation from a surgical emergency to a relatively simple elective procedure in a nontoxic patient.

RENAL ARTERIOGRAPHY. Percutaneous, transfemoral renal arteriography is useful in the evaluation of possible renal vascular hypertension. The technique can demonstrate vascular lesions and thus direct the surgical approach. With congenital anomalies of the kidney arteriography is also helpful, since vascular anomalies frequently coexist and have an important bearing on surgical treat-

ment. Arteriography is also applied to the differential diagnosis of renal masses; a characteristic pooling of opaque is noted in tumor vessels within the parenchyma.

VENA CAVAGRAPHY. Percutaneous catheterization of the femoral vein with instillation of contrast material provides adequate visualization of the inferior vena cava. This study is particularly helpful in evaluating patients with carcinoma of the kidney and testicular neoplasms. Intrinsic involvement and obstruction of the vena cava and renal veins may be present with carcinoma of the kidney, and extrinsic compression of the vena cava may accompany enlargement of the periaortic nodes associated with metastatic testicular cancer. Preoperative evaluation with this study may help determine the most suitable type of surgical procedure for the patient.

LYMPHANGIOGRAPHY. Pedal lymphangiography may provide adequate visualization of the periaortic nodal drainage system as well as nodes of the pelvis. This study is usually employed in evaluation of patients with testicular, bladder, or prostatic carcinomas. A more adequate staging of the patient's disease may be possible with this technique.

RENOGRAPHY. The ^{131}I hippurate renogram provides an isotopic evaluation of the function of the individual kidneys. Dehydration, sodium depletion, and tubular blocking agents may alter the curves, and technical factors such as placement of detectors, dose of isotope, and paravenous injection may complicate interpretation. When properly performed, the renogram can be helpful in recognizing nonfunction or reduced function and delayed excretion, and in ureteral obstruction. It is also applied to differentiate between acute tubular necrosis and dehydration oliguria. Following renal arterial surgical procedures or homotransplantation, renography provides a simple and dependable method of evaluating the vascular status of the organ. Illustrative curves are shown in Figs. 40-7 to 40-10. The use of properly selected isotopes may provide further information regarding renal perfusion, drainage, and morphology.

ULTRASONOGRAPHY. This technique is useful in the differentiation of renal masses. Cystic lesions and hydronephrosis may be readily distinguished from solid masses of the kidney. Percutaneous needle aspiration of cystic masses may be carried out, providing drainage. The instillation of contrast material offers information as to the nature of the lesion. The noninvasive character of the

Fig. 40-7. [131]I hippurate renograms. Both curves are normal.

◀ Fig. 40-6. *A* and *B.* Excretory urogram in complete left ureteral reduplication with ectopic ureteral orifice of nonvisualizing upper segment. Axis of the left kidney *BB* is abnormal. *C* and *D.* Left retrograde pyelogram demonstrating the upper segment. Note the correct axis of the right kidney *AA.* There is a ureterocele at the lower end of the ectopic ureter to the upper left renal segment.

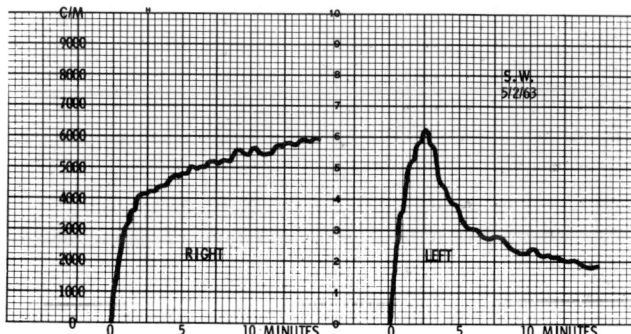

Fig. 40-8. ^{131}I hippurate renograms. Left renogram is normal. Delayed excretion on the right is due to obstructing ureteral calculus.

procedure and the lack of radiation exposure make it a useful screening, outpatient procedure, especially in children.

COMPUTED TOMOGRAPHY. The use of computed tomography for the evaluation of abdominal lesions is becoming a more common procedure. It is performed with and without contrast material. Lesions of the kidneys can be readily identified as to size, location, and consistency. Cystic lesions can be differentiated from solid lesions. The extent of tumor involvement with adjacent structures can be defined, allowing for improved staging of disease. As more experience is gained with this method, it will assume its proper place in the format of evaluation of patients with genitourinary disease.

CYSTOMETRICS, URETHRAL PRESSURE PROFILES, AND SPHINCTER ELECTROMYOGRAPHY. These studies are useful diagnostic tools for the evaluation of patients with micturition dysfunction, including problems which are due to obstruction, neurologic disease, functional disturbances, and dyssynergia.

PERCUTANEOUS RENAL CYST PUNCTURE. Under satisfactory local anesthesia and with fluoroscopic control, selected renal masses may be punctured. Fluid may be obtained for examination. Contrast material may be inserted into the cavity, and the differential diagnosis between cyst and tumor may be accurately determined.

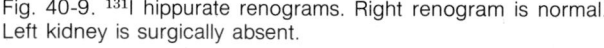

Fig. 40-9. ^{131}I hippurate renograms. Right renogram is normal. Left kidney is surgically absent.

BLADDER FUNCTION

PHYSIOLOGY OF MICTURITION. As the empty bladder fills, the detrusor muscle stretches to accommodate the gradually increasing volume of urine. Normally, the pressure within the bladder is not significantly greater than intraabdominal pressure during the filling stage. When the volume of urine is sufficient, the pressure increases until it stimulates a spinal cord reflex which is under the control of cortical centers and leads to the contraction of the detrusor. This muscular contraction shortens the urethra and opens the bladder neck so that it resembles a funnel. Intravesical pressure at the initiation of voiding ranges between 15 and 30 cm of water. Voiding is resisted by the contraction of the striated muscles of the perineum and external sphincter, which overcome the tendency of the detrusor to effect urination.

In patients with obstructive uropathy, the pressure required to empty the bladder exceeds normal. This results in muscular hypertrophy of the detrusor and an increase in the pressure at the time of voiding so as to compensate for the obstruction. As long as the degree of the obstruction is counterbalanced by detrusor hypertrophy, the patient is able to empty the bladder with minimal amounts of residual urine. With overstretching of the detrusor muscle, the fibers lose their mechanical advantage and are unable to contract and empty the bladder effectively. Overdistension of the bladder occurs with obstruction, under the influence of certain drugs, and also in anesthetized patients with diuresis accompanying large amounts of intravenous therapy. This detrusor atonia is of short duration, disappearing rapidly following emptying of the bladder, while prolonged overdistension, such as occurs with chronic obstructive prostatic hypertrophy, may require several weeks of catheter drainage to effect complete recovery of function.

BLADDER INNERVATION. Sensations, including perception of heat and cold and pain of distension, are mediated by sensory fibers accompanying the sympathetic and parasympathetic nerves. They arise from T_9 to L_2 segments of the spinal cord. Motor pathways originate in the S_2 to S_4 segments and reach the bladder via the pelvic nerves. These parasympathetic nerves are responsible for the reflex contraction of the detrusor. The motor nerves of the external sphincter also originate in the S_2 to S_4 segments but travel via the pudendal nerves. The bladder is also richly supplied by sympathetic nerves which play a major role in detrusor function and outlet resistance.

Motor pathways may be evaluated by the bulbocavernosis reflex, which is elicited by gentle compression of the glans penis evoking contraction of the anal sphincter. *Cystometry* is the best method of evaluating motor function. This can be accomplished either by means of a recording gas or water cystometer or by an improvised system consisting of a reservoir with a drip chamber permitting regulation of fluid flow into the bladder. A Y tube connected to the indwelling urethral catheter and a graded column of fluid completes the system. The zero level of the column of fluid is positioned at the level of the symphysis, and warm saline solution is instilled into the bladder at the rate of 50 ml/minute. There is usually an increase of 10 to 15 cm of water pressure when flow is initiated. The normal cystometrogram shows a gradual increment in pressure during instillation of 400 ml of fluid, and at the end of this instillation the pressure rarely exceeds 20 cm. When bladder capacity is reached, there is a sudden increase in pressure as a result of detrusor response to the stretch reflex. Further information can be gained by combining cystometry with urethral pressure profile studies and a recording of sphincter electromyographic responses.

Neurogenic Bladder Dysfunction

Bladder dysfunction resulting from deficient innervation reflects the degree and type of nerve damage rather than the etiologic factor.

Uninhibited Neurogenic Bladder. Dysfunction is similar to that of the bladder of an infant in whom cortical integration is lacking. Etiology includes cerebral vascular accidents with cortical destruction, multiple sclerosis, and taboparesis. The condition presents as urgent voiding which is almost without voluntary control. A cystometrogram reveals many abrupt increases in pressure during filling, even at low volumes. Treatment with parasympatholytic drugs such as methantheline (Banthine), 50 mg four times daily, frequently produces a dramatic improvement in symptomatology by inhibiting the premature contractions.

Reflex (Automatic) Neurogenic Bladder. Dysfunction results from traumatic transection of the spinal cord. When the area between T_7 and C_7 is involved, a well-functioning reflex bladder usually results. In contrast, lesions above C_7 are often associated with extensive atrophy of the cord below the site of transection and may prevent the development of a reflex arc. The bladder with reflex function can frequently be rehabilitated to provide adequate emptying. This type of dysfunction is commonly associated with intense trabeculation of the bladder and, characteristically, produces a positive urecholine test result. Control pressure measurements are made through a urethral catheter with the bladder filled to 100 ml. Thirty minutes after the subcutaneous injection of 2.5 mg of urecholine, measurements are repeated. With upper motor neuron interruption, increased sensitivity of the neuromuscular junction and ganglionic synapses result in pressures which exceed 15 cm of water greater than control.

Centrally Denervated Neurogenic Bladder. Dysfunction is the result of traumatic, neoplastic, or congenital lesions of the sacral segments or cauda equina. Meningomyelocele or occult spina bifida are the most frequent lesions. The symptoms are overflow incontinence and recurring infections. Diagnosis is established by observing a large smooth-walled bladder containing a large amount of residual urine. Cystometry reveals large capacity associated with low pressures. Conservative management includes encouragement of the patient to strain and empty his bladder at frequent intervals, coupled with the administration of antibacterial agents to prevent the consequences of infection, namely, chronic pyelonephritis. Surgical treatment is directed at balancing the detrusor function

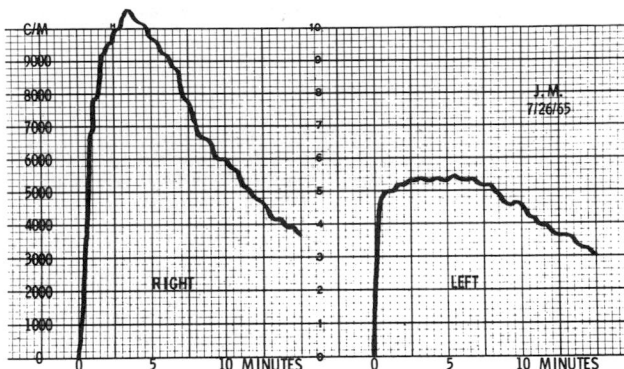

Fig. 40-10. ^{131}I hippurate renograms. Reduced left renal function with low urine volume is due to left renal artery stenosis with hypertension. Right renogram indicates functional hypertrophy.

with the resistance of the normal urethra by transurethral resection of the bladder neck or sphincterotomy. This results in improved emptying of the bladder and increased resistance to secondary infection. Long-term antibacterial therapy, however, is usually required. Intermittent self-catheterization may be required to maintain satisfactory emptying of the bladder at periodic intervals, which will decrease the incidence of infection and protect the upper urinary tract. Further balance between detrusor activity and peripheral resistance may be brought about by the proper use of drugs which will increase detrusor tone (cholinergic) and decrease bladder neck and proximal urethral resistance (sympatholytic).

Sensory Paralytic Bladder. Dysfunction results from the loss of sensory components of bladder innervation, such as in tabes dorsalis or combined cord degeneration. This leads to a huge bladder capacity and overflow incontinence. The patient is unaware of bladder filling. A cystometrogram shows a large capacity with lack of sensation and small response of pressure to volume change. Treatment is similar to that described above for the centrally denervated neurogenic bladder. The patient is then educated to void at regular intervals, since he never senses the need.

Motor Paralytic Bladder. Dysfunction may accompany poliomyelitis or infectious polyneuritis. Loss of motor activity is demonstrated on cystometry, and a large residual urine results. As the patient recovers from disease, bladder function returns to normal, but an indwelling catheter or intermittent catheterization may be required for a period of time.

MANAGEMENT OF POSTTRAUMATIC PARAPLEGIA WITH NEUROGENIC BLADDER DYSFUNCTION. A variety of methods have been utilized to establish bladder drainage in the initial paralytic, atonic phase. Multiple suprapubic aspirations, suprapubic cystostomy, and surgically constructed vesicocutaneous fistulas have been used. The indwelling urethral catheter is most commonly employed. A # 16 or # 18 indwelling balloon type is most practical and should be inserted in accordance with the previously proposed technique. The catheter should be attached to drainage in such a fashion that it can be irrigated by a closed system with a reservoir which is changed periodically. A

100-ml aliquot of sterile saline may be introduced into the bladder several times daily. Irrigations with $\frac{1}{4}$ percent acetic acid, mixtures of antibacterial drugs, and stone-dissolving agents have been proposed. It is seldom necessary to use irrigation to dissolve concretions, but if the situation arises, modified solution G (32.5 Gm of citric acid, 3.84 Gm of magnesium oxide, 8.84 Gm of sodium carbonate at a pH of 5) is useful.

Ascending infection around the catheter can be minimized by cleaning the meatus and surrounding tissue and by promoting the egress of urethral secretions. The latter can be accomplished by taping the penis parallel to the inguinal crease. The most important aspect of catheter care is the ingestion of sufficient fluids to produce an excess of 2 liters of urine daily. In addition to maintaining volume, the pH should be below 6, since an acid pH decreases the incidence of encrustation. The use of an acid-ash diet or ascorbic acid will result in an acid urine. Since paraplegic patients mobilize calcium from the bones and excrete it in the urine, multiple determinations of the 24-hour urinary calcium levels are indicated. If the urinary calcium excretion exceeds 300 mg/day, the patient should be placed on a low-calcium diet. Anabolic agents are also useful in reducing the urinary calcium excretion.

Periodic cultures of the urine and microscopic examination are directed at evaluating urinary infection. Methenamine mandelate is frequently useful to maintain an environment unfavorable for bacterial growth. High fever in a paraplegic is generally related to urinary tract infection. The specific complications of catheter drainage in these patients include acute cystitis and pyelonephritis, acute epididymitis, suppurative urethritis, periurethral abscess with fistula formation, and bladder or kidney stones.

A regimen of intermittent catheterization should be established as soon as possible in the early phase, so that the indwelling catheter can be removed. This can be carried out by self-catheterization, if the patient is able to learn this technique and has the necessary motor power in the upper extremities, or by trained personnel in the hospital ward or rehabilitation center.

Rehabilitation of Bladder. During the first 3 to 4 months of stabilizing a fracture, attention is directed at preventing infection and permanent damage to the urinary tract. Stabilization of the fracture permits the patient to assume an upright position and allows attempts at rehabilitation of the urinary tract. This should be initiated by cystometric and cystoscopic evaluation followed by a trial of catheter removal, if the patient has been on indwelling catheter drainage. In at least 70 percent of patients it is possible to reach a catheter-free state. Prior to and for several days subsequent to catheter removal, appropriate antibiotic therapy is directed at any organisms present. The patient's voiding habits and volume and character of urine should be noted. Success is anticipated when large volumes are voided at infrequent intervals. Frequent voiding of small volumes may precede total cessation of voiding, in which case the catheter is reinserted. A trial of urecholine is occasionally beneficial and may precede catheter reinsertion. If self-catheterization has not been instituted earlier

and the patient is not able to empty the bladder satisfactorily, it can be taught at this time.

If necessary, a reinserted catheter should be left in place for an additional period of time during which reassessment of the anatomic status of the bladder by cystourethroscopy is performed. Over half the patients with upper motor neuron bladder dysfunction require resection of the bladder neck to relieve obstruction. Subsequent to surgical operations, such as sphincterotomy, the majority of patients void satisfactorily. The patients requiring prolonged or permanent catheter drainage are instructed in catheter care and the maintenance of a large urinary volume. Suppressive therapy with agents such as nitrofurantoin and methenamine mandelate is helpful in reducing the problem of chronic infection.

In females, incontinence may persist. If it is of the overflow type, self-catheterization may also be of value. In neglected patients with neurologic disturbance of bladder function, the resultant damage to the upper urinary tract requires a supravesical diversion. The cutaneous ureteroileostomy may resolve the problem, but attention must be given to watertight sealing of the collecting appliance.

ACUTE INFECTIONS

PATHOGENESIS. The most common portal of entry for urinary tract infection is the urethra. *Ascending infection* is potentiated by obstructive uropathy, foreign bodies, and also bladder tumor and papillary necrosis. The normal bladder possesses defense mechanisms which are capable of coping with introduced infection. In the obstructed, inflamed, or ulcerated organ, however, these mechanisms are rendered ineffective. In the presence of obstructive uropathy, the increased pressure required for evacuation frequently leads to retrograde infection by means of reflux of infected urine into the ureter and kidney. Voiding cystourethrograms document this occurrence. Ninety-six percent of pediatric urinary infections occur in the female, because of the shortness of the urethra. Many children who have recurrent urinary infections also have obstructive uropathy. In the adult, 65 percent of urinary infections are in females and are related to the trauma of sexual intercourse, childbirth, and gynecologic procedures. In older age groups, urinary tract infections increase in the male because of the incidence of obstructive uropathy secondary to prostatic hypertrophy.

Urinary tract infections also result from *hematogenous* spread, such as metastatic staphylococcal infection from cutaneous abscesses. This produces the entity known as staphylococcal kidney, or renal carbuncle. Severe hydronephrosis and renal calculi predispose to hematogenous infection. *Lymphatic transmission* of infection from the bowel and lower urinary tract via periureteral lymphatics is also proposed as a cause of pyelonephritis. Urinary tract infections are an infrequent result of spread from contiguous infections such as diverticulitis of the colon, regional enteritis, and appendiceal abscess.

BACTERIOLOGY. The most common organism causing

acute urinary tract infections is *E. coli,* which is responsible in 37 percent of the cases. Other commonly involved pathogens are *Proteus mirabilis, Klebsiella,* the enterococci, and *Pseudomonas.* Other organisms, encountered less frequently, include *Proteus vulgaris, morgagni* and *rettgeri* and the staphylococci. Most of these organisms are normal inhabitants of the fecal flora. With acute urinary tract infection, hundreds of thousands to millions of organisms per milliliter are present in the voided urine, and pure cultures are more prevalent in acute infections than in chronic infections.

TREATMENT. The ability to treat urinary tract infections with drugs is enhanced by the unique ability of normally functioning kidneys to concentrate a variety of antibacterial agents in the urine. Treatment involves proper selection of the right drug or drugs which can be adequately delivered to the urine, tissues, or blood. Drug selection is facilitated by culture and determination of sensitivities. However, these are usually not possible in the early stages of treatment. Further considerations include the age and general health of the patient, kidney function, history of allergy, previous drug therapy, relative cost of therapy, nature of the preparation, and possible complications of the drug to be administered.

Sulfonamides, which are rapidly excreted by the kidney in high concentration, are ideally suited to the treatment of urinary tract infections. Most acute urinary tract infections due to *E. coli* will respond to these drugs administered as 1 Gm four times daily for 7 to 10 days. In acute uncomplicated infections without upper tract involvement, this usually constitutes adequate therapy, but the urine should be reexamined microscopically and cultured at the end of 1 week. In the patient with manifestations of pyelonephritis, such as flank pain, chills, fever, malaise, nausea, vomiting, and leukocytosis, a more prolonged course of therapy is indicated. Other useful antibacterial agents are ampicillin, tetracycline, cephalexin, nitrofurantoin, nalidixic acid, and trimethoprim-sulfamethoxizole. The aminoglycosides, such as gentamicin, tobramycin, and amikacin, are particularly useful for the treatment of *Pseudomonas* infections. Antispasmodics and dye substances which relieve symptoms should be used only in conjunction with antibacterial agents.

The acute infection is sometimes secondary to an important factor which requires correction in order to prevent recurrence. Therefore, although it is justifiable to treat acutely ill patients before the diagnosis is made, complete investigation should be carried out as soon as possible. If the infection is related to defloration cystitis, vaginitis, diarrhea, or poor hygiene, simultaneous treatment of the two conditions will effect a cure. If the infection is secondary to obstruction, the obstruction must be eliminated.

Following subsidence of the acute episode, repeated urinalyses should be performed at 1-month intervals if the patient is asymptomatic and sooner if symptoms recur. Complete urologic evaluation should be performed in all patients who have had attacks of acute pyelonephritis or multiple attacks of cystitis. In the male, since the bladder is protected by a longer urethra, a single attack of cystitis warrants investigation. If recurrent infections occur, long-term therapy for 3 to 12 months may succeed where short courses fail. Drugs useful for long-term therapy include nitrofurantoin, methenamine mandelate, methenamine hippurate, and trimethoprim-sulfamethoxizole. Patients receiving these medications should have periodic blood cell counts to detect granulocytopenia and anemia. Allergic and hypersensitive responses to these medicines are also relatively common.

GRAM-NEGATIVE BACTEREMIA. The syndrome is considered with urologic diseases, since in over half the patients with gram-negative bacteremia the urinary tract provides the portal of entry. Frequently the bacteremia follows instrumentation in the presence of preexisting urinary tract infection which has been ineffectively treated. The patients experience a shaking chill followed by high fever, peripheral vasodilatation, and hypotension. The organisms responsible are frequently resistant to the usual drugs and require large doses of parenterally administered antibacterial agents. Drugs which are bactericidal are preferable, in order to prevent liberation of additional quantities of the endotoxin by the multiplying bacteria. An aminoglycoside, such as gentamicin and ampicillin, or a similar drug used in combination has proved to be quite effective for the management of gram-negative bacteremia. Drug dosage is carefully regulated according to renal function and, when available, culture and sensitivities reports. The treatment of schock is discussed in Chap. 4.

Acute Staphylococcal Infections of the Kidney

Staphylococcal pyelonephritis or abscess is of hematogenous origin and usually the result of metastatic infection from furuncles. The symptoms include fever, flank pain, frequency, and dysuria. On examination, the patient is very ill, with marked tenderness over the kidney and leukocytosis. Urinalysis may reveal staphylococci on stain or culture. In the very acute phase, the urine may be negative, since the organisms are located in the cortex of the kidney and have not found their way into the urine. *Staphylococcus aureus* is the most common offending organism. Treatment consists of parenteral therapy with the appropriate antibacterial agent. Complications include renal carbuncle, which represents liquefaction necrosis, or perinephric abscess resulting from perforation of a renal carbuncle. *Renal carbuncle* usually occurs in patients who are ineffectively treated for the acute staphylococcal pyelonephritis. Clinical manifestations include flank pain and relapsing fever with enlargement and tenderness of the involved portion of the kidney. Treatment of the carbuncle with antibacterial agents is rarely effective, and surgical drainage is mandatory. Occasionally nephrectomy is necessary because of extensive involvement of the kidney with multiple abscesses.

PERINEPHRIC ABSCESS. This usually follows perforation of a renal abscess into the perinephric tissues. In some instances perinephric abscess may result from direct hematogenous spread or from a microabscess in the kidney which is not apparent. The patients present with an extremely high fever and boardlike rigidity of the abdominal wall. Roentgenograms reveal nonvisualization of the psoas shadow and concavity of the spine to the side of the lesion. If one takes a film during breathing, the involved kidney is fixed and does not blur. Nephrotomography, ultrasound, and percutaneous aspiration of the perinephric space may establish the diagnosis when conventional diagnostic procedures fail. Treatment requires prompt drainage and appropriate antibiotics.

Acute Papillary Necrosis

Necrosis of renal papillae occurs in patients with diabetes, sickle cell disease, tuberculosis, and excessive ingestion of phenacetin. In addition to the symptoms related to the associated acute infection of the kidney, renal colic may result from ureteral obstruction by the sloughed papillae. Diagnosis is made by demonstrating sloughed papillae or by characteristic appearance of the intravenous pyelogram showing loss of one or more of the papillae (Fig. 40-11). Loss of renal function may attend papillary necrosis, but recovery usually occurs, and initial measures are directed toward supporting the patient during the acute episode. Specific treatment for the involved organism is administered. If the patient remains febrile and there is ureteral obstruction, surgical intervention may be required to remove the obstructing soft tissue.

Acute Urethritis

Acute urethritis is usually ascending and venereal in origin. Included in the acute types of urethritis are those caused by gonorrhea, mycobacteria, *Chlamydia,* and *Trichomonas vaginalis.* Diagnosis is established by microscopy of the Gram-stained discharge and confirmed by adequate culture techniques. Reiter's syndrome, consisting of the

Fig. 40-11. Renal papillary necrosis. *A.* Retrograde pyelography in diabetic renal papillary necrosis. *B.* Necrotic papillae are indicated by arrows.

triad of arthritis, nongonococcal urethritis, and conjunctivitis, is considered by many to be of venereal origin and should be included in the differential diagnosis.

Gonorrhea is the most common venereal disease of man. The incubation period is 7 to 9 days, after which the symptoms of acute urethritis are manifest. Urethral stricture is a common sequela if the original infection is not adequately treated. Metastatic gonococcal infections include arthritis, tenosynovitis, bursitis, ophthalmitis, perihepatitis, and endocarditis. Gonococcal arthritis, which represents the only common manifestation of metastatic involvement, is polyarticular in 80 percent of the cases and accompanied by tenosynovitis in 50 percent of the cases. The diagnosis of gonococcal infection is established by demonstration of *Neisseria gonorrhoeae,* Gram-negative diplococci, intracellularly in a discharge. Since both syphilis and gonorrhea are contracted by the same exposure in about 3 percent of cases, the latter should be excluded by serologic tests at regular intervals for 6 months. Gonococcal urethral infections are best treated by adequate dosage of penicillin-type drugs. Oral tetracycline could be used for patients allergic to penicillin.

Penicillin therapy is also effective for mimae infection, while *Trichomonas* urethritis and prostatitis are best treated with metronidazole (Flagyl, 250 mg orally twice daily for men and three times daily for women for a period of 10 days). The tetracyclines are effective in the treatment of *Chlamydia* and mycobacteria.

Acute Infections of the Prostate

Acute prostatitis is commonly a complication of untreated or ineffectively treated acute urethritis. Acute prostatitis is particularly common in young or mature males in whom vigorous exertion or exposure may lead to spread of infection from the urethra. Retrograde instrumental trauma in the presence of urethral infection may cause prostatitis at any age. Formerly prostatitis was predominantly of gonococcal origin, but now it is more often associated with a mixed veneral flora including *Streptococcus fecalis, E. coli,* or *Corynebacterium hofmannii,* or exerosis. Acute prostatitis secondary to metastatic spread from furunculosis and caused by *Staphylococcus aureus* or *Staphylococcus albus* occurs less commonly.

Initial symptoms may be mild and consist of perineal discomfort with increasing frequency, initial hematuria, dysuria, and occasional retention. With progression, the perineal pain becomes continuous and severe and is attended by chills, high fever, malaise, and prostration. Leukocytosis is characteristic, and bacteremia is common. In extreme cases, the gram-negative bacteremia may be associated with endotoxin shock. Liquefaction necrosis of the local infection results in the formation of abscesses which may spontaneously or as a result of catheterization rupture into the urethra.

Culture of the urethral discharge should precede administration of antibacterial agents, but these should not be withheld until the culture reports are available. If necessary, the drug may be changed at a later date. Patients with retention should be catheterized gently with a small indwelling catheter. Rectal examination should be performed infrequently and with great care to avoid dissemination of the infection. Several days of treatment should result in symptomatic improvement and return of temperature to normal. Persistence of symptoms and fever suggests the presence of an abscess which will require drainage. The acutely ill patient should be at bed rest, hydrated, and treated with antibiotics until the acute phase of the process subsides. Warm sitz baths and prostatic massage are used to obviate the subacute and chronic phases. Prostatic abscesses occasionally occur with inadequate therapy and are treated by drainage performed either transurethrally with a resectoscope or perineally through a prostatectomy incision.

CHRONIC INFECTIONS

Chronic Prostatitis

"Chronic prostatitis" refers to a syndrome which causes genital discomfort, is associated with purulent prostatic secretion, and responds favorably to prostatic massage and antibacterial agents. It occurs most frequently in men over forty-five, and 35 to 50 percent in this age group are said to be affected. Thirty percent of normal asymptomatic males of military age have purulent prostatic secretions, and this is also present in some prepubertal males. An autopsy incidence of 6.3 percent has been reported by Moore. A variety of factors including gonorrhea, pyogenic urethritis, instrumentation, urethral stricture, prostatic hypertrophy, distant foci of infection, congestion, stasis, and postalcoholic changes have all been implicated as, but not proved to be, predisposing factors.

Chronic prostatitis is frequently caused by retrograde infection from the urethra. This is particularly true in those cases following acute urethritis and instrumentation. Hematogenous spread from distant foci has also been implicated as a cause, particularly in staphylococcal infection. The role of infection in chronic prostatitis has not been completely defined. Since the nonpathogenic bacterial flora of the urethra include staphylococci, streptococci, and diphtheroids, positive cultures from prostatic fluid collected at the urethral meatus are anticipated. In a series of patients with chronic prostatitis, 99 percent of prostatic fluid cultures demonstrated growth, but only 36 percent of the organisms were considered to be the pathogens. In contrast, prostatic secretions obtained through the urethroscope in patients with chronic prostatitis yield pathogens in only 4 percent of the specimens. The organisms include *E. coli, Streptococcus fecalis, A. aerogenes, P. aeruginosa, Staphylococcus aureus,* pleuropneumonia organisms, and *T. vaginalis.*

The pathologic changes in chronic prostatitis are minimal. Microscopically, the gland shows fibrosis and purulent secretions, interstitial fibroplasia, and lymphocytic infiltrations. Dilated acini and prostatic ducts are often filled with obstructing masses of cellular debris and leukocytes. The acini are frequently smaller than normal, and the epithelium may undergo metaplasia, becoming cuboidal or squamous. Associated seminal vesiculitis is seen infrequently, and therefore the term "prostatovesiculitis" is inappropriate.

Symptomatology includes discomfort in the lower abdomen or back and genitalia. In young men, the main complaint is a scanty mucoid urethral discharge. In middle-aged men the more common complaint is that of genital discomfort, while in older men symptoms suggesting obstruction such as nocturia, frequency, and dysuria are often elicited. On rectal examination, the prostate may be boggy or indurated but is of normal consistency in over half the patients.

Prostatic secretion for microscopic examination is obtained by prostatic massage. The normal secretion contains three to five white blood cells per high-powered field. Chronic prostatitis may be accompanied by an increase in number of white cells and a clumping of the leukocytes. However, in half the patients there is no abnormality in the number of white cells in the fluid. Also, no relationship has been demonstrated between changes in prostatic secretion during therapy and the remission or exacerbation of symptoms. The urine frequently contains shreds and leukocytes in the first portion of the voided specimen. Occasional red cells may be seen. The second glass of voided urine is usually normal, but 25 percent have pyuria. This finding is indicative of urinary tract infection, and the patient should be evaluated for obstructive uropathy and other urinary disease.

Treatment of chronic nonspecific prostatitis includes prostatic massage, warm baths, and antibacterial agents when indicated. The usual course includes increasingly vigorous massages at weekly intervals for 3 to 4 weeks, following which the intervals are extended, and finally the patient is advised to return only if recurrent symptoms do not respond to hot tubs. The prognosis for symptomatic improvement is excellent for a given episode, but there is a tendency toward recurrence. Antibacterial treatment is applicable in patients with urethritis or urinary tract infection. Hormones do not appear to be indicated. Instillations and irrigations have afforded symptomatic relief, and sedatives may be of benefit to the patient with psychogenic frequency of urination. Alcoholic beverages and highly seasoned foods are traditionally withheld. Normal frequency of sexual intercourse is not considered harmful, since it promotes emptying of the prostate.

The complications of chronic nonspecific prostatitis are also poorly defined. Acute cystitis, urethritis, epididymitis, and pyelonephritis have occurred during or following an episode of chronic nonspecific prostatitis. Benign prostatic hypertrophy and carcinoma of the prostate do not occur more frequently in the gland involved with chronic nonspecific prostatitis. Similarly, squamous metaplasia and squamous carcinoma have no increased incidence. A relationship between chronic prostatitis and associated arthritis or uveitis is questionable. Chronic prostatitis associated with prostatic calculi usually fails to respond to prostatic massage and may require operative removal of the calculi, with consideration of the fact that this operation interferes with potency.

Comparable infections of the urethra occur in the female. Treatment for acute urethritis of gonococcal origin is similar to that already outlined for the male. *Trichomonas* infestation may require higher doses of the drugs used. Chronic urethritis in the female has been referred to as the "female urethral syndrome" and is probably the result of local inflammation or recurrent attacks of cystitis. The patients generally complain of frequency, nocturia, dysuria, and backache. Marked urgency and dyspareunia are also common symptoms. On examination, the urethra is enlarged, indurated, and tender; urethroscopy demonstrates injection, edema, and cystic changes. Injection and inflammation of the trigone may be an associated finding. A urine specimen obtained by catheterization rarely shows more than a few epithelial cells and occasional white cells. Progressive dilatation of the urethra to the size of #34 F may be helpful. Instillation of nitrofurazone (1:1,000) may prevent ascending cystitis. The prognosis for improvement is good, but, as in the male, the condition tends to recur. Complications include acute cystitis, pyelonephritis, and the development of a urethral caruncle.

Urinary Tuberculosis

Renal tuberculosis is the result of hematogenous spread from primary pulmonary or intestinal lesions. Although the involvement is probably bilateral and cortical in most individuals, some lesions progress to healing, while others assume clinical significance. Renal tuberculosis is generally undetected and asymptomatic until it ulcerates into the collecting system of the kidney. At that time the symptoms include gross hematuria, dysuria, frequency, and pyuria with an absence of bacteria on Gram stain. Many of the symptoms are a consequence of cystitis arising from organisms localizing in the bladder secondary to the renal involvement.

Special culture techniques will reveal the presence of *Mycobacterium tuberculosis*. Intravenous pyelography demonstrates calcification of caseous abscesses, ulceration of calyces, and failure of visualization of calyces filled with caseous debris (Fig. 40-12). Treatment consists of 1 to 2

Fig. 40-12. Renal tuberculosis. *A* and *B*. Left upper pole ulcerative renal tuberculosis. *C* and *D*. Chronic suppurative left pyelonephritis with atrophy.

A

C

B

D

years of isoniazid (0.1 Gm three times daily), cycloserine (0.250 Gm twice daily), and sodium para-aminosalicylic acid (6 to 12 Gm daily). The patient is followed by repeated urine cultures and repeated pyelography, which should be performed at 3-month intervals during the first year.

Genital tuberculosis may accompany renal tuberculosis or may exist independently as a result of hematogenous spread. The epididymis is most frequently involved, and spread may take place from this source up the vas deferens to the prostate or through the scrotum in the form of a fistula. The vas deferens may become beaded with involvement. Epididymal tuberculosis may be successfully managed by chemotherapy, and epididymectomy is held in reserve.

URINARY CALCULI

The consequences of urinary calculi are responsible for 10 percent of the urologic hospital admissions in many parts of the world. An etiologic factor can be defined in only half the patients. Primary metabolic stones result from hyperexcretion of an offending substance. Cystine and uric acid stones form only in those individuals with excessive urinary excretion of these substances. In hyperparathyroidism, increased calcium and phosphorus excretion is responsible for the formation of the triple-phosphate stones. It is questionable whether the calcium oxalate stone is related to an excess excretion of oxalate.

Secondary stones arise as a result of foreign bodies, obstruction, or prolonged recumbency and consequent decalcification of bone with hyperexcretion of calcium salts in the urine. Infections with urea-splitting organisms result in ammonium-magnesium phosphate calculi, while chronic pyelonephritis and ulcerative processes lead to a suitable nidus for the deposition of encrustations and eventual stone formation.

COMPOSITION. Urinary calculi can often be identified by their external appearance. The calcium oxalate stones, which constitute 73 percent of calculi, are frequently small, under 50 mg, dark-colored, and have an external surface which is covered with sharp spicules. Ammonium-magnesium phosphate calculi account for 15.7 percent and are commonly found in infected urine. These stones are characteristically porous, soft, and either tan or white. Uric acid stones, which constitute 7.6 percent of all calculi, are commonly yellowish, orange, or pink. They are porous and easily broken. Cystine stones have been likened to maple sugar and represent only 1 percent of large series.

DIAGNOSIS. Calculi within the ureter usually present with typical renal colic. However, staghorn calculi and bladder stones associated with obstruction may be asymptomatic, except for a history of recurrent infection. Urinalysis may be negative during an attack of colic if the ureter is completely obstructed. As the colic subsides, the first voided urine may show copious quantities of red cells and crystals. The crystals are commonly similar to the constituents of the calculi, and albuminuria, when present, is frequently proportionate to the number of red cells. Pyuria and bacteriuria are present in only 15 percent of the patients.

Ninety-five percent of urinary calculi are radiopaque. Most opaque stones contain calcium, but both ammonium-magnesium phosphate and cystine stones are sufficiently radiopaque to be detectable. Uric acid stones are usually nonopaque, and calculi, which are opaque, may be masked by overlying bony structures. Intravenous pyelograms may reveal the calculi, the point of obstruction, or delayed visualization of the obstructed side. When the latter obtains, delayed films taken up to 24 hours after injection may demonstrate the point of obstruction, since the opaque eventually mixes with the urine in the delayed collecting system (Fig. 40-13A to D). Roentgenographic examination, without adequate preparation, during acute renal colic may be less than satisfactory because of the gas in the colon secondary to reflex ileus. However, early x-ray examination in the differential diagnosis of flank pain is so important that the emergency pyelogram is indicated. Calculi which lie in the segment of ureter within the bony pelvis may be confused with phleboliths. Tomography may be helpful in this situation. However, the majority of calculi lie above a line drawn through the spinous processes of the ischium, and phleboliths have a characteristic spherical smooth configuration and, frequently, nonopaque centers. Occasionally, it is necessary to resort to retrograde ureteral catheterization to determine whether or not a given opacity lies within the ureter. In this circumstance, the combination of anteroposterior and oblique films, which demonstrate the opacity in contact with the catheter, is diagnostic of a calculus. Roentgenographic studies of the phalanges and lamina dura are useful in detecting the presence of bone changes associated with hyperparathyroidism.

MANAGEMENT. Symptomatic relief of the severe pain frequently must be initiated before the diagnosis is established. Narcotics are usually necessary to relieve severe renal colic, while moderate pain is improved by the application of heat. Roentgenographic determination of the size of the calculus and the nature of the urinary passages through which the calculus must pass is critical. The dilated ureter following pregnancy will permit passage of a larger stone than the normal ureter. Recognizable obstructive changes at the ureteropelvic junction may make passage of a small stone unlikely. Ninety-three percent of calculi less than 4 mm pass spontaneously, while only 20 percent of calculi greater than 6 mm in greatest dimension will pass. The patient who is followed expectantly should have renal function assessed at regular intervals, and the isotopic renogram has provided an excellent means for evaluating changes.

Indications for Removal. Although some surgeons feel that the presence of a stone indicates the need for surgical intervention, it seems unlikely that all calculi produce sufficient damage to warrant it. A small stone lodged in the calyx causes no marked loss of renal function, and there may be no alteration in size and no symptoms for

Fig. 40-13. Ureteral calculi. *A* and *B*. Excretory urogram showing left hydronephrosis with nonvisualization of left ureter on early films, calculus in region of left ureteral orifice. *C* and *D*. Excretory urogram, 2-hour delayed film, shows visualization of a dilated left ureter down to ureteral calculus in intravesical portion of ureter, thus establishing the diagnosis.

many years. The following are accepted indications for surgical treatment:

1. Nonfunction of the kidney on intravenous pyelogram or renogram, indicating severe obstruction. Loss of the kidney is inevitable if the obstruction persists.
2. Persistent hydronephrosis above an obstructing stone which fails to pass within a reasonable period of time. This may lead to pyelonephritis and irreparable renal damage.
3. Frequent episodes of incapacitating colic even in the presence of normal renal function.
4. An obstructing stone associated with infection, since the infection usually will not respond to medication.
5. Recurrent infections related to a calculus.

Following surgical or manipulative removal of stones, it is important to ensure that the passages are well flushed by a copious diuresis and that urinary infection is treated with appropriate antibacterial agents.

Surgery. Prior to surgical intervention, it is important to visualize the collecting system to determine if any abnormalities are present and require correction at the time of lithotomy. Calculi of small size may be removed from the lower ureter by means of transurethral instruments which snare the stone. These are referred to as "baskets" and consist of a special catheter with filaments attached so that when the catheter is passed beyond the stone and gradually withdrawn, the stone becomes entangled in the filaments. As peristalsis of the ureter expels the instrument, both the catheter and the stone are moved downward so that the stone passes into the urinary bladder, from which it can be removed easily. Bladder stones, especially soft magnesium-ammonium phosphate calculi, may be crushed and removed by the process of lithotripsy. Manipulative surgical treatment is usually not performed for calculi which lie in the ureter above the pelvic brim. Lithotomy may provide the least traumatic method for removing some stones. The high incidence of success is accompanied by an advantage over lithotripsy in that no fragments are left behind.

Urinary calculi sometimes can be dissolved by alkalinization or by irrigation through ureteral catheters. The latter technique is particularly applicable for some magnesium-ammonium phosphate and uric acid stones. The magnesium-ammonium phosphate stones may be dissolved in a modified solution G, while the uric acid stones are solubilized best by alkaline solutions such as 1% sodium bicarbonate. Although bladder stones may respond to modified solution G, litholapaxy is preferable, because these calculi are readily accessible.

Prevention of Recurrence. Even in the absence of obvious obstructive uropathy, stones tend to recur. In a series of patients presenting with renal colic due to calculi, 39 percent had previously passed stones.

Obstruction and infection must be treated, since stones in the kidney are associated with infection in half the cases. Treatment of infection and elimination of obstruction are particularly important in the stones of the magnesium-ammonium phosphate group and oxalate calculi. Ureteral calculi are associated with infection in only 8 percent of cases.

Hydration should be prescribed, since many patients with recurrent calculi are poor water drinkers and an adequate intake of fluids can prevent, or even result in the dissolution of, stones. The patient classified as a "chronic stone former" should imbibe 4,000 ml of fluid daily.

Urinary pH should be adjusted to favor solution of the components of the stone involved. This requires analysis of the calculus, since adjusting the pH of the urine in the wrong direction may be harmful. Uric acid and cystine stones form only in an acid urine. Changing the pH from 5 to 8 leads to a sixfold increase in the solubility of these substances in urine. This alkalinization may be accomplished by taking 1 tsp of sodium bicarbonate three to four times daily. Potassium citrate may also be used, and the alkalinity of the urine can be assessed by the patient with pH paper. Forty percent of uric acid stones dissolve when an alkaline urine is maintained. Calcium phosphate and magnesium-ammonium phosphate calculi are solubilized in an acid urine. Three to six grams daily of potassium acid phosphate are sufficient to acidify the urine, and the administration of the phosphate ion is also useful in binding calcium within the intestine and in reducing excretion in the urine. When urinary infection is present, the urea-splitting organisms may lead to the formation of ammonia and an intensely alkaline urine. This situation is difficult to handle with acid salts alone and requires active treatment of the infection. As the solubility of oxalate salts in the urine is not pH-dependent, manipulation of urinary pH is not useful for this variety.

Diet regulation is particularly pertinent for certain calculi. A low-protein diet plus anabolic agents is useful in decreasing the quantity of uric acid excreted in the urine. However, adjusting the urinary pH may be more successful and better tolerated. A diet which minimizes the amounts of amino acids containing sulfur may reduce the quantity of cystine excreted in the urine. The administration of penicillamine is also directed toward the cystine calculi, since it leads to the excretion of more soluble conjugates. Pyridoxine (vitamin B_6) has been prescribed to prevent an excess excretion of oxalate in the urine, but the evidence has not been convincing. Diets low in oxalate are available. However, oxalate stones are not necessarily associated with an excess excretion in the urine. For calcium-containing stones, a low-calcium diet which excludes dairy products can be combined with urinary acidifiers and chelating agents. Thiazides also decrease the urinary calcium excretion.

Treatment of acute gout with uricosuric agents may lead to uric acid calculi. Allopurinol, 0.1 Gm three times a day, reduces uric acid production, which lowers serum uric acid without dangers of urinary calculus.

HYPERPARATHYROIDISM. Eighty-four percent of patients with hyperparathyroidism (see Chap. 38) present with renal calculi or nephrocalcinosis, thus making the disease an important urologic consideration. The incidence of hyperparathyroidism among chronic stone formers varies considerably from one report to another. It may be as low as 1 percent and as high as 15 percent of the patients with recurrent renal calculi. The urinary symptoms include polydipsia, polyuria, recurrent renal colic due to calculi, and symptoms of hypertension. In patients with multiple recurrent urinary calculi the serum should be investigated for increased calcium ion and alkaline phosphatase and decreased phosphorus. Treatment consists of surgical removal of the hyperfunctioning parathyroid tissue followed by treatment of the urinary pathologic condition. In untreated patients, a renal death is common.

RENAL FAILURE

Renal failure is characterized by increased blood levels of certain products of metabolism normally excreted in the urine. These include urea, creatinine, potassium, phosphates, phenols, and aromatic oxyacids. The syndrome which accompanies this state has often been called "uremia," though properly this term refers only to an elevated level of blood urea. Since some of the metabolic end products are toxic in high concentrations, a series of symptoms develop. Mental confusion, restlessness, headache, fatigue, muscular twitching, convulsions, anorexia, nausea and vomiting, constipation changing to diarrhea, Kussmaul's breathing, pale dry yellowish skin, pruritis, anemia, anasarca, gastrointestinal bleeding, epistaxis, and heart failure may all be present in varying combinations. Although the specific factors responsible for some of these symptoms are known, the exact etiology of others remains in doubt.

Acute Failure

Acute renal failure is usually accompanied by an oliguria of less than 20 ml/hour or complete anuria. The blood metabolite level may become rapidly elevated, because acute renal failure often arises in association with several catabolic states. The acute changes in these metabolites are less well tolerated than the gradual changes which accompany chronic renal failure. One of the most common causes of oliguria and renal failure is decreased renal blood flow. Congestive heart failure, acute hypovolemia due to blood loss, severe dehydration, circulatory failure in association with overwhelming sepsis, marked fluid and electrolyte loss from the gastrointestinal tract associated with vomiting or diarrhea, tubular or cortical necrosis, nephritis, poisoning, and collagen diseases involving the kidney may all result in oliguria. Complete anuria usually indicates total ureteral or urethral obstruction or bilateral renal artery occlusion. Whenever anuria is present and the patient is not in clinical shock, obstruction should be suspected. The patients in clinical shock with a systolic blood pressure of less than 80 mm Hg cannot be expected to excrete much urine, and no further diagnostic studies are indicated until the hypovolemic shock is adequately treated. When a decreased renal blood flow is present, the urine proceeds through the renal tubule at a slow rate, so that reabsorption of electrolytes and water tends to produce a small volume with a high specific gravity and a low sodium concentration. Characteristically, the urine osmolarity exceeds that of plasma by a factor of two or three times. The urine sodium is usually less than 20 mEq/L.

In toxic nephropathies, the urine osmolarity is similar to that of plasma, and the urinary sodium exceeds 60 mEq/L. The differentiation of tubular necrosis from decreased renal blood flow and dehydration can also be elucidated by means of the PSP test with an indwelling catheter. The patient with marked oliguria and a urinary output of only 10 to 15 ml/hour will still excrete a significant amount of PSP if the oliguria is secondary to decreased renal blood flow but not if the primary lesion is acute tubular necrosis. Mannitol and water load (25 Gm of mannitol in 300 ml of fluid given intravenously over 30 minutes) will usually produce a diuresis if the patient has reduced renal blood flow or dehydration. In contrast, failure to respond to this infusion suggests acute tubular necrosis or toxic nephropathy.

LABORATORY FINDINGS. The serum generally shows an elevation of urea nitrogen, creatinine, phosphorus, and potassium levels, and a reduction in carbon dioxide, sodium chloride, and calcium. Prerenal azotemia is usually accompanied by an elevation of the serum urea nitrogen level combined with a normal serum creatinine level (Fig. 40-14). Dehydration, gastrointestinal bleeding, and catabolic processes associated with the administration of tetracycline, corticosteroids, and thiazide diuretics may produce prerenal azotemia.

With acute tubular necrosis, the urine specific gravity is usually fixed at 1.007 to 1.010. This is referred to as "isothenuria," which indicates that the specific gravity of urine is similar to that of plasma. In this situation, urine also often demonstrates red cell casts, albumin, and, occasionally, sugar in the presence of tubular necrosis.

Incipient or high-output renal failure is frequently undetected when estimations of renal function are based primarily on "adequate urinary volume." A simple method of detection is to perform a spot check of urinary and blood urea in milligrams per milliliter. A ratio of 20 : 1 or greater suggests extrarenal azotemia, while a ratio of 10 : 1 is borderline failure. A ratio as low as 5 : 1 or less, even in the presence of normal urinary volume, is indicative of incipient failure, usually on the basis of acute tubular necrosis.

TREATMENT. The treatment of acute renal failure consists of maintaining the patient in the best possible state until the function of the kidney returns. Therapeutic measures are directed along three main lines: (1) reducing toxic protein moieties in the blood, (2) correcting electrolyte imbalance including hyperkalemia, hyponatremia, and

acidosis, and (3) preventing fluid overload. The first is accomplished by reducing or stopping protein intake, reducing catabolism by treating infection and/or draining an abscess, correcting other tissue injury, the use of anti-catabolic agents, the administration of hypertonic intravenous glucose to spare protein breakdown, and the application of dialysis to decrease the blood and tissue levels. During this period, the patient's caloric requirements can be satisfied by carbohydrates and fats.

The electrolyte management requires frequent measurements of serum levels and serial electrocardiograms. Electrolyte replacement during oliguria or anuria is best managed conservatively. If there is significant loss from gastric aspiration, equivalent amounts of chloride should be administered. Hyperkalemia necessitates early correction to avoid cardiac asystole. Acute hyperkalemia with characteristic spiking T waves on the electrocardiogram may be treated with the intravenous administration of 25% glucose and 1 unit of regular insulin for each 2 Gm of glucose. Forty to eighty milliequivalents of sodium bicarbonate rapidly given intravenously may also temporarily avert an impending cardiac crisis due to hyperkalemia. The elimination of potassium intake, the administration of sodium exchange resins (Kayexalate) orally (30 to 90 Gm in 15 to 45 ml of sorbitol to reduce the constipating effect) or rectally (200 to 500 ml of a 10% solution two to three times daily) results in temporary reduction of the serum potassium level, but this can be effected more directly with dialysis. Hypocalcemia in patients with oliguria may lead to tetany, especially when efforts are directed toward correction of acidosis. Therefore, calcium gluconate (0.5 to 1 Gm daily) should be administered intravenously with alkalinizing agents. In the digitalized patient, the administration of calcium gluconate may be dangerous, since the calcium ion potentiates the effect of digitalis on the myocardium.

Perhaps the foremost therapeutic measure in patients with acute renal failure is fluid restriction. Death from pulmonary edema and congestive failure is not an unusual circumstance. The daily fluid intake should be limited to 400 ml (600 ml insensible loss minus 200 ml of water gained through oxidation) plus replacement of any fluid loss from urine or gastrointestinal tract. If the patient is febrile or if the air temperature and humidity are high, replacement of fluids should be increased slightly. The most valuable single means for estimating fluid requirements is an accurate daily weight. The anticipated weight loss by the starving patient is $\frac{1}{2}$ to 1 lb/day.

Frequent dialysis during the period of renal shutdown represents the most effective treatment, especially when catabolism is marked. In reversible acute renal failure, the salvage rate with extracorporeal hemodialysis should exceed 50 percent.

When patients have been successfully sustained through the acute oliguric failure, a period of polyuria may ensue. Electrolyte losses during this stage may be dangerously high, since the kidney is temporarily incapable of reabsorbing sodium and potassium. Replacement of these anions is indicated. If the patient has been digitalized during acute renal failure, digitalis intoxication may result

Fig. 40-14. Prerenal azotemia due to gastrointestinal hemorrhage.

when serum potassium is reduced either during the polyuric phase or by dialysis. Digitalis intoxication should be prevented by using half the usual dose, removing potassium slowly, and replacing potassium losses during the polyuria.

Chronic Failure

Although complete recovery or death frequently occurs, acute renal failure may progress to chronic failure. Chronic failure may also be the end result of a variety of renal diseases including glomerulonephritis, pyelonephritis, nephrosclerosis, congenital polycystic disease, obstructive uropathy, primary hyperparathyroidism, vitamin D poisoning, gout, collagen diseases, vascular diseases, diabetic nephropathy, medullary necrosis, and various nephrotoxic poisons including phenacetin.

Diagnosis is suspected on the basis of clinical signs and symptoms and confirmed by laboratory evaluation. Since progressive uremia is often well tolerated, the urea level may be higher than the patient's condition indicates. The presence of anemia and acidosis is reflected clinically in a patient's ease of fatigability. Hyponatremia, which leads to further reduction in the glomerular filtration rate, may result from the inability of the kidney to preserve sodium because of tubular damage. The diagnosis of salt depletion is based on examination of intake and sodium loss in urine rather than the serum sodium levels.

Treatment of chronic renal failure includes the same modalities mentioned above for acute failure. Urinary infections must be eradicated and intercurrent infections promptly recognized and treated. Drugs which are excreted by the kidney should be administered in reduced doses, but penicillin may be given in usual doses to patients with oliguria and in half doses when complete anuria is present. Tetracycline and streptomycin, which are excreted predominantly by the kidney, should be given in usual doses at intervals of 2 to 4 days rather than daily. Chloramphenicol, which is detoxified by the liver, may be administered in usual doses over short periods of time. Kanamycin is given in half the usual dose with oliguria, and if anuria is present, this should be administered every 3 days rather than daily. Colistin can be given at the rate of half the usual dose every 2 days in oliguria and every 5 days in anuria. Aminoglycosides must also be given in altered dosage in the presence of renal failure.

Correction of acidosis by oral sodium bicarbonate or citrate therapy often gives marked symptomatic relief. However, increasing the serum pH decreases the ionizable calcium and may result in hypocalcemic tetany. In this circumstance, parenteral calcium gluconate or oral calcium lactate can be used, while calcium chloride is contraindicated.

A high-carbohydrate, low-protein ($\frac{1}{2}$ Gm/kg of body weight daily), low-potassium (less than 15 mEq/L), low-sodium (200 to 500 mg) diet is applicable to prevent tissue catabolism and electrolyte imbalance. Norethandrolone (50 mg three times daily), an anabolic agent, may also have a protein-sparing effect.

Accurate daily weights are valuable for determining the optimal amount of water to be taken daily. A gain of weight denotes an excess intake and may presage pulmonary edema. Optimal urinary volume may be ascertained by gradually increasing fluid intake in these patients. Sodium intake must be reduced to control water metabolism unless the patient has a salt-losing nephropathy with normal or increased volumes of urine. Under these circumstances, large amounts of sodium bicarbonate may be required.

Chronic dialysis and renal homotransplantation are therapeutic modalities available at certain medical centers. They are discussed in Chap. 10. Increasing experience with these methods establishes their merit for relatively stable uremic patients. Periodic dialysis may support the patient through episodes of intercurrent infection associated with diarrhea and vomiting which cause a temporary exacerbation of the uremic state. Peritoneal dialysis or extracorporeal dialysis may reverse the course in such patients for a period of time. Dialysis also may be helpful in preparing the patient with obstructive uropathy for supravesical diversionary surgical treatment.

PEDIATRIC UROLOGY

Both congenital abnormalities of the urinary tract and tumors in children demand prompt and thorough investigation because of their significant incidence and consequences. The genitourinary system should be evaluated in all instances of "failure to thrive" syndrome, undiagnosed febrile illnesses, externally apparent congenital anomalies, and abdominal masses. Sixty-seven percent of surgically correctable abdominal masses in children involve the adrenals or kidneys. Wilms' tumor of the kidney and neuroblastoma of the adrenal are the most common solid tumors in children and are of equal prevalence. Hydronephrosis constitutes 40 percent of renal masses.

Wilms' Tumor (Adenomyosarcoma)

Neoplastic degeneration of embryonal rests has been implicated in the evolution of this tumor. The lesion is often present at birth and frequently becomes clinically recognizable when the patient is under the age of two. The patients most commonly present with a unilateral flank mass recognized by the parent. Hematuria, weight loss, and pain are unusual manifestations and occur late in the course of the disease. On examination, the flank mass is firm and nontender. The blood pressure may be elevated because of renal artery compression, and the urine is usually negative.

Abdominal radiograms show displacement of the intestinal gas shadows and obliteration of the psoas shadow on the side of the lesion. Chest films may demonstrate spherical densities of metastases. Excretory urography is frequently difficult to interpret because of the small rim of displaced functioning renal tissue, which visualizes poorly. In general, since the renal tumor is focal and protrudes from the kidney, some portion of normal kidney is usually visualized (Fig. 40-15). When the tumor invades the renal

Fig. 40-15. Wilms' tumor of the left kidney in a one-year-old male deforming calyces of the left kidney and displacing left abdominal gas shadows.

vein causing occlusion, the kidney on the side of the lesion may not be visualized by intravenous pyelogram. In this circumstance, a retrograde pyelogram should establish the diagnosis. Five percent of Wilms' tumors are bilateral, and it is important preoperatively to estimate the function of the apparently uninvolved kidney.

Differential diagnosis includes adrenal neuroblastoma, hydronephrosis, and renal cystic disease. Neuroblastoma is usually more medial in location. It frequently displaces but does not deform the adjacent kidney, and interstitial calcification may be noted on x-ray. Hydronephrosis with nonvisualization on the excretory pyelogram may be differentiated by retrograde pyelography. Renal cystic disease can be recognized on nephrotomograms or renal arteriograms, but these techniques are not usually required.

The treatment of Wilms' tumor usually consists of immediate transperitoneal surgical excision. This may be followed by postoperative radiation therapy or chemotherapy, or both. Postoperative chemotherapy consists of intravenous actinomycin D (15 μg/kg daily for 5 days). Radiation to the tumor bed (3000 r) is usually adequate when administered in conjunction with actinomycin. There is indication that cyclic courses of actinomycin may double the survival rate. Vincristine, used alone or in combination with actinomycin, has also proved to be a valuable chemotherapeutic adjunct.

The prognosis of Wilms' tumor is related to the patient's age. When the lesions are removed from children under the age of two, the survival rate is 73 percent, whereas over the age of two it is 18 percent according to Lattimer et al. The presence of metastases in lungs, bones, or at the site of surgical treatment is associated with an unfavorable prognosis, and both chemotherapy and radiation therapy are less effective in this situation. However, chemotherapy has been demonstrated to be of significant value in lengthening the survival of patients with proved metastatic Wilms' tumor.

Congenital Anomalies

PHIMOSIS (REDUNDANT PREPUCE) This condition predisposes to difficulty secondary to poor hygiene, infection, and carcinoma of the glans penis. Circumcision is usually performed during the neonatal period. If it is not performed at this time, it can be done when medically indicated or when requested electively by the patient or his family. Risk of anesthesia and psychologic implications should be considered in the selection of cases and timing of the operation.

MEATAL OR DISTAL URETHRAL STENOSIS. This is the most common cause of impaired voiding in children, occurring more frequently in girls. Boys may present with recognizable impairment of the urinary stream or distress during voiding. However, since the longer male urethra offers protection against secondary urinary infection, obstructive changes, such as enlargement of the bladder and ureteral dilatation, may result before the condition is suspected. In girls, urinary infection is a more frequent accompaniment of stenosis and leads to earlier appreciation of the pathologic condition. Girls commonly present with high fever related to pyelonephritis. Other symptoms include enuresis, urgency, diurnal incontinence, and urethral distress. Anorexia and weight loss may accompany chronic or recurrent infections.

The diagnosis is established with acorn-tipped bougies à boule under anesthesia. Insertion and, more particularly, withdrawal of the bougie is accompanied by a sensation of passage through a constriction. With a stenosis in the distal urethra or at the meatus the constricting fibromuscular ring can be visualized as the bougie is withdrawn. Urethral stenosis may also be recognized by a "hang." In the first two years of life a #14 French bougie should pass easily. Between the ages of two and six the normal female urethra should accept a #18, while from six to thirteen years of age a #22 French can be passed. Over the age of thirteen a #26 French should pass easily.

Cystourethroscopy may be indicated to disclose secondary consequences of urethral obstruction such as bladder trabeculation, diverticula, calculi, vesicoureteral incompetence (reflux), and any ureteral obstruction. Radiologic examination, such as voiding cystourethrograms and excretory urograms, are also helpful in establishing the degree of urethral obstruction and the presence of sequelae (Fig. 40-16). Voiding studies have definite limitations.

Treatment of urethral meatal stenosis is dependent upon the extent of secondary involvement. Uncomplicated cases will be satisfactorily treated by meatotomy or dilatations. Most patients with accompanying infection require continuation of antimicrobial treatment followed by suppressive therapy with sulfonamides or nitrofurantoin for 3 or more months. Growth and development are allies in the rehabilitation of pediatric urologic patients. Where morphologic abnormalities are recognized on initial evaluation, follow-up examinations are necessary to determine the course.

About 10 percent of girls with urethral obstruction either fail to respond to conservative therapy or have advanced secondary upper tract damage at the time the condition is recognized. In these cases, corrective procedures are necessary to prevent progressive damage to the kidneys. These are directed at reducing resistance to voiding, preventing reflux of urine (ureteral reimplantation), and diversion of the urine from poorly functioning excretory passages (nephrostomy, ureterostomy, or cutaneous ureteroileostomy). These are to be considered as lifesaving procedures, since they are associated with difficulties. In the female who has had surgical enlargement of the bladder neck (Y–V-plasty), urinary incontinence may develop following pregnancy. The male who has had bladder neck surgical treatment may experience infertility due to retrograde ejaculation. The patient who undergoes a ureterostomy or cutaneous ureteroileostomy requires a permanent appliance.

URETHRAL VALVES. Unlike distal urethral and meatal stenosis, these are more commonly seen in boys. The length of the male urethra serves as protection from secondary infection. The symptoms leading to diagnosis of membranous posterior urethral valves are related to uremia and hypertension. Diagnosis is made by voiding cystourethrography, which clearly depicts the site of obstruction. Dilatation of the proximal urethra and bladder is commonly noted, and marked hydroureteronephrosis is frequent. This advanced degree of secondary dilatation of the bladder, ureter, and calyces necessitates diversion of the urine. Operative excision of the urethral valves may not afford adequate treatment. Cutaneous pyeloileostomy, nephrostomy, or loop cutaneous ureterostomies may be required to bypass the tortuous dilated atonic ureters. Nephrostomy has the disadvantage of periodic need for tube changes and the constant threat of ascending infection. The prognosis for restoration of normal urinary function is dependent upon the degree of secondary changes in the proximal collecting system and the renal function at the time of diagnosis. Since males usually present with more advanced renal deterioration, their prognosis is usually less favorable.

NEUROGENIC BLADDER. This is usually due to autonomic dysfunction accompanying meningomyelocele. Impaired sensation of filling leads to a large residual urine with overflow incontinence. The patient may present with symptoms of infection, diurnal incontinence, or impaired voiding. Diagnosis is established by excretory urography, voiding cystourethrogram, and cystometry. The latter study reveals a large residual urine with low-pressure high-volume tracing and lack of sensation of filling until large volumes have been instilled. Treatment for mild dysfunction may be manual assistance in voiding, coupled with therapy for infection. With moderately severe involvement, treatment is directed at eliminating the residual urine. This may be accomplished by transurethral resection of the bladder neck. If the children are reminded to void at intervals of 2 hours, many become continent. Children may be taught intermittent catheterization when they reach six to eight years of age. For severely compromised urinary tracts with marked loss of renal function, urinary diversion may be indicated.

URETEROCELE. This is a consequence of a stenotic ureteral orifice. As the intravesical ureter dilates, it forms a cystic intravesical mass which may become sufficiently

A

B

Fig. 40-16. Urethral stenosis. Voiding cystourethrogram in distal urethral stenosis. Proximal urethra is markedly dilated. The bladder is irregularly trabeculated. Reflux of contrast is seen in the markedly dilated right ureter. Arrow in *B* indicates the bladder neck.

large to obstruct the bladder neck during voiding. Occasionally, the ureterocele prolapses through the urethra. Diagnosis is established by means of delayed films during intravenous pyelography (Fig. 40-17). The opaque-filled intravesical mass has a thin, nonopaque rim (the ureterocele wall) which contrasts with the opacity of the bladder content, giving the appearance of "cobra head deformity." Many ureteroceles cause sufficient ureteral obstruction to warrant surgical treatment. Small lesions may be removed by endoscopic incision or excision. Prolapsing ureteroceles with urethral obstruction require transvesical excision. In children, ureterocele is often associated with ureteral duplication.

HYDRONEPHROSIS. This is often the result of a congenital stenosis at the ureteropelvic junction. Although narrowing may not be severe, impaired passage of urine through this area leads to dilatation of the renal pelvis and

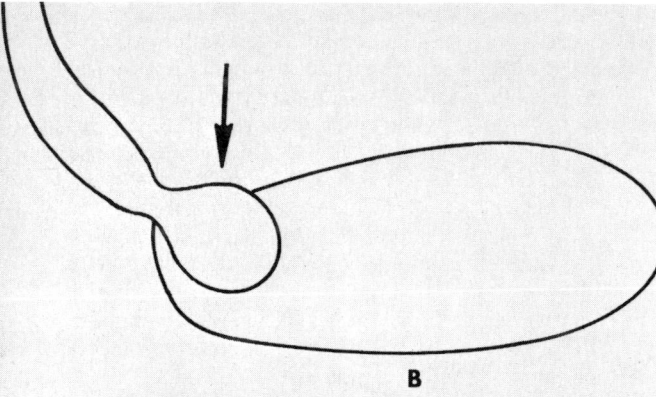

Fig. 40-17. Ureterocele. *A.* Excretory urogram of right ureterocele bulging into bladder. Ureter is obstructed and dilated. *B.* Ureterocele is indicated by arrow.

calyces (Fig. 40-18). Pressure atrophy results in severe loss of renal function. Patients most frequently complain of pain which, on occasion, may mimic the pain of appendicitis. Gastrointestinal symptoms such as nausea and vomiting are common. Abdominal mass represents another presenting finding. A familial history may be present. Diagnosis is established by means of excretory pyelography with delayed films demonstrating an impairment in renal excretion of contrast material. Pyeloplasty should be attempted whenever renal function is not too seriously compromised. With contralateral compensatory hypertrophy noted on the pyelogram, the pyeloplasty may not improve kidney function. Since there is a distinct tendency for hydronephrosis to be manifest on one side and incipient on the other, the patients should be followed with repeated pyelograms until they reach their maximal longitudinal growth in order to determine the presence of progression in the less involved kidney.

CONGENITAL NONOBSTRUCTIVE RENAL DISEASE. The disease may be suspected when kidneys fail to be visualized on intravenous pyelography and the BUN is normal. Congenital or neonatal glomerular disease, which represents a histologic diagnosis, is usually fatal. Cystic disease

Fig. 40-18. Hydronephrosis. This was due to intrinsic ureteral stenosis indicated by arrow in *B.*

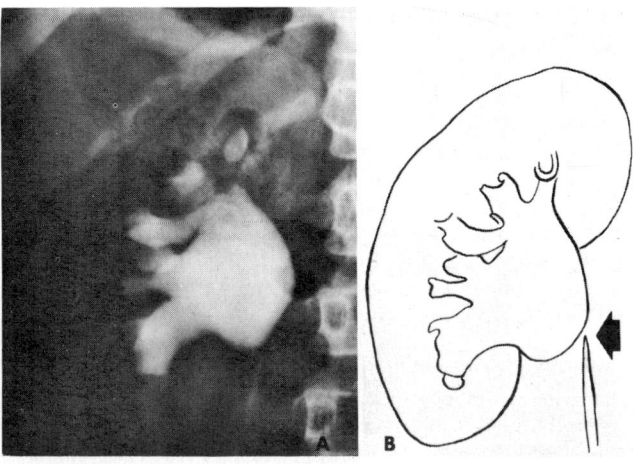

of the kidney has a broad spectrum. The collecting ducts may be ectatic, as in *medullary cystic disease.* There may be failure of communication between tubules and glomeruli, as in *polycystic disease.* Failure of development of the metanephric blastema accounts for *nonfunctioning multicystic renal disease.* Clinically recognizable *simple renal cysts* are infrequently seen in children. Failure to visualize the kidneys on intravenous pyelography in any of these disease states is indication for retrograde pyelography to assess long-term prognosis.

CRYPTORCHIDISM (UNDESCENDED TESTIS). This is the result of a congenital arrest of testicular descent. About 4 percent of full-term infant males have undescended testes at birth. Twenty-one percent of premature males have undescended testes. If the testis fails to reach a scrotal position within 6 weeks (3 months for the premature), it rarely descends in later life. When the testis lies in a position other than the normal scrotal location, it is subjected to a 2.5° increase in temperature, which is injurious to the seminiferous tubules. The normal testis may begin to show active differentiation of the spermatocytic series when the patient is five years old. This does not occur in the cryptorchid. With bilateral cryptorchidism, which is present in 24 percent of the cases, spermatogenesis never develops, and the individual is infertile. After the age of fourteen, the undescended testis may be damaged beyond recovery. Testicular tumors are more common in undescended testes. These tumors occur fifty times more frequently in the abdominal testis and eleven times more often in the inguinal testis than in the normally located organs. Following orchiopexy the tendency to neoplasm is not altered, but examination is more feasible. Orchiopexy should be performed prior to puberty, and it is an advantage to operate before the patient is of school age. Ninety percent of undescended testes are associated with indirect inguinal hernia, and simultaneous repair of the defect should be performed. Nonsurgical treatment with chorionic gonadotropin is occasionally effective but does nothing for the associated hernia.

HYPOSPADIAS. This is the most frequent fusion defect of the urethra. It occurs in approximately 1 of 900 pediatric hospital admissions. The abnormality consists of a dorsal hood (absent ventral foreskin), chordee (ventral curvature of the glans penis on the shaft), and proximal location of the urethral meatus. The urethral meatus may be located anywhere from the coronary sulcus to the perineum but is more frequently distal. Multiple urethral orifices may be present, but only one communicates with the urethra per se.

Hypospadias results in an abnormal urinary stream. The downward deformity of the glans penis causes the urine issuing from the urethral meatus to be deflected. Infertility is frequently associated with a scrotal or perineal meatus. Hypospadias with urethral meatus in the scrotal area is often accompanied by bilateral undescended testes and must be differentiated from adrenogenital syndrome and pseudohermaphroditism. Before performing urethroplasty on such a patient, determination of the genetic sex by karyotyping and adrenal function by determination of 17-oxysteroids and 17-ketosteroids is indicated. Visualization of the lower urinary tract by means of retrograde opaque studies may disclose the presence of a vagina and abdominal exploration may reveal that the child's sex organs are more female than male, in which case excision of the hypertrophied clitoris should be performed.

Treatment of hypospadias may be by staged operations. First the chordee is corrected, and then the urethra is reconstructed. In some cases, stenosis of the original urethral meatus may require meatotomy before the definitive operations are undertaken. One-stage hypospadias repairs are also performed, with simultaneous chordee repair and urethroplasty. Postoperative urethral fistula formation may require further surgical correction. A minimum period of 6 months should be allowed for adequate healing between stages or before a fistula is excised. (See Chap. 51.)

EPISPADIAS. A dorsally cleft urethra is only one-fifth as common as hypospadias. It is the consequence of failure of dorsal fusion and in its most marked form involves the urethral sphincter and may be associated with urinary incontinence. Surgical repair is indicated.

EXSTROPHY OF THE BLADDER. This represents an extremely rare advanced stage of epispadias. Although techniques have been devised to reconstruct the bladder, function is seldom normal. Therefore, a supravesical diversion of urine by cutaneous ureteroileostomy or ureterosigmoidostomy and cystectomy is advisable. The urethra can be reconstructed in the male to permit siring of offspring.

ECTOPIC URETERAL ORIFICE. The ectopic ureteral orifice usually drains the upper part of a double kidney, with complete duplication of the ureters. The condition is four times more prevalent in females. In order to be manifest symptomatically, the ectopic ureteral orifice must empty outside the urethral sphincter in the urethra or vagina. The characteristic complaint is of urinary incontinence despite normal voiding habits. The ureteral segment drained by the ectopic ureter is frequently severely hydroephrotic and may not be visualized on the excretory pyelogram (Fig. 40-6). Treatment is excision of the upper renal segment and ureter in most instances, but at times it is possible to reimplant the ureter into the bladder.

ENURESIS. Nocturnal loss of urine is normal until the age of three. After that age a normal child may occasionally wet the bed. Habitual bed wetting after the age of three may be associated with organic lesions of the bladder or urethra; the presence of additional urinary symptoms suggests such a lesion, and investigation is indicated before ascribing the enuresis to psychogenic factors.

NEOPLASMS

Renal Tumors

INCIDENCE AND ETIOLOGY. Renal tumors account for approximately 3 percent of cancer deaths. The frequency in males is twice that in females. The histologic origin of most carcinomas in males is probably from the renal tubular cell. Experimentally, renal tumors occur in male hamsters treated with estrogens. A virus has been implicated as the cause of the Lücke renal adenocarcinoma in frogs. The intrarenal injection of zinc chloride or Thorotrast has also been observed to produce renal tumors in animals. None of these factors has been implicated in the formation of human renal tumors, and the cause remains unknown.

PATHOLOGY. There are three major types of malignant tumors of the renal parenchyma. The foamy or granular cell carcinoma and tubular adenocarcinomas constitute 60 percent. Wilms' tumor (adenomyosarcoma), which characteristically occurs in children, accounts for 14 percent. Renal sarcoma, originating from the interstitial renal tissue, the renal capsule, and blood vessels, is defined in 6 percent while tumors of the collecting system constitute 14 percent of the total. Benign renal tumors (adenomas) are frequent postmortem findings but are not commonly associated with clinical manifestations.

CLINICAL MANIFESTATIONS. The classic triad of pain, mass, and hematuria occurs late and is seen in its entirety in less than half the patients. Marked variations in the prevalence of these symptoms have been noted in reported series: gross hematuria, 31 to 76 percent; pain, 24 to 75 percent; mass, 6 to 50 percent; fever, 16 percent; metastatic pain, 6 percent. Hematuria is a late manifestation which represents erosion of the tumor into the collecting system. A palpable mass is more frequently present if the tumor involves the lower pole of the right kidney. Pain has been related to the stretching of the renal capsule, in which instance it is usually mild but persistent. Sudden severe flank pain may accompany bleeding into the tumor. The passage of blood clots mimics colic from a ureteral stone. Fever is probably caused by necrosis of a tumor. Although adult parenchymal tumors are usually not associated with hypertension, this is a frequent accompaniment of Wilms' tumor. Hypertension has been related to compression of the renal artery with resultant renal ischemia.

Utz described an interesting group of 27 patients with hepatosplenomegaly and renal tumors. They presented with fatigue, anemia, and fever but had no pain, mass, or hematuria. The sedimentation rate exceeded 100 mm/hour, and the prothrombin time, α-2-globulin, alkaline phosphatase, and Bromsulphalein retention were all increased. Both the hepatosplenomegaly and laboratory

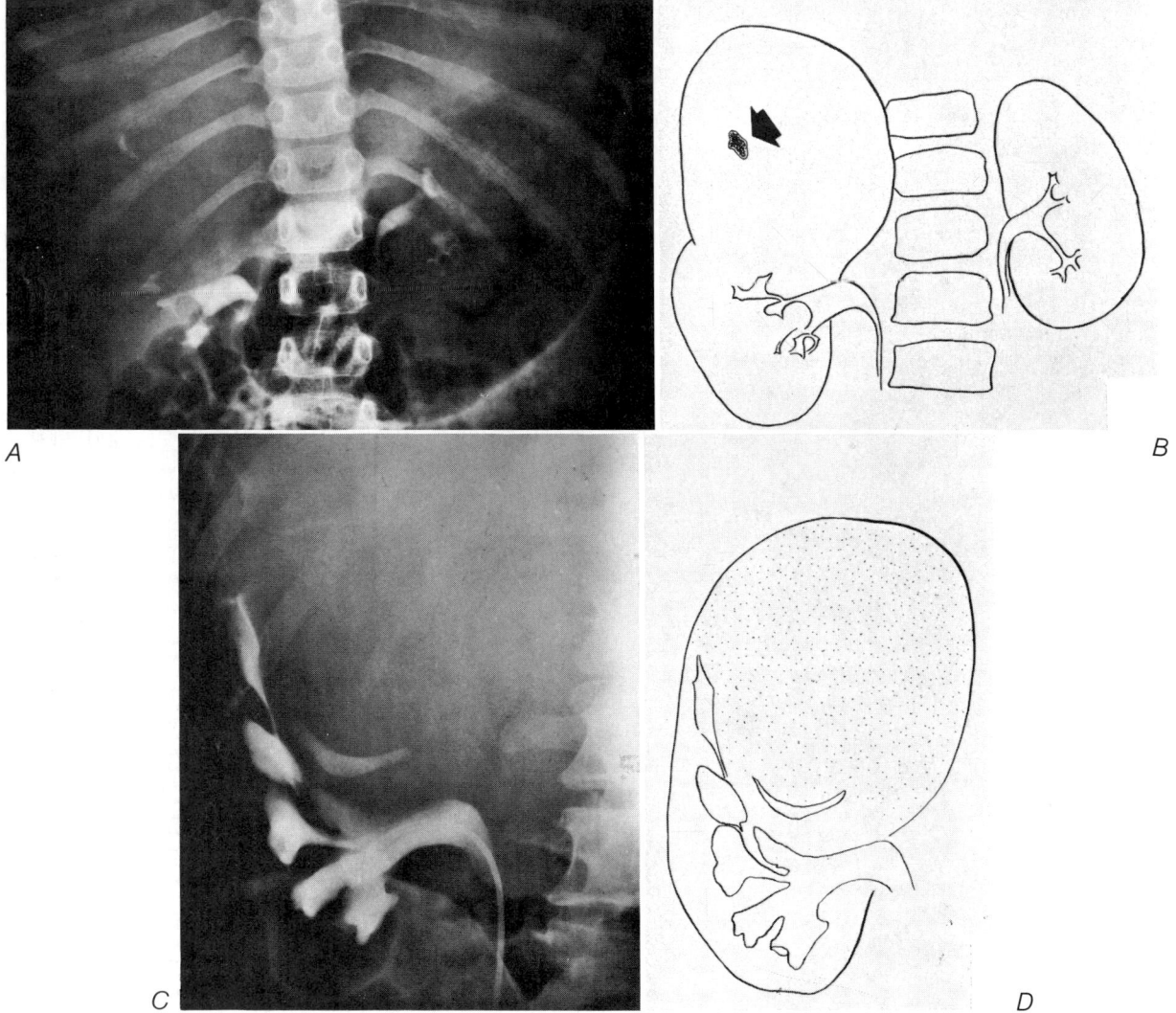

Fig. 40-19. Renal tumor. *A* and *B*. Right upper pole renal cell carcinoma (hypernephroma) deforms calyces on excretory urogram. Calcification is indicated by the arrow on *B*. *C* and *D*. Retrograde pyelogram of a large renal tumor (stippled on *D*) deforming upper calyces.

abnormalities reverted to normal when the tumor was curatively excised. It is thought that the syndrome is caused by a glycoprotein present in the tumor. Erythrocytemia is present in 2 percent of cases with hypernephroma, which accounts for 7 percent of patients evaluated for polycythemia. Erythropoietin has been extracted from these renal tumors.

Despite the nature of the symptoms, the delay between onset and medical consultation has been long, averaging 23 months from the onset of hematuria and 14 months from the onset of pain in one series. Metastases were demonstrated in 37 percent of patients at the time of diagnosis and included involvement of the hip, shoulder, back, and lungs. Skull metastases simulating sebaceous cyst are not uncommon.

DIAGNOSIS. Excretory pyelography is frequently diagnostic. Since the renal tumor is focal, the uninvolved portion of the kidney is usually visualized. The exception to this rule is the presence of renal vein occlusion. Charac-

teristically, there is enlargement of the renal silhouette with deformity of the calyces in the area of the mass (Fig. 40-19). On early films, the renal neoplasm opacifies because of vascularity of the tumor. This may distinguish an opacifying tumor from a nonopacifying cyst (Fig. 40-20). Approximately 30 percent of renal lesions are neoplasms, while 58 percent are cysts and 12 percent represent polycystic disease (Fig. 40-21). Nephrotomography is helpful in differentiating cyst from tumor. While tumors usually opacify, with hemorrhage or necrosis the opacification may be impaired and a false diagnosis of cyst made. The presence of calcium at the edge of the mass is more suggestive of tumor than cyst, with the exception of the echinococcal renal cyst. Ultrasonography is helpful in the differentiation between cystic and solid tumors. Percutaneous cyst aspira-

Fig. 40-20. Renal cyst. Nephrotomogram disclosing a nonopacifying lower pole cyst indicated by arrow on *B*.

tion with analysis of the fluid extracted and instillation of contrast material may offer a definitive diagnosis. Renal arteriography (Fig. 40-22) is indicated for solid lesions, followed by vena cavagraphy (Fig. 40-23) for evaluation of venous involvement. Computed tomography may prove valuable in determining the nature and extent of a kidney lesion (Fig. 40-24). Metastatic series, including chest films and isotopic scans, should be routine for the evaluation of patients with suspected malignant disease (Figs. 40-25 and 40-26).

Abnormalities in serum electrolytes or proteins are rarely noted. If the total renal function is compromised, preoperative evaluation of the uninvolved kidney's function is imperative. The individual renal creatinine clearances and isotopic perfusion studies will aid in the assessment of the situation prior to therapy.

TREATMENT. In some instances it is necessary to explore the renal fossa. The operative approach to renal tumor may be through the flank, chest, or abdomen. Removal of the perinephric fat with the kidney provides the best margin. Early ligation of the renal vessels minimizes venous tumor spread and blood loss. Preoperative radiation therapy and chemotherapy are rarely prescribed, but postoperative radiation may be of some benefit when adequate local resection is compromised. Removal of primary renal tumor has been observed to be followed by regression of metastases in lung and bone. Also, in a few cases, resection of metastatic lesions in the lung or extremities has been associated with prolonged survival.

PROGNOSIS. This depends on the histologic type, the presence of local extension into the renal vein, perinephric tissues, or lymph nodes, and distant metastases. For patients with low-grade local lesions, the survival rate equals the actuarial life expectancy. The overall survival rate for renal tumors without metastases is about 50 percent for 5 years and 33 percent for 10 years.

CARCINOMA OF THE RENAL PELVIS

Tumors of the renal pelvis constitute 14 percent of kidney tumors. Half of these are epidermoid and have been associated with infection or calculus-induced metaplasia of the transitional epithelium of the pelvis. The associated infection or calculus frequently masks the tumor. The patients characteristically have no gross hematuria, flank pain, or mass and frequently present with a resistant urinary infection and markedly reduced function noted on

Fig. 40-21. Polycystic disease. Excretory urogram of a nineteen-year-old girl with congenital polycystic renal disease. Huge left kidney shows classic deformity of calyces and elongation of infundibula by multiple cysts.

A   *B*   *C*

Fig. 40-22. Renal neoplasm and renal cyst. *A*. Selective right renal arteriogram showing avascular lesion which, on needle aspiration, proved to be cyst. *B*. Nephrotomogram showing right renal cyst and left upper pole renal carcinoma. *C*. Selective left renal arteriogram demonstrating vascular renal neoplasm. Diagrams below demonstrate the pathology.

intravenous pyelography. Ureteral urinary cytology may demonstrate epithelial pearls. The treatment for squamous carcinoma is surgical excision, but the prognosis is exceedingly poor because of late diagnosis. Adjuvant radiation therapy and chemotherapy are ineffective.

Transitional cell tumors of the renal pelvis and ureter are histologically similar to the vesical counterparts. They occur more frequently in the male and are seldom seen in patients under the age of fifty. Gross hematuria and renal colic due to the passage of blood clots are common presenting symptoms. Lesions usually become manifest before a tumor is palpable. Intravenous pyelography frequently establishes the diagnosis, showing a filling defect in the portion of the pelvis or ureter (Fig. 40-27). Differential diagnosis of the filling defects include blood clot and nonopaque (uric acid) calculi. Urine obtained by ureteral catheter lavage or brushing may demonstrate clusters of transitional cells. Transitional cell tumors of the pelvis tend to be multiple, and frequently there are ureteral implants involving the distal ureter or the bladder. Treatment therefore consists of removing the kidney, the ureter, and a margin of the bladder around the ureteral orifice. The prognosis for survival is markedly reduced when the tumor infiltrates the adjacent parenchyma. Postoperative radiation therapy and chemotherapy have not been demonstrated to be of value in improving the statistics.

Tumors of the Urinary Bladder

INCIDENCE AND ETIOLOGY. Although tumors of the bladder cause only 3 percent of all cancer deaths, the estimated incidence in the general population is 0.02 percent. The peak age incidence is fifty to seventy years of age.

In 1978, the estimated number of deaths from cancer of the bladder was reported as 6,900 for men and 3,000 for women.

Papillary bladder tumors have been related to the inadvertent ingestion of chemicals which are excreted in the urine as conjugated orthoaminophenols. These include beta-naphthylamine and para-aminobiphenyl. Prolonged periods of exposure are apparently necessary. Certain carcinogenic tryptophan metabolites are present in higher concentrations in the urine of patients with recurring bladder tumors. Tobacco tar applied to the oral mucosa in mice produces vesical papillomas, and there appears to be a prevalence of heavy cigarette smokers among the group with bladder tumors. Chronic infection with schistosomiasis and mechanical trauma due to calculus may cause metaplasia and neoplasia of the bladder epithelium.

CLINICAL MANIFESTATIONS. The patients usually present with gross painless hematuria secondary to partial infarction of a tumor. Hematuria is the initial symptom in 75 percent of cases and is present in 95 percent of cases at the time of diagnosis. Frequency and painful urination are late symptoms which result from sloughing of the tumor and secondary infection.

The physical findings in early cases are minimal, since the tumor remains within the confines of the bladder. Metastases and local extension occur quite late in the course of disease; in one series at the time of death 80 percent of the tumors were confined to the bladder. In

Fig. 40-23. Tumor involvement of vena cava. *A*. Renal vein tumor extending into lumen of vena cava. *B*. Direct extension of renal tumor into vena cava.

untreated cases, the neoplasm may occlude the ureter and lead to uremia. Local extension of the tumor may result in a stony nodular induration at the base of the bladder with fixation to the wall of the pelvis. Lymphatic spread may involve the pelvic and periaortic nodes. Osseous lesions are usually osteolytic and may cause nerve root pain.

Laboratory studies may be normal in early cases but may reveal anemia and uremia in late cases. Urinalysis usually demonstrates red blood cells. White blood cells are seen at times if there is associated infection and necrosis, and clusters of abnormal transitional cells may occasionally be identified. Tumor biopsies provide tissue for histologic diagnosis, and deeper biopsies offer information regarding depth of penetration (staging).

TREATMENT AND PROGNOSIS. Endoscopic resection and electrodesiccation are suitable for superficial small tumors. Many patients have survived for prolonged periods of time with recurring superficial bladder tumors requiring periodic endoscopic treatment. Others demonstrate more rapid recurrences with change toward anaplastic and invasive characteristics. The most satisfactory treatment for locally invasive, resectable carcinoma of the bladder is preoperative radiation therapy followed by cystectomy,

with supravesical diversion of the urine by means of the cutaneous ureteroileostomy (ileal loop) or cutaneous ureterocolostomy (colon loop). Experience with combinations of chemotherapeutic agents and radiation therapy followed by cystectomy has not demonstrated improved survival.

For patients with nonresectable disease, urinary diversion may relieve frequency and reduce hemorrhage. Palliative radiation therapy may also reduce the bleeding. No systemic chemotherapeutic agent warrants enthusiastic recommendation. Thiotepa instilled at weekly intervals for a month has destroyed superficial tumors. The prognosis of bladder tumor depends on the nature and extent of the tumor. When there is no invasion of muscle, the 5-year survival is 77 percent. With deep invasion of the muscle, 5-year survival is less than 10 percent.

Fig. 42-24. *A.* Computed tomography demonstrating cyst of the left renal pelvis. *B.* Diagram for orientation.

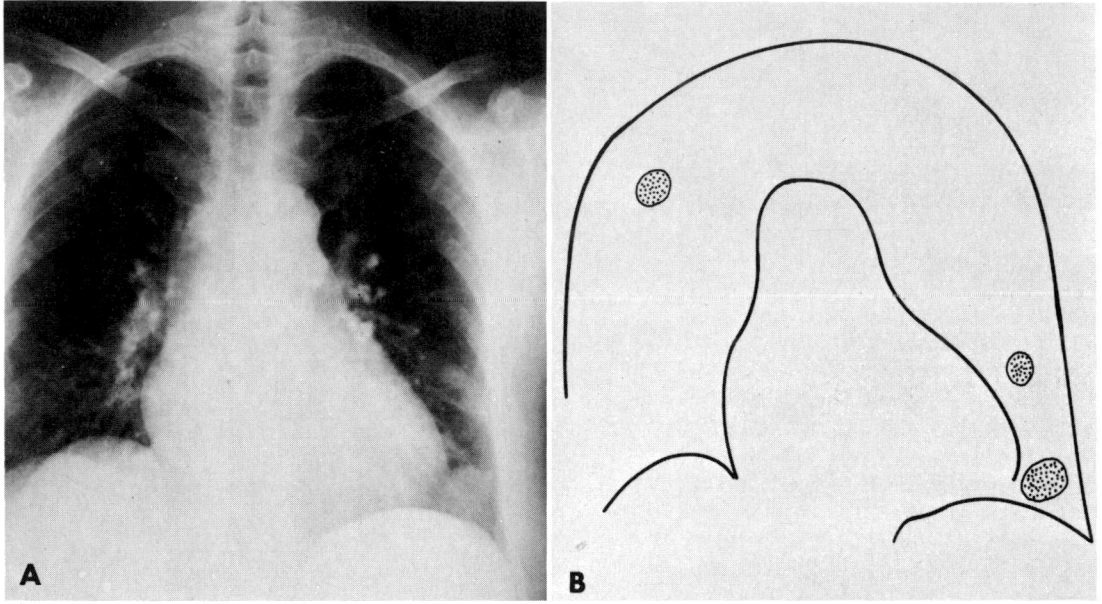

Fig. 40-25. Typical "cannonball" pulmonary metastases from renal carcinoma.

Prostatic Tumors

BENIGN PROSTATIC HYPERTROPHY

INCIDENCE AND ETIOLOGY. Benign prostatic hypertrophy is a benign tumor, adenoleiomyofibromatosis, which originates from the periurethral tissues. The lesion is rare before the age of forty and does not occur in eunuchs. After the age of forty, 55 percent of males manifest typical lesions histologically, and after the age of eighty, 75 percent of males are so affected. However, Chinese males living in their native land have an incidence of only 6 percent after the age of forty.

CLINICAL MANIFESTATIONS. The symptoms are related to mechanical obstruction. Although the initial symptoms consisting of diminished forcefulness and projection of the stream may be apparent, the onset of obstruction is usually so insidious that most patients are unaware of difficulty until it becomes more pronounced. Nocturia is a frequent symptom and is usually due to residual urine, but in the early stages the bladder capacity may be functionally reduced because of compensatory detrusor hypertrophy. Hematuria may result from straining to void. However,

Fig. 40-26. Typical osteolytic metastasis to the calvarium from clear cell renal carcinoma (hypernephroma).

Fig. 40-27. Carcinoma of renal pelvis. *A.* Excretory urogram pyelogram showing a filling defect in the renal pelvis due to papillary carcinoma. *B.* Tumor is indicated by arrow.

other causes of hematuria such as bladder tumor and vesical calculus should be excluded cystoscopically before a prostatic cause is accepted. Acute retention of urine is the ultimate consequence of detrusor decompensation and frequently is the symptom for which the patient first seeks medical assistance.

On examination, 90 percent of patients demonstrate a smooth symmetrical enlargement of the prostate which has the consistency of the thenar eminence. Ten percent of the patients with intravesical enlargement or median bar prostatic hypertrophy have a normal gland on rectal examination. A palpable percussible bladder is indicative of retention of urine. Presence of bilateral direct inguinal hernia and/or external hemorrhoids of recent origin is often an indication of the degree of straining that the patient has experienced to pass his urine. Observation of the urinary stream will evaluate the degree of difficulty. A self-activating flowmeter may be used to estimate the degree of obstruction. Normally, when more than 200 ml is voided, the flow rate will be 20 ml/second. In patients with prostatic obstruction, rates of less than 5 ml/second are common. Cytoscopic and roentgenographic evidences of benign prostatic hypertrophy include trabeculation and thickening of the bladder wall, formation of pulsion diverticula (Fig. 40-28), vesical calculi, ureteral dilatation, hydronephrosis, and a smooth filling defect (the prostate) at the base of the bladder on films made with the patient upright.

RESIDUAL URINE. The amount of residual urine may be determined directly by catheterization or by indirect methods. Following voiding, the bladder is normally empty except for a few drops of urine. A postvoiding film after an intravenous pyelogram may also determine the presence of residual urine.

The mechanism of prostatic obstruction includes functional reduction in the cross-sectional area of the prostatic urethra, attenuation of the muscle fibers which normally open the vesical neck, decreased mechanical advantage of these muscles by virtue of a longer course overlying the adenoma, and increased tissue resistance to opening of the vesical outlet.

Residual urine is the result of stretching of the detrusor muscle when the ability of the bladder to compensate and expel urine against an increased resistance is exceeded. As the degree of obstruction reduces the flow rate with maximal bladder pressures, the percent of bladder volume emptied with each voiding decreases. Thus, the residual urine volume increases. The formation of vesical diverticula and vesicoureteral reflux, which are consequences of the obstructive uropathy, also increase the amount of residual urine. The functionally reduced bladder capacity becomes manifest by the need for multiple voiding, particularly early in the morning. The patient soon learns that it is wiser to void when the need first becomes apparent, since procrastination compounds the difficulty. The patient

Fig. 40-28. Vesical diverticulum. Cystogram showing a large vesical diverticulum (arrow), an important cause of residual urine and persistent infection associated with prostatic hypertrophy.

with residual urine secondary to benign prostatic hypertrophy is always in danger of acute retention if he defers urination until the bladder is so distended that a detrusor contraction cannot be initiated. The diuretic and analgesic responses to alcohol and the effects of anesthesia and of anticholinergic and sympathomimetic drugs also increase the likelihood of acute retention.

The presence of residual urine favors formation of vesical calculi (Fig. 40-29). These may be associated with sharp twinges of pain, the "curbstone" symptom, when the patient descends a stairway or steps down from the curb. This is related to the calculi bouncing on the trigone. Following voiding, the patient may have severe strangury and terminal gross hematuria. Residual urine also predisposes to infection. The normally functioning bladder is capable of eliminating a heavy inoculum of bacteria, while the obstructed bladder remains infected.

TREATMENT. The patient who is a good operative risk with a reasonable life expectancy is best treated by prostatectomy. However, circumstances may dictate a nonsurgical or an altered surgical management. Patients with significant residual urine but without compromised renal function can often be managed without an indwelling catheter. Specific treatment of infection followed by longterm suppressive therapy with mandelic acid or nitrofurantoin is indicated. The patient should be instructed to avoid overdistension of the bladder and to void at the first indication of need. Caution against long automobile trips and ingestion of alcoholic beverages, anticholinergic medications, and diuretics is indicated. Hot tub baths and prostatic massages effect symptomatic relief.

Fig. 40-29. Vesical calculus secondary to long-standing benign prostatic hypertrophy. Note intravesical intrusion of huge middle lobe.

CALCULUS   PROSTATE

The patient with compromised renal function can be managed with an indwelling retention catheter, but if prolonged treatment is anticipated, bilateral partial vasectomy to prevent descending epididymitis should be performed. Patients who fail to tolerate the urethral catheter may be more comfortable with a suprapubic cystostomy performed under local or regional anesthesia. In either situation, the catheter care outlined previously should be adhered to. A leg bag for collection is convenient while the patient ambulates, whereas a floor bottle is preferred for night collection.

The indications for surgical intervention include significant residual urine, difficulty in voiding, and annoying frequency and nocturia, as well as the secondary effects of obstruction such as vesical diverticula, calculi, hydroureteronephrosis, and persistent infection. Presence of benign prostatic hypertrophy per se and symptoms of prostatitis do not constitute indications. As the size of the adenomatous mass increases, the normal prostate is compressed into a 0.5-cm-thick surgical capsule. This portion remains after simple prostatectomy for benign prostatic hypertrophy. Although it is appreciated that carcinoma of the prostate may subsequently arise in the remaining gland, simple prostatectomy is most appropriate, since it is attended by a low morbidity and mortality, and secondary recurrences and neoplasms are infrequent.

Transurethral Prostatectomy. This is performed by application of a high-frequency current to a tungsten wire loop. Multiple fragments of the obstructive tissue are removed by successive cuts under direct endoscopic vision. Hemostasis is effected by sealing the vessels with the coagulating current. Because of low mortality and morbidity, transurethral resection is favored in the elderly patient. It represents an excellent operation for the young patient who values sexual potency. Transurethral resection is particularly adaptable to a median bar prostatic hypertrophy and the removal of small or inflamed glands which do not enucleate easily by the open route. The procedure can be combined with lithotripsy (crushing and removal of a vesical calculus). The technique is also applicable for the relief of urinary obstruction due to surgically incurable carcinoma of the prostate. Transurethral prostatectomy may be precluded by hip disease which interferes with the lithotomy position.

Open Prostatectomy. Whether performed through a suprapubic bladder incision, retropubically, or perineally, it employs similar techniques. Cleavage is developed with fingers or instruments so that the adenomas and attached prostatic urethra are removed. This leaves the entire prostatic cavity to reepithelialize from the bladder neck and urethral epithelium and from ducts of the acinar glands in the remaining surgical capsule. The transvesical suprapubic approach is particularly applicable to the removal of large vesical diverticula and calculi. The retropubic approach is **ideal** for coping with inguinal hernia at the time of **suprapubic** prostatectomy.

Open **prostatectomy** is associated with a four times greater **mortality** rate than transurethral resection. This is related to the increased bleeding problems, wound healing, and urinary fistulae. The catheter drainage for open prostatectomy usually extends over 5 days, as compared with 2 to 3 days for transurethral prostatectomy. The attendant increase in the risk of ascending epididymitis makes bilateral prophylactic vasectomy at the time of open prostatectomy advisable. The postoperative stay with transurethral resection is usually 5 days in contrast to approximately 9 days for open prostatectomy.

With either approach, adequate drainage of the catheter and appropriate antibacterial agents are indicated. Early ambulation should be encouraged and constipation prevented by oral laxatives. Enemas are usually best avoided, since they may initiate bleeding. Upon discharge, the patient should be cautioned that long, bumpy automobile trips, heavy lifting, straining during defecation, and inadequate hydration may lead to bleeding. Oral antibacterial agents are continued when urine cultures are positive. The patient is seen at intervals to evaluate the character and frequency of voiding. A thin stream may be due to metal stricture resulting from the indwelling catheter, a situation which can be corrected by dilation. The majority of patients who do office work may return to their work at 4 weeks. Laborers should not resume work for 2 to 3 months.

PROGNOSIS. Ninety percent of patients have improvement or relief of symptoms. Ten percent develop urethral stricture which must be treated. Many patients have persisting low-grade pyuria which is difficult to eradicate and require continued suppressive therapy until reepithelization is complete. Five-year results indicate that recurrent obstruction requiring additional surgical treatment develops in about 10 to 25 percent. It is important to appreciate the fact that carcinoma may develop in the remaining tissue.

CARCINOMA OF THE PROSTATE

INCIDENCE AND ETIOLOGY. Although the cause of prostatic carcinoma is unknown, it seems to be related to long-standing androgen stimulation. It does not occur in eunuchs and is rare below the age of thirty. However, administration of testosterone to the elderly does not appear to significantly increase the incidence. The new case rate is estimated at 57,000 per year, with approximately 20,600 deaths per year. It is further estimated that approximately 5 million men are living with histologic cancer of the prostate. Although the autopsy rate has doubled recently, the tumor accounts for only 3.5 percent of deaths in males. For each decade over fifty years, the death per 100,000 doubles, reaching 400 at age eighty (Fig. 40-30). Carcinoma of the prostate represents the most frequent malignant tumor in males over the age of sixty-five, but many men die *with* carcinoma of the prostate and not *of* it.

EARLY CARCINOMA. This represents the stage in which prostatic carcinoma is potentially curable. In most series, less than 10 percent of patients present as early cases, and a vast majority are completely asymptomatic with the tumors detected on routine physical examination. Over 50 percent of prostatic nodules palpated on rectal examination are positive for carcinoma on biopsy. Following a positive biopsy, the patient should be evaluated for total prostatoseminal vesiculectomy. This operation is more demanding on the patient's general condition than the simple prosta-

tectomy. During the radical operation, the bladder neck is sutured to the urethra, and the postoperative course is frequently less eventful than that following simple prostatectomy. An indwelling urethral catheter is necessary for 10 days, and constipation should be avoided to prevent straining and bleeding. An adequate operation abolishes sexual function.

An alternative method of treatment for the patient with early carcinoma is radiation therapy. If the patient is not a candidate for either radical surgery or radiation therapy, he may be treated with estrogen therapy or orchiectomy, or in some instances followed without any specific therapy. However, only surgical excision or radical radiation therapy can offer a cure for this disease, and the 5- and 10-year rates associated with these forms of treatment are fairly similar in several series of cases. One can hope to achieve better than a 50 percent 5-year cure in selected cases.

ADVANCED CARCINOMA. The average age of the symptomatic patient who presents with advanced prostatic cancer is seventy-two. Typically, the symptoms are of a few months' duration with rapid progression of frequency and nocturia leading to acute retention in 28 percent. Weight loss is common, severe back pain occurs in 14 percent, and sciatica in 56 percent. Gross hematuria occurs in only 8 percent of patients, and lymphedema secondary to lymphatic obstruction is present in 4 percent.

Rectal examination characteristically demonstrates a fixed, enlarged, nodular, stony hard prostate. Virchow's node and axillary and inguinal nodes may be palpable. The serum acid and alkaline phosphatase levels are elevated in 72 percent of the patients. Combined osteoblastic and osteolytic bony metastases are present in 60 percent, while isolated osteolytic metastases are rare. Pulmonary metastases occur in 1 percent of patients and are usually miliary in appearance.

The diagnosis is established by transperineal or transrectal needle biopsy. Indurations of the prostate also are observed in tuberculosis, prostatitis, calculus, benign prostatic hypertrophy, and carcinoma of the bladder and rec-

Fig. 40-30. Prostatic cancer death rate versus age.

Fig. 40-31. Multiple focal osteoblastic metastatic carcinoma lesions in the pelvis.

tum with prostatic extension. The differential diagnosis of the osseous lesions (Fig. 40-31) is primarily concerned with Paget's disease. The latter is more diffuse, while the bony lesions of carcinoma of the prostate are usually focal and multiple. The wavy, coarsened, trabecular pattern associated with cystic lesions is characteristic of Paget's disease. Elevation of the serum acid phosphatase level is also associated with myeloma and other bony tumors. Hemolysis of the blood and the drawing of blood within 24 hours subsequent to vigorous rectal examination may also raise this level. The alkaline phosphatase level is also elevated in other bone diseases such as Paget's, multiple myeloma, osteogenic sarcoma, and metastatic tumor. Obstructive lesions of the common bile duct also cause an increase in the serum alkaline phosphatase.

Histopathologically, prostatic malignant tumors are adenocarcinomas, and the majority are highly differentiated. Local extension of the tumor into perineural spaces is present in 92 percent of the cases. The prognosis is particularly dependent upon the extent of differentiation of the tumor; with highly differentiated tumors, the life expectancy approaches actuarial levels. Five- and ten-year survival rates also depend on the stage of the disease. If metastatic carcinoma is present, the figures are 20 and 10 percent, respectively. If the prostatic cancer is localized without evident metastases, 5- and 10-year survival rates are 56 and 26 percent.

Fig. 40-32. Age incidence of testicular tumors.

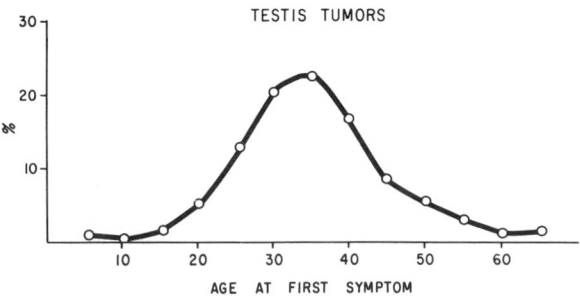

Treatment of advanced carcinoma consists of estrogen therapy and/or orchiectomy. This treatment rapidly improves pain and anorexia and gradually relieves the obstructive urinary symptoms. If a large residual urine persists, transurethral prostatic resection may be indicated. The endocrine therapy is accompanied by palliation in about 90 percent of patients. Diethylstilbestrol (1 mg daily) is generally adequate for long-term therapy and is not associated with significant thromboembolic complications. Increased dosage of stilbestrol may be necessary in the patient who has not had an orchiectomy. Recurrence of symptoms is attended by a poor prognosis. Symptomatic relief may be achieved by large doses of diethylstilbestrol diphosphate administered intravenously. X-ray therapy to isolated metastatic lesions is also palliative. ^{32}P, which localizes in prostatic cancer cells, may relieve metastatic bone pain but is associated with adverse effects on the hemopoietic tissues. Antiandrogen therapy and treatment with compounds such as estramurine phosphate (Estracyt) have proved to be of some value in treatment. The latter drug has been shown to be effective in some patients who are no longer estrogen-responsive. Corticosteroids in large doses are symptomatically beneficial but have no direct effect on the tumor. Hypophysectomy may offer dramatic relief to 10 percent of patients. Five- and ten-year survival rates depend on the stage of disease at the time of institution of therapy. With metastatic carcinoma present, the figures are 20 and 10 percent, respectively.

Testicular Tumors

INCIDENCE AND ETIOLOGY. Testicular tumors account for 2 percent of cancers in the male, and the average age at diagnosis is thirty-two years (Fig. 40-32). The cause of human testicular tumors is unknown, but they occur eleven times more frequently in undescended testes and fifty times more often in abdominal undescended testes. Therefore, they may be related to imperfect embryogenesis. Experimentally, intratesticular injections of zinc chloride result in teratomas, and systemic administration of estrogen produces Leydig cell tumors.

CLINICAL MANIFESTATIONS. Patients usually present with a nonpainful "lump" in the testis. On examination, the lesion is hard, nontender, and solid, and does not transilluminate. About 20 percent of tumors are misdiagnosed as simple hydroceles because of the formation of a secondary hydrocele. The diagnosis of epididymitis may be made erroneously in some situations and delay the appropriate diagnostic surgical intervention. In the patient with a testicular tumor a large scrotal mass may also develop as a result of laceration of the tumor with formation of a hematocele. Late symptoms of metastatic disease include weight loss, fatigue, hemoptysis, and enlargement of the regional lymph nodes.

DIAGNOSIS AND TREATMENT. If a testicular tumor is suspected, surgical exploration is indicated. Measurement of urinary gonadotropins, radioimmunoassay of HCG and AFP markers, may be useful, but surgical treatment should not be delayed. If the lesion is confined to the testis on physical examination, an inguinal surgical approach is preferred. The spermatic vessels are occluded before the testis is exteriorized for inspection, in order to prevent the spread of tumor. Palpation of induration in the testis is indication for orchiectomy, and there is essentially no place for biopsy, since over 90 percent of solid lesions of the testis in this age group are malignant. In patients with apparent lymphatic or pulmonary spread, the primary tumor should be resected for pathologic evaluation. About one-third of the tumors are seminoma, and another third are embryonal cell tumors. The remainder are made up of teratocarcinoma, with 4 percent choriocarcinoma, 5 percent teratoma, and 1 percent interstitial tumors.

Subsequent therapy is dependent upon the histologic diagnosis. Additional surgical treatment is of little use with choriocarcinoma, since this tumor is associated with pulmonary metastases in 81 percent of cases. Pulmonary lesions are present in only 19 percent of cases with seminoma, but bilateral retroperitoneal lymph node resection appears unnecessary for this lesion, since it is extremely radiosensitive. As little as 100 r may sterilize seminomatous lymph node metastases. Lymph node resection is not indicated for benign teratomas but usually is performed for embryonal carcinoma and teratocarcinoma without supradiaphragmatic spread. Lymphadenectomy in such patients increases the 5-year survival significantly.

The use of such chemotherapeutic agents as vinblastine, actinomycin, bleomycin, cisplatinum, and other drugs in combinations has markedly increased the survival of patients with advanced metastatic testicular tumors. These agents may cause severe hemopoietic changes, especially when combined with x-ray therapy. The overall 5-year survival depends on the cell type and stage of disease at the time of diagnosis.

Carcinoma of the Penis

Carcinoma of the penis develops in the squamous epithelium of the glans and foreskin. The risk of squamous carcinoma of the penis is prevented by circumcision in infancy, but the incidence is not altered when the procedure is carried out in adulthood. The lesion is uncommon in the United States, and the average age of onset is over sixty. Patients characteristically present with a sore that does not heal or a palpable nodule under the nonretractable foreskin (phimosis). Because of poor hygiene and associated infection the diagnosis may be difficult. Biopsy provides a definitive diagnosis. Squamous carcinoma of the glans is slow-growing, and local excision or x-ray therapy is associated with a 90 percent 5-year cure rate when no distant spread is present. With nodes involved by tumor, the 5-year survival is reduced to 32 percent, and excision of both inguinal and femoral nodes is attended by improved survival.

GENITOURINARY TRACT INJURIES

Renal Injury

A direct blow or crushing injury to the renal area represents the most frequent type of trauma. Knife and bullet wounds are less common. Change in momentum, such as accompanies a fall from a height, may result in a tear of the renal vessels. The patient frequently indicates pain in the renal area. Physical findings include local cutaneous ecchymoses, guarding, mass, and tenderness. Gross hematuria or microhematuria indicates a need for urologic evaluation; if either occurs without local findings or after trivial hematuria, a predisposing renal lesion should be suspected. In children, 21 percent of renal injuries occur in abnormal kidneys involved with hydronephrosis or tumors and enlarged to the extent that they are not protected by the rib cage.

Diagnosis of renal injury is confirmed by excretory pyelography. The preinjection film may show obliteration of the psoas shadow, scoliosis with the concavity to the side of the injury, and displacement of intestinal gas. Postinjection films may demonstrate delayed, absent, or partial visualization of the injured kidney or extravasation of the opaque medium. The uninjured kidney should be evaluated particularly if nephrectomy is entertained. Arteriography and retrograde pyelography may be applicable and are of definite value if the kidney is not visualized.

Patients with renal contusions and lacerations which do not result in extravasation of urine may be treated by bed rest for 10 days and avoidance of strenuous activity for 3 weeks. When significant segments of the kidney fail to visualize on pyelography and arteriography or when there is extravasation, surgical treatment is considered. Preoperative evaluation of multiplicity of injuries is important. At the time of surgical treatment, perinephric hematoma and necrotic renal parenchyma should be removed. The kidney can be reconstructed by suturing its torn capsule, and the perinephric tissues should be well drained. The transperitoneal approach facilitates exploration and early pedicle control. With massive trauma to the kidney, nephrectomy may be indicated to control the immediate situation and because hypertension due to perinephric scarring may result. Delayed bleeding, urinary extravasation, abscesses, and calculus may require surgical attention.

Bladder Injury

The full bladder is vulnerable to trauma. This situation often prevails in the patient who has recently had an excessive alcohol intake. Direct blows, penetrating injury by spicules of bone associated with pelvic fractures, stab wounds, and gunshot wounds may all result in rupture of the bladder. Direct blows without bony fracture usually cause intraperitoneal rupture, while pelvic fractures are more often associated with an extraperitoneal rupture. The patient may be unable to void, and either a low abdominal or anterior rectal mass may be palpable. The urine obtained by voiding or catheterization is grossly or microscopically bloody. If catheterization is not possible, this suggests that the urethra may have been avulsed from the bladder. Cystography with postevacuation films define the site of extravasation.

Treatment usually consists of surgical repair of the bladder and cystostomy drainage, which should be maintained for a minimum of 10 days. Occasionally, conservative management without an operation may prove satisfactory. This is especially true in the extraperitoneal rupture of the bladder, where catheter drainage may be all that is required in certain circumstances. If the urethra is avulsed, a splinting urethral catheter is also inserted. Perivesical and perineal hematomas should be drained. When trauma is extensive and the patient's condition poor, cystostomy under local anesthesia may be adequate to allow the sites of rupture to heal themselves. Differences of opinion exist regarding the surgical management. Some authors advocate simple suprapubic cystostomy drainage, while others suggest more extensive primary repair of the ruptured urethra.

Ureteral Trauma

Injuries to the ureter occur mainly as the result of trauma during operation. If the injury is recognized at the time of the operation, a direct repair over an indwelling catheter should be performed. If the condition is not recognized at operation, it may become manifest by anuria in the case of bilateral ligation or, more frequently, a urinary tract fistula or an expanding urinoma. Excretory pyelography frequently demonstrates obstructive changes in the site of the ureteral fistula or urinoma. Treatment of the sequelae of ureteral trauma consists of surgical repair. The ureter occasionally may be injured by penetrating objects such as bullets and knives. This situation must be suspected when the patient who has sustained such an injury has microhematuria. There is a definite strong indication for an excretory urogram on a patient who sustains a penetrating injury of the abdomen.

OPERATIONS ON GENITOURINARY ORGANS

Lumbar Nephrectomy

The retroperitoneal approach to the kidney is the traditional route, since in the preantibiotic era a major proportion of renal operations were performed for pyogenic disease and the avoidance of contamination of the peritoneum with urine was considered advantageous. Today, the lumbar renal approach (Fig. 40-33) remains popular but is supplanted on many occasions by the transabdominal route when early access to the renal vessels is required, as in renal tumor, trauma, or renal vascular disease.

Indications for the lumbar approach include inflammatory renal disease, calculi, tumor (especially of the upper pole), pyelonephritis, hydronephrosis, renal trauma, and renal cystic disease. Since it offers a most expeditious exposure, it is frequently used in poor-risk patients or for secondary nephrectomy. The disadvantages are a limited exposure for abdominal exploration, the fact that it may be poorly tolerated by the patient, and that it precludes bilateral renal or adrenal exploration. In addition, the lumbar approach makes early control of the renal pedicle without manipulation of the kidney difficult and therefore should not be applied for certain renal tumors.

The procedure is carried out with the patient in the lateral flexed position, with the involved side on stretch. The incision extends from the lumbar triangle (just below the twelfth rib) to a point 4 cm above the anterior superior

Fig. 40-33. Lumbar nephrectomy. (See text.)

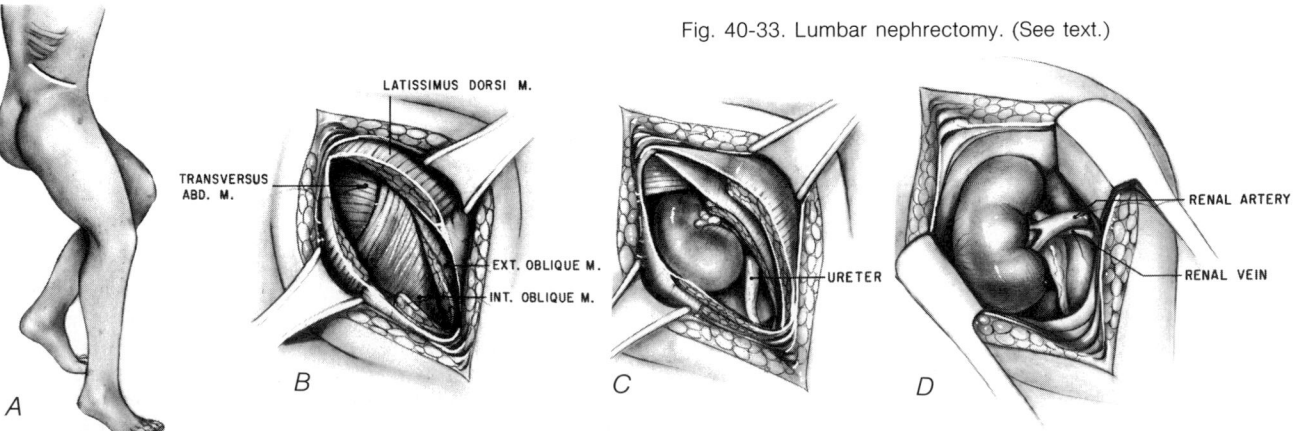

spine of the ileum. The latissimus dorsi and the external and internal oblique muscles are divided in the line of the incision. The transversus muscle is separated, and the aponeurosis of the transversus and the costovertebral ligament to the twelfth rib are divided. At the level of the internal oblique muscle, the large ilioinguinal nerve is encountered. After separating the transversus abdominis muscle in the line of its fibers, the retroperitoneum is exposed, and the peritoneum is displaced toward the midline. The fascia of Gerota is opened, thus exposing the kidney and the perinephric fatty tissue. The important structures within the renal pedicle are located anteriorly (ventrally). During mobilization of the kidney, particular care is necessary in the region of the upper pole because of the adrenal vessels and in the region of the lower pole because of aberrant arteries. Usually the renal artery and vein can be dissected free of fatty areolar tissue, so that individual ligation may be applied. Under adverse circumstances, a renal pedicle clamp can be used to control bleeding and permit transection of the hilus. Suture ligature of the renal pedicle en masse may fail to control the bleeding and can lead to arteriovenous fistula. Absorbable sutures are often used when wound infection is present. Whenever the urinary conductive passages are opened, it is advisable to institute drainage, and a latex tissue drain has been effective. The incision is closed in layers with chromic catgut with the exception of the skin, which is closed with nonabsorbable suture. Nonabsorbable sutures with increased tensile strength, such as Prolene, may be used in the fascia to increase the strength of closure in debilitated patients or those in whom poor wound healing is expected. The drain may be conveniently advanced so that it is removed on the fifth postoperative day.

Cutaneous Ureteroileostomy (Ileal Conduit)

Currently, the most popular method of supravesical urinary diversion for pelvic malignant tumors, neurogenic bladder dysfunction, and chronic lower urinary tract obstruction or infection with deterioration of renal function is cutaneous ureteroileostomy (Fig. 40-34). The major indications for this form of diversion are (1) required removal of the bladder and (2) poor urinary conduction from the kidney with accompanying reduced renal function. The disadvantages of the procedure are the extent of the operation and an increased incidence of postoperative complications compared to cutaneous ureterostomy or nephrostomy. Additional minor disadvantages include reabsorption of urea by the ileum and the requirement of a meticulously applied collection device. These disadvantages are counteracted by the advantages of the ileal conduit in providing a continuous unobstructed drainage of urine and its versatility in coping with varying requirements. The use of colon instead of ileum offers some advantages and is being utilized with increasing frequency (colon conduit).

Preoperative preparation is an integral part of the procedure and the blood volume, cardiac, pulmonary, and renal status should be optimal. Treatment of preexisting infections or metabolic disturbances should be instituted at this time. Antibacterial preparation of the intestinal tract is not necessary, but adequate deflation should be accomplished by a low-residue diet for 3 to 4 days. The urinary appliance should be worn by the patient preoperatively in order to determine his tolerance to adhesive and identify the optimal location of the stoma.

This procedure is best performed through a midline abdominal incision. Prior to making this incision, it is preferable to create the abdominal wall defect for the ileostomy. This results in the creation of a tract through muscles which have not been distorted by the major incision and avoids the problem of mechanical obstruction of the ileostomy. The abdomen is then entered. Appendectomy is performed. A segment of the ileum approximately 20 cm in length is selected for the formation of the conduit. A segment supplied by two arteries is preferred. The ileum is divided at the selected sites, and the isolated segment is irrigated with saline solution. The continuity of the ileum is restored, and the isolated ileal segment is positioned posterior to the ileoileal anastomosis. The proximal end of the ileal segment to be utilized for the conduit is closed with a continuous inverting chromic catgut suture. The left ureter is brought through the sigmoid mesentery and mobilized to provide length and eliminate the possibility of kinking or obstruction. The full thickness of ureter is sutured to the ileal mucosa. If the left ureter is markedly dilated, an end-to-end ureteroileostomy is performed. Calibrated catheters may be used to splint the anastomosis for a few days and to encourage good position of the ureters. The right ureter is anastomosed in a similar fashion over a catheter stent. The isolated segment of ileum and its mesentery are sutured to the posterior peritoneum to prevent an internal hernia. The distal end of the ileal conduit is brought to the previously prepared abdominal opening. The peritoneum or fascia is secured to the serosa of the ileum to prevent hernia. The ileostomy is everted and sutured to the skin and itself. A 1-cm protuberant cuff under no tension is considered optimal. Stay sutures may be used to reduce the tension on the wound, which is closed with catgut for the fascial layers and silk for the skin. A nasogastric tube is necessary postoperatively for 3 to 5 days. Another variation of the procedure involves the joining of both ureters together with one large stoma, which is then anastomosed to the proximal end of the ileal loop as a "cap." This may provide a larger anastomotic opening between the ureters and the segment of ileum and decrease the incidence of the complication of stricture at this vital site.

Cystostomy, Cystolithotomy

Surgical treatment of the bladder (Fig. 40-35) is facilitated by filling the organ, since this elevation the peritoneum out of the line of the incision. A low transverse abdominal incision 4 cm above the pubis is carried through the skin, subcutaneous tissue, and rectus abdominis fascia. The recti are mobilized from their midline attachments and separated. The bladder is easily recognized by its characteristic muscular and vascular pattern. The bladder

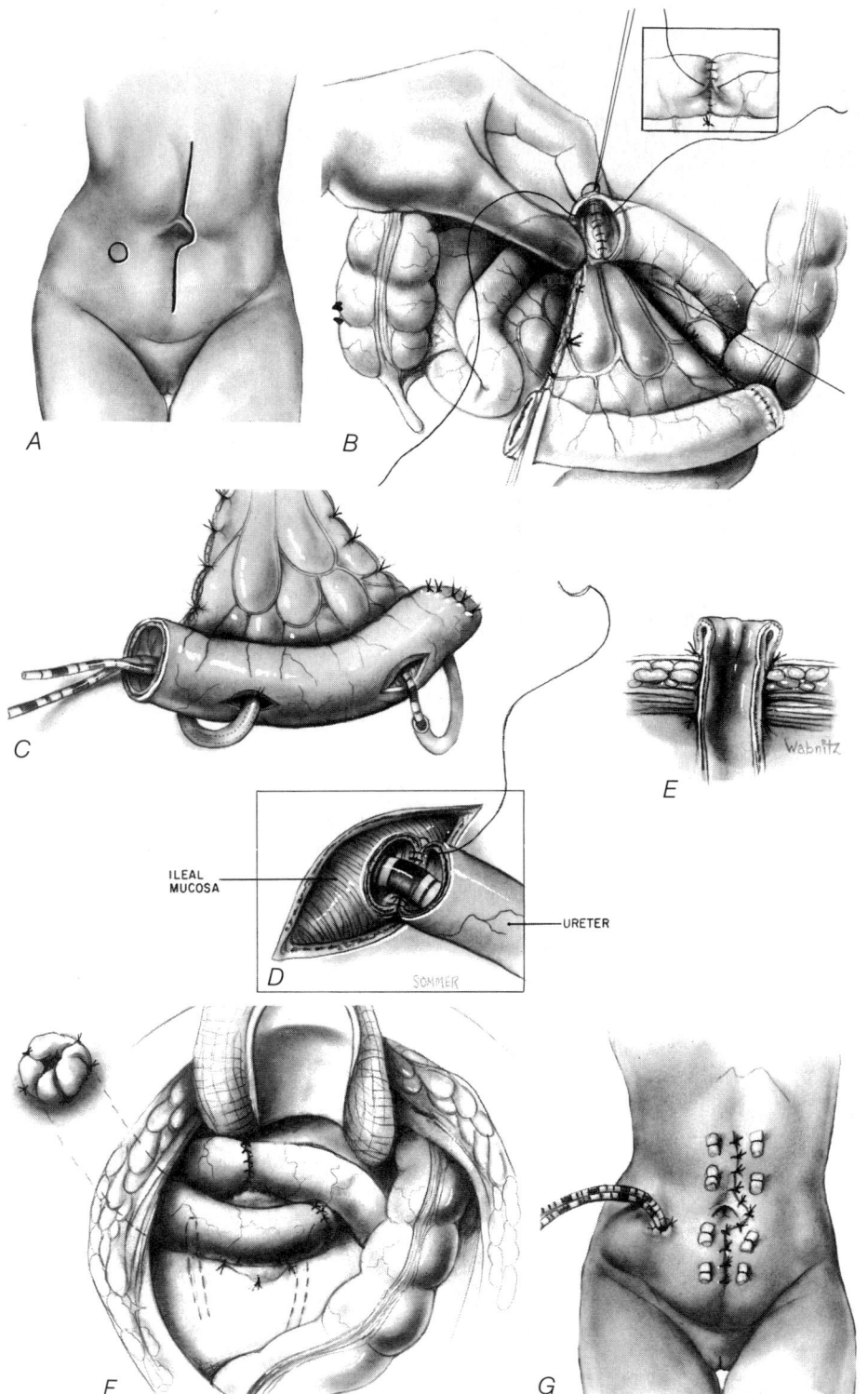

ILEAL
MUCOSA

URETER

Fig. 40-34. Cutaneous ureteroileostomy (ileal conduit).

Fig. 40-35. Cystostomy, cystolithotomy. (See text.)

is entered longitudinally, and if calculi are present, they can be removed digitally or with stone forceps. Thorough digital and visual exploration is indicated. Drainage is best provided by a de Pezzer or Malecot cystostomy catheter brought out through a stab wound above the incision. A prevesical tissue drain should be used and brought out through a separate stab wound below the incision. The bladder is closed with a one-layer continuous zero chromic catgut suture which incorporates the seromuscular wall of the bladder. The rectus fascia is approximated with interrupted zero chromic catgut sutures. The subcutaneous fat may be approximated with 3-0 interrupted plain catgut sutures and the skin edges with nonabsorbable suture material, such as 4-0 silk or nylon.

Prostatectomy (Fig. 40-36)

TRANSURETHRAL PROSTATECTOMY. The most commonly employed operation for removal of prostatic obstruction is the endoscopic approach. Following adequate dilatation of the urethra, the resectoscope sheath is inserted. Excellent visualization through the resectoscope allows for identification of the ureteral orifices, verumontanum, and external sphincter. With a cutting loop, the prostatic tissue is resected and hemostasis is secured with electrocoagulation. A catheter is inserted at the end of the procedure, and further hemostasis may be obtained by pulling the catheter bag against the bladder neck and prostatic fossa. This procedure is well tolerated by the patient, with minimal postoperative discomfort and early removal of the catheter. Contraindications to the transurethral resection are an excessively enlarged prostate gland and the presence of other intravesical pathologic conditions which warrant open exploration. The skilled operator is able to avoid the complications of excessive bleeding, ureteral orifice injury, perforation, and injury to the external sphincter. The results of this procedure are gratifying, and it can be performed on elderly, debilitated patients with minimal morbidity and mortality.

SUPRAPUBIC PROSTATECTOMY (Fig. 40-36C and D). This is performed through the cystostomy approach previously described. The compressed normal prostate represents the surgical capsule from which adenomatous tissue is mobilized by finger dissection. The prostatic urethra and adenomas are removed together. The distal urethral attachment is transected, and the prostatic fossa is packed while the prostatic arteries which are located on either side of the posterior bladder neck are suture ligated. Redundant mucosal fragments or small adenomas may be removed by sharp dissection. After the pack is removed, a #22, 30-cc urethral retention catheter is inserted. If oozing from the bladder neck or prostatic fossa occurs, gentle traction on the urethral catheter may effect hemostasis. A de Pezzer or Malecot catheter and tissue drain are employed in a similar fashion to that described for suprapubic cystostomy.

RETROPUBIC PROSTATECTOMY. This is also accomplished through the incision described for cystostomy. After the bladder wall is identified, the bladder is decompressed, and a 5-cm transverse incision is made 1.5 cm distal to the bladder neck. An alternative approach, known as a vesicocapsular prostatectomy, employs a vertical incision in line with the urethra and into the bladder and has the advantages of easier closure and avoidance of the anterior prostatic venous plexus. After the prostatic capsule is incised, the adenomas are mobilized by finger dissection. The distal urethra and bladder neck attachments are transected, and hemostasis is effected by suture ligature. The prostatic capsule is closed with interrupted catgut sutures, and a watertight closure is desirable. The bladder is drained by a retention catheter. Traction on the catheter following retropubic prostatectomy is not as effective for hemostasis as it is following transvesical prostatectomy and

may interfere with closure of the capsule. If additional security against catheter obstruction is desired, a suprapubic cystostomy can be performed.

PERINEAL PROSTATECTOMY (Fig. 40-36B). A curvilinear perineal incision extending from the two ischiorectal fossae is employed. The prostate is approached by dissecting along the anterior wall of the rectal ampulla. The central tendon is divided, and the portion of the levator ani which is attached to the membranous urethra is separated and reflected posteriorly. During this dissection, it is helpful to insert a urethral sound in order to identify the urethra. When the prostatic capsule is identified, a Young prostatic tractor is used to present the prostate into the perineal incision. After the apex has been carefully identified, two incisions extending laterally and superiorly in the shape of an inverted V prepare for the enucleation of the adenomas. Downward traction with a short Lowsley tractor which replaces the urethral tractor faciltates enucleation of the adenomas. Hemostasis is effected by suture of the bladder neck. A #22, 30-cc urethral retention catheter is inserted, and the prostatic capsule is closed with interrupted 2-0 chromic catgut sutures. A space between the prostate and the rectal ampulla is left open, and the levator ani muscles are brought together in the midline with interrupted chromic catgut. Subcutaneous tissues are closed with plain catgut, and a latex tissue drain is brought out through one corner of the incision. The skin is closed with nonabsorbable sutures.

Fig. 40-36. *A.* Types of open prostatectomy. *B.* Perineal prostatectomy. *C* and *D.* Suprapubic prostatectomy.

Fig. 40-37. Hydrocelectomy. (See text.)

Postoperative patency of the catheter is maintained by induction of osmotic diuresis. The suprapubic cystostomy catheter is usually removed in 24 to 48 hours, while the urethral catheter is usually not necessary after the fifth day.

POSTOPERATIVE MANAGEMENT. Postoperative patency of the catheter or catheters is maintained by irrigation. This may be carried out manually or by continuous drip irrigation. Continuous irrigation may be performed through a three-way catheter if there is no suprapubic tube present. If a suprapubic tube is present, the continuous irrigation flows from the urethral catheter through the bladder and out the suprapubic tube. The suprapubic cystostomy catheter is usually removed in 24 to 48 hours if good hemostasis is present. The urethral catheter is usually removed by the seventh postoperative day, and sooner if the retropubic or perineal approach has been used.

Hydrocelectomy (Fig. 40-37)

A vertical scrotal incision is usually employed. It is carried through the skin, dartos fascia, and overlying coverings of the hydrocele sac. It is desirable to avoid opening the hydrocele until the sac is totally mobilized. The tunica vaginalis is then opened and the excess tunica excised. Hemostasis is secured with multiple ligatures or electrocoagulation of the small bleeders in the cut edge. The edges of the tunica may be sutured together behind the testis with a continuous 3-0 chromic suture. If hemostasis is satisfactory, this may not be necessary. A drain may be brought out through a stab wound in a dependent portion of the scrotum if the hydrocele is excessively large, but in most instances a drain is not required. The incision is then closed in layers. A scrotal suspensory provides an excellent dressing in the postoperative period, and the use of an ice bag decreases the swelling. Hydrocelectomy in children is car-

Fig. 40-38. Inguinal orchiectomy. (See text.)

ried out through an inguinal incision so that an associated hernia can be repaired at the same time.

Inguinal Orchiectomy (Fig. 40-38)

This approach is utilized when a testicular tumor is suspected. It provides access to the spermatic vessels prior to manipulation of the testis. The incision is identical to that performed for repair of a hernia, and the spermatic cord is identified at the external inguinal ring. After a rubber-shod or bulldog clamp has been applied to the cord at this level, the testis is mobilized from its scrotal attachments and exteriorized through the inguinal incision. The tunica vaginalis is opened to permit examination of the testis, and if the lesion looks neoplastic, the cord is ligated and transected. Any solid lesion within the testis is considered potentially malignant, and biopsy is seldom performed. A metal clip is placed in the end of the remaining cord as a marker for future surgery or radiation therapy localization. After the testis has been removed, the inguinal incision is closed. The incision is *not* drained.

Transseptal Orchiopexy
(Fig. 40-39)

This has largely replaced the Thorek and Bevan procedures. The testis is identified through an inguinal incision which permits mobilization of the spermatic cord and correction of an indirect hernia which usually accompanies the undescended testis. After sufficient cord structures have been mobilized to permit placement of the testis in the scrotum, a small incision is made in the contralateral scrotum and a subdartos pouch is prepared to receive the cryptorchid testis. The scrotal septum is incised over a clamp, and traction is applied to the gubernaculum so that the testis is brought down through the scrotal septum into the contralateral scrotum. The septal defect may require a partial closure to prevent the testis from pulling back but should not be closed too tightly, since strangulation of the cord could occur. The scrotal and inguinal incisions are closed, and the patient is usually able to leave the hospital in 24 to 48 hours.

Bilateral Vasectomy (Fig. 40-40)

This male sterilization procedure usually is carried out under local anesthesia in an outpatient setting. Previous consultation with the patient and his wife has allowed for careful selection, instructions to the patient, and the signing of the required papers for sterilization and informed consent. The patient or his wife has been instructed to shave the scrotum on the night before the procedure, and the patient brings a scrotal suspensory with him to the office. The procedure is carried out with the patient in the lithotomy or supine position. The vas on one side is isolated between the thumb and index finger of the operator, and the overlying skin is infiltrated with 1% lidocaine or a similar local anesthetic agent. The underlying cord is also infiltrated. A towel clip is then used to isolate the vas. A small incision is made over the vas and it is delivered into the incision. An Allis clamp is then used to pick up the vas and separate it from the surrounding cord structures. The vas is then mobilized for approximately 3 cm. A segment measuring approximately 1 to 2 cm is excised between clamps. The edges of the vas are then transfixed with sutures. Another suture is placed approximately 1 cm below the previous suture and tied. The end of that suture is then passed through the end of the vas and tied, produc-

Fig. 40-39. Transseptal orchiopexy. (See text.)

Fig. 40-40. Vasectomy. *A.* Scrotal incision. *B.* Double ligation of vasa.

ing a means of bending the vas back on itself so that the ends are no longer in close proximity. One of the ends can also be buried in the adjacent tissues to prevent recanalization. An alternative technique involving electrocoagulation of the lumen of each end is commonly employed. After satisfactory hemostasis has been secured, the ends of the vas are dropped back into the incision. The edges of the skin and underlying dartos are then approximated. A similar procedure is then carried out on the other side. Incorporating the underlying dartos in the skin closure provides excellent hemostasis. A collodion dressing is then applied, and the patient uses the scrotal suspensory over a small gauze dressing. He is instructed to use an ice bag on that area for the remainder of the day and returns to work wearing the scrotal suspensory the following day. He is advised to expect a minimal amount of discomfort, swelling, and ecchymosis. When he resumes intercourse, he

continues contraception until an examination of his semen reveals no sperm. This usually requires a period of 6 weeks or at least 10 ejaculations to evacuate the remaining sperm which are distal to the anastomotic sites.

Vasovasostomy (Fig. 40-41)

This procedure is usually carried out on an in-hospital basis and with the patient under general anesthesia. An incision is made in the scrotum, and the underlying cord structures are delivered into view. The previous site of vasectomy is usually palpable unless a large segment of the vas has been excised. Magnifying lenses, or the use of the operating microscope, facilitate the operation and improve the results. Once the ends of the vas have been isolated, they are excised back to a normal-appearing vas deferens. The ends are then carefully approximated and sutured with 6-0 Prolene sutures. Finer suture material may be utilized when the operating microscope is employed. The lumen is usually reestablished by passage of some of the sutures through it. Care must be taken to prevent excessive tension on the completed anastomosis. Bleeding is minimal, and the reconstituted vas is then dropped back into the scrotum and the skin and dartos approximated. A similar procedure is then carried out on the other side. The patient is often able to leave the hospital the following day. Sperm may begin to appear in the ejaculate as early as 1 month following the procedure, but most often this does not occur until 2 or 3 months following the procedure, at which time the edema may subside enough to allow for passage of sperm through the small lumen of the vas deferens. Satisfactory reconstitution with sperm in the ejaculate occurs in

Fig. 40-41. Vasovasostomy. *A.* Scrotal incision. *B.* Excision of ligated (scarred) ends. *C.* Reanastomosis of ends, restoring continuity.

approximately 50 percent of cases. A higher percentage of success is reported when microsurgery is used. A satisfactory surgical result does not ensure that a pregnancy will result; other factors such as sperm quality and antisperm antibodies may play a role in persistent infertility.

References

Bagshaw, M. A., Ray, G. R., Pistenma, D. A., Castelino, R. A., and Meares, E. M., Jr.: External Beam Radiation Therapy of Primary Carcinoma of the Prostate, *Cancer,* **36:**723, 1975.

Bars, E., and Comarr, A. E.: "Neurological Urology," University Park Press, Baltimore, 1971.

Byar, D. R.: The Veterans Administration Cooperative Urological Research Group's Studies of Cancer of the Prostate, *Cancer,* **32:**1126, 1973.

Campbell, M. F., and Harrison, J. H. (eds.): "Urology," 3d ed., W. B. Saunders Company, Philadelphia, 1970.

Creevy, C. D.: The Correction of Hypospadias: A Review, *Urol Surv,* **8:**2, 1958.

D'Angio, G. J., Evans, A., et al.: Treatment of Wilms' Tumor: Results of the National Wilms' Tumor Study, *Cancer,* **38:**633, 1976.

Einhorn, L. H., and Donahue, J.: Cis-diaminodichloroplatinum, Vinblastine, and Bleomycin Combination Chemotherapy in Disseminated Testicular Cancer, *Ann Int Med,* **87:**293, 1977.

Farber, S.: Chemotherapy in Leukemia and Wilms' Tumor, *JAMA,* **198:**826, 1966.

Flocks, R. H.: Clinical Cancer of the Prostate: A Study of 4,000 Cases, *JAMA,* **193:**559, 1965.

Gartman, E.: The Significance of Hematuria in Young Men, *J Urol,* **75:**135, 1956.

Glenn, J. F. (ed.): "Urologic Surgery," 2d ed., Harper & Row, Hagerstown, 1975.

Herring, L. C.: Analysis of Ten Thousand Urinary Calculi, *J Urol,* **88:**545, 1962.

Hinman, F., Jr.: Vesical Defense against Infection, *Postgrad Med,* **37:**397, 1965.

Horton, C. E., and Devine, C. J.: Hypospadias and Epispadias, *Ciba Found Clin Symp,* vol. 24, no. 3, 1972.

Javadpour, N., and Scardino, P. T.: Recent Advances in Immunobiology of Genito-urinary Cancer, *Urology,* **9:**377, 1977.

Jewett, H. J., et al.: The Palpable Nodule of Prostatic Cancer: Results 15 Years after Radical Excision, *JAMA,* **203:**403, 1968.

Kelalis, P. P., King, L. R., and Belman, A. B. (eds.): "Clinical Pediatric Urology," W. B. Saunders Company, Philadelphia, 1976.

Lindberg, B.: Treatment of Rapidly Progressing Prostatic Carcinoma with Estracyt, *J Urol,* **108:**303, 1972.

Melicow, M., and Uson, A. C.: Palpable Masses in Infants and Children: A Report Based on a Review of 653 Cases, *J Urol,* **81:**705, 1959.

Symposium on Renal Lithiasis, William H. Boyce (guest editor), *Urol Clin North Am,* Vol 1(2) June, 1974.

Robson, C. J., Churchill, B. M., and Anderson, W.: Results of Radical Nephrectomy for Renal Cell Carcinoma, *Trans Am Assoc Genitourin Surg,* **60:**122, 1968.

Rubin, P. (ed.): "Current Concepts in Cancer," pts. IX–XX: Cancer of the Urogenital Tract, p. 117, American Medical Association, Chicago, 1974.

Skinner, D. G.: Non-seminomatous Testis Tumors: A Plan of Management Based on 96 Patients to Improve Survival in All Stages by Combined Therapeutic Modalities, *J Urol,* **115:**65, 1976.

Symposium on Urinary Calculi, *Am J Med,* vol. 45, November, 1968.

Van der Werf-Messing, B.: Carcinoma of the Bladder Treated by Preoperative Irradiation Followed by Cystectomy: Second Report, *Cancer,* **32:**1084, 1973.

Wax, S. H., and Frank, I. N.: A Retrospective Study of Upper Urinary Tract Calculi, *J Urol,* **94:**28, 1965.

Whitmore, W. F., Jr., et al.: Preoperative Irradiation with Cystectomy in the Management of Bladder Cancer, *Am J Roentgenol,* **102:**570, 1962.

Yendt, E. R., Gagne, R. J. A., and Cohanim, M.: The Effects of Thiazides in Idiopathic Hypercalcuria, *Am J Med Sci,* **251:**449, 1966.

Chapter 41

Gynecology

by **Arthur L. Herbst, Howard Ulfelder and Donald R. Tredway**

FEMALE REPRODUCTIVE TRACT

Embryologic Development

Fertilization of the ovum by a sperm carrying the X chromosome initiates the development of a feminine individual, but it is not before the eighth week that the structures specific for this sex attain noticeable dominance. These are the primordial ovaries and the Müllerian ducts. The latter drift medially and become fused throughout their lower two-thirds before the eleventh week of gestation; from this evolves the adult internal genital apparatus (Fig. 41-1). At the lower end it establishes communication with an entodermal derivative, the urogenital sinus, which, when fully differentiated, provides distinct and separate orifices for the urethra and vagina. The distal colon and anus lie well posterior.

The external genitalia begin as folds of ectoderm from the genital tubercle (clitoris), passing back on either side of the orifices and eventually forming the vulva with its major and minor labia (Fig. 41-2). The hymenal membrane partially occludes the vaginal canal at the level of the urogenital diaphragm, below the point of juncture between the urogenital sinus and the Müllerian ducts. Although the male structures (Wolffian ducts) normally regress, remnants can often be seen as small cystic swellings near the ovaries (parovarian cysts), as histologically recognizable rests in the broad ligaments or cervix, or as cystic tumors of the vagina (Gärtner's duct cysts).

A variety of anomalies of the tubes, uterus, cervix, and vagina have been described (Fig. 41-3). All are easily

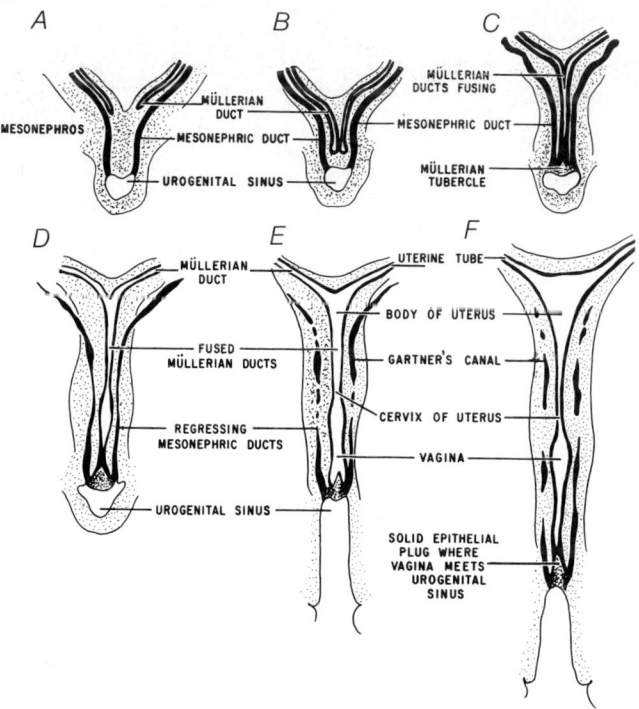

Fig. 41-1. Fusion of the Müllerian ducts to form the uterus and vagina. (*Redrawn after Koff, Carnegie Contributions to Embryology, vol. 24, 1933.*) *A.* 23 mm. *B.* 25 mm. *C.* 32.9 mm. *D.* 48 mm. *E.* 63 mm. *F.* 69 mm.

Fig. 41-2. Schematic diagram showing plan of developing female reproductive system. (*After B. M. Patton, "Human Embryology," 2d ed., McGraw-Hill Book Company, New York, 1953.*)

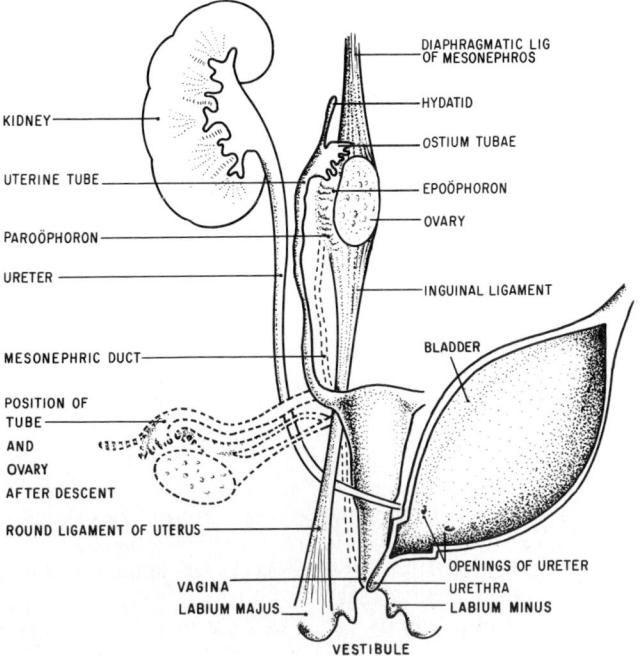

explained as improper Müllerian duct development, by partial or complete failure to fuse, by asymmetrical growth, or by unilateral or bilateral failure to develop at all. These Müllerian anomalies are frequently accompanied by renal (Wolffian) abnormalities, including absent or malformed kidneys; therefore an intravenous pyelogram (IVP) should be performed in individuals with these congenital uterine abnormalities. Abnormal development of the external genital structures usually takes the form of some degree of masculinization. There is enlargement of the clitoris and occasionally fusion of the labial folds caused by excessive androgen stimulation of the fetus in utero. When the hymen is imperforate, there is complete mechanical obstruction of the outlet of the vagina, usually resulting in a blood-filled pelvic mass, a "hematocolpos," first noted months or years after menstruation should have started. Transverse fibrous ridges of the vagina and cervix, as well as distortions of the cavity of the uterus, have been described in association with intrauterine exposure to diethylstilbestrol (DES) and similar compounds. These presumably result from a disturbance in the development of the Müllerian ducts; in the case of vaginal ridges, the urogenital sinus development may have been affected.

Morphologic Anatomy

EXTERNAL GENITALIA. The external genitalia are shown in Fig. 41-4. The entrance to the vagina (introitus) is bounded laterally by two folds of skin, the external labia majora and the internal labia minora. The labia majora form the lateral boundary of the vulva. They meet anteriorly toward the lower abdomen and fuse in an area over the pubis known as the "mons veneris." The posterior extensions of the labia meet in an area known as the "posterior commissure." Just above the posterior commissure is the caudal part of the vaginal opening known as the "posterior fourchette." The "vestibule" consists of that area into which the vagina and the urethra open and which is bounded laterally by the labia. The vulva includes both labia, the vestibular structures, and the clitoris. The clitoris lies immediately above the urethral meatus and is the analog of the male phallus. The "perineum" refers to the area between the rectum and the vagina, and it is through the tissues of this area that obstetric episiotomies are made.

Two types of glands can be considered with the external genitalia of the female. Skene's glands are located about the urethra and are important as a site of infection in cases of gonorrhea. Bartholin's glands supply lubrication to the vagina during times of sexual excitement and are located immediately deep to the labia majora. These glands can be invaded by bacterial organisms resulting in acute bartholinitis and Bartholin's abscesses.

INTERNAL GENITALIA. The internal genitalia and surrounding structures are demonstrated in Fig. 41-5. The uterus is divided into its main body (fundus) and lower portion (cervix). The fallopian tubes open into either side of the endometrial cavity of the uterus, traversing the wall of the uterus at the interstitial, or cornual, end of the tube. The tube widens throughout its course laterally to its ampullary, or infundibular, end. The ovaries are suspended

UTERUS SUBSEPTUS UNICOLLIS

UTERUS SEPTUS DUPLEX

UTERUS BICORNIS SEPTUS

UTERUS DIDELPHYS WITH DOUBLE VAGINA

UTERUS SEPTUS DUPLEX WITH DOUBLE VAGINA

ATRESIA AT LEVEL OF CERVIX

UTERUS BICORNIS UNICOLLIS WITH ONE
UNCONNECTED RUDIMENTARY HORN

UTERUS BICORNIS UNICOLLIS

Fig. 41-3. Schematic diagram of various types of abnormal uteri.

immediately posterior to the tubes by a mesentery (meso-varium). The round ligaments run laterally from the uterus through the inguinal ring in the anterior abdominal wall and end in the labia majora. They lie anteriorly to the fallopian tubes, a fact that is useful in orienting surgical specimens. The round ligament forms the apex for the folds of peritoneum that contain the uterine blood supply (broad ligament). At the base of the broad ligament, running from the cervix to the lateral pelvic wall, are important supporting structures known as the "cardinal" (Mackenrodt) ligaments. Posterior to these and running from the cervix to the sacrum are the uterosacral ligaments. These ligaments and the relationship of the cervix to the bladder and the rectum with the spaces surrounding these structures are shown in Fig. 41-6.

The blood supply to the female pelvis is illustrated in Fig. 41-7, which shows the distribution of the common iliac, external iliac, and internal iliac arteries (hypogastric arteries). It should be noted that the posterior division of the internal iliac artery gives off its superior gluteal branch and then continues further to split into its varying visceral branches. The remainder of the hypogastric artery continues inferiorly into the pelvis and gives off the obturator artery and the obliterated internal iliac artery distal to the superior vesical branch, which runs to the bladder; other branches, including the uterine artery, run to the central pelvic organs. Each ureter enters the pelvis near the bifurcation of a common iliac artery. It passes medial to the

internal iliac artery and runs immediately beneath the uterine artery, an important landmark in the anatomy of pelvic dissection (Fig. 41-32). The ureter then passes forward over the lateral aspect of the cervix and vagina to reach the bladder.

THE PELVIC ENVIRONMENT. Between the uterosacral ligaments anterior to the rectum and posterior to the cervix is a space known as the cul-de-sac, or pouch of Douglas, the most dependent extension of the free peritoneal cavity. This important area can be used for diagnostic exploration of the pelvis via the vagina. The uterosacral and cardinal ligaments form important stays for preventing prolapse of the uterus by helping to fix the position of the cervix back toward the hollow of the sacrum. Their effects can be

Fig. 41-4. External genitalia of the female.

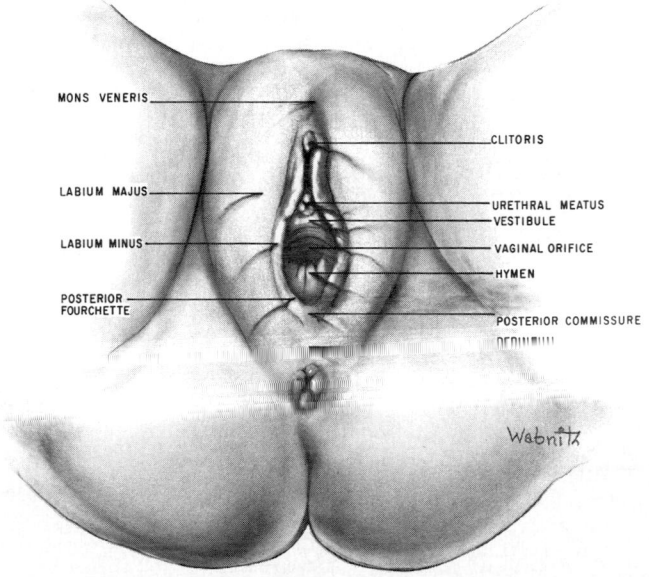

MONS VENERIS

CLITORIS

LABIUM MAJUS

URETHRAL MEATUS
VESTIBULE

LABIUM MINUS

VAGINAL ORIFICE

HYMEN

POSTERIOR
FOURCHETTE

POSTERIOR COMMISSURE
PERINEUM

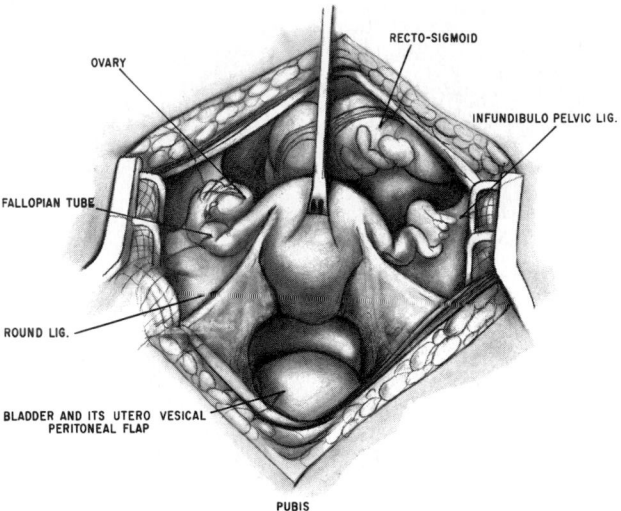

Fig. 41-5. Internal genitalia and surrounding structures.

demonstrated at the operating table by the great increase in mobility of the uterus and cervix after these ligaments are cut. The round ligament, though a firm structure, does not prevent descensus, i.e., downward motion of the uterus and cervix in the plane of the vagina. Changes in the length of the round ligaments do appear to accompany changes in the anterior or posterior orientation of the uterus and cervix. Posterior displacement of the fundus is termed "retroversion," a common finding in females during their reproductive years, especially following pregnancy. It is, in fact, so common that one should be extremely cautious before ascribing any pain or pelvic complaint to the existence of a retroverted uterus.

In addition to the ligamentous supports noted above, a firm and strong supportive shelf is provided by the levator ani muscles, as shown in Fig. 41-8. In the female this muscular complex is pierced by the urethra, vagina, and

Fig. 41-6. Diagrammatic cross section of the pelvis to show the concentration of connective tissue forming ligamentous bands, the junction with the cardinal ligament (Mackenrodt's ligament), and the spaces and tissue planes. (*From Peham and Amreich.*)

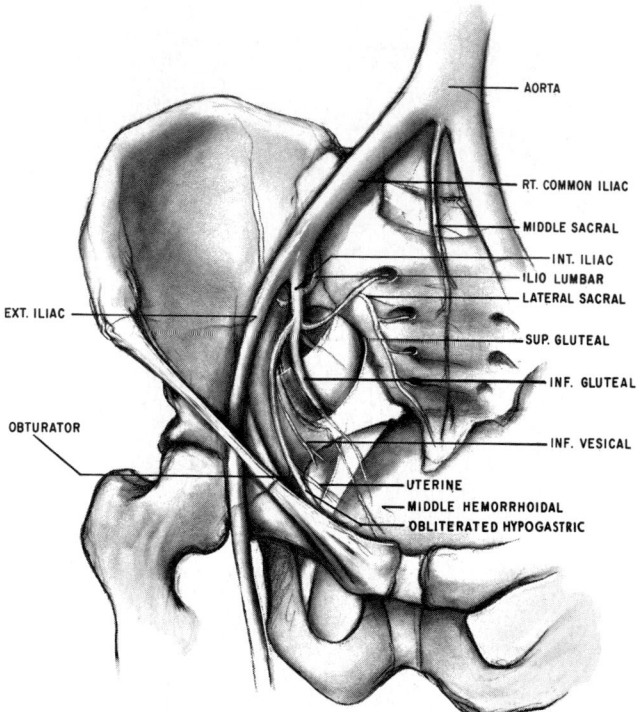

Fig. 41-7. Anterior and superior view of the arterial system of the pelvis showing the named primary arteries and their relationships to the bony and ligamentous structures.

rectum, and these orifices provide a structural weakness for the start of herniation that may be seen in adult life. A second layer of reinforcement beyond the shelf of the levator ani muscles is provided by the muscles of the urogenital diaphragm, which is located between the ischial tuberosities and the pubis, as shown in Fig. 41-9. This secondary layer provides muscular support anteriorly to the main mass of the levator ani muscle. Thus it can be

Fig. 41-8. Components of the levator muscles viewed from below.

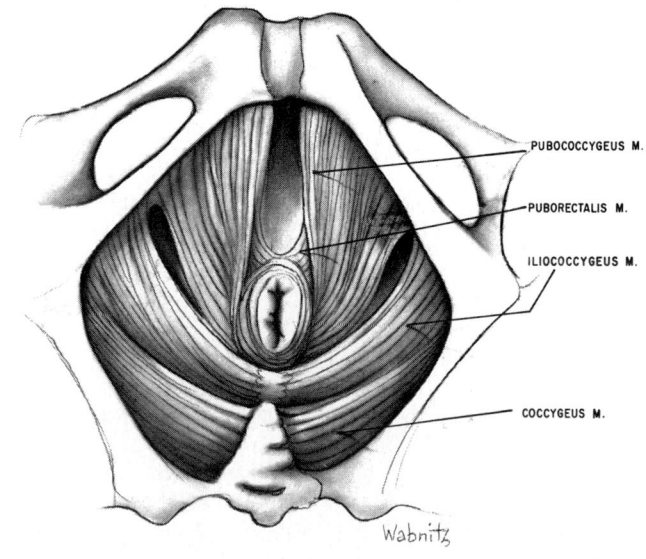

seen that in addition to the bony pelvis, the main support to the pelvic organs in the erect human female is provided by striated muscle, mainly of the levator ani complex, and partially by the urogenital diaphragm. The firm ligamentous attachments at the base of the cervix (the cardinal and uterosacral ligaments) stabilize the uterus at the apex of the vagina.

Weaknesses which give rise to various forms of herniation can occur in this area. Protrusion of the anterior vaginal wall, which includes the bladder, is referred to as a "cystocele," while protrusion of the posterior vaginal wall, which includes the rectum, is referred to as a "rectocele." The latter will occur especially after separation of the levator muscles following childbirth. If weakness develops in the area of the cul-de-sac, then this portion of the vaginal wall descends, occasionally accompanied by the small bowel, resulting in an "enterocele." A weakness can occur in the distal anterior vaginal wall with a bulging of the urethra. This occurs after destruction of the fascial support of the urethra and the bladder neck, and usually urinary incontinence accompanies the hernia in these patients. Weakness can develop in the ligamentous support of the uterus as well as in the muscular support, and this results in varying degrees of uterine and cervical prolapse, as illustrated in Fig. 41-10.

ENDOCRINOLOGY

Hypothalamic Releasing Factors and Gonadotropic Hormones

Releasing factors are polypeptides that originate from the base of the brain (hypothalamus) near the pituitary gland and affect secretion of all the various pituitary hormones. A decapeptide, luteinizing hormone releasing factor (LRF), has been identified and seems to control gonadotropin synthesis and release.

Gonadotropins, polypeptide hormones associated with carbohydrates (glycoproteins), stimulate the gonads. The gonadotropins of pituitary origin are follicle-stimulating hormone (FSH) and luteinizing hormone (LH). The development of sensitive radioimmunoassays for these hormones permits their measurement in human serum, allowing new and more precise investigation of their circulating levels in various physiologic as well as pathologic conditions.

FOLLICLE-STIMULATING HORMONE (FSH). In the female, in the presence of small amounts of LH, this hormone stimulates the immature ovarian follicle to antral formation (Fig. 41-11). In the male, FSH stimulates the cells of the seminiferous tubules and increases spermatogenesis.

LUTEINIZING HORMONE (LH, ICSH). This is the ovulatory hormone. Ovulation occurs after the midcycle LH surge (Fig. 41-11), and luteinization of the ovarian theca cells occurs following the rupture of the graafian follicle. Although another stimulant, luteotropic hormone (LTH), maintains corpus luteum function in rats, only LH appears to have any relation to corpus luteum activity in man. In

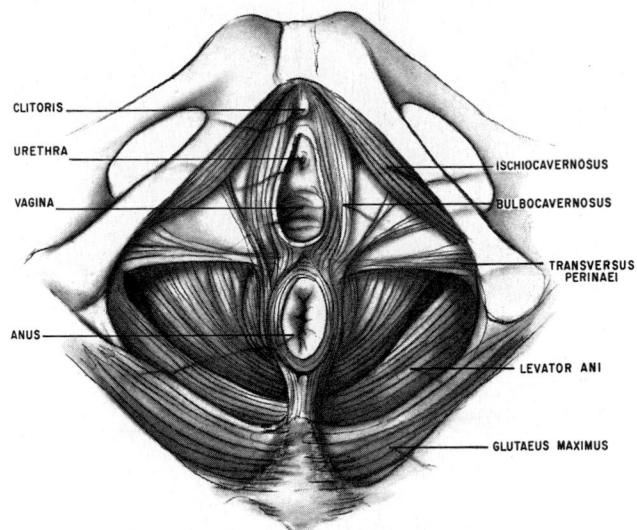

Fig. 41-9. Superficial layer of the urogenital diaphragm in the female.

the male LH stimulates the Leydig cells (interstitial cells), causing androgen secretion. Administration of ovulatory-suppressing oral contraceptives abolishes this peak.

HUMAN CHORIONIC GONADOTROPIN (HCG). This hormone is normally secreted in the human being by the placenta during pregnancy. It is occasionally elaborated by testicular or ovarian tumors. In the pregnant female, it can be detected in the second week of pregnancy or at about the time of the missed period, when it appears in the urine as well as other body fluids. This hormone is secreted maximally in about the third month of pregnancy and then decreases. It rapidly disappears approximately 2 weeks after delivery. Excessive quantities of HCG are secreted by patients with trophoblastic disease (hydatidiform mole and choriocarcinoma). The hormone has primarily a luteinizing effect, although it is not chemically identical with LH from the anterior pituitary. Its biologic action in various animals has formed the basis of many pregnancy tests. HCG causes hemorrhagic follicles and corpora lutea formation in immature mice (Aschheim-Zondek test) and in mature female rabbits (Friedman test).

Fig. 41-10. Diagrammatic representation of first- and second-degree prolapses of the uterus.

NORMAL POSITION

COMPLETE PROLAPSE

The Menstrual Cycle

Fig. 41-11. Hormonal changes during the menstrual cycle.

It also causes spermiation in the toad and frog, making possible the highly sensitive biologic *Rana pipiens* test. Although chorionic gonadotropin is secreted and is detectable by the time of the first missed period, most of these biologic tests do not become positive until 1 or 2 weeks after the first missed period and occasionally even later. The biologic tests now are rarely used clinically. They have been replaced by immunologic assays which are usually based on agglutination of sensitized red cells or latex particles. These immunologic assays are sensitive and clinically useful tools, although false-positive and false-negative reactions can result with these as well as with biologic assays. Radioimmunoassays permit precise and sensitive measurement of HCG and β-HCG in serum and urine and are useful for monitoring patients who have been treated for trophoblastic disease.

Clinical Gonadotropic Estimation. Many clinical studies dealing with problems of reproduction have noted altered gonadotropic activities in terms of the bioassays and radioimmunoassays. Low levels suggest lack of gonadotropic secretion from the anterior pituitary. Very high levels are detected during the menopause and in cases of premature ovarian failure due to excessive gonadotropin production from the pituitary. The urine bioassays are much less accurate than serum assays, which permit measurement of FSH and LH.

Steroid Hormones

A schema of steroid metabolism, starting with cholesterol and ending with estrogen, is shown in Fig. 41-12. However, for simplicity alternative pathways and many steps are omitted.

ESTROGENS

These are female sex hormones secreted primarily from the ovary with a small contribution from the adrenal. In the pregnant female the placenta is a major source of both estrogen and progesterone. Estrogens occur in many chemical forms but in the urine they are usually measured as estrone, estradiol, and estriol. Recent development of sensitive competitive binding assays has allowed their measurement in serum. They are secreted throughout the menstrual cycle, with greater quantities detected after ovulation (Fig. 41-11). These hormones cause an increase in the size of genital tissues, i.e., of the uterus, fallopian tubes, and breasts. Under their stimulation, there is increased mitotic activity in both the myometrium and endometrium. The vaginal mucosa thickens with proliferation of vaginal epithelium and cornification of surface cells. With increased glycogen deposition in the vaginal cells and under the action of the Döderlein bacilli, lactic acid is formed, decreasing the pH of the vagina and providing some protection against vaginal infection.

In addition to the effect on the myometrium, estrogens may cause a growth in the size of fibroids (leiomyomas), a fact that should be remembered when giving patients estrogen-containing oral contraceptives.

PROGESTERONE

This hormone is secreted throughout the cycle but is released in significant quantities mainly from the corpus luteum after the rupture of the graafian follicle (Fig. 41-11). Therefore, changes induced by this increase in progesterone are taken to be reasonable circumstantial evidence for the occurrence of ovulation. However, the only proof of ovulation in the human being is pregnancy, since progesterone can be secreted from an ovary which has undergone theca luteinization without corpus luteum formation.

Progesterone is thermogenic and, as a result, causes a rise of $\frac{1}{2}$ to 1°F in body temperature. This is the basis of the use of a monthly basal body temperature chart as an indirect indication of ovulation. Progesterone can be measured chemically in serum by competitive binding radioimmunoassays available in research laboratories and more recently in commercial laboratories. It can be indirectly measured in the urine in the form of its metabolite, pregnanediol, and 5 to 10 mg/24 hours are usually excreted during the secretory phase of the menstrual cycle.

ANDROGENS

The normal ovary secretes a small amount of androgens during the normal cycle, with a small midcycle peak. As one follicle develops, the other follicles become atretic and stromal cells are formed. These stromal cells secrete prin-

Fig. 41-12. Abbreviated schema of steroid metabolism.

cipally the 17 β-hydroxysteroids (androstenedione, testosterone, etc.).

17-Ketosteroid determinations have been used as an assessment of androgen function. These metabolic products of adrenal and testicular secretion are measurable in the urine. There is only a small contribution from the ovary in the female. Although 17-ketosteroid output may be elevated in certain masculinizing conditions, it is not necessarily a good guide to androgenic function in the female. For example, doubled secretion of testosterone, a potent androgenic hormone, from the adrenal or the ovary would cause very noticeable masculinizing effects. However, because of the small amount of this hormone that would be chemically present, there would not be any detectable change in the 17-ketosteroid output. The recent availability of sensitive radioimmunoassays to measure serum testosterone and other androgens permits more precise investigation of masculinizing conditions.

Hormonal Events in the Menstrual Cycle

At this point it is important to note the dynamic relationship of these hormones during the menstrual cycle. The menstrual cycle can be described in three phases: the follicular, ovulatory, and luteal phases. These phases are determined by the steroid, gonadotropin, and hypothalamic feedback mechanisms.

During the reproductive life of the female, a certain number of follicles begin to grow. The mechanisms that determine which follicles or how many will grow per cycle are undetermined. This selection is probably a matter of timing and morphologic characteristic. Shortly before menses, a rise in FSH (Fig. 41-11) results in stimulation of a follicle or follicles. This rise in FSH probably represents an escape from the negative feedback of estradiol during the previous luteal phase. However, the estradiol level never becomes low enough in the normal menstrual cycle to allow a negative feedback escape for LH. Consequently LH is probably not essential in initiation of the menstrual cycle.

As the follicle grows there is a concomitant rise in estradiol level. The source of estradiol seems to be predominantly the thecal cells surrounding the follicle. With a rise in level of estradiol the negative feedback of FSH occurs and FSH levels begin to drop. The little amount of FSH that remains probably is selectively bound in the developing follicle as a result of the high follicular levels of estradiol. Thus the follicle continues to develop, and this mechanism ensures that only one follicle will reach ovulation. As midcycle approaches, the lesser follicles begin to undergo atresia.

At midcycle a surge of estradiol triggers a midcycle surge of LH and also a small surge of FSH. The actual release of the egg occurs approximately 24 hours after this LH peak. The LH surge also results in the beginning luteinization of the follicle. Consequently, at midcycle the progesterone level begins to rise and remains elevated during the luteal phase.

During the luteal phase, progesterone has a negative effect on LH, especially in the presence of estradiol. FSH is also suppressed because of the high estradiol levels. Although suppressed, small amounts of gonadotropins, especially LH, are necessary for normal corpus luteum function. Also for the first few days after ovulation the granulosa cells enlarge and capillaries penetrate into the granulosa layer, often filling the central cavity with blood. The peak of vascularization occurs by day 8 or 9 after ovulation and is usually associated with the peak serum levels of progesterone and estradiol. After this the corpus luteum enters a period of regression, as noted by decreasing progesterone levels. This life-span for the corpus luteum is consistently 14 days. At the end of this time the steroid levels fall and the whole cycle begins again with menses.

Fig. 41-13. *A.* Proliferative endometrium. *B.* Secretory endometrium.

With pregnancy, survival of the corpus luteum is prolonged by the trophoblastic production of HCG. This new stimulus first appears at the peak of corpus luteum development, just in time to prevent luteal regression. HCG then maintains the corpus luteum until 8 to 10 weeks of gestation, by which time placental steroidogenesis is established.

The gonadotropins are under the control of hypothlamic releasing factors. LRF seems to control both FSH and LH functions. The control of the reproductive cycle seems to depend upon the level of LRF at any given moment. This function, in turn, seems to depend upon complex and coordinated interrelationships among the releasing factor(s), other neurohormones, pituitary gonadotropins, and gonadal steroids. These relationships are governed by feedback mechanisms of both stimulatory and inhibitory nature.

CHRONOLOGIC DEVELOPMENTAL FEMALE PHYSIOLOGY

The normal female infant is born with a small uterus, most of which consists of cervix. The ovaries and fallopian tubes are present but much smaller than in the adult. A small vagina opens to the exterior through the folds of the hymenal ring. Except for the effects of maternal hormones that may be present immediately after birth, the female infant has little, if any, gonadotropin or ovarian hormone present.

Normally puberty will begin between the ages of nine and seventeen (average at twelve and one-half) years of age. If menstruation occurs prior to age nine, precocious puberty is diagnosed, while menstruation after age seventeen warrants the diagnosis of delayed puberty. It appears that menstrual function begins earlier in Western populations, possibly as the result of improved hygiene and nutrition.

The first anatomic evidence of puberty is development of breast budding and then of pubic hair at about the age of ten or eleven. In addition there is an increase in the size of the internal and external genitalia. The uterine fundus increases in volume at a greater rate than the cervix, and in the adult the uterine fundus is approximately twice the size of the cervix. Axillary hair also develops during puberty, but this usually does not take place until after breast and pubic hair development. The adolescent growth spurt is also occurring at this time.

Menstrual bleeding usually follows the development of the secondary sexual characteristics already described. Initial bleeding is usually anovulatory and irregular. Ovulatory cycles, which may occur at 4- to 6-week intervals, begin in about 1 year. Their onset is often heralded by pelvic pain occurring at the time of menses. The characteristic hormonal changes which occur during the menstrual cycle are illustrated in Fig. 41-11. By definition the first day of menstrual bleeding is considered to be day 1 of the cycle. The average volume of blood loss during a normal menstrual cycle is estimated to be from 35 to 150 ml, and it will usually last from 3 to 6 days, with much individual variation. An interval between menses of 6 to 8 weeks is not uncommon.

During menstruation the superficial layers of endometrium are cast off, leaving the stratum basalis and much of the stratum spongiosum, which lies superficial to the basalis, in situ and ready to begin regeneration during the cycle. Estrogen stimulation during the first part of the menstrual cycle causes mitoses in the endometrial glands and stroma, resulting in a proliferative endometrial pattern (Fig. 41-13A). During this proliferative phase of the cycle the endometrium increases in thickness. As the middle of the cycle approaches, estrogen output from the ovary increases (Fig. 41-11). Ovulation occurs, and corpus luteum formation resulting in progesterone secretion follows. Progesterone stimulates coiling of the glands of the endometrium, which become filled with fluid, resulting in a secretory pattern (Fig. 41-13B).

The cervical mucus and vaginal cytologic features are also altered during the menstrual cycle. In the proliferative phase the cervical mucus forms a fernlike pattern when it is allowed to dry. At ovulation the volume of cervical mucus greatly increases. It becomes tenacious and can be drawn into a long thread (*Spinn barkheit* phenomenon). At this time the mucus is maximally receptive to sperm and thus ideally suited to fertilization of the recently released ovum. The cervical mucus then decreases in volume, and because of the influence of progesterone, loses its ability to fern. Serial examination of the vaginal smear during the proliferative phase of the cycle shows a gradual increase in the number of superficial cornified cells. After ovulation these cells are less prevalent because of the influence of progesterone. Thus, a rough estimate of hormonal status can be gained by examining the cervical mucus and vaginal smear during the menstrual cycle.

As menopause approaches, anovulatory periods begin to occur with increased frequency. Occasionally a period will be missed or will come later than expected. Menopausal bleeding is characterized by skips and delays. If menses are absent for more than 6 months, any subsequent vaginal bleeding should be considered abnormal and deserves further investigation. With the decrease in hormonal function and drop in estrogen output, there is a concomitant rise in gonadotropin secretion. The vaginal pH becomes more alkaline, because of decrease in glycogenation of the vaginal epithelium and decreased action of the Döderlein bacillus. The vaginal mucosa becomes thinner and is more prone to secondary infection. The patient may complain of sudden and sharp feelings of heat (hot flashes), which can usually be controlled by small doses of oral estrogen.

GYNECOLOGIC EXAMINATION

The gynecologic history includes careful attention to all the details of menstrual and reproductive function such as onset and frequency of menstruation, length and amount of menstrual bleeding, and the dates of the two most recent menstrual periods. If pain is a problem, when does it occur? Is it related to the menstrual cycle? Where

is it? How severe is it? Does it radiate? What relieves it, and what, if anything, makes it worse? Are there any urinary or gastrointestinal symptoms? Physical examination includes pelvic examination, which is most comfortably done with the patient in the lithotomy position, suitably draped and always accompanied by a nurse chaperone. The external genitalia are first visualized, special note being made of hair distribution, the size of the clitoris, the patency of the hymen, and any enlargements or inflammations, such as may be associated with Bartholin's glands. Skin lesions, such as may be seen with venereal infection, and vaginal discharges are also noted. The cervix is exposed with a water-lubricated speculum. Surgical jelly is not used because it will interfere with cytologic sampling (PAP smear). After cytologic sampling is complete, a bimanual examination is carried out and palpation performed, as illustrated in Fig. 41-14. First the fundus is felt; its position, its size, and the contour of the surface are noted. Leiomyomas (fibroids) cause smooth irregularities in the uterine surface which may vary in size from a few millimeters to several centimeters. A smooth indentation at the apex of the fundus may suggest a bicornuate or arcuate uterus. The left and right adnexal regions are then carefully palpated bimanually. The patient is asked to cough, and the support of the pelvis is carefully noted. If there is a weakness in the anterior wall (cystocele), the support of the urethra is carefully examined, and the patient is evaluated for stress incontinence. Separation of the levators will develop a weakness and herniation of the posterior vaginal wall (rectocele), and occasionally these may become sufficiently severe to cause constipation. Herniation near the apex of the vagina between the uterosacral ligaments usually contains small bowel (enterocele) and frequently is seen in patients with pelvic relaxation. If the ligamentous attachment and levator supports of the uterus and cervix should become weakened, descensus will be noted, and occasionally the cervix may even be seen to protrude through the introitus. Finally a rectal examination is performed, both to confirm the findings of the vaginal examination and also to palpate carefully the uterosacral ligaments, the back of the cervix and uterus, and the contents

Fig. 41-14. *A*. Bimanual abdominovaginal palpation of the uterus. *B*. Bimanual abdominovaginal palpation of the adnexa.

A   B

of the cul-de-sac (pouch of Douglas). These areas are often sites of nodularity and tenderness in cases of endometriosis and are important areas to be checked for spread in cases of cervical carcinoma.

SYMPTOMS

Pain

Cyclic pain associated with the menstrual cycle is known as *"dysmenorrhea."* When no demonstrable pathologic condition is present, the diagnosis is "primary, or idiopathic, dysmenorrhea." This is thought to occur only at the end of the ovulatory cycle. It would appear that some of the pain associated with menstrual bleeding is caused by the dilatation of the cervix due to mechanical stretching of the endocervical canal that accompanies the passage of blood and clot. This pain sensation is believed to be transmitted to the cervicouterine ganglion (Frankenhäuser's plexus) which is located on the posterior wall of the uterus near the uterosacral ligaments. Pain is then transmitted via the hypogastric presacral plexus to the spinal cord, to enter at the level of approximately T_{11} and T_{12}. The pain is usually sharp and may occasionally be colicky. It is usually confined to the lower abdomen and can radiate to the back and sides. The patient often complains of a dull, heavy ache and may also have nausea and a feeling of bloating. In severe cases there may even be vomiting.

The pain may begin prior to, or just with, the onset of menstruation, but as a rule the worst pain occurs early during the menstrual flow. It may be that some of the menstrual pain is due to hyperirritability and irregular contractions of the uterine musculature in addition to the dilatation of the cervix. Constriction of the spiral arterioles in the uterine musculature may result in ischemic pain, which could contribute to the discomfort noted at the time of the menstrual flow.

In dealing with primary dysmenorrhea and premenstrual tension, conservative measures are usually the best. Simple analgesics, such as aspirin and occasionally codeine, are helpful. Sympathomimetic drugs are helpful for menstrual cramps. For those patients who complain of premenstrual tension and the feeling of bloating prior to the onset of menses, salt restriction and even diuretics for approximately a week prior to the onset of menses and for the first few days of the cycle may give symptomatic relief. Since these symptoms are noted with ovulatory cycles, a severe case can be treated by the administration of cyclic oral contraceptives. If all these measures fail and the patient is either incapacitated by pain or requires long-term narcotics for its control, then surgical therapy can be tried. In such cases, removal of the hypogastric plexus, i.e., a presacral neurectomy, is indicated. Care should be taken to remove all the nerve tissue located anterior to the sacrum, which means a complete dissection between the hypogastric vessels and identification of both ureters. It is almost never necessary to undertake this procedure for primary dysmenorrhea.

In cases where there is demonstrable pathology, the term "secondary dysmenorrhea" is applied to the menstrual pain. It is treated by attempts to correct the specific cause. One of the most common causes is endometriosis. The patients complain of severe and increasing menstrual discomfort that progressively becomes worse. A few patients have an extremely tight cervical os, either on a congenital basis or as the result of extensive cauterization or cryosurgical treatment, and nulliparous females are especially prone to stenosis. In such cases, dilation of the stenosed cervix may occasionally help. Some patients will have acute pain and some fever, with diffuse abdominal symptoms at the time of menses. These patients are often previous victims of pelvic inflammation, and their pain during menstruation is believed to be associated with the residual effects of chronic pelvic inflammatory disease (PID). Occasionally, pain is related to an endometrial polyp or an intraluminal fibroid (leiomyoma) which is being extruded from the uterine cavity.

Lower abdominal pain may occur at times other than during menstruation. Chronic pelvic inflammation and adhesions can cause diffuse nonmenstrual abdominal pain. These patients have vague and continuous symptoms of pelvic pain. Pain coming in the middle of the cycle at about the tenth or fourteenth day of the period should suggest ovulation pain (mittelschmerz) or a ruptured ovarian cyst. Ectopic pregnancy should be considered in patients with midcycle pain, especially if the previous period is scanty or of an irregular nature.

Both the gastrointestinal and genitourinary tract can cause pelvic symptoms, and it is important to consider the kidney, ureters, the appendix, and the lower bowel in any evaluation of pelvic pain.

GYNECOLOGIC EVALUATION OF ACUTE ABDOMINAL PAIN. An assessment of the female patient with acute lower abdominal pain necessitates separation of those problems which require operative intervention from cases in which surgical treatment is unnecessary or even undesirable. Ectopic pregnancy, twisted ovarian cyst, ruptured tubo-ovarian abscess, and appendicitis all require surgical intervention, while a ruptured corpus luteum cyst usually requires no therapy and acute pelvic inflammation is preferably treated without surgical intervention. The character and location of the pain combined with the patient's history and physical findings usually provide sufficient clues to lead to a reasonable therapeutic course.

Pregnancy symptoms combined with an adnexal mass suggest ectopic pregnancy. Pain, when present, is often unilateral. Bilateral lower abdominal pain intensified by cervical motion and accompanied by fever is usually seen in patients with acute pelvic inflammatory disease. A tender adnexal mass may be an ovarian cyst, an ectopic pregnancy, or an inflammatory mass. An accompanying high fever and high white blood cell count suggest tuboovarian abscess or pyosalpinx. Further details to be considered in the differential diagnosis of lower abdominal pain in the female patient are discussed in the sections on pelvic inflammatory disease and ectopic pregnancy.

When a pathologic condition of the tube or ovary is suspected (ectopic pregnancy, ruptured ovarian cyst), direct visualization of the internal genitalia through the laparoscope (Fig. 41-15) can provide an accurate diagnosis. The procedure is carried out in the operating room under general and occasionally local anesthesia. The laparoscope is usually introduced through a small subumbilical incision after carbon dioxide has been introduced to distend the peritoneal cavity. The laparoscope provides an excellent view of the pelvis and intraabdominal contents. Laparoscopy is usually performed with the patient in the Trendelenburg position. A second small probe introduced a few centimeters above the symphysis aids in manipulation and helps to provide a complete evaluation of the internal genitalia.

Disorders of Support—Pelvic Hernias and Urinary Incontinence

The involuntary loss of urine is termed "incontinence." If this follows coughing, sneezing, or straining, the term "stress incontinence" applies. Stress incontinence is secondary to inadequate pelvic support and must be differentiated from other causes of incontinence. "Urgency incontinence" is characterized by an involuntary loss of urine accompanied by a frequent urge to urinate. This suggests

Fig. 41-15. *A.* Method of transparietal laparoscopy. (*After Steploes.*) *B.* View of laparoscopy of normal uterus and adnexa with minimal endometriosis. (*After M. R. Cohen.*) Figure reprinted from Gynecological Laparoscopy, Symposia Specialists, P.O. Box 610397, Miami, Fl. 33161.

a urinary tract infection, nonspecific inflammation at the base of the bladder (trigonitis), or occasionally bladder sphincteric spasm. "Overflow incontinence" is due to persistently large, retained urinary volumes which occur in neurogenic atonic bladders of diabetics and are associated with large cystoceles. The involuntary loss of urine unassociated with stress is a characteristic of neurologic disease, such as multiple sclerosis. Involuntary loss of urine occurs with vesicovaginal or urethrovaginal fistulas.

Once it has been established that the patient has stress incontinence requiring correction, further evaluation should include urine culture to rule out urinary tract infection, cystoscopy to rule out trigonitis, a demonstration of stress incontinence at the time of pelvic examination and correction of this when the examiner elevates the bladder neck in such a way as to restore the posterior urethrovesical angle to prevent the loss of urine (Marshall test). Finally, a cystometrogram and measurement of postvoiding residual urine are important to rule out neurogenic causes of urinary complaints. Some investigators find x-ray definition of the posterior urethrovesical angle helpful in evaluating the extent of anatomic derangement.

CONSIDERATIONS IN THE THERAPY OF PELVIC RELAXATION AND URINARY STRESS INCONTINENCE. In certain cases, the amount of stress incontinence is mild. The patient can be helped by practicing starting and stopping her urinary stream during the course of voiding (Kegel exercises). If the patient is found to have urinary frequency and urgency, then conservative therapy of antispasmodics is occasionally helpful. Dilation of the vesical sphincter may give symptomatic relief, especially in elderly patients

A

CUL-DE-SAC
ENDOMETRIOSIS

L. ADNEXA   OVARY

TUBE

L. UTEROSACRAL
LIG.

UTERUS

R. ADNEXA

R. UTEROSACRAL
LIG.

BOWEL

B

troubled with nocturia. Surgical intervention is indicated for those patients who are wet much of the time and suffer social embarrassment or limitation as a result of urinary stress incontinence. If there is simple loss of the posterior urethrovesical angle without a change in the angle of the urethra with respect to the horizontal axis when the patient strains, then the patient is said to have Type I stress incontinence. If, in addition to the loss of the posterior urethrovesical angle, there is rotational descent of the urethra with respect to the horizontal axis, then Type II stress incontinence exists.

If a patient complains of stress incontinence and is noted to have a cystocele and rectocele without descent of the uterus and cervix, then an anterior and posterior colporrhaphy should usually provide a good repair. In deciding whether or not to repair a cystocele, not only is the size of the hernia important but also the degree to which the patient is bothered by it, including prior urinary symptoms. If she has not had stress incontinence but appears to have had recurrent urinary tract infection or overflow incontinence due to a persistently large residual urine as a result of the cystocele, then a repair is also indicated. However, surgical repair is not indicated if the cystocele is asymptomatic and there have been no prior related complaints.

During the repair, the posterior urethrovesical angle is supported, and a sharp angulation of approximately 90° is reconstructed in this area. This is necessary not only to repair the causes of stress incontinence but also to avoid a flattening of the angle at the time of routine cystocele repair, which can lead to post-cystocele-repair stress incontinence. Support of the posterior vaginal wall must be achieved at the time of perineal repair by approximating the pubococcygeus muscle, which reconstitutes the muscular support of the pelvic floor. It is probably wise to avoid repairs in patients wishing to have more children.

If in addition to the above complaints, the patient has descensus of the uterus, then a vaginal hysterectomy may be combined with the repair. When a vaginal hysterectomy is done, the uterosacral ligaments should be used for apical vaginal supports, both to support the vagina and to prevent future enterocele. In certain cases, there is elongation of the cervix with moderately good support of the fundus, in which case a cervicectomy (Manchester-Fothergill operation) can be performed. This operation is also used in cases where there is a severe symptomatic pelvic hernia in patients who wish to preserve childbearing function. Although vaginal hysterectomy can usually be accomplished at the time of most repairs, there are certain relative contraindications:

1. A greatly enlarged uterus, since it is unwise to attempt vaginal hysterectomy if the uterus is much larger than 10 or 12 cm. In many cases an enlarged descended uterus may be removed by splitting it into many small pieces during dissection (morcellation).
2. Extensive pelvic adhesions from previous infection or surgical treatment.
3. A previous abdominal uterine suspension, since the fundus is firmly adherent to the anterior abdominal wall.

If severe stress incontinence exists, especially without uterine descensus, it is less likely that a good repair can be obtained by the vaginal approach. However, in certain obese patients, this approach still can be used with hope of success. In most cases, a Marshall-Marchetti procedure is accomplished by a dissection of the retropubic space of Retzius. The urethra and bladder neck are supported anteriorly toward the symphysis by paraurethral sutures which restore the posterior urethrovesical angle. This operation is also used to treat recurrent stress incontinence previously treated by vaginal repair. If there is failure following Marshall-Marchetti repair, then a second Marshall-Marchetti procedure is occasionally attempted or a sling procedure may be carried out. The latter consists of a repeat dissection of the space of Retzius and also the urethra A strip of anterior rectus abdominis fascia is passed under the urethra and tied to the opposite rectus abdominis fascia in order to suspend the posterior urethrovesical angle.

Prolapse of the vagina following hysterectomy may be corrected through an abdominal or vaginal approach, depending upon the patient's health as well as upon her desire to keep a functioning vagina. In elderly patients, a complete obliteration of the vagina can be carried out to eliminate space for future potential hernias. In patients who desire to keep a functioning vagina, the abdominal route can be used to fix the vaginal apex to the periosteum of the presacral area, thus providing the vagina with permanent support.

The use of a vaginal pessary should be considered, especially in the elderly patient who is not a good surgical candidate. This is particularly useful when the posterior vaginal wall is adequate to support the pessary. Three commonly used pessaries are shown in Fig. 41-16. The pessary used will depend upon the size of the vaginal opening and the comfort of the patient. The Smith-Hodge pessary is useful in younger patients where retroversion exists and where trial replacement of the uterus in an anterior position is desired.

Disorders of Bleeding

In the neonatal period, bleeding can occur secondary to withdrawal of maternal hormone stimulation. Bleeding in the infant and child is exceedingly rare and is usually a sign of vaginal foreign body, a hormonally functional tumor, or a genital tract tumor. Heavy vaginal bleeding may appear in the female with the onset of puberty. During this time, ovulation is not occurring, and partial development of ovarian follicles may result in low estrogen production. The endometrium fails to proliferate and may be atrophic. Surface necrosis appears to occur, and instead of the sharp disintegration that accompanies menstruation, there is a slow and prolonged surface oozing. The resulting bleeding can vary from a slight stain to a severe hemorrhage, and it can be sufficiently severe to require blood transfusion. Since estrogen lack is the cause, high doses of intravenous estrogen can be excellent therapy. Occasionally, prolonged estrogen stimulation without progesterone interaction leads to endometrial hyperplasia and menorrhagia. The bleeding and clotting factors should also be checked, since blood dyscrasia (idiopathic thrombocytopenia) can also be the cause of heavy vaginal bleeding

SMITH-HODGE PESSARY FOR RETROVERSION OF UTERUS

GELLHORN PESSARY

SIMPLE RING PESSARY

Fig. 41-16. Types of vaginal pessaries.

in this age group. Heavy or intermenstrual bleeding during puberty also may be caused by adenocarcinomas of the lower genital tract. Many of these tumors have been shown to arise in young girls whose mothers took nonsteroidal synthetic estrogens, primarily diethylstilbestrol, during pregnancy. Although rare, these tumors increasingly are being reported. Thus, excessive bleeding in puberty should be investigated by vaginal examination.

During the reproductive years, there can be great variation in the menstrual pattern. It is not unusual for a normal, healthy female to have two menstrual periods in a month or to miss a menstrual period without any underlying pathologic condition. Cyclic bleeding at midcycle, corresponding to the time of ovulation, is frequently seen. Changes in the menstrual pattern for which no pathologic explanation is readily available are referred to as "dysfunctional" bleeding. When this is diagnosed, simple observation for a few months is often sufficient.

During the reproductive years, ovulation probably does not occur every month, so that even in the normal individual there may be a few cycles during the year which are anovulatory. These cycles provide the variations in length of flow or intervals between flow that many healthy women occasionally notice. In addition, emotional stimuli can result in anovulation, delaying or changing the menstrual pattern. The bleeding can become extremely heavy and cause anemia. Anovulatory bleeding may be a consequence of old pelvic inflammation. Ovaries encased in adhesions have fewer ovulations as judged by histologic criteria.

Submucous fibroids may cause prolonged and heavy bleeding at the time of menstruation. A similar menstrual pattern is often seen in association with an enlarged uterus in which the myometrium is greatly thickened. The cause of such heavy bleeding may be the large surface of endometrium which is shed at the time of menstruation. Adenomyosis, referring to the condition in which glands of the endometrium grow into the myometrium, may, on rare occasions, be responsible for heavy bleeding. Blood dyscrasias and endocrine imbalance such as hypothyroidism are also very rare causes of heavy menstrual bleeding. Heavy menstrual bleeding may be associated with or produce iron deficiency anemia, which is corrected by oral iron therapy.

Postmenstrual staining is commonly due to endometrial or endocervical polyps, which are usually benign polypoid masses. A severe vaginitis or cervicitis may also be found to be the cause of this symptom. In addition, postmenstrual staining is seen with abnormalities of the secretory phase of the cycle. The syndrome, known as "irregular shedding of endometrium," appears to be caused by a slow shedding of the secretory endometrium, associated with prolonged progesterone secretion extending into the subsequent cycle. The diagnosis is made by performing an endometrial biopsy or a dilation and curettage on the fifth or sixth day of the cycle.

Intermenstrual bleeding can occur at the time of ovulation. Premenstrual staining may result when there is an inadequate luteal phase with a premature drop in progesterone output.

Bleeding unrelated to the menstrual cycle may be due to carcinoma of the cervix, which is the most common malignant condition in women in the reproductive years. The bleeding associated with this lesion is characteristically irregular, consists of postmenstrual staining, and often is accompanied by intermenstrual bleeding and staining. There may be postcoital staining or bleeding. Carcinoma of the ovary does not usually cause nonmenstrual bleeding unless hormonally functional tumors are present.

Tumors of the fallopian tubes rarely cause intermenstrual bleeding. There may be an intermittent mucous or serous discharge with the bleeding or staining, "hydrops tubae profluens." This occurs presumably as a result of blockage of the tube by a tumor. The tumor can occur at any age but is usually seen in older women and often occurs postmenopausally. Similarly, carcinoma of the endometrium is primarily a disease of postmenopausal women but may cause nonmenstrual bleeding in a younger woman.

Brisk bleeding can occur in early pregnancy. It may accompany implantation of the blastocyst a few days after fertilization. It is not unusual to have a small amount of bleeding or staining during the first few weeks of pregnancy. If the patient has bleeding during early pregnancy, then the diagnosis is "threatened abortion." If, however, tissue is passed, then abortion is considered to have taken place. Ectopic pregnancy can cause irregular bleeding early in pregnancy. *Although there is no characteristic history obtained with an ectopic pregnancy,* many patients will complain of a delay in menses followed by scanty bleeding or staining, often in association with pelvic pain. There may or may not be symptoms of pregnancy. Finally, irregular bleeding early in pregnancy, especially if the uterus is larger than anticipated by the menstrual history, suggests trophoblastic disease.

Postmenopausal bleeding frequently is caused by an endometrial or endocervical polyp or atrophic vaginitis. Carcinoma of any part of the reproductive tract or premalignant change in the endometrium may exist in the postmenopausal female. In all cases of vaginal bleeding, the bladder and rectum must be ruled out as origins of the blood.

AMENORRHEA

Primary amenorrhea is the failure to initiate menstruation prior to age eighteen. Secondary amenorrhea is diagnosed in a patient who has menstruated monthly but then fails to bleed for at least 6 months. Primary amenorrhea can result from anatomic abnormalities such as imperforate hymen, atresia of the vagina, and other congenital defects. However, there are numerous nonanatomic conditions which occur with either primary or secondary amenorrhea. In a few patients with recent weight gain and marked obesity, infrequent periods and finally amenorrhea may develop. Often simple diet and weight control will result in a resumption of menstruation. Emotional stimuli also serve as an important cause of amenorrhea.

Although emotional factors certainly must be considered in evaluating any patient, this is a diagnosis of exclusion since there are many endocrine causes of amenorrhea. Pituitary tumors, such as chromophobe adenoma or, in the young person, craniopharyngioma, can cause amenorrhea. In such cases, there may often be signs of failure of other endocrine systems due to the loss of pituitary function. Severe thyroid disturbance may be responsible for amenorrhea, and hyperthyroidism can be involved in varieties of menstrual dysfunction. Overactivity of the adrenal gland, as with adrenocortical hyperplasia or adrenal tumor with excessive hormone production, can result in disorders of ovulatory function and amenorrhea, and occasionally masculinization.

The ovary, itself, rarely can be the hormonal source causing amenorrhea. Functioning ovarian tumors can produce large amounts of estrogen or androgen. On occasion the ovary fails to function even in the early twenties, and the diagnosis of primary ovarian failure or premature menopause can be made in these cases by noting the abnormally high gonadotropin level. Oligomenorrhea or amenorrhea in the presence of polycystic ovaries with thickened capsules represent the Stein-Leventhal syndrome. Such patients may have increased production of ovarian androgens, and in some cases hirsutism and obesity are noted.

Pregnancy per se is the most common cause of amenorrhea in the reproductive age group. The sequelae of pregnancy are often pathologic causes of amenorrhea. Usually menstruation will recur within a month or two following pregnancy, with menses occurring later in patients who breast-feed. However, occasionally patients who undergo severe hemorrhage or shock during delivery do not have recovery of menstrual function and are unable to lactate. This is caused by pituitary insufficiency and is known as "Sheehan's syndrome." In this group of patients the tropic hormones associated with thyroid and adrenal function may or may not be impaired, while gonadotropic hormone is lost.

After delivery, persistent amenorrhea and milk production for a period of at least 6 months suggests the "Chiari-Frommel syndrome." Amenorrhea and galactorrhea not associated with pregnancy is known as "Del Castillo syndrome." In all patients with amenorrhea and persistent lactation, a pituitary tumor must be ruled out.

Occasionally, a patient bleeds following delivery due to retained products of conception and requires a dilatation and curettage. In a few instances, especially with repeated curettage, the lining of the endometrial cavity is so extensively removed that intrauterine synechiae result. This will cause a mechanical and persistent amenorrhea known as "Asherman's syndrome."

Anatomic defects, such as an imperforate hymen or absence of the uterus, are often apparent on physical examination. Evaluation of the pituitary-gonadal axis can be initiated by testing the amenorrheic person with an injection of progesterone. If there is estrogen priming of the endometrium, withdrawal flow will ensue. Similarly, one can examine the cervical mucus; ferning suggests adequate ovarian estrogen secretion and an intact pituitary with gonadotropin function capable of stimulating the ovary.

Thyroid function can be evaluated by one of the serum tests (protein-bound iodine concentration [PBI], resin-T3 uptake, serum thyroxine level). Any recent injections of iodine (uterotubogram, intravenous pyelogram) can alter the PBI. In addition, estrogen administration and oral contraceptives alter the protein binding of thyroid hormones and the results of serum thyroid tests. However, free thyroxine concentration (Free-T4), or T3, can be a useful determination since this substance is not bound to plasma proteins, and the concentration will remain unchanged in euthyroid patients receiving exogenous estrogen.

Adrenal function can be estimated by 24-hour urinary determination of 17-ketosteroid or 17-hydrocorticosteroid concentrations. Radioimmunoassays have become available to measure the plasma testosterone level as well as levels of other androgens such as dehydroepiandrosterone sulfate and androstenedione. Plasma cortisol (hydrocortisone) concentration also can be measured by these techniques.

If the 17-ketosteroid or 17-hydroxycorticosteroid levels are elevated, suppression can be attempted by administering one of the adrenocortical hormones or their analogs. Dexamethasone, 0.5 mg given four times a day, will cause suppression in cases of adrenocortical hyperplasia but not in cases of adrenal tumor. Low urinary steroid levels suggest adrenocortical or pituitary insufficiency. These can usually be differentiated by an ACTH stimulation test and a metyrapone (SU-4885) test. The patient is hospitalized, and 40 I.U. of ACTH is given intravenously over an 8-hour period on two successive days; serial 24-hour urine specimens are collected. A patient with normal adrenocortical function will at least double base-line 17-ketosteroid and 17-hydroxycorticosteroid outputs on the day following ACTH infusion.

If there is adrenocortical insufficiency, a low urinary steroid level will be followed by a small increase in response to ACTH infusion. Since metyrapone blocks 11-β-hydroxylation, its administration inhibits the conversion of progesterone to hydrocortisone. Thus, the normal inhibition of ACTH secretion from the pituitary by hydrocortisone is prevented when metyrapone is given. This results in an outpouring of pituitary ACTH and a concomitant increase in adrenocortical secretion. In patients with normal pituitary reserve, a doubling or tripling of 17-hydroxycorticosteroids follows metyrapone administration. With pituitary insufficiency, the decrease in hydrocortisone formation is unable to evoke an increase in ACTH secretion, and the rise in adrenocortical output and 17-hydroxycorticosteroids does not occur.

Hormonally active tumors should be removed. In cases of adrenal hyperfunction, therapy with 30 to 40 mg/day of cortisone can be tried. Hirsute patients may note a decrease in hair with this therapy. Some amenorrheic patients have been helped by clomiphene citrate (Clomid), which is a potent agent for the induction of ovulation. The drug has been particularly helpful in patients with intact pituitary function as indicated by normal gonadotropin excretion. Patients with the Stein-Leventhal syndrome have been successfully treated with this drug. For an occasional patient who truly fits the category of the Stein-Leventhal syndrome and cannot be treated successfully with clomiphene bilateral wedge resection of the ovary has also proved successful. Finally, there is a group of patients who will not respond to any of the above measures. For them, human menopausal gonadotropin has been useful, especially in cases with pituitary failure or removal due to tumor. These gonadotropins are potent and frequently may cause multiple pregnancies and large ovarian cysts.

A small number of twenty- to thirty-year-old patients are amenorrheic with high gonadotropin values. These patients have premature menopause or primary ovarian failure. Their menopausal symptoms can be controlled by small doses of cyclic estrogen therapy.

If a patient has Asherman's syndrome, attempts can be made surgically to break up the synechiae, which may re-form. In general, therapy of this condition has been disappointing, probably partly because of the necessary retention of residual endometrial tissue, which is capable of regenerating, in order to achieve an effective, new endometrial cavity.

Hirsutism and Masculinization

The amount of hair will vary with the individual's coloring and the family patterns. The amount to be expected on a young female may be estimated by examining the patient's parents. There is an increase in hair over the body, including the trunk, legs, and face, through menarche. Any significant increase in the amount or distribution of hair after the age of twenty-five is unusual.

Although hirsutism may be an early sign of virilization, in most cases it is usually a variant for the individual and not amenable to therapy. Excessive hairiness due to the virilization syndrome may be due to overactivity of the adrenal cortex such as is seen in Cushing's disease, a tumor of the adrenal, or masculinizing tumor of the ovary. Hirsutism is also seen with the Stein-Leventhal syndrome. Adrenal hyperactivity may be diagnosed by tests outlined in the previous section. Cortisone administration suppresses elevated 17-ketosteroid levels in cases of excessive adrenal activity. However, unlike cases of adrenal hyperplasia, functioning tumors will not respond to exogenous hormonal stimulation. Direct visualization of the ovary via the laparoscope (Fig. 41-15) permits diagnosis of the ovarian tumor of Stein-Leventhal syndrome.

Inherited Reproductive Defects

Genetic material is transmitted via the chromosomes, of which the normal human complement is 46, i.e., 23 pairs. These can be studied morphologically and arranged according to size in a karyotype. There are 22 autosomes and two sex chromosomes designated X and Y. The presence of two or more chromosome complements in an individual is termed a "mosaic." In the female there are normally two X chromosomes, and one of these chromosomes is believed to be the basis of a discrete bit of chromatin material in the nucleus of many female cells. This is referred to as the "Barr body" (Fig. 41-17). In general, the number of X chromosomes is one greater than the number of Barr bodies seen. Thus, if there are three X chromosomes, there would be two Barr bodies present in most cells examined. In the normal male (X-Y), no Barr bodies are present. Some of the common chromosomal abnormalities are as follows:

GONADAL DYSGENESIS (TURNER'S SYNDROME). These patients are characteristically short and have primary amenorrhea with high urinary gonadotropins and low estrogen. They are usually of the X-O chromosomal type and thus are negative for Barr bodies. The ovaries are absent or of the so-called streak variety.

MALE PSEUDOHERMAPHRODITISM. A pseudohermaphrodite is defined by the sex which is the true genetic pattern; i.e., the presence of a testicle would result in a male classification, but the patient would be phenotypically female. Thus, a patient with the syndrome of testicular feminization is a male pseudohermaphrodite. These patients are always chromosomally X-Y. The abnormal testis secretes androgen, but there appears to be "target insensitivity," and the patients have breast development with sparse axillary and pubic hair. The testes should be surgically removed, usually in the late teens, because of the high danger of malignancy. This should be followed by female sex hormone replacement, since the patients are psychologically adjusted to female life.

FEMALE PSEUDOHERMAPHRODITISM. In this condition a female patient with an ovary and X-X chromosomal complement develops male external characteristics. Many of these patients present as newborn females who were masculinized in utero from androgens or progestational

Fig. 41-17. Sex chromatin masses in cells of human skin (left) and vaginal mucosa (right). *A.* Normal female: XX. *B.* Klinefelter's syndrome with mental deficiency: XXXY. *C.* Eunuch with microorchism and mental deficiency: XXXXY. The finding of duplicate Barr bodies suggests the presence of a mosaic of an undetected third stem line, such as XXX or XXXY. (*After A. R. Sohval, Am J Med, 31:397, 1961, and M. L. Barr and D. H. Carr, Canad Med Assoc J, 83:979, 1960.*)

hormones administered to the mother during pregnancy. This syndrome can also develop from overactivity of the female adrenal cortex, which produces androgen and thus masculinization, such as in congenital adrenal hyperplasia and the adrenogenital syndrome.

THE POLY-X SYNDROME. This is a syndrome in which females have more than two X chromosomes, such as 47-XXX or 48-XXX. These are referred to as "superfemales." They are usually mentally deficient with underdeveloped female secondary sex characteristics.

TRUE HERMAPHRODITES. This is rare in the human being, although patients have been reported with both testicular and ovarian tissue. It is important to determine early how the patient would function best as an adult. As a rule, it is simpler to create a functioning vagina than to reconstruct the phallus.

FAULTY DEVELOPMENT OF GENITALIA. Patients are

encountered with faulty development of the external genitalia. The two most commonly encountered situations are the imperforate hymen and complete absence of the vagina. In the case of the imperforate hymen, a pelvic mass is usually noted in either the pubertal or newborn female. In the newborn infant such a tumor may be produced by secretions trapped behind the hymen. The infant should be catheterized to rule out bladder distension. Before any newborn female is explored abdominally for a pelvic mass, an imperforate hymen or transverse vaginal septum should be ruled out, for these conditions can be treated quite simply by a hymenotomy or incision of the septum with release of the trapped fluid. Abdominal exploration can result in destruction of the small female pelvic organs with lifelong consequences.

If no vagina exists, one can be constructed. After an adequate space is created, split-thickness skin grafts are placed and held with a vaginal mold. This is usually carried out in the patient's late teens or early twenties when she has sufficient psychosexual maturity and also is able to keep the mold in situ and change it by herself. The mold must be used unless the patient is having frequent intercourse. Delaying this procedure until the patient is ready to marry can result in severe emotional problems for her and her fiancé.

Disorders of Reproductive Capacity

A couple is not usually evaluated for infertility unless there has been 1 year of deliberate effort to conceive. The diagnostic scheme can be divided into four parts as follows (Fig. 41-18).

PROOF OF OVULATION. Since there is no proof except pregnancy, circumstantial evidence is used. A biphasic basal body temperature, an elevated serum progesterone level, and a secretory endometrial biopsy obtained in the luteal phase of the cycle, can be considered as a reasonable indication of ovulation.

THE TUBAL FACTOR. The patency of the tubes must be established. The passage of CO_2 through the tubes (Rubin's test) is recorded by alterations in CO_2 pressure during the test. Confirmation of passage of CO_2 is noted by shoulder pain in the erect patient a few minutes after the completion of the procedure. Since the test does not permit visualization of the tubes, it is possible that only one tube could be open. Direct visualization of the tubes can be obtained radiologically by a uterotubogram (hysterosalpingogram). In such cases the endometrial cavity is outlined, and tubal patency is established. Laparoscopy (Fig. 41-15) is an essential step in the evaluation. When laparoscopy is performed, the tubes can be lavaged with a dye, such as indigo carmine, at the time of the surgical procedure; efflux of the dye through the fimbriate ends of both tubes proves patency. At the same time the pelvic organs are inspected for other pathologic changes, including peritubal adhesions, endometriosis, etc.

PROBLEM OF IMPLANTATION. This includes an evaluation of the adequacy of the size and shape of the uterus, particularly in patients who have repeated first trimester

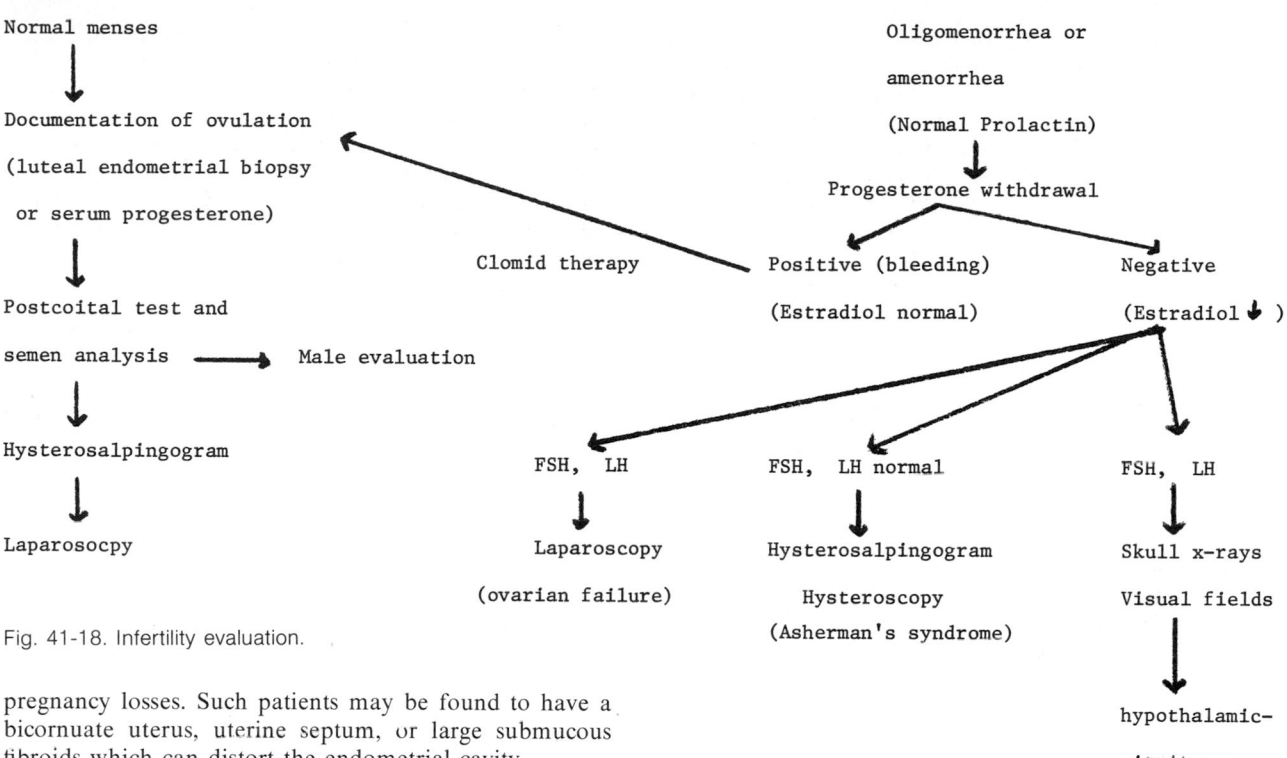

Fig. 41-18. Infertility evaluation.

pregnancy losses. Such patients may be found to have a bicornuate uterus, uterine septum, or large submucous fibroids which can distort the endometrial cavity.

THE MALE FACTOR. The postcoital (PCT, PK, or Huhner's) test evaluates this factor. The patient is instructed to have coitus with her husband about the time of midcycle, because it is at this time that the cervical mucus is most plentiful and most receptive to sperm. The mucus is then examined, optimally within 2 hours after coitus, at which time there should be numerous motile active sperm in a high-powered field (hpf). The number will vary depending upon the time the test is done and the amount of cervical mucus present. Usually 15 or more active sperm per hpf are seen. When the PCT contains this many sperm per hpf, the semen analysis will usually be at least 30 million sperm per cubic milliliter. When the PCT is less than that, repeated semen analyses should be done. The minimum accepted value is 20 million sperm per cubic milliliter, and a normal range is 40 million to 100 million sperm per cubic milliliter. A few pregnancies have been conceived by patients with counts as low as 10 million sperm per cubic millimeter. If a period of continence is followed by frequent intercourse, a gradual lowering of the sperm count can result.

Therapy of the infertile couple depends on the causative factor. If anovulation is the problem, then this should be treated according to the previously mentioned outline. In cases of uterine distortion, a myomectomy, reunification of a bicornuate uterus (Strassmann procedure), or removal of the uterine septum is usually necessary to achieve term pregnancy. If pelvic adhesions are present, chances for pregnancy can be improved if they are lysed, providing ovulatory and sperm functions are normal. Areas of endometriosis should be resected. Although the value of a ventral suspension is unproved, it is usually performed to improve theoretically the cervical exposure to the vaginal pool of semen. Tuboplastic procedures are performed to correct occlusion of the tube. Such surgical procedures should be avoided in cases of severe tubal destruction and are contraindicated in the cases of tuberculosis. A few pregnancies will result from tuboplasty procedures, but in most cases the results have been disappointing.

Pregnancy and Its Disorders

Amenorrhea in the reproductive years is most frequently caused by pregnancy. During the first weeks of normal pregnancy, the cervix becomes blue and soft. The cervico-uterine junction softens, and the fundus of the uterus becomes boggy, especially near implantation site. The cervical vessels enlarge and are easy to palpate. Enlargement of the uterus may be noted as early as 2 to 3 weeks after the first missed menstrual period. Uterine enlargement continues, and by the tenth week the fundus can be felt just above the symphysis. Usually the patient will notice fetal movement (quickening) by the sixteenth to eighteenth week of gestation. The examiner may hear the fetal heart as early as the seventeenth to twentieth week of gestation, depending upon the size of the patient. The fundus reaches the umbilicus by about the twentieth week of gestation and extends to the xiphoid of the sternum by the thirty-sixth week.

A small amount of staining early in the first trimester of pregnancy is not uncommon. However, if bleeding is severe and is unaccompanied by the passage of tissue or dilatation of the os, then the diagnosis of *threatened abortion* is made. The uterine size is usually consistent with the dates of gestation. The urinary test for chorionic gonadotropin remains positive. If tissue has been passed through a dilated cervical os, then usually some products of conception remain in the uterus. Under such circumstances, the diagnosis of *incomplete abortion* is made, and a curettage, usually performed with a suction apparatus, is indicated to prevent further hemorrhage and also to prevent infection from the retained products of conception. Occasionally, in the first trimester of pregnancy, the entire products of conception are passed, and the complete sac of the total pregnancy can be identified. These complete abortions do not require further surgical therapy.

Induced (therapeutic) abortions are frequently performed for a variety of indications, including the preference of the patient. Usually, under local anesthesia, the products of conception are removed by suction curettage after the cervix has been dilated. It is preferable to perform the procedure prior to the twelfth week of pregnancy.

Some first trimester pregnancy losses are complicated by infection. These are almost invariably due to instrumentation to induce abortion. The patient usually presents with lower abdominal pain, fever, and occasionally cervical discharge. The uterus is tender, and there is pain on cervical motion. The white cell count is elevated. In severe cases, septicemia and septic shock may ensue. The patient becomes moribund and is unable to maintain her blood pressure. There is then decreased or absent urinary output.

Therapy of septic abortion is initiated by high doses of intravenous antibiotics. Hyperbaric oxygen has been used for clostridial infections. The treatment of septic shock is discussed in Chap. 4. Once the infection appears controlled and the patient stabilized, gentle evacuation of the uterus is carried out. A vigorous curettage should not be done, as bacteremia and septic shock can result from excessive surgical manipulation. If the patient does not respond to gentle evacuation of the uterus, or if there is persistent shock and decreased urinary output, or if there is a history of the intrauterine injection of a powerful chemical toxin such as soap, detergent, or lysol, then a hysterectomy may be required as a lifesaving procedure. In such cases it is important to remove both the tubes and ovaries, since these are often areas of microabscesses and toxic products which have accumulated as a result of sepsis.

A diagnosis of *missed abortion* is applied if the fetus does not remain viable and there is no sign of external bleeding or loss of the pregnancy. The uterus shrinks in size, and there is necrosis of the fetus and placenta. The chorionic gonadotropin test becomes negative. If the uterus is smaller than a 12-week size, it can usually be safely evacuated by a curettage. In very rare cases, a hysterotomy is necessary.

ECTOPIC PREGNANCY. Implantation of the fertilized ovum outside the endometrial cavity, usually in the tube or, occasionally, on the surface of the ovary or in the abdomen, results in an ectopic pregnancy. It occurs in less than 1 percent of pregnancies. Tubal ectopic pregnancy is believed to result from the improper transport of the fertilized ovum through the tube, either because of a congenital defect in the tube or as the sequela of infection. It has been noted in many cases of ectopic pregnancies that the corpus luteum of pregnancy will exist in one ovary while the ectopic pregnancy is found to exist in the tube on the opposite side. Thus, there may have been transmigration of the fertilized ovum from one ovary to the contralateral tube; the time involved in this passage resulted in abnormal implantation into the tube rather than into the endometrial cavity. Patients who have had an ectopic pregnancy on one side are predisposed to the same problem in the opposite tube.

This is a disease of diagnostic surprises. There may be symptoms associated with early pregnancy such as breast tenderness, nausea, vomiting, and a delay in menses. There may be some bleeding or staining which follows a previously scanty period. The uterus often grows, but if an increase in size is noted, it will usually be less than expected for pregnancy, the duration of which is estimated from the menstrual history. Pain and cramps are often present. On physical examination, in addition to change in uterine size, an adnexal mass is occasionally palpable but may not be felt. Pain on cervical motion does occur and is usually localized to the side of the ectopic pregnancy. The pregnancy test may be positive or negative and often is not useful.

Occasionally, a patient will present with the pregnancy ruptured from the tube or extruded from the tip of the tube into the peritoneal cavity. The symptoms will then be of local peritoneal irritation due to the presence of blood. Characteristically, the patient complains of pain in the shoulder due to diaphragmatic irritation. In advanced cases, shock occurs because of heavy blood loss. Most ectopic pregnancies should be diagnosed before a vascular emergency occurs, but shock is seen in approximately 10 percent.

Ruptured ovarian cysts and pelvic inflammatory disease present with similar findings. Culdocentesis may aid in establishing the correct diagnosis. In most cases, the diagnosis can be made by laparoscopy. If this procedure is not feasible, an abdominal exploration is indicated.

The treatment of ectopic pregnancy consists of removal of the products of conception at the time of laparotomy. In certain cases, this measure can be followed by a tuboplastic procedure, which can preserve tubal patency. However, the tube is usually destroyed, and in such cases a salpingectomy must be performed. It is important to resect the cornual end of the tube to prevent the development of a future ectopic pregnancy in this site. Some authors recommend the removal of the ovary on the same side as the ectopic pregnancy in order to prevent future transmigration into the opposite tube, but such therapy should be reserved for patients in their later reproductive years.

ABNORMAL PREGNANCY GROWTH

Occasionally the products of conception will undergo abnormal growth and even malignant degeneration.

Trophoblastic Disease

Most cases of trophoblastic disease are benign *hydatidiform moles* which can be removed by curettage or hysterotomy. Locally invasive trophoblastic disease is usually referred to as "chorioadenoma destruens"; a truly malignant tumor is referred to as "choriocarcinoma." One cannot accurately predict the malignancy of trophoblastic disease from histologic appearance, but Hertig has devised a useful diagnostic categorization which divides trophoblastic disease into six groups: group I, benign; group VI, malignant; and the intervening groups ranging from the obviously benign to the obviously malignant. The disease occurs rarely and in the United States appears in approximately 1 out of every 2,000 pregnancies. There is a higher incidence in Asia, where there is approximately 1 case per 200 to 250 deliveries. The clinical picture is one of persistent bleeding and staining in early pregnancy with a uterus that is much larger than indicated by the menstrual history. Multiple pregnancies can be confused with this disease. Chorionic gonadotropin determinations often reveal levels higher than seen in normal pregnancy, while human placental lactogen (HPL) titers are lower. These can be measured in the patient's serum by radioimmunoassay. The use of ultrasonography aids in establishing the diagnosis of a normal or an abnormal pregnancy.

Placental polyp is not a true polyp but a focally retained part of the placenta. There is necrosis, inflammation, and occasional bleeding. Hertig classifies a placental polyp as being potentially malignant. It may have neoplastic trophoblast at its base. On the other hand, *syncytial endometritis,* which histologically can be confused with choriocarcinoma, is probably a benign lesion from the placental site that contains many inflammatory cells.

Trophoblastic disease can metastasize, and the most common sites of metastases are the lungs, vagina, brain, and liver, in decreasing order of occurrence. Antitumor agents provide excellent treatment. Methotrexate, actinomycin D, and Velban have been the most commonly used chemotherapeutic agents. It has been estimated that there is complete remission in approximately 50 percent of cases following the use of methotrexate or actinomycin D in the treatment of trophoblastic disease. In certain cases, surgical intervention is necessary, either to control hemorrhage or infection or to irradicate a solitary site which has been refractive to chemotherapy. However, primary surgical treatment of malignant trophoblastic disease does not appear to offer the patient as much benefit as chemotherapeutic agents.

SPECIFIC GYNECOLOGIC DISEASES

Infections and Discharges

During childhood, a whitish discharge, leukorrhea, may develop. At birth this increased vaginal secretion is usually due to maternal hormones and is entirely physiologic. A similar discharge may be seen in the pubertal female with the onset of estrogen stimulation. Severe leukorrhea during childhood is usually the result of infection caused by a foreign body in the vagina. The majority of vaginal discharges of children are caused by coliform organisms. Occasionally pinworm infection is the cause. The correct diagnosis can be established by direct visualization of the foreign body and culturing for pathologic organisms, or by doing a Scotch tape test for pinworms (*Enterobius vermicularis*). With the onset of menarche, various organisms can be implicated as the cause of a discharge.

The most common of these conditions caused by organisms follow.

TRICHOMONAS VAGINALIS INFECTION. This discharge is caused by a parasite. The trichomonad can be identified by its very active flagella, which can be seen beating, when the vaginal discharge mixed with a drop of saline solution is examined microscopically. The parasite flourishes in an alkaline pH. It often causes a strawberry red inflammatory reaction of the cervix and is usually accompanied by a green and extremely odorous discharge that is often worse at the time of menstruation, because of the alkalinity of the menstrual discharge. Treatment is carried out with a trichomonacidal drug, metronidazole (Flagyl). Vinegar douches are occasionally of symptomatic help. The male carries the infection asymptomatically and occasionally must be treated when there is recurrent infection in the female.

MONILIA VAGINITIS (*CANDIDA ALBICANS*). This fungus infection can occur at any time but is often seen during pregnancy, after the use of antibiotics, and frequently in diabetics. It flourishes in an acid environment. The fungus can be cultured on Nickerson's medium. Mycelial budding can be seen on direct examination of the vaginal secretion which has previously been treated with 10 percent potassium hydroxide to lyse epithelial cells. Grossly, the discharge looks like a thick white cottage cheese. It is extremely irritating, and the patients usually complain of marked itching. Local antifungal agents are effective, and it is usually wise to treat the gastrointestinal tract at the same time to eradicate the fungus. Alkaline douches occasionally help, and gentian violet staining of the vagina may also provide relief. Anti-inflammatory agents such as cortisone can be used for the irritated vulva.

NONSPECIFIC VAGINITIS. This discharge is due to bacteria, generally *H. vaginalis,* and is not associated with either *Trichomonas* or *Candida* infections. A purulent discharge is present, and polymorphonuclear cells as well as many bacteria can be seen on examination of the vaginal secretion. Specific bacterial cultures occasionally are done, but usually a gram-negative organism is the offender. There is often secondary infection of a chronically eroded cervix. Triplesulfa creams are effective, and if chronic cervicitis exists, improvement can often be obtained by cauterization of the erosion.

ATROPHIC VAGINITIS. This occurs in the elderly female or in the young patient after removal of the ovaries. The vaginitis is usually of a bacterial origin and results from secondary invasion of the atrophic vaginal tissues which have lost their thickness as well as acid protection. Vinegar douches are occasionally helpful, and small doses of estrogen either locally or orally can restore the integrity of the vaginal mucosa.

BARTHOLINITIS. Infection of Bartholin's duct may lead to obstruction and eventual dilatation, with the formation of a Bartholin's cyst. Occasionally these are asymptomatic and require no treatment. If the cyst is acutely inflamed, drainage by marsupialization is usually successful; in cases of recurrent infection, removal of the cyst and gland may become necessary.

VENEREAL INFECTIONS AND PELVIC INFLAMMATORY DISEASE

SYPHILIS. This disease should be suspected in any genital lesion. Serologic screening (VDRL) tests can be done. Definitive diagnosis is made by dark-field examination of scrapings of ulcers to demonstrate the spirochetes or fluorescent treponema antibody absorption (FTA-ABS) blood tests. The diagnosis may be made by examination of the spinal fluid in more advanced cases. Treatment is with penicillin.

CHANCROID. This is a painful ulcer of the vulva caused by the organism *Hemophilus ducreyi,* which can be cultured from the ulcer and responds to sulfonamide or streptomycin therapy.

GRANULOMA INGUINALE. This is a chronic inflammatory disease. The offending *Klebsiella* bacteria cause inclusion bodies to occur in the cells obtained from the ulcerating area (Donovan bodies). There are usually nontender ulcers, and streptomycin therapy is usually effective.

LYMPHOPATHIA VENEREUM. This is a viral disease which infiltrates the lymphatics and spreads to regional nodes, causing a severe adenitis. The groins, perineum, and lower gastrointestinal tract can be involved. The diagnosis is made by a skin test (Frei test), and therapy is effective with chloramphenicol or sulfonamide. Scarring in the region of the anorectum can become so severe that colostomy may be necessary.

CONDYLOMA ACCUMINATUM. These venereal warts are not truly venereal but often occur secondarily to vaginal discharges. Viruses have been implicated. If the primary cause can be found and the discharge corrected, the condylomas may disappear. They may be removed by hot cautery or chemically with podophyllin, but they frequently recur.

GONORRHEA. This common disease is caused by bacteria of the genus *Neisseria gonococcus.* The diagnosis can be established by examining the purulent discharge from the cervix, urethra, or Skene's glands. Polymorphonuclear leukocytes are present, containing gram-negative intracellular diplococci. The organisms can be cultured from the secretions, but the culture must be done immediately, since the organisms die soon after exposure to air, and a false-negative culture can result. There has been a recent sharp increase in the number of cases treated, and changes in sexual behavior patterns are resulting in continuing spread of the disease to individuals in all socioeconomic categories. Penicillin is the primary mode of therapy, but resistant strains of the organism are being detected. For the female, 4.8 million units of aqueous procaine penicillin plus 1 Gm of probenecid usually are given, and the dosage is repeated if the culture remains positive. For patients allergic to penicillin, tetracycline can be used, although it is usually less effective than penicillin. Tetracycline can be given orally; after a loading dose of 1.5 Gm, 0.5 Gm is given four times daily for 4 additional days. Ampicillin, 3.5 Gm

given orally as one dose, or spectinomycin, 4 Gm intramuscularly, may be used.

PELVIC INFLAMMATORY DISEASE. Neisserian infection is frequently the initial cause of pelvic inflammatory disease in many patients. However, nongonoccal infection of the adnexa and pelvic tissue can follow abortion or pregnancy and has been reported with the use of intrauterine devices (IUD). The patients characteristically present with acute diffuse lower abdominal pain and a high fever, which may reach 103 to 104°F. There is severe pain on even slight motion of the cervix. The vagina is hyperemic and extremely warm. The tenderness noted on pelvic examination usually is bilateral because of the presence of a diffuse cellulitis. There may be some minor gastrointestinal complaints, but normal bowel sounds are usually present. The white blood cell count is elevated out of proportion to the degree of morbidity. In many cases, it is not possible to culture the pathogenic organism, but certainly an attempt should be made to rule out gonorrhea. Acute lower abdominal pain may also suggest appendicitis, ectopic pregnancy, twisted or ruptured ovarian cyst, or occasionally involvement of the urinary tract or the lower gastrointestinal tract.

Therapy. Treatment consists of antibiotics and bed rest. The response is usually rapid. If an IUD is present, it should be removed. There is danger that a focus of chronic infection will exist in the pelvis and that repeated attacks will predispose to infertility. Therefore, complete and adequate therapy, which in many cases may require hospitalization, is necessary. Occasionally, acute attacks are followed by scarring in the pelvis. This may then result in chronic pain and menstrual irregularity. In such patients blocked tubes, sterility, and adnexal adhesions may then develop. In certain cases, the secretions from the lining of the tube are trapped in the tube, and hydrosalpinx develops. In more advanced cases, an abscess develops between the tube and the ovary. These tuboovarian abscesses are best treated by surgical removal. If the abscess has leaked or ruptured, there will be signs of generalized peritonitis. If prompt surgical therapy is not instituted, a significant percentage of these patients will be lost. Total hysterectomy with bilateral salpingo-oophorectomy is the treatment of choice for ruptured tuboovarian abscesses. Occasionally, massive doses of antibiotics and supportive therapy with blood replacement and plasma must precede surgical procedures in order to bring the patient into optimal preoperative condition.

TUBERCULOUS PELVIC INFECTION

Tuberculosis is an uncommon cause of chronic pelvic inflammatory disease in the United States. It is generally associated with irreversible infertility. Tuberculosis is usually not a primary infection of the genital tract and is either of pulmonary or gastrointestinal origin. The diagnosis is made by curettings obtained at the time of menstruation and stained, cultured, and inoculated into guinea pigs. Chemotherapy with antituberculous drugs is the preferred treatment. Attempts to restore fertility by corrective surgical procedures in these cases have uniformly met with poor results.

Endometriosis

The growth of endometrial glands and stroma in areas outside the uterus is known as endometriosis. Such areas may undergo cyclic changes during the menstrual cycle, although histologically the changes do not necessarily mimic that of the endometrium. The sites of occurrence are wide and varied, and may be anywhere in the pelvis. The uterosacral ligaments are typical locations for this disease, and tender nodularity felt along these ligaments is diagnostic. Endometriosis may also be found on the ovaries, where it exists as large chocolate cysts, or endometriomas. Posterior cul-de-sac peritoneal implants are very common, and multiple 2- to 3-mm nodules are often seen in this area. Endometriosis may be on the vulva or vagina and may undergo cyclic changes during the menstrual cycle which can be directly observed. Endometrial implants on the bowel can be the cause of cyclic lower gastrointestinal tract bleeding, and cases of cyclic hemoptysis have been reported from lesions in the lung.

Many theories have been proposed to explain the origin of endometriosis. None has been proved. One widely held theory postulates that implantation of endometrium occurs at the time of menstruation as a result of reflux of endometrial tissue into the peritoneal cavity through the fallopian tubes. The reflux theory is given some support by the fact that implantation of endometrial tissue can occur in cesarean section scars. Embryologic changes have also been suggested as a cause for endometriosis. It has been postulated that a change occurs in the coelomic epithelium, which gives rise to endometrial cell nests. This assumes that the cells with the potential of undergoing change to endometriosis are present at birth and transform during the reproductive years. Such a theory is given strength by endometrial implants found, not only on the bowel, but also in the lung and in other places in the body at a distance from the pelvis. Other theories have been advanced, but none can claim any greater acceptability.

A patient with endometriosis may have no symptoms or may complain of severe dysmenorrhea that becomes increasingly debilitating with the passage of time. Severe dysmenorrhea is usually seen in a patient in her late twenties who has never been pregnant, although endometriosis can occur in an older patient who has not been pregnant for years. The origin of the pain is uncertain but is probably due, in part, to cyclic bleeding into the sites of endometriosis at the time of menstruation. Large endometrial implants are often asymptomatic, while millimeter-size nodules are often associated with severe pain. Although it cannot be stated that endometriosis per se will cause infertility, it is generally accepted that patients with endometriosis will have a smaller chance of becoming pregnant than the general population.

Clinically, the diagnosis can be confirmed by direct visualization of the endometriosis either at laparotomy, laparoscopy, or culdoscopy. However endometriosis often causes obliteration of the cul-de-sac, and culdoscopy can lead to rectal perforation. Therefore, it should not be attempted in those cases where marked uterosacral or cul-de-sac scarring exists. In order to make a microscopic diagnosis of endometriosis, endometrial glands, endometrial stroma, or blood should be demonstrated. The blood may appear in the form of hemosiderin. If two of these three diagnostic criteria are present, then the histologic diagnosis of endometriosis is justified.

Many patients with endometriosis have no symptoms and require no special therapy. Since there is an increased incidence of infertility in these patients, pregnancy preferably should not be delayed. If this is not possible, hormonal treatment with progestational agents accompanied by estrogen (pseudopregnancy) has been suggested to induce long periods of amenorrhea. This may decrease the size of endometrial nodules, but endometriosis may recur following such long-term therapy. Danocrine, a new but expensive hormonal treatment, has been reported to be very successful. However, primate studies have suggested that artificially induced endometriosis lesions do not disappear following hormonal therapy but remain functional. Small doses of methyltestosterone can be given on a cyclic basis for a short period of time for relief of pain. It should be avoided in dark-skinned or hirsute people, since they can become masculinized by androgen therapy.

In certain cases, surgical treatment must be performed. Conservative surgical measures consist of complete removal of as much of the endometriosis as possible, taking care to preserve normal anatomic structures, especially in the areas of the tubes and ovaries. A presacral neurectomy, as outlined in the section on pelvic pain, is also usually performed. In cases where the endometriosis can be completely excised, excellent results are obtained, and the patients usually remain pain-free. If symptomatic endometriosis exists in an older patient who no longer desires to have children, then a total hysterectomy with bilateral salpingo-oophorectomy can be considered. By surgical castration, the endogenous hormonal support of the endometriosis is removed, and the disease is cured.

Intrauterine (DES) Exposure

Clear-cell adenocarcinomas of the vagina and cervix have been observed in young women whose mothers were treated with DES and similar compounds during pregnancy. Fortunately these cancers are rare among the exposed. They have been noted to occur primarily after puberty, with a peak incidence at age nineteen. Through age twenty-four the risk of cancer is estimated to be 1:1,000 or less. Since most of the exposed population is under thirty years of age, it is not known what effect, if any, the exposure may have on these women as they age.

In spite of the low risk of malignancy, DES-exposed females should have a complete gynecologic evaluation once they begin to menstruate or reach the age of fourteen, in order to rule out the presence of malignancy as well as to detect the common nonneoplastic changes that have been found in their vaginas and cervices. These changes include vaginal adenosis, the presence of columnar tissue or its mucinous products in the vagina; cervical eversion (or ectropion), the presence of columnar epithelium or its mucinous products on the cervix; and transverse vaginal and cervical fibrous ridges. The ridges are found in about

20 percent of the exposed; while vaginal adenosis occurs in about one-half (depending upon the time in pregnancy when DES was started), and cervical eversion occurs commonly among the unexposed population, vaginal adenosis and transverse ridges are rare in the absence of intrauterine DES exposure.

Adenosis appears to be a benign lesion that is usually found near the vaginal clear-cell adenocarcinoma. Current evidence suggests that adenosis does not require therapy. The columnar epithelium of vaginal adenosis and cervical eversion is usually physiologically replaced by squamous epithelium (metaplasia). Occasionally neoplastic, squamous epithelium develops (dysplasia, carcinoma in situ), as is discussed in the section on the cervix. The degree to which squamous malignancies may be a problem in the DES-exposed female is unknown at present.

The complete evaluation consists of careful palpation, direct visualization, and cytologic sampling of the vagina and cervix. This is usually followed by colposcopy to study transformation areas of metaplasia, followed by an iodine stain to delineate the extent of the nonglycogenated epithelium. Biopsies are taken from the areas which are markedly abnormal on colposcopic examination or from nodules that are suggestive of malignancy.

Fig. 41-19. Uterine fibroids. *A.* Types. *B.* Various locations.

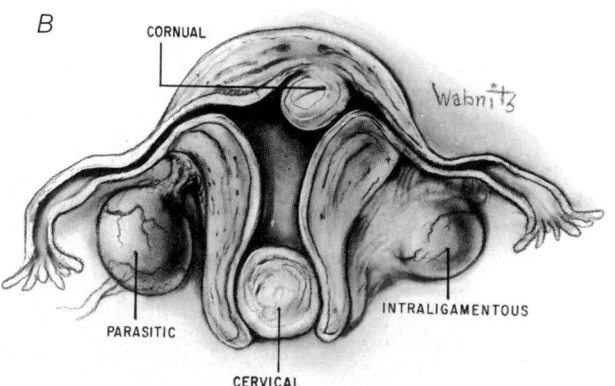

Benign Disorders of the Uterus

FUNDUS

Fibroids

Fibroids (leiomyoma) are extremely common, occurring in perhaps 50 percent of women. They are collections of whorls of interlacing, smooth muscle fibers. Fibroids vary tremendously in size, being as small as a few millimeters or growing sufficiently large to fill the entire pelvis. They are usually named by their location, as shown in Fig. 41-19, where subserosal, intramural, and submucous fibroids are illustrated. Occasionally, a subserosal fibroid develops with a large stalk attached to the fundus of the uterus, in which case it is referred to as a "pedunculated fibroid." This is easily confused on physical examination with an adnexal mass or ovarian tumor. The origin of these benign tumors is unknown, but there appears to be a definite hormonal influence, as the tumors are rarely seen prior to the age of twenty and are known to involute after the menopause. In addition, leiomyomas can be stimulated to grow by administering estrogens. Therefore estrogen-containing medication, such as oral contraceptives, must be used judiciously in the presence of these tumors.

Their presence is not in itself an indication for any therapy. The therapy of leiomyomas is dependent upon the symptoms and problems which are associated with them. Fibroids are associated with four major problems. These are bleeding, pain, increase in size, and infertility.

Bleeding. An increase in menstrual flow or prolongation of the menstrual period sufficient to cause anemia can be associated with submucous fibroids. The endometrial cavity is markedly enlarged and distorted, and there is incomplete endometrial regeneration over the surface of the fibroid, leading to continuous oozing or bleeding and sometimes hemorrhage.

Pain. This is not a common symptom. It occurs primarily when there is degeneration, which usually results when one of these large tumors outgrows its blood supply. It may also occur when a pedunculated fibroid twists and becomes infarcted. Rarely pain is associated with a large leiomyoma that has impinged or caused pressure on local adjacent viscera, and the discomfort would be referred to the involved organ.

Growth. Fibroids do grow during the reproductive years. Usually the growth is at a slow rate, unless there is excessive hormonal stimulation as a result of medication or in association with pregnancy. Since malignancy occurring in a fibroid is an exceedingly rare event, malignant change need only be considered if the growth of the fibroid is extremely rapid, especially during the menopausal years.

Infertility. Many patients who present with problems in conception and infertility are found to have fibroids. Usually fibroids interfering with conception cause distortion of the endometrial cavity and can interfere with implantation. They also can distort the fallopian tube and by their size interfere with the transport of the ovum. Small subserosal fibroids, which do not distort the endometrial cavity and are not in a position to interfere with tubal transport, probably are not related to a patient's infertility problem.

A submucous fibroid will occasionally extrude through the cervix and present as a bleeding and infected mass attached by a stalk to the endometrial cavity. These fibroids are safely treated by removing the stalk, followed by a few weeks' rest period to allow infection to clear from the pelvic lymphatics prior to undertaking further surgical treatment. Attempts at surgical procedures without this waiting period usually result in a high incidence of post-operative complications and wound sepsis. In general, the surgical therapy of fibroids consists of either hysterectomy or myomectomy.

Adenomyosis

Adenomyosis is a growth of endometrial tissue in the myometrium of the uterus and is sometimes referred to as "endometriosis of the uterine corpus." The condition occurs primarily during the reproductive years and leads to a thickening of the myometrial wall with subsequent uterine enlargement. Adenomyosis usually occurs in women who have had a number of pregnancies. Occasionally patients with adenomyosis will complain of dysmenorrhea, and some present with increased uterine bleeding and heavy menstrual flow. However, a number of patients with adenomyosis in hysterectomy specimens have been asymptomatic. Therefore, the association of adenomyosis with heavy menstrual bleeding and dysmenorrhea is questionable.

Polyps

Endometrial polyps can occur at any time after puberty. A polyp is a local hyperplastic growth of endometrial tissue which usually causes postmenstrual or postmenopausal bleeding or staining. The polyps are usually benign, but rare cases of malignant tumor of the endometrium arising in a polyp have been reported. Removal of polyps at the time of curettage is generally curative, although they can recur.

Endometritis

Occasionally patients with menstrual irregularity and postmenstrual staining are found to have endometritis. Histologically, the lesion demonstrates massive inflammatory cell infiltration of the stroma of the endometrium. The infiltration is greater than that normally seen at the time of menstruation and is usually accompanied by plasma cells. Antibiotics and curettage usually are sufficient treatment. Instrumentation or procedure such as obtaining a tubogram should not be performed in the presence of endometritis, since a severe exacerbation of diffuse pelvic inflammation could result.

CERVIX

Common benign conditions of the uterine cervix include inflammation, Nabothian cysts, and polyps. *Cervical polyps* cause the same symptoms as endometrial polyps. Since they are often quite small and are visible at the external os, they often can be removed as an outpatient procedure followed by cauterization of the base of the polyp. *Nabothian cysts* are mucous inclusion cysts of the cervix. They are occasionally associated with chronic inflamma-

tion and can easily be removed with a cautery. However, they are harmless, usually asymptomatic, and generally do not require therapy.

During reproductive years the portio of the cervix is covered primarily with glycogenated squamous epithelium, and columnar epithelium is normally found centrally near the external os in most women. This exposed columnar epithelium is termed *ectropion* or *eversion* and usually is bright red. Unless accompanied by inflammation and a purulent discharge (cervicitis), it requires no treatment. During adult life, the columnar epithelium is usually replaced by squamous metaplasia, and this physiologic process occurs in the transformation zone at the interface of squamous and columnar epithelium. After menopause the squamous columnar junction is usually in the endocervical canal.

Malignant Disease of the Uterus

CARCINOMA OF THE CERVIX

Carcinoma of the cervix is the most common malignant tumor of the female reproductive tract, although recently carcinoma of the endometrium appears to have become almost as common. Carcinoma of the cervix comprises 40 to 50 percent of genital tract cancers. Most of the tumors are epithelial cell or squamous cell carcinomas, while approximately 5 percent are adenocarcinomas. The tumor occurs more frequently in women who have started to bear children at an early age. The malignant change develops at the squamocolumnar junction, and this area is also involved with inflammatory changes following pregnancy. These tumors are not often seen in the virgin female. There is a possibility that a male factor may be etiologically related, and it has been suggested that the disease is less common in women married to circumcised males.

SYMPTOMS. Carcinoma of the cervix may be discovered in a patient who has no symptoms or complaints. She may have intermenstrual bleeding or staining and may complain of bleeding which occurs following douching or intercourse. Any bleeding of an irregular nature which is not associated with menstruation is a danger signal in the female of reproductive years. Postmenopausal bleeding also may be caused by cervical carcinoma, but it occurs more commonly with endometrial malignancy. Pain is a late manifestation of this disease, as is general malaise.

DETECTION AND DIAGNOSIS. The advent of the Papanicolaou smear has offered the possibility of screening large segments of the population for cervical tumor by methods that are approximately 95 percent accurate. The smear may be taken as a vaginal aspiration or by direct aspiration or scraping from the cervix. The stained smear can then be categorized as showing normal, suspicious, or malignant changes. Although malignancy can be suggested by the Papanicolaou smear, the diagnosis of cervical carcinoma can be made *only* on biopsy. Even in the presence of malignant disease, a benign smear may be obtained, especially where there is a great deal of secondary infection accompanying the tumor. Therefore, a malignant tumor of the cervix is not definitely ruled out by a benign Papanicolaou smear, and grossly suspicious areas should be biopsied. A suspicious Papanicolaou smear or report of malignant cells in the smear also require further investigation by biopsy.

By helping the examiner identify abnormal epithelial and vascular patterns in the transformation zone, the col-

Fig. 41-20. *A.* Cervical dysplasia. *B.* Carcinoma in situ of cervix. *C.* Invasive squamous cell carcinoma of cervix.

poscope aids in directed biopsy of the most suggestive areas. It is important that the entire transformation zone be visible on the portio of the cervix for a satisfactory colposcopy to be performed. If colposcopy is unsatisfactory, a diagnostic conization of the cervix will usually be necessary to rule out the presence of invasive carcinoma. Schiller's or Lugol's iodine stain can also be used as a nonspecific guide for biopsy. Nonglycogenated epithelium will usually appear grossly normal but does not stain with iodine. These suggestive areas are then biopsied, although such areas may contain only nonneoplastic or inflammatory changes.

The Papanicolaou smear is particularly important in that it not only can detect the cells of a frankly malignant condition but also can detect changes in the cervical epithelium which are potentially malignant. These changes are termed "anaplasia" (dysplasia) and "carcinoma in situ," depending upon the severity of the alterations in the cervical epithelium.

Colposcopy, which consists of the examination of the cervix with a low-power microscope and built-in light source, has recently gained popularity. It is a technique which aids in differentiating pathologic processes and other atypical lesions.

Dysplasia. Figure 41-20*A* shows an area of dysplasia of the cervix in which the architecture of the squamous epithelium has been disturbed and there is progressive loss of differentiation of the squamous epithelial cells. Dysplasia is in itself not a malignant change and can be treated successfully by cauterization. However, patients with dysplasia must be thoroughly investigated and followed to make sure that a more serious cervical change does not exist or develop in the future.

Carcinoma In Situ. The lesion consists of malignant epithelium that is confined to the surface of the cervix (Fig. 41-20*B*). There is no invasion of the deep layers of the cervix by malignant cells. In spite of its malignant potential, the lesion is benign. Carcinoma in situ is considered a precursor of invasive carcinoma for the following reasons:

1. The peak rate of occurrence of carcinoma in situ precedes by approximately 10 years in age distribution the peak occurrence of invasive carcinoma of the cervix. In situ lesions are seen at about the age of thirty-eight, while invasive carcinoma occurs most frequently at age forty-eight, and both diseases occur at approximately the same rate with the 10-year span separating them.
2. There is a similar racial and ethnic distribution. The disease is uncommon in Jewish women when compared to non Jewish women and is more frequently seen in Negroes than in whites.
3. It is common in cases of carcinoma of the cervix to note microscopically coexisting, adjacent areas of carcinoma in situ.
4. A few patients with carcinoma in situ have been known to develop invasive carcinoma later.

Once the question of malignancy of the cervix has been raised, either by Papanicolaou smear or by biopsy, carcinoma in situ must be differentiated from invasive carcinoma of the cervix, since these lesions can coexist. Colposcopy is used to identify the most abnormal areas, but iodine stain with multiple biopsies and an endocervical curettage can be effectively used by competent examiners. It is vital to rule out invasive cancer, and hospitalization for diagnostic conization of the cervix is occasionally required.

THERAPY. Treatment is determined by the nature of the lesion and most particularly by the extent of involvement.

Carcinoma In Situ. If the diagnosis of carcinoma in situ without invasion can be made, adequate therapy consists of a total abdominal hysterectomy with removal of at least 1 cm of vaginal cuff. The cervix and vagina may be stained with Schiller's solution prior to surgical treatment to detect any parts which do not take Schiller's stain, and these parts are included with the specimen.

All patients treated for carcinoma in situ should be followed by yearly vaginal smears, since the remaining squamous epithelium of the vagina can undergo malignant changes in future years. Patients with carcinoma in situ in whom preservation of reproductive function is desired can be treated by a therapeutic conization of the cervix. Some investigators have utilized locally destructive procedures such as cryosurgery or cauterization to treat carcinoma in situ, with apparently good results, but such treatment is generally performed for dysplasia of the cervix. The follow-up of these patients is particularly important, since future epithelial change can occur in both the vagina and retained cervix.

Invasive Carcinoma. Carcinoma of the cervix is a slow-growing tumor (Fig. 41-20C). It spreads over the surface of the adjacent epithelium of the cervix and may invade the underlying muscular walls and disseminate via lymph channels. Parametrial areas and paracervical areas are prime sites for the spread of the disease. The first metastases are usually found in the lymph nodes of the pelvis and often in the parametrium and paracervical tissues. The tumor spreads to the pelvic wall along the hypogastric vessels and then to the areas of the external and common iliac arteries. The tumor will extend outside the true pelvis as a late manifestation. In untreated cases, death can result from hemorrhage due to major vessel erosion or from urinary tract obstruction which leads to subsequent uremia while the disease may be confined to the pelvic cavity.

STAGING. In order to determine the proper therapy of carcinoma of the cervix, the precise extent of the disease must be defined. This is accomplished by diagnostic x-rays, sigmoidoscopy, cystoscopy, and pelvic examination under general anesthesia. The tumor spread is classified according to international agreement which divides the various categories into the stages depicted in Fig. 41-21.

Stage I refers to invasive carcinoma which is confined to the cervix. If invasive tumor is not clinically evident and a small focus is discovered microscopically, microinvasion or preclinical carcinoma is diagnosed and assigned to Stage I-A. The diagnosis of microinvasive carcinoma is made if invasion is 3 mm or less and vascular or lymphatic involvement is absent. All other Stage I carcinomas then are assigned to Stage I-B. *Stage II* refers to carcinoma that extends beyond the cervix but has not yet reached the pelvic wall and is confined to the upper two-thirds of the vagina. The stage is subdivided by most clinics into Stage II-A, which indicates involvement only of the vagina, and Stage II-B, which indicates involvement beyond the vagina, into the parametrial and paracervical areas. *Stage III* refers to involvement of either the lower third of the vagina or the extension of tumor to the pelvic

wall. If tumor has caused hydronephrosis or a nonfunctioning kidney as determined by intravenous pyelogram, the tumor is assigned to Stage III. *Stage IV* represents either spread of tumor outside the pelvis or invasion of the mucosa of the bladder or rectum by malignant disease.

CHOICE OF THERAPY. Radical surgical procedures and radiation therapy both provide effective treatment for carcinoma of the cervix. The modality of therapy will depend upon the extent of the tumor, the condition of the patient, and the capabilities of the clinic. There are a large number of cases that can be treated successfully by either method with similar likelihood of cure. Although attempts have been made to measure the patient's responsiveness to radiation by studying the histology of cervical tumor following external radiation and by examining the cellular components of the smear, there is no available test which permits one to separate those cases that will best respond to surgical treatment from those that will do better with radiation.

Stage I and II-A. Most young patients with Stage I carcinoma of the cervix or early Stage II-A lesions can be treated equally satisfactorily by either radical surgery or radiation. If radical surgery is performed, ovarian function occasionally can be preserved. Patients with local inflammation or pelvic infection should be treated surgically, since massive sepsis can result if radiotherapy is undertaken. The development of a wide en bloc dissection is an integral part of adequate surgical therapy for this disease, and the extent to which an adequate dissection can be done is illustrated in Fig. 41-22. It can be seen that wide areas of the parametrial and paracervical tissues can be removed. Many investigators feel that microinvasive carcinoma can be effectively treated with total (extrafascial) hysterectomy.

RADIATION CONSIDERATIONS. Adequate radiation therapy requires the delivery of tumoricidal doses of radiation to all areas that either are or can be affected by tumor. The dose of radiation delivered is inversely proportional to the distance between the source and the point being treated. In addition, the tissue absorption of radiation is inversely proportional to the wavelength of the administered dose. Thus, by lowering the wavelength, one increases penetration of the radiation. This can be done by raising the therapeutic voltage, as for example, with the million-electron-volt machines, or it can be accomplished by using filters to eliminate the longer wavelengths. Time and volume factors are important. When a given dose is administered over a long period of time, the tissue reaction is less than if it is given in a short interval. Similarly, a dose which is distributed throughout a large volume causes greater tissue damage than one which is confined to a small volume. The unit of exposure in radiation is usually expressed as the rad, which is equivalent to the transfer of 100 ergs of energy/Gm of tissue. For practical purposes, this is equivalent to 1 r. Thus, 10,000 r given to the cervix is a dose that can be tolerated, while the same dose given to the entire pelvis would cause necrosis of normal tissue. Occasionally, radium doses are expressed in terms of milligram-hours, a quantity determined by multiplying the milligrams of radium used by the number

STAGE I

STAGE II

STAGE III

STAGE IV

Fig. 41-21. Clinical stages of cervical cancer (International Classification).

of hours it is in place. However, this gives no indication of the overall effect or distribution of the dose in relation to surrounding tissue. For convenience, two standard reference points, identified as A and B, are used to specify the dose of radiation given. Point A is 2 cm superior to

Fig. 41-22. Radical hysterectomy section.

Fig. 41-21. Clinical stages of cervical cancer (International Classification).

the fornix and 2 cm lateral to the uterine canal. Point B lies in the same plane but is located 5 cm laterally.

The radiosensitivity of a tissue is proportional to its reproductive capacity and degree of differentiation. Since neoplastic tissues are generally poorly differentiated and have increased mitotic activity, they are, as a rule, more sensitive to radiation than normal tissue. The radiosensitivity of a tumor is an expression of its ability to respond to radiation, and this is not necessarily the same as its ability to be cured by radiation. The radiocurability of a tumor depends upon the ability to deliver sufficient radiation to destroy the tumor completely and eliminate it from the host. The presence in the pelvis of vital structures immediately adjacent to the anatomic distribution of the tumor limits the amount and dose of radiation that can be given, just as it limits surgical treatment.

A useful method of applying radium consists of a stem and box (Stockholm), as demonstrated in Fig. 41-23, where various types of applications are shown. The stem and box are usually applied in two applications, separated by a 3-week interval. By dividing the application, the tumor is given a chance to shrink following the first local application, and a better radium application can be accomplished the second time. The radium treatments are then supplemented with external therapy to the entire pelvis, usually with shielding of the midline. As a rule, 6000 to 8000 r are delivered to Point A and approximately 5000 r to Point B. Afterloading devices, utilizing a central stem and side ovoids (Fletcher-Suit applicator), permit the appliance without radiation exposure to medical personnel. An x-ray film of the application is taken and dosemetry calculated on a computer, depending upon the arrangement of stem and ovoids.

Stages II-B, III, and IV. In cases of extensive Stage II-B carcinomas of the cervix or in Stage III or IV lesions, external radiation is usually initially employed. Since radium is effective only for local cervical disease, external therapy permits treatment of the entire bulk of the tumor before concentrating on the small central part. Following preliminary external radiotherapy, radium application usually can be more effectively completed. If Stage IV lesions involve the bladder or rectum but not the pelvic wall, then a radical surgical procedure removing the bladder (anterior exenteration) or rectum (posterior exenteration) is used, since radiation cure of these lesions is usually less than 5 percent and fistulas can result from radiation treatment. However, preliminary external radiotherapy can be useful to reduce the size of the tumor as well as secondary infection. Smaller doses of radiotherapy are used when future surgical therapy is planned.

PROBLEMS OF SURGERY AND RADIATION. The immediate problems concerned with radiation therapy relate to discomfort of the patient as a result of gastrointestinal upset. Nausea, vomiting, or diarrhea are frequently encountered. However, long-term complications can also occur, and these usually relate to bleeding or inflammation of the lower bowel or chronic irritation of the bladder. Radiation proctitis or cystitis can occasionally become extremely debilitating. Fistulas may result either between the bowel and the vagina or between the bladder and the vagina, especially where extremely heavy doses of radiation have to be used. With recent refinements in radiation techniques, these complications are occurring less frequently.

Surgical complications usually occur early and relate to damage of either the genitourinary tract or the bowel. Urinary fistula is the most common complication and occurs in approximately 1 to 2 percent of cases treated by radical hysterectomy. Many of these close spontaneously, but a few require further surgical treatment, such as repair of a damaged ureter or removal of the affected kidney.

RESULTS OF THERAPY. The curability of carcinoma of the cervix is directly related to the extent of the disease at the time therapy is initiated. Comparable results have been obtained following the effective use of surgical and radiation therapy. Average approximate 5 year survival rates for the various stages are as follows: Stage I, 75 percent; Stage II, 50 percent; Stage III, 25 percent; Stage IV, 10 percent. In Stage I lesions with negative nodes, the 5-year survival approaches 90 percent. When the nodes are positive, the rates drop to 45 percent. In Stage II lesions

Fig. 41-23. Various types of radium applicators employed in radiation therapy of cervical cancer.

the comparable figures for negative and positive nodes are approximately 75 and 20 percent, respectively.

Recurrent Cervical Carcinoma. Carcinoma of the cervix can metastasize to any part of the body, but most recurrences are found in the pelvis. If the patient has pelvic recurrence after primary surgical therapy, then radiation can be tried to treat local disease. If recurrence occurs after primary therapy with radiation, then only by radical removal of the contents of the pelvis is there hope of curing the patient. This usually requires removal of both the lower bowel and bladder (total exenteration), and this procedure is reserved only for those cases where there is some hope of cure. It is occasionally done for palliation. In properly selected cases, a 20 to 30 percent 5-year survival can be obtained by using exenteration for therapy of recurrent carcinoma of the cervix.

Carcinoma of the Cervix in Pregnancy. In general, the therapy of carcinoma of the cervix which occurs during a pregnancy follows the same principles that would pertain if the patient were not pregnant. Consideration for the viability of the fetus is important only in the latter stages of pregnancy and should not be allowed to change treatment in a way that will diminish the chances of curing the mother. In the first trimester of pregnancy, therapy for early Stage I lesions can be accomplished either by radical hysterectomy or by radiation therapy. The latter is followed by spontaneous delivery of the products of conception about 2 weeks after radium therapy. In the second and third trimesters the fetus has become sufficiently large that the size of the uterus becomes a technical problem. It is usually necessary to empty the uterus by hysterotomy before proceeding with either surgical or radiation therapy, but once hysterotomy has been performed, a radical hysterectomy can usually be accomplished at the same time.

Frequently it is advisable to precede surgical exploration with a course of 2000 r external therapy prior to abdominal exploration. Then either radical hysterectomy or further radiation therapy can be accomplished, depending upon the extent of the lesion. For the advanced Stage II and III cases, radiation therapy remains the treatment of

choice. Results of therapy indicate that for each stage the survival following treatment for carcinoma of the cervix in pregnancy is much the same as it is in the nonpregnant patient.

TUMORS OF THE FUNDUS OF THE UTERUS

Endometrial Carcinoma

Most malignant tumors of the fundus of the uterus arise in the glands of the endometrium. Adenocarcinoma (Fig. 41-24C) is the most frequently found tumor, although a few adenocarcinomas with squamous tissue elements (adenoacanthoma) are seen. These tumors are histologically different but appear to have a similar clinical behavior.

Carcinomas of the endometrium are less common than malignant tumors in the cervix. They constitute approximately 20 percent of the tumors seen in the female reproductive tract. Most cases occur in the sixth decade of life and are associated with nulliparity or late childbirth. There is also an increased incidence of endometrial carcinoma in patients who are obese, diabetic, and hypertensive. Thus, these patients will generally present a markedly different social history, reproductive history, and somatic appearance than patients with carcinoma of the cervix.

The endometrium is exquisitely sensitive to hormonal stimulation, and it appears that abnormal stimulation of the endometrium could play a part in the development of certain endometrial carcinomas. It has been observed that there is an increased incidence of endometrial carcinomas in cases of prolonged and excessive estrogen stimulation, such as with estrogen-secreting tumors.

A scheme of development of malignancy has been suggested which begins with a local hyperplastic growth of endometrial glands in the form of an endometrial polyp; then cystic hyperplasia develops, followed by both cystic and adenomatous hyperplasia (Fig. 41-24A) and finally carcinoma in situ (Fig. 41-24B) of the endometrium. This sequence of changes might occur in a fashion similar to that already described for carcinoma of the cervix, although the stimuli are evidently quite different. Patients who have had prolonged anovulatory cycles and continuous estrogen stimulation without progesterone appear to be prime candidates for the development of hyperplastic changes and endometrial carcinoma.

Corpus carcinoma can be staged as follows:

Stage I—the carcinoma is confined to the corpus.
    Ia—the uterus sounds to 8 cm or less.
Stage II—the carcinoma involves the corpus and cervix.
    Ib—the uterus sounds to more than 8 cm.
Stage III—the carcinoma extends outside the uterus but is confined to the true pelvis.
Stage IV—the carcinoma extends outside the true pelvis or involves the mucosa of the bladder or rectum.

The grade of endometrial carcinoma is also important. Three grades (G1, G2, G3) are usually assigned, with the latter identifying the least differentiated lesion.

Initially, carcinoma of the endometrium invades the myometrium and then the lymphatics. When the tumor

Fig. 41-24. *A.* Endometrial hyperplasia (cystic and adenomatous). *B.* Carcinoma in situ. *C.* Adenocarcinoma of endometrium.

is low in the uterus and involves the cervix, the paths of spread are the same as those for cervical carcinoma. In contrast, spread of tumor from the upper part of the fundus goes directly to the aortic or inguinal nodes, which are sites outside the limits of radical pelvic surgical therapy.

THERAPY. The primary method for carcinoma of the endometrium is surgical therapy. This consists of a simple total hysterectomy when the carcinoma is well differentiated and confined to the fundus. To reduce the incidence of vaginal recurrence, a postoperative vaginal radium application is usually done in 4 to 6 weeks. In those cases where the cervix also is involved, therapy is best carried out in accordance with the principles outlined under the discussion of carcinoma of the cervix. External radiation therapy is employed preoperatively in cases where there is a large uterus filled with tumor or if the tumor is poorly differentiated on microscopic examination. Radiotherapy alone is used for patients who are unable to tolerate surgical therapy. These patients are then given additional radium therapy.

RESULTS OF THERAPY. The results of therapy in cases of carcinoma of the endometrium will vary with the extent of the lesion originally treated. For tumors confined to the fundus and treatable by surgical methods, approximately 70 to 80 percent will be alive and free of disease 5 years following treatment. For those who are not, because of medical reasons or spread of tumor, able to be treated by primary surgical procedures, the 5-year survival is markedly reduced. The overall salvage is approximately 50 to 60 percent.

PROBLEMS OF RECURRENCES. Recurrences of carcinoma of the endometrium are most frequently seen in the vagina, especially in the suburethral area or at the vaginal apex. They occasionally occur in the pelvis. Distant metastases are most commonly found in the lung and in the liver. Occasionally, there are intraperitoneal, nonpelvic sites of metastatic disease, but these are less common. Therapy for recurrence of endometrial carcinoma depends upon its location and extent of tumor. In cases where there is a local recurrence in the pelvis, either in the vagina or intraperitoneally, radiation is the treatment of choice. Occasionally, local vaginal radium applications are possible. If there is a large recurrence located centrally within the pelvis and especially if there has been prior radiation therapy, then radical pelvic surgical therapy should be considered. However, as in the case of carcinoma of the cervix, exenteration is generally considered for cure of a patient who is in good medical condition. Distant metastases of carcinoma of the endometrium have been successfully treated by high doses of progestational agents. Delalutin (17-hydroxyprogesterone caproate), Depo-Provera (medroxyprogesterone), and Megace (megestrol acetate) have been employed and in some cases have resulted in regression of metastatic nodules particularly in the lung. Well-differentiated tumors respond most favorably, while highly undifferentiated tumors or those which have been previously irradiated have a less satisfactory response. A response rate of about 25 percent has been obtained.

Sarcomas

These are rare tumors, comprising less than 5 percent of uterine malignant disease. They primarily occur in the postmenopausal female. The following types are those most frequently encountered.

Carcinosarcoma. This is a mixed tumor, probably of endometrial origin, which contains carcinomatous elements which probably arise from Müllerian structures and also have a sarcomatous stroma.

Endolymphatic Stromal Myosis. This refers to an endometrial tissue infiltration into the myometrium. It is a form of low-grade stromal sarcoma. The more mitoses noted in these tumors, the more malignant is the behavior.

Leiomyosarcoma. This category is the most common variety of sarcoma. These tumors generally arise from the myometrium and may be either smooth muscle leiomyosarcomas or may contain more fibrous tissues in the form of fibrosarcoma. Occasionally, one encounters malignant degeneration in a fibroid, but this is a rare occurrence. The prognosis is believed to be better if the sarcomatous change is confined to a leiomyoma.

Stromal Sarcoma. This is a sarcoma which arises from a stromal cell of the endometrium, which then invades the myometrium. It is the more malignant expression of endolymphatic stromal myosis. There are pleomorphic endometrial cells with occasional giant cell formation present inside the tumor. Many of these tumors appear to arise in patients who have had previous radiation. These tumors are usually found in the older age group and are seen primarily in the postmenopausal female. Many of them are associated with pyometrium, since the endocervix becomes closed and there is some accumulated secretion and infection behind it developing into purulent contents contained within the endometrial cavity. It has been estimated that approximately 2 to 4 percent of all patients with uterine cancer, regardless of the histologic features, may be found to have pyometrium.

THERAPY. The primary therapy of sarcoma of the fundus is surgery, consisting of total simple hysterectomy. In general, the prognosis for all these tumors is poor unless they are detected early and confined to the uterus. Radical surgical treatment generally has not been successful. Although some sarcomas have been found to be radiosensitive, they have not, as a rule, been radiocurable. Some additional palliation has been obtained by the use of chemotherapeutic agents.

Disorders of the Vulva

BENIGN AND PREMALIGNANT CHANGES

The vulva is an area which is readily accessible to examination and treatment. Therefore, much attention has been focused on the local changes which precede the development of malignancy. Whitish areas have been noted to coexist with vulvar malignancy, and in many cases these white areas have existed prior to tumor development. Such areas have been termed "leukoplakia" (white patch). However, confusion has arisen, since many white areas of

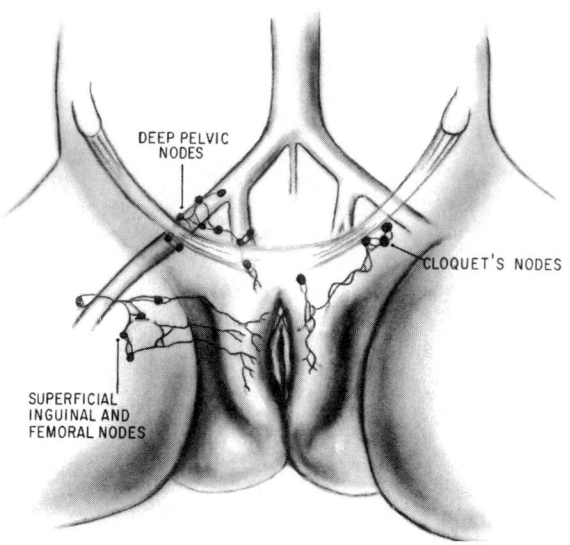

Fig. 41-25. Routes of lymphatic spread in carcinoma of the vulva.

Fig. 41-26. Radical surgical treatment for carcinoma of the vulva. *A.* Incision for a one-stage approach to radical vulvectomy in continuity with bilateral groin and deep pelvic lymph node dissections. *B.* Final operative specimen.

A

B

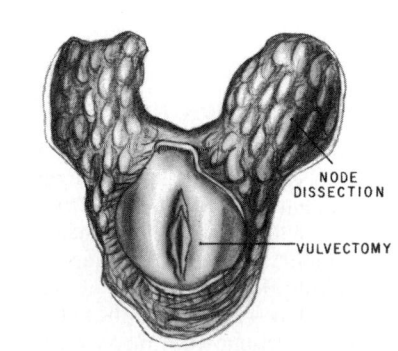

the vulva are associated with pruritic irritations that bear no relationship to malignancy and are without malignant potential. The correct diagnosis of a white vulvar lesion can be made only by biopsy, and this examination should be performed for lesions which are not temporary irritations.

Although the term leukoplakia is often used for any white patch of the vulva, it is properly reserved for areas which show histologically atypical epithelial activity. These alterations may precede the development of malignant changes. In many instances, chronically irritated and itchy white areas of the vulva will show sclerosing atrophy of the skin (lichen sclerosus et atrophicus). The term "kraurosis" is applied when hyperkeratinization becomes part of the sclerosing picture. Lichen sclerosus et atrophicans and kraurosis are pruritic lesions which do not appear to be premalignant. They are chronic problems for which transient relief can occasionally be obtained by the local application of cortisone or some other anti-inflammatory agent. Rarely, however, in severe cases, simple vulvectomy has been used to provide relief.

Noninvasive malignant change of the surface squamous epithelium of the vulva occurs in the same way that has been described for the cervix. Carcinoma in situ of the vulva, both histologically and clinically, behaves like carcinoma in situ of the cervix. The changes are confined to the squamous elements of the vulva, and the condition is sometimes referred to as "Bowen's disease." In certain instances, the apocrine glandular elements of the vulva are involved in association with an intensely pruritic area. Histologically, large, foamy Paget's cells are seen, similar to those noted in the breast, although invasive carcinoma occasionally can accompany Paget cells. Both Bowen's disease and usually Paget's disease are considered part of the carcinoma in situ complex of the vulva and are adequately treated by wide local surgical excision which consists of a simple vulvectomy.

VULVAR MALIGNANCY

Most malignant tumors of the vulva are of the squamous cell variety. These tumors comprise approximately 5 percent of all gynecologic malignant tumors and occur primarily in elderly patients. The average age of a patient treated for this disease is about sixty-one years, and the incidence of vulvar carcinoma increases in each decade. As with carcinoma of the endometrium, vulvar carcinoma tends to occur in obese patients and in nulliparous patients, and the incidence of diabetes is increased in those with this disease. In addition, as many as 10 percent of these patients may have malignant tumors at other sites.

As a rule, the carcinoma arises unilaterally and may be present on any part of the vulva. It may be multicentric in origin. The disease spreads via the lymphatics and in spite of the unilaterality of the primary lesion the lymphatics carry the tumor to both sides. Initially, metastases occur from the vulva to the superficial inguinal and femoral nodes. Then spread progresses to the deep pelvic nodes of the external iliac group (Fig. 41-25). Vulvar carcinomas tend to be slow-growing, locally spreading tumors with distant metastases occurring as late manifestations of the disease.

The rate of cure of this tumor formerly was poor because of attempts at treatment by simple local excision. The recent advent of a wide surgical en bloc resection (Fig. 41-26) has markedly improved the survival rate of these patients. Adequate therapy consists of a radical vulvectomy combined with bilateral superficial and deep groin node dissection (Fig. 41-26B). Dissection includes both groins, even though the tumor is confined to one side of the vulva, because of the high incidence of bilateral spread through the rich supply of anastomosing vulvar lymphatics. In certain cases where the patient is considered not to be an optimal surgical risk and where the upper femoral node (Cloquet's node) is found to be free of tumor, the deep iliac node dissection is omitted.

Approximately half the patients treated in this fashion are cured of the carcinoma. If the lymph nodes are uninvolved with tumor, the cure rate rises to 80 or 90 percent. Even if the lymph nodes are involved, almost half the patients treated by radical vulvectomy and bilateral node dissection can be salvaged. Involvement of the deep nodes markedly diminishes the prognosis. Radiotherapy has not proved to be as satisfactory a method as surgical therapy, especially since the vulvar skin becomes chronically irritated and pruritic after treatment.

Tumors other than epithelial carcinomas can occur in the vulva. Basal cell carcinomas are treated by simple excision. The vulva is a common site for malignant melanoma, and approximately 8 percent of melanomas that occur in females are noted in this region. However, they constitute only about 2 percent of all vulvar malignant tumors. Melanomas occur at any time but are usually noted in later years. Vulvar melanoma is treated similarly to epithelial cell carcinoma by radical vulvectomy and bilateral superficial and deep node dissection.

Carcinomas of Bartholin's glands have been reported, but these are exceedingly rare. Since the tumors are often diagnosed late in the course of the disease, they have generally disseminated through lymphatics. The results of therapy have been poor, although a wide local resection with node dissection would appear to offer the best opportunity for eradication.

Finally, tumors of sweat gland origin are seen in the vulva. These are referred to as "hidradenomas." There is some disagreement as to whether or not these tumors can occur as carcinomas. However, they are locally invasive, and therefore minimum adequate therapy consists of wide local excision.

Malignant Tumors of the Vagina

Although the vagina is frequently a site of extension from vulvar, cervical, or endometrial tumors, it is the rarest site for the origin of a malignant tumor in the female genital tract, with the exception of the fallopian tube. Usually vaginal malignant tumors occur in postmenopausal females around the age of sixty. One exception to this is the sarcoma botryoides, which is a tumor of young children. This malignant sarcoma usually presents as a mass in young infants. It is a bulky, polypoid tumor which is radiation-resistant, and the only hope of cure lies with radical surgical therapy.

Most primary cancers of the vagina are squamous cell carcinomas. Their clinical behavior depends upon the location in the vagina. Those that occur in the upper vagina usually behave as cervical tumors and therefore are treated by the same criteria used in therapy of carcinoma of the cervix. If a squamous cell carcinoma appears to be primarily occupying the vagina but is also on the cervix, it must be classified as a primary cervical tumor. For tumors located in the anterior vagina, either radiotherapy or an anterior exenteration will provide adequate therapy. For those lying in the posterior or upper vagina, either a posterior exenteration or radiotherapy must be considered. The tumors involving the lower vagina are treated as vulvar tumors, since the lymphatic spread in these instances is similar to that noted for vulvar carcinoma.

Recently, adenocarcinomas of the vagina and cervix have been noted in young girls in their late teens and early twenties, many of whose mothers took diethylstilbestrol and similar hormones during pregnancy (see section on disorders of bleeding). Histologically, the tumors consist of clear cells containing glycogen and so-called "hobnail cells." Therefore, they are called "clear cell carcinomas," although they also have been called "mesonephromas." Benign glandular infiltration of the vagina (vaginal adenosis) often accompanies these tumors, and transverse vaginal septa occasionally are seen, presumably resulting from in utero exposure to diethylstilbestrol. Diagnosis is made by vaginal examination. Although vaginal cytology occasionally can detect the tumor, the smear sometimes is negative with tumor present. Thus a complete pelvic examination including inspection of the walls of the vagina is necessary to rule out this malignancy. Therapy is accomplished by the usual considerations governing the treatment of malignancy in this area. Both operative resection and irradiation have been effective in eradicating these tumors. The operative approach is favored for young patients with early resectable lesions. When recurrences occur, they are most frequently noted locally, in the lungs, and in supraclavicular nodes. The results with chemotherapy have been disappointing.

Ovarian Tumors

DIAGNOSIS. Many types of ovarian tumors can occur in both benign and malignant forms, and a few tumors cannot be classified until their clinical behavior has been clarified by following the patient for a number of years. This multipotential behavior of ovarian tumors necessitates the consideration of benign and malignant lesions together. Ovarian malignant tumors occur less frequently than those from either the cervix or the endometrium. In general, there is an increased incidence of malignancy in ovarian tumors with advancing age.

In an infant or child, ovarian tumors may present as large pelvic masses. Adequate evaluation requires an intravenous pyelogram to rule out the urinary tract as the cause of the mass (Wilms' tumor). Patency of the hymen and vagina should be checked to rule out hydrocolpos, and the patient should be catheterized to be sure the mass is not a urine-filled bladder. An ovarian tumor in these young patients is most likely to be a teratoma, usually of the cystic variety (dermoid), or a follicle cyst. Ovarian malignant tumors do occur in the young age group, but they are rare.

During puberty and the reproductive years, ovarian tumors become more common. There is little need for concern about an enlargement unless it has become 5 cm or larger. Most 5-cm tumors in this age group are benign follicle cysts and may be followed through two menstrual periods. If the lesion persists for this length of time or appears to be enlarging, then diagnosis through direct visualization is indicated. Depending upon the size and location of the mass and the age of the patient, this may be accomplished by laparoscopy or abdominal exploration. For patients who are over age forty or in the menopausal years, the ovarian masses estimated to be 5 cm or larger should be explored.

Since ovarian enlargements are often asymptomatic, there can be significant spread of an ovarian tumor before the diagnosis is made. Common subjective symptoms consist of lower abdominal discomfort occasionally accompanied by the feeling of distension. Pain is rare unless there is advanced disease. In about one-third of the cases, the patient may complain of abnormal vaginal bleeding, and in a few cases urinary or intestinal complaints may be elicited.

NONNEOPLASTIC CYSTS

By definition a cystic enlargement of the ovary should be at least 2.5 cm in diameter to be termed a cyst. Some of the more common cysts are as follows.

FOLLICULAR CYSTS. These are unruptured, enlarged graafian follicles. They may grossly resemble true cystomas which are described in the following section. They can rupture, causing acute peritoneal irritation, but more commonly they are associated with torsion and infarction of the ovary or infarction of the tube and ovary.

CORPUS LUTEUM CYSTS. At times these cysts may become as large as 10 to 11 cm. They can rupture and lead to severe hemorrhage and occasionally vascular collapse from blood loss. The symptoms and physical findings of these cysts may mimic those of ectopic pregnancy, and they are thought by some to be associated with delayed menses and spotting.

ENDOMETRIOMAS. These account for most "chocolate cysts" and are simply cystic forms of endometriosis of the ovary.

WOLFFIAN DUCT REMNANTS. These are not ovarian cysts but often cannot be distinguished clinically from tumors of the ovary. They are small unilocular cysts. Occasionally, they enlarge and may twist and infarct. In most instances, they are incidental findings at laparotomy and cause no difficulties or symptoms.

MÜLLERIAN DUCT REMNANTS. These can appear as paraovarian cysts or as small cystic swellings at the fimbriated end of the fallopian tube (hydatids of Morgagni).

NONFUNCTIONING TUMORS

Cystadenomas

Many of the common, benign, cystic tumors of the ovary are believed to arise from the surface germinal epithelium. Some of these tumors, referred to as "serous cystadenomas," appear as cysts with thin, translucent walls containing clear fluid and lined by simple ciliated epithelium. They frequently are on a pedicle and may undergo torsion leading to pain and infarction. When encountered surgically, they are adequately treated by simple excision. Many serum-containing cystic tumors of the ovary are also accompanied by papillary projections and are known as papillary serous cystadenomas. Because of epithelial variation in these tumors, it is often difficult to be sure where they fit in the spectrum of benign to malignant disease. A similar problem of malignant potential exists for the mucinous cystadenoma, which is a cystic tumor containing sticky, gelatinous material. These mucinous tumors are less likely to be malignant than the serous cystadenomas. About 20 percent of the serous tumors and 5 percent of the mucinous tumors are bilateral.

It is not always possible to be sure by gross inspection whether cystic tumors with solid components are benign or malignant. It is usually necessary to excise the involved ovary completely, even though there is no definite evidence of malignancy. The malignant potential of the cystoma is then determined by histologic examination. Frozen-section examination of the tumor at the time of surgical intervention is necessary to determine the proper course of therapy for patients in the reproductive age group. The opposite ovary should be examined for a lesion and may be bivalved.

Occasionally, a condition is encountered known as "pseudomyxoma peritonei," which is a locally infiltrating tumor composed of multiple cysts containing thick mucin. These tumors arise either from ovarian mucinous cystadenomas or from mucoceles of the appendix, both of which commonly coexist. Histologically, they are benign, but by local spread and infiltration they compromise surrounding vital structures. Localized tumors should be completely excised, if possible. Both ovaries and the appendix are removed even though they grossly appear to be normal.

Primary Carcinomas

Primary carcinomas of the ovary most commonly are serous, mucinous, or endometroid cystadenocarcinomas. These are malignant variations of the previously discussed cystadenomas and of endometriosis. A useful method of staging these tumors is as follows:

Stage I—tumor confined to the ovaries
Stage II—tumor confined to the true pelvis
Stage III—tumor extends to peritoneum outside pelvis
Stage IV—spread beyond the abdominal cavity or intrahepatic metastases.

The Stage III and IV tumors have a markedly poorer prognosis than in those cases with malignancy confined to the ovary.

Malignant tumors of the ovary usually spread locally,

and it is common to see seedings on both peritoneum and serosal surfaces of bowel. Giant masses can develop and slowly spread to fill the entire peritoneal cavity encasing the bowel but rarely invading the lumen. Fluid retention occurs, and both ascites and hydrothorax may be present. Lower leg edema may be seen secondary to abdominal lymphatic obstruction. The patient may experience an increase in abdominal girth and, possibly, weight gain accompanied by wasting of the extremities, loss of appetite, and reduction in muscle mass. Increase in fluid retention and in the size of the abdomen continues with the growth of the intraabdominal tumor.

Surgical intervention is the primary therapy for ovarian malignancy and consists of hysterectomy and bilateral salpingo-oophorectomy. If ascites is present, ascitic fluid is examined cytologically for malignant cells. If there is no obvious extension of tumor outside the ovaries, peritoneal saline washings are examined for malignant cells. The omentum is also sampled or excised. An attempt should be made to remove all sites of the tumor, including local peritoneal metastases. However, in widespread cases radical pelvic surgical treatment with removal of the bladder or the rectum has generally not proved to be helpful. Therefore, if a few discrete peritoneal metastases exist, it is wise to remove them and it is generally accepted that maximum tumor reduction surgery is beneficial if it does not seriously expose the patient to the risk of life-threatening complications. Reduction of tumor mass appears to be helpful in improving the response to chemotherapy or irradiation.

When complete surgical removal cannot be accomplished, it has been customary to treat the residual tumor with radiotherapy. Usually there is sufficient response to produce an interval without symptoms during which the patient is comfortable and active. Rarely this is of long duration, but cure is so unlikely that most clinics now prefer to treat patients with known or suspected residual cancer of the ovary with one or another program of systemic chemotherapy.

Chemotherapy has also been effective in treatment of metastatic tumors and has been used with increasing frequency. The alkylating agents Cytoxan, chlorambucil, and phenylalanine mustard have been the most effective drugs. They have radiomimetic effects. These potent agents interfere with rapidly growing cells and thus particularly affect the bone marrow and gastrointestinal tract as well as the tumor. Nausea, vomiting, diarrhea, and loss of hair can accompany their use. Blood indices must be carefully observed since leukopenia and thrombocytopenia may occur, especially in patients who have received radiotherapy. Cytoxan, chlorambucil, and phenylalanine mustard can be taken orally; the dosage is adjusted to maintain a slight leukocyte depression with the white blood cell count kept in the range of 3,500 to 5,000 cells per cubic millimeter. The antimetabolite 5-fluorouracil (5-FU) also is used but is less effective than the alkylating agents. Efforts have been made to improve results by administration of a number of agents at reduced dosages simultaneously.

In addition, another alkylating agent, thiotepa, can be instilled into the peritoneal cavity to help to control the growth of the tumor and ascites formation. Radioactive gold has been used in a similar fashion. One must be careful in using intraperitoneal instillations, since there is often loculation of fluid between areas of tumor and bowel which can cause a high local concentration of the chemotherapeutic agent or the radioactive gold. Bowel perforation can result.

Radiation therapy is useful in situations in which regression can be assessed. It is offered for the relief of ascites when all other modalities have failed. It is also used as adjuvant therapy when the pelvis is contaminated with tumor cells or when there are external papillary projections or cytologically positive peritoneal fluid. In the latter situation, alkylating agents are frequently used.

The ovary is a site for metastases from tumors originating elsewhere in the body. Solid ovarian tumors containing malignant disease which is usually metastatic from the stomach are known as "Krukenberg tumors," identified histologically by the presence of signet cells. However, ovarian metastases from other intestinal malignant tumors are more common. In cases where a Krukenberg tumor can be diagnosed, it is felt by some that oophorectomy may offer a palliation to the patient, even though the primary malignant tumor cannot be found. The ovary is also a common site for metastases from breast carcinoma.

Dysgerminoma

This rare tumor is most often seen in females in the age group of ten to thirty. It often occurs in pseudohermaphrodites. Dysgerminomas are often found during pregnancy, perhaps because they occur most frequently during the reproductive years. Histologically (Fig. 41-27C), the tumors contain masses of germ cells infiltrated with lymphocytes. If the tumor is unilateral and has not broken through its capsule, then a simple oophorectomy is usually sufficient therapy. If it has broken through its capsule but has not spread beyond the ovary and the contralateral ovary is normal, then preservation of the contralateral ovary with radiation to the side of the surgically removed specimen may be considered. If the tumor has spread or metastasized locally in the pelvis, then the prognosis is poorer. The tumor is sensitive to radiation, resembling the seminoma of the male, but is frequently not radiocurable.

Teratoma

These tumors are thought to arise from the totipotential germ cells of the ovary. The tumors often contain calcified masses, and occasionally either teeth or pieces of bone can be seen on abdominal x-rays. Teratomas occur at any age but are more frequent in patients between twenty and forty years. They are usually benign dermoid cysts but occasionally are solid and then are usually malignant (solid malignant teratomas; teratocarcinomas). The embryonal carcinoma is thought to be an undifferentiated form of teratocarcinoma, and the prognosis associated with these tumors is exceedingly poor even if there is complete excision with no apparent tumor extension at the time of surgical treatment.

If a cystic teratoma (dermoid) is encountered in a young woman, it is preferable to shell it out from the ovarian stroma, preserving functioning tissue in the affected ovary.

Fig. 41-27. *A*. Granulosa-theca cell tumor. *B*. Arrhenoblastoma. *C*. Dysgerminoma.

Usually these cysts contain ectodermal, mesodermal, and entodermal tissues, in addition to a thick, greasy, fatty material. If this material is spilled during surgery, a chemical peritonitis may result, and, therefore, it is important to remove these tumors intact. The opposite ovary should be inspected and bivalved at the time of removal of cystic teratomas, because in approximately 12 percent of the cases these tumors are bilateral. Malignant teratomas are treated as a carcinoma of the ovary by hysterectomy and bilateral salpingo-oophorectomy.

Brenner Tumor

These are fibroepithelial tumors which are rare and usually do not secrete hormones. Histologically, the epithelial elements are similar to Walthard rests and are believed to arise from these. These tumors occur primarily in later life and have a small malignant potential. Simple oophorectomy is usually sufficient therapy, and the prognosis is excellent.

Clear Cell Carcinomas

These account for as many as 5 percent of primary carcinomas of the ovary. Histologically they consist of clear cells containing glycogen and "hobnail" cells. In most cases the ovaries and uterus are removed since the tumors predominantly occur in older women.

Meigs' Syndrome

This pertains to ascites with hydrothorax, seen in association with benign ovarian tumors with fibrous elements, usually fibromas. It is more common to see fluid accumulation with ovarian fibromas that are more than 6 cm in size. The cause of the condition is unknown, but the ascitic fluid may originate from the tumor, as a result of lymphatic obstruction of the ovary. Frequently, this clinical picture is encountered with other ovarian tumors, especially ovarian malignancy, which can produce a cytologically benign plural effusion; in such cases it is termed a "pseudo-Meigs" syndrome. Meigs' syndrome can be cured by excising the fibroma.

FUNCTIONING TUMORS

Granulosa-Theca Cell Tumor

Pure theca cell tumors (thecomas) are benign, but those with granulosa cell elements may be malignant. It is often impossible to predict their behavior from the histologic features (Fig. 41-27*A*), and prolonged followup is necessary in order to judge the nature. Usually, granulosa cell tumors elaborate estrogen, but some of these tumors have no hormone production. In the young girl they are characteristically manifested by precocious puberty, and in the elderly female they are sometimes associated with endometrial carcinoma. The tumor can occur at all ages from childhood to the postmenopausal period but are most common in later life, with maximal occurrence between the ages of forty and sixty. If the tumor is discovered in the reproductive years and confined to one ovary without signs of surface spread or dissemination, a simple oophorectomy may be sufficient therapy. If it is discovered in later life, then removal of both ovaries with the uterus is indicated.

Sertoli-Leydig Cell Tumors (Arrhenoblastomas)

These are rare but potentially malignant tumors which are associated with androgen output and masculinization. Rarely, they elaborate estrogen. They usually occur in the reproductive age group and appear to contain tubular structures as well as Leydig-type cells (Fig. 41-27*B*). In young patients with a singly involved ovary, unilateral oophorectomy is adequate therapy, provided there is no extension of the tumor. For older patients or for those with bilateral involvement, total hysterectomy and bilateral salpingo-oophorectomy are performed.

Hilus Cell Tumors

These are also rare tumors and consist of nests of cells resembling the hilus cells of the ovary. They are characteristically associated with masculinization. They occur primarily in the later years of life and often in the menopausal female. None of the reported cases was malignant.

Struma Ovarii

This term refers to the presence of grossly detectable thyroid tissue in the ovary, usually as the predominant element in dermoid cysts. This tissue occasionally may produce the clinical picture of hyperthyroidism.

Choriocarcinoma

These very rare primary tumors of the ovary elaborate chorionic gonadotropin, and the therapy follows similar considerations already outlined for trophoblastic disease, but the therapeutic results for the ovarian tumors have been disappointing.

Adrenal Rest Tumors

These are also very rare tumors of the ovary which may occur at any age and are not always associated with hormonal activity. Those with adrenal tissue usually show masculinization and are, as a rule, benign. Although most of the signs of masculinization regress after surgical therapy, some of the effects, such as enlarged clitoris, may remain.

Tumors of the Fallopian Tube

BENIGN TUMORS

Tumors of the fallopian tube are rare. Occasionally one sees a tube with thick nodularities at its proximal end. This benign condition is referred to as "salpingitis isthmica nodosa," and although its origin is not definitely known, it is thought to be a sequela of tubal inflammation. It is associated with infertility due to blockage of the tubes. In cases of infertility, a tuboplastic procedure can be attempted in the hope of restoring tubal patency, but the prognosis is poor.

Another type of benign lesion is referred to as "adenomatoid tumor." These are small gland-containing enlargements of the tube which are usually located in the tubal muscularis and are often incidental findings at the time of surgical intervention. Other enlargements of the tube secondary to inflammation or associated with pregnancy are discussed in previous sections of the chapter.

MALIGNANT TUMORS

Primary malignant tumors of the tube are the least frequently seen cancers of the female genital tract. There may be an association between previous tubal inflammation and subsequent development of carcinoma in the tube. Usually these tumors are papillary adenocarcinomas. They may present as a pelvic mass. Occasionally, the tumors block the distal end of the fallopian tube and cause a bloody, mucous vaginal discharge. These tumors are occasionally seen during the reproductive years but occur more often in the postmenopausal age group. Because of the paucity of symptoms and physical findings associated with them, tumors of the fallopian tube are difficult to diagnose early. They may metastasize locally and occa-

sionally spread to the inguinal nodes. Primary therapy is by surgical excision, preferably removal of the tumor and of the uterus and opposite tube and ovary as well. In cases where there appears to be some lymphatic spread of the tumor in the area of the cervix, a radical hysterectomy may effect a cure. The 5-year survival ranges between 10 and 40 percent. Radiotherapy may be tried as palliation or as adjunctive therapy.

TECHNICAL CONSIDERATIONS OF GYNECOLOGIC OPERATIONS

Dilatation and Curettage

Dilatation and curettage (D and C) are frequently indicated in a variety of clinical problems. In patients of reproductive age it is often advisable to perform a curettage after a first-trimester pregnancy loss. In such circumstances, as has been noted in this chapter, an incomplete abortion may have occurred, and curettage is advisable both to prevent further blood loss and to reduce the incidence of postabortal infection. These considerations apply only to cases of spontaneous noninfected abortion. In those cases where instrumentation or sepsis have supervened, a curettage should not be carried out until the patient is adequately treated with antibiotics. Any manipulation of a pregnant uterus should be carried out with extreme care because of the high risk of uterine perforation. In addition, only the major products of conception need be removed. Excessively vigorous curettage at this time can denude the uterine cavity of regenerative tissue, which may result in postcurettage intrauterine synechiae (Asherman's syndrome).

A curettage may also be indicated during reproductive years for excessive bleeding and hemorrhage not associated with pregnancy. In such instances, it is important to carry out a meticulous exploration of the endometrial cavity to be sure that neither endometrial polyps nor submucous fibroids are present. During the menopause, excessive bleeding may necessitate a curettage for diagnostic as well as therapeutic reasons. In these circumstances, a thorough curettage of the endometrial cavity is mandatory, not only to remove all foci that might harbor malignancy, but also to denude the cavity of excess endometrial tissue which may be the cause of the bleeding. A thorough curettage is also required in cases of postmenopausal bleeding. In such cases, a "fractional" curettage is accomplished by first curetting the cervix and then dilating the cervix and curetting the uterine fundus. In this way separate endocervical and endometrial specimens are submitted for pathologic examination. If endometrial carcinoma is discovered, the presence or absence of endocervical involvement is immediately determined, and therapy is planned accordingly (see section on therapy of endometrial carcinoma). In all cases a thorough pelvic examination should be performed, since the anesthetized patients provide the physician with an excellent opportunity to find previously unsuspected intrapelvic pathologic conditions.

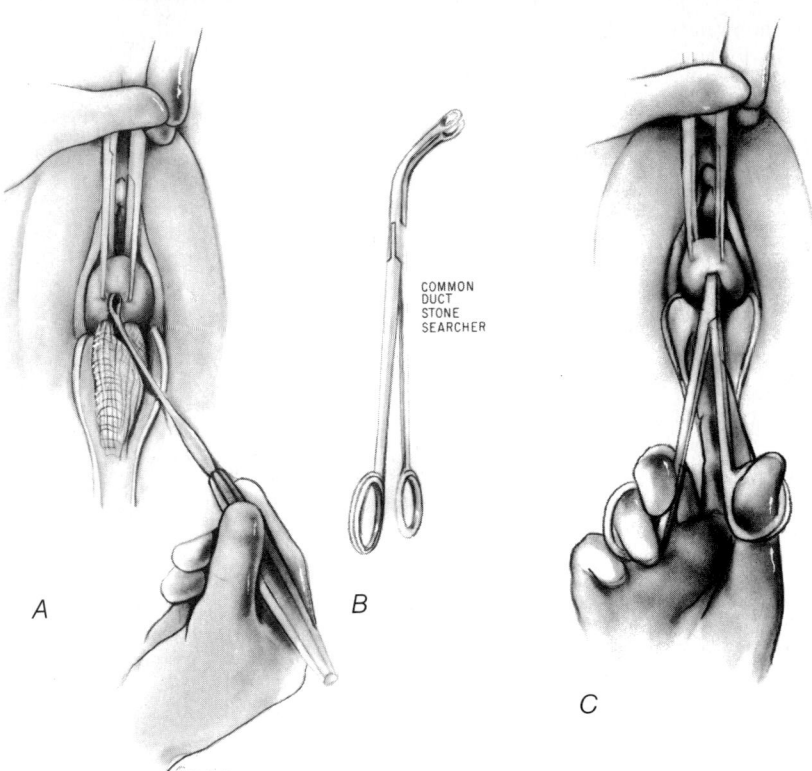

COMMON
DUCT
STONE
SEARCHER

A

B

C

Fig. 41-28. Dilatation and curettage. (See description in text.)

TECHNIQUE (Fig. 41-28). The cervix is grasped with a tenaculum. Dilatation of the cervix following abortion is not necessary, and in other cases a dilatation is carried out with graduated dilators of increasing diameter. The Goodell dilator, which can cause great pressure on the endocervix, should not be used as it can split the cervix. A blunt curet is gently introduced into the cervix and endometrial cavity using only minimal force. Extra pressure on the curet is avoided during this time. The curet is then withdrawn, scraping sharply against the sidewalls of the uterus. Firm pressure on the curet is applied during the withdrawal stroke. The cavity is further explored with a common duct stone searcher in order to remove any large masses of tissue. A sharp curet is often unnecessary in cases associated with pregnancy but is used routinely when a diagnostic or therapeutic curettage is being performed in the nonpregnant uterus.

There are numerous surgical procedures that can be performed vaginally. The uterus can be removed by this route in cases of pelvic relaxation, and many disorders of pelvic support can be corrected by a vaginal operation. A few general guidelines are worth considering: exposure at all times should be adequate, small bites of tissue should be taken under direct vision, and a meticulous dissection should be carried out. An enlarged uterus or adnexal mass may preclude a safe vaginal dissection; under these circumstances the abdominal route is used. The excess blood loss that all too frequently accompanies vaginal surgical procedures must be avoided. Damage to surrounding structures, including bladder, ureter, and rectum, can be prevented by adhering to these principles.

Abdominal Gynecologic Procedures

Incisions

The lower abdomen may be conveniently entered through a transverse or vertical incision. For most gynecologic procedures, either a midline or paramedian incision will provide good exposure. The right paramedian incision is frequently used when there is a pathologic condition in the right lower quadrant, especially in cases where the appendix or right adnexal structures could be involved. If a paramedian incision is used, the rectus abdominis muscle is retracted laterally away from the midline. If a midline approach is used, both the right and left rectus sheaths are opened and then resutured at the close of the procedure, since approximation prevents postoperative diastasis and adds to the long-term strength of the wound. Permanent suture material or heavy absorbable suture material can be used to reapproximate the anterior rectus fascia, since this is the layer that provides the main strength of the wound closure.

In certain instances, where surgical treatment is performed on young patients, a Pfannenstiel incision may be used. This incision provides a better cosmetic result, and although there may be slight decrease in exposure, this usually poses no problem. The incision can provide adequate exposure for operations confined to the uterus or to the adnexa. The risk of hematoma formation and subsequent sepsis is somewhat higher in a Pfannenstiel incision. The incision is placed transversely just above the pubic hairline and extends beyond the border of both rectus abdominis muscles (Fig. 41-29A). The subcutaneous tissue is divided, and the rectus fascia is split transversely (Fig. 41-29B). With traction placed on the lower rectus fascia it is separated from the rectus muscle, and the pyramidalis muscle is preserved on its fascial attachment. After the inferior border of the incision has been delineated, the upper segment of the incision of the anterior rectus fascia is also freed from the underlying muscles (Fig. 41-29C). The rectus abdominis muscles are separated in the midline, and the peritoneum is entered in a vertical fashion (Fig. 41-29D). After the conclusion of the procedure, the peritoneum is reapproximated in the midline. The muscles are then reapproximated with loose interrupted sutures, and then the rectus sheath is reapproximated in a transverse direction. The skin and subcutaneous tissues are closed in routine fashion.

OPERATION FOR ECTOPIC PREGNANCY

Death from intraperitoneal hemorrhage can occur, and rapid entry into the abdomen through a vertical incision may be necessary. In most cases, the architecture of the tube is destroyed. In rare circumstances the tube may be left in situ. Unfortunately a second ectopic pregnancy is a significant risk in these patients, and thus the tube usually is removed.

The question of prophylactic removal of the ipsilateral ovary with the tube in cases of ectopic pregnancy has received a great deal of attention due to the introduction of the theory of transmigration, discussed previously in this chapter. Therefore, it has been suggested that the removal of both the tube and the ovary on the same side may prevent a future ectopic pregnancy in the remaining opposite tube. However, this practice is not routinely adopted in younger patients whose reproductive life is just beginning and who do run the risk of a pathologic condition developing in the opposite ovary. This is consistent with the general concept of retaining normal tissue in conservative operations on the reproductive tract.

TECHNIQUE. A traction suture is placed on the uterus, which is retracted to the side opposite the tube. The tube is brought up into view, and the mesentery of the tube is divided (Fig. 41-30A). After the tube has been freed from its mesentery, it is placed on traction, elevated and dissected free at its base, in order to be sure that the cornual end of the tube is removed (Fig. 41-30B). This prevents the occurrence of future cornual pregnancy. A mattress suture placed in the cornual end of the tube prior to cornual resection helps control hemorrhage. The uterus is repaired, and the mesentery of the ovary is brought to the posterior edge of the broad ligament in order to cover any remaining raw surface (Fig. 41-30C).

Fig. 41-29. Pfannenstiel incision. (See description in text.)

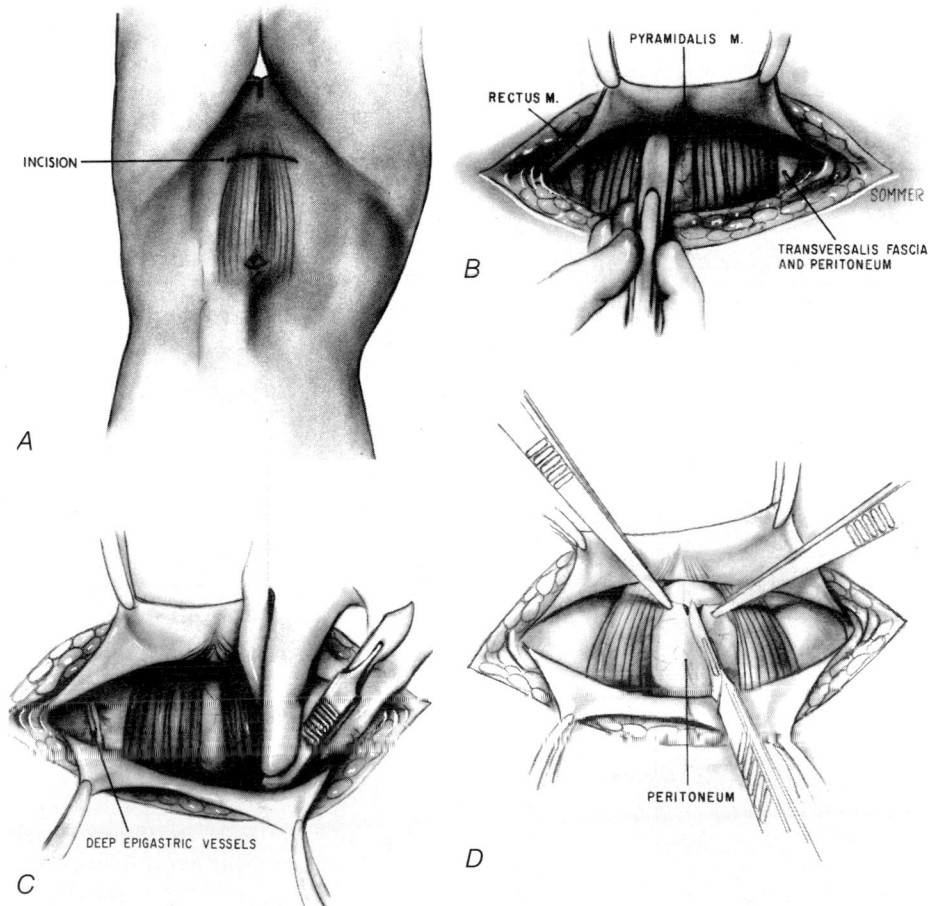

SALPINGO-OOPHORECTOMY

In cases of large ovarian tumors or with torsion of the adnexa, the architecture of the tube and ovary may be destroyed. In this instance, unilateral removal of both is performed. First the infundibulopelvic ligament is divided after the ovarian vessels are sutured (Fig. 41-31*A*). The

Fig. 41-30. Salpingectomy. (See description in text.)

A

B

C

broad ligament is divided and dissection carried to the insertion of the tube into the uterus near the origin of the round ligament (Fig. 41-31*B*). The ovarian branch of the uterine artery is ligated (Fig. 41-31*C*). The cornual end of the tube is excised (as in Fig. 41-30*B*), and the defect in the peritoneum is closed (Fig. 41-31*D*).

ABDOMINAL HYSTERECTOMY

In cases of ovarian or endometrial malignancy, the ovaries and tubes are removed with the hysterectomy specimen. In younger patients who are undergoing surgical treatment for other diseases, ovarian conservation may be practiced. The ureter, bladder, and adjacent intestine can be injured during the course of hysterectomy unless careful surgical technique and adequate exposure are maintained (Fig. 41-32). The ureters are particularly prone to injury in the areas of uterosacral ligaments and the uterine artery, since they pass close to these structures. In cases where there is any doubt, the ureter should be visually identified.

TECHNIQUE. The uterus is placed on tension by a tenaculum in the fundus. The anterior leaf of the broad ligament is opened (Fig. 41-33*A*), and the peritoneum above the bladder is separated away from the anterior portion of the uterus (Fig. 41-33*B*). The bladder is then advanced off the uterus and cervix (Fig. 41-33*C*), with the peritoneal sheath kept on tension during the course of this dissection in order not to injure the dome of the bladder.

If the ovaries are to be preserved, the ovarian vessels with the fallopian tube are ligated approximately 1 in. lateral to the uterus (Fig. 41-33*D*). If the ovaries are to be removed, the technique is similar to that shown in Fig. 41-31. The round ligament is then divided, and the anterior and posterior leaves of the broad ligaments are separated. The uterine vessels lie at the base of the broad ligament, and the ureter can be palpated as it passes beneath the uterine vessels (Fig. 41-33*E*). The uterosacral ligaments are next divided, and once again careful attention should be paid to the location of the ureter (Fig. 41-33*F*). After both uterosacral ligaments have been divided, the posterior peritoneum is separated from the back of the specimen, and care is taken to ensure that the rectosigmoid is separated from the posterior part of the dissection. In this fashion, the posterior wall of the vagina is exposed, and the uterus is separated from its peritoneal attachment.

The uterine vessels are then secured. Clamps should be applied under direct vision (Fig. 41-33*G*). The branches of the uterine artery and vein run close to the cervix and cervicouterine junction, and hemostasis must be obtained at the lateral edge of the cervix and lower portion of the uterus. Traction is placed on the fundus, and the uterine vessels are clamped. A second clamp is added to protect against back-bleeding. The vessels are divided, and an additional clamp is placed to ensure against loss of control of the uterine vessel pedicle. The vessels are ligated, removing the lateral clamp first, following which a second suture is placed.

The bladder is mobilized anteriorly to free it completely from the vagina in the area of the cervix. The cardinal ligament is divided and sutured (Fig. 41-33*H*). It may be necessary to accomplish this step in a number of small bites. The vagina is then entered. This can be accomplished by elevating the uterus and placing clamps at the lateral corners of the vagina. The tissue above the clamps is then divided (Fig. 41-33*I*). The specimen is removed by dividing the vaginal tissue under direct vision. Sutures are placed at each angle of the vagina to ensure hemostasis, and the vaginal tissue is then repaired by a running atraumatic chromic catgut suture placed around the apex, which is then left open for improved drainage (Fig. 41-33*J*).

The pelvis is reconstructed by suturing the uterosacral ligaments to the posterior vaginal wall (Fig. 41-33*K*). This provides important support to the vagina. The round ligaments are then brought to the corners of the vagina (Fig. 41-33*L*). Although this maneuver does not add to the permanent support of the vagina, it does aid in reperito-

nealization of the pelvis. The procedure is completed by bringing together the edges of the remaining peritoneum in order to leave a smooth operative field (Fig. 41-33*L*).

Wertheim Hysterectomy with Pelvic Lymphadenectomy

This operation is performed primarily for cancer of the cervix when the disease appears to be confined to the cervix itself or the immediately adjacent vaginal wall. It has also been performed for treatment of cancer of the endometrium. The operation removes the contents of the pelvis from one obturator fossa to the other, including the lymph nodes in the common iliac, hypogastric, external iliac, and obturator artery areas. The ureters are identified through their entire course from bifurcation of the aorta to entrance into the bladder. Complete mobilization of the bladder and ureters from the vagina permits removal of all the tissue extending from the side wall of the pelvis

Fig. 41-31. Salpingo-oophorectomy. (See description in text.)

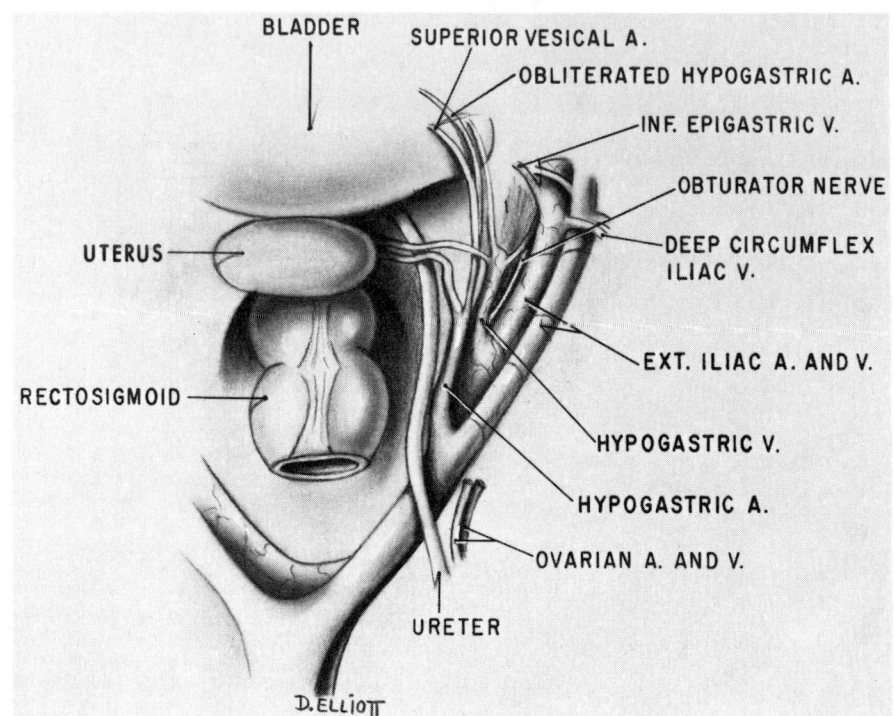

BLADDER   SUPERIOR VESICAL A.

OBLITERATED HYPOGASTRIC A.

INF. EPIGASTRIC V.

OBTURATOR NERVE

DEEP CIRCUMFLEX
ILIAC V.

UTERUS

EXT. ILIAC A. AND V.

RECTOSIGMOID

HYPOGASTRIC V.

HYPOGASTRIC A.

OVARIAN A. AND V.

URETER

D. ELLIOTT

Fig. 41-32. Surgical anatomy of pelvis.

to the paracervical and paravaginal area. The entire uterus, the adnexa, and a wide block of lymphatic tissue are removed in one piece, together with a large segment of vagina.

TECHNIQUE. The operation is performed through a low abdominal vertical incision. Most of the points of technique enumerated for hysterectomy apply; those specifically applicable to the Wertheim hysterectomy are outlined in this discussion. The ureter is initially identified at a point where it crosses the common iliac artery (Fig. 41-34A); the ovarian arteries are dissected free of the ureter and underlying common iliac artery. The ovarian vessels are then divided. The bladder flap is then developed as in the technique of total hysterectomy. The round ligament and broad ligament are transected. The uterus is then retracted medially to permit exposure of the areolar tissue overlying the external and internal iliac arteries. Dissection begins lateral to the artery on the psoas muscle and continues down along its medial surface to enter the upper portion of the obturator space. The genitofemoral nerve lies on the psoas and should be preserved. This dissection exposes the lateral and inferior surface of the external iliac vein and mobilizes all areolar tissue toward the midline (Fig. 41-34B). The common iliac lymph nodes and the external iliac lymph nodes are freed. Dissection of this areolar tissue mass permits exposure of the pubic ramus. The obturator and internal iliac nodes are also dissected free. In the course of this dissection, the obturator nerve is identified and spared. The uterine vein is identified at a point where it enters the internal iliac vein and is transected (Fig. 41-34C). The same dissection is carried out on the opposite side up to this point.

Attention is next directed to the original side, and freeing of the ureter continues. The ureter is dissected down to its entrance into the bladder. The ureter must be cleared from its tunnel along the anterior vaginal wall to permit excision of the paracervical and paravaginal lymphatics. A plexus of vaginal veins lies above and below it, and these must be transected (Fig. 41-34D). The ureter is now completely free from its bed, and the junction with the bladder can be identified. This permits dissection of an adequate length of vagina and paravaginal tissue.

The rectum is then separated from the posterior vaginal wall. All posterior attachments of the uterus are transected, and attention is directed to the anterolateral attachments. The uterus is drawn sharply back toward the promontory of the sacrum, and the bladder and ureters are carefully elevated so that dissection can begin beneath the bladder, freeing it laterally first on one side and then on the other. This represents the most important area of dissection; in order to avoid risk of recurrence, it is imperative that a wide block of tissue containing the paravaginal lymphatics be removed (Fig. 41-34E). This maneuver permits demonstration of the vaginal wall and allows transection and removal of one-half of the vagina. Complete dissection clears both iliac areas and the obturator fossa of all intervening lymphatic tissue. The bladder and ureters lie mobile above the closed vaginal stump (Fig. 41-34F). The vaginal cuff is oversewn, and the area is reperitonealized.

Fig. 41-33. Hysterectomy. (See description in text.)

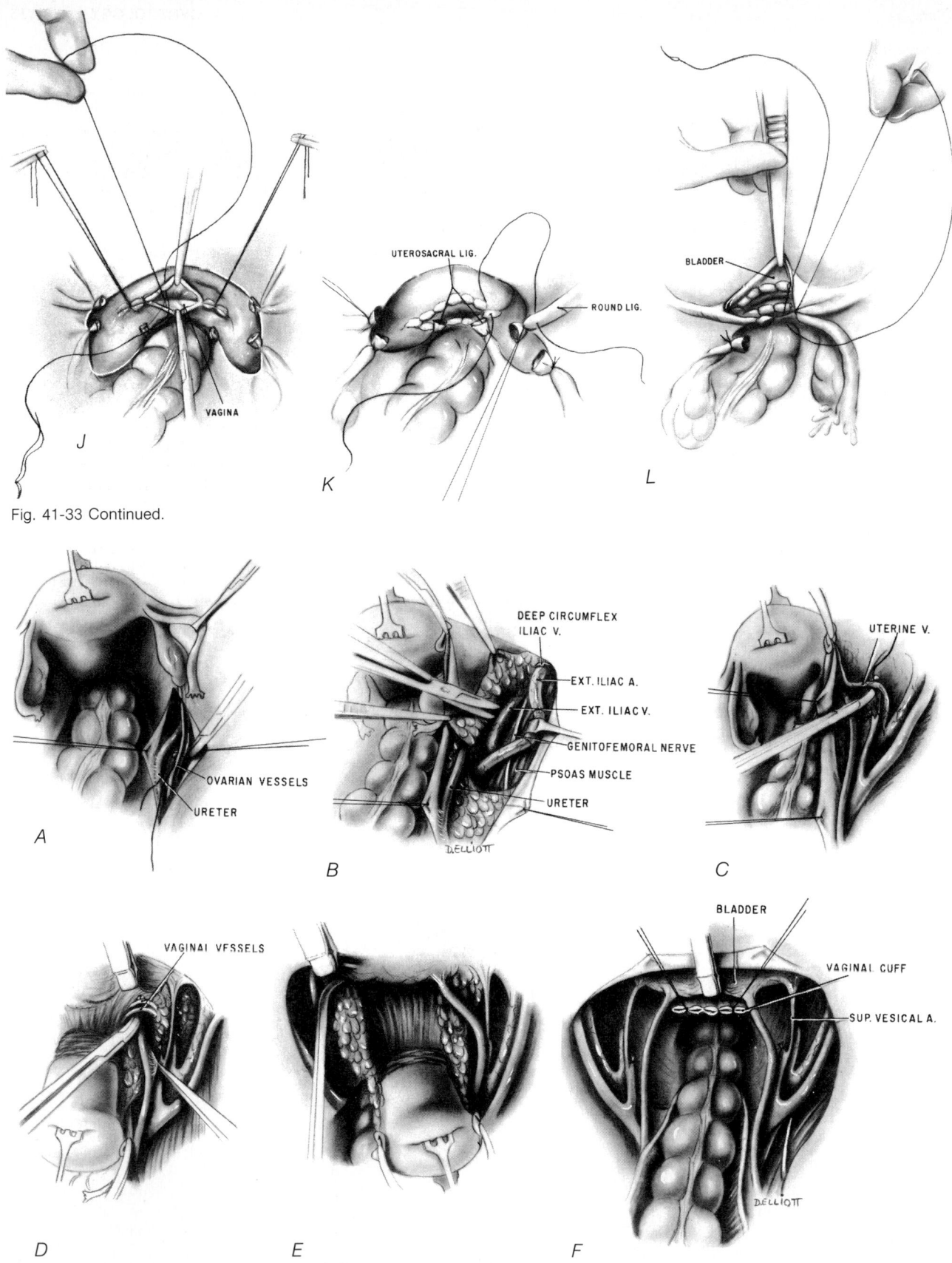

Fig. 41-33 Continued.

J VAGINA

K UTEROSACRAL LIG. ROUND LIG.

L BLADDER

A OVARIAN VESSELS / URETER

B DEEP CIRCUMFLEX ILIAC V. / EXT. ILIAC A. / EXT. ILIAC V. / GENITOFEMORAL NERVE / PSOAS MUSCLE / URETER / DELLIOTT

C UTERINE V.

D VAGINAL VESSELS

E

F BLADDER / VAGINAL CUFF / SUP. VESICAL A. / DELLIOTT

Fig. 41-34. Wertheim hysterectomy with pelvic lymphadenectomy. (See description in text.)

References

General

Glass, R.: "Office Gynecology," Williams & Wilkins Company, Baltimore, 1976.

Green, T. H., Jr.: "Gynecology: Essentials of Clinical Practice," 3d ed., Little, Brown and Company, Boston, 1977.

Herbst, A. L. (ed.): "Intrauterine Exposure to Diethylstilbestrol in the Human," American College of Obstetrics and Gynecology, 1978.

Kistner, R. W.: "Gynecology: Principles and Practice," 2d ed., Year Book Medical Publishers, Inc., Chicago, 1971.

Novak, E. R., Jones, G. S., and Jones, H. W., Jr.: "Textbook of Gynecology," 9th ed., The Williams & Wilkins Company, Baltimore, 1975.

Parsons, L., and Sommers, S. C.: "Gynecology," W. B. Saunders Company, Philadelphia, 1977.

Taynor, M. L., and Green, T. H.: "Progress in Gynecology," vol. VI, Grune & Stratton, Inc., New York, 1975.

Wynn, R.: "Obstetrics and Gynecology: The Clinical Care," Lea & Febiger, Philadelphia, 1974.

Gynecologic Procedures and Techniques

Coppleson, M., Pixley, E., and Reid, B.: Colposcopy: A Scientific and Practical Approach to the Cervix in Health and Disease, in "American Lectures in Gynecology and Obstetrics," American Lecture Series, no. 799, Charles C Thomas, Publishers, Springfield, Ill., 1971.

Kolstad, P. and Stafl, A.: "Atlas of Colposcopy," Scandinavian University Books, Oslo, 1972.

Mattingly, R. F.: "TeLinde's Operative Gynecology," 5th ed., J. B. Lippincott Company, Philadelphia, 1977.

Parsons, L., and Ulfelder, H.: "An Atlas of Pelvic Operations," 2d ed., W. B. Saunders Company, Philadelphia, 1968.

Related Texts of Special Interest

Behrman, S. J., and Kistner, R. W.: "Progress in Infertility," 2d ed., Little, Brown and Company, Boston, 1975.

Gold, J. J.: "Gynecologic Endocrinology," 2d ed., Harper & Row, Publishers, Incorporated, New York, 1975.

Jones, H. W., Jr., and Scott, W.: "Hermaphroditism; Genital Anomalies and Related Endocrine Disorders," 3d ed., The Williams & Wilkins Company, Baltimore, 1971.

Moore, K. L.: "The Developing Human: Clinically Oriented Embryology," W. B. Saunders Company, Philadelphia, 1973.

Morris, J. M., and Scully, R. E.: "Endocrine Pathology of the Ovary," The C. V. Mosby Company, St. Louis, 1958.

Reid, E. D., Ryan, K. J., and Berdirschke, K.: "Principles and Management of Human Reproduction," W. B. Saunders Company, Philadelphia, 1972.

Speroff, L., Glass, R. H., and Kage, N. G.: "Clinical Gynecologic Endocrinology and Infertility," The Williams & Wilkins Company, Baltimore, 1973.

Chapter 42

Neurologic Surgery

by **William F. Collins, Jr., Joan L. Venes, Franklin C. Wagner, Jr., and Dennis D. Spencer**

GENERAL CONSIDERATIONS

Neurologic surgery includes the surgical treatment of diseases of the nervous system, correction of malformations of the nervous system, the care and repair of traumatic lesions of the nervous system, and the surgical palliation of pain and abnormal motor movements. Anatomy and physiology of the nervous system, the pathophysiology of neurologic disease, and surgery in the broadest sense constitute the foundations of neurologic surgery. The goal is to preserve or restore the maximal degree of neurologic function possible within the disease state. This section will discuss a few salient concepts that provide insight into the surgical therapy of nervous system disease.

Consciousness is a prime sign of the working brain, and loss of consciousness can result from many conditions, for the function of the brain not only is dependent upon controlled excitability in many interrelated and interconnected neurons and the integrity of their supporting glia but also upon adequate function in the rest of the organism. Normal central nervous system function presupposes adequate cardiac output of oxygenated blood with normal ionic and molecular constituents and intact vascular channels for perfusion. Loss of consciousness as a presenting symptom requires not only consideration of central nervous system pathology but evaluations of cardiac output, competence of blood vessels, causes of aberrant serum chemistries, possible circulating toxic substances alterations in body temperature, and the myriad causes of each.

One of the important insights into the physiology of the

brain in recent years has been the definition of the relationship of the reticular formation of the brainstem to overall function of the nervous system. Small lesions placed in the mesencephalic reticular formation of experimental animals produce a state of coma. Sudden isolation of the spinal cord from descending influences of the reticular core of the brainstem by transsection at the cervical medullary junction or more caudad in the spinal cord produces areflexic paralysis or spinal shock distal to the section, followed by mass withdrawal reflexes when spinal shock ceases. Isolation of the brainstem reticular formation from descending hemispheric impulses by a section at the upper midbrain produces facilitation of antigravity musculature, or the state known as *decerebrate rigidity*. Removal of the cerebellum in the midbrain-sectioned animal decreases the extensor tone, while sensory stimuli of any sort enhance it.

Electrophysiologic studies have shown that the reticular core is activated by all sensory stimuli and, conversely, that with total sensory deprivation, that is, section of all sensory nerves, a sleep record is obtained from the electroencephalogram that is altered or "activated" by stimulation within the reticular core. For this reason the ascending cortical influences of the reticular core of the brainstem have been called the *reticular activating system.* The reticular core is more than this. Its reticulum, or network of neurons, influences cortical and subcortical function in the broadest sense in that consciousness and gnosis (recognition of sensation), and motor function are all dependent upon its integrity. For these reasons small lesions in the reticular core of the brainstem can cause loss of consciousness, as seen with contusions of the brainstem or infarcts following thrombosis of perforating branches of the basilar artery. These lesions also can alter motor function and motor tone and muscle tone from areflexic paralysis to decerebrate rigidity.

Surgical diseases of the nervous system are manifestations of space-occupying lesions, be they tumor, hemorrhage, abscess, edema, spinal fluid, or foreign body. The technique of their removal or the control of their effects, as well as an understanding of the mechanisms involved in their producing malfunction in the nervous system, makes neurologic surgery a specialty. The fact that the intracranial space and the spinal canal are nearly closed boxes determines a set of mechanical conditions basic to many considerations of the effect of mass lesions on the nervous system. The intracranial space, compartmentalized by the falx and tentorium cerebri, has communication to the spinal space through the incisura of the tentorium and the foramen magnum of the skull. This represents its only major extracranial communication. The brainstem passes through these areas of communication, i.e., from the incisura of the tentorium through the posterior fossa to the foramen magnum. Rostrally it is continuous with the diencephalon and the internal capsule of each hemisphere, where the medial portion of the temporal lobes have immediate lateral relation to the upper brainstem, with a portion of the circle of Willis, the subarachnoid space, and the oculomotor, or third cranial, nerve between them. Caudad it is continuous with the cervical spinal cord,

where at the foramen magnum it lies immediately anterior to the inferior portion of the ansiform lobes of the cerebellum, more commonly known as the *cerebellar tonsils.*

Central nervous system tissue has many of the properties of a fluid; that is, it is deformable but not compressible, and when deformed it flows in the course of least resistance. Deformation over months or years causes "internal" flows, or loss of substance, mainly of myelin, but rapid deformation varying with the imposed pressure causes flow toward sites of decompression, the incisura of the tentorium and the foramen magnum. While the tissue is not compressible, the lumen of its blood supply is, and obstruction of veins, capillaries, and arteries occurs with deformation. The lethal factors of the flow toward decompression areas are in part the limitation of the accommodation allowed by the semirigid infolded meningeal structures of the falx and the tentorium and the sheer stress at their edges, and the unyielding character of the bony rim of the foramen magnum. In addition, the axial as well as lateral shift of the brainstem is functionally limited by the mobility of the circle of Willis, fixed by the carotid arteries where they pierce the dura. The circle of Willis plus the basilar arteries (Fig. 42-1) supply blood to the brainstem by vessels that enter perpendicular to its surface. With progressive axial shift the normally lax vessels become straightened and eventually tether the brain. With continuing shift there is collapse of the vessels with infarction and rupture of the smaller vessels with hemorrhage. At the foramen magnum compression of the medulla by the decompressing (herniating) cerebellar tonsils causes the same phenomena, but failure of perfusion of this area more commonly causes death before gross visible changes occur.

The situation of a noncompressible tissue nurtured by vessels whose lumens are compressible allows the compressing force to set in motion a cycle that includes production of further mass by edema with consequent increase of the size and compressing force of the original mass. The incisural syndrome of altered consciousness followed by loss of function of the oculomotor nerve, decerebrate rigidity, and death reflects the cycle in supratentorial mass lesions. At the foramen magnum, altered consciousness, followed by depression of respiration requiring the stimulus of increased blood CO_2, or Cheyne-Stokes respiration, depression of reflexes, cessation of respiration, and death represent progression of the cycle. The early recognition of any portion of these patterns is necessary if the lethal effects of intracranial masses are to be reversed. Their recognition and treatment is a sine qua non of neurologic surgery.

It is beyond the scope of this section to review all the neurodiagnostic techniques (and their indications) that can or should be used to investigate neurological diseases requiring neurosurgical intervention. With the recognition that the central nervous system requires a degree of homeostasis in the patient in order to function normally, it becomes obvious that a complete history, physical examination, neurological examination, and basic laboratory studies are requisites for any evaluation of neurological disease. The history should be carefully done, since there is a high probability of its indicating the cause of the condition being studied. In contrast, neurological examination indicates the area or areas of the central nervous system involved and when combined with the history will define questions that can be answered by special diagnostic studies.

DIAGNOSTIC STUDIES. These studies may be benign, that is, of no significant risk to the patient, as with skull x-rays or electroencephalogram, or they can be dangerous enough to require the immediate availability of an operating room, as with pneumoencephalography. The accuracy of the special studies depends not only on the technical skill with which they are performed but also on knowing what question is being asked of the test and what answers can be gained. This latter aspect, as well as knowing what the risks of the test are, is why as much knowledge of the patient as a whole should be gained before using the tests and why their use in neurological evaluation is restricted to physicians knowledgeable in nervous system disease.

X-rays of the skull can be helpful in the diagnosis of neurological disorders, for increased intracranial pressure may be reflected in springing of the sutures in the infant or decalcification of the sella turcica in the adult. A calcified pineal gland that defines the posterior position of the third ventricle may be shifted from its usual midline position by a supratentorial mass. Many tumors contain radiopaque calcification which may be visible in skull x-rays. Meningiomas may contain calcification but usually are recognized, because they evoke hyperostosis in the adjacent bones of the skull. Other stigmata of brain tumor in skull x-rays are erosions of the internal auditory meatus with an eighth nerve tumor or erosion of the optic foramen or anterior clinoid with an optic nerve tumor.

Special diagnostic studies can indicate the position, the size, and the blood supply of the tumor, and also may give information as to the amount of brain shift. The studies that involve no risk to the patient are electroencephalography, echo encephalography, brain scan, and computerized axial tomography (CT scan).

Electroencephalography. The electroencephalogram, or EEG, is the recording of electrical activity of the brain from amplification of the cerebral potentials recorded from the scalp. Alterations in cortical cellular excitability are reflected in the electroencephalogram. The most common abnormalities seen with mass lesions are focal slowing or focal paroxysmal activity. Since this is a record of the surface activity of the cerebral hemispheres, lesions not affecting cortical function directly by metabolic changes, by interrupting subcortical projection, or by pressure will not cause alteration in the electroencephalogram.

Echo Encephalography. The echo encephalogram uses the reflection of ultrasonic waves from intracranial structures to locate them within the skull. The third ventricle has a fairly constant ultrasonic echo, and therefore its position can often be determined. As with the pineal gland, shift of this structure by a supratentorial mass is not uncommon. An echo also occurs at any tissue density interphase, and with special equipment solid tumors as well as the lateral ventricles of the hemispheres at times can be located.

Fig. 42-1. Angiograms of thick longitudinal sections of the midline brainstem. *A.* Normal specimen with demonstration of the basilar artery and its paramedian branches. *B.* Specimen from a case with an expanding supratentorial mass. Caudal displacement of the brainstem has occurred with longitudinal shortening of the brainstem and an increase in the anteroposterior dimension. There are several paramedian arteries which have been ruptured with the demonstration of parenchymal hemorrhages. (*From O. Hassler, Neurology, 17:368, 1967.*)

Radioactive Brain Scan. The brain scan uses radioactive materials such as mercury 203 or technetium 99 that will not cross the intact blood-brain barrier. Since most brain tumors are not included within the barrier, an abnormal amount of radioactive material will be present in the area of the tumor and can be localized by counting this radioactive material with a scintillation counter. This counter localizes the abnormal activity through the intact skull, producing a graphic display. Since there are many causes for breakdown of the blood-brain barrier, positive brain scans can be found in conditions which are not caused by tumors, such as in vascular occlusion, infection, or trauma. The problem of false-negative studies of lesions contained within the blood-brain barrier further limits the value of the study.

Computerized Axial Tomography. Computerized axial tomography (Fig. 42-2) is a major advance in radiological diagnosis whose unique attributes are particularly advantageous for diagnosis of intracranial disease. Conventional x-rays use photographic film to measure the relative amount of x-ray absorbed by the structures through which the beam has passed. Limitations of conventional x-ray include the fact that with photographic film, quantitative definition of the amount of x-ray absorbed is poor and slanted towards high-absorption matter such as bone, and the resulting image is only two-dimensional. In the early 1970s, Geoffrey Houndsfield, a British engineer, developed

Fig. 42-2. Computerized axial tomography of a right temporal parietal tumor. The breakdown in the blood-brain barrier is enhanced by use of radiopaque intravenous material (Renografin). Note central area of decreased density (necrosis), surrounded by area of no blood-brain barrier, surrounded by edema (lower density). The mass has also shifted the ventricles. The tumor was a glioblastoma.

a technique of a carefully controlled small beam of x-ray, a focused crystal scintillation counter, to measure accurately the amount of x-ray remaining after the beam passed through an object, and computer technology along with matrix mathematics and pattern storage techniques to produce a three-dimensional array in a computer of the object being studied, which he called *computerized axial tomography.* The small x-ray beam is passed through the object being studied through multiple directions, and the matrix is formed in the computer so that by simultaneously solving a number of equations, the amount of x-ray absorbed in each portion of the matrix is determined. The size of the area in each point is determined by the size of the matrix; with recent scanners, the image resolution is approximately 1 mm in diameter. Since brain, cerebrospinal fluid, and bone have different x-ray absorption coefficients, with the technique of computerized axial tomography, the amount and position of each of these structures can be determined, and with the use of radiopaque compounds, areas of abnormal vascularity or breakdown in the blood-brain barrier can be accurately determined. The ability to show enlarged ventricles, altered cortical surfaces, tumors, and abscesses has allowed accurate diagnosis of many neurological conditions without any significant risk to the patient. By 1974, Ambrose at the Atkinson Morley Hospital in England had demonstrated both the value and the accuracy of the technique. In the past few years, it has become a standard neuroradiological diagnostic technique.

Pneumoencephalography. Pneumoencephalography, or the x-ray study of the brain with air, utilizes the difference in the absorption of x-rays between air, brain, and fluid. Air studies are done in one of two ways and in general outline

the ventricles, the basal cisterns, and a portion of the subarachnoid spaces around the cerebral hemispheres. A patient who is suspected of a major shift of the cerebral hemispheres or who has significant symptoms from intracranial pressure is not a candidate for a lumbar puncture, and therefore the air study is usually done by a technique known as ventriculography. This consists of making openings in the skull, usually in the posterior parietal bone, tapping the lateral ventricles directly, and replacing fluid in the ventricle with air. A series of x-ray films is then taken with the head manipulated to move the air around to show the different portions of the ventricle and to fill the basal cisterns and subarachnoid spaces.

Pneumoencephalography also may be performed with the patient in the upright position. In this position a lumbar puncture is performed, and small increments of air are placed in the lumbar subarachnoid space. The head is positioned so that the ascending air will fill the different portions of the subarachnoid space. Since both studies alter the cerebrospinal fluid circulation and may precipitate sudden shifting of the intracranial contents with possible sudden loss of brainstem function, it is always best to have an operating room and neurosurgeon available at the start of such studies; rapid decompression of the intracranial pressure and/or removal of a tumor or mass can be accomplished if the patient's condition starts to deteriorate. Computerized axial tomography has decreased the need for pneumoencephalography in many conditions, but one of the problems with computerized axial tomography is the difficulty of separating lesions which are close to the bone, so that pneumoencephalography remains an important diagnostic tool for conditions along the base of the skull, particularly pituitary tumors, useful in determining if the tumor has extended past the confines of the sella.

Cerebral Angiography. Cerebral angiography, or what is more commonly called carotid or vertebral arteriography, is the x-ray study of the intracranial circulation as demonstrated by the injection of contrast material. These studies can define the position of the arteries and the presence or absence of abnormal vasculature, and thereby often define not only the presence of a brain tumor but also its blood supply and how it has affected the adjacent structures. Angiography is the main method of demonstrating vascular lesions such as arteriovenous malformations, aneurysms, and vascular occlusive disease. These studies are usually done by injecting the contrast material into the common carotid artery, the subclavian artery, or the arch of the aorta, so that the material is carried into the intracranial vessels; films to demonstrate the arterial or capillary and venous spaces can then be taken.

HEAD INJURY

Included within the term "head injury" are injuries of the scalp, skull, and brain. The immediate care of patients with head injury is no different from that of any injured patient. Primary consideration must be given to the establishment of adequate respiratory exchange, control of hemorrhage, and maintenance of peripheral vascular circulation. Physicians caring for the patient with traumatic injury to the nervous system too often forget these cardinal necessities or blame apparent respiratory difficulty or peripheral vascular collapse on central nervous system factors that they feel unable to alter. During the initial period of treatment of a patient with head injury, as measures are instituted for the control of the vital functions, a preliminary evaluation of the nervous system function is essential and should be followed as soon as possible by careful repetitive neurologic examinations. The reason for repetitive neurologic examinations will become clear as complications of head-injured patients are discussed, but it suffices to state that the care of patients with traumatic lesions of the nervous system is mainly based on the detection of deterioration or improvement in neurologic function.

Scalp

Although the scalp consists of five layers, from a surgical point of view its two important layers are the dermis and the galea. The principles in the care of scalp lacerations are the same as in the care of any laceration, that is, to change a contaminated open wound into a closed clean wound, but some unique problems arise because of the structure of the scalp and its anatomic relationships. The unyielding character of the scalp with its major blood supply lying between the galea and the dermis has a tendency to hold blood vessels open following laceration with the possibility of considerable loss of blood. Hemostasis of the scalp is easily obtained, if the skull is intact, by compression of the scalp against the skull either in a circumferential fashion at the base of the scalp or by direct pressure on the wound edges. When the skull is not intact, traction on the galea by a clamp which grasps the galea, pulling it back over the dermis, will usually control the hemorrhage. The minor hemorrhage of contusions lying between the galea and the skin rarely causes any significant difficulty, but hematomas of the scalp which lie beneath the galea can attain considerable size, causing elevation of a major portion of the scalp from the skull. Early control of such hemorrhage sometimes can be accomplished by pressure and a firm dressing. Such subgaleal hematomas may take weeks to absorb, but with intact skin over them they are best treated by allowing natural absorption to occur. However, if the hematoma is of significant size to embarrass circulation of the scalp or if there is a question of infection as manifested by heat, swelling, and fever, evacuation of the hematoma is indicated. This should be done under sterile conditions, the hematoma totally evacuated, and any dead space obliterated by a compression dressing.

The approximation of the scalp to the skull not only allows lacerations to occur with blunt injury but also causes increased morbidity with infections of the scalp. Infections of the scalp may spread into the intracranial epidural space through the connecting emissary veins in the diploic spaces of the skull and into the veins on the surface of the brain. With these channels for spread of infection, epidural abscess, subdural abscess, cerebral thrombophlebitis, cerebritis, or brain abscess can occur.

Finally the galea is not only a strong fascial layer that is firmly attached to the skin by numerous fascial bands but is also the attachment of the occipitalis and frontalis muscles. These muscles tend by their contraction to separate any weak area of the galea. The problem of such contraction is that any laceration of more than a few centimeters in size will have a tendency to pull open unless the galea is closed at the time that the dermis is closed; any large laceration of the scalp which is allowed to remain open for more than 5 to 6 days may show a significant amount of contraction with fibrosis, so that it cannot be closed without special plastic techniques.

Thus, the toilet of a scalp wound must be thorough and include shaving of hair in the immediate vicinity, debridement of all the devitalized tissue, and removal of any foreign body. The wound closure must include closure of the galea, either as a separate layer or as a layer included within the dermis. If the laceration is of a large size with separation of a major portion of the galea from the subgaleal tissue, a compression dressing will make the patient more comfortable and decrease the chances of a subgaleal hematoma and infection.

Skull

ANATOMY. The skull is divided into the cranium, which contains and protects the brain, and the facial bones. The cranium consists of eight bones: two parietal and temporal bones and one frontal, occipital, ethmoid, and sphenoid bone. The superior, or rounded, portion of the skull is called the *vault,* and its bones are formed as membranous bone. In the adult the bone consists of firm inner and outer tables with cancellous bone, or diploë, lying between them. The skull contains within the frontal, ethmoid, and sphenoid bones mucous membrane-lined sinuses which connect to the nasal cavities. The basilar, or petrous, portion of the temporal bones contains the middle ear and mastoid air cells, which also connect to the nasopharynx via the eustachian tube.

CLASSIFICATION OF SKULL FRACTURE

The clinical term "skull fracture" is used for fractures of the cranium. Such fractures are described by using a term describing the pattern of the fracture (linear, stellate, comminuted), by using the term "depressed" to denote an inward displacement of a portion of the vault, by naming the bone involved, by including the term "basilar" for fractures traversing the base of the skull, and by describing a break in the scalp or mucous membrane over such a fracture with the term "compound fracture." Thus, a compound comminuted depressed fracture of the left parietal bone states that there is a scalp laceration over a fracture of the parietal bone on the left that consists of multiple fragments of bone driven beneath the surface of the cranial vault.

Fractures of the skull may occur in any area of the skull and have a tendency to radiate from the point of contact into the weaker areas of the skull, e.g., basilar or temporal areas. Most skull fractures require no treatment in themselves, but compound and depressed fractures must be treated. A compound fracture of the cranial vault should be cleansed and debrided, and the wound closed. Replacement of large skull fragments in the area of a compound fracture requires surgical judgment and depends upon the degree of contamination, intactness of the dura, the area of the skull involved, and the ability to watch the patient closely after injury. If the surgeon is in doubt in any of these respects, it is always wisest to remove all fragments of a compound fracture.

With depressed fractures the rule is to elevate all of them, but again this should be based on surgical judgment of the size of the depressed segment, the depth to which it is depressed, and the area of the skull depressed, and the ability to be certain that the dura has not been torn. Any fragment which has been depressed more than a centimeter, a fragment which is over the motor strip, and most small fragments that appear sharp on x-ray usually should be elevated, since they may tear the dura and cause damage to the brain. The combination of a depressed and compound fracture will always require elevation to be certain that contamination has not been driven through the dura into the subarachnoid space or the brain.

Another type of compound skull injury, one that is not as obvious as a penetrating injury, is the injury in which a fracture of the skull traverses one or more of the paranasal sinuses, the mastoid air cells, or the middle ear. The indication that this type of open head injury has occurred is the presence of cerebrospinal fluid drainage from the nose or ear. It signifies a rupture of the protective meningeal coverings of the brain and requires observation and prophylactic antibiotics to be certain that infection of the subarachnoid space or brain does not occur. The posttraumatic cerebrospinal fluid fistula of the ear almost always heals within a few days, but healing of rhinorrhea may be more difficult. It is important in both injuries that the patient remain under medical supervision until such drainage ceases, and usually if either otorrhea or rhinorrhea continues for more than 10 to 14 days, surgical repair of the dural tear is necessary.

Brain

MECHANISMS OF INJURY

The most critical aspect of head trauma is what happens to the brain. The immediate brain damage that results from head trauma is dependent upon the force applied to the head, the area of its application, and whether the head is fixed or freely movable. The damage can be caused by the injuring object or a portion of the skull lacerating the brain, the effects of force transmitted to the brain, and the effects of acceleration and deceleration of the head on the brain confined by the semirigid dura and rigid skull. Delayed brain damage is mainly caused by the reactions of the tissues within the skull. When viable tissue receives an application of force strong enough to be injurious, it responds by alteration in intracellular and extracellular fluid content, by extravasation of blood, by increasing blood supply to the local area, and by mobilization of cells

capable of removing cellular debris and repairing any disruption. The same mechanisms occur in injuries of the brain, and these mechanisms, as well as alteration of vasomotor control or autoregulation of cerebral circulation, may have secondary deleterious effects on the brain because of the unique anatomic position of the brain within the skull and the brain's unique dependency on a constant supply of oxygen and glucose.

It is simplest and easiest to consider the initial brain injury of head trauma as being caused in one of two ways: by the application of a focal, or local, force to the skull or by the application of a generalized, or diffuse, force to the skull. There is considerable overlap between the two, since a patient may have both types of injuries at the same time, but the mechanisms and results of the two types of injury are different. In focal injury, a sharp object of low velocity strikes the head and may cause disruption of the scalp, fracture of the skull, and laceration of the brain, either directly or by driving fragments of the skull through the dura mater. The resulting neurologic dysfunction relates to the area of the brain involved, since no significant force is transmitted to the skull or brain generally. There is usually brief loss or no loss of consciousness, and the main problem is the care of the local wound.

Following the application of a more generalized force to the skull, there are three other mechanisms that may cause brain injury and complicate or amplify any focal injury that has occurred. Such an application of force may occur following high-velocity missile injuries, such as a gunshot wound, but is most commonly seen in blunt head injuries or injuries in which the freely movable head is struck by a heavy object or when the head is propelled against a solid structure as seen in a high-speed vehicle accident. These mechanisms of brain injury in the more generalized application of force to the skull are injury caused by the direct transmission of energy to the brain, injury caused by the inertia and momentum of the brain when the head is accelerated and decelerated causing the brain to strike against the skull and edges of the dura, injury caused by the torque or compressive force applied to the relatively fixed upper brainstem with the rotation of the cerebral hemispheres during such acceleration and deceleration, and the stretching effect of this movement on the various tissues of the intracranial content.

The effects of transmitted energy to the brain relate to the amount of force applied minus the amount of energy dissipated by disruption of the scalp or skull. The force dissipated in fracturing the skull can be considerable and in part accounts for the paradoxic situation in which brain injury appears inversely related to the skull injury. The remaining energy after disruption of scalp and skull can either be transmitted through the skull or be directly applied to the brain, if the injuring object penetrates the skull. The energy spreads concentrically from the point of application with maximal transmission in the primary direction in which the force was applied. As this energy passes through the tissues of the brain, and particularly through the interphases of the vascular channels and cerebral spinal fluid spaces, a change in direction of the force occurs and may cause disruption or damage to the tissue.

This type of damage will usually be most marked at cortical and ventricular surfaces and adjacent to blood vessels within the hemispheres, since these are areas of major changes in tissue density and tensile strength.

The other mechanisms of brain injury following head trauma are more commonly the cause of severe brain damage and neurologic dysfunction in the head-injury patient and therefore are more frequently the cause for major difficulty in the care of these patients. The mechanisms relate to induced acceleration and deceleration of the head, the inertia of the brain at the moment of acceleration, and the momentum of the brain at the time of deceleration. These forces cause motion of the head and its contents, forcing the brain against the inner surface of the skull where the force has been applied, as well as against the opposite inner surface of the skull (contrecoup injury). Such contact may cause damage to any surface of the brain but is usually most severe when it involves a motion which throws the brain against the sphenoid ridges and/or the free edges of the tentorium cerebelli. This latter action is most likely to occur when the head is struck in such a way as to produce rotation of the skull. The areas of the brain most likely to receive severe damage are the anterior portions of the frontal and temporal lobes, the posterior portions of the occipital lobes, and the upper portions of the midbrain. The intrinsic movement of the brain tissue with the varying degrees of resistance to such movement of blood vessel, fiber tracts, glia, and neurons results in stretching and rupture of the tissue, with maximum effect on the perivascular tissue and the white matter of the hemispheres and brainstem. The torque effect on the upper brainstem is also most easily obtained in the freely movable head that is struck in a manner to cause marked rotation. The effects of such torque applied to the upper brainstem cause almost instant alteration in neuronal function with resulting change in consciousness. This loss of function is probably the cause of the immediate loss of consciousness seen with "concussion." The leverage of a blow applied to the point of the jaw easily gives this rotational effect to the skull and may explain the "knockout" effect of the uppercut in boxing.

In summary, a force applied to the skull may have a local effect of laceration of the scalp, fracture of the skull, and laceration and contusion of the brain, or it may have a more generalized effect caused by the effect of energy transmitted through a semisolid substance, a contusing and lacerating effect when the brain is driven against the inner portion of the skull and edges of the dura, the stretching and tearing effect of the resulting internal movement of tissue, and the loss of function by the compressive effect of the torque or stress applied to the upper portion of the midbrain with rotational movement of the brain. These mechanisms result in the clinical conditions of cerebral concussion, cerebral contusion, and cerebral laceration. They, plus the effect of alteration in total function of the nervous system, the alterations in cerebral circulation, the changes in respiration and vasomotor control, and the reaction of the nervous system tissue to injury, are the main reasons for the clinical syndromes seen in the head-injured patient.

Care of the Head-injured Patient

The care of the head-injured patient can be divided into temporally sequential aspects. These are first aid; evaluation; protection from the loss of nervous system function; protection from the response of injured nervous system tissue; prevention, recognition, and treatment of complications; and rehabilitation. The eventual morbidity and mortality of the head-injured patient can be markedly improved by knowledgeable and effective care throughout the course of the illness. In general, hospitals with specialized centers for neurosurgical patients and for rehabilitation for neurologically disabled patients should be utilized as soon as it is feasible to move the patient. As a rule the patient is best transferred to such an area for definitive care as early as possible, since with few exceptions the patient is most capable of transport immediately after first aid and evaluation have been completed.

FIRST AID. The basic principles for first aid of the head-injured patient have already been discussed in the opening paragraphs of this section on head trauma. They consist of maintenance of respiration, control of hemorrhage, and maintenance of peripheral vascular circulation. The importance of such measures cannot be stressed too much, since any failure of these vital functions not only is a significant factor in the mortality of head injury but can be significant in increasing eventual morbidity. The addition of anoxia or loss of circulation, either from respiratory obstruction or peripheral vascular collapse, can cause a marked increase in neuronal damage and may contribute to the degree of reaction the brain has to the original injury.

Another aspect of first aid is the transport of the patient, either from the scene of the accident or to a hospital for definitive therapy. The unconscious head-injured patient should always be accompanied by an attendant who can clear the nasopharynx and assist respiration. The patient is most safely transported in a two-thirds prone position with his head slightly elevated by a firm roll or his arm above a firm surface. This allows secretions from the nasopharynx and vomitus to drain onto the stretcher rather than be aspirated into the trachea.

EVALUATION. Evaluation of a head-injured patient includes careful examination for other injuries. Visible lacerations and obvious deformities of the extremities signify lesions which must be treated, but internal injury to the thorax, abdomen, or pelvis may be difficult to diagnose in the unconscious patient. Continued hypotension and tachycardia are the most consistent signs of such injuries and should always indicate further investigation, since peripheral vascular collapse from central nervous system damage is seen only as a terminal event. Injury to the cervical spine may occur in head injury, and x-rays of the cervical spine may be necessary to rule out such injuries.

A complete neurologic examination should be recorded as soon as possible, and this must include an accurate evaluation of the state of consciousness. The most common neurologic deficit that occurs with head injury is altered consciousness. Accurate evaluation of the state of consciousness and comparison of the initial examination with subsequent examinations are the most reliable means for evaluating the progress of the head-injured patient. Terms such as "comatose," "semicomatose," and "stuporous" that are commonly used to describe states of consciousness have little meaning and are best used, if used at all, as a means of introducing descriptions that have objective findings as their method of evaluation. The evaluation of the state of consciousness is done by utilizing the response of the patient to various stimuli. If the stimulus and the response are described, the evaluation can be repeated and compared later by the same examiner or others. Table 42-1 offers a general description of the levels of consciousness to be determined by this method. Levels between those described can be easily devised when required.

By utilizing objective responses to stimuli it is not difficult to recognize progressive neurologic deficit. The difference in neurologic function between the confused patient who follows commands and the patient who responds to painful stimuli with nonpurposeful movements is obvious, and the time it takes for such neurologic deficit to develop indicates how rapidly definitive treatment must be started. Decerebrate posturing as a description of a level of consciousness is the posture assumed by a patient with physiologic or anatomic section of the upper brainstem. It is basically the posture assumed when there is facilitation of all antigravity musculature. The patient therefore extends and internally rotates his extremities, extends his neck, and arches his back. Fragments of decerebrated posturing usually appear first with thrusting of the lower extremities. Since it signifies failure of function of the upper brainstem, it is an ominous sign that requires immediate definitive therapy. It is seen with shift of the brain by a supratentorial mass and therefore is often the preterminal event in the patient with untreated posttraumatic intracranial hemorrhage.

Jennett and coworkers over the past decade have utilized a simple scale to assess the level of severe head injuries in order to study and compare various forms of therapy. Though the outcome of the study comparing various forms of therapy is not complete, the reliability of the "Glasgow Coma Scale" in predicting the outcome of severely traumatized patients who have received good neurosurgical treatment in various clinics and countries has been demonstrated. The scale (Table 42-2) is applied to a patient who has been unconscious for more than 6 hours, thus eliminating relatively minor head trauma. The score is the sum of the highest numbers obtained in each section of the scale, i.e., motor response, verbal response, and eye opening. Jennett has demonstrated that patients with less than 5 on the scale have an overall mortality rate of over 50 percent. The scale basically shows that the levels of consciousness and brainstem function closely parallel the severity of the injury and thus the mortality rate. It further points out how evaluation of general function of the brain, i.e., consciousness and a portion of the brain that responds to shift and flow of intracranial contents, the midbrain, can give a fairly accurate picture of the amount or progression in amount of injury to the central nervous system.

OBSERVATION AND DIAGNOSTIC STUDIES. Therapy is dependent upon the evaluation of the initial and repeated neurologic examinations. Most patients can be observed over a short period of time, 30 minutes to a few hours, while first aid is given and other areas of the body evaluated; following observation a more accurate decision can be made as to what is necessary for treatment. Studies other than observation and neurologic examination are helpful but are never indicated if they remove a seriously ill patient from medical and nursing observation.

Roentgenograms of the skull can be helpful especially if the pineal gland is calcified, since shift of its midline position in the anteroposterior view will signify a mass lesion. The skull roentgenograms may show depressed fractures or fractures that traverse arterial vessel grooves in the skull (middle meningeal artery), indicating a possible source for bleeding (epidural hematoma). They may demonstrate air within the skull, indicating a tear in the coverings of the brain, or they may show a foreign body. Computerized axial tomography has altered the evaluation of acute head problems since it can demonstrate recent

Table 42-1. LEVELS OF CONSCIOUSNESS

Responds to spoken word, is alert, cooperative, and oriented.
Responds to spoken word, is confused, and obeys simple commands.
Responds to spoken word only after receiving painful stimuli of supraorbital pressure; obeys commands only while receiving painful stimuli.
Does not respond to auditory stimuli before or while receiving painful stimuli but has purposeful, effective motor response to painful supraorbital and sternal pressure.
Responds to painful supraorbital and sternal pressure with purposeful but noneffective motor movements.
Responds to painful supraorbital and sternal pressure with nonpurposeful movement.
Responds to painful stimuli only with alteration in pulse and respiratory rate or with decerebrate posturing.
No response to painful stimuli, but cough and gag reflexes are present.
No response to stimuli.
Lowest level is unconsciousness; the only step below this is death.

Table 42-2. GLASGOW COMA SCALE

Best motor response	Obeys	M6
	Localizes	5
	Withdraws	4
	Abnormal flexion	3
	Extensor response	2
	Nil	1
Verbal response	Oriented	V5
	Confused conversation	4
	Inappropriate words	3
	Incomprehensible sounds	2
	Nil	1
Eye opening	Spontaneous	E4
	To speech	3
	To pain	2
	Nil	1

NOTE: The coma scale score is the sum of the sectional scores. See text for details.

intracranial hemorrhage quite accurately and indicate both its size and location. The scanner can also define shift of intracranial contents, as well as areas of localized edema. No diagnostic procedure should displace clinical observation, but in the critically ill, head-injured patient, the accurate knowledge that intracranial hemorrhage or mass exists or does not exist allows more accurate control of intracranial pressure and cerebrovascular perfusion pressure without invasive x-ray procedures such as angiography and ventriculography, and quickly defines the need or lack of need for surgical excision of intracranial masses from the injury. If a scanner is not available, further studies such as carotid arteriography or exploratory perforator openings of the skull are indicated only when the patient's condition precludes serial evaluations or a course of progressive neurologic deficit has been established.

During and following the period of initial evaluation frequent recording of the blood pressure, pulse rate, and respiratory rate is indicated, since elevation of blood pressure and decrease in pulse and respiratory rate are seen with increasing intracranial pressure and may indicate impending medullary failure. As these changes in vital signs are less sensitive and usually occur later than alteration in levels of consciousness, they are helpful but not as accurate in defining the need for active intervention.

Lumbar puncture has little place in the early evaluation of head trauma. The risk involved in altering spinal fluid pressure when the possibility exists of mass lesion in the calvarium far outweighs any information gained. The presence or absence of blood in the spinal fluid or the presence or absence of increased spinal fluid pressure do not signify the need for, or the contraindication for, any form of therapy. Lumbar puncture can at times be helpful in deciding that an unconscious patient without history has had a subarachnoid hemorrhage or meningeal infection before, or instead of, head trauma.

SUPPORTIVE THERAPY. During the entire period of treatment of the head-injured patient measures must be instituted to provide substitutes for the protective nervous system reflexes that may have been lost. Any obstruction to the airway or any difficulty with keeping clear the pharynx, larynx, or trachea should be handled by tracheostomy. This is usually best done as an elective procedure within 24 hours after intubation with a cuffed endotracheal tube. At times with facial or cervical spine injuries an emergency tracheostomy may have to be done. Gastric suction through a nasogastric tube is helpful not only in preventing gastric dilatation and the resulting respiratory difficulty but also in preventing the regurgitation of gastric contents into the nasopharynx and trachea. A Foley catheter for bladder drainage allows accurate measuring of urinary output and prevents overdistension of the urinary bladder.

Control of water balance may be altered so that diabetes insipidus or lack of antidiuretic hormone release may occur. Accurate recording of urinary output, the replacement of fluid, and the use of Pitressin tannate in oil can control this. The opposite effect or the inappropriate secretion of antidiuretic hormone is more common and may cause water retention despite decreasing serum osmolarity.

Water restriction is necessary to avert the complications of water intoxication that will ensue.

Temperature regulation may be deficient with head trauma; most commonly the deficiency is in the heat-loss mechanism, that is loss of superficial vasodilation and sweating. The resulting hyperthermia can contribute to the central nervous system damage and to central nervous system response to damage. Frequent rectal or esophageal temperature should be taken. If fever ensues, exposure of major portions of the body, tepid-water sponging, and water-cooled mattresses should be used to control the fever.

PREVENTION AND TREATMENT OF CEREBRAL EDEMA. The nervous system tissue, like other tissue, responds to injury by formation of edema. Since the brain is encased within the skull and dura, the formation of edema causes increased intracranial pressure which may become of such magnitude that it equals systemic arterial pressure. At that point circulation through the brain ceases, and death of tissue ensues. When this happens, the situation is usually irreversible, because relief of pressure must be accomplished within 4 to 5 minutes in order to avert neuronal death. Since the formation of edema is gradual, starting a few hours after injury and reaching its maximum in 36 to 48 hours, protective measures instituted promptly can have considerable value.

Intracranial pressure in the head-injured patient is dependent upon a number of factors. One of the main ones is the volume of fluid in each of the intracranial compartments, i.e., cerebrospinal fluid and fluid in vascular, intracellular, and extracellular spaces. The extracellular space is small, and its contribution to brain swelling is open to argument; the increase in intracranial pressure appears to relate to alteration in volume of the vascular bed, intracellular space, and the cerebrospinal fluid space. Modification in the reaction of the brain to injury is dependent upon modifying the volume responses of these spaces.

The vascular bed volume is dependent upon venous pressure, CO_2 content of the circulating blood, and arterial pressure. It is generally unwise to alter arterial pressure except to raise it toward normal. The blood CO_2 level and venous pressure can be reduced by making certain there is no obstruction to the airway, by assisting respiration with a short positive and longer negative cycle respirator, and by elevating the head of the bed 15 to 20°. The intracellular response depends on breakdown of the blood-brain barrier, the metabolism of the cells, the osmolarity of the blood, and the availability of free water. Keeping the head-injured patient at normothermic or slightly hypothermic temperature (34 to 37°C) decreases metabolism and protects cells that may have regionally poor perfusion.

Removal of fluid in the hydrated or overhydrated patient with solute diuretics such as mannitol or urea, plus limitation of fluid intake to insensible water loss and urinary output, are helpful for the control of intracellular edema. The fluid intake to accomplish this usually is 1,800 to 2,000 ml/24 hours and should include at least 150 mEq of sodium chloride. One-half normal saline solution and $2\frac{1}{2}$% glucose approximates these requirements for intravenous fluids. The inflammatory response may be decreased and the blood-brain barrier protected by the use of glucocorticosteroid compounds. Dexamethasone is commonly used in intravenous doses of 10 mg shortly after injury and 4 mg every 6 hours for the first 36 to 72 hours. The dose is later tapered at a rate dependent upon the course of the patient. Fluid restriction also helps control the volume of the cerebrospinal fluid compartment.

Lumbar puncture would appear to be of help, but since the possibility of a mass lesion (hemorrhage) always exists and since asymmetric contusion and swelling frequently exists in the head-injured patient, drainage of spinal fluid via the lumbar route is too dangerous. Such drainage may cause herniation of the temporal lobe into the incisura of the tentorium and compression of the upper brainstem or herniation of the cerebellum through the foramen magnum and compression of the lower brainstem.

Recent studies have shown that although posttraumatic edema of the brain can cause such raised intracranial pressure that cerebral perfusion ceases, it is rare, and that most cases of "malignant" posttraumatic edema after head trauma are caused by repetitive episodes of inadequate cerebral perfusion that relate to transient waves of intracranial pressure. These "plateau waves," first described by Lundberg and coworkers, have been shown to relate to dilatation and later constriction of the cerebrovascular resistant vessels. In the injured brain, such changes in cerebrovascular resistance cause changes in blood flow and blood volume, and since the brain has lost its compliance or ability to tolerate small changes in volume without major changes in pressure, these waves of pressure are seen if intraventricular recording of pressure is done. Since cerebral blood flow relates directly to systemic arterial pressure minus intracranial pressure and inversely to the cerebrovascular resistance $\left[CBF = \dfrac{K(SAP - ICP)}{VR} \right]$, during episodes of plateau waves, effective cerebral perfusion is impaired and repetitive inadequate perfusion of the brain occurs. With each occurrence, further damage to the blood-brain barrier, neurons, and glia occurs. When these episodes have caused enough damage or when there is vasomotor paralysis from injury, the increased intracranial pressure causes bradycardia and hypertension systemically or the Cushing effect, which then causes further increase in intracranial pressure from the effect of increased blood volume and pressure intracranially. As mentioned above, this is often a late sign and in the head-injured patient may be the initial sign of impending respiratory arrest and total loss of effective intracranial vascular perfusion.

Since it has been demonstrated that effective cerebral perfusion pressure requires that systemic arterial pressure be at least 50 mmHg greater than intracranial pressure, in the severely injured patient, direct measure of intracranial pressure by placing a catheter in the frontal horn of the lateral ventricle makes it possible, when systemic arterial pressure is also monitored, not only to recognize the presence of plateau waves and inadequate cerebral perfusion pressure but also to undertake treatment to control the pressure and thus avert these transient episodes. The measures described above to control respirations and thus levels of CO_2, the use of solute diuretics such as mannitol or urea, and, since there is a catheter in the ventricle, drainage of spinal fluid can markedly protect the brain against this secondary injury. Many neurosurgical services routinely monitor intracranial pressure in all patients in whom there is major impairment of levels of consciousness for more than 6 to 10 hours and in all patients whose function on the Glasgow Coma Scale is 6 or less. With these techniques, malignant cerebral edema following trauma is rare and protection of the brain against secondary injury from inadequate cerebral perfusion allows a better functional result, although the mortality rate of severely head-injured patients has not been significantly altered.

INTRACRANIAL HEMORRHAGE

Progressive neurologic deficit, the most common being progressive loss of consciousness, following head trauma should always be assumed to be due to intracranial hemorrhage until proved otherwise. The patterns of neurologic change vary with the type of hemorrhage, but all have as a major component the neurologic deficit of progressive loss of consciousness.

The most common intracranial hemorrhage following head trauma is subarachnoid hemorrhage. It has little surgical significance and usually causes signs of meningismus or stiff neck and headache. It may, in the young male, produce maniacal behavior. It has little significance surgically, because the blood is rapidly diluted by the cerebrospinal fluid and flows throughout the subarachnoid space, so that no significant localized mass effect occurs. It may have significance as a late complication of head injury, namely, progressive communicating hydrocephalus. This complication is rare, occurring weeks or months after injury, and presents as a progressive dementia with motor apraxia, usually most marked as a gait disturbance. The mechanism is thought to be obstruction of the arachnoid villi and/or basal cisterns so that the absorption of cerebrospinal fluid is altered. The treatment is the same as for infantile hydrocephalus with the construction of an artificial path for the absorption of cerebrospinal fluid. Most commonly this is done with a shunt from the lateral ventricle to the superior vena cava, using a Holter or Pudenz valve to prevent blood reflux and to stabilize the pressure in the ventricle at 50 to 70 mm of water.

Surgically significant intracranial hemorrhages are best classified by their anatomic positions, i.e., subdural hematoma, epidural hematoma, and intracerebral hematoma. While they are relatively rare, unrecognized and untreated posttraumatic intracranial hematomas have almost a 100 percent mortality rate. Since most of this mortality can be averted by surgical treatment, early and accurate diagnosis is important.

SUBDURAL HEMATOMA

One of the most common types of posttraumatic intracranial hemorrhage is subdural hematoma. It is caused by either rupture of the veins traversing the subdural space from the brain to the dural sinuses or by a laceration of the brain that has torn the overlying piarachnoid. The symptoms may appear as early as within the first few minutes or as late as 6 to 8 weeks after injury. The pattern of symptoms, the findings, the treatment, and the prognosis vary with the rapidity of formation of the hematoma, so that it is logical to consider the syndrome of subdural hematoma as three different types: acute subdural, subacute subdural, and chronic subdural. Subdural hematomas plus epidural and intracerebral hematomas are the common surgically important intracranial hemorrhagic complications of trauma. Although each has a different symptom pattern, all have somewhere in their history the finding of decreased level of consciousness out of proportion to focal neurologic deficit. Portions of the basic patterns are usually present in all patients with subdural hematoma, but at times discovering them can tax the most astute clinician. The following descriptions are to be taken as outlines of patterns commonly presented by the patient with the different types of intracranial hematoma, but the reader should always keep in mind the protean signs and symptoms possible in a patient with intracranial hematoma.

Acute Subdural Hematoma

Acute subdural hematomas are defined as hematomas that cause significant progressive neurologic deficit within 48 hours of injury. They almost always occur following severe head trauma, and since they may have both arterial and venous sources for bleeding, the progression of the neurologic deficit can be rapid, often in terms of minutes or hours. The source of the arterial bleeding is frequently a laceration of the brain, and therefore focal neurologic deficit such as a hemiparesis is common.

Clinical Manifestations. When first seen the patient is usually unresponsive with a focal neurologic deficit. Progressive decrease in sensorium with or without progressive focal neurologic deficit is the warning of increasing intracranial mass. Without treatment the brainstem will be compressed by hemorrhage, edema, and herniation until death results. Death may occur within hours, with cessation of respiration, maintenance of pulse and blood pressure for a short time, and then peripheral vascular collapse as the medulla fails. Diagnosis is made by always considering the possibility of acute subdural hematoma in the severely head-injured patient who shows any deterioration in neurologic status. Aid in the diagnosis and in determining the side of major hemorrhage can be gained by the localization of any focal neurologic deficit, the presence of a lateral shift of a calcified pineal gland, and shift of the midline in the echo encephalogram. As mentioned above, computerized axial tomography is accurate in defining the position and size of recent intracranial hemorrhage and therefore, is the best method, if there is time, of diagnosing acute subdural hematomas. It also can define adjacent intracerebral hematomas, a common concomitant of acute subdural hematomas, making surgical approach to the hemorrhage more accurate and effective. More than half of acute subdural hematomas are bilateral, so that evaluation by either perforator openings or arteriograms of both subdural spaces is indicated.

Treatment. Treatment consists of removal of the hematoma through a large craniotomy with control of bleeding areas, decompression by excision of large areas of the skull and relaxation of the compressing dura, and, when necessary, internal decompression by excision of portions of the frontal or temporal lobes. The methods for controlling edema and secondary injury from loss of effective cerebral perfusion pressure, as outlined in a preceding section, have decreased the necessity for excising large areas of the skull and, therefore, decreased both the problem of shift of the brain and the damage that can occur as an area of brain protrudes through a decompression site, as well as the later need for repair of surgical defect in the skull. Drainage of the hematoma through perforator openings is never satisfactory, since the major portion of the hematoma is solid clot and the problem is a combination of mass from clot and reaction of the brain to severe trauma. Without prompt surgical care mortality is 100 percent, and even with the best care it can be as high as 80 to 90 percent.

Subacute Subdural Hematoma

Subacute subdural hematomas are complications of head trauma that cause significant neurologic deficit more than 48 hours but less than 2 weeks after injury. They are usually caused by venous bleeding into the subdural space.

Clinical Manifestations. The basic pattern of symptoms and signs is a history of head trauma with unconsciousness, gradual improvement in the first few days followed by lack of improvement, fluctuation in levels of consciousness, and then decompensation with progressive loss of consciousness and often partial loss of hemispheric function. The patients are usually not as severely injured as are the patients with acute subdural hematomas. The phase of fluctuation in level of consciousness often heralds that significant shift of the intracranial contents has occurred, and the patient may change from relatively alert to difficult to arouse even with painful stimuli and back to his alert status within a few hours. Herniation of the medial temporal lobe through the incisura of the tentorium and compensation of the midbrain to the pressure of such herniation is a possible mechanism of such fluctuation in levels of consciousness. The presence of a third nerve paresis with dilatation of the pupil is often a warning that midbrain decompensation is imminent. The computerized scanner may not identify subacute subdural hematomas, since they can become isodense within the first 10 to 12 days after injury (i.e., the x-ray absorbed is approximately the same as brain). If the hematoma is unilateral or asymmetrical, the shift of the ventricular system as seen on computerized scanning will suggest the location of the hematoma. If the clinical history and signs suggest subdural hematoma, the diagnosis is better made by multiple perforator openings or by angiography.

Treatment. Treatment is dependent upon how critical the patient's condition is, how much liquid clot there is, and whether significant temporal lobe herniation has occurred. The patient with solid clot, unresponsive from uncal herniation, requires craniotomy, removal of the clot, and elevation of the temporal lobe herniation with or without incision of the tentorial edge. In the less critically ill patient and in the patient with considerable liquefaction of the hematoma the removal of a major portion of the clot through a small craniectomy and multiple perforator openings followed by external drainage of the subdural space may be all that is required. As with acute subdural hematomas, these hematomas are commonly bilateral, and exploration of both subdural spaces is always indicated unless bilateral angiograms have ruled out the presence of bilateral hematomas.

Chronic Subdural Hematoma

Although the initial cause of the chronic subdural hematoma is usually rupture by head trauma of one of the veins traversing the subdural space, the symptoms are caused by the increasing mass effect of the hematoma surrounded by a semipermeable membrane. Within 7 to 10 days after bleeding has occurred in the subdural space the blood is surrounded by a fibrous membrane. As the blood cells within the membrane break down, fluid is osmotically pulled into the hematoma, causing an increase in its volume. This may cause further bleeding from tears in the membrane or by rupturing other traversing veins with the reestablishment of the same process and an increasing size of the semiliquid-filled membrane.

Clinical Manifestations. Chronic subdural hematomas may occur at any age but are most frequent in the infant or the elderly. The causative trauma, particularly in the elderly, may be so slight that the patient does not remember it and gives no history of trauma. The symptoms and signs are best classified as a progressive alteration in mentation and level of consciousness of 4 to 6 weeks' duration out of proportion to the focal neurologic deficit. Therefore, any patient presenting with a progressive change in mental faculties and fluctuation or decreasing level of consciousness should be considered a subdural hematoma suspect.

Treatment. Since the hematoma is liquid, drainage through perforator openings is usually all that is required. In the past many neurosurgeons have felt that removal of the membranes is required, since they may be quite thick. However, experience has shown that there is increased mortality and morbidity from craniotomy removal of membranes and no improvement in the long-term results over those achieved by simple drainage of chronic subdural hematomas.

Subdural Hygroma

Although subdural hygromas are not a part of intracranial hemorrhage, they can produce similar symptoms. Subdural hygroma is usually caused by a tear in the piarachnoid that acts as a one-way valve with leakage of cerebrospinal fluid into the subdural space. The hygroma can increase in size quite rapidly and therefore can mimic an acute or subacute subdural hematoma. Perforator openings of the skull with external drainage is the treatment of choice, but at times formation of an artificial fistula between the subarachnoid space and the subdural space must be made in order to control continued formation of the hygroma.

EPIDURAL HEMATOMA

Epidural hematomas may be caused by either venous or arterial bleeding. They lie between the skull and the dura. The most common cause is venous bleeding, but the surgically important epidural hematomas most frequently are formed by arterial bleeding. Occasionally the patient with a skull fracture may have a significant venous epidural, the removal of which allows decrease in intracranial pressure or release of focal compression of the brain, but generally venous epidural hematomas are limited by the firm adherence of the dura to the inner surface of the skull. The central point of the venous epidural is almost always at the site of a fracture.

The epidural hematoma from arterial bleeding commonly occurs from rupture of the middle meningeal artery. This may be caused by a fracture of the temporal bone where the artery is in close proximity to the bone or by a tear of the middle meningeal artery when a blow causes angular acceleration of the head or sudden decrease or increase in any diameter of the skull. The tear may occur at the foramen spinosum, where the artery enters the skull, or anywhere along its branches.

CLINICAL MANIFESTATIONS. The basic historical pattern of the epidural hematoma is a young adult who has received a relatively minor blow causing momentary alteration in consciousness, followed by a lucid interval extending from a few minutes to a few hours. This interval terminates by rapid progressive loss of consciousness, dilatation of the pupil on the side of the epidural hematoma, evidence of compression of the upper midbrain, either by the production of a hemiparesis or decerebrate rigidity, and then evidence of compromise of the entire brainstem and death. The frequency of the hematoma being over the temporal area, the direct pressure onto the temporal lobe and therefore the maximal chance of herniation of the medial temporal lobe through the incisura, plus the arterial pressure as a source of bleeding are the main reasons for the rapidity with which the entire syndrome can be completed.

TREATMENT. Treatment consists of early recognition, a temporal craniectomy, evacuation of the hemorrhage, and control of the bleeding artery either at the foramen spinosum or at the point of tear in the dura. The mortality from epidural hematoma remains approximately 50 percent, partly because of the difficulty in recognizing the syndrome and partly because even upon recognition rapid control of the hemorrhage is necessary to avert a fatal outcome.

INTRACEREBRAL HEMATOMA

Posttraumatic intracerebral hematomas are most often seen in patients with severe head trauma, often mimic the symptom patterns of an acute or subacute subdural hematoma, and frequently are found in conjunction with them. In some series of posttraumatic intracranial hemorrhage intracerebral hematomas are as frequent as subdural hematomas, especially if the series includes many patients injured in high-speed vehicle accidents. The hematoma usually presents either beneath a cortical laceration or as a confluence of small hemorrhages in a contused area of the brain. Intracerebral hematomas are most commonly found in the anterior third of the temporal lobe where the temporal lobe may strike the sphenoid bone, and less frequently in the tips of the frontal or occipital lobes. They can be seen in any area of the cerebrum. The symptoms of clinically significant posttraumatic intracerebral hematomas are similar to the symptoms of an acute or subacute subdural hematoma. There are many intracerebral hematomas that do not alter the clinical course of a patient, are not diagnosed, and resolve by liquefaction, phagocytosis, and gliosis. The surgically significant intracerebral hematomas present with progressive decrease in consciousness and/or progressive focal neurologic deficit. Most frequently, focal deficits are third nerve palsy and hemiparesis. These symptoms may develop within a few hours or a few days of the injury. An important concept is the fact that these hematomas can cause significant neurologic deficit and, therefore, may explain progressive neurologic deficits in the head-injured patient in whom exploratory trephines have failed to reveal subdural hematoma. As with acute subdural hematomas, computerized axial tomography accurately diagnoses, localizes, and determines the extent of intracerebral hematomas. If a scanner is not available, arteriography is usually the best method to localize the hematoma, and ventriculography the next best. Occasionally an intracerebral hematoma is an incidental finding in surgery for acute subdural hematoma or is diagnosed by exploring the areas where occurrence is anticipated.

TREATMENT. The only effective treatment of surgically significant posttraumatic intracerebral hematomas is craniotomy or craniectomy with incision of the hemisphere at the most superficial area of the hematoma and evacuation of the clot. Simple aspiration of the lesion is not adequate since the majority of the hemorrhage is usually solid clot. The evacuation often must include excision of part of the lobe involved in order to remove devitalized brain and to obtain effective decompression of the injured cerebrum.

REHABILITATION. Rehabilitation of the head-injured patient starts with his initial care and finishes when his function is stabilized at its highest possible level. The rehabilitation of the brain-injured patient is a specialty in itself, but fortunately few patients require retraining or reconstructive surgical procedures to overcome their neurologic deficits. A majority of head-injured patients require only the support and care of a knowledgeable physician. Special problems of the head-injured patient during convalescence fall within three categories: psychologic problems, convulsions, and problems with cerebrospinal fluid circulation.

Psychologic Problems. Changes in personality and mood during the period of convalescence are one of the most common and often one of the most difficult symptoms for both patient and physician. The symptoms usually fall into the broad psychiatric category of a reactive depression with an overlay of anxiety. Complaints of headache, fatigue, loss of memory, excessive difficulty with performing tasks, transient despondency, and overreaction to emotional stimuli demonstrate a mixture of possible organic and psychologic bases for the symptoms. On the organic side is the suggestion of temporal and frontal lobe malfunction, while on the psychologic side is the reaction to physical and mental fatigue with a superimposed anxiety from the fear that the change may be permanent.

Gradually increasing physical activity in a planned fashion with limited goals that can be reached in reasonable periods of time and a planned return to increasingly difficult mental tasks is usually the best method for overcoming the problem. The settlement of any pending litigation is important when psychologic problems become paramount, for unnecessary delay can make a psychologic cripple of the patient. The physician should not abandon these patients or allow them to become dependent but rather insist that they get psychiatric help when necessary and that they work toward any physical and mental goals that seem possible. The best method of giving such support is for the physician to see the patient at planned intervals and during the visits to evaluate the neurologic progress of the patient to be certain that a portion of the problem is not coming from seizures or altered cerebrospinal fluid circulation.

Convulsions. Approximately 30 to 45 percent of patients with a compound injury that involves a laceration of the brain will have seizures if they are not on anticonvulsive medication. In contrast, the incidence of convulsions in the closed-head-injury patient is much lower. It is difficult to obtain any significant figures on the incidence of convulsion in the closed-head-injury patient, for in large series it varies from 0.5 percent to as high as 10 percent. In general it is safe to assume that a patient who has had less than 4 hours of either markedly altered consciousness or focal neurologic deficit will have no significant chance of convulsions' developing late in the convalescence that relate to the head injury. In the group with more serious head injuries there remains a small but persistent percentage in whom convulsions will develop that appear to relate to the head injury. The period in which convulsions may develop extends over many years. It is often difficult to recognize that focal or partial seizures are occurring, but they always should be considered when any paroxysmal symptoms occur, that is, symptoms of relatively brief duration that end with excessive fatigue. Electroencephalograms may be of help in diagnosing the cause of such symptoms as seizures, but at times trials of anticonvulsants are necessary to rule them out. Control of posttraumatic seizures with Dilantin and phenobarbital is usually sufficient, but occasionally resection of the damaged area is necessary for control with anticonvulsant drugs.

Problems of Cerebrospinal Fluid. Alteration in cerebrospinal fluid circulation is probably common in the early convalescence after head injury and may account for some of the complaints of headache, postural vertigo, and feeling of lightheadedness. These symptoms usually require no therapy other than the passage of time. Occasionally mild elevation of cerebrospinal fluid pressure continues and requires investigation by arteriography or air study. If no mass lesion is found to explain the increased pressure, intermittent lumbar spinal drainage over a few days will often control this. Prolonged elevation of cerebrospinal fluid pressure with enlargement of ventricles is a rare but serious complication. Its cause is probably obstruction of the arachnoid villi or basal cisterns by blood. It usually presents weeks or months after the injury with a gradual dementia and motor apraxia or loss of complex coordinated motor movements. The treatment is to shunt the cerebrospinal fluid from the lateral ventricles to the superior vena cava via a Holter or Pudenz valve to maintain the cerebrospinal pressure at 50 to 70 mm of water.

In general, with patience, support, and guidance the head-injured patient will recover and return to useful existence. This may take many months and requires that both the physician and the patient not become discouraged. The degree of recovery of even the very seriously injured patients will justify for the physician the amount of effort and time that he must give to this group of patients.

SPINAL CORD INJURIES

In the treatment of spinal cord injuries the prime objectives are the preservation of neural function and, when

Fig. 42-3. Fracture-dislocation with anterior displacement of C_5 on C_6 and unilateral locking of the left facets in a twenty-year-old man who, following a fall from a horse, presented with signs of weakness and sensory loss in his arms and legs. Radicular (local) signs were weakness of the muscles innervated by the C_6 root, i.e., biceps and brachioradialis muscles. Tract signs were weakness of both lower extremities, the left more than the right, with bilateral plantar extensor responses. Following reduction his neurologic recovery was complete except for residual weakness of the left biceps.

possible, restoration of neural function, followed by the reestablishment of the integrity of the vertebral column and the rehabilitation of the patient.

MECHANISMS OF INJURY. In contrast to skull injuries, in which fracture and brain damage may have an inverse relationship, bony vertebral damage and spinal cord injury have a high correlation, for the bony vertebrae and their attached soft tissue are usually the agents directly causing the spinal cord injury. The construction of the vertebral column with its circumferential bony ring provides ideal protection for low-velocity penetrating injuries or concussive blows, but the intervertebral articulations are weak points for flexion, extension, or rotary stresses. Dislocation and fractures that do not break the vertebral ring allow the vertebrae above and below the area of injury to act as a fulcrum for another vertebra and its attached soft tissue to concuss, stretch, contuse, or disrupt the spinal cord. The rarer fracture-dislocation that separates the posterior arch from the vertebral body demonstrates how much dislocation of the body can occur without permanent spinal cord damage and suggests methods of protecting the damaged cord, namely, laminectomy or removal of the posterior segments of the vertebrae. The stress of flexion, extension, and rotation and the relative weakness of the articulations of the vertebrae operate to make fractures and dislocations most common at points of junction between mobile and relatively fixed segments of the spinal column. These are the lower cervical region (Fig. 42-3) and the upper lumbar region related to the thoracic spine, that is relatively fixed by the ribs.

Most of the spinal cord damage occurs at the time of injury. However, recent studies of experimental spinal cord trauma in animals suggest a progressive hemorrhagic destruction of the central gray matter followed by edema in the white matter. Progressive damage to the white matter may occur during the first 4 to 6 hours after injury and plays a role in eventual spinal cord dysfunction. The mechanism of the pathophysiology is not clear, but in the experimental animal cooling of the injured segment, steroids, and myelotomy have protective value and alter this progressive posttraumatic process. This suggests possible therapeutic approaches to the problem of spinal cord injury, and clinical studies are in progress. Secondary spinal cord damage can occur from further movement of the unstable vertebral column, the movement of the spinal cord against sharp fragments of bone in the canal, and continued compression of the spinal cord. Therapy to prevent any secondary damage to the spinal cord requires stabilization of the vertebral column, removal of any foreign body or fragments of bone from the spinal canal, and decompression of the spinal cord when necessary.

REDUCTION AND STABILIZATION OF VERTEBRAL COLUMN. In the cervical region stabilization of the vertebral column is most effectively obtained by skeletal traction, using skull tongs (Barton, Vinke, or Crutchfield tongs). Stabilization is achieved by anatomic reduction and by tension of the spinal ligaments and soft tissue of the cervical region. Slight extension of the neck will give tension to the anterior spinal ligament, the strongest of the spinal ligaments, and therefore is preferred unless there is evidence of rupture of the ligament. This is usually apparent from an x-ray that shows avulsion of the anterior lip of a vertebral body, the site of insertion of the ligament. Stabilization is promoted by placing the patient on a firm surface. A Stryker or Foster frame bed makes an excellent support, since the patient can be turned from the prone to supine position without changing the relative position of the spinal column.

Reduction of fracture-dislocations of the thoracic or lumbar spine should not be done unless the spinal cord or cauda equina is exposed by laminectomy before the reduction, since the force necessary for such closed reduction carries too high a risk of further damage to the spinal cord or cauda equina. Simple compression fractures of the body of the vertebra, with flexion angulation of the spine but without spinal cord deficit, may be gently extended by positioning in a Foster frame, utilizing extension to stretch the anterior spinal ligament and expand the vertebral body. A foreign body or bone fragment in the canal is a contraindication for any manipulative maneuver, since it may act as a disrupting agent during such maneuvers. The presence of foreign bodies adjacent to or in the spinal cord also allows possible continuing damage from any body movement or from the natural movements of the spinal cord with respirations and pulse. If any continuity of spinal cord function remains across such an area, laminectomy and removal of the fragments is indicated.

DECOMPRESSION OF SPINAL CORD. The most difficult judgment in the early care of spinal cord injury is the decision to decompress the spinal cord. Some surgeons have solved this problem by always doing a laminectomy in any severe spinal cord injury, while others are firmly convinced that it is of value in only the rare case with later progression of neurologic deficit. The first group base their judgment on the concept that there is always edema and swelling of the spinal cord and surrounding tissue and therefore laminectomy with decompression is always of some potential value. Complications of such therapy have to be considered, and in unskilled hands they may be considerable. An argument used by the latter group is that severe injury of the spinal cord rarely can be reversed, since neuronal loss is complete within a short time of the injury and the life of the patient is placed in jeopardy by surgical therapy with little chance of helping spinal cord function.

Experimental evidence in animals demonstrates that the tracts of the spinal cord can tolerate many hours of anoxic compression and recover, even though the neurons within the anoxic area cannot. Since the total functional result is mainly dependent upon the tracts traversing the segment, preservation of viability in these tracts is worthwhile. Evidence that there is compression consists of any progression in neurologic deficit, or a block of cerebrospinal fluid circulation. The Queckenstedt test consists of a measurement of lumbar cerebrospinal fluid pressure before and after compression of the jugular veins of the neck by a blood pressure cuff. If rapid rise and fall in the lumbar pressure does not occur with the compression and release of the neck veins, the test shows evidence of a block in the cerebrospinal fluid circulation between the foramen mag-

num and the lumbar puncture needle. The Queckenstedt test is both inaccurate and dangerous, since an opening at the site of compression just larger than a spinal needle may give a negative test (no evidence of block) despite considerable compression, and increasing cerebrospinal fluid pressure above a block of the spinal canal can cause further spinal cord damage. For these reasons, when a compressive block is suspected, contrast myelography with air or Pantopaque, usually placed in the spinal canal through a lateral C_1-C_2 spinal puncture, is indicated. With such evidence of block in cerebrospinal fluid circulation, laminectomy with opening of the dura is indicated unless rapid improvement in neurologic function is occurring. With trained neurosurgeons the morbidity and mortality of the procedure is far below the risk of allowing progressive spinal cord damage from further compression of the cord.

COMPOUND INJURIES. Trauma to the spinal cord may also result in open or compound injuries. The principles for the care of both closed and open injuries are not substantially different except that compound injuries require debridement and closure of the wound and they rarely have vertebral instability. Compound wounds of the spinal cord may occur from sharp penetrating objects but are most commonly from gunshot wounds. The concussive force of the bullet causes widespread damage and therefore more widespread reactive edema. If there is any possibility of cord continuity, early exploration, wide decompression, and removal of devitalized tissues both within and around the spinal cord are indicated in order to give the patient any significant chance of recovery. Without such surgical measures secondary compressive anoxia of the tracts is certain to occur.

BONY UNION. Reestablishment of vertebral integrity requires time for bony union. If instability is marked, fusion is usually indicated. Marked instability occurs when the articulating facets and ligaments are disrupted or when there is some combination of injury to the vertebral body, pedicles, and facets. If open fusion is indicated, it is best to allow 2 to 3 weeks for reaction of injury within the cord to subside before performing a spinal fusion, since further reaction within the surrounding tissue occurs with such a procedure. Total immobilization of at least 6 weeks is indicated in most cervical injuries, with 6 to 8 weeks of support following this to ensure firm union. In other areas of the spinal column where weight-bearing stresses are greater, the time for sufficient union varies with the area and the type of bony injury but in general is longer than in the cervical area.

REHABILITATION. Rehabilitation of the patient with a spinal cord injury is a specialty by itself. The early care of the skin and bladder, however, can be as important for the time required for rehabilitation as any factor other than neurologic deficit. Following cord injury, spinal shock of varying degree occurs, and protective skin and bladder reflexes are lost. Support of the body is necessary so that the pressure points, such as the sacrum and the heels, take as little weight as possible. A dry smooth covering against any weight-bearing skin, good nutrition, cleanliness, and, most important, turning the patient at least every 2 hours are the necessary nursing measures to protect the skin of the cord-injured patient. Initial constant catheter drainage of the bladder should be followed by intermittent catheter drainage plus high fluid intake to protect the urinary tract from distension and infection.

Illustrative Case

Perhaps the easiest way to summarize the acute neurosurgical care of the cord-injured patient is to review the care of a patient who, immediately following an automobile accident, entered the hospital with weakness and sensory loss from the arms down. Initial examination revealed normal movement of the deltoid and biceps muscles, weakness of both triceps muscles, and only slight movement of the fingers, legs, and toes. Sensory examination showed preservation of deep pain and some touch sensation in both lower extremities but marked hypesthesia and hypalgesia from the ulnar side of the hands and arms caudad bilaterally. There were absent deep tendon and superficial reflexes except for the biceps reflexes. X-rays of the cervical spine were reported as negative.

The history and the examination indicated a C_6-C_7 or C_7-T_1 vertebral column injury, and with this knowledge the x-rays were found to be not negative but inadequate, since they showed only the upper portion of C_6 and more cephalad vertebrae. Further x-rays showed a fracture dislocation with the C_6 vertebra anteriorly displaced on the C_7 vertebra. The patient was placed on a Stryker frame; the bladder was catheterized and connected to constant drainage. Barton tongs were applied to the skull, slightly anterior to the coronal plane traversing the mastoid tips, and 15 lb of weight was applied. Neurologic examination showed no change in function. X-rays showed no evidence of reduction. Five more pounds of weight was applied. Neurologic examination remained unchanged, and x-rays showed slight reduction of the dislocation. Five more pounds, or a total of twenty-five pounds, was applied, and neurologic examination remained unchanged, but x-rays showed reduction of the dislocation. Because of the lack of improvement, a myelogram was done and showed posterior and anterior compression of the spinal cord at approximately the C_6 level. The patient was taken to the operating room for laminectomy, and at operation the laminae and facets of C_6 and C_7 were found to be fractured. The laminae and spinous processes of C_5, C_6, and C_7 were removed, and the dura was opened. The spinal cord appeared posteriorly displaced and swollen. Because closure of the dura appeared to cause constriction of the spinal cord, a fascial graft was placed for dural relaxation, and the dura, muscles, fascia, and skin were sutured with interrupted silk sutures.

The patient showed gradual improvement for approximately 1 week, at which time over a 2-day period the strength of his finger flexors gradually decreased. The Pantopaque that had been left in the canal at the previous myelogram was repositioned into the cervical canal under fluoroscopy, and an anterior filling defect was demonstrated at the C_6-C_7 interspace. The patient was returned to the operating room, and the C_6-C_7 interspace was approached anteriorly. The interspace was exposed and the remains of damaged nucleus pulposus were removed along with the cartilaginous end plates. A fragment of nucleus pulposus was found free in the anterior part of the spinal canal and removed. A piece of bone taken from the ileum was wedged into the hole for stability and future bony fusion. The patient made a gradual recovery over the next 6 months.

The points illustrated are the same as those discussed in the initial portion of this section. It is important that the area of damage be identified from the neurologic examination, so that the examiner is certain that x-rays of the spinal column include the area. When any manipulation is done, both the x-rays and the neurologic function should be checked. If despite reduction there remains evidence of cerebrospinal fluid circulation obstruction and there is no sign of neurologic improvement, decompressive laminectomy is indicated at that time, and the decompression should be complete, so that not even the dura binds the spinal cord. In the case reviewed above, even though there was a question of something displacing the spinal cord when it was seen at laminectomy, it was felt that further manipulation of the cord in order to expose the anterior surface was not indicated, since the spinal cord had already sustained significant trauma. The signs of progressive neurologic deficit even in the late postoperative period indicated either further compression of the spinal cord or instability of the vertebral column despite the traction. When a myelogram demonstrated a filling defect in the anterior portion of the spinal canal, both problems were definitively treated by ventral exposure of the damaged intervertebral space, removal of the free fragment of nucleus pulposus, and placement of an interbody bone graft to allow fusion.

PERIPHERAL NERVE INJURIES

The common types of peripheral nerve injuries are laceration, contusion, and stretch or compression, with or without disruption. The agents causing such injuries are numerous but from a therapeutic view can be divided into those causing a focal injury, such as a knife or a piece of glass; those causing relatively localized injury but imparting force to adjacent areas, such as a gunshot wound; and those causing damage to long segments of the nerve, as with stretch following a dislocation of extremity or compression from swelling under a rigid cast or dressing. Evaluation of nerve injuries includes accurate knowledge of the anatomy and function of the nerve suspected of injury, identification of the agent causing the injury, and recognition of the type of injury resulting. Treatment is based on the evaluation as well as knowledge of the factors influencing the comparative prognosis of the different forms of therapy available and the skill of the surgeon, not only to repair the nerve involved and the adjacent tissues, but also to utilize all reconstructive measures available.

EVALUATION. The evaluation of peripheral nerve injuries is in part similar to the evaluation of central nervous system injuries, for comparison of serial observations and recognition of progressive neurologic deficit or improvement often determine the type of therapy required. The treatment differs from that for central nervous system injuries in that regeneration and reinnervation can occur and therefore the treatment of peripheral nerve injury includes neurorrhaphy, or the surgical repair of the nerve. Since comparison of later examinations with the initial one is important in therapy, it is essential to have an accurate examination that includes the sensory and motor function of all nerves thought to be injured. Peripheral nerve injuries often occur as part of more extensive injuries, and since an accurate examination can be done only on a cooperative patient, all patients suspected of nerve injury should be reexamined when well enough to cooperate.

Accurate knowledge of the anatomy and function of the nerve suspected of injury is a minimal requirement for a competent examination and evaluation. Nerve injuries are a relatively rare experience for the average physician; since the accuracy of even an experienced neurosurgeon can be enhanced by reviewing the anatomy and functions of nerves suspected of injury, the physician making the initial examination or treating the patient at any time should not hesitate to consult an anatomy book and review the anatomic relations and the motor and sensory function of the nerves involved. With this help accurate localization and accurate definition of the neurologic deficit can usually be made.

TREATMENT. The problem after diagnosis is what to do and when to do it. There are only a few alternatives for treatment of peripheral nerve injury: suture of the nerve, resection of damaged areas and resuture, or no treatment of the nerve but reestablishment of function of the part by utilizing other muscles and internal or external support.

A few axioms should be kept in mind. Complete functional loss in a nerve can occur without anatomic disruption, and functional return can occur within 60 to 90 days. This segmental loss of conduction in the nerve following trauma is caused by alteration in the ability of the axons to reestablish their membrane potential and is called *neuronapraxis.* The mechanism of recovery is not known, but the nerve recovers its function in all segments distal to the injury at approximately the same time, and therefore the recovery cannot be secondary to regrowth of the axons.

Although immediate repair gives the best functional results, little is lost by a delay of 3 to 5 weeks. After disruption and reapproximation of a nerve the axons require about 3 weeks to grow across the suture line and then grow at about 2 cm/month. In general, counting the delay across the suture line and the time for reinnervation of the muscle end plates or peripheral end organs, an estimated functional growth of 1 in./month is usually accurate. Following denervation, muscle end plates atrophy and muscle fibers progressively degenerate, so that within 20 to 24 months no significant muscle contraction can be expected from reinnervation. While muscle tone reappears and some movement will occur up to that time, significant strength in a muscle rarely can be regained past 15 months. Since functional nerve regeneration proceeds at approximately 1 in./month, a nerve suture that is more than 15 in. from the denervated muscle cannot be expected

to give significant motor return, and tendon transplants, joint fixation, or bracing should be considered as the treatment for the motor loss. Tone in facial muscles will return up to 24 months past denervation, but as the end of the 24-month period approaches, no movement of expression can be expected.

All nerve injuries are painful, and the pain will continue with varying intensity for many months. Narcotics have no place in the treatment of chronic pain and therefore should not be used after the immediate wound pain has ceased. Functional use of the extremity is the best therapy for the pain and is an important reason for using passive and active motion and functional bracing as soon as possible. It is also a major reason for not waiting for an improbable result, such as reinnervation of a muscle too distant from the point of suture, before using other reconstructive methods.

In contrast to the time limits on return of motor function, sensory function of a significant degree can return whenever reinnervation of the part occurs and often is of help in relieving the discomfort as well as in providing protection of an extremity. This is especially true of the protection offered by sensory reinnervation of the foot.

In general, nerve grafts have not been successful as a method of bridging areas of nerve loss in order to restore function. The delay in crossing two suture lines, the loss and mixing of fibers at each suture line, and the associated tissue damage that usually occurs when grafts have been required have been suggested as the main reasons for functional failures. In almost all nerves, gaps of 8 to 10 cm can be bridged by proximal and distal dissection to release the nerve from surrounding tissue and by positioning of the nerve or the extremity to minimize the distance across joints. This may require wide dissection and positioning of more than one joint of the extremity. When neurorrhaphy is planned, skin preparation and draping should allow for such maneuvers. The problems with these maneuvers are that they may not allow closure of the ends of the nerve without tension, or may, after initial healing of the neurorrhaphy, allow tension and interference with blood supply of the regenerating nerve as the joints are extended. A recent microsurgical technique of perineural suture, i.e., approximation of the perifascicular tissue of the nerve rather than closure of the epineural tissue, suggests improved distal growth both in number and rate of regenerating axons. The technique allows no tension at the site of closure, since very fine suture and low-tensile-strength tissue are used in the approximation. Interfascicular grafts, composed of homologous nerve, usually the sural nerve of the patient, interposed in a defect and sutured by these techniques, are reported to give better results than end-to-end epineural neurorrhaphy under tension. These grafts, by averting the mixture of interfascicular fibers and altered blood supply of a nerve under tension, appear to be an advance in nerve repair and have improved the expected results from some neurorrhaphies that had been done under tension and from some nerve grafts that had been required because of a long area of deficit. Interfascicular (perineural) neurorrhaphy allows better approximation and has reactivated interest in homologous nerve grafts.

EVALUATION OF FUNCTIONAL RECOVERY. In the evaluation of the injured nerve, evidence for functional recovery of the nerve is important, for it determines the success or failure of the therapy. Evidence that the nerve functions is not the same as functional recovery, for nerve function means only that some portion of the nerve has anatomic continuity. Definite evidence of functional recovery consists of:

1.   Voluntary motor function of a muscle innervated by the nerve distal to the injury. This means that a major number of the motor fibers have reinnervated the muscle and that with time increase in strength will occur, either through increased strength of the individual reinnervated muscle fibers or by further innervation.

2.   Muscle contraction on electrical stimulation of the nerve distal to the point of injury when performed more than 7 days after injury. Since the distal segment of a divided nerve will conduct impulses for only 5 to 6 days, evidence of ability to conduct later than 7 days after injury indicates functional continuity or regeneration. Muscle contraction following the stimulation means a major portion of the motor fibers are conducting. Direct electrical stimulation of the muscle does not give evidence of functional recovery, since contraction with this type of stimulation will occur until atrophy of the muscle is complete.

3.   Recovery of sensation in an autogenous area of innervation. There are few such areas for individual nerves. The distal phalanx of the index finger for the median nerve and the distal phalanx of the little finger for the ulnar nerve are the only two in the upper extremity. The distal phalanges of the middle three toes of the foot are autogenous for the sciatic nerve but only if both peroneal and tibial divisions are involved.

Evidence of anatomic continuity but not of prognostic significance for functional recovery consists of:

1.   Tinel's sign distal to the site of injury. Tinel's sign is elicited by percussing the nerve and obtaining paresthesias referred to the superficial area of skin innervation. It requires activation of only a small percentage of the fibers, far less than is required for functional recovery.

2.   Alteration in electromyographic activity with attempted voluntary motion or nerve stimulation. As with Tinel's sign, the activation of far fewer fibers than is necessary for functional return of a muscle is required to elicit alteration in the recorded electromyographic activity.

Evidence that indicates neither anatomic nor functional continuity of an injured nerve consists of:

1.   Shrinkage of the area of sensory loss. The marked overlap of sensory innervation in all areas of the body has been alluded to with the description of the very few autogenous zones of peripheral nerve innervation. Decrease in an area of sensory loss after nerve injury can occur from recovery of the nerve function, but even without reinnervation adjacent nerves reestablish sensation in the area. The mechanism appears to be both utilization of fibers which function with the damaged nerve but which without the spatial summation of the damaged nerve activity do not reach consciousness, and branching of the superficial nerve fibers of the remaining nerves with growth into the denervated area.

2.   Improved use of the extremity. The adaptability of the child to use any remaining function to accomplish coordinated tasks is a major example, but use of gravity, momentum, and muscles with remaining function to simulate the lost function must not be confused with reinnervation.

Illustrative Cases

The application of these concepts is most easily understood in relation to examples of the three major groups of peripheral nerve injury, laceration, or focal sharp injury, focal contusion, and compression or stretch injury.

Focal Laceration. An example of focal sharp injury is a knife wound of the upper extremity at approximately the midhumeral level, resulting in loss of median nerve function. Motor loss would consist of paralysis of all flexors of the wrist and fingers except the flexor carpi ulnaris and the ulnar portion of the flexor digitorum profundus. These latter two muscles would give wrist flexion with ulnar deviation and flexion of the ring and little fingers. Sensory loss would consist of loss of superficial sensation of the palmar surface of the hand extending to the thumb and first two fingers and the radial half of the ring finger. Deep as well as superficial sensation would be lost in the distal phalanx of the index finger.

Immediate repair is indicated *except* when any of the following apply: (1) The nerve appears contused for more than a few millimeters on either side of the injury. (2) There is blood loss from arterial injury that would jeopardize the life of the patient in undergoing a long (2- to 3-hour) operation for repair of the artery and nerve. (3) The wound is older than 5 to 6 hours, and dissection might spread contamination. (4) The surgeon is not certain of his ability to perform adequate neurorrhaphy.

If inadequate repair is done so that regeneration does not occur (no matter what the reason), it will take approximately 6 months, or the time it takes the nerve to grow 6 in. to the flexor muscles of the forearm, before the inadequacy of the repair is recognized. Since the opponens of the thumb is beyond the distance where significant strength can be expected to be regained, as soon as the flexor muscles of the forearm are reinnervated, tendon transplant of one of the flexors to strengthen the apposition of the thumb is indicated.

Focal Contusion. The most common focal contusion of nerve is that secondary to a gunshot wound, and the treatment of a gunshot wound of the midthigh resulting in loss of sciatic nerve function is an example of such an injury. Immediate repair of the nerve is not indicated, since the damage extending up and down the nerve cannot be determined by inspection and after a high-velocity-missile injury it is always present in varying degrees.

The wound is treated to prevent infection, and the patient is fitted with a short leg brace for stabilization of the ankle. Stabilization is necessary, since motor function in all flexors, extensors, evertors, and invertors of the foot, as well as in the intrinsic muscles of the foot, will be lost. The patient is ambulated with a brace as soon as possible and taught to inspect the skin of the foot three or four times a day in order to protect it from unrecognized injury in the anesthetic area. Four to five weeks later, if no function has returned or if only minimal function in one portion of the sciatic nerve has returned, exploration is indicated. By this time fibrosis or neuroma formation will define the area of injury. Resection and resuture may be indicated. Three weeks after repair, when the anastomosis is secure, active use of the leg with the same precautions that were observed preoperatively should be started. Fifteen months later the stability of the ankle should be evaluated, and internal stabilization or arthrodesis may be indicated because of failure of adequate reinnervation.

Stretch or Compression Injury. The problem of the nerve with stretch or compression injury is more difficult. The segment of injury is often longer than can be bridged by any technique, and the loss is usually incomplete, so that even if the area might be bridged by surgical technique, comparison of the deficit from the injury with what might be obtained by resection and suture is essential in the decision for treatment. A common area of stretch injury is the brachial plexus, as might be seen following a shoulder injury. Careful recording of all sensory and motor loss is necessary, and if the pattern of loss suggests a radicular pattern, that is, loss of root function such as at C_5 and C_6, myelography or the fluoroscopic study of the spinal arachnoid space with radiopaque substance is indicated. Rupture of the arachnoid root sleeve with formation of a traumatic meningocele or pouching of the arachnoid through the intervertebral foramen may be demonstrated, indicating avulsion of the roots from the cord. Root avulsions are not repairable, and reconstructive measures such as fusion of the shoulder and triceps transplantation for elbow flexion are indicated rather than surgical exploration of the area of injury.

The possibility of surgical repair of compression or stretch injury is slight, since the area of injury is so long, and 2 to 3 months of evaluation are indicated to determine that the loss is not due to neuronapraxis, with spontaneous recovery occurring. In the brachial plexus injury loss of motion in the forearm would not be significantly improved by resection and suture, and loss of intrinsic muscles in the hands is not an indication for surgical intervention, since return of function cannot be expected. The usual early treatment indicated is protection of the denervated muscles from overstretching by a supporting brace, while later functional bracing, fusion of joints, and transplantation of remaining functioning muscles are the appropriate means of gaining maximum possible function.

BRAIN TUMORS

Although uncommon in the experience of the average physician, brain tumors are not rare. As a clinical entity they are best brought into perspective by realizing that brain tumors constitute almost 10 percent of all benign and malignant tumors requiring hospitalization for surgical removal and that just under 1 percent of all deaths are caused by primary intracranial neoplasm. One reason that brain tumors seem to be uncommon in the experience of physicians is that they are not suspected as the cause of the patient's complaints, for the presenting symptoms are diverse and confusing, and their recognition can be difficult.

CLASSIFICATION AND CHARACTERISTICS. The classifications of brain tumors are at best confusing, partly because the naming of tumors has usually been on the basis of cellular characteristics. The difficulties of such classifications arise not only from the many different names that can be applied to the same tumor in different situations

but also from the difficulty of describing the different characteristics of even the same cell type within a tumor. Clinically a useful classification of brain tumors is the one proposed by Kernohan and Sayre based on naming the tumors for the cells present in the adult nervous system, vascular tissue, and developmental defects, combined with a grading of the malignancy of the tumor from grade I to grade IV, with IV the most malignant (Table 42-3).

Certain types of tumors are more frequent at certain ages and occur with greater frequency in those ages in different areas of the brain. For example, 70 percent of adult tumors are supratentorial, that is, in the middle or anterior fossa, while 75 percent of childhood tumors occur in the posterior fossa. The most common primary tumor of the brain in the middle-aged and elderly is a grade III or grade IV astrocytoma (glioblastoma multiforme), while the most common tumor of childhood is the grade I and II astrocytoma of the cerebellum. Malignant astrocytomas are by far the most common primary brain tumor in adults, followed by meningiomas, pituitary tumors, and neurilemomas, while in childhood the most common tumors are the relatively benign astrocytomas of the posterior fossa, followed very closely by the highly malignant medulloblastomas, and then by ependymomas and craniopharyngiomas. Tumors of childhood occur characteristically near the midline of the brain, as with the tumors of developmental defects, the medulloblastomas, and the astrocytomas of the brainstem and cerebellum. Gliomas in adults occur at a frequency that is related to the volume of the brain itself and therefore are more common in the cerebral hemispheres. Meningiomas have a predilection for areas of arachnoid villi and arachnoid invaginations that contain cells similar to those seen in the meningioma. These areas of predilection are along the sagittal sinus, the sella, the olfactory groove, the tentorium, and the petrous ridges.

Table 42-3. BRAIN TUMORS

	Percent
Gliomas	40–50
Astrocytoma, grade I	5–10
Astrocytoma, grade II	2–5
Astrocytoma, grades III and IV	
(glioblastoma multiforme)	20–30
Medulloblastoma	3–5
Oligodendroglioma	1–4
Ependymoma, grades I–IV	1–3
Meningioma	12–20
Pituitary tumors	5–15
Neurolemmomas (mainly eighth nerve)	3–10
Metastatic tumors	5–10
Blood vessel tumors	
Arteriovenous malformations	
Hemangioblastomas	
Endotheliomas	0.1–1
Tumors of developmental defects	2–3
Dermoids, epidermoids, teratomas	
Chordomas, paraphyseal cysts	
Craniopharyngiomas	3–8
Pinealomas	0.5–0.8
Miscellaneous	
Sarcomas, papillomas of the choroid plexus, lipomas,	
unclassified, etc	1–3

PATHOPHYSIOLOGY. This difficulty is minimized if the physician has a concept of the basic pathophysiology of brain tumors. The basic pattern is one of progressive neurologic deficit. This deficit can be a progressive focal deficit or a progression in the neurologic dysfunction that occurs secondary to increased intracranial pressure. Since these clinical patterns are a continuum, the historical examination of the patient must include the factor of time and its relationship to the development of the symptoms and signs. Their development may vary within the basic patterns because of the different mechanisms by which tumors disturb normal function, the different positions the tumor may occupy within the skull, and the diverse growth potentials of the different tumor types. These variables, when combined with the concepts discussed in the opening portion of this chapter, namely, the anatomic confinement within compartments of the skull of a deformable but relatively noncompressible brain and the changes in neural function that occur from compression of the brainstem passing through the incisura of the tentorium and the foramen magnum, explain in part the diversity of the presenting symptoms produced by brain tumors. With so many combinations of variables possible, learning the symptoms for the different types of tumors in their different clinical stages is almost an endless task unless it is related to functional anatomy of the brain, the mechanisms used by tumors in producing signs and symptoms, and a classification of the tumors by frequency of occurrence and growth potential.

Tumors of the central nervous system manifest themselves most frequently by effects caused by one or more of the following mechanisms:

1. Compression of neural tissue, either direct or secondary to displacement of the brain
2. Infiltration or direct invasion with destruction of neural tissue
3. Alteration in the blood supply to neurons
4. Alteration in neuronal excitability
5. Increase in mass within the skull
6. Alteration in cerebrospinal fluid circulation

CLINICAL MANIFESTATIONS. Direct compression of neural tissue produces a progressive focal neurologic deficit which is the most easily recognized sign of brain tumor. The deficit will vary depending upon the area of the brain involved and is usually partial rather than complete. Thus, hemiparesis rather than hemiplegia is more frequently seen, and sensory loss is more commonly a partial rather than a total deficit.

Progressive focal neurologic deficit can be produced by other mechanisms, such as direct destruction of neural tissue by malignant cells and loss of neural function by alteration in local blood supply. Direct destruction of neural tissue by involvement of malignant cells is uncommon, but alteration in local blood supply does occur and particularly may be seen in the older patient with a highly malignant glioma. Interference with arterial blood supply by tumor usually manifests itself as an acute loss of function, suggesting primary vascular disease, and only the later focal progression from increasing mass effects, or further involvement of local blood supply, completes the pattern of progressive focal neurologic deficit, indicating the diagnosis of brain tumor.

Compression, invasion, and altered blood supply may also cause altered neuronal excitability which is manifested by convulsions. Convulsions are paroxysmal episodes of uncontrolled neural activity, and since the neurons of the cerebral cortex have the lowest threshold for such paroxysmal activity, seizures caused by tumors are most commonly seen in lesions adjacent to or within the cerebral cortex. A focal or a Jacksonian seizure and especially a postictal neurologic loss (Todd's paralysis) indicate the localization of the lesion, and progression in either frequency or severity of the seizures or in the postictal neurologic deficit is strongly suggestive of a brain tumor.

The signs and symptoms of generalized increase in pressure are cloudy mentation and consciousness, headache, papilledema, vomiting, bradycardia, and systolic hypertension. It is rare to have all these findings except as terminal events. Increased pressure can also produce abducens, or sixth cranial nerve palsy, which may have no localizing value, for the abducens nerve is particularly prone to loss of function secondary to increased intracranial pressure. Increased intracranial pressure from brain tumors can result from mass, impaired cerebrospinal fluid circulation, or a combination of these.

The increase in mass may result from a number of factors. There is the neoplastic growth itself and edema formation. Malignant tumors especially produce edema in the adjacent brain. The cause of this edema is not understood, but it can result in massive swelling at considerable distances from the tumor. Some tumors form cysts that have osmotic gradients that cause an enlargement of the cyst by absorption of fluid. Infrequently rapid enlargement may result from hemorrhage within a tumor. Changes may occur in the surrounding nervous tissue, such as edema from venous obstruction or edema from breakdown of the integrity of the blood-brain barrier, secondary to either arterial or venous insufficiency.

The increased intracranial pressure caused by alteration in cerebrospinal fluid circulation usually occurs from obstruction of the passage of cerebrospinal fluid from the lateral ventricles to the subarachnoid space. This can occur when tumors arise within the ventricular system. Obstruction in the flow of cerebrospinal fluid may also occur when there is a shift of the brainstem so that the aqueduct of Sylvius is compressed or the outlets of the fourth ventricle are blocked. Tumors in the basal cisterns may also obstruct cerebrospinal fluid flow.

There are compensatory intracranial mechanisms for altering the effects of increased mass and pressure. Most of them require days or months to be effective and therefore are best utilized in controlling pressure from a slowly growing, benign tumor. These mechanisms include decreases in intracranial blood volume, cerebrospinal fluid volume, intracellular fluid contents, and parenchymal cell numbers.

EVALUATION. The primary necessity in the diagnosis of brain tumor is the suspicion which should be initiated by the patient's history of a progressive neurologic deficit. The more knowledgeable the physician is of the functional anatomy of the brain, the more accurately he will recognize progressive neurologic deficit. While hemiparesis and hemisensory loss or lack of motor function in a cranial nerve are easily recognizable, slow progressive dementia, decrease in pituitary function, or progression in the severity of seizures are more difficult neurologic deficits to recognize as indicating brain tumor.

It is beyond the scope of this section to review the diagnostic investigation that should be completed in evaluating a patient suspected of having a brain tumor, but complete physical and neurologic examinations are the minimal requisites to the use of special diagnostic tests that have been described in the opening section of this chapter. The dangers of alteration in intracranial pressure by some of the studies, such as pneumoencephalography, and the dangers inherent in angiography must be weighed against the benefit of obtaining information needed for treatment, realizing that these special diagnostic studies such as brain scan, computerized axial tomography, echo encephalogram, air study, and arteriography have a high degree of accuracy and aid considerably in the final judgment as to what should be done with a brain tumor.

TREATMENT. The primary goal of tumor therapy is cure, and surgical excision is the method most likely to accomplish a cure. Unfortunately, in the case of brain tumor surgical removal is not always possible or even desirable, since the resulting neurologic deficit may leave the patient so impaired that saving his life is of no significance. The treatment of brain tumors therefore is not just their surgical removal, and it requires experience and knowledge combined with surgical skill in order to obtain the maximal functional result. At times the repetitive use of these special diagnostic tests and evaluation over a period of time are necessary to be certain of what would be the optimal therapy. As often as possible total removal is attempted, but when this is deemed impossible, palliation by partial removal of the tumor for internal decompression, relief of intracranial pressure by shunting of blocked spinal fluid, or treatment of the tumor by x-ray therapy and/or chemotherapy may control the tumor or give significant relief and allow the patient extended periods of normal existence. Combinations of these palliative and curative techniques allow a large percentage of patients to obtain significant relief of symptoms or cure of the brain tumor.

SUMMATION. In summary, it is the evidence of a progressive neurologic deficit that should raise the suspicion of diagnosis of a brain tumor, for progressive neurologic deficit is the most common presenting symptom of brain tumor. This deficit may be of a focal nature which varies according to the area of the brain involved or may be a more generalized type secondary to increased intracranial pressure. The focal neurologic deficit may be a loss of function or can be altered excitability. Loss of neural function secondary to brain tumor is most frequently incomplete, and altered excitability usually presents as a convulsion. The effects of generalized increased intracranial pressure can be secondary to increased mass, alteration in cerebrospinal fluid circulation, or a combination

of these. The deficits seen in brain tumor have a common denominator, that is, evidence of progression in symptomatology and signs over a period of time. A knowledge of the functional anatomy of the brain, classification of brain tumors, their frequency of occurrence and growth potential, and the mechanisms by which tumors manifest themselves will facilitate a high degree of accuracy in suspecting brain tumors, thereby allowing the physician to have the aid of the specialist in diagnosing and treating the tumor.

SPINAL CORD TUMORS

The term *spinal tumors* includes all tumors encroaching on the spinal cord. Primary tumors of the spine are approximately one-sixth as common as intracranial tumors but have a much better prognosis, since almost 60 percent are benign and a high percentage of the remainder respond to therapy, so that prolonged functional palliation can be expected. Metastatic spinal tumors are reported to present as often as primary spinal tumors. Any malignant tumor may metastasize to the bones of the spinal column or to the spinal epidural space, but the most common are from lung, breast, lymphoid tissue, prostate, kidney, and thyroid. Metastatic spinal tumors usually cause pain, followed by neurologic deficit. Since these tumors rarely cause death, palliation by surgical and radiation therapy is indicated in order to preserve neurologic function and decrease suffering during a terminal illness.

CLASSIFICATION AND CHARACTERISTICS. The symptoms, the type of tumor, and the prognosis correlate with where the tumor is in relation to the dura and spinal cord. Therefore, the classification of tumors into extradural and intradural groups and the subdivision of the intradural group into extramedullary and intramedullary has significance from both a clinical and pathologic point of view. Ninety percent of extradural tumors are malignant, while sixty percent of intradural tumors are benign. Seventy-five to eighty percent of extradural tumors are metastatic, while ninety-eight percent of intradural tumors are primary tumors. The common clinical course of extradural tumors is one of rapid compression of the spinal cord, either by the tumor itself or from collapse of involved vertebrae. The patient may present with rapidly progressing flaccid paraparesis and sensory loss that requires rapid recognition and surgical decompression in order to have significant palliative effect. The common clinical course of the intradural tumor is usually much slower and may extend over months or years with the patient presenting with spastic paraparesis and partial sensory loss.

Knowledge of the types of tumors, their potential for growth, and their mechanisms of production of symptoms is the means by which the finer aspects of diagnosis of spinal cord tumor are best attained, but the clinician should always consider the diagnosis of spinal cord tumor when any bilateral progressive neurologic loss occurs below any transverse level of the body. The value of such constant suspicion is the high degree of functional return and the high percentage of cure or palliation of symptoms resulting from the early surgical treatment.

EVALUATION. A suspected spinal cord tumor is localized by utilizing the findings of the neurologic examination, the bony changes in spinal x-rays, and the results of spinal contrast studies, or myelography.

CLINICAL MANIFESTATIONS. The diagnostic neurologic examination findings are of two types, local signs and tract signs. The local signs are segmental changes and localize the lesion along the rostral-caudal axis. The local motor signs are weakness and loss of reflexes with normal above and normal or hyperactive reflexes below the level, fasciculations over a segmental distribution, and atrophy in a myotome pattern. These indicate involvement of the anterior motor horn cells or the anterior spinal roots. Local sensory signs are localized pain and spinal tenderness, radicular or radiating pain, and loss of sensation over a dermatome pattern, indicating involvement of the dorsal root or dorsal root entry zone. Segmental loss of pain and temperature with preservation of touch (sensory dissociation) is also a local sign and indicates involvement of the crossing fibers in the anterior commissure of the spinal cord from a central lesion of the cord.

Tract signs only indicate that the lesion must be cephalad to the highest point of involvement, and the motor changes may vary from increased tone and reflexes to flaccidity with absent reflexes. The difference usually relates to the rapidness of onset, since with rapid loss of spinal cord function spinal shock with flaccid, areflexic paralysis may result whereas spastic paraparesis is more common with the slow, progressive loss of motor function. The other tract signs may relate to involvement of any portion of the spinal cord and thus can consist of loss of pain and temperature (anterolateral fasciculus); loss of position and vibratory sense (dorsal column); weakness, spasticity, hyperreflexia, and Babinski signs (posterolateral fasciculus).

DIAGNOSTIC STUDIES. Roentgenograms are of diagnostic aid if they are taken of the correct area. When doubt exists or when there is a question of multiple levels, the entire spinal column should be visualized. Diagnostic findings in the roentgenograms relate to the type of tumor present. With malignant tumors areas of invasion and destruction, particularly of the vertebral body and pedicles, may give localization. With benign or slowly growing tumors widening of the interpedicular and anteroposterior diameter of the neural canal, erosion of a pedicle or of a body, and enlargement of the intervertebral foramina are diagnostic.

Definitive localization, however, is done by myelography. It is usually best to do the lumbar puncture and obtain fluid, at the time that myelography is done. Prompt surgical intervention may be required with lumbar puncture or myelography, since increase in deficit may follow removal of spinal fluid below the level of the lesion. For this reason none of these should be done unless the patient is in an area where definitive neurosurgical care is available and the patient is under the observation or care of a neurosurgeon.

Extradural Tumors

The different types of patterns of symptoms and the local and tract signs are best remembered in relation to the different types of spinal cord tumors, namely, extradural, intradural-extramedullary, and intradural-intramedullary.

Aside from a rare extradural meningioma, neurofibroma, and benign osteoma of the vertebra, extradural tumors are malignant with rapid growth and a tendency to destroy the spinal column. The symptom pattern of the extradural tumor is one of pain, both localized to the area of involvement and radiating over the dermatome level of the adjacent spinal roots (local sign). This is followed by rapidly progressive transverse loss of spinal cord function (tract sign). The local pain is frequently more severe at night and at rest, while the radicular pain relates to movement, coughing, and straining. Both types of pain may be present for weeks or months before spinal cord involvement. The progressive transverse loss of spinal cord function can be as rapid as a few hours or as slow as a few days, and effective palliation is possible only if surgical decompression is done before total loss of spinal cord function has occurred.

Since these tumors frequently involve the adjacent vertebrae, x-rays of the spine with particular attention to the integrity of the vertebral body and pedicles will often suggest the diagnosis before as well as after the onset of progressive neurologic deficit in the spinal cord. Decompression by removing the posterior neural arch or laminectomy followed by x-ray therapy gives the best palliative result in this malignant group of tumors, and laminectomy with excision of the lesion is the treatment of choice for the few benign tumors.

Intradural-Extramedullary Tumors

Approximately 65 percent of all intradural tumors are extramedullary, and 90 percent are either neurofibromas or meningiomas. Neurofibromas are slightly more common and often are multiple. They have no sex predilection and are more common in the cervical and thoracic areas, while meningiomas are more frequent in females and more common in the thoracic region. It has been stated that the frequency of occurrence of both these tumors in the thoracic areas is in the same ratio as the length of the thoracic spine to the length of the spinal column.

Angiomas are also common in the thoracic area. They are arteriovenous malformations and not true tumors but may at times present like an extramedullary tumor. This is particularly true during the last trimester of pregnancy. Other tumors that occur in the extramedullary-intradural area are epidermoids, dermoids, and lipomas. The basic pattern of symptoms of the extramedullary-intradural tumor is similar to the extradural tumors, namely, local pain and radicular pain (local sign), followed by progressive spinal cord malfunction (tract sign). The course is slower, and the development of the spinal cord deficit is often prolonged so that partial patterns of loss are seen. A common partial pattern is the modified Brown-Séquard pattern in which loss to temperature and pinprick is more marked on one side below the level of the lesion and weakness and spasticity are more marked on the opposite side (tract signs).

Intramedullary Tumors

Over 95 percent of intramedullary tumors are gliomas. In contrast to intracranial gliomas they tend to be more benign histologically and to have a more benign course. This is in part because of the low grade of their malignancy and in part because of their frequently nonlethal position in the spinal cord. Except for the preponderance of ependymomas occurring in the conus medullaris and the filum terminale, they occur equally frequently in all areas of the spinal cord. Approximately one-half of intramedullary tumors are ependymomas, and 45 percent are astrocytomas, with a few oligodendrogliomas, hemangioblastomas, and ganglioneuromas making up the remainder. Arterial venous malformations and syringomyelia may present as intramedullary spinal cord tumors but are developmental abnormalities and not neoplasms.

The basic pattern of symptoms for the intramedullary tumor is different from the extradural and extramedullary tumor in that radicular or radiating pain is rare and the complaint of local pain is uncommon. These tumors tend to grow into the central part of the spinal cord and to destroy crossing fibers and neurons of the gray matter. The destruction of crossing fibers causes segmental loss of pain and temperature sensation with preservation of touch (sensory dissociation), resulting in damage to peripheral skin areas because of lack of protection of pain and temperature sensation (local sign). Trophic changes with alteration in vasomotor control and sweating may cause symptoms that resemble Raynaud's phenomenon or erythromelalgia. Alteration in the function of descending motor pathways or ascending sensory pathways is usually late in appearance, but alteration in sexual function and bladder function may occur early (tract sign). Segmental lower motor neuron destruction is common, and the signs of such destruction, namely, weakness, atrophy, loss of reflex, and fasciculations, should always be searched for in these patients, since they have localizing value (local sign).

Summation

In summary, spinal cord tumors have a good prognosis if treated early. It is important to keep in mind that a progressive decrease in spinal cord function must always be considered to indicate a spinal cord tumor until proved otherwise. Early diagnosis, accurate localization, and surgical therapy can be expected to give a large percentage of cures with good functional result and in the remainder to give considerable and prolonged palliation of symptoms.

MALFORMATIONS OF THE NERVOUS SYSTEM

More than one-half of all congenital defects involve the central nervous system or its coverings. Some anomalies such as anencephaly are lethal; many, such as mongolism and micrencephaly, preclude development of normal intellectual function, while others, such as spina bifida occulta, cause no disturbance of neurologic function. Within the diverse group of prenatal malformations affecting the nervous system directly or indirectly there exist some which necessitate surgical treatment for several reasons: they may provide an actual or potential communication to the body surface, produce compression of neural structures, impede normal circulation of cerebrospinal fluid, restrict normal growth of the nervous system, or act as a source of bleeding or seizures. The more common malformations in this category include the overt forms of cranium and spina bifida, dermal sinus tracts, congenital forms of hydrocephalus, craniosynostosis, congenital tumors, and vascular malformations. Some anomalies such as the leaking myelomeningocele have to be dealt with within hours after birth; others, as for example, vascular malformations of the brain and spinal cord, may not become symptomatic until late in life; most, however, require attention during infancy or early childhood.

Many prenatal defects affecting the nervous system produce or are associated with external evidence of their presence, and a diagnosis often can be made on inspection. Once seen, one is unlikely to forget the enlarged head, bulging fontanel, and prominent scalp veins of the infant with hydrocephalus, the misshapen head of the child with craniosynostosis, or the midline hair-containing dimple in the lumbar or occipital region indicating a dermal sinus tract. By the simple maneuver of transillumination with a strong flashlight in a dark room it is frequently possible in young infants to diagnose abnormal cystic cavities within the cranium and to make the important clinical distinction between a meningocele containing only cerebrospinal fluid and a myelomeningocele or encephalocele which contains nervous tissue as well.

Because of frequently associated bony anomalies, typical locations of certain lesions, and ease of deformation of the growing skull and spine, plain x-rays are fruitful in the diagnosis of congenital abnormalities. Contrast x-ray studies such as ventriculography, angiography, and myelography are, however, often necessary for diagnosis of the occult lesion as well as for better definition of the extent of those that are more obvious.

It is not possible surgically to repair damaged or abnormally constituted portions of the brain or spinal cord. One can only restore the integrity of the protective coverings; relieve pressure caused by space-occupying lesions, compressing bone, or impaired cerebrospinal fluid circulation; repair or occlude abnormalities of the vessels, or destroy malfunctioning nervous tissue when it interferes with normal neurophysiologic processes. In many instances, operations for congenital defects should be carried out early in life to allow unimpeded development of the growing nervous system. Thus, the dermal sinus tract should be recognized and excised before the first attack of meningitis and the fused coronal suture opened before the onset of increased intracranial pressure. The results of such prophylactic surgical measures are often undramatic but are obviously more valuable than if done after the nervous system is compromised.

EMBRYOLOGY. Malformations of the nervous system may result from failure of initial development, from incomplete or aberrant development, or from destruction of already formed tissues by intrauterine infection or infarction. Teratologic studies in animals have revealed that dissimilar insults to the embryo, if delivered at the same stage of development, may produce the same malformation, making it extremely difficult to classify most central nervous system malformations on the basis of etiology.

A better understanding of a number of surgically important prenatal defects can be obtained from a knowledge of the basic details of embryology of the nervous system. The neurons and supporting glia of the brain, spinal cord, and peripheral ganglia are derivatives of the ectoderm. The nervous system begins as a proliferation of ectodermal cells in the craniocaudal axis of the embryo dorsal to the notochord. Growth proceeds in the neural plate so that a longitudinally oriented groove, flanked on either side by a crest, is formed on its dorsal aspect. This process of invagination continues until the dorsal lips of the groove meet and fuse to form a hollow tube extending the length of the embryo. Normally the neural tube which represents the primitive brain and spinal cord completely separates from the cutaneous ectoderm which comes to overlie it, from the underlying notochord around which the vertebral bodies are formed, and from the entodermal structures beneath the notochord. The spinal and peripheral ganglia are formed from cells of the neural crest. Local concentrations of mesoderm give rise to the vascular structures of the nervous system and to its coverings, both meningeal and bony.

Closure of the dorsad situated neural groove and separation of the neural elements from the cutaneous ectoderm commences in its midportion and progresses craniad and caudad. This process occurs during the third and fourth weeks of gestation and if not completed, either because of an insult to the embryo during this period or because of a genetic abnormality, results in a group of malformations characterized by a local defect in any of or all the coverings of the central nervous system. Such defects can occur anywhere in the dorsal midline along the neuroaxis but are most common at its extremes, namely, the lumbosacral and occipital regions.

Spina Bifida and Cranium Bifida

The common denominator in these lesions is a midline bony defect; hence the general terms *spina bifida* (cleft spine) and *cranium bifida* are useful. The spectrum encountered ranges from (1) spina bifida occulta, or incomplete fusion of the two halves of the neural arch of one or two lumbar or sacral vertebrae with intact skin and meninges, present in about 20 percent of the population,

through (2) the meningoceles, in which there is protrusion of the meninges through a defect in the skull or spine to form a sac filled with cerebrospinal fluid, and (3) the myelomeningoceles and their cranial counterparts, the encephaloceles, in which nervous tissue, usually malformed, is present within the sac, to (4) the unclosed neural plate bare of coverings. Closure defects of the spine far outnumber those of the cranium, and myelomeningoceles are many times more common than spinal meningoceles. Rarely herniation of the meninges and sometimes nervous tissue as well occur through ventral bony defects to present in the nasal cavity, thorax, abdomen, or pelvis.

SPINA BIFIDA OCCULTA

Spina bifida occulta most commonly is hidden (occulta) or unable to be diagnosed from examination of the surface over the spine. It is most commonly picked up in adults from an x-ray examination. These lesser degrees of spinal closure defects, however, often have associated cutaneous stigmata, e.g., midline skin angioma, or pigmentation, or tufts of hair. The presence of these superficial lesions should alert one to the possibility of a closure defect of the spine beneath them. Although the closure defect of spina bifida occulta is usually asymptomatic, its presence in a child suspected of neurologic dysfunction or with enuresis should lead one to suspect an underlying lesion of the neural tube. Not uncommonly, in these circumstances, one may find a hamartoma, frequently lipomatous, or a "tethered" filum terminale. Both these lesions may lend themselves to surgical correction with gratifying results. Every child with enuresis in whom the diagnosis of neurogenic bladder is suspected should have careful neurologic examination, plain films of the spine, and positive contrast myelography when indicated. Many of these children have subtle neurologic deficits that can be elicited only by thorough and repeated examinations.

Diastematomyelia (separation of the cord) is often associated with similar midline skin stigmata. In this anomaly, the cord is divided into two halves, each of which undergoes normal maturation. The two parallel spinal cords are often separated from one another by a bony projection or fibrous band arising from the dorsal surface of the body of the vertebra dividing the intradural space into two separate compartments. Because of the high incidence of vertebral abnormality, diagnosis often can be made from the spinal column x-rays. These children usually present with sphincter dysfunction, difficulty in walking, and/or deformities of the feet. When the diagnosis is made in infancy, removal of the bony or fibrous spur is indicated, since with growth there is often traction on the spinal cord and insidious loss of bladder and bowel function may go unsuspected. In the older child, removal is indicated when progressive neurologic deficit ensues.

Dermal Sinus Tracts

This closure defect apparently results from incomplete separation of the neural ectoderm from either the cutaneous ectoderm or the entoderm. These epithelial-lined tracts may provide a direct communication between the skin surface and the subarachnoid space. The opening at the skin, which consists of a small midline pore located in the lumbar or occipital region, is usually inconspicuous and may be completely hidden by surrounding hair. In the occipital region the tract penetrates the skull through a small midline opening that may or may not be apparent on x-rays and is directed caudad toward the posterior fossa. In the lumbar region, the tract may begin as low as the gluteal cleft but always extends in a cephalic direction toward the conus medullaris. In either location the tract may extend for varying distances. It may end at or above the dura, or it may continue through the subarachnoid space to end in the pia or even penetrate nervous tissue. The tract may expand at any point along its course into a dermoid cyst. This lesion therefore not only may be responsible for meningitis but also may cause dysfunction by compression of nervous tissue. In any case of meningitis due to *Escherichia coli,* caused by a mixture of skin organisms, or in infants with recurrent meningitis, a sinus tract should be sought. This includes shaving the occiput and taking x-rays of the skull and spine. It is advised that all sinus tracts be excised before the infant is six weeks of age. This is best done by a neurosurgeon, since, on occasion, laminectomy and intradural exploration are indicated.

Neurenteric cysts are extremely rare lesions that present as a spinal cord tumor. They represent incomplete separation of the neural tube and the underlying entoderm. They usually occur in the upper thoracic region and may be suspected if x-rays reveal vertebral anomalies. The lesion consists of a cyst or solid tumor adherent to the anterior surface of the spinal cord and is lined with, or composed of, entodermal derivatives. A stalk may traverse the opening in the vertebra and connect with a similar mass in the thorax.

MENINGOCELES

Meningoceles are often completely covered by skin at birth, and the communication with the subarachnoid space at the neck of the sac is frequently quite small. Treatment consists of excision of the sac and closure of the dura, fascia, and skin. Surgical intervention should be considered urgent if the sac is extremely thin, is ulcerated, or is leaking cerebrospinal fluid. Patients with meningoceles alone do not have neurologic dysfunction and do not usually develop hydrocephalus. They are at risk for the later development of neurological dysfunction as a result of other anomalies, e.g., tethered filum terminale are often found in association with an initially asymptomatic meningocele.

ENCEPHALOCELES

The majority of encephaloceles occur in the occipital region and are often associated with malformation of the occipital lobes or cerebellum, and either portion of the brain may be present within the sac. These lesions can be huge, often approaching the size of the baby's head. However, size of the encephalocele is not correlated with the degree of neural dysgenesis. Arteriography is of value in

differentiating meningocele from encephalocele and in determining the position of the venous sinuses in preparation for surgical repair. Ideal treatment consists of replacing the herniated brain within the cranium, removing the sac, and effecting a tight closure of dura and skin. Unfortunately, amputation of the herniated nervous tissue often must be carried out, because it is grossly malformed or infarcted or because the cranium is too small to allow its return. Hydrocephalus occurs commonly in infants with encephalocele, including those patients with only a meningocele. It most commonly results from adhesions in the posterior fossa but may include all the causes of hydrocephalus. The hydrocephalus may not become apparent until some weeks following surgical repair. The prognosis in many of these children is quite good, although there is an increased incidence of learning disability and mental retardation. The presence of neural tissue in the sac is associated with a poor prognosis, and the greater the amount of tissue, the poorer the prognosis.

MYELOMENINGOCELES

Myelomeningoceles are the most common of the closure defects. The incidence in United States is about 2.5 per 1,000 live births. All these children have neurologic deficit, the vast majority have hydrocephalus, and many have associated congenital anomalies of other systems, mainly skeletal and urinary. Most myelomeningoceles occur in the lumbosacral region. The bony defect, best seen on x-ray, usually extends over three or more segments, and the spinal canal is often widened. Although the sac is occasionally covered by skin, its dorsum is usually formed of arachnoid. The dysplastic cord can often be seen through this membrane attached to its undersurface. Frequently an unclosed neural plate with both posterior and anterior roots emerging from its ventral surface lies at, or just below, the surface at the cephalic end of the sac. The central canal of the spinal cord may be dilated and may open directly into the sac. If spinal cord is present below the lesion, it too is usually grossly malformed. Duplication of the cord (diplomyelia) extending for various distances proximally is commonly seen with large lesions. The dorsal nerve roots and peripheral nerves are well formed but may not be in continuity with the affected portions of the spinal cord.

Neurologic deficit attributable to the spinal cord lesion is both motor and sensory; its degree depends upon the site and severity of the malformation as well as secondary factors such as infection and infarction of the exposed cord. Most patients have a flaccid paraparesis, the sensory level usually being somewhat lower than the motor level. Virtually all patients have urinary incontinence. Occasionally because of partial lesions of the spinal cord, there is a mixed upper and lower motor neuron deficit in the lower extremities.

Malformations of the nervous system in patients with myelomeningocele are not confined to the spinal cord but are frequently present in the hindbrain, midbrain, and forebrain. The almost constant presence of the Chiari II malformation and frequent occurrence of aqueductal malformation lead to the almost uniform presence of hydrocephalus. The Chiari II malformation consists of an elongation of the medulla and cerebellar tonsils and vermis with displacement of these structures including the fourth ventricle through the foramen magnum into the upper cervical spine canal. Careful pathologic studies have demonstrated that these patients also often have malformations of the cerebrum including an enlarged massa intermedia, heterotropias, and agenesis of the corpus callosum.

In addition to spina bifida, other anomalies of the spine, such as hemivertebrae, are often present. Other structural abnormalities due to muscular hypotonicity and imbalance, including scoliosis, kyphosis, dislocation of the hips, and clubfoot, are common. Disorders of the urinary tract are mainly secondary to neurogenic vesicular dysfunction. No definite correlation has been made between these lesions and intellectual performance, although many of these children have visuomotor perceptual difficulties. There is also an increased incidence of mental retardation within the group as a whole.

TREATMENT. Treatment of patients with myelomeningoceles can be divided into acute and chronic phases. The immediate problems relate to the myelomeningocele and altered cerebrospinal fluid circulation. Long-term problems are the continuing treatment of hydrocephalus, the musculoskeletal abnormalities, and problems associated with bladder dysfunction, including hydronephrosis and infection. Whenever possible an excision of the membranous sac, replacement of the herniated spinal cord within the spinal canal, and closure of the dura, fascia, and skin should be carried out. There is now good evidence to suggest that this operation should be done within the first few hours of life. At this time the sac is smaller and the skin more pliable; there are fewer adhesions between the nervous tissue and the sac; and the risk of infection is lower, because the skin flora have not yet become established. The major advantage in early closure is that neurologic deficit can be reduced to a minimum by surgical intervention before the spinal cord is exposed to infection.

Although the head circumference measurement at birth may be normal, the ventricular system is usually enlarged, and overt evidence of hydrocephalus frequently occurs within the first few weeks of life. Occasionally the hydrocephalus is arrested spontaneously, but all patients should be closely followed by serial head measurements and cerebrospinal fluid shunting procedures carried out if there is progressive ventricular enlargement.

X-rays of the skull, entire spine, and hips, intravenous pyelogram, urinalysis and urine cultures, as well as urologic and orthopedic consultations should be obtained as a base line before discharge and repeated as necessary during follow-up. Long-term care involves multiple disciplines, including neurosurgery, orthopedic surgery, urology, and physical therapy.

Infantile Hydrocephalus

The central canal in that portion of the neural tube which becomes the spinal cord progressively decreases in size and in the adult is seldom patent, its position usually marked only by a collection of ependymal cells. The central canal at the cephalic end of the neural tube, however, ultimately forms the interconnecting ventricular system. Although a small amount of cerebrospinal fluid, considered to be identical with the extracellular fluid of the brain, is formed outside the ventricles as well as within them, there is apparently a net production of fluid secreted by the choroid plexuses. This excess fluid must exit through the openings in the fourth ventricle and through the foramina of Luschka and Magendie, and pass into the subarachnoid cisterns surrounding the brainstem which communicate through the tentorial notch with the subarachnoid space over the cerebral hemispheres. The fluid is finally absorbed by passing into the lumen of the venous sinuses via the arachnoid villi. Major obstruction to this flow at any point in the pathway results in progressive enlargement of the ventricles proximal to the obstruction. With the possible exception of one rare tumor (papilloma of the choroid plexus), in which the production of cerebrospinal fluid may exceed the resorptive capacity of the system, all hydrocephalus can be considered as an obstructive phenomenon, having, however, a diversity of causes including congenital or acquired, neoplastic, and inflammatory.

Confusion frequently exists in regard to the term "communicating hydrocephalus." This means only that there is communication between the lateral ventricles and the lumbar subarachnoid space, tested traditionally by inserting a dye in one of these two compartments and recovering it in the other. The obstruction in communicating hydrocephalus is usually in the subarachnoid cisterns in the posterior fossa or at the base of the cerebrum. Known causes are adhesions following meningitis or subarachnoid bleeding. Hydrocephalus from basal arachnoiditis is quite common in infancy and, although the cause can rarely be determined, is presumably secondary to subarachnoid bleeding from birth trauma or intrauterine or neonatal subclinical meningitis. The prognosis for normal mental development is poor in those instances where hydrocephalus is associated with anoxia, meningitis, or brain trauma, i.e., concomitant with brain injury.

There are several congenital malformations that result in hydrocephalus. Two congenital defects, the Chiari II malformation and malformations of the aqueduct, are common causes of hydrocephalus in infancy. Both are frequently associated with myelomeningocele, but aqueductal malformations are also a common cause of an isolated hydrocephalus in early life. With the Chiari malformation, passage of cerebrospinal fluid around the dislocated brainstem is impeded by the abnormal mass of tissue in the foramen magnum and by surrounding adhesions. The pathology in congenital aqueductal obstruction is more varied; obstruction usually occurs in the upper portion of the aqueduct. The commonest abnormality causing obstruction of the aqueduct in this upper portion is forking or lack of development of a single tube. Although the term "stenosis" is used, it is misleading since it implies constriction rather than the more common failure of development. A glial septum may occlude the lumen at its junction with the fourth ventricle. Progressive gliosis (scarring) of the aqueduct of unknown cause may be responsible for hydrocephalus arising at a later age; it may become symptomatic as late as the second or third decade.

Other malformations are also occasionally responsible for hydrocephalus. Failure of development of the foramina of the fourth ventricle (Dandy-Walker syndrome) results in massive cystic dilatation of the fourth ventricle. The posterior fossa is markedly enlarged, and the cerebellum is reduced to small atrophic remnants on either side of the cyst. The vermis is usually completely atrophied. Congenital cysts within the arachnoid of the posterior fossa may result in a similar picture.

Tumors are a rare but possible cause of hydrocephalus in the infant. These include intraventricular tumors such as ependymomas, medulloblastomas occurring in the fourth ventricle, and tumors adjacent to the ventricular system such as cerebellar astrocytomas, craniopharyngiomas, meningiomas, or pinealomas. Most of these tumors cause hydrocephalus by blocking the cerebrospinal fluid pathways or by compressing the aqueduct.

EVALUATION. The diagnosis of hydrocephalus is to a large extent clinical. Accurate measurement of head circumference and plotting on a chart of normal distribution of head size and palpation of the fontanel should be a routine part of the examination during the first few years of life. Any child with a head circumference outside the normal range should be evaluated by a neurosurgeon.

For years the only adequate means of visualizing the ventricular system was by air encephalography. The advent of computerized axial tomography has replaced ventriculography as the diagnostic procedure of choice in those institutions in which it is available. The advantages of this method are that it is noninvasive, does not alter cerebrospinal fluid dynamics, and may identify associated tumors and/or hematoma. The major disadvantage is that is does not give any information concerning communication between the various cerebrospinal fluid compartments. For this reason, a limited or "bubble" ventriculogram is performed. In infants this is best carried out by introducing a spinal needle into the ventricular system through the coronal suture. Preliminary bilateral subdural taps are carried out to rule out the other most common cause of an enlarged head in infancy, namely, subdural hematoma. The primary aim of the ventriculogram is to demonstrate the site and cause of the block in the cerebrospinal fluid pathways and to determine if the hydrocephalus is communicating or noncommunicating. Communication is verified by the demonstration of air passing into the subarachnoid space. Cerebrospinal fluid is also obtained for aerobic and anaerobic cultures, protein and glucose determination, and cell count. Indolent meningitis or ventriculitis may be the cause of hydrocephalus in infants even in the absence of fever or other clinical signs and symptoms.

More recently, angiography has been used for diagnosing hydrocephalus. It also appears to have value in prognosis, since the presence of normal vasculature, allowing for the distortion from the hydrocephalus, has been associated with a better prognosis than when arteriography shows absence of major arterial branches. This latter may indicate atrophy or lack of development of areas of the brain.

TREATMENT. The treatment of infantile hydrocephalus depends on etiology. There is a small but important group of patients who may be cured by a single operation. These include those in whom hydrocephalus is caused by choroid plexus papillomas, benign tumors obstructing the cerebrospinal fluid pathways, posterior fossa cysts, and occlusion of the aqueduct by thin glial septa. The remainder of the patients require procedures which shunt the cerebrospinal fluid around the obstruction within the cranium, into another body cavity, or into the bloodstream.

The procedure for shunting spinal fluid around an obstruction of the posterior third ventricle or the aqueduct is known as the Torkildsen procedure. It consists of placing a tube from the lateral ventricle to the cisterna magna or cervical subarachnoid space. Although it is an effective method of therapy in many cases of hydrocephalus, it is dependent upon patent subarachnoid spaces with normal absorptive mechanisms. In the infant, these conditions are frequently absent, and in ventricular or midbrain tumors the subarachnoid spaces may be blocked at the incisura of the tentorium. With the development of pliable, nonreactive materials, such as silastic, it has become possible to utilize shunts between the ventricles or the subarachnoid space and the pleural and peritoneal cavities for absorption of spinal fluid. These can be maintained for prolonged periods. Although reactive scarring may occur and, at times, significant effusion develops in some patients following immunization or mild viral illnesses, these shunts have an advantage over the vascular shunting in that there is no foreign body in the venous system, and they are simpler and require less frequent revision for growth in the young infant.

By far the most successful treatment of hydrocephalus has been the ventriculoatrial shunt. A catheter is placed in one lateral ventricle, and a second via the internal jugular vein into the right cardiac atrium. A one-way valve is incorporated between the two catheters so that cerebrospinal fluid at normal pressures can pass into the vascular system but blood cannot reflux. There are three major problems with the ventriculoatrial shunt: The first is the chronic presence of a foreign body within the vascular system that may act as a nidus for infection, especially if the cardiac catheter impinges on the tricuspid valve. The most common organism causing the septicemia is *Staphylococcus albus*. The infection can develop at any time after the shunt has been inserted and should be suspected if there is intermittent or persistent unexplained fever, anemia, and/or splenomegaly. If infection is proved by blood culture, removal of the shunt and antibiotic treatment are indicated. Treatment with antibiotics alone almost invariably fails. The second problem results from progressive upward displacement of the atrial catheter with growth. Once the tip of the catheter reaches the upper superior vena cava, it often becomes obstructed. Periodic chest x-rays are necessary to determine the position of the radiopaque catheter, so that elective lengthening can be done before the shunt obstructs. The third problem, common to all shunts, is obstruction of the ventricular catheter by inspissated protein, brain, or choroid plexus.

Children with hydrocephalus require close and knowledgeable follow-up, and parents should be taught to recognize signs of increased intracranial pressure. Increasing head circumference is a useful guide in evaluating hydrocephalus in the infant, but a gradual fall in psychometric level or school performance may be the only sign of progressive hydrocephalus in an older child. Although hydrocephalus presents a difficult and often frustrating problem, an increasing number of patients with hydrocephalus beginning in infancy are growing up to be useful individuals. It is apparent that many of these patients if adequately treated can develop intellectual capacity to superior levels.

Craniosynostosis

The normal stimulus for growth of the skull is provided by expansion of the growing brain. This fact is easily demonstrable in cases of micrencephaly, in which there is a head size comparable to the size of the brain, and in hemiatrophy of the cerebrum of infancy, in which the hemicranium on the affected side is smaller than on the side with the normal hemisphere. To a large extent, increase in the size of the cranial bones proceeds by incremental growth at the sutural margin. Fifty percent of the brain growth occurs in the first six months and 85 percent by the first year. The major sutures remain open until the growing brain has achieved its maximal volume in the middle of the second decade. Premature closure of a suture (craniosynostosis) therefore results in skull deformities and may also restrict the capacity of the cranium to such an extent that there is compression of the growing brain and a generalized increase in intracranial pressure.

INCIDENCE. The cause of craniosynostosis is unknown. Some cases are clearly familial, but many are sporadic. There is a sexual predilection in some types of craniosynostosis. Isolated closure of the sagittal suture occurs predominantly in males in a ratio of about 4:1, but isolated coronal synostosis is more common in females. In the majority of patients with premature closure of a single suture, no other abnormalities exist. In isolated coronal suture synostosis, an increased incidence of congenital anomalies of the brain, such as agenesis of the corpus callosum, has been reported. In the familial, multiple, or even complete synostosis, such as Apert's syndrome, there is the coexistence of the synostosis, syndactyly, and craniofacial dysostosis; in Crouzon's disease, along with the cranial synostosis, there is facial bone dysostosis with maxillary hypoplasia. In both these conditions, early operative opening of the cranial sutures and decompression of the orbit are indicated to preserve mental functions and vision. Later, cosmetic surgery for the face is often indicated.

The incidence of the different sutures involved in craniosynostosis varies. Isolated sagittal synostosis is the most common, followed in order by premature closure of the coronal sutures, closure of three or more cranial sutures, the metopic suture alone, and finally various combinations of sagittal, coronal, and lambdoid sutures. Closure of the coronal and lambdoid sutures may be unilateral or bilateral.

CLINICAL MANIFESTATIONS. The resulting shape of the head depends on the suture involved and at what age it closes. Deficiency in skull growth with synostosis occurs in a direction perpendicular to the involved suture. Premature closure of the sagittal suture results in a long, narrow head and that of the coronal in a wide, short skull. Total synostosis produces a high vertex with an abnormally small circumference. This entity must be distinguished from micrencephaly, in which the sutures are fused early because there is little or no brain growth. Unilateral synostosis of the coronal suture produces a flat forehead on the involved side. The metopic suture, normally closed at birth, may be involved, giving a characteristic prow-shaped deformity of the forehead, indicating craniosynostosis in utero. Most of these deformities are obvious within a few weeks following birth. Any child with an abnormally shaped head after the effects of molding have subsided should have skull x-rays. Even though accurate diagnosis by x-ray is difficult, it is important to have a base-line determination of the sutures involved. The diagnosis is usually apparent from head shape alone and verified by palpation of a ridge along the involved suture.

TREATMENT. Treatment of craniosynostosis consists of creating an artificial suture at the site of, or parallel to, the natural suture by cutting out a strip of skull. To retard fusion, the periosteum is widely removed from the exposed bone, and strips of plastic, e.g., polyethylene film, are fastened to the margins of the craniectomy. There is little evidence to suggest that brain growth is compromised in metopic, sagittal, and lambdoid or unilateral coronal synostosis. The very significant deformity and negligible operative risk nevertheless justify surgical intervention for cosmetic reasons alone in these types of synostosis. In these conditions, early surgical intervention is indicated to achieve a good cosmetic result.

Surgical treatment for total synostosis and bilateral coronal synostosis must be carried out early to prevent brain damage and visual dysfunction. In these conditions, reoperation at periodic intervals into the early teens may be necessary to keep the artificial sutures patent. In operations of this type, both cosmetic and therapeutic results are better the earlier the operations are done. The optimal time for surgical repair of total and bicoronal synostosis is in the neonatal period. Cosmetic results of any synostectomy are better before four months of age, since the growing brain molds the skull. There is little likelihood that significant change in appearance can be achieved after one year of age. Surgical treatment after the age of eighteen to twenty-four months should be restricted to those patients with symptomatic varieties of synostosis.

VASCULAR DISEASES OF THE NERVOUS SYSTEM

ETIOLOGY. Vascular disease constitutes a set of major causes of neurologic morbidity and mortality spanning several pathologic categories. Congenital lesions are represented by saccular aneurysms which appear and enlarge consequent to defective muscular and elastic layers at vessel bifurcations, and by arteriovenous malformations that result from failure of formation of a capillary bed between segments of the arterial and venous circulations. Infectious and inflammatory conditions of the vessels of the central nervous system occur. These include arteritis and phlebitis accompanying chronic meningitis, thrombophlebitis or dural venous sinus thrombosis accompanying subdural and epidural infections, mycotic aneurysms secondary to septic emboli, and the less specific arteritis as exemplified by temporal arteritis. The degenerative or metabolic disease complex subsumed by the term "atherosclerosis" constitutes one of the characteristic afflictions of the twentieth-century man. Brain ischemia or infarction due to thrombosis of involved vessels or their occlusion by emboli from vessels more proximal with diseased endothelium constitutes a frequent form of this disease. A less frequent but even more catastrophic form of the disease is the intracerebral hemorrhage that can occur with the same basic set of conditions upon which has been superimposed an elevation in blood pressure.

ANATOMY. The major arterial supply to the brain consists of paired internal carotid and vertebral arteries. The internal carotid arteries begin in the neck at the division of the common carotid artery into the external and internal carotid arteries. The internal carotid arteries can be divided into cervical, petrous, cavernous, and intradural portions. The cervical portion has no branches, but the remaining portions have branches that can be significant in collateral blood supply to the brain following obstruction in the internal or common carotid artery. Branches of the petrous portion that anastomose with the internal maxillary artery are the caroticotympanic and pterygoid canal arteries. These are relatively small branches and rarely have significant anastomotic capacity. In the cavernous portion are branches to the cavernous sinus, the hypophysis, semilunar ganglion, meninges, and orbit. The semilunar and meningeal arteries can have significant anastomosis with the meningeal branches of the internal maxillary artery, and the ophthalmic artery is commonly a significant anastomotic channel with the terminal branches of the external maxillary artery. The cavernous sinus branches may be a source of communication between the carotid artery and the cavernous sinus, a carotid cavernous fistula, when they are ruptured by trauma or disease. The intradural branches of the internal carotid artery are the anterior cerebral, the middle cerebral, the posterior communicating, and the choroid arteries. The posterior communicating artery forms an anastomosis with the posterior cerebral artery, and the anterior cerebral artery with the anterior communicating and the opposite anterior cerebral artery to complete the anterior portion of the circle of Willis. The vertebral arteries in their cervical or extradural portion have anastomotic branches with the thyrocervical trunk of the subclavian artery and with the posterior branches of the external carotid. After traversing the dura, they join to form the basilar artery giving branches to the brainstem. The division of the basilar artery into the posterior cerebral arteries completes the posterior portion of the circle of Willis.

There are, therefore, extensive anastomoses between the vertebral basilar system and the carotid system. The collateral circulation can be divided into the extracranial, extracranial-intracranial, and intracranial. The extracranial anastomoses have been described in the paragraph above but, in general, consist of posterior branches of the external carotid and the vertebral and the thyrocervical trunk of the subclavian, the internal maxillary branch of the carotid through the meningeal branches of the internal carotid, and between terminal branches of both external carotid arteries. Most of these anastomoses are normally small but have the capacity to enlarge following proximal or distal occlusion of a carotid or vertebral artery. For example, after obstruction of the cervical common carotid artery below the bifurcation, anastomosis through the external carotid arteries can result in retrograde flow in the ipsilateral external carotid artery to its origin and consequent forward flow in the external carotid artery to the brain, bypassing the obstruction. Extracranial-intracranial collaterals are principally by anastomosis of the external carotid artery to the intracranial circulation by the ophthalmic artery and by collaterals developed between meningeal vessels and the intracranial arteries of the pia on the convexity of the cerebral hemispheres. The major intracranial anastomosis is the circle of Willis described above. In only 18 percent of brains is the circle of Willis fully developed, there being various degrees of hypoplasia in one or more vessels in the majority of cases. Extensive end-to-end anastomoses of arterial branches of the anterior, middle, and posterior cervical arteries have been demonstrated by arteriography following occlusion of major intracerebral vessels. Although these anastomoses are, in general, not present in the normal state, they develop rapidly following vascular compromise and may be, in part, the reason for neurologic recovery following cerebrovascular accidents secondary to occlusion of a major vessel. All the anastomoses, but particularly the larger extracranial-intracranial and intracranial anastomoses, play a significant role in the protection of the brain against neurologic dysfunction in vascular disease and major occlusion.

PHYSIOLOGY. Intracranial circulation is dependent upon many factors, but the main determinants are arterial and venous pressure at the level of the brain, intracranial pressure, blood viscosity, and the state of the vascular bed and its resultant resistance. The brain is one of the most metabolically active organs in the body, requiring a constant supply of oxygen and glucose and, therefore, constant blood flow containing these substances. Intracerebral blood flow has been calculated by several techniques with variations between 44 and 80 ml/100 Gm of brain/minute, but the generally accepted value in the adult normal brain is approximately 50 to 55 ml/100 Gm of brain/minute, or approximately 750 ml of blood/minute in the adult. Thus, the brain, representing only 2 percent of the body weight, ordinarily receives between 17 to 18 percent of the heart's output and consumes nearly 20 percent of the oxygen supply of the body. Gray matter blood flow has been measured at 80 ml/100 Gm of brain/minute, while that of the white matter is 20 ml/100 Gm of brain/minute or roughly one-fourth of the gray matter, indicating further the metabolic activity of the two areas.

There are several intrinsic factors regulating the cerebral blood flow which are unique to the cerebral vasculature, and extrinsic factors which relate to blood flow and its constituents, both of which tend to keep cerebral blood flow and availability of oxygen and glucose constant despite wide variation in systemic flow to other areas of the body. The intrinsic factors are referred to by the term *autoregulation*. In experimental animals with normal autoregulation of the cerebral vessels if the parameters of P_{CO_2}, P_{O_2}, and body temperature are kept constant, cerebral blood flow remains constant between systolic pressures of 80 to 180 mm Hg. Not all the factors affecting autoregulation are clear, but two are well substantiated and a third has been suggested by recent experimental work. Evidence of a local myogenic factor is based on the demonstration that the intrinsic smooth muscle cells of intracranial arteries and arterioles respond to change in intraluminal pressure by contracting with increasing pressure and dilating with decreasing pressure. It has also been demonstrated that intracranial arteries constrict in response to increased levels of oxygen and to decreased levels of P_{CO_2} and expand to the opposite changes in these gases. Alteration in pH cause similar changes to P_{CO_2} alteration, i.e., vasodilation with increase and vasoconstriction with decrease in level of pH. A neurogenic basis for intrinsic control of the intracerebral arteries has been proposed based on physiologic experiments demonstrating areas of the brainstem, whose stimulation or ablation affects the autoregulation of the arteries and larger arterioles of the cerebral circulation.

Loss of autoregulation is seen in toxic states, following injury, and after hypoxia or hypotension; if autoregulation is lost, hypertension or hypotension can in itself be a factor for further brain injury. Methods for determining the intactness of autoregulation are available in the experimental animal and may be estimated in the clinical situation when intracranial pressure (ICP) is being monitored. It has been demonstrated that ICP will passively follow a change in mean arterial blood pressure (MABP) in animals and humans who have lost cerebral autoregulation. Thus, one may observe simultaneously recorded ICP and MABP during physiological fluctuations, or the physician may artificially lower or raise the MABP, noting the effect on ICP. The importance of these measurements is rapidly becoming more apparent in clinical problems such as head trauma or vascular disease.

Extrinsic factors for control of cerebral circulation are intracranial pressure, and vasomotor and cardiac reflexes from special receptors in the carotid artery, the aortic arch, pulmonary arch, vena cava, and splenic artery, via brainstem nuclei to raise or lower systemic pressure toward adequate cerebral perfusion. Elevated P_{CO_2} levels or reduction in oxygen tension via these receptors tend to raise systemic blood pressure. Hypoxia or decrease in blood flow in the hindbrain by direct effect on the muscle causes slowing of the heart, peripheral constriction, and, therefore, relative increase in available circulation to the brain.

In the past, knowledge of the action of autoregulation and reflex activity have been used for diagnosis and prognosis of disease states. More accurate methods of determining their intactness and functions and pharmacologic agents now have therapeutic possibilities.

CLINICAL MANIFESTATIONS. The history of neurologic dysfunction in the patient with vascular disease is one whose course in time is characterized by an abrupt change in neurological function. There may be sudden deterioration, followed by relatively immediate or full recovery, called *transient ischemic attacks* (TIA). The term *stroke* denotes sudden loss of perfusion to a portion of the brain, which may be followed by a prolonged return to the premorbid state (reversible ischemic neurological deficit) or leave the patient with residual deficit (completed stroke). The vascular accident of intracerebral hematoma often results in progressive neurological dysfunction and a decreasing level of consciousness as the mass expands. This same abrupt onset is seen with the subarachnoid hemorrhage as sudden headache, alteration in consciousness, and changes in neurologic function occurring in a very few moments. The symptomatology resulting from vascular disease infrequently can be quite nonspecific, but more commonly the gradual loss of function in the cerebral hemisphere thought to be caused by "little strokes" is found at postmortem not to be vascular but to be a neuronal degeneration. Changes in function of the spinal cord considered to be vascular are rarely proved to be so unless the vascular compromise is secondary to mechanical factors involving the blood supply passing through the intervertebral foramen or mechanical factors in the canal, such as hypertrophic osteoarthritic spurs at the intervertebral spaces causing both vascular and nervous system tissue compression.

Occasionally the patient with a history typical of cerebrovascular disease, on more complete work-up, proves to have a tumor. Conversely, the progressive neurologic deficit which has caused a patient to be suspected of having a tumor turns out to be recurrent transient ischemic attacks, secondary to extracranial vascular disease.

Surgically significant lesions of the cranial vasculature, that is, lesions in which surgical therapy can improve the prognosis for life or can decrease morbidity, are relatively rare compared with the common occurrence of cerebrovascular accidents or strokes. However, since surgery may decrease the morbidity and mortality of cerebrovascular disease and since there is relatively little other than supportive therapy, it is important to keep in mind the possibility of surgical intervention whenever cerebrovascular disease cases are seen. Surgical lesions fall into four groups of conditions with overlapping categories, such as infarction from congenital lesions and hematomas with infarcts. The groups are:

Transient ischemic attacks
Cerebral infarctions
Cerebral and cerebellar hematomas
Congenital lesions
    Aneurysms
    Arteriovenous malformations

Cerebral Ischemia and Infarction

Cerebral ischemia is a multifaceted problem which may originate with progressive atherosclerosis and which encompasses cerebral thrombosis, embolism, altered metabolic substrates, and hypoxia. Its ultimate pathological end point, a stroke, is the third leading cause of death and disability in the United States and accounts for the disability of some 2 million persons today. The logic of surgical intervention in this disease is predicated upon the reversibility of the process and demonstration of statistically significant prophylaxis.

The sites of atherosclerosis are generally bifurcations of major vessels. In decreasing order they are the carotid bifurcation in the neck; the vertebral basilar junction; the middle cerebral (MCA), posterior cerebral (PCA), and anterior cerebral (ACA) arteries; and the major ascending vessels from the aorta. Hypertension increases the predilection for atherosclerosis at each of these sites. Embolic phenomena are generally fibrin-platelet aggregates, and most of them arise in the heart, but many originate from one of the "local" vessels mentioned above. Embolic episodes usually affect the more distant vessels of the intracranial circulation, such as MCA and PCA, while the internal carotid artery (ICA) and vertebral are more subject to thrombosis.

The diagnosis of an occluded artery based on focal neurologic deficit was accepted for a long time, though it rarely was proved to be accurate at postmortem. Since arteriography, the assignment of the site of vascular disease on the basis of neurologic dysfunction has become even more insecure. A wide range of capability for adequate perfusion of the brain is maintained by the anastomoses described above, and these can alter the resulting neurologic dysfunction following occlusion of any of the major vessels.

The syndrome of "middle cerebral artery occlusion," described as a hemiparesis most severe in the arm with cortical sensory dysfunction, a partial visual field defect, and, if the hemisphere involved is the dominant hemisphere, dysphasia, does not necessarily require occlusion of the middle cerebral artery. It may result from narrowing of proximal vessels, the common sites being in the internal carotid artery at its origin in the neck or intracranially in its cavernous portion. In contrast, an individual may have a clinically silent carotid occlusion with maintenance of normal cerebral function distal to it because of adequate perfusion of the vessels by segments of the circle of Willis. Such a patient may eventually present with a "middle cerebral artery" syndrome when his opposite internal carotid has become sufficiently narrowed by atheromas to impair the adequacy of collateral flow. Thus, the effects of ischemia may be first apparent in the most distant reaches of the circulation on the side of the originally silent carotid occlusion. Anomalies and imperfections of the circle of Willis may remove its safety factor for some and make them early victims of arteriosclerosis, for they are less likely to have been protected from the effects of the loss of individual vessels.

The premorbid recognition of cerebrovascular disease often begins with an awareness of marginal cerebral blood flow presenting as transient ischemic attacks (TIAs), defined as focal neurological signs or symptoms of less than 24 hours in duration which have a tendency to recur. In the region of carotid perfusion, they are associated with local embolic phenomenon and herald a completed stroke in one-third of patients within 5 years. Some patients progress to stroke after only one or two warning TIAs. Symptoms include hemiparesis, hemisensory disturbance, and, commonly, decrease or loss of vision in the eye of the involved side (amaurosis fugax). Vertebrobasilar TIAs less frequently progress to stroke with statistical predictability; symptoms include vertigo, dysarthria, facial paresthesia, diplopia, sometimes paresis, and drop attacks. Immediate mortality rates from intracerebral hemorrhage, embolism, and thrombosis are approximately 93 percent, 60 percent, and 37 percent respectively. For those that survive, death rates from 16 to 18 percent per annum should be expected. A portion of this group with TIAs and more major infarctions may have a focal problem amenable to surgical treatment.

Identification of this group which may be helped by surgery is difficult, but a few guidelines are apparent. The workup of patients with TIAs should begin with a physical examination, including auscultation for a focal bruit over the suspected vessel—the carotid in hemispheric lesions, the subclavian or vertebral in brainstem disease. Next, regional cerebral blood flow is ascertained either with conventional nuclear brain scans or with more accurate xenon washout techniques that quantitate cerebral blood flow in milliliters per minute per 100 Gm cerebral tissue. Numerous Doppler systems now available are also able to pinpoint stenotic extracranial vessel disease and determine flow direction. Arch and cerebral angiography, however, must be performed to delineate accurately all the vascular pathologic change. There is a 5 to 7 percent morbidity from angiography in most series. It is important, therefore, to choose those patients in whom the chance of finding a remedial lesion is high enough to warrant this risk. If a stenotic or ulcerative lesion is localized, surgery may be appropriate. Treatment involves excision of the ulcerative or stenotic plaque, with or without vascular reconstruction or bypass around the obstruction. The most ideal patient for extracranial vascular surgery has TIAs, an isolated lesion, and no neurological deficit. In Ojemann's endarterectomy series, 104 patients with TIAs had a 1/104 mortality, 2/104 had neurological morbidity, and 101/104 resumed normal function. Fifty patients with persistent neurological deficit before surgery showed a 45/50 recovery, 2/45 mortality, and 5/45 neurological morbidity. A low surgical morbidity and mortality are dependent upon preoperative blood flow studies to identify the patient with borderline cerebral ischemia. At Yale, intraoperative distal internal carotid artery pressures are obtained and correlated with EEG and evoked cortical response recordings. Temporary bypass shunts are placed when the EEG or cortical evoked responses indicate inadequate perfusion.

Extracranial focal vascular lesions are accessible to direct intervention, however, a joint study of extracranial arterial occlusion concluded that about 33 percent of patients suffered from a surgically inaccessible lesion such as intracranial ICA stenosis, MCA occlusion, or complete ICA occlusion. In 1967, Donaghy and Yasargil successfully anastomosed the superficial temporal artery to a cortical branch of the MCA in two patients with inaccessible vascular disease. Since then, this operation has been performed in hundreds of patients, with low morbidity and mortality rates but without long-enough follow-up for statistical analysis of results. Recently, not only has the STA-MCA bypass been utilized but also occipital to posterior inferior cerebellar artery anastomoses have appeared in the treatment of vertebral basilar disease. At this time, indications for bypass procedures may include low-perfusion syndromes which are accompanied by ICA occlusion, carotid siphon stenosis, and MCA stenosis or occlusion. It has also been successfully employed as an additional source of flow to cerebral regions perfused by major intracranial vessels which may require occlusion during the treatment of another primary disease such as aneurysm, carotid cavernous fistulas, or neoplasms.

The other indication for surgical therapy for patients with cerebrovascular occlusion is in those patients with completed infarcts in whom symptoms of progressive focal neurologic deficit and brainstem involvement occur. The progression most commonly occurs from 12 to 36 hours after the stroke; it consists of increase in the initial focal deficit, such as hemiparesis to hemiplegia; decreasing levels of consciousness; and signs of third nerve paresis (dilated pupil) and midbrain dysfunction. This progression occurs since occasionally a major infarct constitutes a mass because of the volume of swollen edematous and, at times, hemorrhagic brain. In such circumstances, it behaves like other cerebral tumors in producing clinical signs and symptoms of progressive focal neurologic deficit and progressive brainstem involvement. The condition may be amenable to surgical removal or internal decompression of the swollen brain by craniotomy for relief of the pressure.

Cerebral and Cerebellar Hemorrhage

Although intracranial hemorrhage may result from any structural cause of an abnormality in the blood vessels or circulating blood, the most common cause of intracranial hematoma is hypertensive arteriosclerotic vascular disease. In patients succumbing to hypertensive intracranial hemorrhage, the larger arteries show hypertrophic and degenerative changes in their media and intima; the arterioles demonstrate thickness of the vessel walls and reduction in lumen caliber secondary to hypertrophy of the intimal lining; and only minor structural changes are present in the capillaries. The pathogenesis of hypertensive hemorrhage is unclear and thought to involve many factors. The blood pressure fluctuates in hypertension and, during periods of decreased systolic pressure, ischemia of tissue supplied by these diseased vessels and/or the arteries themselves may occur. The lack of arterial support from surrounding tissue (evidenced by "état lacunaire") and weakness in the vessel wall result in hemorrhage when the increased intraluminal pressure returns to the damaged segment. Arterial spasm with distal ischemia and decreased tonus may be significant mechanisms with hemorrhage resulting at the devitalized or necrotic channel after relaxation of the spasm.

The commonest sites of hypertensive hemorrhages are in the regions of the lentiform nucleus, deep white matter or cerebellar hemispheres, pons, and midbrain. Hemorrhage into the basal ganglion can be divided into lateral and medial involvement. The latter arises medial to the putamen and destroys the hypothalamus, usually resulting in death; however, the lateral group are in the putamen, external capsule, and claustrum and often are compatible with survival. In contrast to hemorrhagic infarction in which all tissue in the area is destroyed, hemorrhage has a tendency to track along tissue planes, separating rather than destroying the nervous tissue. This phenomenon is especially true when the hematoma has its origin in white matter and may result in relatively minor permanent neurologic deficit.

CLINICAL MANIFESTATIONS. Initial symptoms of intracranial hemorrhage may be nonspecific and include headache, dizziness, paresthesias, or mild speech disturbances. These symptoms are followed by a sudden "strokelike" syndrome of paresis, severe headache, severe speech disturbances, vomiting and/or loss of consciousness. The space-occupying hemorrhage may continue to enlarge and result in herniation of brain, secondary brainstem hemorrhage, and death. In instances where hemorrhage is situated in the medial basal ganglia, hypothalamus, brainstem, and dominant hemisphere temporal parietal speech areas in patients over fifty-five years of age, surgical intervention is probably not indicated because of the severe mortality and morbidity. However, intracranial hemorrhage at other sites may be surgically evacuated, frequently with little or no neurologic residual.

Approximate localization of the surgically accessible hematomas in the cerebral hemispheres is not difficult, since the patients present with neurologic dysfunction of the area involved. Usually carotid angiography is necessary to accurately localize the lesion in order to minimize surgical trauma. Hematomas of the cerebellar hemisphere are more difficult to recognize. A history suggestive of acute cerebellar dysfunction is most helpful but frequently not obtained, since initial loss of consciousness in patients with cerebellar hemorrhage is not uncommon. Cerebellar dysfunction with altered consciousness followed by progressive lower brainstem dysfunction, but without the pupillary signs and deep unconsciousness seen with pontine hemorrhages, should raise the suspicion of cerebellar hematoma. The brainstem signs most frequently seen in these conditions are slow respiratory rate, often with Cheyne-Stokes characteristics, slow pulse, hiccups, and difficulty with swallowing secretions. Early recognition of a cerebellar hematoma before major compromise of the lower brainstem occurs is necessary if a favorable outcome is to be achieved with surgical intervention.

Congenital Lesions

The vascular diseases most amenable to surgical intervention are those due to congenital lesions, namely, the saccular, or berry, aneurysm and the arteriovenous malformation.

ANEURYSMS

Most cerebral aneurysms are silent lesions that do not cause clinical disease and are often therefore incidental findings at autopsy. However, rupture of an aneurysm initiates a distinctly morbid train of events. The natural history of patients with ruptured aneurysms is still the subject of brisk controversy, since the reported mortality during the initial hemorrhage and during subsequent therapy varies from 20 to 75 percent. It is fair to state that there is a high initial mortality and that some of the lower figures do not take into account patients who never arrived at a surgical service. Although the prognosis is directly related to the degree of neurologic deficit following subarachnoid hemorrhage, approximately 27 percent of patients will die in the first week subsequent to ruptured aneurysm, the percentage declining thereafter. A second hemorrhage has a mortality of 42 percent, the incidence having its peak between 7 and 12 days following the initial hemorrhage. The likelihood of rebleeding then decreases through the ensuing 4 weeks to drop off sharply after 6 weeks; however, 10 percent of patients will rehemorrhage after 1 year. From the onset of the rupture to the second or third month after the rupture there appears to be a mortality between 30 and 40 percent.

The majority of intracranial aneurysms arise from the larger intracranial arteries of the circle of Willis and at the origin of large vessels from the vertebrobasilar system. Intracranial arteries have a thin, poorly developed, adventitial layer, a media which is partially or completely devoid of elastic fibers, and an intima consisting of an elastic lamella and thin collagenous tissue covered by an endothelial lining. Aneurysms develop at the arterial bifurcation and are probably caused by the effect of hemodynamic factors on defects in the medial musculature and elastic layers of the artery.

The most common sites of intracranial aneurysms are the internal carotid artery (42 percent), anterior cerebral artery (43 percent), and middle cerebral arteries (20 percent), with 6 percent of aneurysms arising from the vertebrobasilar system in the posterior fossae. The majority of aneurysms are single; however, there is a 20 percent incidence of multiple aneurysms. When two aneurysms are present, they have a proclivity either for being symmetric in location or for arising from the same parent vessel.

The immediate cause of rupture of aneurysms usually cannot be determined, but the coincidence of hypertension and a congenital aneurysm appears to increase the possibility of rupture no matter what the cause of hypertension. Thus, in young patients with coarctation of the aorta with hypertension in the cerebral circulation ruptured aneurysms are common. There also seems to be a correlation between systolic hypertension and rupture of the aneurysm. Silent aneurysms are seen with approximately the same incidence in patients with or without hypertension, while rupture is more frequent in patients with hypertension.

CLINICAL MANIFESTATIONS. The syndrome of nontraumatic subarachnoid hemorrhage is one of sudden onset of headache followed by altered consciousness. Focal neurologic deficit may occur, but, in contrast to the occlusion of a major intracranial vessel, headache, meningeal signs, and altered consciousness are usually much more prominent and the focal neurologic deficit less prominent. The most common cause of this syndrome is a ruptured berry aneurysm. Other possible causes are hypertensive hemorrhage and a bleeding arteriovenous malformation.

The most benign syndrome of subarachnoid hemorrhage occurring from aneurysm is a sudden headache; maintenance of, or perhaps only transient loss of, consciousness; and the absence of any objective neurologic signs. The presence of the stiff neck and perhaps photophobia, reflecting the presence of blood in the cerebrospinal fluid, are the only signs that a major pathologic vascular syndrome has occurred. A patient with this syndrome is considered to be grade I in each of several schemas for evaluating patients with subarachnoid hemorrhage and presents an excellent opportunity for surgical intervention to alter the natural course of the disease. On the other end of the spectrum of subarachnoid hemorrhage, when a large amount of bleeding occurs in a short period of time, the basal cisterns may be filled with clotted blood, or dissection of the hematoma into the hemispheres may occur. At this time the patient is unconscious, and therapeutic manipulation or angiography has a high probability of increasing morbidity or mortality.

TREATMENT. A major factor in the mortality and morbidity of subarachnoid hemorrhage is vasospasm of the branches of the circle of Willis due to an irritating effect of the blood on the vessels. This may produce neurologic deficit without the presence of mass and has been considered by most surgeons to be a contraindication to early surgical treatment, since it is associated with a high operative mortality. The goal of the treatment is to remove the aneurysm from the force of systolic blood pressure; since recent evidence suggests that the probability of a second hemorrhage increases in a linear manner with time, the earliest possible accomplishment of this is indicated. The most favorable lesion is one in which the aneurysm has a narrow neck which can be occluded without interference of the parent vessel circulation. Not all aneurysms can be so treated; some may be coated with synthetic plastics to reinforce their walls, and others may be treated by occlusion of parent vessels, such as the common or internal carotid artery in the neck, to decrease the pulse pressure applied to an aneurysm of the internal carotid artery intracranially.

ARTERIOVENOUS MALFORMATIONS

A second major type of congenital vascular disease is arteriovenous malformation, which results from replacement of the capillary bed by clusters of abnormal vessels interposed between arterial and venous systems in a segment of the circulation. Such malformations tend to enlarge with time and may present in a variety of ways. Because the contiguous cerebral tissue may be chronically ischemic, neurologic symptoms and signs will include focal loss of neurologic function and altered excitability. For this reason focal neurologic deficits of a minor or major nature and seizures are frequently seen in these patients. Arteriovenous malformations also are causes of subarachnoid hemorrhage and intracerebral hematoma.

Subarachnoid hemorrhage due to arteriovenous malformation occurs generally at a younger age than that due to aneurysm. The majority of cases occur between twenty and forty-nine years of age without a peak incidence, whereas with aneurysm the majority occur between forty and sixty-four years of age with a peak incidence between fifty and fifty-four years.

Intracerebral hematoma resulting from "cryptic" vascular malformations is probably more common than generally appreciated and is frequently mistaken for hypertensive hemorrhage. These small arteriovenous malformations, measuring less than 3 cm maximum size, are usually clinically silent and may be more common than the classic arteriovenous anomaly. The cryptic anomaly may be destroyed by the hematoma and its pathogenesis impossible to determine. In contrast to hypertensive hemorrhage, hematoma secondary to arteriovenous anomalies tend to occur outside the basal ganglion in the cerebral hemisphere white matter and may be present in the cerebellum, spinal cord, and brainstem.

TREATMENT. Because of the possibility of increase in size of the malformation with increased shunting of blood to impair further the oxygenation of surrounding tissue, the continued problem of seizures, and the constant possibility of hemorrhage, surgical excision of the malformation is indicated whenever it is feasible. Feasibility of resection relates to size, position, and source of arterial supply. Arteriovenous malformations that are deep in the hemisphere are in general nonresectable, since according to their natural history they would have a lower morbidity than would be expected from surgical treatment. Excision of arteriovenous malformations in the tip of the occipital, frontal, or temporal lobe not only may be lifesaving in the face of hemorrhage but may control seizures and improve circulation in the involved hemisphere.

THE SURGERY OF EPILEPSY

Epilepsy is perhaps the oldest recorded neurological disorder. Its history traces a fascinating path from mysticism to accurate descriptions of cortical physiology and pathology. Although its study has provided insight into cerebral pathways and cortical functional localization, the cure or control of this disorder continues to frustrate the physician devoted to caring for seizure victims. There is controversy surrounding the incidence of convulsive disorders because of the lack of a universally accepted classification. Most studies place the incidence of epilepsy between 3.7 and 6.2 per 1,000 population. Two-thirds of patients with seizures have their initial seizure before the age of twenty. The older the patient, however, at the onset of epilepsy, the more likely a focal etiological cause will be found. In patients presenting with their first seizure after age twenty, between 10 and 25 percent will have a focal lesion (such as a tumor or arteriovenous malformation) demonstrated on a complete neurological workup.

The cornerstone of seizure control is medical therapy for those patients without obvious cerebral pathologic change. Anticonvulsant drugs will control seizures in more than half of the patients with epilepsy and achieve partial to almost complete control in another 25 percent. Surgical therapy is reserved for patients whose seizures are not well controlled with medication and whose history, description of the seizures, neurological examination, or electroencephalogram suggests a focal cerebral origin. Success of surgical treatment correlates best with accurate identification of these patients with focal seizures, precise localization of the point of origin, and careful surgical excision of the area. Accurate localization of the area and identification of any motor, sensory, or intellectual deficit that may be caused by excision of the focus require a team approach, utilizing the neurosurgeon, neurologist, electroencephalographer, neuroradiologist, and neuropsychologist, as well as the proper electrophysiological equipment and techniques.

The preliminary workup for a patient being considered for surgery includes a careful general physical and neurological examination, with evaluation of past medication and dosages and an additional medical trial if medication has not been used adequately. If the decision is to continue the presurgical workup, continuous electroencephalographic monitoring with scalp electrodes is begun, since the most accurate method of identifying the area of seizure onset is to record the electrical activity of spontaneously occurring seizures. To enhance the opportunity of recording spontaneous seizures, the anticonvulsant medication of the patient is often stopped or markedly decreased. This in itself can be dangerous because it may precipitate a series of seizures or even status epilepticus; therefore, constant observation by specially trained nursing and medical personnel is required. If the candidate's electroencephalogram is not so diffusely abnormal as to obviate further consideration, his workup continues. In search of a focal lesion, x-rays of the skull and computerized axial tomography are usually the first of the special tests. Additional neuroradiographic tests, such as pneumoencephalogram and arteriogram, are usually necessary. At the time of arteriography, with EEG surveillance, a short-acting barbiturate is injected selectively into each internal carotid artery and behavioral testing is carried out to determine speech dominance and the memory capacity of each temporal lobe (Wada test). Extensive neuropsychological testing is always indicated but is often difficult to evaluate because of the sedative effect of the anticonvulsant medication. If the scalp electrode electroencephalography and the special neuroradiological procedures have not identified an epileptic focus but suggest focality in one hemisphere or portion of a hemisphere, depth electrodes are implanted, especially in the deep medial frontal temporal regions where the majority of focal resectable lesions are located. With depth electrodes in place, the patient's condition is again monitored in a special nursing unit and medication again withdrawn if necessary to precipitate typical clinical and subclinical seizures.

A review of cerebral focal pathologic change in patients with intractable seizures was undertaken at the Montreal Neurological Institute. Among patients with intractable seizures, focal resectable lesions were found in the following distribution: temporal lobe, 60 percent; frontal lobe, 9 percent; combined frontal and temporal, 10 percent; parietal, 3 percent; central, 7 percent; occipital, 1 percent; and multilobular, 10 percent. This series does not imply that the majority of intractable seizures arise in the temporal lobe, although it has been well recognized for years that temporal lobe seizures are difficult to control medically and may respond to surgical excision of lesions. The series implies that a majority of potentially resectable lesions will lie in the temporal lobe. The Montreal Neurological Institute's most common findings were medial temporal sclerosis or the scarring secondary to injury of the medial temporal lobe, low-grade gliomas, and a few focal lesions including meningocerebral cicatrix, granulomatous disease, parasitic disease, tuberous sclerosis, vascular abnormalities, and scarring from an infarct. The follow-up of 1,145 patients surgically treated at the Montreal Neurological Institute for intractable epilepsy revealed at the end of 10 years that 36 percent remained seizure-free and 28 percent had rare attacks or reduction to less than 1 percent of their preoperative frequency. However, almost all patients required continuation of their anticonvulsive medication. Thus, 64 percent have almost complete control of their seizures while 36 percent continue to have seizures at variably reduced rates. These results certainly indicate the efficacy of surgical treatment in selected patients with intractable epilepsy. They point out, however, that despite careful evaluation, multiple areas of epileptogenic activity occur in almost one-third of the patients who appear to have a focal seizure disorder, and suggest either the failure of the evaluation techniques or generalized altered neuronal excitability in patients with intractable seizures.

Electrophysiological studies in animals have indicated that subcortical structures alter the excitability of the cortex. Much work has been done in an attempt to utilize this information clinically. As yet, such therapeutic trials are experimental and require further evaluation. The technique which appears most likely to be of value is stimulation of the cerebellum, and surgical and electronic techniques for doing this are well developed. The results are controversial, but the concepts offer the possibility that in the future some patients with diffuse or multicentric origin of seizures may be returned to a more normal existence.

INTRACRANIAL INFECTIONS

Infections of the central nervous system and its coverings have surgical significance if they produce a mass, hydrocephalus, or osteomyelitis, or are the result of a break in, or absence of, continuity of the nervous system coverings.

A mass can be caused by pus, as in abscess or empyema, by the edema of the reaction of the nervous system to infection, by the edema of venous occlusion, or by an effusion in the subdural space. Hydrocephalus may be caused by the interruption of cerebrospinal fluid flow by blockage at the villi or basal cisterns, or within the ventricular system. Osteomyelitis of the skull and spine has surgical significance because of the propensity for the

infected bone to become necrotic and sequester, forming the nidus for chronic inflammation, abscess, and progressive infection of adjacent bone and intracranial contents.

Surgical therapy of infections of the nervous system falls into one or more of the following categories: excision of infected bone, drainage or excision of abscess or empyema, decompression to relieve the effects of edema, shunting to relieve obstruction of cerebrospinal fluid circulation, and the repair or establishment of anatomic barriers to infection. This last category may involve surgical procedures as diverse as repair of a congenital heart lesion, eradication of a chronic middle ear infection, or removal of a pituitary tumor that has eroded into the sphenoid sinus.

Osteomyelitis of the Skull

Infections of the skull are relatively rare. The pathogenesis of osteomyelitis of the skull includes three major avenues of origin: (1) direct extension of preexisting infection in a paranasal sinus, middle ear, or mastoid air cells; (2) infection from a wound of the scalp that extends into or below the subgaleal space; and (3) hematogenous spread from elsewhere in the body. Any organism can be the causative agent, but by far the most common are *S. aureus* and the gram-negative contaminants of ear infection, such as *Bacillus proteus* and *B. pyocyaneus*. Once the infection is established, it usually spreads through the diploic spaces and the epidural space. Although spread under the outer periosteal layer or pericranium does occur, the pericranium is so firmly attached to the skull that it limits this as an important avenue of spread. This same attachment of the pericranium sometimes gives a false impression of the extent of the skull infection. Part of the mechanism of spread of the infection includes damage to the blood supply of the skull, and therefore necrosis and sequestration of the bone is common.

CLINICAL MANIFESTATIONS. The signs and symptoms of pyogenic infection of the skull are those of generalized infection, that is, fever, malaise, and leukocytosis, with focal tenderness and swelling. At times the infection can be indolent and manifest itself first by drainage through an area of the scalp, but more often it is highly virulent with spread into the intracranial structures, resulting in irritation and inflammation of the brain.

TREATMENT. The only effective treatment is excision of the involved bone and drainage of the area. Care must be taken to be certain that no infection remains in the epidural space to strip away the dura or in the diploic spaces to further necrose and infect adjacent bone. Appropriate antibiotics are helpful in protecting the bone edges and epidural space from further spread of the infection but are of little help without surgical excision of infected necrotic bone.

Epidural Abscess

Intracranial epidural abscesses are most commonly seen adjacent to infections of the skull and therefore are common near the middle ear, mastoid air cells, and nasal sinuses. Although the dura is a good protective barrier against inward spread of infection and although many epidural abscesses are discovered as incidental findings of surgical treatment for mastoid and sinus infection, they should not be considered benign processes. The infection can and often does break through the dural barrier, meningitis being the most common result and brain abscess the next most common. As already mentioned, the epidural space is an avenue for progression of osteomyelitis of the skull.

CLINICAL MANIFESTATIONS. The symptoms of epidural abscess are quite similar to skull infections, except that seizures and focal neurologic deficits are more common. These are commonly secondary to thrombophlebitis of superficial cortical veins.

TREATMENT. Treatment of epidural abscess is trephination, drainage, excision of infected bone, and the use of appropriate antibiotics. The excision of any infected bone and the drainage of any infected sinus or mastoid air cells are mandatory if the infection is not to recur.

Subdural Empyema

Although intracranial spread of paranasal sinus, ear, and mastoid infections to the epidural and subarachnoid spaces is more common, the high rate of morbidity and mortality seen with delayed or inadequate treatment with spread to the subdural space requires that this possibility always be kept in mind. Infections of the paranasal sinuses are the most common source of subdural empyema, and the spread of the infection to the subdural space is felt to include direct extension along emissary veins and via dural sinuses.

CLINICAL MANIFESTATIONS. The symptom complex of subdural empyema is related to five factors: First is the pathogenicity of the organism. Although staphylococci, *B. proteus,* and *B. pyocyaneus* are common chronic infecting agents of the sinus, ear, and mastoid areas and may cause subdural empyema, the infection is more often caused by staphylococci or streptococci that are acutely superimposed on a chronic infection. With these highly pathogenic organisms the course of subdural empyema may proceed to serious neurologic deficit in hours and to death within days. Second, there is no natural barrier to spread of the infection within the subdural space. Because of this the surface of an entire hemisphere may be involved within a very short period of time, and progression beneath the falx to the opposite hemisphere may occur as soon as significant pus has accumulated. Third, the veins traversing the subdural space from cortex to the dural sinuses are particularly vulnerable to inflammatory response from the infection, with progressive thrombosis of the cortical veins and dural sinuses resulting. Fourth, the reaction in the subarachnoid space and surface of the hemisphere through the thin piarachnoid causes a sterile meningitis and an acute encephalitis. Finally, there is the mass effect, mainly secondary to the inflammatory reaction and the occlusion in venous drainage but also in part secondary to the volume of pus.

The first factors relate to rapidity of onset and the in-

volvement of the entire hemisphere within a short period of time, while the last three explain in part the high incidence of seizures, signs of meningitis, neurologic deficit, and massive edema. Thus the symptom pattern of a patient with subdural empyema may vary but is best characterized as follows: A patient with a history of chronic sinusitis or chronic ear infection has an acute upper respiratory tract infection. Two or three days later when he should be making an uneventful recovery, he has a sudden secondary rise in temperature, shaking chills, and a convulsion. On regaining consciousness he complains of severe lateralized headache and of mild weakness or numbness on the opposite side of the body. Within a short period of time, a few moments to a few hours, he has another convulsion and then progressive decrease in his sensorium. At this point he is frequently either brought to a hospital or seen by a physician. Initial examination reveals an acutely ill patient with signs of meningitis. Lumbar puncture shows increased cellular response, but the spinal fluid sugar is within normal limits, and the microscopic smears fail to reveal any evidence of bacteria.

Within a few hours the patient can be in severe difficulty, often with total loss of function in the involved hemisphere, evidence of herniation of the temporal lobe with a dilated pupil on the side involved, and the beginning of decerebration.

TREATMENT. Treatment varies with the severity of the symptoms at the time that the patient is seen and the rapidity with which they have progressed. However, early trephination and drainage alone would be a satisfactory treatment only if the patient shows no signs of increased intracranial pressure, major alteration of conscious level, or shift of the midline structures. If the patient already shows any of these signs, drainage of the subdural space, external decompression by removal of a major portion of the skull on the side involved, and opening of the dura to allow expansion of the hemisphere are mandatory if the patient is to survive with good neurologic function. Although this appears to be a rather heroic treatment, the fact that the major deficit is secondary to inflammation and venous occlusion allows a degree of recovery to occur that is most gratifying, provided the treatment is started before the upper brainstem becomes irreversibly damaged.

Brain Abscess

Intracerebral pyogenic infection can be categorized as acute, subacute, or chronic. The symptoms and signs of suppuration within the brain encompass a range that extends from rapidly progressive focal neurologic deficit with a systemic response indicative of severe infection to evidence of an expanding intracranial mass with no suggestion of infection. In the former, the symptoms usually relate to a focal pyogenic encephalitis with little or no frank pus that will either resolve into an abscess or cause death if it continues to spread unchecked, while in the latter the abscess has a well-formed capsule of fibrous tissue and glial reaction.

The brain is resistant to infection by bacteria. Experimentally it is difficult to produce an abscess or focal en-

Fig. 42-4. Roentgenograms of brain abscess. A middle-aged man with a neurologic syndrome compatible with an expanding parenchymal mass in the dominant hemisphere. Diagnosis of brain abscess was established by carotid arteriography and ventriculography. The abscess cavity was tapped, producing 30 ml of pus. One milliliter of microbarium sulfate and several milliliters of air were injected into the cavity to mark the lesion before these x-rays were taken.

cephalitis within the brain unless the area in which bacteria are placed is damaged beforehand, as by trauma, hemorrhage, or anoxia. Although the brain initially responds to infection in the same fashion as any tissue, its ability to wall off the infection by granulation and glial tissue is so effective that it often isolates the infection not only from the brain but even from significant contact with the systemic blood supply. For this reason the contents of a localized brain abscess usually cannot be sterilized by systemic antibiotics.

The pathogenesis of brain abscess includes, in the order of frequency of occurrence, three main routes of entry of the infecting organism: by direct extension from middle ear, mastoid, and paranasal sinus infections; through the blood supply to the central nervous system; and by direct traumatic penetration. Posttraumatic brain abscess is now rare, since adequate surgical care of the wound and antibiotic protection are excellent preventives. The ear is three or four times more common as a source of the infection for brain abscess than are the sinuses, and the temporal lobe and cerebellar hemispheres are the more common sites for abscesses secondary to these infections. Hematogenous abscesses can occur following any bacteremia but are more commonly seen with lung abscess, infected bronchiectasis, and cyanotic heart disease. In the patient with cyanotic heart disease the presence of a right-to-left heart

shunt with the loss of the lung as a filter to remove blood-borne bacteria is felt to be the mechanism responsible for the high frequency of occurrence of brain abscess. The organisms commonly seen in brain abscess are streptococci, pneumococci, and staphylococci. The most common streptococci are the anaerobic strains.

CLINICAL MANIFESTATIONS. The symptom complex of brain abscess will vary according to whether the infection is acute, subacute, or chronic. As was noted earlier, in the chronic walled-off brain abscess there may be no signs of systemic reaction to infection, that is, no fever or leukocytosis. Brain abscess should be considered as a possible diagnosis in any patient with progressive focal neurologic deficit and increasing mass with a short, that is a 2- to 3-week, history. Often with questioning a source of possible brain abscess or an episode suggestive of bacteremia can be found in the recent past. Acute pyogenic encephalitis has a course quite similar to a subdural abscess, from which it is often difficult to differentiate.

The subacute abscess varies between these two extremes, so that the combination of signs of inflammation, progressive focal neurologic deficit, and increasing mass effect not only suggests the presence of a brain abscess but also frequently from the neurologic signs localizes it. Further studies that help in localizing the brain abscess are skull films (Fig. 42-4), which may show shift of the pineal; electroencephalogram, which characteristically has a very high incidence of marked slow-wave activity over the area of abscess; brain scan; and computerized axial tomography. The fibrous tissue and breakdown of the blood-brain barrier around an abscess cause a high uptake of the radioactive material with good localization in the brain scan, but CT scan has become the best method of identifying the presence of one or more brain abscesses, accurately localizing them and demonstrating the presence or absence of a capsule.

TREATMENT. Although in the past it was taught that suppurative intracranial encephalitis could not be treated surgically, decompression, removal of portions of the infected brain, and the use of antibiotics may be lifesaving and function-saving when applied to the critically ill patient in the acute stage. Usually the patient can be carried through the acute stage by the use of antibiotics and anti-inflammatory agents, such as steroids, and by careful control of fluids. Within 10 to 12 days the abscess usually is walled off and can be localized by combining the findings on neurologic examination, electroencephalography, radioactive brain scan, and arteriography. Occasionally ventriculography is necessary.

Once localization has been accomplished, drainage of the abscess by intermittent tapping through a perforator opening, by constant drainage, or by excision of the abscess will give a high percentage of cures. In hematogenous abscesses more than half will be multiple, and care must be taken to be certain that an abscess is not missed. The major dangers to the patient with abscess of the brain are (1) the early acute edematous response the brain has to pyogenic infection, (2) the continued problem of a mass lesion from both the edema and the suppuration itself, and (3) the continued possibility of rupture of the abscess into the ventricular system. This latter complication can be rapidly fatal. With the advent of antibiotics and anti-inflammatory agents such as steroids, brain abscess should have low mortality and, depending upon its location, low morbidity rates. However, failure to diagnose its presence until late in its course, failure to realize the dangers of mass effects from the abscess, the surrounding reaction of the brain, and the concurrence of cardiac disease and systemic infection have kept the mortality rate in most reported series between 35 and 45 percent.

PAIN

Pain, the symptom that most commonly brings a patient to a physician, can be simultaneously the protector and the debilitator. As a protector it calls for diagnostic inquiry, but when it no longer has protective value, it can be a disease in itself. The best treatment of pain is the removal of its cause. When this is not possible or must be delayed, drugs, and particularly opiates and their derivatives, can be used for relief. All potent analgesics, however, have addicting qualities and therefore decreasing effectiveness with continued use, so that if more than a few months of pain relief is required, drugs not only are ineffective but also can contribute to physical deterioration and mental depression. The need for prolonged effective control has been the impetus for surgeons to devise surgical means for relieving pain. Horsley's resection of the gasserian ganglion (1891), section of dorsal roots by Bennett and Abbe (1889), and Martin's incision into the anterolateral portion of the spinal cord (1911) were milestones in this quest, but further success has been limited by the same lack of information that has limited the control of pain by any method. This lack of knowledge exists not only in the spheres of anatomy and physiology but even in defining pain. Is pain a sensory modality with its own anatomic and physiologic correlates, or is it a learned response to environmental alteration which threatens the organism? Is pain an emotional reaction evoked with or without stimuli, or is it the recognition that a central nervous system pathway or area has been activated, indicating that a portion of the organism has reached or exceeded its functional limits? There is justification for the concept that pain contains some or all of these attributes.

ANATOMY AND PHYSIOLOGY. There are many theories concerning the anatomy and physiology of pain, but they usually fall within two extremes: on the one hand pain is considered a sensory modality with specific end organs, peripheral nerve fibers, and central nervous system pathways, while on the other hand pain is regarded as a learned response to patterns of nervous system activity that denotes damage or threatened damage to the body. There is evidence in support of both theories, and there are phenomena that cannot be explained by either. It has been shown that the smaller peripheral nerve fibers and their free endings must be activated to recognize a stimulus as painful, but these fibers and endings have also been shown to be activated by nonpainful stimuli, and with such activation touch, hot, and cold can be recognized. A lesion of the anterolateral spinal cord causes loss of pain and temperature sensation on the opposite side of the body, but return of pain perception in the area occurs over many months or years without evidence of regeneration. Section of several adjacent dorsal roots causes loss of all sensation, including recognition of noxious stimuli over their peripheral distribution, but often is associated with paresthesias that are described as "unbearable" pain in the anesthetic area. Although the expression of pain contains many attributes of learned processes, the person with congenitally absent pain sensation learns to protect his body only from the effects of visible damage, and the newborn infant without significant periods of learning responds to painful stimuli with effective movement and characteristic vocalization.

The diversity of these theories not only reflects the incompleteness of basic knowledge but foretells the difficulties of ablative control of pain. According to theories at the first extreme a correctly placed surgical lesion should always relieve pain, while it would follow from theories at the opposite extreme that a procedure should rarely relieve pain. Neither is the case, nor do the theories at either extreme explain the problems encountered in the surgical relief of pain.

The analogies of the physiology of pain comparing experimental findings in animals and human beings with observations in human beings can be a basis for understanding pain in patients, but the concept must include suffering and its treatment. In the patient pain causes suffering, but suffering alone can be expressed as pain. In the former the removal of the cause of the pain or a lesion to block the conduction of pain from the area will relieve the suffering, but in the latter, since pain is not caused by physical stimuli but is the expression of an emotional problem, alteration in pain perception may increase the suffering and therefore the expressed pain. Differentiating the part each plays in the clinical situation is difficult and at times impossible, but failure to recognize that both exist is probably the most common reason for failure to relieve pain by surgical means.

Studies of the anatomy and physiology of pain encompass many techniques and have engendered much controversy, but despite the lack of a solution as to what is pain, they have indicated directions for conceptualization of pain. Classically, or at least since Edinger's description of the crossed afferent pathway, the spinothalamic tract has been considered to be the pain pathway. Its anatomy consists of a primary neuron in the dorsal root ganglion with its central axon entering the spinal cord in the lateral portion of the dorsal root synapsing on cells of the dorsal root entry zone. The axons of these cells ascend three to four segments and then cross in the anterior commissure of the cord. Its cephalad course continues through the anterior and lateral funiculi of the cord into the lateral portion of the reticular formation of the medulla, through the pons just lateral to the medial lemniscus and ventral to the lateral lemniscus, continuing adjacent to the lateral side of the medial lemniscus in the midbrain, and ending in the nucleus ventralis posterolateralis of the thalamus.

The pathway was defined by staining the altered myelin of wallerian degeneration after section of the dorsal roots and after lesions in the dorsal root entry zone and anterolateral quadrant of the spinal cord. Its function was suggested from the animal experimentation of Schiff, Voroschilov, and Sherrington, and the clinical observations of Gowers, Brown-Séquard, and Spiller. These suggestions were confirmed by the operative section of the anterolateral portion of the spinal cord by Martin and Frazier. The first central ablative procedure for pain, anterolateral chordotomy, has continued to the present to be one of the most effective methods of relieving pain in the lower portions of the body.

Is the spinothalamic tract the pain pathway? As was mentioned above, activation of smaller fibers (less than 6 μ diameter) of peripheral nerve appears necessary for the appreciation of noxious stimuli, and these smaller fibers have been shown to project to central pathways composed of similar or smaller-sized fibers. The Marchi stain, used for staining degenerating myelin in the central nervous system, only stains fibers 6 μ or larger, and a pathway defined by this technique would only coincidentally define a pain pathway. Of the thousands of fibers lying in the anterior and lateral funiculi of the spinal cord only a small percentage can be traced to the posterior ventral nucleus of the thalamus in human beings, and in subprimates none can. Lesions placed in the spinothalamic tract as outlined by the Marchi degeneration at the midbrain level often cause burning dysesthesias rather than relief of pain, and lesions placed anywhere in the tract not only do not give permanent loss of pain but cause only a relative even though marked analgesia.

The Nauta-Glees method of staining degenerating axons also has been used to trace degeneration following a lesion in the anterolateral funiculi of the spinal cord. This method not only allows the smaller fibers to be followed but shows terminal degeneration, i.e., degeneration at synaptic junctions. The technique has shown that in human beings there is little evidence of synaptic transfer as the axons ascend to the cervical medullary junction. It is a lesion of this portion of the central nervous system, that is, the anterolateral quadrant of the spinal cord, that produces marked analgesia. In subprimates there is considerable loss of stainable fibers as each segment of the spinal cord is passed, and there is also degeneration signifying synapses in the gray matter of the cord. This agrees in part with the impression of Brown-Séquard that pain may travel in the central gray matter of the cord. In primates the loss of fibers is less until the medulla is reached, but even these few fibers may explain the gradual decrease in analgesia seen after chordotomy. In both primates and subprimates a major synaptic area is seen at the lower end of the brainstem in the medial portion of the reticular core with many fibers turning into, and projecting to, this area.

Comparison of the findings of the Nauta-Glees technique with the Marchi technique shows major differences. With the Nauta-Glees technique the fibers are more widely disseminated at each level of observation within the central nervous system, and major areas of synapse are seen at the cervical medullary junction, in the midpontine level at the oral pole of the nucleus gigantocellularis, and in the tegmentum. The fibers appear to be more dorsally placed at the level of the colliculus, and in the thalamus only a very few fibers go to the posterior ventral nucleus, more being seen medially approaching the centramedian and parafascicularis nuclei.

The concept that there are specific peripheral nerve fibers and central nervous system neurons responsive only to pain has recently been reexamined; evidence for peripheral receptor units uniquely responsive to noxious stimuli have been demonstrated by Perl and his coworkers, and neurons uniquely responsive to strong mechanical stimuli in the dorsal root entry zone and trigeminal system also have been identified. The fibers have been small myelinated or unmyelinated fibers, and the anatomic characteristics of the receptors are not known. Although this recent evidence further dilutes a basis for the pattern theory of pain, that an isolated receptor or fiber can be stimulated and produce pain has not been demonstrated. The demonstration of such structures uniquely responsive to noxious stimuli still does not explain some of the pain syndromes seen clinically, e.g., causalgia, postherpetic neuralgia, and thalamic pain. These all have the common finding that usually nonpainful stimuli, such as light touch, are painful and that the pain continues after the stimulus and spreads to contiguous areas. This indicates an altered excitability has occurred with a peripheral nerve lesion in the first condition, a peripheral nerve and dorsal root ganglion lesion in the second, and a central nervous system lesion in the third. Little is known concerning the control of excitability of afferent pathways and even less concerning pain. Melzack and Wall, elaborating on experimental studies in animals, suggested that activity in larger peripheral nerve fibers alters excitabilities of the cells upon which the smaller fibers synapse. This suggests an inhibitory influence of the large fibers on pain conduction. Since the peripheral nerve lesion in causalgia and herpetic neuralgia is mainly damage to large fibers, Melzack and Wall offered both pain syndromes as examples of loss of peripheral control. They further postulated that descending influences from upper centers impose control at each synaptic junction.

Anatomical and physiological studies have demonstrated significant evidence for direct and indirect descending cortical, subcortical, and brainstem control of afferent input at various levels of the neuro axis from the dorsal root entry zone to the midbrain. Although this evidence might a priori be assumed to apply to modulation of the afferent input of noxious stimuli, more specific information concerning modulation of the input from noxious stimuli has been gathered from diverse experimental approaches, a portion of which has included activation of spinal descending pathways. The evidence includes a demonstration of effective analgesia in rats from electrical stimulation in the brainstem, the presence of opiate receptors in the paraventricular and brainstem gray matter in vertebrates, and the isolation of endogenous polypeptides from the brain and pituitary gland with opiate properties. Other studies have shown that minute amounts of opiates injected into areas with opiate receptors produce analgesic effects without significant systemic levels of the opiate compound, and that opiate antagonists such as naloxone can reverse the opiate effects of brainstem stimulation in areas of opiate receptors, the opiate effect of focally injected opiates, and some of the analgesic effects of paraventricular stimulation in humans. In rats, analgesic effects from systemic opiates, from brainstem injection of opiates, and from stimulation of the brainstem have been shown to be markedly reduced below lesions sectioning the dorsolateral funiculus of the spinal cord. This information has not only altered some concepts of analgesic actions of opiates but, because of the correlation of many of the sites of opiate receptors and brainstem analgesic responses with what has been designated as a limbic system and its input, has also brought forth hypotheses for unifying some pain states and affective disorders. The combination of the demonstration of specific opiate receptors and peptide ligands that interact with these receptors to produce opiate effects has further melded the anatomy and pharmacology of pain and opened significant new avenues for its study.

Surgical Relief of Pain

Despite the paucity of knowledge concerning pain, empiric observations combined with physiologic studies have given neurosurgeons effective methods for surgically relieving pain. They fall into one of five different categories:

1. Section of the peripheral nerve pathway: neurectomy, sphlanchnicectomy, dorsal rhizotomy
2. Section of central nervous system pathways: anterior lateral chordotomy, and trigeminal tractotomy
3. Procedures to alter affective response to pain: thalamotomy, lobotomy, cingulumotomy
4. Section of the efferent arc of the vasomotor reflex: sympathectomy
5. Suppression by stimulation

Despite many variations in technique and many claims for various procedures, clinical experience has demonstrated that all the procedures for relief of pain from lesions of the nervous system fall into one of the first four categories and that each category has its area of application, its inherent rate of success, and its complications. Experience with suppression of pain by stimulation, if related to acupuncture, has accumulated for centuries. However, there is still too little objective evidence to determine the extent of its usefulness and its long-term effectiveness. Application of the correct procedure at the correct time to a suitable patient is the most difficult aspect of the surgery for pain.

SECTION OF THE PERIPHERAL PATHWAY

Section of the peripheral pathway for pain causes loss of all sensation distal to the area of section. Permanent loss occurs only when the pathway is sectioned proximal to the sensory ganglion, that is, section of the dorsal roots, termed *rhizotomy*. Any procedure that damages primary sensory neurons gives subjective sensory loss, which has as a complication painful paresthesias or spontaneous pain in the anesthetic area in 5 to 8 percent of cases. The explanation for this pain may be altered excitability of the dorsal root entry zone neurons. However, since further pain pathway interruption usually intensifies the pain, a more logical explanation appears to be that in this group of patients the subjective sensation of sensory loss signifies something wrong with the area and is painful. Any further alteration in sensation increases the pain. The psychologic basis of this may be that anything painful is abnormal, and therefore anything abnormal is painful. Stressing the lack of significance of such feelings at times helps, but alteration in affective response either by psychotherapeutic drugs or surgical intervention sometimes is the only recourse when the paresthesias become unbearable.

Section of multiple dorsal roots is seldom considered for relief of pain in a functioning limb, since loss of position sense, gamma afferents, and sense of touch leave the limb useless. It is of value in the thoracic area or where only one root is directly involved. In the former, touch and position senses are not of functional significance, and in the latter, sensory overlap of adjacent roots makes the peripheral sensory loss minimal. This sensory overlap of adjacent roots makes section of at least two and usually three roots necessary for significant deafferentation of any peripheral area.

Rhizotomy of the trigeminal nerve is used to control pain of malignant tumors of the face and trigeminal neuralgia. Trigeminal neuralgia, or tic douloureux, is a painful condition of the trigeminal nerve of unknown cause, characterized by paroxysms of pain over one or two adjacent divisions of the fifth cranial nerve. The paroxysms are often initiated by any stimulus in localized areas of the division involved, known as "trigger zones." Section of the preganglionic fibers of the trigeminal nerve or of the descending trigeminal tract in the brainstem permanently controls the pain, but as with other peripheral nerve section painful paresthesias may arise.

An observation by Jennett that patients with trigeminal neuralgia frequently have vascular compression of the trigeminal rootlets as they exit from the pons suggests altered conduction and excitability at the root entry zone of the brainstem as the cause of the syndrome of trigeminal neuralgia. Jennett also has suggested that other paroxysmal disorders of cranial nerves, such as glossopharyngeal neuralgia and facial tic, have the same cause. Compression of the trigeminal nerve more distally does not correlate with the syndrome, and decompression of the compressing vessels from the trigeminal rootlets has achieved a high percentage of relief without significant sensory loss.

Peripheral pathway section was the first procedure used for relief of pain, but because of the annoyance of the feeling of numbness, the incidence of paresthesias, nerve regeneration, and the availability of other procedures, it is now rarely used except for denervating trigger areas in the control of trigeminal pain by avulsion of either the supraorbital or infraorbital nerve.

Sphlanchnicectomy effectively denervates the upper abdominal viscera and is used for relief of intractable pain of the upper abdomen. Although the sphlanchnic nerves are part of the sympathetic nervous system, it is the interruption of the visceral afferent fibers coursing within the sympathetic nerves that gives the relief of pain. Their cells of origin are in the dorsal root ganglion, as are the cells of all peripheral sensory nerves, but since they have no surface innervation and paresthesias of denervation are always referred to the surface, painful paresthesias are not seen following their interruption. Since at times with malignant disease of the upper abdomen somatic sensory fibers in the intercostal nerves are involved, dorsal root section or chordotomy may be more effective than sphlanchnicectomy.

SECTION OF CENTRAL NERVOUS SYSTEM PATHWAYS

When Martin in 1911 made an incision in the anterolateral quadrant of a patient's spinal cord, the era of surgical control of intractable pain commenced. Anterolateral chordotomy has remained an effective means of controlling intractable pain, and many surgeons have contributed their skill and knowledge to modify Martin's original procedure so that it is a simple and reliable method for production of analgesia. Section of the tract in the spinal cord causes no subjective sensory loss and therefore rarely causes dysesthesias or paresthesias, but it has limitations. Since the fibers projecting to the anterolateral quadrant of the spinal cord ascend three to four segments before crossing in the spinal cord, incision of the quadrant gives loss of pain and temperature sensation on the opposite side of the body three or more segments below the level of the chordotomy. Thus, even a perfectly performed high cervical chordotomy fails to block pain in the upper arm, shoulder, or neck; therefore the procedure is best used for control of pain below the upper thoracic level. The loss of pain, although marked, can be demonstrated to be incomplete, and with time islands of pain perception appear, and with them the original pain usually returns. This may take a year or more to occur and limits in part the usefulness of the procedure for pain from benign conditions.

Lesions further cephalad in the spinothalamic tract, that is, at the midbrain, although causing loss of pain without subjective sensory loss, may also cause dysesthesias or the sensation of pain from nonpainful stimuli. The cause of this dysesthesia is unknown.

Section of the descending, or spinal, tract of the trigeminal nerve in the medulla causes loss of pain and temperature sensation in the ipsilateral face. It is used to control pain in the face, but since the operation has a higher morbidity and mortality than preganglionic section of the trigeminal nerve in the middle fossa, it is usually used only when it is feared a patient would not tolerate anesthesia of the face or when paralysis of the motor portion of the trigeminal on the opposite side is already present. In this latter condition the danger of bilateral paralysis of the muscles of mastication by approaching the nerve distad is higher than the morbidity of medullary tractotomy.

Stereotaxic lesions have been placed in the posterior medial thalamus in the area of the centramedian and nucleus parafascicularis, structures suggested by electrophysiologic and axonal degeneration studies as projections of the medial spinal reticular tracts. These procedures have been reported to relieve pain without any loss of pinprick or temperature sensation in the periphery, but their effectiveness is short-lived. It can be hoped, however, that with more basic information lesions for control will be devised that either interrupt major projections of the impulses defining a stimulus as noxious or increase the blockade of such impulses as they attempt to pass each controlled synaptic junction.

PROCEDURES TO ALTER AFFECTIVE RESPONSE TO PAIN

On a basis of the work in primates of Fulton and Jacobson, Egas Moniz in 1935 persuaded his neurosurgical colleague Lima to perform a prefrontal lobotomy on a psychiatric patient with marked anxiety as part of the basis for the psychiatric problem. The success of the procedure prompted many other surgeons to try prefrontal lobotomy for psychiatric illness. Altered affect, particularly in response to peripheral stimuli, and relief of anxiety was seen in the patients as it had been seen in the animals, and it seemed probable that the reaction of the patients to pain might be similarly altered. Van Wagenen in 1942 performed bilateral prefrontal lobotomies on a mentally ill patient who had phantom limb pain, and his success in altering the patient's complaint prompted other surgeons to use the same procedure in patients with intractable pain. Experience with the procedure of prefrontal lobotomy has shown that the lobotomy patient is unconcerned with the pain but when questioned still reports the pain as present. This lack of concern is no different for pain than it is for other stimuli, and therefore the procedure alters not only the response to pain but the entire affect of the patient. Lesions of the nonspecific nuclei of the thalamus, as in the dorsal median nucleus, lesions of the limbic system, such as cingulumotomy, or excisions of gyri in the prefrontal cortex all produce the same response with varying degrees of affective change.

The major limitation of these procedures is this change in personality. The same effect can be obtained with psychotherapeutic drugs, such as chlorpromazine, but with drugs it can be reversed. For this reason, the procedures for altering affective response to pain are rarely used but still should remain a part of the physician's armamentarium for care of the terminally ill patient whose fears make the situation and the pain unbearable for the patient and the family alike, and for the occasional patient where relief of anxiety will make it possible to resume a more normal life.

SECTION OF THE EFFERENT ARC OF THE VASOMOTOR REFLEX

Pain that occurs in diseases which cause alteration in blood flow of an extremity, such as Raynaud's syndrome or erythromelalgia, or conditions which cause marked vasospasm, such as causalgia following nerve injury, and the pain of obstruction of the major vessels in an extremity where circulation can be reestablished by dilatation of collateral vessels will respond to sympathectomy. Much has been written about possible sensory function in the sympathetic nervous system; however, aside from the visceral afferent fibers in the sphlanchnic nerves, no evidence of sensory function has been demonstrated. The clinical experience that sympathectomy does not relieve pain unless evidence of altered blood flow is present before sympathectomy bears this out. The occasional exception experienced by surgeons is more likely related to the placebo effect of any form of therapy rather than to alteration in peripheral afferent pathways.

Surgical treatment for pain is a useful adjunct to the care of patients and can be effective in prolonging useful life in many situations. An understanding of what it can and cannot do and an awareness of its limitations is an important aspect of its use. The striking relief afforded a patient with intractable pain of malignant pelvic tumor and the return of such a patient to normal interpersonal relationships is an experience that can demonstrate to any physician the effectiveness of chordotomy. The failure of ablative surgical procedures for pain in the patient using pain as a means of removing himself from an intolerable situation should demonstrate just as strikingly to the physician that no therapy should be applied just because a symptom is present.

SUPPRESSION OF PAIN BY STIMULATION

Counterstimulation based on theories foreign to most Western neurophysiologic concepts has been used for centuries. Unfortunately, scientific evaluation of the results is not available, and allegorical reports not recognizing placebo effects, emotional factors, and the striking immediate effect of one pain to suppress a less severe pain are the only evidence available for evaluation. More recently, electrical stimulation applied to peripheral nerves, dorsal columns of the spinal cord, and various subcortical cerebral structures have been used for a variety of intractably painful states with varying clinical results.

Although the initial rationale for using these techniques was based on physiologic concepts, the development of the techniques appears to be more empirically than theoretically based. Stimulation of peripheral nerves is done for painful dysesthesias limited to an area innervated by a single nerve. The technique is based on electrophysiologic evidence mentioned in the introduction of this section that the larger nonpainful fibers of peripheral nerves inhibit the subsequent spinal cord activity secondary to smaller fibers, the latter being essential for pain conduction. Stimulation of nonpainful myelinated fibers by implanted cuff electrodes on peripheral nerve has had limited success in alleviation of pain, and the method is limited to painful entities in a single nerve distribution. It has been more effective in the upper extremity than in the lower extremity.

Electrical stimulation of the spinal cord dorsal column by implanted electrodes has been used for more diffuse intractable pain, particularly of the lower extremities. A theoretic basis for this type of stimulation includes increasing descending inhibition in the dorsal root entry zone, and experimental evidence that such stimulation inhibits the central conduction of smaller fiber activity has been demonstrated. Using nonpainful paresthesias to determine the threshold, implanted dorsal column stimulators have had effective short-term results for relief of intractable pain in many patients.

Electrical stimulation of the thalamus, amygdaloid body, caudate nucleus, and hypothalamus, regions in which lesions have been placed for controlled affective states, has been shown to have varying beneficial effects on some painful syndromes. Although none of these techniques have been universally effective for the control of pain, with further understanding of its etiology by experimental patient and clinical investigation, perhaps newer knowledge in the treatment of pain will be forthcoming.

STRUCTURAL ABNORMALITIES OF AXIAL SKELETON

General Considerations

ANATOMY. The vertebral column with its ligaments and musculature serves two functions: the support of body weight and protection of the neuraxis. The same dual role is played by the basiocciput, which may be considered from an embryologic and functional standpoint as an extension of the spine. In health, the spine is a sturdy yet flexible weight-bearing structure. Most of its weight-bearing property is provided by the vertebral bodies and intervertebral discs. The neural arch formed by the pedicles and laminae complete a bony ring at each vertebral level defining the vertebral canal, while the articular processes and attached facets bridge the intervertebral spaces posterolaterally, providing further support and protection. The spinous and transverse processes of the neural arch serve as attachments for the spinal musculature. The ligamentum flavum and the posterior atlantooccipital ligament, both thick elastic structures, complete the bony and ligamentous tube which extends from the foramen magnum to the lowest part of the sacrum. In the normal skeleton there is ample room within the foramen magnum and the vertebral canal for the contained neural and vascular elements, and the intervertebral foramina provide unrestricted passage of the nerve roots and blood vessels.

There is a considerable discrepancy between the cross-sectional area of the vertebral canal and that of the spinal cord at all levels, the additional space being occupied by the cerebrospinal fluid-filled subarachnoid space and the fat-filled epidural space. The fluid and fat suspend and cushion the neuraxis and, because they are displaceable, provide room for lateral and anteroposterior movement of the neuraxis that must take place with normal motion of the axial skeleton. Radiologic and postmortem studies have shown that the spinal cord and nerve roots also undergo grossly perceptible axial movement when the spine is flexed or extended. The spinal cord and roots must, therefore, be free to move up and down the vertebral canal, and the stress applied to the nerve roots through the movement of the peripheral nerves must be relieved by movement within the intervertebral foramina.

PATHOPHYSIOLOGY. Structural abnormalities which markedly decrease the dimensions of the foramen magnum, the vertebral canal, or the intervertebral foramina may result in damage to the nervous system. The mechanism of injury is primarily that of direct compression of nervous tissue, although in some instances concomitant interference with blood supply may be a factor. Injury to the nervous system may be caused by acute angulation of the vertebral axis, subluxation of one part of the axial skeleton upon another, or encroachment of a mass upon the vertebral canal or intervertebral foramina. Not only the degree but the rate of compression is important. Angulation of the spine, for example, in idiopathic scoliosis may be extremely severe but rarely causes neurologic deficit because of the ability of the cord and roots to accommodate to their distorted position. In contrast, less pronounced angulation from an acute process such as collapse of vertebra in an osteoporotic spine may result in complete destruction of the spinal cord.

The causes of structural abnormalities of the spine which affect the nervous system are extremely diverse. The bones, joints, and associated muscles of the axial skeleton are subject to the same diseases as they are elsewhere in the body. They may be congenital or acquired, local or diffuse. Symptomatic abnormalities often result from a combination of these factors. As an example, the foramen magnum and the vertebral canal in achondroplasia is malformed and disproportionately small as compared with the normal size of the spinal cord. A relatively minor degree of disc protrusion or scoliosis in these patients often causes severe neurologic deficit. It is becoming increasingly apparent as careful measurement of the spinal canal becomes more prevalent that individual differences in response to structural disease in the general population can, at least in part, be accounted for by differences in the size of the vertebral canal. Those persons with congenitally small but undistorted vertebral canals are much more liable to major neurologic deficit in response to degenerative disc disease or relatively minor spine trauma.

It is not the intention of this section to discuss all the etiologic agents that may result in structural abnormalities of the spine. What will be emphasized are the often misunderstood structural lesions occurring at the craniovertebral border and the common lesions resulting from disease of the intervertebral discs.

Abnormalities of the Craniovertebral Border

Structural abnormalities involving the basiocciput and the cephalic portion of the cervical spine are uncommon as compared to those of the remainder of the axial skeleton. Their importance lies in the fact that they may produce profound neurologic dysfunction, which is not infrequently misinterpreted as the result of other causes. Craniovertebral abnormalities are usually congenital but may be acquired. Anatomically these lesions divide into two basic categories, those which affect the basiocciput and those which primarily involve the first and second cervical vertebrae. Both limit the space available for the cervicomedullary junction and can produce similar neurologic dysfunction.

PATHOLOGY. Maldevelopment of the occipital bone resulting in an abnormally small and irregularly shaped foramen magnum occurs in achondroplasia and occasionally in craniosynostosis. More common deformities of the basiocciput are those termed *platybasia* (*platys,* flat) and *basilar impression*. To accommodate the cerebellum and the brainstem, which lie in approximately the same axis as the spinal cord, the level of the floor of the posterior fossa is normally well below that of the anterior and middle fossae. In platybasia, the entire floor of the posterior fossa appears elevated. As seen in a lateral x-ray of the skull, the angle formed by the floor of the anterior fossa and the posterior border of the clivus approaches 180°, and the posterior fossa is therefore extremely shallow. In basilar impression the margins of the foramen magnum are indented as if the weight of the head had caused it to sink toward the vertebral column. This may be the case in acquired basilar impression associated with rickets and Paget's disease. In both platybasia and basilar impression the capacity of the posterior fossa is reduced, and the dimensions of the foramen magnum, especially the anteroposterior diameter, are decreased. In accommodating to the small and abnormally shaped posterior fossa, the hindbrain may be distorted with resulting pressure applied, especially to its ventral surface. Thus the lower cranial nerves and the cervicomedullary junction may be compressed directly or stretched, and hydrocephalus can result from local obstruction to cerebrospinal fluid pathways.

The most significant structural abnormality of the upper cervical spine is atlantoaxial dislocation. This can occur for a variety of reasons. As with dislocations at other levels, it may be the result of trauma, infection, or degenerative bone disease. It most commonly, however, occurs in association with maldevelopment of the atlas. The atlas may be fused to the base of the occiput, and the odontoid, which represents the body of the atlas, may be maldeveloped. Failure of fusion of the odontoid process to the body of the axis may occur without other abnormalities. In occipitalization of the atlas, the head can no longer nod at the atlantooccipital joint, and the added stress on the ligaments holding the odontoid process in place may eventually produce a dislocation. The same ventral dislocation of the atlas on the axis may occur if the odontoid process is rudimentary or ununited to the atlas. With atlantoaxial dislocation the upper cervical spinal cord may be compressed between the odontoid process and the posterior arch of the atlas. The lower medulla may become compromised as well, presumably by resulting angulation at its junction with the posteriorly displaced spinal cord.

CLINICAL MANIFESTATIONS. Structural abnormalities of the craniovertebral border frequently remain asymptomatic until adult life and then frequently are in response to relatively minor trauma. Cranial nerve signs include disassociated sensory loss over the face (descending trigeminal tract) and palatal and vocal cord weakness. Nystagmus and spastic weakness of the extremities are common, and the patient may have loss of position sense, ataxia, bladder dysfunction, and atrophy of the shoulder musculature and small muscles of the hand. Although examination may reveal a short neck and restriction of head movement, diagnosis is confirmed by x-ray studies. Myelography in questionable cases usually reveals a partial or complete obstruction of passage of the contrast agent.

TREATMENT. Immobilization of the neck is indicated for patients with minor degrees of impairment. If the dysfunction is progressive or is already severe, decompression of the craniovertebral border is indicated. The mechanisms of continued compression, however, must be demonstrated. Most frequently, the mechanism is occlusion of the outlet of the cerebrospinal fluid from the fourth ventricle, causing hydrocephalus and increased intracranial pressure. A shunt from the ventricle to the venous system, as described earlier under Infantile Hydrocephalus, will often reverse this process and allow a return toward normal neurological function. If hydrocephalus is not found, air myelography or Pantopaque myelography will demonstrate, in most cases, the direction of the compression of the cervical medullary junction and thus indicate either anterior or posterior decompression of the area. In atlantoaxial dislocation, surgical procedures should be done with the patient in skeletal traction and stabilization obtained by bony fusion.

Degenerative Disease of the Intervertebral Disc

Degenerative disease of the intervertebral disc is one of the most common, yet one of the least understood and often one of the most mistreated, disorders of the spine (see Chap. 43). Although many patients have benefited from removal of herniated portions of an intervertebral disc compressing neural tissue, too many have been crippled by ill-advised operation for symptoms mistakenly interpreted as being due to this same cause. Just as not all right lower quadrant abdominal pain is caused by appendicitis, not all neck and low back pain is caused by surgical disease of the intervertebral disc.

ANATOMY. The intervertebral disc is well suited for its task of supporting considerable weight while still allowing mobility of the spine. It is classically and practically described as consisting of two parts: a tough yet slightly flexible outer ring, the annulus fibrosis, which joins the periphery of adjacent vertebral bodies to one another, and a semisolid plastic center, the nucleus pulposus, interposed between the hyaline cartilage faces of the vertebral bodies.

The joint is further reinforced by the anterior and posterior longitudinal ligaments, which extend the length of the spine. Actually, the intervertebral disc is a composite structure in which three zones grading into one another may be recognized. The outer zone, which may be regarded as the joint capsule, is composed of lamellae of interlacing bundles of fibrous tissue that blend with the longitudinal ligaments. Beneath this fibrous capsule and intimately adherent to it lies a thick envelope of fibrocartilage that in turn surrounds and attaches to the less dense nucleus pulposus. This latter substance is composed primarily of collagenous fibrils and cartilage cells suspended in a fluid matrix. In younger persons remnants of the notochord may be found here as well. Motion between vertebral bodies is allowed by the flexibility of the outer layers, the more fluid center responding to variations in weight distribution by flowing into areas of least pressure within the confines of the annulus.

ETIOLOGY AND PATHOLOGY. Although the intervertebral disc may be damaged by infection, collagen disease, and severe trauma, it is, in comparison with other weight-bearing structures, particularly liable to early degenerative changes. Knowledge of the basic cause of this deterioration, which secondarily involves surrounding bone as well, is uncertain, but it is at least presumably in part a response to the trauma of daily normal activity. It is more prevalent in men than in women and in laborers than in sedentary workers. Degenerative changes occur most frequently in portions of the spine where there is a transition between a relatively mobile segment and a less mobile one, namely, in the lower cervical and lower lumbar region. This distribution again implicates trauma as a causative factor, since there is relatively more motion and therefore more stress at these levels.

Pathologically there is thinning of the fibrous layers of the annulus, destruction of fibrocartilage, and dehydration of the nucleus pulposus. The interspace becomes narrowed and, presumably because of loss of normal joint function, there is frequently new bone formation (osteoarthritis) at the margins of the interspace. These changes are often relatively asymptomatic, producing only transient local pain and the progressive loss of spine mobility usually taken as a matter of course with advancing age. Under certain circumstances, however, essentially the same degenerative processes may have more serious consequences. The nucleus pulposus may herniate through the weakened annulus, and/or large bony spurs may develop to project into the vertebral canal or intervertebral foramina. Of the two processes, herniation of the nucleus pulposus is a much more common cause of neurologic dysfunction and occurs at an earlier age. Approximately three-quarters of symptomatic herniations of the nucleus pulposus occur between the ages of thirty and fifty years. Neurologic disability resulting from osteoarthritis occurs predominantly in the individuals fifty years of age or older.

The effects of herniation of the nucleus pulposus depend on its location, both in respect to the transverse plane and the disc involved, its size, rate of development, and individual differences in surrounding structures. The most common type of herniation of the nucleus pulposus is not through the annulus but rather into the cancellous portion of the vertebral bodies, the so-called "Schmorl's nodules." Such herniation produces no neurologic deficit but by impairing joint function often results in reactive bone formation at the disc margins. Herniation of the nucleus pulposus through the annulus may likewise be asymptomatic. It most commonly occurs at its weakest portion just lateral to the posterior longitudinal ligament near the intervertebral foramen. Herniation into the center of the vertebral canal is relatively uncommon. When it does occur, however, it may result in compression of the spinal cord or of multiple nerve roots if it is below the conus medullaris. The size of the herniated mass varies considerably; it ranges from a protrusion still covered by thinned-out annulus to complete extrusion of the nucleus pulposus as well as the fibrocartilage layers of the annulus into the vertebral canal. The largest intervertebral discs are those in the lumbar region, and, as might be expected, the largest herniated masses occur there. Herniations of the same size are better tolerated in the lumbar area than in other regions, since the spinal cord ends at the thoracolumbar junction, and the lumbar vertebral canal and the intervertebral foramina are larger.

Occasionally in response to severe trauma, especially flexion injuries, an acute rupture of the annulus occurs with massive herniation of the nucleus pulposus and immediate onset of severe neurologic deficit. In the vast majority of patients, however, signs and symptoms resulting from herniation of the nucleus pulposus are more chronic. Although patients often relate their disability to a recent event, such as bending, turning, or lifting, they almost invariably also give a history of past neck or back pain with or without symptoms of nerve root compression. Herniation of the nucleus pulposus is therefore usually a gradual and intermittent process. Signs and symptoms appear when surrounding pain-sensitive structures, such as the annulus, longitudinal ligaments, and dura, are stimulated or nervous tissue, usually roots, is compressed. Anatomic and pathologic adjustments then often occur, and the symptoms regress, perhaps to reappear when the mass enlarges or anatomic relationships change.

CLINICAL MANIFESTATIONS. The clinical picture produced by the common posterolateral disc herniation is characteristic. Diagnosis often can be made by history alone. Signs and symptoms are primarily those of extradural mass: pain over the distribution of the nerve root involved and evidence of lower motor neuron functional loss. Complaints of sensory disturbance over the peripheral distribution of the nerve root involved is commonly of a "pins and needles" type or just a slightly numb feeling. While weakness may be a symptom, it is much less common. The other root signs are loss or decrease in the deep tendon reflex and weakness and atrophy. Examination of the involved area of the spine reveals muscle spasm that may cause loss of normal lumbar or cervical lordosis. In lumbar lesions scoliosis is frequently present, the convexity usually occurring on the side of the lesion. Motion in the affected portion of the spine is limited and painful, especially on lateral flexion toward the lesion. Palpation over the corresponding spinous process and along the major nerve trunks produces pain. Maneuvers such as straight-leg raising which increase the tension of the nerve roots are painful.

DIAGNOSTIC FINDINGS. Plain x-rays may be normal or reveal distortion of alignment of the spine produced by muscle spasm. They may, however, show narrowing of the interspace, lipping of the margins of the vertebral bodies bordering on the disc, and osteoarthritic spurs. X-rays also serve to rule out bone erosion that may be present with spinal neoplasms and congenital bony anomalies such as spondylolisthesis. Computerized axial tomography has recently been used as an adjunct to plain x-ray when stenosis of the spinal canal is suspected. Most commonly caused by hypertrophy of the articular facets, impingement of the neural canal is readily identified by this method. Myelography is often used as final verification of a herniated disc, especially in the cervical and thoracic region. This procedure is best carried out after making the decision to operate based on the course of the disease and the findings on examination.

HERNIATED LUMBAR DISC

The highest incidence of symptomatic herniation of the intervertebral disc is in the lumbar region. Ninety-five percent of lumbar herniations occur at the last two interspaces. The relative frequencies of herniations at these two interspaces are approximately equal. Most of the remainder of the herniated lumbar intervertebral discs occur at the third lumbar interspace. The vast majority of herniations in the lumbar as well as in other locations are unilateral. The disposition of the nerve roots in the lumbar space is such that posterolateral herniation does not compress the nerve exiting at the corresponding intervertebral foramen but rather impinges on the set of anterior and posterior nerve roots, contained in a single dural sleeve, which cross the disc in their course to the foramen immediately caudad.

CLINICAL MANIFESTATIONS. Herniation at the interspace between the fourth and fifth lumbar vertebral bodies usually compresses the fifth lumbar roots, and herniation at the disc located at the lumbosacral junction produces signs and symptoms referable to the first sacral roots. The fifth lumbar anterior root serves as a major supply to the anterior crural muscles, which dorsiflex the foot, and the peroneal muscles, which evert and plantar-flex the foot. The dermatome served by the fifth lumbar posterior root includes the anterolateral aspect of the leg and crosses anteriorly at the ankle to supply the medial aspect of the foot including its dorsum. Compression of the fifth nerve root by a herniated nucleus pulposus occasionally produces a foot drop. The motor deficit, however, is usually less severe; the most common finding is weakness of dorsiflexion of the great toe. Hypesthesia and hypalgesia are usually most evident on the dorsum of the foot between the great and second toes. The motor root of the first sacral nerve supplies some innervation to the gluteal and hamstring muscles but gives a larger supply to the muscles of the calf and the small muscles of the foot. Its sensory distribution covers a narrow strip on the posterior aspect of the leg and the lateral aspect of the foot. The most common motor deficit in patients with herniation at the lumbosacral interspace is weakness of plantar flexion. Minor degrees of weakness may be brought out by having the patient attempt to walk on his toes. In addition, the ankle reflex is diminished or absent, and sensory deficit is found on the lateral aspect of the foot.

TREATMENT. For the majority of patients with herniated lumbar intervertebral discs the appropriate treatment includes a regimen of strict bed rest on a firm mattress, local heat, and analgesics. Pain usually subsides in 1 to 2 weeks, and the patient may then be started on a graded program of exercises designed to strengthen the back musculature. The patient should be instructed to refrain from heavy lifting and from activities that involve sudden bending or twisting of the lumbar spine. Early operation is reserved for those patients who have evidence of major neurologic dysfunction such as a foot drop or bowel and bladder disturbances which indicate a massive disc protrusion. If the patient has not responded to conservative management in a few weeks or is losing considerable time from work each year from repetitive episodes, operation should probably be carried out. Back pain alone is not an indication for operation. The aim of the operation, done through a limited hemilaminectomy, is to relieve nerve root compression by excision of the mass of herniated nucleus pulposus. Relief of signs and symptoms referable to such compression is usual, but many of the patients have residual low back pain. In our experience fusion of the vertebrae does not often solve this latter problem.

HERNIATED CERVICAL DISC

The lower cervical region is the next most common site of herniated discs. Approximately 90 percent of the herniations in this region occur at the interspaces between C_5 and C_6 and between C_6 and C_7 with the lower level predominating. In contrast with the lower lumbar region, cervical nerve roots are short and almost horizontal.

CLINICAL MANIFESTATIONS. Relatively small herniations are often symptomatic, usually lying just beneath the corresponding roots as they enter the intervertebral foramen. It is fortunate that large or medially placed herniations are rare, for when they do occur, they often result in quadriparesis.

With lateral herniations at the lower cervical levels, patients complain of neck pain radiating into the corresponding shoulder and arm. Referred interscapular pain is also common. Localization of the compressed roots by physical signs is somewhat less precise than in the lumbar area. Compression of the sixth cervical roots by posterolateral herniation at the C_5—C_6 interspace usually results in clinically evident weakness of the biceps muscle, depression or absence of the biceps tendon reflex, and sensory loss on the dorsal and lateral aspect of the thumb and radial aspect of the hand often including the index finger. The syndrome of the seventh cervical roots includes weakness of the triceps muscle, decrease or absence of the triceps reflex, and sensory deficit of the distal portions of the corresponding dermatome, which is medial to that of the sixth cervical dermatome. It usually includes both the dorsal and palmar aspects of the index and middle fingers.

TREATMENT. The rationale of treatment of cervical disc herniation is similar to that in the lumbar region. Signs and symptoms in the majority of patients will regress with conservative management. Neck traction is especially useful. Operation is indicated only in patients with evidence of spinal cord compression and those not responding to conservative measures. Central herniations are best removed through the interspace from the anterior aspect of the spine. The common lateral herniations can be removed effectively either from the same anterior approach or by hemilaminectomy.

HERNIATED THORACIC DISC

Disc herniation in the thoracic region is rare. When it does occur, it is usually in the lower thoracic spine and is apt to produce major neurologic deficit, often with little associated pain. This lesion may be suspected on the basis of a past history of trauma to the thoracic spine, but it is usually clinically indistinguishable from the more common neoplasms occurring in this region. Diagnosis is made by x-ray studies. There may be narrowing of an interspace and, in contrast to disc disease in other regions, calcification in the interspace. Myelography is essential for diagnosis. Results of operation by the classic approach, i.e., laminectomy, are in general poor with no improvement or with increased deficit in about one-half of the patients reported in larger series. The reasons for these poor results include the fact that most of these lesions are anterior to the cord and are firm and partially calcified. Their removal with a posterior exposure therefore often necessitates major retraction of an already compressed spinal cord. Removal of the herniated disc by approach through the interspace, either by removing the adjacent ribs and transverse processes or by going through the chest cavity, has been more effective in relieving the myelopathy without causing further neurological deficit.

SPONDYLOSIS

Hypertrophic bone changes are not infrequently associated with disc herniation even in younger individuals. They are especially prevalent in cervical herniations in which spurs of bone projecting into the intervertebral foramina are often a contributing cause of nerve root compression. In relation to its almost uniform presence in the elderly, hypertrophic bony change alone as a cause of significant neurologic dysfunction is uncommon. However, in some patients with advanced hypertrophic bone disease of the cervical spine, often termed *spondylosis,* major spinal cord and nerve root dysfunction develop. This entity, which usually affects two or more lower cervical interspaces, is characterized by narrowing of the interspaces and extensive bony proliferation on the lips of the vertebral bodies adjacent to the discs, producing transverse ridges which project into the vertebral canal. The corresponding intervertebral foramina are narrowed, and in advanced disease minor degrees of subluxation of one vertebra on another may exist.

Why many persons tolerate advanced cervical spondylosis without significant disability while in others a severe spastic quadriparesis may develop is largely unknown. It has been demonstrated that a greater number of patients with symptomatic spondylosis have congenitally narrow cervical vertebral canals than those without spinal cord signs. A simple compressive mechanism, however, does not entirely suffice to explain the problem, since return of function often does not follow seemingly adequate decompression which includes extensive laminectomy combined with removal of bony spurs and fusion from the anterior approach. Chronic vascular insufficiency resulting from a combination of such factors as arteriosclerosis, compression of a long segment of spinal cord, and compression of the arterial supply entering through the intervertebral foramina may explain the difference in the results of surgical therapy for cervical spondylosis as compared with more localized mass lesions in the same region.

CLINICAL MANIFESTATIONS. The clinical picture of symptomatic cervical spondylosis varies considerably. Neck pain radiating bilaterally into the shoulders is frequently but not invariably present. Examination reveals evidence of compression of multiple cervical nerve roots and signs of cervical spinal cord compression. The course of the disease is also variable. Occasionally there is rapid progression which may lead to a severe spastic quadriparesis within a year or less. More often the onset of signs is insidious, and progression is slow. Spontaneous regression of neurologic deficit is rare, but on the other hand progression of deficit may halt at any point.

TREATMENT. The variability of the course makes it difficult to evaluate the effectiveness of operative procedures. In the early stages of the disease immobilization of the cervical spine by a well-fitted collar brace may be of benefit. Traction occasionally may reduce root pain but often is not successful. Operation early in the course of the disease should probably be reserved for those patients with involvement of only one or two interspaces and those with obviously small vertebral canals. With severe and seemingly unrelenting progression of neurologic deficit associated with widespread bony changes, the patient should be informed that a halt in progression may be all that can be hoped for from operation.

References

General Considerations

Jefferson, G.: "Selected Papers," Pitman Medical Publications, London, 1960.
Mullan, S.: "Essentials of Neurosurgery," Springer Publishing Co., Inc., New York, 1961.
Plum, F., and Posner, J.: "The Diagnosis of Stupor and Coma," F. A. Davis Company, Philadelphia, 1972.

Head Injury, Mechanisms of Injury, Care of Head-injured Patient

Adams, J. H.: "The Neuropathology of Head Trauma: Handbook of Clinical Neurology," pp. 35–65, North-Holland Publishing Company, Amsterdam, 1975.
Browder, E. J., and Cook, A. W.: Indications for Surgical Intervention in Head Injuries, *Surg Clin North Am*, **35**:577, 1955.

Ingraham, F., and Matson, D.: "Neurosurgery of Infancy and Childhood," pt. III, chap. 5, Charles C Thomas, Publisher, Springfield, Ill., 1954.
Jennett, B., Teasdale, G., Galbraith, S., Pickard, J., Grant, H., Braakman, R., Avezaat, C., Maas, A., Minderhound, J., Vecht, C. J., Herden, J., Small, R., Caton, W., and Kurze, T.: Severe Head Injuries in Three Countries, *J Neurol Neurosurg Psychiatry*, **40**:291, 1977.
Johnson, R. T., and Yates, P. O.: Brain Stem Haemorrhages in Expanding Supratentorial Conditions, *Acta Radiol (Stockh)*, **46**:250, 1956.
Lewin, W.: Factors in the Mortality of Closed Head Injuries, *Br Med J*, **1**:1239, 1953.
Lindenberg, R.: Compression of Brain Arteries as a Pathogenetic Factor for Tissue Necroses and Their Areas of Predilection, *J Neuropathol Exp Neurol*, **14**:223, 1955.
Schneider, R. C., and Tytus, J. S.: Extradural Hemorrhage: Factors Responsible for the High Mortality Rate, *Ann Surg*, **142**:938, 1955.
Walker, A. E.: Practical Considerations in the Treatment of Head Injuries, *Neurology*, **1**:75, 1951.
Ward, A. A.: Physiological Basis of Concussion, *J Neurosurg*, **15**:129, 1958.

Spinal Cord Injuries

Holdsworth, F.: Review Article. Fractures, Dislocations, and Fracture-Dislocations of the Spine, *J Bone Joint Surg*, **52-A:** 1534, 1970.
Schneider, R. C., Crosby, E. C., Russo, R. H., and Gosch, H. H.: Traumatic Spinal Cord Syndromes and Their Management, *Clin Neurosurg*, **20**:424, 1973.
Symonds, C. P.: The Interrelation of Trauma and Cervical Spondylosis in Compression of the Cervical Cord, *Lancet*, **1**:451, 1953.
Tarlov, I. M.: Spinal Cord Compression Studies: III, *Arch Neurol Psychiatry*, **71**:588, 1954.
——— and Herz, E.: Spinal Cord Compression Studies: IV, *Arch Neurol Psychiatry*, **72**:43, 1954.
Wagner, F. C.: Management of Acute Spinal Cord Injury, *Surg Neurol*, **7**:346, 1977.

Peripheral Nerve Injuries

Lyons, W. R., and Woodhall, B.: "Atlas of Peripheral Nerve Injuries," W. B. Saunders Company, Philadelphia, 1949.
Millese, H., Meissl, G., and Berger, A.: Further Experiences with Interfascicular Grafting of the Median, Ulnar and Radial Nerves, *J Bone Joint Surg*, **58-A**:209, 1976.
Smith, J. W.: Microsurgery of Peripheral Nerves, *Plast Reconstr Surg*, **33**:317, 1964.
Woodhall, B.: Surgical Repair of Acute Peripheral Nerve Injury, *Surg Clin North Am*, **30**:1369, 1951.
Young, J. Z.: The Functional Repair of Nervous Tissue, *Physiol Rev*, **22**:318, 1942.

Brain Tumors

Bailey, P.: "Intracranial Tumors," Charles C Thomas, Publisher, Springfield, Ill., 1948.
Kernohan, J. W., and Sayre, G. P.: "Tumors of the Central Nervous System," sec. X, fasicles 35, 37, Armed Forces Institute of Pathology, Washington, 1952.

Russell, D., and Rubenstein, L.: "Pathology of Tumors of the Nervous System," The Williams & Wilkins Company, Baltimore, 1963.

Spinal Tumors

Dodge, H. W., Jr., Keith, H. M., and Campagna, M. J.: Intraspinal Tumors in Infants and Children, *J Int Coll Surg*, **26:**199, 1957.

Kennady, J. C., and Stern, W. E.: Metastatic Neoplasms of the Vertebral Column Producing Compression of the Spinal Cord, *Am J Surg*, **104:**155, 1962.

Woltman, H. W., Kernohan, J. W., Adson, A. W., and Craig, W. M.: Intramedullary Tumors of Spinal Cord and Gliomas of Intradural Portion of Filum Terminale, *Arch Neurol Psychiatry*, **65:**378, 1951.

Congenital Malformations of the Nervous System

Bunch, W. H., Cass, A. S., Bensman, A. S., and Long, D. M.: "Modern Management of Myelomeningocele," Warren H. Green, Publisher, St. Louis, 1972.

Forrest, D. M., Hale, R., and Wynne, J. M.: Treatment of Infantile Hydrocephalus Using Holter Valve: An Analysis of 152 Consecutive Cases. *Dev Med Child Neurol Suppl*, **11:**27, 1966.

Lorber, J., and De, N. C.: Family History of Congenital Hydrocephalus, *Dev Med Child Neurol Suppl*, **22:**94, 1969.

Matson, D. D.: "Neurosurgery of Infancy and Childhood," chaps. 1–14, Charles C Thomas, Publisher, Springfield, Ill., 1969.

Mealey, J., Dzenitus, A. J., and Hockey, A. A.: The Prognosis of Encephaloceles, *J Neurosurg*, **32:**209, 1970.

Norman, R. M.: Malformation of the Nervous System, in W. Blackwood et al. (eds.), "Greenfield's Neuropathology," chap. 6, The Williams & Wilkins Company, Baltimore, 1967.

Raimondi, A.: Angiographic Diagnosis of Hydrocephalus in the Newborn, *J Neurosurg*, **31:**550, 1969.

Russell, D. S.: Observations on the Pathology of Hydrocephalus, Her Majesty's Stationery Office, London, 1949.

Scarff, J. E.: Treatment of Hydrocephalus: An Historical and Critical Review of Methods and Results, *J Neurol Neurosurg Psychiatry*, **26:**1, 1963.

Shilleto, J.: Craniosynostosis: Review of 519 Cases, *Pediatrics*, **41:**829, 1968.

Surgical Aspects of Central Nervous System Infections

Evans, W.: The Pathology and Aetiology of Brain Abscess, *Lancet*, **1:**1231, 1931.

Irsigler, F. J.: "The Neurosurgical Approach to Intracranial Infections," Springer-Verlag OHG, Berlin, 1961.

Kerr, F. W. L., King, R. B., and Meagher, J. N.: Brain Abscess, *JAMA*, **168:**868, 1958.

Lewin, W.: Cerebrospinal Fluid Rhinorrhea in Closed Head Injuries, *Br J Surg*, **62:**1, 1954.

Matson, D. D., and Salvin, M.: Brain Abscess in Congenital Heart Disease, *Pediatrics*, **27:**772, 1961.

Vascular Disease of the Nervous System

Blackwood, W., et al. (eds.): "Greenfield's Neuropathology," chap. 2, The Williams & Wilkins Company, Baltimore, 1963.

Crawford, T.: Some Observations on the Pathogenesis and Natural History of Intracranial Aneurysms, *J Neurol Neurosurg Psychiatry*, **22:**259, 1959.

Hamby, W. B.: "Intracranial Aneurysms," Charles C Thomas, Publisher, Springfield, Ill., 1952.

Jefferson, G.: Subarachnoid Hemorrhage from Angiomas and Aneurysms in the Young, *Rev Neurol (Paris)*, **80:**413, 1948.

Report on the Cooperative Study of Intracranial Aneurysms, *J Neurosurg*, **24:**782, **24:**789, **24:**792, **24:**807, **24:**922, **24:**1034, **25:**98, **25:**219, **25:**321, **25:**467, **25:**574, **25:**593, **25:**660, **25:**683, 1966.

Russell, D. S.: The Pathology of Spontaneous Intracranial Hemorrhage, *Proc R Soc Med*, **47:**689, 1954.

Yasargil, M. D.: "Microneurosurgery Applied to Neurosurgery," Academic Press, Inc., New York, 1969.

The Surgery of Epilepsy

Blaisdell, W. F., Clauss, R. H., Galbraith, J. G., et al.: Joint Study of Extracranial Arterial Occlusions: IV. A Review of Surgical Considerations, *JAMA*, **209:**12, 1969.

Earle, K. M., Baldwin, M., and Penfield, W.: Incisural Sclerosis and Temporal Lobe Seizures Produced by Hippocampal Herniation at Birth, *Arch Neurol Psychiatry*, **69:**27, 1953.

Hassler, O.: Arterial Pattern of Human Brain Stem, *Neurology*, **17:**368, 1967.

Marshall, J.: The Natural History of Cerebrovascular Diseases, in "Modern Concepts of Cerebrovascular Disease," Spectrum Publications, Inc., New York, 1975.

Ojemann, R. G., Crowell, R. M., Roberson, G. H., and Fisher, C. M.: Surgical Treatment of Extracranial Carotid Occlusive Disease, in "Clinical Neurosurgery," vol. 21, 1976.

Penfield, W., and Jasper, H.: "Epilepsy and the Functional Anatomy of the Human Brain," Little, Brown and Company, Boston, 1954.

Pond, D. A., Bidwell, B. H., and Stein, L.: A Survey of Epilepsy in 14 General Practices: I. Demographic and Medical Data, *Psychiatr Neurol Neurochir*, **63:**217, 1960.

Purpura, D. P., Perry, J. K., and Walter, R. D.: Neurosurgical Management of the Epilepsies, p. 44 in "Advances in Neurology," vol. 8, Raven Press Publishers, New York, 1975.

Yasargil, M. G.: "Experimental Small Vessel Surgery in the Dog Including Patching and Grafting of Cerebral Vessels and the Formation of Functional Extra-intracranial Shunts," The C. V. Mosby Company, St. Louis, 1967.

Pain

Bessou, P., and Perl, E. R.: Response of Cutaneous Sensory Units with Unmyelinated Fibers to Noxious Stimuli, *J Neurophysiol*, **32:**1025, 1969.

Bowsher, D.: Termination of the Central Pain Pathway in Man: The Conscious Appreciation of Pain, *Brain*, **80:**606, 1957.

Keele, K. D.: "Anatomies of Pain," Blackwell Scientific Publications, Ltd., Oxford, 1957.

Knighton, R. S., and Dumke, P. R.: "Pain," Little, Brown and Company, Boston, 1966.

Melzack, R., and Wall, P.: Pain Mechanisms in a New Theory, *Science*, **150:**971, 1965.

Stookey, B., and Ransohoff, J.: "Trigeminal Neuralgia: Its History and Treatment," Charles C Thomas, Publisher, Springfield, Ill., 1959.

White, J. C., and Sweet, W. H.: "Pain: Its Mechanisms and Neurosurgical Control," Charles C Thomas, Publisher, Springfield, Ill., 1955.

Structural Abnormalities of Axial Skeleton

Hinck, V. C., and Sachdev, N. S.: Developmental Stenosis of the Cervical Spinal Canal, *Brain,* **89:**27, 1966.

List, C. F.: Clinical Syndromes of Craniovertebral Anomalies, *Arch Neurol Psychiatry,* **45:**577, 1941.

Spurling, R. G.: "Lesions of the Lumbar Intervertebral Disc," Charles C Thomas, Publisher, Springfield, Ill., 1953.

———: "Lesions of the Cervical Intervertebral Disc," Charles C Thomas, Publisher, Springfield, Ill., 1956.

Wilkinson, M.: The Morbid Anatomy of Cervical Spondylosis and Myelopathy, *Brain,* **83:**589, 1960.

Chapter 43

Manifestations of Musculoskeletal Disorders

by **Robert B. Duthie and Franklin T. Hoaglund**

PAIN

Since pain is the major manifestation of many orthopedic disorders, careful evaluation of its character and properties is essential in the diagnosis, treatment, and understanding of such conditions.

Pain, defined by Sherrington as "the physical adjunct of an imperative protective reflex," is a sensation one feels when injured. Because it appears to vary in quality with each individual, its precise definition is very difficult.

The afferent nociceptive impulses produced by injurious agents stream into the central nervous system, where they are given meaning by the emotional state of the individual based upon the past and present experience. Pain is, therefore, an *experience* rather than a sensory modality in a strict neurologic sense, and psychologic events play an essential role in determining the quality and quantity of its ultimate perception.

Anatomy and Physiology

PAINFUL STIMULUS. The old theory which postulated that pain was the result of stimuli exceeding the intensity threshold for sensory nerve endings can no longer be accepted in the light of modern anatomic and physiologic studies. Woddell has suggested that stimulation of peripheral receptors by noxious agents produces a spatiotemporal pattern of nervous impulses which is interpreted as pain within the higher cerebral centers. Such patterns of nervous activity may be produced by many physical phenomena such as pressure, puncturing, squeezing, and tension;

by alteration in temperature; or by chemical effects, such as the alteration in pH or the concentration of histamine-like substances, serotonin, bradykinin, and other polypeptide compounds. Tissue changes in inflammation are accompanied by a local acidosis. Pus formation, and fibrosis, by virtue of pH changes or internal pressure effects, may convert normal stimuli into stimuli with certain patterns of nervous activity which will be interpreted as pain.

SENSORY END ORGANS. Specialized end organs for pressure and stress do occur in skin and tendons, respectively. However, the old concept of absolute *specificity* of end organs for pressure (Pacini), cold (Krause), and traction (Meissner and Ruffini) requires revision. Weddell and others have demonstrated that most cutaneous sensory nerve endings are unmyelinated fibers forming a dense dermal network. These, when stimulated, may produce sensations of pressure, touch, or pain, depending upon the impulse pattern invoked, rather than the excitation of specific fibers beyond their normal threshold. Similar networks of unmyelinated nerve fibers are found in the walls of blood vessels, particularly arteries, in periosteum, in bone, in synovium, and in joint capsule. In muscles, a similar role is conducted by small myelinated fibers. Cartilage has no sensory end organs.

Specialized end organs, i.e., Pacinian for pressure, can be seen occasionally within the dermis. End organs of Golgi can be identified in ligaments and tendons, where they act as stretch receptors, for muscle control, and perhaps for pain. Bone and periosteum respond to pressure, percussion, or tension. Capsule responds to both tension and traction and is certainly the most sensitive of all joint structures. Although synovium contains scattered free nerve endings, it is difficult to elicit their function experimentally because of the proximity of synovium to capsule.

SENSORY PATHWAYS. The conduction velocity and frequency of impulses in afferent nerve fibers is dependent upon fiber diameter (Table 43-1). The afferent fibers are carried within the peripheral nerves to spinal root ganglia and then to the cord, where they synapse within one or two segments of the dorsal column before crossing the midline to form the contralateral lateral spinothalamic tract. At the site of dorsal column synapse, the pathway

of pain fibers is regulated by fibers descending in the ipsilateral corticospinal tract. There is a controlling mechanism acting at every junction at which nerve impulses are relayed from one neuron to the next on their cerebral ascent. Melzack described this as the mechanism by which psychologic or emotional events determine the quality and quantity of ultimate perception of pain. There are five links in the path by which pain reaches the cerebrum (Fig. 43-1):

1. The spinothalamic tract, excitatory in function and carrying the majority of pain impulses.
2. The central tegmental tract, inhibitory in function. Division increases pain sensitivity.
3. The central gray pathway. Division decreases pain sensitivity.
4. The ascending reticular system, which alerts the entire brain.
5. The medial lemniscal tract, for proprioception and light touch.

The first three of these pathways are depressed by analgesic agents, while the fifth maintains the function of spatial awareness.

Livingston explained the *phantom limb syndrome* in amputees as a disturbance of neural activity in the posterior horn internuncial pool, which produces reverberatory patterns of neural activity. These may be aggravated by minor cutaneous irritations, stimulations of nerve stumps, and emotional upset.

Characteristics

Pain may be expressed in many ways. A deep boring ache is characteristic of tension, whereas a "burning" pain with paresthesias, especially if accompanied by vasomotor phenomena (sweating or redness), indicates a sympathetic as well as a somatic sensory involvement.

Sites

Pain may be described as localized, diffuse, radicular, or referred.

Local pain. Local pain is felt at the site of pathologic processes in superficial structures and is usually associated with local tenderness on palpation or percussion.

Diffuse pain. Diffuse pain appears to be more characteristic of deep-lying tissues and has a more or less segmental distribution.

Radicular pain. Radicular pain, as seen in sciatica and brachialgia, is characterized by its radiation from the center to the periphery in a strict anatomic sense. It is often associated with paresthesia and tenderness along the nerve root. Clinical examination frequently reveals neurologic deficits such as sensory loss, reflex depression, and muscle paresis or paralysis.

Referred pain. Referred pain occurs with injury to, or disease affecting, deep structures such as the spine or the viscera and is a result of misplaced pain projection caused by cortical misrepresentation. For this to occur, sensory pathways must converge on a single cell within the cord or higher centers. Gaze and Gordon and McLeod demonstrated confluence of visceral and cutaneous impulses in the thalamus of the cat. Whitty and Hockaday indicate that there is possible influence upon such convergence

Table 43-1.

Type	Velocity	Fiber diameter	Fiber function
A	120 m/sec	15–25 μ	Proprioceptive afferents from the skin and joints
B		Less than 2 μ	Unmyelinated pain afferents accompanying sympathetic fibers from muscle and bone
C	10 m/sec	5–15 μ	Afferents from muscle and tendon
D			Myelinated fibers in association with visceral nerves

points of stored "pain experience," from cells within the brain, rather than only at the spinal cord level.

The experiments of Kellgren and Samuel have helped to define some characteristics of referred pain in different body tissues (Fig. 43-2). Pain resulting from the injection of 6% saline solution into muscle was diffuse and referred into the spinal segments from which the muscle receives its motor innervation, and it varied with the individual. Pain resulting from injection into deep fascia, periosteum, ligament, or tendon was more accurately localized when these tissues were close to the body surface (Fig. 43-3). When the structures were deeper, the pain was more diffuse and had minimal segmental distribution.

Feinstein et al. demonstrated that similar injection of muscle and intervertebral articulations produced gripping, boring, and cramplike pain, often accompanied by muscle spasm and autonomic effects such as hypotension, nausea, and bradycardia. There was less segmental distribution of pain because of extensive arborization of nerve endings and excitation within the internuncial pools, which resulted in extensive overflow into neighboring segments.

Tissue Patterns

BONE PAIN. Pain originating in bone is carried by small myelinated and unmyelinated fibers from the periosteum and small blood vessels. It has a characteristic deep, boring quality usually attributable to the stimulus of internal tension. Such pain is characteristic of osteomyelitis, tumors, and vascular lesions of bone such as those of Paget's disease.

The deep, boring night pain of osteoarthritis is probably of vascular origin. However, this type of pain in osteoarthritis must be differentiated from that due to capsular fibrosis and muscle spasm often aggravated by unguarded movements. Pain of a similar boring nature but of a somewhat diffuse character occurs in generalized osseous diseases such as osteomalacia, osteoporosis, and hyperparathyroidism or metastatic lesions (myelomatosis, carcinomatosis) of the vertebral column, ribs, and pelvic and shoulder girdles. These conditions may have more severe acute pain superimposed as a result of pathologic fractures.

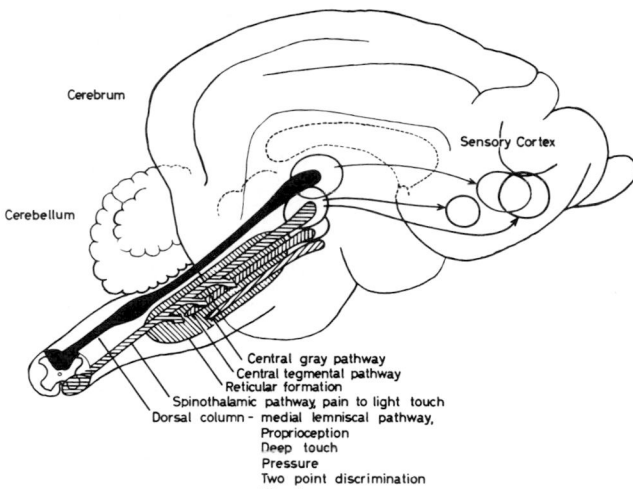

Fig. 43-1. Major pathways along which pain reaches the brain. (*After Melzack, 1961. Taken with permission from Scientific American, 1961.*)

Bone pain associated with fracture has quite a different character. It is often described as sharp or piercing and is characteristically relieved by rest. Pain which is unrelieved by rest is ominous and points toward serious disease processes.

MUSCLE AND TENDON PAIN. Muscle contains many unmyelinated nerve fibers, especially related to its rich blood supply. Many efferent motor fibers to the muscle end plate may subserve a sensory function by virtue of their control over muscle contraction, which, when abnormal, is experienced as pain.

Muscle pain may be the result of direct injury or the effect of chemical irritants such as lactic acid and other products of tissue anoxia. That due to direct injury is usually described as "tearing" and is followed by a soreness aggravated by movement, whereas that consequent upon anoxia is described as a "cramplike" pain. Such a cramplike pain is characteristic of intermittent claudication secondary to atherosclerosis, Volkmann's ischemia, and the anterior tibial syndrome. The pain is aggravated by muscle movement, either passive or active. It is the result of edema secondary to tissue necrosis and the release of chemical irritants which in turn alter the circulation.

Muscle spasm refers to sustained muscular contraction

Fig. 43-2. *A.* Characteristics of muscle pain when stimulated by injected saline solution. *B.* Characteristics of ligament pain when stimulated. (*After Kellgren, 1943. Taken with permission from Mercer and Duthie [eds.], "Orthopaedic Surgery," Edward Arnold [Publishers] Ltd., London, 1972.*)

Fig. 43-3. Distribution of pain in the trunk when the interspinous ligaments between various vertebrae were stimulated. *B.* Distribution of pain in the lower extremities when interspinous ligaments were stimulated. (*After Kellgren, 1943. Taken with permission from Mercer and Duthie [eds.], "Orthopaedic Surgery," Edward Arnold [Publishers] Ltd., London, 1972.*)

and is felt as deep, diffuse, persistent pain often described as "like a toothache." Characteristically, in sciatica it produces a scoliosis and in brachialgia a torticollis due to lumbar and cervical nerve root irritation. It is accompanied by local tenderness and a feeling of hardness of the muscles.

The mode of production of painful symptoms by root compression has been clarified by Frykholm, who stimulated nerve roots in patients under local anesthesia. He found that compression of the motor root produced deep, boring ache which could be abolished by blocking the related sensory root. Then stimulation of the motor root continued to produce contraction but did not produce pain. Stimulation of the sensory root, on the other hand, produced sharp, shocklike pain radiating in a peripheral fashion into the appropriate dermatome. Referred pain also may occur when muscle spasm is associated with visceral disorder, e.g., peptic ulceration, appendicitis, and peritonitis.

Paroxysmal cramplike pain accompanied by rigidity or excessive muscle spasm is seen in tetany, which is due to increased sensitivity of the neuromuscular unit consequent upon hypocalcemia or alkalosis. Muscle cramps are also noted with sodium depletion due to hypermotility of muscle cells, a condition rapidly reversed by restoration of the electrolyte balance. Peripheral neuritis may also present cramping of muscle masses as well as paresthesias. The pain and accompanying tenderness of fibrositis is related

to a specific muscle group, but its pathology is not understood.

JOINT PAIN. It is difficult to define joint pain because of the complexity and number of tissues involved in its structure.

The synovium contains two plexuses of nerve fibers, a superficial plexus lying in close proximity to the capsule and a deeper one in the synovial villi. This plexus is intimately related to blood vessels which carry within their tunica media many unmyelinated sensory fibers.

The capsule has a rich supply of somatic sensory fibers and proprioceptive fibers in the form of specialized Golgi apparatus, Vater-Pacini corpuscles, and Ruffini-like endings. Its connection with joint pain appreciation was demonstrated by Leriche, who showed that local anesthetic injected into the capsule was more effective than a simple intraarticular injection.

Coomes produced patterns of pain around the hip, depending upon the aspect of the capsule stimulated. Stimulation of the anterior capsule produced pain in the groin, buttock, anterior thigh, and knee, whereas posterior capsule stimulation produced pain in the buttock, posterior aspect of the thigh, and heel.

Cartilage is avascular and aneural and, therefore, insensitive to stimuli.

There are many sensory endings in the periosteum and accompanying the blood vessels in bone. Bone pain appears to be commonly associated with increased internal tension.

Thus, pain in joints may be attributable to a number of factors:

1. Hyperemia, both of the synovium and bone
2. Joint effusion, producing capsular distension and ligamentous laxity
3. Joint instability, producing traction on capsular structures
4. Asymmetry of the joint surfaces, particularly in the presence of exposed subchondral bone or cyst formation with tension
5. Muscle spasm

PERIPHERAL NERVE PAIN. Peripheral nerve fibers may be subject to:

1. External pressure—neuralgia
2. Ischemia
3. Infection—herpes zoster
4. Metabolic disturbance—avitaminosis ⎫ neuritis
5. Toxins—lead or arsenic ⎭

The pain of neuralgia is usually paroxysmal and radicular in type. Paresthesia is common, and examination frequently reveals changes in reflexes, loss of sensation, muscle atrophy, etc. The pain of neuritis, however, tends to be continuous until relief of the disease process or total destruction of neural tissue ensues. The special pain of herpes zoster or Guillain-Barré syndrome due to viral involvement of the internuncial element is accompanied by hyperesthesias, with or without sympathetic vasomotor changes.

PAIN ARISING FROM THE VERTEBRAL COLUMN AND/OR ITS CONTENTS. Lesions of the Cord. *Intraspinal Tumors.* To differentiate between vertebral tumors proper and intraspinal soft tissue tumors with their common symptoms of backache and root pain and occasional signs of spinal block is not always possible. However, intraspinal lesions tend to be progressive without periods of remission. The pain is not relieved by rest, and any progression of the intramedullary compression will produce a rapid loss of motor power in the extremities and loss of sphincter control.

Benign nerve sheath tumors and meningiomas are much more common than tumors of the spinal cord itself, i.e., metastatic carcinoma, glial and ependymal tumors, and more rarely connective tissue tumors.

Infection. Infections involving the spinal cord such as poliomyelitis, meningitis, and the Guillain-Barré syndrome tend to produce lancinating peripheral pain due to the involvement of the internuncial pool cells by the virus. In Guillain-Barré disease the peripheral sensory neurons outside the spinal cord are primarily involved rather than those within the spinal ganglia.

Ischemic and Degenerative Lesions. The conditions of amyotrophic lateral sclerosis, multiple sclerosis, subacute combined degeneration of the cord, and tabes dorsalis will all present with lancinating pain radiating to the extremities. Loss of reflexes are commonly found. Syringomyelia can usually be diagnosed by the loss of both pain and temperature sensations.

Lesions of the Vertebrae and/or Joints. Primary and secondary neoplasms, osteoporosis with pathologic fractures, and tuberculous and pyogenic infections affecting bones of the spine will produce severe local pain with local tenderness on palpation and percussion. Radicular pain does not occur unless the peripheral nerves are involved by the lesion. Carcinoma metastases to the skeletal structures from the prostate, breast, kidney, gastrointestinal tract, female genital organs, thyroid, or lung may produce significant symptoms before there are visible radiographic changes. Determination of the acid and alkaline phosphatase levels are indicated. Sternal puncture may demonstrate myeloma cells, and biopsy of the involved area may reveal the lesion.

Coccygodynia is deep, throbbing pain in the vicinity of the lower end of the sacrum and coccyx aggravated by sitting. It tends to be progressive and to last several months, but without any radicular expression or involvement of sphincteric function. It can be traumatic in origin, from arthritis involving the sacrococcygeal joint or from a disc protrusion at the lumbosacral junction. Localized tenderness on rectal examination is present, and radiographic changes of the joint may be noted. Treatment is usually conservative and consists of application of local heat and cushioned sitting. Rarely does the patient require excision of the coccyx.

Lesions Involving Peripheral Nerves. Peripheral nerves may be compressed in the intervertebral foramina by such conditions as neurofibromas, trauma, osteophyte formation associated with osteoarthrosis, and intervertebral disc protrusions. The pain is usually radicular over the area supplied by the nerve roots involved. Pain also may be referred to the back and limbs from visceral involvement as seen in mediastinitis, esophagitis, and diseases of the kidney, stomach, or gonads.

Pain in the Upper Limbs

The diagnosis of the cause of pain in the neck, head, shoulder, and upper limb requires understanding of anatomic, mechanical, and pathologic factors. In the cervical spine, the thoracic outlet region, and the upper extremities there are numerous soft tissues, e.g., muscles ligaments, and capsules around joints, all of which are plentifully supplied with pain nerve endings. Moreover, all these tissues are compressed into small areas and subjected to numerous stresses and strains in relation to movement. Any decrease in the dimensions of these spaces can result in pain and possible loss of function. Pain is more likely to occur if the pressure is acute and transient, whereas loss in function is more likely if pressure is prolonged and continuous.

DIFFERENTIAL DIAGNOSIS OF PAIN IN THE UPPER LIMB, BASED UPON ANATOMIC REGIONS. Pain in the Shoulder-Scapular Area. This will arise from cervical disc protrusion, diseases of the cervical vertebrae, and affections of the shoulder joint, e.g., supraspinatus tendinitis and subacromial bursitis, or it may be referred visceral pain arising from disease of the heart, lungs, or pleura.

Pain in the Vicinity of the Elbow. This may result from local conditions such as arthritis of the radiohumeral articulations or lateral epicondylitis ("tennis elbow"), or it may be referred pain with involvement of the fifth, sixth, or seventh cervical vertebrae or associated discs.

Pain in the Wrist and Hand. This may be the result of local lesions such as tendon sheath disease, e.g., Quervain's disease, radiocarpal arthritis, neoplastic or infective diseases of the bones, or compression of the median nerve within the carpal tunnel. Radicular pain may be due to compression of the ulnar nerve at the elbow or of the brachial plexus at any point from the roots at the intervertebral foramina or in the thoracic outlet; these conditions will be accompanied by other signs of neurologic deficit such as paresthesias, muscle atrophy, reflex changes, and overlying skin changes. Associated vasomotor trophic changes suggest Sudeck's atrophy or the shoulder-hand syndrome.

BRACHIALGIA (BRACHIAL NEURALGIA)

This pain involves the neck, shoulder, or upper extremity; i.e., it is distributed within the brachial plexus dermatome and sclerotome. It may be characterized by:

Upper extremity pain, either unilateral or bilateral
Paresthesias, in a dermatome with altered sensation
Deep tendon reflex changes in the jaw and/or in the upper extremity
Muscle weakness, with atrophy and possibly fibrillation
Vertebral artery or sympathetic plexus disturbance with giddiness or tinnitus or visual disturbance

The disease process may involve the motor neuron, the pyramidal tract, the root, or the surrounding vertebrae. Muscle pain which can be temporarily relieved by physical therapy is unlikely to be due to true nerve root involvement. These features, which are found in the upper extremity, may also involve the lower. Therefore, examination should be made of the reflexes, vibratory sense, and proprioceptive sense in the lower extremities as well as in the abdominal wall.

Radiography (AP and lateral, as well as oblique views), lumbar puncture to show the presence of some degree of block on jugular compression, examination of cerebrospinal fluid for changes in protein and other chemical constituents, and a cell count should be carried out. The differential diagnosis of brachialgia includes:

1. Tumors of the cord and its membranes or of the vertebral column, e.g., ependymoma, neurofibroma, or neurolemmoma
2. Infections, such as acute tuberculosis, osteomyelitis, actinomycosis
3. Prolapsing intervertebral disc, or degenerative disc with arthritis
4. Pancoast's tumor of the apex of lung
5. Congenital anomalies of the cord, e.g., syringomyelia
6. Atlantoaxial dislocation

CERVICAL COMPRESSION SYNDROME (CERVICAL DISC DISEASE)

Maximal movement of flexion or extension and static curvature occur at the level of C_4 to C_6. Maximal stress is to be expected at this level, and this is the most common site for herniations of the cervical intervertebral discs (Fig. 43-4). In addition, the cervical spinal canal contains a relatively immobile and thick spinal cord anchored

Fig. 43-4. Lateral radiograph of the cervical spine to show narrowing of disc spaces between C_4–C_5 and C_5–C_6 with osteophyte formation.

through the meninges by the denticular ligament and by the short, almost transversely directed nerve roots. These nerve roots continue their short horizontal course outside the thecal sac, remaining intradural, to the region of the intervertebral foramina, where they lie close to the intervertebral bodies opposite the intervertebral discs.

The precise situation of the disc protrusion or the osteophytic compression is important, because it determines whether the spinal cord and/or the nerve root will be affected. A prominence in the midline will compress the whole spinal cord and the anterior nerve roots which emerge at this level, but a bulge to one side of the midline will cause unilateral cord compression with a Brown-Séquard type of syndrome. The most common variety of protrusion, however, is that arising from the lateral portion of the disc in relation to the nerve root and is either dorsolateral or intraforaminal in location. An intraforaminal lesion may also be the result of narrowing of an already small intervertebral foramen by osteophytic lipping of the margins of the neurocentral joints of Luschka. These "neurocentral" joints are set at the lateral margins of the vertebrae facing into the intervertebral foramina and lie anteromedial to the nerve roots but posteromedial to the vertebral arteries and veins.

Protrusion of a cervical intervertebral disc can produce:

1. Nerve root compression alone, with pain down the arm
2. Compression of the spinal cord structures
3. A combination of both
4. Local and referred pain in the absence of nerve root compression

When there is nerve root compression, there are additional local symptoms in and about the neck resulting from local disease process in the cervical spine.

CLINICAL MANIFESTATIONS. Symptoms of nerve root compression, when present, usually constitute the chief complaint. However, the majority of patients have only symptoms of local and referred pain as a consequence of the disc degeneration. Occasionally, there is a history of trauma, but usually it is minor in nature. A form of precipitating injury may be an unexpected and abrupt forward jerk of the head as with sudden acceleration or deceleration of an automobile when hit from behind or in a head-on collision. The patient may sometimes notice restriction of neck movement.

The predominant feature of nerve root compression from a laterally placed protrusion is pain distributed according to the level of the disc lesion and the nerve root involved. There are eight cervical nerve roots, the first leaving the canal between the occiput and the atlas, where there is no disc. Therefore, a disc herniation at a particular level will compress the nerve root immediately below it; e.g., a sixth cervical disc will compress a seventh cervical nerve root. Lesions of the sixth cervical nerve produce pain and paresthesia over the radial aspect of the forearm, thumb, and index finger. There is wasting, weakness, and loss of biceps reflex. Involvement of the seventh cervical nerve root will produce pain and paresthesia referred to the dorsal aspect of the forearm and wrist and to one or all of the three middle fingers. On the left side, involvement of the seventh cervical nerve root frequently produces chest pain, which may be misdiagnosed as a coronary thrombosis.

The pain has the usual persistent aching quality associated with nerve root compression, lasting from weeks to months. Attacks tend to recur, and the intervals of relief become shortened until the pain in the upper limb becomes intractable. However, in general, the root symptoms are of a subacute or chronic nature, permitting the patient to carry on with mild restricted activity in spite of some persistent paresthesia of the fingers.

The mode of production of symptoms by nerve compression, as described by Frykholm, has been referred to. Nerve root compression results in pain in the myotome, sclerotome, and dermatome with a wide and diffuse distribution proximally but a more narrow and more localized radiation distally.

There is usually a reduction of mobility in the cervical spine in both lateral and anteroposterior flexion, but any limitation in extension tends to be obscured by free movement of the head at the atlantoaxooccipital articulations. However, even in the presence of marked neurologic signs, cervical movements may sometimes be quite unrestricted.

The compression test of steady downward pressure on the vertex of the skull or forehead from behind with flexion and extension toward the affected side will often produce severe radicular pain, whereas suspension of the head may relieve the pain. Localized tenderness in muscle at the affected level is common, as is tenderness in areas of the shoulder girdle and the upper limb secondary to localized muscle spasm caused by anterior rami irritation.

Neurologic signs such as selective wasting of muscles, reduction or abolition of deep tendon reflexes, e.g., the biceps, triceps, or brachioradialis, and sensory changes in an area of dermatome distribution may be present.

Radiologic examination will reveal absence of the normal cervical lordosis and narrowing of the involved intervertebral space. Oblique views of the cervical spine may reveal narrowing of the anteroposterior diameter of the intervertebral foramina by osteophytes or by osteoarthritic changes of the lateral articulations.

In uncomplicated nerve root compression, examination of the cerebrospinal fluid and/or myelography are usually unnecessary. However, myelography may show a partial block, and the protein content of the cerebrospinal fluid may be increased.

Cervical Myelopathy

This condition will present as weakness and spasticity in one or both legs, with associated exaggerated reflexes and an extensor plantar response. Sensory changes in the legs and trunk are less common and usually are paresthesias, patchy in distribution and rarely with a sharp upper level. In the upper limbs a more complex picture may result from the relative balance of spinal cord versus peripheral nerve root involvement. There may be weakness and wasting, which may be limited to a single root distribution or confined to the small muscles of the hand on one side or both or may be generalized throughout the arm with fasciculation.

Sphincter disturbances occur in about a third of the patients but are not severe and consist mainly of hesitancy or urgency of micturition. Incontinence is unusual.

ETIOLOGY. Simple compression of the spinal cord and its fibers is not the only mechanism responsible for neurologic signs in cervical myelopathy. A purely mechanical cause in the nature of a tethering effect of the dentate ligament which, in preventing backward displacement of the cord, compresses the pyramidal fibers lying beneath its attachments against the osteophyte has been suggested. O'Connell believed that the myelopathy did not result from any sustained compression of the nerve tissues but rather from compression by the discs of the anterior spinal arteries during movement, particularly between C_5-C_6, and C_6-C_7. Changes in the vascular supply also have been implicated, since demyelination is greatest in the territory of supply of the anterior spinal artery and its branches.

Most probably the cause of cord damage is interference with the blood flow in the anterior spinal artery and branches brought about either by intermittent compression or by frictional injuries of the vessel during neck movement.

DIFFERENTIAL DIAGNOSIS OF CERVICAL COMPRESSION OR IRRITATIVE LESIONS. Spinal Cord Tumors and Syringomyelia. In the former, absence of trauma in the history, a slow progressive course, negative clinical tests and radiographs for protrusion, and finally a positive myelogram will aid diagnosis.

In syringomyelia, there is segmental sensory loss over the neck, shoulders, and arms, amyotrophy, and thoracic scoliosis. Symptoms usually begin in late childhood, adolescence, or adult life and progress irregularly, being arrested for long periods of time.

Osteoarthritis of the Cervical Spine. This occurs in middle age groups and affects the spine over more than one segment. It has a slow, episodic, chronic course, with stiffness and sometimes diffuse tenderness on palpation of the cervical spine. Irritative symptoms are sometimes present, but objective neurologic signs from root compression as a rule are absent. X-rays, apart from the usual features of osteoarthritis, may show osteophytes adjacent to the vertebral foramina giving rise to radicular pain and paresthesias.

Direct Injury Producing Laminar Fractures. There is a history of trauma. At times only exploration will establish the diagnosis if the radiographs are negative.

Thoracic Inlet Syndrome. Cervical Rib. The rudimentary rib, although usually symptomless, may affect the lowest trunk of the plexus composed of C_8 and T_1 nerve roots. The course is gradual, without remissions or exacerbations. Motor signs usually involve the median or ulnar nerves, and sensory findings are within the C_8 dermatome. Vasomotor symptoms may be present.

Scalenus Anticus Syndrome. This is due to an abnormal insertion and can simulate the above findings.

Pancoast Tumor (Superior Pulmonary Sulcus Tumor). This is an unusual involvement of the apex of the lung parenchyma in the supraclavicular area by a pleomorphic adenocarcinoma. Radicular pain into one of the extremities, paresthesias, and sensory loss involving the dermatomes of C_5 and C_6 in the forearm and hand or of the C_8 and

T_1 roots are seen. Horner's syndrome of the eye with ptosis and constriction of the pupil may be produced by involvement of the sympathetic inferior cervical ganglion. On radiography, the tumor may be seen as an opacity in the apical area with or without destruction of the ribs, particularly the second thoracic rib, or of the vertebral column itself.

TREATMENT OF THE CERVICAL COMPRESSION SYNDROME. In the most acute case, particularly if the pain persists for more than a few weeks, strict recumbency and immobilization of the neck in cervical traction are indicated with adequate sedation and physiotherapy. Once the pain has subsided and in less severe attacks, the patient may be placed in a cervical collar during the period of the spasm.

Active resistance exercises should be carried out to elongate the soft tissues within their normal range and reduce periarticular fibrous contracture. The accompanying increased circulation to the deep neck tissues improves flexibility, muscle tone, and neck posture.

If there is progression of the neurologic deficit or cord structure compression, surgical intervention is indicated.

Occasionally it may be found that a lateral protrusion produces symptoms of cord compression due to interference with the vascular supply of a segment of the cord. In cases with a more centrally situated lesion, laminectomy is necessary, and, to facilitate the safe retraction of the cord in its coverings, mobilization of the cord by division of several slips of denticulate ligament is advisable prior to removal of the herniation.

Fusion of the spine may be required, particularly if an extensive laminectomy has been necessary. Smith and Robinson have noted that when symptoms are bilateral, disc removal and fusion of the cervical spine by the anterior approach are indicated. This procedure produces less morbidity and less disturbance of the spinal cord than the posterior exposure.

However, Campbell and Phillips, as a result of experience with 60 cases of myelopathy of the spinal cord or radiculitis due to cervical intervertebral disc lesions and spondylosis, believe that brachial neuritis and true disc prolapse with cord compression have a good prognosis. They recommend the use of a light Minerva plastic jacket with both chest and back pieces extending up to form a head halter.

Low Back Pain

Low back pain has a multiplicity of causes, and although few of them result in mortality, this complaint is associated with high morbidity, great inconvenience, and severe economic burden. "Low back syndrome" refers to a disease or injury of the lumbosacral spine with or without an underlying predisposing condition. The condition may be acute, producing a temporary or permanent change in the physical state of the individual, or may be a chronic condition exhibiting variable degrees of frequency, duration of symptoms, and degrees of physical deterioration.

Rowe described the varying conditions which can produce the low back syndrome. These are presented in Table

Table 43-2. CAUSES OF LOW BACK PAIN

A. Structural defects
  1. Segmentation defects
    a. Six lumbar vertebrae
    b. Four lumbar vertebrae
    c. Transitional lumbosacral junction
  2. Ossification defects
    a. Spina bifida
    b. Spondylolysis
    c. Spondylolisthesis
  3. Facet abnormalities
    a. Asymmetry (tropism)
    b. Anteroposterior lumbosacral facets
  4. Increased lumbosacral angle
B. Functional defects
  1. Lateral imbalance (leg-length discrepancy, scoliosis, work or postural attitudes, etc.)
  2. Anteroposterior imbalance (pregnancy, potbelly, flexion contracture of hips and knees, etc.)
C. Infections
  1. Bone and joint
    a. Arthritis
    b. Tuberculosis
    c. Brucellosis
    d. Osteomyelitis
  2. Soft tissue
    a. "Myositis"
    b. "Fibrositis"
D. Degenerative processes
  1. Osteoarthritis
  2. Senile osteoporosis
  3. Degenerative disc disease
E. Neoplastic processes
  1. Primary
    a. Multiple myeloma
    b. Hemangioma
    c. Giant cell tumor, eosinophilic granuloma, osteogenic sarcoma
  2. Metastatic
    a. Prostate and breast
    b. Lung, kidney, thyroid, gastrointestinal tract
F. Traumatic
  1. Compression fracture
  2. Vertebral process fracture (facet, transverse, and spinous process)
  3. Sprain and strain
  4. Ruptured disc

SOURCE: From M. L. Rowe, *J Occup Med*, 2:219, 1960.

43-2, which does not include lumbosacral pain consequent to visceral disease or psychosomatic disorder.

The low back syndrome usually occurs in the third, fourth, or fifth decades of life as an acute low back pain associated with muscle spasm. The pain may be aggravated by coughing, sneezing, defecation, or any other maneuver which raises the intrathecal pressure, but it is rarely of true radicular nature and is usually relieved by lying down with the knees flexed.

On examination, there may be tenderness in the lumbosacral angle or of the spinous processes and interspinous ligaments. There is frequently limitation of vertebral movement with or without spasm of the paravertebral muscles, and very occasionally nerve root involvement may be found. Radiologic examination may show narrowing of the L_4, L_5, or S_1 disc spaces with some associated lumbar spondylosis or posterior facet joint subluxation (Fig. 43-5). However, radiographic evidence of such underlying lesions should not be taken as necessarily indicative of the causative pathologic condition. Rumbold noted that routine preemployment x-rays of the lumbar spine of 1,000 consecutive applicants for work revealed specific conditions such as narrowing of the intervertebral disc or acute lumbosacral angles in 660 of the individuals. Similarly, Splithoff compared the radiographs of the lumbosacral spines of 100 so-called "normal" people with 100 patients complaining of "backache." He found that such conditions as spina bifida, spondylosis, and osteoarthritis occurred just as frequently in the "normal" as in the "backache" group.

ETIOLOGIC FACTORS. Rowe has emphasized the concept of degenerative disc disease as an etiologic factor in the low back syndrome. During the normal aging process, the mechanical stresses in the lumbar spine fall primarily on the posterior aspect of the annulus fibrosus, particularly at L_4 and L_5, so that multiple, though minor, traumas produce gradual loss of disc material. This may result in irritation of the adjacent nerve roots to give the clinical manifestations of a "lumbosacral strain," "lumbago," "myositis," or "sacroiliac strain." Narrowing of the intervertebral space may progress so that the intervertebral foramen becomes smaller and distorted, and spondylosis or even a reverse spondylolisthesis may occur with further narrowing of this intervertebral foramen. Involvement of the nerve root results in a pain-spasm reflex, which may produce some degree of ischemia of muscle tissue and further pain.

Another condition contributing to the low back syndrome was described by Morgan and King, namely, instability in the anteroposterior plane of the adjacent vertebrae, during flexion and extension, presumably due to incomplete tears of the posterior aspects of the annulus fibrosus. This may produce severe low back pain with pain radiating down the thighs, but not of a truly radicular nature. Morgan and King believe that this condition of an "unstable back" makes up nearly 30 percent of all cases of low back pain in the middle age range. They advise educating the patient to avoid forward flexion and lifting strains, and exclusion of other pathologic causes.

CLINICAL HISTORY. In evaluating the clinical history of low back pain, it is important to assess the type of pain, its site, whether it is referred, its duration, its mode of onset, its relationship to activity and to rest, and its association with symptoms relevant to other systems such as the genitourinary, gynecologic, and alimentary organs.

In disease processes such as neoplasm, tuberculosis, and various types of osteomyelitis of the spine, the pain is usually severe, localized, and not relieved by rest. In mechanical lesions, rest usually relieves the pain, except in the presence of severe root irritation. Diurnal variation of the pain and associated stiffness are important. Ankylosing spondylitis is characterized by early morning pain, relieved as activity increases. Pain due to intervertebral disc lesions or lumbar spondylosis is usually relieved by bed rest and aggravated by activity.

CLINICAL EXAMINATION. First, the patient is examined standing; posture, weight, muscular development, the state

A   *B*

Fig. 43-5. Narrowing of lumbar disc space with a reversed spondylosis and deformation of the peripheral nerve. (*After Rowe, 1960. Taken with permission from Mercer and Duthie [eds.], "Orthopaedic Surgery," Edward Arnold [Publishers] Ltd., London, 1972.*)

of lumbar lordotic curve, and the presence of any structural or "discogenic" scoliosis are noted (Fig. 43-6). Ranges of flexion, extension, and lateral flexion of the lumbar spine are determined, especially if there is restriction because of spasm or pain.

The patient is then examined supine. The abdomen is palpated for any mass or tenderness. Particular attention is paid to the presence or absence of peripheral pulses. Joints of the lower limbs are put through the range of movement, and then the straight-leg-raising test is carried out. In this test the patient's straight leg is flexed at the hip and can, under normal circumstances, be lifted to almost 90° depending on the tightness of the hamstrings. Limitation of this movement is usually present in low back pain and sciatica. When dorsiflexion of the foot (Bragard's test) is superimposed upon straight-leg raising, the pull on

Fig. 43-6. Exaggeration of a "discogenic" scoliosis (left) by forward flexion (right) which is restricted in range. (*Taken with permission from Mercer and Duthie [eds.], "Orthopaedic Surgery," Edward Arnold [Publishers] Ltd., London, 1972.*)

the sciatic produces sciatic pain. With straight-leg raising, there is a 4-mm excursion of the L_4, L_5, S_1, and S_2 nerve roots within the intervertebral foramen. This is restricted by adhesion formation, by tumor, or by prolapse of an intervertebral disc.

Finally, a comprehensive neurologic examination is carried out, with assessment of the reflexes, the presence of sensation, and motor power.

A rectal and prostatic examination of the male and a gynecologic examination of the female are essential.

ANCILLARY TESTS. Anteroposterior, lateral, and oblique views of the lumbosacral spine including cone views of the lumbosacral junction are necessary in a patient complaining of back pain. In certain circumstances, it is necessary to carry out detailed examinations of the urine, the blood, and cerebrospinal fluid, and a Wassermann test.

TREATMENT OF LOW BACK SYNDROME. The treatment of low back syndrome should be essentially conservative, with adequate bed rest in a low Fowler position, sedation, and some type of superficial heat to relieve the muscle spasm. Some authorities believe that when the pain improves, knee-to-chest flexion exercises or lumbar flexion and hanging exercises and, in some cases, the restriction of back movements by the use of a corset or brace will help both to relieve symptoms and to prevent recurrence.

SPONDYLOLISTHESIS AND SPONDYLOLYSIS

The term "spondylolisthesis" was first used by Kilian in 1853 and is derived from the Greek word *olisthesis,* meaning a "slipping" or a "falling," and is used to describe the condition of forward subluxation of one vertebral body upon another. The condition is not limited to any specific segment of the vertebral column, but most commonly the term refers to displacement of the fifth lumbar vertebra on the body of the first sacral vertebra. The term "spondylolysis" is used to describe a bony defect of the neural arch, a condition which is felt to be one of the predisposing factors in the production of spondylolisthesis.

There is some evidence that this condition is genetically inherited with an increased penetrance caused by inbreed-

Fig. 43-7. *A.* Normal lumbosacral vertebrae. *B.* Defect at the pars interarticularis with forward slip of the body of the fifth lumbar vertebra upon the sacrum. This is particularly seen on aligning the posterior surface of the bodies of the fifth lumbar and first sacral vertebrae.

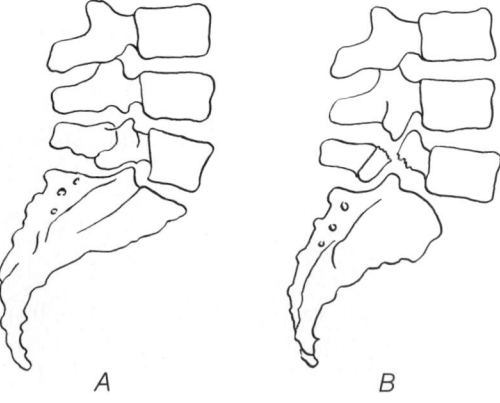

A   *B*

ing. Baker and McHolick examined the x-rays of the lumbosacral region of 400 school children between the ages of six and seven and found an incidence of arch defect in 4.5 percent. Upon examination of the parents of these children it was found that the incidences of arch defect was 27.6 percent, which is more than five times greater than the incidence in the general population.

The incidence obviously varies throughout the world and is higher in certain races or occupations. Roche and Rowe, in an extensive study of 4,000 skeletons, found that white and Negro incidences varied as follows:

White   male : female :: 6.4 : 2.3 percent
Negro   male : female :: 2.8 : 2.3 percent

Stewart described an incidence of 50 percent in the Alaskan Eskimos, a finding which may result from inbreeding.

PATHOLOGY. Spondylolisthesis usually results from a structural defect in the fifth lumbar vertebra, the defective vertebra being divided into two separate parts by a deep bilateral defect in the pars interarticularis of the neural arch. The anterior segment of the vertebra is composed of the body, pedicles, transverse processes, and superior articular facets, while the posterior fragment includes the spinous process, the laminae, and the inferior articular facets (Fig. 43-7).

There is no certainty as to the manner by which the defect develops, although it does not appear to be congenital. None of the series of examinations carried out upon the spines of the newborn has yet yielded a single example of spondylolisthesis or any defect in normal ossification. There are three primary centers of ossification for a vertebra, i.e., one for the body and one for each half of the neural arch from the point where the base of the pedicle is attached to the vertebral body to the tip of the spinous process. Each lateral center forms a pedicle, superior articular facets, pars interarticularis, inferior articular facets, laminae, and half the spinous process.

Wiltse described the etiology of spondylolisthesis as resulting from a defect in the pars interarticularis due to:

1. An inherited dysplasia in the cartilaginous arch of the affected vertebra.
2. The physical forces resulting from the erect position and the curvature of the lumbar spine acting on a weakened pars interarticularis. He believes that bone reabsorption results rather than any new bone formation defect. In his series, the condition was never present at birth and seldom present below the age of four, and the greatest incidence of slipping was seen between the ages of ten and fifteen years.

Spondylolysis, however, is not the only cause of spondylolisthesis, which can occur in the absence of any defect of the neural arch. Newman has described the following types of spondylolisthesis:

1. Infantile spondylolisthesis
   a. Facet deficiency or subluxation
   b. Attenuation of the pars interarticularis
   c. Loss of continuity of the pars interarticularis (spondylolysis)
2. Adult spondylolisthesis
   a. Stress fracture in mature bone
   b. Facet deficiency due to degenerative joint disease

CLINICAL MANIFESTATIONS. In children the condition is usually painless, although the parents may notice an unduly prominent abdomen and buttock. In adolescents and adults, backache may be the presenting symptom. It is usually intermittent, coming on after exercise or strain, and in some cases there may be sciatica as a consequence of root pressure. There are two mechanisms for this root pressure: the first occurs when the displacement of the intervertebral body is marked, producing distortion and narrowing of the intervertebral foramina with root pressure; the second mechanism, producing first sacral root pressure, is the result of a protrusion of the disc or pressure by an irregular osteophytic margin about the defect in the neural arch. Probably the most commonly experienced pain is that which arises in the disc adjacent to the unstable vertebrae as a consequence of altered spine mechanics and increased forces on the disc.

Spondylolisthesis can be completely asymptomatic and may be found during examination for other complaints. It would be difficult otherwise to explain the discrepancy between the 5 percent incidence of the defect in adult skeletons in anatomic museums and the much smaller numbers of the general population who present for treatment. Many patients first appear for treatment in the middle or late decades of life, but they have probably had the defect since early childhood.

Spondylolisthesis may be seen as a characteristic deformity which is the result of forward displacement of the involved vertebra and the vertebrae above. The spinous process above forms a "step" kyphosis in contrast to the "angular" kyphosis of tuberculous disease.

The pelvis is rotated about a transverse axis passing through the hip joints so that the anterosuperior iliac spines are raised to the same level as the posterosuperior iliac spines. This rotation may be so great that the thighs are not in a straight line with the trunk even when they are fully extended. Consequently the patient must stand with his trunk thrust forward if the legs are vertical or with the hips and knees flexed if the trunk is held erect. As the trunk is shortened by the downward displacement accompanying the forward slip, the ribs overlap or approach the iliac crest, and transverse creases appear above the waist.

RADIOLOGIC DIAGNOSIS. In the early stages of disease, especially in cases of simple spondylolysis, a simple translucency may be seen in the pars interarticularis. The lateral radiograph will show the presence of any spondylolisthesis (Fig. 43-8), but doubtful cases are best shown by an oblique view of the pars interarticularis. Under normal circumstances the pars interarticularis and the superior articular facet forms the outline of a "Scottish terrier." In the condition of spondylolysis without slip, the terrier is seen to wear a collar of translucency as compared with the rest of the bone, whereas in spondylolisthesis, when there has been movement forward of the superior articular facet, the terrier is seen to be decapitated.

TREATMENT. The surgical treatment of spondylolisthesis consists of fixing the involved segment by bony fusion, but this is a major undertaking. Therefore, consideration must be given to the age, sex of the patient, severity of the

Fig. 43-8. Radiograph showing a spondylolisthesis of the fifth lumbar upon the first sacral vertebra, with an obvious defect in the pars interarticularis.

deformity, and physical occupation of the individual as well as the severity of his symptoms.

Younger patients are best treated by lumbosacral fusion, but in older people this approach is open to question. A successful fusion will relieve them of all their symptoms, but because the operation is a major one, these patients are probably best treated by the use of spinal brace or corset, combined with sleeping on a firm mattress.

The actual method of lumbosacral fusion is still controversial. Ideally the fusion should be a posterior or posterolateral one uniting the spinous processes, laminas, and transverse processes of the involved vertebrae to the normal vertebrae above and below. Other types of fusion such as anterior, transperitoneal, extraperitoneal, and posterior interbody fusions have been used, but these operations have limited application.

SCIATICA

Sciatica is a symptom and not a disease. It is a term used to describe pain of a radicular nature occurring in one or both lower limbs consequent to inflammation or pressure on one or more nerve roots involved in the formation of the lumbosacral plexus.

Causes of Sciatica

A. Nerve root compression
　1. Intraspinal compression. This may be due to a prolapsed intervertebral disc, an intraspinal tumor, or an intraspinal abscess.
　2. Compression within the intervertebral foramen. This may arise through a tumor of the nerve roots, such as neurofibroma, or a narrowing of the foramen due to a spondylolisthesis, spondylosis, or osteoarthritis of the posterior apophyseal joints.
　3. Compression within the pelvis or buttock. This may arise as a result of intrapelvic or gluteal abscess, or a tumor in one or the other of these sites.
B. Inflammation of nerve and nerve roots
　1. Toxic
　　a. Alcoholism
　　b. Diabetic neuritis
　　c. Arsenical poisoning
　　d. Lead poisoning
　2. "Infective"
　　a. Focal sepsis
　　b. Rheumatism
　　c. Syphilis

Of all the causes of sciatica listed above intervertebral disc protrusion is by far the most common.

LUMBAR AND INTERVERTEBRAL DISC PROTRUSION

ANATOMY. Intervertebral discs, which unite the bodies of successive vertebras from the second cervical vertebra to the sacrum, form a series of amphiarthrotic, or slightly movable, joints with no synovial cavity. Structurally, intervertebral discs consist of three parts: the cartilage end plate, the annulus fibrosus, and the nucleus pulposus.

The cartilaginous end plate is a thin layer of hyaline cartilage adherent to the trabeculae of cancellous bone comprising the major portion of the vertebral body.

Nucleus Pulposus. The nucleus pulposus comprises the central portion of the intervertebral disc; it is a soft, semifluid mass containing over 80 percent water by weight, the water being bound to mucopolysaccharides as in myxoid tissue. Because it contains so much water, the nucleus is virtually incompressible and inelastic, although subject to a great range of changing pressures.

Annulus Fibrosus. Surrounding the nucleus pulposus is the annulus fibrosus, comprised of laminas, fibrocartilage, and fibrous tissue, and containing more cells, a greater abundance of collagen, and a lesser amount of mucopolysaccharide ground substance than the nucleus. The annulus is somewhat elastic; it bends with the overlying spinal ligaments, its fibers running obliquely from vertebra to vertebra, continuous with the fibrils in the cartilaginous end plates and ossified epiphyseal rings in the vertebral bodies. The function of the annulus fibrosus would appear to be twofold: to restrict and regulate movements of the vertebral column and to enclose and retain the nucleus pulposus.

The two components of the intervertebral discs, the annulus fibrosus and the nucleus pulposus, are avascular except for the most peripheral fibers of the annulus, which receive a small blood supply from adjacent vessels. The nutrition of the intervertebral disc therefore would appear to be dependent on the diffusion of fluid into it from the vertebral bodies and the vessels of the peripheral portion of the annulus.

With respect to nerve supply, fine unmyelinated nerve fibers have been found in the posterior longitudinal ligament and a lesser number in the annulus fibrosus. None are in the nucleus pulposus. The ligamentous and articular structures of the vertebral column have a considerable sensory innervation from the nervus sinuvertebralis of Luschka.

MECHANISM OF HERNIATIONS AND PROTRUSIONS OF THE INTERVERTEBRAL DISC. With aging, the collagen increases and becomes coarser. The mucopolysaccharides decrease, with the ratio of karatan sulfate to chondroitin sulfate increasing. The proteoglycans become smaller in molecular size and more firmly adherent to the collagen fibrils. The elasticity, viscosity, and water-binding capacity of the ground substance decrease. The proportion of water decreases from 90 percent in childhood to less than 70 percent in old age.

The nucleus is constantly under compression, and the turgid nucleus of a living person, bounded laterally by the strong elastic laminas of the annulus and vertically by the cartilaginous end plate, may burst through either one of these barriers. Spontaneous herniation of an intervertebral disc may take place either vertically into the spongiosa of the vertebral body or horizontally. Prolapse of nuclear substance can take place only when the nucleus retains its turgescence. This cannot occur in older people whose nuclei pulposi have undergone desiccation.

Vertical prolapse of an intervertebral disc into the vertebral bodies produces the phenomenon known as "Schmorl's nodes." It cannot be detected radiologically until it becomes outlined by a shell of reactive bone. It is of no clinical importance.

On the other hand, horizontal prolapse is of considerable clinical importance. Two forms of horizontal prolapse may occur, namely, nuclear herniation and annular protrusion (Fig. 43-9). In nuclear herniation the nucleus usually displaces posteriorly, but in annular prolapse there is convex bulging of the relaxed annulus fibers in all directions.

Posterior herniation of the nucleus pulposus is seldom accompanied by any gross breach of the annulus, and the semifluid material seems to escape by dissecting its way through the annulus. Most of these posterior herniations lie to one side of the midline, because the posterior longitudinal ligament prevents direct posterior herniation. Consequently, neurologic symptoms caused by direct pressure on the neural tissues tend to be unilateral.

Annular protrusions follow the narrowing of the disc space resulting from desiccation or vertebral prolapse of the nucleus, and the relaxed annulus fibers are squeezed outward. It is these anterolateral protrusions of the fibers of the annulus that account for the common and well-known form of osteophytosis or spondylosis of the vertebral column.

PATHOLOGY OF NUCLEAR PROTRUSIONS. As stated

above, the most common site for posterior herniation of nuclear material is posterolateral. This herniation may enlarge and may impinge on neighboring nerve roots, producing symptoms and signs similar to any other space-occupying lesion in the intraspinal canal. There may be irritation of the nerve root by compression, by stretching, or by friction, an occlusion of its vasa nervorum, or a combination of all these factors. The compressed nerve root becomes edematous, enlarged, and later adherent to the protrusion.

A nerve root may be stretched tautly over a nuclear protrusion in close proximity to the ligamentum flavum. On straight-leg raising there is an excursion of 4 mm of spinal roots at L_4–L_5 and S_1–S_2. Therefore any pressure from a nuclear protrusion on such a nerve root will interfere with its range of movement. This is the basis of the restricted straight-leg raising test. Of course, if the pressure is severe and prolonged, impairment of axonal conductivity will occur in the nerve root, producing symptoms and signs of motor and sensory loss in the lower limb.

CLINICAL MANIFESTATIONS. Fifty percent of cases of intervertebral disc protrusion present initially as low backache followed later by radicular sciatic pain, whereas about one-third of patients may give a history of sciatica preceding the backache and in the remainder sciatica and backache commence simultaneously.

The onset may be acute following a minor degree of trauma such as a fall in the sitting position or the lifting of a heavy weight in the stooping position, but in many cases there is absolutely no evidence of any traumatic incident. In some cases the first attack may be the most severe one, followed by a series of perhaps minor but annoying exacerbations, but in others the reverse sequence of presentation may be the case. The reason for spontaneous remissions in this condition is not clearly understood, but they may occur by degeneration of compressed nerve fibers and the adjustment of the nerve root to its displaced position. Again, there may be diminution of the swelling associated with the herniation and reduction of edema of the nerve root.

Characteristically the pain of sciatica is usually described as a "dull ache," "like a toothache," a "dragging" pain, or a "shooting" pain radiating from the lower lumbar region to the buttock and farther distally into the lower limb. It is important to assess the actual distribution of pain, since it is referred to the dermatome of the involved nerve root and is a valuable method of localizing the site of the occlusion.

It is most important also to ask the patient whether there is any loss of sensation or motor power. It is quite common to find that there is subjective loss of motor power when no such loss is detectable on clinical examination. Inquiry as to urgency or frequency of micturition is most important, since this is an early sign of the rare but serious condition of central protrusion which embarrasses the cauda equina.

The patient is usually an adult male found to be in relatively good health, and in the majority of cases urine examination and rectal examination will be completely normal. It is essential never to omit a general examination

Fig. 43-9. Posterolateral herniation, or prolapse, with deformation of the peripheral nerve. (*Taken with permission from Mercer and Duthie [eds.], "Orthopaedic Surgery," Edward Arnold [Publishers] Ltd., London, 1972.*)

of the patient, however, because back pain and sciatica can have sinister significance.

Examination of the patient is first carried out with the patient standing and undressed. Special note is taken of the presence of any alterations of the spinal curvature with respect to both lumbar lordosis and the presence of any discogenic scoliosis, and then movements of flexion, extension, and lateral flexion to either side are assessed. Where these initially appear to be normal, attention should be paid to the rhythm of flexion and extension of the lumbar spine. It is also important to make sure that what appears to be relatively normal lateral flexion on one side or the other is actually being carried out at the lumbar spine and not at the thoracolumbar junction.

The patient is then asked to assume the supine position, and attention paid to the degree of difficulty he has in mounting the couch. With the patient in the supine position the abdomen can be palpated and the range of movement of the hips and knees examined.

The effects of straight-leg raising or the possible presence of a positive Lasègue sign is then assessed. In the presence of a protrusion, the straight-leg-raising test will aggravate the pain and may actually aggravate the radiation to the extremity. The greater the restriction of straight-leg raising, the larger the protrusion. Such symptoms are aggravated in the straight-leg-raising position by forced dorsiflexion of the foot and then are known as Lasègue's sign.

Finally, a neurologic assessment with respect to reflexes, motor power, and sensation is carried out on the lower limbs. Impairment of sensation may be found along the dermatome of the nerve root involved, especially along the outer thigh, the calf, and the foot. Examination for motor power may reveal weakness of the long extensor or flexor of the great toe and occasionally of the gluteal muscles, where of course the symptom must be assessed with the patient in the prone position. In the presence of a severe protrusion at the L_5 S_1 disc space the ankle jerk may well be diminished. The absence of a knee jerk indicates a higher prolapse than usual.

SPECIAL EXAMINATIONS. Radiography. Anteroposterior and lateral views of the lumbosacral spine and similar cone views of the lumbosacral junction are taken routinely. The major purpose of these x-rays is to exclude diseases of a more sinister nature. They also help to assess the possible presence of discogenic scoliosis and the state of the intervertebral discs (Fig. 43-10). The lumbar disc spaces normally show progressive widening in a caudal direction, the space between L_2 and L_3 being wider than the one above. The lateral view may show diminished disc spaces, but a normal space does not always exclude a small disc protrusion at this level.

Myelography. Myelography is a valuable additional radiologic investigation to exclude other conditions and to help

Fig. 43-10. Lateral radiograph of lumbar spine to show narrowing of the disc space between L_4 and L_5 due to a disc prolapse.

localize the site of the intervertebral disc protrusion (Fig. 43-11). It is especially valuable where the diagnosis is in doubt, as in the presence of an intraspinal tumor. But it is not always necessary as a preliminary to operative removal of the disc protrusion, because neurologic assessment of the level of the herniation, even without myelography, is highly reliable.

Three methods of myelography are available, namely, gas, water-soluble medium, and oily contrast medium.

Since the process of myelography involves lumbar puncture, the opportunity should be taken to test the dynamics of the cerebrospinal fluid as well as to obtain a specimen for biochemical assessment.

DIFFERENTIAL DIAGNOSIS. Although most cases of backache and sciatica are a result of a prolapsed intervertebral disc, it is most important in all cases to exclude the possibility of tuberculosis or tumors of the vertebral column, meninges, or nerve roots, and especially secondary deposits.

In a prolapsed intervertebral disc the complaint is usually episodic, whereas in most other conditions of tumor or infection the symptoms and signs tend to be constant and progressive. When a case of herniated intervertebral disc is examined, the patient is obviously well, whereas in more serious conditions he may be obviously ill or cachectic and the limitation of back movement is usually far more restricted than in an intervertebral disc lesion.

On radiologic examination tuberculous foci and primary or secondary deposits in the vertebral bodies are easily detectable, and other conditions such as spondylolisthesis, spondylosis, or old fractures are also clearly seen. In cases of doubt, myelography should be performed as indicated above.

TREATMENT. Conservative Treatment. With few exceptions conservative treatment is recommended initially in all cases of prolapsed intervertebral discs; in about 80 percent of cases this may effect complete and permanent relief.

The ideal method of instituting conservative treatment is to advise strict recumbency for a period of at least 3 weeks, and if the attack is severe, up to 6 weeks. This forced bed rest should be accompanied by adequate sedation, simple analgesics, and the use of heat. When the symptoms have subsided to some degree, and in some cases as a primary method of treatment, immobilization of the lumbar spine in a plaster jacket which permits the patient to remain mobile is useful. Recurrence of the intervertebral disc protrusion may be prevented by instructing the patient to avoid stooping and lifting as far as possible. A Knight back brace or a lumbosacral corset is of value in limiting motion of the lumbosacral spine, decreasing lordosis and providing counter pressure for the abdominal wall when abdominal muscles are weak. Patients are instructed in Williams' exercises to strengthen the lumbar spine flexors, especially the abdominal muscles and the gluteus maximus.

Surgical Treatment. Operative removal of a herniated intervertebral disc is indicated if the attacks are severe, disabling, frequent, or persisting in spite of a well-planned conservative regimen of treatment. In a few cases, a sudden paraplegia or very severe nerve root compression with paralysis or paresis of muscle groups demands an emergency operation.

The operative procedure for removal of the herniated nucleus pulposus is one of laminectomy in which a small portion of the lamina and ligamentum flavum is removed at the site of the protrusion, the embarrassed nerve root retracted, and the prolapsed and herniating nucleus material removed. Concomitant spinal fusion is necessary only if there has been an extensive laminectomy, if there is associated degenerative disease of the intervertebral column or a congenital malformation, or when the patient is to return to very heavy manual labor.

DISORDERS OF THE LUMBOSACRAL JUNCTION

The lumbosacral junction is an unstable anatomic region because:

1. It is the junction of mobile and fixed portions of the vertebral column.
2. It is more suited to the quadriped position and is a disadvantage in the upright position of man.
3. It is the site of rotary movements which are often asymmetrical.
4. It is the site of great shearing strains.

Lumbosacral Strain

Lumbosacral strain occurs in both acute and chronic forms.

ACUTE. Acute lumbosacral strain may be precipitated by a sudden blow or fall which forces the joints of the lumbosacral region into positions beyond their normal range of movement. In such cases there may be severe pain in the back and occasionally root pressure, sciatic pain, and a sciatic scoliosis. Most patients, however, exhibit pain and tenderness at the lumbosacral junction with restriction of movement.

CHRONIC. Chronic lumbosacral strain is usually insidious in onset but may follow an acute strain which has been unrecognized or unsatisfactorily treated. The middle-aged woman with an obese abdomen and the tall, asthenic individual with poor musculature are both at risk. In the chronic cases symptoms vary from complaints of a "weak back," tiring easily, to others with very acute pain and real disability, although episodic in nature.

TREATMENT. Rest in bed for a period of 1 to 3 weeks is indicated, and as the symptoms subside, spinal and postural exercises are introduced. For those with chronic pain and particularly those with pendulous abdomens or poor musculature a lumbosacral support is advisable.

"Sprung Back"

"Sprung back" is a term devised by Newman to describe the syndrome of chronic low lumbar strain.

The patient is usually a female in the latter half of the second decade or in the third or fourth decade of life complaining of pain across the top of the sacrum often radiating to both buttocks and thighs as far as the knees. The pain is described as dull and nagging and becoming more severe toward the end of the day. There may be a history of a fall, a blow on the back, strain while lifting, difficulty with childbirth, or violent activity during adolescence.

Fig. 43-11. Myelograph to show the deformed outline on the side due to a disc prolapse.

Characteristically, the pain is increased by lumbar flexion exaggerated by the slouch position, sleeping on a soft mattress, bending, stooping, lifting, or leaning forward over low objects as in washing, ironing, or cooking.

Clinical examination of these patients is mainly negative, although occasionally there may be restriction of active flexion with tenderness in the midline of the lower lumbar spine. There may be some widening of the spinous processes with deficiency of the supraspinous ligament. Indeed, it has been suggested that this condition is due to rupture or strain of the posterior ligaments, including perhaps the posterior longitudinal ligament and the annulus fibrosus.

Newman has advised against any temptation to label the condition as psychogenic. Treatment should consist of reassurance and the use of palliative measures such as heat, sedation, postural exercises, and lumbosacral support.

Sacralization of the Fifth Lumbar Vertebra

The lumbosacral region is liable to developmental disorders which diminish its strength and mobility. Small imperfections in this region may cause severe low back pain and sciatica following degenerative changes.

Sacralization of the last lumbar vertebra may vary in that the transverse processes, pedicles, and inferior facets may be transformed into the lateral masses of the sacral vertebra on one side or both. When both sides are sacralized and the vertebra is completely fused to the sacrum, the sacrum is lengthened by an extra vertebra at its upper end. This type of anomaly seldom produces symptoms.

Sacralization of the last lumbar vertebra gives rise to much more trouble when it is unilateral and incomplete (Fig. 43-12). The syndesmosis attaching the sacralized portion of the fifth lumbar vertebra to the sacrum allows some asymmetrical movement with wear and tear in the lateral articulation and the intervertebral disc. The symptoms tend to develop most frequently on the side which is not sacralized, where there is greater movement and a greater susceptibility to injury.

SPINAL OSTEOARTHRITIS AND SPONDYLOSIS

Osteoarthritis is a disease of synovial diarthrodial joints such as the posterior apophyseal joints of the vertebral column. It must be distinguished from spondylosis, which depends upon degeneration of the intervertebral discs, which are amphiarthrotic, and less movable joints possessing no synovial cavity of synovial membrane. Osteoarthritis of the facette joints can occur in the absence of disc disease or in association with it. The processes of osteoarthritis and degenerative disc disease are separate but frequently may coexist in the older patient.

Fig. 43-12. Radiograph of the left side of the fifth lumbar vertebra and the sacrum, showing unilateral sacralization with sclerosis around the abnormal syndesmosis.

FIBROSITIS (LUMBAGO)

Fibrositis refers to cases of low backache in which there may be one or more tender nodules lying fairly superficially in the erector spinae or its attachments, or in the region of the muscular attachments to the crest of the ilium. Lumbago can be caused by some internal derangement of a low lumbar intervertebral joint. The pain comes on suddenly while the patient bends his back and is so severe that the lumbar region is at once immobilized by muscular spasm. After this acute phase, examination shows that lumbar extension is impossible. Treatment consists of rest in bed with heat and sedation.

TUMORS OF THE VERTEBRAL COLUMN

The vertebral column differs from other parts of the skeleton in reference to the relative incidence of various neoplastic lesions. Certain types of primary bone tumors including aneurysmal bone cysts and benign osteoblastomas predominate in the vertebral column, and one primary bone tumor, i.e., the chordoma, occurs exclusively in the axial skeleton. However, most types of primary bone tumors, including giant cell tumor, osteogenic sarcoma, chondrosarcoma, and fibrosarcoma occur less frequently in the spine than in other parts of the skeleton. Metastatic tumors commonly involve the spine and account for the majority of cases in any series of vertebral tumors in adults. Guri reported that the most common primary tumors affecting the vertebral column were multiple myeloma, fibrosarcoma, Hodgkin's disease, hemangioma, giant cell tumor, chondroma, and chondrosarcoma. In 50 cases of destruction of vertebrae by metastasis, 32 lesions were osteolytic lesions from carcinoma of the breast, 7 from carcinoma of the prostate, 3 from hypernephroma, and 1 from each of the following: Ewing's tumor, chondrosarcoma, bronchiogenic tumor, carcinoma of skin, rectum, and cervix, osteogenic sarcoma, and fibrosarcoma.

A classification of tumors of the vertebral column includes:

A. Primary tumors
   1. Malignant
      a. Myelomatosis
      b. Chordoma
      c. Giant cell tumor
      d. Ewing's tumor
      e. Chondrosarcoma
      f. Osteogenic sarcoma
      g. Fibrosarcoma
      h. Hodgkin's disease
   2. Benign
      a. Angioma
      b. Aneurysmal bone cyst
      c. Benign osteoblastoma
B. Secondary tumors
   1. Metastatic carcinoma

The symptoms produced by vertebral tumors depend upon their site, the speed of their growth, and the degree of involvement of cord and/or of nerve roots. In the early stages back pain is the most common symptom, and clinical signs may be restricted to tenderness over the area in which the disease process is present. Later, when the nerve roots or cord are involved, neurologic signs become manifest. It is important to look for signs of both upper and lower motor neuron involvement in any case in which vertebral tumor is suspected. Evidence of the *lower motor neuron* lesion is weakness or paralysis of individual muscles, decrease in muscle tone, reduction in tendon and cutaneous reflexes, which help to delineate the level of involvement, and wasting of muscle. *Upper motor neuron* disease of the pyramidal tract is characterized by loss of voluntary movement with spasticity, increased tendon reflexes, sensory changes, and an increased plantar reflex or a positive Babinski sign. The posterior columns of the posterior nerve roots or the peripheral nerve may also be involved.

Alteration of the spinal cord contents results from direct pressure on the tissues or, secondarily, because of a change in the blood supply to produce edema, hemorrhage, and degeneration. Autonomic system involvement may be evidenced by increased sweating with vasomotor and pilomotor reactions as well as a Horner syndrome when the inferior cervical ganglion is involved. The function of the sphincters must be carefully examined, since either incontinence or retention of urine or constipation or incontinence of feces may be present.

As with all bone tumors, radiologic examination and biopsy are important aids to diagnosis. Biochemical investigations are also important in recognizing myelomatosis, which has an abnormal electrophoretic pattern of the serum proteins, with a Bence Jones proteinuria. In metastatic prostatic carcinoma the serum acid phosphatase level may be elevated. Occasionally in osteoblastic lesions, such as a metastatic carcinoma of the prostate or of the lung, the serum alkaline phosphatase level may be elevated.

With circumscribed and presumably benign lesions, surgical excision is usually the treatment of choice, and this is a procedure which provides the histologic diagnosis. When, however, there is clinical uncertainty about the possibility of malignancy and when some other treatment such as radiotherapy is contemplated, elective biopsy must be undertaken in order to establish the nature of the lesion. Open surgical biopsy is the most desirable procedure, but this is not always possible, because of inaccessibility of the deep-seated vertebrae. In such cases, aspiration biopsy by the special techniques described by Ottolenghi and by Schajowicz may be used.

PYOGENIC OSTEOMYELITIS OF THE VERTEBRAL COLUMN

The most common organism responsible for this condition is *Staphylococcus aureus,* which spreads hematogenously from infective foci, such as boils, septic teeth, tonsillitis, or otitis media.

Pyogenic osteomyelitis in the vertebral column may occur at any age, but it is most common during adolescence and in young adulthood and considerably more common in males than females.

PATHOLOGY. Henson and Coventry and others have drawn attention to the urinary tract as a source of secondary spinal infection by hematogenous spread from the pelvic and abdominal viscera via the vertebral venous plexus described by Batson. However, vascular anatomy studies in relation to this condition by Wiley and Trueta indicate that although this venous plexus does exist, it is unlikely to be the route by which infection reaches the vertebrae.

The levels most commonly affected are the lumbar, thoracic, and cervical regions, in that order, and the actual site of infection is usually in the metaphyseal portion of the vertebra. It often rapidly spreads across the periphery of the disc to involve the metaphysis of the adjacent vertebra above or below, and sometimes two separate pairs of vertebrae are affected, or even three in succession. Wiley and Trueta maintain that this indicates arterial spread via ascending and descending nutrient branches of the posterior spinal arteries.

Marked collapse of the bodies with gibbus formation as in tuberculosis is quite uncommon in pyogenic vertebral osteomyelitis, as is large paravertebral abscess formation. Pus will spread along normal cleavage planes in the tissues to present in the retropharyngeal space in the cervical region, the mediastinum in the thoracic region, and the retroperitoneal space in the lumbar region with perirenal, psoas, and pelvic abscess formation. Occasionally the pus may track backward to form an epidural abscess with compression of the spinal cord.

CLINICAL MANIFESTATIONS. The acute fulminating type is most common in young patients and may be accompanied by very severe and intense toxemia. In the past the mortality rate in these cases was very high. The chronic type, which seems to be somewhat more common in the adult, usually presents as malaise, fever, and very severe spinal pain, which is aggravated by movement and not relieved by rest. Unrelieved or increasing back pain after posterior laminectomy should immediately raise the question of a disc space infection. Examination of these patients reveals marked tenderness over the spinous processes of the involved vertebrae and severe muscle spasm and rigidity of the vertebral column. If the symptoms are of long standing, an abscess may be detected, and if there has been involvement of the spinal cord, signs of partial or complete paraplegia may be evident.

It may be difficult to distinguish this condition, particularly in the subacute or chronic form, from tuberculosis. However, both in acute and chronic vertebral osteomyelitis there is a marked polymorphonuclear leukocytosis and a raised sedimentation rate. A positive blood culture is helpful both for obtaining the organism and determining its sensitivity. The staphylococcal antihemolysin titer may be elevated in osteomyelitis but is normal in tuberculosis.

RADIOLOGIC FEATURES. Radiologic evidence of the lesion may take from 10 days to 2 weeks to appear, although a small paravertebral abscess may be apparent before evidence of bony destruction. One of the earliest signs is slight haziness and loss of definition of bone structure in the end plates adjacent to the disc space. Later a more localized lesion becomes visible with destruction of adjacent vertebral bodies, new bone formation, and disc-space narrowing.

TREATMENT. This is based upon the three principles of treating bone infection, i.e., immobilization of the patient, both local and general, the use of the appropriate antibiotic, and surgical drainage of abscesses with debridement if at all possible.

Immobilization is best achieved by means of a plaster bed. Chemotherapy is selected from the results of culture of blood, urine, or pus aspirated from any localized abscess. The technique of surgical drainage varies, naturally, with the site of the abscess. In general, when surgical debridement is indicated, it is best carried out by an anterior approach to the spine with or without bone grafting.

Pain in the Chest Wall

Such pain may be referred or from local disease of the thoracic structures, i.e.,

1. In the spinal cord and its membranes from tumors or inflammation
2. In the posterior root ganglion from herpes zoster or tabes dorsalis
3. From disease of the vertebrae, such as tumor, tuberculosis, spondylolysis, osteophyte formation
4. From peripheral nerve lesions
5. From visceral disease of underlying lung, pleura, mediastinum, heart
6. Tietze's syndrome involving the costochondral junctions

DISORDERS OF MUSCLE

Anatomy

A single skeletal muscle consists of long cylindrical fibers collected together in many bundles, collections of which form the muscle as a whole. The muscle fibers are supported by fibrous connective tissue containing capillaries, nerve fibers, fibroblasts, histiocytes, and mast cells. A supporting fibrous connective tissue surrounds each individual muscle as the endomysium, from which it extends to enclose fiber bundles as the perimysium, and finally it extends to ensheathe the entire muscle to become the epimysium (Fig. 43-13).

The muscle fibers, which vary in length from 1 to 40 mm and in thickness from 50 to 100 μ, are enclosed in a structureless membrane known as the sarcolemma, which has four to eight nuclei arranged along its surface. Within

Fig. 43-13. The various parts of muscle mass, a muscle fiber, and a myofibril. (*Taken with permission from Mercer and Duthie* [eds.], *"Orthopaedic Surgery," Edward Arnold* [*Publishers*] *Ltd., London, 1972.*)

PERIMYSIUM   SARCOPLASM
EPIMYSIUM   ENDOMYSIUM   SARCOLEMMA

X 200   X 400   X 1200
MUSCLE MASS   MUSCLE FIBRE   MYOFIBRIL

the sarcolemmic membrane lie many myofibrils, 1 to 2 μ in diameter, which form the basic internal unit of the muscle fiber and which are connected together by the sarcoplasm. The sarcoplasm contains numerous inclusion bodies such as glycogen and lipid granules. It also contains reticulum which provides the connecting link for the transmission of excitation impulses from the sarcolemmic membrane to the myofibrils as well as playing some part in the electrolytic exchanges across the sarcolemmic membrane. Chemical analysis of the sarcoplasm reveals that it is made up of a myogen fraction and several enzymes, i.e., zymohexase, phosphorylase, and dehydrogenase.

Biophysics of Muscular Contraction

Striated muscle is so named because of periodic cross striations lying perpendicular to the long axis of the fibers. When viewed under magnification with ordinary transmitted light, these striations are seen to be made up of alternate bands of A, or anisotropic (birefringent), and I, or isotropic, refringency. In the center of each A band is found a slightly less refractile region named the "H band," after Henson, and in the center of the I band is a narrow line of highly refractile material, which therefore looks dark on focusing, called the "Z line" from the German *Zwischenscheibe,* meaning "between disks." The basic unit of the muscle fiber has long been regarded as that area lying between two Z lines; this is called a "sarcomere."

Interference microscopy has been used to measure the relative amount of protein present in the A and I bands of the myofibrils, which consist of two basic protein filaments, myosin and actin. The myosin is confined to the A band, whereas the actin filaments stretch from the Z line through the I band into the A band, terminating at the H zone (Fig. 43-14).

Electron microscopy has shown that these structural proteins, actin and myosin, are arranged in longitudinal filaments spaced out a few hundred angstrom units apart. The myosin filaments, 100 to 110 Å thick and about 450 Å apart, extend from one end of the A band to the other. The actin filaments are thinner, 40 to 50 Å in diameter, and stretch from the Z line to the edge of the H zone. In the A band, each of the myosin filaments is arranged hexagonally and surrounded by six actin filaments, which it shares with its nearest neighboring myosin filament. This observation suggests that striated muscle is built up of two overlapping sets of filaments.

Muscle contraction and shortening occurs as the result of filaments interdigitating, i.e., according to the sliding filament theory of Huxley, who described two interdigitating sets of filaments. His electron microscope pictures of muscle fibers at resting length, contracted, or stretched confirm that the A band remains the same width but that the H zone changes in width according to alteration of the distance between the Z lines. Hence, both the I, or actin filaments, in the A, or myosin filaments, remain at constant length. The actual change in length of the sarcomere during contraction or during applied stretch is achieved by the two filaments sliding over each other. Cross bridges attached to the myosin with active groups at their ends are thought to physically attach to sites on the actin filaments and by some type of configurational change at the cross bridges mechanically translate one type of filament along adjacent filaments of the other type. This mechanical link is thought to accompany the enzymatic splitting of ATP (adenosine triphosphate).

Definitions of Function

The following are some of the definitions used when describing muscle function:

1. A *motor unit* consists of a single motor neuron, its axon, and a group of muscle fibers innervated by this single axon.
2. A *twitch response* is a brief phasic contraction of a muscle fiber or fibers of a muscle unit resulting from a single impulse. It is followed by depolarization of these muscle fibers.
3. *Tetanus* is maximal contraction in the fibers of a motor unit resulting from a series of stimuli or summation of responses from a single stimulus.
4. An *isotonic contraction* is one in which there is shortening of the fibers of the muscle under a constant tension and work is done.
5. An *isometric contraction* is one in which there is no shortening of the muscle fibers and in which no external work is done but tension is maintained.
6. The *equilibrium length* of a muscle is the length of the relaxed muscle at which the resting tension is zero.
7. The *resting, or optimal, length* of a muscle is that length at which maximal contraction tension develops.
8. *Latency relaxation* is the period between the stimulus and the contraction.
9. *Stress relaxation* is the slow loss of tension after a muscle is suddenly stressed and placed under a constant strain. The accompanying slow lengthening is called "creep."

MECHANICAL ASPECTS OF MUSCULAR CONTRACTION. Tension is related to the length of the muscle fiber. Curve 1 in Fig. 43-15 shows the exponential development of tension in a resting muscle which is being passively stretched to increased percentages of its resting length. The resting tension develops almost immediately and is due to the sarcolemma, whereas later other components of the elastic series come into play. The peak tension which then develops is the same as the maximal isometric tetanic contraction.

For practical purposes, the equilibrium length and the optimal, or resting, length are considered the same, and in the resting state no tension is produced when the muscle is passively reduced to a shorter length. In curve 2 of Fig. 43-15 the developing tension is produced by contraction of the muscle after stretch, and the twitch response is maximal at 105 to 110 percent of equilibrium length, whereas tetany is maximal at 100 to 105 percent of optimal length. It is obvious, therefore, that the tetanic stimulation will allow better correlation with the maximum when nearest to the equilibrium length.

"Developed" tension represents the tension over and above the resting tension at a given length with one stimulus. It is dependent upon the number of sites available for cross-bridge formation and the status of elastic elements when the external load is imposed. The sum of these curves is the total tension, which is maximal at optimal length.

Fig. 43-14. Two primary protein filaments—myosin, in the A band, and actin, stretching from the Z line through the I band to terminate in the H zone. On contraction, the two filaments slide over each other. (*After Huxley. Taken with permission from Mercer and Duthie [eds.], "Orthopaedic Surgery," Edward Arnold [Publishers] Ltd., London, 1972.*)

There is a maximal length to which a muscle can be already stretched and then activated before the tension becomes zero. In maximally stretched fibers, the tension rises quite slowly, and a variant of this basic tension-length curve pattern can be demonstrated by adding the entity of an intact tendon, which introduces the phenomenon of stress relaxation and creep. As the tendon slowly lengthens, it allows a slight increase in the overlap of filaments and shows an earlier fall than that noted without tension.

Two further factors which correlate with tension and shortening are those of speed and load. Load can be compared to the tension of an isotonic contraction when the relation of force and speed of shortening is exponential. With a greater load, the muscles shorten much less and

Fig. 43-15. Relationship of tension of a muscle fiber during passive stretch (curve 1) and buildup of developing tension (curve 2) by contraction of muscle after stretch. (*Taken with permission from Mercer and Duthie [eds.], "Orthopaedic Surgery," Edward Arnold [Publishers] Ltd., London, 1972.*)

Fig. 43-16. Muscle length: comparing the speed or velocity of shortening against the load. (*Taken with permission from Mercer and Duthie [eds.], "Orthopaedic Surgery," Edward Arnold [Publishers] Ltd., London, 1972.*)

much more slowly. Of course, if a muscle were purely an elastic body, the velocity curve would be a straight line, but as seen in Fig. 43-16, the velocity is maximal with a zero load. With a load which a muscle just fails to lift and at zero velocity the maximal isometric tension is developed.

A. V. Hill has described isotonic contraction with increased load as follows:

1. There is an increased latent period equal to the time taken for the muscle to develop isometric tension equal to the isotonic load.
2. There is a decrease in maximal shortening.
3. There is a decrease in the initial velocity of shortening.

THE NEUROMUSCULAR JUNCTION (Fig. 43-17). A motor unit consists of a single anterior horn cell, its axon, and a variable number of muscle fibers which it supplies. The muscle fibers in the large motor units are supplied by thick fibers of $15\,\mu$ and the smaller by fine fibers of $4\,\mu$. The

Fig. 43-17. Anatomy of the neuromuscular junction. (*Taken with permission from Mercer and Duthie [eds.], "Orthopaedic Surgery," Edward Arnold [Publishers] Ltd., London, 1972.*)

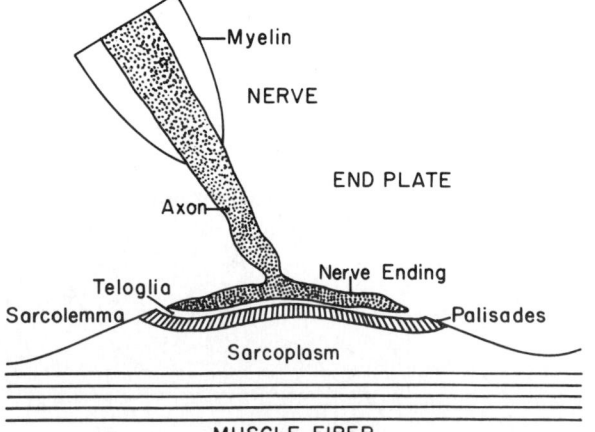

size of a motor unit varies inversely with the precision of the movements performed by the part; e.g., in the limb muscles, the unit may contain 150 muscle fibers, whereas in the eye it may contain fewer than five.

As the motor nerve fiber approaches a striated muscle fiber, it loses its medullary sheath, and the naked axis cylinder breaks up into terminal ramifications which make close and extensive contact with a specialized part of the muscle sarcoplasm known as the "motor end plate."

When an impulse arrives at the motor nerve terminal, there is released from the nerve terminal acetylcholine, which diffuses toward the motor end plate. The acetyl choline attaches to end plate receptors and produces a local end plate potential which alters the permeability of the membrane, allowing a free exchange of sodium and potassium. This process is known as "depolarization."

When the end plate potential reaches a certain critical magnitude, it depolarizes the surface membrane of the muscle fiber. When this local depolarization exceeds 30 to 40 mV, a spike potential in the muscle fiber is initiated which, when it attains an amplitude of 120 to 130 mV, results in muscular contraction.

After the acetylcholine is liberated at the end plate, it is rapidly hydrolized to choline and acetate by the enzyme cholinesterase. This enables the muscle fiber to become repolarized and to respond by contraction to further nervous stimuli. Certain extraneous factors may interfere with this chemical transmission of the nervous impulse, e.g., drugs, such as neostigmine or physostigmine, which are anticholinesterase compounds. These prevent the destruction of acetylcholine pooling, which results in the continued depolarization of the end plate and thus a failure to respond to further nervous stimuli. On the other hand substances such as curare will compete with receptor substances on the end plate for acetylcholine and counteract its effect, reducing the size of the end plate potential so that it can no longer excite the neighboring muscle membrane.

Muscle Paralysis and Spasticity

BASIC CONSIDERATIONS

Motor paralysis is the loss of voluntary muscle power either resulting from interruption of the motor or lower motor neuron pathways controlling it or due to some deficiency of the muscle itself, making it incapable of responding to nervous control. As a result of muscle paralysis, there will be changes in muscle tone, tendon reflexes, and the physical mass of the muscle or muscles involved.

MUSCLE TONE. The term "muscle tone" is used differently by the physiologist and the clinician. The physiologist defines it as a state of partial tetanus of the muscle which is maintained by an asynchronous discharge of impulses in motor neurons supplying it. It is reflexly produced from afferent nerve endings situated within the muscle itself and profoundly influenced by supraspinal mechanisms. Muscle tone provides the background of posture in which active movements occur and is an important element in the coordination of movement.

The clinician commonly estimates tone by the passive manipulation of limbs. This gives him a sense of the degree of tension, or elastic resistance, in the muscle. In lesions of the lower motor neuron muscle tone is abolished; this condition is called "flaccidity," or "flaccid paralysis." In lesions of the upper motor neuron muscle tone is increased, a condition of spasticity which occurs when the pyramidal tract is involved; when there is rigidity, the extrapyramidal tract is involved.

TENDON REFLEXES. The tendon reflexes are short-lived stretch reflexes elicited by tapping the tendon of the muscle, which evokes stimulation of the intrafusal muscle fibers of the muscle spindles. When muscle tone is increased, as in lesions of the upper motor neuron, the response to the tendon tap is increased, and the tendon jerk is thus increased in both amplitude and duration. Sometimes sudden stretching of the muscle will result in a repetitive jerk known as "clonus." The tendon reflex will be completely abolished by any interruption of the lower motor neuron reflex arc system on either the afferent or efferent loop.

PHYSICAL MASS OF MUSCLE. In upper motor neuron lesions the actual physical mass of the muscle remains unchanged, but in lower motor neuron lesions rapid wasting of the affected muscles will occur.

ATAXIA. "Ataxia" may be defined as imperfectly controlled or uncoordinated voluntary movements. It may be due to lesions of the cerebellum or the vestibular system. A sensory ataxia may arise from involvement of the pathways of proprioceptive and position sense, i.e., as seen in tabes dorsalis and in Friedreich's ataxia.

ELECTRICAL DIAGNOSIS AND ASSESSMENT OF MUSCLE DENERVATION. The method of obtaining the electrical "reaction" of muscle by faradic or galvanic stimulation applied to a muscle and its motor nerve has given place to more precise methods of greater complexity such as the intensity duration curve, electromyography, and nerve conduction velocity tests.

Intensity Duration Curve. Intensity duration curves (Fig. 43-18) are obtained by stimulating the muscle mass with pulses of known duration and intensity which produce characteristic patterns of contraction.

Electromyography. Electromyography (Fig. 43-19) is carried out with needle electrodes inserted into a muscle by means of which recordings are made of action potentials picked up within the muscles. The potential patterns reveal the presence or absence of denervation and of certain stages of regeneration of nerve.

Nerve Conduction Tests. Nerve conduction velocity tests are chiefly of value in defining peripheral nerve conduction interruption and together with electromyography form a useful basis in distinguishing among true motor neuron disease, peripheral nerve disease, and myopathy.

INTRINSIC DISEASES OF MUSCLE

Classification

A. Muscular dystrophies
 1. Progressive muscular dystrophy of Duchenne
 2. Fasciascapulohumeral dystrophy of Landouzy-Déjerine
 3. Dystrophia myotonica, or Steinert's disease

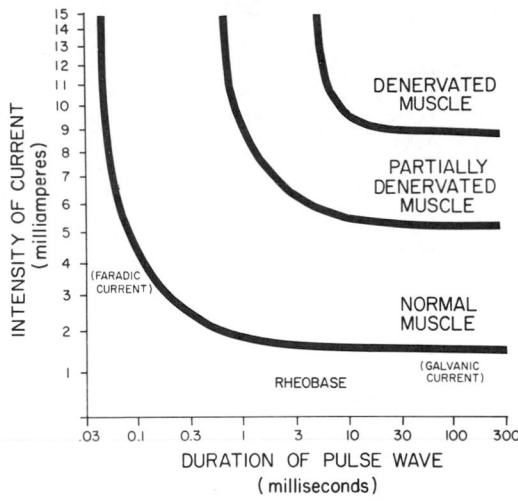

Fig. 43-18. Three common types of intensity duration curves. (*Taken with permission from Mercer and Duthie* [eds.], *"Orthopaedic Surgery," Edward Arnold* [*Publishers*] *Ltd., London, 1972.*)

B. Periodic diseases
 1. Myasthenia gravis
 2. Familial periodic paralysis
C. Other diseases of muscle
 1. Benign congenital hypotonia of Oppenheim-Walton
 2. Glycogen storage diseases of muscle
  a. Type 5, or McArdle-Schmid-Pearson disease
  b. Type 6, or Hers' disease
 3. Myotonia congenita, or Thomsen's disease
 4. Central core disease
D. Developmental defects of muscle
 1. Hypoplasia and aplasia
 2. Arthrogryposis
E. Constitutional disorders of muscle
 1. Neuromuscular atrophies
  a. Poliomyelitis
  b. Progressive muscular atrophy of Duchenne-Aran
  c. Infantile muscular atrophy of Hoffmann-Werdnig
  d. Peroneal muscular atrophy (Charcot-Marie-Tooth disease)

Fig. 43-19. Three electromyographic patterns of muscle fiber action potential showing normal potential curves (left), a myopathic lesion (middle), and lower motor neuron disease (right). (*Taken with permission from Mercer and Duthie* [eds.], *"Orthopaedic Surgery," Edward Arnold* [*Publishers*] *Ltd., London, 1972.*)

   e. Amyotrophic lateral sclerosis
   f. Syringomyelia
   g. Myelodysplasia
  2. Endocrine and metabolic disturbances
   a. Thyrotoxic myopathy
   b. Adrenal insufficiency
   c. Cushing's syndrome
   d. Hyperinsulinism
   e. Hyperkalemia and hypokalemia

In distinguishing the true myopathies from other causes of muscular paralysis, one must take into consideration the early age of onset, the familial history, and the progressive wasting of muscle groups without anatomic relation to any particular nerve supply. Other factors are the absence of fibrillation and the presence of normal tendon reflexes in the face of severe muscle wasting, and if necessary more specific data can be obtained by electromyography, muscle biopsy, and biochemical tests for serum aldolase and urine creatinine levels.

Muscular Dystrophies

PSEUDOHYPERTROPHIC MUSCULAR DYSTROPHY (DUCHENNE). The Duchenne type of muscular dystrophy is a progressive muscular disease which is usually manifested during the first three to six years, although it may be present in infancy or not recognized until adolescence. It affects boys primarily and is genetically determined by a sex-linked recessive gene. The presenting complaint is difficulty or instability in standing or walking. There may be an awkward waddling gait. The child gets up from the floor in a characteristic manner using his arms to get up on his legs to attain the upright posture. The child stands with increased lordosis, is weak, and usually has enlarged bulky muscles. The enlargement is conspicuous in the calves, the deltoids, and the quadriceps. The hands and the forearms usually are not involved. With progression, the pelvic musculature, erector spinae, and intercostals may be involved. Contractures occur early in the course of the disease and are first seen as equinovarus deformity of the foot. The cardiac muscle may be involved late in the course of the disease and may be responsible for death. Most patients are dead by the age of twenty years.

FASCIOSCAPULOHUMERAL TYPE OF MUSCULAR DYSTROPHY (LANDOUZY-DÉJERINE). This type of muscular dystrophy presents with facial and shoulder girdle involvement and is the most common form of muscular dystrophy in adults.

The facial muscles are involved early and may present in childhood or late adolescence. The cheeks droop, the lips pout, and the facies are immobile. Shoulder girdle involvement causes abnormal shoulder posture and difficulty in raising arms. Pelvic musculature is rarely involved. The heart may be affected, but life span is usually not shortened. It is transmitted by an autosomal dominant gene and may affect either sex.

LIMB GIRDLE TYPE OF MUSCULAR DYSTROPHY (ERB). This type of muscular dystrophy is much less common than Duchenne's and occurs later in life, usually in the second decade. Pseudohypertrophy is uncommon. The involvement begins first about the shoulder and pelvic girdles with involvement of the upper arm and thigh. The atrophy of the involved muscles produces striking contrast in the size of the arm, forearm, thigh, and leg in a typical case. The course is progressively downhill until there is involvement of all muscles and is more rapid, with earlier onset. Both sexes are involved. Inheritance is by an autosomal recessive gene.

OCULAR MUSCULAR DYSTROPHY. This is a dystrophic process involving first the levator palpebrae superioris and later the external ocular muscles. There may be weakness and wasting of other muscles about the face, head, and neck. Sexes are affected equally. Inheritance is by autosomal dominant gene.

PATHOLOGY OF MUSCULAR DYSTROPHY. The pathologic features of the various forms of muscular dystrophy are similar. The involved muscle is pink or gray and more whitish than normal. Microscopically there is greater variation of individual fiber size, from 10 to 200 mμ. On cross section fibers are rounded instead of polygonal, lose striation, and appear hyalinized in longitudinal section. There is no attempt at muscle regeneration. Fat and connective tissue replace degenerating muscle fibers. Sarcolemmic nuclei may be increased.

DIAGNOSIS. Early in the course of the disease, the diagnosis may be confused with polymyositis, since it may respond to medication. Serum enzymes, electromyography, and muscle biopsy are helpful in making the diagnosis of dystrophy, although the clinical features must be considered to distinguish the type of dystrophy.

In the Duchenne type of muscular dystrophy, the serum aldolase or creatine phosphokinase levels are invariably extremely high. Late in the disease, they may approach normal after muscle destruction has been complete. In the other dystrophies serum aldolase and creatine phosphokinase levels are raised according to the degree of muscle involvement, and the elevations are usually much lower than in the Duchenne type. Levels of creatine in the urine are increased above normal, while there is a reduction in the urinary excretion of creatinine which is probably related to a decrease in muscle mass. Urinary excretion of amino acid is also increased.

Electromyography of an involved muscle shows lower potentials and polyphasic pattern during voluntary contraction.

Muscle biopsy may be necessary in other dystrophies, but the diagnosis of Duchenne's dystrophy can be made on clinical grounds and on the basis of markedly elevated enzyme levels. The value of the muscle biopsy depends upon the selection of abnormal muscle, careful technique, and adequate tissue preparation. The selected muscle should be a muscle that is abnormal but not severely involved. The site of biopsy should be away from the insertion of the muscle where there is variation in the fiber size. A specimen at least $1\frac{1}{2}$ cm long and 1 cm wide is required for adequate study. The specimen should be gently stretched to the necessary length with ends fastened on a card or held in a special muscle clamp and placed in saline solution for 30 minutes and then fixed in formalin.

TREATMENT. There is no specific curative therapy for muscular dystrophy. Treatment is symptomatic. Vignos has shown that exercise is valuable in maintaining the patient's ability to ambulate and remain functional. The orthopedist should be aware that procedures which confine a patient to bed rest tend to accelerate the muscle weakness. Patients should not be confined to a wheelchair prematurely. Parents are instructed in stretching exercises of the lower extremities, hamstrings, spinal extensors, and gastrocnemius, and encouraged in a program of muscle strengthening exercises against active resistance.

Short and long leg braces for the lower extremities are used to keep the child standing and ambulating as long as possible. When equinus contractures are severe, heel cord lengthening may be carried out. The child should be fitted with a brace postoperatively and encouraged to ambulate within a few days. When spinal extensor and abdominal flexor weakness is severe and a wheelchair is required, the application of a torso body plaster may be of value in maintaining sitting posture.

Myotonias

MYOTONIC DYSTROPHY. This is a rare disorder in which there is a myopathy in combination with other abnormalities. The disorder is inherited as an autosomal dominant. The onset may be at any time during the first three decades of life. The onset commonly starts with dystrophy in the distal musculature and the muscles of the face and neck. Myopathic facies are common. Progress is slow, and proximal muscles may be involved much later. Percussion of a muscle or electric stimulation results in prolonged contraction of the muscle. Gonadal atrophy, cataracts, and frontal baldness occur in males with this disorder.

MYOTONIA CONGENITA, OR THOMSEN'S DISEASE. This is a rare hereditary disorder transmitted as an autosomal recessive or dominant gene. In all voluntary muscles there is difficulty in starting movement following rest. Symptoms may begin at infancy but usually appear between the ages of five and ten years. The patient gives the appearance of excessive muscle mass and muscular overdevelopment. Following repeated motion, the initial weakness improves to where muscle strength may be normal. Percussion of the muscle results in a myotonic sustained contraction. The disease is compatible with normal life expectancy.

PATHOLOGY AND DIAGNOSIS OF MYOTONIA. Histologic examination of a myotonic muscle reveals the presence of long chains of centrally placed nuclei in otherwise intact muscle fibers. Characteristically, some muscle fibers are enlarged. On cross section, the peripheral myofibrils have degenerated and surround a central group of normal fibrils. There is no regeneration, and connective tissue does not replace the muscle, thus accounting for the absence of contractures.

On electromyography, a characteristic shower of electrical activity occurs spontaneously after stimulation. Serum enzyme levels may be similar to those in the dystrophies other than Duchenne's, which has a marked elevation of creatine phosphokinase and serum aldolase levels.

TREATMENT. There is no effective treatment for myotonic dystrophy. However, patients with Thomsen's disease can be improved by the use of procaine amide, prednisone and quinine.

Inflammatory Disease

Myositis, or inflammation in muscles, may be due to specific etiologic agents such as a virus, parasite, bacterium, or spirochete. Myositis occurs in diseases of unknown cause such as the collagen vascular diseases, dermatomyositis, lupus, scleroderma, and rheumatoid arthritis. The term "polymyositis" is used to describe the changes in muscle associated with these conditions as well as those found in association with malignant tumors.

The clinical course of polymyositis is variable and may present as an insidious chronic muscle weakness, or it may begin with acute symptoms of high fever, marked muscle pain, spasm, and weakness. The heart muscle may be involved in any of these conditions. Skin changes associated with the primary diagnosis, i.e., lupus or scleroderma, will assist in making the diagnosis. The course of the disease is variable and may be rapidly progressive, resulting in death, or it may persist with episodes of remission and exacerbation. Spontaneous arrest may occur.

PATHOLOGY. Histologic examination of muscles reveals degeneration and necrosis of muscle fibers associated with infiltration by chronic inflammatory cells, both interstitially and about blood vessels. Serum enzyme studies are of little value in the diagnosis. Electromyography of the involved muscle reveals spontaneous fibrillation potential in the relaxed muscle, distinguishing polymyositis from muscular dystrophy.

TREATMENT. The treatment of polymyositis is directed at diagnosis of the primary condition. In elderly patients presenting with polymyositis, an unrecognized malignant tumor should be suspected. Most patients with polymyositis may be controlled dramatically with the use of cortisone preparations or ACTH. General treatment requires supportive care, physiotherapy in the form of exercise to maintain existing muscle power, appropriate bracing, and occasionally surgical treatment for contractures.

Orthopedic treatment is directed at control of deformities by appropriate bracing or surgical arthrodesis of neurotrophic joints.

POLIOMYELITIS

Poliomyelitis is an acute infectious disease caused by the poliomyelitis virus. The virus is present in the pharynx and feces of infected patients during the preparalytic and postparalytic stages. Invasion of the central nervous system is thought to take place by virus traveling proximally along the peripheral nerve to the spinal cord. Once established in the central nervous system, the virus causes anterior horn cell destruction, which results in a flaccid paralysis. With loss of innervation, the motor unit muscle fibers atrophy. Paralysis or deformity and leg-length discrepancies are the result.

CLINICAL COURSE OF THE DISEASE. In about one-third of patients with poliomyelitis infection an initial febrile illness develops consisting of headache, malaise, and low-grade fever, lasting 48 hours. Such a patient may recover completely or go on to a second, acute phase after 4 or 5 days of apparent good health. The acute phase may develop in the absence of the initial symptoms.

The acute phase lasts from a few days to a week and also may resolve without paralysis. The illness is characterized by meningeal symptoms including headache, fever, stiff neck, and muscle spasms in the spine or extremities. "Nonparalytic poliomyelitis" describes those patients who do not progress to the paralytic stage.

About the third or fourth day of the acute illness, paralysis may develop. There may be loss of deep reflexes, muscle spasm of the erector spinae, and even signs of bulbar paralysis. The lower limbs are involved twice as frequently as the upper extremities. Death may result from bulbar paralysis, due to respiratory insufficiency.

The convalescent stage begins after the acute illness and ends up to 2 years later at a point where there is no significant recovery in muscle power.

The residual stage occurs following changes in muscle recovery. Children will continue to improve in the residual stage because of their improved coordination.

TREATMENT. In the acute stage, treatment is directed at isolation of patients with the disease, general nursing care, and the treatment of respiratory difficulty by the use of mechanical respirators.

Treatment in the Recovery Stage. In the early stages of convalescence, treatment is directed at eliminating deforming tendencies, restoring joint motion, and training and protection of recovering muscles. Later on, the patient is fitted with suitable protective braces and taught resistance exercises to develop residual muscle power.

Muscle spasm is treated to prevent asymmetrical muscle tightness and soft tissue contractures. Trained therapists apply hot packs and give passive range-of-motion exercises. The patients must be nursed in the proper position, to prevent overstretching of paralyzed muscles and joint contractures. Appropriate splints are utilized, depending upon muscle weakness.

The patient is taught muscle reeducation to reestablish control of the extremities and joints as early as possible, when acute symptoms subside. When the patient is ambulatory, orthotic devices to protect and assist control of his paralyzed extremities are utilized.

Treatment in the Residual Stage. Treatment in the residual stage requires orthopedic surgical procedures to correct joint contractures, to improve joint power and function by appropriate muscle and tendon transfers, to stabilize joints by arthrodesis, and to correct leg-length inequality. The following surgical procedures are those most commonly used in poliomyelitis. The reader is referred to *Orthopaedic Surgery,* by Mercer and Duthie, and *Campbell's Operative Orthopedics,* edited by Crenshaw, for detailed discussion of these and other surgical procedures.

Principles of Reconstructive Surgery

TENDON TRANSFER. Tendon transfer is utilized to restore muscle balance to a joint, to restore lost function, and to increase active power of joint motions. Before undertaking tendon transfer, an expendable muscle of suitable strength and excursion must be available for transfer about a joint with a normal passive range of motion. Specific muscle power is graded on the Medical Research Council (MRC) scale, which is a clinical evaluation of muscle strength:

Grade	Muscle power
0	Complete paralysis
1	Flicker of contraction without joint excursion
2	Muscle power to effect partial range of motion
3	Muscle power to effect a full range of joint motion against gravity
4	Less than normal strength but full range of joint motion against resistance
5	Normal muscle strength

A muscle will lose one grade of strength following transfer, so that its power must be grade 4 or better. The muscle selected should have sufficient excursion to replace the lost function. Muscles from synergistic groups provide better results by making muscle reeducation more complete. Joint contractures should be corrected and a passive range of joint motion established prior to tendon transfer. Circulation to, and sensation in, the muscle should not be damaged during transfer. The tendon connecting the new origin and insertion should be as straight as possible to improve the efficiency of muscle action and should be placed in an area where gliding is possible.

BONY STABILIZATION. When muscle power is insufficient to protect or move the joint or when sufficiently expendable muscles are not available for transfer, arthrodesis of the joint will provide stability, prevent deformity, and even permit transfer of local muscles for other functions. A prerequisite of arthrodesis is the presence of adjacent mobile joints to compensate for the lost motion.

JOINT CONTRACTURES. Joint contractures are corrected by judicious stretching by a physiotherapist or by braces incorporating dynamic stretching. The joints may be gradually stretched into the corrected position by successive plaster-cast changes or plaster-cast wedging.

LEG-LENGTH EQUALIZATION. Leg-length discrepancy may be corrected by bone lengthening or shortening procedures. A 1-in. difference in leg length is usually of no practical significance. For patients with significant paralysis about the hip, moderate degrees of shortening facilitate bony stability by the motion of abduction. Before undertaking corrective surgical procedures of any type, the surgeon should be familiar with the patient's progress in reference to the rate of leg-length discrepancy and have an understanding of the degrees of shortening produced by such procedures as ankle arthrodesis and knee arthrodesis in flexion.

Treatment of Deformities

FOOT PARALYSIS. Paralysis from poliomyelitis may cause a wide variety of foot deformities (Fig. 43-20). Deformities are treated by proper bracing to maintain stability and prevent deformity until maximal recovery has occurred. When maximal recovery has occurred, tendon transfers or bony stabilization procedures are indicated. Bony stabilization other than the Grice extraarticular arthrodesis of the subtalar joint is not performed until bony maturity is achieved at age twelve to fifteen. Each foot deformity must be evaluated specifically, taking into consideration many factors including joint motion, other joints involved, and muscles available and their strength.

Valgus deformity is due to muscle imbalance from weakness or absence of functioning invertors which results in pronation of the forefoot and eversion of the calcaneus. The extraarticular arthrodesis of the subtalar joint (Grice) is an effective means of controlling this until bony maturity. A strut of tibial bone graft is wedged between the talus and the calcaneus, between the anterior and posterior components of the subtalar joint (Fig. 43-21A).

Varus deformity is due to muscle imbalance with paralysis of the peroneal muscles. Treatment is directed at restoring eversion power and strength. The anterior tibial may be transferred laterally to reduce its varus deforming force and improve eversion. The posterior tibial tendon may be released from its tendon sheath and allowed to ride in front of the medial malleolus. This effectively releases some inversion force. The posterior tibial tendon also may be transferred laterally through the interosseous membrane.

Calcaneus Deformity. Calcaneus deformity is the result of paralysis of the calf muscles. The unopposed dorsiflexors pull the foot into dorsiflexion, and the calcaneal foot results. This is a difficult deformity to control with bracing. The posterior or peroneal tendons may be transferred into the calcaneus, effecting partial improvement in plantar flexion power. Alternatives are tenodesis of the Achilles tendon, which will provide the fulcrum for push-off. At age twelve to fifteen years, triple arthrodesis may be required (Fig. 43-21B).

Equinus Deformity. Equinus deformity results from paralysis of the anterior tibial tendon, causing foot drop. This deformity may be controlled with a foot drop short leg brace. Forward transfer of the peroneals for dorsiflexion, combined with triple arthrodesis, may be accomplished at bony maturity A Lambrinudi triple arthrodesis or Hoke triple arthrodesis may be effective in the absence of functioning peroneal muscles.

Claw Hallux Deformity. Extension of the metatarsophalangeal (MP) joint of the great toe with flexion of the interphalangeal (IP) joint commonly occurs with paralysis of the tibialis anterior. The overpull of the extensor hallucis longus results in dorsiflexion of the MP joint and clawing. Depression of the first metatarsal shaft is due to the unbalanced pull of the peroneus longus. This deformity can be effectively treated by the Jones procedure. This consists of transplantation of the extensor hallucis longus into the neck of the first metatarsal shaft, combined with stabilization of the IP joint by arthrodesis.

PARALYSIS ABOUT THE KNEE JOINT. Patients with isolated paralysis of the quadriceps get along satisfactorily if there is adequate power in the gastronemius and gluteus maximus to stabilize the knee in extension. Transplantation of the biceps combined with semitendinosis transfer to the patella may be indicated. However, the indications must be individualized and are based on the prerequisite of adequate posterior stability of the knee, including gastrocnemius power and gluteus maximus function.

PARALYSIS ABOUT THE HIP. Paralytic deformity of the hip results in severe disability through the disturbance of gait. The indications for treatment depend upon the avail-

Fig. 43-20. Paralytic deformities of the foot. *A.* Calcaneal deformity. *B.* Cavus (claw) foot. *C.* Valgus deformity. *D.* Varus deformity.

Fig. 43-21. *A.* Grice procedure with a strut of tibial bone graft wedged between talus and calcaneus. *B.* Triple arthrodesis.

ability of function in adjacent muscles and the degree of disability. A posterior transfer of extensor fascia lata, lateral transfer of the iliopsoas (Mustard procedure), or erector spinae transfer for gluteus maximus paralysis give variable results. In the properly selected patients, a small gain in stability may result in great benefit by relieving fatigability of gait and pelvic stabilization. If a painful hip, subluxation, or frank dislocation due to muscle imbalance develops, arthrodesis may be necessary. Careful analysis of the paralysis in other joints, leg-length discrepancy, etc., in each patient must be considered before surgical treatment is undertaken.

PARALYSIS IN THE UPPER EXTREMITY. Shoulder. Paralysis of the deltoid and rotator cuff in the presence of remaining power in the scapular stabilizing muscles— trapezius, rhomboids, serratus anterior—may be treated by arthrodesis of the glenohumeral joint in the appropriate position. The resulting stabilization allows shoulder stability, adequate motion, and power from the function of scapulothoracic muscles.

Elbow. Surgical procedures to improve power across the elbow are directed primarily at restoring elbow flexion in paralysis of the biceps and brachialis. If normal power exists in the flexors of the wrist and fingers, Steindler's operation, which is the proximal transfer of the common flexor origin, will improve elbow flexion power. Alternative methods include transfer of the inferior portion of the pectoralis major or the sternocleidomastoideus attached to a free tendon graft.

Paralytic Hand. Paralysis of wrist extensors may be treated by dorsal transfer of the flexor carpi ulnaris or pronator teres into the extensor carpi radialis longus and brevis. Loss of thumb extension is treated by insertion of the flexor carpi radialis into the abductor pollicis longus and extensor pollicis brevis. The palmaris longus may be inserted into the extensor pollicis longus. Paralysis of the extensor digitorum communis may be treated by transfer of the flexor carpi ulnaris dorsally.

Loss of opposition of the thumb is a common finding in the paralytic hand due to poliomyelitis. Various procedures are available to restore opposition, including Bunnell's transfer of the flexor digitorum superficialis to the ring finger routed about a pulley on the flexor carpi ulnaris and inserted into the base of the thumb.

Wrist arthrodesis may provide stability of the hand and make available expendable tendons for transfer (see Chap. 50).

CEREBRAL PALSY

Cerebral palsy is a neurologic diagnosis of a condition in which there are nonprogressive but permanent upper motor neuron lesions occurring in children. The diagnosis excludes children with active or progressive disease. On examination, there may be disturbance of special senses, including sight, hearing, and peripheral sensation. Mental retardation alone is not cerebral palsy, but it may accompany upper motor neuron abnormalities.

INCIDENCE. Phelps estimated that cerebral palsy occurs in seven births for every 100,000 population. Of the seven patients, one will die within the first year, one will have subclinical involvement and pass unnoticed in the community, two will have such severe involvement as to require custodial care, and the remaining three will require orthopedic treatment.

ETIOLOGY. Cerebral palsy may be caused by a number of factors including head trauma at birth, head injury in childhood, anoxic brain damage, vascular accidents following treatment of brain tumor, involvement of the central nervous system from encephalitis, and other viral diseases, e.g., measles, cytomegalic inclusion body.

The pathologic lesions in the brain have not been well documented, and little information has been correlated between pathology and symptoms. Developmental defects, such as absence of the cerebellum or basal ganglia, may be responsible.

CLINICAL MANIFESTATIONS. Zuck estimates that 50 percent of all new patients are spastic, 25 percent are athetoid, 5 percent are ataxic, 5 percent are rigid, and the remainder have the mixed-type lesion.

Spasticity is due to an upper motor neuron lesion, involving the pyramidal tract. Clinical examination reveals hyperactive stretch reflexes. Sudden passive motion of a joint produced by spastic muscles activates this reflex, and clonus results. Weakness may be present in antagonistic muscle groups and contributes to the development of joint flexion contractures.

Cerebral spastic patients are of four types: sixty percent of all spastics are hemiplegic with paralysis of ipsilateral arm and leg; the patient with left-sided hemiplegia is more likely to have better preservation of intellectual function. The second most common type is the diplegic with symmetrical spastic involvement in the lower extremities and less severe involvement in the upper extremities. Paraplegic patients are uncommon, having involvement only of the lower extremities. The quadriplegic patient tends to have symmetrical involvement of all four extremities.

Athetosis is characterized by involuntary repetitive motion of a muscle group or extremity resulting in severe dysfunction. Athetotic motions may be worsened by sudden stress, tension, weight bearing, and even sudden changes of light. The defect is thought to be in the basal ganglia. Joint contractures are rare with this manifestation.

Ataxia is related to lesions of the cerebellum, causing deficient postural reflexes. There is commonly a voluntary tremor, hypotonia, and easy fatigability. The child walks with a staggering, broad-based gait. Reflexes are decreased and contractures uncommon.

Rigidity results from diffuse cerebral involvement, commonly from birth ataxia.

In *mixed types of cerebral palsy* spasticity commonly coexists with athetosis. Not infrequently, a child at age two to four with spasticity shows evidence of coexisting athetosis as he grows older.

Diagnosis can usually be made by an experienced physician during the first year of life. A history of difficult pregnancy, prolonged labor, delayed respiration, neonatal jaundice, postnatal irritability, or muscle twitching is suggestive.

Stiffness of extremities, weakness, or asymmetrical use of the limbs, retarded motor development, or athetoid movements may be evident in the history. Clinical examination should detect signs of spasticity, purposeless movements, delayed motor development, or incoordination. Any joint contractures should arouse the suspicion of spasticity.

TREATMENT. Adequate treatment of cerebral palsy requires a multidisciplined approach. The pediatrician, the orthopedic surgeon, the neurologist should collaborate with the social worker, psychologist, and teachers trained in the instruction of handicapped children. The total program of care requires understanding and participation by the parents.

Successful treatment is directly related to the intelligence of the child. About two-thirds of cerebral palsied children have IQs below 70, making education and treatment more difficult. There is a close correlation between motor ability and IQ. Motor ability is evaluated by the motor age test. The motor age test is a numerical expression of motor performance expressed as a percentage of age. The normal child would have a score of 100, the motor-handicapped child less than 100. By totaling the motor age and IQ a total is reached to which treatment results can be compared. When the total is below 130, intensive prolonged therapy is usually unrewarding. When the total of motor age and IQ is between 130 and 160, satisfactory results from a complete treatment program can be expected. Physiotherapy for muscle strengthening, gait training, and effective bracing are needed. Orthopedic surgical correction of deformities is important but is the least frequently required therapeutic approach.

Physiotherapy. Physiotherapy is directed at achieving controlled muscle function, which requires muscle relaxation and control of purposeless movements. Physiotherapy is applied under the guidance of the physiotherapist and carried out at home by the mother. Daily passive stretching is required to prevent flexion deformities. The child is taught through repetitive exercises and supervised play to obtain muscle relaxation and strengthen weakened muscles.

Bracing. Braces are necessary:

1. To prevent contractures from muscle imbalance and spasticity
2. To provide stability in the lower extremities, because of muscle weakness
3. To minimize purposeless motion
4. To provide evaluation prior to performing stabilization procedures

Braces have their greatest application to the lower extremities. A double upright, short leg caliper, with added T straps, will help to control varus or valgus deformities of the foot, provide stability in walking and standing, and assist in preventing contractures.

In the spastic child with the tendency to equinus contractures of the foot or flexion deformities of the knees, posterior plaster splints or bivalved plaster casts will assist in overcoming these deformities.

Long leg braces are applied to assist in preventing knee flexion contractures and valgus deformities and provide stability in the upright position. Bilateral long leg braces with a pelvic band provide additional stability at the hip joint.

Upper extremity bracing takes the form of plaster or metal splints to assist in holding the hand in the position of function and preventing flexion contractures at the wrists and fingers or adduction deformities of the thumb.

THERAPY FOR SPECIFIC AREAS. Hip. The effect of adductor spasticity with weakened abductors results in a valgus deformity of the femoral neck. With severe adduction, lateral displacement of the hips and increasing acetabular index develop. If these are not controlled with soft tissue procedure, tenotomy, and neurectomy, a subtrochanteric varus osteotomy with internal fixation is necessary (Fig. 43-22). Rotational deformity is corrected at the same time.

Knee. The knee develops flexion contractures because of isolated or combined problems of hip flexion deformity, spastic hamstrings, and equinus feet. Contractures can be

Fig. 43-22. Hip subluxation in spastic diplegia. *A.* AP of the pelvis showing lateral displacement of the right hip. *B.* AP of the pelvis showing maintenance of the head in the acetabulum following varus derotation osteotomy.

prevented by appropriate plaster night splints, bracing, and exercises. If a contracture has developed, it may be corrected by plaster-cast wedging. When this is unsuccessful, posterior capsulotomy or hamstring lengthening by Z-plasty may effectively relieve the contracture.

In the child walking in a crouched position with hips and knees flexed, surgical release of the hamstrings as described and modified by Eggers and Evans will assist in bringing both hip and knee to extension and improve the erect posture and gait. If there has been long-standing stretching of the anterior patellar retinacula and lengthening of the patellar ligament, effective quadriceps power can be improved by division of the posterior component of the patellar retinácula which allows any quadriceps power to be applied effectively to the stretched patellar ligaments.

Foot. Although any deformity may develop as the result of muscle weakness and spasticity in cerebral palsy, the equinovarus foot is most common. If an equinovarus contracture can be demonstrated with the knee extended but not with the knee flexed, contracture of the gastrocnemius is the cause, and its release is required. The Strayer procedure divides the gastrocnemius at its musculotendinous junction, effectively lengthening it, and does not disturb the underlying soleus.

Orthopedic Surgical Treatment

Orthopedic surgical treatment is used for:

1. Weakening spastic muscles by tendon lengthening
2. Improving joint motion by tendon transplantation
3. Stabilizing deformed or contracted joints by arthrodesis
4. Correcting deformity by osteotomy and correction of leg-length inequality

If children with cerebral palsy are put to bed for surgical procedures, their motor abilities deteriorate at least temporarily. For the athetoid child, surgical intervention is rarely indicated. As Phelps has shown, correction of the deformity at one level results in expression of the disorder at a more proximal level. Most surgical procedures are applied in the treatment of the spastic. Procedures which require stabilization are more likely to be successful, since muscle reeducation and patient cooperation are not required. When tendon transfers are indicated, a higher IQ and higher motor age are prerequisites.

UPPER EXTREMITY. Surgical treatment of the upper extremity is rarely indicated and is done to improve appearance and position of the hand, wrist, and forearm. The functional benefits are uncertain. The common deformity of the upper extremity spastic hemiplegic patient is an elbow in flexion with a forearm pronation contracture with wrist and fingers in flexion and the thumb closely opposed or adducted.

Arthrodesis of the wrist is done in extension and moderate ulnar deviation in order passively to improve thumb abduction. By eliminating wrist motion, finger power and control are improved.

An alternative method is transfer of the flexor carpi ulnaris tendon around the ulnar side of the forearm and insertion into radial wrist extensor tendons. This will improve wrist extension, though there is little effect on supination power.

Stabilization of the thumb by an iliac bone graft between the first two metacarpals may be necessary. Other procedures such as the flexor digitorum superficiallis tenodesis of Swanson and flexor carpi ulnaris transfers to the finger extensors following wrist fusion are rarely indicated.

LOWER EXTREMITY. The flexion adduction deformity of the hip is common in spasticity and requires treatment. The infant is splinted with an abduction splint, and daily passive stretching is carried out, to minimize deformity. When the child begins to walk, scissoring due to adductor spasticity may seriously interfere with gait.

Adductor tenotomy is done by surgical division of the major adductor origins from the pelvis. Postoperatively, abduction should be maintained by splints while abductor power is strengthened by exercise. When there is marked scissoring during attempts at walking, with little or no permanent contracture, obturator neurectomy is done, if tenotomy fails.

Internal rotation, which frequently accompanies adduction and flexion, may be treated by derotational osteotomy in the supracondylar or subtrochanteric areas. However, incision of the tendons of the gluteus medius and mimimus from the anterior portion of the greater trochanter followed by 6 months of immobilization in plaster is generally preferable.

Flexion deformity of the knee due to muscle spasm may be corrected by plaster wedging. When contracture is established and there is a weakened quadriceps or an overstretched patellar tendon with upward migration of the patella, the best procedure is posterior capsulotomy of the knee and Z-plasty lengthening of the hamstrings. The patellar tendon may be advanced, in addition, to aid the quadriceps to reach optimal length. Other procedures free the gastrocnemius from its femoral attachment or release the patellar retinaculum and transfer the hamstrings into the distal femur.

In the foot, the common equinus deformity may be treated by division of the nerve supply to the gastrocnemius or soleus muscles or by lengthening of the Achilles tendon or gastrocnemius. When the equinus deformity is present with knee flexed and extended, then lengthening of the Achilles tendon by Z-plasty with or without posterior ankle capsulotomy is necessary. Release of the posterior tibial tendon to allow it to ride forward of the medial malleolus will assist in overcoming the varus deformity. When bony maturity is reached, varus and valgus deformities may be treated by triple arthrodesis.

MYELODYSPLASIA (Spinal Dysraphism)

Myelodysplasia describes a developmental defect in the vertebral column with associated peripheral neurologic lesions. Lichtenstein used the term "spinal dysraphism" for congenital defects of the lumbosacral regions with failure of fusion of midline structures. The vertebral lesion may be present without involvement of the cord, i.e., as spina bifida occulta. However, spina bifida may be associated with meningocele, myelomeningocele, or myeloschisis, an open neural plate. Hydrocephalus is frequently associated with these lesions.

CLINICAL MANIFESTATIONS. Spina bifida occulta is frequently an incidental finding detected by x-ray and is not usually associated with neurologic abnormality. An occasional patient may have detectable muscle imbalance or sensory abnormalities of the foot which are quite localized.

Meningoceles (cystic enlargement of the lower meninges), myelomeningoceles (cystic enlargement of meninges and intradural contents), or myeloschisis (a frank open neural plate) may occur with spina bifida resulting in severe deformities of the lower extremity. Sharrard et al. have shown that when myelocele, myelomeningocele, or myeloschisis is present at birth, early surgical closure will prevent deterioration of the distal neurologic function. The neural sac is closed by mobilization of fascial flaps and full-thickness skin coverage. Associated hydrocephalus, which occurs in 80 percent of these patients, should be treated simultaneously. The prognosis for a child with these developmental abnormalities of the central nervous system will depend upon the degree of resultant lower extremity paralysis as well as neurologic abnormalities of the bladder and urinary tract.

ORTHOPEDIC MANAGEMENT. The deformities of the lower extremities are related to the level of spinal involvement, which may be complete or spotty in distribution. Neurologic evaluation should be repeated, as functional loss may increase with growth. If a complete lesion occurs at the first lumbar segment, flaccid paralysis is the result; treatment is directed at obtaining weight-bearing attitude in the lower extremities. When the level is between L_3 and L_4, hip adduction and flexion is present, whereas hip abduction and extension are absent, with resulting potential paralytic hip dislocation. The management of such paralytic deformities is similar to that of deformities which occur as a result of flaccid paralysis of poliomyelitis.

Foot and Ankle. Talipes equinovarus is the most common foot deformity resulting from muscle imbalance, although calcaneal valgus or varus also may occur. Management is directed at maintaining the weight-bearing position. If deformity is already present, plaster-cast correction of the foot is carried out and followed by short leg braces to control the muscle imbalance. Lack of sensation makes the possibility of pressure sores a chronic problem for these patients. For the valgus foot, the Grice procedure may be required. When bony maturity has been reached, triple arthrodesis is performed to stabilize the foot.

Knee Deformities. When a complete lesion occurs at the levels of L_3 and L_4, quadriceps function remains in the absence of the hamstring function, and hyperextension of the knee results. In such a patient, the deformity is managed by plaster casts, splints, and long leg braces to prevent recurvation of the knee. Osteotomy may be necessary to correct rotational deformities.

Hip. When a complete lesion occurs between L_3 and L_4 coxa valga and subluxation of the hip occur. It is important to recognize this deformity before actual dislocation results. Management is directed at restoring the muscle bal-

ance responsible for the deformity. Sharrard's lateral transfer of the iliopsoas through the wing of the ilium will improve hip abduction and extension and has given satisfactory results. Varus osteotomy and derotational osteotomy of the femur may also be necessary.

All the principles utilized in the treatment of paralytic poliomyelitis including correction of joint contractures by stretching, plaster-cast wedging, reinforcement of weak muscles by tendon transfers, arthrodesis of unstable joints, and correction of leg-length inequality are applicable in the treatment of deformities due to spinal dysraphism.

DEGENERATIVE DISEASES OF THE NERVOUS SYSTEM WITH SKELETAL DEFORMITY

Peroneal Muscle Atrophy (Charcot-Marie-Tooth Muscular Atrophy)

Peroneal muscular atrophy is a hereditary degenerative process beginning in the peroneal nerve and resulting in peroneal muscular weakness. As the disease progresses, nerve trunks supplying the distal parts of the extremities are involved. Degenerative changes may occur in the spinal nerve roots in pyramidal tracts.

CLINICAL MANIFESTATIONS. The disease usually manifests itself in the first or second decade and may occur as late as the third. The initial complaint is varus deformity of the feet, such that the child walks on the outer borders of his feet. With progressive involvement of the anterior tibial group and foot drop, the patient develops a slapping gait.

Neurologic examination reveals a decrease in reflexes of muscles supplied by involved nerve roots. Anesthesia may accompany the muscle atrophy. The disease is found in several generations and is transmitted as a dominant, recessive, or sex-linked recessive.

Treatment does not affect the slow progressive changes. Short leg braces may control the varus deformity.

Friedreich's Ataxia

Friedreich's cerebellar ataxia is a familial disease in which there is degeneration of spinocerebellar tracts, corticospinal tracts, and posterior columns of the cord.

CLINICAL MANIFESTATIONS. There is usually evidence of the disease in previous generations. It affects males more commonly than females. The onset is usually insidious in childhood, the first abnormality being one of gait or a tendency to fall easily. Later on, there is incoordination, followed by nystagmus, and speech disturbances. Thoracic scoliosis and pes cavus with claw toes are seen very commonly. The disease runs a steadily downhill course. Early in the course of this disease, orthopedic bracing procedures or even tendon transfers or bony stabilization may be indicated to maintain ambulation.

Syringomyelia

Syringomyelia is a degenerative condition of the spinal cord in which there is destruction of neurons in the central portion and proliferation of glial elements resulting in the formation of a cavity. It is usually related to defective development, but similar cavities may occur following vascular processes or trauma.

The sexes are affected with equal frequency. The onset usually is in the second or third decade. Rarely are symptoms severe before the age of twenty. The small muscles of the hands are frequently involved early in the course, with deformity and wasting of the hands as a result. Disturbances in sensibility with loss of pain sense result in trophic disturbances about the hands and upper extremities. There is progressive atrophy of the muscle supplied by the area of the cord, commonly the cervical area, less commonly the bulbar or lumbar area. Skeletal deformities such as kyphosis, scoliosis, and pes cavus may be evident. The diagnosis depends on finding the associated anesthesia with muscle wasting and skeletal deformity.

Fig. 43-23. Atrophy of the intrinsic muscles of the hand.

1   Central Nervous System

   A   Cerebral Palsy
   B   Tumour
   C   Trauma
   D   Cerebral Vascular Accident

11   Spinal Cord- Anterior Horn Cells

   A   Anterior Poliomyelitis
   B   Progressive Muscle Atrophy
   C   Amyotrophic Lateral Sclerosis
   D   Syringomyelia
   E   Vascular Lesions
   F   Tumour

111   Anterior Root- Leptomeningitis of Syphilis

1V   Brachial Plexus

   A   Cervical Disc Prolapse
   B   Klumpke's Obstretical Palsy
   C   Scalenus Anticus Syndrome
   D   Cervical Rib
   E   Pancoast's Tumour

V   Ulnar Nerve

   A   Cubitis Valgus--Tardy Palsy
   B   Ganglion, Deep Branch of Ulnar Nerve

V1   Median Nerve--Carpal Tunnel Syndrome

V11   Median and/or Ulnar Nerve

   A   Ganglion
   B   Leprosy
   C   Polyneuritis
   D   Trauma

V111   Vascular and Ischemia

   A   Volkmann's Contracture
   B   Arteriosclerotic Disease
   C   Buerger's Disease
   D   Raynaud's Phenomenon

1V   Disuse Atrophy

   A   Arthritis
     1.   Rheumatoid
     2.   Gouty

   B   Dupuytren's Contracture

If the disease occurs early in life, the prognosis is relatively serious. The disease may progress very slowly, and the patient may function for many years.

Orthopedic treatment is directed at control of deformities by appropriate bracing or surgical arthrodesis of neuropathic joints. Laminectomy may be required to relieve rapidly expanding cavities of the spinal cord.

See also Chap. 42.

ATROPHY AND WASTING OF INTRINSIC MUSCLES OF THE HAND

Atrophy and wasting of the intrinsic muscles of the hand may be due to involvement of the central nervous system, spinal cord, anterior horn cells, lesions of the brachial plexus or peripheral nerves, or vascular and ischemic disorders (Fig. 43-23).

ORTHOPEDIC MANAGEMENT OF STROKE

This field requires the same type of combined team approach as has been used with good effect in rehabilitation following poliomyelitis and following the more aggressive surgical treatment of meningomyelocele. However, the place of surgery in the management of the stroke patient is limited.

EARLY TREATMENT. The early general medical management of the stroke patient is well known, such as the maintenance of an adequate airway, the introduction of urinary catheter drainage with antibiotics if necessary, and attention to other general medical problems such as unrecognized coronary artery disease, pulmonary disease, or complications, etc. Rehabilitation of the stroke patient begins at the earliest possible time, usually on the third or fourth day after the stroke.

In the flaccid state the patient is in urgent need of external stimuli, to replace the proprioceptive impulses produced by movement of limbs. This deficiency of motion may be replaced by a trained physical therapist. Placing the patient in a wheelchair is far preferable to a horizontal view of the world.

Nursing care is of vital importance in preventing deformity. Correct positioning in bed by the use of a foot board may prevent equinus, and the use of a rolled blanket beneath the greater trochanters to roll the legs may prevent external rotation deformity and flexion of the knees. Correct support of the upper limbs by the use of a pillow in the axilla will maintain shoulder abduction and prevent "frozen shoulder."

Frequent change of position is also of vital importance to prevent hypostatic pneumonia and pressure sores. At each change of position the joints of the limbs are placed through a range of motion and positioned to maintain or increase their range of movement. The prone position should also be used to provide good drainage of secretions and to prevent hip flexion and knee flexion deformities.

ASSESSMENT. Pseudomotor changes are of value in assessing motor control deficits, and it may be possible to predict whether the involvement is bilateral or not.

The involvement of the extrapyramidal system is of importance, because of its potential reversibility. The classical signs of facial immobility, failure of accommodation, and flexor rigidity in the neck muscles are much later occurrences. In the early stages the most reliable sign of cog wheel rigidity is the test of internal/external rotation of the shoulder and, to a lesser extent, of the hip joint.

Difficulties in balance are often overlooked; it is essential to evaluate the patient in the upright position when attempting to assess his ability to walk. Only very occasionally does a stroke disturb the central control of balance. More frequently the inability to stand erect is related to a disturbance of the patient's body image, resulting from a lesion in the nondominant hemisphere of the brain.

The patient with a distorted body image will make no attempt to support or otherwise accommodate for the weight of that side and thus falls toward the involved side without making any effort to protect himself. Techniques to stimulate body awareness, walking aids, and braces are possible means of overcoming this inadequacy.

CONTROL OF SPASTICITY. The ideal method of controlling spasticity would decrease excessive muscle tone permanently without associated loss of motor control and without loss of sensation. Such a method is not yet available; the most useful clinical method is peripheral muscle release. However this has the disadvantage of causing associated muscle weakness, and the procedure cannot be undone. Because of this, a variety of techniques have evolved.

Peripheral nerve block to control spasticity by dilute phenol injections was reported by Khalili et al. Further results also have been reported by Mooney et al. With phenol, spasticity is reduced or abolished for a comparatively short period of time and begins to return at the second or third month.

A simpler technique for the reduction of spasticity has been described using intramuscular alcohol injection in the approximate locus of the motor point. This is an extremely simple technique involving the local infiltration of the affected muscle belly with 45 percent alcohol solution. The reduction of spasticity is comparable to that obtained using phenol. Its effect lasts about 3 months, but reinjection may be used with results similar to those obtained by the first injection.

SURGICAL CORRECTION OF DISABILITIES. Lower Limb Problems. The most common site of deformity in the stroke patient is the foot and ankle equinus. A reliable standing base is most important, and even a patient with very minimal motor control can achieve stability at the knee and hip provided a stable plantigrade position is obtainable at the foot. This deformity, whether due to actual contracture or to spasticity, is relieved by elongation of the tendon Achilles. The patient is encouraged to walk and stand 3 to 5 days following the surgery.

In order to control the varus deformity of the foot which is frequently associated with spasticity or contracture of the gastrocnemius and soleus, the tibialis anterior tendon transfer is a useful adjunct.

Knee flexion deformity is favored by a persistence of the primitive flexor pattern and lack of early stimulation of extensor patterns. Usually the flexed knee deformity is equally accountable to lack of quadriceps muscle tone as to excessive hamstring spasticity. Release of the hamstrings

by sectioning at the musculotendinous junction corrects this deformity.

Disability at the hip joint may arise from three causes:

1. Abductor and extensor weakness
2. Persistent hip flexion deformity
3. Excessive adductor motor tone

Abductor and extensor weakness often may be improved by the use of a walking stick carried in the opposite hand. Hip adduction contracture may be released by adductor division, or in the case of spasticity by obturator neurectomy.

Hip flexion deformity may be released. However it is important to demonstrate spasticity so severe and contractural deformity so marked that the subsequent weakness of hip flexion will be a less severe problem than the preexisting one.

Upper Limb. Surgical procedures in the upper limbs are usually carried out for problems of painful contracture, severe spasticity, or mechanical impairment of function.

The painful frozen shoulder is a major impairment to rehabilitation. Mild spasticity in the internal rotator adductor group at the shoulder is noted frequently in the third and fourth months following a stroke. Active assisted exercises combined with a positioning program may maintain or help regain a good range of shoulder movement.

The Flexed Spastic Elbow. Severe spasticity of the flexors of the elbow does not respond to exercising and positioning programs and may result in a flexion contracture. The deformity is unsightly and prevents the patient from positioning his hand. The contracture is frequently associated with a symptomatic adducted shoulder; both areas may be treated simultaneously during shoulder release surgery. Release procedures in the antecubital fossa are rarely called for, and the surgeon must be prepared to release or lengthen the biceps tendon, brachialis, brachioradialis, the forearm flexor muscles, and the elbow joint capsule.

The Spastic Forearm and Hand. Spasticity and poor motor control are common in the hemiplegic forearm and hand. Procedures to improve these may be considered when the general state of the patient is good and there is intact sensation associated with some selective motor control in the arm. If a patient with an apparent flexion deformity of the wrist and fingers is able to extend the wrist and fingers selectively following a nerve block, then a flexor slide procedure will be of value to weaken the spastic flexor pronators. However, when there is significant fixed flexion contracture in wrist and fingers, a simple muscle origin release procedure will not be sufficient.

POSTURE

Posture is the basis of all movement. All movements start from, and end in, posture. The regulation of normal posture in an intact animal depends upon the integrated activity of many reflex mechanisms. The anterior horn cell forms a convergent point for fibers from many dorsal nerve roots and for fibers from all levels of the brain and spinal cord. Only when the activity of all these converging pathways are properly coordinated does normal posture result.

In the spinal cord there are reflex mechanisms that subserve a variety of movements, but the maintenance of posture is thought to be exclusively a function of reflex arcs that have centers in the pons, medulla, and midbrain. The organization of movement is more complex. In the motor control involving posture and movement, the final common pathways from the anterior horn cells in the cord to the muscles have been found to contain both large alpha neurons, which directly innervate the muscle fibers, and small gamma fibers, which innervate only the intrafusal muscles of the sensory end organs in the muscle spindle. Excitation of these does not produce muscle contraction in the ordinary sense but, by producing contraction of the muscle within the spindles, sets up afferent impulses which return to the cord via the dorsal roots to produce a tonic facilitation of the large alpha neurons. This facilitation is essential to the development of the stretch reflex.

The gamma neurons may be stimulated to activity from the motor cortex, particularly from the tegmentum of the brain stem. There is also evidence that the gamma system of neurons may pass from higher levels of the central nervous system by many routes, one of which is probably the pyramidal or corticospinal system. Afferents which modify the discharge of centers giving rise to the long propriospinal or the reticulospinal tracts are responsible for the adjustments of posture produced by neck reflexes, labyrinthine reflexes, and righting reflexes.

Tonic neck reflexes appear in infants between the fourth and twelfth week, but it is not until the twenty-eighth week that an infant is able to raise his head and control it. By the fifth month the child can roll over, but is usually only creeping or moving forward in the prone position by the tenth month. By the thirty-sixth week he will be able to stand still for a short while without support but usually will not walk unaided before the age of twelve months.

The sensory end organs of ligaments play a significant role in maintaining the stability and position of joints. These act by limiting extreme ranges of movement as well as by indicating the actual position of the joint via proprioceptive pathways.

When assessing any disturbance of posture, one must inspect the child while he is standing, sitting, and lying and determine the presence or absence of any abnormal movements or response to movements. In addition, one should look for any laxity of joints or hypertonia of muscles. When the child stands erect, changes in the spinal column occur with the development of a cervical lordosis, a thoracic kyphosis, and a lumbar lordosis. In the standing position, the gravitational forces lie along lines passing through the mastoid processes, the greater trochanters, and the tibial tubercles, to reach the ground in line with the bases of the fifth metatarsals. A state of equilibrium between these forces occurs when a vertical line passes along the center of gravity but falls within the boundary of the supporting base of both feet.

Postural deformities resulting from habit, occupational attitudes, or body carriage in movement must be differentiated from static forces, which are concerned with bodies at rest, or the equilibrium of weights which are not moving. A postural deformity is dynamic in orgin, whereas a static deformity occurs because of weakened musculature.

Disturbances in Gait (Limping)

In normal gait there are three major phases through which the lower limbs alternate. These are the phases of stance, swing-through, and propulsion.

PHASE I—STANCE. When one leg is moving forward, the body is maintained in an upright position on the other supporting foot, and the center of gravity is balanced high at the level of the superior border of the sacrum. Under these conditions, the static forces passing through the lower extremity joints are immense. Denham has shown that the hip joint of the adult male may be subject to pressures of 350 ft-lb/in.[2]

Stability during this stance phase demands a locking mechanism in both the hip and knee. For the hip joint, Walmsley described this locking mechanism as internal rotation with some abduction in full extension so that the largest diameter of the femoral head will be accommodated within the acetabular socket, whereas Gilmour attributed the stability of the femoral head to a gripping mechanism served by the acetabular labrum, the capsule of the hip joint, and a cushion of synovial fluid.

Structural abnormalities can be aggravated by forces of gravity in all age groups. Postural abnormalities are usually correctible by changing the deforming force, whereas in static deformities the originating disease must be corrected as well.

The knee joint is stabilized and locked in full extension by the contraction of the vastus medialis and the popliteus muscle, which internally rotates the femoral condyle on the tibial plateau.

PHASE II—THE PENDULUM, OR SWING-THROUGH, PHASE. The swing-through phase of gait is characterized by dorsiflexion of the foot and toes and flexion of the knee and the hip. At the same time, a certain proportion of the total body weight is moved forward by means of hip abduction, external rotation of the leg, and rotation of the pelvis.

PHASE III—PROPULSION. The propulsion phase of gait is one of forward movement in which the body leans forward. At the same time the supporting limb is pushing off with plantar-flexed foot, extended toes, extended knee, and extended hip. These dynamic forces of propulsion are contributed to by those of body weight added to those of the muscular contraction.

REQUIREMENTS FOR EFFICIENT LOCOMOTION. These are:

1. Stability of joints, normal bone length, normal skeletal relationships
2. Normal joint range of movement and normal muscle power
3. Cortical control of voluntary muscle action
4. Normal muscle tone, including coordination as well as postural tone
5. Normal sensory modalities
6. Cerebellar control of muscle action, and intact ocular and auditory balance mechanism

Abnormal, or disturbed, gait of mechanical origin must be clearly distinguished from ataxic and other gait patterns of neurologic origin. This requires examination of the joints to determine normal range of motion and detect fixed flexion contractures. Abnormalities of the foot and ankle should be searched for and neurologic disorders evaluated.

NEUROLOGIC DISORDERS

Ataxic gait consists of an uncoordinated, awkward, unbalanced, wide-based gait with poor symmetry and repetition pattern. It may result from:

1. Disturbances of the cerebellum, such as thrombosis of the cerebellar artery, or tumors of the posterior cranial fossa
2. Lesions involving the posterior columns such as disseminated sclerosis, the Guillain-Barré syndrome, and Friedreich's ataxia
3. Lesions involving peripheral sensation and proprioceptive modalities, such as tabes dorsalis, or neuritis and subacute combined degeneration of the cord, which give a characteristic high-stepping gait

A spastic paraplegic gait is characterized by scissoring of the legs, which are held stiff in extension and adducted. If adduction deformity, which is common in cerebral palsy, is severe, the degree of pelvic rotation and elevation may be markedly exaggerated.

In hemiplegia the flail, or spastic, leg is used as a prop until the good leg can be brought forward for the propulsion phase.

MECHANICAL DISORDERS

JOINT DISORDERS. Among the numerous joint abnormalities which may produce gait disturbances are congenital dysplasia, congenital dislocation of the hip, slipped upper femoral epiphysis, Legg-Calvé-Perthes disease, and knee conditions such as juvenile arthritis, osteochondritis dissecans, discoid menisci, congenital genu valgum or varus, and congenital metatarsus varus, flatfoot, or congenital talipes equinovarus (clubfoot).

LEG-LENGTH DISCREPANCY. This may be the result of congenital or acquired shortening of the femur or tibia or soft tissue contractures of the hip or knee joint, secondary to joint or primary muscular disease.

MUSCULAR DISORDERS. Among the muscular disorders resulting in abnormal gait are those secondary to anterior poliomyelitis, cerebral palsy, nerve injury, spina bifida, myelodysplasia, primary motor neuron disease, and muscular dystrophy.

Spinal Deformities

The convexity of the thoracic and sacral curves, the primary curves of the vertebral column, result from the shape of the vertebral bodies, whereas the secondary, lordotic curves of the cervical and lumbar regions are due more to the shape of the intervertebral discs, which are wider anteriorly than posteriorly. In addition, the contour of the vertebral column is dependent upon the integrity of its supporting ligaments and the sacrospinalis and anterior abdominal musculatures.

The intervertebral discs, like arterial walls, reflect the age and tone of the body tissues. With increasing age, the nucleus pulposus loses its elasticity and fluid content, and the fibers of the annulus fibrosus lose their definition. These changes are very marked in those engaged in heavy work, but they are a feature of all aging spines.

Alterations in the normal anterorposterior curvature of the spine occur in both the young and the old and are the consequence of affections of bones, intervertebral discs, or spinal muscles.

KYPHOSIS

The term "kyphosis" refers to an increase in the normal posterior convexity of the thoracic spine, involving a number of vertebral bodies, if not the entire thoracic column. On the other hand, "gibbus" refers to an acute angular deformity resulting from a disease such as tuberculosis or a fractured vertebral body.

Kyphosis of Adolescence

MUSCULAR TYPE. The muscular type of adolescent kyphosis is seen in children of poor physical development and is characterized by a thoracic kyphosis, or "round shoulders." Such children are often slow and clumsy in their movements, i.e., uncoordinated. In the early stages, spinal movements are normal, but later the mobility of the spine decreases, and the kyphosis becomes fixed. Pain is not a common feature of the condition, but postural strain on ligaments may produce backache or pain in the feet or legs.

Early treatment aimed at improving musculature by exercise, swimming, deep breathing, and posture training produces dramatic improvement. External support by braces is not recommended.

OSSEOUS TYPE. This usually results from developmental disturbances such as arachnodactyly, osteochondral dystrophy, or acquired lesions such as tuberculosis. Tuberculosis as a result of bony destruction tends to produce an acute gibbus rather than a smooth kyphosis.

DISCOGENIC TYPE, OR TRUE ADOLESCENT KYPHOSIS (SCHEUERMANN'S DISEASE; VERTEBRAL EPIPHYSITIS). This condition occurs in both sexes between the ages of twelve and seventeen and is seen as marked thoracic kyphosis with round, drooping shoulders and a flat, narrow chest with prominent scapulae.

The cause of this condition, which is familial, is unknown, but possible factors are:

1. Circulatory disturbances affecting the nutrition of the vertebral epiphysis, with fragmentation and irregularities as seen on radiography (Fig. 43-24). Permanent wedging of the vertebral bodies may result.
2. Early disc degeneration consequent upon:
   a. A rapid increase in body weight.
   b. Multiple minor traumas.
   c. Shortening of the hamstrings, which produces hyperflexion strains at the thoracolumbar junction on stooping, or forward flexion

Early active treatment in the form of spinal traction followed by hyperextension and spinal exercises can limit the progress of this deformity. Once spinal growth is complete at the age of sixteen to eighteen years, no further progression will occur.

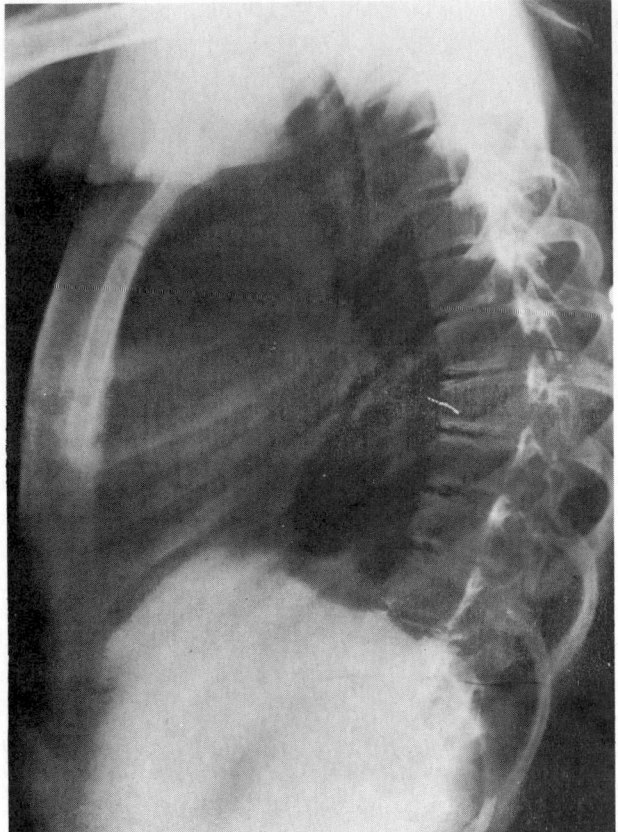

Fig. 43-24. Lateral radiograph showing fragmentation of the vertebral epiphysis in the thoracic spine in Scheuermann's disease.

Increasing spinal kyphosis is a common accompaniment of advancing years. It may result from a variety of pathologic changes affecting the different components of the spinal column.

"TRUE" SENILE KYPHOSIS. Especially in those engaged in heavy occupations, degeneration of the anterior portion of the annulus fibrosus leads to final disintegration of the intervertebral discs. This results in wedging of the anterior aspects of the vertebral bodies until they touch, by osteophyte formation as well as bony absorption.

SENILE OR POSTMENOPAUSAL OSTEOPOROSIS. In this condition, although the degree of osteoporosis of the vertebral bodies varies, it is evenly distributed throughout the vertebral column. There is absorption of the bony trabeculae, but the intervertebral discs remain normal or even tend to bulge into the atrophied spongy tissue of the vertebral body.

In the earliest phase the patient has great difficulty in carrying out extremes of movement, and there is often a history of attacks of "lumbago." Pain may never completely disappear. The individual loses his stature and carries himself stooping, the head and shoulders thrust forward. This loss in height must be differentiated from Paget's disease, Kümmel's disease, multiple myeloma, and secondary malignant deposits.

SCOLIOSIS

When viewed from the back any deviation from the normally straight spine to one side or the other, i.e., a lateral deviation, constitutes scoliosis.

CLASSIFICATION. There are many classifications, but the most simple and practicable is that suggested by Cobb and modified by Ponsetti and Freedman:

Classification of Scoliosis

I. Postural scoliosis
II. Structural scoliosis
   A. Idiopathic
     1. Cervicothoracic
     2. Thoracic
       a. Infantile—age of onset birth to three years
       b. Juvenile—age of onset four to nine years
       c. Adolescence—age of onset ten years to the end of growth
     3. Thoracolumbar
     4. Lumbar
     5. Combined thoracic and lumbar
   B. Osteopathic
     1. Congenital vertebral anomalies
     2. Thoracogenic following thoracoplasty or empyema
     3. Osteochondrodystrophy
   C. Neuropathic
     1. Congenital
     2. Postpoliomyelitis
     3. Neurofibromatosis
     4. Other neuropathies
       a. Syringomyelia
       b. Charcot-Marie-Tooth syndrome
       c. Friedreich's ataxia
       d. Cerebral palsy
   D. Myopathic
     1. Congenital scoliosis
     2. Muscular dystrophies

Postural Scoliosis

Postural scoliosis is seen most commonly in adolescent girls. The curve is usually slight, single, and characteristically a long left thoracolumbar scoliosis, without vertebral rotation, which disappears when the child hangs from a bar or bends forward. In recumbency, the spine appears straight, and when tested for lateral flexion it will bend equally well to both sides.

A short leg will cause a compensatory scoliosis convex to the side of the depressed pelvis, but correcting the shortening with a lift under the shoe, thus leveling the pelvis, will correct the scoliosis.

Treatment of postural scoliosis is the same as for poor posture in general, i.e., improvement in musculature by general spinal exercises.

Structural Scoliosis

CONGENITAL SCOLIOSIS. Congenital scoliosis is associated with demonstrable vertebral anomalies. There may be one hemivertebra or more involved with congenital absence of discs or fusions of vertebral bodies and ribs. In general, isolated vertebral anomalies have a good prognosis, but there are cases, particularly in the thoracic region, in which a long vertebral segment is involved and in which a gross scoliosis develops. Unfortunately, it is not easy initially to recognize which type is present.

It is preferable to determine and to treat surgically at a young age those with an anomalous vertebral development in association with undifferentiated posterolateral bony bars. Congenital scoliosis is more likely than other forms of scoliosis to lead to paraplegia, usually in the later years of growth, and for this reason must remain under observation until the end of the growth period.

PARALYTIC SCOLIOSIS. This most commonly results after anterior poliomyelitis and can be prevented or minimized by adequate initial management. In the young patient with paralytic poliomyelitis and asymmetrical involvement of trunk musculature, asymmetrical soft tissue contractures and subsequent disturbances of vertebral growth may develop.

The various curve patterns of paralytic scoliosis have been divided into high thoracic, thoracic, thoracolumbar, lumbar, and combined thoracic and lumbar scoliosis, and a telescoping spine.

The prognosis in paralytic scoliosis is less dependent on the localization of the primary curve than in idiopathic scoliosis. A more important prognostic factor is the age at which the disease first occurs, because the longer the imbalance of muscle affects vertebral growth, the more the distortion.

Idiopathic Scoliosis

PATHOLOGY. The true pathologic basis of idiopathic scoliosis is still unknown, but interesting animal experiments point the way toward the possible causes. Langerskiold and Michelsson produced a progressive scoliosis in rabbits by removing the posterior ends of five or six ribs as well as by hemilaminectomy of five of the thoracic vertebrae. The common factor was the loss of function of the posterior costotransverse ligaments, and cutting these ligaments alone produced similar deformities. Ponsetti and Shepard produced scoliosis by inducing lathyrism in rats. The skeletal deformities which resulted were due to lesions of the epiphyseal plates with loosening and detachments of the tendinous and ligamentous insertions.

NATURAL HISTORY. Idiopathic scoliosis will progress during growth in the majority of cases. Therefore the two important factors in deciding the prognosis of this condition are the *age of onset* and the *site of the curve*.

Risser and Ferguson first noticed the relationship between spinal growth and the increase of the deformity and also its cessation when the bony structure matured at the age of seventeen in boys and sixteen in girls. Later Risser observed that the completion of ossification of the iliac apophysis coincides with completion of spinal growth. Therefore any growth after this is minimal, as is deterioration in the curve. Thoracic curves beginning before the age of ten years carry a very poor prognosis and usually result in a severe deformity. Steindler, quoted by Crowe, noted that the maximal deterioration of scoliosis generally occurred between the ages of one and two years, between five and ten years, and at puberty when there was rapid growth of the spine. The author of the present chapter,

from a longitudinal growth study of 10 cases of infantile idiopathic scoliosis, found that there was deterioration during two main periods: first, shortly after diagnosis at the age of two to four years, when it was related to the midgrowth spurt, and, second, at the age of six to nine in boys and six to ten in girls. This latter deterioration followed the midgrowth spurt closely. The adolescent growth spurt had little influence on this particular form of scoliosis. Although the infantile idiopathic scoliosis makes up only 10 percent of all cases of scoliosis, it is exposed to the total effects of growth throughout its natural history and because of this has an extremely poor prognosis, producing the most progressive and severe of all curvatures.

In general, to prognosticate for any particular case of idiopathic scoliosis the following observations are required:

1. The site of the curve
2. The age of onset
3. The skeletal or physiologic age rather than the chronological age
4. The state of ossification of the iliac apophysis
5. The developmental age in relation to puberty

CLINICAL FEATURES OF IDIOPATHIC AND OTHER FORMS OF STRUCTURAL SCOLIOSIS. Medical attention is usually sought because of trunk asymmetry, a prominent hip, a prominent shoulder, or a hump on the back. There is occasionally a complaint of backache and fatigue, but severe pain is an unusual complaint. However, in adult life, particularly in lumbar scoliosis, pain due to secondary degenerative changes may produce symptoms.

Later complications of severe scoliosis include reductions in the vital capacity of the lungs and the development of cor pulmonale. Bergofsky et al. have described the correlation of cardiopulmonary pathologic changes in relation to the severity of the curvature.

The most common type of idiopathic scoliosis is a right thoracic curve, which occurs predominantly in girls (Fig. 43-25). The curvature of congenital scoliosis due to abnormal vertebral development is usually a short, sharp curve which is rigid and associated with much less rotational prominence of the posterior rib cage or lumbar area than the idiopathic and paralytic curves. An angular but short scoliosis in the presence of café au lait spots and subcutaneous nevi indicates neurofibromatosis.

Fig. 43-25. Features of an idiopathic scoliosis in a girl with a right thoracic curve.

When a patient with scoliosis is examined, the shoulder girdles, the thoracic and lumbar areas of the trunk, and the iliac crests are assessed for asymmetry. The height of the iliac crest and the posterosuperior iliac spines is determined to note whether the pelvis is level. It is necessary to measure leg length in recumbency to exclude secondary scoliosis due to leg-length discrepancy. On forward flexion of the spine a rotational prominence of the transverse processes will be noted, particularly on the convex side of the curve.

The mobility of the spine is tested by traction applied to the head manually as well as by lateral bending in the erect position and lateral bending in the recumbent position. It will be noted that thoracic curves are usually more rigid than lumbar curves.

Finally a complete radiologic survey of the entire spine is essential including an anteroposterior view with the patient standing and recumbent views with the patient bending to the right and to the left. Lateral views of the spine are also required to assess any degree of congenital anomaly. From these it is possible to assess the site and degree of both the primary and secondary curves.

The primary curve is defined as:

1. The longest curve with the greatest degree of angulation
2. The least flexible curve as determined by clinical and radiologic examination
3. The curve toward which the trunk lists

The degree of angulation is measured on the radiograph in the manner described by Cobb. Perpendicular lines are erected to the superior surface of the proximal vertebra and the inferior surface of the distal vertebra involved. The angle formed by these two intersecting lines is the angle of the curve (Fig. 43-26).

Treatment of Scoliosis

CONSERVATIVE TREATMENT. The object of treatment is to obtain correction and to prevent any further increase in the deformity. In idiopathic scoliosis in particular, treatment requires regular clinical, radiographic, and photographic examination to observe and to record progress of the curvature during growth. General exercises are prescribed to obtain good posture and to maintain mobility of the spine.

With respect to external supports, the Moe brace (Fig. 43-27), which relieves pressure of the vertebral epiphyses on the concave side of the curve, is the most efficient appliance available. The efficient use of this brace permits the postponement of surgical treatment until final correction, and spinal fusion can be carried out at the age of ten years or more.

Paralytic scoliosis is treated more aggressively than idiopathic curvatures during development of the deformity. Initially in the very young child prolonged recumbency is advocated, and stretching exercises are instituted to maintain good spinal mobility and to prevent soft tissue contractures. Bent plaster shells such as the Murk-Jansen bed are used intermittently to counteract any deforming attitude in recumbency, and once correction is obtained, the vertebral column must be supported with a removable plaster jacket or a Milwaukee brace.

SURGICAL TREATMENT. Surgical treatment is required when the deformity cannot be controlled in the growing

Fig. 43-26. Idiopathic scoliosis treated by Harrington rod and massive bone graft. Goldstein technique. *A.* 85° right thoracic primary curve between T_5 and T_{12}. *B.* Lateral bend to the right corrects curve to 56°. *C.* Postoperative correction following Harrington rod instrumentation and bone grafting with massive autogenous cancellous bone. The curve is corrected to 37° and is fused to T_1.

child by the use of the Milwaukee brace and in the case of any correctable deformity at or after maturity which is accompanied by pain. As a general rule, curves under 40° can be controlled by the Milwaukee brace, but when progression of the curve occurs, correction and spinal fusion is indicated. With progression of a paralytic scoliotic curve and instability of the trunk due to muscle imbalance, stabilization of the spine is indicated. In cases of congenital scoliosis where there is a definite undifferentiated bony bar in the concavity of the curve, early fusion over a short segment of the involved vertebrae is mandatory, since the curve will relentlessly progress without it. Congenital curves should be watched closely and fused early if there is progression. Specific indications for operation include curves over 60° and those involving the thoracic or thoracolumbar spine. A more conservative approach may be adopted for double major curves, which are usually balanced. Pain is rare in the adolescent scoliosis patient. Operative intervention is rarely required in adults unless there is severe pain.

The usual operative measures are those of posterior spinal fusion utilizing cancellous bone and some form of internal and external splintage after adequate correction has been obtained. The Harrington rod has added greatly to the ability to improve correction and, when utilized with sound spine fusion techniques, has lowered the rate of pseudarthrosis and loss of correction postoperatively. The Dwyer technique involves an anterior approach to the vertebral bodies, interbody fusion, and correction of the curve by the swadged cable fixed to screws attached to the vertebral bodies. For some types of rigid curves and severe thoracolumbar curves this technique is a definite advantage. When Harrington rod and posterior spine fusions are carried out, patients are immobilized postoperatively in a plaster cast extending from the chin and occiput to at least the groin and occasionally to include both thighs. Plaster cast immobilization is usually required for 4 to 6 months after surgery (Fig. 43-28).

Knee Deformities

GENU VALGUM

This deformity is characterized by an abnormal increase in the distance between the two medial malleoli when the extended knees are just touching each other. It may arise from disturbances of the epiphyseal plate, epiphysis, or ligamentous structures of the knee joint and after fractures of the lateral tibial or the lateral femoral condyle. A common cause used to be deficiency rickets with disturbance of the mineralization process in endochondral ossification. Rachitic deformities may still arise from congenital renal insufficiency such as Fanconi's syndrome or vitamin D–resistant rickets. Genu valgum is not an uncommon complication of rheumatoid arthritis, in which there is gradual attenuation of the medial ligament and collapse of the lateral tibial condyle. Similarly it may complicate postmenopausal osteoporosis.

However, the most common type of genu valgum, or knock-knee, is that seen in young children and is consid-

Fig. 43-27. Moe brace treatment of idiopathic scoliosis.

ered to be postural, or idiopathic, in type (Fig. 43-29). Indeed, it is so common during infancy that it might be considered a normal phase of development. Morley found that 22 percent of children of three to three and one-half years of age had genu valgum with an intermaleolar distance of 2 in. or more, whereas only 1 to 2 percent of children aged seven and over had an equivalent degree of genu valgum. The deformity arises because the line of weight transmission from the femur falls within the lateral side of the center of the knee joint, so that the lateral condyles of both the femur and the tibia bear more weight than their medial counterparts.

TREATMENT. Genu valgum in infants and children below the age of seven can be safely ignored if not excessive and in the absence of underlying causes. It may be advisable in certain cases to raise the inner edge of the heel by $\frac{1}{8}$ to $\frac{3}{16}$ in., especially as a measure of reassurance to the anxious parents.

Fig. 43-28. Localizer cast with windows cut allowing surgical exposure. *A.* Windows in place. *B.* Windows removed, showing access to the iliac crest and spine.

Fig. 43-29. Idiopathic genu valgum deformity.

Active treatment is occasionally necessary in the form of Jones walking genu valgum braces or mermaid night splints. In severe cases, some of which commence posturally and have been aggravated by obesity, operative correction in the form of supracondylar femoral osteotomy may be required.

Fig. 43-30. Genu varum deformity in an infant boy mainly arising from the tibiae.

GENU VARUM

The pathogenesis of genu varum is similar to that outlined above for genu valgum. The idiopathic, or postural, variety in infancy is the most common clinical form of presentation.

A minor degree of the deformity is quite common in children up to three years of age, and the deformity is usually restricted to the tibia (Fig. 43-30). Occasionally, the deformity may be more apparent than real and is really a manifestation of an abnormal arc of rotation in the hips or persistent fetal alignment, in which there is excess of internal rotation over external rotation, due to marked anteversion of the femoral neck.

TREATMENT. As in genu valgum, most postural, idiopathic types without any evidence of underlying metabolic or congenital epiphyseal disorders regress spontaneously and require no treatment.

Foot and Ankle Deformities

In spite of its lightness and elasticity, the foot possesses tremendous strength. The architectural arrangement of its bones and joints into multiple elastic arches and levers provides two main functions: a stable support for the body's weight in standing and a resilient spring, or lever, for propulsion in walking.

The arch configuration of the foot is characteristic of man. Most textbooks describe three arches, two longitudinal and one transverse. The calcaneus forms the common posterior pillar for both the lateral and the medial longitudinal arches. The lateral longitudinal arch is completed by the cuboid and the lateral two metatarsals. The medial is completed by the talus, the cuneiform, and the inner three metatarsals. The third metatarsal, though a component of the medial arch, serves both longitudinal arches physiologically. Also, in forming the anterior pillar of the essential arch, it acts as a pivot to assist in shifting body weight from the lateral to the medial longitudinal arch during locomotion. The transverse arch usually refers to the anterior metatarsal arch, the existence of which as a functional element was denied by Morton, who demonstrated by means of special apparatus that all five metatarsal heads participate in weight bearing and that the foot does *not* distribute its weight like a tripod. Morton's experiment can be verified by standing barefoot on five slips of paper, one under each metatarsal head. If an assistant then attempts to pull out the strips, he soon discovers that the foot is no tripod.

The characteristically human, archlike structure of the foot is obvious in the cartilaginous skeleton at birth, but when the child begins to stand, the arch tends to flatten, and it is not for some years that it develops the ability to resist the forces of weight bearing. Postural tone of the leg muscles, which occurs somewhat late in human development, is essential in assisting the arch of the foot to resist these forces; should the development of this postural tone fail, the inherent bony arches of the foot become flattened, producing variable degrees and types of so-called "flatfoot."

MECHANICS OF THE FOOT. The function of muscles and ligaments in the control of the arch of the foot is much disputed, some emphasizing the ligaments and others favoring the muscles as the prime factor. Keith is largely responsible for the concept that muscles maintain the arch by their dynamic pull. However, many deny this, and Hicks, in an anatomic, electromyographic study of the foot, demonstrated that the leg muscles play no part in the configuration of the foot and are indeed inactive during standing. The arch of the foot should be considered as an inherent and characteristic structure based upon the architectural configuration of the skeletal elements aided by the numerous ligaments joining them and stabilized by the muscles acting upon them.

Hicks described the weight-bearing unit of the foot as a combination of beam action and arch action. An arch-shaped structure has its ends thrust apart when a weight is applied to it. Therefore the strength peculiar to a true arch is only acquired when the ends are prevented from coming farther apart. In the foot this function of the tie between the piers is produced by the plantar aponeurosis. However, when the ends of an archlike structure are not prevented from spreading farther apart, the structure cannot behave as an arch and behaves as a beam. A beam is subject to bending strain, and its strength depends upon the resistance of the material to being broken by bending. The concept of the foot, which is a structure composed of several pieces, as a beam is not acceptable unless there are tense intersegmental ties on the undersurface, the joints being at their limit of extension. In considering the weight-bearing unit of the foot, a distinction must be made between the beam action and the arch action. In the beam action there is bending strain in the bones which produces tension in the intersegmental ligaments, whereas in the arch action there is compression strain in the bones and a tension strain in the plantar aponeurosis.

In the flat standing position, the arch-flattening effect of body weight produces tension in the plantar aponeurosis, and the foot behaves as an arch, but when the line of weight moves forward through the foot as the heel begins to rise, the arch-flattening effect is resisted by both beam and arch mechanisms acting together. In the tiptoe standing position or the push-off phase of walking, the arch mechanism takes over from the beam action by virtue of the fact that the extension of the toes at the metatarsophalangeal (MP) joints "winds up the windlass" of the plantar aponeurosis. The strain on the beam action therefore lessens, and in the extreme raised-heel position the arch mechanism assumes the whole load, and the arch rises.

FLATFOOT (Pes Planus; Pes Valgus)

Congenital Convex Pes Valgus (Congenital Vertical Talus)

See Chap. 44 on Congenital Orthopedic Deformities.

Peroneal Spastic Flatfoot

Although this condition may be produced by inflammatory and traumatic affections of the tarsal joints, Harris has shown that the most common cause is an abnormal

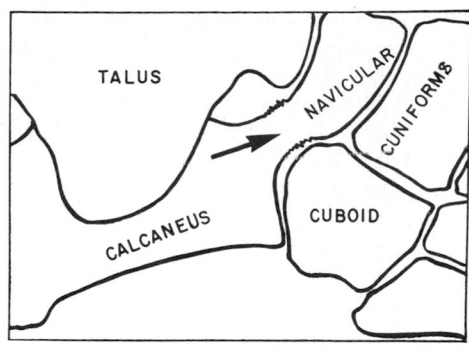

Fig. 43-31. Calcaneonavicular bar.

coalescence between two or more of the tarsal bones. This is in effect a congenital ankylosis which may be either complete or incomplete and may be osseous, cartilaginous, or fibrous.

In young children tarsal coalescence cannot be seen on x-ray, because it is cartilaginous and ossification does not occur until the age of nine or ten. Even in adulthood, special x-ray views and techniques such as tomograms are necessary to demonstrate the abnormal osseous anatomy. There are three common sites for such osseous coalescence between tarsal bones:

1. A calcaneonavicular bar (Fig. 43-31)
2. A talocalcaneal bar (Fig. 43-32)
3. A calcaneocuboid bar

Conservative treatment in the form of manipulation and the use of braces offer little chance of success. An operation is usually indicated. In young children if a bar can be demonstrated, simple resection may be successful, but usually the diagnosis is not made until adolescence or early adulthood when tarsal arthritis supervenes, necessitating triple arthrodesis.

Acquired Flatfoot

Acquired flatfoot may be divided into three pathologic types:

1. Osseous type, due to bony distortion produced by trauma or disease processes
2. Ligamentous type, which may follow rupture or avulsion of the ligamentous attachments of the foot, or sprain
3. Muscular imbalance, as in anterior poliomyelitis and cerebral palsy

Fig. 43-32. Talocalcaneal bar.

A.   B.

Flatfoot will arise whenever the muscles or ligaments fail to support the integral bony architecture of the arch. In the first efforts of walking a child usually walks with his feet flat and abducted. A good deal of this appears to be due to large deposits of fat over the medial aspect of the sole, but it is, in part, really due to inability of the leg muscles to support the arch. As postural tone develops, this deformity gradually disappears.

In an initially normal foot, there are certain predisposing extrinsic and intrinsic factors which may tend to transform it into a flat foot. All these factors will be considered under the following headings: Muscle Hypotonia, Excess of Muscular Fatigue, Footwear.

MUSCLE HYPOTONIA. The muscle hypotonia following recumbency accompanying long illness places the full strain of weight bearing and walking upon the bony and ligamentous structure of the arch. Stretching of these ligaments, which form the segmental ties of the archlike structure, will result in flattening of the foot.

EXCESS OF MUSCULAR FATIGUE. This is commonly an occupational hazard of nurses, policemen, and soldiers, and may also follow excessive exercises after a period of relative disuse. Relative muscular insufficiency as another factor in the development of acquired flatfoot is seen with sudden increases in body weight, a common occurrence in postmenopausal women accounting for much of the foot strain in this group.

FOOTWEAR. It has frequently been implied that unsuitable footwear is a basis of many of our foot troubles, but Hyman considered that this is unlikely, i.e., that ". . . most deformities of the foot and toes are developmental and it would be necessary to alter the genes rather than the children's footwear in order to prevent them."

Fig. 43-33. *A.* Line drawing of the lateral aspect of the foot to show the break occurring at the talonavicular and naviculocuneiform joints. *B.* Line drawing of the lateral aspect of the foot showing the correction of the talonavicular and naviculocuneiform joints, so that a straight line can be drawn through the axes of the talus, navicular, medial cuneiform, and metatarsals. (*After Jack, 1953.*)

An extensive survey of school children's feet revealed that, between the ages of five and fifteen, hallux valgus was much more common in girls than in boys. In girls at the age of five the incidence of hallux valgus was 1.6 percent and by fifteen years had risen to 54 percent. In boys, on the other hand, at five years the incidence was 5.2 percent and at fifteen years had risen to only 14.8 percent. Therefore, the accelerated acquisition of this deformity must have begun before the age of nine, when there is virtually no difference in the footwear of the two sexes. However, Lam and Hodgson have shown significant increase in deformities in shoe-wearing populations in Hong Kong when compared with the unshod. Although there is no simple correlation between foot defects and unsatisfactory footwear, it is accepted that proper footwear is essential for the normal growth and development of the foot.

PATHOLOGY. If the calcaneonavicular ligament gives way, the talus deviates downward and mediad, and its body glides forward on the upper surface of the calcaneus. The calcaneus itself swings mediad, and its anterior end is depressed, with the result that the sustentaculum tali, the head of the talus, and the tuberosity of the navicular come to form prominences on the medial aspect of the foot.

Jack reviewed the anatomic types of flatfoot and pointed out that in lateral radiographs of the normal weight-bearing foot a straight line could be drawn through the axis of the talus, the middle of the navicular, the medial cuneiform, and the metatarsals. He described how a break would produce an unstable and everted foot of varying types depending upon the site of the break. A break may be at the talonavicular joint, producing the so-called "vertical talus deformity" or at the naviculocuneiform joint, or at both these joints combined (Fig. 43-33*A*). He demonstrated that dorsiflexion of the great toe restored the arch, particularly in cases of navicular cuneiform break, but not when the break occurred at other joints (Fig. 43-33*B*).

In time the displaced bones gradually alter in shape, and the navicular and cuneiform bones may become shaped like wedges with their apices situated dorsad. There is then permanent alteration in the architecture of the entire tarsus.

CLINICAL MANIFESTATIONS. The patient first notices that the feet become hot and uncomfortable after walking and standing. Later, they become stiff, especially after resting, and walking becomes increasingly painful. The gait becomes inelastic, clumsy, and "flatfooted," with no heel-and-toe rhythm, and severe pain and tenderness develop in the region of the navicular, the inferior calcaneonavicular ligament, the medial aspect of the sole, and the head of the first metatarsal. Finally, the awkward stiff, non-resilient gait results in abnormal weight distribution and the development of pressure points on the sole.

Four types of flatfoot may present themselves:

1. Foot Strain, or Incipient Flatfoot. This is the earliest stage, the period when pressure is first being exerted upon the ligaments. There is no evidence of deformity but simply symptoms of tenderness and pain.

2. Mobile Flatfoot.
    a. *Due to Faulty Postural Activity of Muscles.* This is seen in the very young child in whom there has been no development of postural tone.
    b. *Due to Short Calcaneus Tendon.* In these patients, the malalignment disappears on tiptoeing, but when the foot is correctly aligned, it is noted to be in planus.
3. Voluntary Flatfoot. This corresponds to the stage in which flattening of the arch has occurred but secondary adaptive changes have not yet ensued and the leg muscles, though they have lost their postural tone, can be used for volitional restoration of the arch.
4. Rigid Flatfoot. In these cases marked degenerative changes have occurred in the subtaloid and midtarsal joints, and the deformity has become fixed.

TREATMENT. The absolute indications for treatment are pain and impaired function. The existence of flatfoot per se does not necessarily mean that treatment is required. Many people with completely flat feet are able to go about their ordinary occupations without the slightest discomfort. Rigid flat feet are more likely to be symptomatic.

The ideal objectives of treatment, if indicated, are:

1. To correct the abnormal center of gravity in the foot so that the body weight is transferred to the outer side
2. To remove pressure symptoms

Treatment of Acute Foot Strain. Treatment of acute foot strain usually resolves itself into palliative measures, such as contrast footbaths, faradic footbaths, and foot exercises. Attention should also be directed toward the use of correct footwear, some features of which are outlined below.

The ideal shoe has a slightly concave inner border and a deep toe cap, and its width should be equal to, or a little greater than, that of the weight-bearing portion of the foot on standing. The sole should be firm over the heel and flexible over the forefoot, and the upper part must be made so as to form a well-fitting counter to support the heel and the high vamp over the instep.

For a short time following acute foot strain it is useful to thicken the medial portion of the sole of the shoe by about $\frac{1}{4}$ in., which deflects the body weight to the lateral side and spares the medial longitudinal arch. Special attention should be given to the fitting of correct footwear in children, but this is not always easy, as children rapidly outgrow rather than outwear their shoes. They should be fitted with Thomas heels, in which the medial border extends $\frac{1}{2}$ in. farther forward than the lateral, thus transferring the body weight to the lateral border of the foot.

Gait instruction and foot exercises are usual adjuncts in the management of foot strain from any cause. The patient should be taught to walk with the feet parallel, as the muscles supporting the arch are then activated and facilitate correction of the arch. Moreover, the heel-and-toe gait also brings into play the strong leg muscles which indirectly support the bony architecture of the foot.

Exercises, both active and against resistance, should be carried out twice daily. The rationale of these exercises is to stretch shortened structures such as the Achilles tendon and the soft parts of the lateral side of the foot and to strengthen relaxed muscles so that they are in a better condition to play their part in supporting the arch.

At the stage of voluntary flatfoot, in which there is still some possibility of volitional correction of the arch by muscle strength, exercises play a great part. While the muscles are being redeveloped, arch supports are often helpful in relieving symptoms. In the rigid and permanent types, however, the degenerative changes in the tarsal joints necessitate either triple arthrodesis or less extensive talonavicular fusions.

CONTRACTURE

The seventeenth-century term "contracture" means "a drawing together or becoming smaller." It implies, in pathologic terms, a permanent shortening and rigidity of muscles, joints, and fascial structures.

Contracture is a common sequel to joint immobility consequent upon disease, pain, etc. Experimental work in rats by Evans et al. has demonstrated that significant structural and progressive changes occur in muscle and intercapsular connective tissue planes after immobilization. Evans noted that these changes were partly reversible providing immobilization did not exceed 30 days, for beyond this time articular cartilage showed many irreversible changes such as matrix fibrillation, cleft separation, and subchondral bone destruction.

Contractures may be congenital or acquired.

CONGENITAL CONTRACTURES. Characteristic examples of congenital contractures are talipes equinovarus (clubfoot), sternocleidomastoid tumor (congenital torticollis), and the deformities associated with arthrogryposis multiplex congenita.

ACQUIRED CONTRACTURES. Acquired contractures of muscle, fascia, and ligaments involve disturbances of many tissue types, and it is therefore best to consider acquired contractures as primary or secondary with respect to their pathogenesis and tissue involvement.

Primary. *Muscle Contracture.* This includes primary muscular disorders such as progressive muscular dystrophy, the ischemia of Volkmann's contracture, and posttraumatic fibrosis.

Fascia. The classic primary, fascial type of contracture is that of Dupuytren's deformity affecting the palmar fascia and producing contractures of the fingers. It is occasionally seen in association with chronic barbiturism and may involve the plantar aponeurosis.

Joints. Many types of arthritic disorders such as rheumatoid arthritis, osteoarthritis, hemophilic arthropathy and infective and traumatic disorders of joints may result in contractures involving the intraarticular or periarticular structures, or both.

Secondary Contractures. These may be defined as contractures of muscles and joints as the result of primary disorders of nervous tissue such as anterior poliomyelitis, cerebral palsy, and many other types of neurologic disorders which produce paresis of muscle groups and unbalanced muscular activity. The skin may also develop severe contractures as a result of scarring, trauma, burns, and primary connective tissue disorders such as dermatomyositis and scleroderma.

Dupuytren's Contracture

This condition was first described in 1832 by Dupuytren, who demonstrated that it was caused by contracture of the palmar aponeurosis. Sir Astley Cooper had suggested the same cause some 10 years earlier.

INCIDENCE AND ETIOLOGY. Dupuytren's contracture chiefly affects people of European origin, and males are affected about twice as often as women. There is an increasing frequency with age. Inheritance of Dupuytren's contracture is well accepted, and family histories have been reported extending back for seven generations. It would appear that there is an autosomal inheritance with almost total penetrance in males, but to assume a single gene for Dupuytren's contracture is probably too simple an approach.

The ethnologic differences in incidence may simply indicate that the frequencies of certain autosomal characteristics are different in different racial groups.

The 40 percent incidence of Dupuytren's contracture demonstrated by Early and by Ling among Anglo-Saxon populations indicates that an autosomal system for Dupuytren's contractures among these populations is al-

Fig. 43-34. Pulling down of the ring finger by Dupuytren's contracture.

ways present but its expression is determined by other undetermined endogenous factors and less often exogenous factors such as injury, alcoholism, and pulmonary disease. It has been shown that there is a very strong association with epilepsy and a very high incidence among chronic invalids, particularly those with chronic pulmonary tuberculosis and alcoholism. On the other hand, no association can be demonstrated between Dupuytren's contracture and occupation, and indeed there is evidence suggesting that the condition might be aggravated by lack of, rather than excessive, manual activity.

PATHOLOGY. The earliest changes of palmar nodules, multifocal in distribution, arise within the palmar connective tissue on the anterior aspect of the palmar aponeurosis. Fibrosis of the nodule results in fixation of the skin and aponeurosis with contraction and thickening of the nodules and bands in the lines of maximal tension. Microscopically, there appears to be an increased vascularity of the palmar fibrofatty tissue. Perivascular cellular infiltration replaces the fat globules, and these hyperplastic foci finally mature into collagen bands. This process appears to commence on the palmar aspect of the aponeurosis and to extend along the formed fibrous elements of the palm including the aponeurosis and its intertendinous septums and the fine septums extending to the palmar skin and fingers. A similar process may occur in the plantar aponeurosis.

Factors such as epilepsy and alcoholism are often associated with severe local disease as well as with poor surgical results. Cases of fibrosis involving the dermal structures in the palm or overlying the proximal interphalangeal joint and "knuckle pads," or in the penis (Peyronie's disease), are examples of the extensive changes which can occur.

CLINICAL MANIFESTATIONS. Hueston described four clinical types:

1. Senile type. This consists of single discrete bands and a very slowly progressive deformity.
2. Middle-age type. This type often has multifocal proliferate nodules and slowly developing bands in one or both palms (Fig. 43-34).
3. Young fulminating type. This type has a tender palmar or digital thickening with pink, warm, and often sweaty skin and knuckle pads. Palmar lesions and sometimes deposits related to the palmaris longus and the insertion of the flexor carpi ulnaris may be found. The prognosis for this type is poor.
4. Feminine. This type demonstrates long-standing localized palmar plaques without deformity. There may be, however, slender bands in relation to these plaques, often very superficially placed and producing very minimal digital deformity. This "feminine" type is occasionally seen in men with delicate hand structure.

TREATMENT. Conservative Treatment. Good results have been claimed for many types of nonoperative treatment including the injection of fibrinolytic substances, cortisone, and radiotherapy, but apart from exercise aimed at hyperextension of the fingers, there is no real alternative to surgical treatment.

Surgical Treatment. The ultimate choice of procedure will depend upon the nature and the severity of the contracture and on the patient's general condition. Minor operations such as fasciotomy are useful where the main distribution of the contracture is limited to single fingers and especially where age or the circumstances of the patient prohibit more extensive procedures.

Radical excision of palmar fascia has the virtue of completely disposing of the affected tissue and must still be considered the method of choice in severe cases.

The ultimate result depends as much on postoperative treatment as on the actual operative procedure. The former involves protective splinting and physiotherapy.

Volkmann's Ischemic Contracture

In 1875 Volkmann described a contracture of the forearm muscles following the tight bandaging of an arm after fracturing the bones of the elbow. Such a contracture is due to ischemia of the muscles and is a common hazard in children following injuries about the elbow, particularly supracondylar fracture. Simultaneous damage to the brachial artery by inducing spasm or by thrombosis may produce segmental arterial spasm with severe ischemia of both muscle and nerves.

PATHOLOGY. The gross pathologic picture is one of muscle infarction in an elliptoid zone which has its axis near the anterior interosseous artery and its central point a little above the middle of the forearm. The greatest damage is usually to the flexor digitorum profundus and flexor pollicis longus, these being the deepest muscles lying in close relation to the anterior interosseous artery. The median nerve running near the anterior interosseous artery may also be involved in the ischemic process, and in very severe cases the ulnar nerve may be involved as well.

In the center of the ischemic mass the muscle fibers lose their nuclei and cross striations, and fuse into a homogeneous mass with little more than a defining membrane separating them. This picture is in contrast to muscle degeneration from other causes such as denervation and sepsis in which the appearance is one of diffuse interfibrillar fibrosis.

Seddon described some reversible changes following vascular ischemia in which dead muscle is removed and replaced by new. Hence, although it might appear initially that destruction is total, often after 2 or 3 months some of the muscles, particularly the extensor group, will recover. During this time, when recovery is occurring, treatment should be aimed at splinting to minimize contractures.

CLINICAL MANIFESTATIONS. The symptoms of pain, pallor, paralysis, and loss of radial pulse occur within a few hours of the injury, and usually intense pain is associated with either passive or active attempts to extend the fingers. Active and passive finger extension should be specifically checked in every patient with an elbow or forearm injury, since inability to extend in association with pain is the earliest sign of a Volkmann's ischemic contracture. Ultimately all voluntary motion is lost. Most of the damage occurs within the first few hours, so that initial treatment is urgent. After this period swelling gradually subsides, the muscles become hard and fibrotic, and as the fibrosis in-

creases, a characteristic deformity of the wrist and hand develops. When the wrist is flexed, extension occurs at the MP joints and flexion at the IP joints, while the forearm is often pronated and the elbow flexed.

PROPHYLAXIS. The circulatory and neurologic condition of the forearm and hand must be carefully watched in the early stage of treatment of all injuries or fractures about the elbow or forearm. It is inadvisable to treat fractures about the elbow, such as supracondylar fractures in children, with splints or bandages applied in a circular fashion.

TREATMENT. In the acute stage it is important to reestablish circulation before irreparable damage is done. The limb must be elevated, any circular bandages removed, and mild external warmth applied. Successful relief of spasm can sometimes be induced by ganglionic injection of the cervical sympathetic chain, but if this is unsuccessful, the artery should be exposed and papaverine applied to its surface. If this proves unsuccessful, complete interruption of the sympathetic reflex arc inducing spasm may be achieved by arteriectomy with resection of the artery and vein graft.

In established cases, prevention of contracture and maintenance of joint mobility can be obtained by splintage and physiotherapy of the fingers and thumb. Once maximal recovery is attained, operative procedures are necessary to remove the fibrotic muscular tissue. Such procedures have been described by Seddon and are preferable to indirect methods of correction such as shortening of forearm bones or carpal bone excision. Occasionally if the median nerve has been irreparably damaged and the ulnar nerve is intact, the latter has been used successfully as a pedicle nerve graft to restore maximal sensation to the hand.

EPIPHYSEAL DISORDERS (OSTEOCHONDRITIS)

General Considerations

The epiphysis is concerned with the growth in length of a bone. It also forms a part of joints and acts as an attachment for muscles and tendons. There are three types of epiphysis: (1) pressure epiphysis, which transmits weight from one bone to another, (2) traction epiphysis, or apophysis, which is situated at the point of attachment of muscles, and (3) atavistic epiphysis, which represents a part of the skeleton that has lost its function.

The epiphysis develops from a secondary center of ossification and is initially separated from the main bone by an area of unossified cartilage. Later, it joins the shaft to make the adult bone. The cartilage lying between the bony tissue and the diaphysis is known as the "epiphyseal cartilage." It does not ossify until bone growth has ceased, nor does the epiphysis become joined to the body of the bone until that time.

The term "osteochondritis," or "epiphysitis," is used to signify a derangement of growth at various ossification centers. The same pathologic process can underlie most epiphyses, though the particular location modifies its clinical manifestation. Unfortunately, in most instances, the lesions have come to be known by a series of eponyms (see the classification that follows).

Areas Involved with Epiphysitis

Primary centers of ossification:
    Vertebral body (Calvé, 1925)
    Carpal scaphoid (Preoser)
    Semilunar, adult (Kienböck, 1910)
    Patella (Köhler, 1908)
    Talus (Mouchet, 1928)
    Tarsal navicular (Köhler, 1908)
Secondary centers of ossification:
    Vertebral epiphysis (Scheuermann, 1921)
    Head of humerus (Hass, 1921)
    Capitellum of humerus (Panner, 1927)
    Head of radius (Brailsford, 1935)
    Pubic symphysis (Van Neck, 1924)
    Ischiopubic junction (Oldsberg, 1924)
    Head of femur (Legg, 1910)
    Patella (Sinding-Larsen, 1921)
    Tubercle of tibia (Osgood-Schlatter, 1903)
    Calcaneus (Sever, 1912)
    Metatarsals (Freiberg, 1914)

ETIOLOGY. The causes of epiphysitis have not been agreed upon; many causes, including genetic, infective, and hormonal, have been suggested. The theory presently favored is that a vascular disturbance, possibly following trauma, results in an avascular necrosis. Legg, in his early description, stated: "As a result of injury, there is an obliteration of a portion of the vascular supply of the epiphysis, which consequently undergoes the atrophy of anemia. A compensatory hyperemia of the adjacent portions of the diaphysis is the natural response, and is the starting-point of these hypertrophic changes which have been noted in the occurrence of broadening."

The traumatic factor is supported by a frequent history of injury, by the greater frequency of the condition in boys, and by the more usual location either in weight-bearing joints such as the hip or in epiphyses which are subjected to great strain, such as in the tibial tubercle. Legg-Calvé-Perthes disease has developed in a hip which was the site of congenital dislocation which had been reduced shortly prior to the manifestation of the disease. Minor degrees of Legg-Calvé-Perthes disease are common radiologic findings in old manipulated congenital hips.

A relationship between osteochondritis and skeletal growth has been described (see Table 43-3). It should be noted that the condition appears clinically (1) soon after the appearance of ossification, e.g., Legg-Calvé-Perthes disease at four years and Osgood-Schlatter disease at eleven years; (2) during or immediately after the mid-growth, or adolescent spurt, e.g., Scheuermann's disease, which is aggravated by adolescent growth spurt; and (3) earlier in girls than in boys, because the latter are slower in maturation.

PATHOLOGY. The pathologic changes in epiphyseal disorders are poorly described because of the paucity of operative material. Histologic sections have demonstrated avascular necrosis of the epiphyses with fibrosis in the metaphyseal region.

CLINICAL MANIFESTATIONS. The affection may be bilateral or unilateral. The onset is usually gradual in a patient with good general health who may offer a history of trauma. The local effects of the disease are similar to those of early tuberculosis and include slight pain, limp in a weight-bearing joint, limitation of the movement, and at times muscle spasm. The symptoms are usually mild. Many cases are asymptomatic and discovered only when deformities develop.

ROENTGENOGRAPHIC FINDINGS. The roentgenographic appearance is usually much more severe than the clinical picture would suggest. There is early osteoporosis with subsequent signs of repair. The epiphysis becomes fissured, fragmented, broadened, and irregular in outline. Areas of dense necrotic bone become evident. The process may involve both the epiphysis and metaphysis, and the former may be compressed and flattened. In the stage of regeneration, there is a gradual loss of osteoporosis with absorption of the dense necrotic bone in the epiphysis. This is fol-

Table 43-3. RELATIONSHIP BETWEEN EPIPHYSITIS DIAGNOSIS AND TIME OF APPEARANCE OF EPIPHYSIS

Site of osteochondritis	Usual age at diagnosis	Range of age incidence	Sex incidence	Year of appearance of epiphysis	
				Male	Female
Upper femoral epiphysis (Legg-Calvé-Perthes disease)	5–9	$3\frac{1}{2}$–15	M > F	1	$\frac{1}{2}$
Tuberosity of tibia (Osgood-Schlatter disease)	12–15	10–23	M > F	11	11
Navicular bone (Köhler's disease)	3–8	$2\frac{1}{2}$–10	M > F	2–4	2–4
Calcanean apophysis (Haglund's disease)	$8\frac{1}{2}$–15	8–22	M > F	10	8
Head of second metatarsal bone (Freiberg's disease)	10–18	10–45	F > M	3	2
Upper and lower epiphyses of vertebrae (Scheuermann's disease)	10–21	. . .	M > F	10	10

SOURCE: From R. B. Duthie, 1959.

lowed by slowly advancing replacement of the necrotic bone by new bone until there is complete bony restitution. The amount of eventual deformity of restored bone depends on the stage at which the disease is first recognized and the nature of treatment applied.

Legg-Calvé-Perthes Disease

Osteochondritis of the hip, also known as "coxa plana," is essentially a disease of boys, occurring usually between the ages of five and nine, but may become manifest between two and eighteen years of age. It is bilateral in about 10 percent of the cases.

CLINICAL MANIFESTATIONS. There are three main stages: (1) the prodromal stage, (2) the active stage, and (3) the restoration stage. During the prodromal stage, the most constant early sign is a limp, which may or may not be accompanied by pain. Muscular spasm may be present in early stages of the disease. During the active stage, the spasm tends to disappear but leaves a residual limitation of mobility. The pain and tenderness also usually disappear. The limping may remit for short periods or may be marked with a completely fixed and painless hip in a position of slight flexion and adduction. The affected hip joint shows limitation of abduction, medial rotation, and flexion, initially because of spasm of adductive muscles and at a later stage because of true shortening of these muscles. Still later, the deformation of the femoral head results in a mechanical condition which prevents full degree of motion. The muscles on the affected side are usually atrophied, but, in spite of the considerable degree of deformity at the head of the femur, there is little if any shortening.

During the restoration stage, the subjective and objective signs gradually diminish, until the function of the hip is restored. Trochanteric thickening and limitation of range of abduction, however, persist through life.

It is usually not difficult to recognize the fully developed disease, particularly if roentgenograms are available. In the early stages, however, there are points of similarity with early tuberculosis involving bone. The distinguishing features between the two are that Legg-Calvé-Perthes disease usually affects boys from five to ten years of age, pain is an inconspicuous feature, extension and sometimes flexion are fairly free, and the patient is usually a healthy child. Tuberculosis may affect either sex at any age, though the subject is often young; all movements of the joints are usually limited, and the child is usually ill.

ROENTGENOGRAPHIC FINDINGS. Roentgenograms (Fig. 43-35) of the femoral head progressively demonstrate flattening, flattening plus fragmentation, flattening with fusion in the disorganized nucleus, and finally an expanded flattened head. The head is at first slightly reduced in its vertical diameter with no appreciable increase in its lateral extent. Later, there is a uniform increased radiodensity of the nucleus with irregular calcification. As fragmentation develops, there is some breaking up of the bony nucleus of the epiphysis with radiolucency apparent. At the same time, the head usually becomes more flattened and expands out of the acetabulum. The onset of the healing

Fig. 43-35. Legg-Calvé-Perthes disease.

stage is marked with fusion changes. The bony fragments join, and the density of the epiphysis diminishes until the shadow becomes not only uniform but comparable to that of the other side. The head, however, remains flattened. Even after the lesion has healed, deformity of the head persists, usually throughout life. In rare cases in which there has been no weight bearing on the joint, the normal contour may be preserved.

In the neck of the femur, deformity can develop early in the disease, even before the head has demonstrated osteoporosis. The upper part of the neck is expanded, and its metaphyseal ends become rounded off. At the same time, the neck becomes progressively shorter. In the acetabular cavity, the distance between the medial pole of the head and the floor of the socket increases early in the disease. This may reach such a degree that the shadows of the head and the ischial bone no longer overlap but leave a gap. This sign may be caused by a grossly swollen ligamentum teres resulting in excavation of the acetabular roof by pressure.

An arthrogram may show whether the cartilaginous outline is nearly normal and can be used to determine the efficacy of treatment.

TREATMENT. It is generally agreed that no systemic measures are successful in modifying the pathologic process. The aim of treatment is to protect the weight-bearing area from pressure and preserve the normal contour of the femoral head. When first seen, if the patient has considerable spasm of hip musculature, a preliminary period of skin traction is indicated. After 5 to 10 days of bed rest and skin traction, the patient is usually comfortable. The patient may then be placed in bilateral, long-leg walking cast fixed with two transverse bars to maintain both hips in 45° of abduction and 5° to 10° of internal rotation as described by Petrie and Bitenc.

The child is allowed to walk with crutches, bearing full weight on the two casts. Plaster casts are changed at intervals of 3 to 4 months and continued until radiographs indicate that mature bone has replaced the avascular epiphysis. Total plaster time averages 19 months. A similar approach can be carried out using the Toronto brace described by Bobetchko et al. In order to reduce the long period of abduction immobilization to provide covering of the femoral head, a rotational-varus osteotomy of the upper femoral component may be performed.

COMPLICATIONS AND PROGNOSIS. Prognosis depends upon the degree of involvement of the femoral epiphysis, as well as the age and sex of the child. In general, with less involvement of the epiphysis, children under four and boys have a better prognosis. Catterall has called attention to specific radiographic signs, including (1) Gage's sign, (2) calcification lateral to the epiphysis, (3) lateral subluxation of the head, and (4) inclination of the growth plate to the horizontal as indicating a worse prognosis.

Ratliffe found that in patients followed into adult life, the overall results of treatment have been disappointing. Only 38 percent achieve good results, 38 percent fair results, and in 24 percent the results were poor. Although a high percentage of patients had no pain and good func-tion, only 40 percent had a good hip roentgenographically, and there was evidence of arthritis in 51 percent. Failure of growth of the femoral neck with resultant shortening also may be a complication.

Osgood-Schlatter Disease (Tibial Tubercle Epiphysitis)

PATHOLOGY. The tibia is developed from four centers: one for the shaft, one for the lower epiphysis, and two for the upper epiphysis. The tuberosity usually arises as a tonguelike protrusion from the lower end of the upper epiphysis, but it may have two centers of ossification, one extending down from the epiphysis and the other reaching up from the shaft. While the center of ossification for the head appears first, it unites with the shaft last. Johnson has shown that the pathology of Osgood-Schlatter disease is comparable to a slipped epiphysis in which excessive traction on the growing epiphysis results in detachment of the epiphyseal plate and increased height of the tibial tubercle.

CLINICAL MANIFESTATIONS. Osgood-Schlatter disease occurs usually in patients from thirteen to fifteen years of age, and the history may suggest injury as a causative factor. The onset of pain and local tenderness is insidious. The patient first complains of some aching in the front of the knee after exercise. In many cases, the overexertion is the only history of trauma obtained. The pain is increased by full voluntary extension of the joint, since the affected epiphysis is pulled on by the contracted quadriceps muscle. There is also pain on passive complete flexion, because the epiphysis is dragged by the quadriceps stretch. The epiphysis itself is tender, and in many cases there is localized swelling and increased temperature.

The roentgenographic appearance is characteristic (Fig. 43-36). The tibial tubercle is irregular in contour and even fragmented. There may be localized haziness in the adjacent tibial metaphysis.

Osgood-Schlatter disease must be differentiated from osteomyelitis, sarcoma of the head of the tibia, bone cysts, and infrapatellar bursitis. It must also be differentiated from partial separation of the tuberosity associated with trauma, which is mainly caused by violent contraction of the quadriceps muscles in males between the age of sixteen and eighteen. In this instance, there is immediate pain over the affected site, and the pain is aggravated by attempts to straighten the knee. The tuberosity is tender and swollen, and the roentgenogram shows detachment of the tonguelike epiphysis.

TREATMENT. The condition is treated in a fashion similar to that used for an epiphyseal separation with severe symptoms. A cylinder plaster cast is applied initially for 6 weeks, during which time weight bearing is permitted. Following removal of the cast the knee is mobilized and the patient's activities modified, i.e., no contact sports or hard running are allowed for a number of months. When symptoms are mild, simple restriction of heavy athletic activity and running are usually sufficient to get the patient through the growth period without immobilization of the extremity.

PROGNOSIS. The end result of Osgood-Schlatter disease

Fig. 43-36. Osgood-Schlatter disease: tibial tubercle osteochondritis.

Fig. 43-37. Osteochondritis of the tarsal navicular: Köhler's disease.

is usually a prominent tibial tubercle which persists into adulthood. A rare complication is that of genu recurvatum. This results from early fusion of the anterior part of the upper tibial epiphysis such that, with continuing growth of the posterior part, recurvatum results.

Köhler's Disease
of the Tarsal Navicular

As is true of the other forms of epiphysitis, Köhler's disease is probably an osteochondritis, but the cause has not been definitely established. It is analogous to Kienböck's disease, which affects the semilunar bone of adults. The navicular is the last bone of the foot to ossify, and since it forms the keystone of the long arch, it is subjected to considerable strain while in the cartilaginous state. Köhler's disease usually occurs in young children, especially between the ages of three and six.

CLINICAL MANIFESTATIONS. The symptoms and signs are often minimal, usually consisting of pain and swelling in the region of the tarsal navicular. The pain is exaggerated by weight bearing, and the affected region is sensitive to movement and may be tender. The condition is usually diagnosed by roentgenograms which reveal definite changes in the bone (Fig. 43-27). These consist of sclerotic narrowing in the anteroposterior diameter with no fragmentation of the bony nucleus. The joint spaces remain clear, and the neighboring tarsal and metatarsal bones are normal in appearance.

TREATMENT. The treatment is relatively simple, and symptomatic recovery usually occurs in a few months. A plaster cast should be applied to hold the foot in a slight varus position, and weight bearing is prevented by the use of crutches. After a few weeks the plaster is removed, and adhesive strapping is used to support the ankle and midtarsal region. The shoe is then fitted with a Thomas heel, i.e., with the medial half of the heel extended forward toward the sole, and sponge-rubber pads are inserted to relieve strain on the longitudinal arch, and, more particularly, on the navicular.

References

Pain

Adams, P., and Muir, H.: Qualitative Changes with Age of Proteoglycans of Human Lumbar Discs, *Ann Rheum Dis,* **35**:289, 1976.

Baker, D. R., and McHolick, W.: Spondyloschisis and Spondylosisthesis in Children (Demonstration), *J Bone Joint Surg* [*Am*], **38A**:933, 1956.

Batson, O. V.: The Role of the Vertebral Veins in Metastatic Processes, *Ann Intern Med,* **16**:38, 1942.

Campbell, A. M. and Phillips, D. G.: Cervical Disk Lesions with Neurological Disorder. Differential Diagnosis, Treatment, and Prognosis, *Br Med J,* **5197**:481, 1960.

Coomes, E. N.: Experimental Pain from the Hip Joint, *Ann Phys Med,* **7**:100, 1963.

Feinstein, B., Langton, J. W. K., Jamieson, R. M., and Schiller, F.: Experiments on Pain (Produced by Intervertebral Injection) Referred from Deep Somatic Tissue, *J Bone Joint Surg,* **36A:**981, 1954.

Frykholm, R.: Mechanism of Cervical Radicular Lesions Resulting from Friction or Forceful Traction, *Acta Chir Scand,* **102:**93, 1951.

Gaze, R. M., and Gordon, G.: Representation of Cutaneous Sense in Thalamus of Cat and Monkey, *Q J Exp Physiol,* **39:**279, 1954.

Guri, J. P.: Tumors of the Vertebral Column, *Surg Gynecol Obstet,* **87:**583, 1948.

Henson, S. W., Jr., and Coventry, M. B.: Osteomyelitis of Vertebrae as Result of Infection of Urinary Tract, *Surg Gynecol Obstet,* **102:**207, 1956.

Hueston, J. T., and Wilson, W. F.: Knuckle Pads, *Aust NZ J Surg,* **42:**274, 1973.

Killgren, J. H., and Samuel, E. P.: The Sensitivity and Innervation of the Articular Capsule, *J Bone Joint Surg [Br],* **32B:**84, 1950.

Livingston, W. K.: Phantom Limb Pain, *Arch Surg,* **37:**353, 1938.

McLeod, J. G.: The Representation of the Splanchnic Afferent Pathways in the Thalamus of the Cat, *J Physiol,* **140:**462, 1958.

Melzack, R.: The Perception of Pain, *Sci Am,* **204:**41, 1961.

Morgan, F. P., and King, T.: Primary Instability of Lumbar Vertebrae as a Common Cause of Low Back Pain, *J Bone Joint Surg [Br],* **39B:**6, 1957.

Newman, P. H.: Sprung Back, *J Bone Joint Surg [Br],* **30B:**30, 1952.

————: Spondylolisthesis: Its Cause and Effect, *Ann R Coll Surg Engl,* **16:**305, 1955.

O'Connell, J. E. A.: Discussion on Cervical Spondylosis, *Procr Soc Med,* **49:**202, 1956.

Ottolenghi, C. E.: Diagnosis of Orthopaedic Lesions by Aspiration Biopsy: Results of 1061 Punctures, *J Bone Joint Surg [Am],* **37A:**443, 1955.

Roche, M. B., and Rowe, G. G.: Incidence of Separate Neural Arch and Coincident Bone Variations: Survey of 4200 Skeletons, *Anat Rec,* **109:**233, 1951.

Rumbold, C.: Industrial Back Prevention, *J Occup Med,* **2:**132, 1960.

Rowe, M. L.: Newer Concepts of Low Back Pain, *J Occup Med,* **2:**219, 1960.

Schajowicz, F.: Aspiration Biopsy in Bone Lesions: Cytological and Histological Techniques, *J Bone Joint Surg [Am],* **37A:**465, 1955.

Smith, G. W., and Robinson, R. A.: The Treatment of Certain Cervical-spine Disorders by Anterior Removal of the Intervertebral Disc and Interbody Fusion, *J Bone Joint Surg [Am],* **40A:**3, 607, 1958.

Splithoff, C. A.: Lumbo-sacral Junction: Roentgenographic Comparison of Patients with and without Backaches, *JAMA,* **152:**1610, 1953.

Stewart, T. D.: Age Incidence of Neural-arch Defects in Alaskan Natives, Considered from Standpoint of Etiology, *J Bone Joint Surg [Am],* **35A:**937, 1953.

Weddell, A. G. M.: Observations on the Anatomy of Pain Sensibility, p. 47, in C. A. Keele and R. Smith (eds.), "The Assessment of Pain in Man and Animals," *Proc Intern Symp UFAW,* E. & S. Livingstone Ltd., Edinburgh, 1962.

————: Normal and Abnormal Sensory Patterns: Pain. II. "Activity Pattern" Hypothesis for Sensation of Pain in R. G.

Grenell (ed.), "Progress in Neurobiology," vol. 5, "Neural Physiology: Some Relationships of Normal to Altered Nervous System Activity," p. 134, Cassell & Co., Ltd., London, 1963.

Whitty, C. W. M., and Hockaday, J. M.: Patterns of Referred Pain in the Normal Subject, *Brain,* **90:**481, 1967.

Wiley, A. M., and Trueta, J.: The Vascular Anatomy of the Spine and Its Relationship to Pyogenic Vertebral Osteomyelitis, *J Bone Joint Surg [Br],* **41B:**796, 1959.

Wiltse, L. L.: The Etiology of Spondylolisthesis, *J Bone Joint Surg [Am],* **44A:**539, 1962.

Disorders of Muscle

Adams, R. D., Brown, D., and Pearson, C.: "Diseases of Muscles," Hansen and Broether, New York, 1962.

Baker, L. D., and Hill, L. M.: Foot Alignment in Cerebral Palsy Patient, *J Bone Joint Surg [Am],* **46A:**1, 1964.

Buchthal, F., Knappies, G. G., and Lindhard, J.: Bie Struktur der quergestreisten, legenden Muskelfaser des Frosches in Ruhe und wahrend der Kontraktion, *Scand Arch Physiol,* **73:**163, 1936.

Crenshaw, A. H. (ed.): "Campbell's Operative Orthopaedics," The C. V. Mosby Company, St. Louis, 1963.

Eggers, G. W. N., and Evans, E. B.: Surgery in Cerebral Palsy, instructional course lecture, American Academy of Orthopaedic Surgeons, *J Bone Joint Surg [Am],* **45A:**1275, 1963.

Elftman, H.: Biomechanics of Muscle with Particular Application to Studies of Gait, *J Bone Joint Surg [Am],* **48A:**363, 1966.

Goldner, J. L.: Reconstructive Surgery of the Hand in Cerebral Palsy and Spastic Paralysis Resulting from Injuries of the Spinal Cord, *J Bone Joint Surg [Am],* **37A:**1141, 1955.

Green, W. T., and Banks, H. H.: Flexor Carpi Ulnaris Transplant and Its Use in Cerebral Palsy, *J Bone Joint Surg [Am],* **44A:**1343, 1962.

Grice, D. S.: An Extra-articular Arthrodesis of the Subastragalar Joint for Correction of Paralytic Flat Feet in Children, *J Bone Joint Surg [Am],* **34A:**92, 1952.

————: Further experience with Extra-articular Arthrodesis of the Subtalar Joint, *J Bone Joint Surg [Am],* **37A:**246, 1955.

Hayes, J. T., Gross, H. P., and Dow, S.: Surgery for Paralytic Defects Secondary to Meningomyelocele and Myelodysplasia, instructional course lecture, American Academy of Orthopaedic Surgeons, *J Bone Joint Surg [Am],* **46A:**1577, 1964.

Hill, A. V.: Development of Active State of Muscle during Latent Period, *Proc R Soc Lond,* ser. B, **137:**320, 1950.

————: Does Heat Production Precede Mechanical Response in Muscular Contraction? *Proc R Soc Lond,* ser. B, **137:**268, 1950.

————: Is Muscular Relaxation Active Progress? *Nature,* **166:**646, 1950.

————: Mechanics of Contractile Element of Muscle, *Nature,* **166:**415, 1950.

————: Note on Heat of Activation in Muscle Twitch, *Proc R Soc Lond,* ser. B, **137:**330, 1950.

————: Series Elastic Component of Muscle, *Proc R Soc Lond,* ser. B, **137:**273, 1950.

Huxley, A. F.: Local Activation of Muscle, *NY Acad Sci,* **81:**446, 1959.

Lichtenstein, B. W.: Spinal Dysraphism and Spina Bifida and Myelodysplasia, *AMA Arch Neurol Psychiatr,* **44:**792, 1940.

Mercer, Sir W., and Duthie, R. B. (eds.): "Orthopaedic Surgery," Edward Arnold (Publishers) Ltd., London, 1972.

Phelps, W. M.: Prevention of Acquired Dislocation of the Hip in Cerebral Palsy, *J Bone Joint Surg* [*Am*], **41A:**440, 1959.

Sharrard, W. J. W.: Posterior Ilio-psoas Transplantation in Treatment of Paralytic Dislocation of the Hip, *J Bone Joint Surg* [*Br*], **46B:**426, 1965.

———, Zackary, R. B., Lorber, J., and Bruce, A. M.: A Controlled Trial of Immediate and Delayed Closure in Spina Bifida Cystica, *Arch Dis Child*, **38:**18, 1963.

Stamp, W. G.: Bracing in Cerebral Palsy, instructional course lecture, American Academy of Orthopaedic Surgeons, *J Bone Joint Surg* [*Am*], **44A:**1457, 1962.

Strayer, L. M.: Gastrocnemius Resection Five Year Report of Cases, *J Bone Joint Surg* [*Am*], **40A:**1019, 1959.

Thomasen, E.: "Myotonia: Thomsen's Disease, Paramyotonia, Dystrophia, Myotonia," Universities Forloget, Aarhus, Denmark, 1948.

Thompson, C. F.: Fusion of the Metacarpals to the Thumb and Index Finger to Maintain Functional Position of the Thumb, *J Bone Joint Surg*, **24:**907, 1942.

Vignos, P. J., and Watkins, M. P.: The Effect of Exercise in Muscular Dystrophy, *JAMA*, **197:**843, 1966.

Zuck, F. N.: *Proc U Cerebral Palsy Assoc*, Washington, 1957.

———: Cerebral Palsy, in Sir W. Mercer and R. B. Duthie (eds.), "Orthopaedic Surgery," chap. 10, Paralysis, Edward Arnold (Publishers) Ltd., London, 1964.

Orthopedic Management of Stroke

Khalili, A. A., and Betts, H. G.: Peripheral Nerve Block with Phenol in the Management of Spasticity, *JAMA*, **200:**1155, 1968.

Mooney, V., Frykman, G., and McLamb, J.: Present Status of Intra-neurol Phenol Injections, *Clin Orthop*, **63:**122, 1969.

Posture

Bergofsky, E. H., Turino, G. M., and Fishman, A. P.: Cardiorespiratory Failure in Kyphoscoliosis, *Medicine*, **38:**263, 1959.

Cobb, J. R.: Outline for the Study of Scoliosis, *Am Acad Orthop Surg Lect*, **5:**261, 1948.

Denham, R. A.: Hip Mechanics, *J Bone Joint Surg* [*Br*], **41B:**3, 550, 1959.

Duthie, R. B.: The Significance of Growth in Orthopaedic Surgery, *Clin Orthop*, **14:**7, 1959.

Gilmour, J.: The Relationship of Acetabular Deformity to Spontaneous Osteo-arthritis of the Hip Joint: An Investigation of the Intra-articular Factors Which Predispose to Osteoarthritic Degeneration, *Br J Surg*, **26:**700, 1938.

Harris, R. I., and Beath, T.: Etiology of Peroneal Spastic Flat Foot, *J Bone Joint Surg* [*Br*], **30B:**624, 1948.

Hicks, J. H.: Foot as Support, *Acta Anat* (*Basel*), **25:**34, 1955.

Hyman, G.: Children's Footwear, *Br Med J*, **1:**1189, 1959.

Jack, E. A.: Naviculo-cuneiform Fusion in the Treatment of Flat Foot, *J Bone Joint Surg* [*Br*], **35B:**75, 1953.

James, J. I. P.: Idiopathic Scoliosis: Prognosis, Diagnosis, and Operative Indications Related to Curve Patterns and Age at Onset, *J Bone Joint Surg* [*Br*], **36B:**36, 1954.

Keith, A.: Bone Growth and Bone Repair, *Br J Surg*, **5:**685, 1918.

Lam, S. F., and Hodgson, A. R.: A Comparison of Foot Form among the Non-shoe- and Shoe-wearing Chinese Population, *J Bone Joint Surg* (*Am*), **40A:**1058, 1958.

Langenskiöld, A., and Michelsson, J. E.: Experimental Progressive Scoliosis in the Rabbit, *J Bone Joint Surg*, **43B:**116, 1961.

Mair, W. G. P., and Druckman, R.: Aberrant Regenerating Nerve Fibres in Injury to Spinal Cord, *Brain*, **6:**448, 1953.

Morley, A. J. M.: Knock-knee in Children, *Br Med J*, **2:**976, 1957.

Outland, T., and Sherk, H. H.: Congenital Vertical Talus, *Clin Orthop*, **16:**214, 1960.

Ponsetti, I. V., and Friedman, B.: Prognosis in Idiopathic Scoliosis, *J Bone Joint Surg* [*Am*], **32A:**381, 1950.

——— and Shepard, R. S.: Lesions of the Skeleton and of Other Mesodermal Tissues in Rats Fed Sweet-pea (*Lathyrus odoratus*) Seeds, *J Bone Joint Surg* [*Am*], **36A:**1031, 1954.

Risser, J. C., and Ferguson, A. B.: Scoliosis: Its Prognosis, *J Bone Joint Surg*, **18:**667, 1936.

Walmsley, T.: The Articular Mechanics of Diarthrosis, *J Bone Joint Surg*, **10:**40, 1928.

Contracture

Early, P. F.: Population Studies in Dupuytren's Contracture, *J Bone Joint Surg* [*Br*], **44B:**602, 1962.

Evans, E. B., Eggers, G. W. N., Butler, J. K., and Blumel, J.: Experimental Immobilisation and Remobilisation of Rat Knee Joints, *J Bone Joint Surg* [*Am*], **42A:**737, 1960.

Hueston, J. T.: "Dupuytren's Contracture," E. & S. Livingstone Ltd., Edinburgh, 1963.

Ling, R. S. M.: Genetic Factors in Dupuytren's Disease, *J Bone Joint Surg* [*Br*], **44B:**219, 1962.

Seddon, H. J.: Volkmann's Contracture: Treatment by Excision of Infarct, *J Bone Joint Surg* [*Br*], **38B:**152, 1956.

Epiphyseal Disorders (Osteochondritis)

Bobetchko, W. P., McLaurin, C. A., and Motloch, W. M.: Toronto Orthosis for Legg-Perthes' Disease, *Artif Limbs*, **12:**36–41, 1968.

Cameron, J. M., and Izatt, M. M.: Legg-Calvé-Perthes Disease, *Scott Med J*, **5:**148, 1960.

Catterall, A.: The Natural History of Perthes' Disease, *J Bone Joint Surg* [*Br*], **53B:**37, 1971.

Duthie, R. B.: The Significance of Growth in Orthopaedic Surgery, *Clin Orthop*, **14:**7, 1959.

Haythorn, S. R.: Pathological Changes Found in Material Removed at Operation in Legg-Calvé-Perthes Disease, *J Bone Joint Surg* [*Am*], **31A:**599, 1949.

Johnson, L. C.: Histogenesis of Avascular Necrosis, Proceedings of the Conference on Aseptic Necrosis of the Femoral Head, St. Louis, Missouri, United States Public Health Service, p. 55.

King, E. S. L.: Localized Rarefying Conditions of Bone as Exemplified by Legg-Perthes Disease, Osgood-Schlatter Disease, Kümmell's Disease and Related Conditions, Edward Arnold (Publishers) Ltd., London, 1935.

Petrie, J. G., and Bitenc, I.: The Abduction Weight Bearing Treatment in Legg-Perthes' Disease, *J Bone Joint Surg* [*Br*], **53B:**54, 1971.

Ratliff, A. H. C.: Pseudocoxalgia: A Study of Late Results in the Adult, *J Bone Joint Surg* [*Br*], **38B:**498, 1956.

Chapter 44

Congenital Orthopedic Deformities

by Robert B. Duthie and Franklin T. Hoaglund

Deformities Resulting from In Utero Position

Congenital Dysplasia and Dislocation of the Hip

Congenital Dislocation of the Knee (Congenital Genu Recurvatum)

Congenital Pseudoarthrosis of the Tibia

Congenital Talipes Equinovarus (Clubfoot)

Congenital Convex Pes Valgus (Vertical Talus)

Arthrogryposis Multiplex Congenita (Myodystrophia Fetalis)

Congenital High Scapula

Congenital Short Neck (Klippel-Feil Syndrome: Brevicollis)

Cleidocranial Dysostosis Syndrome

Congenital Wryneck (Torticollis)

Congenital Radioulnar Synostosis

Madelung's Deformity

Congenital Aplasia and/or Dysplasia of Long Bones
Absence of the Radius
Absence of the Ulna
Absence or Dysplasia of the Fibula
Shortening of the Femur

A congenital malformation is present at or before birth, which implies that it is an inherited or genetically determined disorder. However, it may be difficult to determine whether it is truly of genetic or of environmental (intrauterine) origin. Carter described congenital conditions as resulting from (1) an abnormal genetic constitution, e.g., achondroplasia (a dominant mutant) and Morquio's disease (a recessive mutant); (2) environmental factors, e.g., cretinism; or (3) an interplay of both, such as is seen in congenital dislocation of the hip or talipes equinovarus deformity. Genes produce these effects by influencing either metabolic processes, e.g., in ochronosis, or the endocrine system, e.g., in the hypopituitary dwarf.

Stevenson has described three categories of congenital and/or hereditary disorders: (1) those malformations which are seen at birth but which have arisen during intrauterine life, i.e., true congenital malformations; (2) disorders or diseases determined by a single gene substitution or mutation; and (3) diseases in which the genetic contribution is made more complex by the presence of environmental factors or prenatal influences. Malformations due only to environmental causes are infrequent, e.g., viral infection of rubella or syphilis and the use of aminopyrine (amidopyrine) drugs and thalidomide. These produce teratogenic changes in the fetus, particularly during the first 4 weeks of pregnancy when the fetus is undergoing marked cellular differentiation and the mother's hormonal and nutritional milieu is also changing markedly. By considering embryonic development and its susceptibility to multiple factors it is possible to make a timetable (Fig. 44-1) of the appearance of various congenital malformations.

In a survey of 56,760 live births, McKeown and Record noted a total incidence of malformations 5 years after birth of 23.08 per 1,000. Talipes was found in 4.44 per 1,000, spina bifida and other spinal defects were noted in 3 per 1,000, and dislocation of the hip appeared in 0.67 per 1,000. Gentry et al. reported on congenital malformations found in 1,242,744 children born alive between 1948 and 1955. Malformations of the skeletal system and bones and joints were noted in 3,737 children.

DEFORMITIES RESULTING FROM IN UTERO POSITION

The in utero position has often been implicated as a deforming force, particularly of the lower extremities. Several moderately severe conditions are seen shortly after birth, but these can usually be treated by simple conservative measures:

1. Metatarsus adductus of one or both feet (Fig. 44-2).
2. Everted, or valgus, foot.
3. Talipes equinovarus deformity with one or more of four characteristics: forefoot adduction, inversion of the hind part of the foot, equinus of the whole foot at the ankle joint, and/or torsion of the tibia.
4. Unilateral externally rotated leg with an everted foot, the other leg being either in a neutral position or in internal rotation.
5. Bilateral internally rotated tibiae, which are aggravated by the prone position.
6. Adducted thigh and hip with some external rotation of the leg as a whole. This type of deformity has to be closely differentiated from congenital dysplasia or dislocation of the hip.

These conditions are often aggravated by the sleeping

COMPOSITE TIMETABLE FOR DEVELOPMENT OF
CONGENITAL LIMB ANOMALIES

Fig. 44-1. Etiological timetable of some congential malformations.

or lying position of the child, e.g., the internally rotated leg and varus foot.

Resistance to achieving the full range of passive movements of the hip, knee, ankle, or midtarsal joints must be corrected by passive stretching exercises and by corrective appliances such as straight-last or reversed-last shoes, Denis-Browne splints with adjustable foot pieces, a pillow splint, or double diapers.

The postural deformity must be treated before the development of a static deformity with a structural disorder.

Fig. 44-2. Bilateral metatarsus adductus with medial displacement of the first rays.

If soft tissue contractures develop and passive stretching cannot produce an anatomic position after about 6 weeks of treatment, corrective plaster of paris casting may be necessary, and the diagnosis of in utero position deformities may require revision.

On examining 5,000 newborn infants, Bick found 430 with some form of musculoskeletal malformation. Tibial torsion was seen in 30 children per 1,000 live births, subluxation of the hip in 17, metatarsus varus in 14, clubfeet in 8, deformity of the toes in 3, "bow legs" in 2, and other conditions such as polydactylism, birth fractures, birth palsy, and frank dislocation of the hip. The optimal time for a detailed musculoskeletal examination is between the third and fourth week.

CONGENITAL DYSPLASIA AND DISLOCATION OF THE HIP

Congenital dislocation of the hip consists of a partial or complete displacement of the femoral head from the acetabulum. It is very common, particularly in certain racial and ethnic groups such as the Northern Italian, the American Navaho Indian, and the Japanese. It is distinctly uncommon in the Hong Kong Chinese. Statistics vary depending upon criteria for detection but can be expected once in a thousand births in the Caucasian male, with a higher incidence in the Caucasian female. Its genetic and/or environmental causation has been reviewed by Carter and by Duthie and Townes.

PATHOGENESIS. The acetabulum appears as a condensation of mesoderm at the end of the fourth week of intrauterine life. It begins as a shallow socket, and later the socket is deepened by the progressive development of the posterosuperior rim, or buttress, in response to the head. A constant defect in congenital dislocation of the hip is an aplastic development of this osseous buttress and cartilage. Ossific hypoplasia of the capital femoral epiphysis may also be apparent at an early stage and is a constant feature of the later stage. Haas has classified this condition into a typical and an atypical group—the typical with its postnatal appearance, the atypical with its absence of prenatal development in association with other congenital anomalies such as arthrogryposis and intrauterine muscular dystrophy.

Complete dislocation of the hip in the typical group is seldom found in the immediate postnatal period. Haas found that the socket was only slightly reduced in circumference but corresponded in shape and depth to normal. The soft parts showed no abnormal change except for laxity of the capsule and iliofemoral ligament, permitting subluxation, which then became a frank dislocation.

Bone Changes. The acetabulum is shallower than normal; later its rounded shape disappears, and it becomes triangular with the base in front and below and the apex above and behind. X-ray examination shows that the outer surface of the ilium and the floor of the acetabulum lie in an almost straight line. Instead of containing the head of the femur, the acetabulum becomes occupied by an overgrowth of fibrocartilage, the remains of the ligamentum teres, and is covered over by adherent capsule. Above the acetabulum there is a depression on the ilium—a false acetabulum lined with periosteum—in which the head of the femur lies with a fold of the capsule intervening between the ilium and the head.

Ossification of the *head of the femur* is delayed, and there is marked discrepancy between the size of the cartilage head and the smaller acetabulum.

There is shortening of the *neck of the femur,* which is sometimes anteverted, so that the normal anteversion of 12° is increased until, in late cases, it may be almost 90°; i.e., the neck appears to project straight forward from the shaft.

When there is a bilateral dislocation, the *pelvis* is tilted forward and the normal lumbosacral lordosis increased.

Soft Part Changes. The *capsule* often becomes hourglass-shaped, one cavity containing the head, the other covering the acetabulum; the constriction is caused by the crossing iliopsoas tendon. The capsule becomes a hypertrophied suspensory ligament for the pelvis and supports most of the weight of the body. The ligamentum teres is usually attenuated and may be altogether absent, although in certain cases hypertrophy of the ligamentum teres occurs and blocks reduction.

There is considerable alteration in the *muscles.* There is shortening of the adductors, the hamstrings, and the gracilis, sartorius, tensor fasciae latae, pectineus, and the rectus femoris muscles. There is elongation of the obturators, the quadratus femoris, and the psoas tendon, with alteration in the function of the gluteal group.

In the development of congenital dislocation, subluxation is regarded as an intermediate stage from primary dysplasia to complete dislocation and is frequently associated with either predislocation or dislocation of the other hip.

The exact features responsible for migration of the femoral head from the predislocation stage to subluxation and dislocation are not known. The degree of primary hypoplasia affecting the cartilaginous roof of the acetabulum is probably the most important etiologic factor. Its ability to contain the head and to ossify in response to a correctly reduced head will determine the final result. Badgely considered that the primary dysplasia was produced by increased anteversion with an anterior primary position of the head and subsequent development of a flat socket.

In the early subluxated position the anteverted head can be palpated anteriorly when the legs are extended. The extension thrusts of the limb from the flexed position, which are a feature in the normal development of the growing infant, augment the pressure effect of the anteverted head. In the dysplastic hip, increased anteversion may stretch the capsule and fibrocartilaginous limbus and precipitate displacement.

In more advanced stages of subluxation, the head flattens the limbus and exerts a deforming pressure on the cartilaginous roof, causing further inhibition of ossification and actual flattening of the socket.

Dislocation occurs when the femoral head loses contact with the original acetabulum and rides up over the fibrocartilaginous rim. Arthrography demonstrates that in complete dislocation the fibrocartilaginous lip, or limbus, is inverted, as compared with the eversion which accompanies subluxation.

DIFFERENTIAL DIAGNOSIS. Coxa Vara. In this situation the limp is less severe, the head is not palpable in an abnormal position, nor is there any "telescoping." The x-ray appearance is characteristic.

Pathologic Dislocation. In these patients, there is usually a history of some previous hip joint trouble that developed after birth. There is general limitation of hip movements. The x-ray examination shows greater deformity and absorption of the head, while the acetabulum is usually well developed.

Paralytic Dislocation of Poliomyelitis. This condition simulates congenital dislocation in the waddling gait and shortness of the limb, but the hip joints are normal. There is obvious muscular paralysis.

Other Disorders. Cerebral palsy and septic arthritis must also be differentiated from congenital dysplasia and dislocation of the hip.

CONGENITAL HIP. Prognosis. Symptoms of congenital hip dysplasia depend upon the degree of acetabular dysplasia and whether the hip is subluxed or frankly dislocated. Patients with minor degrees of acetabular dysplasia might not be recognized at birth and only develop symptoms at age forty or fifty when a secondary osteoarthritis supervenes. Hirsch and Scheller have shown that when a positive Ortolani click sign is detected at birth, if the hips are appropriately splinted, clinical examination and x-ray findings on all hips are normal at age five. It is likely that these hips will be protected against osteoarthritis in later years as well.

At the other end of the scale, patients with untreated dislocated hips will carry the stigmata of the deformity throughout life. These patients walk with a short-leg-flexed-hip gait and are likely to have symptoms related to the hip in early adult life and certainly in the forties and fifties. They have diminished exercise tolerance and are more likely to complain of back symptoms as a result of their altered gait.

Symptoms attributable to hip joint with moderate dysplasia and a chronically subluxing hip resulting from inadequate diagnosis or treatment may appear in the early teens, depending upon the degree of anatomic distortion. The results of closed reduction depend upon the ability to restore a congruent stable hip joint relationship, and this depends upon age at which treatment is started. Muller and Sedden reported 50 percent excellent late results following closed reduction in children under three years of age. Platou, in a similar under-three age group, reported good short-term results in 80 percent and good anatomic results in 68 percent. Fourteen years later 68 percent of patients still had good functional results and 58 percent good anatomic results. Smith et al, analyzing patients up to 30 years after treatment of congenital hip dislocation, noted only 25 percent of patients normal in terms of symptoms, clinical examination, and x-ray evaluation. It is clear that maximal short-term and late results of congenital hip dysplasia depend upon early diagnosis and adequate treatment.

Fig. 44-3. Infant with congenital dislocation of the hips showing limitation of abduction on the right as compared with the normal left side. Examination is carried out with the hips in flexion and with an attempt to press the lateral aspect of the thigh on the examining table.

TREATMENT. The treatment of congenital dislocation of the hip depends on the degree of dislocation and the interpretation of the underlying pathology. The preliminary consideration in treatment is the accurate replacement of the femoral head in the acetabulum. Radiographic evidence of reduction, however, does not necessarily imply that development of the joint will proceed satisfactorily to form a normal articulation.

Fig. 44-4. *A.* Trendelenburg sign: left buttock rises slightly when the patient stands on her good right leg and the trunk is vertical. *B.* Same patient, standing on the side of the dislocated left hip. Right buttock drops, and the trunk now leans over the dislocated hip.

Reduction of a dislocation is complicated by secondary changes in the socket, the nature and significance of which remain the subject of much controversy. The secondary changes reported at operation will depend not only on individual interpretation but on the age of the patient, the duration of the dislocation stage, and the influence of preoperative attempts at closed reduction. Scaglietti and Calandriello found one or more of the following factors which prevented reduction of dislocated hips:

In 25 percent of cases—the iliopsoas muscle
In 31 percent of cases—an inverted limbus
In 33 percent of cases—a pericephalic insertion of the capsule
In 32 percent of cases—the ligamentum teres
In 16 percent of cases—capsular adhesions

CLINICAL MANIFESTATIONS. All babies must be examined at birth to determine the presence of congenital hip dysplasia, as successful treatment depends upon immediate diagnosis. If there is a family history of congenital hip dysplasia, difficult labor, or a breech presentation, the incidence of this defect is increased. In Sweden, where 99 percent of children are born in hospitals and examined by pediatricians, the rate of detection is extremely high. Over 600 new cases are diagnosed during the neonatal period, and only about 25 cases per year are detected after the newborn period. If the condition is not diagnosed until the head has dislocated from the acetabulum, the prognosis is much worse. Diagnosis at birth depends upon detection of the snap or click (Ortolani's sign) which is elicited when the head rides over the acetabular rim by abducting the flexed hip (Fig. 44-3). Hart has described the classic signs of dysplasia as being (1) Ortolani's sign, (2) limitation of hip abduction with the knees and hips flexed to 90° with the child on his back, and (3) apparent shortening of the thigh with the hip and knees flexed to 90°.

All children at follow-up examinations at six weeks and three months should be specifically examined for congenital hip dysplasia. If the click sign is no longer present, the only positive finding may be limitation of the symmetric abduction of both hips. If both hips are dysplastic, symmetric abduction may be present, in which case one should suspect dysplasia if adduction is limited to 75° or less. Minor degrees of acetabular dysplasia may go unnoticed throughout life until such time as a secondary osteoarthritis supervenes in the forties or fifties. If the hip progresses to a dislocation, the diagnosis will be apparent when the child begins to walk. The gait becomes abnormal, i.e., a ducklike waddle. The limb is particularly unstable, the trochanter ascending whenever the body weight is transmitted through the leg of the affected side. In a unilateral case, the child lurches toward the affected side. The gait results from inefficiency of the hip abductor muscles, which do not have the acetabular fulcrum. Leg shortening is evident, and lordosis often is noticeable, especially in bilateral cases. A Trendelenburg sign is seen when the child stands first on one foot and then on the other. In unilateral cases, when the child stands on the sound side, the buttock of the opposite side rises slightly, for the gluteus medius contracts in order to raise the pelvis and bring the trunk more directly above the limb which is sustaining the body

Fig. 44-5. Congenital dislocation of the hip. A. The right hip is held in the position of adduction compared with the left. The line parallel with the roof of the acetabulum intersecting Hilgenreiner's line indicates an acetabular index of 38° on the right and acetabular dysplasia. The dotted perpendicular line dropped from the outer margin of the acetabulum shows the proximal capital femoral epiphysis to be laterally displaced, indicating dislocation. The normal right side shows the dotted line at the outer margin of the proximal capital femoral epiphysis. B. Right proximal capital femoral epiphysis is much smaller than the left and is laterally displaced.

weight (Fig. 44-4A). When the child stands on the dislocated side, the opposite buttock drops, for the gluteus medius is relatively inefficient and the pelvis therefore cannot be raised or even be kept horizontal (Fig. 44-4B). In bilateral cases, the phenomenon is present on both sides.

The Trendelenburg test is not pathognomonic of congenital dislocation of the hip but occurs whenever the action of the gluteus medius is interfered with—e.g., in poliomyelitis and in coxa vara. Other signs are the position of the femoral artery, buttock creases, etc.

X-ray Appearance. X-ray examination is essential to establish the diagnosis, but in the young baby it must be realized that the cartilaginous structures involved are not visible on radiographs.

The relation of the head to the acetabulum can be established by Hilgenreiner's lines: the epiphyseal nucleus should be inside a vertical line drawn from the acetabular margin (Perkins line) and below the horizontal line drawn through the Y cartilages (Fig. 44-5A).

The slope of the osseous roof may be measured from the acetabular angle; the normal inclination is 22°, but in congenital dislocation it may be increased to 30 or 40°.

The outline of the femoral head should be noted, and it will be seen that the femur is displaced outward and upward. The epiphyseal shadow is usually smaller than normal and displaced outward in relation to the neck (Fig. 44-5B). The neck is foreshortened and may be anteverted. Anteversion is investigated by taking two plates, one with the patella pointing straight forward, the other with the leg in full medial rotation. Any anteversion is noted by the superimposition of the head on the trochanter in the first plate, while the second shows the outline of the head quite distant from the trochanter.

Arthrography of the hip gives further information of the underlying pathology in the different types of dislocation

and is of occasional value in deciding the appropriate treatment. The arthrogram reveals the extent of the cartilaginous roof in subluxation and in dislocations confirms the interposition of the limbus between the head and socket.

Predislocation. Infants with congenital hip dysplasia without subluxation or with initial subluxation stages diagnosed in the neonatal period of life are treated by simple abduction in a Freijka pillow splint or Von Rosen splint (Fig. 44-6). Hips recognized at birth usually need only 3 to 6 months of splinting until x-rays show normal acetabular and hip joint development.

Frame Reduction of Displacement. If the femoral head is

Fig. 44-6. Abduction splint maintaining the hip of a child with congenital hip dysplasia in the position of abduction.

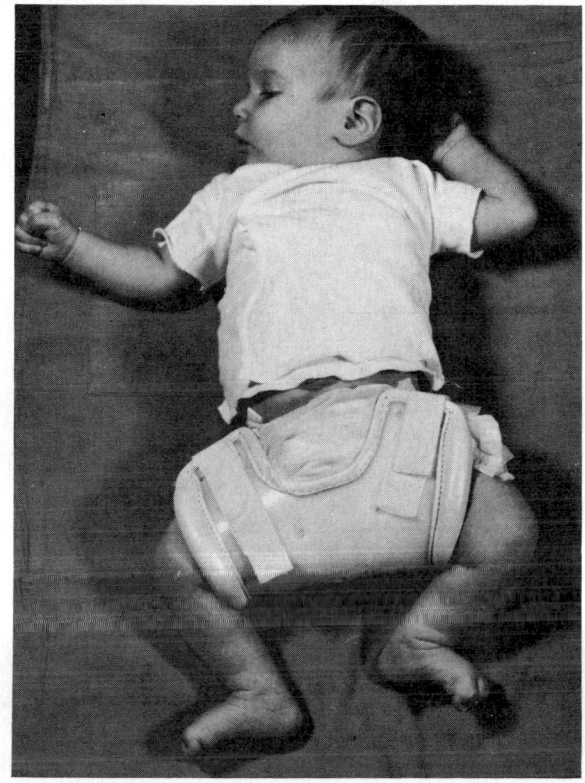

badly subluxated or dislocated, there is associated tightness of the adductor muscles which must be overcome before reduction is possible. Reduction by overhead traction or traction on a modified abduction frame followed by retention in a Batchelor-type plaster is preferred to manipulation under anesthesia and immobilization in the frog position in a plaster spica.

Osteochondritis or avascularity of the femoral head is more liable to follow manipulation than frame reduction. This may be due to the force necessary to overcome the tight adductors or to torsion of capsular vessels in the extreme frog position.

Frame reduction is a gradual process, but in the average case the head can be brought down and opposite the acetabulum in less than 3 weeks.

The child is placed on the frame and skin traction applied to the legs in slight abduction with the foot of the bed elevated. Fixed traction is sufficient in young children, but pulley traction may be necessary in the older child. After 1 week of preliminary traction, abduction is commenced by advancing each leg one opening of the abduction bar on alternate days. Abduction is increased, depending on relaxation of the adductors and the descent of the head as observed on x-ray. When the head arrives opposite the acetabulum, the leg traction is reduced to allow the head to sink into the socket (Fig. 44-7).

Failure of concentric reduction of the head in a correctly treated case usually indicates an obstruction to reduction which will not be affected by continued use of the frame.

Children under six years of age may be treated on the abduction frame, but reduction becomes increasingly difficult after the age of four. The indication for operative measures will depend on the degree of reduction achieved.

Abduction Plaster

Following successful reduction on the frame the hips must be protected until ossification of the acetabular roof provides a more stable socket. Plaster is applied under general anesthesia, and hips are flexed to more than 90°

Fig. 44-7. Abduction frame with a lateral pull on the dislocated right hip.

and in a position of about 45° abduction, the so-called "human position." Neutral rotation appears to be the safest position to maintain the hip, although some degree of external or internal rotation may be indicated depending upon stability. The duration of treatment depends upon the development of the acetabulum but is usually less than 1 year. Children are readmitted for plaster changes under anesthesia at 2 to 3 month intervals.

Subluxation. Subluxation presents no problem at initial reduction provided treatment is commenced before the development of irreversible secondary changes in the joint. In children who have borne weight for several years, the head may be enlarged and the cartilaginous roof of the acetabulum permanently deformed (Figs. 44-8A and B).

In younger children the subluxation is reduced on the frame and the reduction maintained by abduction plaster until ossification of the cartilaginous roof increases. Mobilization is then permitted, unless a marked degree of anteversion persists, in which case correction by derotation osteotomy of the femur should be carried out in order to maintain reduction and provide concentric stimulus to development of the osseous roof.

Dislocation. Dislocation implies complete displacement of the head and loss of contact with the articular surface of the original cartilaginous acetabulum.

Treatment even of the young child is difficult, because in complete dislocation, interposition of soft tissue may complicate reduction and subsequent joint development.

Differentiation between subluxation and dislocation may prove difficult in some cases without the aid of arthrography. Dislocation should be treated by conservative methods, provided the head appears accurately centered following frame reduction and application of abduction plasters. Any tendency for the head to stand out from the acetabulum after reduction or when freedom is permitted indicates the probable presence of an obstruction and requires open reduction.

OPERATIVE TREATMENT OF THE CONGENITAL HIP. Open Reductions. Open reduction of the dislocated hip is usually not required before the age of one year. As a separate operative procedure, it is contraindicated after the age of five or six, at which time other reconstructive operations are necessary.

In the series of 137 cases reported by MacKenzie et al., 58 percent of children under the age of three responded well to open reduction for failure of conservative treatment. Any soft tissue mass within the acetabulum such as an inverted limbus, hypertrophied ligamentum teres, or fibrofatty pad is looked for and, if found, turned outward and upward. The head is then rotated inward and the limb abducted to locate the head concentrically. The wound is closed and the leg placed in a plaster hip spica in a position in which maximal stability is attained. Open reduction is usually carried out in association with procedures to improve coverage of the head by some type of acetabuloplasty or redirection of the acetabulum.

Innominate Osteotomy. The acetabulum is not only deficient in size in congenital hip dysplasia but is maldirected, being open anteriorly and laterally. The procedure described by Salter of innominate osteotomy involves cutting the innominate bone immediately above the acetabulum with a Gigli saw and levering down (anteriorly and laterally) the acetabulum with its attached rami. The point of fulcrum for this rotation is at the symphysis pubis and not at the triradiate cartilage. A wedge of bone from the anterior crest of the ilium is wedged into the osteotomy defect between the upper ilium bone graft and acetabular portion of the innominate bone and fixed with two K wires. The procedure is usually carried out in conjunction with open reduction. Innominate osteotomy may be done without opening the hip joint when the hip is reduced but with significant degrees of persisting acetabular dysplasia. A similar procedure described by Pemberton involves levering down the roof of the acetabulum with an osteotomy and maintaining the position with an iliac bone graft. The Pemberton osteotomy obtains its correction at the triradiate cartilage.

Derotation Osteotomy of the Femur. In an attempt to restore a congruent relationship between the femoral head and the acetabulum in the presence of anteversion of the proximal femur, a derotation osteotomy of the femur is occasionally indicated. This may be carried out in association with an open reduction of the hip as an isolated procedure for severe anteversion and following acetabular surgery when severe anteversion has not been corrected.

The most suitable site for osteotomy is the subtrochanteric region. The lower fragment is externally rotated to the required angle as judged by rotational markers. The position is maintained by a four-hole Vitallium plate and screws. The femur is immobilized in hip spica for approximately 6 weeks.

The Chiari iliac osteotomy for the treatment of the irreducible hip subluxation in the child six years and older is an excellent alternative procedure.

Complications. Certain complications may follow the treatment of congenital dislocation of the hip. Some of these result from the operation itself, while others may be merely coincidental. As a direct result of the manipulative treatment, the femur sometimes is fractured, and occasionally the sciatic nerve may be traumatized.

Osteochondritis deformans juvenilis, which is due to avascular necrosis of the femoral head, may develop after reduction of a dislocated hip, but its occurrence in the normal hip in unilateral cases has also been recorded. Lima et al. studied 184 previously congenitally dislocated hips for vascularity and osteochondritis. He showed that the incidence was highest among patients treated by manipulation rather than frame reduction and also was related to the patient's age at start of treatment and completeness of reduction.

Pain and stiffness of the hip due to arthritis frequently follow manipulative reduction, particularly where the manipulation has been carried out with considerable force.

Palliative Operations. These are reserved for cases in which reduction is no longer possible either by closed or open methods. They are designed to improve stability, decrease lordosis, and control pain arising from the hip or lower back. The advisability of palliative procedures in the young patient with symptomless displacement of the hip is doubtful.

Fig. 44-8. Congenital hip dysplasia, diagnosed at age five. *A.* Position of abduction showing left acetabular dysplasia and subluxation of the femoral head. *B.* Ten weeks after innominate osteotomy with Steinmann's pin in place. *C.* One year following surgical treatment with maintenance of the head in the acetabulum and satisfactory acetabular coverage.

Palliative procedures fall into two categories: (1) arthrodesis and (2) osteotomy.

Arthrodesis. Hip fusion is a satisfactory procedure for relief of arthritic pain in the older patient with unilateral displacement. Arthritic pain occurs more commonly in subluxation than in dislocation unless there is a well-formed acetabulum.

Osteotomy. The primary object of osteotomy is deflection of weight bearing by angulation of the femur to bring the axis of the femoral shaft more in line with the direction of weight transmission.

Angulation osteotomy of the Schanz type is preferred to the bifurcation osteotomy of Lorenz, in which the upper end of the lower fragment is abducted and inserted into the acetabulum. The Lorenz procedure has the relative disadvantage of increased shortening, less mobility, and a greater likelihood of arthritic pain.

Total Hip Reconstruction. This procedure may be considered in middle-aged patients with pain as the main presenting feature. Special small acetabular cup and femoral prosthesis are usually required.

CONGENITAL DISLOCATION OF THE KNEE (CONGENITAL GENU RECURVATUM)

There are three types:

1. The developmental type, which is the most common and is considered to be due to malposition in utero. The legs may be caught by the chin or axilla with the knees extended.
2. A primary embryonic defect, accompanied by other defects, such as harelip, cardiac defects, spina bifida, and congenital dislocation of the hip. It is fortunate that this type is uncommon, since it is much more difficult to treat and usually requires operation.
3. Contracture of the quadriceps extensor muscle due to arthrogryposis.

CLINICAL MANIFESTATIONS. The knee is fixed in hyperextension with a varying degree of subluxation or dislocation of the tibia forward on the femoral condyles, and the skin over the anterior aspect of the joint shows several transverse creases. The patella is small or absent. On the posterior aspect of the joint, the hamstring muscles are palpable as tense cords, and the femoral condyles are felt projecting in the popliteal fossa.

TREATMENT. It may be possible to stretch the shortened quadriceps and replace the tibia in mild cases at birth. In more severe cases manipulation will be insufficient to overcome the contracture. Operative division or lengthening of the quadriceps and its lateral expansion—and occasionally of the iliotibial tract—will permit replacement.

Fig. 44-9. Characteristic deformities of talipes equinovarus, or clubfoot.

After operation, the corrected position is maintained by a splint or light plaster cast.

CONGENITAL PSEUDOARTHROSIS OF THE TIBIA

This is situated at the junction of the middle and lower thirds of the tibia, with sclerosis of bone ends and a gap between the fragments occupied by fibrous tissue. The leg is shorter. This lesion results from aplasia of a portion of the tibial shaft. A definite association with neurofibromatosis has been described.

TREATMENT. This is usually unsatisfactory, especially since the child may present after several attempts to obtain union and may never have walked on the limb. Leg discrepancy is marked, and the bones are markedly osteoporotic and underdeveloped, although the fibula is often intact.

Short of amputation, there are two possible methods of treatment: (1) by shortening the leg sufficiently to get good approximation and side-to-side apposition of the fragments and (2) by some method of bone grafting.

CONGENITAL TALIPES EQUINOVARUS (CLUBFOOT)

Congenital talipes equinovarus is a deformity involving four elements: flexion of the ankle, inversion of the foot, adduction of the forefoot, and medial rotation of the tibia (Fig. 44-9).

1. The "idiopathic" type may arise from such environmental factors as:
    a. Increased intrauterine compression because of change in the size of the uterus or reduction in the amount of amniotic fluid, e.g., oligohydramnios. Surprisingly little is known about intrauterine body mechanisms.
    b. Intrinsic anatomic disturbances in the talocalcaneal joint and in the innervation of the peroneal muscles with segmental changes in the spinal cord. Other factors have been described.
2. Genetic factors:
    a. Wynne-Davies has studied over 100 patients and their first-degree relatives. This deformity occurred in 2.9 percent of siblings, whereas in the general population there were 1.2 per 1,000 cases. No significant observations were possible concerning consanguinity, age of parents, birth order, etc.
    b. In the classic twin studies of Idelberger there was a 32.5 percent concordance in monozygous twins and only 2.9 percent in the dizygotic—the latter having the same incidence as that found in the nontwin sibling.

There is really no recognizable or acceptable inheritance pattern available as yet. However, there is a

1:800 chance of any individual having this deformity
1:35 chance of having it if any siblings have the deformity
1:3 chance if an identical twin is involved

There is real difficulty in defining this disease entity in detail, although from clinical experience two types can be recognized:

1. Those responding well to conservative management
2. A smaller percentage requiring operative therapy

PATHOLOGIC ANATOMY. The essential features are plantar flexion of the talus, inversion of the calcaneus (and with it the other tarsal bones), and adduction of the forefoot. At birth the bones of the foot are normal in shape but altered in position. Over the skin on the outer part of the foot there are usually dimples which may be so marked as to resemble scars. The lateral malleolus is prominent; the medial malleolus appears flattened and poorly developed.

Muscles and Tendons. The tendocalcaneus passes downward and inward to its insertion into the tilted calcaneus, while the plantar muscles, especially on the medial side, are contracted. The anterior muscles of the leg are elongated.

Ligaments. The ligaments on the medial and inferior surfaces of the talocalcaneonavicular joints are contracted, the plantar calcaneonavicular ligament being very small and short. The deltoid ligament of the ankle joint is similarly affected.

Bones. Bony changes appear as a result of the long-continued contraction of the soft parts. They are at first confined to the talus, but subsequently the calcaneus, the navicular, and the cuboid become appreciably altered.

At birth a small inverted heel and reduced calf muscles, suggesting a primary myodysplasia, may be seen. This type is difficult to correct and to maintain in correction.

In unilateral cases the deformity is never very severe, but the leg is obviously smaller and less well developed than on the healthy side.

DIAGNOSIS. The diagnosis is usually easy, but it is well to remember that an inverted position of the feet is frequently assumed by young infants. If this can be easily overcorrected by gentle manipulation and the foot can be dorsiflexed so that it touches the anterior shin without deviation, clubfoot can be excluded. In all cases search should be made for spina bifida and for evidence of poliomyelitis. Varying degrees of clubfoot should cause one to consider cerebral palsy or an arthrogryposis.

PROGNOSIS. Without treatment, the deformity increases, the gait becomes more unsightly, and the foot becomes more troublesome on account of calluses and ulceration. With early, effective, and continued treatment, all cases of clubfoot should be cured and a useful and properly shaped foot obtained. In older children the condition should be greatly improved.

TREATMENT. There are two objects of successful treatment: correction of the deformity and development of sufficient muscular power of the limb to maintain the correction. This implies constant supervision until the period of growth is over, since there is a distinct tendency to retrogression. The mode of treatment varies with the age and the extent of the deformity. The deformity of the hind part of the foot, which is the keystone to the function of such a deformed foot, must be brought into a vertical plane before the equinus deformity is corrected.

Treatment in an Early Case. Treatment of a clubfoot should begin while the child is still in the newborn nursery. The most effective treatment is application of serial corrective plaster casts to include the leg and foot, as described by Kite. It is extremely important to correct the forefoot adduction first, then the hindfoot varus, and not begin to dorsiflex the foot at the ankle until both forefoot adduction and hindfoot varus are completely corrected. Attempts at dorsiflexing the uncorrected hindfoot will result in the production of a rocker-bottom foot.

A single layer of sheet wadding or webril is applied to the leg and foot. On the very first cast, attention is directed at correcting the forefoot adduction, maintaining the foot in equinus, and correcting as much hindfoot varus as is possible. The cast is left on a few days to a week and then changed. At subsequent cast changes the forefoot adduction, hindfoot varus, and then equinus are further corrected. The duration of casting will depend upon the severity of the deformity. Most clubfeet can be corrected within a few weeks.

An alternative method is to manipulate the foot and then strap the foot in some type of L splint. A light lateral splint of aluminum covered with lint is applied to the outer side of the leg and foot, e.g., a Denis-Browne splint (Fig. 44-10). This allows full correction of the deformity and at the same time encourages the activity which is so important for muscular development. When the patient is capable of holding the feet naturally in the corrected position and the feet have full range of movement, the adhesive plaster and aluminum splint are discarded and replaced by a pair of boots riveted to the aluminum crosspiece to hold the feet in the same position as in the splint. These boots have open toes and unlace completely from one end to the other.

If it becomes apparent after some months that the equinus deformity has not been completely overcome, it is occasionally necessary to do a heel cord lengthening and a posterior capsulotomy of the ankle joint. After such operations the foot and leg are encased in plaster of paris with the foot in the slightly overcorrected position, the knee flexed, and plaster extended to the midthigh [Kite]. All children with clubfeet must be followed until bony maturation has taken place and usually require some type of corrective shoe or splint to maintain correction.

Treatment of Old and Relapsed Cases. However early and thoroughly congenital clubfoot is treated, in a certain percentage of cases, because of rigidity or a constant tendency to relapse, manipulative treatment will not suffice. Although a plantigrade foot may still be obtained by manipulation, the heel will remain inverted, and the navicular will still be in close contact with the medial malleolus. Any correction that takes place is between the cuneiform and the navicular, instead of between the navicular and the sustentaculum tali. To ensure a good result in this type of case, an operation is necessary to release the contracted ligaments between the tarsal bones, especially on the medial side of the foot. Goldner has recently called attention to the necessity of releasing the talus in the ankle joint in addition to extensive medial release of fascia and ligaments on the medial side of the foot.

Lateral transfer of the tibialis anterior tendon insertion has been recommended in addition to ligamentous and soft tissue release in order to remove a deforming force.

Fig. 44-10. Clubfeet immobilized in a Denis-Browne splint.

Heyman and colleagues have described a very satisfactory soft tissue release operation for the resistant forefoot adduction deformity. An incision is made across the dorsum of the foot, and the dorsal interosseous and intermetatarsal ligaments as well as the joint capsules are extensively dissected.

If the talipes equinovarus is due to arthrogryposis, the only consistently successful procedure to overcome this deformity is an astragalectomy, which allows positioning of a plantigrade foot.

Treatment in the Adult Patient. In the adult, no manipulation, tenotomy, or muscle operation is likely to be of benefit; operation on the bone is necessary in most cases. Cuneiform tarsectomy is the more certain and satisfactory operation.

In some cases, the best result will be obtained by stabilizing the foot as in the triple arthrodesis of Dunn. Here the midtarsal and subtaloid joints are arthrodesed as in some forms of flail foot.

CONGENITAL CONVEX PES VALGUS (VERTICAL TALUS)

This condition goes under a variety of names, including *congenital vertical talus* and *congenital rocker-bottom flatfoot*. It is thought to develop during pregnancy, but the cause is unknown. The pathology involves a primary dislocation of the talonavicular joint. The navicular articulates with the dorsal aspect of the talus, which is in a plantar-flexed or vertical position. The dorsal talonavicular ligament and the anterior aspect of the deltoid are both contracted, as is the calcaneal cuboid ligament. The muscles of the anterior compartment, peroneus brevis, and triceps surae are contracted.

CLINICAL FINDINGS. The deformity can be diagnosed at birth because of a rigid flatfoot. The sole of the foot has a rocker-bottom configuration. The head of the talus can be palpated on the medial plantar aspect of the foot.

The forefoot is abducted. The hindfoot is in equinovalgus, and the heel cord is tight. The child is able to walk on the foot without pain, although the gait may be awkward.

TREATMENT. Treatment is directed at early manipulative stretching and plaster correction of the forefoot into plantar flexion, inversion, and adduction. If manipulation and plaster cast immobilization can reduce the talonavicular dislocation, it is pinned with percutaneous K wires. If this is unsuccessful, open reduction is indicated at three months of age with a simultaneous tendoachilles lengthening. The calcaneal fibular ligament is also sectioned and posterior capsulotomy of the ankle and subtalar ligaments performed as necessary. Triple arthrodesis may be necessary in the older child.

ARTHROGRYPOSIS MULTIPLEX CONGENITA (MYODYSTROPHIA FETALIS)

There is marked muscular wasting with loss of mass, increased fibrous tissue around the joints, loss of mobility, and characteristic deformities. Bone changes are usually secondary to the overlying soft tissue changes. There may be unilateral or bilateral clubfoot and clubhand with marked rigidity of joints. In the lower limbs, there are also contractures of the knee and the hip, with occasional congenital dislocation.

PATHOGENESIS. Middleton first drew attention to the importance of muscular derangement in this disease. During the growth of the limb bud, before the bone skeleton is evolved, a bar of condensed mesenchyme becomes apparent at the situation where the skeleton subsequently appears. Gradually the mesodermal cells composing it are differentiated into cartilage and, later, into bone. At the same time, surrounding mesenchymal cells become differentiated to form muscle cells, the cells becoming oval and acquiring longitudinal striations, i.e., myoblasts. The transition from the myoblastic stage to the stage of fully developed muscle cell occurs at about the third month. After this there is progressive elongation to keep pace with the growth of the related skeletal tissues.

Middleton divided the pathology of the muscular derangement into three types:

1. There may be an arrest of development at the myoblastic stage.
2. The muscles may develop normally but fail to elongate.
3. The muscles, fully formed, may be the site of intrauterine degeneration, with progressive conversion into scar tissue (myodystrophia fetalis).

Many theories have been suggested, such as amyoplasia, abnormal intrauterine conditions, virus infection, developmental disturbance of the embryonic nervous system. Pathologically fibrous infiltration of the nerve bundles and peripheral nerves has been described. Microscopically the muscle is variable in appearance with greatly hypertrophied muscle fibers lying adjacent to hypoplastic fibers and infiltrated by fat. There is no systemic disturbance of biochemistry.

For the characteristics and treatment of the individual lesions which arise in myodystrophia fetalis see the discussions of congenital dislocation of the hip, congenital dislocation of the knee, and congenital talipes equinovarus earlier in the chapter.

CONGENITAL HIGH SCAPULA

Congenital high scapula (Sprengel's shoulder) was first described in 1863 by Eulenburg. It consists of an abnormally high and permanent elevation of the shoulder and is frequently associated with other deformities, such as congenital scoliosis, absence of vertebrae, fusion of ribs, or cervical rib, bony bridge to the spine, and errors in segmentation or position of the cervical spine.

PATHOGENESIS. This deformity is the result of deranged descent of the shoulder girdle, which first appears as a cervical appendage but normally descends by the end of the third month to the level of the upper part of the thorax.

The muscles suffer in their normal development, undergoing degeneration and necrosis at an early embryonic stage and becoming fibrous. This accounts for secondary contractures in the trapezius, levator scapulae, and rhomboidal group of muscles.

The scapula may be of normal shape or broadened. It lies at an unusually high level and may be attached to the vertebral column or the occipital bone by a band of imperfect muscle tissue or by fibrous tissue, or even by a bar of cartilage called the *omovertebral mass.* This mass is analogous to the suprascapular bone of the lower vertebrae, between the fourth cervical and the third dorsal vertebrae. The atlas may be in two halves, one or both of which may be fused to the occipital condyles.

CLINICAL MANIFESTATIONS. The scapula on one or both sides is 1 to 4 in. higher than usual. It is also tilted forward, so that the shoulder appears to be displaced upward and forward. When the arm is raised, the scapula does not move laterally, nor does its lower angle rotate when the arm is raised above the horizontal.

The deformity of the shoulders rather than any func-

tional disability of the arm attracts attention. There is only occasional weakness of the limb. All movements of the arm are complete except abduction and elevation to the vertical position. The neck frequently appears to be short, though the shortness is often more apparent than real, being caused or accentuated by the high position of the shoulder girdle. Torticollis is present in about 10 percent of cases. Cranium bifidum and spina bifida are often present. Congenital kyphosis affecting the thoracic region almost invariably accompanies the deformity, while scoliosis is quite frequently present as well. This deformity causes cosmetic disturbance or functional impairment, and it can cause pain.

The x-ray appearances are characteristic, the films showing the unduly high situation of the scapula. Other congenital defects in the neighborhood may also be apparent (Fig. 44-11).

PROGNOSIS. Prognosis depends upon the severity of the deformity. Mild cases need no surgery, although more severe cases can be improved at least cosmetically by surgery. Surgery is usually not done until the patient is three years old. Best results occur in the three-to-six age group, when associated deformities about the shoulder are fewer and there is a longer period of growth to adjust to the new position of the scapula.

TREATMENT. The omovertebral bone is removed and the band of fascia to the scapula tenotomized or excised. In severe deformities release of the multiple muscles attached to the scapula is necessary. The Woodward procedure

Fig. 44-11. Radiograph showing the abnormal high situation of the right scapula in Sprengel's deformity.

involves release of all the scapular stabilizing muscles, the trapezius, and the rhomboid major and minor from their origins on spinous processes. In addition to resection of the omovertebral bone, the levator scapula is released at its insertion. The aponeurosis of the trapezius and rhomboids are resutured to the spinous processes at a more distal level after the scapula has been displaced in a caudal direction.

CONGENITAL SHORT NECK (KLIPPEL-FEIL SYNDROME: BREVICOLLIS)

Klippel, in 1912, described the first such case with (1) short neck or absence of neck, (2) absence or limitation of movement of the head, (3) lowered hairline, and (4) often, an expressionless mongoloid type of face.

The neck is froglike and so short that the individual may appear to have no neck at all. Movement of the head is limited. The trapezius muscles are tense and produce a winglike appearance, which has given rise to the name *congenital webbed neck,* with a torticollis of muscular or bony origin. The posterior hairline of the scalp is so low that it reaches the upper part of the thoracic wall. Scoliosis, elevation of the scapula, and other congenital anomalies may be present.

Varying degrees of the deformity occur. In the slighter cases the cervical shortening is not marked. In the typical extreme case there is a fusion of the lower cervical vertebrae and usually the thoracic vertebrae into a solid mass. Less extreme cases vary from simple atlantooccipital fusion to all possible combinations of fusions of different vertebrae. Thus there is a considerable deformity of the cervical spine and usually numerical reduction of its component elements. Cervical spina bifida is usually present. As with other congenital defects, there are frequently associated defects in other parts of the body. Occasionally mental retardation is present. A few patients have shown functional impairment of the upper extremities suggestive of a common neurogenic origin.

This condition has to be differentiated from congenital torticollis, Pott's disease, and elevation of the scapula.

Treatment as a general rule is not indicated, but for patients with an extensive fold of skin a plastic operation may produce marked improvement.

CLEIDOCRANIAL DYSOSTOSIS SYNDROME

The syndrome was described by Marie and Fenton in 1897 and consists of (1) aplasia of the clavicles, (2) exaggerated development of the transverse diameter of the cranium, and (3) delayed closure of the fontanelles. Hereditary transmission is by a dominant expression affecting both sexes equally, although several cases have been reported with neither a familial nor a hereditary history.

Where the scapula is absent in addition, the deformity must be regarded as an aplasia of the whole shoulder girdle rather than a dysostosis. The deformities of the clavicles are always accompanied by variations in the muscles. Little or nothing is known of the cause of this condition.

CLINICAL MANIFESTATIONS. The patient usually presents with a coincidental pathologic condition or injury, but frequently no such history is obtained. Examination usually shows an apparently ununited fracture, defect in the midclavicle, or complete absence of the clavicle, and the patient can usually approximate the tips of his shoulders to each other below the chin. As a rule there is little or no disability or discomfort with abnormal mobility.

CONGENITAL WRYNECK (TORTICOLLIS)

This is a deformity characterized by lateral inclination of the head toward the shoulder, accompanied by torsion of the neck and dysplasia of the face. It is caused by unilateral contracture of the sternocleidomastoid, with secondary shortening of the fasciae and the other muscles of that side of the neck.

ETIOLOGY. Nové-Josserand and Vianny described how the middle part of the sternocleidomastoid muscle is supplied by an "end artery"—a branch of the superior thyroid—and they have noted how this sternocleidomastoid artery has been obliterated. It is generally believed that trauma is the primary cause of this deformity, producing a temporary acute obstruction of the veins followed by patchy intravascular clotting in the obstructed venous tree. In the early months of life this clotting is evidenced by the development of the sternocleidomastoid tumor of infancy, which eventually disappears, to be replaced by fibrous tissue which later contracts, very similarly to the so-called ischemic contracture of the flexor muscles of the forearm (Volkmann's contracture).

CLINICAL MANIFESTATIONS. The condition first becomes evident in the early months of life, when the mother notices an elongated swelling in the lower half of the sternocleidomastoid muscle. This swelling is at first tender, especially if the muscle is stretched. Gradually the swelling and the tenderness subside, but by the end of the first year of life the muscle becomes tense, pulling the head into the characteristic attitude, so that the ear on the affected side appears to be pulled down toward the sternoclavicular joint of the same side while the face is rotated toward the opposite side. If the deformity is not corrected, a gradual atrophy of the face on the affected side becomes increasingly evident with the growth of the child (Fig. 44-12).

PATHOLOGY. A sternocleidomastoid tumor appears about 2 or 3 weeks after birth as a spindle-shaped swelling affecting either the sternal head or frequently both heads. On microscopic examination it is found to consist of young cellular fibrous tissue, containing remnants of the original muscle fibers, which are seen to be undergoing degeneration.

The recognition of congenital wryneck should, theoretically, present no difficulty, but some cases are obscure. Every patient should be x-rayed to exclude any vertebral anomaly which may be the primary error. There is often a history of difficult birth. The early fusiform swelling may have escaped notice, but the later cordlike contraction of the sternocleidomastoid is characteristic. Hummer and MacEwen have pointed out that 20 percent of such patients have an associated congenital hip dysplasia, and this should be specifically looked for.

TREATMENT. The treatment should be begun at an early stage, as the development of the deformity can be arrested in mild cases. It is unwise to manipulate and stretch the sternocleidomastoid muscle when the tumor is tender; in these cases it may be better to excise the tumor as soon as the child will tolerate surgical treatment. The cause of the condition is thus removed, and further changes are prevented.

In later and mild cases, however, manipulation and exercises are sufficient. The head, having been grasped by the hand, is moved into a position in which the deformity is overcorrected, the object being to stretch the affected sternocleidomastoid. The manipulation must be performed gently. If this is carried out daily, there will probably be little or no evidence of contracture at the end of a few months.

When the child is not seen until the age of two or three years, operation is usually indicated. It can be performed through a comparatively short incision, so that the scar is insignificant. The muscular heads are defined and divided. When the muscle has retracted, the deep cervical fascia is divided and, if necessary, the carotid sheath and the scalenus anterior, as well. During the operation the head is gradually manipulated into the correct position, in order to bring any shortened structures into prominence.

The aftertreatment, which is of great importance, should be continued for about 6 months. It consists of active and passive movements to prevent any recurrence of the deformity.

CONGENITAL RADIOULNAR SYNOSTOSIS

One or both forearms are fixed at birth in a position midway between pronation and supination as a result of fusion of the proximal ends of the radius and ulna. In some cases the condition is inherited, and it is equally common in both sexes.

In the *true congenital radioulnar synostosis,* the upper end of the radius is imperfectly formed, being fused by bone to the ulna for a distance of several centimeters, and appears to grow from its upper end. The shaft of the radius angles forward more than usual and is longer and stouter than that of the ulna. The lower ends of the bones are almost invariably separate. Primary synostosis is usually bilateral; in over 80 percent of the recorded cases both forearms have been affected.

There may be congenital dislocation of an ill-formed head of the radius, the radius and ulna being anchored at some point a short way distal to their upper extremities, usually in the region of the coronoid process, by a short, thick interosseous ligament.

CLINICAL MANIFESTATIONS. The main feature is fixa-

Fig. 44-12. Congenital wryneck on the left side with the head pulled down toward the shoulder, atrophy of the left face structure, and prominence of the shortened sternocleidomastoid muscle.

tion of the forearm in a position of midpronation. Extension of the elbow joint may be limited. Wrist movements are often unduly free.

TREATMENT. Although operation on the bony bridge would seem to be the obvious treatment, the soft tissues are not normally developed, and because of this the recorded results of operation are disappointing. In the type of condition associated with dislocation of the head of the radius, where the soft parts are more normal, the prospect of intervention is more hopeful. However, in any case prognosis should be guarded. If the pronation is extreme, it can be reduced by osteotomy.

MADELUNG'S DEFORMITY

Congenital subluxation of the wrist is due to defective development of the inner third of the growth cartilage at the lower end of the radius. This results in stunted growth of the epiphysis and diaphysis on the inner side. Growth of the outer two-thirds continues, and as a result the radial shaft is bowed backward, the interosseous space is increased, and the lower end of the ulna is subluxated backward.

The deformity is often bilateral, is most common in females, and appears frequently for the first time in adolescence. The hand and wrist are weak, and while flexion may be increased, other movements are restricted and may be painful.

The wrist appears enlarged, and dorsiflexion of the hand is impaired. In severe cases pronation and supination are limited.

TREATMENT. Operation is occasionally indicated and consists of an osteotomy of the lower end of the radius.

Darrach advocates the simpler operation of subperiosteal resection of the lower end of the ulna, since this gives as satisfactory a result as the more elaborate procedures.

CONGENITAL APLASIA AND/OR DYSPLASIA OF LONG BONES

These uncommon deformities, consisting of absence of an organ or part, are not recognized as inherited. Various maternal disturbances, e.g., thalidomide toxicity or rubella, can produce such changes. Also, Sanders, by extirpation procedures on the preaxial and postaxial parts of the early wing buds of chicks, has produced absence of the radius and radial half of the carpal and metacarpal bone and agenesis of the ulnar half, respectively.

Frantz and O'Rahilly have classified these various complex and poorly named abnormalities under the general heading of "congenital skeletal limb deficiencies," using a combination of the following terms:

melia, limb
podia, foot
dactylia, finger
preaxial, the thumb or big toe border of the limb
postaxial, the opposite border
terminal, either transverse or longitudinal

For example, an absence of the fibula and distal ray of the foot would be called *preaxial fibular hemimelia,* and the absence of the radius would be *radial preaxial hemimelia.*

Absence of the Radius

Absence of the radius is a rare developmental error but important because it is the commonest cause of clubhand, in which the hand is permanently deviated from the normal axis of the forearm. In less than half the cases the deformity is bilateral. The condition is sometimes hereditary and frequently coexists with other forms of congenital anomaly, notably harelip, cleft palate, and certain forms of congenital clubfoot. Riordin has also described an associated aplasia of the lung as well as Fanconi's syndrome with anemia.

PATHOLOGY. Usually the whole radius is absent, but occasionally, when the defect is only partial, a small portion of it remains generally at the upper end. When a small fragment of radius is present, the ulna may be fused to it, giving rise to a form of radioulnar synostosis. The ulna, which may attain a considerable size in many cases, is short, thick, and curved, and the concavity of its curvature

is nearly always directed toward the radial side of the forearm.

The carpus often shows associated abnormalities, including absence of the scaphoid or fusion of that bone with neighboring carpal bones. More rarely the lunate is absent.

When the radius is totally absent, the biceps is usually inserted into the lacertus fibrosus, though in some cases the muscle is either completely absent or fused with the brachialis anterior or the coracobrachialis. Other disturbances in the brachialis, the extensor carpi radialis longus and brevis, the extensor digitorum communis, the extensor pollicis longus, the flexor pollicis longus, and the pronator quadratus are frequently seen. The radial nerve usually terminates at the elbow, and there is often no radial artery.

CLINICAL MANIFESTATIONS. Generally the affected arm shows some degree of atrophy, but this is most marked in the forearm, which is invariably short, stubby, and bowed with a posterior convexity. The hand is small and atrophic. It is also deviated to the radial side and slightly palmar-flexed—"radiopalmar clubhand." The thumb is occasionally absent. Despite these deformities the limb may retain a surprisingly good function, although grasping power is usually impaired.

TREATMENT. The treatment is aimed at relieving the deformity, weakness, inability to use the arm, and limitation of certain movements, such as dorsiflexion.

Riordin has pointed out that the aim should be to overcome the deformity as early as possible by splintage or by operative removal of the bony anlage which is producing the bowing defect as well as growth disturbance of the intact ulnar bone. Every attempt should be made to stabilize the carpus and hand to the ulnar bone in order to obtain stretching of muscle and any available growth.

Absence of the Ulna

This is a much more uncommon lesion than the absence of the radius and is most difficult to differentiate from the latter lesion.

Absence or Dysplasia of the Fibula

This is a relatively uncommon condition. The whole limb is seen to be shortened in length and reduced in girth. The tibia appears bowed in an anterior direction with the hind part of the foot in the equinovalgus position, and there may be absence of part of the lateral forefoot and toes. There is obvious soft tissue atrophy and development of contractures, e.g., tightness of the tendocalcaneous and peroneus muscles, as well as the lateral ligaments around the ankle. There may be bilateral involvement in about 30 percent of the cases. Radiography will show varying degrees of hypoplosia throughout the bones with delay in the appearance of their ossification centers.

TREATMENT. Because manipulation, casting, tendon lengthening, osteotomy of the tibia, etc., have not been very successful, early amputation, such as a Syme amputation of the foot, with fitting of a below-knee prosthesis, may be preferred.

Shortening of the Femur

Unlike the fibula, the dysplasia appears to affect mainly the proximal end of the femur rather than its center aspect. Steindler has described four types: (1) those with only rudimentary development of the upper third of femur and marked coxa vara, (2) coxa vara with a normal shaft, (3) overall shortening of shaft but a normal upper third component, and (4) dysplasia of the lower third with synostosis at the knee. As growth proceeds, the deformity becomes more severe with marked leg length discrepancy due to disturbance in all bones of the lower extremity. Often these children never put weight on the involved limb.

Treatment is directed toward providing some means of ambulation through an ischial-bearing, weight-relieving brace. Although bracing allows ambulation, it does not provide for the normal stimulation to growth or weight bearing, and, therefore, as well as the aplastic or dysplastic elements, the remaining "normal" components of bone fail to grow and develop. Thus, if the main disturbance is in the more distal components, early amputation with a prosthesis is indicated.

References

Congenital Disorders

Bick, E. M.: Congenital Deformities of the Musculo-skeletal System Noted in the Newborn, *Am J Dis Child,* **100:**861, 1960.

Denis-Browne, R.: Congenital Postural Scoliosis, *Proc R Soc Med,* **49:**395, 1956.

Fuller, D. J., and Duthie, R. B.: The Timed Appearance of Some Congenital Malformations and Orthopaedic Abnormalities, Am. Acad. Orthop. Surg., Instructional Course Lectures, The C. V. Mosby Company, St. Louis, **23:**53, 1974.

Gentry, J. T., Parkhurst, E., and Bulin, G. V., Jr.: An Epidemiological Study of Congenital Malformations in New York State, *Am J Public Health,* **49:**497, 1959.

McKeown, J., and Record, R. G.: Malformations in a Population Observed for Five Years after Birth, in G. E. W. Wolstenholme and C. M. O'Connor (eds.), *Ciba Found Symp Congenital Malformations,* p. 2, 1960.

Norton, P. L.: Pediatric Orthopedics, *Med Clin North Am,* **37:**1427, 1953.

Stevenson, A. C.: Frequency of Congenital and Hereditary Disease: With Special Reference to Maturation, *Br Med Bull,* **17:**3, 254, 1961.

Congenital Dislocation of the Hip

Badgely, C. E.: Etiology of Congenital Dislocation of the Hip, *J Bone Joint Surg [Am],* **31A:**341, 1949.

Carter, C.: Genetics in Orthopaedics, *J Bone Joint Surg [Br],* **39B:**4, 1957.

Duthie, R. B., and Townes, P. L.: The Genetics of Orthopaedic Conditions, *J Bone Joint Surg [Br],* **49B:**2, 1967.

Gill, A. B.: End Results of Bloodless Reduction of Congenital Dislocation of the Hip, *J Bone Joint Surg [Am],* **25:**1, 1943.

Haas, J.: "Congenital Dislocation of the Hip," Charles C Thomas, Publisher, Springfield, Ill., 1951.

Hirsch, C., and Scheller, S.: Result of Treatment from Birth of Unstable Hips: a Clinical and Radiographic Five-year Follow-up, *Clin Orthop,* **62:**162, 1969.

Hummer, C.D., and MacEwen, G.D.: The Coexistence of Torticollis and Congenital Dysplasia of the Hip, *J. Bone Joint Surg [Am],* **54A:**1255, 1972.

Lima, C., Esteve, R., and Trueta, J.: Osteochondritis in Congenital Dislocation of the Hip: A Clinical and Radiographic Study, *Acta Orthop Scand,* **29:**218, 1960.

MacKenzie, I. G., Seddon, H. J., and Trevor, D.: Congenital Dislocation of the Hip, *J Bone Joint Surg [Br],* **42B:**689, 1960.

Muller, G. M., and Seddon, H. J.: Late Results of Treatment of Congenital Dislocation of the Hip, *J Bone Joint Surg [Am],* **35B:**342, 1953.

Pemberton, P. A.: Osteotomy of the Ilium with Rotation of the Acetabular Roof for Congenital Dislocation of the Hip, *J Bone Joint Surg [Am],* **40A:**724, 1958.

Platou, E.: Luxatio Coxae Congenita: A Follow-up Study of Four Hundred and Six Cases of Closed Reduction, *J Bone Joint Surg [Am],* **35A:**843, 1953.

Record, R. G., and Edwards, J. H.: Environmental Influences Related to the Aetiology of Congenital Dislocation of the Hip, *Br J Prevent Social Med,* **12:**8, 1958.

Salter, R. B.: Innominate Osteotomy in the Treatment of Congenital Dislocation and Subluxation of the Hip, *J Bone Joint Surg [Br],* **34B:**518, 1961.

Salvati, E. A., and Wilson, P. D., Jr.: Treatment of Irreducible Hip Subluxation by Chiari's Iliac Osteotomy, *Rev Hosp Spec Surg,* **1:**49, 1971.

Scaglietti, C., and Calandriello, B.: Open Reduction of Congenital Dislocation of the Hip, *J Bone Joint Surg [Br],* **44B:**257, 1962.

Scott, J. C.: Frame Reduction in Congenital Dislocation of the Hip, *J Bone Joint Surg [Br],* **35B:**372, 1953.

Smith, W. S., Badgley, C. E., Orwig, J. B., and Harper, J. M.: Correlation of Post-reduction Roentgenograms and 31-Year Followup in Congenital Dislocation of the Hip, *J Bone Joint Surg [Am],* **50A:**1081, 1968.

Symposium of the Swedish Orthopaedic Association; Prevention of Congenital Dislocation of the Hip Joint in Sweden: Efficiency of Early Diagnosis and Treatment, *Acta Orthop Scand Suppl* 130, 1970.

Wynne-Davies, R.: Acetabular Dysplasia and Familial Joint Laxity: Two Etiological Factors in Congenital Dislocation of the Hip, A Review of 589 Patients and Their Families, *J Bone Joint Surg [Br],* **52B:**704, 1970.

Congenital Talipes Equinovarus (Clubfoot)

Crabbe, W. A.: Aetiology of Congenital Talipes, *Br Med J,* **2:**1060, 1960.

Dunn, N.: Suggestions Based on Ten Years' Experience of Arthrodesis of the Tarsus in the Treatment of Deformities of the Foot, in "Robert Jones' Birthday Volume." Oxford University Press, London, 1928.

Goldner, J. L.: Congenital Talipes Equinovarus: Fifteen Years of Surgical Treatment, in J. P. Adams (ed.), "Current Practice in Orthopaedic Surgery," p. 61, vol. 4, The C. V. Mosby Company, St. Louis, 1969.

Heyman, C. H., Herndon, C. H., and Strong, J. M.: Mobilization of the Tarsometatarsal and Intermetatarsal Joints for the Correction of Resistant Adduction of the Fore Part of the

Foot in Congenital Club-foot or Congenital Metatarsus Varus, *J Bone Joint Surg* [*Am*], **40A:**299, 1958.

Kite, J. H.: "The Clubfoot," Grune and Stratton, New York, 1964.

Steindler, A.: "Orthopaedic Operations, Indications, Techniques, and End Results," Charles C Thomas, Publisher, Springfield, Ill., 1940.

Wynne-Davies, R.: Family Studies and the Cause of Congenital Clubfoot: Talipes Equinovarus, Talipes Calcaneovalgus and Metatarsus Varus, *J Bone Joint Surg* [*Br*], **46B:**445, 1964.

Congenital Convex Pes Valgus

Tachdjian, M. O.: Congenital Convex Pes Valgus, in "Symposium on Current Pediatric Problems," *Orthop Clin North Am,* **3:**131, 1972.

Congenital Limb Dysplasias

Darrach, W.: Colles Fracture, *N Engl J Med,* **226:**594, 1942.

Frantz, C. G., and O'Rahilly, R.: Congenital Skeletal Limb Deficiencies, *J Bone Joint Surg* [*Am*], **43A:**1202, 1961.

Riordin, D. C.: Congenital Absence of the Radius, *J Bone Joint Surg* [*Am*], **37A:**1129, 1955.

Sanders, J. W.: The Proximo-distal Sequence of Origin of the Parts of the Chick Wing and the Role of the Ectoderm, *J Exp Zool,* **108:**363, 1948.

Thompson, T. C., Straub, L. R., and Arnold, W. D.: Congenital Absence of the Fibula, *J Bone Joint Surg* [*Am*], **39A:**1229, 1957.

Other Congenital Lesions

Green, W. T.: The Surgical Correction of Congenital Elevation of the Scapula (Sprengel's Deformity), *J Bone Joint Surg* [*Am*], **39A:**1439, 1957.

——— and Rudo, N.: Pseudoarthrosis and Neurofibromatosis, *Arch Surg,* **46:**639, 1943.

McFarland, B. L.: Pseudarthrosis of the Tibia in Childhood, *J Bone Joint Surg* [*Br*], **33B:**36, 1951.

Neibauer, J. J., and King, D. E.: Congenital Dislocation of the Knee, *J Bone Joint Surg* [*Am*], **42A:**2, 1960.

Chapter 45

Generalized Bone Disorders

by **Robert B. Duthie and Franklin T. Hoaglund**

Bone

Composition
Ossification
Remodeling

Radiologic Diagnosis of Bone Disorders

Classification of Generalized Bone Disorders

Developmental Disorders of Bone

Achondroplasia
Dyschondroplasia
Multiple Enchondromas
Metaphyseal Aclasis
Polyostotic Fibrous Dysplasia
    Monostotic Fibrous Dysplasia
Osteogenesis Imperfecta
Osteopetrosis
    Melorheostosis
    Osteopathia Striata
Osteopoikilosis

Metabolic Diseases

Metabolism of Calcium and Phosphorus
Calcification
Scurvy
Rickets
    Celiac Rickets
    Renal Osteodystrophy
    Hypophosphatasia
Osteomalacia
Parathyroid Osteodystrophy
Osteoporosis
Pituitary Disturbances
    Pituitary Dwarfism
    Hyperpituitary Syndromes
Congenital Hypothyroidism
Mucopolysaccharidoses

Osteitis Deformans

Reticuloses

Hodgkin's Disease
    Histiocytic Granulomatosis
    Lipoid Granulomatosis
    Eosinophilic Granulomatosis
    Letterer-Siwe Disease

Hematopoietic System

Leukemia
Multiple Myeloma
Hemolytic Anemia

BONE

Composition

Bone is made up of organic and inorganic materials, and water.

ORGANIC PHASE. This is made up of osteogenic cells—i.e., the osteoblast, the osteocyte, and the osteoclast—the cartilage cell, or chondroblast, and the intercellular matrix, as well, which consists of approximately 89 percent collagen, 1 percent amorphous mucopolysaccharide complexes, and other proteins (Fig. 45-1). Collagen is a crystalline fibroprotein with a characteristic x-ray diffraction and electron microscopic pattern, having a periodicity of about 680 Å. Its length, diameter, and density vary with age; e.g., when old, its diameter may be over 1000 Å. Chemically it consists of a number of amino acids, such as alanine, leucine, glycine, arginine, glutamic acid, proline, and hydroxyproline with a total nitrogen content of 18.45 percent (glycine, proline, and hydroxyproline making up almost 60 percent of the total weight of collagen). Hydroxyproline is excreted in almost constant amounts in the urine of man at about 70 to 80 mg/24 hours and indicates collagen turnover.

Reticulin, present in small quantities, is a glycoprotein made up of polysaccharides such as glucose, mannose, and galactose combined with amino acids.

The intercellular matrix, or ground substance, which is sometimes called *osseomucoid,* is common to all connective tissues and contains protein, crystalloids, metabolites, and gases similar to plasma. Therefore, it forms the final diffusion or circulatory pathway for the exchange of nutritional substances from blood to the osteogenic cells through the various lacunae and canalicular systems. Osseous mucoid substance consists of (1) proteoglycans and (2) glycoproteins containing chondroitin sulfate, all having a great capacity for binding metal with various radionuclides and possibly calcium. In addition, plasma proteins, lipids, and peptides can be isolated from bone.

In certain inherited connective tissue diseases, these mucopolysaccharides are found in urine in increased amounts, e.g., Hurler's disease—chondroitin sulfate B and

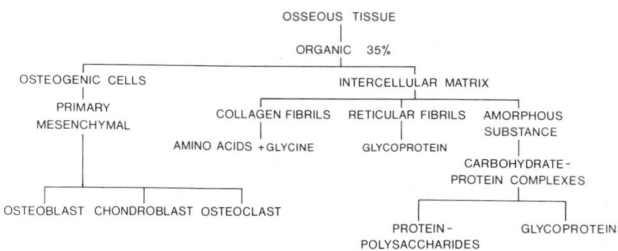

Fig. 45-1. Organic components of bone. (*Taken with permission from Mercer and Duthie, "Orthopaedic Surgery," London, 1974.*)

heparitin sulfate; Morquio's disease—keratosulfate; multiple exostoses—chondroitin sulfate A and C.

INORGANIC PHASE. In this phase, bone contains 99 percent of the total calcium and 90 percent of the phosphorus of the human body. It is made up of calcium, phosphate, hydroxyl, carbonates, and magnesium. The actual chemical composition of the bone crystal has not been fully determined but may be considered a hydroxyapatite crystal with the possible formulas of $Ca_{10}(PO_4)_6OH$ or $3Ca_3(PO_4)_2 \cdot Ca(OH)_2$. It is a single crystalline type with a molar calcium/phosphorus ratio of 1.3 : 2.1. The crystals are very small, and they are generally considered to be rod-shaped: 220 Å × 65 Å. However, Robinson has described them as being approximately 400 Å × 500 Å in thickness with the shape of a hexagonal plate. The solution surrounding the crystal consists of many different ions and is in continuity with the body serum. The serum adjacent to a crystal is normally supersaturated with calcium and hypophosphate ions.

The chemical reactivity of the osteon is determined by the age of crystallization of its contents. Newly deposited crystals are highly hydrated and very imperfect in construction, with ion spaces in the crystal unfilled. Therefore, nearly all their ions are capable of rapid displacement. As aging proceeds, the crystals become larger, less hydrated, and more nearly perfect, with water displaced by mineral. This produces a reduction in the rate and extent of diffusion exchange and crystallization.

WATER OF BONE. Robinson has determined that 8 to 9 percent of the bone matrix, even in the fully mineralized state, is water in the form of either interstitial or extracellular fluid, or within the hydration shell of the apatite crystals. There is much water in the organic phase of mucopolysaccharide complexes, in collagen, in the inorganic component of bone, and in the marrow and osteocytic spaces of bone. Robinson has postulated that, as calcification of osteoid tissue takes place, water is displaced from the matrix, with reduction in the space between the crystals and other solids.

Also ions, such as calcium, sodium, phosphate, potassium, and chloride, require hydration for their movement or diffusion, and as the matrix calcifies, the rate of diffusion or exchange of calcium ions is reduced with slowing of crystallization. This calcification of matrix with reduction in diffusion is also seen in the zone of the mature chondroblasts in phase IV of the epiphyseal plate, where calcium is deposited with death of the chondroblasts and their disintegration into calcifying trabeculae.

CITRATE IN BONE. This represents 70 percent of the total body citrate in animals. It appears to be mainly on the surface of the apatite crystal but may be bound primarily to the calcium ion. As well as being concerned with the metabolic, oxidative processes of carbohydrate, fat, and protein in mammals, it forms soluble but complex compounds with calcium to facilitate absorption from the intestine, diffusion, and hence deposition of calcium into bone. It may also be concerned with making calcium in bone more soluble and, therefore, facilitating its removal without significant change in the local pH.

Not only does the citrate content of the serum parallel the calcium content but also there is a transport function performed by citrate in the cell membrane. Vitamin D in therapeutic doses causes a rise in serum citrate levels, which is also seen in hyperparathyroidism and hypercalcemic states. Normal serum citrate levels are decreased in conditions of hypoparathyroidism, rickets, and osteomalacia. Ordinarily excretion of citrate varies between 200 and 1,000 mg/day and reflects accurately the serum citrate levels.

In vitamin D deficiency rickets, the serum citrate level is low even when the calcium level remains normal; the administration of citrate as the sodium salt is followed by healing of the rachitic lesion of bone.

BONE ENZYMES. Bone cells contain the normal complement of enzymes similar, for example, to those found in liver cells. Bone cells have an active metabolism, the rate of oxygen consumption reaching 50 percent of that of liver cells. However, bone differs from other tissues in relying largely on glycolysis for energy production. Certain enzymes and enzyme systems have special importance in bone tissue:

Glycolytic Enzymes in Osteoclasts. These enzymes transform glucose into pyruvate with concomitant formation of adenosine triphosphate (ATP), which is used by the cell in various synthetic reactions. The pyruvate can then be metabolized further to lactate or to citrate. The production of lactic acid is an important factor in bone resorption, and the metabolism of osteoclasts is primarily glycolytic or anaerobic, which promotes lactate formation.

Acid Hydrolases. An example is cathepsin D, a protease with optimal activity at a pH of 3.6. The acid hydrolases are normally found within the lysosome. Thus, the extrusion or breakdown of the lysosomes in cells leads to the digestion of cells and their surrounding matrix when bone is resorbed by osteoblasts.

Collagenases. Bone contains enzymes that will specifically degrade collagen, a property that few proteases exhibit. Such enzymes are important in the breakdown of the organic matrix of bone during resorption, but little is known about them at present.

Alkaline Phosphatase. This is a phosphomonoesterase which is nonspecific and catalyzes orthophosphoric monoesters of phenol, alcohol, and sugars, and has an optimal activity at a pH of about 9. Its role is uncertain, but the serum level is altered in certain disorders of the skeletal and hepatobiliary systems (see Table 45-1). It is considered to be concerned with the preosseous cellular metabolism and with the subsequent elaboration of bone matrix before

Table 45-1. ALKALINE PHOSPHATASE LEVELS

Alkaline phosphatase levels	Skeletal disease	Hepatobiliary disease
Increased	Rickets and osteomalacia 　In calcifying cartilage Paget's disease Osteosarcoma 　At site of disease Carcinoma, osteoblastic 　metastases	Intra- and extra- 　hepatobiliary 　obstructions
Normal	Osteoporosis Osteopetrosis Healing fracture 　Increase in phosphatase 　　locally Osteosclerosis Fibrous dysplasia 　Variable level	Metastases Thorazine tox- 　icity
Decreased. . . .	Achondroplasia Deposition of radioactive 　substances in bone Hypophosphatasia 　Arrest of skeletal growth 　　with decreased osteo- 　　blastic activity Cretinism Scurvy	

Fig. 45-2. Enzymes participating in endochondral ossification. (*Taken with permission from Mercer and Duthie, "Orthopaedic Surgery," London, 1974.*)

the crystallization of calcium and phosphate ions. It is detectable in the serum of adults with normal levels of 35 to 80 I.U./liter and is also present in bone, calcifying cartilage, intestinal mucosa, liver, and kidneys.

Phosphorylase and Glycolytic Enzyme Systems. These are concerned with converting glycogen via the hexophospho-pyruvates into excess phosphate ions.

Acid Phosphatase. This is present in high levels in the osteoclasts and cells of the prostate. Serum levels in both sexes are very low under normal conditions. The enzyme is distinguished from alkaline phosphatase in that it has an optimal activity at a pH of 5.

Ossification

Much of the skeleton in the embryo is formed in the cartilage model by endochondral ossification, although some is formed in connective tissue by intramembranous ossification.

ENDOCHONDRAL OSSIFICATION. The long bones of the skeleton, with the exception of the clavicle, are all laid down primarily as hyaline cartilage in recognizable anatomic form. In the center of this cartilage model, at a certain stage depending upon cellular age and model mass, the cells undergo hypertrophy and accumulate glycogen. Phosphorylases and other enzymes with their glycolytic action appear in the cells and cartilage matrix to form the osseous centrum (Fig. 45-2).

Such changes in the cartilage are accompanied by ossification in the perichondrium and an ingrowth of vascular

connective tissue which replaces the hypertrophied cartilage cells. Osteoblasts derived from this connective tissue then begin to lay down osteoid and fetal bone on the cartilage matrix. Hematopoietic cells appear from the invading tissues, and red marrow is soon identified.

The process extends up and down the shaft until the level of the future growth plates is reached at the epiphyseal-metaphyseal junction. Here the replacement of the cartilage model ceases, and the cartilage organizes into the proliferative epiphyseal growth plate.

During fetal and childhood osteogenesis, the endochondral growth of bone continues in the epiphyseal plate areas, as well as within the epiphysis. To maintain growth in length, further cartilage cells are added to the epiphysis from the juxtaepiphyseal apparatus or the perichondral ring of Lacroix. Streeter has described the classic five phases of the epiphyseal plate with the characteristic appearance of the cartilage cells (Fig. 45-3).

Accompanying such longitudinal and accretional growth there is remodeling to produce the tubular shape of bone as a result of cellular activity. Follis described how in the five normal processes of endochondral ossification there are three main phases which can undergo disturbance:

1. Disturbance in the actual growth and differentiation of cartilage, such as in achondroplasia
2. Disturbance in the osteogenic-osteolytic balance, such as in osteoporosis, osteosclerosis, and osteitis fibrosis
3. Disturbance in the deposition of the calcium phosphate crystals in the cartilage matrix and/or osteoid, such as in rickets or osteomalacia

INTRAMEMBRANOUS OSSIFICATION. This form of ossification occurs without any preformed cartilage model and is seen particularly in the development of the calvarium. The cells are developed from the germinal layers, and at a certain stage of differentiation the mesodermal cells condense and begin to proliferate in the area where bone will be formed. In this area the cells elaborate increased cytoplasm with an eosinophilic staining reaction and, at the same time, begin to secrete a metachromatic intercellular substance, as well as collagen fibrils. These cells soon become osteoblasts which continue to secrete much intracellular substance, or osteoid, which mineralizes to

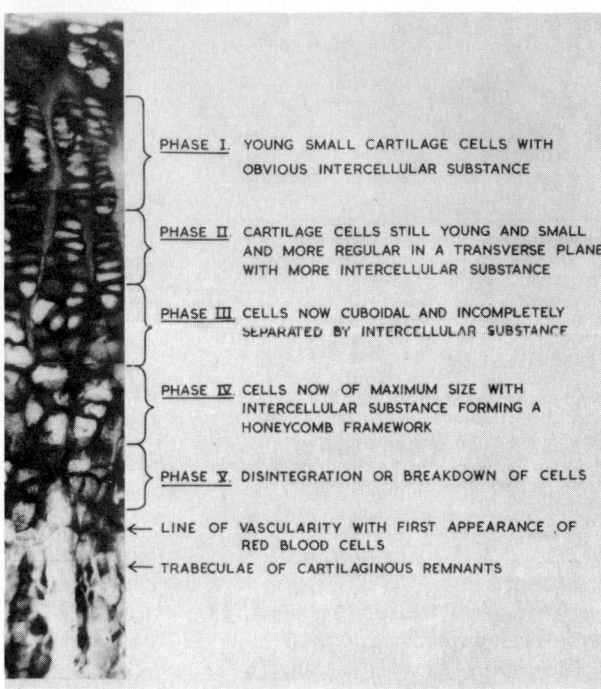

PHASE I. YOUNG SMALL CARTILAGE CELLS WITH OBVIOUS INTERCELLULAR SUBSTANCE

PHASE II. CARTILAGE CELLS STILL YOUNG AND SMALL AND MORE REGULAR IN A TRANSVERSE PLANE WITH MORE INTERCELLULAR SUBSTANCE

PHASE III. CELLS NOW CUBOIDAL AND INCOMPLETELY SEPARATED BY INTERCELLULAR SUBSTANCE

PHASE IV. CELLS NOW OF MAXIMUM SIZE WITH INTERCELLULAR SUBSTANCE FORMING A HONEYCOMB FRAMEWORK

PHASE V. DISINTEGRATION OR BREAKDOWN OF CELLS

← LINE OF VASCULARITY WITH FIRST APPEARANCE OF RED BLOOD CELLS
← TRABECULAE OF CARTILAGINOUS REMNANTS

Fig. 45-3. Photomicrograph of the epiphyseal plate and its division into Streeter's five phases. (*Taken with permission from Mercer and Duthie, "Orthopaedic Surgery," London, 1974.*)

form bone. From such centers of ossification the process spreads.

Remodeling

This consists of extensive but constructive resorption and deposition of new bone which, although most marked during growth and development, continues in the mature skeleton. With resorption there is the shift of both mineral and organic matrix into a fluid phase. During growth at the epiphyseal plate area the remodeling process is essential to change the shape and function of the bones, both in the longitudinal and in the circumferential planes and within the spongiosa of the medullary cavity (Fig. 45-4) in order to produce the normal tubular shape of the shaft. There is a morphologic remodeling process in the periosteal area, adjacent to the juxtaepiphyseal area or the perichondral ring of Lacroix, which contains large numbers of osteoclasts. However, there is a constant remodeling process taking place within the basic structure of bone, i.e., in the osteon itself. Vincent and Haumont have described how bone and its unit—the osteon—is one of two major reactive types, i.e., *metabolic,* undergoing continuous resorption because of its close relationship to the fluid phase or extracellular fluid with accretion, and *structural,* in which there is little exchange of state, because it is completely calcified and stable.

The marrow cavity is also widened during remodeling by osteoclastic activity on the endosteal surfaces of cortex and spongiosa.

RADIOLOGIC DIAGNOSIS OF BONE DISORDERS

The varying densities which may be seen on a radiograph are:

1. Background density of the film
2. Subcutaneous tissue
3. Fatty tissue
4. Fluids, edema, hemorrhage, joint effusion
5. Muscle (similar in consistency to that of water)
6. Cartilage
7. Bone—cancellous being less dense than cortical bone

The cortex encloses the cancellous bone and the medulla and may make interpretation within these structures difficult.

The following tissues are examined:

SOFT TISSUES. It is important to distinguish a soft tissue *swelling* from a soft tissue *mass.* A *soft tissue swelling* has a poorly defined expanded limit which is caused by extracellular fluid infiltrating the area and obscuring the normal soft tissue outlines. A *soft tissue mass* is clearly delineated, obscuring by its own density the normal anatomy of vessel and fat lines. A cyst or tumor would also produce such a finding. The shape of the mass may be significant, e.g., when gravity enlarges its inferior portion because of its fluid or purulent content.

Calcification or Ossification in Soft Tissues. Calcification is characterized by its uniform amorphous appearance, whereas ossification may be mature enough in formation and even remodeled to show cortex and trabecular pattern. Both may be seen in muscle (myositis ossificans), tendon (supraspinal calcification), joint capsule or ligament, or joint.

BONE. *"Apparent" expansion of bone* may be caused by destruction of the cortex followed by the deposition of new bone around the lesion. Thus, a simple bone cyst is never wider than the epiphyseal line. "Apparent" expansion is caused by remodeling above and below the lesion to such an extent that the lesion appears wider than normally remodeled bone.

Generalized decrease in bone radiodensity is seen as a diffuse decrease in bone density by narrowing the width of the diaphyseal cortices or by decreasing the width of the trabeculae or their number, as in osteoporosis, Sudeck's atrophy, and disuse atrophy of immobilization around a joint.

Increased radiodensity usually is seen in an area or segment of bone. It implies new bone formation on cortical bone or on trabecular bone, or an increase in the number of trabeculae in any unit area or compaction of trabecular bone, or a relative increase in density due to a surrounding area's losing its blood supply with decrease of its density, as in developmental osteopetrosis, fluorosis, and Paget's disease.

In *new bone formation,* trabecular bone can be laid down within the bone structure on preexisting trabeculae or filling between these structures. The amount of physical mass which is produced reflects the cause. For example, a staphylococcal infection will produce a much greater amount than a streptococcal infection. The disorganized deposition of new bone in a neuropathic joint, such as in Charcot's or Paget's diseases, will often completely obliterate the original trabecular pattern with a dense amorphous-appearing bone. The new bone pattern must be carefully examined for its degree of organization into trabeculae of normal shape, size, and amount, and the overlying cortex must be searched for evidence of osteon formation. It is important to differentiate *reactive new bone,* which is organized, and *tumor new bone,* which lacks this property. Periosteum will produce new bone in response to growth, infection, tumor, or vascular disturbances. Edeiken and Hodes have described two types of periosteal reactions. The first type is solid reaction of a single uniform layer more than 1 cm thick, which persists unchanged for weeks. It can be thin (eosinophilic granuloma), dense and undulating (vascular), dense and elliptical (malignant tumor or fracture), or Codman's triangle (malignant tumor or hemorrhage).

The second type is an interrupted reaction, either lamellated (onion skin) or perpendicular to the surface (sunburst). This occurs in active aggressive malignant tumors, infections, or subperiosteal hemorrhages or finally amorphous calcific densities lying between periosteal new bone and its adjacent bone cortex—and denoting malignant disease of bone. A localized bony protruberance arising from the surface of the cortex as an exostosis may be found in one or more bones.

Ossification must be distinguished from *calcification.* Ossification implies a cellular activity of depositing calcium phosphate complex crystals with an organized framework to form the structure of bone. Calcification is a chemical activity of laying down calcium phosphate crystals without structure or organization and usually is seen in soft tissue planes of tendons, bursae, etc.

Dysplasia is a disturbance of growth or metabolism without reaction of adjacent bone or periosteum to suggest an inflammatory or neoplastic process. Its location in the epiphyseal, metaphyseal, and diaphyseal areas of several bones suggests its multifocal origin. This may be an arrest of growth or a remodeling defect to produce alteration in shape and size of bones, as in developmental disorders.

JOINT TISSUES. Skin, subcutaneous tissues, and other soft tissue masses (ligaments, capsule) can be identified. Particular attention is given to the ballooning out of the normal layers by an effusion. Comparison should be made with the opposite joint for such soft tissue changes and for observing the normal width of the joint "space" which is formed by the adjacent articular cartilage surfaces or by the menisci of the knees, etc. The relationship of the bones making up the joint is studied, and rotational abnormalities around the hip joint, for example, can be noted by comparing how much of the lesser trochanter profile is visible or how far away the joint lines are displaced. The quality of these bones as regards their density, the presence of subchondral cyst formation in osteoarthritis, or subchondral erosion in rheumatoid arthritis should be noted. The symmetry or lack of it regarding the adjacent bone surfaces should be noted especially when destroyed

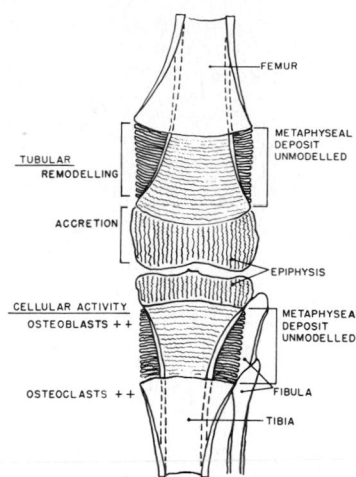

Fig. 45-4. Tubular remodeling and accretion of a long bone. (*After Keith. Taken with permission from Mercer and Duthie, "Orthopaedic Surgery," London, 1974.*)

by bone loss, resorption, or fragmentation of the growing epiphysis (Perthes' disease) or of the adult femoral head (avascular necrosis), or in the relationship of the upper femoral epiphysis to the femoral neck (Table 45-2).

CLASSIFICATION OF GENERALIZED BONE DISORDERS

I. *Developmental disorders* involving the organic phase of bone, i.e., collagen and cartilage matrix formation, calcification, and remodeling
   A. Achondroplasia
   B. Chondroosteodystrophy
   C. Dyschondroplasia
   D. Multiple enchondromas
   E. Metaphyseal aclasis
   F. Osteogenesis imperfecta
   G. Polyostotic fibrous dysplasia
   H. Osteopetrosis
II. *Metabolic disorders*
   A. Deficiency in inorganic constituents of bone
     1. Insufficient absorption of calcium or phosphates
       a. Low intake
         (1) Starvation
         (2) Rickets
         (3) Osteomalacia
       b. Defective absorption
         (1) Vitamin D deficiency
         (2) Defective fat absorption
           (*a*) Biliary deficiency
           (*b*) Pancreatic deficiency
           (*c*) Celiac disease
         (3) Chronic diarrhea
     2. Excessive secretion of calcium or phosphates
       a. Renal rickets, or osteodystrophy
         (1) Total renal insufficiency
         (2) Tubular insufficiency
           (*a*) Lignac-Fanconi syndrome
           (*b*) Hyperchloremic acidosis
           (*c*) Vitamin D-resistant rickets, or "phosphate rickets"

  b. During pregnancy, via placenta and breast
    (1) Osteomalacia
  c. Hyperparathyroidism
3. Decreased phosphate excretion
  a. Hypoparathyroidism
B. Deficiency in organic constituents of bone
  1. Decreased intake
    a. Starvation
    b. Chronic diarrhea
  2. Excessive utilization or loss
    a. Chronic infection
    b. Renal disease
    c. Liver disease
    d. Hormonal
      (1) Hyperthyroidism
      (2) Postmenopausal osteoporosis
      (3) Disuse atrophy
      (4) Stress
      (5) Cushing's disease
III. *Hormonal disorders*—normal, excessive, or deficient secretion, the effect being seen in a *child* as altered rate of epiphyseal growth and skeletal maturation and in an *adult* as alteration in the balance of osteolytic and osteoblastic activity
  A. Pituitary
  B. Sex glands
  C. Thyroid
  D. Adrenals
  E. Parathyroids
IV. *Reticulosis*—disease of bone marrow constituents such as
  A. Reticuloendothelial system
    1. Histiocytic granulomatosis
      a. Letterer-Siwe disease
      b. Eosinophilic granuloma
      c. Hand-Schüller-Christian disease
    2. Lipoid granulomatosis
      a. Gaucher's disease
      b. Niemann-Pick disease
      c. Xanthomatosis with hypercholesterolemia
  B. Lymphatic system
    1. Hodgkin's disease
    2. Lymphosarcoma
  C. Hematopoietic system
    1. Leukemia
      a. Lymphoblastic
      b. Myeloblastic
    2. Multiple myeloma
    3. Hemolytic anemia
      a. Mediterranean, or Cooley's, anemia
      b. Sickle cell anemia
      c. Erythroblastosis foetalis
V. *Vascular disorders*
  A. Paget's disease
  B. Osteodystrophy or Sudeck's atrophy
  C. Massive osteolysis, or "disappearing bones"

In the examination and diagnosis of these conditions Shearer said:

  If a bone lesion as seen radiographically does not show reactive change in the adjacent bone or periosteum, which suggests an inflammatory process or the invasive character of a neoplastic process, you should then have in mind the possibility of a dysplasia. Study then the localization; is it involving primarily metaphyseal bone or does it, in some conditions, involve only the epiphyses or only the small bones? Study then the nature of the abnormal process. Is it merely an arrest of growth; does the appearance suggest a cartilage dysplasia or a fibrous dysplasia? Then proceed to carry out a survey of the skeleton to show the distribu-

Table 45-2. RADIOGRAPHIC DIFFERENTIAL DIAGNOSIS OF GENERALIZED BONE DISORDERS

I. Reaction of adjacent bone and/or periosteum
  A. Tumor
  B. Inflammation
II. Normal adjacent bone and/or periosteum: dysplasia (disturbance of growth or metabolism) occurring in the
  A. Epiphysis
    1. Chondroosteodystrophy
    2. Gargoylism
    3. Epiphyseal dysplasia
    4. Achondroplasia
  B. Metaphysis
    1. Dyschondroplasia
    2. Multiple enchondromata
    3. Metaphyseal aclasia
    4. Polyostotic fibrous dysplasia
    5. Neurofibromatosis
  C. Diaphysis
    1. Engelmann's disease
    2. Dyschondroplasia
    3. Melorheostosis
  D. Marrow
    1. Leukemia
    2. Multiple myelomatosis
    3. Lymphadenoma—Hodgkin's disease
    4. Histiocytic granulomatosis
      a. Hand-Schüller-Christian disease
      b. Eosinophilic granuloma
      c. Letterer-Siwe disease
    5. Gaucher's disease
  E. Whole bone
    1. Porosis (decreased osteoblastic activity)
      a. Osteogenesis imperfecta
      b. Osteomalacia—rickets
      c. Sudeck's atrophy
      d. Osteoporosis
      e. Endocrine
        (1) Hyperparathyroidism
        (2) Hyperthyroidism
    2. Sclerosis (increased osteoblastic activity)
      a. Osteopetrosis
      b. Osteopathia striata
      c. Osteopoikilosis
      d. Melorheostosis
      e. Osteitis deformans
      f. Hypertrophic osteoarthropathy

tion of the abnormal bone. Do not forget to note whether the condition is associated with a generalized osteoporosis or whether bone, apart from the involved area, is normal. Then consider the findings in relation to the full history and clinical examination as well as biochemical blood analysis. Having done this I think you will at least make an intelligent approach to the correct diagnosis, and will usually reach a satisfactory conclusion.

DEVELOPMENTAL DISORDERS OF BONE

The common developmental diseases of bone apart from the obvious endocrine errors can all be arranged in two groups:

1. Errors in the proliferation and calcification of the cartilage model
   a. Achondroplasia
   b. Chondroosteodystrophy
   c. Dyschondroplasia
   d. Metaphyseal aclasis
   e. Multiple enchondromas
   f. Polyostotic fibrous dysplasia
2. Errors in the collagen and matrix formation
   a. Osteogenesis imperfecta
   b. Osteopetrosis

The epiphyseal cartilage proliferates normally in columnar fashion and in due course undergoes maturation, degeneration, and calcification. If the chondroblast is defective, multiple pathologic lesions may occur as a result of failure or irregularity in the maturation and calcification of the cartilage cells. If the failure of maturation and calcification is diffuse, the lack of the zone of preliminary calcification will result in delay of epiphyseal ossification and dwarfism.

A central chondroblast, if it continues to proliferate, will form an enchondroma which gives the bone a cystic appearance; if peripheral, this will result in an ecchondroma, or an exostosis may result instead of calcification to give a fibrous tissue mass. In general the following conditions are produced:

Achondroplasia—dwarfism
Metaphyseal aclasia—exostoses
Dyschondroplasia—cyst formation
Multiple chondromas—enchondromas
Chondroosteodystrophy—combination of all

Achondroplasia (Chondrodystrophia Fetalis)

The basic disturbance is in the calcification and remodeling of cartilage. Membranous bones, e.g., ribs and sternum, are formed, and all develop normally. The disease has been known since the earliest times, the Egyptian goddess Ptah having been pictured as achondroplastic. The severity can vary, and in very severe cases the fetus dies in utero. Achondroplasia is inherited as a dominant expression in the majority of those individuals who survive and reproduce.

The most evident histologic feature is the absence of cartilage proliferation and the columnar formation of cartilage. Ossification is irregular. Bone accretion at the periosteal surface is attached to the growth cartilage and may deposit a layer of compact bone over part of the metaphysis.

CLINICAL MANIFESTATIONS (Fig. 45-5). At birth, the typical infant with achondroplasia has a normal-sized body, very short, fat, flabby limbs, and a large head, with a characteristic depression at the root of the nose. Smallness in stature due to the absence of growth of the extremities becomes increasingly evident during childhood. A dwarf results. Walking occurs at the usual age, and dentition is normal.

When the patient stands erect, the tips of the fingers may only reach the great trochanter or the iliac crests, instead of normally reaching the lower part of the thigh. The achondroplastic hand is short and broad, with the fingers

Fig. 45-5. Achondroplastic girl showing the decreased limb growth with foreshortening of the stature but normal trunk height.

of equal length, e.g., *main en trident.* The short limbs, especially the lower, are often curved, in contrast to the trunk, which is virtually normal. The sacrum is tilted, and, as a consequence, contracture of the pelvic inlet follows.

The head is enlarged, rounded, and markedly brachycephalic. The face is broad, and at the root of the short nose is a characteristic depression or indentation. The upper alveolar processes protrude, and prominence of the lower jaw results in prognathism.

Persons with achondroplasia usually have normal intelligence.

The *"long"* bones of the limbs are very short and curved with a "broadened" shaft. The epiphyses may be disproportionately large and roughly shaped.

The portion of the *skull* developed in cartilage—the base—is grossly abnormal and reduced, especially the presphenoid and postsphenoid and the basiocciput. The vault is more globular in form, and the fontanels are correspondingly enlarged.

Although the vertebral column is of normal length, the centers of ossification of the bodies may be smaller than normal. Often there is a long regular kyphosis at the lumbodorsal region. The most striking feature is the early synostosis between the body and the arch, which in some cases is so severe as to lead to marked diminution in the caliber of the vertebral canal.

Differential Diagnosis. This disorder has to be differentiated from rickets. Radiographically the epiphyseal outline is present with normal ossification in the abnormal epiphysis. In rickets, on the other hand, the epiphyseal outline is blurred and ossification delayed.

Achondroplasia may be confused with cretinism, but in the latter mental deficiency and retardation are evident. In cretinism the essential feature is delay in ossification. In some cases it is associated with stippling of the epiphyses and calcium deposits.

The achondroplastic person is a "dwarfed" individual

in whom the trunk length (crown to pubis) is normal, leg length (pubis to heel) is reduced, and the hand span (fingertip to fingertip) is reduced.

This form of dwarfism has to be differentiated from other forms of stunting in which there is a decrease in the trunk length while the leg length and hand span may or may not be normal, e.g., (1) osteogenesis imperfecta, (2) osteomalacia and rickets, (3) osteoporosis, (4) developmental diseases such as chondroosteodystrophy, metaphyseal aclasis, and (5) in adults, Paget's disease, spondylolisthesis, Charcot spine, neoplasia.

The prognosis varies with the degree of the affection, but an achondroplastic individual may live to a considerable age.

No known treatment is available.

Dyschondroplasia (Ollier's Disease)

In 1899, Ollier first described this condition of varying degrees of ossification of abnormal metaphyseal cartilage formation. The diagnosis can be made in early childhood.

Dyschondroplasia is more commonly diffusely unilateral or bilateral, but occasionally it may be confined to a single bone.

PATHOLOGY. The typical changes are in the ends of the diaphysis of long bones—humerus, femur, radius, etc.—or in the long bones of the hands and feet, where growth is most rapid. The metaphysis is usually broadened and cystic with trabeculae running in parallel lines in the long axis of the bone. Occasionally small exostoses project from the surface, and foreshortening is evident. In the short long bones, multiple enchondromas may form. The ilium, ischium, and pubis may appear stippled and varying in bone density because of the presence of small rounded areas of cartilage.

The differential diagnosis includes metaphyseal aclasis, multiple enchondromas, osteopathia striata, and osteopoikilosis. Dyschondroplasia may be associated with cavernous hemangiomas and phleboliths of the soft tissue, a syndrome described by Maffucci.

The prognosis for normal life expectancy appears to be good, but deformity and secondary arthritis are constant sequelae. Surgical intervention is indicated only when there is mechanical interference with joint function and after epiphyseal growth has ceased.

Multiple Enchondromas

This is a disturbance of growth in which multiple cartilaginous tumors are present in the shafts of the short long bones of the hands and feet. The lesion may be a variant of dyschondroplasia.

The bone may be grossly expanded, and the expansion may be regular, with faint bony striations along the periphery of the expanded area. As the chondromatous tissue grows, more and more of the bone is destroyed, until little of the affected bone may remain save a few scattered bony fragments embedded in irregular striped masses of exuberant chondromatous tissue. Pathologic fractures may occur and require bone grafting.

Metaphyseal Aclasis (Multiple Exostoses, Diaphyseal Aclasis, Hereditary Deforming Dyschondroplasia)

The disease affects only those bones arising from cartilage and from membrane. It is inherited in an autosomal dominant form.

The basic defect is in a failure of remodeling of the metaphysis with the formation of multiple outgrowths or exostoses from the surface of the shaft of long bones, leading to some stunting of skeletal growth (Fig. 45-6).

PATHOLOGY. The membranous bones of the skeleton, the tarsal and carpal bones, are not involved. The condition affects those parts of the long bones in which tubular remodeling is active, i.e., the distal end of the femur, the proximal ends of the tibia and fibula, the distal ends of the radius and ulna, and the proximal end of the humerus. It is also seen at the medial and lateral ends of the clavicle, the vertebral border of the scapula, and occasionally at the neurocentral synchondroses of the vertebrae.

The diaphysis is usually of normal cylindrical form and of normal caliber. The metaphysis is increased in diameter, with roughly parallel sides. Irregular projections— exostoses—appear on the surface.

Exostoses comprise the most singular feature. Normally most marked at the ends of the bone, they may be found at virtually any part of the shaft. Frequently an exostosis marks the junction of normal shaft and the expanded extremity. As the shaft increases in length, the exostoses which were initially near the epiphyseal cartilage are displaced farther up the shaft. In addition they may become obliquely disposed to the shaft, directed away from the extremity of the bone, and they are irregular in shape. The exostoses are composed of poorly trabeculated bone in direct continuity with the bone of the shaft. During the years of growth the exostosis is surmounted by a cap of cartilage, from which progressive growth in size of the exostosis may take place.

There is usually well-marked interference with growth in length of the affected bones with irregularity of the ossification at the epiphyseal plate. It is essentially a failure of maturation of the cartilage cells. In the leg, growth of the fibula lags behind that of the tibia. Adjacent exostoses may produce absorption of the adjacent surface of the neighboring bones.

Two occasional complications of metaphyseal aclasis occur:

1. Formation of a *chondroma* which projects from the surface of the bone near the epiphyseal cartilage and can become chondrosarcomatous
2. *Osteogenic sarcoma* or *chondrosarcoma,* which may arise in one of the exostoses

CLINICAL MANIFESTATIONS. In the diffuse type there may be extensive distortion. The stature is short or even dwarfed. In addition the limbs may show deformities of the nature of bowing or genu valgum. Fracture from slight trauma is common, but the fragments unite as readily as in normal individuals.

The most typical feature is the presence of numerous exostoses. These are most common at sites of active growth, such as the knee and shoulder. The projections are hard, the skin overlying them is normal, and the soft tissues move easily on them. They may be associated with pain if the tumor presses on a peripheral nerve or a nerve root or if the process is inadvertently fractured. They are also liable to interfere with the free play of associated tendons or may even act as a mechanical obstruction to joint movement, in which event they may give rise to considerable disability. A bursa may form over the projection and from time to time become inflamed.

Radiologic examination shows an irregularly expanded metaphyseal mass, with little or no compact cortical bone. The architecture of the interior is altered. The normal cancellous tissue is replaced by a mass of less dense tissue, in which islands of normal ossification may be observed. The exostoses appear as definite projections from the metaphyseal region. Their structure is similar to that of the metaphysis—a clear interior, with a thin shell of cortical bone.

PROGNOSIS AND TREATMENT. The disease has no effect on the general health, but there may be disability as a result of nerve pressure or interference with joint movement. The only treatment indicated is the removal of exostoses which are giving rise to symptoms or which have become malignant.

Polyostotic Fibrous Dysplasia (Osteodystrophy Fibrosa, Unilateral Recklinghausen's Disease, Albright's Syndrome)

The disease usually appears in childhood or puberty as cyst formation in the diaphysis or metaphysis, but rarely in the epiphysis, of long bones. The bones most frequently involved are the femur, tibia, humerus, and radius. Bending deformities of the weight-bearing bones and pathologic fractures with slow union or nonunion are frequent occurrences. On biopsy, there is usually a distinctive appearance of bony trabeculae formation in a stroma of fibrous tissue. Giant cells are not a usual feature except when the lesion has been traumatized. Blood calcium and phosphates are usually normal, and occasionally the alkaline phosphatase is raised, probably denoting compensatory osteogenesis.

The x-ray shows expansion of the bone and thinning of the cortex with numerous trabeculated cystic areas which contain giant cell collections, fibrous tissue, and collections of cartilaginous tissue. It is usually a unilateral disease affecting multiple long bones. When it affects only one bone, it is known as *monostotic fibrous dysplasia.*

This differential diagnosis includes hyperparathyroidism, which rarely occurs in the adolescent. The blood calcium and phosphate changes of hyperparathyroidism are absent, and on x-ray the unaffected parts of the bones have a normal appearance and do not present the diffuse osteomalacic appearance of hyperparathyroidism.

The treatment is of the deformities, and prognosis is good, as this is a self-limiting disease. However, certain lesions may require curettage and autogenous grafting.

Albright's syndrome is a variation of polyostotic fibrous dysplasia occurring in a female and accompanied by sexual precocity and flat pigmented areas of skin. This is thought by some to be due to excessive hormonal secretion.

Fig. 45-6. AP radiograph of the knee joint showing bony spurring in the metaphyseal-diaphyseal area with minimal cap formation.

MONOSTOTIC FIBROUS DYSPLASIA

In this condition a single bone is the site of partial replacement of its substance by fibrous tissue, with or without the additional presence of osteoid. If present, osteoid is occasionally calcified, and cysts are occasionally formed. Any bone may be involved. The blood chemistry is within normal limits. The clinical findings are local swelling where the bone is superficial and pain if the lesion is near a joint. It has been suggested that the condition may represent a disturbance of the normal bone reparative process following trauma.

Osteogenesis Imperfecta

Osteogenesis imperfecta (fragilitas ossium, or Vrölich's disease), in which extreme fragility of bones is present, originates in fetal life. Dwarfism with micromelia occurs, and the patient's general condition is poor.

The classification of *brittle* bones includes:

A. Hereditary type—hereditary hypoplasia of the mesenchyme. Although this type is described as being congenital, it probably is inherited as a gene mutant, but this has been difficult to determine because of its lethal nature.

B. Nonhereditary congenital type—osteogenesis imperfecta (fragilitas ossium, osteopsathyrosis congenita of Vrölich): fetal, infantile, and adolescent (osteogenesis imperfecta tarda).
   1. Osteogenesis imperfecta with white sclera
   2. Osteogenesis imperfecta with blue sclera
C. Acquired type.
   1. Idiopathic
      a. Osteosclerosis fragilis generalisata (marble bone, or Albers-Schönberg disease)
   2. Osteoporosis
      a. Disuse
      b. Trophic
      c. Local disease
      d. Pressure
   3. Endocrine—hyperparathyroidism
   4. Vitamin deficiency
      a. Rickets
      b. Osteomalacia
      c. Scurvy

In the autosomal, dominant inherited form the stature is stunted, the joints are hypermobile, the sclera is blue, and deafness frequently appears after adolescence. Among adults with blue sclera 60 percent have associated fragile bones, and 60 percent have associated deafness.

PATHOLOGY. Knaggs has shown that in osteogenesis imperfecta the epiphyseal cartilage is normal, and the zone of calcified cartilage appears normal. However, in the zone of ossification the trabeculae are slender and delicate and widely separated by interstices filled with cellular connective tissue or fibrous marrow. No cross trabeculae are present as a general rule. The periosteum is thick, and

Fig. 45-7. Photomicrograph of tissue from osteogenesis imperfecta, in which there are numerous mesenchymal cells with poorly organized endochondral ossification, so that trabeculae are widely separated. (×150.)

there is no compact cortical layer of bone, but there are delicate and discrete subperiosteal trabeculae.

The bones are usually shorter and thinner than corresponding bones of normal individuals at a comparable age, so that the general skeletal development tends to be stunted.

In most cases there are many healed fractures, frequently in bad position. The consequent deformity, producing as it does shortening of the affected bones, adds to the dwarfing already present from the feeble osteogenesis.

The basic defect of osteogenesis imperfecta is a diffuse defect of the primitive mesenchymal cells, which fail to produce normal collagen. Studies have shown a deficiency or immaturity in the cross linkages. These abnormal cells enlarge to resemble cartilage cells in appearance. The endochondral arrangement and the Haversian systems are irregular (Fig. 45-7). A similar pathologic differentiation of the primitive mesenchymal cells occurs in the subperiosteal region, where there is no normal compact bone.

The bones are extremely fragile, because of the absence of a well-formed cortex, the sparse and widely separated trabeculae, and the nature of the osseous substance, which is less compact than the ordinary laminated bone. The bone is liable to undergo osteoclastic absorption and also, in late cases, appears to undergo spontaneous disintegration.

The raised serum alkaline phosphatase level, which is a frequent finding, is probably due to compensatory activity of bone repair.

CLINICAL MANIFESTATIONS. In the *fetal form,* the disease is severe, and the child is stillborn or survives only a very short time as a result of brain injury. There are multiple fractures, some healed at birth, while the cranium shows grossly imperfect ossification and consists merely of a membranous bag with a few plaques of poor bone embedded in it.

In the *infantile form,* the disease is less severe. At birth there may be some stunting and evidence of fractures, but the ossification of the skull is more advanced. The child survives for a year or two, but the bones are fragile and break at a touch. The skull may assume a globular shape and may appear large in proportion to the rest of the body. True hydrocephalus may develop and again may be related to intracranial damage at birth.

In the *adolescent type,* often called *osteogenesis imperfecta tarda,* the child may appear normal at birth and during childhood. The only disturbance observed may be a special liability to fractures from comparatively minor injuries. The ossification of the skull may be normal, but one or two soft areas may be found on examination. As time passes, the tendency to fracture decreases.

The disease may on rare occasions be encountered first in adult life, when a case which was slight at birth and during adolescence becomes active or when a case which has regressed spontaneously is reactivated.

Prominent features are:

1. Stunting of growth.
2. Fractures from trivial trauma. The fractures are often subperiosteal and unite readily, often more so than in normal bone,

and the callus is often more dense than in normal bone. The fractures are distinctive in that they cause little or no pain or tenderness—largely because they are subperiosteal. It is largely for this reason that so many are allowed to heal with deformity.
3. Blue sclera. This has been observed in the infantile and late types of fragility and is a result of increased visibility of the pigmented choroid through an abnormally translucent sclera due to alteration in the mucopolysaccharide content.
4. Characteristic skull, showing broadening of the forehead, angular projections above the zygoma, a downward tilting of the axis of the orbit, the ear, and the auditory canals, and an underhung jaw.

Radiologic Findings. In severe types the bones may show almost complete absence of cancellous texture, the cortex appearing as a faintly penciled line. The bones are shorter than normal and occasionally broader. In less severe types the long bones are stunted, are diffusely rarefied, and may have expanded club-shaped extremities. Fractures or old deformities following fractures are often apparent. In adult cases the shafts of the bones appear to shrink and have a dense, relatively thick cortex with no medulla. The ends of the bones are expanded and contain coarse cancellation with poor density. Ultimately the long bones may appear as two poorly calcified end bulbs joined by a slender rod of denser bone.

The ribs are usually bent sharply downward at their angles, and the thorax is therefore greatly deformed. This may be accentuated by scoliosis. The pelvis is asymmetric with irregular deformity. The skull has irregular ossification, with islands of denser bone in a poorly calcified matrix—the so-called Wormian bones.

Differential Diagnosis. The diagnosis is usually evident, but occasionally rickets may have to be excluded, especially since fractures are common. In rickets, however, the radiologic picture is characteristic: the epiphyseal cartilage is broad and fuzzy, the edge of the metaphysis to the zone of calcified cartilage is irregular and poorly defined, and the metaphysis itself is cup-shaped and expanded. On the other hand, the rarefaction of the rest of the bone is considerably less than in osteogenesis imperfecta.

PROGNOSIS AND TREATMENT. In the majority of cases early death is the outcome. Occasionally adult life is reached, but the constant occurrence of fractures and the repeated confinement to bed produce real disability.

No specific treatment is known. Dietetic and other measures to promote the general well-being are indicated. Care should be exercised in handling children, but when fractures occur, they are treated along the usual lines. When healing takes place with deformity, osteotomy may be carried out. Sofield and Millar have described how the limb bones when badly bowed and deformed can be realigned and reinforced by multiple osteotomies and intramedullary rod fixation.

Osteopetrosis (Albers-Schönberg Disease, Marble Bones, Osteosclerosis Fragilis Generalisata, Congenital Osteosclerosis)

Albers-Schönberg, in 1904, described this rare bone disease associated with increased density of the skeleton. Fewer than 40 cases have been described. The condition

Table 45-3. CLASSIFICATION OF OSTEOSCLEROSIS (INCREASE IN BONE DENSITY)

Generalized	Localized
Hypoparathyroidism	Infection—syphilis
Fluorosis	Chronic osteomyelitis
Osteopetrosis	Degenerative—arthritis
Osteopoikilosis	Mechanical—stress
Engelmann's disease	Ischemia
	Neoplasia—osteoblastic
	Metastasis—malignant tumor

has occasionally affected several members of a family as an autosomal recessive inheritance. A classification of osteosclerosis appears in Table 45-3.

PATHOLOGY. The characteristic change is the increased density and thickness with loss of trabeculation of the affected bone, in symmetric fashion, most commonly in the metaphysis. The increased thickness of the bone indicates that the condition affects not only the bone developed from the epiphyseal cartilage but that growing by accretion from the periosteum.

The most marked changes are found in the most rapidly growing extremities of the long bones—the lower end of the femur and radius, and the upper end of the tibia and humerus.

The ribs are similarly affected—thick, dense, and apparently structureless (Fig. 45-8). The vertebrae may be uniformly dense, or a dense zone at the upper and lower thirds of the body may be separated by a zone of normal density in the middle, indicating that the process is affecting the bone laid down from the cartilage end plates of the body. The skull may be so dense that no detail of its architecture can be made out. The bones of the carpus and tarsus are ringed by layers of dense bone, the result of peripheral accretions.

It is well known that so-called marble bones are liable to fractures, especially in the adolescent. It is said to be

Fig. 45-8. X-ray of a chest showing the thick, dense, structureless bones of the thorax characteristic of osteopetrosis, or marble bones.

Fig. 45-9. Photomicrograph of tissue from osteopetrosis showing disorganized cartilage mass, abnormal bone, and fibrous tissue. (×200.)

possible to cut a so-called marble bone with a knife, the sensation experienced being similar to that on cutting chalk.

Microscopically the affected areas are seen to consist of a mixture of calcified cartilage masses, sclerotic bone, necrotic bone, and fibrous tissue (Fig. 45-9). It is noticeable that the tissues are avascular, the marrow spaces being filled with sclerotic tissue with very few capillaries. There, in the absence of true ossification or any lamellar system by osteoblastic activity, much of the sclerosis is due to excessive calcification of osteoid tissues.

The progressive sclerosis of the long bones gradually reduces the medullary cavity and the bone marrow to a degree incompatible with normal hematopoiesis, producing a true aplastic anemia, sometimes with enlargement of the liver and spleen.

In the skull the thickening is apt to restrict the size of the foramina, leading to pressure on, and paralysis of, the cranial nerves, to give blindness, nystagmus and ocular palsies, hydrocephalus, and occasionally signs of hypopituitarism.

MELORHEOSTOSIS

The condition was first reported by Léri in 1922. Its distinguishing features are (1) that the sclerotic changes are confined to one limb, (2) that the outline of an affected bone is definitely distorted, (3) the presence of pain, often severe, and (4) limitation of movement in the joints formed by the affected bone. The affection is usually limited to one limb and occasionally to one bone of a limb.

A portion of the cortex of one of the limb bones is irregularly enlarged, sufficiently to give rise to a swelling with an undulating surface. Between one undulation and another, a linear band of increased density may extend which has been likened to a "flow" of hyperostosis resembling "candle drippings."

OSTEOPATHIA STRIATA

In this condition, zones or striae of dense bone are found in the long axis of a long bone or in the ilium. The condition gives rise to a characteristic x-ray appearance. This is, perhaps, its main significance, for there is no clinical evidence, nor are there secondary pathologic changes.

Osteopoikilosis (Osteopathia Condensans Disseminata, or Spotted Bones)

This condition was described by Albers-Schönberg in 1915 and is characterized by the presence of dense spots in large numbers in the long and short bones but not in the skull, vertebrae, and ribs. The spots are usually uniformly dense but may have clear centers and are grouped toward the end of the bone in the epiphysis. They give rise to no symptoms and are usually discovered by chance. Schmorl found that they consisted of numerous closely packed trabeculae in the lamellae lying mostly in a longitudinal direction.

METABOLIC DISEASES

See "Metabolic disorders," in the Classification of Generalized Bone Disorders.

Metabolism of Calcium and Phosphorus

CALCIUM METABOLISM. Calcium is required in the processes of (1) blood coagulation, (2) transmission of neuromuscular impulses, (3) muscular excitability, (4) maintaining osmotic reactions in cellular permeabilities, (5) maintaining acid-base equilibrium, and (6) providing the mechanical strength of the skeleton.

Mitchell and his coworkers showed that a normal 70-kg adult male had over 1,000 Gm of calcium in his skeleton, over 10 Gm in the soft tissues, and less than 1 Gm in the blood and extracellular fluids. Calcium is readily absorbed from the intestine, particularly in the presence of vitamin D or a high-protein diet, or in any state of calcium demand, such as growth, pregnancy, or lactation (Fig. 45-10). For children, an adequate daily intake is approximately 1 Gm; adults require less, except during states of increased demand. Calcium is excreted in the urine, approximately 100 to 150 mg/day, and in feces, approximately 500 to 700 mg, during a balanced exchange reaction with normal bone accretion (i.e., positive balance) and bone resorption (i.e., negative balance). Neuman and Neuman have shown that over 99 percent of calcium going through the glomeruli is resorbed by the tubules. Serum calcium level is rigidly maintained at approximately 10 mg/100 ml, of which 70 percent is diffusible, the remainder being bound to protein.

Calcium metabolism is influenced by:

1. Thyroid extract. Thyrotoxicosis is characterized by increased urinary and fecal losses of calcium with the development of osteoporosis or a localized osteofibrosis. In myxedema there may be retention of calcium.
2. Growth hormone. Increase in total body mass is seen, and in

the active acromegalic individual serum inorganic phosphorus levels may be increased.

3. Adrenosteroids. In Addison's disease there may be an increased fecal and urinary loss of calcium with osteoporosis in the bone. This may be secondary to breakdown of the protein matrix.

Parathormone. Although Albright and Reifenstein suggested that the primary effect of this hormone was to increase the renal excretion of the phosphate with a resultant decrease in the serum phosphate level, this explanation can no longer be accepted.

The parathormone influences the levels of both serum calcium and serum phosphorus as well as the rate of bone absorption. In addition, it has some control over the urinary excretion of phosphate and through this controls the excretion of urinary calcium.

It should be emphasized that increased serum calcium levels can be obtained in animals after nephrectomy by giving parathyroid extracts. Parathyroid extracts may produce increased glomerular filtration, but decreased renal tubular resorption or increased renal tubular secretion is thought to be the primary mechanism.

Barnicot has demonstrated the direct local resorption of bone by crystals of parathyroid extract and grafts of parathyroid tissue placed in a rat's calvaria.

During hyperparathyroidism there is marked osteoclastic activity in bone, so that hypercalcemia and hypophosphatemia result, in spite of marked hypercalcinuria. Tetany or hypocalcinemia will present as neuromuscular hyperirritability, convulsions, etc.

Talmage has emphasized the important role of the parathyroid gland in maintaining a constant level of ionic calcium in all tissue fluids of the body. A state of equilibrium between the calcium and phosphate concentrations is maintained between the liquid phase and the solid phase of bone, by removing ions from the fluid state and depositing them in bone. Talmage considers that the parathormone is acting in opposition to this equilibration gradient by removing calcium and phosphate from bone to return them to the fluid state and to maintain concentrations which are normal for the host.

McLean and Urist have proposed a feedback mechanism for the homeostatic regulation of serum calcium, in which the parathormone is particularly concerned with the regulation of calcium concentration in blood. Their mechanism consists of two parts: first, there is a compartment containing calcium in perfect chemical equilibrium with both the serum and labile fraction of bone minerals, i.e., approximately 70 percent of the total serum calcium content. Second, there is the feedback mechanism in which any fall in the serum calcium level results in an increased output of the parathormone. This in turn produces resorption in bone from the labile storage pool in the hydration shell of the surface of the crystal, the mobilization of additional calcium causing a rise in the calcium serum level back to the normal level of 10 mg/100 ml.

Parathyroidectomy produces a lowering of the calcium ion in the blood to about 7 mg/100 ml with the clinical evidence of tetany. Increase in parathormone causes increased bone calcium resorption with increased fibrous tissue formation and the condition of osteitis fibrosa.

Fig. 45-10. Intake, homeostasis mechanism, and excretion of calcium. (*Taken with permission from Mercer and Duthie, "Orthopaedic Surgery," London, 1974.*)

Vitamin D deficiency is seen as hypocalcinemia and hypophosphatemia, with the development of rickets or osteomalacia, as well as retardation of growth. The action of vitamin D in rickets may be through suppressing the activity of the parathyroid gland.

Calcitonin. Calcitonin is a polypeptide secreted by the C cells of the human thyroid and other mammals and from the ultimobranchial glands of other vertebrates. It inhibits cell-mediated release of calcium from bone and directly inhibits resorption. It is thus important in controlling induced hypercalcemia, e.g., in Paget's disease and in bony metastases. This effect is of value in diagnosing osteolytic bone disease and controlling associated hypercalcemia of hyperparathyroidism, bone tumors, immobilization osteoporosis, and Paget's disease. Relief of bone pain in Paget's disease is an important therapeutic use of calcitonin.

PHOSPHORUS METABOLISM. Ninety percent of the body phosphorus is found in the skeleton, ten percent being found in the intracellular tissues and blood. An intake of less than 1 Gm/day is required by an adult, although more is required by growing children and pregnant women. Absorption is favored by the presence of calcium, and almost 60 percent of the intake is excreted in the urine. There does not appear to be any homeostatic control of the plasma levels, which in young children is 5 to 6 mg/100 ml and in adults is only 3 to 4 mg/100 ml. Almost all of the phosphorus is inorganic, in the form of orthophosphate with some pyrophosphate radicals, but some is found as phospholipid. Vitamin D may play a part in renal tubular reabsorption of phosphorus.

Serum inorganic phosphorus appears to be under the control of the parathyroids (which affect the resorption of phosphorus in limits, the pituitary and the thyroid. It is influenced by the level of circulating calcium and the excretion mechanism of the kidneys. The level is remarkably labile in a large number of pathologic and disease conditions.

Its serum level can be decreased by hyperparathyroidism, vitamin D deficiency, diabetes, and vitamin D–resistant rickets. They all tend to produce hyperphosphaturia and hypophosphatemia.

Vitamin D. Vitamin D is essential for the absorption of calcium and secondarily for the absorption of phosphorus from the intestine. Knowledge of the mechanism of action of vitamin D has expanded dramatically in the past few years as new metabolites of the vitamin have been identified. Vitamin D stimulates absorption of dietary calcium from the intestine and induces mobilization of bone mineral. Both effects supersaturate the plasma with calcium and phosphate, which allow normal mineralization.

Vitamin D produced from ultraviolet irradiation of 7-dehydrocholesterol in the skin is converted to 25-hydroxycholecalciferol in the liver and is secreted into the plasma. Current evidence suggests that the 25-hydroxycholecalciferol is converted to a polar metabolite in the kidney and passes into the systemic circulation and is involved in calcium transport by the mucosal cells of the small intestine. At physiologic levels, vitamin D is involved with mobilization of bone mineral and perhaps the uptake of calcium by the bone matrix. Current investigation suggests that various metabolites including 25-hydroxycholecalciferol; 21, 25-dihydrocholecalciferol; and other polar metabolites are present in bony extracts, although the active metabolite for mineral mobilization has not been delineated.

Calcification

This process consists of two phases, or systems: first, cellular differentiation to form a suitable medium of matrix osteoid, collagen fibrils, etc., and, second, the process of mineralization.

COLLAGEN AND MATRIX FORMATION. Osteoblasts secrete the organic matrix, or *osteoid,* which is made up of collagen fibers and an interfibrillar cement substance.

Jackson has demonstrated granules which pair within the osteoblast during the secretion of collagen and are thought to be an aminopolysaccharide and alkaline phosphatase, which is essential for developing calcifiable matrix. Sulfation first appears at the cell membrane along with prefibrillar collagen formation, and then the matrix contains the sulfated mucopolysaccharide chondroitin sulfate. This sulfation is defective in vitamin C scurvy, as noted by Reddi and Nörstrom. Any failure of alkaline phosphatase, of sulfation, or of vitamin C may alter the formation of osteoid and hence its calcification.

MINERALIZATION. Calcification involves the precipitation of mineral salts, i.e., calcium phosphate. The deposition of bone mineral requires two distinct steps: first, the grouping of a minimal number of ions capable of survival and growth (nucleation) and, second, the continued growth of these ions. Various theories are presented to explain this complicated process.

Bone cells, by increasing the local concentrations of calcium and phosphate ions, would precipitate the mineral. Robinson first proposed such a theory, suggesting that the local concentration of phosphate ions was elevated by the action of alkaline phosphatase on the phosphate esters. It is thought that these phosphate esters might arise from the phosphorolysis of glycogen. These theories are inadequate because bone is never the sole site of this reaction, and alkaline phosphatase is also abundant in tissues that do not calcify.

The components of matrix may contain specific mechanisms which create nucleating sites or remove barriers to these local calcification areas. It was shown by electron microscope that collagen fibrils are principally responsible for nucleation of bone mineral. The phosphorylation of collagen may be the important chemical reaction that enables nucleation to be initiated by the collagen. Histochemical and chemical analyses on the changes in the organic matrix on calcification indicate that the proteoglycan and phospholipid components may also be involved in mineralization.

Fleisch and his associates have suggested that the inorganic anion pyrophosphate present in bone and other tissues is an important controlling element in calcification. Pyrophosphate is the anhydride formed by condensation and removal of water from two molecules of orthophosphate. These investigations have suggested that calcification or mineral resorption is initiated by specific enzymes known as pyrophosphatases which remove inhibiting pyrophosphate by splitting it into two molecules of orthophosphate. Pyrophosphate in the concentrations found in bone and the body fluids will inhibit both the formation of hydroxyapatite and crystal growth from solutions containing calcium and phosphate ions at concentrations which otherwise spontaneously form hydroxyapatite. It will also prevent the transformation of amorphous calcium phosphate to crystalline hydroxyapatites.

The pyrophosphate theory could account for the absence of calcification, under normal circumstances, in tissues other than bone and cartilage. All these tissues contain concentrations of pyrophosphate sufficient to prevent spontaneous calcification. It is only bone and cartilage that contain the enzymes which remove these inhibiting concentrations of pyrophosphate.

It is suggested that, initially, there is a precipitate of calcium phosphate less basic than hydroxyapatite which is only subsequently converted to hydroxyapatite. There is evidence that this amorphous phase of calcium phosphate may be formed as packets within cells and be excreted into the matrix to form a nucleation center.

It is increasingly appreciated that proper calcification requires the coordinate activity in time and space of several distinct systems. Humoral factors are essential for the continuing supply of calcium and phosphate to the calcification sites. The activities of bone cells are involved both in the elaboration of the organic matrix and in its further transformations to a system that both permits and enhances calcification.

Scurvy

The antiscorbutic vitamin C is found in the majority of fresh foodstuffs—fruit juices, green vegetables, and to a lesser extent in potatoes, milk, and raw meat. Since it is destroyed by heating at 100°C, it is absent in dried, canned, and preserved foods, and in vegetables subjected to prolonged boiling. The absence of vitamin C from the diet gives rise to the clinical condition of scurvy.

The disease occurs most commonly in infants from six to eight months of age who have been fed exclusively on artificial food which has had its vitamin content destroyed. It also occurs in adults who are deprived of fresh food.

A diet deficient in vitamin C need not of necessity be deficient in the other vitamins. However, with a deficiency in vitamin D, a rachitic element may be added to the scorbutic in the case of the growing child, while in the adult there may be some evidence of osteomalacia.

PATHOLOGY. The cardinal feature of scurvy is a defect in the formation of intercellular substances which results in hemorrhage—from the gums, from the alimentary tract, from the subcutaneous tissues, and in bone. The hemorrhage is capillary in origin and occurs at sites at which new capillaries are sprouting, e.g., in bone, at the most actively growing metaphyses and beneath the periosteum (Fig. 45-11). Vitamin C controls the nutrition of capillary endothelium, or the amount of intercellular cement which binds the endothelial cells together.

From the capillary loops there occurs an irregular and patchy oozing of blood, so that small pools of blood collect and disrupt the newly forming bone, the calcified cartilaginous strata, and even the proliferating cartilaginous palisades. The blood clots and is replaced by fibrous tissue or by bone.

In very extreme cases, the hemorrhage may be sufficient to disrupt the growing area, with separation of the epiphyses. The subperiosteal hemorrhages are often extensive, the periosteum being stripped from the shaft for a considerable distance, with abnormal ossification.

CLINICAL MANIFESTATIONS. The child may or may not appear ill-nourished. The earliest features are restlessness and fretfulness, with one or more of the extremities not used. Handling of the parts produces extreme pain.

On examination there may be obvious swelling, fluid in character, in relation to the shaft of one or more of the long bones. The joints may appear swollen and are exquisitely sensitive to touch, appearing like an infective condition. On the other hand, the immobility of the parts may simulate paralysis, and this feature is often known as the *pseudoparalysis of scurvy.* Hemorrhages may also occur into and beneath the skin, and the gums may be swollen and spongy.

DIAGNOSIS. The conditions most liable to cause confusion in the early stages are anterior poliomyelitis, injury to joint, bone, and nerve, osteomyelitis, arthritis, and syphilitic osteochondritis—the latter being more common in the short long bones of hand and foot, the proximal end of the femur, and the distal end of the tibia.

The response to treatment in scurvy is dramatic, in sharp distinction to the other conditions enumerated.

The typical x-ray appearances are seen in Fig. 45-12.

TREATMENT. The administration of vitamin C in any of its forms leads to rapid cure. Within 24 hours pain and crying cease, and in a few days hemorrhages are beginning to heal. It is some months, however, before the bone remodeling occurs.

Rest in bed is indicated in the early stages, and, later,

Fig. 45-11. Photomicrograph of tissue from the vicinity of an epiphysis in a seven-month-old child suffering from scurvy. It shows the irregular cartilage columns, abnormal new bone formation, and increased cellularity. (×200.)

exercises may be usefully employed to augment muscle tone. Unprotected weight bearing should be relieved by caliper until there is radiographic evidence of a return of bony structure, to prevent deformities.

Rickets

Rickets was formerly a disease of the lower classes and was common in industrial districts where poor housing, malnutrition, smoky atmosphere, and lack of sunlight were common. These factors favored a lack of vitamins, and it was generally assumed that rickets was a deficiency disease due to lack of vitamin D. However, Dent and Harris, in a classic description of inherited rickets and osteomalacia, have emphasized that rickets and osteomalacia in modern civilizations are usually due to primary metabolic abnormalities which are genetically determined. Most of the cases now appearing, although clinically similar to environmental or nutritional rickets, are vitamin D–resistant rickets, with or without an abnormality of renal tubular function but requiring massive dosages of vitamin D for cure. The primary defect of vitamin D deficiency intake or effect leads to a state of hypophosphatemia because of the decreased renal tubular resorption of phosphate.

The commonest type of the disease begins during the early years of infancy and is extremely rare after the age of four. It is known as *infantile rickets.* Comparable disturbances may arise at other age periods and are known as *late rickets and osteomalacia.*

Fig. 45-12. X-ray of the lower limbs of a baby with scurvy showing the epiphyseal disturbance and calcifying periosteal hematoma formation.

PATHOLOGY. The normal epiphyseal line is a well-defined narrow strip of cartilage 2 mm deep, but in rickets it forms a wide irregular band, and the metaphysis is broad and irregular from excessive proliferation of the cells of the epiphyseal line. Mineralization is patchy in distribution and uniformly deficient.

The cartilage in the proliferating zone is hyperplastic, but instead of the normal palisade arrangement of the cells, the proliferated cells are arranged irregularly. Associated with this is a poor development of the bone marrow.

In the metaphysis the bony trabeculae are thinned with connective tissue hyperplasia, so that the extremity of the bone appears misshapen and unmodeled—particularly in the costochondral junctions, the lower end of the radius, etc. These changes are most marked in the most actively growing part of the bones. Bone formed before that is normal, while bone formed after the active phase of the disease is also normal.

When the child is able to crawl or to walk, the femur becomes bowed anteriorly and to the lateral side. The neck-shaft angle of the femur may be diminished (coxa vara), the tibia may be bowed, or the knee may assume a valgus attitude (Fig. 45-13). The whole pelvis may be flattened, or it may assume a trefoil shape as in osteomalacia causing obstetric difficulties. The skull is broad-ened, the forehead square, and bosses of new bone may form in the parietal and frontal regions. The vertebral column may assume exaggerated curvatures.

CLINICAL MANIFESTATIONS. Cardinal manifestations include (1) restlessness associated with fear on moving limbs, (2) recurrent diarrhea and constipation, (3) evidences of irritability of the central nervous system, such as convulsions, laryngismus, or other types of spasmophilia, (4) large head, open fontanels, and craniotabes, (5) prominent abdomen, (6) narrow chest and rachitic rosary of costochondral junctions, (7) enlarged and tender epiphyses, (8) bowing of the long bones, (9) delayed dentition, with irregular, soft, decaying teeth, and (10) poorly developed muscles, with delay in walking.

Radiologic Findings. In the *acute stage,* the epiphysis is widened and lacks radiodensity, with delay in appearance of centers of ossification. The metaphysis is splayed out (Fig. 45-14). The periosteum is thickened, with fractures of the long bones frequently seen.

In the *chronic stage,* bowing occurs with the cortical part of the affected bone thickened on the side of the concavity (Fig. 45-15).

DIAGNOSIS. The disease is to be differentiated from congenital syphilis and infantile scurvy. The congenitally syphilitic child usually has other signs of syphilis, but occasionally the chief lesion may be a syphilitic osteochondritis. The epiphyseal region is tender, hot, and swollen; there is loosening and separation of the epiphysis, which can usually be moved on the shaft, with the production of muffled crepitus.

In infantile scurvy, swelling also occurs; it is not limited to the region of the epiphysis but encroaches on the shaft. There are usually hemorrhages in other situations, and the general signs of scurvy are present.

TREATMENT. Nutritional, or vitamin D deficiency, rickets may be cured by administration of one of the vitamin D–containing foods or by one of the standard preparations of the vitamin (e.g., calciferol, 3,000 I.U./day). The effect of this is enhanced by the addition of a calcium preparation (calcium carbonate or calcium phosphate).

Prevention of Deformity. When the bones are so soft, the child's movements should be so controlled that little or no pressure is exerted upon the limbs. He should not be allowed to stand or walk but should have physiotherapy in bed. For difficult children it is often advisable to fit rickets splints.

Treatment of the Established Deformity. Deformity is usually corrected by splints or by osteotomy.

Correction by Splinting. This method is used where the deformity is slight and the disease still active. It is employed particularly for young children, especially those below the age of four, and is most useful for deformities of the lower limb. The method is slow and requires continual supervision to ensure a good result and to prevent the formation of sores.

Correction by Osteotomy. Osteotomy should never be carried out until the radiograph shows eburnation, clearness, and regularity of outline. If corrective operations are attempted before this period, nonunion is likely to occur.

CELIAC RICKETS

Bone changes appear only in late and long-established cases, i.e., after the age of seven years, and are similar to those of rickets. The metaphysis is broad and irregular, the palisade arrangement of cartilage cells is lost, and instead there is an irregular hypertrophy of the cells. The zone of calcified cartilage is narrow, with poor calcification and ossification.

CLINICAL MANIFESTATIONS. In association with the characteristic appearances of celiac disease—pallor, cachexia, muscular hypotonicity, and abdominal swelling—there is lack of body development—stunting. In addition there may be skeletal deformity. Genu valgum is a common feature. Enlargement of the distal ends of the radius and ulna are also frequent signs, but occasionally still more extensive deformation may be present—enlarged costochondral junctions, Harrison's sulcus, kyphosis, coxa vara, bowleg, etc. Fractures may occur with mild trauma.

In celiac rickets there is invariably a lowered serum calcium content. Impaired fat digestion results in insoluble calcium soaps with decreased fat absorption.

The x-ray appearances are very variable, but the whole bone is usually fragile and porotic. The epiphyseal cartilage is broad and irregular with transverse striations of denser bone.

With celiac disease there is inadequate utilization of the fat of the diet and reduction in the source of vitamin D. The excess of free fatty acid leads to precipitation of the calcium in the diet as insoluble soaps, leading to a deficient absorption of these minerals from the alimentary tract. The absorption of calcium, though greatly diminished, appears to be sufficient to calcify the fragile bones of celiac disease so long as there is little or no growth, but when considerable growth appears, this defective absorption results in the development of rickets.

TREATMENT. Treatment is based upon high dosages of vitamin D and special diets.

RENAL OSTEODYSTROPHY

PATHOLOGY. The kidney lesions are mainly of two types:

1. Total renal insufficiency as found in chronic glomerulonephritis, focal nephritis, congenital cystic disease where there is a reduced glomerular function with failure to excrete phosphorus, as well as general uremia and acidosis. The main skeletal change accompanying this lesion is an osteitis fibrosis, with little osteoid formation, either as rickets or osteomalacia.

2. Tubular insufficiency. The resorption of phosphorus, amino acids, glucose, electrolytes, and water is impaired, particularly from the proximal convoluted tubules. If there is disease of the distal tubules, there is disturbance of potassium and creatinine secretion into the urine. As well as these defects of resorption or secretion, there is a marked disturbance in the general acid-base regulation of the body by alteration in the concentrations of bicarbonate, ammonium, and hydrogen ion, which are usually added to the urine to achieve the acid-base equilibrium.

CLINICAL MANIFESTATIONS. In a number of patients, symptoms are present from early days of life; in others, the child is normal for a few years before symptoms arise. *Features of the renal lesion* are polydipsia and polyuria,

Fig. 45-13. Rachitic child showing the valgus deformity of the knees.

Fig. 45-14. X-ray of the hand and wrist of a three-year-old rachitic child showing the delay in the appearance of the carpal ossification center and the widening of the epiphysis with loss of bone density. (*Courtesy of Dr. R. C. Aicheson.*)

Fig. 45-15. X-ray of both knee areas during the healing phase of rickets showing the increasing ossification of the epiphyses but obvious valgus deformity of the knees and a tibia vara deformity.

with thirst. The urine is of low specific gravity, with an output of 1,200 to 3,700 ml daily. Albumin and casts are usually present at some stage of the disease, and cardiovascular symptoms of renal origin may appear. Ultimately, signs of kidney failure—headache, drowsiness, and gastrointestinal disturbance—arise, and death occurs from uremia. From the time of onset of the disease, tests of urinary function show a marked lowering of renal efficiency. The blood urea level is constantly raised, to 73 to 300 mg/100 ml.

Features of disturbance in growth include stunting in growth, often to a degree not equaled by any other form of infantilism. The body weight is correspondingly small, though malnutrition is not present, and the mental development is normal. The secondary sex characteristics do not develop.

Bone Changes. Genu valgum is common with enlargement of the epiphyses at the wrist and ankles, a costochondral rosary, Harrison's sulcus, or bowleg. The average age of recognition of deformity is between five and seven years.

Patients have been described with associated hyperplasia of the parathyroid glands, and these cases were interpreted as a composite picture of osteitis fibrosa and true rickets. The parathyroid hyperplasia may have resulted from the inability of the kidneys to secrete phosphorus and the parathyroid hyperplasia in turn responsible for the bone lesions.

Fanconi's Syndrome. Fanconi in 1931 described a case of renal diabetes in which there was retardation of growth. The features of Fanconi's syndrome are resistant and intractable rickets, hypophosphatemia, renal glycosuria, acidosis, and in some cases calcinosis. It is an affection of early life usually beginning within the first two years. Early signs are retarded development, loss of appetite, gastrointestinal disturbances, bouts of fever, and albumin and casts in the urine. The plasma phosphatase level is raised, and the excretion of calcium and phosphorus is excessive. Rachitic bowing of the legs and fractures may occur. Fanconi suggested that the condition is tubular renal rickets as opposed to glomerular renal rickets and results from hereditary inadequacy of the tubular epithelium, due to an autosomal recessive gene.

The Lignac-Fanconi Syndrome. This consists of a proximal tubular deficiency, with polydipsia, polyuria, anorexia, and vomiting. The children exhibit rickets as well as dwarfism and usually die before puberty. There is hyperphosphaturia with a low serum phosphate level but a normal calcium level, glycosuria which is sometimes accompanied by a mild ketonuria, and marked aminoaciduria, as well. The primary lesion appears to be an impaired resorption of glucose and phosphate because of some failure of phosphorylation in the tubules. Massive dosages of vitamin D may improve the skeletal disorder. Abnormal deposition of cystine crystals in the cornea, spleen, and lymph nodes gives the syndrome the name *cystinosis*.

Renal, or Hyperchloremic, Acidosis. In this condition, the primary defect is in the distal tubules, which fail to resorb water and to secrete ammonium. As well as excreting large amounts of water containing sodium, potassium, and calcium, there is a marked disturbance in the acid-base mechanism of the body with severe loss of bicarbonate and a corresponding retention of chlorides. The skeletal changes of either osteitis fibrosa or rickets are caused by the excessive mobilization of calcium from bone in response to the acidosis. This condition can be improved by administering excessive alkalizing salts, such as ammonium or calcium chlorides, and vitamin D.

Vitamin D–resistant Rickets, or "Phosphate Diabetes." As described by Fanconi and Girardet, this is characterized by a failure of phosphate resorption with a marked hyperphosphaturia and hypophosphatemia. Accompanying this, there is also excessive fecal loss of calcium leading to the typical changes of rickets in children or osteomalacia in adults. There appears to be some relationship between the resorption of bone as seen in von Recklinghausen's neurofibromatosis and that seen in this entity. Unlike vitamin D deficiency rickets, this form requires massive doses of vitamin D (i.e., 50,000 to 100,000 units) daily, which are thought to potentiate the diminished alkaline phosphatase required for transport of the phosphate ions within the tubules. These children tend to survive into adulthood, when they can present features of osteomalacia with reduction in the intestinal absorption of calcium and phosphates and, therefore, the possibility of a disturbed vitamin D metabolism.

Radiologic Findings. The diaphysis is osteoporotic, with the epiphysis broad and irregular. The metaphysis is broadened and its extremity uneven and ragged, like those seen in rickets.

In other forms the metaphysis is grossly enlarged, irregularly honeycombed or stippled or woolly, with subperiosteal resorption.

Calcification occurs in the kidneys with irregularities of the renal pelvis and ureters noted on pyelography. Calcium deposits in the kidney, with or without calculus formation, are usually more common in hyperparathyroidism than in chronic nephritis.

HYPOPHOSPHATASIA

This is an inherited rachitic disease which was first described by Rathbun in 1948 as a markedly impaired mineralization of the long bones and skull. The blood shows increased calcium, phosphorus, and nonprotein nitrogen levels, but a reduced alkaline phosphatase level. McCance et al. and Fraser et al. have shown that there is a large urinary excretion of phosphoethanoline without the other amino acids commonly seen in renal rickets.

Radiologically and pathologically, the lesion suggests severe rickets.

The metabolic defect lies in the osteoblast, which fails to secrete alkaline phosphatase. Severe metabolic disturbances are less marked after the age of sixteen or seventeen, with less liability to tetany, because the demand for calcium in ossification is much reduced. There may be remissions associated with improvement in kidney function and better excretion of phosphate. However, the ultimate prognosis for life depends on the renal pathologic condition, because of the liability of these patients to intercurrent infections. The occurrence of bone deformities is itself grave, and the average duration of life after their appearance is said to be less than 2 years. Therefore operative interference is directed toward restoring kidney function.

Where there is a congenital lesion of the renal tract, such as a posterior urethral valve, early surgical removal of the obstruction may be lifesaving. Surgical intervention, if it is to be successful, must be undertaken before puberty.

In hyperchloremic renal acidosis and nephrocalcinosis, an organic acid such as citric acid should be given in conjunction with sodium citrate to aid absorption of calcium from the intestines. Vitamin D should also be given in those cases to help calcification of the skeleton. In the active stage of the osteodystrophy, weight bearing should be prevented, and splints may be applied to limit deformity until spontaneous remission of the disease occurs.

Osteomalacia

Osteomalacia is a metabolic disease of adult bone in which there is a deficient mineralization of the bony matrix due to the lowered concentration of calcium or phosphorus or both in the body fluids. The diagnosis should be suspected in any patient with radiographic changes of osteoporosis or reduced skeletal mass. Reduced serum calcium or phosphorus may result from reduced dietary intake, impaired absorption from the gastrointestinal tract, increased renal excretion, or lack of vitamin D. Accompanying such change there is a generalized increase in the amount of osteoid, i.e., uncalcified, tissue.

PATHOLOGY. All the bones of the skeleton show decrease in bone density and strength. Frequently the bones are grossly deformed. The trabeculae are attenuated or absent, and the interstices of the spongy bone are filled with vascular or fibrofatty connective tissue, or osteoid tissue. Osteoclastic activity is marked and Howship's lacunae enlarged. The skeleton may become deformed, but bones subjected to muscular strains or to the influence of posture or gravity are the most grossly disturbed. The lower limb bones are therefore more affected than the arm bones, and curvatures of the femur and tibia, i.e., coxa vara, are common. Kyphosis is also frequent. Changes in the pelvis result from pressure of the femoral heads medially with displacement of the acetabula. The angle of the pubic symphysis therefore becomes more acute, and the pubis projects as a sharp beak. The sacral promontory rotates forward under the body weight to assume a trefoil shape. The rib deformities are similar to those of rickets. In some cases multiple almost symmetric radiotranslucent bands of diminished density resembling fractures appear in the cortex of the bone. A characteristic x-ray finding is that of Looser's zones or pseudofractures which are commonly seen in the tibia, in the ribs, or in the pelvic rami as translucent lines extending a short distance through the cortex.

The blood chemistry examination usually shows little deviation from normal values for calcium, but there may be reduced serum phosphorus as well as increased serum alkaline phosphatase.

OSTEOMALACIA OF PREGNANCY. In the late months of pregnancy large amounts of calcium are required for the fetal skeleton, and during lactation there is added excretion of calcium in the milk. However, the essential causative factors are a lack of sufficient calcium in the diet to supply the additional requirements or insufficient amount of vitamin D to permit the absorption of sufficient calcium.

STARVATION OSTEOMALACIA. This form is occasionally observed in circumstances of great food deprivation. It is due partly to an absolute lack of calcium in the diet and partly to avitaminosis.

OSTEOMALACIA OF IDIOPATHIC STEATORRHEA. In this disease there are fatty stools, dilatation of the colon, and anemia. Beginning in infancy, there is disturbance of skeletal development, i.e., celiac rickets with inability to absorb calcium as a result of the excess of free fatty acid in the bowel. At any time in the course of the disease, if the supply of calcium for absorption is insufficient for general requirements, the deficiency may be made good by withdrawing calcium from the bones, so that increased bone absorption occurs, resulting in osteomalacia.

The most common symptom is backache in association with a reduction in height from spinal collapse. There is also great muscular weakness, which may simulate paresis, especially where atrophy is present as well. The muscular hypotonicity may lead to an uncertain, feeble gait.

X-ray appearances of the vertebrae show wedge-shaped bodies or, more characteristically, fishtail-shaped bodies with marked biconcavity and enlarged disks. The vertebrae are most compressed in the lumbar region.

MILKMAN'S SYNDROME. Multiple spontaneous idiopathic symmetric fractures were described by Milkman in 1931. These are now considered not to be a disease entity but rather a clinical description of a condition revealed by x-ray examination and encountered in cases of demineralization of the skeleton. It occurs in association with osteomalacia, hunger osteopathies, celiac disease, idiopathic steatorrhea, and even severe rickets.

The syndrome is more common in females and occurs in adult life from ages twenty to sixty. The cause is usually osteomalacia. The onset is slow and insidious with periods of intermission. The patient suffers from back pain and tenderness before there is any x-ray evidence.

The bones are less dense than normal. The pseudofractures are inclined to be symmetric and have special and distinctive features. In addition to being seen in the long bones they are found at sites seldom if ever affected by fracture except from trauma, e.g., the rami of the pubis and ischium and the scapulae. In a typical Looser zone the clear band is not a mere line but one of considerable width, even as much as 1 cm. There is no callus and no sclerosis.

Parathyroid Osteodystrophy (Osteitis Fibrosa, or Von Recklinghausen's Disease)

The disease is caused by an increased secretion of parathormone, which stimulates the excretion of phosphate so that the serum phosphate level falls and the serum calcium level rises with mobilization of calcium phosphate from the bones. The excess of calcium is excreted along with the phosphate in the urine, and more calcium phosphate is resorbed from the bones. Parathormone also acts directly on the osteoclastic activity of bone. Many of the clinical features of hyperparathyroidism are discussed in Chap. 38, but certain aspects of the skeletal involvement will be discussed in this section.

PATHOLOGY. Skeletal changes consist of progressive absorption of the bones, and deformity, along with new bone formation. There are also collections of giant cells (osteoclastomas) and the formation of cysts containing a thin, brownish fluid.

Histologically, the significant change is the osteoclastic activity. The Haversian canals are enlarged into big irregular spaces lined by a zone of osteoclasts lying in lacunae in close apposition to the bone they are eroding. The spaces are filled with vascular tissue, with many capillaries, and endothelial cells, and as the bone is destroyed, spindle-shaped fibroblasts appear. Adjacent spaces eventually come to communicate with each other (Fig. 45-16).

New bone formation occurs in the mass of fibrous tissue, to form laminae of bone and osteoid.

Macroscopically, there are large reddish brown lesions which are made up of masses of giant cells, or osteoclasts, in a matrix of connective tissue. The distribution of the giant cell areas is of some significance. They are arranged in clusters around areas of hemorrhage or in relation to unabsorbed bony spicules, and their cytoplasm frequently contains red blood cells and hemosiderin.

It appears that in the stage of decalcification, the rapid removal of calcium is attended by marrow hemorrhages, probably as a result of damage to the capillary endothelium from the local concentration of calcium in the capillary vessels of the bone. It is only after the occurrence of the hemorrhage that the connective tissue proliferation and the giant cell accumulation are seen.

CLINICAL MANIFESTATIONS. The most common initial skeletal feature is increasing bone pain and tenderness felt especially in the lower limbs and back. Usually the pain is associated with general weakness and accompanied by pallor and debility. Hypotonia and muscular weakness are common. There may be a fracture from trivial injury, taking a long time to heal, often in a position of deformity. Occasionally, the development of a "brown tumor," in the maxilla or the mandible, may be the earliest evidence. Anorexia and nausea, vomiting, and abdominal cramps are common, and occasionally renal colic due to the development of a renal calculus may occur.

Radiologic Findings. The radiologic appearance consists chiefly of irregular diffuse osteoporosis with absorption of the compact bone and cystlike degeneration (Fig. 45-17). In the skull the bones show a well-marked stippling, but the opaque areas are pinhead in size, distinguishing them from the grosser mottling of Paget's disease. The vertebrae are less dense and show central collapse, the upper and lower surfaces being concave, and bulging of the intervertebral discs. The pelvis shows coarse striations among which large, clear cystlike spaces are usually visible. The earliest changes occur in the hand, the skull, and the outer end of the clavicle.

Fig. 45-16. Photomicrograph from a bone biopsy of a patient, showing the attenuated trabecular patterns with increased filling of the opened-up spaces by fibroblasts, capillaries, and endothelial cells. (×25.)

The femur shows loss of trabeculation. Deformity is common—coxa vara, bowing, and cystlike spaces may be present at the extremities and in the middle of the shaft. Over the cysts the bone may show a slight fusiform enlargement in the long as well as the short bones of the hand and foot.

Loss of the lamina dura around the teeth and severe demineralization of the distal ends of the clavicles, and tufts of the fingers are characteristic though not irreversible changes.

DIFFERENTIAL DIAGNOSIS OF BONE LESIONS (Table 45-4). **Senile Osteoporosis.** In this condition, the blood calcium level is normal, and the age of onset is late, in contradistinction to fibrocystic disease. Nevertheless, the tendency to fracture, deformity, and bone pain may lead to some confusion, and the radiographic bone changes are not dissimilar to the changes of the milder forms of hyperparathyroidism.

Osteitis Deformans. The occasional occurrence of cysts and of hypercalcemia may render it difficult to distinguish from parathyroid osteodystrophy. The radiologic appearances, the age of onset, and the absence of blood changes will lead to a correct diagnosis.

Osteomalacia. In this disease there is deformity of the bones rather than fracture, the serum calcium level is low, and there is rapid response to vitamin D therapy.

Multiple Myeloma. The radiologic appearance of multiple myeloma may simulate closely the appearance of parathyroid osteodystrophy, especially in the collapse of the vertebrae, the occurrence of punctate areas of diminished density in the skull and long bones, and fine mottling of the pelvic bones. The blood calcium/phosphorus ratio is

Table 45-4. POINTS IN DIFFERENTIAL DIAGNOSIS BETWEEN HYPERPARATHYROIDISM AND OTHER BONE DISEASES

| Disease | Differential points | | | Serum | | Alkaline phosphatase‡ | Miscellaneous |
	Symptoms	X-ray appearance	Biopsy	Calcium*	Phosphorus†		
Hyperparathyroidism with bone involvement	Bone pain, deformity, fracture, tumor; polyuria; symptoms related to stones	Increased radiability; generalized deformity; cysts; tumors; fractures; stones	Rarified bone; fibrosis of marrow; osteoclasts + + +; osteoid tissue only slightly increased; osteoblasts + + +	High	Low	High	All age groups
"Senile" osteoporosis	No bone tumor, polyuria, or stones	No cysts, tumors, or stones	No fibrosis of marrow; osteoclasts normal; osteoid tissue normal or decreased; osteoblasts decreased	Normal	Normal or low	Normal	Old age
Paget's disease	Bones enlarged; no polyuria; stones infrequent	Polyostotic but not generalized; bones hypertrophied, e.g., thickened skull	May occasionally be difficult or impossible to differentiate	Normal or slightly high	Normal or slightly high	Very high	Runs in families; predilection for weight-bearing bones; seldom seen in patients under 40; arteriosclerosis + + +
Osteomalacia	No bone tumor, polyuria, or stones	No tumors or stones; bending deformities + + +	Osteoid tissue + + + osteoblasts + +; osteoclasts decreased	Normal or low	Low	High	Virtually absent in this country except with fatty diarrhea
"Solitary" cysts	Confined to cysts	No generalized changes; cysts may be multiple	Cannot differentiate if taken from lesion	Normal	Normal	Normal	
Solitary benign giant cell tumor	Confined to tumor	No generalized changes	Cannot differentiate if taken from lesion	Normal	Normal	Normal	
Osteogenesis imperfecta	Fractures + + +; no bone tumor, polyuria, or stones	Cysts rare; no tumors or stones	No fibrosis of marrow; osteoclasts normal	Normal	Normal	Normal or very slightly elevated	Hereditary, often coupled with blue sclera and deafness; improves after cessation of growth
Multiple myeloma	Can cause some bone symptoms and renal symptoms	Can be almost indistinguishable	Tumor tissue	Normal or high	Normal or high	Normal	Bence Jones proteinuria

* Normal values for calcium 9–11 mg/100 ml.
† Normal values for phosphorus 2.5–5 mg/100 ml.
‡ Normal values for alkaline phosphates 35–80 I.U./liter.
SOURCE: After Albright. Taken with permission from W. Mercer and R. B. Duthie, "Orthopaedic Surgery," 7th ed., Edward Arnold (Publishers) Ltd., London, 1974.

Fig. 45-17. *A.* X-ray of pelvis and upper femur of a middle-aged woman who presented with a stress fracture of the femoral neck and a serum calcium level of 12 mg/100 ml. *B.* X-ray of the same patient after internal fixation of pathologic fracture with three Knowles pins.

as a rule normal, while an abnormal protein—the Bence Jones proteose—may appear in the urine. A raised blood protein level frequently results in a raised total blood calcium level, but the diffusible fraction is usually normal. A biopsy may be required.

Diagnosis of parathyroid osteodystrophy depends upon the demonstration of hypercalcemia and hypophosphatemia in association with characteristic bone changes. In late hyperparathyroidism, renal damage may result in a rise in the renal phosphate threshold and a consequent rise in the blood phosphate level with a lowering of the blood calcium level. Hypercalcinuria also frequently accompanies parathyroid osteodystrophy but may also be seen in osteolysis of bone in malignant conditions, multiple myeloma, and sarcoidosis, in immobilization for chronic diseases, in hypervitaminosis D, and in renal rickets.

TREATMENT. Parathyroidectomy is the treatment of the basic disorder. Following this procedure the prognosis is generally good with immediate relief of bone pain and gain in weight and in strength of the bones. Orthopedic treatment is directed toward adequate protection of the softened bones with reduction in all deforming stresses and strains. After the disease has been arrested and recalcification of bone has taken place, any established deformity can be corrected by osteotomy or other measures.

Osteoporosis

This condition has been defined by Sissons as a structural change in bone whereby the supporting tissue is reduced in amount but remains highly mineralized. Albright and Reifenstein have pointed out that it is a disorder of protein metabolism which is reflected in abnormal trabeculae formation, but the metabolism of calcium is normal, and the trabeculae present are normally calcified.

Because of this definition Cooke, in a complete review of this subject, has emphasized how osteoporosis must be clearly differentiated from such terms as "decalcification," in which the radiologic or postmortem appearance of the bones is deficient in minerals, or "halisteresis," in which the bone mineral is removed to leave only a proteinlike structure in osteoid tissue, or "uncalcified matrix," an artificial state which does not occur naturally.

ETIOLOGY. Osteoporosis is a response of the bony skeleton to a variety of factors.

Mechanical Factors. Mechanical factors are those of immobilization of the whole body or a part of it for the treatment of fractures, prolonged postoperative bed rest, tuberculosis, etc. Osteoporosis can result from conditions such as anterior poliomyelitis, rheumatoid arthritis, and traumatic paraplegia. The condition is general or local. Accompanying muscle loss and osteoporosis is a negative nitrogen balance, resulting from an increased urinary excretion of nitrogen.

Nutritional Factors. Severe protein deficiency resulting from malnutrition or failure in absorption or abnormal protein excretion can result in osteoporosis. With such a deficiency, the calcium and phosphorus intake is reduced and forms part of the circumstances leading to senile osteoporosis. Scurvy due to deficiency in vitamin C can also produce osteoporosis.

Endocrine Factors. Osteoporosis is a common complication in Cushing's syndrome, of a basophil adenoma of the pituitary, or in disease of the adrenal cortex. These give rise to an excess of the antianabolic S hormone, or glucocorticoid hormone, which also acts on sugar metabolism. The adrenal corticoids are considered to withdraw amino acids from protein synthesis, during glyconeogenesis, with disturbance in *matrix formation.* Accompanying the generalized osteoporosis are other endocrine changes such as sexual characteristics, obesity, and diabetes mellitus.

In von Recklinghausen's disease, with hyperparathyroidism resulting from an adenoma, as an early manifestation there may be osteoporosis of the skull and spine, before the appearance of the fibrocystic lesions, osteoclastomas, and stone formation.

Postmenopausal osteoporosis may result from ovarian insufficiency with diminution in estrogen secretion. That there is some sex hormonal factor in this condition may be inferred from the much higher incidence for women.

In other endocrine diseases, such as acromegaly and gigantism, or in the hypothyroidism of cretinism or myxedema in which there is excessive utilization of nitrogen-containing substances for caloric needs, reduction in matrix formation and osteoporosis occur.

Thyrotoxic Osteoporosis. In thyrotoxicosis there is a marked increase in the general metabolism with an associated nitrogen loss to produce osteoporosis. Krane et al., by radioactive calcium studies, have shown both increased bone resorption and increased bone formation in this state. Biochemically, there is hypercalcinuria with a negative calcium balance and increased serum phosphorus and alkaline phosphatase concentrations. In hyperthyroidism, the serum calcium and phosphorus levels are normal, but there is exaggerated excretion, sometimes to as much as eight times the normal. In association with this, the bones undergo marked rarefaction, through increased osteoclastic activity, and eventually become so weak that spontaneous fractures occur. Apart from definite fractures, deformities may arise from weight bearing or from muscular action. Thus kyphosis or scoliosis and pelvic asymmetry may be present. Deformity is less common in the long bones.

Other Factors. Other pathologic conditions in which the normal bone architecture is replaced, e.g., myelomatosis and tumor invasion, are etiologic factors in osteoporosis.

PATHOLOGY. There is reduction in the thickness of the cortex, especially of the endosteal surfaces, the intermedullary contents being made up of a yellow and fatty cancellous bone tissue. On microradiography of undecalcified bone specimens, a reduction is seen in the number and size of the trabeculae and in the number of osteoblasts present. This results in a marked reduction in the mechanical strength of the involved bone, which therefore is fractured or crushed by minor trauma.

Fundamentally, there appears to be a disturbance of the normal balance between *bone formation* (osteoblastic activity) and bone resorption (osteoclastic activity). Osteoblastic activity is greatest during growth and repair of bone but is also stimulated by physical activity. However, in osteoporosis there appears to be a decrease in osteoblastic activity with the usual bone resorption of the osteons, leading to a state of imbalance. Nordin describes how there is a mineral loss as well as resorption of matrix to give a negative calcium balance but no real evidence of impaired osteoblastic activity. This negative calcium balance is seen in calcium intake deficiency, faulty resorption, faulty mobilization and transport of calcium, or excessive loss of phosphorus. It also may be accompanied by a negative nitrogen balance.

CLINICAL MANIFESTATIONS. Most patients are in the senile and postmenopausal groups. The other forms of osteoporosis are usually discovered incidentally to the main disease process, by radiology. Pathologic fractures, especially of the femoral neck, commonly arise because of this condition.

Pain is in the nature of a lumbar backache which radiates around the trunk or down the lower limbs. It is aggravated by movement or jarring, and although suggestive of a nerve root compression, this is rarely seen. Acute sudden onset of pain with localized tenderness in the chest or back is most suggestive of a pathologic fracture of a rib or vertebral body.

Loss of height may have been noted by the patient, with the appearance of a thoracic kyphosis and an approximation of the rib margin to the iliac crests.

Radiologic Findings. The involved bone has a "ground glass" appearance (a late manifestation) because of loss of definition of the trabeculae. In the spine, the vertebral bodies become flattened but biconcave with increase in the intervertebral spaces, varying degrees of collapse and wedging may be seen (Fig. 45-18). Healing of the pathologic fracture is usually accompanied by little callus formation.

Biochemistry. The serum calcium, phosphorus, and alkaline phosphatase levels are within normal limits. The total

Fig. 45-18. X-ray of the spine of a patient with osteoporosis. Note the "ground glass" appearance, biconcavity of vertebral bodies, and increase in the intervertebral spaces.

plasma protein and plasma albumin levels may be low, but this is of little value from the diagnostic aspect. A measurement of urinary calcium excretion over a 24-hour period may be of some help, particularly if the daily intake can be estimated.

Biopsy. Specimens can be obtained by trephining from the iliac crest or the spinous processes of the lumbar vertebrae and are of value.

DIFFERENTIAL DIAGNOSIS. *Osteomalacia* is a condition of hypocalcification which radiologically may resemble osteoporosis but results from a failure in calcification of the bone matrix due to a calcium and vitamin D deficiency. The plasma phosphorus level is lowered with an increase in the serum alkaline phosphatase.

As a general rule, osteoporosis is seen in the spine and pelvis with frequent pathologic fracturing, whereas osteomalacia is more commonly seen in the extremities, with more deformity than fractures and osteofibritis. Osteitis fibrosa is particularly common in the skull.

Secondary osteoporosis of other diseases such as hyperparathyroidism, either primary or secondary, Cushing's syndrome, and acromegaly can be identified by the features of the primary disease. Metastatic carcinoma, multiple myeloma, and rheumatoid arthritis with excessive corticoid therapy are also included in the differential diagnosis.

TREATMENT. *Ambulation* must be encouraged and support given to the diseased spine in the form of a light plaster jacket or a brace, or to the pathologic fracture of the femur by a walking non-weight-bearing caliper. Internal fixation is sound in principle because of the loss in mechanical strength of the surrounding bone. A high-protein-high-calcium diet should be prescribed.

Hormonal Therapy. Estrogen therapy has been shown to produce hyperossification in animals. It can be given as 1 mg/day orally or by injection as estrogen dipropionate, 2 mg/day, for a period of 4 weeks with a following rest of 2 weeks before recommencing the drug. This may produce uterine bleeding, which is an indication to stop treatment.

Androgen therapy has been shown to produce an increase in the bone matrix, body weight, and musculature. Because of this Cooke recommends administering testosterone propionate, 10 to 20 mg/day, by injection or methyl-testosterone, 30 mg/day, by mouth in combination with the estrogens. The latter combination may prevent the masculinizing effects of the androgen.

Hormonal administration can induce both a positive nitrogen and calcium balance and improvement in matrix and bone formation, but the side effects have proved to be difficult and disturbing. A more recent anabolic hormone—methandrostenolane, or Dianabol, appears to have greater potency in doses as low as 2.5 to 5 mg/day. A weekly measurement of the body weight is recommended to check for edema. Therapy is still very controversial but is required to decrease bone resorption and/or increase bone formation. Calcitonin and the diphosphonates have not proved useful. The estrogens, synthetic anabolic hormones, calcium, and any such combinations are believed only to slow the progression of bone loss. Combinations of fluorides, calcium, and vitamin D may enhance bone formation.

Pituitary Disturbances

The anterior lobe of the pituitary gland, by its secretion of the thyrotropic, adrenocorticotropic, and gonadotropic hormones, "controls" the activity of the thyroid, adrenal cortex, and sex glands. However, there is the reciprocal relationship of feedback, or control by the amount of circulating hormone, as well as indirect relationships of the hormones to each other. In addition to this endocrine control there is the integration of the endocrines with the nervous system by the hypothalamus.

The *anterior lobe* of the pituitary is made up of:

Clear chromophobe cells ⟶   Acidophil cells   Basophil cells
            ↓   ╱   ╲ |
Hypopituitarism (by pressure) Hypersecretion   Hyposecretion Hypersecretion
                                    | | |
                               Gigantism or   Infantilism Cushing's syndrome
                               acromegaly | |
                                        Lorain's or Froehlich's syndrome
                                              |
                                       Simmonds' disease

The *posterior lobe* is made up of neurologic cells and fibers which are connected to the supraoptic nuclei of the hypothalamus. Secretion of oxytocin or vasopressin from the posterior lobe of the pituitary does not appear to have any direct effect upon osseous tissues.

PITUITARY DWARFISM

The term *dwarf* is applied to an individual whose physical dimensions are less than those peculiar to his race.
There are two main types:

1. *Froehlich's adiposogenital type,* in which skeletal stunting is associated with general obesity, genital hypoplasia, and often stupidity or idiocy.
2. The *Lorain type,* in which there is no mental change and no physical change except lack of skeletal growth; i.e., children with Lorain's syndrome are "attractive and graceful children."

The usual cause of hypopituitarism is a tumor or cyst (suprasellar cyst) compressing and destroying the gland. In some cases where the dwarfing is already present at birth, there is said to be aplasia of the gland, or a failure of differentiation of the eosinophil cells.

PATHOLOGY. The growth of all parts of the skeleton is delayed or arrested. The epiphyses remain ununited for a prolonged period, and the metaphysis terminates in a line of dense bone. The histologic change is an absence of division of the cartilage cells in endochondral bone and absence of division of the primitive connective tissue cells in the membrane bones.

DIAGNOSIS. The differential diagnosis of dwarfism, or reduction in all structural diameters, which can be made before the age of five years includes (1) achondroplasia (usually inherited and present at birth), (2) osteogenesis imperfecta, (3) chondroosteodystrophy, (4) pituitary dwarfism, (5) renal dwarfism, (6) nutritional dwarfism—steatorrhea, rickets, and (7) cretinism.

HYPERPITUITARY SYNDROMES

Gigantism

This condition begins before the epiphyses have closed, and there is an increase both in the rate of epiphyseal growth and in the maturation of the skeleton. The mental development is subnormal and the body strength often surprisingly slight. In the majority of cases some of the features of acromegaly develop later.

Pathology. The bones of the skeleton show increased thickness and length; the membrane bones are also hypertrophied.

At the epiphyseal cartilage growth of the cartilage cells is active, but the orderly palisade arrangement is lost, the cells being arranged in irregular groups. The amount of matrix is increased. The number of vascular buds and of advancing osteogenic cells is increased.

Acromegaly

The manifestations of acromegaly appear after skeletal growth has ceased, and the disease is characterized by an unevenly distributed exaggeration of ossification, due to the effects of local pressure and traction.

Acromegaly results from abnormal secretion of the eosinophil cells of the anterior lobe of the pituitary, with either hyperplasia or a tumor—an eosinophil adenoma.

Pathology. Abnormal bone formation occurs in the alveolar margins of the jaws, leading to great elongation of the face and projection of the chin, but the ramus of the jaw is narrow and elongated. The malar bones and the vault of the skull may be thickened. The skull change begins or is most marked in the frontal bone, and the deposits or osteomas grow from the inner table of the skull. The foramen magnum is usually displaced forward and the pituitary fossa enlarged from the presence of the adenoma.

The thorax is massive, because of the increased length of the ribs, which is partly the result of the exaggerated bone growth and partly the result of the hypertrophy of the lungs.

In the long bones the most obvious changes are found toward the extremities, which are more massive than normal and less well modeled. Muscular insertions and tuberosities and ridges are usually accentuated.

The short long bones are thick and usually elongated. Muscular and tendinous insertions are again prominent, and at the articular ends lipping may be pronounced.

In the vertebral column there is new subperiosteal bone, which is thickest on the anterior surface of the body and gradually diminishes as the body is traced around to the vertebral canal. This phenomenon is occasionally referred to as *acromegalic spondylitis*.

Acromegalic arthritis may affect any of the limb or spinal joints. In osteoarthrosis the earliest change consists of attenuation and ultimate disappearance of the articular cartilage at the points of greatest pressure. In acromegaly, articular cartilage thickens under the stimulus of growth hormone and subsequently degenerates.

Congenital Hypothyroidism (Cretinism)

When the thyroid gland is completely absent (athyrosis) or is destroyed in early infancy by disease, cretinism with decrease in cartilage proliferation and osteoblastic activity is produced.

The prominent features of cretinism are signs of mental deficiency, anomalies in genital growth, and generalized growth disturbances.

The cretin is a dwarf because of delayed ossification and retardation in growth and skeletal maturation. The long bones are short, while the ossification of the skull is delayed, and the fontanel closes late—as late, sometimes, as at twenty years. The root of the nose is depressed, from defective growth of the base of the skull. The vault of the skull may appear large in comparison with the body.

The principal skeletal changes are the late appearance of the epiphyses and of bones whose ossific nuclei develop after birth, e.g., the carpal and the tarsal bones, and delayed union of the epiphyses.

The shafts of the long bones appear short, with a thick cortex, but their caliber is diminished. Toward the extremities of the bones the size more nearly approximates the normal. The epiphyses are not only late in appearing but are small and often irregular in ossification, appear fragmented, and show a superficial resemblance to those of a patient with osteochondritis.

There may be delay or arrest in fusion between the two halves of the neural arch or the neurocentral synchondrosis, with disturbance of normal ossification of the vertebral bodies.

The administration of thyroid extract is curative if treatment is begun in infancy. It is interesting to note that since epiphyseal fusion is delayed, the administration of thyroid may produce growth in stature even of the adult.

Mucopolysaccharidoses

Abnormalities of mucopolysaccharide metabolism result in skeletal deformities in addition to involvement of other systems including the central nervous, cardiovascular, and reticuloendothelial systems. McKusick has reviewed the inheritance of the various disorders and correlated the clinical findings with the biochemical abnormalities (Table 45-5).

DIAGNOSIS. Chondroitin sulfate A accounts for 80 percent of normally excreted urinary mucopolysaccharide; chondroitin sulfate B, 10 percent; and heparitin sulfate, 10 percent. Approximately 3 to 15 mg is excreted each 24 hours. Excessive excretion of any of the above or the presence of keratosulfaturia is abnormal.

Metachromatic granules may be present in circulating leukocytes, lymphocytes, and bone marrow cells and should be investigated.

Mucopolysaccharidosis I (Hurler Syndrome). This rare condition, inherited as an autosomal recessive trait, is recognizable in infancy or early childhood. There is severe mental deterioration, dwarfism, and clouding of the corneas. Hepatosplenomegaly is present. The skull is large with a saddle-like nose. The tongue is large and lips are patulous with mouth open (gargoyle facies). The neck is short, and the dorsal spine has a kyphosis with a gibbus at the dorsal lumbar area. The abdomen is protuberant and the lower thorax flared as a result of the hepatosplenomegaly. X-ray examination of the spine shows wedge-shaped bodies with anterior beaking. Varus or valgus knees and foot deformities are frequently present, and joints are stiff. Radiographic changes in the extremities include expansion of the medullary cavity, cortical thinning, and shortened phalanges. The fundamental defect is an abnormality of metabolism of heparitin sulfate and chondroitin sulfate B.

Mucopolysaccharidosis II (Hunter Syndrome). The Hunter syndrome is inherited as a sex-linked recessive trait with abnormality of mucopolysaccharide metabolism similar to that of the Hurler syndrome. The disease is clinically similar although less severe in all aspects including dwarfing, hepatosplenomegaly, and the gargoyle facies.

Table 45-5. THE GENETIC MUCOPOLYSACCHARIDOSES (as classified in 1972)

Designation	Clinical features	Genetics	Excessive urinary MPS	Substance deficient
MPS I H Hurler syndrome	Early clouding of cornea, grave manifestations, death usually before age 10	Homozygous for MPS I H gene	Dermatan sulfate Heparan sulfate	α-L-iduronidase (formerly called Hurler corrective factor)
MPS I S Scheie syndrome	Stiff joints, cloudy cornea, aortic regurgitation, normal intelligence, normal life span	Homozygous for MPS I S gene	Dermatan sulfate Heparan sulfate	α-L-iduronidase
MPS I H/S Hurler-Scheie compound	Phenotype intermediate between Hurler and Scheie	Genetic compound of MPS I H and I S genes	Dermatan sulfate Heparan sulfate	α-L-iduronidase
MPS II A Hunter syndrome, severe	No clouding of cornea, milder course than in MPS I H but death usually before age 15	Hemizygous for X-linked gene	Dermatan sulfate Heparan sulfate	Hunter corrective factor
MPS II B Hunter syndrome, mild	Survival to 30's to 50's, fair intelligence	Hemizygous for X-linked allele for mild form	Dermatan sulfate Heparan sulfate	Hunter corrective factor
MPS III A Sanfilippo syndrome A	Identical phenotype: Mild somatic, severe nervous system effects	Homozygous for Sanfilippo A gene	Heparan sulfate	Heparan sulfate sulfatase
MPS III B Sanfilippo syndrome B		Homozygous for Sanfilippo B (at different locus)	Heparan sulfate	N-acetyl-α-D-glucosaminidase
MPS IV Morquio syndrome (probably more than one allelic form)	Severe bone changes of distinctive type, cloudy cornea, aortic regurgitation	Homozygous for Morquio gene	Keratan sulfate	Unknown
MPS V Vacant				
MPS VI A Maroteaux-Lamy syndrome, classic form	Severe osseous and corneal change, normal intellect	Homozygous for M-L gene	Dermatan sulfate	Maroteaux-Lamy corrective factor
MPS VI B Maroteaux-Lamy syndrome, mild form	Severe osseous and corneal change, normal intellect	Homozygous for allele at M-L locus	Dermatan sulfate	Maroteaux-Lamy corrective factor
MPS VII β-glucoronidase deficiency (more than one allelic form?)	Hepatosplenomegaly, dysostosis multiplex, white cell inclusions, mental retardation	Homozygous for mutant gene at β-glucoronidase locus	Dermatan sulfate	β-glucoronidase

SOURCE: Taken with permission from V. A. McKusick, "Heritable Disorders of Connective Tissue," 4th ed., The C. V. Mosby Company, St. Louis, 1972.

Mental deterioration is slower, and there is neither the lumbar gibbus nor the clouding of the cornea. Patients may survive well into the thirties.

Mucopolysaccharidosis III (Sanfilippo Syndrome). This syndrome is rare, inherited as an autosomal recessive trait, and associated with excessive production of urinary heparitin sulfate. Severe mental retardation is the predominant finding, although skeletal changes may be present. Stiffness in the joints occurs, but dwarfing may be mild. Corneal clouding has not been reported.

Mucopolysaccharidosis IV (Morquio-Brailsford Syndrome, Chondroosteodystrophy). This syndrome, inherited as an autosomal recessive trait, was described independently in 1929 by both Morquio and Brailsford. The defect is an abnormality in keratosulfate metabolism.

The patient appears normal at birth, but dwarfism becomes apparent within the first two years of life. Lumbar spinal changes are similar to those of the Hurler syndrome, are recognizable within the first year of life, and progress to flat or platyspondylitic vertebrae. Wrists are enlarged, and a pigeon-breasted thorax develops. Clouding of the cornea is progressive.

Radiographs of the long bones reveal shortening and wide metaphyses with increase in the thickness of epiphyseal and articular cartilages. Epiphyseal centers of ossification begin as multiple foci and become distorted, resulting in joint incongruity. Genu valgum and flatfoot with a posture of hip and knee flexion are common.

Mucopolysaccharidosis V (Scheie Syndrome). This is a rare variant of the Hurler syndrome, transmitted as an autosomal recessive and related to a defect in mucopolysaccharide metabolism of chondroitin sulfate B. Height is usually low-normal to normal, joints are stiff, and corneal clouding is the most striking finding. Intellect is normal or above normal.

Mucopolysaccharidosis VI (Maroteaux-Lamy Syndrome, Polydystrophic Dwarfism). In this syndrome the dominant findings are severe osseous abnormalities in the presence of normal intellect. Metaphyses are irregular and epiphyses deformed. Vertebral bodies are flattened and may be wedge-shaped. Hepatosplenomegaly, deafness, and corneal clouding are common.

It is apparent that there are other abnormalities of mucopolysaccharide metabolism, and as the biochemistry is clarified, other syndromes will be recognized and correlated. Current treatment for these conditions is based on empiric treatment of orthopedic deformities, although progress rests upon an exact understanding of the biochemical defect.

OSTEITIS DEFORMANS

Osteitis deformans was described in detail by Sir James Paget in 1876 and is often known as *Paget's disease.* The disease has a universal distribution in the human race but has also been identified in horses and monkeys.

ETIOLOGY. The origin of Paget's disease is not known. Paget believed it to be inflammatory in origin.

Brailsford regarded the disease as a primary localized vascular disturbance with a secondary adverse effect on the bone. Mercer and Duthie consider that the vascular disturbance is produced by some form of an arteriovenous malformation not yet demonstrated. They found an increase in the bone blood flow sufficient to produce circulatory disturbances compatible with those resulting from an arteriovenous shunt and high blood pressure. In such cases death from congestive heart failure is not an unusual occurrence. The basic lesion appears to be an acceleration of bone turnover with an associated increase in urinary hydroxyproline.

PATHOLOGY. The *bone changes* are characterized by thickening, softening, and deformity, and later by ossification. Knaggs described three stages in the pathology of the skull changes: In the first, or *vascular,* stage, there is a deposit of finely porous bone beneath the pericranium with permeation of a very vascular connective tissue. In the second stage, that of *advancing sclerosis,* the thickness of the skull is increased and the calvarial sutures obliterated. In the stage of *diffuse complete sclerosis* the condensed type of bone is present for the most part throughout the whole thickness of the calvaria.

In the *spine* there is thickening, with osteoporosis of the various parts, and as a consequence of the weight-bearing function some of the bodies may collapse. Secondary

changes—synostosis of adjacent bodies, even ankylosis of a segment of the spine—are common. These changes may lead to marked reduction in stature. The thickening of the neural arch leads to a reduction in the caliber of the vertebral canal, which may reach a sufficient degree to give rise to evidence of spinal cord compression.

In the *long bones* there are marked resorption of bone and ingrowth of vascular connective tissue, which subsequently ossifies. The periosteum is normal. The thickening of the bone leads to irregularity on the surface, with marked reduction in the medullary cavity. In the stage of softening and enlargement the bone is apt to become deformed, partly because the soft bone yields to normal gravitational weight bearing or muscular stresses and partly, in the forearm and leg, because one bone may be more involved than its neighbor.

In the early stages of the disease there is a diffuse infiltration by young granulation tissue, and the trabeculae of the bone are attenuated. Howship's lacunae are enlarged and occupied by granulation tissue cells or osteoclasts. In the stage of osteogenic activity the sections show numerous trabeculae of new bone containing an irregular lamellar system which appears typically as a mosaic pattern (Fig. 45-19). These are elaborated from the connective tissue and are irregular in their distribution. They are so numerous that adjacent struts may fuse to enclose an irregular space, or lacuna, containing connective tissue.

CLINICAL MANIFESTATIONS. The disease usually begins between the ages of thirty-six and fifty years. Incidence in the sexes is equal. Pain in the lower limbs, thighs, or hips is often the initial feature and present in 30 percent of patients with this disease. It may be aggravated by exercise or be more pronounced at night. Gradual bowing of the legs and/or the development of a spinal curvature are common, with gait abnormality.

The circumference of the head may gradually increase. Headache and vertigo may result from the cranial thickening. Compression of the cranial nerves in the foramina appears when the lumen of the foramen is encroached upon with resulting auditory and visual disturbances. Spi-

Fig. 45-19. Microscopic section in Paget's disease (see text).

Fig. 45-20. X-ray of the pelvis and femur of a patient with Paget's disease.

coarse striae are apparent throughout the cortex (Fig. 45-20).

The *long bones* are thickened from enlargement of the cortex. The natural curves of the bone are accentuated, but sometimes the deformities are more bizarre.

Fairbank has described four typical radiologic appearances which can be seen in most bones: (1) a honeycomb, or spongy, appearance, which is the commonest and most widespread manifestation; (2) a striated appearance, as seen in the pelvis, sacrum, and calcaneum; (3) a uniform and increased density, which is most frequently seen in the vertebrae; and (4) true cystic areas, as seen in the pelvis or long bones.

Laboratory Findings. The serum calcium and the serum phosphorus levels are usually normal, but there is a very high serum alkaline phosphatase content. The urinary excretion of calcium and phosphorus is on occasion increased, and pathologic calcification may occur in arterial walls and in the interventricular septum of the heart.

TREATMENT. No curative treatment of Paget's disease is known, and the most that can be done in the usual case is to relieve the pain. Radiotherapy is of benefit in alleviating the bone pain. Recently three drugs have been used for the relief of bone pain: (1) fluorides, which are effective only in doses producing other severe skeletal changes; (2) diphosphonates, which have been shown to produce rickets by blocking vitamin D metabolism; and (3) the calcitonins (porcine, salmon or human), which markedly reduce bone turnover, with minimal side effects.

Internal fixation by some form of intramedullary nailing for all fractures is worthwhile to relieve pain. Resection of sarcomas should be attempted and the area replaced by some form of prosthesis.

RETICULOSES

The cells forming the lining of the minute blood vascular channels of the bone marrow are part of the reticuloendothelial system. The other cellular elements of the system are certain adult connective tissue cells (fibrocytes), the endothelium lining blood and lymph vessels, the reticulum cells of the spleen, and certain of the large mononuclear cells of the blood.

The cells of the reticuloendothelial system are believed to be the scavengers of the body, and their activity is concerned mainly with the removal from the circulating fluid of dead and damaged cells, bacteria, and other foreign or noxious material. They are also energetic in the disposal of such metabolic substances as hemoglobin and cholesterol.

Red bone marrow consists of blood-forming cells as well as reticuloendothelial cells. Affections of any of these resulting in increased volume or vascularity will result in absorption of the adjacent bony trabeculae. In response to continued strain new bone is laid down to buttress the weak site. Hodgkin's disease usually affects the spine, skull, and pelvis; leukemia, the long bones; and chloroma, usually bones of the orbit.

In the adult the red marrow is confined to irregular or

nal cord compressions producing paraplegia have also been reported in a number of instances.

Trivial violence can result in spontaneous fractures, especially in the femur and the tibia. Development of osteogenic sarcoma in one of the affected bones may present as increased pain or pathologic fracturing.

Osteitis deformans usually begins in the monostotic form, most commonly in the tibia, but in 75 percent of cases this will progress to give the generalized, or polyostotic, form.

Radiologic Findings. The bones most commonly involved, in order of frequency, are the skull, tibia, femur, pelvis, radius, bones of the hand, bones of the foot, humerus, and ulna.

The earliest change in the *skull* is blurring of its surface outline, together with some flattening. New bone formation is irregular and appears as irregular islands of dense bone, giving the calvaria a mottled or coarsely piebald appearance. The base of the skull may show comparable changes.

Changes in the spine consist of a woolly appearance of the bodies, with coarse striae at the periphery and horizontal striae near the upper and lower surfaces. The bodies may be fatter and squatter than normal, and abnormal curvatures may be present.

The *pelvis* tends to assume a trefoil shape, as a result of the pressure of the femoral heads. The bone appears thick and massive, but the texture of the bone is altered; it now appears mottled and blurred, while occasionally flat bones or to the ends of long bones. It is here that malignant involvement and bony changes first occur.

The reticuloendothelial tissue of bone is found mainly at the ends of the long bones and in the spongy bone of the flat and short bones, and it is here that any affections occur most markedly.

RETICULOSES—DISEASES OF BONE MARROW CONSTITUENTS

A. Reticuloendothelial system
  1. Histiocytic granulomatosis
    a. Letterer-Siwe disease
    b. Eosinophilic granuloma
    c. Hand-Schüller-Christian disease
  2. Lipoid granulomatosis
    a. Gaucher's disease
    b. Niemann-Pick disease
    c. Xanthomatosis with hypercholesterolemia
B. Lymphatic system
  1. Hodgkin's disease
  2. Lymphosarcoma
C. Hematopoietic system
  1. Leukemia
    a. Lymphoblastic
    b. Myeloblastic
  2. Multiple myeloma
  3. Hemolytic anemia
    a. Mediterranean, or Cooley's, anemia
    b. Sickle cell anemia
    c. Erythroblastosis foetalis

Hodgkin's Disease

Autopsy records show that involvement of the bone marrow in Hodgkin's disease is more frequent than clinical studies would lead one to suspect.

PATHOLOGY. The bodies of the vertebral column and pelvis are the bones most often involved. The cancellous tissue of the upper end of the femur is also a common site. Of the other bones, the diploë of the skull, the ends of the tibia, the lower end of the femur, and the ends of the humerus are less commonly affected.

In the cancellous tissue and red marrow of the affected bone, an infiltrating mass of tissue with destruction of bone develops. In the vertebrae the destruction is usually so extreme that collapse of one or more of the bodies occurs. In the pelvis, areas of rarefaction are surrounded by areas of sclerosis, while in the skull the infiltration is predominantly osteolytic. In the ribs, complete destruction of the affected segment is the rule and is pathognomic. In the long bones there is often subperiosteal new bone formation which may be so marked that the lesion resembles chronic osteomyelitis. In other cases the lesion resembles a lymphosarcoma in which the lesions are purely osteolytic with invasion throughout bone.

CLINICAL MANIFESTATIONS. The sexes are equally liable, and age bears no relationship to the severity or the frequency of the bone changes. In most cases pain is the first indication of the osseous spread with delay in radiologic evidence. The pain is of a dull aching or lancinating character and may be so severe as to interfere with the function of the neighboring joints. In the spine there may be girdle pains, and in some cases evidences of cord compression have subsequently arisen. The bone changes have little or no effect on the constitutional course of the disease. Differential diagnosis includes lymphogranuloma of bone.

TREATMENT. In common with the other lesions of Hodgkin's disease the bone changes appear to respond to x-ray therapy. The pain is relieved, and in some cases reparative changes appear in the affected bones.

HISTIOCYTIC GRANULOMATOSIS

A combined syndrome is a more appropriate consideration, because the permanent and constant pathologic feature is the presence of numerous histiocytes and granulomatous tissue (Table 45-6). Anatomically the underlying lesion in eosinophilic granuloma is related to the lesion of Hand-Schüller-Christian disease and that of Letterer-Siwe disease. These three conditions have been described as different clinicoanatomic expressions of the same disorder.

LIPOID GRANULOMATOSIS

Disturbances in lipoid metabolism may give rise to a specific pathologic change in the reticuloendothelial system involving the spongy skeleton. In Gaucher's disease a lipoprotein of the cerebroside type is at fault; in Niemann-Pick disease, a phosphatid lipoid; in Tay-Sachs syndrome, a cerebroside protein; and in Hand-Schüller-Christian disease, cholesterol. In all these, bone changes have been reported or observed, though the main effects of the disease are found in the extraosseous portions of the reticuloendothelium. Hand-Schüller-Christian disease has particular orthopedic importance.

PATHOLOGY. There is an increased lipoid content of the circulating body fluids with the reticuloendothelial cells absorbing and depositing the substance. It is suggested that a congenital or acquired deficiency of liver and lungs increases the reticuloendothelium elsewhere—especially in bone. In the skeleton, the diploë of the skull, cancellous tissue of the mandible, clavicle, ribs, pelvis, and vertebrae are affected. In addition, the pleura, the lungs, the liver, and the cerebellum have been the sites of typical deposits. In this situation, the deposits appear as multiple circumscribed, rounded tumors, golden yellow or brownish yellow.

These "tumors" are composed of large, often multinucleated reticuloendothelial cells, with small nuclei and a finely reticulated cytoplasm. The cytoplasm contains for the most part innumerable globules of lipoid which give the cell a "foamy" appearance. The largest foam cells are found away from the vessels; around the vessels are arranged smaller reticuloendothelial cells. The presence of the deposits of lipoid produces granulation tissue around the deposits. This causes destruction of the bone without new bone reaction, to give rise to large defects with irregular margins (Fig. 45-21).

The condition in a typical case is marked on the skull base in the vicinity of the sella turcica. The pituitary gland may be compressed or obliterated, and the lipogranulomatous tissue may extend through the superior orbital fissure to collect behind the globe of the eye and push it forward.

Table 45-6. DIFFERENTIAL DIAGNOSIS BETWEEN HAND-SCHÜLLER-CHRISTIAN DISEASE,
EOSINOPHILIC GRANULOMA, AND LETTERER-SIWE DISEASE

	Hand-Schüller-Christian disease	*Eosinophilic granuloma*	*Letterer-Siwe disease*
Age	Early childhood but occasionally in adults	Older children, adolescents, and young adults	Infants
Clinical features	Triad of exophthalmos, polyuria, polydipsia, swelling; N.B.: other pituitary dysfunction	Pain, swelling, and local tenderness; systemic manifestations of fever, loss in weight	Low fever, pain and swelling; low-grade anemia; short and rapidly fatal course in most cases
Localization	Base of skull, spine, ilium, mandible—most common in "membranous bones"; liver and spleen sometimes	72%—solitary lesion involving all bones but mainly ribs, skull, femur, pelvis, humerus; soft tissues rare	Multiple lesions of liver, spleen, glands, skin, lungs, and mainly skull
Pathology	Secondary deposition of cholesterol in "foam cells" following formation of granuloma; (?) unknown infection	Granuloma formation with histiocytes, eosinophils in large numbers, multinucleated cells and areas of necrosis	Eosinophils + +; foam cells sometimes present; true reticuloendotheliosis
Radiology		Cannot be differentiated	
Blood picture and biochemistry	Normal; hypercholesteremia in most cases	"Circulating" eosinophilia; normal	Anemia; normal
Prognosis	Slow and benign except in 25% of cases	Good but guarded in multiple lesions	Fatal

SOURCE: Taken with permission from W. Mercer and R. B. Duthie, "Orthopaedic Surgery," 7th ed., Edward Arnold (Publishers) Ltd., London, 1974.

CLINICAL MANIFESTATIONS. The disease as originally described consisted of a distinctive syndrome—defects in the membranous bones, exophthalmos, with thirst and polyuria (diabetes insipidus). It is to this triad of effects that the term Hand-Schüller-Christian syndrome is given. The exophthalmos is the result of the retrobulbar accumulation of lipoid-laden reticuloendothelial cells, while the diabetes insipidus is the sequel to the distortion of the hypothalamus.

Thus interference with the pituitary may lead to retardation of growth, and the irritation or tension on the dura mater to irritability and restlessness. Should the extraosseous reticuloendothelium be affected, splenomegaly or hepatic enlargement may be present, and in the latter case jaundice may be observed. The blood shows a cholesterol content which may be increased to 280 mg/100 ml. Biopsy with histologic examination will give an accurate diagnosis.

TREATMENT. The disease tends to be progressive, and in many published cases death has resulted. An attempt is made to reduce the hypercholesteremia by dietetic means. Deep radiotherapy is employed to control the deposits, while in the event of polyuria and thirst from dia-

Fig. 45-21. Lipoid granulomatosis demonstrating destruction of bone with large defects, irregular margins, and absence of new bone reaction.

betes insipidus pituitary extract may be given. Any pathologic fractures should be immobilized by internal fixation devices.

EOSINOPHILIC GRANULOMATOSIS

This is an affection of the young, 64 percent of patients being under twenty years of age. The cause is unknown, though it is believed to be an infection or toxin of some sort. The lesions, usually multiple, affect the skeleton almost exclusively, although in some cases lymph glands and the lungs may also be involved. The local lesion, though frequently silent, may give rise to local pain and tenderness and even swelling. The illness may be initiated by fever. Where the skull is affected, headache is often a complaint. Blood examination is not characteristic, although eosinophilia may be present.

The radiologic appearance varies and may simulate other types of disease. Most commonly the lesion is oval or circular, translucent, and cystlike. It may be accompanied by some periostitis adjacent to the osteolytic area. The confluences of the translucent areas, particularly in the skull, sometimes gives the appearance of the "geographic" skull. In the long bones the lesions are endosteal and usually affect the shafts; only occasionally is a lesion seen in the epiphysis. Vertebra plana due to eosinophilic granuloma has been described by Compere et al. Biopsy was carried out in their four cases and demonstrated the typical eosinophilic granulomatosis lesion. However, an inflammatory lesion must be excluded, in which case rest and splinting will cause the symptoms to disappear, and even the deformed and flattened vertebral body may reossify.

The lesion may resolve spontaneously; it may heal after curettage without the aid of radiotherapy or after radiotherapy alone.

The contents of a relatively early lesion consist of soft brownish granulation tissue which may be streaked with yellow necrotic material. Patches of hemorrhage may be present. Histologically it shows histiocytes, eosinophils in large numbers, and leukocytes, and large multinuclear giant cells, especially near hemorrhage or necrosis.

Diagnosis must differentiate this condition from Hand-Schüller-Christian disease (Table 45-6), in which there is often exophthalmos, diabetes insipidus, and a characteristic histologic appearance, and from myelomatosis by the lesions in the skull, which are larger and less numerous, and by the absence of Bence Jones protein in the urine. Polyostotic fibrous dysplasia also has to be excluded.

LETTERER-SIWE DISEASE

This very rare condition, a reticuloendotheliosis, occurs in infants up to the age of three or four and is regarded as an acute form of Hand-Schüller-Christian disease. It usually runs a short and rapidly fatal course without the secondary deposits of cholesterol esters in the cells of the granulomas. The soft tissues, particularly of the viscera, are chiefly affected, although in most cases destructive lesions are found in the skeleton. There is a low and progressive anemia, and lesions are found in the liver and spleen (which are usually enlarged) as well as in glands, lungs, skin, and the bones of the skull. The x-ray picture closely resembles that of the Hand-Schüller-Christian disease. If the base of the skull is involved, the characteristic symptoms of Hand-Schüller-Christian disease—exophthalmos and diabetes insipidus—may develop, although the lesions are without foam cells. Histologically there is difficulty in distinguishing the condition from the other two forms of histiocytic granulomatosis. (See Table 45-6.)

In most cases death ensues within a few weeks.

HEMATOPOIETIC SYSTEM

Leukemia

Lymphoblastic leukemia most commonly produces bony changes. Myeloblastic leukemia has a lower incidence of bony changes because of its shorter acute course. In aleukemic leukemia bony changes do occur in spite of its very rapid course.

These lesions can be found in any part of the skeleton, although they most commonly occur in the knee and shoulder regions around the metaphysis. The skull is rarely involved.

On x-rays, the characteristic lesion is a translucent zone adjacent to the metaphysis, but there may be a diffuse spotty osteolysis with vertebral collapse and deformity as well as abnormal periosteal ossification. The metaphyseal translucent zone is not specific for these diseases but is seen in numerous unrelated conditions such as prolonged immobilization of the limb or scurvy.

The main differentiation is from juvenile rheumatism; both may present as a polyarticular "arthritis" with pain, swelling, and loss of movement.

Treatment with ACTH and folic acid antagonists has been successful in some of these diseases.

Multiple Myeloma

Marrow develops from the primitive undifferentiated mesenchyme cell, and in the process of differentiation progeny of distinctive characteristics are produced. There are the reticulum cell with its fibrils, the plasma cell with its typical cartwheel nucleus eccentrically placed and showing in the basophilic cytoplasm a characteristic clear area, the cells of the lymphocyte series, and the forerunners of the polymorphonuclear cells and erythrocytes of the blood. Tumors arising in the marrow can therefore exhibit a wide variation in cell type, resembling in greater or lesser detail the cells normally found and affording ample opportunity for complex classification. Such discussion, however, is of little clinical significance.

PATHOLOGY. The affected bones show replacement of their marrow and the bone trabeculae without reactive new bone formation, so that the tumors bear a close resemblance—on inspection as well as on radiologic examination—to diffuse carcinomatosis. Hemorrhage with cyst formation is common, and pathologic fracture is frequent. When the disease is extensive, there may be gross restriction of the absolute amount of red marrow, with anemia.

Myelogenous tumors are most commonly encountered

Fig. 45-22. Skull x-ray of a patient with hemolytic anemia, demonstrating the "brush" appearance.

in the skull and vertebrae, ribs, pelvis, femur, and humerus, but the bones of the peripheral parts of the limbs are only occasionally the site of disease. The sternum frequently contains tumors, and sternal puncture in consequence may be a valuable diagnostic procedure. The disease is closely related to the leukemias except that in myelomatosis the plasma cell is the predominant cell type.

In myelomatosis metabolic disturbance is common, the blood calcium level is raised, and there is hyperproteinemia, the globulin being raised. In 50 percent of patients, globulin (Bence Jones protein) is present in the urine, a fact which, however, can also occur in leukemia, skeletal carcinomatosis, and rarely in nephritis.

Amyloid deposits in muscles and joints have been described in 10 percent of cases of myelomatosis and are particularly common when large amounts of globulin are present in the urine. Renal insufficiency is another frequent complication. This is believed to be due to plugging of the renal tubules by globulin casts, and the cortex may be eroded from the marrow surface.

In certain myelomas, when the tumor is sectioned, the cut surface is bright green, which is due to a pigment the character of which is not fully understood. The color rapidly fades. To this group of tumors the name *chloroma* has been given.

CLINICAL MANIFESTATIONS. The disease is one of adult life and chiefly affects men between the ages of forty and sixty years. A history of trauma preceding the development of individual local lesions is often obtained. Pain is a common initial symptom, but pathologic fracture or paraplegia have frequently been the presenting symptoms. Multiple myeloma, Paget's disease, and metastasis constitute the commonest causes of pathologic fracture. Backache as an initial symptom is noteworthy, and the condition should be borne in mind as the cause of such symptoms in the elderly, especially in the presence of osteoporosis and where the pain is not relieved by rest. Fever may be observed in the course of the disease, and pathologic fracture is not infrequent; eggshell crackling may be noted on examining the individual lesion.

The tumors appear as multiple circumscribed areas of destruction in which all parts of the bone are involved.

DIFFERENTIAL DIAGNOSIS. Radiologic examination of the skull, ribs, and vertebrae, estimation of the total serum proteins and serum albumin and globulin, examination of the urine for Bence Jones protein, and sternal marrow puncture are necessary.

The multiple nature of the lesions, the absence of pulmonary metastases, the late age period, and the osteolytic character of the radiologic picture are the significant features. The most likely error is a diagnosis of diffuse secondary carcinomatosis, and a thorough investigation for a demonstrable focus in breast, thyroid, prostate, or uterus must be undertaken.

TREATMENT. When the disease is generalized, with pyrexia, loss of weight, and pain, the administration of such alkylating agents as phenylalanine, nitrogen mustard, and cyclophosphamides may produce bone marrow depression with regression of the disease. When there is thrombocytopenia, hypercalcemia, or renal failure, prednisolone will improve the blood counts.

Solitary Myeloma

Rarely, cases have been described of solitary lesions of bone in which on careful examination the histologic picture has been that of a myeloma typical of the plasmacyte type and in which other lesions have not been demonstrated. Patients with a condition of this character in which the local lesion has been resected or treated by radiation have survived without evidence of recurrence or of other foci developing elsewhere in the skeleton. Accordingly it is now accepted that solitary myeloma constitutes a definite disease entity. Curettage is contraindicated, since it may disseminate disease.

Hemolytic Anemia

Both Mediterranean, or Cooley's, anemia and sickle cell anemia produce bone marrow changes in the vertebral bodies and, most prominently, in the bones of the skull and face. The skull shows a striking picture similar to periosteal "sun ray" formation and is called the "brush skull" (Fig. 45-22); avascular necrosis of the femoral head is also common.

References

Anatomy and Physiology of Bone

Albright, F., and Reifenstein, E. C.: "The Parathyroid Glands and Metabolic Bone Disease," The Williams & Wilkins Company, Baltimore, 1948.

Barnicot, N. A.: Local Action of Parathyroid and Other Tissues on Bone in Intracerebral Grafts, *J Anat,* **82:**233, 1948.

Bourne, G. H.: "The Biochemistry and Physiology of Bone," vol. 1, "Structure," 2d ed., Academic Press, Inc., New York, 1972.

———: "The Biochemistry and Physiology of Bone" vol. 2, "Physiology and Pathology," 2d ed., Academic Press, Inc., New York, 1972.

———: "The Biochemistry and Physiology of Bone," vol. 3, "Development and Growth," 2d ed., Academic Press, Inc., New York, 1972.

Brailsford, J. F.: "The Radiology of Bones and Joints," J. & A. Churchill Ltd., London, 1944.

Dixon, T. F., and Perkins, H. R.: The Chemistry of Calcification, chap. 10 in G. H. Bourne (ed.), "Biochemistry and Physiology of Bone," Academic Press, Inc., New York, 1956.

Duthie, R. B., and Barker, A. N.: Autoradiographic Study of Mucopolysaccharide and Phosphate Complexes in Bone Growth and Repair, J Bone Joint Surg [Br], 38B:304, 1955.

Edeiken, J., and Hodes, P. J.: "Roentgen Diagnosis of Diseases of Bone," The Williams and Wilkins Company, Baltimore, 1967.

Fleisch, H.: Mechanism of Calcification: Inhibitory Role of Pyrophosphate, Nature, 195:911, 1962.

Follis, R. H.: A Survey of Bone Disease, Am J Med, 22:469, 1957.

Freeman, S., and Chang, T. S.: Role of Kidney and of Citric Acid in Production of Transient Hypercalcemia following Nephrectomy, Am J Physiol, 160:335, 1950.

Glimcher, M. J.: Calcification in Biological Systems, Symp Am Assoc Adv Sci Washington 1958, vol. 64, p. 421, 1960.

Gutman, A. B., and Yü, T. F.: A Concept of the Role of Enzymes in Endochondral Calcification, Metab Interrelations Trans Conf 2d, vol. 2, p. 167, 1950.

Harrison, H. E.: The Interrelation of Citrate and Calcium Metabolism, Am J Med, 20:1, 1956.

Hass, G. M.: Studies of Cartilage: Morphologic and Chemical Analysis of Aging Human Costal Cartilage, Arch Pathol, 35:275, 1943.

Heinz, E., Müller, E., and Rominger, E.: Citronensäure und Rachitis, Z Kinderheilkd, 65:101, 1947.

Jackson, S. F.: The Fine Structure of Developing Bone in the Embryonic Owl, Proc R Soc Lond [Biol], 146:270, 1957.

Keith, A.: Bone Growth and Bone Repair, Br J Surg, 5:685, 1918.

Knaggs, R. L.: "Inflammatory and Toxic Diseases of Bone," Wright, Bristol, England, 1926.

Lacroix, P.: "Radiocalcium and Radiosulphur in the Study of Bone Metabolism at the Histological Level," Proc Radioisotope Conf 2d, Oxford Engl, 1:134, 1954.

McLean, F. C., and Urist, M. R.: "Bone: An Introduction to the Physiology of the Skeletal Tissue," The University of Chicago Press, 1972.

Neuman, W. F., and Neuman, M. W.: The Nature of the Mineral Phase of Bone, Chem Rev, 53:1, 1953.

Reddi, K. K., and Nörstrom, A.: Influence of Vitamin C on Utilization of Sulphate Labelled with Sulphur-35 in Synthesis of Chondroitin Sulphate of Costal Cartilage of Guinea Pig, Nature (Lond), 173:1232, 1954.

Robinson, R. A.: Crystal-Collagen-Water Relationships in Bone Matrix, Clin Orthop, 17:69, 1960.

Shearer, W. S.: Review of Radiographic Features of Bone General Affections of Skeleton, Edinburgh Med J, 61:101, 1954.

Sheldon, H., and Robinson, R. A.: Electron Microscope Studies of Crystal Collagen Relationships in Bone. IV. The Occurrence of Crystals within Collagen Fibres, J Biophys Biochem Cytol, 3:1011, 1957.

Siffert, R. S.: Role of Alkaline Phosphatase in Osteogenesis, J Exp Med, 93:415, 1951.

Talmage, R. V.: "Action of Parathyroids on Bone Studied with Radio-isotopes," Blackwell Scientific Publications, Ltd., Oxford, 1962.

Vincent, Y. J., and Haumont, S.: Autoradiographic Identification of Metabolic Osteones after the Administration of Ca 45, Rev Fr Etud Clin Biol, 5:348, 1960.

Metabolic Bone Disorders

Bauer, C. C. H., Carlsson, A., and Lindquist, B.: Bone Salt Metabolism in Human Rickets Studied with Radioactive Phosphorus, Metabolism, 5:573, 1956.

Dent, C. E.: Some Problems of Hyperparathyroidism, Br Med J, 2:1495, 1962.

——— and Harris, H.: Hereditary Forms of Rickets and Osteomalacia, J Bone Joint Surg [Br], 38B:204, 1956.

Fanconi, G., and Girardet, P.: Familiärer persistierender Phosphatdiabetes mit D-Vitamin-resistenter Rachitis, Helv Paediatr Acta, 7:14, 1952.

Fleisch, H., Russell, R. G. G., Bisaz, S., Termine, J. D., and Posner, A. S.: Influence of Pyrophosphate on the Transformation of Amorphous to Crystalline Calcium Phosphate, Calcif Tissue Res, 2:49, 1968.

Fraser, D., Leeming, J. M., Cerwerka, E. A., and Kenyers, K.: Studies of the Pathogenesis of the High Renal Clearance of Phosphate in Hypophosphatemic Vitamin-D Refractory Rickets of the Simple Type, Am J Dis Child, 98:586, 1959.

Gutman, A. B., and Yü, T. F.: Metab Int 2d Conf, 1950, 1967.

McCance, R. A., Morrison, A. B., and Dent, C. E.: Excretion of Phosphoethanolomine and Hypophosphatasia: Preliminary Communication, Lancet, 1:131, 1955.

McKusick, V. A.: "Heritable Disorders of Connective Tissue," 3d ed., The C. V. Mosby Company, St. Louis, 1966.

Rathbun, J. C.: "Hypophosphatasia": New Developmental Anomaly, Am J Dis Child, 75:822, 1948.

Snapper, I., and Nathan, D. J.: Rickets and Osteomalacia, Am J Med, 22:939, 1957.

Osteoporosis

Cooke, A. M.: Osteoporosis, Lancet, 1:877, 1955.

Krane, S. M., Brownell, G. L., Stanbury, J. B., and Corrigan, H.: Effect of Thyroid Disease on Calcium Metabolism in Man, J Clin Invest, 35:874, 1956.

Nordin, B. E. C.: Osteomalacia, Osteoporosis and Calcium Deficiency, Clin Orthop, 17:235, 1960.

Sissons, H. A.: Osteoporosis and Epiphyseal Arrest in Joint Tuberculosis, J Bone Joint Surg [Br], 34B:275, 1952.

Reticuloendothelial Disturbances in Bone

Compere, E. L., Johnson, W. E., and Coventry, M. B.: Vertebra Plana (Calvé's Disease) Due to Eosinophilic Granuloma, J Bone Joint Surg [Am], 36A:969, 1954.

Griffith, D. L.: "Modern Trends in Blood Diseases," Butterworth & Co. (Publishers), Ltd., London, 1955.

Mercer, W., and Duthie, R. B.: Histiocytic Granulomatosis, J Bone Joint Surg [Br], 38B:279, 1956.

Meyer, K., Grumbach, M. M., Linker, A., and Hoffman, P.: Excretion of Sulfated Mucopolysaccharides in Gargoylism (Hurler's Syndrome), Proc Soc Exp Biol Med, 97:275, 1958.

Generalized Bone Disorders

Albers-Schönberg, W.: Roentgenbildung einer seltenen Knochen-
erkrakung, *Munch Med Wochenschr,* **51:**365, 1904.
———: Einer seltener bisher nicht Bekannter Structuranomalie des
Skellets, *Fortschr Geb Roentgenstr Nuklearmed,* **23:**174, 1915.
Bailey, J. A.: Orthopedic Aspects of Achondroplasia, *J Bone Joint
Surg [Am],* **52A:**1285, 1970.
Brailsford, J. F.: "The Radiology of Bones and Joints," J. & A.
Churchill Ltd., London, 1944.

Knaggs, R. L.: "Inflammatory and Toxic Diseases of Bone,"
Wright, Bristol, England, 1926.
Milkman, L. A.: Pseudofractures (Hunger Osteopathy, Late Rick-
ets, Osteomalacia): Report of Case, *Am J Roentgenol,* **24:**29,
1930.
Sofield, H. A., and Millar, E. A.: Fragmentation, Realignment and
Intramedullary Rod Fixation of Deformities of the Long
Bones in Children, *J Bone Joint Surg [Am],* **41A:**8, 1371,
1959.

Chapter 46

Tumors of the Musculoskeletal System

by Robert B. Duthie and Franklin T. Hoaglund

Biologic Properties

Classification of Bone Tumors

True Bone Tumors

Osteoma
Osteoid Osteoma
Osteosarcoma (Osteogenic Sarcoma)
Chondroma
Benign Chondroblastoma (Codman's Tumor)
Chondrosarcoma
Fibroma
Fibrosarcoma
Osteoclastoma (Giant Cell Tumor)

Nonosteogenic Tumors of Bone

Unicameral (Solitary) or Juvenile Bone Cyst
Periosteal Fibrosarcoma
Ewing's Tumor
Reticulum Cell Sarcoma

Blood Vessel Tumors

Aneurysmal Bone Cyst
Hemangioma
Angiosarcoma (Angioendothelioma)

Tumors Arising from Included Tissues

Adamantinoma
Neurilemmoma
Chordoma

Malignant Tumors of Soft Tissues

Metastatic Tumor of Bone

In response to injury, infection, or hormonal disturbance, localized overgrowth of bone, cartilage, or fibrous tissue may occur to give rise to a bony swelling, or "tumor," but these are not neoplasms. In bone there are not only "osteogenic" tissues but many other tissues, i.e., hematopoietic tissue, fat, nerves, blood vessels, which give rise to tumors within bone.

New bone formation may result during malignant ossification, i.e., bone formed by malignant osteoblasts, and *benign* ossification, i.e., bone formed by normal osteoblastic activity in malignantly formed cartilage, osteoid, or collagenous tissues or as reactive bone by normal tissue response to the adjacent malignant process.

Destruction or resorption of bone may result from increased vascularity, by pressure of the tumor or by mechanical compression of the blood vessels with consequent ischemic necrosis and sequestrum formation.

BIOLOGIC PROPERTIES

In relating the site of origin of musculoskeletal tumors to the cellular activity in that area (Fig. 46-1), Johnson has shown that the giant cell tumor commonly arises in the juxtametaphyseal area, where there is much osteoclastic activity, required for remodeling; the osteogenic-osteolytic sarcoma is seen just below this area, whereas the fibrosarcoma is in relation to the endosteum and the round cell sarcoma occurs within the medullary cavity.

The terms "benign" and "malignant" are relative terms; Foulds emphasized that it is the tumor's response to its environment, or any change in this environment, which should be used as a guide to the subsequent behavior of the tumor and, hence, prognosis.

The relative age incidence shows the first peak of mortality between the ages of fifteen and twenty years and a secondary peak from the age of thirty years up to about seventy-five years. The first peak is due mainly to the primary malignant tumors of bone, e.g., osteogenic sarcoma, whereas the second peak is due to malignant neoplasia in such preexisting conditions as Paget's disease.

In the development of a malignant condition there may be either (1) chromosomal or genetic factors or (2) extrachromosomal factors. At the present time, no one single etiologic agent has yet been determined, and probably there are a number of etiologic factors taking part. In studying skeletal neoplasia there are only four known examples of premalignant change:

1. Diaphyseal aclasis (rare) $\longrightarrow$ chondrosarcoma
2. Fibrous dysplasia (few) $\longrightarrow$ fibrosarcoma
3. Irradiated tissues $\longrightarrow$ osteogenic sarcoma
4. Paget's disease (10–20%) $\longrightarrow$ multiple sarcomas (both osteogenic sarcomas and chondrosarcomas)

In diaphyseal aclasis, which is inherited from a dominant mutant gene, lesions rarely undergo chondrosarcomatous changes. In Paget's disease, which is present in about 3 to 4 percent of the European population over the age of forty years, 10 to 20 percent of the patients have been observed postmortem to have developed sarcomas.

Growth patterns and their hormonal backgrounds may have some significance in the development of osteogenic

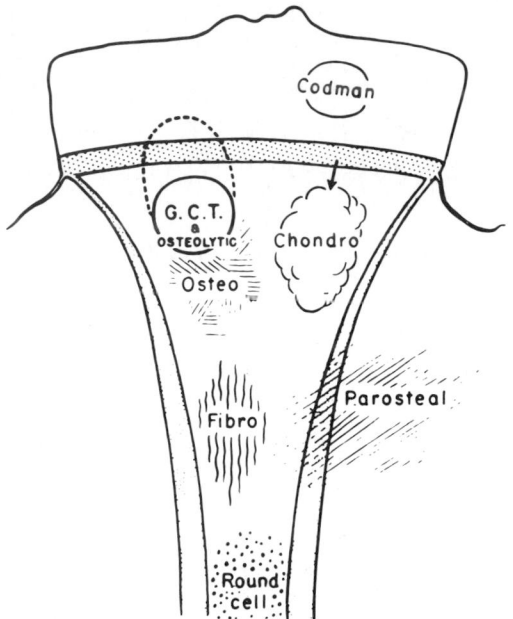

Fig. 46-1. Common sites of origin of bone tumors. (*Used with permission of L. C. Johnson, 1953.*)

sarcoma in males and females. Price has shown that the greatest incidence in females occurs between the ages of five and fourteen years, whereas in males it is between the ages of fifteen and twenty-four years, because males grow longer and larger and, therefore, there are more cells available to undergo malignant change. Extraneous carcinogenic agents are now well recognized; e.g., hydrocarbons, aromatic and azo dyes which can produce fibrosarcoma, and radiation both from internal sources—e.g., plutonium, radium, yttrium, strontium—and from external sources of x-radiation are also well known etiologic factors in osteosarcoma.

CLASSIFICATION OF BONE TUMORS

A. *True bone tumors*—neoplasms arising from cells of mesenchymal origin, whose function is primarily skeletal bone formation. These tumors fall into four main groups according to the predominant cell type present:

B. *Tumors arising from tissues normally found in bone but not participating in bone formation:*
    1. Tumors arising from fibrous tissue
        a. Periosteal fibroma
        b. Periosteal fibrosarcoma
    2. Tumors arising from bone marrow
        a. Myeloma
        b. Reticulum cell sarcoma
        c. Hodgkin's disease of bone
        d. Lymphosarcoma
        e. Ewing's tumor
    3. Tumors from blood vessels
        a. Hemangioma
        b. Hemangioblastoma
        c. Aneurysmal bone cyst
        d. Angiosarcoma
    4. Tumors arising from adipose tissue
        a. Lipoma
        b. Liposarcoma
    5. Tumors arising from nerves
        a. Neurilemmoma
        b. Neurofibroma
C. *Tumors arising from included tissue:*
        a. Chordoma
        b. Adamantinoma
D. *Metastatic tumors*

TRUE BONE TUMORS

Osteoma

This small, sessile, rare tumor is found in the orbit, nasal sinuses, external auditory meatus, and oral side of the mandible. The tumor is dense and hard and is termed *ivory exostosis.*

Bone may form from abnormal growth or imperfect remodeling, and a variety of names have been given depending on the site and etiology.

Irritative exostosis results from lesions causing a proliferation of fibroblasts or granulation tissue with ossification.

Traumatic osteomas are most frequently seen on the femur in relation to the adductor magnus (the so-called "rider's bone") or in relation to the medial collateral ligament of the knee joint (Pellegrini-Stieda disease).

Osteoid Osteoma

This lesion occurs in young males between the ages of ten and thirty years, particularly in the bones of the lower

Cell type predominating	Simple tumor types	Malignant

1. Osteoblast: tumor cells show active ossification.	Osteoma
	  Osteoid osteoma
	  Benign osteoblastoma
		Osteosarcoma
		  Primary
		  Parosteal

2. Chondroblast: tumor cells show active cartilage formation.	Chondroma
	  Benign chondroblastoma
	  Chondromyxoid fibroma
		Chondrosarcoma
		  Primary
		  Secondary

3. Fibroblast: tumor cells show active collagen formation.	Fibroma
	  (?) Solitary bone cyst
	  Nonosteogenic fibroma
		Fibrosarcoma
		
		Rhabdomyosarcoma

4. Osteoclast: tumor cells show active bone destruction by giant cells.	Osteoclastoma	Malignant osteoclastoma

extremities. There is doubt as to whether this is a true tumor.

The patient presents with pain, frequently felt during the night and not aggravated by exercise or position but often relieved specifically, although empirically, by salicylates.

On radiography, a zone of bony sclerosis is seen surrounding a radiolucent nidus (Fig. 46-2).

This condition has to be distinguished from (1) the sclerosing nonsuppurative osteomyelitis of Garre, (2) Brodie's abscess, (3) osteogenic sarcoma, (4) Ewing's tumor, (5) nonossifying fibroma.

Three characteristic regions have been described by Jaffe: (1) an inner region of vascular granulation tissue containing osteoblasts and (2) a zone of calcification and osteoid formation which is surrounded by (3) a zone of trabecular formation of bone in various stages of reorganization (Fig. 46-3).

Complete resection, if possible, will provide cure, but partial removal of the sclerotic bone and the nidus is often sufficient for symptomatic improvement.

Ossifying fibroma is almost exclusively seen in the jawbones of adolescents. It is often asymptomatic, being discovered during dental examinations. Histologically it consists of dense fibroblastic proliferation within compact bone.

Osteosarcoma (Osteogenic Sarcoma)

These tumors arise from cells concerned with bone formation. There are various forms, or types, including myxosarcoma, pseudomyxoma, and osteochondrosarcoma.

Osteosarcoma is rare, about 1 in 75,000 of the population, with a predilection for the second decade.

The tumor occurs in the metaphysis of the femur (52 percent), in the upper end of the tibia (20 percent), and in the humerus (9 percent). Less usual sites are the radius, the ulna, the ilium, and the scapula. The short long bones are rarely affected.

The tumor may originate beneath the periosteum or more centrally in the shaft of the bone and extend in two directions: (1) toward the medulla and (2) to the subperiosteal area, with destruction of bone trabeculae. Initially the periosteum is a barrier and is raised off the bone with new bone formation to produce a fusiform swelling. The intramedullary part of the tumor rarely transgresses the cartilage of the epiphysis.

The tumor may be soft, fleshy, vascular, and destructive, or it may be grayish white, containing cartilage or bone. The new bone may be arranged as scattered islands throughout the tumor which impart a gritty sensation on cutting, and in the form of spicules radiating from the periosteum, giving the "sun ray" appearance on radiography. On the diaphyseal side of the tumor the periosteum is often raised for a short distance, with new bone formation, triangular in shape, and is called Codman's triangle. Pathologic fractures may occur.

Histologically, cells are small and spindle-shaped, with hyperchromatic nuclei with great variation in cell form and shape. The degree of pleomorphism is most marked in the

Fig. 46-2. Tomographs of a patella showing an osteoid osteoma in the right upper quadrant. (*Used with permission from Mercer and Duthie, "Orthopaedic Surgery," 1974.*)

extremely anaplastic tumors in which there are often giant multinucleated cells of bizarre shapes. Mitosis is evident. The intercellular substance may be scanty in amount and in character, being myxomatous, cartilaginous, osteoid, or osseous, according to the degree of differentiation and metaplasia taking place (Fig. 46-4). Blood vessels are thin-walled and numerous.

Pain, especially at night, is usually the first symptom and is caused by periosteal irritation. Such pain in the long bone of a young adult should arouse suspicion of sarcoma. The clinical history of trauma is unreliable. The general

Fig. 46-3. Photomicrograph to show zone 3 of an osteoid osteoma with trabecular bone formation and numerous osteoblasts. (×300.)

Fig. 46-4. Photomicrograph showing numerous "malignant" osteoblasts and pleomorphic cells of an osteogenic sarcoma with new bone formation. (×300.)

condition is good until a late stage with spread when rapid deterioration occurs.

Later, general dissemination of the tumor takes place. While the lymphatic stream occasionally plays a definite role, spread by the blood vessels is predominant. Pulmonary metastases are the most frequent. The first clinical signs of these lesions are usually those of a diffuse bronchitis, but occasionally the cough, dullness, fever, and leukocytosis suggest a diagnosis of pneumonia. Dilated veins may be evident at an early stage.

Pathologic fracture is not typical of osteogenic sarcoma, since the swelling and pain usually keep the patient off his feet. There may be some initial pain and effusion into the nearest joint, but movement is free and painless.

The x-ray appearances (Fig. 46-5) have been categorized:

1. The sclerotic type, usually found at puberty, where dense new irregular bone occurs in the metaphysis and there may be a few spicules projecting from its surface.

Fig. 46-5. Osteogenic sarcoma of the femur. The films show characteristic bone destruction, soft tissue mass, new bone formation, and sclerosis limited to the metaphysis of the lower femur.

2. The osteolytic type, usually metaphyseal. An eccentric translucent gap is found and at its edges a gradual increase of density compared to that of the normal bone.
3. The radiating spicule type, the least common, usually found at puberty in the metaphyseal region.

The radiologic diagnosis may be obvious in the early lesion, but histologic evidence is required and biopsy is indicated. The added risk of any biopsy in view of the already grave prognosis appears justified when compared with the chance that amputation may be carried out unnecessarily on equivocal clinical and radiologic findings.

Until recently the standard treatment has been intensive irradiation with delayed amputation, giving a 5-year survival of about 20 percent. However, with the discovery of Doxorubicin (adriamycin) in 1970, Cortez et al. demonstrated a marked regression in patients with pulmonary metastases. In 1972 Jaffe reported similar results with the use of high-dose methotrexate and citrovorum, hemopoietic tissue-rescue factor. Following these successes, primary amputation with chemotherapy is now producing over 50 percent survivals.

Osteogenic sarcoma has been shown to possess specific tumor-associated antigens. Therefore, attempts are now being made to enhance the host's immune mechanisms either by specific antibodies to the tumor-specific antigen or by sensitized lymphocytes.

Recently Morton et al. reported management of extremity, skeletal, and soft tissue sarcomas with preoperative intraarterial adriamycin and radiation therapy, radical surgical resection, and postoperative chemotherapy or immunotherapy. Some patients in whom bone was resected and replaced with cadaver allografts remained free of disease with functional extremity for as long as 34 months.

OSTEOSARCOMA IN PAGET'S DISEASE. In 10 percent of cases of Paget's disease sarcomatous changes occur. The histologic appearance is similar to that arising de novo in younger patients but appears at a much later age—usually over fifty years. The tumor is more diffuse in character and can arise simultaneously at multiple sites; i.e., it can be polyostotic. Osteosarcoma in Paget's disease has the lowest rate of survival of any of the tumors of the sarcoma series.

PAROSTEAL SARCOMA. This occurs in older age groups and presents as a painful tumor mass, near the knee joint. It is juxtacortical and usually is densely ossified with areas of less ossified or calcified cartilage. There are usually no periosteal reactions, or "sun rays." Growth is slow, but eventual destruction of the cortex with invasion of the medullary cavity by malignant bone and osteoid tissue with malignant connective tissue stroma occurs. Parosteal sarcoma has a better progress than osteosarcoma, particularly when treated with a primary amputation.

Chondroma

Chondroma is a benign tumor arising from the cartilaginous elements of developing bone with slow growth. Calcification frequently occurs in the fibrous septums dividing the lobules. Microscopically there is a chondroid matrix containing cartilage cells; encapsulation and lobulation are present. When ossification does occur, the lesion is known as *osteochondroma*.

If malignancy develops, it does so after the age of thirty-five and occurs most commonly in tumors of the large long bones. If this type of tumor presents as a centrally placed mass of such a bone or of a flat bone, e.g., the ilium or scapula, one must seriously consider a low-grade chondrosarcoma.

When a chondroma occurs in the small bones of the hand or foot, it is known as a *solitary cystic chondroma,* and when it occurs elsewhere within a bone, as a *single enchondroma.* Radiologic features are characteristic. There is a dense shadow, with a feathery outline composed of calcified spicules.

SOLITARY CYSTIC ENCHONDROMA. This occurs in the short long bones of the hand and foot in the metaphyseal region of a proximal phalanx or metacarpal. The tumor arises asymptomatically and is brought to attention by trauma or even a pathologic fracture. If cortical expansion or pathologic fracture occurs, the cyst should be curetted with bone grafting. When the cyst wall is thick and asymptomatic, it should be left alone.

CARTILAGINOUS HYPERTROPHY. This always arises from existing cartilage; when it occurs mainly in the confines of bone, it is known as *enchondroma* and when on the surface, *ecchondroma.*

The common sites are the epiphyseal plates, the cartilaginous parts of ribs (Fig. 46-6), and the symphysis pubis. Such lesions may be part of a generalized chondroosteodystrophy. They rarely, if ever, become malignant and may be multiple, especially in the short long bones of the hand and foot. The well-formed fibrous capsule enables the tumor in most cases to be cleanly excised.

MULTIPLE ENCHONDROMAS. Multiple enchondromas occur in childhood and affect the short long bones of the hand and foot, so that the part may be distorted and appear to be of excessive size. They arise in the center of the shaft as a collection of cartilage cells which, in the process of growth, gradually expand the surrounding cortex (Fig. 46-7).

Operative treatment is indicated when the tumors are rapidly growing and have become unsightly or a source of inconvenience. Complete excision, with curettage and autogenous bone grafting, is the treatment of choice.

Benign Chondroblastoma (Codman's Tumor)

The lesion occurs in an earlier age group, i.e., in the first and second decades, in which the epiphyseal line has not yet closed, and its origin may be from a primitive cartilage cell type.

There is often a long history of a painful swelling with loss of joint function. On x-rays (Fig. 46-8) the typical lesion in the epiphysis is an osteolytic one which contains calcium deposits. Extension into the metaphysis and articular cartilage may occur, but the margin is always discrete and demarcated by a zone of sclerotic or condensed bone. This tumor is most commonly confused with a sarcoma or an inflammatory process such as tuberculosis.

On biopsy, the lesion is found to be very vascular and

Fig. 46-6. Chondroma of the rib.

gritty. Histology shows much chondroid material with "chondroblastic"-appearing cells, which exhibit strong metachromasia and a positive periodic acid–Schiff reaction. Osteoid tissue and calcified areas are seen.

Treatment consisting of adequate curettage and cancellous bone grafting gives excellent results.

Fig. 46-7. Multiple enchondromas of the hand.

Fig. 46-8. Benign chondroblastoma (Codman's tumor) of the humerus.

Chondrosarcoma

This tumor occurs mainly between the ages of twenty and sixty years. It occurs as a primary malignant tumor in the earlier age groups but as secondary malignant change in such conditions as an osteochondroma, in Paget's disease, or diaphyseal aclasia.

The bones most commonly involved are the pelvis, the

Fig. 46-9. Chondrosarcoma of the upper femur showing an expanding lesion with irregular mottling of calcified tissue. No definite periosteal reaction or spiculation is seen.

ribs and sternum, and the femur. Dahlin and Henderson have stated that the nearer a cartilaginous tumor is to the axial skeleton and the larger it is, the more likely it is to be malignant.

On x-ray (Fig. 46-9), there is often frank destruction of trabecular bone and cortex with an expanding lesion which contains irregular flecking or mottling of calcified tissue. With this tumor periosteal new bone formation may be present, in which case it often extends outward.

On biopsy, the sarcomatous mass appears as grayish, translucent, fairly vascular tissue. Histologically, varying degrees of pleomorphism, hyperchromatism, mitotic figures of cartilage cells, and chondroid formation with calcification and ossification are seen (Fig. 46-10).

Thomson and Turner-Warwick have divided this tumor into three types of malignancy:

1. *Low-grade,* a well-differentiated tumor, in which the cells are cartilaginous in type although increased in number, with the matrix well formed. Nearly three-quarters of these patients were alive 10 years after treatment.
2. *Average-grade,* in which there is a reduction in the amount of matrix and an increase in the cellularity, the cells varying in size and shape with nuclear irregularities. Less than half the patients were alive at 5 years, and only one-third were alive at 10 years.
3. *High-grade,* a poorly differentiated cartilaginous pattern with anaplastic cells common, frequent mitoses, and only occasional islands of cartilage seen. This type of tumor behaves similarly to osteosarcoma; i.e., only 1 of 10 patients survived 3 years. Treatment should be excision, using a wide margin, or amputation, especially if recurrence takes place after resection.

Secondary chondrosarcoma arises in a preexisting chondroma, osteochondroma, multiple exostoses, and Ollier's disease, occurring mainly in the pelvis, the vertebrae, the femora, and the humeri.

Fibroma

Benign fibrous tumors of bone are rare lesions and closely allied to the fibrous dysplasias.

The cellular and collagenous fibrous content varies but is usually arranged in whorls. Growth is slow and unlimited with mucoid or necrotic degeneration. Ossification is also common but differs in that the bone is laid down in an irregular manner without the organized compact bone of a true osteoma (Fig. 46-11).

Included in this group is the *nonosteogenic fibroma* (nonossifying fibroma) (Fig. 46-12).

These lesions are usually discovered incidentally by x-rays in children. Roentgenographically, they present as small cortical areas of translucency in the metaphysis. During growth some will disappear. However, a few are displaced toward the center of the bone, where they may grow large, with thinning of the sclerotic cortex.

On biopsy, the tissue is fibrous, containing both fibroblasts and "small" giant cells in a relatively large amount of collagenous fibrous tissue in which rarely there are delicate trabeculae of bone which help to differentiate these lesions from fibrous dysplasia.

Curettage or local resection is indicated.

Fig. 46-10. *A*. Photomicrograph of a chondrosarcoma showing the pleomorphism of the "cartilage" cells with chondroid formation. (×250.) *B*. Photomicrograph of the same tissue showing the characteristics of the malignant cartilage cells. (×500.)

Fibrosarcoma

Medullary fibrosarcomas are characterized by definite collagen formation as the predominant feature, and early destruction of bone. These tumors appear to have a much more favorable prognosis than osteosarcoma, with a 25 percent 5-year survival rate by radical surgical treatment or x-radiation and local excision. Among the patients of Thomson and Turner-Warwick, over 50 percent of those who died had pulmonary metastasis, and a few had malignant deposits in lymph nodes. Thomson and Turner-Warwick differentiate fibrosarcoma from a spindle cell sarcoma, which is distinguished by the complete lack of intercellular substance, by its occurrence in a younger age group, and by its greater radiosensitivity.

Fibrosarcomas have been reported at all ages and as a secondary malignant degeneration in Paget's disease of the

Fig. 46-11. Ossifying fibroma of the mandible in a fourteen-year-old boy with a 1-year history of gradual, painless swelling.

Fig. 46-12. Nonossifying fibroma of the left fourth rib. The patient was asymptomatic, the lesion having been detected on routine chest x-ray.

Fig. 46-13. Fibrosarcoma of the lower femur. The films show a lytic lesion apparently of medullary origin on the distal end of the femur. The lesion is destroying cortex. There is no evidence of sclerosis and new bone formation or any definite soft tissue mass.

skull, etc. They usually occur in long bones around the knee joint, as a central lesion which expands and partially destroys the cortex (Fig. 46-13).

Osteoclastoma (Giant Cell Tumor)

The typical osteoclast is a large cell containing a variable number of centrally placed but distinct nuclei, which are identical in vesicular appearance, ovoid, and basophilic on staining with hematoxylin and eosin. Its cell of origin is unknown, since it is found in many states and conditions of bone. For example, these cells are commonly found in areas where bone is being remodeled, in recesses named *Howship's lacunae*. They also follow hemorrhage into the marrow or during cyst formation and are particularly prominent in hyperparathyroidism or osteitis fibrosa cystica during the formation of the "brown tumor." They are also found in such bone lesions as nonosteogenic fibroma, unicameral bone cysts, aneurysmal bone cyst, fibrous dysplasia, chondroblastoma, osteosarcoma, and histocytic granulomatosis, but these must be clearly differentiated from a giant cell tumor.

The critical feature of this tumor is the vascular and cellular stroma, which is made up of oval-shaped cells containing a small, elongated, darkly stained nucleus with little eosinophilic cytoplasm on staining with hematoxylin and eosin. The stroma cells show a varying degree of

malignancy with the typical features of mitotic activity, pleomorphism, and hyperchromatism (Fig. 46-14). In the more frankly malignant giant cell tumors, the giant cells become anaplastic, with areas of necrotic material and hemorrhage. These true neoplasms occur primarily in the second and third decades with an equal sex distribution. They are seen mainly in the ends of long bones, particularly in the vicinity of the knee and at the lower end of the radius. They commonly arise in the metaphyseoepiphyseal area and are related to the usual osteoclastic activity of remodeling in this area.

On x-rays, the metaphyseoepiphyseal areas are seen to be enlarged and occupied by a clear cystic tumor (Fig. 46-15). The cortex is thin and may sharply limit the tumor from the surrounding soft tissues, with a sharp line of demarcation between the tumor and the unaffected shaft in contradistinction to sarcomas and bone cysts. The expanding osteolytic lesion can continue to destroy the

Fig. 46-14. *A*. Photomicrograph of tissue from a giant cell tumor containing numerous giant cells and scanty stroma. (×300.) *B*. Photomicrograph of the same tissue showing that the nuclei of the stroma appear similar to those of the giant cells. (×500.)

cortex, although usually it leaves some external rim. The tumor grows eccentrically to destroy the epiphyseal cartilage, and it may penetrate the articular cartilage, but rarely does it extend into a joint. Pathologic fractures occur.

Clinically these patients present because of pain and loss of function around the joint, which may even suggest a possible inflammatory lesion or a swelling of an asymmetric nature.

Although in the past these tumors have been regarded as relatively benign, up to 30 percent behave with malignant characteristics despite a benign histologic appearance. There are varying degrees of malignancy of this tumor; because of this, excision is indicated. With curettage there is up to a 50 percent local recurrence rate. Treatment is therefore directed to a complete and total local resection if at all possible. Amputation is occasionally indicated. Radiotherapy has not been shown by Dahlin's group to decrease the recurrence rate, and 10 percent of tumors given such treatment underwent sarcomatous degeneration.

Malignant giant cells are found in osteosarcomas. These are found especially in the more anaplastic lesions and contain a variable number of nuclei but seldom so many as in the osteoclast. The cells and nuclei are irregular in form and size. These features serve to differentiate such malignant giant cells from the osteoclast.

NONOSTEOGENIC TUMORS OF BONE

Unicameral (Solitary) or Juvenile Bone Cyst

This lesion occurs during the years of active bone growth, particularly in the metaphyseal area of long bones, such as the upper end of the humerus and femur. It usually presents because of a pathologic fracture without previous symptoms except for a minor injury.

On x-ray (Fig. 46-16) a characteristic expanding lesion is seen in the metaphysis with thinning of the cortex, as a shell, but it rarely, if ever, penetrates or passes through the still open epiphysis like a giant cell tumor. It is loculated with relatively large cystlike areas.

On biopsy, these cysts are seen to contain a clear, glary fluid with a fine fibrous framework which is relatively avascular. Histologically, the thin fibrous framework is in continuity with the fibrous wall, but there is little cellular activity unless a pathologic fracture has occurred (Fig. 46-17).

This lesion must be differentiated from:

1. *Osteitis fibrosa cystica,* either the generalized form of von Recklinghausen's disease or the localized form. The latter usually occurs during adolescence in the metaphysis, but it tends to spread down the shaft more often. On biopsy, the obvious feature of vascular connective tissue invading cortex and cancellous bone, with degeneration and cyst formation, is obtained.
2. *Hydatid disease.* This usually occurs in the long bones of adults, in which there are localized "solid" masses of hydatid material replacing the marrow, cancellous, and cortical components of bone to extend into the soft tissues.
3. *Tumors.* Giant cell tumors occur in older age groups, and al-

Fig. 46-15. Benign giant cell tumor of the lower femur. The films show a sharply demarcated area of decreased density in the lateral condyle of the femur, extending through the cortex. Some soft tissue swelling around the lesion is visible.

Fig. 46-16. Simple bone cyst of the humerus.

Fig. 46-17. Photomicrograph of the wall of a unicameral bone cyst which is lined with relatively acellular fibrous tissue above the trabeculae of the bone. (×200.)

though the x-ray appearance may be similar, the histologic character is obviously different. Chondromas, myelomas, sarcomas, neurofibromatosis, and secondary metastases must also be differentiated. In sarcoidosis, also to be considered, the tumors are usually multiple, involving the short, miniature bones, such as the metacarpals or phalanges.

Treatment is surgical and directed toward total obliteration of the cavity by a guttering and curetting procedure or collapsing down of the surrounding and thinned cortex by compression. Bone grafting, to restore continuity, is then carried out both with autogenous cancellous bone and overlying cortical matchstick grafts.

Periosteal Fibrosarcoma

This tumor originates in the outer nonosteogenic fibrous layer of the periosteum. It is a fascial sarcoma and similar in character to those arising in other sites in the soft tissues. It is extracortical and neither invades nor infiltrates the bone. The tumor remains encapsulated for a long time; as it grows, it pushes aside the soft tissues but rarely infiltrates them.

Secondary changes eventually appear in the underlying bone, but they result from the pressure and the contact of the tumor. Saucer-shaped erosions may occur where the cortex is in contact with the tumor and areas of new periosteal bone formation at the periphery.

The tumor may appear to be encapsulated, but the capsule merely consists of the condensed surrounding tissues. It remains localized for a considerable time, but ultimately, as the vascularity and cellularity increase, it becomes more malignant. At this stage secondary metastases usually occur in the lungs.

Histologically the tumor is a spindle cell fibrosarcoma with a variable degree of collagen formation. There is no true ossification, but calcification can occur.

Radical removal of the tumor is the operation of choice, with a favorable prognosis when the tumor is encapsulated. If the operation is incomplete, it may be followed by local recurrence and general metastases. The operation should be supplemented by a prolonged course of deep x-ray therapy, although its beneficial effects are questionable.

Ewing's Tumor

In 1921 Ewing described a rare lesion of bone characterized by the development of a tumor from the endothelial marrow of the diaphysis of the long bones, occurring in childhood and associated with febrile attacks. The tumor rapidly involved other parts of the skeleton and was radiosensitive. Willis demonstrated that many of the cases diagnosed clinically and radiologically as "Ewing's tumor," because the histologic pattern demonstrated a rosette formation, were really neuroblastomas, and a primary tumor could be found in the adrenal. Ewing's tumor must also be differentiated from reticulum cell sarcoma (Table 46-1) and from chronic osteomyelitis.

Ewing's tumor usually appears between the ages of five and fifteen. The bones most commonly affected are the tibia, the fibula, the humerus, and the femur. Regional lymph glands may be involved, and polyostotic lesions may be present.

The tumor begins in the diaphyseal marrow; it is grayish white with areas of necrosis and hemorrhage causing destruction of trabeculae and suggesting osteomyelitis. From the medulla the tumor extends to the periosteum, where new bone formation occurs. This has been aptly described as "onion layers."

The tumor is very cellular; the cells are small, round or polyhedral, and arranged in solid cords or sheets with little intercellular substance. The nuclei are always prominent, and mitosis is frequent (Fig. 46-18).

Many tumors show a rosette arrangement, and within the center of the rosette, by special staining methods, fibrils can sometimes be demonstrated, similar to those of a

Table 46-1. DIFFERENTIAL DIAGNOSIS OF EWING'S TUMOR AND RETICULUM CELL SARCOMA

Ewing's tumor	Reticulum cell sarcoma
1. Under 20 years	1. 35–40 years
2. Much periosteal reaction with some bone destruction	2. Little periosteal reaction, but destructive and expanding lesion
3. Small cells with compact chromatin and less well-defined cytoplasm	3. Larger, round, or oval cells with indented, or kidney-shaped, nucleus but poorly defined and stained cytoplasm; delicate framework of interlacing fibers with pattern
4. Radiosensitive	4. Radiosensitive
5. No 5-year survivors	5. 50% 5-year survivors

SOURCE: From W. Mercer and R. B. Duthie, "Orthopaedic Surgery," 7th ed., Edward Arnold (Publishers) Ltd., London, 1974.

Fig. 46-18. Photomicrograph of tissue from the Ewing's tumor of the scapula, to show the marked cellularity with small round cells and little intercellular substance. (×250.)

neuroblastoma. The vessels of both the tumor and the lymphatics may contain obvious emboli, for the tumor spreads by the blood and lymphatic systems.

CLINICAL MANIFESTATIONS. A history of trauma may be elicited, and chronic pain may occur. There may be febrile attacks and leukocytosis. X-rays demonstrate a circumscribed osteoporotic area in the center of the shaft, extending for a considerable distance. Later, the periosteum shows onion-skin layers parallel to the shaft and rather like osteomyclitis, or more commonly small spicules appear (Fig. 46-19). Pathologic fracture seldom occurs. When the vertebrae are involved, there is severe root pain or paralysis. Death usually results from metastatic involvement of the lungs.

TREATMENT. Deep x-ray therapy may cause the local lesion to disappear, but subsequent local recurrence is the rule. Accordingly it has been the practice to follow primary radiation with amputation. Such treatment will not affect the ultimate prognosis in those cases where the tumor has metastasized. Survival is usually about 2 years, and it is commonly stated that the lesions of the so-called 5-year survivors have been misdiagnosed and have really been reticulum cell sarcoma. Dahlin et al. reviewed their experience of Ewing's sarcoma treated at the Mayo Clinic and emphasized that the 5-year survival rate of 133 patients was only 15 percent, 95 patients having died within 2 years of the time of diagnosis.

Reticulum Cell Sarcoma

This tumor occurs in patients between twenty and forty years of age and particularly affects the femur, tibia, and humerus. Pain is often the first complaint, preceding the formation of a tumor which may invade a large part of the shaft.

Radiologically there is an osteolytic lesion in the end of the diaphysis which later extends throughout the length, and pathologic fracture may occur.

Fig. 46-19. Ewing's tumor of the tibia. The films show diffuse bone reaction with periosteal lifting and onion-skin thickening of the cortex plus some spiculation.

The tumor is made up of a pinkish gray granulation tissue, and the cells are larger than a lymphocyte and have round, oval, indented, or lobulated nuclei with considerable cytoplasm. Delicate reticulum fibers pass between the cells, which often show a large number of mitotic figures (Fig. 46-20).

Although the initial response to radiation is good, local recurrence may take place, and therefore radiation should be followed by amputation or radical resection.

BLOOD VESSEL TUMORS

Aneurysmal Bone Cyst

This lesion occurs in the metaphyses of long bones in young people. X-rays show a characteristic lesion of an eccentrically placed osteolytic expansion of the cortex, with some extension into the surrounding soft tissues, and periosteal new bone formation. On biopsy, there is a mass of blood spaces filled with frank blood. Histologically, the characteristic feature consists of cavernous spaces built by fibrous tissue containing some osteoid tissue, but rarely an

Fig. 46-20. Photomicrograph of tissue from a reticulum cell sarcoma showing the rounded or indented cells with large numbers of mitotic figures. (×300.)

endothelial lining. Giant cells may be present, particularly in the more cellular areas of the tumor. Stroma cells are usually fibroblastic and have to be differentiated from those of a giant cell tumor. Local curettage, with or without bone grafting, will give an adequate result.

Hemangioma

Vascular tumors of bone are rare, but the most common sites for these lesions are in the skull and vertebral column. In the vertebral column when the body is affected, the appearance may suggest tuberculosis, secondary neoplasm, or Paget's disease. Collapse of the vertebral body occurs with pressure on the cord.

These tumors are benign in a majority of instances. Treatment is difficult on account of the location of the tumor, but should the lesion be peripheral, radical excision has been advised.

Angiosarcoma (Angioendothelioma)

This is *extremely* rare and must be differentiated from the reticulosarcoma, which may mimic it closely because of the potential endothelial function of reticular cells.

TUMORS ARISING FROM INCLUDED TISSUES

Adamantinoma

Adamantinoma, or adamantine epithelioma, occurs in the jaw and more rarely in the tibia. The long-bone tumors may not be related to adamantinomas of the jaw, since no enamel has been found in them. Pain accompanied by tenderness is commonly the first symptom.

It is a slow-growing tumor the origin of which is unknown. This epithelial tumor may be a basal cell or squamous cell carcinoma. Microscopically it consists of solid strands, sheets, or whorls of dark-staining polygonal or spindle-shaped cells, often with a tendency toward a syncytial character. It shows a tendency to form clefts and cysts, and in most cases there are collections of cuboidal cells arranged in irregular acini. The treatment of choice is amputation, preferably through the more proximal bone. Metastasis has been proved by biopsy in several cases, further emphasizing the need for radical surgical treatment, especially with local bone destruction.

Neurilemmoma

This is a type of nerve sheath tumor which may grow in bone. Clinically the tumor may present as a cystic swelling, and the x-rays show a destruction of the bone. The common and often only symptom is the physical presence of a tumor. This is always single and circumscribed. The clinical course appears to be benign, and local removal appears to be adequate.

Chordoma

Chordoma is a rare malignant neoplasm found at either end of the spinal axis. It is generally accepted as originating from embryonic remnants of the notochord. Although in the adult remnants of the notochord persist in the intervertebral disks in the form of the nucleus pulposus, the majority of chordomas arise in either the sphenooccipital or sacrococcygeal region. Sixty percent occur in the latter area. The physical presence of a tumor is usually the first symptom, though there is often pain in the back with sacral tumors. The tumors are locally invasive and tend to recur after removal.

The radiogram usually shows destruction of bone with an expanding soft tissue shadow (Fig. 46-21). There is nothing characteristic in the bony erosion, and the diagnosis, though it may be guessed at from the site, is usually made by biopsy. The tumor is slow-growing but malignant and kills by invasion of vital structures.

Microscopically chordomas are distinguished with difficulty from atypical chondromas and mucoid, or signet-ring cell, carcinomas arising in the gastrointestinal tract. Myeloblastomas originating in the sacrococcygeal region are usually interpreted as chordomas. The chordoma cells are more epithelial in appearance than cartilage and more variable in size. There is a great tendency for vacuolization and variability in the size of the nuclei.

An attempt at complete surgical extirpation must be made, since these growths are radioresistant.

MALIGNANT TUMORS OF SOFT TISSUES

FIBROSARCOMA OF MUSCLE. These are of two types: differentiated fibrosarcoma with malignant fibroblasts and malignant fibrosarcoma with anaplastic cells. Both usually infiltrate widely, and the patient presents with a painful and large tumor mass, particularly in the thigh.

Fig. 46-21. Chordoma destroying the coccyx of an infant.

Fig. 46-22. Photomicrograph of tissue from a rhabdomyosarcoma to show the giant rhabdomyoblasts with multiple nuclei. (× 350.)

MALIGNANT GIANT CELL TUMORS. These tumors can arise in subcutaneous tissues as well as joint structures, tendons, and tendon sheaths. Their malignancy is variable and can be evaluated by their histologic pattern.

DESMOID TUMOR. This appears to be a very low-grade fibrosarcoma which is locally invasive but does not tend to metastasize by blood. It occurs in the deep muscle masses as a painful tumor or swelling. It has a much better prognosis than a fibrosarcoma, even though it occurs in young people, but it can recur following inadequate resection. Therefore, it is advisable to remove the involved muscle mass in its entirety.

GENERAL PRINCIPLES OF TREATMENT OF SOFT TISSUE MALIGNANT TUMORS. Bowden and Booher have pointed out that usually no capsule surrounds the malignant cells but by rapid growth the surrounding soft tissues may be

Fig. 46-23. Photomicrograph of tissue from a synovial sarcoma to show the large synovioblastic cells forming a villuslike structure. (×350.)

LIPOSARCOMA. This occurs in the soft tissues of the extremities and is one of the more common malignant soft tissue tumors. It presents in the middle age groups with little difference between the sexes. It occurs commonly in the thigh, in the popliteal area as well as in the inguinal and gluteal regions. It does not appear to arise in simple lipomas. Like the fibrosarcoma, these tumors are of two types, well-differentiated and anaplastic. Curative treatment is directed toward wide surgical excision, because their radiosensitivity varies.

RHABDOMYOSARCOMA. This is a malignant tumor involving the striated muscle cells. It occurs commonly in infants and young adults. It has a high incidence of blood metastasis with rapid growth and fungation. Histologically it is characterized by giant rhabdomyoblasts with multiple nuclei which attempt to form myofibrils (Fig. 46-22). It is rarely radiosensitive.

SYNOVIAL SARCOMAS. These occur in subcutaneous tissue as well as in deeply placed muscle layers and have no obvious continuity with joint tissue, although it is supposed that they arise from embryologically sequestered "synovioblastic cells" (Fig. 46-23). They infiltrate and spread locally. Total radical local excision should be carried out and should include the main muscle mass involved.

RETICULUM CELL SARCOMA. This also arises in subcutaneous as well as in muscle layers and develops at any age, growing rapidly and infiltrating widely with metastasis via the bloodstream to the lungs. These tumors have to be differentiated from Ewing's sarcoma.

compressed to form a pseudocapsule. More often this capsule is made up of the peripherally situated neoplastic cells. Therefore, if the malignant tumor is only enucleated, a shell of neoplastic cells will be left behind. The entire muscle bundle surrounding the sarcoma must be removed from its point of origin to its insertion, by sharp dissection as well as ligation of all major tributaries. Amputation is indicated when the anatomic location requires it.

Although in recent decades heroic attempts have been made to reduce the mortality and morbidity of malignant tumors in the upper aspect of both extremities, by such operations as the forequarter and hindquarter amputations, for such tumors as osteosarcoma, Ewing's tumor, etc., these procedures have proved of little value in prolonging life. Their main indication appears to be the need to prevent fungation or ulceration and to relieve local symptoms, except in malignant tumors of soft tissues arising high in the buttock or thigh, such as liposarcoma, fibrosarcoma, or secondary chondrosarcoma. Modification of the classic hemipelvectomy has been described by Sherman and Duthie in which there is less deformity and dysfunction but still an adequate tumor excision. With operation it is possible to obtain a 30 to 40 percent 5-year survival rate.

METASTATIC TUMORS OF BONE

The skeleton is one of the most common sites for metastases, accounting for more than half the cases of malignant bone tumors. Their actual incidence is probably higher than that recorded, since the skeleton is inadequately examined at necropsy. Abrams and his colleagues, in 1,000 consecutive autopsies on patients with carcinoma, described metastases in 27 to 84 percent from prostatic carcinomas, 73 percent from breast, 50 percent from thyroid, and 32 percent from bronchogenic carcinomas. The carcinomas which commonly metastasize to bone arise in the

Fig. 46-24. Osteoblastic metastases from carcinoma of the breast.

breast (about 30 percent; Fig. 46-24), prostate, thyroid, kidney, and lung, as well as from adrenal neuroblastoma. However, skeletal metastases have been found in virtually all types of malignant tumors including melanomas, carcinoids, and testicular, ovarian, and intestinal tumors.

METHOD OF SPREAD. Bone may be involved as a result of direct spread from an overlying tumor such as from squamous carcinoma of the skin in the facial bones and in the calvarium and in the ribs from bronchogenic and mammary carcinoma. However, the usual route is via the bloodstream. This may be by the systemic circulation with the cells entering veins in the tumor, passing through the pulmonary circulation to the arterial bloodstream, and then to the capillary beds. This does not explain the selective distribution of skeletal metastases in the dorsal and lumbar spine, pelvis, rib cage, skull, and proximal end of the femur.

In an attempt to explain the high incidence of metastases in the axial skeleton, Batson has described an alternative route for the dissemination of malignant cells. He has shown that the vertebral venous system, which contains no valves, communicates freely with venous channels of the chest wall and the intrathoracic and abdominal viscera. When the intrathoracic or intraabdominal pressure rises as in coughing or sneezing, the flow of blood in the venous vertebral system can be reversed. By this method malignant cells may be carried into the bodies of the vertebrae or reach the central nervous system.

DIAGNOSIS. Conventional methods of diagnosing skeletal metastases are inaccurate. Of 86 patients with advanced mammary carcinoma, all of whom had skeletal metastases evident on x-ray, only 65.1 percent complained of pain at any stage of the disease, tenderness was elicited in only 16 percent, and the alkaline phosphatase level was raised in only 66 percent. Pain may be localized to a few sites and is not associated with every metastasis.

The serum phosphorus level is raised only when there is associated renal failure with phosphate retention. The serum acid phosphatase concentration is usually elevated in patients with skeletal metastases from prostatic carcinoma.

X-rays also are unreliable. Metastases start growing in the medulla and from there involve the cortex. It has been shown that at least 50 percent of the medulla must be destroyed before a lesion will be seen radiologically. Tomograms are more sensitive.

There is now evidence which indicates that radioisotopes may be more sensitive than x-rays for the early detection of skeletal metastases. Of the bone-seeking isotopes available, the most sensitive would appear to be fluorine 18, although good results have been obtained with ^{47}Ca ^{85}Sr, and ^{87}Sr.

The vast majority of skeletal metastases evoke an osteoid reaction by the invaded bone. The degree of osteoid and new bone formation varies from tumor to tumor. It is most marked in prostatic carcinoma. Because this osteoid has an increased avidity for the bone-seeking isotopes, they can be used for the early detection of skeletal metastases.

The separation of skeletal metastases into lytic or sclerotic, depending on their radiologic appearance, is reinforced by histologic examination. In all metastases there is a combination of destruction due to the tumor and new bone formation caused by the reaction of the bone to the lesion.

Hypercalcemia is found particularly in association with bronchogenic and mammary carcinoma. It is usually produced as a result of the destruction of the skeleton by metastases. As the bone is destroyed, the calcium is released into the circulation. If the kidneys are functioning, the calcium is excreted in the urine as a hypercalcinuria. However, if the kidneys are unable to excrete the increased load, the serum calcium level rises to produce hypercalcemia. Hypercalcemia may also be caused by the secretion of a parathormone-like or parathyrotropic principle by the tumor, which is sometimes found in a bronchogenic carcinoma, by the excretion of a vitamin D–like principle, or by the excretion of specific osteolytic sterols which have been isolated from mammary carcinoma.

TREATMENT. Treatment of skeletal metastases is essentially palliative, although there have been cases described where a solitary metastasis from a hypernephroma has been removed, after the primary tumor was treated, with apparent cure (Fig. 46-25). As many patients may live for months or years with skeletal metastases, it is important to relieve their symptoms.

Pain may occur only in association with hypercalcemia. Once the hypercalcemia has been treated, the pain will be relieved. It may be associated with a pathologic fracture; again, the pathologic fracture must be treated. Large lytic metastases with impending fracture may also produce pain and require treatment. If the patient has a hormonally dependent tumor such as carcinoma of the breast or prostate, the pain is often relieved by hormonal therapy. In carcinoma of the prostate, therapy with diethylstilbestrol diphosphate (stilbestrol), orchidectomy, or a combination of both frequently relieves pain. In mammary carcinoma approximately 27 percent of patients respond objectively to hormonal therapy. In the premenopausal woman this usually consists of an oophorectomy. In the postmenopausal woman diethylstilbestrol is usually given. In both groups when the primary treatment fails to produce a remission, androgens, progestogens, or corticosteroids have been tried; if these fail, endocrine ablative surgery is usually indicated. This includes procedures such as adrenalectomy, hypophysectomy, or pituitary ablation using rods of ^{90}yttrium.

Where hormonal therapy is not indicated or not effective, radiotherapy to a localized area of pain will frequently produce relief. Where the pain is not controlled by radiotherapy or hormonal therapy, analgesics must be given without concern over drug addiction. Interruption of the nerve supply to the painful area is sometimes indicated. This may take the form of phenol blocks, rhizotomies, and even a spinothalamic tactotomy.

Large lytic lesions with impending fracture should be internally fixed. They usually occur in the shafts of the femur or humerus or in the neck of the femur. Lesions in the shafts should be fixed with a closed nailing using a Küntschner nail. For lesions in the neck of the femur a Massie nail pin and plate are required. Following inter-

Fig. 46-25. Solitary metastasis in the radius from hypernephroma. The lesion characteristically involves the more proximal bones such as the humerus and femur.

nal fixation the area is irradiated. Where radiotherapy is given prior to internal fixation, a pathologic fracture may occur, making treatment more difficult.

More than 50 percent of patients in whom a pathologic fracture occurs die of the disease within 3 months, although survivals of 6 years or more after pathologic fracture have been known. Without treatment the fracture will not heal. Since the most common site is the femur, the patient will become bedridden.

When several vertebrae have collapsed, some form of brace may be required. Occasionally compression fractures may be associated with involvement of the spinal cord or cauda equina with sensory, motor, or bladder disturbances. Laminectomy and decompression is urgently indicated, since once paraplegia is established, it is very rarely relieved by surgery. Radiotherapy is very useful for treating pain but usually does not improve an established paraplegia. However, a laminectomy can be carried out only if there is sufficient bone in the vertebral body to prevent complete collapse and instability of the spinal column.

References

Abrams, H. L.: Skeletal Metastases in Carcinoma, *Radiology,* **55:**534, 1950.

———, Spiro, R., and Goldstein, N.: Metastases in Carcinoma: Analysis of 1000 Autopsied Cases, *Cancer,* **3:**74, 1950.

Batson, O. V.: The Role of the Vertebral Veins in Metastatic Processes, *Ann Intern Med,* **16:**38, 1942.

Bowden, L., and Booher, R. J.: The Principles and Technique of Resection of Soft Parts for Sarcoma, *Surgery,* **44:**6, 1958.

Collins, D.: Paget's Disease of Bone: Incidence and Subclinical Forms, *Lancet,* **2:**51, 1956.

Cortez, E. P., Holland, J. F., and Wang, J. J.: Doxorubicin in Disseminated Osteogenic Sarcoma, *JAMA,* **221:**1132, 1972.

Dahlin, D. C.: "Bone Tumours," Charles C Thomas, Publisher, Springfield, Ill., 1957.

———, Coventry, M. B., and Scanlon, P. W.: Ewing's Sarcoma: A Critical Analysis of 165 Cases, *J Bone Joint Surg [Am],* **43A:**185, 1961.

——— and Henderson, E. D.: Chondrosarcoma, A Surgical and Pathological Problem: Review of 212 Cases, *J Bone Joint Surg [Am]* **38A:**5, 1956.

Edelstyn, G. A., Gillespie, P. J., and Grebbell, F. S.: The Radiological Demonstration of Osseous Metastases: Experimental Observations, *Clin Radiol,* **18:**158, 1967.

Foulds, L.: Experimental Study of Tumour Progression: Review, *Cancer Res,* **14:**327, 1954.

Gordan, G. S.: Medical Staff Conference: Hypercalcemia of Malignant Disease, *Calif Med,* **107:**54, 1967.

Grimes, B. J., Fisher, B., Finn, F., and Danowski, T. S.: Steroid-resistant Hypercalcemia and Parathyroid Hyperplasia in Non-osseous Cancer, *Acta Endocrinol (Kbb),* **56:**510, 1967.

Guri, J. P.: Tumors of the Vertebral Column, *J Surg Gynecol Obstet,* **87:**583, 1948.

Jaffe, H. L.: "Osteoid-osteoma": Benign Osteoblastic Tumour Composed of Osteoid and Atypical Bone, *Arch Surg,* **31:**709, 1935.

———: "Tumors and Tumorous Conditions of the Bones and Joints," Lea & Febiger, Philadelphia, 1958.

Jaffe, N.: Recent Advances in the Chemotherapy of Metastatic Osteosarcoma, *Cancer,* **30:**1627, 1972.

Johnson, L. C.: A General Theory of Bone Tumours, *Bull NY Acad Med,* **29:**2, 1953.

Lichtenstein, L.: "Bone Tumors," 3d ed., The C. V. Mosby Company, St. Louis, 1965.

McKenna, R. J, Schwinn, C. P., Soong, K. Y., and Higinbotham, N. L.: Sarcomata of the Osteogenic Series (Osteosarcoma, Fibrosarcoma, Chondrosarcoma, Parosteal Osteogenic Sarcoma, and Sarcomata Arising in Abnormal Bone): An Analysis of 552 Cases, *J Bone Joint Surg [Am],* **48A:**1, 1966.

Marcove, R. C., Miké, V., Hajek, J. V., Levin, A. G., and Hutter, R. V. P.: Osteogenic Sarcoma under the Age of 21: A Review of 145 Operative Cases, *J Bone Joint Surg [Am],* **52A:**411, 1970.

Marsh, B., Flynn, L., and Enneking, W.: Immunological Aspects of Osteosarcoma and Their Relationship to Therapy, *J Bone Joint Surg [Am],* **54A,** 1367, 1972.

Milch, R. A., and Changus, G. W.: Response of Bone to Tumor Invasion, *Cancer,* **9:**340, 1956.

Morton, D. L., Eilber, F. R., Townsend, C. M., Jr., Grant, T. T., Mirra, J., and Weisenburger, T. H.: Limb Salvage from a Multidisciplinary Treatment Approach for Skeletal and Soft Tissue Sarcomas of the Extremity, *Ann Surg,* **184:**268, 1976.

Plimpton, C. H., and Gelhorn, A.: Hypercalcemia in Malignant Disease without Evidence of Bone Destruction, *Am J Med,* **21:**5, 1956.

Price, C. H. G.: Primary Bone-forming Tumours and Their Relationship to Skeletal Growth, *J Bone Joint Surg [Br],* **40B:**574, 1958.

Sherman, C. D., and Duthie, R. B.: Modified Hemipelvectomy, *Cancer,* **13:**1, 1960.

Sissons, H. A., and Duthie, R. B.: "British Surgical Practice: Surgical Progress," Butterworth & Co. (Publishers), Ltd., London, 1959.

Spjut, H. J., Dorfman, H., Feckner, R., and Ackerman, L.: "Tumors of Bone and Cartilage," ser. 2, Armed Forces Institute of Pathology, Washington, 1971.

Thomson, A. D., and Turner-Warwick, R. T.: Skeletal Sarcomata and Giant-cell Tumour, *J Bone Joint Surg [Br],* **37B:**266, 1955.

Willis, R. A.: "Pathology of Tumours," 2d ed., Butterworth & Co. (Publishers), Ltd., London, 1953.

Chapter 47

Fractures and Joint Injuries

by **Franklin T. Hoaglund and Robert B. Duthie**

Fig. 47-1. Types of fractures. Top row, segmental, comminuted, and spiral; bottom row, oblique and transverse.

GENERAL CONSIDERATIONS

Definitions

A fracture is a linear deformation or discontinuity of bone produced by forces exceeding the modulus of elasticity of the bone. The strength of bone may be below normal because of pathologic conditions such as tumor, infection, or metabolic bone disease, which impair its normal viscoelastic properties. If bone is normal, excessive force will cause a fracture. The force applied to the bone may be direct, as when a car bumper strikes a tibia causing a fracture at the site of impact. The force may be applied indirectly by torsional stress, resulting in fracture occurring at a distance from the area of force application.

Fractures are classified anatomically as to location in the bone, e.g., epiphyseal, metaphyseal, or diaphyseal. Fractures are also characterized according to the plane of the fracture surface (Fig. 47-1). In a transverse fracture the plane of the fracture surface is perpendicular to the long axis of the bone. A spiral fracture is one in which the fracture surface is spiral and is produced by torsional stress which fractures the bone along the line of maximal sheer. In an oblique fracture the fracture surface forms an angle with the axis of the shaft. Comminution indicates more than two fragments or potential fragments are present.

A fracture is undisplaced when a plane of cleavage exists in the bone, without angulation or displacement. If separation of bone fragments exists, the fracture is said to be displaced. The direction of displacement is described by the relationship of the distal fragment with respect to the proximal fragments as medial, lateral, posterior, etc. Displacement is measured in terms of the thickness of the shaft; e.g., the distal fragment is displaced laterally one-half the diameter of the shaft. Angulation indicates angular deformity between the axes of the major fragments. It is also described by the position of the distal fragment with respect to the proximal one. Rotational deformity is expressed in similar fashion.

A *closed,* or simple, fracture is one in which the fracture surface does not communicate with the skin or mucous membranes. An *open,* or compound, fracture is one with communication between the fracture surface and the skin or mucous membrane. A *pathologic* fracture is a discontinuity occurring in the bone at an area of weakness caused by pathologic processes including tumor, infection, or metabolic bone disease. A *stress,* or fatigue, fracture is the response of bone to repeated stress, none of which by itself is sufficient to cause a fracture. The earliest pathologic process in stress fracture is osteoclastic resorption, followed by periosteal callus, in an attempt to repair and strengthen the bone. If the repeated stress is halted in time, actual discontinuity of the bone does not occur. A *compression* fracture results when a compression force causes compaction of bone trabeculae, resulting in decreased length or width of a portion of the bone, e.g., compression wedging in thoracic spine fractures. A *greenstick* fracture is an incomplete fracture with the opposite cortex intact. A *torus* fracture is one in which one cortex is intact with buckling or compaction of the opposite cortex (Fig. 47-2).

Diagnosis

The clinical manifestations of fracture are (1) pain, (2) swelling, (3) deformity, (4) ecchymosis, (5) instability, (6) crepitus. The most reliable diagnostic signs are instability and crepitus. Crepitus should not be tested for specifically, since it increases the local soft tissue injury. A specific diagnosis requires two plane film x-rays at right angles to each other, taken at the level of the fracture site. When the patient is examined a few minutes after injury, swelling and ecchymosis may not be present. In such situations, reexamination and/or x-ray diagnosis is necessary. The surgeon should not place absolute faith in the x-rays in ruling out undisplaced or chip fractures. When the patient has significant symptoms and the x-rays are negative, the patient should be treated with splints and re-x-rayed at 14 to 21 days, when sufficient resorption or periosteal new bone formation is present about the fracture site.

Evaluation of the Injured Patient

The immediate threat to a patient's life from an injured extremity is rare but does occur. Associated injuries to the thoracic, peritoneal, and cranial cavities are potentially more serious and should be immediately evaluated and receive priority for treatment. Shock is not usually caused by one injured extremity, although multiple fractures including pelvic fractures may be responsible. Shock is treated by replacement therapy, while splinting of the fractures continues. It is imperative to determine the presence of a fractured spine and prevent subsequent spinal cord injury by proper handling of the patient. At the scene of the accident and/or when the patient arrives in the emergency room, the spine is carefully palpated for tenderness. Before allowing the patient to sit, stand, or be turned, appropriate spine x-rays should be obtained to determine its stability.

Evaluation of the Injured Extremity

The injured extremity is examined immediately for neurovascular, soft tissue, and bone injury. The presence of peripheral pulsations, capillary flow, and peripheral muscle and nerve function are evaluated to determine vascular competence. Neurologic function is determined by evaluating motor power, as well as skin sensation of touch and pinprick. It may be difficult to get the patient to contract muscles which are injured at a fracture site, but with proper splinting a determination of function, based on an accurate knowledge of peripheral nerves, can usually be made.

The presence of intact skin indicates a closed fracture. However, if the skin is severely damaged or abraded and is nonviable, subsequent skin loss may convert a closed fracture to an open wound. Proximity of sharp bone spicules in relation to the skin should be observed and attempts made to prevent further skin damage from the underlying bone. If there is sufficient skin damage and open-fracture surgical treatment cannot be given within the first 6 hours, it may have to be delayed until the skin is healed.

Emergency Splinting of Fractures

After close scrutiny and evaluation of neurovascular injuries and local skin trauma, splinting of the fracture is carried out to minimize further soft tissue or neurovascular injury. If the wound is compound, exposed bone which has been contaminated is not replaced into the depths of the wound until debridement is complete. Splinting of fractures of the knee or distal to the knee or elbow is done with an air splint if available (Fig. 47-3). A pillow splint may be used to bind an injured ankle, or folded magazines bound with loose mesh gauze may be used on forearm fractures. Fractures involving the humerus or shoulder girdle can be splinted by the use of a sling and a swath bandage. Fractures involving the femur require the application of traction over a Thomas splint.

Fig. 47-2. Torus, or buckle, fracture. *A.* AP x-ray, on which the radiolucent line is visible proximal to the distal radial epiphysis. *B.* Lateral x-ray, showing a buckling of the distal cortex of the radius.

Anesthesia for Fracture Reductions

When reduction of fractures is indicated, anesthesia is usually required. An exception to this is the dorsally angulated distal radius in a child, which may be reduced with deft manipulation.

The use of local infiltration anesthesia to the fracture site hematoma can be effective, safe, and minimally hazardous to the patient.

TECHNIQUE. The area overlying the fracture site is cleansed with 2% aqueous iodine and alcohol. An area of undamaged skin is infiltrated with local 2% Xylocaine; a sensitivity to Xylocaine must be determined by the history. The fracture site is entered and infiltrated with a few milliliters of 2% Xylocaine. The hematoma is partially evacuated to accommodate the increased volume of local anesthetic solution. In the case of fractures of both bones of the forearm or bimalleolar fractures both fracture sites

Fig. 47-3. Long leg air splint about the lower extremity.

must be anesthetized. Manipulation of the fracture is not carried out until at least 10 to 30 minutes following fracture site injection.

Peripheral nerve block, spinal anesthesia, general anesthesia, or intravenously administered procaine plus a tourniquet may be required in some closed fractures and is invariably necessary for open wounds.

Open Fractures

An open, or compound, fracture has a direct pathway of communication through the skin or mucous membrane. Regardless of how the injury is sustained, there is resultant contamination of the fracture site and potential infection, i.e., osteomyelitis. Less than adequate treatment by the initial surgeon may result in delayed union, skin loss, loss of joint motion, chronic osteomyelitis, and even amputation. The degree of initial injury to the bone and surrounding soft tissue with its attendant circulation to the bone determines the end result. The union of fractures requires adequate circulation to the bone fragments. When the periosteum, muscle, and skin have been severely traumatized by injury or further devitalized by ill-advised and ill-applied surgical technique, complications, from nonunion to infection, are the end result. Once infection complicates a fracture, adjacent bone may be rendered avascular, which interferes with or prevents union. When circulation to an area of infected bone is still present, the normal response of the bone is to lay osteoid seams about the contaminating bacteria. In so doing, the bacteria are contained, but normal mechanisms of bacterial destruction by phagocytosis are prevented, and chronic osteomyelitis may result.

The major aim in the treatment of open fractures is to prevent infection and provide an environment for bone union. This is accomplished by excising sources of contamination and devitalized tissue without further compromise to local, viable, uninjured tissue. Since all open wounds are contaminated from the instant the bone comes in contact with skin, antibiotic therapy is always indicated. This should in no way be construed as prophylactic antibiotic treatment. However, the umbrella of antibiotic coverage is not a substitute for meticulous, complete, surgical debridement of the wound. Both antibiotic treatment and debridement are basic necessities in the proper management of open fractures. Immobilization of the fragments is needed to prevent further soft tissue devitalization and promote union.

Debridement of open wounds is optimally done within the first 6 hours after injury. In some wounds it may be possible to cover these structures with muscle or skin and to institute appropriate drainage at a distance from tendons, nerves, and blood vessels. Primary closure of open wounds is hazardous and rarely indicated. Secondary closure at 5 to 7 days is preferable.

TECHNIQUE. The following technique is outlined for the treatment of an open tibial shaft fracture with a 6-in. wound over the medial subcutaneous surface of the tibia. Steps in treatment of this wound apply generally to most open fractures.

1. The wound is covered with a sterile bandage and placed in a long leg air splint, as soon as evaluation of the injury is complete.
2. Intravenously administered penicillin, 2 million units, and 1,000 ml of glucose and water are started as soon as the patient arrives in the emergency room (after questioning as to penicillin sensitivity). One gram of streptomycin is given intramuscularly. A booster dose of tetanus toxoid is given, or appropriate human tetanus antitoxin. If the patient does not have an adequate blood level at the time of surgical intervention, 1 Gm of crystalline local penicillin is instilled into the wound prior to closure.
3. In the operating room, under regional or general anesthesia, a sterile sponge is placed over the wound and skin, which has been shaved and prepared with antiseptic, taking care not to contaminate the wound further.
4. Skin edges of the wound are excised, taking only those amounts of tissue necessary to remove avascular and contaminated skin. Relatively clean areas require only a 1- to 2-mm excision. The first set of instruments is then discarded. The leg is then carefully redraped and all devitalized tissue debrided from the depths of the wound. Avascular muscle is recognized by noncontractility, blue or black color, and soft fish-flesh consistency.
5. If necessary, the skin incision is enlarged to expose the fracture site properly. Careful evaluation of damaged skin and a basic knowledge of circulation to skin flaps are required to prevent further devitalization of skin adjacent to the wound.
6. The ends of the bone are exposed with a bone hook, and the fracture surface is gently curetted to remove all sources of debris. Small, detached fragments are removed. Larger fragments are curetted and left in place as judgment indicates.
7. The fracture is aligned and the skin approximated over exposed bone if possible. As a rule, some area of the wound is left open; if there is any question about adequate debridement, the entire wound is left open. Only under optimal conditions should the wound be closed tightly.
8. The leg is immobilized in a well-molded plaster cast over two thicknesses of sheet wadding. If there is a question of viability of the foot or difficulties with position of fracture fragments, skeletal traction through the os calcis, with the leg on a Böhler-Braun frame, may be used.
9. Intravenous Keflin or another appropriate antibiotic is administered prior to and during debridement in order to have therapeutic levels at the fracture site hematoma. Antibiotics are continued for a minimum of 10 to 14 days postinjury. The cast is split to relieve swelling of the leg, as necessary. The wound is inspected at 5 to 7 days, and secondary closure carried out. If the wound is not sufficiently clean at that time, the wound may be left open and early weight bearing started.

In an occasional fractured tibia with a 1-mm puncture wound caused by penetrating bone from the inside with good evidence that it did not penetrate the pants leg of the patient, surgical exposure of the bone may not be necessary. In the rare case where these conditions prevail, antibiotics are indicated and continued for a minimum of 2 weeks.

Vascular Injury

Major arterial injury should be suspected with any fracture-dislocation or trauma to an extremity. The first diagnostic consideration must be the determination of vascular competence. A maximal time limit for irreversible change from complete muscle ischemia is 6 to 8 hours, and delay in diagnosis may result in ultimate amputation. Arterial injury may accompany any fracture or dislocation, although certain fractures or dislocations, such as supracondylar fractures of the humerus or femur, femoral shaft fractures, and knee dislocations, carry a higher incidence. Gunshot wounds and open fractures have the highest incidence.

The diagnosis of vascular compromise may be difficult. One should never hesitate to seek experienced consultation when the diagnosis is in doubt. Diagnosis depends on evaluation of skin color, warmth, capillary return, ischemic pain, motor and sensory nerve function, and the presence of arterial pulsations. In the upper extremity, the ability of the patient to extend the fingers actively or passively in the absence of pain and in the presence of good capillary return is good evidence for adequate circulation. The absence of a radial pulse in the presence of these findings is not in itself an indication for vessel exploration. However, the hand must be normal in all aspects. If the radial pulse is absent and hand circulation is in doubt, because of associated local injury, exploration of the proximal arterial supply is indicated.

In the lower extremity, the determinations of pedal pulsations may be difficult. Oscillometric or Doppler determinations will aid in the diagnosis and assist in localization of pulsatile arterial flow. Capillary flow, skin color, warmth, and sensation are difficult to evaluate. Pain due to ischemia is characteristically severe and unrelenting, and continues after the fracture is splinted, reduced, or immobilized. Most patients show marked improvement in comfort when a fracture is immobilized. This is not true of the patient with a fracture and associated arterial insufficiency. Glovelike anesthesia is an important early sign of ischemia.

Griffiths has categorized the signs of vascular compromise by the four P's: pain, pallor, pulselessness, and paralysis, either sensory or motor. When two of these signs are present and vascular insufficiency cannot be ruled out, exploration is indicated. It must be emphasized that the injured limb must be evaluated and reexamined at intervals. Initial injury may produce only intimal trauma, resulting in delayed thrombosis with delayed onset of signs of vascular compromise.

Hypoxemia and the Fat Embolism Syndrome

Tachakra and Sevitt have shown that 50 to 60 percent of patients with femoral shaft fractures will have reduced arterial blood oxygen concentrations either immediately or within 2 to 3 days post injury. Fat macroglobules from the marrow or other sources occluding the pulmonary circulation are the most likely cause. About 10 to 20 percent of patients with femoral shaft fractures will also develop skin petechiae and/or central nervous system depression in addition to hypoxemia within 3 days post injury. This combination of signs is referred to as the fat embolism syndrome. The incidence is greatest in patients with femoral shaft involvement, occurs not infrequently with tibial fractures, and may occur with any fracture or other conditions such as sepsis where bone has not been injured. The diagnosis is a clinical one. Tests for urinary and sputum fat or serum lipase have not proved specific.

All patients with femoral shaft fractures should have their arterial blood gas tested on admission to hospital; if it is low, the patient should be given oxygen and his or her condition should be carefully monitored both for clinical signs of fat embolism and for subsequent changes in arterial blood oxygen concentration. In patients not responding to oxygen administration, corticosteroids may be of some benefit. Other therapeutic agents include the use of dextran to improve microcirculatory flow and decrease platelet adhesiveness, low-dose heparin for its plasma-clearing effect, and Lasix, especially if there is any question of fluid overload.

Peripheral Nerve Injuries

Soft tissue injuries and fractures of the extremities are not infrequently accompanied by injuries to the peripheral nerves (see Chap. 42). The clinical manifestations and course depend on the degree of injury. With the least severe of nerve injuries, which has been referred to as "neurapraxia," there is a physiologic interruption of nerve conduction manifested by a transient incomplete or complete paralysis and associated with recovery within a 10-week period postinjury. This type of lesion occurs with minor stretch injuries and contusions, and as a result of local continuous pressure on the nerve. With severe stretch injuries, as in brachial plexus stress, or trauma associated with fractures Wallerian degeneration of the axon may occur while the Schwann sheath remains intact, i.e., axonotmesis takes place. In this circumstance, there may be axonal regeneration, and the prognosis is good. The most severe lesion is complete division of the nerve, neurotmesis, which can accompany violent stretch in open or closed fractures.

The axiom that closed soft tissue wounds and fractures cause nerve injuries in continuity, i.e., neurapraxia or axonotmesis, is generally reliable. Peripheral nerve injuries associated with open wounds are more likely to result in actual division of the nerve. Peripheral nerve injuries in continuity should be allowed to heal spontaneously, while transected nerves require nerve suture at a time when surgical repair is feasible. The conservative treatment of a closed fracture should not be altered because of associated peripheral nerve injury. However, attention should be given to splinting the limb in order to maintain the function of unopposed paralyzed muscles and avoid contractures. If treatment of the fracture requires open reduction, this affords an opportunity to inspect the nerve. It is not always possible to recognize the extent of local nerve injury at the initial surgical procedure, since local inflammation, which persists for about 10 days, interferes with determination of the junction between injured and normal nerve.

Neurotmesis, or division of the nerve, requires exact approximation of the nerve ends, so that regeneration of the axon can proceed into the distal portion of the severed tube. Peripheral nerve injuries which should be repaired primarily are sharp lacerations without adjacent stretch, a situation which does not commonly pertain when there are associated soft tissue injuries or fractures. Divided digital nerves are difficult to repair secondarily if length is a problem and do well with primary repair because of their pure sensory character.

At the time of debridement for open fractures, the nerve should be inspected and, if in continuity, should be left undisturbed. If transected, the nerve ends may be loosely approximated and this procedure followed by early delayed repair when the extent of the lesion can be accurately defined. The operative microscope can facilitate examination of the extent of injury and allow primary repair in some situations. It may be necessary to delay repair until the fracture is healed. In general, nerve suture is technically easier after 10 days, at which time the sheath has thickened. Following nerve injury and/or nerve repair, continued critical evaluation by physical examination and a variety of specific tests is necessary to determine the progress of healing.

Injury to Bone

After injury to bone there are three main morphologic sequences that overlap in time and space. These are concerned with actual injury to cells and tissues, with defense and demolition, and with healing and regeneration.

IMMEDIATE INJURY. The immediate injury results in structural and chemical changes in cells and tissues, which may or may not die; vascular changes (hemorrhage, clotting, and exudation); and neurogenic changes. Miles has described two early phases: an early phase, mediated by the local release of histamine from mast cells, platelets, and other blood cells, and a delayed phase, in which there is activation of peptide systems to form plasma kinins, as well as the globulin permeability factor of Spector and Willoughby. The vasoconstrictor amine epinephrine may also be inactivated locally.

Wilhelm has characterized permeability factors as belonging to three main groups: (1) the proteases, e.g., plasmin (fibrolytic), kallikrein (vasodepressor), and the globulin permeability factor; (2) the polypeptides, e.g., leukotaxine, bradykinin, and kallidin; and (3) the amines, e.g., histamine, 5-hydroxytryptamine, epinephrine, and norepinephrine. These substances are believed to produce increased permeability, cellular migration, small vessel dilation (similar to the triple response of Lewis), and alteration in the diffusion mechanisms of the intercellular matrix or ground substance.

From damaged capillaries or from increased capillary permeability, protein-rich plasma and numerous cells—lymphocytes, neutrophils, and eosinophils—leak out. Plasmacytes are thought to be derived from these lymphocytes and are believed to hold or synthesize within their cytoplasm nucleoproteins liberated by the autolysis of cells, the necrosis of tissues, and protein leak.

Following this, a clot of insoluble fibrin forms. This protein is derived from the circulating soluble fibrinogen by the addition of two amino acids—phenylalanine and lysine—in the presence of thrombin, calcium, platelets, and other clotting factors. The amino acids are derived from serum albumin, γ-globulin, and the globulin of red blood cells from the extravasated blood. Fibrinogenesis provides a screen, or framework, of fibrin fibers to collect plasma proteins and extravasated cells. This framework is invaded by reticuloendothelial cells, e.g., macrophages, round cells, and histiocytes; by endothelial cells, which undergo mitosis to form capillaries; and finally by fibroblasts. The fibrin filaments are oriented to provide a framework for the fibroblasts and capillaries to follow along definite patterns. The fibroblasts arise from undifferentiated mesenchymal cells and synthesize acid mucopolysaccharides, which are used later in collagen formation. Although mast cells contain acid mucopolysaccharides in their cytoplasmic granules, they are not the direct source of this material for collagen synthesis.

DEFENSE AND DEMOLITION. In the defense-and-demolition stage there are significant vascular reactions that affect inflow of tissue fluids and cellular infiltration. The arterioles and efferent veins particularly are involved. There is redistribution of blood flow through capillary channels by shunt mechanisms under poorly understood neurogenic reflexes.

Wray and Lynch have shown a quantitative increase in vascular volume of fractures by enlargement of existing vessels, as well as formation of new ones. Rhinelander and Baragry, in bone microangiographic studies, saw a marked opening of the existing medullary arterial tree within the first day, but it was not until the fourth day that periosteal vessels were seen entering the fracture site. Accompanying these changes was a marked infiltration of polymorphonuclear leukocytes, lymphocytes, and monocytes. This infiltration alters the physical state of the ground substance from a solution to a gel and produces autolysis, phagocytosis, and digestion of debris. Plasmin, with its fibrinolytic and permeability effects, is formed from the circulating but inactive serum protein plasminogen. Plasmin is considered to be able to digest necrotic mesodermal tissues and to release further active substances. Lack has demonstrated its autolytic digestion of articular cartilage. Mast cells may influence white cell migration because of their heparin content and stimulate phagocytic activity because of their 5-hydroxytryptamine content, but these actions have not yet been clearly demonstrated.

HEALING AND REGENERATION. Blastema formation results from hyperplasia and proliferation of undifferentiated mesenchymal cells, from monocytes, from lymphocytes, and from pseudolymphocytes, which form fibroblasts. The phylogenic characterization, or specific naming of cells, is much more certain in this stage, because their functions and environments are more clearly understood; e.g., fibroblasts form collagen, myxoblasts form ground substance, chondroblasts form cartilage, and osteoblasts form bone. Such changes are very rapid. Tonna and Cronkite have demonstrated marked proliferation of local mesenchymal cells making up the periosteum within 16 hours of wounding. Within 3 days the proliferative reaction spreads some distance along the shaft away from the fracture site.

There have been many attempts to determine the stimulus for such proliferation. Abercrombie reviewed various "wound hormones" and suggested that increased mitosis and increased migration of cells are produced by one chemical stimulus. A possible factor which accelerated the healing of skin wounds has been demonstrated in cell-free extract of human granulation tissue. A wound factor in amphibian tissues produced by damaged tissue at the time and site of wounding has been proposed. It also has been demonstrated that injured cells liberate a growth-promoting factor in the inflammatory exudate. The stimulation factor also had been thought to be present in the organized blood clot of the fracture hematoma, and to promote new bone formation by the "chronic irritation of the necrosis and hemorrhage."

During a study of fracture repair in rats, Duthie and Barker noted the accumulation of mast cells in greater numbers than those seen in the opposite (control) leg within 48 hours of the fracture, which persisted for the next 7 days. Because of this, it was suggested that mast cell appearance was related to the trauma, and that these cells might function in the ensuing regeneration processes, especially because of their cytoplasmic content of histamine, heparin, and 5-hydroxytryptamine. Mast cells subsequently were observed during the response of standard fractures to various systemic and hormonal change, as well as to locally applied drugs.

The result of the hyperplasia and proliferation of mesenchymal cells is the callus which obliterates the medullary cavity and connects the two ends of bone by irregularly surrounding the fracture defect. With sufficient organization of this callus the fracture site becomes clinically stable. The early bone of the callus is fiber bone which has spicules perpendicular to the cortical surface. This is gradually replaced and remodeled with osteonal bone. Conversion and remodeling continue up to 3 years following an acute fracture. Motion plays a role in the amount of cartilaginous tissue formed. Anderson has shown that when fractures are initially fixed with compression, eliminating motion, there is little callus from the endosteum and none from the periosteum. There is direct bridging of the fracture site by endosteal callus and bone formation.

The use of weight-bearing treatment for fractures of long bones has raised questions about the need for strict immobilization to achieve union. When patients bear weight on a healing fracture, motion at the fracture site results. Despite this, the stability of the callus formation is greater sooner, resulting in more rapid union. It is possible that rapidity of union is explained by better approximation of bone ends and compression forces across the fractured surfaces, but it seems likely that altered circulation either from rhythmic contraction of muscles or from changes in medullary blood flow as a result of this are responsible. Further experimental work in this area is needed.

All processes involved in fracture healing occur much more rapidly in children, accounting for the rate of fracture union and the almost unheard of nonunion in this age group.

Delayed Union and Nonunion

Delayed union is an ill-defined term arbitrarily applied to fractures taking longer than average to heal. It should be defined in relation to the specific fracture for which it is used.

Nonunion refers to a fracture in which healing cannot be expected even with prolonged immobilization. X-ray examination of a nonunion will reveal sclerosis of bone ends, plugging off of the medullary canal with sclerotic bone, rounding of the adjacent fracture surfaces, and a definite defect between the fragments, consisting of fibrous tissue, cartilage, etc.

Wray has pointed out that the normal contribution of fracture callus is primarily from the surrounding soft tissues and vascularization of the callus occurs from the same soft tissues. Most nonunions are of local origin and are the result of inadequate callus or vascularization of this fracture callus. They frequently occur in young adults in whom there has been excessive soft tissue destruction or infection.

Inadequate reduction of a fracture may result in, or be caused by, interposition of soft tissue between the bone ends, interfering with callus formation. Inadequate immobilization predisposes to the formation of fibrous or cartilaginous tissue instead of osteoid or bone. The most common cause of nonunion is local damage to the soft tissues surrounding the fracture. A frequent cause is ill-advised operative reduction of fractures. When open reduction of fractures is done, every attempt should be made to minimize periosteal stripping and devitalization of the fracture area. Local infection, destroying adjacent soft tissue, may contribute to delay or nonunion, but the possibility exists for healing in the presence of infection.

Pathologic Fractures

Fractures occurring through abnormal bone which has been weakened by a preexisting pathologic condition is considered a pathologic fracture (Fig. 47-4). Whenever fractures occur with minor trauma, consideration should be given to generalized or local bone disease.

In children, developmental diseases such as osteogenesis imperfecta, osteopetrosis, or nutritional deficiencies such as rickets or scurvy may result in pathologic fractures. Unicameral bone cysts, aneurysmal bone cysts, eosinophilic granulomas, fibrous dysplasia, and any of the primary or secondary malignant processes also may weaken a bone sufficiently to cause pathologic fracture.

Idiopathic osteoporosis in the adult is a common cause of pathologic fractures, as is osteoporosis associated with prolonged cortisone therapy. Hyperparathyroidism should always be considered, since it is a correctable lesion.

Patients with slow-growing metastatic bone tumors, for example, from breast or kidney, should be carefully followed in an attempt to prevent pathologic fractures. Sizable bone lesions occurring in the femoral or humeral shafts should be prophylactically nailed, since this may save the patient considerable morbidity.

Stress Fractures

Stress fractures occur in characteristic locations in specific age groups and certain occupational situations. Stress or fatigue fractures are the end result of repeated stress to a bone which would not be injured by isolated forces

Fig. 47-4. Pathologic fracture. Metastatic carcinoma with pathologic subtrochanteric fracture of the femur. There is diffuse involvement of the adjacent pelvis.

of the same magnitude. Johnson et al. have shown that repeated stress causes accelerated osteoclastic remodeling in areas of bone which have not yet been converted to osteonal bone. Following osteoclastic resorption, with a loss of normal structural mass, there is new periosteal bone formation in an attempt to strengthen the weakened area. If the repeated stress is discontinued, the bone may not go on to fracture. Patients complain of aching pain following unusual activity during the early phases of this process and go on to complete fracture if the stress activity is not discontinued.

Stress fractures commonly occur in young soldiers required to force-march. The second and third distal metatarsal shafts, proximal tibia, distal fibula, and calcaneus are common sites (Fig. 47-5). Early in the course of the symptomatology, x-ray findings may reveal only subtle osteoporosis at the stressed area, but later new periosteal bone formation occurs with incomplete or complete fracture.

Treatment of stress fracture is immobilization and discontinuance of the fatiguing activity.

Epiphyseal Plate Injuries

Longitudinal growth of bone occurs by cartilaginous growth at the epiphyseal plate and conversion to bone by endochondral ossification. Interference with normal epiphyseal growth will result in abnormalities of length of the affected bone or deformity. Epiphyseal separations occur consistently between the uncalcified hypertrophying cells and the zone of provisional calcification, which is the weakest area through the plate. In such an injury, normal growth will continue, since the proliferating cells are still attached to their blood supply in the bony epiphysis. Any injury which damages the proliferating cells or interferes with circulation may cause growth disturbance.

Salter and Harris have devised a classification of epiphyseal plate injuries, with a rationale for treatment. Type I is a complete separation of the epiphysis from the me-

Fig. 47-5. Stress fracture of the distal second metatarsal shaft. Note periosteal new bone formation about the transverse defect proximal to the second metatarsal head.

Fig. 47-6. Salter and Harris classification of epiphyseal injury Type I. See text for description. *A.* Types I to III. *B.* Types IV to V.

Fig. 47-7. Type II epiphyseal separation at the distal radius. Distal radial epiphysis is displaced dorsad and ulnarward with a fragment of the metaphysis.

taphysis without bone fracture (Fig. 47-6). Such injuries occur at birth or in early childhood in scorbutic bones. Treatment is by closed reduction, and the prognosis is excellent, since the proliferating cells and blood supply have not been damaged.

Type II is a separation along part of the epiphyseal plate with a fracture through the metaphysis (Fig. 47-7). It commonly occurs at the distal radial epiphysis or distal tibial epiphysis. Treatment is closed reduction, and the prognosis is excellent, even though reduction is not anatomic (Fig. 47-8).

Type III, epiphyseal plate injury, is an intraarticular

Fig. 47-8. *A* and *B.* AP and lateral x-rays showing lateral displacement of the distal tibial epiphysis with the fracture line extending into the distal metaphysis and also through the medial malleolus with fracture of the distal fibular shaft. *C* and *D.* Oblique and lateral x-rays in plaster following successful closed manipulation.

fracture, extending from the joint surface through the bony epiphysis to the plate and then along the plate to the periphery.

Accurate reduction is necessary to minimize articular deformity. The prognosis is good if the blood supply to the fractured portion has not been compromised.

Type IV is also an intraarticular epiphyseal injury. The fracture line extends through the joint surface across the bony epiphyseal plate and through a portion of the metaphysis. The commonest Type IV injury is a fracture of the lateral condyle of the humerus. Anatomic reduction and usually open reduction are required to prevent union across the epiphyseal plate at the fracture site and growth abnormality.

Type V epiphyseal plate injuries are those in which severe crushing damages the epiphyseal plate. Displacement is not common, and the initial severity may go unrecognized. Because of crushing injury to the proliferating cartilage cells, growth disturbances may occur.

With any injury or suspected injury to an epiphyseal plate, the parent of the child should be cautioned that growth abnormalities are possible. Type IV and Type V injuries are more likely to cause growth disturbances. Injuries which interfere with the blood supply to the epiphysis or damage proliferating cells will result in greater deformity in the young child. However, if neither of these occurs, the younger child has greater remodeling potential where accurate reduction cannot be obtained.

Fractures in Children

A fracture in a child presents different problems from those of a similar fracture in the adult. Compound fractures are much less common than in the adult. Nonunion is almost unheard of in children. Fracture healing is more rapid with the younger patient.

The challenge in handling children's fractures is in recognizing and understanding what degree of fracture site angulation, displacement, and shortening will be corrected, in relation to remaining growth potential. The presence of healing fracture callus in the neighborhood of an epiphysis causes epiphyseal stimulation. If a displaced femoral shaft fracture is reduced anatomically, overgrowth and leg length inequality will ensue. If rotational deformity at a fracture site involving a long bone is not corrected, permanent deformity results. However, certain degrees of angulation, displacement, and shortening will be corrected and remodeled depending upon the age of the child. Shaft fractures in the long bones must not be opened because of the hazard of infection or epiphyseal growth disturbance and deformity. However, certain articular and epiphyseal fractures must be recognized and anatomically reduced.

Closed Reduction versus Open Reduction

The optimal method for handling a specific fracture should (1) permit rapid union, (2) reestablish length and alignment of the injured extremity, (3) restore complete painless range of motion of adjacent joints, and (4) return the patient to gainful functional activity, with as little morbidity and hazard to the patient as possible.

The closed treatment of fractures has the advantages of little or no risk of infection or subsequent interference with local blood supply to the fracture site. However, closed treatment requires prolonged traction or immobilization which may cause restriction of joint motion, and accurate anatomic restoration of length and alignment may not be possible.

In order to obviate the difficulties of prolonged immobilization and overcome the problems of inaccurate reduction, open reduction and internal fixation have been proposed. However, open reduction carries the risks of local infection and delayed union resulting from compromise of local blood supply to fracture fragments. Also, internal fixation may not provide sufficient immobilization of fracture fragments to permit early motion of adjacent joints.

Despite the disadvantages of each technique, closed treatment is frequently indicated for some situations, while open reduction is mandatory for others. The system of internal fixation devices has been developed by Muller and colleagues; it provides stainless steel plates fixed to bone with a modified bone screw and employs the principle of compression across fracture surfaces. This technique has allowed early joint motion when sufficient stabilization of the fracture site has been accomplished, which may allow earlier and more complete return of joint function. Surgeons using this technique should bear in mind the hazards of open reduction outlined above.

Application of Plaster Casts

External immobilization for fractures and dislocations is obtained by the application of plaster casts. Plaster consists of anhydrous calcium sulfate, which solidifies with hydration. Plaster, to which water is added, sets up in minutes but does not completely dry for 36 to 48 hours. It comes in rolls or strips of crinoline bandage to which anhydrous calcium sulfate has been added.

Plaster in rolls is applied circumferentially to make a cast but never wrapped directly on the skin. Strips are used to construct splints by applying a strip of plaster to one surface of an extremity without intervening padding. When plaster is applied for an acute injury, sufficient padding should be employed to accommodate the anticipated swelling. As a general rule, one layer of stockinet and one layer of sheet wadding or webril is sufficient with extra padding for bony prominences. The cast is applied smoothly and molded over bony prominences and articulations. In order to permit evaluation of peripheral circulation, the toes or digits are never completely enclosed with plaster.

Postinjury patients in plaster casts should be placed in bed with the extremity elevated. The nursing staff and house staff should be completely familiar with cast complications and signs of impending vascular insufficiency. The patient should never be sent home when the possibility of circulatory compromise exists.

COMPLICATIONS OF PLASTER CAST TREATMENT. The most serious complication associated with plaster casts is the development of vascular insufficiency due to unrelieved swelling. The cast will not shrink, but it may restrict soft tissue swelling to the point of gangrenous necrosis. Unrelieved pain, pulselessness, pallor, and sensory or motor paralysis are signs of this complication. Unrelenting pain should be investigated immediately and not allowed to progress to the point where other signs are present. Narcotics are administered with great caution to patients in plaster. Unrelieved pain beneath the cast should be treated by splitting the cast with parallel cuts on the opposite sides of the extremity, to allow anteroposterior swelling. The cast is split down to include the underlying padding, since blood-soaked padding may be as resistant as plaster and not allow sufficient expansion. Leg casts are split medially and laterally in their entirety, and forearm

Fig. 47-9. Long leg cast.

Fig. 47-11. A 1½ hip spica.

Fig. 47-12. Short arm cast.

Fig. 47-13. Gauntlet cast.

casts split along the radial and ulnar borders of the arm.

Patients who complain of burning pain at a localized site in the cast should be suspected of a pressure point from the plaster. This commonly occurs over the site of a bony prominence. This is investigated by cutting an appropriate window and inspecting the underlying skin. Skin necrosis may result and be associated with pain relief due to damage of sensory receptors. When a point of pressure is detected, the cast window should be hollowed out and sufficient padding applied to relieve the pressure. Windows in the cast should always be replaced, or local swelling will occur through the window and cause pressure on the skin at the window margins.

TYPES OF PLASTER CASTS. Casts for fractures should immobilize the joint above and the joint below the fracture. Plasters which include the ankle are extended to the bases of the toes to prevent swelling, edema, and irritation of the forefoot. A long leg cast extends from the bases of the toes to include the knee and thigh as high as possible (Fig. 47-9). A boot cast extends to the level of the tibial tubercle (Fig. 47-10). A cylinder cast is a circular cast which extends from just above the ankle to include leg, knee, and thigh. It is used for immobilization of the knee.

A hip spica is a plaster designed to immobilize the hip. A single hip spica extends from the nipple line or upper abdomen to include the pelvis and one thigh and lower leg. A double hip spica immobilizes the pelvis and extends to include both thighs and lower legs. A 1½ hip spica extends only as far as the knee on one side (Fig. 47-11).

A short arm cast extends from below the elbow to the proximal palmar crease, leaving the entire thumb free (Fig. 47-12). A gauntlet cast is similar but includes the thumb (Fig. 47-13). A long arm cast extends from the proximal palmar crease, leaving the thumb free to include the elbow and arm as far as the axilla (Fig. 47-14). A shoulder spica is a body jacket with the plaster immobilizing the shoulder and elbow.

Body casts are applied for immobilization of the spine

Fig. 47-10. Boot cast.

Fig. 47-14. Long arm cast.

Fig. 47-15. Buck's traction.

and extend to the groin and as high as the sternum, anteriorly. They may be applied with plaster straps across the shoulders. A scoliosis plaster, or localizer plaster for scoliosis correction, extends to the groin anteriorly, to the sacrum posteriorly, and as far proximally as to provide a distracting force on the chin and occiput. Distally, the distracting force is applied by well-molded pressure areas across the crest of the ilia.

Traction

Traction is used in orthopedics:

1. To overcome muscle spasm and apply reducing force in fractures of the long bones
2. To provide immobilization of long bone fractures
3. To provide immobilization and distracting force for painful and diseased joints
4. To correct joint deformities or contractures

Skin traction is applied by tapes attached to the skin and skeletal traction by pins or screws affixed to bone. The maximal weight tolerated by adhesive tapes to the skin is about 10 lb. In children, skin traction is usually sufficient to overcome muscle pull in the reduction and treatment of fractures. The most common form of skin traction is Buck's traction, in which tapes with attached weights are applied to the leg and thigh (Fig. 47-15). This is commonly used prior to surgical treatment in the immobilization of intertrochanteric hip fractures. Skin traction is used with Russell's traction (Fig. 47-16), which is designed to apply traction to the femoral shaft with the knee flexed. A fem-

Fig. 47-16. Russell's traction.

oral shaft fracture in a small child may be treated with Bryant's traction. In this technique, skin traction is attached to both legs, which are suspended from the bed.

Skeletal traction (Fig. 47-17) is usually applied to a Steinmann pin or Kirschner wire driven percutaneously across the distal femoral shaft or proximal tibia. A traction bow is affixed to the metal wire and weight applied. Kirschner wires drilled across the olecranon may be used for supracondylar or humeral shaft fractures. Crutchfield tongs affixed to the outer table of the skull and the halo device, which has a similar purchase on the skull, are other forms of skeletal traction.

FRACTURES AND JOINT INJURIES IN THE UPPER EXTREMITY

SHOULDER MOTION. The act of moving the hand from the anatomic position to a position of full abduction requires normal function in the glenohumeral joint, the acromioclavicular joint, the sternoclavicular joint, and the scapulothoracic joint. Interference with any of these joints will limit full shoulder motion.

Inman and colleagues have worked out the ranges of motion occurring at these joints during normal shoulder function. During the first 30° of abduction or 60° of forward flexion, the scapula seeks a position of stability with the humerus. This occurs by lateral or medial motion of the scapula on the chest wall or by motion at the glenohumeral joint, with the scapula remaining fixed. When the position of 30° of abduction or 60° of forward flexion has occurred, there is a simultaneous 10° of glenohumeral joint motion for each 5° of scapula rotation on the thorax during the continued elevation of the arm.

The rotation of the scapula involves motion of the sternoclavicular and the acromioclavicular joints. As the arm is elevated, elevation of the clavicle occurs at the sternoclavicular joint. It is almost complete during the first 90° of arm elevation. For every 10° of elevation of the arm, there are 4° of elevation of the clavicle. Motion at the acromioclavicular joint is approximately 20° and occurs during the first 30° of abduction and after 135° of elevation. On the long axis of the acromioclavicular joint during the position of 60 to 180° of elevation of the arm, 40° of clavicular rotation occurs. It is apparent, from this anatomic description, that fusion or disruption of any one joint will interfere with the elevation of the arm.

Sternoclavicular Joint Injuries

Injuries to the sternoclavicular joint occur from direct lateral force to the shoulder applied in an axial direction to the clavicle. Dislocations are commonly anterior, but in some cases, when posterior and lateral forces are applied, retrosternal dislocation of the sternoclavicular joint occurs.

Reduction is necessary in retrosternal dislocations, because of compression of neurovascular structures. When closed manipulation and lateral traction are not sufficient, open reduction is indicated. With interior dislocation, reduction is not critical. However, for best results, closed reduction and maintenance of position are required. Old, unreduced dislocations, if symptomatic, require excision of the proximal end of the clavicle.

Fractures of the Clavicle

Fractures of the clavicle occur at any age from direct downward force to the shoulder or from forces applied indirectly as in falling on the extended arm. Fractures may occur at any level but are most common at the junction of the middle and distal thirds (Fig. 47-18). In older age groups, fractures of the distal tip of the clavicle are more common.

CLINICAL MANIFESTATIONS. The patient presents supporting the affected extremity by his opposite hand, with his head tilted to the affected side, and chin rotated away. There is local swelling and direct tenderness at the site of the fracture. Any motion of the extremity causes pain. The diagnosis is confirmed by x-ray.

TREATMENT. The clavicle is difficult to immobilize, because of its anatomic location and muscle attachments. In spite of this, nonunion is rare (about $\frac{1}{2}$ percent) with conservative treatment. The weight of the shoulder causes the distal fragment to be inferiorly angulated or depressed, while the proximal fragment is superiorly angulated by the pull of the sternocleidomastoid and upper fibers of the trapezius.

Treatment in Children. Both shoulders are drawn back and elevated by a figure-of-eight apparatus, which may be constructed of felt padding covered with stockinet (Fig. 47-19). The axillae are padded with large gauze pads to prevent irritation of the skin and compression of the neurovascular bundle. The figure-of-eight should be maintained in a taut position by frequent adjustment by the parents. Warning is given about swelling in the hands from venostasis. This is relieved by having the patient lie supine while elevating the arms overhead. Fracture reduction in children is not important. Bayonet overriding is accepted and will remodel with age. The figure-of-eight is left in place for 2 weeks in infants and until the fracture is clinically solid in older children, 4 to 6 weeks if necessary.

Fig. 47-17. Skeletal traction. Traction bow is attached to a transverse Steinmann pin through the tibial tubercle for a supracondylar or femoral shaft fracture.

Treatment in Adults. When growth of the clavicle has been completed, accurate reduction and maintenance of position is required to prevent cosmetic deformity. It is difficult to maintain a displaced fractured clavicle in the reduced position with any ambulatory apparatus. However, in men and older women, a figure-of-eight apparatus for 6 weeks would provide sufficient immobilization for union but may leave a cosmetic deformity. In women who desire a cosmetic result, supine bed rest with a small sandbag placed in the interscapular area and lateral traction on the abducted arm are required for 4 to 6 weeks. Open surgical reduction with intramedullary fixation will minimize angular deformity at the fracture site but leaves a scar and may result in nonunion.

Acromioclavicular Injuries

The acromioclavicular joint is injured by forces applied downward from the point of the shoulder. Such injuries occur frequently during blocking and tackling in football (Fig. 47-20) and in all contact sports. The age incidence coincides with that of people participating in sports, usually the latter part of the second decade or the third or fourth decades. Acromioclavicular joint injuries may occur

Fig. 47-18. *A.* Fracture of the middle third of the clavicle with complete displacement and overriding. *B.* Healing of a clavicle fracture in 6 weeks with internal callus formation.

Fig. 47-19. Figure-of-eight for treatment of a fractured clavicle. The axillae are padded with gauze pads over which a figure-of-eight of felt and stockinet is applied.

in the elderly, but fractures of the distal third of the clavicle are more common in this age group, with the same type of trauma. The integrity of the acromioclavicular joint is primarily dependent upon the coracoclavicular ligaments, the conoid and trapezoid, which run upward, backward, and laterally from the base of the coracoid process to the inferior surface of the clavicle. Superior and inferior acromioclavicular ligaments contribute little to the stability of the joint.

CLINICAL MANIFESTATIONS. Signs of acromioclavicular joint injury include local swelling and tenderness over the acromioclavicular joint and palpable deformity. The patient cocks his head to the affected side to relax the sterno-

Fig. 47-20. Acromioclavicular dislocation incurred from a direct fall on the shoulder while playing football.

cleidomastoid and supports his arm with the opposite hand to relieve the weight of the shoulder distracting the joint.

When the patient is examined lying supine, a subluxation may reduce spontaneously, making diagnosis difficult. In the upright position or in the obese patient, or with sufficient local swelling, the diagnosis may not be readily apparent. The diagnosis is made by obtaining comparable AP x-rays of both acromioclavicular joints with the patient standing. With a subluxation, it may be necessary to have the patient suspend a 10-lb weight in the affected hand to distract a partially disrupted acromioclavicular articulation.

TREATMENT. The treatment of minor sprains or subluxations is symptomatic. It is accomplished by a sling on the affected side, supporting the weight of the arm. Complete dislocation of the acromioclavicular joint will not be held with less than open reduction or the suspension cast of Stubbins and McGaw, which applies relocation pressure to the clavicle.

In treating complete dislocations of the acromioclavicular joint, consideration should be given to the patient's age and occupation. Jacobs and Wade have shown that there is no significant improvement in results whether conservative treatment (sling) or open surgical reduction is used. For young men with the desire to continue sports activities and reacquire maximal strength, surgical treatment of the type described by Neviaser or Weaver and Dunn may be indicated. Open reduction is also indicated for young women who will accept the surgical scar in the place of a permanent high-riding clavicle. However, for older patients symptomatic treatment for the initial dislocation is all that is necessary. In any patient with persistent symptoms from a subluxed or painful acromioclavicular joint, excision of the distal end of the clavicle generally provides good results.

Technique of Open Reduction. A curved incision is made over the outer half of the clavicle at its anterior border and extends to the outer border of the acromion. The deltoid fibers attaching to the clavicle are stripped subperiosteally. The coracoacromial ligament and the acromioclavicular joint are exposed. No attempt is made to repair the coracoclavicular or acromioclavicular ligaments. The dislocation is reduced and maintained with a Kirschner wire, transfixing the acromion and the clavicle but placed behind the acromioclavicular joint. The tip of the wire extending lateral to the acromion is bent to prevent inward migration.

The coracoacromial ligament is detached from its coracoid attachment by reflecting a small piece of bone from the coracoid process. With the normal attachment of ligament distad to the undersurface of the acromion, the proximal end is then reflected over the acromion, where it is sutured with catgut sutures and turned back across the acromioclavicular joint and affixed to the clavicle by catgut sutures passing through the drill holes in the clavicle.

The patient's shoulder is immobilized in a sling and swath for 4 to 6 weeks. The pin is then removed and motion begun.

Fractures of the Scapula

Fractures of the body of the scapula and glenoid are invariably the result of severe trauma, either to pedestrians or automobile occupants. Such injuries are usually associated with injuries to the brachial plexus, fractured ribs, and cardiopulmonary trauma. Treatment of such patients is aimed primarily at the associated injuries. Symptomatic immobilization of the shoulder is preferable to open reduction.

Dislocations of the Shoulder

ACUTE ANTERIOR DISLOCATIONS

The humeral head may be dislocated from the glenoid in any direction. For superior dislocation to occur, fracture of the overlying acromion must be present. Anterior dislocations include subglenoid and subcoracoid dislocations. The humeral head is dislocated anteriorly when an extension force is applied to the abducted arm. The initial injury is typically one involving a fall with the arm in the abducted position or direct trauma to the abducted arm as may occur with football injuries. Less force is required to dislocate the shoulder when there is a congenital defect in the labrum or with paralysis of shoulder musculature. The humeral head is driven anteriorly, tearing the anterior shoulder joint capsule and detaching the labrum from the glenoid, producing a compression fracture in the posterior lateral aspect of the humeral head, as it is wedged between the anterior-lying subscapularis tendon and the anterior rim of the glenoid.

CLINICAL MANIFESTATIONS. The patient holds his arm in slight abduction and is unable to bring his elbow to the side. There is flattening of the normal deltoid prominence with a depression laterally beneath the acromion. The humeral head creates a prominence anteriorly, although in the obese person these findings may be difficult to define. Any attempt at arm motion causes severe pain. In a small percentage of cases, injury to the axillary nerve is incurred, as it is stretched around the neck of the humerus. This diagnosis may be made before reduction by localizing an area of sensory loss overlying the deltoid muscles and supplied by the superficial branch of the axillary nerve. Postreduction, weakness, or loss of power in the deltoid may be demonstrable.

Anteroposterior x-rays of the shoulder will reveal the head displaced medially into the subcoracoid or subglenoid position (Fig. 47-21).

TREATMENT. The dislocation should be reduced immediately. Closed reduction can be accomplished within the first 2 to 3 weeks, but open reduction may be required when dislocations are neglected for longer periods.

Over 90 percent of acute anterior dislocations may be reduced by a modification of the Milch maneuver (Fig. 47-22). Under mild analgesia, the patient is placed supine on a stretcher with his elbow extended and the arm in the position of 90° forward flexion, hanging off the side of the stretcher. A pail of water is attached to the arm

Fig. 47-21. Anterior subcoracoid dislocation of the shoulder. The articular surface of the humeral head can be seen medial to the glenoid fossa and inferior to the coracoid process.

Fig. 47-22. Reduction technique for anterior dislocation of the shoulder. With the patient in the prone position and the arm in the position of forward flexion, water is added to the bucket, and traction is gradually increased.

with an Ace bandage. Water can gradually be added to the bucket and traction increased. A few minutes of this traction is sufficient for the shoulder to reduce gradually, but in more muscular individuals 30 minutes may be required. In some instances, it is necessary to rotate the humeral head internally while maintaining traction. In the few instances where this treatment is insufficient, general anesthesia and a Hippocratic maneuver is accomplished by applying manual traction with countertraction applied by the stockinged foot of the operator to the axilla.

Postoperative management is as important as the closed reduction. The arm is bound to the side with the elbow flexed at 90° across the abdomen. A sling and swath are applied and are not disturbed for 6 weeks in young individuals. In patients over fifty, 4 weeks is sufficient, and in elderly patients mobilization of the shoulder is begun after 2 or 3 weeks.

RECURRENT ANTERIOR DISLOCATIONS

With adequate initial treatment and postreduction immobilization, the majority of patients will not redislocate unless subjected to significant trauma. However, redislocations occur when the initial dislocation is not immobilized in sufficient time and may do so with minor trauma. Some patients abducting the arm in getting dressed or reaching out to open a door may incur a recurrent dislocation.

TREATMENT. A number of surgical repairs are used in the treatment of recurrent dislocations, including the methods of Magnuson and Stack, Eden, Hybbinette,

Fig. 47-23. Posterior dislocation of the shoulder. AP x-ray shows an indistinct border of the humeral head, superimposed upon the glenoid rim. There is also compression fracture in the region of the lesser tubercle.

Bankhart, and Bristow. Before instituting any of these, it is mandatory to document the direction of the dislocation. Excellent results have been obtained using the Putti-Platt procedure.

Technique. The shoulder is exposed through a standard deltopectoral incision. The clavicular origin of the deltoid is incised, leaving a $\frac{1}{2}$-cm attachment to the clavicle, in order to make resuture easier. The coracoid process is osteotomized at its tip and muscle origins of the pectoralis minor, and coracobrachialis retracted, medially. The axillary approach, as proposed by Leslie and Ryan, dividing the pectoralis major insertion is also used and has the advantage of leaving a less disfiguring scar.

The veins delineating the lower borders of the subscapularis tendon are located and ligated. The subscapularis tendon is divided 1 in. medial to its insertion on the lesser tuberosity. The capsule is divided vertically at the same level of the incision in the subscapularis tendon. The lateral capsule and subscapularis tendon are sutured to the inferior surface of the medial capsule and glenoid rim with interrupted heavy silk sutures. The medial capsule is then sutured anterior to this. The distal end of the proximal stump of the scapularis is then reattached to the lesser tuberosity to limit external rotation beyond neutral. A reefed shoulder capsule with a shortened subscapularis tendon limits external rotation and assists retention of the humeral head. The patient is immobilized with sling and swath, or Velpeau bandage, for 6 weeks, and then mobilization is begun. The results of this treatment are excellent in preventing repeated dislocation.

CHRONIC DISLOCATIONS. In patients with chronic complete anterior dislocation, arthrodesis of the shoulder at 45° of abduction, 15° of internal rotation, and 20° of forward flexion will eliminate pain and restore shoulder function.

POSTERIOR DISLOCATIONS

The shoulder dislocates posteriorly during epileptiform convulsions, during electroshock therapy, and in automobile accidents in which the arm is axially loaded in the position of forward flexion. Any patient complaining of shoulder pain following a convulsion should be considered to have a dislocated shoulder until proved otherwise.

Clinical findings on examination reveal prominence of the humeral head posteriorly, loss of the anterior shoulder contour, limitation of full abduction, and complete loss of external rotation.

Routine AP x-rays may reveal the diagnosis, but an axillary x-ray will confirm the location of the humeral head posterior to the glenoid fossa. On the AP x-ray, the humeral head will appear smaller than the opposite side, since it is closer to the x-ray film (Fig. 47-23). In the normal shoulder, there is an overlap of the shadow of the humeral head on the posterior lip of the glenoid, which gives a *sharp* half-moon shadow. When the head is dislocated posteriorly, this half-moon shadow will be blurred or absent. Proof of posterior dislocation is by an axillary x-ray. Frequently, the lesser tuberosity is fractured at the time of the dislocation. The presence of this finding should

Fig. 47-24. Fracture of the proximal humerus in a twelve-year-old girl. The fracture is an epiphyseal separation with a large metaphyseal fragment attached to the epiphysis. *A*. Initial fracture position. *B*. Slight improvement after closed reduction. *C*. Healed fracture with remodeling changes at 1 year postinjury. The patient has a normal range of shoulder motion.

suggest a posterior dislocation or a reduced posterior dislocation.

TREATMENT. Reduction is accomplished by the modified Milch maneuver under analgesia or general anesthesia or by direct traction. Following reduction, the shoulder is immobilized in 30° of abduction, in external rotation, with a modified shoulder spica. This permits adequate healing of the posterior capsule in the shortened position.

A few posterior dislocations are recurrent. Treatment of posterior recurrent dislocations is accomplished by a bone block applied to the posterior glenoid or reefing of the infraspinatus tendon, which is the posterior analog of a Putti-Platt procedure.

FRACTURE DISLOCATIONS OF THE SHOULDER

A fracture of the neck of the humerus may occur in combination with an anterior dislocation. The initial treatment is the same but generally requires closed reduction and manipulation under general anesthesia. Traction is applied in the long axis of the shaft of the humerus in the position in which it lies. Direct counterpressure is applied in a posterior direction over the head of the humerus. If the dislocation can be reduced, subsequent treatment is the same as for fractures of the humeral neck. In the young, when it is not possible to reduce such fracture dislocations, open reduction and internal fixation of the fracture are indicated.

Fractures of the Proximal Humerus

The most common fracture of the proximal humerus is a fracture of the surgical neck. It is prevalent in older individuals but may occur at any age. In children, a similar injury results in a fracture of the anatomic neck, with epiphyseal displacement, usually of Type II of the Salter and Harris classification (Fig. 47-24). The treatment of

such an injury in a child is by closed reduction with manual traction, followed by hanging cast immobilization. Moderate degrees of displacement may be accepted if there is sufficient growth potential remaining in the epiphysis. It may be necessary to place the arm at full abduction in a shoulder spica, to hold position.

Fractures of the surgical neck of the humerus have a varus deformity at the fracture site. A hanging cast or sling and swath are sufficient to hold reduction of most fractures of the surgical neck. When manual reduction and sling and swath are unsuccessful in maintaining reduction, skin traction applied to the adducted arm will maintain position. However, in some patients, open reduction with blade plate fixation, staples or screws, or Rush pinning may be necessary. Neer has described an excellent system for classification and treatment of proximal humeral fractures.

Fractures of the greater tuberosity should be reduced anatomically to maintain normal function. If this cannot be obtained by closed means, open reduction and screw fixation of the fragment are necessary. In all fractures of the humerus, it is necessary to begin early shoulder motion as soon as stability at the fracture site can be ascertained. With fractures of the surgical neck in elderly patients, shoulder motion and gentle pendulum exercises may be started as early as 7 to 10 days to minimize shoulder stiffness. In younger individuals with displaced fractures, motion is not started before 3 to 4 weeks.

Fractures of the Humeral Shaft

Fractures of the humeral shaft (Fig. 47-25) occur from direct blows to the humerus, which cause transverse or comminuted fractures, or by indirect force, i.e., torsional stress, as in falling on the elbow. On physical examination, there is swelling, ecchymosis, and deformity, with inability to elevate the arm because of painful instability. It is necessary to determine the presence or absence of associated neurovascular injuries, which are common, especially with serious traumatic forces. The radial nerve is the most commonly injured nerve, but any of or all the major nerves may be stretched or interrupted with either closed or open

Fig. 47-25. Spiral fracture at the junction of the middle and distal thirds of the humeral shaft. *A*. Lateral x-ray showing displacement with angulation. *B*. AP x-ray. *C* and *D*. AP and lateral x-rays showing postreduction positions after closed reduction and the application of coaptation splints. The patient had a complete radial nerve palsy (axonotmesis) from which there was complete recovery in 8 months.

fractures. Holstein and Lewis have described an oblique fracture at the junction of the middle and distal thirds of the humerus, in which radial nerve injury is commonly encountered.

TREATMENT. Various methods of treatment have been devised for this injury, but the most successful has been to reduce the fracture with gentle longitudinal traction, injecting 2% Xylocaine at the fracture site as necessary. With the patient in a sitting position, a coaptation plaster splint is applied to the medial surface of the arm, as high in the axilla as possible, encompassing the elbow and continuing over the lateral surface of the arm with a small extension of the plaster over the superior surface of the shoulder. While the plaster is hardening, it is circumferentially wrapped to the arm with a soft bandage roll. The elbow is flexed 90° across the abdomen, and the entire arm is bound to the side with a Velpeau, or sling and swath, dressing. The weight of the arm in this situation acts like a hanging cast to apply gentle traction for the fracture. This method of coaptation is superior to the hanging cast, because it provides more immobilization and comfort with less hazard of distraction from overweighted plaster.

In individuals with multiple injuries who require bed rest, the reduction may be maintained with skin traction applied to the arm. Two or three pounds is sufficient for lateral traction; when greater weight is added, the hazard of distraction is likely. With either method, when the fracture is clinically stable, the arm is placed in a sling and active elbow and shoulder motion started.

Spontaneous recovery ensues in over 95 percent of the patients with associated traction injuries to the radial nerve. The presence of such a lesion is not an indication for open reduction or primary exploration of the nerve.

When primary repair of a brachial artery is required, internal fixation of the humeral shaft is necessary. This is accomplished by plate and screw fixation of the AOI type but may also be effected by intramedullary fixation.

Primary open reduction of the closed humeral shaft fracture is indicated when it is not possible to get bony apposition because of marked displacement or interposition of soft tissue.

In all humeral shaft fractures, it is necessary to get biplanar check x-rays at intervals during the first 3 weeks and make traction or plaster adjustments as necessary.

Fractures and Dislocations about the Elbow

The motions at the elbow joint are flexion and extension from the hinge joint between the distal end of the humerus and the proximal radius and ulna, and pronation and supination of the forearm, which requires motion of the proximal radioulnar joint and radiohumeral joint. Significant injury to any area of these articulations may interfere with both forearm motion and elbow flexion and extension. Because of this complex articulation, the elbow is less able to withstand minor degrees of anatomic distortion. Injuries involving this articulation have a propensity for stiffness if immobilized too long and for production of new periosteal bone or myositis ossificans if irritated during the immediate postinjury period. Because rather minor injuries can produce subtle fractures, it is imperative not only to have standard AP and lateral x-ray views of the elbow joint but also oblique x-rays; in difficult diagnostic situations comparable views of the opposite normal side should be obtained. With children, in the presence of incompletely or unossified bony epiphyses, interpretation of x-rays following trauma is difficult, making it mandatory to have comparably positioned x-rays of the normal side.

Fractures of the Radial Head and Neck

Fractures of the head of the radius usually occur from falls on the outstretched hand. This force drives the head of the radius against the capitellum, which causes various degrees of cartilage contusion on the capitellum or head of the radius or fractures of the radial head.

CLINICAL MANIFESTATIONS. Patients with isolated fractures of the radial head may notice immediate stiffness of the elbow. As the hematoma and effusion increase, further limitation is noted, and pain becomes constant and severe. On examination, there is localized tenderness over the radial head, with painful limitation of motion.

TREATMENT. Successful treatment of radial head fractures is dependent upon the establishment of early joint motion. The initial treatment consists of aspiration of the joint hematoma and instillation of 2 to 3 ml of 2% Xylocaine. Following this, the patient should have improved motion and comfort. The patient is treated with a sling, and active motion within the range of pain tolerance is encouraged. After 3 weeks, the sling is discarded, but the patient is instructed to refrain from lifting heavy objects for 6 weeks. If the patient is still unable to pronate and supinate in the midrange of joint motion, excision of the radial head is indicated, because of mechanical block. Immediate range of motion is started following excision of all fragments of the radial head.

FRACTURES OF THE RADIAL NECK IN CHILDREN

The mechanism of injury causing a fracture of the radial head in adults produces a fracture of the radial neck (Fig. 47-26) in young children. This fracture is reduced by manipulation. The elbow is angulated into varus, while direct digital pressure is applied to the valgus-angulated radial head.

Fig. 47-26. AP and lateral x-rays of a fracture of the radial neck in a child.

Blount states that if less than 45° of angulation is present, the end result will be excellent. However, if residual angulation is more than 45°, open reduction during the first week is indicated. After 3 weeks open reduction is not justified. The radial head should never be excised in a child, because of the resultant shortening which will develop from loss of the proximal radial epiphysis.

Fractures of the Proximal Ulna

Isolated fractures of the olecranon occur most commonly in adults and are very infrequent in children. They are caused by forced flexion of the elbow against the actively contracting triceps, as when a patient falls on an outstretched hand. The olecranon is avulsed by the triceps.

In children, the fractures are, as a rule, undisplaced and can be treated with immobilization in extension.

When the fracture is displaced in adults, operation is invariably indicated if local skin condition is satisfactory. For noncomminuted fractures, open reduction and internal fixation of the fracture with a rigid olecranon screw is the treatment of choice. For very comminuted fractures, it may be necessary to excise the olecranon fragments and resuture the triceps aponeurosis to restore active extension.

Supracondylar Fractures of the Humerus

The supracondylar fracture (Fig. 47-27) accounts for the majority of fractures sustained about the elbow in children. The same injury occurs in adults but is rare in comparison with its incidence in children. It is usually caused by a fall upon the extended elbow; a small percentage of these fractures occur with the elbow flexed and should be recognized, so that the treatment and immobilization can be applied in extension.

A supracondylar fracture is the most hazardous fracture treated by the orthopedist, because of the vascular com-

Fig. 47-27. Displaced supracondylar fractures of the humerus in a child. *A.* AP and lateral x-rays on initial examination. *B* and *C.* AP and lateral x-rays obtained following closed manipulation after the local instillation of 2% Xylocaine.

plication of Volkmann's ischemic contracture. As the humeral condyles are driven back into extension, the brachial artery may be stretched, contused, or lacerated over the distal end of the proximal fragment during the initial injury. An injury to the brachial artery may cause collateral vasospasm, producing ischemia to the flexor forearm muscles and resulting Volkmann's contractures.

Fig. 47-28. Position of skeletal traction (Smith) for supracondylar fracture of the humerus.

CLINICAL MANIFESTATIONS. Children with displaced supracondylar fractures present with marked swelling about the elbow, deformity, and ecchymosis when initially seen. Undisplaced fractures may have considerable swelling and symptoms of pain, but without deformity. Before instituting treatment, it is necessary to determine the presence of circulation to the hand and the presence or absence of a radial pulse. A small percentage have injuries to the radial or median nerves in the presence of normal circulation. If the radial pulse is absent, it is imperative to reduce the fracture immediately.

TREATMENT. Manipulation reduction can be accomplished after local anesthetic infiltration of the fracture site with 2% Xylocaine or using general anesthesia. With countertraction applied to the axilla, one hand of the operator grasps the biceps, placing the thumb over the distal fragment. Traction is applied to the forearm with the opposite hand, and when the fracture fragments have been disengaged by slight hyperextension, the elbow is brought into the position of maximal flexion. While holding the elbow in maximal flexion, x-rays are obtained to determine the accuracy of reduction. If reduction is satisfactory and the radial pulse is present or has returned, the arm is immobilized at 90° with the forearm in neutral or slight pronation, in a collar and cuff, with plaster splints. All patients with supracondylar fractures should be hospitalized so that possible changes in circulation can be monitored.

If the radial pulse disappears with maximal flexion, the elbow is brought toward a right angle into a position in which the pulse is present but with as much flexion as possible. If the pulse does not return and there is good capillary circulation to the hand, the patient has no pain, and he can fully extend the fingers without discomfort, it is sufficient to temporize and evaluate these findings each 1 or 2 hours. If at any time circulation to the hand is in doubt in the presence of pain or if inability to extend the fingers painlessly develops, exploration of the brachial artery where it crosses the fracture site is indicated, along with release of the antebrachial fascia.

If fracture reduction and its maintenance are not possible, the patient should be placed in a traction device described by Smith (Fig. 47-28). A $\frac{3}{32}$-in. Kirschner wire is driven across the crest of the ulna, 1 in. distal to the tip of the olecranon process, and a traction bow is attached. With the patient lying supine in bed and the arm in forward flexion of 90°, enough weight is suspended overhead to reduce the fracture with the elbow at 90° of flexion and the forearm suspended in an overhead sling. The accuracy of reduction is determined by aligning the bony prominences with the distal humerus and comparing it with the opposite side. X-ray check is made to determine the degree of apposition and rotation of fracture sites, but alignment is best determined by the visual method of Smith. Traction is removed at 14 days, and the arm is placed in a long arm cast.

Reversal of the carrying angle, or so-called gunstock deformity, results when medial angulation of the distal fragment is not corrected. It also may be due to stimulation of the lateral condylar epiphyses from the fracture itself, since deformities have been noted following undisplaced fractures.

FRACTURES OF THE LATERAL EPICONDYLE IN CHILDREN

These injuries occur from hyperextension of the elbow with a valgus force. The child complains of pain with minimal swelling. If adequate x-rays are not taken and compared with the opposite side, this fracture may be overlooked. The fracture is either undisplaced or pulled from its normal location (Fig. 47-29) and rotated into the joint by the extensor muscles of the forearm attached to the fragment.

TREATMENT. This is a Type IV epiphyseal injury of the Salter and Harris classification, and requires anatomic reduction. Even if reduction is successful and the elbow is placed in acute flexion, when muscle tone is recovered following anesthesia, the fragment will be displaced again. As a rule, only undisplaced fractures do not require surgical treatment.

The elbow is exposed through a Kocher incision. The fracture fragment is anatomically reduced and fixed with two small Kirschner wires or by periosteal suture. The elbow is immobilized in neutral position at 90° flexion for 3 weeks, after which the pins are removed. Unreduced fractures may be opened up to 3 or 4 months postinjury. Beyond this time it is best to accept the nonunion, limitation of motion, and cubitus valgus which occurs.

FRACTURES OF THE MEDIAL EPICONDYLE IN CHILDREN

A sudden valgus strain of the elbow in a child may avulse the medial epicondylar apophysis. Minor degrees of displacement need not be anatomically reduced. If there has been a temporary dislocation of the joint with avulsion and incarceration of fragments in the joint or if ulnar nerve symptoms are present, open reduction and pinning of the fragments are required.

Fig. 47-29. AP, lateral, and oblique x-rays showing Type IV epiphyseal fracture of the lateral epicondyle with displacement and rotation.

COMMINUTED FRACTURES OF THE DISTAL HUMERUS

Comminuted fractures of the distal end of the humerus are uncommon and usually result from a direct fall on the elbow or automobile collisions. Open reduction and internal fixation carried out through a posterior approach is the treatment of choice. If sound fixation can be obtained, early elbow motion at 7 to 10 days is started. If secure internal fixation cannot be anticipated, traction through an olecranon pin is used, followed with motion as soon as callus can be demonstrated. Residual disability from such an injury is painless loss of motion.

Dislocations of the Elbow

A posterior dislocation of the elbow without associated fracture is more likely to occur in a child than an adult but is not a common injury. The injury is caused by falling on an outstretched arm with extension confined by adduction or abduction forces applied across the joint. The entire

Fig. 47-30. Posterolateral dislocation of the elbow with a fracture of the radial head. *A* and *B*. AP and lateral x-rays prior to reduction. *C* and *D*. Postreduction x-rays showing satisfactory reduction with a minimally displaced small fracture of the radial head.

anterior capsule is torn with damage to medial and lateral ligaments of the elbow.

These patients have severe pain and marked swelling. In contrast to fractures of the supracondylar region, the dislocation is quite stable.

TREATMENT. The treatment is immediate reduction. The reduction may be carried out under local anesthesia into the joint or by use of analgesics. In large muscular individuals, general anesthesia may be necessary. Traction is applied to the axis of the forearm in the position in which it lies, maintaining countertraction on the humerus. When reduction has been accomplished, the elbow is brought to

a 90° flexion, and check x-rays are obtained. The arm is then immobilized in a collar and cuff in maximal flexion; active exercises are started in 3 weeks in children.

Adults are put in a posterior splint at 90° in neutral rotation. The splint is discarded at 10 days, and the arm is placed in a sling. Active motion is begun within the tolerance of pain. The treatment of lateral dislocations is the same.

FRACTURE-DISLOCATIONS OF THE ELBOW

In addition to a posterior dislocation of the elbow, there may be a fracture of the coronoid process, the head of the radius (Fig. 47-30), or the lateral condyle. In the coronoid process it is usually a small chip fracture and is caused by the insertion of the brachialis, avulsing this portion of the bone during the dislocation. Its significance is that postreduction position of the elbow is more unstable, and immobilization is continued for a longer interval (3 weeks). If the radial head is fractured, the elbow is treated in the same manner as a posterior dislocation (reduction and immobilization). If motion does not return, radial head excision is indicated.

Monteggia's Deformity

Monteggia described deformity in which there was a dislocation of the radial head with a fracture of the proximal third of the ulna (Fig. 47-31). In 85 percent of the cases the radial head is dislocated anteriorly, and in 15 percent, posteriorly. The deformity may be caused by a direct blow on the ulna, fracturing it and driving the radial head anteriorly. Evans has shown that the injury is usually caused by a forced pronation and that reduction can be accomplished by closed methods.

Whenever an x-ray reveals a fracture of one bone of the arm or dislocation of one end, the concomitant injury

Fig. 47-31. Monteggia's deformity. *A*. Midshaft ulna fracture with anterior bowing and anterior dislocation of the radial head. *B*. Midshaft ulna fracture with posterior bowing and posterior dislocation of the radial head (most common).

to the adjacent bone should be ruled out by x-rays of the entire forearm.

If reduction of the ulna can be maintained, closed reduction of the radial head is usually possible by maintaining the arm in supination. If the ulnar fracture is displaced, intramedullary fixation (except in children) is required. After stabilization of the ulna, supination of the forearm and direct pressure over the radial head will accomplish its reduction. If the radial head is still not reduced, open reduction and suture of the annular ligament are carried out. If the radial head is anterior, the elbow is reduced and maintained in flexion. If the radial head is posterior, reduction and immobilization are carried out in full extension with the forearm in supination. Following reduction, immobilization is maintained with a circular plaster cast.

SUBLUXATION OF THE RADIAL HEAD IN CHILDREN

One of the most common injuries of children under the age of five is the "nursemaid's elbow," or "pulled elbow." The usual history is that the child's hand is suddenly pulled, forcing the elbow into extension and causing the sudden onset of pain in the elbow. The child avoids motion of the arm. Passive, painless elbow flexion is possible from 30 to 120°. X-rays of the elbow are negative.

Salter has demonstrated that the thin distal attachment of the annular ligament to the periosteum of the radial neck is torn when traction is applied to the pronated radius. The radial head escapes beneath the anterior part of the annular ligament, which is caught between the joint surfaces.

Treatment is effected by the deft maneuver of firm supination with the elbow held at 90° flexion. The arm may be in a sling 1 week, and the parents should be cautioned against repeated traction injury to the elbow.

Fractures of the Capitellum

Fractures of the capitellum may occur in the same manner as fractures of the radial head. The patient complains of pain with any attempt at motion, and flexion is limited, depending upon the degree of displacement of the fracture.

TREATMENT. In some cases, closed reduction is sufficient. This is accomplished by extending the elbow while applying adduction force to the elbow joint. While traction is maintained, local digital pressure is applied to the fragment. The elbow is then maintained in marked flexion for 3 to 4 weeks, at the end of which time active motion is begun.

If closed manipulation fails, the elbow is exposed through a lateral Kocher approach. If the fragment is small, it is excised; if large, it is reattached with a Kirschner wire or screw fixation. When the capitellar fracture is recognized after 4 weeks, excision and early motion are necessary.

Fractures of the Forearm

Fractures of the forearm are most common in children, but occur at any age from falls on the outstretched arm

or direct trauma. Clinical findings include deformity, local swelling, tenderness and instability. Anteroposterior and lateral x-rays are obtained of both bones and should include views of the elbow and wrist. If only one bone is fractured, dislocation of the proximal or distal joint should be suspected.

ANATOMIC CONSIDERATIONS. The radius has both a slight lateral bow and a posterior bow. The ulna has less medial bow but also has a slight dorsal curve. Any loss of this anatomic feature or compression of the interosseous space will interfere with rotation.

The pronator quadratus attached to the distal radius tends to pull it ulnaward and encroach upon the interosseous space. Both supinators act upon the proximal radial fragment. In fractures of the proximal third, the proximal radius will usually be in supination. The attachments of the pronator teres and the brachioradialis act to shorten the deformity and increase the lateral bow of the radius. Interference with the interosseous membrane from scarring will interfere with rotation.

In other diaphyseal fractures, alignment is the only consideration. However, in fractures of both bones of the forearm, because of the interrelationship required for rotation, anatomic restoration is required for normal function. If this can be accomplished by the closed method, there will be less scarring from surgical trauma, and the patient is more likely to have normal function. However, if the anatomic features cannot be restored by closed means, open reduction is indicated.

METHODS OF CLOSED REDUCTION. General anesthesia or axillary block anesthesia is required for reduction of forearm fractures. With the elbow flexed 90°, traction is applied to the long axis of the forearm by grasping the thumb and index finger of the patient and applying countertraction to the humerus. This may be done with the help of an assistant or by suspending the thumb and index finger with traction and adding weight over the humerus proximal to the flexed elbow as countertraction. When length has been regained, the fracture fragments are grasped by the operator, angulation increased, displacement corrected, and the fracture reduced.

If there is more than one fracture, reduction of the transverse fracture is accomplished first. Using the length gained from this reduction, reduction of the adjacent bone is then effected. The arm is immobilized in a position in which stability is greatest. For proximal-third fractures, this is supination, and for distal-third fractures, pronation, although there are exceptions to this rule. A well-molded, minimally padded plaster from the proximal palmar crease to the axilla, with the elbow at 90° flexion, is used. X-rays are obtained to determine accuracy of reduction. Interpretation may require comparison with the normal side. It is necessary to take check x-rays at intervals during the first 3 weeks to be certain that position is maintained. When position is lost, open reduction may be necessary.

The fractures most often requiring open reduction are displaced fractures of the proximal third and oblique fractures of the radius. Segmental fractures also require open reduction and internal fixation.

Fig. 47-32. Fracture of both bones of the forearm with open reduction and internal fixation. *A.* AP and lateral x-rays following closed reduction, showing displacement of distal radial fragment. *B.* AP and lateral x-rays showing anatomic position following open reduction and fixation with compression plates.

Fig. 47-33. *A.* Greenstick fracture of the radius with torus fracture of the ulna. *B.* Satisfactory position following manipulation and application of plaster.

Open reduction of the radius is carried out through the approach of Henry. The ulna is exposed through a separate incision, along its subcutaneous border. A compression plate is an ideal means of internal fixation for open reduction, although both bones may be fixed with intramedullary nails (Fig. 47-32).

Postoperative immobilization is continued until union has occurred. The approximate time is 10 to 12 weeks, but a considerably longer period may be required. Open fractures, if clean and treated immediately after injury, may be fixed with internal fixation, although we prefer debridement, closure, and skeletal pin fixation. Skeletal fixation is accomplished with a Kirschner wire through the bases of the second and third metacarpals, incorporated in plaster.

FOREARM SHAFT FRACTURES IN CHILDREN

Operative reduction of shafts of both bones is almost never indicated in the young child. Treatment of these injuries is by closed reduction and immobilization in plaster. However, in children twelve years of age and older (i.e., close to epiphyseal maturity), there will be minimal remodeling, and operative reduction may be required.

TREATMENT. Greenstick fractures with angulation (Fig. 47-33) should be manipulated to correct the deformity and at the same time break the unbroken cortex. Otherwise, deformity will occur in the cast. The apex of the deformity is deftly snapped over the operator's knee, a maneuver which will usually correct the deformity.

The principles of reduction of displaced fractures in children are the same as for displaced fractures in adults. If both bones are displaced, one bone is reduced, and using this as a lever the adjacent bone is reduced. The forearm is then immobilized with the elbow at 90° and in the position of greatest stability: supination for proximal-third, pronation for distal-third, and neutral position for midshaft fractures. Check x-rays are obtained immediately post-reduction and at 7 to 10 days to be certain that reduction is maintained. If it is not possible to hold both bones reduced, fixed traction as outlined by Blount, in which skin traction is applied to the fingers and attached to an outrigger splint from the cast, is necessary. Experience is required in judging what degrees of angulation will be corrected with remodeling. The closer the fracture to the growing epiphysis, the greater remodeling possible. In general, 30° of shaft angulation in an infant will correct itself. However, this should not be accepted in the older child.

Fractures of the Distal Radius

COLLES FRACTURE

A fracture of the distal radius with dorsal angulation produces a typical silver fork deformity, as was described by Abraham Colles in 1814. Since Colles was describing a clinical deformity before the use of x-ray, the use of the term *Colles fracture* has come to mean dorsally angulated fractures of the distal radial metaphysis with an associated fracture of the ulnar styloid (Fig. 47-34) and not fracture of the distal ulnar shaft, which occurs in children.

CLINICAL MANIFESTATIONS. Distal radial fractures usually occur in patients over the age of fifty, more commonly in women, and are produced by a fall on the outstretched hand. The term "silver fork" offers an appropriate clinical description. Depending upon the degree of comminution, there may be considerable instability, tenderness, and swelling about the wrist. Palpation of the wrist will reveal a more proximal position of the tip of the radial styloid. On examination, it is important to rule out the presence or absence of a concomitant median nerve injury. X-ray examination should include AP, lateral, and both oblique views. A carpal dislocation can clinically simulate this deformity.

TREATMENT. The aim of treatment of this injury is to obtain a functional hand and wrist and, secondly, to minimize cosmetic deformity. In the past, many operative skeletal traction methods have been used in an attempt to improve the cosmetic deformity. Unfortunately, immobilization of the hand required of these methods compromises hand function. The best results in this fracture have been obtained by closed reduction and plaster immobilization.

Manipulation Technique. With an assistant applying countertraction to the humerus and with the elbow flexed, traction is applied to the radial side of the hand for disimpaction of the distal radial fragment, which is displaced and angulated in a radial and dorsal direction.

Fig. 47-34. Colles fracture in a twenty-five-year-old woman. *A*. AP and lateral x-rays postinjury. *B*. AP and lateral x-rays after closed reduction under local anesthesia and cast immobilization.

While traction is maintained, the operator grasps the distal radial fragment between thumb and index finger and displaces it anteriorly to correct the displacement. At the same time, counterpressure is applied in a dorsal direction, with the opposite hand applied to the anterior surface of the forearm. Simultaneously, the wrist is brought into maximal flexion and ulnar deviation while pronating the forearm.

If reduction has been accomplished, there will be palpable dorsal step, and the tip of the radial styloid will be at least 1 cm distal to the ulnar styloid. It may be necessary to repeat the manipulation.

Over two layers of sheet wadding a well-molded plaster cast is applied which includes the elbow, with the wrist in maximal ulnar deviation, 30° of palmar flexion. Check x-rays are obtained immediately and at 7 to 10 days to be certain that reduction has been maintained.

The patient should be encouraged to keep the hand elevated for 2 or 3 days or until swelling has subsided. The patient is instructed in exercises to maintain a full range of motion of all interphalangeal (IP) and metaphalangeal (MP) joints. The patient should maximally flex the IP joints with the MP joints in extension and flex the MP joints with the IP joints in extension. Patients who are able to do this have little difficulty in mobilizing the wrist following 6 weeks of plaster immobilization. Patients should do range-of-motion shoulder exercises daily. This prevents the occasional episodes of shoulder stiffness that accompany Colles fractures. Shoulder stiffness may be due to traction on the shoulder joint from the weight of the cast or from a primary capsular injury at the time of initial injury. If the wrist is placed in maximal palmar flexion, median nerve compression in the carpal tunnel may ensue. If median nerve paresthesias occur, decrease in the amount of wrist flexion is necessary. If unrelieved, the flexor retinaculum is incised surgically.

SMITH FRACTURE

A fall on the dorsum of the wrist may cause a reverse Colles or Smith fracture. In such fractures position is difficult to maintain (Fig. 47-35) because of comminution.

Fig. 47-35. Smith fracture. *A*. Lateral x-ray. *B*. Oblique x-rays showing minimal anterior angulation and displacement of the distal fragments.

Plaster immobilization in the position of dorsiflexion of the wrist is required. If this will not maintain position, continuous skeletal traction to the thumb metacarpal or open reduction and screw fixation are necessary.

Injuries to the Wrist

A person falling on the outstretched wrist may sprain the anterior radial carpal ligament, with resulting synovial effusion and wrist pain, and limitation of motion. It is important to distinguish this from a fractured navicular or dislocation of the lunate, which have similar signs.

FRACTURES OF THE NAVICULAR

Young adults who fall on the outstretched hand frequently fracture the navicular (Fig. 47-36) against the unyielding anterior radial carpal ligament. In elderly patients, a Colles fracture occurs, because the distal radius is the point of least resistance. There is tenderness to direct pressure over the tuberosity of the navicular, with limitation of wrist flexion and extension. With any wrist injury, it is imperative to rule out a fractured navicular by x-ray examination.

In addition to AP, lateral, and oblique x-rays of the carpal bones, with the wrist in neutral position, a special 17° angled AP x-ray view of the wrist is needed. If the patient has tenderness over the tuberosity of the navicular and x-ray examination is negative, the patient is presumed to have a fractured navicular, treated as such, and then re-x-rayed when there has been some resorption at the fracture site (3 weeks). At 3 weeks, if clinical and x-ray examination are still negative, the wrist is mobilized.

There is little or no displacement with fractures of the navicular. Arterial supply enters the distal third of the bone constantly. The proximal-third blood supply may be only by communication in the bone from the vessels entering distad. Fractures transecting the waist or proximal third may interrupt the entire circulation to the proximal third. Because of this, nonunion or avascular necrosis of the proximal fragments is not uncommon.

TREATMENT. When there is little or no displacement and the injury is diagnosed accurately, the optimal treatment is by plaster cast immobilization. Plaster is applied from the tip of the thumb to include the elbow. By immobilizing the elbow, pronation-supination, which causes motion at the fracture site, is prevented.

Most navicular fractures require 16 weeks of adequate plaster immobilization. The patient is seen at monthly intervals and the cast replaced, if loose, without disturbing the position of the wrist. X-rays out of plaster are obtained at 8 weeks and at subsequent 4-week intervals. When all tenderness from direct pressure over the tuberosity of the navicular has disappeared and x-rays show obliteration of the fracture site, plaster immobilization is discontinued. In some situations, 6 months or longer is necessary.

When a patient has an acute fracture in which displacement cannot be corrected, the best treatment is open reduction and the insertion of a McLaughlin lag screw. This is preferable to accepting a possible nonunion or the long delay necessary for union of the displaced fracture. Displaced fractures usually occur as the result of, and in combination with, perilunar dislocation of the carpus.

When the interval between trauma and diagnosis is less than 6 months, prolonged plaster immobilization (6 to 9 months) will usually result in union.

NONUNION OF NAVICULAR FRACTURES. With a simple nonunion of navicular fractures, without avascular necrosis and without degenerative arthritis at the wrist, an autogenous bone graft is indicated. In patients with significant degenerative changes adjacent to the nonunion, excision of the radial styloid gives satisfactory pain relief and maintenance of wrist power. When the proximal fragment is small and avascular, excision will give satisfactory results. However, if large, bone grafting is the procedure of choice.

DISLOCATIONS OF THE LUNATE

Dislocations of the lunate are uncommon but occur from trauma causing hyperextension of the wrist. Patients complain of pain, swelling, and limitation of motion. Median nerve symptoms are frequent. The diagnosis is made by AP and lateral x-rays. On the lateral x-ray of the wrist, the semilunar shape of the lunate is displaced anterior to the distal radial articular surface. On the AP x-ray, the normal quadrilateral shape of the lunate appears triangular and larger than on the opposite side.

TREATMENT. Treatment is by closed reduction and plaster immobilization. Reduction is accomplished by hyperextending the wrist and applying direct pressure of the operator's thumb over the dislocated lunate. After it is reduced, the wrist is brought into the flexed position. There is a high incidence of avascular necrosis following this injury, for which lunate excision is indicated. Kienböck's disease, which is avascular necrosis of the lunate, may occur without known trauma. The onset of symptoms, which include wrist pain, stiffness, and local swelling, is insidious. Treatment is excision of the avascular lunate.

A similar mechanism of injury may produce a perilunar

dislocation of the carpus with or without fracture of the scaphoid or rotatory subluxation of the scaphoid—so-called traumatic instability of the wrist. The diagnosis of the former is obvious radiographically, but attention should always be directed at the scaphoid-lunate relationship to detect subtle signs of scaphoid subluxation. The reader is referred to the work of Linscheid et al. for discussion of therapy.

Fractures and Dislocations in the Hand

METACARPAL FRACTURES

Metacarpal fractures occur from direct violence to the hand, as in crushing injuries, although the most common mechanism is by striking the hand against an opponent (Fig. 47-37). Fractures of the necks of fourth and fifth metacarpals invariably occur in young men as a result of altercations. There is local swelling involving the fracture site which minimizes the actual degree of anterior angulation of the head of the metacarpal. Therefore, the degree of angulation can be determined only by x-ray. Rotational deformity of such a fracture must be determined clinically. Each finger, when flexed individually into the palm, points to the navicular, and any deviation from this is an indication of rotational deformity of the finger or its metacarpal shaft.

TREATMENT. Treatment of the acute metacarpal neck fractures is by closed manipulation, making certain that rotational deformity is corrected. The finger is then splinted with the MP and the IP joints in 45° of flexion and with the tip pointing toward the navicular. It is not always possible to hold the fracture by this method, and some cosmetic deformity of the knuckle may persist. However, since there is mobility at the carpometacarpal joints of the fourth and fifth fingers, the grip will not be compromised. It is preferable to accept some degree of anterior angulation without rotation rather than immobilize the MP joint at 90° with pressure on a fully flexed IP joint, as has been described.

Fig. 47-36. Fracture of the carpal navicular. *A.* AP x-ray 1 day postinjury is negative for fracture. *B.* Patient was persistently tender over the navicular tuberosity. X-ray at 3 weeks reveals fracture at the junction of the proximal and middle thirds. Fracture subsequently healed without avascular necrosis.

Fig. 47-37. AP and oblique x-rays of a fracture of the neck of the fifth metacarpal which occurred during an altercation.

Fig. 47-38. Bennett's fracture. Two views showing intraarticular fracture of the base of the proximal first phalanx with displacement. Such an injury requires reduction and maintenance of position by plaster or open reduction.

Metacarpal shaft fractures which are oblique or spiral usually require nothing more than anterior splinting for 2 to 3 weeks. Anterior angulated fractures of the second and third metacarpals which do not have carpometacarpal mobility must be protected against anterior angulation, or interference with grasp will result. Multiple fractures of metacarpal shafts may require intramedullary fixation. This is done by inserting a single intramedullary wire percutaneously from distal to proximal direction, starting on the lip of the metacarpal head and avoiding the articular surface. Comminuted fractures of the metacarpal heads involving the articular surface are difficult to treat because

Fig. 47-39. *A.* Lateral x-ray of the dorsal dislocation of the proximal interphalangeal joint of an index finger. *B.* After closed reduction under local anesthesia, postreduction position was maintained on a metal splint in the position of function.

of the extensive damage to the articular surface. Such fractures should be immobilized in a position of function over a metal splint and motion started at 2 to 3 weeks.

Fracture dislocations of the carpometacarpal joint occur very rarely. A typical mechanism of injury is severe force applied to a hyperextended wrist. If possible, it is preferable to maintain closed reduction of a carpometacarpal fracture dislocation. However, there may be interposition of tendons and soft tissue, necessitating open reduction. Kirschner wire fixation across the carpometacarpal junction is used to maintain the reduction.

BENNETT'S FRACTURE

Bennett's fracture is an intraarticular fracture involving the base of the carpometacarpal joint of the thumb (Fig. 47-38). Such an injury is the result of forcible abduction on the thumb. There is an oblique fracture which involves the base of the metacarpal and which transects the proximal articular surface. The resulting instability causes subluxation of the shaft and the remaining articular surface. If such a fracture is unreduced, the normal range of abduction and carpometacarpal joint motion will be compromised.

Closed methods may hold reduction of minimally displaced and undisplaced fractures. Traction is applied to the axis of the shaft of the metacarpal, which is then brought into abduction, while direct adduction pressure is applied over the base of the carpometacarpal joint. If displacement persists, closed reduction and percutaneous wire fixation of the first carpometacarpal joint will hold the fracture. If this is not sufficient, open reduction and Kirschner wire fixation across the fracture is indicated.

PHALANGEAL FRACTURES

Undisplaced fractures of phalangeal shafts require splinting with the MP joints in 70° flexion and IP joints in slight flexion. The finger is placed on a metal splint and taped in this position without traction. If the fracture is displaced, it is manipulated into position and placed on a metal splint as for undisplaced fractures.

A small chip fracture involving an IP joint is treated symptomatically by the use of a splint for 2 weeks followed by early motion. Interphalangeal dislocations (Fig. 47-39) require closed reduction and splinting in a position of function. Open reduction is rarely necessary.

Distal Phalanx

A crushed fingertip with resultant fracture of the distal phalanx is one of the most common injuries seen in an emergency room. Initial treatment is aimed at cleansing the skin and relieving the pain by splinting the finger. There is usually no intraarticular involvement, and position of fragments is rarely a consideration.

Mallet Finger

When the distal phalanx is forcibly flexed against the taut extensor tendon, avulsion of the extensor tendon may occur with or without a fragment of bone from its insertion on the distal phalanx. This causes a characteristic dropped finger; the last 15 to 20° of active extension is lost, although full passive extension is possible. There is local tenderness and swelling over the dorsal aspect of the distal interphalangeal (DIP) joint.

Many types of treatment have been tried for this lesion. If the tendon has been avulsed without a bone fragment, the finger is splinted over a metal splint with the DIP joint in maximal extension or hyperextension and with the proximal interphalangeal (PIP) joint in 60° of flexion. The splint needs to be repeatedly inspected and adjusted. Care should be taken not to cause excessive pressure over the DIP joint. If active extension is not gained in 6 weeks, splinting should be continued for another 2 or 3 weeks. Incomplete extension is not always associated with disability. However, if the patient shows symptoms, surgical reefing of the lengthened extensor tendon is indicated.

When avulsion occurs with a fragment of bone (Fig. 47-40) involving one-third of the distal articular surface, open reduction and Bunnell pullout wire fixation are required. If the bone chip is small or does not involve the articular surface, the treatment may be the same as with a pure tendon avulsion.

In crush injuries of any IP joint with severe comminution of articular surface the phalanges should be splinted in a position of function at 45° of flexion and consideration given to early arthrodesis, if symptoms are evident.

Compound fractures involving the hand invoke the same principles as those applied to other compound fractures.

FRACTURES AND JOINT INJURIES IN THE LOWER EXTREMITY

Fractures of the Proximal Femur

Fractures of the proximal femur are a challenge to everyone responsible for the care of patients with such injuries. The hospital mortality of 25 percent encountered with this injury, as reported by Horowitz, is an indication of the severity of the problem. Prior to the introduction of internal fixation, such fractures were treated by bed rest and traction, with a much higher mortality rate. The age of most patients with fractures of the proximal femur is in the sixties or seventies. Complications of immobility imposed by this fracture in this elderly age group are responsible for the high mortality. Operative fixation will allow early mobility and relief of pain and is the treatment of choice. Only in the occasional younger individual with this injury can bed rest and traction be tolerated.

FEMORAL NECK FRACTURES

Femoral neck fractures usually occur in the elderly but may occur in young adults or children when severe trauma is involved. Fractures are commonly produced by a fall, although the history may suggest that the fracture occurred from a twist or indirect type of force and the patient fell as the fractured femoral neck gave way.

CLINICAL MANIFESTATIONS. The patient is usually unable to stand on the side of the affected hip and has increasing pain as a tense hemarthrosis develops. On clinical examination, the affected leg may be slightly shorter

Fig. 47-40. Mallet finger. Lateral x-ray of a finger with avulsion of the extensor tendon at its bony insertion. There is minimal subluxation, and open reduction and direct suture of the fragment are indicated.

and held in a position of external rotation of 30 to 40°. Attempts at motion cause excruciating pain. There may be ecchymosis over the trochanter, but local swelling is not prominent.

Anteroposterior and tube lateral x-rays demonstrate interruption between the trabeculae of the head and neck. The head is rotated into varus with posterior angulation. There are varying degrees of comminution of the posterior neck at the fracture site.

CLASSIFICATION. Garden has classified femoral neck fractures according to displacement and comminution (Fig. 47-41): Type I fractures are incomplete fractures; Type II, complete fractures without displacement; Type III, partially displaced fractures; and Type IV, complete displacement. This classification is useful in evaluating therapy, since displaced fractures have a higher rate of nonunion and avascular necrosis.

Fig. 47-41. Types of subcapital fracture (Garden; see text).

MEISENZAHL

TREATMENT. The prognosis of this fracture depends upon the attainment of union, without development of avascular necrosis. In adults, the blood supply to the femoral head is via the metaphyseal vessels (which are interrupted by the fracture), the artery of the ligamentum teres, and the lateral epiphyseal vessels. The location of a fracture site high on the neck with associated displacement may damage the lateral epiphyseal vessels. If the artery of the ligamentum teres provides insufficient circulation, avascular necrosis may ensue.

The periosteum on the neck has no cambium layer, so that external callus does not develop. The absence of external callus and the precarious circulation contribute to the high incidence of nonunion.

Massie and Deyerle have shown that early reduction and adequate immobilization of the fracture site can overcome these difficulties. Despite the apparent medical contraindication for surgical treatment in these patients, internal fixation will relieve pain, allow mobilization, and at the same time facilitate union and minimize the incidence of avascular necrosis.

Impacted Femoral Neck Fractures

Type I (Garden) subcapital fractures or Type II fractures which are impacted may be treated conservatively. Some patients have walked with the fracture by the time of examination. If the fracture is impacted in slight valgus with less than 15 to 20° of anterior angulation at the fracture site, it is worthwhile to attempt nonoperative management, as outlined by Crawford. The patient is instructed not to bear weight or use leverage with the leg. The patient is kept in bed until he can actively control the leg without discomfort. This usually takes from a few days to a week. In Crawford's series, the few impacted

Fig. 47-42. Subcapital fracture fixed with Deyerle plate and pins.

fractures, which subsequently were displaced, all occurred within the first 10 days. If displacement occurs, closed reduction and internal fixation are indicated.

Displaced Fractures of the Femoral Neck

Treatment. Pain, associated with such fractures, causes rapid deterioration in the patient's condition, making the treatment of this fracture a surgical emergency. If a patient is in congestive heart failure, diabetic acidosis, or a state of dehydration, i.e., in a condition which can be alleviated within 24 hours, this time should be invested for correction of the condition. Mortality rates are lower when such fractures are fixed immediately. It is not sufficient to place the patient in traction, expecting his condition to improve for surgical treatment, because this does not relieve the pain, and the complications of pneumonia, pulmonary emboli, decubitus ulcer, urinary tract infection, or paralytic ileus will occur.

Technique of Reduction and Fixation. *Reduction.* Under spinal or general anesthesia, the patient is placed on a standard fracture table equipped for AP and lateral x-rays to be taken during surgical procedures.

Closed reduction is done by manipulation. The affected leg is grasped in both hands, and with the knee flexed traction is applied in the long axis of the thigh with the hip in 20 to 30° of abduction and 30 to 40° of external rotation. As part of the same motion, the hip is flexed about 45°, internally rotated 15°, and then slowly brought toward extension to a position of 15° of flexion. While traction is maintained manually, the foot is taped to the foot plate of the fracture table in 30 to 45° of internal rotation, in 10° of abduction, and with sufficient tension to hold the reduction.

Check x-rays are obtained to determine the adequacy of reduction. If reduction is not satisfactory, repeat manipulation is carried out. A satisfactory reduction is one in which the head is in a position of a few degrees of valgus, with the medial point of the proximal fracture surface displaced a millimeter or two lateral to the calcar on the distal fragment. On the lateral x-ray, the head should be anatomically aligned with the neck.

*Internal Fixation (**Deyerle Method.**)* A lateral incision is used to expose the lateral aspect of the proximal femur. The skin, subcutaneous tissue, and fascia lata are divided in line with the incision. The vastus lateralis is separated by muscle-splitting incisions close to the linea aspera. The intermedius and periosteum are separated from the proximal femoral shaft, exposing the base of the greater trochanter. A guide pin is inserted in a $\frac{1}{4}$-in. drill hole placed $1\frac{1}{4}$ in. below the flare of the greater trochanter and at a point midway between the anterior and posterior cortices. The guide pin is inserted through the bone across the fracture site into the head. A Deyerle guide plate (Fig. 47-42) is then passed over the guide pin and affixed to the shaft. The appropriate nine holes using the guide plate are predrilled with a $\frac{9}{64}$ drill. The guide plate is then removed and the regular plate affixed to the shaft with the screw. Nine Deyerle pins of appropriate length to give secure fixation of the femoral head are inserted. Selection of pins is monitored by biplane check x-rays. After all pins have been inserted, traction is removed from the extremity, and the fracture site is impacted using the impactor applied to the plate.

Although superior results have been reported with the Deyerle procedure, the Massie nail technique is also suitable. The Smith-Petersen nail is no longer recommended, because it does not control rotation satisfactorily.

When closed reduction is not satisfactory for routine fractures, open reduction, through either a Watson-Jones or Smith-Petersen incision, is required prior to internal fixation. Primary insertion of a femoral head prosthesis may also be used.

Postoperative Management. Postoperatively, patients are mobilized as rapidly as possible. They are allowed out of bed the following day and mobilized to use crutches without weight bearing as soon as possible. Check x-rays are obtained at monthly intervals to follow the progress of healing. Approximately 4 to 6 months is required for sufficient healing across the fracture site. Unprotected weight bearing is not allowed until union is solid.

If nonunion exists in the presence of a viable head, reconstructive surgical treatment, with bone grafts, or osteotomy may be required. In elderly patients, excision of the femoral head and insertion of a prosthesis is a satisfactory solution when this complication occurs.

Insertion of Femoral Head Prosthesis

Because nonunion and avascular necrosis are problems, attempts have been made to obviate these difficulties by the insertion of a primary femoral head prosthesis (Fig. 47-43). Such measures taken on a routine basis do not give as good results as hip nailing. Hinchey and Day list spastic hemiplegia, severe arthritis of the fractured hip, pathologic fracture, the need for ambulatory care because of blindness, extreme age, or poor general health contraindicating a second operation as indications for a primary prosthesis. If the complications of avascular necrosis or nonunion develop in the aged patient, a femoral head replacement prosthesis is indicated.

Technique. The prosthesis may be inserted from anterior or posterior approaches, although we have found the posteroinferior exposure of Austin Moore to be satisfactory.

The patient is placed in a lateral or semiprone position, lying on the normal side. An incision is started 2 to 3 in. lateral to the posteroinferior spine of the ilium and is extended across, and parallel with, the fibers of the gluteus maximus to the tip of the great trochanter and then approximately 4 in. distad along the lateral aspect of the trochanter. Fibers of the gluteus maximus are separated at the junction of the superior three-quarters and inferior one-quarter of the muscle. Sharp dissection is used to split the fascia lata where the inferior fibers of the gluteus maximus are inserted. If necessary, the gluteus maximus insertion on the gluteal tubercle may be partially divided. The sciatic nerve is next located, identified, and retracted medially. The short external rotators, piriformis, gemellus inferior and superior, and obturator internus are divided just proximal to the insertion on the femur. If necessary, the upper fibers of the quadratus femoris are divided also.

The hip capsule is exposed and incised. The detached

Fig. 47-43. Austin Moore's appliance inserted for displaced fracture of the femoral neck.

femoral head is then gently levered from the joint. The neck is fashioned to accept the Austin Moore prosthesis, and the medullary cavity is reamed with an Austin Moore rasp. Care should be taken to insert the reamer accurately in the proper position of 20° of anteversion and also to seat the prosthesis sufficiently laterally. Excessive reaming may result in a loose prosthesis with pain.

An Austin Moore or Thompson prosthesis which matches the size of the excised femoral head is driven into the proximal femur. If it is not possible to match it exactly, a slightly smaller prosthesis is accepted, in order to reduce the hazard of postoperative dislocation. If the femoral canal is large and osteoporotic, the prosthesis may be fixed with methyl methacrylate to minimize subsequent loosening.

The head of the Austin Moore prosthesis, which is securely driven into the femoral shaft, is then relocated in the acetabulum. The capsule is closed, if possible, and the short external rotators reapproximated.

Postoperative care is extremely important. Nursing care should prevent adduction, flexion, and internal rotation, which is the position in which dislocation occurs. The patient is allowed out of bed in 2 or 3 days. Protected

Fig. 47-44. *A.* Fracture of the femoral neck in a nine-year-old boy with varus deformity. *B.* AP x-ray showing united fracture 1 year postinjury in satisfactory position. Russell's traction was the method of treatment.

weight bearing (50 percent) is started early using crutches or a walker. Patients may progress to a cane held in the opposite hand at 3 months if able to walk painlessly and without a limp.

Femoral Neck Fractures in Children

Fractures of the femoral neck occur in children (Fig. 47-44) only after severe trauma, such as in pedestrian injuries or in falls from a great height. Since there are usually associated injuries, operative treatment is not always possible. If satisfactory reduction can be obtained by Russell's traction, it is continued until union is sound, usually for 10 to 16 weeks, depending upon the age of the child. If union is not sound, a hip spica will not protect against loss of position into varus. If closed reduction is not satisfactory, operative internal fixation treatment, as

in adults, is indicated. The fracture should be pinned with three parallel Knowles pins. There is a high incidence of avascular necrosis of both the head and neck in children.

INTERTROCHANTERIC AND SUBTROCHANTERIC FRACTURES

Intertrochanteric and subtrochanteric fractures occur very commonly in the elderly from a direct fall onto the hip. They also occur from severe traumatic forces in younger individuals as in automobile accidents or crush injury.

There is considerably more instability to this type of fracture than intracapsular fractures of the femoral neck. On clinical examination there is shortening and external rotation, which may be 90°, and swelling about the anterior and proximal thigh.

In treatment of this type of fracture in the elderly patient indications for open reduction are the same as in intracapsular fractures. The main aim of treatment is to relieve pain and mobilize the elderly patient to prevent the complications of immobility. In younger individuals who can tolerate bed rest, the conservative treatment, such as Russell's traction or skeletal traction and balanced suspension, will maintain reduction if there are contraindications to surgical treatment. If traction is decided upon, it must continue until union is solid, which may require 16 weeks or longer with bed rest. Surgical treatment involves closed or open reduction on a fracture table, combined with internal fixation (Fig. 47-45). A Jewett blade plate appliance or Richards compression screw will provide satisfactory internal fixation.

Subtrochanteric fractures should have a sufficiently longer fixation on the shaft than intertrochanteric fractures. There should be at least 3 to 4 screw holes below the lowest point of the subtrochanteric fracture (Fig. 47-46). An ex-

Fig. 47-45. Intertrochanteric hip fracture. *A.* AP x-ray postinjury. *B* and *C.* AP and lateral x-rays showing postoperative fracture position with a Jewett plate in satisfactory position.

Fig. 47-46. Comminuted fracture of the femoral shaft incurred in automobile accident. *A* and *B*. AP and lateral x-ray before treatment. *C* and *D*. AP and lateral x-rays at 9 months showing union with a Jewett appliance in place.

cellent device for subtrochanteric fractures, especially in younger patients, is the Zickel nail.

The patient is placed in bed for 2 or 3 days and then mobilized from chair to non-weight-bearing crutch walking. Four months is the average time for union. Weight bearing should not be allowed until union has occurred.

Postoperative care should include attention to proper hydration and pulmonary hygiene. Prophylactic anticoagulation or dextran (which have been shown to prevent embolic complication) is indicated. The medical aspects of the patient's condition are a challenge to the surgeon and are at least as important as the technique and insertion of internal fixation devices.

Fractures of the Femoral Shaft

Femoral shaft fractures occur at any age, from severe violence, but injuries in children may occur from less severe indirect torsional stress applied to the leg. When major trauma is involved, associated injuries of the chest, head, and abdomen are common and should be the first consideration. When a patient with a fractured femur is in shock, other injuries requiring immediate attention should be suspected, although hemorrhage into a thigh may produce severe hypotension.

CLINICAL MANIFESTATIONS. Patients with a fractured femoral shaft have severe pain with any attempt at motion of the extremity. There is usually rotational deformity, shortening of the affected leg, with prominent swelling of the thigh.

The most important immediate local consideration with fractures of the femoral shaft is whether there has been damage to the femoral or popliteal vessels. If the patient has good pedal pulses, with normal sensation and motor power in the foot, major arterial injury is unlikely. However, when signs of ischemia are present or cannot be ruled out, arteriography and/or exploration of the vessels are indicated. This may be a difficult judgment, and consultation with the most experienced surgeon should be obtained.

TREATMENT. Emergency treatment at the scene of the accident should include splinting the leg to the adjacent extremity or, optimally, traction applied to the foot over a Thomas splint. If the wound is compound and the bones are protruding, they should not be repositioned until proper debridement has been carried out.

Femoral shaft fractures in children are treated exclusively by closed methods. Internal fixation is contraindicated because of potential damage to the epiphyseal plate and growth disturbances of the femur. Anatomic reduction is not required (Fig. 47-47). With a displaced femoral shaft fracture in a child, 1 cm of overriding is acceptable as long as there are no more than a few degrees of angulation and rotational deformity has been completely corrected. The epiphyseal stimulation provided by the presence of healing callus will make up 1 cm of shortening. In the very young child, where a maximum of 2 lb can be used to reduce the fracture, Bryant's traction provides an effective means for reduction. However, the child's ability to dorsiflex his great toe should be repeatedly inspected to be certain that an anterior compartment syndrome or vascular compromise is not developing in either lower extremity. Russell's traction is used for older children. Repeat check x-rays are obtained at intervals to be certain that position and reduction are maintained. It is imperative that reduction be accomplished in a few days, because by 10 days most fractures in children are clinically firm. When the fracture is clinically stable and nontender and callus

Fig. 47-47. Femoral shaft fracture in a child treated by traction. *A* and *B*. AP and lateral x-rays in satisfactory position in skin traction. *C* and *D*. AP and lateral x-rays of healed fracture showing satisfactory position. The anterior angulation at the fracture site will remodel itself.

is present by x-ray, the child is placed in a 1½ hip spica. Progressive weight bearing between crutches is started when bony union is solid.

Treatment of shaft fractures in adults may be accomplished by either closed methods or open reduction. Methods employing intramedullary fixation or plate reduction have been used, at times with disastrous results. If a shaft fracture is transverse or of a short oblique type without comminution and occurs at the narrowest portion of the medullary cavity, intramedullary fixation may be indicated provided the skin is normal and the patient is in optimal condition for operative intervention. Intramedullary fixation requiring an open reduction of the fracture site has a high incidence of wound sepsis (6 percent) and an increased incidence of delayed union. An infection at the site of an intramedullary nail means 3 to 4 years of treatment, stiff joints, and the possibility of chronic osteomyelitis.

Closed intramedullary nailing using the technique of Küntscher is superior to that in which the fracture site must be opened. Küntscher's technique relies upon reaming of the medullary cavity, allowing good fixation of both fracture fragments when the fracture site is not at the narrowest portion of the medullary canal. The incidence of infection with blind nailing is much less than with exposure of the fracture site. This may be nearly as safe as the treatment with skeletal traction. It is imperative that the operator be familiar with the technique and be equipped with a fracture table as well as an image intensifier for accomplishing the closed reduction and blind nailing.

Femoral shaft fractures, by virtue of the surrounding muscle mass, require skeletal traction to maintain length and alignment. Traction is applied to a threaded Steinmann pin placed across the supracondylar area or proximal tibia. When there is associated knee injury, it is best to insert the Steinmann pin through the supracondylar area and not to apply skeletal traction across the injured knee.

Technique of Insertion of the Steinmann Pin. The supracondylar region is prepared and draped under aseptic conditions. Local anesthesia is infiltrated to the skin and periosteum both medially and laterally, at a point just proximal to the femoral condyles. A threaded Steinmann pin is then drilled across the supracondylar region from medial to lateral, making certain that the pin is placed as far posterior as possible, to prevent crossing the suprapatellar pouch.

If the fracture is in the distal femoral shaft, the Steinmann pin is inserted from lateral to medial at the level of the tibial tubercle in order to prevent damage to the lateral popliteal nerve. The leg is placed in a balanced suspension apparatus with weight applied to the skeletal traction bow on the Steinmann pin. If conditions permit, the fracture is manipulated into position and held there with skeletal traction.

Repeat AP and lateral x-rays are obtained in traction, and skeletal traction is adjusted accordingly. When the fracture is stable and firm, i.e., with no tenderness at the fracture site, and shortening does not occur when traction is removed, the patient is ready for immobilization in a 1½ hip spica if the fracture is high at the junction of the upper and middle thirds. A cast brace is applied and weight-bearing treatment instituted if the fracture is in the middle or distal third of the femur.

Cast Brace Treatment (Fig. 47-48). Cast brace treatment for fractures of the midshaft and distal one-third of the femur treated initially with skeletal traction allows more rapid mobilization of the patient and results in more rapid union and better functional return of knee motion than with spica cast immobilization. It may be possible to mobilize some fractures in a cast brace as early as the first or second week postinjury.

Technique of Cast Brace Application. A well-molded total contact plaster cast is applied to the thigh. An elastic Spandex sock is placed over the thigh, over which one layer of webril is wrapped snugly about the thigh. Elastic plaster of paris is wrapped over these layers, following which standard plaster, which has greater strength, is applied. The proximal rim is fashioned with an adjustable plastic quadrilateral rim or constructed in standard fashion. An elastic bandage is applied about the knee, following which a well-molded short leg cast is applied with the ankle at 90° and the foot in neutral position. When both plasters have dried, a single axis or polycentric knee joint hinges are applied medially and laterally connecting the two plasters with the knee hinge.

The patient is instructed in quadriceps exercises and knee range-of-motion exercises in the cast brace. He is allowed to bear increasing weight on the fractured extremity between crutches as tolerated. The brace is changed if it loosens and is discontinued when the patient can bear full weight painlessly without crutches, usually an additional 6 to 8 weeks from the time of its application. Mooney et al. have reported the mean healing time of $14\frac{1}{2}$ weeks for fractures in the distal femur treated with skeletal traction and the cast brace technique.

Delayed union when the cast brace technique is used is uncommon. However, if it occurs, it requires a reinforcing bone graft of circumferential iliac autogenous cancellous bone strips tied in place with catgut as indicated. In some instances it may be necessary to use internal plate fixation or intramedullary rod fixation in addition to autogenous iliac bone graft. Restriction of knee motion with the method of cast brace mobilization is uncommon but may occur when a $1\frac{1}{2}$ hip spica is applied.

Supracondylar Fractures

Supracondylar fractures of the femur and Y or T intracondylar fractures occur in all age groups from trauma occurring in automobile accidents, pedestrian injuries, falls, and various other accidents. Patients with this injury present with the usual signs of fracture, i.e., local swelling, instability, deformity. In some cases, the patient will appear to have only a knee effusion. Supracondylar fractures are intraarticular fractures, since they communicate with the suprapatellar pouch of the knee. Scarring in this region may obliterate the suprapatellar pouch and interfere with knee motion.

The supracondylar fragment is angulated posteriorly from the pull on the gastrocnemius muscle, attached to the posterior aspect of the femoral condyles. The pull of the quadriceps and hamstrings acts to increase shortening and the posterior angulation. The supracondylar fragment may have a valgus deformity produced by the strong pull of the adductors on the proximal femoral fragment. In T

Fig. 47-48. Ischial weight-bearing brace, quadrilateral plaster thigh socket for fractured femur.

or Y condylar fractures, the proximal fragment tends to be wedged between the condylar fragments by the existing muscle pull.

TREATMENT. Results of treatment of fractures in this region have been discouraging. With optimal treatment, a third of patients have significant restriction of knee motion. In attempting to overcome the poor results, open reduction and internal fixation have been tried, but the results are still inferior to conservative traction treatment.

A Steinmann pin is inserted through the tibial tubercle, and through this skeletal traction is applied. If persistent posterior angulation at the fracture site occurs, a transsupracondylar Steinmann pin is inserted and 3 to 5 lb of additional traction applied at right angles to the shaft of the femur. Reduction is monitored by check x-rays.

Quadriceps exercises are begun at 10 days and are continued in the traction apparatus until clinical stability is attained, at approximately 6 weeks. The cast brace technique of Mooney may be used when the fracture is stable.

TRAUMATIC EPIPHYSEAL SEPARATION OF THE DISTAL FEMUR

This injury occurs from forced hyperextension of the knee, in the adolescent child. Treatment should be immediate closed reduction and plaster immobilization. Open reduction of this injury is indicated only when the fracture is causing circulatory embarrassment.

Ligamentous Injuries of the Knee Joint

Injuries to the ligamentous supporting structures of the knee occur in all types of athletic endeavors but are especially common in sports utilizing cleats where the foot becomes fixed to the ground and direct or indirect force is applied to the knee joint. A similar mechanism occurs in skiing, where the long lever arm of the ski applies torque or stress to the knee joint, resulting in ligamentous damage. It must be emphasized that determination of ligamentous damage is dependent upon clinical examination and that routine x-rays add little information.

MEDIAL COLLATERAL LIGAMENT

The medial collateral ligament consists of a superficial portion which originates from the medial femoral epicondyle proximally and is attached distally a handbreadth below the knee joint on the medial aspect of the tibia beneath the pes anserinus. In addition to the medial collateral ligament are capsular ligaments which form a half-sleeve medially extending from the popliteal space behind to the patellar tendon in front. The anterior portion is represented by the anterior knee capsule with a contri-

Fig. 47-49. Knee ligament injuries from valgus force. Anterior cruciate is interrupted near its femoral origin. Medial collateral may avulse at the upper and lower ends of rupture in the middle as well as be disrupted from its meniscal attachment. (*After O'Donoghue.*)

bution from the vastus medialis retinaculum. The anterior capsular ligament is tight when the knee is flexed and relaxes as the knee is extended. The middle portion of the capsular ligament is also referred to as the deep layer of the medial ligament or the short internal lateral ligament. The upper part of the middle portion of the capsular ligament is attached to the medial femoral condyle slightly forward of the superficial tibial collateral ligament and is fixed to the middle third of the medial meniscus (the meniscal femoral ligament). The lower portion continues distally from the meniscus and is attached to the tibia just below the articular margin (the meniscal tibial ligament). The middle one-third is taut in all positions of flexion. The posterior part of the medial capsular ligament is a portion of the posterior capsule. When the knee is extended, the posterior ligament tightens; it slackens as the knee is flexed.

With increasing valgus stress to the knee and usually with simultaneous external rotation of the tibia upon the femur, medial capsular ligaments rupture, followed by rupture of the tibial collateral ligament. If the force continues, rupture of the anterior cruciate may occur (Fig. 47-49).

CLINICAL MANIFESTATIONS. With an acute injury to the medial ligamentous structures, symptoms and findings will vary according to the degree of damage. With a mild sprain without complete disruption of any of the components, the patient may only complain of pain and have a mild hemarthrosis. Occasionally, there is no hemarthrosis as the bleeding is external to the capsule. If clinical examination of the knee does not reveal instability or increased motion as compared with the opposite knee, the injury can be treated as a sprain with temporary immobilization and restriction of activity. When the force results in complete disruption of the ligaments, the findings are usually obvious, and there is no difficulty in deciding upon the need for surgical repair.

The real difficulty lies in moderate degrees of instability on clinical examination. If there is any doubt as to the integrity of the ligaments on clinical examination, the examination should be repeated under anesthesia and surgical exploration carried out as necessary. The uninjured knee is examined first and all examinations repeated on the injured side and compared with the normal.

The knee joint is flexed 20° to relax the posterior capsule, and valgus stress is applied to the knee. Opening up of the medial joint space is abnormal and indicates ligamentous discontinuity. The knee is then flexed to 90° and AP stability tested by pulling the tibia forward on the femur. This is carried out with the tibia in internal rotation, external rotation, and neutral rotation. Motion of the medial tibial condyle greater than 5 mm is abnormal and is a sign of rotational instability with damage to the medial capsular ligament. Forward motion of both condyles is an indication of anterior cruciate damage. When varus stress applied to the knee in 20° of flexion causes greater opening up of the lateral joint than the normal, it indicates lateral collateral and iliotibial band disruption. Valgus and varus testing is carried out on the extended knee to determine the integrity of the posterior capsule. Instability in this position indicates posterior capsule damage in addition to medial or lateral collateral ligament injury.

ANTERIOR CRUCIATE LIGAMENT RUPTURE

The anterior cruciate ligament may be ruptured in association with complete tears of the medial collateral ligaments. Isolated tears occur as the result of hyperextension or internal rotation of the tibia on the femur but may be due to a direct blow on a flexed knee. Determination of anterior cruciate rupture depends upon demonstrating forward displacement of both tibial condyles on the femur usually of more than 5 mm when compared with the opposite uninjured knee. This test is best carried out with the knee in near-extension. Interpretation of the findings is subjective, and great experience is necessary in this examination.

TREATMENT OF MEDIAL COLLATERAL AND CRUCIATE LIGAMENT INJURIES. Mild sprains of the medial collateral ligament when there is no evidence of instability are treated symptomatically. A tense hemarthrosis may be aspirated with considerable relief. The limb is splinted in a position of extension with a compression bandage or a posterior plaster splint. The patient is started on immediate isometric quadriceps exercises performed hourly. He may bear partial weight between crutches with the quadriceps set and the knee in full extension. It is helpful to reevaluate the knee in a few days in order to confirm the findings of stability.

Complete tears of the medial collateral ligaments, medial capsular ligaments, or anterior cruciate require surgical repair. This should be carried out as soon as possible but certainly within 2 weeks. A detached ligament may be retracted from its attachment with resultant healing in a lengthened or lax position. At the present time, there is no way to determine this without surgical exploration.

Operative Technique. The knee is exposed through an incision overlying the medial collateral ligament. When the subcutaneous tissue is entered, the site of ligamentous rupture will be marked by localized ecchymosis if surgical treatment is carried out within 24 hours of the time of injury. After ligamentous damage has been assessed, the knee joint is entered through a separate peripatellar incision in the capsule, and the anterior cruciate and menisci are evaluated. If the meniscus is torn, it is excised. Ruptures of the anterior cruciate ligament occurring in its substance are irreparable, and its remaining portion should be excised with attention then directed to an accurate repair of the medial ligamentous structures. If the anterior cruciate is pulled from its bony attachment, it is reattached with silk sutures passing through the substance of the femoral condyle or tibial condyle.

The medial collateral ligament is reattached to bone with silk sutures passed through drill holes in bone, and ruptures in the substance are repaired with silk approximating the two ends. Postoperatively the leg is immobilized in a long leg plaster cast from toes to groin with the ankle at neutral position and the knee in 40° flexion and maximal internal rotation. The cast is changed if there is sufficient loosening. Plaster immobilization is continued 6 to 8 weeks. The knee is mobilized gradually, with active motion strengthening both quadriceps and hamstrings. Protection against weight bearing is continued until full extension is possible and power of the quadriceps is near normal.

INJURIES TO THE LATERAL COLLATERAL LIGAMENT

The lateral collateral ligament is interrupted when a varus force is applied to the knee. The lateral popliteal nerve, by virtue of its location and fixation as it winds around the neck of the fibula, is commonly stretched by the same injury. The treatment of this acute injury requires open exploration repair of the avulsed ligament from the femoral condyle or head of the fibula. The iliotibial band crossing the knee joint is commonly ruptured and requires repair. The nerve should be examined at the time of surgical treatment, but since this is usually a stretch injury, delayed repair depending upon follow-up evaluation is necessary. Injuries to the posterior cruciate ligament occur rarely as isolated injury but may accompany medial lateral collateral ligamentous injuries. Repair of the posterior cruciate is similar to the repair of the anterior cruciate, i.e., by utilizing drill holes through the femur or tibia.

CHRONIC LIGAMENTOUS INJURIES TO THE KNEE

Persistent laxity of the collateral ligamentous structures or cruciate ligaments results in knee joint instability. Such injuries, if severe, are disabling and may require the competitive athlete to discontinue competition. With minor degrees of instability, symptoms may be apparent only with vigorous athletics. When severe, the knee may be chronically effused, painful, and unstable with normal activity. Patients give a history of pain, locking, sudden giving way, or feeling of instability.

Reconstruction of the chronically unstable knee is difficult and is not always successful in returning a patient to athletics. Reefing the posterior medial capsule, shortening the medial collateral structures, and pes anserinus transfer are of value for medial collateral instability. Similar procedures are available for the lateral side. It is occasionally difficult to separate medial from lateral instability in the chronically unstable knee, in which case stress x-rays should be obtained.

INJURIES OF KNEE MENISCI

The tibia rotates laterally upon the femur as the knee joint goes from flexion to extension, and medial with the opposite motion. If this simultaneous rotation is interfered with or forcibly reversed, the semilunar cartilage may be injured. A common injury occurs when the football player catches his cleated shoe while weight is applied to the flexed knee. Similarly, a person squatting with the knees fully flexed and suddenly twisting his knee without simultaneous movement into extension will suffer an acute meniscus tear. Helfet believes that only the fibrotic medial meniscus of the elderly is actually torn by pressure grinding between the femoral and tibial surfaces.

In the young adult, rotation without flexion or extension causes the cartilage to straighten out. If the force is excessive, the cartilage is unable to accommodate, and a tear occurs at its inner free border, usually about the midpoint.

The cartilage may be detached from its attachment to the anterior cruciate or be split longitudinally to produce a bucket-handle tear, or it may be injured in its posterior portion by detachment from its posterior capsular attachments (Fig. 47-50). The medial meniscus is injured at least nine times as commonly as the lateral in the Caucasian, although lateral meniscal tears are more common in the Oriental. The medial meniscus is fixed to the capsule and is relatively immobile, whereas the lateral meniscus is not fixed to the capsule and has the popliteus muscle to assist in controlling its position.

CLINICAL MANIFESTATIONS. Meniscal injuries are commonly found in the young male individual who is using his knee vigorously, either for athletics or vocationally. Such injuries are less common in women.

The injury causes acute pain, which may subside rapidly. If the cartilage is undisplaced, there may be no immediate interference with motion. A joint effusion, with associated discomfort and stiffness, gradually develops in response to the injury. This will occur sooner and more severely if the meniscal damage is at its peripheral attachment, where blood vessels may be interrupted.

The diagnosis of a torn meniscus will depend on an accurate history, which should include the position of the knee and the direction of the rotational force at the time of the injury. The patient should be questioned about locking, instability, episodes of giving way or buckling, and previous injuries to the knee.

Examination of the knee after an acute injury may reveal varying degrees of joint effusion. There is local tenderness over the meniscus, which is greatest at the site of injury. Stability of the knee ligaments should be examined by valgus, varus, and anteroposterior stress.

The knee motion is examined with special emphasis on testing for synchronous rotation as the knee goes into full extension. By grasping both heels, both knees are passively brought to full extension and any limitation determined. Normally, the tibial tubercle in full extension aligns with

Fig. 47-50. Types of meniscal injuries. Top left, complete bucket-handle tear; top right, complete detachment of the meniscus from its peripheral margin; lower left, posterior tab tear; lower right, anterior tab tear of the medial meniscus.

the lateral border of the patella. If rotation has been compromised, the tibial tubercle will align with the central axis of the patella. In carrying out extension motions, there is localization of pain to medial or lateral aspects of the joint, at the site of the injury to the meniscus. Palpation of the joint line may indicate displacement of the meniscus. The test described by McMurray to delineate meniscal tears is occasionally helpful. The maneuver is elicited by passively flexing hip and knee of the supine patient. The foot is gradually externally rotated, while abduction stress is applied to the knee as it is gradually brought into extension. A displaced portion of the medial meniscus, catching between the femur and tibia, will cause a definite click and pain.

The diagnosis of acute meniscus injury may be difficult. Unless there is definite evidence of locking or displacement of the meniscus, the patient should be treated conservatively and reevaluated when the acute symptoms subside. Knee effusion, if severe, is aspirated, and the knee is brought to maximal extension and immobilized in a splint or compression bandage. The patient is allowed to bear weight between crutches with his quadriceps taut. The patient is reevaluated at weekly intervals and meniscectomy carried out only when the diagnosis is certain.

Arthrography is extremely helpful when the diagnosis is not absolutely certain. It is also of value in ruling out damage to the opposite meniscus. The technique of arthrography is demanding and requires exact positioning of the knee at the time of x-ray and experience in interpreting the arthrograms. The technique of Fryberger involves injection of air and absorbable contrast media into the joint. The x-ray beam is centered on the meniscus, and x-rays are taken in various positions of rotation for both medial and lateral menisci. The technique of arthroscopy increases the accuracy of the diagnosis when it is questionable. Even in patients with locked knees, when arthrotomy cannot be avoided, arthroscopy will delineate pathologic change in the other meniscus.

TREATMENT. When the diagnosis is established, meniscectomy is indicated to prevent the further cartilage and ligamentous damage associated with displaced menisci.

Technique. If injury to the patella is suspected, meniscectomy should be carried out through a median parapatellar incision, so that better exposure of the patella can be obtained. If the diagnosis can be localized to the meniscus, a transverse incision is used. A transverse incision is made parallel to, and immediately above, the medial meniscus between the patellar ligament and the anterior border of the medial collateral ligament. The anterior capsule is split vertically above the meniscus, and the joint is inspected through this incision.

The anterior horn of the meniscus is detached from its attachment to the cruciate and upper tibial plateau and the peripheral edge incised by sharp dissection as far posteriorly as possible. The interval of dissection is in the most peripheral portion of the meniscus and not between the capsule and meniscus, which would cause hemorrhage. By externally rotating the tibia on the femur, it is possible to view the posterior attachment of the meniscus. However, in some instances, it may be necessary to make a second vertical incision posterior to the medial collateral ligament in order to define the posterior third attachment. When the meniscus has been detached peripherally, it is displaced into the intracondylar notch, and the posterior attachment to the tibial surface is divided under direct vision. The wound is closed in routine fashion.

Postoperatively, the leg is immobilized in a position of full extension and the patient started on hourly quadriceps exercises. He is allowed out of bed when he can control his leg without pain and can bear partial weight between crutches with his quadriceps taut. Gradual knee flexion is started between 2 and 3 weeks, and the patient should be back to full activity in 6 weeks.

Injuries to the lateral meniscus are much less common and are handled in similar fashion. Discoid meniscus and cysts of the lateral meniscus also require meniscectomy.

Fractures of the Patella

Patellar fractures are usually due to direct trauma to the patella but also occur with sudden forced flexion of an actively contracting quadriceps. Fractures are more commonly transverse or comminuted but may take any direction. As the patella is an integral part of the extensor mechanism, separation at the fracture site is an indication that the adjacent patellar retinacula have been interrupted and active extension will not be possible (Fig. 47-51). Treatment is aimed at restoring a smoothly gliding extensor mechanism.

TREATMENT. Undisplaced fractures require a plaster cylinder cast for 6 to 8 weeks to prevent separation of the fragments. Check x-rays in plaster should be obtained at 7 to 10 days to be certain that displacement has not occurred. The patient is instructed in quadriceps exercises and may bear partial weight between crutches.

Transverse fractures with separation of the fragments require operative intervention to restore continuity of the extensor mechanism. Although some surgeons advocate circumferential wire suture to hold the fragments together, there is usually enough comminution in the region of the subchondral surface of the patella that an irregular articular surface of the patella will remain. For this reason, excision of the smaller fragments, usually the lower half, is indicated, combined with reattachment of the patellar ligament through drill holes on the raw fracture surface of the proximal fragment. At the same time, the patellar retinaculum is surgically repaired.

For grossly comminuted fractures of the patella, immediate excision of all fragments is carried out and the quadriceps mechanism repaired. Postoperatively, the limb is maintained in extension, and quadriceps exercises are immediately instituted. At 4 weeks, the cast is removed and beginning range of motion exercises started. At 6 weeks, active flexion is begun.

The same principles apply to open fractures of the patella.

The quadriceps may be ruptured or the patellar ligament avulsed from its insertion on the patella when acute flexion

Fig. 47-51. Comminuted fracture of patella. AP and lateral x-rays showing comminuted patella with separation of the upper and lower major fragments indicating interruption of the extensor mechanism.

forces are applied to the contracting extensor mechanism. Immediate diagnosis and surgical repair are required.

Recurrent Dislocation of the Patella

The patella may be dislocated in any direction. Upward dislocation is the result of rupture of the patellar ligament. Medial dislocation is uncommon but may occur from severe injury or, rarely, after poliomyelitis. Lateral dislocation is the most common type. This may occur with severe injury or poliomyelitis but is most commonly seen in young women or girls after minor trauma. It is related to the increased valgus angle of the female knee but may also be the result of hypoplastic development of the external condyle of the femur, congenital abnormalities of the patella, or congenital contractures of the vastus intermedius.

The patient complains of the knee's giving way as the patella momentarily slips laterally over the lateral femoral condyle and spontaneously reduces. In more severe cases the patella may become lodged lateral to the femoral condyle, requiring manipulative reduction. Following spontaneous relocation of the patella, the patient has symptoms of mild synovitis and effusion.

Treatment for the acutely dislocated patella is manual reduction followed by immobilization of the knee in full extension in plaster and rehabilitation of quadriceps muscle power. It is necessary to treat the initial dislocation by plaster immobilization of the knee, or the medial patellar retinaculum will heal with capsular laxity, allowing subsequent dislocation. By maintaining the tone of the vastus medialis, there may be sufficient muscle power to prevent subsequent dislocation. With recurrent dislocations, surgical treatment is usually necessary. Before epiphyseal closure, the Roux-Goldthwait operation may be done. This consists of transposing the lateral half of the patellar ligament at its insertion medially beneath the undisturbed medial insertion. At the same time, an ellipse of capsule and medial patella retinaculum is excised and the capsule reefed to hold the patella medially. After the age of fourteen, the Hauser procedure, a medial transposition of a block of bone encompassing the attachment of the patellar ligament, is utilized. With recurrent dislocation the progression of chondromalacia to severe damage to the undersurface of the patella may necessitate patellectomy and quadricepsplasty.

Fractures of the Tibial Plateau

Fractures of the tibial plateau occur at any age but are more common in the middle-aged or elderly. Fractures of the lateral tibial plateau occur when there is a sudden valgus stress to the knee joint, when there is an axial load applied to the femoral shaft. Common causes involve an automobile bumper striking the knee joint of a pedestrian or a worker falling from a scaffolding. The medial collateral ligament may be ruptured, concomitantly.

Types of fractures are (1) a simple split fracture of the lateral tibial plateau, (2) severe comminution of the lateral tibial plateau, and (3) fractures of both condyles with a vertical fracture line into the region of the tibial spines.

TREATMENT. If the medial collateral ligament is ruptured, surgical repair is indicated. If there is severe displacement of the lateral tibial plateau, open reduction in an attempt at elevation of the depression may be required.

However, most fractures can be handled with best results by the method of Weissman and Harold. Large hemarthroses are aspirated. The knee is splinted in extension for 1 week during which time hourly quadriceps and straight-leg-raising exercises are instituted. When normal quadriceps muscle power has been regained, flexion exercises are started; a posterior splint is reapplied between exercises. The splint is gradually discontinued as power and motion improve. Partial weight bearing is permitted between 4 and 6 weeks, and full weight bearing at about 8 to 10 weeks. Despite the apparent severity of these fractures as seen by x-ray, good results usually can be obtained.

Tibial Shaft Fractures

Fractures of the tibial shaft occur from direct trauma and may occur when an automobile passenger strikes his leg against the dashboard or when the leg of a pedestrian is struck by a car bumper (Fig. 47-52). Fractures also may occur by indirect torsional forces as with sports injuries, such as in skiing. In falling, the skier applies torsional force to the shaft of the tibia, via the long lever of the attached ski. Some fractures of the tibia occur from simple falls.

Tibial shaft fractures occur at any age. About 70 percent of such fractures are closed and 30 percent open. Indirect torsional forces cause oblique or spiral fractures, whereas direct trauma may result in transverse, segmental, or comminuted fractures of the tibial shaft. There is no difference in the rate of healing of tibial shaft fractures according to the location of the fracture or the plane of the fracture surface. Rate of healing is correlated with the severity of trauma. Fractures caused by high-energy trauma from automobile accidents with or without open wounds have the longest rate of healing. The presence of an intact fibula results in a more rapid rate of union.

CLINICAL MANIFESTATIONS. Undisplaced fractures may

Fig. 47-52. Fracture of the proximal tibia shaft with fracture of the neck of the fibula incurred by an automobile bumper's striking a pedestrian. A and B. AP and lateral x-rays postinjury. C and D. AP and lateral x-rays showing postreduction position in a long leg cast.

Fig. 47-53. Fracture of the distal tibia and fibula shafts. *A* and *B*. AP and lateral x-rays postinjury. *C* and *D*. AP and lateral x-rays showing healed fracture in satisfactory position.

have only tenderness and swelling at the site of fracture, but patients are unable to put weight on the affected extremity. Undisplaced spiral fractures occur in the very young. Such fractures may be quite stable, and diagnosis is suggested by the fact that the child will not use the affected leg.

Displaced fractures result in deformity with swelling and ecchymosis. Anteroposterior and lateral x-rays will characterize the fracture.

TREATMENT. Closed tibial shaft fractures are best handled by closed conservative measures (Fig. 47-53). Dehne et al. and Sarmiento, using plaster methods and allowing early weight bearing, have achieved rapid union with no infection and a low incidence of delayed union.

Technique of Closed Reduction

With the patient under analgesia or local anesthesia to the fracture site and lying supine with both legs flexed at the knees, hanging over the end of the table, most tibial shaft fractures can be realigned and deformity corrected by gentle manipulation. The opposite leg is used as a guide to determine correction of rotation and deformity.

Over one layer of stockinet and one layer of sheet wadding, a well-molded plaster cast is applied to the knee with the foot in 10 to 15° of plantar flexion or, if possible, at a right angle. When the plaster has hardened, the knee is brought to full extension and the plaster extended to include the thigh. The reduction is checked by AP and lateral x-rays. The patient is hospitalized with the leg elevated and ice applied over the region of the fracture site. Circulation to the foot and the patient's ability to dorsiflex and plantar flex toes comfortably is checked every 2 hours to be certain that vascular insufficiency or com-

partment syndromes are not occurring. If necessary, the cast is split to relieve swelling.

When the patient is comfortable and can actively control the affected extremity, he is allowed up on crutches to bear as much weight as pain tolerates. The patient may continue in the long leg cast until union is complete, or at 3 weeks the plaster may be changed to a below-knee cast appropriately molded about the tibial condyles and patellar ligament to control rotation, as described by Sarmiento.

Any type of fracture including transverse, comminuted, or oblique spiral fractures may be treated in this fashion. Approximately a $\frac{1}{2}$-cm shortening can be anticipated from the weight-bearing treatment in addition to whatever shortening is present at the time of the closed reduction. If this seems unacceptable, pins may be placed above and below the fracture site to control length and weight bearing not allowed. The weight-bearing method of treating tibial shaft fractures is clearly the best method available with the lowest incidence of complication. The average time until plaster removal is about 13 weeks.

Management of Compound Fractures. Compound fractures must be immediately debrided and fractures immobilized. Depending upon the kind of wound and adequacy of debridement, the skin may be closed, but the indications for this are extremely rare. Secondary closure of the wound may be carried out or the wound left open to granulate beneath a weight-bearing plaster cast as described by Brown and Urban. The use of internal fixation in open fractures is not justified because of the hazard of infection, skin loss, and nonunion.

Administration of antibiotics is continued until the wound is healed and followed with appropriate check x-rays during the first month to make certain that position is being maintained. Cast wedging or remanipulation may be required to restore alignment.

Compartment Syndromes

After fractures, soft tissue injury, prolonged limb compression (as in drug-overdosed patients), and arterial operations, progressive muscle ischemia may occur in any of the fascial compartments of the limbs. In the upper extremity this includes the anterior compartments of the forearm, and in the lower extremity the four anterior and posterior compartments. The mechanism involved is unrelieved swelling in the tight osseofascial compartments. The arteries may continue to pulsate while the ischemia is developing, since the latter occurs when the capillary filling pressure is exceeded. Hence the clinical signs depend upon detection of change in muscle function, i.e., loss of motor power or extreme pain with passive stretch. Patients should also be observed for ischemic pain (severe pain at rest) or pain not responding to analgesics. Distal pulses of the extremity are usually present early in the course and may persist until complete and irreversible necrosis has occurred.

Prevention of sequelae depends upon early recognition and surgical decompression of the individual compartments. Compartment pressures can be determined by direct measurement, as with the Wick catheter, but when in doubt surgical exploration (and decompression) is indicated. It is important to consider the possibility that compartment syndromes may develop after open fractures or during elective tibial osteotomies. In those instances compartments should be decompressed prophylactically.

Ankle Injuries

ANATOMY. Motion of the tibiotalar joint is pure flexion and extension. Inversion and eversion of the foot is accomplished at the subtalar and midtarsal joints. The upper surface of the talus is dome-shaped in the anteroposterior plane, with a narrower articular surface, posteriorly. The talus is without muscular origin or insertion and is attached to its related articulations by capsule and ligaments. The ankle mortise is formed by the downward medial and lateral projections of malleoli grasping the dome of the talus. Maintenance of the normal mortise is a prerequisite for painless ankle motion. Stability of the talus in the mortise is dependent on the distal tibiofibular ligaments and interosseous membrane, as well as the anterior and posterior talofibular ligaments, calcaneofibular ligaments laterally, and a strong deltoid ligament medially.

MECHANISMS OF INJURY. Ankle injuries are caused by a sudden application of force which exceeds the strength of the ligaments or malleoli. Applied across the ankle joint, the force rotates the foot into inversion-eversion, or adduction-abduction in relation to the tibia, or rotates the tibia similarly in relation to the fixed foot. Athletic injuries account for a large proportion of ankle injuries, although a simple fall or sudden misstep may be sufficient to cause a severe fracture-dislocation. All combinations of ligamentous injuries and fractures are possible, depending upon the severity and direction of force.

The injured ankle should be carefully examined for the location of tenderness, swelling, and deformity. If the patient was able to walk on the ankle immediately after the injury, this indicates stability but does not rule out undisplaced fracture. Caution should be applied in diagnosing injuries on the football field before all signs have had time to develop.

The ankle should be splinted with an air splint or with a pillow splint until x-ray examination is complete. Three x-ray views are necessary for x-ray evaluation of the ankle joint. Standard AP and lateral x-rays are required and, in addition, a 30° medial oblique view to determine the competence of the mortise.

LIGAMENTOUS INJURIES

The most common ankle injury which involves portions of the lateral collateral ligaments is caused by a sudden inversion force applied to the foot. The anterior talofibular ligament is usually involved. On examination, there is local tenderness and ecchymosis at the midpoint or attachments of the anterior talofibular ligament or calcaneofibular or posterior talofibular ligaments.

If the patient has minimal swelling and tenderness on examination, can walk with minimal discomfort, and x-rays are normal, it is sufficient to treat the injury as a sprain by adhesive strapping for 2 to 4 weeks. Tenderness on the medial side of the joint immediately after the injury is an indication of sufficient lateral damage to allow subluxation to produce stretch or injury to the deltoid ligament. If there has been complete division of any component of the lateral collateral ligament, stress films are indicated, for which the ankle is anesthetized under local or general anesthesia and the foot brought into maximal inversion. X-rays taken with the foot in this position will reveal tilting of the talus in the mortise, if there is discontinuity of any portion of the lateral collateral ligaments. If a talar tilt is present, immobilization in a short leg plaster with the foot in neutral position and the ankle at a 90° angle is required for 6 weeks. Plaster immobilization may be elected in the absence of stress films. With any ankle injury requiring plaster, it is necessary to obtain check films immediately after reduction and also at 10 to 14 days to ensure maintenance of position. If patients continue to have instability after conservative treatment, secondary open repair of the involved lateral ligaments can be performed.

Distal Tibiofibular Diastasis

With eversion injuries to the ankle, there may be interruption of the ligamentous continuity of the distal tibiofibular joint, resulting in a diastasis of the ankle mortise. The patient's ankle is unable to bear weight, and marked swelling occurs in the region of the tibiofibular joint.

It is rarely possible to maintain reduction without operative intervention. A 1½-in. vertical incision is made over the distal fibula and the periosteum elevated from the fibula, proximal to the level of the tibiotalar articulation. A lag screw is inserted across an overdrilled hole in the fibula to close the diastasis. This is accomplished with the ankle at 90° and not with the foot in plantar flexion. When the foot is in plantar flexion, the narrowest portion of the talus is in contact with the tibia, and permanent limitation

Fig. 47-54. Compound fracture-dislocation of the ankle. *A, B,* and *C.* AP, lateral, and oblique x-rays postinjury showing comminuted fracture of the distal fibula and posterior dislocation of the ankle. The deltoid ligament was avulsed from the medial malleolus, which protruded through the skin. *D* and *E.* AP and lateral x-rays following debridement and closed reduction.

of dorsiflexion will result. At 8 weeks, the cast is removed and the screw excised at a second operation.

FRACTURES AND DISLOCATIONS (Fig. 47-54)

Undisplaced fractures of malleoli require immobilization in plaster for 8 weeks. The most common isolated malleolar fracture is an oblique fracture of the lateral malleolus caused by an external rotation injury. If the ankle mortise is not involved, a well-molded plaster cast is applied with the foot in neutral varus-valgus position and maintained for 6 weeks. Check x-rays are obtained to be certain that reduction has not been lost. If there is a fracture of the lateral malleolus with lateral displacement of the talus, this is corrected by manipulation under local or general anesthesia and the hind part of the foot placed in maximal inversion with the ankle at 90° of dorsiflexion.

Medial Malleolar Fractures

Undisplaced fractures of the medial malleolus with an intact mortise are treated by plaster immobilization. Bimalleolar ankle fractures with dislocation require accurate reduction until union is solid. The usual mechanism of injury of a bimalleolar fracture is by external rotation and eversion. If the talus is displaced laterally, reduction is necessary. Most fractures can be handled by closed reduction.

Technique of Closed Reduction. With local or general anesthesia and the leg hanging over the end of the table, traction is applied to the hind part of the foot in the long axis of the leg. With traction maintained, the hind part of the foot is gradually brought into inversion, to correct the lateral displacement, while lateral countertraction is applied to the medial subcutaneous surface of the tibia. Simultaneously, the foot, which is resting on the knee of the operator, is brought into 90° of dorsiflexion. The reduction should be stable when the foot is held at 90° of dorsiflexion at maximal inversion. A well-molded cast is applied over one thickness of stockinet and one thickness of sheet wadding. The cast is then extended to include the knee. Check x-rays are obtained and the patient admitted to the hospital for evaluation of circulation. If the medial malleolus fracture extends to the point where the vertical and horizontal articular cartilage meet at the distal end of the tibia, sufficient medial buttress will not be present to hold a closed reduction, and open reduction will be required.

Technique of Open Reduction. A 2-in. vertical incision is centered over the medial malleolus. The fracture site is exposed, and the medial malleolar fragment retracted distad by hinging it upon its deltoid attachment, thus exposing the joint. Intraarticular fragments are removed. Soft tissue dissection, for inspection of the joint, is minimized. The fragment is reduced anatomically, held with a towel clip, and fixed with a 2-in. standard bone screw. Using a reconstituted medial malleolar buttress, closed reduction is carried out and the foot held in maximal inversion. X-rays are obtained to determine reduction, and a well-molded long leg cast is applied with the knee at 20° of flexion, the ankle at 90° of dorsiflexion, and the foot in maximal inversion. Plaster immobilization is continued for 8 weeks, and weight bearing is not allowed before 12 weeks.

Posterior Malleolar Fractures

The posterior malleolus is usually fractured in combination with medial or lateral malleolar fractures. The importance of the posterior malleolus is to maintain anteroposterior stability of the ankle joint. When 30 percent of the tibial articular surface is involved in the posterior malleolar fracture, instability will ensue if anatomic reduction is not obtained.

Anatomic reduction of a large posterior malleolar fragment can be maintained only with internal fixation. The posterior malleolar fragment is exposed through a posteromedial or posterolateral incision and fixed with a screw to the major tibial fragment. Trimalleolar fractures with small posterior fragments and good anteroposterior stabil-

A   B   C

Fig. 47-55. Trimalleolar ankle fracture-dislocation. AP, lateral, and oblique x-rays showing posterior dislocation of the talus and fractures of the medial malleolus, the lateral malleolus, and a small fragment from the posterior malleolus.

ity require maintenance of reduction of the mortise, and the posterior fragment can be disregarded (Fig. 47-55).

Fractures involving the anterior articular surface occur from severe trauma, as in falls from heights and in automobile injuries. The anterior portion of the distal tibial articular surface may be fractured or crushed, but usually this is in association with adjacent malleolar fractures. Such injuries are serious, because there is an associated crush injury to the articular cartilage which may cause difficulty, regardless of the reduction.

Attempts should be made to realign the articular surface by closed manipulation. In some cases, it may be possible to perform open reduction, although when comminution is severe, subsequent ankle arthrodesis may be necessary.

Fractures and Dislocations of the Foot

FRACTURES AND DISLOCATIONS OF THE TALUS

The talus is fractured in its distal portion, through the neck or body. Neck fractures account for the majority of talus injuries. Fractures of the neck occur from forcible dorsiflexion of the foot, such that the neck is driven against the anterior margin of the distal tibia.

If the vertical force continues, a subtalar dislocation may complicate the fracture. Still greater force is associated with fractures of the neck of the talus, subtalar dislocation, and posterior displacement of the body from the ankle joint. Such fracture-dislocations are commonly compound. In some cases, the patient presents with the posterior body of the talus having been driven out through the wound and left at the scene of the accident.

The subtalar joint may be dislocated by maximal inversion stress in the position of plantar flexion. In such a case, the foot is dislocated medially, beneath the body of the talus. Greater force results in dislocation of the talus from the ankle joint, resulting in total dislocation of the talus.

If there is sufficient damage across the neck of the talus, avascular necrosis of the body may ensue. In the series by Dunne et al., avascular necrosis developed in 69 percent of neck fracture-dislocations and 50 percent of body fractures.

TREATMENT. Fractures of the neck are treated by closed reduction and plaster cast immobilization until bony union is complete. Displaced fractures with dislocation are reduced by closed manipulation carried out with the foot in the talipes equinus position. If accurate closed reduction cannot be accomplished, open reduction through a lateral approach is indicated. Care is taken not to devitalize soft tissue attachments. Kirschner wires are used for internal fixation. Postoperative plaster immobilization is continued until union is evident (3 months or longer).

Undisplaced fractures of the body of the talus may be treated by immobilization in neutral position. For severe compression fractures, primary tibial-talar fusion using the method of Blair may be indicated. Avascular necrosis, which develops in the majority of cases, is not a deterrent to a good result if immobilization is continued until union is solid and weight bearing is prevented until revascularization occurs.

Complete talar dislocations or subtalar dislocations are reduced by placing the foot in maximal inversion and, with direct pressure over the talus, bringing the calcaneus and forefoot into eversion. Considerable force and general anesthesia may be necessary to accomplish reduction of the completely dislocated talus. The foot is then immobilized until soft tissue healing is complete.

FRACTURES OF THE CALCANEUS

Fractures of the calcaneus commonly occur from falls in which the maximal force is applied to the calcaneus.

It has been shown experimentally by Thoren that the type of fracture is related to the position of the subtalar joint at the time of impact. Involvement of the posterior articular facet is least likely to occur when the foot is in maximal pronation. The main fracture line is oblique, creating two major fragments, an anteromedial fragment and a posterolateral fragment. Fractures of the anterior portion of the calcaneus or the tuberosity also may occur.

A suitable classification of fractures of the calcaneus has been described by Dart and Graham (Fig. 47-56). Type I isolated fractures include beak fractures of the tuberosity or fractures of the anterior part of the calcaneus with minimal calcaneocuboid joint involvement. Type II includes fractures of the body without joint surface involvement. Type IIIa consists of depressed fractures of the posterior facet with minimal depression of Böhler's angle. Böhler's angle (tuberosity joint angle) is the angle formed by the axis of the subtalar joint and the superior surface of the tuberosity. Type IIIb is severe depression of Böhler's angle. Type IV fractures are grossly comminuted fractures (Fig. 47-57), involving subtalar and calcaneocuboid joints. Type V consists of avulsions of the tendocalcaneus with a portion of bone from the posterior portion of the calcaneus.

Approximately 25 percent of patients presenting with fractures of the calcaneus have associated injuries, including compression fractures of the spine, pelvic fractures, or fractures in the lower extremities.

TREATMENT. Treatment of severely comminuted calcaneus fractures is difficult because of the associated soft tissue injury, which contributes to chronic swelling as well as to interference of subtalar joint motion. Compression of the cancellous calcaneus makes stable reduction difficult. The patient should be hospitalized; regardless of what course of treatment is decided upon, the limb must be immediately elevated to prevent swelling and minimize hematoma formation. Types I and II are treated by bed rest, elevation, and early range-of-motion exercises. Patients are allowed to ambulate with crutches after 2 to 3 weeks, and weight bearing is prevented for 3 months. In Type III fractures, Böhler's angle should be corrected by the method of Essex-Lopresti. This involves the insertion of a Steinmann pin through the tendocalcaneus and posterior fragment, which is then forcibly depressed, correcting the tuberosity-joint angle. The pin is then driven across the anterior fragment and/or calcaneocuboid joint. Any significant widening of the calcaneus is corrected by manual compression. The foot and protruding Steinmann pin are immobilized in plaster for 6 weeks. At 6 weeks, range-of-motion exercises are started, and weight bearing is allowed at 3 months.

One may elect the same type of treatment for Type IV fractures, although triple arthrodesis may be indicated when the acute swelling has subsided, approximately 6 weeks after injury.

For Type V fractures, the fragment should have open reduction and screw fixation of the tendocalcaneus insertion.

Many patients, in spite of early active motion and physiotherapy, will have stiffness, chronic swelling of the foot,

Fig. 47-56. Types of fracture of the calcaneus (after Dart and Graham).

and broadening of the heel. If the early active motion can be instituted, there will be less difficulty due to swelling and less restriction of motion.

METATARSAL FRACTURES

Fractures of the Fifth Metatarsal

The base of the fifth metatarsal may be fractured during inversion injuries of the foot (Fig. 47-58). The attachment of the peroneus brevis to the base of the fifth metatarsal avulses this portion of the bone during sudden, forceful inversion. The patient may sustain an associated sprain of the anterior talofibular ligament at the same time. On examination, there is local tenderness over the base of the fifth metatarsal. The patient may be unable to bear weight because of discomfort.

Fig. 47-57. Comminuted (Type IV) fracture of the calcaneus incurred from a fall from a two-story window. A. Lateral x-ray. B. Axial view of calcaneus and subtalar joint.

Fig. 47-58. Avulsion fracture of the base of the fifth metatarsal. Lateral and oblique x-rays showing undisplaced fracture. Treatment was by boot walking cast for 6 weeks.

Treatment of this injury is symptomatic. For some individuals, taping of the foot and ankle to provide immobilization in the position of eversion is all that is necessary. Most patients, however, are best managed with a short leg walking plaster which will provide stability and comfort for a 4- to 6-week period.

Multiple Metatarsal Fractures

Fractures of the metatarsal shafts may occur with severe traumatic or crush injuries to the foot. Isolated fractures of the necks of fourth and fifth metatarsals may also occur. Stress fractures of the shafts of the second and third metatarsals should be suspected when the patient complains of insidious pain, without acute injury.

Fracture-dislocations occur at the tarsometatarsal junction, with associated fractures of the bases of metatarsals. Such injuries occur from severe trauma, such as cycling injuries or crush injuries to the feet. There is commonly associated severe soft tissue damage with or without compounding. In closed fractures, reduction should be accomplished by closed efforts, but in some instances Kirschner wire fixation is required. The handling of multiple fractures of the metatarsal shafts should include an attempt at alignment to restore painless weight bearing.

PHALANGEAL FRACTURES

Fractures of the phalanges of the toes may occur at any age from direct trauma to the forefoot, as in the dropping of heavy objects upon the toes or striking the toes against a door or foot of the bed. Such an injury may dislocate MP or IP joints as well.

Treatment of phalangeal fractures is directed at alignment and relief of pain. Reduction should be accomplished and the toes splinted to adjacent toes with adhesive tape. The patient may be allowed to walk if symptoms are tolerated.

PELVIC AND SPINE INJURIES

Acetabular Fractures and Hip Dislocations

Dislocation of the hip with or without associated fracture of the acetabulum is caused by force applied to the proximal femur. Such injuries may result from automobile collisions, pedestrian injuries, or falls from a great height. The type of fracture and dislocation is dependent upon the position of the hip and the direction of the force at the moment of impact. Force applied to an abducted femur may result in an anterior hip dislocation without fracture. Striking the knee on a dashboard of a car with the hip in a position of adduction and flexed at 90° may result in a posterior dislocation (Fig. 47-59) with or without a fracture of the posterior acetabular rim. Direct trauma to the trochanter with the hip in various positions will result in inner wall or bursting fractures of the acetabulum, including central dislocation.

Patients with fracture-dislocations about the hip may have other, more serious injuries, as with any fractures of the pelvis. Regardless of the type of dislocation, reduction should be accomplished as soon as possible, to minimize the change of avascular necrosis of the femoral head.

ANTERIOR HIP DISLOCATIONS

Such injuries occur from extreme abduction or trauma applied anteroposteriorly to an abducted thigh. Patients with this dislocation have the thigh held in abduction, flexion, and external rotation. Reduction is accomplished by applying force to the anesthetized patient in the direction of the deformity. When muscle resistance has been overcome and the femoral head has been pulled laterally to the rim of the acetabulum, the leg is adducted in flexion and internally rotated. Check x-rays are obtained to be certain that bone fragments are not displaced into the acetabulum. If bone fragments are obstructing reduction, open excision of the fragments must be accomplished.

The patient is maintained in traction, with the hip in extension for 10 to 14 days, following which active range of motion is carried out. Crutch walking with partial weight bearing is continued for 6 weeks, and then full weight bearing is allowed.

POSTERIOR HIP DISLOCATIONS

Posterior hip dislocations occur when axial force is applied to the flexed, adducted femur. The hip may be dislocated through a rent in the posterior capsule or with the posterior rim of the acetabulum driven off by the femoral head (Fig. 47-60). The diagnosis is usually apparent on clinical examination. The clinical deformity reveals the hip in a position of flexion, adduction, and internal rotation. Attempts to lower the limb to the table are met with severe resistance and anguish from the patient. Reduction of a dislocation should be accomplished immediately, but not before x-rays define the lesion. A standard AP x-ray of the pelvis is required, but a lateral x-ray of the hip joint may be necessary to demonstrate the dislocation accurately.

TREATMENT. Before moving the patient from the x-ray

table, reduction should be accomplished by the method of Bigelow. Most patients can be reduced under mild analgesia or with local anesthesia to the hip joint, but a few require general anesthesia. The basic principle is to pull the dislocated femoral head back through the rent in the capsule. If a large fragment has been fractured from the acetabulum, reduction may not be difficult.

Technique of Reduction. With the patient lying supine and with countertraction exerted across the pelvis, traction is applied to the long axis of the femoral shaft, with the knee flexed, and with the hip in a position of flexion, adduction, and internal rotation. When the femoral head has been brought to the level of the posterior acetabular rim, the femur is then gradually abducted, externally rotated, and placed in extension. If this cannot be accomplished gently or if the hip does not reduce with a sudden click, it should not be forced, or fracture of the femoral neck may occur. The stability or tendency to redislocation should be estimated after reduction, to decide whether screw fixation of this fragment is indicated. Anteroposterior, oblique, and lateral check x-rays are obtained to delineate the position of the posterior rim of the acetabulum to be certain that fragments are not displaced intraarticularly and that the posterior acetabular rim has been satisfactorily reduced. As a general rule, the acetabular rim requires open reduction. It is important to reduce the dislocation promptly and carry out open reduction of the acetabular rim when the patient's condition warrants, usually within the first week.

The uncomplicated dislocation is reduced, and the patient is placed in skin traction of 10 lb for 10 to 14 days, and weight bearing is prevented for an additional 4 weeks. Aspirin is administered to minimize progression of the cartilage injury sustained at the time of dislocation. All patients with hip dislocations should be followed indefinitely after this injury, because of the incidence of avascular necrosis and degenerative arthritis. Avascular necrosis,

Fig. 47-59. Posterior dislocation of the hip with fracture of the posterior acetabular rim. Axial force applied to the femur drives the femoral head from the acetabulum and the posterior rim of the acetabulum along with it. Such injuries are common to automobile passengers.

the incidence of which is directly related to the delay of reduction, develops in about 20 percent of patients and is usually clinically apparent by the 2-year interval. Traumatic arthritis occurs in about 50 percent of patients and may occur as late as 5 years postreduction.

Technique of Open Reduction of Acetabular Rim Fractures. The patient is placed in a semiprone position with the affected hip close to the edge of the table. The posterior approach of Osborne or Austin Moore will expose the hip joint. The short external rotators of the hip are divided just proximal to their insertion and reflected medially, pro-

Fig. 47-60. Posterior dislocation of the hip with fracture of the acetabular rim. *A.* AP x-ray postinjury showing the femoral head, which appears smaller than that of the opposite side and is superiorly displaced. *B.* AP x-ray showing the relocation of the femoral head with persistent displacement of the acetabular fragment. *C.* AP x-ray following open reduction and screw fixation of the acetabular fragment.

Fig. 47-61. Undisplaced fracture of both pubic rami.

tecting the sciatic nerve. The hip joint may be inspected through the fracture defect, which commonly consists of a large fragment of the posterosuperior rim of the acetabulum. The joint is inspected and any small, loose fragments removed. Compression of articular cartilage and underlying cancellous bone in the acetabulum are gently elevated with a periosteal elevator. Large fragments are accurately reduced and fixed with screws inserted at an angle and directed toward the midcrest of the ilium. The wound is closed, and skeletal traction of 10 lb is maintained for about 6 to 8 weeks, followed by plaster spica immobilization for another 6 weeks. Weight bearing is not allowed before 4 months or until union of the fragment has occurred.

FRACTURES OF THE INNER WALL OF THE ACETABULUM

Fractures of the inner wall of the acetabulum represent the most common type. If there is a central dislocation of the femoral head and the superior dome of the acetabulum is intact, reduction of the dislocation should be ac-

Fig. 47-62. Displaced fracture of all pubic rami, suggesting injury to the pelvic viscera.

complished by manipulation and maintained with skeletal traction for 8 weeks. It is important to reduce the femoral head into a normal relationship with the intact superior weight-bearing portion of the acetabulum. Active motion of the hip is then begun. Protected weight bearing between crutches is not allowed until the fractures are consolidated, about 4 months after injury.

Fractures of the Superior Acetabulum

Bursting or superior wall fractures have the worst prognosis of acetabular fractures. The ultimate result will depend upon the severity of comminution of the superior dome, as well as the restoration of the superior dome relationship to the femoral head. Attempts should be made to restore this relationship by closed or conservative methods. However, in some instances, open reduction through an anterior approach or even a combined anterior and posterior approach is necessary.

Pelvic Fractures

The pelvic ring, composed of the coxae and sacrum, provides protection for the pelvic viscera, attachments of muscles, and the transmission of weight-bearing forces from the lower extremities. Only the posterolateral wings, which connect the acetabula with the sacrum, function in the transmission of weight.

Injuries to the pelvic ring may occur at any age and from various types of violence. Elderly patients with osteoporosis who fall may sustain isolated fractures of the pubic rami (Fig. 47-61) or undisplaced fractures of the acetabula, the coccyx, or even the sacrum but usually do not have disruptions of the weight-bearing segments. The most common cause of the pelvic fracture is automobile collision. Passengers, drivers, pedestrians, and cyclists sustain pelvic injuries by direct crushing of the pelvis and combinations of rotational stress on the iliac wings.

CLINICAL MANIFESTATIONS. Patients with an acute fracture of the pelvis are unable to bear weight without discomfort. If this is an isolated fracture of the pubic ramus, weight bearing on the affected side causes pain in the groin. There may be local tenderness and swelling at the site of the fractured pubic ramus.

The examiner should test the stability of the pelvis by anterior compression with direct pressure over the symphysis and should determine lateral stability by compressing the pelvis in a frontal plane and applying direct pressure over both iliac wings. Both hips should be put through a range of motion. Any pain associated with these maneuvers requires AP, lateral, and oblique x-ray views of the pelvis to delineate fractures and displacement.

TREATMENT. The treatment of the acute pelvic fracture is first directed at the detection and treatment of associated injuries to the pelvic viscera or abdominal viscera, as well as treatment for shock. One-third of patients with pelvic fractures die as a result of local hemorrhage. Patients with severe retroperitoneal or pelvic hemorrhage complain of abdominal or back pain. There may be signs of hemorrhage into the scrotum or buttocks. If there is any doubt of intraabdominal hemorrhage, laparotomy is indicated.

The risk of laparotomy is far outweighed by the hazard associated with missing an intraabdominal lesion. Ten to twelve percent of patients with pelvic fractures, especially bilateral pubic rami fractures, have an associated injury to the bladder or urethra. Therefore a large indwelling catheter should be inserted immediately and retrograde cystograms obtained. Lesions of the lumbosacral plexus also should be suspected.

Isolated fractures occurring in elderly patients from a single fall are treated by bed rest for a few days, until acute symptoms subside. The patient is then gradually mobilized, and weight bearing is allowed as it is tolerated. Since the anterior arch is not contributing to weight bearing, there is no problem of pelvic stability. Thrombophlebitis and ileus with urinary retention are common complications.

Bilateral fractures of the pubic rami (Fig. 47-62) have the highest incidence of associated injuries and mortality of any pelvic fractures. Some degree of immobilization of bilateral pubic rami fractures can be obtained by bed rest and a pelvic sling.

Symphysis pubis separations account for a small percentage of all pelvic fractures. The main complication is damage to the urethra and bladder. There may be an associated subluxation or dislocation of one sacroiliac joint (Fig. 47-63). Reduction is accomplished by placing the patient in the lateral position on the sound side and, with direct downward and forward pressure, rotating the displaced hemipelvis into position. The patient may then be nursed in a pelvic sling, or if there is an isolated injury, a double hip pantaloon spica may be applied, with the patient lying on his side. If there is an upward displacement of the hemipelvis, skeletal traction to the femur may be required to hold the reduction. All combinations of fracture, including unilateral pubic rami fracture with separation of the sacroiliac joint or separation of the symphysis with a fracture through the wing of the ilium, are handled in similar fashion.

It is not always possible to reduce these fractures anatomically. Every attempt should be made to restore the pelvic outlet in young women of childbearing age. Open reduction is rarely indicated.

Isolated fractures of the iliac wing are usually the result of a direct blow to the crest of the ilium. If the major portion of the iliac wing is intact, weight bearing will not be affected. Fractures of the sacrum (Fig. 47-64) may occur from direct trauma or in association with fractures of the hemipelvis. Fractures of the coccyx occur from a direct blow to the coccyx as in a fall to a sitting position. The patient is treated by having him sit on a support beneath his thighs to take the direct pressure from the coccyx. In refractory situations, the coccyx may be excised.

Fractures and Dislocations of the Spine

Fractures and dislocations involving the cervical, thoracic, or lumbar spine are most commonly the result of injuries sustained by pedestrians, motorcyclists, or automobile occupants but may occur with any severe trauma. The prognosis in these injuries is dependent on whether

Fig. 47-63. Disruption of the hemipelvis by separation of symphysis pubis and sacroiliac joint.

there is associated cord injury. Fractures or dislocations without cord damage can result in normal function.

MANAGEMENT OF THE ACUTE INJURY. Everyone responsible for the first-aid care of patients at the scene of an accident should be well versed in the hazards of spine injuries and well informed in the transportation of these patients, to prevent or minimize neurologic damage.

Any patient complaining of neck or back pain from an automobile collision or serious fall should be presumed to have an unstable spine until completely examined both clinically and radiologically by a competent physician. Patients sustaining a neck injury with or without acute cord damage should be placed supine on a stretcher with sandbags beside the head to hold it in neutral position. Since half of the cervical spine fractures occur from hyperextension, the neck should be positioned midway between flexion and extension.

Patients with thoracic or lumbar spine injuries should be transported in a position to minimize motion of the spine. The patient is placed supine or prone on a board

Fig. 47-64. Vertical fracture through the sacrum at the neural foramina.

Fig. 47-65. Fracture-dislocation of C_5 upon C_6. Lateral x-rays show complete displacement of C_5 with fracture of the neural arch. The patient was paraplegic immediately following his injury.

or rigid stretcher, which can be moved to the x-ray table so that repositioning is not necessary. If the patient has other injuries, including chest, head, or abdominal hemorrhage, these should be treated first with the establishment of airway, resuscitation, and blood replacement.

A neurologic examination is accomplished as soon as possible. Appropriate AP and lateral x-rays of the cervical, thoracic, or lumbar spine are obtained before moving the patient from the stretcher. If x-rays indicate stability of the spine, oblique x-rays of the cervical spine may be obtained to supplement the AP and lateral x-rays. Immediate and continued immobilization is indicated if there is any question of instability.

CERVICAL FRACTURES AND DISLOCATIONS

Flexion injuries of the cervical spine occur when there is acute forcible flexion of the head upon the neck. With this type of injury, the first lesion to occur is compression of the vertebral body, resulting in an anterior wedge compression fracture of the vertebral body. The common areas are the lower three cervical vertebrae. For this reason, it is imperative to be sure that x-ray diagnosis includes the entire cervical spine and the relationship between C_7 and T_1.

As the flexion force continues, the posterior longitudinal ligament may be ruptured, and one or both facets may be subluxated or dislocated. Beatson has shown that a unilateral facet dislocation results in only forward displacement of less than one-fifth the anteroposterior diameter of the vertebra. With bilateral facet dislocations, forward displacement may be greater than one-half the anteroposterior diameter. Cord injuries occur when the neural canal is compromised by forward dislocation and are more common with bilateral dislocations of the facets.

When a compression force (vertical load) is applied to the cervical spine, a bursting fracture of a vertebral body may occur. This may result in backward displacement of the posterior portion of the vertebral body, resulting in impingement upon, and damage to, the spinal cord. Combinations of flexion, compression, and rotation may occur, resulting in pedicle or lamina fractures, causing dislocation with or without cord damage (Fig. 47-65).

Forsythe has called attention to the hyperextension injury of the cervical spine. Patients from automobile accidents may present with a contusion of the forehead, and x-rays may reveal forward displacement of an upper vertebra upon the one below it. As the upper cervical spine is driven into extension, the anterior longitudinal ligament is ruptured, causing a compression force at the facet joints. As the force continues and the head is driven back, secondary flexion and forward displacement of an upper vertebra occurs upon the adjacent lower vertebra. Lateral x-rays reveal horizontal facet fracture or fracture of the anteroinferior border of the cervical spine body. Care must be taken in these injuries not to hyperextend the neck, or subsequent cord damage may result. Hyperextension injuries may result without a facet or body fracture and spontaneously be reduced. The cord is driven back against the sharp edge of the lamina, resulting in cord damage. With the head brought into neutral position, the dislocation may be spontaneously reduced, and the x-rays may appear normal, although the patient is paraplegic.

Injuries of the transverse process in the cervical spine are rare and represent avulsion fractures. Fractures of the spinous processes may also occur and have been characterized as the clay shoveler's fracture. A sudden stress on the supraspinous ligament pulls off the tip of the spinous process. Also, a direct blow to the spinous process may cause fracture.

Fractures of the atlas occur when compression force is applied to a thin posterior ring by downward force on the head (Jefferson's fracture).

Fractures of C_2, involving the odontoid or posterior elements, may occur from flexion and extension or rotational forces. In children under the age of six, injuries to the odontoid result in an epiphyseal displacement and associated subluxation or dislocation of atlas upon the axis.

MANAGEMENT OF CERVICAL SPINE FRACTURES AND DISLOCATIONS WITHOUT NEUROLOGIC INJURY. Unstable fractures must be immobilized and dislocations or subluxations reduced. Patients arriving at the emergency room are placed in a cervical halter traction, which will provide immediate stability, while appropriate x-rays or associated conditions are managed. For the long-term immobilization of these injuries, skeletal traction is required. This is accomplished by the use of a halo apparatus. The halo purchases with four pins inserted under local anesthesia onto the outer table of the skull. To this skeletal traction device 5 lb is added for upper cervical lesions and as much as 30 lb for lower cervical lesions.

Dislocations and fractures are reduced with skeletal traction. When the dislocation or fracture is reduced, the halo device is connected to a body plaster jacket molded over the iliac crests and the patient is allowed to walk until stability has ensued, a period of approximately 12 weeks. The patient is then immobilized in a four-poster cervical brace for an additional period. Before immobilization is discontinued, flexion and extension films are obtained to determine stability. When stability cannot be anticipated with immobilization alone, spine fusion is carried out after a 6-week interval.

In some undisplaced fractures, such as a pedicle or lamina fracture, where stability is certain, an initial Minerva plaster jacket may be elected. However, if there is uncertainty about stability, skeletal traction, followed by Minerva plaster, is the safest procedure.

Rogers reported an incidence of 12 percent recurrent instability following the conservative management of unstable fractures and dislocations. For this reason, he and Forsythe have recommended early posterior spine fusion with wiring of spinous processes. Their procedure is to resolve the acute general injuries, during which time skeletal traction is maintained and is then continued during posterior spine fusion. Spine fusion in the face of instability is not recommended before 6 weeks, until ligamentous healing has added some stability. Anesthesia will relieve the protective muscle spasm of the unstable spine, and the very act of positioning such a patient at surgery is not without hazard. The technique is to wire together the spinous process of the affected adjacent vertebrae.

Fig. 47-66. Wedge compression fracture L$_2$. *A.* Lateral x-ray shows compression wedging of the upper portion of L$_2$. *B.* AP x-rays do not demonstrate the fracture.

Autogenous iliac bone is applied to the roughened posterior lamina and spinous processes. If satisfactory stability is obtained by wiring, the patient is kept in a four-poster cervical spine brace until bone union is solid (12 to 16 weeks).

CERVICAL FRACTURES AND DISLOCATIONS WITH ASSOCIATED NEUROLOGIC INJURY. There is disagreement about the indications for open laminectomy and decompression of acute fracture-dislocations of the cervical spine with associated cord injury. There is little disagreement that patients who present with minimal neurologic findings and have progressive neurologic deficits require immediate laminectomy and exploration. Another indication is unsuccessful reduction and persistence of bone fragments in the spinal canal. Proponents of the nonexploration attitude argue that irreparable damage has been done from the time of the initial injury and will not be influenced by decompression and subsequent exploration, which in themselves are life-threatening procedures. Also, if the lesion is partial, surgical procedures may further endanger the cord. The operative school base their indications on the fact that occasionally a displaced disc or fragment of bone will compress the cord and unrelieved swelling may further damage a cord capable of recovery.

THORACOLUMBAR FRACTURES AND DISLOCATIONS

Fractures and dislocations involving the upper thoracic and midthoracic regions are uncommon because of the stability afforded by the adjacent rib cage. The principles involved in treatment of such injuries are the same as in thoracolumbar spine fractures.

Holdsworth has clearly shown that flexion force applied to the thoracolumbar spine results in anterior wedge compression fractures which are stable by virtue of intact posterior structures and longitudinal ligaments (Fig. 47-66). Wedge compression fractures may occur in any osteoporotic spine from relatively minor trauma. Wedge compression fractures also occur in normal spines from severe flexion forces common in mine cave-ins, automobile collisions, and falls from a height.

When rotation is combined with flexion, the posterior

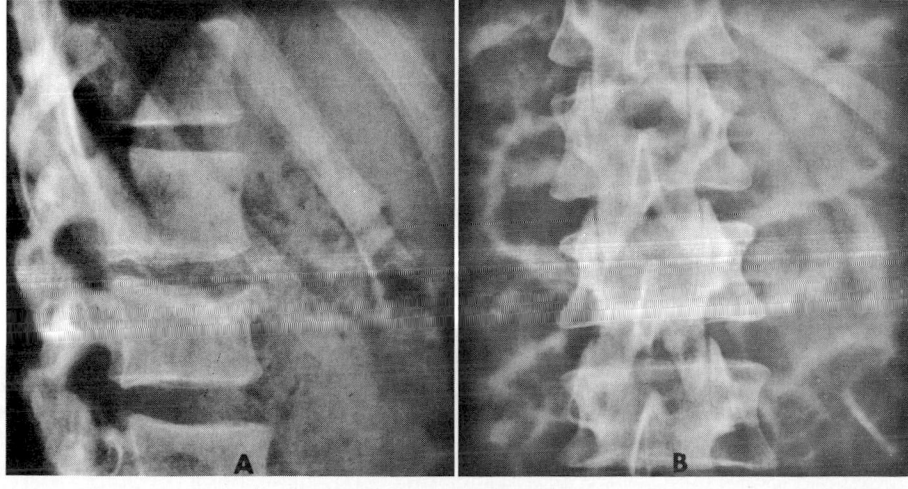

ligaments rupture or the articular processes fracture, and a wedge-shaped fracture may occur through the upper border of the lower vertebral body, resulting in a fracture-dislocation (Fig. 47-67). Extension injuries may cause dislocation with rupture of the anterior longitudinal ligaments and may cause posterior dislocation. This is rare in the lumbar region. When compression force (vertical load) is applied to the line of vertebral bodies, especially at the thoracolumbar area and upper lumbar spine, the result is a bursting fracture with the posterior fragments displaced into the spinal canal.

MANAGEMENT OF ACUTE INJURIES OF THE THORACO-LUMBAR SPINE. Patients with acute traumatic injury to the spine should be presumed to have an unstable situation and potential paraplegia until proved otherwise. They should be placed prone or supine on a stretcher and not moved until AP and lateral x-rays delineate the lesion.

Clinical examination will give some indication of the extent of the lesion. The patient should be inspected for signs of impact, abrasion over one shoulder causing flexion and rotation, etc. If the supraspinous ligaments are ruptured, a defect between the spinous processes will be evident. With any compression fracture, there is tenderness over the affected vertebrae.

Interpretation of the AP and lateral x-rays is important. Flexion injury causing compression wedging will be evident on the lateral x-ray but not on the AP x-ray.

When the "slice wedge" fracture of the upper part of the lower vertebrae is seen on both AP and lateral x-rays without dislocation, instability should be suspected. Such

Fig. 47-67. Posterior fracture-dislocation of the thoracic spine. Lateral x-rays show backward displacement of T_7 upon T_8 with fracture involvement of the neural arch. Patient was paraplegic upon arrival.

fractures are so unstable that they are reduced just by placing the patient supine. Any displacement in the lumbar spine is an indication of instability.

Treatment of fractures of the thoracolumbar spine will depend on the degree of instability caused by the trauma. Wedge compression fractures are usually stable. Patients are confined to bed rest until symptoms allow mobilization. The patient should be watched for paralytic ileus. Prescribing a liquid diet for a few days to minimize these problems is worthwhile. When patients are comfortable, they are taught hyperextension exercises, which are continued for 6 to 12 weeks. No reduction for a stable wedge compression fracture is necessary, since the deformity rarely causes disability. Bursting fractures are usually stable but may not be. Stable fractures are immobilized in plaster, and spontaneous fusion across the involved disc will usually result. If instability is present or questionable, the patient should be treated on a Foster frame and spine fusion performed at 6 weeks.

Pure dislocations in the thoracolumbar region are rare; when they occur, they require spine fusion.

Fracture-dislocations without injury to the cord may be handled by immobilization on a Foster frame for 6 to 8 weeks and then plaster cast immobilization for another 6 to 8 weeks. Union across adjacent involved vertebrae usually occurs.

A different situation exists when injury to the cauda equina is associated with this rotational fracture-dislocation. The fracture must be adequately reduced to free the nerve roots from pressure. Immobilization must be maintained to prevent recurrent injury during the early postfracture period. For this reason, Holdsworth employs early stabilization above and below the site of injury. The best method for stabilization is the use of Harrington rods. Others feel that exploration is not indicated and Foster frame reduction and immobilization are sufficient.

MANAGEMENT OF SPINAL CORD INJURY. See Chaps. 42 and 52.

References

Evaluation

Griffiths, L. L.: The Management of Acute Circulatory Failure in an Injured Limb, *J Bone Joint Surg* [*Br*], **30B**:280, 1948.

Mercer, W., and Duthie, R. B.: "Orthopaedic Surgery," 6th ed., Edward Arnold (Publishers) Ltd., London, 1964.

Seddon, H. J.: Three Types of Nerve Injury, *Brain*, **66**:237, 1943.

Tachakra, S. S., and Sevitt, S.: Hypoaxemia after Fractures, *J Bone Joint Surg*, **57B**:197, 1975.

Healing and General Treatment

Abercrombie, M.: "Advances in Biology of Skin: V. Wound Healing," Pergamon Press, New York, 1964.

Aegerter, E., and Kirkpatrick, J. A.: "Orthopaedic Diseases," W. B. Saunders Company, Philadelphia, 1964.

Anderson, L. D.: Compression Plate Fixation and the Effect of Different Types of Internal Fixation on Fracture Healing, instructional course lecture, American Academy of Orthopaedic Surgeons, *J Bone Joint Surg* [*Am*], **47A**:191, 1965.

Bier, A.: Beabactungen über Regeneration beim Menschen, *Dtsch Med Wochenschr,* **43:**705, 1917.

Duthie, R. B., and Barker, A. N.: An Autoradiographic Study of Mucopolysaccharide and Phosphate Complexes in Bone Growth and Repair, *J Bone Joint Surg [Br],* **37B:**304, 1955.

Johnson, L. C., Stradford, H. T., Geis, R. W., Dineen, H. R., and Kerley, E. R.: Histogenesis of Stress Fractures, *Armed Forces Inst Pathol Annu Lec,* 1963.

Lack, C. H.: Increased Vascular Permeability, Chondrolysis and Cortisone, *Proc R Soc Med,* **55:**113, 1962.

Miles, A. A.: Local and Systemic Factors in Shock, *Fed Proc,* **20**(*Suppl* 9):141, 1961.

Muller, M. E., Allgower, M., and Willenegger, H.: "Technique of Internal Fixation of Fractures," Springer-Verlag, Inc., New York, 1965.

Ray, R. D., Sankaran, B., and Fetro, K. O.: Delayed Union in Non-union Fractures, instructional course lecture, American Academy of Orthopaedic Surgeons, *J Bone Joint Surg [Am],* **46A:**627, 1964.

Rhinelander, F. W., and Baragry, R. A.: Microangiography in Bone Healing, *J Bone Joint Surg [Am],* **44A:**1273, 1962.

Salter, R. B., and Harris, R. W.: Injuries Involving the Epiphyseal Plate, instructional course lecture, American Academy of Orthopaedic Surgeons, *J Bone Joint Surg [Am],* **45A:**587, 1963.

Tonna, E. A., and Cronkite, E. P.: Cellular Response to Fracture Studied with Tritiated Thymidine, *J Bone Joint Surg [Am],* **43A:**352, 1961.

Wilhelm, D. L.: "The Inflammatory Process," Academic Press, Inc., New York, 1965.

Wray, J. B.: Factors in the Pathogenesis of Non-union, instructional course lecture, American Academy of Orthopedic Surgeons, *J Bone Joint Surg [Am],* **47A:**168, 1965.

—— and Lynch, C. J.: The Vascular Response to Fracture of the Tibia in the Rat, *J Bone Joint Surg [Am],* **41A:**1143, 1959.

Fractures and Joint Injuries to the Shoulder and Girdle

Bankart, A. S. B.: Recurrence of Habitual Dislocation of the Shoulder Joint, *Br Med J,* **2:**1132, 1923.

"Campbell's Operative Orthopaedics," chap. 5, p. 366, The C. V. Mosby Company, St. Louis, 1963.

Inman, V. T., Saunders, J. B., and Abbott, L. C.: Observations on the Function of the Shoulder Joint, *J Bone Joint Surg [Am],* **26A:**1, 1944.

Jacobs, B., and Wade, P. A.: Acromioclavicular Joint Injury and End Result Study, *J Bone Joint Surg [Am],* **48A:**475, 1966.

Lacey, T., III, and Crawford, H. B.: Reduction of Anterior Dislocation of the Shoulder by Means of Milch Abduction Techniques, *J Bone Joint Surg [Am],* **34A:**108, 1952.

Leslie, J. T., and Ryan, T. J.: The Axillary Incision to Approach the Shoulder Joint, *J Bone Joint Surg [Am],* **44A:**1193, 1962.

Neviaser, J. S.: Acromioclavicular Dislocations Treated by Transference of the Coraco-acromio Ligaments, *Arch Surg,* **64:**292, 1952.

Nobel, W.: Post-traumatic Dislocation of the Shoulder, *J Bone Joint Surg [Am],* **44A:**523, 1962.

Osmond-Clark, H.: Habitual Dislocation of the Shoulder: The Putti-Platt Operation, *J Bone Joint Surg [Br],* **30B:**19, 1948.

Rowe, C. R.: Symposium on Dislocation of the Shoulder, instruc-
tional course lecture, American Academy of Orthopaedic Surgeons, *J Bone Joint Surg [Am],* **44A:**998, 1962.

Stubbins, S. G., and McGaw, W. H.: Suspension Casts for Acromioclavicular Separation and Clavicle Traction, *JAMA,* **169:**672, 1959.

Weaver, J. K., and Dunn, H. K.: Treatment of Acromioclavicular Injuries, Especially Complete Acromioclavicular Separation, *J Bone Joint Surg,* **54A:**1187, 1972.

Fractures and Joint Injuries to the Humerus, Elbow, and Forearm

Adler, J. B., and Shaftan, G. W.: Radial Head Fractures: Is Excision Necessary? *J Trauma,* **4:**115, 1964.

Blount, W. P.: "Fractures in Children," The C. V. Mosby Company, St. Louis, 1955.

Cave, E. F.: "Fractures and Other Injuries," Year Book Medical Publishers, Inc., Chicago, 1961.

Darrach, W.: Colle's Fracture, *N Engl J Med,* **226:**594, 1942.

Evans, E. M.: Pronation Injuries of the Forearm with Special Reference to the Anterior Monteggia Fracture, *J Bone Joint Surg [Br],* **31B:**578, 1949.

Gould, N.: Early Mobilization of the Joint in Intra-articular Fractures with Special Attention to the Elbow Joint, *Surg Gynecol Obstet,* **115:**575, 1962.

Holstein, A., and Lewis, G. B.: Fractures of Humerus with Radial Nerve Paralysis, *J Bone Joint Surg [Am],* **45A:**1382, 1963.

Hughston, J. C.: Fracture of the Forearm in Children, instructional course lecture, American Academy of Orthopaedic Surgeons, *J Bone Joint Surg [Am],* **44A:**1678, 1962.

Miller, W. E.: Comminuted Fractures of the Humerus in the Adult, instructional course lecture, American Academy of Orthopaedic Surgeons, *J Bone Joint Surg [Am],* **46A:**644, 1964.

Neer, C. S.: Displaced Proximal Humeral Fractures: Part 1. Classification and Evaluation, *J Bone Joint Surg,* **52A:**1077, 1970.

——: Displaced Proximal Humeral Fractures: Part II. Treatment of Three Part and Four Part Displacements, *J Bone Joint Surg,* **52A:**1090, 1970.

Neviaser, J. S.: Complicated Fractures and Dislocations about the Shoulder Joint, instructional course lecture, American Academy of Orthopaedic Surgeons, *J Bone Joint Surg [Am],* **44A:** 984, 1962.

Salter, R. B., and Harris, R. W.: Injuries Involving the Shoulder Joint, instructional course lecture, American Academy of Orthopaedic Surgeons, *J Bone Joint Surg [Am],* **45A:**587, 1963.

—— and Zaltz, C.: Anatomic Investigations of the Mechanism of Injury and Pathologic Anatomy of "Pulled Elbow" in Young Children, *Clin Orthop,* **77:**134, 1971.

Scuderi, C. S.: Operative Indications in Fractures of Both Bones of the Forearm, instructional course lecture, American Academy of Orthopaedic Surgeons, *J Bone Joint Surg [Am],* **44A:** 1671, 1962.

Smith, L.: Deformity following Supracondylar Fractures of the Humerus, *J Bone Joint Surg [Am],* **42A:**235, 1960.

Fractures and Joint Injuries to the Wrist and Hand

Barnard, L., and Stubbins, S. G.: Styloidectomy of the Radius in the Surgical Treatment of Non-union of the Carpal Navicular: A Preliminary Report, *J Bone Joint Surg [Am],* **30A:**98, 1948.

Boyes, J. H.: "Bunnel's Surgery of the Hand," J. B. Lippincott Company, Philadelphia, 1964.

Linscheid, R. L., Dobyns, J. H., Beabout, J. W., and Bryan, R. S.: Traumatic Instability of the Wrist. Diagnosis, Classification and Pathomechanics, J Bone Joint Surg, 54A:1612, 1972.

Fractures of the Hip and Femur

Banks, H. H.: Healing of Femoral Neck Fractures, Proc Conf Aseptic Necrosis Femoral Head, St. Louis, 1964.

"Campbell's Operative Orthopaedics," The C. V. Mosby Company, St. Louis, 1963.

Clawson, D. K.: Trochanteric Fractures Treated by the Sliding Screw Plate Fixation Method, J Trauma, 4:737, 1964.

———, Smith, R. F., and Hausen, S. T.: Closed Intramedullary Nailing of the Femur, J Bone Joint Surg [Am], 53A:681, 1971.

Crawford, H. B.: Conservative Treatment of Impacted Fractures of the Femoral Neck: A Report of 50 Cases, J Bone Joint Surg [Am], 42A:471, 1960.

Deyerle, W. M.: Multiple Pin Peripheral Fixation in Fractures of the Neck of the Femur: Immediate Weight Bearing, Clin Orthop, 39:135, 1965.

Dimon, J. H., and Hughston, J. C.: Unstable Intertrochanteric Fractures of the Hip, J Bone Joint Surg [Am], 49A:440, 1967.

Furuya, M., Harrison-Stubbs, M. O., and Freiberger, R. H.: Arthrography of the Knee: Analysis of 2101 Arthrograms and 623 Surgical Findings, Rev Hosp Spec Surg, 2:11, 1972.

Garden, R. S.: Stability and Union in Subcapital Fractures of the Femur, J Bone Joint Surg [Br], 46B:630, 1964.

Harris, W. H., Salzman, E. W., and Desanctis, R. W.: The Prevention of Thromboembolic Disease by Prophylactic Anticoagulation: A Controlled Study in Elective Hip Surgery, J Bone Joint Surg [Am], 49A:81, 1967.

Hinchey, J. J., and Day, P. L.: Primary Prosthetic Replacement in Fresh Femoral Neck Fractures, J Bone Joint Surg [Am], 46A:223, 1964.

Horowitz, B. G.: Retrospective Analysis of Hip Fractures, Surg Gynecol Obstet, 123:565, 1966.

Lowell, J. D.: Fractures of the Hip, N Engl J Med, 275:1418, 1966.

Massie, W. K.: Avascular Sequelae of Femoral Neck, Studied by a Radioisotope Technique, Proc Conf Aseptic Necrosis Femoral Head, St. Louis, 1964.

———: Fractures of the Hip, instructional course lecture, American Academy of Orthopaedic Surgeons, J Bone Joint Surg [Am], 46A:658, 1964.

Stewart, M. J., Sisk, D., and Wallace, S. L.: Fractures of the Distal Third of the Femur, instructional course lecture, American Academy of Orthopaedic Surgeons, J Bone Joint Surg [Am], 48A:784, 1966.

Trueta, J., and Harrison, M. H.: The Normal Vascular Anatomy of the Femoral Head in Adult Man, J Bone Joint Surg [Br], 35B:442, 1953.

Zickel, R. E.: A New Fixation Device for Subtrochanteric Fractures of the Femur. A Preliminary Report, Clin Orthop, 54:115, 1957.

Fractures and Injuries of the Knee Joint, Patella, Tibia, and Fibula

Brown, P. W., and Urban, J. G.: Early Weight-Bearing Treatment of Open Fractures of the Tibia: An End-Result Study of 63 Cases, J Bone Joint Surg [Am], 51A:59, 1969.

Dehne, E., Metz, C. W., Deffer, P. A., and Hale, R. M.: Nonoperative Treatment of the Fractured Tibia by Immediate Weightbearing, J Trauma, 1:514, 1961.

Goldthwait, J. E.: Slipping or Recurrent Dislocation of the Patella with Report of Eleven Cases, Boston Med Surg J, 150:169, 1904.

Hauser, E. D. W.: Total Tendon Transplant for Slipping Patella: New Operation for Recurrent Dislocation of the Patella, Surg Gynecol Obstet, 66:199, 1938.

Helfet, A. J.: "The Management of Internal Derangements of the Knee," J. B. Lippincott Company, Philadelphia, 1963.

Hoagland, F. T., and States, J. D.: Factors Influencing Rate of Healing in Tibial Shaft Fractures, Surg Gynecol Obstet, 124:71, 1967.

Karlen, A.: Congenital Fibrosis of the Vastus Intermedius Muscle, J Bone Joint Surg [Br], 46B:488, 1964.

Kennedy, J. C., and Fowler, P. J.: Medial and Anterior Instability of the Knee: An Anatomical and Clinical Study Using Stress Machines, J Bone Joint Surg [Am], 53A:1257, 1971.

Mooney, V., Nickel, V. L., Harvey, J. P., Jr., and Snelson, R.: Cast-Brace Treatment for Fractures of the Distal Part of the Femur, J Bone Joint Surg [Am], 52A:1563, 1970.

Nicoll, E. H.: Fractures of the Tibial Shaft: A Survey of 705 Cases, J Bone Joint Surg [Am], 46B:373, 1964.

O'Donoghue, D. H.: Surgical Treatment of Fresh Injuries to the Major Ligaments of the Knee, J Bone Joint Surg [Am], 32A:721, 1950.

Sarmiento, A.: A Functional Below-the-Knee Cast for Tibial Fractures, J Bone Joint Surg [Am], 49A:885, 1967.

Slocum, D. B., and Larson, R. L.: Rotatory Instability of the Knee: Its Pathogenesis and a Clinical Test to Demonstrate Its Presence, J Bone Joint Surg [Am], 50A:211, 1968.

Weissman, S. L., and Harold, Z. H.: Fractures of the Tibial Plateau, Clin Orthop, 33:194, 1964.

Ankle Injuries, Fractures, and Dislocations of the Foot

Dart, D. E., and Graham, W. D.: Treatment of the Fractured Calcaneum, J Trauma, 6:362, 1966.

Dunne, L. R., Jacobs, B., and Campbell, R. D.: Fractures of the Talus, J Trauma, 6:443, 1966.

Morris, H. D., Hand, W. L., and Dunn, A. W.: The Modified Blair Fusion for Fractures of the Talus, J Bone Joint Surg [Am], 53A:1289, 1971.

Thoren, O.: Os Calcis Fractures, Acta Orthop Scand Suppl, 70, 1964.

Watson-Jones, Sir Reginald: "Fractures and Joint Injuries," vol. II, chap. 28, p. 813, and chap. 29, p. 862, 4th ed., The Williams & Wilkins Company, Baltimore, 1956.

Pelvic and Spine Injuries

Beatson, T. R.: Fractures and Dislocations of the Cervical Spine, J Bone Joint Surg [Br], 45B:21, 1963.

Flesch, J. R., Leider, L. L., Erickson, D. L., Chou, S. N., and Bradford, D. S.: Harrington Instrumentation and Spine Fusion for Unstable Fractures and Fracture-Dislocation of the Thoracic and Lumbar Spine, J Bone Joint Surg, 59A:143, 1977.

Forsythe, H. F.: Extension Injuries of the Cervical Spine, instructional course lecture, American Academy of Orthopaedic Surgeons, J Bone Joint Surg [Am], 46A:1792, 1964.

Holdsworth, F. W.: Fractures, Dislocations, and Fracture-Dislocations of the Spine, *J Bone Joint Surg [Br]*, **45B:**6, 1963.

McCarroll, J. R., Braunstein, T. W., Cooper, W., Helpren, M., Seremetis, M., Wade, P. A., and Weinberg, S. B.: Fatal Pedestrian Automobile Accidents, *JAMA,* **180:**127, 1962.

Peltier, L. F.: Fractures of the Pelvis, instructional course lecture, American Academy of Orthopaedic Surgeons, *J Bone Joint Surg [Am]*, **47A:**1060, 1965.

Rogers, W. A.: Treatment of Fracture Dislocation of the Cervical Spine, *J Bone Joint Surg [Am]*, **24:**245, 1942.

Rowe, C. R., and Lowell, J. D.: Prognosis of Fractures of the Acetabulum, *J Bone Joint Surg [Am]*, **43A:**30, 1961.

Stewart, M. J., and Milford, L. W.: Prevention of Disability after Traumatic Dislocation of the Hip, and End Result Study, *J Bone Joint Surg [Am]*, **36A:**315, 1964.

Watson-Jones, Sir Reginald: "Fractures and Joint Injuries," vol. II, chap. 32, p. 934, and chap. 33, p. 946, 4th ed., The Williams & Wilkins Company, Baltimore, 1956.

Chapter 48

Diseases of Joints

by Franklin T. Hoaglund and Robert B. Duthie

The problem of joint injury or disease is common. An estimated 2 to 8 percent of the population have rheumatic complaints at some time in their lives. Virtually everyone over the age of fifty years has sufficient degenerative changes in joints to have some restriction of some joint motion, although only a small percentage show symptoms. Injuries frequently involve joints; the immobilization imposed by every fracture or injured extremity results in restriction of joint motion either temporarily or in some cases permanently.

ANATOMY

Joints are either fibrous or cartilaginous. A fibrous joint, or synarthrosis, consists of two bones united by fibrous tissue, such as the syndesmoses or sutures of the skull.

Cartilaginous joints consist of bones united by either hyaline cartilage or fibrocartilage. An example of a primary cartilaginous joint is an epiphyseal plate. Examples of fibrocartilaginous joints are the pubic symphysis and the intervertebral discs.

Diarthrodial joints are movable joints in which the cartilage-covered bone ends are united by a capsule lined with synovium (Fig. 48-1).

The plane or planes of motion occurring in the synovial joint characterize the joints as uniaxial, i.e., ginglymus (hinge), trochoid (pivot), biaxial, or multiaxial. The motion permitted in a diarthrosis depends upon the configuration of the articular surface, adjacent capsule, and supporting musculature, and upon the unique properties of articular cartilage.

ARTICULAR CARTILAGE. Normal articular cartilage is blue-white, has a smooth surface, and is slightly compressible. The thickness of articular cartilage varies in different locations of specific joints.

Articular cartilage is composed of chondrocytes, which

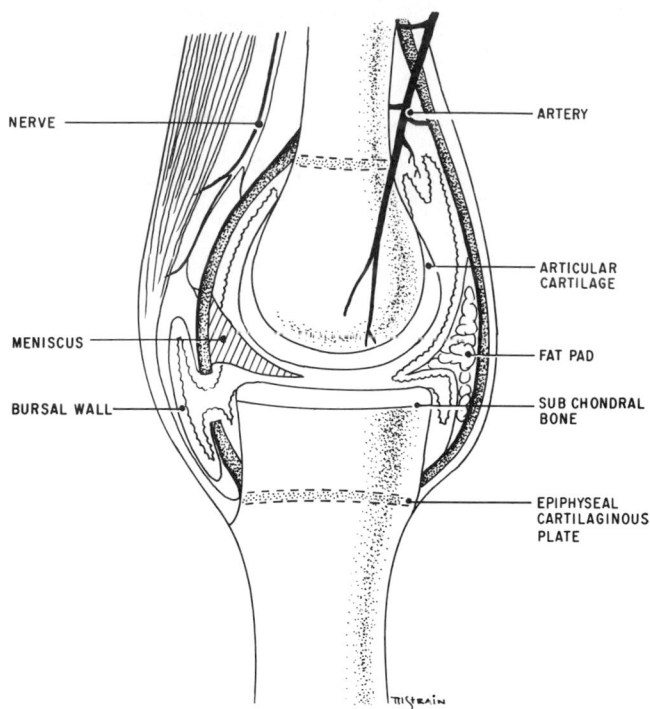

Fig. 48-1. Schematic drawing of synovial joint structures.

are embedded in a network of collagen fibers, surrounded by a matrix of proteoglycans. It is separated from the underlying supporting subchondral bone by a thin layer of calcified cartilage. Histologically, there are four distinct layers of normal cartilage: in the superficial, or surface, layer the cells are numerous, flattened, and smaller than in the deeper layers; the intermediate zone blends imperceptibly with the surface layer, but the cells are larger; the deep zone contains larger cells and lies upon the calcified cartilage. In the immature animal in the deeper layers of the articular cartilage, there are two zones which show evidence of cell reproduction and growth. The deepest layer is responsible for circumferential epiphyseal enlargement, and the more superficial zone is responsible for growth of the articular surface. Cell reproduction does not occur in normal healthy adult articular cartilage. After injury and in degenerative disease of articular cartilage, the rate of deoxyribonucleic acid (DNA) synthesis is increased, indicating cell replication.

CARTILAGE MATRIX. The cartilage cells produce the intercellular substances composed of matrix, or ground substance, and collagen fibers. The matrix, proteoglycan, is a complex substance and contributes to the maintenance of the water content and resiliency of the cartilage. Proteoglycan is composed of a linear protein to which aggregates of chondroitin 6-sulfate, chondroitin 4-sulfate, or keratan sulfate are attached. The amounts of each vary with age; keratan sulfate is present in trace amounts in the young and may reach 50 percent in the elderly.

COLLAGEN. The collagen of articular cartilage is different from that of bone and contains three a_1 (II) chains with more hydroxyline residues and increased glycolosylation of

hydroxylysine. The network of collagen fibrils in normal hyaline cartilage ranges from the normal characteristic banding of 645 to 700 Å down to widths of 50 to 250 Å. The collagen fibers have a definite arrangement. In the depths of the cartilage, the fibers are at right angles to the surface of the subchondral bone. At the articular surface, the fibers curve to run parallel with the surface. The resulting network is called Benninghoff's arcades.

In the adult, cartilage is nourished by diffusion of substances from the synovial fluid on the surface and in the immature animal before the basal layer calcifies, also by diffusion from the underlying capillaries on the subchondral bone.

SYNOVIAL MEMBRANE. The synovial membrane is composed of secretory and phagocytic cells, which are arranged in depths of one to three cells over subsynovial connective tissue. The latter consists of a vascular network surrounded by fibroblasts, macrophages, fat cells, and mast cells. Over ligaments, the synovium is quite thin, while in regions of the fat pads and loose capsule there is considerable areolar tissue beneath the synovium. Circulation to the synovium comes from the main blood vessels about the joint which first supply the fibrous capsule. The synovium is much more vascular, with a large plexus immediately beneath the synovial surface. At the synovial membrane junction with the articular cartilage, the vessels are continued as the circulus articuli vasculosus. The blood vessels in the synovia are continuous and communicate with metaphyseal and epiphyseal blood vessels.

The secretory cells produce the hyaluronate of the synovial fluid. In addition, electrolytes and certain plasma proteins diffuse from the synovial capillaries into the joint space. Normal synovial fluid is a weakly alkaline, viscous, clear, pale yellow nonclottable fluid. The viscosity is dependent upon the presence of hyaluronate, a sulfate-free mucopolysaccharide, containing glucuronic acid and N-acetylglucosamine. When hyaluronate is depolymerized, the viscosity is reduced.

The concentration of α- and β-globulins in synovial fluid is the same as in serum, but α_2- and γ-globulin levels are lower. Albumin accounts for about three-fourths of the total protein in the synovial fluid. The protein molecules with molecular weight greater than 160,000 such as fibrinogen, α- and β-macroglobulin, and β-lipoprotein are absent in normal joint fluid. However, when capillary permeability is increased during inflammation, the clotting proteins will enter the joint space.

Normal synovial fluid contains up to 200 nucleated cells consisting of polymorphonuclear leukocytes, lymphocytes, and monocytes. Electrolytes and glucose are present. Nonprotein nitrogen and uric acid concentrations are approximately the same as in serum.

Joint fluid nourishes cartilage and has the added function of joint lubrication. The coefficient of friction of cartilage on cartilage with synovial fluid as a lubricant is extremely low. There is disagreement as to whether this is an example of hydrodynamic or boundary lubrication. Another theory incorporates the hydrodynamic theory with a "weeping" lubrication in which the synovial fluid oozes from the articular cartilage.

The nerve supply of each synovial joint is by articular twigs from nerves supplying muscles responsible for the control of motion of that joint. The distribution and location of these branches is quite variable, making complete denervation of a joint difficult. The capsule and ligaments are the most pain-sensitive structures in a joint. Synovium also contains free nerve endings, but the areas of pain sensation are variable and ill defined.

Nerve fibers accompany arteries into bone, and this may be the basis for bone pain in certain inflammatory conditions about joints. The pain from the joint is difficult to localize and is often referred distally. There are proprioceptive endings in the capsule and joint ligaments which are sensitive to stretch and are indicators of joint position. Articular cartilage is without sensation.

EXAMINATION

The diagnosis of joint disease is dependent upon:

1. Clinical history of joint symptomatology
2. Clinical examination of all joints
3. X-ray examination
4. Synovial fluid analysis
5. Serologic tests

The patient is questioned about the specific onset of the joint complaint and any relation to trauma. Information about aggravation and relief of pain, and history of previous joint complaints, morning stiffness, locking, giving way, swelling, erythema, and symptoms related to other joints are necessary. Complete clinical history regarding other systems is always required.

CLINICAL EXAMINATION. The involved joint or joints should be inspected for signs of swelling and effusion, and evidence of erythema and local skin temperature increase. In unilateral involvement, the opposite side is used for comparison. The ligaments responsible for stability are examined and ranges of joint motion recorded. Active motion is examined by asking the patient to put the joint through a range of motion. Passive motion is measured by putting the joint through the maximal range of motion with muscles relaxed. The proximal and distal joints are always examined to be certain that the complaint is not due to referred pain. Muscle girth is determined by measurement, and muscle power is graded. Clinical examination is incomplete without evaluation of all joints in both upper and lower extremities, as well as a complete physical examination.

X-RAY EXAMINATION. Standard biplanar x-rays of the involved joints are necessary. The x-rays should clearly show the margins of the joint, as well as the adjacent bone metaphysis. In some situations, oblique x-rays and laminograms are necessary to delineate the adjacent bone and specific lesion. X-rays may be required in positions of flexion and extension to test for subluxation and dislocation. In certain traumatic situations, i.e., ankle and knee injuries, x-rays may be required with stress applied to the joint to determine the continuity of ligaments. Arthrography with the injection of radiopaque dyes is useful in delineating the shoulder capsule and rotator cuff, as well as soft tissue structures involved in congenital dislocation of the hip.

SYNOVIAL FLUID EXAMINATION. The examination of synovial fluid may give a specific diagnosis in pyogenic arthritis, tuberculous arthritis, gout, and pseudogout, and may add valuable diagnostic information in most other types of arthritis, including degenerative and rheumatoid arthritis, and in traumatic injuries. The technique of aspiration of a joint will depend on an accurate knowledge of anatomy of the specific joint to be aspirated. The following technique is suggested for the knee joint in which there are moderate degrees of fluid evident in the suprapatellar pouch (Fig. 48-2):

With the patient lying supine and the knee flexed 20° over a small pillow, the entire knee region is prepared with Betadine. With scrupulous aseptic technique, the skin immediately proximal and lateral to the upper pole of the patella, as well as the underlying capsule, is anesthetized with a few milliliters of 2% lidocaine. Using a #18 needle or larger and with the patella pointing toward the ceiling, the insertion is made with the needle parallel with the floor and just anterior to the anterior surface of the femur at the upper pole of the patella.

A large-bore needle is used, since thick, purulent secretion may not be withdrawn through a smaller needle. The joint is completely evacuated of all fluid by displacing fluid from other areas of the joint to the region of the site of entry of the needle. The fluid is collected in (1) a culture tube, (2) a tube with a few crystals of EDTA, and (3) an empty tube.

The synovial fluid is examined for color, appearance, and viscosity. Bacterial culture, Gram stain examination, mucin clot test, white blood cell count, crystal examination, and glucose concentration determination are made (Fig. 48-3).

Color, Turbidity, and Viscosity. Normal synovial fluid is slightly straw-colored. In gout, the fluid may be white or yellow, depending upon the concentration of urate crystals. Septic joint fluid may be gray, thin, and watery or white, purulent, and thick.

A tube of normal joint fluid is completely clear, and

Fig. 48-2. Site of needle penetration for aspiration of the knee joint effusion.

Fig. 48-3. Synovial fluid analysis.

mucin is very poor, only a turbid suspension of fragments may occur. Poor clots occur in the presence of inflammation such as rheumatoid arthritis, gout, or septic arthritis.

Fluid removed at the bedside should be cultured aerobically and also plated on anaerobic media such as chocolate agar if gonoccocal arthritis is suspected. Aspirates should be cultured in hypertonic growth media in order to detect the presence of atypical bacterial forms. Routine cultures for tuberculosis as well as guinea pig inoculation may be carried out if tuberculous arthritis is suspected.

Cell Count and Other Determinations. A total cell count is carried out on the fluid, to which EDTA has been added. If normal white cell counting solution is used, the acidity will precipitate the mucin and make the count inaccurate. The joint fluid is diluted with saline solution to which a drop of methylene blue is added, and a routine count is done in a white cell counting chamber. A differential white blood cell count is done on smears of this fluid stained with Wright's stain.

Joint fluid is examined for the presence of urate or calcium pyrophosphate crystals. It is important not to perform this on fluid to which oxylate or EDTA has been added. The fluid is first centrifuged to concentrate the white blood cells. Supernatant is removed and the sediment examined under polarized light. Urate crystals will be rod-shaped with rounded ends and exhibit strongly negative birefringence under polarized light. Calcium pyrophosphate crystals are rodlike or rhomboid with sharp ends. Under polarized light, they show weakly positive birefringence. If there is doubt about the type present, uricase is added to dissolve the urate crystals.

Glucose determination is performed on the synovial fluid. At the same time, a fasting blood glucose is determined. In conditions with a high white cell count, such as rheumatoid arthritis or infection, the gradient between blood and joint fluid may be 50 mg/100 ml or greater. In the normal, there is 10 mg/100 ml less glucose in joint fluid than in blood.

PYOGENIC ARTHRITIS

If the diagnosis of septic arthritis can be made very early, the chances of restoring a normal joint are excellent. If the diagnosis is missed and the purulent destructive process goes unchecked, disability due to chronic arthritis is the end result.

PATHOGENESIS. Joints may become infected by:

1. Hematogenous spread from septicemia
2. Direct infection by traumatic wounds or at surgical treatment
3. Extension of an adjacent osteomyelitis

In hematogenous infection, a nidus of bacteria is lodged in the synovium and if not destroyed erupts into the joint space. Inflammatory response results in passage of plasma proteins, fibrinogen and plasminogen, into the joint space because of the increased capillary permeability. Leukocytes are attracted into the joint fluid by chemotaxis. The

newsprint can be read through it. When the white cell count is increased or crystals present, turbidity is increased. Viscosity is tested by spreading a drop of fluid between the thumb and index finger. It is usually possible to spread the stringy viscous fluid for 2 in. before it separates. Viscosity is due to the property of the hyaluronic acid polymerization; in conditions of inflammation, it is depolymerized, and thus viscosity is reduced.

Mucin Clot Test. The mucin clot test is an indication of the character of the protein polysaccharide complex of the synovial fluid. The simplest test is the Ropes test, which is performed by adding a few drops of synovial fluid to a small test tube containing 10 ml of 5% acetic acid. A good clot is a firm, ropey clot which on agitation will not separate or fragment. These characteristics are dependent upon normal polymerization and normal concentration of mucin. A good clot is present in normal joints and with degenerative arthritis. A poor clot is one which is small and fragments immediately with agitation. When the end result of this inflammation is an abscess in the joint space. This abscess is no different from an abscess in other areas of the body, with the exception that the lining or synovial wall may be more permeable to systemic antibiotics.

Proteolytic enzymes from the lysozymes of disintegrating white blood cells and activated plasminogen degrade the proteoglycan of the articular cartilage, exposing collagen fibers. Phemister has pointed out that the white blood cell is necessary for cartilage destruction. The first microscopic change in the articular cartilage is in the central pressure or weight-bearing area where cartilage is in contact with adjacent cartilage. It has been postulated by Curtiss and Klein that the matrix is first lost, exposing the collagen fibers to pressure denaturation. The collagen fibers are then subject to degradation by white blood cell enzymes. The chondrocytes may be killed by bacterial toxins, and, because of poor or absent regenerative capacity, chronic arthritis supervenes.

Staphylococcus aureus and hemolytic streptococci are the two most common organisms producing a pyogenic arthritis. The actual incidence is not important, since the bacterial type in each infection must be determined. Coliform organisms, *Hemophilus influenzae,* pneumococci, meningococci, and *Brucella,* may be the etiologic agents.

CLINICAL MANIFESTATIONS. Septic arthritis may occur at any age but has a higher incidence in patients with debilitating disease and/or on cortisone therapy, or in those with rheumatoid arthritis. Premature infants have a high incidence of septic arthritis of the hip joint.

Patients with hematogenous spread may have more than one joint involved, although localization is commonly confined to one large joint, e.g., knee, hip, shoulder, or elbow; however, any joint may be involved. The patients complain of malaise, chills, fever, and general lassitude. An increase in the white blood cell count with increased polymorphonuclear leukocytes is usually noted. However, in some patients, an elevated sedimentation rate may be the only abnormality.

Examination of the involved joint will reveal the classic signs of inflammation, local tenderness, erythema, swelling, and extreme pain with attempts at motion. The joint will assume a position which is influenced by muscle spasm and pressure/volume relationship. For the knee joint, this is about 20° of flexion. Usually, the patient will not allow complete examination of the joint because of the excruciating pain. In some low-grade infections the range of joint motion may be close to normal early in the course of the disease.

X-rays of a septic joint will show only soft tissue swelling and joint effusion. Bone changes will not be present on the initial x-ray examination (Fig. 48-4). In a child with lax joint capsule and ligaments, the shoulder or hip joint may be subluxed or dislocated as a result of the pressure from the synovial abscess.

DIAGNOSIS. The diagnosis of pyogenic arthritis is made by joint aspiration and synovial fluid analysis. The physician should be cautioned to be reasonably certain that the joint is infected and that the symptoms are not coming

Fig. 48-4. Pyogenic hip joint. *A.* AP x-ray of hip joint taken 48 hours after onset of acute hip pain associated with minor hip injury. Joint space is normal. No bone changes are seen. *B.* Three and one-half weeks later there is complete loss of joint space with no bone changes. Cartilage destruction was due to *Hemophilus influenzae* septic arthritis.

from an overlying cellulitis. This problem occurs in children in whom an infected prepatellar bursitis develops with secondary effusion of the knee joint. If ill-advised aspiration is done through an overlying infection, the joint may be directly inoculated with bacteria. If there is doubt, however, the joint should be aspirated away from the area of superficial infection.

At the time of aspiration, every attempt is made to evacuate the joint completely by compressing fluid into the suprapatellar pouch, from which it is aspirated. The fluid is immediately sent for anaerobic and aerobic cultures, as well as examination for fungus and tuberculosis. A mucin clot test, white blood cell count, and differential and joint fluid glucose determination are carried out on the remainder of the fluid. Blood sugar is drawn simultaneously and the blood sugar synovial fluid gradient determined. An immediate Gram stain examination is carried out on the synovial fluid as well. If organisms are seen in the fluid and the culture is positive, this is diagnostic of sepsis. A poor mucin clot, a white blood cell count between 23,000 and 250,000 with 90 percent polymorphonuclear leukocytes, and a blood/synovial fluid glucose gradient of more than 40 mg/100 ml are consistent with the diagnosis of septic arthritis.

TREATMENT. The treatment of septic arthritis begins with complete aspiration of the joint, which is done for diagnostic purposes. If the Gram stain is positive, immediate antibiotic treatment is instituted. If the Gram stain is negative and the diagnosis is still strongly suspected, antibiotic therapy should be started. Choice of antibiotics will depend upon the suspected organism and the age of the patient. For children, antibiotic coverage for *H. influenzae* should be included; ampicillin is appropriate. For an adult patient with suspected resistant staphylococci, methicillin should be included in the antibiotic regimen.

Surgical Drainage. As soon as the culture report is available, surgical drainage of the involved joint is considered. Surgical drainage is the treatment of choice, but daily aspiration and systemic antibiotic treatment are occasionally indicated. With joints previously damaged by rheumatoid arthritis and where it is possible to evacuate the joint completely by aspiration, or with streptococcal infections where complete daily aspiration is possible, omission of surgical drainage may be appropriate. However, when it is not possible to evacuate the joint completely because of loculated collections of fluid or when biopsy is necessary, surgical drainage should be undertaken as soon as the diagnosis is certain. All infections of the hip must be drained, since the surrounding musculature makes it difficult to monitor the adequacy of needle aspiration drainage. For the knee joint, two parapatellar incisions are necessary, while the hip joint usually requires one well-placed posterior incision. Septic hips of children should always be drained surgically in order to minimize the chance of dislocation from pressure of the intraarticular abscess.

Technique of Posterior Drainage of the Hip Joint. An incision is made parallel with the femoral neck, beginning at the base of the greater trochanter and directed toward the posterior superior iliac spine. The gluteus maximus is split in line with its fibers and the short external rotators divided after retracting the sciatic nerve. The distended capsule is then incised longitudinally and the joint evacuated. Drains are inserted down to the capsule but not into the joint.

Postoperatively, antibiotics are continued, and the patient is nursed supine with the leg in 8 to 10 lb. of Buck's traction.

Adjunctive Measures to Treatment. In addition to surgical drainage and treatment with systemic antibiotics, the patient and joint should be placed at rest. In the case of the knee or hip joint, skin traction is applied to the leg for purposes of immobilization, and an attempt is made to minimize cartilage compression at the point of contact. Where traction is not possible, i.e., for the elbow or wrist, a posterior plaster splint is applied to the joint for immobilization in a position of function.

Antibiotic therapy is continued for a minimum of 4 weeks or until the sedimentation rate returns to normal. If the septic arthritis is an extension of adjacent osteomyelitis, antibiotic treatment is indicated until osteomyelitis has been successfully controlled, i.e., 6 weeks or longer.

Restoration of Joint Motion. If the joint has been treated by closed methods, i.e., aspiration and antibiotics, when the joint remains dry and asymptomatic, early active range-of-motion exercises are started. If treated by surgical drainage, joint motion is not begun until the wounds are granulating or completely closed. Early motion is important in giving a good result.

If damage to the articular cartilage occurs, patients may have residual stiffness, deformity, and a painful joint. Depending upon the severity of symptoms, reconstructive procedures including arthrodesis, arthroplasty, or osteotomy may be necessary.

BONE AND JOINT TUBERCULOSIS

General Considerations

Skeletal tuberculosis is now an uncommon infection in the United States, although it is still a major problem in parts of Asia and Africa. The incidence in the United States has dropped remarkably because of the control of bovine sources, protective measures for infected patients, and the effective use of antituberculous chemotherapy.

Tuberculosis involving the spine or peripheral joints is always secondary to infection elsewhere in the body. The primary infection is usually pulmonary.

PATHOLOGY. The most common site of skeletal involvement with tuberculosis is the spine. The highest incidence occurs in the vertebral bodies opposite the kidney. Hodgson et al. believe that infection is spread via the veins or lymphatics from the kidneys. Once infection starts in a vertebral body, it may spread across the disc space margin to involve the adjacent vertebrae. By tracking beneath the anterior longitudinal ligament, it may spread through Batson's plexus of veins. Infection in the dorsal spine usually is contained beneath the anterior longitudinal ligament, but in the lumbar spine the intimate origin of fibers of the psoas muscle results in spread into the psoas and formation of a psoas abscess.

Peripheral joint tuberculosis involves synovial membrane, bone, and cartilage. It is not certain whether the bone or synovium is infected first, but the result is involvement of both structures. Tuberculous synovitis with tubercle formation and synovial pannus develops, which gradually covers the cartilage and invades the underlying subchondral bone. The cartilage is the last structure to be involved. In contrast to pyogenic joints which have increased leukocytic protease activity, the cartilage in tuberculous joints is destroyed by interference with its underlying circulation. The end result of this process is complete destruction of the joint. Fibrous ankylosis of adjacent surfaces is a common sequel, but spontaneous bony ankylosis is rare.

CLINICAL MANIFESTATIONS. Any chronic monarthritis should be suspected of being tuberculous. There is frequently a history of pulmonary disease, although tuberculous monarthritis may be the first presentation of the systemic illness. Any of the large joints may be infected. Tuberculous arthritis may occur at any age but is more common in children.

The clinical course is insidious, and patients have symptoms for weeks or months prior to seeking consultation. Low-grade pain occurring at night is common. Limitation of joint motion with local synovial swelling is present. Examination of the joint reveals local synovitis out of proportion to the content of synovial fluid. There may be limitation of joint motion and signs of higher local temperature over the joint, but erythema is uncommon. Frequently, in children, the onset of tuberculosis of the hip is suggested by a limp and a history of pain and night crying.

Fig. 48-5. Tuberculosis of the knee joint. *A* and *B*. AP and lateral x-rays of the knee showing erosion of the margins of the medial tibial plateau and medial femoral condyle. There is only minimal joint space narrowing. *C* and *D*. Postsurgical arthrodesis of the knee.

ROENTGENOGRAPHIC FINDINGS. Early in the course of the infection, there may be roentgenographic evidence of soft tissue swelling and adjacent osteoporosis. As the disease progresses, marginal erosion occurring at the cartilage synovial junction may be seen on both sides of the joint (Fig. 48-5). The joint space commonly maintains its integrity because cartilage destruction occurs late in the course of the disease.

In children with long-standing tuberculous synovitis, there may be enlargement of the adjacent growing epiphyses due to chronic inflammation. In long-standing disease in adults, the joint may be completely destroyed with areas of necrosis secondary to undermining, and "kissing" sequestra develop.

DIAGNOSIS. The specific diagnosis of tuberculous arthritis is dependent upon the recovery of organisms from the joint or demonstration of organisms in granulomas on pathologic section. The demonstration of pulmonary lesions or other joint infections as well as positive Mantoux test results are helpful but are not pathognomonic. Joint aspiration, smear, and culture or guinea pig inoculation with the synovial fluid should be carried out in all suspected cases. Synovial fluid analysis will reveal a leukocytic response of less than 20,000 and a poor mucin clot. If the diagnosis cannot be made by joint fluid aspiration, open biopsy should be done without hesitation, since early treatment is mandatory.

TREATMENT. Treatment of skeletal tuberculosis includes (1) general supportive measures, (2) chemotherapy, (3) local treatment of the involved joint or joints, (4) surgical treatment.

General supportive measures include adequate protein and caloric intake, hydration, and proper rest. Patients are started on antituberculous chemotherapy. If the chemotherapy is started before significant necrosis and caseation or walling off has occurred, treatment is associated with a high success rate.

Patients are started on triple-drug therapy until culture reports of the specific organisms are available. Streptomycin is administered in 1-Gm doses daily for 2 or 3 months and then twice weekly for an additional 3 months. Para-aminosalicylic acid (PAS) is administered in doses of 12 Gm/day in three or four divided doses. Isoniazid (INH) is administered at the rate of 3 to 5 mg/kg of body weight, which is about 300 mg for an adult. When the cultures are available and if resistance to one or all of these is present, other agents such as viomycin, Pyrazinamide, oxytetracycline, or cycloserine may be indicated. Tuberculous chemotherapy is continued for at least 18 months.

The treatment of the specific joint involves immobilization by traction, plaster splinting, or casts, combined with bed rest. If the infection is diagnosed early, local immobilization combined with chemotherapy may be sufficient. However, if the joint does not respond to these measures or if the disease has already progressed to involve subchondral bone, surgical joint clearance including synovectomy and excision of tuberculous foci is necessary. Joint debridement with the excision of involved tissues may be quite successful in controlling the local infection and still allow a partially mobile joint. If the joint is totally destroyed, arthrodesis of the involved joint is the treatment of choice.

Tuberculosis of the Spine

Tuberculous spondylitis (Pott's disease) is the most common form of skeletal tuberculosis (Fig. 48-6). The infection is located in the anterior border of the vertebral body, commonly in the thoracic region. Multiple areas may be involved. The infection spreads across the disc space to

Fig. 48-6. Spinal tuberculosis (Pott's disease). *A*. AP x-ray of thoracic spine showing large paravertebral abscess. *B*. Lateral x-ray of thoracic spine showing disruption of the T_7–T_8 interspace with kyphotic deformity.

involve the adjacent upper or lower vertebrae. The disc space is lost because of loss of fluid from the disc. Actual destruction of the disc does not occur early, because of lack of proteolytic enzymes. The disc may be sequestrated into the paraspinal abscess which develops if treatment is delayed.

If there is sufficient destruction of the involved vertebrae, damage to the posterior-lying spinal cord may occur from the pressure of abscess formation or from angular deformity at the site of infection.

Symptoms of Pott's disease include back pain, limitation of spinal motion, paraspinal muscle spasm, and the systemic signs of infection, as well. With cord involvement, the patient will have neurologic signs and symptoms involving the lower extremities.

Treatment requires specific diagnosis. The x-ray findings of tuberculous spondylitis and staphylococcal disc space infection are the same. The diagnosis rests on the recovery of organisms or characteristic histologic evidence from the site of infection. The direct anterior approach to the spine, as described by Hodgson and Stock, provides an effective means for early diagnosis and stabilization of the spine at the same time.

Patients suspected of having spinal tuberculosis are started on triple-drug chemotherapy and bed rest in anterior and posterior plaster shells. After adequate chemotherapy has been established, the spine is exposed by the anterior approach and biopsy material obtained. All infected disc and bone are excised and the adjacent vertebral bodies stabilized with autogenous rib or iliac bone grafts.

Postoperatively patients are nursed in plaster shells or Bradford frames until consolidation has occurred at the site of bone grafting. If paraplegia is present, immediate decompression of the spinal cord is mandatory via the same anterior approach or, occasionally, costotransversectomy. Laminectomy is contraindicated, because it decreases posterior spine stability and allows the anterior-lying abscess, which is not drained, to increase pressure on the dural contents.

Tuberculosis of the Hip

When the diagnosis of tuberculosis of the hip is made early, bed rest with skin traction to the hip, combined with antituberculous chemotherapy, may suffice. If the infection cannot be controlled, open arthrotomy through the Smith-Petersen approach and joint debridement should be carried out to remove the necrotic material. Postoperatively, the patient is kept in traction until the wound is healed. Chemotherapy is continued, and early active motion of the joint is instituted. With severe destruction of the hip joint, surgical arthrodesis by the method of Trumbell or Brittain may be required.

GONOCOCCAL ARTHRITIS

Gonococcal arthritis occurs in females secondary to gonococcal cervicitis or vaginitis. Since the clinical manifestations of the primary cervical infection are relatively occult, treatment may not be effected, and the patient is subject to gonococcal septicemia and gonococcal arthritis. In contrast, the male with gonococcal urethritis has symptoms, seeks early medical treatment, and rarely presents with a gonococcal joint infection.

CLINICAL MANIFESTATIONS. Symptoms usually begin with migratory polyarthralgia, followed by localization in one or two joints. The knee, elbow, and wrist are common sites of infection. A variable febrile course may occur concomitantly with the joint infection.

DIAGNOSIS. The diagnosis is dependent upon the recovery of gonococcal organisms from the septic joint. Cultures of joint fluid are performed on chocolate agar and incubated in 10% carbon dioxide. Aspirates should be cultured in hypertonic broth media to detect the presence of bacterial L forms. It is important to inoculate the culture medium at the bedside and to withhold antibiotics until the culture has been taken.

Synovial fluid analysis will reveal white cell counts in the region of 20,000, with poor mucin and depressed glucose content, which are not in themselves diagnostic of gonococcal infection.

X-rays early in the course of the disease will show only soft tissue swelling.

Cervical smears and cultures should be obtained to prove the primary focus of the infection.

TREATMENT. Intramuscular penicillin G, 1 to 2 million units/day for 2 weeks, is sufficient to eradicate the primary focus and the intraarticular infections completely. With a patient failing to respond to penicillin therapy, other organisms, Reiter's syndrome, or early rheumatoid arthritis should be considered. Local treatment of the joint by immobilization is required and provides additional symptomatic relief. With early adequate penicillin treatment, recovery of a normal joint is the rule.

RHEUMATOID ARTHRITIS

General Considerations

Rheumatoid arthritis is a systemic disease affecting any organ of the body including those of the cardiovascular, respiratory, nervous, and musculoskeletal systems.

PATHOLOGY. The pathologic features of rheumatoid arthritis are found in the diarthrodial joints as well as in adjacent tissues, tendons, tendon sheaths, and bursa.

Articular Changes. The synovitis associated with rheumatoid arthritis is variable and depends on the duration and location of the inflammation. The synovium is congested and edematous with fibrin exudates on the surface or diffusely dispersed throughout the synovium itself. There may be diffuse infiltration of polymorphonuclear leukocytes with localized and nodular collections of small lymphocytes. Plasma cells are commonly arranged about small blood vessels. The end result is thickened hypertrophied villous synovial tissue, covered with fibrin and infiltrated with both acute and chronic inflammatory cells. These changes are not specific for rheumatoid arthritis.

The articular cartilage may be covered by the synovial granulation tissue called pannus (Fig. 48-7). At the cartilage synovial junction, the synovial granulation tissue in-

Fig. 48-7. Pathology of rheumatoid arthritis. Photomicrograph of articular cartilage of the metacarpal head showing synovial pannus on the surface of articular cartilage with pannus invading, destroying, and undermining the articular cartilage in the region of the subchondral bone.

vades the subchondral bone, causing crosive changes, which are visible by x-ray. New periosteal bone formation develops in the region of the capsular attachments, and subchondral bone becomes osteoporotic.

As the granulation tissue and pannus increase, the articular cartilage is eroded. The area of calcified cartilage increases in thickness, effectively diminishing the thickness of the uncalcified cartilage. Roentgenographically, the joint space is narrower, because of the advancement of calcified cartilage as well as the loss of surface contour. The end result of the cartilage destruction and synovial inflammation may be complete disintegration of the joint and instability, with or without superimposed degenerative changes. The joint may undergo fibrous or bony ankylosis.

Subcutaneous Nodules and Other Lesions. In about 25 percent of patients subcutaneous nodules develop commonly over the subcutaneous border of the ulna, olecranon process, dorsal aspects of the fingers, or any area receiving recurrent trauma. There are characteristic histologic findings in the usual subcutaneous nodule consisting of a central area of fibrinoid necrosis surrounded by a second layer of palisading fibroblasts, enveloped by a third layer of diffuse chronic inflammatory cell infiltration. Similar nodules occur in the tenosynovial lining of tendons. Ruptures, due to attrition or invasion by the rheumatoid process, may result.

Skeletal muscle commonly has scattered foci of chronic inflammatory cells. Aggregations of lymphocytes and chronic inflammatory cells may be present in the endoneurium and perineurium of peripheral nerves. The granuloma like lesions resembling the subcutaneous nodules may occur in valve leaflets or any of the layers of the heart. Pericarditis is present in about 40 percent of cases of rheumatoid arthritis. Granulomatous lesions also occur in the lungs. Anthracite-coal miners develop silicotic nodule formation coupled with rheumatoid arthritis. Rheumatoid arthritis patients may demonstrate uveitis or episcleritis. There may be involvement of lacrimal and salivary glands with lymphoid infiltration.

CLINICAL MANIFESTATIONS. Rheumatoid arthritis affects two or three females to one male and occurs at any age with the peak incidence in the thirties and forties. Involvement of joints may be sudden but is usually insidious without antecedent cause. Patients commonly have stiffness of the hands or affected joints in the morning or after inactivity. Muscular weakness and atrophy occur and may be related to the joint pain but are also due to lymphocytic infiltration of the muscles.

DIAGNOSIS. The diagnosis of a patient with long-standing classic rheumatoid arthritis and deformity is not difficult, but in the early stages and with unusual presentations the diagnosis may be quite difficult. There is no specific histopathologic character, since the pathologic findings in the arthritis associated with lupus, dermatomyositis, or periarthritis may be indistinguishable from classic rheumatoid arthritis. Laboratory tests such as the sheep cell agglutination test and latex fixation test are not specific and are positive in other diseases. Because of the difficulty and confusion associated with this diagnosis, the committee on diagnosis of the American Rheumatism Association, under Marion Ropes, set up criteria to aid in this diagnosis. The following features of the disease should be considered:

1. Morning stiffness present for longer than 15 minutes
2. Pain with motion or direct tenderness in at least one joint
3. Swelling unrelated to bony overgrowth of at least one joint for at least 6 weeks
4. Swelling observed in a second joint within a 3-month interval
5. Symmetric joint swelling excluding distal interphalangeal (DIP) joints
6. Presence of subcutaneous nodules over bony prominences
7. X-ray changes consistent with rheumatoid arthritis
8. Positive sheep cell agglutination test or latex fixation test

Fig. 48-8. X-ray findings in rheumatoid arthritis: soft tissue swelling about MP joints and IP joints; erosive changes in the third metacarpal head, right; marked joint space narrowing of the right PIP joint of the index finger; marked destruction and loss of joint space of the carpal bones; erosion of the styloid bilaterally.

9. Poor mucin clot on synovial fluid analysis
10. Characteristic histopathologic changes in the synovial membrane on biopsy
11. Characteristic histopathologic changes in nodules

Classic rheumatoid arthritis would have seven of the above criteria with continuous joint swelling for 6 weeks. A definite diagnosis requires five criteria with continuous joint swelling for at least 6 weeks. A "probable rheumatoid" has three of the above criteria and joint symptoms for at least 4 weeks.

A possible diagnosis of rheumatoid arthritis is suggested if two or more of the following symptoms are present for at least 3 weeks:

1. Morning stiffness
2. Recurrent pain on motion
3. Observed joint swelling
4. Subcutaneous nodules
5. Elevated sedimentation rate
6. Iritis

Rheumatoid arthritis is excluded if a diagnosis of lupus, polyarteritis nodosa, or erythema nodosum can be made. Similarly, rheumatic fever, gout, tuberculous arthritis, Reiter's syndrome, hypertrophic pulmonary osteoarthropathy, ochranosis, multiple myeloma, or lymphomas may simulate the joint findings.

LABORATORY FINDINGS. A normochromic or hyperchromic, normocytic anemia of moderate severity occurs with rheumatoid arthritis. The sedimentation rate is elevated and is a good index of the activity of the disease.

In the serum of 90% of adult patients with rheumatoid arthritis the anti-γ-globulin factor called *rheumatoid factor* is present. Only 20 percent of juvenile patients with rheumatoid arthritis have positive results of tests for rheumatoid factor. Rheumatoid factor is measured by the sheep cell agglutination test or latex fixation test.

Positive lupus erythematosus (LE) cell preparation may be present in less than one-fourth of patients. Serum complement level may be normal or elevated.

Synovial Fluid Analysis. Analysis of synovial fluid from a rheumatoid joint will reveal a poor mucin clot, decrease in synovial fluid glucose, joint fluid leukocytosis reaching 50,000 or more, and decreased viscosity.

ROENTGENOGRAPHIC FINDINGS. The roentgenographic findings (Figs. 48-8, 48-9) in the extremities of early rheumatoid arthritis are related to the presence of destructive influences of the hyperplastic synovia. As the disease progresses, degenerative or responsive changes in the joint may be superimposed upon the rheumatoid process. The earliest x-ray changes are best identified in the involved hands. Similar processes and changes may occur in any joint.

The earliest finding is soft tissue swelling. This fusiform swelling may be about the proximal interphalangeal (PIP) joint, metatarsophalangeal (MP) joints, or radiocarpal joint. The presence of persistent synovial swelling causes osteoporosis in the ends of the bones adjacent to the inflammation. With long-standing arthritis, osteoporosis is a common finding and is in part related to disuse atrophy of the bone.

The presence of synovial and capsular inflammation produces new periosteal bone in the region of capsular attachment. This is noted particularly in the region of capsular attachments about the PIP and MP joints. Proximal to the capsular attachment, there may be cortical involvement with irregularity produced by osteoclastic resorption. The presence of rheumatoid synovium causes erosion at the cartilage synovial junction and on the so-called bare area of bone. Erosions occur commonly on the metacarpal heads, PIP joints, radial margin of the navicular, ulnar styloid, and ulnar aspect of the triquetrum. The damage caused by the synovium when seen in profile appears to be a pseudocyst. The presence of vascular tenosynovium in the region of the radial styloid or on the dorsal aspect of the first metacarpal may cause resorption of bone resulting in irregularity of the bone cortex.

Joint space narrowing may occur quite early in the disease or late. The presence of joint space narrowing in the absence of sclerosis or degenerative changes is indicative of an inflammatory process of the rheumatoid type. With progression of the rheumatoid process, joint subluxations, ulnar deviation at the MP joints (Fig. 48-10), and dislocation may occur. If the patient is actively using this hand, superimposed degenerative changes may occur.

In the juvenile, the presence of rheumatoid synovitis causes soft tissue swelling and osteoporosis. Increased local vascularity results in circumferential enlargement and change in shape of the epiphyses. Leg length inequality may occur as a result of unilateral epiphyseal stimulation. Juvenile rheumatoid arthritis is more likely to go on to ankylosis in comparison with the erosion and instability which predominates in adults.

Management

Treatment of patients with rheumatoid arthritis should be a multidisciplined approach. Ideally, a team should consist of a rheumatologist, orthopedist, physiotherapist, occupational therapist, and social worker. Only by combining the efforts and interests of these individuals can maximal therapy be rendered to the arthritic. The team should strive for early diagnosis and, therefore, early treatment.

By nature of the systemic manifestations of rheumatoid arthritis, it is, at present, a surgical disease only by default. In previous years, many patients with rheumatoid arthritis were treated surgically for established deformity with no attempt at prevention of deformity. The orthopedic surgeon should be involved in the care of every rheumatoid patient. The basic aim of treatment is to halt the progressive destruction caused by this disease, to relieve the patient's pain, and to allow him to continue functioning without the hazard of progressive deformity. This is not possible for all patients, but the progress of the disease usually can be minimized with adequate medical and physical therapy and well-timed surgical intervention.

MEDICAL MANAGEMENT

Medical management includes administration of anti-inflammatory drugs and analgesics, as well as physical and

Fig. 48-9. X-ray changes in rheumatoid arthritis: severe destruction of radiocarpal articulation with subluxation and ulna deviation at the wrist; loss of ulna styloid bilaterally due to the rheumatoid process; dislocation of the PIP joint of the left thumb and dislocation of the right fourth and fifth finger MP joints and left MP joint; diffuse joint space narrowing of many IP joints.

Fig. 48-10. Dorsal and ventral photographs of a rheumatoid arthritic hand showing a mild degree of ulnar deviation with MP joint swelling.

emotional supportive treatment. The drugs now available for treating this form of arthritis are numerous, but Huskisson has suggested a simple classification:

1. Simple analgesics, e.g., aspirin in small doses (2 mg daily), paracetamol, codeine.
2. Analgesics with minor anti-inflammatory properties, e.g., ibuprofen, naproxen, nefenamid acid.
3. Analgesics with major anti-inflammatory properties, e.g., indomethacin, phenylbutazone, aspirin (at least 3.6 Gm daily).
4. Pure anti-inflammatory drugs, e.g., corticosteroids, corticotropin.
5. "Slow-acting" drugs, e.g., gold, penicillamine, the antimalarials, and immunosuppressives.

Corticosteroids have a place in the management of rheumatoid arthritis, especially in life-threatening situations of vasculitis or severe exacerbations of the disease, but are contraindicated as routine treatment.

ORTHOPEDIC MANAGEMENT

PHYSICAL THERAPY. The patient should be informed about deforming forces on inflamed joints. For example, patients with MP joint involvement should understand that grasping heavy objects between thumb and forefingers or grasping objects over long periods which requires excessive force will put undue strain on the inflamed capsule, contributing to subluxation and ulnar drift. Patients with acutely swollen knees should be cautioned about putting excessive stress on the knees when arising from a chair, walking, or standing for long periods. Patients with hip disease should be cautioned to use crutches during acute flare-up of the joint disease.

Inflamed joints should be protected against mechanical trauma that aggravates and complicates the inflammatory destruction. An inflamed joint assumes the position in which the greatest volume of fluid can be accommodated in the joint with the least capsular pressure. In the knee, this is about 20° of flexion. If a contracture in the position of 20° flexion occurs, the patient will have difficulty walking and will superimpose mechanical trauma on the joint inflammation. Wrists go into flexion, which weakens grip. Metatarsophalangeal joints drift into flexion and ulnar deviation, weakening grasp and function.

Anterior plaster shells should be constructed to hold the

Fig. 48-11. Night wrist splint for rheumatoid hand. Wrist is in slight radial deviation, in dorsiflexion with MP joints in extension and IP joints in slight flexion.

wrists in 30° of dorsiflexion, MP joints in extension, and interphalangeal (IP) joints in slight flexion (Fig. 48-11). Posterior plaster shells are constructed to maintain the knees in full extension and the ankles at 90°. Splints are always worn at night and may be worn continuously during the acute episode.

It is extremely important for patients with joint disease to maintain active muscle power. Patients are instructed to carry out daily range-of-motion exercises. This should be done without putting undue force on the capsule of the joint. Knee joints should be exercised while the patient is sitting or lying without body weight applied. Patients should do isometric exercises in a position of function, i.e., full extension for the knees. Patients with cervical spine involvement are urged to maintain a range of full extension. Inflamed hips will develop flexion deformities which can be minimized by passive stretching daily. The patient accomplishes this by lying in a prone position for 15 to 20 minutes twice a day.

The deformities and disabilities from rheumatoid arthritis are insidious. The surgeon should be prepared to fit patients with lower extremity braces as well as wrist splints. The patient who must continue to work and walk with severely involved knees can be helped by the use of a long leg brace with the knee locked in full extension. Valgus and varus deformities involving ankle and subtalar joints can be stabilized by the use of double upright short leg braces.

SURGICAL TREATMENT OF RHEUMATOID ARTHRITIS. The presence of inflamed rheumatoid synovium is intimately associated with joint destruction, but the mechanism has not been defined. When the biochemical processes are understood, it is hoped that systemic or local pharmacologic agents will be developed to interrupt the destructive processes. At the present time, when proper joint rest, modification of activity, and systemic anti-inflammatory medications are unable to control the rheumatoid process, early synovectomy is indicated. If this is carried out before there is significant joint space narrowing and bony collapse, it can protect against joint destruction and effectively relieve pain. As reported in multicenter trials, after 3 years, knees treated by early synovectomy were less painful and tender than those treated by conservative measures and had less effusion. This procedure did not halt the irreversible changes in all treated joints but significantly slowed the development of further pathological changes in some knee joints. However, the results from metacarpophalangeal joints when treated by synovectomy showed no advantage over control joints at 3 years, either clinically or radiographically.

Synovectomy is particularly applicable when synovitis is concentrated in a few joints. However, when the synovitis is generalized, early synovectomy is indicated, especially in the hands and knees.

TECHNIQUE OF KNEE SYNOVECTOMY

Under tourniquet control, a long, curved, median parapatellar incision is made, starting 2 in. proximal to the patella, curving medially over the medial condyle of the femur, and extending distally to end in the region of the tibial tubercle. The capsule and medial patellar retinaculum are divided in line with the incision. The incision is carried across the insertion of the vastus medialis and extends proximally into the quadriceps tendon.

The synovium is excised with meticulous dissection from the suprapatellar pouch en bloc by finding the avascular plane between synovium and capsule or femur. Pannus encroaching upon margins of articular cartilage is wiped off with a sponge or dissected free by sharp dissection. Care is taken to excise all synovium from both lateral and medial recesses. Menisci usually are excised. Synovium invading and surrounding cruciate ligaments is excised. Fibrillated cartilage from the undersurface of the patella is excised with a scalpel. The tourniquet is removed prior to closure, and all bleeders are cauterized. The quadriceps tendon and patellar retinaculum are repaired with interrupted chromic catgut sutures, and the skin is closed in a routine fashion. The knee is splinted in extension for 5 days, during which time the patient does hourly isometric quadriceps exercises. In 5 days the posterior splint is removed and active knee flexion started. The patient is allowed to continue active knee motion within pain tolerance and is allowed out of bed for non-weight-bearing crutch walking. The patient should have 90° of knee flexion by 3 weeks. If not, the knee is manipulated into flexion under general anesthesia.

This technique excises the anterior two-thirds of the synovium. In some instances, it may be necessary at the second operation to excise the posterior one-third through a lateral or posterior incision.

KNEE SURGERY FOR INSTABILITY

If the rheumatoid process has progressed to the point where cartilage substance has been lost, there is concomitant relative lengthening of the collateral ligaments and, therefore, instability. There may be a varus or valgus deformity associated with the cartilage destruction. Synovectomy alone at this stage of the disease is not sufficient to relieve pain and provide knee stability. Such patients require total knee arthroplasty (Fig. 48-12), in which the femoral surface is replaced with metal and the tibial surface with high-density polyethylene. If collateral ligament damage or bone destruction is severe or marked flexion contractures are present, total knee prosthesis with built-in stability (constrained or semiconstrained) is necessary. In rare situations the problem will require the use of a hinge prosthesis.

As a salvage procedure, arthrodesis of the knee is an effective means for controlling pain and relieving instability. However, the patient should have a good ipsilateral hip joint and a mobile functioning contralateral knee joint.

Total knee arthroplasty presently is being used for patients with severe damage to the knee joint as an alternative to arthrodesis. The principle is similar to that used in total hip arthroplasty in which the components are fixed to the bone with acrylic cement. This procedure is in an early period of development but promises to be a significant advance for the unstable knee.

Fig. 48-12. *A*. Internal x-ray of Murray-Shaw total knee prosthesis. *B*. Anteroposterior x-ray of Murray-Shaw total knee prosthesis.

HIP SURGERY

At the present time, there has been insufficient experience with prophylactic synovectomy in the rheumatoid hip with early involvement. However, for the patient with moderate or severe hip disease with disabling pain, total hip replacement is the treatment of choice. (See Total Hip Replacement, under Osteoarthritis.) When there is failure of total hip replacement or infection, the Girdlestone pseudarthrosis will provide pain relief and good hip mobility.

TECHNIQUE FOR GIRDLESTONE PSEUDARTHROSIS

The femoral head is excised at the base of the neck. The lateral portion of the acetabulum is osteotomized and excised to construct a parallel surface to articulate with the osteotomized base of the neck. In selected cases, the iliopsoas tendon may be reinserted distad on the anterior aspect of the femoral shaft to assist in stability. Postoperatively, the patient is maintained in 6 to 8 lb of Buck's traction in a balanced suspension apparatus for 4 weeks. After soft tissue and capsular healing, active exercises including adduction, flexion, and extension are initiated. The patient is allowed on crutches and at 6 to 8 weeks bears weight using an ischial weight-bearing brace. Crutches are converted to a cane as pain is tolerated. Most patients develop sufficient stability about the hip to discard the ischial weight-bearing brace. Most patients achieve improved motion and marked relief in comfort and continue to improve to as long as 3 years postoperation.

ANKLE AND FOOT

Most rheumatoid deformities about the ankle and hind part of the foot can be controlled by adequate bracing techniques. An occasional patient will require bony stabili-

Fig. 48-13. Rheumatoid synovitis involving the hind part of the foot and the forefoot. Note claw toes with lateral deviation of all toes.

zation with correction of deformity at the ankle or subtalar joints. The insertion of a total ankle in which the damaged joint surfaces are replaced with metal and polyethylene may eliminate the need for arthrodesis.

FOREFOOT

The rheumatoid process occurs almost as frequently in the MP joints of the toes (Fig. 48-13) as in the hands. Claw toes with dislocation of the MP joints and flexion of the IP joints is the resultant deformity. The patient is unable to displace forefoot weight between the toes and the metatarsal heads. With the loss of fat pad beneath metatarsal heads and increased weight over this area, painful calluses develop, and difficulty in ambulation occurs. The Hoffman operation, which consists of proximal partial

Fig. 48-14. Hoffman operation used in rheumatoid deformities of the forefoot to relieve metatarsal head pressure and improve toe function and alignment. Metatarsal head and proximal portions of phalanges are excised through transverse dorsal incision.

phalangectomy of all MP joints and excision of the metatarsal heads, will give great relief to the patient and improve gait (Fig. 48-14).

SURGICAL REHABILITATION OF THE RHEUMATOID HAND. The rheumatoid process commonly involves the PIP joints, MP joints, carpal joints, and the tenosynovium of the flexor and extensor tendons about the wrist.

The rheumatoid synovitis of the MP joints causes capsular distension and laxity of collateral ligaments (Fig. 48-10). As the disease progresses, the MP joints sublux anteriorly and ulnarward, causing ulnar drift of the fingers. The extensor tendons are dislocated into the gutters between the metacarpal heads, accentuating the deformity.

Joint involvement of the MP joints as well as rheumatoid disease involvement of the intrinsic muscle mass may produce flexion contracture of the MP joints, hyperextension of the PIP joints, and flexion of the DIP joints. This is the so-called "swan-neck deformity of the intrinsic-plus hand."

Involvement of the PIP joint may result in rupture of the central slip of the extensor tendon crossing the PIP joint, which allows the lateral bands to sublux anteriorly, and a typical boutonnière flexion deformity of the PIP joint develops.

With synovial distension of the MP joint of the thumb, lateral instability occurs, usually with a flexion deformity due to damage or attrition of the extensor pollicis brevis as it inserts into the proximal phalanx. Synovitis may similarly injure the interphalangeal joint of the thumb. Destruction of the carpometacarpal joint may interfere with opposition.

Synovial inflammation of the carpal joints will result in limitation of wrist dorsiflexion and cause anterior subluxation of the wrist. Involvement of the distal radioulnar joint may cause dorsal dislocation of the ulna, interference with wrist rotation, flexion, and extension.

Tenosynovitis occurs about the extensor tendons, and rheumatoid nodules may develop in the tendons themselves. The tendon may stretch or rupture because of the tenosynovial inflammation process or because of mechanical erosion from the involved distal radioulnar joint. The common tendon ruptures occur in those tendons crossing the distal radioulnar joint, the extensor tendons to ring and small finger, and the extensor digiti minimi proprius (Fig. 48-15). The extensor pollicis longus may be involved along its path across the dorsum of the wrist.

Flexor tenosynovitis is commonly overlooked because of the deep position of these structures. With sufficient tenosynovitis, there may be compression of the median nerve in the carpal tunnel. Tenosynovitis of the flexor tendons will cause limitation of active motion of the fingers in the absence of MP or IP joint involvement.

METATARSOPHALANGEAL JOINT SYNOVECTOMY

Metatarsophalangeal joint synovectomy is indicated when the synovitis cannot be controlled by conservative measures. Minimal subluxation can be corrected at the same time, but if severe ulnar drift is present, arthroplasty is required.

TECHNIQUE. Under tourniquet control, a transverse incision is made across the dorsal midpoint of the finger metacarpal heads (Fig. 48-16). Care is taken not to interrupt the veins draining the fingers. A vertical incision is made on the radial side of the MP joint extensor hood, radial to the extensor tendon. A plane is developed between the extensor hood and the underlying capsule and synovium, which are excised en bloc. Pannus is excised from the cartilage as well. The synovial recesses between collateral ligaments and metacarpal heads are also excised.

Ulnar subluxation of the extensor tendons is corrected by reefing the capsule at the time of closure. Involvement of the MP joint of the thumb requires synovectomy through a dorsal curved incision.

Postoperatively, the hand is immobilized in a bulky compression dressing, keeping the MP joints in full extension and neutral position with all IP joints in a position of 45° of flexion. The compression dressing is continued for 3 to 4 weeks and active motion instituted.

If an intrinsic-plus deformity is present, Littler releases in addition to MP joint synovectomy are carried out. Individual dorsal incisions are made over each MP joint, and the lateral triangular bands which represent intrinsic insertions, responsible for extension of the PIP joint, are divided and excised. Postoperatively, the MP joints are kept in extension and the PIPs in 45° flexion.

ARTHROPLASTY

When there is subluxation or dislocation of the MP joint which cannot be corrected by crossed intrinsic muscle transfer, MP arthroplasties are indicated. The technique of arthroplasty using an implant described by Swanson or Niebauer is recommended.

FLEXIBLE IMPLANT ARTHROPLASTY (SWANSON). A transverse incision is made across the necks of the metacarpals. Dorsal veins are retracted but not divided. A longitudinal incision is made on the ulnar aspect of each extensor hood. The neck of the metacarpal is divided, and the metacarpal head, lateral ligaments, synovium, and capsule removed. Appropriate soft tissue releases are carried out in order to reduce and displace the proximal phalanx dorsal to the metacarpal. Osteophytes are removed from the base of the proximal phalanx. The intramedullary canal of the metacarpal and phalanx are curetted out to accept the stems of a Swanson silastic prosthesis. After insertion of silastic prostheses, the radial aspects of the extensor hoods are reefed so that the extensor tendon is displaced slightly to the radial side of the center of the joint. After closing the skin, a bulky hand dressing is applied to splint the MP joints in extension and the IP joints in flexion. A dynamic brace is applied on the fourth or fifth postoperative day, and active motion is started. A similar procedure may be carried out on the proximal interphalangeal joints, appropriately modified if the deformity is of the boutonniere or swan neck type.

TENOSYNOVIAL INVOLVEMENT OF EXTENSOR TENDONS

Unrelieved tenosynovitis of the dorsum of the wrist will result in attrition or destruction of tendons. Early dorsal

Fig. 48-15. Rupture of extensor tendon on the ring finger and small finger from direct invasion of rheumatoid synovium about the distal radial ulnar joint. Note inability to extend ring and small finger at the MP joint and a prominent ulna styloid which is dorsally subluxed.

tenosynovectomy should be carried out when possible. At the same time, the distal $\frac{3}{4}$ in. of the ulnar shaft and styloid should be excised with adjacent diseased synovium of the distal radioulnar joint.

TREATMENT OF TENDON RUPTURES

The extensor tendons of the ring and small fingers are commonly ruptured with any long-standing process in the

Fig. 48-16. Synovectomy of MP joints for rheumatoid arthritis. *A.* Transverse incision is made over the dorsal aspect of the MP joints. *B.* Incision is made on the radial side of the ulnar deviated extensor tendon, and the synovium is excised. *C* and *D.* Extensor hood is reefed in a radial direction to improve tendon alignment over metacarpal heads.

dorsum of the wrist. The extensor pollicis longus may also rupture. When rupture has occurred, tenosynovectomy is indicated, during the repair of the tendons. The tendons are repaired by attaching the distal stumps to the intact extensors of the index and long fingers. In the case of the extensor pollicis longus, a new motor tendon is attached to the distal stump. This is best supplied by the extensor indicis proprius, if available.

FLEXOR TENOSYNOVITIS
AND THE CARPAL TUNNEL SYNDROME

In rheumatoid arthritic patients, flexor tenosynovitis may encroach on the available space for the median nerve as it passes through the carpal tunnel. The patient complains of pain in the thumb, index finger, or long finger with weakness of grasp due to thenar muscle weakness. The patient is commonly awakened at night and shakes his hand in an attempt to relieve the discomfort. On examination, there may only be minimal swelling due to the flexor tenosynovitis. A positive Tinel sign, thenar weakness, and atrophy and numbness in the median nerve distribution may be present in varying degrees. Frequently there is only a history of night pain with paresthesias in the median distribution.

Flexor tenosynovitis may limit active flexion of the fingers with or without median nerve compression. The patient should always be examined for his ability to flex fingers actively to the same degree as that achieved in passive motion. When passive motion is significantly increased over active, flexor tenosynovitis is the diagnosis.

THUMB DEFORMITIES

With sufficient destruction of the MP or IP joint, the functioning of the hand may be severely limited. Instability is corrected by MP arthrodesis (Fig. 48-17) in the position of 15 to 20° of flexion. The pulp of the thumb should be rotated into the position of opposition. In some instances, it may be necessary to fuse the IP joint. Painful involve-

ment of the carpometacarpal joint with subluxation or limitation of motion will require an arthroplasty by excision of the trapezium.

OTHER RHEUMATOID DEFORMITIES
IN THE UPPER EXTREMITY

The rheumatoid process may cause severe painful instability of the elbow. Pain is controlled by proper splinting of the elbow, which is usually sufficient. If ankylosis of the elbow occurs bilaterally or flexion is limited bilaterally, so that the patient cannot feed himself, an arthroplasty may be necessary. This is carried out by excision of the distal humerus and proximal ulna and radius with interposition of fascia lata.

Acromioclavicular involvement which is painful may require excision of the distal clavicle. Rheumatoid disease of the glenohumeral joints is quite difficult to manage. Local injection of cortisone may be helpful in managing the acute stage. These problems are best handled by physical therapy to maintain shoulder motion.

OSTEOARTHRITIS

Osteoarthritis is a term used to describe degenerative changes in diarthrodial joints. The primary change is in the articular cartilage, which is characterized by softening, fibrillation, and abrasion of the articular surface. Since inflammation is not a primary mechanism, *osteoarthrosis* or *degenerative joint diseases* are, perhaps, more accurate terms. Degenerative joint changes occur secondarily in joints previously damaged by inflammation or trauma.

Fig. 48-17. Flexion deformity of the thumb in a patient with long-standing juvenile rheumatoid arthritis, treated by arthrodesis of the MP joint. *A.* Joint space narrowing of the MP joint with inability to extend the thumb beyond 45° flexion. *B.* Crossed Kirschner wire fixation following excision of articular surfaces. *C.* Eight months postfusion with solid arthrodesis in functional position.

PATHOLOGY. The first recognizable changes in osteoarthritic joints occur in the articular cartilage. There is a loss of metachromasia followed by fissuring in the surface of the cartilage. On gross examination, the cartilage appears softer and yellower than its normal blue-gray color.

As the process progresses, flaking of the articular cartilage and fibrillation of its surface occur. Chondroitin sulfate is decreased in osteoarthritic cartilage, although turnover of matrix is actually increased, as indicated by sulfate utilization. Thymidine uptake indicates increased synthesis of DNA and thus an attempt at cell replication. The earliest changes, since they are present only in the articular cartilage, are not demonstrable by x-ray until there has been some joint space narrowing.

With loss of cartilage, the underlying subchondral bone may be exposed and eburnated. Osteophytes occur at the margins of the articular surfaces or in the capsule and ligamentous attachments at the joint margins. The osteophytes on the joint margins are usually covered with a layer of hyalin or fibrocartilage. The earliest roentgenographic change may be sharpening of the normally smooth, rounded marginal contours of the subchondral bone. Bone proliferates in the area below cartilage fibrillation and accounts for sclerosis, which is manifested roentgenographically by increased density in the subchondral region.

Cysts may develop in the subchondral bone. In this situation, the marrow has undergone mucoid degeneration; trabeculae are lost, and sclerotic new bone encircles the cystic rarefied area. The zone of calcification of the base of the articular cartilage advances into the uncalcified cartilage, which accounts for further loss of joint space seen by x-ray.

Concomitant with changes in the underlying bone, the subsynovial layers develop increasing amounts of fibrous tissue with capsular scarring. There may be moderate degrees of villous synovitis if the joint has been repeatedly injured.

PRIMARY AND SECONDARY OSTEOARTHRITIS. Joints deranged by any process will develop secondary osteoarthritic changes. Secondary osteoarthritis is particularly common in the hip following congenital dysplasia, Legg-Calvé-Perthes disease, slipped capital femoral epiphysis, aseptic necrosis of the femoral head, or fractures involving the acetabulum. In joints damaged by crystal deposition, such as in gout or pseudogout, by ochronosis, or by hemophilia and neurogenic lesions, secondary osteoarthritis develops.

When there is no predisposing cause for the articular cartilage change, the osteoarthritis is considered primary. There is no known cause of primary osteoarthritis and no known reason for the basic change in the cartilage. The majority of persons over forty have some changes compatible with the diagnosis of primary osteoarthritis. Whether these changes are attritional and associated with age or represent a primary disease entity is still under discussion. In a postmortem study of hip joints, Byers et al. were able to separate aging changes from the progressive changes of osteoarthritis.

Kellgren and Moore have described an entity called *primary generalized osteoarthritis*. It occurs mainly in females, with onset during menopause, and involves multiple joints to include the DIP, in which Heberden's nodes develop. Heberden's nodes are osteophytic growths on the proximal aspects of the distal finger phalanges. The symptoms in this type of arthritis tend to be more acute, with clinical evidence of local inflammation at the articular sites.

Certain factors predispose to specific joint osteoarthritis. Trauma or repetitive stress to a joint may be a contributing factor, but hereditary factors as yet unknown are also implicated. Patients with obesity have a significantly higher incidence of osteoarthritis of the knees. The carpometacarpal joints of seamstresses and manual workers are involved with greater frequency than those of other workers. Elbows of pneumatic drill operators are frequently involved. Population and genetic studies indicate a higher incidence of affected relatives with osteoarthritis in patients who have Heberden's nodes.

CLINICAL MANIFESTATIONS. Although radiologic and pathologic studies indicate that the incidence of osteoarthritic joints increases with age, only a small percentage have symptoms related to the joint pathology. It is estimated that only 5 percent of all individuals past fifty have clinical symptoms, and the percentage increases to 20 to 30 percent after the age of sixty. Clinical manifestations are more common in women, although pathologic changes are found with equal incidence in both sexes.

Secondary osteoarthritis may affect any joint in which there is an underlying pathologic condition; i.e., a previously injured hip joint or knee joint may be the only symptomatic joint. Primary osteoarthritis tends to affect the large weight-bearing joints—hips or knees (Fig. 48-18). Osteoarthritis without underlying trauma or other inflammatory joint disease only rarely involves elbows, wrists, or MP joints.

The onset of osteoarthritis symptoms is commonly in-

Fig. 48-18. Primary osteoarthritis of the knee. AP and lateral x-rays showing varus deformity of the knee with joint space narrowing, osteophyte production on medial, lateral, and posterior aspects of the tibia, on anterior aspects of femoral condyles, and on both upper and lower poles of the patella. There is minimal cyst formation and sclerosis of subchondral bone of the medial joint space.

sidious; at the time of presentation the x-ray changes indicate that bone and joint abnormality has long been present. Except in the primary generalized osteoarthritis of Kellgren and Moore, there are no systemic manifestations. Local symptoms include pain with motion, relieved by rest. Stiffness occurs after rest and resolves after the joint has been repetitively exercised. Muscle atrophy is not common. On examination, there is restriction of joint motion.

There are no specific laboratory examinations to prove the diagnosis. All blood tests including latex fixation are normal. Occasionally, the sedimentation rate may be slightly elevated. The synovial fluid contains a white blood cell count below 2,000, a good mucin clot, and a normal synovial fluid/blood glucose gradient.

X-ray findings may be quite normal in the very early stages of cartilage change. As the disease progresses, joint space narrowing, subchondral bone sclerosis, osteophyte formation, and subchondral bone cysts are present in varying degrees (Fig. 48-19). The presence of such x-ray signs should not be interpreted as the cause of the patient's symptoms, since these x-ray findings may exist without symptoms. The patient may have underlying rheumatoid disease, gout, or even septic arthritis, superimposed on a degenerative joint.

Conservative Treatment

Most patients with osteoarthritis can be treated by conservative measures. The pain in an osteoarthritic joint is probably due to irritation of the capsular and ligamentous structures of the joint. The abnormal articular surface and incongruous articulation predisposes to minor sprains of the joint capsule and ligaments. In later stages, underlying vascular change in the bone may account for the local and referred pain which persists following rest of the affected joint.

Conservative measures should be attempted and can be successful for the relief of pain.

Fig. 48-19. Bilateral osteoarthritis of the hips showing marked osteophyte formation, sclerosis, acetabular cysts, obliteration of joint space, and partial subluxation.

Immobilization of a painful osteoarthritic joint is dramatic in its relief of pain. Frequently, protection of a painful joint for a few days or weeks is sufficient to alleviate symptoms, and the patient can return to his previous activity. Since most symptoms are due to minor strains on the mechanically abnormal joint, the patient should be instructed in ways to minimize further injury. The patient should understand the differences between osteoarthritis and rheumatoid arthritis, etc., and be given reassurance of his good prognosis.

All factors adding to stress across the symptomatic joint or joints should be minimized or eliminated. Obese patients should be put on a reducing diet. Muscle power which will stabilize the damaged joint should be strengthened. The patient should be instructed to rest the joint when minor symptoms return so as to prevent the pain–muscle-spasm–limitation-of-motion cycle. In some situations, weight-relieving calipers or braces or splints will effectively protect the joint. Daily and occupational activities should be evaluated and activities modified, if possible. Range-of-motion and muscle-strengthening exercises may be helpful because of the protective stabilizing effect to a deranged joint.

Analgesic drugs are helpful in controlling symptoms, but under no circumstances should the patient be started on narcotic or habit-forming drugs. Aspirin, in addition to its analgesic action, has a direct anti-inflammatory effect on cartilage, as well as on periarticular structures. Phenylbutazone and indomethacin are also helpful. The local instillation of hydrocortisone into a painful joint may afford relief if conservative splinting and local rest measures fail. Although there have been reports of neurotropic joints developing following excessive injections, Hollander has had good results and minimal complications with local cortisone.

Orthopedic Management

Surgical treatment of osteoarthritis is indicated when conservative measures fail to control pain or when joint motion is significantly limited and symptomatic. Procedures available for relief of pain of an osteoarthritic joint include arthrodesis, arthroplasty, osteotomy, pseudarthrosis, and neurectomy.

Arthrodesis eliminates motion and relieves the irritation of pain-producing structures. Arthroplasty and pseudarthrosis provide increased mobility of a joint but may be less effective in relieving the discomfort. Osteotomy is effective in correcting deformity and realigning joints and has the added benefit of pain relief by mechanisms incompletely understood at the present time. Neurectomy is indicated in rare situations, but because of the gross overlap of articular innervation, complete denervation of a joint is difficult.

SPECIFIC JOINT INVOLVEMENT

THUMB CARPOMETACARPAL JOINT OSTEOARTHRITIS.
In clothing workers, seamstresses, and surgeons osteoarthritis of the carpometacarpal joint of the thumb may develop. The patients have pain with any motion of the

thumb and marked interference with grasp, due to pain.

Painful DIP joints afflicted with osteoarthritis are rarely unstable. Conservative treatment will usually suffice, and rarely arthrodesis or flexible implant arthroplasty of one of these joints may be indicated.

WRIST, ELBOW, AND SHOULDER. Surgical treatment is infrequently required for wrist, elbow, and shoulder osteoarthritis, which usually result from injuries. Wrist pain due to posttraumatic arthritis not responding to conservative measures may be treated by arthrodesis of the radiocarpal and intercarpal joints. Management of the painful posttraumatic elbow may require excision of the radial head, because of radiohumeral joint subluxation. In sedentary individuals and office workers, a fascia lata arthroplasty will allow motion, although it will increase instability. For laborers who are unable to change occupations, arthrodesis of the elbow in the correct position will provide pain relief and stability. Posttraumatic symptomatic acromioclavicular and sternoclavicular joints may be treated by arthroplasty. In the case of the acromioclavicular joint, the distal 1 in. of the clavicle is removed, and for the sternoclavicular joint, the proximal 1 in. of the clavicle is excised.

OSTEOARTHRITIS OF THE HIP. Osteoarthritis of the hip may be primary or secondary as a result of abnormalities of the acetabulum or shape and alignment of femoral head and neck. Patients with significant acetabular dysplasia, post-Legg-Calvé-Perthes disease with femoral head enlargement, and slipped epiphyses tend to become symptomatic a decade sooner, in their forties and fifties, than patients with primary osteoarthritis of the hip.

In primary osteoarthritis of the hip, two patterns develop: In the *adduction–external-rotation type* the only remaining mobility is usually that of flexion. The most severe bony changes of cyst formation and sclerosis occur in the superior part of the joint with marked osteophyte formation and a valgus position of the neck. In the *non-adducted type,* although the only mobility may be flexion with external rotation, the femur is in a neutral or abducted position. The most severe bony changes occur in the deepest part of the joint.

Clinical Manifestations

The presenting complaint with osteoarthritis of the hip is invariably pain. In the early symptomatic stages, pain is intermittent with episodes occurring after excessive activity and followed by asymptomatic remissions. Pain is aching in character, referred to the groin, the lateral aspect of the thigh, and frequently as far distally as the medial aspect of the knee. Pain is more severe with activity following joint rest, either in the morning or after sitting. With increased activity, the symptoms are less severe. Later in the course of the disease, pain may be severely aggravated by activity, followed by rest pain lasting a few hours.

The origin of pain in an osteoarthritic hip is still conjectural, but it can arise from (1) disease in the subchondral bone, which contains blood vessels and their nerve fibers; (2) muscle spasm and contractures of the muscles around the diseased joint, i.e., the adductors, iliopsoas, and rectus femoris; (3) disease within the sensitive capsule, which is particularly sensitive to the stimulus of tension and trac-

tion; (4) disease in the synovium, although it is unknown whether this tissue is sensitive to painful stimuli or whether transmission is from adjacent joint capsule; or (5) disease in the periosteum.

Patients with osteoarthritis of the hip are usually unaware of restriction of motion early in the disease. As the disease progresses, restriction may be severe. The earliest loss of motion is that of internal rotation but also with associated loss of abduction and extension. Patients may present with an adduction–external-rotation flexion contracture.

The loss of mobility results from (1) articular cartilage destruction with marked loss of joint space and incongruity of the joint surfaces, (2) muscle spasm and contractures with fibrosis of overlying fascia and their musculotendonous junctions, (3) capsular contracture, or (4) mechanical blocking by loose bodies or from large osteophytes. Patients walk with a characteristic hip limp of the Trendelenburg type or an abductor lurch, because they spend less time on the involved hip during the stance phase of gait.

Treatment

Conservative treatment should be attempted. It may be sufficient to allow the patient to continue activities with modification, and while conservative treatment is in progress, the physician can evaluate the patient's cooperation and motivation prior to undertaking reconstructive surgical procedures.

Rest in bed with skin traction to the leg or non-weight-bearing crutch walking during acute episodes are helpful when the pain is severe. The simple maneuver of having the patient carry a cane in the opposite hand to relieve weight load across the contralateral hip may dramatically relieve symptoms. Salicylates are administered. Often, modification of the patient's activities and job requirements will allow him to continue working. If conservative measures fail, surgical procedures are available, each with advantages and disadvantages but all requiring a patient who is a good operative risk (Fig. 48-20).

Arthrodesis. For the young individual who experiences repetitive stress to a hip and who must stand for long periods, hip arthrodesis (Fig. 48-20*A*) may be the procedure of choice. The most frequent indications are sepsis (pyogenic or tuberculous) and cases in which implant arthroplasty is contraindicated. Surgical arthrodesis requires a patient who is physiologically young enough to undergo this treatment, and who will tolerate the plaster cast immobilization and bedrest for 3 to 6 months. Patients with previous back injuries or disease are not suitable candidates for this procedure because of the added stress to the lumbar spine. Patients with bilateral hip disease or involvement of other joints in the lower extremities should be considered for other surgical procedures.

Femoral Osteotomy. The displacement osteotomy (Fig. 48-20*B*) described by McMurray may provide dramatic pain relief and allow hip joint mobility. In young patients with early osteoarthritis, before bone collapse, and with 90° of hip flexion, displacement osteotomy is a good procedure with a high rate of pain relief and minimal risk to

Fig. 48-20. Surgical treatment of hip disease. *A.* Arthrodesis. *B.* Displacement osteotomy. *C.* Cup arthroplasty. *D.* Femoral head replacement arthroplasty.

the patient. In the early stages of osteoarthritis, this procedure can provide complete pain relief and a mobile hip, which can be expected to last for many years. Compared with hip arthrodesis or cup arthroplasty, there is less risk to the patient in this procedure, and if unsuccessful (10 to 20 percent of patients) anatomy is not distorted, and other procedures may be undertaken. The femoral shaft is divided immediately above the lesser trochanter and displaced mediad about one-half the width of the shaft. It is then affixed to the proximal fragment in abduction or adduction, depending upon preoperative joint motion and x-ray studies which show the best seating of the head in the acetabulum. The reason for pain relief, improvement in joint motion, and reestablishment of the joint space is not understood. Possible explanations have to do with changing the vascular bed of the underlying subchondral bone and decreasing the force of tight muscles about the hip. The indications for displacement osteotomy require an osteoarthritic joint in its early stages, before joint motion is severely restricted and before bone collapse.

Cup Arthroplasty. Cup arthroplasty employs the interposition of a well-fitting metal cup between the femoral head and acetabulum (Fig. 48-20*C*), which are shaped to accommodate the cup. The healing process covers the raw bone surfaces with a regenerated arthroplasty surface resembling articular cartilage. Insertion of the cup requires precision, and patients must be willing to have the cup modified by a second surgical procedure if satisfactory results are not obtained. The postoperative management is complicated and requires experienced physiotherapists and a well-motivated patient to continue the exercises. This operation can be done in severely involved hips or even ankylosed joints. The best results are obtained in patients with good preoperative ranges of motion. One can expect relief of disabling pain in about 85 percent of patients including 25 percent with complete relief, unlimited walking in 25 percent, walking without support in 30 percent, and walking with a cane or stick in 55 percent. Since the advent of total hip replacement, the need for cup arthroplasty is rare.

Femoral Head Replacement Arthroplasty. This operation (Fig. 48-20*D*) is used when there is severe damage to the

femoral head in the presence of a normal acetabulum. The indications include nonunion of the femoral neck or avascular necrosis of the femoral head secondary to fracture or other causes. The operation should not be considered in primary or even secondary degenerative arthritis where there are abnormalities on both sides of the articulation.

Total Hip Replacement. All reconstructive procedures on the adult hip must be evaluated in the light of the superior results being obtained with total hip replacement arthroplasty. The total hip arthroplasty replaces both sides of the joint with a prosthetic femoral head and prosthetic acetabular component (Fig. 48-21). The concept for this is not new, dating to 1938 when Wiles designed a stainless steel femoral head with a matching acetabulum, both of which were fixed mechanically to bone. Charnley, and McKee and Watson-Farrar, who began work in the early 1950s, must receive the credit for the current state of total hip replacement arthroplasty.

Indications for Total Hip Arthroplasty. Total hip replacement surgery has been utilized for various types of disabling hip diseases such as osteoarthritis, primary or secondary, and rheumatoid arthritis. It is also used for reconstruction of previously unsuccessful hip surgery such as osteotomy or cup arthroplasty and in any type of joint disorder where infection is not present. Since component-part wear can be expected and loosening may occur in patients who put high demands and excessive forces on their hips, the operation is currently limited to older patients or younger patients with shortened life expectancy or diminished physical capacity. The operation has the best short- or medium-term results of any type of hip reconstructive operation. The uncertainties, of course, are whether the fixation of the component parts to bone can be maintained, how long the bearing surfaces will wear, and whether there is any long-term toxicity to the cement or wear debris. If a patient develops an infection following total hip arthroplasty, either acutely or as a delayed phenomenon, removal of the prosthesis will likely be necessary. The loss of stock results in a Girdlestone pseudarthrosis. In essence, the patient is gambling on an operation

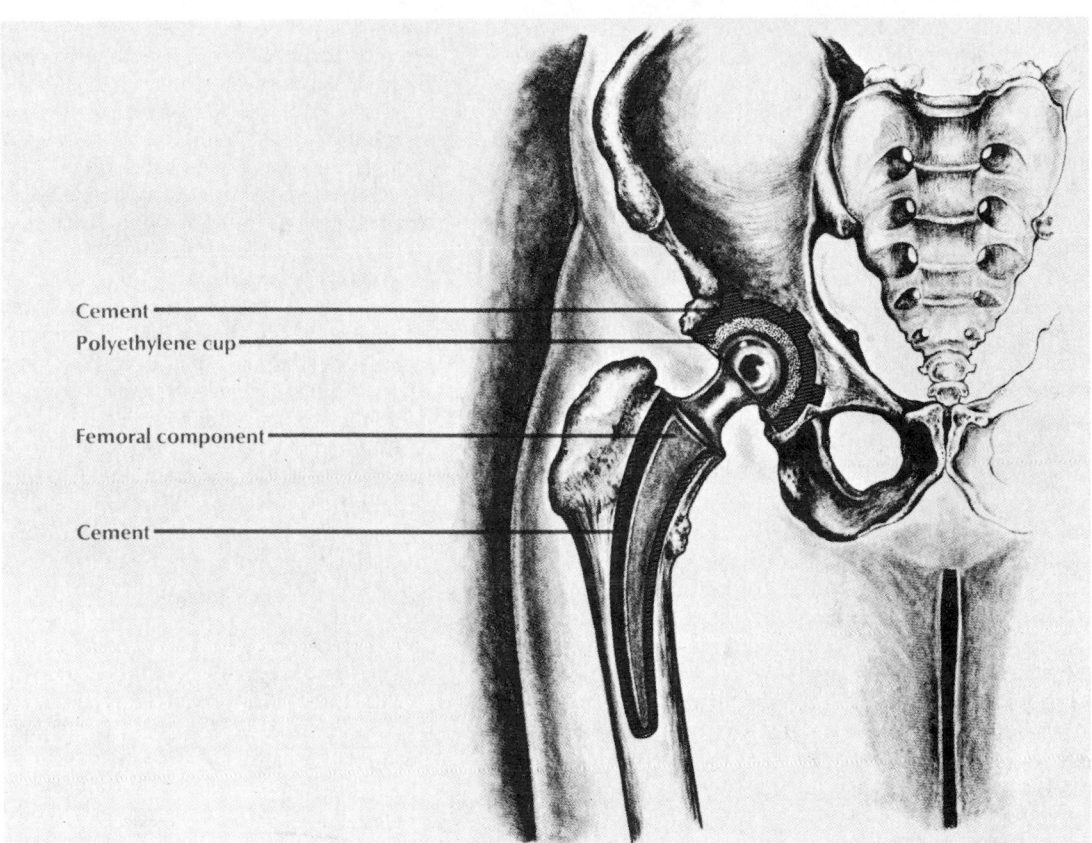

Cement
Polyethylene cup
Femoral component
Cement

Fig. 48-21. Schema of total hip replacement (Charnley-Muller prosthesis). (*From S. Graves et al., RN Magazine, 34:35, 1971.*)

which has a high rate of success but severe disability if complications due to infection develop. The operation has the advantage that severely damaged joints can be reconstructed; there is no urgency in early timing of the procedure as there is, for example, with displacement osteotomy.

Bioengineering Considerations. Total hip replacement requires (1) an understanding of forces across the prosthesis or hip joint, as well as of friction, wear, and lubrication of the component parts of the prosthesis; (2) fixation of the prosthesis to bone; and (3) biologic acceptance of the prosthetic materials.

Forces across the Hip. In the normal walking cycle it has been shown that loads across the hip joint vary between zero and four times the body weight. With the patient standing on one foot, the weight of the body is balanced by the simultaneous contraction of the abductor muscles of the hip in the stance phase. Since the body weight is working on a lever arm, about three times the length of the lever arm across which abductor muscles have their force application, the multiplication of forces about the hip can be accounted for. Recognition of these lever arm forces demands attention to prosthetic materials capable of withstanding the loads. Because of the leverage applied to the hip joint, the acetabular component of the total hip must be placed as mediad as possible, with a corresponding lateral displacement of the greater trochanter. This requires reaming of the acetabulum and osteo-

phytes on the medial acetabulum in order to displace the center of the total hip device mediad. Increasing the length of the prosthetic neck will necessarily displace the greater trochanter laterally, thereby increasing the leverage of the abductor muscles and reducing the force across the joint.

Friction, Wear, and Lubrication of the Total Hip Appliance. The introduction of an appliance system into the body in which there is motion between two components involves considerations of friction, wear, and lubrication between the parts. Bearing material utilized in total hip replacement is of two types, metal on metal and metal on plastic. To prevent corrosion arising in the biologic system, similar metals are necessary. Alloys of cobalt, chromium, and molybdenum as are used in the McKee-Farrar prosthesis have been shown to be suitable for this. Motion between similar metals in either the dry or lubricated state has a higher coefficient of friction than in the metal-plastic type of prosthesis used in the Charnley or T-28 types. In the Charnley prosthesis, a stainless steel femoral head is in contact with a high-density polyethylene acetabular component. Reducing the size of the femoral head component reduces the frictional resistance between the surfaces and minimizes the tendency of the components to separate from bone. The optimal femoral head size should be one which is small enough to minimize the volume of wear debris and at the same time maintain sufficient mechanical strength. Characteristics of the fluid lubricating the surfaces of a total hip replacement in vivo are not known but may correspond closely to normal synovial fluid. Wear of the metallic surfaces in a metal-to-metal prosthesis is of the adhesive wear type in which separation of welded asperities results in metal transfer and loose wear particles. Abrasive wear, in which a harder surface such as the metal erodes through the softer surface of the plastic, occurs in the metal-plastic type. Information on the tribiologic characteristics of total hip replacement is incomplete. The reader is referred to the work of Dowson and Wright and Scales and Lowe.

Fixation of the Prostheses to Bone. The marked long-term relief of pain with a total hip replacement is attributed to the optimal mechanical relationship and stability between prosthesis and the bone. This is accomplished by the use of cold curing acrylic cement, methyl methacrylate, which acts as a force diffuser between the stem of the prosthesis and the bone or between the acetabular prosthesis and the pelvis. The methacrylate does not adhere to the bone but acts only by mechanical interdigitation. Force across the prosthesis is transmitted to a much greater surface area of bone by the interposition of the acrylic. Thus, the force on any given area of bone is insufficient to cause resorption, and stability is maintained.

The acrylic cement is prepared by mixing liquid methyl methacrylate monomer and dimethyl-*p*-toluidine stabilized with hydroquinone and a fine powder of polymethyl methacrylate and 2% benzoyl peroxide. After a few minutes of mixing, a doughlike substance is obtained which increases its viscosity over the next few minutes. When the doughy consistency is reached, the material is pushed into the roughened medullary canal or acetabulum. When the cavity has been filled, the stem of the prosthesis, or acetabular prosthesis, is inserted and excess cement removed. Total curing time is about 8 minutes for Surgical Simplex. Depending upon the mass of acrylic used, temperatures of 90°C may be attained. There is concern for the amount of tissue damage resulting from the exothermic reaction. Just prior to the acute rise in temperature, expansion of the Simplex occurs by $1\frac{1}{2}$ percent, and during the cooling period contraction of 1 percent occurs.

Biologic Acceptance of the Prosthetic Materials. Within the time frame of methacrylate use, there has been no evidence of carcinogenic or toxic reactions of the acrylic. Absorption of methacrylate constituents at the time of surgery may result in hypotension. At the bone cement interface, both experimentally and in prostheses removed at postmortem, there is a fibrous layer of tissue between cement and bone. Wear debris from a metal-to-metal prosthesis can be seen as particulate material in macrophages in the regenerated capsule. There is little information about the fate of wear debris from high-density polyethylene.

Types of Total Hip Joint Replacement. *McKee-Farrar Prosthesis.* The McKee-Farrar prosthesis is a metal-to-metal prosthetic design in which both femoral head and acetabular components are made of a cobalt chrome alloy and designed so that the components are fixed with methyl methacrylate. Two head sizes are in standard use, $1\frac{3}{8}$ and $1\frac{5}{8}$. The acetabular cup has a rim with multiple studs for fixation with acrylic cement. The large size adds stability to the articulation, making the technique of insertion less

demanding. The rate of loosening with this device is greater than when the acetabular component is made of high-density polyethylene.

Charnley Prosthesis. The Charnley prosthesis consists of a stainless steel femoral component with a head of 22.25 mm fabricated of surgical stainless steel. The acetabular cup is made of high-density polyethylene with an external diameter of 42 mm. Varying stem sizes are available as well as smaller external diameters of the cup. The cup contains a reference wire for radiographic determination of wear. This device generates less frictional torque due to the smaller head size and the improved frictional characteristics of metal on plastic. The smaller head size and the wide cup thickness demand exacting surgical technique to minimize dislocation.

Charnley-Muller Prosthesis. The Charnley-Muller prosthesis is a modification of the Charnley and consists of a cobalt chrome femoral component with a head size of 28 mm with standard long and short necks available. The acetabular component is made of high-density polyethylene. The possibility of dislocation is less with the larger head size.

Other modifications of the metal-on-metal and metal-on-plastic designs are available and include the Amstutz, T-28, Harris, and Stanmore types.

Ring Prosthesis. The Ring prosthesis is a metal-on-metal prosthesis which is designed to be used without cement or acrylic fixation. The femoral component is a modification of Austin Moore's prosthesis. The acetabular component consists of a cup with a long threaded stem for fixation into the weight-bearing line of the ilium. The design has eliminated cement. It is anticipated that loosening of the components will be increased with this design.

Technique of Insertion of a T-28 Prosthesis. With the patient lying in the lateral position, a standard Harris approach to the hip is carried out. A gently curved incision is centered at the posterior border of the trochanter and extending to $1\frac{1}{2}$ in. posterior and distal to the anterior spine of the ilium, the distal limb being symmetric with the proximal. The greater trochanter is osteotomized and retracted proximally with its attached abductors. The short external rotators are divided from the greater trochanter and retracted posteriorly. The exposed capsule of the hip joint is excised and the femoral head dislocated by flexing, adducting, and externally rotating the hip. Using an oscillating saw, the femoral head and neck are removed at a point just above the lesser trochanter. The iliopsoas is divided for better mobility of the proximal femur as necessary. The acetabulum is then reamed, taking care to remove acetabular debris and osteophytes from the medial acetabulum in order to attain medial cup displacement. Two $\frac{1}{2}$-in.-diameter holes are drilled into the iliac portion of the acetabulum. Two additional holes are drilled through the acetabulum into the superior ramus of the pubis as it joins the acetabulum and also the ischial ramus. The holes are undercut with a curet. Hemostasis is maintained by gel foam packs into the holes.

Methyl methacrylate cement is mixed; when it becomes of doughy consistency, it is inserted as a mass into the acetabulum and drill holes. A T-28 acetabular component is then inserted as far medially as possible and held in a position of 45° abduction and 10° anteversion. Excess cement is removed. Acrylic cement projecting around the rim of the cup after hardening is trimmed with an osteotome. The proximal femur is then reamed using an appropriate rasp. The femoral component with the correct neck length is then inserted into the femur without cement and a trial reduction carried out. If this is satisfactory, the prosthesis is cemented into the proximal femur in a position of 10 to 15° anteversion using acrylic cement. The greater trochanter is reattached with steel wire through two drill holes across the lateral cortex of the proximal femur. Closed suction drainage is applied to the wound. Postoperative management includes bed rest in balanced suspension followed by early partial weight bearing between crutches. Protected weight bearing is continued until union of the trochanter has occurred.

Complications of Total Hip Replacement. The dread complication of total hip replacement is a wound infection. This may occur as an acute postoperative complication or as a delayed phenomenon months or years after primary wound healing. Prevention of wound infection from total hip replacement requires scrupulous operative technique on the part of operating personnel. Surgery is often carried out in operating theaters equipped with positive-pressure rapid air changes with high-efficiency particle filters. Penicillinase-resistant antibiotics are administered preoperatively, intraoperatively, and postoperatively. Infection rates in total hip replacement series vary from as low as less than 1 percent to as high as 10 percent.

Thrombophlebitis and pulmonary embolism are complications of any type of hip surgery, and total hip replacement is no exception. Prophylactic measures against thrombophlebitis are indicated, such as administration of Coumadin or low-molecular-weight dextran. Both lower extremities should be elevated postoperatively. Patients should be cautioned against sitting for even short periods until hip motion and activity have been restored.

The prosthesis can be dislocated. The incidence of this is low and can be minimized by accurate positioning of the prosthetic components and positioning of the operative extremity until soft tissue healing has occurred.

Loosening of the prosthetic components is a late complication and may be evident if the patient begins to experience pain in the characteristic hip distribution. Loosening can be determined by unusual resorption of bone at the bone-cement interphase. It may be necessary to do an arthrogram or bone scan for diagnosis.

Charnley has reported follow-up results on 379 hips followed between 4 and 7 years postoperatively. Ninety percent of the patients maintained excellent results. Late mechanical failure occurred in 1.3 percent of patients. The overall infection rate was 3.8 percent, 2.2 percent being late infections. The average degree of acetabular prosthesis wear varied from 1 mm in 5 years to absence of wear at 7 years postsurgery. Preoperative range of motion was improved in all patients, and there was no tendency to decrease motion with increasing time of follow-up.

CHONDROMALACIA OF THE PATELLA. Chondromalacia of the patella represents degeneration, or the first stage

of osteoarthritis, involving the cartilage surface of the patella. Changes in this cartilage are common by the age of thirty, although symptomatology is infrequent in terms of incidence of the pathologic change. The earliest changes occur on the medial facet of the patella. The cause of chondromalacia is unknown, but trauma, such as striking the knee on the dashboard of a car, and mechanical factors of an incongruent relationship of the patella with the femoral condyle may play a role. In teen-agers, especially girls, mild degrees of recurvatum and valgus knees are associated with subluxing patella with attendant chondromalacia. Chondromalacia is not uncommon with clinical symptoms after immobilization of a fractured femur for prolonged periods.

Clinical Manifestations. The onset may be insidious; the patient is aware only of minor discomfort in the knee with acute flexion or in descending stairs or kneeling. Often the onset is acute following a direct blow to the knee. Chondromalacia frequently presents with symptoms of subluxation or even frank dislocation of the patella. The patient may be aware of crepitus. Synovial effusion, although uncommon, does occur. Physical examination will demonstrate tenderness if the patella is pressed distad in its groove while the quadriceps is actively contracted. By displacing the patella, mediad, the undersurface can be palpated and also may reveal tenderness. Atrophy of the vastus medialis is uncommon.

Radiographs are negative early in the course of the disease but are taken to rule out other causes for discomfort. With progressive change, osteophytes may be present on the proximal and distal pole of the patella, progressing to frank osteoarthritis of the entire knee joint. Other causes of knee pain must be excluded, i.e., rheumatoid arthritis, loose bodies, and meniscal injuries, some of which have patellar symptoms in addition to the primary condition.

Treatment. The majority of patients with symptoms are managed by conservative treatment. The patient is taught quadriceps-strengthening exercises. He is cautioned to sit with his knee extended and to avoid flexion until symptoms subside (1 to 3 weeks). In some cases, crutches or posterior plaster splints are necessary.

Surgical Treatment of Chondromalacia. Patients not responding to conservative treatment or having persistent recurrent episodes may require excision of the diseased cartilage, realignment of the quadriceps patellar mechanism by tibial tubercle transfer or similar procedures, or even patellectomy when the condition has progressed to severe osteoarthritis of the patellofemoral joint.

The knee is explored through a median parapatellar transverse incision, and the undersurface of the patella is examined. If the cartilage destruction is not severe or less than one-third of the undersurface is involved, the diseased cartilage is excised. If there are clinical findings of patellar subluxation, a tibial tubercle transfer may be carried out. If involvement is greater or large osteophytes are present, patellectomy may be necessary (Fig. 48-22).

Postoperative treatment requires an initial period of immobilization and quadriceps-strengthening exercises. The knee is placed in a posterior splint or circular plaster cylinder, and hourly quadriceps exercises are instituted. In

Fig. 48-22. Patellectomy. Patella exposed through transverse skin incision and excised through vertical incision in its tendinous envelope.

the case of cartilage excision, active knee flexion and range-of-motion exercises are started at 2 to 3 weeks. The patient is allowed to bear full weight when range of motion and quadriceps power are normal.

For postpatellectomy management, a cylinder is applied for 3 to 4 weeks, and then gradual active flexion within pain tolerance is begun within 4 to 6 weeks. Weight bearing is allowed when there is 90° of knee flexion and quadriceps power is normal.

OSTEOARTHRITIS OF THE KNEE. Osteoarthritis of the knee does not commonly require surgical intervention. Patients are reassured and activity is modified. Salicylates and quadriceps-strengthening exercises are usually sufficient to overcome discomfort.

If symptoms can be localized to the patellofemoral joint, patellectomy is indicated. If symptoms do not respond to conservative treatment and there is a mild varus or valgus

Fig. 48-23. Charnley compression arthrodesis of the knee.

deformity of the knee, realignment by proximal tibial osteotomy may afford dramatic relief. The mechanism by which osteotomy is beneficial is not understood. Part of the value lies in realignment of the knee joint, although the change in vascularity to the subchondral bone may be of importance. In severe osteoarthritis of the knee of posttraumatic causation, arthrodesis may be indicated when other joints are normal (Fig. 48-23). Total knee joint replacement appears to be a significant advance in osteoarthritis of the knee in older patients and should be considered when osteotomy is contraindicated. An alternative procedure is the insertion of MacIntosh prostheses.

OSTEOARTHRITIS OF THE ANKLE AND FOOT. Osteoarthritis of the ankle is usually the result of injury. Attempts at modifying discomfort or deformity should be made with a short leg brace, the ankle fixed in appropriate position to minimize medial-lateral and flexion-extension forces. Arthrodesis may be required. Similarly, subtalar joint problems requiring treatment are more likely the result of posttraumatic osteoarthritis. Again, arthrodesis may be indicated.

Hallux Valgus (Bunion)

Hallux valgus, or lateral deviation of the great toe, is a disease of the shoe-wearing population. Hodgson has shown that foot deformities have a much greater incidence in the shoe-wearing population in Hong Kong than in those without shoes. The incidence of hallux valgus is much greater in the female than in the male and is certainly precipitated by improper shoe wear. A short first metatarsal or metatarsus primus varus may contribute to or initiate deformity. Once the great toe starts to deviate laterally, there is little conservative treatment can do to overcome deformity. With lateral deviation of the great toe, the long flexor and extensor tendons are bow-stringed laterally across the joint and maintain and increase the deformity.

Traction on the capsule of the MP joint at its attachment to the metatarsal head, as well as local shoe pressure over the medial aspect of the metatarsal head, contribute to the development of a large exostosis with an overlying soft tissue bursa, a bunion. Contracture in the adductor hallucis contributes to hallux valgus with further displacement of the first metatarsal mediad. The lateral sesamoid may become displaced in the direction of the lateral side of the foot. Changes occur in the articular cartilage which resemble the early stages of osteoarthritis. The end result is an osteoarthritic MP joint. Hallux rigidus is a stiff MP joint and is associated with pain during attempts to bear weight and during the push-off phase of walking.

Clinical Manifestations. Hallux valgus is a common deformity, although few are symptomatic. The most common complaint is the inability to wear the modern shoe with its narrow forefoot. Patients may complain intermittently of pain over the bunion due to acute bursitis from local shoe pressure. Such patients wear old shoes and commonly take their shoes off after a day's work.

With sufficient deformity and lateral deviation and rotation of the great toe, there is less distribution of weight between metatarsal heads and toes. The result is increased pressure on metatarsal heads during the push-off phase of gait. Callosities develop over the second and third metatarsal heads because of this increased pressure.

Treatment. If hallux valgus has already developed, symptoms from the bursa and osteophyte over the metatarsal head can be minimized with appropriate modification of shoes. Symptoms due to metatarsalgia from abnormal weight distribution from the malaligned great toe may be handled with insoles and metatarsal arches to distribute the weight proximally away from the metatarsal head pressure area. A metatarsal bar on the external surface of the sole may assist in accomplishing the same changes in weight distribution. There are over 100 different operations for bunions and hallux valgus which attest to the inefficiency of the various procedures. The most common surgical procedure for bunions is the Keller arthroplasty (Fig. 48-24). This consists of excision of the proximal one-half of the proximal phalanx of the great toe and excision of the osteophyte on the medial dorsal surface of the metatarsal head. Following this surgical procedure, the great toe is shorter, but long tendons take up the slack, restoring function to the great toe. This procedure is applicable to any degree of hallux valgus and has a high rate of success.

In the young female with minimal osteoarthritic changes and essentially normal joint flexion and extension, the McBride procedure or a modification of it will give a satisfactory result. The procedure involves a dorsal incision between the first and second metatarsal heads in which the fibular sesamoid is excised. This interrupts the adductor insertion on the great toe. Through a second incision over the dorsal medial aspect of the MP joint, the osteophyte is excised, and the abductor tendon and capsule insertion are reefed to hold the toe in neutral, but not varus, position. McBride reattaches the adductor to the first metatarsal neck to assist in controlling the varus of the first metatarsal shaft. The capsules of the first and second metatarsal heads are sutured together to assist in controlling the metatarsus primus varus.

The end result of this procedure is realignment of the toe with function and normal length maintained. Another approach is to osteotomize the adducted, or varus, first metatarsal. This should be done before significant MP joint changes have occurred. The procedures which excise only the bursa overlying the metatarsal head or its exostosis do not usually result in relief of symptoms.

GOUT

Gout is a metabolic disease in which crystals of sodium urate monohydrate are deposited in and about joints. Patients with gout have an increase in serum uric acid concentration. Patients may have complicating renal diseases due to urate deposition.

Gout is said to be primary when it is due to an inborn error of metabolism. Secondary gout may be due to other diseases such as myeloproliferative disorders, leukemia, hemolytic anemias, or glycogen storage disease. It is generally accepted that the hyperuricemia of primary gout has a hereditary transmission. However, the hyperuricemic rela-

Fig. 48-24. Keller arthroplasty. *A.* Exostosis and proximal phalangectomy carried out through dorsal medial incision. *B.* Postoperative position.

tives of patients with gout have an incidence of gout symptoms of only 20 percent, suggesting that there are other factors than hyperuricemia determining the clinical condition.

Hyperuricemia must be defined for each laboratory. With colorometric methods, the upper limit of normal in the male is about 6.4 mg/100 ml and 5.8 in females. Population studies indicate that hyperuricemia may be transmitted by an autosomal dominant or sex-linked dominants. Other information suggests that polygenic transmission is also operative. Hyperuricemic patients of primary gout both overproduce and underexcrete uric acid. Both processes may operate in varying degree in patients with clinical gout.

The incidence of gout is less than 1 percent in Europe and the United States. It is much higher in Filipinos and reaches the incidence of 8.2 percent in the Chamorros of the Mariana Islands and Carolinians of the Caroline Islands. In most series only 3 to 7 percent of cases of primary gout occur in the female. The clinical onset is rare before the third decade. The mechanism by which an acute attack is precipitated is still unknown. When crystals of sodium urate are injected experimentally into animals or human beings, acute arthritis will ensue whether the patient has hyperuricemia or is normal. Following injection of urate crystals, joint pressure increases, and the pH of synovial fluid drops. The change in pH is related to lactic acid produced by leukocytes. Leukocytes ingest the urate crystals, a mechanism which is blocked by treatment with colchicine.

Seegmiller and Howell propose a cycle of crystallization of sodium urate from supersaturated body fluids. Once crystals enter the joint, leukocytosis increases lactate production, causing a fall in local pH and a tendency for further crystal deposition. The mechanism of initiation of deposit of the crystals in the joint is not known. Certain clinical situations such as trauma, stress, and ACTH withdrawal are associated with a high incidence of acute gout in the hyperuricemic.

PATHOLOGY. Urate crystals are deposited in cartilage, subchondral bone, and the periarticular structures and kidneys, as well. The tophaceous deposit consists of urate crystals surrounded by an inflammatory granuloma. The crystalline deposit may calcify and be detectable on roentgenograms.

Tophi may occur anywhere in the body but are common in the external ear, in the olecranon, and about tendons and bursae. Secondary degenerative joint changes occur in response to urate deposits. Urate crystals may be deposited in the kidney and be surrounded by giant cell granulomas.

CLINICAL MANIFESTATIONS. The classic presentation of an acute attack is in a male over the age of thirty who experiences sudden onset of a monarticular arthritis, usually involving the MP joint of the great toe (Fig. 48-25). The onset is dramatically acute with swelling, erythema, and tenderness about the affected joint. Untreated, an attack lasts from a few days to 2 weeks. The initial attack is most common in the big toe but may involve any of the weight-bearing joints of the foot, ankle, or knee. Occasionally, an olecranon bursa is the location for the first attack.

Following an acute attack, the patient may be completely asymptomatic for many months or years. However, subsequent attacks may involve other joints and follow a longer and febrile course. In less than half the patients

with recurrent attacks chronic gouty arthritis develops. Chronic gouty arthritis may develop gradually without preceding acute symptoms in a specific joint. Tophi may ulcerate and drain urate material intermittently. Acute gonococcal arthritis, acute rheumatoid arthritis, or acute rheumatic fever may simulate an acute gouty arthritis. In less typical situations, gout may resemble any of the chronic arthritides.

The diagnosis is confirmed when urate crystals can be detected by polarized light microscopy of fluid aspirated from an acutely affected joint. The serum uric acid level is commonly elevated during an acute attack but during the interval stage may be within normal limits. Patients with an acute attack may have leukocytosis and an increased sedimentation rate. The presence of tophi aids in the diagnosis, and aspiration will reveal urate crystals. In chronic tophaceous gout, characteristic punched-out lesions in the regions of the subchondral bone and at capsular attachments of involved joints are found. Such findings, however, may be seen in rheumatoid arthritis, sarcoid, hyperparathyroidism, and other conditions, making x-ray interpretation nonspecific.

TREATMENT. Management of the Acute Attack. Colchicine has been known to be effective since the days of Hippocrates. Recently, it has been shown that colchicine interferes with the metabolic activity of leukocytes. Colchicine in a dose of 0.65 mg is given each hour or 2 hours, until acute symptoms subside or until diarrhea or vomiting results. The response to colchicine is quite often dramatic and diagnostic of acute gout. Phenylbutazone, 200 mg, two or three times daily during the acute stage, is an alternative. Indomethacin will also result in rapid resolution of symptoms.

The acutely inflamed joint should be immobilized and the patient put at bed rest.

Subsequent Management. Since not all uric acid is derived from exogenous sources but much of it is synthesized in the body, a strict dietary limitation of purines will not prevent subsequent attacks. However, the diet should be limited in this respect, although even with complete abstinence from purines attacks will recur.

Patients should be maintained on continued colchicine dosage in attempts to reduce the frequency of recurrences of acute symptoms. Most patients are managed with one or two colchicine tablets per day, increasing the dosage at the first signs of recurrence.

The formation of new tophi and recurrent attacks can be reduced by uricosuric agents: probenecid and salicylates. Allopurinol, a xanthine oxidase blocking agent, will reduce serum uric acid concentration and is effective in reducing chronic tophaceous deposits.

Chronic Gouty Arthritis. Treatment of chronic gouty arthritis is almost exclusively by medical measures. When severe joint destruction has occurred, surgical reconstruction including arthrodesis and arthroplasty may be required. Large tophaceous deposits causing irritation of overlying skin about joints may be excised with considerable benefit to the patient. Tophaceous deposits requiring excision have also been responsible for median nerve compression in the carpal tunnel.

Fig. 48-25. Severe gouty arthritis involving the MP joint of right toe with destruction of the metatarsal head. Proximal phalanx with joint space narrowing. Note large soft tissue gouty tophus.

Pseudogout (Chondrocalcinosis, or Crystal Deposition Disease)

McCarty has called our attention to the condition of calcium pyrophosphate crystal deposition disease. Prior to the characterization of articular chondrocalcinosis and the discovery that calcium pyrophosphate crystals could induce an acute arthritis, these patients were thought to have a type of gout. The incidence of pseudogout may be more common than gout, but it is not as well recognized. It occurs in males $1\frac{1}{2}$ times as commonly as females. The age of onset is commonly in the middle or the late decades but may be in the twenties.

CLINICAL MANIFESTATIONS. An acute attack may be similar to gout and occurs frequently after joint trauma or in postoperative patients. The onset may be acute, with symptoms increasing in a joint over 1 to 2 days in contrast to the more abrupt onset of gout. The joint most commonly involved is the knee joint. It is quite uncommon in the MP joint of the great toe. Patients with acute attacks have asymptomatic intervals. One-third of such patients have an elevation of the serum uric acid level.

A small percentage of patients will have continuous acute attacks, but the most frequent pattern is that of progressive chronic arthritis of large joints. Hypertension and diabetes are associated with one-fourth to one-half of patients with pseudogout.

The patients complain of acute pain in the involved joint with stiffness, local swelling, tenderness, and erythema overlying the joint. In the chronic presentation, the joint may resemble a degenerative arthritis.

The diagnosis is dependent upon finding calcium pyrophosphate crystals in the synovial fluid or in leukocytes of synovial fluid. Polarized light microscopy reveals the crystals to show weakly positive birefringence. X-rays reveal crystalline deposits in the articular cartilage (Fig. 48-26) as well as in fibrocartilaginous structures as menisci (Fig. 48-27) and ligaments in joint capsules. The distal radioulnar nerve and symphysis pubis, as well as glenoid and acetabular labra, may show calcification. The calcification of the articular cartilage is in the midzonal layer and appears as a radiopaque line, paralleling the subchondral bone.

Treatment of an acute attack is by aspiration of the synovial effusion and the local injection of cortisone. Systemic phenylbutazone and salicylates may be helpful, but colchicine is not. At present, there is no means of halting the progressive deposition in joints.

HEMOPHILIC ARTHRITIS

The major problem confronting the hemophiliac between episodes of acute bleeding is his disability due to hemophilic arthropathy. Duthie et al. have shown spontaneous bleeding occurs only with 0 percent circulating Factor VIII; severe bleeding after minor injury occurs when Factor VIII is between 1 to 5 percent, and excessive bleeding after minor injury or operation at 5 to 25 percent of normal (Fig. 48-28). Classic hemophilia is due to Factor

Fig. 48-26. Pseudogout chondrocalcinosis. Note calcification of the articular cartilage of the humeral head.

Fig. 48-27. Calcification of knee menisci in a patient with pseudogout.

Factor VIII level (% average normal)	Haemorrhagic manifestations
50 - 100	None
25 - 50	Excessive bleeding occasionally after serious injury or major operation
5 - 25	Excessive bleeding after minor injury or surgery
1 - 5	Severe bleeding after minor injury. Occasional haemarthrosis and spontaneous bleeding
0	Severe haemophilia with spontaneous bleeding into muscles and joints.

Fig. 48-28. Relationships of blood Factor VIII levels to hemorrhagic manifestations.

VIII deficiency, while Christmas disease is due to a deficiency of Factor IX.

Synovia and capsule have no tissue thromboplastin. In the hemophiliac with inability to generate circulating thromboplastin, the absence of tissue thromboplastin allows hemorrhage due to injury or spontaneous hemorrhage to occur and go unchecked in joint cavities. Repeated hemorrhage into growing joints results in progressive deterioration and chronic arthritis.

PATHOLOGY. The synovium is thickened with hyperplasia of the synovial lining cells. There are diffuse areas of chronic and acute inflammatory cells with hemosiderin deposition in the surface and the depths of the synovial tissue. New blood vessels and fibrous tissue increase in the subintimal synovial tissue.

The adjacent growing epiphyses enlarge and change shape, findings which are demonstrated by x-ray. There is osteoporosis of the adjacent epiphyses and metaphyses. Cartilage destruction occurs in varying degrees and increases with severity and chronicity of the joint hemorrhage. Cysts may occur in the subchondral bone in longstanding cases. Degenerative changes are superimposed if the patient survives.

CLINICAL MANIFESTATIONS. In the severe hemophiliac, bleeding into one of the large joints occurs spontaneously or with mild trauma. The most common joint of involvement is the knee, followed by elbow, ankle, and shoulder, with joint hemorrhage in any joint a possibility. If unchecked by coagulation therapy, hemarthrosis becomes acute, and the joint assumes that position which accommodates the greatest volume of fluid and comfort, i.e., 20° of flexion for the knee or adduction and external rotation for the hip joint. The patient will not move the joint because of pain and associated muscle spasm.

The hemorrhage tends to run in cycles, one or two joints being repeatedly affected, followed by other joints with recurrent episodes. In the chronic stage, with sufficient joint destruction and arthritis, there is limitation of motion, fixed contracture, and deformity.

In the acutely involved joint, x-ray findings may show only soft tissue swelling and the presence of effusion. With repeated hemorrhage, adjacent epiphyses enlarge and change the configuration. The characteristic findings in the knee joint (Fig. 48-29) are a squared-off lower pole of the patella, enlargement of femoral condyles, and increase in size of the intercondylar notch. Osteoporosis may be marked, and joint space is narrow. In the chronic state, the residual changes in epiphyseal configuration are super-

Fig. 48-29. Hemophilic arthritis. AP and lateral x-rays of the knee joint showing enlargement of epiphyses of the knee, joint space narrowing, with irregularity and squaring of the lower end of the patella. Note also the soft tissue swelling about the knee. *A.* AP x-rays. *B.* Lateral x-rays.

imposed with sclerosis and osteophytes of degenerative change.

TREATMENT. If joint hemorrhage can be minimized, the chronic arthritis will not ensue. Patients with the first sign of hemorrhage into the joint should be treated with appropriate coagulation factors, i.e., Factor VIII. The joint is splinted with a compression bandage until effective blood clotting ensues. Weight-bearing joints are protected with crutches until the range of motion of the joint returns and the joint effusion resolves. Joints subjected to repeated hemorrhage must be protected with bracing to limit motion and prevent recurrence. The short leg brace preventing ankle motion is used for the ankle, and a light plastic splint is used for repeated hemorrhage into the knee.

If contractures have developed, these are corrected by reversal dynamic traction. When the contracture has been corrected, an immobilizing brace is applied. A Quingle-type cast may be used for severe degrees of subluxation of the knee. Ischial weight-bearing braces may be required for serious involvement of the hip joints. With adequate prophylaxis and early treatment, severe deformity can be prevented. Reconstructive surgery for joint deformities is now being carried out in specialized centers where the clotting factor deficiency can be reversed for the healing and rehabilitation phases.

SYNOVIAL LESIONS

Pigmented Villonodular Synovitis

Pigmented villonodular synovitis is an inflammatory process of unknown cause which occurs in monarticular form in young adults. The peak incidence of this condition is in the thirties, with men more frequently involved than women.

Patients present with symptoms of pain and swelling which may be intermittent and are frequently of long duration. The most commonly involved joint is the knee, but any single large joint may be involved. On examination there is usually evidence of synovial thickening with effusion. Joint aspiration characteristically reveals bloody or dark brown sanguineous fluid. X-ray evaluation may reveal soft tissue swelling and occasionally cystic erosion of joint margins.

The pathologic finding is a villous, thickened, brownish proliferation of synovial tissue which has nodules and pedicles of synovium projecting into the joint. Microscopic examination reveals proliferated synovial cells with large, round, stromal connective cells beneath the surface. Hemosiderin and cholesterol are diffused throughout the synovium in the intercellular space and in multinucleated giant cells.

Treatment of this condition depends upon its early recognition and removal by synovectomy. If there is recurrence after synovectomy, repeat surgical treatment is required and is usually successful. The same process may occur as a localized nodular form, and a similar pathologic condition may occur in a bursa or as a localized nodular tenosynovitis.

Synovial Chondromatosis

Synovial chondromatosis is a condition occurring in synovium, bursa, or tendon sheaths in which metaplastic cartilage growth occurs. Such growths may ossify and persist in the synovium or become detached and displaced into the joint cavity as a loose body. The condition occurs as a monarticular arthritis in middle-aged adults. The knee is most commonly involved, but any large joint may be affected. Clinical examination reveals signs of inflammation with effusion. X-rays show evidence of calcified bodies in the synovium or joint space. The remainder of the joint may be normal or secondarily degenerative because of mechanical trauma from the loose body. Synovectomy is the treatment of choice.

Acute Synovitis of the Hip in Childhood

Children in the Legg-Calvé-Perthes age group, age three to ten years, may present with an acutely painful hip. The mother may note a hip limp of several days' duration in the child. In other situations, the discomfort is acute enough so that the child will not bear weight. X-rays of the hip may reveal soft tissue swelling of the hip in the absence of bone changes of the capital femoral epiphyses.

Immediate evaluation should attempt to rule out acute septic arthritis by hip joint aspiration. Acute synovitis of the hip is a diagnosis of exclusion. If an initial sepsis can be ruled out, the child is placed at bed rest with the leg in Buck's traction. When the acute symptoms resolve, he is allowed to ambulate with non-weight-bearing crutch walking. Repeat x-rays are obtained in 6 weeks to be certain that Legg-Calvé-Perthes disease is not developing. In the absence of signs of Legg-Calvé-Perthes disease, the child is allowed weight-bearing ambulation.

HYPERTROPHIC PULMONARY OSTEOARTHROPATHY

Hypertrophic pulmonary osteoarthropathy is a syndrome affecting bone and joints of the extremities and occurring in association with intrathoracic pathologic conditions. Patients develop insidious asymptomatic clubbing of the fingers, which is an increased nail bed convexity with loss of the normal angle between the proximal nail beds and the distal covering of the dorsal surface of the phalanx. The nail may be brittle and striated with an underlying vascular engorgement. Associated with the clubbing may be a synovitis of a peripheral joint. X-ray examination of the extremities may reveal new periosteal bone along the shafts, including distal phalanges. This is responsible for the clubbing effect.

When clubbing is noted, a thoracic pathologic condition should be immediately suspected. Bronchiectasis, chronic emphysema, tuberculosis, valvular disease of the heart, and, especially, pulmonary malignant tumors are possible causes.

The exact cause is unknown, but is thought to be associated with changes in tissue oxygenation or arteriolar blood flow as a consequence of lung disease. Treatment depends upon diagnosis and treatment of the underlying lung condition. It is not uncommon to excise a pulmonary neoplasm and have peripheral joint symptoms completely resolve.

NEUROPATHIC, OR CHARCOT, JOINTS

A neuropathic joint, or Charcot joint, is a condition which occurs as a consequence of various neurologic diseases. Tabes dorsalis, syringomyelia, leprosy, or diabetes may be associated with the development of neuropathic joints. Neuropathic joints have also been described in association with insensitivity due to peripheral nerve lesions and in rare situations where no neurologic lesion is evident.

The prevailing opinion as to the mechanism of destruction in such joints has been repeated trauma on structures rendered insensitive by sensory interruption. However, some patients do have pain associated with these lesions, suggesting that other factors may be responsible.

CLINICAL MANIFESTATIONS. The onset is commonly insidious with the patient unaware of the degree of joint disability developing. There may be minor discomfort in a weight-bearing joint—hip, knee, ankle, or tarsus—with diffuse swelling about the joint, but medical aid may not be sought until gross instability and deformity are present. The knee joint may have a massive effusion with gross instability of all ligamentous supporting structures. Associated with this may be varying degrees of edema and swelling involving the leg. In the case of the tarsal joints, swelling with erythema and valgus or varus deformity are common presentations.

Radiographic findings (Fig. 48-30) include extreme dissolution of bone ends with frank dislocation, enlarged joint space, and large collections of bone fragments deposited

Fig. 48-30. Neuropathic knee due to tabes dorsalis showing marked destruction of medial femoral condyle. Clinically there was marked synovial swelling and effusion with marked instability due to the loss of bone substances.

in the enlarged synovial cavity. A rapid rate of change by x-ray, with bone loss and destruction, is suggestive of a neuropathic joint. Infection frequently complicates the diagnosis of neuropathic joints, due to diabetes.

TREATMENT. The rate and degree of destruction of bone ends with marked ligamentous instability make conservative treatment difficult. A well-fitting ischial weight-bearing brace may benefit a patient with a Charcot knee or hip joint. If this is not tolerated, surgical arthrodesis of the knee, using the principles of Charnley or hip arthrodesis, is indicated.

In the insensitive foot of the diabetic, plaster cast immobilization has resulted in spontaneous fusion. Molded orthopedic shoes with contoured arch supports and metatarsal bars have been used for diabetics and lepers with severe neurotropic destruction of the tarsal joints. The end result in the diabetic is usually below-knee amputation.

PAINFUL SHOULDER

Spontaneous pain or pain after minor strains of the shoulder are extremely common after the age of thirty-five. The most common lesion responsible for shoulder pain in this age group is that of lesions of the rotator cuff, bicipital tendonitis, or subacromial bursitis. Before ascribing the diagnosis to a local lesion, it is mandatory to rule out disease of the cervical spine and central nervous system, as well as lesions of the brachial plexus, caused by Pancost's tumor, and referred pain from the heart, lungs, or gastrointestinal tract.

Lesions of the Rotator Cuff

The rotator cuff consists of the common tendinous insertion of supraspinatus, infraspinatus, and teres minor muscles as well as the subscapularis tendon. These tendons form a continuous fibrous sheath, which is intimately adherent to the underlying shoulder capsule. When the shoulder is moved from the anatomic position to the position of full elevation or abduction, the rotator cuff comes in contact with the undersurface of the coracoacromial ligament and is subject to mechanical irritation, and degenerative change occurs. With sufficient degeneration, bursitis may develop in the intervening subacromial bursa, which separates the undersurface of the acromion and coracoacromial ligament from the rotator cuff. With changes in the tendon, deposition of calcium occurs in the worn and degenerative tendon, as well as in the subacromial bursa.

CLINICAL MANIFESTATIONS. In the absence of preexisting symptomatology, a patient may note the spontaneous acute onset of severe unrelenting pain in the shoulder and in the region of the glenohumeral joint, occasionally referred into the arm and elbow. The onset may occur after unusual vigorous exercise or sports activities in the patient over thirty-five years. The patient may awaken with minor discomfort in the shoulder, which gradually increases in severity. The pain is unimproved by position and may require narcotics for relief.

On examination, there is local tenderness over the greater tuberosity of the humerus. Any motion of the shoulder causes pain. Routine x-rays of the shoulder may be negative or show a calcium deposit in the subacromial bursa or supraspinatus tendon.

TREATMENT. Untreated, the lesion will take about 5 to 10 days for relief of symptoms. If the patient is seen when symptoms are resolving, sling immobilization combined with analgesia may be sufficient. In the acutely painful situation, the bursa should be needled, 2% Xylocaine injected, and an aspiration of the bursa contents attempted. One milliliter of cortisone is then introduced. The results of this treatment are often dramatic. After injection, the shoulder is immobilized until pain relief is complete; then gradual shoulder-motion exercises of the pendulum type are instituted.

If the shoulder symptoms do not completely resolve, repeat cortisone injection is considered.

CHRONIC SUPRASPINATUS TENDONITIS

The presentation of degenerative lesions of the rotator cuff are often insidious. The patient complains of low-grade discomfort in the shoulder with sudden motion and with certain positions, such as full internal rotation and the extremes of abduction. These may be aggravated by increase in shoulder activity.

X-ray examination in such instances is more likely to show evidence of calcification in the supraspinatus tendon (Fig. 48-31). The treatment of this lesion should start with conservative therapy. The shoulder is immobilized in a sling and swathe for 10 days to 2 weeks until relief from pain is complete. Then gradual range-of-motion exercises are started. If this does not produce a response, cortisone is injected into the shoulder, or the shoulder is treated with diathermy or ultrasound.

RUPTURES OF THE ROTATOR CUFF

A rupture of the rotator cuff occurs commonly in middle age but may also occur in late adolescence and in the elderly. Occupation has no relationship to incidence. Minor strain or injury will cause a rupture in a previously degenerative tendon. The patient may have had preexisting chronic low-grade shoulder symptoms. The patient has difficulty in achieving full active shoulder motion, although there is no contracture on examination.

If radiopaque solution is injected into the shoulder, the solution will enter the subdeltoid bursa if there is discontinuity in the rotator cuff. X-ray evidence of fracture of the greater tuberosity indicates that the tendon has been avulsed. If the rupture has been present for a few weeks, the muscles involved, such as the supraspinatus, may show evidence of atrophy. If a calcium deposit is present, it is unlikely that rupture has occurred.

TREATMENT OF ROTATOR CUFF RUPTURES. Since 25 percent of shoulders at postmortem, in the absence of previous symptoms, have had evidence of tear or degenerated cuffs, immediate surgical treatment is not indicated. Most patients will recover with conservative treatment. The acute symptoms are treated by immobilization in a sling. When pain is resolved, gradual range-of-motion

Fig. 48-31. Calcific supraspinatus tendonitis. *A.* AP x-ray of the shoulder with internal rotation shows calcium deposit in the region of the supraspinatus tendon. *B.* External rotation shows calcific shadow superimposed over the greater tuberosity.

exercises are instituted. If symptoms do not resolve within a few months with this type of treatment, open surgical repair, as described by McLaughlin, is done.

BICIPITAL TENDONITIS

Shoulder symptoms resembling supraspinatus tendonitis may be due to a bicipital tendon which has become irritated and inflamed in its groove and long passage through the shoulder joint. The symptoms are quite similar, but differentiation may be made on the basis of pain and tenderness extending farther distad over the bicipital groove. Treatment is by conservative means—cortisone, short-wave diathermy, immobilization—followed by return of motion. An occasional patient will require surgical exploration.

References

Anatomy

Barnett, C. H., Davies, D. V., and MacConaill, M. A.: "Synovial Joints: Their Structure and Mechanics," Charles C Thomas, Publisher, Springfield, Ill., 1961.

Curtiss, R. H.: Changes Produced in the Synovial Membrane and Synovial Fluid by Disease, instructional course lecture, American Academy of Orthopaedic Surgeons, *J Bone Joint Surg [Am]*, **46A:**873, 1964.

Examination

Hollander, J. L.: "Arthritis and Allied Conditions," Lea & Febiger, Philadelphia, 1966.

Pyogenic Arthritis

Clawson, B. K., and Dunn, A. W.: Management of Common Bacterial Infections of Bones and Joints, instructional course lecture, American Academy of Orthopaedic Surgeons, *J Bone Joint Surg [Am]*, **49A:**164, 1967.

Curtiss, P. H., and Klein, L.: Destruction of Articular Surfaces in Septic Arthritis. I. In Vitro Studies, *J Bone Joint Surg [Am]*, **45A:**797, 1963.

Hollander, J. L. (ed.): "Arthritis and Allied Conditions," Lea & Febiger, Philadelphia, 1966.

Phemister, D. B.: The Effect of Pressure on Articular Surfaces in Pyogenic and Tuberculosis Arthritides and Its Bearing on Treatment, *Ann Surg,* **80:**481, 1924.

Bone and Joint Tuberculosis

Henderson, M. S.: Tuberculosis of Joints with Special Reference to Knee, *Aust NZ J Surg,* **6:**27, 1936.

Hodgson, A. R., and Stuck, F. E.: Anterior Spine Fusion for the Treatment of Tuberculosis of the Spine, *J Bone Joint Surg* [*Am*], **42A:**295, 1960.

———, Wong, W., and Yau, A.: "X-ray Appearances of Tuberculosis of the Spine," Charles C Thomas, Publisher, Springfield, Ill., 1969.

Somerville, E. W., and Wilkinson, M. C.: "Girdlestone's Tuberculosis of Bone and Joint," Oxford University Press, London, 1965.

Gonococcal Arthritis

Ford, D. K.: Gonorrheal Arthritis, in J. L. Hollander (ed.), "Arthritis and Allied Conditions," Lea & Febiger, Philadelphia, 1966.

Rheumatoid Arthritis

Arthritis and Rheumatism Council and British Orthopaedic Association: Controlled Trial of Synovectomy of Knee and Metacarpophalangeal Joints in Rheumatoid Arthritis, *Ann Rheum Dis,* **35:**437, 1976.

Casagrande, P.: Surgical Rehabilitation of the Upper Extremities in Rheumatoid Arthritis, in Dixon, A. S. (ed.), "Progress in Clinical Rheumatology," chap. 6, Little, Brown and Company, Boston, 1965.

Clayton, M. L.: Surgery of the Thumb in Rheumatoid Arthritis, *J Bone Joint Surg* [*Am*], **44A:**1376, 1962.

———: Surgery of the Lower Extremity in Rheumatoid Arthritis, instructional course lecture, American Academy of Orthopaedic Surgeons, *J Bone Joint Surg* [*Am*], **45A:**1517, 1963.

Flatt, A. E.: "Care of the Rheumatoid Hand," The C. V. Mosby Company, St. Louis, 1963.

Hoffman, P.: An Operation for Severe Grades of Contracted or Claw Toes, *J Orthop Surg,* **9:**441, 1916.

Huskisson, E. C.: Report on Rheumatic Diseases, No. 54, Arthritis and Rheumatism Council, London, 1974.

Littler, J. W.: Basic Principles of Reconstructive Surgery of the Hand, *Surg Clin North Am,* **40:**383, 1960.

MacIntosh, D. L., and Hunter, J. B.: The Use of Hemiarthroplasty Prosthesis for Advanced Osteoarthritis and Rheumatoid Arthritis of the Knee, *J Bone Joint Surg* [*Br*], **54B:**244, 1972.

Mercer, S. W., and Duthie, R. B.: "Orthopaedic Surgery," Edward Arnold (Publishers) Ltd., London, 1972.

Murray, W. R., Lucas, D. B., and Inman, V. T.: Femoral Head and Neck Resection, *J Bone Joint Surg* [*Am*], **46A:**1184, 1964.

Niebauer, J. J., Shaw, J. L., and Doren, W. W.: Silicone-Dacron Hinge Prosthesis. Design, Evaluation, and Application, in J. S. Calnan and P. J. L. Holt (eds.): "Workshop on Artificial Finger Joints," vol. 28, pp. 56–58, British Medical Association, London, 1969.

Sokoloff, L.: Pathology of Rheumatoid Arthritis and Allied Diseases, in J. L. Hollander, "Arthritis and Allied Conditions," Lea & Febiger, Philadelphia, 1966.

Swanson, A. B.: Flexible Implant Arthroplasty for Arthritic Finger

Joints: Rationale, Technique, and Results of Treatment, *J Bone Joint Surg* [*Am*], **54A:**435, 1972.

Osteoarthritis

Aufranc, O. E.: "Constructive Surgery of the Hip," The C. V. Mosby Company, St. Louis, 1962.

———: Mould Arthroplasty of the Hip, in W. D. Graham (ed.), "Modern Trends in Orthopaedics," vol. 5, p. 23, Appleton Century Crofts, New York, 1967.

Byers, P. D., Contepomi, C. A., and Farkas, T. A.: A Post Mortem Study of the Hip Joint, Including the Prevalence of the Features of the Right Side, *Ann Rheum Dis,* **29:**15, 1970.

Charnley, J.: The Long-Term Results of Low Friction Arthroplasty of the Hip Performed as a Primary Intervention, *J Bone Joint Surg* [*Br*], **54B:**61, 1972.

Copeman, W. S. C.: Osteoarthrosis, in W. S. C. Copeman (ed.), "Textbook of the Rheumatic Diseases," E. & S. Livingstone Ltd., Edinburgh, 1964.

Denham, R. A.: Hip Mechanics, *J Bone Joint Surg* [*Br*], **41B:**550, 1959.

Dowson, D., and Wright, V.: Lubrication, Friction and Wear of Total Hip Replacements, in M. Jayson (ed.), "Total Hip Replacement," J. B. Lippincott Company, Philadelphia, 1971.

Girdlestone, G. R.: Acute Pyogenic Arthritis of the Hip, *Lancet,* **1:**419, 1943.

Harris, N. H., and Kirwan, E.: The Results of Osteotomy for Early Primary Osteoarthritis of the Hip, *J Bone Joint Surg* [*Br*], **46B:**477, 1964.

Hoaglund, F. T.: Osteoarthritis, *Orthop Clin North Am,* **2:**3, 1970.

Jackson, P., and Waugh, W.: Tibial Osteotomy for Osteoarthritis of the Knee, *J Bone Joint Surg* [*Br*], **45B:**618, 1963.

Jayson, M.: "Total Hip Replacement," J. B. Lippincott Company, Philadelphia, 1971.

Keller, W. L.: Surgical Treatment of Bunions and Hallux Valgus, *NY Med J,* **80:**741, 1904.

Kellgren, J. H., and Moore, R.: Generalized Osteoarthritis and Heberden's Nodes, *Br Med J,* **1:**181, 1952.

Kettelkamp, D. B., Wenger, D. R., Chao, E. Y. S., and Thompson, C.: Results of Proximal Tibial Osteotomy: The Effects of Tibiofemoral Angle, Stance-Phase Flexion-Extension and Medial Plateau Force, *J Bone Joint Surg,* **58A:**952, 1976.

McBride, E. D.: Hallux Valgus, Bunion Deformity: Its Treatment in Mild, Moderate, and Severe Stages, *J Int Coll Surg,* **21:**99, 1954.

McKee, G. K., and Watson-Farrar, J.: Replacement of Arthritic Hips by the McKee-Farrar Prosthesis, *J Bone Joint Surg* [*Br*], **48B:**245, 1966.

Mankin, H. J.: Biochemical and Metabolic Aspects of Osteoarthritis, *Orthop Clin North Am,* **2:**19, 1971.

Pearson, J. R., and Riddell, D. M.: Idiopathic Osteoarthritis of the Hip, *Ann Rheum Dis,* **21:**31, 1962.

Scales, J. T., and Lowe, S. A.: Some Factors Influencing Bone and Joint Replacement: With Special Reference to the Stanmore Total Hip Replacement, in M. Jayson (ed.), "Total Hip Replacement," J. B. Lippincott Company, Philadelphia, 1971.

Sokoloff, L.: The Pathology and Pathogenesis of Orthoarthritis, chap. 51, in J. L. Hollander (ed.), "Arthritis and Allied Conditions," Lea & Febiger, Philadelphia, 1966.

Walker, P. S., and Bienenstock, M.: Fixation Properties of Acrylic Cement, *Rev Hosp Spec Surg,* **1:**27, 1971.

West, F. E., and Soto-Hall, R.: Recurrent Dislocation of the Patella in the Adult: End Results of Patellectomy and Quadriceps Plasty, *J Bone Joint Surg [Am]*, **40A:**386, 1958.

Wiles, P., Andrews, T. S., and Bevas, M. B.: Chondromalacia of the Patella, *J Bone Joint Surg [Br]*, **38B:**95, 1956.

Gout

Burch, T. A., O'Brian, W. M., Kurland, L. T., Need, R., and Bunim, J. J.: Hyperuricemia and Gout in the Marianas Islands, *Arthritis Rheum,* **7:**296, 1964.

McCarty, D. J.: Pseudogout: Articular Chondrocalcinosis Calcium Pyrophosphate Crystal Deposition Disease, chap. 56, in J. L. Hollander (ed.), "Arthritis and Allied Conditions," Lea & Febiger, Philadelphia, 1966.

———, and Hollander, J. L.: Identification of Urate Crystals in Gouty Synovial Fluid, *Ann Intern Med,* **54:**452, 1961.

Seegmiller, J. E., and Howell, R. R.: The Old and New Concepts of Acute Gouty Arthritis, *Arthritis Rheum,* **5:**616, 1962.

———, ———, and Malowista, S. E.: The Inflammatory Reaction to Sodium Urate: Its Possible Relationship to the Genesis of Acute Gouty Arthritis, *JAMA,* **180:**469, 1962.

Smyth, C. J.: Hereditary Factors in Gout: A Review of Recent Literature, *Metabolism,* **6:**218, 1957.

Stecher, R. M., Hersh, A. H., and Solomon, W. M.: The Heredity of Gout and Its Relationship to Familial Hyperuricemia, *Ann Intern Med,* **31:**595, 1949.

Wyngaarden, J. B.: Etiology and Pathogenesis of Gout, chap. 54, in J. L. Hollander (ed.), "Arthritis and Allied Conditions," Lea & Febiger, Philadelphia, 1966.

———, Rundles, R. W., Silberman, H. R., and Hunter, S.: Control of Hyperuricemia and Hydroxypyrazolopyrimidine, a Purine Analogue Which Inhibits Uric Acid Synthesis, *Arthritis Rheum,* **6:**306, 1963.

Hemophilic Arthritis

Atprup, T., and Sjolini, K. E.: Thromboplastic and Fibrinolytic Activity of Human Synovial Membrane in Fibrous Capsular Tissue, *Proc Soc Exp Biol,* **92:**852, 1958.

Duthie, R. B., Matthews, J. M., Rizza, C. R., and Steel, W. M.:

"The Musculoskeletal Problems in the Haemophilics," Blackwell Scientific Publications, Oxford, England, 1972.

Synovial Lesions

Chung, S. M. K., and James, J. M.: Diffuse Pigmented Villonodular Synovitis of the Hip Joint, *J Bone Joint Surg [Am]*, **47A:**239, 1965.

Jaffe, H. L., Lichtenstein, L., and Seutro, C. J.: Pigmented Villonodular Synovitis, Bursitis, and Tenosynovitis, *Arch Pathol,* **31:**731, 1941.

McIvor, R. R., and King, D.: Osteochondromatosis of the Hip Joint, *J Bone Joint Surg [Am]*, **44A:**87, 1962.

Murphy, A. F., and Wilson, J. N.: Tenosynovial Osteochondroma in the Hand, *J Bone Joint Surg [Am]*, **40A:**1236, 1958.

Hypertrophic Pulmonary Osteoarthropathy

Smyth, C. J.: Rheumatism and Arthritis: Sixteenth Rheumatism Review, *Ann Intern Med,* **61**(*Suppl* 6):3, 1964.

Neuropathic or Charcot Joints

Charnley, J., and Baker, S. L.: Compression Arthrodesis of the Knee: A Clinical and Histological Study, *J Bone Joint Surg [Am]*, **34A:**187, 1952.

Johnson, J. T. H.: Neuropathic Fractures and Joint Injuries: Pathogenesis and Rationale of Prevention and Treatment, *J Bone Joint Surg [Am]*, **49A:**1, 1967.

King, E. J. S.: On Some Aspects of the Pathology of Hypertrophic Charcot's Joints, *Br J Surg,* **18:**113, 1930.

Mooney, V., and Mankin, H. J.: A Case of Congenital Insensitivity to Pain with Neurotrophic Arthropathy, *Arthritis Rheum,* **9:**821, 1966.

Painful Shoulder

McLaughlin, H.: Rupture of the Rotator Cuff, instructional course lecture, American Academy of Orthopaedic Surgeons, *J Bone Joint Surg [Am]*, **44A:**979, 1962.

Milone, F. P., and Copeland, M. M.: Calcific Tendonitis of the Shoulder Joint: Presentation of 136 Cases Treated by Irradiation, *Am J Roentgenol Radium Ther Nucl Med,* **85:**901, 1961.

Chapter 49

Amputations

by **Seymour I. Schwartz**

GENERAL CONSIDERATIONS

Indications

The indications for amputation of part or all of an extremity include (1) trauma which is sufficiently extensive to preclude repair; (2) tumor of the bone, soft tissue, muscles, blood vessels, or nerves, (3) extensive infection which does not respond to conservative measures or contributes to septicemia; and (4) a variety of peripheral vascular diseases. Refinement in surgical technique as applied to blood vessels and peripheral nerves has markedly reduced the indications for amputation following trauma and has permitted reimplantation of totally amputated extremities.

Amputations accounted for 2 percent of all operations performed in Veterans Administration hospitals in 1964. Presently, more than two-thirds of the amputations on civilians in Western society are performed for peripheral vascular disease in patients over the age of fifty.

AMPUTATION OF ISCHEMIC LIMBS

Amputations are performed for four main categories of vascular disease: (1) arteriosclerosis obliterans, (2) arteriosclerosis obliterans with diabetes, (3) thromboangiitis obliterans, and (4) miscellaneous conditions such as embolic occlusion, peripheral aneurysm, vascular trauma, and venous obstruction. The specific indications for amputation in these patients are severe arterial insufficiency with necrosis of all or part of an extremity, intractable and severe pain which disables the patient, and infection which is spreading or unresponsive to therapy. In a few patients, extrarenal azotemia and hyperkalemia secondary to tissue necrosis constitute specific indications for amputation.

Amputation performed on a patient with compromised circulation requires special consideration. The patients are generally more brittle and require more intensive preoperative preparation. The compromised vascular supply within the limb necessitates meticulous and somewhat refined techniques, as described below. It is more difficult to achieve healing of the stump, and even after it has healed, breakdown related to the trauma of a prosthesis may occur. Finally, the patients are generally less vigorous and less adept at handling prostheses.

Selection of Site

Several factors contribute to the decision concerning level of amputation. When amputation is performed for malignant disease, the principal factor is wide excision of grossly apparent tumor. In the case of amputation subsequent to trauma or for peripheral vascular disease, the major factor determining the optimal level is usually the extent of healthy tissue. Other factors include the length of the stump sufficient for function of a prosthesis, the cosmetic effect of a prosthesis, and the placement of the scar so that it will neither break down nor compromise the fitting of the prosthesis.

In general, the longer the amputation stump, the more functional the limb and the better control the patient has of his prosthesis. For traumatic amputations with irregular damage to the skin, grafting procedures and mobilization of flaps are indicated to maintain as much of the bony length as possible. Regarding the upper extremity, as much length as possible should always be saved, even if there is only a very short below-elbow or humeral stump. There are exceptions to the general rule of "the longer, the better." For the lower extremity, proximal to the Syme amputation, the best level below the knee as far as prosthetic fitting is concerned is at the gastrocnemius musculotendinous junction. Proximal to knee disarticulation, an amputation which removes at least 4 in. of the distal femur is indicated, so that a prosthetic knee joint can be fitted with less difficulty. For children, disarticulation is frequently the procedure of choice in order to save the growing epiphysis and minimize the problem of distal bone overgrowth.

Other factors which contribute to selection of amputation site are the patient's general condition and, particularly, the feasibility of rehabilitation. More proximal amputations are indicated for bedridden patients who require nursing care, since these procedures are associated with a higher incidence of primary healing. If there is established contracture, it is usually preferable to plan to amputate above the level of contracture, to permit rehabilitation.

Factors which influence selection of the level of amputation in patients with peripheral vascular disease vary with the region. At all levels, healing ability is a function of nutritional skin blood flow. The status of the skin circulation may be evidenced by the extent of skin circulation. More recently, the clearance of radioxenon, measured at the anterior incision line, has been shown to correlate well with the healing of amputations. In one series no patient with a flow exceeding 0.6 ml/100 Gm tissue per minute failed to heal because of ischemia, and no patient with a lower flow was able to heal a BK amputation.

A correlation has been reported between the healing of both digital and transmetatarsal amputations and the presence of peripheral pulses. In patients with a palpable popliteal pulse, healing at this level occurred twice as effectively as in those in whom only femoral pulse was demonstrated. Potential for healing minor forefoot amputations has been predicted by determining ankle pressures using Doppler Ultrasound. No amputations in this region healed with a pressure of less than 60 mmHg. Although the presence of a palpable popliteal pulse generally ensures adequate circulation below the knee, several series have reported that the presence or absence of the pulse did not affect the healing of a BK amputation. Oscillometry may be applied to determine the level of pulsatile circulation, and arteriography is helpful in determining the patency of major vessels in significant collateral circulation around the knee.

The recent advances in rehabilitation and the application of the immediate prosthetic fitting have increased the indications for BK amputations and reduced the incidence of AK amputations. In selecting between these two sites, there are two additional factors which have to be assessed, viz., the patient's general condition and the prospect for rehabilitation.

Preoperative Management

Amputations for massive trauma should be performed early to reduce the extent of contamination and the potential for infection. When an amputation is being considered for ischemia, care of the patient and the involved and uninvolved extremities is critical. Atelectasis, pneumonia, and decubiti must be prevented in elderly bedridden patients. This can be accomplished by frequently turning the patients and providing them with a trapeze which can also be used to condition muscles to be used postoperatively. If the patient is diabetic, it is generally preferable to revert to a regimen of crystalline insulin rather than long-acting medications, since this is easier to regulate on the day of the operation and postoperatively.

Care of the ischemic extremity and also the contralateral extremity, which is frequently compromised, involves strict avoidance of injuries to areas of deficient circulation. The strength of wasted muscles and the motion of the critical joints must be preserved or, frequently, restored. Efforts should be made to heal necrotic or infected lesions, and only after direct arterial reconstruction and occasionally sympathectomy have failed to evidence improvement of the lesion is amputation indicated. The leg is usually kept in a slightly dependent position, and Buerger's exercises may be applied to improve the circulation. In the face of infection, drainage and local wet dressings of warm saline solution coupled with the appropriate antibiotic are employed. Intense heat and soaks are contraindicated, and if no infection is apparent and there is dry gangrene, wet dressings should not be used. Injury to ischemic areas is avoided by moving the patient frequently and preventing pressure to the heel by placing the foot on a pillow or lambskin mat. Foot care is administered to all areas without open lesions and to the uninvolved extremity. In some instances of digital gangrene, spontaneous amputation will occur, and this is frequently preferable to an operative procedure.

Refrigeration may be used preliminary to amputation to improve the condition of the patient by decreasing the metabolic by-products of the necrotic limb and also decreasing the absorption of these products and infectious material. Refrigeration also relieves pain, but the technique should not be employed if there is any hope of salvaging the extremity. The technique involves the placement of ice bags below the proposed level of amputation and may require use of mild narcotics.

Wrapping of the extremity in towels impregnated with antiseptic materials such as hexachlorophene for 12 hours prior to operation has been advised as a method of reducing the incidence of wound infection. Either spinal or inhalation anesthesia may be used for lower extremity amputations, while regional block may be applicable for distal upper extremity amputations.

Principles of Technique

The three general classes of amputations are (1) the standard or conventional amputation, (2) the osteomyoplastic or myodesis amputation, and (3) the provisional, or open (guillotine), amputation.

The conventional amputation is performed by constructing curved skin and fascial flaps which have their base at the level of amputation. The muscles, major blood vessels, and bone are divided at the level of amputation, while the major nerves are put on slight stretch and transected so that they retract approximately 1 in. proximal to the level of amputation. The muscles may be tapered so that not too much soft tissue remains over the bone end, and the distal inch of periosteum may be removed to avoid leaving a detached segment which can cause bone spur formation. After the amputation has been completed, the deep and superficial fascia are approximated over the bone, and the skin is loosely closed. The wound may be closed without drainage, or drainage may be established by soft rubber tubes or preferably a catheter connected to a closed section suction apparatus.

The osteomyoplastic amputations and myodesis provide for improved function and have been employed with increasing frequency when immediate postsurgical prosthetics (IPOP) are applied. Skin and fascial flaps are prepared in a manner similar to that used during conventional amputation, and the nerves and blood vessels are also divided in a routine fashion. In the osteomyoplastic technique, the muscles are divided 2 in. distal to the level of bone transection, and, prior to amputation of the bone, an osteoperiosteal flap is developed so that it may be sutured to the opposing periosteum in order to cover the bone and plug the marrow cavity. Then, with the remaining extremity in neutral position, i.e., extension for BK amputation and hip extension for AK amputation, the antagonistic muscles are sutured across the bone ends. Closure and drainage is similar to that employed in conventional amputations. In the case of myodesis, the distal ends of the transected muscle are attached to the bone by suturing through drill holes through the distal end. The muscles should be attached at a point that will put them under moderate tension so that they will become fixed along their normal pathway in a position slightly beyond rest length and therefore capable of providing maximal function.

Open, or provisional (guillotine), amputations should be regarded as drainage procedures and are rarely indicated. They are of historical interest in that they represent the most commonly employed procedures prior to the age of modern surgery. The procedure is still employed to release a person whose extremity is caught under an immovable object and is used for severely ill and toxic patients who are considered unable to tolerate a definitive amputation. All tissues are cut circularly, but the bone is transected higher than the fascia, which, in turn, is cut higher than the skin, in the hope that the soft tissue will ultimately cover the bone end with the help of traction. The results are generally poor, and a large scar, which adheres to bone, often results. The operation is frequently followed by a long healing period, exuberant granulation tissue, fibrosis, muscle retraction, prolonged drainage, reinfection, and exposure of the bone; definitive reamputation is frequently required.

AMPUTATIONS FOR PERIPHERAL VASCULAR DISEASE

Under no circumstance should a tourniquet or constricting bandage be applied, and throughout the procedure undue trauma should be avoided. Short skin and fascial flaps with minimal undermining are employed.

For patients who are to be fitted with an IPOP, the technique is modified. The anterior incision is made at the level of the anticipated bone division, and no anterior flap is constructed. Skin coverage is achieved with a thick posterior flap which includes subcutaneous tissue and fascia. Extreme gentleness is used throughout the procedure. Careful hemostasis is necessary to prevent hematoma formation and subsequent infection. If there is any question of compromised blood supply at the level of amputation, that site of amputation is abandoned and a higher site immediately used. In the case of midthigh amputation for peripheral vascular disease, some surgeons have advised routine ligation of the ipsilateral common femoral vein to obviate embolism.

Postoperative Management

The conventional postoperative care has been directed toward providing an adequate period of rest for tissues by splinting, firm compression over the injured tissue to prevent postoperative edema, exercises and positioning to prevent contracture, and rehabilitation (see Chap. 52) to provide the patient ultimately with a prosthesis compatible with both his vocational demands and ability.

A lightly compressive dressing is applied to the stump immediately after the operation and until the sutures are removed. Following this, elastic bandages are repeatedly applied to minimize the postoperative edema. Contractures are prevented by stump exercises and stretching the proximal joint in the hope of achieving full motion of the remaining joints of the amputated extremity. Rehabilitation requires the services of an experienced physiotherapist, occupational therapist, and prosthetist. In the case of lower extremity amputees, the sequence progresses from balance to crutch walking to use of temporary prosthesis with eventual application of permanent prosthesis. The upper extremity amputee frequently requires intensive training in the activities of daily living and of his specific vocation.

IPOP have recently achieved popularity in the management of extremity amputees. In this situation, a rigid dressing is applied at the operating table. This is accomplished by covering the stump with a sterilized sock and elastic plaster of paris bandages. Relief is provided for areas sensitive to pressure, and a prosthetic unit which includes socket attachment flaps may be applied immediately after the rigid dressing has dried. The patient is then encouraged to walk between parallel bars 24 hours after the operation, and weight bearing is increased daily. At 48 hours, a window may be cut in the plaster of paris to permit removal of the drain, and the material removed to provide the window is immediately replaced with plaster bandage. The rigid dressing is kept in place for approximately 2 weeks, at which time the sutures are removed and a new socket is applied without delay. Ten days later the second socket is removed, and at that time stump measurements and a cast are made for permanent prosthesis. Another temporary socket is provided until the permanent prosthesis is available. With both IPOP and the conventional management, shrinkage of the stump occurs in time and may necessitate a new socket for use with a permanent prosthesis.

Prognosis, Morbidity, and Mortality

Mortality and morbidity statistics and the incidence of rehabilitation are frequently difficult to evaluate, since many amputations have been performed by general surgeons with minimal training in postoperative rehabilitation, by orthopedic surgeons who are not experienced in the principles of operating on ischemic tissue, or all too often the most junior resident with the least training. The operative mortality for amputations performed for isolated tumor, trauma, or infection is less than 3 percent. By contrast, the mortality for amputations performed for peripheral vascular disease has been reported to be 22 and 29 percent in two large series. The mortality rate was doubled in patients who exhibited signs of arteriosclerotic disease of other systems and was increased twofold by postoperative complications. Diabetes did not apparently influence the mortality rate. The mortality rates were generally higher for more proximal amputations in the lower extremity; e.g., the mortality rate for AK amputations was 28 percent as compared with 10 percent for BK amputations. This could be related to the greater frailty of patients subjected to more proximal procedures. The results of recent series are more encouraging, with mortality rates of 3 percent and failure rates of 4 percent reported.

In a recent series reported by Couch and associates the operative mortality rate was 13 percent, with the most frequent causes being cardiac (52 percent) and pulmonary (26 percent) complications. Dale and Capps noted that pulmonary embolism caused 39 percent of deaths in their series. The high incidence of pulmonary embolism and other embolic phenomena has been stressed by Thompson and associates, who reported that in 4 percent of amputees pulmonary infarcts developed, 3 percent had myocardial infarctions, and 3 percent experienced cerebrovascular accidents in the postoperative period.

Phantom limb pain occurred relatively infrequently in most series, and the incidence has been reduced by avoiding the incorporation of nerve in scar tissue of the stump and by IPOP.

The median hospital stay for upper extremity amputees is between 2 and 3 weeks, whereas the average stay for lower extremity amputees was 11 weeks.

In a recent series of 130 patients with unilateral amputation, 70 received prostheses and 84 percent of these had successful rehabilitation. However, of the total group of those receiving unilateral amputations, only 30 percent of the AK group were successfully rehabilitated, while 66 percent of the BK group walked on prosthesis. In those patients with bilateral amputations, 30 percent have had successful rehabilitation, and this required that at least one of the amputation sites be at the BK level. Moore and associates compared the results of amputation and IPOP with the standard procedure. The IPOP group had a lower mortality, a higher primary healing rate, a reduction of time from amputation to fitting of a permanent prosthetic, and an increased rate of rehabilitation.

AMPUTATIONS OF THE LOWER EXTREMITY

The overwhelming majority of amputations in the lower extremity (Fig. 49-1) are performed for ischemia. A variety of eponyms have been applied to specific levels of amputations and refinements of technique, but the most commonly employed procedures are AK and BK amputations. Transmetatarsal and digital amputations are less frequently applicable in patients with peripheral vascular disease. The Syme amputation, knee disarticulation, hip disarticulation, and hemipelvectomy are usually reserved for malignant and traumatic lesions. At each level, the operative procedure and postoperative management are directed at achieving primary healing, a painless stump which will withstand the pressures of a prosthesis, and relatively unrestricted ambulation.

Toe Amputations

Amputations of one or more toes may be performed for gangrene or osteomyelitis. The procedure is rarely indicated for deformity, because excision of a toe results in deviation of adjacent toes. A transphalangeal level may be used if necrosis is distal to the proximal interphalangeal (PIP) joint and if there is absence of cellulitis, necrosis, and edema in the skin to be used for the flaps. If a more proximal amputation is required, transmetatarsal resection with removal of the head is preferable to disarticulation. The latter is associated with an increased incidence of breakdown, since the stump is bulky, and in the face of infection or poor vascular supply the exposed cartilage resists infection less effectively than bone. The incidence of healing at both the transphalangeal and transmetatarsal level has been relatively poor, with reports ranging from 40 to 60 percent. A direct relationship has been demonstrated between healing at these levels and the presence of popliteal and pedal pulses, suggesting that the poor results have been related to poor selection of amputation sites. Holden reported that digital amputations led to major amputations in 37 percent of cases and reported a mortality rate of 23 percent for these patients.

Transphalangeal Amputation

Either lateral or anteroposterior flaps may be used, and in either instance they should be sufficiently long to cover anticipated bone length. If an anteroposterior flap is employed, the plantar flap should be longer, so that the scar is placed dorsad. After the flaps have been established, the tendons and nerves are placed under slight tension and transected to permit retraction. The bone is transected and the skin and subcutaneous tissue closed loosely.

oped, and the head and neck of the metatarsal is amputated. Excessive skin is removed, and a closure without tension is accomplished.

The foot should be elevated in the immediate postoperative period, and ambulation may begin as soon as the incision is healed. There is no need for a special shoe.

Transmetatarsal Foot Amputations

The indications for this procedure include necrosis proximal to the PIP joint but distal to the level of the transmetatarsal incision. Necrosis in the interdigital creases constitutes a relatively frequent indication. Although Bradham and Smoak reported a failure rate of 66 percent in patients with atherosclerosis, the combined statistics reported by Warren et al. indicated that between two-thirds and three-fourths of the patients achieved healing, which in 10 to 50 percent of the instances was delayed. In one series, primary healing was achieved in 54 percent of patients with absent pedal pulses. Prior lumbar sympathectomy apparently did not alter the rate of healing.

TECHNIQUE (Fig. 49-3). Skin incisions and subcutaneous flaps are established so that the plantar flap is longer than the dorsal flap in order to maintain the thicker skin and permit placement of the scar on the distal surface. The plantar incision extends to within a centimeter of the crease between the base of the toes and the ball of the foot, and this flap is left as thick as possible, while the dorsal incision is developed directly to the bone and not established as a flap. Metatarsals are divided just proximal to the level of the dorsal incision, the specimen is removed, and the skin and fascia are closed in layers.

POSTOPERATIVE MANAGEMENT. The amputation provides a good stump, and preservation of the tibialis anterior tendon and intrinsic flexors and the fat pad help to maintain the short arch. The patients generally walk within 3 weeks after the operation, using a shoe with a pad of cotton in the toe.

Syme Amputations

This procedure is usually performed when most of the foot has been destroyed by trauma. Terminal arterial disease involving the distal part of the foot constitutes one of the few peripheral vascular disorders for which the Syme amputation is indicated. Functionally, it represents an excellent level for amputation since it maintains the length of the extremity, and preservation of the heel skin provides an excellent weight-bearing stump. However, the prosthesis is more difficult to fit, and because it is bulky, a BK amputation is preferable for females.

TECHNIQUE (Fig. 49-4). The incision extends from the anteroinferior border of the medial malleolus around the sole to the lateral malleolus and thence around the anterior aspect of the ankle to complete the circumference. The soft tissue is incised in a line down to the bone, avoiding trauma to the posterior tibial artery and its branches. The calcaneus is dissected from the skin and shelled from its attachments to permit removal of the foot. The tibia and fibula are then cleared and transected proximal to the flare

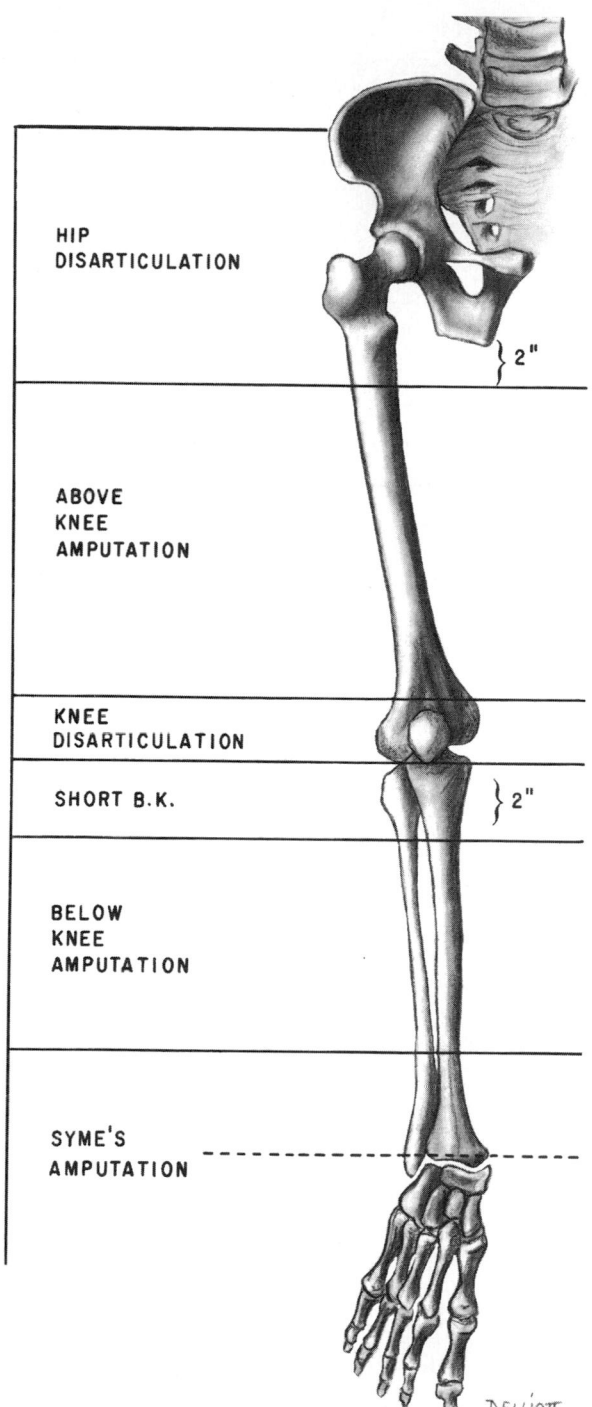

HIP
DISARTICULATION

2"

ABOVE
KNEE
AMPUTATION

KNEE
DISARTICULATION

SHORT B.K.

2"

BELOW
KNEE
AMPUTATION

SYME'S
AMPUTATION

DELLIOTT

Fig. 49-1. Levels of amputations in the lower extremity.

Transmetatarsal Amputation (Fig. 49-2)

A racquet incision is usually employed. In the case of a second, third, and fourth toe, the long limb is positioned on the dorsum of the foot, whereas it is placed on the medial and lateral surface for the great and small toes, respectively. Skin and subcutaneous tissue flaps are devel-

Fig. 49-2. Transmetatarsal toe amputation. *A*. Technique for amputation of any of the middle three toes. 1. Racquet incision made. 2. Toe disarticulated and line of transection of the head of the metatarsal indicated. 3. Skin closure. *B*. Transmetatarsal amputation of the great or little toe. 1. Racquet incision with long limb on the side of the foot. 2. Toe disarticulated and the head of the metatarsal resected. 3. Lateral skin closure.

of the tibial malleolus. The long plantar flap is sutured to the anterior portion of the incision, with care to center the heel flap.

POSTOPERATIVE MANAGEMENT. In the conventional approach, the position of the heel pad is supported by tape. Since weight bearing occurs at the end of the stump, healing should be advanced and the heel flap firmly fixed to the end of the stump before the patient is permitted to walk either on the stump or on the prosthesis. The Canadian Syme prosthesis, which incorporates a SACH (solid ankle cushion heel) foot and ankle and an end-bearing socket on foam rubber, is one which is frequently employed. Excellent results have been obtained with immediate fitting of a prosthesis following the Syme procedure. Some of the weight-bearing load is transferred to the patellar tendon and the flares of the tibial condyles, and it is not necessary to immobilize the knee joint. Weight bearing is then begun within 24 hours when the stump is mature and stable, measurements for a permanent prosthesis are made, and the stump is replaced in a plaster bandage until the prosthesis is available. The permanent prosthesis is usually applied earlier with this approach than with the conventional management.

Below-the-Knee Amputations (BK)

This level is being employed with increasing frequency since the advent of IPOP. Major functional advantages of

the BK amputation over the AK level are the ability to provide a more functional prosthesis for complete rehabilitation, the ability of the patient to move more easily in and out of bed, and a reduction in the incidence of phantom limb pain. Even a BK stump which is too short to accept a BK prosthesis is superior to an AK stump and can be fitted with a bent-knee prosthesis. BK amputations constitute the level of choice for ischemic lesions of the foot which do not extend above the malleoli but are generally not applicable if the gangrene extends in continuity above the ankle. Ischemic rigor of the calf muscles is another contraindication. Contracture of the knee or hip represents a relative contraindication, since it negates the functional advantages of this level.

The choice between the BK and AK amputation is determined by the patient's general health and potential for rehabilitation and an evaluation of the vascular status at the proposed level of amputation. No essential difference in healing rate was noted when patients with or without palpable popliteal pulses were evaluated, and, similarly, healing was not influenced by the presence or

Fig. 49-3. Transmetatarsal foot amputation. *A.* Skin incision is outlined. Note the short dorsal flap and longer plantar flap. *B.* Distal part of the foot has been removed, and the head of the metatarsals have all been amputated. *C.* Fascia and skin have been closed so that the scar is located dorsad.

absence of diabetes. Healing of BK amputations has been reported in 68 to 90 percent of cases in large series as compared with healing rates of 82 and 98 percent, respectively, for AK amputations. By contrast, considering the relative general status of the patients, a higher percentage of BK amputees walk on prosthetics. Precise figures are difficult to evaluate since they reflect the efforts and aggressiveness of the rehabilitation team. The range of reported figures for rehabilitation of BK amputations in patients with ischemia is from 50 to 90 percent.

TECHNIQUE (Fig. 49-5). The amputation should be performed proximal to the lower third of the tibia, since the preponderance of tendinous structures distal to this area predisposes to poor circulation and an unstable, painful

stump. Equally short anterior and posterior flaps may be made, or a longer posterior flap may be combined with a short anterior flap or only a longer posterior flap made with no anterior flap. When possible, the skin flaps are fashioned so that they are longer to permit an even closure, but if there is compromised circulation, short skin and subcutaneous flaps are reflected together. The posterior incision is beveled to reduce the bulk of muscle in order to provide a better stump. The tibia is usually transected 2 in. above the distal level of the skin flap, and the fibula is transected approximately 1 in. above the tibial level. The tibia may be beveled approximately 45° both anteriorly and mediad to provide a better stump. The nerves are pulled down gently and transected so that they are allowed to retract, and the vessels are ligated above the level of the end of the tibia. If a myodesis is performed (see Fig. 49-5*B*), the muscles are sutured to the tibia by drilling small holes through the bone into the marrow and suturing the muscles so that they are attached under moderate tension along their normal pathways, in a position slightly beyond rest length. The fascia and skin are loosely closed, and either a through-and-through drain or a catheter which will be connected to suction apparatus may be used for 2 days.

Fig. 49-4. Syme amputation. *A.* Incision is outlined. *B.* Foot has been amputated by disarticulating the calcaneus. Tibia and fibula are transected proximal to the flare of the tibial malleolus. *C.* The long plantar flap is sutured to the anterior part of the incision, with care to center the heel flap.

Fig. 49-5. BK amputation. *A.* Equally short anterior and posterior flaps have been made (a long posterior flap may be combined with a very short anterior flap). The muscles have been beveled, and the fibula is transected approximately 1 in. above the tibia. The periosteum has been removed from the distal portion of the bones. *B.* Myodesis: individual muscle fibers are sutured to the tibia through small drill holes. *C.* Fascia and skin are closed (dotted lines indicate skin closure when a long posterior flap is used).

POSTOPERATIVE MANAGEMENT (Fig. 49-6). With the conventional management, a small splint is applied in the operating room to prevent flexion of the knee joint. The splint is usually removed on the second day, and joint motion is then begun. Measurements for a temporary prosthesis may be made on the second day, and walking on this temporary prosthesis, with which the weight is borne on the ischium, may be performed within 3 days. When the patient is physically capable and the stump is well healed, a permanent prosthesis with which the weight is borne on the patellar tendon and tibial flares is provided. Walking on this permanent prosthesis should be possible about the fourth postoperative week.

IPOP may be applied, in which case the patient is encouraged to stand and bear weight on the first postoperative day and activity is rapidly increased. A permanent prosthesis can usually be applied at the time of the second cast change, i.e., at 3 weeks when the stump is sufficiently mature. In a series of cases, the use of IPOP at this level has not been associated with a single incidence of sustained phantom limb pain.

Knee Disarticulation

This is most commonly employed in children in whom there is a reason for maintaining the epiphysis for bone growth. Other advantages of the disarticulation are that it provides maximal length and good weight bearing and lends itself to a good fit between stump and socket. The disadvantages are that the end of the stump is bulky and has bony prominences which may result in skin breakdown. The procedure is rarely indicated when there is impaired circulation.

TECHNIQUE. The skin incision is placed about 1 in. above the stump end posteriorly, and the anterior flap is fashioned approximately 4 in. distal to the inferior border of the patella. The skin and subcutaneous tissue are re-

flected together. The femoral condyles and patella are usually not disturbed. If the patella is displaced or damaged by disease, it should be excised, leaving the quadriceps tendon or patellar ligament intact. Myodesis is easy to perform at this level. If the patella has been left in place, the patellar tendon is then sutured to the cruciate ligaments posteriorly. If the patella has been removed, the remaining tendon and quadriceps tendon are brought down through the intercondylar notch and sutured to the cruciate ligaments posteriorly. The hamstring tendons may also be brought down through this notch and sewn to the cruciate ligaments.

POSTOPERATIVE MANAGEMENT. The postoperative care and the application of a prosthesis is similar to that which is described below for the AK amputations.

Above-the-Knee Amputations (AK)

This level has generally been selected when gangrene extends above the level of the malleoli. Absolute indications for the procedure include extension of skin gangrene above a level which would permit BK amputation and rigor of the calf muscles. Peripheral gangrene coupled with contracture of the knee or hip constitutes a relative indication, since there is no advantage to a BK amputation.

The AK amputation is associated with the highest healing rate in patients with peripheral vascular disease; in series reviewed by Warren and Kihn this ranged between 84 and 100 percent. The rate of reamputation is lower, which is an important consideration in elderly and debilitated patients. These characteristics contribute to the fact that the mortality rate is higher than that reported for other levels of amputation of the lower extremity. The procedure has been associated with a relatively high incidence of pulmonary embolism, and some have advised routine anticoagulation or ligation of the ipsilateral femoral vein.

TECHNIQUE (Fig. 49-7). Anterior and posterior skin flaps are fashioned of equal length, and if there is any question of compromised vascular supply, as is frequently the case, short skin flaps are used. The skin and subcutaneous tissue are reflected together, taking care not to compromise the circulatory status. When possible, the adductor and hamstring muscles are beveled to provide a cylindrical stump rather than a bulbous one, but if there is a severe vascular problem, beveling is contraindicated. The vascular bundles are divided individually at the level of proposed transection of the femur, and gentle traction is applied to the sciatic nerve. Ligature of the nerve may be required if there is a significant vessel within, and the nerve is transected so that it retracts proximal to the stump of the femur. The periosteum of the femur is incised circularly and scraped to avoid leaving detached periosteum in the stump and consequent bone formation. The femur is transected at a level proximal to the condyles at a distance approximately equal to one-half the anteroposterior diameter of the thigh proximal to the most distal point of the skin flap. The edge of the bone is beveled to provide a smooth radius.

If myodesis is performed (see Fig. 49-5B), the muscles are attached through several small holes extending through the bone to the marrow, approximately 1 in. proximal to the distal end of the bone. Slight tension is applied to the anterior, medial, and posterior muscle groups, and these are sutured individually to the bone. The muscle should be able to effect maximal contraction and provide good function for the use of a prosthesis. Subcutaneous tissue and skin flaps are loosely approximated.

POSTOPERATIVE MANAGEMENT. With conventional management, a small dressing and stockinet are employed. The patient is positioned in bed so that there is no hip flexion and is turned frequently to the prone position. He is not allowed to sit in a chair or bed until he is able to hyperextend the stump. Measurements may be performed for a temporary prosthesis as early as the second day, since the weight is borne on the ischium, gluteal region, and thigh. The weight of the permanent prosthesis is borne either on the end of the stump, if it is end-bearing, but more usually on the ischial tuberosity, gluteal, and thigh regions. Fitting of the permanent prosthesis may take several months because of stump shrinkage but may occur as early as 4 to 6 weeks after amputation. A suction contact may be used for young patients with long stumps, but a suspension apparatus (Fig. 49-8) with a purchase across the iliac crest is more frequently employed. The incorporation of a single-action friction knee or a hydraulic mechanism which incorporates swing phase control depends upon the degree of rehabilitation required. A SACH foot and ankle are usually incorporated.

If an IPOP is used, a rigid dressing is applied in the

Fig. 49-6. Postoperative rehabilitation for BK amputation. Left. BK stump. Right. Prosthesis fitted.

operating room in such a fashion that the ischial tuberosity is resting on the posterior brim incorporating a waist belt and harness for suspension. The patient is encouraged to stand as soon as possible after the first postoperative day and to progress rapidly toward ambulation. Rehabilitation toward ambulation usually requires more time than with BK amputations.

Hip Disarticulation

The indications usually include bone tumors, soft tissue tumors, and extensive traumatic injuries. Flaps are fashioned so that they will come together anteriorly, and the posterior flap is constructed so that it forms a unit of skin, fascia, and muscle to swing forward in order that the patient may sit comfortably in the socket of his prosthesis. The femoral vessels are ligated anteriorly, and after the posterior dissection is completed, the femur is disarticulated. The sciatic nerve is cut high and tied in order to prevent bleeding from vasa nervorum. The undersurface of the gluteal muscle is tapered to facilitate approximation of the structures to the lower abdominal wall. Prostheses are available to permit ambulation, and have been applied to this level. A specially constructed Canadian prosthesis is used for these patients (Fig. 49-9).

Hemipelvectomy

This procedure has been used in the treatment of malignant tumors of the upper thigh, particularly those of soft tissue and bone, when it is felt that hip disarticulation

SCIATIC NERVE
(RETRACTED)

Fig. 49-7. AK amputation. *A.* Outline of short anterior and posterior flaps. *B.* Amputation completed with muscles beveled. Note that the sciatic nerve has been cut after tension had been applied in order that it retract proximal to the bone end. *C.* Skin closure which does not interfere with fitting of prosthesis.

would give a questionable margin of clearance around tumor. Soft tissue sarcomas have a predilection for extension along tissue planes between the muscles, and they continue to the muscular attachment in the pelvis. Hemipelvectomy or a modification thereof avoids local recurrence to a greater extent in these cases. Modification of the classic procedure by dividing the ileum through the greater sciatic notch requires less surgical manipulation and results in less shock. The adjustment to a prosthesis is better when a leaf of the ileum and pubic rami are left as supporting points for the socket. Following this procedure, patients have also been permitted to ambulate with a special Canadian prosthesis.

AMPUTATIONS OF THE UPPER EXTREMITY

In most instances, upper extremity amputations (Fig. 49-10) are performed for trauma. Malignant disease represents the second most common indication. Peripheral vascular disease, particularly thromboangiitis obliterans, constitutes a rare indication.

In all circumstances, the treatment is directed at conserving as much viable tissue as possible and, with more distal amputations, maintaining the function of the hand

as a grasping organ. The latter requires preservation of intrinsic muscle-tendon systems of the hand and the longer and more powerful flexors and extensors originating in the arm. The technique employed for amputations in the upper extremity is directed at producing minimal scar tissue, and the procedure is planned so that the scar is in an area as far removed as possible from bones, tendons, nerves, and points of external contact. Above the level of the metacarpals, opposing tendons should be fixed in order to preserve muscle length and tone.

In view of the precise nature of surgical technique, tourniquets are frequently employed to provide a bloodless field and facilitate identification of critical structures. They are best tolerated high in the upper arm with the cuff inflated to 280 mm Hg. Digital tourniquets, such as rubber bands, should not be used, because of the danger of thrombosis. Anesthesia is frequently best accomplished by the use of regional block, particularly since many of the patients present with multiple injuries and a full stomach and cannot tolerate general anesthesia at the preferred time for operation.

Fig. 49-8. Rehabilitation for AK amputation. *A.* Healed AK stump. *B.* Prosthesis for AK amputation. Note that the weight is not borne on the end of the stump.

Amputations in the Hand (See Chap. 50)

AMPUTATION OF DIGITS

When part or all of the distal phalanx requires amputation, an attempt should be made to create a longer volar flap and a shorter dorsal flap, so that the scar may be positioned dorsad away from pressure. Neither bone nor

Fig. 49-9. Rehabilitation following hip disarticulation. *A.* Healed amputation site. *B.* Patient fitted with special Canadian prosthesis.

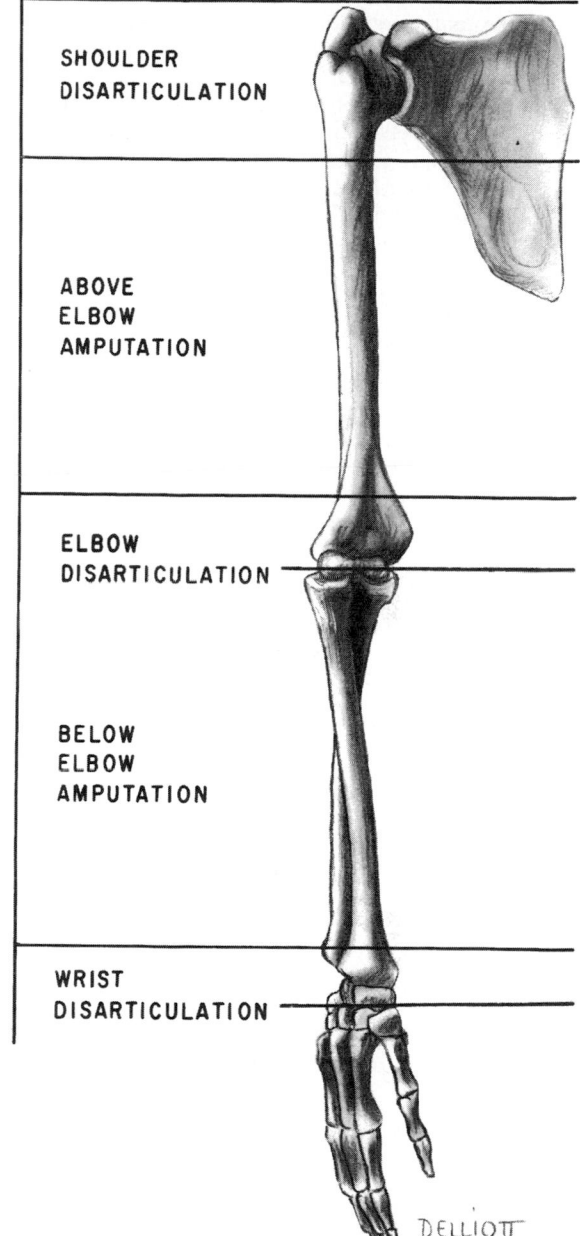

Fig. 49-10. Levels of amputation in the upper extremity.

viable soft tissue should be sacrificed to produce an ideal flap. If the amputation removes less than one-half the nail, it is preferable to retain the nail bed, but if more than half the nail is removed, the entire root should be excised. When it is necessary to disarticulate at the distal interphalangeal joint, the cartilage should be removed from the head of the middle phalanx, and the flexor digitorum profundus tendon should be withdrawn, transected, and allowed to retract.

Amputations of fingers distal to the PIP joint leave function which is useful for pinching and finer movements.

Amputations through the middle phalanx result in little alteration of extension when only the more distal portion of the dorsal expansion of the extensor digitorum communis tendon is cut. By contrast, the flexor digitorum superficialis tendon has a long insertion on either side of the phalanx, and if a significant portion of this insertion cannot be left intact, disarticulation may be necessary. Whenever possible, amputation through the proximal phalanx is preferable to disarticulation at the metacarpophalangeal joint, since the stump, however short, has function.

When one or more fingers must be removed in entirety, attention should be directed at the hand as a working unit. When the long and ring fingers are both removed, the adjoining fingers may continue to function perfectly, or they may deviate toward each other, and deviation weakens flexion. If only the long or ring finger is removed, it is best also to remove the head of its metacarpal to allow the adjoining metacarpals to approximate each other. This tends to prevent adjoining fingers from rotating and crossing toward each other. As a secondary procedure, the index (in the case of amputation of the long finger) or the little finger (in the case of amputation of the ring finger) may be moved over by resecting the metacarpal of the missing finger through the proximal third of its shaft and shifting the adjoining finger on to the stump (Fig. 49-11).

When the middle finger plus either the index or little finger are removed together, the heads of the metacarpals should be obliqued to produce a smooth contour. When the index finger has been disarticulated, the metacarpal should be partially excised to improve the final appearance of the hand and to avoid interference with function. In the case of the little finger, it is preferable to resect the whole metacarpal.

The thumb is the most important of the digits, and every bit should be saved, since even the smallest stump is preferable to a prosthesis. When only the thumb and small finger remain, a rotation osteotomy of the metacarpal of the thumb may be performed to permit approximation and grasping.

A variety of prostheses are available for more major amputations of the digits. These include functional terminal devices, such as hooks and cosmetically acceptable plastic hands. The selection of the prosthesis is dependent upon the patient's individual needs.

AMPUTATION THROUGH THE CARPOMETACARPAL LEVEL

After dorsal and volar skin and subcutaneous tissue flaps have been established, the digital extensor tendons are pulled down, transected, and allowed to retract, while the tendons of the carpal extensors are separated from their attachments to the metacarpal bases and left long so that they may be inserted into the carpal bone. The thenar and hypothenar muscles are tapered to make a smoothly rounded stump. The long flexor tendons are transected after applying gentle traction so that they will retract. After the metacarpals have been disarticulated from the carpals and the synovial cartilage has been removed from the distal carpals, the flexor carpi radialis and the tendons of carpal extension are sutured to the carpal bones. The skin and subcutaneous tissue then must be closed.

Fig. 49-11. Shifting of finger. *A.* Middle finger has been amputated at a transmetacarpal level. *B.* The remaining portion of the shaft of the middle finger metacarpal has been resected, and the metacarpal of the index finger has been transected and the distal portion secured to the base of the metacarpal of the middle finger by means of a Kirschner wire.

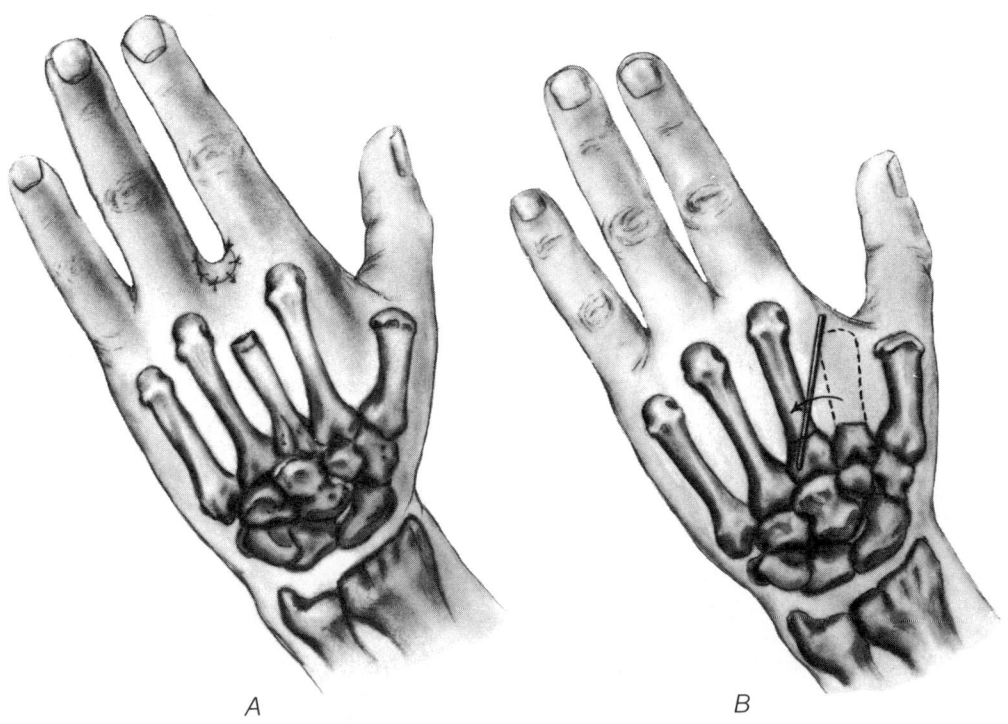

A   *B*

The stump is capable of more motion than a forearm stump, since there is more pronation and supination and good flexion and extension at the wrist. It accepts prostheses to provide a cosmetic hand and also more versatile and functional hooks.

Wrist Disarticulation

This level preserves greater length and provides better prosthetic control than amputations proximal to the wrist joint. The tendons of the hand should be transected with the muscles at rest length, so that they may be sutured to the ligaments and periosteum in order to prevent retraction and atrophy. The brachioradialis should not be disturbed. The styloid processes should be removed to permit a smoother fit for the prosthesis. The articular cartilage should also be removed and covered with a fascial flap to prevent limitation of pronation and supination by scar formation.

Although the stump is less strong and less versatile than when the carpal bones are left in, a less conspicuous prosthesis can be used. In women, amputations are generally carried a little higher in order to reduce the size of the prosthetic wrist by removal of the bulbous mass of bone at the end.

Forearm Amputations

In order to avoid excessive scarring and immobility of skin, skin flaps should not be dissected extensively from the fascia. The long flexor and extensor muscles and tendons are dissected and tapered so that they adhere to underlying tissue. After the bones have been transected, about $\frac{1}{2}$ in. of periosteum should be removed to prevent spur formation, and the fascia should be closed over the end so that muscle length is maintained.

With longer stumps, the actions of pronation and supination should be preserved, and the tendinous muscles and bones are therefore treated atraumatically to prevent fibrosis. Even if only a short stump can be achieved, this is superior to an above-elbow amputation. The formation of a functioning stump through the upper forearm can be successful if there is only a short segment of either radius or ulna which may be preserved distal to the tuberosity. This can be lengthened secondarily with a bone graft or flap.

The biceps and pectoralis muscles have been used in cineplastic operations as prime movers of artificial limbs in this situation. The plastic procedure is usually performed secondarily after the stump has healed. An inverted skin flap is formed and sutured into a tube and drawn through a tunnel of muscle in the biceps. The biceps tendon is divided at the midpoint and skin graft applied to cover the defect from the inverted flap (Fig. 49-12). The biceps can then transmit its force externally, while the brachialis muscle remains as a flexor of the forearm. The transmission of force is accomplished by attaching the rod through a muscle to a cable which exercises power over a hook.

The Krukenberg operation may be used in the forearm

Fig. 49-12. Cineplastic procedure for forearm amputation. *A.* Amputation has healed, and an inverted skin flap has been fashioned into a tube. *B.* Dermal tube has been brought through a tunnel of biceps muscle, and the biceps tendon is divided at the midpoint. A skin graft is then applied to cover the defect on the inverted flap. *C.* Prosthesis fitted. The transmission of force is accomplished from the biceps muscle to the cable which powers the hook.

when amputation is performed on a blind patient. With this procedure, a cleft is constructed between the radius and ulna to provide a grasping terminus which possesses tactile sensation.

Elbow Disarticulation

Flaps are created as in the case of forearm amputations so that the closure of skin and fat will not lie directly over the fascial incision. In order to obviate a bulky stump, the epicondyles are removed, and the cartilage is excised from the end of the bone. The tendons of the biceps, brachialis, and triceps muscles are sutured over the end at rest length. A cineplastic procedure to develop power for a functional terminal device may be performed secondarily.

Amputation through the Humerus

Every attempt should be made to preserve as long a stump as possible, since the longer the stump, the greater the applicability of subsequent cineplastic procedures for functional prosthesis. If a high amputation is necessary, it is preferable to preserve the head of the humerus, since this maintains the width of the shoulder and acts as a support for a prosthesis.

After anterior and posterior flaps are developed, the muscles are transected so that there is sufficient length of biceps and brachialis tendons and triceps muscle so that these muscles can be joined over the end of the bone to avoid retraction. In the case of shorter stumps, the biceps and triceps may be fixed to the humerus in a fashion similar to that described for myodesis procedures in the lower extremity. The skin and muscles are then closed loosely.

As soon as the stump is mature, it can be fitted with a prosthesis with a terminal device operated by a shoulder cable and with an elbow which can be fixed at varying degrees of flexion. The type of elbow joint utilized depends upon the type of function required by the patient. The most functional terminal devices are hooks which may be voluntarily opened. In the case of the adult unilateral amputee, the prosthesis usually functions only as an aid for the contralateral hand.

Disarticulation of the Humerus and Forequarter Amputation

The former procedure is usually performed for extensive trauma, whereas the latter operation may be indicated for malignant disease of the proximal upper extremity.

In most instances, care must be taken in individually ligating the vessels and nerves. In the case of disarticulation of the humerus, the flaps are fashioned to provide covering of the glenoid fossa, and the deltoid muscle is retained to be incorporated in this closure. Forequarter amputation includes excision of the scapula and clavicle followed by closure of the chest and back muscles over the chest wall and coverage with previously established skin flaps. A prosthetic device operated by the opposite shoulder may be applied.

LIMB REPLACEMENT

A 1970 review limited to replacement of the arm transected at or above the wrist revealed sufficiently detailed data on 51 patients, including 15 with complete amputa-

tions, 24 with near-complete amputations, and 12 failures in replacement. Only 23 of the 39 successful replacements were evaluated as to long-term result. Full functional recovery was not achieved.

References

General Considerations

Aitken, G. T.: Surgical Amputations in Children, *J Bone Joint Surg [Am]*, **45A:**1735, 1963.

Burgess, E. M., and Romano, R. L.: Immediate Postsurgical Prosthesis Fitting, *Bull Prosthetic Res,* vol. 10, no. 4, 1965.

Jansen, K.: Amputation: Principles and Methods, *Bull Prosthetic Res,* vol. 10, no. 4, 1965.

Warren, R., and Record, E. E.: "Lower Extremity Amputations for Arterial Insufficiency," Little, Brown and Company, Boston, 1967.

Amputations of the Lower Extremity

Baker, W. H., and Barnes, R. W.: Minor Forefoot Amputation in Patients with Low Ankle Pressure, *Am J Surg,* **133:**331, 1977.

Couch, N. P., David, J. K., Tilney, N. L., and Crane, C.: Natural History of the Leg Amputee, *Am J Surg,* **133:**469, 1977.

Dale, W. A., and Capps, W., Jr.: Major Leg and Thigh Amputations, *Surgery,* **46:**333, 1959.

Hansson, J.: The Leg Amputee: A Clinical Follow-up Study, *Acta Orthop Scand Suppl* 69,1964.

Harris, P. D., Schwartz, S. I., and DeWeese, J. A.: Midcalf Amputation for Peripheral Vascular Disease, *Arch Surg,* **82:**381, 1961.

Holden, W. D.: Arteriosclerotic Ischemic Necrosis of the Lower Extremities, *Surgery,* **22:**125, 1947.

Moore, W. S.: Determination of Amputation Level: Measurement of Skin Blood Flow with Xenon-133, *Arch Surg,* **107:**798, 1973.

————, Hall, A. D., and Lim, R. C., Jr.: Below the Knee Amputation for Ischemic Gangrene, *Am J Surg,* **124:**127, 1972.

Nagendran, T., Johnson, G., Jr., McDaniel, W. J., Mandel, S. R., and Proctor, H. J.: Amputation of the Leg: An Improved Outlook, *Ann Surg,* **175:**994, 1972.

Sherman, C. D., and Duthie, R. B.: Modified Hemipelvectomy, *Cancer,* **13:**51, 1960.

Stahlgren, L. H., and Otteman, M. G.: Review of Criteria for the Selection of the Level for Lower Extremity Amputation of Arteriosclerosis, *Ann Surg,* **162:**886, 1965.

Warren, R., Crawford, E. S., Hardy, I. B., and McKittrick, J. B.: The Transmetatarsal Amputation in Arterial Deficiency of the Lower Extremity, *Surgery,* **31:**132, 1952.

———— and Kihn, R. B.: A Survey of Lower Extremity Amputations for Ischemia, *Surgery,* **63:**107, 1968.

———— and Record, E. E.: "Lower Extremity Amputations for Arterial Insufficiency," Little, Brown and Company, Boston, 1967.

Amputations of the Upper Extremity

Burnham, P. J.: Regional Block of the Great Nerves of the Upper Arm, *Anesthesiology,* **19:**281, 1958.

———: Amputation of the Upper Extremity, *Clin Symp,* **11:**107, 1959.

———: Regional Block at the Wrist of the Great Nerves of the Hand, *JAMA,* **167:**847, 1958.

Chase, R. A., and Laub, D. R.: The Hand: Therapeutic Strategy for Acute Problems, *Curr Probl Surg,* 1966.

Limb Replacement

McNeill, R. E., and Wilson, J. S. P.: Problems of Limb Replacement, *Br J Surg,* **57:**365, 1970.

Malt, R. A., Remensnyder, J. P., and Harris, W. H.: Long-Term Utility of Replanted Arms, *Ann Surg,* **176:**334, 1972.

Chapter 50

Hand

by **Robert A. Chase and Lester M. Cramer**

Congenital Abnormalities
Syndactyly
Polydactyly
Circumferential Grooves and Amputations
Missing Parts
Macrodactyly

Hand Infection
Subcutaneous Abscess
Paronychia
Felon
Bacterial Tenosynovitis
Palmar Space Infections
Acute Suppurative Arthritis
Unusual Infections

Hand Injuries
Hand Amputation
Replantation of Amputated Digits

Elective Incisions

Postoperative Care
Unusual Pain Syndromes

The philosophic exaltation of the hand by scholars of antiquity is equaled by the profound regard for its complexity and versatility held by functional anatomists and surgeons. Its capabilities depend on the intricate relationships between its architectural, motor, and sensory elements with the brain and its peripheral linkages. Therefore, an understanding of the anatomy and unique healing capacities of nerves, tendons, bone, skin, and blood vessels is not the only prerequisite essential for the hand surgeon. He also must understand the functional contribution of each part of the hand in order to be able to judge what the expectations for function may be if parts in various combinations are rendered functionless.

Diseases and injuries of the hand covered in other chapters are burns of the hand (Chap. 7), diseases of muscle and Dupuytren's contracture (Chap. 43), tumors (Chap. 46), fractures and joint injuries (Chap. 47), and diseases of joints (Chap. 48).

CONGENITAL ABNORMALITIES

The genetic and environmental factors cited as etiologic agents in other congenital anomalies also apply in upper limb abnormalities. Anomalies fall into no fixed pattern, but generally they consist of specific deficits, supernumerary parts, fusions, clefts, or hypertrophy or atrophy.

Syndactyly

Webbing of the fingers is the most common of all congenital hand abnormalities. The condition varies from a thin web between otherwise normal digits to fusion of skeletal elements as well as soft tissues. It is characterized by phenotypic variability and genetic heterogeneity. However, in many of the families reported, there has been dominant autosomal inheritance. A dominant gene may give various expressions of syndactyly in association with preaxial and/or postaxial polydactyly. Syndactyly is also an integral part of many different syndromes such as anhidrotic ectodermal dysplasia, Laurence-Moon-Bardet-Biedl syndrome, Poland syndactyly, oculodentodigital dysplasia, and acrocephalosyndactyly (Apert's Syndrome). Very frequently, both the hands and the feet are involved at the same time.

Digits are not separated in fetal life until about the sixth week. The arrest of digital separation at this stage creates this abnormality. The incidence is variously reported as 1 in 1,000 to 1 in 3,000 births. Males are affected more frequently than females in a ratio of about 2:1. Roentgenographic examination is helpful in assessing the nature of skeletal involvement.

TREATMENT. The timing of surgical intervention has been a subject of debate. When digits of different growth rates are involved, separation of the bony junctures is recommended prior to age one year, to prevent growth retardation of the larger digit and progressive deviation of the connected ones. After this has been attended to or if there has been no concern with the growth problem, it is advisable to wait until the end of the second year of life for surgical intervention. Surgical correction must be planned to avoid compounding the problem by creating scar contractures. Because there is inadequate local skin to achieve complete closure and a functioning web space, a combination of local flap tissue supplemented by free skin grafting is essential.

The operation (Fig. 50-1) involves creation of geometric interdigitating skin flaps on the adjacent sides of the two involved digits. If more than two digits are involved, the procedures should be staged; working on both sides of any single digit would endanger its vascular supply. The interdigitating flaps with the grafts will avoid linear closure

Fig. 50-1. Congenital syndactyly. *A.* Incisions outlined to create interdigitating flap and web space pedicle. *B.* Palmar incision. *C.* Result after syndactyly correction.

which would result in scar contracture. The web requires special attention to avoid scar fixation of the digits in a position of adduction toward one another. The flaps of skin and subcutaneous tissue of both dorsal and palmar skin are designed to interdigitate within the web cleft for this purpose. The areas of skin deficit at the time of exposure are covered with free full-thickness skin grafts obtained either from the inguinal crease or from the arch of the plantar surface of the foot.

Polydactyly

Extra digits are a manifestation of embryologic duplication. They may appear as supernumerary phalanges, duplications of whole extremities, or any degree of variation between these extremes. The most common form of polydactyly consists of a rudimentary digit without its own tendons. It may be associated with an extra metacarpal, or it may extend from another metacarpal which is Y-shaped. Fortunately, the supernumerary digit is usually on the radial or ulnar margin of the hand, where it may be removed without difficulty. Duplications of the thumb are most common. When duplication involves the whole thumb, it is occasionally difficult to tell which is the prime digit and which is vestigial. Supernumerary digits must be amputated precisely, with care to preserve tendons and sensory nerves to the digit left in situ.

Circumferential Grooves and Amputations

Shallow or deep circumferential grooves in the extremities are not uncommon congenital anomalies. There is controversy as to whether the defect is a result of intrauterine environmental factors such as amniotic bands or of influences transmitted genetically. It seems most reasonable (although admittedly on incomplete evidence) that circumferential grooves and congenital amputations are influenced by growth and developmental changes determined genetically.

If the grooves do not threaten survival of the part, they may be ignored or treated by Z-plasty for cosmetic im-

provement. Rarely, the constriction is so severe that the survival of the extremity or part is threatened. Surgical release and Z-plasty then become more urgent.

Missing Parts

Children born with specific parts of the hand and arm totally absent or represented by a small vestige may have numerous combinations of deformities. There are, however, a few common combinations of absences. Parts of digits or whole rays (phalangeal and metacarpal) may be absent. Absence of the thumb or a vestigial first ray preventing good prehensile grasp is very disabling. Missing central rays result in a cleft or lobster-claw-like hand. Congenital absence of the whole hand is an obvious disaster. Absence of segments of the forearm, much more commonly the radius than the ulna, are found in combination with hand losses or as an independent anomaly. Total absence of the extremity or an extremity nub with vestigial hand is recognizable as the phocomelia deformity, such as was seen in the thalidomide cases.

Surgical reconstruction is individualized for each specific deformity. For example, the child born with absence of the first ray may have four normal digits, or there may be five fingers with no opposable thumb unit. Surgical reconstruction is planned after careful study of the deformity, including level of function of each of the digits, and roentgenograms. When four normal fingers exist but the thumb ray is totally absent, pollicization of the index digit is a reasonable procedure (Fig. 50-2). This is best and most safely performed at the age of four to five years, before the child enters school. Some surgeons prefer to carry out the procedure in the first year of life.

Macrodactyly

Digital gigantism, localized symmetric enlargement of one or more digits, is most common in the index finger, most often unilateral, more common in the male, and

Fig. 50-2. Congenital absence of thumb. *A*. Incision outlined for transfer of index digit to thumb position. *B*. Preoperative x-ray. *C*. Postoperative x-ray. *D*. Index digit pollicized.

frequently accompanied by such other congenital anomalies as syndactyly, café au lait spots, neurofibromas arteriovenous fistulae, nevi, polydactyly, and hemangiomas. Commonly this is a form of neurofibromatosis. Treatment is difficult. Obviously, if there is a single, functionless, grotesque digit, amputation of the finger or the ray would be the treatment of choice. If it is a functional single digit, particularly in children, multiple operations of bone remodeling, epiphyseal arrest, and excision of the excessive soft tissues including longitudinal excision of hypertrophic nerves constitute a reasonable approach.

HAND INFECTION

The vulnerability of the hand to frequent wounding makes the hand a common portal of entry for bacterial invasion. This, coupled with the concentration of tendons (with their poor blood supply), as well as the difficulty in sustaining natural immobilization, sets the stage for grave local infections. The hand is so important in every form of activity that one is not likely to protect or immobilize it when early infection occurs. The potential spaces and moist synovial sheaths are a fine environment for bacterial growth, particularly because of constant massaging motion and lack of luxuriant blood supply so important in mobilizing local resistance to infection.

A succinct but specific history and general physical examination must precede the examination of the hand. In addition to noting influencing diseases, such as diabetes, arthritis, cardiopulmonary or renal disorders, and drug addiction, the infection symptomatology of fever, tachycardia, nausea, vomiting, malaise, and polycytosis should be sought. The amount and quality of pain is important. Severe pain is ominous, but the absence of pain can be misleading. Local signs of spread along the lymphatic system, ascending lymphangitis or lymphadenopathy, must be examined for. The three primary lymph node drainage sites are the epitrochlear nodes for the ring and little fingers, the axillary nodes for the thumb and index finger, and the deltopectoral nodes for the middle finger. Inspection of the suspected infection will reveal erythema, edema, tenderness, and perhaps purulent drainage; gentle palpation can reveal fluctuance.

Injuries that are particularly susceptible to subsequent infection are those where crushing is a factor, those occurring in a filthy environment (some meatcutting plants, farmyards, some types of manual labor, city streets), puncture wounds involving a contaminated or irritating foreign body (plant thorns, fish hooks) or the injection of human or animal saliva (bites, fights), and the drug addict's self-inflictions (needles, glass droppers). There is an ever-increasing incidence of severe and exotic hand infections in the drug culture. As the proximal veins become obstructed or thrombosed, brawny edema of the hand develops, causing addicts to use digital veins as a portal of entry. At this site extravasation of contaminated materials will lead to disastrous infections and sloughing of chemically injured, contaminated tissues.

Many of the common and less serious infections can be treated on an ambulatory basis. A position-of-function splint and a brachial sling are used for rest and elevation, appropriate antibiotics and pain medications are given, and multiple soakings are advised. If pus is localized, many subcutaneous abscesses and most paronychiae can be drained in the emergency department or office. Narcotics, sedatives, and/or tranquilizers may be needed. The patient should always be lying down, his arm on a side table, sterility assured, and a brachial tourniquet in place. In the office or emergency room, a blood pressure cuff can be used to record the blood pressure and then left on the arm to act as the tourniquet, subsequently being inflated just prior to incision. During the cleansing of the skin and the application of the sterile drape, the arm is kept elevated so that when the cuff is inflated to 280 mm Hg, there will be a minimum of congestion in the hand. The need for a bloodless field to assure accuracy is critical, even for the most seemingly insignificant drainage procedure. The brachial cuff for a tourniquet is preferred in all situations, but there are some surgeons and emergency physicians who feel that a digital tourniquet suffices for fingertip procedures. A rubber band should never be used as a digital tourniquet, as pressure is difficult to control, it may injure the digital nerves, and it might easily be left in place accidentally. Soft rubber tubing held in place by an artery clamp is preferred. Inducing hand ischemia by distal-to-proximal wrapping as is done in elective, clean surgery is contraindicated, since this can encourage proximal spread via synovial sheaths or lymphatics, enhancing the spread of infection.

Postoperative care consists of rest, constant elevation of the hand higher than the heart, an absorptive and non-constricting dressing with a position-of-function splint incorporated, pain control with narcotics, and sedatives for sleep.

For the more seriously ill, immediate hospitalization may be needed, and antibacterial therapy should be instituted immediately by the intravenous route. All incision and drainage operations should be done in the operating room, except for the few exceptions noted above.

The judicious use of antibiotics is important, and urgency may justify initiating the appropriate agent on the basis of a smear or characteristics of the clinical picture prior to receipt of culture and sensitivity reports. Empiric selection of a proper antibiotic is guided by the following considerations:

1. Familiarity with the usual pattern of infection, since the pathophysiology of the lesion makes diagnosis more definitive (Fig. 50-3)
2. The local and systemic response to the lesion
3. Knowledge of the local bacterial ecology
4. Gram stain, if material is available
5. Total health picture of the patient
6. The properties of the antibiotic agent

Staphylococci are present in nearly 80 percent of hand infections. Over one-half are penicillinase-producing. Beta-hemolytic streptococci, *Escherichiq coli, Proteus* species, and *Pseudomonas* species account for the remaining. Over one-third of all infections have a mixed flora; the most frequent combination is *Staphyloccus aureus,* beta-hemolytic streptococci, and *E. coli.* Fungal superinfection may develop after several days of high doses of antibiotics, especially if used in combinations.

When an area shows the signs of early inflammation and possible infection, the differential diagnosis must include chemical or metabolic synovitis, gout, rheumatoid arthritis, Reiter's syndrome, and nonspecific tenosynovitis. If these are not prime suspects, the inflammatory lesion should be treated promptly, although the antibiotic is difficult to select as usually there is no area to culture. Systemic antibiotics often can be supplemented by local instillation or topical applications of antibiotic solutions or ointments. If the process subsequently progresses to one requiring incision

Fig. 50-3. *A.* Diagram of the locations of common infections showing spreading and pointing. 1. Dorsal subcutaneous abscess. 2. Paronychia. 3. A vesicle or pustule indicative of felon beneath. 4. Felon. 5. Abscess in volar fat pad; this can point in a palmar direction or track to the dorsum before pointing; the flexion creases frequently act as barriers to spread. 6. Abscess in palmar fat pad may spread by perforating dorsad, by passing the flexion crease barrier through bacterial action and going proximally to the subcutaneous tissue in the palm, or by spreading via the lumbrical canal to a palmar space. *B.* The collar-button abscess. This advanced lesion, with abscess cavities on both the palmar and dorsal aspects, is common in the area of the metacarpophalangeal joint. It has the potential for spreading beneath the palmar fascia or into the dorsal compartment opposite the web space, or it may fill the web space and extend along the tendons into the midpalmar space or to the thenar space.

and drainage or if purulence is already apparent at the initial examination, prompt surgery is recommended.

When an infection is not hospital-acquired, a penicillin is the best choice of antibiotic at the outset. For ambulatory outpatients or for lesions of apparent staphylococcus infections to which there is good body response, oral dicloxacillin may be used. If the lesion is not localizing well and lymphangitis is prominent, penicillin should be added, since it is so much more effective against the nonpenicillinase-producing staphylococci and against beta-hemolytic streptococci. If the patient is allergic to penicillin and needs antistaphylococcal treatment, either gentamicin or lincomycin is recommended. Daily evaluation at 24 and 48 hours is essential to assess the response and the patient's compatibility with the antibiotic. The specific cultural sensitivities will determine subsequent continuation or change of drug. If more than one antibiotic is being used, only the best one needs to be continued.

When severe infection has supervened, intravenous administration of antibiotics must be begun immediately and a hospital surgical procedure performed when there is adequate antibiotic within the patient's system.

For the gram-positive cocci, methicillin or nafcillin are recommended as intravenous therapy; if the infection appears to be less well localized or mixed, cephalothin is added.

If there is an impending tenosynovitis in a critically ill patient, the treatment is cephalothin or carbenicillin to which are added methicillin or nafcillin. In a compromised host, e.g., a diabetic or drug addict, and especially if the infection is mixed, either gentamicin or ampicillin may be added. Ampicillin is not commonly recommended for treating hand infections unless there is specific positive cultural information. Despite the possibility of encouraging a superinfection, it is best to slightly "overtreat" a severe infection initially and be able to withdraw a *possibly* unnecessary antibiotic when the culture information is available rather than have the infection progress rapidly because of a delay. Special note should be made of infections from human bites or those caused when the fist strikes the tooth of an opponent. In the latter situation there is often some crush of tissue plus the injection of organisms into tendon sheaths or joints. Early aggressive antibiotic therapy with penicillin and tetracycline is indicated.

Subcutaneous Abscess

These abscesses are quite common, accounting for about 15 percent of all infections of the hand. Most of them are situated on the palmar aspects of the middle and proximal segments of the fingers or in the palm; only a few will occur on the dorsal surfaces of the fingers or hand. They frequently follow a needle or thorn prick and thus are very common in gardeners. Other cases may follow blistering from hard manual work. They usually present in the stage of cellulitis with diffuse redness and swelling of the fingers, which must be differentiated from some of the deeper and more dangerous infections. The tenderness generally is confined to the small area at the site of the abscess, although all have the potential for spreading out laterally or

deeply to become the initiating sites for deeper infections. Treatment with rest, elevation, and antibiotics sometimes will abort the process, but most abscesses will localize and require drainage. Abscesses may point in a palmar direction or at the side of the finger, but even a palmar lesion may point to the dorsum. This situation, if not treated promptly by antibiotics and drainage, can lead to acute suppurative tenosynovitis, acute suppurative arthritis, osteomyelitis, and occasionally gangrene.

Paronychia

Infection around the nail bed occurs because the area is frequently subject to injury which creates a portal of entry for bacteria, and also because the nail juncture with soft tissues is a weak area of defense against local invasive infection. The initiating cause may be hangnails, ingrowing nails, manicure trauma, unclean subungual areas, steel wool slivers, or other foreign bodies. Once the paronychia is established, the cornified nail acts as an intrinsic foreign body, perpetuating the infection. Staphylococcus is usually the offending organism. Combined infection with staphylococcus and streptococcus is resistant to treatment and requires not only incision and drainage but appropriate antibiotics and intensive soaking. Frequently a portion of the nail must be removed (Fig. 50-4), since the pathologic process has progressed. Occasionally a chronic paronychia may need long-term treatment with frequent applications of antifungal agents.

Felon

Infection of the digit pulp has certain important characteristics. The fibrous septa to the skin limit swelling of the part, and pressure builds up in the pulp space. This gives rise to deep ischemic necrosis. Thus more culture medium is created, and severe deep infection with osteomyelitis of the distal phalanx may result. All this occurs before pointing and spontaneous external drainage. Erythema, pain, and tenderness characterize the felon. The pulp space should be incised and drained before deep necrosis occurs (Fig. 50-5).

Bacterial Tenosynovitis

As bacteria invade the more proximal areas in the digit, they find a receptive site for growth in the slippery synovial sheaths around the flexor tendons. The area is characterized by poor natural resistance to infection and the presence of nearly avascular tendon. It takes little disruption to convert living tendon into a collagenous foreign body with its tendency to augment the infectious process.

The anatomy in the tendon sheaths varies significantly, but the general pattern should be known in order to predict routes of natural extension of the infection (Fig. 50-6). For example, a single felon in the pulp of the little finger may extend to the flexor tendon sheath, then along a natural anatomic route to the ulnar bursa. From this site in the hand it may readily extend to the radial bursa and into the thumb flexor tendon sheath. Where the anatomy is of

A

B

Fig. 50-4. *A.* Surgical drainage of the paronychial abscess is best performed through an incision proximal to the corner of the involved nail. *B.* If the abscess extends around the nail base or lateral margin, the base or margin should be excised to assure adequate drainage and removal of nonviable nail which serves as a foreign body. The fingernail will regenerate from the nail bed.

the classic pattern, the little finger infection would be more likely to extend to the thumb than to the adjacent ring finger or the middle or index fingers.

When the flexor tendon sheath is infected, the posture assumed by the involved digit is one of mild flexion at all points. Active or passive attempts to extend the finger elicits local pain. Swelling, inflammation, and local temperature elevation may not be striking but are observed on close examination. The differential diagnosis between true bacterial tenosynovitis and acute rheumatoid or nonspecific tenosynovitis can be difficult. Roentgenograms for calcium deposits may be helpful in diagnosing a reactive chemical (nonbacterial) local inflammation. A history of previous episodes of tenosynovitis, rheumatoid disease, gout, recent local or systemic infection, injury, or excessive use of the part may provide the clue for the correct diagnosis. Aspiration of the tendon sheath for smears and culture may be helpful.

Proper therapy (Fig. 50-7) for established bacterial tenosynovitis is surgical drainage and administration of appropriate antibiotics. The tendon sheath must be adequately opened with a midaxial (ulnar or radial side of digit along joint axes) incision. Once drainage is performed, vigorous treatment is required to achieve early wound closure to preserve the flexor tendons.

Palmar Space Infections

The deep spaces in the hand between the deep flexor tendons and the metacarpals with their interposed interosseous muscles are potential receptive pockets (Fig. 50-6). The subtendinous palmar area is divided into a thenar space and midpalmar space by a thick vertical septum from the palmar fascia to the third metacarpal. Frequently one of these deep spaces becomes the seat of grave infection without involvement of the other. The localized swelling, redness, and tenderness make diagnosis quite straightforward. These spaces may be surgically drained through any of a variety of incisions, with care to avoid violating the general principle of not crossing areas of flexion (Fig. 50-8).

Fig. 50-5. *A.* Incision and drainage of felon with preservation of sensory digit pulp. (*From R. A. Chase and D. R. Laub, The Hand: Therapeutic Strategy for Acute Problems, in "Current Problems in Surgery," Year Book Medical Publishers, Inc., Chicago, 1966. By permission of Year Book Medical Publishers, Inc.) B.* A centrally located incision permits excellent drainage and decompression. This alternate incision lies between innervation areas but does leave a scar in the finger pad.

A

B

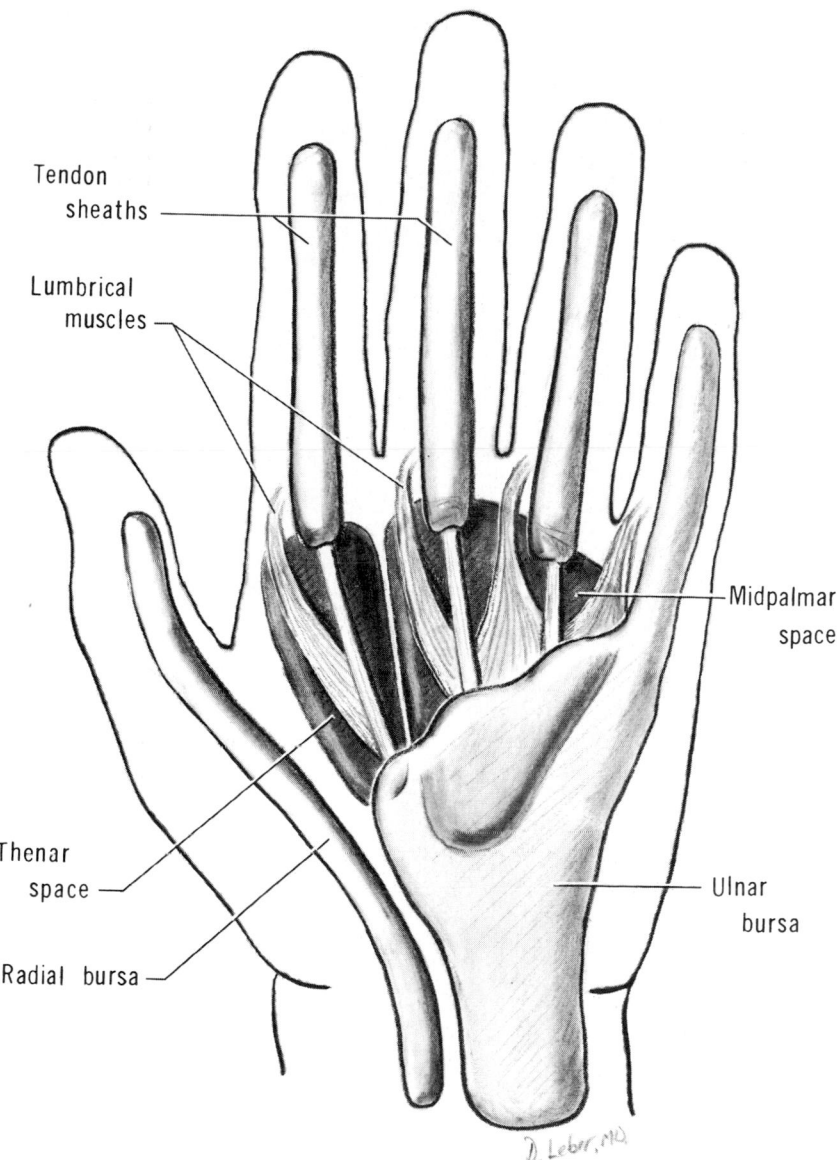

Tendon sheaths

Lumbrical muscles

Midpalmar space

Thenar space

Ulnar bursa

Radial bursa

D. Leber, MD

Fig. 50-6. The anatomy of the synovial sheaths and deep spaces in the hand.

Acute Suppurative Arthritis

When the joints are involved with a purulent disease, they are most commonly secondarily affected from a penetrating wound or from the direct spread from a neighboring abscess. Also, with the increasing incidence of venereal disease, monarticular gonococcal arthritis is becoming more common. Early surgery supplemented by both systemic and articular infusion antibiotics (Fig. 50-9) may preserve function, but prognosis for a normal joint is always guarded.

Unusual Infections

A group of severe infections which must be watched for carefully includes acute streptococcal hemolytic gangrene, necrotizing fasciitis, streptococcal myositis, clostridial cellulitis, gram-negative anaerobic cutaneous gangrene, and progressive bacterial synergistic gangrene. Although these severe soft tissue infections occur infrequently, early recognition is important to prevent progressive destruction secondary either to continuing bacterial action or to ischemic necrosis from pressure produced by swelling. The diagnosis should be entertained for a hand or forearm that has had recent trauma or surgery and presents with extensive swelling and systemic toxicity without the usual signs of local acute inflammatory process. Figure 50-10 presents a brief summary of the differential diagnostic characteristics of common hand infections.

HAND INJURIES

A large proportion of accidental injuries in industry, at home, or in automobile accidents involve the forearm and

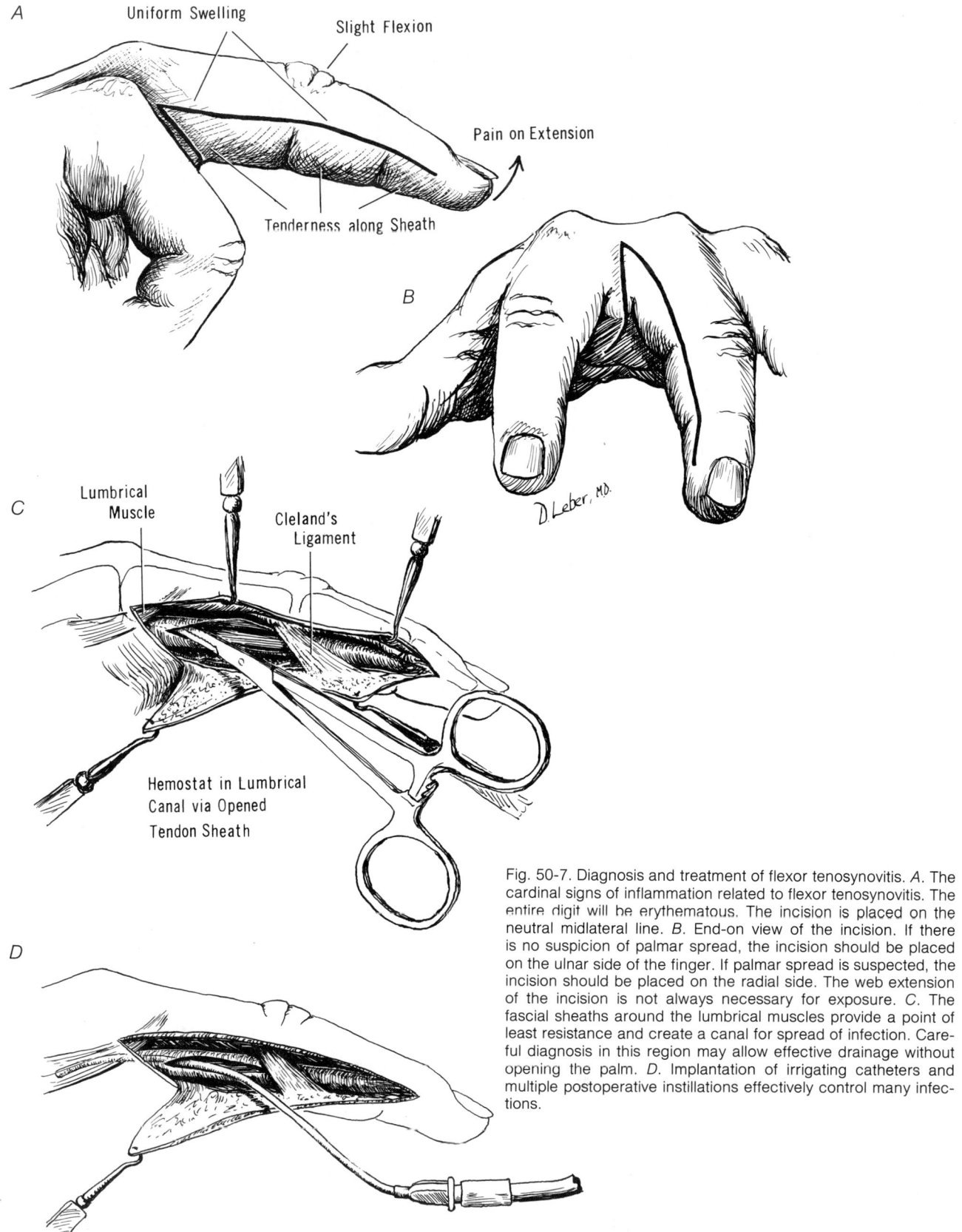

A

Uniform Swelling

Slight Flexion

Pain on Extension

Tenderness along Sheath

B

D Leber, M.D.

C

Lumbrical Muscle

Cleland's Ligament

Hemostat in Lumbrical Canal via Opened Tendon Sheath

D

Fig. 50-7. Diagnosis and treatment of flexor tenosynovitis. *A.* The cardinal signs of inflammation related to flexor tenosynovitis. The entire digit will be erythematous. The incision is placed on the neutral midlateral line. *B.* End-on view of the incision. If there is no suspicion of palmar spread, the incision should be placed on the ulnar side of the finger. If palmar spread is suspected, the incision should be placed on the radial side. The web extension of the incision is not always necessary for exposure. *C.* The fascial sheaths around the lumbrical muscles provide a point of least resistance and create a canal for spread of infection. Careful diagnosis in this region may allow effective drainage without opening the palm. *D.* Implantation of irrigating catheters and multiple postoperative instillations effectively control many infections.

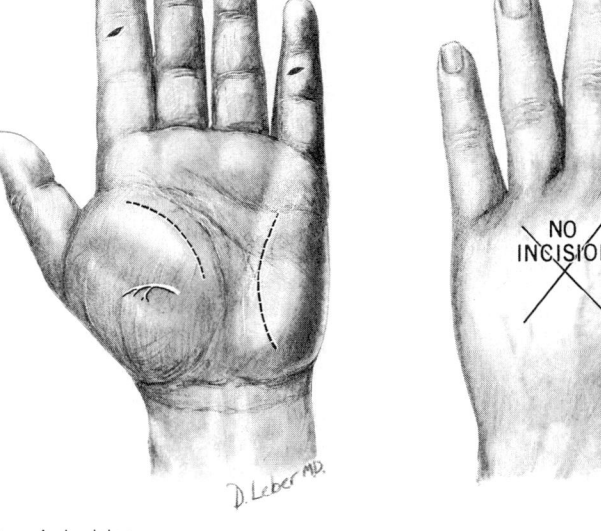

A

B

C

NO INCISION

D. Leber MD.

Fig. 50-8. Spread of digital infection into the palm. *A.* Incision for drainage of the midpalmar space. *B.* Incisions for drainage of the radial bursa and the ulnar bursa. *C.* Palmar digital infections frequently create extremely swollen regions on the dorsum of the hand, because the lymphatic drainage runs from the palmar to dorsal aspects. A common error is to expect to drain such a lesion at this lymphadenitis point. When there are dorsal infections, incision and drainage will be performed dorsally. *D.* The incision for drainage of the thenar space.

D

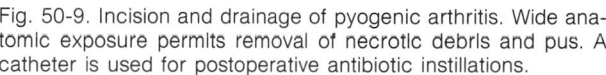

Fig. 50-9. Incision and drainage of pyogenic arthritis. Wide anatomic exposure permits removal of necrotic debris and pus. A catheter is used for postoperative antibiotic instillations.

Extensor Tendon
Retracted

D. Leber, MD.

	Paronychia	Terminal pulp infection	Acute cellulitis
Time of presentation from onset	2–5 days	4–5 days	12–24 hours
Cause	Nail biting. Manicuring.	Puncture wound	Prick or not known
Organism	Mixed	Staphylococcus	Streptococcus
Symptoms	Tender swelling round nail fold.	Throbbing pain confined to the end of the finger increasing daily and preventing sleep.	Hot red finger. Malaise shivering and tenderness up arm to axilla.
Physical Signs	Fluctuant swelling of nail fold. Often subcuticular pus.	Hot red tense and tender pulp. Often subcuticular pus. Rest of the finger normal.	Hot red finger. Not very swollen.
Movements	Full. Painless.	Full. Painless.	Practically full. Painless.
Temperature	Normal	Normal	Raised
Lymphagitis	No	No	Yes
Differential diagnosis	1 Early acute cellulitis 2 Lateral pulp infection 3 Late subungual haematoma	1 Acute cellulitis 2 Early paronychia 3 Haematoma of pulp following trauma	Early pulp infection especially apical infection

Fig. 50-10. Differential diagnosis of hand infection. (*From J. Sneddon, The Care of Hand Infections, The Williams & Wilkins Company, Baltimore, 1970.*)

hand. The hand is frequently used as a protective shield, it is generally unclothed, and it is the probe with which man explores his environment. It is no surprise that it is frequently subject to trauma. The complexity of its anatomy and the compact proximity of all its elements set the stage for every injury to be a threat to subsequent normal function, and the surgeon must be alert to subtle functional losses when specific nerves, tendons, or architectural elements are compromised. Systematic, precise examination of the hand is necessary even when the injury appears to be minor.

CLINICAL MANIFESTATIONS. History. One must know the circumstances leading to the injury in order to outline and execute an optimal program of treatment. Knowledge of the time elapsed since the injury, the character of the wounding agent, the nature of first-aid care, and the patient's general health are important; an elderly patient on steroid therapy for an unrelated disease who sustained a laceration while working with a garden tool several hours before being seen presents an entirely different problem from a healthy teen-ager brought directly to an emergency suite with a cut from broken glass.

Sensibility. The distribution of sensory nerves in the hand is such that they are subject to frequent injury. In adults it is simple to assess areas of anesthesia by simple touch and pinprick testing. If there is doubt about the patient's response or if one is dealing with a small child, peripheral nerve injury may be assessed by a more objective test: Using Ninhydrin as a reagent, one may demonstrate presence or absence of sudomotor (sweating) function in the digits. Fingerprints are made on test paper and processed with the reagent. When sensory nerves are transected, there is loss not only of sensibility but also of sympathetic sweating function. The patterns of anesthesia clearly document which of the sensory nerves has been injured. Testing for sensibility must be done before local anesthetic agents are used and before any wound exploration is done.

Tendon sheath infection	Boil or carbuncle	Palmar and web infection	Infective arthritis
6–36 hours	2–3 days	2–3 days	1–3 days from onset infection Up to 3 wks from time of original injury
Midline injury with sharp instrument	Often not known	Puncture wound—often splinter	Cut or puncture over dorsum of the joint
Streptococcus	Staphylococcus	Staphylococcus	Mixed
Hot red swollen finger. Extremely painful especially on movement. Malaise. Tenderness up arm to axilla.	Painful swelling on the back of the hand or fingers. History of previous boils.	Throbbing pain in the palm and gross swelling of the back of the hand.	Painful swelling all round the infected joint and discharging wound on the dorsum
Whole finger hot, red and swollen. Maximal on dorsum. Tenderness along course of the sheath maximal in proximal compartment in the palm.	Cellulitis and oedema of dorsum, with triangular spread to the wrist. Later, discharging lesion.	Infected puncture wound in palm brawny, red and tender. Swelling and pitting oedema of dorsum. In web infections fingers separated. Best seen from the dorsum.	Cellulitis of whole finger. Swelling tenderness maximal all round the infected joint. Discharging wound on dorsum.
Extremely painful, especially extension.	Full	Slight limitation by pain in fingers.	Flexion and extension limited and painful. Lateral movement increased and crepitus present.
Raised	Slightly raised	Slightly raised	Normal
Yes	Sometimes	Sometimes	No
1 Acute cellulitis *2* Middle or proximal space infection *3* Fascial infection	Palmar or web infection	*1* Early carbuncle *2* Tendon sheath infection involving proximal compartment	*1* Infected laceration not involving the joint *2* Neglected acute paronychia *3* Mallet finger

Extrinsic Muscular Function. *Distal Interphalangeal (DIP) Joint Flexors.* The tendons of the profundus muscles and the flexor pollicis longus insert on the distal phalanges of the fingers and thumb, respectively. Inability actively to flex the distal phalanx means loss of functional integrity of the tendon, the muscle, or its innervation (Fig. 50-11A).

Superficialis Muscles. The superficialis flexors primarily flex the proximal interphalangeal (PIP) joints. They operate independently of one another and thus are responsible for independent interphalangeal flexion of a single finger. If one checkreins the profundus tendon by holding other fingers in extension, the ability to flex the finger at the interphalangeal level is dependent upon the integrity of the superficialis mechanism (Fig. 50-11B).

Long Extensors. The extensor digitorum, the extensor digiti minimi, and the extensor indicis are prime extensors of the metacarpophalangeal joints of the fingers. Transection of the extensors to a single digit results in a flexion drop of the finger at the metacarpophalangeal joint and inability actively to extend it. The presence of intertendinous bridges leads to diagnostic errors by masking a proximal injury of a solitary extensor, since some extension will be retained. Independent extension exists only in the index and little fingers. Loss of this independence is diagnostic of transection or paralysis of the extensor indicis or extensor digiti minimi.

Intrinsic Muscular Function. Although there is considerable minor variation in the patterns of innervations of the intrinsic muscles of the hand, the classic pattern is generally reliable for proper diagnosis of nerve injuries.

The thenar muscles on the radial side of the flexor pollicis longus (abductor pollicis brevis, opponens pollicis, and superficial head of the flexor pollicis brevis), and the first two lumbrical muscles are innervated by the median nerve. The test for function of the thenar muscles is palmar abduction of the thumb into position for pulp-to-pulp opposition with the fingers (Fig. 50-12). One may readily observe tensing of the abductor pollicis brevis, the most superficial muscle in the thenar group.

The ulnar nerve innervates all the hypothenar and inter-

Fig. 50-11. Test for long digital flexors. *A*. Flexion of distal interphalangeal joint dependent upon profundus tendon. *B*. Flexion of proximal interphalangeal joint with remaining fingers checkreined is dependent upon an intact superficialis tendon. (*From R. A. Chase and D. R. Laub, The Hand: Therapeutic Strategy for Acute Problems, in "Current Problems in Surgery," Year Book Medical Publishers, Inc., Chicago, 1966. By permission of Year Book Medical Publishers, Inc.*)

osseous muscles and the third and fourth lumbricals. If innervation is lost to these muscles, the patient cannot abduct or adduct his fingers (Fig. 50-13*A*). This is particularly obvious when he attempts to abduct (radially) the index finger. One may readily observe tensing of the prominent first dorsal interosseous muscle in the first web space when ulnar nerve function is intact. The ulnar-innervated intrinsic muscles are responsible also for primary flexion of the metacarpophalangeal joints. If these joints can be held in flexion while the interphalangeal joints are in extension, ulnar-innervated intrinsic muscles are intact (Fig. 50-13*B*).

Retaining Ligaments. In recent years excellent descriptions of the structure and function of the retaining ligaments of the hand have been presented by Landsmeer, Kaplan, and Milford. These ligaments are dense, fibrous

Fig. 50-12. Test for median nerve–innervated intrinsic muscles in the thenar eminence. Palmar abduction of the thumb for pulp-to-pulp opposition of thumb with other digits is possible only with these muscles. (*From R. A. Chase and D. R. Laub, Therapeutic Strategy for Acute Problems, in "Current Problems in Surgery," Year Book Medical Publishers, Inc., Chicago, 1966. By permission of Year Book Medical Publishers, Inc.*)

MEDIAN INTRINSIC

Fig. 50-13. Testing for ulnar nerve–innervated intrinsic muscles of the hand. *A*. Abduction and adduction of the fingers. *B*. Flexion of the metacarpophalangeal joints with the interphalangeal joints in extension. (*From R. A. Chase and D. R. Laub, The Hand: Therapeutic Strategy for Acute Problems, in "Current Problems in Surgery," Year Book Medical Publishers, Inc., Chicago, 1966. By permission of Year Book Medical Publishers, Inc.*)

bundles that retain either the skin (Cleland's ligaments, Grayson's ligament, peritendinous ligaments) or the extensor mechanism (oblique retinacular ligament, transverse retinacular ligament, and the sagittal bands).

Cleland's cutaneous ligaments radiate in two planes on either side of the interphalangeal joints of each digit, connecting the joints to the skin. They lie dorsal to the digital neurovascular bundle; palmar to the bundle are similar fibers. Together, these fibers form a protective tunnel for the neurovascular structures. They are excellent surgical landmarks in finger exploration and are used in some reconstructions. The peritendinous fibers hold the skin creases in position over the respective interphalangeal joint.

The retaining ligaments of the extensor mechanism have more functional significance. The transverse retinacular ligament originates from the palmar aspect of the PIP joint capsule and flexor tendon sheath, passes superficial to the fibers of Cleland's ligament (acting as a sling for them), and inserts mainly on the lateral margin of the lateral tendon of the extensor mechanism. Its major function is to act as a stabilizer for the lateral tendon of the extensor mechanism. The oblique retinacular ligament is more tenuous in character. Its fibers arise from the bone of the distal fourth of the proximal phalanx and pass lateral to the lateral extensor tendon palmar to the axis of rotation of the

PIP joint when the joint is flexed. The fibers traverse distad along the palmar portion of the lateral bands and insert dorsal to the axis of rotation of the DIP joint. Because of its relation to these axes, this ligament does not allow easy flexion, either active or passive, of the DIP joint when the PIP joint is in extension. Contraction of this ligament, either in cases of arthritis or secondary to trauma, can cause constant hyperextension of the DIP joint when the PIP joint is partially extended; if the PIP joint becomes fully extended, it may prevent flexion of the DIP joint.

The sagittal bands originate from the deep transverse intermetacarpal ligament, project perpendicular to the long axis of the finger, and insert on the lateral margin of the extensor tendons. They actually continue over the dorsum of the tendon on the dorsum of the hand to become continuous with the sagittal bands of the opposite side of the digit. As pointed out by Tubiana, these structures are important in helping to balance the extensor and flexor mechanisms.

X-rays. X-rays should be considered for every major hand injury, not only to assess bone and joint injury but also to reveal radiopaque foreign bodies.

Vascular Integrity. The simple notation of color, capillary emptying and filling, peripheral pulses, bleeding, and temperature of the hand may require refinement by Allen's test for determining the integrity of vascular arches, and tourniquet blushing for evaluating blood supply to flaps of soft tissue or whole composite units of the hand. If the arm is emptied of blood by elevation and a pneumatic tourniquet is inflated to a level above systolic blood pressure, reactive hyperemia results when the tourniquet is released after 5 minutes of ischemia. This hyperemia may help demarcate the vascularized from the nonvascularized parts. Ultrasonic probes are also useful.

TREATMENT. The Wound. Initial wound care has been discussed in Chap. 8. Cleansing and debridement are particularly important, since the achievement of a closed wound at the earliest possible date is crucial to salvaging functional parts of the hand.

Exploration of Acute Wounds. When there is suspicion that deeper structures are injured, probing is contraindicated, because it may cause further injury and inoculate the wound with organisms which produce infection; functional testing can accurately determine the extent of injury. The wound is immediately and thoroughly cleansed and covered with a sterile protective dressing. Figure 50-14 shows the most common approaches for enlarging hand wounds to provide maximal exposure with minimal secondary scar or contracture.

Control of Hemorrhage. Vigorous bleeding rarely calls for clamping, since indiscriminate and/or successful efforts to clamp arteries can lead to median nerve (radial artery) or ulnar nerve (ulnar artery) injury. Furthermore, the artery itself should not be injured until decision for or against arterial repair is made. With the patient supine and the hand and extremity maximally elevated, external pressure should be applied. This will control bleeding in almost all situations. If not, a brachial tourniquet is applied after the limb is rendered ischemic, and under sterile conditions the bleeding vessel is clamped and ligated or the artery is

Fig. 50-14. Incisions for exploration of laceration following acute trauma. Flexion creases should not be traversed; if the laceration has traversed the crease, a Z-plasty should be created. Following the natural creases of the hand will give the best final scar. Incisions should be long enough to provide adequate exposure. When curved, the curve should be gradual to prevent long flaps. In the forearm, incisions should be transverse when possible; to provide exposure, a gently curved vertical component is required.

repaired; ×2 magnification is recommended to ensure nerve protection.

Principle of Delayed Closure. Most civilian injuries will qualify as "tidy" wounds for which primary closure of the skin with maximal repair of the tendons, nerves, and bones is indicated. Experiences with military injuries as well as with crushing injuries caused by farm instruments and industrial machines have shown that not all hand wounds should be closed immediately after injury. Staged closure is indicated for explosive injuries of the hand, considerable foreign body contamination, delay of initial treatment, or significant crush injury. In these situations, an initial debridement is accomplished and the hand reevaluated for closure 72 to 96 hours later. It is well to reemphasize that most civilian hand injuries should be closed primarily; only the unusual, difficult, and/or contaminated wounds should be considered for staged management.

Wringer Injuries. A very common injury, particularly of the very young or very old, is crushing of a hand and upper limb by the wringer of a washing machine. This must be differentiated from the severe crushes seen from industrial or farm machinery in which there is frequently complicating deep tissue destruction, impending ischemia, and severe burns. Most victims of home wringer injuries will require only the wound care and/or suturing needed at the initial examination. Even though 25 percent of the patients will need surgery later, this is commonly a small skin graft to replace the skin lost by the friction burns; the need for subsequent grafting can almost always be determined reliably at the time of the initial examination. Less frequently will there be nerve injury, hematoma or edema leading to vascular occlusion or nerve pressure. This may require fasciotomy of the hand or forearm. Dislocation of joints and fractures may result during more severe wringer injuries. The possibility of a developing Volkmann's ischemic contracture must not be overlooked, but the occurrence after a home wringer injury is not common.

Recommended treatment involves evaluation of the history and experienced examination of the skin, nerves, and pulse; x-rays only if there are signs of fractures; suture of lacerations; and application of an absorptive noncompressive dressing with an incorporated splint to keep the elbow straight and the wrist extended. Hospitalization is recommended for those patients in whom there is doubt raised by the physical findings or by the judgment that the parents cannot assume the responsibility for reliable outpatient care.

Patients with complex wringer injuries obviously will need to be hospitalized and will probably require early debridement and either prompt or staged skin coverage by grafting or by flaps. Fasciotomies may be necessary. Definitive nerve, tendon, or bone surgery is delayed except for stabilization of obviously unstable bone fragments. If blood vessels are damaged, they must be repaired initially, either by suture or by graft, or be ligated.

Crush Syndrome after Limb Compression. An increasing and easily overlooked problem produced by the growing number of drug addicts is the appearance of the crush syndrome in a comatose patient. The weight of the patient's body upon an extremity compromises the vascularity, resulting in erythema, induration, ulceration, vesiculation, and paralysis. Swelling of the limb may not be seen early but always develops subsequently. An early reliable sign of impending muscle damage is increased turgor involving a muscle compartment, with pain on passive muscle stretch. Myoglobinemia and myoglobinuria should be tested for as evidence of muscle necrosis. Nerve involve-

ment will be indicated by both sensory and motor loss. The peripheral pulse will frequently be normal upon palpation. Recognition of the crush syndrome is critical because prompt replacement of fluid deficits and careful renal management will diminish the threat of renal shutdown and early fasciotomy may preserve the function of the involved limb by decreasing the severity of damage to nerves and muscles.

The Injured Fingertip. Lacerations should be meticulously debrided and closed as soon as possible. If the nail bed is injured, it should be approximated carefully. When crush injury is involved, conservative amputation may be indicated. In some people, a crush injury will produce a secondarily painful fingertip; however, a secondary amputation in a few months is preferable to an immediate amputation unless there is loss of viability immediately after the injury. Distal transverse amputations are best treated with a thin split-thickness skin graft on the end of the tip. If the absent tissue contained the pulp and the bone or a tendon is exposed, a cross finger flap should be considered. If the pulp injury preserves the pad, a free full-thickness skin graft is satisfactory. Fractures of the tuft of the distal phalanx rarely require internal fixation. If they are badly comminuted and lack sufficient tissue cover, shortening them and covering them with available local tissues or covering the stump with a free skin graft are the procedures of choice. If the bone is not fractured but is uncovered by loss of soft tissues at the fingertip, flap tissue either from an adjoining finger or from the palm will preserve the length of the finger and give it a protective covering with reasonable sensibility.

Nerve Injury. Injury to peripheral nerves results in a specific pattern of sensory and motor loss. Ultimate recovery may depend upon proper surgical management of the injured nerve.

Nerve Transection. There has been much debate over whether peripheral nerves should be repaired at the time of initial wound therapy or secondarily after a short delay. In sharp transections a precise repair should be done primarily in any wound clean enough to close primarily. Careful realignment of funiculi is aided by realigning the tiny blood vessels found on the nerve surface. Fine nonabsorbable sutures placed only in the nerve sheath should be used (Fig. 50-15).

Nerves may be successfully repaired as far distally as the proximal third of the distal phalanges. Arborization of digital nerves beyond this point makes nerve repair difficult. Adequate regeneration for protective sensibility occurs with precise wound closure alone. Microsurgery, using extremely small nylon suture material, improves the repair significantly by allowing accurate separate suture of major funiculi in a large mixed peripheral nerve.

Purposeful or unintentional delay in repairing a peripheral nerve does not measurably alter the ultimate result unless the delay interval is extensive; delayed repair in the first 3 months after nerve transection may achieve a result indistinguishable from that following primary repair. The axons at the proximal cut end of the nerve sprout and attempt to regrow distally. In a receptive distal nerve sheath where wallerian axonal degeneration occurs, the

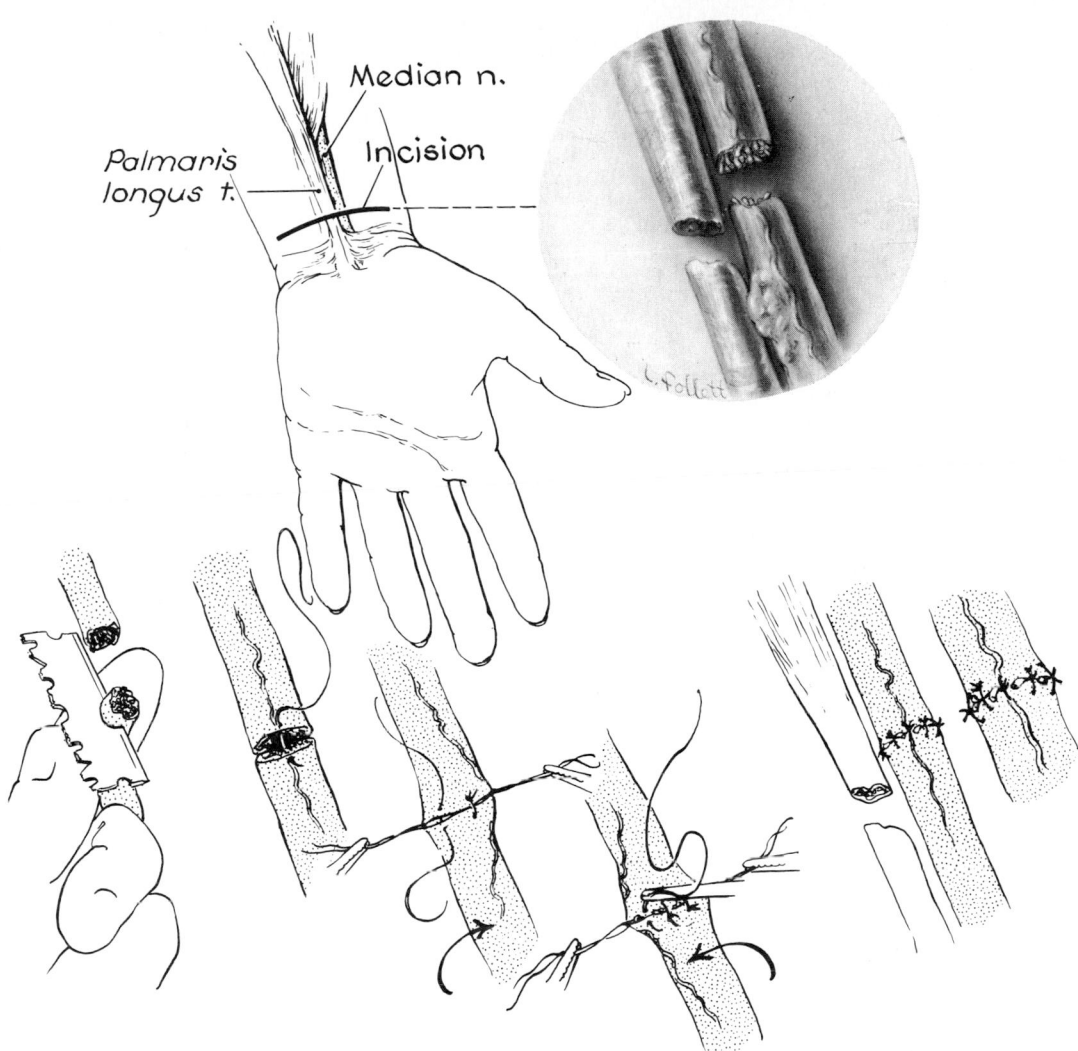

Fig. 50-15. Technique of nerve repair, showing sharp retransection, sutures in the sheath only, and careful axial alignment using surface blood vessel as a guide. (*From R. A. Chase and D. R. Laub, The Hand: Therapeutic Strategy for Acute Problems, in "Current Problems in Surgery," Year Book Medical Publishers, Inc., Chicago, 1966. By permission of Year Book Medical Publishers, Inc.*)

regrowing axons are directed to peripheral sensory end organs and motor end plates. As time passes, the peripheral sheath becomes less receptive, and denervation atrophy in peripheral muscles makes them nonreceptive to reinnervation. The time scale is variable, but generally nerve repair is progressively less effective after 6 months after injury. After 2 years results are generally poor, but there are enough exceptions to make late repair worthwhile.

Recovery after nerve repair progresses in a predictable manner. Sensibility return starts at the proximal area of anesthesia and moves distally as the axons regenerate and grow down the sheath. Nerve regeneration proceeds, on the average, at the rate of 1 mm/day, but this varies depending on the site (proximal regeneration is faster than peripheral) and the age of the patient (regeneration is faster and more complete in young children than in adults). Regeneration may be followed clinically by observation of the distal progress of Tinel's sign, an electric-shock-like sensation on percussion over the regenerating nerve; specific sensibility testing; motor return observation; electromyography; and sudomotor testing (Fig. 50-16).

Nerve Stretching or Compression. Injuries which do not transect the nerve have a better prognosis and faster recovery than those involving nerve transection. Electromyography may be very helpful in assessing the nature of a closed injury to a peripheral nerve. If compression can be released and stretching relaxed by appropriate surgical treatment and splinting, no direct nerve operation is necessary.

Nerve Gaps. Millesi et al. have made a major recent contribution by demonstrating that when injury results in a loss of nerve substance, the best results are achieved if the nerve gap is overcome by accurate interposition of fascicular nerve autografts. The key to his successes, corroborated by the authors and others, is the absence of any tension

ELECTROMYOGRAPHY

RETURN OF
MOTOR FUNCTION

SUDOMOTOR FUNCTION
(MOBERG)

NERVE BLOCK

POSITIVE TINEL'S SIGN

RETURN OF SENSATION

ELECTRICAL STIMULATION

Fig. 50-16. Methods of assessment of recovery following nerve injury. (*From R. A. Chase and D. R. Laub, The Hand: Therapeutic Strategy for Acute Problems, in "Current Problems in Surgery," Year Book Medical Publishers, Inc., Chicago, 1966. By permission of Year Book Medical Publishers, Inc.*)

upon the proximal or distal suture lines. The results are much superior to those previously achieved by rerouting the peripheral nerve and positioning joints to gain enough length in the nerve to overcome the nerve gap. Unfortunately, nerve homografts (allografts) are not successful. Thus, the patient exchanges one deficit for another, since a donor nerve must be used with resulting loss of its prime function. The best donor for nerve is the sural. Allografts of nerve, notoriously unsuccessful in the past, remain so despite efforts to decrease their antigenicity by immunosuppressive agents.

Neuroma. When a peripheral nerve is left unrepaired, the sprouting axons at the proximal cut end form a tumor mass with local fibroblasts. This neuroma is tender to palpation and percussion, and electric-shock-like sensations interpreted as coming from the area previously innervated are bothersome. The best treatment is nerve repair, directing the axons peripherally. When this cannot be done, the cut nerve end should be placed deep in soft tissue away from the superficial scar. Protection from repeated trauma may serve to relieve the symptoms.

Substitution after Nerve Injury. Where peripheral nerve function is permanently lost, sensibility reorientation peripherally, appropriate tendon transfers, and selected arthrodeses may be substituted.

Restoration of Sensibility. When peripheral nerve repair or grafting is impossible, alternative measures for restoring sensibility may be considered. Nerve crossing by transfer of a digital nerve from a secondary digit to a prime digit has been used. The restored sensibility is not as normal or exact as that resulting from transfer of the nerve together with a patch of its innervated soft tissue on a vascular pedicle. The versatility of such innervated and vascularized islands of skin and subcutaneous tissue is great. The radial arrangement of the digital vessels and nerves

lends itself to this method. A prime digit such as the thumb may be restored by simultaneous correction of skin and sensory deficit, using an island pedicle flap from the protected sides of the long or ring fingers. The transferred sensibility is precise and immediate, although the switch does result in misidentification of the source of a stimulus; i.e., a touch stimulus on the thumb resurfaced by an island pedicle from the long finger will be interpreted as a touch on the long finger in the early period after transfer and sometimes permanently.

Substitution for Irreversible Motor Paralysis. When there is irreversible paralysis of muscles innervated by a peripheral nerve, muscles innervated by intact motor nerves may be transferred to overcome lost function. For example, when the median nerve is irreversibly damaged, usable muscles innervated by the radial and ulnar nerves are transferred to substitute for the paralyzed muscles. There are several standard patterns of tendon transfers and many additional individually tailored transfers.

Median Nerve Palsy. Low median nerve loss (wrist level) results in paralysis of the thenar thumb-positioning muscles (abductor pollicis brevis, opponens pollicis, and superficial head of the flexor pollicis brevis) and the radial two lumbricals. The important functional deficit is inability to position the thumb for proper pulp-to-pulp opposition with the fingers. Transfer of the tendon of an unparalyzed muscle (e.g., ring finger superficialis) to the insertion of the abductor pollicis brevis will substitute its pull for that of the median-innervated thenar muscles.

High median nerve palsy produces the same pattern of

peripheral intrinsic muscular paralysis plus paralysis of the flexor carpi radialis, all superficialis muscles, the flexor pollicis longus, the profundus muscles to the index finger, and the pronators (teres and quadratus). The serious functional deficit is loss of phalangeal flexion in the thumb and index finger and diminished strength and independence of flexion in all fingers. The ulnar-innervated abductor digiti minimi may be swung across the palm as an opponens substitute. The index finger profundus tendon and even the flexor pollicis longus may be sutured side-to-side to the intact ulnar-innervated profundus tendons above the wrist.

Ulnar Nerve Palsy. All the intrinsic muscles of the hand except the thenar thumb-positioning muscles and the radial two lumbricals are paralyzed by interruption of the ulnar nerve at the wrist. If the ulnar nerve is interrupted before it enters the forearm, the flexor carpi ulnaris and the ulnar two or three profundus muscles are also paralyzed. Functionally, the important loss is in the hand, with paralysis of the intrinsic muscles as evidenced by loss of isolated flexion of the metacarpophalangeal joints of the fingers and strong side pinch between the thumb and fingers. Claw deformity results, because the metacarpophalangeal extensors are unopposed. As the metacarpophalangeal joints are pulled into extension and hyperextension, the effect of the long flexors on the interphalangeal joints is accentuated, and clawing (intrinsic minus) position is assumed. This is less marked with high ulnar nerve paralysis, since the profundus flexors are also paralyzed.

Any procedure which restricts hyperextension of the metacarpophalangeal joints is helpful (volar plate advancement, or tenodesis). One of several specific muscle substitutions is the Brand operation, which substitutes a major wrist extensor (extensor carpi radialis longus) for the interossei. In this operation a tendon graft divided into four separate tails routed below the intermetacarpal ligaments and inserted into the lateral bands of the fingers creates a dynamic substitute for the digital intrinsic function. An abductor pollicis substitution using a superficialis tendon from a finger with an intact profundus is commonly done in combination with the Brand operation.

Radial Nerve Palsy. Radial nerve interruption at the axilla or interruption of its motor branches in the proximal half of the arm results in paralysis of the triceps muscle. The radial nerve passes through the spiral groove of the humerus and enters the forearm adjacent to the brachioradialis, which it innervates. It then passes through the supinator muscle to innervate it as well as the wrist and digital extensors. Thus if the radial nerve itself is interrupted, the extensor-supinator group of muscles in the forearm is paralyzed.

The most serious disability results from paralysis of the major wrist extensors (extensor carpi radialis longus and brevis). This may be overcome by releasing the pronator teres from its insertion on the radius and transferring it to the wrist extensors. These are immediately superficial to the pronator insertion and need not be interrupted for the surgical insertion of the tendinous portion of the pronator teres.

Other muscles available for transfer as substitutes for muscles paralyzed by radial nerve interruption are the median- and ulnar-innervated superficial palmar forearm muscles. A variety of transfers of the flexor carpi radialis, flexor carpi ulnaris, palmaris longus, and superficialis tendons can supply motor power to the finger and thumb extensors.

Tendon Injuries. The healing of a tendon is a dynamic event dependent upon local cellular activity. In this respect there is no basic difference initially from the healing of any other injured structure. Because of the relative avascular nature of tendons, the slow metabolism of the very few cells within the tendon substance, and the great reactivity of the vascular pedicle (mesotendon) and the layering covering structures, later phases of tendon healing are somewhat different. Later healing is further influenced by the physicochemical nature of the milieu, remodeling of the tendon callus, and differential development of tendon healing and gliding capability (see Chap. 8). Atraumatic repair must bring cut tendon ends into precise coaptation without interfering seriously with the physiologic elements important for healing and callus differentiation (Fig. 50-17). Technical finesse will contribute to the final result by minimizing scar formation. However, there remain many situations where unavoidable adhesions negate good results. Many efforts are being aimed at systemic control of scar tissue (see Chap. 8). In addition, the local use of silicone rods to create channels for tendon sliding has proved useful in special circumstances. Specific treatment for individual tendon injuries varies greatly because of differences in anatomy and functional demands on each tendon or group of tendons in the hand.

Extensor Tendon Injuries. The relatively short excursion of the long extensors of the digits and their location in loose areolar tissue favors a good prognosis after injury and repair. Adhesions between the tendon at its site of injury and the overlying skin wound rarely restrict function significantly, because the mobility of the dorsal hand and

Fig. 50-17. Technique of end-to-end tendon repair using double-armed, single nonabsorbable suture with final knot away from repair site. (*From R. A. Chase and D. R. Laub, The Hand: Therapeutic Strategy for Acute Problems, in "Current Problems in Surgery," Year Book Medical Publishers, Inc., Chicago, 1966. By permission of Year Book Medical Publishers, Inc.*)

Fig. 50-18. X-ray of mallet finger deformity. Because a significant surface of the DIP joint is fractured, open reduction of this closed fracture is indicated. Most situations are handled by closed reduction and internal fixation.

finger skin is as great as the physiologic excursion of the extensor tendons.

Injuries to the Extensor Mechanism on the Hand. The technique of repair can be that shown in Figure 50-17 or the figure-of-eight pullout technique using wire or other nonabsorbable suture material (Fig. 50-18). The latter uses the skin as a backing, thus avoiding the pulling of sutures through the longitudinally aligned extensor tendon fibers. Postoperative splinting is for 5 weeks with the wrist and metacarpophalangeal joints in extension the entire time. The PIP joint should be held in extension for 2 weeks and then placed in 15° of flexion.

Fig. 50-19. Closed reduction and internal fixation of mallet finger deformity. The PIP joint is kept in mild flexion by a dorsal splint.

Injuries to the Extensor Mechanism in the Finger

Boutonniere Deformity. Transection of the central extensor tendon near its insertion into the middle phalanx is frequently accompanied by a tear in its lateral extension into the lateral bands. This results in displacement of the lateral bands palmar to the axis of rotation of the PIP joint, causing the bands to lose their extensor function at this joint and to actually become PIP joint flexors. The joint loses both its extrinsic and its intrinsic extensors and assumes an attitude of flexion. Attempts to extend the joint actively accentuate its flexion and are transmitted to the DIP joint through the lateral bands and the oblique retinacular ligament, causing hyperextension of the DIP joint. The defect in the digital extensor apparatus assumes the shape of a buttonhole, through which the PIP joint protrudes.

The injury creating this acute boutonniere deformity is usually a laceration but may be a closed injury. In the closed injuries, immobilization of the PIP joint in extension and usually the whole finger and wrist as well for a 5-week period will avoid the chronic progressive deformity. If the injury is a laceration, the extensor mechanism should be repaired and the same immobilization schedule followed.

Dropped Tip, or Mallet, Finger. Injuries of the extensor insertion into the distal phalanx are common and challenging. The closed injury, such as a baseball finger or the pressure of a football or other object on the end of the finger, causes an avulsion of the insertion of the extensor mechanism. X-rays must be taken to determine the presence or absence of an associated avulsion fracture of the distal phalanx. The configuration of the associated fracture may determine proper management. If a minimal amount of the joint surface is involved, closed reduction and correct joint positioning is the treatment of choice. The PIP joint should be kept flexed for 2 weeks, using an external splint (Fig. 50-19). The DIP joint should be kept at 0°, not in hyperextension; a temporary internal fixation using a Kirschner wire across this joint for 6 weeks is the most secure means of immobilization. After 2 weeks DIP joint fixation by the wire is supplemented with a volar splint, and splinting of the PIP joint is discontinued and mild active and passive flexion begun. After 6 weeks the wire is removed and graded exercise begun for the DIP joint.

Flexor Tendon Injuries. The management of lacerations of flexor tendons of the forearm, wrist, hand, and fingers has been the subject of debate for many years. There are no absolute rules for correct treatment, but several facts should be considered. An injury which involves several tendons, nerves, vessels, surrounding fascia, joints, and soft tissues heals as a single wound. Tendons with repairs in contact with one another are very likely to become adherent to one another as healing progresses. Wherever a tendon repair is adjacent to a fixed fibrous structure, it may become fixed to it by scar tissue. The flexor tendon anatomy is such that there are certain sites where the functional success following primary repair is poor. Better understanding of anatomy and physiology and technical advances during the past several years have improved the prognosis for these situations.

The long flexor tendons (superficialis and profundus) in each digit pass through a rigid tunnel of fascia which extends from the distal palmar crease to the middle phalanx, providing the necessary mechanical action to prevent ventral bowstringing during flexion. In addition there is a major pulley mechanism at the wrist, where the thick, resistant, fibrous flexor retinaculum constitutes the roof of the carpal tunnel.

Forearm lacerations involving multiple tendons will commonly lacerate the median or ulnar nerves, or both. All the involved structures should be repaired primarily. In the wrist portion, because of the unyielding nature of the fibrous retinaculum, rarely are all the tendons within the carpal tunnel actually sectioned. If all these tendons are lacerated, only the profundus tendons and flexor pollicus longus should be repaired. Elimination of repair of the superficialis tendons gives more space within the tight tunnel and better functional results.

Verdan (Fig. 50-20) has designated six zones of the hand correlated with prognosis. Zone 1, distal to the digital tunnel, is an area where prognosis is good. Repair of the profundus tendon should be performed primarily at this level. In zone 6, the wrist area, only the profundus tendon should be repaired. In zone 5, in the palm, both the superficial and profundus tendons should be repaired. Tendon lacerations in zone 2, "no-man's-land," the region of the fibrous digital tunnel, remain controversial in terms of treatment. For children, all surgeons agree on primary repair of the profundus tendon or the flexor pollicis longus. In adults, the trend appears to be toward immediate repair of the profundus tendon in the digit provided the laceration is clean, there is minimal associated injury (at least one digital nerve intact), and treatment is prompt. Proper attention to technique, good wound care, and early and intensive physiotherapy seem to produce adequate results in the hands of some surgeons following primary repair at this level. An alternative procedure, thorough wound toilet and only primary skin closure and digital nerve repair as necessary initially, may be performed when there has been a jagged laceration, if treatment is delayed, or by the surgeon's preference. After the digit has been mobilized passively and after a suitable delay for wound healing, a free or attached tendon graft is performed. One anastomosis then is placed in the palm, where there is no fixed fibrous sheath, and the other is at the site of insertion on the distal phalanx. In this circumstance, anastomosis is usually made by end-to-end suturing (Fig. 50-17). The distal anastomosis is made at the site of tendon insertion in the distal phalanx, where there is no need for sliding (Fig. 50-21, 50-22).

Hand Amputation

Hand amputations should follow careful assessment of critical levels of function and appearance for each digit (Fig. 50-23). Preservation of bony architecture to encourage stronger grasp is preferable for manual laborers (Fig. 50-24A), while people who require finer movements and/or are predominantly concerned with appearance have different functional and aesthetic needs (Fig. 50-24B).

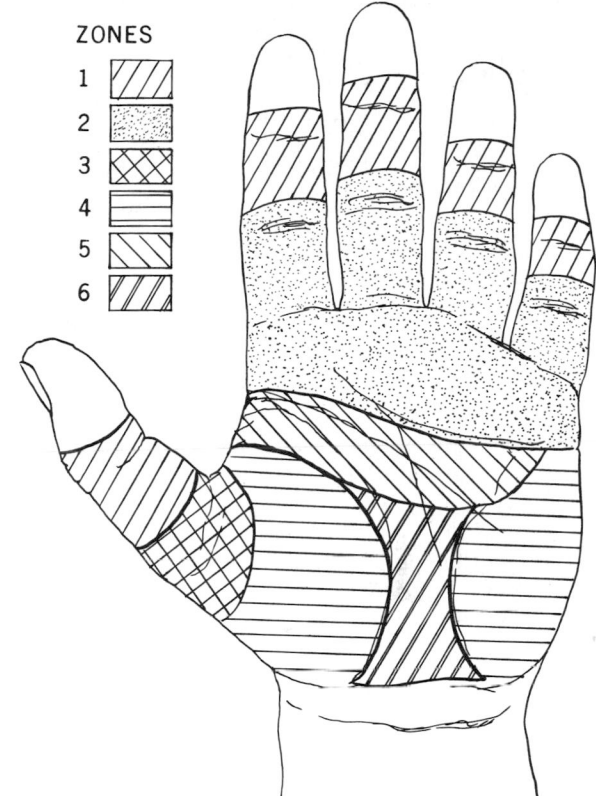

ZONES
1
2
3
4
5
6

Fig. 50-20. Verdan's zones of flexor injury.

With injuries to many digits, normally unimportant digits or partial digit lengths attain prime importance after partial or complete amputation of the damaged digits.

The thumb is the most important digit by virtue of being the opposable unit for all the fingers. Any length which can be salvaged by conservative surgical treatment should be preserved. When an injury results in loss of soft tissue in excess of bone, the protruding bone should be preserved by immediate coverage with vascularized soft tissue, using a local or distant pedicle flap or even a primary vascularized island pedicle flap.

The peripheral fingers (index and little fingers), if foreshortened seriously, may be best treated by ray amputation (amputation through the proximal metacarpal), particularly if there is associated metacarpophalangeal joint injury. The index finger is very important and versatile. It functions primarily by pinching and manipulating with its pulp opposing the pulp of the thumb. Any amputation of the index finger proximal to the PIP joint leaves insufficient length for useful pinching. It then becomes an impinging nub in the new web space between the thumb and the middle finger, which assumes the role of primary pinching finger. Therefore, all length possible should be saved in amputations distal to the PIP joint, but when amputation is proximal to this joint, immediate closure by further shortening may be done. Within the first few months after injury, an index finger may become stiff and painful or may lack sensation, deterring rehabilitation of the rest of the hand. Early amputation of an index finger, including

Fig. 50-21. Atraumatic, removable suture technique for distal attachment of profundus tendon or a tendon graft. A flexible, strong, and slippery material has replaced wire; this simplifies the placement of the suture and allows distal removal in a more efficient and painless manner.

the second metacarpal, may well result in the best final cosmetic and functional result.

Even when the central fingers (the middle and ring) are amputated, they can contribute to efficient handling of small objects as long as some of the proximal phalanx remains. Thus any salvage of length beyond the metacarpophalangeal joint is helpful. If the injury is confined to a central finger, there is no reason to use complicated procedures to preserve length. The traumatic amputation may be immediately revised and closed. Amputation at the metacarpophalangeal joint leaves a space between digits with the hand cupped or in a fist. If this creates palmar incontinence, allowing small objects to fall through the resulting space, transfer of the adjacent peripheral finger and its metacarpal should be considered.

Amputation of all fingers and the thumb at the metacarpophalangeal joint level leaves an endpiece for a hand which has little function. Later reconstruction to increase

function should include deepening of the space between the thumb metacarpal and the rest of the hand.

Replantation of Amputated Digits

With the advent of blood vessel repair and more recently with refinement of microsurgical repair of vessels, many reports have appeared of replantation of amputated portions of the upper limb. Initially, replantation of whole arms or of arms amputated through the forearm was reported. This has been followed in the last several years by reports of replantation of digits or parts of digits. These technical triumphs have opened up new opportunities to salvage hand elements that heretofore were irreversibly lost.

Whenever new technology develops, there follows a period during which sensible indications for use of that technology settle in place. In the case of replantation it is particularly important that sound reasoning be applied to indications and more significantly to contraindications for its application. To achieve survival of a part which is useless or even detrimental can represent a serious breach of the doctrine, "first, do no harm."

Some principles in replantation surgery are well established.

1. The replantable part must be important enough to balance the risk of the procedure.
2. The prospect of subsequent useful function after replantation must be adequate to make the part worthy of replantation.
3. The risks of the procedure must be assessed by carefully noting the patient's general health and associated injuries or disorders requiring simultaneous treatment.
4. All the technical requisites must be met including (*a*) the condition of the amputated part, (*b*) nature of the wound, (*c*) time elapsed since amputation, (*d*) status of the amputation site, (*e*) facilities and professional team.

Fig. 50-22. A variation of distal profundus tendon or graft insertion.

In general the farther distal the amputation occurs with a replantable part, the better the final return of sensibility and function will be. Except under unusual circumstances, replantation of single fingers in the absence of other digital losses is not indicated. Amputation of the thumb is an indication for surgical replantation when it is technically possible. Amputation through the hand and wrist or low forearm is an ideal level in terms of indication for replantation, all other things being equal. Amputations above the elbow may be an indication for replantation, particularly in children. Even if hand function fails to return and distal sensibility is lost to the point that elective amputation and prosthesis replacement are decided upon, salvage of a functional elbow by replantation makes rehabilitation by prosthesis far better than amputation at the original level.

With replantation at its present level of reliability, it behooves the surgeon who first sees the patient suffering an amputation to know how to handle the wound and amputated part prior to transfer of the patient to the replantation team for decision and definitive treatment. The wound should be treated with as little manipulation as possible to avoid further injury to the cut vessels and nerves. A tourniquet or pressure dressing is preferable to instrumentation of the wound for hemostasis. The amputated part should be kept clean in sterile dressings and when possible it should be placed in a plastic bag and kept in a cool atmosphere (4°C) but not a freezing one. Placing the watertight, wrapped part on ice is appropriate, but the part should not be immersed in fluid unprotected.

If decision of the replantation team is to attempt replantation, veins, arteries, nerves, and selected tendons will be repaired after skeletal fixation is achieved. Sometimes repeated procedures must be done in the first several days if vessel occlusion occurs.

ELECTIVE INCISIONS

Elective incisions in the hand must be planned to avoid contractures and to avoid scars in an area of importance for sensory perception.

Scars lack elasticity and have a tendency to heal by contraction. Any scar which ends up where stretching of its length is important for full function will cause disability. Thus scars on the palmar surface of the hand where the skin is tethered to the underlying palmar fascia should not cross the hand creases without changing direction. When the fingers are fully flexed there are areas where palm skin from one phalanx contacts that of another like the pages of a book. The diamond-shaped area of contact is like similar areas at all major palmar creases (see Fig. 50-25). Any incision crossing from one-half of the diamond to the other across the crease may result in contracture as the wound heals. One may elect freely to make incisions which do not violate this principle.

POSTOPERATIVE CARE

Success following surgery or trauma to the hand is facilitated by the control of pain, principally by appropriate

Save all possible length, unless crushed

Can be shortened for good coverage

Fig. 50-23. The recommended levels for elective amputations or for completion of traumatic amputations.

rest and elevation. Comfortable elevation of the traumatized hand by a compressive nonconstricting immobilization dressing is a cardinal principle. Supportive drugs (analgesics, narcotics, tranquilizers, and sedatives) should be administered to ensure rest, relieve anxiety, and control pain. Activity of adjacent parts that do not need rest is extremely important in reducing sensitivity to pain; exercise of the shoulder and elbow can be most helpful for early rehabilitation. Patient motivation, including preoperative, operative, and postoperative encouragement and reassurance, is another key to rapid and successful rehabilitation.

Early hand motion is important. The earliest day to start active motion, guarded passive motion, energetic passive motion, dynamic splinting, or whirlpool manipulations is determined by the injury received and the procedure per-

A

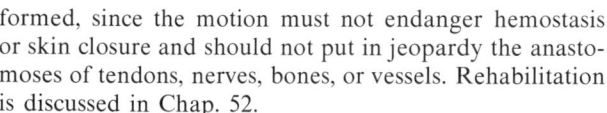

Preserve

Less important

Amputate

B

Fig. 50-24. Recommended levels for amputation in the hand, showing the bony architecture. *A.* For those requiring heavy-labor strength. *B.* This variation may be more critical for patients who need fine motion or for whom appearance is of paramount importance. Efforts to maintain extra digital length must be correlated to the sensation possible in the covering skin.

formed, since the motion must not endanger hemostasis or skin closure and should not put in jeopardy the anastomoses of tendons, nerves, bones, or vessels. Rehabilitation is discussed in Chap. 52.

Unusual Pain Syndromes

Some discomfort is to be expected after operations on the hand. Since it is used to perceive and evaluate the environment, the hand has a concentration of sensory nerves and end organs. It is sensitive to ischemia resulting from swelling or compression; thus when pain occurs postoperatively, the surgeon must examine the hand sufficiently to assure himself that there is no impending or existing complication.

When pain persists or appears after healing is complete, thorough diagnostic evaluation is mandatory. Pain may be a result of continuing ischemia, as when marginal blood supply remains after a severe injury. Nerve injuries with resulting neuroma at the injury site may give rise to pain from repeated trauma to the neuroma site.

Very trying for the patient and the surgeon are the sympathetic dystrophies which occur after hand injuries or operations. True causalgia (burning pain) generally follows partial nerve injuries in the limb. This is a disabling syndrome consisting of severe burning pain set off by motion of the part, touching the part, and even emotional trials. Sympathetic outflow touches off the pain, and it is commonly relieved by sympathetic stellate ganglion block. Such treatment and even sympathectomy should be instituted early.

Other forms of reflex sympathetic dystrophy may occur after hand and arm injuries. Vascular syndromes with coldness, cyanosis, and atrophic changes in the skin and nails may predominate, or osseous atrophy (Sudeck's atrophy) may be prominent in sympathetic dystrophies. Elements within the healing wound which might trigger such reflex dystrophies should be corrected as the first therapeu-

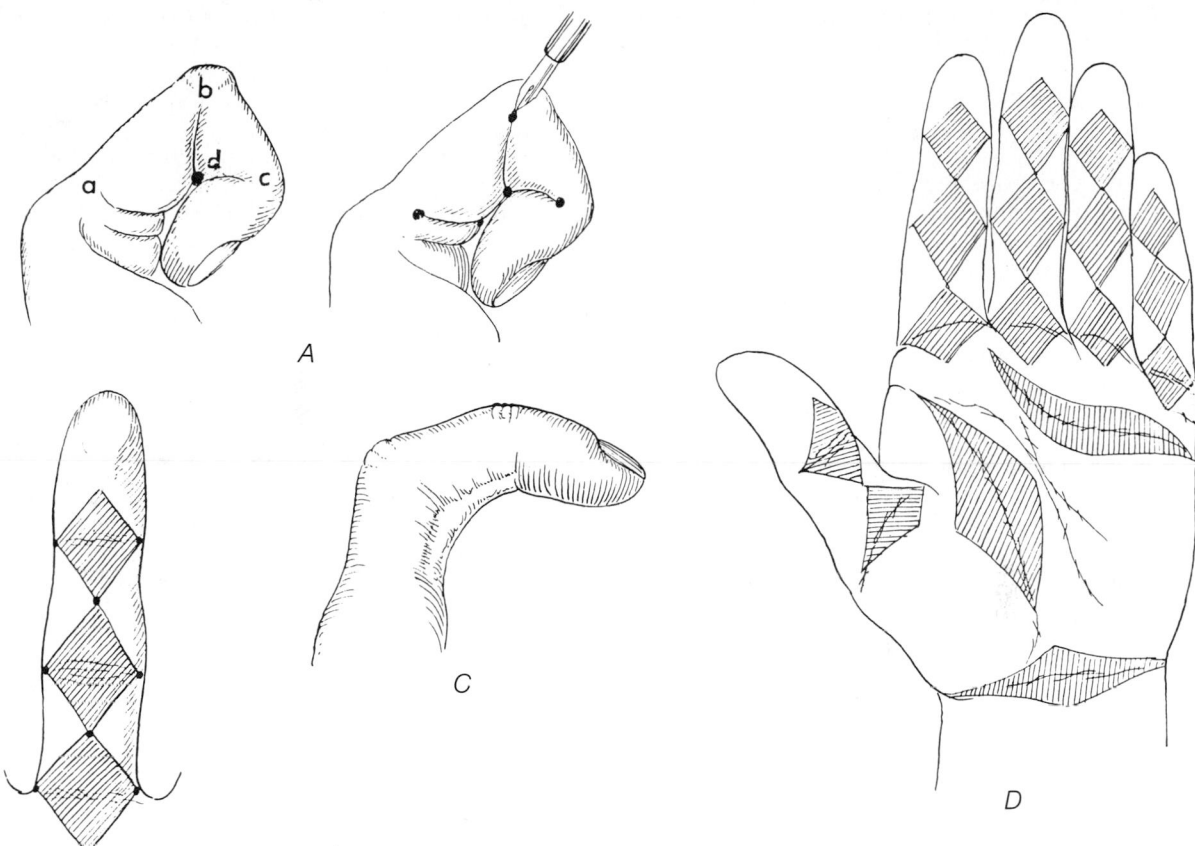

Fig. 50-25. In maximum flexion, skin folding results in skin-to-skin contact in diamond-shaped areas. Any incision which crosses from one-half of the diamond to its contact area in the other half may result in flexion contracture as the wound heals. *A.* In each of the fingers the contact areas may be seen by flexing the finger, marking the dorsal extent of each skin crease (*a, b,* and *c*), and marking the point of contact in the palmar midline where skin from all three finger segments meets. *B.* Extension of the finger and connection of these marks by lines makes visible the contact triangles. *C.* Any longitudinal incision crossing from proximal to distal triangle across flexion creases may result in flexion contracture. *D.* The same incision principles must be adhered to in contact areas at flexion creases in the hand and wrist if contracture and concomitant scar hypertrophy are to be avoided. Free choice of incision may then be made as long as none of the diamonds resulting are crossed from contact surface to contact surface.

tic approach. For example, neuromas should be excised, unhealed areas should be covered with skin, crushed useless finger parts should be amputated, and irreversible ischemic elements should be removed.

Some of the persistent pain syndromes may be amenable to psychotherapy, transcutaneous sensory counterstimulation, or physiotherapy; some are relieved simply by time.

References

Babcock, W. W.: Standard Techniques for Operations of Peripheral Nerves with Special Reference to Closure of Large Gaps, *Surg Gynecol Obstet,* **45:**364, 1927.

Bailey, D. A.: "The Infected Hand," Harper & Row, Publishers, Incorporated, New York, 1963.

Barsky, A. J.: "Congenital Anomalies of the Hand and Their Surgical Treatment," Charles C Thomas, Publisher, Springfield, Ill., 1958.

Baxter, C. R.: Surgical Management of Soft Tissue Infections, *Surg Clin North Am,* **52:**1483, 1972.

Bonica, J.: Regional Anesthesia for Surgery, *Clin Anesth,* **2:**123, 1969.

Boyes, J. H.: "Bunnell's Surgery of the Hand," 5th ed., J. B. Lippincott Company, Philadelphia, 1970.

—— and Stark, H. H.: Flexor-Tendon Grafts in the Fingers and Thumb: A Study of Factors Influencing Results in 1000 Cases, *J Bone Joint Surg [Am],* **53A:**1332, 1971.

Chase, R. A.: "Atlas of Hand Surgery," W. B. Saunders Company, Philadelphia, 1973.

—— and Laub, D. R.: The Hand: Therapeutic Strategy for Acute Problems, June, *Curr Probl Surg,* 1966.

Chong, J. K., Cramer, L. M., and Culf, N. K.: Combined Two-Stage Tenoplasty with Silicone Rods for Multiple Flexor-Tendon Injuries in "No-Man's-Land," *J Trauma,* **12:**104, 1972.

Cramer, L. M., and Chase, R. A.: "Symposium on the Hand," The C. V. Mosby Company, St. Louis, 1971.

Edshage, S.: Peripheral Nerve Suture, *Acta Chir Scand [Suppl],* **3:**31, 1964.

El Shami, I. N.: Congenital Partial Gigantism, *J Surg,* **65:**683, 1969.

Guth, L.: Degeneration in Mammalian Peripheral Nervous System, *Physiol Rev,* **36:**441, 1956.

Hunter, J. M., and Salisbury, R. E.: Flexor-Tendon Reconstruction in Severely Damaged Hands, *J Bone Joint Surg [Am]*, **53A:**829, 1971.

Kanavel, A. B.: "Infections of the Hand," Lea & Febiger, Philadelphia, 1912.

Kaplan, E. B.: "Functional and Surgical Anatomy of the Hand," 2d ed., J. B. Lippincott Company, Philadelphia, 1965.

Landsmeer, J.: The Anatomy of the Dorsal Aponeurosis of the Human Finger and Its Functional Significance, *Anat Rec,* **104:**31, 1949.

Lendvay, P., and Owen, E.: Microvascular Repair of Completely Severed Digits, *Med J Aust,* **2:**818, 1970.

Lucas, G. L.: "Examination of the Hand," Charles C Thomas, Publisher, Springfield, Ill., 1972.

Milford, L. W.: "Retaining Ligaments of the Digits of the Hand," W. B. Saunders Company, Philadelphia, 1968.

————: "The Hand," The C. V. Mosby Company, St. Louis, 1971.

Millesi, H., Meissl, G., and Berger, A.: The Interfascicular Nerve-Grafting of the Median and Ulnar Nerves, *J Bone Joint Surg [Am]*, **54A:**727, 1972.

Minkowitz, S., and Minkowitz, F.: A Morphological Study of Macrodactylism, *J Pathol,* **90:**323, 1965.

Moberg, E.: Objective Methods for Determining the Functional Value of Sensibility in the Skin, *J Bone Joint Surg [Am]*, **37A:**2, 1955.

Peacock, E. E.: Treatment of Finger Tip Injuries, *Ann Surg,* **173:**812, 1971.

Schreiber, S. N., Leibowitz, R., and Bernstein, L.: Limb Compression and Renal Impairment (Crust Syndrome) following Narcotic and Sedative Overdose, *J Bone Joint Surg [Am]*, **54A:**1683, 1972.

Seddon, H. J.: Practical Value of Peripheral Nerve Repair, *Proc R Soc Med,* **42:**427, 1949.

Simeone, F. A. (ed.): Symposium on Operative Nerve Injuries and Their Repair, *Surg Clin North Am,* vol. 52, no. 5, October 1972.

Smith, J. W.: Microsurgery of Peripheral Nerves, *Plast Reconstr Surg,* **33:**317, 1964.

Sneddon, J.: "The Care of Hand Infections," The Williams & Wilkins Company, Baltimore, 1970.

Stenstrom, S. J.: Functional Determination of the Flexor-Tendon Graft Length, *Plast Reconstr Surg,* **43:**633, 1969.

Stone, N. H., Hursch, H., Humphrey, C. R., and Boswick, J. A., Jr.: Empirical Selection of Antibiotics for Hand Infections, *J Bone Joint Surg [Am]*, **51A:**899, 1969.

Symonds, F. C.: Pitfalls in Management of Penetrating Wounds of the Forearm, *J Trauma,* **11:**47, 1971.

Temtamy, S., and McKusick, V. A.: Synopsis of Hand Malformations with Particular Emphasis on Genetic Factors in "The First Conference on the Clinical Delineation of Birth Defects," pt. III, "Limb Malformations: Birth Defects," Original Article Ser, vol 5, no. 3, pp. 125–184, The National Foundation—March of Dimes, New York, 1969.

Tsuge, K.: Treatment of Megalodactyly, *Plast Reconstr Surg,* **39:**590, 1967.

Tubiana, R.: Surgical Repair of the Extensor Apparatus of the Fingers, *Surg Clin North Am,* **48:**1015, 1968.

———— and Valentin, P.: The Anatomy of the Extensor Apparatus of the Fingers, *Surg Clin North Am,* **44:**897, 1964.

Verdan, C.: Basic Principles of Surgery of the Hand, *Surg Clin North Am,* **47:**355, 1967.

White, W. L.: Secondary Restoration of Finger Flexion by Digital Tendon Grafts: An Evaluation of 76 Cases, *Am J Surg,* **91:**662, 1956.

————: Restoration of Function and Balance of the Wrist and Hand by Tendon Transfers, *Surg Clin North Am,* **41:**427, 1960.

Williams, S. B.: New Dynamic Concepts in the Grafting of Flexor-Tendons, *Plast Reconstr Surg,* **36:**377, 1965.

Woodhall, B., and Beebe, G. W.: "Peripheral Nerve Regeneration: A Follow-up Study of 3,656 World War II Injuries," Veterans Administration Medical Monograph, 1956.

Woolf, C. M., and Woolf, R. M.: A Genetic Study of Polydactyly in Utah, *Am J Hum Genet,* **22:**75, 1970.

Zancolli, E.: "Structural and Dynamic Bases of Hand Surgery," J. B. Lippincott Company, Philadelphia, 1968.

Chapter 51

Plastic and Reconstructive Surgery

by **Lester M. Cramer** and **Thomas J. Brobyn**

HISTORICAL BACKGROUND

Surgery had its origin in procedures which are traditionally considered in the field of plastic surgery today. Many of the initial thrusts were attempts by man to correct deformity, since, in the centuries before anesthesia and asepsis, surgical procedures were limited to the body surface.

Among the earliest operations performed were those by Hindu surgeons for restoration of missing parts. Our present day approach to total and subtotal nose reconstruction does not differ in principle from that of at least 4,000 years ago. An account of Hindu manners and customs written in 1800 mentions punishment of highway robbers by amputation of the right hand and nose, and amputation of the noses of conquered warriors as well as those of women who incurred their husbands' jealousy. Susruta, about 600 B.C., repaired the injured nose with a patch of "living flesh slided off the region of the cheek." This popular procedure employed by the Hindus now bears the name "Indian method." This technique for nose construction migrated from East to West. The Brancas, a family of Sicilian laymen, became prominent around 1430, when it was learned that they could repair noses, ears, and lips with flaps from the cheek or forehead. Antonius, the youngest of the Brancas, perfected the method now referred to as the "Italian method" for nose reconstruction by using a skin flap taken from the arm.

In the fifteenth century, the renowned Gasparo Tagliacozzi produced his classic volume on reconstruction of the nose and other parts by pedicle flap surgical methods. Having the advantage of the printing press, Tagliacozzi disseminated knowledge of the details of the techniques of reconstruction. However, following this era, operations for reconstruction of missing parts fell into disrepute for about 200 years. The procedures once again appeared in the eighteenth century in England. Carpue of London gave a detailed account of the restoration of lost noses. In the nineteenth century, von Graefe and Dieffenbach recorded several techniques for reconstruction of missing parts.

In the twentieth century, Gillies in England, Davis, Ivy, and Kazanjian in the United States, and Filatov in Russia were stimulated by World War I tragedies to pioneer newer methods of wound closure and tissue transfer. The next generation of pioneers, McIndoe, Mowlem, and Kilner in England, Wallace in Scotland, and Blair, Brown, Cannon, Bunnell, Webster, and Pierce in the United States received impetus for further development from problems raised by World War II injuries.

WOUND HEALING

The principles and the specifics discussed in Chap. 8 are especially important for plastic and reconstructive surgery.

Fig. 51-1. The final result of suturing lacerations is greatly improved if careful wound toilet and debridement is supplemented by fastidious skin management. Technically, three-point fixation of the skin facilitates accurate excision, permitting straight-line execution and cutting of tissues at right angles to the surface. The assistant holds the skin hooks under moderate tension, and the operator varies the amount of tension needed with the pickup.

Metabolic and genetic characteristics greatly influence the final outcome of surgical wounds, and the knowledge and ability of the surgeon are even more critical in determining most results. Attention to detail and meticulous wound closures have become identified with plastic and reconstructive surgery. Halsted's principles and those outlined by Esmarch in 1877 have become self-evident requirements in proper wound care. Techniques are critical in avoiding excessive scar formation but are not the only factors.

Abnormalities of wound healing leading to hypertrophic scars, mismatched scars, and large secondary iatrogenic markings (crosshatches from large suture material tied too tightly) are mainly avoidable by the critical attention to known facts. Scar tissue can be further controlled either by the systemic use of biochemical antagonists or by the local injection of steroids. Keloid scar, as differentiated from hypertrophic scar, is a true metabolic anarchy of scar tissue. It is much more difficult to control but can be judiciously handled by working totally within the keloid lesion and by the intralesional injection of steroids at the time of surgery.

The implantation of prosthetic materials is increasingly applied. There are two types, according to the surface presented. The first is totally inert, a smooth *macro* surface such as that presented by silicone or Teflon. The body reacts minimally, but walling-off by a lining membrane does occur. This membrane, a mesothelia-like surface, allows these implanted substances to remain in situ for long periods of time, perhaps indefinitely, but infection is a hazard. Smooth-surfaced prostheses also can be used to create tissue channels, the prosthesis later being electively removed in order to insert moving surfaces, such as tendons, through these channels (see Chap. 50). The second type of tissue implant works on the principle of capture. These implants are purposely felted or veloured, in the case of materials such as Dacron or polypropylene, or sintered, in the case of ceramics. By presenting *micro* surfaces to the body, membrane formation is avoided, and a true tissue-prosthetic interface without walling off is created. This type of implant has a better opportunity for long life, since it is less liable to become infected.

TECHNICAL CONSIDERATIONS

Wound Closure

The principles outlined in this section pertain to all wounds, but their importance in achieving a cosmetically acceptable result is magnified in the face and neck regions and usually the extremities. The wound should be thoroughly cleaned; if the edges are ragged, they should be revised (Fig. 51-1). Subcutaneous undermining to achieve closure without tension is essential. The dermal and subcutaneous tissue trimming should be fashioned so that subcuticular sutures will hold the skin edges in approximation. Fine absorbable subcutaneous sutures positioned so that the knots are tied in the depth of the wound lend strength to the wound closure during the critical first weeks

D. Leber, MD.

Fig. 51-2. Examples of wound closure. The elimination of dead space and the approximation of the corresponding layers (or levels) of tissue are desirable. The transcutaneous suture is best placed by ensuring that the deeper portion of the suture (y) is wider than the superficial portion (x). This causes the wound pressures to encourage slight edge eversion (curved arrow), an excellent way of preventing edge inversion. Inversion would delay wound healing and result in a wider cutaneous scar. With all these closure methods, the cutaneous perforation should never exceed 3 mm from the wound edge, and it should be appropriately closer on the face. A suture should never be tied tightly. *A.* Simple conventional suture. *B.* Vertical mattress suture. *C.* Horizontal mattress suture. *D.* Half-buried mattress suture, the preferred method on most flaps. This is especially useful on the corners of lacerations or on Z-plasties because of its slight interference with the blood supply. *E.* Running lockstitch, infrequently indicated. *F.* Running subcuticular stitch of Halsted, the recommended method of wound closure and the one most commonly employed by the authors. *G.* Nonsuture closure of wounds with nonallergic, porous tape.

of healing. Fine-caliber skin sutures have been employed to achieve accurate epidermal and dermal coaption and to diminish the skin wound interface. The use of subcuticular running pullout sutures accomplishes the same tissue coaption without having extra external markings across the wound. In many instances accurate placement of the subcuticular and subcutaneous closure requires approximation only with porous, nonallergic tape, completely obviating skin sutures (Fig. 51-2). Early removal of sutures is not necessary, particularly if they have been placed carefully and have been loosely tied for the wound approximation. Since suture support of the scar can improve

the final result and since a subcuticular pullout suture causes less tissue reaction both at the surface and in the depth because it does not cross the dermal-subcutaneous juncture, the use of subcuticular pullout sutures takes on added importance.

Skin Grafting

Skin which is completely removed from its donor site and transplanted into a recipient area is a *graft*. A graft is composed of epidermal and dermal tissue whose survival in the recipient bed is via a plasmatic circulation until capillary juncture occurs. A graft differs from a *skin flap*, which is composed of epidermal, dermal, and subcutaneous tissue whose survival in the recipient bed is via a well-maintained or surgically reestablished vasculature. A skin flap is never devoid of its blood supply. Transplantation by graft or flap has become a commonplace and practical surgical procedure for covering open wounds or for replacing the skin after surgical excision of scars or tumors.

HISTORICAL BACKGROUND. Aulus Cornelius Celsus in 30 A.D. wrote of eyelid surgery and mentioned the possibility of free skin grafts in his *De re medica,* Book VII. During the Middle Ages, there were few references to free transplantation of tissue, although isolated instances were recorded. Sancassani described a female street vendor, who, in order to prove the efficacy of a certain salve, removed a piece of skin from her leg, passed it around the audience on a plate, replaced it in its original position, and covered it with the salve. The subsequent reunion was such that the site of operation was described as "scarcely discernible." In the nineteenth century, Baronio carried out a series of successful experiments on animals, mainly sheep, in which he transplanted pieces of skin. Reverdin and Guyon independently reported the use of pinch grafts to achieve healing on human granulating wound surfaces, although Frank Hamilton of New York initially suggested the implantation of a piece of skin 20 years prior to Reverdin's report. Hamilton's presentation concerned a patient on whom Reverdin had successfully carried out skin grafting with "two small bits of epidermis raised with the point of a lancet from the patient's right arm." The work was ridiculed by many, including David Page, then president of the Royal Medical Society of Edinburgh, who remarked, "It is not likely to occupy a permanent position in minor surgery." In 1870, in a paper entitled "On the Transplantation of Portions of Skin for the Closure of Large Granulating Surfaces," Lawson laid down the following dicta, which are still applicable: (1) that the new skin should be applied to a healthy granulating surface, (2) that only skin which is devoid of fat should be taken, (3) that the portion of skin should be accurately and firmly applied to the granulating surface, and (4) that the new skin should be kept in its new position without interruption.

In 1872, Ollier announced his new method of skin grafting in which he transplanted large squares of epidermis, up to 8 cm long, as free grafts. Shortly thereafter, Thiersch suggested using a razor to cut thin skin grafts, which were actually very thin split-thickness grafts devoid of dermal elements.

In 1875, Wolfe, an oculist in Glasgow, suggested grafting full-thickness segments of skin for correction of ectropion deformity. He also pointed out the importance of removing fat beneath the skin to be transferred and emphasized that "after a lapse of a fortnight, massage should be started with lanolin or cold cream," exactly the orders one would give today. Although skin grafting was rarely employed in World War I, with the development of the Padgett dermatome the technique became established in the 1930s. With the use of electric dermatomes developed by Brown and McDowell, and facilitated by the techniques developed in World War II, grafting become a routinely used operative procedure.

SKIN STRUCTURE (Fig. 51-3). The skin is a complex organ, varying in thickness, elasticity, color, and texture.

Fig. 51-3. Diagrammatic representation of the skin with correlation for use as graft donor sites. Split-thickness skin grafting is possible because the epithelial appendages in the donor dermis allow healing by proliferation and migration of the epithelial cells left behind. Healing is faster when there are more of these cells, as when the site is hairy or the donor graft is thin, and when the cells are metabolically active, as in young and healthy patients. When the graft contains more of the donor dermis, it probably is more serviceable and cosmetically superior. But the thicker the graft removed, the more epithelial cells removed; the fewer cells remaining at the donor site will determine slower healing. When the full thickness of the skin is removed, the wound is usually closed by undermining the skin and approximating it by sutures. If the wound is extremely large, a split-thickness skin graft would be needed.

Epidermis
Dermis
Subcutaneous tissue

Thin
Medium
Thick
Split thickness
Full thickness

D. Leber, MD.

These traits are influenced by age, sex, and state of nutrition. Use of a portion of skin as a donor to be transplanted elsewhere involves donor site selection based on the function and appearance of the skin in its recipient site and the proclivity of the donor site to heal. The latter is determined by the character of the remaining dermis, its thickness, and the number of epithelial appendages remaining. Because donor site healing may leave some scarring, it is advisable to remove the skin from an area that will be socially inconspicuous. The donor sites should also be selected to match the recipient area in texture and color when possible, e.g., grafting to the face mandates a donor site from the blush area (skin above the level of the nipples, on the ventral aspect of the body).

SPLIT-THICKNESS GRAFTS

A skin graft in which the epidermis and a partial thickness of the dermis is employed is referred to as a *split-thickness graft*. There are several advantages in this procedure. The donor site will heal spontaneously by reepithelialization through retained epidermal appendages such as sweat glands and hair follicles. Also the likelihood of graft survival, or "take," is high, because the thin skin can survive on the plasmatic nutrition while the blood supply is being restored by capillary juncture.

Indications for split-thickness skin graft are many and varied: Whenever there is a large wound with a well-vascularized bed which cannot be readily closed by suture or local flaps, a split-thickness skin graft is appropriate, although a local flap is superior to free skin grafts. The skin deficit may exist as a result of trauma, surgical excision, a burn wound healing by secondary intention, or skin loss from infection now under control. The recipient site must be cleaned and well vascularized to be receptive to split-thickness skin grafting. The selection of the donor site and thickness of split-thickness skin graft to be used is dependent upon the need at the recipient site. For example, if a skin graft is to be used as permanent skin coverage in an area of wear where contraction of the wound is undesirable, a thick (0.018- to 0.025-in.) split-thickness graft should be used. In an area where circumstances are not perfect for skin graft application, a slightly thinner, or moderate-thickness, split-thickness skin graft 0.012 to 0.018 in. thick may take more reliably and yet be thick enough to prevent contraction of the wound at the graft site. Skin grafts thinner than 0.01 in. are thin split-thickness skin grafts. These provide excellent early coverage for large granulating burn wounds, and the donor site can be used two or three times because the healing is more rapid. It is important to achieve the proper color match between the skin graft and its recipient site, particularly on the face and hands. When color match is not important, skin grafts are taken from the inconspicuous places, usually from the high thigh, buttock, or abdominal areas.

Split-thickness skin grafts are commonly taken with mechanical dermatomes which precisely control thickness. There are many varieties of drum dermatomes which pick up skin with a mechanically attached blade, controlling thickness by adjustment of the blade. Electrified or air-driven mechanical dermatomes are useful in rapidly procuring large lengths of split-thickness skin for coverage of burned areas requiring grafting. Special knives are also used, either with or without mechanical guards to determine thickness, to take freehand grafts. Large sheets can be obtained with all these techniques.

The split-thickness skin graft is carefully fitted to the recipient site and under most circumstances is best sutured in place with nonabsorbable suture. Usually the peripheral stitches are left long so that they can be tied over a dressing to immobilize it upon the graft site to apply pressure and prevent motion. In some wounds, particularly granulating ones, the split-thickness skin graft is best left unsutured and exposed during the early phases of healing. It must be protected in place by proper splinting. Exposure will allow meticulous postoperative wound care, such as removal of fluid accumulated beneath the graft, to facilitate the graft take.

FULL-THICKNESS GRAFTS

A full-thickness skin graft, as the name implies, consists of the full thickness of both epidermis and dermis (Fig. 51-4). There are several advantages in using the full thickness of skin. The donor site may be closed; when small grafts are required, a sutured donor site is less bothersome than a raw healing split-graft donor area. There is no limitation on the area which may be used for the donor site, a situation which does not pertain to grafts taken with a freehand knife or a dermatome. The postauricular area, upper eyelid, flank, groin, arm, and wrist are examples of the areas which are excellent sources of full-thickness grafts (Fig. 51-5). No special instrument is required to procure the graft, and skin appendages remain intact. Although the take is somewhat less reliable, once the survival is secure, the full-thickness graft is much more

Fig. 51-4. Full-thickness free skin grafts. Removal from donor site free of subcutaneous fat and areolar tissue.

Fig. 51-5. Because full-thickness grafts are cosmetically superior on the face, the appropriate donor sites must be determined according to availability, color match, and texture. *A*. Correct design on the upper eyelid, retroauricular area, and supraclavicular region allow closure with a linear scar and minimal noticeable defect. *B* and *C*. Nonfacial full-thickness-graft donor sites, primarily for use on the hands and occasionally on the feet. These allow maximal availability and a linear closure with minimal discomfort and an inconspicuous scar.

durable and more acceptable in consistency and color. Because of these attributes, full-thickness grafts may be employed for cosmetic reasons in some areas and are particularly applicable in areas in which the skin must withstand pressure or repeated trauma such as the fingers and palm.

COMPOSITE GRAFTS

A composite graft consists of skin, in combination with other tissue, which is transferred without its blood supply as a free graft from the donor to the recipient area. As rapid vascularization is needed for survival of the composite graft, its use is restricted to recipient areas of good blood supply. Under optimal circumstances and for relatively small defects, it is a reliable graft.

The classic composite graft is a free graft of skin, subcutaneous tissue, and cartilage from the ear to the nose (Fig. 51-6). This is applicable for through-and-through defects in the nose, especially those involving the alar edge. The composite graft which matches the defect is procured from the edge of the ear incorporating both anterior and posterior ear skin and interposed cartilage.

Free composite grafts from the hair-bearing scalp have been employed for eyebrow reconstruction for many years (Fig. 51-7). In recent years, the treatment of male pattern baldness has become popularized. Multiple circular grafts of hair follicles, each graft containing approximately six hairs, are transferred from the posterior region to the anterior bald portion. These are interspersed with short linear segments of 8 to 10 hairs apiece. Eventual luxuriant growth of these hairs can camouflage the bald region effectively. Transfer of total-thickness segments of lip, usually from the lower lip to the upper lip without a pedicle, also illustrates the use of composite grafts.

Fig. 51-6. Composite graft from ear to furnish both lining and alar skin.

PEDICLE TISSUE TRANSFERS

The salient feature in the technique of pedicle transfer of tissue is that the tissue being transferred is never devoid of blood supply; the pedicle is the handle by which the tissue maintains its attachment and blood supply during the first stage of the transfer. Once the transferred tissue heals to the recipient site, its nourishment is supplied by the recipient site, and the pedicle may be severed. A better final result can be achieved if the pedicle is a permanent one, maintaining its original blood and nerve supply for better trophism. Thus, local pedicle flaps are the best tissue, and if they can be geometrically devised, they become the best replacement.

Knowledge of the blood supply of the skin allows correct design. Tracing this blood supply from the aorta out to the dermal capillaries categorizes the vessels into the following groups: (1) segmental, (2) perforator, and (3) cutaneous.

Segmental branches are direct branches of the aorta, such as the internal mammary or the inferior epigastric systems, which lie deep to the muscles.

Perforators are the branches from the segmental vessels, connecting to the cutaneous vessels and supplying muscles as they pass through them. Examples are the thoracoacromial or the anterior and posterior humeral circumflex.

Cutaneous branches represent the third level and are most important to understand for flap design. They supply the skin directly and are the principal determinants of flap survival. They are the musculocutaneous arteries and the direct cutaneous arteries. The musculocutaneous arteries individually supply a small area, but collectively are the predominant blood supply to the skin. The direct cutaneous arteries run parallel to the skin surface, each perfusing a much greater area, but are quite limited in number and location throughout the body. A summation of the characteristics of cutaneous arteries is presented in Table 51-1.

Excellent examples of named direct cutaneous arteries upon which well-conceived flaps have been designed are the following: (1) superficial temporal, (2) superficial inferior epigastric, (3) superior thoracic, (4) superficial external pudendal, (5) lateral thoracic, (6) intercostal–internal mammary (Bakamjian et al.), (7) superficial circumflex iliac artery (McGregor), (8) dorsal artery of the penis.

Table 51-1. CHARACTERISTICS OF CUTANEOUS ARTERIES

Musculocutaneous	Direct
Dominant	Supplementary
Ubiquitous	Fixed
Regional variations	Anatomic variations
perpendicular	Parallel, deep subcutaneous
Single vein	Paired venae comitantes + associated subdermal veins

SOURCE: Classification of Williams and Daniel.

Fig. 51-7. Composite free graft from hair-bearing scalp for eyebrow reconstruction. Note that the graft is split and interposed in the recipient area so that the hairs interdigitate and give an eyebrow effect.

Flap Design. Flap design based on specific length/width ratios have clinical application, on a statistical basis, for the different parts of the body. They are positively influenced when there are major named direct cutaneous arterial systems. In the head and neck region, length/width ratios as high as 3:1 or even 4:1 can be safely used; in other regions such as the deltopectoral or the ilioinguinal, such high ratios or higher have been accomplished on the named systems, giving long lengths of tissues on relatively narrow bases. However, in most parts of the body it is difficult to make a flap of a higher ratio than 2:1, and below the knee rarely is the safe limit for a primary transfer any higher than 1:1. It is important to understand that the viable lengths of such skin flaps are really only indirectly related to their widths. Flaps of varying widths all survive to the same length provided they have similar conditions of blood supply; decreasing the width will decrease the chance of the pedicle's containing large vessels.

Delay. The principle of delay allows safer transfer when a larger amount of tissue is needed than can be supplied by designing a flap from the local region. When this would exceed the safety factor of the vasculature, the dimensions of the flap needed can be augmented by one or more preliminary operations which consist of incising portions of the flap periphery or depth in stages. This old concept is based on the observation that the blood supply of a part is better after it has been previously partially separated from its blood supply.

Reinisch has done much to help explain the incompletely understood pathophysiology of the delay phenomenon. His experimental model shows substantial blood supply in the distal ends of flaps which are designed to be longer than their predicted surviving length. This circulation is contained in thick, nonnutritive arteriovenous channels, controlled by the sympathetic nervous system. Elevation of a flap denervates it, allowing the arteriovenous

Fig. 51-8. The V-Y advancement principle, allowing the apex of the V to advance along the axis of a scar to facilitate lengthening.

shunts to open, thus causing lethal bypassing of nutrient capillaries in areas of decreased circulation. Delay of the flap causes denervation and retains enough residual blood supply to provide adequate flow through both capillaries and dilated shunts. Because the difference between an ischemic flap (leading to a successful delay) and a necrotic flap is frequently very small, judgment and experience in delay design and execution are critical.

LOCAL PEDICLE FLAPS. A local pedicle, as differentiated from a distal pedicle, involves tissue with its blood supply intact reaching the recipient area without moving the recipient area or without intervening stages of donor area movement. These most useful reconstructive procedures include the following:

V-Y advancement
Z-plasty
Rotation
Advancement
Transposition
Interpolation
Bilobed
Bipedicle
Island
Microvascular

Fig. 51-9. The clinical application of a V-Y advancement.

Potentially bewildering, this array of local tissue shifts is easily understood and should receive primary consideration for all wounds that cannot be closed by direct suture. When they can be used, they are superior to free graft, because of more reliable healing, easier wound management, and better cosmetic and functional results. In addition an avascular recipient site, e.g., the cortical bone devoid of its periosteum, cartilage devoid of its perichondrium, or a previously heavily irradiated area, will be unable to support a free graft.

The V-Y advancement (Fig. 51-8) obtains small amounts of length along a correct axis when the apex of the V-flap is placed on that axis. It is useful in a few highly selected instances of scar revision, particularly at free borders (Fig. 51-9).

Much more useful, perhaps the most commonly employed reconstructive procedure, is the Z-plasty (Fig. 51-10). By changing the direction of a laceration or a scar, using the geometric principles of a parallelogram, great advantage is gained in added length.

Transposition (Fig. 51-11), rotation (Fig. 51-12), and interpolation flaps (Figs. 51-13, 51-14) all use the attached local tissues, widely undermined, to close the wound.

The bipetal, or bilobed, flap, popularized by Zimany, has been a useful modification, because it eliminates the need for grafting the donor site defect when it might otherwise have been necessary to employ such a skin graft to close the donor site (Fig. 51-15).

The bipedicle flap is still a very useful maneuver, despite notoriety gained from lack of understanding of its design. It is commonly employed in the pretibial region to cover compound fractures on the night of injury. The donor site of this flap must always be grafted, and the correct proportions of the flap accurately maintained by a curved incision allowing two wide bases (Fig. 51-16).

The island pedicle flap diminishes the size of the pedicle which carries nourishment so that it incorporates only the major blood vessels and allows movement of composite tissue blocks without a skin bridge, the bridge being these blood vessels and some surrounding subcutaneous and dermal tissue. Since the introduction of this technique by Gersuny, Monks, and Esser, its versatility has encouraged increasing use, particularly as knowledge of direct cutaneous arteries and microsurgical technique improve, so that the principle of vascularized island pedicle transfer is now widely applied. Loops of bowel are shifted to areas well away from their normal residence on a pedicle of mesenteric vessels alone. Esophageal substitution and bladder substitution with bowel are classic examples. Composite tissue carried on the temporal vessels has great value in facial reconstruction (Fig. 51-17). Total eyebrow reconstruction may be carried out using composite hair-bearing scalp shifted on a pedicle of the temporal vessels. Vascular pedicle grafts which incorporate digital nerves have been useful in hand surgery to transfer tissue to the critical area of denervation of the thumb and index finger.

DISTANT PEDICLE FLAPS. These include *jump flaps*, either direct or via a carrier, and *tubed flaps*.

Direct jump flaps are those which are elevated and left attached to their nourishing pedicle while the recipient site

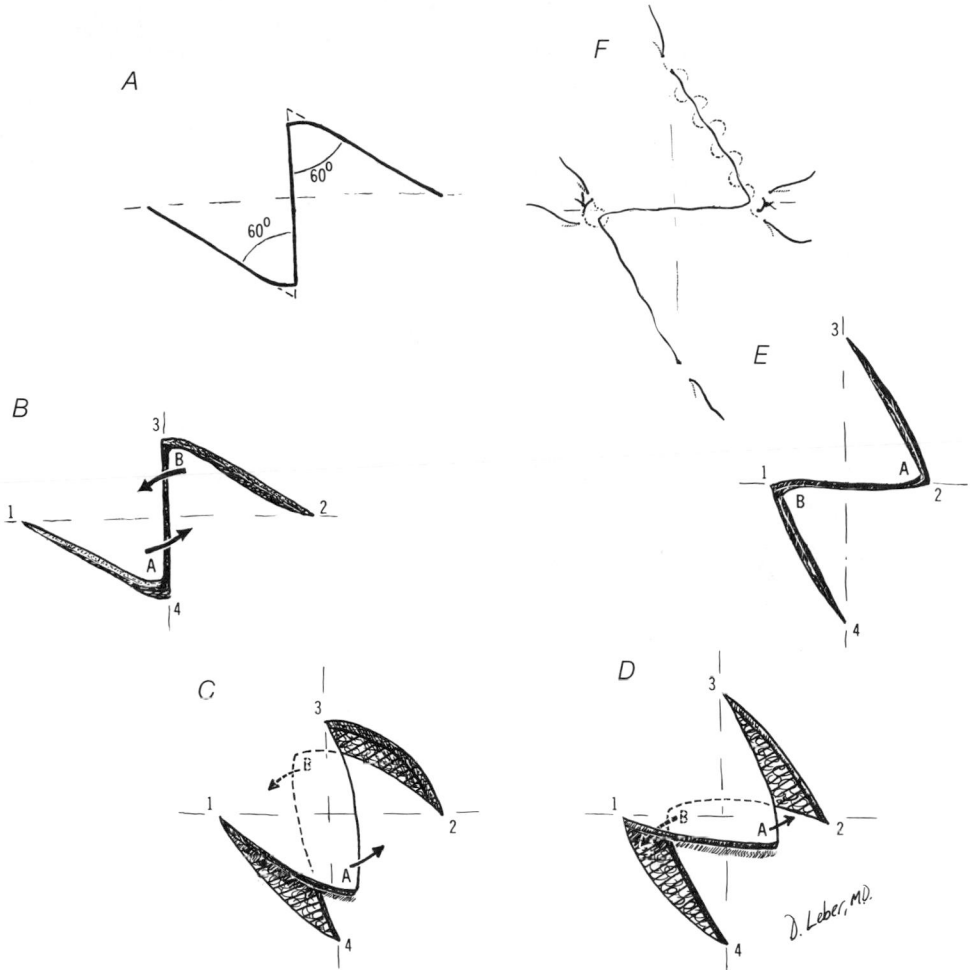

Fig. 51-10. Principles of the Z-plasty. Construction of two identical equilateral triangles based on any scar line makes two triangular flaps which together constitute a parallelogram. Interchanging these two flaps will lengthen the original line by 50 percent. This is easy to understand by noting that the short leg of a parallelogram is exchanged for the long leg.

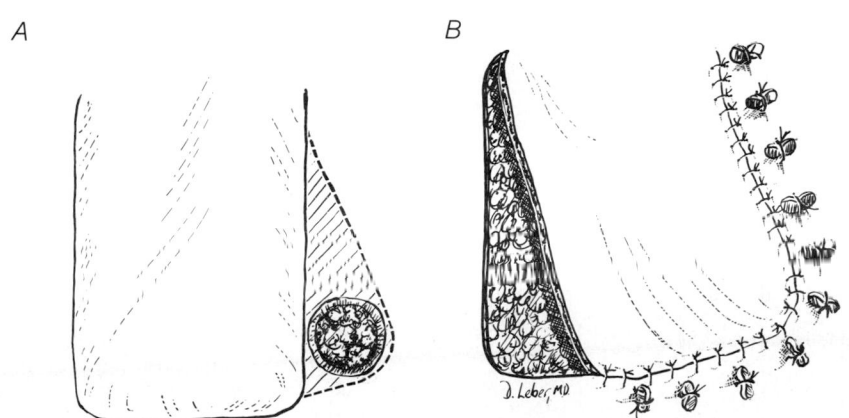

Fig. 51-11. A transposition flap.

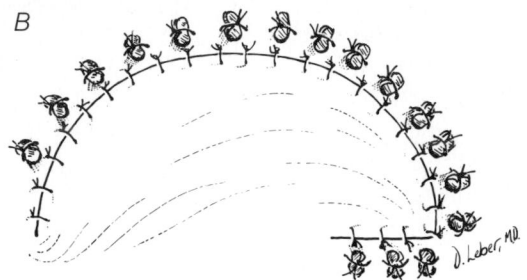

Fig. 51-12. A rotation flap.

is moved to an adjacent position. These may be of many sizes and shapes. Some involve only small amounts of tissue being brought to a critical area, such as a cross finger flap (Fig. 51-18). They may involve massive tissue shifts, such as truncal flaps to the hand from the abdominal wall (Fig. 51-19), or the shoulder region (Fig. 51-20).

When the tissue cannot be made to reach the place for which it is intended, a carrier can be devised, such as attachment to the wrist, as an intermediate phase. A series of operations then will be performed to eventually transfer the tissue to the recipient site.

Tubed flaps are used less frequently as better designs of local or jump flaps become available, because tubed flaps involve more inherent complications and many more operations in sequence. However, when tissue must be transferred over a considerable distance, the tubed flap,

despite the possible complications, must be considered because of the provision for constant tissue nourishment and the reliability of a completely closed wound. Gillies has been generally credited with popularizing this technique, but it was probably initially reported by Filatov in 1917.

The tubed pedicle is created by fashioning two parallel incisions and closing the pedicle edge to edge, resulting in a handle effect (Fig. 51-21). This creates the closed wound, which incorporates the blood supply and the soft tissue in addition to the skin. Later the pedicle is transferred to a new site (Fig. 51-22). One end of the pedicle is initially transected and positioned over the recipient site about 3 or 4 weeks later. After another 3 or 4 weeks, the opposite end also may be transected, so that the entire tube pedicle now has been moved to the distant site. During

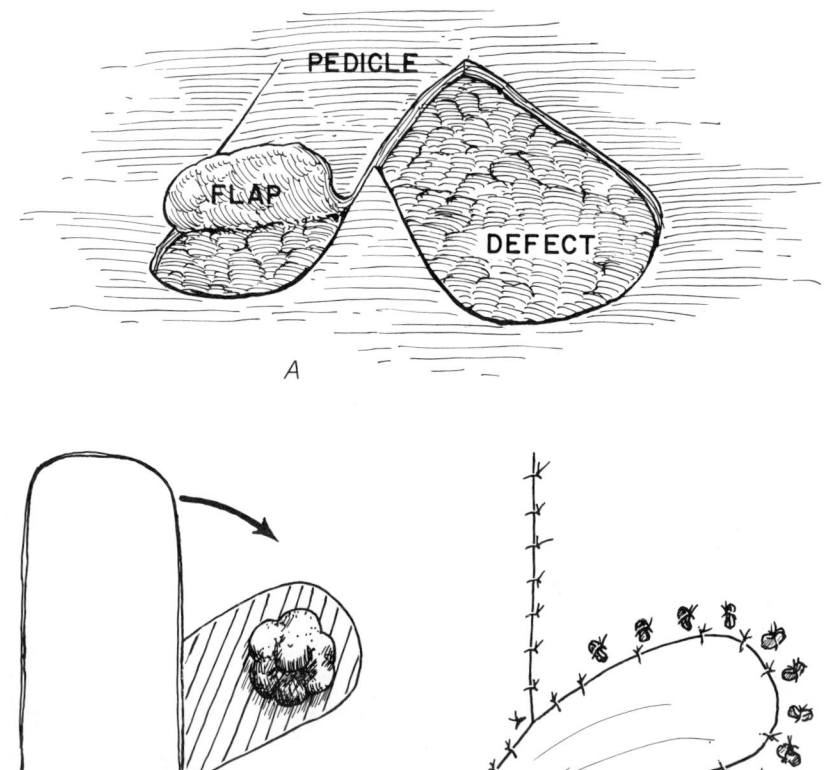

Fig. 51-13. Interpolation pedicle flap.

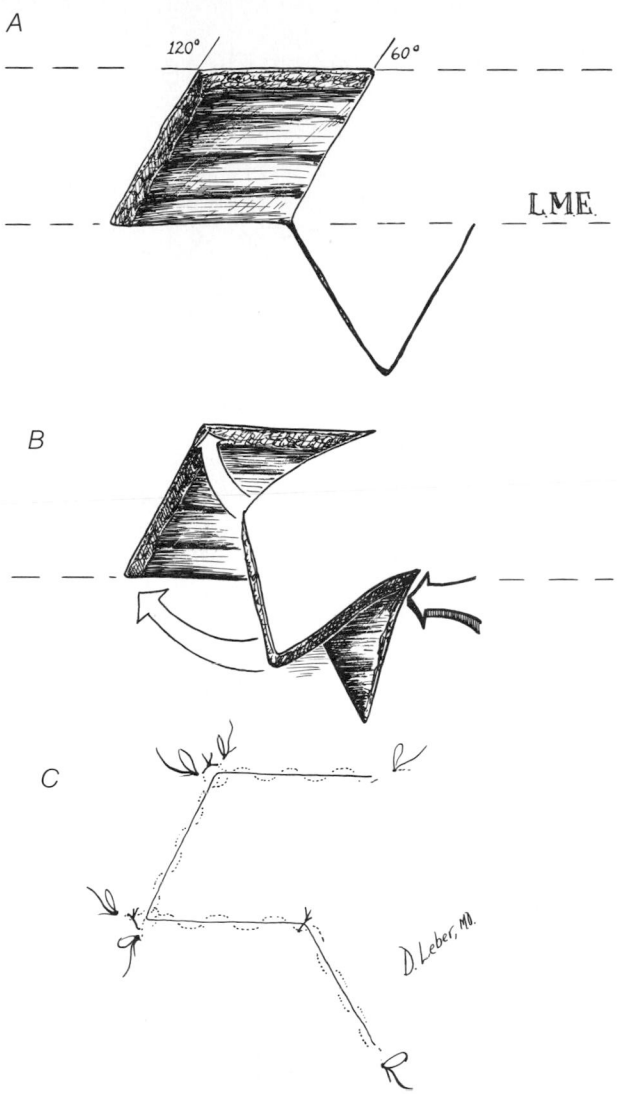

A

120°   60°

L.ME.

B

C

D. Leber, M.D.

Fig. 51-14. Limberg flap. This is designed as shown by excision of a 60° rhomboid, oriented correctly in relation to the lines of maximum extensibility (LME) of the skin. *A.* Excision of the 60° rhomboid, showing correct orientation with regard to the LME. The flap is constructed by extending the short diagonal (short axis) by its own length and constructing a third side arranged at a 60° angle to the extended short diagonal and equal in length to any side. *B.* Elevation and transposition of the Limberg flap. The heavy arrow emphasizes the closure of the donor defect parallel to the LME, a critical consideration in the design and execution of this flap. *C.* Completed closure.

Fig. 51-15. A bipetal (bilobed) flap.

D. Leber, M.D.

Fig. 51-16. A bipedicle flap.

Fig. 51-17. Island pedicle graft. Vascularized islands of composite tissues may be transferred over a wide area of the face when carried solely on temporal vessels. This allows the surgeon to pass the tissue and its pedicle to the recipient area through a subcutaneous tunnel. The blood supply is permanently retained, and there is no need for a second stage to cut the carrying pedicle and set the composite graft in place.

Fig. 51-18. The cross finger flap. *A.* The dorsum of the next digit in the ulnar direction is the usual donor site. *B.* The donor site and some of the carrier are grafted with a medium split-thickness skin graft so that there will be a closed wound system. *C.* An example of the tie-over dressing to maintain pressure and immobilization on a split-thickness skin graft. The material best suited is sponge rubber. *D.* The flap replacing the defect. *E.* When the replacement area is the touch strip on the volar aspect of the thumb, the best donor site is not on the index finger but on the middle finger, because the position of the thumb in relation to the index finger creates acute angles in the joints, leading to pain and potential stiffness.

Fig. 51-19. An extremely large abdominal pedicle flap can be constructed without delay because of the inferior epigastric system. The major disadvantage of using this flap to resurface the hand is that the dependent position of the hand increases edema. The donor site and flap carrier portion are skin-grafted. The deltopectoral flap popularized by Bakamjian for reconstruction in the head and neck area is also excellent for hand coverage, because it makes available a large amount of tissue without delay while allowing the hand to be in a position for dependent drainage. This flap is based on the internal mammary vasculature. Its only disadvantage is that the donor site is left with a more visible scar.

these intervals, the transferred tissue becomes nourished by the recipient site and no longer requires its original vascular supply.

Myocutaneous Flaps. The use of multiple large, compound muscle-skin flaps has recently been described in detail by McCraw et al. Utilization of these flaps provides new avenues of approach to reconstruction problems, with definite advantages. They provide a blood supply to an avascular area and bulk for filling defects or covering bone grafts, and they make possible the creation of longer viable flaps. Delay procedures may be decreased or avoided.

Myocutaneous flaps consist of a "carrier" muscle segment and the overlying skin and subcutaneous tissues. Vascularity is provided to the carrier muscle by a dominant pedicle and its segmental blood supply. This pedicle will support a large muscle segment even when the remaining pedicles are ligated. Complete detachment of the myo-

cutaneous flap except for its blood supply is possible, providing an increase in its effectiveness for reconstruction.

Independent myocutaneous vascular territories which have been described include the sternomastoid, upper trapezius, latissimus, lower sacrospinalis, upper and lower rectus abdominus, thoracoepigastric, upper and lower sartorius, rectus femoris, gracilis, biceps femoris, and gastrocnemius.

The viable muscle length, location of the dominant vascular pedicle, and functional expendability of the muscle are among the essential considerations.

Muscle Flaps. The reconstructive problems of the lower extremities, such as nonunion of the tibia, soft tissue loss with exposed bone, chronic tibial osteomyelitis, or venous stasis ulcers, have long been appreciated. Correction has required prolonged hospitalization and carries significant morbidity. The use of available lower extremity muscle flaps, popularized by Ger, has greatly facilitated the treatment of these conditions.

The principle is transposition of an available muscle with its intact neurovascular bundle to provide soft tissue coverage and an immediately suitable bed for split-thickness skin grafting. This bed is not dependent on surrounding pathologic tissue for vascularity.

Muscles suitable for transposition must be of adequate length and must have a vascular pedicle located near the muscle origin to provide satisfactory rotation. If there are

D. Leber, M.D.

Fig. 51-20. The deltopectoral flap (Bakamjian). A direct cutaneous internal system provides a large amount of tissue in one stage.

multiple vascular pedicles, delay may be necessary. Also, synergistic muscles must be present to replace the lost function of the transposed muscle.

The muscles most suitable for transposition have been cataloged into areas: (1) tibia (upper third)—medial head gastrocnemius; (2) tibia (middle third)—soleus and flexor digitorum longus; (3) tibia (lower third)—peroneus and flexor digitorum longus; (4) tibia (upper two-thirds)—gastrocnemius, soleus, peroneus, flexor digitorum longus; (5) medial malleolus—abductor hallucis; (6) lateral malleolus—abductor digiti minimi; (7) calcaneus—flexor digitorum brevis.

In addition to the lower extremity flaps, muscles flaps for tissue defects in other areas have been used. Vasconez et al. described use of the deltoid for scapular coverage, abductor digiti quinti for the wrist, sartorius for the pubis, and paravertebral muscles for the ilium.

Bone Flaps. Osteocutaneous flaps consisting of all or part of the clavicle in a tubed flap have been described for mandibular reconstruction. The flap is transferred in stages, and there is evidence to show that the bone remains viable in the tube. Preservation of the periosteal circulation maintains bone viability.

Omental Flaps. Large defects in the chest wall can be corrected by combined use of the greater omentum and split-thickness skin grafting. The omentum can be freed from the stomach and, utilizing either the right or the left gastroepiploic vessels, transposed to the chest wall. Choice of the pedicle depends on whether the right or left chest wall is to be reconstructed. Segments of omentum have been transferred to repair skull defects and hemifacial atrophy.

Free Flaps. Successful one-stage distant transfer of an island flap using microvascular anastomosis was first reported a few years ago. This *free flap* has since become well established as a feasible alternative to multistaged flap transfer. A high level of microvascular expertise is required to successfully perform this procedure, since anastomosis of vessels less than 1 mm in diameter may be necessary. Also, there must be a predictable vascular supply in the donor flap and suitable recipient vessels. Use of the free flap technique carries a higher risk of failure than other methods of tissue transfer. The technique is not limited to flaps of skin and subcutaneous tissue but has been described for direct transfer of lower extremity muscle to

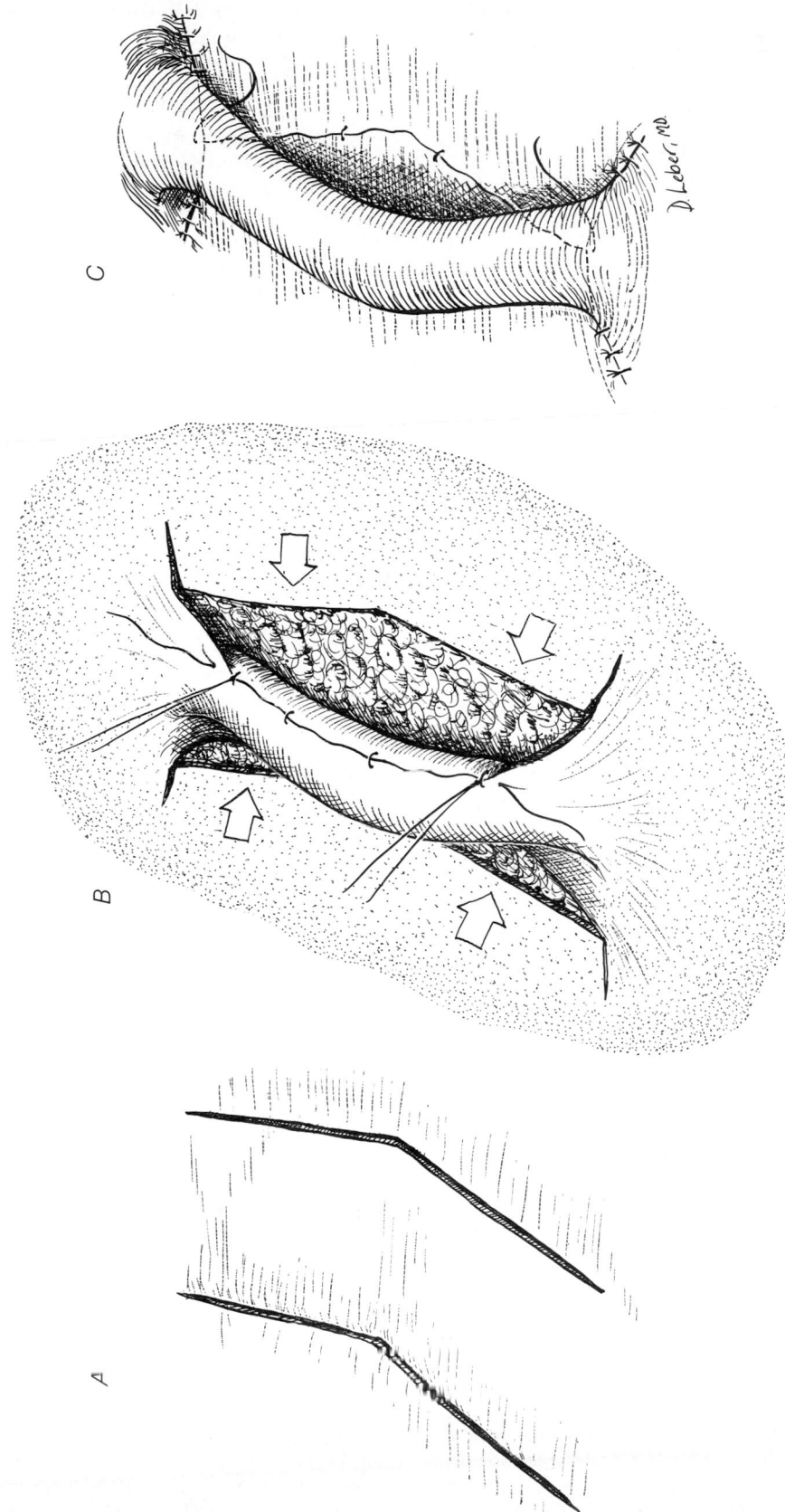

Fig. 51-21. Tubed pedicles are used much less frequently than in the past because of better understanding of direct tissue transfer possibilities. Their construction necessitates careful adherence to length/width ratio (A) and meticulous, atraumatic technique. Proper undermining and advancement (B) allow direct closure of nearby tube pedicle donor site.

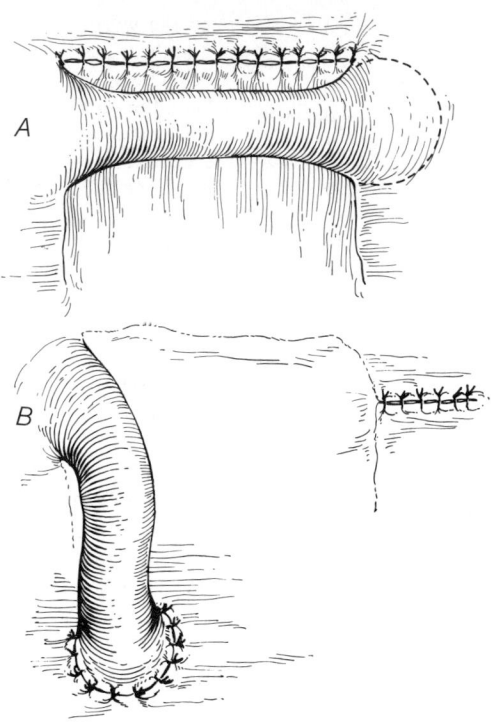

Fig. 51-22. Transfer of tubed pedicle flap. *A*. Tubed pedicle constructed. *B*. After healing, the tissue at one end of the tube may be transferred, retaining its blood supply through the tube.

reanimate the face in selected cases of facial nerve paralysis.

Although several donor sites have been described for free skin flaps, the best is one based on the superficial circumflex iliac and superficial inferior epigastric systems—the "regional" iliofemoral flap. Flaps as large as 15 by 24 cm may be transferred in one stage. This flap has the disadvantage of a short pedicle and excess bulk in obese patients. A satisfactory alternative is a free deltopectoral flap based on the second and third perforators of the internal mammary vessels. Skin flaps based on the dorsalis pedis vessel can also be taken from the dorsum of the foot.

Microsurgery

Magnification techniques have made possible the abundant transfer of composite units by vascular restoration. Microsurgery has extended the use of tissue transfer to whole organs and composite units whose vascular supply is from small vessels, allowing successful anastomosis of blood vessels less than 1 mm in diameter with rather predictable reliability. The reconstructive surgery that has developed with these improved techniques has been exciting and imaginative. Previously unmanageable problems can now be solved by the use of microsurgical anastomoses of arteries, veins, and nerves. Approximately seven to nine interrupted sutures of monofilament nylon are required for an artery 1 mm in external diameter, while six to seven sutures are needed for a 1 mm vein. The flap vasculature is not irrigated, but the vascular stumps are washed out with diluted heparin solution. Postoperative systemic heparinization is not used, but dextran, aspirin, and Persantin may be employed. In the first 12 to 24 hours postoperatively, it is mandatory to monitor the patient closely by Doppler radar, for an embarrassed flap may be saved by early thrombectomy.

Large units of skin can be transferred by using donor sites from the groin (superficial circumflex iliac artery and vein or superficial epigastric artery and vein), the scalp (superficial temporal artery and vein), the deltopectoral region (second perforating branch of internal mammary artery and vein), the dorsum of the foot (dorsalis pedis artery and vein), and the skin of the lateral chest wall (the thoracodorsal artery and vein).

Large segments of omentum utilizing vascular stalks of the gastroepiploic vessels have been transferred to repair skull defects, chest wall defects, and hemifacial atrophy.

Reconstruction of the thumb by free total toe transplantation is now a reality, utilizing neurovascular anastomosis. Replantations of digits and extremities have been reported with increasing frequency. Successful replantation after total scalp or penile avulsion also is now possible with these techniques.

Free transplantation of muscle by microneurovascular techniques has been successful in treatment of Volkmann's contracture, using the pectoralis major, and in facial palsy, using the gracilis. Free bone transplantation has also been done by making pedicles of the ribs and the intercostal vessels.

It is now possible to determine units of the body from which the muscle and the overlying skin can be transplanted as a unit. The most reliable unit is the rectus femoris muscle and its skin; others that have been employed are the gracilis and skin and the latissimus and skin.

Skin Banking

At the time of the creation of a surgical defect (e.g., the large donor site of a deltopectoral flap being used for a pharyngoesophageal reconstruction) or the grafting of an already existing wound (e.g., debridement of a granulating wound or a burn), one may wish to postpone the grafting procedure for a few days. Such postponements are occasioned by such specific factors as inadequate hemostasis, unhealthy wound bacteriology, or poor patient condition necessitating termination of the operation. The split-thickness skin graft preserved for usage within the next week, by either in vitro or in vivo banking, is an *autograft*. In the past in vitro preservation has been best accomplished by maintaining the tissue in a balanced salt solution containing antibiotics at 4°C. More recently, it has become apparent that skin replaced upon its donor site is better preserved, as there is less chance for infection and improved opportunity for a more satisfactory take when the skin is eventually used. Skin banked in this way can be easily removed at the bedside without anesthesia, using narcotic sedation, in the first few days. It is still readily removed up to 10 days, although after 6 days it is much more firmly attached and causes more pain and increased bleeding on removal.

Allograft skin is being used much less frequently at present. However, as tissue typing procedures become more sophisticated and are more extensively applied by national and international computer systems, the uses for allografts will resurge.

Currently, the most commonly used nonautograft of skin is the pig *xenograft*. It has become readily commercially available and has assumed a very important place in wound management. As these xenografts do not take in the classic sense, they do not evoke classic immunologic responses and their sequential re-use is possible. They effectively combat fluid loss and wound organisms, and successfully prepare granulating wounds for early subsequent autografting. They may be used fresh, lyophilized, or freeze-dried with nearly equal success, although the fresh product appears to have some slight advantage.

Scar Placement and Correction

Every area in the body has lines of least skin tension (Fig. 51-23). The placement of incisions or the redirection of lacerations or scars should be guided by these antitension lines. In the face (Fig. 51-24) these natural lines created by animation should never be electively crossed by incisions. When incorrectly oriented wounds are created by

trauma, it may be wise to revise and alter the wounds by Z-plasty or other geometrically conceived techniques (Fig. 51-10). The wound in the new direction can be predicted by placing points along the desired line in the face and dropping parallel lines to the scar or laceration, creating a Z for interchange of flaps. If a scar or laceration crosses the nasolabial fold, the segment which crosses the fold can be altered to fall in the fold itself (Fig. 51-25*A*). Notches in borders are likewise easily corrected by Z-plasty technique (Fig. 51-25*B*).

In order to correctly orient scars or to aid in planning for flap rotation, knowledge of the lines of skin extensibility is essential. It is possible to determine a line of maximum extensibility (LME) and a line of minimum extensibility perpendicular to it. In the face, skin crease lines and the lines of minimum extensibility are the same. If elliptical facial excisions are oriented with the long axis of the ellipse parallel to the skin crease lines, excision of the maximum amount of tissue that allows direct wound closure is possible.

When an elliptical incision is employed to remove a lesion, "dog ears" may be obviated by planning adjustment excisions at the ends of the wound. These adjustments can be avoided if the ellipse is made four times as long as its greatest central width. When this is not feasible, the adjustments can be made at the ends of the wound by geometric excisions (Fig. 51-26*A*).

Fig. 51-23. In nearly every area of the body the line of least tension is readily discernible. It is generally related to the direction of the muscle fibers beneath and to the orientation of the collagen in the dermis, appearing to be at right angles to these determining factors. The correct lines for the presternal, deltoid, and interscapular regions are difficult to determine. Except for these areas, placing incisions in the direction of the line will enhance the chance of an excellent scar.

Fig. 51-24. The relation of the elective lines of tension in the face to the underlying mimetic musculature. Only in the lower eyelid are these lines not perpendicular to the muscles. The left side of the drawing shows the use of this principle when excising common facial lesions.

Other methods of scar control are either mechanical or biochemical. Early and continuous pressure can prevent scar contracture as demonstrated by Cronin and by Larson et al.; this has important application in the treatment of the scars following burns. The biologic control of scars by chemical or metabolic means is a promising frontier. The experimental uses of beta-aminoproprionitrile, D-penicillamine, and *cis*-hydroxyproline all may lead to effective scar control in the clinical situation.

Dermabrasion

The casual observation that lacerated wounds accompanied by traumatic abrasions over their surfaces seemed to heal with less perceptible scars stimulated the elective use of dermabrasion. Purposeful abrasion of the skin using air-driven carborundum wheels planes the skin to remove pitted scars, deep wrinkles, and superficially embedded dirt. Perhaps the most frequent use of dermabrasion is in the treatment of the face pitted by previous acne. The sharp edges of the acne pit are abraded down to diminish the shadow cast in the pits, making them less perceptible. The technique is particularly useful when the acne pits do not have acutely angled borders.

Dermabrasion is also important in treating traumatic wounds containing particulate matter, efficiently removing

this matter to prevent permanent tattooing. It can also remove some embedded pieces secondarily.

Dermabrasion is useful in abrading a scar revision to help camouflage.

Tattooing

Skin tattooing has been used to establish proper color match between facial skin and that transferred to the face from an alien donor site. It can also provide stippling over a non-hair-bearing skin graft implanted on the bearded area in the male to make the repair less conspicuous. Camouflage in the area of an eyebrow graft with poor hair growth can be provided, and the lip vermilion can be evened by the use of tattooing pigment.

Perhaps its most widespread use has been to cover a facial capillary hemangioma (port wine stain), although it is still very difficult to mix the pigments to obtain the correct color match.

Cartilage Grafts

Reconstruction of the ear, the nasal tip, and the eyelid will frequently require the use of cartilage to ensure proper

Fig. 51-25. Common clinical applications of Z-plasty.

size and consistency. Free cartilage grafting is most successful when autografting is performed, although irradiated homografts have been successful in many instances. The best donor sites are the ribs and the concha of the nonaffected ear.

Bone Grafts

The ribs and the iliac crest are the best sources for bone when large amounts are needed for stability. Cancellous bone has a higher survival rate but may need cortical struts for the necessary strength. Alternate methods include using small bone chips or mechanically pulverized bone dust which will act as a nidus for new bone formation. Urothelium can also form bone in ectopic placement but has not been useful clinically as a graft. The newest pedicle methods include placement of the bone at the end of a muscle pedicle and transfer of a segment of rib as a free graft, utilizing microvascular anastomosis of the intercostal vessels.

Muscle Grafts

Muscle can be transplanted by free grafting (without vessel and nerve anastomosis). To function successfully, the muscle must be small in volume, the recipient bed must be very vascular, and the environment must be favorable to motor neurotization by ingrowth. Preliminary denervation of the donor muscle a few weeks prior to transplantation is recommended. Grafting of muscle as a free flap, utilizing microneurovascular anastomoses, is now feasible, its major applications being the treatment of Volkmann's contracture and the correction of facial palsy.

FACIAL TRAUMA

General Considerations

In the management of injuries to the head and neck, top priority is assigned to the control of the life-threatening problems of airway obstruction and hemorrhage. Tracheotomy is frequently necessary in severe facial injuries,

A

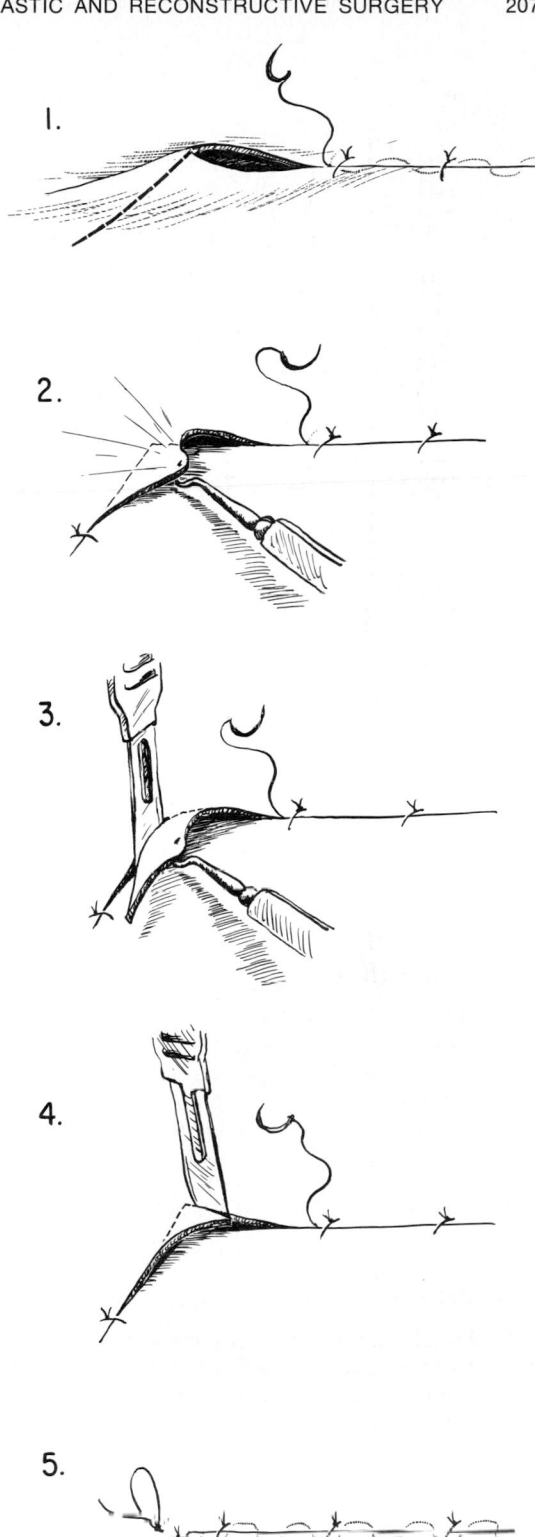

B

Fig. 51-26. Adjustment for wound dog ears by appropriate geometric excision.

Fig. 51-27. Surface projection of the parotid duct on a line between the earlobe and nasal alar origin. The oral entry is found at the bisection of this line by a vertical line from the lateral canthus of the eye.

particularly when both the maxilla and mandible are fractured or when there is an associated injury to the trachea, larynx, or chest. Even though a fractured, and thus flail, mandible removes support from the tongue and the floor of the mouth tracheotomy for the airway obstruction resulting from a fracture of the mandible alone may be obviated by clearing the air passages of mucus, blood, dirt, and dentition and providing judicious support of the mandible. Tracheal intubation via the nose or mouth for sev-

Fig. 51-28. Facial nerve laceration. *A.* Small superficial laceration. Note marginal (mandibular) branch paralysis of facial nerve. *B.* Stab wound below mastoid. Note total facial paralysis.

eral hours may also make tracheotomy unnecessary. In general, hemorrhage is best managed initially by pressure until the injured structures are carefully assessed.

Meticulous closure and primary revision of traumatic wounds should be performed only if there are no life-threatening injuries of higher priority. The liberal use of free skin grafts and tissue shifts to achieve the objective of early wound closure is very important at the time of primary care. However, before any specific efforts at skin closure are undertaken, a careful examination must assess injury to anatomic structures which cross the site of the wound. Injuries to the facial nerve, parotid duct, salivary glands, and facial bones represent some of the situations which must be evaluated. The parotid duct may be probed transorally to determine its integrity if the wound falls across a line from earlobe to alar cartilage posterior to a vertical line dropped from the lateral canthus of the eye (Fig. 51-27). Before any local anesthesia is administered, the function of the facial nerve should be evaluated for the integrity of its multiple branches, and sensation should also be assessed (Fig. 51-28).

When the face is abraded on a roadway or dirty surface, the dark particles are frequently ground deeply into the skin; retention will result in permanent tattooing. Treatment consists of thorough irrigation and cleansing with a stiff brush, followed by abrading with fine carborundum. This procedure must be carried out at the time of primary wound care, since secondary removal is much more difficult and not as successful.

Facial Fractures

Facial fractures, themselves, do not constitute life-threatening injuries and therefore are not assigned top priority in the patient with multiple wounds. However, facial fractures are frequently associated with serious head trauma and central nervous system injury. Under these circumstances, treatment of the fracture is deferred until the patient is stable, in order to avoid the additional hazard of anesthesia, but temporary wound approximation frequently can be accomplished with a few well-placed sutures and microporous tape.

DIAGNOSIS. The clinical diagnosis of facial fractures incorporates careful examination for a variety of specific physical findings (Fig. 51-29).

Deformity or Depression. Shortly after injury, there may be obvious evidence of architectural abnormality when one looks down on the face from above. Depression of the zygoma or zygomatic arch with asymmetry is frequently apparent.

Anesthesia or Paresthesia. An area of numbness over a major branch of the trigeminal nerve suggests fracture involving specific bones through which branches of this nerve pass. Anesthesia or hypesthesia over the distribution of the mental nerve suggests mandibular fracture, whereas the same finding over the distribution of the infraorbital nerve should arouse suspicion of a fracture of the zygoma or of the orbitomaxillary complex.

Ocular Disparity. Enophthalmos, depression of the globe, incomplete extraocular movement, double vision, and oc-

DEFORMITY

FACIAL FRACTURE DIAGNOSIS

(CLINICAL)

OCULAR DISPARITY

FALSE MOTION

MALOCCLUSION

Fig. 51-29. Common physical findings in facial fractures.

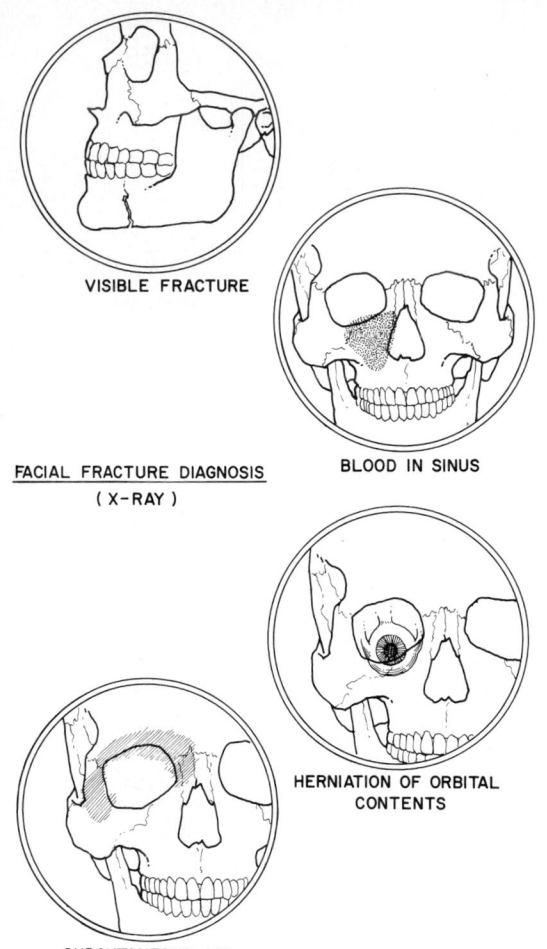

VISIBLE FRACTURE

FACIAL FRACTURE DIAGNOSIS
(X-RAY)

BLOOD IN SINUS

HERNIATION OF ORBITAL
CONTENTS

SUBCUTANEOUS AIR

Fig. 51-30. Common roentgenographic findings in facial fractures.

casionally exophthalmos all suggest facial fracture involving the orbit.

False Motion. Palpable crepitation and demonstrable false motion are diagnostic of facial fracture. These signs should be very gently elicited.

Malocclusion. This finding is characteristic of fractures of the mandible or maxilla or both with displacement. It is a reliable sign of architectural disruption in the normal maxilla-to-mandible relationship and also provides later evaluation of the reduction of major maxillary and mandibular fractures.

RADIOLOGIC FINDINGS (Fig. 51-30). Although careful clinical examination, even of an uncooperative patient, usually allows quite accurate diagnosis, very specific roentgenograms taken at very specific angles supplement the clinical diagnosis by defining the exact location, direction, and nature of the facial fracture (Fig. 51-31). The gymnastic positions needed to take roentgenograms that are capable of interpretation contraindicate these studies until the patient is stable and cooperative. Because of the intricate picture produced by multiple superimposed facial bones, stereo views or laminography may be necessary for final specific diagnosis in some instances. In addition to direct visual evidence of interruption of osseous continuity, other features which may be demonstrated on roentgenogram include hemorrhage into sinuses, herniation of orbital contents or teeth into the sinuses, foreign bodies, and subcutaneous air indicative of fracture into the nose or sinus.

TREATMENT. If an open wound exposes the fracture sites and the patient's condition is satisfactory, immediate fracture reduction and fixation are recommended. In all other cases, *early* reduction and fixation are the procedures of choice, usually a few days following the injury when the patient's status has been completely evaluated. If an extremely serious accompanying injury necessitates a long

Fig. 51-31. Chart for x-ray for facial bone fractures.

Bone	X-Ray
Mandible	
Condylar and coronoid processes Ascending ramus and body	Right and left lateral obliques of mandible
Symphysis, parasymphyseal Body and ascending rami	Posterior–anterior of mandible
Condyle and condylar neck	Towne's (modified) Anterior–posterior of base of skull
Anterior arch	Occlusal of anterior mandible
Maxilla & Zygoma	Water's (posterior-anterior oblique) Anterior–posterior of face Lateral of face
Zygomatic arch	Submental–vertex
Orbital Floor	Water's Stereo Water's Laminography
Nasal Bone	Superior–inferior of nose Lateral of nose

waiting period, this should be no longer than 2 weeks. After this, successful reduction is difficult to achieve, and severe cosmetic and functional deformity, nonunion, or osteomyelitis may ensue.

Attaining preinjury occlusion is the prime goal if either the maxilla or mandible is fractured, and restoration of vision, airway, and cosmesis are the aims of treatment of the other fractures. Cerebrospinal fluid rhinorrhea, diagnosed by testing for glucose in the nasal secretions, is usually successfully managed by exact reduction. Occasionally a delayed dural repair or graft may be needed.

Fixation is accomplished by applying wires, bars, or splints to the teeth, reestablishing occlusion, and fixing one jaw to the other by attaching the appliances to each other. Open reduction and internal fixation by wires, bars, or clamps across the fracture site frequently is necessary, particularly if muscle or fat interposed between the fracture fragments prevents their reduction by external means or if the direction of the fracture and the muscle pull will make a closed reduction unstable. External splints with wires or pins inserted transcutaneously may also be helpful in securing final fixation.

ZYGOMA

The prominence of the cheek, formed by the zygoma, may be depressed by a blow to the side of the face fracturing the zygoma. This usually manifests itself in one of three ways: (1) fracture of the arch of the zygoma (Fig. 51-32), (2) crushing of the bone of the cheek, or (3) fracture-dislocation with rotation of the zygoma in a downward and outward or downward and inward direction (Fig. 51-33).

Frequently the result of a fight or a fall, the isolated zygoma fracture is very common, or it may be accompanied only by associated nasal bone injury. When it is the result of high-speed trauma, an increasing occurrence, it is one of a group of facial and skull fractures and is accompanied by fracture of the maxilla, frontal bone, temporal bone, nasoethmoidal complex, and mandible. Common findings are disparities of the eye level, palpable notches in the inferior orbital rim (zygomaticomaxillary suture) and at the lateral rim (zygomaticofrontal suture), anesthesia in the distribution of the infraorbital nerve, and a characteristic lateral subscleral hemorrhage (Fig. 51-34). The diplopia present is predominantly horizontal, with images side by side, because of the direction of the displacement and the injury to the lateral rectus muscle. If the eye level drops because of injury to Lockwood's ligament, there will be a concomitant vertical aspect accompanying this horizontal diplopia. However, when vertical diplopia is the predominant or only finding, it usually indicates injury to the inferior rectus muscle, perhaps injury to the inferior oblique muscle, and trapping of these muscles by an injured orbital floor. Trismus may occur as a fragment of the zygomatic arch impinges on the temporalis muscle and coronoid process of the mandible. Techniques for treatment include completely closed reduction, a closed reduction through small incisions, and open reductions with internal fixation. For reduction employing an elevator inserted from small incisions, temporal, oral,

Fig. 51-32. *A.* A depressed fracture of the zygomatic arch, which may impinge upon the mandible and prevent opening or closing (trismus). *B.* The "tripod," or "tripartite," fracture of the zygoma which will dislocate when separated at its three suture lines where the fractures manifest: the zygomaticofrontal, zygomaticotemporal, and zygomaticomaxillary. The orbital floor and wall are always injured with this fracture, sometimes in a linear fashion and at other times by being comminuted or disrupted.

or antral insertion approaches will be employed, each with specific indications. If the zygomatic fracture is displaced and/or rotated, open reduction and fixation using interosseous wiring are usually necessary. If, in addition, the orbital floor is so crushed and sagging that it can be supported only from below, packing the sinus may aid in its reduction, but this is not usually necessary. A portion of the orbital floor may be missing; this allows herniation of the orbital contents into the maxillary antrum and may result in trapping of the inferior rectus and inferior oblique muscles within the defect. These injuries may also occur in the absence of other fractures of the zygomatic maxillary complex, such as following a direct blow to the globe. When occurring in this pure form, these classic "blowout" fractures may be inapparent unless the clinician is alert. They are manifested by *vertical* diplopia (one image above the other image), particularly on upward gaze; enophthal-

Fig. 51-33. Fracture-dislocation of the zygoma with rotation, disparity of eye level, lateral subscleral hematoma, and a surface representation of anesthesia of the infraorbital nerve.

Fig. 51-35. Blowout fracture. *A.* Blowout fracture of orbital floor. Note depression of globe. *B.* Upward gaze shows incarceration of inferior rectus.

pending upon the magnitude, direction, and site of the blow (Fig. 51-37). The upper dentition, the maxillary sinus, the orbital floor, and the maxillary division of the fifth cranial nerve are important anatomic structures to be considered in the diagnosis and therapy of maxillary fractures.

A displaced maxillary fracture is characteristically manifested by gross malocclusion. Anesthesia over the cheek and upper lip, which are areas innervated by the infraorbital nerve, may be demonstrable. Enophthalmos with

mos; and depression of the globe (Figs. 51-35 and 51-36). Such fractures require open reduction, deliverance of the orbital contents back into the orbit, and primary orbital floor reconstitution with the fracture fragments, prosthetic implants, or a bone or cartilage graft. Only occasionally must this treatment be supplemented by packing of maxillary antrum.

MAXILLA

Maxillary fractures frequently result from a direct anteroposterior blow to the middle third of the face, de-

Fig. 51-36. A blowout fracture of the orbital floor with characteristic hanging drop sign.

Fig 51-34. *A.* A lateral, subscleral hematoma confined anteriorly, due to direct trauma. White sclera is visible behind the hematoma when the patient moves the globe in the opposite direction. *B.* The lateral subscleral hematoma secondary to zygomatic fracture or frontal bone trauma does not allow visualization of white sclera behind it, because the blood has dissected forward subperiosteally and subconjunctivally.

A   *B*

fluid or herniation of orbital contents into the maxillary sinus.

Fixation may be accomplished by wiring the maxillary and mandibular teeth in occlusion or by open reduction, intraosseous wiring, and packing the maxillary antrum. In true craniofacial dysjunction, the entire maxillary complex must be wired to the frontal bone, since this represents the only adjacent fixed skeletal unit.

MANDIBLE

The mandible is the most frequently fractured bone within the facial complex. Knowledge of the sites and frequencies aids the diagnosis immensely (Fig. 51-38). About 60 percent of mandibular fractures are bilateral. The powerful muscles of mastication inserting on the mandible may account for continuing displacement of the fractures unless fixation is achieved by treatment. The complex temporomandibular joint, lower teeth, and mandibular division of the fifth cranial nerve are important anatomic structures related to fractures of the mandible. Examination may reveal deformity or malocclusion, with crepitation and swelling as characteristic signs. Anesthesia over the chin and lower lip suggests injury to the inferior alveolar nerve.

Accuracy of reduction and immobilization are important to avoid nonunion and also the late development of temporomandibular joint symptoms resulting from malocclusion. The majority of mandibular fractures may be successfully treated by wired fixation of the teeth in occlusion. Some fractures must be treated by the addition of open reduction to remove interposed muscle and fat and replace the bones in anatomic position; this reduction is maintained by interosseous wires, plates, or compression devices. When there are not enough teeth present, the occlusal fixation can be supplemented by imaginative dental prostheses which are attached either to the teeth or to the bones themselves. When the mandible is completely edentulous and the patient is elderly, a direct approach to the mandible under local anesthesia is indicated, fixing the parts securely with internal, interosseous wires or compression.

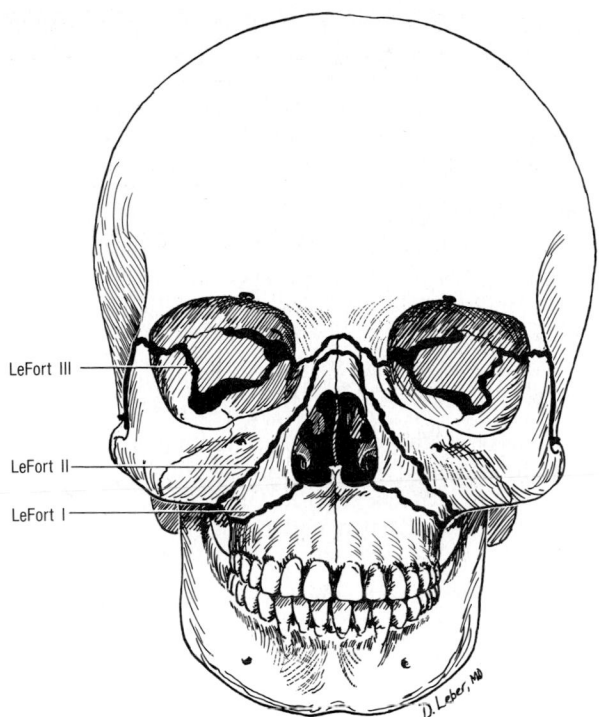

Fig. 51-37. The common levels of fracture of the middle and upper face, based on the work of LeFort. (*After R. LeFort, Experimental Study of Fractures of the Upper Jaw, Rev Chir* [*Paris*], *23:208, 23:360, 1901.*)

depression of the globe is an important diagnostic finding. Subcutaneous emphysema with palpable crepitus over the cheek suggests communication between the antrum and subcutaneous space through the fracture site. False motion may be demonstrated by palpation or grasping of the upper teeth and noting movements separate from the cranium. With marked displacement and true craniofacial disjunction, the patient may present a "long-faced" appearance. Roentgenograms are indicated to confirm the presence of maxillary fractures and may demonstrate

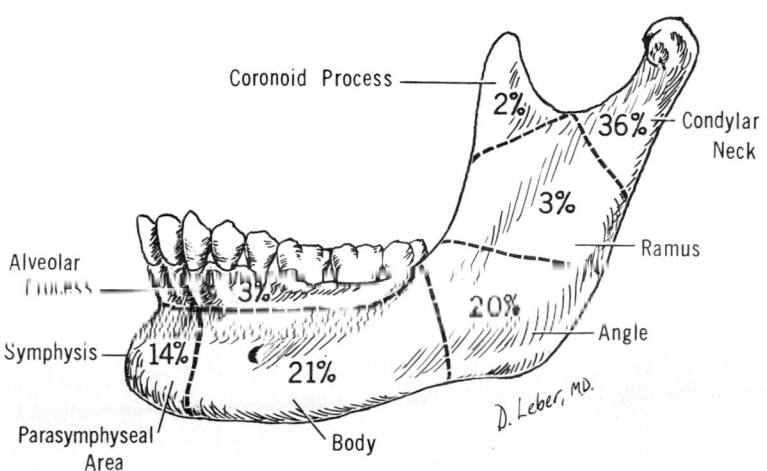

Fig. 51-38. The common mandibular fracture sites. (*After R. O. Dingman, and P. Natvig, "Surgery of Facial Fractures," W. B. Saunders Company, Philadelphia, 1964.*)

NOSE (Fig. 51-39)

Nasal fractures are very common but assume clinical significance only if they are displaced. Immediate reduction of the nasal bones and septum is generally achieved without difficulty under local anesthesia. The crushed and depressed nasal bridge may be elevated with intranasal manipulation at the same time that the bones are manipulated from the external nasal surface.

It must be emphasized that straightforward nasal fractures may be accompanied by major injuries to the septum or contiguous structures. The septum may be grossly displaced laterally, or it may be telescoped up under the dorsum. With any injury to the nose, the septum must be carefully inspected for a submucosal hematoma. If not evacuated, this may lead to pressure necrosis and secondary infection causing septal perforation. Associated injuries to adjacent structures will include disruption of the medial canthal ligament or injury to the base of the skull resulting in cerebrospinal fluid leak. These need to be treated in the operating room under general anesthesia.

The nose can be properly splinted by using individually fashioned splints made from dental compounds, plaster of paris, or plastic-impregnated gauze. Intranasal packing can help maintain the parts in proper reduction.

Soft Tissue Facial Injuries

Soft tissue injuries of the face may be associated with considerable deficits in function in addition to disturbance in a normal appearance. A simple laceration is "simple" only if it does not involve important ingredients of normal facial, ocular, aerodigestive, and aesthetic function. Therefore, a careful assessment of function of structures in anatomic proximity to a facial injury is essential prior to any instrumentation or injection of an anesthetic agent.

FACIAL NERVE

The wide distribution and relatively superficial position of the branches of the facial nerve in the face and upper neck make these structures vulnerable to injury with even small lacerations (Fig. 51-28). To administer anesthetic agents prior to careful assessment of function of this purely motor nerve is to eliminate the only possibility of assuring that the injury and not the treatment is responsible for partial facial motor deficit. A sterile pressure dressing should be used to control hemorrhage during assessment of facial nerve function, since the indiscriminate application of hemostats may in itself result in nerve injury (Fig. 51-40).

Fig. 51-39. The severity of fractures of the nose varies from simple (*A, B*) to the more complex (*C, D, E*). *A* will need no treatment, and *B* can be successfully reduced under local anesthesia in the office or emergency department. *C, D,* and *E* require adequate sedation and anesthesia to allow the manipulations necessary to prevent secondary cosmetic defects or obstructed breathing. In addition, the more severe fractures may need additional treatment to the ethmoid region or the medial canthal ligament.

Fig. 51-40. Facial nerve trauma. *A.* Laceration of temple with arterial hemorrhage. Note multiple hemostats. *B.* Forehead branch facial palsy secondary to injury (?) or instrumentation (?).

Branches of the facial nerve should be repaired if significant motor deficits exist. Microsurgical techniques have increased the successes of such repairs. If facial nerve injury results in paralysis of the orbicularis oculi muscle, the eye must be protected during the postoperative period. Temporary tarsorrhaphy, i.e., surgical attachment of the upper lid to the lower lid, in the region of the lateral canthus may be necessary if ointments, external support by tape, and glasses cannot protect the eye from exposure keratitis.

TRIGEMINAL NERVE

Trauma to the trigeminal nerve interferes with sensation in the face, and, as in the case of facial nerve injuries, evaluation of the areas of sensory loss must be carried out prior to any manipulation or treatment. The losses of sensation are of diagnostic significance in localizing fractures and soft tissue injuries. Anesthesia of the chin and lower lip on one side suggests injury of the mandibular division. If the loss of sensation is localized to this area, the injury is peripheral at the mental foramen. However, if the lower teeth are also anesthetic, this indicates that the inferior alveolar nerve has been injured more proximally or by a mandibular fracture. Anesthesia in the ear region and detectable weakness in mastication or tongue anesthesia are suggestive of even more proximal injury of the mandibular division.

PAROTID

The parotid duct lies caudad to a line drawn from earlobe to the nasal ala and enters the mouth at a point where this line is bisected by an imaginary vertical line from the lateral canthus of the eye (Fig. 51-27). Transection of the parotid duct usually occurs in its superficial portion where it lies over the masseter; this is frequently associated with injury of the buccal branches of the facial nerve. Repair of the duct over a polyethylene tube represents optimal therapy, but ligation may be indicated in the case of severe injury. Lacerations through the parotid gland substance per se are best treated by careful repair of the gland capsule and simple drainage of the wound. Postoperatively, parotitis and temporary salivary drainage are the rule, but spontaneous remission and closure generally occur. The postoperative management should include the avoidance of gustatory stimulation by diet and the use of anticholinergic drugs to reduce secretion.

LACRIMAL DUCTS

Lacerations in the region of the medial canthus of the eye must be carefully evaluated for lacrimal duct injury. The ducts should be probed to assure their integrity. Lacerations are best repaired over a small polyethylene stent carried from the punctum to the nasal cavity.

AREAS OF AESTHETIC IMPORTANCE

HAIRLINE. Injuries and surgical procedures which involve the forehead hairline require careful consideration. Local flaps of hair-bearing skin may be used to construct the hairline in its proper position. Conversely, if hair-bearing scalp is initially used to cover a traumatically or surgically created defect in a non-hair-bearing area close to the scalp hairline, it should be removed later and restored with non-hair-bearing skin to avoid grossly noticeable deformity.

EYEBROW. Precise realignment of the eyebrow which has been divided is important, since a 1- or 2-mm stepwise offset is noticeable at conversational distance. Sharp lacerations which are closed simply may leave an area of alopecia in the eyebrow. This occurs because of the obliquity of the hair roots which are transected by the laceration. Retrimming wound edges parallel to hair follicles prior to closure will avoid this problem (Fig. 51-41). When lacerations cross the eyebrow, the eyebrow should be repaired first, and the remaining portion of the laceration

Fig. 51-41. Avoidance of alopecia during repair of eyebrow laceration. *A.* Oblique projection of eyebrow hairs creates eyebrow alopecia at the laceration site unless the wound is revised parallel to hair follicles. *B.* Laceration crossing the eyebrow. *C.* Precise realignment of eyebrow elements is important.

Fig. 51-42. Estlander flap. *A.* Lines of incision for removal of lower lip lesion and establishment of flap. *B.* Lower lip lesion is excised and flap established. *C.* Flap transferred and upper lip reconstructed.

may then be shifted or revised to conform with the eyebrow repair.

EYELID. The healing and normal wound contraction associated with vertical lacerations of the eyelid result in a predictable contracture. The incisional direction may be altered by performing a primary Z-plasty to avoid this contracture and ugly, uncontrolled exposure of the eye. When soft tissue has been lost by avulsion, primary skin grafting may be essential. Potential donor sites for eyelid skin include the contralateral eyelid, the posterior auricular area, low cervical supraclavicular areas, and the prepuce. These sites furnish skin which is pliable and of appropriate color.

NASOLABIAL FOLD. Hypertrophic bridging scars occur when a laceration crosses this fold. Such lacerations should be altered to place part of the scar within the nasolabial fold per se, employing the technique of Z-plasty (Fig. 51-25).

VERMILION BORDER OF LIP. An offset in this area produces an abnormal step which is apparent at conversational distance. Therefore, precise coaptation of this important landmark deserves primary attention at the time of initial repair. During the repair, the first suture should be placed at this ridge; adjustments of the rest of the wound then can be made accordingly.

HEAD AND NECK TUMORS

Since head and neck tumor therapy (see Chap. 16) may result in functional and/or cosmetic deformity, principles of reconstructive surgery are particularly applicable in this area.

Lip

A small lesion up to 1 cm can generally be readily excised by a shield-shaped resection, and the wound closed with minimal deformity. However, larger tumors which require removal of half or more of the lower lip should have restorative surgical treatment using local soft tissue in various geometric shifts. Such an example is the Estlander flap (Fig. 51-42), which makes use of a segment of the upper lip rotated around at the commissure, with the marginal vessels (coronary vessels) preserved for blood supply. The Abbe modification of the Estlander flap also takes tissue from the upper lip to fill the lower lip deficit (Fig. 51-43). In this instance, the upper lip wedge is connected to the upper lip by a vascular pedicle which crosses the opening of the mouth, preserving the commissure. This results in a double oral stoma which is reconverted to the single stoma about 2 weeks later. Preserving the commissure is a major advantage, because commissure reconstruction is so difficult.

The Bernard procedure (Fig. 51-44) has been applied to allow movement of cheek skin mediad in order to reconstruct larger defects of the lower lip. A similar procedure devised by Webster can be used to reconstruct the upper lip. Nasolabial triangles are the key to the tissue

Fig. 51-43. Abbe modification of Estlander flap. *A.* Incisions outlined. *B.* Tumor excised from lower lip, and upper lip flap established. *C.* Upper lip flap turned down to fill defect in lower lip. Note double oral stoma. *D.* Upper-to-lower lip pedicle transected, with single stoma as a result.

Fig. 51-44. Bernard procedure. *A.* Outline of skin incisions for removal of tumor and skin plus mucosal incision for removal of nasolabial triangles. *B.* Tumors and nasolabial triangles excised and buccal mucosa turned down to enlarge lower lip. *C.* Incisions closed.

movement; their removal allows the advancement of full thicknesses of the cheek into the medial position to make a lip. For the lower lip, cheek rotations of the mucosa are used for the vermilion reconstruction.

Tongue

If the lesion is small, adequate excision may be accomplished by a wedge resection, if this is located in the free margin of the tongue. This is applicable to very few malignant tumors (Fig. 51-45). Most tumors of the anterior portion of the tongue are best treated by a combination of supervoltage radiation followed by hemiglossectomy, partial mandibulectomy, and cervical node dissection. Selecting the proper combinations of radiation, surgery, and adjunctive chemotherapy, for each situation is critical. Proper dental splinting to control mandibular fragments and the imaginative use of flaps of the forehead, neck, or chest will help control the cosmetic and functional deformity.

Fig. 51-46. *A.* Carcinoma of the nose. *B.* Wide through-and-through resection of tumor. *C.* Forehead flap reconstruction. *D.* Result after healing.

Nose

Reconstructive surgical treatment is frequently indicated for the cosmetic deformity which results from removal of a tumor. The procedures generally employ a forehead, a cheek, or occasionally a distant pedicle flap to replace the resected tissue (Fig. 51-46).

Fig. 51-45. Wedge excision of small anterior tongue lesion and primary closure.

Eyelid

The functional and cosmetic deficit created by excision of eyelid tumors must usually be reconstructed immediately. Loss of function, if not corrected, may result in

A

B

Fig. 51-47. Five months after composite resection including a large portion of the tongue and pharynx, rehabilitation is accomplished by only two operations: (1) the original extirpation and reconstruction with deltopectoral flap, and (2) insetting of the flap and return of its base to the chest wall. *A.* A deltopectoral flap has been raised from the right shoulder and chest, rotated upward, tubed upon itself, and used to reconstruct the pharynx and esophagus. The large clamp is in this skin-lined tube; the end of the clamp is in the mouth. This has accomplished the reconstruction at the time of the resection. Only one further procedure will be needed approximately 10 weeks later to transect the flap, close the fistula, and return the base of the flap to its original position. *B.* Note that there are no vertical scars on the neck (use of the MacFee incisions) or the shoulder donor site of the pharyngeal wall. *C.* The lip-splitting incision leaves a permanent but not objectionable scar. Forty percent of the mandible has been removed from the right side. *D.* Deviation is controlled by the special dental metal outrigger on the right, attached to an acrylic splint. The lighter area on the left is the upper end of the shoulder tissue forming the lateral pharyngeal wall. (*Source: R. Goldwyn (ed.), "The Unfavorable Result in Plastic Surgery: Avoidance and Treatment," Little, Brown and Company, Boston, 1972.*)

permanent damage to vision. Local flaps, utilizing available skin, and full-thickness skin grafts are the most common methods of repair. Large cheek rotation flaps or eyelid flaps may be required in some cases.

Soft Tissue Losses

Excision of large tumors of the head and neck frequently results in major losses of soft tissue and consequent contour defects. The lining of the mouth and pharynx, as well as the cutaneous surfaces, are generally best replaced by pedicle flap reconstruction, although split-thickness skin grafts are serviceable in certain regions. When flaps are used, they are preferably obtained locally from the head, neck, or chest, unless all the donor sites have been subjected to irradiation or are otherwise compromised. When this occurs, pedicle flaps from distant sites may be carried on the upper extremity or may be moved end over end in stages, as popularized by Gillies. These multiple transfer flaps have been mainly replaced by the newer flap techniques (Fig. 51-47), which usually close defects by primary reconstruction. If the reconstruction cannot be accomplished early, a defect may present secondarily. Before any secondary defect is closed, all necrotic bone and cartilage must be removed from the depths of the wound, since they

D

C

Fig. 51-47. (*continued*).

Fig. 51-48. (See Fig. 51-17.) Repair of orocutaneous fistula in irradiated area. *A.* Note osteoradionecrosis of mandible. *B.* Some time after mandibular resection. Fistula closure started. *C.* Island pedicle flap taken from the forehead carried solely on the temporal vessels prepared to be passed subcutaneously to the fistula site where vascularized soft tissue is needed. *D.* Healing with the island pedicle flap furnishing skin and subcutaneous tissue with blood supply from the temporal vessels, which now course subcutaneously from the temporal area to the large composite skin patch.

represent nonviable active foreign bodies which will perpetuate draining and interfere with healing. Orocutaneous, pharyngocutaneous, or esophagocutaneous fistulas may be covered and closed with flaps such as a forehead tissue flap transferred to the area on a pedicle of temporal vessels (island pedicle flap) (Fig. 51-48). This same type of technique is particularly applicable to the covering of defects in heavily irradiated areas, because the flap provides its own permanent blood supply. Free skin grafts (Fig. 51-49) are also frequently used for closing defects left after excision of cancer of the head and neck. Care must be taken to match color, consistency, and hair-bearing characteristics.

Bone Losses

The major areas of loss of bone are from the calvarium, maxilla, mandible, or nose. Each of these areas has its own particular specifications for replacement. The calvarium is best replaced by rib grafts, split longitudinally, or by plates made of metal or plastic. The maxilla is best replaced by soft prosthesis, preferably sponges made from silicone. The mandible may be replaced either with bone grafts or by an implanted synthetic prosthesis. The best donor site for a mandible graft is the ilium, since autogenous cancellous

Fig. 51-49. Free skin grafts to cover soft tissue losses. *A*. Face skin graft with poor color match. Donor site, abdomen. *B*. Skin graft of face with good color match. Donor site chosen for proper match. *C*. Full-thickness graft to face from supraclavicular area. Note good color match and texture.

bone appears to have the best chance for survival. Problems of immobilization of the jaws are challenging and require the ingenious use of dental wiring or splints, external fixation appliances, and bone carpentry with internal fixation by means of wires, plates, or compression devices. Defects of nasal losses can be replaced by cancellous bone, cartilage, or a solid silicone prothesis. In all these situations it is critical that adequate soft tissue coverage and lining is provided to prevent secondary extrusion.

CONGENITAL ANOMALIES OF THE HEAD AND NECK

Cleft Lip and Palate

One in eight hundred living neonates has cleft deformity of the lip and/or palate. Today, children with this defect may be completely rehabilitated through combined surgical, orthodontic, otologic, psychologic, and speech therapy. Although the treatment is very individualized, each patient benefits greatly if the specialists in these many disciplines are closely allied as a diagnostic and therapeutic team.

CLASSIFICATION. Clefts of the palate and lip are classified by various criteria according to whether the primary palate (lip and alveolar ridge) or the secondary palate (hard and soft palate), or both, are involved in the fusion failure. Clefts of the primary palate may be incomplete (Fig. 51-50*A* and *B*), involving only part of the vertical lip dimension, or they may extend into the nostril (Fig. 51-50*C*). The clefts may be bilateral or unilateral, and they may or may not involve the alveolar bone (tooth-bearing alveolus). Clefts of the lip and alveolar ridge may extend to involve the hard and soft palate (secondary palate); these are classified as complete unilateral clefts of the lip and palate (Fig. 51-50*C* and *F*) and complete bilateral clefts of the lip and palate (Fig. 51-50*D* and *G*). The fusion defect may be limited to the secondary palate, in which case it is termed an incomplete cleft of the palate (Fig. 51-50*E*).

TREATMENT. Prior to any surgery, the dental specialist and the surgeon evaluate the patient. This applies to the neonate, since appropriate neonatal dental obturators may be important in preventing subsequent arch deformity. The newborn patient with a cleft lip and palate is a true emergency for both the plastic surgeon and the dentist. The plastic surgeon's therapy begins as soon after birth as is feasible, even though no surgery may be planned for several weeks. Counseling of parents can be best accomplished by the plastic surgeon who has the longitudinal depth of knowledge of this problem.

Timing of Surgery. There is little disagreement that our knowledge to date supports the notion that cleft lip should be repaired early (i.e., during the first three months of life,) and that the cleft palate should be repaired a little later (i.e., when the patient is 1 to 1½ years of age). Whether the lip should be repaired at birth or at age three months depends on the individual preference of the surgeon, since the results are equivalent. The authors prefer to carry out the definitive repair when the baby is approximately ten to twelve weeks of age; when general anesthesia may be used with greater safety, the repair can be technically more precise, since the lip elements are larger, and conversion to cup or dropper feeding in the postoperative period is somewhat easier. When the lip has been repaired at birth prior to the baby's exposure to the parents, they may not adequately appreciate the severity and problems of this deformity and thus may not be as gratified by the surgical repair. This is important because the parents' satisfaction or dissatisfaction may be transmitted to the child.

It is customary to repair the palate when the child is between 1 and 1½ years of age, and the younger the better,

Fig. 51-50. Classification of cleft lip and palate. *A*. Minimal incomplete cleft of the lip (primary palate). Note nostril asymmetry. *B*. Moderately severe incomplete cleft of the lip (primary palate). Note nostril asymmetry. *C*. Complete unilateral cleft lip and palate (primary and secondary palate). *D*. Complete bilateral cleft lip and palate (primary and secondary palate). *E*. Incomplete cleft of the palate (secondary palate). *F*. Unilateral complete cleft of lip and palate (primary and secondary palate). *G*. Bilateral complete cleft of lip and palate (primary and secondary palate).

so that there will be a repaired palate during a major initial speech effort. However, repair earlier than at one year is hazardous, because blood loss may represent a significant percentage of the child's blood volume. Blood transfusions are rarely indicated or necessary in these operations. It also has been noted that repairs of the cleft palate prior to the age of eighteen months result in a much higher percentage of children with normal speech, greater than 70 percent. If the procedure is delayed to three or more years after

birth, the speech is not as good.

Techniques. The unilateral incomplete cleft of the primary palate (lip) may be repaired so that the defect is barely perceptible. The goal is to achieve adequate length from the nostril floor to the vermilion ridge, to match precisely the contralateral side of the lip. The usual techniques for closure of the cleft lip are variations of a Z-plasty. The various methods proposed by Skoog, Tennison, LeMesurier, Millard and Pigott, Randall, and Wynn differ in the vertical level at which the Z-plasty is performed, but all represent the application of surgical geometry with an interdigitation of flaps. The type of Z-plasty repair selected (occasionally a straight-line, i.e., Rose-Thompson repair) is determined by the anatomy of the defect. The authors of this chapter generally employ the Millard infranasal Z-plasty (Fig. 51-51), since it places the primary scar along the normal philtrum line. The Millard technique is applicable to all types of clefts, but is most suitable when there is a large infraalar portion of white lip on the cleft side. When the lip cleft is a complete one and is

Fig. 51-51. Millard infranasal Z-plasty. *A*. Lines of incision outlined. *B*. Closure demonstrated. *C*. Preoperative photograph. *D*. Postoperative photograph.

Fig. 51-52. Tennison Z-plasty. *A.* Lines of incision outlined. *B.* Closure demonstrated. *C.* Preoperative photograph. *D.* Postoperative photograph.

particularly wide, even though primary closure can be accomplished, it may be desirable to perform a preliminary operation, or "lip adhesions." This procedure is performed 8 weeks prior to definitive cheiloplasty, best at age four to six weeks. The cleft is bridged by two matching quadrangular flaps designed from the tissues on the borders of the cleft that eventually would have been discarded. This operation achieves four important goals: (1) it molds anterior alveolus, (2) it directs nasal ala to correct direction, (3) it stimulates local growth processes, and (4) it increases the amount of tissues available for subsequent repair.

When the local pathologic anatomy is such that the rotation-advancement technique of Millard will encounter a difficulty in adding vertical length, the authors favor the supravermilion triangular flap Z-plasty, described by Tennison and modified by Randall (Fig. 51-52).

Occasionally, the nostril deformity common to all clefts is minor and can be corrected completely at the primary operation. The distortions of the nostril can be corrected considerably during these early operations, to lessen the deformity during the growing years. However, most nostril distortions will require corrective procedures at secondary operations when the child is older, at age five, age eight, and finally a definitive rhinoplasty just prior to the teens.

Bilateral clefts of the lip and palate are an even greater challenge. Repair of the lip may be performed in one or two stages, care being taken to preserve the prolabium (central portion of the lip between the clefts), because it

becomes the central segment of the reconstructed lip and will grow in an amazing fashion when it has been connected to the lateral segments. This creates an intact muscular lip arch which will help mold the alveolar ridge into the correct position, with adjunctive orthodontic devices guiding the ridge. The repaired lip itself is acting as an orthodontic traction to bring elements of the alveolar dental arch into the proper relation (Fig. 51-53).

Additional orthodontic methods are required for complete clefts of the palate in order to mold the alveolar arch and prevent its collapse. Although early orthodontic treatment remains popular, the early grafting of bone across the cleft is decreasing in applicability, since the long-term benefits have not been forthcoming, and there is perhaps less growth in the area where bone grafting has been done. However, after the age of five there are many instances when only bone grafting can obtain the proper arch and facial configuration. The clefts of the soft and hard palate are closed by a modification of the Kilner operation (Fig. 51-54) or by the Langenbeck technique.

All patients with cleft palate have drainage problems

Fig. 51-53. Effects of lip closure on alveolar dental arch. *A.* Complete cleft of lip and palate. *B.* Closure of defect of lip brings alveolar segment in anatomic position. *C.* Note correction of alveolar arch. Guidance of the parts by intraoral appliances may be necessary to enhance correct positioning.

A   *B*   *C*

Fig. 51-54. Common types of palatal lengthening operations. Retropositioning during the repair of a cleft is a logical means of improving speech. 1. Long flaps are designed; note the anterior shape and the incisions along the cleft and laterally. 2. The mucoperiosteal flaps are elevated, with isolation and preservation of the greater palatine vessels and nerves. The nasal mucosa is widely undermined from the hard palate on the nasal side. 3. The handling of the nasal mucosa (a) in a palate that is long; the mucosa does not need to be transected, only widely mobilized; the soft palate aponeurosis is separated from the posterior edge of the hard palate, and the levator palati muscles are repositioned posteriorly. (b) When the palate is short, the nasal mucosa is sectioned obliquely; these angled incisions form a Z-plasty which lengthens the palate and prevents linear contracture from tension. (c) If the palate is short and the cleft wide, a turned-over island flap to bridge the gap is useful, although necessary only occasionally. 4. (a and b) The second and third layers of the closure are now completed using a row of buried sutures to approximate the muscles, in addition to the row of mucosal sutures already present. The only raw surfaces left are overlying the bony palate. (c) The method of closure when an anterior island flap has been used for closing the nasal surface superiorly.

of the middle ear. These frequently require drainage at an early age, usually supplemented with insertion of tubes for more permanent drainage. Upper respiratory tract infections must be even more closely monitored and promptly treated with decongestants, anti-inflammatory agents, and antibiotics guided by appropriate cultures.

The appearance of the patients and their dental occlusion is important, but of equal or more significance is their communication, as the speech results are intimately intertwined with hearing and motivation. Speech therapy is helpful for all patients. Careful assessment clinically, aerodynamically, and radiographically is imperative. Both static roentgenograms (Fig. 51-55) and cineradiography in lateral, frontal, and superoinferior planes are helpful. Secondary procedures include methods of adding length to the palate itself, reinforcing the elevation properties of the palate, occlusion of the space by attachment of a flap of the posterior pharyngeal wall to the palate, or techniques to make the pharyngeal port smaller either by retropharyngeal implantation or by procedures to decrease the size of the opening by protrusion of the pharyngeal muscle and mucosa.

A

B

Fig. 51-55. Cephalometric speech studies. *A.* The head-holding cephalostat which is used so that the film can have its exact parameters duplicated at any subsequent time. Note that during a maximal effort at stimulating the palate it hangs loosely so that there is a wide gap in the pharynx communicating to the nose. This patient will have excessive escape of air and unintelligible speech, and will need a surgical procedure of the pharyngeal flap type. *B.* In marked contrast is this soft palate which has elevated excellently, although a gap between it and the posterior pharyngeal wall can still be noticed. For a palate such as this a lengthening procedure or a pharyngeoplasty procedure would be effective, and a pharyngeal flap is not needed.

Congenital Microtia

Severe hypoplastic malformations of the ear, which occur in 1 of 15,000 births, represent branchial arch deformities. There may be partial or complete absence of the external, middle, and/or inner parts of the ear. Frequently, the external auditory meatus and canal are totally absent, and there may be associated anomalies of the facial

nerve, the temporomandibular joint, and the mandible. The unilateral situation is about six times as frequent as bilateral.

TREATMENT. When radiologic and audiologic examination reveals a functioning hearing apparatus and the patient has bilateral atresia of the canals, surgery on one side should be attempted to alleviate the total deafness. In unilateral situations, no surgery is recommended to improve the hearing on the affected side.

Reconstruction of the absent or nearly absent external ear is usually recommended, because of the great improvement in the surgical techniques of cartilage reconstruction. As prosthetic techniques improve, both in the materials to design the prostheses and the glues used to attach them, there is a growing feeling that surgery can be replaced by an excellent prosthesis. However, at this date the authors still recommend surgical reconstruction. Cartilage is still preferred. The initial successes with prosthetic implanted ears described by Cronin and others have had to be modified, as long-term results indicate that the implants become extruded, although autogenous fascia lata coverage has improved the retention rate. Even though a perfect ear is not reproduced, the results of cartilage reconstructions seem to be more reliable and satisfactory.

Any of these ear reconstructions require multiple operations. They are best performed when ear growth is nearly complete, so that further contralateral growth will not cause a size disparity, and when the child is old enough to have well-developed costal cartilages. This usually means that the first stage should be deferred until the child is approximately six or seven years old. The first-stage operation is designed to place the remaining visible ear elements in their proper relationship, so that they will accept the supporting material at a later date in the correct position. This initial operation is also the time when unsightly, nonusable tags of skin and fragments of cartilage may be discarded. At the second stage the supporting material is obtained from the ribs and carved. It is inserted beneath the mastoid skin as the architectural framework. At a third stage, the posterior surface of a reconstructed ear is grafted with skin after it has been elevated from its mastoid bed (Fig. 51-56).

Thyroglossal Anomalies

About 6 percent of the masses found in the neck are of congenital origin. The most common lesions, which represent two-thirds of the total, are cysts or sinuses of the thyroglossal duct. The thyroid gland has its embryonic origin in the middle of the anterior pharynx in an area which later becomes the tongue. The thyroid anlage migrates into the neck but remains attached at the foramen cecum by the thyroglossal duct. Normally, this connection becomes obliterated early in embryonic life, but occasionally it may persist as a sinus tract, which becomes enclosed by the fused elements of the hyoid bone, or as a cyst (Fig. 51-57).

The lesions appear in the midline or just off the midline of the neck at some point between the isthmus of the thyroid gland and the hyoid bone. The cystic lesions may

Fig. 51-56. A multistaged ear reconstruction in microtia. *A.* The original defect—congenital absence of normal ear cartilage and malposition of the lobule. *B.* The first stage. Repositioning of the lobule has been accomplished by the use of a Z-plasty. The marks indicate the correct size and angle for reconstruction. Measurement of the opposite normal ear, acrylic models, and photography are essential to correct placement. *C.* The completed ear. Costochondral cartilage is used to form the structure.

be identified by their position and rubbery characteristics. These may become infected and rupture spontaneously or require surgical incision. Once the cyst has become infected, it will persist with repeated episodes of abscess formation and drainage until the entire cyst and its tract are removed. A midline sinus, which is diagnostic of a persistent thyroglossal duct, should also be surgically excised.

Incomplete removal represents the most common error in treatment of thyroglossal anomalies. Removal of either cyst or sinus requires excision of the central hyoid segment if recurrence is to be avoided (Sistrunk procedure). If the mass is of significant size, the presence of thyroid tissue in its normal position should be demonstrated in order to avoid the possibility of removing the patient's only functioning thyroid from the base of the tongue.

Branchial Anomalies

Abnormalities in the cervicofacial complex result from arrest and alteration of the developing branchial arches and clefts. Congenital cysts, sinuses, fistulas, and growth alterations in the head and neck fall into a pattern which is specific for each branchial cleft and arch. As a group, these represent the second most common congenital lesion of the neck.

EMBRYOLOGY. Each of the five branchial arches seen in early embryonic life (Fig. 51-58) is separated from the adjacent arch by a cleft. Normally, the clefts close and disappear, and the arches coalesce to create a smooth continuity of the face and neck tissues. The first arch provides the building blocks for the maxillomandibular complex and part of the auricle. The second arch gives rise to the cervical structures and part of the auricle. Between these two arches is the first branchial cleft, which

is the embryonic origin of the eustachian apparatus and auditory canal. The third branchial arch derivatives are neck structures in the hyoid region. The second cleft anatomically runs from the tonsillar fossa anteriorly to the lower neck. It normally closes prior to birth. Parts of the larynx and cervical vascular structure have their origin in the fourth and fifth arches. Anomalies in the fourth and fifth arches rarely cause abnormalities and will not be considered in this section.

FIRST BRANCHIAL ARCH ANOMALIES. These become manifest as abnormal development confined to the mouth, mandible, and anterior parts of the ear, referred to as the *oromandibuloauricular syndrome.* More frequently, the anomalies are not confined, and parts derived from the second arch are also abnormal.

FIRST BRANCHIAL CLEFT ANOMALIES. A cyst, sinus, or fistula which lies between the external auditory canal and

Fig. 51-57. Sagittal section indicating tract of thyroglossal duct. Originating at the foramen cecum, it passes through the hyoid bone in the midline and continues to the skin at the suprasternal notch.

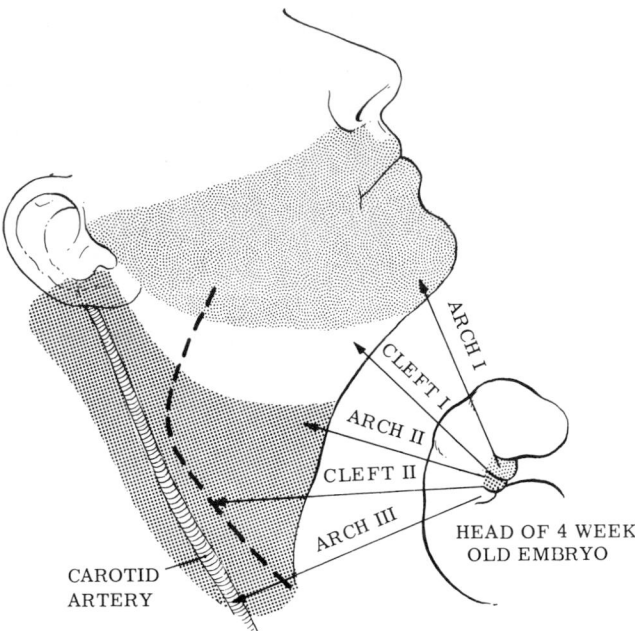

Fig. 51-58. Contribution of the embryonic branchial arches to the parts of the adult face. (*Modified from Knute Berger.*)

the submandibular area originates from the first branchial cleft. Proximity of such sinuses to the facial nerve may make removal difficult (Fig. 51-59).

SECOND BRANCHIAL CLEFT ANOMALIES. The vast majority of branchial anomalies represent remnants of the second branchial cleft. These commonly present as a cyst

Fig. 51-59. Pathologic consequences of incomplete embryonic dissolution of the first and second branchial grooves and clefts. (*Modified from Knute Berger.*)

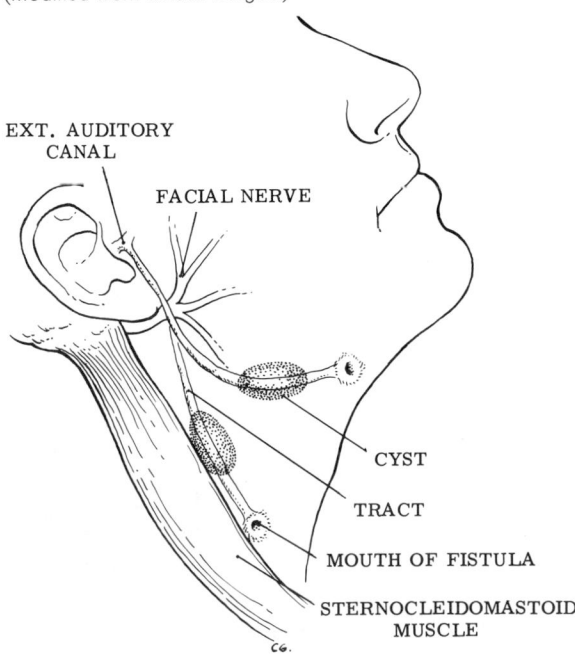

which is located anterior to the sternocleidomastoid muscle in the middle third of the anterior triangle of the neck (Fig. 51-59). The cyst is lined with squamous or columnar epithelial tissue and contains a greenish mucuslike detritus, which accumulates in the lumen and gradually causes the cyst to increase in size. It may become secondarily infected or may cause pressure symptoms by sudden increase in size. The original internal opening of the branchial cleft is in the tonsillar fossa, and sinuses can connect to the tonsillar fossa from the cyst or extend all the way to the skin. Treatment is by excision of the cyst and its tract. Since the tract descends between the internal and external branches of the carotid artery, care must be taken during the surgical procedure.

COSMETIC SURGERY

Scar Revision

Facial scars resulting from trauma, infection, previous surgical treatment, chemical and radiation therapy, or dermatologic disorders frequently are dramatically improved by surgical renovation. Not all scars can be eliminated completely, but improvement is accomplished by excision and precise closure to achieve the best per primam healing. The lines of the scar may be altered by geometric reorientation to avoid crossing normal facial lines of tension. Scar characteristics such as pigmentation, depigmentation, depression, hypertrophy, improper alignment, tattooing, and ragged edges are correctible by excision, reclosure with or without Z-plasty, or other geometric reorientation techniques.

Distorting contractures and unsightly hypertrophy may necessitate excision and replacement with skin graft. If no contour defect exists, free skin grafts are employed. These should be obtained from areas with the same characteristics, i.e., color, texture, hairlessness, and thickness, as the area of skin to be grafted (Fig. 51-49). Small defects on the face may be successfully and inconspicuously covered with free full-thickness grafts from the postauricular area or the supraclavicular region. The thin eyelid skin is best replaced by contralateral lid skin or from the prepuce in the uncircumcised male.

If the facial scar is accompanied by an abnormality in contour, pedicle flap reconstruction is essential. A graft fashioned from local tissue is superior, because it creates the least conspicuous correction as far as color and texture are concerned. The copious blood supply in the head and neck assures the success of local pedicle flaps even when the pedicle is reduced to a vascular bundle. If local tissue is not available, pedicles may be carried from a distant site, in which case multiple stages of advancement may be required.

Eyebrow Reconstruction

An eyebrow which has been destroyed by trauma, leprosy, radiation, or another cause creates a noticeable defect. The hair-bearing eyebrow may be replaced by a free

Fig. 51-60. Eyebrow restoration using a vascularized hair-bearing scalp island carried on the temporal vessels.

composite graft from the scalp (Fig. 51-7) or contralateral eyebrow or, even more reliably, by using a temporal vascular island pedicle flap from the scalp (Fig. 51-60). Since the replaced eyebrow hair maintains the characteristics of the donor site, it must be clipped regularly, just as one cuts the hair on his head.

Prominent Ears

Prominent ears with no antihelix fold and, frequently, overdevelopment of the concha occur in both sexes. Corrective surgical procedures consist of weakening the cartilage on its anterior surface, resecting a portion of the hypertrophic conchal wall, suture fixating the antihelix fold, and removing excesses of helix tail and retroauricular skin excisions. This can result in near-perfect restoration. The optimal age for correction is not determined, but it is best done the summer before entering school, either under local or general anesthesia (Fig. 51-61).

Rhinoplasty

Nasal size and contour are largely dependent upon the bony and cartilaginous framework. Occasionally the skin and soft tissue over this underlying architecture may be the cause of the deformity, as in rhinophyma. Deformities may result from trauma to the nasal skeleton, previous surgical treatment, infection, or simple inherited characteristics.

Rhinoplasty represents the most frequently considered cosmetic surgical procedure. With today's reliable, safe, and simple procedures to overcome nasal deformity, whether congenital or traumatic, it seems unduly conservative to consider rhinoplasty as unnecessary surgical treatment. In some individuals, these deformities, even though purely cosmetic, are psychically disturbing. The psychosocial readjustment that frequently follows the op-

eration is most rewarding in patients who have been carefully selected and assessed prior to operation (Fig. 51-62).

The usual cosmetic nasal deformities are correctible by revision of the bony and cartilaginous architecture, allowing the soft tissues to readjust naturally. The nasal bones, like the roof of a house, support one another at the midline of the nose. They are joined at this point by the nasal septum. When a permanent nasal hump is removed, the nasal bones and septum remain as three separate elements creating a broad nasal bridge. During rhinoplasty, the hump is removed and the nasal bones are fractured through lateral osteotomies in the nasal processes of the maxilla, so that the bridge of the nose may be made narrow at the same time.

The nasal tip and septal support are entirely cartilaginous, and they may be reshaped by trimming the alar, upper lateral, and septal cartilages appropriately.

Very frequently deformity of the septum causes obstruction to breathing. The majority of septal resections may

Fig. 51-61. A. Congenital prominence of ears. B. After otoplasty.

Fig. 51-62. Cosmetic rhinoplasty. *A.* Preoperative photograph. *B.* Postoperative photograph.

accompany the rhinoplasty. However, if the septal removal will compromise support of the dorsum of the nose, the combined septal resection and rhinoplasty should not be done and either one or the other electively deferred for a few months.

Rhytidectomy (Face-lifting) and Blepharoplasty

The aging face may create significant problems among people whose occupations depend upon their appearance. Premature looseness of facial tissues or wrinkling of facial skin and eyelid skin can be a psychologic barrier impossible to overcome; surgical correction may be urgently indicated. Although this type of aesthetic surgery occupies an extremely important place in American medical practice, it is poorly understood by many physicians who must be supportive toward their patients and recognize their need when making the difficult preoperative decisions. The gratifying results to such a high percentage of patients are eloquent testimony to the fulfillment of *realistic* needs.

The fine wrinkles and grooves in the skin are best treated by chemical peeling or dermabrasion. Looseness and ptosis of the skin are corrected by excising excessive skin at a site where the residual scar is not readily visible. From these incisions in the hairline and around the ear, there is wide undermining of the facial and cervical skin, allowing it to be rotated upward and backward to permit the excess to be removed in order to accomplish tightening by this overlapping at the incision site. In the eyelids, age expresses itself by sagging and wrinkling of the eyelid skin and also weakening of the lids' orbital septums, allowing protrusion of the intraorbital fat into the lids. This will give the appearance of constant tiredness, or even a deceptive look of debauchery. Resections of the excessive eyelid skin and removal of the fat herniations, a procedure known

as blepharoplasty, may precede, accompany, or follow a face-lifting procedure.

FACIAL CONTOUR DEFECTS

Loss of soft tissue substances or skeletal support results in facial contour defects which are cosmetically unattractive and occasionally grotesque. A number of useful techniques are available to restore facial contour and symmetry. Free autogenous grafts of bone, cartilage, dermis, and fat have been employed in the standard techniques for many years. Nonreactive plastic materials recently have been refined to the extent that they are now being used with increasing frequency as contour-restoring tissue substitutes.

FREE GRAFTS. Autogenous bone grafts are useful in correcting defects in the orbital margins, over a depressed zygoma, and over the mandible where the support beneath the skin and subcutaneous tissue is normally firm. In the cheek areas, defects are better corrected with soft tissue grafts of dermis and fat, or with prostheses. During vascularization of free autogenous grafts, some atrophy and loss of fat occurs; for this reason the graft should overcorrect the deformity initially. Spontaneous readjustment generally takes place 6 months to 1 year after operation.

PEDICLE GRAFTS. Subcutaneous tissue and dermis may be transferred from a local area or a distant site using a tubed pedicle in order to fill contour defects. Since the transfer tissue is never devoid of blood supply, atrophy does not occur to the same extent as noted in free grafts. Therefore, overcorrection is not essential with this technique.

PLASTIC MATERIALS. Of the various plastic materials available for implantation, silicones have proved to be the most useful. Dacron, Teflon, polyethylene, and acrylics each have many specific indications. Medical-grade silicone is chemically inert, readily fabricated, easily sterilized, and noncarcinogenic. It can be manufactured in a wide variety of consistencies from semiliquid to sponge to rigid. Studies of the tissue reactions both to silicone and to the other materials mentioned suggest that there is minimal foreign body response, although a bursal separation is common around the smoother types. The smaller the fiber presented to the patient's tissues, the less the total reaction. Studies are still in progress to determine the total longevity of these materials. Injectable liquid silicone is still experimental.

Distorted Maxillomandibular Relationship

Distortion of the anatomic relationship of the maxillary and mandibular units may be associated with minimal abnormality of aesthetic significance or severe disproportion of a disfiguring nature. Disproportion may be due to congenital malformation, growth abnormality, infection, trauma, or surgical procedures. Skeletal aberration may or may not be associated with dental occlusion. Conversely, malocclusion in itself may be responsible for distorted facial patterns. In the latter case, orthodontic therapy alone is sufficient.

MANDIBULAR RETRUSION

Inadequate mandibular substance with foreshortening of the mandible is called *micrognathia*. This may be congenital or may result from injury to the condylar epiphysis. With unilateral mandibular growth disturbance, there are asymmetry and problems with lateral occlusion. With temporomandibular joint disease, ankylosis of this joint is the problem.

Surgical relief of ankylosis is achieved by osteotomy and removal of sufficient bone of the condyle to allow free motion of the mandible. Interposition of soft tissue or silicone aids in preventing recurrent ankylosis. To achieve appropriate correction of the mandibular retrusion, precise measurements must be made roentgenographically, photographically, and with dental models. Correction is accomplished by osteotomy with or without bone grafting, which may produce dramatic results. Both the abnormal occlusal relationship and the cosmetic aberration can be corrected. When the deformity is severe and there is no major occlusion problem, a bone graft or sponge silicone implant over the point of the chin is corrective.

MANDIBULAR PROTRUSION

Prognathism, or protrusion of the mandible, represents another disproportion between the mandible and maxilla. Malocclusion usually occurs, and osteotomy and recession of the mandible are the preferable approach. Vertical, sagittal, and horizontal osteotomies applied in many geometric variations are used. Once the bilateral osteotomy has been performed, the teeth are brought into proper occlusal relation, maintained there by an interdental acrylic occlusal wafer, and then immobilized by intermaxillary fixation for 10 to 12 weeks so that proper healing will ensue.

MAXILLARY RETRUSION

Flattening and depression of the middle third of the face, referred to as the "dish-face deformity," may represent a familial trait and is commonly associated with congenital cleft palate. Trauma may also result in maxillary retrusion. Correction of maxillary retrusion by osteotomy and adjustment of occlusion is more difficult than correction of the distortions of the mandible. Substitution for the cosmetically important flattened area can be achieved by onlay grafts or silicone implantation. Prosthetic devices as part of an upper denture also may be helpful.

Craniofacial Anomalies

Severe craniofacial anomalies such as those seen in Apert's syndrome, Crouzon's disease, and hypertelorism are now amenable to correction. Pioneer surgery by Tessier et al., Converse et al., Dingman and Natvig, Edgerton et al., and Murray and Swanson has proved the worth of the combined intracranial-transfacial approach to correct the abnormal facies by complicated osteotomies and bone grafts. These are extremely complex and exacting procedures, requiring a well-trained team of plastic surgeons, neurosurgeons, anesthesiologists, and dental specialists.

FACIAL PARALYSIS

The causes of facial nerve palsy vary from the incompletely understood Bell's palsy to complete or partial transection of the nerve by trauma or surgical procedure. The proximal intratemporal portion of the nerve is characterized by a lengthy and circuitous passage through the temporal bone. The nerve emerges via the stylomastoid foramen, enters the parotid gland, and arborizes with considerable variability as it passes anteriorly through the gland. The peripheral motor branches, i.e., temporal, zygomatic, buccal, mandibular, and cervical, lie just deep to the very superficial facial musculature. The diffuse spread of these branches coupled with their superficial position makes them subject to injury in face lacerations. Operations in the parotid region, middle ear, or intracranially in the auditofacial area may all result in facial nerve injury.

Localization of the lesion requires a knowledge of nerve anatomy and an appreciation of the function of individual branches. Central (supranuclear) palsy characteristically presents with paralysis of the facial muscles with the exception of the forehead and eyelid musculature. The paralysis is contralateral to the site of the lesion. The intratemporal portion of the nerve gives rise to the chorda tympani nerve and therefore may be assessed by testing taste from the anterior two-thirds of the tongue. The nerve to the stapedius is difficult to test, but the greater superficial petrosal nerve supplies taste to the soft palate. All muscles of facial expression, the platysma, and the buccinator are supplied by the intraparotid portion of the nerve. Except for a few sensory fibers to the ear carried in the posterior auricular branch, the extratemporal facial nerve is purely motor.

Facial Nerve Repair

Paralysis of the facial nerve may pose two separate problems for reconstruction: one involves a direct approach to the nerve itself, while the other consists of methods to overcome the functional and cosmetic disability which results from irreversible paralysis.

Intratemporal nerve decompression and repair of the nerve with grafting techniques are procedures which are now performed regularly with acceptable success. The extratemporal nerve should be repaired as soon as the diagnosis is established, and studies of nerve conduction, chronaxie, and electromyography are all helpful in this regard. The application of an operating microscope has facilitated precise repair of small facial nerve branches.

When gaps exist as a result of loss of nerve substance, nerve grafts may be used. For many years surgeons have experimented with nerve crossings using proximal ends of the spinal accessory, hypoglossal, phrenic, glossopharyngeal, and descendens hypoglossi nerves sutured to the distal end of the transected facial nerve. These techniques have resulted in diminished atrophy and improved tone of the facial muscles. The most satisfactory results have been achieved with the hypoglossal nerve (Fig. 51-63). In this case, the anticipated paralysis of one-half of the tongue

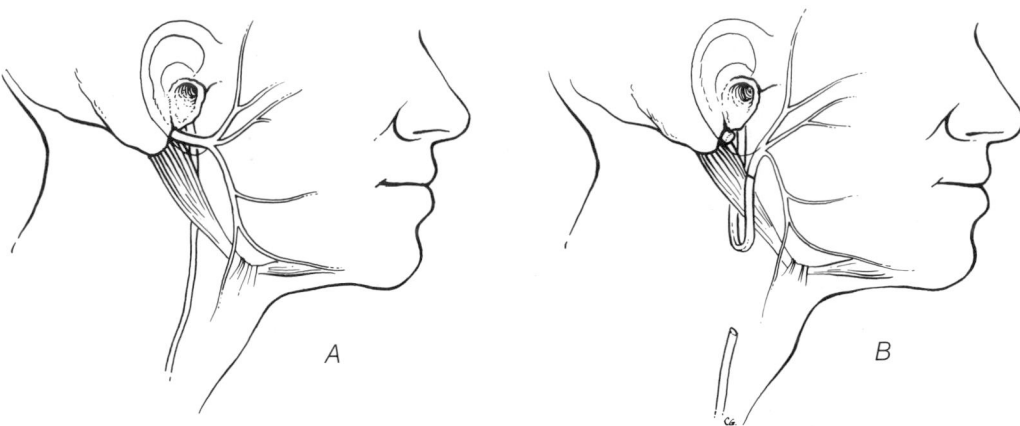

Fig. 51-63. Facial nerve graft using hypoglossal nerve. *A.* Normal relationship between descendens hypoglossi and facial nerves. *B.* Nerve graft from proximal descendens hypoglossi to distal facial nerves.

and occasional difficulty in swallowing, unless the descendens hypoglossi is preserved, should be explained to the patient prior to the operation. Substitution via the trigeminal nerve has been less effective. Spontaneous return of some function has been noted after complete transection of the facial nerve without subsequent repair.

Reconstructive Procedures

EYE. The loss of the protective function of the eyelid musculature is the most pressing problem associated with total irreversible facial paralysis. Exposure keratitis and epiphora not only are troublesome but may result in severe corneal damage and ultimate blindness (Fig. 51-64). If nerve recovery is anticipated, the patient must be taught to protect the eye from exposure by wearing glasses, using ophthalmic ointments, and, at times, applying a patch to the eye. The best surgical procedure for ocular protection is lateral tarsorrhaphy, i.e., attaching the upper lid to the lower lid by tissue overlapping. A medial canthoplasty is

Fig. 51-64. Exposure keratitis and leukoma formation as a result of facial nerve paralysis.

the procedure used to tighten the loose lower lid and turn the punctum in against the globe to diminish epiphora.

Transfer of intact motor power to the eyelids may be achieved by the Gillies operation (Fig. 51-65). This procedure consists of turning down the central portion of the temporalis muscle, which is innervated by the fifth nerve, from the temporal fossa and extending temporalis fascial strips from the lateral canthus through the upper and lower lids. The strips are attached at the medial canthal ligament. The procedure allows dynamic function of the eyelids and supplies enough tone to keep the lower lid against the globe.

Another useful palliative procedure for the paralyzed eyelid is the insertion of a palpebral spring as advocated by Morel-Fatio and Lalardrie. This can be done through small incisions with minimal scarring under local anesthesia in the outpatient clinic.

FACE. The contorted appearance of the face creates a great deal of anxiety for the patient with total unilateral facial palsy. The marked asymmetry is contributed to by excessive activity of facial muscles on the contralateral unparalyzed side. Surgical measures to overcome asymmetry consist of operations to substitute for paralyzed muscles, to diminish the pull of antagonistic muscles, or to excise skin in order to overcome redundancy.

Muscle substitution may be static, using slings of fascia or tendon extending from the temporalis fascia down into the lips and eyelids (Fig. 51-66). Dynamic substitution may be achieved by attaching these slings to muscles of mastication, such as the temporalis or masseter, which have been diverted from their primary function. Segments of muscles may be redistributed into the facial muscles directly as in the Gillies procedure. For example, the anterior one-half of the masseter may be reflected forward into the orbicularis oris as a dynamic support (Fig. 51-67).

Thompson has reported on the successful free graft of skeletal muscle in man. Using the muscle bellies of the extensor digitorum brevis muscles applied directly to the temporalis muscle, the tendons are passed subcutaneously

Fig. 51-65. Gillies' procedure to establish motor power for eyelids. *A* and *B*. Temporalis muscle reflected forward with strips of its own fascia passed through the upper and lower lids to the medial canthal ligament. *C* and *D*. Preoperative eyelid paralysis. *E* and *F*. After Gillies' operation.

along the eyelid margins and are anchored to the medial palpebral ligament. Neurotization of the free graft occurred, as proved by clinical motion and electromyography. In dogs, this has been corroborated by cholinesterase staining of motor end plates.

Facial Nerve Surgery. The two newest methods of reinnervating the face both show great promise. One of these is the previously mentioned transplantation of the gracilis muscle by microneurovascular anastomosis. The other, also a microsurgical technique, has been popularized by J. W. Smith. It incorporates the use of extremely long sural nerve grafts, anastomosed to fascicles on the normal side and passed subcutaneously to the paralyzed side, where they

Fig. 51-66. Facial palsy treated with slings of fascia lata.

Fig. 51-67. Facial palsy treated with transfers of portions of muscles of mastication and a static sling to the zygomatic arch.

are tagged to be identified 6 months later, when they are anastomosed to their respective facial nerve branches.

The antagonistic, unparalyzed muscles on the contralateral side of the face may be surgically paralyzed or excised to diminish asymmetry. Selective neurectomy after preoperative trial with nerve blocks is useful in creating proper facial balance. The mandibular and the temporal branches of the facial nerve are most frequently transected surgically to overcome specific asymmetry in the face with unilateral facial palsy. Excision of segments of muscle on the unparalyzed side of the face selectively weakens these muscles without creating paralysis and an expressionless appearance.

Removal of redundant skin by "face-lifting" techniques is helpful in overcoming gross asymmetry. In general, a combination of slings, muscle transfers, myectomy, neurectomy, and removal of redundant skin produces the best results in patients with this difficult problem.

MISCELLANEOUS PROCEDURES

Surgery for Decubitus Ulcer

Skin and soft tissue defects in the trunk and extremities are frequently the result of pressure necrosis from prolonged pressure because of lack of sensation or because of inability to move secondary to unconsciousness or debility. Any disease or trauma which destroys sensation removes the protective barrier against destruction by pressure. The ulceration and ultimate loss of fingers and toes in leprosy, diabetic neuropathy, familial sensory neuropathy, and peripheral nerve injuries are all attributable to loss of pain sensitivity. It is also this pathway which is implicated in the formation of decubiti in patients with spinal cord injury. The majority of decubitus ulcers occur in elderly patients who are confined to bed for long periods of time.

Restoration of soft tissue and skin losses usually requires pedicle flaps. In the paraplegic, particularly, these operations are difficult to plan and tedious to execute, and necessitate meticulous and time-consuming wound care both pre- and postoperatively. The flap donor sites invariably need a skin graft for closure, creating even another wound, the skin donor site, which also may need very special attention for healing. The skeletal prominences in the base of the pressure ulcers, most frequently the greater trochanter, the ischial tuberosity, or the posterior surface of the sacrum, must be resected along with the infected bursae overlying them. In addition to the skin flaps that will cover them they frequently can best be protected by the local rotation of muscle flaps. Well-conceived plans can often secure healing and diminish the likelihood of reulceration, but constant vigilance by the patient, the families, attendants, and paramedical as well as medical personnel may be unable to ward off recurrences.

Surgery of the Breast

MALIGNANT AND PREMALIGNANT DISEASE

Cooperation between general and oncologic surgeons and the reconstructive surgeon can benefit the patient with breast disease. Too few women are given the opportunity to benefit from reconstruction after they have been cured of this malignant breast disease. Reconstruction of the

Fig. 51-68. Breast reconstruction after mastectomy. *A.* The patient had had a modified radical mastectomy through a transverse incision; good skin flaps and pectoralis bulk were present. *B.* Postoperative appearance, showing the breast mound recreated.

missing breast can be accomplished readily in most instances, particularly if a transverse incision has been used for the extirpation. If a modified radical mastectomy has been performed, the reconstruction is done in one stage. The result is cosmetically superior, and the pectoralis muscle may provide excellent protective covering for the prosthesis that is implanted (Fig. 51-68). If the surgical cure necessitated a more extensive procedure so that there is less skin, more scar, and perhaps an irradiated field, the reconstruction may be more complicated, entailing preliminary flap rotation procedures. These results are still gratifying, even though they are not as cosmetically good as the reconstruction after the modified extirpation.

Patients who do not have breast cancer but are at high risk should be considered for breast removal. This may be performed by a subcutaneous mastectomy with immediate or delayed prosthesis implantation. If a total mastectomy is done, the nipple is left attached to the specimen and the areola is removed to be grafted to the skin covering the prosthetic implants.

Of special note is the patient who has had a breast involved and is at high risk for contralateral breast involvement. If this patient is young and the breast texture or the radiograph is difficult to interpret, or if the patient is excessively bothered by the situation, prophylactic total mastectomy with implantation of a prosthesis and free areola graft is recommended.

REDUCTION MAMMOPLASTY

FEMALE. Enlargement of the female breasts is a much misunderstood clinical problem. It can occur in adolescence and become quite massive, or it can occur gradually through the developmental years and then with loss of support and the addition of ptosis become even more of a problem. The psychologic strains associated with this deformity are great. In addition the physical symptoms of postural deformity, backache, shoulder pain and ulceration from brassiere straps, inframammary skin eruptions, and mastodynia are all most bothersome and frequently incapacitating. Surgical correction will handle both the physical and psychologic problems, and the functional result is also aesthetically pleasing. Many varieties of procedure have been proposed. Rarely is it necessary to resort to an amputation of the breast with subsequent free transplantation of the nipple and areola. This must be reserved only for the most massive of breasts. Usually the technique can retain the nipple-areolar complex on a dermal pedicle to preserve its sensation and function. The geometric design is not complex but does take understanding and planning (Fig. 51-69).

MALE. In approximately 10 percent of the normal male population adolescent gynecomastia will occur. The great majority recede spontaneously. For those which do not, a subcutaneous mastectomy performed through a circumareolar incision is recommended to remove the breast with a minimal scar.

AUGMENTATION MAMMOPLASTY

The augmentation of breast size for cosmetic purposes has become an acceptable procedure in carefully selected patients. A multiplicity of prosthetic breasts are available. The silicone breasts devised by Cronin and Greenberg have been used most and have the greatest longevity of clinical experience. Recently other materials such as polyurethanes have been recommended. In addition inflatable prostheses are now being investigated.

The operation consists of implanting the prosthesis in a plane beneath the breast tissue if any is present. Most surgeons prefer to place the prosthesis upon the superficial surface of the fascia overlying the pectoralis muscles, although there are some who prefer placing it behind the pectoralis muscle.

When patients have extensive cystic disease of the breast which has been painful and recurrent and for which a simple mastectomy is indicated, a subcutaneous mastectomy is a good alternative. Either at the same procedure or several weeks later, a breast prosthesis is implanted so the woman does not feel neutered. The aesthetic result is good, but the complication rate is 10 to 15 percent.

Hypospadias

The congenital hypospadias deformity, incomplete masculinization of the external genitalia, occurs once in every 300 to 400 boys born in the United States. Chromosomal studies have shown no consistent abnormalities associated with hypospadias. Failure of the embryonic fusion during the second month of development gives rise to this deformity, which is often minimal. A useful clinical classification is the following: glans, distal penile, midpenile, penoscrotal junction, scrotal, and perineal. The more distal lesions, i.e., glans, distal penile, and midpenile, usually do not have any associated anomalies. Those situated more proximally need more extensive work-up, since they are more likely to be associated with abnormalities of the upper urinary tract.

All varieties of hypospadias are frequently accompanied by chordee, a ventral curvature of the penis caused by the replacement of the dartos fascia, Buck's fascia, and corpus spongiosum by a band of tough fibrous tissue in a triangular area extending from the urethral meatus to the edge of the hooded prepuce.

When a newborn infant is seen with a hypospadias, two important steps must be taken at once: The first is to evaluate the urethral opening to determine whether it is constricted, necessitating a meatotomy. The second is to prevent circumcision, even that required by ritual. All patients should eventually have cystoscopy, intravenous pyelography, and sex chromatin studies. Surgery is best performed during the latter portion of the second year, with the ultimate goals of providing (1) a straight penis, (2) the urethral opening at the tip of the penis, (3) normal voiding, (4) normal appearance, and (5) normal erection.

Reconstruction of the urethra and release of the chordee can be accomplished in simultaneous operations, although most surgeons will precede the urethroplasty by the chordee release (Fig. 51-70A to D). During the stage of the urethral reconstruction, urinary diversion is accomplished, usually through a perineal urethrostomy although occasionally by a suprapubic drainage procedure. Of the many procedures that have been advocated, the authors favor either the buried-strip method proposed by Denis-Browne (Fig. 51-70*E* and *F*) or the free skin graft (Fig. 51-71). Success is usually possible without fistula formation (Fig. 51-72).

Body Contouring

Abdominoplasty, thigh lift, and reduction of upper arm skin redundancy are most frequently considered in patients who have undergone massive weight loss after years of obesity. Frequent pregnancies with resulting flaccid abdominal skin and diastasis recti, surgically denervated abdominal wall musculature, or lipodystrophy are also indications. Surgical correction requires extensive mobilization of tissues and will cause scars of great length. The surgeon must carefully plan scar placement to provide the best aesthetic result.

Vaginal Reconstruction

Successful construction of a vagina for agenesis is best accomplished by creation of a perineal pocket lined with a skin graft. After vaginectomy or pelvic exenteration for malignant disease, however, lack of sufficient bony coverage makes skin grafting less satisfactory. Local flaps, distant flaps, and colonic interposition have been utilized with only limited success. Use of myocutaneous flaps based on the gracilis muscle, as described by McGraw et al., provides an excellent reconstructive modality. The procedure can be performed in one stage, resulting in primary wound healing and decreased morbidity. Good sensibility and successful intercourse are reported.

Transsexual Surgery

Transsexual surgery has received increasing publicity since its popularization in 1952. Increasing numbers of patients are requesting sexual reassignment, and several medical centers have formed interdisciplinary medical teams for the evaluation, diagnosis, and treatment of this difficult problem. Although the primary modality of diagnosis is psychiatric, an adequate medical team should include plastic surgery, gynecology, urology, endocrinology, genetics, neuropsychiatry, and psychology.

TECHNIQUES: MALE TO FEMALE. After exhaustive psychiatric evaluation and cross-gender role adaptation with hormonal therapy, selected patients are started on a course of operative procedures. In addition to removal of testes and penis and construction of a vagina, this may also include adjunctive procedures such as breast augmentation, rhinoplasty, and reduction of thyroid cartilage. The most satisfactory method of vaginal construction utilizes the skin and subcutaneous tissue of the penis as an inverted pedicle for a surgically created perineal pocket. The glans is used as a clitoral substitute, and labia are constructed from scrotal skin. "Normal" sexual intercourse has been reported in many patients.

TECHNIQUES: FEMALE TO MALE. This conversion is more difficult but far less common. Most often, a phallus is

A

B

C

D

Fig. 51-69. Reduction mammaplasty. *A.* Correct location of the new nipple site is determined by measuring from the midclavicular line and the sternal notch. An equilateral triangle is recommended, extending from the sternal notch to both nipples, each side measuring between 20 and 23 cm according to height and torso. *B.* The crosshatched area is deepithelialized to preserve the vasculature just beneath the dermis; this dermal pedicle ensures survival of the nipple and areola. The circumference of the area demarcated by a line from *A* to *B* to *B'* to *A* must be approximately 13 cm to accommodate the areolar area, which has a diameter (*A'B''*) of 4 cm. The line *B'C'* must equal the *BC* and measure 4.5 to 6.5 cm; these lines are joined to form the new vertical dimension of the inferior breast. The wedge resected beneath the areola and between lines *C'C''* and *CC''* frequently may weigh as much as 1,500 Gm. *C.* Repositioning the breast tissues: The suspending suture at *A* for the top of the areola and the reconstructions beneath the areola at *BB'*, *CC'*, and *C''* give the new breast its size and shape. Additional breast tissue, the two triangles on either side of the sagittal closure, is resected just above the inframammary fold. *D.* Before and after breast reduction and reconstruction.

Fig. 51-70. *A.* Hypospadias of the midpenile area with chordee. *B.* Release of the chordee in a preliminary operation always drops the urethral opening back to a more proximal position. Circumcision now can be accomplished but without discarding any skin. *C.* The dorsal hooded prepuce is rearranged by moving it to the ventral surface to cover the defect left by the straightening. *D.* The Denis-Browne technique: The perineal urethrostomy has been accomplished. The parallel lines are made from the tip of the glans and extend proximally around the urethral orifice. This buried strip of skin accomplishes tubing without suturing. It is necessary to have good skin closure over this strip. *E* and *F.* Reliable closure is accomplished with running pullout sutures in three layers, the dartos fascia, Buck's fascia, and the skin.

Fig. 51-71. Urethroplasty by the free skin graft method. *A.* The inner surface of the prepuce is removed and made into a tube around a catheter, the skin side against the catheter. If the patient has been previously circumcised, hairless skin from the inner arm is substituted. *B.* The catheter is placed within the urethra and the skin graft sutured to the distal portion of the urethra. Coverage is accomplished by using the hooded prepuce, moving it to the ventral surface. *C.* The completed procedure. In this case the diversion is accomplished by the catheter, obviating a perineal urethrostomy.

A

B

C

Fig. 51-72. Urethroplasty by the Denis-Browne method. *A.* The chordee has been released 3 months previously; the design of the buried strip is shown. *B.* Wide undermining is necessary to accomplish good closure to prevent fistula formation. *C.* The functional result.

constructed from a midline abdominal tube flap, with a urethra formed from a section of ilium. A silicone rod may be implanted to increase rigidity, and testes may be simulated with inflatable prostheses. Adjunctive procedures may include subcutaneous mastectomy to improve body contour. Liquid silicone has been injected into the vocal cords to deepen the voice.

References

Historical Background

Esser, J. F. S.. Island Flaps, *NY Med J,* **106:**264, 1917.

Gersuny, R.: Platischer ersatz der Wangenschleimhaut, *Zentrlbl Chir,* **14:**706, 1887.

Gillies, H. D.: The Tubed Pedicle in Plastic Surgery, *NY Med J,* **111:**1, 1920.

Lawson, G.: On the Successful Transplantation of Portions of Skin for the Closure of Large Granulating Surfaces, *Lancet,* **2:**708, 1870.

Maltz, M.: "Evolution of Plastic Surgery," Froben Press, New York, 1946.

Ollier, Leopold Louis Xavier Edouard: Sur les greffes cutanées ou autoplastiques, *Bull Acad Med Paris,* **1:**243, 1872.

Rogers, P. O.: Historical Development of Free Skin Grafting, *Surg Clin North Am,* **39:**289, 1959.

Tagliacozzi, Gasparo: "De curtorum chirugia per insitionem," libri duo, Gaspari Bindonus, Jr., Venice, 1597.

Thiersch, C.: Über Hautverpflanzung, *Verh Dtsh Ges Chir,* **15:**17, 1886.

Von Graefe, C. F.: "Rhinoplastik, oder die Kunst den Verlust der Nase organisch zu ersetzen in ihren früheren Verhaltnissen erforscht und durch neue Verfahrungsweisen zur hoheren Vollkommenheit gefordert," Berlin, 1818.

Wolfe, J. R.: A New Method of Performing Plastic Operations, *Br Med J,* **2:**360, 1875.

Technical Considerations

Bakamjian, V. Y., Culf, N. K., and Bales, H. W.: The Versatility of the Medially Based Delto-pectoral Skin Flap in Primary Reconstruction in Head and Neck Surgery, *Trans 4th Int Cong Plast Surg (1967) Amsterdam,* Excerpta Medica Foundation, New York, 1969, p. 808.

Barron, J. H., and Emmett, J. J.: "Subcutaneous Pedicle Flaps," *Br J Plast Surg,* **18:**51, 1965.

Brobyn, T. J., Cramer, L. M., Hulnick, S. J., and Kodsi, M. S.: Facial Resurfacing with the Limberg Flap, *Clin Plast Surg,* **3:**481, 1976.

Brown, J. B., and McDowell, F.: "Skin Grafting," 3d ed., J. B. Lippincott Company, Philadelphia, 1958.

Cronin, T. D.: The Use of a Molded Splint to Prevent Contracture after Split Skin Grafting on the Neck, *Plast Reconstr Surg,* **27:**7, 1961.

Daniel, R. K., and Taylor, G. I.: Distant Transfer of an Island Flap by Microvascular Anastomoses, *Plast Reconstr Surg,* **52:**111, 1973.

———, and Williams, H. B.: The Free Transfer of Skin Flaps by Microvascular Anastomoses, *Plast Reconstr Surg,* **52:**16, 1973.

Ger, R.: Surgical Management of Ulcerative Lesions of the Leg, *Curr Probl Surg,* p. 1, March, 1972.

Grabb, W. C., and Myers, M. B.: "Skin Flaps," Little, Brown and Company, Boston, 1975.

————, and Smith, J.: Plastic Surgery: A Concise Guide to Clinical Practice, Little, Brown and Company, Boston, 1968.

————, Ohmori, K., and Ohmori, S.: Successful Clinical Transfer of Ten Free Flaps by Microvascular Anastomosis, *Plast Reconstr Surg,* **53:**259, 1974.

————, ————, and Shuhei, T.: Free Gracilis Muscle Transplantation, with Microneurovascular Anastomosis for the Treatment of Facial Paralysis, *Plast Reconstr Surg,* **57:**133, 1976.

Ikuta, Y., et al.: Free Muscle Transplantation by Microsurgical Technique to Treat Severe Volkmann's Contracture, *Plast Reconstr Surg,* **58:**407, 1976.

Kubacek, V.: Transposition of Flaps on the Face on a Subcutaneous Pedicle, *Acta Chir Plast (Praha),* **2:**108, 1960.

Larson, D. L., Abston, S., Evans, E. B., Dobrkovsky, M., and Linares, H. A.: Techniques for Decreasing Scar Formation and Contractures in the Burned Patient, *J Trauma,* **11:**807, 1971.

Lewis, J. R., Jr.: "The Surgery of Scars," McGraw-Hill Book Company, New York, 1963.

Longacre, J. J.: "Scar Tissue: Its Use and Abuse," Charles C Thomas, Springfield, Ill., 1972.

McCraw, J. B., et al.: Vaginal Reconstruction with Gracilis Myocutaneous Flaps, *Plast Reconstr Surg,* **58:**176, 1976.

————, Dibbel, D. G., and Carroway, J. H.: Clinical Definition of Independent Myocutaneous Vascular Territories, *Plast Reconstr Surg,* **60:**341, 1977.

McFarlane, R. M., Heagy, R. M. R., Aust, J. C., and Wermuth, R. E.: A Study of the Delay Phenomenon in Experimental Flaps, *Plast Reconstr Surg,* **35:**245, 1965.

McGregor, I. A.: Fundamental Techniques of Plastic Surgery, 4th ed., The Williams & Wilkins Company, Baltimore, 1968.

Mathes, S. T., McCraw, J. B., and Vasconez, L. O.: Muscle Transposition Flaps for Coverage of Lower Extremity Defects: Anatomic Considerations, *Surg Clin North Am,* **54:**1337, December, 1974.

Milton, S. H.: Pedicled Skin-Flaps: The Fallacy of the Length: Width Ratio, *Br J Surg,* **57:**502, 1970.

Myers, M. B., and Cherry, G.: Augmentation of Tissue Survival by Delay, *Plast Reconstr Surg,* **39:**397, 1967.

———— and ————: Mechanism of the Delay Phenomenon, *Plast Reconstr Surg,* **44:**52, 1969.

Ohmori, S. (ed.): Microsurgery, in *Trans 6th Int Cong Plast Reconstr Surg,* Sec. 2, p. 33, Masson et Cie, Paris, 1976.

Peacock, E., and Van Winkle, W: Surgery and Biology of Wound Repair, W. B. Saunders Company, Philadelphia, 1970.

Peet, E. W., and Patterson, T. J. S.: The Essentials of Plastic Surgery, F. A. Davis Company, Philadelphia, 1963.

Reinisch, J. F.: The Role of Arteriovenous Anastomosis in Skin Flaps, in W. C. Grabb and M. B. Myers (eds.), "Skin Flaps," p. 81, Little, Brown and Company, Boston, 1975.

Smith, P. J., Foley, B., McGregor, I. A., and Jackson, I, T.: The Anatomical Basis of the Groin Flap, *Plas Reconstr Surg,* **49:**41, 1972.

Taylor, G. I., and Daniel, R. K.: The Anatomy of Several Free Flaps Donor Sites, *Plast Reconstr Surg,* **56:**243, 1975.

Thompson, N.: A Review of Autogenous Muscle Grafts and Their Clinical Applications, *Clin Plast Surg,* **1:**349, 1974.

Vasconez, L. C., Bostwick, J., and McCraw, J. B.: Coverage of Exposed Bone by Muscle Transposition and Skin Grafting, *Plast Reconstr Surg,* **53:**526, 1974.

Facial Trauma

Dingman, R. O., and Natvig, P.: Surgery of Facial Fractures, W. B. Saunders Company, Philadelphia, 1964.

Georgiade, N. G., (ed.): "Plastic and Maxillofacial Trauma Symposium," vol. 1, The C. V. Mosby Company, St. Louis, 1969.

Grabb, W. C.: Emergency Department Facial Injuries, in "Techniques in Surgery." Ethicon, Inc., New Jersey, 1972.

LeFort, R.: Experimental Study of Fractures of the Upper Jaw, *Rev Chir Paris,* **23:**208, 1901; reprinted in *Plast Reconstr Surg,* **50:**497, 1972.

Rowe, N. L., and Killey, H. C.: Fractures of the Facial Skeleton, 2d ed., The Williams & Wilkins Company, Baltimore, 1968.

Mustarde, J. C.: Repair and Reconstruction in the Orbital Region, The Williams & Wilkins Company, Baltimore, 1966.

Head and Neck

Bakamjian, V. Y.: A Two-Stage Method for Pharyngoesophageal Reconstruction with a Primary Pectoral Skin Flap, *Plast Reconstr Surg,* **36:**173, 1965.

————, Culf, N. K., and Bales, H. W.: The Versatility of the Medially Based Delto-pectoral Skin Flap in Primary Reconstruction in Head and Neck Surgery, *Trans 4th Cong Plast Surg (1967) Amsterdam,* Excerpta Medica Foundation, New York, 1969, p. 808.

Bromberg, B. E., Song, I. C., and Craig, G. T.: Split-Rib Mandibular Reconstruction, *Plast Reconstr Surg,* **50:**357, 1972.

Cramer, L. M., and Culf, N. K.: Complications of Radical Neck Dissection, in R. Goldwyn, "The Unfavorable Result in Plastic Surgery: Avoidance and Treatment," Little, Brown and Company, Boston, 1972.

Elliott, R. A.: Rotation Flaps of the Nose, *Plast Reconstr Surg,* **44:**147, 1969.

Gaisford, J. C.: Symposium on Cancer of the Head and Neck, The C. V. Mosby Company, St. Louis, 1969.

MacComb, W. S., and Fletcher, G.: Cancer of the Head and Neck, The Williams & Wilkins Company, Baltimore, 1967.

Rappaport, I., Boyne, P. V., and Nethery, J.: The Particulate Graft in Tumor Surgery, *Am J Surg,* **122:**748, 1971.

Webster, J. P.: Crescentic Peri-alar Cheek Excision for Upper Lip Flap Advancement, *Plast Reconstr Surg,* **16:**434, 1955.

Congenital Anomalies

Bill, A. H.: Branchiogenic Cysts and Sinuses, in C. D. Benson, W. T. Mustand, M. M.: Ravitch, W. H. Snyder, Jr., and K. J. Welch (eds.), "Pediatric Surgery," vol. 1, Year Book Medical Publishers, Inc., Chicago, 1962.

Converse, J. M., Horowitz, S. L., Valauri, A. J., and Montandon, D.: The Treatment of Nasal Maxillary Hypoplasia. A New Pyramidal Naso-orbital Maxillary Osteotomy, *Plast Reconstr Surg,* **45:**527, 1970.

Cronin, T. D., Greenberg, R. L., and Brauer, R. O.: Follow-up Study of Silastic Frame for Reconstruction of External Ear, **42:**522, 1968.

LeMesurier, A. B.: A Method of Cutting and Suturing the Lip

in the Treatment of Complete Unilateral Clefts, *Plast Reconstr Surg,* **4:**1, 1949.

Millard, D. R., Jr., and Pigott, R. W.: Rotation-Advancement in Wide Unilateral Lip Clefts, *Trans 4th Int Cong Plast Surg Rome 1967,* Excerpta Medica Foundation, Amsterdam, 1969, pp. 349–355.

Murray, J. E., and Swanson, L. T.: Mid-Face Osteotomy and Advancement for Cranio-synostosis, *Plast Reconstr Surg,* **41:** 299, 1968.

Obwegeser, H. L.: Surgical Correction of Small or Retrodisplaced Maxillae, *Plast Reconstr Surg,* **43:**351, 1969.

Randall, P.: A Triangular Flap Operation for the Primary Repair of Unilateral Clefts of the Lip, *Plast Reconstr Surg,* **23:**331, 1959.

————: A Lip Adhesion Operation in Cleft Lip Surgery, *Plast Reconstr Surg,* **35:**371, 1965.

Skoog, T.: Repair of Unilateral Cleft Lip Deformity: Maxilla, Nose and Lip, *Scand J Plast Reconstr Surg,* **3:**109, 1969.

Tanzer, R., and Converse, J. M.: Deformities of the Auricle, in J. M. Converse (ed.), "Reconstructive Plastic Surgery," vol. II, W. B. Saunders Company, Philadelphia, 1964.

Tennison, C. W.: The Repair of the Unilateral Cleft Lip by Stencil Method, *Plast Reconstr Surg,* **9:**115, 1952.

Tessier, P., Guiot, G., Rogerie, J., et al.: Ostéotomies cranio-naso-orbito-faciales: Hypertélorisme, *Ann Chir Plast,* **12:**103, 1967.

————: Ostéotomies totales de la face. *Ann Chir Plast,* **12:**273, 1967.

Wynn, S. K.: Lateral Flap Cleft Lip Surgery Technique, *Plast Reconstr Surg,* **26:**509, 1960.

Cosmetic Surgery

Brown, J. B., and McDowell, F.: "Plastic Surgery of the Nose," Charles C Thomas Company, Springfield, Ill., 1965.

Denecke, H. J., and Meyer, R.: "Plastic Surgery of Head and Neck," vol. 1, "Corrective and Reconstructive Rhinoplasty," Springer-Verlag New York Inc., New York, 1967.

Edgerton, M. T., Knorr, N., and Hoopes, J.: Psychiatric-Surgical Approach to Adolescent Disturbance in Self Image, **41:**248, 1968.

Webb, W. L., Slaughter, R., Meyer, E., and Edgerton, M. T.: Psychosomatic Medicine: Mechanism of Psychosocial Adjustment in Patients Seeking "Face-Lift" Operation, **27:**183, 1965.

Facial Paralysis

Babcock, W. W.: Standard Techniques for Operations of Peripheral Nerves in Special References to Closure of Large Gaps, **45:**364, 1927.

Beahrs, O. H.: Use of Nerve Grafts for Repair of Defects in the Facial Nerve, *Ann Surg,* **153:**433, 1944.

Conley, J. J.: Treatment of Facial Paralysis, *Surg Clin North Am,* **51:**403, 1971.

Edgerton, M. T.: Surgical Correction of Facial Paralysis, *Am J Surg,* **120:**82, 1970.

Freeman, B. S.: Facial Palsy, in J. M. Converse (ed.), "Reconstructive Plastic Surgery," vol. III, W. B. Saunders Company, Philadelphia, 1964.

Hanna, D. C., and Gaisford, J. C.: Facial Nerve Management in Tumors, *Plast Reconstr Surg,* **35:**445, 1965.

Kessler, L.: Twelfth Nerve to Seventh Nerve Anastomosis for Treatment of Facial Paralysis, *Neurology,* **9:**118, 1959.

Morel-Fatio, D. (ed.): Facial Palsy, in *Trans 6th Int Cong Plast Reconstr Surg,* Sec. 6, p. 330, Masson et Cie, Paris, 1976.

————, and Lalardrie, J. P.: Palliative Surgical Treatment of Facial Paralysis: The Palpebral Spring. *Plast Reconstr Surg,* **33:**446, 1964.

Niklison, J.: Contribution to the Subject of Facial Paralysis, *Plast Reconstr Surg,* **16:**276, 1956.

Rees, T. D., Rhodes, R. D., and Converse, J. M.: The Palliation of Facial Paresis, *Am J Surg,* **120:**82, 1970.

Smith, J. W.: Advances in Facial Nerve Repair, *Surg Clin North Am,* **52:**1287, 1972.

Sunderland, S., and Cossar, D. F.: The Structure of the Facial Nerve, *Anat Rec,* **116:**147, 1953.

Thompson, N.: Autogenous Free Grafts of Skeletal Muscle, *Plast Reconstr Surg,* **48:**11, 1971.

————: Investigation of Autogenous Skeletal Muscle Free Grafts in the Dog: With a Report on a Successful Free Graft of Skeletal Muscle in Man, *Transplantation,* **12:**353, 1971.

————: Treatment of Facial Paralysis by Free Skeletal Muscle Grafts, *Trans 5th Int Cong Plast Reconstr Surg Aust 1971,* Butterworth Scientific Publications, London, p. 660.

Miscellaneous Procedures

Broadbent, T. R., and Woolf, R. M.: Augmentation Mammoplasty, *Plast Reconstr Surg,* **40:**517, 1967.

————, ————, and Toksu, E.: Hypospadias: One-Stage Repair, *Plast Reconstr Surg,* **27:**154, 1961.

Browne, D.: An Operation for Hypospadias, *Proc R Soc Med,* **42:**466, 1949.

Conway, H., and Smith, J. W.: Breast Plastic Surgery: Reduction Mammoplasty, Mastopexy, Augmentation Mammoplasty and Mammary Construction, *Plast Reconstr Surg,* **21:**8, 1958.

Cronin, T. D., and Greenberg, R. L.: Our Experiences with Silastic Gel Breast Prosthesis, *Plast Reconstr Surg,* **46:**1, 1970.

Edgerton, M. T., and Meyer, J. K.: Surgical and Psychiatric Aspects of Transexualism, in C. Horton (ed.), "Plastic and Reconstructive Surgery of the Genital Area," p. 117, Little, Brown and Company, Boston, 1973.

Griffith, B. H., and Schultz, R. C.: Prevention and Surgical Treatment of Recurrent Decubitus Ulcers in Patients with Paraplegia, *Plast Reconstr Surg,* **27:**248, 1964.

Hoopes, J. E., Edgerton, M. T., and Shelley, W.: Organic Synthetics for Augmentation Mammoplasty: Their Relation to Breast Cancer, *Plast Reconstr Surg,* **39:**263, 1967.

Horton, C. E., and Devine, C. J.: Hypospadias and Epispadias, *Ciba Found Symp,* **24:**2, 1972.

Maliniac, J. W.: "Breast Deformities and Their Repair," Grune & Stratton, Inc., New York, 1950.

McCormack, R. M.: Simultaneous Chordee Repair and Urethral Reconstruction for Hypospadias, *Plast Reconstr Surg,* **13:**257, 1954.

Strombeck, J. O.: Breast Reconstruction: I. Reduction Mammoplasty, *Mod Trends Plast Surg,* **1:**237, 1964.

Webster, J. P.: Mastectomy for Gynecomastia through a Semicircular Intra-areolar Incision, *J Surg,* **124:**557, 1946.

Chapter 52

Rehabilitation

by J. Herbert Dietz, Jr., and Howard A. Rusk

PRINCIPLES OF REHABILITATION

The principles of rehabilitation are those of readaptation of each disabled individual to the situation and the setting in which he or she must survive, with maximum independent function, comfort, and emotional support, for whatever time of life is allowed. This entails the setting of an appropriate goal—whether preventive, restorative, supportive, or palliative—for each person. All patients are candidates for appropriate effort directed toward adaptation to disability or distress. Rehabilitation is a dynamic concept and active program.

Following severe trauma or surgical treatment, there is an increased nitrogen loss in peripheral skeletal muscles, the principal nitrogen donor, resulting in a decrease in muscle mass. Since much of physical therapy is directed toward use or reeducation of muscle, nitrogen intake during this phase is important. Planning and regulation of oral or parenteral nutrition may become an essential part of the rehabilitation process.

Disabilities result from the interference by disease with bodily functioning and control, or they may follow trauma or result from surgical procedures, radiation therapy, chemotherapy, or immunotherapy.

Disabilities may be primary or secondary. Primary disability is a direct result, while secondary disability arises from restrictions and conditions which evolve in the course of treatment and convalescence. Primary disabilities include loss of limb, sensory perception, motor function, or communication; restriction in cardiopulmonary reserve; impaired vision; or alterations in organ function. Secondary disabilities include muscle atrophy, joint contraction, osteoporosis, urinary calculi, phlebothrombosis, pneumonia, decubitus ulcers, and psychologic deterioration.

Inactivity in bed results in 3 percent loss of strength and endurance daily. The value of early postoperative mobilization was demonstrated in 1893 by Emil Ries and reconfirmed by John H. Powers in the light of modern science. Nutritional intake during inactivity is converted primarily to fat, while under the influence of programmed exercising, muscle-mass improvement results.

TECHNIQUES OF REHABILITATION

Rehabilitation should begin at the earliest possible opportunity, at times in the preoperative period, and should continue throughout the entire course of care until maximal benefit is achieved. Treatment measures should be directed toward appropriate care for any disability, as soon as recognized, and toward the reduction or prevention of predictable disability, whenever possible. Prompt assessment of the entire clinical picture of the disabled patient will permit the setting of an appropriate rehabilitation goal of prevention, restoration, support, or palliation. Rehabilitation of the patient is best conducted by a team which may include physicians, surgeons, physiatrists, psychiatrists, nurses, physical therapists, social workers, orthotists or prosthetists, and volunteers. The family should be involved, whenever appropriate, in the acceptance of and assistance to the patient with emotional, cosmetic, or physical disability.

Basic techniques include (1) physical therapy; (2) occupational therapy; (3) training in activities of daily living (A.D.L.); (4) application of mechanical devices including splints, braces, prostheses, and ortheses; (5) educational, vocational, and psychosocial services.

Physical Therapy

EXERCISES AND MUSCLE REEDUCATION

1. Objectives of exercise:
    a. Power. Exercises for power are based on maximal active effort with few repetitions and are especially helpful where atrophy is the result of disease.
    b. Endurance. Exercises for endurance are designed to increase tolerance. They are based on submaximal effort with many repetitions and are especially useful following a period of convalescence.
    c. Coordination. Exercises for coordination are designed to develop an efficient pattern of function. They are based on the principle that practice and repetition lead to precision in performance.
    d. Range of motion. Exercises designed for maintaining or increasing range of motion are of value whenever there is limitation or potential limitation of normal range from any cause.
    e. Speed. Exercises for speed are designed to shorten activity time. Speed is attained by frequent repetition of functional activities during the final phase of the rehabilitation program.
2. Types of exercise:
    a. Passive. Exercise accomplished by the therapist or apparatus with no active participation by the patient. The main purpose is to prevent contractures by maintaining the normal range of joint motion.
    b. Active assistive. Exercise accomplished by active voluntary movement by the patient with the assistance of the therapist or mechanical device. This is the first step in a program of muscle reeducation. The use of mechanical or hydrotherapeutic modalities is often prescribed during this phase of treatment.
    c. Active. Free exercise accomplished by the patient without either assistance or resistance.
    d. Resistive active. Exercise accomplished by the patient against added resistance, either manual on the part of the therapist or by the use of mechanical resistance. Resistive exercises are usually given when a muscle is rated "good" to "normal." The major effect of any resistive exercise program is the development of strength, and the exercises must be graduated to the patient's tolerance.
    e. Stretching. Exercises accomplished by applied force, either vigorous and of short duration or moderate and prolonged. The therapeutic use of stretching is designed to restore the normal range of motion where limitation of this range is due to loss of elasticity of the soft tissue.
    f. Functional. Exercises that are the foundation for a training program in functional performance. They may be done in the patient's bed, on an exercise mat, on a training apparatus unit, on parallel bars, or on crutches and include techniques of ambulation.
    g. Special exercises. Included are breathing exercises and coughing, which are useful to correct or minimize respiratory function deficit, eliminate secretions, improve alveolar ventilation, and maintain a clear airway. The patient is taught to put forth repeated slow and gentle maximal effort during inspiration and to utilize the diaphragm to full extent. Strengthening exercises for the abdominal muscles are of help in the presence of restrictive or obstructive lung disease. Proper voluntary coughing, with appropriate splinting, and regional costal expansion are taught, with consideration given to the patient's functional needs and restrictions and to whether it is before or after the operation. When the patient requires the assistance of a respirator, he can be taught to perform glossopharyngeal breathing for use during periods when he must be off the respirator. The patient who has been given a tracheostomy should be instructed in adequate "huffing" to clear secretions.

AMBULATION

Training in adequate ambulation with or without supportive devices such as crutches, walker, or canes and with or without bracing is part of physical therapy. Ambulation training is necessary for patients with neuromuscular dysfunction, including ataxia, and for those who have lost the use of a leg, either temporarily due to injury or local surgery or permanently due to amputation. If there is leg-length discrepancy following trauma or surgery, or if the patient cannot clear a cast or splint, a lift under the shoe on the uninvolved side will facilitate walking.

HEAT

Heat may be used to relieve pain, increase circulation, or increase the local metabolic activity. The physiologic effects of heat are most applicable in lesions affecting the musculoskeletal system such as bursitis, arthritis, myositis, tenosynovitis, tendinitis, fractures, dislocations, contusions, sprains, and strains. Externally applied heat causes vasodilatation and an increase in circulation. Sedation, relief of pain, and reduction in muscular tension may also result.

Heat is not used in acute inflammation or acute trauma until the initial reaction has subsided. Obstructed venous or arterial circulation present definite contraindications, and heat must be cautiously applied when the circulation is even partially impaired. The increase in circulation and capillary engorgement associated with heat therapy creates a tendency toward the formation of edema. Heat alone is not used over areas involved by neoplastic disease, except in conjunction with radiation therapy. The use of thermotherapy in cancer treatment is still under investigation. Heat is contraindicated in the presence of noninflammatory edema. Special precautions should be taken when sensation is absent or impaired and when an infant or psychotic patient is unable to report the onset of unpleasant sensation of heat. The therapeutic application of heat usually involves radiant, conductive, or conversive mechanisms.

SUPERFICIAL HEAT. The increase in temperature is maximal in the skin, with no significant rise in temperature occurring beyond 1 to 2 cm depth of tissue. Most sources of superficial heat require from 20 to 30 minutes to produce the desired effect. Commonly used means of therapeutic application include luminous or nonluminous radiation and various forms of dry or moist heat. Effects are superficial and topical or reflex.

Infrared Radiation. A simple and safe device for applying infrared radiation to fairly large areas, such as the back or both thighs, is the luminous heat "baker." The baker consists of several luminous bulbs mounted in the center of a semicircular metal reflector on adjustable legs. The intensity can be varied by changing the distance from the lamp to the skin. The patient should feel comfortably warm, and at the end of the treatment period, the skin should be warm, pink, and moist.

Hydrotherapy. Heat given by immersion in warmed water has some advantages over radiant heat. The buoyancy of the water provides gentle support without hindering movement.

Whirlpool Bath. The usual temperature ranges from 102 to 104°F except where there is an impairment of circulation, in which case the water temperature should not exceed 100°F. It is indicated principally for the treatment of extremities and can be used where there are open wounds and denervated areas. One disadvantage is that the immersed extremity is dependent and edema may develop.

Whirlpool provides heat, gentle massage, relief of pain, muscular relaxation, and assists in debridement. When used with a large tub, it is useful in the treatment of burns and decubitus and other ulcers, and in facilitating performance of range of joint motion exercises.

Hubbard Tank. All of the body except the head and neck is immersed in heated water at a temperature of 98 to 104°F. The water is usually agitated gently like the whirlpool. It provides a means of giving heat and gentle exercise and is especially useful where disease or disability affects many joints of the body or where burns, ulcerations, or denervated areas exist.

Hot Packs. These are effective in the relief of tenderness and muscle spasm, for localized areas, and for reflex vasodilation in the lower extremities from lumbar region application. Moist rather than dry heat is used.

Paraffin. Application is especially useful in localized or chronic joint diseases such as arthritis.

DEEP HEAT. Deep heat sources include ultrasound, microwave, and ultra-short-wave diathermy. The most effective agent for heating of periarticular tissues is ultrasound, and because of its characteristics it is safe to use in the presence of implanted metallic pins, plates, or prostheses. Muscle heating is obtained through use of microwave or short-wave diathermy.

Deep heat is contraindicated when there is a bleeding tendency, over a pregnant uterus, and over a fracture site before callus has formed. Microwave therapy should not be used over superficial accumulations of fluid and should be applied cautiously over growing or superficial bones, over eyes and testes, and when metal is present in the area. Ultrasound is contraindicated in or about the brain, eyes, ears, nasal sinuses, heart, reproductive organs, and epiphyses of growing bones. It should be used with caution over large nerves.

COLD THERAPY. Ice bags, cold-water bags, and cold compresses are used to minimize the initial reaction of tissues to local traumatic injuries such as contusions and sprains. It has been suggested that the beneficial effects of ethyl chloride spray for painful joints and muscles are due to direct and reflex effects of the change in tissue temperature produced by the spray. Induced hypothermia and refrigeration anesthesia for surgical purposes are widely used, but these phases of cold therapy are not within the scope of this chapter.

ULTRAVIOLET. Decubitus ulcers and some indolent ulcers respond favorably to ultraviolet, especially with the use of cold quartz mercury lamps. Ulcers resulting from Raynaud's disease, thromboangiitis obliterans, and chronic varicosities do not respond. Specific contraindications to this therapy are photogenic diseases of the skin, such as pellagra, lupus erythematosus, hydroa aestivale, and xeroderma pigmentosum. Certain antibiotics and other medications result in a photosensitivity which also contraindicates ultraviolet therapy. It has been suggested that ultraviolet should not be used in patients with hyperthyroidism, diabetes, advanced cachexia or inanition, nephritis, or myocarditis.

ELECTROTHERAPY

A variety of currents can be used to stimulate motor and sensory nerves. The interrupted direct and the faradic currents are used mainly for electrodiagnosis. Interrupted direct current may also be used for stimulation of denervated muscles. The therapeutic objective of stimulation for temporarily denervated muscles is to maintain the muscle in as normal a state as possible during the period of nerve recovery. Conduction deficit without denervation (neurapraxia) is usually a temporary condition but may last for several weeks, and stimulation during this period may be of definite benefit. The best results have been obtained with frequent brief periods of stimulation; 25 to 50 contractions a session, four times a day, can be performed by the patient with his own portable battery unit, when he is properly instructed.

MASSAGE

Manual massage exerts the effect of direct displacement of fluid in vascular and lymphatic channels. There is also direct and reflex dilation of the smaller vessels leading to an increase in rate of flow and interchange of substances between bloodstream and tissue cells. Lymphatic flow is assisted and edema is reduced. Mechanical stretching and disruption of connective tissue fibers can be effectively accomplished by the friction type of massage where undesirable fibrosis has occurred in subcutaneous and superficial muscle layers. Light stroking massage results in relaxation of involuntary muscular contraction.

Pain threshold can be increased by slowly increasing stimuli to the central nervous system beginning with light stroking movement and slowly increasing the intensity of the massage. Massage may be used to assist in the accommodation of tissue to pressure, for example, the preparation of an amputation stump prior to the use of a prosthesis. The effect is obtained by progressing from gentle kneading and tapping to firm pounding and weight bearing. Massage will not prevent atrophy or loss of strength

Fig. 52-1. Plastic splint, molded directly or to a positive cast of the patient's hand, maintains the spastic hand in a functional position, preventing flexion contractures of the fingers or thumb.

due to inactivity or denervation, nor will it increase muscular strength. Only active exercise will strengthen muscles. Even the most vigorous massage will not reduce local deposition of fat.

Massage is indicated where the following effects are sought: (1) relief of pain, (2) relaxation of muscle tension, (3) improvement of circulation, (4) reduction of induration or edema, and (5) stretching of adhesions. Local application of heat is commonly used prior to massage, because it enhances the desired effects. Both heat and massage are frequently used prior to active or passive exercise, because the combined effects enable a patient to get maximal benefit from the exercise.

Contraindications for massage include (1) acute inflammation, since massage may result in systemic spread; (2) skin lesions; (3) malignant tumors; (4) acute circulatory disturbances such as phlebitis, thrombosis, or lymphangitis.

Occupational Therapy

Occupational therapy has been described as functional (physical or kinetic), vocational (prevocational therapy or work adjustment), and supportive (psychiatric or diversional). The goals of therapy are (1) to assist in the increase of range of motion of affected joints; (2) to assist in the increase of muscle strength; and (3) to develop motor coordination, skills, and work tolerance.

Fig. 52-2. Molded plastic cuff with a spring-steel pencil clip compensates for loss of opposition in writing. A small extension on the ulnar side permits dialing a telephone or operating a keypunch.

Functions of the upper extremities are concentrated upon. Training is given also to patients with upper extremity prostheses or orthoses in the proper use of the particular device and its application to the activities of daily living and of work.

The purposes of vocationally oriented occupational therapy are (1) prevocational evaluation for the patient who has never had a vocation or vocational objective; (2) a vocational exploration utilizing present physical capacities for the patient who may need to consider changing vocations because of his disability; (3) work adjustment for the patient needing to regain lost work skills, habits, or tolerance; and (4) development of skills for the patient who is considering a further academic career.

ACTIVITIES OF DAILY LIVING

The purpose of an A.D.L. program is to train the patient to perform his maximum in the daily activities inherent in his life. The degree to which a patient can carry out these activities determines his level of independence. There are three functional abilities required: (1) self-care, (2) mobility, and (3) communication. Activities in daily living are divided into the following groups: (1) bed activities, (2) wheelchair activities, (3) self-care activities, (4) miscellaneous hand activities, (5) ambulation and elevation activities, (6) traveling activities, and (7) kitchen and household activities.

ORTHOTICS AND PROSTHETICS

This is a field of knowledge relating to orthopedic devices which are either static or dynamic in character. Static units provide support and correction and dynamic units actively aid or provide elements of function. These devices can be helpful in promoting self-sufficiency for the patient with permanent, severe disability. They may be directed toward providing positioning and support for extremities, increasing the function of permanently weakened muscles, replacing the function of muscles, and assisting in the control of incoordination (Figs. 52-1 to 52-5).

SPLINTS AND BRACES. These control the action of specific joints to prevent or decrease motion, provide support, maintain position, and prevent contracture. Splints and braces may be used for flaccidity, spasticity, incoordination, contracture, or protection from pain and trauma. Splints may be classified as (1) static, those designed to support the involved segment, to prevent contracture, and to protect a painful, weakened, or injured part; and (2) dynamic, those designed to add active mechanical assistance to therapeutic exercise and functional use.

MANAGEMENT OF PSYCHIATRIC PROBLEMS AND PAIN

Emotional and motivational attitudes can have a decisive effect on the outcome of the rehabilitation process. In about 50 percent of adults with physical disability such factors are of major importance. In children the figures run considerably higher, approximately 75 percent. Important problems which frequently need psychiatric assistance are management of persistent pain and drug addiction, and sexual problems.

Physical disability may be accompanied by pain. Since

Fig. 52-3. Dorsal cockup splint keeps the wrist in extended position, and the C-bar positions the thumb for better opposition. The lumbrical bar prevents hyperextension of the metacarpophalangeal joints, while the spring-steel outriggers and plastic finger rings encourage finger extension and permit active flexion.

pain can inhibit activities and lead to interpersonal difficulties, its proper management may determine the success or failure of rehabilitation. Pain produces emotional changes even in well-adjusted individuals. It is not a static condition but changes with circumstances. It tends to be exaggerated at night because of fear, aloneness, and absence of diverting interests. Patients vary in their threshold to painful stimuli, and certain disabilities present special problems. In the paraplegic patients, pain *below* the level of the cord lesion is common and can be quite severe, despite total sensory loss below the test level.

Successful management of pain requires accurate medical diagnosis, as well as analysis of psychologic, emotional, and socioeconomic factors. Measures for relief include adequate counseling, the use of nonnarcotic drugs, physical therapy, radiation therapy, anesthetic block, and surgical procedures. The use of acupuncture and transcutaneous neural electrostimulation has been extensively investigated, but dependable, reproducible response has not been documented. Selected patients, especially those with suitable psychological characteristics, may respond to these modalities. Inquiry into the presence of possible sources of painful reaction to life situations should be considered. If methods are properly employed, narcotics can be avoided, and the disabling problem of addiction can be obviated.

In physically disabled persons, sexual function may be interfered with in two ways: (1) local anatomic injury or neurologic deficit, which may make normal sexual functioning impossible, and (2) psychologic changes resulting from the disability, such as doubts about adequacy and attractiveness. A serious problem for both male and female patients is loss of control of bladder and bowel function. When assistance in care is needed from husband or wife, additional sexual problems may result. The presence of a colostomy or the absence of a uterus or breast may cause anxiety and distaste. Maturity and understanding increase adjustive capacity.

SOCIAL SERVICE

The social worker should meet with the patient and his family as soon as feasible following his admission. The

Fig. 52-4. Simple leather and spring-steel dorsal wrist cockup splint has a double dorsal leather strip into which spring-steel bands are inserted. The number required depends on the weight of the hand and the degree of residual wrist extension. A palmar pocket holds standard eating and grooming utensils, typing sticks, or an adapted pencil holder.

Fig. 52-5. Wrist-driven flexor hinge splint utilizes residual wrist power to obtain pincer or three-point grasp between the thumb, index, and middle fingers or gross grasp employing the thumb web space. A rachet on the metal bar locks for static holding and releases with slight pressure.

interview has many purposes: (1) to give the patient and his family information and understanding regarding the services that are available to him; (2) to evaluate from the patient's social history his environmental resources and his abilities to utilize the services; (3) to refer the patient and his family to the appropriate resource, outside the hospital, for alleviating environmental problems.

In permitting the patient to adjust to interpersonal relations and relative independence, vocational evaluation and counseling may be employed. Returning the patient to his home environment as a fully functioning member may necessitate preparation of special home programs.

VOCATIONAL REHABILITATION

Vocational rehabilitation assistance should be sought for any patient whose residual disability limits his capacity to return to his previous occupational activity or potential.

Directly or through the medical social worker, the patient can be referred to the State Vocational Rehabilitation Service counselor for evaluation, guidance, and eligible financial support for definitive treatment, rehabilitation therapy, and any indicated training or retraining for work. This includes driver training for the handicapped driver and provision of needed controls for the car.

REHABILITATION OF PATIENTS WITH SPECIFIC PROBLEMS

Musculoskeletal Problems

Programs are directed at the goals of efficient function with painless and free motion, good alignment and posture, and adequate coordinated muscular control. Deformities are prevented by immobilizing affected parts in optimal position, supervising bed posture, and avoiding unnecessary fixation of the joints. The function of uninvolved parts should be maintained, and this may involve electrical stimulation of the muscles which patients cannot move. Mobilization is carried out as early as possible without jeopardizing healing. This program will retard atrophy, prevent permanent scar formation, preserve joint range of motion, stimulate reciprocal muscle function, and reduce the extent of the disability. Pain should be relieved before performing any therapeutic exercises. The patient's weaknesses should be protected by avoiding activities for which he does not have the required strength and by using splints and braces when needed.

Involved muscles are treated specifically with selective exercise, while involved joints are treated extremely gently, avoiding forced motions and combining complete rest with short periods of motion of the painful joints. The plan is carried out as early as possible. Limited weight bearing may be achieved in deep water in a therapeutic pool or using parallel bars, a walker, or crutches.

FRACTURES

During the period of required fracture immobilization, the major goal of rehabilitation is directed toward the prevention of osteoporosis, atrophy of muscles, contracture

of ligaments, and edema of soft tissue. Immobilization should be limited to include only the joints proximal and distal to the fracture site. All other joints in the involved extremity should be permitted free motion and carried through their full range at least once daily. With time, this activity should increase.

As soon as possible after cast application, active exercises should be carried out at levels proximal and distal to the immobilized area. Pain should be minimal, and severe pain represents an indication for investigation of the cast or fracture position. At all times, the use of narcotics should be minimized.

Control of swelling and edema is particularly important during the first 5 to 7 days of treatment. Elevation of the involved areas should be started immediately postoperatively and maintained for prolonged periods of time. Application of intermittent massage may relieve the discomfort, aid circulation, and reduce edema.

Isometric muscle-setting exercises are effective, especially when extremities cannot be actively moved. They are of great potential value because of their widespread applicability, but their effective use requires careful planning and explanation to the patient. The precaution of instructing each patient in strict avoidance of breath holding (creating a Valsalva maneuver) during muscle-setting exercises must be observed. Such precaution is to prevent impairment of coronary circulation and possible occlusion. Isometric exercises should be followed, after termination of immobilization, by active exercise through full range of motion. In the lower extremity, isometric quadriceps exercises are directed at preventing loss of stability of the knee. In the upper extremities, attention is particularly directed toward hand function and prevention of contracture of the fingers. In all these situations rehabilitation should be initiated within 24 hours after treatment of the injury, sequentially employing passive motion, isometric exercises, and active exercises.

Immediately following cast removal, active exercises should be started with direction toward return of full joint range of motion.

Current concepts of care for patients with metastatic bone cancer with impending or actual pathological fracture have introduced procedures of hip replacement and intramedullary nailing and use of methylmethacrylate which allow the patients to regain activity on a schedule similar to that offered patients after procedures for trauma, arthritis, or aseptic necrosis.

JOINT DISABILITIES

TRAUMATIC ARTHRITIS. Joint damage may result from a single major trauma, such as a fracture extending into the joint space, but more commonly it follows from repeated small traumas. The latter may be related to occupational stresses, joint instability, postural derangement, or torn ligaments. The arthritic joint has a decrease in functional efficiency and range of motion, and movement may be associated with pain and swelling.

Treatment of the traumatic arthritic joint should be directed toward (1) elimination of any residual etiologic factor, (2) relief of pain, (3) therapeutic exercise, and (4) protection of the joint against further wearing. The latter is attained only by reducing the amount of physical work or weight imposed on the damaged joint structure. Definitive therapy includes physical activity, therapeutic exercises to build periarticular muscle power and the dependent joint stability to a maximum, and transfer of stress to other uninvolved joints through the use of such measures as shoe lifts, stabilizing supports, crutches, canes, braces, and energy-saving devices.

INFECTIOUS ARTHRITIS. In the acute active phase of the infection, the objectives of physical medicine are analgesia and the maintenance of motion of the involved joint to prevent deformity. Heat applied locally is usually indicated, and warm, moist heat in the forms of compresses or packs is generally best tolerated. In the less acute phase, hydrotherapy in the form of whirlpool baths or the Hubbard tank may be used more effectively to permit early active exercising. Even in the active phase of a specific infectious arthritis, the involved joint should be carried passively through normal range of motion at least once a day to prevent capsular and tendinous tightening and the development of deformity. Pain sedation with nonnarcotic medications and intermittent rest periods should spell the exercise or movement efforts. As the process subsides, an active exercise program should be initiated to maintain normal range of motion and to prevent muscle atrophy.

Following the eradication of the infection, the problem of physical rehabilitation is contingent upon the degree of muscle weakness which has resulted, the range of motion which may have been lost, and the extent of structural intraarticular damage produced by the infection. The first two conditions should be actively treated with stretching and range-of-motion exercises and progressive resistive exercises. Active range-of-motion exercises or use may prevent intraarticular damage from causing increasing range restriction.

AMPUTATIONS

In the United States, more than 75 percent of lower extremity amputations are performed in treatment for peripheral vascular disease problems on individuals over the age of sixty. Since many people in this age group fail to achieve even the minimal standards of success with the use of prostheses, it is necessary to be selective in the planning of rehabilitation programs. Most of the failures can be directly attributed to medical factors such as (1) coexisting cardiovascular disease or advanced peripheral vascular disease in the unamputated extremity; (2) personal factors such as lack of insight, motivation, or opportunity in the use of a prosthesis; or (3) the prosthesis itself, which may be ill-conceived or improperly prescribed for the patient's individual needs. Diagnoses of cancer and trauma account for about 10 percent each of the remaining amputations performed.

Successful physical and vocational rehabilitation is dependent upon (1) the reason for the amputation, (2) general health and the presence or absence of other disabilities, (3) the level and characteristics of the amputation stump, (4) personal characteristics of the individual,

(5) preparation for function, (6) prescription for the prosthesis, (7) the quality of training with the prosthesis and the nature of rehabilitation facilities available to the patient. Rehabilitation of the amputee is achieved through the following progressive procedures:

PRELIMINARY ORIENTATION. The patient and his family should be informed in general terms regarding the future procedures and estimated timetable.

SURGERY.* The amputation stump in most cases is the key to determining whether or not the patient will be successful in developing skill with a prosthesis. The surgeon is responsible for creating a stump which tapers from above downward and in which all the tissues have been treated in such a manner that the patient can be fitted with conventional prosthetic equipment, leading to a high degree of function.

Each of the tissues encountered in the amputation can be responsible for creating a problem formidable enough to interfere with good function. Flexion contractures are often created by closing amputation stumps with the proximal joint in acute flexion. No tension should exist in the skin closure. Skin flaps which are tightly stretched across the end of the stump remain painful and often break down under conditions of function. The fascia should be used as a barrier between the deep tissues and the skin flaps, so that the skin flaps remain freely movable over the end of the stump. The muscles must be anchored down to, and in some instances in the form of myofascial flaps across, the end of the bone, so that they provide good control and do not retract upon movement of the stump. Such myodesis or myoplasty is particularly mandatory when immediate postoperative application of a prosthesis is planned for the above- or below-knee amputee. The bone requires accurate cutting without piling up the periosteum at the end, since this inevitably will result in the development of exostosis, which may create pain with the use of the prosthesis.

Hemostasis during and after surgical procedures is an extremely important factor. The accumulation of hematoma under the skin flaps not only may jeopardize healing of the wound but may eventually result in a hard, painful scar which can interfere with comfort. Nerves should be pulled down and cut as high as possible, so that they are not incorporated in the scar at the end of the stump. All severed nerves form neuromas, but when a neuroma is in the scar or low in the stump where it may be compressed against the solid wall of a prosthesis, it can become extremely painful and may preclude the possibility of the amputee's developing tolerance for weight bearing. The postoperative dressing is related to hemostasis, and if an efficient compressive dressing or the cast for an immediate prosthesis cannot be applied, drainage should be employed.

The degree of function achieved with a prosthesis is directly proportional to the amount of the functioning limb

---

* Adapted from Allen R. Russek, management of Lower Extremity Amputees, *Arch Phys Med Rehabil,* vol. 42, September, 1961; and E. M. Burgess, R. L. Romano, and J. H. Zettle, "Management of Lower Extremity Amputations," U.S. Government Printing Office, Publication TR10-6, August, 1969.

remaining. In the upper extremity, the general principle holds of saving as much bone length as possible. Myoelectric control units are still experimental, and claims vary, but usefulness is limited to below-elbow-level amputees.

Standard sites of amputations are recognized. In the upper extremity, the most proximal amputation is the interscapulothoracic or forequarter amputation. Below that level there are standard amputations of disarticulation at the shoulder, above-elbow or below-elbow amputations, disarticulation at the wrist, and partial-hand amputations. Amputations of individual digits, especially through the thumb and index finger, may require special surgical reconstructive procedures following the initial surgical procedure. Finger and thumb stumps may be built out and webbed spaces deepened to improve ultimate hand function.

In the lower extremity, the standard amputations are the hemipelvectomy, hip disarticulation, above-knee and below-knee amputations, Syme amputation, and partial foot amputations. Amputations within 2 in. immediately above or below the knee are undesirable. When amputating above the knee it is preferable to sever the bone not closer than 4 in. from the knee joint. This makes it possible to use conventional prosthetic equipment, whereas if the amputation is performed closer to the knee joint, there may be asymmetry of the position and function of the normal and prosthetic knee joints. Very short stumps of less than 2 in. below the knee create frequent interference with anatomic knee function and satisfactory prosthetic fit and function.

Because of the appearance of the prosthesis, the Syme amputation is frequently unacceptable to women. However, it is a good amputation for men. Partial foot amputations result in a complicated weight-bearing stump and have the tendency to break down, particularly following trauma. They are seldom selected, and amputation is more often performed at a Syme level.

Successful translumbar amputation (hemicorporectomy) has been performed by disarticulation at the L_4-L_5 or L_5-S_1 levels, with prosthetic replacement and rehabilitation to complete independence including ability to drive a car.

STUMP AND PREPROSTHETIC STAGE. The muscles of the amputation stump and the remaining limb should be strengthened. It is necessary to make sure that all the joints can be carried through their full range of motion with control. The patient's ability to balance independently on the remaining leg should also be noted. Training should be given with crutches for standing and balance and eventual ambulation on the remaining limb. It is necessary that the patient achieve a safe, stable, and secure crutch-walking gait without pain in the calf of the remaining leg and without the development of dyspnea from effort. The patient's posture on the remaining leg and the stability of his pelvis are very important to develop and control. Excessive weight is a serious problem and requires a positive approach.

Immediate postoperative or early postoperative (within 14 days) application of a lower extremity prosthesis provides excellent concomitant stump conditioning and shaping. The snug cast and early partial weight bearing are positive forces and increase control, utilize proprioception, and limit phantom sensations.

When techniques for the early application of the prosthesis are not used, the stump requires conditioning, shaping, shrinkage, and a full range of motion in the proximal joints. Conditioning of the stump is achieved by a graded program of exercise: at first gentle active, later assistive, and finally resistive exercises. For midthigh amputations it is important to make sure that there is no flexion or abduction contracture at the hip and that all the muscles controlling the amputation stump and the leverage of the stump are strong and reliable. Shrinkage of the tissues and shaping of the stump are accomplished by means of proper wrapping with elastic bandages and/or use of elastic stump-shrinking socks.

Wrapping of the proximal mass of tissues is as important as wrapping the distal tissues, since the anatomic points of fitting are proximal rather than distal and these will shrink rapidly with the use of prosthesis and should be prepared prior to the application of the prosthesis. Most patients are unable to apply the bandage properly by themselves. The repeated encircling of the limb with turns of elastic bandage can actually constitute a tourniquet. Bandaging should be tight, with exertion of pressure only distad. The proximal turns should be relatively loosely applied, as they are used only to hold the wrapping in place. Elastic stump-shrinking socks are preferred. These have a predetermined degree of compression necessary for shaping and shrinkage of the stump and are far superior to bandaging by an inexperienced patient or attendant. Wrapping or shrinker socks must be carried high on the stump to eliminate formation of bulging flesh at the top.

PERSONAL CHARACTERISTICS OF THE AMPUTEE. Throughout the management of the patient, his personal characteristics require understanding. His type of employment should be considered. The age of the patient is an important factor, and his insight, understanding, ability to cooperate, and motivation require detailed attention and a positive approach. When personality problems present themselves, investigation of the psychologic factors associated with this difficulty is essential, if the patient does not emerge from this state voluntarily by gaining confidence.

PRESCRIPTION FOR A PROSTHESIS. The prescription is based upon individual needs. Components prescribed should provide the degree of function and stability needed. Patients with good potentials are given prescriptions which allow unobstructed use of all joints in conventional alignment. Others will need limited function components and added assistive devices. Prescription is best made with the advice of a physiatrist or prosthetist.

TRAINING. Training is a graded procedure and should begin by making the patient familiar with the prosthesis. He then learns to care for the prosthesis and keep it clean, to utilize and wash stump socks, to maintain good hygienic care of the skin, and to avoid stresses on the remaining limb. The achievement of skill requires practice and effort, and the patient should be informed of the need for his participation in the training program. When the prescription for the prosthesis is made, some estimate of the expected achievements of the patient should be established. It is obvious that not all patients reach a safe, acceptable level of function. The classifications of function are important to recognize, and each patient should be informed as to his potential and his individual goal.

Class 1—full restoration. This indicates that the individual has been functionally restored and trained with his prosthesis. Despite his physical handicap, he is able to function maximally. Few people attain such an objective.

Class 2—partial restoration. The patient who achieves this level of function, when trained with a proper artificial limb, will be able to work. He may possibly have to make changes in his job. He lives a normal life, may dance or even play golf, but he has very definite limitations in nonessential areas.

Class 3—self-care plus. While people in this class are disabled and have physical limitations, they are capable of doing everything for themselves in terms of their personal needs. Many are able to work at jobs that do not require much standing and walking. They give up competitive sports and long walking, but they are still able to maintain a satisfactory degree of function, which permits them to live without modification of their normal standards. They may require fairly frequent services of the prosthetist to keep the prosthesis in a satisfactory serviceable condition.

Class 4—self-care minus. People in this category are better off with a prosthesis than they are without one. Their best achievement, however, falls somewhat short of taking care of all their needs. They require the help of another person. They have frequent difficulty in maintaining comfort in the artificial limb. People in this class may be quite functional for short periods and may have a tolerance of several hours of the use of the prosthesis but cannot wear it all day. Others may be quite functional all day but are uncomfortable and need to remove the prosthesis from time to time.

Class 5—cosmetic plus. Amputees in this group are better off with a prosthesis than without one, but the difference is quite small. They do little more than they would without the prosthesis, but for personal reasons and appearance the prosthesis serves a definite function. Also in this class are people for whom the prosthesis serves one single function of personal import, such as getting in and out of a car, or standing when changing from one chair to another, or possibly going to the bathroom unassisted.

Class 6—not feasible. There are some patients for whom no clear objective, not even a cosmetic one, justifies the prescription of a prosthesis. In these instances, the patient should be trained to do as much as he can for himself from a wheelchair.

When prescribing a prosthesis for an amputee, it must be understood that the various medical and psychologic problems which affect amputees may detract from their potential function. The amputee suffers from a summation of problems which affect him. If several factors unrelated to each other each interfere with function, he will not achieve a great degree of skill. For example, a patient without motivation and short, above-knee stump with a flexion contracture has three unrelated problems, each of which, on its own, will interfere with function. Awareness of problems which interfere with function will help establish the class in which each patient falls when the prosthesis is prescribed. Establishment of the goal is important,

since this determines the extent of training. In addition, it is possible to tell the patient in advance how far he may expect to go, so that he does not hope to achieve more than is possible.

IMMEDIATE AND EARLY PROSTHETIC FITTING. Efforts can frequently be directed toward fitting patients with temporary prostheses in the operating room. This is preceded by myoplasty or myodesis in the closure of the amputation stump so that all opposing muscle groups are firmly anchored to opposing fascia or to the end of the bone and the amputation stump is shaped in the operating room to accommodate a total contact socket for weight bearing, quadrilateral for the above-knee and patellar tendon–bearing for the below-knee procedure. This has been highly satisfactory for early weight bearing. It does not jeopardize the healing of the wound and is considered by many to enhance healing. Fitting with temporary prostheses in the operating room has resulted in readiness of the patient to wear a permanent prosthesis at between 4 and 6 weeks following major amputation above or below the knee, and a return to work within 2 months.

Another concept is that of early fitting, when only the elastic plaster of paris dressing cover is applied postoperatively. In the normal uncomplicated case, the dressing and sutures are removed after about 2 weeks, and the patient is measured then for a temporary prosthesis. Conditioning, shaping, and shrinking of the amputation stump are accomplished in the ensuing 3 or 4 weeks with the use of the temporary prosthesis. Thereafter, the patient can be fitted with a permanent prosthesis.

UPPER EXTREMITY AMPUTATIONS. Excellent prostheses are now available for patients with upper extremity amputations at any level. These prostheses consist of plastic laminated sockets made from corrected plaster casts of the amputation stumps. They are harnessed by means of a split figure-of-eight strap, one end of which suspends the prosthesis while the other end operates a cable within a housing. The cable in turn activates the functional terminal device, which may consist of one of the available split hooks or a functional hand. Cosmetic hands are also obtainable and are interchangeable with the other terminal devices. Myoelectric control units are still in the experimental stage and are limited principally to below-elbow amputations. It is more difficult to fit patients with certain partial hand amputations where only part of the palm remains, since there is no satisfactory functional equipment for such an amputation. Whenever such a part of a hand is left, if no practical function is achieved below the wrist, it may then be better to disarticulate at the wrist, making it possible to use commercially available prosthetic equipment.

Application of immediate postoperative prosthesis to the upper extremity is limited. Experience has been gained in both below elbow and above-elbow techniques, however, and the plaster dressing can be fitted with a terminal device with shoulder harness. Rehabilitation is speeded, especially in the case of the double amputee.

AMPUTATIONS IN CHILDREN. Some children are ready to use upper extremity prostheses before three years of age.

Most children learn rapidly and well. The objective for the young child is the achievement of complete physical rehabilitation by the time he enters school. In the management of children who have had an extremity removed because of a malignant tumor, it is generally agreed that the restored function and cosmesis afforded by prosthetic fitting are of practical and psychologic value to both the child and his parents. Data from recent studies indicate that a significant percentage of amputees with malignant tumors survive for 1 to 5 years postoperatively and wear prostheses successfully for 1 year and longer. The majority of these patients are full-time users of their prostheses. If there is no evidence of metastasis and the stump is suitable for fitting, a limb should be provided at the earliest possible date.

HIP-REPLACEMENT SURGERY

Hip-replacement surgery allows postoperative weight-bearing activity earlier than pinning procedures for fractures. Austin-Moore-type prosthetic hips, without an artificial acetabular socket, will allow start of weight bearing by 2 to 3 weeks postsurgery. Acetabular replacement requires an additional 2 to 3 weeks of limited weight bearing. The patient's age, condition of tissues at time of surgery, absence of other diseases, and the basic diagnosis (trauma, osteoarthritis, cancer) need assessment in setting time for progression in activity.

WIDE RESECTION OF EXTREMITY SOFT TISSUE

Wide resection of soft tissue, including muscle groups, fascia, and nerves, creates functional loss directly related to the structures involved. Postoperative rehabilitation, particularly for lower extremity disability, may require prescription of appropriate bracing to stabilize against quadriceps, gastroc-soleus, or anterior tibial muscle deficit. Loss of sensation precludes application of heat and requires attention to foot protection and cover. Forearm soft tissue resections may benefit from supportive static splinting or from a dynamic, functional tenodesis splint to provide grasp through wrist extension, when finger flexors have been lost or resected.

Grafts placed over surgical defects require protection from trauma, particularly during healing in the early postoperative period.

LONG-BONE RESECTION

Long-bone resection, such as total or *en bloc* bone resection for cancer, requires special programming for rehabilitation of the patient. Such a procedure as the Tikhov-Linberg resection of scapula, clavicle, and upper humerus for malignant tumors of the scapular and shoulder region preserves the neurovascular bundle and leaves the patient with a functional forearm, wrist, and hand, limited only by lack of stabilization to the body. Sling and swathe support of the arm and forearm assists the patient in hand use.

The problems which follow long-bone excision and replacement include deficient muscle attachment to the internal prosthetic replacement for movement control and power, minimal cover over the internal prosthesis potenti-

ating infection after skin break, potential fracture of the internal prosthesis, hip joint instability, and prolonged interval prior to allowance of joint activity or weight bearing. These patients can be permitted ambulation, initially without weight bearing and with the support of combined ischial seat and double-bar long leg bracing over a Jordan splint. Subsequent gradual increase in weight bearing in the brace has been successful after 4 to 8 months. Unhandicapped, free use of the limb cannot be expected. Consistent care must be paid toward protection of the skin from injury where it covers the artificial knee joint and the prosthesis.

THE HAND

Rehabilitation of the patient with a poorly functioning hand requires the closest collaboration between the disciplines of surgery and rehabilitation. The benefits of active and passive exercise, heat, massage, and related techniques may not be optimal unless superficial scars, densely adherent tendons, and nerve injuries are repaired. Maximal surgical benefit to the patient will not accrue, in many instances, unless rehabilitation measures are also supplied.

TENDONS AND TENDON TRANSFERS. Freshly lacerated tendons are frequently repaired within the early hours after injury. Should the fear of infection or the loss of superficial tissues dictate delay in repair, such repair may well be postponed for several months. During this time, physiotherapeutic efforts designed to maintain the mobility of the joints and the integrity of the muscles are instituted. Whenever the repair of the involved tendons is carried out, whether early or late, immobilization for about 3 weeks is usually mandatory for the development of firm union at the suture lines. The position of the hand during immobilization will depend in great part upon the nature of the surgical repair, but in general the principle to be followed is to avoid tension at the suture line while keeping the joints, as nearly as possible, in the neutral position of function. Optimal position for immobilization of the hand is in slight dorsiflexion at the wrist, flexion at the metacarpophalangeal joints, minimal flexion of the fingers, and moderate abduction and slight flexion of the thumb. After termination of immobilization, progressive and intensive efforts must be directed toward the reestablishment of function.

In general, the period of rehabilitation following tendon transfer is longer than that following tendon repair or tendon grafting. This is because of (1) the problem of reeducation of the muscles to perform unaccustomed tasks, (2) the usual loss of one grade of power in the muscle of the transferred tendon, and (3) the generally more extensive disability in the patient requiring the tendon transfer.

POSTTRAUMATIC BACK PAIN

Pain in the back may result from single or multiple incidents of external violence, from a pathologic condition of an intervertebral disc, from neoplasm, from excessive effort, and from cumulative prolonged stress and strain. It may develop without apparent cause, perhaps from emotional stress or instability. It is necessary to determine the cause before appropriate treatment can be given.

In the majority of cases of acute strain or sprain of a ligament, the pathologic condition will spontaneously resolve when the local tissue damage has healed. Acute injuries of the back, without damage to the bony structures, usually heal spontaneously under protected conditions of rest and support. When a patient fails to respond to therapy and pain becomes prolonged, detailed reexamination should be performed.

When a positive diagnosis of herniated intervertebral disc has been made, the treatment should be conservative at first, since a significant percentage of cases can be brought under satisfactory control without surgical intervention. If recurrences of pain are frequent or insufficient relief follows conservative treatment, then surgical measures should be considered. Most authorities agree that the best results following surgical treatment are obtained in the patients operated on fairly early. Because of the secondary changes in muscles, posture, habits, and emotional reactions with passage of time, it may be too late for surgical procedures to relieve more than a small part of the complex problem after a case has become chronic.

In general, a patient who has suffered recent back trauma should be placed at rest, muscular spasm released, range of motion of the trunk restored, weight bearing gradually introduced, tolerance to activities developed according to individual needs, and continuous reassurance given to prevent excessive concern. The relief of pain during the treatment period must be achieved in order to permit the patient to cooperate.

The patient should be kept at rest on a firm mattress, preferably on one under which a bed board has been placed. Sedative and analgesic drugs should be used to control pain. Active setting exercises for the gluteal, abdominal, and back muscles should be begun as soon as they can be tolerated. Non-weight-bearing stretching exercises in the bed are sometimes effective in relieving tension from spasm. The use of muscle-relaxant drugs during the acute or chronic stage has not proved effective. When symptoms begin to subside, the use of local heat by means of moist hot packs, tub bath, or Hubbard tank should follow. Focal pain may be relieved by ultrasound application to joint or muscle but not to nerve structures. As the symptoms permit, passive stretching of tight muscles should be attempted. Exercises for 20 minutes in a Hubbard therapeutic tank with the water at 100°F are frequently followed by rapid improvement in range of motion. Occasionally, walking in the deep end of a therapeutic pool restores coordination and elasticity of muscles.

When the patient is capable of resuming activities on a progressive basis, it may be useful to protect the back from the stresses of movement and to support body weight by the use of reinforced belts or braces. The "chair back" and Knight-Taylor types of braces provide best limitation of motion of the thoracic and upper lumbar spine, and a lumbar corset or belt is best for midlumbar and lower lumbar regions (where motion is actually aggravated by the application of a long back brace). The patient should be kept on a sustained program of exercises of increasing intensity, designed to rebalance the supporting musculature of the trunk and pelvis, while he is wearing these supports. The brace or belt may be removed later, when the patient has a muscular corset of his own sufficient to handle the stresses. If symptoms have been severe and the patient's usual work is strenuous, it may be advisable to discuss a change in occupation in order to avoid recurrence under working conditions. If the patient fails to respond to these methods and chronic back pain persists, he may develop numerous psychogenic superimposed symptoms which complicate the picture. Such patients should obtain the supportive therapy of professional personnel such as psychologists, social workers, vocational counselors, and psychiatrists, when necessary. Chronic or recurrent backache is one of the most frequent symptoms of psychologic and emotional disturbances.

Diseases of the Nervous System

FACIAL PARALYSIS

Although facial paralysis is usually due to idiopathic Bell's palsy, it may be the result of tumor, abscess, or cyst, or a consequence of head and parotid trauma or surgical treatment. The majority of patients with a benign process exhibit spontaneous improvement within 6 weeks after the onset of the paralysis.

Initial treatment is primarily symptomatic and includes local application of warmth to the involved muscles, attention to eye hygiene, and protective glasses or a patch. Gentle perioral and periorbital massage several times daily in front of a mirror is prescribed. The massage should be begun at the medial and inferior margins of mouth or eye, gradually stroking upward with a circular motion in the direction of the muscle fibers. Attempts at volitional movement should be made or practiced regularly with the aid of a mirror. The therapeutic use of electrical stimulation is controversial and is usually not recommended beyond the acute stage. It is considered to be of little value when volitional movement has returned. Facial splints and supports of many types have been designed to prevent stretching and asymmetry. A simple one extends over the ear on the affected side and hooks into the angle of the mouth.

There frequently will be transient synkinetic movement of the platysma or other facial musculature, which may distress the patient. Mild sedation and reassurance are commonly all that is required in managing the patient. If there is no improvement within 2 weeks after the onset of the paralysis, electrodiagnostic studies may prove invaluable in prognosticating recovery or permanence of denervation. If no recovery is seen in 6 weeks, surgical intervention should be considered.

PERIPHERAL NEUROPATHY

Peripheral neuropathy may be caused by nerve trauma including complete division, crushing, stretching, and pressure. Although the disability is primarily due to the resultant muscle paralysis, superimposed contractures and atrophic changes complicate the situation. Proper rehabilitation procedures instituted early can do much to prevent or to correct problems.

Following traumatic interruption of a nerve, suture is essential. Proper subsequent treatment requires an accurate diagnosis of the involved nerve and the extent of the pathologic condition, and knowledge of the motor ramifications. Electrodiagnostic testing techniques are invaluable for this purpose, but the examination is best deferred for 2 or 3 weeks, to allow for possible wallerian degeneration and permit detection of denervation potentials and measure nerve conduction velocity change. In occasional instances, nerve blocks are of diagnostic value, and, in specific instances, surgical exploration may be necessary.

Periodic retesting is necessary in many cases to determine the prognosis. Serial changes in the electrical studies frequently presage obvious clinical improvement. Return of function may be measured clinically by the development and progression of Tinel's sign, alteration in the extent and character of the sensory deficit, retrogression of the vasomotor signs, and gradual return of motor function.

The rehabilitation program for the patient with peripheral nerve involvement must frequently be of long duration, in view of the fact that regeneration occurs from the proximal portion of the nerve and is considered to occur at an average of 1.5 mm/day. The initial approaches are preventive. Passive motions are utilized to prevent joint contractures and the development of adhesions between tendons and their sheaths. These exercises and massage may frequently retard but cannot prevent reduction in muscle volume and tone. Electrical stimulation is also useful for this purpose but in no way appears to influence the rate of neuron regeneration. Special splints, slings, casts, or braces may be needed to prevent overstretching of the muscle by the intact antagonist or by gravity. If these are used, they should be so designed as to allow daily passive movements of the involved joints. Attempts to stimulate the circulation of the involved part consist of gentle massage, the cautious administration of heat with padded hot packs or warm baths, with or without whirlpool.

When voluntary motion begins to return, the program is supplemented by intensive muscle reeducation procedures. At first these are performed with gravity eliminated, but they are gradually increased until progressive resistive exercises are employed.

Causalgia is a distressing symptom which is frequently very difficult to treat. The limb may have to be carefully protected from inclement weather and minor trauma by adequate padding and support. Moist heat and gentle massage may be applied. Despite the discomfort, the importance of passive motion must be emphasized in instructions to the patient, and it should be carried out regularly if at all possible. Nerve block to determine the presence of a neuroma may be considered. Psychotherapy may be indicated. Sympathetic block, followed, if successful, by preganglionic sympathectomy, may be needed to relieve causalgic pain.

SPECIFIC PERIPHERAL NEUROPATHIES. The *long thoracic nerve* may be involved by direct injury, surgical procedure, or sudden stretching; the result is paralysis of the serratus anterior muscle. With the lack of scapular fixation

it is difficult or impossible for the patient to raise his arm above the horizontal level. In selected patients, it has been possible to stabilize the scapula and restore a great deal of arm function by the use of a special brace, designed with firm scapular plates and a firmly affixed breast plate. The *axillary nerve* may be involved by injuries or lesions in the region of the neck of the humerus. During treatment the arm is splinted in a shoulder-abducted position while the usual program for peripheral nerve lesions is instituted. The *musculocutaneous nerve* is seldom involved alone, but it may be injured by direct trauma or dislocation of the head of the humerus. The forearm should be supported by a sling during treatment.

The *radial nerve* is commonly damaged by injuries to the humerus, dislocations in the axilla, or a crutch or other pressures (abduction and pressure on the operating table, malpositioning). A splint providing for extension of the wrist and of the fingers with moderate metacarpophalangeal flexion is essential. Spring and elastic extensions for the fingers, extending over the dorsum of the hand and fixed to a rigid wrist support, or a spring-assisted bar to extend the proximal phalanges of the fingers are used to provide active motion at the metacarpophalangeal joints.

The *median nerve* is most commonly injured in civilian life by lacerations of the wrist. In some cases the ulnar nerve may also be damaged. A splint to keep the thumb in a position of abduction and opposition is recommended. Causalgia may be a serious problem and hamper rehabilitation. The *ulnar nerve* may be involved as the result of injuries in the region of the elbow. A splint designed to posture the hand in a position of flexion at the metacarpophalangeal joints with extension of the interphalangeal (IP) joints is of value.

The *femoral nerve,* although vulnerable to many pathologic processes, is most commonly involved with fractures of the pelvis. The resulting weakness of the quadriceps can be compensated for in many individuals by the use of elastic devices running from the waist or upper thigh to the anterior margin of the lower leg, by special knee braces with spring action to retard knee flexion, or by a long leg brace, depending on the degree of weakness.

The *sciatic nerve* terminates as the common peroneal and tibial nerves. It and its many branches are very susceptible to injury, and one of the complicating features is associated causalgia. The *common peroneal nerve* is frequently injured by trauma involving the upper end of the fibula. Compression bandages also represent common causes. Usually the peroneal muscles are more involved than the anterior tibial group. In addition to providing range of motion, it is necessary to prevent and compensate for foot drop and equinovarus deformity. If the patient is bedridden, the foot may be supported by the use of a posterior molded splint or a footboard. In ambulatory patients, the use of a high-topped shoe is frequently all that is necessary to correct a slight foot drop. In others, a posterior spring brace, made of molded, fitted plastic or of metal, inserted into the shoe heel or attached to a foot plate, is needed to provide support. Occasionally, it is necessary to use a short leg brace with either a spring or a 90° plantar flexion stop at the ankle. The *tibial nerve* is less commonly involved. Care must be taken to prevent the common tendency toward the formation of trophic ulcers. Paralysis of the triceps surae muscles creates gait difficulties and calcaneus deformity of the foot. Short leg braces with stirrup attachment and 90° dorsiflexion stop are needed.

PARAPLEGIA OR QUADRIPLEGIA

The patient with paraplegia or quadriplegia needs a coordinated program designed (1) to prevent decubitus ulcers, (2) to maintain range of motion, (3) to prevent contractures, (4) to improve the power of those muscles which are intact, (5) to strengthen weakened muscles to their maximal capacity, (6) to establish a satisfactory bowel and bladder program, and (7) to reestablish independence in activities of daily living.

Any paralyzed patient, either operative or nonoperative, should, at the onset, be kept in an extended neutral position. Special nursing care, with particular attention to nutrition, skin care, and posture, is mandatory.

SKIN CARE. The patient must be turned at least every 2 hours, day and night, in order to prevent decubitus ulcers. Nurses should inspect the skin carefully over the following pressure points: sacrum, trochanters, iliac crests, ischial tuberosities, knees, and heels. As the patient is turned, these areas should be cleansed very carefully with soap and water, dried gently, and massaged lightly, and a bland oil or neutral ointment should be applied.

CONTROL OF DECUBITUS ULCERS. This requires adequate relief of local pressure by application of surrounding polyurethane foam pads or use of alternating pressure mattresses or pads, multiple bolsters, flotation pads or beds, Stryker frames, or Circle beds. Adequate debridement of slough and frequent changes of dry, soft, sterile dressings aid control or healing. Various dressings from sugar to dried plasma or red cells have been used with success. Hyperbaric oxygen may be beneficial to healing, and application of mild electric currents to ulcer surfaces has aided infection control and granulation.

MAINTENANCE OF RANGE OF MOTION. All joints of the affected extremities should be taken through a complete range of motion twice daily. Patients who have residual muscle power but with some weakness should be encouraged to carry through their range of motion actively, as far as possible, and the therapist should then assist the patient or complete the range of motion with passive movement. These patients are prone to develop short heel cords with subsequent equinus deformity. To prevent this, bedclothes should *not* be pulled down tightly over the foot of the bed. The patient's feet must be kept at right angles to the legs at all times, either by means of a footboard and pillow or sandbag support, or by a carefully padded posterior splint.

THERAPEUTIC EXERCISE. Muscle-strengthening exercises should emphasize conditioning the shoulder depressor, including the latissimus dorsi, and the triceps brachii. These are the muscles which the patient with paraplegia must utilize in order to walk with braces and crutches. Exercises for these muscle groups should be started early and increased in intensity as rapidly as possible.

CONTRACTURES. Prevention of contractures is fundamental. To neglect this preventive procedure may delay rehabilitation by weeks or even months. Special care must be given to the hip and knee joints, where flexion contractures are most prone to occur. These can be prevented by full range-of-motion exercises performed passively twice daily and periods of lying on the abdomen. Prolonged sitting should be avoided. A tilt table can be used to elevate the patient with hips and knees kept in extension. Severe spasticity may be relieved by intramuscular or perineural injection of dilute phenol solution.

DRUGS. Habit-forming narcotics should be avoided, except when absolutely necessary during postoperative periods. Most paraplegic pain can be controlled with a mild analgesic. Persistent pain which is not relieved by these drugs may require neurosurgical or orthopedic intervention. It is virtually impossible to rehabilitate the paralyzed patient who has become addicted to drugs.

EARLY STANDING. Quadriplegic or paraplegic patients should be put in a standing position by means of a tiltboard as soon as possible. Usually this can be accomplished 10 days to 2 weeks following surgical treatment, depending on the clinical condition of the patient. Patients without cord transection, with a hope of return of muscle function but with spine injury that remains unstable, must be carefully protected to avoid further cord damage. Here, it is best to be conservative and withhold tilting.

In the absence of abdominal muscle function, the use of a Scultetus binder or canvas corset with stays is recommended during tilting. At the onset the angle of inclination is usually 20 to 30°. The angle of inclination and length of time that the patient can stand are increased rapidly, so that at the end of 2 to 3 weeks the patient should have reestablished circulatory equilibrium and be able to stand in a vertical position for a minimum of 1 hour daily.

It has been pointed out that an hour of standing each day will help retard osteoporosis in the lower extremities and decrease the incidence of urinary calculi and genitourinary infection, which are frequent causes of death in patients with paraplegia and quadriplegia. Circulation and nutrition, as well as morale, are also aided by keeping the patient in an upright position for several hours each day. When maximal physiologic response has been obtained, plastic repair of decubitus ulcers should be performed.

Bladder and bowel care and training for all paraplegic and quadriplegic patients involves careful initial urologic evaluation, appropriate handling of catheter drainage and irrigation, and training in autonomous or automatic reflex emptying. Adequate fluid intake and control of infection are necessary. Bowel training is less complex and usually requires added glycerine suppositories, occasional enemas, stimulant medications by mouth or rectally, and regular digital stimulation as well as removal of scybala or impaction. Neurogenic uropathy is discussed in detail below.

Upon completion of definitive medical and surgical treatment, the rehabilitation program becomes the primary therapeutic regimen. A full day's program, usually extending from 4 to 6 hours, is indicated. General conditioning exercises performed on the mat should be stressed for 2 to 3 hours daily if the physical condition of the patient is satisfactory. Exercises should be designed to strengthen the muscle groups of the upper extremities, particularly the shoulder depressors and triceps brachii, and the abdominal and trunk muscle groups. The patient is also taught sitting balance. Short sawed-off crutches or wooden blocks may be used to practice push-ups on the mat while sitting. These exercises are designed to prepare the patient for training in transfers, in activities of daily living, and for ambulation with braces and crutches where feasible.

BRACES. Patients with lesions at the T_{10} level and above are usually given double-bar long leg braces with a pelvic band and a Knight spinal attachment for back support. These braces are fitted with sliding box-type locks at the hip and knee joints. The ankle joints should have stirrup attachments to the shoes with a 90° plantar-flexion stop. Patients with lesions from T_{10} to L_1 are given double-bar long leg braces with a pelvic band, and those with lesions below L_1, depending upon the specific functioning muscle groups around the hips, are given ordinary long leg braces. It is better, at first, to prescribe too much bracing than too little.

ACTIVITIES OF DAILY LIVING. The program in activities of daily living includes training in bed, toilet, eating, dressing and undressing, hand, wheelchair, elevation, walking, climbing, and traveling activities.

All quadriplegic and paraplegic patients have emotional and social problems as well as physical disability. Each patient should be seen as early as possible by the social service worker and, when indicated, by the psychologist. As the patient becomes more proficient in his activities of daily living, more and more emphasis should be placed on vocational testing, counseling, and training.

QUADRIPLEGIA. Most of these patients have lesions at the C_6 or C_7 level or above. The patient with traumatic quadriplegia resulting from a cervical fracture or dislocation requires immediate skeletal traction, which is continued for approximately 8 weeks. It may be necessary to provide some type of neck support for 2 to 4 months following removal of traction, particularly if cervical laminectomy has been required.

Extremities should be carried through a complete range of motion of all joints twice daily. Extreme care must be taken by the therapist to protect the vertebral traction. Little can be done at this time toward strengthening the remaining muscles. Modified isometric exercises may be started with care. After the patient is released from traction, gradually placing him in a standing position by means of a tiltboard is initiated. Again, as with the patient with paraplegia, standing an hour or more a day with the use of the tiltboard helps prevent urinary infection and calculi. The majority of patients with quadriplegia are not braced for ambulation.

These patients usually need the care of an attendant. Electric devices are available which can be controlled with the pressure of a shoulder, by one functional muscle in the forearm or elbow, by the touch of the chin or the teeth, by breath impulse, and also by reflected light from the corneas of the eyes to the control units. These devices will operate electric wheelchairs, feeder arm supports, special telephones, and other mechanisms.

NEUROGENIC UROPATHY

Urinary tract complications and infections (see Chap. 40) are the most frequent causes of death in quadriplegic and paraplegic patients. In the beginning, there is stasis which is readily followed by infection. Subsequent to infection, calculus formation, renal obstruction, and gradual loss of renal function ensue as part of the vicious cycle.

Following traumatic lesions of the spinal cord with the stage of spinal shock and also with lower motor neuron lesions involving the posterior sacral roots, the bladder immediately becomes atonic. The detrusor reflex is abolished, and the sensation of fullness is absent. As mechanical pressure overcomes the forces of external urethral resistance, small amounts of urine are emptied periodically. In contrast, lesions affecting both afferent and efferent limbs of the reflex arc leave the bladder completely autonomous and capable of exerting expulsive force by myoneural activity of the vesical ganglionic plexuses within the wall. Emptying is by overflow dribbling only.

In quadriplegic and paraplegic patients with upper motor neuron lesions, spastic reflex bladder occurs following the stage of spinal shock. Bladder capacity in these patients is small, and variable amounts of urine are passed without warning. Occasionally, erection, fullness in the head, and autonomic reactions such as transient hypertension, flushing, or sweating may precede involuntary evacuation of the bladder. In addition, spasticity of the external sphincter may cause interruption of the stream at any point.

The uninhibited neurogenic bladder rarely follows traumatic lesions of the cord and is more commonly associated with acquired lesions of the cerebral cortex as an accompaniment of hemiplegia from tumor or following craniotomy. In this situation, sensation is intact, and there is usually great urgency coupled with an inability to control sphincter contraction with resultant incontinence.

MANAGEMENT. Treatment of the flaccid bladder is by catheterization adhering strictly to the principles of catheter management outlined in Chap. 40. In these patients, a low-grade infection is almost always present, and chemotherapy is directed at preventing acute episodes of urinary tract infections rather than eliminating the low-grade infection. The atonic stage may last for a period of several weeks depending on the level of spinal lesion. Cystometric examination helps define the status of detrusor activity.

Urinary tract complications which are encountered in quadriplegics and paraplegics include cystitis, acute pyelonephritis, formation of calculi, hydronephrosis, and epididymitis. Complications require immediate treatment and control, as urinary tract problems are generally the most serious and dangerous which the patient has to face.

BLADDER TRAINING PROGRAM. In the urologic rehabilitation of the patient with quadriplegia or paraplegia, efforts are directed toward achieving complete or nearly complete evacuation of the bladder. This goal is rarely attained in the paraplegic patient, particularly in those individuals with spastic reflex activity of upper motor neuron lesions. The surgical conversion of upper into lower motor neuron lesions usually results in more predictable bladder function. Even though sensation of bladder fullness is seldom present, the patient may aid emptying by straining and Credé maneuvers performed at regular intervals. The functionally adequate spastic reflex bladder has an unpredictable action, and a majority of patients require some type of external collection apparatus. A variety of surgical procedures have been employed and are directed at the elimination of obstruction and consequent residual urine. These include transurethral resection of bladder neck or prostate, pudendal neurectomy, sacral rhizotomy, spinal cordectomy, and intrathecal alcohol injection.

Transurethral resection is best applied in patients with lower motor neuron lesions in whom voiding is accomplished by straining and Credé maneuvers but where an obstructive outlet pathologic condition is found. Pudendal neurectomy is used in patients with upper motor neuron lesions, particularly at the cervical and upper thoracic levels, to effect relaxation of muscles of the pelvic floor and the external urinary sphincter. The potential efficacy of this procedure can be tested by local anesthetic block of the pudendal nerves.

Anterior and posterior sacral rhizotomy converts an upper motor neuron lesion into a lower motor neuron lesion and may be indicated in paraplegic and quadriplegic patients with severe peripheral spasticity and a spastic reflex bladder. Preliminary sacral nerve blocks can be used to determine the potential value of this procedure. Spinal cordectomy or the intraspinal injection of alcohol represent relatively radical procedures to create a more completely autonomous bladder and are indicated only where no motor function return in the lower extremities can be expected.

Pulmonary and Cardiovascular Procedures

The goals of therapy include (1) improvement in ventilation by techniques of proper breathing and coughing; (2) prevention of postural deformity with maintenance of the strength of neck, shoulder girdle, and upper extremity musculature and range of joint motion; (3) facilitation of bronchopulmonary drainage by postural exercises and coughing. Humidification, bronchodilators, mucolytic agents, and incentive spirometers are frequently employed and directed at these aims. The intermittent positive-pressure breathing (IPPB) machine has been found less useful, except for assistance in administration of nebulized medications and as an adjunct when assistance in respiratory function is needed.

During surgical procedures, muscles may be divided or stretched causing resultant dysfunction, progressive structural scoliosis, and alteration in shoulder girdle mobility. The position of the patient during the operative procedure may be attended by unintentional trauma to the subclavicular portion of the brachial plexus, resulting in palsy of one of its branches or of the radial, median, or ulnar nerves.

Rehabilitation of patients undergoing thoracic surgical procedures is initiated preoperatively and continued during the postoperative period. The object of preoperative therapy is to educate the patient with a program of breathing exercises and instruction in coughing which are pertinent to adequate ventilation and maintenance of a clear airway. Preoperative training includes deep breathing with pursed-lip expiratory phase, diaphragmatic breathing, regional costal breathing, and instruction in adequate voluntary productive coughing. Postoperatively the instructions are continued as appropriate, and assistance is given by splinting the chest with hand support. Range-of-motion activity of the shoulder arm and hand on the side operated on are encouraged, as well as frequent change of position while in bed, both to prevent limitation and to promote stimuli to cough.

Radical Mastectomy

Rehabilitation is directed toward aiding psychologic adjustment, restoring external appearance, and maintaining good function of the ipsilateral arm and shoulder. The patient frequently experiences disappointment and depression from the loss of a symbol of femininity and anxiety regarding her future. She is therefore in need of support and encouragement from members of the family, her physicians, and the members of the hospital team. Early return to normal activity affords a significant psychologic boost. Shortly after the wound is healed, a suitable prosthesis should be provided for the patient. A variety of uncomplicated prostheses are available and can usually be obtained in the larger department stores. The nurse, the physical therapist, and the medical social worker can act with teamwork to counsel and instruct the patient. The surgeon's office nurse can afford prime help to the patient both pre- and postoperatively. The American Cancer Society's "Reach to Recovery" program is widely available to provide trained volunteers, who are mastectomy patients themselves, to help and instruct patients in the hospital and at home.

Current concepts of reconstruction potential following mastectomy allow for the consideration for selected patients of silicon prosthetic implants as replacement, as well as cosmetic reconstructive procedures. Implants or procedures may be performed as immediate operations or may follow the mastectomy by a year, depending on the choice of the surgeon. The use of such approaches depends on the attitude and desires of the patient, the type of mastectomy performed, and the status of the chest wall, including the opposite breast. Plastic surgeons are increasingly aware of the potential of reconstruction or prosthetic implant replacement after mastectomy.

In order to prevent adhesions about the shoulder joint, a routine exercise schedule should be instituted in the immediate postoperative period, with emphasis on elevation and abduction of the arm coupled with active exercises of the arm, forearm, and hand.

Postmastectomy lymphedema in the ipsilateral extremity frequently causes concern. It varies markedly among patients and the areas involved. Slight swelling may occur in the immediate postoperative period and then subside. Swelling which occurs weeks or months postoperatively is more likely to be persistent or progressive and may cause disability in addition to disfigurement. Prevention is more effective than treatment. Each patient should be instructed carefully in prevention of injury, burns, and infection, during her work or recreation. Injections or venipuncture should be avoided in the arm on the side operated on. Advice should be given covering proper rest positioning by frequent elevation of arm, forearm, and hand, so as to promote gravity-assisted outflow of tissue fluids. The patient should also avoid exposure to sunburn, to heat, or to hot water, and to the stress of prolonged vigorous work with the arm on the mastectomized side. The patient should be made aware of the need for immediate attention to the slightest sign of infection in a local site.

Once edema occurs and persists, treatment can be less than satisfactory. Use of elastic sleeves and daily, repeated 20- to 30-minute applications of intermittent compression by air sleeve, salt-free diets, diuretics, and mechanical massaging have all been used with varying effect. For severe intractable edema, the transposition of the partially detached omentum as a pedicle graft (Goldsmith procedure) to the axilla and upper arm has afforded relief in selected patients. Also, the insertion of a series of parallel nylon threads down the arm and forearm in the subcutaneous fat has been reported occasionally helpful. Lymphedema which has progressed to cause paralysis, weeping and chronic infection may require high amputation or shoulder disarticulation of the arm.

The patient may be the victim of recurrent attacks of cellulitis of the arm and will require antibiotics as both preventive and definitive treatment. After several years of lymphedema a lymphangiosarcoma may develop, and this possible change must be kept in mind.

Colostomy and Ileostomy

The formation of a colostomy is associated with a variety of problems requiring adjustment. Concern over leakage, noisy expulsion of gas, and the presence of odor results in anxiety. Care of the colostomy usually requires the establishment of a routine. Dietary changes may be required. Impotence occurs in 50 percent of male patients following abdominal perineal resection of the rectum.

Rehabilitation should begin in the preoperative period when the surgical procedure and the immediate and long-term function of the colostomy is described. Initial postoperative care of the colostomy is directed at avoiding massive evacuation or soiling. It is frequently preferable immediately to employ and maintain cover of the stoma with a disposable plastic collecting bag. During the patient's postoperative hospitalization, he should be instructed in self-care, using either the irrigation or nonirrigation technique. Instruction and assistance in irrigation need to be consistent and should be regularly given by the same nurse or the enterostomal therapist. Most patients are more readily managed by irrigation, using a regular enema administered via catheter and bulb syringe. Commercial kits are available. A daily routine enema at any time which is preferable for the given patient should be established and adhered to. In many patients, a small gauze pad is all that is required to cover the colostomy, but some patients gain a sense of security by wearing a disposable plastic bag. The nonirrigation technique is not widely used but may have merit where toilet facilities are not satisfactory or when regulation has not been accomplished with the irrigation method. Assistance may be obtained from "stomal care" clinics and colostomy clubs, which are widespread. The colostomy may require occasional or regular digital dilation. In general, the patient with a well-regulated colostomy may carry out all activities without concern.

In contrast to the colostomy, the ileostomy requires a collecting appliance. The location of the stoma should be determined with consideration for the appliance to be used and prior to performing the abdominal incision, which distorts the abdominal wall. A variety of satisfactory appliances are available. These are secured to the anterior abdominal wall so that there is no leakage. Ileostomy clubs offer help or counseling to the patient. A well-fitted ileostomy appliance should permit the patient normal and unimpeded activities.

Maxillofacial Surgery

Surgical treatment for tumors of the face and mouth may be attended by severe cosmetic problems. Impairment of mastication may result in nutritional deficiency. Resection of the tongue may be followed by difficulties with speech and swallowing. Enucleation of the eye creates a reduction in the total field of vision, changes in accuracy of depth perception, and cosmetic needs for prosthetic replacement, as well. Care should begin in the preoperative period and should include counseling of the patient and family. Careful oral hygiene and dental preparatory care should precede all orofacial surgery and radiation therapy. The anticipated ultimate cosmetic and functional results should be defined, and if staged procedures are to be carried out, a description and timing should be outlined.

Temporary and permanent maxillofacial prostheses may play a significant role in rehabilitation by lessening the disfigurement and restoring function. Reconstructive surgical procedures may be needed to improve appearance and function. Speech therapy can assist most patients in overcoming the major portion of this disability. Frequently, the most difficult problem is the disfigurement itself. Efforts with the patient, his family, and associates are directed toward preventing the patient from assuming an attitude of social withdrawal. Prostheses, prosthodontic procedures, and plastic reconstructive surgery help according to individual indications.

Laryngectomy

While hemilaryngectomy and radiation therapy may permit effective phonation, total laryngectomy is followed by total loss of speech. There is also frequently a temporary loss of the sense of taste, which returns reasonably well as the patient recovers. Speech instruction should be initiated by trained therapists shortly after discharge from the hospital. Esophageal voice training, which is successful in up to 80 percent of cases, is more satisfactory than a prosthetic appliance as far as articulation, intelligibility, and phonation are concerned. Patient "clubs," such as "Lost Chord" and "New Voice" societies, are very helpful in promoting confidence and motivation. When esophageal speech is unsuccessful, the patient may resort to electronic devices such as a hand-held artificial larynx. There also are surgical procedures, such as devised by Asai, with construction of a skin tube from tracheostomy to pharynx, which will vibrate to produce sound when the tracheostomy is covered, and by Taub, to utilize a pharyngostomy to carry the sound created by a reed apparatus applied to the tracheostomy. These have worked well, but in contrast to esophageal speech, they immobilize one of the patient's hands during speech. In care of the permanent tracheostomy, tubes, gauze pads, tape for covering, plastic stoma protectors for showering, disposable bibs, and portable suction apparatus with catheters are employed. The patient should avoid exposure to fumes and dust, and small boating is usually contraindicated because of the tracheostomy-associated danger of drowning.

Radical Neck Dissection

Extensive radical neck dissection may result in shoulder disability in addition to cosmetic defect. Disability is related to section of the spinal accessory nerve, which may result in paralysis of the trapezius muscle and a dropped, painful shoulder with rotation of the scapula. Support of the arm and shoulder in a sling or on a padded roll or bar hand rest may be helpful. Exercises are used to promote fixation of the scapula by the rhomboid and serratus anterior muscles, so that the scapula is stabilized during shoulder activities. The results of these maneuvers are frequently discouraging. A nerve graft may be used to replace the excised segment of the accessory nerve, and electromyographic testing of the trapezius will determine return of innervation. In the interim, supportive passive motion and electrical stimulation of the trapezius are useful. Occasional patients have partial or full direct innervation of the trapezius muscle from C_1, C_2, and C_3 motor roots and sustain less or little disability.

Radiation Therapy

Radiation therapy causes changes in normal tissues. Fibrosis occurs in the lungs and in joint tissues. Patients with respiratory problems need support and understanding. There is little specific therapy other than establishment of good voluntary respiratory patterns and controlled and paced breathing to limit dyspnea on exertion. Joints which are affected need gentle active and assisted range-of-motion exercises. Any forceful stretching is contraindicated.

Radiation necrosis of soft tissue is rare, but interference with wound healing in previously radiated tissue may be encountered, as well as decrease in the resistance of such areas to stress or trauma. Exposure of bone may be followed by aseptic radiation necrosis. All these factors involve limitations when activities involving stress may be ordered or contemplated for the patient. Patients who have had their full tolerance dose of radiation therapy should be protected from any further exposure to diagnostic or therapeutic radiation, except when under the advice and guidance of a radiation therapist.

Exposure of the hospital staff to patients treated with radioactive implants should be monitored by the wearing of radiation monitor badges, regularly checked. Staff exposure to patients treated by after-loading techniques must be kept at a maximum of 2 to 3 minutes, and distance from the patient maintained as appropriate and possible.

Bone Marrow Replacement

The current research in the treatment of myelogenous neoplasia by the use of bone marrow replacement introduces periods of immunodeficient susceptibility for the patients. Protection from exposure to infection by laminar flow and reverse isolation requires that recommended activity programs be provided in limited space areas and by properly trained personnel.

Advanced Disease

To this point our consideration has been for patients whose goals could be set for restoration or long-term support. Care for many other patients requires planning for a course of advanced or terminal disease. This is particularly a need for cancer patients with extended disease and widespread metastases. Such patients must be evaluated for and helped in the maintenance of maximum comfort, independence in physical function, reduction of complications such as pain, lymphedema, or decubiti, and provision of emotional support. Palliation can be accomplished by an active program of adjustment and instruction in activity, recreation therapy, and positive involvement within the capacity of the individual patient. The stabilizing effects of a regular schedule of modified physical and emotional support therapy prevent these patients from feeling isolated and abandoned during the remainder of the life they must live.

References

Brompton Hospital Physiotherapy Department, "Physiotherapy for Medical and Surgical Thoracic Conditions," 3d rev. ed., Brompton Hospital, London, 1967.

Burgess, E. M., Romano, R. L., and Zettle, J. H.: "The Management of Lower Extremity Amputation," TR 10-6, Superintendent of Documents, Government Printing Office, Washington, 1969.

Cicenia, E. F., and Hoberman, M.: Braces and Brace Management, *Am J Phys Med,* **36:**136, 1957.

Dietz, J. H., Jr.: Rehabilitation of the Cancer Patient, *Med Clin North Am,* **53:**607, 1969.

———: Rehabilitation of the Surgical Patient, *Contemp Surg,* **4**(5):22, 1974.

———: Rehabilitation of the Cancer Patient: Its Role in the Scheme of Comprehensive Care, *Clin Bull, Memorial Sloan-Kettering Cancer Center,* **4**(3):104, 1974.

———: Rehabilitation of the Mastectomy Patient, *Breast,* **2**(3):7, 1976.

Druss, R. G., O'Connor, J. P., and Stern, L. O.: Psychologic Response to Colectomy, *Arch Gen Psychiat,* **20:**419, 1969.

Friedmann, L. W.: Rehabilitation of Amputees, in S. Licht (ed.), "Rehabilitation and Medicine," Elizabeth Licht, New Haven, Conn., 1968.

Katona, E. A.: Learning Colostomy Control, *Am J Nurs,* **67:**534, 1967.

Krusen, F. H., Kottke, F. J., and Ellwood, P. M., Jr.: "Handbook of Physical Medicine and Rehabilitation," 2d ed., W. B. Saunders Company, Philadelphia, 1972.

Lauder, E.: "Self Help for the Laryngectomee," 2d ed., Lauder, San Antonio, Texas, 1969.

Moskowitz, E.: "Rehabilitation in Extremity Fractures," Charles C Thomas, Publisher, Springfield, Ill., 1968.

Myers, S. J. (ed.): "An Orientation to Chronic Disease and Disability," The Macmillan Company, New York, 1965.

Rusk, H. A.: "Rehabilitation Medicine," 3d ed., The C. V. Mosby Company, St. Louis, 1977.

Schottstaedt, E. R., and Robinson, G. B.: Functional Bracing of the Arm, *J Bone Joint Surg* [*Am*], **38A:**477, 1956.

Snyderman, R. K. (ed.): "Symposium on Neoplastic and Reconstructive Problems of the Female Breast," vol. 7, Educational Foundation of the American Society of Plastic and Reconstructive Surgeons, The C. V. Mosby Company, St. Louis, 1973.

Turnbull, R. P.: Instructions to the Colostomy Patient, *Cleve Clin Q,* **28:**134, 1961.

——: Construction and Care of the Ileostomy, *Hosp Med,* **2:**145, 1966.

Weiss, A. A.: The Phantom Limb, *Ann Intern Med,* **44:**668, 1956.

Wilson, A. B.: Limb Prosthetics—1970, *Artif Limbs,* **11:**1, 1970.

Name Index

Subject Index